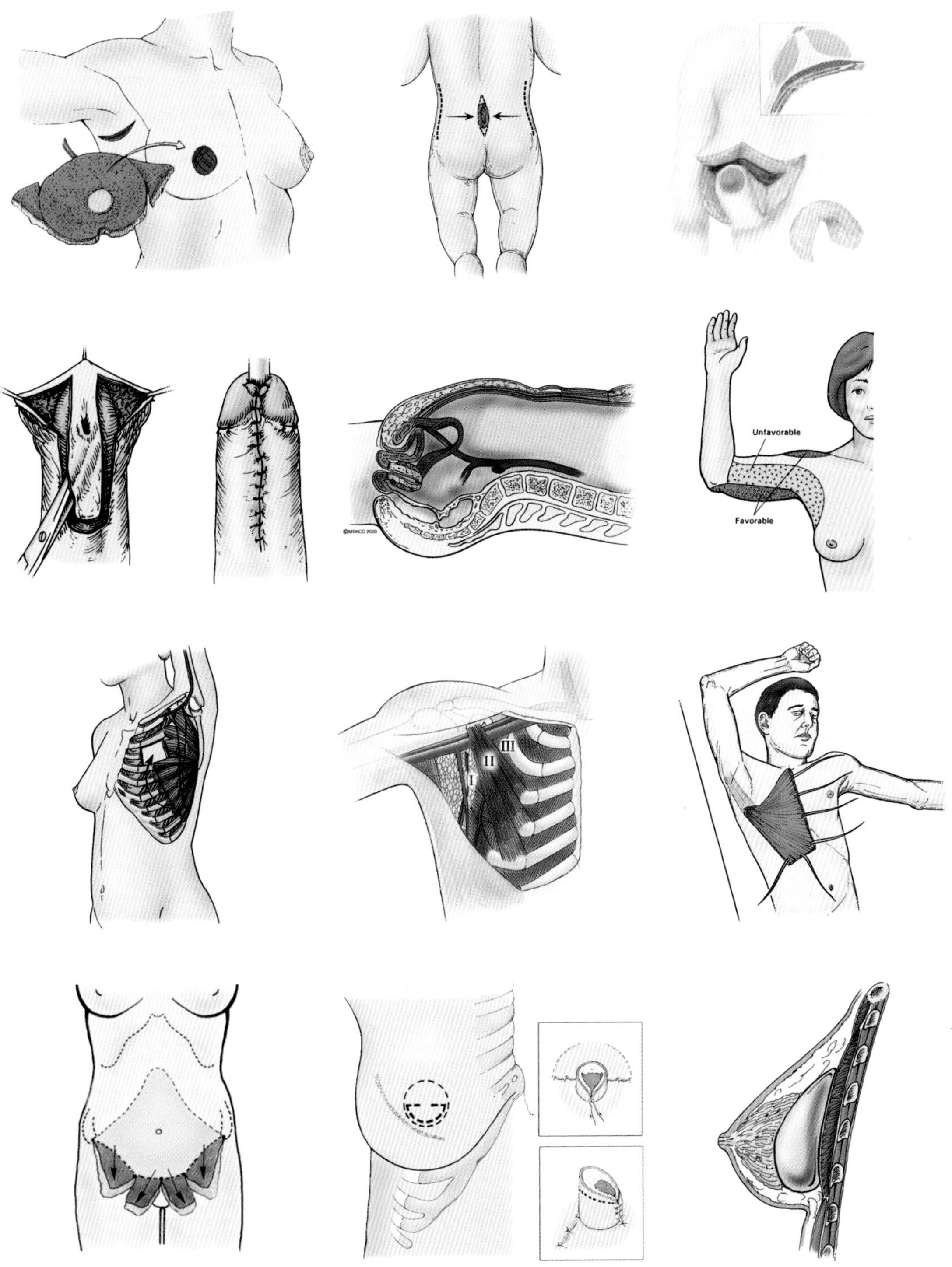
Unfavorable
Favorable
I
II
III

Plastic Surgery

Plastic Surgery

First Edition

Editor:
Joseph G. McCarthy, MD

Editors, Hand Surgery volumes:
James W. May, Jr., MD
J. William Littler, MD

Plastic Surgery

Second Edition

Editor
Stephen J. Mathes, MD
Professor of Surgery
Chief, Division of Plastic Surgery
University of California, San Francisco
School of Medicine
San Francisco, California

Editor, Hand Surgery Volumes
Vincent R. Hentz, MD
Professor of Surgery
Chief, Division of Plastic and Hand Surgery
Stanford University School of Medicine
Stanford, California

With illustrations by Kathy Hirsh and Scott Thorn Barrows, CMI, FAMI

Shireen L. Dunwoody, Editorial Coordinator

VOLUME *VI*

TRUNK AND LOWER EXTREMITY

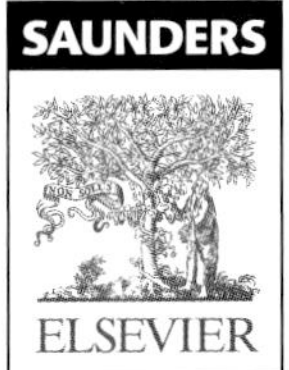

Volume I General Principles
Volume II The Head and Neck, Part 1
Volume III The Head and Neck, Part 2
Volume IV Pediatric Plastic Surgery
Volume V Tumors of the Head, Neck, and Skin
Volume VI Trunk and Lower Extremity
Volume VII The Hand and Upper Limb, Part 1
Volume VIII The Hand and Upper Limb, Part 2

SAUNDERS
ELSEVIER

1600 John F. Kennedy Blvd.
Ste 1800
Philadelphia, PA 19103-2899

PLASTIC SURGERY, 2nd ed.

Volume I 0-7216-8812-8/978-0-7216-8812-1
Volume II 0-7216-8813-6/978-0-7216-8813-8
Volume III 0-7216-8814-4/978-0-7216-8814-5
Volume IV 0-7216-8815-2/978-0-7216-8815-2
Volume V 0-7216-8816-0/978-0-7216-8816-9
Volume VI 0-7216-8817-9/978-0-7216-8817-6
Volume VII 0-7216-8818-7/978-0-7216-8818-3
Volume VIII 0-7216-8819-5/978-0-7216-8819-0
8-Volume Set 0-7216-8811-X/978-0-7216-8811-4

Notice

Knowledge and best practice in this field are constantly changing. As new research and experience broaden our knowledge, changes in practice, treatment and drug therapy may become necessary or appropriate. Readers are advised to check the most current information provided (i) on procedures featured or (ii) by the manufacturer of each product to be administered, to verify the recommended dose or formula, the method and duration of administration, and contraindications. It is the responsibility of the practitioner, relying on his or her own experience and knowledge of the patient, to make diagnoses, to determine dosages and the best treatment for each individual patient, and to take all appropriate safety precautions. To the fullest extent of the law, neither the Publisher nor the Editors assume any liability for any injury and/or damage to persons or property arising out of or related to any use of the material contained in this book.

The Publisher

Previous edition copyrighted 1990.

Library of Congress Cataloging-in-Publication Data
Mathes, Stephen J.
Plastic surgery / Stephen J. Mathes ; editor Vincent R. Hentz.—2nd ed.
p. cm.
ISBN 0–7216–8811–X
1. Surgery, Plastic. I. Hentz, Vincent R. II. Title.
RD118.M388 2006
617.9′5—dc21

2003041541

Acquisitions Editors: Sue Hodgson, Allan Ross, Joe Rusko, Judith Fletcher
Senior Developmental Editor: Ann Ruzycka Anderson
Publishing Services Manager: Tina Rebane
Senior Project Manager: Linda Van Pelt
Design Direction: Steven Stave
Cover Designer: Shireen Dunwoody

Printed in China

Last digit is the print number: 9 8 7 6 5 4 3 2 1

This text is dedicated to Mary H. McGrath, who is my inspiration and a source of joy in our daily life together, our adventures at home and away, and our shared enthusiasm and excitement as plastic surgeons.

✦ CONTRIBUTORS

LEE W. T. ALKUREISHI, MBChB, Bsc (Hons)
Postdoctoral Fellow
University of California, San Francisco, Medical School
San Francisco, California
Senior House Officer in Surgery
Glasgow Royal Infirmary
Glasgow, Scotland

GARY J. ALTER, MD
Assistant Clinical Professor of Plastic Surgery
David Geffen School of Medicine at the University of California, Los Angeles
Staff Surgeon
Cedars-Sinai Medical Center
Century City Hospital
Los Angeles, California

PHILLIP G. ARNOLD, MD, FACS
Professor of Surgery
Mayo Clinic College of Medicine
Division of Plastic and Reconstructive Surgery
Clinical Faculty
Mayo Clinic
Rochester, Minnesota

TANYA A. ATAGI, MD
Staff Surgeon
Grossman Plastic Surgery
Denver, Colorado

PAUL E. BANWELL, BSc, FRCS
Specialist Registrar in Plastic Surgery
Oxford-Wessex Training Rotation
Oxford, United Kingdom

RICARDO BAROUDI, MD
Postgraduate Professor
International Society of Aesthetic Plastic Surgery
Editor, Aesthetic Plastic Surgery
Sao Paulo, Brazil

ELISABETH K. BEAHM, MD, FACS
Associate Professor
Department of Plastic Surgery
University of Texas, MD Anderson Cancer Center
Houston, Texas

MICHAEL S. BECKENSTEIN, MD, FACS
Director, Breast Surgery Center of Alabama
Birmingham, Alabama

PATTI BERGEY, PA-C
Staff, Physician's Assistant
Atlanta Plastic Surgery
Atlanta, Georgia

KRISTIN BOEHM, MD, FACS
Clinical Instructor
Department of Surgery
Mercer University School of Medicine
Attending Surgeon
Medical Center of Central Georgia
Private Practice
Renaissance Plastic Surgery
Macon, Georgia

EUGENE J. CARTER, MD
Former Fellow in Plastic and Reconstructive Surgery
Harbor/University of California, Los Angeles, Medical Center
Torrance, California

TE NING CHANG, MD, PhD
Staff Physician
California Pacific Medical Center
San Francisco, California
Seton Medical Center
Daly City, California
Children's Hospital of Oakland
Oakland, California

STEPHEN M. CHEN, MD
Assistant Professor of Surgery
Division of Plastic Surgery
Virginia Commonwealth University School of Medicine
Medical College of Virginia Campus
Richmond, Virginia

DAVID J. COLEMAN, MS, FRCS (Plast)
Honorary Clinical Senior Lecturer
University of Oxford Faculty of Medicine
Consultant, Plastic and Reconstructive Surgery
The Radcliffe Infirmary
Oxford, United Kingdom

LAWRENCE B. COLEN, MD, FACS
Associate Professor of Surgery (Plastic and Reconstructive)
Eastern Virginia Medical School
Chairman, Department of Plastic Surgery
Sentara Hospitals
Norfolk, Virginia

PETER G. CORDEIRO, MD, FACS
Associate Professor of Surgery
Weill Medical College of Cornell University
Chief and Associate Attending Surgeon
Plastic and Reconstructive Service
Department of Surgery
Memorial Sloan-Kettering Cancer Center
New York, New York

JORGE I. DE LA TORRE, MD, FACS
Associate Professor of Surgery
Division of Plastic Surgery
University of Alabama School of Medicine
Director, Center for Advanced Surgical Aesthetics
Chief, Plastic Surgery Center
Birmingham Veterans Administration Hospital
Birmingham, Alabama

L. FRANKLYN ELLIOTT II, MD, FACS
Clinical Assistant Professor of Surgery
Emory University School of Medicine
President, Atlanta Plastic Surgery
Atlanta, Georgia

JULIUS W. FEW, MD, FACS
Assistant Professor of Surgery
Division of Plastic Surgery
Northwestern University Feinberg School of Medicine
Attending Surgeon
Northwestern Memorial Hospital
Chicago, Illinois

ROBERT D. FOSTER, MD, FACS
Associate Professor of Surgery in Residence
Division of Plastic and Reconstructive Surgery
Department of Surgery
University of California, San Francisco (UCSF), School of Medicine
Attending Surgeon
UCSF Medical Center
San Francisco General Hospital
San Francisco, California

JASON C. GANZ, MD
Chief Resident
Georgetown University Hospital
Washington, D.C.

SHARON Y. GIESE, MD, FACS
Private Practice
New York, New York

DAVID A. GILBERT, MD, FRCS(C), FACS
Associate Professor of Plastic Surgery
Eastern Virginia Medical School
Medical Director
The Hague Center for Cosmetic and Plastic Surgery, Inc.
Norfolk, Virginia

MARY K. GINGRASS, MD, FACS
Assistant Clinical Professor of Surgery
Department of Plastic Surgery
Vanderbilt University School of Medicine
Chief, Department of Plastic Surgery
Baptist Hospital
Nashville, Tennessee

LAUREN GREENBERG, MD
Private Practice
Palo Alto, California

JAMES C. GROTTING, MD, FACS
Clinical Professor of Surgery
Division of Plastic Surgery
University of Alabama School of Medicine
Private Practice
Grotting Plastic Surgery
Birmingham, Alabama

R. WINFIELD HARTLEY, JR., MD
Staff Surgeon
Boulder Community Hospital
Boulder, Colorado
Avista Adventist Hospital
Louisville, Colorado
Longmont United Hospital
Longmont, Colorado

EDWARD J. HARVEY, MD, MSc
Assistant Professor of Surgery
McGill University Faculty of Medicine
Head of Hand and Microvascular Surgery
Chief, Orthopedic Trauma
Medical Director
Bone/Fracture Metabolism
McGill University Health Center
Montreal, Quebec, Canada

JOHN M. HENSEL, JR., MD
Private Practice
Mount Pleasant, South Carolina

CHRISTOPHER L. HESS, MD
Chief Resident in Plastic Surgery
Georgetown University Hospital
Washington, D.C.

TED T. HUANG, MD, FACS
Clinical Professor of Surgery
Division of Plastic Surgery
University of Texas Medical Branch Medical School at Galveston
Staff Surgeon
Shriners Burns Hospital
Galveston, Texas

CRAIG H. JOHNSON, MD
Assistant Professor of Surgery
Mayo Clinic College of Medicine
Chairman, Division of Plastic and Reconstructive Surgery
Consultant, Division of Hand Surgery
Department of Orthopedic Surgery
Mayo Clinic
Rochester, Minnesota

GLYN E. JONES, MD, FACS
Associate Professor of Surgery
Division of Plastic Surgery
Department of Surgery
Emory University School of Medicine
Chief, Department of Plastic Surgery
Emory Crawford Long Hospital
Atlanta, Georgia

GERALD H. JORDAN, MD, FACS
Professor and Chairman
Department of Urology
Eastern Virginia Medical School
Attending Surgeon
Sentara Hospitals
Norfolk, Virginia

DAVID KAUFMAN, MD
Adjunct Clinical Professor of Surgery
Stanford University School of Medicine
Stanford, California
Associate Director, Division of Plastic Surgery
Acting Director, Burn Unit
Santa Clara Valley Medical Center
San Jose, California

JEFFREY M. KENKEL, MD, FACS
Associate Professor and Vice Chairman
Department of Plastic Surgery
University of Texas Southwestern Medical Center at Dallas Medical School
Chief, Plastic Surgery
Dallas Veterans Affairs Medical Center
Dallas, Texas

JAMES KNOETGEN III, MD
Mayo Clinic College of Medicine
Plastic Surgeon
Division of Plastic and Reconstructive Surgery
Mayo Clinic
Rochester, Minnesota

STEPHEN S. KROLL, MD[†]
Professor of Surgery
Department of Plastic Surgery
University of Texas, MD Anderson Cancer Center
Houston, Texas

JULIE LANG, MD
Chief Resident in General Surgery
Department of Surgery
University of California, San Francisco, Medical Center
San Francisco, California

DONALD R. LAUB, SR., MD, FACS
Volunteer Clinical Faculty
Former Chief, Division of Plastic and Reconstructive Surgery
Department of Surgery
Stanford University School of Medicine
Stanford, California
Founder, Interplast
Mountain View, California

MALCOLM ALAN LESAVOY, MD, FACS
Clinical Professor of Plastic and Reconstructive Surgery
David Geffen School of Medicine at the University of California, Los Angeles (UCLA)
Los Angeles, California
Former Chief, Division of Plastic Surgery
Harbor/UCLA Medical Center
Torrance, California
Director, Encino Outpatient Surgery Center
Encino, California

L. SCOTT LEVIN, MD, FACS
Professor of Plastic and Orthopaedic Surgery
Duke University School of Medicine
Chief, Division of Plastic, Reconstructive, Maxillofacial and Oral Surgery
Duke University Medical Center
Durham, North Carolina

TED E. LOCKWOOD, MD, FACS[†]
Clinical Associate Professor of Plastic Surgery
University of Kansas Medical School
Kansas City, Kansas
Private Practice
Overland Park Regional Medical Center
Overland Park, Kansas

[†]Deceased.

ROBERT F. LOHMAN, MD, FACS
Assistant Professor of Clinical Surgery (Plastic Surgery)
Department of Surgery
University of Chicago Pritzken School of Medicine
Chicago, Illinois

DOUGLAS J. MACKENZIE, MD
Private Practice
Pacific Plastic Surgeons
Santa Barbara, California

ANN P. MARX, MD
Private Practice
Women's Institute of Cosmetic and Laser Surgery
DeKalb, Illinois

MARGA MASSEY, MD
Assistant Professor
Director of Clinical and Basic Science Research
Division of Plastic Surgery
Department of Surgery
University of Utah School of Medicine
Attending Surgeon
Huntsman Cancer Institute
Salt Lake City, Utah

STEPHEN J. MATHES, MD, FACS
Professor of Surgery
University of California, San Francisco, School of Medicine
Professor of Growth and Development,
University of California, San Francisco, School of Dentistry
Chief, Division of Plastic Surgery
Department of Surgery
University of California, San Francisco, Medical Center
San Francisco, California

G. PATRICK MAXWELL, MD, FACS
Assistant Clinical Professor of Surgery
Department of Plastic Surgery
Vanderbilt University School of Medicine
Attending Surgeon
Institute for Aesthetic and Reconstructive Surgery at Baptist Hospital
Nashville, Tennessee

EDWARD P. MIRANDA, MD
Resident in Plastic Surgery
University of California, San Francisco, Medical Center
San Francisco, California

STEVEN F. MORRIS, MD, MSc, FRCS(C)
Professor of Surgery
Dalhousie University Faculty of Medicine
Head, Division of Plastic Surgery
Queen Elizabeth II, Health Sciences Centre
Halifax, Nova Scotia, Canada

FOAD NAHAI, MD, FACS
Private Practice
Paces Plastic Surgery and Recovery Center
Atlanta, Georgia

PETER C. NELIGAN, MB, BCh, FRCS(I), FRCS(C), FACS
Professor of Surgery
University of Toronto Faculty of Medicine
Chair, Division of Plastic Surgery
Wharton Chair in Reconstructive Plastic Surgery
University Health Network
Toronto, Ontario, Canada

R. BARRETT NOONE, MD, FACS
Clinical Professor of Surgery
University of Pennsylvania School of Medicine
Philadelphia, Pennsylvania
Chief, Division of Plastic Surgery
Main Line Hospitals Bryn Mawr
Philadelphia, Pennsylvania

MOTOHIRO NOZAKI, MD
Professor and Chairman
Department of Plastic and Reconstructive Surgery
Tokyo Women's Medical University
Tokyo, Japan

GERALD H. PITMAN, MD, PC, FACS
Clinical Associate Professor of Surgery (Plastic)
New York University School of Medicine
New York, New York

ANDREA L. PUSIC, MD, MHS, FRCS(C)
Assistant Professor of Surgery
Weill Medical College of Cornell University
Assistant Attending Surgeon
Memorial Sloan-Kettering Cancer Center
New York, New York

ROD J. ROHRICH, MD, FACS
Crystal Charity Ball Distinguished Chair in Plastic Surgery
Betty and Warren Woodward Chair in Plastic and Reconstructive Surgery
University of Texas Southwestern Medical School
Chairman, Department of Plastic Surgery
University of Texas Southwestern Medical Center
Chief, Plastic Surgery
Zale Lipshy University Hospital
Dallas, Texas

AMER A. SABA, MD
Breast and Cosmetic Surgery Fellow
Division of Plastic Surgery
Georgetown University School of Medicine
Washington, D.C.

KENJI SASAKI, MD
Professor and Chairman
Department of Plastic and Reconstructive Surgery
Nihon University School of Medicine
Tokyo, Japan

WESLEY SCHOOLER, MD
Chief Resident in Plastic Surgery
University of California, San Francisco, Medical Center
San Francisco, California

ALAN E. SEYFER, MD, FACS
Distinguished Professor
Department of Surgery
Department of Anatomy, Physiology and Genetics
Course Director, Gross Anatomy
F. Edward Hébert Uniformed Services University of the Health Sciences
Bethesda, Maryland
Attending Surgeon
Walter Reed Army Medical Center
Washington, D.C.

KENNETH C. SHESTAK, MD, FACS
Associate Professor of Plastic Surgery
University of Pittsburgh School of Medicine
Chief, Plastic Surgery
Magee Women's Hospital
Pittsburgh, Pennsylvania

DAVINDER J. SINGH, MD
Assistant Professor of Surgery
University of Pennsylvania School of Medicine
Attending Surgeon
Hospital of The University of Pennsylvania
Children's Hospital of Philadelphia
Philadelphia, Pennsylvania

SCOTT L. SPEAR, MD, FACS
Professor of Plastic Surgery
Georgetown University School of Medicine
Chief of Plastic Surgery
Georgetown University Hospital
Washington, D.C.

CRISTIANE M. UENO, MD
Postdoctoral Research Fellow in Surgery
University of California, San Francisco, School of Medicine
San Francisco, California

THEODORE UROSKIE, JR., MD, FACS
Assistant Professor of Surgery (Plastic and Reconstructive)
Eastern Virginia Medical School (EVMS)
Staff Surgeon
Plastic Surgery Clinic of EVMS
Norfolk, Virginia

JUDY VAN MAASDAM, MA
Coordinater
Gender Dysphoria Program, Inc.
Palo Alto, California

LUIS O. VÁSCONEZ, MD, FACS
Professor of Surgery
Chief, Division of Plastic Surgery
University of Alabama School of Medicine
Staff Surgeon
Center for Advanced Surgical Aesthetics
Birmingham, Alabama

PETER A. VOGT, MD, FRCS(C), FACS
Lecturer in Plastic Surgery
University of Minnesota Medical School
Mineapolis, Minnesota

KLAUS J. WALGENBACH, MD, FACS
Attending Surgeon
University of Bonn Medical Center
Bonn, Germany
Former Assistant Professor of Surgery
University of Pittsburgh School of Medicine
Pittsburgh, Pennsylvania

ROBERT L. WALTON, MD, FACS
Clinical Professor of Surgery
University of Chicago Pritzker School of Medicine
Chief, Section of Plastic and Reconstructive Surgery
University of Chicago Hospitals
Chicago, Illinois

MARLA E. WATSON, MA
Clinical Research Assistant
Department of Surgery
Washington University School of Medicine
Staff, Body Aesthetic Plastic Surgery
St Louis, Missouri

V. LEROY YOUNG, MD, FACS
Chief of Surgery
Barnes-Jewish West County Hospital
Staff Surgeon
Body Aesthetic Plastic Surgery
St. Louis, Missouri

✦ PREFACE

It is a great thing to start life with a small number of really good books which are your very own. *Through the Magic Door* (1908), Sir Arthur Conan Doyle

My meeting for lunch with Joseph McCarthy in Boston in 1998 during the annual meeting of the Society of Plastic Surgery was arranged to discuss the possibility of my becoming the editor of the new edition of *Plastic Surgery.* I was well aware of the responsibility of assuming this giant project. My admiration of the past editors, including Joseph McCarthy for the 1990 edition of *Plastic Surgery* and John Marquis Converse for the 1964 and 1977 editions of *Reconstructive Plastic Surgery,* was great since these texts in my estimation really defined our specialty of plastic surgery and provided the platform for future advances in treating congenital and acquired deformities. My memory of Converse's first edition started with my residency in plastic surgery on my first rotation at the private practice of William Schatten, John Hartley, and John Griffith in Atlanta, Georgia. There, in moments when I was not involved in patient care activities, I would enjoy reading the pages of clinical advice on all subjects related to plastic surgery in the five volumes of *Reconstructive Plastic Surgery.* Subsequently, in 1977, as a faculty member at Washington University, I was privileged to be able to purchase my own copy of the then six-volume edition of *Reconstructive Plastic Surgery,* again edited by Converse. This time, my reading of the exciting pages was less relaxed, since I was using the text as the reference in preparation for my plastic surgery board examinations.

By 1990, I was able to contribute a chapter to *Plastic Surgery,* edited by Joseph McCarthy, and I personally knew most of the contributors, having witnessed the evolution of many of the new advances and unique contributions contained within the then eight volumes. With this background, I was excited and honored to have been recommended as the next editor of this text, which has so well reflected the greatness of the specialty of plastic surgery. My meeting was punctuated by advice regarding the importance of the text and the selection of experts who would provide both guidance and stimulation to future readers on the many subjects important to physicians involved in plastic surgery. The complexity of orchestrating so many contributors in a timely fashion was also emphasized. I left this luncheon inspired to undertake this project, with the anticipation of capturing the best and most innovative surgeons as contributors to achieve an edition in keeping with the unique traditions of excellence of the past editions of *Plastic Surgery* and *Reconstructive Plastic Surgery.*

My first step was to find an academic hand surgeon to edit the two hand volumes. J. William Littler had served as the editor of the hand and upper extremity volume in Converse's two editions of *Reconstructive Plastic Surgery.* Littler was a master hand surgeon and one of the foremost innovators in hand surgery. McCarthy selected a unique combination of academic hand surgeons, James W. May and J. William Littler, to edit the two volumes dedicated to upper extremity and hand surgery in the 1990 edition of *Plastic Surgery.* With the many new techniques related to microvascular surgery, the space devoted to this important aspect of plastic surgery had been expanded into two volumes. Jim May, like Bill Littler, is a master hand surgeon, a gifted teacher, and an innovator in all aspects of plastic surgery and was able to include both his contributions and those of many other hand surgeons, who all took part in advancing this important discipline.

Fortunately, the decision regarding who should be the hand editor for this edition of *Plastic Surgery* was obvious. Vincent R. Hentz is a master hand surgeon and past president of the American Society of Surgery of the Hand. As an accomplished educator and chief of the division of plastic and hand surgery at Stanford, he is the ideal person to follow in the footsteps of Littler and May. In keeping with the many innovations and new techniques in upper extremity and hand surgery, this edition contains two volumes devoted to hand surgery. Of interest, we have shifted the editorial geography from the East Coast (New York City and Boston) to the West Coast (San Francisco and Palo Alto). Unfortunately, despite the improvement in weather characteristics of the western coastline of the United States, the commitment to continue the excellence of this text has kept the editors mostly indoors during the complex editing process necessary to complete these volumes.

The goal of this edition is to cover the scope of plastic surgery. The key was to select the best contributors to define the problems encountered in plastic surgery, to provide both the most current and the most successful solutions, and to deliver the challenge for future innovation in each area of plastic surgery. In this new edition, there are 219 chapters with 293 contributors. Each of the senior authors of the 219 chapters was carefully selected for his or her recognized expertise in the assigned subject of the chapter. Each author has personally contributed to the advancement in knowledge related to his or her area of expertise in our specialty.

The authors selected are inspirational leaders due to their many innovations toward improvement in the management of the plastic surgery patient. After the manuscripts were submitted, each chapter was carefully reviewed by the editors to ensure that all aspects of the authors' assigned topics were adequately covered and well illustrated so that the reader could readily incorporate the chapter content into the practice of plastic surgery.

In the eight volumes included in this edition, all subjects pertinent to the scope of plastic surgery are covered. Many new topics, 67 in all, have been developed or were enlarged from broader subjects and warranted a new individual chapter. Thirteen of these new chapter topics are included in Volume I: General Principles. The enlargement of the volume containing general principles reflects the continuing expansion of our specialty, the emphasis on experimental and clinical research, and the impact of research on the practice of plastic surgery. In the remaining volumes, devoted to specific clinical topics, two new types of chapter formats were added: 25 technique chapters and 7 secondary chapters. The technique chapters are added to complement the overview chapters and are designed to focus on particular techniques currently in use for a clinical problem. Likewise, the secondary chapters are again an extension of the overview chapters on particular subjects but focus on problems that persist despite the application of primary plastic surgery solutions. These secondary chapters are designed to demonstrate areas where operations may fail related to improper patient or technique selection or technique failures. They also discuss procedures to correct unsatisfactory outcomes following primary plastic surgery.

Volumes II through VII are divided into specific topographical areas of plastic surgery. Volume II: The Head and Neck (Part 1) is devoted to cosmetic procedures and contains six new topic chapters, seven new technique chapters, and three new secondary chapters. This volume now contains color illustrations, which will help the reader evaluate problems and results following cosmetic procedures. Many important subjects are expanded and introduced. For instance, there are now five chapters on the face lift, which provide the reader with the ability to compare techniques and focus on specific aspects of the procedure. Volume III: The Head and Neck (Part 2) is dedicated to reconstructive procedures and contains 10 new topics as well as the traditional subjects used in the previous edition. Volume IV: Pediatric Plastic Surgery contains five new topics and provides multispecialty approaches to children presenting with congenital facial anomalies. Volume V: Tumors of the Head, Neck, and Skin has seven new topics. Along with management principles of head and neck cancer, identification and treatment of melanoma and non-melanoma skin cancer have been added in new topic chapters. Volume VI: Trunk and Lower Extremity contains 34 added topics. For example, in the area of postmastectomy reconstruction, 12 new chapters have been added to provide specific diagnostic, management, and technical information on breast reconstruction issues. Similarly, four new chapter topics have been added on body contouring procedures. With emphasis on bariatric surgery and body contouring procedures, these chapters provide a complete array of information on techniques and outcomes. Volume VII: The Hand and Upper Limb (Part 1) contains introductory and general principles related to diagnosis and management of acquired disorders, both traumatic and nontraumatic. Volume VIII: The Hand and Upper Limb (Part 2) contains three parts: congenital anomalies, paralytic disorders, and rehabilitation. The two volumes on hand and upper extremity surgery contain an additional 22 chapters introducing new subjects to this edition of *Plastic Surgery.*

Education involves the process of observation as well as contact with teachers, mentors, colleagues, and students and the literature. Each component is essential to learning a specialty in medicine and maintaining competence in the specialty over the course of one's career. In plastic surgery, the abundance of master surgeons gives everyone the opportunity to observe excellence in technique, during residency and later through educational programs. Contact with teachers and colleagues must be maintained in order to keep abreast of the new innovations in medicine and to measure one's outcomes in the context of standard of care. Our professional society meetings and symposia, both locally and nationally, provide us with this opportunity. Contact with mentors and students is critical for innovation. The physician must seek out these sources of inspiration and stimulation to improve patient care. Collaboration with professionals is a unique opportunity to allow further growth in our specialty and is available in every medical environment. The literature allows the physician to see where we have been, where we are currently, and what the future holds. The physician can hold a piece of literature in the hand and review its message both in critical times, when patient management decisions must be made on a timely basis, and during leisure times, when a subject is studied and carefully measured against personal experience and knowledge acquired through professional contacts. It is hoped that this edition of *Plastic Surgery,* like its predecessors, can serve the purpose of literature in teaching. Its eight volumes contain more than 6800 pages of information carefully formulated by recognized experts in our specialty in plastic surgery. It is designed, as initially stated, to define the current knowledge of plastic surgery and to serve as a platform for future creativity to benefit the patient we see with congenital and acquired deformities.

Stephen J. Mathes, MD, 2005

✦ ACKNOWLEDGMENTS

So many talented and dedicated professionals are necessary to complete a text of this magnitude. It is impossible to really thank everyone adequately, since there are so many people behind the scenes who were silently working toward the completion of this project. However, I shall endeavor to acknowledge the people who provided scientific, technical, and emotional support to make this edition of *Plastic Surgery* possible.

My first contact with the publisher (Saunders, now Elsevier) started with my meeting with Allan Ross and Ann Ruzycka Anderson. Allan Ross, executive editor, was assigned to guide this text to publication. He is a dedicated publishing executive who was most supportive at the inception of this project. Ann Ruzycka Anderson, senior developmental editor, has been working in medical publishing for 20 years. This text was most fortunate to have Allan and Ann assigned as the guiding forces at the onset. Ann states that working on this text is "something exciting, worthwhile, and important" because she is helping to "produce the largest book in medical publishing history."

Because this book took 5 years to complete, there were changes in the personnel involved in the project. Joe Rusko, medical editor, assumed the responsibilities of guiding the development of the text, with Allan Ross taking on the role of consultant. Joe has great enthusiasm and provided great ideas for the format of this book and for associated advertising. During the past year, the project was turned over to the leadership of Sue Hodgson, currently the publishing director and general manager for Elsevier Ltd. With Sue living in London, the project took on a more international outlook, with Sue flying between London, Philadelphia, New York, and San Francisco to keep the project moving ahead to completion. Both Sue Hodgson and Allan Ross have a great deal of success in guiding complex publications to press. Sue has published highly successful books in dermatology, and now, it is hoped, she will be able to make the same claim for the field of plastic surgery. For sure, she can now lay claim to publishing the largest medical book in existence. Recently, Sue Hodgson summed up her role in the publishing industry as follows: "The opportunity to create new products to answer the market's educational needs and handling high-profile and demanding projects are what get me out of bed in the morning." All plastic surgeons who use this text are indebted to the perseverance and commitment of these publishing leaders: Allan Ross, Joe Rusko, and Sue Hodgson.

"The quality of a person's life is in direct proportion to their commitment to excellence, regardless of their chosen field of endeavor."

—Vince Lombardi

After the authors were selected for the 219 chapters, it was obvious that we needed someone special to serve as the editorial coordinator between the editors and the authors. Thanks to the advice of Allan Ross and Ann Ruzycka Anderson, Shireen Dunwoody was recommended for this position. Shireen is an accomplished computer programmer and musician and has served as a senior medical writer, media programmer/editor, and developmental editor since 1991. Among the high-profile medical texts on which she has worked are *Clinical Oncology* (Martin Abeloff et al., editors), *Surgery of the Liver and Biliary Tract* (Leslie Blumgart, editor), and *Fundamentals of Surgery* (John E. Niederhuber, editor). Shireen has worked closely with the editors and our assigned authors during every step of the process—obtaining the manuscripts (including a multitude of meetings and phone calls with authors), helping find artists when needed, confirming references, discovering historical information as related to the many subjects covered in *Plastic Surgery*, and coordinating all these data with the publishing staff in Philadelphia and New York. When asked to describe what this job was like, she described the process as follows: "At times, this project has been a struggle, but most of the time it has been a joy (kind of like raising eight children). On any given day, working on this project has given me a reason to (1) get up in the morning; (2) stay up all night; (3) despise the morning; (4) stay sober; (5) get drunk; (6) laugh; (7) cry; (8) live; (9) lie; (10) rejoice. Who could ask for anything more? It has certainly kept things interesting!" Shireen credits special members of the publishing staff for helping this immense project move ahead at a fairly steady pace. In Philadelphia, Linda Van Pelt, senior project manager, book production, and RoseMarie Klimowicz, freelance copyeditor, have been with this project since its inception. They have both dedicated vast amounts of blood, sweat, tears, and personal time. Ann Ruzycka Anderson has been dedicated to this project since the onset and has also worked closely with Shireen. Judy Fletcher, publishing director, provided the support needed for timely layouts and served as an advocate for this project even when layout or illustrations were changed to maintain the continuity and artistry of the chapters. Finally, Shireen acknowledges her two amazing assistants in Palm Springs, California, Donna Larson and Carla Parnell, who have helped her scan, copy, crop, sort, mail, and stay sane. Without the dedication and brilliance of Shireen Dunwoody in bringing out the best in the editors, publishers, authors, and artists, this text would not have the quality and completeness it now possesses.

My immediate family was always supportive of this project despite the time-consuming work associated with text preparation. I wish to acknowledge and thank my family for their exciting accomplishments, which are a source of pride and enjoyment: Mary, Norma, Paul, Leslie, Isabelle, Peter, David, Brian, Vasso, Zoe, Ned, Erin, Maggie, and Rick.

In any profession, the support and encouragement of one's colleagues are essential for productivity. I wish to thank the faculty in our division of plastic surgery for their specific contributions to the text and their active roles as outstanding teachers for our residents and students at the University of California in San Francisco. The faculty, both full time and clinical, include the following: Bernard Alpert, Jim Anthony, Ramin Behmand, Kyle Bickel, Greg Buncke, K. Ning Chang, Tancredi D'Amore, Keith Denkler, Issa Eschima, Robert Foster, Roger Friedenthal, Gilbert Gradinger, Ronald Gruber, William Hoffman, Clyde Ikeda, Gabriel Kind, Chen Lee, Pablo Leon, Mahesh Mankani, Robert Markeson, Mary McGrath, Sean Moloney, Douglas Ousterhout, John Owsley, Lorne Rosenfield, Vivian Ting, Bryant Toth, Philip Trabulsy, D. Miller Wise, and David Young.

During the time span in which this book was edited, a group of outstanding residents completed their plastic surgery residencies at UCSF. All these residents contributed to both the care of many of the patients included in the chapters written by our faculty and the development of concepts used in the chapters of this edition. Each resident listed has contributed to the advancement of our knowledge in plastic surgery: Delora Mount, Richard Grossman, Jeff Roth, Laura McMillan, Kenneth Bermudez, Marga Massey, Yngvar Hvistendahl, Duc Bui, Te Ning Chang, Hatem Abou-Sayed, Farzad Nahai, Hop Nguyen Le, Clara Lee, Scott Hansen, Jennifer Newman-Keagle, and Wesley Schooler. General surgery residents, research fellows, and students who participated in the project include Lee Alkureishi, Julie Lang, Edward Miranda, and Cristiane Ueno.

Without the dedication of our staff, the preparation of this text would not have been possible. Crystal Munoz served as our office manager during most of the preparation time. My patient coordinators, Marian Liebow and, later, Skye Ingham, are patient advocates and made the arrangements necessary to treat the patients discussed in our chapters. Our nurses, Janet Tanaka and, later, Ann Hutchinson, were essential to the overall care of patients presenting to our clinical practice. Our staff provides the support needed to allow the faculty to have the time necessary to participate in the creative activities expected in academic plastic surgery.

Plastic surgeons depend on visual assessment of problems; thus, illustrations are an essential part of our scientific literature. Numerous artists were involved in the chapters selected by the individual authors. However, two artists were available to all the contributors and provided outstanding art to accompany many of the chapters. Kathy Hirsh, located in Shanghai, China, and Scott Barrows, in Chicago, have worked diligently to provide accurate artistic interpretations of the surgical procedures recommended throughout this text.

"Mental toughness is many things. It is humility because it behooves all of us to remember that simplicity is the sign of greatness and meekness is the sign of true strength. Mental toughness is spartanism with qualities of sacrifice, self-denial, dedication. It is fearlessness, and it is love."

—Vince Lombardi

All the authors who contributed to these volumes exemplify mental toughness. To complete a chapter for a text is often considered an unappreciated task. However, thanks to the great reputation established by the prior editors of this comprehensive work, John M. Converse and Joseph G. McCarthy, and the previous editors of the hand volumes, William Littler and James May, the top plastic surgeons in their respective fields have given their time and efforts to maintain the excellence associated with past editions of this text. Thanks to these contributors, this book provides information at the forefront of innovation and current practice in the specialty of plastic surgery. The contributors and their families are thanked for their perseverance and sacrifice in the completion of these chapters and for their dedication to our specialty, plastic surgery.

SJM

✦ CONTENTS

✦ VOLUME I
General Principles

✦ VOLUME II

The Head and Neck, Part 1

✦ VOLUME III

THE HEAD AND NECK, PART 2

✦ VOLUME IV

Pediatric Plastic Surgery

✦ VOLUME V

Tumors of the Head, Neck, and Skin

✦ VOLUME VI

Trunk and Lower Extremity

✦ VOLUME VIII

The Hand and Upper Limb, Part 2

CHAPTER

118

Breast Augmentation

G. PATRICK MAXWELL, MD, FACS ✦ R. WINFIELD HARTLEY, Jr., MD

Female glandular hypomastia is a frequently encountered entity that occurs either developmentally or by postpartum involution. Historically, women have long sought breast enlargement to improve physical proportions, to foster a more feminine appearance, or to enhance self-image. Following the introduction of the silicone gel prosthesis in 1962,[1] breast augmentation has become the most frequently performed operation in plastic surgery.[2] It is estimated that more than 1% of the adult female population in the United States (between 1 and 2 million) has undergone breast augmentation.[3] The women undergoing breast implantation have been scientifically scrutinized since its inception and found to range from outgoing healthy individuals with a desire for aesthetic improvement to women with depression, low self-esteem, negative body image, and sexual inhibitions.[4,5] The popularity of the procedure is thought to be based on the satisfaction of the patients' results.[6] Women in general have enhanced self-image, increased self-assurance, improved sexual functioning, and better interpersonal relationships after augmentation.[7]

Czerny[8] reported the first augmentation mammaplasty, in which he transferred a lipoma to the breast, in 1895. Longacre[9] attempted autogenous "flap" augmentations in the 1950s, and the use of various injectable substances such as petroleum jelly, beeswax, shellac, and epoxy resin soon followed.[10] Uchida[11] reported the use of injectable silicone in 1961. Solid materials implanted in the 1950s and early 1960s included polyurethane, Teflon, and polyvinyl alcohol formaldehyde (the Ivalon sponge[10]). Although none of these methods proved satisfactory, the introduction of the silicone gel breast implant in 1962 by Cronin and Gerow[1] began the modern era of breast augmentation.

EVOLUTION OF MAMMARY IMPLANTS

Silicone Gel Implants

The silicone gel implants commercially available in the United States today are a refined and safer device than their predecessors. Silicone development evolved to meet the needs of the aircraft-engineering industry during World War II. Because of its softness and inert nature, it attracted interest from the medical sector and was soon evaluated as an implantable medical device by plastic surgical researchers.[12,13] The Cronin and Gerow mammary implant of the 1960s, which was manufactured by Dow Corning,[1] was composed of a viscous silicone gel contained within a thick silicone shell in the shape of a teardrop. Seams were present at the periphery of the device, and Dacron fixation patches were placed on the posterior surfaces to help ensure proper position (Fig. 118-1). These early devices had such a high incidence of capsular contracture that a new generation of silicone implants was developed by various manufacturers in the mid to late 1970s in an attempt to produce a more natural result. These implants were round and characterized by a seamless, thin, smooth silicone shell. There were no fixation patches, and the

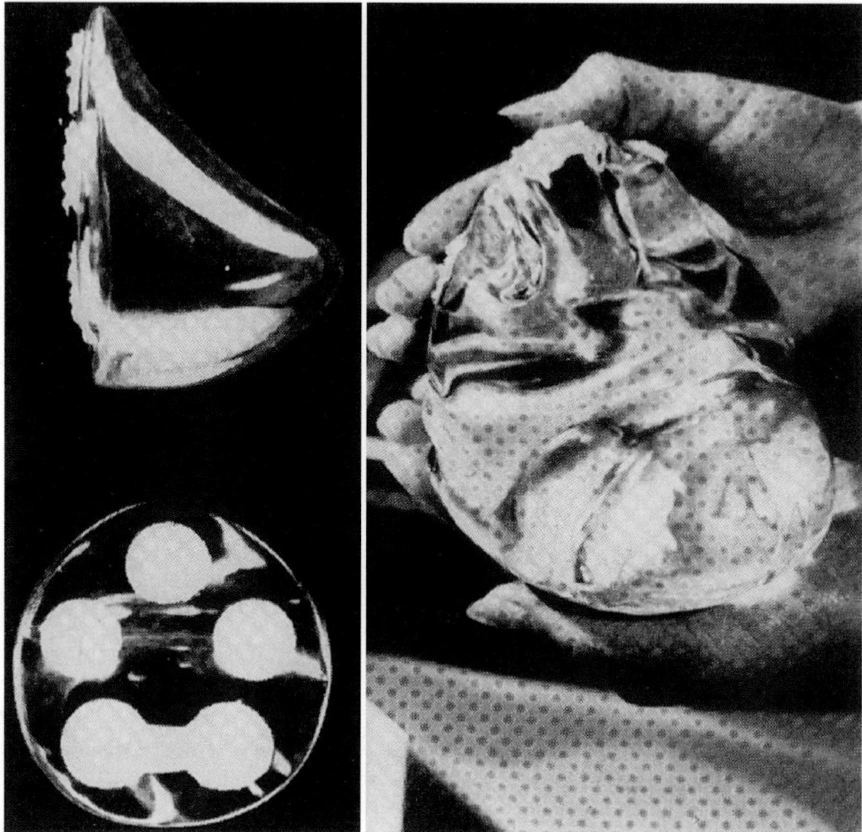

FIGURE 118-1. The original Cronin-Gerow silicone implant introduced in 1962 had an anatomic (teardrop) shape, smooth surface, and posteriorly placed Dacron patches to help maintain the implant's position. (From Cronin TD, Gerow FJ: Augmentation mammoplasty: a new "natural feel" prosthesis. Transactions of the Third International Congress of Plastic Surgery, October 13-18, 1963. Amsterdam, Excerpta Medica Foundation, 1963:41-49.)

silicone gel was less viscous than in first-generation implants. Whereas the incidence of capsular contracture may have been improved somewhat, the incidence of silicone gel "bleed" and shell rupture was enhanced (especially from manufacturers who made very thin shells[14]). Gel bleed is a phenomenon whereby low-molecular-weight particles of silicone gel diffuse or leak through the silicone elastomer shell, giving a sticky feel to the surface. It has been theorized that silicone bleed could promote capsule contracture.[15,16] Whether it is due to silicone bleed or other factors, capsule contracture has been the biggest clinical problem with the use of smooth-surfaced silicone gel implants.

The third generation of smooth-surfaced silicone implants, developed in the early to mid 1980s, focused on improving the strength and integrity of the silicone shell as well as on minimizing the silicone bleed phenomenon.[17,18] This generation of implants was characterized by two layers of "high-performance" elastomer with a thin fluorosilicone "barrier coat" in between (produced by McGhan Medical, Heyer-Schulte, Dow Corning, and Cox-Uphoff). There are data to suggest that these improvements enhanced shell life and lessened capsule contracture. Third-generation silicone gel implants with the application of a textured surface can be considered fourth-generation devices, and cohesive silicone gel–filled implants can be considered fifth-generation devices. These are discussed in the following paragraphs (Table 118-1).

Saline-Filled Implants

The inflatable saline-filled implant was first reported by Arion[19] in France in 1965. The impetus for its development was to allow smaller incisions through which a noninflated device could be inserted and then inflated with its liquid filler material. Saline implants were subsequently developed by American manufacturers and underwent clinical evaluation in the early 1970s.[20,21] The emphasis for the inception of and interest in these devices was focused on their inflatable

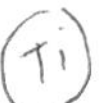

TABLE 118-1 ✦ DEVELOPMENT AND CHARACTERIZATION OF SILICONE GEL BREAST IMPLANT

First Generation (1962-1970)
Thick shells Thick gel Dacron patches Teardrop shape
Second Generation (1970-1982)
Thin shells Thin gel No patches (smooth) Round shape
Third Generation (1982-present)
Thicker (stronger) shells "Barrier coat" ("low-bleed") shells Thicker gel No patches Round shape
Fourth Generation (1986-present)
Third-generation technology Textured silicone surfaces Round and anatomic shapes
Fifth Generation (1993-present)
Enhanced cohesive silicone gel Textured silicone surface Diverse anatomic and round shapes

nature, allowing smaller incisions, not on the character or safety of the liquid filler or an attempt to lessen the rates of capsular contracture.

Although it is generally accepted that the contracture rate with saline implants is relatively low, two qualities of these devices have plagued their clinical use. The foremost was their deflation rate. The original French implant manufactured by Simaplast was found to have a deflation rate near 75% at 3 years and was withdrawn from the market. Heyer-Schulte developed an American saline implant in 1968. Whereas silicone gel implant shells are high-temperature vulcanized (HTV) platinum cured, the shells for saline-filled implants were made thicker and cured by a room-temperature vulcanized (RTV) process. This significantly decreased the deflation rate, and all American-made saline implants have since had shells cured by this process.[22]

A second factor found to increase deflation rates was valve failure.[23] The original Heyer-Schulte prosthesis had a retention (leaflet) valve, which was subsequently replaced by a diaphragm valve. Saline implants currently manufactured in the United States by Mentor (which purchased Heyer-Schulte) and INAMED (formerly McGhan Medical) have diaphragm valves and RTV-cured shells.

The other characteristic of saline implants that has been a problem relates to the saline itself, which may transmit visible surface wrinkles and a knuckle-like feel in volumetrically underfilled devices. When the device is overfilled, it may feel and look like a firm ball and transmit a peripheral "scalloping" look. For these reasons, saline implants historically perform better under thicker tissue, and surgeons generally fill implants to the recommended volume or just beyond. Saline implants are also heavier than silicone gel implants on a volumetric basis and may cause more tissue thinning with inferior displacement of the implant over time.

Double-Lumen Implants

The original double-lumen implant was developed by Hartley[24] as a means of countering capsular contracture. It was constructed of an inner silicone gel–filled lumen surrounded by an outer saline inflatable shell. The conceptual use of the device employed the initial inflation of the outer saline shell to make a larger pocket, with subsequent percutaneous deflation to leave the smaller silicone gel–filled shell within a larger pocket. The device became popular without going through these machinations as a fixed-volume, two-chamber device or as a drug delivery device, which allowed the addition of steroids or antibiotics to the outer saline-filled chamber.

Cox-Uphoff developed a "reverse double-lumen" implant,[25] which had an outer silicone gel–filled shell surrounding an inner inflatable shell. Today, the only double-lumen device on the U.S. market is the Mentor Becker, an expander-implant used primarily for reconstruction.[26] This device was originally developed as a saline device but subsequently converted to a reverse gel and saline double-lumen design to minimize deflation rates. INAMED (McGhan) makes a similar round design and additionally has an anatomic version in which the postoperative addition of saline selectively enhances only breast projection. The McGhan style 153 anatomic silicone gel implant is also structurally composed of two lumens with different shapes to enhance its anatomic form.

Textured-Surface Implants

Early attempts at augmentation with polyurethane sponge were not successful, but in 1970, Ashley[27] reported the favorable use of a silicone gel implant covered with a thin layer of polyurethane foam.

Although the foam was placed on the implant primarily to maintain its position, clinical use seemed to show a lessened incidence of capsular contracture.[28,29] Throughout the 1980s, increasing numbers of plastic surgeons found polyurethane-covered silicone gel implants to produce aesthetically pleasing results with low capsular contracture rates.[30-32] The polyurethane surface adhered to the surrounding tissues, subsequently delaminated, and created a relatively noncontractible capsule.[33] Unlike smooth-surfaced implants that had to be mobile within their pocket, polyurethane-covered implants could be immobile yet soft. These devices had reached a zenith of popularity by 1990, when questions of the safety of polyurethane foam breakdown products caused Bristol-Myers Squibb, which owned Surgitek (the company manufacturing the implants), to withdraw from the breast implant market.[34]

The favorable clinical outcomes and commercial success of polyurethane-covered implants (Fig. 118-2) led American implant manufacturers to develop textured silicone surfaces in the hope of achieving similar results. In 1986, McGhan Medical introduced Biocell textured implants and expanders, and Mentor introduced Siltex textured implants. These remain the two textured surfaces available in the United States today. Dow Corning subsequently introduced its MSI "structured surface" in 1990, but the company withdrew from the market in 1992.

Biocell is an aggressive open-pore textured silicone surface composed of irregular pores having an average density of 3.1 pores/mm^2 with a mean pore size of 289 μm (range, 37 μm to 648 μm) (see Fig. 118-2). Created by a lost-salt technique, these interconnected pores promote adherence to the surrounding, developing capsule through an "adhesive effect."[35-37] This tissue adherence, which is clinically similar to that seen with the polyurethane foam surface, differs in that there is no delamination of the texture as occurs with polyurethane. The adhesive effect and tissue adherence are enhanced in Biocell-covered expanders; these have the added mechanical advantage of expansion pressure, which pushes the textured surface into the developing capsule and imparts its mirror image into the surrounding tissue.[38] Whereas adherence may not occur around the entire device or with all Biocell breast implants, there is a high friction coefficient around these devices, making them relatively immobile. Thus, similar to the polyurethane implants, "immobility with softness" characterizes Biocell-covered implants. Prospective clinical studies have demonstrated that Biocell textured implants have a significantly lower incidence of capsule contracture than do their smooth counterparts, whether they are filled with silicone gel[39] or saline.[40]

Siltex is a less aggressive textured silicone surface created as a negative contact imprint off texturing foam (see Fig. 118-2). It is characterized by a raised, dense pattern of irregular nodules ranging in height[36] from 65 to 150 μm and in width from 60 to 275 μm. Siltex does not adhere to the surrounding tissue and thus is not characterized by immobility with softness, as are polyurethane and Biocell.[37] Whereas Siltex-covered implants thus move within their surrounding pocket similar to smooth-walled implants, prospective clinical studies have shown a significantly lower incidence of capsule contracture compared with their smooth counterparts, whether they are filled with silicone gel[41,42] or saline.[43]

Other textured-surface devices that have been available in the past or are currently available outside the United States include the MSI pillar-structured texture previously manufactured by Dow Corning[44] and the polyurethane foam–covered implant manufactured by Silimed in Brazil.[45]

"Alternative Filler Implants"

When safety issues with silicone gel implants became a concern, investigators looked for alternative filler substances. Three actually came to market. Polyvinylpyrrolidone is a low-molecular-weight "bio-oncotic" gel thought to be more radiolucent than silicone. It composed the fill material of the Misti Gold implant introduced in 1991 by Bioplasty.[46] NovaMed purchased this company, and the polyvinylpyrrolidone implant is currently still available outside the United States under the name NovaGold. In December 2000, the British Medical Devices Agency issued a device alert regarding this implant and other alternative filler devices, citing the opinion that studies demonstrating the safety of these devices are lacking.[47]

LipoMatrix manufactured triglyceride-filled implants termed Trilucent implants in 1994. Soybean oil composed the fill material, which was said to be radiolucent. Problems with oil bleed,[48] tissue irritation, and a rancid or foul smell[49] were reported, and the implants were withdrawn from the market in 1999.

Hydrogel implants are implants filled with an organic polymer, which is a mixture of polysaccharide and water. These implants have been manufactured in France by PIP and Arion. There have been reports of swelling of hydrogel (as well as polyvinylpyrrolidone) implants after implantation due to osmotic gradient pressure.[47] The British Medical Devices Agency alert of 2000 also applied to these devices. None of these alternative filler devices is available in the United States.

Enhanced Cohesive Silicone Gel Implants

All silicone gel implants are cross-linked to maintain a gel consistency, and thus all silicone gel has cohe-

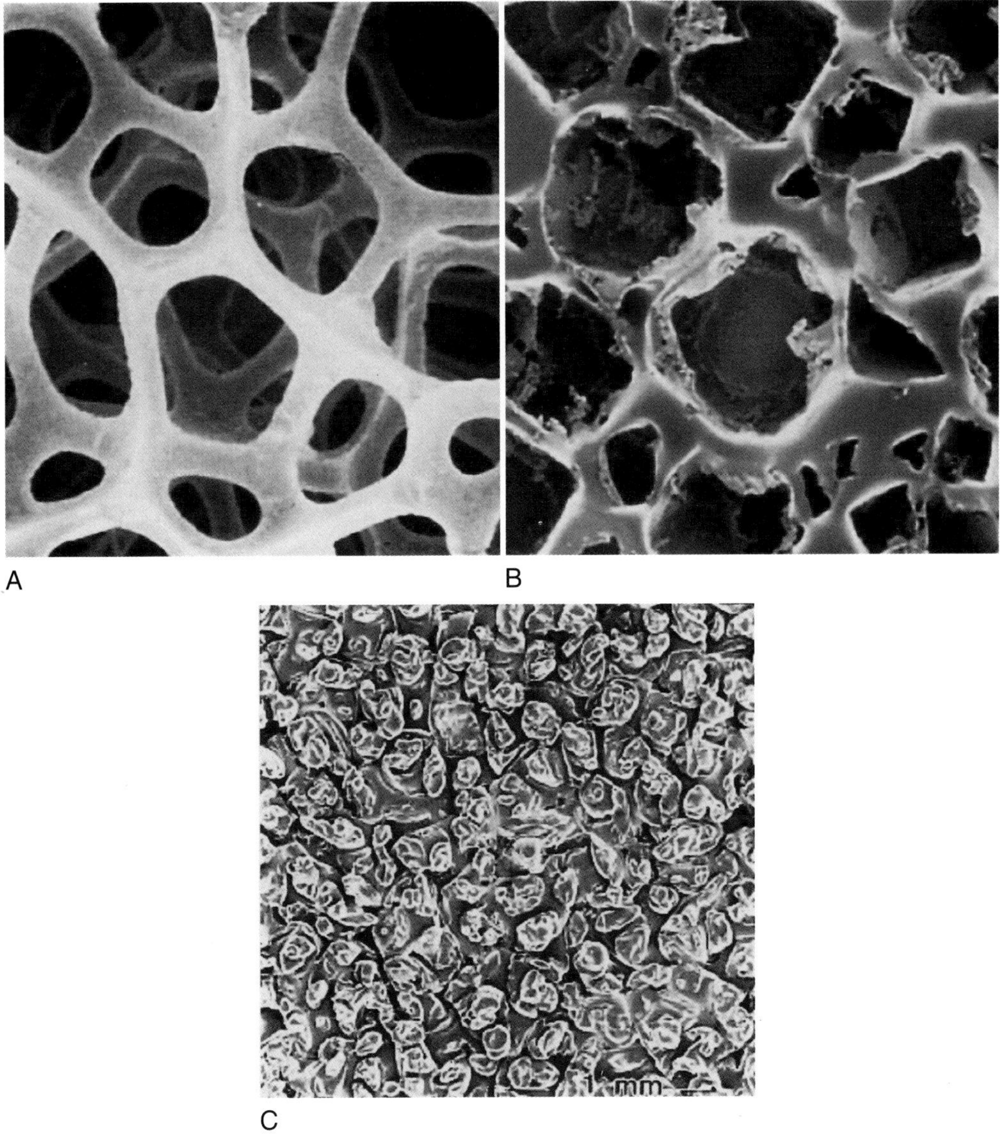

FIGURE 118-2. *A,* Polyurethane foam gains tissue adherence and delaminates from the implant. No longer available in the United States, this texture fostered the development of textured silicone surfaces. *B,* Biocell is an aggressive silicone textured surface that adheres to surrounding tissue by an adhesive effect. *C,* Siltex is a less aggressive silicone textured surface that does not demonstrate any adhesive effect and does not gain tissue adherence. (From Maxwell GP, Hammond DC: Breast implants: smooth vs. textured. Adv Plast Reconstr Surg 1993;9:209.)

sive properties. As the cross-linking is increased, the consistency or firmness of the "liquid-feeling" gel changes to that of a soft cheese. The enhanced cohesive nature of these implants makes them "form stable." This refers to the implant's maintaining its shape in all positions (shape maintenance). These implants are designed in various anatomic dimensions in addition to round shapes and are collectively referred to as cohesive silicone gel implants. These form-stable implants are currently popular worldwide and undergoing Food and Drug Administration (FDA)–approved clinical trials in the United States (Fig. 118-3).[45]

Anatomic-Shaped Implants

The original Cronin and Gerow silicone gel implants had a teardrop shape, as did a number of the early

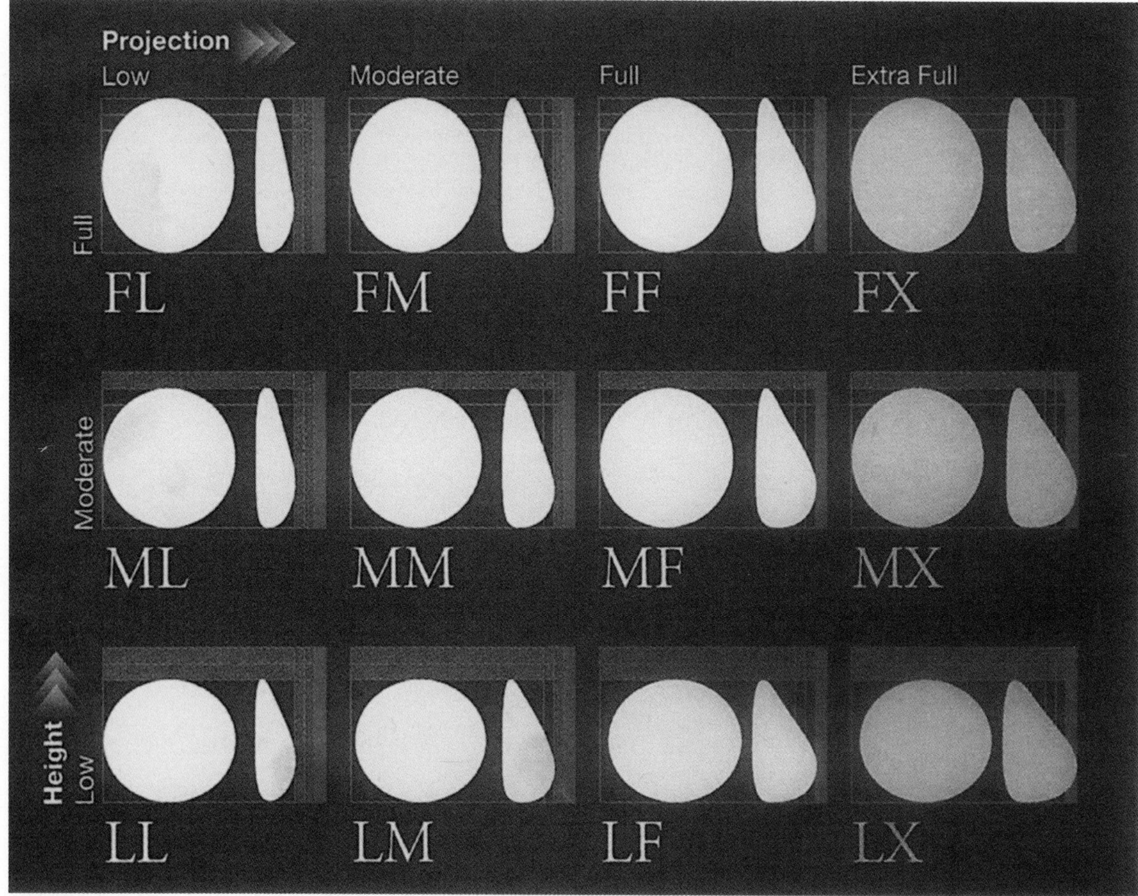

FIGURE 118-3. Style 410 Matrix (INAMED) of enhanced cohesive silicone gel implants offers varying heights and projections of shaped devices for breast augmentation and reconstruction. (L, low; M, moderate; F, full; X, extra). (Courtesy of INAMED Health, Santa Barbara, Calif.)

saline- and gel-filled devices. Problems with capsular contracture, however, led manufacturers to design round, smooth-surfaced low-profile implants, which would move within their surgical pockets. These round, smooth designs dominated the market for nearly 20 years. Only when the phenomenon of immobility with softness was appreciated was the creation of anatomic devices clinically appropriate.[38,51] The polyurethane Optimum and Replicon devices (no longer available) were early-generation anatomic-shaped implants popular in the 1980s.[28,29] The adherence of the polyurethane surface, in fact, lent itself to the "stacking" of these implants, one on top of another, to produce an anatomic shape with enhanced projection.[51]

The tissue adherence observed with tissue expanders that had the Biocell surface led McGhan to develop anatomically shaped expanders and subsequently an internally stacked style 153 gel anatomic-shaped implant.[35,38,51,54] Favorable clinical experience and advanced product design led to a matrix of variable height-to-width ratio anatomic expanders and implants, the Style 133 expanders and Style 410 Matrix cohesive implants (see Fig. 118-3). The latter enjoy widespread international use in aesthetic surgery[45,55] and have completed their initial FDA clinical Investigative Device Exemption study in the United States, awaiting longer follow-up.

Silimed (Brazil) markets polyurethane-covered cohesive silicone gel implants in anatomic shapes.[34] These devices also enjoy international popularity, but to date, no clinical investigative studies have taken place in the United States.

Mentor introduced a midheight Siltex anatomic-shaped tissue expander in 1997 and other height options in 2003. In the fall of 2002, an Investigative Device Exemption study on a midheight anatomic cohesive gel implant was initiated. These "contour"-shaped devices are covered with the Siltex texture. Because tissue adherence does not generally occur, the pocket must be exact and only minimally larger than the footprint of the reduced height device to minimize the possibility of implant rotation.[56]

Anatomic-shaped saline inflatable implants are available in the United States manufactured by both Mentor and INAMED (McGhan), and there is debate among plastic surgeons about the merit of each relative to the resultant breast form.[58-62] This debate seems confined to saline-filled implants alone as virtually all tissue expanders marketed for breast reconstruction in the United States are textured and anatomically shaped. It is predicted that once cohesive gel anatomic implants and other gel implants are available in the United States, the issue will be of less concern as evidenced by surgeons' preferences worldwide.

SAFETY AND REGULATORY ISSUES CONCERNING BREAST IMPLANTS

In 1976, the U.S. Congress passed a Medical Device Amendment to the Food, Drug, and Cosmetic Act that gave the FDA authority over medical devices. Implants on the market at the time or those considered "substantially equivalent" to those marketed before 1976 were "grandfathered" in and allowed to remain in use until the FDA could formally review their safety and efficacy. In 1988, the FDA called for the manufacturers of silicone gel–filled implants to submit their Premarket Approval Applications containing data adequate to substantiate the safety and efficacy of the devices they were marketing. In November 1991, the FDA convened an advisory panel of experts to hold public hearings and evaluate the manufacturers' data. The panel concluded that more research was necessary (to establish safety and efficacy) but recommended continued availability of implants while that research was carried out. In January 1992, however, the FDA Commissioner went against the recommendation of the advisory panel and called for a voluntary moratorium on the use of silicone gel implants. After further evaluation of the situation by the advisory panel (who thought there was a public need for the devices), the FDA Commissioner, in April 1992, ruled that although silicone breast implants were not necessarily unsafe, the law required more data to substantiate safety and efficacy than the manufacturers had supplied.[62,63] The use of silicone gel implants was thus restricted to clinical trials until the data were produced. This was interpreted by the media and the public at large that silicone gel implants were "banned" because they were not safe. This effectively took silicone gel implants off the market for breast augmentation in the United States for the next 12 years.

The "media frenzy" surrounding this issue was further heightened by several lay jury court decisions that found silicone implants to be responsible for women's pathologic conditions. This led to the filing of thousands of product liability lawsuits against the implant manufacturers. This culminated in a class action lawsuit involving more than 400,000 women.[22] Unable to withstand the financial pressure to defend this massive number of cases, Dow Corning filed Chapter 11 and Bristol-Myers Squibb withdrew from the market. Ultimately, a settlement of approximately $4 billion was reached, and Mentor and McGhan were left as the only two American manufacturers of saline and silicone breast implants.

Concerns relating to the safety of foreign materials implanted in the female breast began in Japan in 1964 when the term *human adjuvant disease* was suggested on speculation of an association between paraffin breast injections and connective tissue disease-like symptoms in several women.[64] In the 1980s, several reports questioned a link between silicone gel breast implants and various collagen vascular diseases.[65-67] Questions were raised as to whether silicone "leaked" into the body and caused pathologic conditions. Whereas increased levels of silicone were found within the surrounding tissue capsule[68,69] and axillary lymph nodes, no correlation with symptoms or any disease could be established. Likewise, no specific antibodies to silicone could be found.[70,71]

Amid this background of lawsuits, public concerns, and implant restrictions, the scientific data began to prevail, demonstrating the safety of silicone gel and the lack of its correlation with any disease or pathologic condition. By the late 1990s, approximately 20 epidemiologic studies and other important scientific investigations found no increased risk for development of connective tissue disorders in women with breast implants.[22] In addition, respected independent scientific groups including the Independent Review Group in England,[72] the Institute of Medicine,[73] and the National Science Panel[74] (appointed by the judge of the class action litigation), after carefully reviewing all scientific data available, found no relationship between silicone gel implants and connective tissue disease.

The other health issue that clouded the breast implant arena in the early 1990s was the possibility of a polyurethane foam breakdown product being carcinogenic. Specifically cited was a National Cancer Institute study in which mice fed extremely high doses of 2,4-toluenediamine showed an increased incidence of breast cancer.[75] Since the foam used to cover the Surgitek implant was produced by a mixture of 2,4- and 2,6-toluenediisocyanate, the FDA questioned whether the polyurethane itself or one of its biodegradation products could be carcinogenic in patients after breast implantation. Scientific scrutiny of patients in whom these devices had been implanted found minimal exposure to 2,4-toluenediamine,[76] and the FDA ultimately concluded that it was unlikely any woman with polyurethane-covered implants was at increased risk for development of cancer.[77] Before these scientific findings of safety, however, Bristol-Myers Squibb failed to make premarket approval for the FDA in April of 1991 and withdrew these devices from the market.

Despite this decade of turbulence, the future of silicone gel implants looks bright. No fill material has been found to be as safe and as functional as silicone. Saline clinical inadequacies (in certain situations) are well appreciated by American plastic surgeons. Manufacturing practices of silicone gel implants have been improved and brought into compliance to ensure better-quality products.

CURRENT STATUS OF SILICONE GEL IMPLANTS

The Premarket Approval Application for silicone gel breast implants submitted by INAMED in December 2001 was heard by the FDA expert advising panel in October 2003. After intense scrutiny of the data submitted, as well as public testimony, the panel recommended approval of the application "with conditions," setting the stage for the return to market of silicone gel implants in the United States. The panel found no evidence to support that silicone gel implants cause disease. They did, however, question the adequacy of the length of follow-up on the studies.

In January 2004, the Commissioner of the FDA went against the panel's recommendation and asked for additional data with longer follow-up from all manufacturers on silicone gel implants.* In addition, more information was requested on life expectancy of implants, causes and effects of shell failure, and clinical evaluation of possible "silent rupture" of implants. In light of these requests from the FDA, silicone gel implants will probably not be back on the American market until 2005. They remain available for clinical use (as they have for the last 12 years) under FDA-approved clinical studies.

INFORMED CONSENT/LITIGATION PREVENTION

Because the breast is historically viewed as a symbol of female sexuality and the quality of the surgical result is primarily in the eye of the beholder (and her companion) alone, emotional outcome can on occasion be somewhat volatile. The facts are that almost 40% of aesthetic plastic surgical claims relate to elective breast operations and half of these to breast augmentation.[78] It is thus incumbent on the surgeon to evaluate the patient's emotional state, timing, and appropriateness of the desired outcome. It is the surgeon's responsibility to listen, educate, and evaluate; this process and the communication that takes place between patient and surgeon are documented in the medical record.

Informed consent is not simply the signing of a paper or contract but refers to the entire process between patient and physician as well as physician extenders. To be "informed," the patient must be provided with adequate information about risks, benefits, and treatment alternatives to the proposed procedure. To "consent," the patient must be an adult (by age), be capable of rational communication, and be able to understand the information. The informed consent documentation must be thorough and specific to the operation and preferably the surgeon. A checklist of specifics (which must be initialed by the patient) is considered advisable. "Before and after" photographs may be shown but should be realistic. Photographs of the patient are a necessary form of documentation, requiring appropriate permission. Their confidentiality is essential unless permission is given for any use other than medical review documentation. A male surgeon should be accompanied by a female chaperon during all breast photography and examinations.

Because of the multiple options in breast augmentation surgery, a second office visit is advisable. There must be a clear understanding (which is documented in the medical record) between patient and surgeon of the specific desired outcome (size, shape), the alternative ways by which this can be achieved, and the risk-to-benefit ratio of the chosen "pathway."

SURGICAL GOALS

The conceptual goal of breast augmentation is to enhance the form and volume of the female breast in the most predictable manner with the fewest possible complications. The resultant form of the augmented breast will be determined by dynamic interaction over time between the compliance and character of the soft tissue envelope; the quality and consistency of the breast parenchyma; and the dimensions, volume, and characteristics of the breast prosthesis (Fig. 118-4).[79] To achieve these goals, experience has shown that a surgical approach based on dimensional concepts rather than on volume alone is preferable. This "biodimensional" approach takes into account the patient's existing breast dimensions and tissue characteristics of the form of the patient's desired surgical result.[80,81] A breast implant is then selected of appropriate dimensions, character, and volume to accomplish this goal (Table 118-2).

SURGICAL TREATMENT

Each year, more than 100,000 women in the United States elect to have surgical enhancement of their breasts. Women seeking breast augmentation place considerable emphasis on their physical appearance, and time should be taken to understand their

*http://www.fda.gov/cdrh/ode/guidance/1239.html

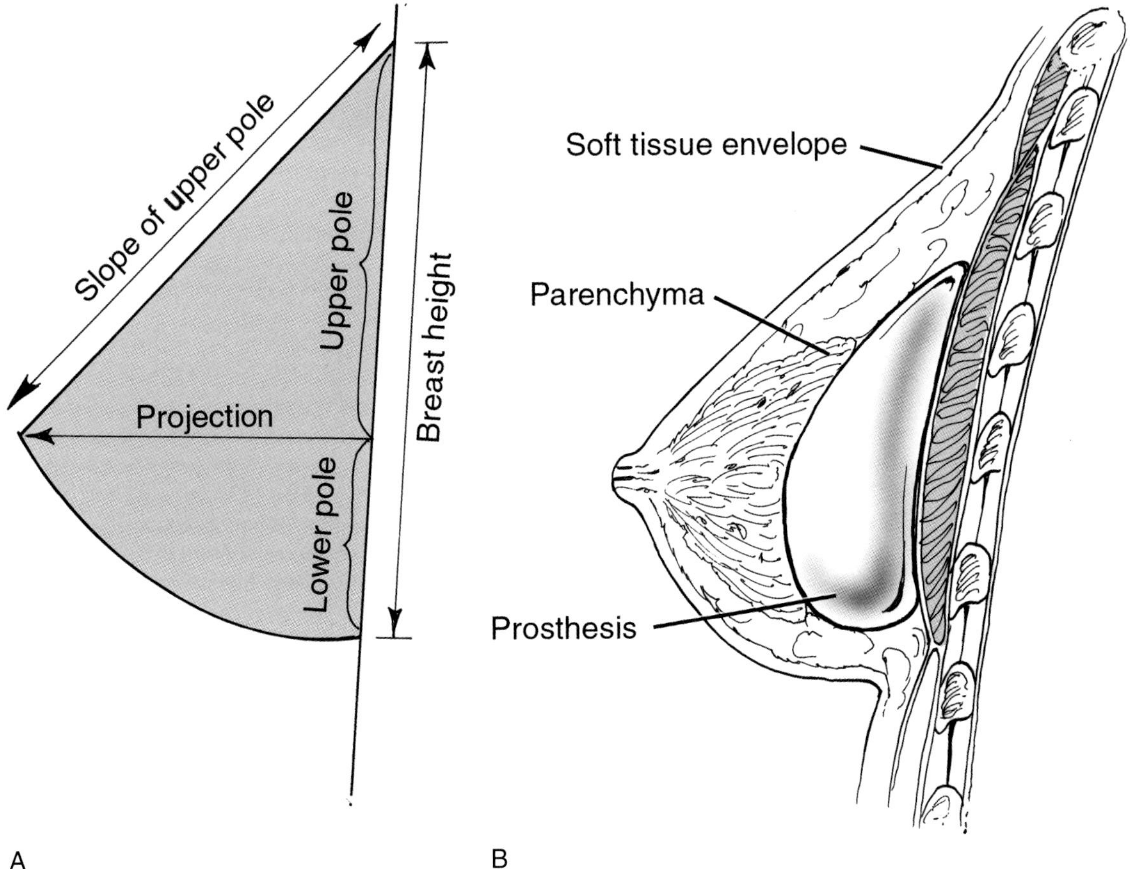

FIGURE 118-4. *A,* The aesthetic breast form is composed of measurable parameters. This form can be attained by the careful planning and surgical performance of a breast augmentation. *B,* The resultant breast form desired after surgical augmentation is determined by the dynamic interaction between the character and compliance of the soft tissue envelope; the quality, volume, and consistency of the breast parenchyma; and the dimensions, volume, and characteristics of the breast implant.

motivations for having surgery. Most patients are properly motivated with realistic goals, but the preoperative visit is the time to identify patients who may have unrealistic expectations or are using surgery as a crutch for other problems. The patient's desires and expectations must be weighed against the predictability of achieving those goals. A high level of satisfaction can be ensured if the patient's aesthetic concerns and expectations are within a predictable and attainable result.

TABLE 118-2 ✦ STEPS IN A BIODIMENSIONAL APPROACH TO BREAST AUGMENTATION

Evaluate existing chest and breast form.
Characterize the soft tissue envelope.
Plan the resultant breast form desired.
Select implant and site location to accomplish this goal.
Select incision and approach.

Whereas individual preferences will affect operative planning and procedural specifics, the goal of breast augmentation is to enhance the form and volume of the female breast. The form of the female breast is determined by the quality, volume, and dimensions of the breast parenchyma and the character and compliance of the soft tissue envelope. The form of the augmented female breast (assuming that capsule contracture is not present) is based on these in dynamic interaction with the dimensions, volume, and consistency of the breast prosthesis (see Fig. 118-4).[79] There must be mutual understanding between the patient and surgeon of the specific resultant breast form that is desired and the predictability (and tradeoffs) of achieving that form.

Assessment

After the patient's goals are determined and reasonable expectations are established with regard to outcome, a thorough physical assessment is

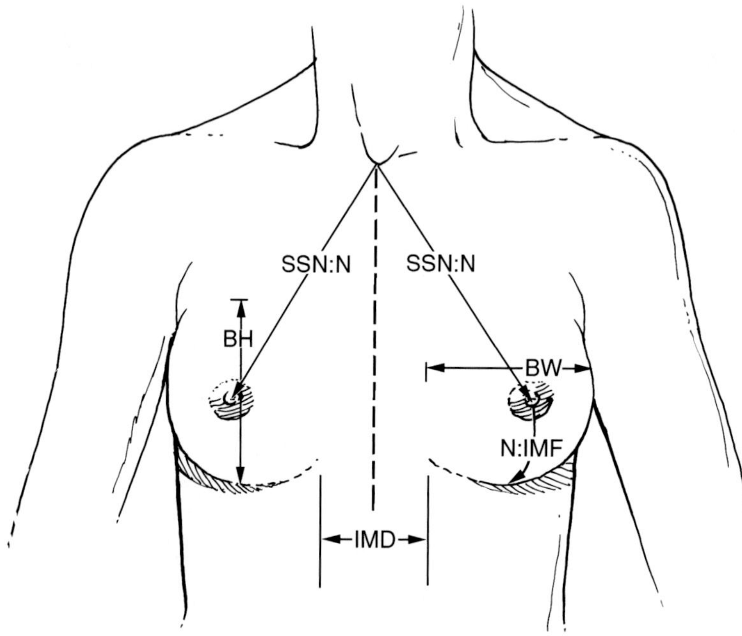

FIGURE 118-5. Preoperative measures (taken before breast augmentation) include SSN to N (suprasternal notch to nipple), N to IMF (nipple to inframammary fold), BW (breast width), BH (breast height), and IMD (intermammary distance).

undertaken. The bone and muscle structural foundation of each breast must be assessed. Note the shape of the thorax as well as whether the patient is "long" or "short" chested.

The majority of women will have some degree of asymmetry when the breast and chest wall are critically evaluated.[82] It is imperative to document and discuss any amount of nipple-areola complex asymmetry as well as chest wall asymmetry with the patient. Precise measurements must be taken (Fig. 118-5). Key measurements include suprasternal notch to nipple distance, nipple to inframammary fold distance, base width or diameter, and breast height.

The compliance of the soft tissue envelope is then assessed. Characterize the elasticity of the skin by noting evidence of poor compliance, such as stretch marks or thin nonelastic dermis. The soft tissue pinch test is a useful measurement; the superior pole of the breast is gathered between the thumb and index finger (skin plus parenchyma), and the distance between the two is measured (Fig. 118-6). A rough estimate for the amount of inherent soft tissue necessary to cover a subglandular implant is 2 cm. A pinch test result of less than 2 cm may lead to subpectoral implant placement. Skin redundancy may also be present.[83] Older patients or those with a history of weight loss may exhibit varying degrees of pseudoptosis or true breast ptosis. These patients may benefit from a concomitant mastopexy.

It is also important to characterize the breast parenchyma itself. Determination of the amount, quality, and distribution of the parenchyma may alter surgical techniques; thus, these should be evaluated and documented. It may be necessary to redistribute, adjust, or reshape the parenchyma to achieve the desired breast mound form.

Operative Planning

IMPLANT SIZE (DIMENSIONS)

The patient's request for a particular breast size and shape will largely determine the dimensions of the

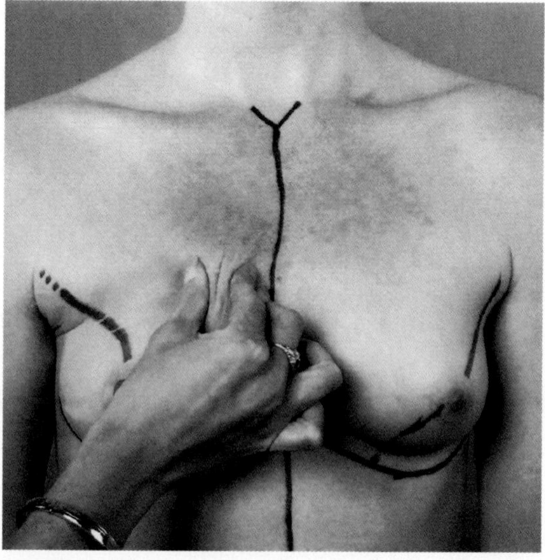

FIGURE 118-6. Soft tissue pinch test. Assessment of the thickness and quality of the soft tissue in the upper pole of the breast preoperatively will help the surgeon in considering pocket location options for implant placement.

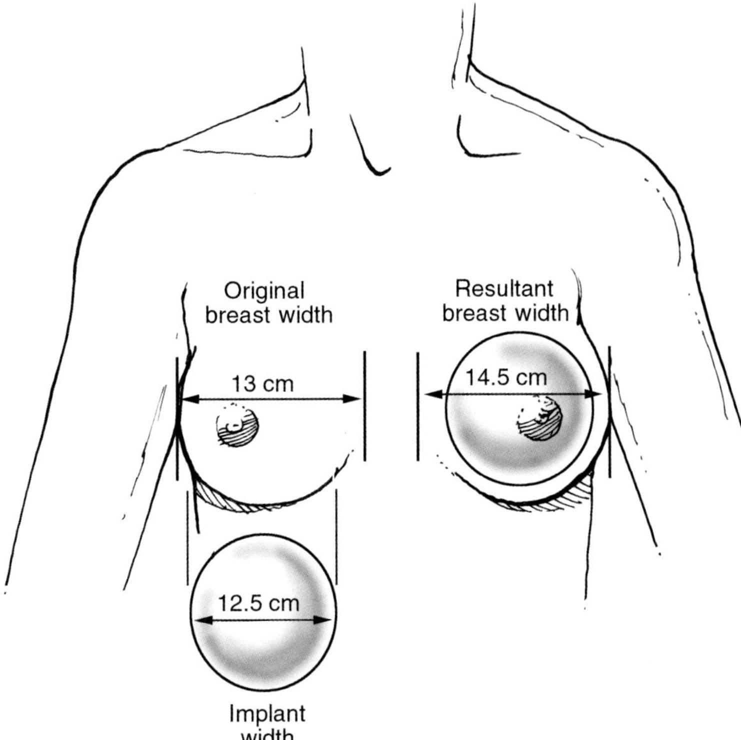

FIGURE 118-7. After the width of the existing breast is measured and the desired resultant breast form is formulated, an implant is selected (generally just narrower than the original breast, shown on the patient's right) that in combination with the preoperative breast tissue will achieve the desired postoperative dimensions and form (shown on the patient's left).

breast implant used. In addition to a thorough discussion with the patient as to her desire for the resultant form and size, it is often helpful to have the patient bring photographs showing the size and shape of breast that she finds appealing.

The most important clinical factor in determining breast prosthesis size is the base width or diameter of the patient's native breast. After measuring the patient, one turns to the manufacturer's published data charts and generally selects an implant slightly less wide than the existing breast. Rarely does the selected implant vary significantly more or less than the measured breast width to avoid an unnatural postoperative appearance (Fig. 118-7). In addition to the desired width of the implant, one also considers height, projection, and volume before making an implant selection. Anatomic-shaped implants allow implant height and projection options to be much more important operative considerations.

SILICONE VERSUS SALINE

The decision between a saline-filled prosthesis and a silicone gel implant is one of the patient's preference after the surgeon's conveyance of information. Experience has shown the results of silicone gel implants in primary breast augmentation to be generally soft and to have a natural feel and appearance, assuming capsule contracture is not present. Although the authors prefer silicone gel implants, saline implants placed in the subpectoral position can produce good results with a low incidence of capsule contracture. The thicker the soft tissue under which a saline implant is placed, the better it performs. Despite our preference for silicone gel, some patients will undoubtedly continue to have concerns about silicone-filled devices, and subpectoral saline implants have proved to be a reasonable alternative (Fig. 118-8). Ultimately, the patient must feel comfortable with the implant device, so the final decision rests with the patient.

TEXTURED VERSUS SMOOTH

The decision between textured and smooth-walled implants is only applicable for round implants. Anatomic implants are all textured by design to minimize malrotation. With round implants, the choice between textured and smooth-walled implants is based primarily on minimizing capsular contracture. For subpectoral augmentation, either implant can probably be used with comparable results. When the device is placed in the subglandular pocket, a smooth-walled implant offers the best protection from visible rippling and palpability but runs a greater risk for development of capsular contracture. A textured implant can be used in the subglandular position, but it should be reserved for those patients with adequate soft tissue coverage such that it will not be visible or easily palpable.

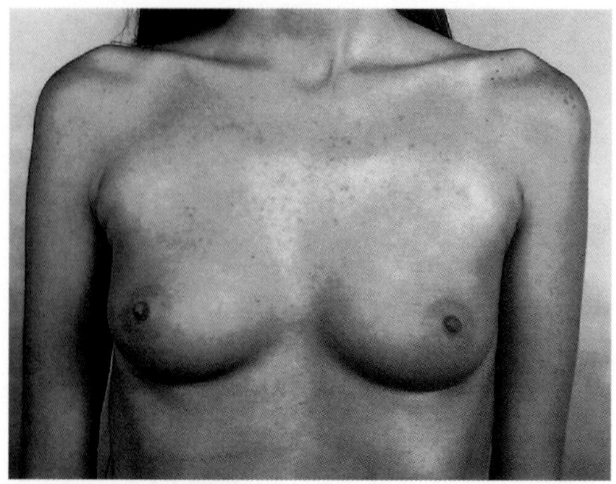

A

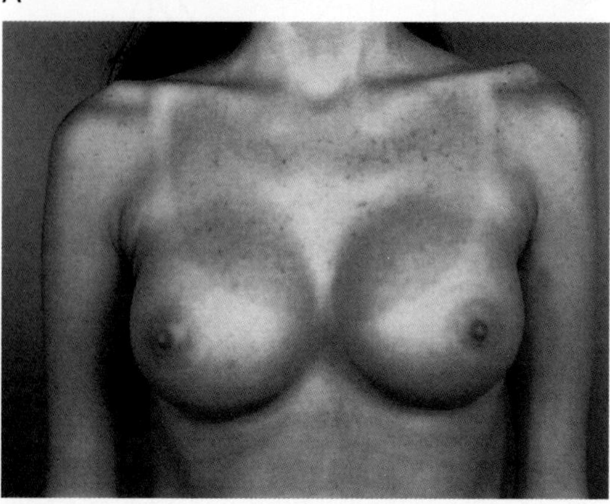

B

FIGURE 118-8. *A,* A typical patient presenting for breast augmentation. *B,* Postoperative result with subpectorally positioned, smooth saline implants (275 mL filled to 300 mL) placed through an inframammary incision.

ANATOMIC VERSUS ROUND

The decision between anatomic implants and round implants is determined by the shape and form of the existing breast. If a patient has hypovolemic breasts with good natural shape, form, and contour, round implants will provide the desired final result with the lowest risk of complications. By augmentation of volume while shape is maintained, a natural result is attainable (Fig 118-9*A*). In a patient who would benefit from having the form and shape of her breasts improved in addition to volumetric enhancement, an anatomic implant is preferable. Breast parenchymal maldistributions can be corrected, with a more aesthetically pleasing result (Fig. 118-9*B*).

POCKET SELECTION

The decision of subglandular or subpectoral implant placement depends on implant selection (fill and texture) and tissue thickness. In theory, the best position for a mammary implant is in the subglandular plane. This is the most anatomically correct position to maintain natural shape and form. The reasons for placement of implants in the subpectoral plane are to minimize the risk of capsular contracture (primarily for gel implants) and to minimize implant visibility and palpability. Other considerations relate to possible effects on mammography and tissue stretch over time. There are benefits and tradeoffs to each site (Table 118-3). In practice, saline implants are predominantly placed in the subpectoral pocket because of their ease of palpability and visibility. Silicone gel implant placement is determined largely by soft tissue adequacy. In patients with a pinch test result of more than 2 cm, the implant can safely be placed in the subglandular plane (Fig. 118-10). Previous data suggest that textured gel implants have a lower rate of capsular contracture when they are placed subglandularly. If one chooses smooth gel implants for the subglandular plane, additional measures to prevent capsular contracture must be taken. These include larger pocket dissections with displacement exercises or possible dilute steroid pocket irrigation (Fig. 118-11*A*). Anatomic-shaped textured implants are placed in the appropriate pocket as determined by soft tissue thickness. Pockets for these implants are made only minimally larger than the footprint of the device to minimize displacement or malrotation (Figs. 118-11*B*, 118-12, and 118-13).

When subpectoral pockets are selected (Fig. 118-14), one generally divides the origin of the pectoralis major muscle just above the inframammary fold to allow better projection in the lower pole of the augmented breast and to maintain a natural inframammary fold. This places the superior portion of the implant in a subpectoral position while the inferior portion is subglandularly located. In constricted breasts (tuberous breasts) or ptotic breasts, for which more parenchymal surgical manipulation is necessary, or when there is a greater need for the implant to fill out the lower soft tissue envelope, more dissection between parenchyma and muscle will allow the muscle to cover less of the implant with a resultant greater subglandular implant coverage. Alternatively, the pectoral muscle can be divided at a higher level to give a similar result. These pocket manipulations have been described as dual-plane maneuvers to allow varying degrees of subpectoral to subglandular implant coverage (Table 118-4).[84]

An additional pocket more recently introduced and advanced by some is the subpectoral fascial pocket. This thin layer of tough tissue is said by some to offer the advantage of subglandular placement with a thicker soft tissue cover.[84a]

Text continued on p. 19

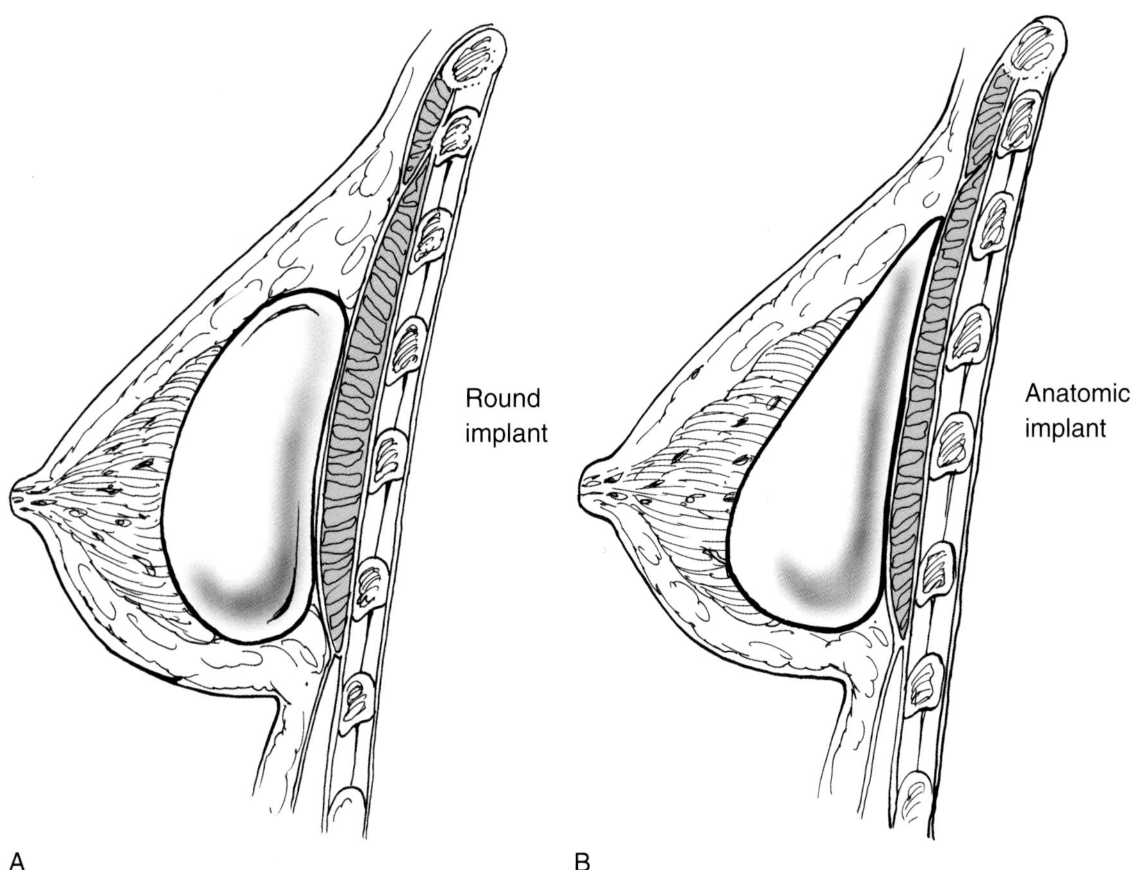

FIGURE 118-9. *A,* When the preoperative breast has an acceptable form and inadequate volume, a round implant may be preferable to achieve the desired result. *B,* When the breast form and volume are inadequate, an anatomic-shaped implant may be preferable.

TABLE 118-3 ✦ ALTERNATIVE POCKET LOCATIONS WITH POTENTIAL TRADEOFFS

Pocket	Tradeoffs	Potential Benefits
Retromammary	Increased risk of edge visibility or palpability Possible increased interference with mammography Possible increased incidence of capsular contracture	Increased control of breast shape Usually a more rapid postoperative recovery Minimal or no distortion with pectoralis contraction Increased control of inframammary fold position and shape
Partial retropectoral (*without* dividing pectoralis origins along the inframammary fold)	Lateral implant displacement over time, widening the space between the breasts Less control of upper medial fill More postoperative tenderness and a more prolonged recovery Distortion of breast shape with pectoralis contraction Less precise control of inframammary fold position, depth, and configuration. This potential tradeoff is minimized or eliminated by division of pectoralis origins along the inframammary fold in patients who have adequate soft tissue coverage. Increased risk of superior implant malposition or displacement (when inferior pectoralis origins across inframammary fold are *not* divided) Longer time required for deepening of the inframammary fold (when pectoralis origins along the inframammary fold are *not* divided)	Muscle coverage mandatory if pinch thickness <2 cm above breast parenchyma Possibly more accurate mammograms Less risk of palpable or visible implant edges Possible decreased risk of capsular contracture (small difference with saline-filled implants, greater difference with silicone gel–filled implants)
Total submuscular	All tradeoffs listed above for partial retropectoral, plus: Highest risk of superior implant displacement or malposition Longer operative time Longest postoperative recovery and morbidity Least accurate and predictable inframammary fold and longest to achieve depth Greatest risk of inframammary fold irregularities, lateral flattening, and fold level inaccuracies	Possible increased coverage inferolaterally but clinically no significant additional cover long term

From Tebbetts JB: Dual plane breast augmentation: optimizing implant–soft tissue relationships in a wide range of breast types. Plast Reconstr Surg 2001;107:1255.

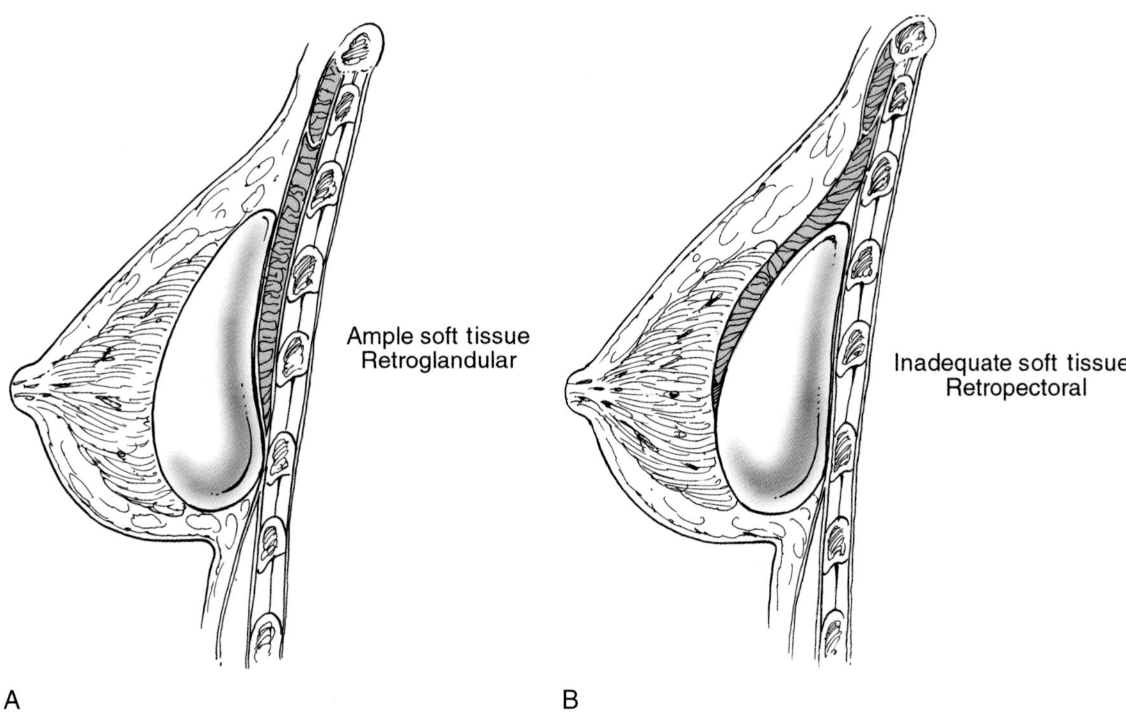

FIGURE 118-10. *A,* When ample soft tissue is present, implants may be placed in the subglandular position. *B,* When there is soft tissue inadequacy, the subpectoral position is generally preferable.

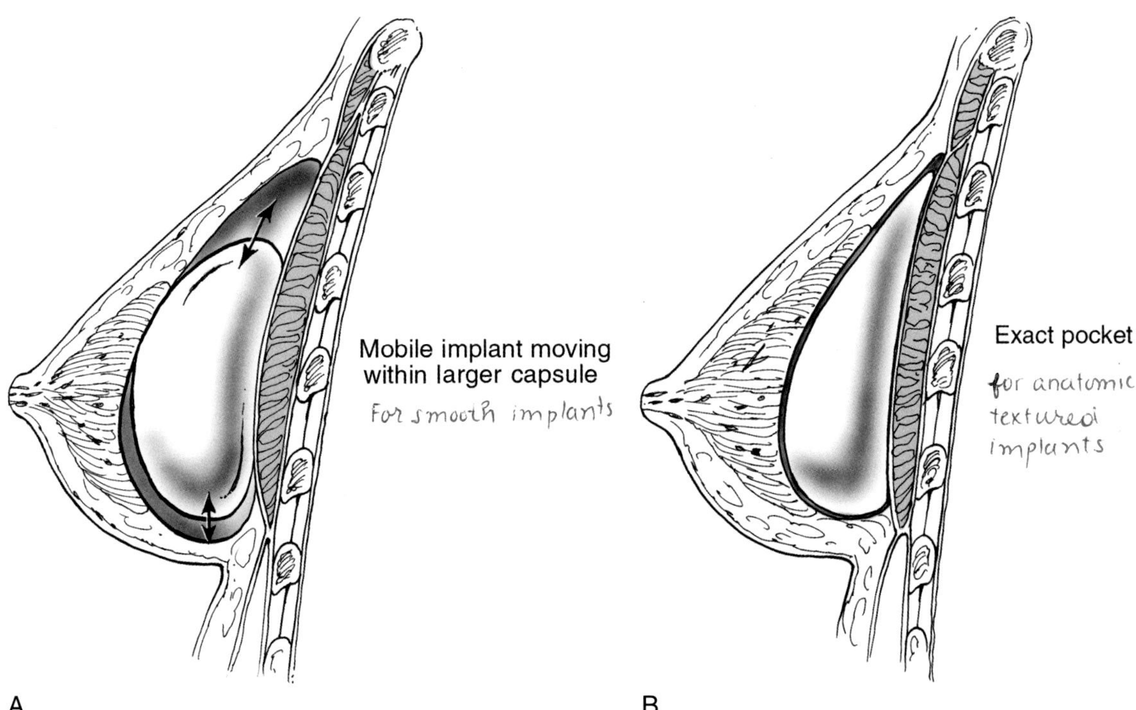

FIGURE 118-11. *A,* Round pocket dissection for smooth-surfaced implants to allow tissue redraping and encourage implant mobility to minimize capsule contracture. *B,* Precise pockets only slightly larger than the base of an anatomic textured implant help maintain implant position. Movement is not desirable when the implant allows immobility with softness.

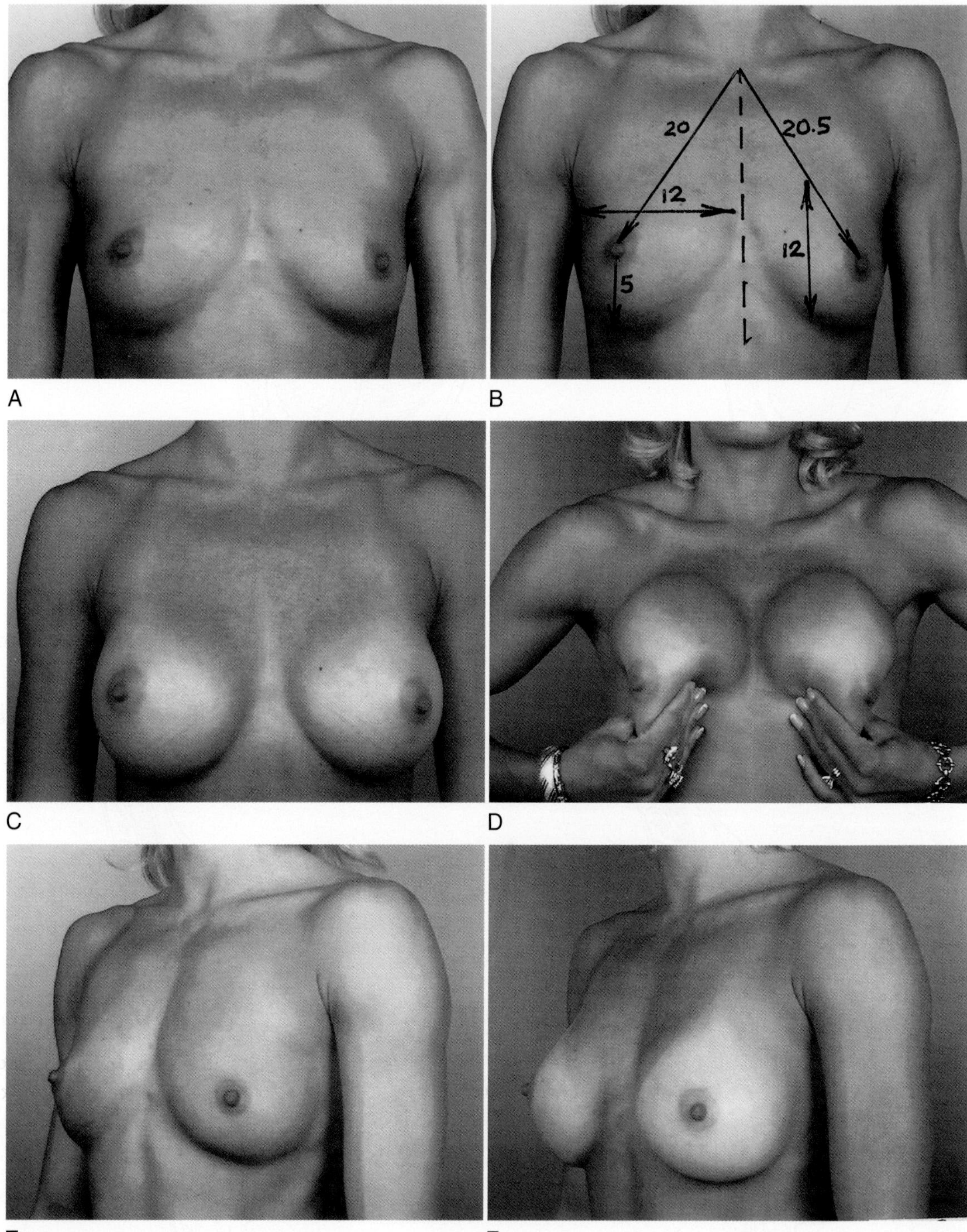

FIGURE 118-12. *A,* The biodimensional approach is demonstrated in this physically fit patient wishing no pectoral flexion distortion. *B,* Minor chest-breast asymmetries are noted on examination. *C,* Result with subglandular placement of smooth, 240-mL (width of 10.5 cm) round, silicone gel implants. *D,* The subglandular pocket selected because of her athleticism requires smooth implant displacement exercises within the large pocket to minimize capsule contracture. *E* and *F,* Oblique preoperative and postoperative appearance.

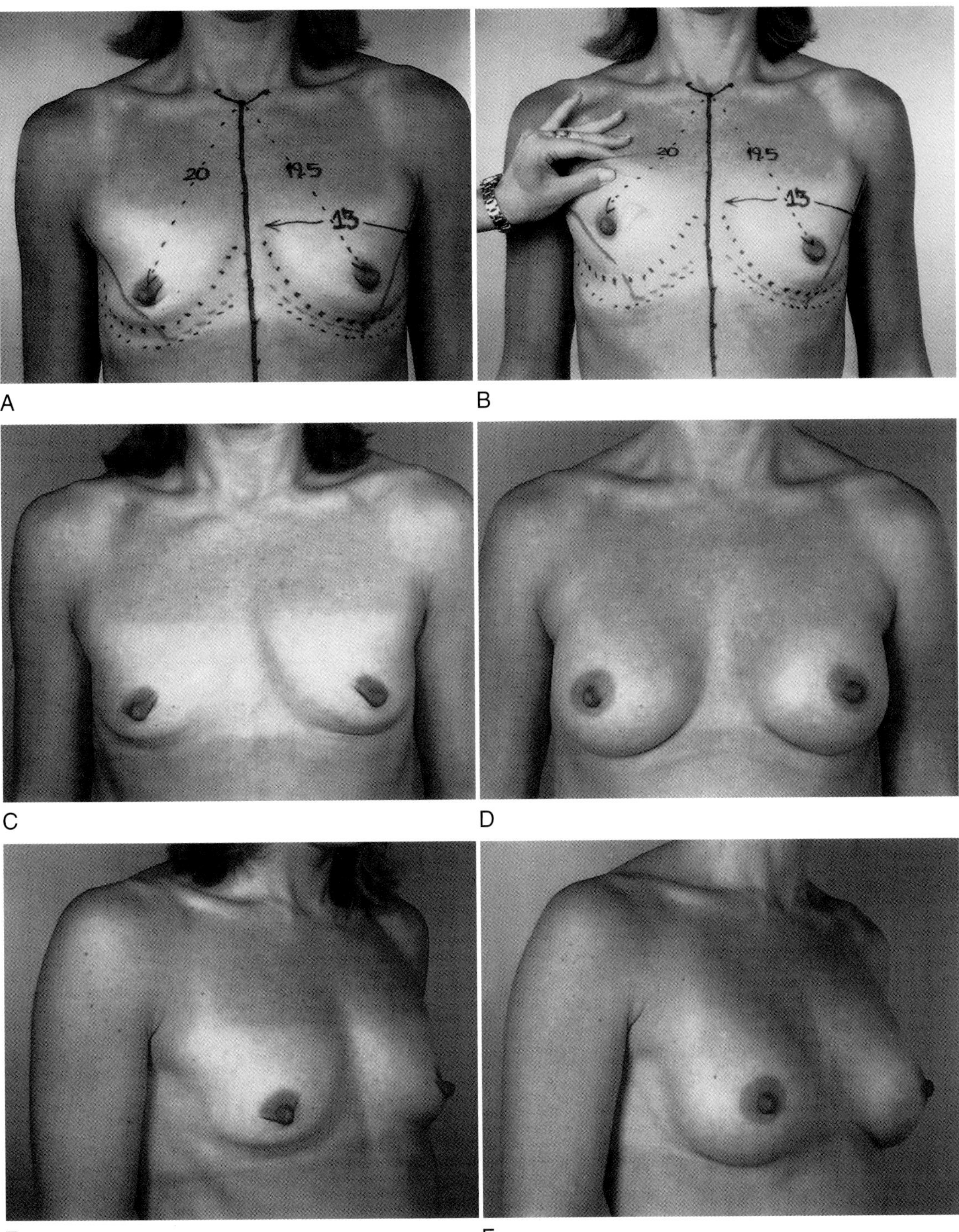

FIGURE 118-13. A biodimensional approach is demonstrated in this postpartum patient desiring a natural proportionate appearance. *A,* N-SSN and BW measurements are noted. *B,* The soft tissue pinch test result is 1.5 cm. *C* and *D,* Preoperative and postoperative photographs; style 410 MM cohesive gel implants were placed in precise subpectoral pockets through an inframammary incision. On the patient's right, a 245-mL implant (11.5-cm width and 10.6-cm height) was used; on the patient's left, a 215-mL implant (11-cm width and 10.1-cm height) was used. *E* and *F,* Oblique views of preoperative and postoperative appearance.

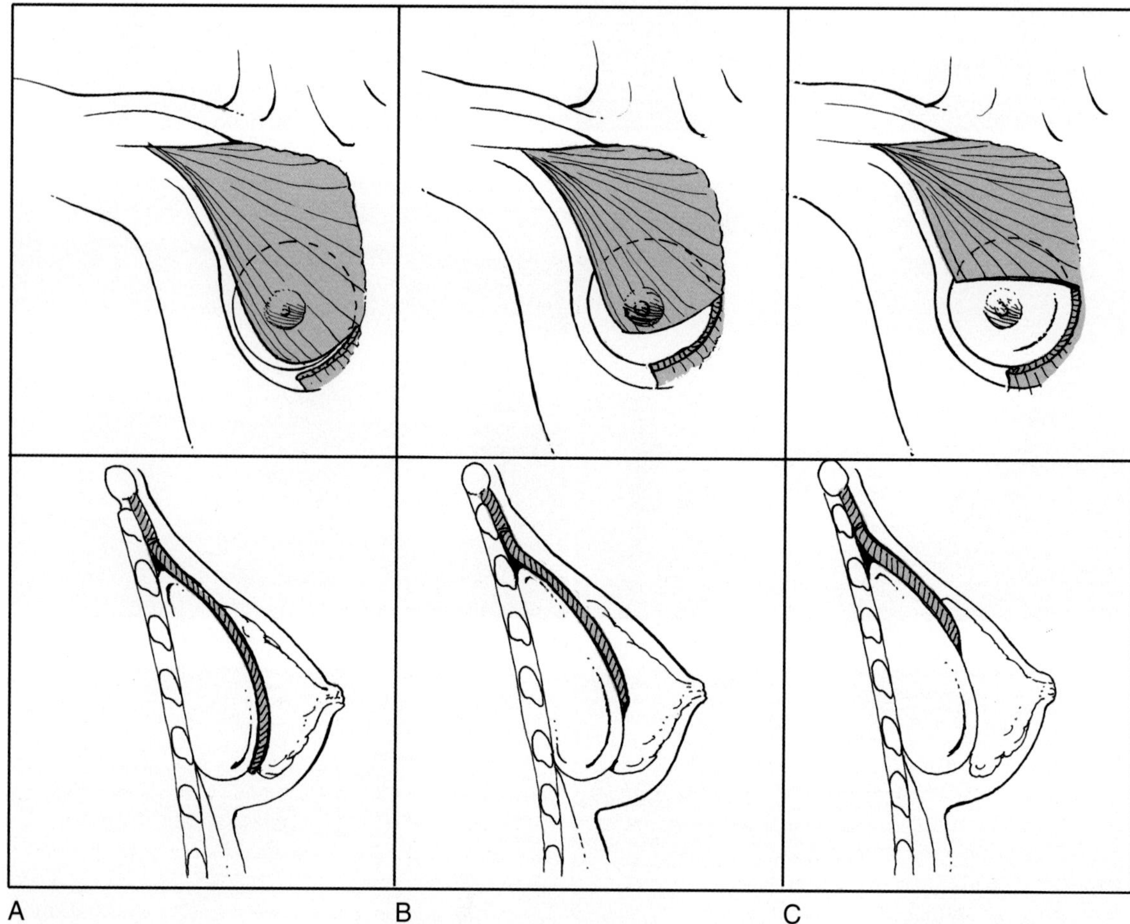

FIGURE 118-14. Subpectoral implant placement generally involves release or division of the pectoralis major muscle, resulting in varying coverage relationships of muscles and parenchyma to implant. *A,* Muscle division near the inframammary fold results in muscle coverage of most of the implant. *B,* Muscle division (or muscle-parenchymal detachment) to the lower areolar level results in muscle coverage of the upper half of the implant. *C,* Muscle division (or muscle-parenchymal detachment) to the upper areolar level results in muscle coverage of the upper third of the implant.

TABLE 118-4 ✦ POTENTIAL BENEFITS AND TRADEOFFS OF THE DUAL-PLANE POCKET LOCATION

Pocket	Tradeoffs	Potential Benefits
Dual plane (compared with retromammary)		Preserves the potential increased control of lower breast shape with retromammary With proper techniques can have similar recovery as with retromammary Reduced risk of edge visibility or palpability of retromammary by providing more upper pole coverage Reduced interference with mammography by retromammary Reduced possibility of capsular contracture of retromammary by reducing contact with parenchyma compared with retromammary
Dual plane (compared with partial retropectoral)	Possible increased risk of palpable or visible implant edges inferiorly	Provides same mandatory muscle coverage if pinch thickness <2 cm above breast parenchyma Reduced risk of lateral implant displacement over time; dividing inferior origins decreases pectoralis pressure on implant Better control of upper medial fill with division of inferior origins to decrease pectoralis tension and pressure on upper pole of implant Reduced postoperative tenderness and recovery period with proper technique Reduced distortion of breast shape with pectoralis contraction Decreased risk of superior implant malposition or displacement by decreasing pressure of pectoralis on lower pole of implant by dividing lower pectoralis origins Increased control of inframammary fold position, depth, and configuration by decreasing pressure of pectoralis on lower pole of implant along inframammary fold Retains possibility of more accurate mammograms, depending on position of muscle Possible decreased risk of capsular contracture (small)

From Tebbetts JB: Dual plane breast augmentation: optimizing implant–soft tissue relationships in a wide range of breast types. Plast Reconstr Surg 2001;107:1255.

INCISIONS

Four types of incision are commonly employed in breast augmentation: transaxillary, inframammary, periareolar, and transumbilical. After implant selection, the decision as to which type of incision is to be used should be made by the patient and surgeon after the options, risks, and benefits of each have been thoroughly explained. Surgeons should offer only the techniques that they are comfortable performing. The final choice should allow the surgeon optimal control and visualization to deliver the desired outcome for the specific patient and the specific implant (Table 118-5).

The inframammary incision permits complete visualization of either the prepectoral or subglandular pocket and allows precise placement of virtually all implants. The technique does leave a visible scar within the inframammary fold. Smaller incisions (<3 cm) can be used for saline-filled implants, but silicone gel implants often require incisions up to 5.5 cm in length. The incision should be placed in the projected inframammary fold rather than in the existing fold to avoid visibility and widening of the subsequent scar (Fig. 118-15).

The periareolar incision is placed at the areolar-cutaneous juncture and generally heals inconspicuously. The dissection allows easy adjustment of the inframammary fold and direct access to the lower parenchyma for scoring and release when a constricted lower pole is present. Disadvantages include limited exposure of the surgical field, transection of the parenchymal ducts (which are often colonized with *Staphylococcus epidermidis*), potentially increased risk of nipple sensitivity changes, and visible scarring on the breast mound. This technique should not routinely be used on patients with an areola diameter less than 40 mm and may not allow introduction of larger gel or enhanced cohesive gel implants.

The transaxillary approach can be performed either bluntly or with the aid of an endoscope. The endoscope allows precise dissection and release of the inferior musculofascial attachments of the pectoralis major as well as direct visualization for hemostasis. This approach avoids any scarring on the breast mound and can be used with both saline and gel

TABLE 118-5 ✦ INCISION OPTIONS IN BREAST AUGMENTATION

Factor	Axillary	Periareolar	Inframammary	Periumbilical*
Implant plane				
Submuscular	+	+	+	–
Subglandular	–	+	+	+
Implant type				
Saline round	+	+	+	+
Saline shaped	–	+	+	–
Silicone round/shaped	–	+	+	–
Preoperative breast volume				
High (>200 g)	+	+	+	+
Low (<200 g)	+	+	–	+
Preoperative breast base position				
High	+	+	+	+
Low	–	+	+	+
Breast shape				
Tubular	–	+	–	–
Glandular ptosis	+	+	+	+
Ptosis (grade I-II)	–	+	–	–
Areolar characteristics				
Small diameter	+	–	+	+
Light/indistinct	+	–	+	+
Inframammary crease				
None	+	+	–	+
High	+	+	–	+
Low	+	+	+	+
Secondary procedure	–	+	+	–

+ indicates applicable; – indicates not generally recommended.
* Included for completeness but not generally recommended.
From Hidalgo DA: Breast augmentation: choosing the optimal incision, implant, and pocket plane. Plast Reconstr Surg 2000;105:2202.

implants in either a subpectoral or subglandular pocket. Disadvantages include difficulty with parenchymal alterations and the probable need for a second incision on the breast mound for revisionary surgery. Precise implant placement can be more difficult with this incision, and enhanced cohesive gel and anatomic implants may be precluded.

Transumbilical breast augmentation has the obvious advantage of a single, well-hidden, remote incision. It can be used only with saline implants, however, and precise pocket dissection requires experience. The pocket is dissected bluntly, and hemostasis can be difficult from the remote access port. As with the transaxillary approach, revisions often necessitate a second incision on the breast mound.

Technique

INFRAMAMMARY INCISION

The patient is marked preoperatively in the standing or seated position, with shoulders even and arms resting comfortably at her sides. The midline of the chest is marked as a point of reference from the sternal notch to the xiphoid process. The existing inframammary folds are marked, as are the proposed limits of the dissection. The incision site is marked along the expected new inframammary fold after augmentation. Frequently, augmentation mammaplasty will lower the existing inframammary fold, and this must be taken into account when the patient is marked. The resultant location of the inframammary fold is determined by the dimensions of the selected implant postoperatively in interaction with the existing tissues. The incision should begin on a straight line dropped from the medial areolar border and extend laterally. For saline implants, a 3-cm incision is often sufficient, whereas silicone gel implants require incisions 4 cm or more in length; enhanced cohesive implants may require 5.5- to 6-cm incisions (Fig. 118-16).

Proper positioning of the patient is important to the outcome of the procedure. The patient is placed in the supine position, well centered on the operating room table. Her arms should be at 90-degree angles to her torso and well secured to fixed arm boards. The patient must be able to flex fully at the waist to 90 degrees during the procedure (Fig. 118-17). Finally, the patient's shoulders must be visible after sterile draping to ensure symmetry when the intraoperative appearance is evaluated. The incision sites are injected with 2 to 3 mL of 1% lidocaine with 1:1000 dilution of epinephrine to aid in hemostasis.

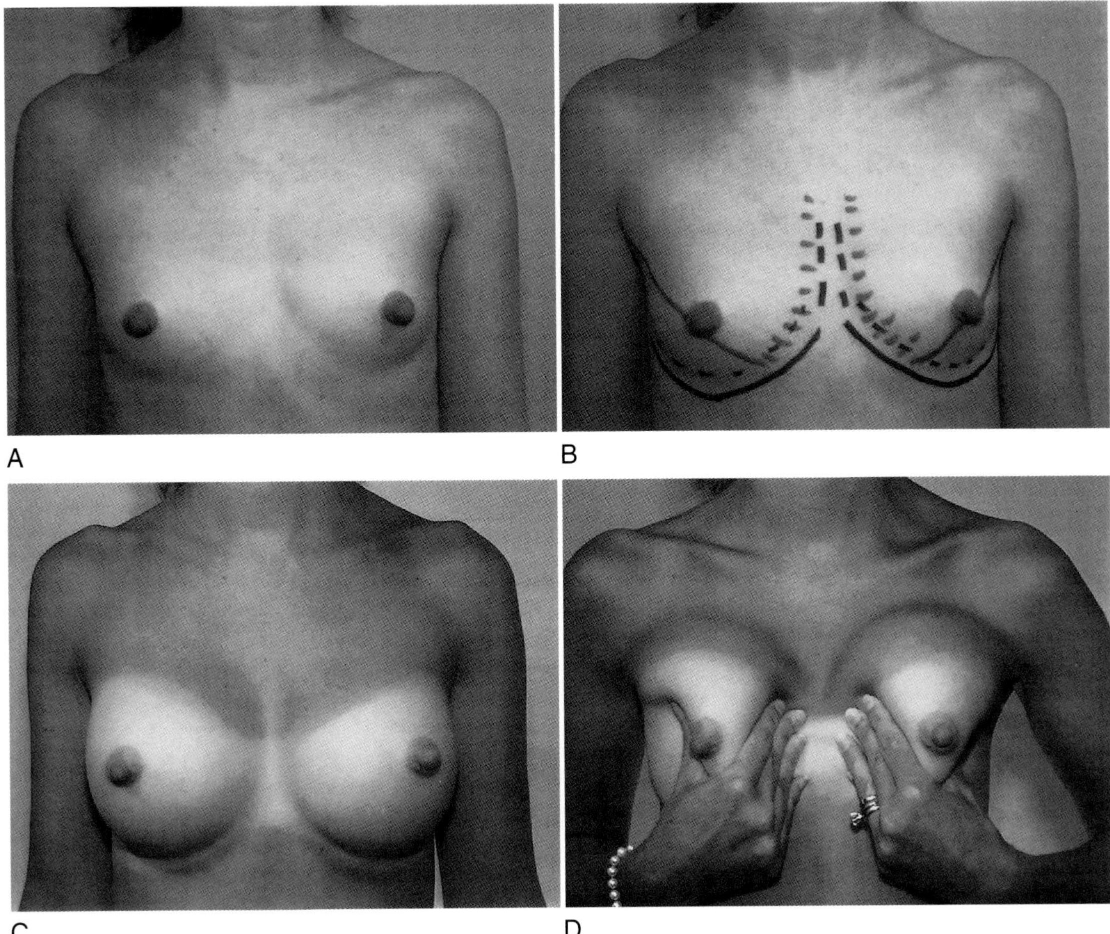

FIGURE 118-15. *A,* A small-breasted woman with a soft tissue pinch test result of less than 2 cm desirous of full, round result. *B,* A 340-mL round, smooth, silicone gel implant is selected, which will be placed in the subpectoral position after the inframammary fold is lowered 1.5 cm. The inframammary incision will be 4.5 cm in length and placed in the new lowered inframammary fold location. *C* and *D,* The patient's postoperative appearance.

The incision is made along the proposed markings, and the dissection is continued with an insulated electrocautery instrument through Scarpa fascia. A fiberoptic headlight is worn throughout the procedure, or a variety of lighted fiberoptic retractors are available to aid illumination and direct visualization within the pocket. If the implant is to be placed in the subglandular pocket, the dissection proceeds above the pectoralis major fascia directly beneath the gland. Meticulous hemostasis can be maintained during the complete dissection with the use of the electrocautery. Several medial intercostal perforating vessels may be encountered. These should be avoided or coagulated with insulated forceps if need be. For smooth-walled implants, a larger pocket is dissected to allow mobility of the implant. For anatomic implants, the pocket is precisely dissected to snugly accommodate the implant. Care should be taken to preserve the lateral intercostal cutaneous nerves, especially the fourth intercostal, which contains the primary sensory innervation of the nipple-areola complex.

If a subpectoral pocket is chosen, the dissection is initially carried out laterally to identify the lateral border of the pectoralis major muscle. The muscle edge can be lifted by forceps to allow easy entry into the submusculofascial plane. This plane is readily identified by the wispy areolar connective tissue and ease of dissection. An extended electrocautery instrument is used to complete the dissection. The inferior origin of the pectoralis major is released from lateral to medial at the level of the inframammary fold. Various slips of origin of the pectoralis major muscle are generally encountered and divided. Division of the pectoralis continues medially to the sternal border. Partial deep division may selectively be carried out 1 to 3 cm above the xiphoid, depending on which implant is to be used.

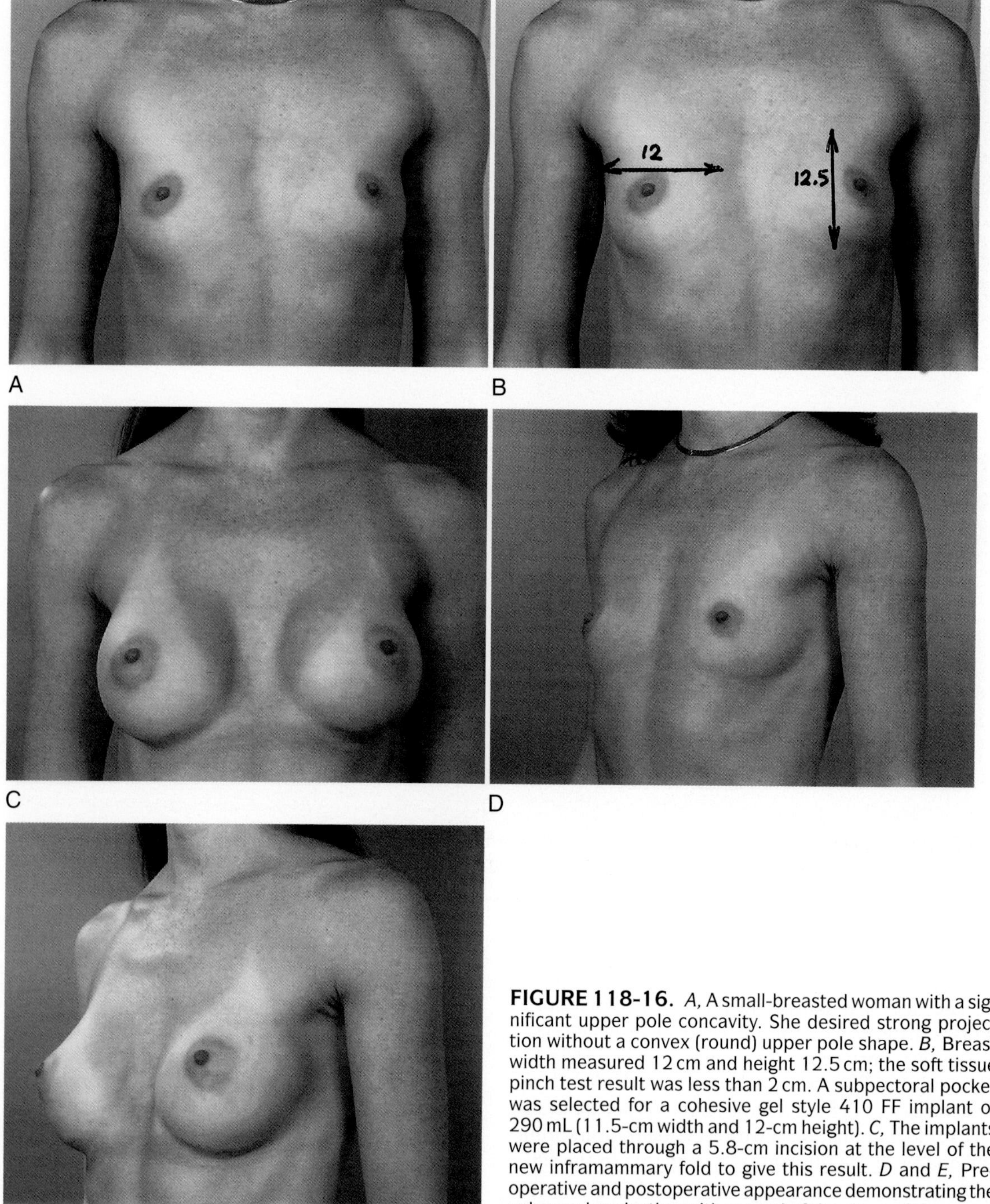

FIGURE 118-16. *A,* A small-breasted woman with a significant upper pole concavity. She desired strong projection without a convex (round) upper pole shape. *B,* Breast width measured 12 cm and height 12.5 cm; the soft tissue pinch test result was less than 2 cm. A subpectoral pocket was selected for a cohesive gel style 410 FF implant of 290 mL (11.5-cm width and 12-cm height). *C,* The implants were placed through a 5.8-cm incision at the level of the new inframammary fold to give this result. *D* and *E,* Preoperative and postoperative appearance demonstrating the enhanced projection with control of the slope of the upper pole.

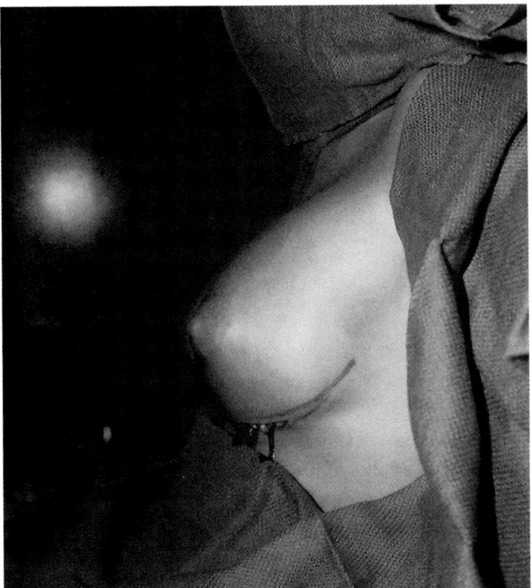

FIGURE 118-17. The operating table is flexed to a 90-degree angle intraoperatively to allow the surgeon to carefully evaluate the patient with the sizer or final implants in position before closure.

Lateral dissection can be done bluntly with a finger to avoid injury to the lateral neurovascular bundles. The nerves can be stretched to accommodate the implant but should be preserved to minimize postoperative sensory changes. When the pectoralis major muscle is elevated, care must be taken to leave the pectoralis minor down on the chest wall. This will minimize bleeding and allow proper placement of the implant.

Exact implant "sizers" (gel or saline) are used when available to evaluate the pockets and resultant breast form. After the sizers are in place, the patient is placed in a 90-degree upright position and evaluated from various perspectives (see Fig. 118-17). Any asymmetry or underdissected areas are marked, and the patient is placed back in the supine position. Once adequate hemostasis is obtained and pocket dimensions are finalized, the pocket is irrigated with an antibiotic-containing solution, and the implants are carefully placed by a minimal-touch technique. The final results are assessed, again with the patient in a sitting position, and a multilayer closure is performed with absorbable suture. It is important to close off the implant pocket with a separate layer of suture before closing the skin. Once closure is complete, SteriStrips are applied along the direction of the incisions.

PERIAREOLAR AUGMENTATION

The markings for a periareolar approach are similar to those for an inframammary augmentation. The patient is marked in a seated or standing position with even shoulder position. The sternal midline is marked as reference. The existing inframammary fold is marked, as are the limits of the dissection and the planned resultant inframammary fold (if it is to be changed). The incision is marked along the junction of the areola and the breast skin. The limits of the incision are the 3-o'clock and 9-o'clock positions.

The positioning of the patient is identical to that for an inframammary approach. It is imperative that the patient be able to fully flex at the waist for evaluation of the intraoperative appearance of the implants.

With the patient prepared and draped and after injection of lidocaine with epinephrine, the precise incision is made. Wound edges are elevated directly up from the chest wall with an opposing pair of small sharp retractors. An insulated electrocautery unit is used to dissect straight down through the breast parenchyma to the pectoralis major fascia. The retractors are repositioned as needed to keep the gland elevated into the wound. For subglandular implant placement, dissection is carried out on top of the pectoralis major and serratus anterior fasciae. Although it is preferable to use a fiberoptic headlight, fiberoptic retractor illumination can also facilitate the dissection by aiding visualization. The dissection is carried out to the extent of the preoperative markings with use of an extended electrocautery instrument, which allows meticulous hemostasis. If the inferior pole of the breast is constricted, radial scoring of the gland in the inferior pole can allow proper redraping of the soft tissue over the implant to correct the deformity (Fig. 118-18).

For subpectoral implant placement, an identical incision is made, but the dissection is carried down through the breast tissue in an oblique plane angled inferiorly, rather than directly through the gland. When the dissection plane approaches the inframammary fold, it is carried directly down to the pectoralis major fascia and continued laterally to identify the lateral border of the muscle. This is an easy area in which to begin the subpectoral dissection and ensure that the dissection planes are correct. The submuscular dissection is done under direct vision with use of the electrocautery, in a lateral to medial direction. The origin of the pectoralis major muscle onto the chest wall can then be divided. This release is done approximately 1 cm above the origin of the muscle fibers and proceeds from lateral to medial to allow adequate redraping of the muscle over the implant. This usually requires division of several medial slips of muscle that often contain perforating vessels. The endpoint of the dissection is adequate release of the pectoralis muscle, usually at the sternal border. Dual-plane techniques differ slightly despite which incision is used.

When the pocket is dry, sizers are used to evaluate the dissection and to determine the final prosthesis to

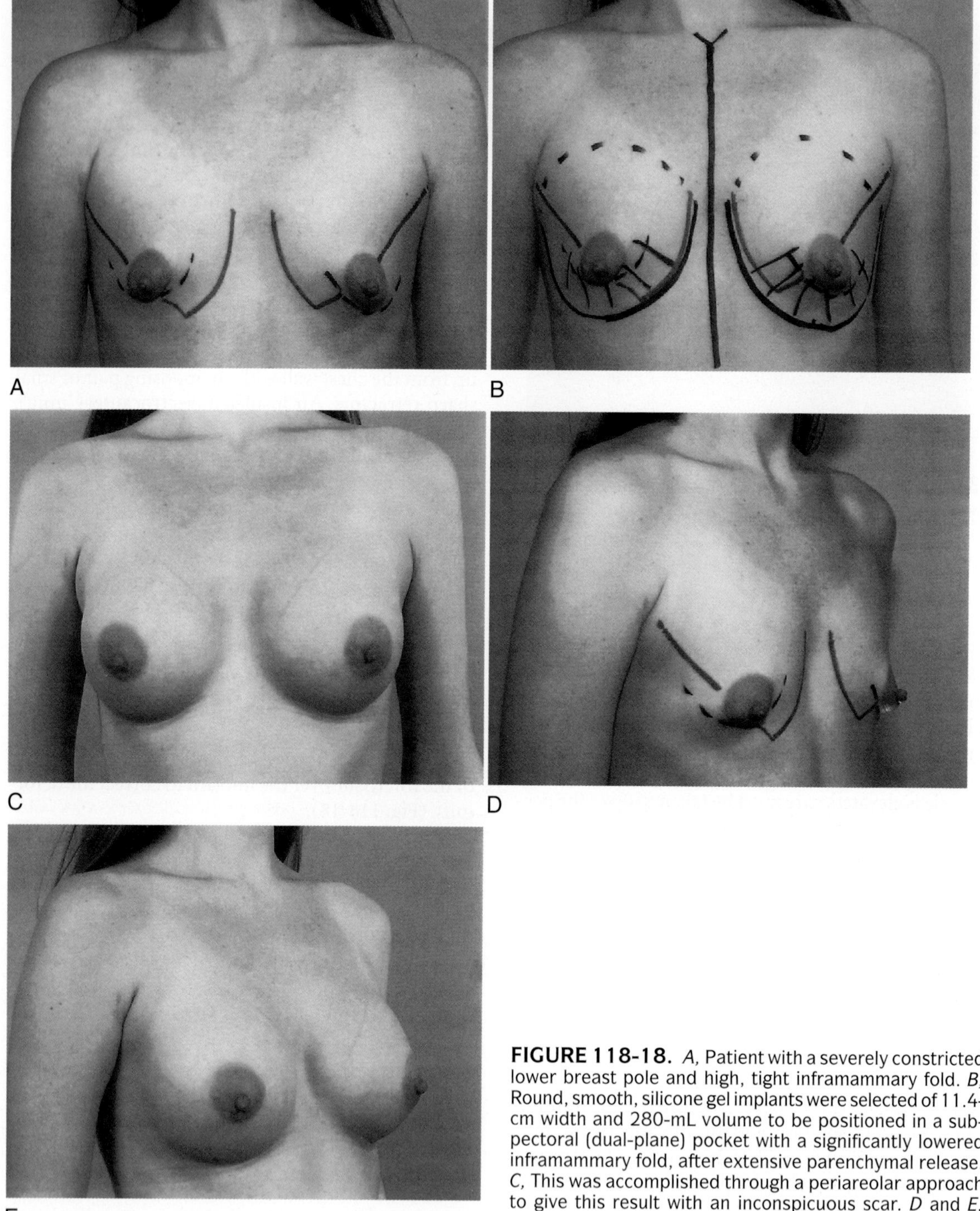

FIGURE 118-18. *A,* Patient with a severely constricted lower breast pole and high, tight inframammary fold. *B,* Round, smooth, silicone gel implants were selected of 11.4-cm width and 280-mL volume to be positioned in a subpectoral (dual-plane) pocket with a significantly lowered inframammary fold, after extensive parenchymal release. *C,* This was accomplished through a periareolar approach to give this result with an inconspicuous scar. *D* and *E,* Preoperative and postoperative appearance.

be implanted. Before final implant placement, the pocket is once again checked for hemostasis and irrigated with an antibiotic solution. The closure is particularly important with this technique. The gland must be precisely reapproximated and closed with several layers of interrupted absorbable sutures to prevent distortion of the nipple-areola complex. The skin is closed with deep everting dermal sutures and a running subcuticular absorbable monofilament. SteriStrips are applied to the closed incision.

TRANSAXILLARY AUGMENTATION

The markings for transaxillary breast augmentation are also made with the patient in the sitting or upright position. The existing and resultant inframammary folds are marked, as are the boundaries of the proposed dissection. To locate and mark the incision, the patient's arm is placed in complete adduction and the most anterior aspect of the axilla is marked. The incision should not extend beyond this line. The arm is then abducted approximately 45 degrees, and a prominent axillary crease is identified. Any fold may be used, but preference is given to one high in the axilla, which aids in instrumentation during the procedure. For saline-filled implants, the incision should generally be 2.5 to 3.5 cm. Silicone implants require larger incisions.

The patient is placed on the operating table in the supine position with arms abducted 90 degrees and secured to arm boards that allow 10- to 15-degree variations in abduction and adduction from 90 degrees. She must be able to flex 90 degrees at the waist during the procedure. After sterile preparation and draping, the incision is infiltrated with 1 to 2 mL of 1% lidocaine containing 1:1000 dilution of epinephrine. The breast parenchyma is then elevated from the chest wall by manual traction, and the inframammary fold and medial sternal border are infiltrated with 10 to 15 mL of the same lidocaine solution to aid hemostasis during the dissection.

The incision is made, and small sharp retractors are used to elevate the medial aspect of the incision. Superficial subcutaneous dissection to the lateral border of the pectoralis major prevents injury to the intercostobrachial nerve. Scissor dissection is employed with use of the electrocautery and insulated forceps to control any bleeding. The fascia of the pectoralis major muscle is visualized at the lateral edge of the muscle, and the dissection is carried deep to this, with care taken to identify the wispy areolar plane between the pectoralis major and the pectoralis minor. One must be certain the correct plane is entered before continuing the dissection further.

The subpectoral space is developed bluntly with either an Agris-Dingman breast dissector or a 36 French urethral sound. For a standard transaxillary augmentation, the origin of the pectoralis major muscle must be avulsed by the dissectors to allow release of the muscle from the chest wall to a point 1 to 2 cm up the medial aspect of the sternum. Complete division of all the muscle fibers is not always necessary.

For an endoscopically assisted augmentation, the endoscope is passed into the transaxillary tunnel, and the subpectoral space is seen under direct vision. This allows a more controlled release of the pectoralis major origin with a long insulated electrocautery instrument. The pectoralis muscle fibers are released approximately 1 cm above their origin along the inferior and inferomedial aspects. Meticulous hemostasis can be confirmed with the electrocautery, and drain tubes are seldom necessary.

On completion of the dissection, implant sizers are used to evaluate the pocket and identify any areas that need final adjustment. This must be done with the patient in the sitting position. The pockets are then irrigated with an antibiotic solution, and the final implants are inserted. Before closure, the patient is once again placed in the sitting position for a final check of the implant position. The pectoralis muscle fascia is repaired with a single absorbable suture, and the incision is closed in one or two layers. SteriStrips are applied to the incision.[85,86]

TRANSUMBILICAL BREAST AUGMENTATION

The markings for transumbilical breast augmentation are similar to those for a standard inframammary fold approach. The patient is marked in the seated or standing position. The existing inframammary fold is marked, as are the limits of the proposed dissection. The midline is marked for reference.

The patient is placed on the operating table in the same manner as for an inframammary augmentation. An additional mark is made with the patient supine: a line is drawn from the umbilicus to the medial border of the areola bilaterally. An incision is made within the umbilicus, large enough to easily accommodate an index finger. An endotube with a blunt obturator is passed just above the rectus fascia along the line from the umbilicus to the areola. Care is taken to constantly palpate the progress of the obturator with the surgeon's other hand, always keeping the force up and away from the abdominal and thoracic cavities. The endotube is advanced over the costal margin. For subglandular implant placement, the force applied to the endotube is directed upward at the inframammary fold to prevent the obturator from slipping beneath the pectoralis major. The tunnel ends just cephalad to the nipple. Subpectoral positioning is possible by careful technique with use of special instruments to enter the fascial plane high laterally.

The obturator is then removed, and an endoscope may be used to verify correct pocket identification. Hemostasis is also ensured. Both the endotube and endoscope are removed from the tunnel, and an expander is rolled up and placed within the incision. The expander is "milked" up the tunnel by manual external pressure. The expander is filled with saline to 150% of the final volume of the implant. Pocket adjustments can be made manually during filling.

When the expansion is complete, the expander is drained and removed from the pocket by traction on the fill tube. The implant is placed and filled in exactly the same manner as the expander. The endotube is then replaced, and an endoscope may be used to verify implant position, valve patency, and hemostasis. The incision is closed with a single layer of absorbable suture. An ABD pad is placed over each breast, and an elastic bandage is wrapped tightly around the upper chest to compress the upper pole of the breast. An abdominal binder is used for compression on the abdominal tunnels.

Postoperative Care

Breast augmentation, when it is performed as a single procedure, is done on an outpatient basis. Patients are discharged with oral analgesics and 3 days of an oral first-generation cephalosporin. They are allowed to take the dressings down (when applied) on the first postoperative day and shower as desired. The first follow-up visit is scheduled for 3 to 5 days after the procedure. If smooth-walled implants were used, implant placement exercises are initiated at this time. If there is any suggestion of the upward implant positioning, a circumferential upper pole elastic wrap is initiated to provide downward pressure.

Patients are usually able to return to work in the first few days after surgery but are not permitted to return to rigorous exercise for 2 to 3 weeks. They are seen again at 4 to 6 weeks, 3 months, and 1 year for follow-up and photographs. Beyond 1 year, visits are scheduled as needed, but patients should be seen every several years.

CLINICAL ISSUES

Capsular Contracture

Capsular contracture results from an exaggerated scar response to a foreign prosthetic material. All surgical implants undergo some degree of encapsulation, but clinical problems arise when this scar formation becomes excessive, much in the same way as hypertrophic and keloid scars represent the unchecked proliferation of the normal healing process. Baker[87] proposed a clinical classification system in 1975 that remains the most commonly used reporting system (Table 118-6).

Capsular contracture remains the most common complication of breast augmentation, with rates reported between 0.5% and 30%. As such, the evolution of breast augmentation mammaplasty has been driven by the need to prevent the development of capsular contracture. The first Dow Corning teardrop-shaped smooth-surfaced silicone implants were found to have an unacceptably high rate of capsular contracture. These implants were placed in a retroglandular position and fixed in place by a Dacron patch on the posterior aspect of the device. The first advancement in prosthetic design was the removal of the Dacron patch with the belief that the Dacron was initiating an inflammatory response resulting in formation of a capsule around the implant. When this failed to sufficiently lower the rate of capsule formation, smooth round devices with thinner shells and less viscous silicone gel were developed. Displacement exercises and implant massage were advocated. Although the rate of capsular contracture was improved, these implants were complicated by high rates of rupture and bleed.

The double-lumen implant was developed with the idea that capsule formation was inevitable. With a larger outer saline-filled lumen, the capsule could be allowed to form and the outer lumen drained, leaving a large pocket for a soft gel implant.[24]

In the late 1970s, the thinking began to shift away from the prosthetic device to the surgical technique. Implant placement moved from the subglandular position to the subpectoral position. This was done in the belief that the active contraction of the pectoralis major muscle would provide internal massage of the implant, maintaining its pocket and ensuring its softness. Subsequent research has confirmed a significant decrease in capsular contracture by this surgical approach.[88-91] With the devices available at the time, the key to maintaining implant softness was to allow implant mobility within the breast pocket. This remained true until the advent of textured surface implants.

In 1970, Ashley[27] introduced the polyurethane-coated silicone breast implant, the use of which became popular in the United States in the 1980s. A dramatic decrease in capsular contracture to less than 3% was noted in multiple studies.[92-94] The polyurethane was found to delaminate from the surface of the implant during the course of the first few months and favorably affect the collagen orientation in the devel-

TABLE 118-6 ✦ BAKER CLASSIFICATION OF CAPSULAR FIRMNESS IN AUGMENTED BREASTS

Grade I	No palpable capsule	The augmented breast feels as soft as a natural one.
Grade II	Minimal firmness	The breast is less soft; the implant can be palpated, but it is not visible.
Grade III	Moderate firmness	The breast is harder; the implant can be palpated easily, and it (or distortion from it) can be seen.
Grade IV	Severe contracture	The breast is hard, tender, painful, and cold. Distortion is often marked.

oping periprosthetic space.[95] This allowed the implant to remain soft in a pocket that does not undergo any significant degree of contracture. Thus, it was possible to have an immobile implant that remained soft in a fixed pocket. A large study demonstrated that there was no statistical significance between the rates of capsular contracture whether the prosthesis was placed in a subpectoral or a subglandular plane.[32] This type of implant became popular with many plastic surgeons until it was removed from the U.S. market in early 1991 because of concerns about the potential toxicity of polyurethane breakdown products.

Another method to alter the tissue interface by use of the prosthetic surface evolved with silicone implant surface texturing. By the application of various methods of surface texturing to silicone implants, thinner and more pliable capsules were formed that had increased resiliency and a lower likelihood of contracture (see section entitled "Evolution of Mammary Implants"). Multiple studies have confirmed that textured surfaces significantly decrease or delay the occurrence of capsular contracture for silicone gel implants placed in a retroglandular position.[96-100] The data are less clear with retroglandular saline-filled devices.[40,43,101,102]

With the restriction of silicone gel implants in 1992, the implant manufacturers made the rapid transition to enhanced production of various saline-filled implants. The silicone implant data were extrapolated to the saline device, and textured saline implants were initially popular. One observed benefit of the saline-filled devices was a significant decrease in rates of capsular contracture[103-106]; however, problems were seen with widespread use of these devices, including palpable shell folding or "knuckling," visible rippling, and palpability. Many of these problems could be minimized by subpectoral implant placement. This resulted in the preferred use by a majority of American surgeons of round, smooth-walled, saline-filled implants placed in a subpectoral pocket. Whereas capsular contracture rates were minimized, so was the surgeon's ability to control shape and form.

ETIOLOGY

Despite extensive research, the cause of capsular contracture remains unknown. Two main theories address the underlying cause: subclinical infection and hypertrophic scarring.

Hypertrophic scarring is thought to be secondary to a hematoma, seroma, or silicone gel bleed. The most likely mechanism involves stimulation of the myofibroblasts, which have been shown to be present in the walls of the capsule.[107] An increase in the myofibroblast activity leads to subsequent scarring and contracture of the capsule. The stimulus may be silicone gel particles that have bled through the shell[108,109] or silicone that is derived from the shell itself.[110] However, despite numerous studies, no correlation has been shown between the number of myofibroblasts or the presence of silicone particles in the capsule and the hardness of the capsule.[111,112] Hematomas and seromas have been implicated in the stimulation of myofibroblast activity. Undrained hematomas have been shown to induce capsular contracture in an animal model[113]; however, the data have not been transferable to human studies. Foreign bodies such as dust, lint, and glove powder may also incite the inflammatory process.

There has been much research into an infectious process leading to capsular contracture. Often, this is secondary to a subclinical infection by normal skin flora, most notably *S. epidermidis*. In a rabbit model, inoculation with *S. epidermidis* was shown to induce thicker capsules than in control animals.[114] Numerous studies have linked subclinical infection with an increased incidence of capsular contracture.[115,116] Further studies showed a reduction in early capsule formation (within the first 3 months of surgery) with the use of local antibacterial agents, suggesting at least an early link to an infectious process.[117]

A theory relating to the infectious process suggests that a biofilm forming on the breast implant surface harbors the causative organism (usually *S. epidermidis*). The agent can be identified only by special techniques, which explains why routine swabs of the encapsulated pocket are frequently culture negative. This theory would suggest appropriate treatment to be total capsulectomy or site drainage and a new mammary prosthesis (not contaminated with the biofilm).[118]

PREVENTION

Much of the history of breast augmentation prosthetics and techniques has centered on prevention of capsular contracture. There is still no definitive solution; however, there are many proposed methods of reducing the risk of capsule formation. Saline implants have been shown to have a significantly lower rate of contracture than silicone gel implants when they are placed in either the subglandular or submuscular position.[119-123] Unfortunately, most of these data relate to older "high-bleed" silicone gel implants, and the data may not extrapolate to the newer more cohesive styles of gel implants.

Textured implants have been used to prevent capsular contracture, but there are conflicting reports throughout the literature as to their efficacy. Clearly, studies have shown the protective effect of texturing on gel implants, but there are conflicting data on the effect of texturing on subglandular saline implants.

Surgical placement of the prosthesis in a retropectoral pocket has repeatedly been proved to decrease the risk of capsular contracture.[88-90] This has led many surgeons to preferentially use the subpectoral plane for both primary augmentations and treatment of established subglandular capsular contracture.

Antibiotic irrigation of the implant pocket arose in response to the infectious theory of the cause of capsular contracture.[117] Betadine (5% povidone-iodine) has been shown to effectively control the bacterial colonization around an implant and to decrease the risk of capsular contracture. However, the FDA issued a caution concerning the use of Betadine irrigation with saline implants in the spring of 2000. Betadine, in direct contact with the implant, was thought to cause weakening of the implant shell, which could lead to higher rates of deflation of saline-filled implants. Critical scrutiny has not supported this claim; however, many surgeons were forced to choose alternative methods of bacterial control in the augmentation pocket. Current recommendations include a solution containing 50,000 units of bacitracin, 1 g of cefazolin, and 80 mg of gentamicin in 500 mL of normal saline.[124]

Other attempts to reduce bacterial contamination include a minimal-touch or "no-touch" technique.[125] In this technique, only the surgeon handles the implant with fresh powder-free gloves. The device is then inserted either through a sterile plastic sleeve or into a pocket where the skin has been prepared again with an antibiotic solution.

In an attempt to control bleeding and fluid formation around the implant, blunt dissection should be avoided when possible, maximizing the amount of dissection done under direct vision with an electrocautery unit and ensuring maximum hemostasis before placement of the implant. Primary augmentation mammaplasty should not routinely require the use of drainage catheters. Copious saline irrigation should be used to flush the pocket when bleeding is encountered during the dissection. Meticulous attention to hemostasis during the dissection is the best prevention against bleeding complications.

Corticosteroids have been used both intraluminally and within the implant pocket, with good results.[126] Rates of capsular contracture have been shown to decrease with both methods of steroid delivery; but at higher doses, steroid-related complications, such as delayed wound healing, implant exposure, and thinning of the overlying dermis, have prevented their widespread use.[127,128] Low-dose pocket irrigation may see a rise in popularity with the return of gel implants to the market for primary augmentation.

With smooth-walled implants, regardless of implant type or product location, the early initiation of implant displacement exercises is recommended. When the implant is allowed to move freely in its pocket, the contractile forces of the capsular collagen are countered, and the implant can remain soft. Motion exercises should begin at the first postoperative visit (usually 4 to 6 days) and emphasize implant displacement both medially and superiorly. If the implants appear to be riding above the intended inframammary fold, downward displacement and the use of superior pole elastic compression wraps can be added to the regimen.

There have been anecdotal breakthroughs with use of immunomodulation in the prevention and treatment of capsular contracture. Leukotriene receptor antagonists, specifically zafirlukast (Accolate) and montelukast (Singulair), two medications developed and used to treat asthma, have been thought to reverse the effects of capsular contracture in women with both conditions.[129] This off-label use has led some physicians to use the medications prophylactically in all their breast augmentation patients, but there are no clinical trials to date to support these claims. Because significant hepatic complications may rarely be associated with zafirlukast, more research needs to be done to establish the safety and efficacy of these medications in the treatment and prevention of capsular contracture. More important, however, by learning to modify the collagen response at the cellular level, the key to prevention of capsular contracture may be found.

TREATMENT

Once a firm capsule has been established, several methods of treatment are available. Historically, closed capsulotomy, in which manual external pressure was placed on the breast in an attempt to rupture the capsule, was popular but probably led to a significant number of implant ruptures; this technique employed both hands to apply force to the capsule until an audible and palpable tear in the capsule was appreciated.[130] Although it is not used today for established capsules, this maneuver may be a useful technique when early capsules (capsules occurring within the first few months of surgery) are identified in established patients. Potential complications requiring operative intervention are well described with this technique, however, and include hematoma, implant rupture, gel migration, "dumbbell" deformity, and incomplete capsular rupture.[131] There is a higher risk for complications in a patient with older implants and long-standing capsules.

As discussed before, there are anecdotal reports in the literature now of pharmacologic interventions for the treatment of capsular contracture. Most notably, the leukotriene receptor antagonists have enjoyed some success; but to date, there have been no scientific data to support their use. The potential risks of the medications should be considered before their initiation.

Several operative strategies are employed to deal with established capsules. Among the options are open capsulotomies, partial or total capsulectomies, surgical site changes, implant exchanges, and implant removal. Open capsulotomy requires opening and scoring of the capsule as required to achieve the desired release. This can range from several circumferential incisions to multiple crosshatchings along the entire capsule. Open capsulotomy is often an effective technique for dealing with early capsules and breast asymmetries due to asymmetric capsule formation. Open capsulotomy may be the only alternative in patients with very thin skin flaps in whom an extensive resection would risk skin perforation or devitalization.

Complete and partial capsulectomies require resection of at least some of the capsule. This technique is effective for very thick fibrous capsules, capsules with a significant degree of calcification, or capsules with silicone granulomas.[136] If the implant is to be replaced or exchanged, a complete capsulectomy is recommended. This allows the re-creation of a "virgin" pocket that is the equivalent of a surgical site change.[132] Whereas open capsulotomies may not require drainage tubes, patients who undergo extensive or total capsulectomies are routinely drained.

Site change surgery has become popular in treatment of established capsule contracture. This allows the newly inserted implant to be positioned in contact with a virgin vascularized tissue pocket.[34] Capsule contractures in the subglandular space are treated by a site change to the subpectoral position after capsulectomy. Capsule contractures in the subpectoral position can be treated by a site change to the subglandular space if adequate soft tissue thickness is present. Other site change options employ planes in front of or behind the capsule itself. If the encapsulated implant has a smooth surface, a switch to a textured surface implant (or a saline implant) in conjunction with a site change (or total capsulectomy) is suggested.

Complications

Augmentation mammaplasty is a highly successful procedure associated with a high degree of satisfaction of patients. As with any procedure, however, complications do arise. In breast augmentation, there are both surgical complications and implant complications.[133] The most frequent surgical complications are hematoma formation, seroma formation, wound infection, alterations in nipple sensation, and Mondor disease. Implant complications include displacement, rippling, deflation (saline), and rupture (gel).[134]

Hematoma development after breast augmentation has both short-term effects (pain, disfigurement, blood loss) and long-term consequences (capsular contracture). The best treatment of hematoma development is prevention. Regardless of the surgical approach, meticulous hemostasis should be obtained under direct vision with an electrocautery unit. Staining of the tissues with blood should be diluted by copious saline irrigation, and drainage tubes should be used as needed. Preoperatively, it is important to discontinue any medications that induce a bleeding diathesis and to provide patients with a list of over-the-counter medications containing aspirin or other compounds that contribute to excessive bleeding. Should a hematoma develop, prompt evacuation and copious irrigation should be instigated. Unfortunately, it is the exception rather than the rule to find an actively bleeding vessel at the time of re-exploration, but every attempt should be made to ensure a dry field before reinsertion of the implant. Postoperative management is the same.

Patients may occasionally present with a delayed hematoma, most often 1 to 2 weeks after surgery but in rare cases as long as several years later. A history of trauma may often be elicited. All expanding hematomas with tight skin envelopes need to be explored regardless of the length of time from the original procedure. Nonoperative management of small nonexpanding hematomas is an option but puts the patient at a higher risk for subsequent capsule formation.

Wound infections can range from mild cellulitis of the breast skin to a purulent periprosthetic space infection. The most frequently identified pathogen is *S. epidermidis.* It is imperative to treat infections early, when they are typically responsive to oral or intravenous antibiotics, rather than to let the infection go unchecked to the point where the implant has to be removed; the breast tissue is allowed to heal by secondary intention. As with hematoma formation, prevention is the best strategy. A single dose of an intravenous first- or second-generation cephalosporin may be used before skin incision followed by 3 days of postoperative oral antibiotics. It is preferable to employ a minimal-touch technique when the implant is handled; clean powder-free gloves are worn for implant insertion, and both the implant and the pocket are irrigated with antibiotic solution. A closed system is used to fill saline implants, and a multiple-layer closure ensures a tight seal around the implant. If there is any question about the proper course of treatment for an infection around an implant, it is always safe to remove the implant, let the body clear the infection, and subsequently replace the implant.

Periprosthetic seroma fluid is usually resorbed by the body within the first week of surgery. Persistent seromas may require ultrasound-guided aspiration or, for refractory cases, placement of drainage catheters. Dilution of antibiotic irrigation and minimal use of the electrocautery may help prevent seroma formation.[124]

Alterations in nipple sensation vary according to the type of approach used. The periareolar approach is generally associated with the highest rate of changes in nipple sensation, and the transumbilical approach is reported to have the lowest. Rates in the literature vary widely, but patients should be advised that the risk of permanent alterations in nipple sensitivity is about 3% to 5% for all approaches. Care must be taken to preserve the third, fourth, and fifth lateral intercostal nerves during the dissection. These nerve branches often run with their concomitant artery and vein and often need to be stretched but should never be divided.

Mondor disease is a superficial thrombophlebitis that usually occurs in the veins on the inferior aspect of the breast. It may occur in up to 1% to 2% of augmentation patients, most frequently after an inframammary incision. Fortunately, it is a self-limited problem that usually resolves with warm compresses during the course of several weeks.

The most common implant-related complication remains implant displacement with subsequent breast asymmetry. This ranks second only to capsular contracture as the major source of dissatisfaction of patients with breast augmentation. If the displacement is seen at the first postoperative visit, taping in the desired position for several weeks will often correct the problem. If the problem goes untreated, it is often necessary to correct it surgically.

Rippling may be caused by either traction or underfilling of a saline implant. Thin soft tissue cover causes upper pole traction wrinkles. The weight of the implant is transmitted to the upper pole skin, causing a visible deformity. Underfilled implants can also cause lower pole knuckling. Rippling can also be a problem with underfilled saline implants, in which there is inadequate fill to prevent shell folding. When either of these problems is present, it is preferable to slightly overfill smooth saline or gel implants placed in a subpectoral plane to correct the deformity.

Deflation of saline implants has been reported to be as high as 5.5%. Risk factors include underfilling of the implant, intraluminal antibiotics, and intraluminal steroids.[94] Deflation can follow trauma or occur spontaneously. The only treatment is to exchange the implant.

The incidence of rupture of silicone gel implants varies greatly according to the type of implant used. The risk factors for implant rupture include age of the implant,[135] type of implant,[136] degree of capsular contracture, history of trauma (including mammography), and symptoms present. The diagnosis can be made by physical examination, mammography, ultrasonography, and magnetic resonance imaging. Most gel failure leads to intracapsular rupture, which can be treated by simple implant exchange. Extracapsular gel extravasation requires debulking, thorough washout, and implant replacement.

REFERENCES

1. Cronin TD, Gerow FJ: Augmentation mammoplasty: a new "natural feel" prosthesis. Transactions of the Third International Congress of Plastic Surgery, October 13-18, 1963. Amsterdam, Excerpta Medica Foundation, 1963:41-49.
2. National Clearing House of Plastic Surgery Statistics, 2001 Data. Arlington Heights, Ill, American Society of Plastic Surgeons.
3. Terry MD, Skovron ML, Garbers S, et al: The estimated frequency of cosmetic breast augmentation among U.S. women 1963 through 1988. Am J Public Health 1995;85:1122.
4. Baker JL Jr, Kolin IS, Bartlett ES: Psychosexual dynamics of patients undergoing mammary augmentation. Plast Reconstr Surg 1974;53:652.
5. Shipley RH, O'Donnell JM, Bader KF: Personality characteristics of women seeking breast augmentation, comparison to small-busted and average-busted controls. Plast Reconstr Surg 1997;60:369.
6. Hetter GP: Satisfaction and dissatisfaction of patients with augmentation mammoplasty. Plast Reconstr Surg 1979; 64:151.
7. Druss R: Changes in body image following augmentation breast surgery. Int J Psychoanal Psychother 1973;2:248.
8. Czerny V: Plastic replacement of the breast with a lipoma. Chir Kong Verhandl 1895;2:216.
9. Longacre JJ: Correction of the hypoplastic breast with special reference to reconstruction of the "nipple type breast" with local dermofat pedicle flaps. Plast Reconstr Surg 1954;14:431.
10. Bondurant S, Ernster V, Herdman R, eds: Safety of Silicone Breast Implants. Washington, DC, National Academy Press, 2000.
11. Uchida J: Clinical application of crosslinked dimethylpolysiloxane, restoration of breast, cheeks, atrophy of infantile paralysis, funnel-shaped chest, etc. Jpn J Plast Reconstr Surg 1961;4:303.
12. Brown JB, Fryer MP, Randall P, et al: Silicones in plastic surgery: laboratory and clinical investigations, a preliminary report. Plast Reconstr Surg 1953;12:374.
13. Marzoni FA, Upchurch SE, Lambert CJ: An experimental study of silicone as a soft tissue substitute. Plast Reconstr Surg 1959;24:600.
14. Feng LJ, Amini SB: Analysis of risk factors associated with rupture of silicone-gel breast implants. Plast Reconstr Surg 1999;104:955.
15. Barker DE, Retsky MI, Schultz S: "Bleeding" of silicone from bag-gel breast implants, and its clinical relation to fibrous capsule reaction. Plast Reconstr Surg 1978;61:836.
16. Caffee HH: The influence of silicone bleed on capsule contracture. Ann Plast Surg 1986;17:284.
17. Price JE Jr, Barker DE: Initial clinical experience with "low bleed" breast implants. Aesthetic Plast Surg 1983;7:255.
18. Barker DE, Retsky MI, Searles SL: New low bleed implant—Silastic II. Aesthetic Plast Surg 1985;9:39.
19. Arion HG: Retromammary prosthesis. C R Soc Fr Gynecol 1965;5.
20. Regnault P, Baker TJ, Gleason MC, et al: Clinical trial and evaluation of a proposed new inflatable mammary prosthesis. Plast Reconstr Surg 1972;50:220.
21. Rees TD, Guy CL, Coburn RJ: The use of inflatable breast implants. Plast Reconstr Surg 1973;52:609.
22. Young VL, Watson ME: Breast implant research. Clin Plast Surg 2001;28:451.
23. Lavine DM: Saline inflatable prostheses: 14 years experience. Aesthetic Plast Surg 1993;17:325.
24. Hartley JH Jr: Specific applications of the double-lumen prosthesis. Clin Plast Surg 1976;3:247.
25. Colon GA: The reverse double-lumen prosthesis—a preliminary report. Ann Plast Surg 1982;4:293.
26. Becker H: The expander mammary implant. Plast Reconstr Surg 1987;76:631.

27. Ashley FL: A new type of breast prosthesis. Preliminary report. Plast Reconstr Surg 1970;45:421.
28. Ashley FL: Further studies on the natural-Y breast prosthesis. Plast Reconstr Surg 1972;49:414.
29. Capozzi A, Pennisi VR: Clinical experience with polyurethane-covered gel-filled mammary prostheses. Plast Reconstr Surg 1981;68:512.
30. Herman S: The Meme implant. Plast Reconstr Surg 1984;73:411.
31. Melmed EP: Polyurethane implants: a 6-year review of 416 patients. Plast Reconstr Surg 1988;82:285.
32. Hester TR Jr, Nahai F, Bostwick J, et al: A 5-year experience with polyurethane-covered mammary prostheses for treatment of capsule contracture, primary augmentation mammoplasty, and breast reconstruction. Clin Plast Surg 1988;15:569.
33. Sinclair TM, Kerrigan CL, Bantic R: Biodegradation of the polyurethane foam covering of breast implants. Plast Reconstr Surg 1993;92:1003.
34. Hester TR Jr, Tebbetts JB, Maxwell GP: The polyurethane-covered mammary prosthesis: facts and fiction. Clin Plast Surg 2001;28:579.
35. Barone FE, Perry L, Maxwell GP, et al: The biomechanical and histopathologic effects of surface texturizing with silicone and polyurethane in tissue implantation and expansion. Plast Reconstr Surg 1992;90:77.
36. Maxwell GP, Hammond DC: Breast implants: smooth versus textured. Adv Plast Reconstr Surg 1993;9:209.
37. Danino AM, Basmacioglu P, Saito S, et al: Comparison of the capsular response to the Biocell RTV and Mentor 1600 Siltex breast implant surface texturing: a scanning electron microscopic study. Plast Reconstr Surg 2001;108:2047.
38. Maxwell GP, Falcone PA: Eighty-four consecutive breast reconstructions using a textured silicone tissue expander. Plast Reconstr Surg 1992;89:1022.
39. Hakelius L, Ohlsen L: Tendency to capsule contracture around smooth and textured gel-filled silicone mammary implants: a 5-year followup. Plast Reconstr Surg 1997;100:1566.
40. Burkhardt B, Eades E: The effect of Biocell texturizing and povidone-iodine irrigation on capsule contracture around saline-inflatable breast implants. Plast Reconstr Surg 1995;96:1317.
41. Coleman DJ, Foo IT, Sharpe DT: Textured or smooth implants for breast augmentation? A prospective controlled trial. Br J Plast Surg 1991;44:444.
42. Malata CM, Felderg L, Coleman DJ, et al: Textured or smooth implants for breast augmentation? Three year followup of a prospective randomized controlled trial. Br J Plast Surg 1997;50:99.
43. Burkhardt BR, Demas CP: The effect of Siltex texturing and povidone-iodine irrigation on capsule contracture around saline inflatable breast implants. Plast Reconstr Surg 1994;93:123.
44. Batra M, Bernard S, Picha G: Histologic comparison of breast implant shells with smooth foam and pillar microstructuring in a rat model. Plast Reconstr Surg 1995;95:354.
45. Heden P, Jernbeck J, Hober M: Breast augmentation with anatomical cohesive-gel implants. Clin Plast Surg 2001;28:531.
46. Ersek RA, Salisbury AV: Textured surface, non-silicone-gel breast implants: four years clinical outcome. Plast Reconstr Surg 1997;100:1729.
47. Spear SL, Mardini S: Alternative filler materials and new implant designs. Clin Plast Surg 2001;28:435.
48. Choudhary S, Cadier MAM: Local tissue reactions to oil-based breast implant bleed. Br J Plast Surg 2000;53:317.
49. Papanastasiou S, Odili J, Newman P, et al: Are triglyceride breast implants really biocompatible? Ann Plast Surg 2000; 45:172.
50. Rohrich RJ, Beran SJ, Ingram AE Jr, et al: Development of alternative breast implant filler material: criteria and horizons. Plast Reconstr Surg 1996;98:455.
51. Hester TR, Cukic J: Use of stacked polyurethane-covered mammary implants in aesthetic and reconstructive breast surgery. Plast Reconstr Surg 1990;10:503.
52. Hammond DC, Perry LC, Maxwell GP, et al: Morphologic analysis of tissue expander shape using a biomechanical model. Plast Reconstr Surg 1993;92:255.
53. Maxwell GP: Breast Reconstruction utilizing subcutaneous tissue expansion followed by polyurethane-covered silicone implants [discussion]. Plast Reconstr Surg 1991;88:640.
54. Maxwell GP, Spear SL: Two-Stage Breast Reconstruction Using BioDimensional System. Santa Barbara, Calif, McGhan Medical Corporation, 1995.
55. Bronz G: A comparison of naturally shaped and round implants. Aesthetic Surg J 2002;22:238.
56. Baeke JL: Breast deformity caused by anatomical or teardrop implant rotation. Plast Reconstr Surg 2002;109:2555.
57. Hamas RS: The postoperative shape of round and teardrop saline-filled breast implants. Aesthetic Surg J 1999;19:369.
58. Hamas RS: The comparative dimensions of round and anatomical saline-filled breast implants. Aesthetic Surg J 2000;20:281.
59. Hobar PC, Gutowski K: Experience with anatomic breast implants. Clin Plast Surg 2001;28:553.
60. Tebbetts JB: Breast augmentation with full-height anatomic saline implants: the pros and cons. Clin Plast Surg 2001;28: 567.
61. Tebbetts JB, Tebbetts TB: The Best Breast: The Ultimate Discriminating Woman's Guide to Breast Augmentation. Dallas, Texas, CosmetXpertise, 1999.
62. Kessler DA, Merkatz RB, Schapiro RA: A call for higher standards for breast implants. JAMA 1993;270:2607.
63. Kessler DA: The basis of the FDA's decision based on breast implants. N Engl J Med 1992;326:1713.
64. Miyoshi K, Miyamura T, Kobayashi Y, et al: Hypergammaglobulinemia by prolonged adjuvanticity in men: disorders developed after augmentation mammoplasty. Jpn Med J 1964;2122:9.
65. Van Nunen SA, Gatenby PA, Basten A: Post-mammoplasty connective tissue disease. Arthritis Rheum 1982;25:694.
66. Spiera H: Scleroderma after silicone augmentation mammoplasty. JAMA 1988;260:236.
67. Endo LP, Edwards NL, Longley S, et al: Silicone and rheumatic diseases. Semin Arthritis Rheum 1987;17:112.
68. Peters W, Smith D, Lugowski S, et al: Analysis of silicon levels in capsules of gel and saline breast implants and of penile prostheses. Ann Plast Surg 1995;34:578.
69. Schnur PL, Weinzweig J, Harris JB, et al: Silicon analysis of breast and periprosthetic capsular tissue from patients with saline- or silicone-gel implants. Plast Reconstr Surg 1996; 98:798.
70. Barnard JJ, Todd EL, Wilson WG, et al: Distribution of organosilicon polymers in augmentation mammoplasties at autopsy. Plast Reconstr Surg 1997;100:197.
71. Rohrich RJ, Hollier LH, Robinson JB Jr: Determining the safety of the silicone envelope: in search of a silicone antibody. Plast Reconstr Surg 1996;98:455.
72. Independent Review Group: Silicone-gel breast implants: The Report of the Independent Review Group. Available at: www.silicone-review.gov.uk.
73. Bondurant S, Ernster V, Herdman R, eds: Safety of Silicone Breast Implants. Washington, DC, National Academy Press, 2000.
74. Diamond BA, Hulka BS, Kerkvliet NI, et al: Silicone breast implants in relation to connective tissue diseases and immunologic dysfunction: a report by a National Science Panel to the Hon. Sam C. Pointer, Jr. (coordinating judge for the Federal Breast Implant Multidistrict Litigation). Birmingham, Ala, Federal Judicial Center, November 1998. Available at: http://www.fjc.gov/BREIMLIT/SCIENCE/report.htm.

75. National Cancer Institute Report: Bioassay of 2,4-Diaminotoluene for Possible Carcinogenicity. Bethesda, Md, National Institutes of Health, 1979. DHEW publication NIH-79-1718.
76. Hester TR, Ford NF, Gale J, et al: Measurement of 2,4-toluenediamine in urine and serum samples from women with Meme and Replicon breast implants. Plast Reconstr Surg 1997;100:1291.
77. MDDI Reports: Polyurethane foam-covered breast implant cancer risk negligible. The Gray Sheet, July 3, 1995.
78. Gorney M: Preventing litigation in breast augmentation. Clin Plast Surg 2001;28:607.
79. Maxwell GP: Breast asymmetry. Aesthetic Plast Surg 2001;21:552.
80. Maxwell GP: Breast Reconstruction Using Textured Tissue Expansion. Santa Barbara, Calif, McGhan Medical Corporation, 1990.
81. Tebbets JB: Dimensional Augmentation Mammaplasty Using the Biodimensional System. Santa Barbara, Calif, McGhan Medical Corporation, 1994.
82. Rohrich RJ, Hartley RW Jr, Brown S: Incidence of breast and chest wall asymmetry in breast augmentation: a retrospective analysis of 100 patients. Plast Reconstr Surg 2003; 111:1513.
83. Tebbetts JB: A system for breast implant selection based on patient tissue characteristics and implant-soft tissue dynamics. Plast Reconstr Surg 2002;109:1396.
84. Tebbetts JB: Dual plane breast augmentation: optimizing implant–soft-tissue relationships in a wide range of breast types. Plast Reconstr Surg 2001;107:1255.
84a. Graf RM, Bernardes A, Rippel R, et al: Subfascial breast implant: a new procedure. Plast Reconstr Surg 2003;111: 904.
85. Tebbetts JB: Transaxillary subpectoral augmentation mammaplasty: long-term follow-up and refinements. Plast Reconstr Surg 1984;74:636.
86. Maxwell GP: Transaxillary subpectoral augmentation mammaplasty: long-term follow-up and refinements [discussion]. Plast Reconstr Surg 1984;74:648.
87. Baker JL Jr: Classification of spherical contractures. Presented at the Aesthetic Breast Symposium, Scottsdale, Arizona, 1975.
88. Biggs TM, Yarish RS: Augmentation mammaplasty: retropectoral versus retromammary implantation. Clin Plast Surg 1988;15:549.
89. Gutowski KA, Mesna GT, Cunningham BL: Saline-filled breast implants: a Plastic Surgery Educational Foundation multicenter outcomes study. Plast Reconstr Surg 1997;100:1019.
90. Puckett CL, Croll GH, Reichel CA, Concannon MJ: A critical look at capsule contracture in subglandular versus subpectoral mammary augmentation. Aesthetic Plast Surg 1987;11:23.
91. Woods JE, Irons GB, Arnold PG: The case for submuscular implantation of prostheses in reconstructive breast surgery. Ann Plast Surg 1980;5:115.
92. Handel N, Silverstein MJ, Jensen JA, et al: Comparative experience with smooth and polyurethane breast implants using the Kaplan-Meier method of survival analysis. Plast Reconstr Surg 1991;88:475.
93. Gasperoni C, Salgarello M, Gargani G: Polyurethane-covered mammary implants: a 12-year experience. Ann Plast Surg 1992;29:303.
94. Penisi VR: Long-term use of polyurethane breast prostheses: a 14-year experience. Plast Reconstr Surg 1990;86:368.
95. Smahel J: Tissue reactions to breast implants coated with polyurethane. Plast Reconstr Surg 1978;61:80.
96. Embrey M, Adams EE, Cunningham B, et al: A review of the literature on the etiology of capsular contracture and a pilot study to determine the outcome of capsular contracture interventions. Aesthetic Plast Surg 1999;23:197.
97. Coleman DJ, Foo ITH, Sharpe DT: Textured or smooth implants for breast augmentation? A prospective controlled trial. Br J Plast Surg 1991;44:444.
98. Ersek RA: Molecular impact surface textured implants (MISTI) alter beneficially breast capsule formation at 36 months. J Long Term Eff Med Implants 1991;1:155.
99. Hakelius L, Ohlsen L: Tendency to capsular contracture around smooth and textured gel-filled silicone mammary implants: a 5-year follow-up. Plast Reconstr Surg 1997; 100:1566.
100. Pollack H: Breast capsular contracture: a retrospective study of textured versus smooth silicone implants. Plast Reconstr Surg 1993;92:404.
101. Tarpila E, Ghassemifor R, Fagrell D, Ander B: Capsular contracture with textured versus smooth saline-filled implants for breast augmentation: a prospective clinical study. Plast Reconstr Surg 1997;99:1934.
102. Fagrell D, Berggren A, Tarpila E: Capsular contracture around saline-filled fine textured and smooth mammary implants: a prospective 7.5-year follow-up. Plast Reconstr Surg 2001; 108:2108.
103. Cairns TS, de Villiers W: Capsular contracture after breast augmentation—a comparison between gel- and saline-filled prosthesis. S Afr Med J 1980;57:951.
104. Gylbert L, Asplund O, Jurell G: Capsular contracture after breast reconstruction with silicone-gel and saline-filled implants: a 6-year follow-up. Plast Reconstr Surg 1990;85:373.
105. McKinney P, Tresley G: Long-term comparison of patients with gel and saline mammary implants. Plast Reconstr Surg 1983;72:27.
106. Reiffel RS, Rees TD, Guy CL, Aston SJ: A comparison of capsule formation following breast augmentation by saline-filled or gel-filled implants. Aesthetic Plast Surg 1983;7:113.
107. Baker JL Jr, Chandler ML, LeVier RR: Occurrence and activity of myofibroblasts in human capsular tissue surrounding mammary implants. Plast Reconstr Surg 1981; 68:905.
108. Winding O, Christensen L, Thomsen JL, et al: Silicone in human breast tissue surrounding silicone gel prostheses. A scanning electron microscopy and energy dispersive x-ray investigation of normal, fibrocystic, and peri-prosthetic breast tissue. Scand J Plast Reconstr Surg Hand Surg 1988;22:127.
109. Thomsen JL, Christensen L, Nielsen M, et al: Histologic changes and silicone concentrations in human breast tissue surrounding silicone breast prostheses. Plast Reconstr Surg 1990;85:38.
110. Gayou RM: A histological comparison of contracted and noncontracted capsules around silicone breast implants. Plast Reconstr Surg 1979;63:700.
111. Rudolph R, Abraham J, Vecchione T, et al: Myofibroblasts and free silicone around breast implants. Plast Reconstr Surg 1978;62:185.
112. Piscatelli SJ, Partington M, Hobar C, et al: Breast capsule contracture: is fibroblast activity associated with severity? Aesthetic Plast Surg 1994;18:75.
113. Williams C, Aston S, Rees TD: The effect of hematoma on the thickness of pseudosheaths around silicone implants. Plast Reconstr Surg 1975;56:194.
114. Shah Z, Lehman JA Jr, Tan J: Does infection play a role in breast capsular contracture? Plast Reconstr Surg 1981;68:34.
115. Virden CP, Dobke MK, Stein P, et al: Subclinical infection of the silicone breast implant surface as a possible cause of capsular contracture. Aesthetic Plast Surg 1992;16:173.
116. Dobke MK, Svahn JK, Vastine VL, et al: Characterization of microbial presence at the surface of silicone mammary implants. Ann Plast Surg 1995;34:563.
117. Burkhardt BR, Dempsey PD, Schnur PL, Tofield JJ: Capsular contracture: a prospective study of the effect of local antibacterial agents. Plast Reconstr Surg 1986;77:919.

118. Panjkos A, Deva AK, Vickery K, et al: Detection of subclinical infection in significant breast implant capsules. Plast Reconstr Surg 2003;111:1605.
119. Burkhardt BR: Supplement to Augmentation Mammaplasty and Capsular Contracture. An Annotated Review and Guide to the Literature. Tucson, Arizona, privately published, 1985.
120. Asplund O: Capsular contracture in silicone gel and saline-filled breast implants after reconstruction. Plast Reconstr Surg 1984;73:270.
121. Gylbert L, Asplund O, Jurell G: Capsular contracture after breast reconstruction with silicone-gel and saline-filled implants: a 6-year follow-up. Plast Reconstr Surg 1990;85:373.
122. Biggs TM, Yarish RS: Augmentation mammaplasty: a comparative analysis. Plast Reconstr Surg 1990;85:368.
123. Puckett CL, Croll GH, Reichel CA, Concannon MJ: A critical look at capsule contracture in subglandular versus subpectoral mammary augmentation. Aesthetic Plast Surg 1987;11:23.
124. Adams WP Jr, Conner WCH, Barton FE Jr, Rohrich RJ: Optimizing breast pocket irrigation: the post-Betadine era. Plast Reconstr Surg 2001;107:1596.
125. Mladick RA: "No-touch" submuscular saline breast augmentation technique. Aesthetic Plast Surg 1993;17:183.
126. Gutowski KA, Mesna GT, Cunningham BL: Saline-filled breast implants: a Plastic Surgery Educational Foundation multicenter outcomes study. Plast Reconstr Surg 1997;100:1019.
127. Ellenberg AH: Marked thinning of the breast skin flaps after the insertion of implants containing triamcinolone. Plast Reconstr Surg 1977;60:755.
128. Carrico TJ, Cohen IK: Capsular contracture and steroid-related complications after augmentation mammaplasty. Plast Reconstr Surg 1979;64:377.
129. Schlesinger LS, Ellenbogen R, Desvigne MN, et al: Zafirlukast (Accolate): a new treatment for capsular contracture. Aesthetic Surg J 2002;22:329.
130. Baker JL, Bartels RJ, Douglas WM: Closed compression technique for rupturing a contracted capsule around a breast implant. Plast Reconstr Surg 1976;58:137.
131. Nelson GD: Complications of closed compression after augmentation mammaplasty. Plast Reconstr Surg 1980;66:71.
132. Young VL: Guidelines and indications for breast implant capsulectomy. Plast Reconstr Surg 1998;102:884.
133. de Cholnoky T: Augmentation mammaplasty: survey of complications in 10,941 patients by 265 surgeons. Plast Reconstr Surg 1970;45:573.
134. Bostwick JB: Augmentation Mammaplasty—Plastic and Reconstructive Breast Surgery. St. Louis, Quality Medical Publishing, 2000.
135. Rohrich RJ, Adams WP Jr, Beran SJ, et al: An analysis of silicone gel–filled breast implants: diagnosis and failure rates. Plast Reconstr Surg 1998;102:2304.
136. Feng LJ, Amini SB: Analysis of risk factors associated with rupture of silicone gel breast implants. Plast Reconstr Surg 1999;104:955.

CHAPTER

119

Breast Augmentation Techniques

MALCOLM ALAN LESAVOY, MD

OPERATIVE TECHNIQUES
COMPLICATIONS
MISCELLANEOUS ISSUES

In today's world, the aesthetic aspect of the female breast is a point of admiration, beauty, function, "womanhood," disparity, conjecture, comparison, and debate. The role of augmentation mammaplasty is, obviously, to increase the size, profile, and projection of the female breast, and decisions have to be made by the patient and the surgeon together, in concert, for the ideal expected outcome.

The average patient who desires augmentation mammaplasty is usually in her early to mid 30s, has had her children, is content with her significant other, and is content with her life but would just like to have an improvement in the size of her breasts. Most patients state that they have always had small breasts, have had difficulty in filling out a bathing suit top, and would like to feel more confident about their breast profile.[1,2] On the contrary, patients who desire an increase in their breast size for business purposes (e.g., entertainment) or to attract or keep a significant other will usually not be satisfied with the outcome and are not good candidates for this procedure. This is also true in many other types of aesthetic surgery, and expectations must be realistic.[3]

The technique of breast augmentation involves placement of an implant behind the breast or the breast and pectoralis major muscle to push the breast forward and to increase its projection and size.[4-8] The implants that are used are either silicone gel or saline filled. Both the saline- and silicone gel-filled implants have an identical silicone shell or envelope and are manufactured with either a smooth surface or a textured surface. The Food and Drug Administration requires the use of saline-filled implants for first-time new patients. Silicone gel-filled implants can be used for first-time patients or secondary procedures in the following circumstances: for the replacement of silicone- or saline-filled implants in breast reconstruction, for women with significant breast asymmetry, and for women who desire a mastopexy and augmentation.[9,10]

As with any operative procedure, a full history is obtained and physical examination is performed. This history includes family history of breast cancer, previous breast biopsies, nipple discharge, bra cup size, and recent growth or atrophy of the breasts due to pregnancy or breast-feeding. In addition, a complete past medical history, including medications and allergies, should be listed. The physical examination includes a comprehensive breast examination to look for various masses, previous scars, nipple position such as retraction, thoracic deformity, and asymmetries. After this, a complete and comprehensive discussion ensues with the patient about the operative techniques and complications and realistic expectations.

If the patient has significant deformity of her breasts, such as tubular breasts, ptosis, marked nodularity, thoracic deformity, or significant asymmetry, it must be addressed. These patients will possibly require discussion of other operative interventions.

OPERATIVE TECHNIQUES

Assuming the patient is a good candidate for augmentation mammaplasty, has realistic expectations, and understands the possible complications, the surgery is scheduled. The patient is first marked preoperatively in the upright position with attention to the inframammary crease; the medial, lateral, and superior aspects of the glandular tissue; and the uppermost axillary fold. Once this is accomplished, the patient is placed in the supine position on the operating table, and intravenous sedation or general anesthesia is commenced. Both breasts and axillae are infiltrated with 0.5% lidocaine with epinephrine.

The choice of operative approach is previously discussed with the patient and usually depends on the surgeon's choice. The three usual approaches are through the inframammary crease, through the periareolar approach, and through the axilla[11-14] (Fig. 119-1).

The most common approach is through the inframammary crease. The incision should be placed 1 or 2 mm above this crease to avoid a visible scar when the patient raises her arms or is wearing a halter top or bikini. The incision is usually 5 cm in length, centered under the areola, and is usually 5.5 cm inferior to the lower border of the areola. Advantages of the inframammary crease approach include the ease and directness, the facility in placing the implant in the subglandular or submuscular plane, and a previous scar if a secondary procedure is needed. The disadvantage is a scar on the chest wall that usually fades nicely but can be hidden by the shadow of the lower portion of the breast. The inframammary approach is thought to be the most common incision by plastic surgeons.

The periareolar approach is performed with an incision along the inferior half of the areola (1 mm within the pigmented skin of the areola) that traverses from the 3-o'clock to the 6-o'clock to the 9-o'clock position. The dissection is carried directly through the breast tissue to the retroglandular space or retropectoral space, and a large pocket is then dissected. Through this same periareolar approach, an inferior subcutaneous dissection can be performed at the inframammary crease. Dissection in the subglandular or submuscular plane can then be accomplished with a careful approach. The advantage of the periareolar approach is a small scar.

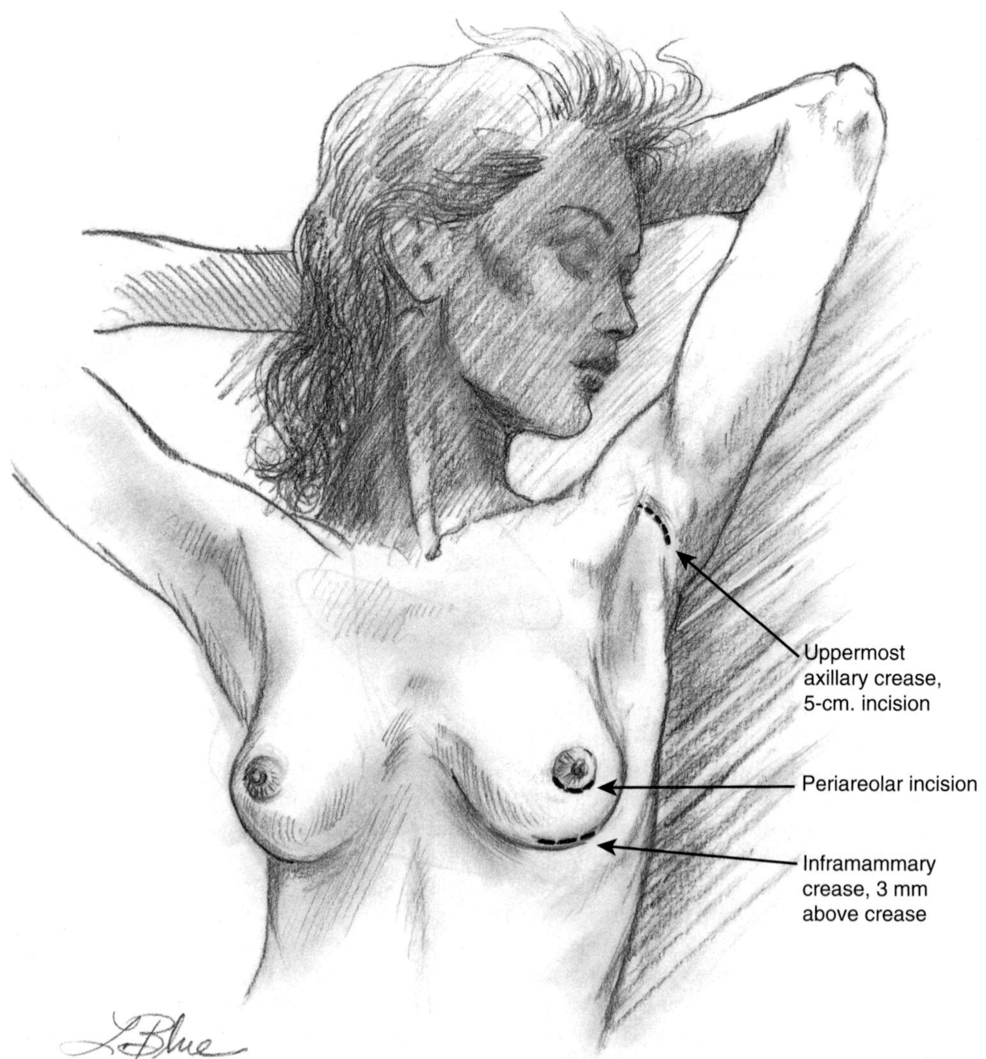

FIGURE 119-1. The most common incisional approaches for augmentation mammaplasty.

The disadvantages can include future breast nodularity from suturing of the bisected breast tissue, induration of the subcutaneous tissues inferior to the areola, possible nipple retraction inferiorly, nipple and areola paresthesias, and future uncertainty of nodularities postoperatively due to the surgical intervention or parenchymal disease. The periareolar approach is thought to be the second most common approach for augmentation mammaplasty.

The transaxillary approach, the least common incision by plastic surgeons, is placed in the uppermost axillary fold and kept within the hair-bearing tissue; it is usually 5 to 6 cm in length. This approach can also easily give access to a subglandular or submuscular placement and has the advantage of a hidden scar within the axilla. A disadvantage is the somewhat "blind" dissection that can frequently result in placement of the implant too high, and hemostasis can be difficult to achieve if the proper planes are not dissected. When secondary revisions are necessary, the inframammary approach is usually more desirable because of direct exposure and easier manipulation.

It is this author's choice to perform most primary augmentation mammaplasties by the transaxillary approach. The patient is placed on the operating table with her arms outstretched at approximately 80 degrees, and a towel is placed under each scapula to raise the operative site from the operating table to allow easier access (Figs. 119-2 and 119-3). Care must be taken not to overextend the shoulder and place traction on the brachial plexus; this is aided by ensuring that the patient's palms are facing toward the floor and not in an exaggerated position. Once the decision has been made to place the implant in a subglandular or submuscular plane, the dissection is carried medially in the subcutaneous plane, avoiding the axillary contents (Fig. 119-4). If the axillary contents are broached, bleeding and subsequent hematoma can ensue.

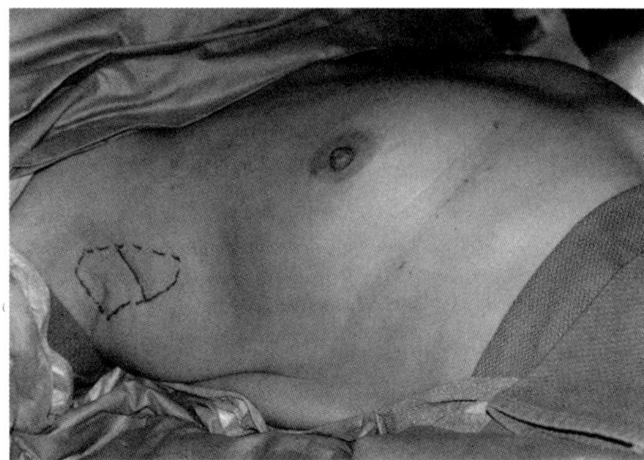

FIGURE 119-3. The dotted line indicates hair-bearing tissue of the axilla; the solid line indicates incision in the uppermost axillary crease.

It is this author's choice to place the implant in the subglandular plane for it is thought that a more natural appearance can ensue. The subglandular placement versus the submuscular placement has been and will continue to be a topic of debate, but it is generally considered the surgeon's choice[15-17] (Fig. 119-5). With submuscular placement of the implant, some think that significant disadvantages occur. First, anatomically, the inferior border of the pectoralis major muscle usually resides at the lower border of the nipple-areola complex. Once the submuscular plane is dissected, the lower third or lower half of the implant is not covered by the pectoralis major muscle. In addition, placement in the submuscular plane may cause the implant to reside in a more lateral position because of the sternal origins of the pectoralis major muscle; with arm motion and flexion of the pectoralis, the implants (and therefore the breasts) move abnormally and do not appear natural. Because the pectoralis major

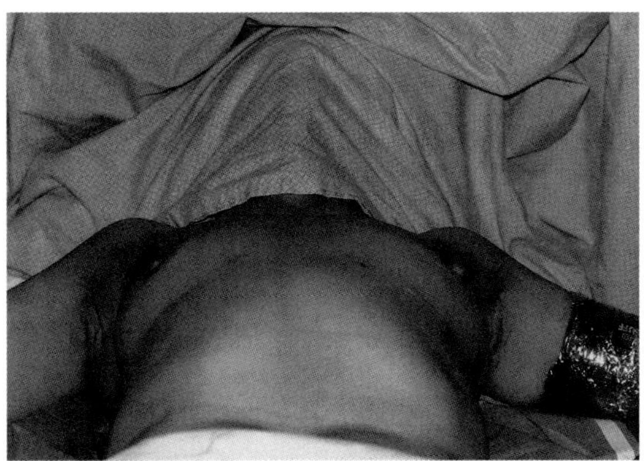

FIGURE 119-2. Transaxillary approach with patient in the supine position with arms outstretched.

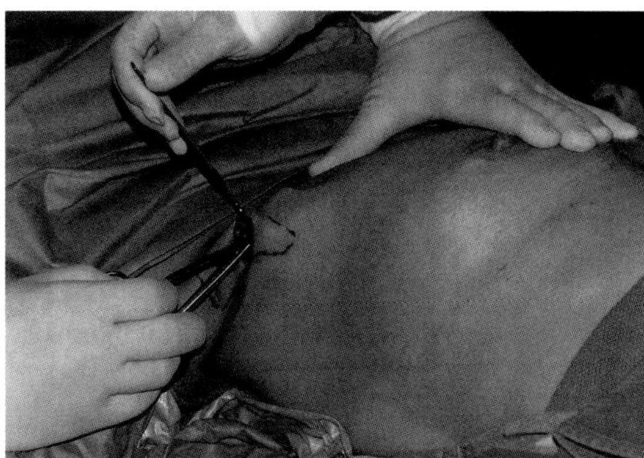

FIGURE 119-4. Subcutaneous dissection medially and horizontally below the clavicle and to the upper pole of the breast parenchyma.

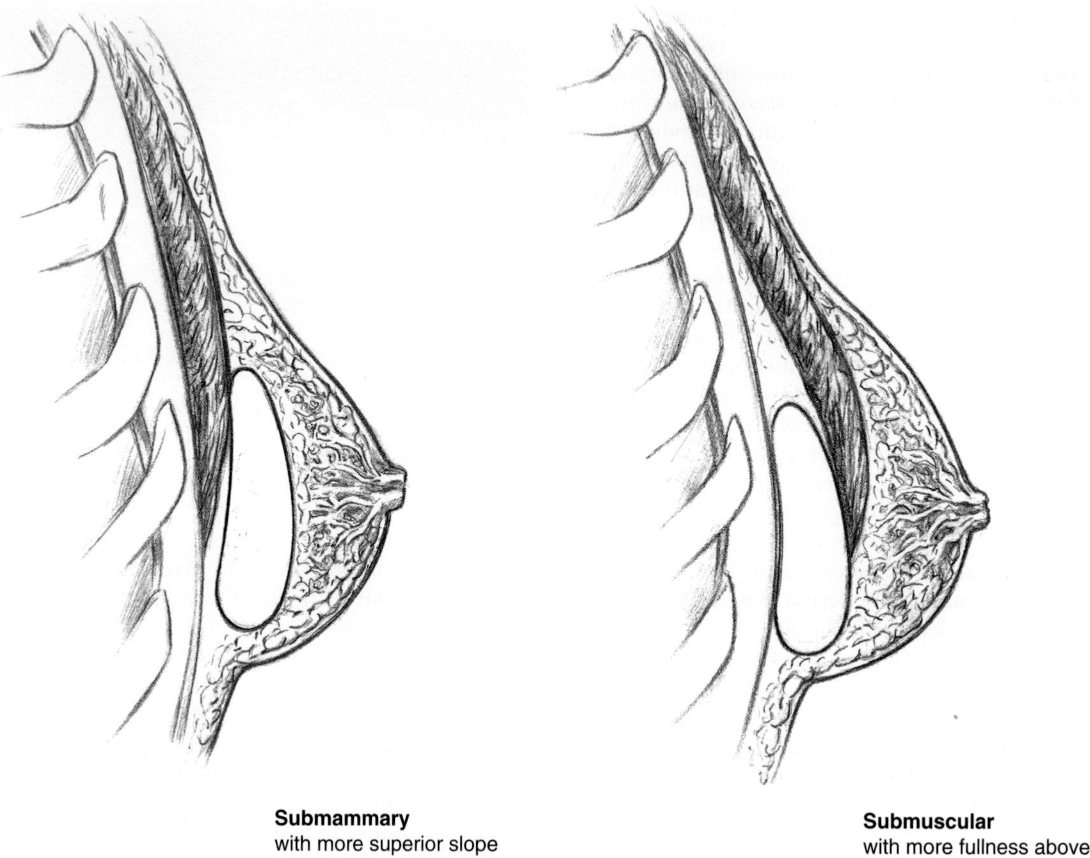

FIGURE 119-5. Submammary versus submuscular placement of breast implant.

muscle resides in the upper half of the breast, more tissue is thrust forward in this area. Therefore, a "fullness" can be seen or felt in the upper pole of the breast. Obviously, the appearance of fullness depends on the firmness and tightness of the pectoralis major muscle in each individual patient. Some surgeons prefer to release the inferior portions of the sternal origins of the pectoralis major muscle to allow a "looser fit" of the implant. However, even less of the implant will then be covered by the muscle, and on occasion, the inferior portion of the pectoralis major muscle will "roll up" like a window shade (from inferior to superior) and cause unevenness. Early on, it was thought that submuscular placement of the implant would allow continuous "massage" of the implant and thereby reduce capsular contracture, similar to manual massage of the implant in the subglandular space. To date, no significant studies have shown that the rate of capsular contracture is decreased by submuscular versus subglandular placement of the implants, but this is still a matter of discussion and debate. One positive aspect of submuscular implant placement is that when the saline-filled implants are used, the degree of rippling is decreased because there is more tissue between the implant and the superficial breast tissue. However, this is effected by more tension or pressure placed on the upper pole of the implant by the pectoralis major muscle, which therefore causes a tighter or firmer envelope inferiorly for the saline implant. Obviously, in breast reconstruction after mastectomy, submuscular placement is the norm because one needs to recruit as much tissue as possible in these patients.

When the axillary subglandular approach is used, after the medial subcutaneous dissection is made above the pectoralis major muscle fascia, a loose areolar plane is bluntly found in the area between the breast and pectoralis major muscle. This area is then bluntly dissected with the fingers, followed by the use of a long, stout object (e.g., a urethral sound, esophageal or thoracic dissecting scissors, various spatulas that have been designed for the axillary approach) (Figs. 119-6 and 119-7). Once dissection has been accomplished, from just below the clavicle to the lateral border of the sternum to just beyond the inframammary crease inferiorly and laterally to the anterior axillary line (Fig. 119-8), hemostasis can be achieved. By placement of various extended gauze dressings into the wound, one can usually blindly assess the degree of bleeding

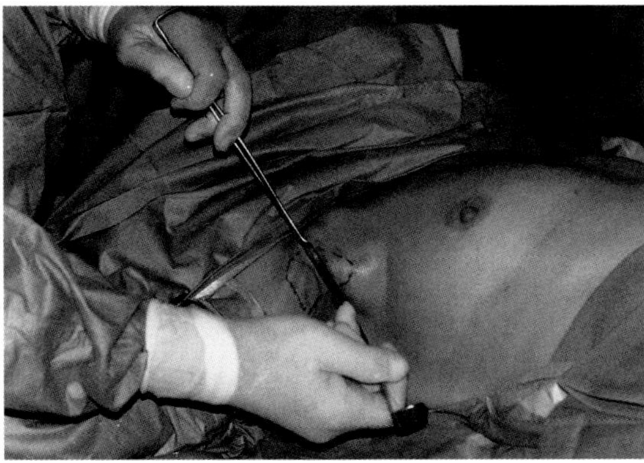

FIGURE 119-6. Blunt and forceful retraction of the incision pocket to expand the access.

(or lack thereof) (Fig. 119-9). On occasion, hemostasis can be aided by fiberoptic retraction and direct cauterization. Once hemostasis is achieved, various implant sizers can be used to assess the permanent implant size (Fig. 119-10). The determination of implant size is a matter of experience, taste, and discussion preoperatively with the patient. However, on the operating table, it is the surgeon's choice.

After hemostasis is achieved, copious irrigation with normal saline should ensure a clean and sterile wound, devoid of particulate matter and fat. This maneuver will also give the surgeon an idea of the degree of hemostasis that has been achieved. Usually, at this time, 30 mL of 0.25% bupivacaine with epinephrine is placed within the pocket to decrease the patient's postoperative discomfort (Fig. 119-11). The saline implant size is chosen, the insert tubing is placed in the implant (Fig. 119-12), and the air is evacuated from the implant as it comes from the manufacturer (Fig. 119-13). The implant is then folded on itself and, with some mild lubrication, inserted through the axilla into the submammary space and seated digitally (Figs. 119-14 and 119-15). The saline implant is then inflated to the desired volume, and placement of the implant, centered behind the breast gland, is assessed. The implant filler tube is then removed (Fig. 119-16), and the valve of the implant is checked digitally to ensure that it is seated properly. The wound is then closed in layers, and attention is given to the contralateral side (Fig. 119-17).

Once both breasts have been augmented and both wounds closed, the operating table is placed in a sitting position so compression dressings can be applied. A surgical bra is placed, and then compression is achieved with either elastic bandages or elastic wraps placed circumferentially around the chest superiorly to keep the implant in its appointed position. The compression dressings are left for 3 or 4 days. On the patient's first postoperative visit, she is examined for hematoma and infection. If there is no evidence of hematoma or infection, the superior compression dressing is then reapplied and maintained for the next 2 to 3 weeks. After surgery, vigorous exercise with use of the upper body is restricted for a period of 3 to 4 weeks. However, the patient can usually resume normal, everyday activity within 4 or 5 days. The sutures are removed at the appropriate time, and patients return every 2 weeks for 1 month and then every 2 months for 4 months. The author prefers to see patients on an annual basis for ongoing evaluation and examination (Figs. 119-18 to 119-22).

COMPLICATIONS

Complications in augmentation mammaplasty are relatively infrequent but can include hematoma, infection, periareolar paresthesias, asymmetries, implant displacement, capsular contracture, implant rippling,

Text continued on p. 45

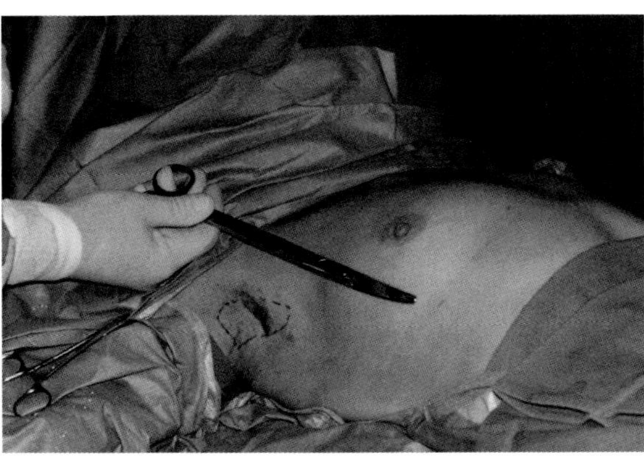

A

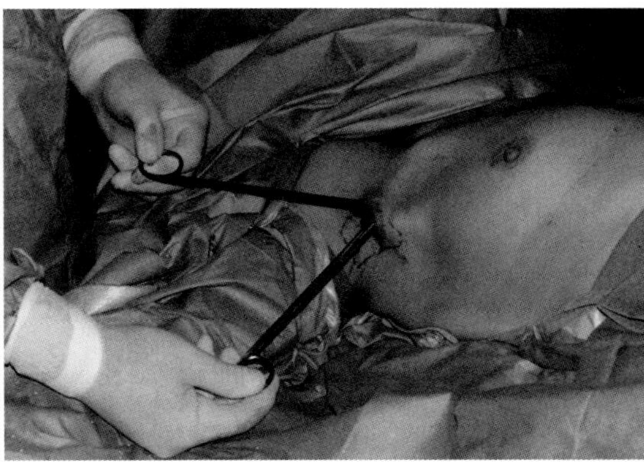

B

FIGURE 119-7. *A* and *B,* The use of a large, blunt thoracic dissecting scissors for spreading and dissection of the subglandular space.

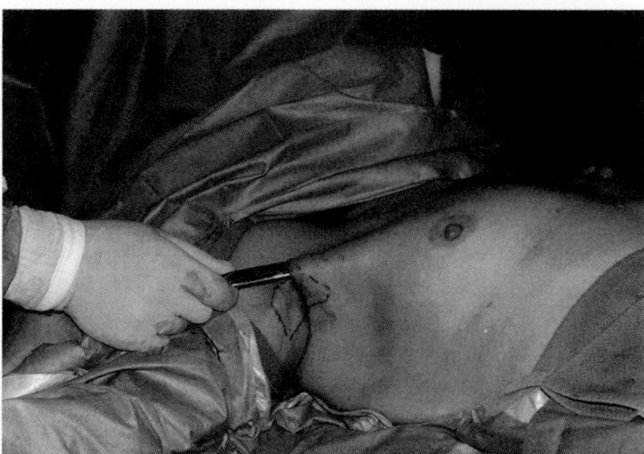

FIGURE 119-8. Blunt dissection medially, inferiorly, and laterally.

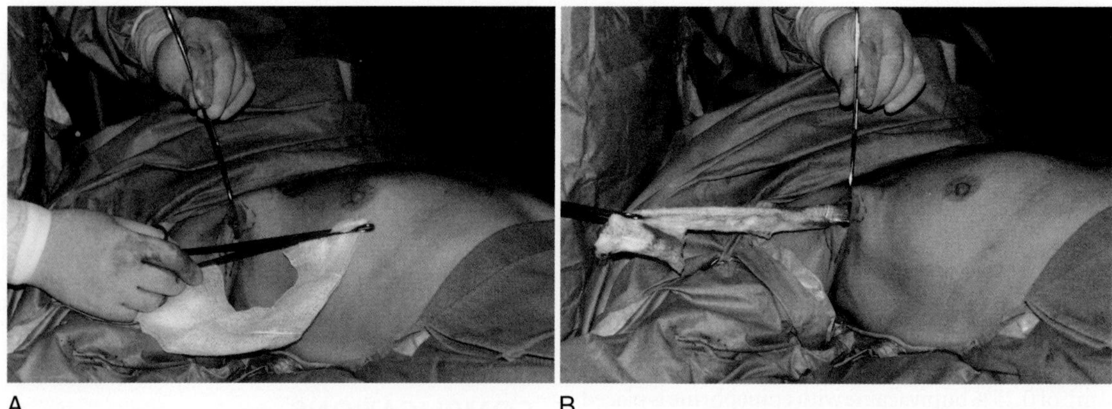

A B

FIGURE 119-9. *A* and *B,* Checking for hemostasis in a relatively dry wound.

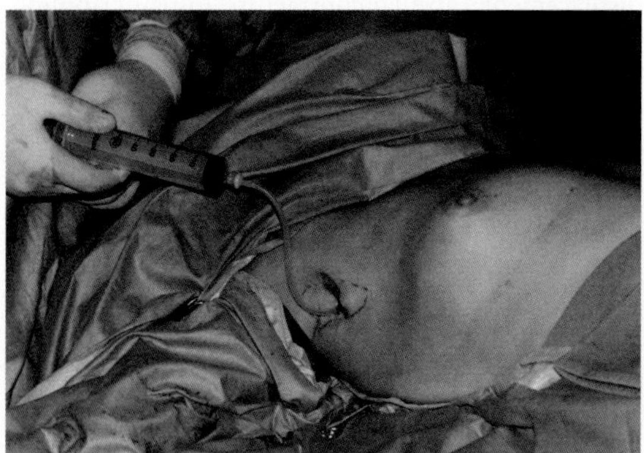

FIGURE 119-10. Insertion of a temporary implant sizer for determination of the permanent volume.

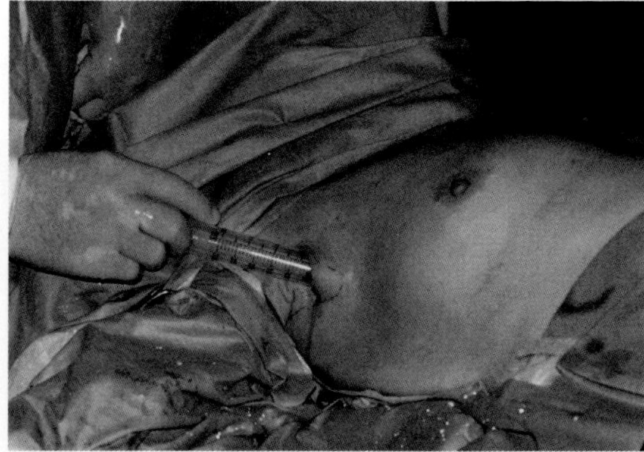

FIGURE 119-11. After removal of the sizer, copious irrigation with normal saline followed by instillation of 0.25% bupivacaine with epinephrine for postoperative pain.

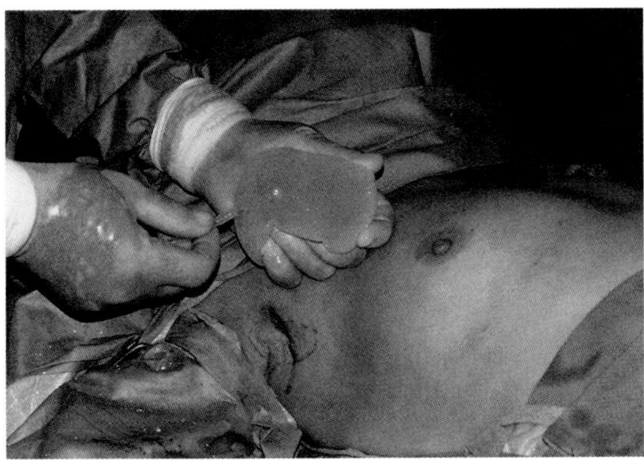

FIGURE 119-12. Permanent saline-filled implant chosen and filled tube inserted.

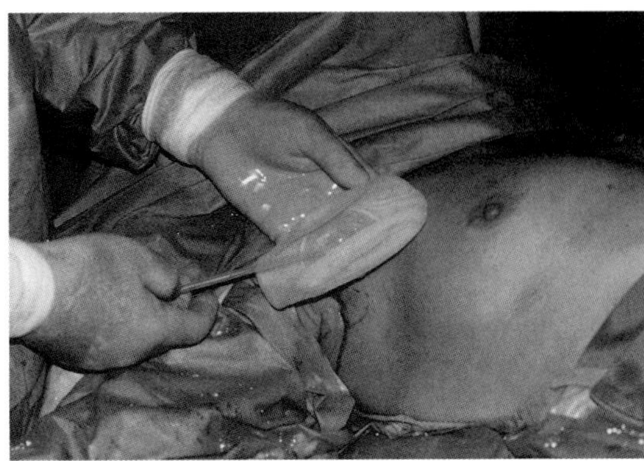

FIGURE 119-13. Evacuation of air from the implant and folding to fit into the incisional access.

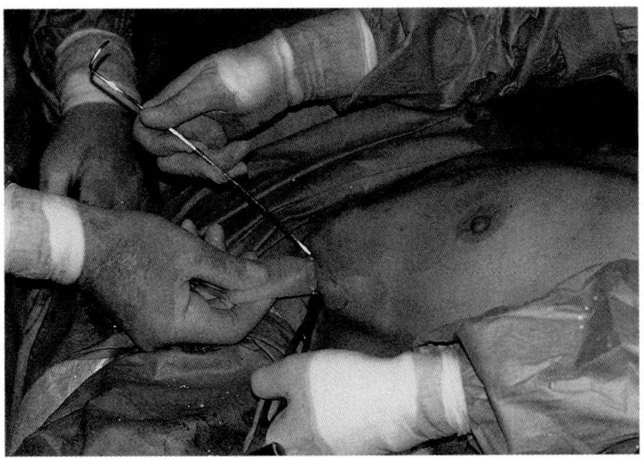

FIGURE 119-14. Insertion of the folded saline implant.

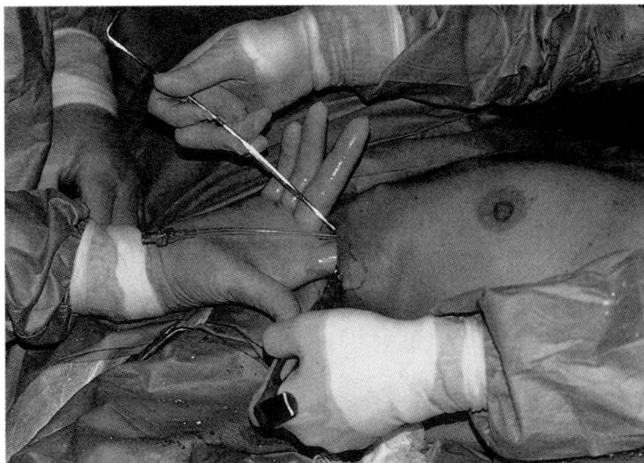

FIGURE 119-15. Digital placement of the implant in the proper submammary space.

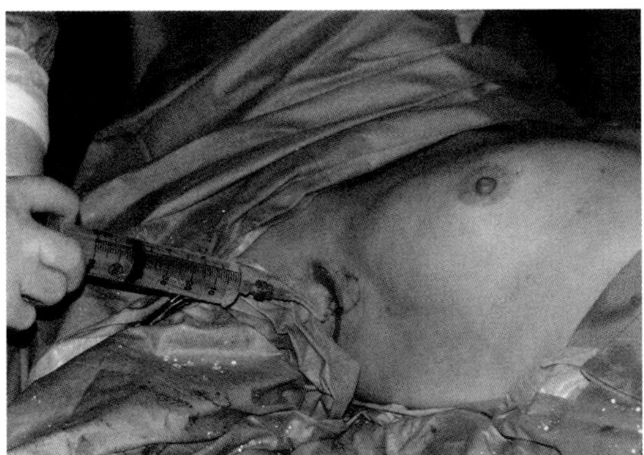

FIGURE 119-16. Filling of saline implant to the manufacturer's implant volume.

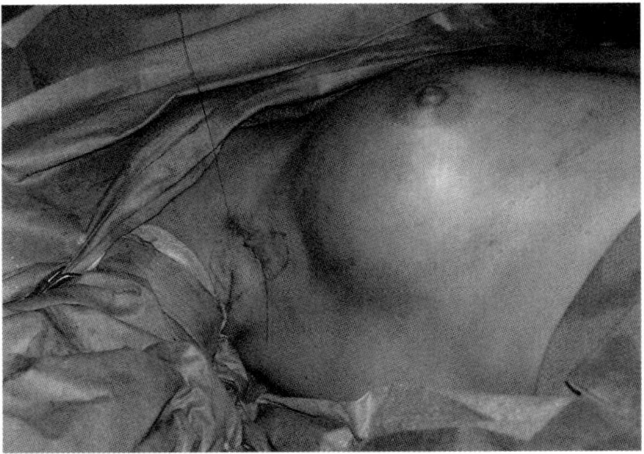

FIGURE 119-17. Closure of the wound in layers and subcuticular suture in the skin.

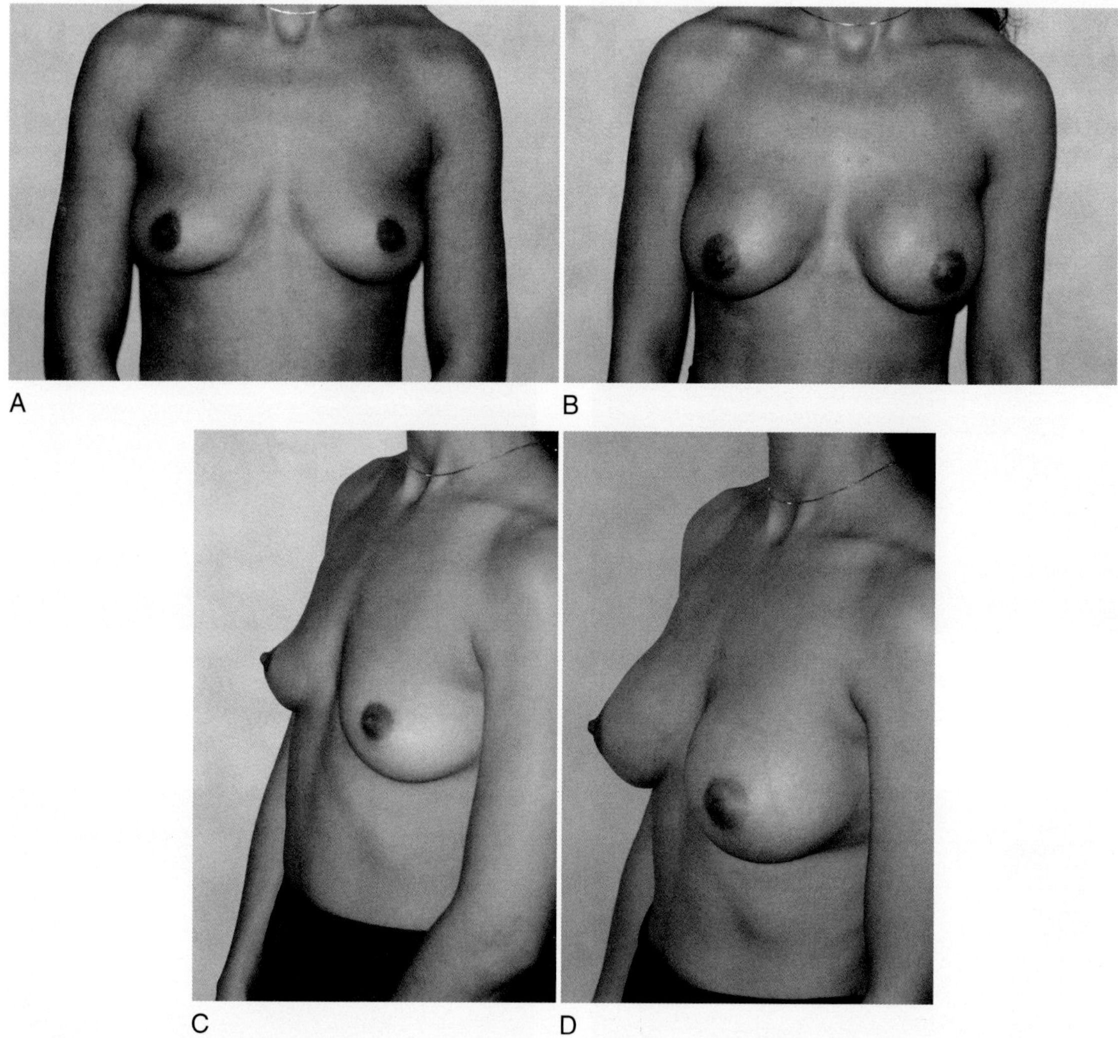

FIGURE 119-18. *A* and *C*, Preoperative views of patient. *B* and *D*, Postoperative views of patient after augmentation mammaplasty.

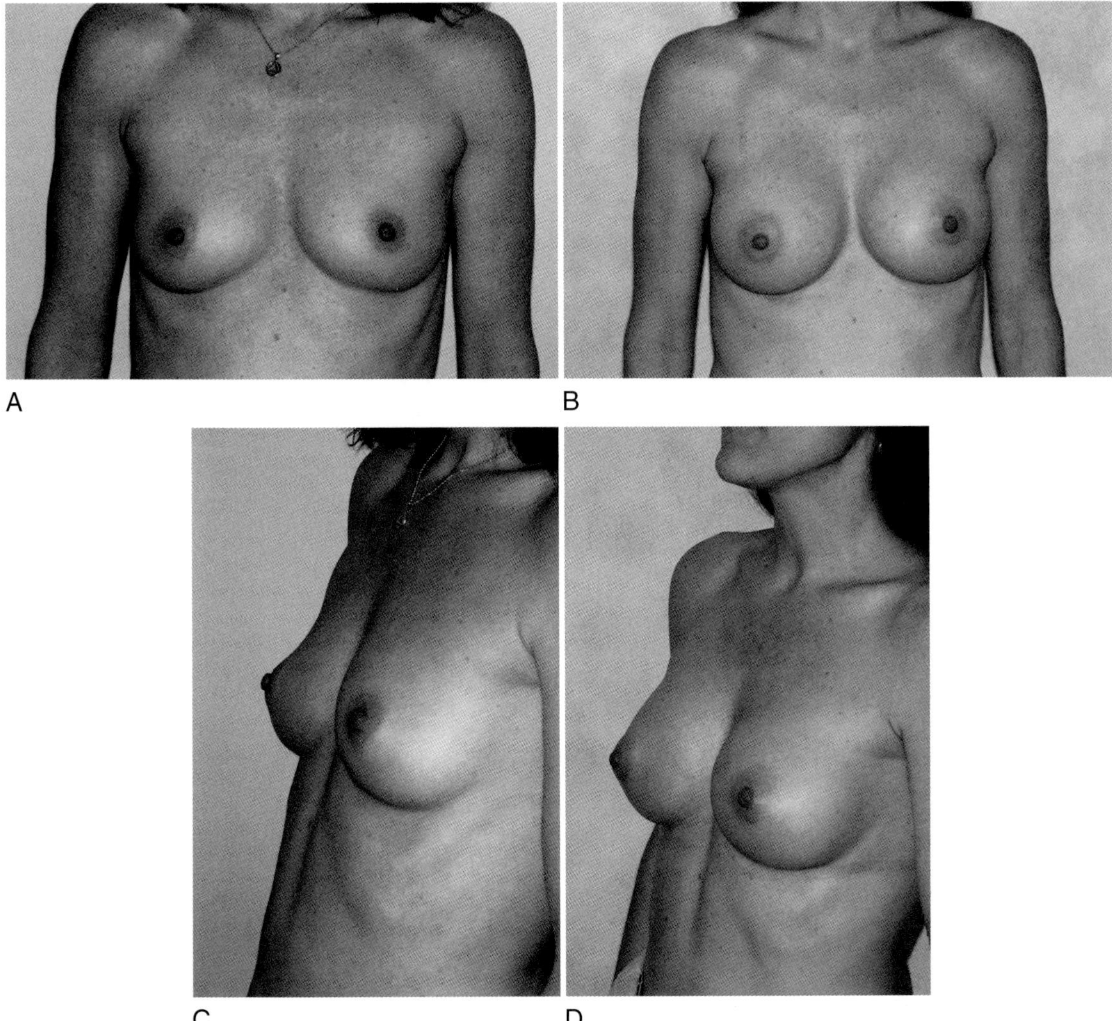

FIGURE 119-19. *A* and *C,* Preoperative views of patient. *B* and *D,* Postoperative views of patient after augmentation mammaplasty.

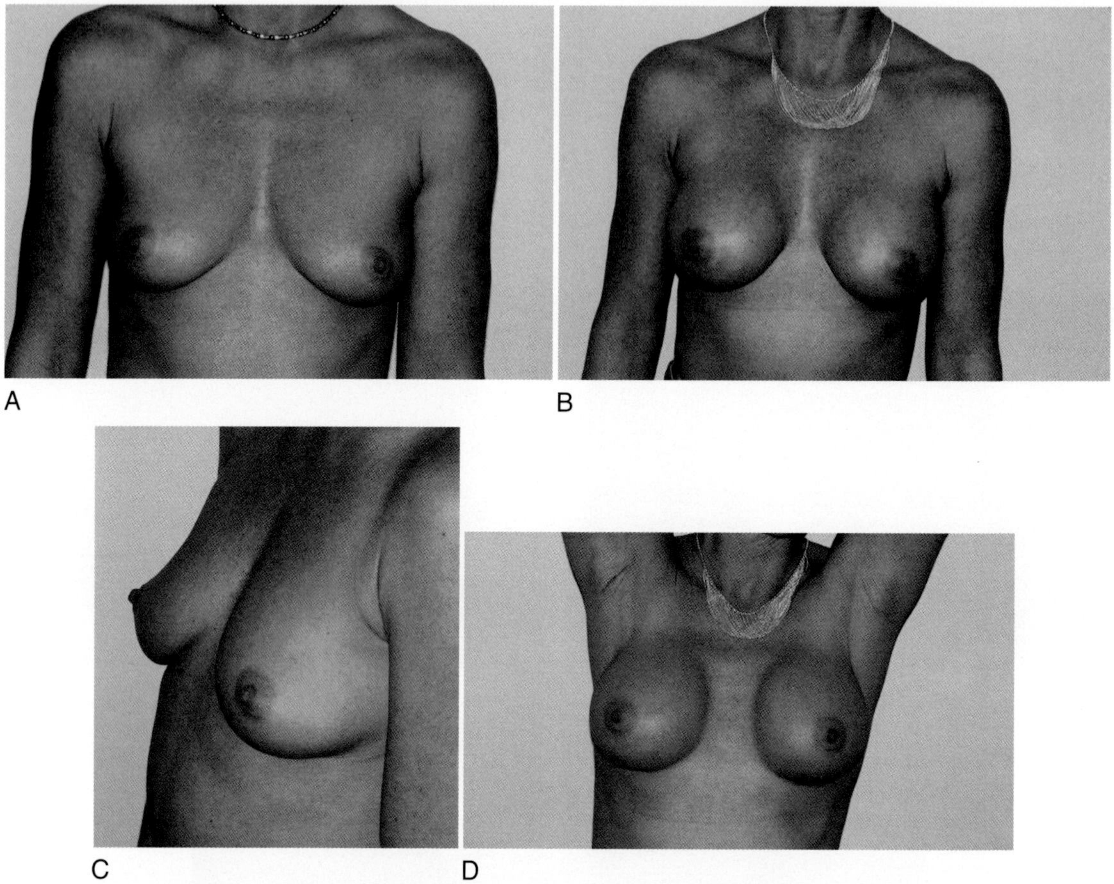

A B

C D

FIGURE 119-20. *A* and *C*, Preoperative views of patient. *B*, Postoperative view of patient after augmentation mammaplasty. *D*, Postoperative view of patient after augmentation mammaplasty with axillary scar.

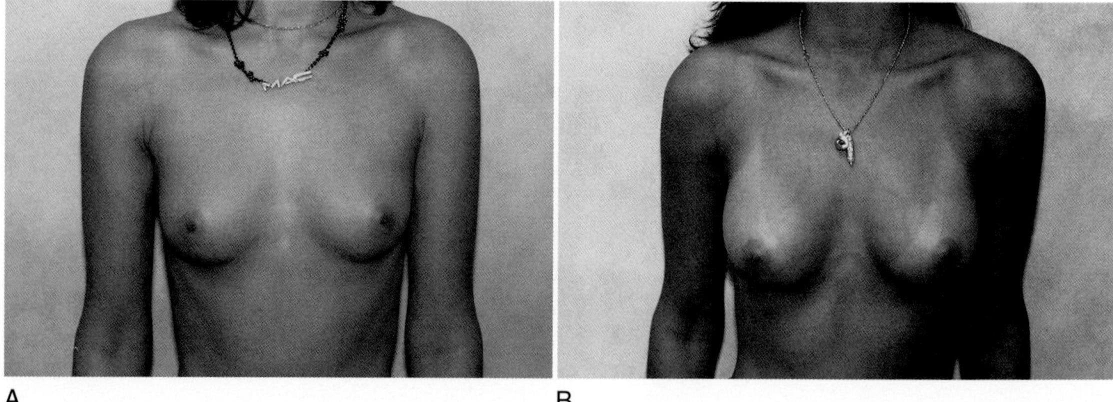

FIGURE 119-21. *A*, Preoperative view of patient. *B*, Postoperative view of patient after augmentation mammaplasty.

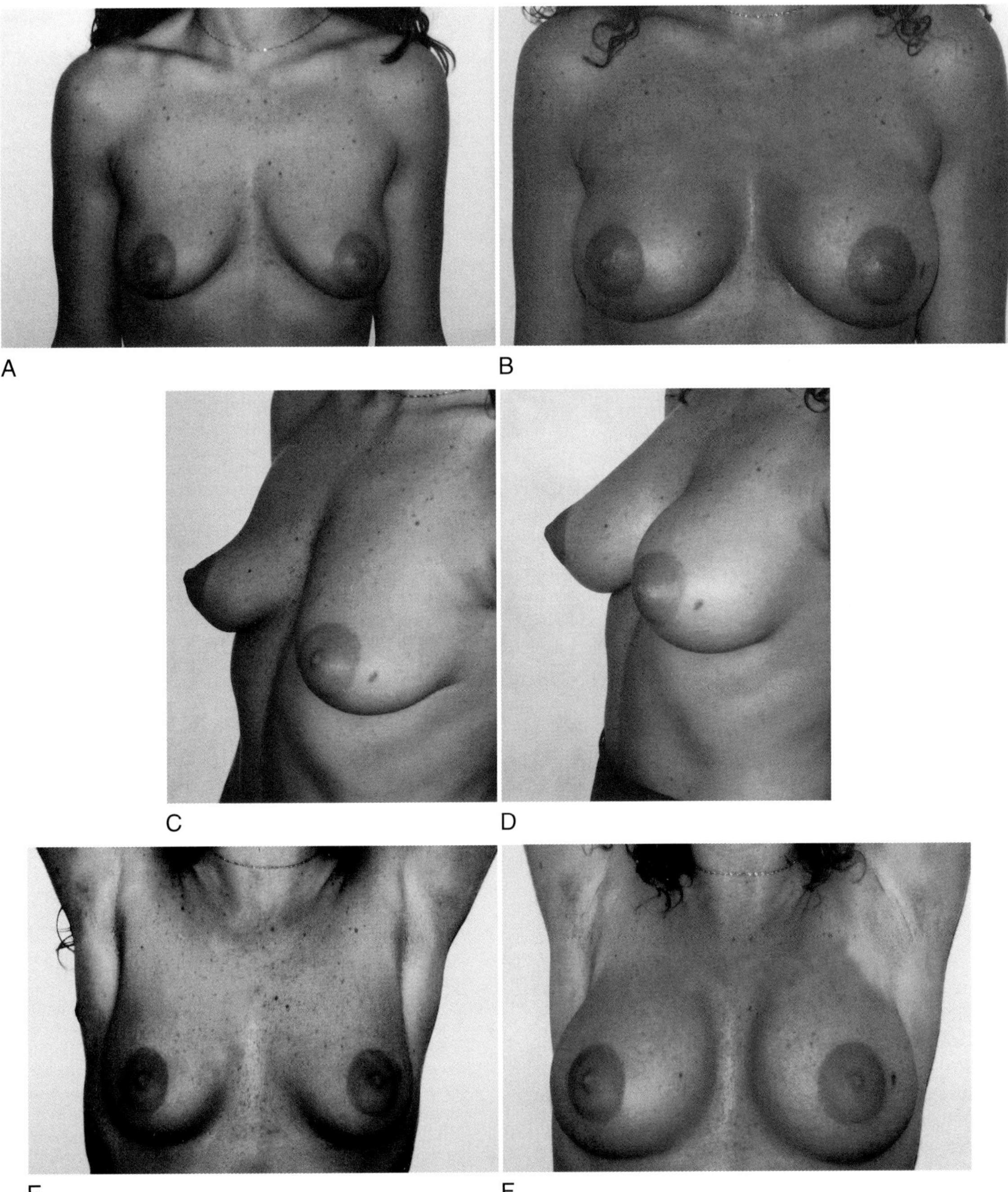

FIGURE 119-22. *A, C,* and *E,* Preoperative views of patient. *B* and *D,* Postoperative views after augmentation mammaplasty. *F,* Postoperative view of patient after augmentation mammaplasty with axillary scar.

and implant rupture.[18,19] These complications are not the purview of this chapter. However, rippling is seen most frequently in the textured saline implant. If the implant is underfilled, there is more of a chance for "fold failure," and eventual leakage of the saline ensues. It is best to fill or slightly overfill the saline implants to the manufacturer's recommended level.

If a hematoma forms postoperatively, immediate attention must obviously be given to this matter, and the inframammary approach is usually desired. Capsular contracture has decreased markedly since the advent of the textured implant; however, in thin women, the smooth-shelled implant is frequently used.[20-23]

The use of drains has largely been abandoned by most surgeons; it can allow egress of fluids, but it may also cause irritation of the implant and ingress of bacteria. Nipple and areolar paresthesias rarely occur but will usually subside in a few weeks.[24]

The use of intraoperative and postoperative antibiotics is usually preferred, but it depends on the surgeon's choice.

MISCELLANEOUS ISSUES

The transumbilical approach to breast augmentation is controversial and still in debate. Advantages include a relatively innocuous periumbilical scar and the endoscopic performance of the procedure. Difficulty in implant placement, hematoma complications, and necessary revisions can ensue, rendering the umbilical approach inappropriate for most patients.[25,26]

Implant shape by the manufacturer is also a matter of controversy.[27] The teardrop or anatomic implant has marketing value but at times can shift and give undesired fullness in areas other than the lower pole of the breast. The round implant, in the upright position, gravitationally becomes teardrop in shape and, in general, is the norm. However, in patients who have very developed pectoralis major musculature, the teardrop-shaped implant may be desirable.

There is still a debate about saline versus silicone implants, and it remains the choice of the patient and surgeon. However, the Food and Drug Administration has mandated (as of 1992) that first-time patients receive only saline implants. The four exceptions are breast reconstruction after mastectomy or trauma, simultaneous mastopexy and augmentation for postpartum mammary atrophy and ptosis, previous placement of either saline or silicone implants, and congenital anomaly of breast asymmetry.[9,10]

A new, nonsurgical technique of breast enlargement has been introduced, the Brava system.[28] The patient wears a bra-like apparatus that applies 20 mm Hg of vacuum distraction to each breast for a period of 10 hours per day for a 10- to 14-week duration. The patients may expect enlargement of one-half to one cup size, which is equivalent to approximately 75 to 100 mL of breast tissue. Patients with tight, relatively immobile breast tissue are not good candidates for this system, but women interested in nonoperative intervention who have relatively small but loose breast tissue are excellent candidates and have been satisfied.

Various herbs and over-the-counter preparations have not been shown to be a viable avenue for breast enlargement.

REFERENCES

1. Baker JL Jr, Kolin IS, Bartlett ES: Psychosexual dynamics of patients undergoing mammary augmentation. Plast Reconstr Surg 1974;53:652.
2. Brody GS: Breast implant size selection and patient satisfaction. Plast Reconstr Surg 1981;68:611.
3. Hetter GP: Satisfactions and dissatisfactions of patients with augmentation mammoplasty. Plast Reconstr Surg 1979;64:151.
4. Biggs TM, Cukier J, Worthing LF: Augmentation mammoplasty: a review of eighteen years. Plast Reconstr Surg 1982;69:445.
5. Bostwick J: Aesthetic and Reconstructive Breast Surgery. St. Louis, CV Mosby, 1983.
6. Goldwyn R: Plastic and Reconstructive Surgery of the Breast. Boston, Little, Brown, 1976.
7. Letterman G, Schurter M: History of augmentation mammoplasty. In Owsley JQ, Peterson RA, eds: Symposium on Aesthetic Surgery of the Breast. St. Louis, CV Mosby, 1978:243-249.
8. Tebbetts JB: The greatest myths in breast augmentation. Plast Reconstr Surg 2001;107:1895.
9. McGrath MG, Burkhardt BR: The safety and efficacy of breast implants for augmentation mammoplasty. Plast Reconstr Surg 1984;74:550.
10. McKinney P, Gilbert T: Long-term comparison of patients with gel and saline mammary implants. Plast Reconstr Surg 1983; 72:27.
11. Jones FR, Tauras AP: A periareolar incision for augmentation mammoplasty. Plast Reconstr Surg 1973;51:641.
12. Tebbetts JB: Transaxillary subpectoral augmentation mammoplasty: long-term follow-up and refinements. Plast Reconstr Surg 1984;74:636.
13. Wilkinson TS: Breast augmentation for periareolar incision. In Georgiade NG, ed: Aesthetic Breast Surgery. Baltimore, Williams & Wilkins, 1983:71.
14. Maxwell GP: Discussion of "Transaxillary subpectoral augmentation mammoplasty: long-term follow-up and refinements." Plast Reconstr Surg 1984;74:648.
15. Truppman ES, Ellenby JD: A thirteen year evaluation of subpectoral augmentation mammoplasty. In Owsley JQ, Peterson RA, eds: Symposium on Aesthetic Surgery of the Breast. St. Louis, CV Mosby, 1978.
16. Mahler D, Ben-Yakar J, Hauben DJ: The retropectoral root for breast augmentation. Aesthetic Plast Surg 1982;6:237.
17. Regnault P: Partially submuscular breast augmentation. Plast Reconstr Surg 1977;59:72.
18. Georgiade NG, Riefkohl R, Georgiade GS: Problems in aesthetic breast surgery and their management. In Georgiade NG, ed: Aesthetic Breast Surgery. Baltimore, Williams & Wilkins, 1983:365.
19. Schmidt GH: Mammary implant shell failure. Ann Plast Surg 1980;5:369.
20. Asplund O: Capsular contracture in silicone gel and saline-filled breast implants after reconstruction. Plast Reconstr Surg 1984;73:270.
21. Baker JL Jr: The effectiveness of alpha-tocopherol (vitamin E) in reducing the incidence of spherical contracture around breast implants. Plast Reconstr Surg 1981;68:696.
22. Baker JL Jr, Chandler ML, LeVier RR: Occurrence and activity of myofibroblasts in human capsular tissue surrounding mammary implants. Plast Reconstr Surg 1981;68:905.
23. Scully SJ: Augmentation mammoplasty without contracture. Ann Plast Surg 1981;6:262.
24. Courtiss EH, Goldwyn RM: Breast sensation before and after plastic surgery. Plast Reconstr Surg 1976;58:1.
25. Dowden RV: Dispelling the myths and misconceptions about transumbilical breast augmentation. Plast Reconstr Surg 2000;106:190.
26. Sudarsky L: Experience with transumbilical breast augmentation. Ann Plast Surg 2001;46:467.
27. Hamas RS: The comparative dimensions of round and anatomical saline-filled breast implants. Aesthetic Surg J 2000;July/August:281.
28. Khouri RK, Schlenz I, Murphy BJ, Baker TJ: Nonsurgical breast enlargement using an external soft tissue expansion system. Plast Reconstr Surg 2000;105:2500.

CHAPTER

120

Mastopexy

JAMES C. GROTTING, MD ✦ ANN P. MARX, MD ✦ STEPHEN M. CHEN, MD

Mastopexy, or breast lift as it is commonly referred to by those seeking the procedure, encompasses a wide array of techniques, depending on the patient's presenting characteristics. The universal complaint among these women is ptosis or "sagging breasts." However, mastopexies are also used to treat congenital and acquired asymmetries as well as congenital deformities, such as a tuberous breast.

Ptosis should not be confused with gigantomastia or massive breast hypertrophy, for which a formal breast reduction mammaplasty with excision of breast parenchyma is the appropriate treatment. Whereas there are some women whose ptosis is exacerbated by excess breast tissue, most women seeking mastopexy have a deficiency of breast tissue in relationship to their skin envelope. Conversely, one can also envision the deformity as having "too much skin" for the amount of parenchyma present. Although some mastopexy procedures necessarily incorporate reduction techniques, and although many women may believe that their breasts are smaller after mastopexy, it is only skin that is excised in the majority of patients and not breast parenchyma.

The degrees of ptosis have been defined by Regnault[1] by the relationship of the nipple to the inframammary fold (Fig. 120-1). In first-degree or mild ptosis, the nipple is within 1 cm of the level of the inframammary fold and above the lower contour of the gland and skin envelope. In second-degree or moderate ptosis, the nipple is 1 to 3 cm below the level of the inframammary fold but above the lower contour of the gland and skin envelope. In third-degree or severe ptosis, the nipple is more than 3 cm below the level of the inframammary fold and below the lower contour of the breast and skin envelope. There is a fourth classification known as pseudoptosis in which the nipple is above or at the level of the inframammary fold with the majority of the breast tissue below, giving the impression of true ptosis.

Brink[2] classifies ptosis by morphologic differences as glandular ptosis, true ptosis, pseudoptosis, and parenchymal maldistribution and proposes a management scheme based on these differences (Table 120-1 and Fig. 120-2).

Ptosis has many causes. The most common are breast parenchyma involution after pregnancy, excess residual skin after weight loss or explantation of a saline or silicone implant, and loss of skin elasticity secondary to aging. Because of the various degrees of ptosis and the different amounts of parenchyma versus skin, it follows that many different mastopexy techniques have evolved to treat the wide array of presenting symptoms.

Whereas there are many techniques for mastopexy, as with most surgical procedures, there are advantages and disadvantages inherent in the employed technique. One almost universal drawback to treatment of the ptotic breast is the visible breast scar that results from the operation. All mastopexy procedures produce scarring, which varies in extent and location according to

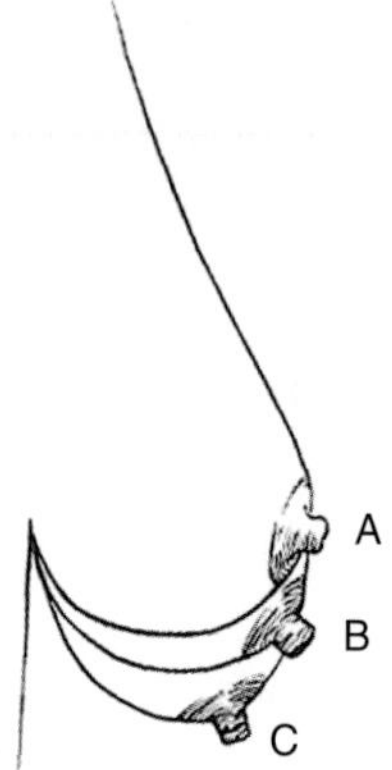

FIGURE 120-1. Breast ptosis classification as described by Regnault. *A,* Minimal ptosis; the nipple is at the level of or just inferior to the inframammary crease. *B,* Moderate ptosis; the nipple is 1 to 3 cm below the inframammary crease. *C,* Severe ptosis; the nipple is more than 3 cm below the inframammary crease. (From Georgiade NG, Georgiade GGS, Riefkohl R: Esthetic breast surgery. In McCarthy JG, ed: Plastic Surgery. Philadelphia, WB Saunders, 1991:3839.)

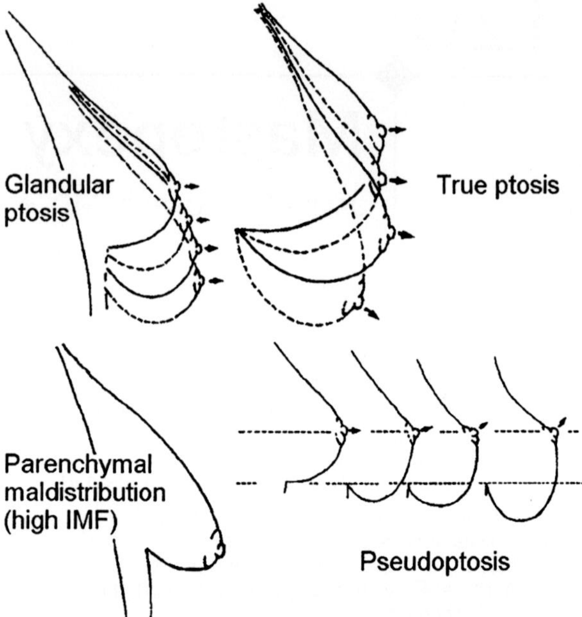

FIGURE 120-2. Different types of breast ptosis. IMF, inframammary fold. (From Brink RR: Management of true ptosis of the breast. Plast Reconstr Surg 1993;91:657.)

the amount of necessary skin resection. The patient must be informed of the extent of the incisions that she can expect from the procedure she will undergo. This can be a major factor in the patient's decision-making process. Many patients will accept a suboptimal result just to avoid excessive scarring. Also, many patients will request to have ptosis treated only with an implant, which is often inappropriate.

An additional trade-off that needs to be considered is that of reducing the breast size concurrently with mastopexy techniques. Whereas many women can obtain the improvement they desire with mastopexy alone, there are those in whom an optimal lift can be achieved only by combining a small reduction with mastopexy. Most women are more than willing to accept this; in fact, many women prefer a slightly smaller uplifted breast. There are those women with large ptotic breasts, however, who resist this compromise and maintain their quest for large uplifted breasts. The

TABLE 120-1 ✦ PROCEDURAL SPECIFICS FOR FORMS OF BREAST PTOSIS

	Inframammary Fold Position	Parenchymal Position	Nipple-Areola Position	Nipple to Fold Distance	Clavicle to Nipple Distance	Clavicle to Fold Distance
True ptosis	Fixed normal	Fixed rotated	Low downward pointing	Unchanged normal	Elongated	Unchanged normal
Glandular ptosis						
Common	Mobile descended	Mobile descended	Low forward pointing	Elongated	Elongated	Elongated
Uncommon	Fixed normal	Mobile descended	Low relative to fold	Elongated	Normal to elongated	Unchanged
	Normal					Normal
Parenchymal maldistribution	Fixed high	Fixed high	Normal downward pointing	Short	Normal	Short
Pseudoptosis*	Variable, usually low*	Mobile redescended	Surgically fixed	Elongated	Surgically fixed	Variable, usually elongated*

* Pseudoptosis is most common after corrective procedures for glandular ptosis where the fold has descended preoperatively.
From Brink RR: Management of true ptosis of the breast. Plast Reconstr Surg 1993;91:657.

operating surgeon must be sure these women understand that without a reduction, a temporary and suboptimal lifting will be all that can be realized with mastopexy techniques alone. Recurrence of some degree of ptosis will be the rule.

Last, the effects of surgery in the formation of a more youthful breast are not permanent. The breast will continue to age, and there will be a recurrence of ptosis.

There are other trade-offs that are specific to certain mastopexy procedures, and these are addressed in the following sections as each procedure is discussed.

SELECTION OF PATIENTS

Each patient must be evaluated in terms of the amount of breast parenchyma, the amount and quality of excess skin, and the scars she is willing to accept. The ideal patient for a mastopexy is one who has a close to normal amount of breast tissue along with a minimal to moderate amount of good-quality excess skin. Breast parenchyma is the scaffolding over which the skin will be draped to shape the breast. When a large excess of breast parenchyma is the cause of the patient's ptosis, a formal reduction mammaplasty may be warranted. If there is minimal breast tissue in the face of ptosis, the patient may best be served by an augmentation procedure with or without skin excision. Before any procedure is undertaken, a thorough and detailed discussion must be carried out with the patient outlining the benefits and limitations of each of the mastopexy techniques being considered.

Many techniques have been developed to improve ptotic breasts. The three most important considerations for deciding the most appropriate procedure are extent of ptosis, amount of glandular tissue versus excess skin, and extent of scars the patient is willing to accept. With such an array of techniques available for mastopexy and with the many modifications that have been developed, the easiest classification system is based on the incisions required by the procedure. The majority of mastopexy procedures fall into one of three incisional patterns: periareolar, vertical or short scar, and inverted T. The procedures in any group can cross treatment boundaries between extent of ptosis and extent of glandular tissue because of various modifications performed after the incisions are made.

PERIAREOLAR TECHNIQUES

When the proper technique is executed, the periareolar technique confines incisions and therefore potential scars to the areola-skin interface. Resulting scars in this area are usually minimally noticeable and acceptable to both the patient and the surgeon. One must be diligent to ensure that the incision is made precisely where the areola and breast skin meet. If the incision varies onto either the areola or the skin, a noticeable and unsatisfactory scar can result and the primary benefit of this technique is lost. Subsequent correction of these poorly positioned scars can be difficult if not impossible.

The periareolar approach is best used in patients with mild to moderate breast ptosis in whom there is adequate gland parenchyma that is firm. If a patient has mild to moderate breast ptosis but minimal gland parenchyma, a small implant may be added in certain periareolar techniques to achieve a pleasing breast shape. The simplest periareolar technique involves excision of skin around the areola. Depending on the degree of ptosis and the shape of the breast, the skin excisions can take the form of a donut or a crescent.

Spear et al[3,4] proposed a series of rules to limit complications.

Rule 1: $D^{outside} \leq D^{original} + (D^{original} - D^{inside})$. The amount of nonpigmented skin excised should be less than the amount of pigmented skin excised. In doing so, there will be no undue tension on the new areola with subsequent widening. The distance from the edge of the areola to the outer diameter located on the normal breast skin should roughly equal the distance to the inner diameter located within the areola.

Rule 2: $D^{outside} \leq 2 \times D^{inside}$. The design of the outside diameter should be no more than two times the inside diameter to minimize the discrepancy in circle sizes and thus reduce tension at the line of closure. Ultimately, some leeway is present if the skin envelope is lax.

Rule 3: $D^{final} = {}^{1}/_{2}\ (D^{outside} + D^{inside})$. The final rule helps predict the final size of the areola. This is especially helpful in patients with asymmetry as well as in those in whom there is no round block stitch (Fig. 120-3).

Small, mildly ptotic breasts with adequate breast parenchyma respond best to this technique. Modifications can be made to this technique, however, to accommodate moderate degrees of ptosis and where adequate breast parenchyma may be lacking. The usual modification is the addition of a small implant to take the place of breast tissue and fill the skin envelope. Nipple position will usually remain low after this augmentation, and a simultaneous removal of skin around the areola allows elevation of the nipple-areola complex to a more anatomically desirable position.

As with all periareolar techniques, the main advantage is a minimal incision with placement where the resulting scar can best be camouflaged. Even if an implant is needed, this can be accomplished through the same periareolar incision used to excise the excess skin.

The primary disadvantages have to do with the requirement for meticulous precision in the placement

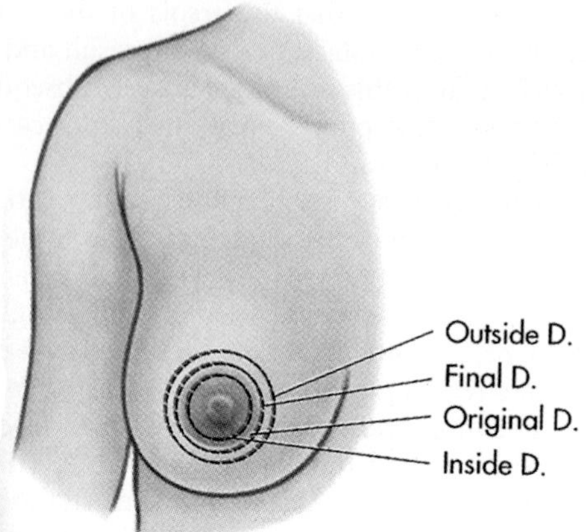

FIGURE 120-3. Periareolar design guides as described by Spear et al[3,4] (D = diameter). Refer to text for guidelines. (Modified from Michelow BJ, Nahai F: Mastopexy. In Achauer BM, Eriksson E, Guyuron B, et al, eds: Plastic Surgery: Indications, Operations, and Outcomes, vol 5. St. Louis, Mosby, 2000.)

of the incision and amount of skin excised. Even with this, the scar can widen because of excessive tension on the closure as the result of either too aggressive of a skin excision or trying to use this procedure on a large ptotic breast. Sometimes, the weight of the implant can put too much tension on the closure. In addition, the patient's skin quality (i.e., thickness and elasticity) can also be a major factor in the final scar. It is not a coincidence that those women with poor skin quality are the same ones most frequently presenting with complaints of ptosis.

Excessive tension on the closure can also result in the breast's assuming a flattened shape with poor projection. This must be guarded against because a good scar loses its value if it is placed on a misshapen breast.

Concentric Mastopexy without Parenchymal Reshaping

TECHNIQUE

The amount of skin to be excised is determined by the position of the nipple-areola complex. One must take care to excise only the amount of skin necessary to raise the nipple-areola complex to the proper level for correction of the ptosis. Consideration must be given to any excess areola that is to be removed. The lines of excision are marked on the breast with the patient in a sitting or standing position in the preoperative area. Symmetry is checked by comparing sternal notch to nipple distance and sternum to nipple distance. In the operating room, the amount of the areola that is to remain is marked on the stretched breast with an areolar marker. The skin between these two marks is infiltrated with 1% lidocaine with 1:100,000 epinephrine to facilitate de-epithelialization. Once the skin is removed, the edge of the dermis can be elevated. At the same time, the remaining skin around the exposed dermis can be elevated off the gland for a short distance superiorly. The freed dermis can then be tacked to the gland under the elevated skin, giving additional support to the breast. A purse-string suture of Gore-Tex or Mersilene is then placed in the deep dermis of the skin edge. This is then cinched to the approximate size of the areola and tied. The areola is then tacked to the skin with half-buried horizontal mattress sutures followed by a running Monocryl or polydioxanone subcuticular stitch.

Periareolar Benelli Mastopexy

The periareolar Benelli mastopexy technique is a logical extension of the donut mastopexy.[5,6] The Benelli modifications allow the periareolar technique to be used to treat larger breasts with increasing degrees of ptosis. This technique can be combined with reduction techniques when necessary to ensure the best possible result while remaining true to the idea of a minimal scar.

The fundamental concept behind the Benelli mastopexy is treatment of the skin and the gland as two separate components. The glandular tissue of the breast is accessed through the periareolar incision and separated from the overlying skin component. The gland is then restructured by an inverted T incision, and excision reduction is performed where necessary. The gland is reassembled, reducing the glandular width and tightening the lower pole. The skin envelope is redraped over this newly formed glandular scaffold. A round block cerclage stitch is used as in the donut mastopexy to help control tension at the areola-skin junction. As can be seen, this technique allows a more precise shaping of the breast by the inverted T incision through the gland while requiring no additional incisions to the skin.

INDICATIONS, ADVANTAGES, AND DISADVANTAGES

Because this technique affords access to the gland and therefore more flexibility in reshaping the gland, the indications for this procedure can be broadened to include patients with larger breasts or greater degrees of ptosis while still satisfying the requirement of minimal scars. It can be used on breasts with minimal glandular tissue by forgoing the glandular incision in favor of plication while simultaneously adding an implant. It can be used as described for larger breasts requiring a modest degree of reduction. This technique, however, is not recommended for breasts that are mainly fat or have a large amount of skin excess, especially if skin is of poor quality. Also, this technique is not indicated in large breasts for which a formal reduction may be the more appropriate procedure.

The main advantages are the improved ability to shape the gland and recontour the breast and the commitment to minimizing the scar. The disadvantages of this technique include those of the donut and crescent mastopexies. In addition, care must be taken on incision and reconstruction of the gland to avoid damage to the vascular supply of the gland and overlying skin.

There is a significant learning curve associated with Benelli's technique. If there is an overresection of skin or inadequate glandular support, the breast has a marked tendency toward a flattened appearance along with widening of the nipple-areola complex.

TECHNIQUE

Preoperative marking is initiated by marking the midline and the estimated meridian of the newly shaped breast with the patient in the upright position. The new meridian is often medial to the breast meridian approximately 6 cm from the midline. The future superior border of the areola, point A, is marked on the meridian approximately 2 cm above the anterior projection of the inframammary fold. The future inferior border of the areola, point B, is marked with the patient supine approximately 5 to 12 cm above the inframammary fold on the basis of the estimated final breast volume and the expected skin retraction. The medial and lateral limits of the new areola, points C and D, are marked on the basis of estimates of the final breast volume. These limits are equal distance from the previously marked meridian; point C averages 8 to 12 cm from the midline (Fig. 120-4).

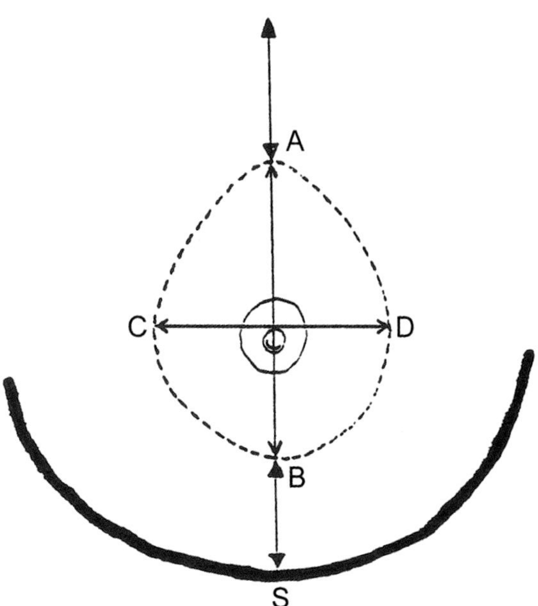

FIGURE 120-4. Markings for Benelli mastopexy: A, future superior point of the nipple; B, future inferior point of the nipple; C, medial limit of the nipple; D, lateral limit of the nipple. Point C averages 8 to 12 cm from the midline. S is the point where the breast meridian intersects the inframammary fold. (Modified from Benelli L: A new periareolar mammaplasty: the "round block" technique. Aesthetic Plast Surg 1990;14:93.)

The opposite breast is marked with reference to the already marked breast. The preoperative markings are verified by pinching together the superior and inferior points and then the medial and lateral points, ensuring that enough skin will remain to adequately cover the breast tissue without tension.

Infiltration with dilute saline (1000 mL), epinephrine (0.25 mg), and lidocaine 2% (20 mL) is performed subcutaneously in the area that will be detached. The ellipse and surrounding 3 cm is not infiltrated to preserve vascularity of the skin edges. The prepectoral area is also infiltrated. The desired areolar diameter is marked, and the periareolar ellipse is de-epithelialized. The de-epithelialized dermis is incised from the 2-o'clock to the 10-o'clock position. The dissection is extended toward the inframammary fold in the subcutaneous plane (Fig. 120-5).

The dissection continues to the upper outer quadrant of the breast and becomes more superficial to preserve the vessels coming from the lateral thoracic artery. Glandular dissection is then initiated with a semicircular incision approximately 3 cm from the inferior areola edge to preserve innervation and blood supply to the areola. Dissection is continued to the prepectoral space in the avascular central space, preserving the peripheral blood supply. The inferior glandular flap is then cut vertically beyond the breast meridian up to the fascia. Four flaps will have thus been formed: a superior dermoglandular flap supporting the areola, a glandular medial flap, a glandular lateral flap, and the detached skin flap (Fig. 120-6).

These glandular flaps will be reassembled and repositioned to decrease the base of the breast, thus promoting the lifted appearance. If necessary, these flaps can be trimmed to reduce unwanted fullness. Volume reduction should be performed at the distal ends of the flaps to limit their length.

Once the appropriate resection is complete, the gland is initially lifted by placing a stitch in the glandular tissue of the superior flap and fixating this to the pectoralis fascia (Fig. 120-7). This should elevate the areola and cause an exaggerated convexity in the superior pole of the breast (Fig. 120-8). This exaggerated convexity will disappear within a few weeks secondary to gravity and the weight of the breast.

Next, the medial and lateral flaps are folded over one another and sutured in place. Because most ptosis

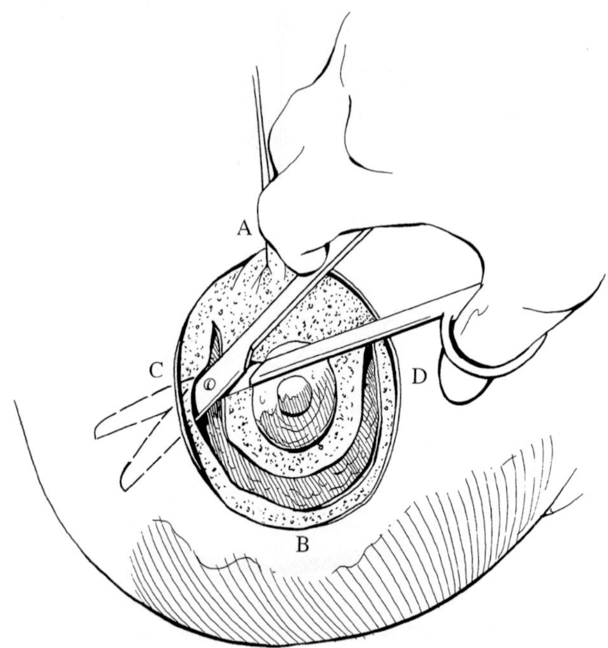

FIGURE 120-5. Dissection of the breast during Benelli mastopexy. Incision of dermis from the 2-o'clock to the 10-o'clock position with dissection to the inframammary fold subcutaneously. (From Benelli LC: Periareolar Benelli mastopexy and reduction. In Spear SL, ed: Surgery of the Breast: Principles and Art. Philadelphia, Lippincott-Raven, 1998:685.)

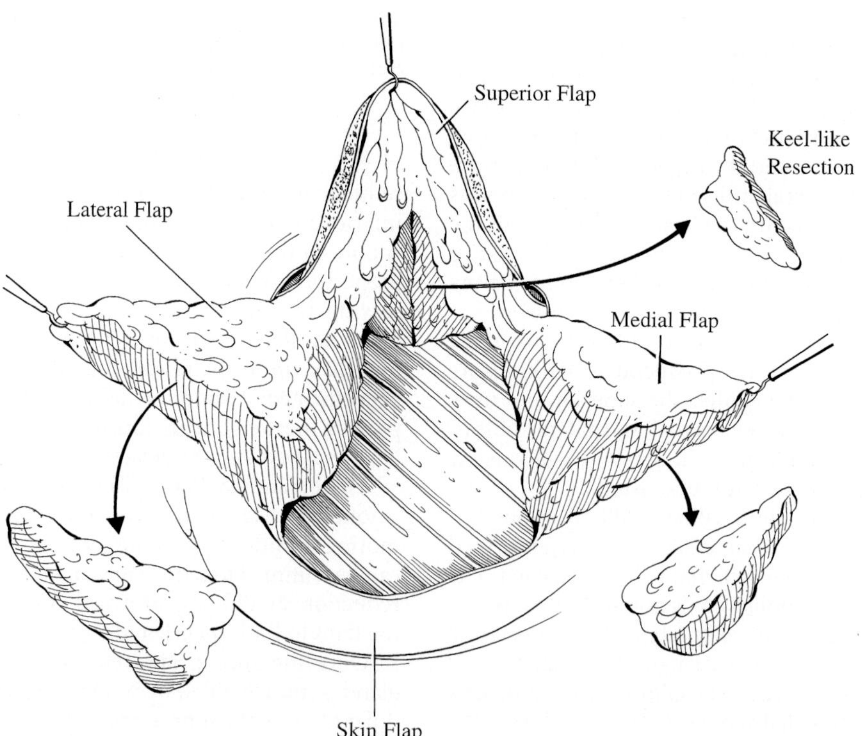

FIGURE 120-6. Four flaps of the Benelli mastopexy: superior dermoglandular flap supporting areola, glandular medial and lateral flaps, and detached skin flap. (From Benelli LC: Periareolar Benelli mastopexy and reduction. In Spear SL, ed: Surgery of the Breast: Principles and Art. Philadelphia, Lippincott-Raven, 1998:685.)

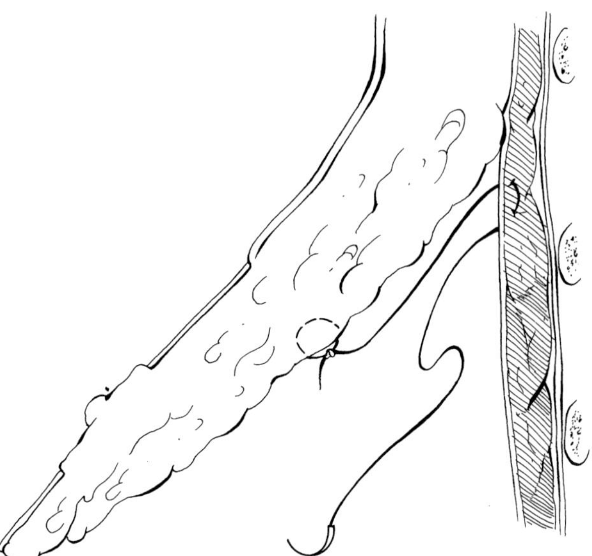

FIGURE 120-7. Benelli mastopexy. Attachment of the superior flap to the chest wall by the pectoralis fascia. (From Benelli LC: Periareolar Benelli mastopexy and reduction. In Spear SL, ed: Surgery of the Breast: Principles and Art. Philadelphia, Lippincott-Raven, 1998:685.)

involves a lateral migration of the breast, the goal here is to medialize the breast. Therefore, the crisscross mastopexy is begun by rotating and folding the medial flap behind the areola, fixing its distal portion to the pectoralis muscle with superficial stitches

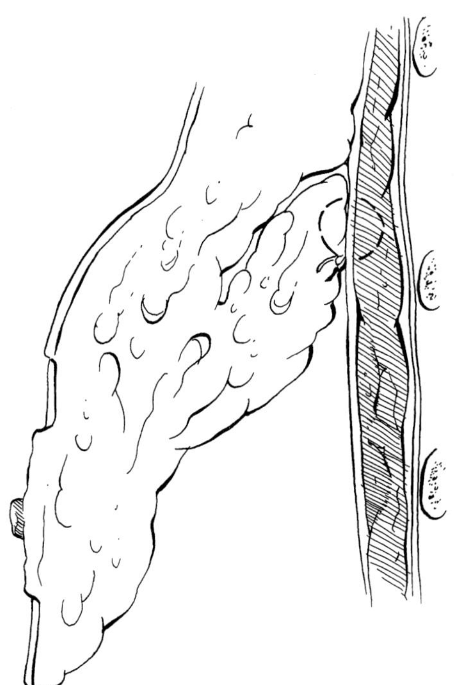

FIGURE 120-8. Benelli mastopexy. Superior flap attached to the chest wall demonstrating areolar elevation and exaggerated convexity of superior pole. (From Benelli LC: Periareolar Benelli mastopexy and reduction. In Spear SL, ed: Surgery of the Breast: Principles and Art. Philadelphia, Lippincott-Raven, 1998:685.)

(Fig. 120-9). The lateral flap is then crossed over and fixed to the medial flap (Fig. 120-10). The movement of these flaps reduces the base of the breast, forming a glandular cone on which to place the areola. If the gland requires no resection, a plication invagination can be performed to achieve an elevated conical breast shape (Fig. 120-11).

The areola is fixated to the superior border of the ellipse through a 1-cm dermal incision made near the superior skin edge. This allows the knot to be buried and the areola to be supported without tension on the skin (Fig. 120-12). Support for the breast shape is achieved by full-breast lacing. Braided polyester suture on a long straight needle is used for the large inverted sutures along the underside of the gland. The superior stitch should pass through the superior dermoglandular flap, allowing control of the anterior projection of the nipple-areola complex. These full-breast lacing sutures should be applied without tension, their goal being to provide passive support of the newly formed conical breast. Tying these lacing sutures overly tight can result in glandular necrosis.

The skin is redraped over the breast. A round block cerclage stitch is passed in the deep dermis in purse-string fashion (Fig. 120-13). It is then cinched around a tube of the desired diameter, ensuring even distribution of the skin pleats. The block stitch is then tied, burying the knot in the previously formed dermal window. Further regulation of the projection of the areola is accomplished by an inverted dermoareolar stitch that takes a large vertical bite in the areola and a large horizontal bite in the dermal ellipse. This helps distribute any remaining deep pleats evenly around the areola.

A diametrical transareolar U suture (point) is placed to serve as a barrier and help prevent areola

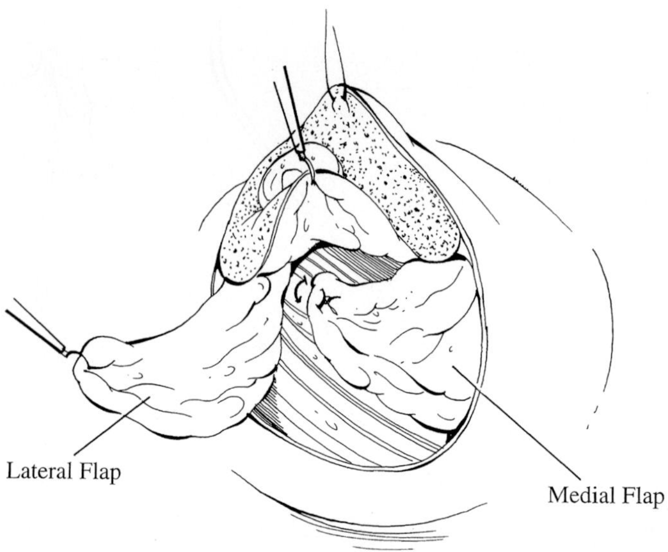

FIGURE 120-9. Benelli mastopexy. Medial glandular flap affixed to the underlying pectoralis muscle. (From Benelli LC: Periareolar Benelli mastopexy and reduction. In Spear SL, ed: Surgery of the Breast: Principles and Art. Philadelphia, Lippincott-Raven, 1998:685.)

protrusion (Fig. 120-14). It can also be used to give a circular shape to the areola in those patients in whom it tends to be ovoid. A 4-0 Vicryl intradermal suture around the areola completes the procedure.

Dressing consists of a wet compress on the areola and dry compresses on the detached skin, held in place by an adhesive bandage of moderate compression to prevent hematoma. These are removed on postoperative day 2 along with any drains and replaced with a sterile, ultrathin, semiocclusive polyurethane foam adhesive pad. This dressing covers the areola and scar and maintains all the detached skin in place. This pad will be changed weekly. The patient wears a mammary support bra for 2 months day and night.

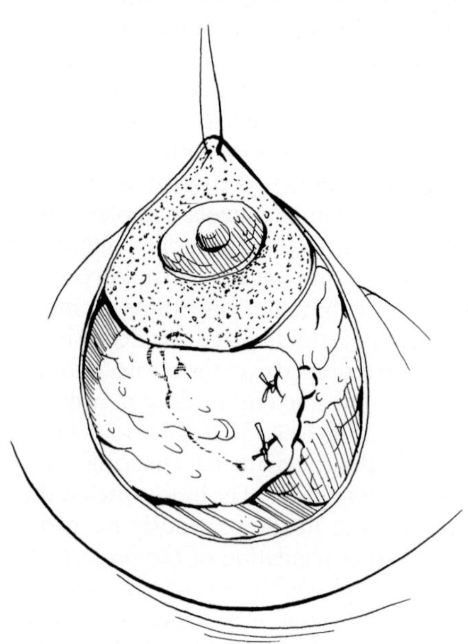

FIGURE 120-10. Benelli mastopexy. Lateral flap is affixed to the medial flap. (From Benelli LC: Periareolar Benelli mastopexy and reduction. In Spear SL, ed: Surgery of the Breast: Principles and Art. Philadelphia, Lippinçott-Raven, 1998:685.)

Goes Periareolar Technique with Mesh Support

Further expanding the indications for the periareolar technique is Joao Carlos Sampaio Goes.[7,8] He introduced the "double skin" technique, in which the basic principle involves formation of a resistant lining of the breast by the use of a layer of prosthetic mesh. This mesh provides increased support of the new breast shape during the healing and skin contraction processes.

Like Benelli, Goes treats the glandular unit separately from the cutaneous lining. This method forms an internal brassiere, making use of the anterior pectoral fascia, the intramammary connective ligaments, a periareolar dermal flap (used as internal skin lining), an absorbable mixed mesh, and the external skin lining.

INDICATIONS, ADVANTAGES, AND DISADVANTAGES

The primary indication for this method is the correction of ptosis or a slight reduction of hypertrophy with or without ptosis. Reduction should be no more than 500 g. Better aesthetic results can be obtained in younger patients with firmer tissue, more elastic skin, and little fatty tissue. Obesity, as in all periareolar techniques, can be regarded as a contraindication.

The main advantages of this technique have much to do with the addition of a specially made mixed mesh.

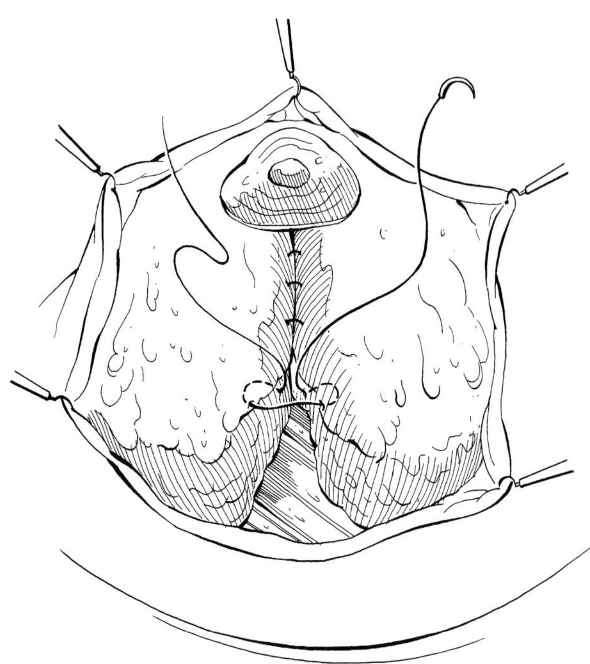

FIGURE 120-11. Benelli mastopexy. Plication invagination of the gland to form a conical shape. (From Benelli LC: Periareolar Benelli mastopexy and reduction. In Spear SL, ed: Surgery of the Breast: Principles and Art. Philadelphia, Lippincott-Raven, 1998:685.)

The mesh causes a fibrotic reaction that serves to support the breast for a longer time during the healing and cicatrization process. Whereas this goal necessitates a more rigid postoperative breast, which can last for up to 2 months, the gland ultimately does regain its elastic consistency and normal movement. By the time the mesh is absorbed, the cicatrization that has occurred is strong enough to enable the breast to maintain its new shape against its own weight and the effects of gravity. Breast palpation is normal, and no mesh can be felt by either patient or physician after healing is complete.

The main disadvantages of this procedure are the increased technical difficulty and the steep learning

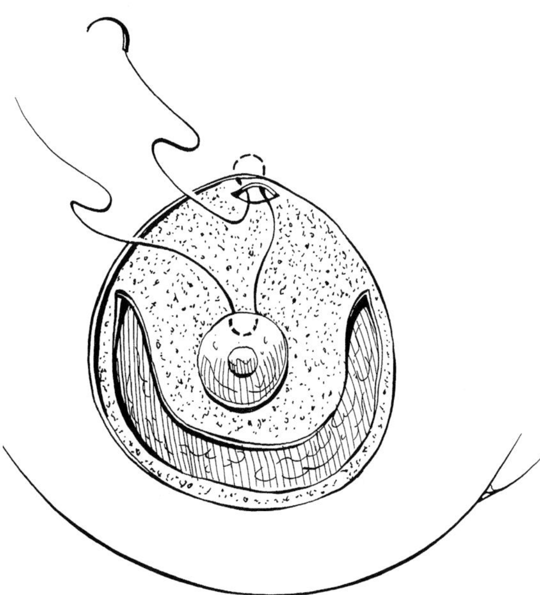

FIGURE 120-12. Benelli mastopexy. Fixation of areola to the superior border of the ellipse. (From Benelli LC: Periareolar Benelli mastopexy and reduction. In Spear SL, ed: Surgery of the Breast: Principles and Art. Philadelphia, Lippincott-Raven, 1998:685.)

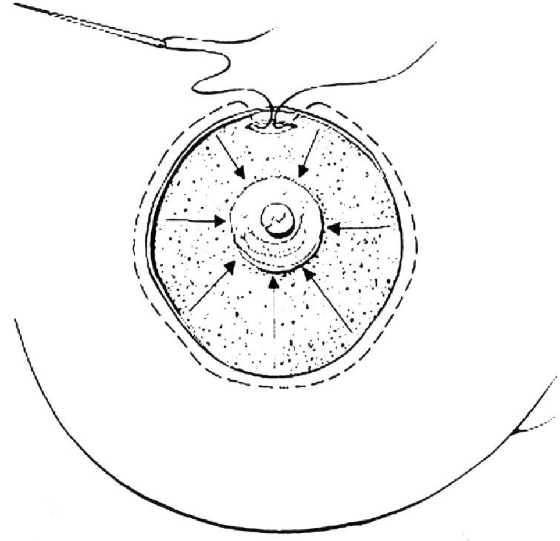

FIGURE 120-13. Benelli mastopexy round block suture. (From Benelli LC: Periareolar Benelli mastopexy and reduction. In Spear SL, ed: Surgery of the Breast: Principles and Art. Philadelphia, Lippincott-Raven, 1998:685.)

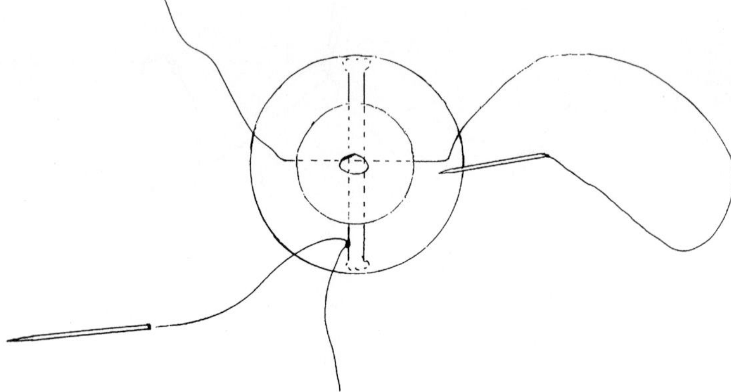

FIGURE 120-14. U stitches to help prevent areolar herniation and aid in producing a round shape in the Benelli mastopexy. (From Benelli LC: Periareolar Benelli mastopexy and reduction. In Spear SL, ed: Surgery of the Breast: Principles and Art. Philadelphia, Lippincott-Raven, 1998:685.)

curve. Although Goes indicates no instances of mesh extrusion, infection, retraction, or skin necrosis, there are many opportunities for the inexperienced surgeon to get into trouble. Extreme vigilance in excising the skin flaps and optimal retraction with meticulous placement and securing of the mesh are imperative to prevent suboptimal results and potentially disastrous outcomes.

TECHNIQUE

The technique is begun with the preoperative marking. Four cardinal points are determined (Fig. 120-15). It is important to ensure that enough skin is left to cover the newly formed breast mound.

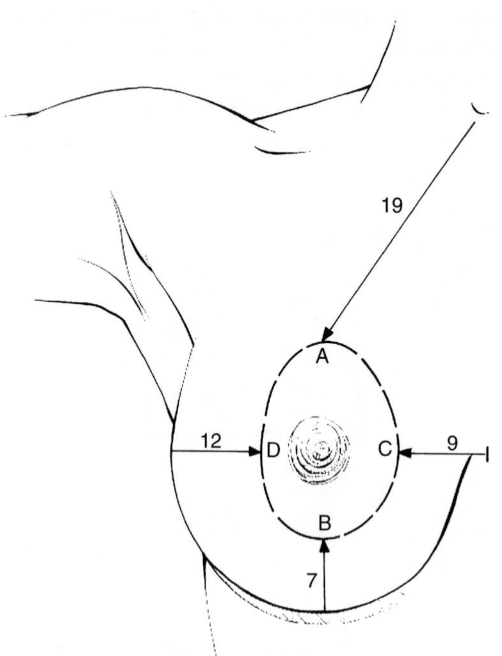

FIGURE 120-15. Four cardinal points for the Goes mammaplasty. (From Goes JCS: Periareolar mastopexy and reduction with mesh support. In Spear SL, ed: Surgery of the Breast: Principles and Art. Philadelphia, Lippincott-Raven, 1998:697.)

The area between the areola and the skin marking is de-epithelialized. An incision is made along the outer ellipse, and the skin flap is developed. The superior dissection proceeds along the base; the thickness of the subcutaneous fat tissue is progressively increased as one gets closer to the base of the breast. Undermining continues over the pectoral fascia for approximately 5 cm superiorly and then inferiorly under the gland approximately one third of the way into the retromammary space. Care should be taken to identify and preserve all perforating vessels (Fig. 120-16).

Once the skin and the gland are separated, wedges of tissue can be removed superiorly and inferiorly to accomplish any needed reduction of breast tissue. The base of the mammary gland should not be disturbed. To reassemble the gland, any superior excisional defect is closed, and the gland is fixed to the thorax in a way that fills and elevates the upper pole of the breast (Fig. 120-17*A*). The lower hemisphere excisional defect is then closed and secured to the intramammary connective ligaments and the anterior pectoral fascia. The dermal flap, which has been undermined to the areola, is gently stretched over the gland; it is attached inferiorly to the anterior pectoral fascia when possible and superiorly to the connective ligaments. This dermal component is the so-called internal skin lining (Fig. 120-17*B* and *C*).

Next, the mixed mesh (Vicryl mesh with Dacron filaments) is applied over the dermal flap as a brassiere. It is used to give an ideal shape to the parenchymal cone and to elevate the breast slightly. It is sutured to the anterior pectoral fascia. Overcorrection of the breast mound is not necessary and in fact is detrimental because there is no postoperative settling of the breast tissue (Fig. 120-18; see also Fig. 120-20).

The external skin lining is brought up over the breast mound and closed around the areola with a circular continuous deep intradermal suture of Mersilene

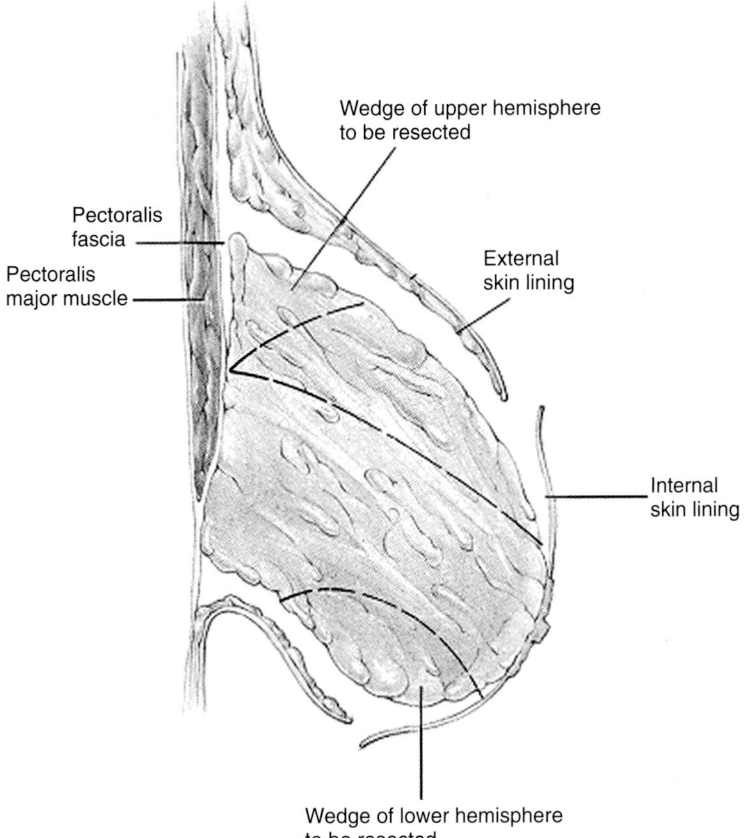

A

B

FIGURE 120-16. Goes technique. *A,* Dissection of the gland to separate it from the skin along with lines of excision of the gland. Note formation of the internal skin lining. (From Goes JCS: Periareolar mastopexy and reduction with mesh support. In Spear SL, ed: Surgery of the Breast: Principles and Art. Philadelphia, Lippincott-Raven, 1998:697.) *B,* Breast dissected free from skin. The skin flaps become slightly thicker with dissection from the periareolar region to the chest wall. Note the internal skin lining that is the de-epithelialized dermis around the nipple.

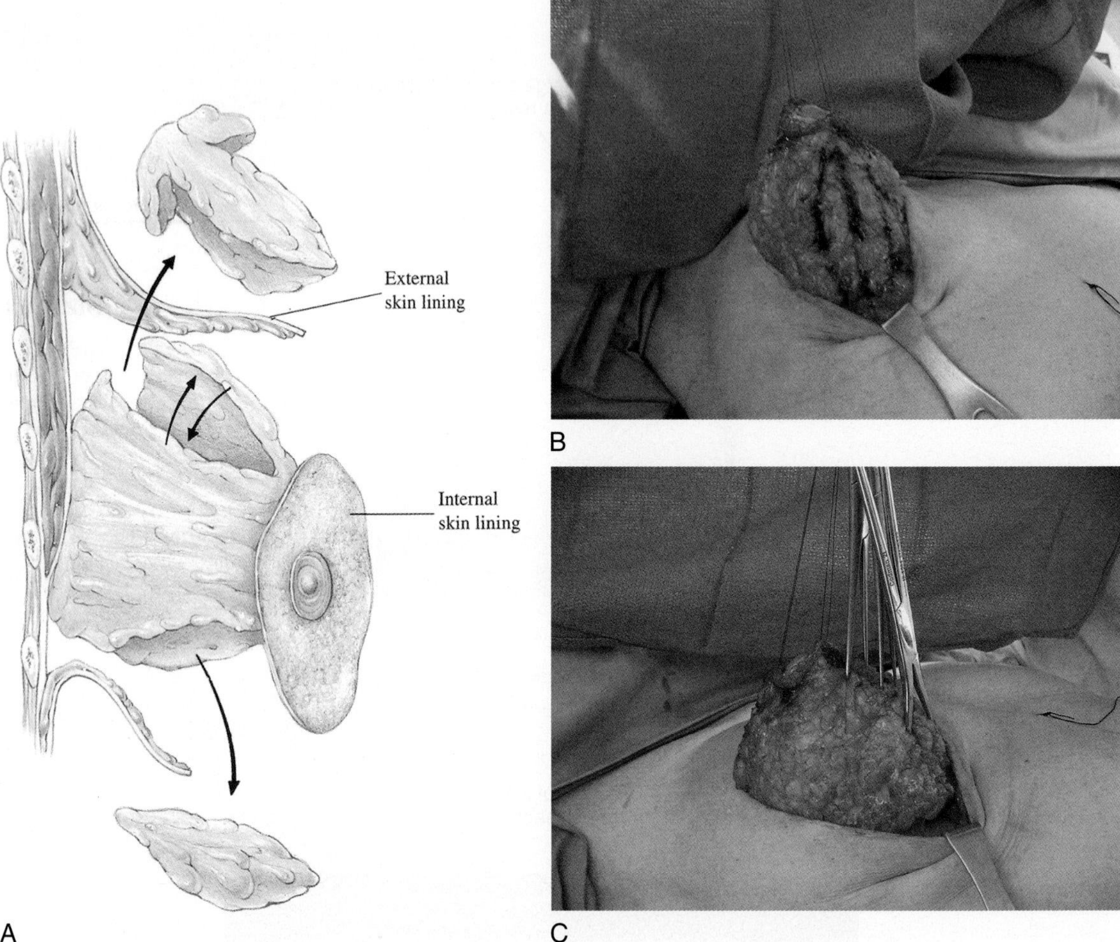

FIGURE 120-17. Goes technique. *A,* Lines of resection from the superior and inferior hemispheres to narrow the base. Note that with mastopexy alone, these regions can simply be imbricated rather than resected. (From Goes JCS: Periareolar mastopexy and reduction with mesh support. In Spear SL, ed: Surgery of the Breast: Principles and Art. Philadelphia, Lippincott-Raven, 1998:697.) *B,* Line of imbrication of the inferior portion of the gland. *C,* The closure of the inferior portion of the gland contributing to its cone shape.

2-0 on a straight needle (Figs. 120-19 and 120-20). A continuous intradermal Monocryl 4-0 suture is used to fix the areola skin to the external skin lining. Dressing consists of triangular pieces of Micropore tape covering the whole gland, which is left in place for 20 days. Tegaderm also works well for this purpose. Suction drains are removed after approximately 5 days (Fig. 120-21).

VERTICAL OR SHORT-SCAR TECHNIQUES

As the degree of the breast ptosis increases, so does the total length of the incision necessary to correct it. The logical extension of the periareolar scar is the addition of a vertical component.

Lassus Vertical Scar Technique

Claude Lassus[9-12] developed a technique for reduction and mastopexy combining four principles: a central wedge resection to reduce the size of the breast, if needed; transposition of the areola on a superiorly based flap; no undermining of the skin; and addition of a vertical scar component.

INDICATIONS, ADVANTAGES, AND DISADVANTAGES

The best candidate for this procedure is a young woman with good skin elasticity, a firm glandular breast, and breasts that are not excessively large or ptotic.

Lassus cites numerous advantages of this technique. First, the central vertical wedge resection, when

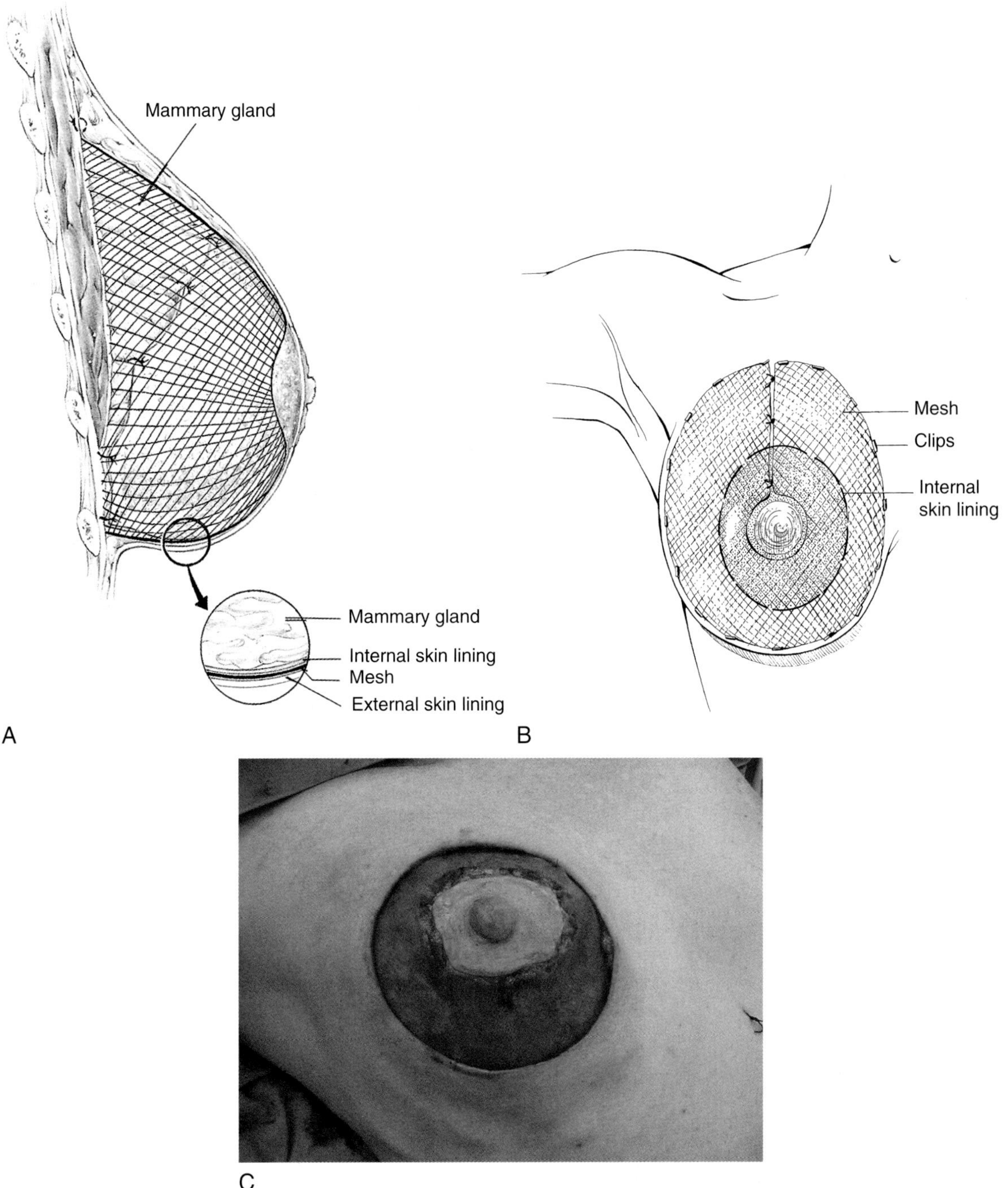

FIGURE 120-18. Goes technique. *A,* The breast projects anteriorly and superiorly after formation of the cone and reinforcement of the breast with mesh. *B,* Schematic for the placement of mesh. The polyglactin-Dacron composite mesh of Goes' original description is replaced with a Vicryl-Prolene composite. (From Goes JCS: Periareolar mastopexy and reduction with mesh support. In Spear SL, ed: Surgery of the Breast: Principles and Art. Philadelphia, Lippincott-Raven, 1998:697.) *C,* Intraoperative photograph of mesh placement.

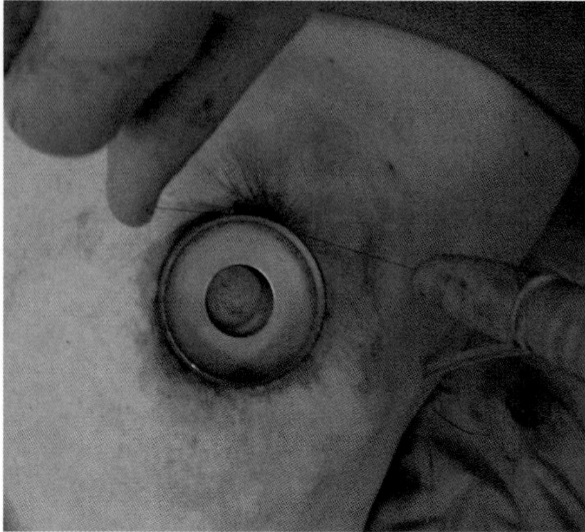

FIGURE 120-19. Goes technique. Closure of the areola.

necessary, does not impair the blood supply to the gland. Because there is no undermining of the skin from the gland or the gland from the muscle, the vascular perforators are not disturbed, theoretically eliminating the possibility of skin or glandular necrosis. In addition, the use of a superiorly based pedicle to transpose the nipple-areola complex preserves most of the neurovascular supply of the areola, thereby reducing the occurrence of necrosis or decreased nipple sensation. If, however, the nipple-areola complex has to be elevated more than 10 cm, a lateral pedicle as advocated by Skoog[13] is used. A superior pedicled flap would necessarily have to be folded over onto itself, increasing the risk for venous congestion and possible areolar necrosis.

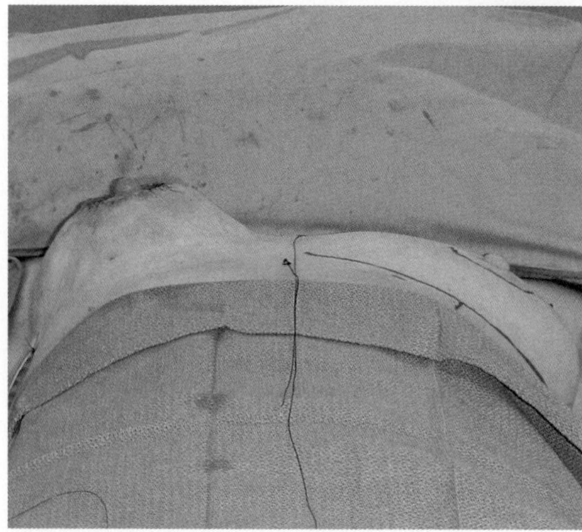

FIGURE 120-20. Goes technique. Demonstration of the anterior projection of the breast.

Because no undermining is performed, the risk for necrosis of skin and areola is decreased. By the joining together of composite blocks of skin, fat, and gland to shape the breast, subsequent healing produces a solid fibrous band the thickness of the breast. This becomes the main support to ensure projection of the breast and helps achieve long-lasting results. Also because there is no undermining, drains are usually not necessary.

A disadvantage of the procedure is the visible vertical scar. Although some would argue that a vertical scar in the standing position may be hidden and that most of the time it vanishes over the years, it is still a scar on the breast and many woman are not willing to accept this. The patient must also be made aware that the early postoperative breast shape will be less than aesthetically pleasing and that it may take several months for the breasts to obtain their final shape. Some women may not be psychologically able to wait 3 months or more to obtain a result they can accept.

In addition, an important aspect of the procedure is an "adjust as you go" philosophy. Inherent in this is the necessity of removing sutures and revising the breast shape by multiple excisions. Some surgeons may find this removal and replacement of suture lines frustrating. Also, one must be careful not to handle the tissue too aggressively while making these fine adjustments, which can result in problems with wound healing.

TECHNIQUE

Lassus does not advocate exact preoperative markings because he prefers to make adjustments intraoperatively. Instead, he uses two key landmarks. Point A is the new nipple position; this is determined as a point 2 cm below the midpoint of the acromion-olecranon distance in line vertically with the nipple. Point B, the second key point, is 4.5 cm above the inframammary fold also in vertical alignment with the nipple (Fig. 120-22).

The lateral and medial boundaries of resection are estimated either by pushing the breast medially, then laterally, or by pinching the breast with the fingers. These markings thus delineate the area to be de-epithelialized over the superior flap and the skin resection to be carried out in the lower portion of the breast.

The patient is placed on the operating room table in the semisitting position. The area within the preoperative markings is de-epithelialized. The lateral markings below the nipple flap are incised to pectoralis fascia. The lower central portion of the breast is elevated from the chest wall at the level of the inframammary fold extending to the upper pole. The

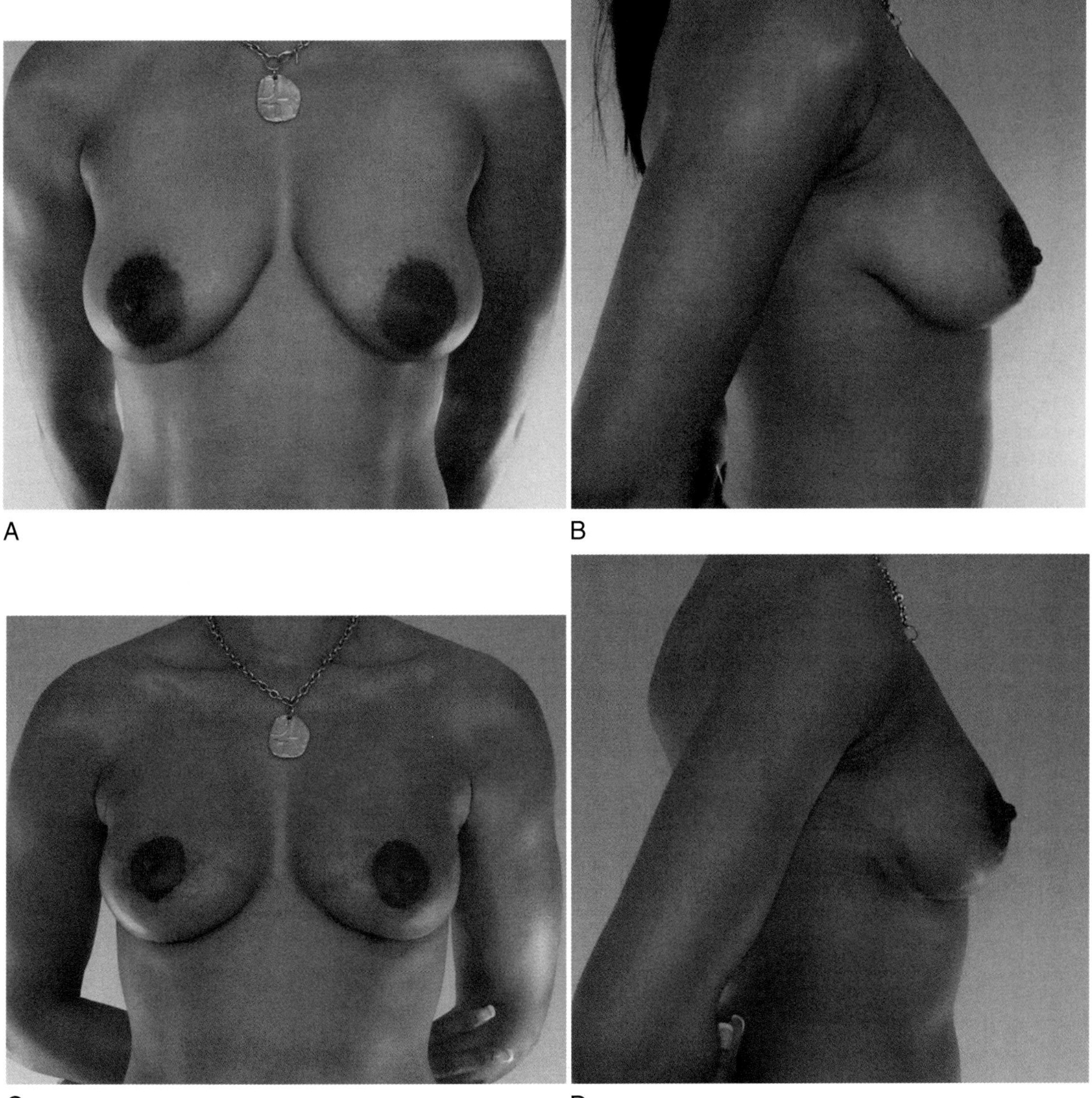

FIGURE 120-21. Goes technique. *A,* A 37-year-old patient with mild ptosis who requested rounder, more youthful breasts without an increase in overall size. *B,* Preoperative lateral view. *C,* Six months after Goes mastopexy with Vicryl mesh. *D,* Lateral view at 6 months.

superior flap is then elevated at a thickness of approximately 7 to 8 mm, leaving a glandular lining to the areola and continuing to point A. The inferior portion of the glandular flap is folded back on itself and anchored to the pectoralis muscle. If resection is needed, it is accomplished by cutting the lateral margins of the glandular tissue under the areolar flap, thereby completing the central wedge resection, which inferiorly is composed of skin, fat, and gland and superiorly consists only of fat and gland. This leaves the remaining skin attached to the gland and the remaining gland attached to the pectoralis muscle (Fig. 120-23).

The breast is reshaped by approximating the lateral and medial portions of the remaining tissues from bottom to top, checking volume and shape as sutures are placed. If more resection is needed, the sutures are removed and excision is performed. The remaining tissue is again reapproximated as before. This allows generalized shaping and a volume check. Because the breast shape at this point is suboptimal, skin stitches are used to form a satisfactory breast shape. This new

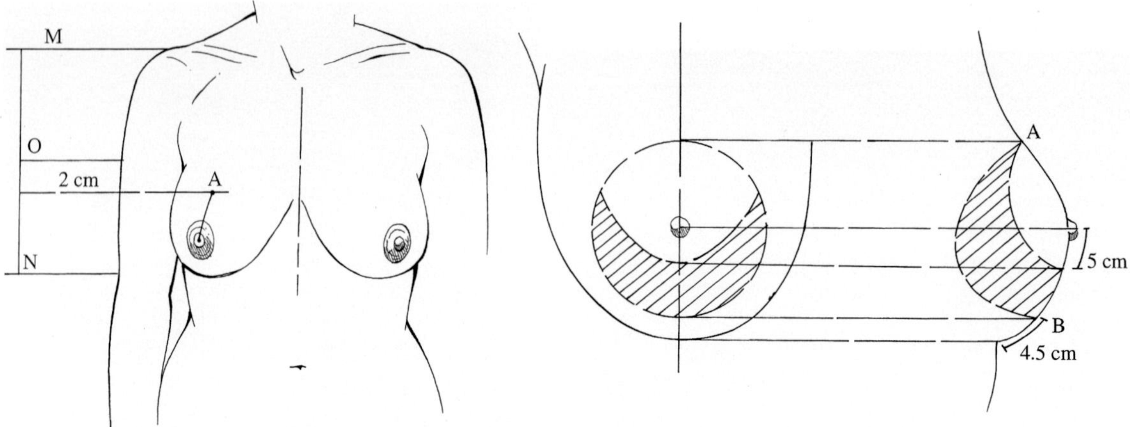

FIGURE 120-22. Lassus technique, preoperative markings. Point A is the new nipple position 2 cm below the midpoint of the olecranon-acromion distance. Point B is 4.5 cm above the inframammary fold in a vertical line with the nipple. (From Lassus C: Vertical scar breast reduction and mastopexy without undermining. In Spear SL, ed: Surgery of the Breast: Principles and Art. Philadelphia, Lippincott-Raven, 1998:717.)

suture line is marked with methylene blue along with three or four horizontal lines to allow ease in reapproximation of the tissues. The sutures are removed, and the necessary resection as marked is performed. The skin edges are reapproximated by use of the horizontal markings to aid in lining up the tissues. Sutures are then placed in the deep dermis and the superficial subcutaneous tissues, followed by a row of subcutaneous running suture. The intradermal running sutures are removed 2 weeks postoperatively. No brassiere is worn for at least 3 months while the breasts take on their final appearance.

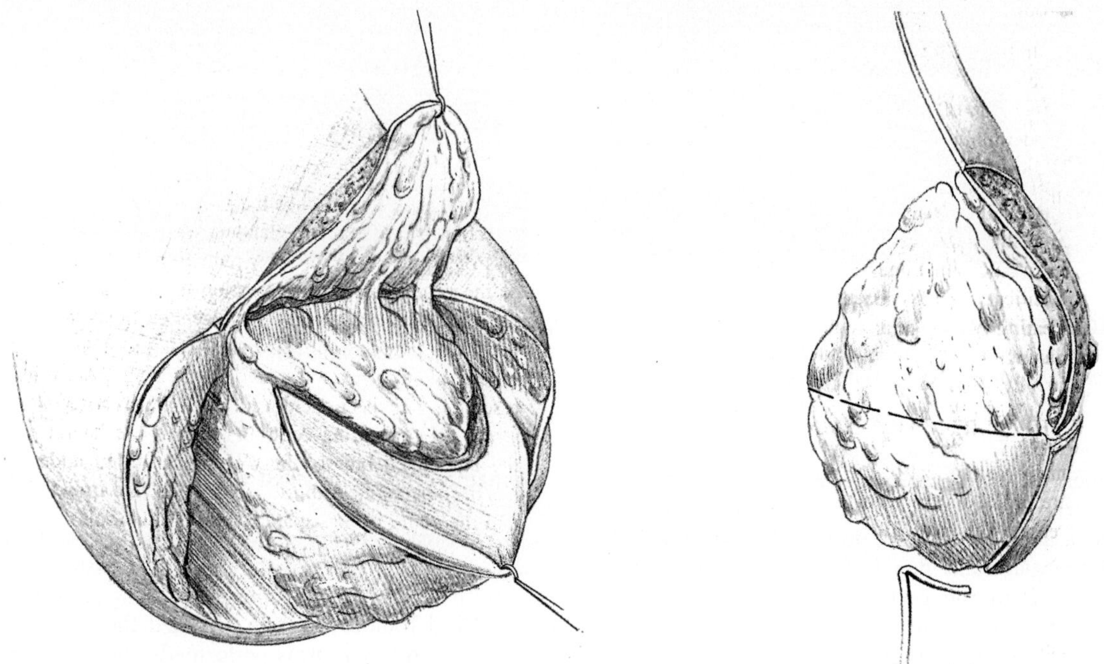

FIGURE 120-23. Lassus technique. En bloc resection of the lower pole of the breast encompassing skin, fat, and gland beneath the areola and fat and gland beneath the areolar flap. (From Lassus C: Vertical scar breast reduction and mastopexy without undermining. In Spear SL, ed: Surgery of the Breast: Principles and Art. Philadelphia, Lippincott-Raven, 1998:717.)

Lejour Vertical Scar with Undermining

Madeleine Lejour[14-16] derived her variation of the vertical scar technique by modifying concepts from Lassus,[9,10] Marchac,[24] Arie,[17] and Pitanguy.[18] This technique uses adjustable markings, a superior pedicle for the areola, and central pedicle reduction where necessary with lower skin undermining. Her modifications can be described by the following three principles: wide lower skin undermining to promote skin retraction and to reduce the amount of scarring; overcorrection of the deformity to promote better late results; and liposuction of the breast to facilitate molding and to remove unnecessary fat tissue, which has a tendency to resorb if the patient loses weight, thereby contributing to recurrence of ptosis.

INDICATIONS, ADVANTAGES, AND DISADVANTAGES

The Lejour technique can be used either as a reduction technique or as a mastopexy technique; therefore, it is applicable to many breast sizes and skin qualities. The author points to many advantages of this technique.[19]

First, by detachment of the skin from the lower portion of the breast and use of strong subglandular sutures to reshape the gland, postoperative stability is enhanced. Also, the redraped skin can retract over the gland without pressure from the weight of the gland acting against the contraction forces. By performing minimal skin excision, one can avoid overresection, which can lead to widening of scars and wound complications. The remaining skin is gathered into fine wrinkles to reduce the length of the closure. These wrinkles flatten within a few weeks to months. The resulting scar is limited to the periareolar region with a vertical limb that does not cross the inframammary fold. Nipple sensitivity is preserved by superior pedicle techniques, especially when the base of the upper pedicle is large (as with this technique).

Liposuction, which is used when volume reduction of the breast is necessary, is considered by Lejour to be advantageous because it helps make the breast softer, more pliable, and easier to shape. It protects nerves, vessels, parenchyma, and connective tissue while removing breast volume. Suction can be used at the end of the procedure to decrease any tension on the closure. Any noted asymmetry can be corrected before leaving the operating room. Finally, because liposuction removes more fat than other tissue, the resulting breast is less susceptible to recurrent ptosis should the patient experience subsequent weight loss. This contributes to the stability of the final breast shape.

As with the Lassus technique, the major drawback is the amount of time postoperatively before the final result can be realized and appreciated. Both the surgeon and the patient must have patience while the skin retracts, the wrinkles flatten, and the overcorrected breast, with its superior bulge and inferior flatness, evolves to an aesthetically pleasing breast. The author notes that some skin redundancy occasionally remains, which necessitates excision by a horizontal approach. Although this horizontal incision is small, it does add a horizontal component to the resulting scar.

TECHNIQUE

The preoperative markings show only skin resection and not gland excision. The same sets of markings are used whether or not simultaneous reduction is needed. With the patient in an upright position, the midline, inframammary fold, and vertical axis of the breast below the inframammary fold are marked. This vertical axis averages approximately 10 to 12 cm from midline. It will serve as a reference for the marking of the medial and lateral aspects of the skin excision. The breast is pushed superior-medial and then superior-lateral. Two lines are drawn on the breast in continuity with the vertical axis. These lines are joined inferiorly by a curved line placed slightly above the inframammary fold. Another curved line is used to join these lines superiorly. It is drawn to curve around the future site of the nipple, this being chosen on the basis of the preferred method of the surgeon. The superior portion of the periareolar marking is placed 2 cm above the future nipple site. This periareolar marking is joined perpendicularly to the two previously marked vertical lines. The distance between these connection points usually averages 14 to 16 cm. The markings thus drawn indicate the area to be de-epithelialized (Fig. 120-24).

The patient is brought to the operating room and placed in a semisitting position. If reduction is to be performed, 0.5% lidocaine with 1 : 100,000 epinephrine is infiltrated into the lower half of the breast. The skin excision is performed. If reduction is necessary, de-epithelialization is stopped approximately 2 to 3 cm below the areola. Liposuction is then performed through an incision inferior to the areola. If no reduction is necessary, the entire marked area is de-epithelialized and no liposuction is performed at this time. The medial and lateral markings are incised, and the skin outside these markings is dissected from the underlying gland down to the inframammary fold, leaving 0.5 cm of fat under the skin. The lower central portion of the breast is elevated from the chest wall beginning at the inframammary fold and continuing superiorly to approximately the level of the third intercostal space. Any necessary reduction is performed at this time. Tissue is excised in an oblique fashion, leaving lateral and medial pillars. The remaining breast tissue is elevated centrally by a suture

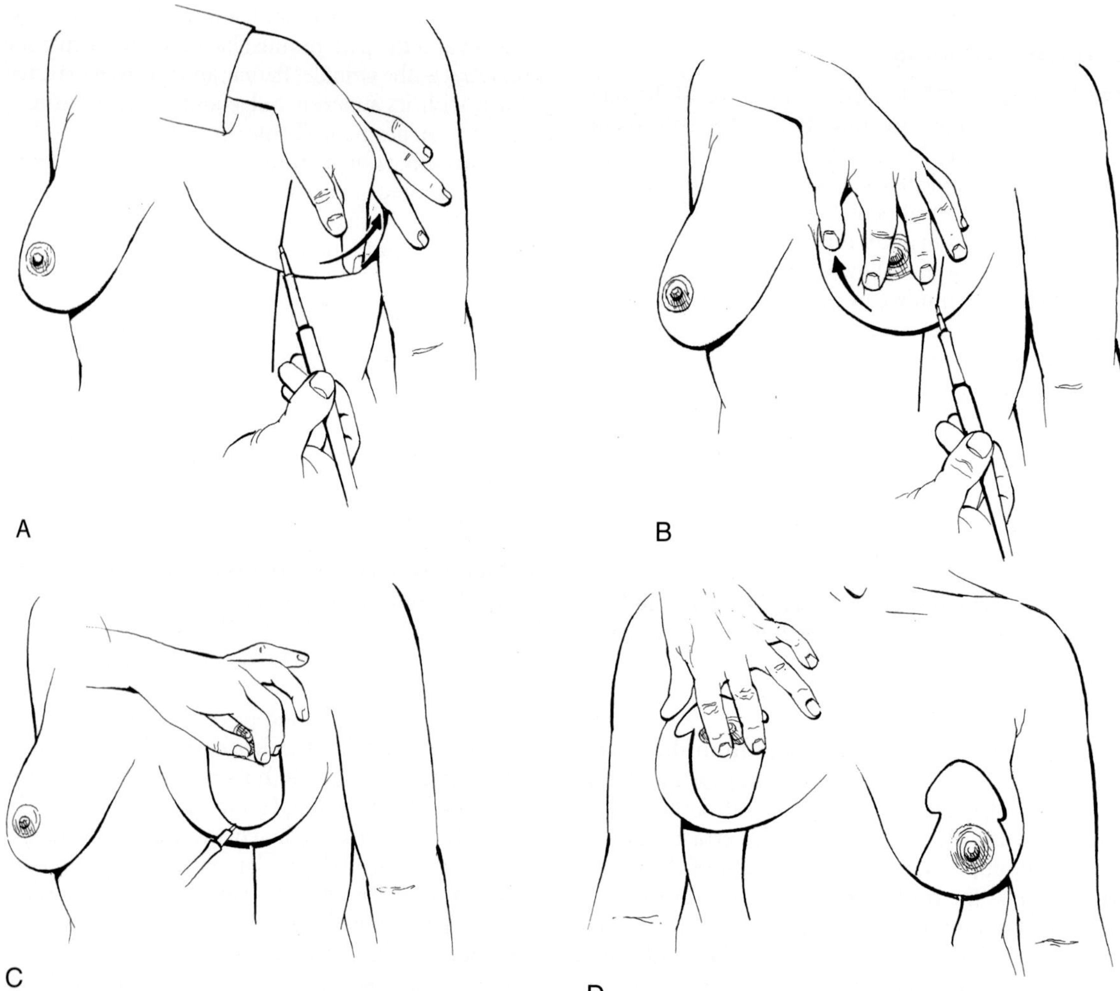

FIGURE 120-24. Skin markings for the Lejour vertical mammaplasty. *A* and *B*, Medial and lateral markings in line with the vertical axis of the breast projected on the chest wall. *C*, Curved line joining the medial and lateral limbs above the inframammary fold. *D*, Upper marking of the future nipple site, generally 14 to 16 cm in length. (From Lejour M: Vertical mammaplasty for breast reduction and mastopexy. In Spear SL, ed: Surgery of the Breast: Principles and Art. Philadelphia, Lippincott-Raven, 1998:735.)

securing the gland to the pectoralis musculature. The medial and lateral pillars are then approximated (Fig. 120-25).

If no glandular excision is needed, the centrally elevated tissue is pexied to the pectoralis musculature. The resulting folds in the gland become the medial and lateral pillars and are sutured together, forming the cone shape of the breast. The breast should be overcorrected with superior pole bulging and inferior pole flattening. The skin is redraped and sutured in two layers. First, a 3-0 slowly absorbable running stitch is placed in the subcutaneous tissue, resulting in wrinkling of the skin, greatly reducing its length. This suture line should remain above the inframammary fold in its entirety. Next, a 4-0 nylon subcuticular running suture is placed (Fig. 120-26). This further gathers the skin. Drains are placed, and the lower breast is molded with Micropore tape on a few compresses supporting the breast upward. A sport brassiere is worn for the next 2 months.

The drains are removed on postoperative day 1. The dressing is removed in 1 week and new Micropore tape placed. Sutures are removed in 2 weeks. The final result should be seen between 1 and 6 months, depending on the amount of resection and the quality of the skin.

Authors' Preferred Variation of the Vertical Technique

With increasingly better results being shown with the vertical techniques of mastopexy and reduction,

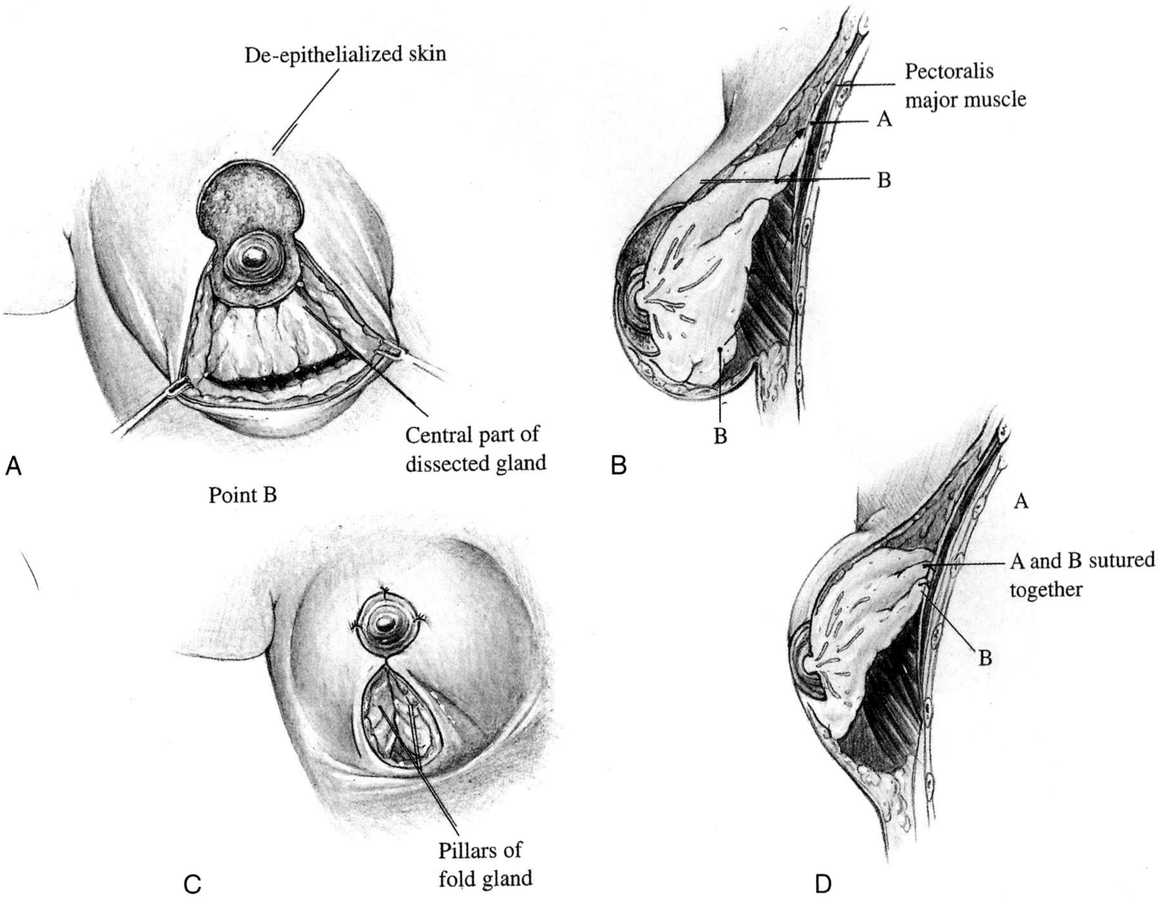

De-epithelialized skin

Central part of dissected gland

A

Pectoralis major muscle

A

B

B

B

Point B

A

A and B sutured together

B

Pillars of fold gland

C

D

FIGURE 120-25. Lejour mastopexy technique. *A,* Elevation of the skin and separation of the central portion of the gland from the pectoralis fascia. *B,* Schematic showing path of fixation for point B to the most cephalad portion of the subglandular dissection, point A. *C,* Suturing of the medial and lateral edges of the gland. *D,* Schematic of the gland pexied and elevated. (From Lejour M: Vertical mammaplasty for breast reduction and mastopexy. In Spear SL, ed: Surgery of the Breast: Principles and Art. Philadelphia, Lippincott-Raven, 1998:735.)

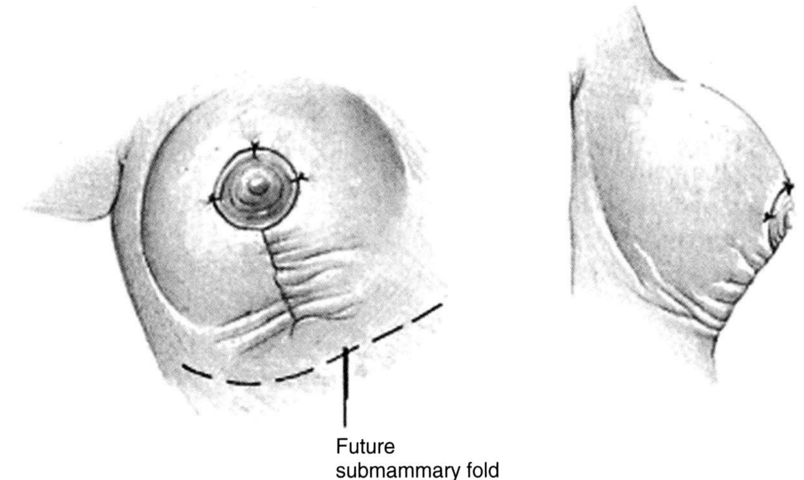

FIGURE 120-26. Lejour mastopexy technique. After completion of suturing, the skin should have wrinkling along the portion inferior to the areola. Note the overcorrection in the superior pole and the flat appearance of the inferior pole.

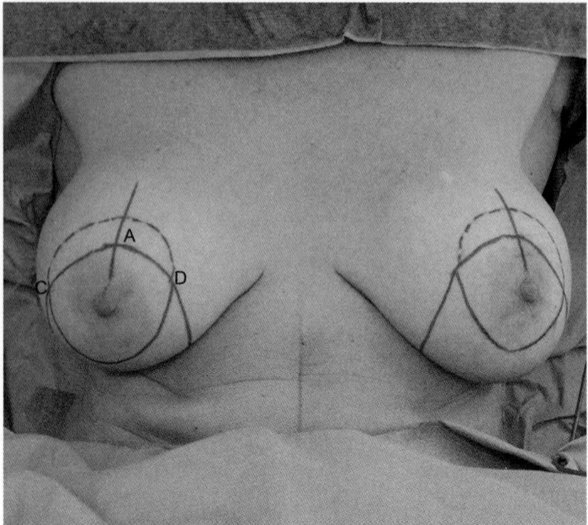

FIGURE 120-27. Authors' preferred modification of vertical technique, preoperative markings. Point A is the location of the new nipple. Points C and D will become the bottom of the new areola. The dashed line represents the new areola boundary and is usually 12 to 14 cm in length.

the authors developed a modification of the vertical technique to produce a beautiful shape with short scars that also minimized complications. The current preferred method has the latitude to allow resection of glandular tissue, if desired, and also the insertion of an implant in either the subglandular or the subpectoral plane if more volume is required.

The markings are performed with the patient in the standing position (Fig. 120-27). The future nipple position is determined right at the reflection of the inframammary fold on the anterior surface of the breast. Typically, this point is about 2 cm lower than the point chosen for inverted T techniques. It is preferable to use the standard superior pedicle for the nipple-areola complex, but if the density of the gland or distance of elevation appears restrictive, the superomedial pedicle recommended by Elizabeth Hall-Findlay[20,21] is used.

The medial and lateral pillar lines are drawn by manually distracting the breast tissue medially and laterally and approximating the volume to be left behind as well as visualizing the shape (Fig. 120-28). If tissue is to be removed, the lines should anticipate that, but similarly, if an implant is to be added, the final tension on the closure is a critical factor. The lines are adjusted in or out on the basis of those factors. Inferiorly, the bottom of the V should be at least 2 to 3 cm above the native inframammary fold (Fig. 120-29).

It is also preferable to mark on the skin surface any inferior glandular tissue that will be resected much the same way as one would mark this in an inverted T reduction. Local anesthesia with epinephrine is used in the intended lines of incision as well as beneath the gland. In straightforward mastopexy, the superiorly based inferior flap will be completely de-epithelialized and folded underneath the nipple-areola complex to fill the upper pole. It is often necessary to resect the base of the pillars at a level that measures approximately 6 cm from the top of the vertical limb down

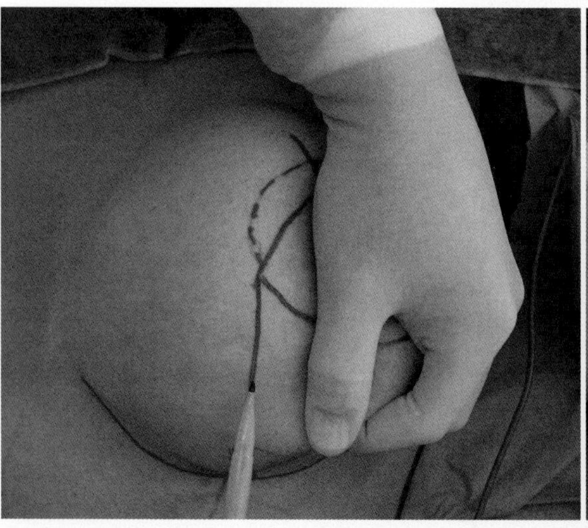
A

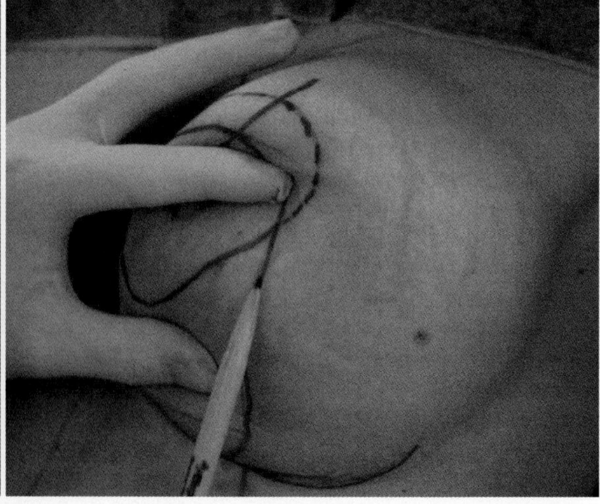
B

FIGURE 120-28. *A* and *B,* Medial and lateral limbs are formed by distracting the breast medially and laterally and connecting point A with the midmammary line of the breast projected on the chest wall.

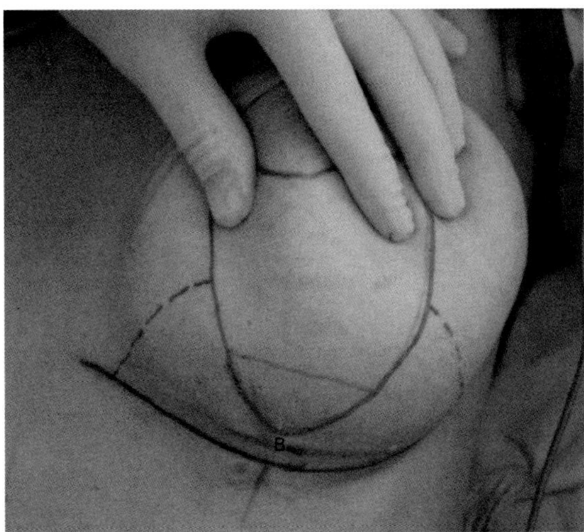

FIGURE 120-29. Note the bottom of the incision line coming to a V approximately 2 to 3 cm above the inframammary fold (point B). The hatched lines show the location of the glandular resection or the superiorly based inferior flap if it is retained for upper pole fill.

to the pectoral muscle beneath it. Appropriate projection of the gland left behind prevents recurrence of ptosis.

After de-epithelialization, the lower pole of the breast is undermined in the subcutaneous plane over that portion of the breast to be resected inferiorly, if any (Fig. 120-30). The gland is then undermined up to the superior pole to establish space into which to fold the superiorly based inferior flap. The flap is sutured into an appropriate position. If no flap is used and the tissue is resected between the medial and lateral pillars, a suture is used from the undersurface of the gland beneath the nipple-areola complex to the pectoral fascia as high up in the upper pole as possible. This gives a roundness and fullness to the upper pole.

Laterally, a "shaping suture" is used to bring the lateral parenchyma at the anterior axillary fold toward the midline of the breast to form an aesthetic curve to the lateral portion of the breast. The medial and lateral pillars are then simply reapproximated with 2-0 Vicryl sutures in the parenchyma and 3-0 polydioxanone as a layered and running skin closure. The nipple-areola complex is exteriorized in its virtual position with the patient sitting up in the operating room (Fig. 120-31). The "on the table" shape is usually one of a flattened lower pole and a rounded upper pole with the nipple pointing slightly inferiorly, the so-called upside-down breast (Fig. 120-32). It is recommended that a drain be left overnight.

The use of Tegaderm to support the final shape is an important aspect of postoperative care (Fig. 120-33). It should be left on for up to 2 weeks, at which

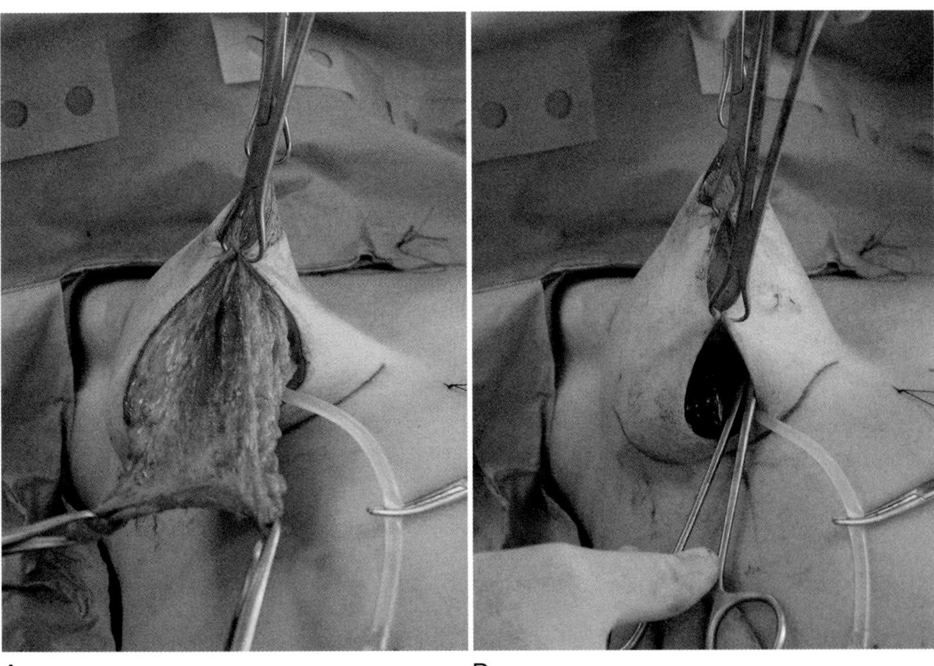

A B

FIGURE 120-30. *A,* The lower pole of the breast has been detached. *B,* The flap is transposed underneath for added projection and superior pole fill. A subpectoral saline implant was also used for added volume.

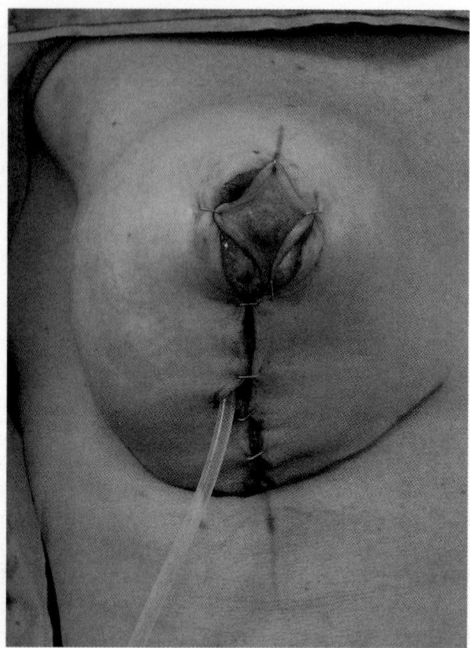

FIGURE 120-31. Temporary closure of the breast.

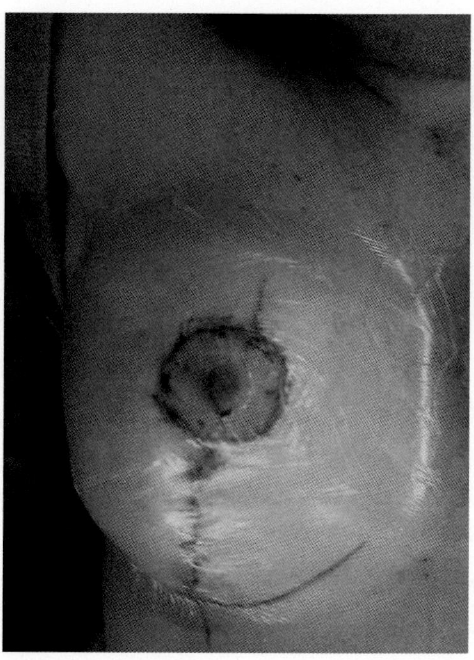

FIGURE 120-33. Final closure and cover with Tegaderm dressing.

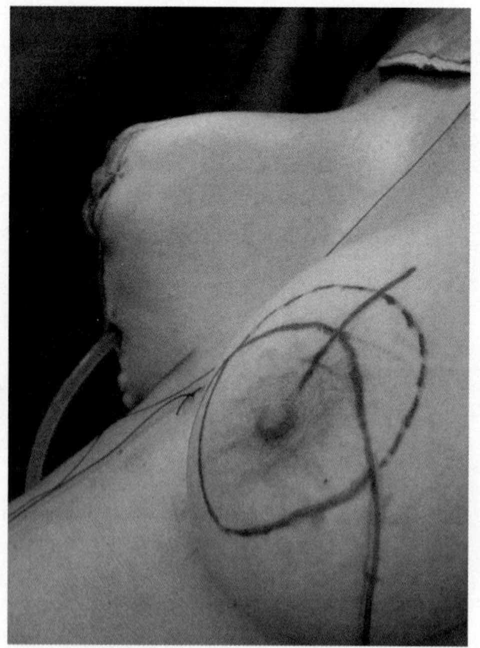

FIGURE 120-32. Authors' preferred technique. Rounded superior pole, flat lower pole, and slightly downward-pointing nipple.

point a bra should be used day and night for 6 to 8 weeks (Figs. 120-34 and 120-35).

Chiari L Short-Scar Mammaplasty

Another short-scar technique is proposed by Chiari et al.[22,23] This procedure adds a lateral horizontal component to the vertical incision, resulting in an L-shaped scar (or J-shaped scar for the right breast). It is more commonly used for breast reduction with resection of skin and breast tissue from the inferior and deep central portions of the breast while the main ductal system and the third, fourth, and fifth lateral intercostal nerves are preserved. It can, however, also be adapted to mastopexy by taking the tissue that would normally be resected in a breast reduction and folding it to provide superior pole fullness.

INDICATIONS, ADVANTAGES, AND DISADVANTAGES

Chiari's guiding principle is "that which remains is more important than that which is removed." For this reason, one of the most important indications for this procedure is the correction of asymmetry. It is most useful as a reduction technique in patients with mild to moderate breast hypertrophy (up to 600 g) and as a mastopexy technique for those patients with loose skin causing a moderate ptosis but otherwise adequate amount of breast tissue.

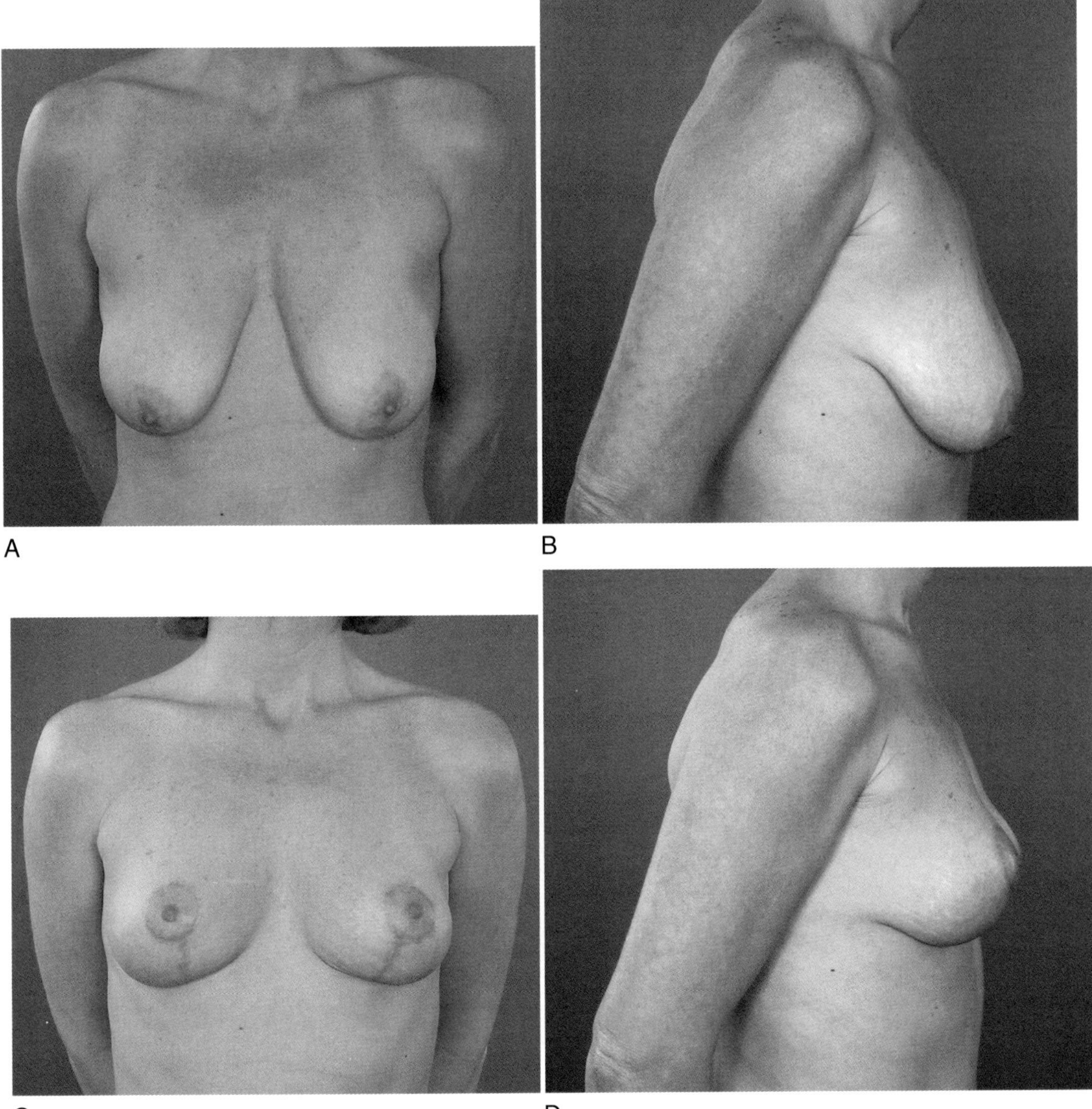

FIGURE 120-34. *A* and *B*, Preoperative anteroposterior and lateral views of a 42-year-old patient with moderate to severe ptosis. *C* and *D*, Patient seen 6 months postoperatively from vertical mastopexy with use of the authors' modifications.

The advantage of this technique lies primarily in the scar, which has no medial horizontal component and a shortened (compared with the inverted T incision techniques) lateral horizontal component. The authors note the ability to obtain a good breast shape with an undistorted areola, good projection, and preservation of innervation secondary to the formation of a broad-based superior pedicle as other advantages. Also, unlike with the vertical scar techniques discussed previously, the breast has an immediate postoperative shape that is acceptable to the patient.

The main drawback to this procedure is the preoperative markings, which can be daunting to the novice when first attempted. With experience and perseverance, the surgeon can and should make the Chiari procedure a part of his or her surgical repertoire.

TECHNIQUE

The preoperative markings are the major obstacle to this procedure. In an attempt to avoid confusion, they are listed in stepwise fashion.

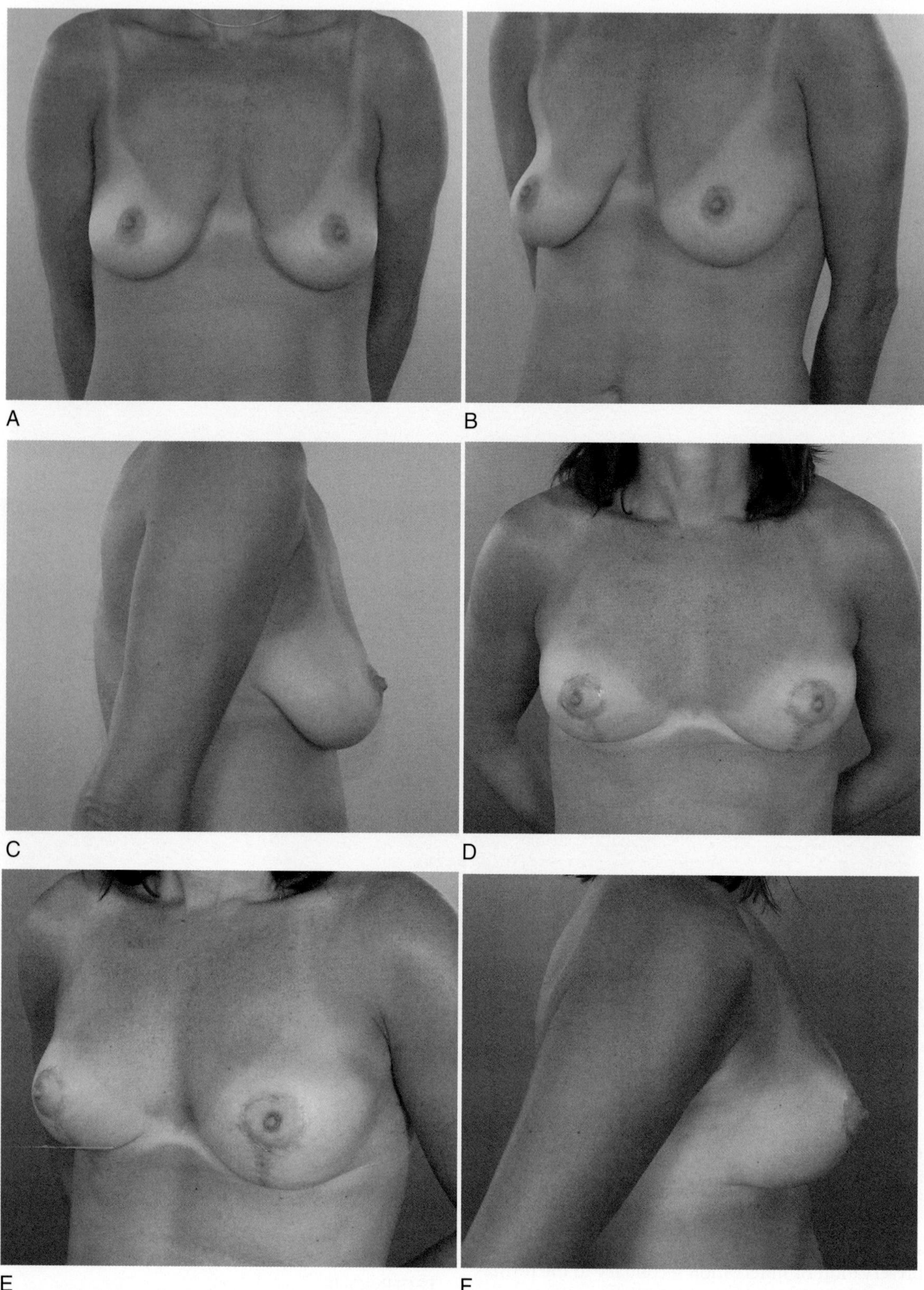

FIGURE 120-35. *A* to *C*, A 37-year-old patient with pseudoptosis. *D* to *F*, Patient seen 6 months postoperatively after vertical mastopexy.

With the patient in a standing position, the midsternal line, the anterior axillary lines, and the midmammary lines are marked. The chest width, x, is determined by dividing the distance between axillary folds by 4. This value averages approximately 8.5 cm. Point A is determined by finding the anterior projection of the inframammary fold along the midmammary line. Point A′ is marked 2 cm above point A, also on the midmammary line. The medial markings come next. Point C is 1 cm above the inframammary fold at x distance from the midsternal line. Point B is 7 cm above point C and $x + 2$ cm from the midsternal line. Next, the lateral markings are made. Point B′ is at the same horizontal level as point A, $x + 4$ cm from the anterior axillary line. C′ is placed 6 cm below B′, $x + 2$ cm from the anterior axillary line. The markings are then checked by manual approximation of BC to B′C′ to ensure that adequate tissue will remain. If necessary, a second line b′c′, inferior and parallel to B′C′, is drawn; b′ is always situated below the level of point A. Finally, point D is drawn 1.5 cm above the inframammary fold at the lateral edge of the skinfold formed when BC is opposed to B′C′ (or b′c′). By connecting BC, C, B′C′ (or b′c′), and D, a distorted trapezoid is obtained. When united, BC and B′C′ (or b′c′) will form the vertical limb, and joining C′D (or c′D) to CD will form the lateral horizontal limb (Figs. 120-36 and 120-37).

The patient is then brought to the operating room. The area bounded by B, A, B′ (or b′) and outside the areola skin, which will be preserved, is deepithelialized. Incisions are made on lines CD and

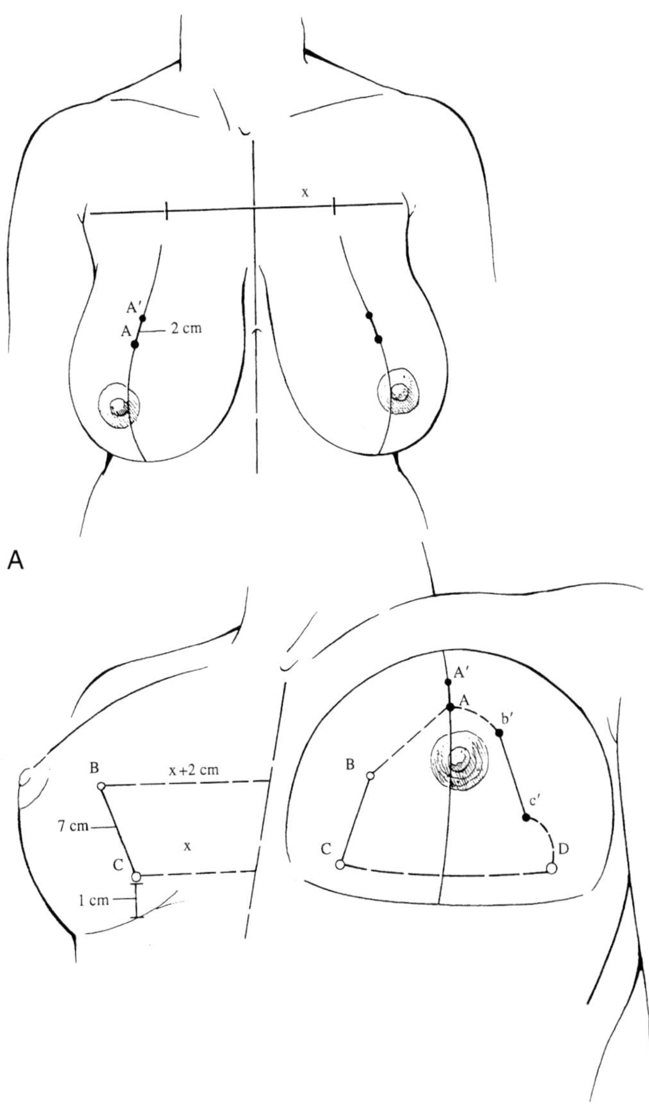

FIGURE 120-36. Chiari mastopexy technique. *A,* In the standing position, the chest is divided into fourths from anterior axillary line to anterior axillary line. This measurement is now *x* cm. Point A is the anterior projection of the inframammary fold onto the midmammary line. *B,* In the supine position with the skin under tension, the medial markings are made in reference to the length of *x,* the midsternal line, and the midmammary lines. (From Seidel SP, Chiari A, Grotting JC: The L short-scar mammaplasty. In Spear SL, ed: Surgery of the Breast: Principles and Art. Philadelphia, Lippincott-Raven, 1998:793.)

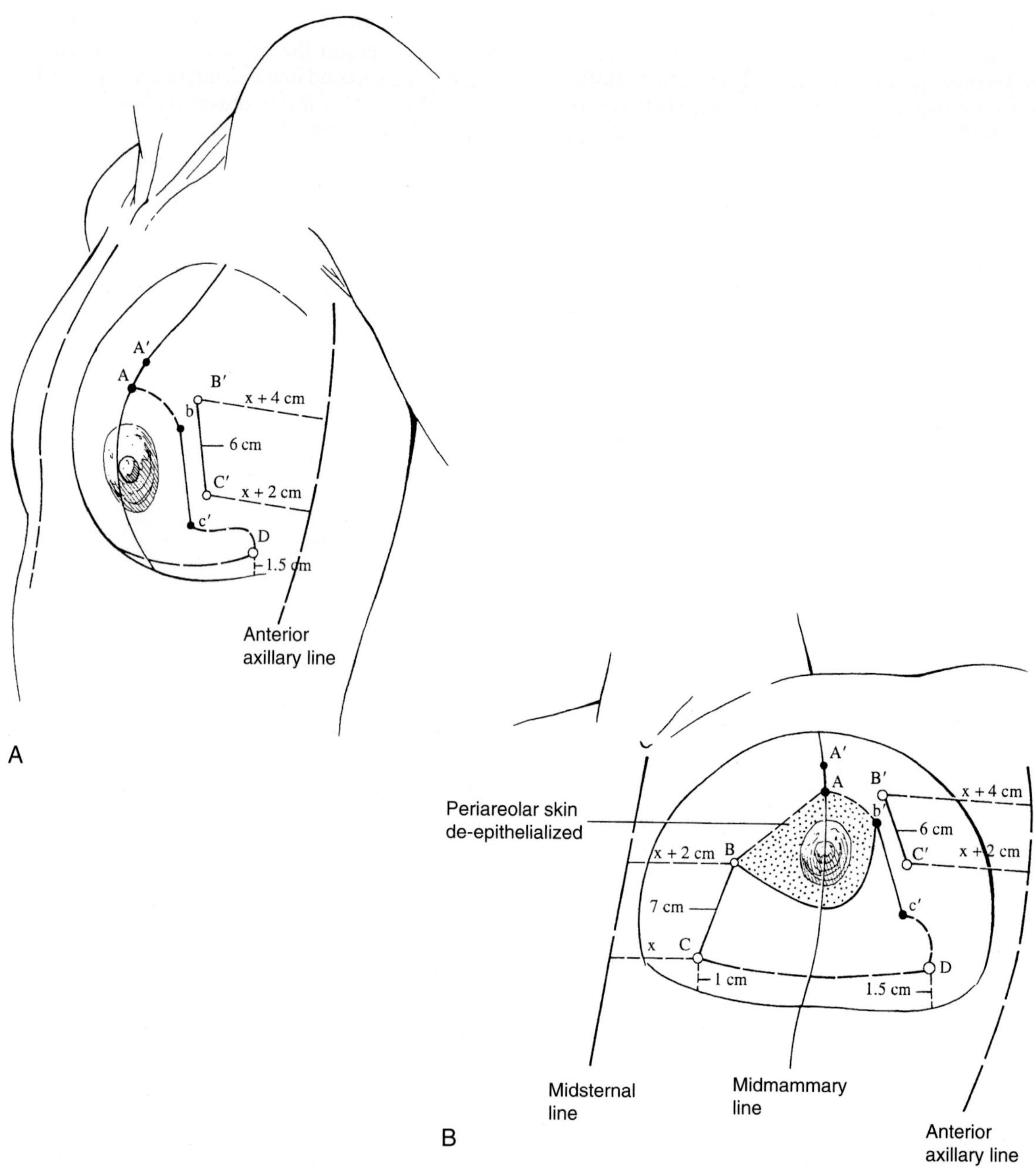

FIGURE 120-37. Chiari mastopexy technique. *A* and *B*, The lateral markings are made. B′ is at the level of point A, $x + 4$ cm from the anterior axillary line. C′ is 6 cm below B′ at a distance $x + 2$ cm from the anterior axillary line. The markings are then manually checked to see if one can approximate B to B′ and C to C′. If needed, a secondary line b′c′ can be drawn to lessen the tension of closure. The last mark is D, which is the point 1.5 cm above the inframammary fold formed at the lateral edge of the skinfold established by approximating BC to B′C′ or b′c′. (From Seidel SP, Chiari A, Grotting JC: The L short-scar mammaplasty. In Spear SL, ed: Surgery of the Breast: Principles and Art. Philadelphia, Lippincott-Raven, 1998:793.)

C′D (or c′D). The lower breast border is dissected from the skin to the level of the inframammary fold. Undermining of the breast gland is performed from the inferior margin of the pectoralis major muscle to the superior breast border. The dissection continues laterally to the third, fourth, and fifth intercostal nerves and medially to the level of the anterior cutaneous branches of the same intercostal nerves, with care taken to preserve these nerves. With the breast retracted upward at point A, the parenchyma is divided along C′D (or c′D) perpendicular to the skin. BC and B′C′ (or b′c′) are incised at a 60-degree angle, meeting at the pectoralis fascia along the midmammary line. If a reduction is being performed, this wedge of tissue is removed. If not, this superior-based flap is de-epithelialized, folded, and secured to the pectoralis fascia to provide superior pole fullness to the breast. A final incision of parenchyma only is made from B′ (or b′) toward the ipsilateral axilla lateral to the ductal system. This cut is made from the undersurface of the parenchyma upward until the subcutaneous fat is reached. This will facilitate rotation of the lateral tissue toward the midline. In breasts with soft parenchyma, this maneuver may not be necessary.

These incisions completed, two "pillars" of tissue remain, a medial pillar and a lateral pillar (Fig. 120-38). Beginning at the base, the medial and lateral pillars are approximated with deep sutures. The new areola position is marked and de-epithelialized with A′ as the vertex. The vertical scar should measure 3.5 to 5 cm. The lateral edge of the horizontal incision may need to be adjusted superiorly by excision of a small laterally based skin triangle. The skin is closed in two layers, and the nipple-areola complex is sutured into place (Fig. 120-39).

Vertical Mammaplasty with Short Horizontal Scar

In an attempt to avoid the prolonged contraction phase required by the vertical scar techniques, Marchac[24,25] devised a technique adding a short horizontal incision to remove the excess skin. He introduced the concept of upper glandular plication with suspension to the pectoralis fascia, conical gland reconstruction, and lower support of the gland by suturing together the lateral and medial pillars. These concepts were later used and modified by Lejour[14] to develop her vertical mammaplasty technique. Marchac's technique relies on three main principles: vertical incision (or excision when reduction is required) of skin and glandular tissue, conical reconstruction of the gland along with suspension to the pectoralis fascia, and formation of a short horizontal scar obtained by limiting the vertical skin resection to above the inframammary

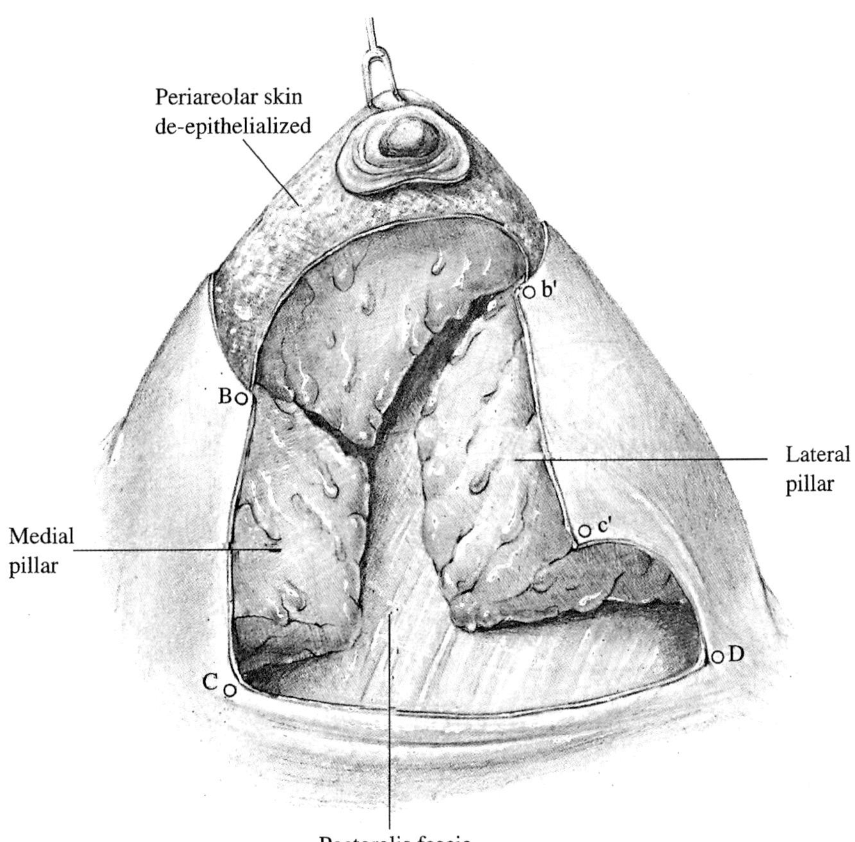

FIGURE 120-38. Perioperative illustration of the Chiari mastopexy technique. (From Seidel SP, Chiari A, Grotting JC: The L short-scar mammaplasty. In Spear SL, ed: Surgery of the Breast: Principles and Art. Philadelphia, Lippincott-Raven, 1998:793.)

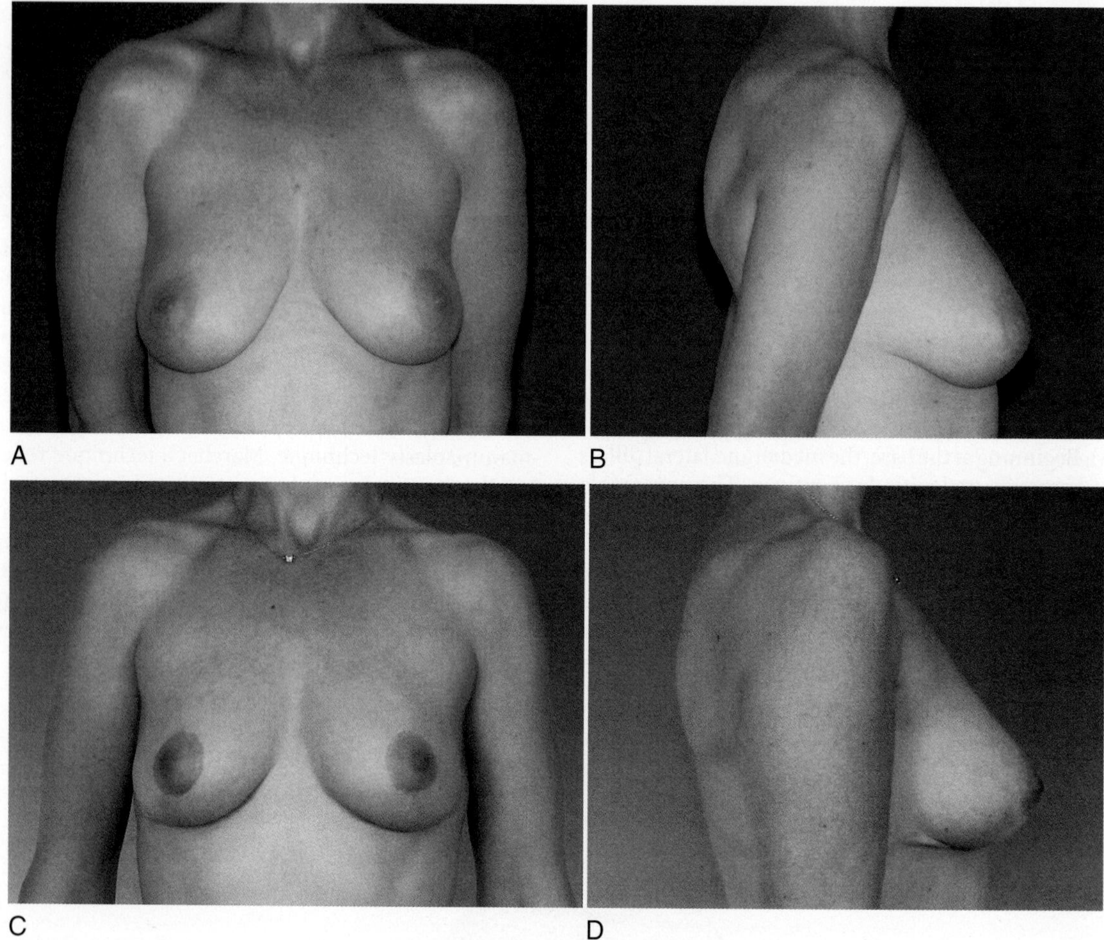

FIGURE 120-39. *A* and *B*, A 42-year-old patient with mild ptosis. *C* and *D*, One year after Chiari mastopexy.

fold and converting the lower strip of mammary skin into thoracic skin.

INDICATIONS, ADVANTAGES, AND DISADVANTAGES

This procedure is best suited for those women with adequate or moderately excessive glandular tissue in relation to the skin envelope. Also, they should be willing to accept a small horizontal scar.

One of the advantages of this procedure over the vertical scar procedures lies in the resection of the excess lower pole skin intraoperatively rather than waiting for the contraction process or a secondary skin excision procedure. Another advantage is the broad superior pedicle with limited undermining, thereby decreasing the risk for skin and areolar necrosis. This enables protection of nipple and areola sensitivity by preservation of the upper and lateral connections of the areola to the superficial sensory nerves. The superior pedicle technique combined with a central or vertical glandular resection allows a great deal of intraoperative flexibility and is therefore particularly useful in patients with glandular asymmetry. The glandular reconstruction of a cone by approximation of the vertical pillars and suspension of the gland to the pectoralis fascia produces an aesthetically pleasing and stable result.

A potential disadvantage of this procedure is the horizontal scar. Whereas it does allow a predictable, attractive result that is immediately visible after surgery and the scars generally become acceptable over time, an additional scar is produced. Some women are adamant about the minimization of their scars and would therefore consider this procedure unacceptable.

TECHNIQUE

Preoperative markings are made with the patient in a standing position. Point A is the projection of the inframammary fold onto the anterior surface of the breast. The symmetry of these markings is checked. The axis of each breast, the line on which to place the nipple-areola complex and the vertical scar, is then marked. A vertical line is then drawn on the thorax beginning at the inframammary fold. This line is usually 8 to 10 cm from the midline. Again, symmetry is verified.

The area of de-epithelialization or, in reduction, the vertical wedge excision is marked by gently pushing the breast medially, then laterally, being sure to retain adequate fullness. A line is drawn in continuity with the thoracic axis on the breast medially and laterally. The lower portions of these vertical lines are pinched together, and a horizontal line connecting them is drawn, indicating the site of the new inframammary fold. This line is usually approximately 3 to 4 cm above the original inframammary fold. The length of the vertical incision is determined by measuring up from the new inframammary fold 4, 5, or 6 cm, depending on the size of the breast. At this superior point, a 0.8-cm indent is marked to diminish tension below the areola (points B and C). The periareolar line is then drawn by connecting point A with points B and C, making a gentle semicircular curve. Finally, the superior extent of the pectoral undermining is marked. Again, symmetry is checked (Fig. 120-40).

The patient is taken to the operating room and placed in the semisitting position. The key points are marked with methylene blue. Lidocaine (0.5%) with epinephrine (1%) is used to infiltrate the periareolar area, the vertical and horizontal incision lines, the lower portion of the breast along the inframammary fold, and the retroglandular space. The areola is marked, and the area outside this but inside the previous markings is de-epithelialized. If a reduction is to be performed, the de-epithelialization will stop approximately 2 cm below the areola.

The horizontal incision is made and the skin is undermined to the inframammary fold. The undermining is continued under the lower pole of the breast until the pectoralis fascia is reached. The glandular tissue is freed from the pectoralis fascia posteriorly to the upper limit of the breast. Laterally, care is taken to avoid injury to the intercostal nerves.

A vertical incision is made up to the areola. The dermis is incised at the border of the skin medially and laterally to allow mobilization of the dermoglandular component. A heavy absorbable suture is passed through the pectoralis fascia at the upper limit of the superior undermining and through the posterior portion of the gland approximately 2 cm above the areola, in line with the breast axis. This stitch plicates the upper portion of the breast and gives fill to the superior pole to lift the entire breast. The lower dermoglandular flaps are then crisscrossed (lateral to medial, then medial to lateral) and sutured in place (Fig. 120-41).

In patients with glandular hypertrophy, a wedge resection is performed. Vertical incisions through skin and gland are made along the preoperative markings

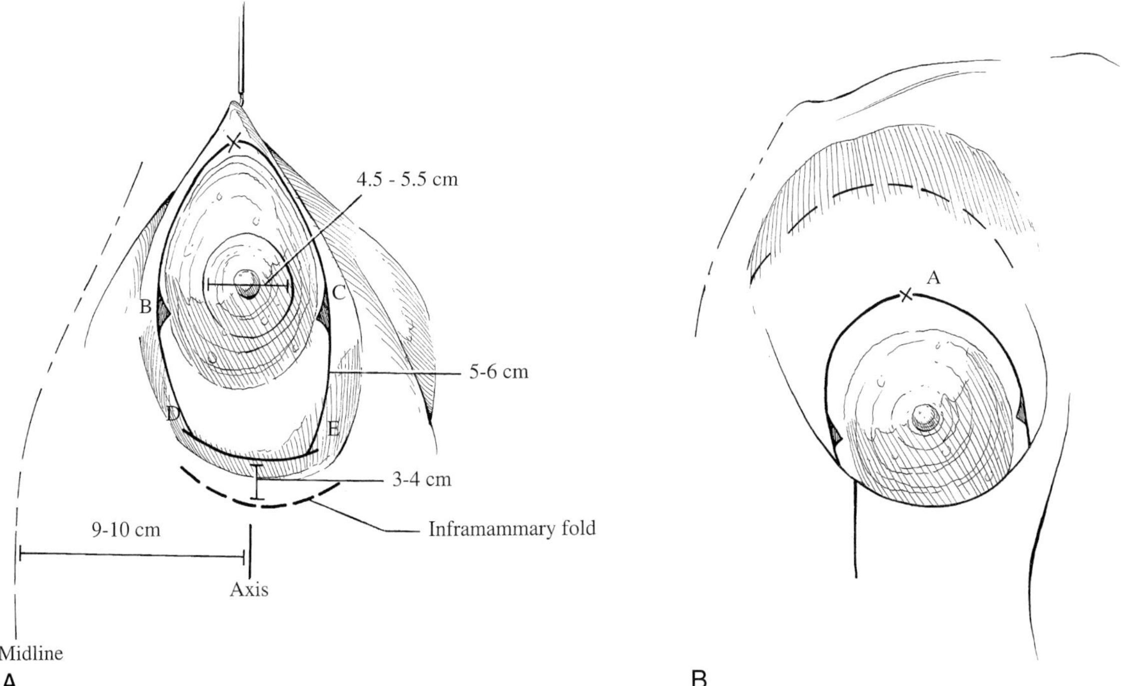

FIGURE 120-40. Skin markings of Marchac technique. Line DE is usually 3 to 4 cm above the inframammary fold. (From Marchac DA: Vertical mammaplasty with a short horizontal scar. In Spear SL, ed: Surgery of the Breast: Principles and Art. Philadelphia, Lippincott-Raven, 1998:749.)

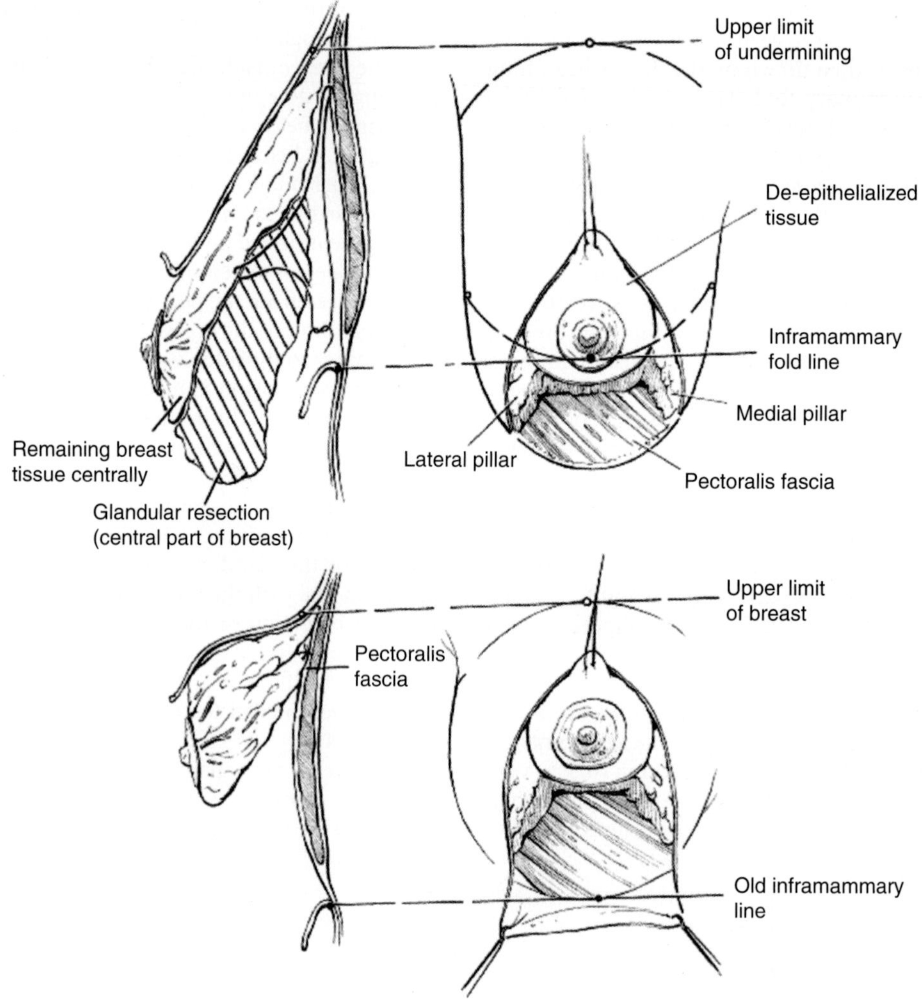

FIGURE 120-41. Plication of the superiorly based flap to the pectoralis to establish superior fill with the Marchac technique. (From Marchac DA: Vertical mammaplasty with a short horizontal scar. In Spear SL, ed: Surgery of the Breast: Principles and Art. Philadelphia, Lippincott-Raven, 1998:749.)

laterally and medially. Superiorly, an incision is made in the central portion of the breast, leaving approximately 1.5 cm of tissue under the areola. A vertical and central resection is thus performed. If additional glandular resection is necessary, a circumferential excision at the base of the breast can be performed. The remaining breast tissue is suspended in the manner already described.

The medial and lateral pillars are approximated with several layers of heavy absorbable suture. The glandular cone is thus reconstructed and the new higher inframammary fold is visible, usually approximately 1.5 cm above the old inframammary fold (Fig. 120-42).

A skin dog-ear has been formed in the lower portion of the breast. A horizontal incision is made at the level of the new inframammary fold long enough to allow excision of the dog-ear. It is important to defat carefully on each side of the horizontal incision to help define the new inframammary fold (Fig. 120-43).

At this point, the areola can usually be sutured in place with no further adjustments. If an excess of skin remains superiorly, a new areola opening can be marked with additional de-epithelialization performed. If necessary, a slowly absorbable periareolar deep dermal suture may be placed to alleviate tension on the areola-skin closure.

Postoperatively, a brassiere with a wide lower band is placed. This band helps flatten the pocket between the old and new inframammary folds. This brassiere is worn day and night for 2 weeks and daily for another month.

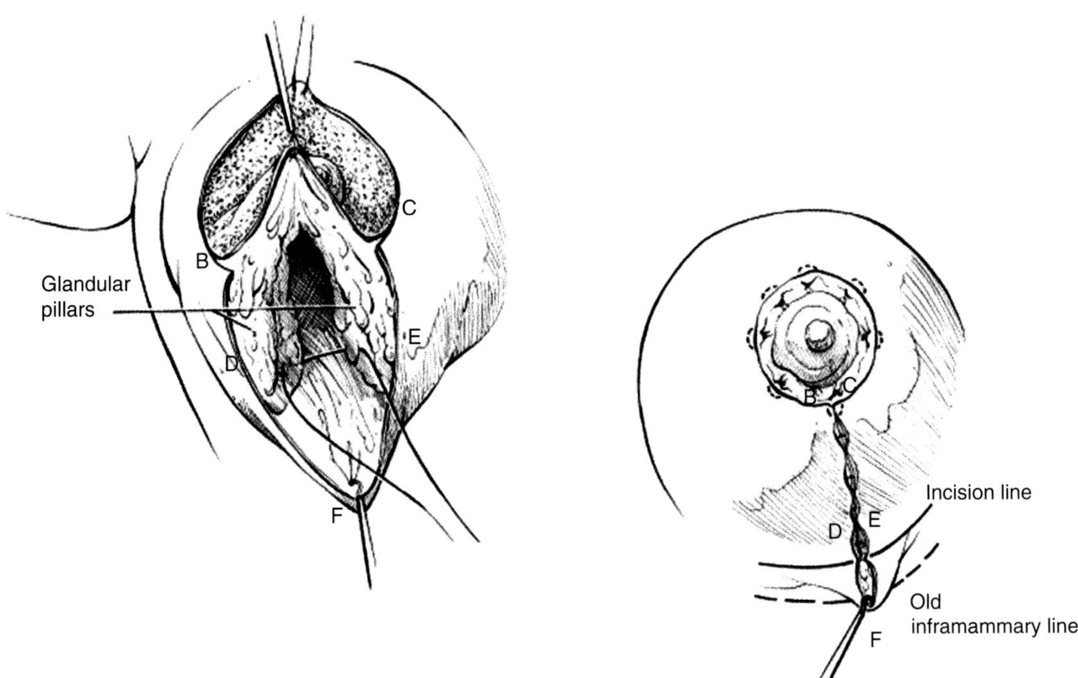

FIGURE 120-42. Reapproximation of medial and lateral pillars. Note how the new inframammary fold is above the old at approximately the same level as DE. (From Marchac DA: Vertical mammaplasty with a short horizontal scar. In Spear SL, ed: Surgery of the Breast: Principles and Art. Philadelphia, Lippincott-Raven, 1998:749.)

Inverted T Skin Closure

The inverted T or keyhole closure is the technique most familiar to plastic surgeons trained in the United States.[17,26] The Wise[27-29] vertical scar with long horizontal scar is based on the reduction technique of the same name. Regardless of the name, the long horizontal component allows adequate resection of the skin envelope in extremely ptotic breasts.

INDICATIONS, ADVANTAGES, AND DISADVANTAGES

The inverted T scar technique is reserved for those women with moderate to severe breast ptosis with a large excess of skin and a moderate amount of glandular tissue. This technique uses the same markings as traditional reduction techniques do; however, a reduction procedure is usually not required for mastopexy in these patients.

The advantages of this technique are the ability to excise all excess skin and the ability to see the final shape of the breast while the patient is still on the operating table. This allows final adjustments to shape and symmetry to be made before the end of the procedure and decreases the chance that a subsequent revision will be necessary.

The major disadvantage of this procedure is the increased length of the incisions, which increases the length of subsequent scars. The horizontal component usually runs from the most medial aspect of the breast to the most lateral aspect. In no patient should the medial incisions meet or be within 1 to 2 cm of midline. The risk for hypertrophic scarring is greatly increased in this area, and extension of the medial leg of these incisions should be avoided.

Another potential disadvantage is that the shape of the new breast is supported mainly by the skin envelope. There are no pillars or intraglandular sutures to help support the newly formed breast shape. This lack of internal support increases the chance of recurrent ptosis during the subsequent months and years.

TECHNIQUE

Markings proceed with the standard Wise pattern. First, the meridian line of the breast is marked. The new position of the nipple is marked along this line at the anterior projection of the inframammary fold. A wire keyhole pattern is spread to allow it to just encompass the original areola. The superior aspect of the pattern is placed approximately 2 cm above the location of the projected nipple position. These markings can be checked by bringing these points together with infolding of the central and inferior skin and assessing tension. Some tension is necessary to compensate for the inevitable postoperative relaxation of skin

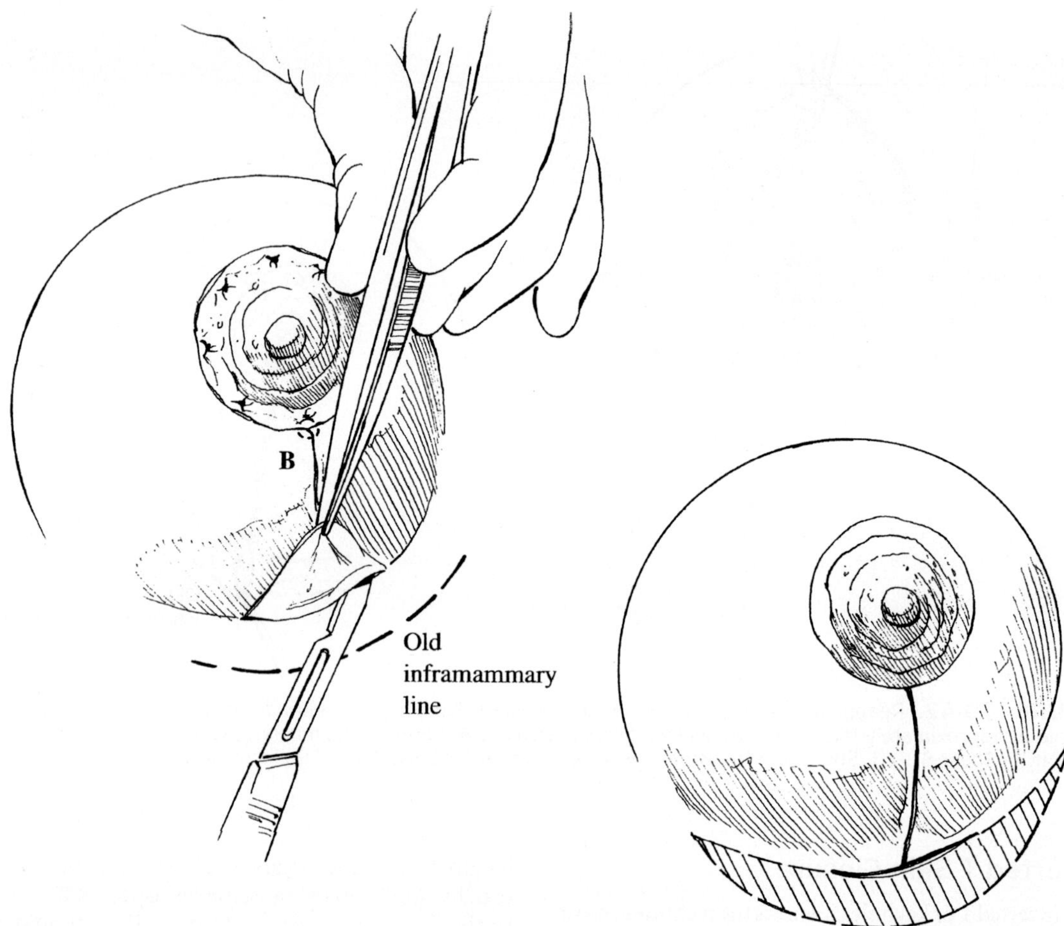

FIGURE 120-43. Tailoring of the short horizontal incision. Note that the new fold is above the old. (From Marchac DA: Vertical mammaplasty with a short horizontal scar. In Spear SL, ed: Surgery of the Breast: Principles and Art. Philadelphia, Lippincott-Raven, 1998:749.)

support; however, it should not be so great as to risk ischemia or wound problems or to cause an unnatural tightness to the base of the breast. These vertically oriented markings are extended laterally and medially on the breast to converge with the inframammary fold.

In the operating room, the portion of the areola to be preserved is marked with an areolar marking device of the appropriate diameter. The area within the marks is de-epithelialized. Transdermal incisions are made along the upper portion of what would be the vertical bipedicle flap of a reduction mammaplasty on either side of the nipple-areola complex. If there is an abundance of de-epithelialized breast tissue below the inframammary fold, dissection of the gland off the pectoralis muscle is undertaken starting from the inframammary fold and proceeding upward to establish a superiorly based dermoglandular pedicle. The dissection continues until the pocket can accept the excess inferior glandular tissue. This tissue is folded behind the breast and attached to the pectoralis fascia high enough to eliminate gross glandular redundancy. Skin closure is accomplished in standard fashion with little or no further undermining. The nipple-areola complex is positioned and sutured into place (Fig. 120-44).

Suction

In the never-ending quest to reduce the length of scars, liposuction has been proposed as a method not only to reduce the size of the breast but also to raise the nipple-areola complex slightly while reducing its size.[30-33] Most of the substance removed from the breast with liposuction is fatty tissue, and this plays a role in selection of patients. In addition, the raising of the nipple-areola complex with its reduction in size is a function of removal of tissue from the breast, which thereby decreases the weight and subsequently decreases the tension on this structure. This allows the

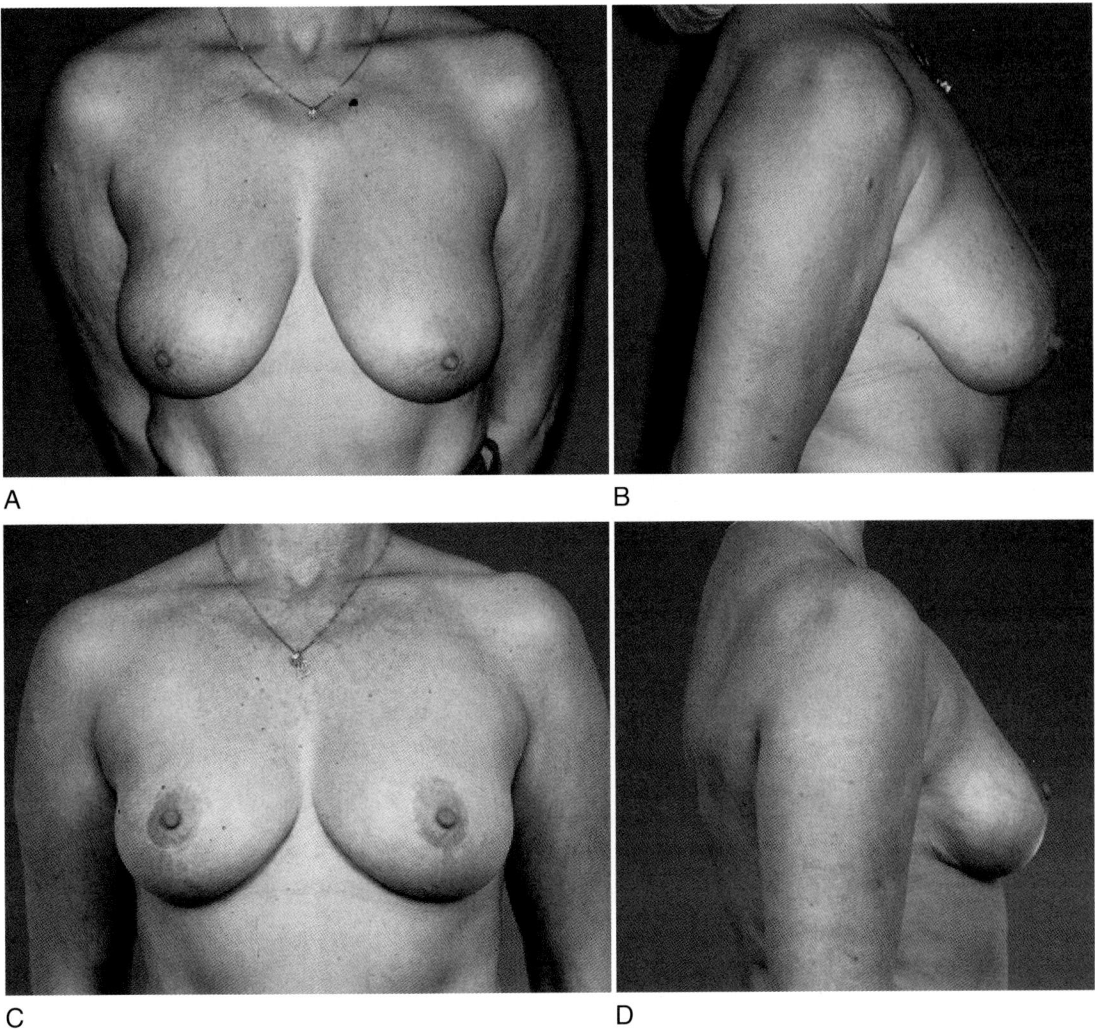

FIGURE 120-44. *A* and *B*, A 45-year-old woman with moderate ptosis. *C*, Patient seen 1 year after mastopexy and small reduction with inverted T technique.

slight raising of the complex and its similarly slight reduction in size.

Originally, this technique used suction-assisted lipectomy methods. However, with the advent of ultrasound-assisted lipectomy techniques, there has been application of ultrasound-assisted lipectomy to try to improve the results that can be achieved. This is mainly by virtue of the ability of ultrasound-assisted lipectomy to enhance skin retraction and nipple-areola complex elevation.

INDICATIONS, ADVANTAGES, AND DISADVANTAGES

This technique has limited application. It is best suited for women who require minimal reduction, whose hypertrophy is mainly due to fat, whose ptosis is not extreme (i.e., mild to moderate), and with good skin quality.

Another indication for this technique is for those patients who have had previous reduction mammaplasty and wish further reduction. Because the previously designed pedicle may already have partially compromised vascular and nerve supply to the nipple-areola complex, further reduction by a transposition technique may further risk the viability and sensitivity of this complex. Reduction by liposuction minimizes the risk to these structures while reducing the residual fat content of the breast.

This technique has two main advantages, minimal scarring and minimal risk to vascular and sensory structures. This procedure is accomplished by two or three stab incisions; two are placed just above the inframammary fold medially and laterally, and the third, an intra-areolar incision, can be used if necessary to reach the upper aspects of the breast. The other advantage has to do with protection of the neurovascular supply of the nipple-areola complex. Liposuction cannulas, when chosen and used properly, preserve neurovascular supplies to the tissues, thereby reducing the risk for nipple-areola complex necrosis and loss of sensitivity.

The main disadvantage of this treatment is its limited application. Only a small subset of women fit the strict criteria this procedure necessitates. If it is used on the wrong patient, this technique will produce suboptimal results that may be difficult to correct.

TECHNIQUE

The breast is marked with the patient in the standing position. The standard concentric circle pattern is used to indicate the location of the greatest protrusion. If local anesthesia is to be used, the breast can be injected with up to 100 mL of 0.25% bupivacaine with 1:400,000 fresh epinephrine and 300 units of hyaluronidase. If general anesthesia is to be used, a standard tumescent solution may be used to infiltrate the breast (1 ampule epinephrine, 50 mL of 0.5% lidocaine in 1 liter of lactated Ringer solution).

Stab incisions are made as previously described. The placement of these incisions allows a crisscross pattern of suction that will facilitate an even reduction of tissue from the breast (Fig. 120-45).

Cannula selection usually depends on the experience of the surgeon. Inexperienced surgeons may be wise to use a smaller cannula at first to “get a feel” of the patient’s tissues and then switch to a larger cannula for major tissue removal. Pretunneling is not required. Care should be taken not to inadvertently enter the chest cavity.

Suctioning is performed in a manner to produce a symmetric breast. Suctioning of the base of the breast can also be included to reduce its volume and to help encourage retraction of the entire breast mound against the chest wall. Tissue removal should be enough to correct the hypertrophy and reduce the weight. The overall volume of the remaining tissue should be checked frequently. This will determine when suction should be stopped. Overresection should be avoided. One can always redo the procedure if necessary, but replacement is impossible.

No drains or sutures are used. Absorbent pads are used to catch the drainage. Paper tape is applied horizontally from the bottom of the breast toward the nipple-areola complex, forming a sling under the lower

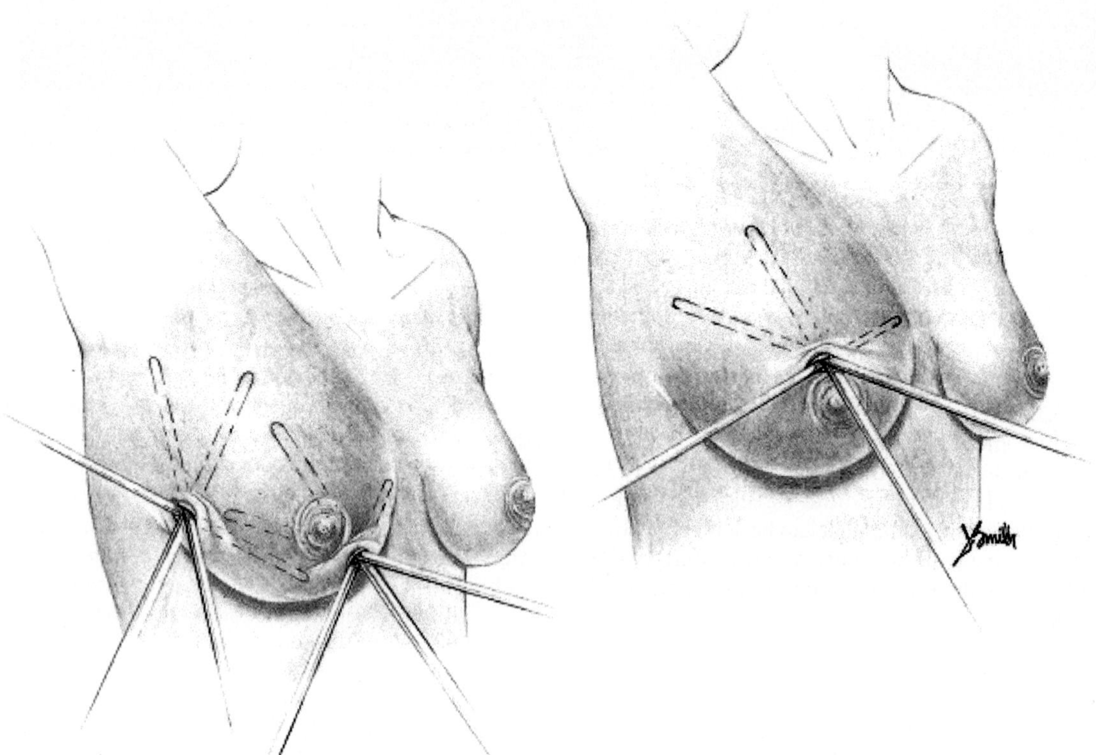

FIGURE 120-45. Access points for the suction cannulas. (From Courtiss EH: Breast reduction by suction alone. In Spear SL, ed: Surgery of the Breast: Principles and Art. Philadelphia, Lippincott-Raven, 1998:709.)

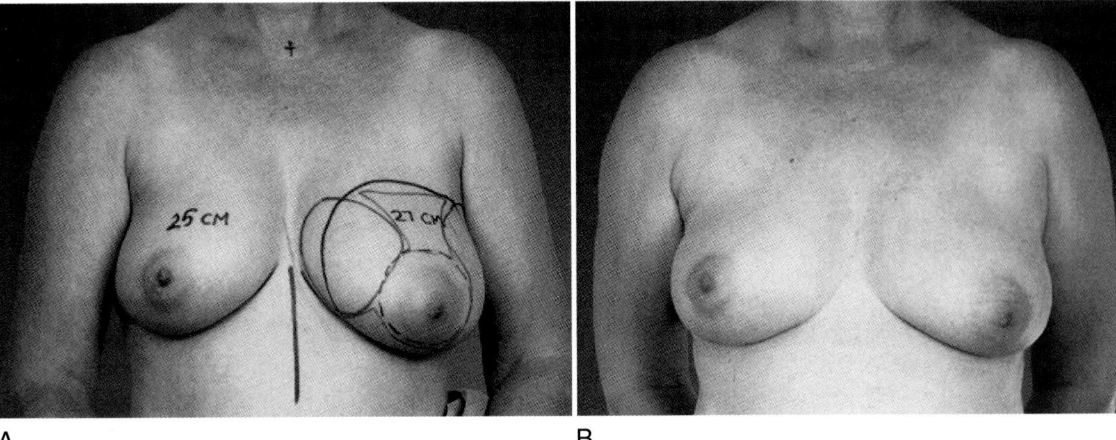

FIGURE 120-46. Reduction with suction alone in a patient with asymmetry. *A*, Patient seen preoperatively. *B*, Patient seen 6 months postoperatively.

portion of the breast. Horizontal pieces of paper tape are then applied from the superior portion of the breast downward toward the nipple-areola complex. A Reston sponge is applied in half-moon shapes followed by a snug bra. Firm supportive pressure on the breast is the goal of these dressings. The dressings are removed at 1 week, and the patient's bra is changed. To help combat any persistent edema, the patient is instructed to wear the bra day and night for up to 6 months (Fig. 120-46).

ADDITIONAL TECHNIQUES

Augmentation Mastopexy

Augmentation mastopexy is the combination of augmentation techniques with mastopexy techniques for the correction of ptosis. Because ptosis is the result of deficient glandular tissue, excess skin with nipple malposition, or more commonly a combination of both, it makes sense that correction of this deformity would combine a technique that increases breast volume (augmentation) with a technique that decreases the skin envelope and allows repositioning of the nipple-areola complex (mastopexy). These techniques are by no means for everyone, but they should be included in the plastic surgeon's choice of techniques for the correction of breast ptosis.

INDICATIONS, ADVANTAGES, AND DISADVANTAGES

Any of the previously discussed mastopexy techniques can be combined with augmentation. The chosen combination will depend on the patient's presenting complaints and anatomy. In general, this technique is most useful for those women with a deficit of glandular tissue regardless of the size of the skin envelope. Another good indication is asymmetry when one breast is hypoplastic and the other is ptotic.

The advantages and disadvantages of the mastopexy techniques remain the same as already noted; however, the added benefits and risks of augmentation mammaplasty must now be considered. Advantages include better fill of the skin envelope by virtue of the implant. The risks include an increased chance of wound problems and dehiscence because of the added weight of the implant and increased tension on the suture lines, especially in the face of overresection of the skin flaps by the surgeon's incorrectly estimating the final breast volume in light of the implant.

The increased risk for wound problems and dehiscence can be lessened if the surgeon is vigilant and keeps skin resection to a minimum at the beginning of the procedure. Additional skin resection can always be performed at the end of the procedure on the basis of the final volume of the breast with the implant in place.

There are also the inherent risks of the implants (malpositioning, leakage, rupture, capsular contracture) and the patient's perceived risks of silicone.[34] In the United States at this time, the patient has the choice of silicone gel or saline implants if concurrent mastopexy is to be performed. Although no conclusive evidence has been found linking silicone to systemic illness, there are those women who would not be comfortable with a silicone gel implant and some who will not accept a saline implant secondary to its silicone outer shell. These women, obviously, are not candidates for augmentation mastopexy.

TECHNIQUE

Augmentation mammaplasty proceeds with marking and incisions according to the mastopexy technique chosen. Once the breast tissue or muscle is exposed, the pocket for the implant, either submuscular or subglandular, can be formed and the implant inserted. The mastopexy can then be completed. Choosing an implant (textured versus smooth, silicone gel versus saline) and choosing where to place the implant (submuscular versus subglandular) are decided in the same manner as for augmentation mammaplasty without mastopexy and will not be discussed here.

There is one final point that should be carefully considered before proceeding with augmentation mastopexy, especially in those women with severe ptosis when a formal Wise-pattern mastopexy is to be performed, and that is the blood supply to the nipple-areola complex and the skin flaps. In their zeal to correct a woman's severe ptosis deformity, surgeons must remain vigilant of the blood and nerve supply in relation to the incisions made for both the augmentation and the mastopexy portions of the procedure. Whereas the neurovascular supply is usually not compromised by formal mastopexy alone, the addition of the augmentation procedure may cause significant alteration in blood supply. Any mastopexy technique that requires wide undermining of skin flaps should not be combined with subglandular augmentation because this would almost certainly result in glandular necrosis. With combination of these two procedures, there is the possibility of a denervated or devascularized nipple-areola complex, breast tissue, or skin flap. One should undermine judiciously and carefully evaluate the mastopexy technique as it is being performed to help avoid these potential complications.

Should there be a suggestion of nipple or skin flap compromise at the conclusion of the procedure, there are steps that can be taken in an attempt to reverse this process. These include removing the periareolar skin sutures to allow relaxation of the tissues and increased blood supply to the nipple-areola complex. Removal of the implant is sometimes necessary to reduce tension on both the skin flaps and the nipple-areola complex. This too can sometimes allow increased blood flow to the tissues. Loss of the nipple is a devastating complication for both the patient and the surgeon, and aggressive measures must be undertaken when there is concern about its viability.

Nerve damage is difficult to assess immediately postoperatively. Therefore, one must perform careful and well thought out dissection in an attempt to minimize damage to these structures.

In one's enthusiasm to treat severe degrees of ptosis, one should not lose sight of the main goal, which is the formation of a well-shaped, well-proportioned, viable breast with intact sensation. Most of the time, this goal can be achieved with proper selection of patients and careful planning and execution of the surgical technique, much to the delight of the patient and the satisfaction of the surgeon (Fig. 120-47).

Mastopexy After Explantation

A woman may request explantation of her breast implants for many reasons.[35] Some women have concerns with the recent silicone controversy, some have implants that have ruptured or leaked, some have disfiguring or painful capsular contractures, some have malpositioned implants that have not responded to subsequent attempts at correction, and some have implants that have become infected. Finally, there are those women who after many years no longer wish to be as large as they are.

INDICATIONS, ADVANTAGES, AND DISADVANTAGES

When an implant is removed, the breast may assume an excessively lax and ptotic position. Often, there will also be a maldistribution of glandular tissue with inferior pole deformities. The potential for this post-explantation result should be included when the explantation procedure is discussed with a patient. The surgeon should also be prepared to discuss procedures that are available to help reshape the remaining breast tissue. This discussion should include realistic expectations of what can be accomplished along with the possibility of needing additional scars to achieve an optimal breast shape. If additional scarring is not acceptable, the patient must be made aware of the probability of a suboptimal result.

The surgeon should ascertain the patient's motivation for removal and post-removal expectations. If a patient is happy with her implants and is having no problems with them but is concerned with the silicone gel filling, she may be a candidate for a simple removal of the silicone implant and replacement with a saline implant. If a woman has had an implant rupture, whether it is silicone or saline, she may merely wish to have it replaced with the same type of implant; if she had silicone implants, she may wish to have both implants removed and replaced with saline.

Those women with capsular contractures may opt for replacement, but there are those who just want the implants removed. This is similar to those women with malpositioned implants that have not responded to secondary or even tertiary procedures. Then there are those women who for one reason or another, mostly because of changes in body image, decide after many years to have their implants removed.

These women all have the option of explantation alone, explantation with replacement, or explantation with some type of concurrent mastopexy procedure. The women with only one option are those with an infected implant. These women require explantation, irrigation, and drainage. Implant replacement or pexy procedures must be postponed until the infection has resolved and the tissues have healed.

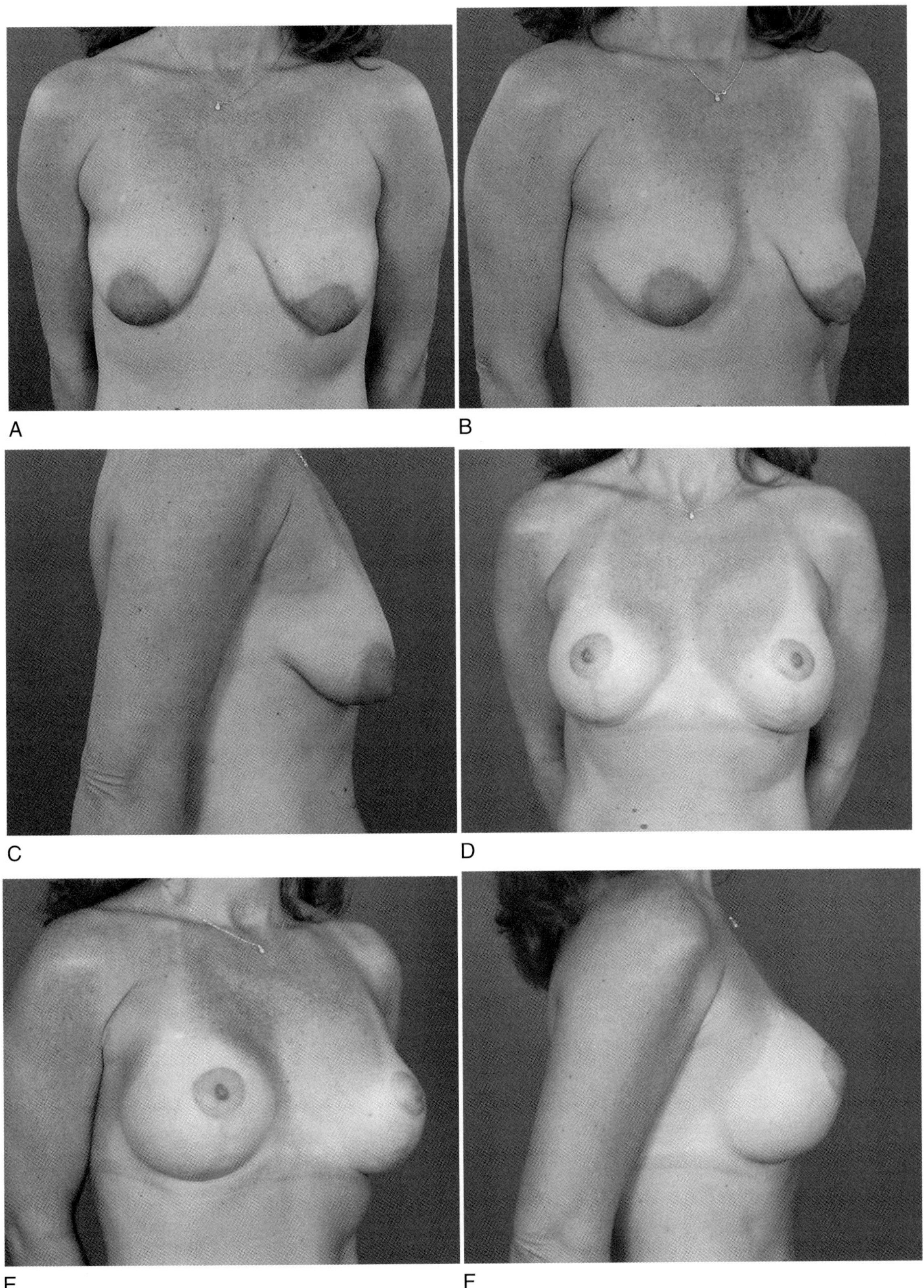

FIGURE 120-47. Vertical mastopexy by the authors' modified technique with subpectoral augmentation in a 39-year-old patient. *A* to *C*, Preoperative photographs demonstrating parenchymal maldistribution and ptosis. *D* to *F*, Patient seen 1 year postoperatively.

One other group of women needs to be mentioned here, and these are women who have had implants placed secondary to reconstruction after mastectomy. These women have one other option on explantation, that being reconstruction with autologous tissue (e.g., latissimus dorsi flap, TRAM flap). This subject is beyond the scope of this chapter and is not discussed. The reader is referred to the chapters on breast reconstruction in this book. Our discussion here focuses on those women who wish explantation with mastopexy.

As with mastopexy procedures in general, the most important component in determining the ability to reshape the gland is the amount of glandular tissue available. In those women with minimal glandular tissue, explantation followed by mastopexy procedures alone will produce a suboptimal result. These women may best be served by some type of augmentation mastopexy procedure. Another option would be just to perform the explantation and then allow the skin envelope to contract. Some of these women may obtain significant improvement after contraction is allowed to take place. For them, a simple nipple-areola complex repositioning procedure may be all that is required to achieve a satisfactory result. Whichever procedure is chosen for reshaping, the neurovascular supply for the nipple-areola complex must always be considered. The mastopexy procedure chosen must always take into consideration possible alterations to the nerves and vessels secondary to the original augmentation. In some patients, especially when there is little native breast tissue, it may be prudent to perform mastopexy as a delayed event.

The next issue that needs to be addressed is whether to perform capsulectomy or capsulotomy. Although there are many differing opinions among surgeons and many special situations, in general, capsulectomy should be performed in patients with ruptured silicone gel implants, in patients with severe capsular contracture, or when the capsule contains large amounts of calcium deposits. Otherwise, the capsule, with or without additional capsulotomy incisions, may be left in place to add bulk to the glandular reconstruction.

TECHNIQUE

Before removal of the implant, the new areolar border is marked. De-epithelialization is performed on the basis of the mastopexy technique. Any of the previously discussed mastopexy procedures may be used. It is usually easier to perform the initial mastopexy maneuvers with the implant in place.

An incision is usually made in the inframammary fold, but a periareolar incision can occasionally be used to gain access to the implant or capsule. If the implant to be removed is silicone and there is suspected leakage of the implant, the capsule is left intact. Dissection proceeds on its anterior surface followed by posterior release from the pectoralis muscle or chest wall, depending on where the implant was originally placed. Dissection is with a combination of cautery and blunt technique. In dissecting anteriorly over the capsule in a submuscularly placed implant, one should take care to avoid the thoracoacromial artery because cautery-induced muscle contraction brings the artery close to the dissection plane.

Once the capsule is freed, it is removed totally and intact. The pocket is then visualized and palpated. Any lumps or irregularities are excised for biopsy. The pocket is then irrigated, and the mastopexy portion of the procedure is begun.

If the implant to be removed is silicone without evidence of leakage or if it is a saline implant, a total capsulectomy is usually not necessary. An exception to this is the silicone implant that is subsequently found to be ruptured. In addition, if the capsule is calcified to such an extent that leaving it in place would distort the subsequent breast reshaping, a partial capsulectomy is in order.

If the capsule is to be left in place, dissection should proceed through the tissues to the capsule. The capsule can be opened and the implant delivered. The capsule should be palpated for calcifications and irregularities; if these are found, a partial capsulectomy can be performed. Reshaping of the gland can then be accomplished. Drains are placed and the skin envelope is closed. The nipple is repositioned and sutured in place. When sufficient glandular tissue is available, mastopexy after explantation often yields an aesthetically pleasing breast shape. This is most often accomplished by use of a superiorly based dermoglandular flap that is folded back on itself to establish projection and upper pole fill.

COMPLICATIONS

Although most mastopexy procedures produce a higher positioned and shapely breast that pleases most patients, there are complications that may require revision procedures. These include nipple loss, unacceptable scars, flap necrosis, nipple malposition, and cosmetic disappointments. In the event of any of these, revision procedures to correct any shortcomings should be made available to the patient. The primary goal, however, is the avoidance of any of these sequelae.

Nipple Loss

Nipple loss is one of the most devastating complications that can happen to both patient and surgeon. The incidence of nipple loss by various techniques is reported to be less than 10%, usually in the range of 0% to 5%. In addition to technical errors, nipple loss can be predicted by a variety of patient factors including smoking, diabetes, obesity, and hypertension.

Avoidance of this complication begins with proper selection of patients and technique. In high-risk patients (i.e., smokers, diabetics, patients weighing more than 200 pounds, or those with severe ptosis), a free nipple graft technique is an option that can be considered. This is also a possibility intraoperatively or postoperatively if the viability of the transposed nipple appears compromised. Up until approximately 12 hours postoperatively, the compromised nipple-areola complex may be converted to a free nipple graft. This, of course, assumes that a satisfactory dermal bed can be found to accept the nipple graft. After 12 hours, conservative treatment of any nipple necrosis should be undertaken, including release of sutures, topical nitropaste or leeches, greasy dressings, hyperbaric oxygen therapy (if available), and appropriate antibiotic therapy. Many times, conservative treatment and closure by secondary intention produce a satisfactory result. Whereas the usual rule with ischemic tissues is early sharp débridement, in nipple necrosis, débridement should be delayed as long as possible.

If healing does not produce a satisfactory result, the nipple-areola complex can be reconstructed by standard reconstruction techniques ranging from simple tattooing of the areola to flap reconstructions of the nipple itself.

Scars

Although scars are an inherent part of any surgical procedure, their final quality cannot be predicted. Ironically, those who are the least concerned with scarring (i.e., elderly women with thin skin) tend to have scars of the best quality, whereas those who are most concerned with their scars (i.e., young women 16 to 25 years of age, especially those with darker, thick, acne-prone skin) tend to have the worst scarring results. Obviously, the best way to minimize the occurrence of bad scars is to minimize the incision. The surgeon can help with this by choosing the proper mastopexy technique, by proper execution with gentle skin handling, by minimal or no tension on the wound, and by minimizing the incisions where appropriate. Once healed, prominent scars may first receive a trial of vitamin E, compression with tape or silicone sheeting, laser treatment, or intralesional triamcinolone (Kenalog) injections. In some situations, particularly bad scars can be resected, followed by a precise and careful closure. It is preferable to assess patients for scar revision after 1 year.

Flap Necrosis

Flap necrosis can occur by virtue of the flaps used, especially when the inverted T or Wise-pattern mastopexy technique is used. The lateral flap is most commonly affected secondary to the substantial undermining required in this region to allow proper shaping of the breast. Although excessive tension is thought occasionally to play a small role, most flap loss is primarily ischemic. Treatment is similar to that of the ischemic nipple—greasy dressings, hyperbaric oxygen, or antibiotics. Débridement of large areas of flap necrosis should be undertaken when they are clearly demarcated. Delayed closure can be performed, thereby avoiding weeks or months of caring for an open breast wound. Small areas of skin necrosis (1 to 2 cm) may be treated conservatively, especially along the inframammary fold.

Nipple Malposition

Although there are many formulas and methods to determine nipple position (i.e., sternal notch to nipple distance, inframammary fold to nipple distance, nipple to sternal distance, and midhumeral position), none is perfect and nipple malposition may occur. This type of result can cause a patient's disappointment with the procedure no matter how well shaped the newly constructed breast is or how well the incisions have healed.

The nipple should be properly situated on the breast, at or near the point of greatest projection, with ample but not an excessive amount of tissue underneath it. When malposition of the nipple occurs, one can attempt to reposition it; however, one should wait at least several months to allow complete healing of the breast and nipple-areola complex. The tissues should be soft and supple. It is easier to raise the nipple-areola complex than to lower it. If the nipple-areola complex is too low, a small crescent of skin can be removed above it and the complex raised. More often, all the incisions must be reopened and the skin envelope tightened.

Nipples that appear too high can be caused by one of two situations. The breast may have bottomed out inferiorly; if this has occurred, a simple tissue resection can be performed inferiorly with use of the already present vertical and horizontal incision sites. If a high-riding nipple is the result of incorrect positioning, this is a more complex problem. One can attempt to lower the nipple by one of a series of maneuvers including V-Y advancement inferiorly, transposition as a flap, or transfer as a graft. Regardless of the method used, a scar superior to the areola will be produced. This scar will be subject to the same potential problems as are other breast scars. In addition, a scar above the nipple-areola complex, regardless of how well it heals, is not particularly aesthetic and will not be well accepted by the patient.

Cosmetic Disappointments

Regardless of the technique, the goal of mastopexy is to produce attractive, symmetric, higher positioned, fuller breasts. In some instances, this goal is not reached.

Overresection, underresection, and healing complications can contribute to cosmetic disappointments.

Underresection can easily be corrected by additional tissue excision. Overresection, however, presents a more disturbing problem that may require placement of an implant for correction. Residual tissue deformities secondary to infection, hematoma, or fat necrosis may require additional surgery for excision of resultant lumps and bumps to produce a breast with a soft, smooth contour.

Cosmetic problems may be apparent immediately postoperatively, or they may take weeks and even months to become evident. Although it is not always possible to avoid these cosmetic disappointments, one should do everything one can to keep them from occurring. In the majority of patients, mastopexy is a useful and rewarding procedure for both the patient and the surgeon.

THE FUTURE

Currently, mastopexy procedures are usually predictable and well accepted by most patients. The future lies in developing methods to correct greater degrees of ptosis with smaller scars. Today, the smallest scars are produced with liposuction. The major obstacle to these current liposuction procedures is the inability to control contraction of the skin envelope. If skin contraction could be mediated, liposuction procedures would become applicable to a large number of patients, and, perhaps in some, skin resection would no longer be required at all.

Short of controlling skin contraction, treatments that could render improved or even invisible scarring would be invaluable for this as well as for all surgical procedures. Research is under way to determine factors that might one day make this a reality. Until then, it is the surgeon's responsibility to match the patient to the appropriate procedure and to execute that procedure to the best of his or her ability.

REFERENCES

1. Regnault P: Breast ptosis. Definition and treatment. Clin Plast Surg 1976;3:193.
2. Brink RR: Management of true ptosis of the breast. Plast Reconstr Surg 1993;91:657.
3. Spear SL, Kassan M, Little JW: Guidelines in concentric mastopexy. Plast Reconstr Surg 1990;85:961.
4. Spear SL, Giese SY, Ducic I: Concentric mastopexy revisited. Plast Reconstr Surg 2001;107:1294.
5. Benelli L: A new periareolar mammaplasty: the "round block" technique. Aesthetic Plast Surg 1990;14:93.
6. Benelli LC: Periareolar Benelli mastopexy and reduction. In Spear SL, ed: Surgery of the Breast: Principles and Art. Philadelphia, Lippincott-Raven, 1998:685.
7. Goes JCS: Periareolar mammaplasty: double skin technique with application of polyglactine or mixed mesh. Plast Reconstr Surg 1996;97:959.
8. Goes JCS: Periareolar mastopexy and reduction with mesh support. In Spear SL, ed: Surgery of the Breast: Principles and Art. Philadelphia, Lippincott-Raven, 1998:697.
9. Lassus C: Breast reduction: evolution of a technique. A single vertical scar. Aesthetic Plast Surg 1987;11:107.
10. Lassus C: A 30 year experience with vertical mammaplasty. Plast Reconstr Surg 1996;97:373.
11. Lassus C: Update on vertical mammaplasty. Plast Reconstr Surg 1999;104:2289.
12. Lassus C: Vertical scar breast reduction and mastopexy without undermining. In Spear SL, ed: Surgery of the Breast: Principles and Art. Philadelphia, Lippincott-Raven, 1998:717.
13. Skoog T: A technique of breast reduction. Acta Chir Scand 1963;126:453.
14. Lejour M: Vertical mammaplasty and liposuction of the breast. Plast Reconstr Surg 1994;94:100.
15. Lejour M: Vertical mammaplasty for breast hypertrophy and ptosis. Operative Techniques Plast Surg 1996;3:189.
16. Lejour M: Vertical mammaplasty for breast reduction and mastopexy. In Spear SL, ed: Surgery of the Breast: Principles and Art. Philadelphia, Lippincott-Raven, 1998:735.
17. Arie G: Una nueva tecnica de mastoplastia. Rev Iber Latino Am Cir Plast 1957;3:28.
18. Pitanguy I: Surgical correction of breast hypertrophy. Br J Plast Surg 1967;20:78.
19. Lejour M: Vertical mammaplasty: update and appraisal of late results. Plast Reconstr Surg 1999;104:771.
20. Hall-Findlay EJ: A simplified vertical reduction mammaplasty: shortening the learning curve. Plast Reconstr Surg 1999;104:748.
21. Hall-Findlay EJ: Pedicles in vertical breast reduction and mastopexy. Clin Plast Surg 2002;29:379.
22. Chiari AJ: The L short scar mammaplasty: a new approach. Plast Reconstr Surg 1992;90:233.
23. Seidel SP, Chiari A, Grotting JC: The L short-scar mammaplasty. In Spear SL, ed: Surgery of the Breast: Principles and Art. Philadelphia, Lippincott-Raven, 1998:793.
24. Marchac D, Olarte G: Reduction mammaplasty and correction of ptosis with a short inframammary scar. Plast Reconstr Surg 1982;69:45.
25. Marchac DA: Vertical mammaplasty with a short horizontal scar. In Spear SL, ed: Surgery of the Breast: Principles and Art. Philadelphia, Lippincott-Raven, 1998:749.
26. McKissock PK: Reduction mammaplasty with a vertical dermal flap. Plast Reconstr Surg 1972;49:245.
27. Wise RJ: A preliminary report on a method of planning the mammaplasty. Plast Reconstr Surg 1956;17:367.
28. Wise RJ, Gannon JP, Hill JR: Further experience with reduction mammaplasty. Plast Reconstr Surg 1963;32:12.
29. Courtiss EH, Goldwyn RM: Reduction mammaplasty by the inferior pedicle technique. Plast Reconstr Surg 1977;59:500.
30. Matarasso A, Courtiss EH: Suction mammaplasty. The use of suction lipectomy to reduce large breasts. Plast Reconstr Surg 1991;87:709.
31. Courtiss EH: Reduction mammaplasty by suction alone. Plast Reconstr Surg 1993;92:1276.
32. Courtiss EH: Breast reduction by suction alone. In Spear SL, ed: Surgery of the Breast: Principles and Art. Philadelphia, Lippincott-Raven, 1998:709.
33. Matarasso A: Suction mammaplasty: the use of suction lipectomy to reduce large breasts. Plast Reconstr Surg 2000;105:2604.
34. Handel N: Managing local implant-related problems. In Spear SL, ed: Surgery of the Breast: Principles and Art. Philadelphia, Lippincott-Raven, 1998:953.
35. Friedman RJ: Secondary cases; managing the implant patient. In Spear SL, ed: Surgery of the Breast: Principles and Art. Philadelphia, Lippincott-Raven, 1998:938.

CHAPTER

121

Abdominoplasty

Luis O. Vásconez, MD ✦ Jorge I. de la Torre, MD

The abdominoplasty encompasses not only aesthetic body contouring but also reconstruction of structural integrity. The aesthetic goals of an abdominoplasty are to improve contour of the abdominal wall, to minimize scarring, and to maintain a natural-appearing umbilicus. The reconstructive goals are to re-establish the appropriate anatomy of the muscular layer and to prevent recurrence of hernias or diastasis. Both reconstructive and aesthetic goals should be incorporated in any abdominoplasty procedure. Ideally, maximal resection of excess skin and sufficient reduction of subcutaneous adipose tissue volume can be achieved. In addition, closure of musculoaponeurotic laxity improves the overall contour and restores the structural integrity of the abdominal wall. As with all elective procedures, minimizing morbidity and postoperative disability is important.

HISTORY

Abdominal wall surgery as it was described in the 19th century focused on the removal of redundant skin for repair of large umbilical hernias. Kelly[1] published one of the first reports on the use of abdominoplasty in this country. He described the use of a large horizontal midabdominal incision in 1899; Babcock,[2] in 1916, proposed a vertical midline incision. A variety of incisions were described during the next 4 decades, including the lower abdominal transverse incision advocated by Thorek[3] in 1924 (Fig. 121-1). Despite a multitude of variations, the lower abdominal incision became the approach of choice.

The abdominoplasty as a distinct procedure did not gain popularity until 1957, when the modern version, including umbilical transposition and musculoaponeurotic plication, was described by Vernon.[4] Subsequent refinement came with the reports of Pitanguy's series of 300 patients, Regnault's W technique, and Psillakis' understanding of the approach to aponeurotic musculature.[5-7] The advent of suction-assisted lipectomy in the early 1980s allowed further evolution in body-contouring techniques.[8] Minimal incisions can be employed to remove redundant skin while liposuction contours the areas of lipodystrophy. External ultrasonic liposuction and endoscopic surgery have minimized the approach to the abdomen even further.

During the past several years, the popularity of abdominoplasty as an aesthetic procedure has grown. More than 46,000 abdominoplasties were performed in 1998 according to the American Society of Plastic Surgeons. This represents an increase of 36% since 1996 and 177% since 1992, making abdominoplasty the eighth most common cosmetic surgical procedure.

EMBRYOLOGY

The abdominal wall is embryonically derived in a segmental, metameric manner, and this is reflected in blood supply and innervation. These sections—two lateral, one superior, and one inferior—develop and merge to form the embryonic abdominal wall. The transition of the embryo from a trilaminar disk to a three-dimensional structure on the 22nd day of gestation initiates formation of the abdominal wall; however,

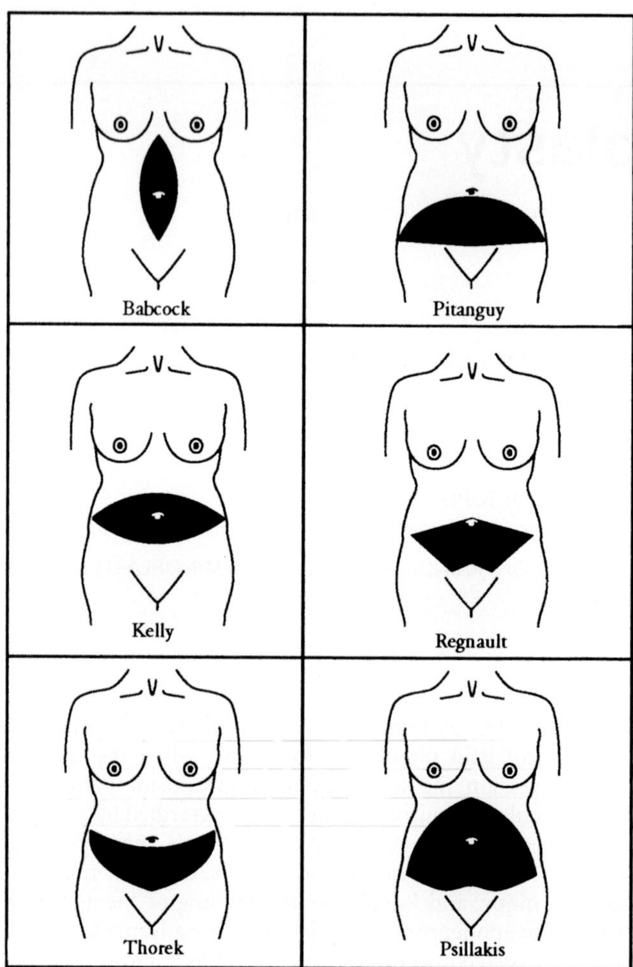

FIGURE 121-1. Historical incisions and evolution of the abdominoplasty procedures.

the abdominal wall does not achieve its definitive structure until birth, when the umbilical cord separates from the fetus.[9]

The primitive abdominal wall consists of ectoderm and mesoderm without musculature, vasculature, or innervation. This somatopleure is eventually invaded by mesoderm from the myotomes that develop on either side of the vertebral column. Migration of four abdominal wall folds—the cephalic, caudal, and two lateral folds—forms the anterior abdominal wall (Fig. 121-2). Problems with folding will result in such anomalies as omphalocele, gastroschisis, pentalogy of Cantrell, and cloacal exstrophy.[10] With elongation of the midgut during the sixth week of gestation, a physiologic herniation of the abdominal contents occurs through the umbilicus.

By the seventh week, the mesodermal mass has migrated ventrally and laterally as a sheet, and the leading edges forming the rectus abdominis muscles and the lateral portion split into three layers, which can be recognized as the external oblique, internal oblique, and transversalis layers. The midgut returns to the abdomen during week 10 to allow closure and development of the abdominal wall to continue. Closure of the midline proceeds from both caudal and cranial directions as the two rectus abdominis muscles meet in the midline. Although this process is complete by week 12 of gestation, final closure of the umbilical ring does not occur until separation of the cord at birth.

ANATOMY

The landmarks of the abdomen include the umbilicus, the anterior and lateral contour, and the surface appearance of the underlying structural components. Fat distribution and abdominal contour vary between the genders.[11] The female body habitus follows a gynoid or "hourglass" shape. It is narrow at the waist and wider at the hips with fat accumulation in the lower trunk, hips, thighs, and buttocks. Ideally, the female waist-to-hip ratio is approximately 0.7.[12] There

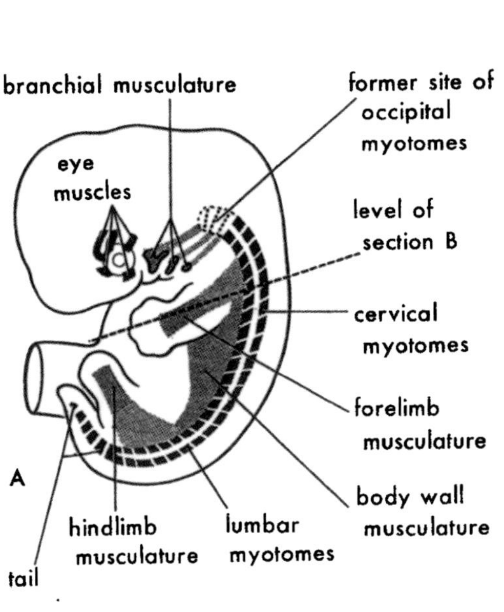

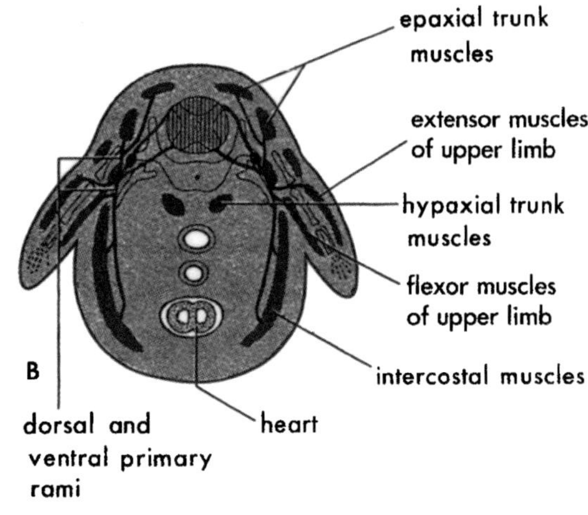

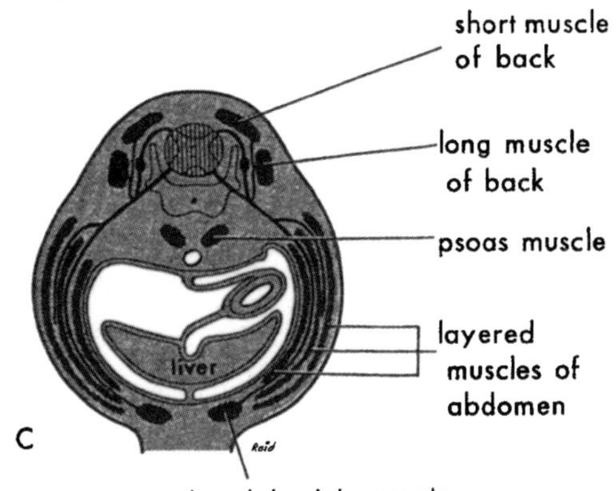

FIGURE 121-2. Development of the abdominal wall at 41 days of gestation showing the myotomes and developing musculature. (From Moore KL, Persaud TVN: The Developing Human: Clinically Oriented Embryology. Philadelphia, WB Saunders, 1993:371.)

is a small fullness just above the pubis with a scaphoid contour from just below the umbilicus to the costal margin. The umbilicus is inset with slight hooding superiorly. The ideal male trunk contour has an android pattern, becoming narrower with descent from the chest to the hips in a V shape. The anterior abdomen is flat with indentations visible at the transcriptions and along the midline. Fat accumulation tends to occur circumferentially around the abdomen and flanks.

The umbilicus lies in the midline, midway between the xiphoid and pubis at the level of the superior iliac crest. There is a slight depression in the periumbilical area that is approximately 4 to 6 cm in diameter. Ideally, the youthful umbilicus is hooded superiorly and attached tightly to the midline fascia.

The layers of the abdominal wall include the skin, subcutaneous tissue, musculofascial layer, and underlying peritoneum. The dermis of the abdomen is relatively thick. The subcutaneous tissue consists of two distinct layers of adipose tissue, separated by Scarpa fascia. The superficial layer is typically dense and fibrous in nature, whereas the deeper layer is looser with a less organized septum.[13] Scarpa fascia, a fibrous layer of connective and adipose tissue, forms a discrete layer in the lower abdominal wall. Although it does not offer much strength in wound closure, proper approximation helps to make an aesthetic hairline scar.

The musculature of the abdomen includes the paired rectus abdominis, which meet in the midline at the linea alba (Figs. 121-3 and 121-4). These two long muscles originate at the infracostal margin and attach at the pubis. The muscle bellies are enclosed in a fascial sheath formed by the lateral abdominal wall aponeurotic layers. In the upper two thirds of the abdomen, the anterior sheath is formed by the external and internal oblique aponeurosis and the posterior sheath by the internal oblique and transversalis aponeurosis. Inferior to this level, the posterior sheath is absent and all three aponeurotic layers pass anterior to the rectus muscle, except the internal lamina of the transversus abdominis, the transversalis fascia, and the peritoneum, which pass posterior. This transition, known

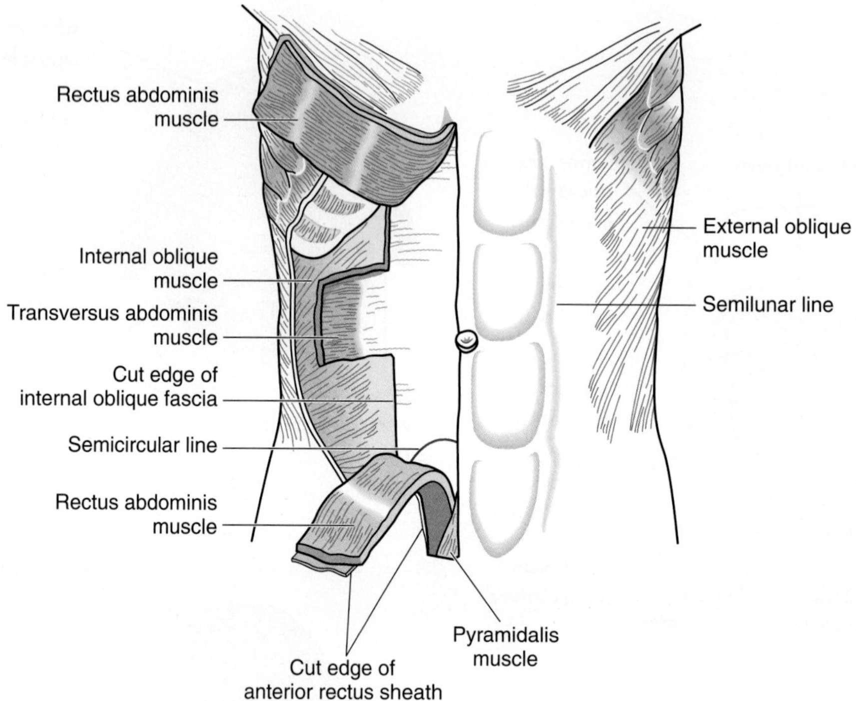

FIGURE 121-3. Anatomy of the musculature of the anterior abdominal wall. (Redrawn from Mathes SJ, Krizek TJ, Ariyan S, et al: Plastic Surgery: Principles and Practice. St. Louis, Mosby, 1990:1149.)

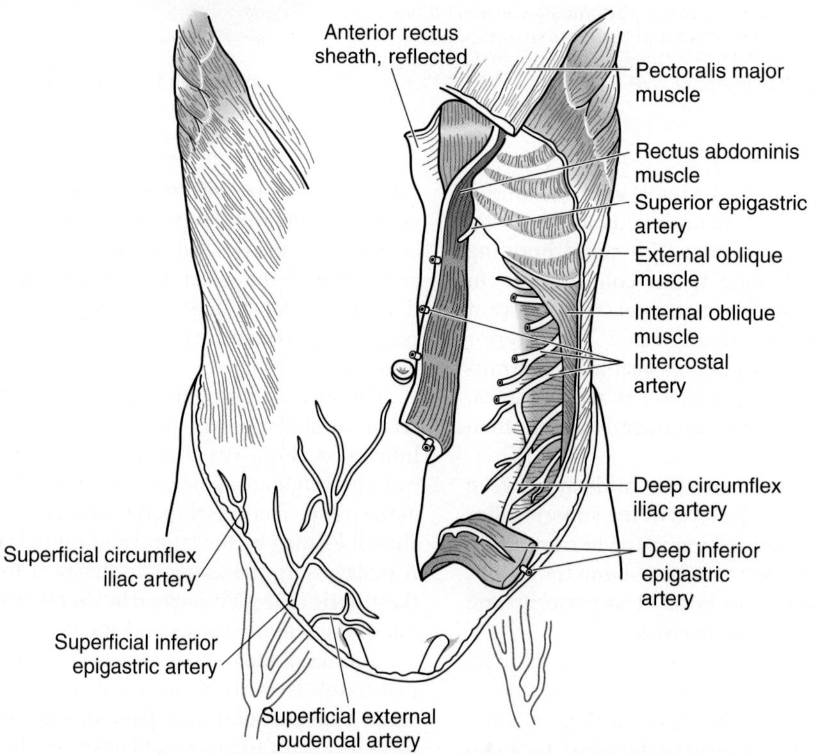

FIGURE 121-4. Anatomy of the musculature of the anterior abdominal wall with arterial supply. (Redrawn from Mathes SJ, Krizek TJ, Ariyan S, et al: Plastic Surgery: Principles and Practice. St. Louis, Mosby, 1990:1151.)

as the arcuate line, the linea semicircularis, or the semicircular line of Douglas, is present halfway between the umbilicus and pubic symphysis. The inferior epigastric artery enters the rectus sheath below the arcuate line, where there is not a true posterior rectus sheath. There are several inscriptions, or fascial condensations, that improve the mechanical advantage of the rectus muscle to flex the abdominal wall. The linea semilunaris corresponds to the lateral border of the rectus. The lateral abdominal wall consists of three layers of muscle, the external oblique, the internal oblique, and the transverse rectus. At the caudal aspect of the rectus muscles, the pyramidalis muscles are present in 80% to 90% of patients.

The muscular layer of the lateral abdominal wall is composed of three flat muscles. All three originate from the costal margin, thoracolumbar fascia, iliac crest, and inguinal ligament. The external abdominal oblique muscle is the largest and thickest of these abdominal muscles. The fascicles of the external oblique muscle are directed from superolateral to inferomedial. The external oblique aponeurosis passes anterior to the sheath of the rectus abdominis.

The internal abdominal oblique muscle is deep to the external oblique, and its fibers course in the opposite direction. The internal oblique aponeurosis splits to envelop the rectus muscle and reunites in the midline to form the linea alba. Fibers from the lateral half of the inguinal ligament pass through the abdominal wall at the inguinal ring to form the cremasteric muscle.

The transversus abdominis muscle is the deepest and smallest of the muscles of the abdomen. It has an origin similar to that of the oblique muscles and forms a flat aponeurosis that inserts into the linea alba. This aponeurosis passes behind the rectus sheath in its upper two thirds. The fibers of the transversus abdominis are directed in a transverse direction. Deep to the muscular layer is the transversalis fascia. This fascial layer forms a continuous lining of the abdominal cavity. A disruption in this layer is by definition a hernia. Therefore, a successful hernia repair requires re-establishment of the integrity of the transversalis fascia.

The abdomen is divided into three vascular zones (Fig. 121-5). The midabdomen is supplied by the deep epigastric arcade (zone I), the lower abdomen is supplied by the external iliac artery (zone II), and the lateral abdomen is supplied by the intercostal and subcostal arteries (zone III). The deep inferior epigastric artery, a branch of the external iliac artery, is the dominant arterial supply of the rectus muscles. The superior epigastric artery is the continuation of the internal mammary artery. It extends inferiorly to an anastomosis with the inferior epigastric artery in the region of the umbilicus. Several perforators extend through the anterior fascial sheath to supply the overlying skin. The intercostal arteries originate from the thoracic aorta and extend to the internal mammary. They pass between the external and internal oblique muscles. The superficial external pudendal artery, the superficial epigastric artery, and the superficial and deep circumflex iliac arteries are branches of the femoral artery that pass through the femoral triangle to supply the lower abdominal wall skin.

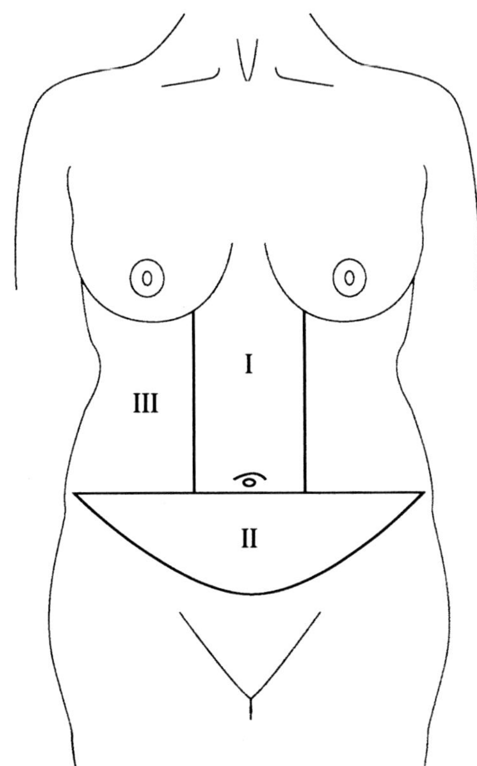

FIGURE 121-5. Vascular zones of the abdominal wall.

Venous drainage is parallel to the arterial supply. The lymphatic drainage of the abdominal wall is divided by the umbilicus. Above it, drainage is to the ipsilateral axillary lymph nodes. Below the umbilicus, lymphatics flow to the ipsilateral superficial inguinal lymph nodes.

The nerve supply of the abdomen is predominantly from the intercostal nerves. A neurovascular plane exists between the internal oblique and the transversus abdominis muscles. Through this plane pass the nerves as well as the blood vessels that supply the abdominal wall. The main trunks of the anterior cutaneous rami nerves are found in the neurovascular plane as they pass anteriorly to provide sensation to the anterior skin. There is significant overlap of these sensory dermatomes. Motor innervation of the abdominal oblique and transversalis muscles is from the lower thoracic and lumbar dorsal rami. Innervation to the rectus abdominis is by the 5th through 12th intercostal nerves.

The ilioinguinal and iliohypogastric nerves pass between the internal oblique and the transversus abdominis muscles as they extend from the lateral costal margin to the pubic area. Although they do not supply innervation to the abdomen, their course can be disrupted with dissection, particularly in the lateral abdomen. Loss of function results in a sensory defect in the medial thigh and the groin.

PATHOLOGY

Fat accumulates when calorie intake exceeds expenditure. It occurs in two patterns, cell hypertrophy and, less commonly, cell hyperplasia. The pattern of accumulation varies according to gender. With rapid weight gain or pregnancy, significant abdominal wall stretching can occur, leaving striae in locations where the dermis has been disrupted (Fig. 121-6). Post partum or after weight loss, the skin may remain flaccid with a significant loss of elasticity. Moderate weight gain results in hypertrophy of the existing adipocytes.[14] Pronounced weight gain results in hyperplasia of these cells in a distribution pattern that differs between men and women (Figs. 121-7 and 121-8). Women demonstrate weight gain in the region of the lower trunk and hips; in men, excess fat is seen primarily with an increase in abdominal girth.

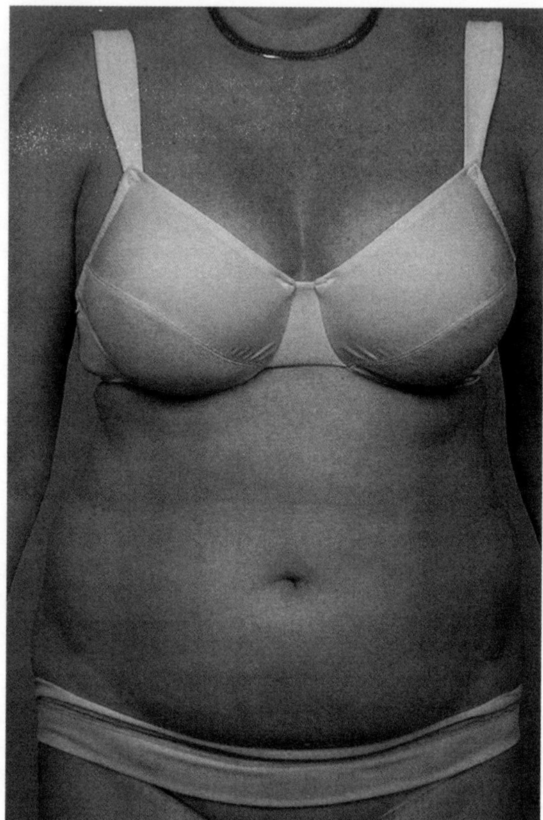

FIGURE 121-7. Typical female fat accumulation pattern in the lower abdomen and hips.

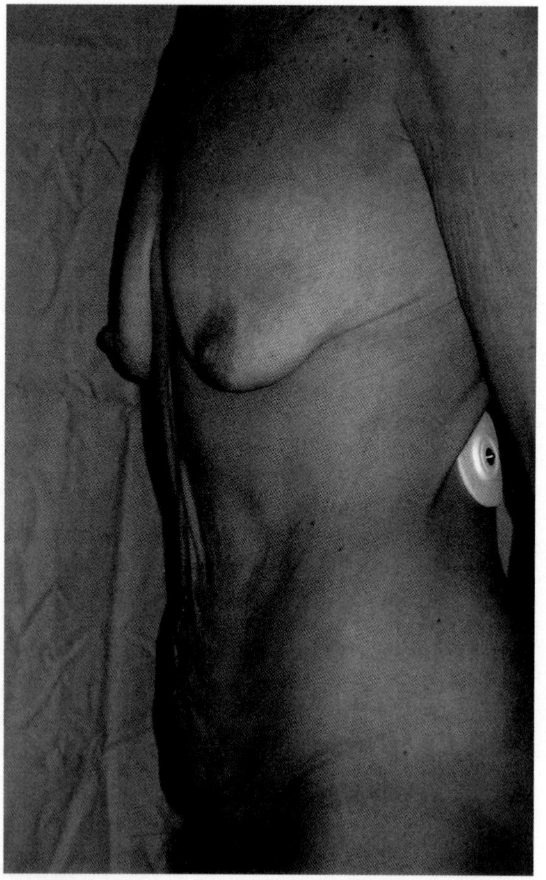

FIGURE 121-6. Example of flaccid, redundant skin that can follow weight loss of pregnancy.

Fat accumulation can result not only in an undesirable contour but also in a change in the quality of the skin, referred to as cellulite. This dimpling of the skin is more common in women and is frequently seen in the region of the posterior thigh. Analysis of this tissue has indicated that fibrous septa within the subcutaneous adipose tissue cause indentations visible on the skin surface.[15] Histologic changes also include extrusion of underlying adipose tissue into the reticular dermis.[16]

Diastasis recti represents a weakness of the linea alba and presents as an upper midline protrusion of the abdominal wall between the right and left rectus abdominis muscles. Whereas this is the most common variant of normal anatomy seen in the abdominal wall, it can present after increased intra-abdominal volume. Although it is not a true hernia, this weakness can occur in conjunction with an epigastric hernia. Identification of epigastric hernia is important to allow proper

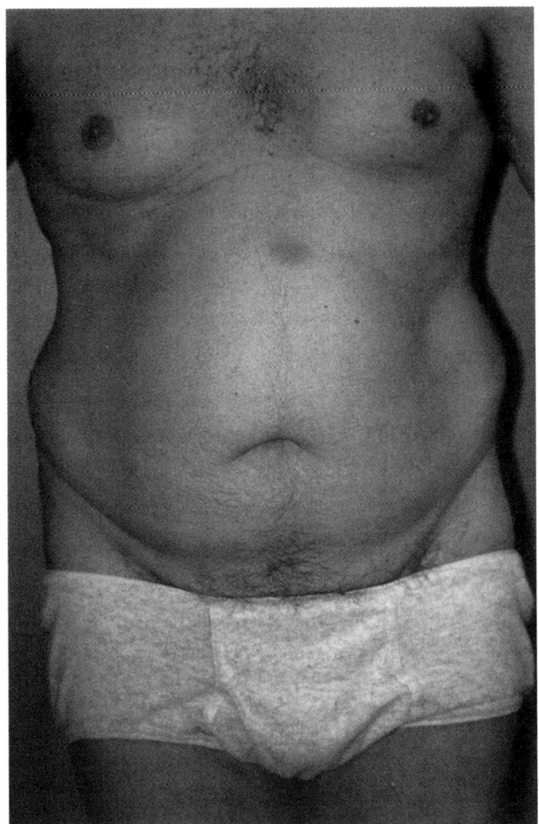

FIGURE 121-8. Typical male fat accumulation pattern in flanks and through abdominal wall.

surgical management. In addition, if it is present, it should be identified before any aesthetic procedures to prevent enteral injury or hernia sac perforation. True ventral hernia includes the formation of postoperative incisional hernias and exacerbation of congenital epigastric and umbilical hernias. Preoperative evaluation should include examination for respiratory, urinary, and bowel diseases because these can contribute to the formation of acquired hernias.

Additional pathologic processes that can result in soft tissue and structural defects of the abdominal wall include infectious processes such as bacterial gangrene and necrotizing fasciitis. These are life-threatening infections that require early radical débridement and proper antibiotic therapy. Omphalitis is generally an innocuous disease that results from poor hygiene and resolves with cleaning and local care of the umbilicus.

Both benign and malignant tumors can result in abdominal wall defects. Benign tumors of the abdominal wall may arise from any of the elements contained within the abdominal wall itself and are treated like any other benign tumor. Desmoid tumors are benign fibrous tumors that arise from the musculoaponeurotic abdominal wall. Because they are locally invasive and are likely to recur, wide excision is necessary to prevent local recurrence. Primary malignant neoplasms of the abdominal wall, such as cutaneous neoplasms and sarcomas, are uncommon. They are best treated by surgical excision. The abdominal wall is only occasionally the site of metastasis from primary malignant neoplasms located elsewhere.

Congenital defects include those that involve a structural defect of the abdominal wall and those that result from persistent fetal ducts. Omphalocele, a defect in the closure of the umbilical ring, results in herniated viscera covered by amnion. Closure that is nearly complete results in congenital periumbilical herniation. Because closure of the umbilical ring is not complete until birth, it is not unusual to have this finding in newborn infants; however, it resolves spontaneously in 80% of patients by 1 year of age.[17] Gastroschisis is located lateral to the umbilicus and is caused by failure of closure of the body wall. The abdominal viscera protrude through the defect, but unlike omphalocele, there is not a sac to cover the intestine. Remnants of the omphalomesenteric duct may present as abnormalities related to the abdominal wall. Umbilical polyps or sinuses and persistence of the entire omphalomesenteric duct or urachus require total excision and closure to prevent recurrent sinus track formation.

PREOPERATIVE CLASSIFICATION SYSTEM

Patients seeking abdominoplasty can be classified on the basis of physical examination findings and plan for operative management.[18,19] A type I patient is typically younger, with good skin elasticity and isolated lipodystrophy (Figs. 121-9 and 121-10). There is good muscle tone and no diastasis. A type II patient is one who usually has had at least one pregnancy. There is mild lower abdominal laxity and diastasis recti (Figs. 121-11 and 121-12). Lipodystrophy is mild to moderate and most notable inferior to the umbilicus. Patients classified as type III have muscle wall laxity including diastasis of the rectus muscles. Redundant skin and lipodystrophy are significant, particularly below the umbilicus (Figs. 121-13 and 121-14). There are often significant striae after multiple pregnancies. A type IV patient has severe upper and lower flaccidity of skin and muscle with excess fat throughout (Figs. 121-15 and 121-16). Diastasis recti is significant to severe, and the patient is often mildly to moderately obese. The umbilicus may be located below the ideal location with relationship to the iliac crest.

AESTHETIC ABDOMINAL PROCEDURES

Operative management for aesthetic improvement of the abdomen involves a continuum of procedures

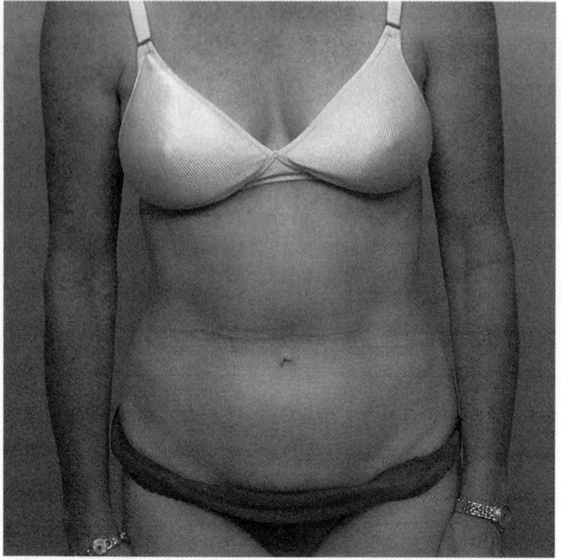

FIGURE 121-9. Type I patient, preoperative anterior view with minimal abdominal fullness and no skin laxity.

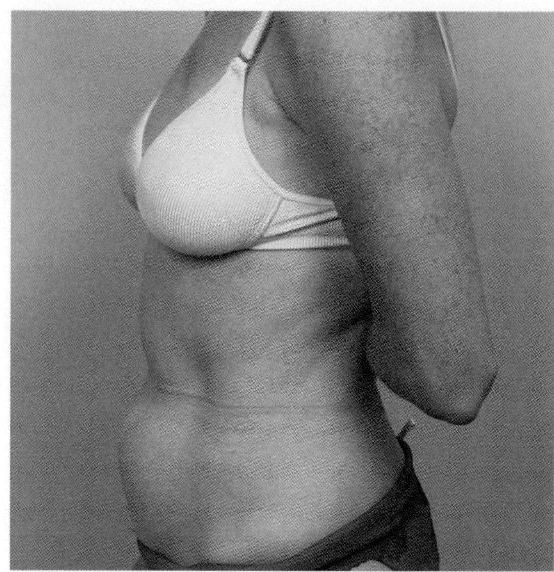

FIGURE 121-10. Type I patient, preoperative lateral view.

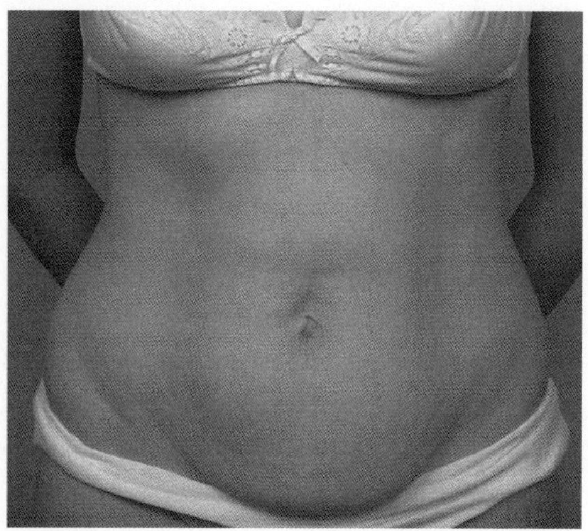

FIGURE 121-11. Type II patient, preoperative anterior view with limited lower abdominal fullness and minimal skin laxity.

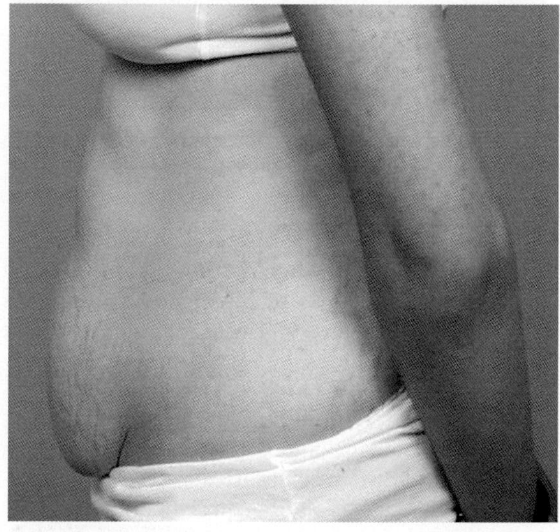

FIGURE 121-12. Type II patient, preoperative lateral view.

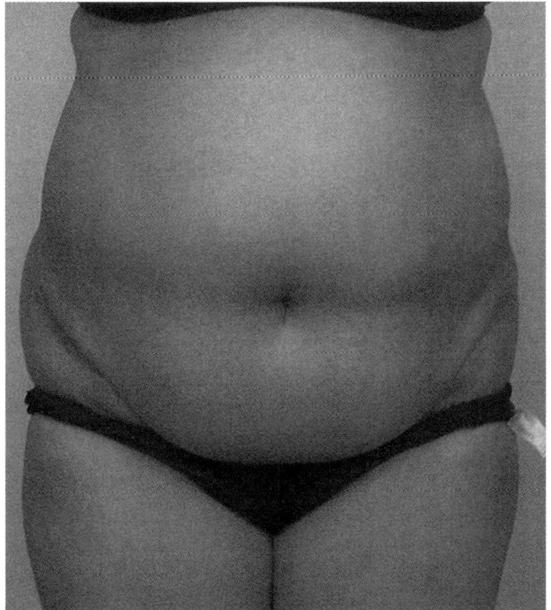

FIGURE 121-13. Type III patient, preoperative anterior view with lower abdominal fullness and skin laxity.

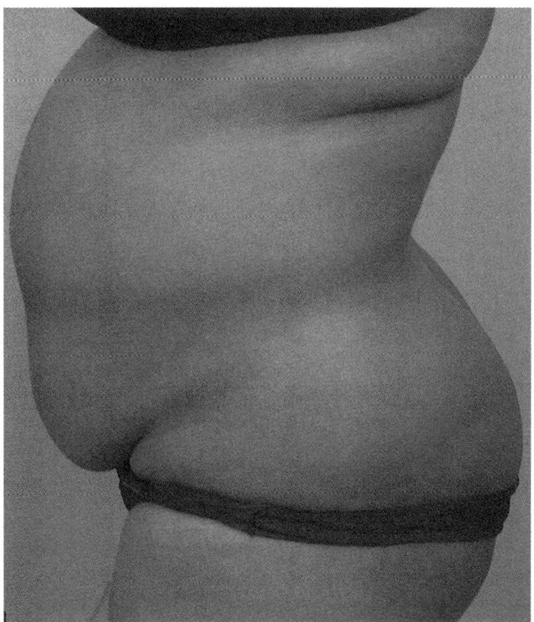

FIGURE 121-14. Type III patient, preoperative lateral view.

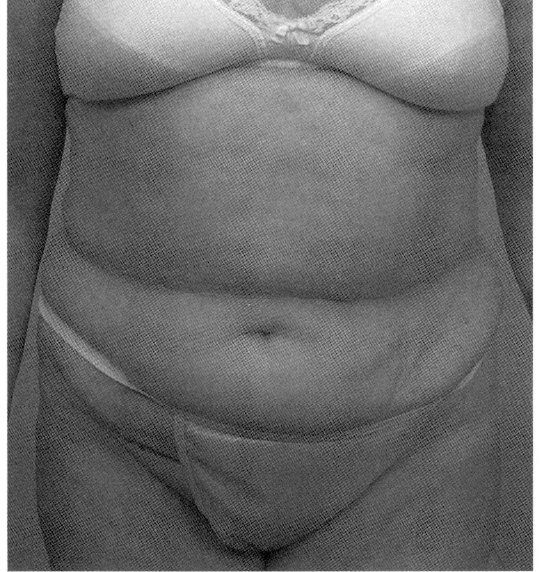

FIGURE 121-15. Type IV patient, preoperative anterior view with upper and lower abdominal fullness and skin laxity.

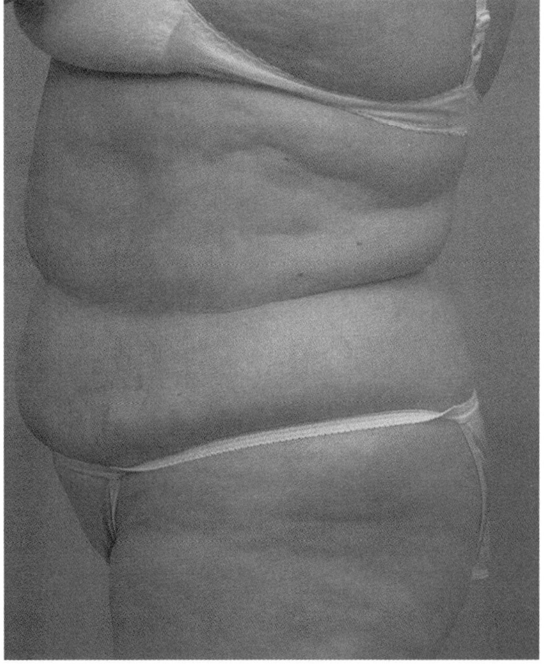

FIGURE 121-16. Type IV patient, preoperative lateral view.

ranging from suction-assisted liposuction alone to multistaged belt lipectomy with tightening of the musculofascial elements. Patients with a type I deformity can usually be treated with liposuction alone. No repair of the musculoaponeurotic layer is needed. Liposuction alone uses several small access incisions in the umbilicus, at the top of the pubic hairline, and laterally within the bikini or underwear line. This technique allows abdominal contouring with the least amount of visible scarring. Unfortunately, if the quality of skin elasticity is inadequate, redundant skin will remain. Placement of access incisions should be liberal; avoiding a small scar is less important than obtaining a smooth, symmetric contour. Care is taken to remove fat from the superficial adipose layer and to avoid intra-abdominal penetration. In addition to standard liposuction, ultrasonic suction and power-assisted suction can be used.

The mini-abdominoplasty combines minimal-length abdominal incisions to allow resection of redundant infraumbilical skin (Fig. 121-17). This procedure is suitable for type II deformities and includes conservative liposuction with resection of the lower abdominal skin. Variable sharp resection can be combined with liposuction to remove fat. Exposure of the midline below the umbilicus allows tightening of muscle laxity. The umbilical stalk is preserved.

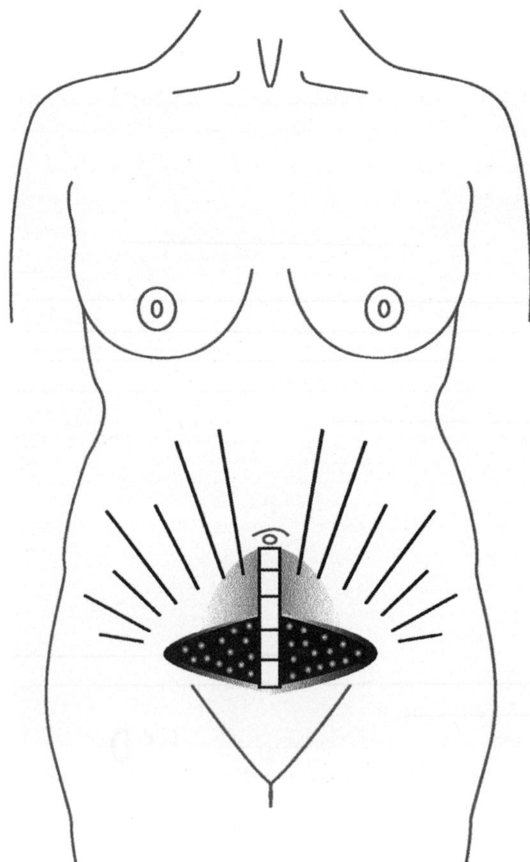

FIGURE 121-17. Diagram of mini-abdominoplasty; stippled areas represent resection, and dashed lines indicate infraumbilical plication. Liposuction can be performed along the radiating lines.

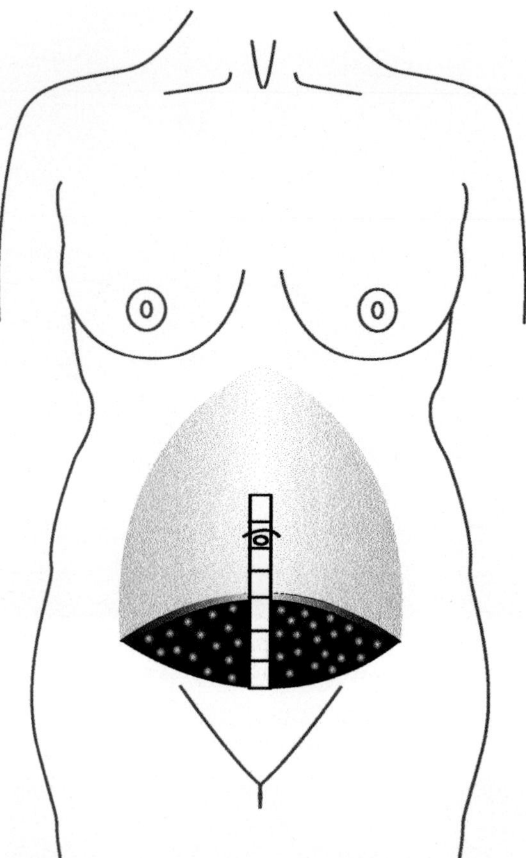

FIGURE 121-18. Diagram of modified abdominoplasty; stippled areas represent resection, dashed lines indicate plication, and shaded areas represent upper flap elevation.

The modified abdominoplasty involves elevation of a skin flap from the pubis to the subcostal margin (Fig. 121-18). It is indicated for type III patients. The umbilicus is detached from the fascial midline, and the upper abdominal laxity is removed. The umbilicus is lowered, but care must be taken to avoid lowering it to an unnaturally inferior location. The redundant lower skin margin is resected. Fat resection is performed sharply rather than by liposuction. The fascial midline is tightened to address muscle laxity both above and below the umbilicus. The wound is closed in layers with the patient in the semi-Fowler position to avoid any tension at closure. Closed suction drains and compressive dressings are used.

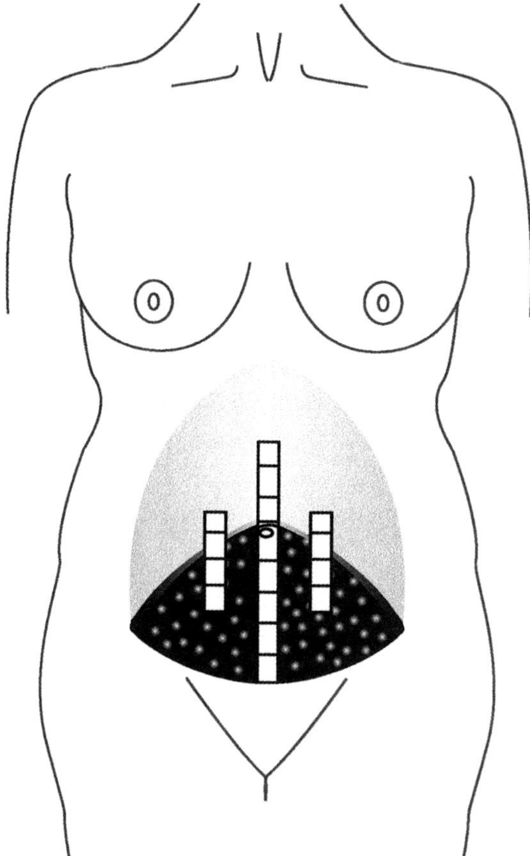

FIGURE 121-19. Diagram of standard abdominoplasty; stippled areas represent resection, dashed lines indicate infraumbilical plication, and shaded areas represent the upper flap elevation.

Standard abdominoplasty requires aggressive elevation of the upper abdominal flap to the level of the subcostal margin (Fig. 121-19). It is well suited for patients with a type IV deformity and those with concomitant ventral or umbilical hernias. Management involves wide undermining of the superior flap to the costal margin. This is necessary to allow resection of the entire skin flap inferior to the umbilicus. Liposuction is avoided because the risk for flap necrosis is greatly increased. The umbilicus must be transposed. It is detached from the abdominal skin and left attached to the underlying fascia. Resection of the redundant skin is to the level of the umbilical window. The patient can be placed in semi-Fowler sitting position to facilitate resection of the skin up to the level of the original umbilicus. Care is taken to preserve a layer of subcutaneous lymphatic tissue over the fascia to decrease the incidence of seroma formation. Exposure is more than adequate to allow repair of diastasis recti and significant tightening of muscle flaccidity.

Once the musculofascial layer is tightened and the redundant skin is resected, the new umbilical location can be determined. The skin is temporarily closed with staples, leaving enough room to palpate the umbilical stalk and transpose its location to the umbilical wall. A mark is placed, and the location of the new umbilical window is checked to ensure that it is in the midline and that it is properly positioned in relationship to the iliac crest, xiphoid, and pubis.

Flap elevation is usually employed without the use of suction-assisted lipectomy. The significant flap elevation compromises the vascularity of zone III. With the liposuction and the potential injury to zone II, the superiorly based upper abdominal flap is dependent on one vascular zone and at risk for vascular insufficiency. If liposuction is performed, it should be done conservatively and with caution (Figs. 121-20 and 121-21).

For the majority of patients, including those who are type II and type III and even some type IV, appropriate management can be obtained with the modern abdominoplasty (Figs. 121-22 to 121-32). This

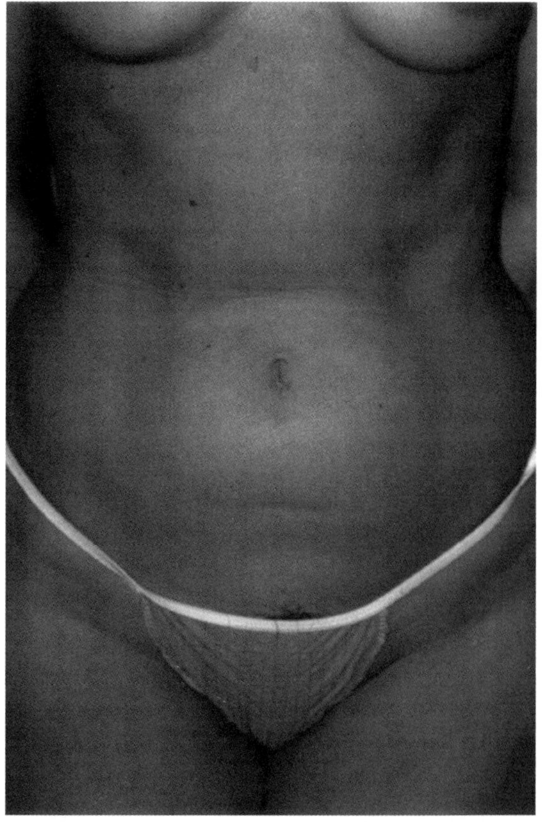

FIGURE 121-20. Preoperative view of a patient for whom an inverted T incision, standard abdominoplasty, is planned.

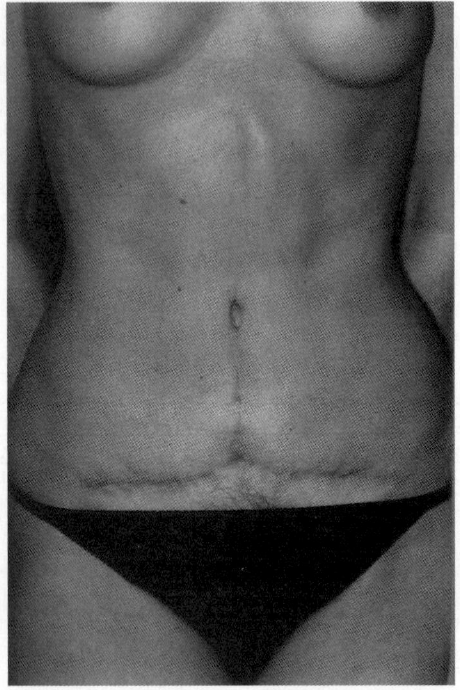

FIGURE 121-21. Postoperative view of a patient with an inverted T incision, standard abdominoplasty.

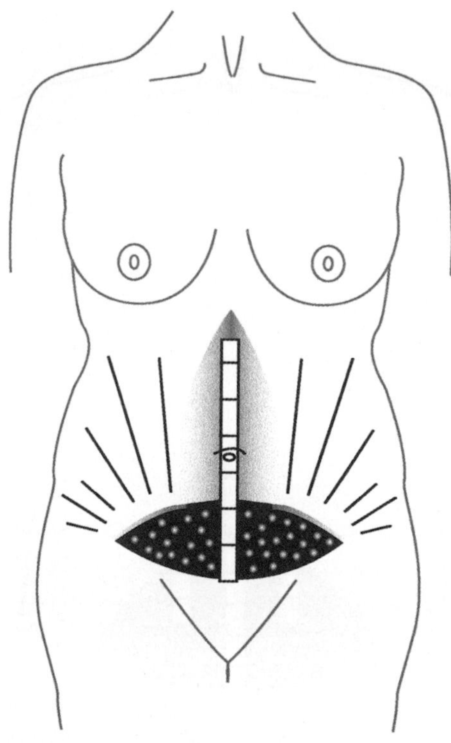

FIGURE 121-22. Diagram of modern abdominoplasty; stippled areas represent resection, dashed lines indicate plication, shaded areas represent the limited upper flap elevation, and radiating lines indicate area of liposuction.

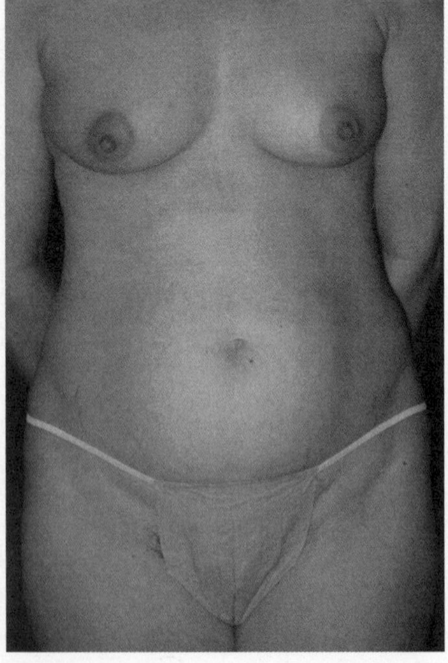

FIGURE 121-23. Example of a candidate for modern abdominoplasty technique, preoperative anterior view.

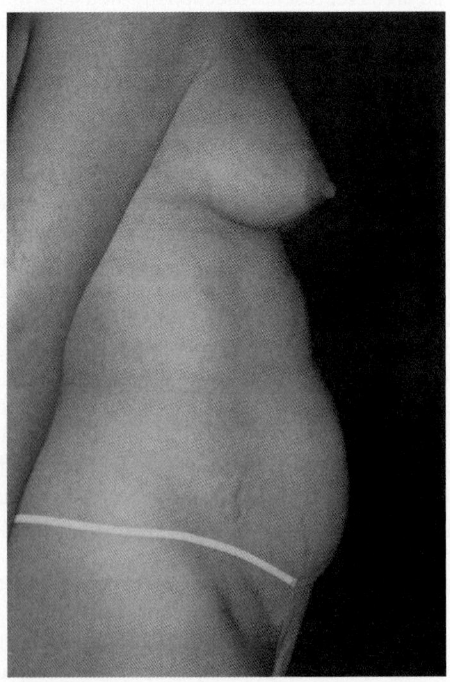

FIGURE 121-24. Modern abdominoplasty technique, preoperative lateral view.

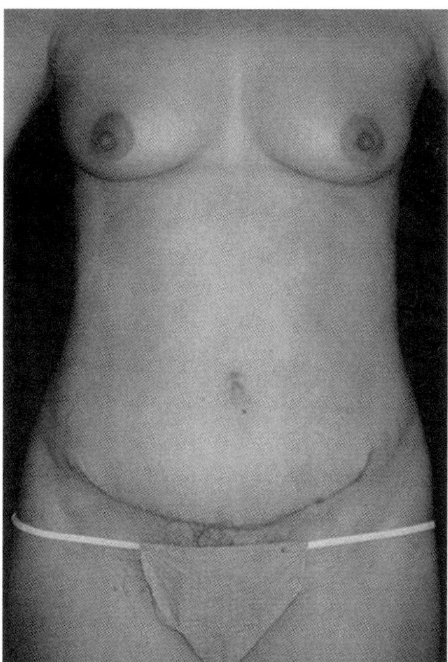

FIGURE 121-25. Modern abdominoplasty technique, postoperative anterior view.

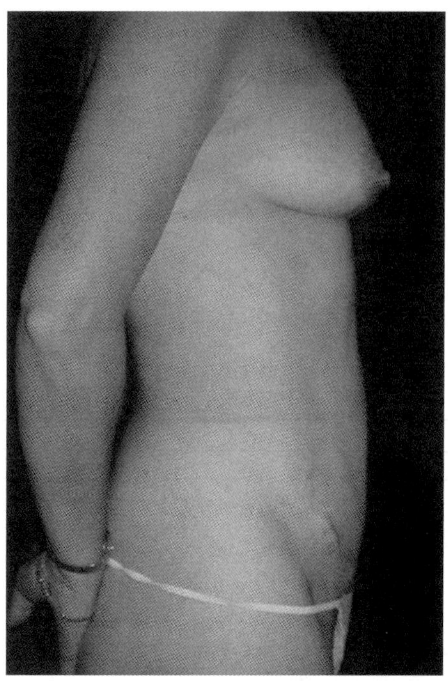

FIGURE 121-26. Modern abdominoplasty technique, postoperative lateral view.

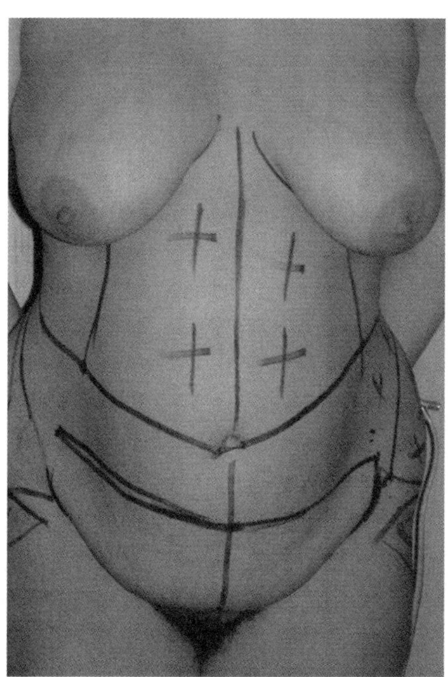

FIGURE 121-27. Modern abdominoplasty technique, preoperative anterior view to indicate lower abdominal resection and areas for aggressive liposuction.

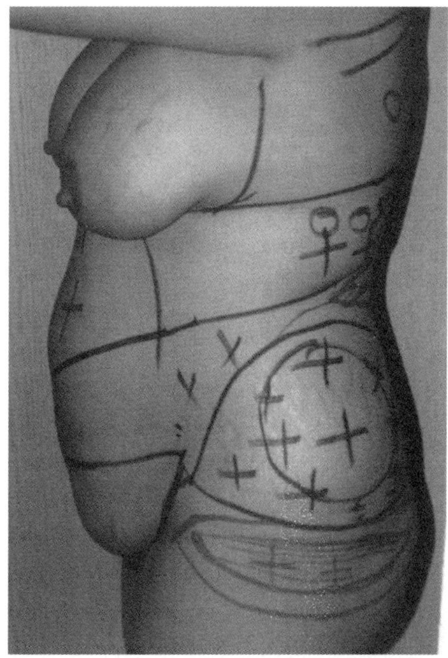

FIGURE 121-28. Modern abdominoplasty technique, preoperative lateral view to indicate lower abdominal resection and areas for aggressive liposuction.

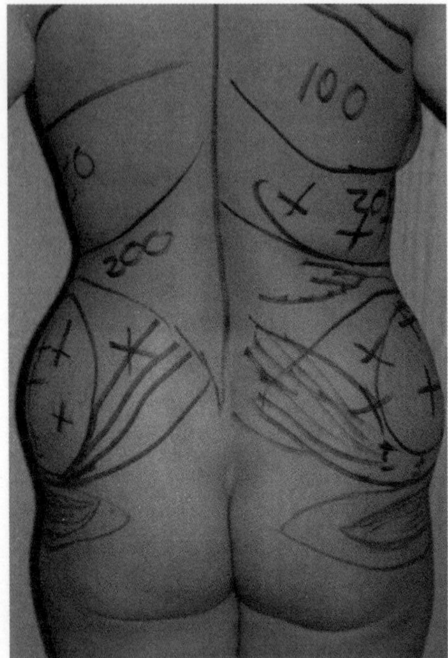

FIGURE 121-29. Modern abdominoplasty technique, preoperative posterior view to indicate lower abdominal resection and areas for aggressive liposuction.

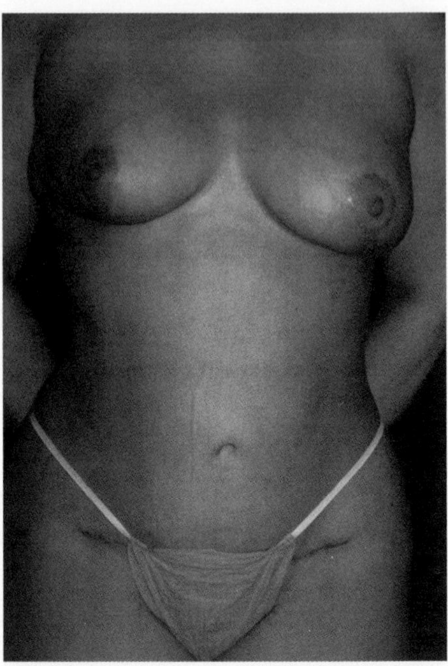

FIGURE 121-30. Modern abdominoplasty technique, postoperative anterior view demonstrating improved contour with shorter scar.

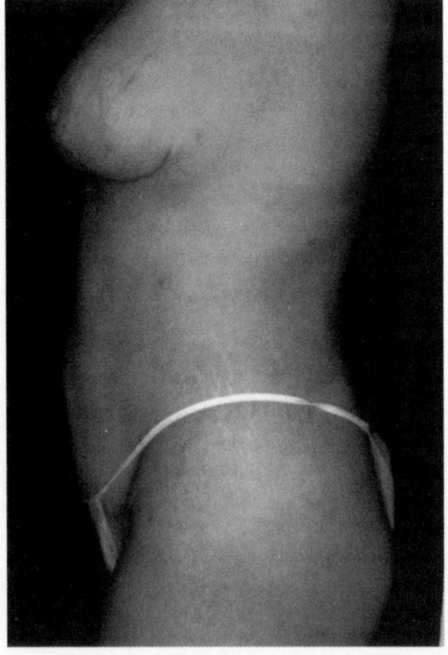

FIGURE 121-31. Modern abdominoplasty technique, lateral view.

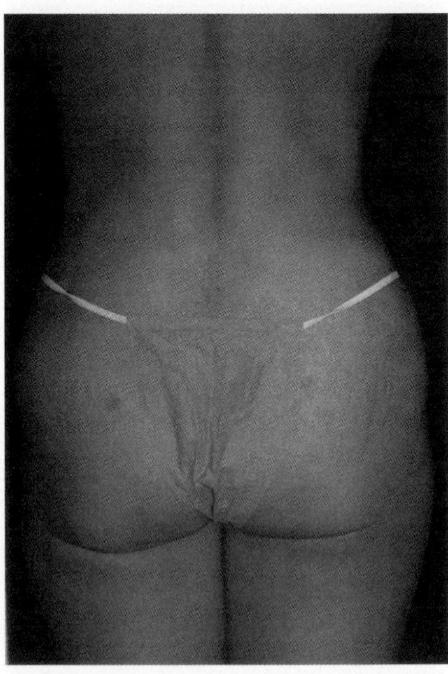

FIGURE 121-32. Modern abdominoplasty technique, posterior view.

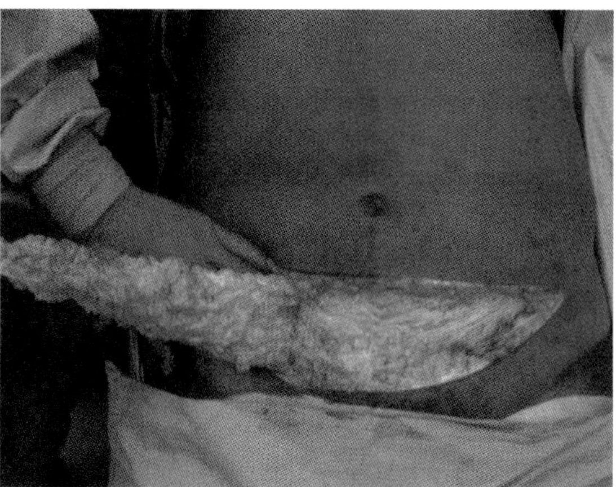

FIGURE 121-33. Modern abdominoplasty, lower abdominoplasty lipectomy by avulsion technique to remove the fat and skin above Scarpa fascia.

incorporates aggressive liposuction of the abdomen and flanks, including the infraumbilical region. Resection is performed in a small area below the umbilicus. Undermining is limited to the midline in a 4- to 5-cm region from the upper portion of the resection to the xiphoid. The umbilical attachments can be preserved or released, depending on the location of the umbilicus and the exposure required. Resection of the skin is limited to a small area above the pubis.

After aggressive liposuction deep to the planned skin resection, the skin is incised with a scalpel along the preoperative markings. Sharp Mayo scissors are used to complete the incision to Scarpa fascia. Each end of the skin paddle is grasped with a clamp, and the segment is avulsed (Fig. 121-33). With adequate liposuction, the resection will leave some of the adipose tissue deep to Scarpa fascia (Fig. 121-34). When the wound is closed, the superior and inferior edges will align because the flaps are of similar thickness. The skin edges are checked to ensure that primary closure can be obtained without aggressive undermining. With use of a lighted retractor or endoscope, the fascial plication (see later) and repair of the diastasis can be performed (Fig. 121-35). The umbilicus is rarely released from the abdominal wall, but if this is necessary, it can be reattached.

Patients who have had massive weight loss require special attention. These patients have excess skin in addition to excess adipose tissues. Significant changes occur in the excess skin, resulting in a loss of the dermal elasticity. For the large amount of lax, redundant skin to be resected adequately, standard excisions must be extended. It is not unusual for these patients to have symptoms such as back pain, intertriginous skin changes, and difficulty with daily activities.

Simple panniculectomy is effective to address the lower abdomen, particularly in patients who have medical comorbidities that prohibit lengthy surgery (Figs. 121-36 to 121-39). In patients who have undergone bariatric surgery, the midline scar can be used to make a vertical midline incision to tighten the upper waist and flanks in the horizontal direction (Figs. 121-40 to 121-45). This provides improved aesthetic results, and contouring avoids the need to reposition

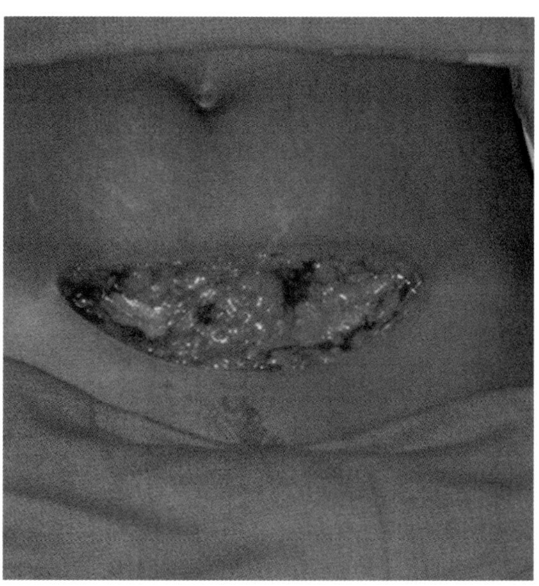

FIGURE 121-34. After lipectomy by avulsion technique.

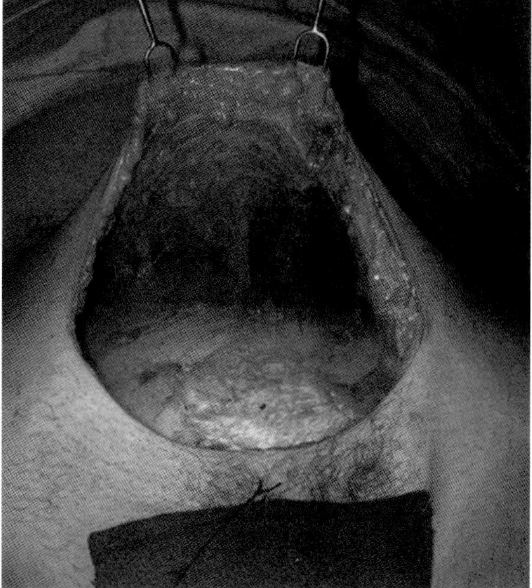

FIGURE 121-35. Intraoperative view of limited upper flap elevation for placement of plication sutures during modern abdominoplasty.

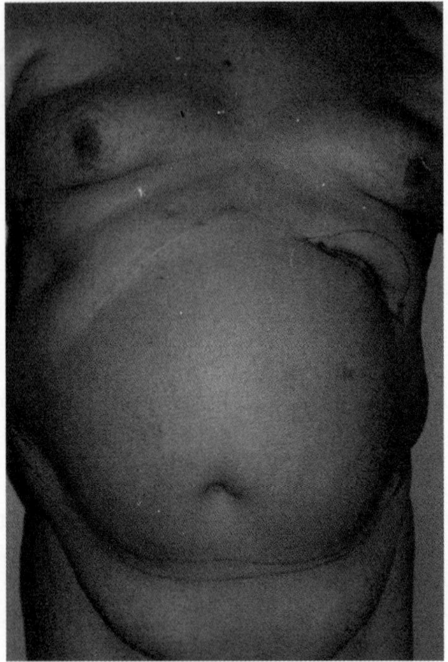

FIGURE 121-36. Pannus in an obese male patient, preoperative anterior view (note subcostal incision).

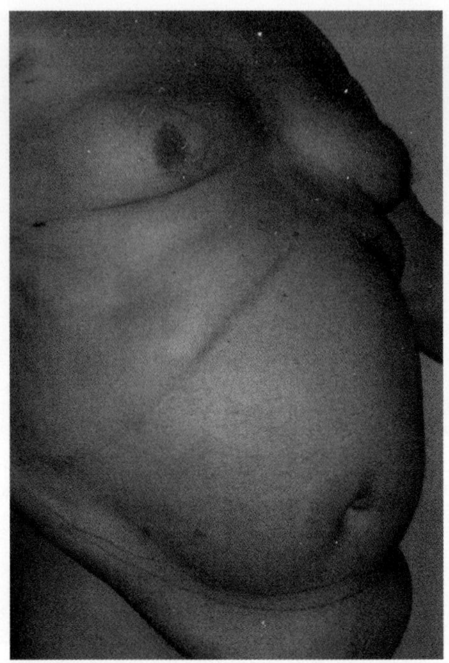

FIGURE 121-37. Pannus in an obese male patient, preoperative oblique view.

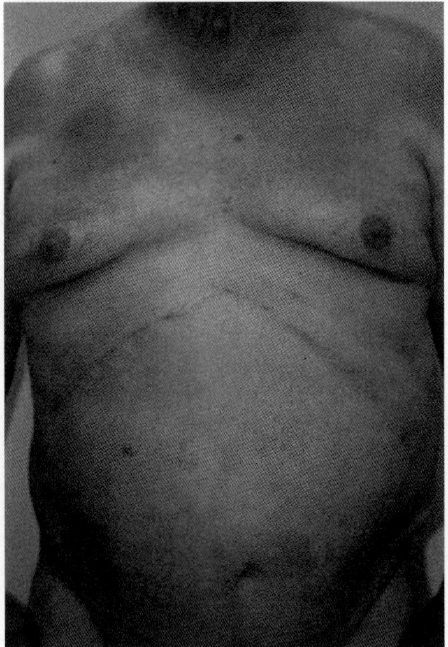

FIGURE 121-38. Simple panniculectomy in an obese male patient, postoperative anterior view (note subcostal incision).

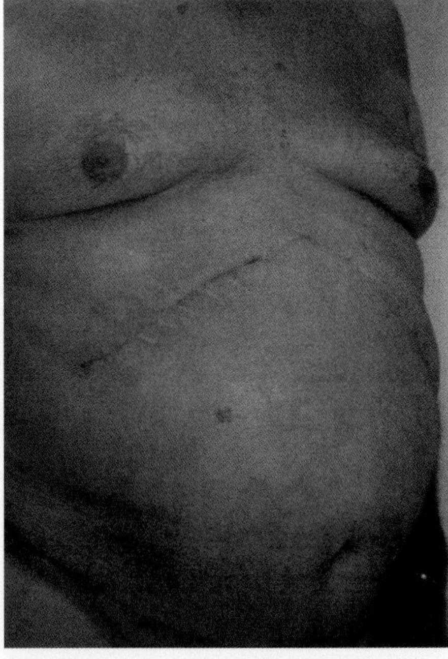

FIGURE 121-39. Simple panniculectomy in an obese male patient, postoperative oblique view.

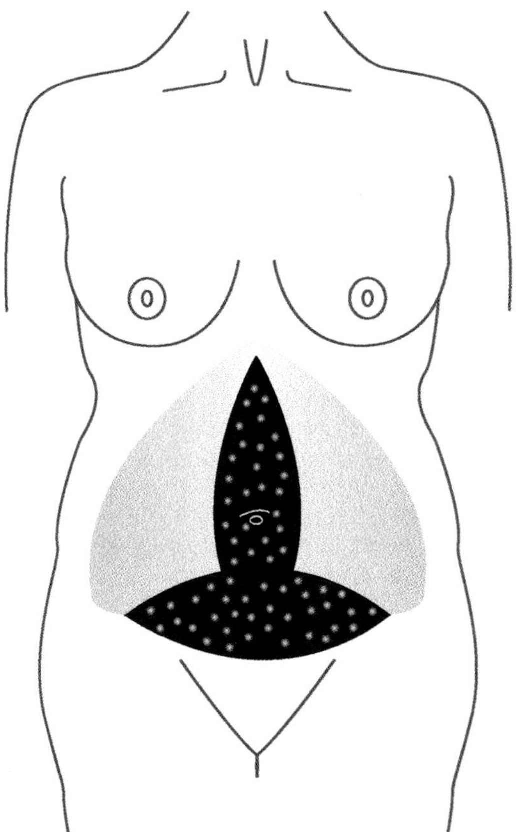

FIGURE 121-40. Diagram of inverted T resection; stippled area represents resection, and shaded area represents undermined area.

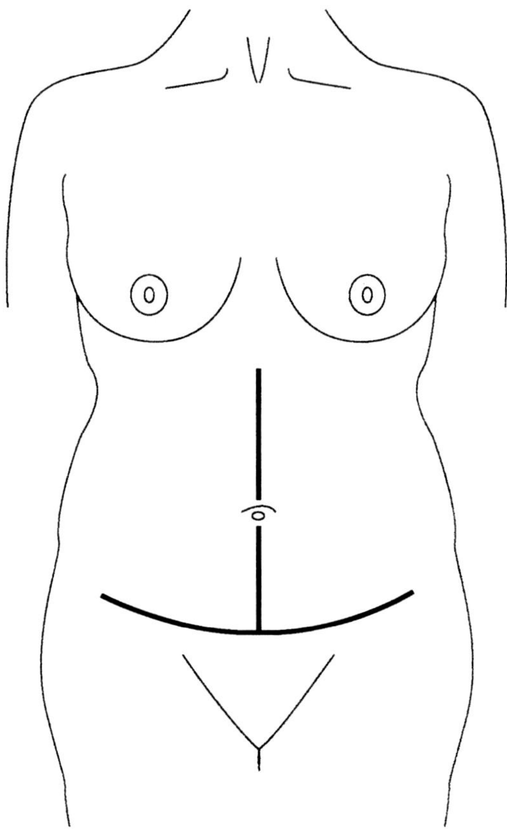

FIGURE 121-41. Diagram of inverted T postoperative scar location.

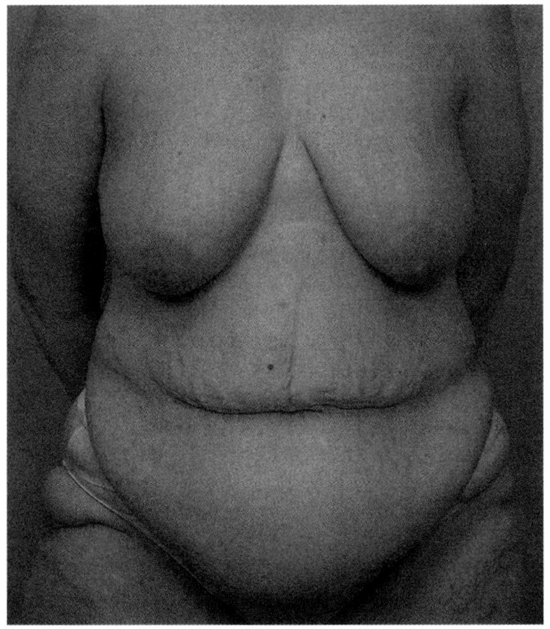

FIGURE 121-42. Pannus after gastric bypass and massive weight loss, anterior view.

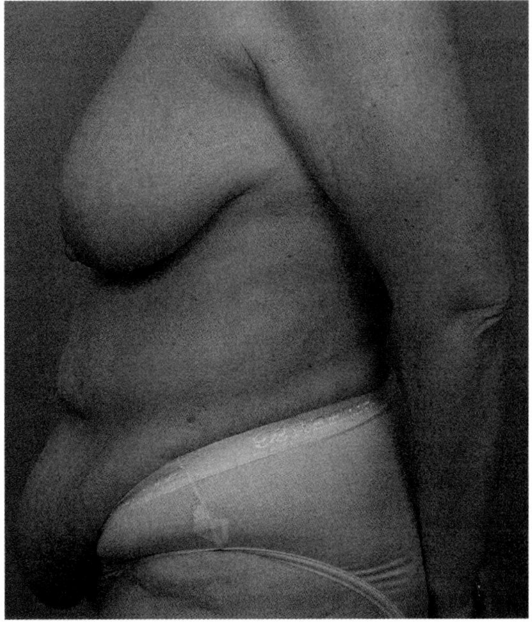

FIGURE 121-43. Pannus after gastric bypass and massive weight loss, lateral view.

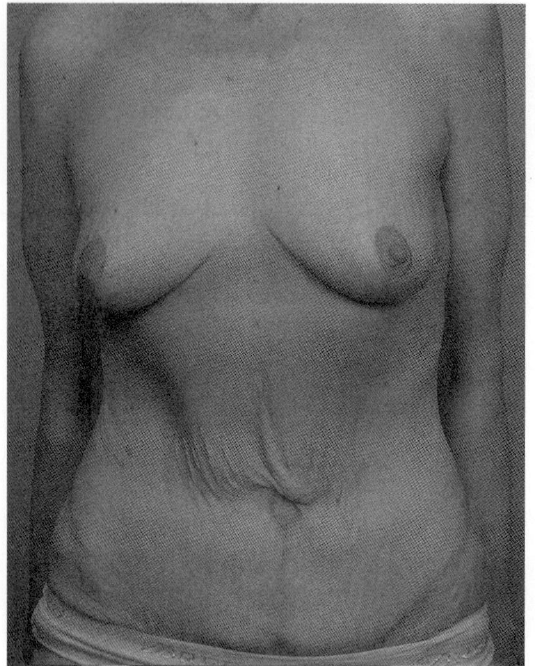

FIGURE 121-44. Panniculectomy abdominoplasty by inverted T approach, anterior view.

the patient intraoperatively. Vertical tightening can be obtained by use of the circumferential belt dermolipectomy. The patient must be turned over on the table, but circumferential resection improves the upper thigh, buttock, and upper abdomen. Particular care is needed to address the umbilicus because the umbilical stalk can be long. With circumferential dissection, the umbilical blood supply can be compromised.

MALE ABDOMINOPLASTY

The male abdominoplasty patient has specific needs.[20] Male patients tend to have less realistic goals and are more frequently dissatisfied with the final outcome of their body contour procedures (Figs. 121-46 to 121-49). The thicker male skin has less elasticity and is less likely to have cellulite. The male pubic hair distribution is different and requires the transverse abdominal incision to be placed higher. The fat distribution is different, as is the skin. Accumulation of intra-abdominal fat, rather than subcutaneous fat, is likely to contribute to the bulging abdominal contour. In addition, the accumulation of adipose tissue in the flanks (love handles) may require direct incision in some patients. Incision planning should be appropriate for male clothing.

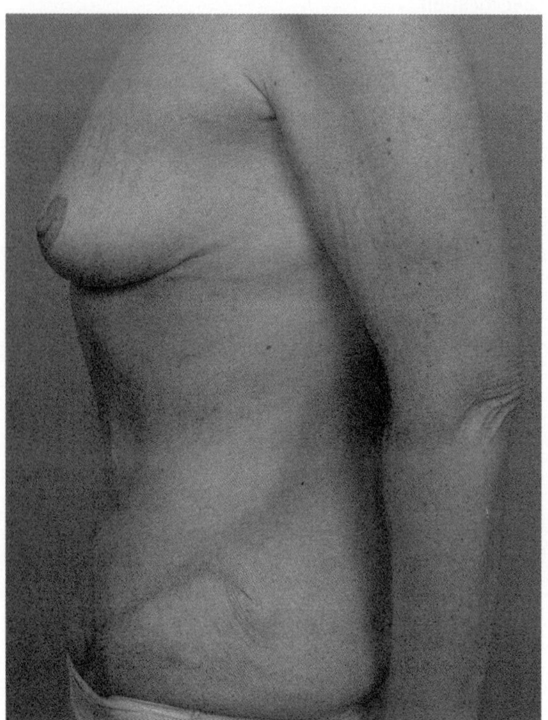

FIGURE 121-45. Panniculectomy abdominoplasty by inverted T approach, lateral view.

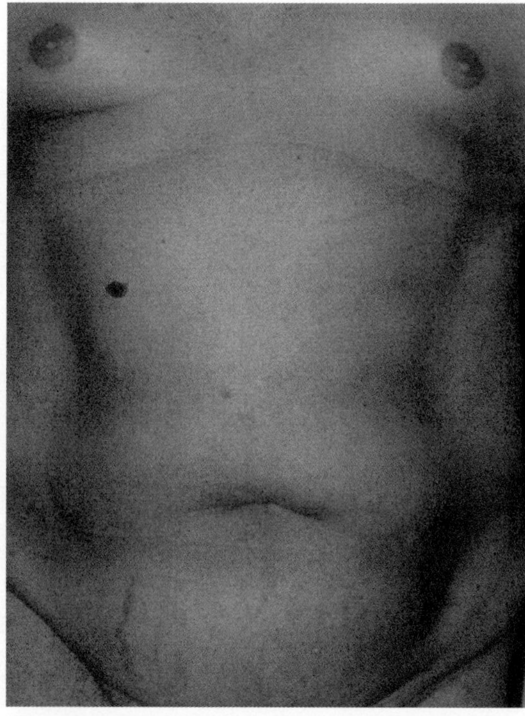

FIGURE 121-46. Male abdominoplasty, preoperative anterior view.

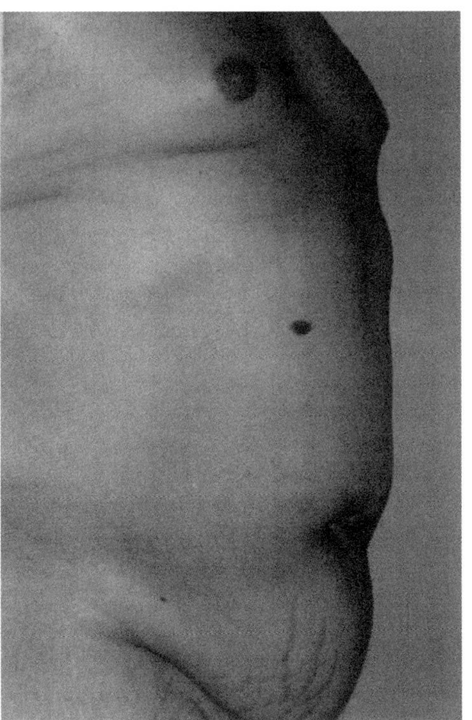

FIGURE 121-47. Male abdominoplasty, preoperative lateral view.

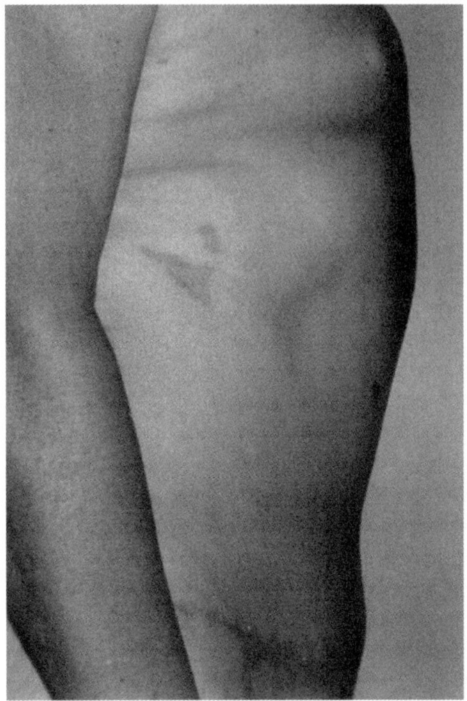

FIGURE 121-49. Male abdominoplasty, postoperative lateral view.

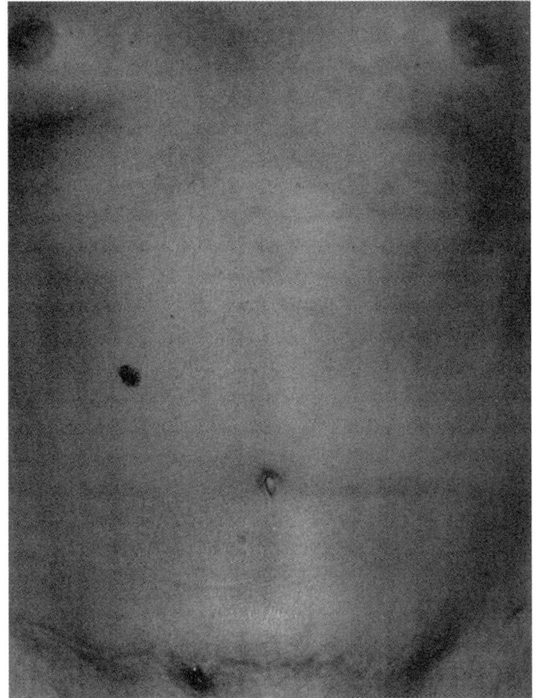

FIGURE 121-48. Male abdominoplasty, postoperative anterior view.

UMBILICOPLASTY

Many techniques have been described to preserve or recreate the aesthetic appearance of the umbilicus. At the time of abdominoplasty, an area of subcutaneous fat surrounding the umbilicus can be removed by either liposuction or direct excision. The goal is to make a periumbilical dimple approximately 5 cm in diameter. Tacking sutures can be used to attach the umbilicus carefully to the fascial midline to further emphasize this depression (Fig. 121-50). In patients who undergo full abdominoplasty with umbilical transposition, half-buried horizontal mattress sutures can be used to approximate the skin edges properly and to minimize suture marks (Figs. 121-51 to 121-54). Care must be taken to make an umbilical window of sufficient size or the contracting scar will leave an abnormally small umbilicus, which is unnatural and presents a hygienic problem. Several incision patterns have been used. The horizontal crescent-shaped incision with the convexity either up (sad face) or down (smiley face) is used most frequently. In addition, the V inverted incision and a diamond pattern are described (Figs. 121-55 and 121-56). The goal is to make an opening of sufficient size and additionally to permit some superior hooding to occur (Fig. 121-57). The modified and modern abdominoplasties leave

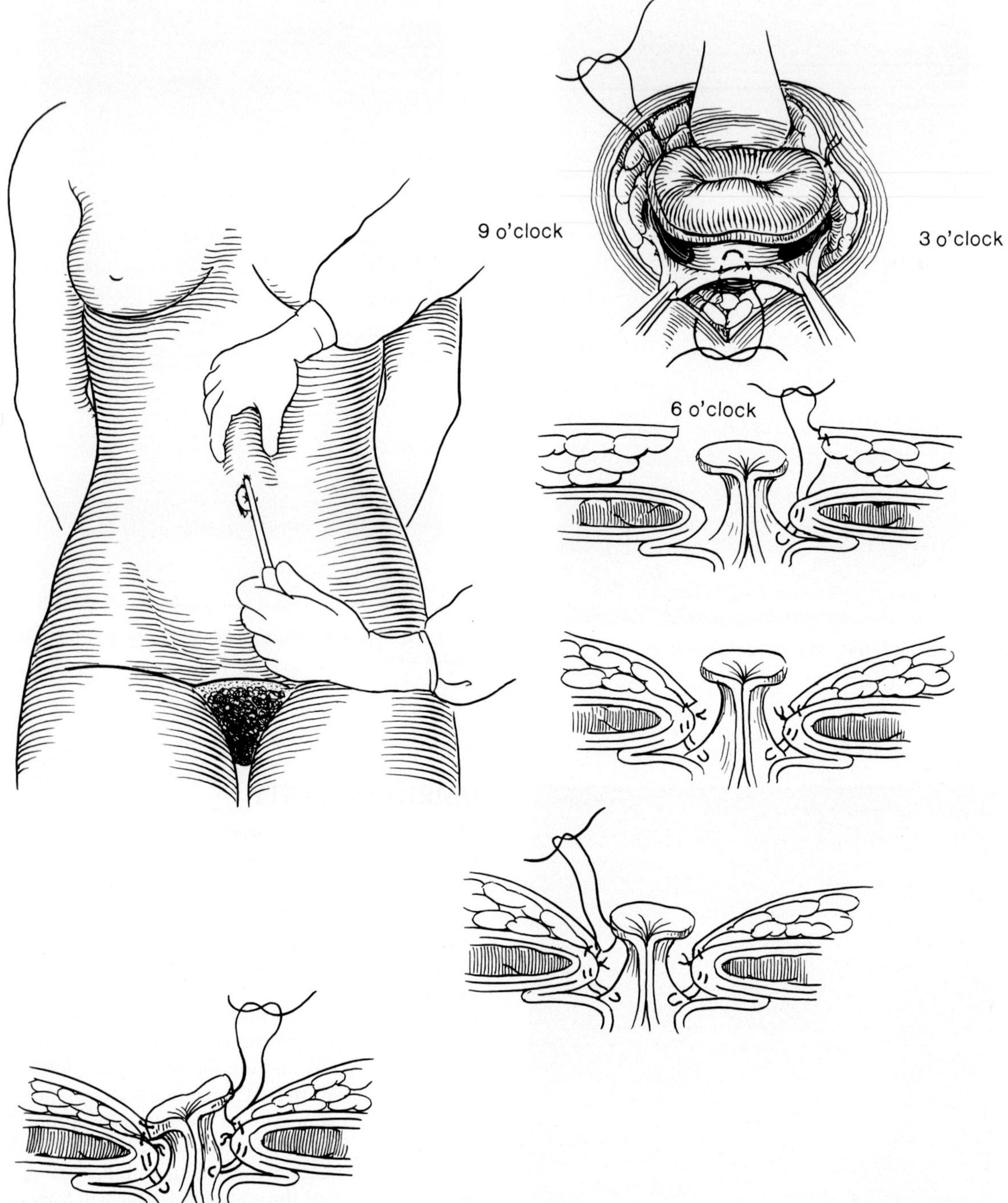

FIGURE 121-50. Suturing of the umbilical stalk at 3-, 6-, and 9-o'clock positions down to the fascia layer to make a periumbilical depression. (From Grazer FM: Abdominoplasty. In McCarthy JG, ed: Plastic Surgery. Philadelphia, WB Saunders, 1990:3929.)

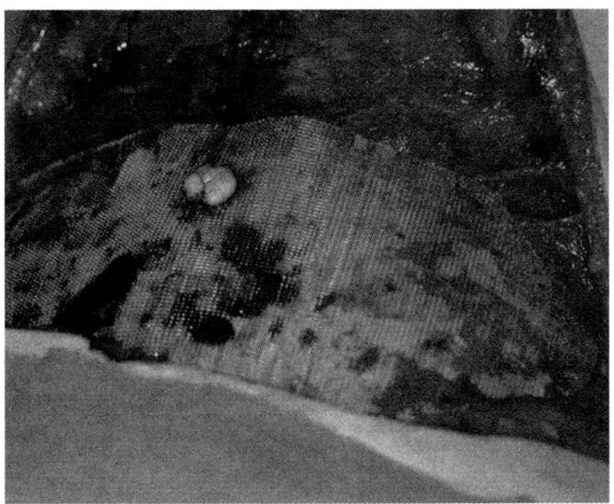

FIGURE 121-51. Umbilical stalk delivered through Marlex mesh repair.

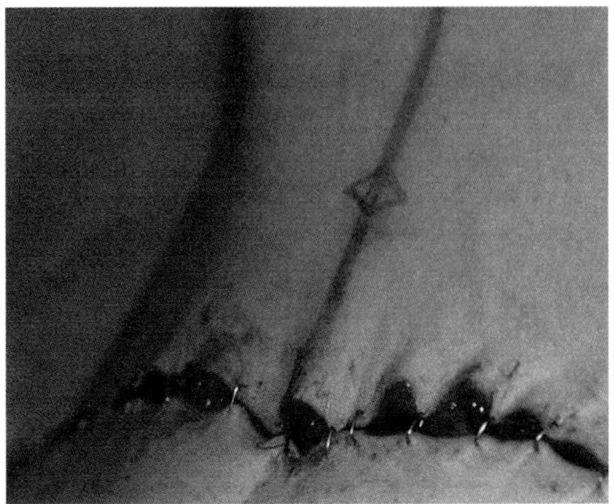

FIGURE 121-52. Umbilical window markings.

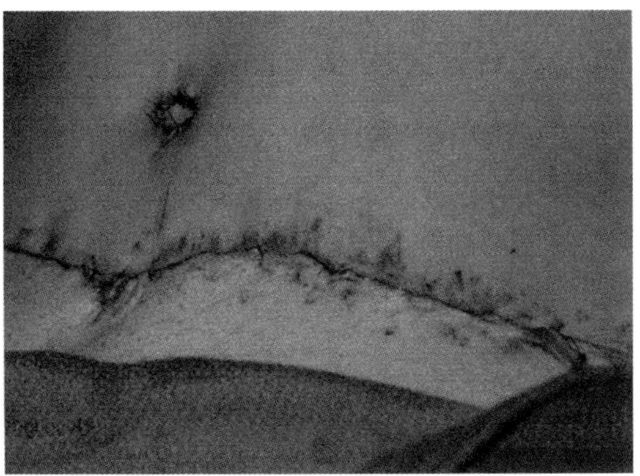

FIGURE 121-53. Umbilical window with stalk inset and periumbilical depression.

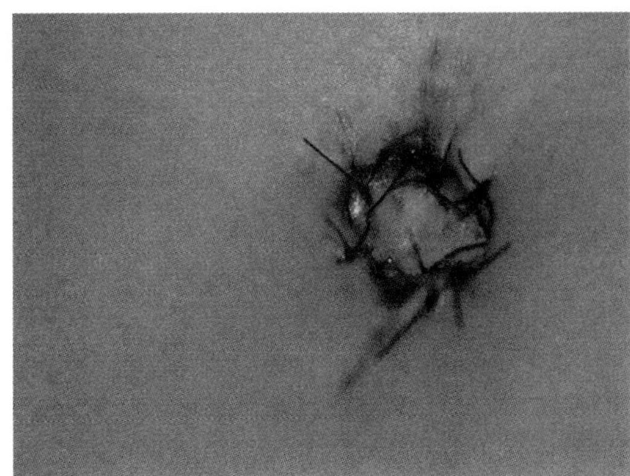

FIGURE 121-54. Umbilical closure, close-up view.

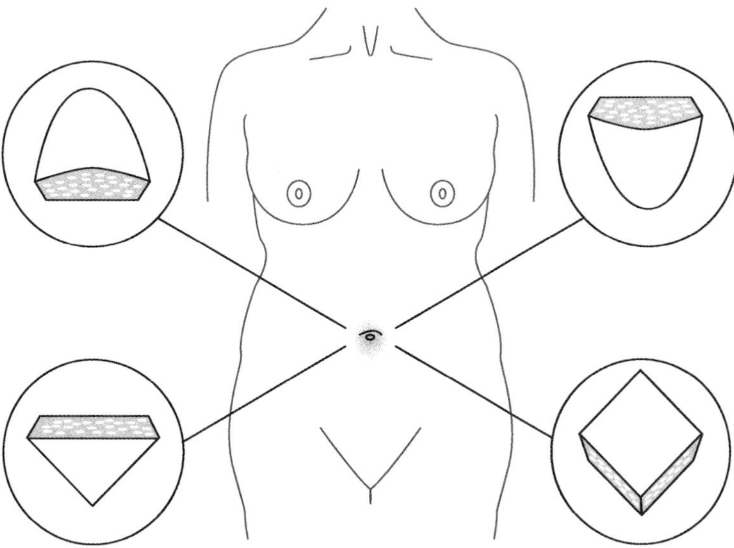

FIGURE 121-55. Various umbilical window markings: crescent up, crescent down, V-shaped, and diamond.

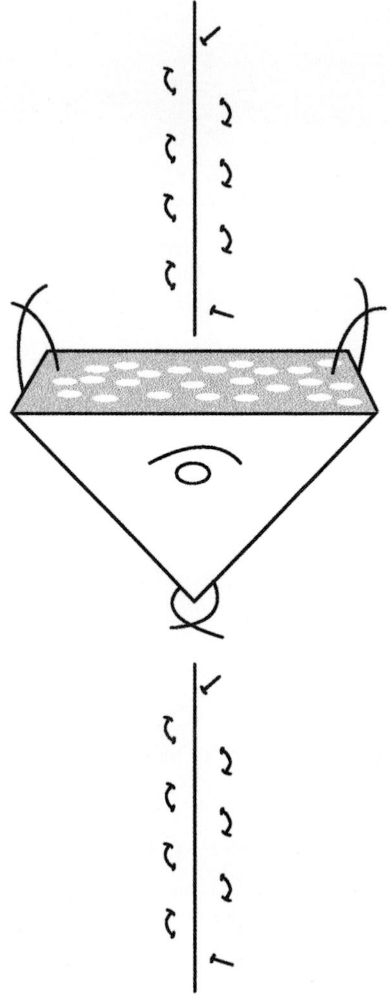

FIGURE 121-56. Suture location for inset of umbilical stalk into a triangular window, the preferred technique of the authors.

the umbilicus attached to the overlying skin. It is important to check the location of the umbilicus (Fig. 121-58). In the modified abdominoplasty, which detaches the umbilical stalk from the fascia and reattaches it, the umbilicus can be reset to a noticeably low position.

One technique that allows proper location of the umbilicus without any visible scarring has been reported.[21] The umbilicus is freed from the surrounding tissue of the superior abdominal flap. It is then completely de-epithelialized. When the new umbilical location is determined, a section of the abdominal flap is defatted. The intact umbilical stalk is then applied to the overlying skin as a skin graft. The resulting umbilicus maintains adequate form without the apparent scars.

ABDOMINAL FASCIAL MANAGEMENT

Management of the fascia is particularly important when limited skin undermining is performed. Tightening in the midline as well as along paramedian lines is often necessary (Figs. 121-59 and 121-60). The authors have also more recently used a transverse plication to tighten the fascia.

With any approach, the fascia should be marked at the anticipated closure to avoid any confusion of the degree of tightening to be provided as the sutures are being placed. The midline is closed with several 0 Prolene simple interrupted sutures both above and below the umbilicus. Use of interrupted sutures offers more control over the degree of plication obtained. When necessary, a lighted retractor or endoscope will facilitate placement of the most cephalad sutures. A running suture of 2-0 looped nylon is placed as a second layer to further imbricate the midline (Fig. 121-61).

Aggressive plication around the umbilical stalk will result in necrosis and should be avoided. The plication can be discontinued just above the

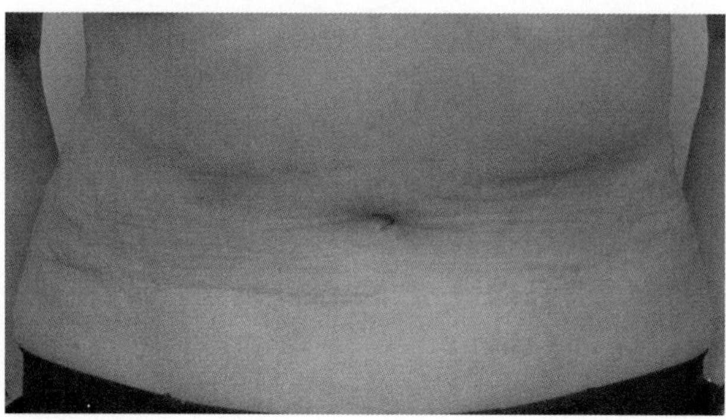

FIGURE 121-57. Long-term follow-up of umbilical inset with use of the triangular window. Note superior hooding.

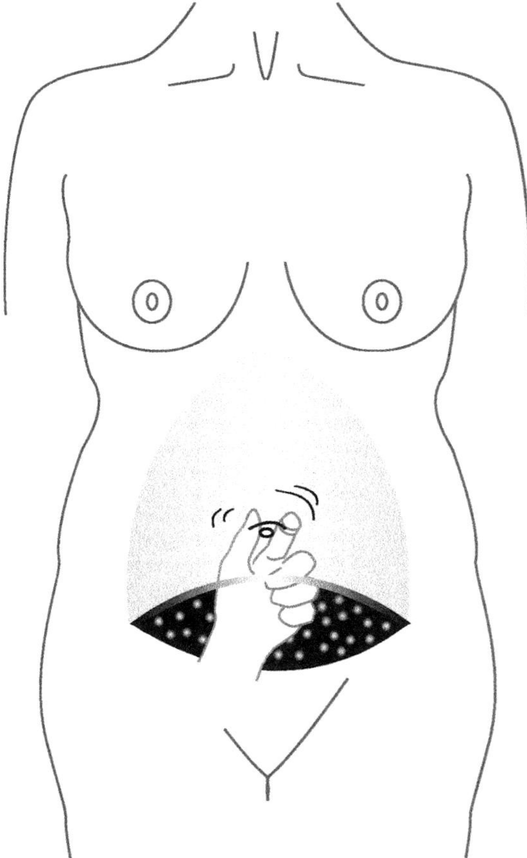

FIGURE 121-58. Transposing the location of the umbilical stalk to the abdominal wall for creation of the window.

umbilicus and restarted below it (Figs. 121-62 and 121-63). Alternatively, a continuous suture can be continued around the umbilicus, passing to one side of the stalk for approximately 2 cm. Large palpable, permanent knots should be buried with

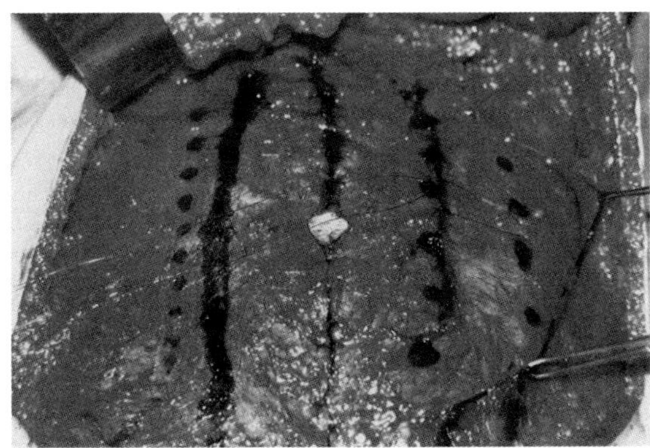

FIGURE 121-59. Intraoperative view after midline plication with markings for the lateral plication.

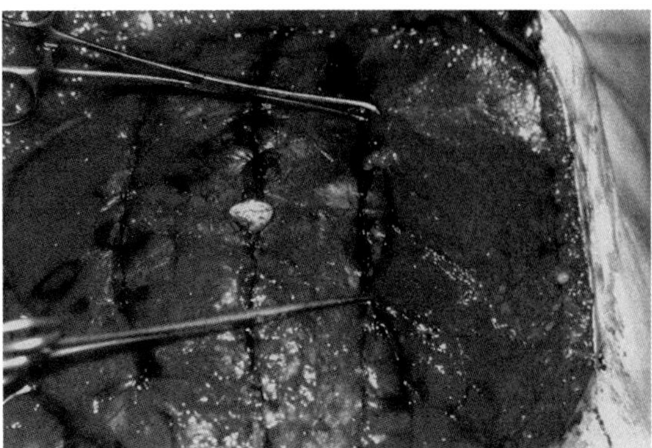

FIGURE 121-60. Intraoperative view of the midline and lateral plication.

use of smaller slow-absorbing suture such as Vicryl or PDS.

To accentuate the hourglass figure and further tighten the waist, paramedian plication can be performed by a similar technique. The paramedian plication also permits correction of an asymmetrically located umbilical stalk. In addition, a transverse plication inferior and lateral to the location of the umbilicus is helpful to further emphasize the desirable contour of both the lateral and anterior aspects of the lower abdomen. Although this method avoids undermining the superior flap and does tighten the abdomen in a longitudinal direction, it is not indicated to correct diastasis recti (Fig. 121-64).

If a ventral hernia repair is performed, the same incision and skin resection are performed

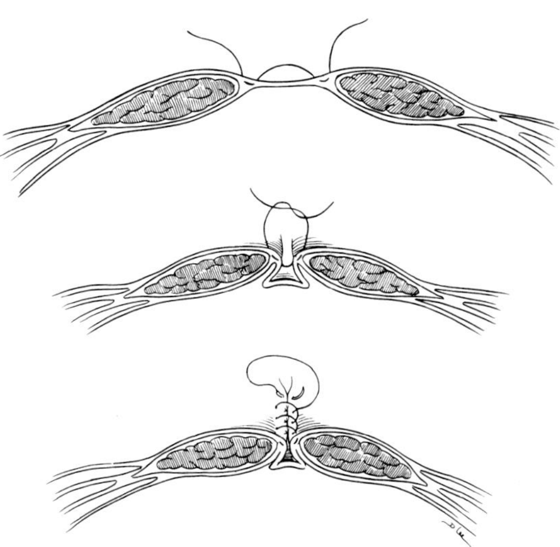

FIGURE 121-61. Diagram of midline plication of diastasis recti in two layers. (From Grazer FM: Abdominoplasty. In McCarthy JG, ed: Plastic Surgery. Philadelphia, WB Saunders, 1990:3929.)

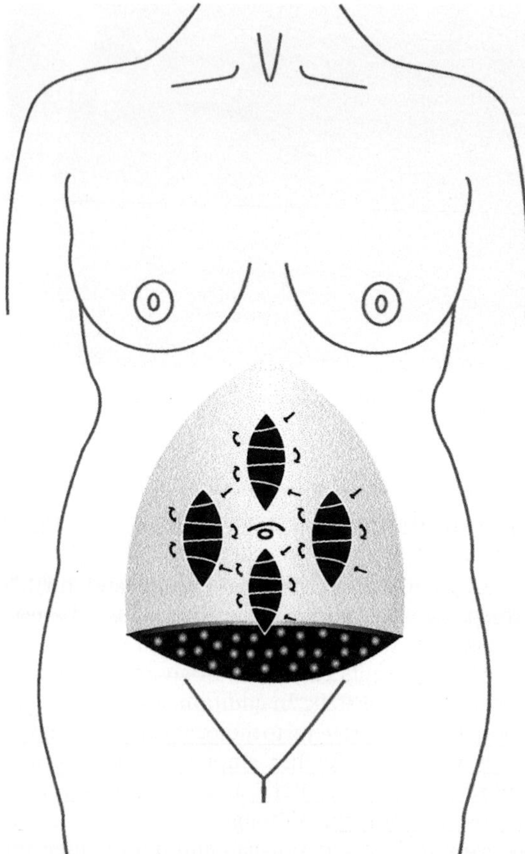

FIGURE 121-62. Diagram indicating markings for plication in the midline above and below the umbilicus and laterally on each side.

(Figs. 121-65 to 121-68). The location of the skin incision allows dissection from the normal tissue planes around the hernia, minimizing the risk of enteric injury. In addition, if permanent mesh is used, the skin incision will be away from the mesh. The skin resection is easily performed in almost all of the patients. It permits wider exposure for the hernia repair.

With small defects, hernia reduction and primary approximation can be performed. Larger hernias may require the use of mesh. When primary approximation of the fascial defect is obtained under tension, a layer of absorbable Vicryl mesh is placed in an onlay fashion to release tension of the fascial repair. Large defects may require either tension-releasing incisions or the use of permanent mesh as a preperitoneal patch. If the patch must be placed intraperitoneally, it is advisable to separate it from the underlying viscera with omentum or an alloplastic material, such as AlloDerm or Seprafilm, to minimize severe intra-abdominal adhesions (Figs. 121-69 to 121-73).

SPECIAL CONSIDERATIONS

Endoscopic abdominoplasty offers an option to address patients who have diastasis recti but require minimal fat resection.[22] Minimal incisions can be used to tighten the midline fascia. In combination with liposuction, contour improvement can be significant. Selection of patients should be limited to those with minimal skin laxity or good skin tone or to allow skin retraction after liposuction. Lateral skin abnormalities must be addressed separately with either direct resection or liposuction.

Extended liposuction can be helpful in contouring procedures. The use of dilute local anesthesia is helpful. Large amounts (35 mg/kg) can safely be used in the subcutaneous tissue. Ultrasonic liposuction uses sonic energy to break up fat cells. Power-assisted liposuction uses a small rotating blade within the cannula. Either technique can be helpful in areas with dense fibrous septa, such as the back and male breast, but it provides less of an advantage over standard suction-assisted lipectomy in the abdomen.

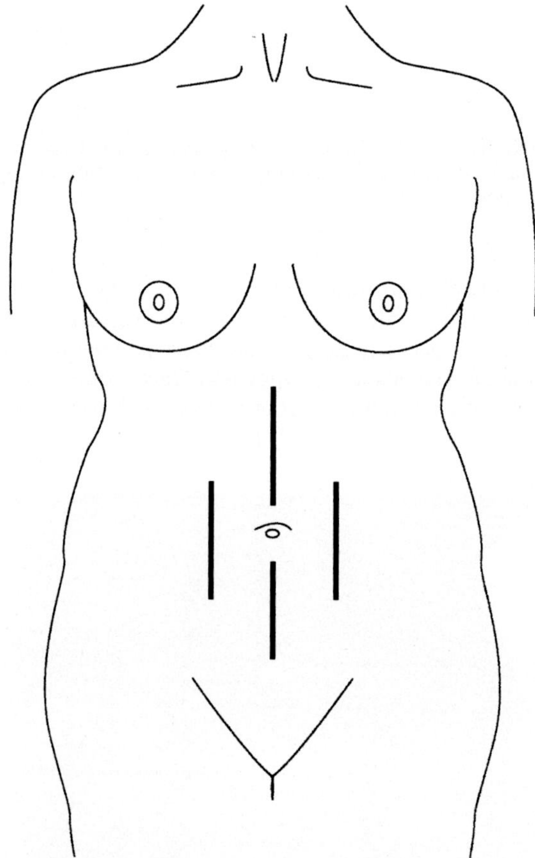

FIGURE 121-63. Diagram after standard plication in the midline and laterally.

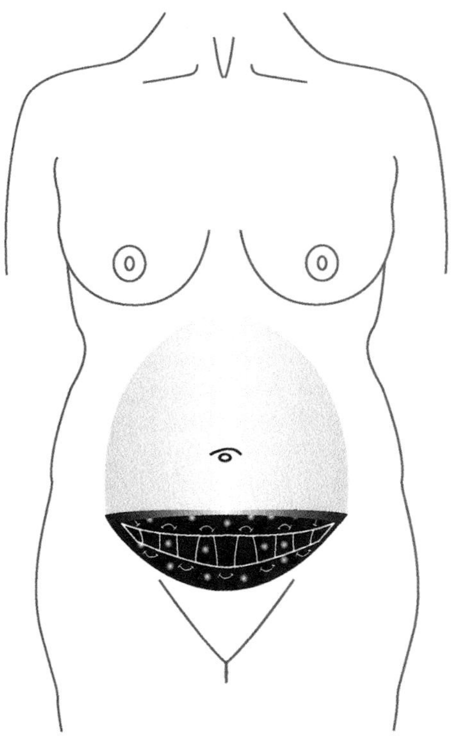

FIGURE 121-64. Diagram of transverse plication, which tightens the waistline and requires no flap elevation.

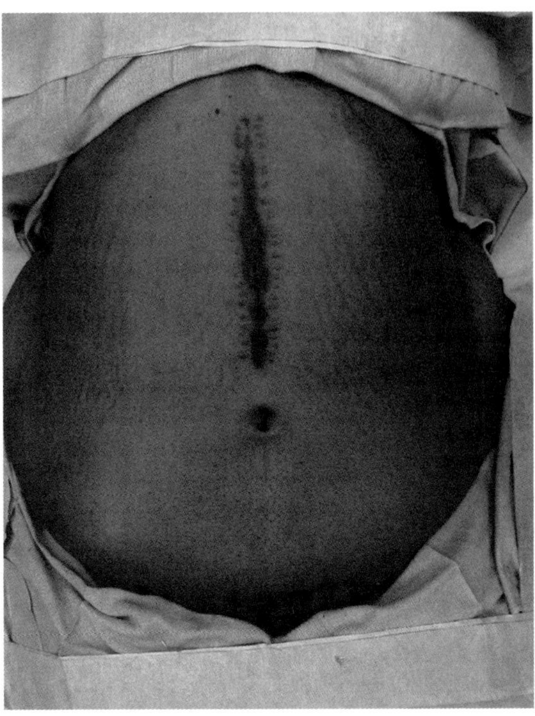

FIGURE 121-65. Abdominoplasty approach to ventral hernia repair, preoperative view.

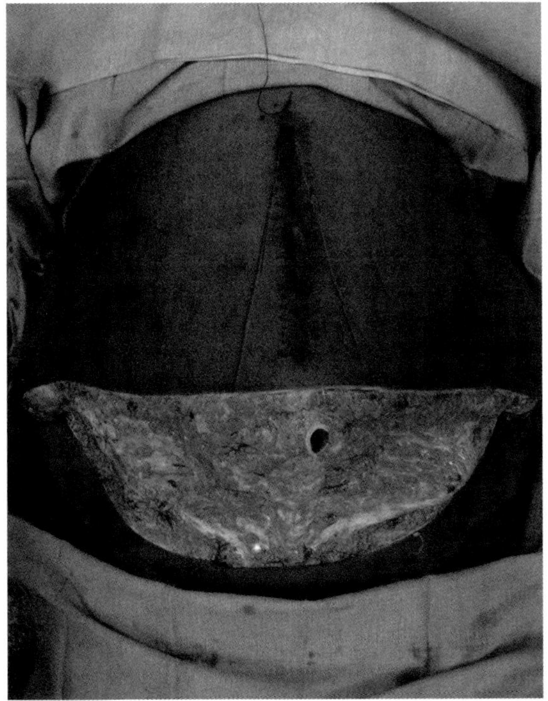

FIGURE 121-66. Abdominoplasty approach to hernia repair for skin avulsion.

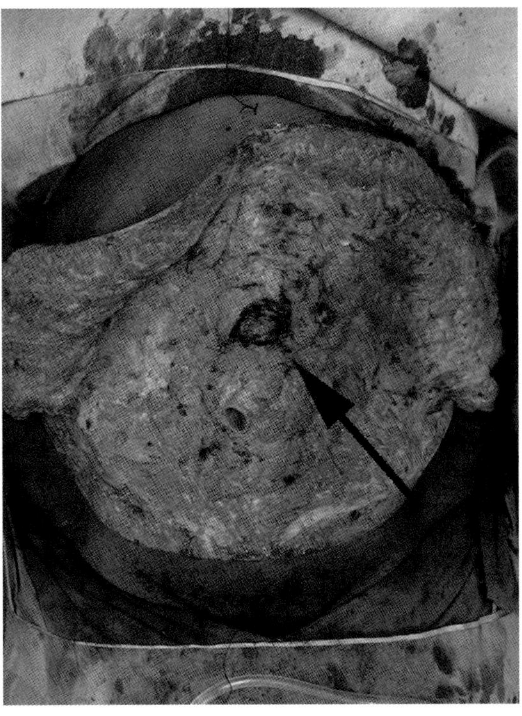

FIGURE 121-67. Abdominoplasty approach to hernia repair: demonstration of the hernia.

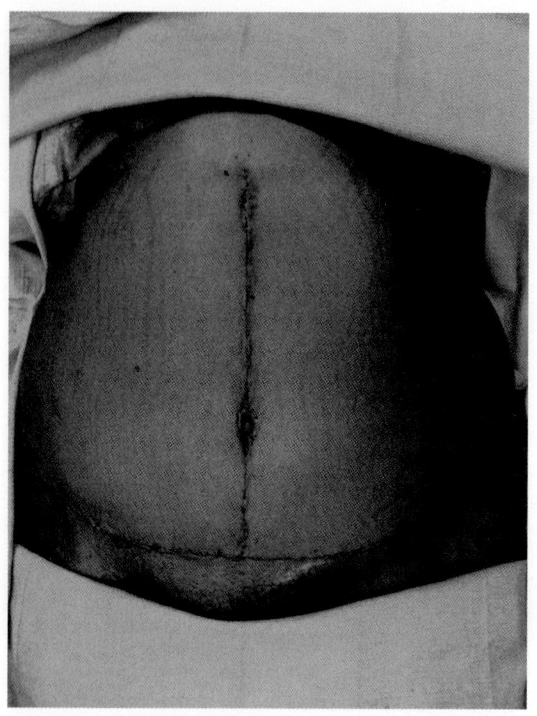

FIGURE 121-68. Abdominoplasty approach to hernia repair: after repair and skin closure.

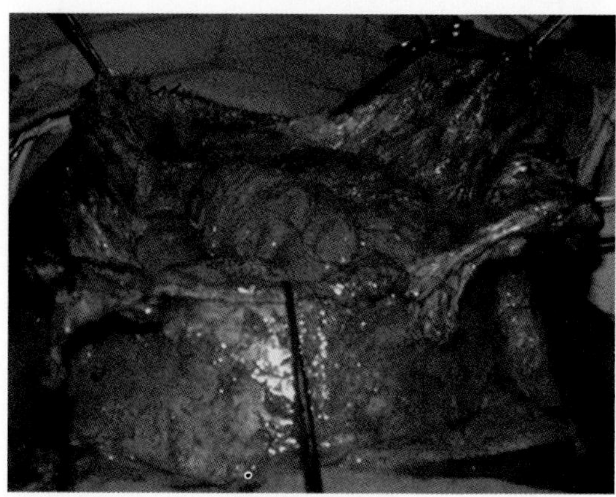

FIGURE 121-69. Large abdominal hernia exposed by the abdominoplasty approach.

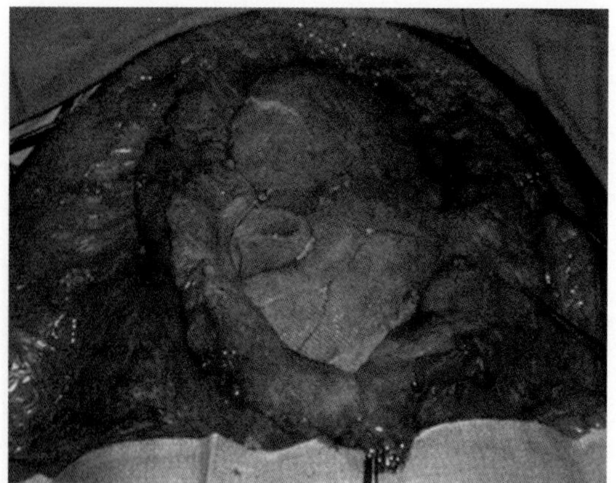

FIGURE 121-70. Large abdominal hernia exposed with placement of Marlex mesh under the fascia.

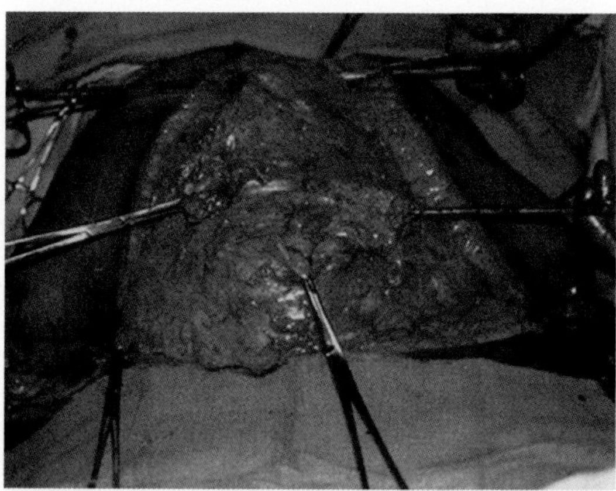

FIGURE 121-71. Large abdominal hernia with approximation of the fascial edges with clamps.

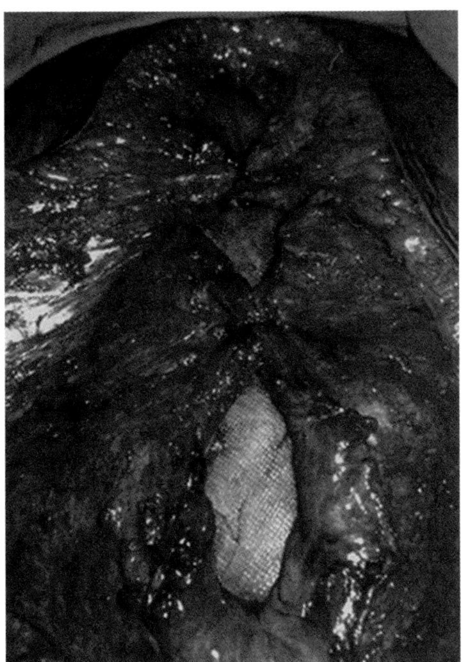

FIGURE 121-72. Large abdominal hernia after resection of redundant hernia sac and partial closure of the fascia.

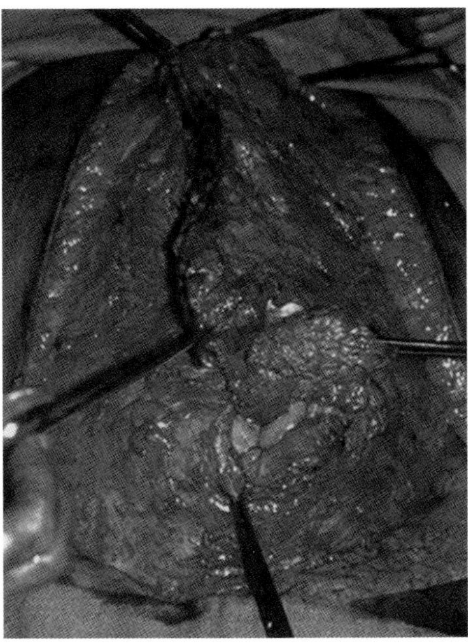

FIGURE 121-73. Large abdominal hernia after the fascia has been closed completely.

The reverse abdominoplasty is ideal to address redundant adipose tissue and skin isolated to the upper abdomen (Fig. 121-74). A W-shaped incision is placed under the inframammary fold at the upper portion of the abdomen. Undermining is performed above the level of the fascia. The redundant tissue can be advanced in a cephalad direction and resected.

Resection of the inferior ribs in conjunction with abdominoplasty can improve some of the bone alterations in the upper abdomen after pregnancy. This technique has been described, particularly in the South American literature, to address asymmetry or to increase diameter of the costal margin.[23] The potential morbidity associated with this procedure and the refinement of other adjuncts to abdominoplasty relegate it largely to historical interest in the authors' opinions.

Abdominoplasty procedures performed in conjunction with intra-abdominal surgery reduce length of anesthesia, hospitalization, and recovery time. Most

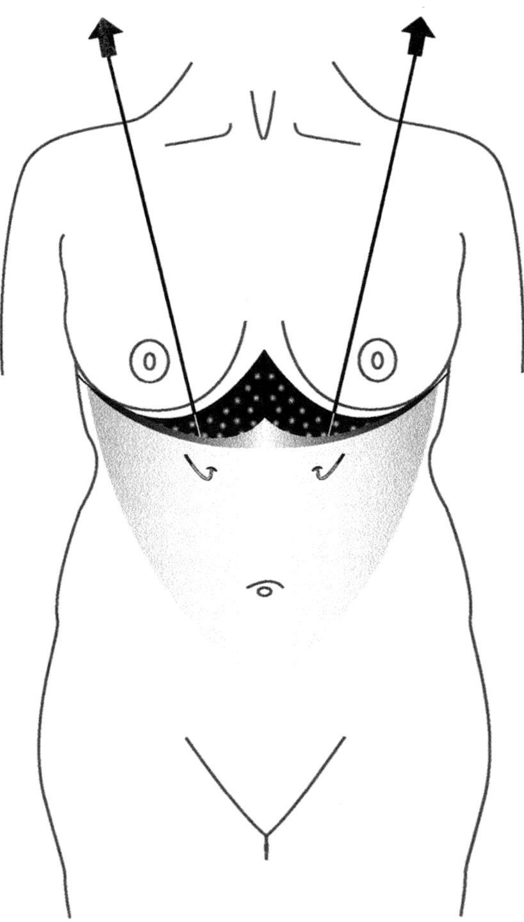

FIGURE 121-74. Diagram of incision and undermining for reverse abdominoplasty to tighten only the upper abdomen.

often, these include elective gynecologic surgeries, such as hysterectomies and tubal ligations. Multiple studies have demonstrated the safety of combining these clean elective procedures.[24,25]

Preexisting abdominal scars are found in well above half of all patients who seek abdominoplasty procedures and can present special difficulties in planning abdominal contour or reconstructive surgery (Figs. 121-75 and 121-76). Scar tissue can make the dissection more difficult and distort tissue planes. Infracostal or supraumbilical incisions pose increased risk of fat necrosis and skin necrosis. With proper planning, infraumbilical incisions can be removed with resection of the redundant skin. Supraumbilical scars, particularly the Kocher type incisions, contribute to a significant increase in rate of complications. Fat necrosis is the most common complication compared with severe complications such as skin necrosis and wound dehiscence, which occur rarely.[26]

These complications can be avoided by clearly understanding how various abdominal scars affect blood flow to the skin and subcutaneous tissue.

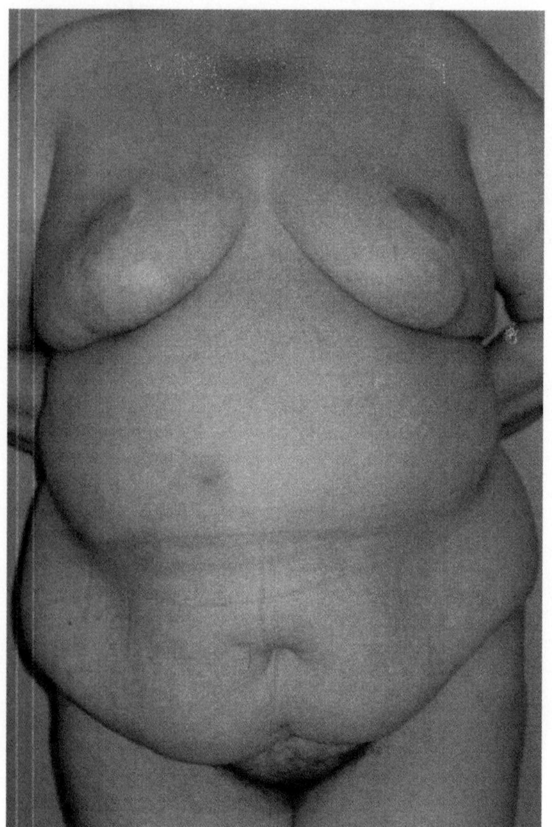

FIGURE 121-75. Standard abdominoplasty with aggressive undermining and umbilical transposition in a patient who has had prior subcostal incision for cholecystectomy, preoperative view.

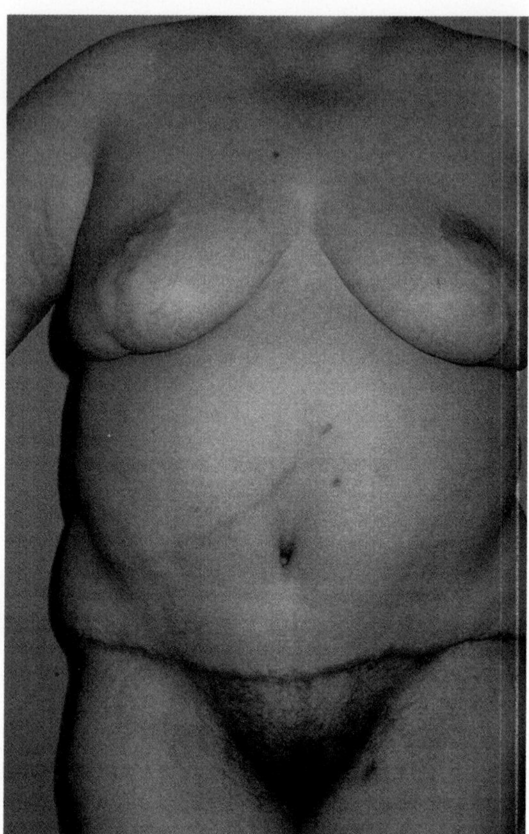

FIGURE 121-76. Standard abdominoplasty with aggressive undermining and umbilical transposition in a patient who has had prior subcostal incision for cholecystectomy, postoperative view.

Secondary abdominoplasties can also be complicated by scar tissue, which can make subsequent operations difficult. Scarring in the subcutaneous layer tethers the skin, which prevents mobilization and makes resection of skin difficult. Most secondary abdominoplasty surgeries involve correction of either contour irregularities or asymmetry and require minimal skin resection.

ANESTHESIA

General anesthesia is preferred when significant fascial tightening is to be performed; however, resection of redundant skin and liposuction can be performed under sedation with the use of local anesthesia. Dilute local anesthetic solution (35 mL of 1% lidocaine, 1 mL of 1 : 1000 epinephrine per liter of lactated Ringer solution) is employed even when general anesthesia is administered. This allows a decreased amount of general anesthesia to be used as well as offering hemostasis. Studies have indicated that 35 mg/kg of lidocaine, when it is administered in the subcutaneous tissue, is without any adverse effects on the patient.[27]

After elevation of the superior flap and the fascial tightening have been performed, placement of the patient in the semi-Fowler position will facilitate closure of the transverse incision.

POSTOPERATIVE MANAGEMENT

Closed suction drains are brought out through the lateral aspect of the incision and secured. The wound is closed, and rarely must the patient remain in semi-Fowler position postoperatively.

Compression garments play an important role in postoperative management, particularly when extensive liposuction is required. A standard operative abdominal binder can be placed directly over a light dressing immediately after surgery (Fig. 121-77). This not only provides compression to decrease seroma formation and maximize contouring results but also acts to hold the dressings in place without the need for tape.

Starting at approximately 48 hours, this binder can be removed to allow the patient to shower and the garment to be cleaned; however, it is critical that it otherwise remain in place continuously for the first week. After the first week, the patient can be given the opportunity to select a compression garment, a variety of which are available through specialty equipment providers or retail stores. The specific garment is not critical as long as the patient will wear it nearly continuously and it provides moderate compression to the affected areas. From 3 to 6 weeks, compression garment use is semielective because it offers only minimal advantage in outcome, but it can increase the patient's comfort and minimize postoperative edema.

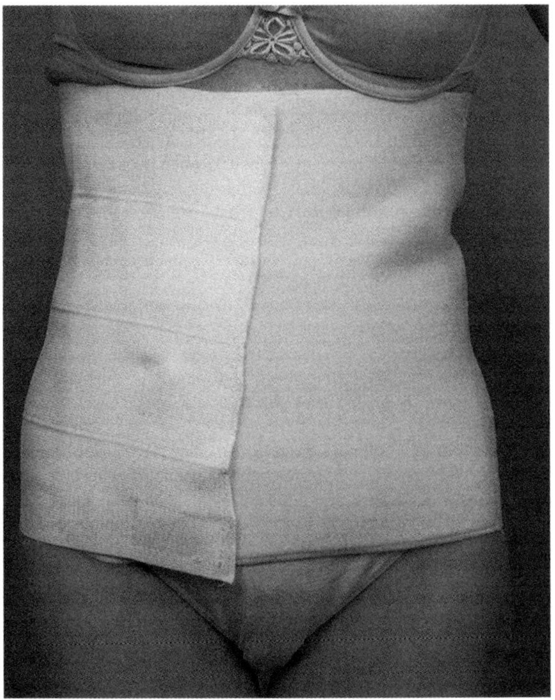

FIGURE 121-77. Abdominal binder in place.

COMPLICATIONS

After abdominoplasty, complications can be minor or serious, even life-threatening problems. Minor complications include seroma, hematoma, wound separation, wound infection, umbilical necrosis, asymmetry, and contour irregularities. The most frequently described postoperative complications are wound separation (24%), seroma (24%), and infection (11%).[28] These are usually relatively minor in nature and can be addressed nonoperatively. Postoperative skin necrosis (7%), scar dehiscence (2%), dog-ears, and above-scar fat folds (28%) frequently require revision procedures (30%) to correct unsatisfactory scars.[29] Injuries to the lateral cutaneous nerve of the thigh occur in as many as 10% of patients.[30]

Local complications can be prevented with meticulous technique and careful tissue handling. Placing all tension in the fascial layer and avoiding tension on the skin closure prevent wound breakdown. It is also important to maintain adequate thickness of any elevated skin flaps. Liberal use of drains is advisable because the risk of seromas is otherwise high. Perioperative antibiotics are helpful in prevention of wound infections.

Fatal pulmonary embolism is uncommon, but prophylaxis is prudent. Pneumatic compression devices are effective and can be used without increasing the risk of postoperative bleeding. Patients are encouraged to ambulate the day of surgery in most cases. Low-molecular-weight heparin can be administered to patients who are at higher risk for deep venous thrombosis and pulmonary embolism. In addition, fat embolism has been reported when liposuction is added to abdominoplasty procedures.[31]

Large quantities of tumescent fluid when liposuction is performed in conjunction with abdominoplasty can lead to complications. In addition to lidocaine toxicity, significant fluid shifts can lead to pulmonary edema. Prevention of these problems comes from careful control of tumescent fluid and intravenous fluid administration.

The most common complication of hernia repair is recurrence. This can occur in 30% to 40% of cases, depending on which technique is used. The use of permanent suture for the midline plication will avoid the high rate of recurrence seen with the use of absorbable mesh.[32] Enterocutaneous fistulas occur less frequently but can result in a mortality rate of 60%. In addition, an increased infection rate (15% to 45%) is a particular risk for this population of patients. Treatment includes the use of antibiotics, bowel rest, and parenteral nutrition for 6 weeks to stabilize the fistula.

Complications can occur more frequently (7% to 33%) when prosthetic material is used to repair incisional hernias.[33] Early complications can range from cellulitis and postoperative ileus to hematomas, seromas, and pulmonary complications. Long-term complications in these patients include recurrences in almost 20% as well as chronic infection, draining sinus tracks, small bowel obstruction, and enterocutaneous fistula. The risk of repair failure is increased fourfold in patients who have recurrent hernias, and it is doubled in patients who are actively smoking cigarettes. Providing stable soft tissue coverage can significantly reduce the rate of complications related to permanent mesh, particularly in recurrent and complex abdominal wall reconstructions.[34]

CONTRAINDICATIONS TO ABDOMINOPLASTY

Patients with primary contraindications to elective aesthetic abdominal procedures are those who have significantly elevated operative health risks and those who have unrealistic surgical goals. All patients should undergo thorough preoperative evaluation. Aesthetic surgery patients should be emotionally stable and self-motivated. Both aesthetic and reconstructive procedures may require operative revisions, and all patients should be aware of this.

Scars from previous abdominal surgery may compromise flap viability and require thorough consideration.[35] Medical contraindications that specifically affect outcomes after abdominoplasty include pulmonary problems, pregnancy, and abdominal disease. Significant pulmonary insufficiency can be further compromised when the abdomen is tightened. Patients who anticipate future pregnancy are at risk not only of complications during pregnancy but of less than desirable aesthetic outcomes. Patients who are obese and seeking a weight loss procedure must understand that abdominoplasty is a body contour procedure.

REFERENCES

1. Kelly HA: Report of gynecological cases. Johns Hopkins Med J 1899;10:197.
2. Babcock WW: The correction of the obese and relaxed abdominal wall with special reference to the use of buried silver chain. Am J Obstet Gynecol 1916;74:596.
3. Thorek M: Plastic Surgery of Breast and Abdominal Wall. Springfield, Ill, Charles C Thomas, 1924.
4. Vernon G: Umbilical transplantation upward and abdominal contouring in lipectomy. Am J Surg 1957;94:490.
5. Pitanguy I: Abdominal lipectomy: an approach to it through an analysis of 300 consecutive cases. Plast Reconstr Surg 1967;40:384.
6. Regnault P: Abdominoplasty by the W technique. Plast Reconstr Surg 1975;55:265.
7. Psillakis JM: Plastic surgery of the abdomen with improvement in the body contour: physiopathology and treatment of the aponeurotic musculature. Clin Plast Surg 1984;11:465.
8. Illouz Y-G: Body contouring by lipolysis: a 5-year experience with over 3000 cases. Plast Reconstr Surg 1983;72:591.
9. Sadler TW: Langman's Medical Embryology. Baltimore, Williams & Wilkins, 1985.
10. Kline MD, Herzler JH: Congenital defects of the abdominal wall. Surg Gynecol Obstet 1981;152:805.
11. Vague G, Finasse R: Comparative anatomy of adipose tissue. In Renold AE, Cahill GF, eds: Handbook of Physiology. Washington, DC, American Physiological Society, 1965:25-35.
12. Singh D: Adaptive significance of female physical attractiveness: role of waist-to-hip ratio. J Pers Soc Psychol 1993;65:293.
13. Markman B, Barton FE Jr: Anatomy of the subcutaneous tissue of the trunk and lower extremity. Plast Reconstr Surg 1987;80:248.
14. Salans LB, Cushman SW, Weismann RE: Studies of human adipose tissue, adipose cell size and number in nonobese and obese patients. J Clin Invest 1973;52:929.
15. Querleux B, Cornillon C, Jolivet O, Bitoun J: Anatomy and physiology of subcutaneous adipose tissue by in vivo magnetic resonance imaging and spectroscopy: relationships with sex and presence of cellulite. Skin Res Technol 2002;8:118.
16. Rosenbaum M, Prieto V, Hellmer J, et al: An exploratory investigation of the morphology and biochemistry of cellulite. Plast Reconstr Surg 1998;101:1934.
17. Grosfeld JL: Pediatric surgery. In Sabiston DC, ed: Textbook of Surgery: The Biologic Basis of Modern Surgical Practice, 14th ed. Philadelphia, WB Saunders, 1991:1167.
18. Matarasso A: Abdominoplasty. Clin Plast Surg 1989;16:289.
19. Bozola AR, Psillakis JM: Abdominoplasty: a new concept and classification for treatment. Plast Reconstr Surg 1988;82: 983.
20. Mladick RA: Male body contouring. Clin Plast Surg 1991;18:797.
21. Schoeller T, Wechselberger G, Otto A, et al: New technique for scarless umbilical reinsertion in abdominoplasty procedures. Plast Reconstr Surg 1998;102:1720.
22. Matarasso A: Minimal-access variations in abdominoplasty. Ann Plast Surg 1995;34:255.
23. Psillakis JM: Plastic surgery of the abdomen with improvement in the body contour. Physiopathology and treatment of the aponeurotic musculature. Clin Plast Surg 1984;11:465.
24. Hester TR Jr, Baird W, Bostwick J 3rd, et al: Abdominoplasty combined with other major surgical procedures: safe or sorry? Plast Reconstr Surg 1989;83:997.
25. Pitanguy I, Ceravolo MP: Our experience with combined procedures in aesthetic plastic surgery. Plast Reconstr Surg 1983;71:56.
26. de Castro CC, Aboudib Junior JH, Salema R, et al: How to deal with abdominoplasty in an abdomen with a scar. Aesthetic Plast Surg 1993;17:67.
27. Burk RW III, Guzman-Stein G, Vasconez LO: Lidocaine and epinephrine levels in tumescent technique liposuction. Plast Reconstr Surg 1996;97:1379.
28. Hensel JM, Lehman JA, Tantri MP, et al: An outcomes analysis and satisfaction survey of 199 consecutive abdominoplasties. Ann Plast Surg 2001;46:357.
29. Chaouat M, Levan P, Lalanne B, et al: Abdominal dermolipectomies: early postoperative complications and long-term unfavorable results. Plast Reconstr Surg 2000;106:1614.
30. von Uchelen JH, Werker PM, Kon M: Complications of abdominoplasty in 86 patients. Plast Reconstr Surg 2001;107: 1869.

31. Scroggins C, Barson PK: Fat embolism syndrome in a case of abdominoplasty lipectomy with liposuction. Md Med J 1999;48:116.
32. von Uchelen JH, Kon M, Werker PM: The long-term durability of the anterior rectus sheath assessed by ultrasonography. Plast Reconstr Surg 2001;107:1578.
33. Girotto JA, Ko MJ, Redett R, et al: Closure of chronic abdominal wall defects: a long-term evaluation of components separation. Ann Plast Surg 1999;42:394.
34. Mathes SJ, Steinwals PM, Foster RD, et al: Complex abdominal wall reconstruction: a comparison of flap and mesh closure. Ann Surg 2000;232:586.
35. Nahai F, Brown RG, Vasconez LO: Blood supply to the abdominal wall as related to planning abdominal incisions. Am Surg 1976;42:691.

CHAPTER

122

Abdominoplasty Techniques

TE NING CHANG, MD, PhD ✦ RICARDO BAROUDI, MD

The well-contoured abdomen is attractive because it reflects health and reproductive fitness. Both increasing waist circumference and a greater waist-to-hip ratio (Fig. 122-1) correlate with increasing risk for diabetes, hypertension, and cardiovascular disease.[1,2] Women with larger breasts and narrower waists have been shown to have higher levels of hormones of conception, signaling reproductive fitness.[3] Studies show that both male and female physicians[4] as well as college-age men[5] give a higher rating of attractiveness, healthiness, and reproductive potential to female images with a smaller waist-to-hip ratio. The association of a narrow waist and attractiveness is true in men as well.[6] It is no wonder, then, that improving the contour of the abdomen is a primary concern for many patients seeking aesthetic surgery.

Since the first published description of dermolipectomy by Kelly[7] in 1899, modern abdominoplasty has undergone three major phases of development. Until the 1960s, abdominoplasty focused on optimizing tissue resection and included numerous variations of transverse, vertical, and combined vertical with transverse incisions. The designs were often central, with no attempt to hide the incision; the umbilicus was often sacrificed (Fig. 122-2*A* to *C*).[8-15]

In the mid-1940s, the two-piece "bikini" swimsuit (its design so explosive it was named after the nuclear test site, the Bikini Atoll) was introduced. The growing popularity of the bikini paralleled the new focus in abdominoplasty on hiding the scars by lowering the incision toward the pubis, tightening lax abdominal muscles, and improving the umbilicoplasty.[16] A low transverse incision became common in the 1960s,[17] designed to cover the hip-slung St. Tropez bikini. The lateral borders of the incision crept up in parallel with the changing shape of the bikini line.[18,19] The mid-1980s saw the popularization of the French-line bikini, cut high at the hips and low centrally; the bicycle handlebar incision was designed to be hidden under this new style (Fig. 122-2*D*).[20]

The introduction of liposuction in 1980 by Illouz[21] heralded a new emphasis on reducing the length of the incision or degree of undermining while improving circumferential contour of the abdomen and trunk through a combination of tissue resection and lipocontouring.[22-30]

While incisions have changed, the components of the full abdominoplasty, which include a low transverse incision, abdominal skin undermining, and umbilical transposition to allow flap advancement and plication,[16] remain the same. Variations that include techniques for manipulating the umbilicus allow shorter scars and more limited undermining. Refinements in liposuction techniques used adjunctively with abdominoplasty have improved overall contouring. More recently, extensive liposuction in conjunction with abdominoplasty with minimal or no undermining has been used to reduce the risk of flap necrosis. The term *abdominoplasty* now covers a wide spectrum of techniques from simple lower abdomi-

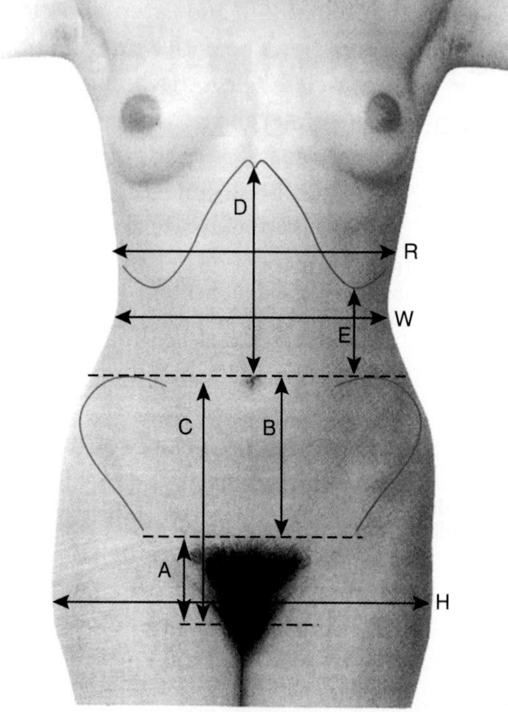

FIGURE 122-1. Normal abdominal anatomic proportions. The approximate measurements for an average female abdomen are listed. These vary according to individual height and bone structure. The umbilicus is located in line with the most superior point of the iliac crest in 99% of patients. A, Distance between top of mons and anterior vulvar commissure. Average height is 5 to 7 cm. B, Distance between umbilicus and top of mons. Average height is 11 to 13 cm. C (= A + B), Distance between umbilicus and top of anterior vulvar commissure. Average height is 16 to 20 cm. D, Distance between sternal notch and umbilicus. This is approximately equal to the distance between umbilicus and anterior vulvar commissure (C = D). E, Distance between the costal margin and the iliac crest. The proportion of this distance to the width of the base of the rib cage (R) determines whether the patient is long waisted or short waisted. The normal proportion (E:R) is roughly 1:3 (long waisted approaches 1:2, short waisted approaches 1:3). The rib cage tapers inferiorly. A more narrow lower rib cage relative to the width under the armpits helps to emphasize the waist by creating a subtle V. H, hip width. A wider pelvis than rib cage emphasizes the waist; the waist is more defined when R < H. W, Natural waist—the narrowest point on the torso. (Note that the umbilicus usually sits below the natural waist by about 1 to 4 cm.) Relative to the hips, this waist-to-hip (W:H) ratio in healthy women is roughly 0.72:1; in healthy men, it is roughly 0.83:1. Note that the natural contour of the healthy abdomen reveals a subtle epigastric sagittal depression transitioning to a mild infraumbilical convexity. A subtle vertical sulcus at the lateral rectus border, which is more distinct in a muscular person, may also be seen.

nal elliptical skin resection for mild skin laxity to comprehensive treatment of skin, musculofascial, and adipose contour deformities of the abdomen.

There are now many alternatives to the traditional full abdominoplasty that may, in the appropriate patient, produce excellent results with less prominent scars. The following discussion emphasizes evaluation of the patient, selection of abdominoplasty technique, and technical variations. The classic abdominoplasty is described. Surgical refinements and alternatives that may improve contour, permit smaller incisions, result in improved scars, or require less undermining and options for treatment of the umbilicus are discussed. The prevention and treatment of complications are also reviewed.

ETIOLOGY

The etiology of abdominal contour deformity amenable to abdominoplasty includes congenital fascial weakness or skin laxity, postsurgical scars and fascial defects, and sequelae of significant weight fluctuations. A classic and common example is the postpartum woman. Pregnancy, especially multiple pregnancies, can stretch the skin and musculofascial system beyond their biomechanical capacity; stretching and thinning of these structures lead to pannus formation and rectus muscle diastasis. Further skin retraction and fascial contraction are less likely to occur more than 1 year after baseline weight is achieved.

The other increasingly common presentation with skin and muscle laxity is the post–bariatric surgery patient. The American Society for Bariatric Surgery reports that bariatric surgery more than doubled between 2002 and 2004, with more than 144,000 operations projected in 2004 (*http://www.asbs.org*). These patients often seek treatment of the significant skin excess that results from rapid and large-volume weight loss. Based on the annual survey by the American Society for Aesthetic Surgery, this population of patients has contributed largely to the 42% increase in abdominoplasties performed from 2002 to 2003 to more than 117,000 operations in 2003 (*http://www.surgery.org*).

FIGURE 122-2. Abdominoplasty: development of incisions and techniques. *A* to *C*, Early incisions were central. *A*, Transverse incisions. *B*, Vertical incisions. *C*, Combined incisions. *D*, Low transverse incisions. By the mid-1960s, incisions were placed closer to the pubis. As the bikini bottom became smaller and higher laterally, the lateral abdominoplasty incision was similarly elevated so the scar could be hidden. (Modified from Moufarrege R: The Moufarrege horseshoe abdominoplasty. Aesthetic Surg J 1997;17:91. Reproduced with permission from The American Society for Aesthetic Plastic Surgery, Inc.)

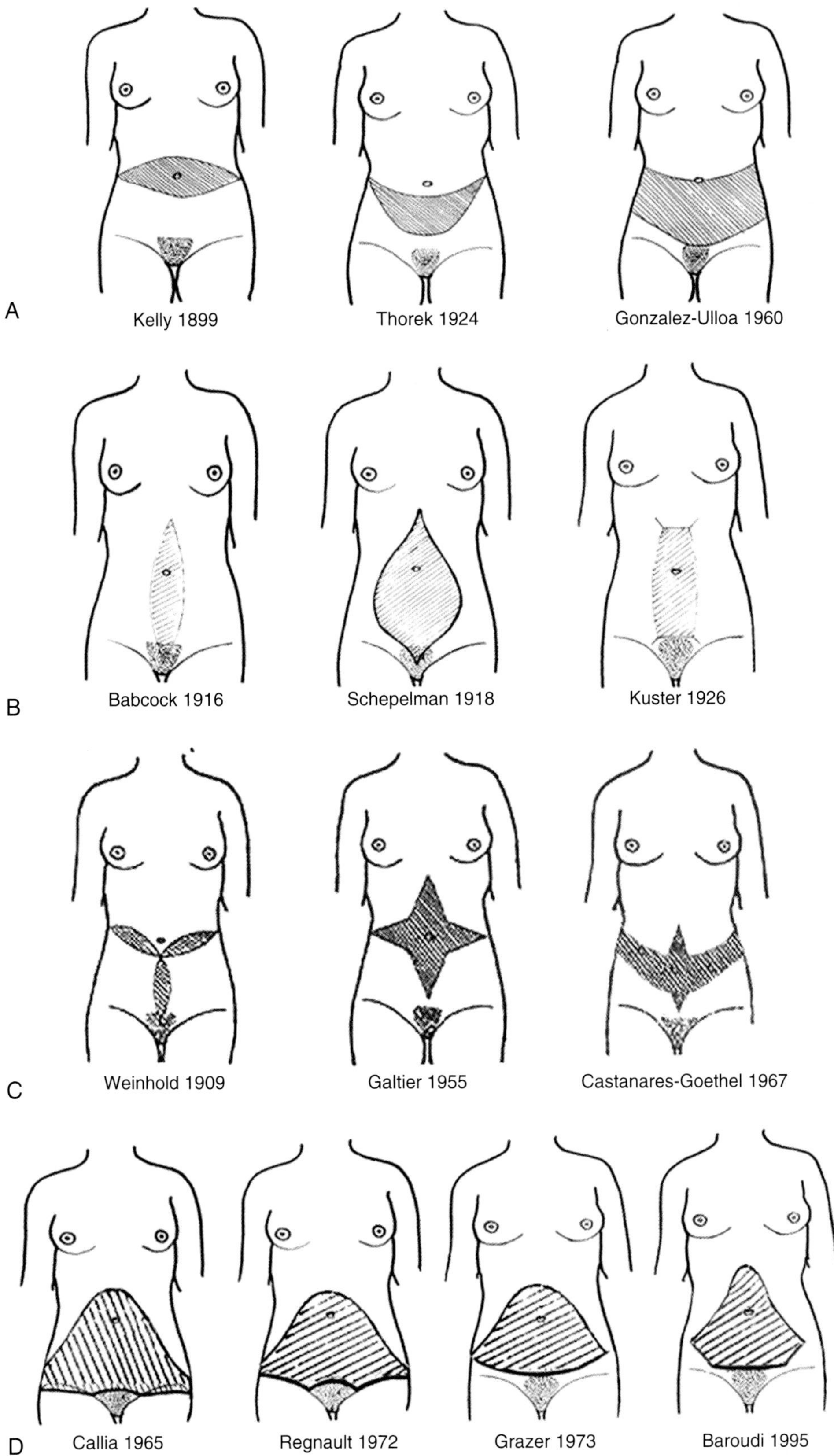
A
Kelly 1899
Thorek 1924
Gonzalez-Ulloa 1960
B
Babcock 1916
Schepelman 1918
Kuster 1926
C
Weinhold 1909
Galtier 1955
Castanares-Goethel 1967
D
Callia 1965
Regnault 1972
Grazer 1973
Baroudi 1995

INDICATIONS AND PATIENT SELECTION

Abdominal skin excess with or without musculofascial laxity is the primary indication for abdominoplasty. Adipose tissue excess may be addressed as well during abdominoplasty, but isolated adipose deposits without skin or musculofascial deformity should be treated with liposuction alone. A thorough preoperative examination (see "Physical Examination") will help clarify the appropriate procedure or combination of procedures to achieve the best outcome. Some patients who qualify for surgery on the basis of physical parameters may not be good surgical candidates for other reasons. A careful preoperative history should reveal comorbid diseases, weight fluctuations, prior surgical incisions, plans for future pregnancy, or unrealistic goals that may alter the surgical plan or preclude surgery altogether (see "Informed Consent").

PREOPERATIVE EVALUATION

Patient's History and Goals

The appropriate surgical procedure for abdominal contouring not only depends on the abdominal deformities discovered during a careful physical examination but also must be tailored to the patient's goals, expectations, and lifestyle. At the preoperative interview, the patient should clearly state his or her chief complaint, whether it be excess adipose tissue, skin laxity, scars, a protuberant abdomen, or an ill-defined waist. A medical history is taken to include the following: comorbid diseases, such as lung disease, cardiovascular disease, or diabetes; history of chronic cough, bleeding, or clotting; prior abdominal surgeries, including liposuction; history of pregnancy or plans for future pregnancy; history of breast cancer or family history of breast cancer; weight fluctuations; and smoking history. Activity level and clothing preferences, especially swimming attire and underwear, should be noted. Baseline height, weight, clothing size, and waist measurements should be recorded, and standardized preoperative photographs are taken.

Physical Examination

The physical examination assesses degree of skin laxity, fascial laxity, and excess adipose tissue. Aspects that cannot be changed by surgery must be noted and discussed with the patient. Neither abdominoplasty nor liposuction will address intra-abdominal fat or a short waist, which is determined by the skeletal framework. The appearance of cellulite or skin irregularity due to adipose tissue bulging between fibrous septa may be diminished but will not be eliminated. If striae are not completely excised, remaining marks may be further widened. Taking the time to discuss physical findings and surgical limitations with the patient during the consultation and preoperative examination will help prevent postoperative disappointment.

BONY FRAMEWORK

On physical examination, the framework of the abdomen should be noted. In the well-contoured woman, the waist will be more defined if the hips are wider than the rib cage, so this relationship will be emphasized by abdominoplasty as bony framework is revealed. In contrast, in the well-contoured man, the rib cage, waist, and hips form a much more subtle indentation. Waist definition is emphasized in men by wide shoulders and muscular thighs.

The lower rib cage is cartilaginous and can splay outward with increased intra-abdominal pressure, such as from intra-abdominal fat, organomegaly, or chronic obstructive pulmonary disease (COPD). A widened lower rib cage changes the normal taper of the ribs from a subtle inverted cone to a cylindrical or even conical shape, giving rise to the "barrel chest." The space between the two bony cages of the torso (the rib cage and the pelvis) defines an area where contouring is not limited by bone, but by the intra-abdominal contents and muscle. In women, palpate and measure the distance between the bottom of the costal margin and top of the iliac crests and note its relationship to the width of the rib cage (see Fig. 122-1). The normal relationship of this bony frame–free distance to the rib cage diameter is roughly 1:3. In a longer waisted person, this proportion is relatively smaller; in the short-waisted person, it is relatively larger. The bony architecture of the barrel-chested short-waisted patient provides less opportunity for waist definition even with the best abdominoplasty, and the patient should understand this.

SKIN

Inspection of the standing patient reveals any skin laxity, ripples, striae, and scars. Note with the patient any irregularities, such as an umbilicus that is off midline. A subcostal or chevron incision is a relative contraindication for traditional abdominoplasty. Vertical midline scars will decrease the amount of flap advancement possible. Note whether scars are mobile or fixed to the underlying fascia; fixed scars are more likely to reflect interrupted flap circulation. Palpation helps assess elasticity and dermal thickness. In general, men tend to have thicker skin with better elasticity and can support significant liposuction with good skin contraction. If the skin appears of good quality with minimal or no laxity and the defect appears to be excess adipose tissue or musculoaponeurotic laxity, a minimal scar procedure may be appropriate. If there is skin laxity, the lower abdominal skin should be pinched to determine the amount that can safely be excised (Fig. 122-3). If the

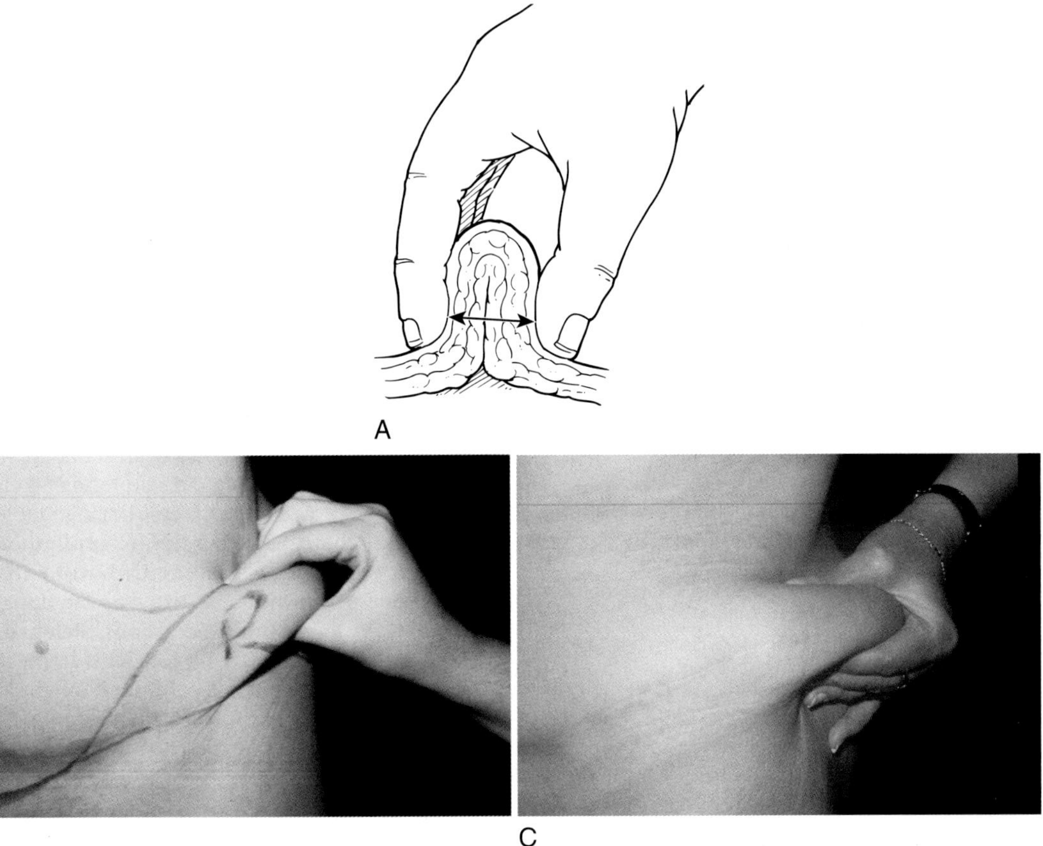

FIGURE 122-3. Pinch test. *A* to *C*, The surgeon grasps the full thickness of skin and subcutaneous fat between thumb and four fingers or, in patients with massive skin excess, between the two hands, pinching the tissues together until the unclasped tissues on either side become taut. This can give an estimate of the amount of tissue that can be resected.

umbilicus is neither mobile nor ptotic and is not distorted by pinching the redundant infraumbilical tissue, the umbilicus usually does not need to be transposed. If the vertical height of skin and subcutaneous tissue equal to the distance between umbilicus and pubis cannot be pinched between thumb and index finger or the surgeon's two hands, a modified technique should be considered. Upper and lower abdominal skin laxity with significant umbilical ptosis should be addressed with full abdominoplasty. The amount of lateral and back skin laxity should also be assessed with the pinch technique to determine whether a high lateral tension abdominoplasty, abdominoplasty with thigh lift, or circumferential torsoplasty would be appropriate.

SUBCUTANEOUS FAT

The location and extent of adipose deposits should be noted to assess whether concurrent or staged liposuction is indicated or whether direct excision alone is preferable. Pinching the subcutaneous tissue between thumb and forefinger in various locations helps assess the differences in thickness of the subcutaneous layer. Note any local deposits or differences between left and right. Distinguishing between intra-abdominal and subcutaneous fat can also be aided by having the patient contract the abdominal wall in the standing and supine positions. The relative contribution of subcutaneous fat and intra-abdominal contents to the abdominal contour defect should be assessed and discussed with the patient if it is relevant to the outcome. The appearance of the fat deposits should also be noted. Significant rippling can be caused either by skin excess ("secondary cellulite") or by the quality of the fibrous septa that encase the fat in the superficial fascial system (resulting in "primary cellulite"). Secondary cellulite may by improved by skin excision. Primary cellulite is a function of the patient's anatomy and may not be improved by surgery.

MUSCULOFASCIAL SYSTEM

The musculofascial system should be evaluated in both the standing and supine positions. Look for midline abdominal protuberance in the standing patient. In this position, gravity helps unmask fascial weakness as intra-abdominal contents press against the abdominal wall. Note whether any prominence is epigastric, infraumbilical, or both. If a lower abdominal prominence is noted, the patient should be asked to strain while the surgeon has the edge of one hand firmly pressed over the lower abdominal midline to simulate surgical fascial plication. Like plication, this can unmask an upper diastasis recti that might need repair. In the supine position, the strength of the abdominal wall musculature as well as diastasis recti and musculoaponeurotic laxity can be further assessed by asking the patient to lift either the shoulders or legs off the examination table without the assistance of the arms. The abdomen should be palpated for masses, organomegaly, and hernias. If a ventral or umbilical hernia is discovered, this must be addressed during operative planning. Note whether abdominal fullness can be attributed more to intra-abdominal contents or to subcutaneous tissue.

Informed Consent

The potential risks and benefits of surgery must be reviewed carefully so the patient has a clear understanding of both the general risks of abdominoplasty and the specific risks in relation to his or her history and physical status. The patient should also be made aware of the postoperative recovery course. The risks of undergoing any operation include anesthesia reaction, pulmonary embolism and deep venous thrombosis, cardiovascular accident, reactions to medications, bleeding, hematoma, and infection. Risks particularly associated with abdominoplasty include seroma, dehiscence, skin necrosis and irregularity, umbilical loss, nerve injury, hypertrophic scar or keloid, slow healing, swelling, and visible scar.

Patients must clearly understand that because of bone structure, intra-abdominal fat, or existing scars, there are limitations to the results that can be achieved. Patients with scars that cross the blood supply to the abdominal skin or with risk factors such as smoking or cardiovascular disease that may compromise flap viability may not be acceptable candidates for surgery. Patients with a history of breast cancer or family history of breast cancer should understand that standard abdominoplasty eliminates one option for autologous breast reconstruction, the transverse rectus abdominis musculocutaneous (TRAM) flap. There have been numerous reports of uncomplicated pregnancy after full abdominoplasty as well as TRAM flap breast reconstruction; however, intended future pregnancy is still a relative contraindication for standard abdominoplasty with muscle plication because of the theoretical concern for increased intra-abdominal pressure and fascial tears during pregnancy.

Before surgery, the patient must understand that he or she must avoid straining the abdominal muscles for at least 6 weeks if fascial plication is performed. In addition, drains may be placed and may remain in place for 1 week or more, and there may be discomfort and bruising for several weeks as well as significant swelling that can mask the final result for several months. The abdominal flap may initially be numb, so care must be taken to avoid extremes of heat or pressure on the flap. Patients must understand that although scars usually fade over time, they are permanent.

An excellent candidate for abdominoplasty is healthy, close to his or her ideal body weight (within 20%), wishes to address lax abdominal tissue that is diet and exercise resistant, has been stable in weight for at least 6 months, has good skin tone and elasticity, has realistic expectations, is emotionally stable, and understands the risks of surgery. Contraindications to surgery include significant comorbid disease, morbid obesity, unwillingness to stop smoking, and the patient's unrealistic expectations. Relative contraindications or indications for considering a less extensive procedure include continued weight loss or weight fluctuation, plans for future pregnancy, and upper abdominal transverse scars.

OPERATIVE PLANNING

The surgical options and refinements for abdominal contour improvement available today allow plastic surgeons to address the entire range of contour deformities from localized fat deposits to severe skin laxity. While the patient seeks cosmetic improvement, it is the surgeon's task to accurately evaluate the cause of the contour deformity and select the optimal technique or combination of techniques to safely achieve the desired aesthetic result.

Anatomic Considerations

It is important to understand the factors that define abdominal contour to assess what types of deformities may be addressed by abdominoplasty. The contour of the abdomen is determined by the drape of fascia and muscle, fat, and skin over the bony framework and internal organs. The relative width of the rib cage and pelvis and their distance from each other define the waist. Unlike the rib cage above and the pelvis below, waist contour and definition depend on circumferential support from abdominal and back muscles of the internal organs and tissues. Waist definition may be blurred or distorted by hypertrophy of the overlying soft tissues or internal structures. Subcutaneous adipose deposits, intra-abdominal fat, organomegaly, lack of abdominal muscle support from atrophy or fascial laxity, skin laxity, or any combination of these factors can contribute to suboptimal abdominal contour.

Abdominoplasty can address skin laxity and scars, excess subcutaneous fat, and musculofascial laxity. It cannot, however, address contour defects due to an unfavorable bony anatomy or intra-abdominal disease, although it may help mask them. These factors must be noted in the preoperative examination and discussed so that the goals of the operation are clear between the surgeon and patient.

The appearance and drape of the skin and subcutaneous fat over the abdominal wall are determined by the relative quantity and quality of the skin, subcutaneous fat, and superficial fascial system. The superficial fascial system is a connective tissue reticular network that forms one or more layers parallel to the skin and connects the dermis to the underlying fascia through fibrous septa.[31] It may be diffuse and indistinct in parts of the body and in patients with significant amounts of subcutaneous fat, or it may be distinct enough to be named, as in Scarpa's fascia in the lower abdomen or Colles' fascia in the perineum. In certain regions of the body, it is more adherent to the underlying muscle fascia or periosteum (called zones of adherence[32]). In the inguinal region, the transition from this tight apposition results in a fold or crease in the obese patient, above which a pannus may form. Above the umbilicus, superficial fascial system adhesion to the linea alba forms a midsagittal depression visible in the slim, muscular patient. At some locations, the zones of adherence are different between men and women. For instance, at the lateral hip, the zone of adherence in men is at the iliac crest, while it is several centimeters lower in women, forming the lateral gluteal depression. Fat deposits above the zone of adherence result in the higher "love handles" above the iliac crest in men, distinct from the "saddlebags" found lateral to the iliac crest in women (Fig. 122-4).

A clear understanding of the arterial supply of the abdominal wall is crucial to operative planning, especially when prior abdominal surgeries have been performed. As defined by Huger,[33] the abdominal wall is fed anteriorly by the vertically oriented deep epigastric arcade (zone I) and laterally by six lateral intercostal and four lumbar arteries (zone III) (Fig. 122-5). The lower abdominal circulation is provided by the

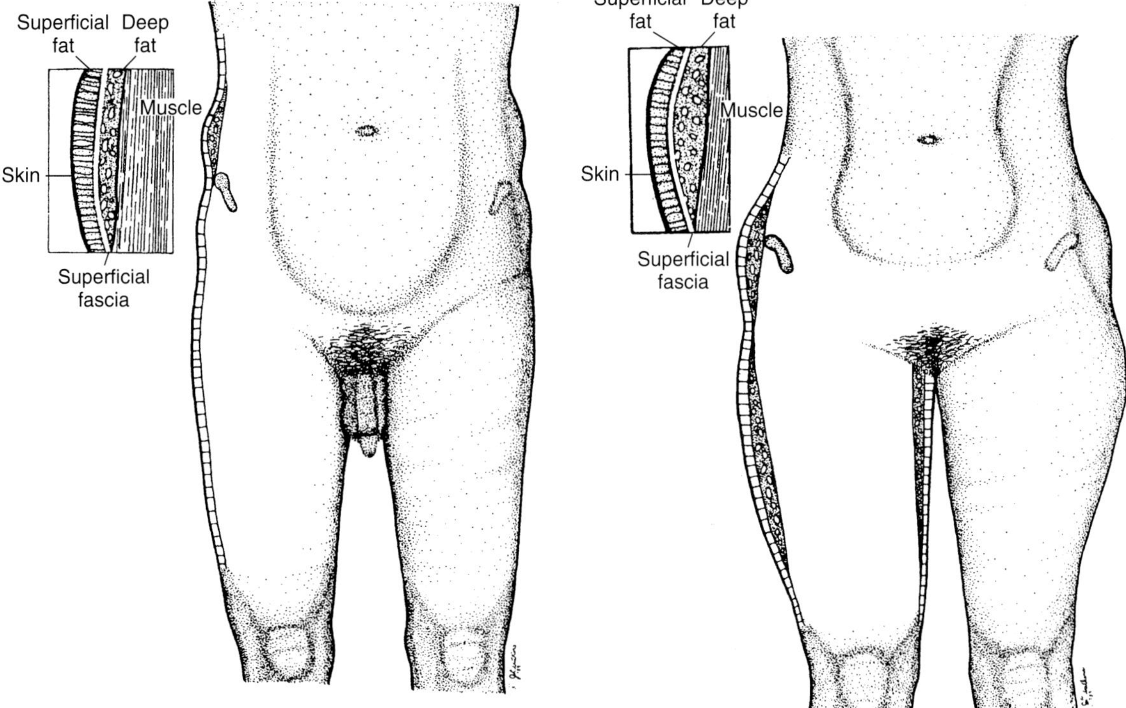

FIGURE 122-4. Superficial fascial system and zones of adherence. The superficial fascial system forms a reticular network that provides support for the subcutaneous tissues. The superficial fascial system should be incorporated in a deep closure to take tension off the skin closure. The superficial fascial system is closely adherent to the underlying structures at specific locations, including the inguinal region and supraumbilical midline, at the iliac crest in men, and several centimeters below the iliac crest in women. Fat tends to accumulate between these adherent areas, resulting in characteristic fat deposits in men and women. (From Lockwood TE: Superficial fascial system [SFS] of the trunk and extremities: a new concept. Plast Reconstr Surg 1991;87:1009.)

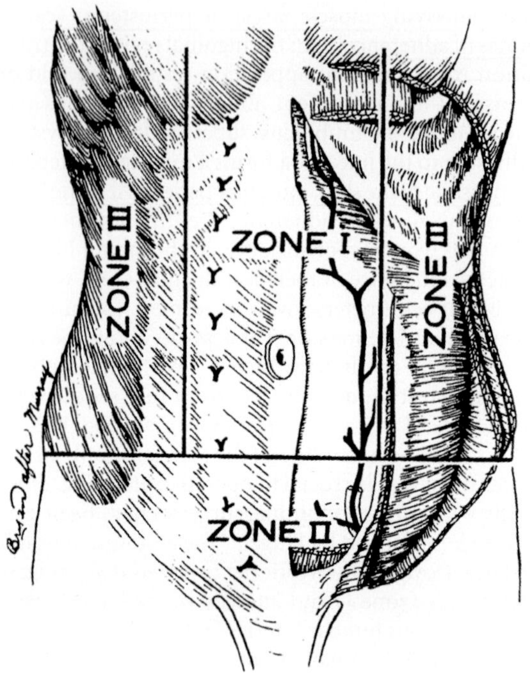

FIGURE 122-5. Three zones of blood supply to the abdominal flap as described by Huger[33] are depicted diagrammatically: zones I, II, and III. (From Huger WE Jr: The anatomic rationale for abdominal lipectomy. Am Surg 1979;45:612.)

superficial epigastric, superficial external pudendal, and superficial circumflex iliac systems (zone II). A rich plexus between these systems allows collateral flow. During abdominoplasty, the cutaneous blood supply to zone I and much of zone II is divided, with the abdominal flap circulation fully dependent on zone III. If a scar, such as a subcostal cholecystectomy incision, crosses the elevated flap, the circulation to the tissue distal to the scar is at jeopardy. A vertical midline incision can further jeopardize flap circulation.

Lastly, an appreciation of the normal proportions of the abdominal wall in men and women aids in establishing a natural, more youthful and aesthetic appearance. For instance, the waist-to-hip ratio in healthy women is approximately 0.72:1, compared with 0.83:1 in men (see Fig. 122-1).[34] Narrowing the waist in the male patient too much relative to the width of the hips would be feminizing. The umbilicus is properly positioned at the level of the superior margin of the iliac crest[35] and usually sits 1 to 4 cm below the natural waist (narrowest circumference of the torso). The youthful umbilicus is either round or slightly ovoid with a vertical orientation (Fig. 122-6). Umbilical hooding arises from supraumbilical skin draping over the fixed umbilical stalk. In the youthful, healthy person, the xiphoid to umbilical distance is approximately equal to the distance from umbilicus to the anterior vulvar commissure. The anterior vulvar commissure to top of the mons is one third to never more than one half of this height. Although actual distances depend on the height of the individual patient, the distance between the top of the mons and the umbilicus should not be less than 11 cm in women in the normal height range. These proportions should be preserved when incisions are designed. The natural contour of the healthy abdomen reveals a subtle epigastric sagittal depression that transitions below the umbilicus to a slight convexity. A subtle lateral depression at the lateral rectus border that is more distinct in a muscular person may also be seen. An attempt should be made to preserve or to develop these natural contours during abdominoplasty. Keeping scars at intersections of aesthetic units provides a more natural appearance. When possible, the transverse incision should be kept at the top of the mons, which should be returned to a nonptotic youthful height, and the lateral scar should sweep toward the iliac crest, following natural contours.

Choice of Technique

A number of different classification schemata have been described to help determine the best procedure for a given abdominal deformity.[36-40] These classifications may help guide the choice of technique, but the actual procedure performed must be individualized for the patient's medical history, physical examination findings, and personal preferences. A useful classification system combines many of the common findings with appropriate surgical options but is

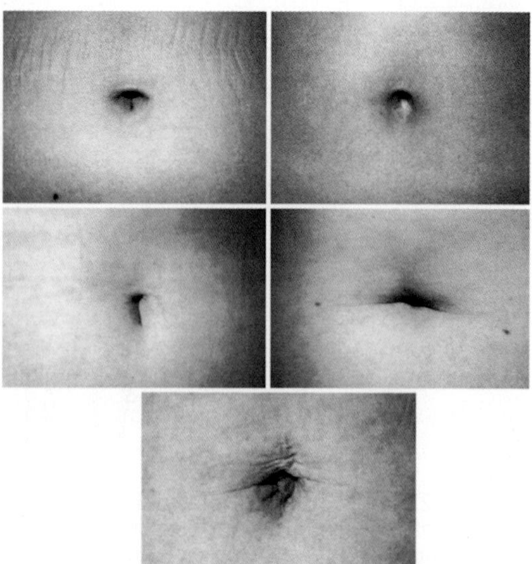

FIGURE 122-6. Normal umbilical variations. (From Craig SB, Faller MS, Puckett CL: In search of the ideal female umbilicus. Plast Reconstr Surg 2000;105:389.)

TABLE 122-1 ✦ CLASSIFICATION OF ABDOMINAL CONTOUR DEFORMITIES

Type	Other Names	Clinical Finding	Treatment	Example
0	Normal contour	No diastasis recti, no lax skin, no excess fat	No indication for surgery	Figure 122-7
1	Excess fat only	Fat deposit Normal musculoaponeurotic layer No excess skin	Suction-assisted lipectomy	Figure 122-8
2	Mini-abdominoplasty	**Infraumbilical skin excess** Normal musculoaponeurotic layer Fat may or may not be in excess	Lower abdominal skin resection Suction-assisted lipectomy or defatting as needed	Figure 122-9
3	Mini-abdominoplasty	**Infraumbilical skin excess** **May have laxity of the infraumbilical musculoaponeurotic layer** Fat may or may not be in excess	Lower abdominal skin resection **Suture of the rectus sheath from the pubis to the umbilicus** as needed Suction-assisted lipectomy or defatting as needed	Figure 122-10
4	Limited, modified, or extended mini-abdominoplasty	Infraumbilical ± mild supraumbilical skin excess May have laxity of the **overall musculoaponeurotic layer** Fat may or may not be in excess	Lower abdominal skin resection **Transection of the umbilical stalk *or* umbilical translocation with closure of donor site** **Suture of the rectus sheath from the pubis to the xiphoid** as needed Suction-assisted lipectomy or defatting as needed	Figure 122-11
5	Full, traditional, classic abdominoplasty	Infraumbilical and supraumbilical **skin excess** May have laxity of the musculoaponeurotic layer Fat may or may not be in excess	Traditional abdominoplasty **Resection of skin from the pubis to the umbilicus** Suture of the rectus sheath from the pubis to the xiphoid as needed **Umbilical translocation** Suction-assisted lipectomy when needed	Figures 122-12 and 122-13
6	Circumferential torsoplasty, belt lipectomy	**Circumferential skin laxity**, usually secondary to massive weight loss, with or without muscle laxity, with or without residual excess fat	**Circumferential torsoplasty** with umbilical translocation	Figures 122-14 and 122-15

subject to modification as new techniques arise (Table 122-1). The Bozola and Psillakis[36] system, one of the most commonly used, categorizes abdominal deformities into five common types. Pitman[38] adds a sixth category for severe circumferential skin laxity requiring circumferential abdominoplasty. Pitman's classification system presents standard options for contour deformities that can be treated with the most commonly used low transverse incision and does not include all surgical options or contour deformity combinations. The classification presented here is a modification of the Bozola-Psillakis[36] and Pitman[38] classification systems. Techniques not listed include the vertical abdominoplasty and reverse abdominoplasty, which are described separately (Figs. 122-7 to 122-15).

The classic abdominoplasty involves a low transverse lenticular resection of abdominal skin and subcutaneous tissue, undermining of the abdominal flap to the costal margin, and reimplantation of the umbilicus in the inferiorly advanced flap, with or without fascial plication. These basic steps have numerous variations and refinements based on the particular contour deformity and the patient's preference. The surgical

Text continued on p. 134

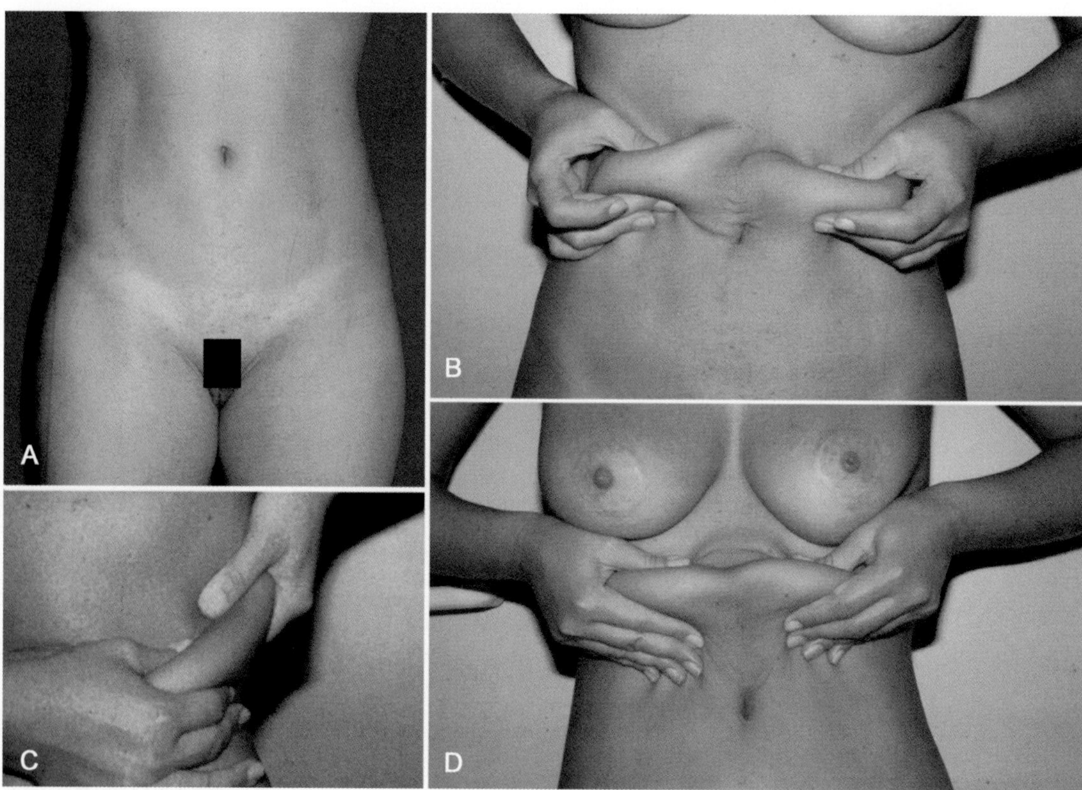

FIGURE 122-7. *A* to *D*, Type 0. Shown is a 26-year-old woman with normal, healthy abdominal contour. The patient requested liposuction using the "pinch test" argument. Surgery was refused.

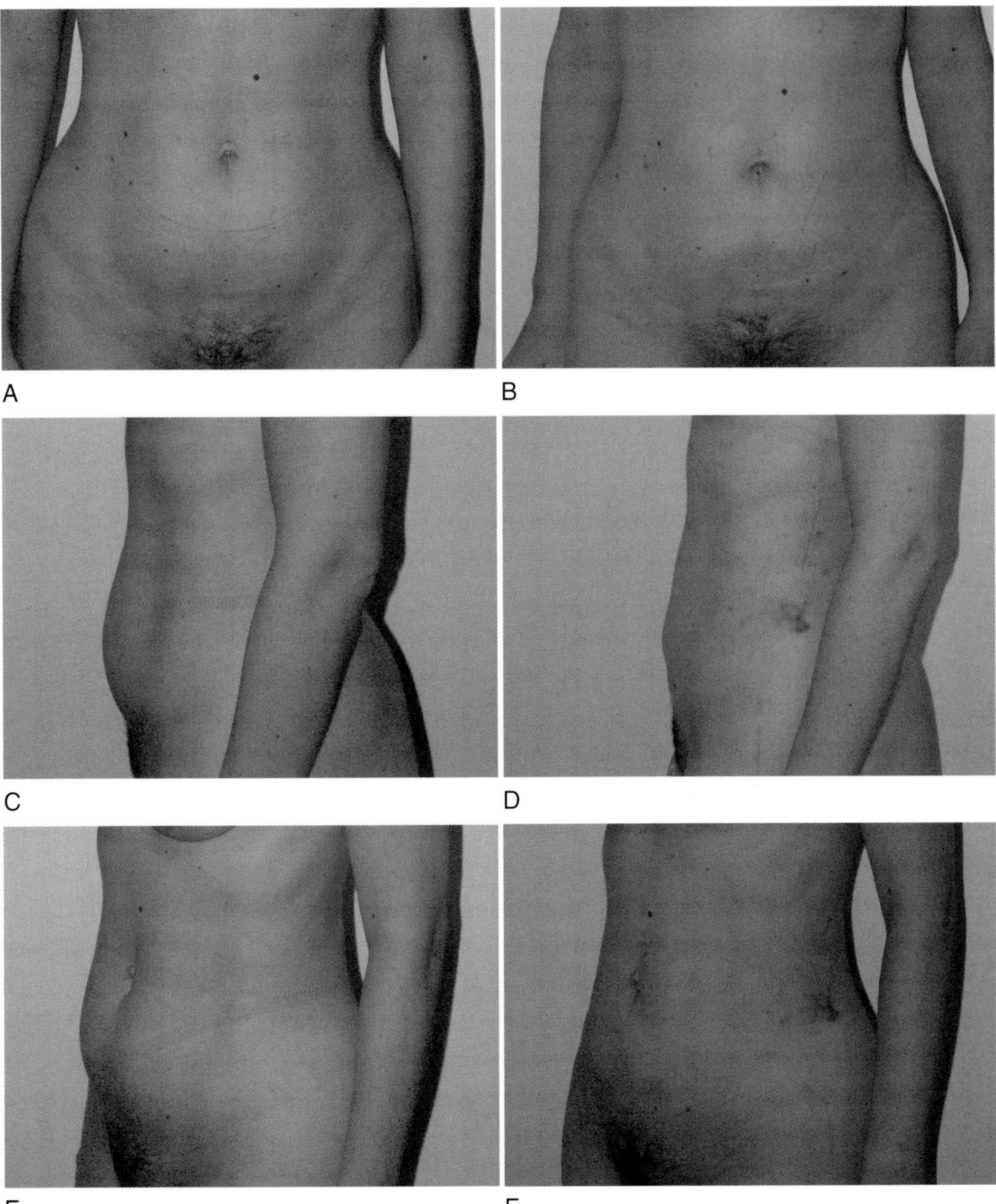

FIGURE 122-8. Type 1, excess fat only, no skin excess and no musculofascial laxity. Liposuction alone is performed to recontour the abdomen. *A, C* and *E,* Preoperative views. *B, D,* and *F,* Postoperative views after liposuction. See Table 122-1.

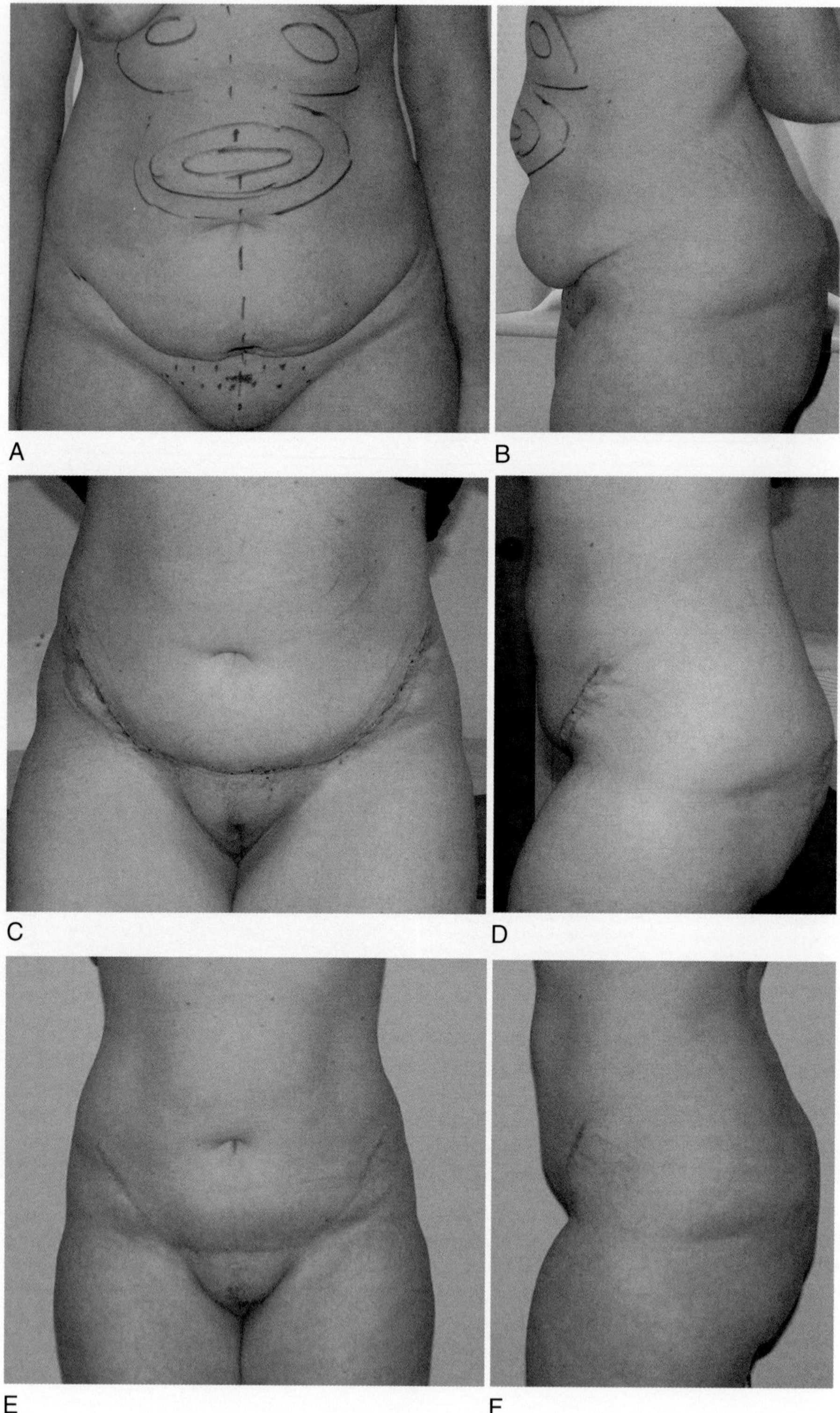

FIGURE 122-9. Type 2, excess fat, significant infraumbilical skin excess (pannus) without musculofascial laxity. *A* and *B*, Preoperative views. *C* and *D*, Early postoperative views after mini-abdominoplasty with a high lateral excision pattern and epigastric liposuction. No umbilical reinset or release or muscle plication was performed. *E* and *F*, Postoperative views at 9 months. Suprapubic edema is resolving. The scar is well hidden within a bikini line. Note the elevation of the mons and the absence of drain scars (drains exited along the pubic incision rather than in separate stab incision in the pubis). See Table 122-1.

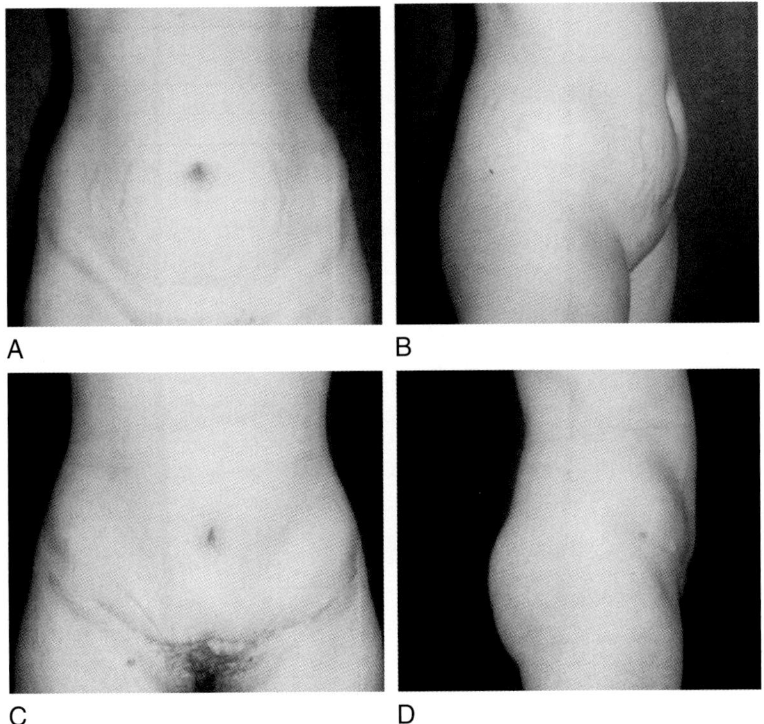

FIGURE 122-10. Type 3, mild skin and fat excess with musculofascial laxity. *A* and *B,* Preoperative views. *C* and *D,* Postoperative views at 1 year after mini-abdominoplasty with infraumbilical rectus plication. See Table 122-1.

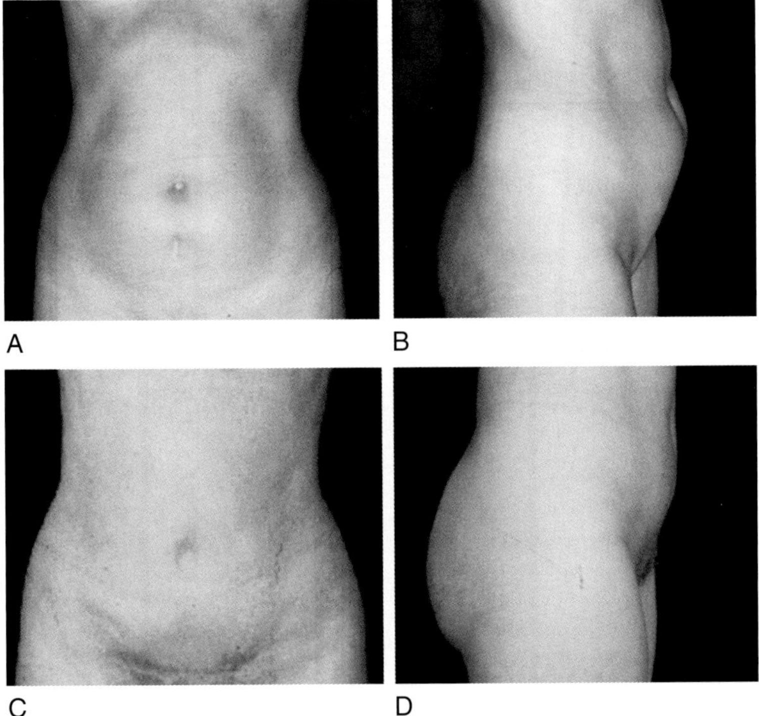

FIGURE 122-11. Type 4, overall musculofascial laxity with mild fat and moderate skin excess. *A* and *B,* Preoperative views. *C* and *D,* Postoperative views at 1 year after extended mini-abdominoplasty. The procedure included liposuction, umbilicus mobilization, rectus plication, and elliptical skin resection. See Table 122-1.

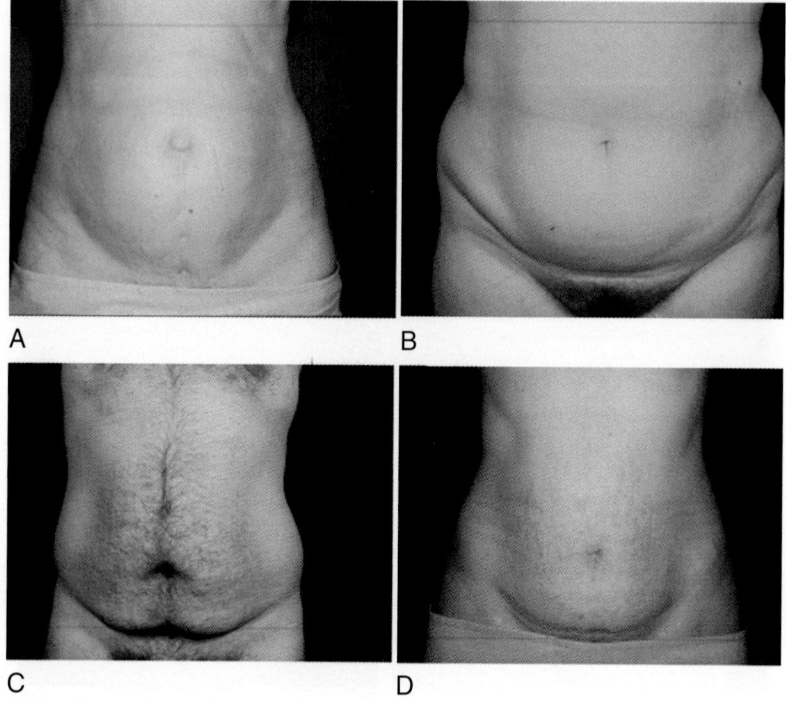

FIGURE 122-12. Type 5. *A* to *D*, Preoperative candidates with supraumbilical and infraumbilical skin excess and differing degrees of myofascial laxity and fat excess. See Table 122-1.

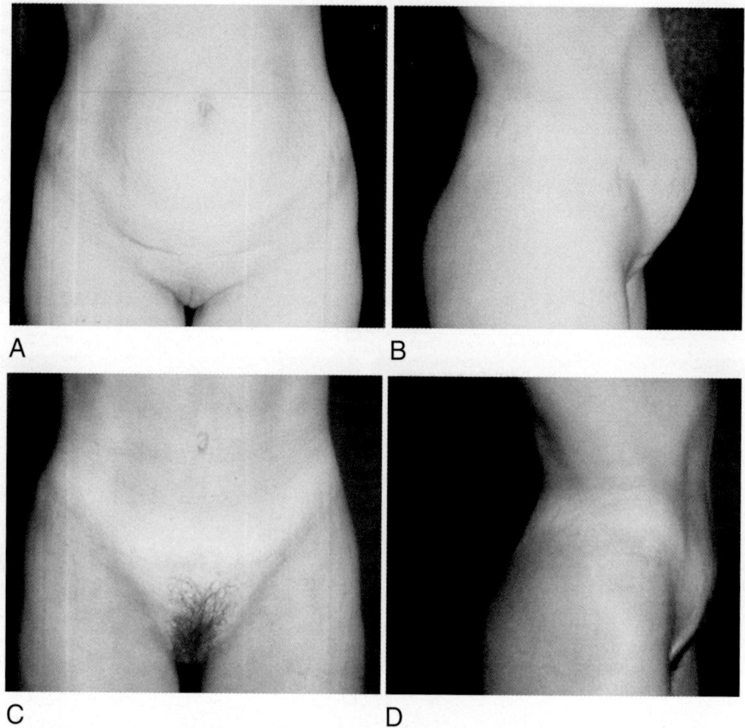

FIGURE 122-13. Type 5, significant musculofascial laxity with mild fat and skin excess. *A* and *B*, Preoperative views. *C* and *D*, Postoperative views 3 years after abdominoplasty through the handlebar incision. See Table 122-1.

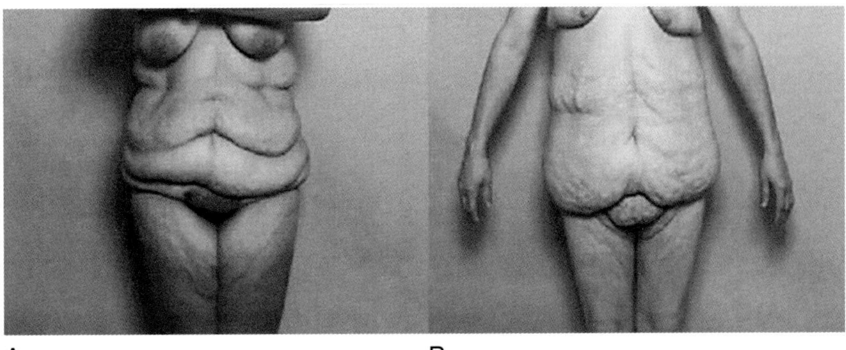

FIGURE 122-14. Type 6. *A* and *B,* Examples of circumferential skin laxity after massive weight loss. (From Aly AS, Cram AE, Heddens C: Truncal contouring surgery in the massive weight loss patient. Clin Plast Surg 2004;31:611.)

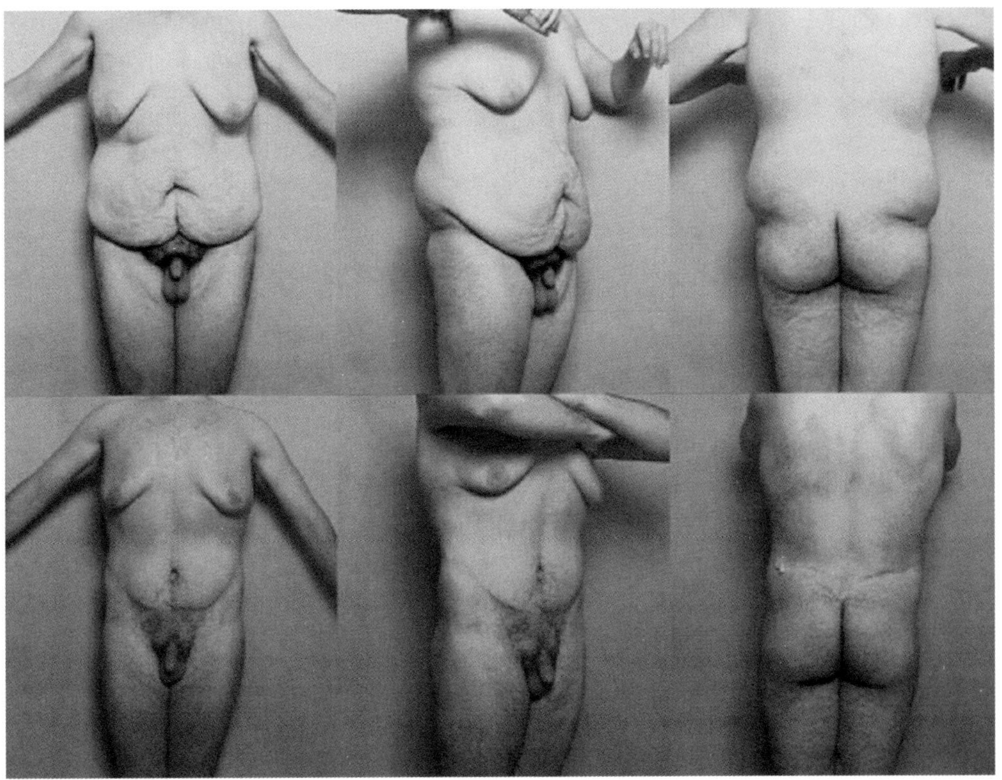

FIGURE 122-15. Type 6. Preoperative (top) and postoperative (bottom) views of patient who underwent circumferential torsoplasty. (From Aly AS, Cram AE, Heddens C: Truncal contouring surgery in the massive weight loss patient. Clin Plast Surg 2004;31:611.)

plan may include skin excision for skin laxity, muscle plication to tighten musculoaponeurotic laxity, and liposuction or fat excision to remove excess adipose tissue. Clinical and aesthetic decisions include incision type, extent of tissue excision, umbilical treatment, plication of the myofascial layer, extent of flap undermining, and extent of any liposuction. At the time of evaluation, other contour deformities, such as in the thighs, buttocks, chest, and arms, should also be discussed because the best result will be obtained from a sequential, balanced plan.

The choice of technique may be limited by the medical profile and priorities of the patient. For instance, if the patient has a cholecystectomy scar, a full abdominoplasty may be contraindicated. A smoker may be offered a procedure with less undermining. The morbidly obese patient may be offered panniculectomy instead of circumferential torsoplasty. If contour is of paramount importance to the patient, a more extensive excision may be chosen. The patient should bring preferred swimwear or lingerie to the preoperative evaluation and on the day of surgery in order to design the final scar to be hidden as much as possible.

Skin Incision and Excision

The contour, location, and length of the incision are determined by the amount of excess skin, the location of the excess, the patient's lingerie and bathing suit preferences, and the existence and placement of preexisting scars that can be incorporated into the excision. The three main types of abdominoplasty incisions are transverse, vertical, and combined. For practical purposes, the isolated vertical incision is reserved for patients who already have a vertical midline incision as it results in a prominent scar without addressing vertical skin excess (Fig. 122-16). It is also used in combined vertical and transverse techniques with concurrent revision of a vertical scar (Fig. 122-17) or for excision of massive skin excess. The low transverse incision is most versatile for allowing a well-hidden scar.

The amount and location of skin excision have produced different names for procedures aimed at direct excision of excess tissue. The modern trend is to "downstage"[37] procedures because much of the contour deformity contributed by subcutaneous fat deposits can be addressed with liposuction. However, redundant, flaccid skin or skin marked with striae will generally not be improved by liposuction, which can make such qualities even more noticeable.

The preferred modern incisions are dictated by the prevailing lingerie and swimsuit fashions, which are low cut anteriorly and high laterally for women and low across the hips for men. Keep in mind that fashions change regularly, so the patient should be consulted as to clothing preferences. For instance, if the patient frequently wears low-cut pants or skirts, the lateral ends of the standard bicycle handlebar incision[20] may be exposed (Fig. 122-18). The lower border of this incision cuts straight across the top of the mons and turns upward at the groin crease at a 60-degree angle toward the iliac crest, extending as far as necessary to achieve a smooth contour. If there is mons ptosis, a moderate upward lift should be applied when the lower incision is marked to mimic the final location of the

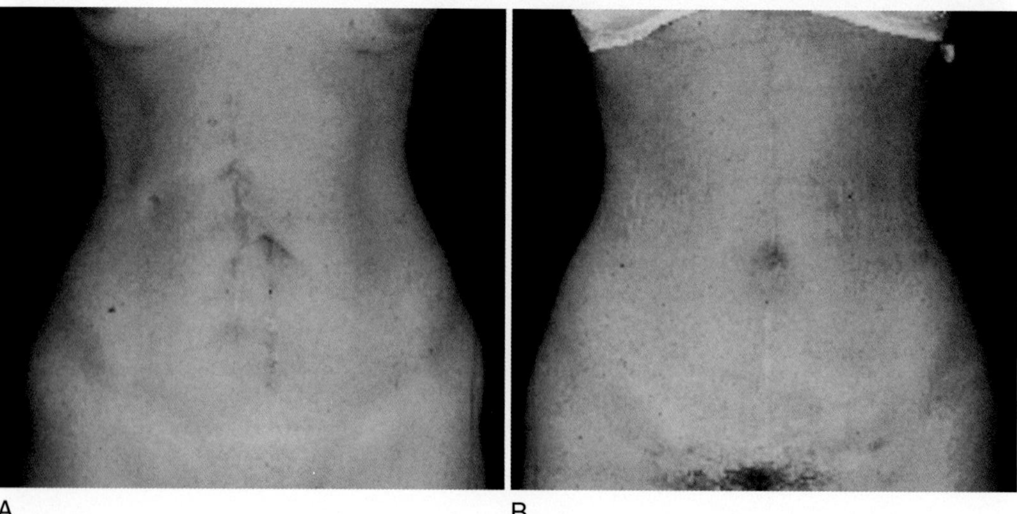

FIGURE 122-16. *A,* Preoperative view in a patient with skin laxity and two vertical and parallel scars at the midline of the abdomen due to previous celiotomy. *B,* Postoperative view 5 years after vertical abdominoplasty with neoumbilicoplasty. The short transverse scar is recent and unrelated.

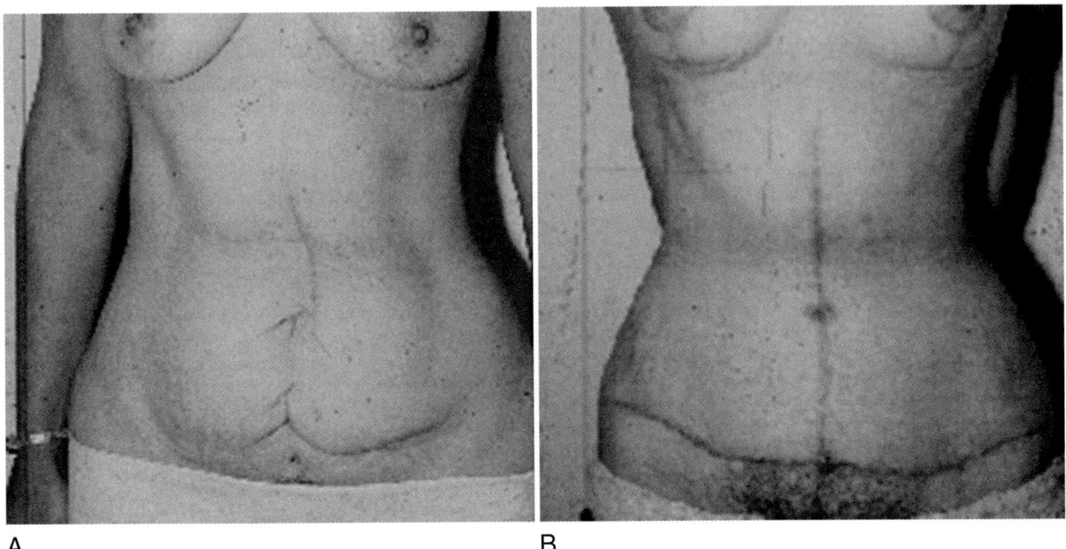

A B

FIGURE 122-17. Preoperative *(A)* and postoperative *(B)* views of a patient with vertical scar at the anterior abdominal wall after a combined vertical and transverse abdominoplasty.

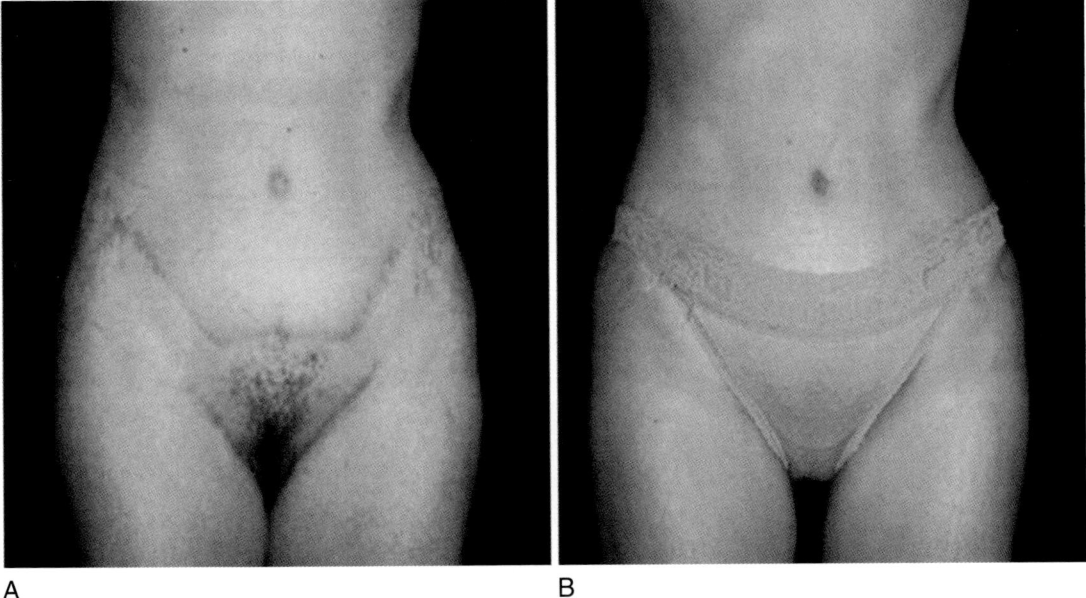

A B

FIGURE 122-18. *A,* Postoperative view following an abdominoplasty with a bicycle handlebar incision. The scar is lower at the pubis and higher at the lateral branches. *B,* The scar is easily hidden.

tissues at closure. This maneuver will avoid an unsightly elevation of the mons and incision at closure. The upper incision is determined by the amount of skin that should be excised and is more variable. The upper incision can be made by intraoperative flap advancement and trimming to fit, or it can be marked preoperatively. Preoperative marking can be made with a pinch technique to determine the amount of skin that can safely be excised (see Fig. 122-3).

Simple skin excision is limited by the umbilicus. The surgeon must assess whether the umbilicus can remain where it is, whether detachment of the umbilicus from the underlying fascia and allowing it to "float" as much as 2 cm inferiorly would allow adequate skin excision, or whether the umbilicus must be circumscribed and reinset into the advanced abdominal flap. If there is no supraumbilical skin laxity, the umbilicus should not be altered. If the supraumbilical skin laxity is minimal (about 2 cm by pinch test) and the native umbilicus is high, consider an umbilical float. When the amount of skin excised would make the umbilicus less than 16 cm from the anterior vulvar commissure if it is advanced with the flap (i.e., the umbilical stalk is divided), the umbilicus should be circumscribed and left attached to the abdominal fascia and reinset in the advanced flap. The surgeon must next decide whether the abdominal flap can be advanced safely past the umbilical excision site (see Fig. 122-13) or whether a vertical closure of the previous umbilical site should be performed (Figs. 122-19 and 122-20). To avoid a vertical closure when there is insufficient excess skin to permit safe flap advancement from supraumbilicus to pubis, some surgeons will place the lower incision above the mons on the infra-abdominal skin. This option should be avoided because it results in a scar that is exposed by normal bikini underwear and crosses the lower abdominal aesthetic unit.

The mini-abdominoplasty and extended mini-abdominoplasty techniques (also known as limited or modified abdominoplasty)[23,42] advocate shorter incisions and less undermining in conjunction with liposuction. The mini-abdominoplasty may be combined with infraumbilical fascial plication. The extended mini-abdominoplasty adds either an umbilical float[17,43] or umbilical reinset with closure of the umbilical donor site to allow resection of an intermediate amount of skin while maintaining appropriate umbilical position (see "Technical Variations and Refinements"). These techniques are appropriate when there is only infraumbilical laxity or minimal supraumbilical laxity and when other factors prohibit wide undermining.

Significant lateral laxity with a prominent vertical scar may be best addressed by adding a midline vertical excision. Otherwise, lateral laxity can be addressed

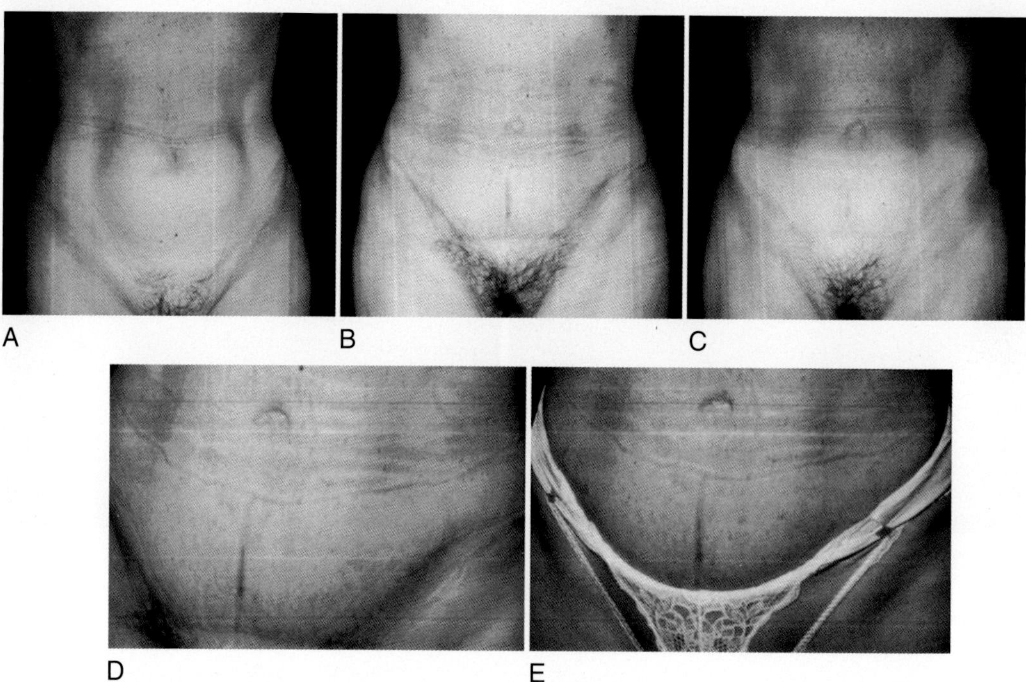

FIGURE 122-19. Preoperative view *(A)* and postoperative views at 6 months *(B)* and 2 years *(C)* in a patient with an umbilical donor site detect that did not advance to the transverse pubic incision. Thus, the patient has a midline scar between the neoumbilicus and the pubic scar. *D* and *E,* Close-up views.

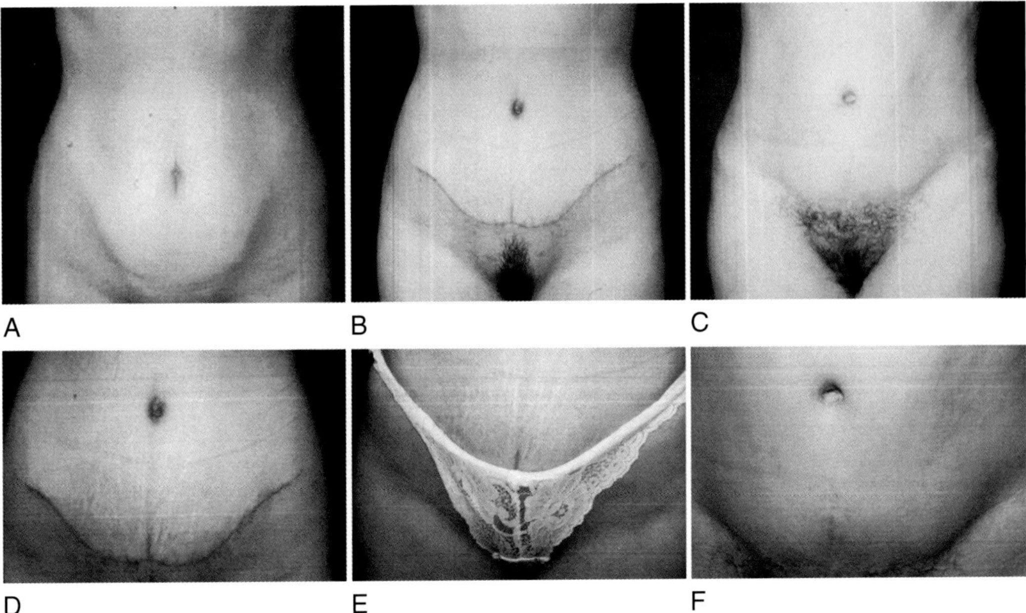

FIGURE 122-20. *A,* Preoperative view of a patient with inadequate skin excess for complete excision of the umbilical donor site. *B,* Postoperative view at 6 months. *C,* Postoperative view at 5 years. *D* to *F,* Close-up views of the abdomen at 6 months (*D* and *E*). The vertical closure is approximately 1 to 4 cm in length. The scar is easily covered (even covered by small underwear, only the upper extremity of the vertical scar is visible). The scar is even less visible at 5 years (*F*).

with a high lateral tension abdominoplasty (see "High Lateral Tension Abdominoplasty"). If the skin laxity is circumferential, circumferential excision is indicated. Depending on the medical condition of the patient and the preference of the surgeon, this may be a staged operation. Finally, reverse abdominoplasty involves skin excision at the inframammary line and is reserved for patients with primarily supraumbilical laxity or preexisting or planned inframammary scars (see "Reverse Abdominoplasty").

Despite the number of options available, the principles of designing the skin excision are straightforward. First, mark the inferior incision while lifting ptotic tissue. Next, determine the amount of skin that can be removed safely with a tension-free closure and whether the excision needs to be extended laterally and posteriorly. Finally, decide whether the umbilicus should be left alone, released, or repositioned.

Flap Undermining

The degree of flap undermining should be determined by the individual needs of a patient, but it should never be more than is absolutely necessary to allow flap advancement or to provide access to the muscle fascia for plication.

If circulation to the skin is in question because of an upper abdominal scar, obesity, smoking, or other comorbidity, a simple panniculectomy should be considered. A panniculectomy is a simple wedge excision of skin and fat, traditionally used for the "fat apron" or pannus (Fig. 122-21). No undermining is performed to avoid disruption of perforating vessels to preserved skin. Judicious discontinuous undermining with the liposuction cannula allows thinning and advancement of the flap while preserving perforators (see "Abdominoplasty Without Undermining"). Classically, the abdominal flap is undermined in an inverted U (wider inferiorly) up to the costal margins. Wider undermining gains flap advancement and contour improvement at the expense of flap circulation, as trans-rectus perforators from the deep epigastric system (zone I) are transected (Fig. 122-22).

Fascial Plication

Musculofascial laxity can be congenital or result from significant weight fluctuations as with pregnancy. If the patient is of childbearing age, fascial plication should be deferred as it may cause an increase in abdominal pressure during pregnancy, and pregnancy will undo or diminish its benefits. Musculofascial deformities have been classified by severity and treatment by Nahas[39] (Table 122-2 and Fig. 122-23). If the fascial laxity is not associated with skin excess, an endoscopic midline rectus plication with or without

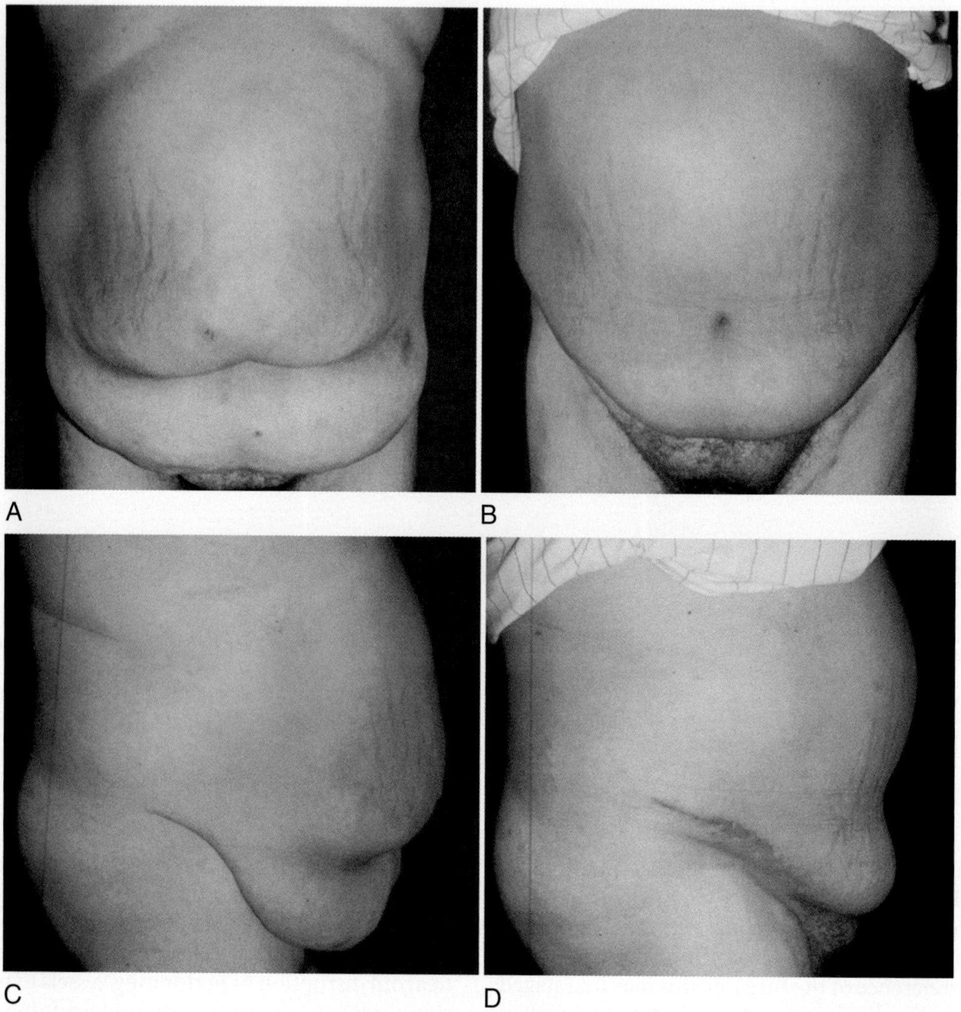

A B C D

FIGURE 122-21. *A* and *C,* Preoperative views of a 45-year-old man. *B* and *D,* Postoperative views after abdominoplasty with skin apron resection without undermining above the level of the umbilicus. Skin flap demonstrated fat pad of approximately 10 cm.

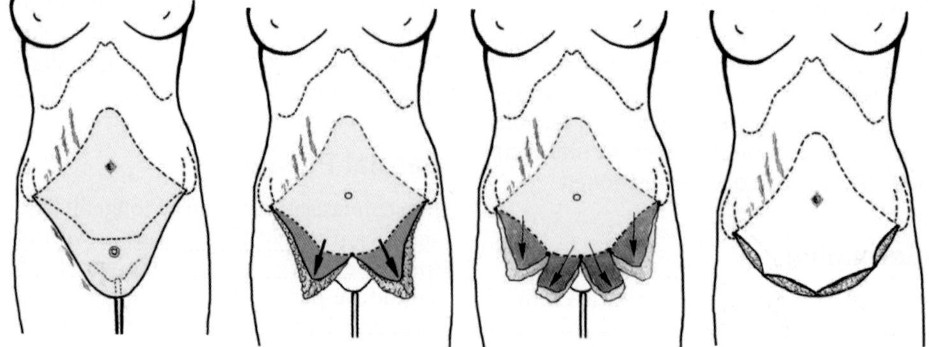

FIGURE 122-22. Schematic of excess skin resection and extent of undermining. After undermining, the patient is placed in flexion on the operating table, and the flap is stretched inferiorly toward the initial incision site. The skin flap is divided up to the point where the flap can reach the lower incision without undue tension and be temporarily sutured in place. Each subsequent flap is similarly divided. Three stay sutures fix the flap in its definitive position for resection of the excess skin.

TABLE 122-2 ✦ CLASSIFICATION AND TREATMENT OF ABDOMINAL WALL DEFORMITIES BASED ON MUSCULOAPONEUROTIC DEFORMITY

Myofascial Deformity Type	Clinical Finding	Treatment
A	RD secondary to pregnancy	PRS
B	RD and laxity of the lateral and infraumbilical aponeurotic layer	PRS + L-shaped plication of the external oblique aponeurosis
C	Congenital lateral insertion of the recti muscles	Release and undermining of the recti muscles from their posterior recti sheaths and advancement of these muscles to the midline
D	RD and poor waistline	PRS and advancement of the external oblique muscles

RD, rectus diastasis; PRS, plication of the anterior rectus sheath.
From Nahas FX: An aesthetic classification of the abdomen based on the myoaponeurotic layer. Plast Reconstr Surg 2001;108:1787.

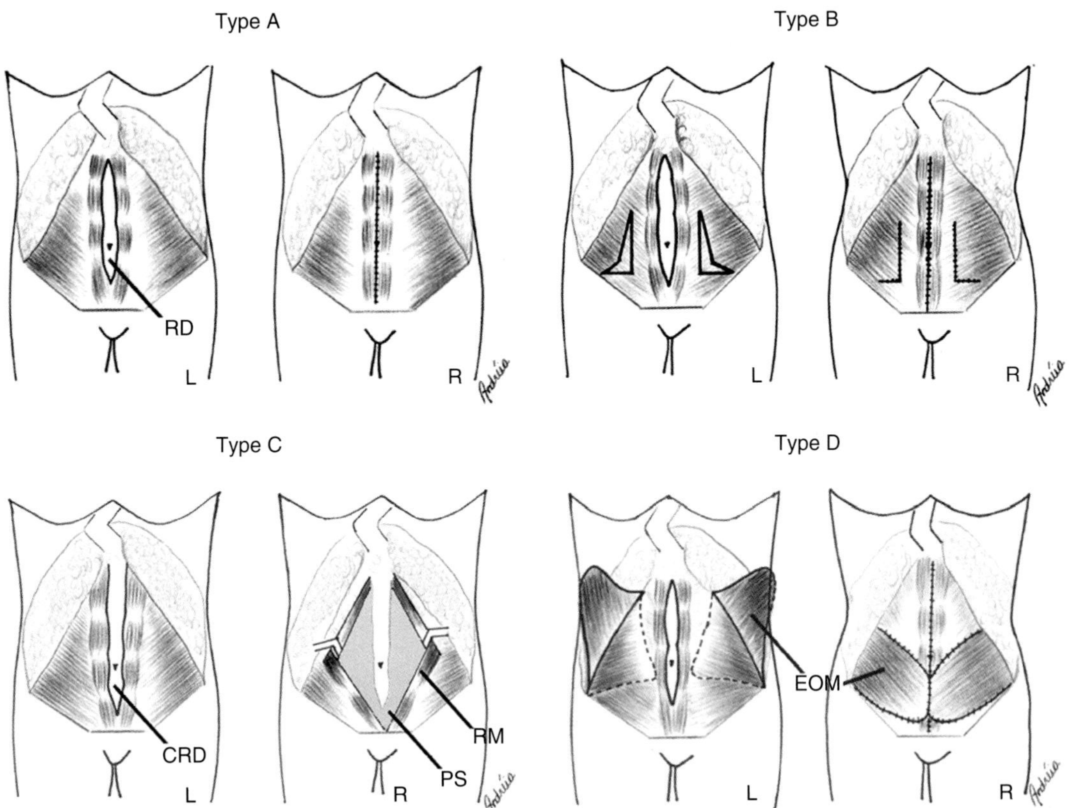

FIGURE 122-23. Types of abdominal deformity and their correction. Type A, Diastasis recti (RD) secondary to pregnancy; correction is by plication of the anterior rectus sheath. Type B, Diastasis recti with laxity of the musculoaponeurotic layer; correction is by plication of the anterior rectus sheath and external oblique aponeurosis. Type C, Congenital lateral insertion of the rectus muscles at the costal margins and probable hernias. Correction is accomplished by undermining the posterior rectus sheath (PS), invagination of the linea alba, and anchoring of the anterior rectus sheath to the midline. CRD, congenital rectus diastasis; RM, rectus muscle. Type D, Diastasis recti and poor waistline definition. Correction is by anterior rectus sheath plication and medial advancement of the external oblique muscles (EOM). (From Nahas FX: An aesthetic classification of the abdomen based on the myoaponeurotic layer. Plast Reconstr Surg 2001;108:1787.)

liposuction can be considered. Severe fascial laxity may be addressed with additional bilateral lenticular plication of the external oblique fascia. Other muscle-tightening procedures that have been described include addition of a transverse plication called the "waistline stitch"[44]; incision of the rectus fascia bilaterally just lateral to the diastasis, and then closing the resultant defect in two layers with the idea that the raw edges will aid in scar adhesion of the plicated fascia[26]; and advancement of the oblique muscles to narrow the waistline[45] (see Fig. 122-23). Plication should establish a naturally taut abdomen without placing the fascia under undue tension to avoid having the sutures pull through the fascia. If the muscle fascia is too weak to support sutures, plication will provide no benefit.

Fat Excision and Concurrent Liposuction

Excess adipose tissue on the flap and at the lateral borders of the incision (the potential "dog-ear") can be addressed with direct excision. Excision of adipose tissue on the flap can be safely performed deep to the superficial fascial system. This excision will provide a smooth layer of subcutaneous tissue to drape over the fascia while preserving the intercostal perforators. If no undermining is performed (as with panniculectomy), liposuction can safely be performed on the anterior abdomen.

The concern over the combination of liposuction with abdominoplasty is due to the division of the main circulation to the abdominal flap (zone I) as well as the inferiorly based blood supply (zone II) during a full abdominoplasty (see Fig. 122-5). The standard inverted U flap undermining from a low transverse incision to the costal margin that is used to advance the flap and to allow a smooth contour divides all vascular supply to the flap except from the laterally arising intercostals. Liposuction on the flap, as well as laterally, can disrupt these perforators along their path, leading to devascularized areas of the flap. There are several ways to reduce the likelihood of flap ischemia from devascularization. Flap undermining should be minimized and liposuction avoided in the central portion of the flap, which is most distant from its vascular supply, or performed only deep to the superficial fascial system. Second, avoid undermining by combining skin resection with extensive deep liposuction to allow advancement of the abdominal skin flap with its epigastric perforators intact (Fig. 122-24). Finally, the procedure can be staged so that liposuction is not performed at the time of abdominoplasty (Fig. 122-25). Whether abdominoplasty or liposuction should be done first depends on which procedure will better address the patient's main concerns.

SURGICAL TECHNIQUES

Abdominoplasty

PREOPERATIVE MANAGEMENT AND MARKINGS

Before surgery, the patient should be told to avoid medications, herbs, and foods that interfere with blood coagulation, such as aspirin products, large doses of garlic, vitamin E, fish oil, gingko, ginger, ginseng, and cayenne, for 2 weeks and to abstain from smoking for at least 4 weeks. If there is any question of fungal or bacterial infection at skinfolds, the infection should be treated and cleared and the patient instructed to shower with antimicrobial soap for 3 consecutive days before surgery.

In the preoperative area, before sedation, the patient should be marked in the standing position. The vertical midline must be marked while the patient is standing. Midaxial vertical lines and a horizontal waistline marking parallel to the floor may be marked to aid in symmetric resection. The lower incision is determined by lifting the mons to the level anticipated at closure and marking the midline 5 to 7 cm above the anterior vulvar commissure (Fig. 122-26). In the ptotic mons, this will cut through the hair-bearing tissue. The mark is extended laterally to just before the groin crease. Under moderate upward and medial tension, the lateral limbs of the inferior incision are drawn to the anterior superior iliac spine and checked for symmetry. An estimate of the upper incision (extent of excision) may also be marked at this time, as a guideline for tissue resection and symmetry, and checked for ease of resection by the pinch test (see Fig. 122-3). Any areas of planned liposuction are marked. Visible diastasis or areas of fascial laxity or bulging should also be marked.

TECHNIQUE

In the operating room, the patient is positioned on the operating table so that he or she can be flexed at the hips and knees ("beach chair" or semi-Fowler position) to take tension off the incision at the time of closure if needed. The arms are placed on arm boards, with the wrists and hands elevated so that the elbow is not hyperextended to prevent neurapraxia, and then cushioned and secured with tape. Antiembolism stockings and sequential compression devices are placed before induction so that venous pooling does not occur. An upper body warm air blanket is used, and the room is kept warm; the anesthesiologist is asked to keep the patient well hydrated to maintain good tissue perfusion. Gram-positive antibiotic coverage is given before incision. The patient is widely prepped and draped, making sure to extend the prep as far laterally as possible to allow dog-ear excision and

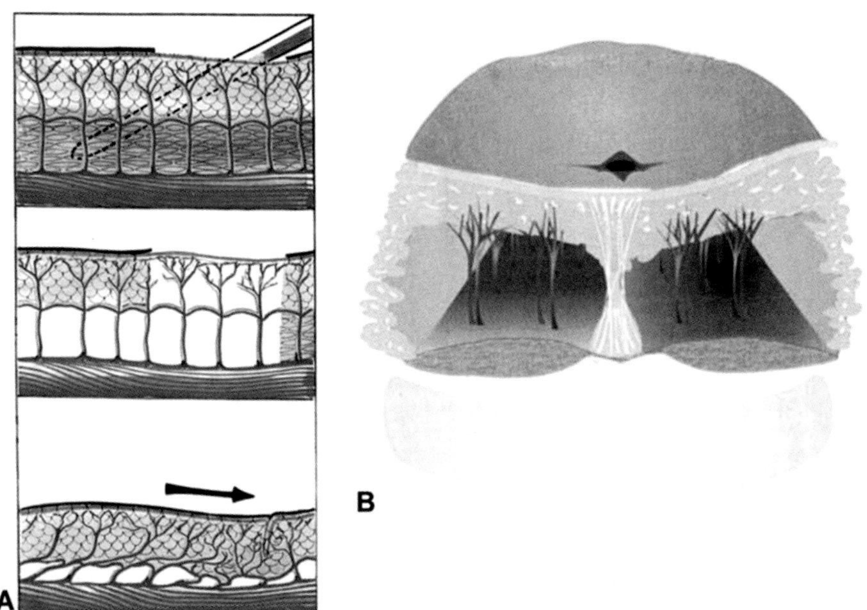

FIGURE 122-24. *A,* Schematic of a section of the abdominal panniculus. *Top,* The cannula was introduced through the subcutaneous tissue after skin resection was performed. *Middle,* View after lipoplasty shows thickness of the skin-resected area and removal of fat (from underneath the fascia superficialis). *Bottom,* After suturing, the panniculus slid downward *(arrow)* while the perforator vessels were preserved. *B,* Architecture of the panniculus after lipoplasty. The perforator vessels originating from the rectus abdominis were preserved. (From Avelar J: Abdominoplasty without panniculus undermining and resection: analysis and 3-year follow-up of 97 cases. Aesthet Surg J 2002;22:17. Reproduced with permission from The American Society for Aesthetic Plastic Surgery, Inc.)

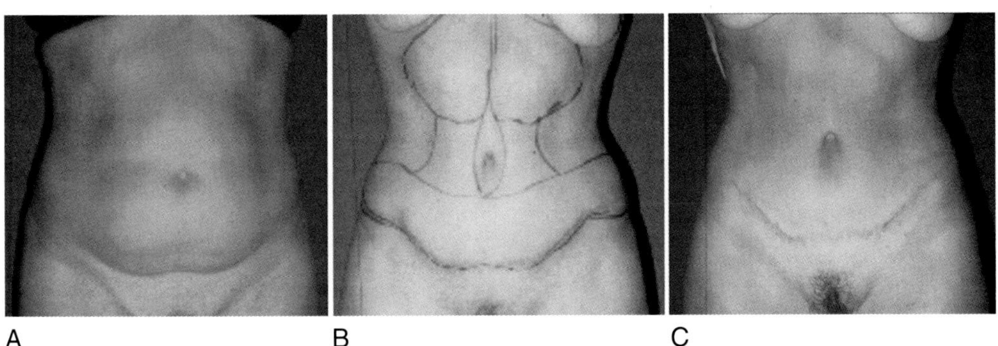

FIGURE 122-25. Preoperative view *(A)* and postoperative view at 6 months after traditional abdominoplasty *(B)*. The residual fat deposits in different regions of the abdomen were outlined (with the patient standing) for secondary liposuction. *C,* Same patient 8 months after liposuction procedure.

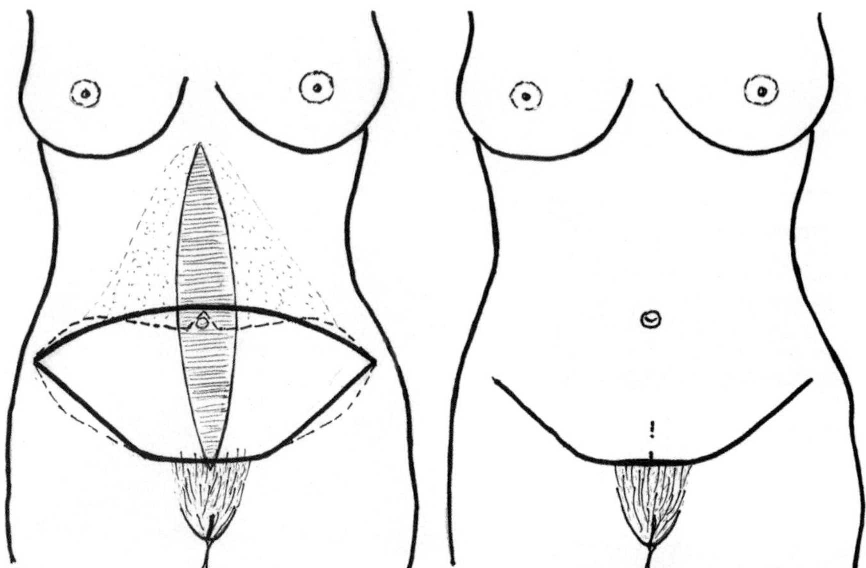

FIGURE 122-26. Full abdominoplasty. *A,* Dark line is traditional abdominoplasty excision pattern. Dotted line shows the high lateral tension variation for lateral laxity. Fusiform hatched area marks the area of rectus diastasis to be plicated. The shaded area indicates extent of undermining. *B,* Resulting scar is low at the pubis and sweeps up to the iliac crests. A circumumbilical scar indicates reinset of the umbilicus into the advanced flap. The umbilical donor site may be fully excised with the excess flap, closed in layers leaving a vertical scar between the umbilicus and pubis, or partially excised leaving a small inverted T (dotted lines).

liposuction. After the patient has been prepped as widely as possible in the supine position, a more extensive lateral prep may be achieved by pulling the patient's torso and pannus laterally while the circulating nurse preps under the patient. The scrub nurse then tucks a sterile half-sheet under the patient's side before the surgeon releases the torso. The same steps are taken on the contralateral side.

The preoperative markings are reviewed and modified if needed. If the planned flap resection is level with or above the umbilicus, the umbilicus is elevated with skin hooks to minimize stalk length and circumscribed sharply (Fig. 122-27). Scissor dissection is taken down to fascia, spreading and dividing in a cone shape away from the umbilical stalk to preserve deep perforators to the umbilicus. Care is taken to ensure that an occult umbilical hernia is not missed; if it is found, it is repaired once the flap is elevated and the fascia defect exposed. At the inferior marking, the skin and subcutaneous tissues are incised down to fascia. The tissue is elevated off the underlying fascia with use of electrocautery along the suprafascial loose areolar plane up to the umbilicus (Fig. 122-28). Care is taken to leave behind the white mesh-like cellular layer overlying the fascia (fascia of Gallaudet), which contains a fine vascular network and can help resorb serous exudate. Dissection advances cephalad. As the dissection approaches the umbilicus, lateral to medial flap elevation will help avoid transection of the umbilical stalk. Once the flap elevation is level with the umbilicus, it is carefully separated from the abdominal flap. The flap may be divided at the vertical midline almost to the level of the upper marking to allow easier elevation of the flap superiorly (Fig. 122-29). Before reaching the superior incision marking, the flap should

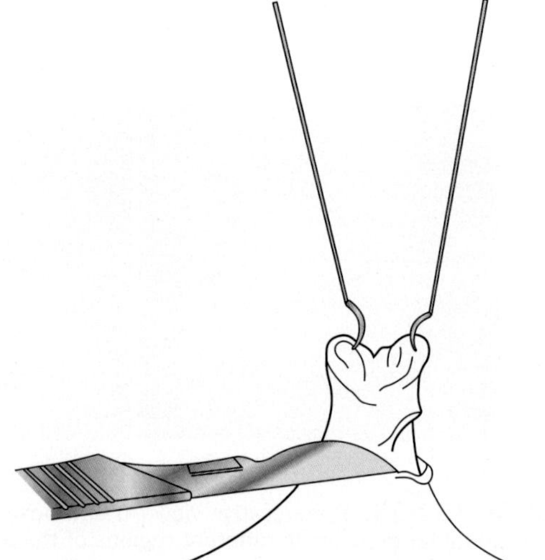

FIGURE 122-27. Circumscribing the umbilicus. The umbilicus is elevated with two skin hooks and the skin divided circumferentially. The double hooks are then used to separate the umbilicus from the abdominal flap, and dissection is taken with Metzenbaum scissor spreading down to fascia to isolate the umbilical stalk from the abdominal flap.

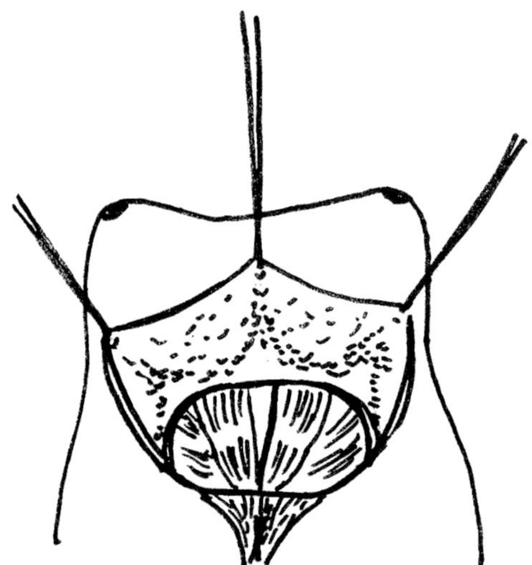

FIGURE 122-28. The lower incision of the abdominoplasty is taken down to fascia. The flap is then elevated cephalad along the suprafascial plane.

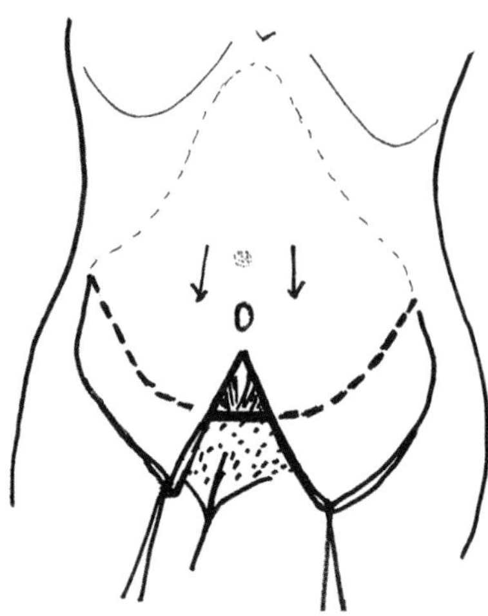

FIGURE 122-29. After circumscribing the umbilicus, the flap can be divided in the midline to improve access to the epigastrium. Do not divide farther than the flap can safely be advanced for closure.

be advanced to check for tension-free reach to the lower incision. Flap advancement is checked regularly to avoid elevating the flap any more than necessary for tension-free closure or access to diastasis recti for plication, so that flap devascularization is minimized. The abdominal flap may be elevated superiorly up to the costal margins as needed, but care should be taken to avoid undermining too widely (Fig. 122-30).

Midline rectus plication is performed if needed. The planned plication is marked as a fusiform vertical band from the xiphoid to the pubis. The width is determined by the degree of diastasis recti and the quality of the fascia. Two running looped No. 1 Prolene sutures are used, one above and one below the umbilicus (Fig. 122-31). Care is taken to bury the knots as these may sometimes be palpated by the patient. Buried figure-of-eight sutures may be added to reinforce the plication. If laxity persists, two additional fusiform plications of the external oblique fascia can be added (see Fig. 122-23). If the umbilical stalk is long, the umbilical dermis may be tacked to the rectus

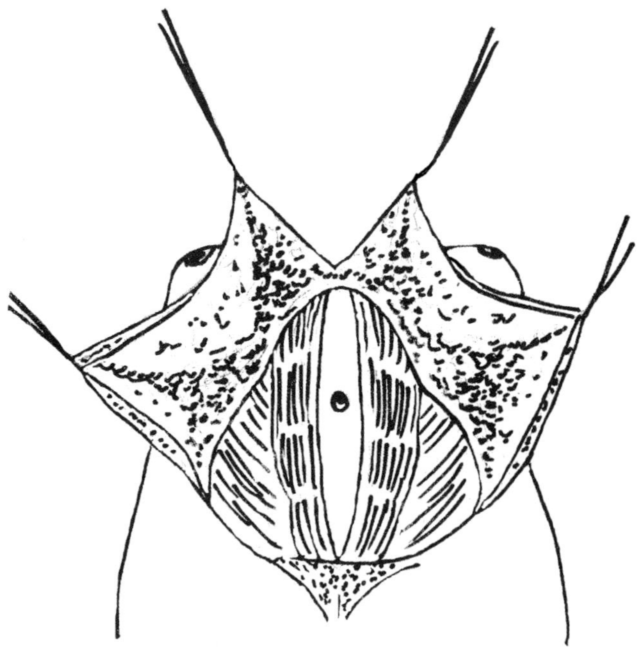

FIGURE 122-30. The flap is elevated to the xiphoid, with care taken not to elevate laterally any more than is necessary for smooth flap advancement to minimize devascularization of the flap.

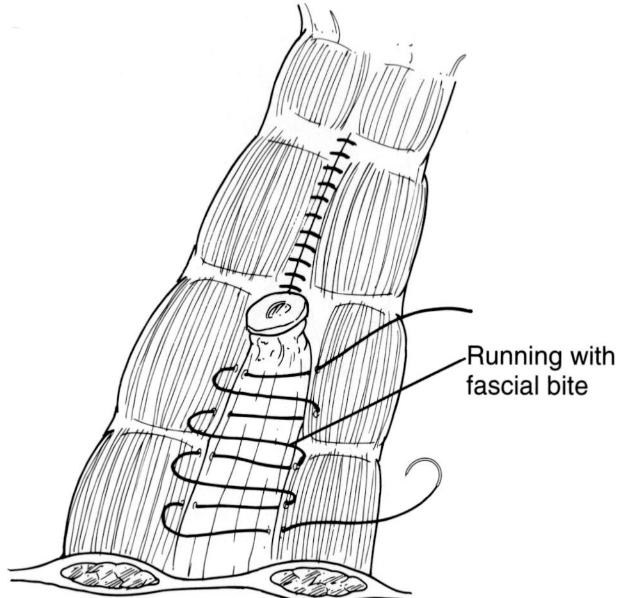

FIGURE 122-31. Fascial laxity or dehiscence is marked with an ellipse and closed with running looped No. 1 Prolene suture, one row above and one below the umbilicus.

fascia so that on closure, there will be an invagination at the umbilicus.

At this point, general thinning of the abdominal flap can be performed if needed by direct excision of the fat deep to the superficial fascia, preserving the blood supply that runs in the superficial fascial system and deep dermal plexus.

To aid in closure, the operating table is placed in beach chair position with about 30 degrees of flexion at the hips. The flap is advanced and checked for smoothness. If there are areas of tension laterally, these are released with blunt dissection, carefully preserving intercostal perforators as they are encountered. The upper marking is checked to confirm adequate reach and symmetry or modified as necessary; the excess tissue is then excised using Pitanguy forceps to confirm the extent of resection (Figs. 122-32 and 122-33). The abdominal flap is then fastened to the fascia with interrupted 2-0 Vicryl sutures at 5-cm intervals from superficial fascia to the abdominal wall, applying progressive tension. Sutures are placed starting from the superior extent of the flap, and tension is applied inferiorly as well as lateral to medial. This technique aids in contouring the waist, takes tension off the inferomedial aspect of the flap and closure, helps tailor any lateral dog-ears medially, and reduces flap shear and dead space. Progressive tension sutures are added at

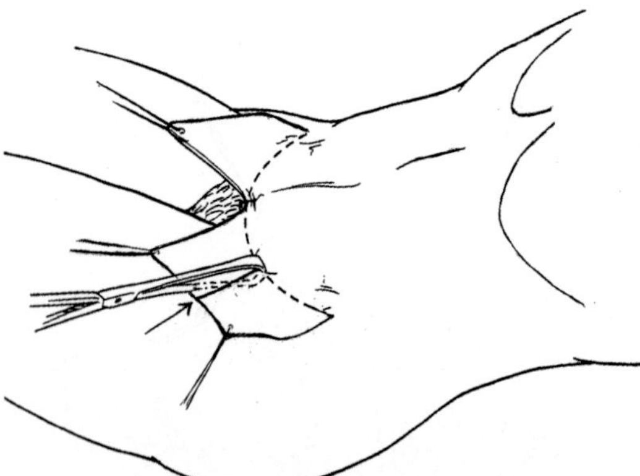

FIGURE 122-32. Flap excision. The operating table is flexed at the hip about 30 degrees. The flaps are adjusted to minimize lateral dog-ears. Pitanguy forceps are used to mark the extent of flap resection at the center of the flap. The flap is divided to the marked point, and the two edges are temporarily stapled in place. This step is repeated as necessary to confirm the upper border for resection. Once the upper resection line is clearly defined, the abdominal flap excess is excised.

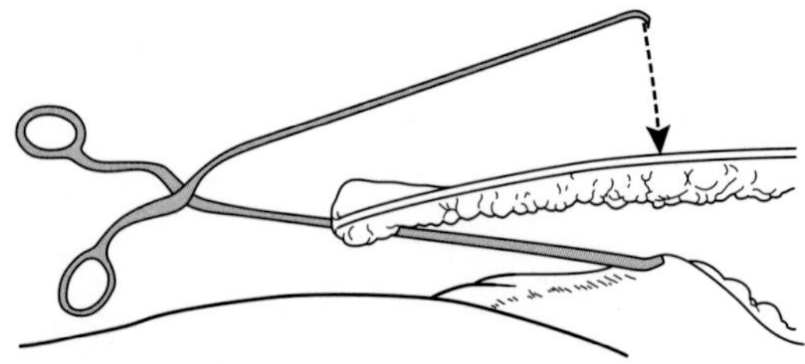

FIGURE 122-33. Pitanguy forceps are placed with the lower prongs abutting the midpoint of the lower border of the incision. It is pushed slightly cephalad to approximate the final closure, and the flap is laid down without tension. The arms are closed, and the point at which the upper prongs touch the flap is marked. The flap is divided up to this point.

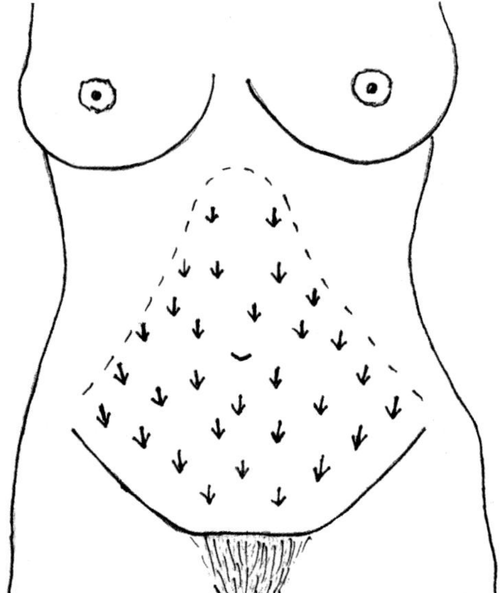

FIGURE 122-34. Progressive tension sutures are placed between the superficial fascia on the flap and the abdominal fascia using progressive inferiomedial tension. Arrows indicate direction of pull. These sutures help to eliminate dead space, to control flap advancement and placement, to prevent flap sliding, and to take tension off the closure.

5-cm intervals along the whole area of the undermined flap, down to the level of the umbilicus (Fig. 122-34).

The midpoint of the flap is now temporarily stapled to the lower incision, and the umbilical stalk location under the flap is reflected to the abdominal flap by the surgeon's nondominant hand (Fig. 122-35). A 2-cm U-shaped incision is placed in the abdominal flap directly over the umbilical stalk. At the new umbilical site, the flap adipose tissue may be judiciously thinned circumferentially if needed to allow the umbilicus to rest in a concavity. The umbilicus is sutured in place with a buried absorbable stitch from rectus fascia to flap dermis to umbilical dermis in four quadrants. Next, progressive tension sutures are placed on the remainder of the flap at 5-cm intervals down to the closure. After accurate flap excision and placement of the progressive tension sutures, the flap and lower incision should sit apposed without tension. Two Blake drains are laid on the fascia (threading them between the quilting sutures as needed) and exited within the pubic hairline. The flap is temporarily approximated with surgical staples, advancing the upper flap medially to place the greatest lift laterally and the least tension medially. If lateral dog-ears are noted, they should be addressed with direct tissue excision. The flap is sutured to the lower border in three layers, superficial fascial, deep dermal, and running subcutaneous, to avoid any tension on the skin closure. Layered closure will help prevent flap thinning and the resulting unsightly depression at the incision as well as scar widening. Liposuction can smooth the contour of the lateral corners of the incision and is relatively safe here. If significant liposuction is required, a staged procedure may be preferable.

The incision is dressed with Steri-Strips and sterile absorbent dressing. Tape is applied loosely, as postoperative edema can cause blistering. An abdominal binder is placed lightly for support without causing undue pressure on the flap. If concurrent liposuction is performed, adhesive foam padding may be used over those areas to reduce edema and bruising. Postoperatively, the patient is transferred to a bed that has been preset in a beach chair position to take tension off the abdominal closure. Immediate mobilization of the patient is encouraged to decrease risk of embolic complications.

POSTOPERATIVE CARE

The patient is encouraged to get out of bed as soon as possible but should continue to use antithrombotic prophylaxis (such as sequential compression devices) until he or she is moving normally. If fascial plication is performed, the patient is instructed in how to avoid use of the abdominal muscles during normal activity and is told to avoid heavy lifting or strenuous exercise for 4 to 6 weeks. The normal hospital stay is 1 to 2 days. The drains are removed when drainage is below 30 mL a day per drain, usually at discharge or at the

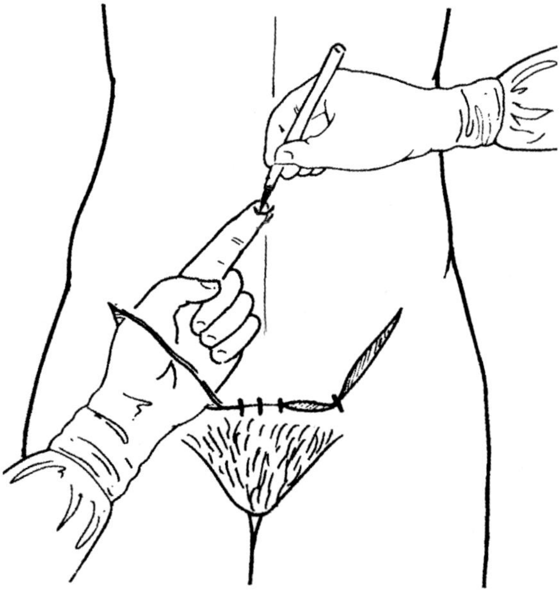

FIGURE 122-35. Locating the new umbilical site. The flap is temporarily stapled in place medially. The surgeon's nondominant hand locates the umbilicus under the flap and palpates the location on the flap directly above it on the midline. The dominant hand marks this location.

first postoperative visit. The patient is allowed to shower after 2 days and is warned to avoid heating pads, hot tubs, sunbathing, tight clothing, or other extremes of temperature or pressure on the abdomen as the flap will be numb for several months. A light abdominal binder may be used postoperatively for support and comfort, but care must be taken to avoid tightening to the point of compromising abdominal flap vascularity. An improperly worn abdominal binder may also form bands of edema on the flap if venous outflow is impaired.

Baroudi Abdominoplasty Technique[20]

General anesthesia with endotracheal intubation and epidural anesthesia are routinely used. After skin marking is completed, the surgical area is infiltrated with saline solution with 1:200,000 epinephrine along the incision line and 1:500,000 in the cutaneous flap that will be undermined. The preoperative infusion is useful when liposuction is planned.

MARKINGS

Skin marking is performed with the patient in the supine position after induction of anesthesia and preparation of the sterile surgical field. The bicycle handlebar demarcation starts with an X-X′ line from the xiphoid to the anterior vulvar commissure to orient the midline and position of the new umbilicus (Fig. 122-36). Two lines perpendicular to X-X′ are placed: one at the pubic level, 5 to 7 cm from the vulvar commissure, and the second at the umbilical upper pole. Points 1 and 2 are equidistant from X′ and placed at the pubic level, bilaterally. The distance between them is 10 to 16 cm, depending on the size of the pubis.

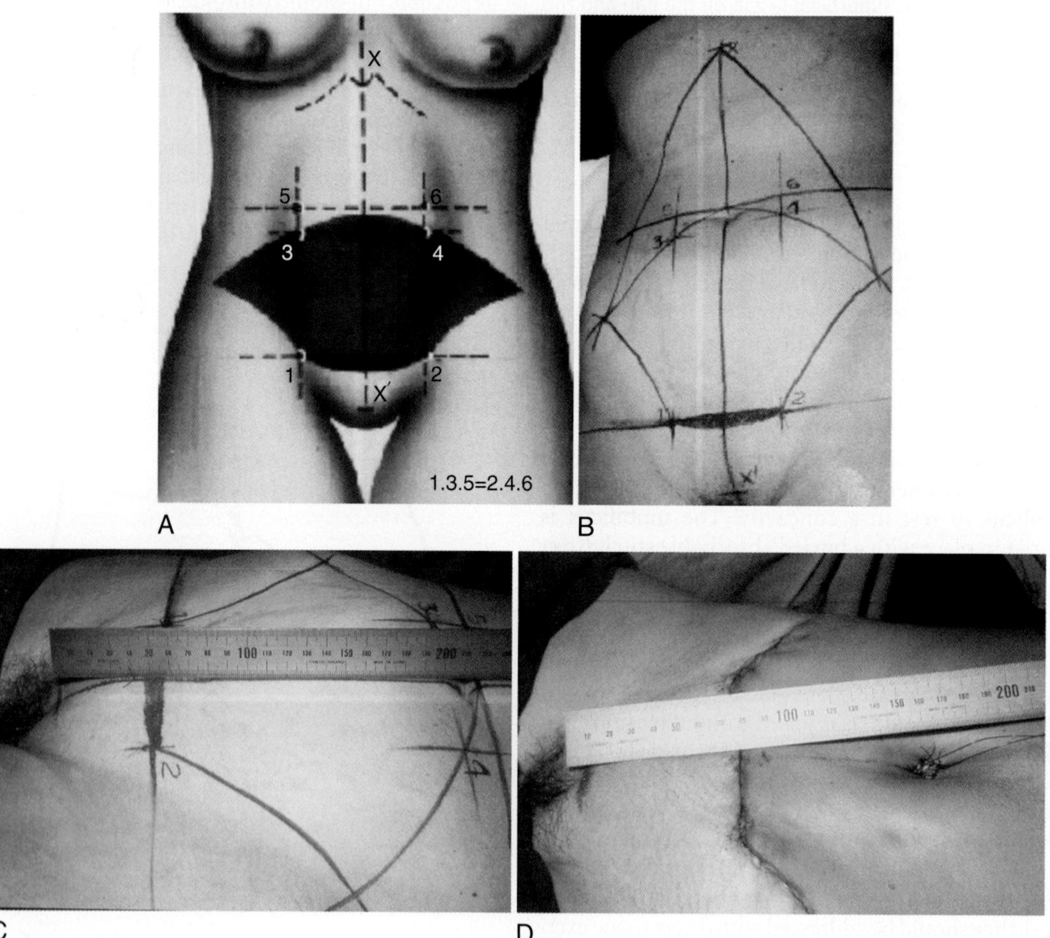

FIGURE 122-36. *A* and *B*, Schematic of patient's marking for traditional abdominoplasty with the bicycle handlebar incision. *C*, Close-up view of the ruler placed along X-X′ to show the distance of 7 cm from the vulvar commissure to the pubic transverse incision line before the surgery. *D*, The same distance measured to the suture line at the end of the procedure.

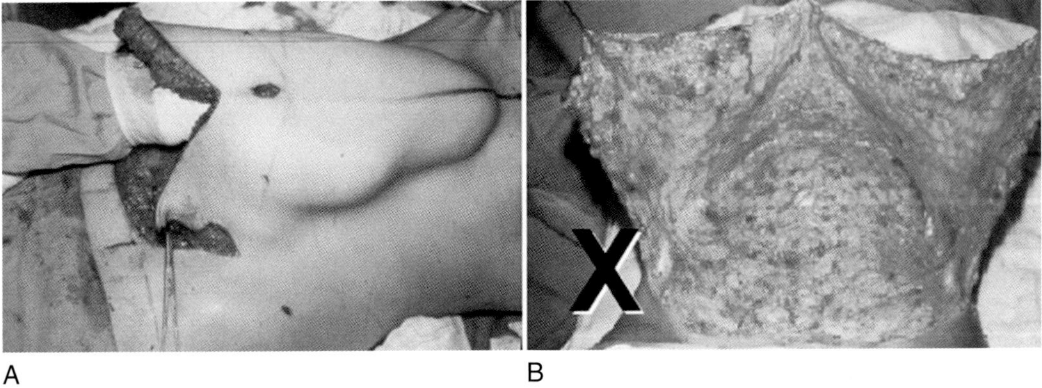

A B

FIGURE 122-37. *A,* The surgeon's hand shows the limited amount of skin flap undermining, mostly located in the epigastrium. *B,* Type of excessive undermining that is no longer recommended.

Points 5 and 6 reproduce points 1 and 2 at the transverse umbilical line. The distance from point 1 to point 5 should be equal to the distance from point 2 to point 6. From points 1 and 2, a concave, curved line is drawn toward the anterior superior iliac spine, bilaterally. The lateral segments and the transverse pubic line together form the bicycle handlebar incision.

From the umbilicus, a concave line is drawn and reaches the extremities of both lateral branches at the iliac spine. From points 5 and 6, a vertical line angled toward points 1 and 2 touches the superior curved lines at points 3 and 4, respectively (1 to 3 to 5 should be equal to 2 to 4 to 6). These reference lines and points are fundamental for symmetric resection of excess skin bilaterally. The superior concave curved line and the inferior handlebar together delineate an elliptical area that is resected from the hypogastric region. From point 1 to point 2 (the darkened, arrow-type segment) is 1 cm wide. This area represents an extra amount of skin resection at the end of the surgery in which the pubic suture can be placed even lower (see Fig. 122-36). Finally, points 1, 2, 3, and 4 receive a provisionary stitch used as a reference point when the skin flap is stretched caudally for the resection of skin excess because the ink markings often fade during the surgery.

INCISION AND UNDERMINING

The skin incision is made along the handlebar line down to the fascial plane. Skin flap undermining is performed along the muscular fascial plane up to the umbilicus (Fig. 122-37). Meticulous hemostasis is maintained. The umbilicus is dissected with its stalk from the surrounding fat, and a circular incision 1 cm in diameter resects the umbilicus from the skin abdominal flap (Fig 122-38). The skin flap is then undermined up to the xiphoid. The undermined portion along with the vertex at the xiphoid and the base of the handlebar forms a triangle. The

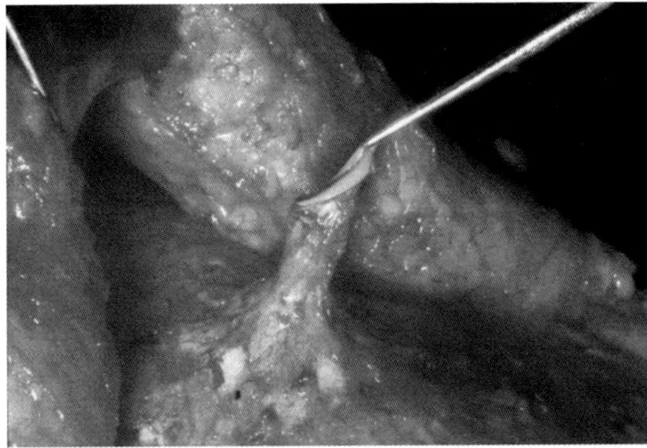

A

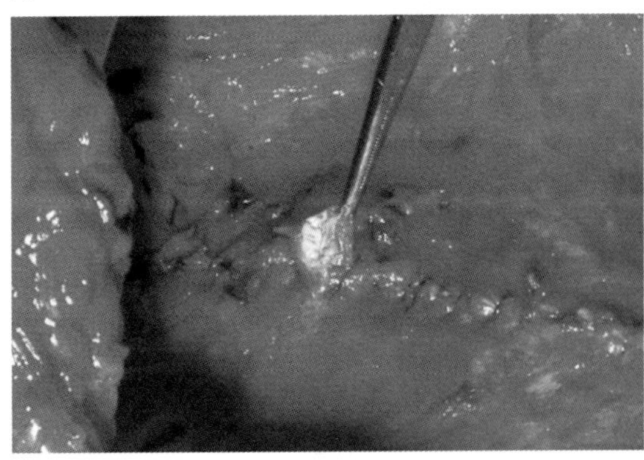

B

FIGURE 122-38. *A* and *B,* Close-up view of the umbilical pedicle dissected; a skin island, 1 cm in diameter, is preserved on the pedicle stalk. After muscle plication, the umbilical skin island is anchored to the flap by sutures placed at the fascial level, shortening the umbilical stalk.

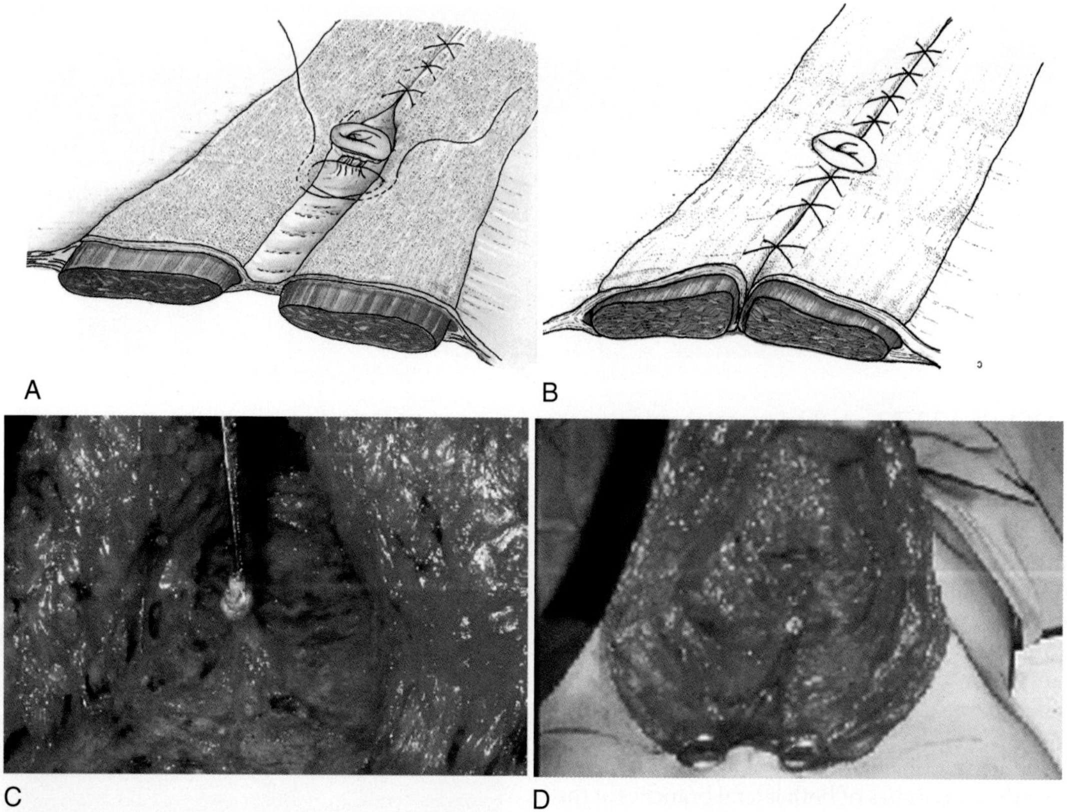

FIGURE 122-39. *A* and *B*, Schematic representation of rectus fascia plication performed in two levels. *C* and *D*, Close-up view of the plication. The umbilical stalk is shortened, and the skin island is placed at the fascial level. The tunnel-like undermining of the epigastrium becomes narrow and frequently bulges, requiring additional undermining laterally.

supraumbilical skin undermining is narrow, staying a few centimeters away from the rectus abdominis external edge limits. Wide lateral undermining is not recommended.

FASCIAL PLICATION

Fascial plication is performed in two layers; the first layer is sutured with interrupted 2-0 nylon stitches and the second with continuous 0 Prolene sutures. The umbilical stalk is telescoped to leave the skin island placed at the fascial level. This maneuver is performed with two stitches, one at the upper and the other at the lower umbilical pole. The stitches bite the fascia on each side and the lower dermis of the skin island. When the stitches are tightened, the skin island remains at the fascial level. The continuous 0 Prolene suture stops 3 cm above the umbilicus and should begin 3 cm below it. Contamination may occur through the umbilicus if this detail is not followed (Fig. 122-39).

EXCESS SKIN RESECTION

Excess skin is resected with the patient placed between 30 and 40 degrees of flexion. When the skin is stretched caudally, the excess flap tissue overlaps the pubis and the lateral incision branches (see Fig. 122-22). Skin wrinkling is often seen along the lateral aspect of the trunk bilaterally because of the limited lateral undermining after fascial plication. In addition, a slight bulging of the epigastrium may be seen. These irregularities are easily removed by additional lateral undermining or by establishing several tunnels by use of scissors oriented transversely along the trunk and parallel to the orientation of the vessels. After this maneuver, the skin flaps are released, the wrinkles disappear, and dead space is minimized. Making several parallel tunnels helps preserve the skin flap blood supply.

Three different situations exist for the skin excess resection as explained in the following discussion.

1. The umbilical donor site on the flap extends beyond the pubic transverse incision. When the skin flap is stretched caudally, the umbilical skin hole extends beyond the pubic transverse incision in around 77% of patients. The skin flap is incised along the line X-X′ up to the desired point for excess resection, whether it reaches the

umbilical hole or not (see Fig. 122-22). A mattress stitch is placed to fix the flap to the pubis. Two half skin flaps are obtained. Each half-flap is also incised vertically up to the desired level where point 3-5 with its provisionary point is used as reference for symmetric future resection. Point 4-6 is also used as reference when the incision reaches that level. Two other mattress stitches are placed from these reference points to points 1 and 2 bilaterally. Four flaps are obtained, and then the excess skin is resected (Fig. 122-40).

2. The umbilical hole partially overlaps the pubic transverse incision. When this situation occurs, the skin flap is incised vertically in the midline to obtain two half-flaps. The extension of the umbilical hole above the transverse pubic incision is estimated, and then a mattress stitch is placed to fix the flap at the level of the future inverted T compensation. After this, each flap is incised according to the previously described procedure and the excess resected. The vertical donor site closure may be 1 to 4 cm in length, according to the residual amount of the skin hole that did not surpass the pubis. The closure of the umbilical donor site is performed in three layers: subcutaneous, intradermal, and cuticular. These sutures avoid dimples and dead space above the pubic line. This vertical closure is done in approximately 17% of patients (Fig. 122-41).
3. The umbilical donor site defect does not reach the pubic incision. In only 6% of patients, the umbilical hole does not reach the pubic incision. This occurs when there is no flaccid skin, in secondary abdominoplasty, and in patients in whom the umbilicus is too high (22 to 25 cm from the anterior vulvar commissure). This possibility should be considered before the median vertical incision is performed. The incision along line X-X′ (i.e., vertical midline) extends cephalad only to the point where the flap can reach the lower incision. The skin hole is closed vertically in three layers. The rest of the skin excess resection is performed routinely. The vertical umbilical donor site closure length varies from 3 to 4 cm (Fig. 122-42; see also Fig. 122-19).

UMBILICOPLASTY[46,47]

Umbilicoplasty is performed after the skin flap excesses are resected and positioned with three mattress sutures. The tip of a Kocher clamp is placed biting the dermis below the umbilical skin island, and the clamp should remain below the skin flap to be used as a reference point for placement of the umbilicus in the correct position. The surgeon should be able to feel the Kocher tip and the umbilicus under the flap. This projection is marked on the skin (Fig. 122-43*A*). The distance between the vulvar commissure and the new umbilical position should measure between 16 and 18 cm. A 2-cm transverse incision is made at the point of the Kocher tip projection. After this incision, the mattress sutures and the Kocher clamp are removed. The skin flap is everted, and a small circular area is defatted around the incision (Fig. 122-43*B*). Four stitches with 2-0 nylon are placed at 12-, 3-, 6-, and 9-o'clock positions. The sutures should be placed near the incision edge, bite the fascia under the skin island, fix the skin island in position, and emerge through the skin hole (Fig. 122-43*C* and *D*). They remain loose until the adhesion sutures are applied and the incision edges are sutured to the deeper fascial layer. Often, an asymmetric suture line and fat thickness are observed. When an asymmetric suture line is observed, fat trimming below Scarpa's fascia

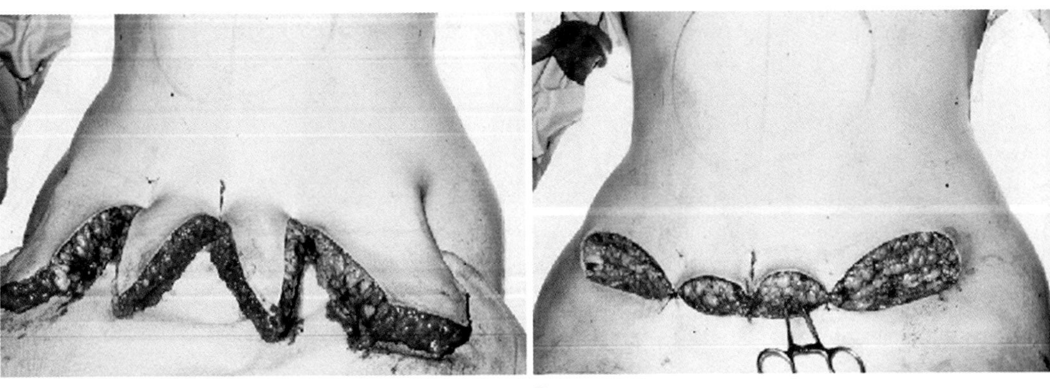

FIGURE 122-40. *A* and *B*, Excess skin resection and placement of stay sutures in preparation for umbilicoplasty procedure.

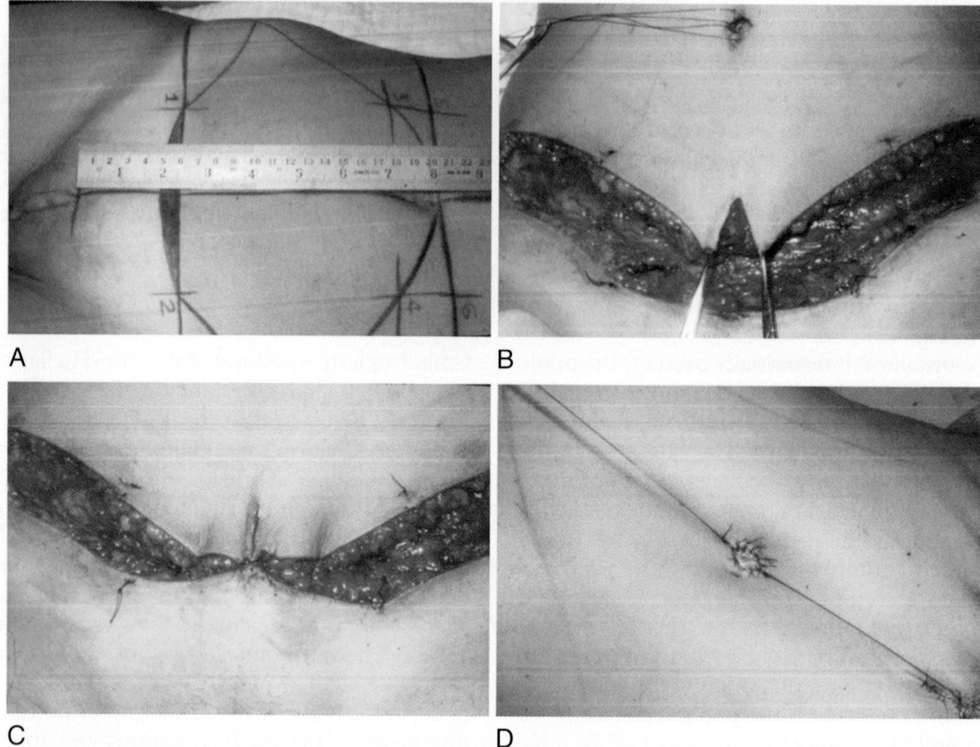

FIGURE 122-41. *A,* The transverse pubic incision is measured with a ruler and placed 7 cm from the vulvar commissure. The closure must also be the same distance from the vulvar commissure. *B* and *C,* The umbilical donor site should be closed in three layers: subcutaneous, dermal, and cuticular. Dead space should be avoided. *D,* After the umbilicus is sutured to the skin flap, two lines of sutures, at 12- and 6-o'clock, remain in place for 2 days and serve as a tie-over bandage. (See Figure 122-20 for preoperative and postoperative views.)

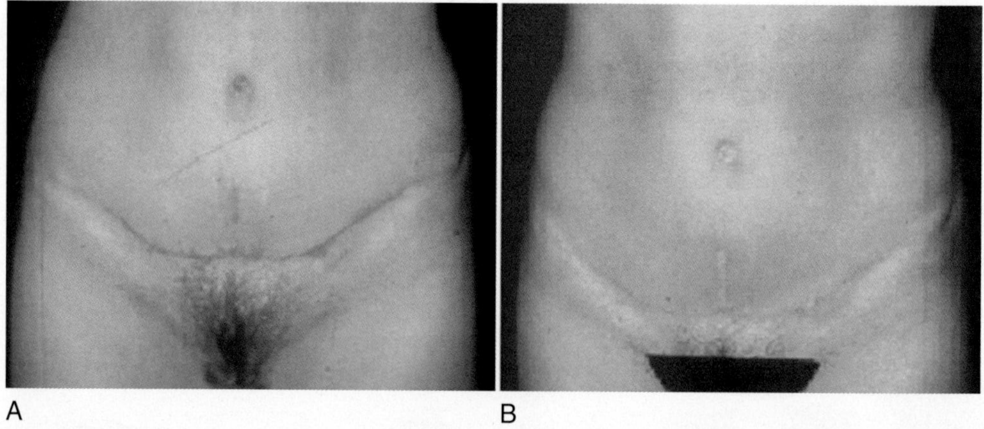

FIGURE 122-42. Postoperative views of similar types of abdominoplasty procedures in which the umbilical scar was placed at the midline between the new umbilicus and the pubic transverse scar. *A,* The patient is seen 6 months postoperatively. *B,* The patient is seen 2 years postoperatively. Note significant fading of scar.

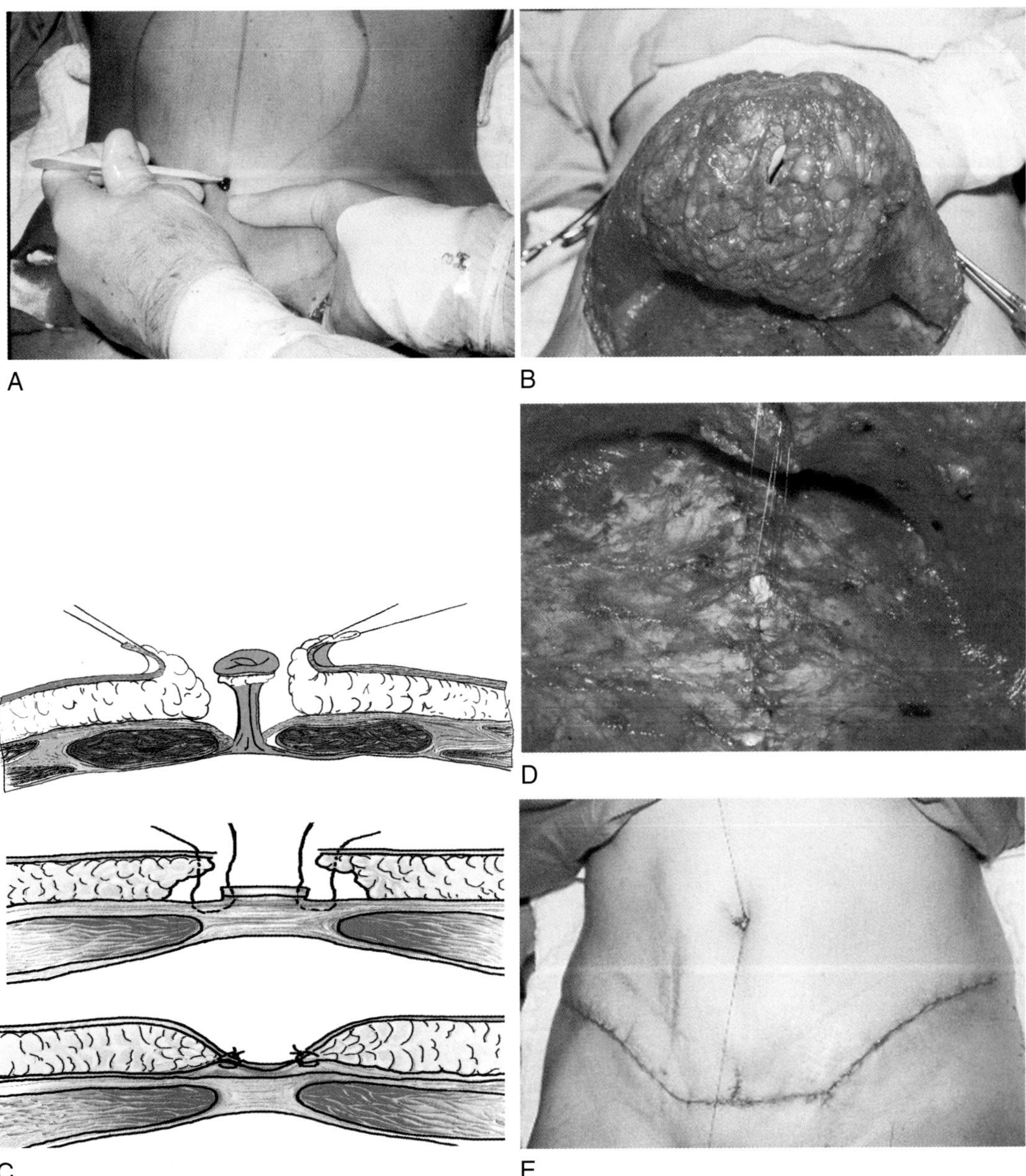

FIGURE 122-43. Umbilicoplasty. *A,* The nondominant hand of the surgeon reaches under the skin flap to touch the umbilical skin projection while the blade in the dominant hand makes the transverse incision (approximately 2 cm in length) on the skin flap. *B,* The flap is everted, and the fat below the incision is resected. *C,* Schematic illustration of umbilical fixation to the skin through the overlying skin island. *D,* Close-up view of the sutures, skin island, and muscular fascia. *E,* Final closure of abdominoplasty site and suturing of umbilical skin island to overlying skin flap. Note the invagination.

with scissors and revision of the incision edges should be performed for symmetry (Fig. 122-44). After this maneuver, the four "cardinal" stitches are tightened. Another six to eight isolated 4-0 nylon stitches complete the suture. Skin invagination of the flap at the umbilical area occurs, establishing a natural-appearing navel (Fig. 122-43*E*). When closure at the handlebar line is completed, a small gauze pad with ointment is placed in the umbilicus and tightened with the lines of the sutures at 12- and 6-o'clock (as a tie-over bolster). The gauze bandage should remain in place for 2 to 3 days.

ADHESION SUTURES

Interrupted sutures with 3-0 Vicryl are applied from the xiphoid down to the handlebar incision. The sutures are placed approximately 4 cm apart and distributed in columns and lines.[48] This procedure requires 30 to 34 sutures and takes approximately 20 minutes to complete. The skin flap becomes completely attached to the fascia. The skin flap should not slide, and there is no dead space. Drains are not required. After the adhesion sutures are placed from the xiphoid to the umbilical level, the umbilicoplasty is performed. After umbilicoplasty, the adhesion stitches are continued to the inferior extent of the flap (Fig. 122-45).

CLOSURE AND DRESSINGS

The suture of the skin to the lower wedge incision is performed in three layers. Deep interrupted subcutaneous 2-0 or 3-0 Vicryl sutures, similar to the adhesion sutures, bite the muscular fascia, fat, and superficial fascia together. No dead space should be left below this suture. A second dermal layer of isolated 3-0 Vicryl sutures is placed to better adjust the edges. Finally, a running cuticular 4-0 Vicryl suture completes the closure.

Dressings include Micropore, which covers the suture line, and abdominal pads placed over the abdominal segment. The patient wears an elastic girdle for 30 days. The girdle is removed only for baths and hygiene. The umbilical stitches are removed after 2 weeks.

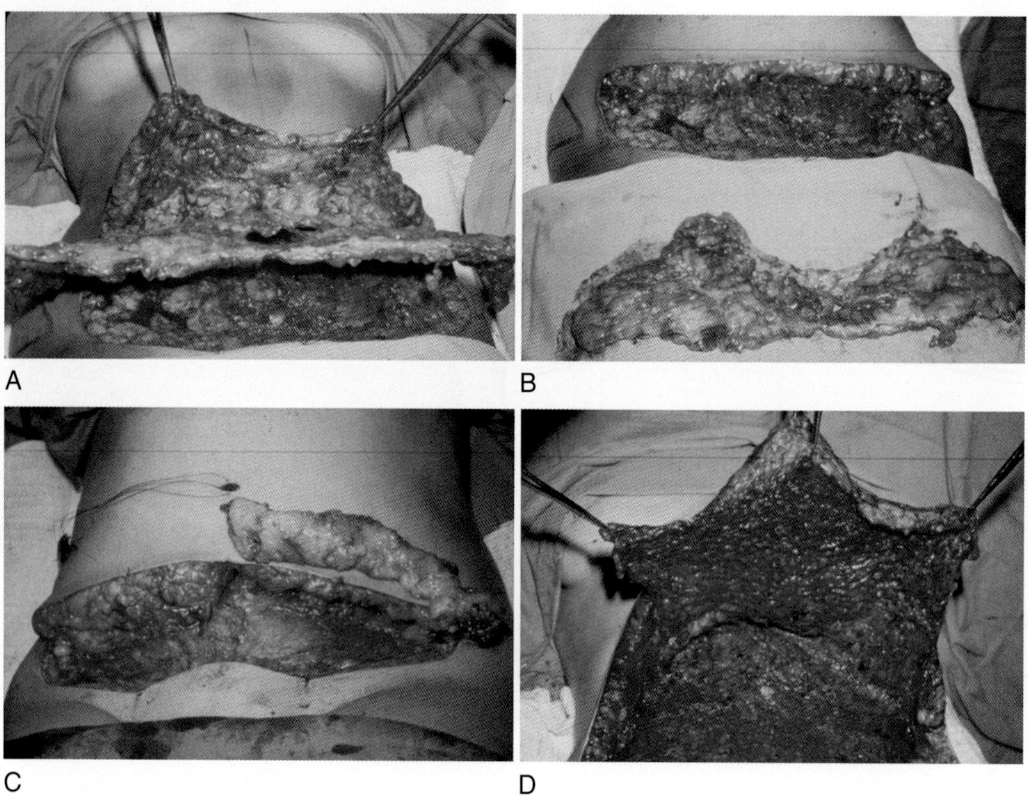

FIGURE 122-44. Fat trimming. *A* to *D*, The abdominal flap can be thinned by trimming the fat deep to Scarpa's fascia with scissors.

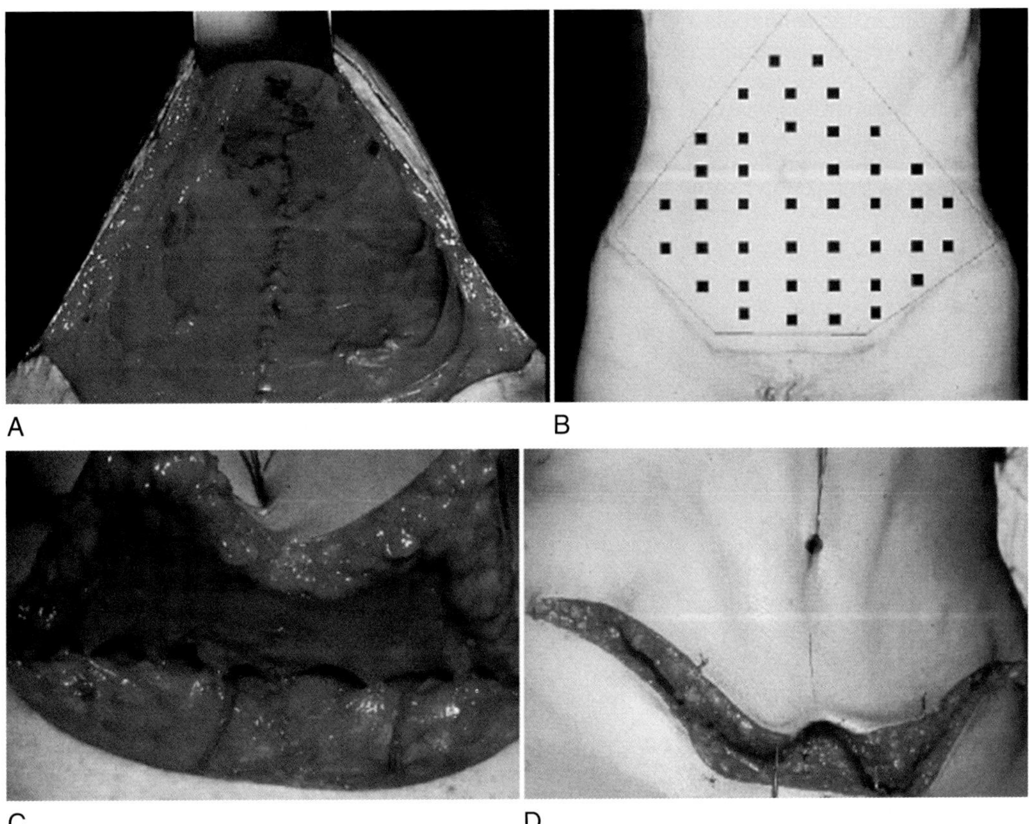

FIGURE 122-45. *A* and *B*, Close-up views of skin flap undermining. *C*, As diagrammed, the dead space is collapsed by adhesion stitches placed in lines and columns. *D*, Intraoperative view of adhesion stitches and closure. Using this technique, Dr. Baroudi has not needed drains since 1998.

Technical Variations and Refinements

HIGH LATERAL TENSION ABDOMINOPLASTY

Lockwood[41] first pointed out that because the linea alba is adherent in the epigastrium, the tissues there resist sagging and are the least lax. Noting the bulging and drape of lax tissue over the horizontal zones of adherence at the hip-thigh junction in women and the flank in men, he suggested that the best contour improvement in abdominoplasty would be achieved by focusing tissue resection laterally rather than medially as in the traditional abdominoplasty. In the classic abdominoplasty, wide undermining is taken to the costal margins to advance tissue sufficiently. With the high lateral tension abdominoplasty, the focus is on resecting the area of laxity, not on avoiding an umbilical closure site through a tight central closure (Fig. 122-46). This technique achieves a number of objectives: it takes tension off the central portion of the flap, which is the most susceptible to ischemia; it resects more of the lax lateral tissue, improving the waistline; and it can provide a noticeable lift to both the medial and lateral thighs. The keys to this technique are limited paramedian epigastric undermining to provide a tunnel for fascial repair; discontinuous undermining with scissor spreading or cannula dissection as needed for smooth draping; tissue excision pattern with emphasis on lateral resection; permanent suture repair of the superficial fascial system along the entire incision; and liberal adjunctive liposuction in the upper abdomen and lateral and posterior trunk.[41] The upper incision is marked preoperatively, but final tissue resection is determined with use of Pitanguy forceps to adjust and mark the flap under moderate inferomedial tension. These techniques together allow safe concurrent abdominoplasty with liposuction,

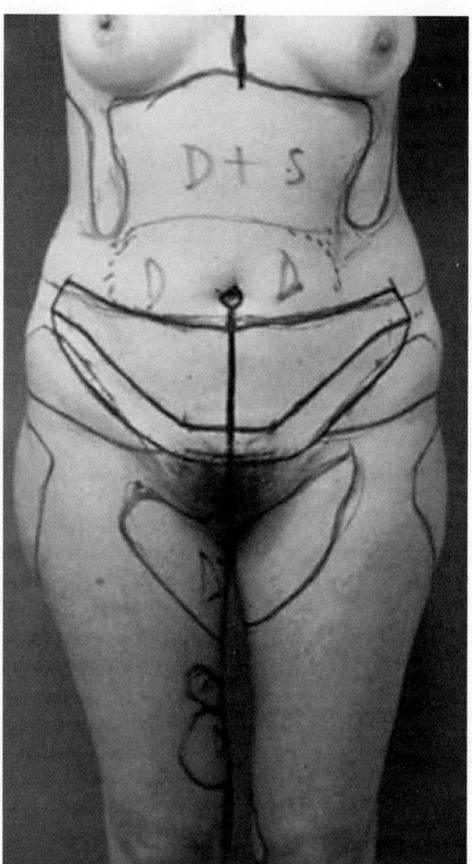

FIGURE 122-46. Typical markings for the high lateral tension abdominoplasty. (From Lockwood TE: Maximizing aesthetics in lateral-tension abdominoplasty and body lifts. Clin Plast Surg 2004;31:523.)

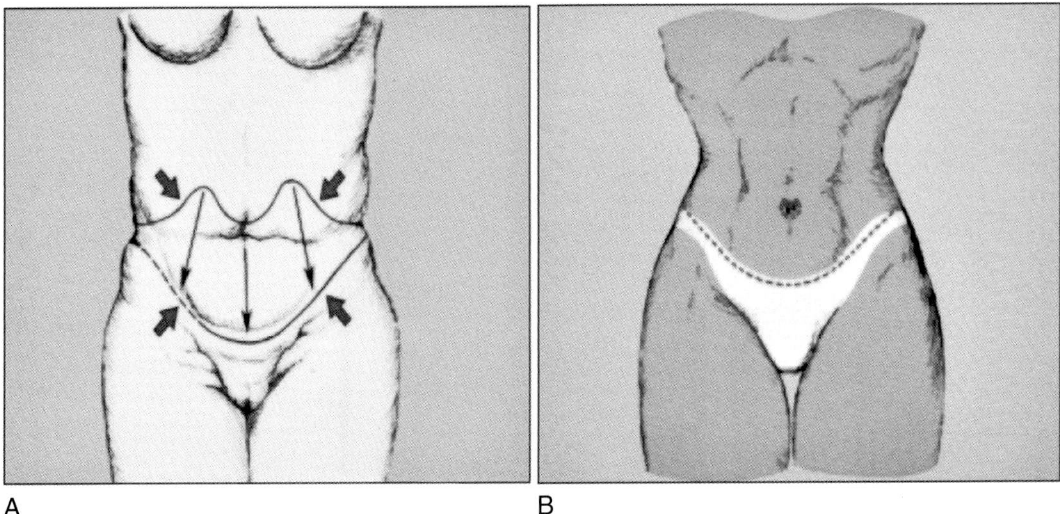

FIGURE 122-47. *A,* Preoperative U-M abdominoplasty markings. The open U starts low in the pubis and is oriented toward the waistline. The lazy M has its highest points around the umbilicus. Large arrows indicate the approximate matching points for closure. Small arrows indicate the orientation of the manual shifting of the upper flaps to decrease tension toward the central flap. *B,* Postoperative result of U-M abdominoplasty. The final incision is inside the bikini line. (From Ramirez OM: U-M abdominoplasty. Aesthetic Surg J 1999;19:279. Reproduced with permission from The American Society for Aesthetic Plastic Surgery, Inc.)

significant tissue resection, and lift while minimizing tension on the dermal closure as well as promoting a thin scar.

The high lateral tension abdominoplasty requires careful marking of the inferior incision while the patient is standing, with elevation of ptotic tissue to the anticipated level at closure to avoid an elevation of the final scar. The superficial fascial system is reapproximated with permanent sutures to reduce tension on the dermis and to prevent spreading of the underlying tissues, which can result in a tissue depression under the scar. As the maximal excision is more lateral than medial, the defect left by the original umbilical site on the flap may not always be excised at flap closure. This former umbilical site should be closed with a vertical slit in layers to avoid a depression at this site.

With the lateral tension abdominoplasty design, it is difficult to avoid lateral tissue dog-ears even with judicious flank liposuction because of the obtuse lateral closure angle. The U-M dermolipectomy, developed by Ramirez,[26] avoids the lateral dog-ear at the expense of a somewhat longer incision, incorporating the high lateral tension concept in an excision pattern that matches upper and lower incision length (Figs. 122-47 and 122-48).

ABDOMINOPLASTY WITHOUT UNDERMINING

The concept behind abdominoplasty without undermining is to allow maximal lipocontouring and abdominal skin resection without risking the abdominal vasculature. The traditional abdominoplasty involves dividing the trans-rectus epigastric perforators, which are the main circulation to the abdominal wall, during elevation of the abdominal flap to the costal margin. The remaining circulation to the flap is from the lateral intercostal vessels, which can be damaged by improper liposuction. Techniques to avoid injury to the intercostal vessels include hyperinfiltration of the tissues before suctioning, suctioning deep to the superficial fascial system, and suctioning parallel to the vessels. The no-undermining technique first described by Illouz[49] avoids this issue by preserving the epigastric blood supply. Liposuction deep to the superficial fascial system preserves the blood supply while allowing the abdominal flap to slide caudally for tension-free closure. Because the entire circulation to the flap is maintained, extensive liposuction can be performed without concern for abdominal skin viability (see Fig. 122-24).

Avelar[29] described a lenticular skin-only resection, followed by deep (below Scarpa's fascia) and superficial suction of the subcutaneous tissue left after resection, and deep-only suctioning of the epigastrium, flanks, and suprapubic region. Fascial plication, if needed, is performed through a circumumbilical incision. The technique aims to preserve the vascular and lymphatic circulation, reducing risk of ischemia and seroma while reducing flap thickness and allowing flap advancement. Epigastric skin laxity is addressed by bilateral inframammary crescentic excisions, thus

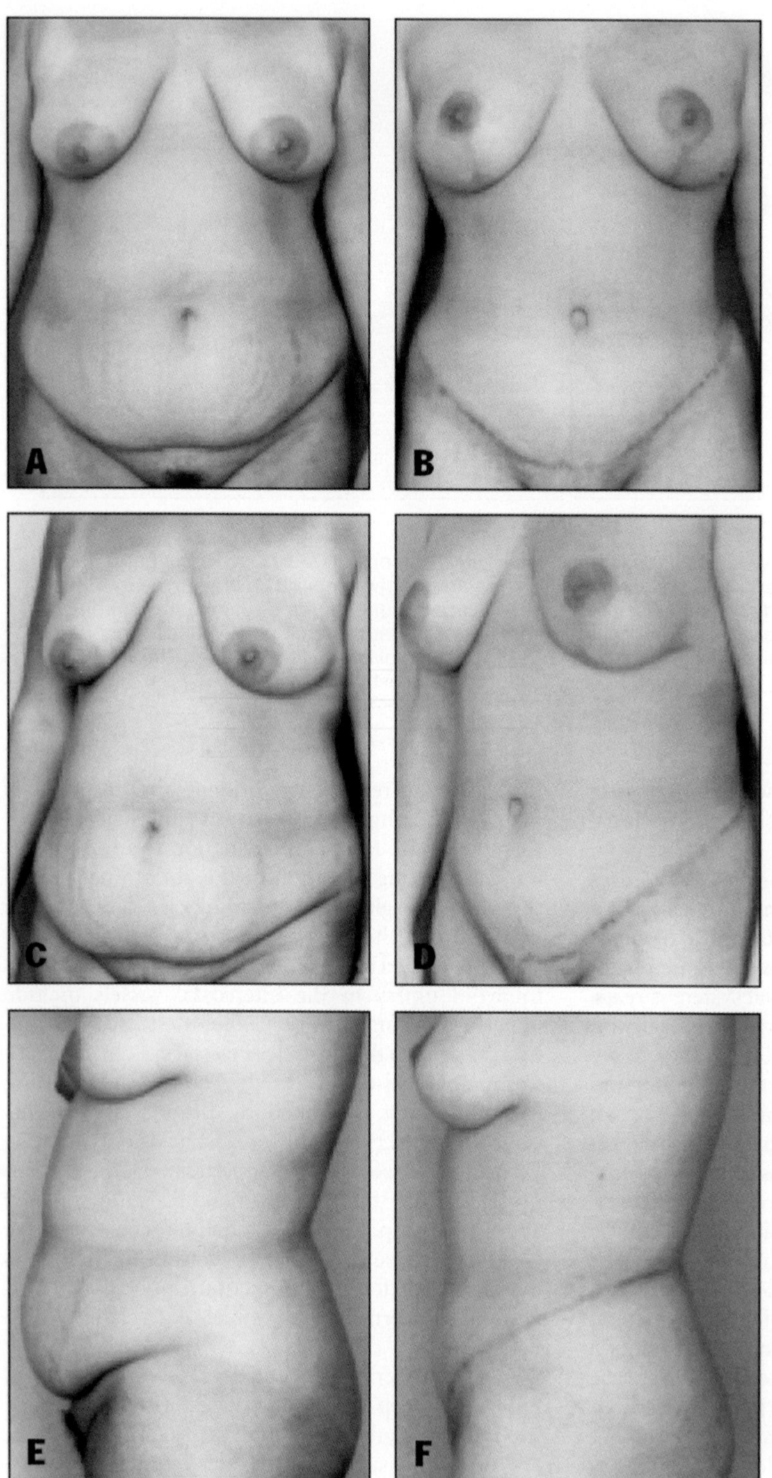

FIGURE 122-48. *A, C,* and *E,* Preoperative views of a 31-year-old woman. Observe the hanging panniculus and hanging abdominal apron over the pubis and groin as well as the loose ptotic pubis. Note also the volume of the abdomen and excess tissue on the upper thighs. *B, D,* and *F,* Postoperative views at 14 months after U-M abdominoplasty. Rectus plication, umbilicoplasty, and suction-assisted liposuction of the entire abdomen and waistline were performed. The patient also had augmentation mastopexy for tuberous hypoplastic breasts. Observe the reduction in the waistline and the orientation of the incisional scars as well as the lifting effect on the pubis and anterolateral thigh. Note the reduction of abdominal volume and reduction of striae. Observe the change in shape of the pubis to a more youthful one. The incision ends on the posterior aspect of the waistline silhouette and does not continue circumferentially. (From Ramirez OM: U-M abdominoplasty. Aesthetic Surg J 1999;19:279. Reproduced with permission from The American Society for Aesthetic Plastic Surgery, Inc.)

allowing the umbilicus to be preserved in its location. A variation of this technique avoids submammary incisions but requires umbilical transposition.[30] The procedure is performed through liposuction of the abdomen and flanks, followed by skin-only resection of the premarked lenticular excision. A 4-cm tunnel is made down the midline, and subcutaneous tissue is resected to reveal the fascia and allow plication. The umbilicus is reinset in the advanced flap (Fig. 122-49).

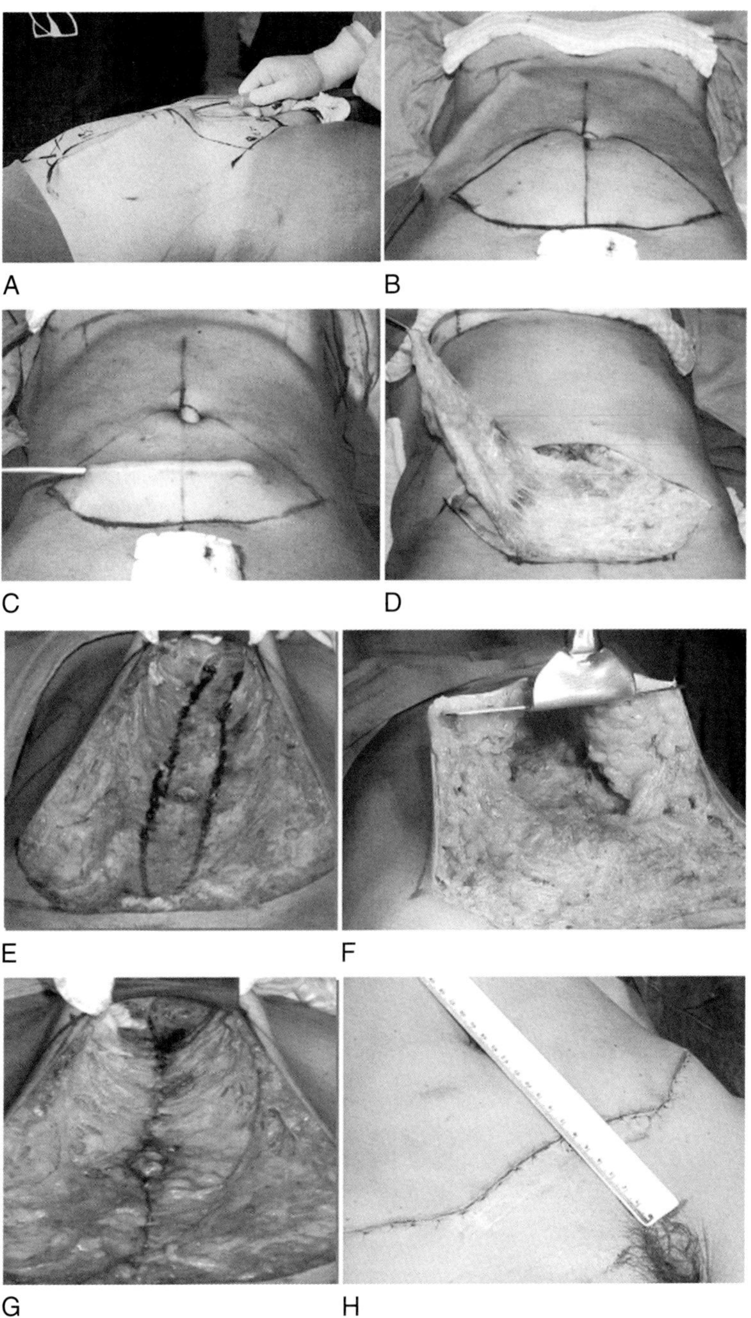

FIGURE 122-49. *A* to *C*, Liposuction proceeds from the region above the umbilicus (*A*) to the flanks (*B*) and the region below the umbilicus (*C*). *D*, Resection of the infraumbilical skin. *E* and *F*, A narrow tunnel is undermined to the sternum for diastasis rectus plication. *G*, After rectus plication, the exposed fascia is obliterated. *H*, The skin slides easily to cover the exposed area. The pubic closure is planed 7 cm from the vulvar commissure.

MINI-ABDOMINOPLASTY

The mini-abdominoplasty involves infraumbilical skin excision, infraumbilical undermining, and a suprapubic incision of varying length (Fig. 122-50). The mini-abdominoplasty is generally limited to those patients with minimal infraumbilical skin laxity without epigastric laxity (type 3) (Fig. 122-51), being originally designed to treat patients with lower abdominal deformities through a smaller incision.[23] Significant infraumbilical laxity, such as an infraumbilical pannus, may be treated with the mini-abdominoplasty in the appropriate patient (see Fig. 122-8). Infraumbilical fascial plication may be performed with this procedure; epigastric fascial laxity must be addressed with a more extensive technique. Some additional lateral flap dissection or midline liposuction is usually needed to avoid an unnatural midline bulge after rectus plication with this technique. Adjunctive procedures are performed as needed.

Baroudi Mini-Abdominoplasty Technique[50]

The mini-abdominoplasty is indicated for patients with moderate fat and excess skin in the hypogastrium. The patient may also have fat deposits and rectus muscle diastasis below the umbilicus. The epigastric muscle should be aesthetically normal, requiring no treatment (Fig. 122-52). The technique involves an elliptical skin resection transversely placed at the pubis, up to 7 cm above the vulvar anterior commissure. The width of the ellipse averages approximately 5 cm; greater amounts of skin resection leave longer scars. When fat deposits are present, the region to be suctioned should be marked while the patient is standing. With use of the pinch test near the pubis, an elliptical transverse area is outlined to evaluate the amount of skin to be resected.

The surgery is performed with the patient in the supine position and under epidural or general anesthesia. Saline solution with 1:500,000 epinephrine is infiltrated into the liposuction areas. Routine liposuction is performed, followed by skin resection. Skin undermining is limited to the amount of resection necessary, to minimize the dead space. Isolated adhesion sutures are applied as needed. The umbilicus remains untouched surgically. Occasionally, the dissection of the hypogastrium is taken up to the umbilical level if rectus muscle diastasis is present. Suction drains are not required. Standard dressings and a girdle are routinely used. The patient may stay in the hospital 24 hours or possibly go home the same day. Swelling in the abdominal area may persist for approximately 2 months postoperatively. Moderate exercises are allowed after postoperative day 45.

EXTENDED MINI-ABDOMINOPLASTY

The extended mini-abdominoplasty and the limited and modified abdominoplasty all lie within a spectrum of procedures used when skin cannot be resected

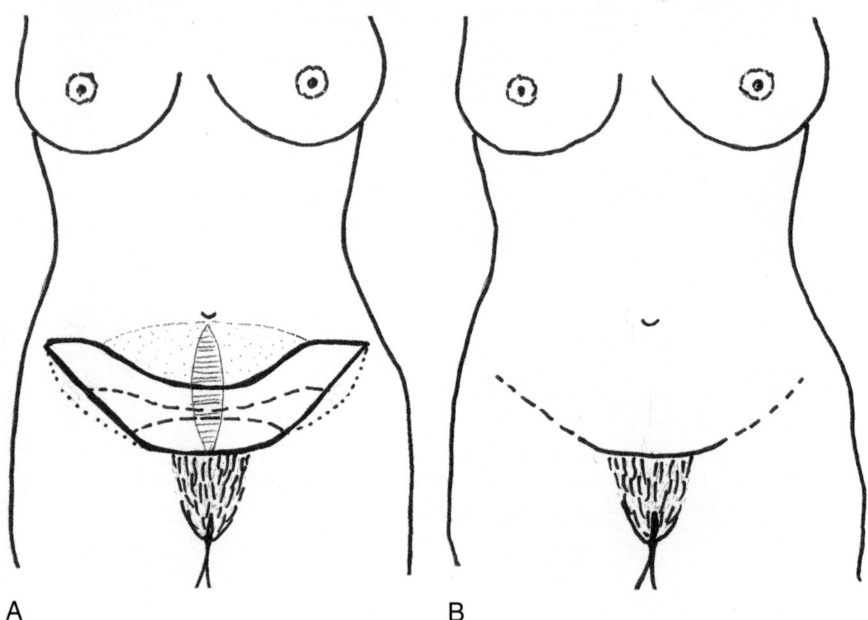

FIGURE 122-50. Mini-abdominoplasty involves tissue resection only in the hypogastrium. *A,* Dark line marks the excision. The dashed lines show lesser tissue excisions with smaller scars. The dotted line adds lateral resection to address lateral laxity. Shaded area is extent of undermining. Hatched area indicates infraumbilical rectus plication, which is performed as needed. *B,* Resulting scar may be of varying lengths. The umbilicus is untouched.

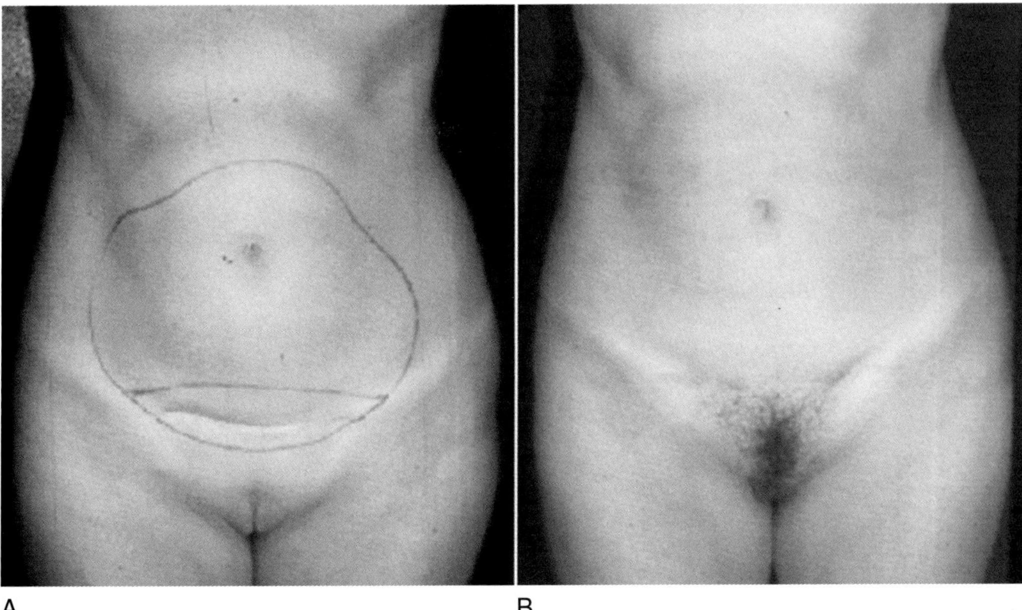

FIGURE 122-51. Preoperative view with markings *(A)* and postoperative view of a patient who underwent a mini-abdominoplasty procedure *(B)*. The transverse incision scar length is less than 18 cm, and surgery involved only liposuction and minor skin ellipse resection (less than 6 cm in width).

to the level of the umbilicus, when a smaller scar or no periumbilical scar is a priority, or when an upper abdominal scar precludes extensive epigastric flap elevation (Fig. 122-53). The procedures are scaled-back versions of the full abdominoplasty, with more limited undermining and often a shorter scar, but can include fascial plication of the epigastrium by use of a narrow midline suprafascial tunnel for access. Adjunctive liposuction is commonly used with the limited abdominoplasty. The umbilicus may be either transected (floated) or circumscribed and reinset on the flap with closure of the donor site. Strictly speaking, the "modified" procedure refers only to the limited abdominoplasty with the umbilical float. If resection of the excess skin will leave 13 cm or more of abdominal skin from the top of the mons to the umbilicus, the umbilicus can be released to gain access to the upper abdomen for plication and then reattached. Minor supraumbilical skin laxity can be aided by affixing the detached umbilical stalk up to 2 cm inferior to its original position, provided its new location is still at least 11 cm from the pubis. This is a good option when the original umbilical position is high. Alternatively, if the mons is high, the lower incision may be made in the hair-bearing skin to maintain an 11-cm hair-free section of lower abdomen while achieving adequate resection. If the original position of the umbilicus is less than 11 cm from the bottom of the flap, it should be left attached to the abdomen, circumscribed, and reinset into the advanced flap as for the full abdominoplasty. The umbilical donor site in the skin flap should be closed vertically in three layers, including the superficial fascia, to avoid a depression at the scar. The result will be a short vertical scar between the new umbilical site and the abdominoplasty closure that may be partially excised during flap advancement, resection, and closure (see Figs. 122-20 and 122-42).

Baroudi Extended Mini-Abdominoplasty Technique[50]

The extended mini-abdominoplasty is indicated for patients with moderate skin flaccidity of the supraumbilical and infraumbilical regions. Very often, rectus muscle diastasis is observed. The anesthesia (saline solution for infiltration) and skin marking for resection are similar to those for the mini-abdominoplasty (Fig. 122-54). Lipoplasty is performed with the patient in the supine position. The lower incision is made and the skin flap is then undermined up to the xiphoid. The umbilicus is amputated at its base. A tunnel-like access, opened by a retractor, allows viewing for muscle plication. After rectus plication and excess skin resection, the tunnel becomes narrow, and more wrinkling and possibly a skin bulge may be observed in the epigastrium and hypogastrium. Additional undermining is usually necessary to eliminate these problems. Isolated adhesion sutures are placed from the xiphoid down to the pubic incision. No drains are required. The umbilicus is sutured back to its original position or perhaps 1 to 3 cm caudad when only

Text continued on p. 165

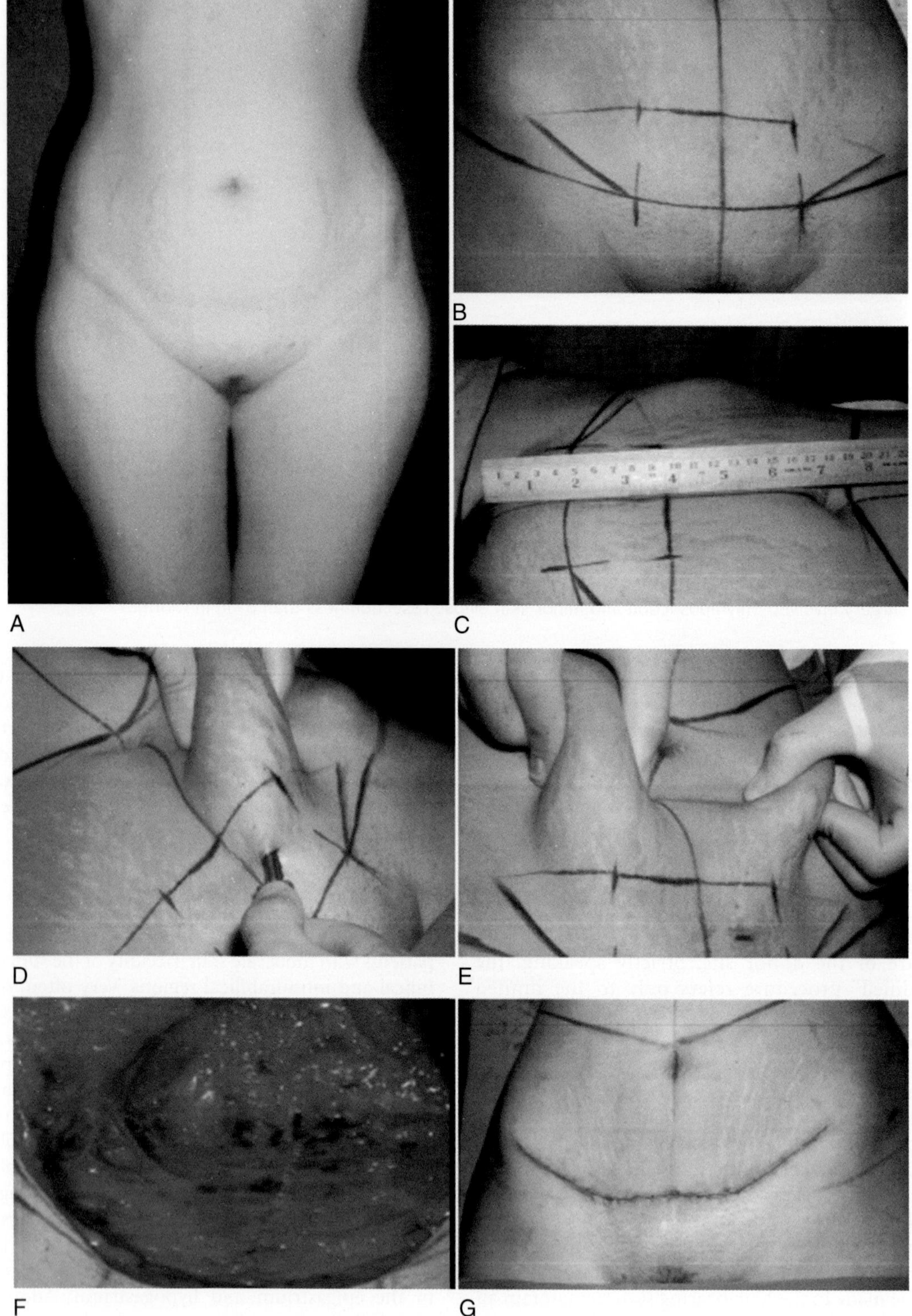

FIGURE 122-52. *A*, Preoperative view of a patient selected for mini-abdominoplasty that was not extended. *B* and *C*, Skin markings for resection and liposuction. *D* and *E*, Liposuction of the hypogastrium. In general, the liposuction stops after 60% of the local fat is removed. *F*, Close-up view of the skin flap dissection up to the umbilicus level; plication of the rectus fascia and placement of adhesion stitches to collapse the dead space. *G*, Curved closed suture line is approximately 18 cm. (See Fig. 122-10 for preoperative and postoperative views.)

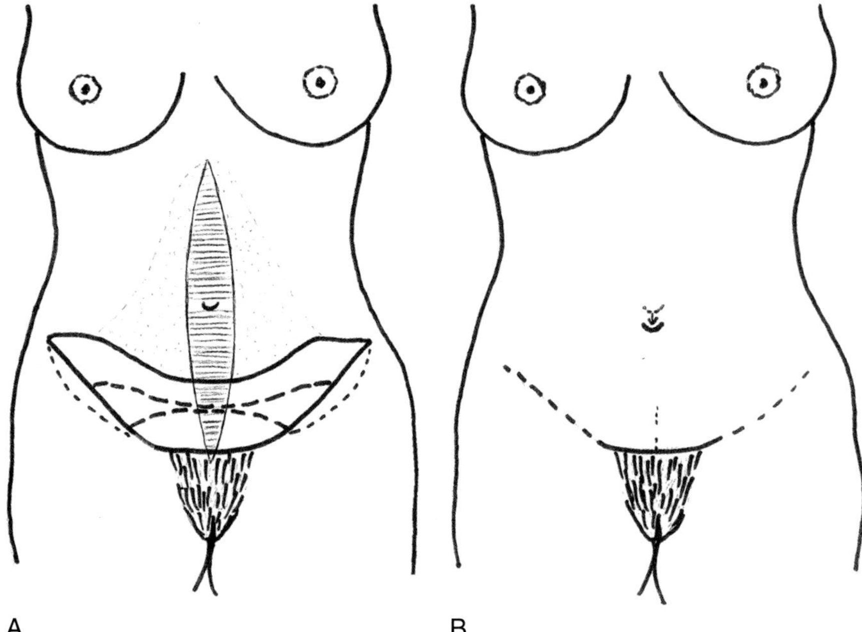

FIGURE 122-53. Extended mini-abdominoplasty manipulates the umbilicus to allow access to the epigastrium. *A,* Dark line marks the excision. The dashed lines show lesser amounts of tissue resection with smaller scars. The dotted line adds lateral resection to address lateral laxity. Shaded area is extent of undermining. Hatched area indicates rectus plication from costal margin to pubis, performed as needed. *B,* The umbilical stalk may be divided and the umbilical skin advanced caudally with the flap up to 2 cm (indicated by *arrow*) and sutured to the fascia. If greater advancement is needed, the umbilicus can be circumscribed and reinset into the advanced flap, as for full abdominoplasty. The resultant donor site defect on the flap is either partially excised and closed vertically in layers when the flap is advanced, or closed in layers as a vertical scar between the umbilicus and the pubic incision (*dotted lines*).

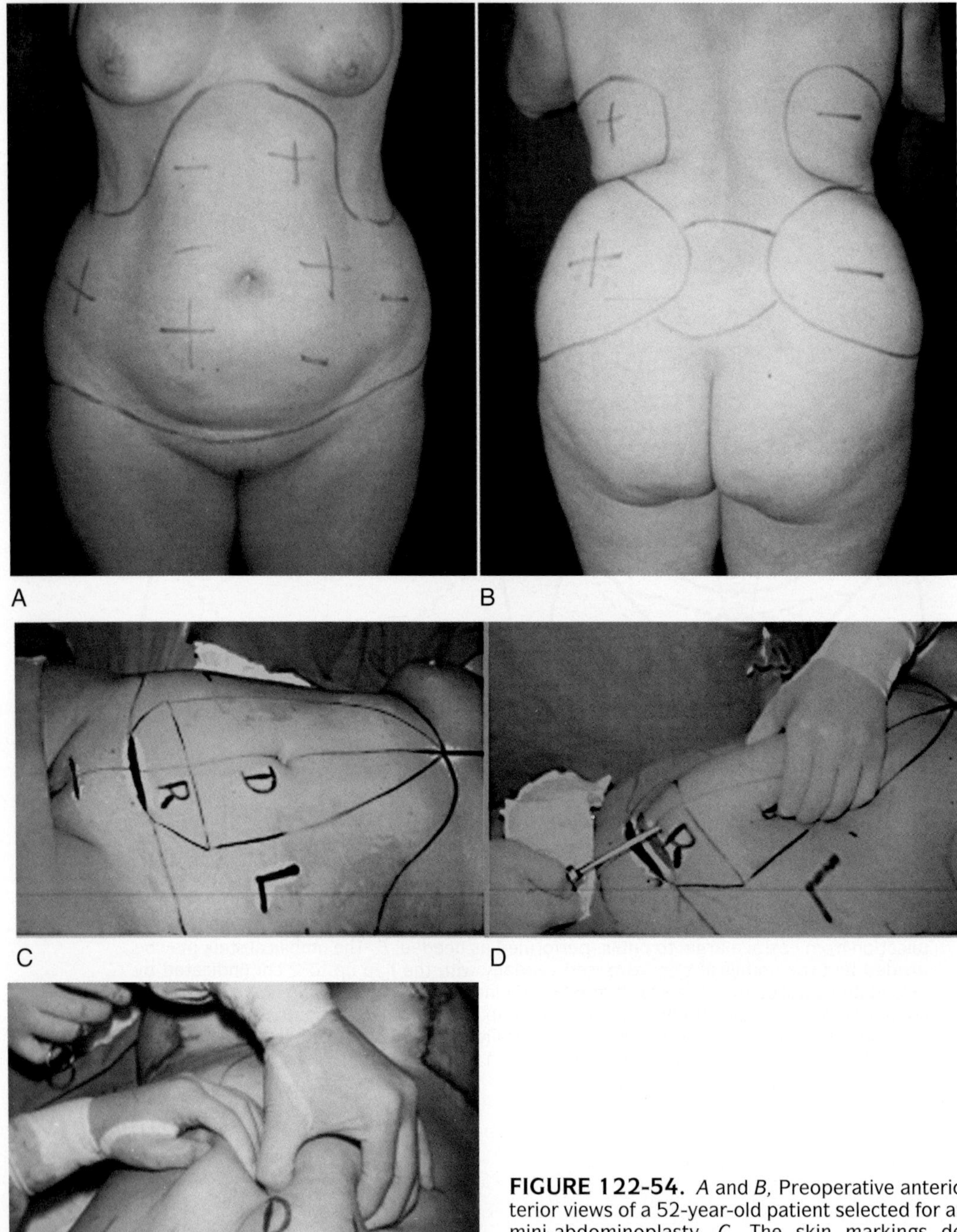

FIGURE 122-54. *A* and *B*, Preoperative anterior and posterior views of a 52-year-old patient selected for an extended mini-abdominoplasty. *C*, The skin markings demonstrate resection of a skin ellipse at the pubis and a triangular xiphoid-pubic area for liposuction, skin undermining, and diastasis recti plication. *D* and *E*, Liposuction stage—determining the excess removed by pinch test.

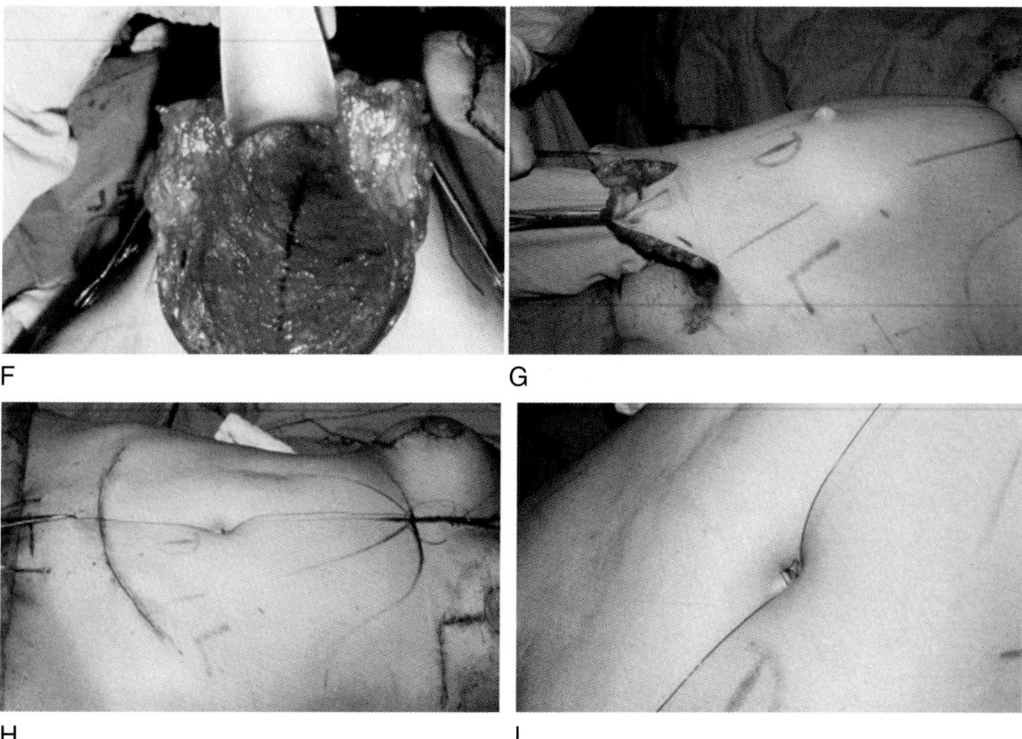

FIGURE 122-54, cont'd. *F,* Tunnel shape, skin undermining, and diastasis recti plication. *G,* The surgeon's hand inside the tunnel demonstrates the extent of the undermining, umbilical skin connection, and its stalk amputation. *H* and *I,* Final view of suture line and reimplantation of the umbilicus. *Continued*

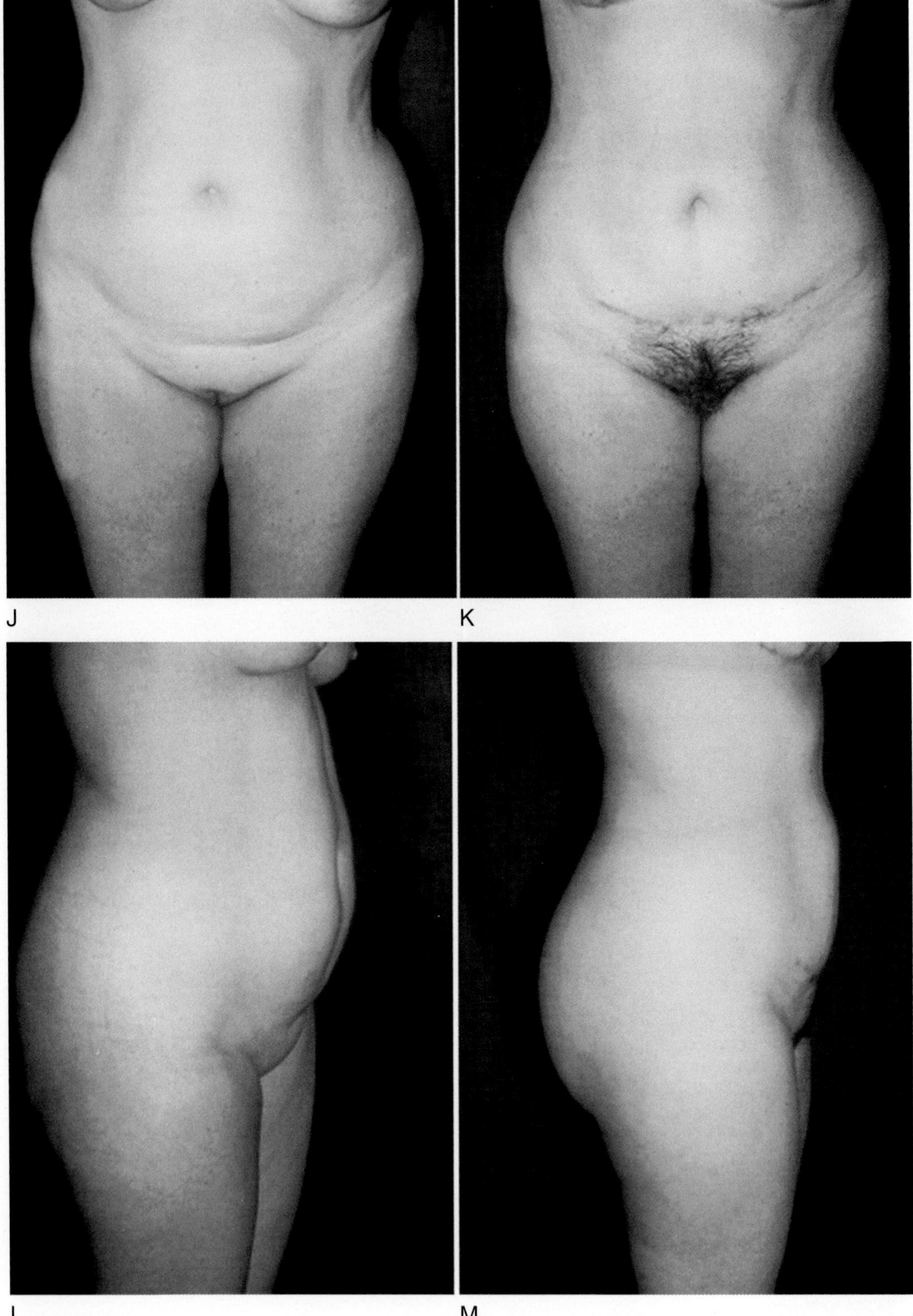

FIGURE 122-54, cont'd. *J* and *K,* Preoperative and postoperative anterior views. *L* and *M,* Preoperative and postoperative lateral views of the same patient.

a small skin ellipse is resected. Two isolated stitches, one at 3-o'clock and the other at 9-o'clock, are placed crossing the umbilicus skin, biting the fascia below and emerging again through the skin. When the stitches are tightened, the umbilical dimple is produced. A small gauze pad with ointment is tightened like a tie-over bolster. The gauze dressing is removed after 3 days, and the umbilical stitches are removed after 14 days. If the umbilicus will be placed in a lower position (less than 16 cm from the vulvar anterior commissure) because of the downward displacement of the flap, the umbilicus is circumscribed and separated from the skin, similar to a full abdominoplasty. The umbilical donor site defect is sutured closed and remains a few centimeters below the new position of the umbilicus. The umbilical stalk is replaced in the correct position as previously described. The closure and postoperative care are similar to those described for the mini-abdominoplasty.

The extended mini-abdominoplasty reduces the waistline and allows a greater amount of skin to be resected without increasing the length of the incision. The procedure is often indicated for patients with problems after parturition by cesarean delivery, secondary abdominoplasty, and limited skin flaccidity.

REVERSE ABDOMINOPLASTY

As its name implies, tissue resection in the reverse abdominoplasty is epigastric and results in inframammary scars (Fig. 122-55). The ideal candidate for reverse abdominoplasty has primarily upper epigastric laxity and either has preexisting epigastric scars from a prior breast reduction or will undergo simultaneous breast reduction or lift at the time of surgery (Fig. 122-56).[51]

The operation begins with an inframammary incision that is marked preoperatively (see Fig. 122-55). The abdominal flap is elevated off the pectoralis fascia, and dissection continues inferiorly to the umbilicus. The flap is pulled upward and the excess skin marked and excised, resulting in excision of a wedge of skin. Care must be taken to affix the superficial fascial system to the inframammary cohesion to prevent descent of the scar and inframammary line. Depending on the degree of laxity, the excision may cross midline or be restricted to bilateral inframammary crescentic excisions. Avelar described a variation in combination with a low transverse resection and no undermining, thereby preserving the position of the umbilicus on the flap.[29]

ENDOSCOPICALLY ASSISTED ABDOMINOPLASTY

The indications for endoscopically assisted abdominoplasty are limited to musculofascial defects without skin excess requiring excision and perhaps extended mini-abdominoplasty, where a limited incision can make access to the upper abdomen under direct vision difficult. An appropriate candidate is the male patient

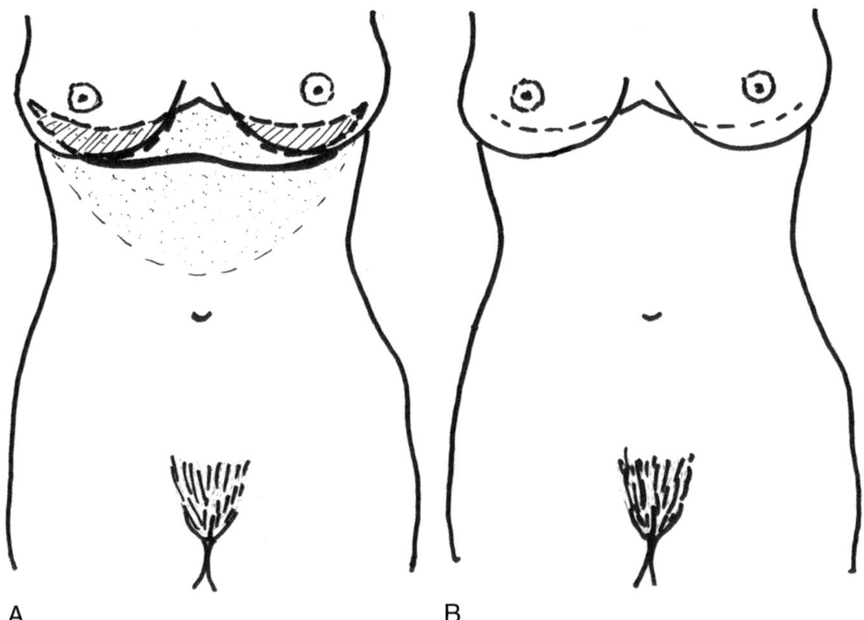

FIGURE 122-55. Reverse abdominoplasty. *A*, Excision pattern. This may be either bilateral crescent-shaped excisions (hatched area) at the inframammary fold for minimal epigastric skin laxity or a cross midline wedge excision, following the natural inframammary lines. *B*, Scar.

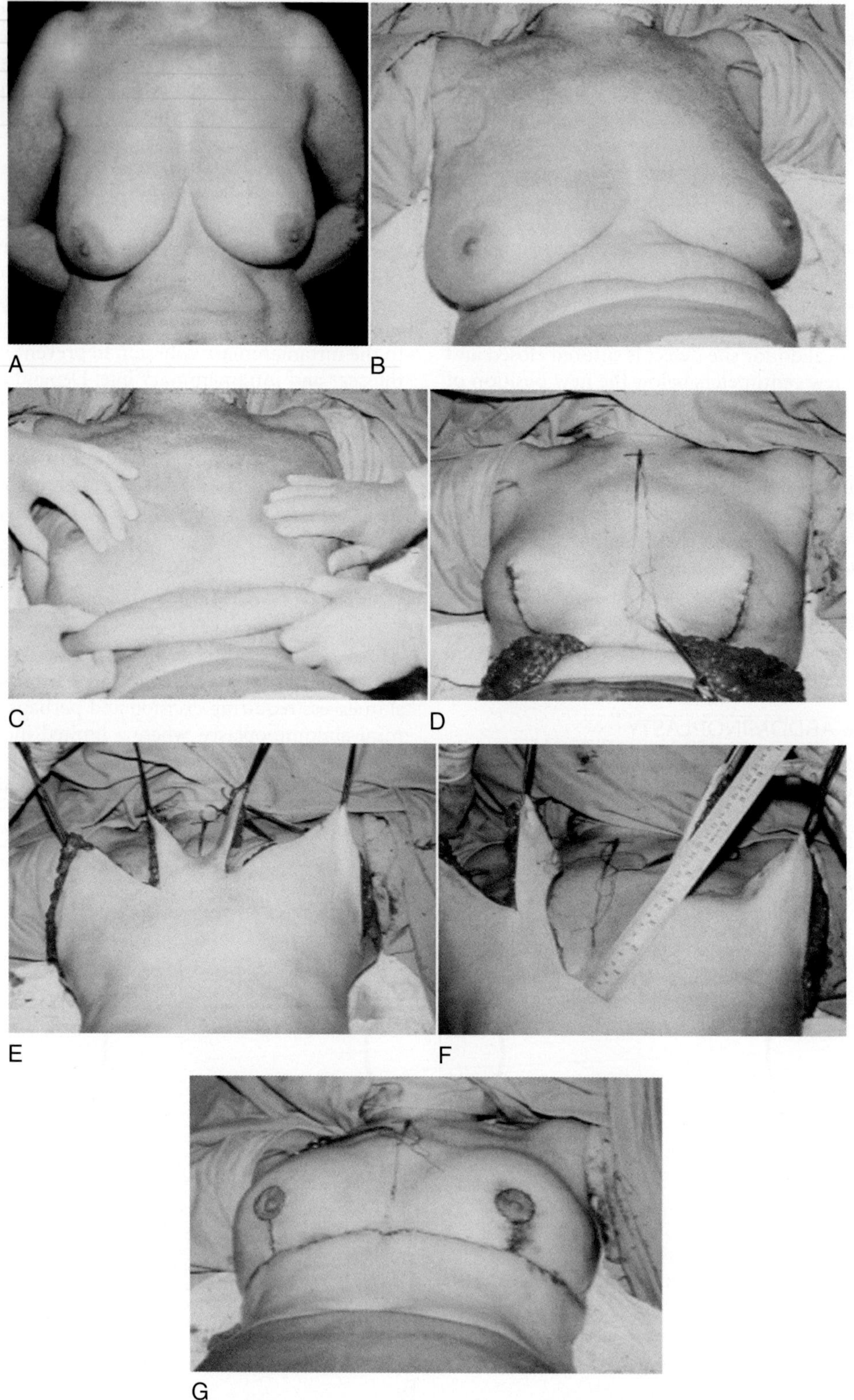

FIGURE 122-56. *A,* Preoperative view of a 55-year-old patient who was an excellent candidate for a reverse abdominoplasty with breast reduction. *B,* The patient in supine position. *C,* The pinch test shows the amount of skin excess. *D,* Reduction of the breast mound bilaterally. *E* and *F,* Evaluation of the amount of skin excess for resection. *G,* Intraoperative view of closure at inframammary line.

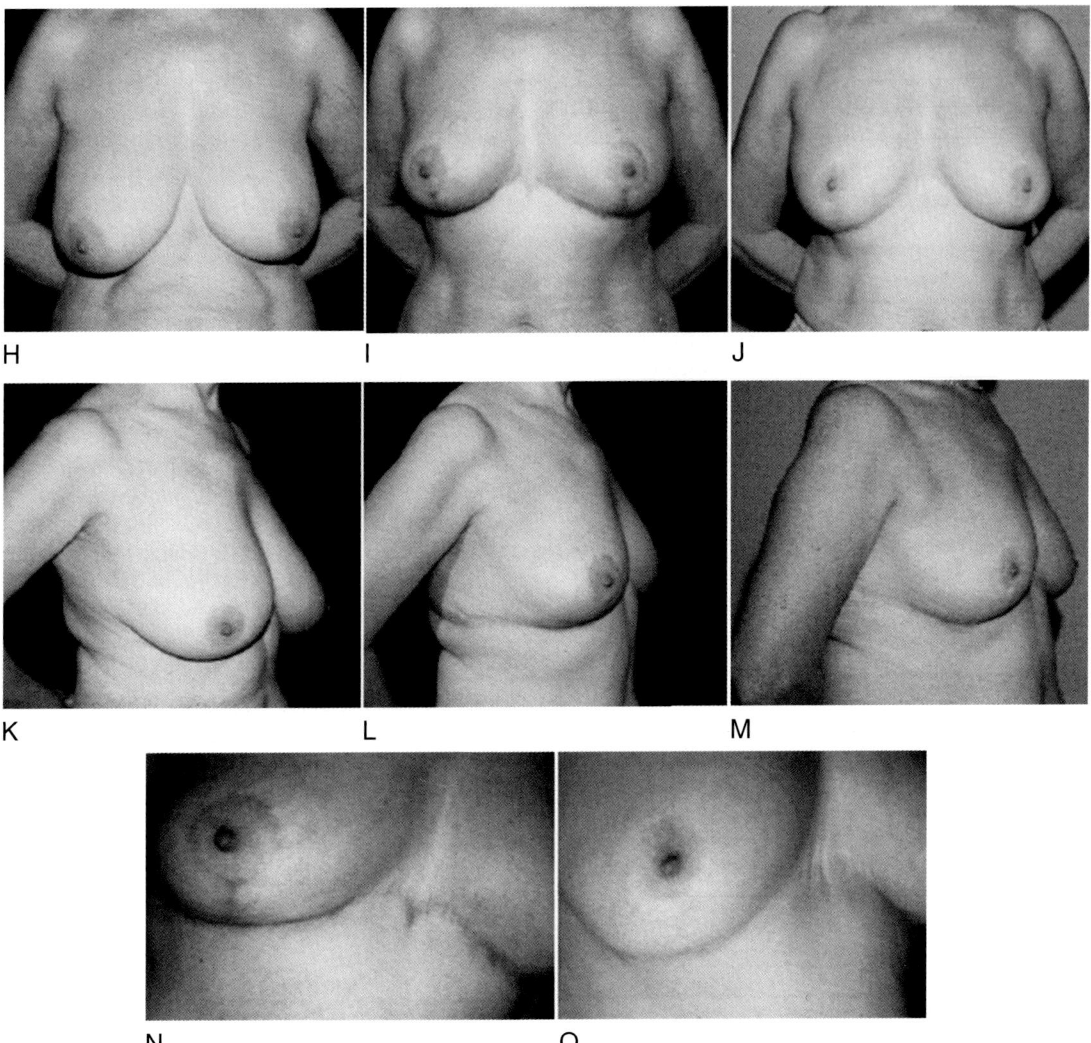

FIGURE 122-56, cont'd. *H,* Preoperative view. *I,* Postoperative result at 6 months. *J,* Postoperative result at 3 years. *K* to *M,* Lateral views of the same patient. *N,* Close-up view of sternal scar at 6 months. *O,* Close-up view of sternal scar at 3 years.

with an epigastric bulge but no skin excess.[52] Endoscopically assisted abdominoplasty is performed with the surgeon placed on the same side of the patient as the surgeon's operating hand, with the assistant opposite the surgeon. The video monitor is placed at the head of the bed. The fascial plication is performed before any planned liposuction to optimize visualization and dissection above the fascial plane. A short transverse suprapubic incision and a periumbilical incision are made for access. Dissection is taken down to the fascia at the lower incision, and a tunnel the width of the bilateral rectus muscles is made under direct vision superiorly as far as possible. Further dissection is performed under endoscopic vision to the umbilicus or to the xiphoid, depending on the myofascial deformity. The midline may be marked temporarily with a suture laid midline from an insertion at the xiphoid to the pubis. The midline is then plicated with either a running over and over permanent suture (switching to horizontal mattress at the umbilicus) or interrupted sutures.[53,54]

ABDOMINOPLASTY AFTER MASSIVE WEIGHT LOSS

With the rising popularity of gastrointestinal bypass surgery, an increasing number of patients are presenting with massive weight loss and large skin excess. These patients represent a population with specialized requirements for body contouring surgery; they often present with circumferential skin laxity of the torso involving the abdomen, chest, sides, upper back, and flanks as well as laxity in the upper arms and medial and lateral thighs. The patient will also often note skin laxity of the face and neck. The patient with massive weight loss is usually a candidate for circumferential torsoplasty. Anterior resection only may be chosen as part of a staged procedure or when circumferential treatment is not an option. To avoid complications due to prolonged surgical time, procedures should be staged if the planned operations cannot be completed within 5 or 6 hours. Discuss with the patient his or her contouring priorities to develop a comprehensive but medically sound plan.

Preoperative Evaluation and Planning

For maximum benefit, contour surgery should not be offered until weight has been stable at least 6 months. In the gastric bypass patient, this generally occurs after $1^1/_2$ to 2 years. In some instances, patients may have undergone significant weight loss yet are still obese. Although excess tissue resection will aid in mobility and further weight loss, the patient should understand that there is an increased risk for wound infection and skin necrosis due to comorbid disease and impaired circulation to the flaps. The obese patient has increased risk for cardiac, pulmonary, and thrombotic complications during and after surgery. To decrease risk, these patients may be offered a panniculectomy with the option of aesthetic abdominoplasty after further weight loss.

There does *not* seem to be an increased complication rate in the nonobese massive weight loss patient.[55] After massive weight loss, patients often have improvements in blood pressure, plasma glucose level, respiratory status, and other physiologic parameters.[56] In addition, the vascular supply to the subcutaneous tissues and skin is relatively robust since the now-decreased tissue volume exerts less perfusion demand on the previously expanded vascular network.[57]

Post–gastric bypass patients have additional considerations. Bypass procedures may be restrictive or malabsorptive or a combination of the two. The Roux-en-Y gastric bypass is the most commonly performed bariatric surgery and combines elements of both. These patients may need nutrient supplementation with iron folate and vitamin B_{12}, and they may be susceptible to electrolyte abnormalities. Thorough blood tests should be performed and imbalances corrected before surgery. Both obesity and prior surgery predispose the patient to development of a ventral or incisional hernia. If the patient has had an open gastric bypass, the vertical midline scar can be incorporated into the operative design. In addition, the formerly obese patient is more likely to have had a cholecystectomy. An open cholecystectomy scar (subcostal) is a contraindication to extensive flap undermining.

Operative Design and Markings

The principle behind safe dermolipectomy for extreme skin laxity is minimal or no undermining to preserve the attenuated circulation to the skin. The epigastric perforator supplying perfusion to a portion of the flap that may be hanging at midthigh might exit the rectus fascia at the periumbilical level. If the skin is lax but the subcutaneous tissues are thin, the flap will advance without undermining. Skin laxity will be evident during the physical examination as it will be mobile over the underlying abdominal wall. Because the skin is mobile relative to the underlying fixed structures, it is crucial in the massive skin excess patient to make meticulous standing markings for reference. Owing to severe skin laxity, ptotic tissues must be lifted against gravity while transverse incisions are marked. Gravity allows plumb determination of the vertical midline, which should be marked from xiphoid to anterior vulvar commissure. Additional full-length truncal sagittal markings should be made; these reference points will otherwise be lost during surgery. Loose abdominal skin tends to move off midline in the supine position, and orientation is further lost after incision. Pay attention during the examination and marking to areas of adhesion where the overlying skin and soft tissue do not slide. These areas are often found along the back and waist, in association with a skinfold and local pannus, and may define areas of attenuated perfusion from the intercostals.[58] Division of primary perforators during flap elevation past these lines of adhesion will jeopardize flap circulation.

Technique

If a transverse excision provides adequate skin reduction, a simple panniculectomy is performed, with wedge excision of the skin and subcutaneous tissue. Tissue excision is beveled away from the incision to maximize the vascular perforators. The final resection should expose very little fascia and divide only the perforators that supply the excised portion of the flap. If umbilical reinset is indicated, perform minimal undermining with a narrow tunnel to provide access. Similarly, if fascial plication is indicated, only sufficient undermining to permit plication is performed.

A midline vertical wedge resection may be undertaken to adjust for lateral excess, but because it causes an additional scar and risk of skin necrosis at the inverted T closure, it should be avoided if possible unless a vertical midline scar already exists or if circumferential torsoplasty is not an option (Fig. 122-57). As with the low transverse incision, resection should bevel toward the midline to preserve epigastric perforators. The umbilicus is circumscribed and sutured into the midline closure. If the umbilicus has tenuous circulation or if aesthetic refinement is necessary, a new umbilicus may be established with rectangular flap extensions from the vertical incisions (Fig. 122-58).

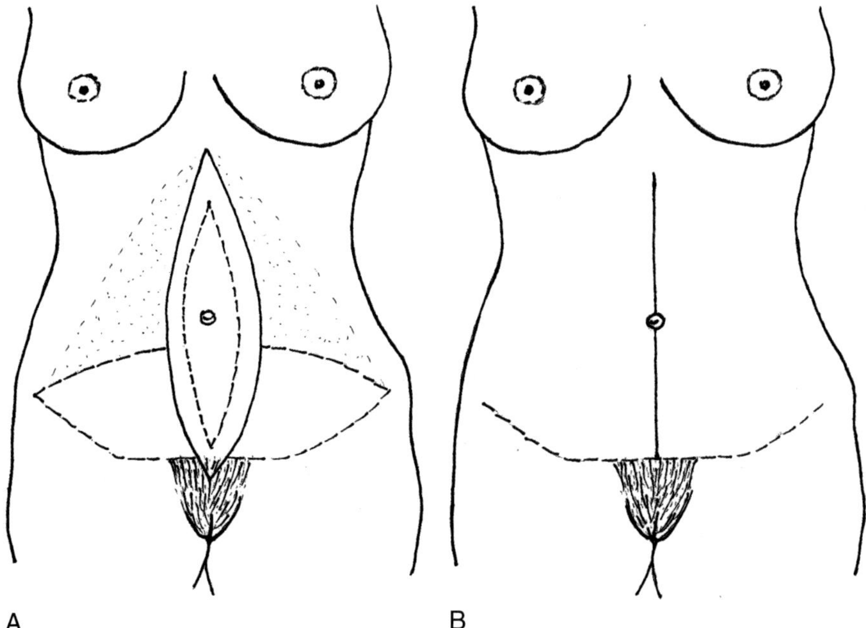

FIGURE 122-57. Vertical or combined abdominoplasty. *A,* Excision pattern. Note that a vertical wedge extension may be made in the mons to reduce mons width. The corners of the inverted T should be kept at a 90-degree angle. The more obtuse the angle, the greater the tension on the trifurcation point at closure. The shaded area indicates possible undermining, which should be avoided if possible to prevent necrosis at the inverted T closure. Rectus plication can be performed as necessary through the vertical incision. *B,* Scar.

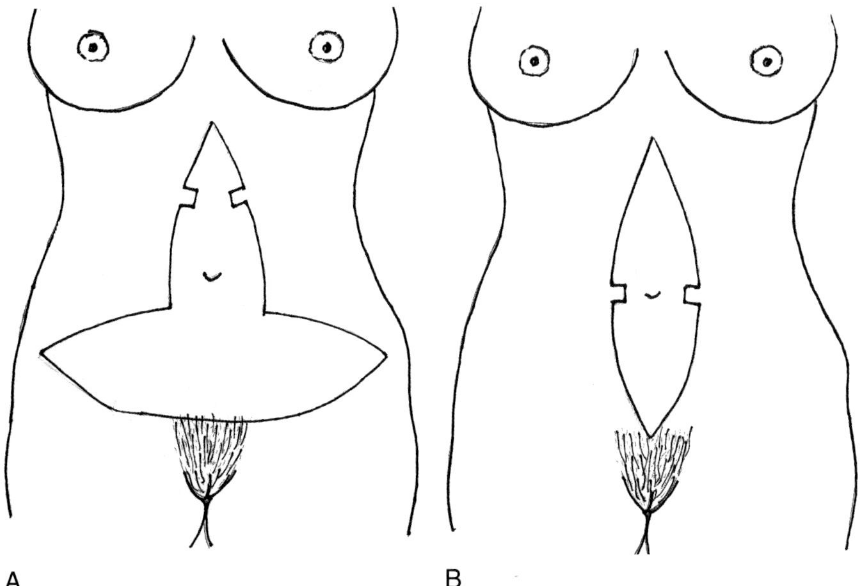

FIGURE 122-58. Umbilical reconstruction. Neoumbilicoplasty along a vertical scar with transverse component *(A)* and vertical incision only *(B)*. The two rectangular neoumbilicoplasty flaps must be designed to lie symmetrically along the vertical border of the excisions so the neoumbilicus is properly located after flap advancement and closure. Proper vertical localization of the neoumbilicoplasty flaps can be made by temporarily approximating the flap inferiorly after transverse excision. (See also Figure 122-59.)

The design of the rectangular flap should be marked before tissue excision. The new umbilical location is determined by pulling the superior marking down to the pubis and finding the horizontal extension of the most superior point of the iliac crest on the redraped abdominal skin. A bilaterally based neoumbilicus avoids a circumferential periumbilical scar and has excellent circulation (Fig. 122-59).

The mons is usually ptotic and should be rejuvenated as part of the abdominoplasty. The lower incision should be placed within the pubic hairline, marking 5 to 7 cm above the vulvar commissure while lifting the skin superiorly under moderate tension so that vertical mons excess can be excised. If necessary, a wedge excision may be taken to decrease width. The ptotic mons tissue should be resuspended to the superficial fascia of the abdominal flap.

Perioperative and Postoperative Care

The deep skinfold in the abdomen of the massive weight loss patient may make hygiene difficult. Patients should be instructed to shower with an antibacterial

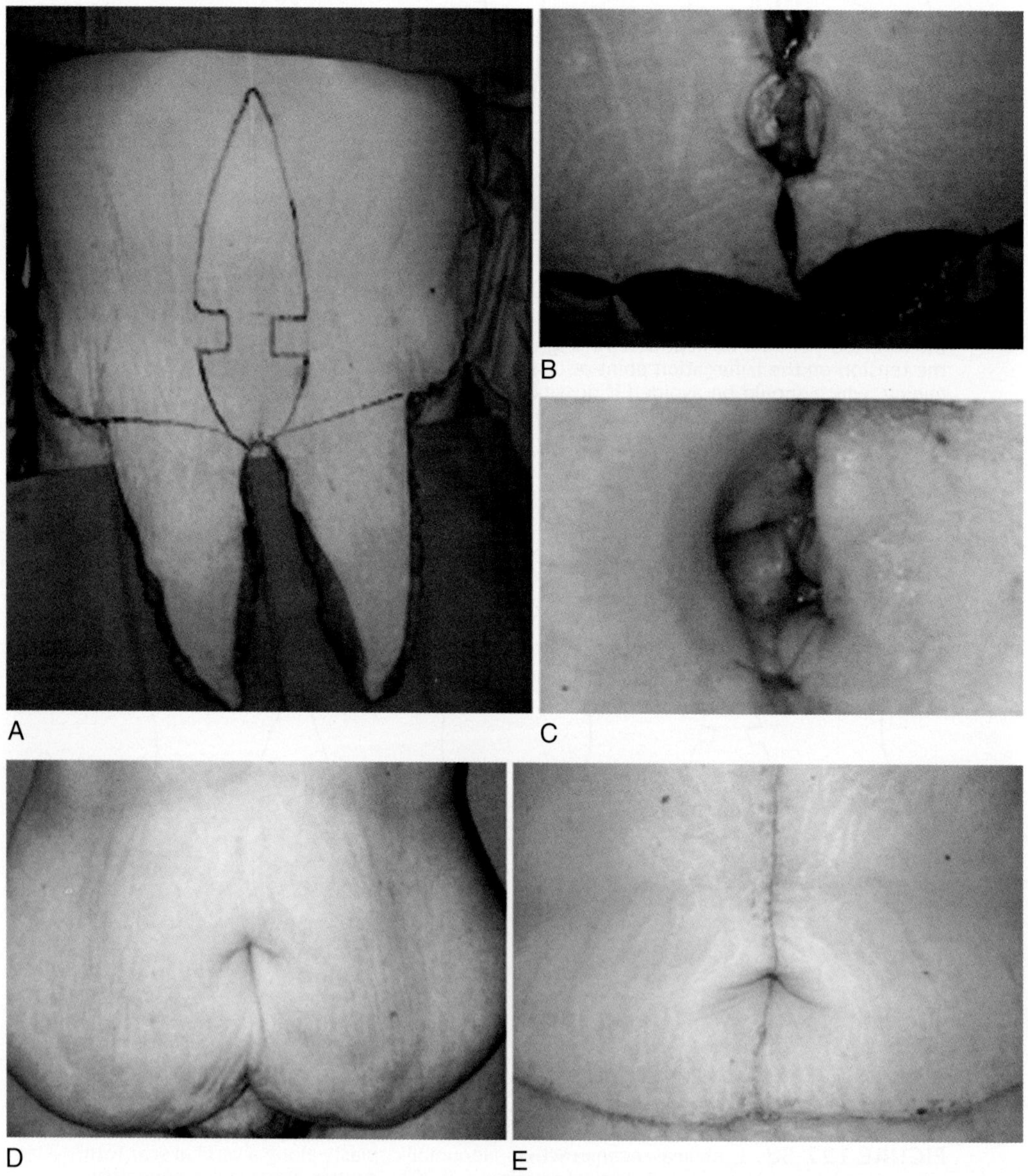

FIGURE 122-59. Umbilical reconstruction with bilateral rectangular flaps. *A,* Design of flaps and extent of resection. *B,* Appearance of neoumbilicus with top and bottom of flaps approximated before inversion. *C,* Appearance after inversion and closure on operating table. *D,* Preoperative appearance. *E,* Late postoperative appearance. Note the absence of a circumferential scar.

soap for 3 days before surgery. Fungal infections should be treated before surgery. As with any abdominoplasty, precautions should be taken against venous thromboembolic complications. Before induction in the operating room as well as during the postoperative recovery, antithromboembolism stockings and sequential compression devices should be used. The room should be kept warm, upper body heating blankets used, and good urine output maintained to maximize tissue perfusion. Subcutaneous heparin or enoxaparin should be considered in the obese patient. Early mobilization is critical. The patient should get out of bed and walk with assistance on the evening of surgery.

CIRCUMFERENTIAL TORSOPLASTY

Circumferential torsoplasty or belt lipectomy involves resection of redundant tissue circumferentially and is indicated in those patients with circumferential skin excess. The procedure can improve laxity and contour in the lateral thighs and buttocks and flanks; it eliminates the problem of lateral dog-ears, which are the inevitable result of limiting lateral resection in a patient with circumferential skin excess. This is commonly indicated in a patient with massive weight loss. The downside of belt lipectomy is that it approximately doubles the operating time as the tissue resection and incision length are doubled, and the patient must be repositioned intraoperatively. If there is any question because of the patient's medical history whether the increased surgical time poses a significant risk, staging the operation into an anterior dermolipectomy or formal abdominoplasty followed by a lateral thigh lift and buttock lift should be considered.

Standard circumferential torsoplasty should be considered distinct from the lower body lift (see Chapter 125), which involves more extensive undermining and aggressive resection. The lower body lift can provide additional benefits to contour and skin appearance and is an excellent option in the appropriate patient. Elements of the lower body lift have been incorporated into an excellent circumferential torsoplasty described by Cormenzana and Samprón,[59] which includes high lateral tension, minimal direct undermining, adjunctive liposuction, discontinuous cannula undermining, and fascial fixation (see Fig. 122-15). Key points in this technique include operating in the prone and then the supine position; ultrasound-assisted lipoplasty of the back, hips, sides, and epigastrium, with more conservative lipoplasty of the subcostal area; rectus fascial incision and double plication to guarantee adhesion; and upper and lower flap superficial fascial system advancement and suture to the underlying muscular fascia to anchor the scar and reduce incisional tension. Aly et al[58] describe a modified form of belt lipectomy with elements of a lower body lift meant to address the massive weight loss patient (Fig. 122-60). Different treatment options and goals are offered, depending on the patient's weight status at the time of surgery. Elements of the procedure include operating in the supine position and both lateral decubitus positions, making the superior incision first, and undermining the inferiorly based flap, including indirect undermining of the lateral thighs. In this consecutive series of 50 patients, 32% developed seroma and 12% had dehiscence. The authors suggest that additional tacking sutures may reduce these complication rates.

Technique

Preoperative preparation should proceed as for abdominoplasty in the massive weight loss patient, with meticulous preoperative skin care and cleaning, careful markings made with the patient in a standing position, and perioperative antiembolic precautions. The anterior and posterior midlines are marked in the standing position. Vertical paramedian reference lines are also drawn. The lower incision should be marked circumferentially while ptotic tissue is elevated with one hand to counter gravity and approximate the pull of the final closure. The anterior lower incision is marked as for abdominoplasty with oblique extensions to bilateral anterior superior iliac spines. The marking is continued in a smooth convex curve over the iliac crest, meeting in the posterior midline in a shallow V. An estimate for the upper incision may be marked by the pinch technique and is used as a reference for symmetry (Fig. 122-61). In the operating room, before any sedation is administered, the standing patient is circumferentially prepped from epigastrium to knee with warmed povidone-iodine (Betadine) solution. The patient is then draped with a sterile half-sheet and asked to lay on the sterilely draped operating table. Alternatively, the patient is placed supine and prepped after induction of anesthesia as for full abdominoplasty, then prepped and draped again when turned prone.

After induction of general anesthesia, the procedure begins in the supine position as with full abdominoplasty. There is no need to tailor the flap medially. Progressive tension sutures are placed, the umbilicus inset is completed, drains are placed, and the anterior incision is sutured completely, including the subcuticular closure, up the lateral border. A large dog-ear on both sides is temporarily stapled closed, and the patient is sterilely turned to the prone position. The patient's positioning is checked for pressure points or neurapraxia and adjusted or padded as necessary before proceeding. The lower incision is made along the skin marking, and resection of the lateral thigh tissue and back is performed with flap undermining only to the upper skin resection line. Pitanguy forceps are used to mark the upper incision on the flap. After flap resection and undermining, any

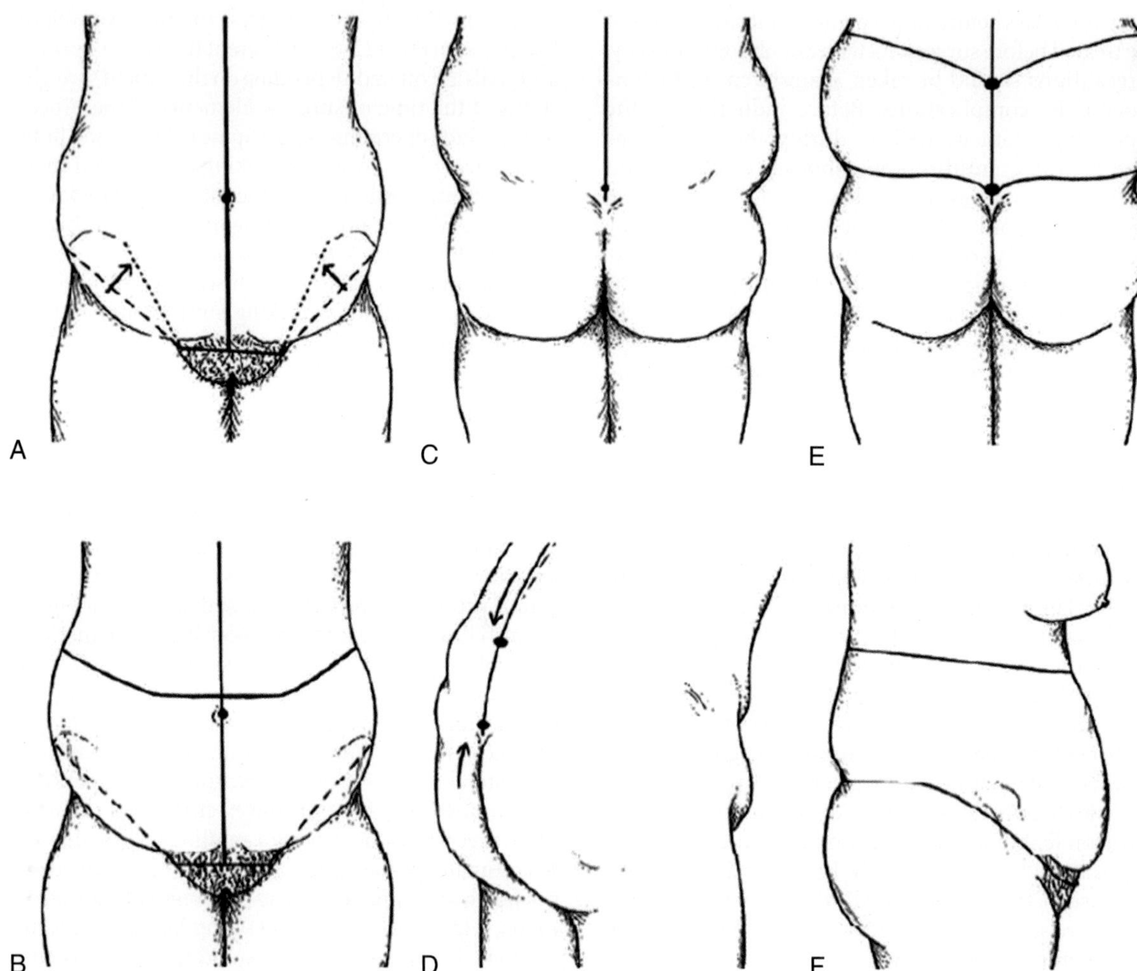

FIGURE 122-60. Diagrammatic representations of markings for circumferential torsoplasty in the gastric bypass patient. *A,* The midline is marked, and the horizontal pubic incision is marked below the natural hairline to allow elevation of a ptotic mons pubis. The arrows between the two sets of dotted lines indicate that tissues of the inguinal area are elevated superiorly and medially before marking from the lateral edge of the pubis to the anterior superior iliac spine. *B,* The superior extent of the anterior resection is marked, and the final position of the inguinal region mark is noted below the anterior superior iliac spine. *C,* The midline of the back is marked, and the inferior mark for the midline back resection is based on the desired level of the resection. This is an arbitrary point, depending on the buttocks deformity. *D,* The upper midline mark is made with the patient bent at the waist by use of the pinch technique represented by the arrows. This maneuver is important for the prevention of dehiscence. *E* and *F,* The remainder of the lateral and back marks. (From Aly AS, Cram AE, Heddens C: Truncal body contouring surgery in the massive weight loss patient. Clin Plast Surg 2004;31:611.)

dead space is closed with quilting sutures and the superficial fascial system is approximated. Drains should be placed bilaterally. As with the anterior flap, the incision is closed in three layers.

UMBILICAL REFINEMENTS

The ideal umbilical shape has variously been described and reconstructed as round, superiorly hooded, or vertical (see Fig. 122-6).[60] Regardless of the configuration, the properly reconstructed umbilicus should be midline and symmetric, form a natural depression, and have an unobtrusive scar. Stretching a suture from xiphoid to anterior vulvar commissure on the standing patient can aid in proper localization of the umbilicus to the true midline. In most nonobese persons, the umbilicus is transected by an imaginary line drawn between the most superior point of the iliac crests.[35] In re-establishing its location on the abdominal flap, the circulation to both the lower portion of the flap and the umbilicus must be considered. The infraumbilical skin is most at risk for

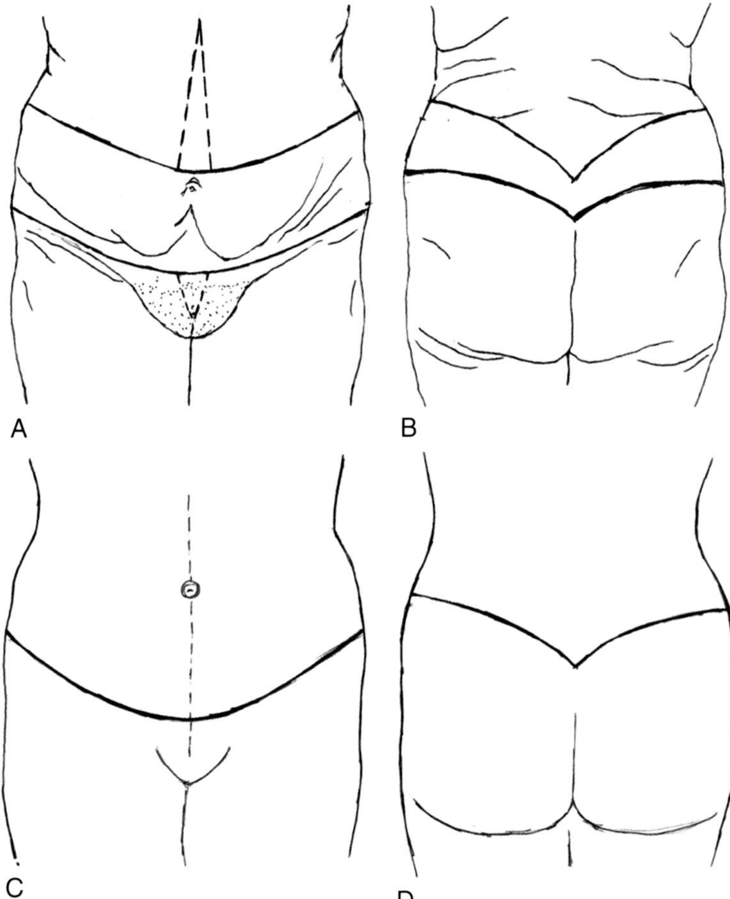

FIGURE 122-61. Circumferential torsoplasty—pattern of excision. With the patient standing, medial and paramedian vertical plumb lines should be drawn for reference (not shown). *A* and *B,* The lower incision is marked circumferentially, lifting the pannus against gravity to approximate the final location of the closure. The marking is curved laterally around the iliac crest and dips slightly in the posterior midline. Possible vertical reduction of the mons and vertical excision of tissue or scar can be marked at this time. *C* and *D,* Location of scar.

ischemia because this is often the location of greatest tension and is the most distal point from the lateral intercostal inflow. If a flap excision that incorporates the former umbilical site would result in a closure under tension, it is preferable to close the original umbilical site on the abdominal flap with a layered closure and retain the abdominal skin lateral to it. The umbilical site closure will become a vertical slit located on the meridian from umbilicus to pubis. The key to avoiding a prominent scar or a divot at the former umbilical site is a multilayered closure including reapproximation of the superficial fascial layer. A multilayered closure will counter lateral forces and prevent both scar widening and tissue thinning, which can result in a depression under the scar.

There are many different options for both the circumumbilical incisions and the abdominal flap incision for umbilical inset, ranging from a simple circular incision to more complex geometric shapes. If the flap umbilical inset incision is too large, the scar will be prominent; if it is too small, the umbilicus may become stenotic, which is unnatural appearing as well as difficult to clean. The circumscribed incision should leave a 1 cm skin island on the umbilical stalk. A 2-cm-diameter incision on the abdominal flap is standard but should be adjusted to best fit the patient. The best way to design the umbilical site on the abdominal flap is to temporarily approximate the flap closure with suture or staples at the midline to properly locate the flap medially as well as at its appropriate height relative to the iliac crests. Depending on the degree of lateral or vertical tension on the flap, the incision may be either a circular or oval excision or a vertical or horizontal slit. On a thick flap, the subcutaneous fat around the new umbilical site should be cored out to form a natural-appearing indentation. Another consideration is whether the umbilical stalk should be fixed to the rectus fascia to promote an indentation. Fixation to the rectus fascia should be performed when the stalk is very long, as after massive weight loss. Fixation can be accomplished by suturing the umbilicus to the fascia in four quadrants with a buried suture from flap dermis to fascia to umbilical dermis. Alternatively, the umbilical stalk can be fixed to the fascia before umbilical inset on the flap. Superior hooding, which has been lauded as a feature of an ideal umbilicus, is the result of skin laxity across a fixed umbilicus. If this is a desired effect, it can be replicated by insetting the umbilicus slightly inferior to its actual projection on the abdominal flap, resulting in an inferiorly oriented (superiorly tethered) umbilicus. In addition, the superior midline (12-o'clock) fascial fixation suture may be eliminated.

Common variations to the technique include the Avelar[61] stellate umbilicoplasty, which uses an inverted Mercedes incision on the flap with matching triangular excision on the umbilical stalk, and the Juri[62] umbilicoplasty, which uses a V-shaped incision on the flap. The Juri umbilicoplasty adds a vertical incision or matching triangular excision at the superior border of the umbilical stalk before inset. The advantages of these techniques include a multiangled incision with less chance for stenosis and a broken line that is better hidden. A scar-free umbilicoplasty has been described[63] that involves defatting of the recipient site on the flap and de-epithelialization of the umbilical stalk; a purse-string suture on the flap is used to establish an indentation, and then the flap is fixed to the umbilical stalk (see also "Umbilical Revision").

MONSPLASTY

The mons pubis undergoes the same effects from skin laxity and excess adipose tissue as the rest of the abdomen does. If the mons is not addressed during abdominoplasty, the result can be unbalanced and emphasize the ptotic or prominent mons. The prominent mons may be reduced by liposuction. The ptotic mons should be reduced and resuspended. The normal height of the mons from anterior vulvar commissure to the top of the pubis is about 5 to 7 cm. Concurrent reduction of the mons can be performed during abdominoplasty by marking the lower incision at this level with the ptotic mons lifted against gravity during marking. If there is extreme skin laxity, a midline V-shaped excision of skin can be taken. The mons will often be thicker than the advanced abdominal flap. To avoid a step-off between the mons and the abdominal flap, the lower abdominal incision can be tapered superiorly, leaving a ramp of subcutaneous tissue on the inferior abdominal fascia that will lie under and supplement the thinned abdominal flap. Closure of the superficial fascial system will help prevent further flap thinning, which can result in a depression at the incision.

COMPLICATIONS

Normal sequelae of abdominoplasty include postoperative swelling, flap numbness, serous drainage, and a permanent incisional scar. Patients can expect some pain or soreness, numbness of the elevated abdominal flap, bruising, and general fatigue lasting, in some instances, several weeks after surgery. These sequelae should be anticipated consequences of abdominoplasty and discussed during the preoperative consultation and informed consent discussion. Proper preoperative counseling can help the patient understand the difference between normal postoperative recovery and an unplanned complication of surgery.

Medical conditions such as cardiovascular disease including hypertension, angina, history of myocardial infarction, lung disease (including asthma and chronic obstructive pulmonary disorder), history of thromboembolism or bleeding, smoking, obesity and diabetes, and prior abdominal surgical scars all impair perfusion and can increase the risk of abdominal flap ischemia. A good preoperative history and physical examination can direct planning toward safer perioperative management and surgical design or screen patients who may be poor candidates for abdominoplasty.

Complications related to the abdominoplasty procedure can be placed roughly into two categories: rare, potentially life-threatening complications and more common complications that prolong recovery or require secondary procedures. The reported incidence of death after abdominoplasty in two large surveys is 0.02%[64] and 0.04%.[65] In the Grazer-Goldwyn series,[64] 6 of the 17 deaths were from pulmonary embolus. Pulmonary embolism occurs in up to 1% of patients undergoing abdominoplasty.[64-66] In contrast, pulmonary embolism and death are 20 times less likely after lipoplasty.[67]

More common complications include seroma, nerve injury, prominent scar or contour irregularity, bleeding, and hematoma. Complications related to local ischemia include tissue necrosis, dehiscence, and wound infection.

Avoidable Risk Factors

SMOKING

Cigarette smoke contains a number of known toxins including nicotine, carbon monoxide, and hydrogen cyanide. Nicotine is a vasoconstrictor that impairs access to oxygen and circulating factors and cells. It also increases platelet adhesiveness and directly injures endothelial cells, increasing risk of thrombotic microvascular occlusion, and impairs function of red blood cells, leukocytes, fibroblasts, and macrophages. Carbon monoxide reduces oxygen-carrying capacity of blood, and hydrogen cyanide inhibits oxidative metabolism. All these mechanisms contribute to impaired wound healing and tissue ischemia. Impaired wound healing or ischemic tissue loss is most evident when tissues are at most risk for interrupted circulation, as in digital replantation and elevated cutaneous flaps, such as TRAM abdominoplasty flaps[68] and full abdominoplasties.[69] Smokers have about a threefold increase in wound healing problems, including partial flap necrosis and wound dehiscence. In the study by Manassa et al,[69] a retrospective survey of the smokers showed that although the patients had been asked to quit smoking for 2 weeks before surgery and 2 weeks after surgery, only 14.7% stopped preoperatively and 41.2% complied postoperatively. In fact, studies point to an abstinence from smoking of at least 4 weeks to achieve statistical benefit.[70-73]

OBESITY

In the United States, the prevalence of obesity increased from 12% in 1991 to 21.3% in 2002.[74] Obesity also substantially increases overall morbidity and contributes to an increased prevalence of type 2 diabetes mellitus, heart disease, high blood cholesterol level, high blood pressure, gallbladder disease, and osteoarthritis.[75] Obesity also increases the complication rate in surgery, including abdominoplasty. To document the weight status of a patient, it is useful to measure body mass index (Table 122-3). This calculation also will provide ranges for ideal body weight for a given height.

Studies consistently show that obese patients undergoing various surgical procedures suffer at least a twofold increase in wound complications, such as infection, wound dehiscence, and tissue necrosis. However, there does not seem to be an increased complication rate in the nonobese post-gastric bypass patient.[55] In some obese patients, removal of excess weight, whether by panniculectomy or liposuction, may improve mobility as well as cardiovascular risk factors.[76,77]

DIETARY SUPPLEMENTS

Dietary supplements include over-the-counter products such as vitamins and minerals, isolated food products, and herbal medications, many of which can influence anesthetic or operative outcome. More than one third of adult men and half of adult women use multivitamins, with the trend being higher in the western United States and with higher education and income.[78,79] Vitamin E increases bleeding time by impairing platelet aggregation and may adversely affect wound healing, and it should be discontinued preoperatively. Surveys show that at least 12% of the population uses herbal medications in the United States, with an almost fourfold increase between 1990 and 1997. Up to 50% of surgical patients admitted to taking herbs when asked specifically; however, more than two thirds of the patients failed to disclose herbal medication use during routine preoperative assessment.[78,79] Many of the most popular supplements (e.g., fish oil, gingko, garlic, ginseng, echinacea, St. John's wort) may influence surgical outcome by various mechanisms, including impairment of platelet function, potentiation of anesthetics, and alteration of cardiovascular function (Table 122-4).

Two supplements with proven positive effects on healing should be considered. Vitamin A is well known to enhance wound healing and immune function. It may be supplemented for 1 week before surgery at 25,000 IU per day. Bromelain has been shown in a placebo-controlled human trial to significantly increase the resorption rate of hematomas.[80] If it is used, bromelain should be ingested on an empty stomach at 500 mg four times a day during the 72 hours before surgery[81] (Table 122-5).

A double-blind trial of marathon runners using homeopathic arnica showed a lower creatine kinase level and less stiffness in the arnica group than in the control group.[82] However, a review of placebo-controlled trials of homeopathic arnica concluded there was no statistically proven benefit.[83] Mention is made here because this is a widely used product with numerous unofficial reports of its benefits for bruising, swelling, and soreness. Keep in mind that arnica is a potent drug with deleterious effects if it is ingested at full strength. According to the tenets of homeopathy, homeopathic benefit increases with greater dilution; at homeopathic dilutions, there is no chemically detectable drug. If it is used, homeopathic arnica is taken before surgery and continued up to 1 week postoperatively.

TABLE 122-3 ✦ BODY MASS INDEX

Body Mass Index*	Ideal Body Weight	Weight Status
<19	<80%	Underweight
19 to <25	100%	Optimal
25 to <30	>110%	Overweight
30 to <40	>120%	Obese
>40	>200%	Morbidly obese
>50	>225%	Super obese

*Body mass index = weight/height^2 (kg/m^2).

Prevention and Treatment of Specific Complications

THROMBOEMBOLISM

Venous thromboembolism is the most common preventable cause of death in surgical patients.[84] Types of risk factors for thromboembolism include certain medical conditions, medications, surgery, and inherited thrombophilia. Risk factors commonly seen in abdominoplasty candidates include obesity, cigarette

TABLE 122-4 ✦ CLINICALLY IMPORTANT EFFECTS AND PERIOPERATIVE CONCERNS OF 8 HERBAL MEDICINES AND RECOMMENDATIONS FOR DISCONTINUATION OF USE BEFORE SURGERY

Herb: Common Name(s)	Relevant Pharmacological Effects	Perioperative Concerns	Preoperative Discontinuation
Echinacea: purple coneflower root	Activation of cell-mediated immunity	Allergic reactions; decreased effectiveness of immunosuppressants; potential for immunosuppression with long-term use	No data
Ephedra: ma huang	Increased heart rate and blood pressure through direct and indirect sympathomimetic effects	Risk of myocardial ischemia and stroke from tachycardia and hypertension; ventricular arrhythmias with halothane; long-term use depletes endogenous catecholamines and may cause intraoperative hemodynamic instability; life-threatening interaction with monoamine oxidase inhibitors	At least 24 hours before surgery
Garlic: ajo	Inhibition of platelet aggregation (may be irreversible); increased fibrinolysis; equivocal antihypertensive activity	Potential to increase risk of bleeding, especially when combined with other medications that inhibit platelet aggregation	At least 7 days before surgery
Ginkgo: duck foot tree, maidenhair tree, silver apricot	Inhibition of platelet-activating factor	Potential to increase risk of bleeding, especially when combined with other medications that inhibit platelet aggregation	At least 36 hours before surgery
Ginseng: American ginseng, Asian ginseng, Chinese ginseng, Korean ginseng	Lowers blood glucose; inhibition of platelet aggregation (may be irreversible); increased PT-PTT in animals; many other diverse effects	Hypoglycemia; potential to increase risk of bleeding; potential to decrease anticoagulation effect of warfarin	At least 7 days before surgery
Kava: awa, intoxicating pepper, kawa	Sedation, anxiolysis	Potential to increase sedative effect of anesthetics; potential for addiction, tolerance, and withdrawal after abstinence unstudied	At least 24 hours before surgery
St John's wort: amber, goat weed, hardhay, Hypericum, klamatheweed	Inhibition of neurotransmitter reuptake, monoamine oxidase inhibition is unlikely	Induction of cytochrome P450 enzymes, affecting cyclosporine, warfarin, steroids, protease inhibitors, and possibly benzodiazepines, calcium channel blockers, and many other drugs; decreased serum digoxin levels	At least 5 days before surgery
Valerian: all heal, garden heliotrope, vandal root	Sedation	Potential to increase sedative effect of anesthetics; benzodiazepine-like acute withdrawal; potential to increase anesthetic requirements with long-term use	No data

PT-PTT indicates prothrombin time–partial thromboplastin time.
From Ang-Lee M, Moss J, Yuan CS: Herbal medicines and perioperative care. JAMA 2001;286;208.

smoking, immobility, oral contraceptive use, and hormone replacement therapy (Table 122-6). Prophylaxis includes use of foot or leg sequential compression devices in every patient undergoing abdominoplasty under general anesthesia, with compression starting before induction. Pneumatic compression devices have been shown to reduce thromboembolic events by more than half without increasing bleeding risk by preventing venous pooling and activating fibrinolysis. An indwelling Foley catheter should be placed if anticipated surgery time is more than 3 hours because the distended bladder can compress the vena cava. In patients with higher risk factors, including genetic thrombophilia and history of prior deep venous thromboembolism (DVT) or pulmonary embolism, consider deferring surgery or using perioperative low-molecular-weight heparin, such as enoxaparin. Low-molecular-weight heparin appears to be at least as effective as heparin in DVT prophylaxis with possibly less bleeding complications.

TABLE 122-5 ✦ SURGICALLY SIGNIFICANT NUTRITIONAL SUPPLEMENTS

Supplement	Blood Coagulation	Wound Healing	Immune Function	Hematoma Resorption	Stop Preoperatively	Start Preoperatively
Garlic	Inhibits platelet aggregation	—	—	—	Yes	—
Vitamin E	Inhibits platelet adhesion	Impairs	—	—	Yes	—
EPA	Inhibits adhesion and aggregation	—	—	—	Yes	—
Vitamin A (25,000 IU qd)	—	Enhances	Enhances	—	—	Yes
Bromelain (500 mg qid)	Insignificant effect	—	—	Enhances	—	Yes, 72 hours (on empty stomach)

From Petry JJ: Surgically significant nutritional supplements. Plast Reconstr Surg 1996;97:233.

The clinical presentation of DVT is nonspecific but may include extremity swelling, tenderness, calf pain on ankle dorsiflexion, and fever. Diagnosis can be made by Doppler ultrasonography. Proximal thrombosis may lead to pulmonary embolism. Clinical signs may include dyspnea, chest pain, hemoptysis, tachycardia, rales, and electrocardiographic changes. Diagnosis is confirmed by pulmonary arteriography. High clinical suspicion due to acute onset of shortness of breath or chest pain without another obvious cause warrants further evaluation. Heart rate may be elevated, a chest radiograph may show an elevated hemidiaphragm or plate-like atelectasis, and blood gas analysis may show decreased oxygen saturation. History of prior pulmonary embolism or DVT or increased age increases risk. Clinical suspicion of thromboembolism should prompt a D-dimer measurement.[84] Patients with D-dimer levels of 500 μg/L or higher should have a lower limb compression ultrasound examination. If a DVT is found, anticoagulant treatment may be initiated without further testing. A patient with a normal ultrasound finding when clinical suspicion is high should

TABLE 122-6 ✦ RISK FACTORS FOR PULMONARY EMBOLISM

Environmental
Long-haul air travel
Obesity
Cigarette smoking
Hypertension
Immobility

Natural
Increasing age

Women's health
Oral contraceptives, including progesterone-only and especially third-generation pills
Pregnancy
Hormone replacement therapy

Medical illness
Previous PE or DVT
Cancer
Congestive heart failure
Chronic obstructive pulmonary disease
Diabetes mellitus
Inflammatory bowel disease
Antipsychotic drug use
Chronic indwelling central venous catheter
Varicose veins

Surgical
Trauma
Orthopaedic surgery, especially total hip replacement, total knee replacement, hip fracture surgery, knee arthroscopy
General surgery, especially for cancer
Gynecological and urological surgery, especially for cancer
Neurosurgery, especially craniotomy for brain tumor

Thrombophilia
Factor V Leiden mutation
Prothrombin gene mutation
Hyperhomocysteinemia (including mutation in methylenetetrahydrofolate reductase)
Antiphospholipid antibody syndrome
Deficiency of antithrombin III, protein C, or protein S
High concentrations of factor VIII or XI
Increased Lipoprotein (a)

PE, pulmonary embolism; DVT, deep venous thrombosis.
From Goldhaber SZ: Pulmonary embolism. Lancet 2004;363:1295.

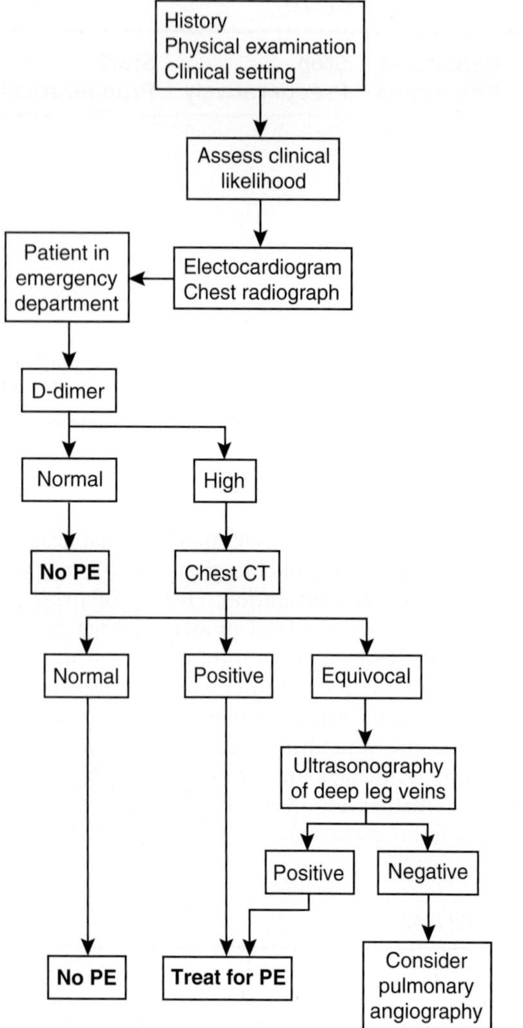

FIGURE 122-62. Diagnostic algorithm for suspected pulmonary embolism (PE). (From Goldhaber SZ: Pulmonary embolism. Lancet 2004;363:1295.)

undergo a helical computed tomographic scan. If the helical computed tomographic scan is normal or inconclusive with high clinical probability, obtain a chest angiogram for definitive diagnosis. An abnormal helical computed tomographic scan or angiogram for pulmonary embolism is an indication for anticoagulation treatment for at least 6 months (Fig. 122-62).[84]

ISCHEMIA

Factors that contribute to tissue ischemia in abdominoplasty include physiologic factors of the patient and factors related to surgical technique. Physiologic factors that preclude surgery or should be remedied before surgery include obesity, which increases the occurrence of wound complications by twofold; smoking, which increases wound complications by at least threefold; and any preexisting cardiovascular or pulmonary disease that can adversely affect tissue perfusion. Smokers should quit for at least 4 weeks before surgery, and obese patients should lose weight to within 30% of their ideal weight. Technical factors that increase the risk of ischemic wound complications include division of vascular supply from undermining or aggressive liposuction, reimplantation of the umbilicus, closure under tension, inverted T closure, flap undermining in the face of an upper abdominal transverse incision, and concurrent liposuction on the undermined flap. Proper surgical design, minimal undermining, progressive tension sutures, and layered closure including reapproximation of the superficial fascial system help prevent these problems. Ischemia and tissue loss can also be due to improper postoperative care resulting in damage or disruption of the tenuous vascular supply to the flap. Causes include excessive pressure from a tight dressing or binder and burns from use of a heating pad or a hot tub while the abdominal flap is still insensate.

If flap circulation appears marginal after elevation, consider marking the umbilical site but delaying externalization for a few days to avoid further compromise of the circulation of the lower flap. If excessive tension at closure results in acute flap ischemia, the flap closure should be released. The open wound may be treated with vacuum-assisted closure (VAC) therapy to prevent flap contracture until the delayed flap is more robust and can be advanced and approximated. Evidence, mainly in rat studies, shows some improvement in survival of ischemic flaps with topical nitroglycerin for vasodilation, enteral calcium channel blocker such as nifedipine to decrease vasospasm, pentoxifylline to improve blood cell conformability, or some combination of therapies.[85-87] These techniques have been variably used clinically but do not have proven benefit.

Tissue Necrosis

If flap ischemia proceeds to necrosis, it is better to treat the wound conservatively with local débridement, dressing changes, or vacuum-assisted closure therapy until the tissues are healed and the viable margins delineated. Early attempt at revision may lead to further tissue trauma and progression of ischemia. The healing wound will often contract, resulting in a smaller defect to close. Once the tissues have demarcated and the flap's viability is certain, the exposed borders should be excised and the flap advanced (Fig. 122-63).

HEMORRHAGE AND HEMATOMA

Factors of the patient that increase the risk of hemorrhage include blood-thinning medications or foods, inherited bleeding disorders, and acquired coagu-

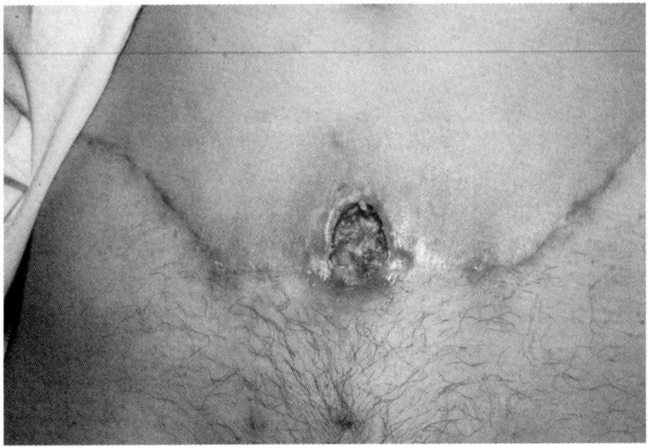
A

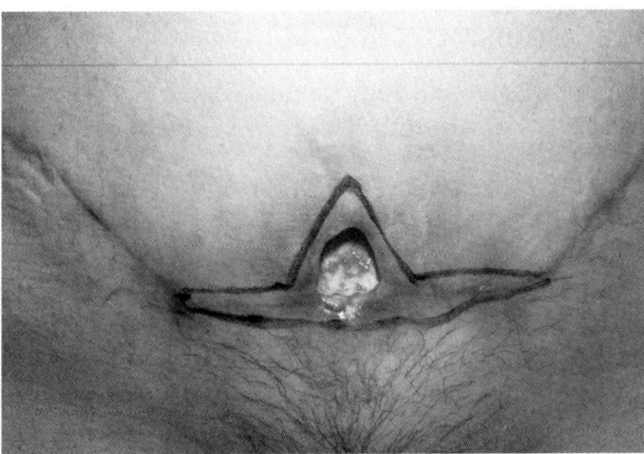
B

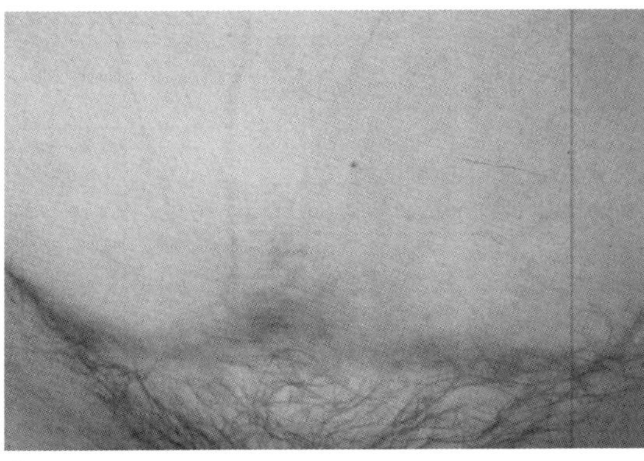
C

FIGURE 122-63. Wound dehiscence with skin and subcutaneous tissue necrosis *(A)*. Demarcated area of necrosis is marked for excision *(B)*. *C*, Postoperative view of incision site after resection and surgical revision.

lopathies. Bleeding disorders should be screened during the routine history. Reversible or avoidable causes include vitamin K deficiency; intraoperative hypothermia; and medications, foods, and herbs that impair coagulation, such as aspirin products, garlic, vitamin E, gingko, and nonhomeopathic arnica (see "Dietary Supplements"). A positive history of bleeding without a clear cause requires further investigation. Whereas some coagulopathies may be reversible for surgery, the risk of blood product transfusion makes surgery a greater risk for the elective patient with a clinical deficiency of a coagulation factor or blood component.

While active bleeding as evidenced by acute swelling under the flap or red blood in the drain is an indication for re-exploration, hematomas may not be immediately apparent postoperatively but may become evident as swelling subsides, presenting as a convex irregularity that may or may not be fluctuant. To better monitor for bleeding, Blake drains are preferable to Jackson-Pratt drains because they are less susceptible to clogging. Small hematomas may be allowed to resorb; however, medium to large hematomas should be drained or evacuated to prevent infection, capsule formation, and contracture scarring.

SEROMA

Persistent seroma is one of the most common postsurgical complications in abdominoplasty, with a reported incidence between 5% and 50%.[48] The etiology of seroma formation involves raw tissue surfaces producing serum in the face of compromised lymphatic drainage combined with prolonged impairment of flap adhesion to the abdominal wall fascia. Flap adhesion is impaired by flap movement as well as by physical separation of the flap from the underlying abdominal wall by undrained fluid; impaired flap adhesion in turn prolongs serous fluid production. Proven methods of decreasing seroma frequency include adequate drainage, with removal of drains only after drainage is less than 30 mL per day, and quilting sutures between the superficial fascia of the flap and abdominal wall fascia to eliminate dead space and prevent flap movement.[48] Use of these sutures, which prevent flap shearing and eliminate dead space, can be so successful that there is no need for drains (see Fig. 122-70). Pitanguy[88] noted a reduction in seroma rate in his clinic from 16% to 0.3% by covering all dissected tissues with moist sterile towels to prevent desiccation, rigorous hemostasis, placement of drains, and use of a plaster shield molded over a thick soft dressing. Care is taken during formation of the shield to avoid the bony protuberances of the costal margin and iliac spines. This anterior abdominal plate is held in place for the first 2 postoperative days with a 2-kg weight placed on top. The thin layer (called the fascia of Gallaudet or innominate fascia) that lies just above the muscular fascia contains a fine vascular plexus. Preservation of this layer aids in lymphatic drainage and flap adhesion.

SCAR FORMATION

Keloid formation is genetic; however, prominent scars can form in anyone and may be minimized by good surgical technique. Clean incisions along natural lines of tension that are closed without dermal tension are least likely to form a widened or hypertrophic scar. Tension must be reduced at a subdermal level, which requires a superficial fascial and deep dermal closure in abdominoplasty. To help prevent formation of raised and widened scars in the postoperative period, hypoallergenic tape or silicone sheets may be used to reduce skin tension and add a slight pressure dressing. Hypertrophic scars that form in spite of preventive measures may be treated with intralesional cortisone injection if they persist beyond 6 to 12 months of conservative treatment.[89] Other treatment modalities include intralesional 5-fluorouracil, pulsed dye laser, and focal irradiation (Fig. 122-64).

Control scar placement with good operative planning by remembering that the final position of the closure depends on the relative pull of the two sides of the incision. The postoperative tension can be approximated by lifting the tissues against gravity before the lower incision is marked. In addition, tension can be adjusted intraoperatively by use of the liposuction cannula or Lockwood elevator inferiorly (see Chapter 125) to release attachments without dividing vessels and by use of progressive tension and flap fixation sutures to control the tension.[90]

NERVE INJURY

Sensory nerve entrapment during closure may cause permanent chronic postoperative pain and may occur in as many as 1 in 10 patients.[91,92] Nerve injury can be prevented by avoiding deep fascial sutures (Fig. 122-65).

SECONDARY ABDOMINOPLASTY

Scar Revision

Even a thin flat scar may be unacceptable if it is malpositioned. The actual scar may be narrow but

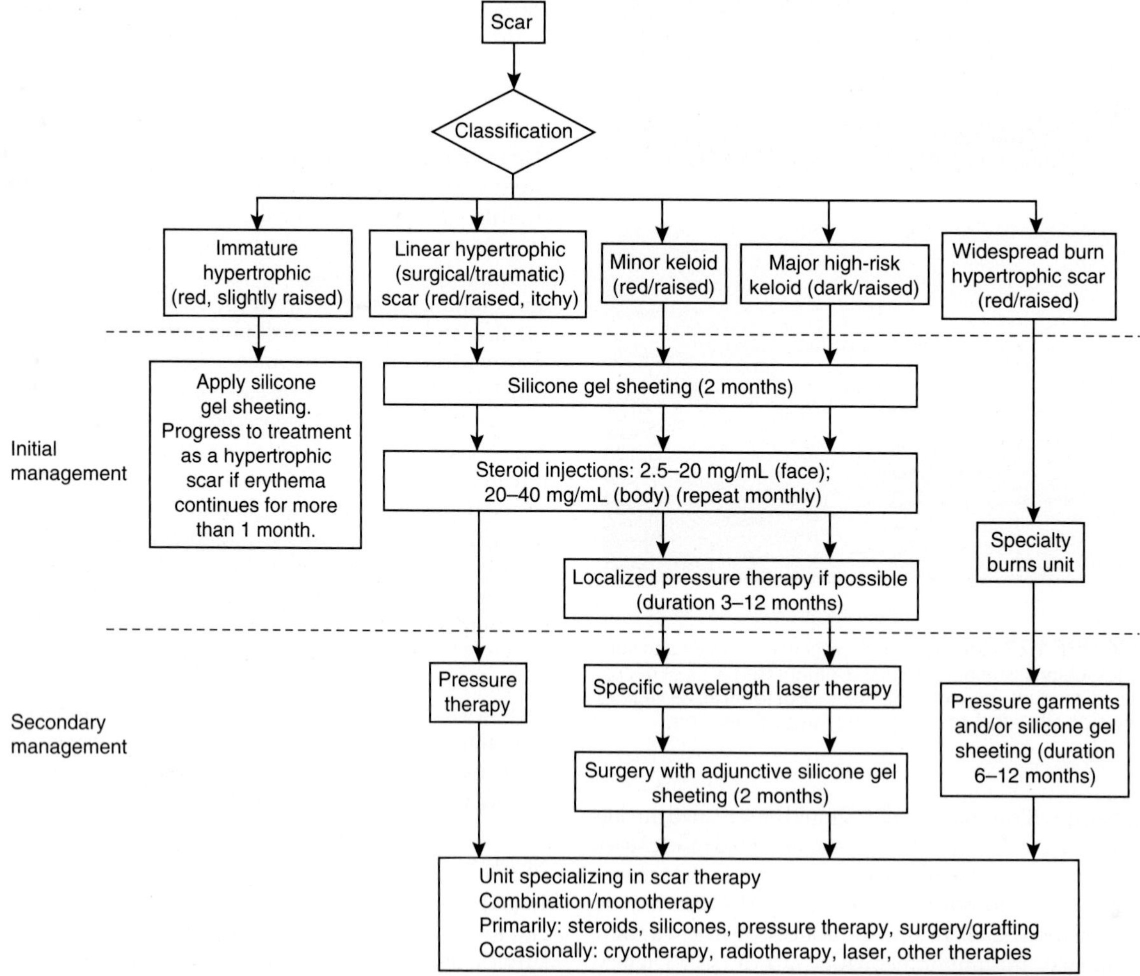

FIGURE 122-64. Scar management algorithm. (Modified from Mustoe TA, Cooter RD, Gold MH, et al, International Advisory Panel on Scar Management: International clinical recommendations on scar management. Plast Reconstr Surg 2002;110:560.)

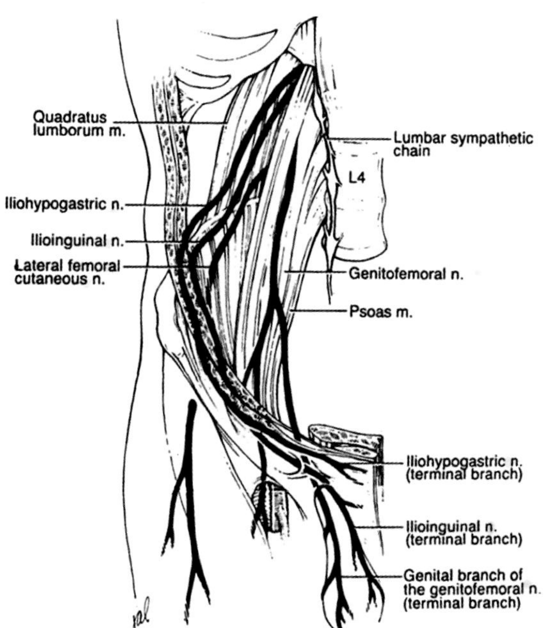

FIGURE 122-65. Superficial nerve trajectory in inguinal region. (From Choi PD, Nath R, Mackinnon SE: Iatrogenic injury to the ilioinguinal and iliohypogastric nerves in the groin: a case report, diagnosis, and management. Ann Plast Surg 1996;37:60.)

depressed, with peri-incisional bulging of soft tissues. The final surgical scar may be high (often centrally), low (especially laterally), or irregular (higher on one side than the other) (Fig. 122-66). Once the flap has been allowed to heal, revision can be performed. For instance, the flap can be advanced centrally to lower the incision at the pubis and excised laterally to raise the lateral scar (e.g., the Baroudi handlebar incision, which is well hidden under high-cut bikinis) (Fig. 122-67).

A widened scar may result from spreading of dermis from inadequate suture support during early scar formation. It may be revised by excising the scar and performing a multilayered closure including Scarpa's fascia and deep dermis. A depressed scar, which can result from inadequate deep tissue approximation and subsequent flap thinning, is similarly treated.

Residual Contour Irregularity

Tissue fullness and bulges following abdominoplasty can result from mismatched thickness of the abdominal flap and lower incision, areas with inadequate flap undermining or tissue excision, flap thinning under the scar resulting in a depression, or postoperative tissue necrosis and contracture. For instance, a midline epigastric bulge may be seen after rectus fascial plication, especially when a narrow tunnel is developed instead of wide flap elevation to minimize devascularization. This epigastric bulge can be reduced at initial surgery by liposuction or blunt scissor dissection that will form tunnels parallel to the intercostal vessels, feathering out the areas of flap adherence. If the flap is thick, fat deep to Scarpa's fascia can be excised directly (see Fig. 122-44). If residual epigastric fullness is not fully resolved by these methods, focal liposuction can be performed after waiting at least 6 months.

The flank and lateral corners of the incision are subject to residual fullness and dog-ears (see Fig. 122-69*A*). Bulges seen at the end of the operation will not flatten or disappear without intervention. Fullness due to residual fat can be excised directly. Focal liposuction at the hips and flanks can safely be performed without compromising the abdominal flap. A dog-ear due to skin excess should be excised; patients generally prefer longer scars over a residual bulge or wrinkled skin.

Tissue irregularity can result from internal tissue contracture and scarring, from fat necrosis, or during gradual resorption of a hematoma or seroma. Prevention is meticulous surgical technique minimizing flap trauma and desiccation and prompt and complete drainage or evacuation of any retained fluid. Repair of the defect may require late re-elevation of the flap with excision of the scarred tissue or seroma or pseudobursa (Fig. 122-68).

Residual abdominal contour deformity can result from performing a lesser operation with inadequate tissue excision. A patient may have undergone a lesser procedure in the interest of a shorter scar and is dissatisfied with the result. These patients undergo a standard evaluation with a clear understanding of any previously divided vasculature. Know the extent of prior flap elevation and whether the umbilical stalk has been divided. If the umbilicus was floated previously, it cannot be circumscribed. If the flap needs to be advanced to a point where the umbilicus will be unnaturally low (less than 16 cm above the anterior vulvar commissure), the umbilicus should be excised, the site closed in layers, and a neoumbilicoplasty performed (see "Umbilical Revision"). A properly designed secondary abdominoplasty can address residual contour deformity as well as revise and reposition scars and the umbilicus as needed (Fig. 122-69).

Umbilical Revision

UMBILICAL DEFORMITY

Umbilical distortions after abdominoplasty include partial or complete umbilical stenosis or an umbilicus that is large, prominent, flat, or malpositioned (Fig. 122-70).[46] The large umbilicus can be reduced by reducing the umbilical stalk to 1 cm in diameter and using

Text continued on p. 188

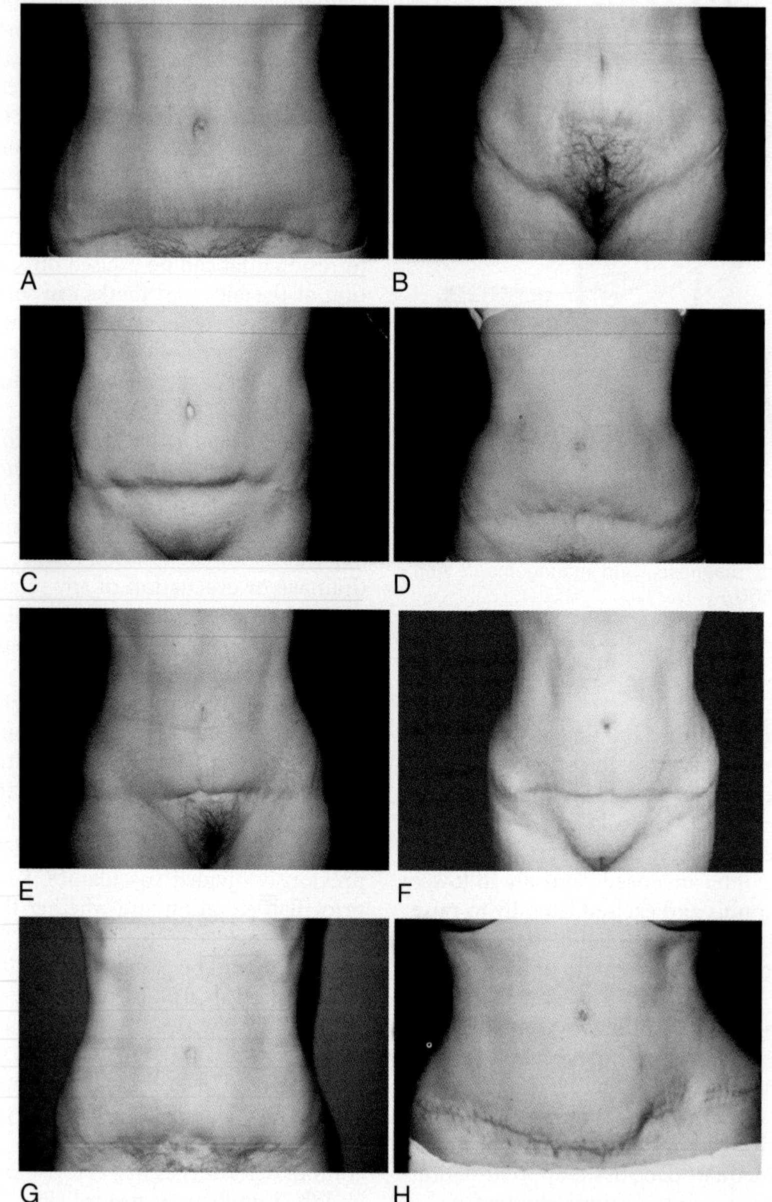

FIGURE 122-66. Unaesthetic scars and contour deformities after abdominoplasty. Scars may be fine but malplaced (*A*, *B*). Scars may be too low laterally (*A*) or too high centrally (*B*, *C*, *D*). They may be depressed owing to tissue thinning under the scar (*C*, *D*, *E*) or wide from dermal thinning and stretching (*D*, *E*) or from secondary healing after ischemia (*G*). Tissue bulges can be due to inadequate scar length, resulting in bunching (*D*) and dog-ears (*F*), or may be the result of soft tissue contracture or necrosis (*G*, *H*).

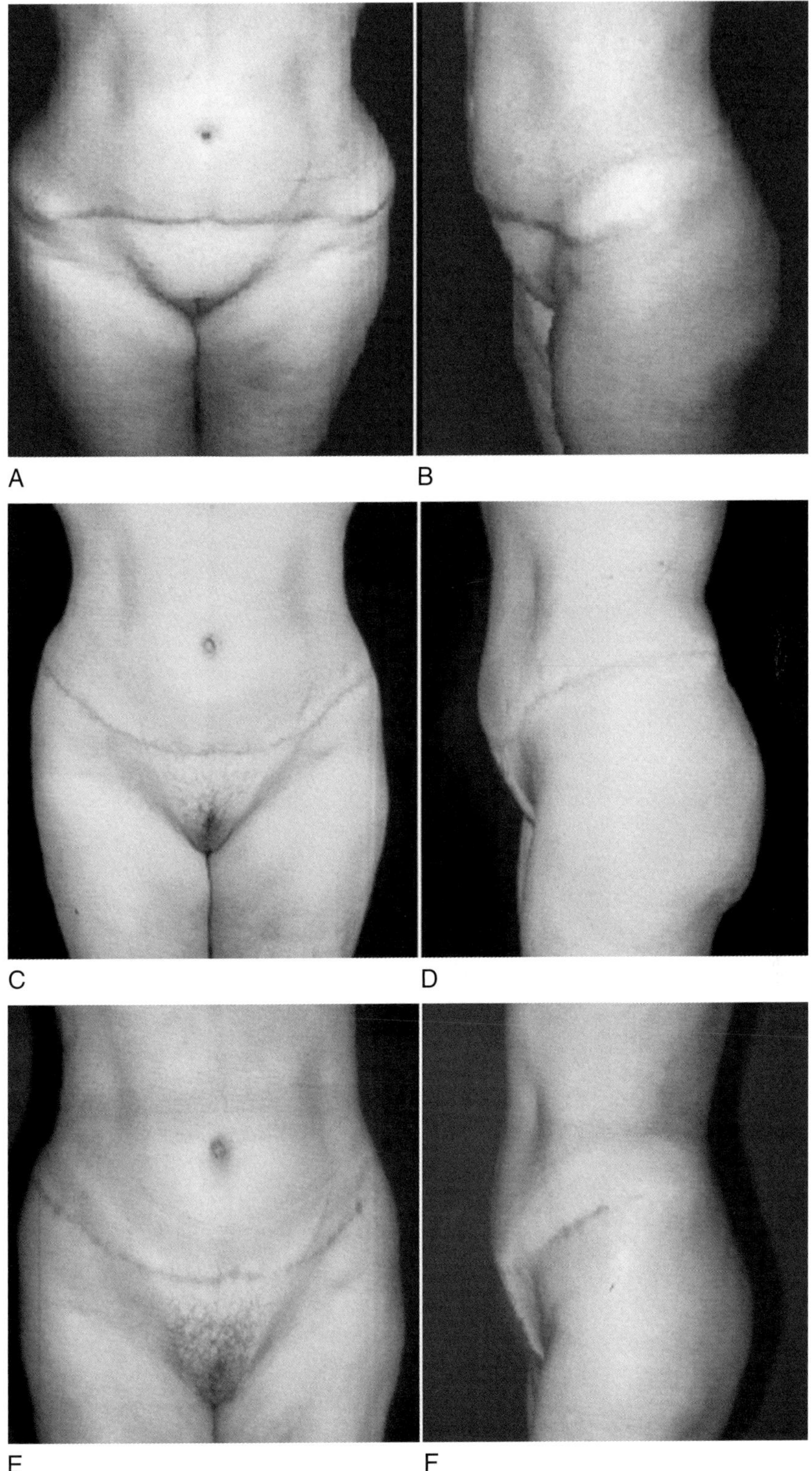

FIGURE 122-67. *A,* Anterior view of a self-explanatory suboptimal abdominoplasty result. *B,* Lateral view. *C,* Postoperative view 6 months after secondary abdominoplasty with the handlebar incision. *D,* Lateral view. *E,* Postoperative view at 6 years. *F,* Lateral view.

Continued

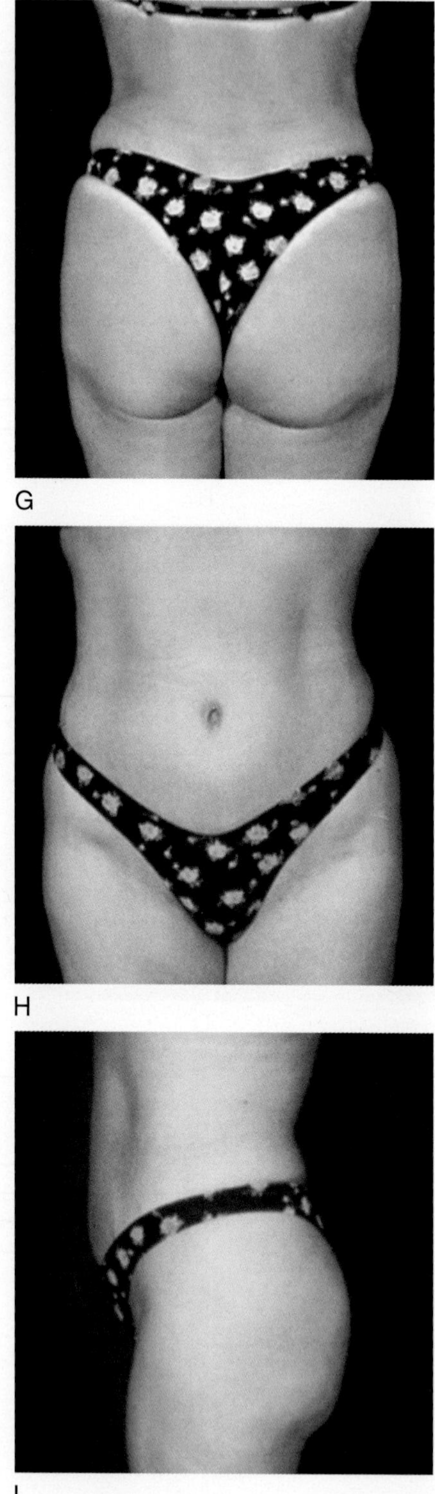

FIGURE 122-67, cont'd. *G* to *I*, Views of patient in small, high-cut bikini; scar is not visible.

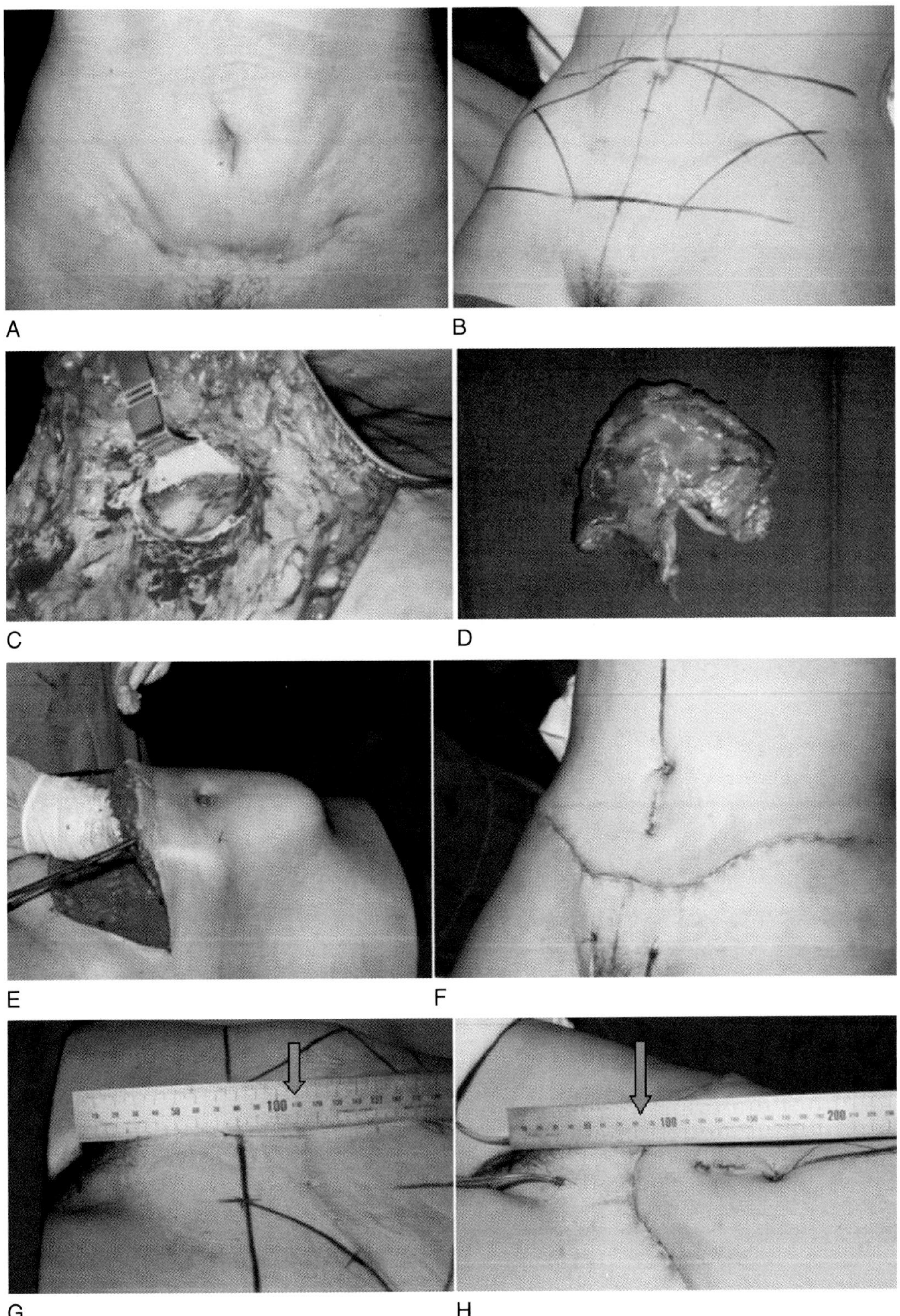

FIGURE 122-68. *A,* Anterior view of a protrusion of the hypogastrium after mini-abdominoplasty due to a localized, hardened seroma. *B,* The patient is marked for secondary abdominoplasty. *C* and *D,* Close-up view of the resected seroma capsule. *E,* Skin undermining. *F,* Final closure of transverse incision site. Note vertical closure of umbilical donor site. *G* and *H,* Preoperative and postoperative measurement of incision site to vulvar commissure. The incision was lowered from 11 cm to 7 cm from the anterior vulvar commissure.

Continued

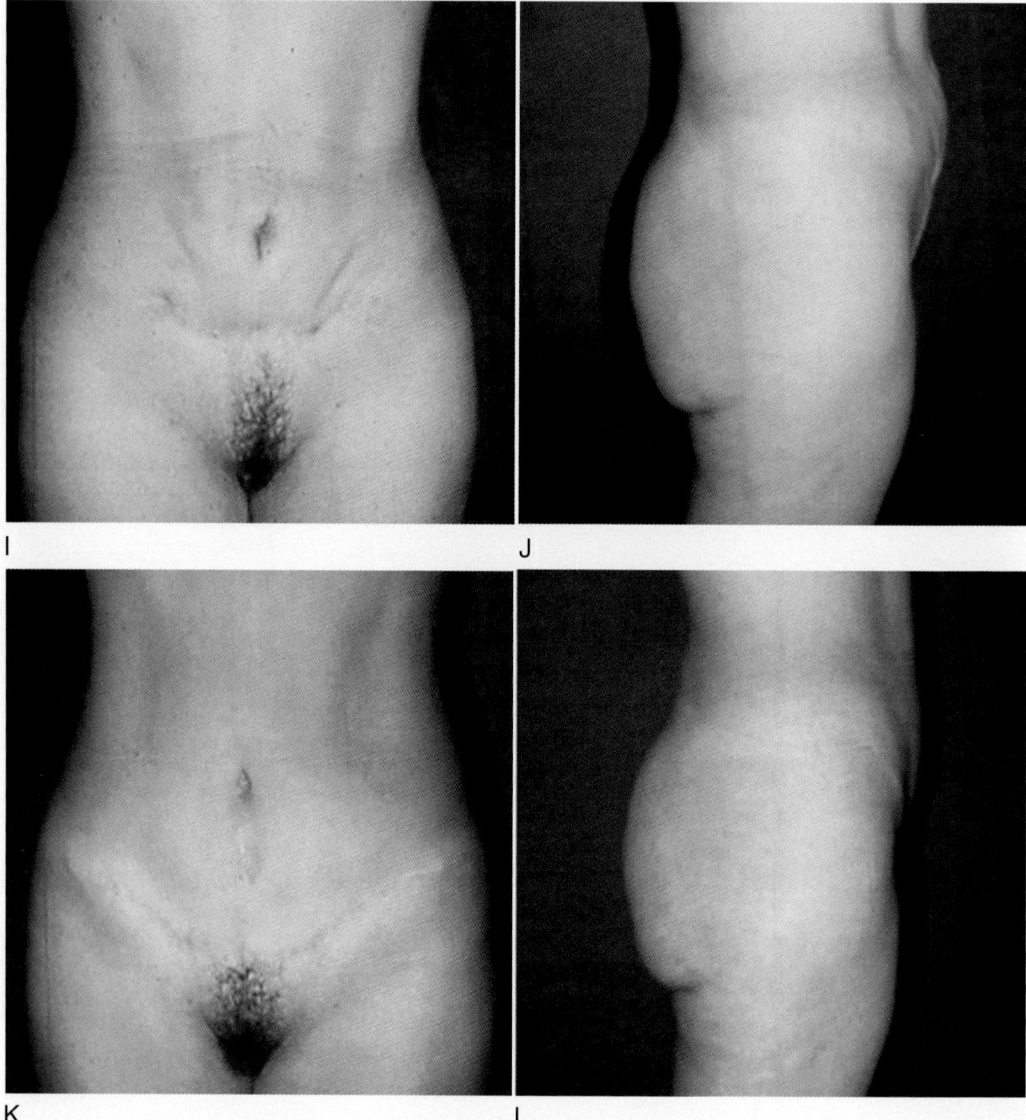

FIGURE 122-68, cont'd. *I* and *J,* Preoperative anterior and lateral views. *K* and *L,* Postoperative anterior and lateral views at 1 year. Note maintenance of lowered closure.

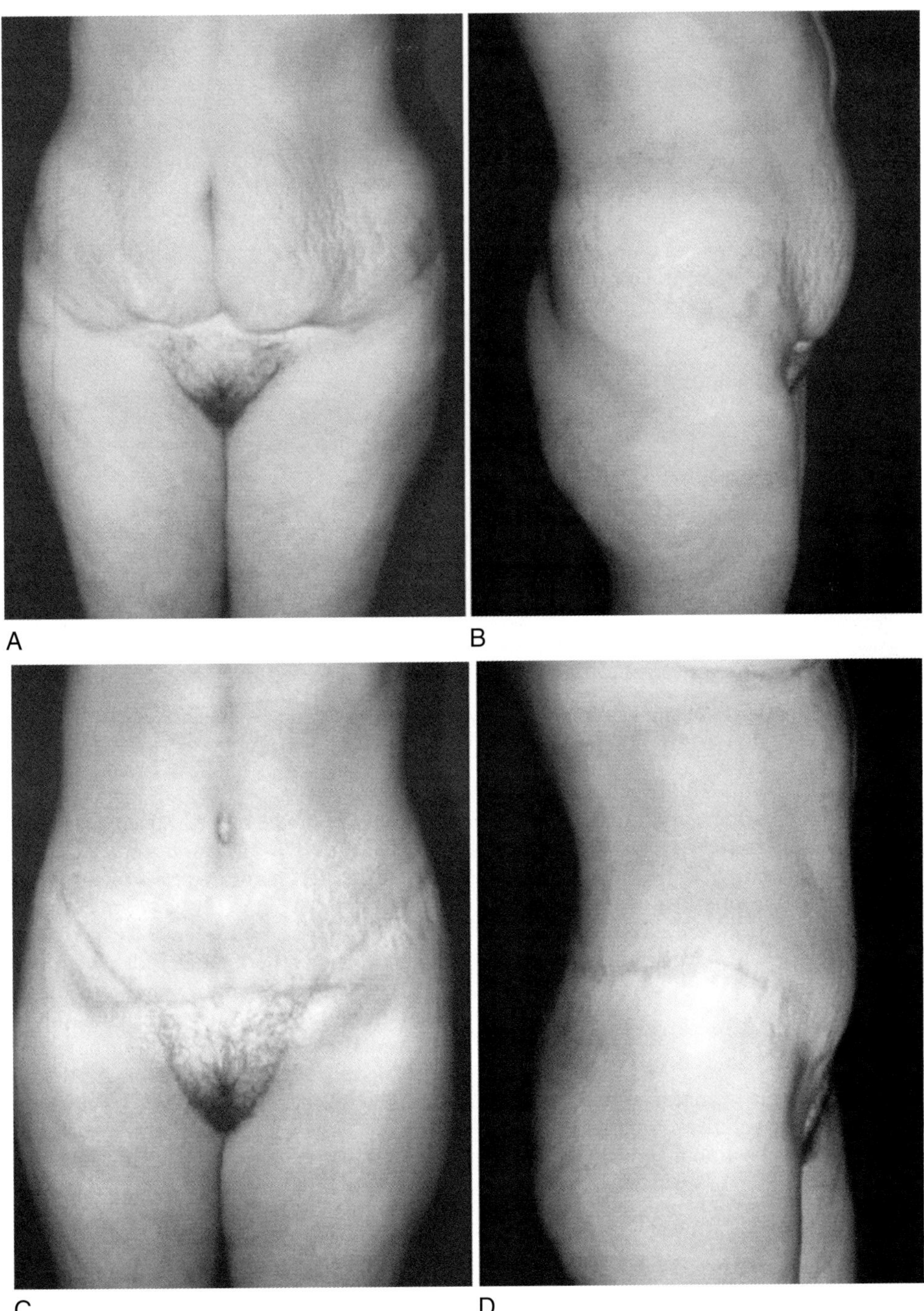

FIGURE 122-69. *A,* Anterior view of patient who underwent an unsuccessful mini-abdominoplasty. *C,* A secondary full abdominoplasty with the handlebar incision was performed to improve the result. The former scar was eliminated. *B* and *D,* Preoperative and postoperative lateral views.

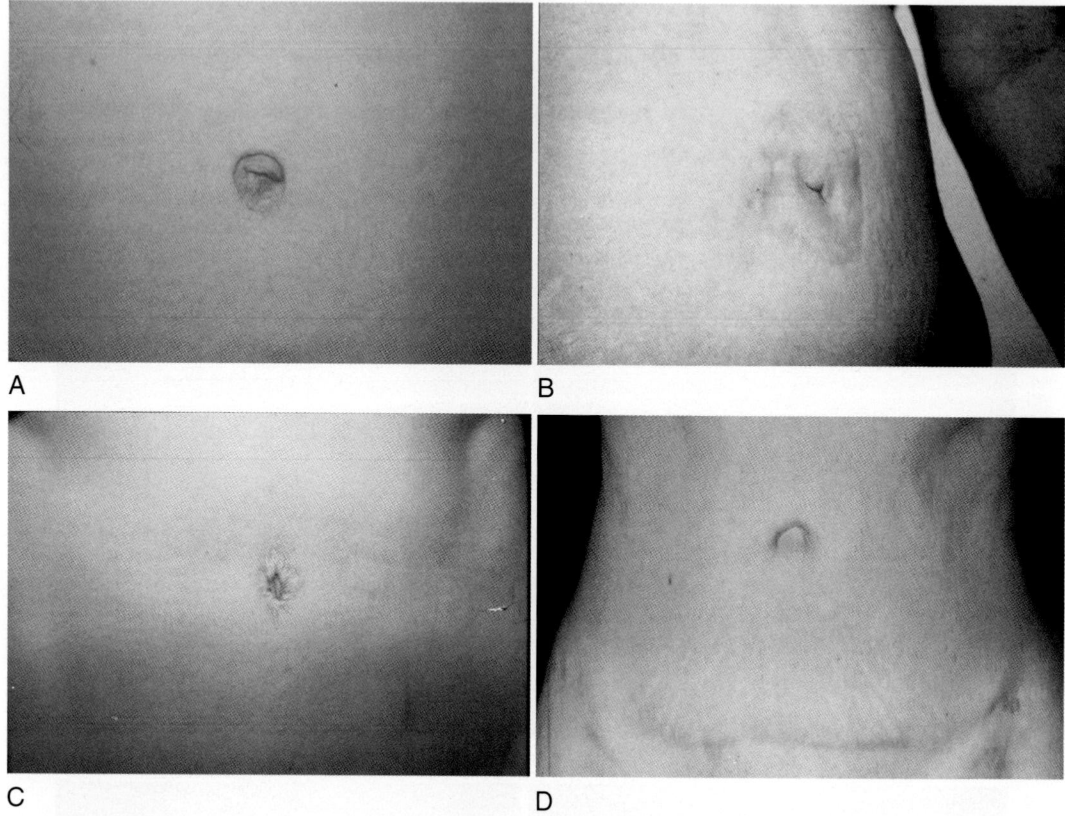

FIGURE 122-70. *A* to *D*, Suboptimal umbilicoplasty results after traditional abdominoplasty. Many of these patients require secondary surgery for an optimal aesthetic outcome.

a pursestring suture on the abdominal flap. The stenotic umbilicus should be released, as with a double Z-plasty[93] or wedge excision at the inferior border of the stenotic scar.[46] If the problem cannot be fixed directly, the umbilical site may be excised and closed meticulously in layers, and a neoumbilicoplasty is performed.

UMBILICAL RECONSTRUCTION

When the umbilicus is missing or malformed because of prior surgery or postoperative complications such as infection or necrosis, the umbilicus must be reconstructed. The ideal umbilical reconstruction is natural appearing, has a well-hidden scar, and is properly located on the skin flap.

Several techniques have been described for establishing a neoumbilicus with use of the abdominal flap as a blank canvas. The subcutaneous tissue on the abdominal flap at the site of the neoumbilicus can be thinned to dermis and the flap sutured to fascia.[63] Various local flaps have been used to establish a natural indentation.[46,93,94]

When a vertical midline incision exists or is planned, a neoumbilicus can be developed with use of bilateral, laterally based rectangular flaps (see Fig. 122-58; also see "Dermolipectomy After Massive Weight Loss"). This procedure is useful in patients with a vertical incision or scar where the original umbilicus is missing, scarred, or at jeopardy because of prior operations or a hernia; it results in a neoumbilicus with a deep sulcus and no circumferential scar (see Fig. 122-59). The vertical extent of the incision is marked. If a transverse excision will be taken, the bilateral laterally based flaps must be designed to sit level with the top of the iliac crest *after flap advancement and inset.* This location may be determined by advancing the flap caudally to its anticipated position at closure. If no transverse component is planned, the umbilicoplasty flaps are designed adjacent to the native umbilical scar. The vertical incision is closed, the umbilicus is inverted, and the base is secured to the abdominal fascia.

Baroudi Neoumbilicoplasty Technique[46,47]

The native umbilicus may be excised and substituted with a neoumbilicus. This procedure involves a mini-abdominoplasty, with skin flap undermining up to the necessary level above the umbilicus. The defect in the skin resulting from excision of the umbilicus is sutured

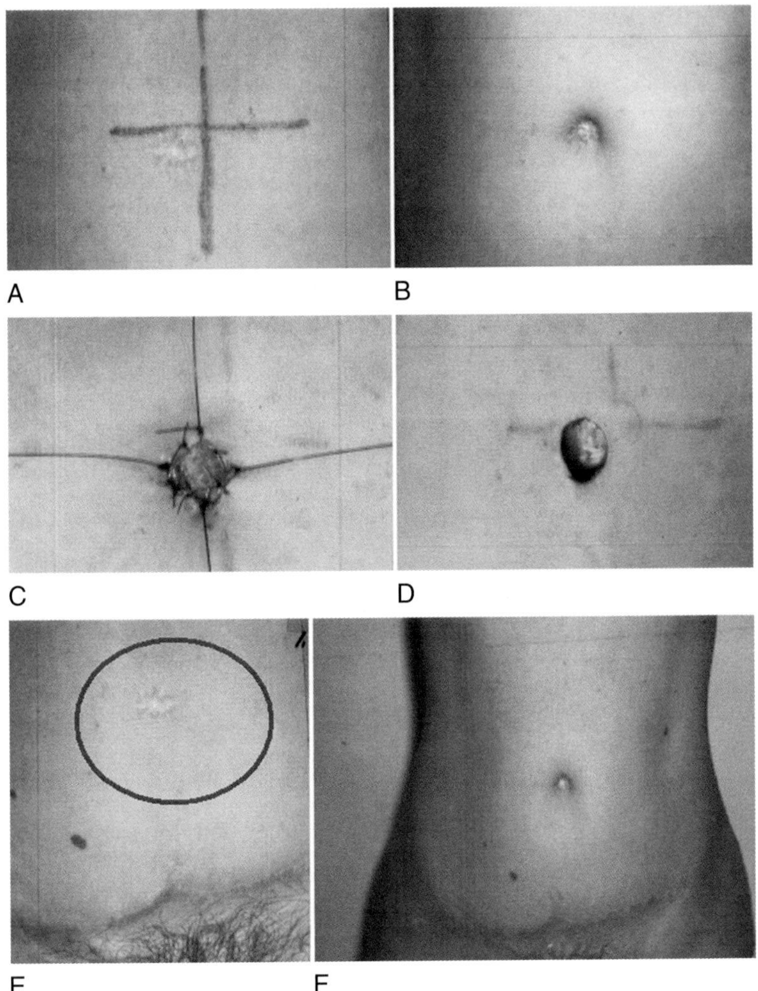

FIGURE 122-71. Baroudi neoumbilicoplasty. *A,* Location marked at midline along the axis of the superior iliac spines. *B,* The umbilical inset site is prepared with a 2-cm incision in the skin flap. The flap is then defatted adjacent to the incision site. *C,* The skin edges are sutured to the underlying fascia with interrupted 4-0 nylon sutures. *D,* Complete healing after 4 weeks. *E,* Preoperative close-up view of umbilicus lost because of necrosis after abdominoplasty. The patient requested an umbilical revision but refused abdominal scar revision. *F,* Same patient after neoumbilicoplasty procedure.

in layers. The skin flap is then moved caudally and anchored with a mattress suture at the pubis level. A neoumbilicoplasty is then performed by making a transverse 2-cm skin incision, with limited defatting below, followed by several interrupted 4-0 nylon sutures that bite the skin edge and fascia below (Fig. 122-71). A small gauze pad with ointment is sutured in place with a tie-over bolster to cover the neoumbilicus. The gauze dressing is left in place for 3 days, then removed. The patient may shower, and the exposed area should be washed twice a day with soap and water and covered with a new gauze pad with ointment. The healing is complete in about 4 weeks through secondary intention.

REFERENCES

1. Cikim AS, Ozbey N, Orhan Y: Relationship between cardiovascular risk indicators and types of obesity in overweight and obese women. J Int Med Res 2004;32:268.
2. Rexrode KM, Carey VJ, Hennekens CH, et al: Abdominal adiposity and coronary heart disease in women. JAMA 1998; 280:1843.
3. Jasienska G, Ziomkiewicz A, Ellison PT, et al: Large breasts and narrow waists indicate high reproductive potential in women. Proc R Soc Lond B Biol Sci 2004;271:1213.
4. Singh D: Waist-to-hip ratio and judgment of attractiveness and healthiness of female figures by male and female physicians. Int J Obes Relat Metab Disord 1994;18:731.
5. Singh D: Adaptive significance of female physical attractiveness: role of waist-to-hip ratio. J Pers Soc Psychol 1993; 65:293.

6. Dixson AF, Halliwell G, East R, et al: Masculine somatotype and hirsuteness as determinants of sexual attractiveness to women. Arch Sex Behav 2003;32:29.
7. Kelly HA: Report of gynecological cases (excessive growth of fat). Bull Johns Hopkins Hosp 1899;19:197.
8. Thorek M: Plastic Surgery of the Breast and Abdominal Wall. Springfield, Ill, Charles C Thomas, 1924.
9. Gonzalez-Ulloa M: Belt lipectomy. Br J Plast Surg 1960;13:179.
10. Babcock WW: The correction of the obese and relaxed abdominal wall with special reference to the use of buried silver chain. Am J Obstet Gynecol 1916;74:596.
11. Schepelmann E: Über Bauchdeckenplastik mit besonderes Berucksichtigung des Hängebauches. Beitr Klin Chir 1918; 111:372.
12. Kuster H: Operation bei Hängebrust und Hängeleib. Monatsschr Geburtsh Gynak 1926;73:316.
13. Weinhold S: Bauchdeckenplastik. Zentralbl Gynak 1909;38:1332.
14. Galtier M: Traitement chirurgical des obésités de la paroi abdominale avec ptose. Mem Acad Chir 1955;81:12.
15. Castanares S, Goethel J: Abdominal lipectomy: a modification in technique. Plast Reconstr Surg 1967;40:373.
16. Pitanguy I: Abdominal lipectomy: an approach to it through an analysis of 300 consecutive cases. Plast Reconstr Surg 1967; 40:384.
17. Callia WEP: Contribuicao para o estudo da correcao cirurgica do abdomen em pendulo e globoso: tecnica original [tese de doutoramento apresentada à Faculdade de Medicina]. Universidade de São Paulo, 1965.
18. Régnault P: Abdominal lipectomy: a low W incision. New York International Society of Aesthetic Plastic Surgery, 1972.
19. Grazer FM: Abdominoplasty. Plast Reconstr Surg 1973;51:167.
20. Baroudi R, Moraes M: A "bicycle-handlebar" type of incision for primary and secondary abdominoplasty. Aesthetic Plast Surg 1995;19:307.
21. Illouz YG: Une nouvelle technique pour les lypodystrophies localisées. La lipectomie selective ou lipolyse. Rev Chir Esthet 1980;4:19.
22. Avelar J: Fat suction versus abdominoplasty. Aesthetic Plast Surg 1985;9:265.
23. Greminger RF: The mini-abdominoplasty. Plast Reconstr Surg 1987;79:356.
24. Ousterhout DK: Combined suction-assisted lipectomy, surgical lipectomy, and surgical abdominoplasty. Ann Plast Surg 1990;24:126.
25. Wilkinson TS: Limited abdominoplasty techniques applied to complete abdominal repair. Aesthetic Plast Surg 1994;18:49.
26. Ramirez OM: U-M abdominoplasty. Aesthetic Surg J 1999;19:279.
27. Shestak KC: Marriage abdominoplasty expands the mini-abdominoplasty concept. Plast Reconstr Surg 1999;103:1020.
28. Matarasso A: Liposuction as an adjunct to a full abdominoplasty revisited. Plast Reconstr Surg 2000;106:1197.
29. Avelar J: Abdominoplasty without panniculus undermining and resection: analysis and 3-year follow-up of 97 cases. Aesthetic Surg J 2002;22:17.
30. Saldanha OR, De Souza Pinto EB, Mattos WN Jr, et al: Lipoabdominoplasty with selective and safe undermining. Aesthetic Plast Surg 2003;27:322.
31. Lockwood TE: Superficial fascial system (SFS) of the trunk and extremities: a new concept. Plast Reconstr Surg 1991;87:1009.
32. Rohrich RJ, Smith PD, Marcantonio D, Kenkel JM: The zones of adherence: role in minimizing and preventing contour deformities in liposuction. Plast Reconstr Surg 2001;107:1562.
33. Huger WE Jr: The anatomic rationale for abdominal lipectomy. Am Surg 1979;45:612.
34. Tahara Y, Tsunawake N, Yukawa K, et al: Sex differences in interrelationships between percent body fat (% fat) and waist-to-hip ratio (WHR) in healthy male and female adults. Ann Physiol Anthropol 1994;13:293.
35. Dubou R, Ousterhout DK: Placement of the umbilicus in an abdominoplasty. Plast Reconstr Surg 1978;61:291.
36. Bozola AR, Psillakis JM: Abdominoplasty: a new concept and classification for treatment. Plast Reconstr Surg 1988;82:983.
37. Matarasso A: Minimal-access variations in abdominoplasty. Ann Plast Surg 1995;34:255.
38. Pitman GH: Liposuction and body contouring. In Aston SJ, Beasley RW, Thorne CHM, eds: Grabb and Smith's Plastic Surgery. Philadelphia, Lippincott-Raven, 1997:669.
39. Nahas FX: An aesthetic classification of the abdomen based on the myoaponeurotic layer. Plast Reconstr Surg 2001;108:1787.
40. Toledo LS: The overlap of lipoplasty and abdominoplasty: indication, classification, and treatment. Clin Plast Surg 2004;31:539.
41. Lockwood TE: High-lateral-tension abdominoplasty with superficial fascial system suspension. Plast Reconstr Surg 1995;96:603.
42. Wilkinson TS, Swartz BE: Individual modifications in body contour surgery: the "limited" abdominoplasty. Plast Reconstr Surg 1986;77:779.
43. Gradel J: Umbilical technical maneuvers to facilitate abdominoplasty with limited incisions. Aesthetic Plast Surg 1991;15:251.
44. Jackson IT, Downie PA: Abdominoplasty—the waistline stitch and other refinements. Plast Reconstr Surg 1978;61:180.
45. Psillakis JM: Plastic surgery of the abdomen with improvement in the body contour. Physiopathology and treatment of the aponeurotic musculature. Clin Plast Surg 1984;11:465.
46. Baroudi R: Umbilicoplasty. Clin Plast Surg 1975;2:431.
47. Baroudi R, Carvalho CG: Neoumbilicaplasty: un procedimiento en el transcorso de las abdominoplastias. Cir Plast Ibero Latinamer 1981;7:391.
48. Baroudi R, Ferreira CA: Seroma: how to avoid it and how to treat it. Aesthetic Surg J 1998;18:439.
49. Illouz YG: A new safe and aesthetic approach to suction abdominoplasty. Aesthetic Plast Surg 1992;16:237.
50. Baroudi R: Abdominoplasty: historical review and personal preferences. Lipoplasty Newslett 1993;10:8.
51. Baroudi R, Keppke EM, Carvalho CG: Mammary reduction combined with reverse abdominoplasty. Ann Plast Surg 1979;2:368.
52. Lockwood TE: Rectus muscle diastasis in males: primary indication for endoscopically assisted abdominoplasty. Plast Reconstr Surg 1998;101:1685.
53. Eaves FF III, Nahai F, Bostwick J III: Endoscopic abdominoplasty and endoscopically assisted miniabdominoplasty. Clin Plast Surg 1996;23:599.
54. Zukowski ML, Ash K, Spencer D, et al: Endoscopic intracorporal abdominoplasty: a review of 85 cases. Plast Reconstr Surg 1998;102:516.
55. Vastine VL, Morgan RF, Williams GS, et al: Wound complications of abdominoplasty in obese patients. Ann Plast Surg 1999;42:34.
56. Van Gaal LF, Wauters MA, De Leeuw IH: The beneficial effects of modest weight loss on cardiovascular risk factors. Int J Obes Relat Metab Disord 1997;21(suppl 1):S5.
57. Rubin JP, Nguyen V, Schwentker A: Perioperative management of the post-gastric-bypass patient presenting for body contour surgery. Clin Plast Surg 2004;31:601.
58. Aly AS, Cram AE, Heddens C: Truncal body contouring surgery in the massive weight loss patient. Clin Plast Surg 2004;31:611.
59. Cormenzana P, Samprón NM: Circumferential approach to contouring of the trunk. Aesthetic Surg J 2004;24:13.
60. Craig SB, Faller MS, Puckett CL: In search of the ideal female umbilicus. Plast Reconstr Surg 2000;105:389.
61. Avelar J: Abdominoplasty—systemization of a technique without external umbilical scar. Aesthetic Plast Surg 1978;2:141.
62. Juri J, Juri C, Raiden G: Reconstruction of the umbilicus in abdominoplasty. Plast Reconstr Surg 1979;63:580.
63. Schoeller T, Wechselberger G, Otto A, et al: New technique for scarless umbilical reinsertion in abdominoplasty procedures. Plast Reconstr Surg 1998;102:1720.

64. Grazer FM, Goldwyn RM: Abdominoplasty assessed by survey, with emphasis on complications. Plast Reconstr Surg 1977; 59:513.
65. Teimourian B, Rogers WB 3rd: A national survey of complications associated with suction lipectomy: a comparative study. Plast Reconstr Surg 1989;84:628.
66. Hester TR Jr, Baird W, Bostwick J 3rd, et al: Abdominoplasty combined with other major surgical procedures: safe or sorry? Plast Reconstr Surg 1989;83:997.
67. Hughes CE: Reduction of lipoplasty risks and mortality: an ASAPS survey. Aesthetic Surg J 2001;21:120.
68. Kroll SS: Necrosis of abdominoplasty and other secondary flaps after TRAM flap breast reconstruction. Plast Reconstr Surg 1994;94:637.
69. Manassa EH, Hertl CH, Olbrisch RR: Wound healing problems in smokers and nonsmokers after 132 abdominoplasties. Plast Reconstr Surg 2003;111:2082.
70. Krueger JK, Rohrich RJ: Clearing the smoke: the scientific rationale for tobacco abstention with plastic surgery. Plast Reconstr Surg 2001;108:1063.
71. Nakagawa M, Tanaka H, Tsukuma H, Kishi Y: Relationship between the duration of the preoperative smoke-free period and the incidence of postoperative pulmonary complications after pulmonary surgery. Chest 2001;120:705.
72. Padubidri AN, Yetman R, Browne E, et al: Complications of postmastectomy breast reconstructions in smokers, ex-smokers, and nonsmokers. Plast Reconstr Surg 2001;107:342.
73. Chang DW, Reece GP, Wang B, et al: Effect of smoking on complications in patients undergoing free TRAM flap breast reconstruction. Plast Reconstr Surg 2000;105:2374.
74. Mensah GA, Mokdad AH, Ford E, et al: Obesity, metabolic syndrome, and type 2 diabetes: emerging epidemics and their cardiovascular implications. Cardiol Clin 2004;22:485.
75. Must A, Spadano J, Coakley EH, et al: The disease burden associated with overweight and obesity. JAMA 1999;282: 1523.
76. Giese SY, Bulan EJ, Commons GW, et al: Improvements in cardiovascular risk profile with large-volume liposuction: a pilot study. Plast Reconstr Surg 2001;108:510.
77. Giugliano G, Nicoletti G, Grella E, et al: Effect of liposuction on insulin resistance and vascular inflammatory markers in obese women. Br J Plast Surg 2004;57:190.
78. Ang-Lee M, Moss J, Yuan CS: Herbal medicines and perioperative care. JAMA 2001;286:208.
79. Adusumilli PS, Ben-Porat L, Pereira M, et al: The prevalence and predictors of herbal medicine use in surgical patients. J Am Coll Surg 2004;198:583.
80. Woolf RM, Snow JW, Walker JH, Broadbent TR: Resolution of an artificially induced haematoma and the influence of a proteolytic enzyme. J Trauma 1965;5:491.
81. Petry JJ: Surgically significant nutritional supplements. Plast Reconstr Surg 1996;97:233.
82. Tveiten D, Bruseth S, Borchgrevink CF, Lohne K: Effect of Arnica D 30 during hard physical exertion. A double-blind randomized trial during the Oslo Marathon 1990 [in Norwegian]. Tidsskr Nor Laegeforen 1991;111:3630.
83. Ernst E, Pittler MH: Efficacy of homeopathic arnica: a systematic review of placebo-controlled clinical trials. Arch Surg 1998;133:1187.
84. Goldhaber SZ: Pulmonary embolism. Lancet 2004;363:1295.
85. Davis RE, Wachholz JH, Jassir D, et al: Comparison of topical anti-ischemic agents in the salvage of failing random-pattern skin flaps in rats. Facial Plast Surg 1999;1:27.
86. Davies BW, Lewis RD, Pennington G: The impact of vasodilators on random-pattern skin flap survival in the rat following mainstream smoke exposure. Ann Plast Surg 1998;40:630.
87. Karacaoglan N, Akbas H: Effect of parenteral pentoxifylline and topical nitroglycerin on skin flap survival. Otolaryngol Head Neck Surg 1999;120:272.
88. Pitanguy I: Evaluation of body contouring surgery today: a 30-year perspective. Plast Reconstr Surg 2000;105:1499.
89. Mustoe TA, Cooter RD, Gold MH, et al, International Advisory Panel on Scar Management: International clinical recommendations on scar management. Plast Reconstr Surg 2002;110:560.
90. Pollock T, Pollock H: Progressive tension sutures in abdominoplasty. Clin Plast Surg 2004;31(4):583.
91. Liszka TG, Dellon AL, Manson PN: Iliohypogastric nerve entrapment following abdominoplasty. Plast Reconstr Surg 1994; 93:181.
92. van Uchelen JH, Werker PM, Kon M: Complications of abdominoplasty in 86 patients. Plast Reconstr Surg 2001; 107:1869.
93. Baack BR, Anson G, Nachbar JM, White DJ: Umbilicoplasty: the construction of a new umbilicus and correction of umbilical stenosis without external scars. Plast Reconstr Surg 1996; 97:227.
94. Kirianoff TG: Making a new umbilicus when none exists. Case report. Plast Reconstr Surg 1978;61:603.

CHAPTER

123

Body Contouring: Comprehensive Liposuction

Gerald H. Pitman, MD ✦ Sharon Y. Giese, MD

Liposuction is the surgical aspiration of subcutaneous fat by use of a cannula attached to a vacuum pump. Lipoplasty, liposculpture, and suction-assisted lipectomy are other terms describing this process. Liposuction is, however, the most commonly used term for this procedure and is universally recognized by surgeons and lay persons as the word meaning vacuum evacuation of fat. In this chapter, the term *liposuction* encompasses the other terminologies.

The essence of liposuction is removal of fat by blunt, discontinuous dissection without interruption of the larger neurovascular bundles coursing to the skin from the deep fascia. Blood supply and innervation to the overlying skin are preserved. Volume reduction of the subcutaneous fat compartment is followed by tissue collapse, healing, and contracture. Contour is diminished as the overlying skin becomes more closely adherent to the underlying musculature (Color Plate 123-1).

Liposuction was initially used for spot reduction of localized fat deposits in patients at or near ideal body weight. More recently, however, liposuction has been used for circumferential treatment of multiple anatomic areas, resulting in more comprehensive reshaping and reduction of the body.[1-3] Notwithstanding the surgeon's ability to remove large volumes of fat, liposuction is not a substitute for a healthy lifestyle.[4] Permanent weight loss requires modification of diet and permanent change in eating habits. Whereas liposuction can change body proportions by surgical removal of adipocytes from a specific location, persistent overeating will result in excess fat deposits in remaining adipocytes, sometimes in areas of the body other than those treated.

INSTRUMENTATION

Liposuction achieves the selective debulking of subcutaneous fatty deposits with use of small-diameter cannulas passed through minimal skin incisions. Each step of the procedure requires specialized instruments.

Infusion

Paramount to achieving an even removal of the underlying fat is the accurate infusion of a wetting solution. Preoperative instillation of dilute lidocaine-epinephrine solution into the fat is performed with infiltration cannulas and pumps. The cannulas have blunt tips and range in diameter from 1 to 3 mm and in length from 10 to 30 cm. Multiple openings near the tip facilitate rapid delivery of fluid in all directions (Fig. 123-1). The infiltrating needle can be mounted onto a syringe filled with the wetting solution or be propelled into the subcutaneous tissue at a faster rate by the following methods:

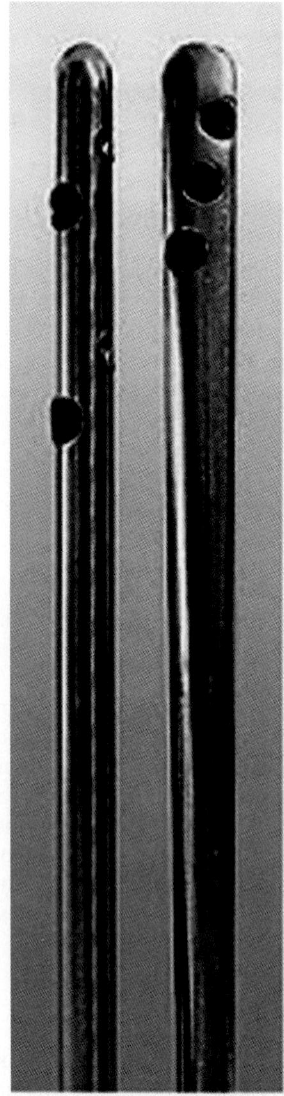

FIGURE 123-1. Infiltrating cannulas. (Courtesy of Wells Johnson Group, Tucson, Arizona.)

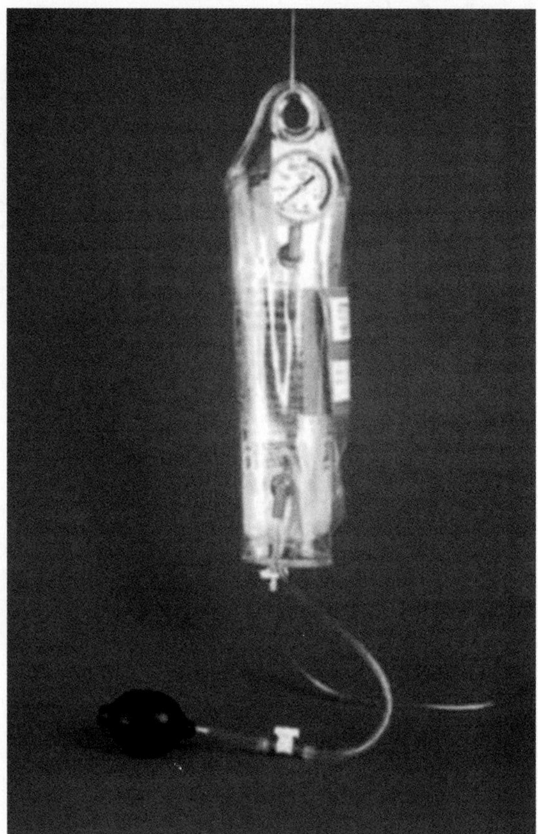

FIGURE 123-2. Pneumatic sleeve for pressurized infusion of wetting solution. (BP Cuff Pressure Infiltrator. Courtesy of Byron Medical, Tucson, Arizona.)

- a pneumatic sleeve surrounding the intravenous bag of wetting solution (Fig. 123-2). The increased pressure forces the fluid into the tubing and out the cannula at a faster rate.
- a roller device, which also forces the fluid through the tubing at a faster rate (Fig. 123-3).
- a level 1 trauma infuser, which holds two 1-liter intravenous bags or a single 3-liter bag of wetting solution in variable pressure chambers (Fig. 123-4). The level 1 device warms the fluid to body temperature before infusion.

Delivery of fluid through large-diameter tubes (up to 3 mm) also increases the rate of infusion.

Evacuation

CANNULAS

Suction of the fat is achieved through small access incisions with hollow tubes (cannulas). Three important features determine the efficiency of a cannula: tip configuration, diameter, and length.

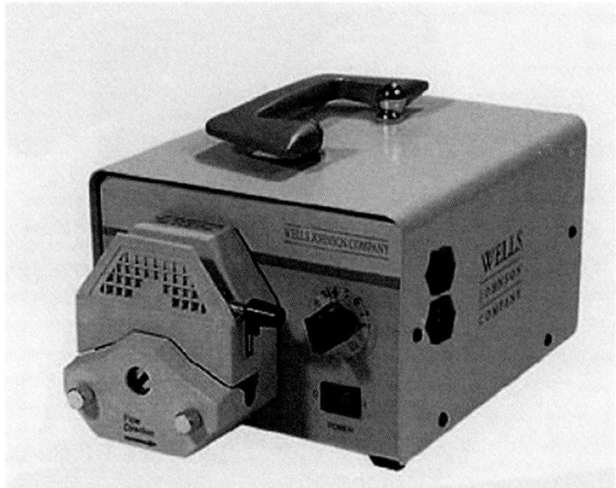

FIGURE 123-3. Roller device for rapid instillation of fluid into the subcutaneous tissues. (Infusion System 20-6000-00. Courtesy of Wells Johnson Group, Tucson, Arizona.)

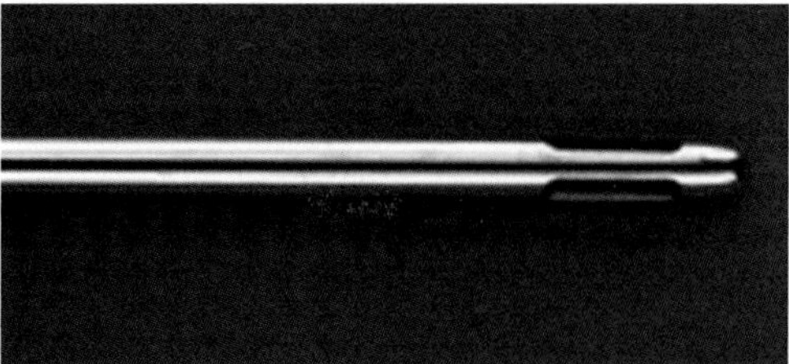

A

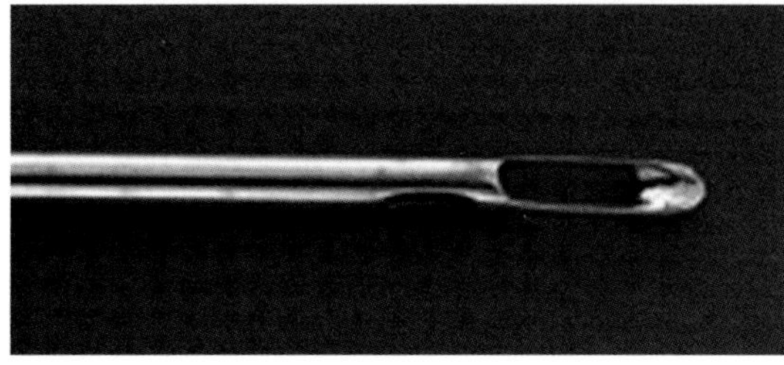

B

FIGURE 123-5. Cannula tip configurations. *A,* The "Mercedes" tip: three apertures at 120 degrees to each other around the circumference of the cannula adjacent to the tip. This is an efficient and moderately fast configuration. *B,* Keel tip: three apertures near a tapered tip. This is a fast, aggressive configuration.

Tip Configuration

The shape of the distal tip of the cannula and the number, configuration, and position of the apertures affect the efficacy and speed of liposuction. Most instruments have a blunt tip with multiple openings placed several millimeters back from the tip of the cannula. A less blunt, more tapered tip will more easily pass through the tissue but is also more likely to penetrate the fascia or skin (Fig. 123-5).

Multiple openings at the cannula tip increase the area from which fat can be suctioned. In addition, the multiple openings can increase shearing of the fat and increase speed of evacuation, resulting in decreased tissue trauma.

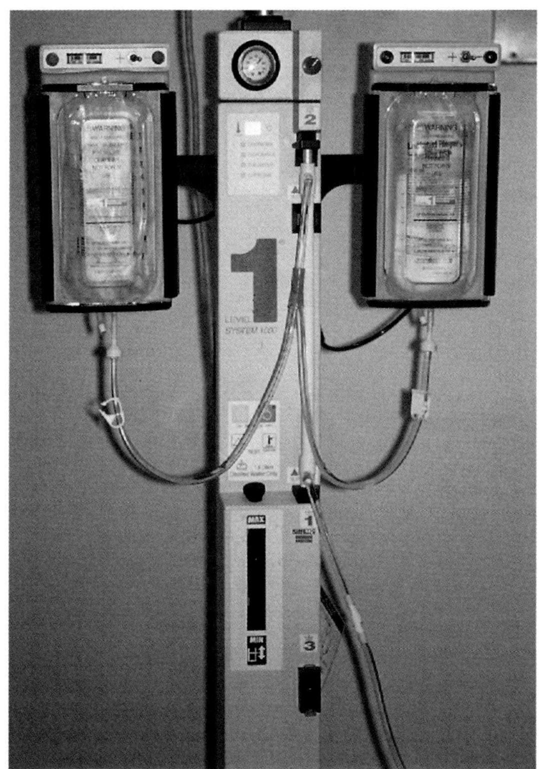

FIGURE 123-4. Level 1 rapid infiltration device also warms fluid to body temperature. (Level 1 H-1200 Fast Flow Fluid Warmer, Smiths Medical, Rockland, Mass.)

Cannula Diameter

Commonly used cannulas range from 1.8 to 5 mm in diameter. The smaller diameter cannulas permit minimal tissue resistance but slower fat evacuation. They are useful for fine, precise fat removal in relatively small fat compartments. Larger diameter cannulas provide increased efficiency of evacuation but require greater force to operate secondary to increased tissue resistance. Care must be taken with any size to achieve smooth, confluent removal of fat. Deeper, larger fatty deposits can be removed with larger cannulas; superficial fat in smaller compartments should be removed with smaller cannulas.

Cannula Length

Shorter cannulas offer better control. Longer cannulas provide access to distant areas with fewer incisions. The most commonly used cannulas are 18 to 23 cm long. Shorter cannulas, 10 to 14 cm in length, are generally used in the face, neck, calves, and ankles.

Handles

Ideally, the handle should be ergonomic and have a comfortable grip. Common shapes are hexagonal and round.

SUCTION PUMPS

The speed of evacuation is increased with high vacuum aspiration, which is essential to efficient liposuction. The minimal requirement is that the pump vaporize water. Vaporized water (gaseous phase) flows 100 times more rapidly than the liquid phase. With vaporization, viscosity is decreased and flow rate is increased, compensating for the reduction in flow rate that occurs when fine cannulas are used.

The aspirator holds a collection bottle for the aspirate, an overflow trap, a biologic filter that removes particles up to 0.3 μm in size, an intake filter that protects the pump from contaminants, the pump itself, and an exhaust filter. The filters protect the machine from contaminating the operating room environment and staff with oil or other vaporized substances and microbes.

Fat can also be evacuated without pumps by a syringe system. Various sizes of syringes are used with specially designed cannulas to fit the syringes. When the cannula is inserted into the fat, a vacuum is established by withdrawing the plunger. This technique is helpful for the removal of smaller amounts of fat, such as for the harvest of fat for autologous fat grafting or for small revision procedures.

Power-Assisted Liposuction

The power assist device, in use since 1999, reciprocates a cannula as it passes through the tissues. The cannula reciprocates in a plane parallel to the length of the cannula over a 2-mm amplitude at a speed of 3000 cycles per second. The power eases passage of the cannula through the tissues and assists in avulsion and evacuation of fat. Power is supplied from an electric console or by a pneumatic hose (Fig. 123-6). The power assist device reduces the surgeon's fatigue.

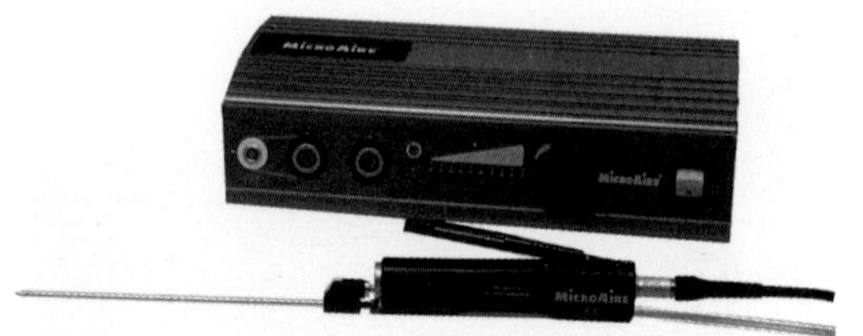

FIGURE 123-6. Electric power-assisted liposuction device. (1025 Electric Control Console shown with PAL-660E Electric PAL Handpiece. Courtesy of MicroAire Surgical Instruments, Charlottesville, Virginia.)

Ultrasonic-Assisted Liposuction

An ultrasonic assist device consists of a handpiece that converts electrical energy to ultrasonic energy and transmits the energy to the tissues through a titanium probe (Fig. 123-7*A*). The tip of the ultrasound device reciprocates at 20,000 to 35,000 cycles per second over an amplitude of 100 μm. The ultrasonic energy at the tip of the probe causes a cavitation effect in the fat cells, which subsequently implode. Ultrasonic probes are solid or hollow. The hollow probes (Fig. 123-7*B*) allow evacuation of a portion of the "liquefied fat." Technical considerations limit the size of the aperture and the hollow core in ultrasonic probes. Therefore, evacuation of fat is slow and incomplete. A conventional cannula is required to evacuate residual fat after ultrasound energy has been applied to the tissues.

VASER is the proprietary name of an ultrasonic assist device that offers the option of intermittent or continuous bursts of energy. The system employs a solid probe that is grooved near the tip, diffusing the energy wave and facilitating tissue fragmentation along the side of the probe (Fig. 123-8).

Ultrasonic-assisted liposuction may be advantageous in fibrous areas or in areas scarred from previ-

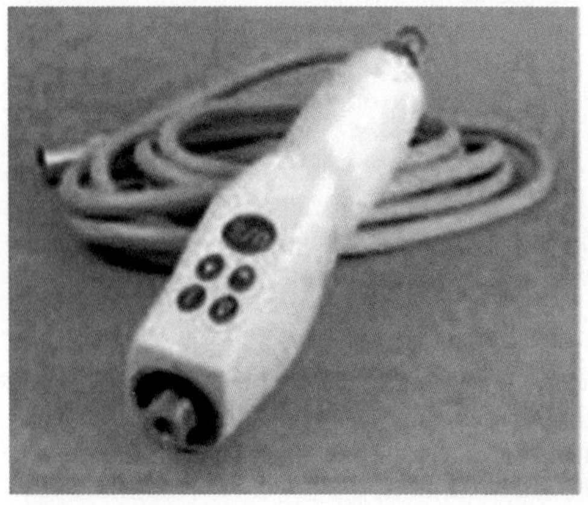

A

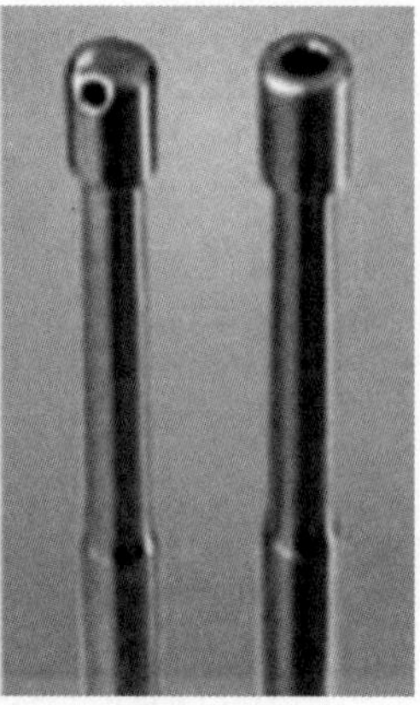

B

FIGURE 123-7. *A,* Handpiece of an ultrasonic device. The handpiece converts electrical energy from a generator to kinetic energy, which is transmitted to a probe as ultrarapid vibrations. The handpiece is connected to a generator by a flexible cord. The probe attaches to the handpiece by a screw mount (Contour Genesis Ultrasonic Handpiece). *B,* Hollow ultrasonic liposuction probe tips. Ultrarapid vibration at the probe tip implodes fat cells. Openings at the tip permit suction evacuation of liquefied fat. (Courtesy of Byron Medical, Tucson, Arizona.)

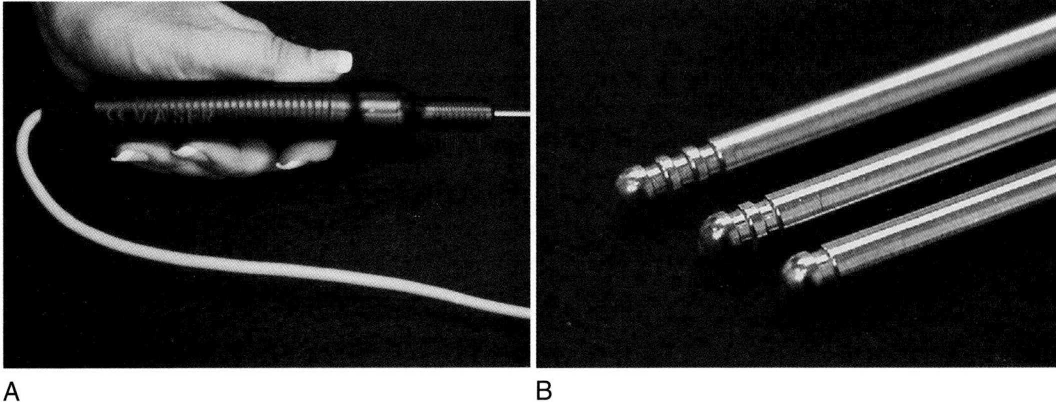

A B

FIGURE 123-8. *A,* The VASER ultrasonic device (Sound Surgical Technologies LLC, Louisville, Colorado). The handpiece is attached to the generator by the power cord. The probe screws into the distal end of the handpiece (right). *B,* The VASER ultrasonic probes. The tips of the probes are grooved to facilitate fragmentation in a lateral direction.

ous liposuction because the ultrasound energy fragments and liquefies some of the subcutaneous fat before suction evacuation. Both ultrasonic-assisted and power-assisted liposuction devices reduce the surgeon's work effort. The ultrasonic assist device, however, adds another step and more time to the procedure. Ultrasonic-assisted liposuction devices can also cause thermal burns.

Although liposuction is a unique surgical procedure requiring specialized instrumentation and techniques, no particular instrument or device will produce a better result than any other instrument or device. Ultimately, the quality of the result is dependent on the skills of the surgeon.

EVALUATION AND ASSESSMENT OF THE PATIENT

Selection of the patient is the first step in achieving a successful result and starts with a complete history of issues related to body shape as well as a general medical history. The physical examination addresses the entire body, not just the particular area in question.

History

The history begins with the initial telephone call from the prospective patient. The scheduling secretary routinely asks each caller for height and weight. The secretary consults a body mass index (BMI) chart* (Fig. 123-9). If BMI is 30 or more, the caller is gently informed that his or her weight is in the obese range and that liposuction is not a proven effective permanent weight loss modality. Referrals are offered to nutritionists, bariatric physicians, and Weight Watchers. The caller is also told what his or her weight should be to achieve a BMI less than 30 and encouraged to call back for an appointment once the goal weight is reached.

At the office consultation, the patient is asked to fill out a complete medical history form before seeing the surgeon. A nurse reviews the form with the patient and has the patient expand on any issues that may influence selection for surgery or perioperative care. The surgeon reviews the history before seeing the patient and also has the patient elaborate on portions of the medical history that may have an impact on the patient's care and recovery.

Medical impairments such as diabetes, hypertension, or coronary vascular disease do not automatically preclude consideration for surgery, but comorbidities will require preoperative notification of the anesthesiologist and evaluation by an internist or other appropriate physician to optimize the patient's care before surgery and to advise on special medical needs in the perioperative period. The scope of the operation may also be limited if the patient has significant medical disease.

The patient is queried about body weight history, exercise patterns, and eating disorders. A past history of bulimia or *anorexia nervosa* does not automatically exclude the patient from consideration for surgery, but evidence of recent eating disorders raises the possibility that liposuction is not in the patient's best interest and may prompt referral for a psychiatric evaluation.

The physician-patient interaction begins with a question to the patient, such as "Please tell me why you are here" or "Please tell me what brings you to the office." The interrogatory is intentionally open-ended. No

*http://www.nhlbi.nih.gov/guidelines/obesity/bmi_tbl.pdf

Body Mass Index Table

	Normal						Overweight					Obese										Extreme obesity														
BMI	19	20	21	22	23	24	25	26	27	28	29	30	31	32	33	34	35	36	37	38	39	40	41	42	43	44	45	46	47	48	49	50	51	52	53	54
Height (inches)	Body weight (pounds)																																			
58	91	96	100	105	110	115	119	124	129	134	138	143	148	153	158	162	167	172	177	181	186	191	196	201	205	210	215	220	224	229	234	239	244	248	253	258
59	94	99	104	109	114	119	124	128	133	138	143	148	153	158	163	168	173	178	183	188	193	198	203	208	212	217	222	227	232	237	242	247	252	257	262	267
60	97	102	107	112	118	123	128	133	138	143	148	153	158	163	168	174	179	184	189	194	199	204	209	215	220	225	230	235	240	245	250	255	261	266	271	276
61	100	106	111	116	122	127	132	137	143	148	153	158	164	169	174	180	185	190	195	201	206	211	217	222	227	232	238	243	248	254	259	264	269	275	280	285
62	104	109	115	120	126	131	136	142	147	153	158	164	169	175	180	186	191	196	202	207	213	218	224	229	235	240	246	251	256	262	267	273	278	284	289	295
63	107	113	118	124	130	135	141	146	152	158	163	169	175	180	186	191	197	203	208	214	220	225	231	237	242	248	254	259	265	270	278	282	287	293	299	304
64	110	116	122	128	134	140	145	151	157	163	169	174	180	186	192	197	204	209	215	221	227	232	238	244	250	256	262	267	273	279	285	291	296	302	308	314
65	114	120	126	132	138	144	150	156	162	168	174	180	186	192	198	204	210	216	222	228	234	240	246	252	258	264	270	276	282	288	294	300	306	312	318	324
66	118	124	130	136	142	148	155	161	167	173	179	186	192	198	204	210	216	223	229	235	241	247	253	260	266	272	278	284	291	297	303	309	315	322	328	334
67	121	127	134	140	146	153	159	166	172	178	185	191	198	204	211	217	223	230	236	242	249	255	261	268	274	280	287	293	299	306	312	319	325	331	338	344
68	125	131	138	144	151	158	164	171	177	184	190	197	203	210	216	223	230	236	243	249	256	262	269	276	282	289	295	302	308	315	322	328	335	341	348	354
69	128	135	142	149	155	162	169	176	182	189	196	203	209	216	223	230	236	243	250	257	263	270	277	284	291	297	304	311	318	324	331	338	345	351	358	365
70	132	139	146	153	160	167	174	181	188	195	202	209	216	222	229	236	243	250	257	264	271	278	285	292	299	306	313	320	327	334	341	348	355	362	369	376
71	136	143	150	157	165	172	179	186	193	200	208	215	222	229	236	243	250	257	265	272	279	286	293	301	308	315	322	329	338	343	351	358	365	372	379	386
72	140	147	154	162	169	177	184	191	199	206	213	221	228	235	242	250	258	265	272	279	287	294	302	309	316	324	331	338	346	353	361	368	375	383	390	397
73	144	151	159	166	174	182	189	197	204	212	219	227	235	242	250	257	265	272	280	288	295	302	310	318	325	333	340	348	355	363	371	378	386	393	401	408
74	148	155	163	171	179	186	194	202	210	218	225	233	241	249	256	264	272	280	287	295	303	311	319	326	334	342	350	358	365	373	381	389	396	404	412	420
75	152	160	168	176	184	192	200	208	216	224	232	240	248	256	264	272	279	287	295	303	311	319	327	335	343	351	359	367	375	383	391	399	407	415	423	431
76	156	164	172	180	189	197	205	213	221	230	238	246	254	263	271	279	287	295	304	312	320	328	336	344	353	361	369	377	385	394	402	410	418	426	435	443

FIGURE 123-9. Body mass index chart for screening patients. (Adapted from Clinical Guidelines on the Identification, Evaluation, and Treatment of Overweight and Obesity in Adults: The Evidence Report. Bethesda, Md, National Heart, Lung, and Blood Institute. NIH publication 98-4083.)

matter how long the reply, the patient is not interrupted until the response is completed.

Physical Examination

Physical examination of body contour patients of the opposite sex is always performed with a chaperone who works for the surgeon and is the same sex as the patient. Some patients are more comfortable being alone with the surgeon, but a chaperone is always necessary for the surgeon's protection.

The examination starts with height and weight and a calculation of BMI. If a patient's BMI is 30 or more, the patient is informed that any offer of surgery is conditional on weight loss to achieve a BMI of less than 30, and a date for surgery is not scheduled until the patient achieves the desired weight. Weight is also recorded at all subsequent visits.

Measured circumferences of selected body areas can be helpful, particularly for surgeons early in their practices as they work to establish judgment, accuracy, and consistency of results. Care must be taken to ensure that target areas are measured at precisely the same location on successive visits.

The most essential part of the examination is a careful, critical inspection and palpation of the entire body. Even if patients inquire about treatment of only one or two areas, they are encouraged to undergo a comprehensive examination. It is insensitive and unwise to insist that a shy or embarrassed patient undergo a complete examination. Most patients, however, welcome a full evaluation that permits the surgeon to better assess disproportionate areas and asymmetries and to recommend treatment of areas the patient may not have considered.

Examination is performed in a rigorous, orderly manner. The patient is observed first from the back to note posture, body proportions, and asymmetries. The relative heights of the right and left shoulders and iliac crests are recorded. Starting with the upper posterior torso, pinch thickness and estimates of fat volume to be aspirated are recorded for the various body areas (back, flanks, hips, thighs, knees, calves, and ankles) (Fig. 123-10). Similar measurements are recorded for the upper arms if the patient requests. The elasticity and laxity of the skin are evaluated, as are striae and fine and coarse irregularities denoting so-called cellulite.

The patient is asked to turn to the right and tighten and pull in the abdominal muscles. The effects of postural changes are noted. A protuberant abdomen may

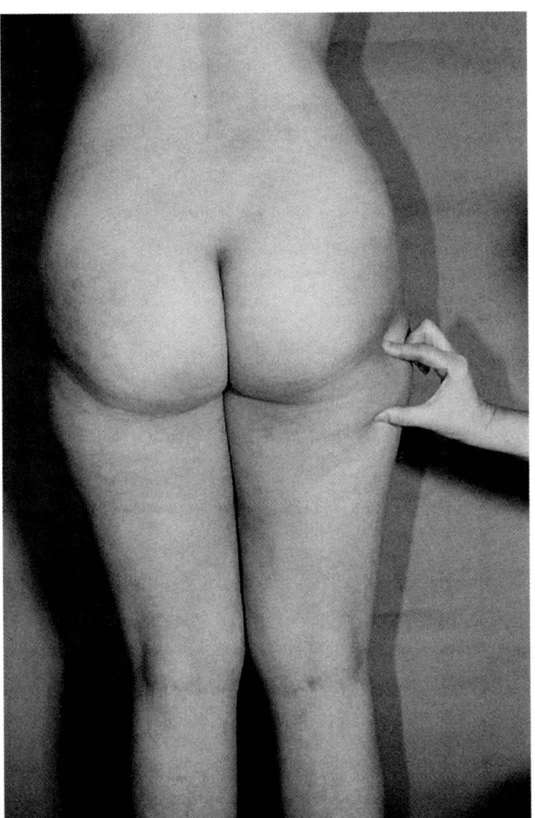

FIGURE 123-10. Assessment of pinch thickness on the outer thigh.

not be due to excess fat but may be caused by poor posture or lack of muscle tone (Fig. 123-11).

Last, the patient faces the examiner, who performs pinch tests and volume estimates for the anterior abdomen and anterior thighs. Abdominal scars and their location are noted. In men, the chest is examined. If abdominoplasty is being considered, the abdomen is also examined with the patient supine to evaluate the musculofascia.

Visual Record of Examination

History and physical findings are recorded on a specially designed form with large-scale drawings of male and female figures, permitting precise and quantitative notes as to fat volumes, skin condition, and tone of the underlying musculature (Fig. 123-12).

Recommendation to Patient

A recommendation is made, and the patient is given the surgeon's estimate of the magnitude of contour change to be anticipated from treatment of each area. Expected results will range from subtle to dramatic. Limitations imposed by skin elasticity and other factors are emphasized. The patient is frequently given a hand-held mirror to view all areas as the surgeon sees them.

Once the examination is complete, the patient is given an explanation of the surgery and perioperative period. Possible complications and alternatives are discussed before the end of the consultation.

Options for the Patient with Skin Laxity

It is common to see patients who request liposuction but who have skin laxity as a significant or dominant factor contributing to figure faults. Many of these patients require skin excision and tightening to produce an optimal result. Such patients, however, are frequently opposed to the more extensive surgery, possible increased morbidity, and longer scars associated with the various abdominoplasties and lower body lifts.

The surgeon needs to take the time to sit down with the patient to explain options. Some patients will obtain a significant improvement from liposuction alone but will clearly benefit more from an abdominoplasty or body lift combined with liposuction. Both options should be offered to these patients, although the surgeon's preference should be expressed clearly.

Other patients will obtain little benefit from liposuction, or their appearance will predictably worsen after aspiration of fat. A lift or abdominoplasty is the only option that will produce a satisfactory result. These patients need to be offered a form of excisional surgery as their only choice. They may refuse surgery or go to another practitioner who is willing to perform liposuction, but the ethical plastic surgeon will resist performing liposuction where there is little fat and much loose skin.

SAFE SUCTION: TUMESCENT METHOD, FLUID MANAGEMENT, AND BLOOD LOSS

Introduction of the tumescent method fundamentally changed liposuction.[5-8] Infiltration of the fat with dilute epinephrine solution (epinephrine in lactated Ringer solution, 1:1,000,000) 20 minutes before liposuction dramatically reduces blood loss and provides total fluid replacement. The swelling and expansion of the target area ease passage of the cannula and promote more efficient evacuation of fat. Bruising and swelling are minimized.

Addition of lidocaine to the infiltrating solution at a concentration of 0.05% to 0.1% can provide complete local anesthesia. If only one or two small areas are being suctioned and the procedure is of short duration, these concentrations will be sufficient to perform liposuction without systemic sedation or narcotics.

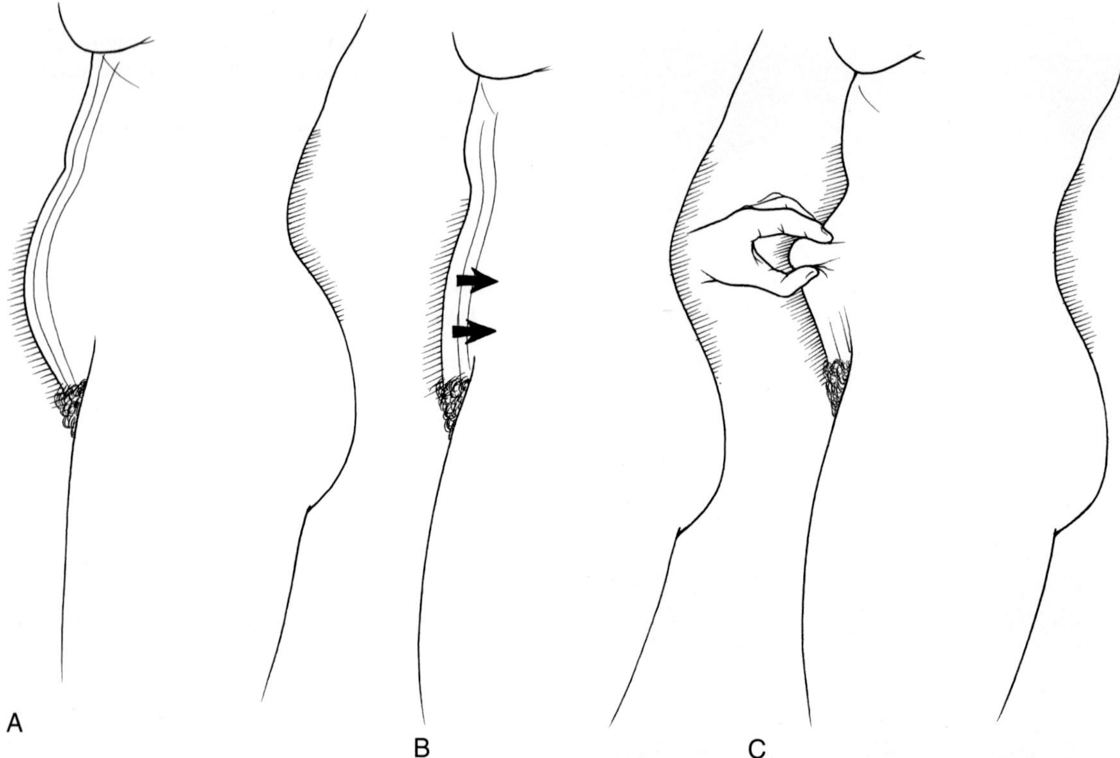

FIGURE 123-11. A patient with a protuberant abdomen with paucity of subcutaneous fat. *A,* The patient's protuberance is due to muscle laxity and poor posture. *B,* When the patient is asked to "pull in" the muscles, protuberance lessens. *C,* Pinch thickness is minimal.

Most patients, however, have multiple areas suctioned in procedures lasting more than 1 hour. These patients require systemic agents for complete comfort. The senior author uses a dilute concentration of lidocaine 0.04% with epinephrine 1:1,000,000 injected into the subcutaneous tissues in combination with general anesthesia administered by an anesthesiologist.

The subcutaneous injection solution is formulated by adding lidocaine and epinephrine to a 1000-mL bag of sterile lactated Ringer solution for injection (Table 123-1). Lidocaine 0.04% does not provide complete intraoperative anesthesia to the target area, but it does give enough analgesia so that the anesthesiologist can reduce the dose of systemic agents. The dilute lidocaine in the tissues also provides excellent postoperative analgesia and reduces the need for postoperative narcotics.

TABLE 123-1 ✦ INJECTION SOLUTION

The following recipe provides 400 mg of lidocaine in each 1000 mL of lactated Ringer solution:

Lidocaine, 2.0%	20 mL
Epinephrine, 1:1000	1 mL
Lactated Ringer solution	1000 mL
Lidocaine 0.04% with epinephrine 1:1,000,000	1021 mL

Fluid Replacement

The primary purpose of the local injection is to provide vasoconstriction and analgesia at the target site. The injected fluid is absorbed, however, and can provide complete and total fluid replacement by hypodermoclysis. The subcutaneous tissue is injected with sufficient volume such that the solution is evenly dispersed throughout the target area, producing slight swelling, or tumescence, and intense vasoconstriction. The exact volume injected into each area varies according to the amount of fat and the elasticity of the skin and subcutaneous tissues.

Total subcutaneous injection for each operation is directly related to total volume of aspirate. Patients undergoing low-volume aspirations (<2000 mL) will usually have subcutaneous injections of fluid in a 3:1 or 2:1 ratio to aspirate; patients undergoing medium-volume aspirations (2000 to 4000 mL) usually have subcutaneous injections of fluid in a 2:1 ratio to

NAME: ______________________________________ DATE: ____/____/____
(Last) (First) (M.I.)

FEMALE BODY CONTOUR CONSULTATION

HX: CONCERNS, PREVIOUS SAL OR OTHER BODY CONTOUR SURGERY: ______________________

WEIGHT HISTORY: ______________________

EXERCISE: ______________________

EATING DISORDERS (anorexia, bulimia, amenorrhea): ______________________

LMP ________ POST MENOPAUSE? Y/N ________ PERIMENOPAUSE? Y/N ________

G ___ P ___ A ___ DRESS SIZE ________ DISPROP? ________ BRA ________

HT: ________ BP: ______/______ SHOULDER: R: ____ L: ____ HIPS: R: ____ L: ____

DATE: consult ___/___/___ ___/___/___ SCOLIOSIS: NONE ____ MOD ____ SEV ____

WT: ________ ________ ________

BMI ________ ________ ________

WAIST ________ ________ ________

HIP ________ ________ ________

THIGH ________ ________ ________

Concentration = g / 100 mL

• Xylo 2% = 20 mg / mL

→ 20 mg → 1 mL ; x → 100 mL] x = 2g

• 2g → 100 mL ; x → 20 mL] x = 400 mg = 0,4g / 20 mL

• 0,4g → 1000 mL LR ; x → 100 mL] x = 0,04%

A

FIGURE 123-12. *A,* Office f… …ultation. *Continued*

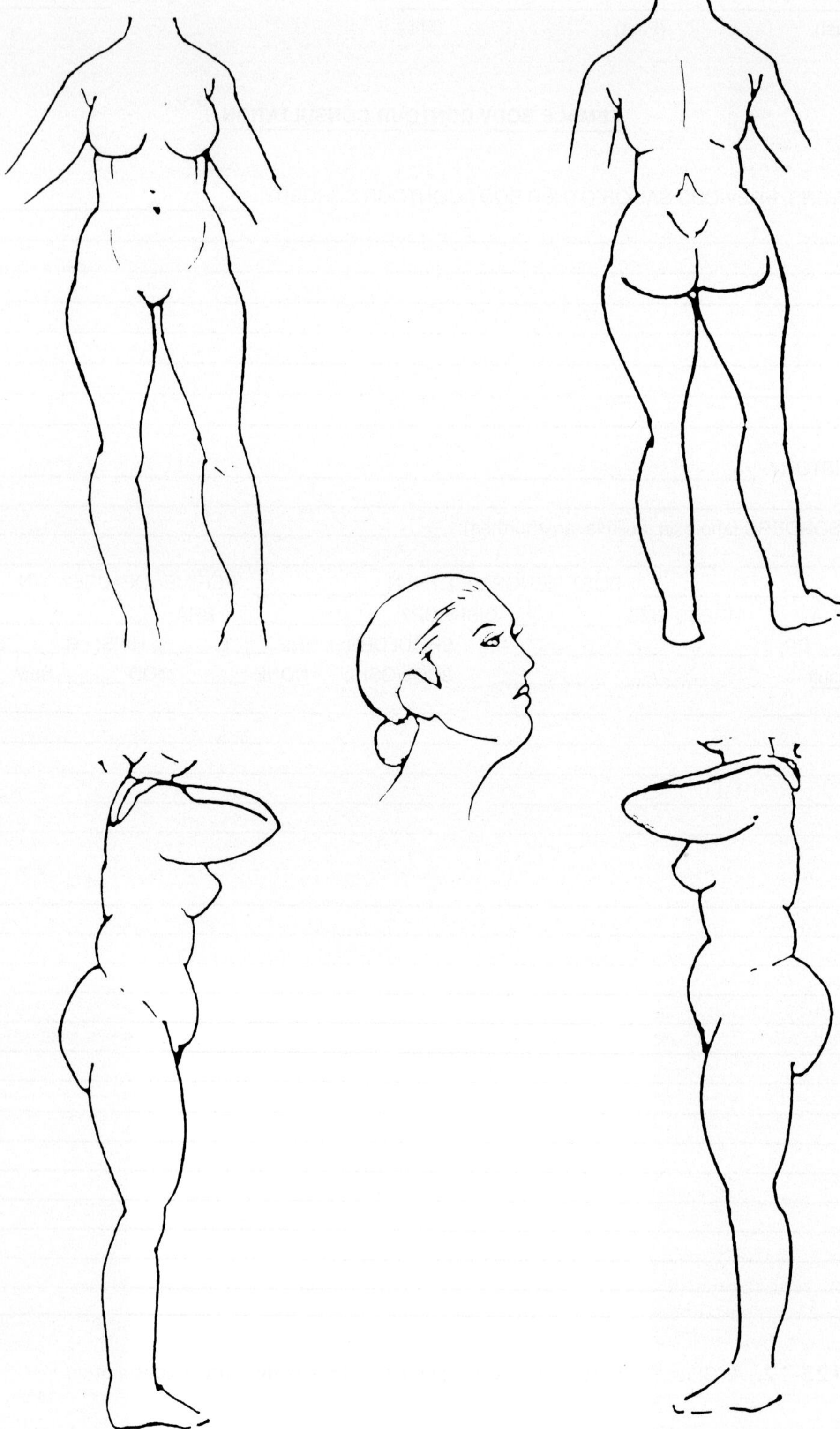

FIGURE 123-12, cont'd. *B,* Drawings are used to record pinch thickness and estimated fat volume from each anatomic area. An estimate of the total volume of fat to be aspirated is also recorded.

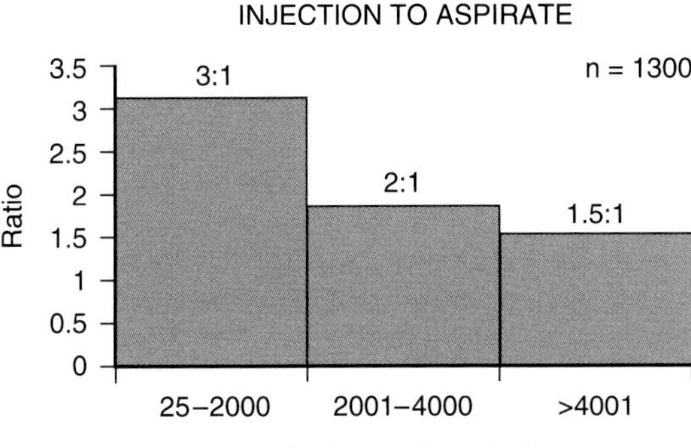

FIGURE 123-13. Ratio of subcutaneous injection to total aspirate in 1300 consecutive operations by the senior author (Pitman). (Data from Pitman GH, Fikry BA: Liposuction: safety issues in 1300 cases. Scientific Presentation at annual meeting of American Society of Aesthetic Plastic Surgery, New York, May 7, 2001.)

aspirate; and patients undergoing large-volume aspirations (>4000 mL) usually have subcutaneous injections of fluid in a 1:1 ratio (Fig. 123-13). A 1:1 ratio of subcutaneous injection to total aspirate usually provides adequate hemostasis and analgesia as well as complete fluid replacement for patients having aspirations of up to 10,000 mL.[2,3]

As larger volumes of fat are removed, correspondingly larger volumes of fluid are infiltrated. The anesthesiologist and surgeon should plan in advance such that the volume of injected subcutaneous fluid plus the volume of intravenous fluid is appropriate to meet the patient's overall fluid requirements. The anesthesiologist limits intravenous injection to the minimum necessary to deliver medication because a large volume of fluid will be delivered to the subcutaneous space by the surgeon and gradually be absorbed by the patient through hypodermoclysis. Additional infusion of fluids through the rapidly absorbed intravenous route can produce fluid overload and pulmonary edema.[9] Absent hemodynamic instability, the anesthesiologist should limit intravenous fluids to the minimum amount necessary to deliver medications and maintain access. This volume is always less than 500 mL during the operation.

At the conclusion of the procedure, the anesthesiologist and surgeon review the patient's fluid balance. For most patients, if total fluid replacement (intravenous plus subcutaneous) is in a 1:1 ratio with total aspirate volume, the patient will have had an adequate fluid resuscitation, and postoperative fluids can be at maintenance levels until such time as the patient is able to take oral fluids.[3] A formula has been devised for postoperative fluid replacement in large-volume liposuctions (>4000 mL).[2] This formula closely approximates a 1:1 ratio of aspirate to total fluid replacement.

Most patients do not require Foley catheters for monitoring of urine output, but catheters should be considered for procedures lasting more than 3 hours and for operations in which liposuction is combined with other surgical procedures.

Reduction of Blood Loss

Intraoperative and postoperative bleeding is minimized by preinfiltration with epinephrine-containing solution and waiting 20 minutes after infiltration before beginning liposuction. In 147 consecutive operations, use of preinfiltration with dilute epinephrine resulted in an average estimated blood loss that was 8% of total aspirate.[8] By extrapolation, average estimated blood loss for a patient undergoing liposuction of 5000 mL would be 400 mL. Therefore, proper planning and execution of even large-volume cases (>5000 mL aspirate) can make transfusion unnecessary.[2,8]

Whereas the average patient loses little blood in a typical liposuction procedure, not all patients are average, and wide variation in the quantity of blood loss during liposuction is the rule. Therefore, aspirate should be monitored continually for the presence of blood. A very red aspirate may necessitate modification of the operative plan, reduction of planned liposuction volume, or termination of the procedure.

Use of the tumescent method has obviated the need for transfusion in almost all patients, but some patients undergoing liposuction may need to be prepared for autologous transfusion. It is incumbent on the responsible surgeon to use the best clinical judgment in deciding whether to prepare the patient for autologous transfusion. Factors such as the estimated volume of liposuction, the performance of simultaneous concomitant procedures, the surgeon's past experience, and other issues will determine the exact nature of the preoperative preparations.

It is the authors' preference to shorten or to abort a procedure rather than to transfuse homologous blood. Nevertheless, if excessive blood loss is not recognized at surgery or occurs in the postoperative period, transfusions of autologous or homologous blood may be necessary and should not be withheld. A rapidly falling hematocrit and hemodynamic instability are urgent indications for transfusion.

Safe Use of Lidocaine for Anesthesia and Analgesia

A maximal dose of 7 mg/kg of lidocaine with epinephrine has been recommended by the principal manufacturer.[10] Multiple studies, however, have demonstrated the safety of higher lidocaine doses for use in liposuction when the lidocaine is delivered to the subcutaneous tissues in hyperdilute concentrations containing epinephrine.[5-8,11-14] Klein[12] has recommended 35 mg/kg as the highest safe dose of lidocaine when the lidocaine is injected into the subcutaneous tissues in a dilution of 0.05% lidocaine with epinephrine 1:1,000,000.

The current practice of the senior author is to limit total lidocaine dose in young, healthy patients to less than 50 mg/kg when using 0.04% lidocaine with epinephrine 1:1,000,000 injected into the subcutaneous tissues of the torso and lower extremity. In a study of 147 operations, doses as high as 50 mg/kg injected subcutaneously at a concentration of 0.05% with epinephrine 1:1,000,000 produced no clinical or chemical lidocaine toxicity.[8] One can infer (although it is not proven) that the same dosing of lidocaine at a lesser concentration (0.04%) would be even less likely to result in toxicity.

Readers are cautioned that use of such high doses of lidocaine is an off-label practice that has proven safe only under the strict conditions described. Use of such high doses of lidocaine may result in unsafe increases in serum concentration levels. Patients with medical impairments, particularly impairments reducing hepatic and renal function, may be at increased risk for lidocaine toxicity. Treatment and dosing should be individualized for each patient's unique medical circumstances.

OPERATIVE PLANNING AND CONDUCT

A methodical order of operation has been developed that facilitates safe and efficient treatment of a wide variety of patients. The planned operative framework accommodates equally well the patient with only one or two localized areas of excess fat deposition and the patient with multiple diffuse areas of circumferential fat deposition.

Marking

Before operation, the surgeon marks areas of fat excess on the standing patient. With a standard surgical marker, protuberant areas are outlined. The drawings are precise and include estimates of expected aspirate volume. At the conclusion of marking, the target area will resemble a topographic map.

Locations of access incisions are also marked. Incisions are planned in Langer lines, skin creases, or hair-bearing areas so that scars will be inconspicuous (Fig. 123-14).

Notwithstanding cosmetic issues, most areas will require at least two access incisions for optimal contouring, and access incisions should be directly adjacent to or overlying the target area. Placement of incisions at a distance from the target area reduces fine control of aspiration and may result in inadvertent and unwanted removal of fat from areas that do not have excess fat. Because the actual incisions are only 3 to 6 mm long, they rarely create a cosmetic issue. The most important goal is to achieve a smooth, aesthetically pleasing contour reduction.

Anesthesia

One or two small areas may be treated under pure local anesthesia without sedation, narcotics, or inhalational agents. Only a small minority of patients are in this category. Most patients undergo treatment of multiple areas, and the awake patient may become uncomfortable and apprehensive as successive areas are injected with local anesthetic. Therefore, an anesthesiologist attends all patients to ensure total freedom from pain and unawareness of the procedure. The exact form of systemic anesthesia is chosen by the anesthesiologist in consultation with the patient and surgeon and ranges from intravenous conscious sedation to general endotracheal anesthesia.

Maintenance of Core Body Temperature

It is desirable to maintain core body temperature at a normal level, both for the patient's comfort and to reduce the incidence of complications.[15] Body temperatures are monitored for all patients and maintained between 96.0°F and 98.0°F during surgery.

The patient wears a heat-retaining cap,* and a forced-air warming blanket† covers exposed parts of the body not in the operative field. Much of the time, however, a warming blanket cannot be used because the entire torso and both lower extremities may be in the sterile operative field. The single most important factor in maintaining core body temperature in liposuction patients then becomes the ambient temperature in the operating room, which is maintained at 80°F.

Quantitative Operative Report

Precise and accurate knowledge of quantitative aspects of the operation is critical, both to ensure the patient's safety and as an aid in achieving the desired aesthetic result. A standard liposuction operative report has been designed that facilitates efficient and accurate reporting (Fig. 123-15). The form includes space to record the following:

- volumes of aspirate as they are removed from each side,
- volumes of subcutaneous and intravenous injection,

*Thermadrape, OR Concepts Inc., Roanoke, Texas.
†Bair Hugger, Augustine Medical Inc., Eden Prairie, Minnesota.

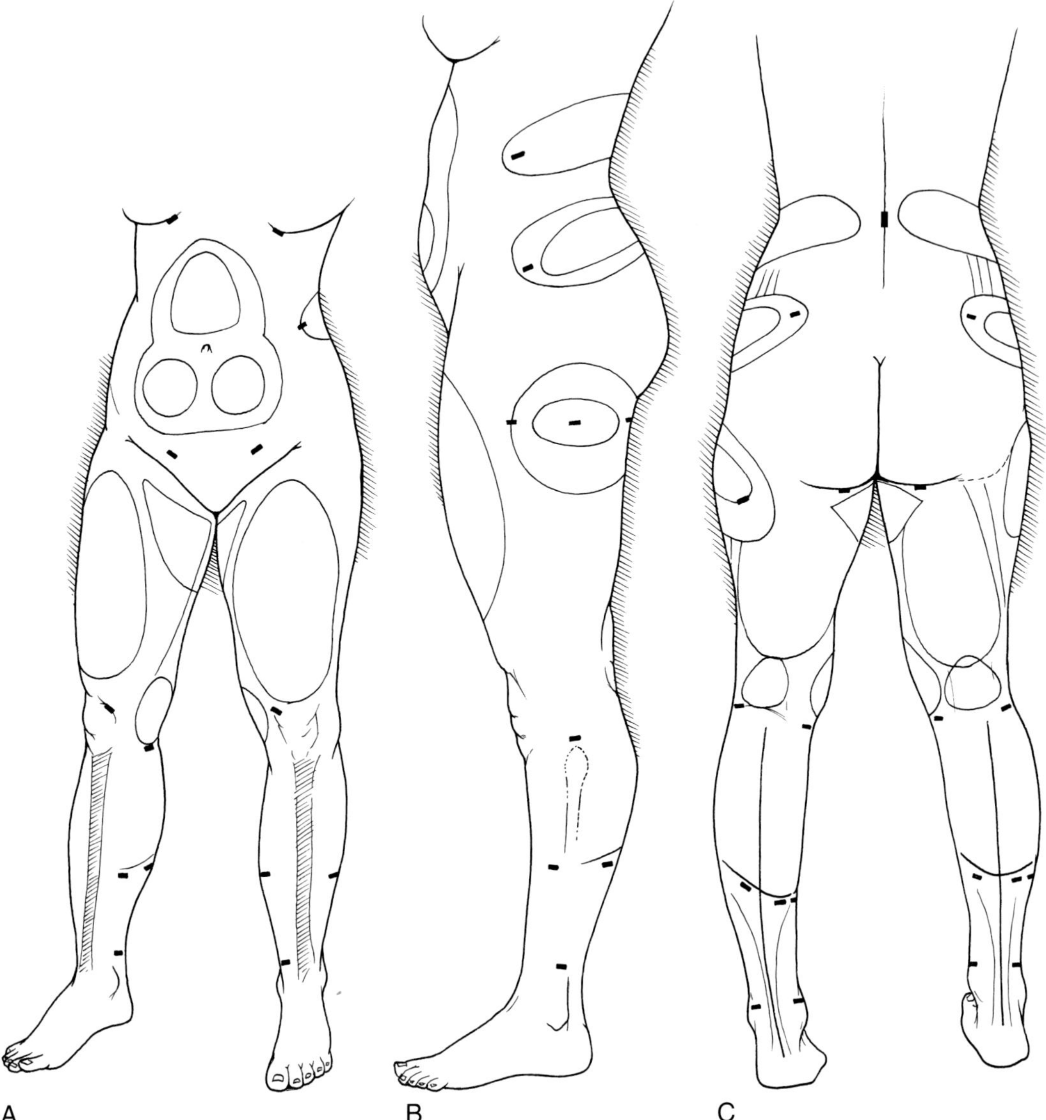

FIGURE 123-14. Schematic of markings. *A*, Anterior view. *B*, Lateral view. *C*, Posterior view.

- lidocaine dosage,
- total volume of aspirate and supranatant fat, and
- ancillary procedures.

The report also includes a line drawing of a typical male or female patient. At the conclusion of the procedure, the surgeon fills in the drawing to provide a graphic as well as a numeric description of the operative procedure.

The anesthesiologist fills out the report as the operation proceeds. The surgeon has ready reference during the procedure to volumes of aspirate from each anatomic area. This information is frequently useful in achieving side-to-side symmetry. At the conclusion of the operation, surgeon and anesthesiologist can refer to the volume of aspirate and the volume of intraoperative fluid administration to plan postoperative fluid orders.

Preparation and Draping

While standing on an absorbent pad, the patient is circumferentially painted from the upper thorax to the feet with a warmed, germicidal solution, usually povidone-iodine (Betadine) (Fig. 123-16). The patient is then helped to lie supine on a sterile-draped operating room table with arms out at 90 degrees. The feet are wrapped in sterile towels. A sterile Mayo stand cover

LIPOSUCTION OPERATIVE REPORT
DATE:______________ NAME:______________
ATTENDING SURGEON: Pitman
ATTENDING ANESTHESIOLOGIST: ______________
ANESTHESIA: ______________
PROCEDURE PERFORMED: Liposuction
PRE-OPERATIVE DX: Localized Adiposity, ICD 278.1
POST-OPERATIVE DX: Same
PATHOLOGY: There was excess fat as listed

	VOL	
FACE		
NECK		
ABDOMEN	200	
SUBTOTAL		
	LEFT	**RIGHT**
ARM		
CHEST		
BACK		
FLANK		
HIP	250	250
BUTTOCK		
MED. TH	100	125
ANT. TH	200	250
LAT. TH	350	450
POST. TH		
KNEE	100	100
LAT. CALF		
LAT. ANKLE		
MED. CALF		
MED. ANKLE		
SUBTOTALS	**1000**	**1175**

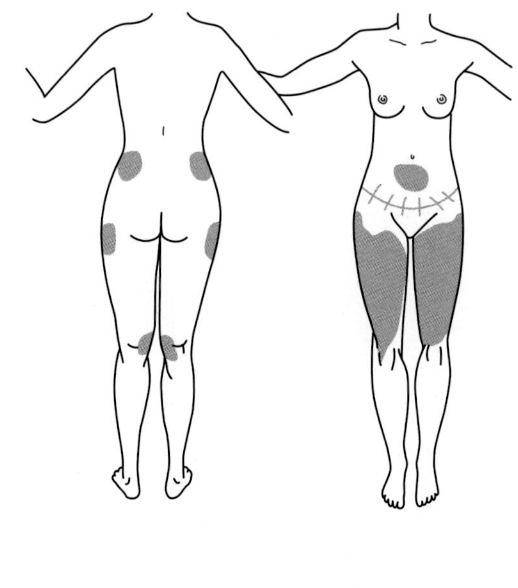

PROCEDURE: Patient prepped, induced, intubated, sedated or given local only. Areas to be treated infiltrated with lidocaine 0.04% with epinephrine 1:1,000,000. Stab incision made at appropriate places. Liposuction carried out. Patient taken from OR in good condition.

FLUIDS:
i.v. 300 ml
s.c. 4300 ml
Total 4600 ml

LIDOCAINE:
400mg/1 x 4.3 l = 1720 mg
Pt. wt. 50 kg
Lidocaine = 1720 / 50 mg/kg
= 34+ mg/kg

CONTAINER	ASPIRATE	WATER	FAT	ADDENDUM
1	1000	200	800	LASSR
2	2600	200	1400	
3				
4				
5				
6				
7				
8				
TOTAL	2600	400	2200	

Gerald H. Pitman, M.D.

FIGURE 123-15. Liposuction operative report form, filled in for a typical patient undergoing liposuction and one ancillary procedure (lower abdominal skin resection).

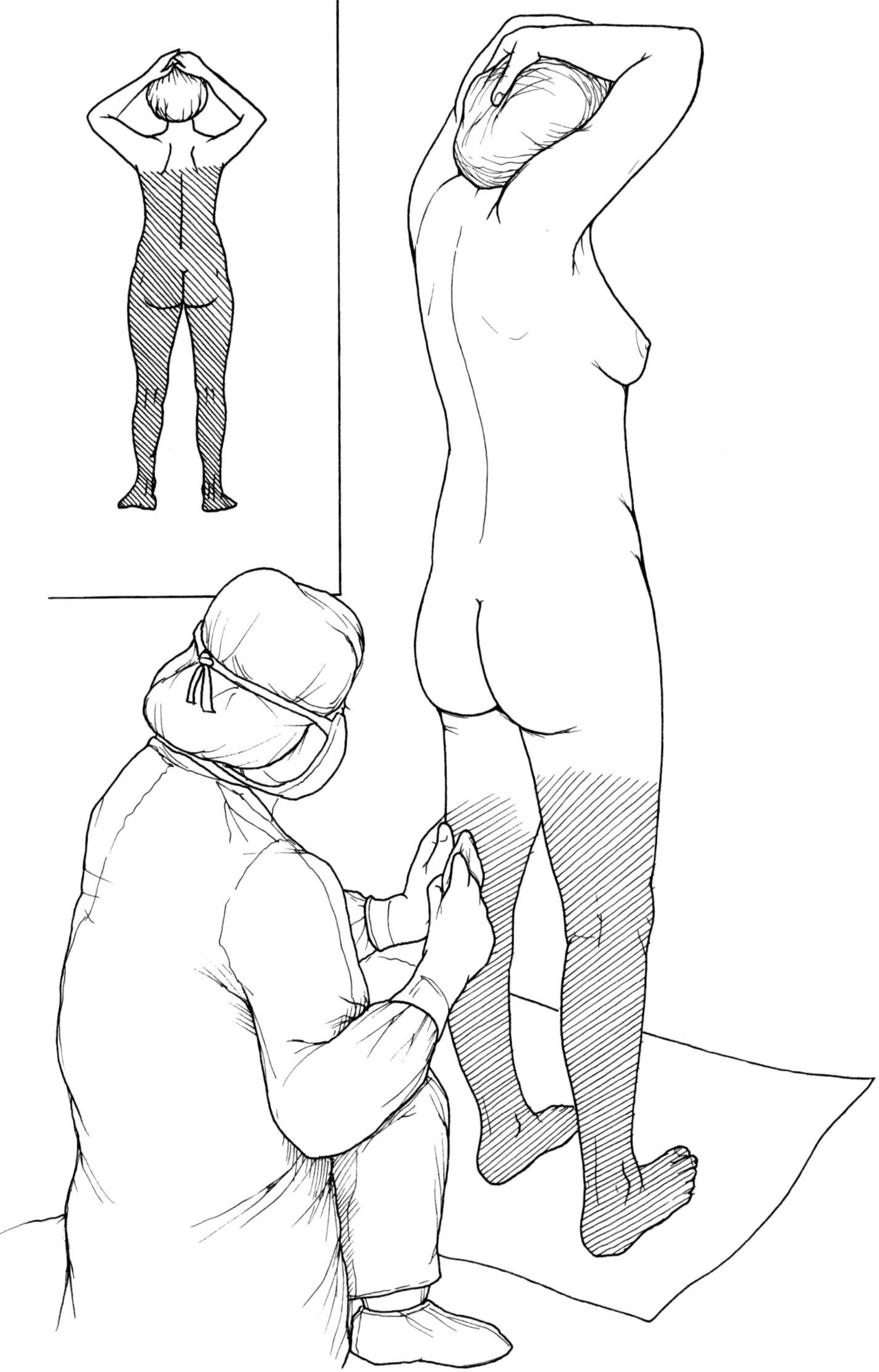

FIGURE 123-16. Patient is painted circumferentially from neck to feet with warm povidone-iodine (Betadine) solution.

is placed beneath the patient to serve as a draw sheet for ease of positioning the patient during surgery. A sterile barrier sheet is placed between the anesthesiologist and the sterile field. One surgical assistant and an operating room technician or nurse usually work with the surgeon.

The patient will be repositioned several times during the course of the operation without need for additional sterile preparation of the skin or redraping. Anesthesiologist, surgeon, and assistants will work in smooth concert to reposition the patient without causing injury.

Infiltration

All areas to be treated are infiltrated with large volumes of dilute lidocaine 0.04% with epinephrine 1:1,000,000 before the start of liposuction. Infiltration volumes vary with the size of the fat deposit and other local factors (e.g., whether the fat is fibrous, presence or absence of scarring). Infiltration fluid should be dispersed evenly throughout the targeted area. Volume of infiltration depends on local factors but in all cases should be sufficient to produce slight swelling and uniform vasoconstriction. Ratios of infiltration volume to aspirate volume range from 1:1 to 3:1.

- The first areas infiltrated will be the first areas aspirated. The operation typically begins by turning the patient into the left lateral decubitus position and infiltrating solution into the posterior and right lateral subcutaneous tissues. The medial and posterior aspects of the left lower extremity are also infiltrated from this position.
- Next, the patient is turned into the right lateral decubitus position, and the left lateral and posterior subcutaneous tissues are infiltrated along with the medial and posterior aspects of the right lower extremity.
- Infiltration of the anterior areas of the torso and lower extremities is completed after the patient is turned supine.

Details of Positioning for Aspiration

A method of treatment is described for circumferential treatment of the entire torso and both lower extremities. Although a complete circumferential treatment is described, the operative plan is similar even if only a limited number of localized fat deposits are treated. Some steps may be eliminated or modified, but the basic operative framework is still followed.

LEFT LATERAL DECUBITUS POSITION. To begin liposuction, the patient is again turned to the left lateral decubitus position, and the right posterolateral aspects of the torso are treated with use of access incisions in the posterior midline and on the anterolateral aspect of the trunk. Areas of the torso treated in this position may include the back, flanks, and hips. Areas of the lower extremities treated in this position include the right buttock, right lateral thigh (Fig. 123-17*A*), right lateral calf, right lateral ankle, left posteromedial proximal thigh, left medial knee, left medial calf, and left medial ankle (Fig. 123-17*B*).

RIGHT LATERAL DECUBITUS POSITION. The patient is then turned into the right lateral decubitus position, and corresponding areas of the left posterolateral torso, left lower extremity, and right lower extremity are treated.

PRONE POSITION. For treatment of the posterior thighs, the patient is turned from the right lateral decubitus position to the supine position. The anesthesiologist deepens the level of anesthesia, and the patient is then turned from supine to prone. The posterior

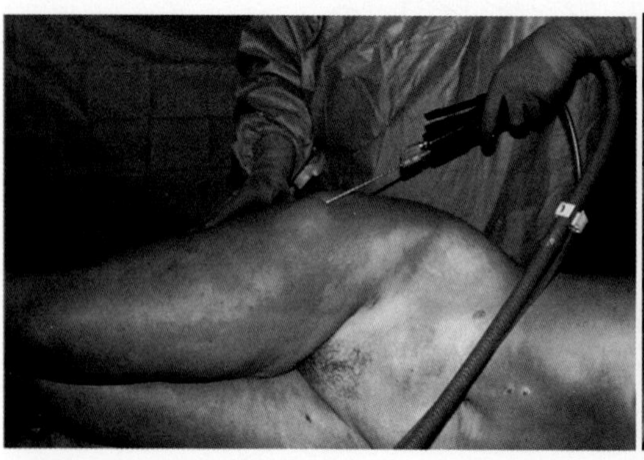

A

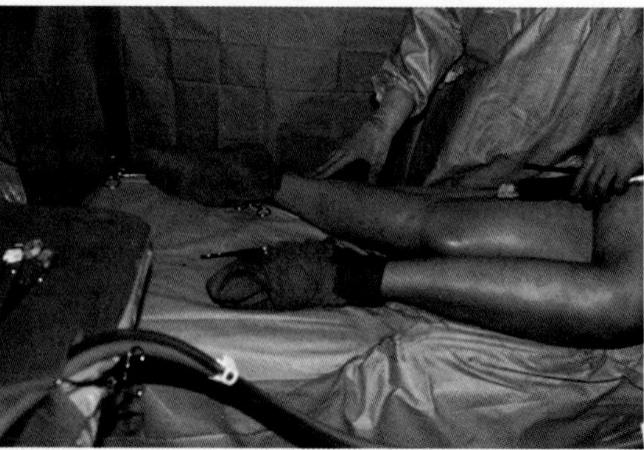

B

FIGURE 123-17. Liposuction of the right lateral thigh *(A)* and the medial aspect of the left calf and ankle *(B)* with the patient in the left lateral decubitus position.

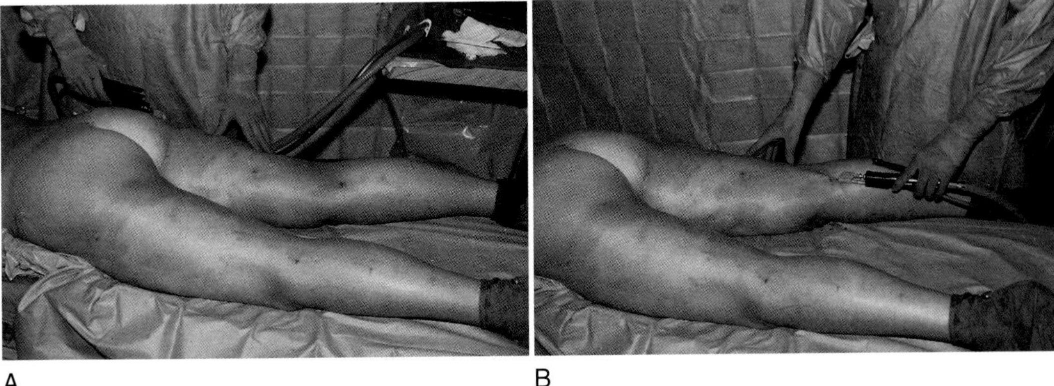

FIGURE 123-18. *A* and *B*, Posterior thighs being treated with patient prone.

aspect of the thigh is aspirated with the patient prone (Fig. 123-18). For larger patients, it is more efficient also to aspirate the back, flanks, hips, buttocks, and lateral thighs with the patient prone (Fig. 123-19). For smaller patients, however, control of fat contouring and judgment of endpoint are more easily accomplished in the lateral decubitus position (see Fig. 123-17*A*).

Supine Position. At the conclusion of aspiration from the posterior areas, the anesthesiologist once again deepens the patient, disconnects lines and monitoring devices, and helps turn the patient to the supine position for treatment of the anterior aspects of the trunk (breasts, abdomen) (Fig. 123-20). The anteromedial thighs are also treated in this position (Fig. 123-21). The operation is completed after treatment of anterior areas.

Choice of Cannula

The preferred cannulas are 3, 4, and 5 mm in diameter. Cannulas range in length from 15 to 30 cm. Because shorter cannulas permit better control, the shortest cannula capable of reaching the entire area is used. Small fat deposits are treated with the 3-mm cannula, and very large fat deposits are treated in their depths by use of a 4- or 5-mm cannula. Whatever the size of the fat deposit, superficial tissues are treated with the 3-mm cannula. Very small fat deposits and calves and ankles may be treated with a 2.4-mm cannula.

Technical Details of Fat Aspiration

A series of tunnels are evacuated of their fat content by reciprocating motion of the cannula as the surgeon directs the cannula back and forth through the tissues. In time, the tunnels collapse, producing a reduced contour. Tunnels in the deeper fat can be larger and more numerous and still preserve smooth surface contour. Evacuation of more superficial fat requires smaller diameter cannulas to avoid surface irregularities (Color Plate 123-2).

Whatever the size of the cannula, the access incision should be large enough to accommodate the cannula easily. An incision that fits tightly around the cannula is more subject to surface abrasion and wound edge necrosis.

Because aspiration tunnels radiate from an access incision, the tunnels are closely spaced near the access incision and farther apart as the distance from the access incision increases. Maximal fat aspiration occurs directly under the access incision and adjacent to it. If all of the fat from a localized fat deposit is removed through one access incision, a depression at the site of the incision is a likely consequence. Therefore, more than one access incision is the rule for aspiration of fat.

Monitoring Aspirate for Blood

The surgeon should closely monitor aspirate color and quality. The color of the aspirate at the beginning of liposuction is almost always bright yellow. As suctioning continues, some bleeding occurs and the aspirate will become blood tinged, turning orange and, eventually, red. Persistent bright red aspirate, especially at the beginning of liposuction, may signify an unrecognized clotting disorder. Early bleeding and excessive bleeding are indications to modify or shorten the operative plan.

Evaluation of Endpoint

It's not what you take out, but what you leave in.
—Anonymous

The most important criteria for determining endpoint are visual assessment of contour, pinch thickness, palpation for smoothness, and volume of aspirate.

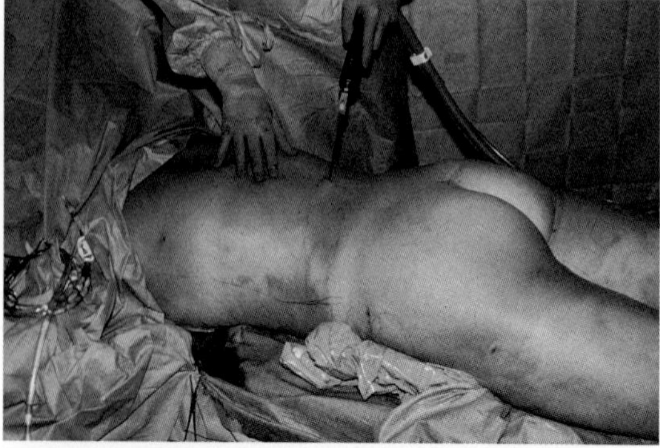

A

B

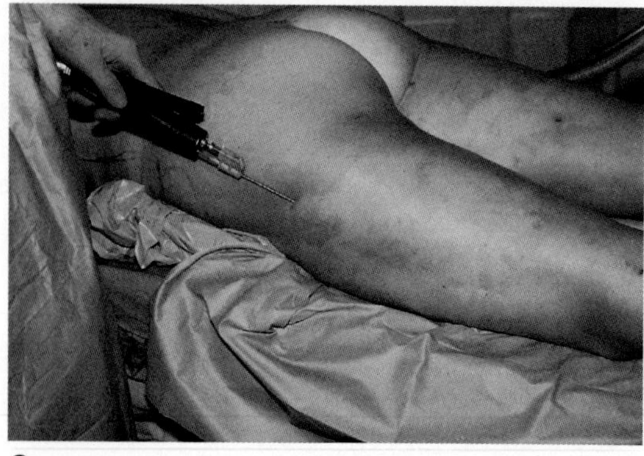

C

FIGURE 123-19. Posterior waist *(A)*, buttocks *(B)*, and lateral thigh *(C)* being treated with the patient prone.

VISUAL ASSESSMENT OF CONTOUR

Visual assessment of contour is the single most important criterion for endpoint evaluation. With few exceptions, the surgeon looks for a smooth reduction of convexity in the treated area. How much of a reduction is a matter of judgment obtained only with experience. If in doubt, err on the side of removing less fat. It is easier to perform a secondary procedure for additional fat aspiration than it is to graft a depressed area.

A few areas, most notably the flanks, are treated to produce concavity. Again, aspirate until a concavity is achieved. Do not overresect.

PINCH THICKNESS

Pinch thickness should be assessed in the operating room before infusion and again as liposuction proceeds. Exact pinch thickness at endpoint will vary from area to area and is dependent on thickness of dermis, thickness of subcutaneous fat, and amount of preaspiration infusion. Most areas that are treated have initial pinch thicknesses in excess of 3 cm. Postaspiration pinch thickness should be 1 to 2 cm less. Endpoint pinch thicknesses are rarely less than 1 to 2 cm but always less than preoperative pinch thickness (Fig. 123-22).

PALPATION FOR SMOOTHNESS

During the course of the liposuction, the surgeon should periodically run the palm of the hand along the surface of the skin to test for smoothness of reduction. Subtle areas of depression or elevation may more easily be felt than seen.

MEASUREMENT OF VOLUME

It is important to make a preoperative estimate of planned aspirate volume from each area. Actual aspiration volume may vary from the estimate, but the estimate is a good starting point for planning fat extraction. The actual volume of aspirate from each area should also be recorded as the operation progresses. The surgeon can review these volumes periodically as an aid to achieving side-to-side symmetry. Notwithstanding the value of comparative side-to-side volume measurements, visual assessment and pinch test are more important determinants of endpoint.

Wound Closure

Most of the access incisions are small and do not need to be closed. Healing and eventual cosmetic result are similar with or without closure. Incisions longer than 7 mm are closed with one or two 5-0 nylon sutures. Sutures are removed within 5 days to prevent leaving permanent marks in the skin.

Garments and Aftercare

Use of compression garments after liposuction is a time-honored custom because the garments minimize early swelling and help achieve the final result more quickly. The eventual cosmetic result is, however, the same whether or not garments are used. The advantages of the garments are the following:

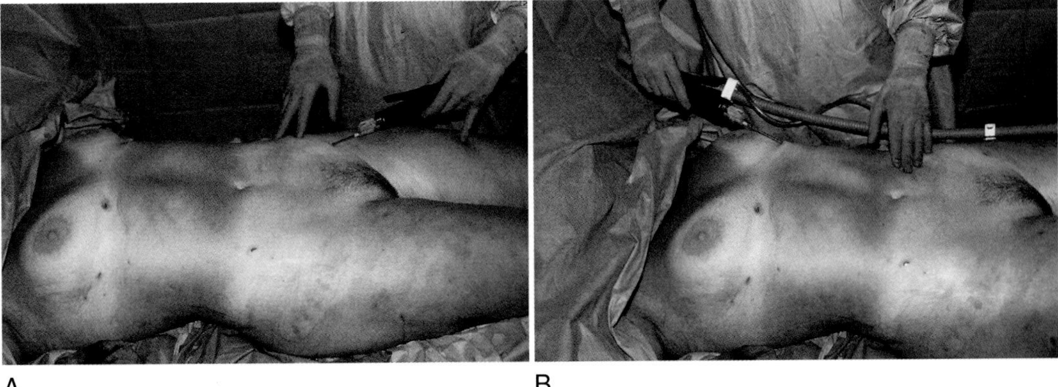

A B

FIGURE 123-20. Patient supine for liposuction of the abdomen from the groin access incision *(A)* and the inframammary crease access incision *(B)*.

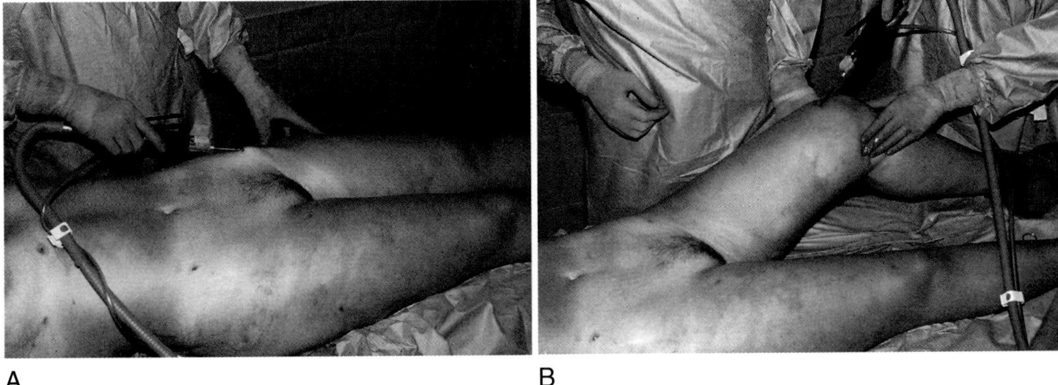

A B

FIGURE 123-21. Patient supine for liposuction of the anteromedial thighs from the groin access incision *(A)* and the suprapatellar access incision *(B)*.

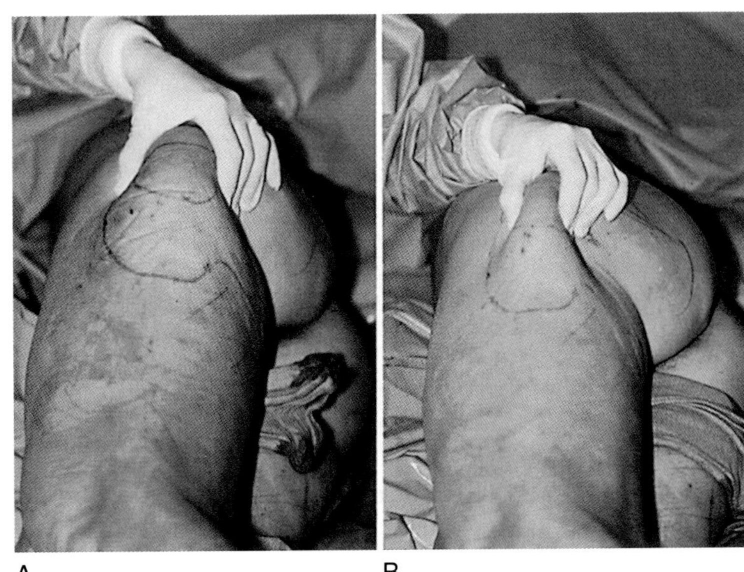

A B

FIGURE 123-22. Pinch thickness before *(A)* and after *(B)* liposuction. (From Pitman GH: Liposuction and Aesthetic Surgery. St. Louis, Quality Medical Publishing, 1993:369.)

- Early swelling and bruising are minimized.
- Reduction of swelling is more rapid, and the final result is achieved earlier.
- Some patients are provided with a greater sense of security.

The disadvantages of the garments are the following:

- They are uncomfortable to wear for many patients.
- They are impossible to wear for severe claustrophobes.
- It is difficult and sometimes painful to change garments or to partially remove garments for bladder and bowel functions and bathing.
- They may create unwanted creases in the skin.
- Some patients are allergic to latex in the garments.
- They are expensive.

Whether to use garments depends on multiple factors: number and anatomic location of treated areas, total volume of aspirate, and desires of the individual patient.

Postoperative compression garments should always be used for the calves and ankles because of the dependency of these areas. Persistent swelling of the ankles may induce trophic changes in the skin and subcutis that may be permanent. All patients having liposuction of the calves and ankles wear support hose during the day for 6 weeks after surgery.

Patients having aspirate volumes of less than 5000 mL are usually treated on an ambulatory basis. Older patients or those with comorbid conditions may benefit from staying overnight in the hospital even if the liposuction volume is less than 5000 mL. Patients spend most of their time in bed and confined to their room in the first 48 hours because of oozing from access incisions and the discomfort associated with the operation.

Most patients are ambulatory after 48 hours and return to usual sedentary activities within 5 to 7 days. Patients return to exercise and sports after 3 weeks. Persons having very high volume liposuctions (>5000 mL) may require longer recovery times, whereas those undergoing minimal liposuctions of one or two areas may fully recover as early as 48 hours after surgery, although these patients are the exception.

Swelling and bruising are the rule. For most patients, the swelling subsides enough by day 5 so that the patient's usual clothing may be worn. Seventy percent to 90% of swelling is gone by 6 weeks. Bruising may last 3 to 4 weeks. Final result is evaluated at 6 months.

TREATMENT OF SPECIFIC AREAS AND POPULATIONS OF PATIENTS

The general principles of evaluation of patients and treatment discussed before apply to all anatomic areas. Therefore, discussion is limited to aspects of care specific to each individual area.

Face

ANATOMY

Two main fat deposits exist in the cheek: superficial and deep. The superficial fat lies between the skin and the superficial musculoaponeurotic system–platysma. The deep fat is largely composed of the buccal fat pad (Color Plate 123-3).

EVALUATION OF THE PATIENT

It is a truism that a round and full face is a sign of youth and good health, whereas a thin and drawn face is a sign of age or illness. Most patients will not benefit from fat removal in the face. Facial fat extraction, therefore, should be limited to patients who have disproportionately full cheeks.

The smoothest results are obtained when the desired contour change is achieved by extraction of fat from both the subcutaneous and deep compartments. Removal of relatively small amounts of fat from each compartment generally gives a better result than trying to make the desired change by removing all of the fat from one compartment, either superficial or deep.

MARKINGS

No external markings are required for removal of the buccal fat pad. For liposuction of the face, areas of cheek protuberance between the malar prominence and body of the mandible are outlined (Fig. 123-23).

ANESTHESIA

Local anesthesia is relatively easy to obtain in the face, and most patients may be treated in this way. Patients having removal of the buccal fat pad who require sedation of any kind are most safely treated with a general endotracheal anesthesia so that the airway is protected from possible intraoral bleeding.

If other areas of the body are not being infiltrated with tumescent solution, local anesthesia to each external cheek is established by subcutaneous infiltration of 20 to 30 mL of 0.25% lidocaine with epinephrine 1:200,000. For intraoral buccal fat pad extraction, infiltration of 5 to 10 mL of solution to the buccal mucosa and directly into the buccal fat pad on each side is sufficient.

All patients are given general anesthesia when undergoing liposuction of multiple areas of the body simultaneously with liposuction of the face or buccal fat pad extraction. If tumescent solution is being used for other areas of the body, the same low-concentration lidocaine solution is used, but sufficient epinephrine is

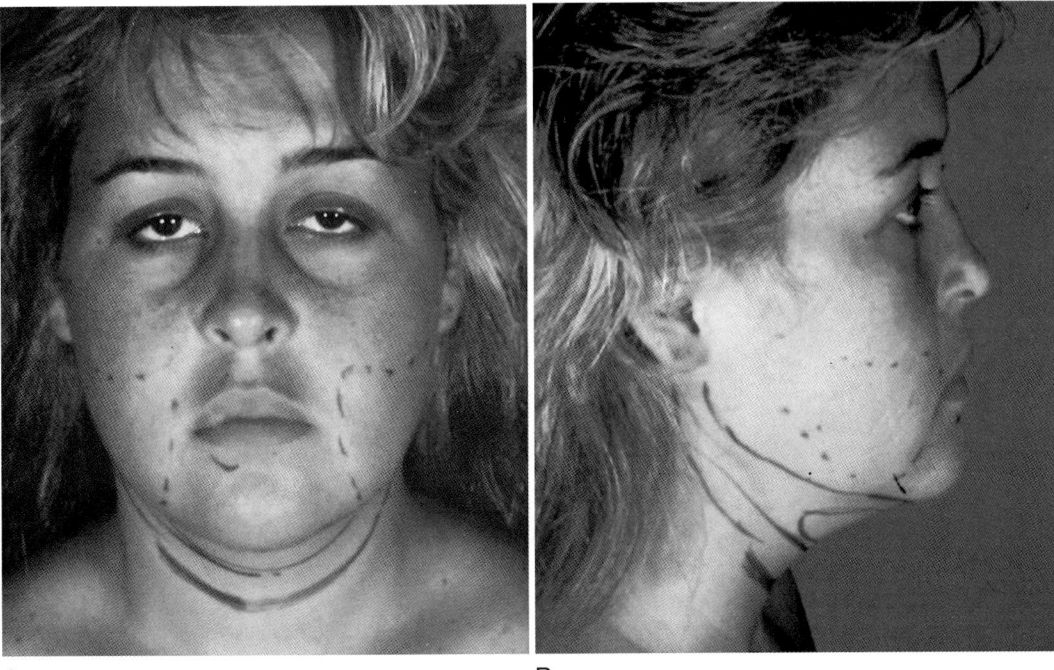

A B

FIGURE 123-23. *A* and *B*, Markings for liposuction of the face. The preparotid area and lower cheek protuberance are marked while the patient is standing or sitting upright. The patient is also marked for liposuction of the neck. (From Pitman GH: Liposuction and Aesthetic Surgery. St. Louis, Quality Medical Publishing, 1993:148.)

added to that portion of the solution being used for the face such that epinephrine concentration is 1:200,000.

OPERATIVE TECHNIQUE

The cheek is suctioned through access incisions in the retrolobular crease and through the nasal vestibule. A 1.8- or 2.4-mm cannula is used (Fig. 123-24). Aspirate volume is usually less than 3 mL per side.

For extraction of the buccal fat pad, a 1.5-cm incision is made in the buccal mucosa halfway between the parotid duct papilla and the gingivobuccal sulcus. The incision is centered on the second molar. By use of a Stevens scissors, the buccinator muscle fibers are spread, and the buccopharyngeal fascia is pierced (Color Plate 123-4). Gentle spreading with the scissors while pushing on the skin of the cheek brings the buccal fat pad through the incision into the mouth. The pad is teased out and excised over a clamp (Color Plate 123-5). The electrocautery is used to secure hemostasis before the clamp is released. The incision is closed with two 4-0 chromic sutures. Removal of 5 to 10 g of tissue usually produces the desired result (Fig. 123-25).

AFTERCARE

The patient should be limited to clear liquids for 24 hours and a soft diet for 3 days. Swelling will begin to recede starting approximately 4 days after surgery. Final result will be apparent in 4 to 6 weeks.

COMPLICATIONS

Hematoma and infection are the most common complications from extraction of the buccal fat pad. Meticulous hemostasis in removal of the buccal fat pad will prevent postoperative hematoma. If a postoperative hematoma does occur, it should be drained promptly through the mouth to avoid development of an abscess. Reaching into the depths of the incision with a hemostat or forceps to pull out fat can potentially result in injury to the facial vein or buccal branches of the facial nerve. The surgeon should remove only the fat that is easily protruded into the mouth.

Neck

ANATOMY

In the neck, the greatest concentration of fat is in the superficial compartment between the skin and the platysma muscle. Additional superficial fat lies deep to the platysma and superficial to the investing fascia of the neck. In the submental area, there is frequently a well-demarcated collection of fat deep to the investing fascia between the anterior heads of the right and left digastric muscles (Color Plate 123-6).

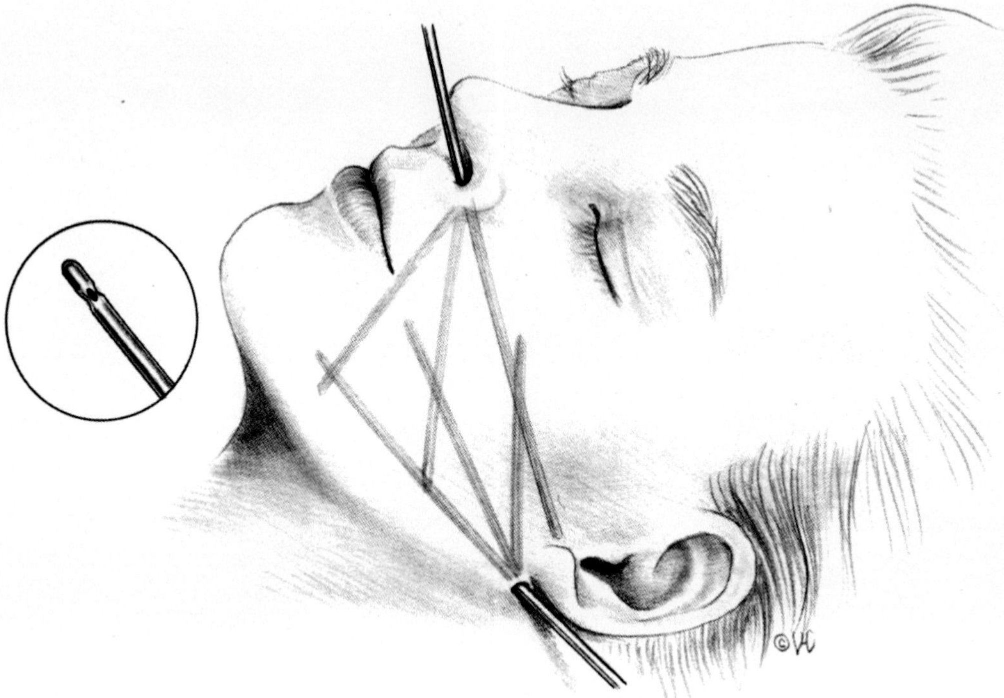

FIGURE 123-24. Liposuction of the cheek. (From Pitman GH: Liposuction and Aesthetic Surgery. St. Louis, Quality Medical Publishing, 1993:145.)

Liposuction of the fat between the skin and platysma will produce the desired results in most patients. Excision of deeper fat requires open access and frequently results in contour depressions, particularly in the submental area.

EVALUATION OF THE PATIENT

An overly full neck is a sign of overweight or aging, and indications for fat extraction in the neck are more liberal than indications for fat extraction in the cheek. The sine qua non of selection of patients for neck liposuction is adequate skin elasticity so that the skin will retract to the reduced contour. Although there are no absolute age limitations, good results from liposuction of the neck are usually confined to patients in early middle age and younger.

Patients with lax anterior platysma bands may benefit from anterior platysma plication in addition to liposuction. This ancillary procedure is more common in men because of the increased bulk of the platysma in men.

MARKINGS

With the patient standing or sitting upright, maximal fat deposition in the submental area is marked. The inferior border of the mandible and the inferior and lateral extent of excess fat are also marked. Access incisions are marked in the submental crease and bilateral retrolobular creases (Fig. 123-26).

ANESTHESIA

If other areas of the body are not treated, pure local anesthesia may be used for liposuction of the neck. Infiltration of 100 to 200 mL of 0.25% lidocaine with epinephrine 1:200,000 will provide adequate anesthesia. All patients undergoing liposuction of multiple areas of the body as well as of the neck are given general anesthesia. If tumescent solution is being used for other areas of the body, the same low-concentration lidocaine solution is used, but sufficient epinephrine is added to that portion of the solution being used for the neck such that epinephrine concentration is 1:200,000.

OPERATIVE TECHNIQUE

The retrolobular skin is tightly adherent to the sternocleidomastoid fascia. Before suctioning through this incision, the surgeon inserts a Stevens scissors and, with a gentle spreading motion, separates the subcutaneous tissues from the fascia (Fig. 123-27). Scissors dissection proceeds in an anteroinferior direction until the scissors enter the preplatysma space in the upper neck. The subcutaneous tissues overlying the platysma are only loosely attached to the subjacent fascia, and once

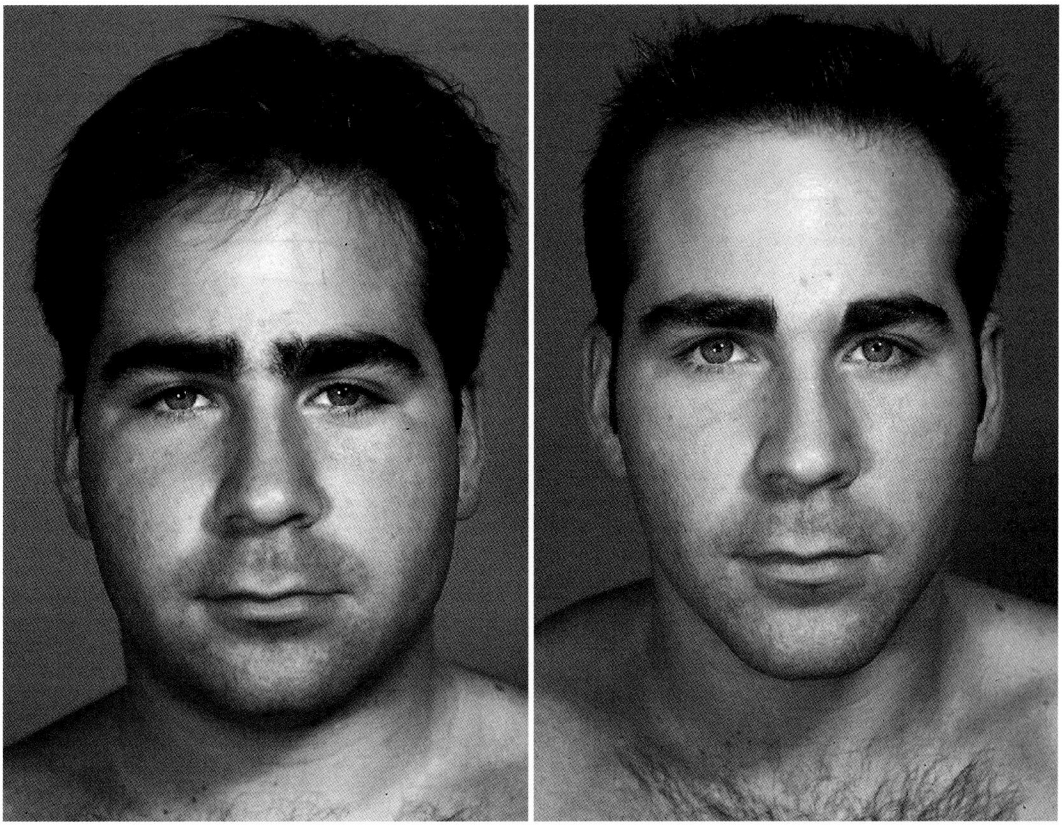

A B

FIGURE 123-25. Patient before *(A)* and after *(B)* liposuction of the face and buccal fat pad excision through the intraoral route.

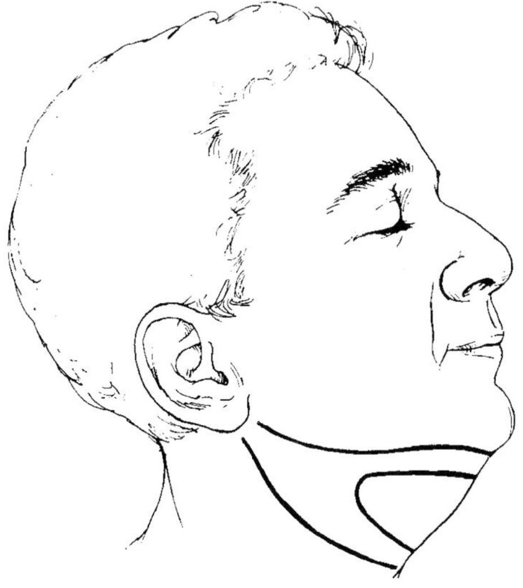

FIGURE 123-26. Markings for liposuction of the neck. (From Pitman GH: Liposuction and Aesthetic Surgery. St. Louis, Quality Medical Publishing, 1993:127.)

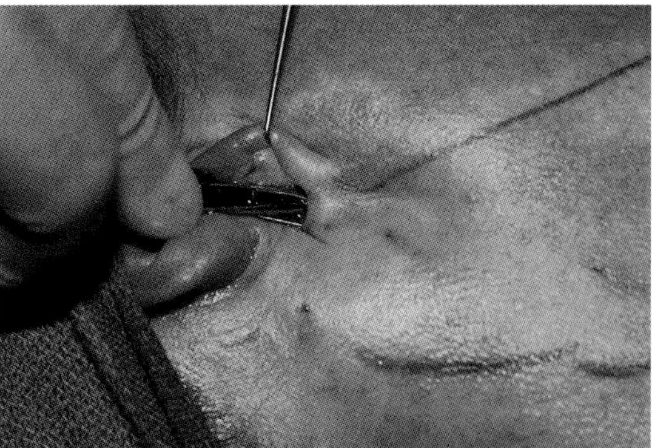

FIGURE 123-27. With Stevens scissors, the skin of the perilobular area is separated from the underlying sternocleidomastoid fascia before insertion of the suction cannula.

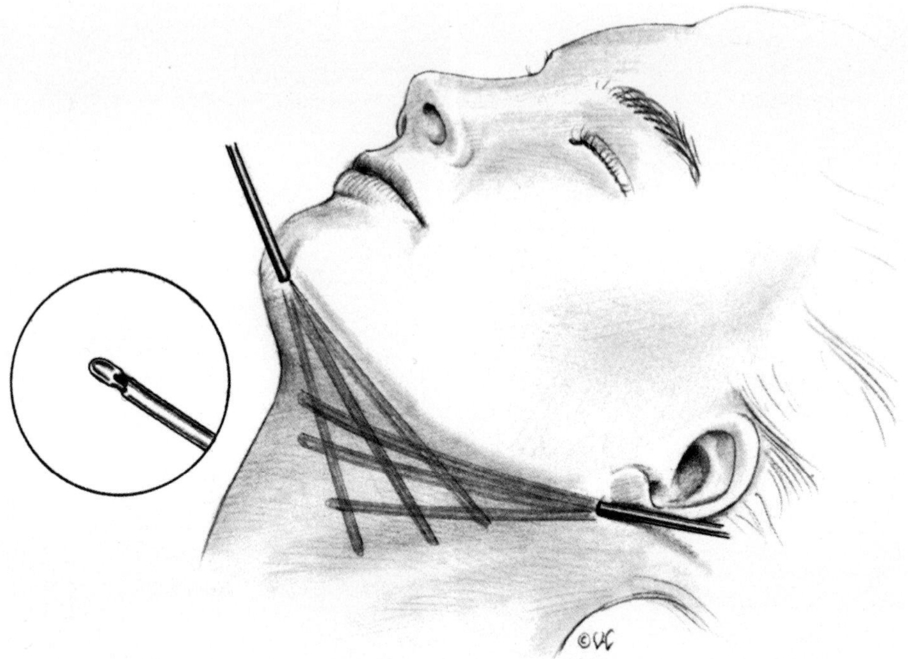

FIGURE 123-28. Liposuction of the neck is performed from a single submental access incision and bilateral retrolobular incisions. (From Pitman GH: Liposuction and Aesthetic Surgery. St. Louis, Quality Medical Publishing, 1993:129.)

the scissors enter the preplatysma space, dissection proceeds easily. The cannula may now be placed into the incision and easily directed into the correct plane.

Liposuction is performed with a 2.4- or 3.0-mm cannula, the larger cannula being used for fuller necks (Fig. 123-28). Young patients with good skin elasticity will have consistently good results (Fig. 123-29).

AFTERCARE

Incisions do not need to be sutured and are simply covered with adhesive bandages. A strip of Reston foam sponge 4 inches wide by $^{1}/_{4}$-inch thick is placed on the neck after completion of the procedure. The Reston foam is removed after 5 days, and the patient is instructed to wear an elastic chin strap at night for 3 weeks after surgery.

COMPLICATIONS

It is possible to injure the marginal mandibular branch of the facial nerve by compressing it against the mandible with the tip of a misdirected cannula. If postoperative weakness of the lower lip does occur, it is almost always the result of a neurapraxic injury and will resolve in 3 to 6 weeks without treatment. As described before, freeing the skin from the underlying sternocleidomastoid fascia before insertion of the cannula through the retrolobular incision permits unrestricted passage of the cannula and makes this complication less likely.

Hematomas are rare and, if small, do not require treatment. A large or expanding hematoma should be drained promptly through a dependent incision. Placement of a small suction catheter after drainage will hasten recovery. The catheter may be removed in 2 to 5 days, depending on how quickly the hematoma cavity is eliminated.

Arms

ANATOMY

Most of the superficial fat on the arm lies in the loose areolar tissue along the posterior aspect (that portion of the arm that faces backward when the hand is resting at the side with the palm facing medially) (Fig. 123-30). Smaller amounts of subcutaneous fat are on the lateral aspect of the arm where the skin is more tightly adherent to the underlying fascia. Absent obesity, there is rarely enough superficial fat to suction in the medial and anterior superficial brachial compartments.

EVALUATION OF THE PATIENT

Patients complain of excess of fullness of the arms, especially noticeable when the arms are at the side and compressed against the chest wall. If the skin is lax, patients will also complain of an unsightly, hanging fullness most noticeable when the arms are abducted (Fig. 123-30).

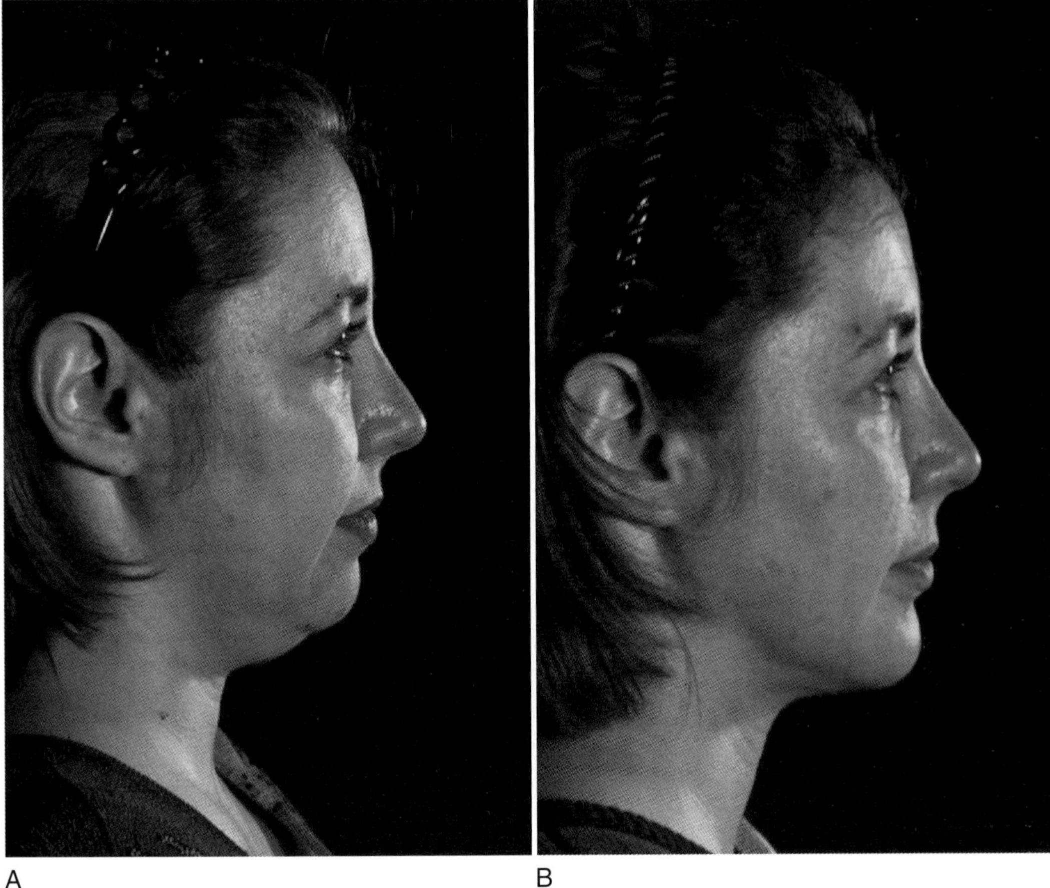

FIGURE 123-29. Patient before *(A)* and after *(B)* liposuction of the neck. The patient also had a chin implant.

If the skin is excessive, brachioplasty is indicated with or without liposuction (see Chapter 127). If pinch thickness is 2 cm or more on the posterior aspect of the arm and the skin is not excessively lax, liposuction will produce a predictable reduction in contour. The overlying skin will usually retract smoothly to envelop the reduced volume.

MARKINGS

The skin of the arm is marked while the patient stands with arms held out 90 degrees laterally. Markings include both the posterior and lateral aspects of the proximal upper extremity (Fig. 123-31).

ANESTHESIA

If only the arms are being treated, tumescent anesthesia with 0.1% lidocaine with epinephrine 1:1,000,000 will provide total anesthesia to the target area. Depending on the size of the patient, 300 to 800 mL of fluid will be required per side.

OPERATIVE TECHNIQUE

With the patient supine, both upper extremities are prepared circumferentially with povidone-iodine solution. The anterior chest and neck are also prepared. The arms are placed on sterile-draped arm boards at 90 degrees to the body, and the hands and wrists are wrapped in sterile towels (Fig. 123-32).

After infiltration of anesthetic solution, liposuction is carried out. A 3- or 4-mm cannula is used on the posterior aspect of the arm (Fig. 123-33). A 2.5- or 3-mm cannula is used on the lateral aspect. Aspirate volumes range from 150 to 450 mL, depending on the size of the patient. Endpoint is determined largely by reduced pinch thickness and, to a lesser degree, by visually apparent diminution in contour (Fig. 123-34).

AFTERCARE

Dressings and garments are not required. Patients usually remain at home in bed with arms elevated on pillows for 48 hours, after which sedentary activities

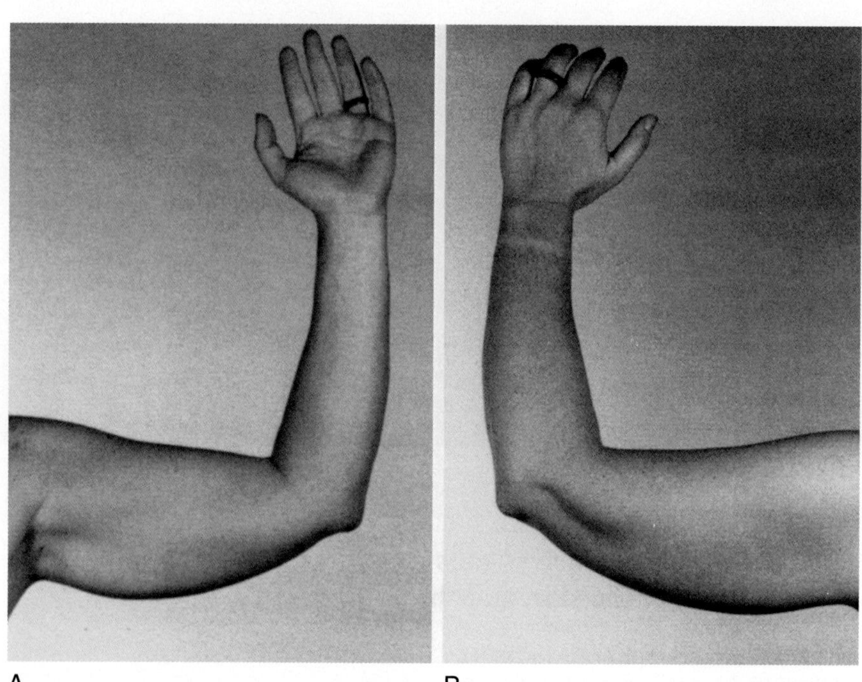

FIGURE 123-30. *A* and *B*, Most of the brachial subcutaneous fat lies on the posterior aspect of the arm in loose, areolar tissue that hangs down when the arm is held out at a 90-degree angle. (From Pitman GH: Liposuction and Aesthetic Surgery. St. Louis, Quality Medical Publishing, 1993:176.)

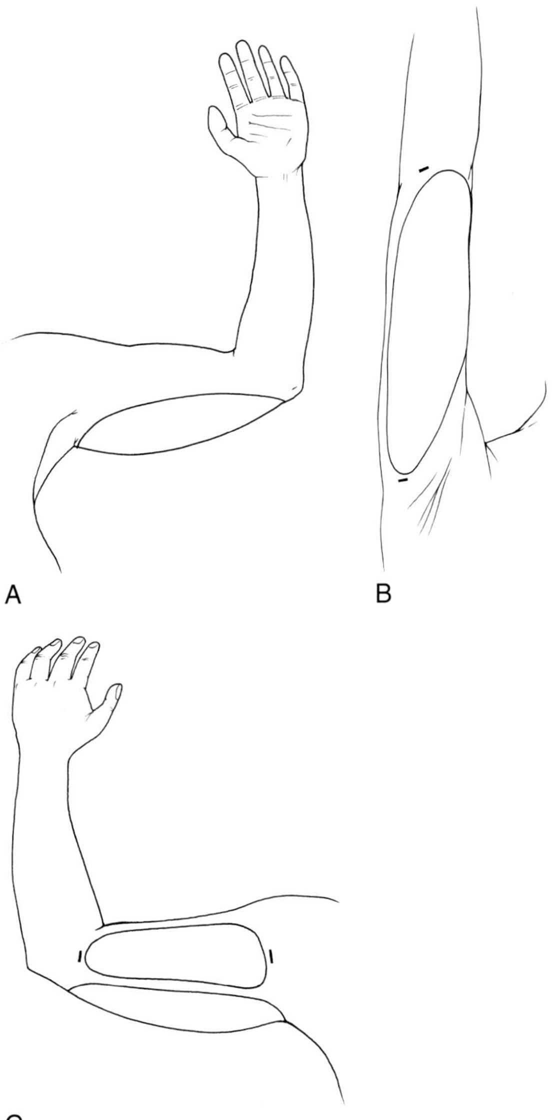

FIGURE 123-31. *A* and *B,* The posterior brachial area is treated most frequently. The patient is marked in a standing position with the arm held out at a 90-degree angle. Areas of fat are outlined as well as two access incisions: one near the medial epicondyle and one in the axilla. *C,* Markings on the lateral aspect. (Modified from Pitman GH: Liposuction and Aesthetic Surgery. St. Louis, Quality Medical Publishing, 1993:179.)

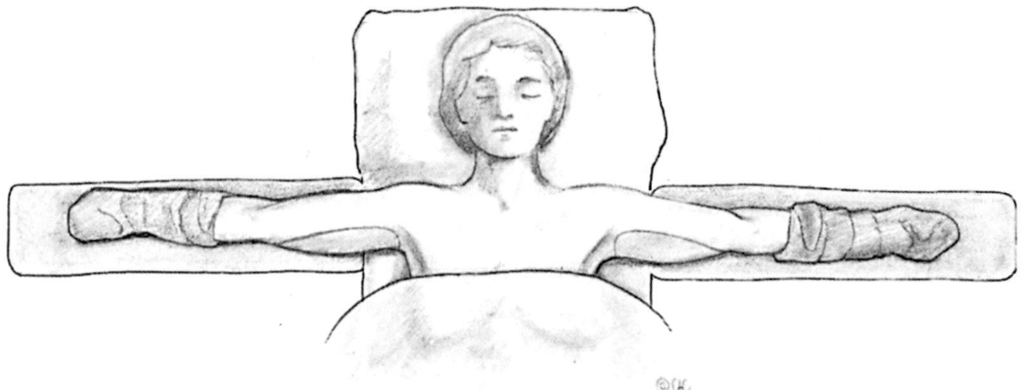

FIGURE 123-32. Sterile draping for treatment of the arms. (From Pitman GH: Liposuction and Aesthetic Surgery. St. Louis, Quality Medical Publishing, 1993:180.)

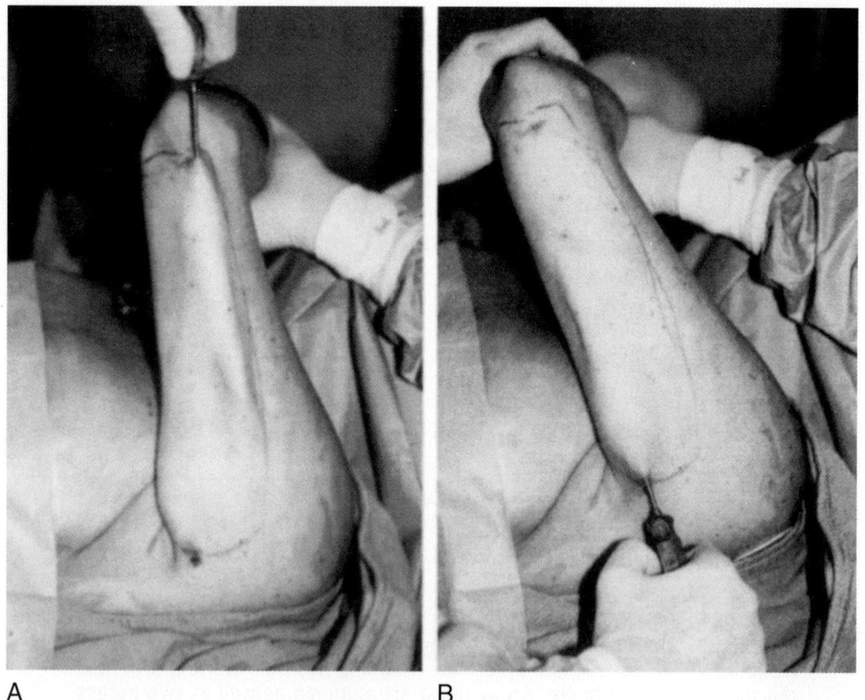

FIGURE 123-33. *A,* Liposuction of the posterior aspect of the arm from the access incision near the elbow. *B,* Liposuction of the posterior aspect of the arm from the access incision near the axilla. (From Pitman GH: Liposuction and Aesthetic Surgery. St. Louis, Quality Medical Publishing, 1993:182.)

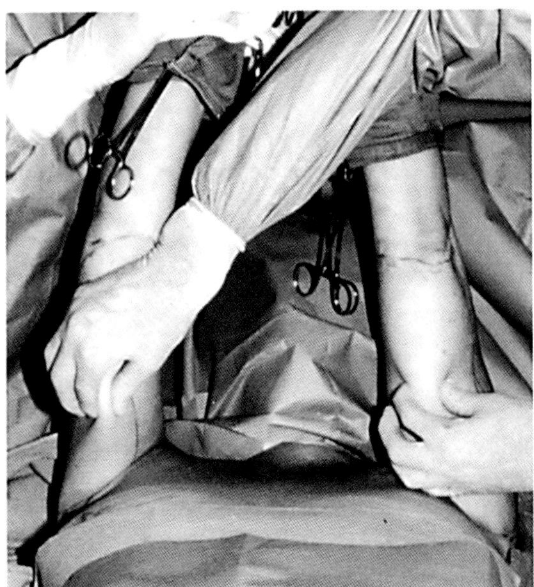

FIGURE 123-34. Reduced pinch thickness in the treated right arm compared with the left. (From Pitman GH: Liposuction and Aesthetic Surgery. St. Louis, Quality Medical Publishing, 1993:183.)

may be resumed. Results are usually apparent within 3 weeks, but subtle improvement continues for 3 to 6 months (Fig. 123-35).

COMPLICATIONS

The most common complication specific to the arms is an aesthetic one: overresection. This complication is more easily avoided than treated. If depressions are severe, autologous fat grafting no sooner than 6 months after initial treatment may improve smoothness. Injury to the ulnar nerve at the elbow has not been reported but is a theoretical possibility, and care should be taken to avoid hitting the nerve with the cannula.

Male Breasts

ANATOMY AND PHYSIOLOGY

Liposuction is the treatment of choice for most cases of male gynecomastia. Glandular breast tissue in men is normally limited to the area deep to the nipple-areola complex and measures 3 to 4 cm in diameter. The glandular disk of tissue may not be palpable in some men, but most men being evaluated for gynecomastia have a readily appreciated, soft or slightly firm glandular mass. Varying amounts of fat contribute to protuberance.

Multiple physiologic conditions, including puberty, senescence, and overweight at any age, may be associated with gynecomastia. Various drugs, legal and illegal, have also been associated with gynecomastia. Medical treatment seeks the underlying cause and treats the condition, but in many patients, the cause remains undiscovered. If the disease has persisted for a long period and the patient is medically asymptomatic, laboratory investigation is usually not fruitful, and etiology may be disregarded in healthy patients.[16]

EVALUATION OF THE PATIENT

Men usually present to the office with persistent, embarrassing breast enlargement. A drug history should be elicited. Transient gynecomastia is relatively common in adolescent boys, but breast enlargement persisting more than 2 years is an indication for surgical treatment.[16] Endocrine work-up for gynecomastia of adolescence is largely fruitless, but counsel from the patient's pediatrician is a good habit to follow. Exogenous steroid use, sometimes illicit, is a common cause of gynecomastia in bodybuilders. Breast enlargement in middle age and beyond is usually associated with testicular involution and weight gain.

Gynecomastia may be unilateral or bilateral. A firm, well-defined mass centered deep to the areola is suggestive of mostly glandular tissue. A softer, more diffuse mass will be mostly fat. A hard or fixed mass may represent a malignant neoplasm, and biopsy should be performed before definitive removal.

A soft, diffuse mass with no palpable glandular disk is fat and will respond to liposuction. A firm, discrete mass in a thin adolescent boy is composed of pure glandular material. It cannot be removed by liposuction and should be excised through an inferior periareola incision. If, on physical examination, the breast mass suggests mixed glandular and fatty components, it is prudent for the surgeon to inform the patient before surgery that the mass will be treated with liposuction, but if a residual mass remains after liposuction, direct excision will be performed. A pinch thickness of 2 to 3 cm usually indicates enough fat for the patient to benefit from liposuction.

Even patients with lax skin will have some skin retraction after liposuction. Unless there is severe ptosis, skin excision is not recommended because scarring in the male chest is usually of poor quality, and most men would like to be able to remove their shirts at a beach or swimming pool.

MARKINGS

With the patient standing, the protuberant area is outlined with ink. The nipple-areola complex generally represents the apex of the protuberance, but more lateral fat excess just caudal to the axilla should also be marked if it is present. Access incisions are well hidden in the inferior areola border and within the axillary hair. An access incision can also be marked in

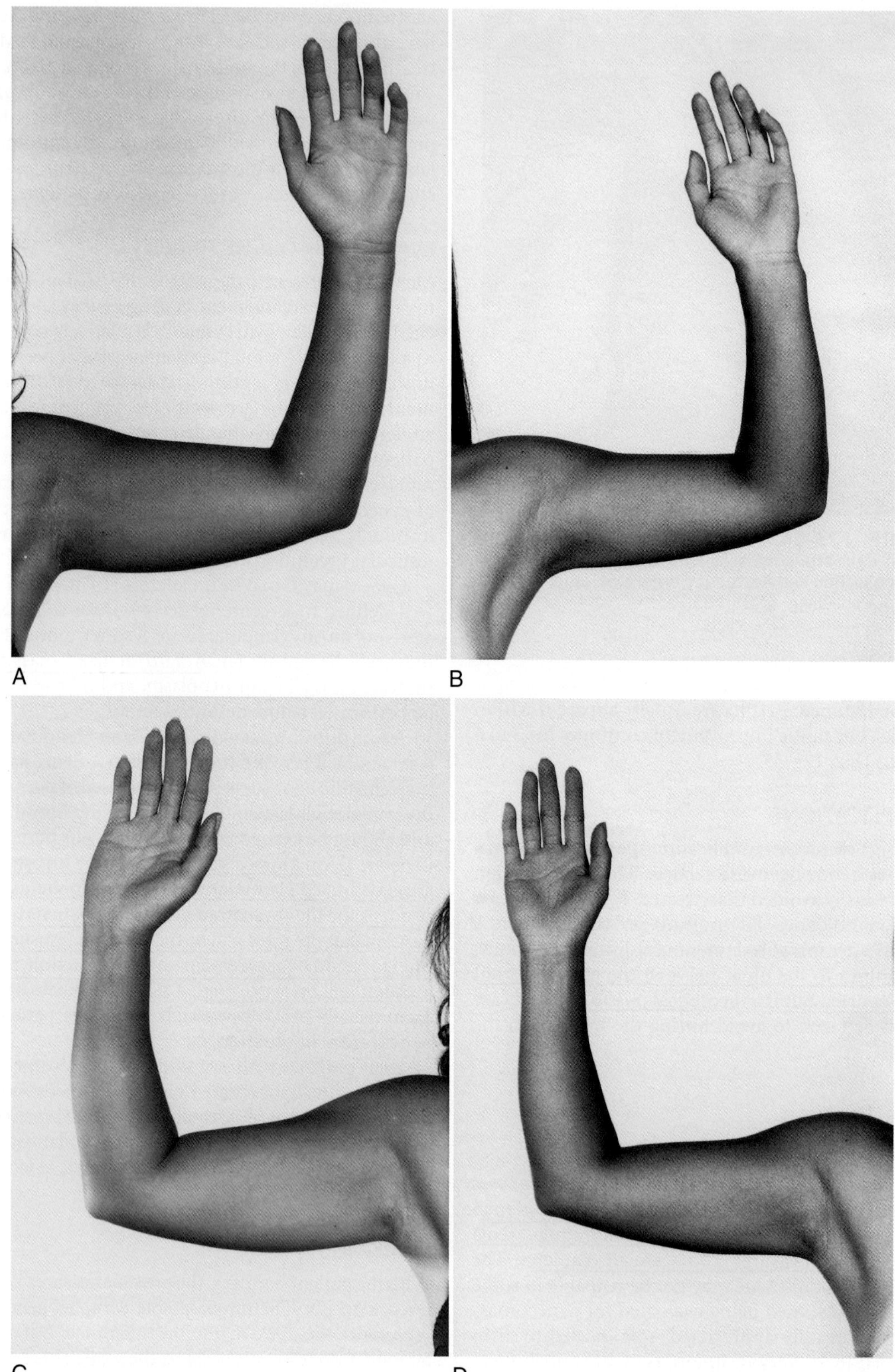

FIGURE 123-35. Anterior view of the left arm before *(A)* and 9 months after *(B)* liposuction of 200 mL. Anterior view of right arm before *(C)* and after *(D)* liposuction.

the inframammary crease if there is sufficient chest hair to camouflage the scar (Fig. 123-36).

ANESTHESIA

Although the procedure can be performed under pure local anesthesia, many patients have simultaneous liposuction of the abdomen or waist. General anesthesia is a better choice when multiple areas are treated.

OPERATIVE TECHNIQUE

With the patient supine, 3- or 4- mm cannulas are used to evacuate the fat. Small amounts are taken from each access incision serially until the desired contour diminution and pinch thickness reduction are achieved (Fig. 123-37). Ultrasound devices and sharpened cannulas have been used in this area in the past but have not improved results and can cause additional complications. Aspirate volumes usually range from 200 to 400 mL per side (Fig. 123-38).

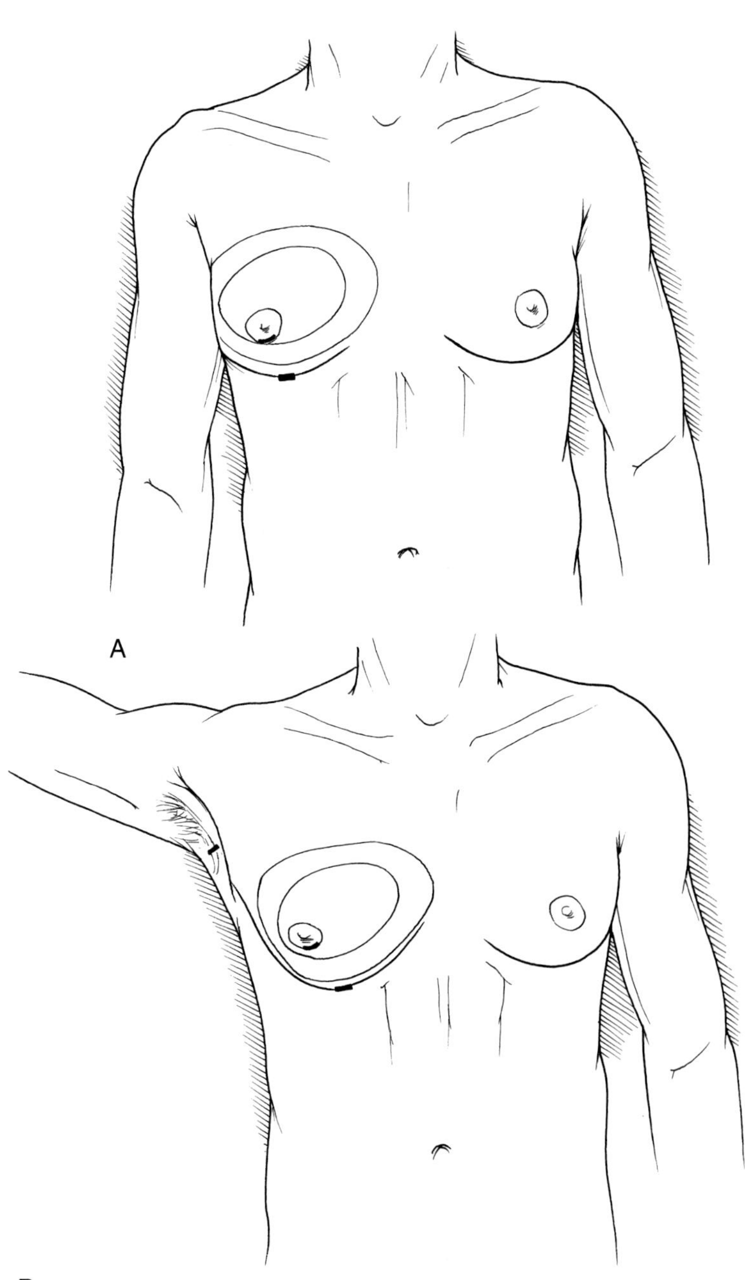

FIGURE 123-36. *A,* Markings for male gynecomastia. The inframammary crease incision is used only in patients with abundant chest hair. *B,* Access incision in the axillary hair.

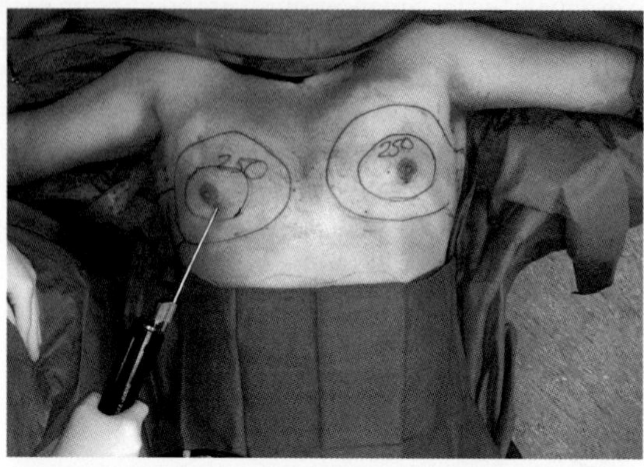

A

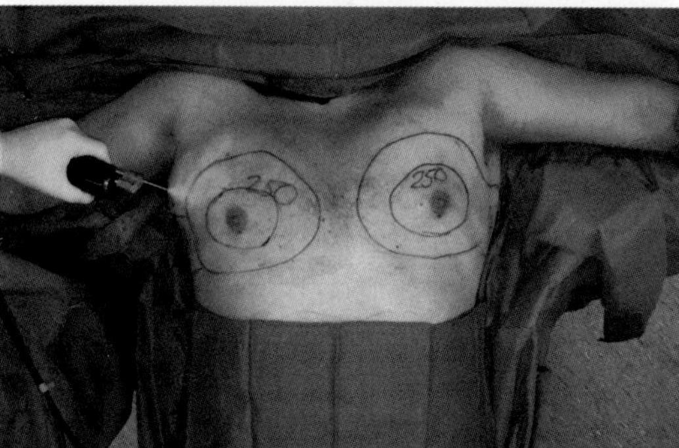

B

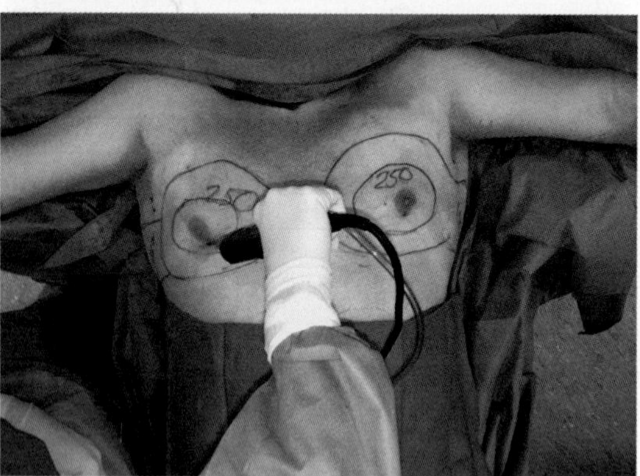

C

FIGURE 123-37. *A,* Liposuction of the male right breast from the inferior periareola access incision. An inframammary crease incision is not used in men who are hairless on the chest. Preoperative estimates of volume of aspirate are noted on the breast (250 mL). *B,* The male breast can also be treated from an axillary access incision within the axillary hair. *C,* Liposuction of the left axilla from the inferior periareola incision. The axilla adjacent to the breast is often a site of excess fat deposition in overweight men seeking treatment for gynecomastia.

AFTERCARE

A chest compression garment is worn for 1 week.

COMPLICATIONS

The most common complications are asymmetry, irregularities from too aggressive resection, and insufficient volume resection.

Female Breasts

The overwhelming appeal of liposuction for breast reduction is the near elimination of scarring on the breasts. A large-volume breast reduction can be performed through two 4-mm incisions in the inframammary crease. Treatment of both breasts can take less than 1 hour and is less physiologically disruptive than traditional breast reduction with scalpel resection of tissue. Whereas liposuction will not produce a reshaping or significant elevation of the breast, it is an effective method of volume reduction in breasts with abundant fat.

ANATOMY AND PHYSIOLOGY

Beneath the skin, breasts are composed of glandular stroma and fat. In adolescence and early adulthood, the predominant tissue is glandular. With advancing age and waning hormone production, glandular stroma is progressively replaced with fat. At any age, breasts of overweight women will contain abundant fat.

EVALUATION OF THE PATIENT

The ideal candidate for breast liposuction is menopausal, is not taking hormone replacement, and has enlarged breasts with little or no ptosis. Excluded as candidates for surgery are women with minimal breast fat. Typically, a thin woman in her late teens or early 20s will have little or no reduction from breast liposuction. A large variety of patients with varying amounts of breast fat and varying degrees of ptosis will present for breast reduction. The presence of abundant fat in the breast is the sine qua non of patient selection.

The history, physical examination, and preoperative testing (including mammography) should be as complete and probing as for any form of breast surgery. In particular, a strong family history of breast cancer and a previous breast cancer in the patient are relative contraindications.

MARKINGS

The main area of breast tissue is outlined with a marker. The mammary crease is marked for two access incisions.

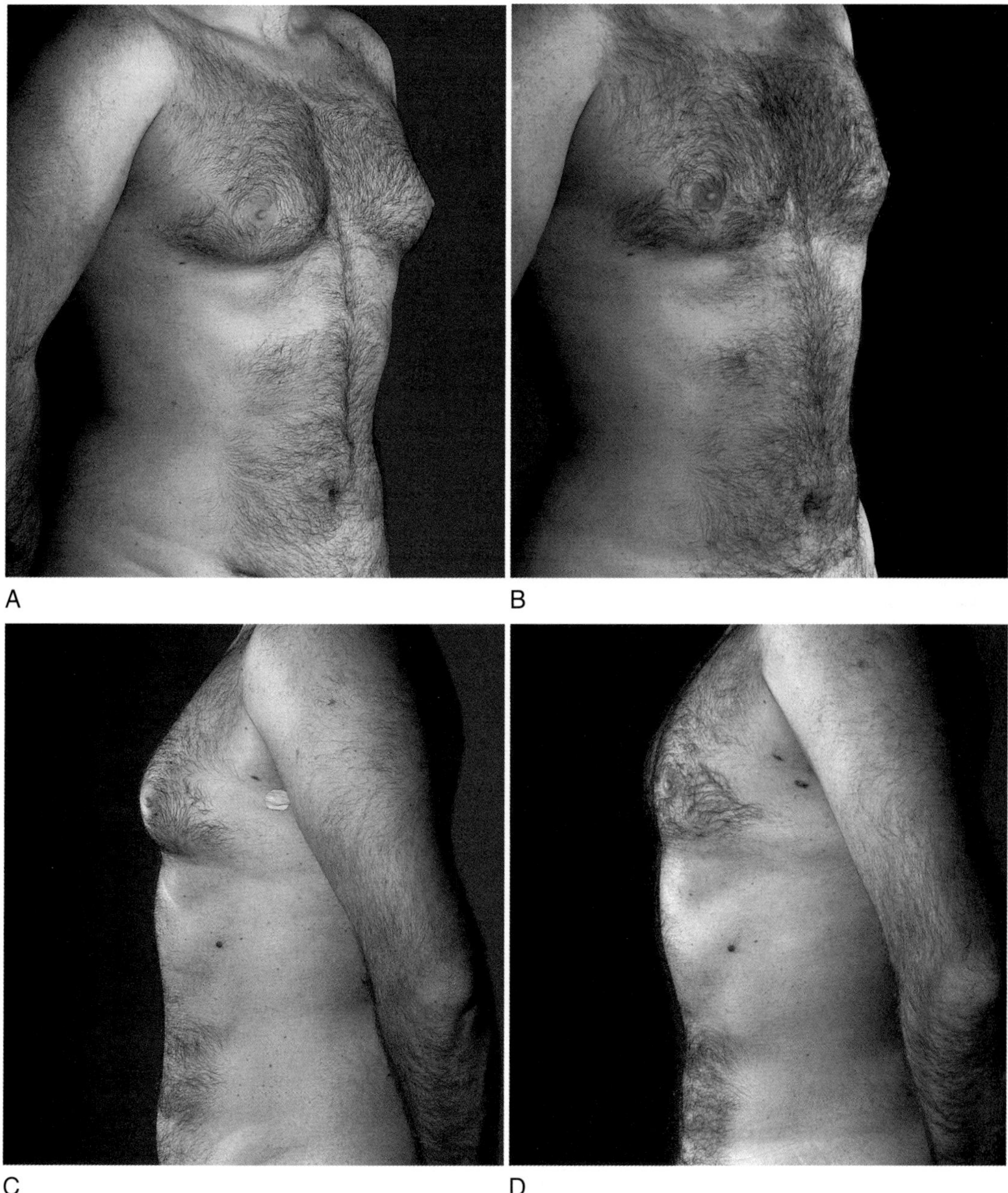

FIGURE 123-38. Right oblique view before *(A)* and 6 months after *(B)* liposuction of the chest; abdomen and flanks also treated. Left lateral view before *(C)* and after *(D)* liposuction.

ANESTHESIA

Most patients are treated under general endotracheal anesthesia so that they can be put safely into a sitting position during the course of the procedure to evaluate shape and size of the breasts.

OPERATIVE TECHNIQUE

Liposuction is performed with 3- and 4-mm cannulas through lateral and medial inframammary crease incisions. Suctioning begins in the depths of the breast, adjacent to the pectoral fascia, and proceeds to the more superficial portions of breast tissue. Aspirate volumes are usually in the range of 200 to 500 mL (Fig. 123-39).

AFTERCARE

Patients are placed in a surgical support bra to be worn for 1 week. Course of recovery is similar to recovery after treatment of other areas.

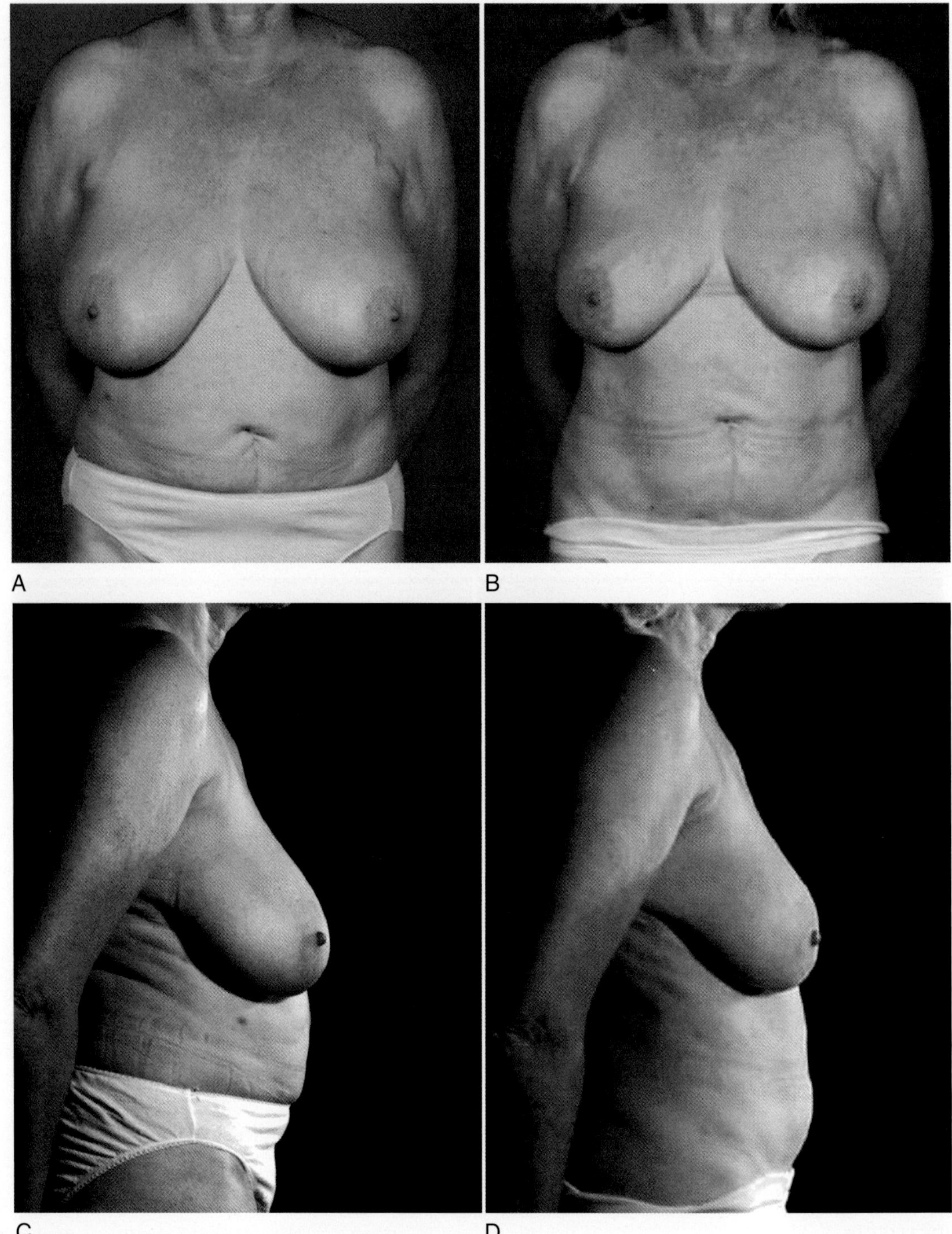

FIGURE 123-39. Frontal view before *(A)* and 6 months after *(B)* liposuction of 625 mL from the left breast and 700 mL from the right. Right lateral view before *(C)* and after *(D)* liposuction of the breasts.

COMPLICATIONS

Complications specific to this area are similar to complications after gynecomastia. Surgery of any type on the breast may result in calcification secondary to fat necrosis. Calcifications after liposuction are common but easily distinguished on mammography from calcification associated with breast cancers.

Abdomen, Hip, Flank, and Back (Lower Torso)

This area comprises the entire circumferential lower torso. Abdomen refers to the lower anterior torso from below the chest to the pubic area. Hip refers to the lateral area overlying the upper ilium and iliac crest. Flank refers to the area cephalad to the hip (posterolateral waist). Back refers to the lower posterior thorax. The lower torso is frequently an area of excess fat deposition due to age-related changes in body composition or excess weight gain.

ANATOMY

Excess superficial fat lies between the skin and the deep fascia. In the anterior abdomen, there is, in addition, a fat deposit deep to the musculofascia. This deep fat in the preperitoneal and intraperitoneal compartments is, of course, inaccessible to liposuction.

EVALUATION OF THE PATIENT

The pinch test in the anterior abdomen will distinguish between abdominal protuberance due to superficial fat that can be suctioned and abdominal protuberance due to fat deep to the muscle fascia. Very loose skin or weakness of the musculofascia is an indication to consider abdominoplasty instead of or in addition to liposuction (see Fig. 123-11).

The hips are frequently the destination of excess fat in women as a result of weight gain or age-related changes in distribution of body fat. In men, excess fat of the posterior lateral torso tends to settle more frequently in the flank or waist area, cephalad to the hips. In both men and women, thickening of the waist is a cardinal sign of aging of the torso.

MARKINGS

On the anterior abdomen, concentric circles are drawn around areas of maximal fat protrusion. Access incisions are usually in or near the pubic hair, in the umbilicus, in the inframammary creases (if the upper abdomen is to be treated), and in the lower lateral abdomen (Fig. 123-40).

The hips are marked bilaterally, and access incisions are placed at the posterior and anterior extents of the protuberant areas (Fig. 123-41). The back and waist area are similarly marked (Fig. 123-42). Usually one or two access incisions in the posterior midline permit treatment of most of the posterolateral waist and back.

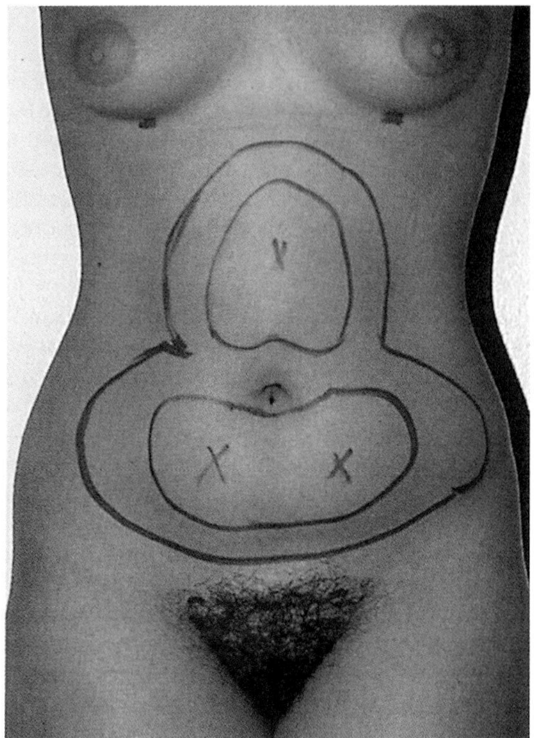

FIGURE 123-40. Markings for the anterior abdomen. (From Pitman GH: Liposuction and Aesthetic Surgery. St. Louis, Quality Medical Publishing, 1993:243.)

ANESTHESIA

If the anterior abdomen alone is treated, local anesthesia with or without sedation is appropriate. Circumferential treatment of the torso usually requires general anesthesia.

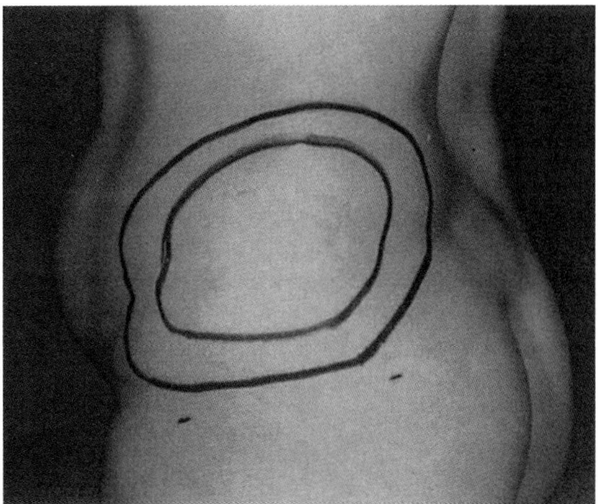

FIGURE 123-41. Typical markings for the hip. (From Pitman GH: Liposuction and Aesthetic Surgery. St. Louis, Quality Medical Publishing, 1993:324.)

OPERATIVE TECHNIQUE

Liposuction of the anterior abdomen is performed in the supine position with use of 3-, 4-, or 5-mm cannulas, depending on the volume of extraction (see Fig. 123-20). Aspirate volumes range widely, but 200 to 2000 mL encompasses most cases. Silicone suction drains are placed in the treated areas and led out the most inferior access incisions when anterior abdominal aspirate volume exceeds 1000 mL. Drains remain in place for 5 days.

Hip, flank, and back areas are usually treated from the lateral decubitus position, rolling the patient slightly anterior or posterior as the respective access incisions are used. Although the lateral decubitus position affords excellent exposure and control for the lower torso, it can be difficult to maintain this position for very large patients. Therefore, larger patients have these areas treated from the prone position. Again, aspirate volumes vary over a wide range. Unilateral aspirate volume is commonly 100 to 400 mL from the hip, 150 to 600 mL from the flank, and 100 to 300 mL from the back (Fig. 123-43).

AFTERCARE

Recovery is similar to recovery from treatment of other areas. Patients having treatment of multiple areas or large-volume extractions will take a longer time to recover.

COMPLICATIONS

Postoperative seromas are more common in the anterior abdomen than in other areas and occur more

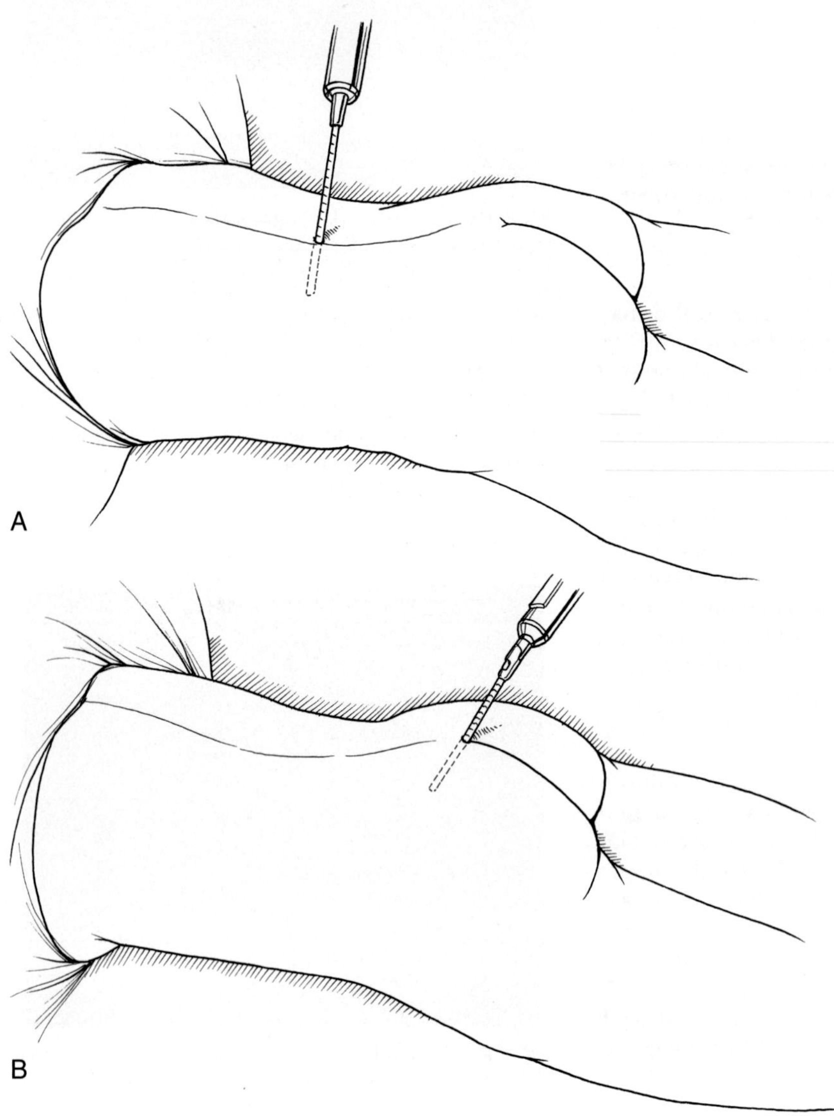

FIGURE 123-42. *A* and *B*, Liposuction of the back. Note access by midline and natal crease incisions.

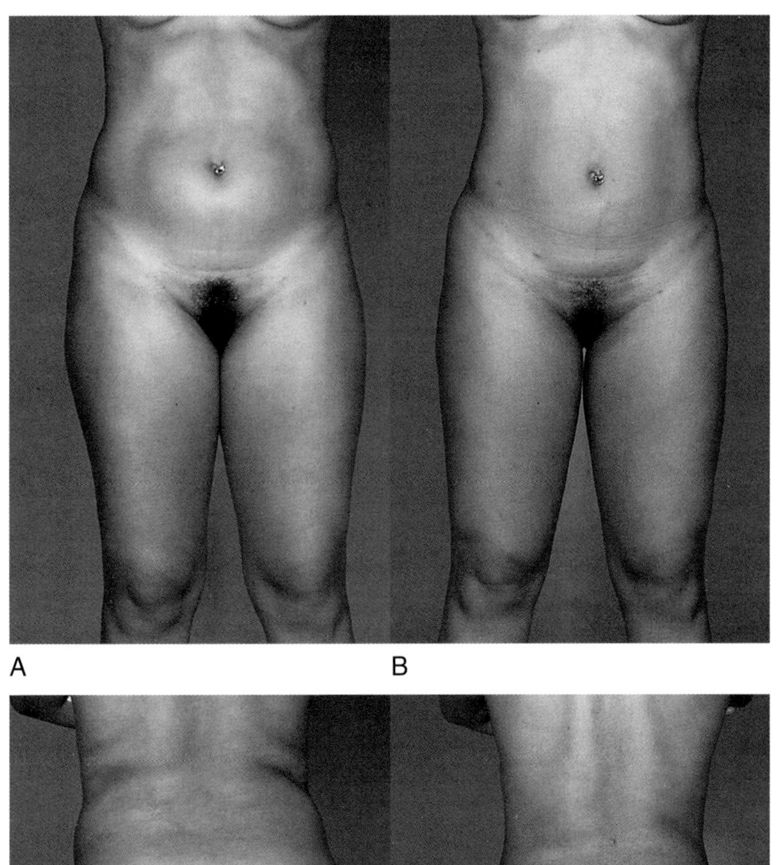

A B

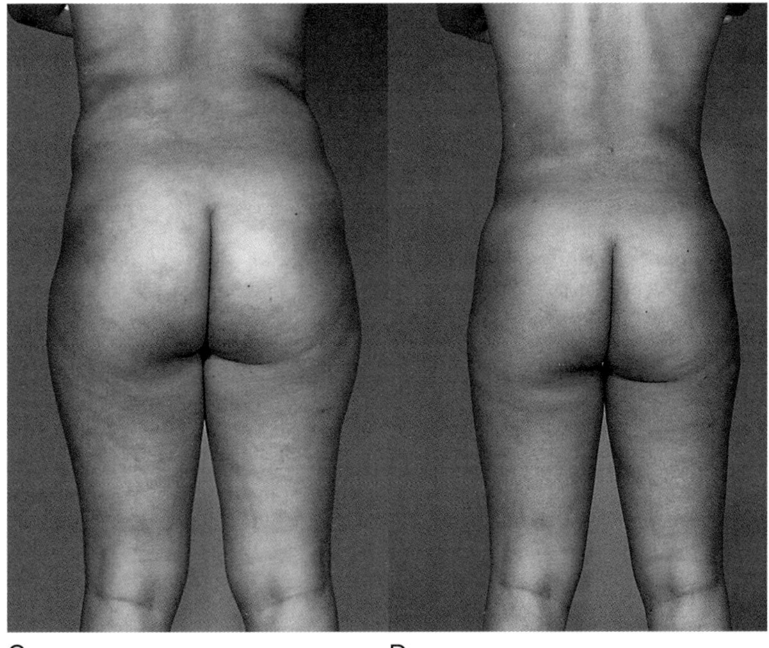

C D

FIGURE 123-43. Patient before (*A, C,* and *E*) and after (*B, D,* and *F*) liposuction of the abdomen (700 mL), flanks (350 mL/side), and hips (150 mL/side). Buttocks, lateral and medial thighs, and knees were also treated.

Continued

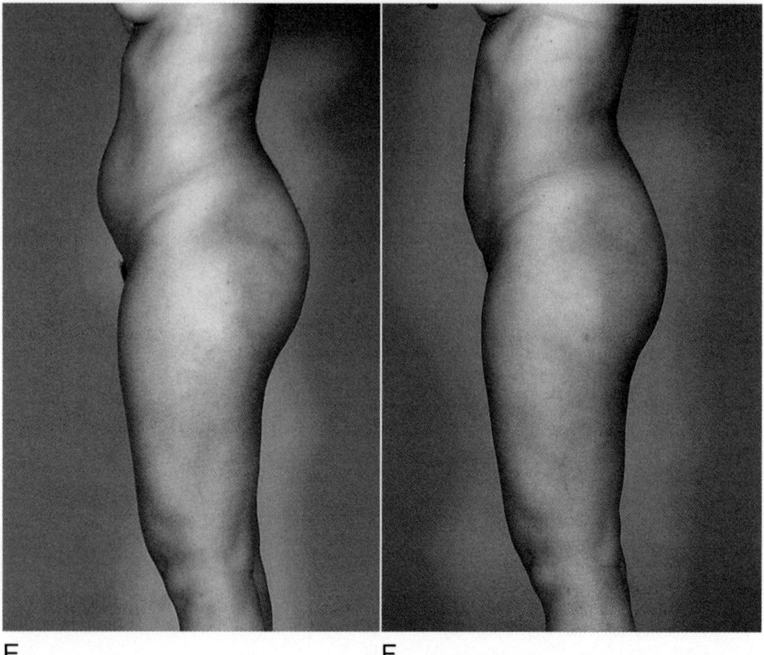

FIGURE 123-43, cont'd.

frequently with high-volume extractions. Such patients are seen frequently in the office in the postoperative period to be examined for seromas, which are usually discovered 10 to 14 days after surgery as discrete, subcutaneous, ballotable masses. Small seromas (<20 mL) are aspirated with a hypodermic syringe and permitted to resorb spontaneously. Larger volumes are drained surgically under local anesthesia. Flat suction drains are placed in the seroma cavity and remain for 5 to 7 days. Whenever possible, the patient is put at bed rest while the drains are in place to promote rapid closure of the seroma cavity.

Buttocks

Whereas overly full buttocks can be a sign of overweight or obesity, very flat buttocks suggest advanced age or illness. High, rounded buttocks are a sign of youth, athleticism, and sexual attractiveness. Desirability in shape and size of the buttocks also reflects ethnic variation. Whatever the wishes of the patient, the surgeon should respect the essential roundness and fullness of a normal, healthy buttock area.

MARKINGS

The patient is marked standing, and areas of excess protuberance are circled. Access incisions are drawn at the top of the natal crease, in the lateral portion of the infragluteal crease, and in the superolateral buttock near the hip.

OPERATIVE TECHNIQUE

The lateral decubitus position is convenient, but the prone position can also be used. Cannulas 3 or 4 mm in diameter are used (Fig. 123-44). Aspirate volumes are usually in the range of 150 to 400 mL, depending on the size of the patient (Fig. 123-45).

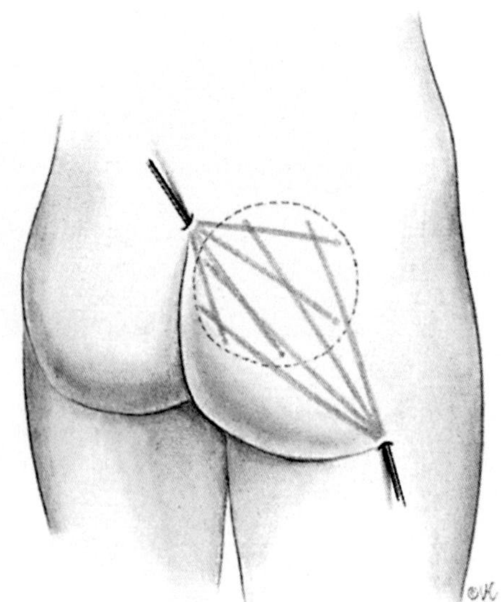

FIGURE 123-44. Liposuction of the buttocks from the natal crease access incision and from the inferior gluteal crease. (From Pitman GH: Liposuction and Aesthetic Surgery. St. Louis, Quality Medical Publishing, 1993:374.)

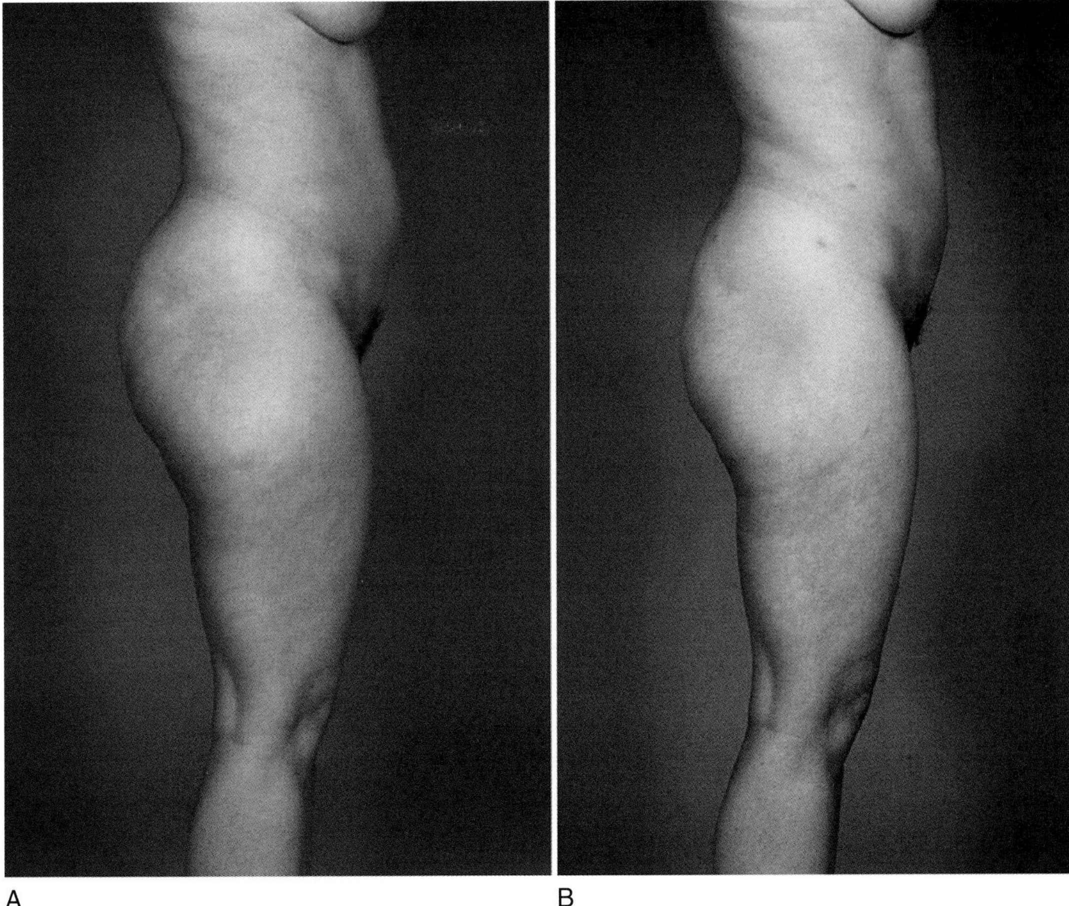

FIGURE 123-45. Before *(A)* and 7 months after *(B)* liposuction of 250 mL from each buttock. The patient also underwent liposuction of the torso and thighs. Total aspirate was 3000 mL.

Thighs

The lateral thighs are the most frequently treated region of the lower extremities. Localized and disproportionate fat deposition is common in this area. Removal of fat from the medial thighs is also desired by many women to achieve a straighter line along the inner thigh. Patients with more diffusely full thighs will benefit from treatment of the anterior and posterior aspects as well.

MARKINGS (see Fig. 123-14)

A circle is drawn around the protuberance of the trochanteric area. Three access incisions are usually marked: a central incision at the point of maximal protuberance and incisions anterior and posterior to the entire fat deposit.

For the medial thigh, the protuberance is usually most pronounced in the upper quarter, and it is marked as a crescent. Access incisions are marked in the anterior and posterior groin creases.

For the anterior thigh, incisions are marked in the anterior groin crease and the suprapatellar crease.

For the posterior thigh, incisions in the posteromedial knee crease and posterolateral upper thigh distal to the infragluteal crease usually suffice for full coverage. More incisions may be added as necessary.

OPERATIVE TECHNIQUE

The trochanteric area is optimally positioned for access and viewing by the surgeon with the patient in the lateral decubitus position (see Fig. 123-17*A*). Typically, small amounts are suctioned from each access incision, with continual checking of contour and pinch as the aspiration proceeds (Fig. 123-46). All of the access incisions are used seriatim, with approximately equal volumes taken from each access incision, until about half the expected aspirate volume has been suctioned.

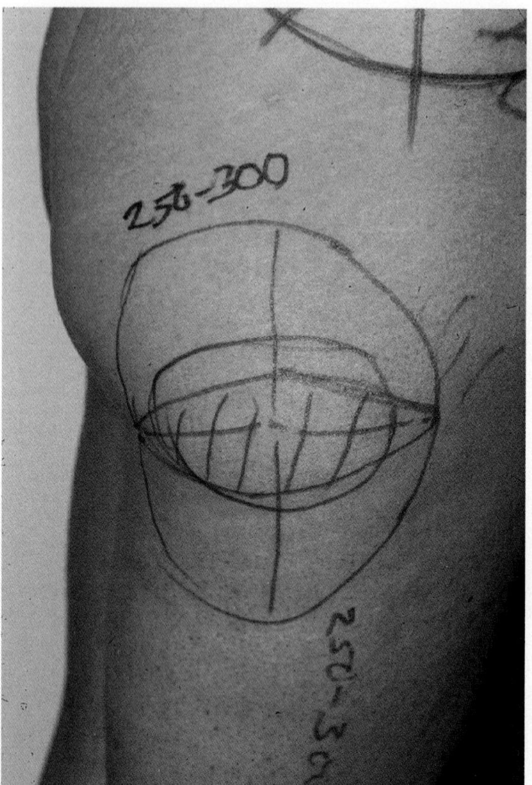

FIGURE 123-46. Lateral thigh area showing markings and access incisions for liposuction. The central access incision is placed at the site of maximal protuberance. Two additional access incisions are used: a posterior incision near the subgluteal crease and an anterior incision at the most anterior extent of the markings. The hatched area denotes the highest density of overlapping tunnels and is hatched as a reminder to the surgeon not to overtreat this area.

The area then undergoes a preliminary evaluation. Additional suctioning is carried out from whichever incisions give the best access until the desired contour and pinch thickness are obtained. The process is methodical and conservative with frequent pauses for checking contour and pinch thickness. Cannulas 3 and 4 mm in diameter and 22 cm long are most frequently used for this area. Aspirate volumes typically range from 200 to 600 mL.

The patient is turned prone for suctioning of the posterior thigh including the medial knee and upper portion of the medial thigh (see Fig. 123-18). Cannulas 3 or 4 mm in diameter and 30 cm long are used to reach all areas from access incisions in the posterolateral upper thigh and medial posterior knee crease. Volumes range from 200 to 500 mL.

Last, the patient is turned supine, and the anterior and anteromedial aspects of the thigh are treated (see Fig. 123-21). Cannulas 3 or 4 mm in diameter and 30 cm long are used through access incisions in the groin and suprapatellar crease. Aspirate volumes are typically 200 to 500 mL (Fig. 123-47).

Calves and Ankles

Liposuction of the calves and ankles can produce dramatic and gratifying results. Successful treatment of this area, however, requires that the surgeon have a well-developed sense of the three-dimensional shape of the calves and ankles and the patience to use fine cannulas in a carefully controlled fat removal.

ANATOMY

The fat layer is relatively thin, and distinction between the superficial and deep subcutaneous fat is clinically nonexistent. The surgeon must assume that much if not all of the fat extraction will be within 1.5 cm of the skin surface and that irregularities can be avoided only by use of fine cannulas.

Although all motor nerves lie deep to the investing fascia, the common peroneal nerve lies in a relatively superficial position as it winds around the neck of the fibula. It is vulnerable to compression against the bone by an errantly directed cannula.

EVALUATION OF THE PATIENT

Thick calves and ankles may be secondary to musculoskeletal enlargement or excess fat. The pinch test is critical in selection of patients, and a minimal pinch thickness of 2 cm is a sine qua non of a successful result.

MARKINGS

Markings are planned to outline the principal anatomic features and to segment each calf and ankle into four quadrants (Fig. 123-48). Each quadrant is treated separately and successively to control volume of aspirate and to ensure right to left symmetry.

With the patient standing flat-footed, the surgeon marks the posterior midline from knee to ankle. The patient is then asked to stand on tiptoe while the surgeon marks the inferior border of the gastrocnemius medial and lateral heads. On the anterior skin surface, the surgeon outlines the tibial face. Last, access incisions are marked: four on the larger lateral surface and three on the smaller medial surface.

OPERATIVE TECHNIQUE

Cannulas 15 or 22 cm long and 2 to 3 mm in diameter are used. All fat extraction is performed with the patient in the lateral decubitus position. The patient is placed first in the left lateral decubitus position to treat the medial aspect of the left calf and ankle and the lateral aspect of the right calf and ankle (Fig. 123-49). Endpoint is determined by visual reduction in

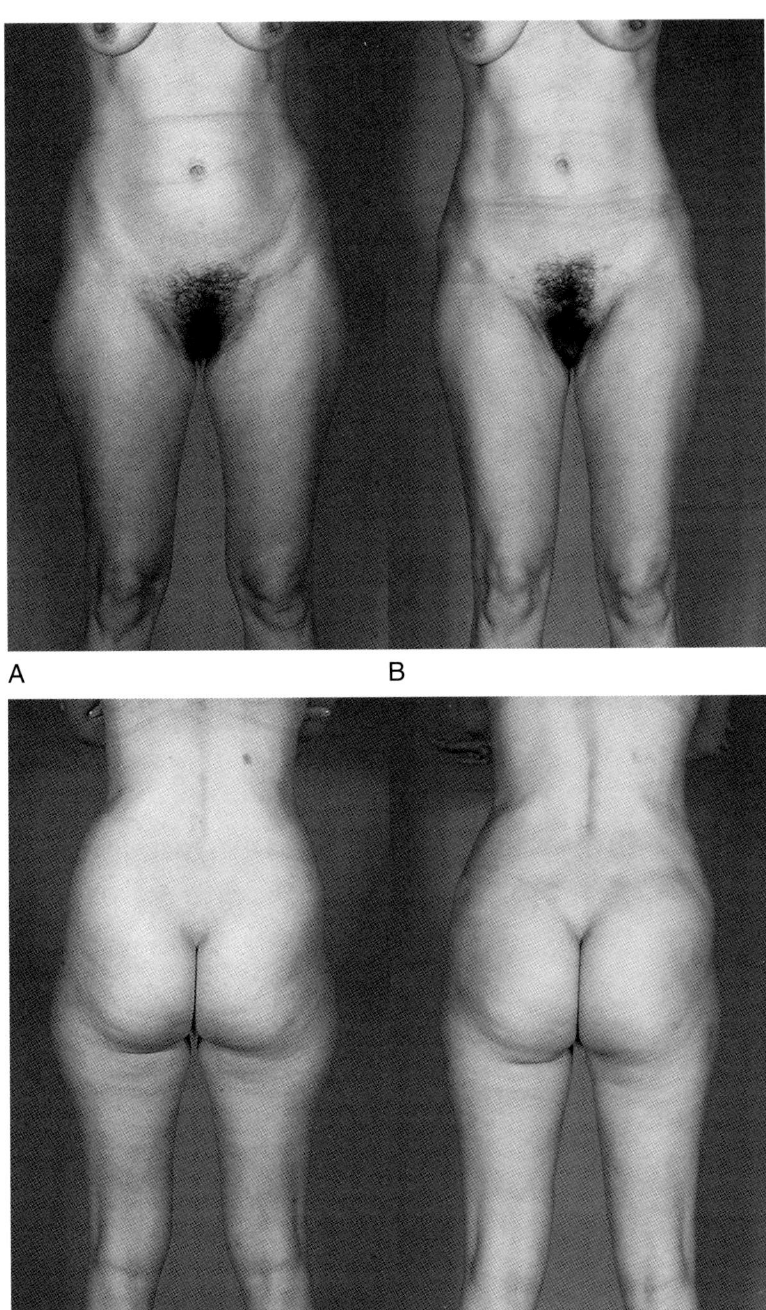

FIGURE 123-47. Before (*A, C,* and *E*) and after (*B, D,* and *F*) liposuction of the lateral thighs (250 mL/side), medial thighs (150 mL/side), and knees (50 mL/side). The abdomen, flanks, and hips were also treated.

Continued

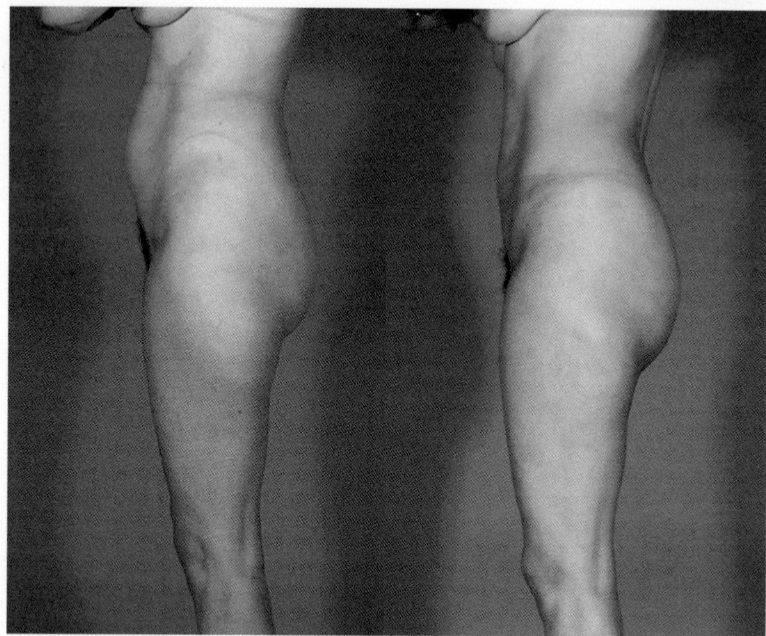

FIGURE 123-47, cont'd.

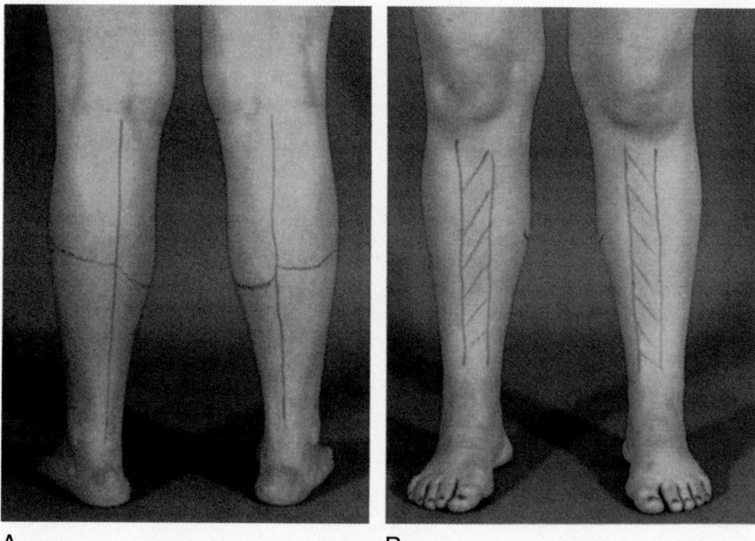

FIGURE 123-48. The calf is marked by having the patient stand on the toes facing away from the kneeling surgeon. This position emphasizes the shape of the gastrocnemius and permits the surgeon to accurately mark the lower borders of this muscle. *A,* A vertical line is drawn down the midline of the posterior leg. The leg is further divided into upper and lower segments by the markings at the lower border of the gastrocnemius. Thus, the leg is divided into four roughly equal quadrants. *B,* The pretibial area is marked with vertical lines on either side of the anterior tibia because there is generally little fat in the pretibial area and suction is rarely necessary. By marking the vertical midline and the anterior tibia, the surgeon divides the leg into medial and lateral halves. (From Pitman GH: Liposuction and Aesthetic Surgery. St. Louis, Quality Medical Publishing, 1993: 431.)

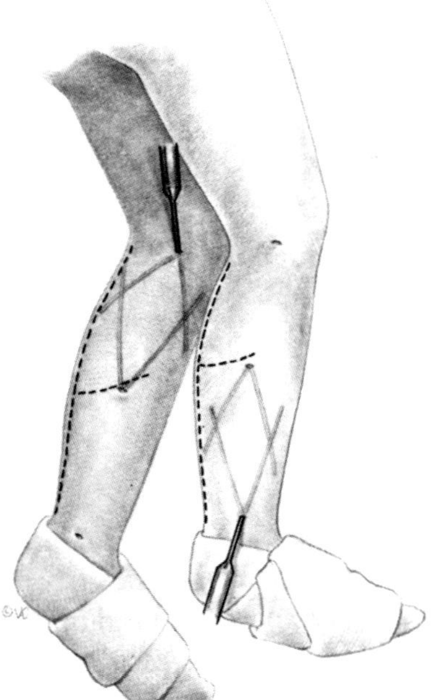

FIGURE 123-49. Artist's schematic of treatment of the left medial calf and ankle. (From Pitman GH: Liposuction and Aesthetic Surgery. St. Louis, Quality Medical Publishing, 1993:432.)

contour and diminished pinch thickness. Volumes are noted individually for the left medial calf, the left medial ankle, the right lateral calf, and the right lateral ankle.

The patient is then turned to the right lateral decubitus position to treat the medial aspect of the right calf and ankle and the lateral aspect of the left calf and ankle. Endpoint is again determined principally by visual reduction in contour and diminished pinch thickness, but comparison of volume extraction from left and right sides becomes a useful secondary determinant (Fig. 123-50).

AFTERCARE

Patients are told to rest at home for 1 week, to sleep with their feet elevated for 6 weeks, and to wear surgical support hose during the day for 6 weeks. Other aspects of recovery are similar to that for liposuction of other areas of the body.

COMPLICATIONS

Complications peculiar to this area include neurapraxic injury to the common peroneal nerve, which can be avoided by careful direction of the cannula near the neck of the fibula. Prolonged ankle swelling is avoided by strict adherence to the aftercare protocol.

COMPLICATIONS

Complications from liposuction can be divided into two broad categories: medical complications resulting in morbidity and aesthetic complications producing undesirable results. Complications may be those common to any plastic surgery procedure or may be specific to liposuction. Becoming a skilled liposuction surgeon requires not only the ability to artistically perform the operation but also an awareness of potential complications and the ability to diagnose and treat them in timely fashion.

Medical Complications

BLEEDING

Excessive blood loss during liposuction can result in localized hematoma, excessive bruising and swelling, postoperative anemia, or shock. Prevention of bleeding begins with a careful history. Patients who report easy bruising or bleeding diatheses should be evaluated by a hematologist before surgery. Patients are instructed to eliminate all drugs that might cause platelet dysfunction or other coagulopathies 2 weeks before surgery. Significant anemias should be corrected before liposuction.

Use of tumescent preinfiltration with dilute epinephrine-containing solutions has largely eliminated the need for transfusions in liposuction.[2,3,8] Keeping the patient warm reduces the likelihood of coagulopathies and bleeding.[15,17]

Diffuse bruising after liposuction does not require treatment. If excessive bleeding is suspected or diagnosed during or after surgery, the patient should be admitted to the hospital, monitored with serial hematocrit determinations and frequent assessment of vital signs, and transfused as necessary. Persistent bleeding requires urgent surgical and medical investigation to discover and correct the source.

Localized hematomas, especially those that are tense or expanding, should be surgically drained and explored. The bleeding has usually stopped at the time of drainage, but continual bleeding at the site of a hematoma mandates sufficient surgical exploration of the operative site to find and control the source, which may be deep to the muscle fascia. Once bleeding is controlled, closed suction drainage should be instituted and maintained for several days.

SEROMAS

Frequency of seromas increases with degree of surgical trauma to the target area. The anterior abdomen has a higher frequency of postoperative seromas, perhaps secondary to the prominence of periumbilical perforators. In the past, ultrasonic liposuction was associated with a high incidence of seromas. Reduction in the duration of treatment with the ultrasonic probe has reduced the incidence of seromas associated

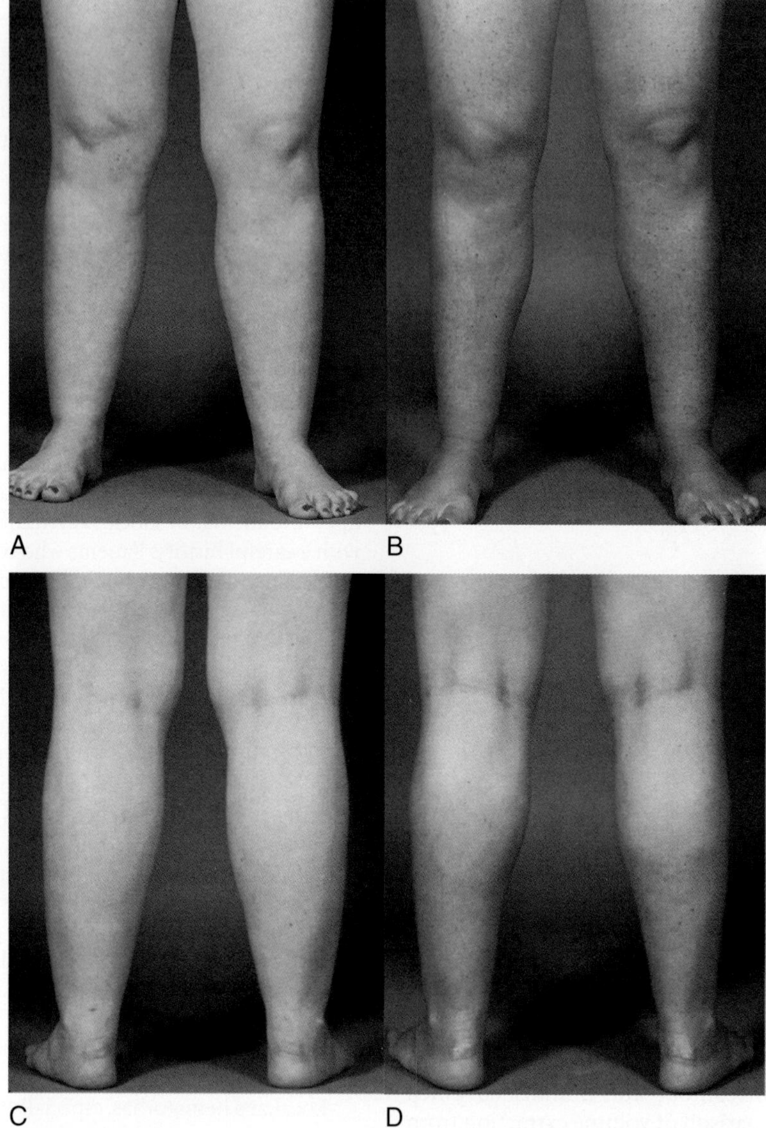

FIGURE 123-50. Before (*A* and *C*) and 6 months after (*B* and *D*) aspiration of 800 mL from each knee, calf, and ankle. (From Pitman GH: Liposuction and Aesthetic Surgery. St. Louis, Quality Medical Publishing, 1993.)

with ultrasonic-assisted liposuction. The senior author places closed suction drains in the anterior abdomen for patients undergoing extensive liposuction of this area. The drains remain in place for 5 days. See the preceding discussion of complications in the section "Abdomen, Hip, Flank, and Back (Lower Torso)" for information on management of seromas.

INFECTION

Serious infections are uncommon given an uncompromised host and strict observance of sterile technique. In 1300 liposuction operations during 5 years, the senior author (Pitman) reported a 0.003 incidence of minor cellulitides requiring outpatient treatment: rest, elevation, and oral antibiotics.[18] In more than 3000 liposuction operations during 20 years, the senior author (Pitman) has had six patients who developed postoperative infections that required hospitalization or open drainage (incidence of less than 0.002).[19] There is no proof that routine use of prophylactic antibiotics reduces these already low infection rates.

Postoperative infections should be evaluated quickly and treated aggressively. Fatal necrotizing fasciitis has occurred after liposuction.[20] Pain at the operative site is a cardinal symptom of necrotizing fasciitis, and patients reporting pain in the postoperative period should be seen by the surgeon without delay. Necrotizing fasciitis is a medical and surgical emergency, with high morbidity and mortality, requiring immediate hospitalization and treatment.

Steps to avoid infection include the use of proper sterile technique, preparation of the patient with antiseptic solution, and proper use and maintenance of the pump filters. Poor hygiene of the patient may be an additional cause of infections, and some surgeons have their patients treated with chlorhexidine scrub showers the night before and morning of surgery.

SKIN NECROSIS

Skin necrosis has been described after any method of liposuction. The strongest contributing factor to skin loss is disruption of the delicate subdermal vasculature by excessive superficial fat evacuation. Ultrasound has the added risk of being able to cause thermal injury of the skin, internally or externally. If internal ultrasound is used, the most important safety precautions include applying the energy to a wet environment and always keeping the ultrasound probe in motion.[21,22]

Pressure necrosis of the skin can also occur after surgery but is almost always attributed to tight compressive garments. The anterior superior iliac spines are particularly susceptible to this type of injury. Properly fitted garments and use of foam padding beneath the garments in the area of bone prominences avoid this problem.[2,23]

FLUID IMBALANCE

Proper fluid balance and replenishment are crucial to safe liposuction (see "Safe Suction: Tumescent Method, Fluid Management, and Blood Loss"). The patient's circulating volume must be maintained without significant blood loss (or dilution) in the presence of a potentially large third space created by the liposuction. Inadequate fluid resuscitation or a large blood loss can result in hypovolemia and shock. Fluid overload can result in pulmonary edema with possible cardiac arrest.[2,3,8,9,24]

LIDOCAINE TOXICITY

Severe lidocaine toxicity is a rare but potentially fatal complication of liposuction.[25] Minor toxic effects can occur at serum concentrations between 3 and 6 μg/mL and include lightheadedness, restlessness, drowsiness, tinnitus, slurred speech, a metallic taste in the mouth, and numbness of the lips and tongue. At plasma levels between 5 and 9 μg/mL, shivering, muscle twitching, and tremors may occur. With yet higher levels, the patient may experience convulsions, central nervous system depression, coma, respiratory depression, and eventually cardiac arrest.[13,14]

Once toxicity is recognized, treatment consists of hyperventilation and administration of benzodiazepines. Both of these therapies are designed to lower the seizure threshold. Airway protection is necessary for loss of consciousness or neuromuscular control secondary to convulsions (see also "Safe Use of Lidocaine for Anesthesia and Analgesia").

DEEP VENOUS THROMBOSIS AND PULMONARY EMBOLUS

Deep venous thrombosis (DVT) and pulmonary embolus (PE) occur infrequently when liposuction is performed as a stand-alone procedure. Embolic phenomena are much more common during abdominoplasty.[26] The goal of the surgeon should be to minimize the risk of occurrence, and the surgeon should have a low threshold of suspicion for postoperative signs or symptoms that may indicate the presence of DVT or PE. Equally important is to identify and not operate on high-risk patients.

Virchow's triad, first described in 1856,[27] is venous stasis, injury to the intimal layer, and subsequent hypercoagulability and can result in DVT and PE. Factors that increase the risk for the development of DVT and PE include age older than 40 years, obesity, diabetes mellitus, prolonged operating time, malignant disease, immobility or paralysis, previous thromboembolism, and protein C deficiency. Oral contraceptive use and hormone replacement therapy are considered potential risks.

Symptoms of DVT and PE include acute lower extremity swelling or pain, sudden chest pain, and shortness of breath. Sometimes there are no warning symptoms, and the presentation may be sudden death. If DVT is suspected, the patient should have immediate Doppler flow studies. If PE is suspected, a ventilation-perfusion scan is the most commonly ordered test. Once a diagnosis is confirmed, anticoagulation therapy should begin.

Several strategies to minimize risk for DVT and PE after liposuction include proper selection of patients, limiting the duration of operations, use of sequential compression devices for longer procedures, and encouragement of early progressive ambulation.

Fatal postoperative PE in patients undergoing elective general surgery is reported to be 0.1% to 0.8% in the absence of any prophylaxis.[28] According to a survey conducted by the American Society for Aesthetic Plastic Surgery,[24] the rates show 1 DVT per 3040 (0.00033%) procedures and 1 PE per 3759 (0.00027%)

procedures, including lipoplasty combination procedures. Others report pulmonary thromboembolism as the major cause of death, accounting for nearly 25% of the fatalities, after liposuction.[29] Reports of the morbidity and mortality of PE and DVT when a procedure is combined with abdominoplasty have been published.[26,29-31]

FAT EMBOLI AND FAT EMBOLISM SYNDROME

Fat embolization probably occurs in all liposuction operations but is of no clinical significance.[32] Fat embolism syndrome with respiratory decompensation occurs rarely in liposuction patients, and most of the literature reports do not withstand critical analysis.[33-35]

Diagnosis of fat emboli is largely clinical and includes the classic triad of respiratory distress, cerebral dysfunction, and petechial rash. Symptoms appear within 48 hours of surgery in 85% of the patients. The clinical presentation can vary from mild shortness of breath with a rash to adult respiratory distress syndrome, coma, and death. Chest radiographs often begin normal and progress to diffuse bilateral infiltrates. Ventilation-perfusion scan may show matching defects.[36] Most important, fat embolism syndrome must be distinguished from PE because treatment is vastly different. In addition, fluid overload, cardiac failure, pulmonary edema, severe postoperative atelectasis, and aspiration pneumonia must be eliminated as causes of respiratory distress.

Initial treatment includes pulmonary support and hemodynamic monitoring. Pharmacologic therapy is high-dose corticosteroids, which are believed to inhibit the inflammatory reaction.

MAJOR ORGAN OR VESSEL PERFORATION, PNEUMONIA, AND DEATH

Perforations of the abdomen and viscera are rarely reported but can occur. Patients at higher risk are those who have abdominal wall or umbilical hernias or have had multiple previous abdominal procedures, including abdominal liposuction. Such patients have poor integrity of the abdominal wall fascia, making inadvertent entry with a cannula easier, and they are also more likely to have intestinal adhesions, making enterotomies more likely if the abdominal cavity is entered. In addition, scar tissue from previous liposuction results in fibrotic tissue planes, again making misdirection of the cannula more likely.

The risk for occurrence of visceral perforation can be diminished with a careful preoperative history and physical examination for previous abdominal surgery or hernias. An ultrasound examination or computed tomographic scan may be used for preoperative screening, or the patient may be determined not to be a good candidate for elective liposuction. Gentle, precise placement of the infiltration and aspiration cannulas will help minimize the occurrence of this potentially fatal complication.

Definitive diagnosis and treatment are obtained by a laparotomy. Patients experiencing severe abdominal pain after liposuction should be evaluated immediately for peritoneal signs. If perforation is suspected, rapid laparoscopic evaluation and exploration can be lifesaving.

Other potential sites of cannula misdirection include the thorax, retroperitoneum, and major vessels (femoral, axillary). Gentle use of blunt cannulas and a bimanual technique with keen awareness of the position of the cannula tip at all times will aid in the avoidance of visceral perforation.

DYSESTHESIA

Temporary numbness of the skin overlying the areas treated with liposuction is normal. Dysesthesia usually resolves the first week after surgery and rarely persists beyond 6 weeks. Hyperesthesia or increased sensitivity is uncommon and usually transient. Animal studies[37] have been conducted to study the effect of ultrasonic energy on the sciatic nerve of a rat model. A direct correlation between the power (amplitude) of the generator settings and number of passes and the degree of injury was noted. A similar clinical study has not been performed, but if safe principles of ultrasound technique are employed (i.e., a wet environment and keeping the probe in motion), such injuries will be avoided.

Dysesthesia and hyperesthesia in all likelihood represent a transient inflammatory neuritis of the sensory nerves. Patients may find relief during this period with oral anti-inflammatory medications, light massage, and garments. As the postoperative swelling diminishes, so will the neuritis.

Cosmetic Complications

CONTOUR ABNORMALITIES

Contour abnormalities are one of the most common complications of liposuction. Typical words to describe contour deformities are dents, waviness, and depressions. It is the most likely reason for dissatisfaction of patients and reoperation. Secondary surgeries to correct contour abnormalities and asymmetries or to remove additional fat are reported at a rate of 5% to 15%.[38]

A contour abnormality results from uneven or overzealous subdermal fat removal and can occur in any area in which liposuction is performed. Performing superficial fat removal more commonly results in contour abnormalities. The arms and medial thighs are particularly unforgiving areas because superficial suction is more commonly performed in these areas and the skin is thinner.

Revision of contour deformities should not be planned for at least 6 months to allow complete healing, resolution of swelling, and softening of tissue. Surgical options include autologous fat grafting[39,40] for depressions and buttock drop and additional liposuction for inadequately treated areas and for asymmetries. Skin laxity is treated with dermatolipectomy.

HYPERPIGMENTATIONS AND SKIN IRRITATIONS

Most skin discolorations that occur after liposuction are temporary. Hyperpigmentation occurs when the pigment heme, a breakdown product of hemoglobin, remains in the subcutaneous tissue after the gross discoloration from bruising has resolved. Resolution can take up to 18 months after surgery. Some color changes may be permanent.

Hyperpigmentation can also result from an internal inflammatory response to constricting band from a compression garment, which tends to occur at the waist, elbows, and knees. An allergic reaction to a garment, if it is used, may also occur and cause hyperpigmentation.

Treatment for established hyperpigmentation is generally ineffective, and avoidance is paramount. Staying in the deep and intermediate fat layers and avoiding prolonged and traumatic liposuction at the dermal level will avoid most hyperpigmentation problems. Frequent checking of the effects of pressure garments on the skin will avoid traumatic or allergic hyperpigmentation from garments.

REFERENCES

1. Rohrich RJ, Beran SJ, Kenkel JM, et al: Extending the role of liposuction in body contouring with ultrasonic assisted liposuction. Plast Reconstr Surg 1998;101:1090.
2. Commons GW, Halperin B, Chang CC: Large-volume liposuction: a review of 631 consecutive cases over 12 years. Plast Reconstr Surg 2001;108:1753.
3. Pitman GH: Discussion of large-volume liposuction: a review of 631 cases over 12 years. Plast Reconstr Surg 2001;108: 1764.
4. Klein S, Fontana L, Young VL, et al: Absence of an effect of liposuction on insulin action and risk factors for coronary heart disease. N Engl J Med 2004;350:2549.
5. Klein JA: The tumescent technique for liposuction surgery. Am J Cosmet Surg 1987;4:263.
6. Klein JA: Tumescent technique for local anesthesia improves safety in large-volume liposuction. Plast Reconstr Surg 1993;92:1085.
7. Pitman GH: Discussion of tumescent technique for local anesthesia improves safety in large-volume liposuction. Plast Reconstr Surg 1993;92:1099.
8. Pitman GH, Aker JS, Tripp ZD: Tumescent liposuction: a surgeon's prospective. Clin Plast Surg 1996;23:633.
9. Gilliland MD, Coates N: Tumescent liposuction complicated by pulmonary edema. Plast Reconstr Surg 1997;99:215.
10. Xylocaine [package insert]. Wilmington, Delaware, Astra Zeneca, 2001.
11. Klein JA: The tumescent technique. Anesthesia and modified liposuction technique [review]. Dermatol Clin 1990; 8:425.
12. Klein JA: Tumescent technique for regional anesthesia permits lidocaine doses of 35 mg/kg for liposuction. J Dermatol Surg Oncol 1990;16:249.
13. Samdal F, Amland PF, Bugge JF: Plasma lidocaine levels during suction-assisted lipectomy using large doses of dilute lidocaine with epinephrine. Plast Reconstr Surg 1994;93:1217.
14. Ostad A, Kageyama N, Moy RL: Tumescent anesthesia with lidocaine dose of 55 mg/kg is safe for liposuction. Dermatol Surg 1996;22:921.
15. Rohrer MJ, Natale AM: Effect of hypothermia on the coagulation cascade. Crit Care Med 1992;20:1402.
16. Carlson HE: Gynecomastia. N Engl J Med 1980;303:795.
17. Doufas AG: Consequences of inadvertent perioperative hypothermia [review]. Best Pract Res Clin Anaesthesiol 2003;17:535.
18. Pitman GH, Fikry BA: Liposuction: safety issues in 1300 cases. Scientific presentation at annual meeting of American Society of Aesthetic Plastic Surgery, New York, May 7, 2001.
19. Pitman GH: Unreported data.
20. Alexander J, Takeda D, Sander G, et al: Fatal necrotizing fasciitis following suction assisted lipectomy. Ann Plast Surg 1988;20:562.
21. Maxwell GP, Gingrass MK: Ultrasonic-assisted lipoplasty: a clinical study of 250 consecutive patients. Plast Reconstr Surg 1998;101:189.
22. Zocchi ML: Ultrasonic assisted lipoplasty. Clin Plast Surg 1996;23:575.
23. Giese SY, Bulan EJ, Commons GW, et al: Improvements in cardiovascular risk profile with large volume liposuction. A pilot study. Plast Reconstr Surg 2001;108:510.
24. Iverson RE, Lynch DJ: Practice advisory on liposuction. Plast Reconstr Surg 2004;113:1478.
25. Rao RB, Ely SF, Hoffman RS: Deaths related to liposuction. N Engl J Med 1999;340:1471.
26. Teimourian B, Rogers WB 3rd: A national survey of complications associated with suction lipectomy: a comparative study. Plast Reconstr Surg 1989;84:628.
27. Virchow R: Gesammelte Abhandlungen zur wissenschaftlichen Medizin. Frankfurt, Germany, Meidinger, 1856.
28. Hull RD, Raskob GE, Firsh J: Prophylaxis of venous thromboembolism: an overview. Chest 1986;89(suppl):374.
29. Grazer FM, de Jong RH: Fatal outcomes from liposuction: census survey of cosmetic surgeons. Plast Reconstr Surg 2000; 105:436.
30. Hetter GP: Closed suction lipoplasty on 1078 patients: Illouz told the truth. Aesthetic Plast Surg 1988;12:183.
31. Dillerud E: Abdominoplasty combined with suction lipoplasty: a study of complications, revisions, and risk factors in 487 cases. Ann Plast Surg 1990;25:333, discussion 339.
32. Hunsstad JP, Withers JP: Pulmonary fat embolism: does it occur following suction-assisted lipectomy? Presented at the 56th annual scientific meeting of the American Society of Plastic and Reconstructive Surgeons, Atlanta, November 13, 1987.
33. Pitman GH: Liposuction and Aesthetic Surgery. St. Louis, Quality Medical Publishing, 1993:466.
34. Laub DR Jr, Laub DR: Fat embolism syndrome after liposuction: a case report and review of the literature [review]. Ann Plast Surg 1990;25:48.
35. Ross R, Johnson G: Fat embolism after liposuction. Chest 1988;93:1294.

36. Skarzynski JJ, Slavin JD Jr, Spencer RP, Karimeddini MK: "Matching" ventilation/perfusion images in fat embolization. Clin Nucl Med 1986;11:40.
37. Howard B, Beran S, Kenkel J, et al: Effects of ultrasound-assisted liposuction on nerve tissue. Presented at 31st annual American Society for Aesthetic Plastic Surgery meeting, Los Angeles, Calif, May 1998.
38. Chang KN: Surgical correction of postliposuction contour irregularities. Plast Reconstr Surg 1994;94:126.
39. Coleman SR: Long term survival of fat transplants: controlled demonstrations. Aesthetic Plast Surg 1995;19:421.
40. Coleman SR: Structural fat grafts: the ideal filler? Clin Plast Surg 2001;28:111.

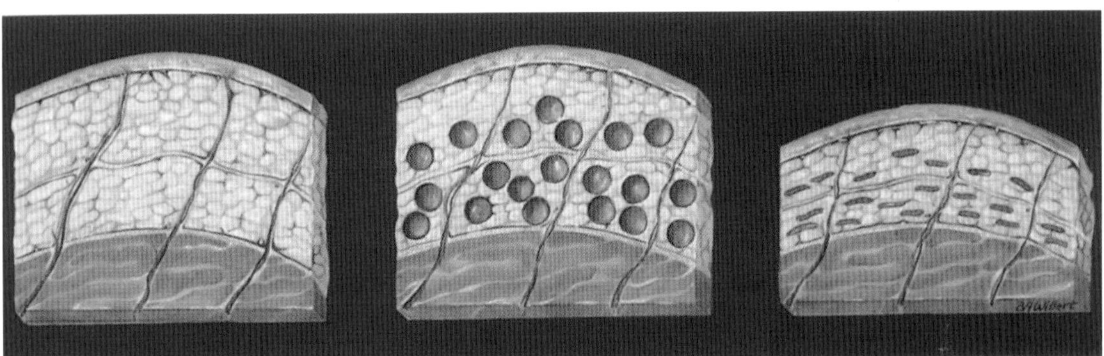

COLOR PLATE 123-1. Artist's schematic of removal of subcutaneous fat by liposuction. Neurovascular elements remain intact as fat is evacuated and contour is reduced. (From Pitman GH: Liposuction and Aesthetic Surgery. St. Louis, Quality Medical Publishing, 1993:60.)

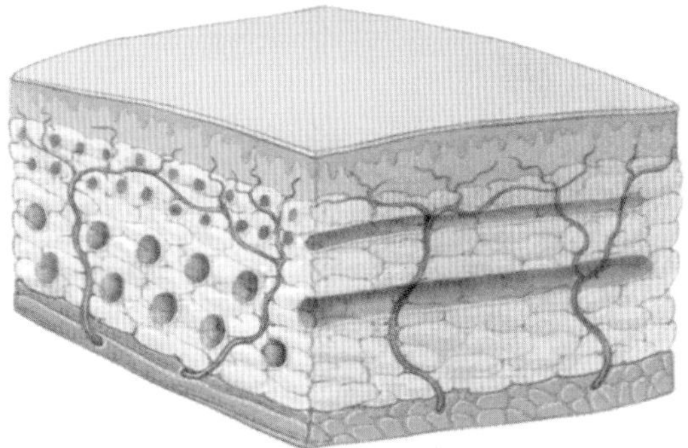

COLOR PLATE 123-2. Larger diameter cannulas can be used in the deep fat, but only narrow-gauge cannulas should be used in the more superficial fat. (From Pitman GH: Liposuction and Aesthetic Surgery. St. Louis, Quality Medical Publishing, 1993:62.)

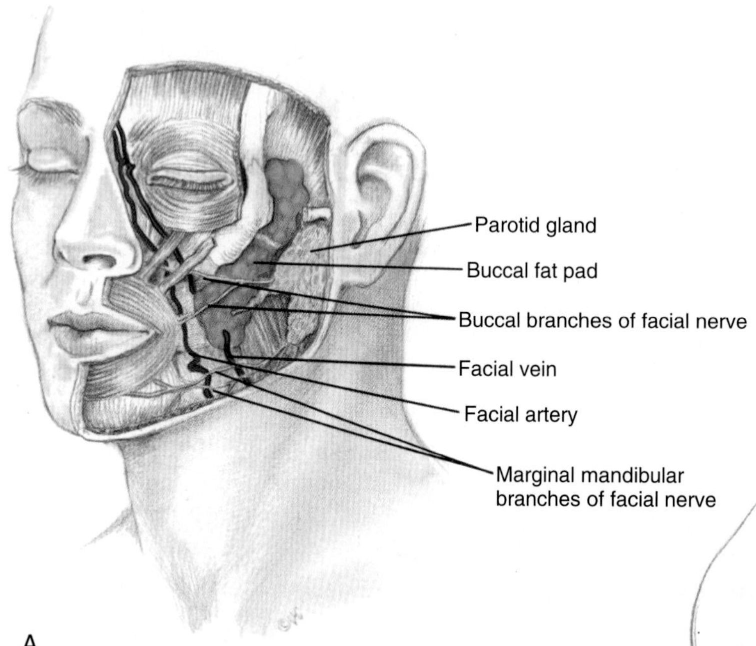

Parotid gland
Buccal fat pad
Buccal branches of facial nerve
Facial vein
Facial artery
Marginal mandibular branches of facial nerve

A

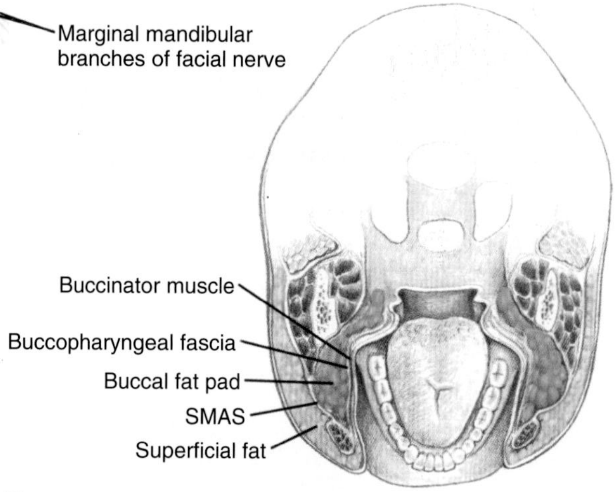

Buccinator muscle
Buccopharyngeal fascia
Buccal fat pad
SMAS
Superficial fat

B

COLOR PLATE 123-3. *A,* Position of the buccal fat pad in the face and temporal area and the anatomic relationships of adjacent structures. *B*, Interdental cross section showing subcutaneous cheek fat and its relationship to the buccal fat pad in producing cheek fullness. Note the proximity of the buccal fat pad to the intraoral buccal mucosa. SMAS, superficial musculoaponeurotic system. (From Pitman GH: Liposuction and Aesthetic Surgery. St. Louis, Quality Medical Publishing, 1993:117.)

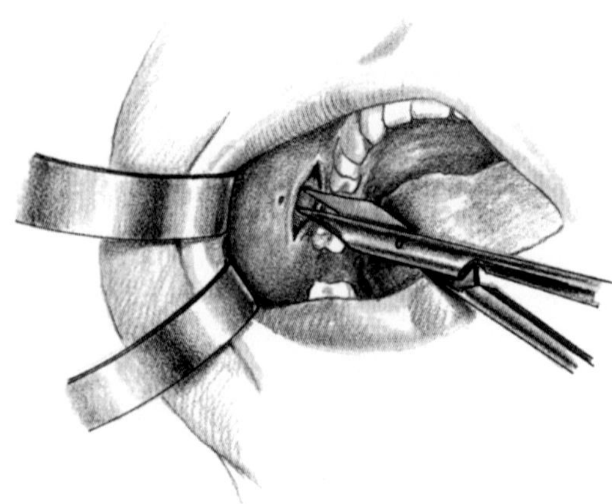

COLOR PLATE 123-4. Mucosal incision used to access buccinator muscle and buccopharyngeal fascia. Muscle fibers are spread with Stevens scissors, which are then used to pierce the buccopharyngeal fascia, exposing the underlying buccal fat pad. (From Pitman GH: Liposuction and Aesthetic Surgery. St. Louis, Quality Medical Publishing, 1993:144.)

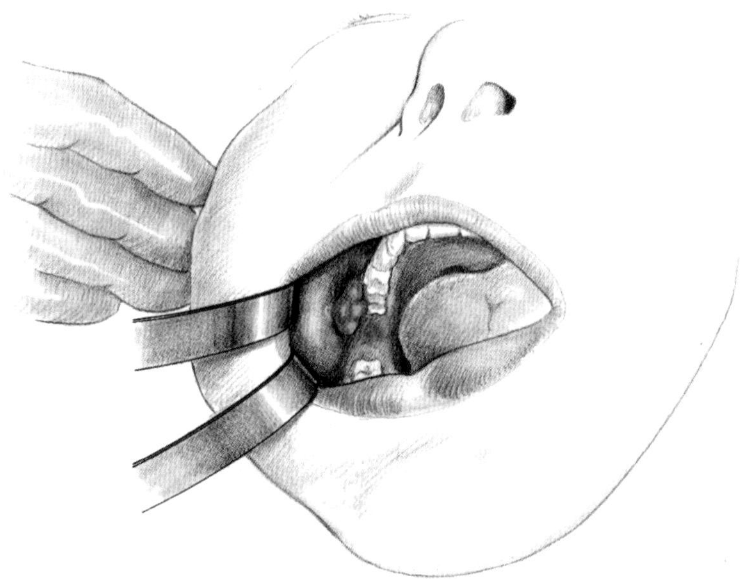

COLOR PLATE 123-5. The buccal fat pad is brought into the mouth by gentle external pressure. Only the fat that can be teased into the oral cavity is excised. Reaching into the wound with an instrument can cause injury to the buccal branches of the facial nerve or the facial vein. (From Pitman GH: Liposuction and Aesthetic Surgery. St. Louis, Quality Medical Publishing, 1993:144.)

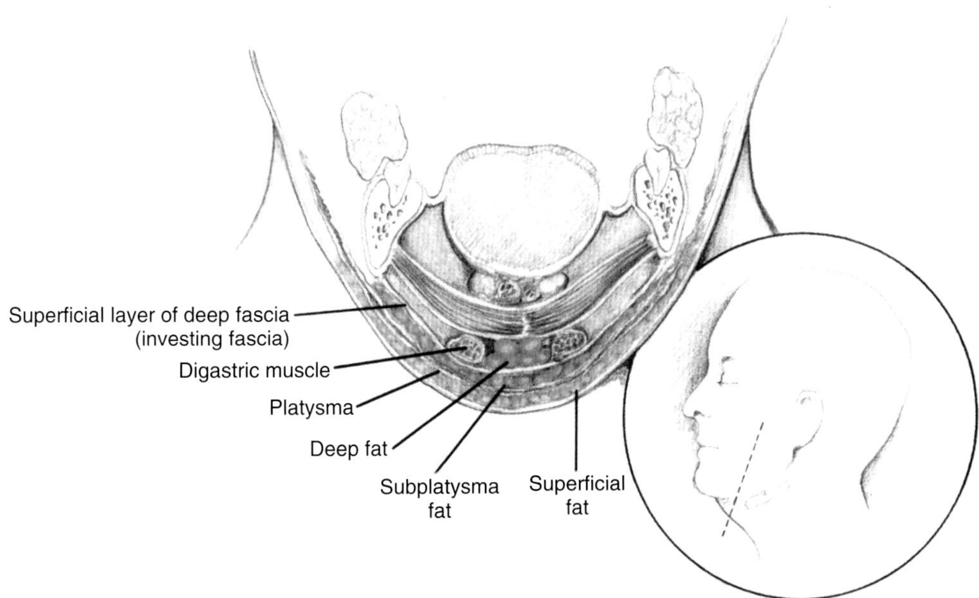

COLOR PLATE 123-6. Coronal section through the submental region showing fatty layers with relationships to the platysma and deep musculofascia. (From Pitman GH: Liposuction and Aesthetic Surgery. St. Louis, Quality Medical Publishing, 1993:116.)

CHAPTER

124

Body Contouring: Large-Volume Liposuction

JEFFREY M. KENKEL, MD, FACS ✦ ROD J. ROHRICH, MD, FACS

The incorporation of ultrasonic liposuction has allowed plastic surgeons to extend the role of liposuction. This technique is no longer limited to small or "spot" reductions. Larger, more circumferential reductions are now commonly performed, allowing greater lipoaspirates and enhanced contouring in patients previously not considered to be candidates for liposuction. As larger volumes are achieved, greater risks are encountered. It is therefore necessary for these procedures to be performed in a facility qualified to handle the associated fluid shifts and by a surgeon and anesthesiologist familiar not only with the surgical technique but also with the proper resuscitation of patients undergoing large-volume liposuction.

The American Society of Plastic Surgeons* defines large-volume liposuction as the removal of more than 5 liters of total aspirate in one setting. This arbitrary distinction between small-volume liposuction and large-volume liposuction has been made to help serve as a useful guide for the preoperative, operative, and postoperative management of the patient. Whereas many of the components of care for patients undergoing small-volume and large-volume liposuction are similar, greater attentiveness and experience are essential to ensure safe and optimal results with large-volume liposuction.

*http://www.plasticsurgery.org

SELECTION OF PATIENTS

Proper selection of patients is foremost in achieving optimal results after body contouring surgery or any other procedure. When patients are subjected to greater physiologic stress, as in a large-volume liposuction case, this becomes all the more important. First and most important is the establishment of good medical health. Patients with cardiopulmonary disease (especially a history of pulmonary problems), neurologic impairment, morbid obesity, insulin-dependent diabetes, history of deep venous thrombosis, or any other significant medical problems should not be considered for large-volume liposuction. In addition, patients with a personal or family history of thromboembolic disease or those taking either oral contraceptives or hormone replacement may be at increased risk for development of perioperative morbidity. Large-volume liposuction should be considered moderate surgical trauma; therefore, each patient must be able to handle the stress imposed from such a procedure.

CONSULTATION

Initially, the consultation establishes the reasons the patient has come to see the plastic surgeon. Open-ended questions allow the patient to voice concerns and help establish the patient's goals of surgery. A priority is given to those areas for which the patient has the most concern. This is useful, particularly in the patient being considered for large-volume liposuction, because staged procedures may be required. A thorough review of the patient's dietary habits and exercise regimen is conducted. Aside from the physical requirements, patients seeking large-volume liposuction must be properly motivated to undergo lifestyle changes that will allow them to achieve the best possible result. Whereas many patients can "commit" to surgery, it is the alteration of lifestyle that is often the greatest hurdle for them to overcome.

Diet: Patients have to commit to a *realistic* diet program so that a stable and reproducible weight may be achieved before surgery and maintained after surgery. This must not include the "fad" and "quick-fix" diets that so often lead to relapse. If it is necessary, patients are referred to appropriate counselors or bariatric physicians to help facilitate this.

Exercise: Equally important is establishing a goal-oriented exercise program that the patient will be able to maintain postoperatively. As with the diet, extreme programs must be avoided because they carry such high failure rates. A trainer may help establish a patient-specific program.

Lifestyle changes: Once proper diet and exercise programs have been established, the patient must commit to the lifestyle changes necessary to maintain these programs. The patient should be shown the "body contouring cycle" (Color Plate 124-1), which is helpful in visualizing what one must do to optimize results with liposuction.

How best to incorporate liposuction with these factors is often difficult to determine and is clearly patient specific. In general, patients who are able to maintain a stable weight and have incorporated diet, exercise, and lifestyle changes are considered for surgery if they are not morbidly obese. Surgery should not be the first step in enhancing body contour because it is likely to lead to failure or only temporary improvement. Some commitment by patients encourages them to invest in their own successful outcome. As a general rule, "jump starting" patients with surgery rarely stimulates radical changes in lifestyle or dietary habits and ultimately results in failure and unhappy patients.

Once the initial discussion is complete, a careful history is obtained; this includes a medical and surgical history, medications (prescription, herbal, and over-the-counter), allergies, and tobacco use. The use of prescription and over-the-counter weight loss medications and nonsteroidal anti-inflammatory drugs (Table 124-1) preoperatively can subject the patient to avoidable risks during surgery, and these should be discontinued at least 2 weeks before surgery. A preoperative evaluation by an internist or cardiologist is performed in select patients, especially if there is a concern about the patient's health issues or a history of cardiac or pulmonary problems.

Before examination, the operative and postoperative course is discussed at length with the patient. Specifically, the details of the operation including access sites, surgical technique, and postoperative course are reviewed. The patient is typically provided with a brochure before the visit so that he or she is somewhat familiar with the procedure. Potential risks and benefits are also discussed with the patient, specifically problems with fluid overload, deep venous thrombosis, pulmonary embolism, and even death. All questions and concerns are addressed and answered. The patient is then given privacy to change for the examination and is thoroughly examined with a chaperone in the room.

Height and weight are recorded routinely. This allows an assessment of the efficacy of the patient's lifestyle changes and provides for a comparison postoperatively. Because these patients do not require "spot" resections, they are assessed circumferentially. Examination of the patients seeking body contouring is done in four positions: posterior, anterior, and right and left lateral. Assessment of the trunk and extremities should not only include an evaluation for lipodystrophy but also assess for skin tone and quality, asymmetries, dimpling, and myofascial support. These components must be addressed particularly in this group of patients because they are often deficient or inadequate and may not be corrected by liposuction alone. Of note, competency of the abdominal wall can be difficult to evaluate in these patients. Any concern for herniation, particularly in patients with prior surgery and in men, should be further evaluated preoperatively with either an ultrasound examination or computed tomographic scan. Detailed evaluation in this area will help prevent potential intra-abdominal injury.

The examination is typically performed in front of a mirror, allowing the patient to visually appreciate the deformity. Areas to be treated as well as those to be avoided (Color Plate 124- 2) are reviewed with the patient. Zones of adherence are areas where contour irregularities occur more commonly and should be treated cautiously.

Standardized photography is performed.[1] Computerized imaging is offered to patients and encouraged. This typically occurs 2 to 3 weeks after the initial consultation. It is an invaluable tool to assist the physician in establishing realistic expectations, especially in the patient being considered for large-volume liposuction. The enhanced images will show not only the potential advantages of contouring but also limitations of the procedures, such as severe asymmetries or skin irregularities that will not be corrected. This second visit also provides the patient with the opportunity to ask the physician more questions directly.

Once the patient has been examined, a decision must be made as to whether the patient is a candidate for circumferential large-volume liposuction. Many of these patients may benefit from excisional surgery in

TABLE 124-1 ✦ MEDICATIONS TO BE AVOIDED BEFORE SURGERY

Patients should notify the physician if they are taking any vitamins, herbal medications, or natural supplements. These can also cause problems during surgery and should not be taken for the 2-week period before surgery.

Section 1

The following drugs either contain aspirin or have undesirable side effects that could cause abnormal bleeding and bruising. These drugs should be avoided for at least 2 weeks before surgery. Patients should be advised to take Tylenol for relief of minor pain.

APC
ASA
ASA Enseals
Advil
Aleve
Alka-Seltzer
Alka-Seltzer Plus
Anacin
Anaprox
Ansaid
Argesic
Arthritis Pain Formula
Arthritis Strength Bufferin
Arthropan liquid
Ascriptin (all types and brands)
Asperbuf
Aspergum
Aspirin (all types and brands)
Atromid
Axotal
BC tablets and powder
Backache Formula
Bayer Children's Cold Tablets
Buf-Tabs
Buff-A Comp
Bufferin (all formulas)
Buffets II
Buffinol
Butazolidin
Cama Arthritis Pain Reliever
Carisoprodol
Clinoril
Congespirin Chewable
Cope tablets
Damason-P
Darvon (all compounds)
Disalcid
Dolobid
Dolprin
Easprin
Ecotrin
Empirin with Codeine
Endep
Equagesic tablets
Etrafon
Excedrin
Feldene
Fiorinal
Fish oil
Flagyl
Four-Way Cold Tablets
Gemnisin
Ginseng (all types and brands)
Gleprin
Goody's
Ibuprofen
Indocin
Indomethacin
Lanorinal
Lioresal
Lortab
Magan
Magsal
Marnal
Marplan
Medomen
Methocarbamol with aspirin
Micrainin
Midol
Mobidin
Mobigesic
Momentum Muscular
Motrin
Nalfon
Naprosyn
Naproxen
Nardil
Nicobid
Norgesic
Norgesic Forte
Nuprin
Orudis
Pabalate-SF
Pamelor
Parnate
Pepto-Bismol (all types)
Percodan
Persantine
Phentermine
Phenylbutazone
Ponstel
Propoxyphene Compound
Robaxisal
Rufen
SAC
Saleto
Salocol
Sine-Aid, Sine-Off, Sinutab
SK-65 Compound
St. John's wort (all types)
St. Joseph Cold Tablets
Sulindac
Synalgos
Tagamet
Talwin Compound
Tenuate Dospan
Tolectin
Tolmetin
Toradol
Triaminicin
Trigesic
Trilisate tablets and liquids
Uracel
Vanquish
Verin
Vitamin C (>1000 mg/day)
Vitamin E (>600 mg/day)
Voltaren
ZORprin

Section 2

These drugs can have undesirable side effects that may affect anesthesia during surgery. Patients should inform the physician if they are taking any of the following medications.

Achromycin
Adapin
Amitriptyline HCL/MCL
Amoxapine
Anafranil
Asendin
Aventyl
Carbamazepine
Co-Tylenol
Comtrex
Desipramine HCL
Desyrel
Imipramine HCL
Isocarboxazid
Limbitrol
Ludiomil
Maprotiline HCL
Matulane
Medipren
Mysteclin-F
Norpramin
Nortriptyline HCL
Novahistine
Omade
Sinequan
Sumycin
Surmontil
Tetracycline
Tofranil
Tranylcypromine
Tri-Cyclen
Triavil
Trimipramine maleate
Vibramycin
Vivactil
Wellbutrin

Continued

TABLE 124-1 ✦ MEDICATIONS TO BE AVOIDED BEFORE SURGERY—cont'd

Dilantin	Perphenazine	Zoloft
Doxepin HCL	Phenelzine sulfate	Zomax
Elavil	Procarbazine HCL	Zovirax
Etrafon	Protriptyline HCL	
Flexeril	Prozac	

Section 3

The following foods contain salicylates, which affect blood clotting. Although these foods do not need to be omitted completely from a patient's diet, they should be kept to a minimum for 2 weeks before surgery.

Almonds	Grapes	Plums
Apricots	Grape juice	Prunes
Berries	Jellies and preserves	Raisins
Cherries	Nectarines	Tomatoes
Cucumbers	Oranges	Tomato products
Currants	Peaches	Vinegar
Curry	Pickles	Wine

combination with large-volume liposuction (Fig. 124-1).[2] The impact this procedure will have on the patient's recovery and proposed scarring must be reviewed. If necessary, planned stages are discussed. If the patient has poor skin tone with excessive skin, it is preferable to perform the excisional central body lift concomitantly with the liposuction. This includes the circumferential extended abdominoplasty with lateral thigh lift in conjunction with ultrasound-assisted liposuction (UAL) to mobilize the lateral flanks, back, and thighs. Total operative time is kept below a maximum of 6 hours at one procedure. Additional stages are performed at 3- to 6-month intervals.

INFORMED CONSENT

Informed consent is necessary to protect both the patient and the physician. The surgeon is required by law to provide sufficient information to the patient so that the patient is able to make an informed decision. This discussion details the proposed procedure, alternatives, potential complications and risks, and financial obligations and establishes the patient's understanding that future surgeries or revisions may need to be performed. The American Society of Plastic Surgeons provides a useful information guide to help ensure that an adequate and complete informed consent is obtained. An additional consent for the use of preoperative and postoperative photographs is also required.

PREOPERATIVE MARKING AND STRATEGY

Consistent and accurate marking is of paramount importance to achieve the proposed goals established between the physician and the patient during preoperative consultations. A four-position stance including anterior, posterior, and left and right lateral is used. Areas to be suctioned are marked with one color of ink; those areas to be avoided are marked differently (Fig. 124-2). These areas typically highlight symmetries, dimpling, indentations, and zones of adherence. Areas that may require autologous fat transfer can also be delineated. It is often helpful to mark the patients in front of a mirror so they can play a role in this important process. Once completed, the marks are reviewed and confirmed with the patient in front of the mirror.

Access incisions are also marked. In the past, access incisions were placed in well-concealed areas because of their excessive length; however, with newer techniques (smaller cannulas, smaller skin protectors), this has become less of a problem. It is unusual to make an incision longer than 5 mm. The sites should be chosen to facilitate treatment in multiple areas from a single site, if possible. An attempt should be made to make these incisions asymmetric or staggered to avoid a surgical appearance. It is important to review the proposed incision sites with the patient preoperatively. Ideal access sites may vary from patient to patient on the basis of fat distribution and areas to be treated.

OPERATIVE CONSIDERATIONS

Anesthesia

A thorough history and physical examination are of paramount importance in surgery of this magnitude. It is important to elicit any history of diet regimens that may have been deleterious to the patient's health. Patients with a history of weight loss medication use should be properly evaluated by their internist or cardiologist before surgery. Specific questions should be directed toward the use of herbal medications; many

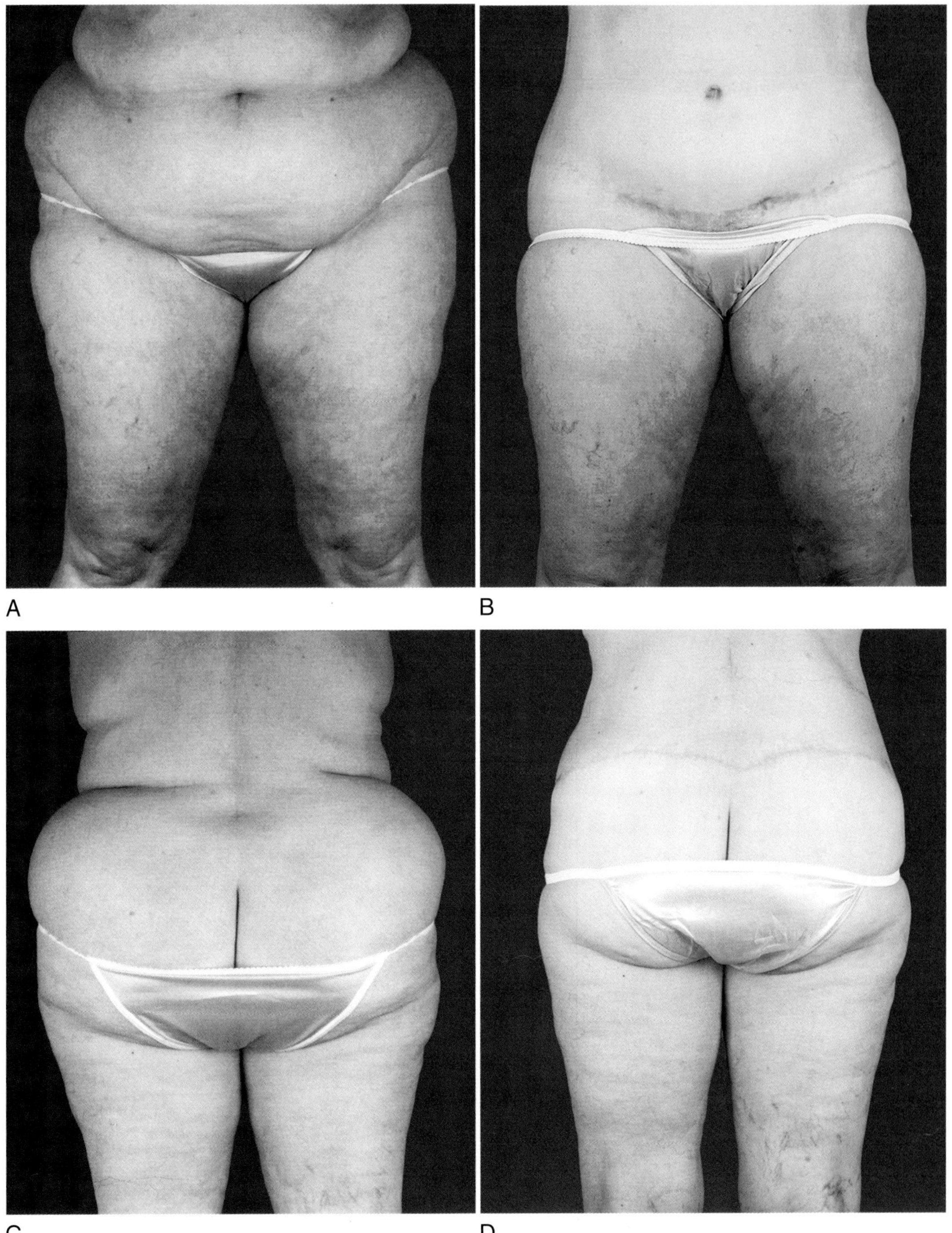

FIGURE 124-1. Example of excisional contouring with liposuction. *A, C,* and *E,* Preoperative views. *B, D,* and *F,* Postoperative views. *Continued*

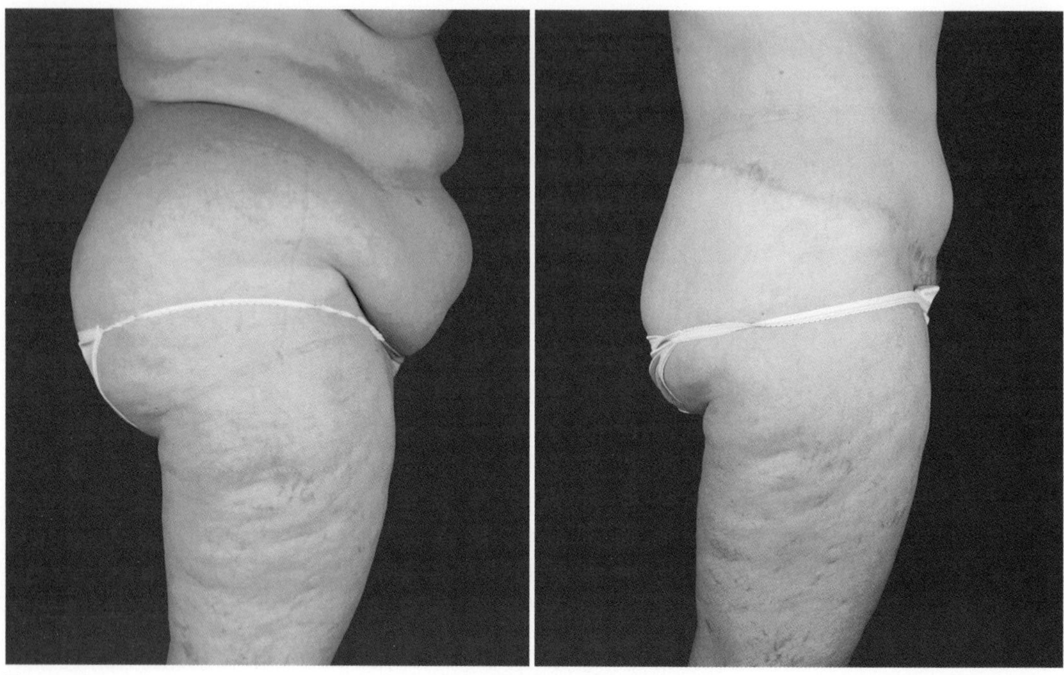

E F

FIGURE 124-1, cont'd.

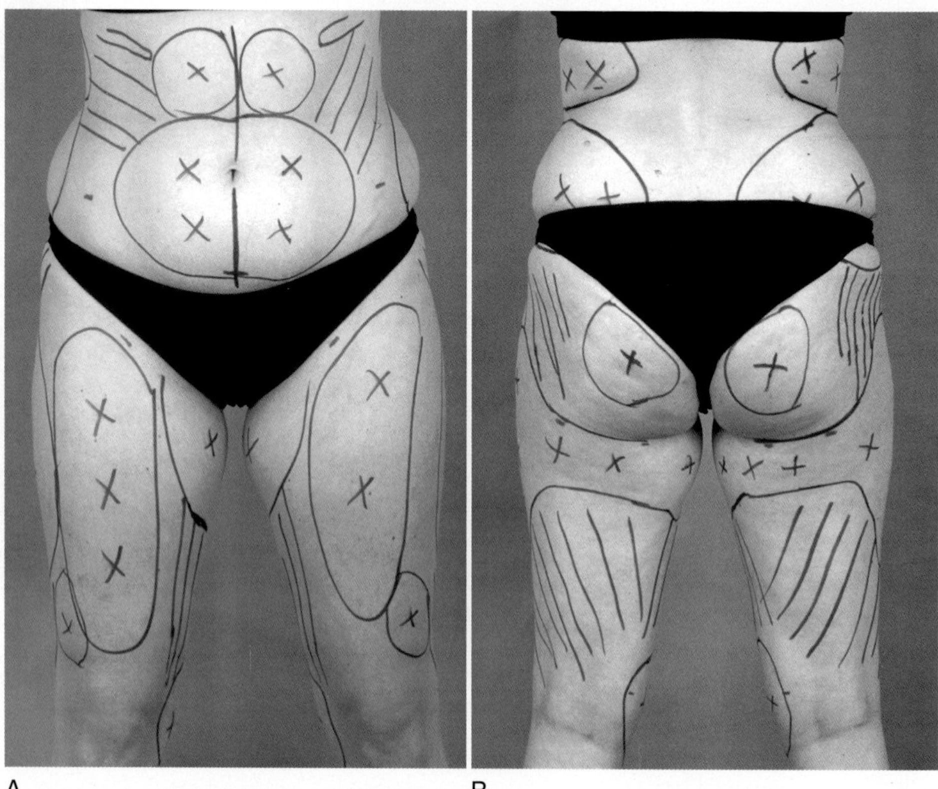

A B

FIGURE 124-2. Preoperative markings and access incisions. *A,* Anterior view. *B,* Posterior view. (From Rohrich RJ, Beran SJ, Kenkel JM: Ultrasound-Assisted Liposuction. St. Louis, Quality Medical Publishing, 1998:130.)

of these substances can negatively react with anesthesia. Most of these drugs should be stopped at least 2 weeks before surgery. Laboratory tests are not routinely obtained unless they are guided by specific findings in the examination. In the setting of large-volume liposuction, a hematocrit is useful because up to one third of premenopausal women do exhibit iron deficiency anemia. These patients benefit from preoperative treatment with iron by use of Niferex, which minimizes constipation versus an over-the-counter iron supplement.

Foot compression or calf compression devices are applied before induction of anesthesia to help prevent deep venous thrombosis. Foot compression devices may be preferable for contouring below the knee. A general anesthetic is routinely administered to ensure the patient's safety and comfort during large-volume liposuction. Hypothermia is common in patients undergoing large-volume liposuction because of the amount of exposed body surface area during the procedure. This is compounded by the vasodilatory effects of general anesthesia and the infiltration of room-temperature wetting solutions.[3] To maximize heat preservation, Bair Huggers should be used, especially in the head and neck areas. It is also advisable to use warmed intravenous solution and warm wetting solution in large-volume liposuction patients.

Hypothermia can result in prolonged bleeding and recovery. Forced air is effective in maintaining core body temperature in this group of patients. Euthermia can be sustained by use of forced air over the head and upper extremities during these procedures.

Positioning

Positioning of the patient ensures optimal surgical exposure, but care must be taken to avoid cardiopulmonary compromise or injury to peripheral nerves or bone prominences (Fig. 124-3). Inspiratory pressures should be less than 30 mm Hg. The prone and supine positions offer the most versatility for treatment, allowing comparison from one side to the other. While the patient is prone, a soft hip roll is placed beneath the iliac crests to elevate the treatment areas off the bed. The bed is typically jackknifed. Longitudinal rolls or pillows should be placed beneath the breasts, positioning them medially, to avoid postoperative discomfort. The arms are extended on padded arm boards parallel to the long axis of the table, ventral to the transverse axis of the shoulders. Appropriate protection of the face is of paramount importance. The cervical spine is placed in neutral position with the orbits protected. The prone position allows contouring of the arms, back, hips and flanks, lateral thighs, posterior thighs, and medial thighs. The remainder of the thigh and abdomen contouring is completed in the supine position.

Fluid Resuscitation

Several factors must be considered in the evaluation of perioperative fluid management: maintenance intravenous fluids, third-space losses, wetting solution, and total lipoaspirate.[4-6] A constant dialogue between the anesthesiologist and the surgeon ensures the safety of the patient and is facilitated by the use of a perioperative data sheet.[7] This data sheet optimally includes visual documentation with a standard graphic (Fig. 124-4) as well as more precise information, including measurements, wetting solution infused, amount of lipoaspirate, and varying techniques. It should be finalized immediately after the completion of surgery to ensure accuracy and serves as a complement to the standard operative note.

Because large-volume liposuction is considered "moderate" surgical trauma, the following resuscitative formula is used:

Replacement of losses from absence of oral intake preoperatively
Crystalloid replacement at 4 to 5 mL/kg per hour, adjusted according to vital signs and urine output

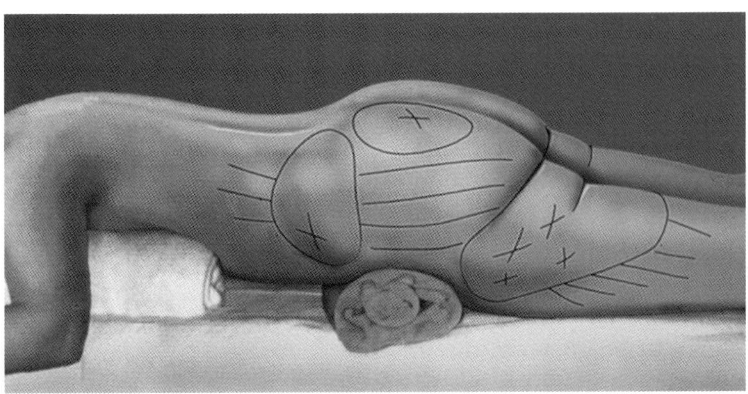

FIGURE 124-3. Proper padding in prone position. (From Rohrich RJ, Beran SJ, Kenkel JM: Ultrasound-Assisted Liposuction. St. Louis, Quality Medical Publishing, 1998:74.)

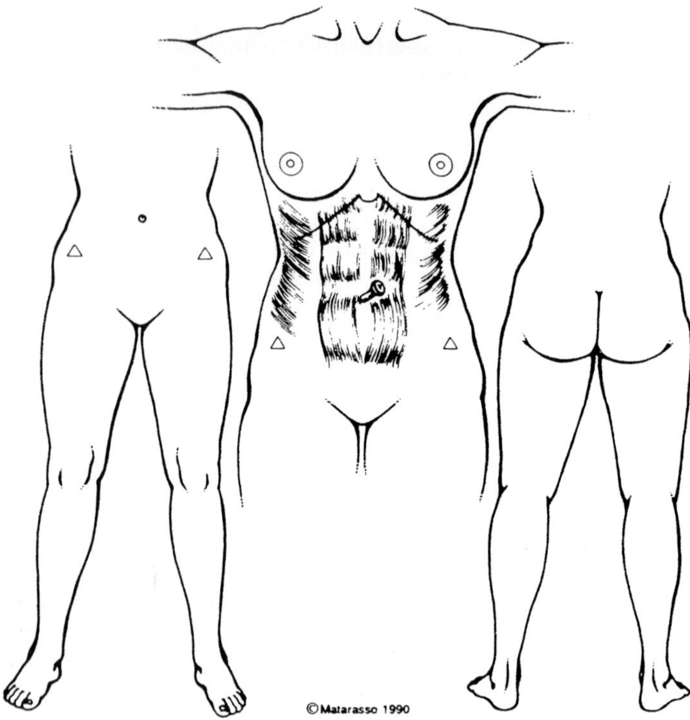

FIGURE 124-4. Standard anatomic drawing for liposuction perioperative data sheet. (Modified from Matarasso A: The anatomic data sheet in plastic surgery: graphic and accurate documentation for standardized evaluation of results. Plast Reconstr Surg 1993;91:734.)

Replacement of 0.25 mL of crystalloid for every milliliter aspirated above 5 liters
Superwet infiltration

Lidocaine is routinely used because its omission has resulted in increased postoperative pain in the authors' experience. The following formula is used for the incorporation of lidocaine in the wetting solution:

<5 L lipoaspirate: 30 mL of 1% lidocaine plain
>5 L lipoaspirate: 15 mL of 1% lidocaine plain

For hemostasis and to prolong the absorption of lidocaine from the subcutaneous space, 1 mL of epinephrine 1 : 1000 is used per liter of wetting solution.

Infiltration

Seventy percent to 80% of body contouring with liposuction can be performed in the prone position. The lateral decubitus position is not preferred because it does not allow comparison of the contralateral side or easy access to the posterior medial thigh. Positioning is as described in the previous section. Once access incisions are determined, infiltration begins.[8] Initially, a 3-mm stab incision is made with a No. 11 blade scalpel. Room-temperature wetting solution is then infiltrated uniformly in the intermediate layer of fat. This is recorded in the perioperative data sheet.

The specific number of treatment areas to be infiltrated at a time is a function of the patient's size and the surgeon's experience. Because the wet environment is so important in ultrasonic liposuction, it is beneficial to treat an area before a significant amount of time elapses between infiltration and UAL. As a general rule, any area that cannot be treated within 30 minutes should be infiltrated later. For example, if it takes 30 minutes to treat arms and hips, the thighs should not be infiltrated. Once UAL and evacuation are completed in the initial areas, the next areas to be treated can be infiltrated.

Ultrasound-Assisted Liposuction[9-12]

After infiltration, the access incision is enlarged to 3 to 5 mm to accommodate a skin protector. Alternatively, it may be enlarged to 4 mm if continuous irrigation is to be used. A wet towel should always be used to protect the skin from thermal injury. Cannula or probe type and tip configuration are specific to each surgeon and beyond the scope of this chapter. With experience, the solid probe becomes more attractive because it is more efficient. Energy application begins from superficial to deep in a parallel, radial manner (Fig. 124-5). Once resistance is lost in a specific plane, a deeper one is approached and treated until a region of resistance is once again lost (Table 124-2).

Most areas have two or three planes that are treated. Stroke rate is similar to that of traditional

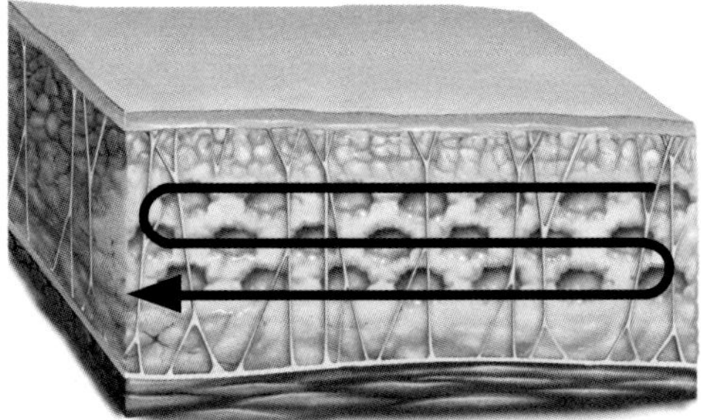

FIGURE 124-5. Ultrasound treatment begins superficially and proceeds to the deeper plane. (From Rohrich RJ, Beran SJ, Kenkel JM: Ultrasound-Assisted Liposuction. St. Louis, Quality Medical Publishing, 1998:139.)

liposuction. The nondominant hand helps guide the cannula tip, providing feedback as to its location. Superficial application of energy is reserved for those patients exhibiting superficial skin irregularities. This is done at lower amplitudes (<30%). Superficial UAL should be performed only with a blunt probe or cannula with the aspiration off.

The most important endpoint for UAL is the loss of tissue resistance. This is appreciated when the cannula or probe easily passes through the tissues. At this point, treatment will stop or the probe will be placed in a different plane. If a cannula is being used with continuous aspiration, more blood-tinged emollient may be seen in addition to the loss of resistance. Useful secondary endpoints are site-specific treatment time and volume (Table 124-3).

UAL of the arms is performed in the prone position. Access is through an incision on the radial aspect of the elbow. If necessary, a second incision can be made along the posterior axillary fold, more proximally (Fig. 124-6). However, this incision may widen and is more noticeable and should be reserved for patients with more extensive proximal lipodystrophy. Energy is applied along the posterior aspect of the arm, staying in an intermediate plane. UAL should be avoided along the ulnar aspect of the arm to prevent injury to the ulnar nerve. Contouring here should be performed with suction-assisted liposuction cannulas.

TABLE 124-2 ✦ ENDPOINTS OF ULTRASOUND-ASSISTED AND SUCTION-ASSISTED LIPOSUCTION

Endpoint	Ultrasound-Assisted Liposuction	Suction-Assisted Liposuction
Primary	Loss of tissue resistance	Final contour
	Blood in aspirate	Symmetric pinch test results
Secondary	Treatment time	Treatment time
	Treatment volume	Treatment volume

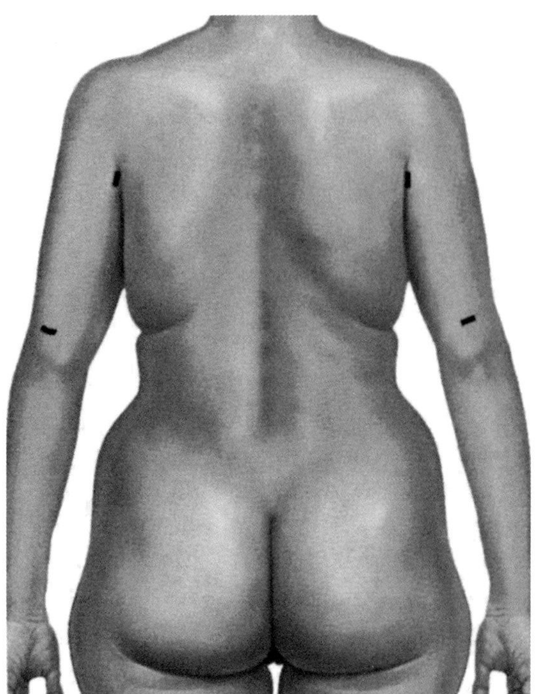

FIGURE 124-6. Access incisions for arms. (From Rohrich RJ, Beran SJ, Kenkel JM: Ultrasound-Assisted Liposuction. St. Louis, Quality Medical Publishing, 1998:246.)

TABLE 124-3 ✦ PREFERRED PLACEMENT OF ACCESS INCISIONS FOR ULTRASOUND-ASSISTED LIPOSUCTION

Anatomic Area	Access Site
Breast (male)	Lateral inframammary fold
Lateral back	Lateral bra line
Vertical back	Midline
Flank-hip	Lateral gluteal fold, lateral lower hip-flank
Abdomen	Lateral lower abdomen, suprapubic region, umbilicus
Buttock	Lateral gluteal fold, hip-flank
Lateral thigh	Lateral gluteal fold
Posterior thigh	Lateral gluteal fold
Medial thigh	Medial gluteal crease (posterior)
Anterior thigh	Inguinal crease
Upper arm	Posterior radial proximal humerus (prone)
	Distal radial humerus (supine)

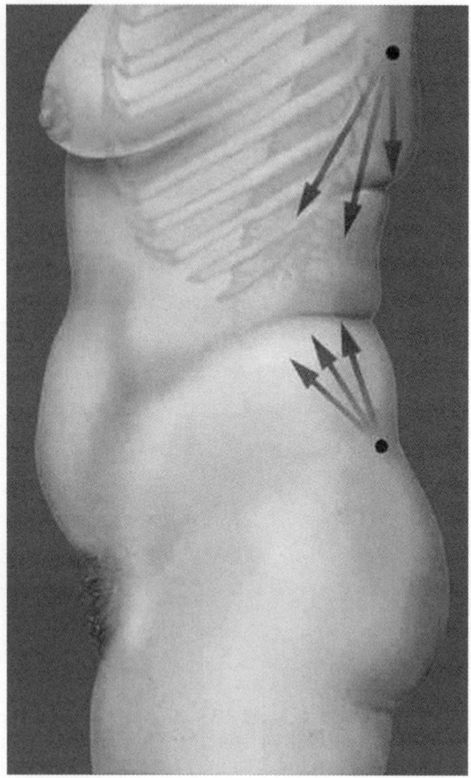

FIGURE 124-7. Concave areas should be treated from adjacent convexities. (From Rohrich RJ, Beran SJ, Kenkel JM: Ultrasound-Assisted Liposuction. St. Louis, Quality Medical Publishing, 1998:237.)

Access incisions for the back are placed either in the midline, if the fat is more posteriorly located, or in a paraspinous position to help facilitate more lateral contouring. It is useful to place these in the bra or bathing suit line to help conceal the scars. If multiple back rolls exist, it is imperative to choose sites that will adequately break each inherent roll. For these patients, upper and lower incisions may be required. Treatment of the upper back from the lower back access incisions should be done with great caution because intrathoracic penetration may occur when convex areas are treated from adjacent concavities (Fig. 124-7). It is important for patients to realize that back scars, in particular, may widen postoperatively. Thus, it is essential to place these incisions in areas that will be concealed by clothing. The placement of a deep dermal suture will decrease skin tension and diminish the risk for widening.

Treatment of the hip roll in women or the flank in men may be accomplished through several different access sites. Classically, two lateral paraspinous incisions have been used that are easily concealed by undergarments or bathing suits. These incisions may be moved more laterally in the man with generous flanks extending more laterally. In women, with more posteriorly oriented fat deposits, a single midline incision may suffice in combination with the lateral gluteal fold access incision. This truly is a utilitarian access site for treatment of the hip and flank, buttock, lateral thigh, posterior thigh, and medial thigh. This site in combination with a single, midline access site allows nice contouring and avoids incisions overlying the buttock area, which have a tendency to dimple. Caution must be used to avoid overzealous resection through the trochanteric adherent zone. In general, the hip-flank region is fairly forgiving and a good place to introduce oneself to UAL (Fig. 124-8).

UAL of the thigh is accomplished through the lateral gluteal site. This allows excellent access to the lateral thigh, the posterior thigh roll, and the medial thigh. A second, more medial incision in the fold may be made in patients with prominent lipodystrophy in the

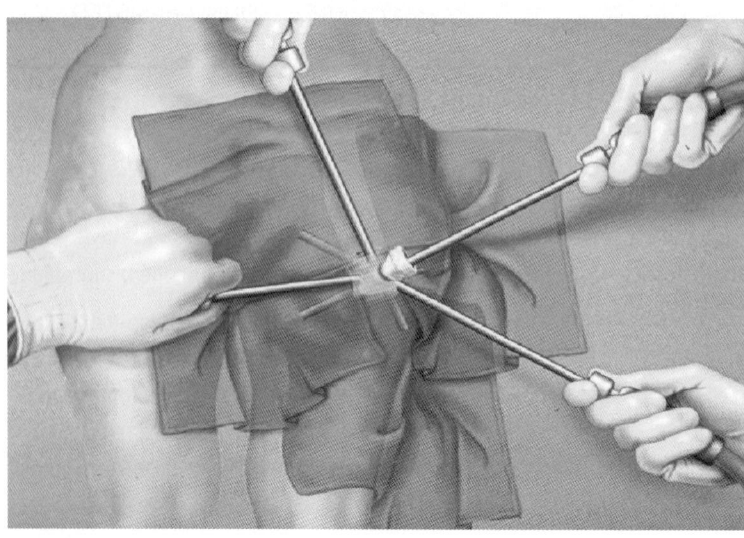

FIGURE 124-8. Gluteal fold access incision. (From Rohrich RJ, Beran SJ, Kenkel JM: Ultrasound-Assisted Liposuction. St. Louis, Quality Medical Publishing, 1998:222.)

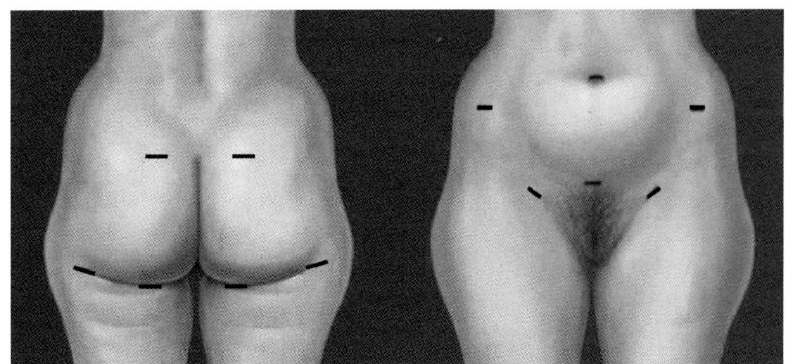

FIGURE 124-9. Extremity access incisions. (From Rohrich RJ, Beran SJ, Kenkel JM: Ultrasound-Assisted Liposuction. St. Louis, Quality Medical Publishing, 1998:221.)

medial thigh region. This additional site is well concealed within the fold and can be used liberally (Fig. 124-9). These access sites allow treatment of the proximal posterior thigh as well. One should be careful not to treat through the gluteal fold adherent zone. Overtreatment may result in buttock ptosis and a poorly defined lower buttock.

In the supine position, UAL on the anterior and medial thigh may be performed through a single incision in the inguinal crease. UAL is not typically done on the knees, which respond nicely to traditional methods. Jackknifing the table will help lower the iliac crests and the pubic bone, which can impede excursion of the operator's hand and the handpiece during treatment of the thighs and abdomen. Treatment of the abdomen is accomplished through a suprapubic incision and umbilical incision. This will allow treatment of the lower and upper abdomen. In larger patients with longer torsos (typically men), bilateral incisions above the anterior spine of the iliac crest will provide adequate access to the entire abdomen and allow continuation of the circumferential contouring begun in the prone position. These access sites are concealed by truncal hair in many male patients. Caution should be used in patients with prominent costal margins. These patients may require an incision at the lower costal margin or inframammary fold for treatment of the epigastrium. Inadvertent fascial perforation can occur when convex areas are treated from adjacent concave areas.

Evacuation and Final Contouring

Once UAL endpoints have been achieved, evacuation can begin (Fig. 124-10). In contrast to SAL, evacuation begins in the deepest layer and works superficially, with gradually decreasing cannula size. This technique allows removal of the emulsified fat, which tends to settle in the deepest plane. In areas where deep fat is removed, a 4.6-mm cannula is used initially for evacuation followed by 3.7- and 3.0-mm cannulas for final contouring. In more superficial areas, evacuation is begun with a 3.7-mm cannula. Contour can then be assessed. Primary endpoints after evacuation are those parameters most are accustomed to use with traditional liposuction. Contour, pinch test, and roll test are all useful for assessment of final shape. Persistent asymmetries or deformities can be addressed with further liposuction or fat injection.

Before skin closure, manual massage is performed to facilitate removal of any remaining fluid within the subcutaneous space. This may also further refine minor irregularities that may persist. Wounds are closed. Very rarely is a drain required in any region treated. The only exception may be in very large male patients in whom abdominal lipoaspirates exceed 2 liters. A nonadherent foam dressing is placed over the areas treated, and the patient is placed in a compression garment.

CONCLUSION

Large-volume liposuction is a safe and effective treatment for patients seeking circumferential contouring changes rather than spot reductions (Figs. 124-11 to 124-13). Establishment of realistic expectations helps the patient understand the limitations of large-volume liposuction. Proper selection of patients is of paramount importance because this technique results in

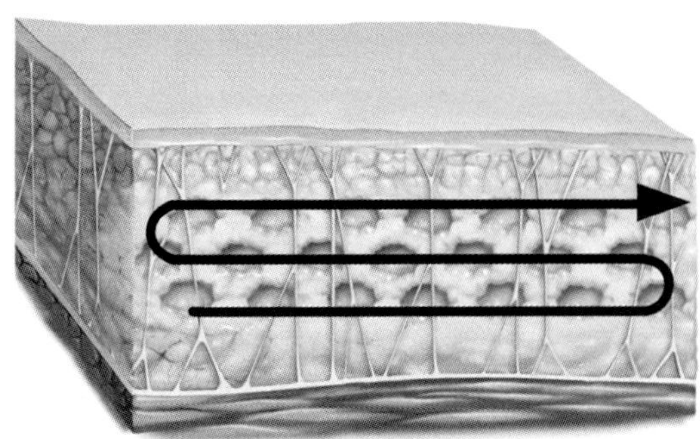

FIGURE 124-10. Evacuation begins in the deep plane and proceeds more superficially.

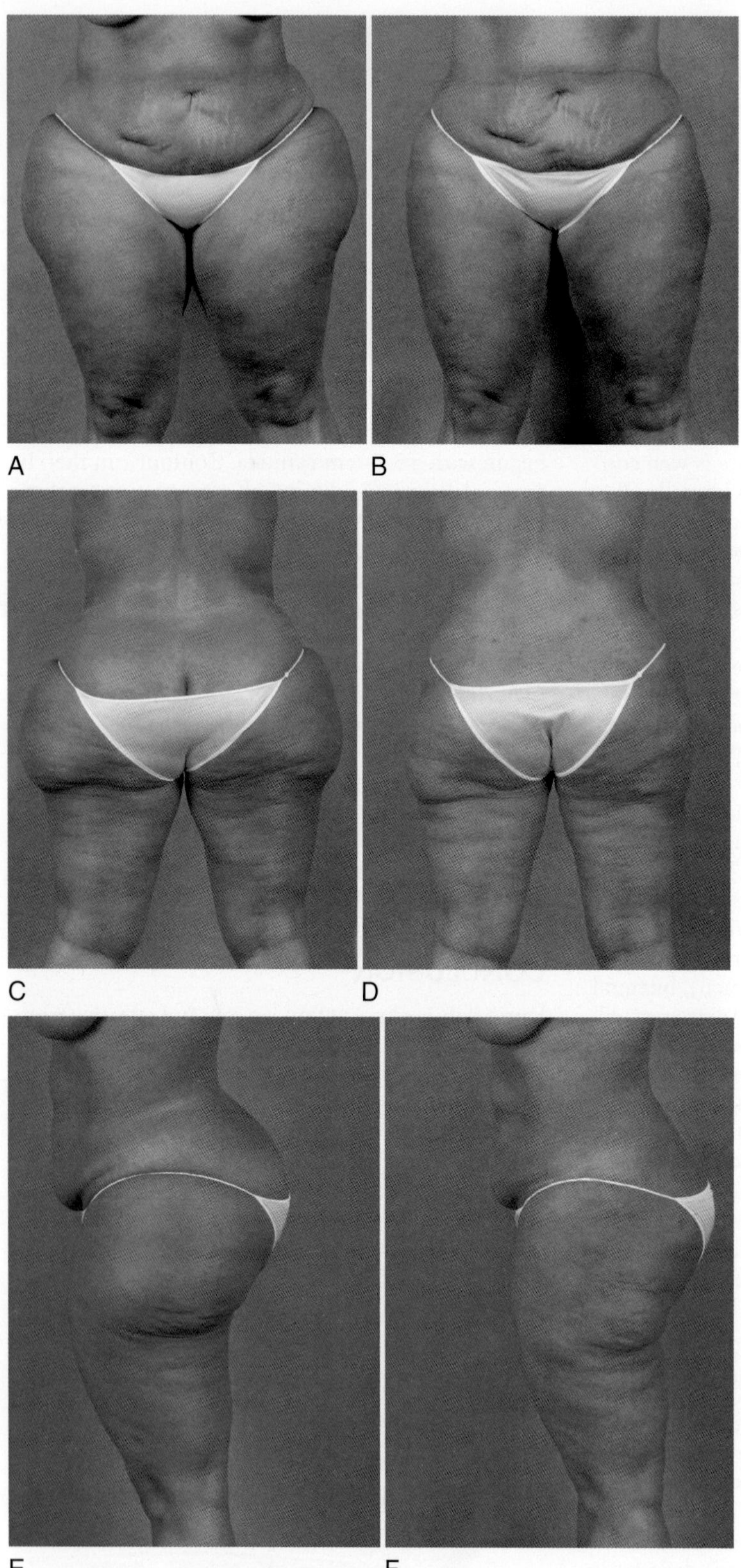

FIGURE 124-11. *A, C,* and *E,* Preoperative views of patient. *B, D,* and *F,* Patient seen 8 months postoperatively. Wetting solution infused, 12,500 mL; lipoaspirate, 15,500 mL. (From Rohrich RJ, Beran SJ, Kenkel JM: Ultrasound-Assisted Liposuction. St. Louis, Quality Medical Publishing, 1998:258.)

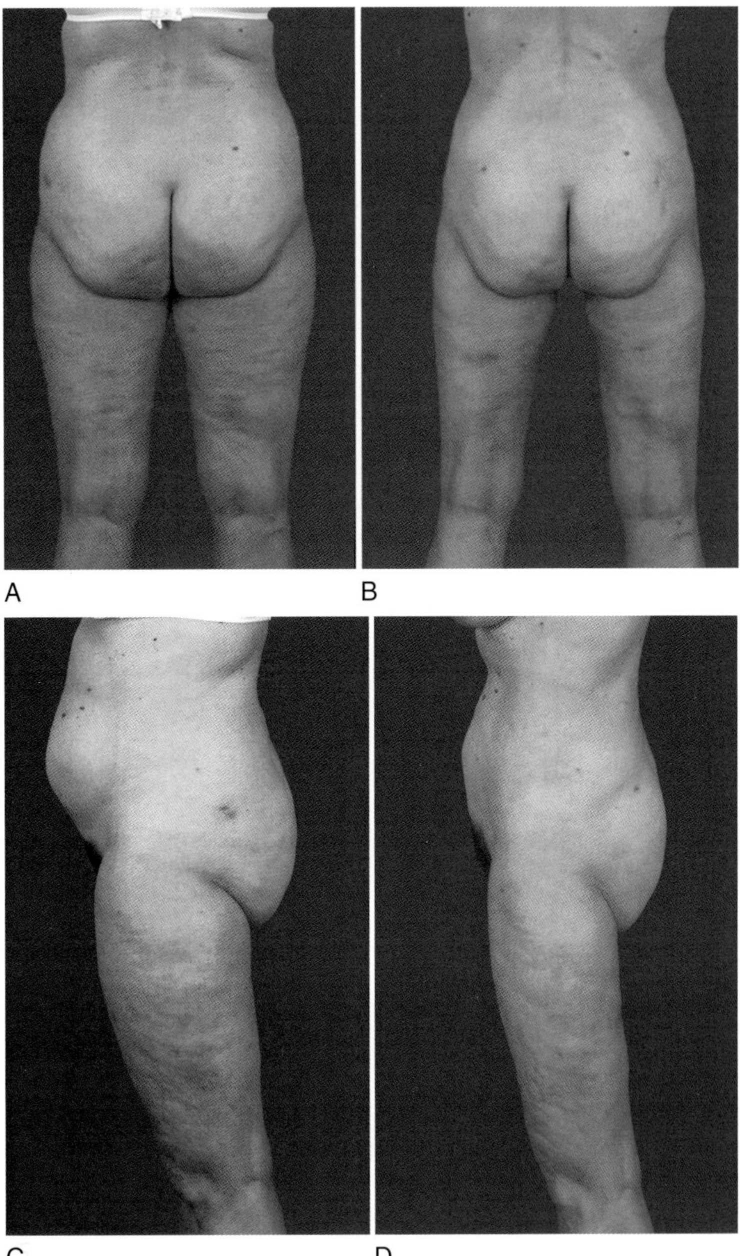

FIGURE 124-12. *A* and *C,* Preoperative views of patient. *B* and *D,* Patient seen 8 months postoperatively. Wetting solution infused, 7150 mL; lipoaspirate, 8390 mL.

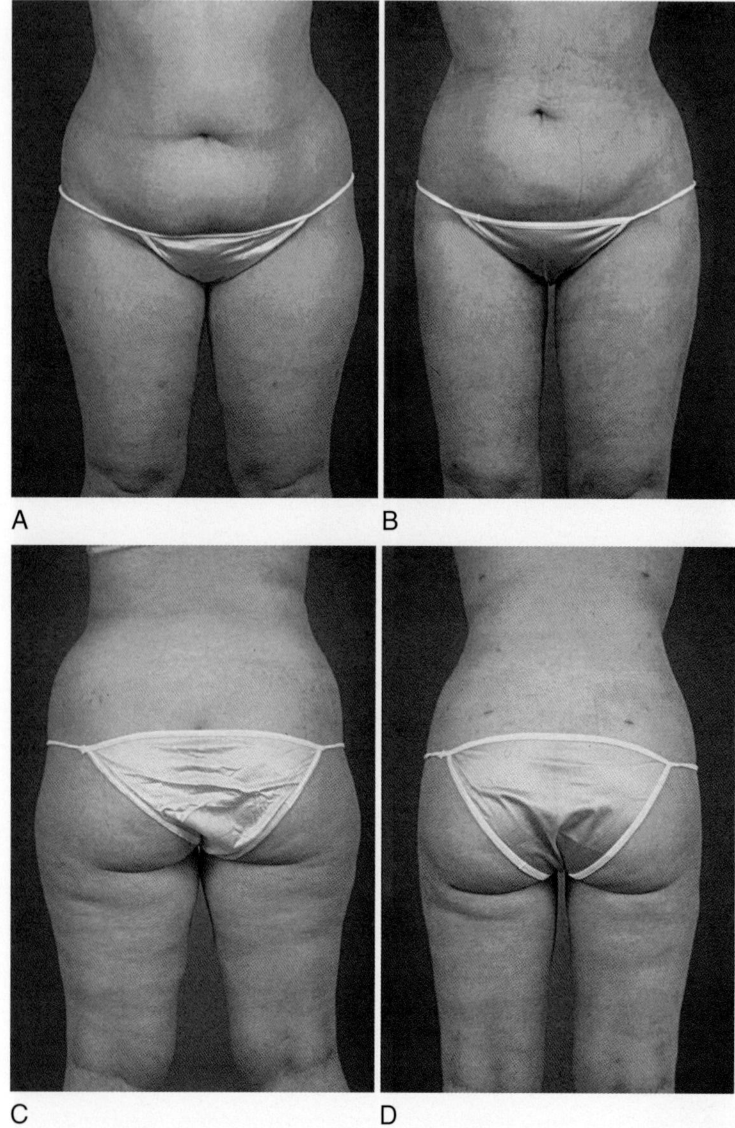

FIGURE 124-13. *A* and *C*, Preoperative views of patient. *B* and *D*, Patient seen 3 months postoperatively. Wetting solution infused, 8500 mL; lipoaspirate, 10,125 mL. (From Rohrich RJ, Beran SJ, Kenkel JM: Ultrasound-Assisted Liposuction. St. Louis, Quality Medical Publishing, 1998:187.)

moderate surgical trauma. Continuous communication during the surgery with the anesthesiologist, proper monitoring of vital signs, and use of a perioperative data sheet will help ensure appropriate resuscitation. After surgery, the patients should be monitored in an overnight facility. A skilled and experienced team including the plastic surgeon, anesthesiologist, ancillary nursing staff, and office personnel will help ensure the patient's safety and a favorable outcome.

REFERENCES

1. Smith H: Photographic standards. In Rohrich RJ, Beran SJ, Kenkel JM: Ultrasound-Assisted Liposuction. St. Louis, Quality Medical Publishing, 1998:100-114.
2. Lockwood T: The role of excisional lifting in body contour surgery. Clin Plast Surg 1996;23:695.
3. Ablaza BJ, Gingrass MK, Perry LC, et al: Tissue temperatures during ultrasound assisted lipoplasty. Plast Reconstr Surg 1998;102:534.
4. Burk RW, Stein G, Vasconez LO: Lidocaine and epinephrine levels in tumescent liposuction. Plast Reconstr Surg 1996;97:1379.
5. Knize DM, Pepper G: Does the tumescent technique require tumescence? Aesthetic Surg Q 1996;16:59.
6. Trott SA, Beran SJ, Rohrich RJ, et al: Safety considerations and fluid resuscitation in liposuction: an analysis of 53 consecutive patients. Plast Reconstr Surg 1998;102:2220.
7. Matarasso A: The anatomic data sheet in plastic surgery: graphic and accurate documentation for standardized evaluation of results. Plast Reconstr Surg 1993;91:734.
8. Rohrich RJ, Beran SJ, Fodor PB: The role of subcutaneous infiltration in suction-assisted lipoplasty: a review. Plast Reconstr Surg 1998;99:514.

9. Maxwell GP, Gingrass MK: Ultrasound-assisted lipoplasty: a clinical study of 250 consecutive patients. Plast Reconstr Surg 1998;101:189.
10. Rohrich RJ, Beran SJ, Kenkel JM, et al: Extending the role of liposuction in body contouring with ultrasound-assisted liposuction. Plast Reconstr Surg 1998;101:1090.
11. Rohrich RJ, Beran SJ, Kenkel JM: Ultrasound-Assisted Liposuction. St. Louis, Quality Medical Publishing, 1998.
12. Zocchi ML: Ultrasound-assisted lipoplasty: technical refinements and clinical evaluations. Clin Plast Surg 1996;23:575.

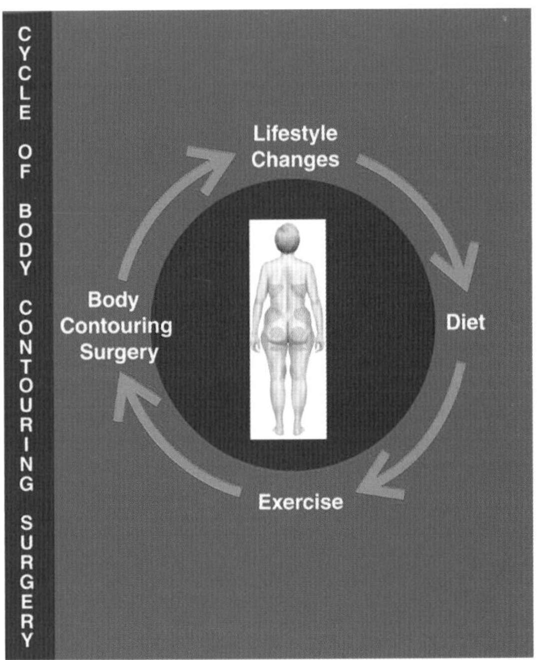

COLOR PLATE 124-1. Components to improve contour.

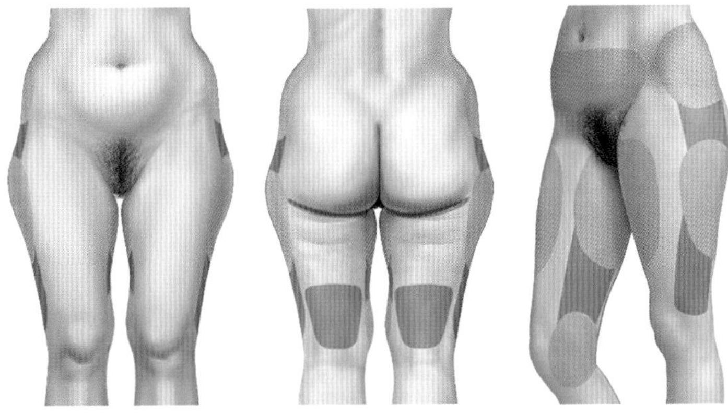

COLOR PLATE 124-2. Zones of adherence. (From Rohrich RJ, Beran SJ, Kenkel JM: Ultrasound-Assisted Liposuction. St. Louis, Quality Medical Publishing, 1998: 125.) = en rouge

CHAPTER

125

Body Contouring: Trunk and Thigh Lifts

TED E. LOCKWOOD, MD, FACS†

THE AESTHETIC DEFORMITY

Aesthetic concerns about trunk and thigh contours are frequent for both women and men. In the past 2 decades, liposuction has revolutionized the treatment of aesthetic contour deformities of the body to the extent that it is now synonymous with body contour surgery. However, liposuction deals with only one element of body aesthetics. Whereas excess fat deposits are the major component of body contour problems, skin laxity and skin contour irregularities (cellulite) are also significant problems for many patients. In addition, rectus muscle diastasis in both women and men may play a role in the aesthetic deformity.

EVALUATION OF THE PATIENT

Consultation

The ultimate success of body contour surgery depends as much on the accuracy of the initial assessment of the patient as it does on the technical expertise of the surgeon. Too often, we immediately categorize a prospective body contour patient by the surgical procedures that might be possible or that are requested by the patient rather than on the basis of careful study of the proportions and aesthetics of the patient's body.

Aesthetic body contour deformities frequently involve multiple areas of the trunk and thighs. The circumferential aesthetic unit of the trunk and thighs extends from the breasts to the knees. Surgery on one part of the aesthetic unit without consideration of its effect on the overall aesthetic balance of the body can lead to mediocre results and an imbalance in body contours. For example, for patients who have aesthetic deformities of both the trunk and thighs, dramatic sculpturing of the trunk aesthetic unit may make the patient appear to have much larger thighs, leading to an imbalance of the trunk-thigh aesthetic unit.

Dealing with the myriad variations of aesthetic body deformities is not only challenging; for many aesthetic surgeons, it may also be the most difficult area in which to obtain consistently superior results. The distances are long, the surface areas are large, and the body aesthetic deformities are extremely varied. Each patient requires a careful artistic analysis of the entire circumferential body for an appropriate and individualized surgical design to be produced.

As the patient's advocate regarding possible body contour surgery, the surgeon must listen carefully to requests of the patient but must also teach the patient about body aesthetics. Patients are often not totally objective about their appearance and usually do not understand the interactions or relationships of various aspects of the body aesthetic. Just as patients requesting a neck lift without a face lift must be warned about producing an aesthetic imbalance, we must also teach patients about the desirability of viewing and treating all aspects of the circumferential trunk and thigh

†Deceased.

TABLE 125-1 ✦ AREAS OF THE MEDICAL HISTORY THAT SHOULD BE EXPLORED

History of generalized or localized obesity, especially in childhood, teenage years, or early adulthood
History of yo-yo dieting, starvation dieting, or dramatic weight loss
History of pregnancies, both the number and the degree of abdominal distention with pregnancies
Skin tone of patient and family members, including early onset of skin laxity and appearance and distribution of striae of the trunk and thighs
History of previous surgery of the trunk and thighs, including liposuction or other body contour surgery, intra-abdominal surgery, or genital surgery
Degree of chronic sun exposure and plans for future sunbathing
History of the patient's aesthetic deformity: when did it start? familial patterns? is it progressive or stable?

aesthetic unit to avoid disproportion of the body contour. Lateral and posterior truncal deformities are commonly associated with abdominal deformities. Abdominoplasty without treatment of other truncal contour deformities will lead to aesthetic disharmony of the body aesthetic unit.

As in all aesthetic surgical consultations, thorough evaluation of the patient's goals, motivations, expectations, and overall medical and psychological status is performed. Specific areas of a patient's medical history that relate to diet, skin tone, previous surgery, and the particular deformity should be explored (Table 125-1). Although specific goals of the patient cannot be developed until after the physical examination and explanation of possible treatment options, general goals can be discussed in the initial interview. Does the patient want to be able to wear a skimpy bikini or just to look better in clothes? Is the patient primarily concerned with fat deposits, skin laxity (including stretch marks), or both fat and skin problems?

A discussion of both short-term goals and long-term goals is important in designing an individualized treatment plan for each patient. Planned weight loss, future pregnancies, desirable lifestyle changes, athletic pursuits, new professional directions, and interpersonal relationships may be factors to consider before body contouring surgery.

Physical Examination

The examination of the female patient should be performed in a warm, well-lit examination room with a supportive, friendly female assistant. The patient is provided an attractive cloth examination gown and is initially instructed to remove all clothing except for lingerie. The examination begins in the standing position in front of a full-length mirror so the patient can follow the examiner's evaluation. Sketching the findings of the examination on line drawings of the human figure is helpful.

Assess the body as a whole before focusing on the aesthetic units. Note overall obesity or lack of it and significant disproportion of the body. The patient should be asked about her aesthetic deformity, what her primary concerns are, and what her secondary concerns are.

The location and size of localized fat deposits of the trunk and thighs are noted. The thickness and elasticity of the skin, the extent and location of cellulite and striae, and the degree and pattern of flaccidity of the skin-subcutaneous tissue unit are observed. In examining patients for laxity of the skin and subcutaneous tissue, we should not only observe the degree of actual laxity but also estimate the degree of potential laxity that would occur if liposuction alone were used to treat the aesthetic deformity. The extent of rectus muscle diastasis and of total musculofascial wall decompensation is determined. Hernial defects and abdominal scars are documented.

Before photography, the patient is weighed without clothes for future reference. The patient should understand that if weight is gained after any body contouring surgery, the contour results could change from the expected postoperative appearance. The patient is responsible for maintaining body weight at an acceptable level.

Photographic Documentation

Documentation of skin quality photographically is particularly challenging but essential in body contour surgery. The most common long-term aesthetic complication of liposuction is skin laxity with surface contour irregularities (cellulite), resulting in an acceleration of the aged appearance of the skin. In body lifts requiring long incisions, an accurate documentation of the degree of skin laxity problems and their improvement postoperatively is necessary to justify long incisional scars.

Several photographic tips have been found helpful. In addition to nude photographs, photograph the patient with the same dark bikini underwear before and after surgery to compress the soft, loose fat and skin, producing "bikini overhang." Use a moderate to dark background with overhead lighting without flash (ASA 400 Ektachrome). Replace fluorescent bulbs with Spectralite bulbs for natural colors. Available-light photography most accurately demonstrates subtleties of skin contour irregularities, whereas flash techniques "fill the shadows," losing surface detail. In addition, avoid light-colored backgrounds and bikinis; the backlighting effect produces loss of surface detail.

SELECTION OF PATIENTS

Appropriate selection of patients is essential to limit unfavorable results. Although liposuction and body lifts are both useful in body contour surgery, the indications for surgery are not the same. Liposuction treats localized fat deposits; lifts treat skin quality problems. It is important to dispel the myth that "liposuction tightens skin." Liposuction does not tighten or lift relaxed skin and fat, but it does allow youthful and elastic skin to retract and conform to smaller contours. This is true for both traditional small-cannula liposuction and ultrasonically assisted liposuction. In patients with flaccid skin, attempts to use liposuction to gain maximum skin retraction often result in significant and permanent skin contour irregularities.

Likewise, excisional lifts should not be used as the primary treatment for localized fat deposits. Because many patients have fat deposit and actual or potential skin laxity problems, body lifts and liposuction can be combined in one or multiple surgical procedures.

Because surgical complication rates are higher for body lifts than for moderate-volume liposuction, patients selected for excisional surgery should have moderate to severe laxity problems and should be well informed of the potential risk for complications and unfavorable results. To reduce the risk of unfavorable results, avoid patients on any form of nicotine and patients with generalized obesity or other medical problems (cardiovascular, respiratory, history of deep venous thrombosis).

OPERATIONS

Indications

Excisional lifts are designed to treat skin quality problems of the aesthetic body contour deformity. Laxity of skin and cellulite will occur in all women with the normal aging process. In the last decade, significant progress has occurred in the understanding of aged aesthetic body deformities, allowing new body lift designs based on modern surgical principles.[1-8] Body lifts are a useful adjunct to liposuction and should be considered when an overall surgical plan is developed for an individual patient. Clear indications for trunk and thigh lifts include skin laxity without significant fat deposits, excessive skin laxity and cellulite, patients in whom skin tightening is the primary goal, aged medial thigh deformities, and significant buttock ptosis.

Lifts may be used at the time of initial liposuction or may be required to treat skin laxity and contour irregularities that appear after liposuction. Patients should be aware of the limitations of liposuction and that subsequent body lifting may be required to gain optimal body contours. This discussion before initial liposuction helps the patient understand that skin tone is the primary determinant of the aesthetic success or failure of liposuction even with the best liposuction technique. Patients who understand this principle rarely have unrealistic expectations about the results of liposuction and are reasonably prepared to consider body lifts in the future if needed.

The excisional lifts presented in this chapter are based on a careful analysis of youthful aesthetic anatomy as well as both youthful and aged body aesthetic deformities. These body lifts have proved to be effective and long-lasting with low risk of significant complications.

Treatment Strategies

Aesthetic body contour deformities frequently involve multiple areas of the trunk and thighs. In these patients, the ideal surgical plan targets the entire circumferential trunk and thigh aesthetic unit in one or several stages.[4,9] With the development of the lateral tension abdominoplasty concept,[5] it has become increasingly clear that the abdomen is the cornerstone of the trunk-thigh aesthetic unit. Relaxation of the abdomen is usually associated with relaxation of the waist, groin, pubis, and upper thighs. A side effect of this relaxation is the mature relaxed posturing caused by the aged pelvic tilt (Fig. 125-1).

Aged pelvic tilt is a term used to describe the anterior rotation of the pelvis that occurs with age in all of us. This leads to more projection of the lower abdomen with a loss of the youthful lordosis of the lower back. There is a flattening of the posterior body contour with loss of the youthful projection of the buttocks. The buttocks flatten and fall.

Postural changes with aging have been solely linked to relaxation of the musculoskeletal framework.[10] A second and perhaps more important cause of aged pelvic tilt is the relaxation of the superficial fascial system (SFS) "body suit" of the trunk and thighs.[2] The SFS is a three-dimensional fibrous meshwork of the subcutaneous tissue that shapes and supports the fat during many decades of life and holds the skin on the body. It is the main support structure of the skin-fat unit. Evidence supporting such an observation is the "buttock lift" effect of lateral tension abdominoplasty that is not seen with classic abdominoplasty (Fig. 125-2).[5] Both procedures include rectus muscle plication, but only the lateral tension abdominoplasty significantly tightens the SFS. In addition to a buttock lift effect, a mild to moderate lifting of the anterior, medial, and lateral thigh occurs with the lateral tension abdominoplasty.

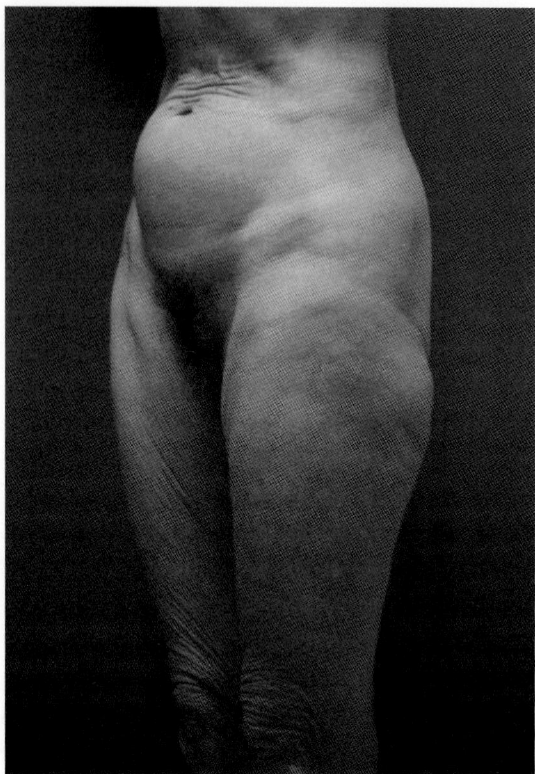

FIGURE 125-1. Example of aged pelvic tilt in a 63-year-old woman. Anterior rotation of the pelvis with age or after pregnancy or major weight loss leads to prominent lower abdomen, flattening of posterior body contours (loss of spinal lordosis), and poor buttock projection with ptosis.

The most common body lift performed in the author's practice is the lateral tension abdominoplasty with liposuction. This provides an excellent rejuvenation for early (mild to moderate) relaxation of the trunk-thigh aesthetic unit. For more significant generalized laxity problems, a lower body lift will be required. The original lower body lift design combined the transverse flank-thigh-buttock lift with the medial thigh lift to treat laxity of the circumferential trunk and thighs (Color Plate 125-1).[1,3,4] In addition, a second lower body lift design, version 2, combines the transverse flank-thigh-buttock lift with the lateral tension abdominoplasty.[3,5,7] The lower body lift, version 2, has become the most commonly performed lower body lift in the author's practice (Color Plate 125-2).

Although both lower body lift techniques deal with laxity of the skin and soft tissues of the trunk and thighs, the patient's goals and specific aesthetic deformity are used to outline an overall treatment plan for each individual. If there is moderate to severe abdominal laxity, either an initial lateral tension abdominoplasty followed by thigh-buttock lifting at a second stage or a lower body lift, version 2, incorporating bilateral transverse flank-thigh-buttock lifts with the lateral tension abdominoplasty is recommended. This latter combination will produce a degree of anteromedial thigh tightening, although if the medial thigh problem is more severe, a second-stage medial thigh lift will be required.[1]

If the patient has had previous abdominoplasty or has a mild to moderate abdominal problem and a moderate to severe medial thigh problem, the original lower body lift procedure (version 1) is recommended.[4] This procedure combines bilateral flank-thigh-buttock lifts with bilateral medial thigh lifts along with a limited suprapubic skin resection. The lower body lift, version 1, produces dramatic lifting of the anterior, medial, and lateral thighs and of the buttocks and flanks along with moderate lifting of the abdomen.

High Lateral Tension Abdominoplasty

SURGICAL DESIGN

Modern abdominoplasty techniques were developed in the 1960s.[11-15] Although many modifications have been presented during the past 30 years,[16-20] the surgical principles for standard abdominoplasty have remained largely the same. These principles include a transverse lower abdominal incision, wide undermining to the costal margins, tightening of the abdominal musculature, resection of the redundant abdominal flap with the maximum resection centrally, umbilical transposition, and skin closure with hips flexed.

Whereas the operation has been standardized, the long-term aesthetic results of standard abdominoplasty have often been inconsistent and disappointing. Common unfavorable features after standard abdominoplasty include initial overtightening of the central abdomen; residual laxity of the inguinal and lateral abdominal regions; late suprapubic scar depression with soft tissue bulges above and below the incisional scar; superior displacement of the pubic hair; poor waist definition; and asymmetric, irregular, and hypertrophic scars.[5]

Standard abdominoplasty techniques are based on faulty principles. Maximal truncal laxity occurs laterally in most patients, not centrally as assumed by standard abdominoplasty designs. The strong midline adherence of the epigastrium to the linea alba limits true vertical descent above the umbilicus. A more effective abdominoplasty design would tighten the lateral abdomen, waist, groin, and upper thighs more than the central abdomen as well as allow circumferential liposculpturing of the trunk and thighs in a single stage.

The high lateral tension abdominoplasty addresses the practical and theoretical faults of standard

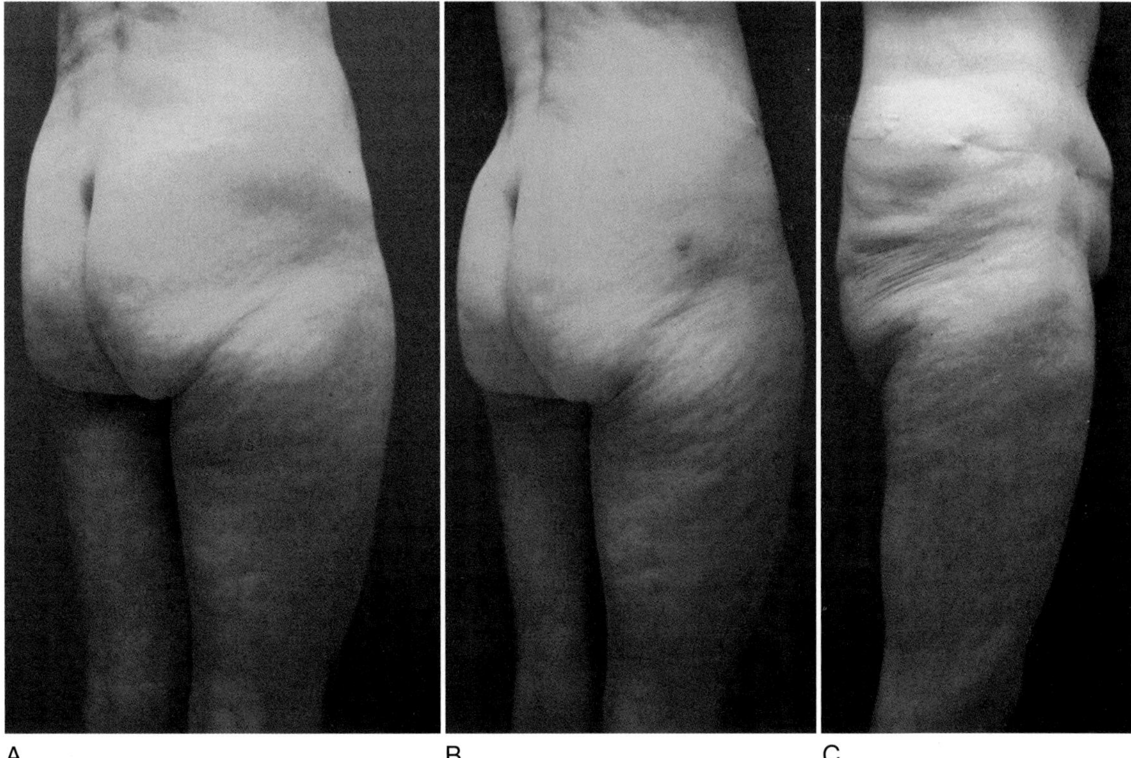

FIGURE 125-2. A 42-year-old patient with mild aged pelvic tilt after pregnancies *(A)* and 9 months after high lateral tension abdominoplasty *(B)*. Note reversal of aged pelvic tilt. The spinal lordosis is restored, resulting in more youthful body posture. The buttock appears lifted with enhanced projection. *C,* A 45-year-old patient after classic abdominoplasty with strong rectus muscle diastasis repair. Note the persistent aged pelvic tilt.

abdominoplasty design.[5] Key features are limited direct undermining, increased lateral skin resection with highest tension wound closure along lateral limbs, two-layer SFS repair, and significant truncal liposuction when it is needed (Color Plate 125-3). The high lateral tension design limits the unfavorable features of standard abdominoplasty and produces balanced natural aesthetic contours (Figs. 125-3 and 125-4).

Resection maximally along the lateral limbs of the abdominoplasty more accurately reverses truncal aging; provides lifting of the waist, inguinal area, and upper thighs; and decreases the tension on the suprapubic wound repair. Less tension centrally reduces the risk for skin necrosis and superior migration of the pubic hair. SFS repair reduces tensions on the skin repair, resulting in improved scars with less late scar depression. Limitation of direct undermining to the diastasis centrally and to the tissues to be resected laterally will reduce the risk for seromas and hematomas and also allow circumferential truncal liposuction in all areas except the new hypogastrium.

INDICATIONS

The high lateral tension abdominoplasty is indicated for moderate to severe, actual or potential laxity of the skin, fat, and muscles of the abdomen. There is often generalized relaxation of the entire trunk and upper thigh regions. For isolated problems of the hypogastrium, a limited abdominoplasty may be indicated. The high lateral tension abdominoplasty rejuvenates the abdomen, lower trunk, and upper thighs while allowing significant liposculpturing of the entire trunk-thigh aesthetic unit in one stage.[5] In contrast, the standard abdominoplasty design produces maximal lifting of the central abdomen, resulting in even more laxity in the lateral trunk. No lifting of the thighs occurs. In addition, the wide undermining required by the standard abdominoplasty design precludes significant circumferential liposuction.

OPERATIVE TECHNIQUE

After general anesthesia, the patient is draped to allow moving from supine to lateral decubitus position

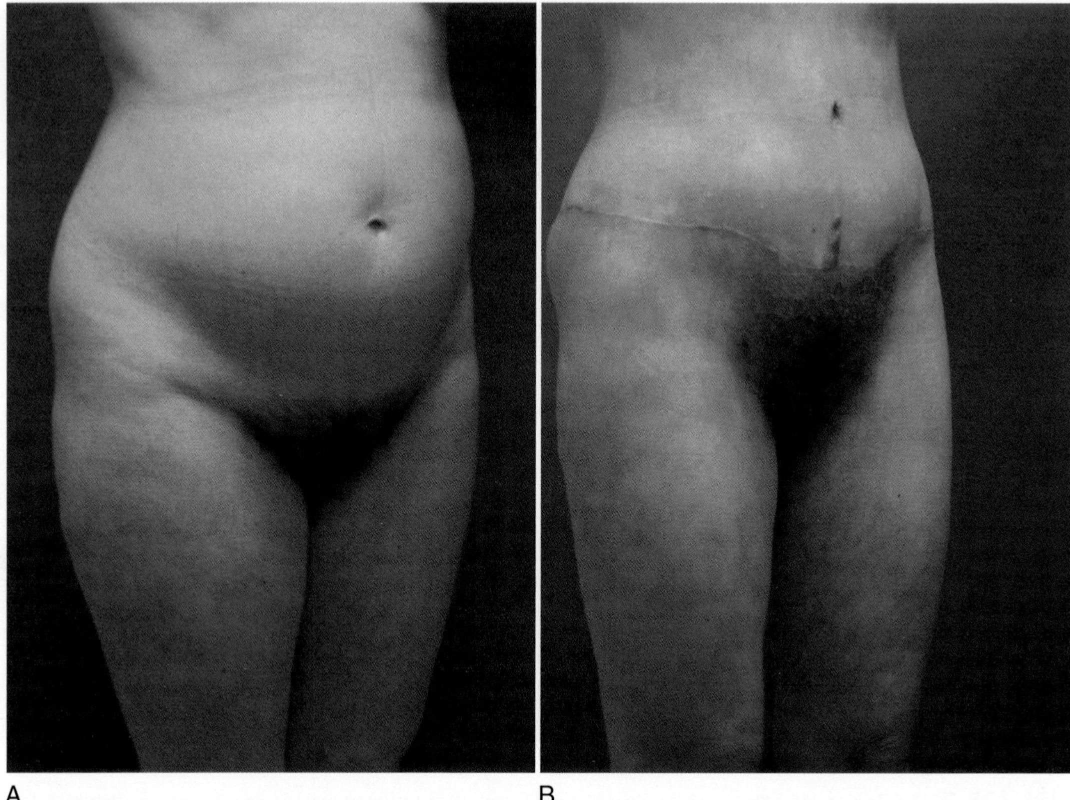

FIGURE 125-3. *A,* Preoperative anterior oblique view. A 35-year-old patient after one pregnancy presented with familial fat deposits and actual and potential laxity of trunk and upper thighs. *B,* Postoperative view. One year after high lateral tension abdominoplasty and liposuction of trunk and upper thighs. Note the relaxed youthful posture, excellent abdominal skin tone, tight waist, lengthened thighs, and fading bikini line scar. The vertical repair of the old umbilicoplasty defect is still mildly hypertrophic. The high lateral tension abdominoplasty is a body lift, not just an abdominoplasty.

during surgery. The inferior resection line is incised, and the inferior abdomen is undermined to the umbilicus. Direct undermining superior to the umbilicus is limited initially to the medial rectus border. The table is flexed 30 to 35 degrees before rectus muscle plication from the xiphoid to pubis in two layers. Midline bunching of the abdominal skin and fat occurs after muscle plication. This may be partially released by discontinuous undermining of the abdominal flap with vertical spreading scissor dissection. Liposuction of epigastric fat after the redundant abdominal flap is resected will resolve residual contour irregularities. In thin patients not requiring abdominal liposuction, wider direct undermining before flap resection may be necessary.

The redundant abdominal flap is resected by use of a Lockwood marking clamp with maximum tension along the lateral thirds of the incision (Fig. 125-5). The SFS is repaired initially with 0 braided nylon on a large taper needle along the entire wound (except near the incision ends), followed by a second SFS suture of 2-0 or 3-0 braided nylon. Deep dermis is repaired with a running 3-0 polydioxanone suture, skin with a running 3-0 polypropylene suture. Three 15 French or 19 French fluted (Blake) silicone drains are brought out through the mons pubis. Drains are removed as drainage decreases; one drain remains for 10 to 12 days on average. The old umbilical defect must be sutured with the same technique to avoid hypertrophy.

A 2.5-cm vertical incision is made over the umbilicus for the umbilicoplasty. After adjunctive truncal liposuction, light gauze dressings are applied without pressure. No compression garment is used initially, but it may be started once all wounds are healed in 2 to 3 weeks.

Transverse Flank-Thigh-Buttock Lift

SURGICAL DESIGN

The thigh-buttock lift of Pitanguy was originally designed in 1964 to allow direct excision of trochanteric fat deposits.[21] For nearly 30 years, the Pitanguy lift was

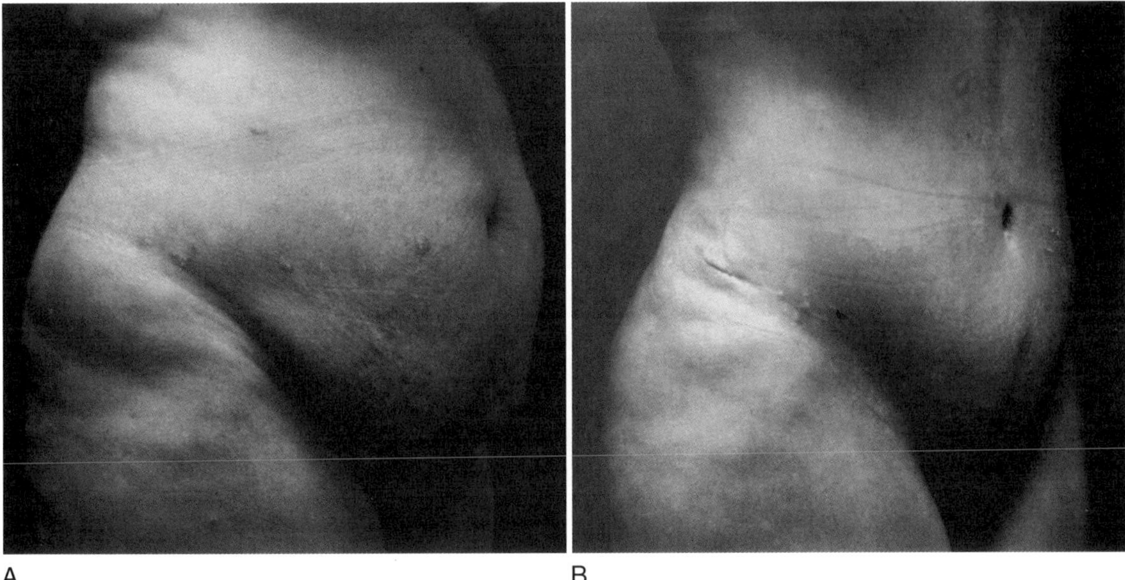

A B

FIGURE 125-4. *A,* Preoperative anterior oblique view. A 33-year-old patient after multiple pregnancies presented with significant familial fat deposits and laxity of the trunk and upper thighs. *B,* Postoperative view. One year after high lateral tension abdominoplasty and liposuction of trunk and upper thighs. Note the harmonious and balanced rejuvenation of the trunk and upper thigh aesthetic unit.

also used as the standard procedure for laxity and cellulite of the lateral thigh and buttock region (Fig. 125-6). However, Pitanguy's procedure was infrequently performed because of problems such as noticeable scars, early recurrence of deformities, unnatural contours, significant wound complications, long operative time, and prolonged postoperative disability.[22]

With the advent of liposuction[23] and a better knowledge of the vascular anatomy of skin and the anatomy of the SFS,[2] a new thigh-buttock lift procedure was designed with a transverse resection of redundant skin and fat of the trunk and an incisional scar within high-cut bikini lines.[3] Although belt lipectomies have been used since the 1940s to treat circumferential laxity of the trunk,[11,14,24] the new transverse thigh-buttock lift produces simultaneous lifting of both the trunk and thigh tissues. With use of appropriate direct and discontinuous cannula undermining as well as SFS suspension with permanent sutures (No. 1 or 0 and 2-0 braided nylon), the transverse thigh-buttock lift provides numerous advantages for truncal contouring. There is improved skin flap vascularity; strong yet dynamic fascial support; simultaneous lifting of the trunk, buttocks, and thigh tissues; and a stable scar that remains hidden in bikini lines (Color Plate 125-4).

INDICATIONS

The transverse flank-thigh-buttock lift is indicated for moderate to severe laxity and cellulite of the trunk and thighs or buttock ptosis. Patients presenting with laxity and cellulite of the flank-lateral thigh-buttock region usually have associated relaxation of the abdomen and medial thighs. Strong lifting of the posterolateral trunk and thighs without concomitant abdominoplasty increases the degree of abdominal relaxation, resulting in marked disharmony of the body aesthetic unit. The transverse thigh-buttock lift is infrequently used alone except as a staged procedure after previous abdominoplasty. Even then, a modified secondary abdominoplasty is often required.

The thigh-buttock lift is most commonly combined with the high lateral tension abdominoplasty (lower body lift, version 2) (see Color Plate 125-2). This combination will produce a mild medial thigh lift. A more significant medial thigh problem will require a staged medial thigh lift. The medial thigh lift is combined with the thigh-buttock lift (lower body lift, version 1) as a primary procedure in patients with minimal abdominal problems (or previous abdominoplasty) and significant medial thigh relaxation.

OPERATIVE TECHNIQUE

Preoperative markings are made in the standing position with the knees 6 to 10 inches apart. After high-cut bikini margins are outlined, the desired position for the final incisional scar is symmetrically drawn within these outlines. The amount of soft tissue laxity superior to the planned line of closure is estimated. This is usually 4 to 5 cm (stretched skin) and

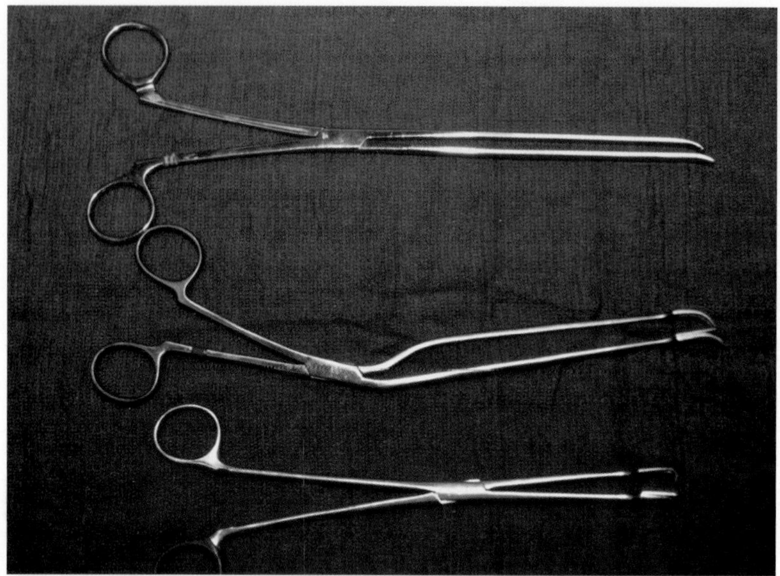

A

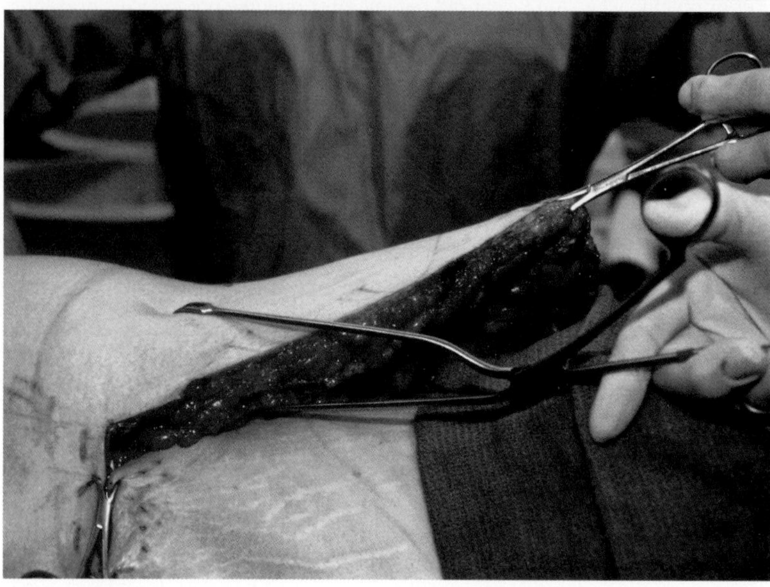

B

FIGURE 125-5. *A,* The Lockwood marking clamp *(center)* is a modification of the Pitanguy *(upper)* and D'Assumpcao *(lower)* clamps. There is an angle at the hinge to accommodate the angled body position with abdominoplasty and thigh-buttock lifts. The arms are longer and are separated by a wider space to accommodate the usual flap thickness. *B,* The Lockwood marking clamp in use. Marking clamps allow more accurate tissue resection and decrease the need to split the flap for resection purposes.

represents about one fourth of the vertical excess along the lateral body. Next, the lax tissue inferior to the line of closure is estimated. This generally ranges from 10 to 18 cm vertically along the lateral contour, producing a total vertical resection of 14 to 23 cm of stretched skin.

After general anesthesia, the patient is placed in the lateral decubitus position on a vacuum beanbag positioner. The hips are flexed 45 degrees; the thighs are abducted with foam blocks to keep the knees 15 to 18 inches apart. Liposuction of the posterolateral trunk and thigh is performed if needed. An incision is made through the superior resection line. Undermining superficial to muscle fascia is begun along the lateral contour anterior to the iliac crest, staying lateral to the femoral triangle lymphatics. The dissection then sweeps posteriorly in the same plane, leaving deep fat posterior to the iliac crest. Direct undermining should extend beneath the flap to be resected. Beyond this, no direct undermining is performed over the buttocks or into the thigh except in the trochanteric region. The SFS fibrous adherence in the trochanteric region must be released to allow distal transmission of the lifting forces.

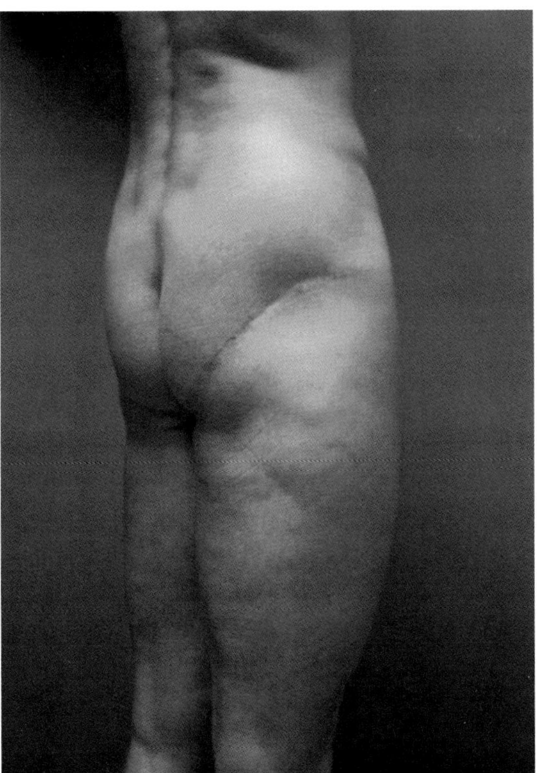

FIGURE 125-6. A 37-year-old patient 4 years after a Pitanguy thigh-buttock lift. There is aged pelvic tilt with loss of lordosis and flattened buttock contour. The supratrochanteric depression is accentuated. The incisional scar would be visible in many current bikini patterns. There are residual fat deposits of the trunk and thighs.

Next, discontinuous cannula undermining is performed more distally if the aesthetic deformity extends into the lower half of the thigh (Fig. 125-7). The redundant soft tissue is resected by flap-splitting techniques and a Lockwood marking clamp, with care taken to leave more skin than underlying SFS. This allows minimal-tension skin repair after SFS anchoring sutures are placed (two-layer, No. 1 and 2-0 braided nylon dipped in antibiotic or povidone-iodine solution, taper needles). The anterior incisions usually meet across the suprapubic area to resect a limited amount of skin excess of the lower abdomen. Any lower abdominal muscle laxity can easily be repaired (in a final supine position). Two 15 or 19 French fluted (Blake) silicone drains are inserted into each thigh as far distally as possible, exiting in the mons pubis anteriorly and near the incision posteriorly. Stacked towels are temporarily sutured superior to the incision to reduce pressure when surgery is performed on the opposite side.

Light dressings are applied; no compression garment is used. Postoperatively, the hips are flexed and the thighs abducted to reduce tension on the wound. At least one drain on each side is left for 14 to 21 days. Antibiotics are continued until all drains are removed.

Medial Thigh Lift

SURGICAL DESIGN

Skin laxity in the medial thigh is frequently the earliest sign of aging in the thighs and is one of the first signs of significant ptosis in the body.[25] The skin of the medial thigh is thin and inelastic, resulting in early relaxation with age and poor retraction after liposuction even by the age of 35 years. Laxity of the medial thighs may occur at even earlier ages when there is a history of obesity or a familial trait of early skin relaxation.

The classic medial thigh lift has been plagued with persistent problems, such as inferior migration and widening of scars, lateral traction deformity of the vulva, and early recurrence of ptosis.[26,27] In an attempt to limit untoward results, the medial thigh lift was modified to allow anchoring of the inferior skin flap to the tough, inelastic deep layer of the superficial fascia of the perineum.[1]

Use of Colles fascia as the central anchor for the medial thigh lift has produced more consistent, long-lasting results, decreasing the risk for problems commonly associated with the classic skin-suspension medial thigh lift (Fig. 125-8). Since the fascial anchoring technique for medial thigh lifts was originally described in 1987, numerous technical refinements have been developed to provide enhanced predictability and aesthetics. The design of the lift has changed owing to a better understanding of thigh aesthetic deformities. Because the majority of skin laxity occurs at the juncture of the anterior and medial thighs, the resectional pattern has rotated anteriorly, allowing the entire procedure to be performed in the supine position (Fig. 125-9). In contrast to previous descriptions, the incision should not extend into the buttock fold posteriorly. The resectional ellipse can be extended to the anterior superior iliac spine for more extensive problems in the anterior thigh and inguinal areas.

INDICATIONS

Significant actual or potential laxity of the medial thigh tissues remains the standard indication for medial thigh lifting. As noted before, the "medial thigh lift" effect of the high lateral tension abdominoplasty has reduced the need for medial thigh lifting in many patients. Also, tightening the medial thigh without first tightening lax tissues of the lower abdomen, pubis, and groin will lead to an unaesthetic appearance of this region.

OPERATIVE TECHNIQUE

Preoperative markings are made in the standing position with the knees apart. The medial thigh fat deposits

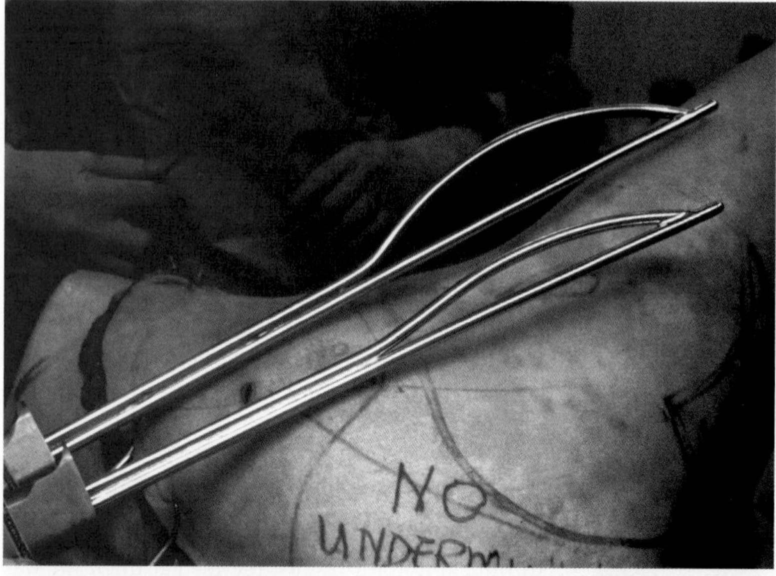

A

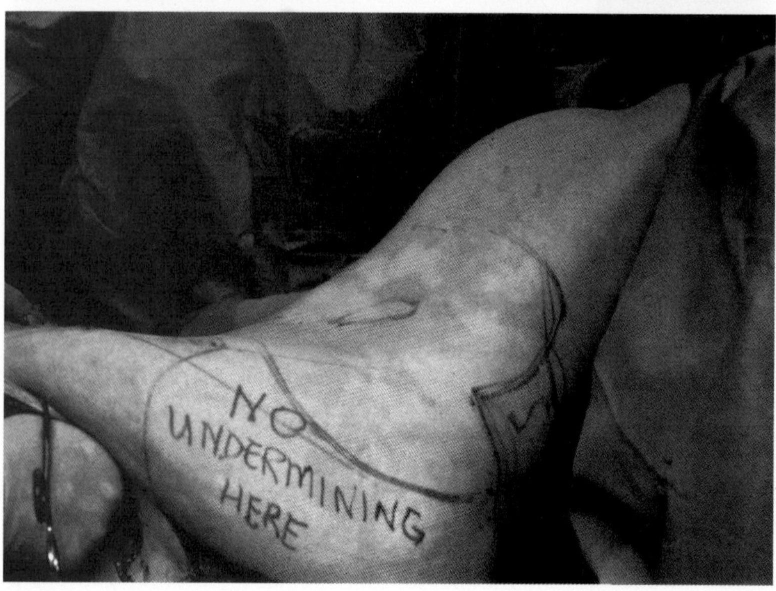

B

FIGURE 125-7. *A,* Similar to vertical spreading scissor dissection, the Lockwood undermining cannula loosens fibrous adhesions at a distance without damaging nerves or vessels. *B,* The cannula slides distally just superficial to the muscle fascia. Always keep the cannula perpendicular to the plane of the muscle fascia and skin.

are marked, and an estimate of the amount of skin redundancy is determined. The actual skin resection has become more conservative over the years, averaging 5 to 7 cm of stretched skin at the anteromedial corner of the thigh. Reanchoring of the perineal-thigh crease into Colles fascia provides an additional 3 to 5 cm of lift.

The patient is placed in the supine position with the hips flexed 30 to 35 degrees. The thighs are prepared and draped to allow repositioning during surgery. The excision of redundant tissue and subsequent repair are performed with the knees shoulder-width apart to avoid undercorrection. The thighs can be abducted for exposure as needed.

Initial deep liposuction is followed by skin-only incision along the superior resection line. Posteriorly, the perineal-thigh crease incision should not extend into the buttocks' fold. Anteriorly, the incision will leave the crease at the origin of the adductor longus muscle (pubic tubercle) and extend vertically along the lateral border of the mons pubis to varying degrees, depending on the aesthetic deformity. A more youthful, narrowed pubic hair pattern should be selected, although I would caution against making the pattern too

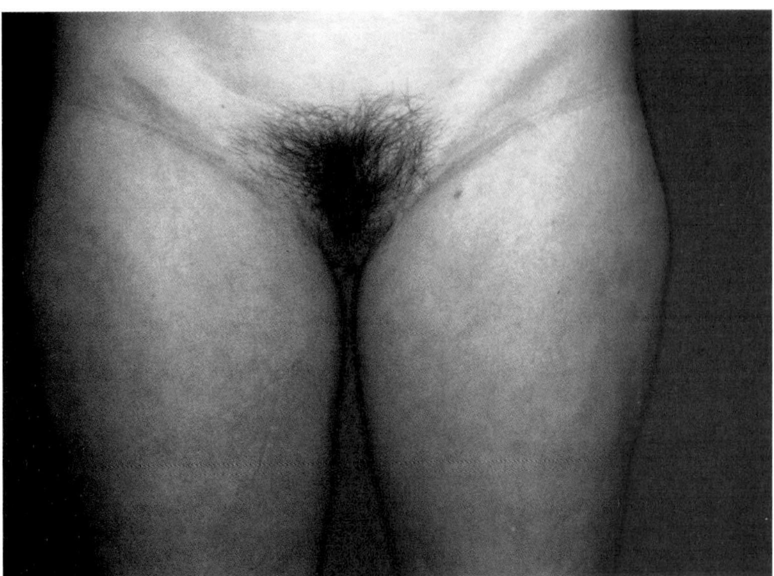

A

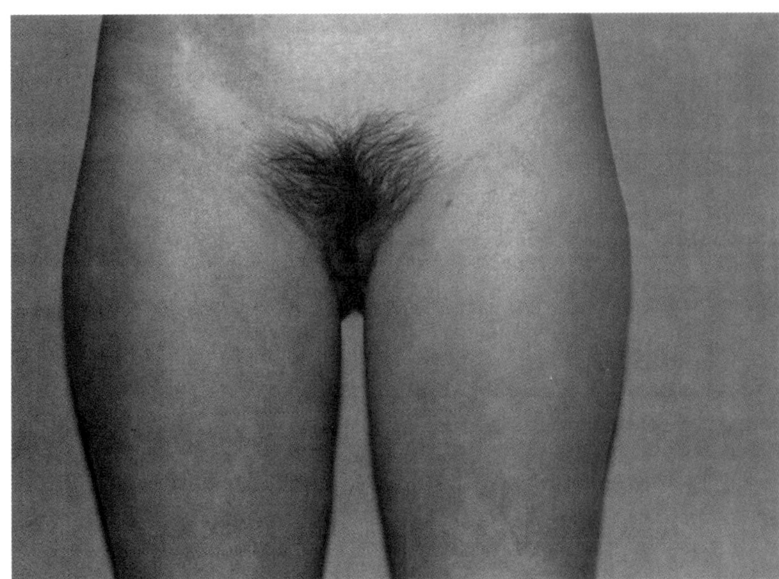

B

FIGURE 125-8. *A,* Preoperative view. A 35-year-old patient with fat deposits and actual and potential laxity of the medial thighs. *B,* Postoperative view. One year after Colles fascial anchoring medial thigh lift and liposuction of medial and lateral thighs. The scars remain hidden in the perineal-thigh crease.

narrow. After skin incision, undermining of the inferior flap posterior to the pubic tubercle is performed superficial to fascia of the adductor muscles.

Anterior to the pubic tubercle, care is taken to leave the soft tissue bundle coursing between the mons pubis and the femoral triangle. Superficial undermining over this bundle (leaving 8 to 10 mm of subdermal fat) preserves the external pudendal blood and lymphatic vessels, reducing the risk of lymphatic complications. Blunt dissection through this soft tissue bundle at the mons pubis exposes Scarpa fascia or muscle fascia, either of which can be used for anchoring of the thigh flap in the pubic region. Once flap undermining is completed, the Colles fascial roll is identified. It is important not to overdissect this fascia because like all superficial fascia, it tends to be somewhat vague and indistinct on gross examination. Attempts to overly define this fascia will lead to disruption of the fibrous connections between Colles fascia and the periosteum of the ischiopubic ramus, jeopardizing the strength of the fascial anchoring technique. Digital dissection with a dry gauze sponge most reliably preserves Colles fascial anatomy. Push superiorly over the adductor muscles until the tendinous muscle origins are seen and the

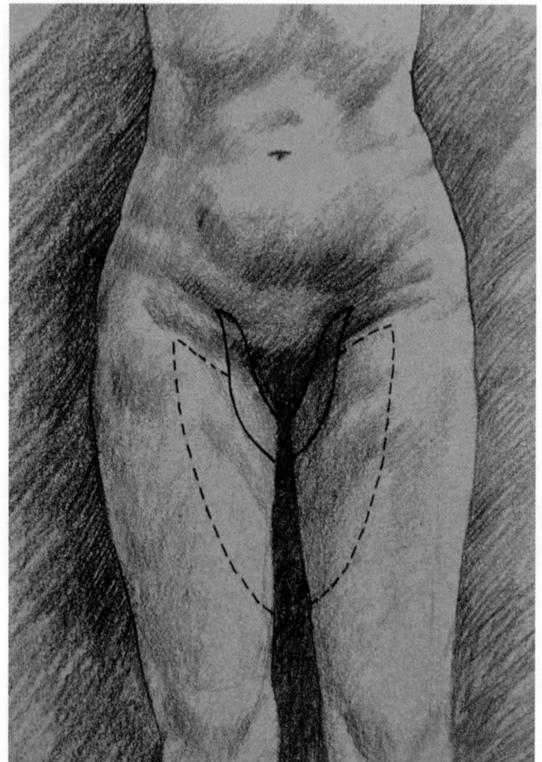

FIGURE 125-9. The current skin resection design for the fascial anchoring medial thigh lift *(solid lines)*. Deep liposuction of any medial thigh fat deposit is performed before the lift *(dashed lines)*.

bony ischiopubic ramus is palpated at fingertip. Retraction of the skin and superficial fat of the vulva medially will expose the Colles fascial roll at the deepest and most lateral aspect of the vulvar soft tissues.

Nonabsorbable anchoring sutures into Colles fascia are used for all patients (0 braided nylon, dipped in antibiotic or povidone-iodine solution) (Fig. 125-10). In addition, Scarpa fascia is used as the anchor anteriorly and the buttock fold SFS posteriorly. Next, the 0 braided nylon sutures are placed into the SFS of the thigh flap. Skin is repaired with 3-0 Vicryl dermal sutures and interrupted 3-0 nylon simple sutures. Light dressings are applied. Drains are generally not used. No compression garments are used.

Lower Body Lifts

SURGICAL DESIGN

Aesthetic body contour deformities frequently involve multiple areas of the trunk and thighs. Whereas isolated relaxation of the abdomen or medial thighs after pregnancy is relatively common, patients presenting with laxity and cellulite of the flank-lateral thigh-buttock region usually have associated relaxation of the abdomen and medial thighs. In these patients, the ideal surgical plan targets the entire circumferential trunk and thigh aesthetic unit in one or several stages.

Lower body lifts using circumferential bikini line incisions lift the trunk and thighs simultaneously. The original lower body lift design combined the transverse thigh-buttock lift and the medial thigh lift along with a limited suprapubic skin resection.[4] Today, this technique is reserved for patients who have had previous abdominoplasty or who have a mild abdominal problem and moderate to severe circumferential thigh laxity and cellulite (Fig. 125-11).

The lower body lift, version 2, combines the high lateral tension abdominoplasty with the transverse flank-thigh-buttock lift.[7] This is the most commonly performed lower body lift in the author's practice. This design is useful for treatment of generalized laxity of the entire trunk-thigh aesthetic unit of moderate to severe degree (Fig. 125-12). Although this technique does produce a modest lifting of the medial thighs, more severe medial thigh laxity will require a second-stage medial thigh lift.

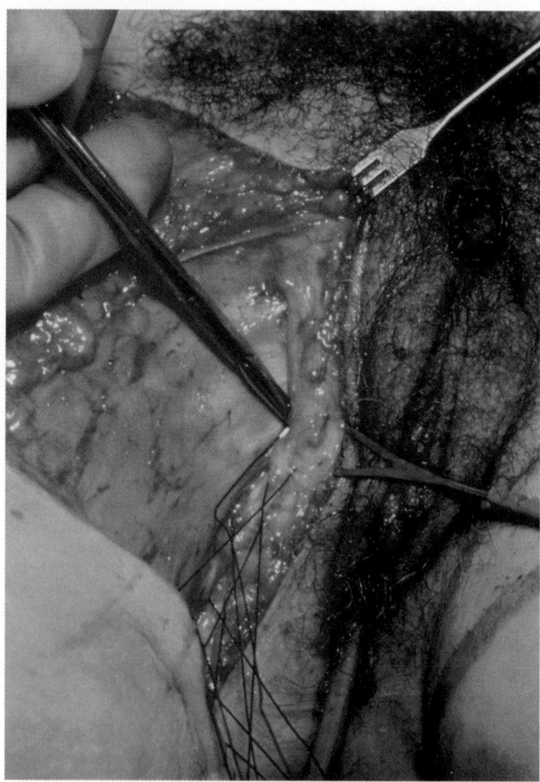

FIGURE 125-10. Permanent 0 braided nylon on a large (CT-1) taper needle is used to anchor the SFS of the medial thigh flap to Colles fascia of the perineal tissues. No distortion of the vulvar tissues should be noted after this first suture layer.

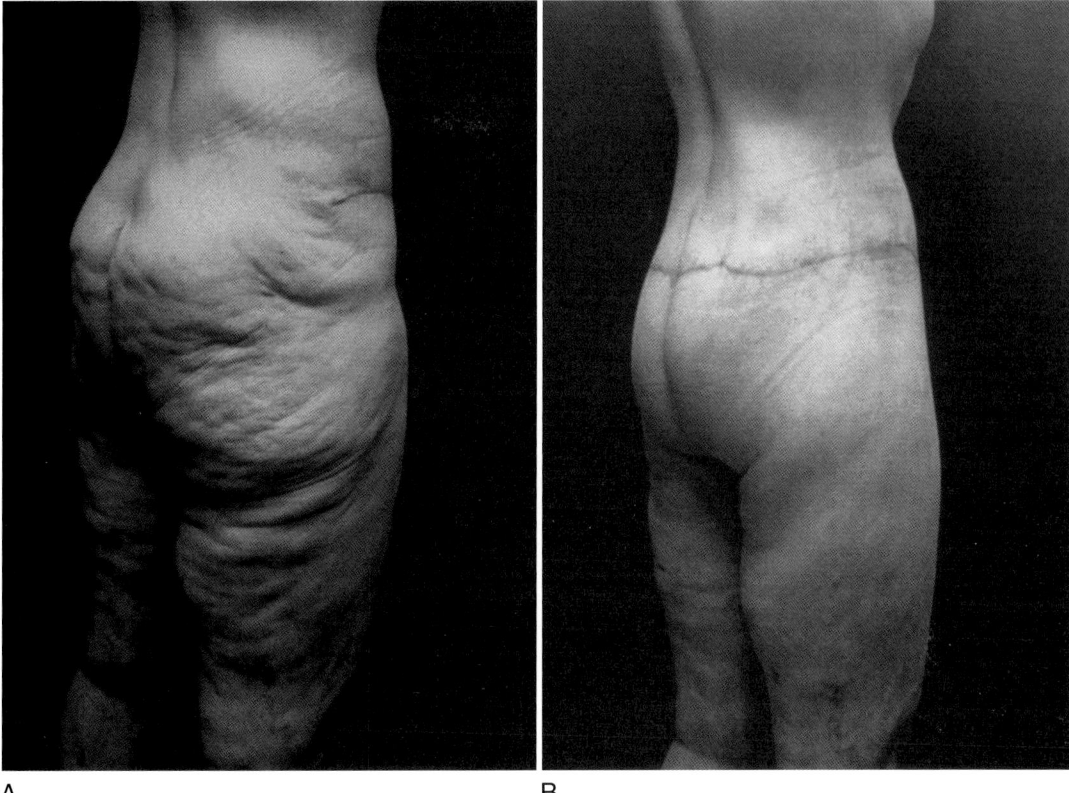

FIGURE 125-11. *A,* Preoperative view. A 41-year-old patient after massive weight loss and previous abdominoplasty. *B,* Postoperative view. Eight months after liposuction and lower body lift combining medial thigh lift and transverse thigh-buttock lift.

INDICATIONS

Lower body lifts are indicated for generalized relaxation of the skin and fat involving the circumferential body from the inframammary fold line to the knees.

OPERATIVE TECHNIQUE

Lower Body Lift, Version 1

After completion of bilateral thigh-buttock lifts in the decubitus position, the patient is placed supine with knees shoulder-width apart and the hips flexed 30 degrees. The medial thigh lift technique described earlier is followed. No undermining is performed over the femoral triangle lymphatics. No compression garment is used.

Lower Body Lift, Version 2

After completion of bilateral thigh-buttock lifts in the decubitus position with incision closure to the anterior superior iliac spine, the patient is placed in the supine position with the hips flexed 30 to 40 degrees with the thighs abducted. The high lateral tension abdominoplasty is performed as described before. No compression garment is used.

POSTOPERATIVE MANAGEMENT

All body lift patients are monitored on an inpatient basis for 3 to 5 days, depending on the degree of liposuction and lifting. Prophylactic antibiotics are begun preoperatively and continued until after the last drain is removed (10 to 20 days). Dressings are removed in 1 to 2 days, then silver sulfadiazine cream is applied to the incision twice daily. Patients stand at the bedside in 24 to 36 hours, then progressively ambulate with a walker. Stool softeners and protein drinks are started the first postoperative day, followed by a high-protein diet. An exercise body suit or leotard is started in 2 to 3 weeks and worn for several weeks for comfort and support.

COMPLICATIONS

Avoidance

In addition to appropriate selection of patients, procedure design, and surgical technique, thoughtful postoperative care is required to limit unfavorable results after major body lifting. The initial 24-hour period is critical to skin flap viability. To ensure adequate

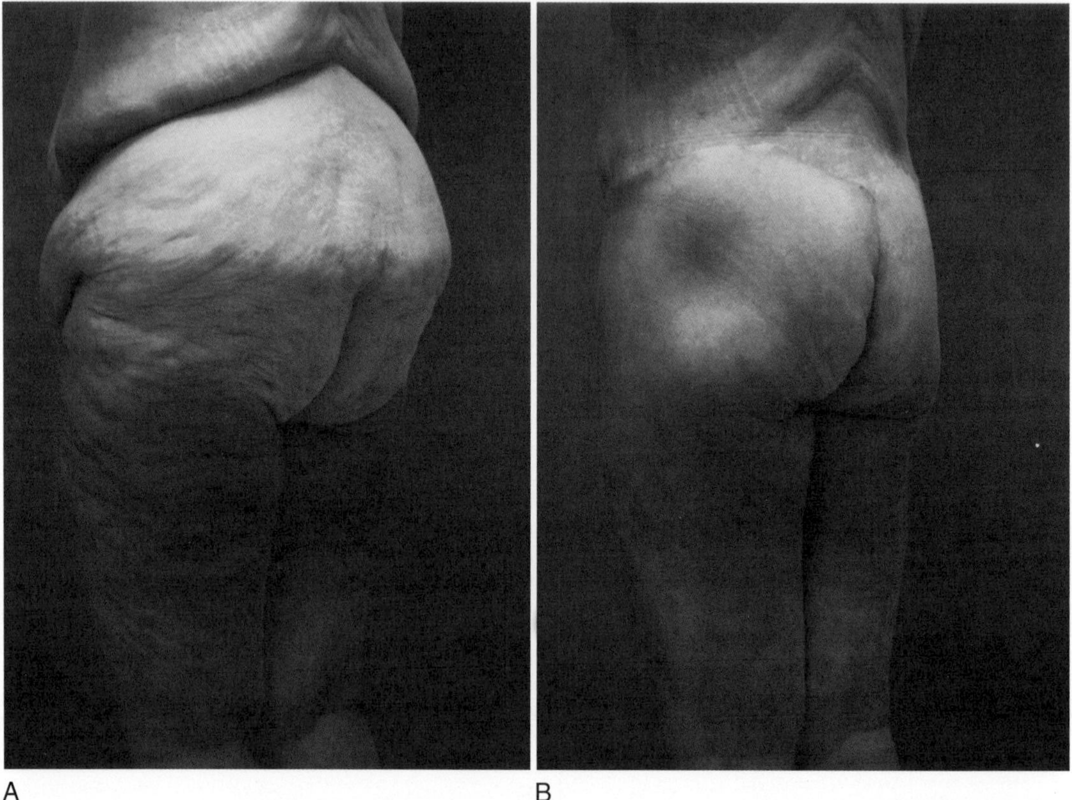

A B

FIGURE 125-12. *A,* Preoperative view. A 51-year-old patient after massive weight loss with generalized severe laxity and familial fat deposits of the trunk and thigh aesthetic unit. *B,* Postoperative view. One year after liposuction and lower body lift combining high lateral tension abdominoplasty and transverse thigh-buttock lift.

cardiac output and tissue perfusion, vigorous intravenous lactated Ringer (nondextrose) fluid resuscitation and frequent urinary output monitoring are performed in the early postoperative period. In addition, a slow intravenous (piggyback) drip of 500 mL of hetastarch (Hespan) is started at the end of the procedure and continued during 5 hours to help stabilize the intravascular blood volume. In addition to adequate fluid resuscitation, proper positioning of the patient reduces postoperative wound tension, enhancing tissue perfusion of the wound edges.

Prophylaxis for deep venous thrombosis in patients without previous disease includes leg elevation, support hose, pulsatile stockings or pneumatic compression boots started before anesthesia, anemia (hemodilution), bed exercises and ambulation, and, in the absence of a significant blood loss problem, enteric-coated aspirin started on the first postoperative day. Performing major body lifts in a hospital setting ensures appropriate nursing care and monitoring. Pulmonary radiographs or scans, pulse oximetry, intensive care, and specialty medical consultants are available in a timely manner should the need arise.

Treatment

Life-threatening complications, such as pulmonary embolus and massive infection, are rare (<0.25% risk). Medical consultation, diagnostic scans, anticoagulation, and intensive care monitoring can successfully treat many pulmonary emboli. Massive infection will also require consultation with an infectious disease specialist, diagnostic wound cultures, antibiotics, surgical drainage as needed, and in-hospital monitoring.

Major skin necrosis is unusual (<3% risk) with new body lift designs and appropriate postoperative care. The risk for lesser complications is more significant (10% to 20% of body lift patients). These include wound infection, delayed healing including wound dehiscence, minor degrees of necrosis, poor scarring, suture reactions and infection, seromas or hematomas, anemia, nonautologous blood transfusion, dog-ears, significant areas of anesthesia or paresthesia, inadequate lifting of tissues, and prolonged hospitalization or recovery.

If skin ischemia is noted after body lifting, initial treatment is application to the ischemic area of either

2% nitroglycerin ointment every 4 to 6 hours or silver sulfadiazine cream twice daily. Either technique is useful in reducing the risk for and extent of full-thickness skin loss. If marginal skin necrosis is minimal, delayed wound healing should occur uneventfully. The silver sulfadiazine cream is continued until healing is complete. If skin necrosis is more significant, conservative débridement is performed once wound healing is stable (2 to 4 weeks). After wound débridement is completed and granulations have appeared, secondary wound repair with antibiotic prophylaxis is frequently successful in treating areas of skin loss or wound dehiscence. For larger wounds, secondary healing during weeks or months will allow wound contraction to reduce the size of the scar for future scar revision. Skin grafting may be necessary for patients who desire rapid wound closure.

Hypertrophic scars are less common with strong two-layer SFS repair but may still occur in a minority of patients. Excessive scars generally require many months or years to be improved. Silicone elastomer sheeting may speed scar maturation. Scar revision after 1 year may be indicated. Suture reaction or infection is somewhat more common when nonabsorbable sutures are used in the subcutaneous tissues. Braided nylon SFS sutures are dipped in povidone-iodine or antibiotic solution before use to help reduce suture complications. Suture granulomas or sinus tracks or exposed sutures will require suture removal for healing to progress.

Hematomas are uncommon after body lifts. Significant hematomas will require surgical drainage. Seromas occur in 3% to 5% of body lift patients. Prevention of seromas begins with surgical technique. Minimizing direct undermining in both abdominoplasty and thigh lifts will decrease the seroma rate. If wider undermining techniques are used, tacking of the undermined flap to muscle fascia with multiple absorbable sutures is recommended. In addition, strong suturing of the SFS with nonabsorbable sutures avoids the subincisional dead space that can occur if the SFS repair separates in the first weeks after surgery. Use of ample drains with slits rather than holes allows the drains to function longer without becoming plugged, even with minimal amounts of drainage. In general, long 15 or 19 French drains are used. Drains should not exit through the incision.

If the diagnosis of seroma is in doubt, ultrasonography can be effective in confirming the diagnosis.[28] Once seroma is diagnosed, it must be treated early with frequent, repetitive external drainage and compression dressing or by the placement of a percutaneous drainage system.* Neglected seromas can evolve into a pseudobursa that requires surgical treatment.

*SeromaCath, Greer Medical, Santa Barbara, Calif.

Widened, asymmetric, misplaced, or hypertrophic scars may occur after body lifting. Careful preoperative planning and avoidance of excessive wound repair tensions reduce scar complications. Treatment of scar complications should generally be delayed for 8 to 12 months. Widened or hypertrophic scars may be improved with simple scar revision. Misplaced scars often require further body lifting.

CONCLUSION

Modern body lifting is an exciting frontier for plastic surgeons. Whereas the results can be dramatic and fulfilling, the surgeries are labor-intensive and challenging. Although life-threatening complications are rare, there is a significant risk for unfavorable results that can be minimized with proper selection of patients; careful surgical design, planning, and execution; and appropriate postoperative care.

REFERENCES

1. Lockwood T: Fascial anchoring in medial thigh lifts. Plast Reconstr Surg 1988;82:299-304.
2. Lockwood T: Superficial fascial system (SFS) of the trunk and extremities: a new concept. Plast Reconstr Surg 1991;87:1009-1018.
3. Lockwood T: Transverse flank-thigh-buttock lift with superficial fascial suspension. Plast Reconstr Surg 1991;87:1019-1027.
4. Lockwood T: Lower body lift with superficial fascial system suspension. Plast Reconstr Surg 1993;92:1112-1122.
5. Lockwood T: High-lateral-tension abdominoplasty with superficial fascial system suspension. Plast Reconstr Surg 1995;96:603-615.
6. Lockwood T: Brachioplasty with superficial fascial system suspension. Plast Reconstr Surg 1995;96:912-920.
7. Lockwood T: Lower body lift. Operative Techniques Plast Reconstr Surg 1996;3:132-144.
8. Lockwood T: Reduction mammaplasty and mastopexy with superficial fascial system (SFS) suspension. Plast Reconstr Surg 1999;103:1411-1419.
9. Baroudi R, Moraes M: Philosophy, technical principles, selection, and indications in body contouring surgery. Aesthetic Plast Surg 1991;15:1-18.
10. Turek S: Orthopedics—Principles and Their Application, vol 2, 4th ed. Philadelphia, JB Lippincott, 1984:1598-1600.
11. Gonzalez-Ulloa M: Belt lipectomy. Br J Plast Surg 1961;13:179-184.
12. Spadafora A: Abdomen pendulo: dermolipectomia anterolateral baja (technica persona). Prensa Med Argent 1962;49:494-503.
13. Callia W: Dermolipectomia Abdominal. São Paulo, Centro de Cinematografia Carlo Erba, 1965.
14. Vilain R, Dubousset J: Techniques et indications de la lipectomie circulaire: a propos de 150 interventions. Ann Chir 1964;18:289-294.
15. Pitanguy I: Abdominal lipectomy: an approach to it through an analysis of 300 consecutive cases. Plast Reconstr Surg 1967;40:384-391.
16. Grazer F: Abdominoplasty. Plast Reconstr Surg 1973;51:617-623.
17. Baroudi R, Keppke E, Tozzi Neto F: Abdominoplasty. Plast Reconstr Surg 1974;54:161-167.
18. Regnault P: Abdominoplasty by the W technique. Plast Reconstr Surg 1975;55:265-274.

19. Planas J: The "vest over pants" abdominoplasty. Plast Reconstr Surg 1978;61:694-700.
20. Guerrerosantos J, Spaillat L, Morales F: Some problems and solutions in abdominoplasty. Aesthetic Plast Surg 1980;4:227-237.
21. Pitanguy I: Trochanteric lipectomy. Plast Reconstr Surg 1964;34:280-286.
22. Regnault P, Daniel R: Secondary thigh-buttock deformities after classical techniques: prevention and treatment. Clin Plast Surg 1984;11:505-513.
23. Illouz YG: Body contouring by lipolysis: a 5-year experience with over 3000 cases. Plast Reconstr Surg 1983;72:591-597.
24. Somalo M: Dermolipectomia circular del tronco. Semana Med 1940;1435-1441.
25. Illouz YG, De Villers Y: Body Sculpturing by Lipoplasty. New York, Churchill Livingstone, 1989.
26. Lewis J: The thigh lift. J Int Coll Surg 1957;27:330-334.
27. Planas J: The "crural meloplasty" for lifting of the thighs. Clin Plast Surg 1975;2:495-503.
28. Mohammad J, Warnke P, Stavraky W: Ultrasound in the diagnosis and management of fluid collection complications following abdominoplasty. Ann Plast Surg 1998;41:498-502.

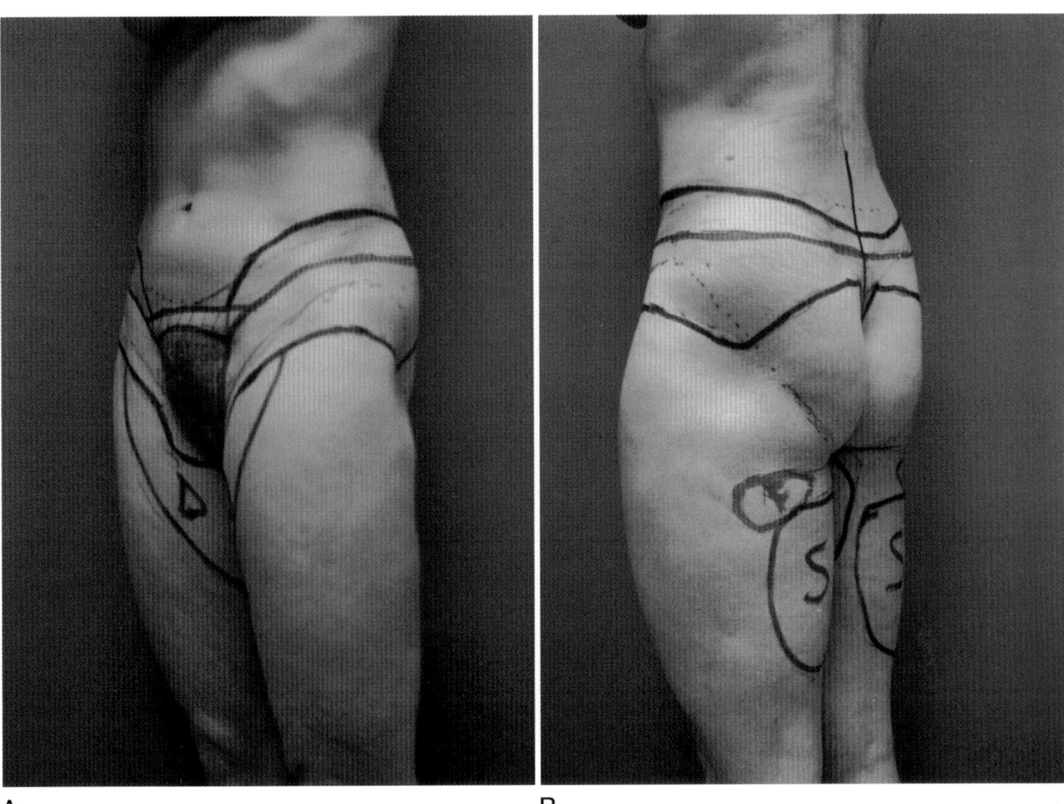

A B

COLOR PLATE 125-1. *A,* Anterior oblique view. The original lower body lift design (1993) combined the transverse flank-thigh-buttock lift with the medial thigh lift to treat laxity of the circumferential trunk and thighs. The patient has had previous Pitanguy thigh-buttock lift and has minimal abdominal laxity. Deep liposuction of medial thighs is planned. The final incisional scar line is marked in red. *B,* Posterior oblique view. The estimated resection margins are marked in blue. Whereas the posterior thigh fat deposit is marked for superficial liposuction, the familial fat deposits of the posterior thigh are deep. Superficial liposuction in the thighs is currently reserved for the infragluteal fat bulge and for the suprapatellar area of the anterior distal thigh.

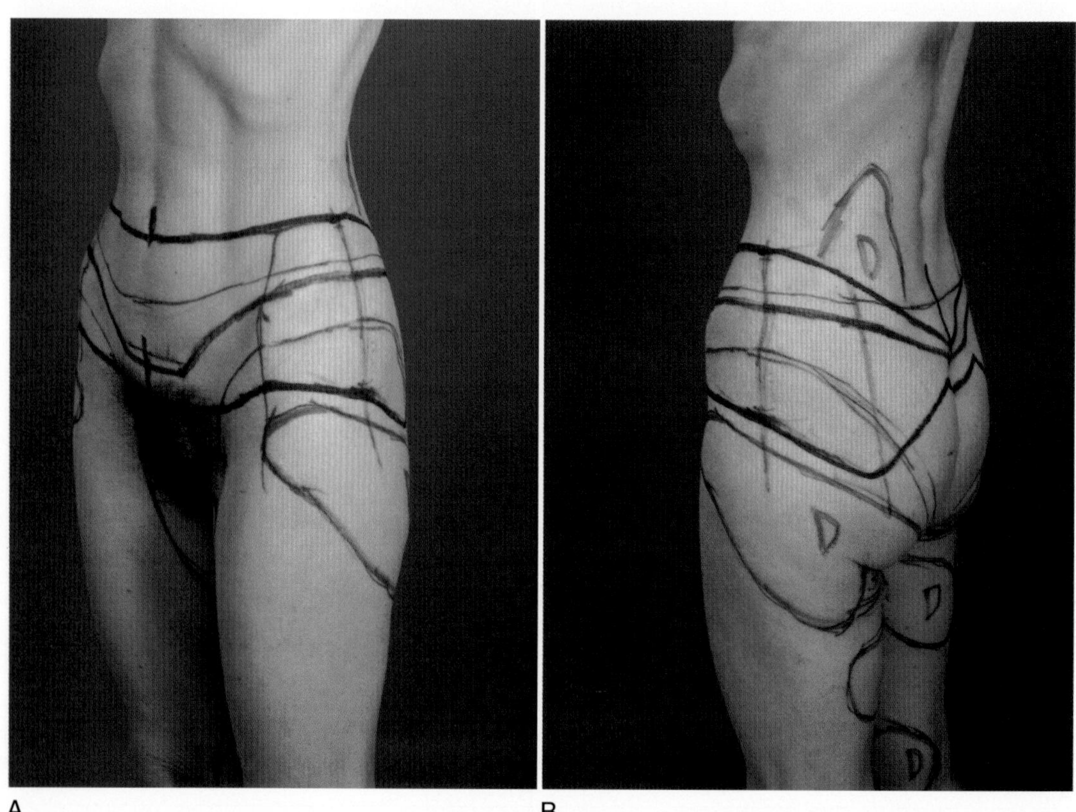

COLOR PLATE 125-2. *A,* Anterior oblique view. A second lower body lift (version 2) design (1996) combines the transverse flank-thigh-buttock lift with the lateral tension abdominoplasty. Bikini outlines are initially marked (purple). The final incisional scar line (red) is within the bikini outlines and is symmetric. *B,* Posterior oblique view. The estimated resection limits are marked in blue, and the fat deposits for liposuction are marked in green.

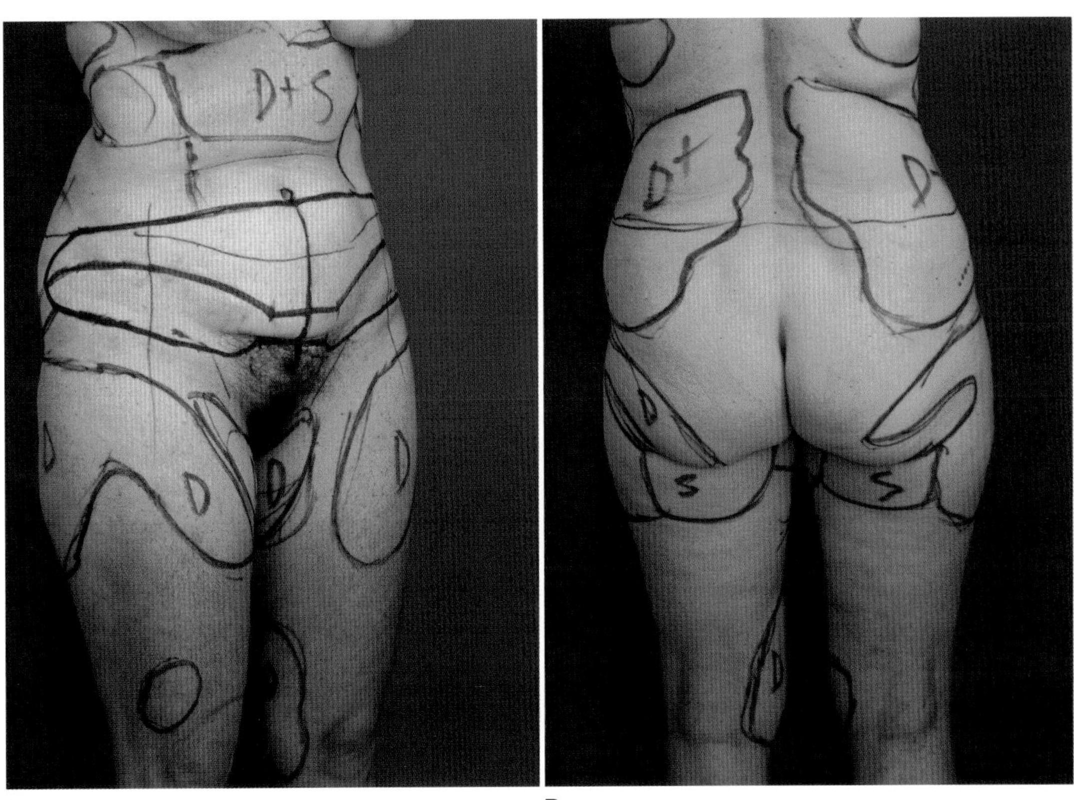

A B

COLOR PLATE 125-3. *A,* Anterior oblique view. Markings for the high lateral tension abdominoplasty (1995) with liposuction of circumferential trunk, upper thighs, and medial knees. The inferior blue line is termed the anchor resection line and is the initial incision line. The superior blue line is only a reference line to help maintain symmetry. The actual extent of tissue resection is determined intraoperatively. *B,* Posterior view. Planned liposuction of fat deposits: deep (D), deep and intermediate (D+), and superficial (S).

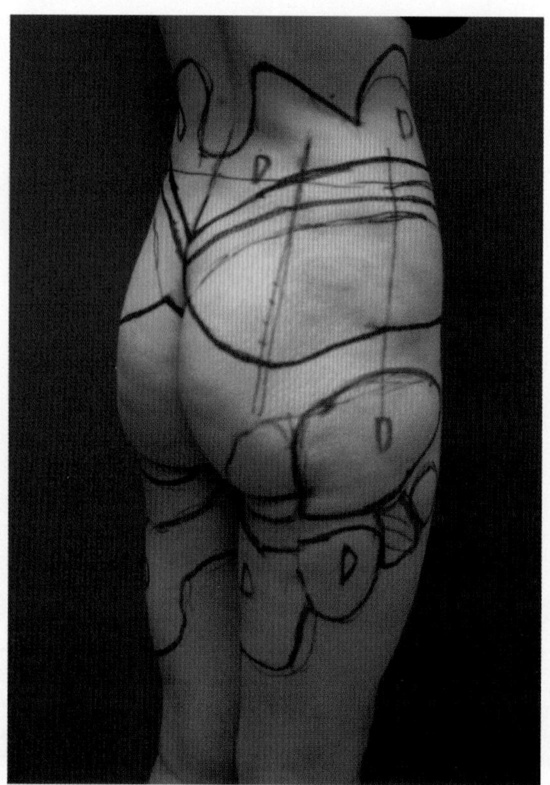

COLOR PLATE 125-4. Example of markings for the transverse flank-thigh-buttock lift and liposuction. The trunk and thighs are simultaneously lifted with this technique. The incisional closure line (red) will be hidden even in thong bikinis.

CHAPTER

126

Liposuction of the Trunk and Lower Extremities

MARY K. GINGRASS, MD, FACS ✦ LAUREN GREENBERG, MD

Liposuction has become the most popular cosmetic procedure performed by board-certified plastic surgeons in the United States.[1] Although liposuction is not a technically difficult procedure, it requires thoughtful planning and an artistic eye to achieve aesthetically pleasing postoperative results. The goal of the liposuction surgeon is to remove "target" fat, leaving the desired body contour and smooth transitions between suctioned and nonsuctioned areas. Careful selection of patients and proper surgical technique will help avoid contour irregularity, and diligent perioperative care of the patient will help avoid postoperative complications.

SELECTION OF PATIENTS

The selection of patients is one of the most important determinants of a good aesthetic surgical result, especially when it comes to body contouring. A liposuction consultation should begin by asking the patient, What would you like to change about your body? It is then up to the surgeon to give the patient a realistic appraisal of what *can* and, at times more important, what *cannot* be accomplished with liposuction. Some patients who present for liposuction consultation may require alternative procedures or liposuction combined with an open surgical procedure to accomplish their goals.

A detailed weight history is an important part of any liposuction consultation. An ideal candidate is at a stable weight and has a working diet and exercise regimen in place (Table 126-1). Patients who have a history of frequent or significant weight fluctuations are at high risk for weight gain after liposuction. Maintaining a stable weight and practicing a diet and exercise regimen for 6 months usually indicate a commitment to lifestyle change.

Liposuction should not be offered as a treatment for obesity. It is best used to remove genetically distributed or diet-resistant fat; however, in practical terms, it is frequently used to remove fat that could be lessened with diet and exercise. Ideal liposuction candidates are within 20% of their ideal body weight[2] or less than 50 pounds above chart weight. In most instances, patients who fall outside these parameters should be encouraged to lose weight first and then address diet-resistant areas with liposuction.

A thorough physical examination is then performed. Although the focus of the examination should be "problem areas," it is important to take the entire body shape into consideration. An overall harmonious body contour is desirable. The patient is examined for areas of disproportionate fat, asymmetry, dimpling or cellulite, varicosities, and zones of adherence. One of the most important physical findings that has significant bearing on final outcome is the skin tone or dermal quality. It is important to pinch and palpate the skin, assessing for the degree of laxity and dermal thickness. A thicker dermis is more likely to retract after liposuction. Thin, stretched out skin with striae (indicating dermal breakage) is unlikely to retract. Loose, thin skin covering soft fat will often look worse after liposuction (Fig. 126-1).

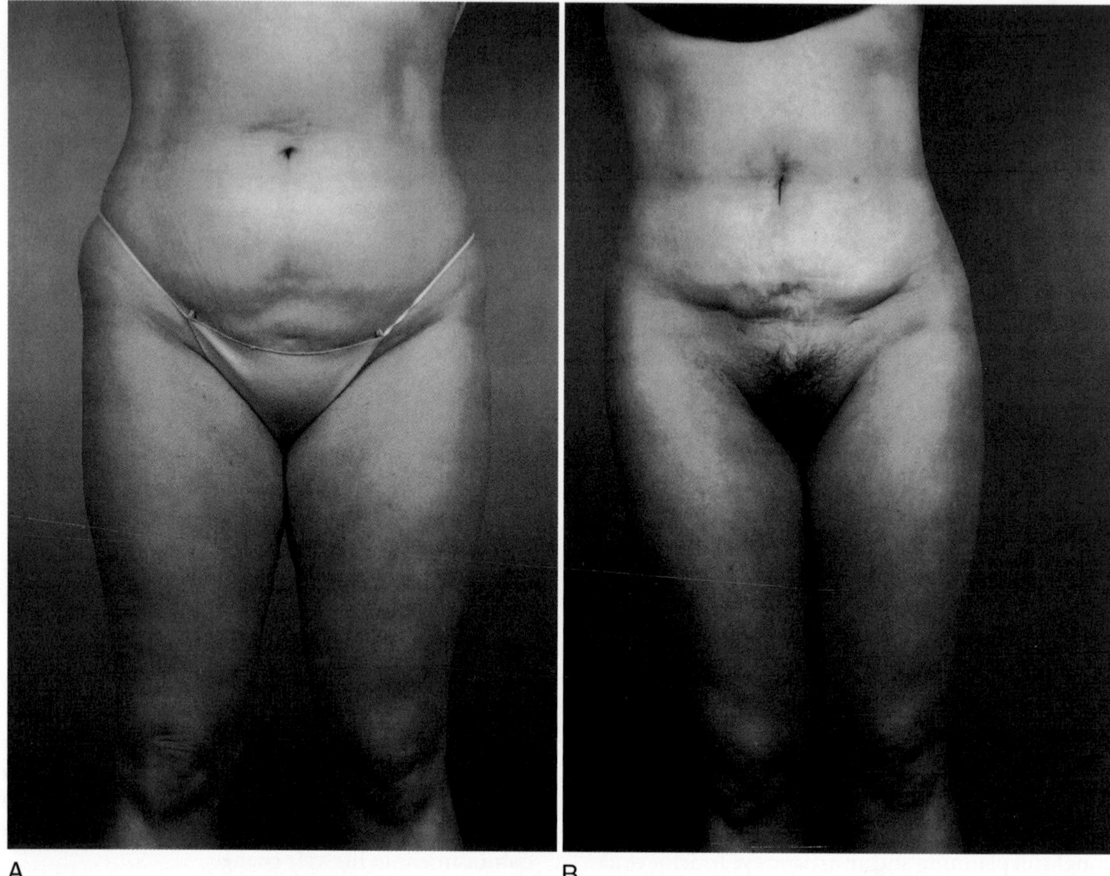

FIGURE 126-1. *A,* Preoperative photograph of a 40-year-old woman with a history of two pregnancies and significant weight fluctuations. Her skin is thin and flaccid; the fat is soft and "loose" on examination. *B,* The same patient is shown 6 months after liposuction of the abdomen and hips. The hips responded well, but the abdominal skin has not retracted. This represents poor selection of patients on the part of the surgeon. The patient required secondary skin excision to correct this contour irregularity.

The quality of the fat should also be assessed because it may also affect the outcome. Generally speaking, thick, fibrous fat is more "forgiving" than soft, loose fat. The softer fat has large lobules with wispy intervening fibroconnective tissue. This type of fat is removed readily and is easy to overresect; as a general rule, the overlying skin is thin. The fibrous type of fat tends to be densely packed between tightly woven intervening fibroconnective tissue. This type of fat is less readily removed. The overlying skin tends to be thicker and can be expected to retract well. The better retraction is theoretically due to the retractile properties in the fibroconnective tissue and in the dermis itself.

TABLE 126-1 ✦ LIPOSUCTION PATIENT HISTORY

What is your current weight?
How long have you been at this weight?
Have you had any significant weight gains or losses?
What is your current diet and exercise regimen?
For how long have you maintained this regimen?
Have you taken any diet pills to assist with weight reduction?
Have you had previous liposuction?

Once it is determined that a patient is a good candidate for liposuction, the procedure itself is explained to the patient. The appropriate type of anesthesia is chosen on the basis of the surgeon's preference, the patient's choice, the estimated volume to be removed, and whether additional surgical procedures are being combined with liposuction. Local anesthesia is generally appropriate for patients with a smaller volume to be removed; general anesthesia is preferable for larger volumes. Incision sites are discussed. Standardized photographs, including anterior, posterior, lateral, and oblique views, should be taken preoperatively.

Risks, possible complications, and the anticipated postoperative course are then reviewed with the patient (Table 126-2). If the patient is scheduled for a

TABLE 126-2 ✦ RISKS AND POSSIBLE COMPLICATIONS ASSOCIATED WITH LIPOSUCTION

Bleeding causing excessive bruising
Infection
Asymmetry
Contour irregularity
Prolonged skin numbness/dysesthesia
Seroma
Dyschromia
Abdominal or thoracic perforation
Lidocaine toxicity

large-volume procedure involving prolonged general anesthesia or a combined open surgical procedure like an abdominoplasty or a thigh lift, it is prudent to discuss additional risks such as deep venous thrombosis and pulmonary embolism.

SURGICAL PLANNING

It is up to the surgeon to decide which surgical tools he or she will use to perform the surgical procedure. A number of tools are available to the liposuction surgeon today. There are advantages and disadvantages, and some surgeons may simply have a preference for one tool or technique over another.

Traditional suction-assisted lipoplasty (SAL) became popular in the United States in the 1980s. It has a long track record and is considered the "gold standard" tool for liposuction. Traditional SAL cannulas are bendable and come in many sizes and tip shapes, and most hospital operating rooms and surgery centers own this type of equipment. SAL is an excellent technique for patients with smaller volume requirements and removal of soft fat; however, it is a less efficient tool for the removal of fat from more fibrous areas and requires a fair amount of physical effort on the part of the surgeon, which becomes a disadvantage in removal of larger volumes. Bruising is expected because of disruption of blood vessels by the suction forces. Cross-tunneling is a necessary step with SAL to avoid contour irregularity, reported to be as high as 20% in one SAL study.[3] The most frequently reported unsatisfactory results in this study were insufficient fat removal and excessive waviness. Asymmetry, excessive fat removal, and unacceptable scarring were less frequent.

Ultrasound-assisted liposuction (UAL) was introduced in the United States in the mid-1990s to address some of the shortcomings of SAL. Ultrasonic energy is produced in a piezoelectric crystal within the UAL surgical handpiece. The ultrasonic energy is transmitted down the attached titanium probe to the instrument tip, where the ultrasonic energy causes emulsification when it is applied to subcutaneous fat. The intervening fibroconnective tissues remain relatively unharmed and therefore available for postoperative skin retraction. The emulsified fat can then be suctioned away with low-power suction. UAL requires much less physical effort on the part of the surgeon compared with SAL because much of the "work" is done by the ultrasonic energy. UAL is an extremely efficient tool in fibrous areas such as the upper back, the hypogastrium, and the breast. UAL has been shown to cause less disruption of vasculature than SAL does.[4] This translates into less bruising. There is energy dissipation in all directions at the tip of the UAL cannula, which gives it a certain "airbrush" effect. Some surgeons think that it is a superior tool for sculpting and find less need for cross-tunneling compared with SAL.

There are also disadvantages to UAL. There is some elevation of tissue temperature with UAL, and if proper technique is not used, thermal injury can occur. There is potential for frictional injury at the skin entry site, so constant irrigation at the incision or a skin protector must be used. Seroma rates can be high with prolonged ultrasound treatment times.

Power-assisted liposuction (PAL) was developed in the late 1990s to address some of the concerns about UAL. PAL is basically traditional SAL instrumentation powered by a reciprocating cannula. The main advantages of PAL over SAL are the efficiency with which it works in fibrous areas and the ease of operation for the surgeon. There is no particular salvage of fibroconnective tissue or neurovascular structures as there is with UAL. The main advantage of PAL over UAL is the lack of heat generation; however, UAL has been shown to be safe and effective when the surgeon is properly trained and the procedure is properly performed.[5] PAL is an excellent tool for surgeons who remain uncomfortable with the potential for heat associated with UAL.

MARKING AND POSITIONING

Preoperative markings provide an important "topographic map" that allows the surgeon to visualize the targeted convexities, to avoid concavities, and to address asymmetries when the patient is lying on the operating table. Markings should be done immediately before surgery with the patient in a standing position. A permanent marking pen is recommended so the markings will not wash off when the patient is prepared. Asymmetries should be carefully marked and brought to the attention of the patient. Depressions and indentations are marked with a different color marker so these areas can be avoided (Fig. 126-2).

Positioning should be planned before the patient enters the operating room and depends on which areas are being suctioned. Most body areas can be suctioned from the prone and supine positions; however, some

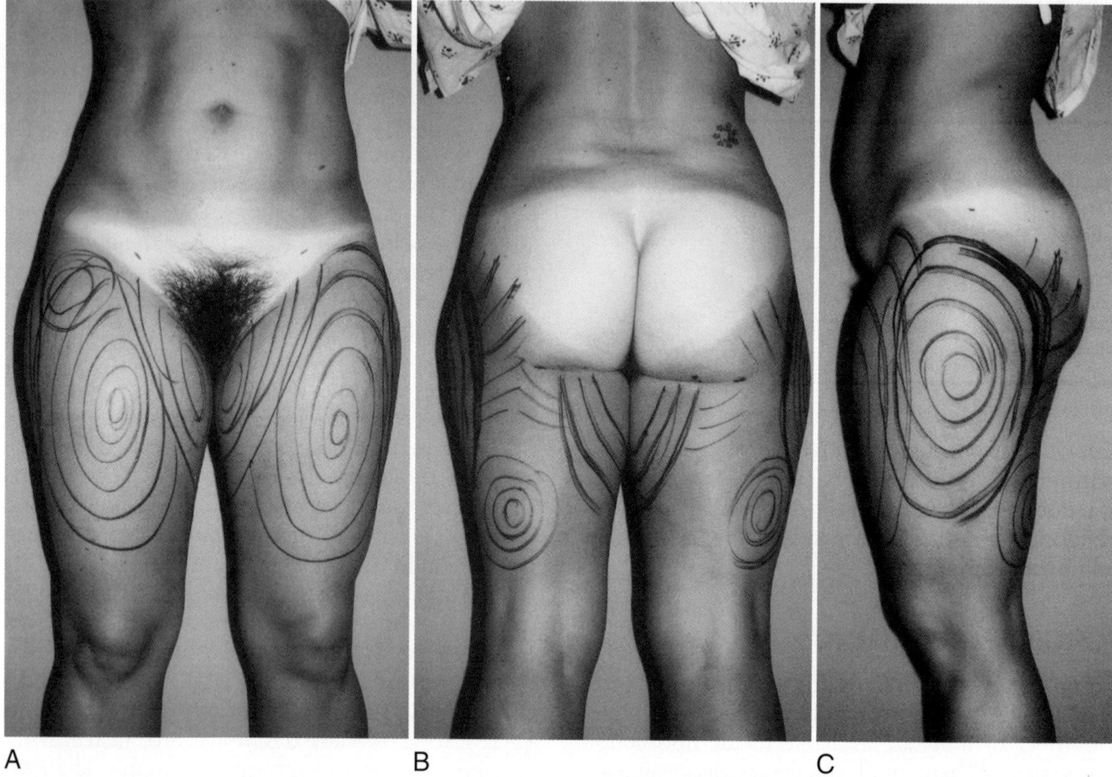

FIGURE 126-2. *A,* Surgical markings for circumferential thigh liposuction. Groin incisions are made about 2 cm more cephalad and more lateral than those usually made for medial thigh liposuction. This allows better access to the anterior thigh (postoperative result is shown in Figure 126-10). *B,* Two incisions are usually required in the gluteal crease, one for the posterior medial thigh area and one for the lateral thigh and posterior thigh. This patient does not have a significant banana roll deformity and does not need a lot of posterior thigh work. *C,* A stab incision for a 3.0- or 3.7-mm SAL cannula is made at the midaxillary line for feathering. This is an important incision to blend the prone and supine "operations."

surgeons prefer the lateral decubitus position for the hips and lateral thighs. When several body areas are being suctioned, an intraoperative position change is often necessary. With use of local anesthesia, it often makes sense to prepare the patient circumferentially in the standing position and then lying down on a sterile drape; the patient is rotated on the operating table as necessary throughout the procedure. With general anesthesia, the patient is first prepared in the prone position, which allows easy access to the back, flanks, buttocks, lateral thighs, and posterior aspect of the entire lower extremity. The patient is then turned to the supine position and re-prepared and draped. The abdomen, breasts, arms, and anterior aspect of the lower extremity can be addressed from this position.

Patients are prepared with a 3-minute povidone-iodine (Betadine) scrub, followed by povidone-iodine paint. Bair Hugger warming blankets are recommended on unexposed body parts, and a Foley catheter should be placed when aspirations of more than 5 liters are planned. When liposuction is combined with an open surgical procedure or when large-volume liposuction is performed, compression hose and sequential compression boots for prophylaxis of deep venous thrombosis are recommended whenever feasible.

WETTING SOLUTION

The importance of infiltration of wetting solution cannot be stressed enough (Table 126-3). The total amount of lidocaine infused per patient should never exceed the maximum recommended subcutaneous dose of 35 mg/kg.[6] The maximum dose for each patient should be calculated at the beginning of the procedure. If more infiltrate is needed once the maximum dose has been reached, lidocaine can be left out of the final bags when general anesthesia is used. Lidocaine is still recommended in addition to general anesthesia because it decreases the general

TABLE 126-3 ✦ STANDARD WETTING SOLUTION

Local Anesthesia	General Anesthesia
1 liter lactated Ringer solution	1 liter lactated Ringer solution
1 ampule epinephrine (1 : 1000)	1 ampule epinephrine (1 : 1000)
50 mL 1% lidocaine	30 mL 1% lidocaine

anesthesia requirements and provides some postoperative analgesia.

Wetting solution can be infused by a superwet or tumescent technique. The superwet technique involves infiltration of approximately 1 mL of wetting solution for every 1 mL of fat plus infiltrate removed. The tumescent technique involves infiltration of 2 or 3 mL for every 1 mL of fat plus infiltrate removed. This technique was originally developed as a method of local anesthesia and works well for this purpose when smaller volumes are removed; however, the risk of pulmonary edema and difficulties with fluid management become issues when larger volume liposuction is performed. Approximately 70% of infiltrated fluid will be absorbed.[7]

The infiltration technique used is especially important. An uneven infiltration of wetting solution increases the chances of an uneven final result. The infiltration process allows the surgeon to "feel" the tissue planes and the thickness of fat. Infiltration is begun in the deepest plane to be suctioned and proceeds in a systematic fashion from deep to superficial. Each layer or plane should be evenly infiltrated before slowly moving a bit more superficial. The infiltrated fat should be evenly firm with no disproportionate bulges in the skin at the end of the infiltration process. "Peau d'orange" infiltration of the subdermal fat is not necessary unless the goal is superficial liposuction.

It is common practice in some operating rooms to warm the wetting solution to body temperature before infiltration. During ultrasonic liposuction, the tissue warms 1° for every minute of ultrasonic energy use[8]; therefore, the fluid should not be warmed before infusion. It has been well documented that when room-temperature wetting solution is infused and proper technique is used, there is no significant elevation of subcutaneous temperature above core body temperature.[5]

More specific details in regard to anatomic variations with gender, selection of patients, positioning, and surgical technique are outlined in the following sections.

TRUNK

Variations with Gender

Men and women differ in their usual fat distribution. Men tend to accumulate fat centrally and generally take on an apple shape with advancing age and weight gain. The ideal male contour has a gradual taper between the lower ribs and the iliac crest, with no flair at the crest. In the midline, men rarely have isolated extra-abdominal convexity below the umbilicus but rather tend to accumulate fat intra-abdominally. The superficial fascial system zone of adherence is at the iliac crest[9] in men, and excess extra-abdominal fat tends to accumulate above this in the "spare-tire" distribution (Fig. 126-3).

It is imperative to assess whether abdominal protuberance is due to extra-abdominal fat, intra-abdominal fat, or a combination of both. Rectus diastasis, generalized fascial weakness, and isolated intra-abdominal fat all occur in men and are not amenable to liposuction. Fascial weakness or diastasis may be due to weightlifting, large weight fluctuations, or genetic predisposition. Extra-abdominal fat is diagnosed by the traditional pinch test. In addition, it is helpful to have the patient lie down to see how much of the abdominal protuberance disappears. The abdomen should be examined for hernia or diastasis with the patient in the supine position. Instruct the patient to raise his feet off the examining table, keeping ankles and knees together with the legs straight. A diastasis or hernia will bulge anteriorly with the increase in intra-abdominal pressure. The diastasis or weakness can sometimes be addressed by an endoscopic plication.[10] When this is combined with liposuction, the patient can sometimes avoid the need for a full abdominoplasty.

Liposuction is an excellent tool for male body contouring. The dermis tends to be thick and generally retracts well. The fatty tissue tends to be more fibrous, making UAL or PAL especially advantageous. Hair on the chest and abdomen hides scars nicely.

Female fat distribution is entirely different from that of the male. Women tend to accumulate fat in the lower abdomen, hips, and thighs, giving them more of a pear shape as opposed to an apple shape. They have a lower superficial fascial system zone of adherence, situated laterally approximately 5 cm below the iliac crest near the greater trochanter of the femur, separating the hip from the lateral thigh[9] (see Fig. 126-3). In the ideal aesthetic female contour, the "waistline" between the lower ribs and the iliac crest is concave. In the midline, there is generally a concavity above and a slight convexity below the umbilicus. In general, women tend to accumulate fat extra-abdominally and more diffusely than men do. The same abdominal examination is recommended to assess fascial integrity, to estimate intra-abdominal fat, and to diagnose the presence of a rectus diastasis.

The female body may also have to bear the added extremes of pregnancy. Some women lose abdominal wall integrity after multiple pregnancies. There may be numerous striae in the periumbilical area due to rapid weight fluctuations. Effective treatment may require a formal abdominoplasty with fascial plication. However, when skin integrity is good, liposuction offers an excellent method for removal of excess or abnormally distributed fat.

Abdomen

Excellent liposuction results are obtainable in the abdomen, but it can be an unforgiving area. Abdominal liposuction may be a poor choice in patients with poor skin quality, excessive or loose skin, or moderate to severe abdominal wall laxity. Patients with a pannus of skin and fat are particularly poor candidates. Although it is sometimes difficult to predict postoperative skin retraction, numerous striae generally indicate poor dermal quality and therefore poor retractile potential.

The abdomen possesses two distinct layers of fat, a superficial layer and a deep layer separated by Scarpa fascia. Below the umbilicus, the deep layer of fat is generally loose. Above the umbilicus, the deep layer of fat tends to be more dense and fibrotic. The superficial layer of fat is generally loose both above and below the umbilicus.

Preoperative marking is done in the usual topographic manner. It is important to discuss the aesthetic ideal with the patient preoperatively. Most patients want the lower abdomen as flat as possible. Some patients desire a sculpted waist with a flare at the iliac crest or hip; others desire a more gradual taper. This information will help guide the surgeon to sculpt the ideal form to suit the patient. Differences between the two sides are marked and demonstrated to the patient.

The patient is positioned supine on the operating table to suction the abdomen. The table can be jackknifed to allow better access to the upper abdomen and to help the surgeon avoid unintended penetration under the costal margins. Incisions are made on either side of the pubic area within the pubic hair and at the upper margin of the umbilicus. The dual suprapubic incisions allow good access, hidden scars, and crosshatching to help smooth the result. Infiltration of wetting solution is then undertaken (see earlier). Infiltration technique is nowhere more important than in the abdomen because penetration into the wrong plane in this area carries a high risk of morbidity. Careful infiltration above the abdominal fascia makes fascial perforation less likely. Starting the infiltration in the deepest plane, just above the fascia, is beneficial to orient the surgeon to the location of the fascia. The surgeon

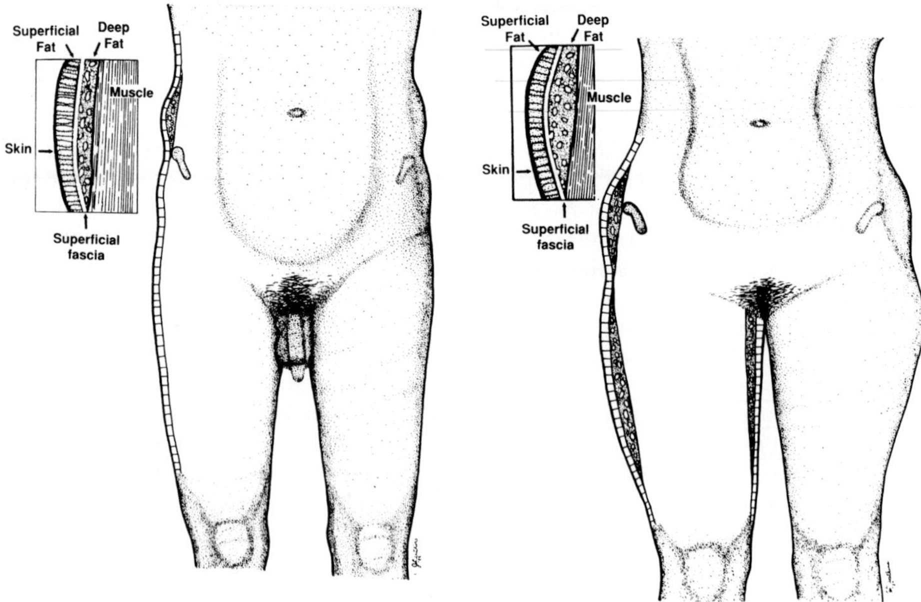

FIGURE 126-3. *A,* Diagram of superficial fascial system anatomic variations in men *(left)* and women *(right)*. The superficial fascial system zone of adherence is at the iliac crest in men and several centimeters inferior to the iliac crest in women. (From Lockwood T: Superficial fascial system [SFS] of the trunk and extremities: a new concept. Plast Reconstr Surg 1991;87:1011.)

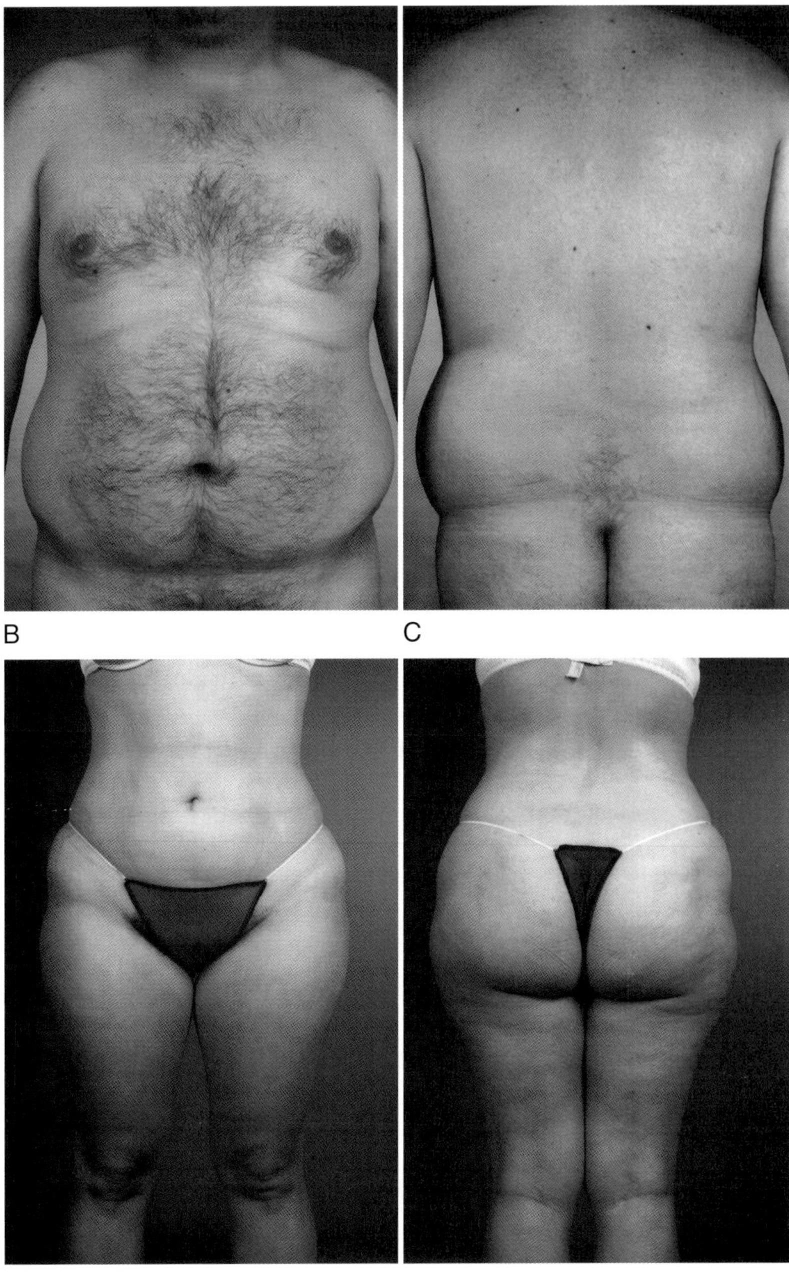

FIGURE 126-3, cont'd. *B* and *C,* Example of the superficial fascial system tightly adherent to the iliac crest in the man, forming the spare-tire body habitus. *D* and *E,* Example of the superficial fascial system that is tightly adherent to the muscle fascia several centimeters below the iliac crest in the woman, in line with the gluteal depression, forming the violin body habitus.

should pick up the skin and fat of the lower abdomen with his or her nondominant hand and insert the infiltration cannula just above the rectus fascia. The fat is then released and the infiltration proceeds in a radial fashion, from deep to superficial. The non-dominant hand rests gently on the surface of the area being infiltrated to guide the process.

Liposuction then proceeds parallel to the deep fascia. Fat is removed from both the deep and the superficial planes (above and below Scarpa fascia) according to the patient's deformity. There is generally significantly more deep fat than superficial fat. Crosshatching is particularly important in the abdomen because it tends to be a relatively large area. The most superficial 5 to 10 mm of subdermal fat should be left intact, except by the most experienced liposuction surgeons. This superficial fat helps maintain skin vascularity and hide contour irregularities.

Once final contouring is accomplished, the incisions are closed with interrupted nylon sutures. This does not provide an airtight closure, thus allowing fluid to egress from the wounds. A drain is sometimes recommended in the abdomen when ultrasonic energy is used for more than 20 to 25 minutes in the abdomen alone or when more than 2 liters of fat is removed from the abdomen.

Hips and Back

The hips (sometimes referred to as flanks) and back respond well to liposuction in both men and women. These are "forgiving" areas because the dermis is thick, the skin retracts well, and the fat tends to be fibrous. All these factors make contour irregularities less common in these areas.

It is important to evaluate the hips for asymmetry, which is not uncommon. If there is gross asymmetry between the two sides, the back should be evaluated for scoliosis because this may be the cause of the asymmetry. Obviously, bone asymmetry cannot be corrected with liposuction, but it can be compensated for or camouflaged. In the ideal posterior male waistline, there is a gradual taper from the ribs to the iliac crest. Fat accumulating above the iliac crest is commonly referred to as a love handle deformity and is a common reason for the male patient to seek a plastic surgery consultation. In the ideal female posterior waistline, there is a concavity between the chest and the hips, that is, the classic hourglass figure.

Moderately overweight women commonly complain about the excess fat along the "bra line" area of the back. Extra fat here bulges around the bra and tends to show through blouses and causes suit coats to pull. This area responds well to liposuction, especially ultrasonic liposuction. The dermis is thick and tolerates superficial liposuction that stimulates skin contraction. Liposuction of this area combined with liposuction of the hips can dramatically alter the body contour (Fig. 126-4).

The posterior hips and back are suctioned from the prone position. Some advocate use of the lateral decubitus position for the hip areas, but this is a matter of the surgeon's preference. The prone position allows intraoperative assessment of symmetry that is especially important to the novice liposuction surgeon. A cylindrical gel padding pillow (or a rolled blanket) placed under the patient's slightly flexed hip joint will raise the buttocks and hips off the table, thereby increasing exposure. Shoulders are extended, and the elbows are flexed (Fig. 126-5). Padding is placed under the axillae, elbows, knees, and feet. A Bair Hugger and antiembolism stockings are used on unexposed areas whenever appropriate. The patient is prepared to the anterior axillary line.

Incisions should be planned preoperatively. Back incisions should be made in the midline whenever possible. A lateral stab incision in the posterior axillary line, within the bra line or where it can be hidden by

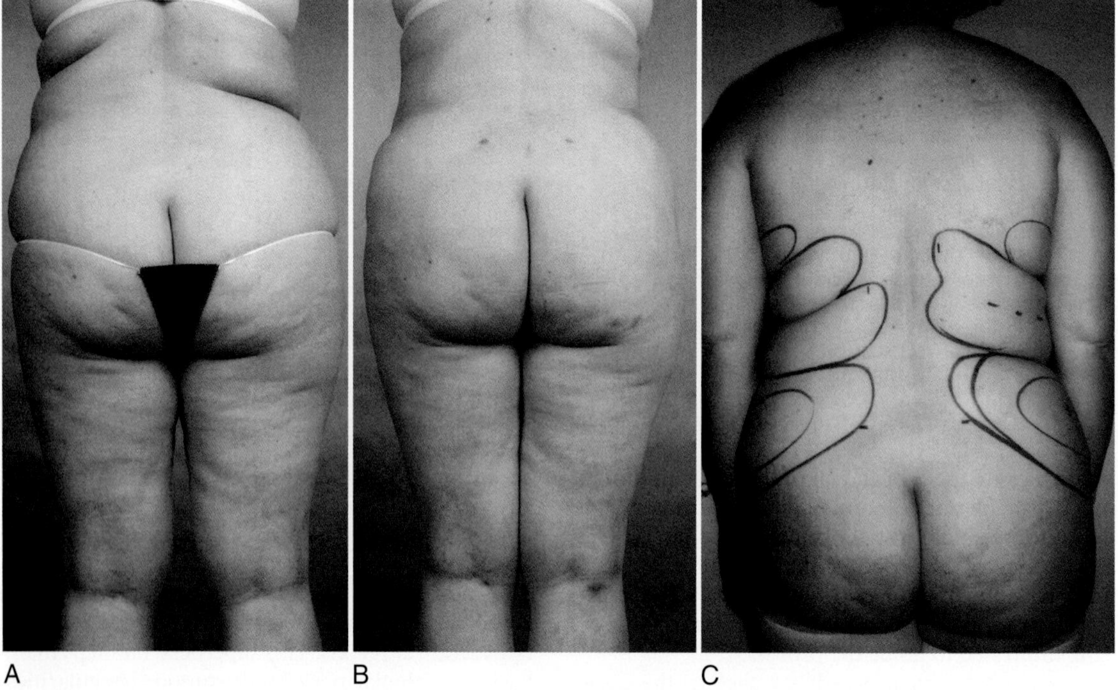

FIGURE 126-4. *A,* A 55-year-old woman shown before UAL. *B,* Postoperative views 4 months after UAL of the posterior hips and back. *C,* Surgical markings on the same patient indicate significant preoperative asymmetries.

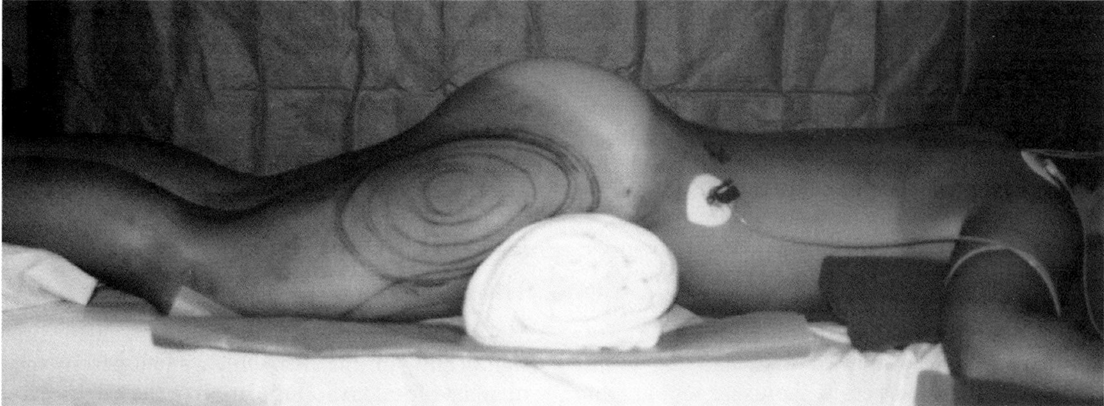

A

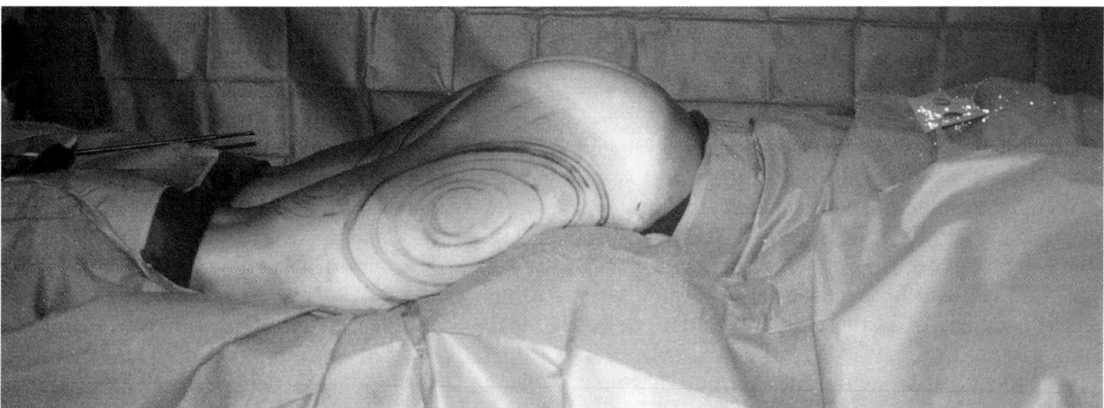

B

FIGURE 126-5. *A,* A rolled blanket or a gel positioning cylinder is placed under the patient's hips to raise them off the table. This allows preparation to the anterior axillary line. The shoulders should be extended and the elbows flexed. Proper padding is imperative. *B,* The patient is shown prepared for liposuction of lateral, posterior, and posterior medial thighs.

a one-piece bathing suit, can assist with lateral "feathering" when necessary. Feathering is the process of making a smooth transition between a treated and an adjacent nontreated area. It is important that the surgeon remember to "feather" his or her wetting solution as well as the liposuction itself. It is easier to blend into the adjacent nontreated areas when the wetting solution and liposuction are feathered.

Female hips can sometimes be approached through a single midline sacral incision, but larger patients usually require two parasacral incisions to achieve harmonious contour laterally. Because male flank lipodystrophy is usually directly above the iliac crest, a more lateral incision is usually required. As long as it is kept within the bathing suit or underwear line, the scar is usually not a problem. A true spare-tire deformity that extends both anterior and posterior to the iliac crest may need to be approached from both a supine and a prone position. One should be cautious not to overresect the male waistline, making it appear "too feminine." The aesthetic male waistline would be almost a straight line between the costal margins and the iliac crests, whereas the ideal female waistline is concave to form the classic female hourglass figure.

Gynecomastia

Gynecomastia describes abnormally large mammary glands in the man. The term derives from the Greek words *gyne,* meaning associated with women, and *mastos,* meaning breast. In true gynecomastia, the tissue present is histologically breast tissue; in pseudogynecomastia, the tissue is fatty in composition. Mixed gynecomastia is a combination of the two. Most patients with either kind of gynecomastia pursue treatment because of embarrassment by their feminine appearance.

Gynecomastia typically presents in three different age groups: neonates, pubertal boys, and adult men between the ages of 50 and 80 years. Breast enlargement occurs when there is a relative imbalance of estrogen and testosterone. Causative factors range from physiologic to endocrine to exogenous. In the majority of patients (25%), the disorder is idiopathic in origin. Exogenous medications may be a causative factor in 10% to 20% of all patients.[11,12] The majority of middle-aged or older men who present to the plastic surgeon for treatment of gynecomastia are simply overweight, whereas the younger population may have true gynecomastia or anabolic steroid-induced gynecomastia.

The breasts should be marked with the patient in the upright sitting position. The midline and the inframammary folds are marked first, and the breast mounds are then marked in the usual topographic manner. Incisions should be planned preoperatively so they can be discussed with the patient. Inframammary fold incisions are easiest for the surgeon, and if the patient has hair on his chest to hide scars, this is the access incision of choice. If the patient has no hair to hide scars or is very scar conscious, the axillary area is the best choice. The arms must be carefully abducted to avoid traction injury during surgery, and a roll between the shoulder blades to extend the shoulders out of the way (as in putting in a central line) is helpful if the patient has big shoulders. The periareolar incision is difficult and not recommended as a primary incision, especially if there is substantial breast parenchyma to be removed from the subareolar area. If the patient has a significant amount of breast parenchyma, it is wise to get a consent for *possible* open excision through a small periareolar incision, although this is rarely necessary.

The breasts are suctioned with the patient in the supine position, with the arms abducted at approximately 90 degrees. It is helpful to sit the patient up during the procedure to assess whether the inframammary folds "redrape" appropriately after the suctioning. Ultrasonic liposuction or power-assisted liposuction is extremely helpful in this setting. The breast parenchyma can be extremely dense and the fibroconnective tissue very tight, making traditional liposuction with a blunt cannula frustrating and inefficient. The squared off "golf tee" titanium cannula with a single distal hole (LySonix) is a relatively aggressive cannula at higher than average ultrasonic generator settings and can be used as a "cutting cannula" to dissect breast tissue in the appropriate clinical setting. In mixed and true gynecomastia, the ultrasonic energy can be increased, allowing controlled destruction and removal of the denser parenchyma. The improved efficiency of UAL in the treatment of dense, fibrous areas requires less physical effort, allowing the surgeon to attend to more precise contouring.

In general, men request that the breast area be made as flat as possible; however, it is important that the contour remain consistent with the overall body habitus. In true and mixed gynecomastia, the densest parenchyma is found under the areola. Overresection of this area can cause what is known as a saucer deformity, which is extremely difficult to revise. Drains should be placed when a large resection (1 liter of fat and fluid removed per side) is performed or when the skin is particularly loose (Fig. 126-6).

LOWER EXTREMITY

Thighs

Male and female fat distribution also differs significantly in this area. Only a small percentage of men have focal fat accumulation in the thighs, except for the rare man with a gynecoid body habitus. In contrast to the woman, the man rarely demonstrates cellulite. Male adipose tissue tends to be more fibrous, with more fibroconnective tissue and tighter connective tissue spaces, so that less fat can bulge between the tight fibrous septa to give the dimpled cellulite appearance. Women, on the other hand, accumulate fat more diffusely in the thigh, either in a circumferential pattern or focally along the medial and lateral thigh.

Common terms used to describe deformities of the thigh area are *saddlebag*, a trochanteric bulge lateral to the gluteal crease; *banana roll*, a preoperative or postoperative roll of fat inferior to the gluteal fold; and *violin deformity*, a particular female contour that includes a narrow waist, full hips, and full lateral thighs with a depression in the zone of adherence between the hips and thighs (Fig. 126-7; see also Fig. 126-3*D* and *E*).

Women commonly form cellulite in the thigh area, and it is often their chief complaint during a liposuction consultation. Lockwood[9] describes two kinds of cellulite. Primary cellulite, or cellulite of adiposity, is attributed to hypertrophied superficial fat. This type of cellulite is generally improved with weight loss but not necessarily with liposuction. Secondary cellulite, or cellulite of laxity, results from laxity of the skin and soft tissues and is correctable with surgical lifting procedures. Unrealistic expectations for cellulite reduction are common. Liposuction can improve contour and soften cellulite by decreasing the fat load within the fibrous connective tissue, but even superficial liposuction cannot "cure" cellulite. It is wise not to promise any improvement in cellulite. If improvement does occur, the patient will be pleased. If there is no improvement, the patient has not been encouraged to have this expectation.

Preoperative marking is accomplished in the usual topographic manner, with particular care taken to mark asymmetries and zones of adherence. Because the thigh is a particularly difficult area to sculpt, with multiple neighboring zones of adherence, it is also helpful to mark areas that may need special attention

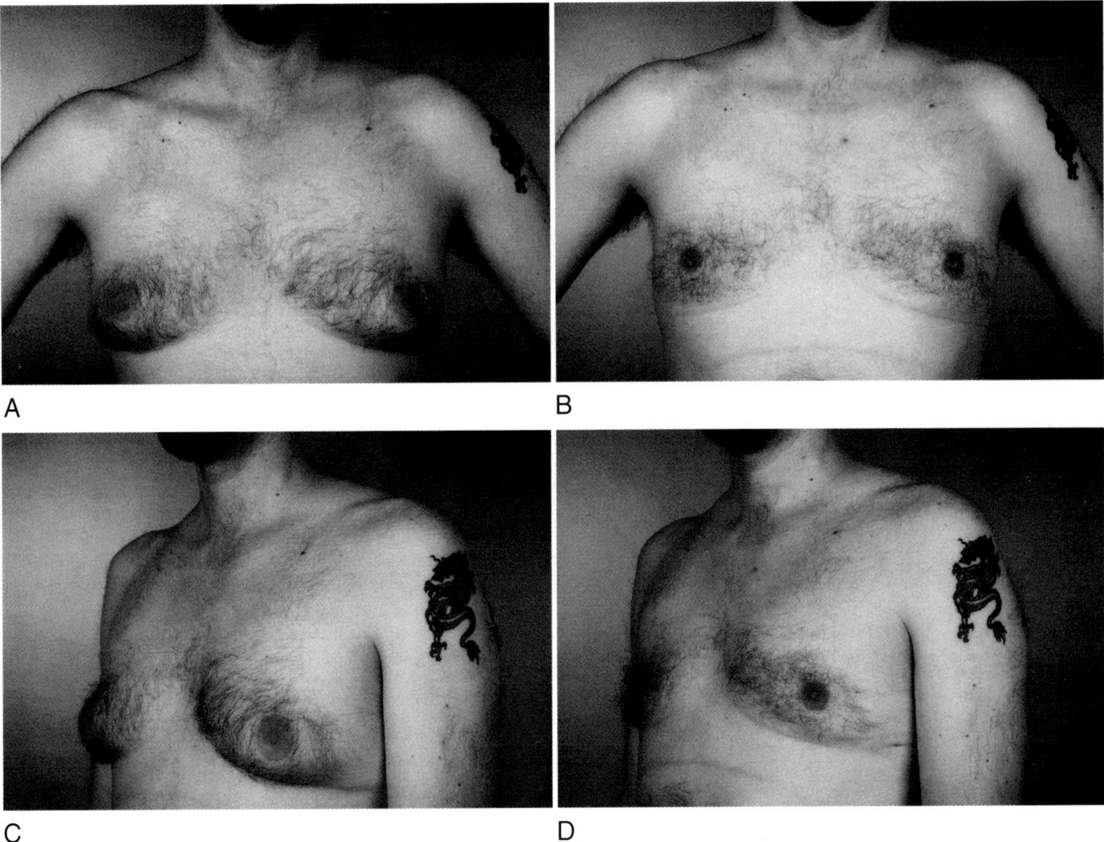

FIGURE 126-6. *A* and *C*, An otherwise healthy man with mixed gynecomastia (deformity consists of breast tissue and fat) shown before UAL. *B* and *D*, Postoperative views 1 year after UAL of both breasts.

to feathering. For example, the lateral thigh must be blended with the adjacent hip, buttocks, and anterior and posterior thigh.

LATERAL AND POSTERIOR THIGH

The lateral thigh can be suctioned from the prone or the lateral decubitus position. The prone position allows intraoperative assessment of symmetry between the two sides while you work, but some think there is encumbrance at the anterior axillary line. The lateral decubitus position gives an unencumbered lateral work area but does not allow the surgeon to see both sides at the same time and usually requires an extra intraoperative position change if the supine position is also necessary. Incisions are placed in the lateral gluteal crease and along the midaxillary line at the level of the fascial adherence (or within the bathing suit line, whichever is more acceptable to the patient). Smaller stab incisions are made to help SAL contouring where needed. UAL is recommended for most moderately sized to large lateral thighs. However, in thinner women, who may lack a lateral gluteal crease, one should consider use of SAL alone to avoid the larger, visible incision. The appropriate plane is intermediate or deep in the lateral thigh, and it should become superficial only when skin retraction is particularly important.

The posterior thigh, especially the banana roll area, should be approached with caution. Most authors recommend that the gluteal crease *not* be crossed with the liposuction cannula. The area of the posterior thigh just under the gluteal fold is a common area for postoperative contour problems caused by overresection. Overresection in this area can lead to secondary gluteal ptosis that is difficult to correct with anything short of a lower body lift. The posterior thigh can, however, be successfully suctioned. The key is to be conservative. It is best to stay superficial in the banana roll area. Suctioning too deep may lead to loss of support and subsequent ptosis of the buttocks.

MEDIAL THIGH

Women commonly accumulate fat along the anteromedial and posteromedial aspects of the upper thighs. Patients complain that their "legs rub together" when they walk or that their "jeans pull" at their inner thighs.

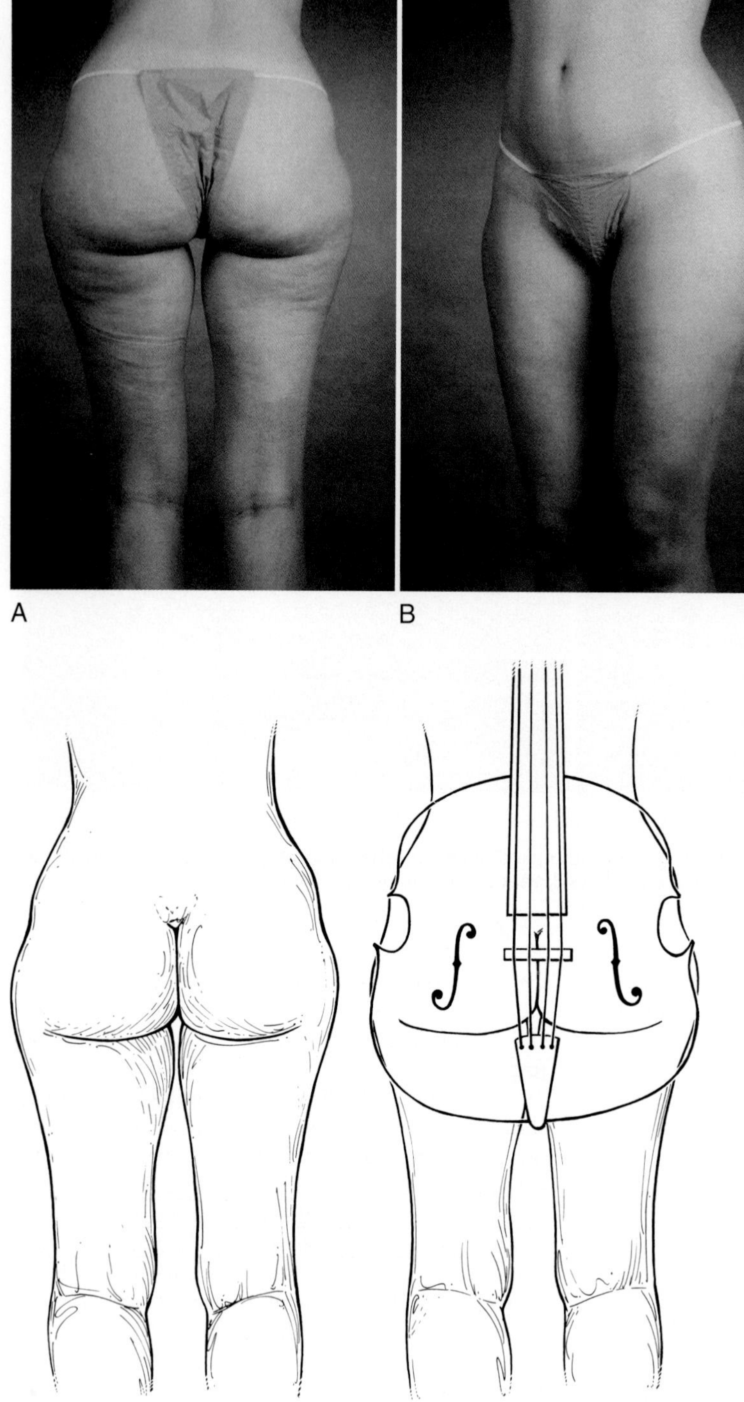

FIGURE 126-7. *A* and *B,* An otherwise healthy woman with classic saddlebag fat distribution. She has disproportionate fat over the trochanter area, just lateral to the gluteal crease. *C* and *D,* She also demonstrates the violin deformity, which refers to a narrow waist, full hips, and full lateral thighs with a depression in the zone of adherence between the hips and thighs.

The fat in this area tends to be soft and the skin is thin, making it easy to overresect. When overresection occurs, fat injection or a medial thigh lift may be necessary. The suction plane in the medial thigh is intermediate to superficial as opposed to deep. The vital structures in the medial thigh (femoral vessels and lymphatics) lie in the deep plane and can be avoided by staying more superficial. The planes here are not defined by any named fascial layers but are "relative" planes. Smaller cannulas such as a 3.0-mm Mercedes tip are used for most work, and a 2.4-mm cannula can be used for feathering.

The medial thigh is suctioned from the supine position. It is helpful to prepare the patient in such a way that the leg can be positioned outstretched and flat on the operating table and also in the frog-leg position (abducted and externally rotated). This usually involves a circumferential preparation with a stockinette on the calf and ankle. The primary incision is made in the upper groin crease, and the suctioning is performed with the leg lying flat as well as in the frog-leg position. An additional incision is made at the distal two thirds of the medial thigh to allow crosshatching and access to the posteromedial thigh lipodystrophy. The posteromedial fat can also be accessed from the prone position through a medial gluteal crease incision (Figs. 126-8 and 126-9).

ANTERIOR AND CIRCUMFERENTIAL THIGH

The anterior thigh has been considered a taboo area for liposuction by many authors, yet it is a fairly common area of lipodystrophy. Although the anterior thigh can be successfully treated as an isolated area, it is most commonly treated as part of circumferential thigh lipodystrophy. The primary indications for circumferential thigh liposuction are circumferential thigh lipodystrophy and the inability to achieve harmony with the upper body by spot liposuction.

The circumferential thighs are suctioned first from the prone and then from the supine position. The

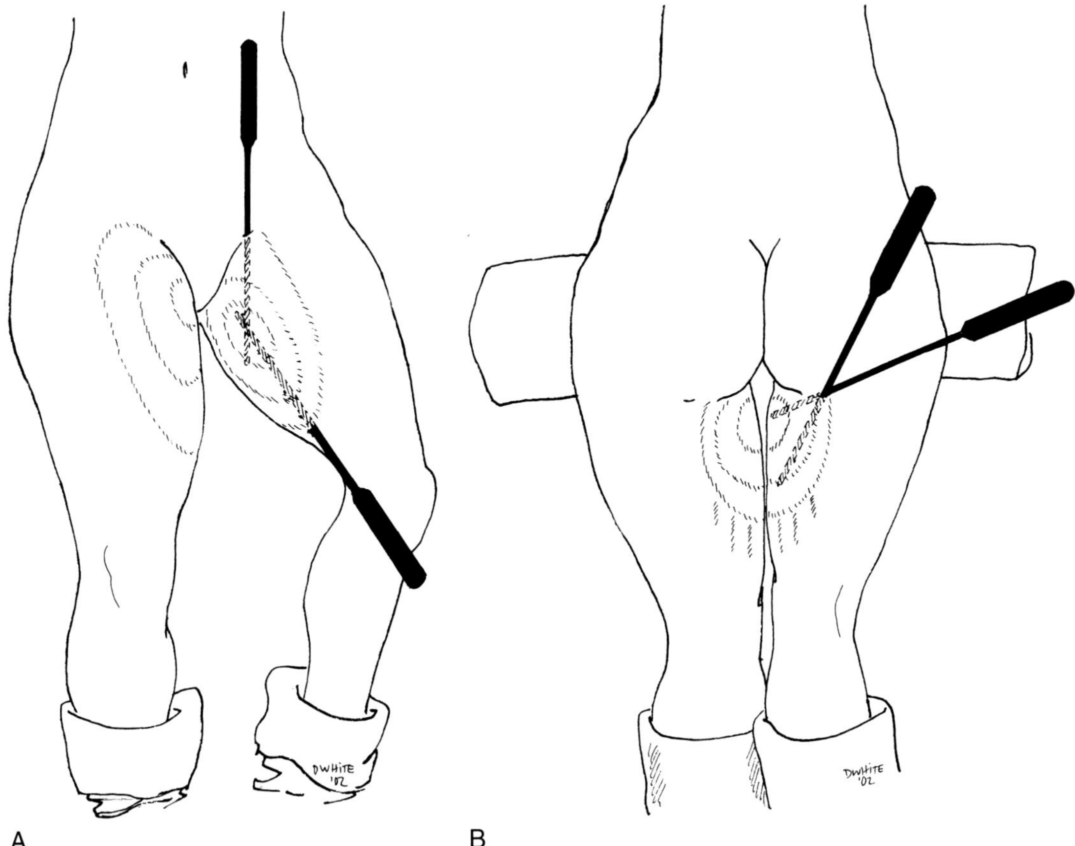

FIGURE 126-8. *A,* The primary access incision for medial thigh liposuction is in the upper groin crease. The patient's legs should be prepared so that they can be abducted and externally rotated. This usually involves a circumferential preparation as shown. An additional incision is made at the distal two thirds of the medial thigh to allow crosshatching and access to the posterior fat. *B,* The posteromedial thigh fat can also be accessed from the prone position through a medial gluteal crease incision.

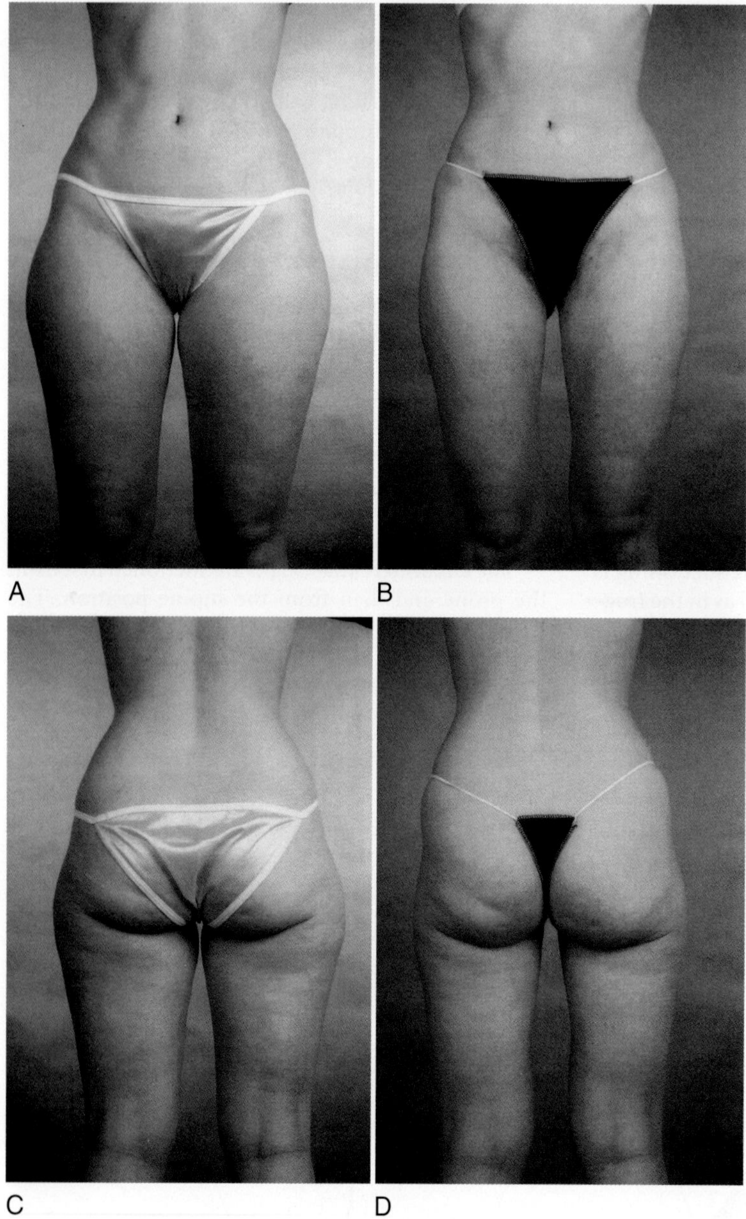

FIGURE 126-9. *A* and *C*, A 30-year-old woman shown before liposuction of the medial and lateral thighs. *B* and *D*, Postoperative views 6 months after traditional SAL of the medial thighs and UAL of the lateral thighs.

lateral, posterior, and posteromedial thighs are suctioned with the patient prone, with a hip roll under the greater trochanters to allow exposure of the lateral thighs (see Fig. 126-5). The patient is then turned to the supine position and re-prepared and draped. Groin incisions to access the anterior thighs are made about 2 cm more cephalad and 2 cm more lateral than the usual access incisions for medial thigh liposuction (see Fig. 126-2). In suctioning the anterior thighs, it may be helpful to jackknife the operating table to move the patient's trunk out of the way of the backstroke of the surgeon's cannula. This allows the surgeon to keep the cannula parallel to the underlying quadriceps musculature. Small stab incisions can be made distally wherever needed to feather from below with a 3.0-mm Mercedes tip cannula (Fig. 126-10).

Although there is no specifically named superficial fascial plane in the thigh analogous to Scarpa fascia in the trunk, the anterior thigh should be suctioned in the "deep" plane, preferably with UAL or a small SAL cannula. The superficial plane is extremely unforgiving, especially in the distal third of the anterior thigh, which should be approached conservatively. Overly aggressive suction here can lead to ptosis of the skin

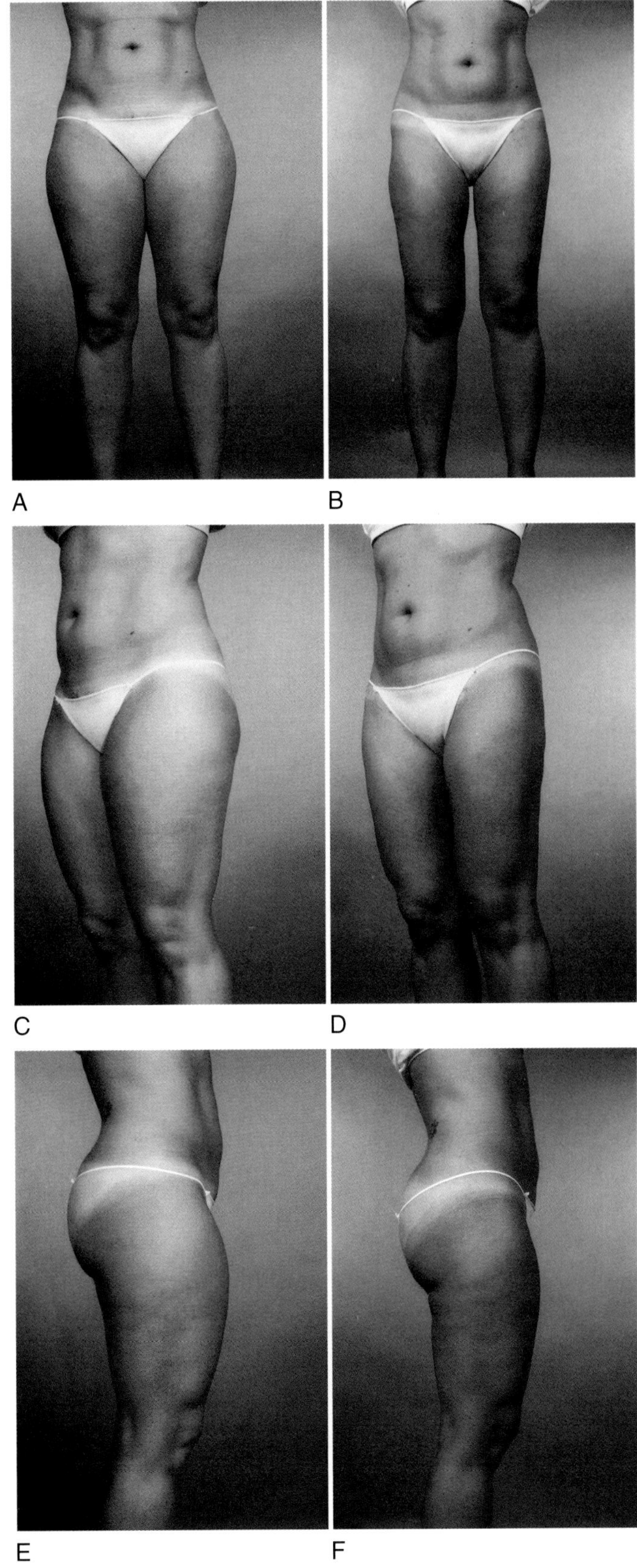

FIGURE 126-10. *A, C,* and *E,* A 26-year-old woman shown before circumferential thigh liposuction. *B, D,* and *F,* Postoperative views 6 months after circumferential thigh UAL. Preoperative markings of this patient are shown in Figure 126-2. Intraoperative positioning photographs of this patient are shown in Figure 126-5.

and rhytids, which are extremely unsightly and not amenable to correction even by aggressive lifting procedures.

Knees, Calves, and Ankles

Women commonly complain of excess fat along the medial and anterior aspects of the knee. The fat here is soft and removed easily. Below the knee, lipodystrophy is less common, and when it does occur, most women report it "runs in the family." Lipodystrophy in the calf and ankle area, like anywhere else on the body, should be diagnosed by physical examination including palpation and the pinch test. One must be certain that "oversized" calves and ankles are not simply well-developed muscles and large bones.

Patients may complain that their lower legs lack definition or that their calves look like "tree trunks" or "sausages." Interestingly, the skin seems to be much more adherent to the underlying musculofascial layers below the knee than above the knee. Although the skin is not particularly thick in this area, it retracts surprisingly well, perhaps because of the relatively dense fibroconnective tissue that encases the fat. This is consistent with the general lack of cellulite below the knee.

Marking is done in the routine topographic manner. If the calves are not being suctioned and there is a fat pad in the medial subpatellar area, suctioning of this area will significantly improve the aesthetics of the knee area (Fig. 126-11). The most common technical error in suctioning the knees is to overresect along the medial knee, making the medial leg contour too straight, with no shape at all.

The knees are suctioned with the patient in the supine position, after the legs have been prepared circumferentially. It is helpful to be able to abduct the legs as well as to place the patient in the frog-leg position during suctioning of this area. Small stab incisions can be made with impunity because they heal well (see Fig. 126-11).

The calves and ankles should be marked with the patient in the standing position. It is the surgeon's job to unmask or to establish definition in lower legs that lack definition. Posteriorly, the medial and lateral heads of the gastrocnemius muscle represent an "anatomic unit" of the calf. In the ankle area, the Achilles tendon may need to be "excavated" from under a fatty layer. Anteromedially, the lower leg is relatively flat over the tibia, whereas anterolaterally, it is smoothly curved over the anterior compartment.

The calves and ankles can be suctioned entirely from the supine position, with the patient prepared and draped circumferentially. When circumferential thighs are being suctioned at the same time, it is advisable to begin the procedure in the prone position and suction the posterior calves from the prone position, then finish the procedure from the supine position.

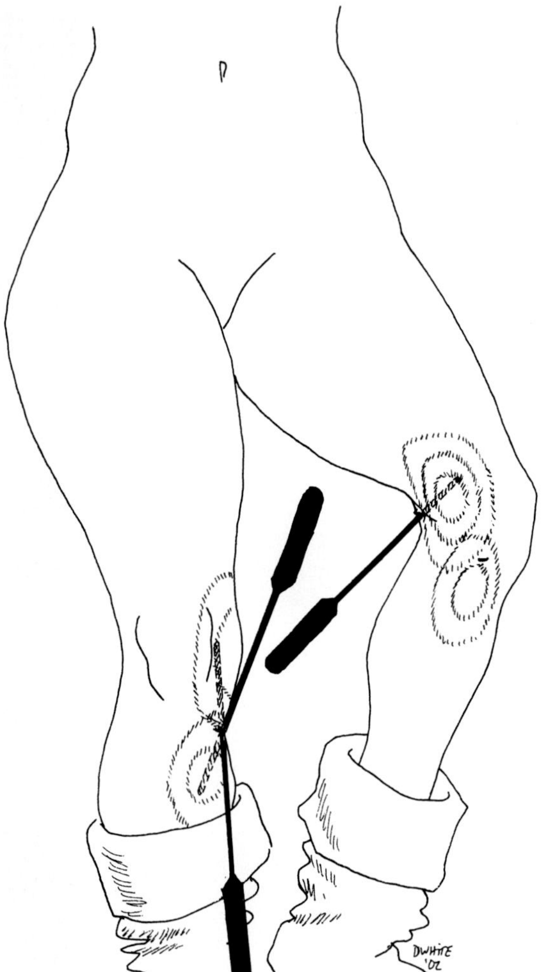

FIGURE 126-11. Small stab incisions can be made at the posteromedial knee or the anteromedial knee as shown. These incisions allow access to the medial knee as well as to the medial subpatellar area. Suctioning of the subpatellar area can significantly improve the aesthetics of the lower leg.

Multiple small incisions will be required, and it is helpful to bend the liposuction cannulas to maneuver around curves. Small traditional liposuction cannulas, such as 3.0- and 2.4-mm Mercedes tip cannulas, are recommended. UAL and PAL are of little added value in the knee, calf, or ankle area. Traditional SAL is the best tool to suction the knees, calves, and ankles.

PERIOPERATIVE PRINCIPLES

The most common question asked by the beginning liposuction surgeon is, How do I know when an area is done? There are signals, other than volume, that indicate completion. Visual cues are the most important:

an area is "done" when optimal contour has been achieved. The area being suctioned must be carefully watched because the surgeon should be aware of the "goal" contour. The infiltration of wetting solution has become a standard tool in almost all forms of lipoplasty, but it does distort the final contour to some degree. The goals of the liposuction surgeon are to remove specifically targeted fat, to leave a smooth body contour without deep or superficial contour irregularity, and to establish a smooth transition between the suctioned and the nonsuctioned areas.

The pinch test is another tool to help assess whether an area is nearing completion. It is important to do the pinch test preoperatively to know the starting thickness. Pinching or rolling the remaining subcutaneous tissue between one's fingers will also assist the surgeon in finding missed adipose pockets or uneven areas of resection.

Final contouring is routinely done at the end of the liposuction procedure. The surgeon may use saline to wet the skin and glide his or her hand over the surface to assist in finding small irregularities. Smaller diameter cannulas (2.5 or 3.0 mm) will usually be chosen to do the final contouring and feathering. The old adage "the enemy of good is better" should be remembered when the final contouring step is completed. Overresection can occur quickly while chasing small contour irregularities.

POSTOPERATIVE COURSE

Once the final contouring is performed, the incisions are closed. Incisions for cannulas larger than 3.0 mm are generally closed with a 5-0 nylon suture. Some surgeons recommend leaving smaller incisions open to allow wetting solution to drain. The patient is dressed in a compression garment that covers the areas that have been suctioned. Compression foam (TopiFoam) under the garment seems to decrease bruising and swelling in the early postoperative period. An abdominal binder and compression foam can be used when the hips and abdomen are suctioned alone. When thigh work is done as well, a girdle is preferable.

When drains are used, they are left in place until drainage is less than 30 mL in a 24-hour period. Foam padding should be left in place for 3 to 5 days. Compression garments are generally encouraged 23 hours per day for 4 weeks. Patients are warned that with larger volume liposuction, some will experience lightheadedness (a vasovagal response) the first time the garment is removed. Therefore, it is important that someone accompany the patient for the first dressing change.

Patients are instructed to remove their garments or foam and to take a shower after 1 to 3 days, depending on the amount of suction performed. When one or two areas are suctioned, the patient can typically replace the foam padding over the liposuctioned areas and replace the garment after the shower. When multiple areas are suctioned, it is often better to perform the first dressing change in the office.

Postoperative follow-up visits are scheduled at 5 days, 2 weeks, 6 weeks, 3 months, and 6 months. The patient will experience red-tinged, serosanguineous drainage from incision sites for the first 24 to 36 hours. Maximal swelling can be expected during postoperative days 3 to 5. If the patient has bruising, it will usually resolve during 7 to 10 days.

The patient is instructed to begin lymphatic massage of the areas suctioned approximately 2 weeks after surgery. This reduces edema and helps reduce small contour irregularities. A referral to a massage therapist trained in Dr. Vodder's manual lymphatic drainage techniques[13] will instruct the patient on proper massage technique, and many patients may choose to continue with the massage therapist. Manual lymphatic drainage is a common technique used to treat lymphedema patients and is useful in the treatment of liposuction patients the first 4 to 6 weeks. Patients can expect approximately 80% of the edema to resolve within 4 to 6 weeks; it takes a full 4 to 6 months for all of the swelling to resolve.

Patients should begin ambulating on the day of surgery. Oral fluids and a high-protein diet should be encouraged. Physical activity should be low for the first week, followed by a gradual increase in activity during the second week, depending on the amount of suction performed. At the end of the first or second week (depending on the amount of suction), the patient should be encouraged to get on a treadmill or walk outside (with compression garments on). Upper body conditioning can also begin. At 4 to 6 weeks, assuming edema and bruising are resolving appropriately, the patient should be advancing to full activity. These guidelines are general and must be tailored to the individual patient.

Return to work depends on many factors: the patient's profession, the amount of liposuction, the patient's general health, the patient's physical and emotional recovery, and the patient's desire to return to work. After an average medium-volume liposuction (2 to 4 liters), most patients return to work in less than 1 week. They feel tired and sore but can function appropriately. For large-volume liposuction (>5 liters), the average patient should schedule 2 weeks off work. Many patients who schedule small-volume liposuction (<2 liters) desire surgery on Friday afternoon and plan to return to work on Monday. This can be done, but anecdotally, those patients who do not plan any "recovery time" seem to have a lot of early swelling and their eventual total recovery time is prolonged.

SUMMARY

Liposuction has become an extremely popular cosmetic procedure in today's body-conscious society. Technically, it is a simple procedure to perform *adequately;* however, true body contouring takes an artistic "eye" and the skill and experience to shape an "artistic vision" into a reality. When liposuction is thought of in the greater context of body contouring, it is truly an art form.

REFERENCES

1. American Society of Plastic Surgeons: 2003 Report of Procedural Statistics. Available at: http://www.plasticsurgery.org
2. Hughes CE 3rd: Patient selection, planning and marking in ultrasound-assisted lipoplasty. Clin Plast Surg 1999;26:279.
3. Pitman GH, Teimourian B: Suction lipectomy: complications and results by survey. Plast Reconstr Surg 1985;76:65.
4. Kenkel JM, Robinson JB Jr, Beran SJ, et al: The tissue effects of ultrasound-assisted lipoplasty. Plast Reconstr Surg 1998;102: 213.
5. Ablaza VJ, Gingrass MK, Perry LC, et al: Tissue temperatures during ultrasound-assisted lipoplasty. Plast Reconstr Surg 1998;102:534.
6. Klein JA: Tumescent technique for regional anesthesia permits lidocaine doses of 35 mg/kg for liposuction. J Dermatol Surg Oncol 1990;16:248.
7. Rohrich RJ, Beran SJ, Kenkel JM: Ultrasound-Assisted Liposuction. St. Louis, Quality Medical Publishing, 1998:80.
8. Commons G, Halperin B: Ultrasound-assisted lipoplasty: a clinical study of 250 consecutive patients [discussion]. Plast Reconstr Surg 1998;101:203.
9. Lockwood T: Superficial fascial system (SFS) of the trunk and extremities: a new concept. Plast Reconstr Surg 1991;87: 1009.
10. Lockwood T: Rectus muscle diastasis in males: primary indications for endoscopically assisted abdominoplasty. Plast Reconstr Surg 1998;101:1685.
11. Braunstein G: Gynecomastia. N Engl J Med 1993;328:490.
12. Carlson J: Gynecomastia. N Engl J Med 1980;303:795.
13. Wittlinger H, Wittlinger G: Textbook of Dr. Vodder's Manual Lymph Drainage, 4th ed. Basic Course, vol 1. Heidelberg, Haug, 1992.

CHAPTER

127

Body Contouring: Upper Extremity

PETER A. VOGT, MD, FRCS(C), FACS

The upper arms have always presented a major challenge to plastic and reconstructive surgeons. Brachial fat deposits and skin laxity are primarily seen in women. Little was published about this area until Gonzalez-Ulloa, Pitanguy, and others[1-9] began writing about skin resection procedures. Baroudi, Regnault, Teimourian, Hallock, and others[10-13] followed with excellent papers in the 1970s and 1980s. Again, these articles largely dealt with skin resections. Baroudi pioneered the principle of using shorter upper arm and axillary incisions, adding a new dimension to the approach in this area. With the introduction of liposuction in the late 1970s and early 1980s, a major new surgical tool became available to those surgeons treating patients with contour defects in the upper arm.

Upper arm fullness can occur at any age. There appears to be a familial tendency and an obvious association with weight gain. Lack of toning exercises may also contribute to fullness in the upper arm or subsequent laxity. Laxity is most commonly seen in people with significant weight loss or through the aging process when fat deposits tend to diminish, leading to development of the "bat wing deformity." Both fullness and laxity of upper arm skin can lead to discomfort when clothing with short sleeves is worn (Table 127-1). As patients (particularly women) reach the fourth and fifth decades of life, even if they have been thin most of their adult life, they can develop laxity of the upper arm that makes them reluctant to wear any garments that reveal it.

In previous reviews,[14-16] it became evident that surgeons had a great deal of discomfort when they were approached by patients requesting correction of upper arm deformities. An effort was made at that time to assist clinicians in the preoperative evaluation of upper arm problems to facilitate the selection of an operative plan. Obviously, upper arm scarring was previously and is still less than completely acceptable, except perhaps in the most extreme instances of upper arm flaccidity. Suction-assisted lipoplasty is obviously a much less invasive procedure and in many patients is effective in reducing upper arm diameter and volume, but it may also lead to increased wrinkling and skin flaccidity due to poor skin contraction. Many investigators (Pitman,[17] Teimourian,[18] Illouz,[19] Lockwood,[20] Gilliland[21,22]) concur that suction-assisted lipoplasty of the upper arm is a useful treatment modality, particularly in the posterior, superior, and deltoid regions, but that the medial portion of the upper arm must be respected for the thin subcutaneous fat layer that exists.

The author proposed the hypothesis in 1995 that in hereditary and idiopathic brachial enlargement, if lipoplasty is performed early enough, volume reduction and skin contraction may be permanent (Fig. 127-1). The hypothesis is proving to be accurate in familial enlargement of the upper arm. Whereas few surgeons performing body contouring would venture into the upper arm in the 1980s, suction-assisted lipoplasty of the upper arm has today become a frequently performed procedure that is not only safe but also effective.

Brachioplasties, however, still cause a great deal of discomfort for the surgeon. When patients arrive and ask for correction of a bat wing deformity, many surgeons may still envision subsequent long scars in the upper arm leading to the surgeon's and patient's dissatisfaction. Plastic surgeons are taught to achieve the best possible result in any operative procedure performed. This principle holds true in brachioplasty as

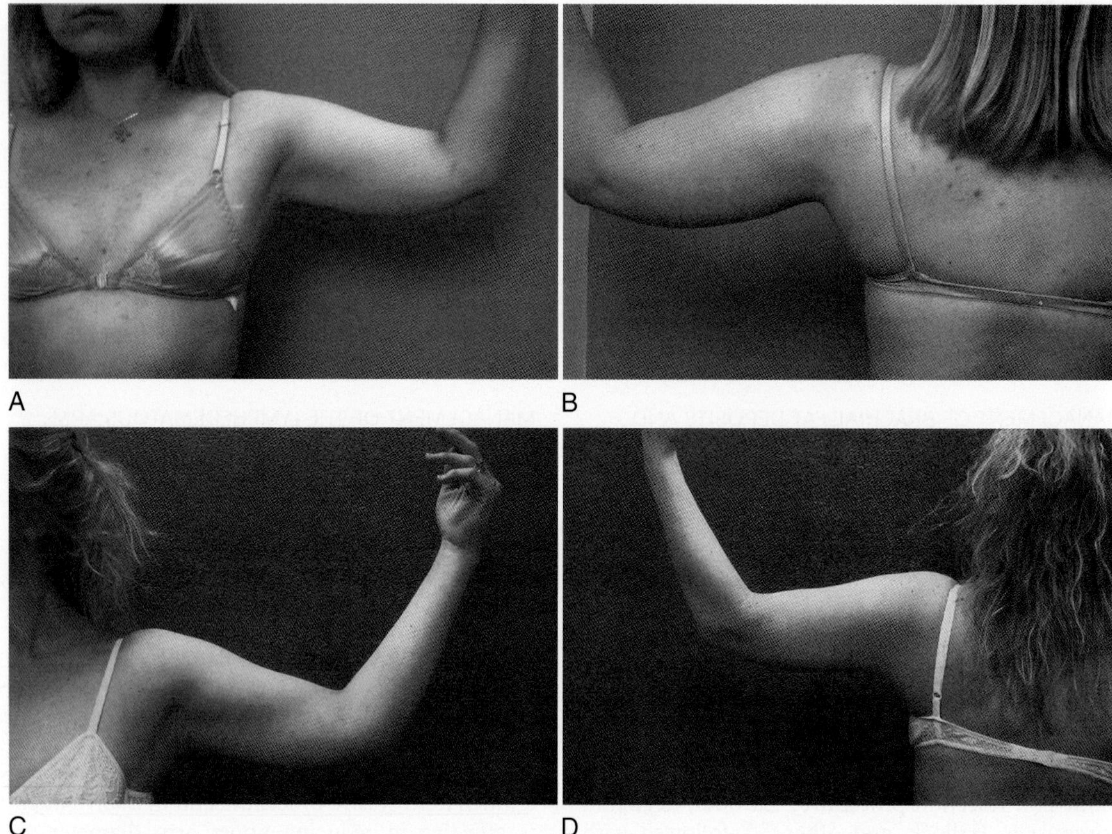

FIGURE 127-1. A 42-year-old woman with 350-mL suction-assisted lipoplasty of each upper arm. *A* and *B*, Preoperative views. *C* and *D*, Six years postoperatively with four pregnancies in the same 6-year interval. Note continued excellent skin contraction.

well; however, there is a need to reduce both the patient's and one's own expectations. By developing a better understanding of the patient's expectations and of which operative procedure to perform and with proper assessment of the upper arm, surgical results can be gratifying, even though they are far from perfect. One should know how to evaluate patients for upper arm surgery and how to devise a good surgical plan.

In most instances, brachial fat deposits and skin laxity are seen in women. Upper arm fat deposits are frequently recognized even in adolescence, particularly in teenagers and women in their 20s. This is commonly seen in women who seek breast reduction surgery (Fig. 127-2). In patients seeking breast reductions, there also appear to be increased fat deposits in the entire chest and upper arm area and shoulder region. When these women are questioned, there is often a hereditary component to the trunk and upper arm obesity.

TABLE 127-1 ✦ CAUSES OF BRACHIAL FAT DEPOSITS AND SKIN LAXITY

Heredity
Obesity
Aging
Postsurgical
Trauma
Medications (e.g., prednisone)
Idiopathic—figure fault

Aging and prolonged sun exposure to the upper arms contribute significantly to laxity of upper arm skin, even in women who have always maintained their weight at a fairly constant level and who have exercised throughout their adult life. This is most evident along the inferior border of the upper arm and in the axillary region as well and leads to frustration in trying to wear sundresses or gowns.

Postsurgical upper arm fullness is still seen despite the performance of fewer radical mastectomies. Brorson and Svensson[23-25] have discussed this extensively and have concluded that liposuction is effective in this population of patients.[14]

The major traumatic cause of brachial fat deposits is blunt trauma, resulting in a hematoma with an

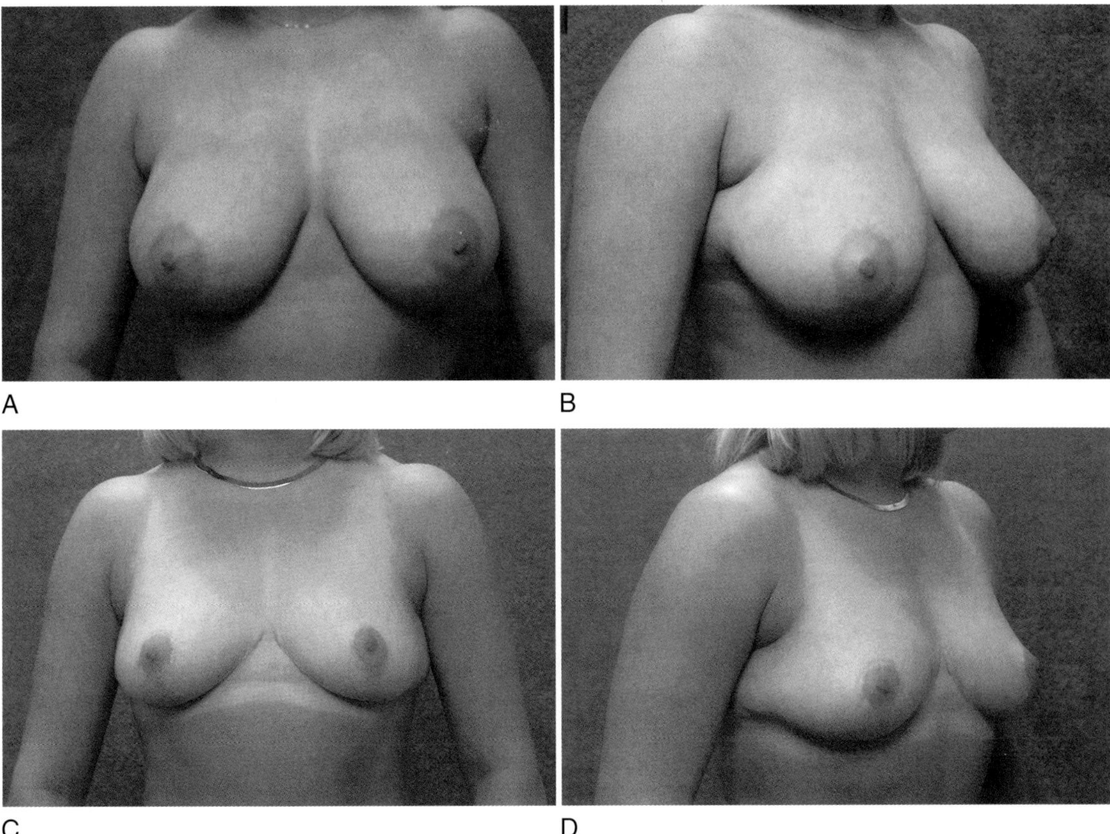

FIGURE 127-2. A 22-year-old woman: height, 5′4″; weight, 128 pounds. *A* and *B*, Preoperative views. *C* and *D*, Reduction mammaplasty. Suction-assisted lipoplasty of 200 mL of each upper arm, 6 months postoperatively. Note anterolateral arm and axillary fat deposits.

organized lipoma. Skin laxity can be caused by neuromuscular disorders, leading to atrophy of upper arm and shoulder girdle muscles.

MANAGEMENT OF BRACHIAL FAT DEPOSITS AND SKIN LAXITY

Classification

Classifications are useful in development of a treatment plan. There are four specific groups of patients who present with aesthetic upper arm complaints (Table 127-2).

Evaluation of the Patient

A good understanding of the proper evaluation of the upper arm is essential to development of a sound surgical plan. This in turn leads to greater comfort for the surgeon and patient. A thorough history is obtained (Table 127-3), and an extensive physical examination is performed.

The arm is observed in the resting position, with particular attention paid to the posterior lateral aspect of the arm, the deltoid region, and the para-axillary regions including the anterior and posterior axillary folds. In addition, the upper arm is examined in the victory position with the arm abducted 90 degrees and flexed 90 degrees at the elbow. In particular, observe the inferior border of the upper arm in this position and laxity in the para-axillary region.

TABLE 127-2 ✦ CLASSIFICATION OF BRACHIAL FAT DEPOSITS AND SKIN LAXITY

Group 1	Minimal to moderate subcutaneous fat with minimal skin laxity
Group 2	Generalized accumulation of subcutaneous fat with moderate skin laxity
Group 3	Generalized obesity and extensive skin laxity
Group 4	Minimal subcutaneous fat and extensive skin laxity

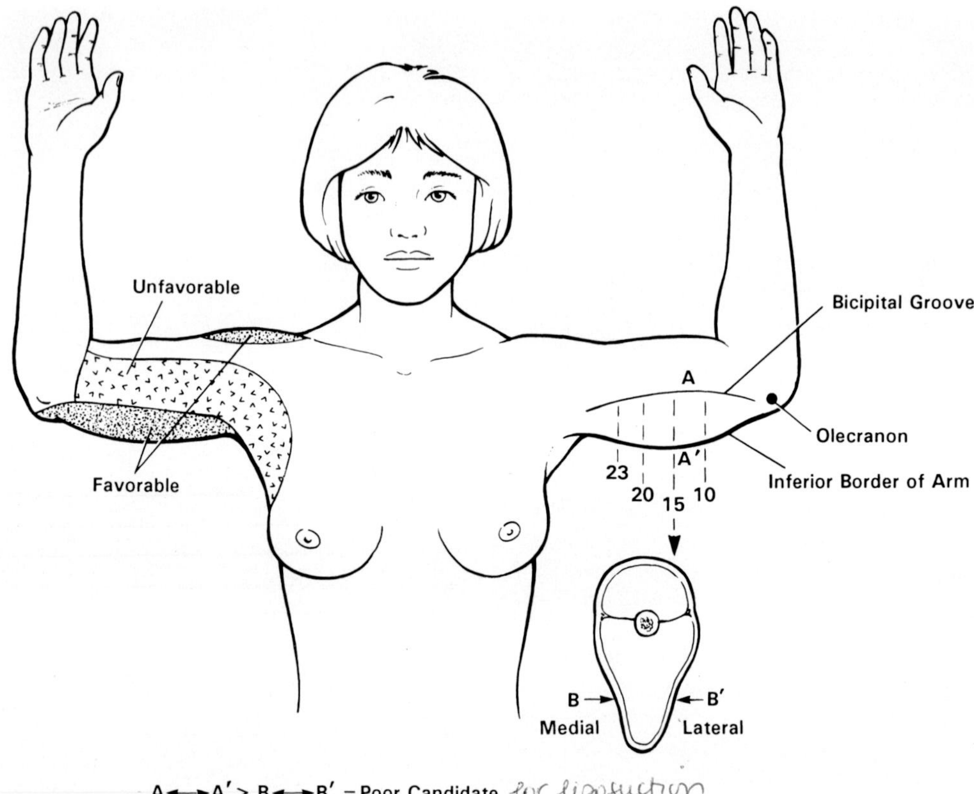

FIGURE 127-3. Preoperative measurements. Left arm: circumferential measurements and A-A' + B-B' at fixed points with use of the olecranon as an anatomic landmark. Right arm: areas of favorable and unfavorable suction-assisted lipoplasty are indicated.

PINCH TEST. The amount of fat in various portions of the shoulder girdle, para-axillary region, and upper arm is evaluated. There is usually little fat present in the medial aspect of the upper arm.

SKIN TONE. A skin retraction test should be performed. The majority of skin laxity is usually noted in the more proximal portion of the inferior border of the upper arm, bordering on the axillary skin.

MUSCLE TONE. The impact of muscle contraction on the overlying skin is carefully assessed.

MEASUREMENTS. The following measurements are obtained.

Circumferential Measurements (Fig. 127-3). These measurements are taken at fixed points on the upper arm with use of the olecranon process as the reference point (e.g., 10 cm, 15 cm, 20 cm proximal to the olecranon process). These measurements are useful for monitoring postoperative results.

Bicipital Groove to Inferior Border and Medial to Lateral Width Measurements (Fig. 127-3). These measurements were initially proposed by Illouz,[19] and the author uses these extensively in the evaluation of patients. These measurements are particularly helpful in determining whether patients fall into group 2 or whether they belong in group 3 or group 4. This determination can, however, be made by good clinical observation after one becomes more comfortable with the evaluation of these patients.

TABLE 127-3 ✦ PATIENT'S HISTORY

Age at onset of upper arm fullness
Family history of upper arm fullness
Weight gain or loss
Pregnancy history: amount of weight gain and loss during pregnancy
Level of physical activity
History of prolonged sun exposure
History of surgery in the upper arm and axillary or chest region
History of radiation therapy to the axillary or chest region
History of trauma (e.g., neuromuscular trauma to the upper arm or shoulder region, brachial plexus injury)
Neurologic disorders (e.g., multiple sclerosis, progressive shoulder girdle–upper arm muscle weakness)
Medication history (e.g., prednisone)

Patient's Weight. The patient's weight must be carefully documented on the chart immediately preoperatively and in subsequent visits. Any significant weight gain will definitely register as fullness in the upper arm despite the surgeon's best efforts.

PHOTOGRAPHIC DOCUMENTATION (Fig. 127-4). Photographs of the patient in the following positions should be taken preoperatively and postoperatively. Whenever possible, standardize the photographs with the same backdrop, same film, and no distracting clothing.

The Victory Position. The arm is abducted 90 degrees at the shoulder and flexed 90 degrees at the elbow. This photograph should include the para-axillary region.

Anteroposterior and Posteroanterior Views of the Arms in a Resting Position. The patient should have the arms at the sides in a resting position. Fat deposits in the anterior and posterior axillary folds and along the posterolateral arm are more readily appreciated in these views (M.K. Gingrass, MD, personal communication, 2002). The upper humeral fat

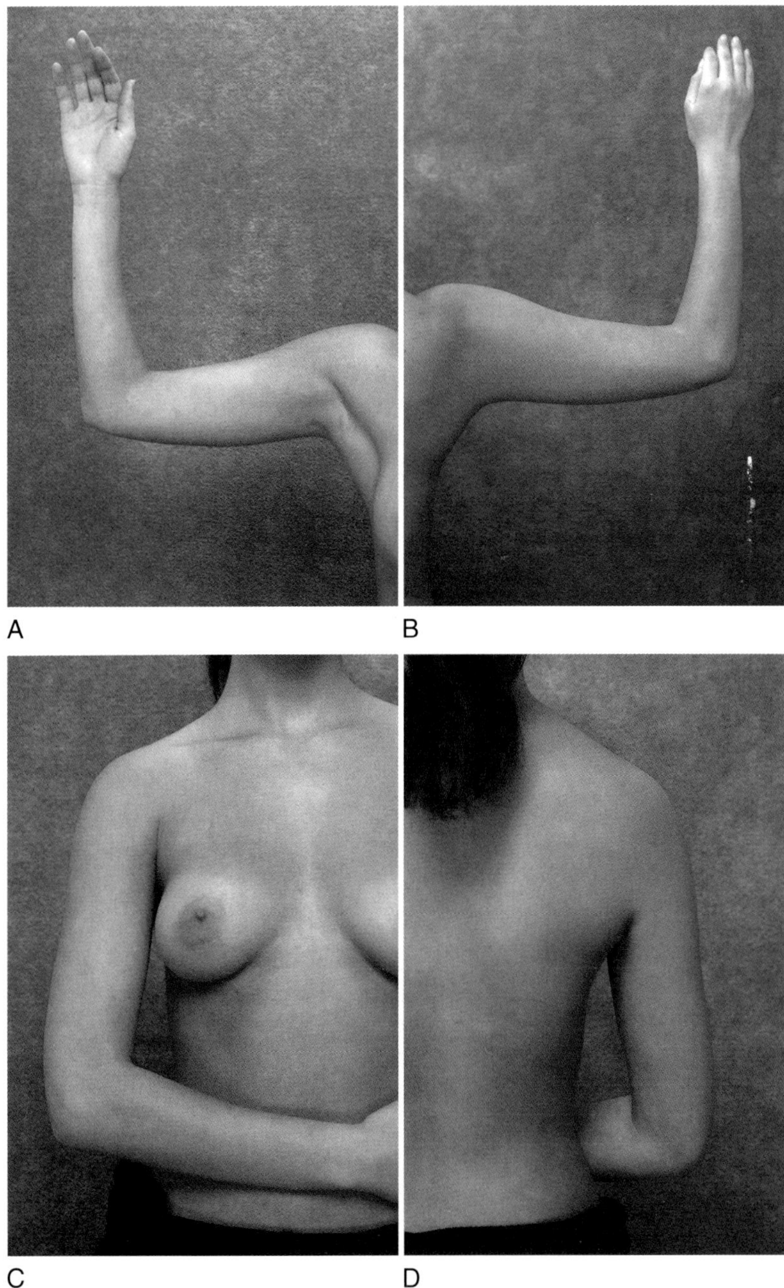

FIGURE 127-4. Photographic documentation. *A* and *B,* Victory position. *C* and *D,* This is how women evaluate themselves.

deposits are particularly troublesome for fitted blouses or jackets.

Treatment

Initially, patients with generalized fat deposits of the upper arm, along with good skin tone, should be encouraged to exercise and lose weight to reduce the overall circumferential diameter. If this fails to produce results, a surgical treatment plan may be proposed. Caution should be exercised in describing possible results one hopes to achieve. One should categorize the upper arm defect as excellent, very good, good, fair, or poor. Let the patient know the current category, and document this in the record. Emphasize that with weight management, exercise, and good genes, the result could be one category higher. Again, be careful what you promise. It is easier to achieve a very good to excellent result in true group 1 patients than it is in the remaining three groups. There must be a clear understanding between the surgeon and the patient that in patients assigned to groups 2 to 4, it may be necessary to undergo a later revision. Equally important is the total understanding on the part of the patient as to what the financial arrangements will be for any revisional surgery. As with any aesthetic procedure, the financial burden of a second surgical procedure can often taint the physician-patient relationship unless this has been clarified preoperatively. This understanding is especially important in procedures on the upper arm, for which one can often anticipate that the final result will be less than optimal.

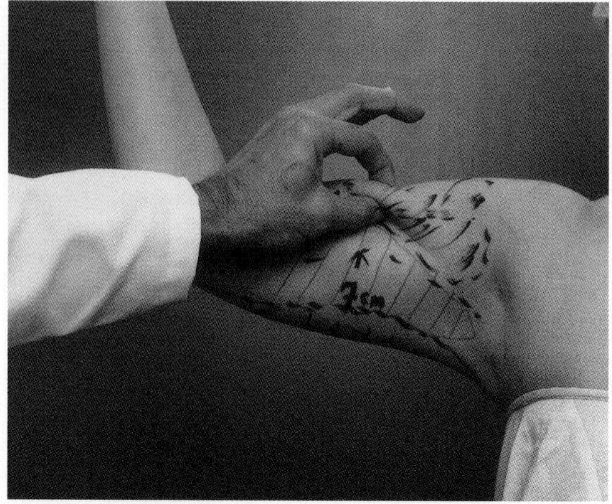

A

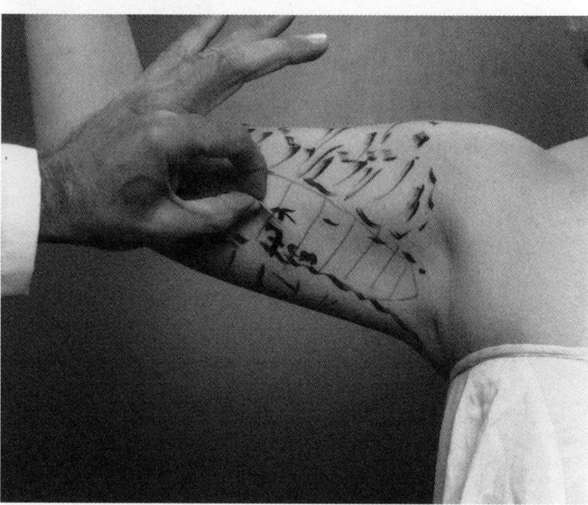

B

FIGURE 127-5. *A,* Pinch test—map out areas of suction-assisted lipoplasty. *B,* Note thin layer of fat in medial aspect of upper arm.

GROUP 1 PATIENTS

Group 1 patients have minimal to moderate subcutaneous fat with minimal skin laxity. These patients will do well with circumferential lipoplasty of the upper arm and para-axillary region. Their skin tone is good and should contract to the new underlying contour. In hereditary and idiopathic brachial enlargement, if lipoplasty is performed early, volume reduction and skin contraction may be permanent (see Fig. 127-1).

The pinch test (Fig. 127-5) is the most critical test to perform in marking the areas of liposuction preoperatively. With the patient in the sitting position and the arm initially at rest, the posterior and anterior axillary folds and the posterior lateral border of the arm are clearly marked. With the arm then held in the victory position (Fig. 127-6), the inferior border and the anterior and medial aspect of the arm and the midportion of the axilla are evaluated. The small incision lines are then carefully marked in the superior portion of the axilla anteriorly and posteriorly and the medial and lateral epicondyle regions.

The treatment of the entire upper arm and the para-axillary region was popularized by several people in the 1980s and 1990s, including Gilliland,[21,22] who proposed the circumferential, para-axillary, superficial, and tumescent technique. In many instances, suction-assisted lipoplasty is extended to the upper back (Fig. 127-7) because of ease of access to this region. One area in which caution should be exercised is the medial portion of the upper arm directly below the bicipital or intermuscular septal groove. The subcutaneous fat layer in this particular area is very thin and can lead to wrinkling and poor skin contraction if suction is performed (see Fig. 127-5*B*).

The age of the patient has been extended in the past 10 years. The best results, of course, are seen in the younger age group. Older women with some skin laxity of the inferior border of the upper arm in the para-axillary region are often willing to undergo suction-assisted lipoplasty only to avoid the scarring of the axillary and medial upper arm region. Moderate

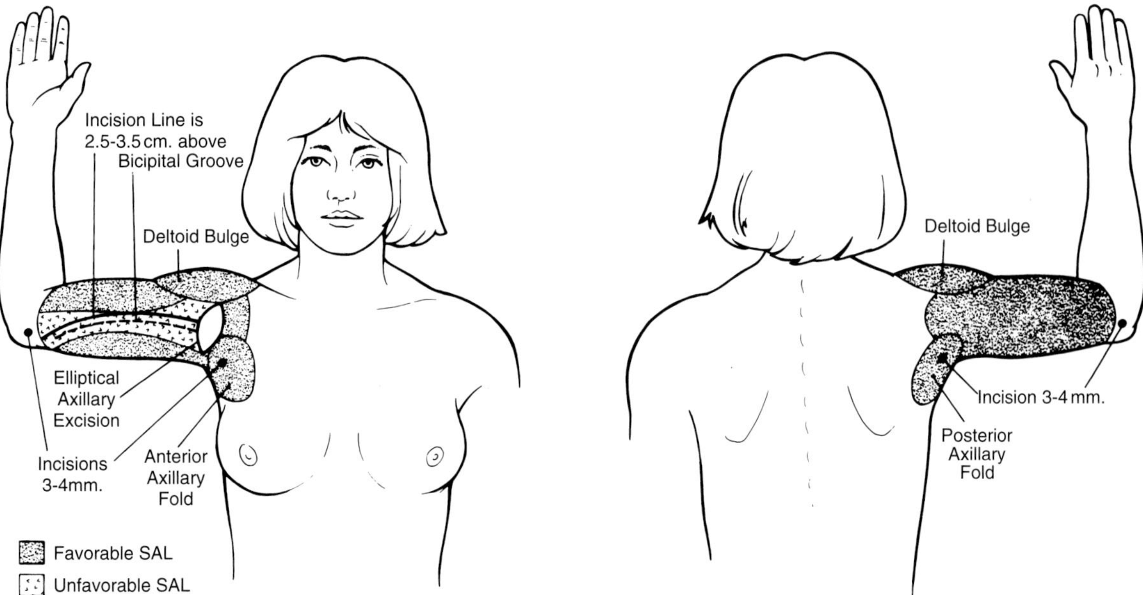

FIGURE 127-6. Favorable and unfavorable areas for suction-assisted lipoplasty (SAL). Para-axillary area and anterior and posterior axillary folds are now routinely treated.

amounts of skin laxity are often viewed as acceptable by the patient. Skin laxity can also be viewed as the first stage in a two- or three-stage procedure in which 6 months to a year is allowed to pass before a determination is made as to whether some skin should be resected after all the skin contraction has occurred.

Suction-assisted lipoplasty in the upper arm is also popular in patients undergoing breast reduction surgery. Portions of the posterior lateral upper arm and the para-axillary region can be suctioned at the time of the breast reduction procedure. This will significantly improve the overall appearance of the upper arm and chest area (see Fig. 127-2). In addition, suction-assisted lipoplasty of the lymphedematous upper arm and forearm can be performed to significantly improve the patient's status when it is combined with compression therapy.[23-25]

Operative Technique

The procedure can be performed under local anesthesia and sedation or under general anesthesia. Either way, the superwet technique discussed in this section is used (Table 127-4). Intravenous antibiotics are administered. The patient is placed in the supine position with the arms abducted at the shoulder and held out on arm boards. The intravenous line is placed in one arm, and a blood pressure cuff can be placed on the forearm of the contralateral arm. After preparation of the arm, shoulder girdle, para-axillary region, and chest, the forearms are wrapped with sterile towels, sterile barrier drapes to form a seal just distal to the elbow, and Kerlix rolls wrapped down around the intravenous lines and the blood pressure cords. With the cooperation of the anesthesia and nursing staff, the arms can then be brought across the chest comfortably to gain access to the para-axillary region and the upper back and to manipulate the arms so that the suction cannulas can be introduced through the various incisions.

The surgical procedure itself can be performed with use of standard liposuction cannulas. One may also choose to use 3- or 4-mm blunt-tipped, single-hole, standard cannulas (Fig. 127-8*A* and *B*) or a combination of standard cannulas and ultrasound-assisted lipoplasty (Fig. 127-8*C* and *D*). It is preferable to use a combination of standard cannulas and power-assisted lipoplasty (Fig. 127-8*E* and *F* and Table 127-5). However, any of these treatment methods is acceptable, depending on the surgeon's expertise.

One should use caution in suctioning the medial upper arm because there is little fat in this area (see Fig. 127-5*B*). Also, avoid superficial suction-assisted lipoplasty in the upper arm and para-axillary areas to

TABLE 127-4 ✦ FORMULA FOR SUPERWET SOLUTION FOR GENERAL ANESTHESIA*

1 liter of lactated Ringer solution
50 mL of 0.5% plain lidocaine
1 mL of epinephrine (1:1000)

*Different formulas are used for local anesthesia and sedation or pure local anesthesia.

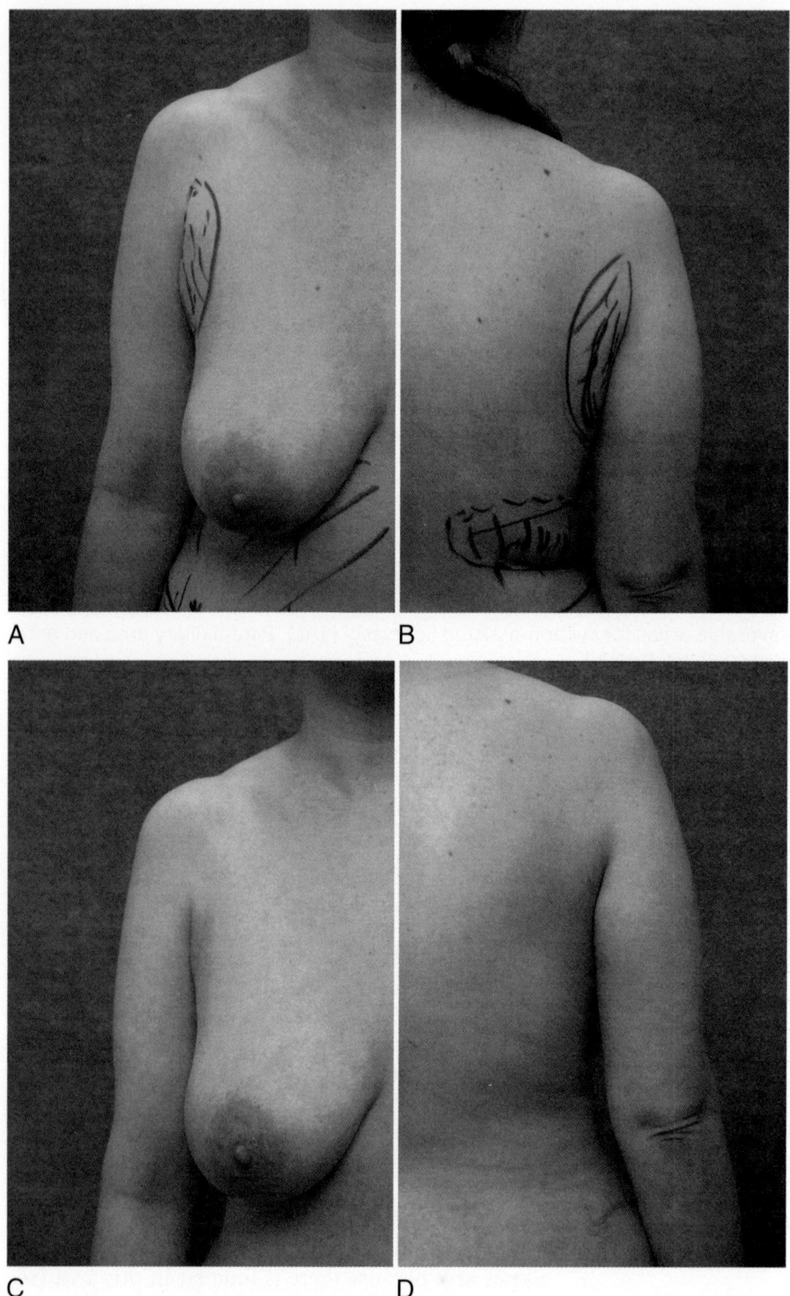

FIGURE 127-7. A 39-year-old woman: height, 5′2″; weight, 123 pounds; suction-assisted lipoplasty of anterior and posterior axillary folds and lower back (right, 170 mL; left, 160 mL). *A* and *B*, Preoperative markings. *C* and *D*, Postoperative views.

diminish irregularities and grooving. Finally, the assistant should hold the arm in the victory position before the end of the procedure; this can reveal irregularities that may not be visualized with the arm in the abducted position.

After completion of removal of the desired amount of fat as shown by the pinch test, the incisions are sutured with 4-0 Monocryl suture material, 5-0 black nylon interrupted, or 5-0 fast-absorbing plain catgut. A compression garment (Fig. 127-9) is used for 1 week to 10 days, with care taken to prevent development of a constriction band at the level of the elbow. If there is swelling of the forearm or hand, the constriction band at the elbow should be released by cutting the garment longitudinally to a point just above the elbow. The arms should also be elevated for a day or two, and movement of the hands and arms should be encouraged to further reduce postoperative edema. Sutures are removed in 3 to 5 days; normal activities are encouraged in a week to 10 days and exercise in 2 weeks. Ultrasound and massage therapy are instituted 10 days postoperatively and used twice

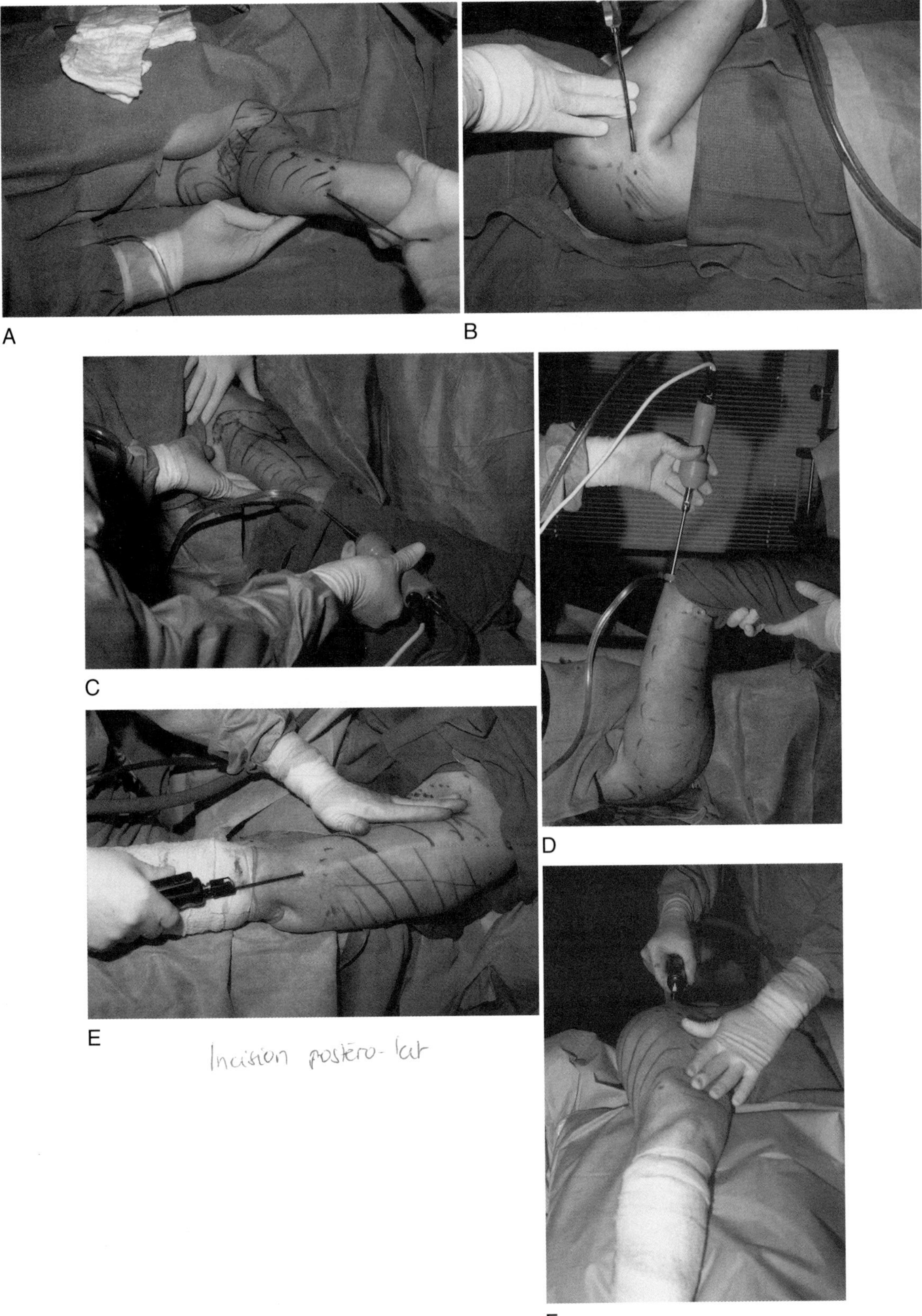

FIGURE 127-8. Suction-assisted lipoplasty techniques. *A* and *B*, Standard cannulas. *C* and *D*, Ultrasound-assisted lipoplasty; slightly larger incisions are made. *E* and *F*, Power-assisted lipoplasty cannulas can be used.

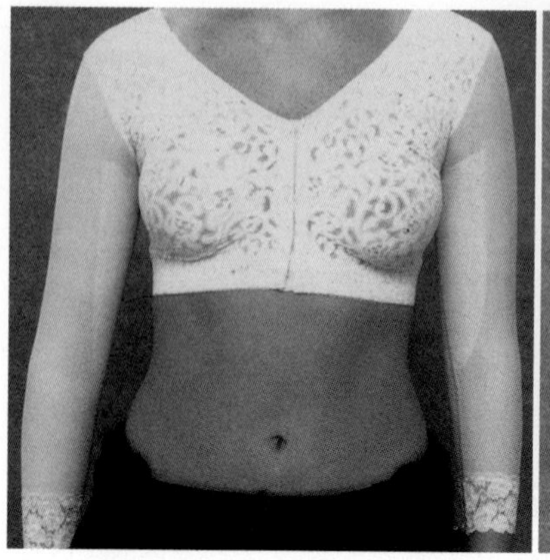

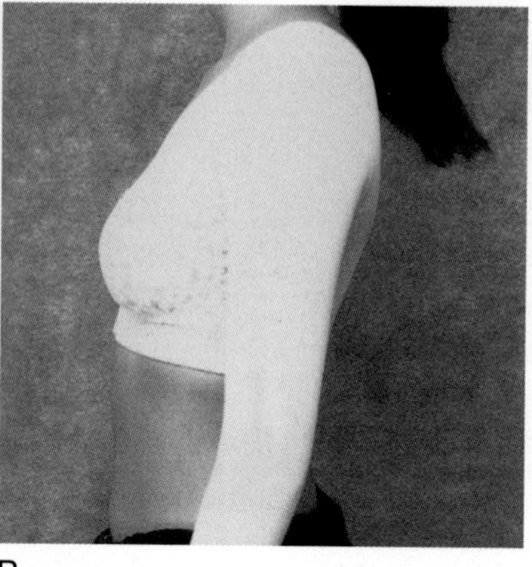

FIGURE 127-9. *A,* Postoperative compression garment. *B,* Smooth compression of para-axillary and upper arm area.

a week for 4 weeks to reduce postoperative swelling and edema.

Results depend on many variables including age, amount of fat removed, level of activity, amount of sun damage, muscle tone, and skin tone. In active, relatively young women, one may observe excellent skin contraction (even when large volumes of fat are removed), decreased circumferential diameters, and improved athletic upper arm contour (Figs. 127-10 and 127-11). In older patients with extensive sun damage and fair skin tone, one may still obtain an adequate result even when large volumes of fat are removed (Fig. 127-12).

GROUP 2 PATIENTS

Patients in group 2 exhibit generalized accumulation of subcutaneous fat with moderate skin laxity. Again, the patient should be marked preoperatively in a sitting position with the arms held comfortably at the side and gently flexed at the elbow. The anterior and posterior axillary folds and upper back areas should be marked with use of the pinch test. The patient is then asked to abduct the arm 90 degrees from the shoulder and to flex the elbow 90 degrees in the victory position. At this time, measurements are made by use of the olecranon process as the reference point along with the skin retraction test and the pinch test to see if any skin resection will be necessary. If only a slight skin tightening is necessary immediately adjacent to the axilla, an axillary ellipse may be all that is required (Fig. 127-13). If there is a little more skin laxity extending along the proximal upper arm, a T excision (Fig. 127-14) may need to be marked. This incision includes the axillary ellipse and an extension above the bicipital groove (medial bicipital sulcus, intermuscular septal groove, medial bicipital groove) of the upper arm (Fig. 127-15). The length of the incision along the medial portion of the upper arm is determined by the surgeon in combining an upward and proximal pull of the skin of the inferior border of the upper arm. It is critical to mark these carefully with ink that is not removed during the surgical preparation.

TABLE 127-5 ✦ ADVANTAGES OF STANDARD CANNULAS COMBINED WITH POWER-ASSISTED LIPOPLASTY OVER STANDARD CANNULAS COMBINED WITH ULTRASOUND-ASSISTED LIPOPLASTY

Ease of fat extraction
Ability to bend cannulas and negotiate curves
Decreased postoperative pain and tingling
Decreased seromas
Lack of postoperative lymphedema, even in combination with aggressive skin resection
Smaller incisions (2 to 3 mm) with few or no friction burns
Lower equipment cost

Operative Technique

The operation is usually performed under general anesthesia, with the same preparation as for patients in group 1. Again, intravenous antibiotics are given. Care should always be exercised not to abduct the arm more than 80 to 85 degrees for any prolonged period to avoid injury to the brachial plexus. Suction-assisted lipoplasty of the upper arm and para-axillary region is performed first. The axillary and upper arm incision is then made, and the axillary and upper arm flaps are elevated. A thin layer of fat is left over the fascia of the medial upper arm musculature to preserve as many of the sensory branches of the medial cutaneous nerve as possible (Fig. 127-16). Also, every effort is made to save the basilic and cephalic veins, which are not usually visualized in the modified procedure. An interesting

Text continued on p. 308

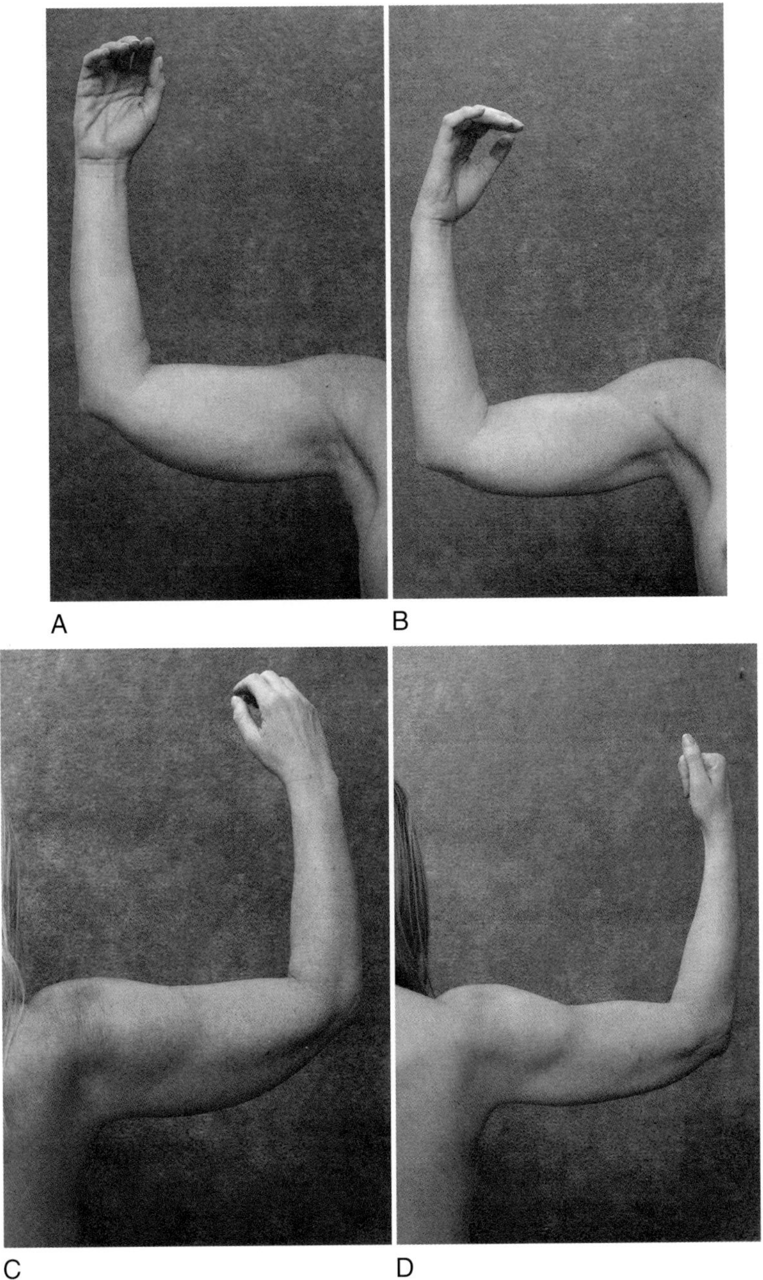

FIGURE 127-10. *A* to *D,* A 38-year-old woman: height, 5′4″; weight, 110 pounds; suction-assisted and power-assisted lipoplasty (volume, 550 mL). Note good skin contraction and muscle definition. *A* and *C*, Preoperative views. *B* and *D*, Postoperative views.

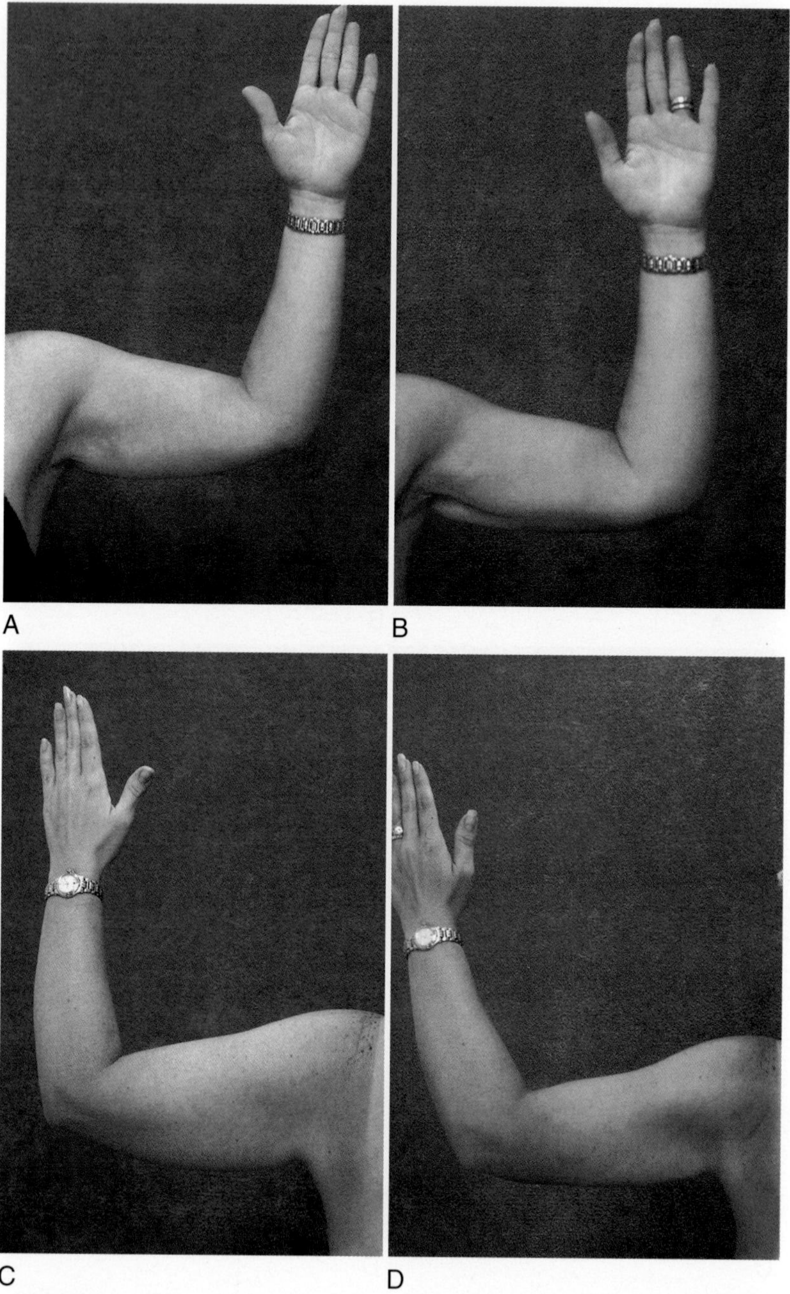

FIGURE 127-11. A 39-year-old woman: height, 5′2″; weight, 130 pounds; power-assisted and suction-assisted lipoplasty of upper arms (volume, 650 mL). Good volume and diameter reduction; fair to good skin contraction. *A* and *C,* Preoperative views. *B* and *D,* Postoperative views.

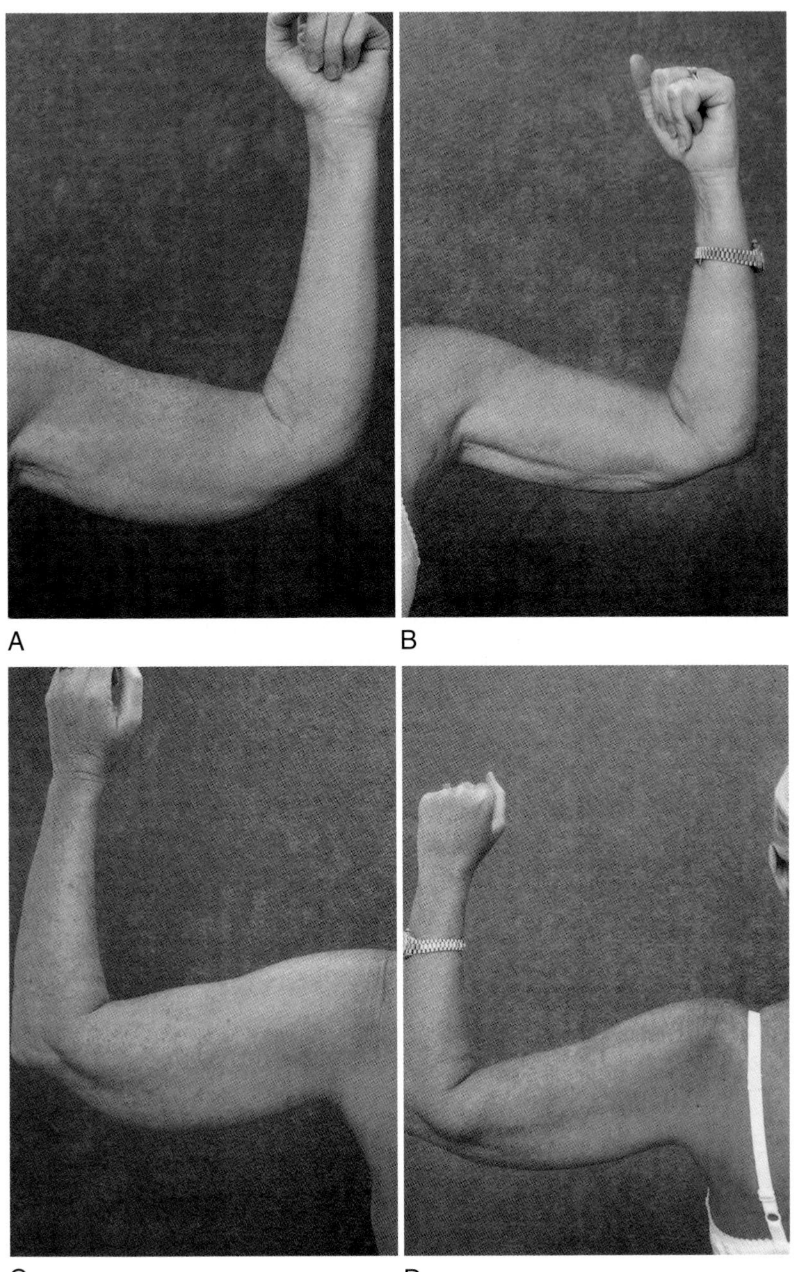

FIGURE 127-12. A 48-year-old woman: height, 5′7″; weight, 131 pounds; ultrasound-assisted and suction-assisted lipoplasty of upper arm and para-axillary area (volume, 600 mL). *A* and *C,* Preoperative views. *B* and *D,* Three years postoperatively; good volume reduction and fair skin contraction on inferior border.

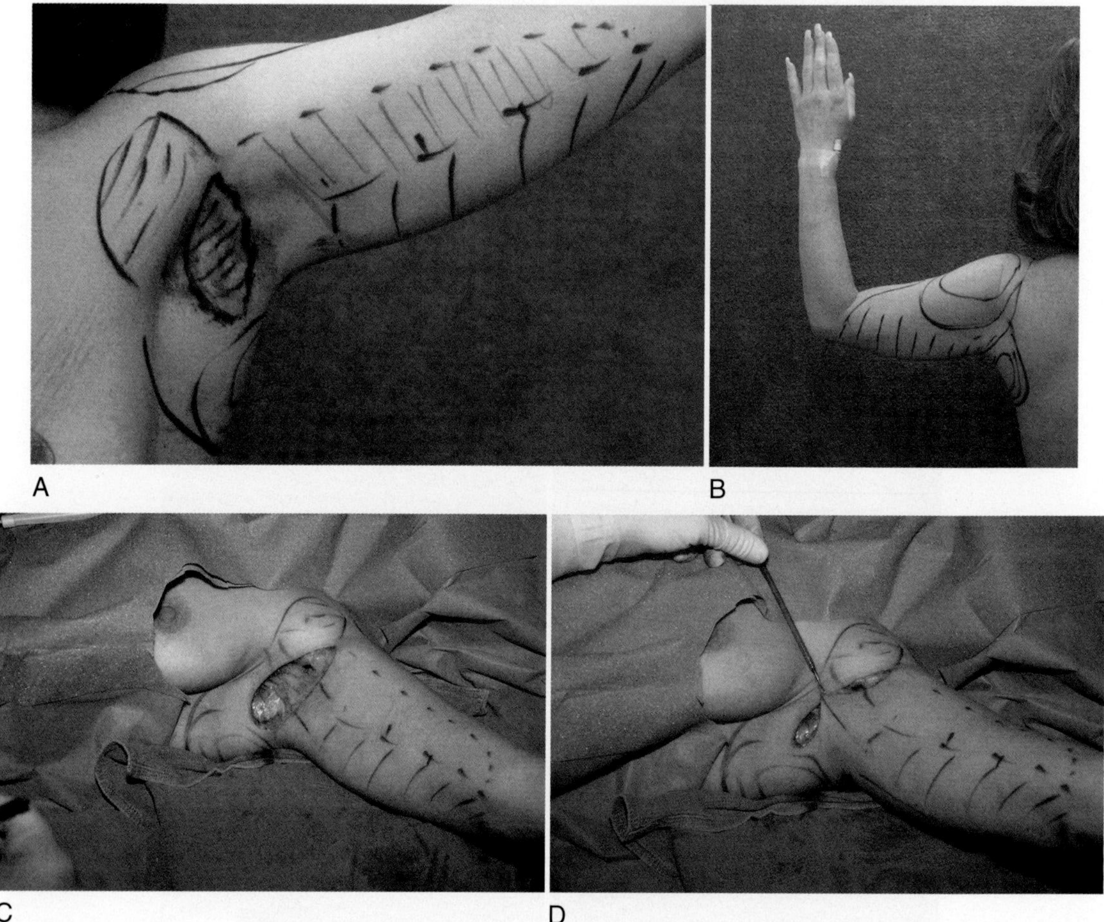

FIGURE 127-13. A 43-year-old woman: height, 5′3″; weight, 120 pounds; axillary ellipse and suction-assisted lipoplasty (right arm: 400 mL, 106-gm excision; left arm: 400 mL, 136-gm excision). *A* and *B,* Preoperative markings, axillary ellipse in apex of axilla. Keep the scar in the axilla. *C,* Suction-assisted lipoplasty first, followed by elliptical excision. *D,* Closure.

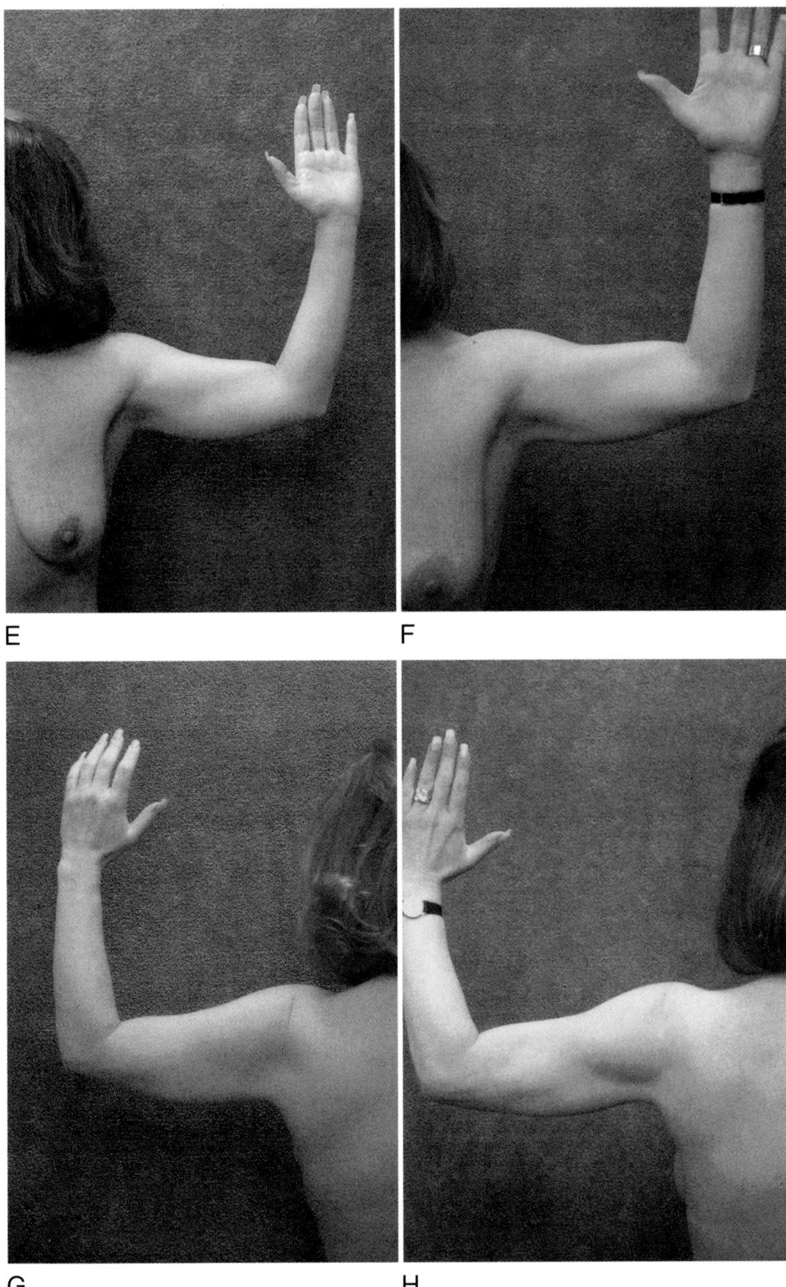

FIGURE 127-13, cont'd. *E,* Anterior preoperative view. *F,* Anterior postoperative view. There is better muscle definition, and the scar is well hidden. *G,* Posterior preoperative view. *H,* Posterior postoperative view. There is improved upper arm definition, and the inferior border is tighter.

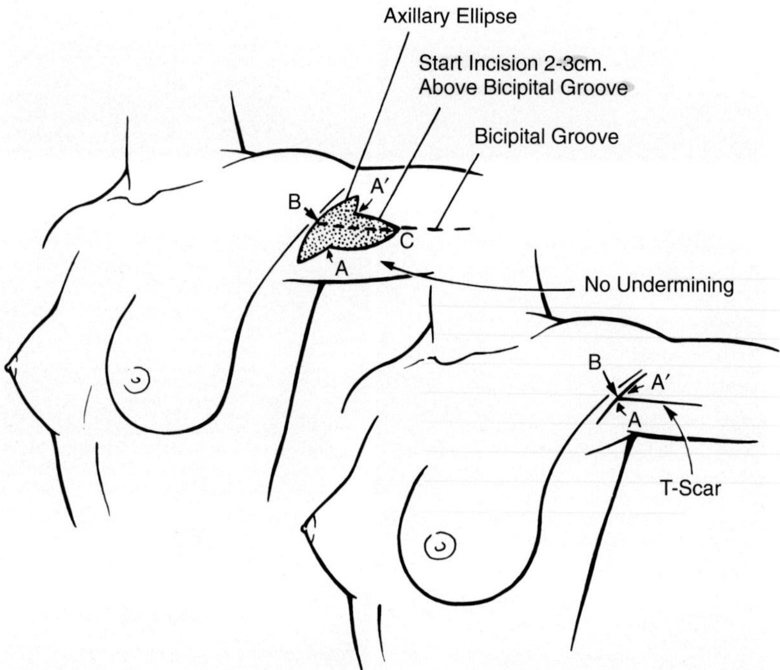

FIGURE 127-14. Modified brachioplasty with T incision: B, central portion of axillary ellipse; A-A′, sutured to central portion of axillary ellipse (B); A-C, length of incision depends on inferior border skin laxity.

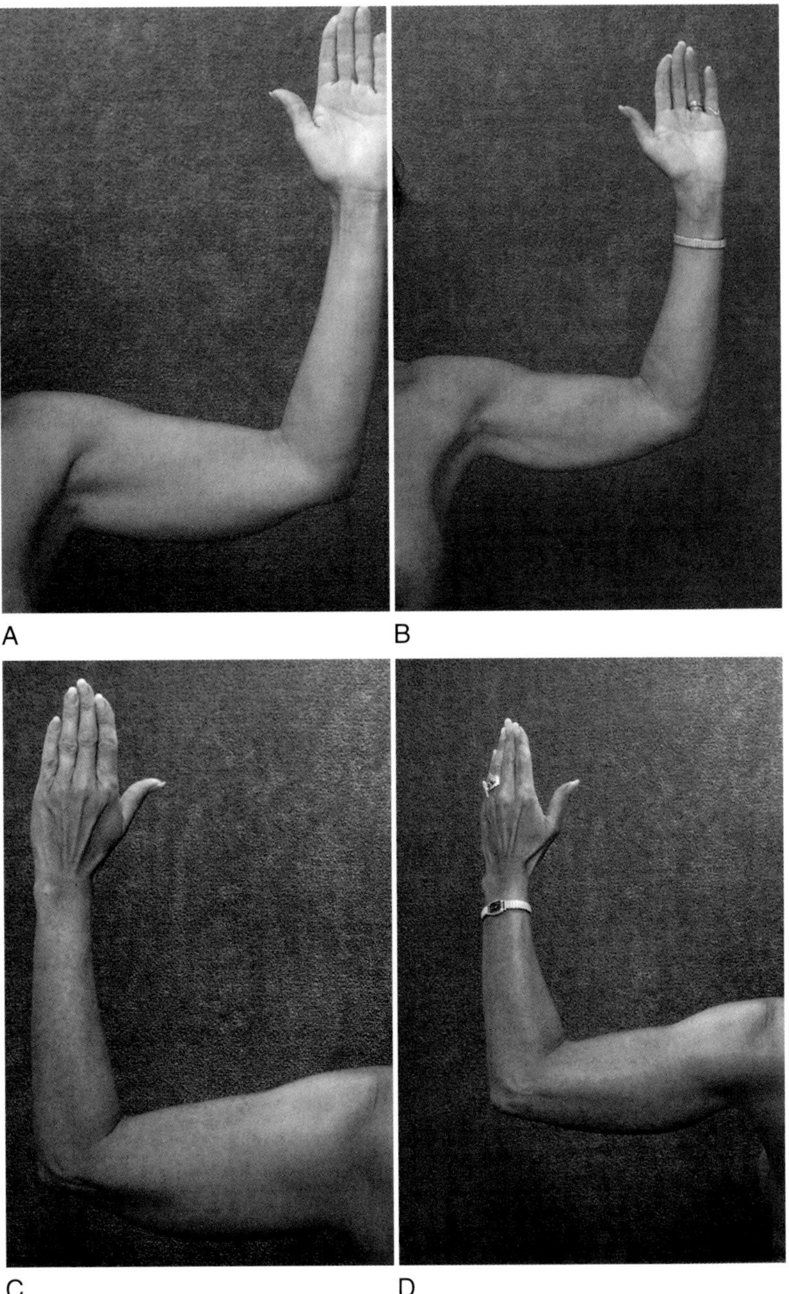

FIGURE 127-15. *A* and *C*, Preoperative views of a 53-year-old woman who underwent axillary ellipse with 8-cm T extension and 475-mL suction-assisted lipoplasty. *B* and *D*, Three years postoperatively.

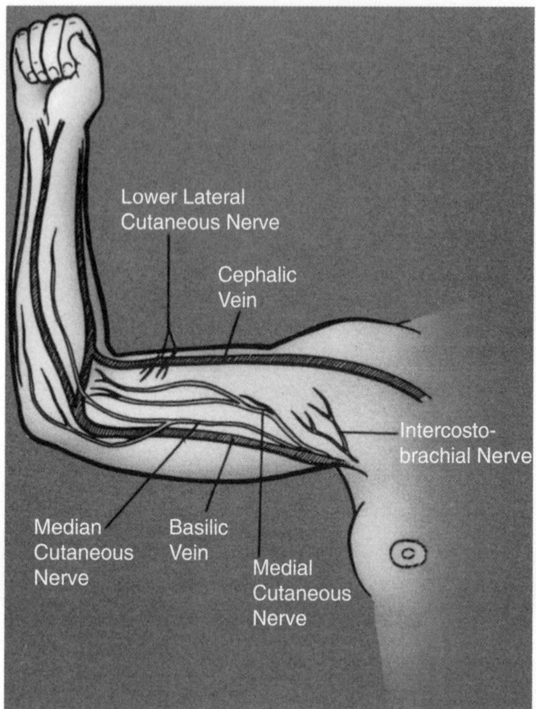

FIGURE 127-16. Sensory nerves and veins of medial upper arm.

variation of elevation of the upper arm flaps was presented by Goddio,[26] in which the flap is de-epithelialized and brought beneath the upper arm skin to design a fullness or a softer contour of the upper arm. This may have some application in the very thin upper arm in which there is a mild to moderate degree of ptosis. Undermining is usually performed only to the extent that the skin flap will be resected. The axillary skin flap and the upper arm flap are elevated repeatedly to evaluate when the desired result has been accomplished. Again, it helps to have the assistant hold the upper arm in the victory position during the operative procedure as the flaps are retracted to evaluate how much skin will be resected. The skin resections must be performed sequentially with placement of tacking sutures to avoid overresection of skin. A drain can be left in place for 24 to 48 hours and brought out through the posterior or inferior portion of the axillary incision line. A compression garment is applied (see Fig. 127-9) and held in place for up to 10 days postoperatively. Postoperative massage and ultrasound therapy are performed by a physical therapist twice weekly for up to 4 to 6 weeks postoperatively.

GROUP 3 AND GROUP 4 PATIENTS

The surgical excision or brachioplasty portion of the operation is similar in both these groups. In the group 3 patients, there is a larger amount of subcutaneous fat and fatty tissue, and more fatty tissue is therefore removed at the same time the skin resection is performed. Markings are identical to those for patients in group 2, with use of the pinch test to determine the amount of fat to be removed. The incision line is marked in the axillary region and above the bicipital groove extending to the elbow (Figs. 127-17 and 127-18*A* and *B;* see also Fig. 127-6). Molds can be used in marking the upper arm.[27] These can be useful for those with less experience with this procedure. If the incision needs to be extended, it is preferable to use an incision posterior to the medial epicondyle in a curvilinear fashion, extending onto the forearm. These markings should all be made with the patient in the sitting position with the arms in the victory position.

If liposuction is necessary, this is performed first (Figs. 127-17 and 127-18*C* and *D*). The skin flaps are then elevated in the axillary region and from above the bicipital groove to the inferior border of the arm medially (Figs. 127-17 and 127-18*E* and *F*), with care taken to avoid injury to the sensory branches of the medial cutaneous nerve and branches of the medial nerve and also to preserve the large basilic and cephalic veins (see Fig. 127-16). Lockwood[20] has studied the axillary fascia and the superficial fascial system of the upper arm in detail and sutures these two fascial systems to reduce the amount of skin resection and to decrease the risk of widening or migration of scars and development of unnatural contours in the area. The risk of this technique is that the fascia sits directly over the axillary vein, and the medial brachial cutaneous nerve is also nearby. The axillary fascia is quite thin, and, in theory, it would seem that tightening of these two fascial systems would be beneficial. However, it may be safer to obtain a similar result by anchoring the flap at the point of the superior portion of the anterior axillary fold followed by a careful, multilayered closure along the longitudinal and axillary incision.

In patients with marked laxity of the skin and muscles of the upper arm, a 2-0 or 3-0 Supramid suture may be used to secure the fascia of the triceps to the fascia of the biceps to further reduce the laxity of the upper arm. This is most effective in complete brachioplasties, particularly in the older patient (Fig. 127-19). Sequential resection of skin with tacking sutures must be used to avoid overresection (see Fig. 127-17 and 127-18*G* and *H*). *A moderate amount of tension* is desirable because postoperative swelling will lead to some recurrence of laxity. After the tacking sutures have been applied, the arm should be held up by the assistant in the victory position. Further suctioning, particularly along the inferior border or the posterior lateral surface of the arm, may be necessary to obtain an optimal final result (see Fig. 127-17 and 127-18*I*). A 3- or 7-mm silicone drain is left in place for 24 to

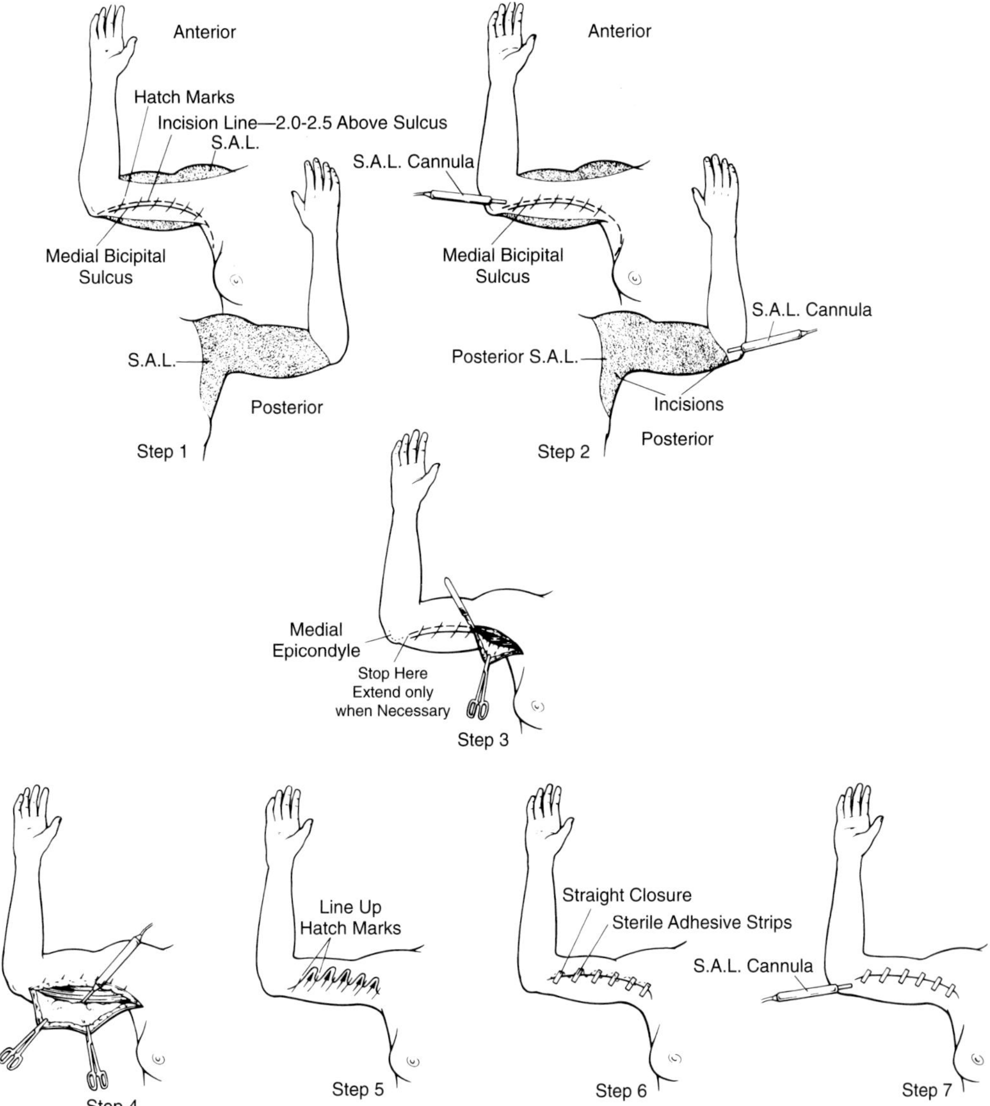

FIGURE 127-17. Surgical technique for patients in group 3 and group 4. S.A.L., suction-assisted lipoplasty.

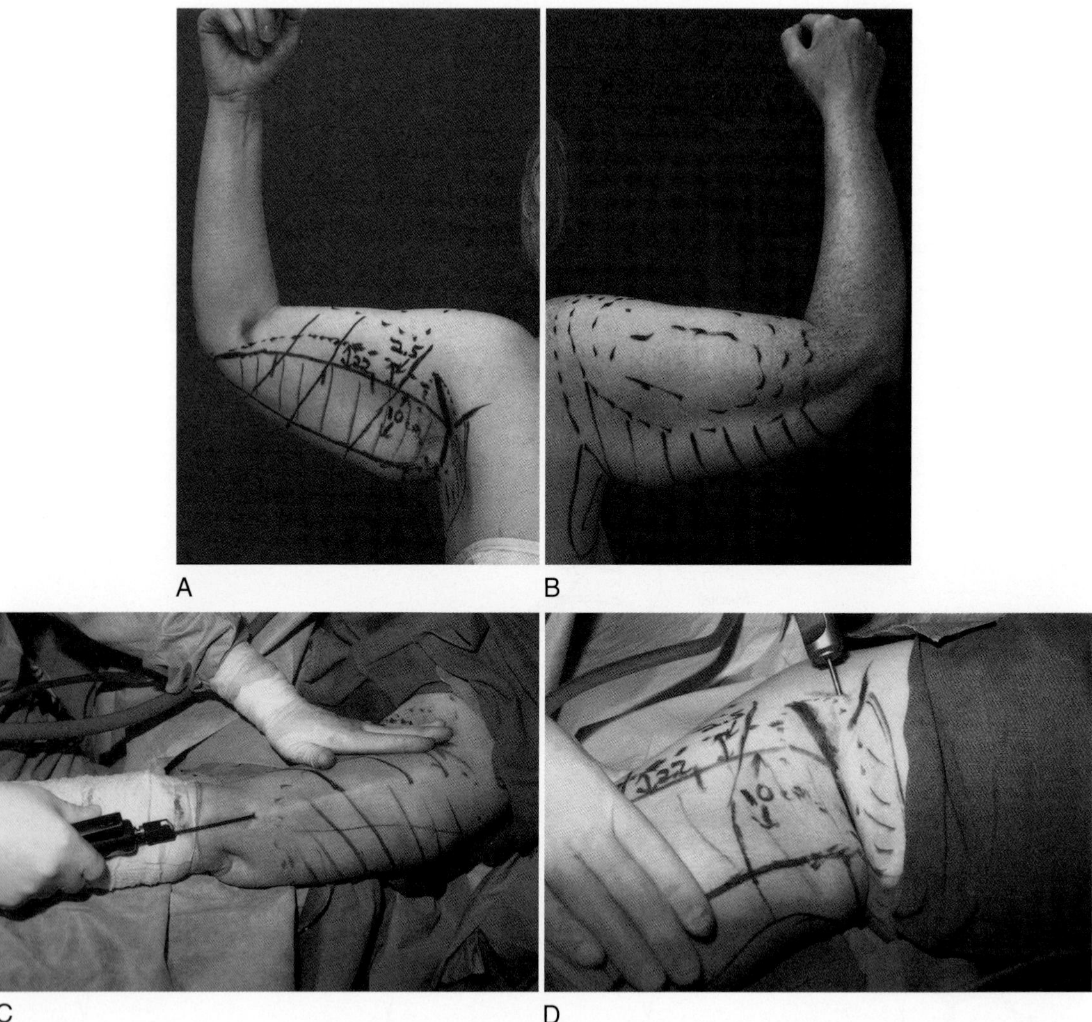

FIGURE 127-18. Clinical demonstration of surgical steps for patients in group 3 and group 4. *A* and *B,* Step 1: axillary ellipse; incision of 2.5 cm above the bicipital groove; marking at the elbow behind the medial condyle; hatch marks—superior proximal. *C* and *D,* Step 2: combination of suction-assisted and power-assisted lipoplasty.

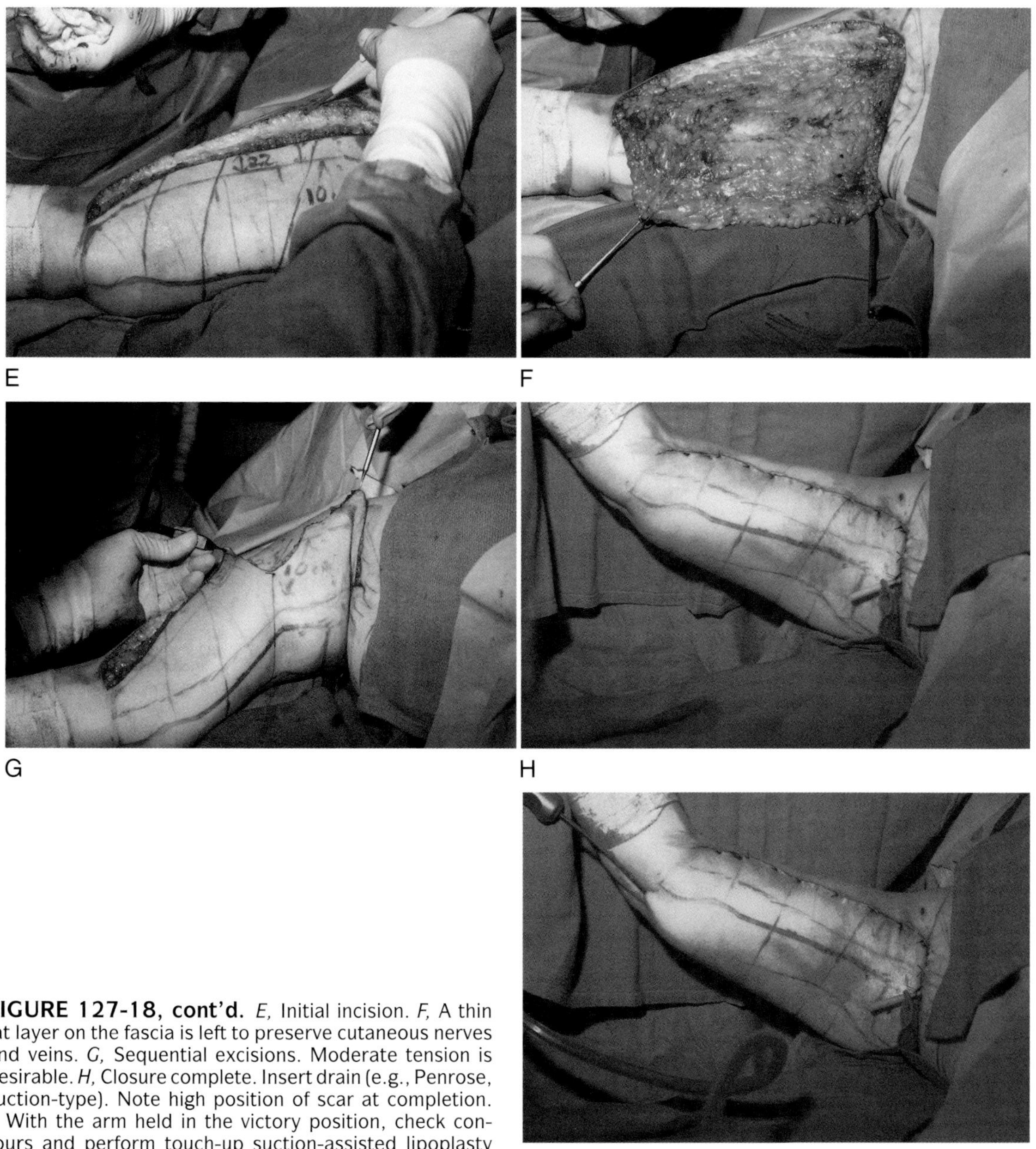

FIGURE 127-18, cont'd. *E,* Initial incision. *F,* A thin fat layer on the fascia is left to preserve cutaneous nerves and veins. *G,* Sequential excisions. Moderate tension is desirable. *H,* Closure complete. Insert drain (e.g., Penrose, suction-type). Note high position of scar at completion. *I,* With the arm held in the victory position, check contours and perform touch-up suction-assisted lipoplasty where needed.

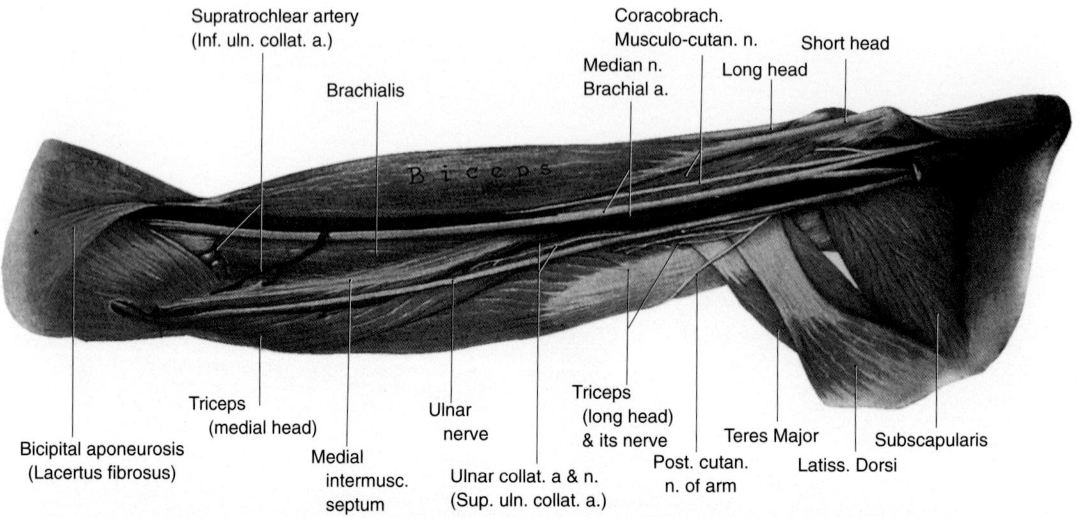

FIGURE 127-19. Muscle suturing of upper arm. In theory, it reduces upper arm flaccidity, and there is tighter redraping of skin. However, in experience, it has not seemed to work except in complete brachioplasties.

48 hours and is brought out through the axillary incision line. A compression garment is applied day and night for 10 days. Compression garments at night are encouraged for up to 3 months to further reduce upper arm edema and decrease the possibility of hypertrophic scar formation. Silicone sheeting is used at the first hint of hypertrophic scar development, and silicone lotions may also be implemented. Dilute (10 mg/mL) cortisone injections of the hypertrophic scar are sometimes beneficial 6 weeks postoperatively if the scar has become painful or itchy (Fig. 127-20).

MANAGEMENT OF THE LYMPHEDEMATOUS ARM

There are now a limited number of patients who present with a lymphedematous arm.[14] Fortunately, radical mastectomies are performed much less frequently, and axillary lymph node dissections are often limited to samplings, preserving lymphatic drainage of the upper extremities. There are still instances, however, in lymph node dissections after melanoma of the upper arm and occasionally when lymph node dissections are combined with radiation that result in lymphedema.

Advances in treatment for the lymphedematous arm were presented by Brorson and Svensson[23-25] of Malmö University Hospital in Malmö, Sweden. They combined lipoplasty with controlled compression therapy and have concluded that liposuction effectively reduces arm lymphedema after breast cancer treatment and also lowers the incidence of cellulitis. They have also concluded that it is important to continue the use of compression garments to maintain the primary surgical outcome.

COMPLICATIONS

Complications during upper arm surgery are extremely rare, but they do occur (Table 127-6). Scars of the upper arm take 6 months to a year to fade or mature adequately. Hypertrophic scars initially develop in as many as 30% to 40% of patients and require compression therapy, silicone sheeting, or mild cortisone injections. Lymphedema has been seen on a few occasions in complete brachioplasties in group 3 patients when liposuction was performed with ultrasound-assisted lipoplasty probes. In group 3 patients, it may be safer to use standard or power-assisted lipoplasty techniques. Malposition of scars can usually be avoided by following the suggested principles of surgery of the upper arm.

CONCLUSION

Upper arm surgery has become far more popular in the past 15 years. This is most likely the result of both surgeons and patients who are better informed. There is also a greater understanding of the indications for

TABLE 127-6 ✦ COMPLICATIONS OF AESTHETIC UPPER ARM SURGERY

Hematoma
Seroma
Infection
Skin necrosis
Wound dehiscence
Sensory loss of the upper arm or forearm
Lymphedema
Prolonged hypertrophic or keloid scars
Malposition of scars

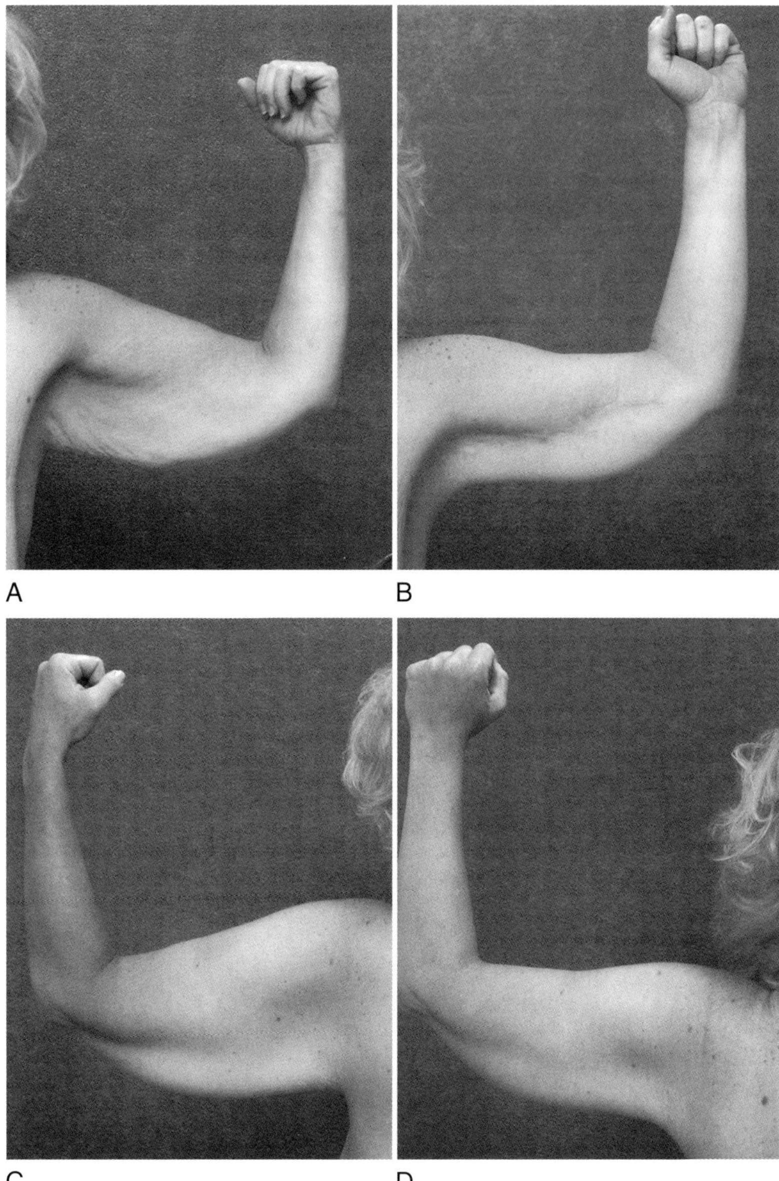

FIGURE 127-20. Group 3 patient, a 37-year-old woman: height, 5′7″; weight, 165 pounds; suction-assisted lipoplasty, 275 mL; resection, 164 g. *A* and *C,* Preoperative views. *B* and *D,* Postoperative views. Note that the scar is in the bicipital groove. The axillary scar is invisible.

and the use of lipoplasty techniques in the upper arm. The use of suction-assisted lipoplasty has been broadened considerably by a better understanding of skin contraction and its promotion by use of postoperative compression.[28-35] Aesthetic surgery of the upper arm is not technically difficult. It is, however, vital to maintain realistic expectations of postoperative results and to inform the patient that revisions may be necessary to achieve an optimal result, particularly in group 2, group 3, and group 4 patients. The physical and financial consequences of revision surgery should also be carefully reviewed before any treatment plan is initiated.

Lymphedema of the upper extremity can be managed by suction-assisted lipoplasty, particularly when it is used in combination with careful compression techniques. This also reduces the amount of postlymphedema cellulitis.

As knowledge of aesthetic procedures is broadened, patients who seek breast reduction surgery may also benefit from para-axillary or para-axillary and shoulder girdle suction-assisted lipoplasty.

The upper arm is an area of concern for many patients, and the degree of its importance should not be underestimated. Improvement in this area often leads to satisfied patients.

REFERENCES

1. Glanz S, Gonzalez-Ulloa M: Aesthetic surgery of the arm. Part 1. Aesthetic Plast Surg 1981;5:1.
2. Pitanguy I: Aesthetic plastic surgery of the upper and lower limbs. Aesthetic Plast Surg 1980;4:363.
3. Pitanguy I: Correction of lipodystrophy of the lateral thoracic aspect and inner side of the arm and elbow dermosenescence. Clin Plast Surg 1975;2:477.
4. Grazer F, Klingbeil J: Body Image: A Surgical Perspective. St. Louis, Mosby, 1980.
5. Franco T: Aesthetic surgery of the upper and lower limbs. Aesthetic Plast Surg 1980;4:245.
6. Lewis JR: Atlas of Plastic Surgery. Boston, Little, Brown, 1984.
7. Juri J, Juri C, Elias JC: Arm dermatolipectomy with quadrangular flap and T-closure. Plast Reconstr Surg 1979;64:521.
8. Baroudi R: Dermatolipectomy of the upper arm. Clin Plast Surg 1975;2:485.
9. Guerrerosantos J: Brachioplasty. Aesthetic Plast Surg 1979;8:1.
10. Baroudi R: Body sculpturing. Clin Plast Surg 1984;11:419.
11. Hallock GG, Altobelli JA: Simultaneous brachioplasty, thoracoplasty, and mammoplasty. Aesthetic Plast Surg 1985;9:233.
12. Regnault P: Brachioplasty, axilloplasty, and pre-axilloplasty. Aesthetic Plast Surg 1983;7:31.
13. Regnault P, Daniel RK: Aesthetic Plastic Surgery. Boston, Little, Brown, 1984.
14. Baroudi R, Vogt P: Brachioplasty and brachial suction-assisted lipectomy. In Cohen M, ed: Mastery of Plastic and Reconstructive Surgery, vol 3. Boston, Little, Brown, 1994:2219.
15. Vogt PA: Brachioplasty. Aesthetic Surg Q 1995;15:13.
16. Vogt PA: Brachial suction-assisted lipoplasty and brachioplasty. Aesthetic Surg J 2001;21:164.
17. Pitman G: Liposuction of the arms. Aesthetic Surg Q 1995;15:12.
18. Teimourian B, Malekzadeh S: Rejuvenation of the upper arm. Plast Reconstr Surg 1998;102:545, discussion 552.
19. Illouz Y, De Villers Y: Body Sculpturing by Lipoplasty. Edinburgh, Churchill Livingstone, 1989.
20. Lockwood T: Brachioplasty with superficial fascial system suspension. Plast Reconstr Surg 1995;96:912.
21. Gilliland MD, Lyos AT: CAST liposuction of the arm improves aesthetic results. Aesthetic Plast Surg 1997;21:225.
22. Gilliland MD, Lyos AT. CAST liposuction: an alternative to brachioplasty. Aesthetic Plast Surg 1997;21:398.
23. Brorson H, Svensson H: Skin blood flow of the lymphedematous arm before and after liposuction. Lymphology 1997; 30:165.
24. Brorson, H, Svensson, H., Norrgren K, Thorsson O: Liposuction reduces arm lymphedema without significantly altering the already impaired lymph transport. Lymphology 1998;31: 156.
25. Brorson H, Svensson H: Liposuction combined with controlled compression therapy reduces arm lymphedema more effectively than controlled compression therapy alone. Plast Reconstr Surg 1998;102:1058, discussion 1068.
26. Goddio AS: A new technique for brachioplasty. Plast Reconstr Surg 1989;84:85.
27. DeSouza-Pinto EB, Erazo PJ, Matsuda CA, et al: Brachioplasty technique with the use of molds. Plast Reconstr Surg 2000;105:1854, discussion 1861.
28. Baroudi R: Dermatolipectomy of the upper arm. Aesthetic Plast Surg 1998;12:251.
29. Hetter G: Lipoplasty: The Theory and Practice of Blunt Suction, 2nd ed. Boston, Little, Brown, 1990.
30. Schlesinger SL: Suction-assisted lipectomy of the upper arm: a four-cannula technique. Aesthetic Plast Surg 1990;14:271.
31. Lillis PJ: Liposuction of the arms, calves, and ankles. Dermatol Surg 1997;23:1161.
32. Lillis PJ: Liposuction of the arms. Dermatol Clin 1999;17:783.
33. Bank DE, Perez ML: Skin retraction after liposuction in patients over the age of 40. Dermatol Surg 1999;25:673.
34. Erni D, Banic A: Body contouring by removal of skin and fatty tissue [in German]. Ther Umsch 1999;56:206.
35. Johnson DS, Cook WR Jr: Advanced techniques in liposuction. Semin Cutan Med Surg 1999;18:139.

CHAPTER

128

Secondary Breast Augmentation

V. LEROY YOUNG, MD, FACS ✦ MARLA E. WATSON, MA ✦ TANYA A. ATAGI, MD

THE FREQUENCY OF SECONDARY SURGERY

The need for revisional surgery after augmentation mammaplasty occurs for a variety of reasons, most of which relate to the implant itself, the body's response to the implant, or the surgical technique. Breast implant patients also request revision because of cosmetic concerns, such as asymmetry, skin wrinkling, implant palpability, or desired size change (Table 128-1).

Most surgeons agree that local and perioperative complications associated with breast implantation as well as factors diminishing the quality of aesthetic results are the primary reasons for reoperation. Unfortunately, revisional procedures to deal with complications have at least the same (perhaps more) risks as primary surgery, including infection, bleeding, altered sensation, and morbidity and discomfort of anesthesia and surgery.

SILICONE GEL IMPLANTS. The frequency of secondary surgery after breast augmentation has not been systematically studied, but Gabriel et al[1] have conducted perhaps the best investigation to date. After receiving their first implants (95% of which were

TABLE 128-1 ✦ REASONS FOR REOPERATIONS IN PATIENTS WITH BREAST IMPLANTS

Fibrous capsular contracture	Implant palpability
Gel implant rupture (intracapsular or extracapsular)	Implant pocket revision
Silicone gel migration or exudation through skin or nipple	Loss of or change in sensation of the breast or nipple
Silicone granuloma	Necrosis of nipple, areola, or flap
Axillary adenopathy	Rash or skin necrosis
Saline implant deflation	Asymmetry of breast size or shape
Implant fill port or valve malfunction	Chronic breast or chest wall pain
Hematoma	Implant extrusion
Seroma	Implant malposition
Periprosthetic (capsule) infection	Implant shifting or displacement
Wound infection or dehiscence	Correction of ptosis
Implant size change (larger or smaller)	Mammography improvement
Skin wrinkling	Capsule calcification
Breast mass, need for biopsy, cancer diagnosis	Patient's request

silicone gel), almost 24% of 749 Mayo Clinic patients required reoperation for a complication, most often capsular contracture. The authors found a statistically significant difference between women who received implants for augmentation and those who received implants for reconstruction. By the 5-year follow-up point, 12% of augmentation patients had developed at least one complication requiring reoperation; this compared with 34% of cancer reconstruction and 30% of prophylactic mastectomy reconstruction patients. Even though secondary surgeries are less common after augmentation than after reconstruction, the need for revisional procedures remains a troubling problem for both patients and surgeons. Nearly every plastic surgery practice has augmentation patients who have had five or more reoperations to deal with complications.

Reports of silicone gel implant complications among augmentation patients have consistently found reoperation frequencies of 15% to 20%,[2-4] and some investigations calculate even higher figures. For example, a prospective study by McGhan Medical (now Inamed Aesthetics) evaluated 583 women who received silicone gel or double-lumen implants, most with textured surfaces, between 1990 and 1992 (AR90 study). During the 5-year follow-up period, explantation or revisional surgery was performed on 23% of augmentation patients because of anxiety about silicone or local complications. In an investigation by the Food and Drug Administration (FDA), 907 women with silicone gel implants who were part of a National Cancer Institute cohort in Alabama were interviewed. One third of these women (303) reported that they had at least one explantation surgery.[5]

Because Inamed's study was conducted during the peak years (1992-1995) of controversy over breast implants, about one third of the explantations were done for safety concerns and not for clinical indications. The same was true for women in the FDA investigation; 30% of the explantation group (92 of 303) cited safety concerns about silicone as the reason. The number of patients requesting removal of silicone gel implants solely because of safety concerns has greatly diminished since the mid-1990s.

Saline-Filled Implants. In its long-term Saline Prospective Study, Mentor Corporation calculated 3-year cumulative complication risk rates for 1264 augmentation patients with 2526 saline-filled implants. Within the first 3 years after implantation, 13% of augmentation patients (10% of implants) required reoperation.[6] Of 358 secondary surgeries performed, 32% involved implant exchange (5.4% of all 2526 implants). Other procedures included capsule modification, scar revision and wound repair, saline fill volume adjustment, and implant repositioning. Inamed's 1995 Augmentation Study (A95) of saline-filled implants has produced data for the 5-year follow-up point. Among the 1800 augmentation implants (in 901 patients), there was a cumulative risk rate that 26% of patients would require additional surgical treatment within 5 years of implantation.[7] The most frequent treatments were a "capsule procedure," scar revision and wound repair, change of saline fill volume, and mastopexy. These two manufacturer studies may reflect expected reoperation frequencies with currently available room-temperature vulcanized saline-filled devices for the short term. Similar to the reoperation frequency for silicone gel implants, the frequency ranges from 13% to 26% of patients.

Older saline implants seem to have a similar reoperation frequency. A multicenter retrospective study involving 504 (mostly augmentation) patients with 995 saline-filled implants was conducted by Gutowski et al.[8] The implants were primarily manufactured by Mentor/HS and placed between 1980 and 1989. Although the number of perioperative complications was low (1.6% for hematoma and ≤0.3% for wound dehiscence, wound infection, and seroma), 21% of patients required reoperation, mainly for explantation with or without implant exchange or for open capsulotomy. In a separate study by the same research group, Cunningham et al[9] reviewed 882 saline-filled breast implants (the majority made by Mentor/HS) placed between January 1980 and mid-1986 in 450 patients. In addition to the removal or exchange of 8% of implants because of deflation, another 26% of the implants required secondary surgery. The most common reason for reoperation was capsular contracture (20.4% of patients); complications such as hematoma, seroma, and wound problems accounted for the other secondary procedures.

The authors have collected data on revisional surgery among patients undergoing augmentation or reconstruction with silicone gel, double-lumen, and saline-filled breast implants. This study population consists of all patients who had a permanent breast implant removed by one surgeon (V.L.Y.) between January 1988 and December 2000, with the exclusion of patients for whom the duration of implantation was unknown. The primary objective of this investigation was to compare the outcome of explantation in patients with ruptured implants with that in patients with intact implants and to determine whether a rupture produces any adverse consequences. The rupture outcome series consists of 299 patients who had 452 explantation surgeries and 778 implants removed (119 saline, 588 silicone gel, 65 double-lumen, and 6 soybean oil). The 217 augmentation patients had 559 implants explanted in 307 surgeries. The 82 reconstruction patients had 219 implants removed in 145 surgeries.

As with other studies, the need for revisional surgery was higher among reconstruction patients in this rupture outcome series. Among the 217 augmentation patients, 24% had more than one explantation. More than one explantation was performed in 43% of reconstruction patients. Many women had more than one indication for explantation (e.g., severe capsular contracture and a rupture diagnosis). In the augmentation group, the top five reasons for explantation were rupture or deflation (n = 132), capsular contracture (n = 78), nonlocal physical symptoms (n = 50), fear of silicone (n = 49), and asymmetry (n = 23). Interestingly, patients' reports of nonlocal symptoms and fear were essentially nonexistent before 1992 and after 1995, the year when several large studies finding no correlation between breast implants and connective tissue disease began to be published.

In addition to explantation surgeries, patients in the authors' rupture outcome series underwent many other revisional procedures without implant removal, primarily in an attempt to deal with capsular contracture (e.g., open capsulotomy) or to improve the aesthetic result (e.g., pocket revision). Some surgeries were planned, such as tissue expander exchange or nipple-areola reconstruction, but most were unforeseen. The 217 augmentation patients underwent 51 unplanned surgeries, and the 145 reconstruction patients had 82.

A new and constantly updated source of data on primary and secondary surgeries is the National Breast Implant Registry, begun in 2000 by the Plastic Surgery Educational Foundation. This project is an ongoing, voluntary, and confidential multicenter registry of patients undergoing breast augmentation, reconstruction, and replacement in the United States. Major purposes of the National Breast Implant Registry are to collect data on the pattern of implant use and clinical outcomes, to establish an identifiable cohort of patients that can be used for future studies, to provide public information about reasonable expectations for implant surgery, and to offer surgeons real-time data so they can compare their results with those of their peers. To enlarge the already substantial database, surgeons are encouraged to submit basic information (by a secure Internet connection or paper/fax) of all their implant patients as surgeries are performed.[10] The registry is designed so that patients can be followed, no matter who the surgeon is, and complications recorded over time.

Data from the studies cited do not permit determination of the incidence rate of reoperation because multiple study designs were employed. Taken together, however, a picture emerges that suggests approximately one of four or five augmentation patients, with silicone gel or saline implants, will undergo more than one implantation surgery. Other implanted medical devices also have considerable reoperation rates, but the frequency of secondary surgeries in augmentation patients seems entirely too high, especially considering that breast augmentation is an elective procedure.

Unfortunately, many of the local complications that most often lead to the need for secondary augmentation are not entirely preventable, at least not with currently available implants. No matter how experienced the surgeon, some devices will still fail, some capsules will still contract, and some infections will still develop. However, there is now more control over other problems that lead to reoperations. For example, one can work with patients to agree on the most desirable and appropriate breast size; understand which patients receiving saline implants are most likely to develop skin wrinkling; and carefully consider the best implant type, volume, and pocket position needed to reduce the risk of implant displacement and breast size or shape asymmetry. All of these reasons for reoperation, plus others, are examined in the remainder of this chapter.

EXPLANTATION AND IMPLANT EXCHANGE

The vast majority of augmentation patients who need to have an implant removed choose to have it replaced. In most instances, the patient who has a complication with one implant (such as rupture, asymmetry, or contracture) will want both implants exchanged, especially if they are more than a few years old. Throughout this chapter, specific surgical details are offered that relate to secondary augmentation in different contexts (e.g., treatment of a malpositioned or extruded implant, revision for asymmetry, removal of a ruptured implant). At this point, however, general guidelines are presented for removal and replacement of implants. For additional information, refer to the appropriate chapter sections that address the particular complication being treated.

Secondary Augmentation Surgical Technique

PREOPERATIVE PLANNING AND DETERMINATION OF IMPLANT SIZE

When it is necessary to remove a breast implant, the surgeon and patient must make a number of decisions together, including the incision site, the need for a capsulectomy, the choice of a new gel or saline implant, the most suitable size for the replacement, and the tissue plane to be used for reimplantation (above or below the muscle). Decisions on such matters largely depend on factors related to the patient and her implants before explantation. For example, does she have severe capsular contracture, rupture, sufficient tissue padding, or ptosis? Are the current implants smooth or textured, filled with silicone gel or saline? Are the patient's breasts symmetric, and is she generally pleased with her appearance before the secondary augmentation? A good outcome that lasts over time is best achieved with careful preoperative planning and consultation with the patient.

Major reasons for secondary augmentation include correction of asymmetry, repositioning of an implant, and changing the size of an implant. These problems are best addressed through prevention. Proper assessment of the patient's anatomy should begin through visual and quantitative examination of the breasts and chest. The degree of ptosis should be recorded for each breast. Visual inspection—including a simple assessment of the size, shape, and position of the two breasts—should be supplemented by measurements, which provide objective documentation of the anatomy (Table 128-2).

Breast augmentation produces significant changes in the breast width, inframammary crease to nipple distance, and circumference of the chest at the nipple line. Minimal changes occur in the other measurements. The breast width measurement is the best surrogate for bra cup size; a 7-inch breast width typically translates to an A cup, an 8-inch to a B cup, a 9-inch to a C cup, and a 10-inch to a D cup. This information is helpful in planning and performing surgery. If a patient wants to be a C cup size, you can usually assume you want to achieve a 9-inch breast width and test this assumption when a sizer is used in surgery and the final implant size and volume are determined. While recording the preoperative measurements, discuss with the patient any differences between the breasts to ensure she understands any asymmetry that exists. Also talk about whether and how you plan to correct or improve it.

TABLE 128-2 ✦ USEFUL MEASUREMENTS OBTAINED DURING EVALUATION OF THE PATIENT

Distance from the suprasternal notch to the nipple
Distance from the midpoint of the inframammary crease to the nipple
Distance between the nipples
Circumference of the chest at the inframammary crease and at the nipple line
Width of the breasts in inches (measure from the lateral breakpoint near the midaxillary line to the medial breakpoint [1 cm lateral to the sternum at the level of the nipple])

In general, patients with wider chests require implants with a wider base diameter. The measured distance from the center of the nipple to the point 1 cm lateral to the midline of the sternum will indicate the implant radius appropriate for the patient. The maximum base diameter can then be selected preoperatively on the basis of this radius measurement. If you try to use an implant with a base diameter too large for the patient, the breast will tend to elongate vertically or to be displaced medially or laterally, all of which are aesthetically abnormal. The base diameter of different implant sizes varies with the nominal volume; thus, the base diameter essentially restricts the fill volume range. Women with narrow chests who need a small base diameter but desire a larger volume may benefit from a high-profile implant, in which the base diameter is smaller in relationship to the volume. However, caution is required so the volume does not exceed the tissue's ability to support it. If the pre-secondary augmentation implant size is appropriate, the same base diameter and size can be used unless the patient requests a change.

EXPLANTATION

In most instances, explantation is performed on an outpatient basis under general anesthesia and usually requires 1 to 2 hours in the operating room, depending on whether an implant has ruptured and whether implants will be exchanged or a mastopexy performed. The patient should be placed on the operating table in the supine position with both arms abducted 90 degrees. Helpful landmarks to be marked include the midline of the sternum, the proposed new inframammary crease, an outline of the proposed implant pocket, and a point 1 cm lateral to the sternum midline at the level of the nipple. To prevent synmastia, pocket dissection should never be carried more medial than this point.

When an implant is placed, the nipple should always be at the center of the breast mound postoperatively. Remembering this can help in determining where the inframammary crease will be after augmentation. In most women without implants, the inframammary crease is typically 5 to 7 cm from the nipple. After augmentation, this distance usually increases to 7 to 10 cm, depending on the base diameter of the implant inserted. In addition, the inframammary crease migrates superiorly (as the increased breast volume recruits tissue from the abdomen to the breasts), and a new inframammary crease develops at the inferior margin of the implant. If an inframammary incision is to be used, this migration must be anticipated or the scar will be too high on the breast mound. In all but the most petite women, the new inframammary crease should be marked at a location 8 cm inferior to the nipple. This marking is tentative, however, as the ultimate goal is to place the nipple at the center of the breast mound.

In general, implants can be removed through the original augmentation incision. Exceptions to this include the patient with a very small original incision who needs a capsulectomy and the patient who has a rupture complication, such as a distant silicone granuloma. In these patients, a larger incision may be required to gain adequate exposure to the capsule and breast tissue. If the patient has a small preexisting inframammary incision, it can be lengthened to gain better exposure. A second incision is rarely required but may be useful for excision of a granuloma in the area of the axilla or distant from the implant. Once the best location has been chosen, deepen the incision to the periprosthetic capsule.

Some surgeons remove an implant and its capsule en bloc, but it is preferable to remove the implant before the capsule is manipulated. An incision into the capsule with a blunt-tipped electrocautery exposes the implant and allows examination of its surface. Use of electrocautery should not damage an implant, and a Teflon-coated cautery further decreases this risk. The integrity status of a saline-filled implant will be known before explantation. If the status of a silicone gel implant is unknown or equivocal preoperatively, the capsule should be carefully opened and the implant inspected. An intact implant may have either a dry or an oily surface. Should the shell appear grossly intact but free silicone gel is evident on the surface, the implant is probably leaking through a pinhole defect. Pulling on or manipulating an implant in this condition may convert a small hole to a large tear. For this reason, it is recommended that an implant be removed before the capsule is manipulated; doing so reduces the chance of changing the integrity status of the implant. Once the implant is removed, the shell should be closely inspected so its status can be correctly classified as intact, leaking, or ruptured. Any implant that ruptures during removal should be noted in the operative report.

Always attempt to remove a silicone gel implant without releasing gel because its slick, sticky consistency makes instruments more difficult to handle. It does not, however, seem to expose the patient to a risk of future granuloma formation unless free gel is left in the implant pocket. If an implant is grossly ruptured, the silicone gel should be expressed into a basin and any residual gel wiped from the capsule with cotton sponges. Because free gel usually gets on the instruments, drapes, and gloves, the instruments should be cleaned and the drapes and gloves changed.

In most instances, an implant with a smooth surface can be removed by grasping it with the thumb and a finger and gently pulling while pressure is applied to the breast. Some older silicone gel implants have Dacron fixation patches or tabs that strongly adhere to the capsular tissue. Unless the patch is detached from the capsule before the implant is removed, the shell will tear. In this situation, en bloc removal of both the capsule and the implant is recommended. The area of adherent tissue is then exposed and the patch incised away from the tissue with the implant to reduce the chance of silicone spillage. There should be minimal adherence or tissue ingrowth with textured implants, and they can usually be freed from the capsule by blunt dissection with a finger. If a polyurethane-covered implant is present, removal of the implant may require some sharp dissection. However, because the polyurethane covering seems to fragment and break down over time and most of these implants have been in place for several years, there is usually minimal polyurethane adherence to the capsule.

Once the implant is removed, a capsulectomy should usually be performed or the retained capsule can fill with fluid to form a seroma or present as a palpable mass or mammographic abnormality (see the section on capsulectomy for more specific guidelines). If a capsule is thin and therefore difficult to remove, a capsulectomy may not be necessary, especially if a new implant will be placed in the same pocket. Saline implants tend to be surrounded by thin capsules; they are therefore less likely to leave palpable masses and pose minimal risk of causing radiographic artifacts, particularly when the capsule is in a submuscular position. Because submuscular capsules are often thin and evanescent, their removal may be difficult and lead to significant blood loss. A partial capsulectomy may be preferable in this context. However, in these instances, a total capsulectomy should be anticipated, with or without reimplantation. This is particularly true when a textured implant is to be inserted; textured devices need a fresh tissue surface with which to interact.

After the capsulectomy, a thorough bimanual examination of the breasts is performed to make certain there are no masses and to look for granulomas if the patient has a history of silicone gel implants. Some women have had multiple sets of implants, and a granuloma may still be present even years after a gel implant was removed. After total or partial capsulectomy and careful examination, the pocket is irrigated with copious amounts of saline and hemostasis achieved.

REIMPLANTATION

Before secondary augmentation, the surgeon and patient should have thoroughly discussed the type of implant to be used (e.g., silicone gel versus saline, textured versus smooth, round versus contoured). Silicone gel is often better for thin women who have small breasts with minimal tissue because they are at greater risk for skin wrinkling and implant palpability. The best solution for women with little padding is submuscular* silicone gel. If gel is not an option, smooth saline placed beneath the muscle is the next best option. Results are generally less than optimal in secondary augmentation patients who receive subglandular saline implants that are textured. However, if a patient with sufficient breast tissue previously had saline implants in the subglandular position and the result was acceptable, a replacement implant in the same position is acceptable.

In most instances, a subpectoral position is preferable for secondary augmentation because previous implants probably compressed the breast tissue and thereby reduced the thickness of available tissue padding. Also, the quality of mammography will be improved. Many women underwent breast augmentation in their 20s or 30s, and as they age, better mammography becomes an important issue. The need for replacement implants often prompts a preference for the subpectoral position.

The surgical technique for reimplantation after implant removal is basically identical to a primary augmentation. Helpful intraoperative steps include proper positioning of the patient, proper marking, referral to the objective measurements obtained preoperatively, and use of a sizer.

After the implant and capsule are removed, the breast is manually examined, and the wound is irrigated. A sizing implant should be inserted to help shape the pocket and to determine the size and volume of implant to be placed. The use of a sizing implant is important, but the base diameter of sizers varies from that of implants, and this difference can have a significant effect on breast projection and shape. Sizer selection should begin in the general size range the patient will need. As the sizer is inflated, a finger or blunt instrument such as a Hegar dilator is used to enlarge and shape the pocket. The lateral margin of the pocket should never extend beyond the midaxillary line.

For submuscular augmentation, the lateral border of the pectoralis major is identified and the muscle freed from the chest wall by blunt dissection. The inferior attachment of the pectoralis major should be detached until fat is visible. The medial extent of this detachment should not go beyond a transverse line down from the inferior border of the areola to the sternum. Detachment superior to this point is not usually necessary and increases the risk that implant shell wrinkling or edges will be visible. A final decision about further release or attenuation of the pectoralis major can be made after the sizer is inflated. If increased cleavage is needed, the muscle can be attenuated medially by blunt dissection with a finger or Hegar dilator. In most instances, the pectoralis fascia should not be divided.

With subglandular placement, use of a sizer to help make the implant pocket is difficult unless the approach is transumbilical. Subglandular pockets must be made primarily with sharp dissection and according to the preplanned landmark markings described earlier. Unfortunately, this sharp dissection makes identification of the nerves at the lateral aspect of the pocket more difficult.

Although some surgeons believe that large pockets diminish the risk of capsular contracture, there is no convincing evidence to support this belief. It is generally acknowledged that large pockets increase the risk of asymmetry by allowing implants to be displaced or rotated (especially anatomically shaped implants). Thus, the pocket should be shaped to fit the implant precisely. Sharp dissection and dissection with electrocautery must not extend lateral to the lateral border of the pectoralis major. The nerve branches providing sensation to the breast (second through sixth) emerge in this area and could be damaged with sharp dissection. Although blunt dissection may stretch or bruise these branches, it should not divide them. These nerves can be palpated as tight bands running vertically. Sometimes these "bands" cause creases in an

*Throughout this chapter, we use the terms *submuscular* and *subpectoral* to refer to an implant placed primarily, but not completely, beneath the pectoralis major muscle. Approximately the upper half of the implant will be covered by the muscle. Total submuscular placement requires elevation of the inferolateral portion of the serratus anterior muscle and a continuous pocket beneath the serratus and pectoralis major. This type of dissection is difficult and rarely performed for augmentation.

implant, but as the nerves stretch over time, the creases disappear.

Both breast pockets should be shaped before the final implant size is chosen for the patient. With both sizers inserted and inflated, observe the patient from all angles (both sides, head, and foot) and in the sitting position. The sitting position is most helpful for assessing the level of the inframammary crease. These precautions allow the surgeon to evaluate the volume, shape, and position of the two breast mounds in a thorough and objective way and help determine whether additional pocket revisions are needed.

If the patient is symmetric or minimally asymmetric preoperatively, use implants of the same size. It is easier to exacerbate minor preexisting asymmetry when differently sized implants (instead of the same size) are used. If implants of different sizes or fill volumes are used and the patient is asymmetric postoperatively, the patient may blame the surgeon. Alternatively, if implants of the same size and volume are used but minor asymmetry is apparent, the patient is more likely to accept that she had a preexisting difference, especially if this was discussed preoperatively. However, differently sized implants are appropriate if the patient has a 50- to 100-mL difference in breast volume.

Once the most appropriate implant size is selected, a fresh towel is placed over the chest, and a sterilized Teflon cutting board is placed on the towel. The inert, smooth surface of the board minimizes the risk of contaminating the wound with towels, blood, and debris. The pocket is irrigated with saline; hemostasis is checked; and moist laparotomy sponges are used to remove all blood and debris from the pocket, incision, and gloves. Some surgeons change gloves at this point. The implant package should not be opened until just before insertion so it is not exposed to potential contamination in the operating room environment. Only the surgeon and first assistant—both wearing clean gloves—should touch the implant that is inserted with as little contact with the wound as possible.

Although the sizer serves as a guide, a permanent saline implant should be one size smaller than the selected sizer. This smaller implant should then be filled to approximately the recommended maximum volume. Overfilling beyond the recommended maximum technically voids the warranty, but implant manufacturers have tended to be liberal in replacing failed implants that were overfilled.

Saline implants are rolled for insertion and filled with a closed filling system to eliminate the risk of introducing microorganisms. The implant is inflated in 50-mL increments with use of a 60-mL syringe. Both the surgeon and scrub nurse should count the number of 50-mL syringes, and the nurse should write down the number as they are instilled; this technique minimizes the chance of adding the wrong saline volume. Protective sleeves for implant placement are usually not necessary but may be a good idea with very small incisions.

After both implants are placed and inflated, observe the patient again from both sides of the table, the foot, and the head. Different viewing angles produce different impressions of the volume, shape, and position. The anatomic measurements described before should be made again to ensure equality of the right and left breasts. The final decision about implant position requires placement of the patient in the sitting position to make sure the inframammary creases are at the same level and the widths of the breast mounds are equal. Push the breasts medially to be sure they are symmetric with respect to the sternal midline. Also check that the breast mounds extend laterally to the same position.

Incisions are closed with two layers of absorbable sutures. The first layer reapproximates the breast parenchyma and closes the deep dermis; the second layer closes the skin. Drains are typically not necessary; however, they should be used if there is concern about hemostasis. Postoperative care usually consists of an incision dressing and a sports bra. In addition, a 5-day course of an antibiotic designed to cover *Staphylococcus* organisms is typically prescribed. No special exercises are necessary after implant removal with or without exchange. If there are no complications, the postoperative recovery period is about 2 weeks.

CAPSULAR CONTRACTURE

Since the early days of breast implantation, severe capsular contracture has persisted as a leading reason for secondary surgery in both augmentation and reconstruction patients. Not only does this complication compromise aesthetic results, but it also undermines the patient's satisfaction to the point that some women request treatment or implant exchange multiple times. The Baker system has remained the standard for classification of capsular contracture (Table 128-3).[11] Even though this system is subjective, experienced examiners agree on capsule grading approximately 85% of the time; agreement rises to 97% for the two major subdivisions of I/II and III/IV.[12] In general, grades I and II are cosmetically acceptable; grades III and IV are not.

At the time of primary augmentation, the surgeon's overall objective is to prevent grade III and grade IV capsular contracture formation. However, prevention is complicated by unknown factors that cause capsular contraction. It most likely involves a combination of local (breast) and patient variables. This is demonstrated in patients with unilateral rather than bilateral capsular contracture, and two patients with identical surgeries and implants do not necessarily have the same outcome with respect to contracture. Even so, bilateral capsular contractures are more common

TABLE 128-3 ✦ THE BAKER SYSTEM FOR CLASSIFICATION OF CAPSULAR CONTRACTURE

Grade I	The augmented breast feels as soft as a natural breast.
Grade II	The breast is not naturally soft, but the shape is normal and the implant is not visible; however, the implant can be palpated. The patient is usually not concerned.
Grade III	The breast is firmer than normal, and the implant is visible and easy to palpate. Some breasts have a normal shape but others are overly round and visibly distorted.
Grade IV	The breast is abnormally hard and, in some cases, cold and tender. The implant is visible, and gross distortion is obvious.

From Baker JL Jr: Classification of spherical contractures. Presented at the Aesthetic Breast Symposium, Scottsdale, Arizona, 1975.

than unilateral, which suggests that a patient's individual response to an implant is an important factor in contracture development. Additional variables that seem to affect the timing and severity of capsular contracture are related to the implant, whereas others may depend on surgical technique. There is no evidence that an immune-mediated response to silicone in general or to breast implants in particular plays a role in the development of contracted capsules.

Unfortunately, much of the literature dealing with capsular contracture suffers from shortcomings, such as failure to use the same grading scale, multiple types of implants, short follow-up durations, and improper or inadequate controls. Nevertheless, a picture has emerged that gives insight into the major variables that seem to contribute to capsular contracture.

Capsule Development and Histology

Development of a capsule around an implanted device is a normal response of the body to a foreign object, and a mature capsule is typically constructed of cells similar to scar tissue. After implant insertion, the body initiates a local inflammatory response characterized by activation of polymorphonuclear leukocytes and mononuclear cells. Within a few days, the polymorphonuclear leukocytes disappear, and the implant is surrounded by lymphocytes, fibroblasts, and monocytes, the last of which differentiate into macrophages and foreign body giant cells.[13] At the same time, the fibroblasts proliferate and produce collagen (types I, III, and V), which is found in higher concentrations in contracted than in noncontracted capsules. When the fibrous tissue of a capsule contracts to the point of a grade III or grade IV contracture, patients may experience pain, and the aesthetic result of breast implantation is seriously compromised.

Capsules around smooth implants generally have the appearance of a smooth, gray, and shiny membrane of varying thickness. When mature, these capsules are relatively acellular and have a flattened unicellular lining or pseudoepithelial cell layer next to the implant; as the capsule merges with the breast tissue, it is composed of linearly oriented dense collagen cells and vascularized connective tissue.[13] Capsules around textured implants tend to be thicker. Next to a textured implant is a phagocytic synovial multicellular layer that lacks a basement membrane; this merges into layers with more disorganized and randomly oriented connective tissue that is more cellular and vascularized than in smooth implant capsules. Synovial metaplasia is relatively common around textured implants (although it is also found around some smooth implants) and may help explain why textured implants produce fewer contracted capsules.[14,15] Capsular synovium is probably caused by the shearing movement of an implant as it rubs against the capsule. The resulting irritation may lubricate the capsule-implant interface through the secretion of proteoglycans, chondroitin 4-sulfate, and keratan sulfate.[16]

Myofibroblasts have been theorized to be an important factor in the process of capsule contraction,[17,18] but researchers are still not certain whether these cells are the cause or result. Myofibroblasts are smooth muscle–like cells derived from fibroblasts that are detected in all implant capsules, although they are more common in contracted capsules than in soft ones and around silicone gel rather than saline implants. Because they tighten and relax like smooth muscle cells, myofibroblasts may provide the force that contracts a capsule. As the capsule matures, fibroblasts deposit more fibrous tissue and the capsule becomes a stable structure.[19,20]

Capsule Thickness

Capsule thickness is highly variable with ranges reported from 0.25 to 4 mm. The average thickness seems to be about 1.3 to 1.4 mm.[13] There is controversy as to whether increased capsule thickness correlates with breast firmness, but thicker capsules are more often found around textured implants. Capsules around saline-filled implants tend to be thinner—and less symptomatic—than those around silicone gel implants, especially those that have ruptured.

Timing of Capsular Contracture

Capsules around breast implants are typically evident within 4 to 6 weeks of implantation. Many investigators believe that approximately 90% of contractures have stabilized by 9 to 12 months after implantation,[21-24] whereas others assert that contractures continue to develop after the first postoperative year.[25,26] Peters et al[27] believe that there is a progressive increase in capsule contraction over time and speculate that the prevalence of grade III and grade IV contracture around gel implants will approach 100% by 25 years, largely because silicone bleed remains a chronic inflammatory stimulus. The authors have seen a few patients with grade I capsules who have had subglandular silicone gel implants for more than 20 years. Regardless of differing study conclusions, it seems wise to inform patients that capsular contracture may very well be a progressive process over time. If so, problematic encapsulation will remain a risk that can require additional treatment, usually implant exchange.

Implant Surface Properties

It is generally agreed that a textured implant surface decreases the prevalence of grade III and grade IV capsular contracture. Texturing of an implant's elastomer shell came about in response to the success of polyurethane-covered implants in reducing severe contracture. The texture may also decrease the tendency of an implant to migrate or be displaced. Different manufacturers have used a variety of methods to produce textured surfaces, ranging from simple surface irregularities to grooves of varying widths and spacing to an open-cell structure. It is still unknown why a roughened surface decreases the prevalence of capsular contracture, although it may be because the textured structure reduces fibroblast proliferation and produces a random orientation of fibroblasts and collagen in the capsule that vectors the contractile forces in many directions.[28] Capsules surrounding smooth implants have a more parallel cellular structure.

In the context of breast augmentation, the routine placement of implants in the subpectoral plane began only around 1990. Consequently, more studies have examined the variable of implant surface in the context of subglandular placement. The frequency of contracture is higher for implants with a smooth surface, no matter what the filler (Table 128-4). Perhaps the longest term data come from Collis and Sharpe,[26] who have followed capsular contracture in a group of subglandular augmentation patients for 10 years. At the 10-year point of their prospective randomized trial, 65% of patients with smooth implants had grade III or grade IV contractures, compared with 11% of patients with textured implants.

The authors' limited research suggests that implant surface characteristics are essentially irrelevant for subpectoral implants, at least those filled with saline. In an ongoing prospective study, 154 primary augmentation patients receiving subpectoral saline implants are being followed. Of 216 patients with smooth saline devices, 1% have a grade III contracture (no grade IV). Among 92 patients with textured saline implants, 8% have grade III contractures, and 1% have grade IV. Statistical significance has not yet been calculated, and the mean follow-up period is only 1 year.

Implant Filler Material

In general, saline-filled and double-lumen implants reportedly produce lower frequencies of grade III and grade IV capsular contracture than do silicone gel implants, especially those with a smooth surface (see Table 128-4). Although it has not been conclusively

TABLE 128-4 ✦ COMPARATIVE STUDIES OF GRADE III AND GRADE IV CAPSULAR CONTRACTURE FREQUENCY WITH SUBGLANDULAR IMPLANTS BY FILLER MATERIAL AND SHELL SURFACE

First Author, Year of Study	Reference	Silicone Gel		Saline		Double Lumen	
		Smooth	*Textured*	*Smooth*	*Textured*	*Smooth*	*Textured*
Cairns, 1980	29	81%†		8%†			
McKinney, 1983	30	31%†		16%†			
Ersek, 1991	25					38%†	3%†
Coleman, 1991	12	58%†	8%†				
Pollock, 1993	31		2%†			7%†	
Burkhardt, 1994	32			40%†	2%†		
Burkhardt, 1995	33			23%†	14%†		
Hakelius, 1992	34	44%†	0†				
Tarpila, 1997	35			38%†	29%†		
Collis, 2000	26	65%*	11%*				

*Frequency by number of patients.
†Frequency by number of implants.

proved, this difference has been attributed to silicone bleed, which may generate a chronic inflammatory reaction that stimulates fibrosis and contributes to contracture.

"Low-bleed" implants were introduced in the 1980s in an effort to decrease or eliminate the bleed of silicone fluid through the shell. Theoretically, adding a barrier layer between two layers of elastomer decreases the fluid bleed across the shell and thereby lowers the frequency of grade III and grade IV contracture, at least in the short term. However, given enough time, perhaps 5 years or so, the barrier loses its effectiveness, and silicone bleed seems to increase gradually. Thus, barrier layers may only delay capsular contracture, not prevent it. Adequately controlled studies with sufficient patients and follow-up have not been conducted to provide definite proof of benefit for low-bleed implants.

Newer breast implants with "cohesive gel" have been commercially available in Europe since the mid-1990s and are currently offered by Inamed and Mentor in their clinical trials in the United States. Cohesive silicone gel is highly cross-linked so it will not migrate out of the shell, even if an implant ruptures. Thus far, these devices seem to produce low frequencies of severe (grade IV) contraction (<0.5% in one Swedish series).[36] This may be explained by the cohesiveness of the silicone gel, which does not seem to "bleed" as standard (liquid) gel implants do.

Implant Position

Many studies of implant surface (smooth or textured) have also looked at the question of implant position (Table 128-5). The prevalence of grade III and grade IV contracture is clearly lower for submuscular placement, with the exception of the study by Moufarrege et al,[23] which found no differences after lengthy follow-up periods of 4 to 10 years. Many researchers speculate that the reduced frequencies of contracture with subpectoral placement result from the pectoralis major muscle's moving the implant around the pocket in the course of daily activity; essentially, the muscle massages the implant.

Not all investigators agree that textured surfaces are better than smooth, that saline filler is better than silicone gel, or that the subpectoral position is better with respect to the prevalence of severe capsular contracture. For example, Asplund[42] detected no significant difference between smooth and textured silicone gel implants (15% versus 9%) in the submuscular position. In an investigation of 167 smooth saline implants placed for reconstruction, augmentation, and replacement, Worseg et al[43] found that 38% of patients had grade III or grade IV contractures. There were no significant differences between contracture grade and the position of the implant or the reason for surgery (augmentation versus reconstruction). Rheingold et al[44] reported on 326 saline implants, 95% of which

TABLE 128-5 ✦ COMPARATIVE STUDIES OF GRADE III AND GRADE IV CAPSULAR CONTRACTURE FREQUENCY BY IMPLANT POSITION

First Author, Year of Study	Reference	Smooth Silicone Gel	Smooth Saline
Vazquez, 1987	37		
Subglandular		58%†	
Submuscular		9%†	
Moufarrege, 1987	23		
Subglandular		35%*	
Submuscular		34%*	
Puckett, 1987	38		
Subglandular		41%†	
Submuscular		8%†	
Biggs, 1990	39		
Subglandular		11%†	
Submuscular		3%†	
Cocke, 1994	40		
Subglandular			44%*
Submuscular			19%*
Mladick, 1993	41		
Subglandular			20%*
Submuscular			1%*
Peters, 1997	27		
Subglandular		81%†	
Submuscular		21%†	

*Frequency by number of patients.
†Frequency by number of implants.

had a smooth surface and 61% of which were placed in a subglandular position. For all the implants, there was a 9.5% frequency of capsule contraction. In another study, Handel et al[45] applied Kaplan-Meier survival analysis to 752 consecutive augmentation, reconstruction, and replacement patients (1655 implants) during a 15-year period. The survival analysis—which factors in follow-up time for each implant variable—found no significant differences in the risk of capsular contracture between textured and smooth implants, between silicone gel and saline versus double-lumen implants, or between subglandular and submuscular position. There was a significant difference when procedures were compared, with contractures being more frequent after reconstruction and implant replacement. This finding may indicate that the risk rises with longer and more difficult surgeries.

Although there may be an advantage for subpectoral placement in terms of capsular contracture, some surgeons believe the subglandular position produces more natural-looking breasts in patients with adequate tissue coverage, better correction of ptosis, and less postoperative pain. The subpectoral operation is also technically more difficult and produces more postoperative discomfort. However, these disadvantages are outweighed by the benefits of submuscular placement—less skin wrinkling and implant palpability with use of saline devices, better mammography, and perhaps a lower prevalence of contracture. Surgeons skilled in the subpectoral technique should be able to achieve aesthetic results equivalent to those with subglandular placement, even in correcting ptosis.

Steroids

Some surgeons have advocated the placement of corticosteroids, primarily triamcinolone and methylprednisolone, either in the periprosthetic pocket or inside saline or double-lumen implants as a possible approach to lowering the frequency of grade III and grade IV capsular contracture.[46,47] However, there is now consensus that addition of steroids to an implant lumen or pocket produces no significant long-term benefits. In fact, some studies have found that breasts receiving periprosthetic steroids had higher frequencies of grade III and grade IV contractures than did untreated breasts.[37,39]

As with all issues related to breast implantation, benefits must be weighed against risks. When steroids are used, patients may have to pay the price of increased complications, such as atrophy and thinning of breast tissue or implant displacement or extrusion, which can occur several years after implantation.[48,49] Steroids may also alter the properties of silicone elastomer; Gutowski et al[8] found that saline implants containing intraluminal steroids were almost $2^1/_2$ times more likely to fail. Because of serious complications, unknown effects on implant shells, and the fact that intraluminal steroids turn an implant into a drug delivery device, steroids are contraindicated.

Bacterial Contamination

Numerous bacterial species are routinely cultured from the breast tissue, the surface of breast implants, and the surrounding capsule. The existence of positive cultures has led numerous authors to speculate that bacterial contamination of an implant or the periprosthetic space may establish a subacute infection, which either causes or contributes to capsule contraction. For example, Virden[50] identified positive cultures around 56% of implants with contractures and 18% of implants without. In addition, 91% of painful contractures were associated with positive cultures. The presence of bacteria may also explain unilateral contractures.

Attempts to reduce microbial contamination of breast implants have produced mixed results. Although perioperative parenteral antibiotics have been found to lower the number of positive cultures from implant pockets, their use seems to have no effect on capsular contracture development.[51] Oral antibiotics are also frequently prescribed before and after surgery, but there are no data to show that this preventive approach makes any difference in capsule contraction.

Some authors have determined that antibiotic solutions for use in pocket irrigation or added to saline or double-lumen implants can reduce the frequency of severe contractures. For example, Burkhardt et al[52] conducted a prospective randomized study using saline-filled subglandular implants with and without pocket irrigation with povidone-iodine (Betadine), antibiotic foam, or intraluminal cephalothin. Grade III and grade IV capsular contractures were more than twice as likely (41% versus 19%) to develop around implants that received no antimicrobial treatment. Gutowski et al[8] also determined that implants with intraluminal antibiotics produce fewer severe contractures. However, those same implants were $2^1/_2$ times more likely to deflate, perhaps because of a chemical interaction with the shell material.

Data on povidone-iodine used for pocket irrigation are inconsistent. One study found no clear advantage with povidone-iodine irrigation,[33] whereas another showed significant benefit.[32] Even if pocket irrigation with povidone-iodine does reduce the prevalence of capsular contracture, an experiment by Mentor Corporation—in which implants were filled with povidone-iodine for prolonged periods—determined that intraluminal iodine (a strong oxidizing agent) can disrupt the glue bond at the patch-shell interface and cause the patch to delaminate. In some of Mentor's clinical studies, a threefold increase in saline deflations was also found when povidone-iodine was used for pocket irrigation. Although the Mentor study designs are flawed, the FDA now maintains that use of povidone-iodine with breast implants is contraindicated, even as an irrigant. More rigorous scientific investigation is needed to determine whether povidone-iodine, as used clinically for irrigation, damages breast implants. The only study thus far conducted on this issue determined that no damage results from extraluminal exposure to breast implants. The investigation tested the mechanical properties of 13 explanted implants known to have been placed in pockets irrigated with povidone-iodine and removed between 1 week and 55 months after implantation. For the Mentor saline implants analyzed, there was no evidence of patch or shell delamination, and the mechanical properties of the smooth-surface explants exceeded ASTM-required standards.[52a] More studies are needed before the FDA's prohibition on povidone-iodine for pocket irrigation can be judged to be unwarranted. (The placement of antibiotics or povidone-iodine inside a breast implant makes it a drug delivery device, and the FDA has not approved implants for this purpose.)

Treatment of Capsular Contracture

CAPSULOTOMY

Closed and open capsulotomies have both been used to treat established capsular contracture and were especially popular with silicone gel implants from the late 1970s through the 1980s. Repeated closed capsulotomies in a single patient were relatively common until around 1990. Today, however, closed capsulotomy is rarely done because of its frequent association with complications. James Baker first introduced the closed capsulotomy technique in 1976.[53] By 1977, surgeons started reporting that closed capsulotomy could cause extracapsular rupture, extrusion of gel into the axilla, and silicone granulomas.[54-56] Other reported complications associated with closed capsulotomy are implant displacement, hematoma, uneven capsule release, and injury to the treating physician.

In a 1980 survey of surgeons, Nelson[57] determined that about 10% of closed capsulotomies result in complications that require surgical intervention. More recently, Robinson et al[58] reported a statistically significant association between rupture and closed capsulotomy ($P < .005$). Similarly, the authors' rupture outcome series revealed a significant association ($P < .0001$) between implant failure and closed capsulotomy. The odds ratio was nearly five times as high for extracapsular rupture with closed capsulotomy than with no closed capsulotomy, regardless of how many times the procedure was performed. In one patient, a subcutaneous mastectomy was required after a closed capsulotomy because the gel extrusion was so widespread. The patient had received the implant only 6 months earlier, so it was assumed the implant was intact before the capsulotomy.

In addition to possible implant rupture, closed capsulotomy rarely provides more than temporary relief of capsular contracture. Reported recurrences of grade III and grade IV contracture are as high as 67% after one closed capsulotomy, 80% after two, and 90% after three.[23] The more times the procedure is attempted, the greater the risk for complications that typically require reoperation.

In short, closed capsulotomy no longer has a role in the management of capsular contracture, and the FDA has stated that this procedure is contraindicated. If a silicone gel implant—particularly one that is 10 years old or more—is in place, the risk of producing an extracapsular rupture with extravasation of gel is too great.

Open capsulotomy, or scoring of a capsule without its removal, has been used for years to treat capsular contracture. However, this procedure is similarly unsuccessful in providing long-term relief, with contracture recurrence found to be approximately 50% after one open capsulotomy.[23,52] Moufarrege et al[23] reported that the odds of recurrence increase with each subsequent open capsulotomy and reach 75% after three procedures. High recurrence rates should not be surprising because nothing is done during open capsulotomy to change the biologic processes involved in capsular contracture development or the implant's surrounding "environment." Furthermore, open capsulotomy without implant exchange subjects the reinserted implant to surgical trauma that may contribute to later failure. In light of the associated complications and the likelihood that a capsular contracture will recur, closed and open capsulotomies are not recommended as effective treatments.

There are a few contexts in which open capsulotomy may be reasonable, including correction of a malpositioned implant (when the breast is soft but the implant is misplaced because of a technical error in pocket formation), modification of the breast mound shape, conversion of a tissue expander to a permanent implant, and insertion of a larger implant. In some instances of implant malposition and shape modification, the same implant is reused if it is intact. Because the package inserts that come with implants state that they are for single use only, implant reuse after capsulectomy or open capsulotomy is technically precluded. Surgeons must be aware of a manufacturer's recommendation, as well as FDA rulings, and be prepared to defend any device reuse.

CAPSULECTOMY

The most effective treatment for grade III and grade IV capsular contracture is usually implant removal,

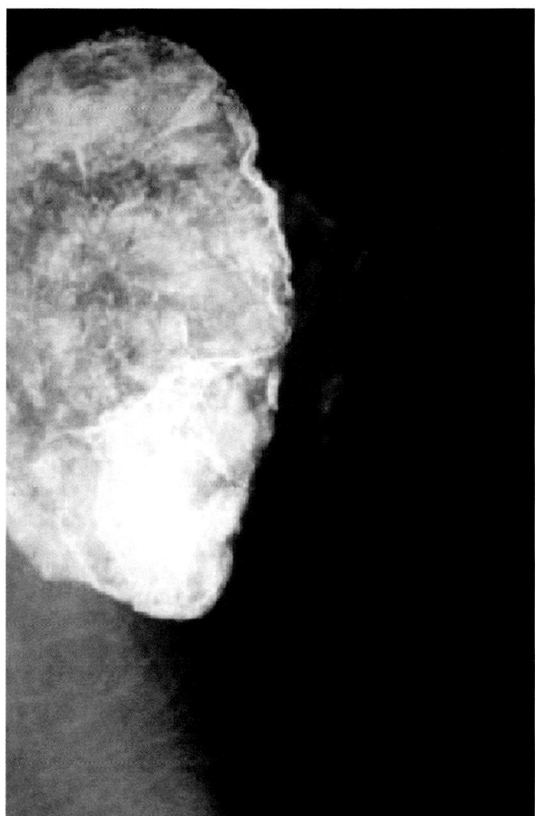

FIGURE 128-1. Mammogram of a patient after explantation of a subglandular silicone gel implant without capsulectomy. The retained capsule is heavily calcified and produces both a palpable mass and this type of mammographic artifact, which makes visualization of the breast tissue nearly impossible.

total capsulectomy, and reimplantation, and this should provide the best chance for reducing the risk of recurrence. The question of contracture recurrence after explantation has not been investigated until recently. In a group of patients undergoing implant exchange for the reason of capsular contracture, Collis and Sharpe[59] compared partial (anterior) and total capsulectomy. Most of the explants had a smooth surface, and all the replacement implants were textured silicone gel. Contractures recurred in 46% of 100 breasts that had only a partial capsulectomy and in 10% of 99 breasts receiving total capsulectomy.

Experience supports the Collis and Sharpe findings. With respect to secondary procedures, any capsule with a Baker grade III or grade IV contracture should be removed, regardless of whether the implant will be replaced. A contracted capsule is often thick; if it is not removed, it can produce breast deformity, a palpable mass, and mammographic artifacts, which may require future biopsies to rule out breast carcinoma. Calcification is an absolute indication for capsulectomy because calcified capsules cause significant mammographic abnormalities (Fig. 128-1). Established grade III or grade IV capsules may also be colonized by bacteria. Their removal decreases the bacterial load and may diminish the likelihood for development of a subsequent capsular contracture when implants are replaced. Furthermore, if a silicone gel implant has ruptured, total capsulectomy allows more complete removal of gel or granulomas.

In some contexts, a partial capsulectomy is preferable (Table 128-6). For example, implants in the subcutaneous plane usually produce capsules that are close to the skin. Because inadvertent injury to or devascularization of the skin may occur, a partial capsulectomy should remove only the posterior portion of the capsule.

Capsulectomy in the submuscular space may also be difficult, especially if the capsule is adherent to the chest wall. Aggressive attempts to totally excise such a capsule may injure the muscle, cause pneumothorax, or produce major blood loss. Thus, partial capsulectomy of only those submuscular capsule portions that can be removed safely with relative ease, usually the anterior segment, is recommended. Thin, flimsy capsules are particularly difficult to remove from the intercostal spaces. Consequently, thin capsules without calcification in the submuscular plane usually do not need to be removed, and they are likely to be resorbed. One exception is the ruptured silicone gel implant; maximum removal of the gel can be difficult without a capsulectomy.

TABLE 128-6 ✦ CONTEXTS IN WHICH CAPSULECTOMY (TOTAL OR PARTIAL) SHOULD USUALLY BE PERFORMED IN CONJUNCTION WITH EXPLANTATION[60]

No replacement of an explanted implant or tissue expander
Exchange of an existing implant in one tissue plane for a new implant in a different tissue plane (e.g., movement from a subglandular to a submuscular position or from a submuscular to a subglandular position)
Capsular contracture (Baker grades III and IV)
Calcified or thick, fibrous capsule
Removal of a ruptured implant, especially one filled with silicone gel
Removal of silicone granulomas
Exchange of an implant for one with a larger volume
Replacement of a smooth implant with a textured implant (regardless of filler material in existing or new implant)
Removal of an implant with a polyurethane-covered shell (with or without implant replacement)
Infection around an implant
Carcinoma in or adjacent to an implant capsule

Sometimes a portion of a capsule, usually one in a subpectoral position, will extend into the axilla; this scenario most often occurs in the context of extracapsular rupture of a silicone gel implant. The superior portion of capsules that extend into the axilla may be near the axillary contents, and attempted removal of this piece risks damage to blood vessels and nerves. This risk is usually too high to warrant complete removal of the capsule. Instead, the free silicone gel should be wiped away, leaving the axillary portion of the capsule in place; it will often be resorbed over time. If resorption does not occur, the capsule fragment in the axilla typically does not interfere with mammography. However, should it be necessary to remove this part of a capsule because of a palpable mass or a patient's insistence, a separate axillary incision should be made to gain adequate exposure and minimize risk to the axillary structures.

A few other contraindications to capsulectomy exist. Patients who need tissue padding to cover a replacement saline-filled implant may benefit from a retained (noncalcified) capsule, which can be used to pad the area and make saline implant wrinkling or palpability less noticeable. This is especially true if there are no strong indications for performing a capsulectomy, such as the presence of a calcified or severely contracted or thick capsule that would leave a palpable mass. Capsular flaps are also sometimes used to modify a malpositioned implant pocket or to improve the aesthetic result after implant exchange. As examples, flaps might be helpful in raising an inframammary crease that is too low, defining the midline in synmastia, or narrowing an implant pocket that extends too far laterally.

Sound clinical judgment must be exercised in deciding whether to perform total, partial, or no capsulectomy. The overriding guideline should be that the potential benefit outweighs the risk. When removal risks a serious complication, the capsule (or the portion that would be a problem to remove) should be left intact. A partial capsulectomy is usually better than no capsulectomy, especially if complete removal cannot be accomplished without jeopardizing surrounding structures.

IMPLANT REMOVAL AND EXCHANGE

Successful treatment of grade III and grade IV capsular contracture usually requires explantation, with or without implant exchange. At the time of secondary augmentation, careful consideration must be given to numerous variables, including implant position, surface characteristics, and filler material,[60] as well as to complications such as infection or hematoma that are believed to contribute to capsule contraction.

Various options are generally available for removal and replacement of implants with grade III or grade IV capsular contractures according to the implant type and position (Table 128-7). In all of these contexts,

TABLE 128-7 ✦ OPTIONS FOR EXCHANGING IMPLANTS WITH GRADE III OR GRADE IV CAPSULAR CONTRACTURES*

Explanted Implant Type and Position	Option	Replacement Implant Type and Position
Smooth silicone gel		
Subglandular	1	Textured silicone gel in same subglandular position
	2	Textured silicone gel in subpectoral position
	3	Smooth or textured saline in subpectoral position
Subpectoral	1	Textured silicone gel in same subpectoral position
	2	Smooth or textured saline in subpectoral position
Textured silicone gel		
Subglandular	1	Textured silicone gel in subpectoral position
	2	Smooth or textured saline in subpectoral position
Subpectoral	1	Smooth or textured saline in subpectoral position
Smooth saline		
Subglandular	1	Smooth or textured saline in subpectoral position
	2	Textured saline in same subglandular position if patient has adequate tissue coverage
Subpectoral	1	Textured saline in same subpectoral position
Textured saline		
Subglandular	1	Smooth or textured saline in subpectoral position
Subpectoral	1	Textured saline in same subpectoral position *(no variable to modify)*

*A total capsulectomy should be performed at the time of explantation for all subglandular implants unless there is a specific reason not to do so. A partial capsulectomy is sometimes more appropriate for subpectoral implants, especially if the capsule is adherent to the chest wall.

another option is explantation only (no replacement), with or without a mastopexy. Saline-filled implants pose some special considerations. As a rule, reaugmentation patients do not do well with subglandular saline implants because they can produce noticeable skin wrinkling and implant palpability, especially if the implant has a textured surface. Unfortunately, patients with saline implants who need a secondary augmentation cannot currently receive silicone gel implants unless they are willing to enroll in and meet criteria for a manufacturer's clinical trial. Thus, saline replacement options are limited. Effective treatment of grade III and grade IV capsular contracture in patients who have either smooth or textured saline implants in the submuscular position is a difficult problem. Unless there is some potential predisposing cause, such as a hematoma or infection, capsular contracture may never be resolved in these patients.

Capsular Contracture After an Infection. In this situation, it seems prudent to change the position of the implant to a new tissue plane as a precaution against possible residual bacterial contamination.

Capsular Contracture After a Hematoma. If a hematoma is associated with a contracted capsule, personal experience suggests that the lowest risk of contracture redevelopment involves a total capsulectomy and a saline-filled implant placed in the submuscular position. However, if the submuscular plane is scarred or the muscle is fibrotic, subglandular placement may be a better choice. No studies have been conducted to substantiate this opinion.

PREVENTION IS THE BEST TREATMENT

Because successful treatment of established capsular contractures is rare without implant exchange, attention should be focused on prevention to minimize the need for reoperation. Experience and much of the literature suggest that implant surface properties, filler material, and position probably play important roles in lowering the risk of contracture development. In the subpectoral plane, smooth and textured saline devices seem to produce similarly low contracture frequencies. In the subglandular position, a textured saline implant is probably less likely to cause capsule contraction, but the risk of implant palpability and skin wrinkling will be greater than with a smooth implant. Although silicone gel implants in general seem to be associated with higher frequencies of capsular contracture than are saline-filled devices, the risk appears lower with textured gel implants, especially when they are placed in the subglandular position.

If grade III and grade IV capsular contractures are not prevented, implant replacement plus capsulectomy is the best treatment and offers the best chance for inhibiting recurrence. However, this is true only if some variable is changed to alter the biologic environment of the replacement implant. There are several variables to work with, including smooth or textured surface, silicone gel or saline filler, and subglandular or submuscular placement. The key to reducing the risk of capsular contracture recurrence is to change at least one of these variables.

Some patients will develop capsular contracture despite efforts at prevention, which suggests that individual biologic responses can indeed play an important role in this common reason for secondary augmentation. If proper steps have been taken to prevent capsular contracture as described and the patient still develops a recurrence, do not fall into the trap of repeated operations. Instead, have a frank discussion with the patient and explain that she will have to live with this complication or have her implants permanently removed with or without mastopexy.

It is wise to be wary of claims that some new texturing process or modification of silicone gel filler has solved the problem of capsular contracture. The likelihood for development of capsular contracture—particularly around silicone gel implants—seems to increase over time, and it may take 5 to 10 years to learn the outcome of an implant modification. Claims of device improvement can be verified only when they are presented as data from scientific studies that have adequate power, statistical significance, lengthy follow-up, and proper controls.

BREAST IMPLANT FAILURE

Before the implant controversy in the early 1990s, explantation of a ruptured breast implant was an occasional event, usually triggered by a woman's discovery of a lump due to a silicone granuloma, a mammogram showing evidence of rupture, or the deflation of a saline implant. A traumatic event (e.g., a blow to the chest) sometimes resulted in a changed breast size or shape and prompted a patient to be evaluated for rupture. In general, though, plastic surgeons believed—and many women were told—that breast implants would last a lifetime. As women grew concerned about the safety of their implants around 1992 and returned for evaluations, it became apparent through imaging studies and explantation series that implant rupture was more common than previously thought. Today, implant failure is one of the leading reasons for secondary augmentation.

In the mid-1990s, several important epidemiologic studies reported no association between breast implants and immune responses. As FDA, physician, and patient worries about autoimmunity began to diminish, the issues that moved to the forefront concerned local complications, including device failure. The lack of information about the frequency and timing of breast implant failure has led to a great deal of speculation about the life span of implants, but a clearer picture has begun to emerge as research progresses. Rupture seems to be time dependent, with the frequency increasing over time, but the issue is difficult to study because of several confounding factors, such as year of manufacture (implant "generation" and material formulations), normal variability in the materials used, design modifications (valves, patches, tabs), and implant exposure to traumatic events (injury, closed capsulotomy, surgical damage). At present, the issue of rupture rate or device life span remains the most important unanswered question regarding breast implants.

Some investigators believe that there is a "survival effect" in breast implant failure data: the defective devices drop out (rupture or deflate) early, leaving the "survivors" to remain intact for prolonged periods. Others theorize that textured implants may be more susceptible to early failure than are smooth devices because the elastomer is stiffer, the irregular surfaces create stress concentrations, and the texturing process may in some instances cause variations in shell thickness. However, there are insufficient data at this point to substantiate these theories.

Definition of Rupture

In engineering, it is important to clearly define death, failure, or the endpoint, but such a definition has been lacking for silicone gel breast implants. Saline implant failure is easy to define; if the integrity of the shell, valve, or patch is compromised, the saline leaks out, and the implant soon empties. Silicone gel implant failure is a more complicated question because "failure" can go undetected for years. The FDA believes that any breach of the implant shell or loss of shell integrity—no matter how small—represents failure. However, approximately 75% to 80% of ruptures are intracapsular, which means the capsule remains intact and confines the gel within it. There is minimal evidence (mostly anecdotal) to suggest that gel migrates to other areas of the body under these conditions. One must ask, then, what is the difference *for a patient* between an intracapsular rupture and "normal" silicone bleed, which is considered an acceptable state? In both instances, the silicone remains encapsulated. If a patient has a silent intracapsular rupture but otherwise a grade I capsule and a good shape, does this represent a failed device? The implant was originally placed to enlarge the breast, produce cleavage, and possibly correct minor ptosis. Even a ruptured implant can accomplish these goals.

This issue of defining failure is clouded by a lack of standard terminology used by investigators reporting implant status in explantation series; for example, a heavy bleed, a small leak, a pinhole, and a rupture are all considered a "failure" by some. An agreed-on standard terminology is needed, and the authors propose one based on the collection and direct examination of hundreds of explants. These explants fall into three categories of integrity status: (1) intact implants with no shell defect, (2) grossly intact implants with a very small pinhole defect (often with free gel on the surface), and (3) overtly ruptured implants with an obvious tear in the shell.

An intact implant need not be perfectly dry and may have an oily film on its surface. This oil is composed of non–cross-linked silicone molecules that exist in a fluid state. Silicone fluid bleed is not a failure because the seepage of silicone oil through the elastomer shell is normal for these materials. A shell with a pinhole defect may appear grossly intact. Implants with free gel on the surface usually have one or more tiny holes (2 to 3 mm in diameter) in the shell, but these defects can be difficult to find without magnification. In this instance, the integrity of the shell has been disrupted, and the implant has technically failed. But is a pinhole defect equivalent to a gross rupture (an immediately visible large hole or tear) or more like silicone bleed? In accordance with FDA guidelines, both pinhole defects and ruptures represent device failure because the shell has lost its integrity. However, this engineering perspective may not be the best clinical definition of failure. In a clinical sense, a pinhole defect is probably more comparable to an intact implant than a ruptured one, at least in the context of silicone gel exposure (Fig. 128-2).

Etiology

Most breast implant failures appear to result from abrasion of the shell that occurs in folds or at the apex of a fold. Even though saline-filled implants seem more susceptible to abrasion because they lack the lubricating effects of silicone gel, scanning electron microscopy examination of pinhole defects and shell folds has demonstrated wear patterns consistent with abrasion in silicone gel devices.[61] Pinhole defects tend to be associated with shell folds, and it is suspected that most of these defects are caused by abrasion. In other instances, pinhole defects present as tiny linear tears and may represent fatigue fracture of the elastomer.

Saline implants can quickly develop permanent folds. Saline cannot lubricate the elastomer shell to reduce abrasive effects, which may help explain why these devices might be more susceptible to early failure. When saline implants are placed in a subglandular position, these shell folds are sometimes visible as wrinkling in the overlying skin and tissue. However, submuscular placement does not necessarily mean that a saline implant shell does not develop folds, although skin wrinkling may not be evident. Additional study is needed to determine whether submuscular

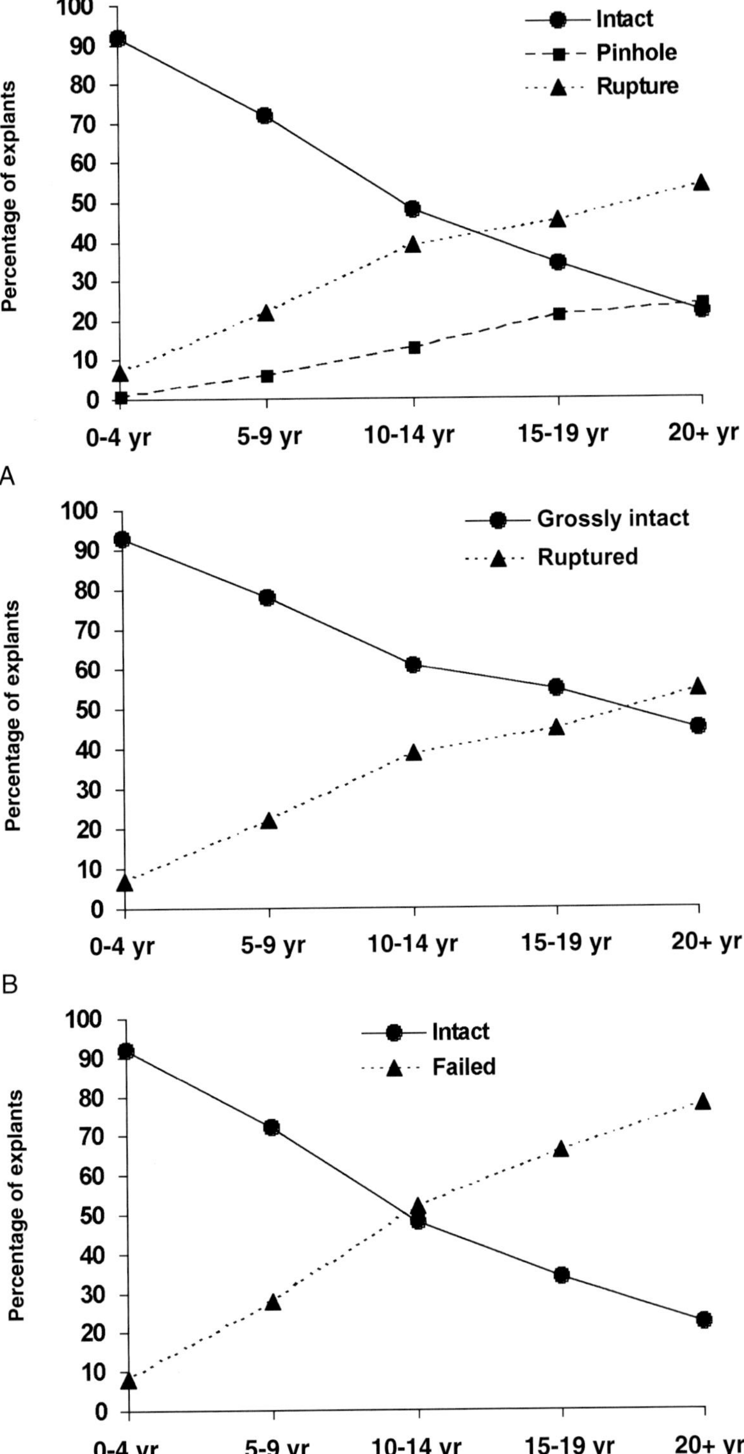

FIGURE 128-2. Status of 653 silicone gel and double-lumen explants according to implantation time and terminology used to classify implant integrity status. The graphs illustrate how failure data can differ from an engineering versus a clinical viewpoint. *A,* Implant status at removal is plotted according to three categories: intact, pinhole defect, and rupture. *B,* Implant status at removal is plotted according to the classifications of "grossly intact" and "ruptured." This probably best represents a clinical perspective, especially in considering exposure to silicone gel. *C,* When implant status at removal is plotted according to "intact" or "failed," pinhole defects are considered a failure. This classification probably best represents an engineering perspective because the shell has experienced some degree of disruption (whether major or minor). The graph lines in *B* and *C* give very different pictures of failure.

placement plays any role in reducing shell collapse and deflation or whether shell folds that contribute to failure are simply hidden beneath the muscle.

Research indicates that most implant failures are likely to begin with a pinhole or linear tear, which subsequently progresses to a gross rupture. The normal daily movements of an implant probably cause the shell surfaces within folds to rub together until a hole or linear tear develops. The hole or tear then propagates into a rupture as compressive forces stress the shell material in the course of everyday activities (e.g., the shell is subjected to gravity loading numerous times throughout a day, and the implant is further stressed by compressive motions such as squeezing, lifting, hugging, and rolling over in bed or injury).

Engineering studies have been conducted at Washington University to examine the multiple material properties of various types of breast implants. In testing elastomer shells to look for changes in material properties that result from implantation, it is not sufficient to examine only explanted devices because the mechanical and chemical properties of implant shells vary according to model and manufacturing lot. For example, Dow Corning Silastic I and Silastic II implants have different strength characteristics, and the material properties of shells can vary within a single lot.[62,63] Thus, engineering investigations have compared explanted implants (with varying durations of implantation) with lot-matched controls obtained from the manufacturers that were never implanted. To date, no evidence has been found that the mechanical or chemical properties of the lot-matched shells significantly degrade over time after implantation.

As discussed earlier, closed capsulotomy appears to be a cause of or contributor to implant rupture. Less extreme compressive loads may also be associated with device failure. Unexpected trauma to a breast implant can be caused by a multitude of events. We have seen ruptures that seem directly connected to falls, motor vehicle accidents, sporting injuries, and chiropractic treatment. Cohen et al[64] found a statistically significant correlation between breast trauma and silicone gel implant failure ($P < .001$). Trauma has also been reported as a known cause of saline implant deflation in two large multicenter studies.[8,9] Even more problematic is the possibility that a traumatic event may lead to an extracapsular rupture or conversion of an intracapsular to an extracapsular rupture. For example, in the authors' rupture outcome series, three individuals were documented in whom breast trauma directly resulted in extrusion of gel into the breast parenchyma or axilla (after a boating accident, a fall off a chair, and a heavy object falling on the chest). One patient required subcutaneous mastectomy to remove all the extruded silicone gel (Fig. 128-3). It is unknown whether any of these women had a preexisting pinhole defect or silent intracapsular rupture or whether the force of the chest trauma by itself was sufficient to cause the extracapsular rupture.

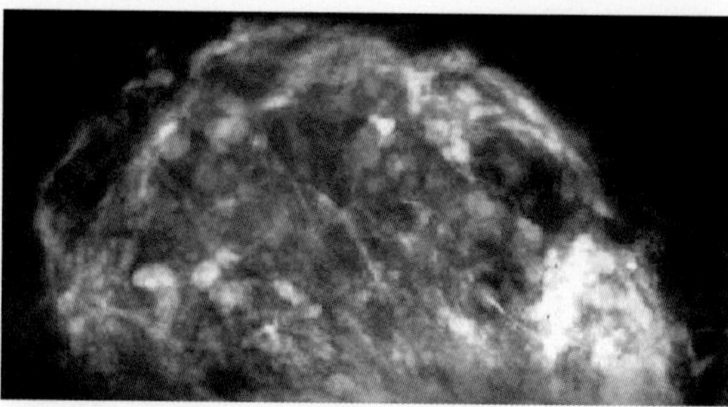

FIGURE 128-3. Mammogram of a patient who required subcutaneous mastectomy because of extensively extruded silicone gel. This extracapsular rupture followed a serious chest trauma (boating accident).

Because it applies a compressive load to the breast, mammography has been suggested as a potential cause of implant rupture. At least two patients in the authors' rupture outcome series suffered intracapsular ruptures during mammography (both implants were in the subglandular position), and others have reported similar events.[65-67] In a multicenter study by Cunningham et al,[9] 10 of 73 saline implant deflations were associated with mammography. Although the potential benefits of mammography far outweigh the risk of device failure, patients should be informed that anecdotal reports suggest an association between implant rupture and mammography.

Other sources of possible device failure are procedures such as needle biopsy and cyst aspiration as well as revisional surgery without implant exchange (such as open capsulotomy or pocket revision). Unintentional surgical damage has been documented.[8] Implants may also be damaged at the time of insertion or removal. In a study of 2844 saline implants that deflated within 6 months of surgery, Rapaport et al[68] found that nearly 7% had been damaged by needles, presumably during wound closure. Instruments are not the only potential source of implantation damage. The authors have studied lot-matched control Dow Corning Silastic II implants to determine the effect of insertion on shell strength properties.[69] Implants placed into the breast of a female cadaver through a 4-cm-long inframammary incision were then removed in atraumatic fashion through a long incision below the clavicle. This study demonstrated local areas of damage to the shells caused by pushing the implant with a finger in a typical implantation procedure. It is theorized that localized damage produces a weakened spot in the shell, which could predispose the device to early failure. The same would apply to implants placed through smaller incisions or a subcutaneous tunnel. Implants may also be damaged during explantation. In one study, Slavin and Goldwyn[70] noted that 11 of 46 patients had their implants broken during removal. If a surgeon does not immediately recognize and record this type of damage, an implant that was intact may be misclassified as ruptured.

Some have suggested that the compressive effects of capsular contracture may contribute to implant failure by inducing folds in the shell.[71] This question has not been examined systematically. However, in the authors' rupture outcome series, implants surrounded by grade III and grade IV contractures were no more likely to be ruptured than those with grade I and grade II capsules (25% versus 24%).

Saline implants have failure mechanisms that do not apply to silicone gel devices. During the last few years, surgeons have recognized that use of a proper fill volume can minimize the deflation frequency of saline implants. Underfilled implants develop more shell folds and are therefore more likely to fail because of abrasion and fatigue fracture. Raj and Wojtanowski[72] analyzed 345 saline implants made by a single manufacturer and found that underfilled implants had the highest failure frequency of 16%. For implants filled to the nominal value, the deflation frequency was somewhat lower, 12%. The frequency was 7% for implants filled within the manufacturer's recommended range, and none filled above the recommended values deflated. In a study of 995 saline implants from multiple centers, Gutowski et al[8] determined that saline implants underfilled by more than 25 mL below the recommended volume were 3.3 times more likely to deflate than were implants filled within 25 mL of the recommended range or overfilled. Lantieri et al[73] also examined the clinical effects of saline implant fill volume for 709 implants. When implants were filled to less than 100% nominal value, the failure frequency was 17%; for implants filled to the nominal value or higher, the frequency was 4%. Clearly, underfilling increases the frequency of saline implant deflation, but unfortunately, the optimal fill volume has not yet been scientifically determined.

Silicone Gel Implant Rupture

PREVALENCE

The incidence rate and prevalence of silicone gel breast implant rupture are currently unknown. Attempts to determine rupture prevalence primarily come from retrospective reviews of explantation patients in whom implant status has been confirmed through surgery. Most series suggest that failure is time dependent and more frequent in devices implanted for 10 years or more, although a more specific correlation between rupture and implant type has also been found (specifically for second-generation devices) (Table 128-8).

Although studies are the primary sources of available information about silicone gel implant rupture, explantation series cannot establish accurate prevalence data, nor can they determine the incidence rate of rupture. First, when a gel implant is removed, its integrity status is known only at that point in time; the timing of rupture is unknown. Second, explantation studies tell us nothing about the whole population of women with breast implants. It is unclear whether the data reflect the condition of gel implants that have not been removed. Third, explantation series are composed of a biased sample of self-selected patients. A large percentage requested explantation because they had a symptom (such as a lump or change in breast size), were worried about silicone gel, had a complication such as severe capsular contracture, or had an imaging study that suggested or diagnosed a rupture.

Establishing an accurate prevalence and incidence rate of rupture for silicone gel breast implants requires starting with a well-defined cohort of augmented women. Defining a proper cohort requires identification of *all* women in a practice or geographic area who have undergone augmentation over a specified time. Good medical records are needed to obtain demographic data plus the duration of implantation, the implant manufacturer and model (to determine implant generation), and other variables such as capsule grade and breast trauma history. From the identified cohort, a representative sample would be recruited to participate in a longitudinal study with use of magnetic resonance imaging (MRI). Study participants would first undergo baseline MRI examination; the number of women with evidence of rupture would yield the prevalence of rupture. Ideally, those implants identified as ruptured would be removed to confirm the diagnosis. The remaining women with intact implants would undergo repeated MRI examination at regular intervals over time. Stratification of implants by duration of implantation, manufacturer, and model compared with serial MRI results would permit determination of the rupture incidence rate and clarify the timing of failure. Because patients will have implantation durations that extend backward in time (up to 20+ years), the study will also help establish whether the failure rate is constant or changes over time as well as whether higher rates are associated with specific manufacturers or implant models.

Part of this investigative approach using MRI was applied in a study conducted in Birmingham, Alabama, that randomly selected patients from a National Cancer Institute cohort of women with breast implants. The study found that 55% of 687 silicone gel breast implants were identified as ruptured on MRI; another 7% were indeterminate.[81] The 55% rupture prevalence figure is somewhat misleading because the majority of women examined had second-generation devices,

TABLE 128-8 ✦ FAILURE PREVALENCE OF SILICONE GEL EXPLANTS WITH KNOWN IMPLANTATION DURATIONS

Author (Year)	Reference	No. of Explants (Patients)	Failure Prevalence of Explants by Implantation Time or Implant Generation	
Cohen (1997)	64	350 (159)	23% "not intact" overall	0-4 yr = 8% not intact 4-8 yr = 14% not intact 8-12 yr = 30% not intact >12 yr = 63% not intact
Collis (2000)	74	282 (162)	33.7% ruptured overall 1st generation = 33% 2nd generation = 65% 3rd generation = 9%	1-5 yr = 6% ruptured 6-10 yr = 19% ruptured 11-15 yr = 53% ruptured 16-20 yr = 56% ruptured ≥21yr = 29% ruptured
Feng (1999)	75	1619 (842)	43% ruptured overall	0-4 yr = 4% ruptured 5-9 yr = 21% ruptured 10-14 yr = 59% ruptured 15-19 yr = 73% ruptured ≥20 yr = 67% ruptured
Malata (1994)	76	83 (51)	12% ruptured 11% localized leaks (pinhole)	Mean age of failed implants = 11.5 yr Mean age of intact implants = 5.5 yr
Netscher (1995)	71	389 (198)	29% ruptured overall	Placed 1961-75 = 54% Placed 1976-80 = 38% Placed 1981-85 = 27% Placed 1986-92 = 13%
Peters (1994)	77	102 (57)	33% ruptured overall	2-5 yr = 4% ruptured, 2% pinhole 6-10 yr = 59% ruptured, 10% pinhole 11-15 yr = 55% ruptured, 15% pinhole
Peters (1996)	78	352 (239)	1st generation = 0% ruptured 2nd generation = 77% ruptured 3rd generation = 3.6% ruptured	
Robinson (1995)	58	592 (300)	36% ruptured overall (mean age = 11.7 yr) [year breakdown data are by patient, not implant]	1-5 yr = 27% ruptured 6-10 yr = 48% ruptured 11-15 yr = 57% ruptured 16-20 yr = 58% ruptured 21-25 yr = 0 ruptured
Rohrich (1998)	79	292 (148)	39% ruptured overall (mean age = 13.4 yr) 26% "leaking" overall (mean age = 10.1 yr)	<10 yr = 18% ruptured, 31% leaking >15 yr = 61% ruptured, 21% leaking
Spear (1998)	80	303 (146)	25% ruptured overall	0-5 yr = 12% ruptured 6-10 yr = 26% ruptured 11-15 yr = 47% ruptured ≥16 yr = 68% ruptured
Young (2001)		653 (270)	28.8% ruptured and 10.6% pinhole overall (mean age of ruptured implants = 13.7 yr)	0-4 yr = 7% ruptured, 1% pinhole 5-9 yr = 22% ruptured, 6% pinhole 10-14 yr = 39% ruptured, 13% pinhole 15-19 yr = 45% ruptured, 21% pinhole ≥20 yr = 55% ruptured, 24% pinhole

which have thin shells and thin gel and are more likely to fail than are thicker-shelled first- and third-generation implants. Furthermore, most women in the Birmingham study had received implants manufactured by Surgitek, which seem to have the highest rupture prevalence among all manufacturers. The integrity status of these implants was not confirmed by surgery, and serial examinations over time were not performed; consequently, the investigation could not address incidence rate or rupture timing.

Investigations designed to determine the incidence rate of silicone gel implant rupture are currently under way in Scandinavia. Scandinavian countries offer several advantages for breast implant studies: a verifiable cohort of women can be identified with implants by manufacturer, generation, and style comparable to those used in the United States; the countries' health care systems maintain centralized, detailed medical records of citizens; and the climate of breast implant litigation and mass media reports of implant-related illness that existed in the United States in the early to middle 1990s was not an issue in Scandinavia. Thus, there is minimal bias among the population. In a Danish study that used MRI examinations performed 2 years apart to identify ruptured silicone gel implants, implant age–adjusted incidence rates of rupture were calculated, and implant survival was estimated.[82] The overall incidence rate for definite rupture of silicone gel implants was 5.3 ruptures per 100 implants per year, with the rate increasing significantly as implant age increased. For modern gel implants that were intact 3 years after implantation, the study estimated rupture-free survival of 98% at 5 years and 83% to 85% at 10 years. A larger study is under way in Finland, where serial MRI examinations will be performed on between 500 and 1000 women with silicone gel implants randomly chosen from all public and most private plastic surgery clinics. Investigators will determine both the prevalence and incidence rate of rupture in the Finnish population.

DIAGNOSIS

Physical findings that are especially suggestive of rupture include a mass directly adjacent to an implant, a diverticulum that seems connected to the implant capsule when the breast is compressed, and a distortion of breast shape. Physical examination is more difficult if a patient has a severely contracted capsule. Symptoms associated with implant rupture include the sudden onset of burning breast pain; a change in the size, shape, or consistency of the breast; and detection of a mass remote from the implant. However, when a breast mass is found, it should not be automatically attributed to a silicone granuloma; it must be adequately evaluated for carcinoma or a benign condition (e.g., cyst, fibroadenoma, scar, retained capsule).

Other important ways of screening patients for rupture of silicone gel implants include history (ask about breast trauma) and imaging studies (mammography and ultrasonography). However, none of these methods is as reliable as MRI, which is recognized as the only technique sufficiently sensitive and specific to reliably diagnose or exclude rupture. When MRI is properly performed with a breast coil using the correct sequence of imaging and interpreted by an experienced radiologist, current estimates are as follows: sensitivity, 74%; specificity, 98%; positive predictive value, 98%; negative predictive value, 79%; and accuracy, 86%.[4] Unfortunately, MRI is too expensive to be used as a standard screening tool, and the examination is time-consuming as well as frightening for claustrophobic patients.

A major problem in evaluating silicone gel implants is deciding when to obtain an MRI examination. If findings from a physical examination, history, mammogram, or ultrasound examination suggest a possible rupture, MRI should be considered. At least 75% of ruptures are "silent" and intracapsular, not associated with symptoms or physical findings, and pose minimal risk to patients. In view of this, it is wise to assess a patient's willingness to tolerate the small risk that an intracapsular rupture might convert to an extracapsular rupture because of a traumatic event. Ordering an MRI examination is prudent if a patient is worried about rupture and would definitely have an implant removed if she knew it was ruptured, even if she believed that a rupture is not harmful. If the patient is not frightened by the idea of rupture, annual physical examination, history, and mammography are acceptable, with the understanding that the patient will call should she develop breast pain, notice a change in size or shape of her breast, or sustain trauma to her chest.

TREATMENT

Most surgeons recommend removal of ruptured silicone gel breast implants. This is certainly true for implants with extracapsular rupture, especially if a granuloma is present. Asymptomatic intracapsular ruptures are somewhat more controversial. First, diagnosis is more difficult than with extracapsular rupture and is best established with MRI. Most women who pursue an MRI examination are so risk aversive that they request removal of an intracapsular rupture. The authors prefer to remove all ruptured implants because of two patients in the rupture outcome series who needed a subcutaneous mastectomy after a traumatic event extruded gel into the breast parenchyma. However, the risk of extracapsular rupture after trauma is so small (3 of 778 implants, or <0.4% in the authors' series) that it is considered acceptable to observe an asymptomatic intracapsular rupture rather than to remove it. As mentioned, follow-up of such patients must be close, and the patients should be instructed to report any changes that could indicate extracapsular rupture.

Patients should be informed that a ruptured silicone gel implant is not an emergency, with the possible exception of a traumatic injury causing widespread gel extrusion. In almost all instances, implant removal can be timed for the patient's convenience and the patient assured that the rupture will not make her systemically ill.

There are no special guidelines for removal of a ruptured implant other than those mentioned earlier in this chapter. The incision should be large enough to gain adequate exposure to the implant, capsule, and any extracapsular silicone gel. Thus, if the original augmentation was done through an axillary incision, a new inframammary or periareolar incision should be used for explantation. In addition, a mastopexy performed at the same time as ruptured implant removal may carry an increased risk of compromised circulation to the nipple-areola complex, especially if the implant was in the subglandular plane. A delayed mastopexy is preferable in this context.

OUTCOMES

The outcome of patients with ruptured silicone gel implants has been incompletely documented. However, the authors' rupture outcome study has collected data to identify any consequences of rupture and to determine whether patients with ruptured implants have a worse outcome than do those with intact implants. The answer to this overriding question is no. There are no statistical differences between patients with intact implants and those with failed implants. By all measures used, patients with a rupture did as well as or better than patients with intact implants in terms of surgical complications, preoperative reporting of symptoms (local, rheumatologic, and nonspecific), postoperative symptom relief, aesthetic outcome, and satisfaction. With respect to both health and aesthetics, a ruptured implant does not seem to cause adverse consequences.

Saline-Filled Implant Failure

Diagnosis of a failed saline implant is simple: any loss of shell integrity causes the saline to leak out, the implant deflates, and the size of the breast decreases. Typically, patients diagnose the failure themselves and seek implant exchange.

PREVALENCE

Saline-filled breast implants have generally been considered to fail after shorter implantation durations than those of silicone gel devices. However, this opinion is largely based on data that include saline implants placed in the 1970s, when these devices had thin, heat-cured shells. At present, there is no proof that modern room-temperature vulcanized (RTV) saline implants, with their thicker shells, are more likely to fail than are silicone gel implants, which have historically had the thinner high-temperature vulcanized (HTV) shells.

Manufacturing era and implant type are important factors in saline implant deflation. In a large study of 2863 saline implants in 1327 augmentation patients, Mladick[41] reported failure prevalences ranging from 1.3% (for RTV shells) to 38% (for HTV shells). A study funded by the Plastic Surgery Educational Foundation looked at saline implant deflation through a multicenter retrospective review of 450 patients with 882 saline implants and at least a 10-year follow-up period.[9] Deflation occurred in 73 implants (8.3%). However, 26 of 74 Surgitek implants failed at one center (more than 35% of the total failures). When these Surgitek implants were excluded from the data analysis, the deflation frequency was 5.8%. The study determined that the type of implant used was the most significant factor for predicting failure. In addition to the Surgitek implant, which was 17 times more likely to fail, the Heyer-Schulte/Mentor model 1800 had a threefold higher risk of deflation.

Studies of currently available saline implants reveal a lower failure prevalence. In the Large Simple Trial conducted by Inamed as part of the pre-market approval application process, deflation was reported in 4% of the 2313 augmentation patients and 2% of implants after 1 year of follow-up.[7] In Inamed's 5-year prospective study (A95) that is observing 901 augmentation patients with 1800 implants, the 5-year cumulative risk rate of deflation is 7%. The Large Simple Trial conducted by Mentor Corporation (which enrolled 2066 augmentation patients) determined the 1-year risk of deflation to be 1% for augmentation implants. Mentor's longer term Saline Prospective Study is observing 1264 augmentation patients. The 3-year cumulative risk rate for deflation is 3%.[6] Unfortunately, none of these studies broke down the data by fill volume or surface type (smooth versus textured).

The incidence rate of saline implant failure over time should be relatively easy to determine because deflation—and therefore its timing—is readily apparent. Within a few more years, several prospective studies now under way, including those by the manufacturers, should provide reliable data about the failure incidence rate and expected lifetime of currently available saline breast implants.

TREATMENT

For cosmetic reasons, patients may view replacement of a deflated saline implant as a greater emergency than silicone gel rupture, which rarely causes a dramatic change in breast size or shape. A deflated saline implant may be noticeable even when the patient is dressed.

With prompt treatment, replacement of a deflated saline implant is simple, and because removal does not always require capsulectomy, it can sometimes be performed under local anesthesia. However, when a deflated saline implant is untreated for more than a week, the capsule may begin to contract, which necessitates a capsulectomy or capsulotomy and therefore more operative time. General anesthesia is recommended for patients with a grade III or grade IV capsular contracture, for those in whom the implant pocket will be moved to a different tissue plane (e.g., subglandular to subpectoral), for women receiving larger implants, and whenever another procedure is planned. If a textured implant will replace a smooth one, a capsulectomy should also be performed to give the textured surface "fresh" tissue with which to interact.

OUTCOMES

For saline implant exchange, morbidity is minimal and recovery prompt. The aesthetic results of removal and replacement of a deflated saline implant are usually comparable to those present before deflation, unless the patient has little tissue padding. In this situation, treatment may be more complicated because of the risks for development of skin wrinkling or implant palpability.

SKIN WRINKLING AND IMPLANT PALPABILITY

The increased use of saline devices since the early 1990s has made skin wrinkling and implant palpability more common reasons for secondary augmentation. There is now a better understanding of why these occur and how they can be prevented. As with capsular contracture, the causes of skin wrinkling and implant palpability are multifactorial; implant position, fill volume, surface type, and characteristics of the individual patient (e.g., the amount of breast tissue) all affect the risk for development of one or both of these complications.

Skin wrinkling is perhaps the major aesthetic drawback of saline-filled implants. It presents as wrinkles, ripples, or grooves caused by folds in the implant shell that are reflected in the overlying skin and soft tissue (Fig. 128-4). Although wrinkling is more common and typically more severe with saline-filled devices, it also occurs with silicone gel implants. Implant palpability refers to an unnatural feel that an implant gives the breast. The presence of an implant can always be detected, but a palpable implant produces an abnormal feel, like a water bag. Whereas skin wrinkling and palpability often occur together, palpability is much more common. It is also better tolerated by patients because implant palpability is a more private problem (few people would be aware of its presence), whereas skin wrinkling may be visible in some clothes.

Etiology

Skin wrinkling and implant palpability both arise from folding of the implant shell, inadequate soft tissue padding, and stiffness of the elastomer. The viscosity of the filler material is an important component of fold formation. Viscous materials such as silicone gel are less responsive to changes in position and therefore less likely to cause wrinkling. In contrast, low-

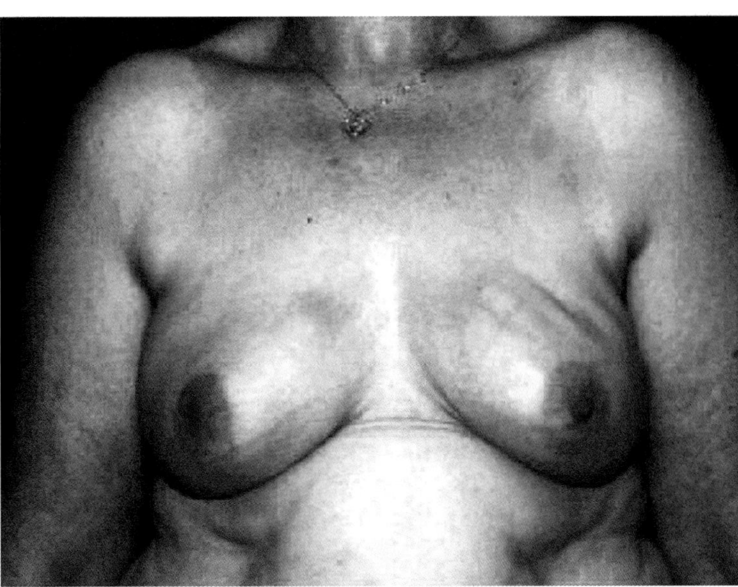

FIGURE 128-4. This photograph illustrates grade III skin wrinkling in a patient with round, textured saline breast implants placed in the subglandular position. Submuscular implant placement would have been a better choice because the patient lacks tissue padding sufficient to reduce skin wrinkling.

viscosity fillers such as saline respond immediately to gravity loading, and shell folds develop as the saline empties from the superior aspect of the shell and the upper pole collapses. The resulting folds translate to the skin as wrinkles, especially when saline implants are filled below the manufacturer's recommended volume. At the same time, shell folds play a major role in implant deflation (discussed in the previous section on implant failure).

Patients who lack sufficient tissue padding are obviously at much higher risk for the translation of shell folds to the overlying skin and tissue. There is presently no widely used method to quantify the amount of soft tissue needed to prevent skin wrinkling and implant palpability. However, Tebbets[83] described a technique for measuring the pinch thickness of the soft tissue superior to the breast parenchyma. He recommends that women with a pinch thickness less than 2 cm have implants placed in a submuscular position to reduce the risk of skin wrinkling.

The stiffness of an elastomer shell also contributes to implant folding and palpability. Texturing the surface of an implant adds to the thickness of the shell and makes it stiffer, which is why textured implants are more palpable and more likely to produce skin wrinkling than are smooth devices. Some types of surface texturing cause capsular tissue to adhere to the implant, and this process seems to reduce the frequency and severity of contraction. However, the textured surface can also cause traction wrinkling, wherein the implant pulls with it the capsule and overlying tissue as the saline filler responds to gravity, the upper pole collapses, and the shape of the implant and its folds are translated to the skin.

Wrinkling and palpability can also be caused by excessive detachment of the medial portion of the pectoralis major muscle. If the muscle prevents the projection needed to produce cleavage, it is better to attenuate the muscle rather than to divide it completely. Rarely should the medial fascia be divided.

Frequency

Skin wrinkling and implant palpability have not been consistently reported in the breast implant literature, although researchers are now paying closer attention to these problems as saline implant use rises. In a large study of complications associated with 1655 breast implants of various types, Handel et al[45] determined that saline implants had a significantly greater risk of producing visible skin wrinkling than did silicone gel implants (7.3% versus 2.1%). Shell surface type was also significantly associated with skin rippling; textured implants caused wrinkles in 2% to 10% of patients (depending on the texturing process) compared with 0.4% of smooth implants. In addition, there was a statistically significant difference between implant procedures, with visible wrinkling occurring in 1.6% of primary augmentations, 3.6% of reconstructions, and 3.7% of implant replacements.

In another large comparative investigation of 1327 primary augmentation patients with 2863 implants, Mladick[41] determined that the skin wrinkling frequency (by patient) with smooth saline implants was 3.3% for subglandular placement and 0.2% for submuscular placement. A comparison of reconstruction patients with different implant fillers found that 26% of women reconstructed with saline devices had implant wrinkles that could be seen and felt, compared with 15% with silicone gel.[51] Mentor's Saline Prospective Study calculated a 3-year risk rate of 21% of patients developing visible skin wrinkling and 2% with implant palpability.[6] In Inamed's A95 study of saline devices, 14% of patients can be expected to have skin wrinkling by 5 years after augmentation, with 12% of implants being palpable.[7] The surface texture and implant position were not detailed in the manufacturers' data.

The authors have been studying the frequency of skin wrinkling and implant palpability in a consecutive series of patients undergoing primary breast augmentation with either smooth or textured saline implants (manufactured by Inamed or Mentor). To quantify the degree of skin wrinkling and implant palpability, two scales have been developed (Tables 128-9 and 128-10). These scales are useful, standard rating for complications. In this ongoing prospective study of saline-filled implants, variables are kept constant as much as possible, including the manner in which fill volume is chosen, insertion of round implants, method of muscle detachment, and use of the "no-touch" implantation technique.[41] All patients are operated on by a single surgeon, all devices are placed in the submuscular position, and all implants are filled to at least the recommended volume.

Thus far, data have been tabulated for 154 patients with 215 smooth and 91 textured saline subpectoral implants. Only 4% of breasts with smooth saline implants had grade II skin wrinkling, and 2% had grade

TABLE 128-9 ✦ SKIN WRINKLING SCALE

Grade I	No visible skin wrinkling in any position
Grade II	Minimal skin wrinkling that is not visible in swimsuit or low-cut clothes Typically seen only in certain positions, such as when the patient leans forward Minimal problem for most patients
Grade III	Skin wrinkling readily visible in the nude when the patient is standing or lying down and in swimsuit or low-cut clothes Major problem for most patients

TABLE 128-10 ✦ IMPLANT PALPABILITY SCALE

Grade I	No implant palpability Neither surgeon nor patient can feel implant
Grade II	The surgeon can feel the implant during examination, but the patient and her partner do not Although not normal, grade II palpability is not a problem for most patients
Grade III	The implant is easily felt by the surgeon, the patient, and her partner Major problem for most patients

III.[84] In the textured implant group, 12% of breasts had grade II wrinkling and another 10% had grade III. Regarding implant palpability, 13% of breasts with smooth implants had grade II palpability and 3% had grade III. With textured devices, 44% of breasts had grade II palpability and 29% had grade III. Thus, there was no detectable palpability (grade I) for 84% of smooth saline implants; this was true for only 27% of textured implants. This study contains fewer patients with textured implants because these devices were used less often once it became evident that they are associated with more severe wrinkling and palpability. In thinner patients with less tissue padding, it seemed unethical to continue placing textured devices when it is known that the cosmetic result would be less than optimal.

Implant palpability and skin wrinkling are not serious complications like infection or grade IV capsular contracture. However, both can compromise aesthetic outcome, diminish the patient's satisfaction, and lead to reoperation, particularly in secondary augmentation patients whose breast tissue has been compressed by previous implantation. Some women also have very low tolerance for these problems, especially skin wrinkling, and may find grade II unacceptable. In fact, some request a change from saline to silicone gel implants solely because the skin wrinkling or palpability evident with saline is so objectionable. These potential complications should be discussed with patients preoperatively as the secondary augmentation is planned.

Treatment

Management of skin wrinkling or implant palpability at the time of secondary augmentation depends on the filler material, surface type, position, and fill volume of the existing implants. In general, both complications are least likely to develop if the replacement implants are silicone gel placed in the submuscular position. Should a patient with grade III skin wrinkling or palpability already have submuscular gel implants, she will probably have to accept and live with the complication or have the implants removed and not replaced. One must also remember that skin wrinkling and palpability can occur with silicone gel implants, so exchanging saline for gel will not always eliminate the problem.

Because silicone gel is not currently a real option for the majority of patients, reliance must be placed on saline-filled implants to solve or to improve the problems of skin wrinkling and implant palpability. In planning a secondary procedure, other factors, such as the amount of existing breast tissue and the risk of other complications (e.g., capsular contracture), should be considered.

The literature and experience indicate that both skin wrinkling and implant palpability are more common in patients with inadequate subcutaneous tissue padding who have implants placed in the subglandular plane. This is why reconstruction and secondary augmentation patients, who usually have less tissue padding than primary augmentation patients do, are at the greatest risk for development of these complications. In patients exchanging their implants, submuscular placement is the better choice (unless there is some reason that this position is contraindicated) because the pectoralis major muscle can add significant padding. This is especially true if saline implants are used. However, excessive detachment of the medial portion of the pectoralis major can produce medial skin wrinkling and palpability; thus, muscle detachment should be approached cautiously.

In thin patients who previously had subpectoral implants but still developed grade II or grade III skin wrinkling or palpability, the area between the implant and skin can be padded with a surgical material that provides a matrix to reinforce soft tissue. AlloDerm* and Surgisis† are two products currently available. An alternative is to use capsular flaps for extra padding.

SALINE FILL VOLUME

Perhaps the most important factor in trying to solve a problem with skin wrinkling or implant palpability is finding the correct volume of saline filler, regardless of implant type (smooth versus textured) or position (subglandular versus submuscular). The volume of saline filler is especially critical when textured implants are used in the subglandular position because both variables exacerbate the risk of skin wrinkling.

Unfortunately, the optimal fill volume for saline implants is currently unknown. Recent research indicates that they should not be filled below the nominal

*LifeCell Corporation, Branchburg, New Jersey.
†Cook Biotech, West Lafayette, Indiana.

volume because underfilling raises the risk of implant deflation as the shell develops folds and abrades. The best approach is to fill the implant to at least the recommended maximum volume. If a sizer indicates the need for a 400-mL implant, the patient will be better off with a 350-mL nominal volume implant that is inflated to 400 mL. Not only will there be a better aesthetic outcome, with less skin wrinkling, but the risk of deflation will also be lower.

Some have suggested that the optimal volume exceed the manufacturer's recommended maximums for most implant styles; thus, the optimal fill lies somewhere between the recommended maximum and the point at which the implant begins to deform.[85] At the absolute upper limit for overfilling, edge scalloping develops and the shell's edge distorts into indentations and protrusions along the periphery. A major drawback to overfilling is that the implant becomes progressively firmer as the volume increases. Overfilled implants also tend to have an unnatural feel and excessive upper pole fullness. Additional research and experience should help surgeons find the best compromise between visible wrinkling (associated with underfilling) and excessive palpability (associated with overfilling). In the meantime, underfilling should be avoided because of its association with saline implant deflation.

BREAST ASYMMETRY

Breast asymmetry is a visible or measurable difference between the two breasts in size, shape, or position. Along with differences in the breast mounds, asymmetry may relate to the diameter or position of the areolae as well as to nipple size and projection. Although it is more common in reconstruction patients, breast asymmetry unrelated to capsular contracture or implant rupture is a major reason for secondary augmentation.

Etiology

Breast asymmetry is typically congenital and may vary from a minor disparity to more than a bra cup size difference, which can be a serious concern for women who have unilateral or asymmetric hypoplasia or hyperplasia. More rarely, the asymmetry is severe, as in aplasia. There may also be other chest wall and upper extremity abnormalities, as with Poland syndrome. In addition, asymmetry may be acquired from trauma, surgery, burns, and irradiation.

Asymmetry after primary augmentation has many possible causes: preexisting asymmetry; technical errors of pocket dissection or implant positioning (see next section on malpositioned and displaced implants); underfilling or overfilling of saline implants; implant migration due to an excessively large implant or pocket; breast or chest trauma; tissue atrophy resulting from pocket or intraluminal steroids; incorrect release of the pectoralis major muscle; distortion from rupture; asymmetric release during closed capsulotomy; and capsular contracture.

Frequency

The incidence of breast asymmetry in the normal population is inadequately documented, but perfect symmetry is probably the exception rather than the rule. Minor degrees of asymmetry (less than one bra cup size) are common, present in perhaps as many as 50% of women. If women with unnoticed landmark measurement discrepancies are added plus those with a visible size or shape difference, the frequency of breast asymmetry increases. Fortunately, the more severe deformities are relatively rare.

Asymmetry after augmentation is also inadequately documented. However, the Inamed A95 prospective study of saline implants calculated a 3-year risk rate of moderate to severe asymmetry in 12% of primary augmentation patients.[7] In Mentor's comparable Saline Prospective Study, the risk of moderate to severe asymmetry after augmentation was 7% of patients after 3 years of follow-up.[6]

Data from the authors' rupture outcome series are similar to those from the manufacturers. Of 307 explantations in augmentation patients with silicone gel or saline implants, 7.5% cited size or shape asymmetry as a reason for explantation. This compares with 22% of 145 reconstruction surgeries. These numbers exclude patients who were asymmetric because of implant rupture or severe capsular contracture. Although data are limited, postoperative asymmetry is an important complication leading to secondary surgeries among implant patients. Consequently, careful attention must be paid to symmetry before and during primary and secondary breast augmentation.

Treatment

Any asymmetry that exists before secondary augmentation should be pointed out to the patient and a frank discussion held as to whether an attempt should be made to correct it. Most patients will request that the surgeon endeavor to correct asymmetry. These women must be informed of the strong likelihood that some degree of asymmetry will persist after implant exchange, unless there is an implant-related reason for the asymmetry (e.g., rupture, capsular contracture, differently sized implants).

Secondary augmentation patients who have asymmetric breasts should be asked which they prefer so the measurements from that breast can be used to match its size and shape during implant exchange. If there is a difference in the levels of the inframammary crease, the patient should be told that lowering the crease is usually easier than raising it. Thus, unless one inframammary crease is abnormally low, the preferred choice is to match the lower crease.

During the physical examination, the inframammary crease should be carefully examined and measured. If the distance from the center of the inframammary crease to the nipple is less than 8 cm and the crease is tight or the lower pole constricted, a fold in the inferior portion of the augmented breast may be evident postoperatively (Fig. 128-5). Pushing the inframammary crease superiorly can help determine how it will respond to the insertion of an implant. If the lower pole of the breast is constricted by this maneuver, the problem will be exacerbated with an implant in place. Illustrate the problem with a drawing and photographs, if available, and carefully document the preoperative discussions.

A frank dialogue with patients can ensure they understand that few women are perfectly symmetric. The different degrees and types of asymmetry should be explained, and the anatomic measurements described earlier are discussed to help patients comprehend why perfection cannot be realistically expected. A well-informed augmentation patient is more receptive to a suboptimal outcome should it occur.

Treatment of asymmetry must be based on an accurate diagnosis of the abnormality and individual analysis of its three components: position, size, and shape. Differences in breast mound position may be medial, lateral, inferior, or superior. (All of these are discussed in the next section.) Differences in breast size can be corrected only by reaugmentation with a larger or smaller implant. If a smaller implant is chosen and the patient has a grade I or grade II capsule, there is no need for a capsulotomy, and surgery can be done under local anesthesia in a cooperative patient. If a larger implant is the solution, a capsulotomy or capsulectomy is likely, and general anesthesia is the better choice.

Differences in shape can involve the breast mound, the areola, or the nipple. Breast mound shape problems due to asymmetric implant pockets can be corrected by enlarging the pocket that is too small or narrowing the pocket that is too large or has a diverticulum. Reshaping procedures should be done through an inframammary or periareolar incision. The best way to narrow or shrink a pocket is to plicate portions of the preexisting implant capsule with a nonabsorbable, running suture to close off the unneeded part of the pocket. Some surgeons recommend reinforcement of suture-plicated areas with tape for 7 to 10 days after surgery to increase support.[86] Close examination from multiple angles, including the sitting position, is especially critical in patients with breast mound shape problems to make sure the breasts are symmetric before wound closure.

Residual asymmetry secondary to inadequately treated constricted or tuberous breast deformities is particularly difficult to manage. A better result on the less severe side may lead the patient to believe something was done wrong on the other side. If the deformity is not severe and does not involve skin deficiency, an attempt can be made to stretch the inferior breast poles by having the patient wear an elastic breast band

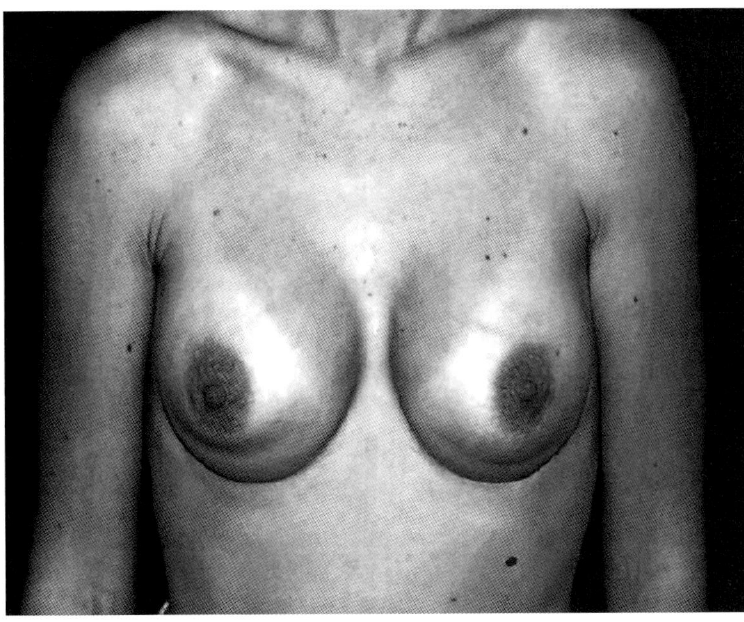

FIGURE 128-5. Patient with a postoperative crease evident in the inferior portion of the augmented breast. She received 350-mL round, textured, saline implants placed in the subpectoral position through an inframammary incision. This deformity can occur when a patient has a short nipple to inframammary fold distance and a tight inframammary crease preoperatively.

over the top of the augmented breasts. This will sometimes produce significant improvement after 3 to 6 months. If the problem persists, it is usually because the parenchyma and fascia of the inferior poles were not properly released during the previous augmentation. In these patients, vertical scoring to release the soft tissue in tethered areas should be done during the secondary augmentation to allow the tissue to drape properly over the implant. Severe constricted breast deformity usually involves a skin deficiency that can be completely corrected only with skin expansion or flap transfer.

Differences in areolar diameter or areolar herniation are best managed by concentric circle mastopexy. Inverted nipples are corrected by dividing the short ducts beneath the nipple and transposing tissue below the nipple to add support. Large or long nipples can be corrected by nipple reduction or shortening.

Asymmetry is a very real pitfall of augmentation mammaplasty because breast implants can make preexisting asymmetry more noticeable, whether the difference is in size, shape, or position of the breast mound or in size and positioning of the areola and nipple. Prevention of breast asymmetry is preferable, but if treatment is needed, it must be based on a detailed preoperative assessment of the patient's anatomy, an accurate diagnosis of the anatomic abnormalities, and, finally, a properly executed operative plan.

MALPOSITIONED AND DISPLACED IMPLANTS

Breast implants may be incorrectly placed at the time of augmentation, or they may become displaced over time. Whenever an implant is not properly centered behind the nipple, the breast looks distorted. Malpositioned or displaced implants may be too high, too medial (synmastia if bilateral), too low, or too lateral. Rarely, an implant may be displaced in a combination of directions, depending on the patient's position or muscle activity.

Etiology

Causes of malpositioned and displaced implants include technical errors in pocket dissection, congenital deformities, implants that are too large for the patient, trauma, closed capsulotomy, rupture, and capsular contracture.

Technical errors that result in implant malposition or displacement include incorrect pocket placement, construction of a pocket with the wrong dimensions, improper pectoralis major muscle detachment, incorrect inframammary crease positioning, and failure to center the pocket and implant behind the nipple. Some surgeons believe that large pockets allow implants to move around and decrease the risk of capsular contracture. However, overdissection of a pocket allows an implant to migrate from the center of the breast mound. Although this may occur only in certain positions (e.g., supine), it can be disconcerting to patients. The pocket should be properly positioned and dissected to fit the implant size accurately. A good pocket-implant fit disrupts the fewest anatomic structures, elicits the least amount of inflammatory response and repair, and minimizes the risk of implant displacement (see technique for pocket dissection described earlier). There are three technical pitfalls of pocket construction that are particularly likely to produce implant position problems: (1) excessive medial dissection, (2) excessive or inadequate inferior dissection, and (3) lateral dissection beyond the midaxillary line. Of these, excessive medial dissection is the most difficult to correct.

Large-volume implants can migrate and produce other shape-related distortions of the breast mound. This is particularly true in thin, small-breasted women with narrow chests. One reason that large implants are more likely to be displaced is their weight, which may be too heavy for the patient's tissues to support. It is important for both patients and surgeons to understand how large is too large. Some guidance can be obtained from the patient's anatomic measurements (described earlier). The radius of the implant base should never be greater than the distance from the nipple to a point 1 cm lateral to the midline of the sternum. The base diameter essentially limits the implant volume, although more volume can be attained with a high-profile implant.

The average patient experiences an increase of two bra sizes after augmentation.[87] This is true even for larger women, who have wider chests and therefore receive implants with a larger base diameter and volume. If more than a two-cup change in breast volume is attempted, the risk of implant displacement is increased. Although there is no absolute cutoff point, placing implants larger than 500 mL in thin, small-breasted women should be avoided. Also beware of women who say, "Make me as big as possible." They almost certainly will not remember their request if a postoperative complication develops.

Frequency

The literature contains few data on the incidence of displaced or malpositioned implants. A study of silicone gel explantations by Beekman et al[88] cited implant "dislocation" as the second most common indication for revisional surgery, with a frequency of 23% for 182 augmentation and reconstruction patients. In Inamed's A95 study of 901 patients with saline implants, the 5-year risk rate for malposition was 9% of implants.[7] Mentor's Saline Prospective Study, involving 1264 patients with saline devices, did not calculate the 3-year risk rate for malpositioning; however, 8% of 358 reoperations performed within 3 years of primary augmentation required repositioning.[6]

The Inamed and Mentor studies reported only 3 to 5 years of follow-up; because implant displacement usually does not occur for several years, the frequency of this complication may not be known for several more years. Even though data are lacking, experienced surgeons know that implant malposition and displacement are not rare complications. Consequently, surgeons need to pay particular attention to the technical details and clinical decisions to prevent this problem.

Treatment

IMPLANT TOO HIGH

DEFORMITY. The center of the implant is above the nipple, and the superior pole of the breast appears too full.

ETIOLOGY. Causes of an implant that is too high include failure to dissect the pocket adequately inferiorly, inadequate detachment of the inferior border of the pectoralis major muscle, malposition of the inframammary crease, failure to properly center the implant beneath the nipple, capsular contracture, and rupture of a silicone gel implant. Most implants that are too high result from technical errors at the time of surgery. Delayed superior displacement is unusual but can result from capsular contracture.

TREATMENT. Because correction of an implant that is too high depends on the cause, an accurate anatomic diagnosis is essential before reoperation. If capsular contracture is the cause and the implant is subglandular, it should be removed, a capsulectomy performed, and the replacement implant placed in a submuscular pocket. If the implant is in a submuscular position, the most likely cause is inadequate detachment of the inferior border of the pectoralis major muscle.

When malpositioning results from an inframammary crease that is too high, the crease must be lowered. If a capsulectomy is needed, the new implant pocket should be dissected lower. If only a capsulotomy is performed, the capsule should be incised inferiorly or scored until the desired inframammary crease level is reached.

Submuscular implants often show superior pole fullness early in the postoperative period, but this is not a problem of implant positioning if the inframammary crease is not too high. The fullness should spontaneously correct in 1 to 4 months as the muscle stretches and the implant settles into its final position. Resolution of this fullness can be accelerated by having the patient wear an elastic band over the superior poles of the breasts.

IMPLANT TOO MEDIAL

DEFORMITY. If the breast mound is too close to the sternum, the implant is malpositioned in the medial direction. In extreme situations, the soft tissues detach from the sternum because of tissue stretching by the implant. When this occurs bilaterally, the deformity is called synmastia.

ETIOLOGY. Medial malpositioning of implants may be evident soon after augmentation, or an implant may become displaced or migrate over time. In both instances, the deformity typically results from dissection of the pocket too close to the midline of the sternum, use of excessively large implants that pull away tissue and skin from the sternum, and trauma, including closed capsulectomy. Proper technique in dissecting the implant pocket can prevent medial malpositioning and displacement in most patients. In particular, the pocket dissection should not extend closer than 1 cm lateral to the midline of the sternum. An attempt to correct pectus excavatum with an alloplastic sternal implant in combination with breast augmentation also produces synmastia.

TREATMENT. Medial displacement—particularly synmastia—is difficult to treat. At the time of secondary augmentation, the simplest treatment is to perform a capsulorrhaphy, in which the existing implant capsule is used to design flaps that are reflected medially and sutured to the sternal or rib periosteum with a nonabsorbable suture such as 3-0 Mersilene. (Absorbable sutures may allow an implant to be displaced again.) The new implant pocket should not extend medially beyond a point 1 cm lateral to the sternal midline. Some patients with medial malpositioning may require a new implant pocket in a different tissue plane (e.g., switch the implant from a subglandular to a subpectoral pocket or vice versa). In severe instances, the deep dermis may need to be tacked down to the presternal periosteum with a few nonabsorbable sutures, although this procedure sometimes leads to a problem with skin dimpling. Patients with recalcitrant synmastia are best treated with explantation and capsulectomy, followed by delayed reaugmentation after the tissues have been allowed to reattach and heal for several months. If the patient has implants larger than her tissues can support, use smaller ones for secondary augmentation. To compensate for the excess of stretched skin, a mastopexy may be needed, which is safest when it is performed at a separate operation.

Many patients with pectus excavatum can be managed by augmentation alone; breast implants inserted in a subpectoral position give the illusion of enhanced cleavage. Never attempt to put an alloplastic implant in the sternal area at the same time implants are placed. This almost always produces synmastia.

IMPLANT TOO LOW

DEFORMITY. When the center of the breast mound is below the nipple, the implant is inferiorly malpositioned and at risk of further inferior displacement over time.

ETIOLOGY. An implant that is too low results from improper placement of the inframammary crease, inadequate tissue support, use of large implants, aggressive release of the inferior capsule during open capsulotomy, and, rarely, trauma. The distance from the midpoint of the inframammary crease to the nipple increases with augmentation. However, if this distance is greater than the radius of the implant, the inframammary crease (and therefore the implant) will be too low. Correctly positioning the inframammary crease can be difficult in submuscular augmentation, particularly if a remote approach is used, such as a transaxillary or transumbilical incision.

TREATMENT. It is critical to properly place the inframammary crease intraoperatively because nonsurgical efforts to change the location will not succeed. For example, the inframammary crease cannot be repositioned postoperatively with tape or bras. No matter what incision location was used for primary augmentation, a secondary procedure will require an inframammary or periareolar incision to correct an implant that is too low.

The simplest treatment for inferior implant displacement or malposition is to plicate the existing capsule with nonabsorbable sutures to close off its inferior portion. This will raise the pocket, reposition the inframammary crease, and secure it permanently. When needed, attach capsular flaps to the rib periosteum with nonabsorbable sutures. Textured implants, some of which adhere to surrounding tissue, may also be part of the remedy for displacement. Patients with recurrent inferior migration usually require an external surgical approach, such as a Ryan procedure, in which the dermis is advanced superiorly and sutured to a rib. Even a Ryan procedure will probably not solve the problem if a large implant is then inserted.

Very large implants are a setup for inferior displacement if the tissues cannot support the weight. Because saline implants are heavier than silicone gel, this scenario is more common with saline-filled devices. It sometimes takes years for the displacement to occur; by then the skin and tissues are stretched, and it is difficult to use a smaller implant for replacement without a mastopexy. If an appropriately sized implant is selected for primary augmentation, this complication should be avoided.

Rarely, a patient may have multiple inferior dislocations that cannot be corrected. If it becomes evident that a patient's tissues simply will not support an implant for some reason, implants should probably be abandoned. Such patients could have autologous tissue augmentation or a mastopexy.

IMPLANT TOO LATERAL

DEFORMITY. If the lateral extent of the breast mound extends beyond the midaxillary line, or if the center of the implant is lateral to the nipple, the implant is laterally malpositioned.

ETIOLOGY. Malpositioning or displacement in the lateral direction is caused by dissection of the implant pocket beyond the midaxillary line, use of implants that are too large, or improper release of the pectoralis major muscle at the time of submuscular augmentation. Other possible causes are inadequate tissue support, trauma, and closed capsulotomy.

TREATMENT. In most patients, a laterally malpositioned or displaced implant is relatively easy to correct with a capsulorrhaphy by plicating the lateral portion of the capsule with nonabsorbable sutures. The pocket must not extend past the midaxillary line, and the implant must be centered beneath the nipple. In performing a secondary augmentation to treat a too-lateral implant, make sure the implant size is appropriate for the patient's body build and tissues and carefully shape the pocket to fit the implant. If the cause of the lateral positioning was an implant that is too large, a smaller one should be used for replacement. Textured implants should also be considered as an option if there is sufficient tissue padding to cover shell wrinkling. For implants placed in the subpectoral plane, the pectoralis major muscle must be correctly released to prevent lateral displacement.

COMBINATION DISPLACEMENT

DEFORMITY. In rare instances, implants may be displaced in multiple directions. Most often, the combination is inferior and lateral.

ETIOLOGY. Combination displacement results from poor selection of patients, poor preoperative planning, poor technique, use of implants that are too large, or trauma. In addition, there are rare patients who simply do not seem to form a sufficient capsule to support an implant. Their capsules are flimsy, evanescent, and of no use in trying to reshape the pocket with capsulorrhaphy. These women obviously do not do well with large implants and may not fare much better with smaller ones.

TREATMENT. When they were available, polyurethane-covered implants were useful for correction of malpositioned or displaced implants because tissue ingrowth fixed the implant in place. Today, textured implants probably still have an advantage over smooth ones because of greater tissue adherence.

Combination displacements usually require multiple techniques as described for each type of displacement. Treatment of patients who suffer multiple displacements after corrections may require starting over with an explantation and capsulectomy, followed by reimplantation several months later after the tissues have healed. Some women simply are not good candidates for implants, and multiple surgeries will not serve them well. These patients should be offered the choice of explantation plus mastopexy or autologous tissue transfer.

CONCLUDING CAUTIONS

Malpositioned and displaced implants are not rare; their treatment can be difficult and the results suboptimal. The causes are multifactorial, including technical errors, improper implant size or base diameter, patient and tissue variables, and poor luck (trauma). Correction of such problems during secondary augmentation and their prevention at the time of primary augmentation require an individualized approach for each patient and an understanding of how her anatomy can affect the final implant position. The cause of malpositioning or displacement must be correctly diagnosed before it can be successfully treated. For all patients, treatment begins by use of the anatomic measurements described earlier to help select implants with the most appropriate volume and base diameter. Equally important is the use of proper technique to construct an implant pocket that fits the implant and centers it behind the nipple.

MAMMARY PTOSIS

Breast ptosis is rarely an indication for secondary augmentation, but this deformity is often addressed at the time of reoperation performed for other reasons. Ptosis exists when the skin envelope is too large for the breast parenchyma; the nipple-areola complex is inferiorly displaced with relation to the clavicle, suprasternal notch, and inframammary crease and therefore not centered on the breast mound. When ptosis is corrected, the overall goal is to tighten the skin envelope and place the nipple in its proper relationship to the breast mound and inframammary crease. This often requires performing a mastopexy, with or without implant exchange (see Chapter 120).

Etiology

Ptosis that follows an augmentation mammaplasty can result from preexisting ptosis (not addressed at the time of primary surgery), weight gain followed by weight loss, or the glandular hypertrophy and subsequent atrophy associated with pregnancy. Ptosis also occurs as a natural process of aging and, in this context, involves a combination of glandular atrophy, changes in skin elasticity, and stretching of the ligamentous supportive structures of the breast parenchyma. In all ptotic breasts, the skin and fascial attachments cannot support the breast mass at its ideal location. Skin stretching may be more pronounced when a breast implant is present because of the added volume and weight. At the time of secondary augmentation, patients older than 40 years often show some degree of ptosis that may need attention.

Frequency

No data could be found on the frequency of ptosis at the time of secondary augmentation, but there are reports on the number of patients undergoing secondary surgery who also have a mastopexy. In one series of 282 patients with silicone gel implants, Rohrich et al[89] performed a breast contouring procedure (with or without an implant) on 59 patients (21%) at the time of explantation. Among the augmentation patients in the authors' rupture outcome series, 15 of 307 explantation surgeries (5%) included a mastopexy plus reimplantation. In the Inamed A95 prospective study of saline implants with 5 years of follow-up, 6% of secondary surgeries involved a mastopexy.[7] Mentor's Saline Prospective Study augmentation patients underwent 358 secondary surgeries, 23 (6%) of which included a mastopexy at the 3-year follow-up point.[6]

Treatment

Minor (grade I) ptosis can almost always be corrected with implants. With moderate (grade II) ptosis, satisfactory results are achieved with implants alone in some patients, but others require tissue resection within either a vertical ellipse or a vertical plus small horizontal ellipse. The correction of major (grade III) ptosis always requires excision of skin and tissue in both the vertical and horizontal directions. The type of mastopexy performed often depends on how far the nipple-areola complex needs to be elevated. No matter which option is chosen, mastopexy results can usually be enhanced by inserting an implant to modify the breast contour and prolong the effects of the procedure.

Correction of grade I—and often grade II—ptosis with implants depends on whether the patient is willing to accept a relatively large implant that may substantially increase the breast size. As discussed throughout this chapter, use of a large implant is appropriate only in patients who have adequate tissue coverage. A thin patient with minimal tissue padding will be better served with a smaller implant and a mastopexy. Proper implant selection (e.g., volume and base diameter) is especially important in correction of ptosis by implant insertion alone. Two objectives need to be addressed,

(1) filling the skin envelope and (2) elevating and increasing the projection of the nipple-areola complex. In some individuals, these two objectives can be met only when some skin and tissue are removed. Choosing the procedure that will produce the best result is not always easy, but the patient's preference should be a major deciding factor. The patient must live with the added scarring associated with mastopexy versus the possible drawbacks of a large implant.

Surgeons must engage patients in frank discussions about the possible options and outcomes of ptosis correction, especially if a patient is reluctant to have her breasts made significantly larger, if a question exists about the degree of correction attainable by implant insertion alone, or if the patient is overly concerned about the amount of scarring that results from a mastopexy. During preoperative discussions and planning, surgeons must inform patients about the appearance of residual ptosis, the double-bubble effect, and the location and extent of scarring associated with different types of mastopexy. Treatment of ptosis often involves a trade-off; a mastopexy plus implant should improve a woman's appearance in clothes, but she may object to the scarring and possible contour deformity visible in the nude. If patients are fully informed of the results attainable with both methods of ptosis treatment as well as the drawbacks, they will be happier with the outcome.

Mastopexy has more potential risks than does reimplantation alone, including scarring, asymmetry, hypertrophy, delayed healing due to skin undermining, distorted breast shape, and necrosis (of skin, fat, or nipple-areola). These risks must be explained to patients in understandable terms. Do not present an overly optimistic picture of mastopexy; instead, use drawings and actual photographs of realistic results to illustrate what should be expected. Women who have unrealistic goals, refuse to believe that scarring might be unsightly, or are perfectionists about their bodies are not good mastopexy candidates. In addition, mastopexy is less successful in obese women because their large epigastric region approaches the inframammary crease area and causes loss of breast definition.

No surgeon wants to inflict the added scarring of mastopexy if correction can be accomplished with an implant alone. If skin and tissue resection is needed, complete education of the patient and careful preoperative planning are essential. Rohrich et al[89] have developed an algorithm to help surgeons decide what type of mastopexy or breast recontouring might best serve patients with pseudoptosis or grades I, II, and III ptosis (e.g., wedge excision at the inframammary crease, periareolar, modified Kiel, or Wise-pattern mastopexy).

The question of whether a mastopexy should be delayed after secondary augmentation is unsettled. The safest course is to postpone a mastopexy until the new implant and tissues have settled before deciding whether the skin envelope actually needs to be resected or the nipple-areola complex elevated.[86,89] A delayed mastopexy is probably wise in women who have minimal breast tissue, require several centimeters of nipple elevation, or are smokers. In addition, a two-stage approach may reduce the incidence of serious complications, such as skin or nipple-areola necrosis.[89] However, most patients probably cannot afford two operations to get a result they can accept. Others are unwilling to wait several months for an implant to settle into its final position and then undergo another surgery to produce an acceptable shape.

If a patient has grade I or grade II ptosis, she may prefer to undergo the secondary augmentation, see the result, and then decide about a mastopexy later. Others give preoperative consent to a mastopexy only if ptosis correction cannot be attained with implants alone. Whenever a mastopexy is planned, it should not be decided whether the actual procedure is needed until the implants are in place. At that point, one is better able to choose what type of mastopexy will produce the best result. With the implants positioned, place tailor tacking sutures or staples to recontour the breast mound; these can subsequently be used to outline the pattern of skin excision.

Some surgeons believe that aesthetic results are superior when ptosis is corrected with implants placed in a subglandular position. This is not true as long as the pectoralis major muscle is properly detached or attenuated and the pocket is shaped appropriately to achieve adequate correction. Consequently, even women with grade II ptosis can be treated with subpectoral augmentation alone if the procedure is done correctly and the patient is willing to accept an implant large enough to fill the skin envelope.

BREAST IMPLANT–RELATED INFECTIONS

Implant-related infections are a relatively rare reason for secondary augmentation, but this complication is serious and usually requires two surgeries for treatment. Infection after breast augmentation may occur early (perioperative) or late. Perioperative infections are defined as those that occur within 30 days of implantation surgery.[90] Delayed or late infections sometimes develop many years after surgery, often for no apparent reason. Superficial infections affect the incision only; deep infections, by definition, involve the periprosthetic space. Periprosthetic infections demand prompt treatment as a serious complication that typically results in loss of the implant.

Implant-related infections should not be confused with the presence of microorganisms on an implant surface, in capsular tissues adjacent to implants, or inside an implant lumen. A number of microbes can survive and even reproduce in the saline filler of an intact saline implant.[91] Contamination of the lumen during filling can be eliminated by use of a closed filling system. Microbes inside an intact implant do not represent an implant-related infection and do not affect the patient because large molecules such as toxins or proteins cannot diffuse through the shell. However, if an implant containing microbes were to leak, a clinical infection could be established, although the literature contains no reports of this scenario.

Etiology

Perioperative implant-related infections, both deep and superficial, are caused by the same microorganisms that frequently have been cultured from the periprosthetic capsule or outer surface of breast implants. Most culture studies tested capsular tissue and implants removed from patients who showed no clinical signs of infection. Those most often identified are *Staphylococcus epidermidis,*[27,50,90,92-98] *Staphylococcus aureus,*[90,92-94] *Propionibacterium acnes,*[27,50,93,96,98] and alpha and beta streptococci.[27,90,92-94] Other microbes have been found less frequently in implant capsules: *Streptococcus intermedius,*[97] *Pseudomonas aeruginosa,*[90,93,94,99] *Bacillus* species,[50,94,98] *Corynebacterium,*[50,92,98] *Mycobacterium* species,[93,100] and *Escherichia coli* and *Klebsiella.*[50,93,98] In a study of implanted women with clinical perioperative infections, Courtiss et al[90] identified *S. aureus* in 76% of drainage specimens cultured from augmentation patients and in 100% of specimens from reconstruction patients. Their cultures of nipple secretions from breasts with postimplantation infections revealed that 67% were positive for *S. epidermidis* and 8% were positive for a *Bacillus* species and for diphtheroids.

All these organisms are "native" to breast tissue. One study of the endogenous flora of the human breast determined that deep breast tissue contains organisms similar to those found on the skin; these organisms are probably carried to the deep tissue through the ductal system.[101] Cultures for aerobic organisms revealed that 53% of the 59 breasts studied were positive for *Staphylococcus* species, but diphtheroids (9%), *Bacillus* species (5%), and *Streptococcus* species (4%) were also found in normal breast tissue. Anaerobic species, primarily *P. acnes,* were present in 44% of the breasts. Another study of natural breast flora produced similar findings.[51]

Delayed periprosthetic infections are not well understood. They may result from *Staphylococcus* organisms, but more unusual and resistant organisms, such as fungi, mycobacteria, and clostridia, have also been implicated.[13] Typically, the reason that a patient develops a delayed infection is never identified. Delayed infections have been known to present after a dental procedure, an upper respiratory infection, a genitourinary infection, or a gastrointestinal problem. Augmentation patients with subglandular implants may develop delayed periprosthetic infections after breastfeeding or even insect bites. Perhaps a breast implant pocket somehow serves as a collection point for microorganisms in certain patients or contexts, such as when the immune system is compromised. Another theory suggests that the presence of a foreign body may reduce the threshold for infection, which means that fewer organisms are required to produce infection.[102]

Although patients with total joint replacements, artificial heart valves, and transplants benefit from prophylactic antibiotics when they undergo minor surgery or teeth cleaning, no data suggest that breast implant patients derive similar benefits. Many surgeons prescribe perioperative prophylactic antibiotics at the time of implant placement; at least as many do not, in part because selection of an antibiotic is complicated by the number of microorganisms implicated in implant-related infections. Furthermore, there are no data to show that prophylactic antibiotics play any role in reducing the frequency of infection.

Factors that increase the likelihood of implant-related infections are prolonged operative time, a break in sterile technique that leads to pocket or implant contamination, and multiple insertions and removals of sizers or implants. To reduce potential sources of microbial contamination, closed filling systems should be used whenever saline is introduced into tissue expanders or breast implants. The saline and all implant components should also remain in their sterile packaging until immediately before implantation. Environmental organisms most commonly isolated from operating room air are *Propionibacterium* species, *S. aureus,* and diphtheroids.[103]

Potential nonpreventable sources of contamination, such as those in a patient's natural flora, are more of a problem than preventable sources. Placing implants in a subpectoral position may reduce the chances of contamination by skin flora carried through the breast ducts. Subpectoral placement has another advantage; because muscle is better vascularized than the breast parenchyma, infection-causing organisms should be less prevalent. Even if all these precautions are taken, it is not difficult to imagine that naturally occurring organisms in the periprosthetic space could collect and produce an infection long after implantation.

Frequency

The literature indicates that infections after breast augmentation are rare, generally below 4%.[1,8,9,30,41,44,88,100] Periprosthetic infections tend to occur more often after breast reconstruction. Handel et al[45] examined several variables to look for any associations between infection and implantation. The only significant finding related to procedure type, with infection twice as common after reconstruction (4.3%) as after primary augmentation (1.9%) or implant replacement (1.5%). No associations were detected between infections and implant filler material, surface type (smooth versus textured versus polyurethane), or implant position (subglandular versus submuscular).

In the Inamed Large Simple Trial of saline implants, the 1-year risk rate for implant-related infection was calculated to be 2% of augmented breasts, 6% of reconstructed breasts, and 3% of breasts undergoing secondary procedures.[7] For 132 augmentation implants removed by the 4-year follow-up point in Inamed's prospective A95 study, infection was the main reason for removal of 1% of implants (compared with 10% of reconstruction implants). The Mentor Saline Prospective Study reported similar results.[6] The 3-year risk rate for infection was 2% of implants placed for augmentation (9% for reconstruction). Through 3 years, 5% of 137 explanted Mentor augmentation implants were removed because of infection (as opposed to 24% of reconstruction implants). In the authors' rupture outcome series, surgery was needed to remove 7 of 559 implants (1.3%) because of infection in augmentation patients. Only one infection was perioperative; the other six were delayed for time frames ranging from 6 months to 4.5 years.

Diagnosis and Treatment

Superficial infections, which are usually perioperative, tend to be limited to the area of the incision and are manifested by localized tenderness, erythema, and occasional drainage. These infections can often be managed by opening the incision, providing local wound care, and treating with antibiotics. Cultures should be obtained to guide antibiotic treatment, but because most are caused by *Staphylococcus* species, the initial antibiotic should be directed at these organisms. In a review of infections associated with implanted devices, Dougherty[94] pointed out that gram-positive bacteria, such as staphylococci and streptococci, are found most frequently; however, infections caused by gram-negative organisms and fungi tend to be more serious and are unlikely to resolve without implant removal.

Deep infections of the periprosthetic space present with breast pain and enlargement, fever, chills, and malaise. In many instances, the incisions will be unremarkable and no erythema will be present. Rare instances of life-threatening infections, including toxic shock, have been reported with breast implants, so serious complications must be considered when patients are evaluated. If a patient with implants presents with breast enlargement, pain, and malaise, an ultrasound examination should be performed to confirm the presence of fluid around the implant.

Antibiotics can be administered, but deep infections almost always require explantation. Infected capsules are often inflamed, and their removal can cause significant bleeding. If the capsule is thin and not calcified, a capsulectomy may be contraindicated. Insertion of a suction drain is usually wise because the inflammation associated with an infection will result in transudation of large amounts of fluid. Infection resolution is usually rapid after removal of the implant, thorough irrigation of the pocket, and administration of antibiotics. Replacement of the implant should always be delayed.

After explantation because of an infection, when can an implant be safely reinserted? Two considerations are involved in this question, an infectious component and a tissue component. Although the overt symptoms of infection may resolve quickly, microorganisms may lie dormant in the tissues for months. Reinsertion of an implant may not lead to a clinical suppurative infection but may predispose to capsular contracture, perhaps because residual organisms establish a subclinical infection. Immediately after explantation for an infection, the tissues are swollen and indurated, and resolution may take 1 to 6 months, depending on the virulence of the infection and the patient's healing characteristics. Reimplantation should be postponed until the tissues are soft and pliable. At a minimum, this will require 1 to 3 months. However, if the infection was severe, the tissues may not be ready for up to 6 months. Do not rush into reaugmentation and experience a second infection and another two operations (for removal and delayed replacement).

Although periprosthetic infections almost always require explantation and delayed replacement, the authors have treated two patients whose infections resolved with intravenous antibiotic therapy. One patient was hospitalized for nearly 2 weeks, and the other underwent intravenous treatment at home. Both women had valid reasons for not wanting to undergo additional surgeries and were willing to try intravenous therapy after oral antibiotics failed. One of the patients ended up with a grade II capsule; the other developed a grade IV contracture, which, for her, was preferable to additional surgery. This treatment approach is not recommended because of the inconvenience and expense, plus there are no data to show how effective intravenous therapy would be for the majority of patients. Even so, for those who are adamantly opposed to additional surgery, intravenous treatment may be worth trying.

IMPLANT EXTRUSION

Extrusion of a breast implant occurs if the overlying skin and tissue erode to such a degree that the implant is exposed. Extrusion typically occurs in the inferior portion of the breast, and gravity no doubt plays a role in this. In addition, tissue is more likely to erode around the incision site where the breast tissue and skin have been disrupted. Although extruded implants are rare, this serious complication inevitably leads to secondary surgery. Most extrusions happen soon after implantation, but delays of several years have been reported.

Etiology

Intraluminal or periprosthetic steroids, large implants, inadequate tissue padding, capsular contracture, closed capsulotomy, implant variables, delayed wound healing, and trauma are potential causes of extruded implants. Although pocket or wound infection can result in implant extrusion, most are sterile, with development of infection secondary to implant exposure.

In an effort to reduce the severity of capsular contracture, some surgeons placed corticosteroids either in the periprosthetic pocket or inside saline or double-lumen implants. As discussed earlier, this approach has been abandoned because it can produce serious complications, including atrophy and thinning of breast tissue that may lead to implant extrusion or displacement as well as implant ptosis. Because these complications are often not evident for several years after augmentation, surgeons may still encounter implants that extruded after steroid treatment.

Large implants placed in thin, small-breasted women or in others with little tissue padding press against the tight overlying skin. Gravity exerts a downward pressure on the subcutaneous tissue and skin that may be sufficient to produce tissue thinning and subsequent implant exposure. Some have speculated that underwire bras or tight garments may generate a "counterpressure" that could exacerbate skin erosion.[104]

As early as the 1960s, researchers noticed that capsular contracture contributes to implant extrusion, especially if the capsule develops a palpable projection that continually applies pressure to the overlying tissue.[105,106] Also implicated are approaches to treat or to prevent capsular contracture, including closed capsulotomy, excessive breast massage, and implants with thick textured surfaces.[104,107] In addition, Derman[104] reported that extrusion of an underfilled saline implant probably related to excessive folding in the implant shell that rubbed against the tissue.

Frequency

Implant extrusion is more common after breast reconstruction than after augmentation, as much as 16% versus 2%, respectively, in a 1970 study.[108] This no doubt relates to the fact that reconstruction patients have so little tissue padding. The patients in the authors' rupture outcome series reflect the same trend; 0.3% of augmentation explantations involved an extruded implant compared with 3.4% of reconstruction explantations. Among this series, the one augmentation patient who had an extruded implant also had a periprosthetic pocket infection. The Mentor Saline Prospective Study reported no extrusions of saline implants among its augmentation patients; in the reconstruction group, 5% of 135 implants removed by the 5-year follow-up point had extruded.[6] Results from the corresponding Inamed 1995 Augmentation (A95) and 1995 Reconstruction (R95) studies were similar; one augmentation implant extruded, compared with 6% of reconstruction implants.[7]

Treatment

Extruded breast implants always require surgical treatment. Some surgeons recommend explantation, capsulectomy if needed, and delayed reaugmentation after the wound and surrounding tissues have completely healed.[104] Others believe an extruded implant that is not associated with an infected pocket or incision can be managed with one surgery.[106] This approach has the obvious advantage of requiring only one surgery instead of the added expense and discomfort to the patient of two. Implant exchange may be necessary in a one-stage procedure but is not always required if the extruded implant is new.

It is doubtful that an extruded implant can be salvaged in a single procedure without adding padding in the thin area through which the implant eroded. This might involve moving the implant from a subglandular to a subpectoral plane, where the muscle can provide additional coverage. Another option is the addition of a surgical padding material between the implant and the skin. At least two products (AlloDerm and Surgisis) that serve as a matrix to reinforce soft tissue are currently available. In extreme instances, padding can be added by transposing the latissimus dorsi muscle to the breast mound; however, this is a much more complicated procedure and produces a scar on the back.

The reason for the implant extrusion should be addressed in the secondary augmentation. For example, if capsular contracture or implant folding is the cause, the reoperation should resolve these problems. If steroids led to atrophy or thinning of the tissues, a new implant without steroids should be inserted. Large implants should not be used for replacement after an extrusion because the risk of recurrence is too great. Problems with wound healing or a periprosthetic infection call for explantation and delayed reaugmentation. No matter what the cause of an extruded implant, every effort should be made to supplement the padding between the implant and the skin. If sufficient padding can be added and a reasonably sized implant without steroids is placed, acceptable results can be obtained after extrusion.

HEMATOMAS AND SEROMAS

Hematoma and seroma are relatively rare indications for secondary augmentation, although they may require surgical evacuation without implant exchange. Their greatest significance is the speculated role they may play in capsular contracture development. Some clinical studies have found statistical associations between hematomas and severe contractures.[45,109,110] Others have detected no association.[12,34,42] Handel's investigation,[45] which used Kaplan-Meier and chi-squared analysis of 1655 implants, discovered no correlation between hematoma or seroma and implant filler material, surface texture, or implant position.

A hematoma is a significant accumulation of blood in the space surrounding an implant or at the incision site. Some blood accumulates around every implant, but clinically significant hematomas present with noticeable breast enlargement, sometimes nearly twice the size of the opposite breast. The breast with a hematoma is also tight, painful, and often bruised. When a patient complains of a swollen breast and increasing unilateral pain, she should be seen promptly to rule out hematoma, which can lead to tissue ischemia if it is not quickly treated. Superficial hematomas in the wound do not result in breast enlargement but produce swelling and pain in the incision area. Hematomas may also occur in the long subcutaneous tunnel developed as part of the transumbilical approach to augmentation. These produce pain, swelling, and bruising along the tunnel.

A seroma is a buildup of body fluids around an implant. No data on the chemical analysis of seroma fluid could be found, but it is generally considered a protein-rich solution. Seromas generally do not generate sufficient pressure to cause tissue ischemia, but they can be a source of breast enlargement and asymmetry. A seroma should be suspected in the early postoperative period when there is breast enlargement. It may be possible to palpate the fluid in the breast, but an ultrasound examination is usually required to establish the diagnosis.

Etiology

HEMATOMA

There is no specific cause of hematomas, although inadequate hemostasis, aspirin consumption, history of easy bruisability, overexertion, and trauma can be contributory. Meticulous hemostasis is essential in all surgery. Patients should stop taking aspirin or any acetylsalicylic acid–containing compounds for a minimum of 2 weeks before surgery and not restart for 2 weeks after surgery. Women with coagulopathy are poor candidates for breast implantation in the first place and are at high risk for hematoma. Because most hematomas occur within the first week after surgery, patients should restrict their activities during that time. Mild exertion may be enough to cause blood vessels to break in the developing capsule.

Late hematomas are extremely rare but may develop years after augmentation or reconstruction. The reason is unknown, but they have been associated with microfractures in severely contracted capsules, closed capsulotomy, and traumatic injuries.[111-113] In all these possibilities, some force that starts bleeding is probably responsible.

Many surgeons employ drains to evacuate blood and tissue fluids after surgery. The literature contains no proof that drains prevent or treat expanding hematomas, although some believe that drains can play a role in preventing seromas and the resultant pseudobursa around textured implants. However, because the efficacy of drains in preventing hematoma and seroma has not been demonstrated and because they are a significant source of discomfort to patients, many surgeons believe the use of drains in routine primary and secondary augmentation is unnecessary.

SEROMA

There is no clear etiology for seromas, but they occur more frequently around textured implants. Irritation of the surrounding tissue by the roughened shell surface, which enhances exudation of fluid, is thought to play a role in seroma formation, although no experimental evidence has confirmed this. Tissue irritation may also explain synovial metaplasia in implant capsules. Synovial metaplasia, which is more common around textured implants, is associated with a slippery, joint-like fluid that resembles the seroma fluid around breast implants.

Frequency

The frequency of hematoma formation after breast implantation ranges from 0% to 6%.[1,8,9,11,39,41,44,114,115] Seromas are reported even more rarely. Most hematomas develop within hours or days of implantation, and most require reoperation. The 5-year risk rate was 2% for hematoma (3% for seroma) in the Inamed A95 study and 1% for hematoma (4% for seroma) in their R95 study.[7] In the Mentor Saline Prospective Study, the 3-year risk rate for hematoma was 2% in augmentation patients and 1% of reconstruction patients; the risk rate for seroma was 6% in reconstruction patients.[6]

Treatment

HEMATOMA

If superficial hematomas do not resolve on their own, they can be managed by evacuation and expression of blood under local anesthesia. Deep expanding hematomas require prompt open evacuation because there is a small risk of ischemic damage from the pressure of the expansion. If a remote incision was used for implant placement, hematoma evacuation should be done through an inframammary incision to reduce the risk of implant damage. When a deep hematoma is treated, the implant should be removed, the blood clots washed out with saline, and hemostasis obtained. There will frequently be diffuse bleeding that requires persistence to control. Topical thrombin may be useful as an adjunct, although there is no clear evidence of its benefit. After hematoma evacuation, insert a suction drain—not to prevent a recurrence but to prevent a seroma. Some surgeons prescribe antibiotics or irrigate with antibiotic solution because of concerns about infection or the belief that hematomas are associated with severe capsular contracture. The literature does not substantiate an increased rate of infection after hematoma evacuation, and the relationship to capsular contracture remains unclear.

Technically, implants are single-use devices and should not be removed and then put back. For practical reasons, however, most surgeons reinsert the same implant, especially if a hematoma is evacuated within a few days of implant placement.

SEROMA

Many small seromas resolve spontaneously without intervention. Larger seromas that produce problematic asymmetry require open evacuation. Although it is possible to drain seromas percutaneously with ultrasound guidance, there is a small risk of damaging the implant. The safest course is to insert a vacuum drain, under direct visualization and sterile conditions, until the fluid drainage is less than 30 mL/day. If a textured implant is present, drainage should be prompt and thorough to prevent pseudocapsule formation.

CHANGE IN BREAST IMPLANT SIZE

A patient's request for a change in implant size is not a complication of implantation but an exclusively cosmetic concern. The size of the implant is sometimes changed at the time of reoperation for another indication, such as breast asymmetry, capsular contracture, or device failure. Too often, though, secondary augmentation is done solely because patients are unhappy with their implant size. Miscommunication between patient and surgeon is probably at fault when women request a size change within a year or so of augmentation. A change request several years after augmentation is more understandable; as women age, their body image may have evolved or they may have developed ptosis that is best treated with a larger implant. Getting the size right at the time of primary augmentation is extremely important because implant size change is a major reason for secondary augmentation that is usually avoidable. It is unfortunate that patients feel the need to undergo a secondary surgery because of dissatisfaction unrelated to a complication.

Frequency of Size Change Requests

Two large multicenter outcome studies of saline-filled breast implants have reported on satisfaction with implant size as part of patients' satisfaction. Although these data do not directly relate to the question of size change frequency because the patients were not requesting another surgery, both studies reported that more than 30% of patients were not satisfied with their implant size.[8,9]

Most women who request a size change want larger implants. In the authors' rupture outcome series, 12 of 307 secondary augmentation surgeries (3.9%) were done to change implant size. Nine patients wanted to be made larger, and three wanted to be smaller. The implantation duration for the 12 size change surgeries ranged from 1.5 months to 18 years; three requests for size change were made within 12 months of augmentation.

The National Breast Implant Registry collects data on numbers of and reasons for implant replacement surgeries. Since the Registry was started in 2000, "change in implant size" has consistently been given as a reason for implant exchange in at least 30% of surgeries.

The frequency of size change is also high in the Mentor and Inamed prospective saline implant studies. For both manufacturers, a requested size change was the most common indication for secondary augmentation at the 3-year follow-up point (43% of Inamed's 132 implant removals[7] and 37% of Mentor's 137 implant removals[6]). Although the frequency of size change requests has not been well documented in the literature, the numbers from the McGhan and Mentor studies seem embarrassingly high and largely unnecessary.

Reducing the Frequency of Size Change Requests

Why do so many augmentation patients request a change in implant size? The cause is rooted in how the first implant and resultant breast size were chosen. Historically, surgeons have asked patients roughly what they want and then selected implants that will produce a breast mound that is pleasing in appearance with good projection and cleavage. In reality, this approach does not always produce the results the patient wanted or needed and, in fact, may generate demands for change. The same is true for having patients try out different sizes of external prostheses inside a bra. This method of sizing does not give a good indication of the final result because it cannot account for tissue compression.

The need for secondary augmentation to change implant size can be almost eliminated if surgeons follow a few simple steps. Begin by having the patient find a photograph of an augmented patient with a body build similar to her own. Several excellent Web sites post hundreds of "before" and "after" photographs of real women (not models) with breast implants. Most patients can find someone similar to themselves (usually they discover several examples of augmented women with body builds like their own). When the patient returns with her photographs, spend some time looking at them with her and explain whether the result she desires is achievable and realistic. If not, look at the Web site with her to illustrate results that are reasonable. Working from photographs of actual augmentations is greatly preferable to having a patient bring in pictures of a model with "ideal" breasts when the rest of the model's body bears little resemblance to the patient's own.

Another important step for reducing the need for a size change reoperation is to follow the suggestions for selecting an appropriately sized implant described early in this chapter. Especially important is measuring the width of the breast at the level of the nipple. Pechter[116] reported an 84% correlation between breast width in inches and bra cup size in the United States; a breast width of 7 inches equates to an A cup, 8 inches to a B cup, 9 inches to a C cup, 10 inches to a D cup, and so on. This information is useful for determining postoperative breast size in both augmentation and reduction patients. The average woman experiences an increase of two bra sizes with breast augmentation,[87] and patients usually have a good idea of what bra cup size they want to be.

Having the patient take an active role in choosing her final appearance and breast size largely eliminates requests for size changes. The first author has been using this approach for several years, and it largely accounts for the disparity between the number of size change requests in the authors' rupture outcome series (3.9% of patients) and those of the manufacturers (43% and 37%). The steps to getting the size right are simple: have the patient find photographs of other patients that illustrate what she wants to look like, ask what cup size she has in mind, discuss whether the result she desires is realistic, measure the breast width as a surrogate of cup size, and try to match the patient with the photographs intraoperatively.

A few cautions are necessary. Changing to a larger implant size is usually a reasonable request but is inadvisable in thin women with a narrow chest and in those who have minimal breast tissue. Also be wary of the patient who wants to be larger than a D cup. Overly large implants are sometimes associated with complications, including inferior or lateral displacement, synmastia, pain, extrusion, palpability, and asymmetry. It is better to say no to a request for larger implants than to be sorry a few years later when problems develop. Changing to a smaller implant size may also be a problem if the skin and breast tissue have stretched in response to the existing implant. A patient who wants smaller implants probably will not be happy if her breasts sag as a result. To move to a smaller size, she may also need a mastopexy.

BREAST PAIN

Mastalgia is the perception of pain in the breast. It is a common symptom in the general population and has been inadequately studied in patients with breast implants. Breast pain has long been viewed as a local complication of breast augmentation and reconstruction that sometimes leads to reoperation, although other indications usually accompany breast pain as reasons for implant removal or exchange.

Etiology

Breast pain is a common complaint among women, with up to 70% suffering from mastalgia at some point in their lives.[117] Mastalgia can be classified as cyclic or noncyclic.[118] Cyclic pain is usually described as dull, burning, or aching; although it is bilateral, one breast is typically more painful than the other. More than two thirds of all women experience cyclic pain, which may be present during the entire menstrual cycle but more often starts 5 to 7 days before the menses. In contrast, noncyclic pain is less frequent, reported by about one quarter of women. It is of short duration, usually unilateral, and not exacerbated premenstrually.

The causes of mastalgia are poorly understood, but its cyclic nature in most women and its tendency to disappear after menopause strongly implicate endocrine effects. Nevertheless, specific hormonal events have been difficult to identify. Some possibilities include high levels of prolactin[119] or estrogen,[120] changes in the progestin-to-estrogen ratio,[121] and unbalanced secretion of follicle-stimulating and luteinizing hormones.[122] Several nonendocrine effects, such as caffeine and saturated fat intake, have also been postulated as contributors to cyclic and noncyclic breast pain.

Frequency

With about 70% of women in the general population reporting some type of breast pain, it is obviously not unique to women with breast implants. However, patients with implants may have additional reasons for mastalgia beyond those in nonimplanted women. Examples include capsular contracture, calcification of capsules, nerve injury or compression, implant rupture, and muscle compression.

Unfortunately, pain associated with breast augmentation and reconstruction has not been studied in a systematic manner, which requires knowing how many patients had breast pain before augmentation, the severity of their preoperative and postoperative pain, and whether it is cyclic or noncyclic. Descriptions of pain after augmentation have generally been poorly characterized, with breast pain reported as one local complication among many in series of explantation patients.

The only prospective data on breast pain and augmentation are those currently being obtained by saline implant manufacturers. Among the 901 augmentation patients in its A95 study of saline implants, Inamed calculates that 16% have a 3-year risk rate for development of breast pain.[7] The 3-year risk rate in the Mentor Saline Prospective Study is 5%.[6] The manufacturers do not address the question of whether these patients had breast pain before receiving implants.

In a retrospective explantation study, Beekman et al[88] reported that localized pain or paresthesia was an indication for reoperation in 19% of 182 patients with silicone gel implants. Another investigation of gel implants by Peters et al[27] cited breast pain as a reason for explantation in 36% of 100 patients, plus another 28% had mastalgia ranging from minimal to severe. Thus, 64% of these women reported some degree of breast pain (similar to the frequency reported for the general population). Peters et al found a significant association between breast pain and capsule calcification or grade III and grade IV contracture. In both the Beekman and Peters reports, breast pain was not always the only indication for explantation, and some reconstruction patients were included in the data.

In a comparative study of breast pain in patients who had undergone mastectomy, mastectomy plus reconstruction, augmentation, or breast reduction, Wallace et al questioned 282 women at least 1 year after surgery. Breast reduction patients reported the lowest frequency of pain (22%) compared with 31% of the mastectomy group, 38% of the augmentation group, and 49% of the mastectomy plus reconstruction patients.[122a] The authors believed that at least some of the breast pain is secondary to implants; 53% of women reconstructed with implants reported pain, in contrast to 30% of patients who had reconstruction without an implant. In all groups, most of the patients had intermittent pain, not constant. The study also found significantly higher frequencies of pain in patients with submuscular implants (50%) than in those with subglandular implants (21%). Although not significant, pain was more common in women who received saline rather than silicone gel implants (33% and 22%, respectively).

In the authors' rupture outcome series, breast pain was an indication for explantation in 17 of 307 surgeries among augmentation patients (5.5%), and mastalgia was reported before another 94 surgeries. This investigation was not designed to focus on breast pain as a complication of implantation, but preliminary data give some insight into this issue (Table 128-11). The percentage of grade III or grade IV contractures is almost identical when the "breast pain" and "no breast pain" groups are compared. In addition, no difference could be found between the two groups with respect to status of the removed implant; ruptured implants were found in approximately the same percentage of surgeries. The only real difference between the two groups relates to replacement implants; women with breast pain were much less likely to request replacement implants than were those with no pain. The variable of "breast pain status after explantation" compares postoperative symptoms according to whether a patient received new implants. It is unclear as to why breast pain was more than twice as likely to remain unchanged after explantation in those who did *not* receive replacement implants.

The issue of localized pain and breast implants needs additional investigation, but the presence of a large percentage of women in the general population who experience breast pain (usually of a cyclic nature) complicates future study designs.

Evaluation and Treatment

Breast pain that affects a patient's quality of life must be seriously addressed. In all women, mastalgia has many possible causes, and those with breast implants may have additional contributing factors. The multiple causes mean that surgeons performing secondary augmentations need to be familiar with the evaluation and management of breast pain to offer their patients the best treatment advice.

EVALUATION

The evaluation of patients with breast pain begins with a thorough history, physical examination, and appropriate imaging studies. It should not be assumed that pain after implantation is due to implants; instead, question patients about any pain they experienced before augmentation. In addition, localized pain is a symptom in 15% of women presenting with breast carcinoma and the only symptom in 7%.[123] Thus, a thorough evaluation is essential in patients presenting with mastalgia, particularly unilateral pain.

During the history, ask whether the pain is localized or diffuse, sharp or dull and aching, and unilat-

TABLE 128-11 ✦ PRE-EXPLANTATION BREAST PAIN IN 292 AUGMENTATION SURGERIES*

	Breast Pain n = 110		No Breast Pain n = 182
Percentage of all augmentation surgeries	38%		62%
Implant status at removal (worst by patient)			
All intact	46% (51)		50% (91)
1 or more pinholes	14% (15)		11% (20)
1 or more ruptures	40% (44)		39% (71)
Pre-explantation implant position			
Subglandular	86% (95)		76% (138)
Submuscular	14% (15)		24% (44)
Capsular contracture grade			
I or II (by patient)	29% (32)		37% (68)
III or IV (by patient)	48% (53)		47% (86)
I/II on one side and III/IV on other	21% (23)		13% (23)
Unknown	2% (2)		3% (5)
Implant replaced	55% (61)		82% (150)
No replacement implant	45% (49)		18% (32)
Breast pain status after explantation	No implant	Implant replaced	
Resolved	51% (25)	71% (43)	N/A
Improved	25% (12)	18% (11)	N/A
Unchanged	20% (10)	8% (5)	N/A
Unknown	4% (2)	3% (2)	N/A

*The number of augmentation surgeries is 292 rather than 307 because we had no information on pre-explantation symptoms for 15 surgeries.

eral or bilateral; assess the degree of severity, its relationship to the menstrual cycle, and the presence of any musculoskeletal component. If patients are vague about their symptoms, encourage them to chart their daily breast pain (noting presence and severity by day) to determine whether a cyclic pattern exists. Also inquire about methylxanthine intake (coffee, chocolate, soft drinks), diet (especially saturated fats), medications (hormone replacement), and stress levels (illness, work, divorce). Potential causes of chest wall or referred pain, such as heart disease, hiatal hernia, and cholelithiasis, should be ruled out.

Physical examination must be thorough and document any localized tenderness (which may suggest nerve injury), areas of altered sensation, the grade of capsular contracture, any palpable implant folds that might act as a source of pain, and fibrocystic changes. Any palpable mass should be evaluated with mammography (which will also show capsule calcification), and ultrasonography can be used to discriminate between solid and cystic masses. Taken together, the history and physical examination should help classify a patient's breast pain as cyclic, noncyclic, chest wall, or implant related.

TREATMENT

Potential advocated treatments of breast pain include aspiration of cysts, elimination of methylxanthines from the diet, decrease of saturated fat intake, dietary supplementation with evening primrose oil, use of medications (anti-inflammatory drugs, danazol, gabapentin, or antidepressants), and removal of symptomatic capsular contracture. Also effective is simple reassurance that breast pain is common in all women. According to Gateley et al,[124] positive responses to treatment can be expected in 92% of women in the general population with cyclic pain and in 64% with noncyclic pain. Thus, implant removal should not be the first line of treatment for breast pain, especially if there are no other indications for explantation. Implant removal will probably not improve a condition unrelated to the implant.

Nutritional Treatments

Some believe that women with breast pain and fibrocystic changes improve within a few months if they abstain from consuming methylxanthine-containing compounds such as coffee, tea, chocolate, cola, stimulants, and cough and cold remedies.[125,126] However, several controlled studies have failed to find a causal link between caffeine and breast pain.[127-129] Another dietary treatment approach is to reduce the intake of fat (particularly saturated fat), which has been found to significantly improve cyclic breast pain,[130] perhaps because of cyclic changes in lipid metabolism.[131,132] Compliance with dietary restrictions may be difficult to achieve, especially if pain reduction is not quickly seen. Still, the reduction of dietary fat is free, has no side effects, probably has healthful benefits, and may eliminate or reduce the severity of cyclic mastalgia.

Some women with cyclic breast pain have abnormal levels of essential fatty acids.[133] Supplementing these fatty acids with evening primrose oil has been found to alleviate symptoms in 45% of patients with cyclic pain and in 27% with noncyclic pain.[134] Because evening primrose oil treatment is cheap and has few side effects, a dosage of 3 g/day is worth trying. Anecdotal reports suggest that vitamin E supplements, at a dosage of 800 IU/day, improve symptoms of fibrocystic conditions and therefore may be useful in treatment of breast pain.

Drug Treatments

Patients who do not respond to simple dietary approaches can try drug therapy. Danazol is the only FDA-approved drug for the treatment of mastalgia. A weak androgen that inhibits estrogen and progesterone receptors, danazol has been found to produce significant relief of breast pain in many women who do not respond to nutritional treatments. For example, danazol response occurred in 57% to 70% of women with cyclic pain and in 25% to 31% of those with noncyclic pain.[134,135] The recommended treatment schedule for danazol is 100 mg twice a day for 2 months. If no response is seen, the dose can be increased to 200 mg twice daily. Danazol can produce unpleasant side effects, including acne, hot flashes, muscle cramps, hair growth, increased libido, nervousness, voice changes, and depression. Thus, some investigators recommend a low-dose maintenance regimen (800 mg/month) taken during the luteal phase of the menstrual cycle.[136] Studies of this low-dose treatment found that side effects were dramatically reduced yet danazol response remained high.

Gabapentin (Neurontin) is another drug that can be effective in treating breast pain. Approved for use in seizure disorders, gabapentin also successfully manages neurogenic pain. Its mechanism of action is unknown, but gabapentin has few side effects and may be used for long periods. With use of the dose of 100 mg three times daily, the authors have seen dramatic improvements in breast implant patients complaining of severe burning pain. Antidepressants have also been successful in treating many types of chronic pain. Reported improvement may simply reflect the fact that the patient was depressed by the pain and treatment of the depression led to a more positive attitude.

For women who have a musculoskeletal (chest wall) component to their mastalgia, nonsteroidal anti-inflammatory drugs can be helpful.

BIOPSY AND CANCER OF THE AUGMENTED BREAST

Several large epidemiologic studies and meta-analyses of existing data have found no causal relationship between breast implants and cancer of the breast or other sites.[137-143] In fact, some studies suggest a decreased risk of breast cancer in women who underwent breast augmentation.[144] Nevertheless, women with breast implants develop both benign and malignant breast masses, and most surgeons will encounter a small percentage of augmentation patients who require biopsy or undergo secondary surgery because of breast cancer. In the authors' rupture outcome series, for example, 3 of 307 explantation surgeries in augmentation patients were performed because of a breast cancer diagnosis. (All three patients had saline implants.)

Plastic surgeons evaluating augmented women must always obtain a thorough history, perform a complete breast examination, and order the appropriate imaging studies to screen for breast carcinoma. It should not be assumed that a palpable mass is a granuloma or postsurgical change without conducting a proper evaluation. Augmented patients should have their first mammogram by the age of 35 years, followed by mammography at least semiannually from the age of 40 to 49 years and annually thereafter. Women with breast implants require diagnostic mammograms performed by personnel experienced in imaging patients with implants. Four views are typical: the standard craniocaudal and oblique views plus two displacement views.[145]

Biopsy of Breast Mass

Any palpable masses should be evaluated by ultrasonography to discriminate between solid and cystic masses. To prevent damage to the implant with a needle, ultrasonography should also be used to guide aspiration of cystic lesions as well as fine-needle aspiration of solid masses. Biopsy should be performed for imaging abnormalities suggestive of carcinoma. In centers equipped with a Mammotome and stereotactic equipment, percutaneous biopsy can be performed. If not, an open biopsy with needle localization will be necessary. All biopsies risk damage to the implant, and the closer the mass lies to the implant, the greater the risk. Any evidence of silicone on or in the instrument usually indicates that the implant has been punctured or a silicone granuloma has been sampled. All patients who undergo percutaneous or open biopsy should be observed closely to rule out implant failure.

Biopsies should be performed by surgeons experienced with breast implants because of the possibility of damage and necessity of replacement. Surgeons who are uncertain what to do or lack the facilities or experience to order necessary imaging studies or to perform a biopsy should consult a surgical oncologist specializing in breast neoplasia.

Treatment of Augmented Patients Who Develop Breast Cancer

Although treatment guidelines for augmentation patients with breast cancer have not been established, the standard of care has been a modified radical mastectomy. However, many surgeons use breast conservation treatment (excision until the margins are microscopically clear, axillary lymph node dissection, and radiation therapy) in patients with small stage I and some stage II tumors.[146-148] As always, treatment of breast cancer in women with implants should be dictated by clinical staging of the tumor. With respect to development of future cancer recurrence, breast conservation treatment seems comparable to mastectomy. However, lumpectomy and irradiation may be contraindicated in augmented patients unless reaugmentation is delayed. A breast-conserving approach requires close follow-up; because an implant may decrease the accuracy of mammography in detecting a local recurrence, subpectoral placement is recommended.[149] More data and longer follow-up times are needed before breast conservation treatment can be recommended as an accepted standard of care comparable to modified radical mastectomy.

Breast implants do not appear to interfere with or to be altered by chemotherapy for breast cancer. In addition, irradiation does not damage implants, and implants do not impair the ability to deliver therapeutic radiation. However, irradiation can cause severe capsular contracture (up to 65% in one series), which degrades the aesthetic outcome.[149] Thus, tissue transfer with a flap is probably a wiser choice for reconstruction in women who need radiotherapy.

REDUCING THE NEED FOR REOPERATION

The frequency of revisional surgery may be as high as 20% to 25% of augmentation patients and 30% to 45% of reconstruction patients. Only a small percentage of these surgeries result from perioperative complications such as infection or hematoma. More often, secondary surgeries are performed to correct local complications (rupture and deflation, capsular contracture, implant displacement or malposition) and for cosmetic revision (size change, asymmetry, skin wrinkling). Requests from patients for implant removal because of anxiety about silicone or systemic symptoms started to decrease in the mid-1990s; as a result, the overall frequency of reoperation has probably already declined. Even so, it is still too high.

Some factors that lead to secondary augmentations are related to the implant—especially implant failure—and can be changed primarily by manufacturer modifications. Other factors are related to the patient (e.g., the biologic response of the individual to an implant) and are beyond the control of the surgeon. However, surgeons can greatly influence the need for revisional surgery. For example, the use of textured silicone gel implants and submuscular placement, both of which began in the late 1980s, has undoubtedly reduced the frequency of symptomatic capsular contracture requiring reoperation. This is partly a matter of improved implant features, but the fact that surgeons gained more experience and got smarter about how to reduce contractures is equally important. As more experience is gained with saline-filled implants, techniques to minimize skin wrinkling are perfected, and results with saline devices are comparable to those with silicone gel implants, the need for reoperation should further decline.

Technical error is another factor related to the need for secondary augmentations. Good technique influences complications such as infection, hematoma, and wound problems, but it is also the most important variable for problems such as implant malposition and poorly designed pockets. The frequency of secondary augmentations can be further reduced with good preoperative planning and proper selection of the most appropriate implant type, position, and volume. Finally, good communication with patients to determine their goals and to agree on postoperative breast size is critical for reducing the high number of reoperations performed because patients are not satisfied with their implant size. If techniques continue to improve, patients are involved in the preoperative planning, experiences are shared, and manufacturers are pressured to improve implants, it should be possible to dramatically reduce the frequency of secondary augmentations in the future.

REFERENCES

1. Gabriel SE, Woods JE, O'Fallon WM, et al: Complications leading to surgery after breast implantation. N Engl J Med 1997;336:677-682.
2. Fiala TGS, Lee WPA, May JW Jr: Augmentation mammoplasty: results of a patient survey. Ann Plast Surg 1993;30: 503-509.
3. Edworthy SM, Martin L, Barr SG, et al: A clinical study of the relationship between silicone breast implants and connective tissue disease. J Rheumatol 1998;25:254-260.
4. Middleton MS: Magnetic resonance evaluation of breast implants and soft-tissue silicone. Top Magn Reson Imaging 1998;9:92-137.
5. Food and Drug Administration: Study of re-operation and self-reported silicone-gel breast implant rupture [interview component]. May 19, 2000. http://www.fda.gov/cdrh/breastimplants/studies/

6. Mentor Corporation: Saline-filled breast implant surgery: making an informed decision [patient brochure]. Santa Barbara, Calif, 2004.
7. Inamed Aesthetics: Saline-filled breast implant surgery: making an informed decision [patient brochure]. Santa Barbara, Calif, 2002.
8. Gutowski KA, Mesna GT, Cunningham BL: Saline-filled breast implants: a Plastic Surgery Educational Foundation multicenter outcomes study. Plast Reconstr Surg 1997;100: 1019-1027.
9. Cunningham BL, Lokeh A, Gutowski KA: Saline-filled breast implant safety and efficacy: a multicenter retrospective review. Plast Reconstr Surg 2000;105:2143-2149.
10. National Breast Implant Registry (NaBIR): www.dataharbor.com
11. Baker JL Jr: Classification of spherical contractures. Presented at the Aesthetic Breast Symposium, Scottsdale, Arizona, 1975.
12. Coleman DJ, Foo ITH, Sharpe DT: Textured or smooth implants for breast augmentation? A prospective controlled trial. Br J Plast Surg 1991;44:444-448.
13. Bondurant S, Ernster V, Herdman R, eds: Safety of Silicone Breast Implants. Washington, DC, National Academy Press, 2000. Available at www.nap.edu.
14. Lin K, Bartlett SP, Matsuo K: Hyaluronic acid–filled mammary implants: an experimental study. Plast Reconstr Surg 1994;94:306-313.
15. Raso DS, Crymes LW, Metcalf JS: Histological assessment of fifty breast capsules from smooth and textured augmentation and reconstruction mammoplasty prostheses with emphasis on the role of synovial metaplasia. Mod Pathol 1994;7:310-316.
16. Vistnes LM, Ksander GA, Isaacs G, Rozner L: Elevated glycosaminoglycans and chondroitin 4-sulfate, and other properties of contracted human prosthesis capsules. Ann Plast Surg 1981;7:195-203.
17. Baker JL Jr: The effectiveness of alpha-tocopherol (vitamin E) in reducing the incidence of spherical contracture around breast implants. Plast Reconstr Surg 1981;68:696-698.
18. Ryan GB, Cliff WJ, Gabbiani G, et al: Myofibroblasts in human granulation tissue. Hum Pathol 1974;5:55-67.
19. Lossing C, Hansson HA: Peptide growth factors and myofibroblasts in capsules around human breast implants. Plast Reconstr Surg 1993;91:1277-1286.
20. Rudolph R, Abraham J, Vecchione T, et al: Myofibroblasts and free silicon around breast implants. Plast Reconstr Surg 1978;62:185-196.
21. Little G, Baker JL Jr: Results of closed compression capsulotomy for treatment of contracted breast implant capsules. Plast Reconstr Surg 1980;65:30-33.
22. Malata CM, Feldberg L, Coleman DJ, et al: Textured or smooth implants for breast augmentation. Br J Plast Surg 1997;50:99-105.
23. Moufarrege R, Beauregard G, Bosse J-P, et al: Outcome of mammary capsulotomies. Ann Plast Surg 1987;19:62-64.
24. Vogt PA, Seider HA, Moufarrege R, et al: Surface-patterned silicone implants decrease contracture for soft breast prostheses. Contemp Surg 1990;37:25-29.
25. Ersek RA: Rate and incidence of capsular contracture: a comparison of smooth and textured silicone double-lumen breast prostheses. Plast Reconstr Surg 1991;87:879-884.
26. Collis N, Sharpe DT: Ten-year review of a prospective randomized controlled trial of textured versus smooth subglandular silicone gel breast implants. Plast Reconstr Surg 2000;106:786-791.
27. Peters W, Smith D, Fornasier V, et al: An outcome analysis of 100 women after explantation of silicone gel breast implants. Ann Plast Surg 1997;39:9-19.
28. Van Kooten TG, Whitesides JF, von Recum AF: Influence of silicone (PDMS) surface texture on human skin fibroblast proliferation as determined by cell cycle analysis. J Biomed Mater Res 1998;43:1-14.
29. Cairns TS, deVilliers W: Capsular contracture after breast augmentation—a comparison between gel- and saline-filled prostheses. S Afr Med J 1980;57:951-953.
30. McKinney P, Tresley G: Long-term comparison of patients with gel and saline mammary implants. Plast Reconstr Surg 1983;72:27-29.
31. Pollock H: Breast capsular contracture: a retrospective study of textured versus smooth silicone implants. Plast Reconstr Surg 1993;91:404-407.
32. Burkhardt BR, Demas CP: The effect of Siltex texturing and povidone-iodine irrigation on capsular contracture around saline inflatable breast implants. Plast Reconstr Surg 1994;93:123-128.
33. Burkhardt BR, Eades E: The effect of Biocell texturing and povidone-iodine irrigation on capsular contracture around saline inflatable breast implants. Plast Reconstr Surg 1995;96:1317-1325.
34. Hakelius L, Ohlsén L: A clinical comparison of the tendency to capsular contracture between smooth and textured gel-filled silicone mammary implants. Plast Reconstr Surg 1992;90:247-254.
35. Tarpila E, Ghassemifar R, Fagrell D, Berggren A: Capsular contracture with textured versus smooth saline-filled implants for breast augmentation: a prospective clinical study. Plast Reconstr Surg 1997;99:1934-1939.
36. Hedén P, Jernbeck J, Hober M: Breast augmentation with anatomical cohesive gel implants: the world's largest current experience. Clin Plast Surg 2001;28:531-552.
37. Vazquez B, Given KS, Houston GC: Breast augmentation: a review of subglandular and submuscular implantation. Aesthetic Plast Surg 1987;11:101-105.
38. Puckett CL, Croll GH, Reichel CA, Concannon MJ: A critical look at capsule contracture in subglandular versus subpectoral mammary augmentation. Aesthetic Plast Surg 1987;11:23-28.
39. Biggs TM, Yarish RS: Augmentation mammaplasty: a comparative analysis. Plast Reconstr Surg 1990;85:368-372.
40. Cocke WM Jr: A critical review of augmentation mammoplasty with saline-filled prostheses. Ann Plast Surg 1994;32:266-269.
41. Mladick RA: "No-touch" submuscular saline breast augmentation technique. Aesthetic Plast Surg 1993;17:183-192.
42. Asplund O, Gylbert L, Jurell G, Ward C: Textured or smooth implants for submuscular breast augmentation: a controlled study. Plast Reconstr Surg 1996;97:1200-1206.
43. Worseg A, Kuzbari R, Tairych G, et al: Long term results of inflatable mammary implants. Br J Plast Surg 1995;48:183-188.
44. Rheingold LM, Yoo RP, Courtiss EH: Experience with 326 inflatable breast implants. Plast Reconstr Surg 1994;93:118-122.
45. Handel N, Jensen JA, Black Q, et al: The fate of breast implants: a critical analysis of complications and outcomes. Plast Reconstr Surg 1995;96:1521-1533.
46. Lemperle G, Exner K: Effect of cortisone on capsular contracture in double-lumen breast implants: ten years' experience. Aesthetic Plast Surg 1993;17:317-323.
47. Spear SL, Matsuba H, Romm S, Little JW: Methyl prednisolone in double-lumen gel-saline submuscular mammary prostheses: a double-blind, prospective, controlled clinical trial. Plast Reconstr Surg 1991;87:483-487.
48. Oneal RM, Argenta LC: Late side effects related to inflatable breast prostheses containing soluble steroids. Plast Reconstr Surg 1982;69:641-645.

49. Ellenberg AH, Braun H: A $3^1/_2$-year experience with double-lumen implants in breast surgery. Plast Reconstr Surg 1980;65:307-313.
50. Virden CP, Dobke MK, Stein P, et al: Subclinical infection of the silicone breast implant surface as a possible cause of capsular contracture. Aesthetic Plast Surg 1992;16:173-179.
51. Gylbert L, Asplund O, Berggren A, et al: Preoperative antibiotics and capsular contracture in augmentation mammaplasty. Plast Reconstr Surg 1990;86:260-267.
52. Burkhardt BR, Dempsey PD, Schnur PL, Tofield JJ: Capsular contracture: a prospective study of the effect of local antibacterial agents. Plast Reconstr Surg 1986;77:919-930.
52a. Brandon HJ, Young VL, Jerina KL, et al: Mechanical analysis of explanted saline-filled breast implants exposed to Betadine pocket irrigation. Aesthetic Surg J 2002;22:438-445.
53. Baker JL Jr., Bartels RJ, Douglas WM: Closed compression technique for rupturing a contracted capsule around a breast implant. Plast Reconstr Surg 1976;58:137-141.
54. Eisenberg HV, Bartels RJ: Rupture of a silicone bag-gel breast implant by closed compression capsulotomy. Plast Reconstr Surg 1977;59:849-850.
55. Goin JM: High-pressure injection of silicone gel into an axilla—a complication of closed compression capsulotomy of the breast. Plast Reconstr Surg 1978;62:891-895.
56. Addington DB, Mallin RE: Closed capsulotomy causing fractures of the scar capsule and the silicone bag of a breast implant. Plast Reconstr Surg 1978;62:300-301.
57. Nelson GD: Complications of closed compression after augmentation mammaplasty. Plast Reconstr Surg 1980;66:71-73.
58. Robinson OG, Bradley EL, Wilson DS: Analysis of explanted silicone implants: a report of 300 patients. Ann Plast Surg 1995;34:1-6.
59. Collis N, Sharpe DT: Recurrence of subglandular breast implant capsular contracture: anterior versus total capsulectomy. Plast Reconstr Surg 2000;106:792-797.
60. Young VL: Guidelines and indications for breast implant capsulectomy. Plast Reconstr Surg 1998;102:884-891.
61. Brandon HJ, Young VL, Jerina KL, Wolf CJ: Scanning electron microscopy characterization of surgical instrument damage to breast implants. Plast Reconstr Surg 2001;108:52-61.
62. Brandon HJ, Young VL, Jerina KL, Wolf CJ: Variability in the properties of silicone gel breast implants. Plast Reconstr Surg 2001;108:647-55.
63. Brandon HJ, Jerina KL, Wolf CJ, Young VL: Ultimate strength properties of explanted and control SILASTIC II silicone gel-filled breast implant shells. Aesthetic Surg J 2000;20:122-132.
64. Cohen BE, Biggs TM, Cronin ED, Collins DR Jr: Assessment and longevity of the silicone gel breast implant. Plast Reconstr Surg 1997;99:1597-1601.
65. de Camara DL, Sheridan JM, Kammer BA: Rupture and aging of silicone gel breast implants. Plast Reconstr Surg 1993;91:828-834.
66. Beraka GJ: Rupture of implants following mammography [letter]. Plast Reconstr Surg 1995;95:936-937.
67. Pickford MA, Webster MHC: Implant rupture by mammography [letter]. Br J Plast Surg 1994;47:512.
68. Rapaport DP, Stadelmann WK, Greenwald DP: Incidence and natural history of saline-filled breast implant deflations: comparison of blunt-tipped versus cutting and tapered needles. Plast Reconstr Surg 1997;100:1028-1032.
69. Wolf CJ, Brandon HJ, Young VL, Jerina KL: Effect of surgical insertion on the local shell properties of SILASTIC II silicone gel breast implants. J Biomater Sci Polym Ed 2000;11:1007-1021.
70. Slavin SA, Goldwyn RM: Silicone gel implant explantation: reasons, results, and admonitions. Plast Reconstr Surg 1995;95:63-69.
71. Netscher DT, Walker LE, Weizer G, et al: A review of 198 patients (389 implants) who had breast implants removed. J Long Term Eff Med Implants 1995;5:11-18.
72. Raj J, Wojtanowski MH: Spontaneous deflation in saline solution–filled breast implants. Aesthetic Surg J 1999;19:24-26.
73. Lantieri LA, Roudot-Thoraval F, Collins ED, et al: Influence of underfilling on breast implant deflation. Plast Reconstr Surg 1997;100:1740-1744.
74. Collis N, Sharpe DT: Silicone gel-filled breast implant integrity: a retrospective review of 478 consecutively explanted implants. Plast Reconstr Surg 2000;105:1979-1985.
75. Feng L-J, Amini SB: Analysis of risk factors associated with rupture of silicone gel breast implants. Plast Reconstr Surg 1999;104:955-963.
76. Malata CM, Varma S, Scott M, et al: Silicone breast implant rupture: common/serious complication? Med Prog Technol 1994;20:251-260.
77. Peters W, Keystone E, Smith D: Factors affecting the rupture of silicone-gel breast implants. Ann Plast Surg 1994;32:449-451.
78. Peters W, Smith D, Lugowski S: Failure properties of 352 explanted silicone-gel breast implants. Can J Plast Surg 1996;4:55-58.
79. Rohrich RJ, Adams WP Jr, Beran SJ, et al: An analysis of silicone gel–filled breast implants: diagnosis and failure rates. Plast Reconstr Surg 1998;102:2304-2308.
80. Spear SL, Bowen DG: Secondary surgery and silicone implants: one center's experience before and after the Food and Drug Administration hearings of 1991 and 1992. Aesthetic Surg J 1998;18:167-174.
81. Brown SL, Pennello G, Berg WA, et al: Silicone gel breast implant rupture, extracapsular silicone, and health status in a population of women. J Rheumatol 2001;28:996-1003.
82. Hölmich LR, Friis S, Fryzek J, et al: Incidence of silicone breast implant rupture. Arch Surg 2003;138:801-806.
83. Tebbets JB: Alternatives and trade-offs in breast augmentation. Clin Plast Surg 2001;28:485-500.
84. Young VL, Watson ME: Breast implant research: where we have been, where we are, where we need to go. Clin Plast Surg 2001;28:451-483.
85. Dowden RV: Saline breast implant fill issues. Clin Plast Surg 2001;28:445-451.
86. Hammond DC, Hidalgo D, Slavin S, et al: Revising the unsatisfactory breast augmentation. Plast Reconstr Surg 1999;104:277-283.
87. Young VL, Nemecek JR, Nemecek DA: The efficacy of breast augmentation: breast size increase, patient satisfaction, and psychological effects. Plast Reconstr Surg 1994;94:958-969.
88. Beekman WH, Feitz R, Hage JJ, Mulder JW: Life span of silicone gel–filled mammary prostheses. Plast Reconstr Surg 1997;100:1723-1726.
89. Rohrich RJ, Beran SJ, Restifo RJ, Copit SE: Aesthetic management of the breast following explantation: evaluation and mastopexy options. Plast Reconstr Surg 1998;101:827-837.
90. Courtiss EH, Goldwyn RM, Anastasi GW: The fate of breast implants with infections around them. Plast Reconstr Surg 1979;63:812-816.
91. Young VL, Hertl C, Murray PR, et al: Microbial growth inside saline-filled breast implants. Plast Reconstr Surg 1997;100:182-196.
92. Burkhardt BR, Fried M, Schnur PL, Tofield JJ: Capsules, infection, and intraluminal antibiotics. Plast Reconstr Surg 1981;68:43-47.
93. Brand KG: Infection of mammary prostheses: a survey and the question of prevention. Ann Plast Surg 1993;30:289-295.
94. Dougherty SH: Pathobiology of infection in prosthetic devices. Rev Infect Dis 1988;10:1102-1117.

95. Shah Z, Lehman JA, Tan J: Does infection play a role in breast capsular contracture? Plast Reconstr Surg 1981;68:34-37.
96. Dowden RV: Periprosthetic bacteria and the breast implant patient with systemic symptoms. Plast Reconstr Surg 1994;94:300-305.
97. Dobke MK, Svahn JK, Vastine VL, et al: Characterization of microbial presence at the surface of silicone mammary implants. Ann Plast Surg 1995;34:563-571.
98. Parsons CL, Stein PC, Dobke MK, et al: Diagnosis and therapy of subclinically infected prostheses. Surg Gynecol Obstet 1993;177:504-506.
99. Liang MD, Narayanan K, Ravilochan K, Roche K: The permeability of tissue expanders to bacteria: an experimental study. Plast Reconstr Surg 1993;92:1294-1297.
100. Clegg HW, Bertagnoll P, Hightower AW, Baine WB: Mammaplasty-associated mycobacterial infection: a survey of plastic surgeons. Plast Reconstr Surg 1983;72:165-169.
101. Thornton JW, Argenta LC, McClatchey KD, Marks MW: Studies on the endogenous flora of the human breast. Ann Plast Surg 1988;20:39-42.
102. Jennings DA, Morykwas MJ, Burns WW, et al: In vitro adhesion of endogenous skin microorganisms to breast prostheses. Ann Plast Surg 1991;27:216-220.
103. Ayliffe GAJ: Review of airborne spread of pathogens in the operating room. Infect Surg 1987;6:39-47.
104. Derman GH, Argenta LC, Grabb WC: Delayed extrusion of inflatable breast prostheses. Ann Plast Surg 1983;10:154-158.
105. Gurdin M, Carlin GA: Complications of breast implantations. Plast Reconstr Surg 1967;40:530-533.
106. Planas J, Carbonell A, Planas J: Salvaging the exposed mammary prosthesis. Aesthetic Plast Surg 1995;19:535-540.
107. Abramo AC, Casas SG, Dorta AA, et al: Late spontaneous extrusion of a textured silicone gel mammary implant. Aesthetic Plast Surg 1999;23:433-436.
108. DeCholnoky T: Augmentation mammoplasty: survey of complications in 10,941 patients by 265 surgeons. Plast Reconstr Surg 1970;45:573-577.
109. Hipps CJ, Raju DR, Straith RE: Influence of some operative and postoperative factors on capsular contracture around breast prostheses. Plast Reconstr Surg 1978;61:384-389.
110. Wagner H, Beller FK, Pfautsch M: Electron and light microscopy examination of capsules around breast implants. Plast Reconstr Surg 1977;60:49-55.
111. Frankel SD, Occhipinti KA, Kaufman L, et al: MRI of a silicone breast implant surrounded by an enlarging hemorrhagic collection. Plast Reconstr Surg 1994;94:865-868.
112. Marques AF, Brenda E, Saldiva PHN, Andrews JM: Capsular hematoma as a late complication in breast reconstruction with silicone gel prosthesis. Plast Reconstr Surg 1992;89:543-545.
113. Cederna JP: Hematoma as a late complication in breast reconstruction with silicone gel prostheses [letter]. Plast Reconstr Surg 1995;96:235-236.
114. Lavine DM: Saline inflatable prostheses: 14 years' experience. Aesthetic Plast Surg 1993;17:325-330.
115. Williams JE: Experiences with a large series of Silastic breast implants. Plast Reconstr Surg 1972;49:253-258.
116. Pechter EA: A new method for determining bra size and predicting postaugmentation breast size. Plast Reconstr Surg 1998;102:1259-1265.
117. Holland PA, Gateley CA: Drug therapy of mastalgia. What are the options? Drugs 1994;48:709-716.
118. Maddox PR, Harrison BJ, Mansel RE, Hughes LE: Non-cyclical mastalgia: an improved classification and treatment. Br J Surg 1989;76:901-904.
119. Cole EM, Sellwood RA, England PC, Griffith K: Serum prolactin concentrations in benign breast disease throughout the menstrual cycle. Eur J Cancer 1977;13:597-603.
120. Fechner RE: Benign breast disease in women on estrogen therapy: a pathologic study. Cancer 1972;29:273-279.
121. Sitruk-Ware R, Clair F, Sterkers N, et al: Prolactin secretion in benign breast diseases. Gynecol Endocrinol 1987;1:195-200.
122. Kumar S, Mansel RE, Scanlon MF, et al: Altered responses of prolactin, luteinizing hormone and follicle stimulating hormone secretion to thyrotrophin releasing hormone/gonadotrophin releasing hormone stimulation in cyclical mastalgia. Br J Surg 1984;71:870-873.
122a. Wallace MS, Wallace AM, Lee J, Dobke MK: Pain after breast surgery: a survey of 282 women. Pain 1996;66:195-205.
123. Preece PE, Baum M, Mansel RE, et al: Importance of mastalgia in operable breast cancer. Br Med J Clin Res Ed 1982;284:1299-1300.
124. Gateley CA, Miers M, Mansel RE, Hughes LE: Drug treatments for mastalgia: 17 years experience in the Cardiff Mastalgia Clinic. J R Soc Med 1992;85:12-15.
125. Minton JP, Abou-Issa H, Reiches N, Roseman JM: Clinical and biochemical studies on methylxanthine-related fibrocystic disease. Surgery 1981;90:299-304.
126. Minton JP, Foecking MK, Webster DJ, Matthews RH: Caffeine, cyclic nucleotides and breast disease. Surgery 1979;86:105-109.
127. Lubin F, Ron E, Wax Y, et al: A case-control study of caffeine and methylxanthines in benign breast disease. JAMA 1985;253:2388-2392.
128. Marshall J, Graham S, Swanson M: Caffeine consumption and benign breast disease: a case control comparison. Am J Public Health 1982;72:610-612.
129. Allen SS, Froberg DG: The effect of decreased caffeine consumption on benign proliferative disease: a randomized clinical trial. Surgery 1987;101:720-730.
130. Boyd NF, McGuire V, Shannon P, et al: Effect of a low-fat high-carbohydrate diet on symptoms of cyclical mastopathy. Lancet 1988;2:128-132.
131. Goodwin PJ, Neelam M, Boyd NF: Cyclical mastopathy: a critical review of therapy. Br J Surg 1988;75:837-844.
132. Sharma AK, Mishra SK, Salila M, et al: Cyclical mastalgia—is it a manifestation of aberration in lipid metabolism? Indian J Physiol Pharmacol 1994;38:267-271.
133. Gateley CA, Maddox PR, Pritchard GA, et al: Plasma fatty acid profiles in benign breast disorders. Br J Surg 1992;79:407-409.
134. Pye JK, Mansel RE, Hughes LE: Clinical experience of drug treatments for mastalgia. Lancet 1985;2:373-377.
135. Gateley CA, Maddox PR, Mansel RE, Hughes LE: Mastalgia refractory to drug treatment. Br J Surg 1990;77:1110-1112.
136. Maddox PR, Harrison BJ, Mansel RE: Low-dose danazol for mastalgia. Br J Clin Pract Suppl 1989;68:43-47.
137. Lamm SH: Silicone breast implants, breast cancer and specific connective tissue diseases: a systematic review of the data in the epidemiological literature. Int J Toxicol 1998;17:497-527.
138. Berkel H, Birdsell DC, Jenkins H: Breast augmentation: a risk factor for breast cancer? N Engl J Med 1992;326:1649-1653.
139. Birdsell DC, Jenkins H, Berkel H: Breast cancer diagnosis and survival in women with and without breast implants. Plast Reconstr Surg 1993;92:795-800.
140. Brinton LA, Brown SL: Breast implants and cancer. J Natl Cancer Inst 1997;89:1341-1349.
141. Bryant H, Brasher P: Breast implants and breast cancer—reanalysis of a linkage study. N Engl J Med 1995;332:1535-1539.
142. Engel A, Lamm SH, Lai SH: Human breast sarcoma and human breast implantation: a time trend analysis based on SEER data (1973-1990). J Clin Epidemiol 1995;48:539-544.

143. Mellemkjaer L, Kjoller K, Friis S, et al: Cancer occurrence after cosmetic breast implantation in Denmark. Int J Cancer 2000;88:301-306.
144. Deapen DM, Bernstein L, Brody GS: Are breast implants anticarcinogenic? A 14-year follow-up of the Los Angeles study. Plast Reconstr Surg 1997;99:1346-1353.
145. Eklund GW, Busby RC, Miller SH, Job JS: Improved imaging of the augmented breast. AJR Am J Roentgenol 1988;151:469-474.
146. Schirber S, Thomas WO, Finley JM, et al: Breast cancer after mammary augmentation. South Med J 1993;86:263-268.
147. Silverstein MJ, Handel N, Gamagami P, et al: Breast cancer diagnosis and prognosis in women following augmentation with silicone gel–filled prostheses. Eur J Cancer 1992;28:635-640.
148. Carlson GW, Curley SA, Martin JE, et al: The detection of breast cancer after augmentation mammaplasty. Plast Reconstr Surg 1993;91:837-840.
149. Handel N, Lewinsky B, Jensen JA, Silverstein MJ: Breast conservation therapy after augmentation mammoplasty: is it appropriate? Plast Reconstr Surg 1996;98:1216-1224.

CHAPTER

129

Secondary Abdominoplasty

KLAUS J. WALGENBACH, MD, FACS ✦ KENNETH C. SHESTAK, MD, FACS

Abdominoplasty is performed to improve abdominal aesthetics by addressing the problems of skin redundancy, adipose tissue excess, and musculoaponeurotic laxity. The scope of procedures varies from limited abdominoplasty or mini-abdominoplasty, which predominantly treats lower abdominal deformities, to full abdominoplasty, which is performed to address imbalances in the skin, fat, and musculoaponeurotic layers of the entire abdominal wall.

The full abdominoplasty operation (see Chapter 121) usually incorporates a long, horizontally oriented incision to achieve access to the musculofascial layer, permitting resection of skin and adipose tissue excess while enabling redraping of the skin on the reshaped muscle layer. Indeed, various modifications have been employed. For certain patients, an inverted T incision (fleur-de-lis) may be performed to address extensive horizontal and vertical skin excess. In full abdominoplasty, liposuction may also be used cautiously to improve flap contour with careful respect for the blood supply of the abdominal advancement flap.[1-4] The mini-abdominoplasty operation most often entails a shorter horizontal incision and is frequently combined with liposuction of all or a portion of the abdominal adipose layer[4,5] and adjacent contours.

Several studies have focused on identifying the rate of complications and secondary procedures after abdominoplasty.[6-11] The rate of secondary procedures varies according to the cited series and ranges between 2%[7,11,12] and 43%.[13] In the authors' experience, the rate of revision procedures has been considerably less and is approximately 5%. No difference has been found in this rate for abdominoplasty with or without liposuction.

Careful preoperative analysis of the patient's deformity, appropriate planning and marking, and consistent surgical technique are important aspects of achieving good results while minimizing the rate of complications. The preoperative assessment and technical details of abdominoplasty procedures are described elsewhere in this volume (see Chapter 121).

It is extremely important to obtain a thorough history, including a survey of the patient's general health and physical activity level, fluctuations of weight, history of any tobacco use, and history of any previous abdominal surgery. In addition, a systematic and thorough examination of the abdomen must be performed, focusing on the amount and location of skin excess or redundancy, the adipose tissue excess, and the location of any musculoaponeurotic laxity along with careful note of the presence and location of previous scars. These components of the abdominal wall must be assessed both in the supine position and with the patient relaxed in the standing position. Only after such an assessment can an optimal preoperative plan be formulated. This plan, whether it is for a full abdominoplasty or a modified abdominoplasty or mini-abdominoplasty, is then explained to the patient. After this communication and the patient's acceptance, the procedure is performed by standard plastic surgery techniques.

Despite adequate planning and good surgical technique, suboptimal outcomes do occur. Some of these postoperative problems are best managed conservatively with the expectation of improvement with "the tincture of time." Other untoward results can be surgically addressed at the appropriate time, that is, when tissues have regained their normal state of softness and when the patient is optimally prepared psychologically. Suboptimal outcomes are related to skin problems such as persistent redundancy, wrinkling, and asymmetry. In addition, problems can be seen with the scar, including hypertrophy, asymmetry, depression, and malposition. Contour abnormalities, which include step-off at the incision line and bulges due to asymmetric excess in the adipose layer and untreated or recurrent musculofascial laxity, constitute the main indications for revision surgery after a previous abdominoplasty. It is important for the surgeon to support the patient with frequent office visits, letters, and telephone conversations while the patient is healing and also before secondary surgery.

GENERAL: COMPLICATIONS

A survey of board-certified plastic surgeons in the United States was conducted in 1989 by Teimourian and Rogers[11] to assess general medical complications after abdominoplasty and to compare them with those seen after dermolipectomy and liposuction. In this study, 26,562 abdominoplasties were retrospectively analyzed for mortality, myocardial infarction, cerebrovascular accident or transient ischemic attack, pulmonary thromboembolism, fat embolism, major skin loss, anesthesia complications, transfusion complications, and deep venous thrombosis. The incidence of these complications was 2.0%. This was higher than with either suction lipectomy (0.1%) or dermatolipectomy (0.9%). Postoperative mortality was reported in abdominoplasty patients, but the overall death rate was low (0.0133%). In 60% of these patients, pulmonary thromboembolism was the causative factor.

In an earlier survey,[9] 10,490 patients undergoing abdominoplasty were analyzed. A total of 17 deaths from all cases were reported (0.02%). Deep venous thrombosis occurred in 1.1%, pulmonary embolism in 0.8%. Six of the 17 deaths were related to pulmonary emboli. A significant postoperative ileus was documented in 15%.

Duration of surgery alone does not seem to be a major determinant of postoperative morbidity[14]; thromboembolic complications were also reported in patients who had abdominoplasty with only 2 hours of operating time.[9] Medical management for these problems and proposals to minimize their occurrence are discussed in the following section.

ANATOMY OF THE UNFAVORABLE OUTCOME IN ABDOMINOPLASTY

Suboptimal aesthetic outcomes can be specifically noted or explained by the various anatomic components of the abdominal wall that are surgically modified during abdominoplasty. This section outlines the most common aesthetic problems as well as specific corresponding anatomic sites and proposes strategies for correction and avoidance.

Skin

In abdominoplasty, "the skin is the thing." The skin provides the most critical finishing touch to the aesthetic appearance of the abdomen. Factors that are most notable include skin tone, appropriate redraping, and position and appearance of the skin scar.

REDUNDANCY

A relatively common problem after abdominoplasty is persistent skin excess. This is usually located in the lower abdomen, but it can also be seen in the upper abdomen. It is important for the operating surgeon to preoperatively recognize and quantitate any skin excess in *both* the upper and lower abdomen. If there is excess skin in the upper abdomen, the patient *must* be treated with undermining and advancement of the upper abdominal tissues in the form of a full abdominoplasty and is not a candidate for a mini-abdominoplasty.

In most instances, the amount of skin resection can be accurately estimated preoperatively with the patient in a standing position. This is true for both lower or limited abdominoplasty (mini-abdominoplasty) and full abdominoplasty. The maneuver that is particularly useful for accurately defining the amount of skin excess is the pinch test. This is carried out by pinching the excess skin between the examiner's fingers with the patient in the standing position. This redundancy is marked, and excision proceeds in standard fashion (Fig. 129-1). Standard maneuvers (flexing the waist and raising the back of the table) for flap redraping should be carried out in every abdominoplasty to achieve the appropriate degree of skin excision.

As in most aesthetic procedures, it is not what you remove but what you leave behind that makes the difference in abdominoplasty. There must be a maintenance of the normal aesthetic relationship between the xiphoid-costal margin region, the umbilicus, and the pubic area (Fig. 129-2).

There is a relatively constant ratio of approximately two-thirds upper abdomen to one-third lower. This varies slightly, depending on whether a patient is long waisted or short waisted. One should not develop a "crowded" appearance between the umbilicus and pubic hair region with an abdominoplasty. To avoid this, it is necessary to maintain at least 11 cm of skin between the umbilicus and pubic hair region (Fig. 129-3). In certain patients, this distance is longer and the absolute number in centimeters is larger. Attempts to resect all of the skin between the umbilicus and pubic area in a patient without significant skin excess can result in shortening of the distance between the umbilicus and pubic hair region and produce an imbalance of the aesthetic appearance of the normal abdomen. The amount of skin excess must be accurately determined preoperatively because it is not

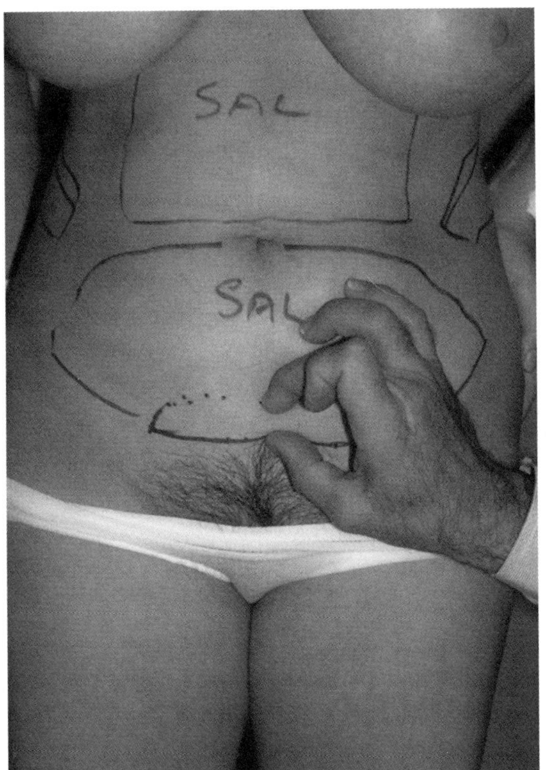

FIGURE 129-1. Pinch test. This test demonstrates the amount of skin that can safely be resected.

possible in many patients to remove the "umbilical cutout" and maintain enough skin. This will result in a short vertical scar between the umbilicus and lower incision. This is especially true for patients who are undergoing the procedure of lateral tension abdominoplasty (see Fig. 129-3).[15] The amount of skin that can be removed depends on the amount of excess in the upper abdomen and the pinch test maneuver (see Fig. 129-1).

POSTOPERATIVE SKIN EXCESS

Not infrequently, there is an area of excess skin above the lower abdominal scar. It is important to allow at least 6 months to elapse after surgery before reoperating to excise this excess. As the edema in the abdominal flap subsides, the exact amount of skin excess often becomes more apparent than it is immediately after surgery. Should such an area be persistently bothersome to the patient, it can be excised in a straightforward manner in an office setting under local or sedative anesthesia.

Skin excess after full abdominoplasty can be seen laterally or centrally. It is most commonly seen laterally, as occurs with the closure of any ellipse where the width of the skin excision would dictate a much longer length of the ellipse or, in this case, the lower abdominal scar. This results in the appearance of dog-ears. Interestingly, dog-ears, or excess skin, at the lateral extremes of the incision are more commonly seen in mini-abdominoplasty (Fig. 129-4). This is the result of a well-intentioned but illogical intent on the part of the surgeon to limit the length of the incisions. A dog-ear will not usually disappear with time, and it should be excised at the time of surgery when the abdominal incision is closed. It is important to "work" the upper abdominal flap skin incision from lateral to medial, trying to minimize or eliminate the skin excess or dog-ear. The trade-off of a longer scar for a smooth contour in the hip area is a good one for the patient (Fig. 129-5). Virtually any dog-ear that persists after surgery can be excised as an outpatient procedure in the office setting at a later time. If the dog-ear is related to a large amount of excess fat, liposuction can be used to improve it significantly.

Skin excess centrally is less common. This is especially true for patients undergoing conventional abdominoplasty or dermolipectomy. However, skin excess in the lower abdomen can occur, and it may

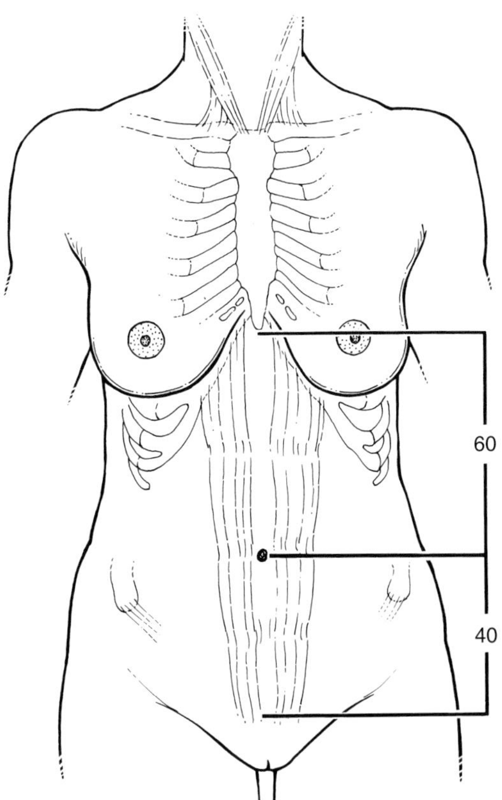

FIGURE 129-2. Aesthetic proportions of the abdomen with an approximately 60/40 relationship of the upper portion to the lower portion.

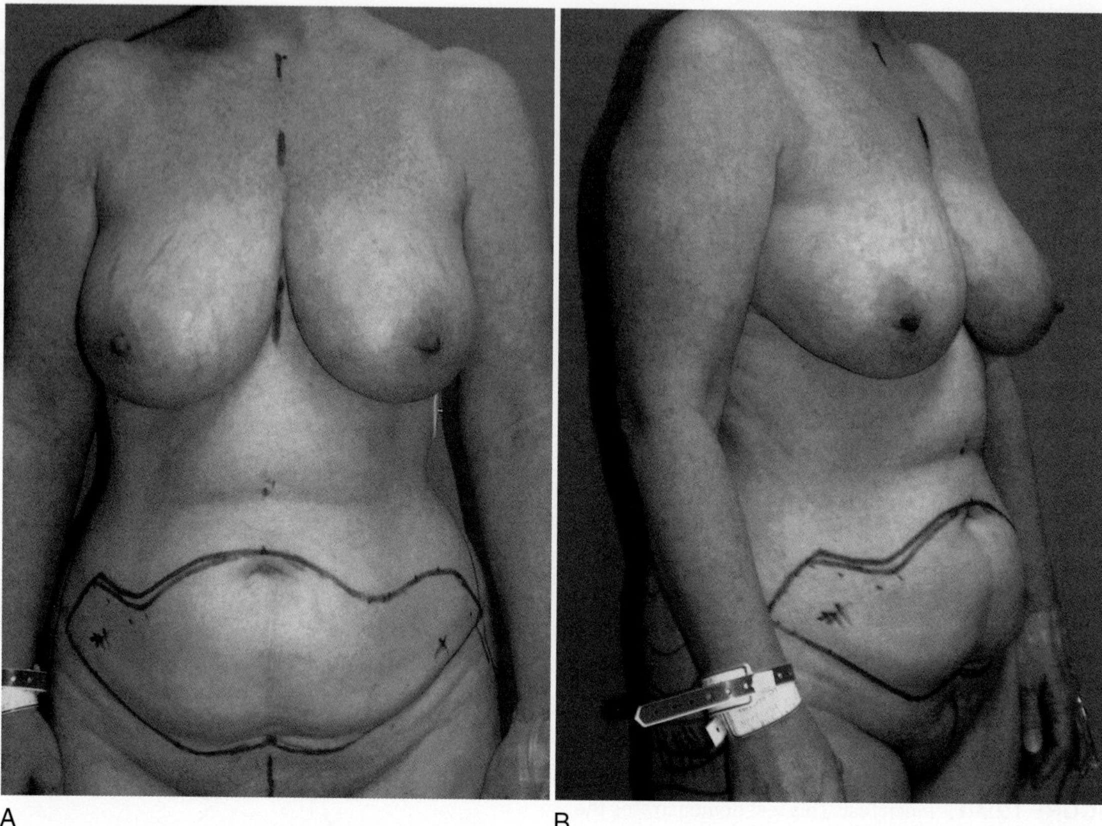

FIGURE 129-3. *A* and *B,* Preoperative markings.

require a secondary excision (Fig. 129-6). This can often be done in the office setting under local anesthesia.

STRETCH MARKS

Stretch marks or striae are common in many patients who request abdominoplasty. They are usually the result of a relatively rapid expansion of the skin, which causes a rupture in the elastin fibers of the skin. This is most commonly seen after pregnancy, but it can also be seen in patients who have undergone massive weight gain and then had subsequent weight loss.

Stretch marks will not disappear after abdominoplasty. This must be discussed with the patient before surgery. Some of these stretch marks can be excised and the appearance of the remaining lines may improve, but they will most often remain after surgery. It is important to point out to the patient which stretch marks will be excised and which will not be excised with an abdominoplasty.

SKIN WRINKLING

Skin wrinkling is most frequently seen in patients who are thin. This usually takes the appearance of "crepe paper" skin in the supraumbilical region. It is characteristically seen in a patient who is fit and almost petite. It is a problem that is seen in patients with thin, inelastic skin. Improvement can be obtained only by undermining the involved skin appropriately and then advancing and tightening it.

Wrinkling of the skin in the upper abdomen is the result of inadequate undermining and improper redraping. Failure to perform adequate undermining and advancement usually results in a recrudescence of the wrinkled skin appearance (Fig. 129-7).

SKIN LOSS

Skin loss after abdominoplasty can be a devastating problem for the patient and the surgeon.[16] Small areas of skin loss are not uncommon. Loss of large areas of skin is preventable in most patients. It is usually the result of excess tension at the site of wound closure in the midline, but other factors may contribute to it. Careful analysis of every patient from the standpoint of comorbidities and the local condition of the abdomen is paramount.[17]

Abdominoplasty should be undertaken only with extreme caution in patients who smoke. Smoking

Text continued on p. 371

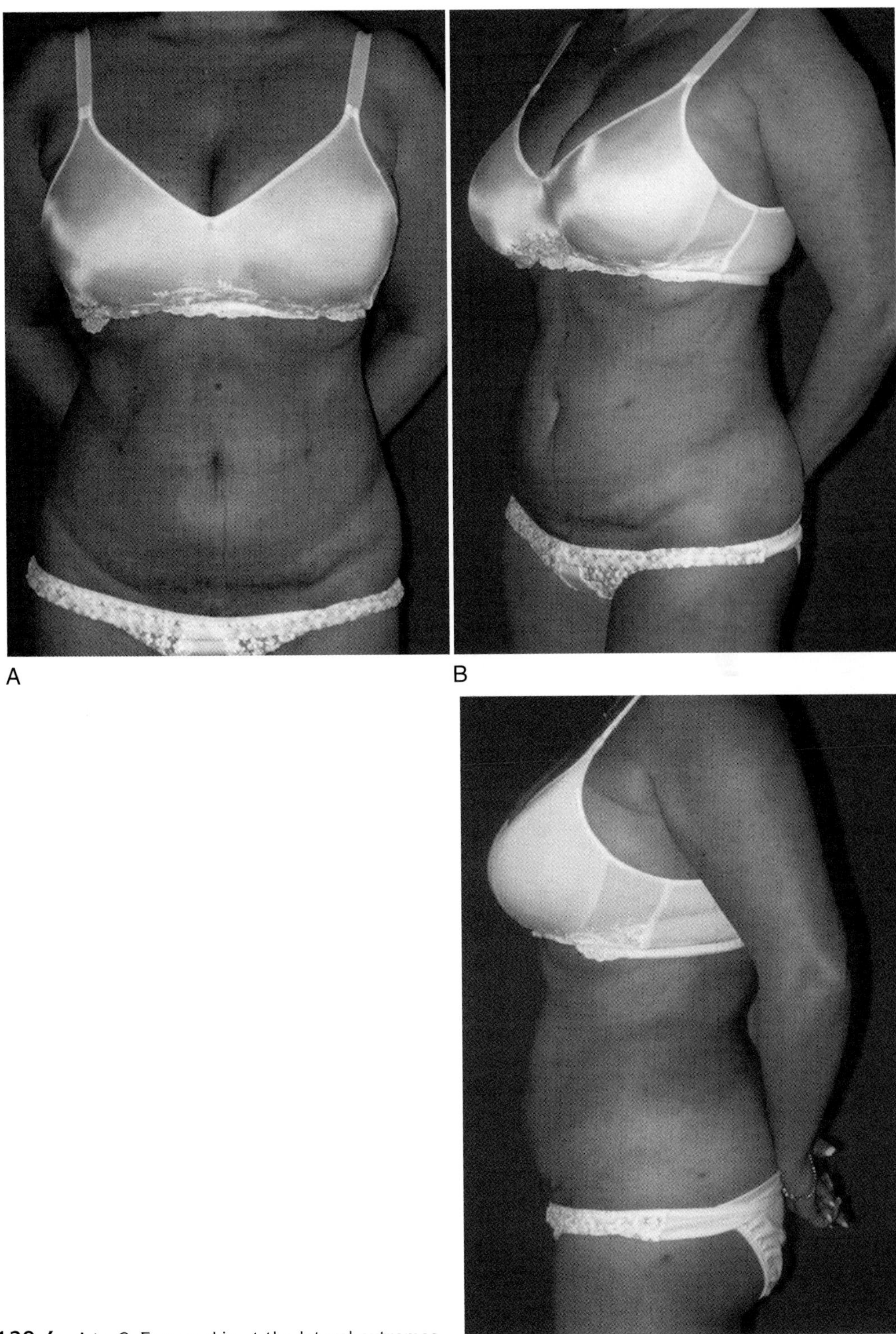

FIGURE 129-4. *A* to *C*, Excess skin at the lateral extremes (especially the left side) of the incision (dog-ears).

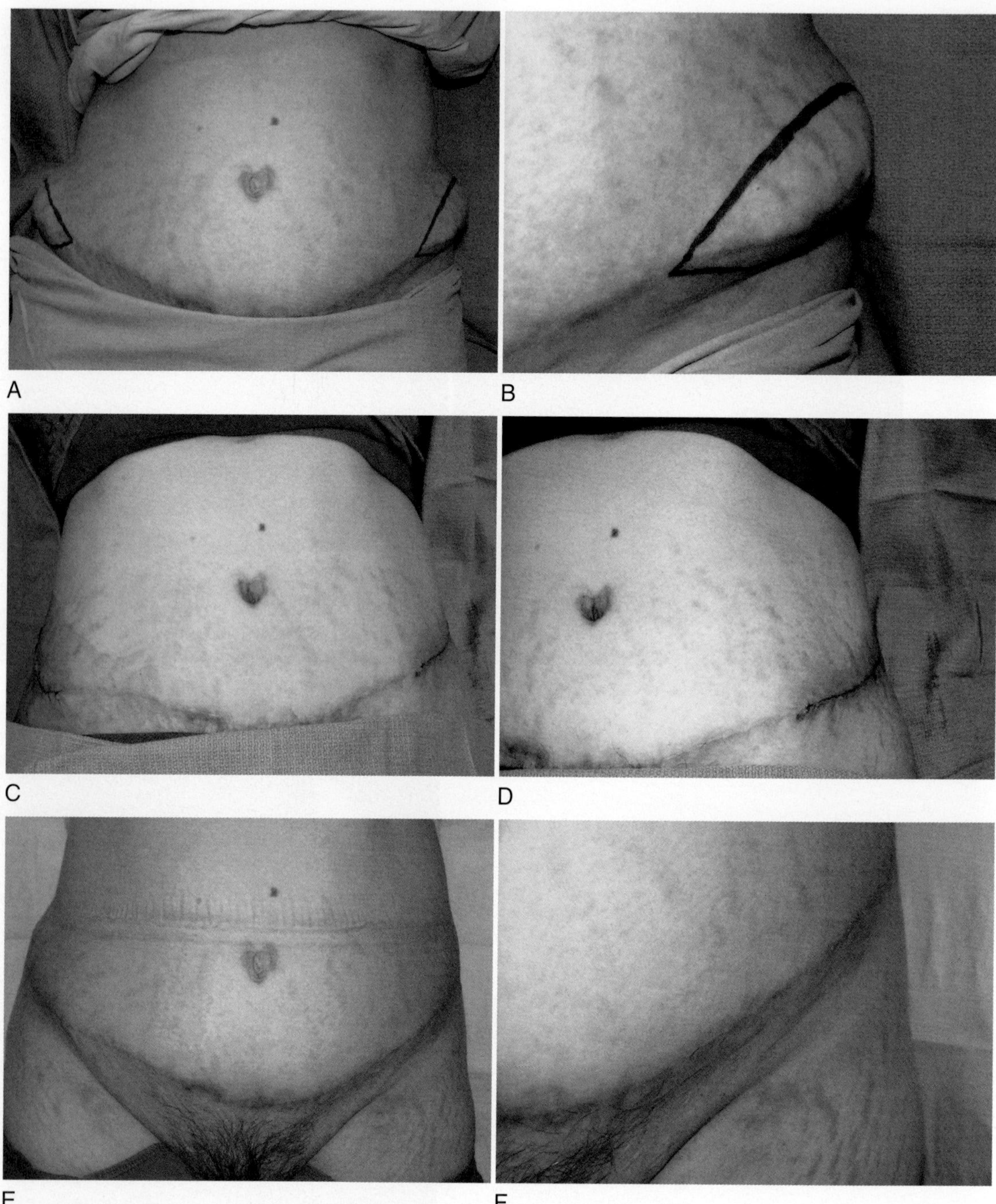

FIGURE 129-5. *A* to *F*, Dog-ears after abdominoplasty and incomplete lateral resection. Before and after bilateral resection.

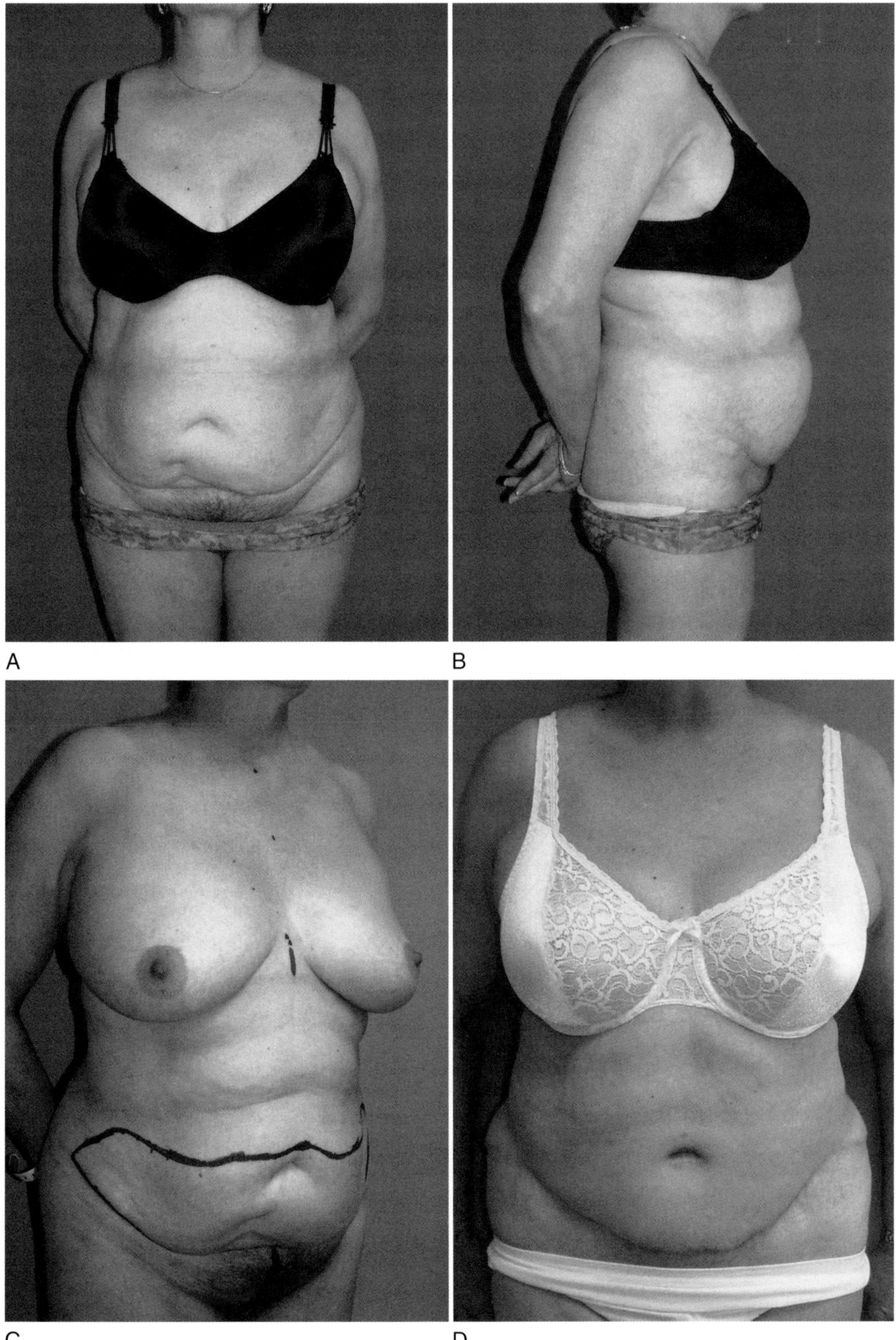

FIGURE 129-6. *A* to *C*, Scar after previous abdominoplasty. *D* and *E*, Significant improvement after revision surgery, bilateral dog-ears still persistent. *Continued*

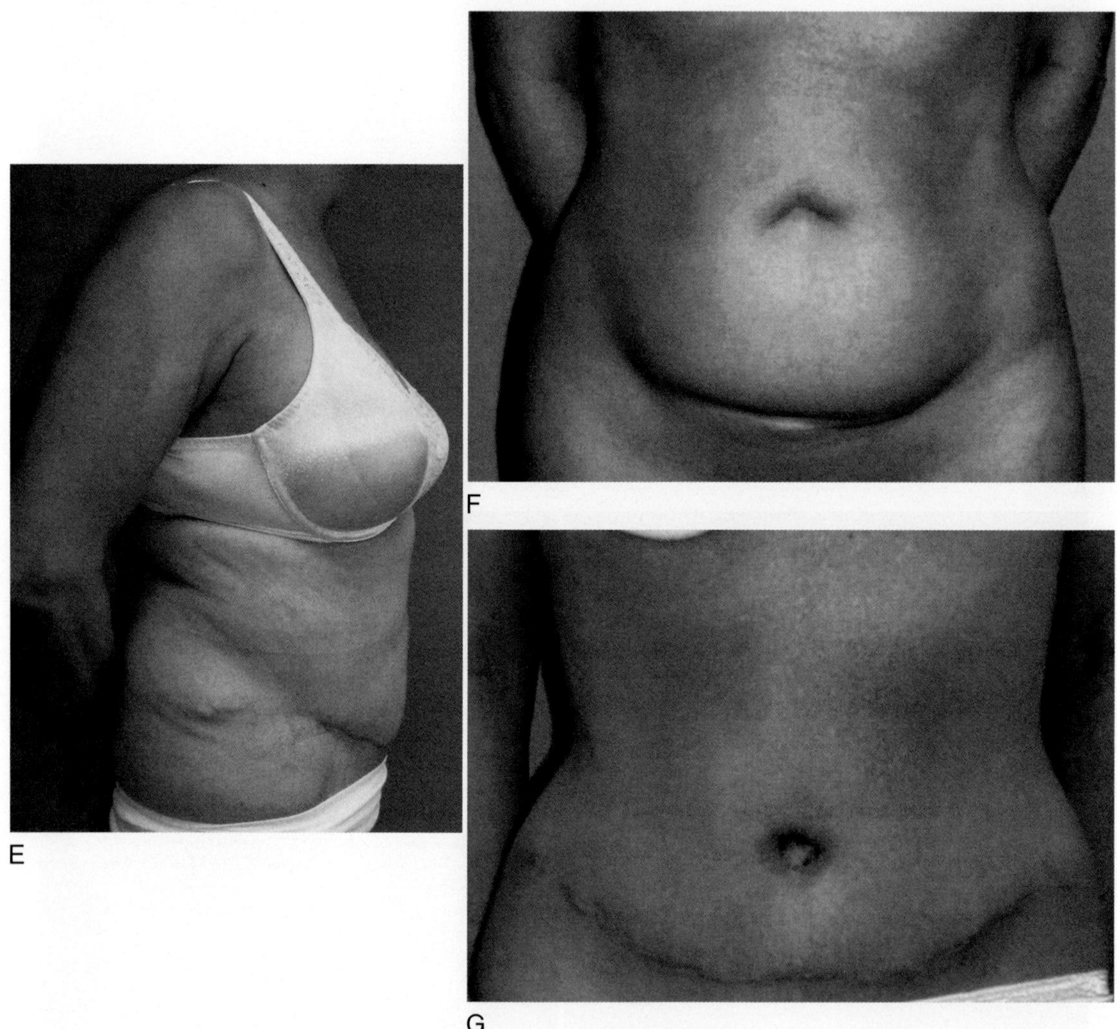

FIGURE 129-6, cont'd. *F* and *G,* Second patient preoperatively and postoperatively.

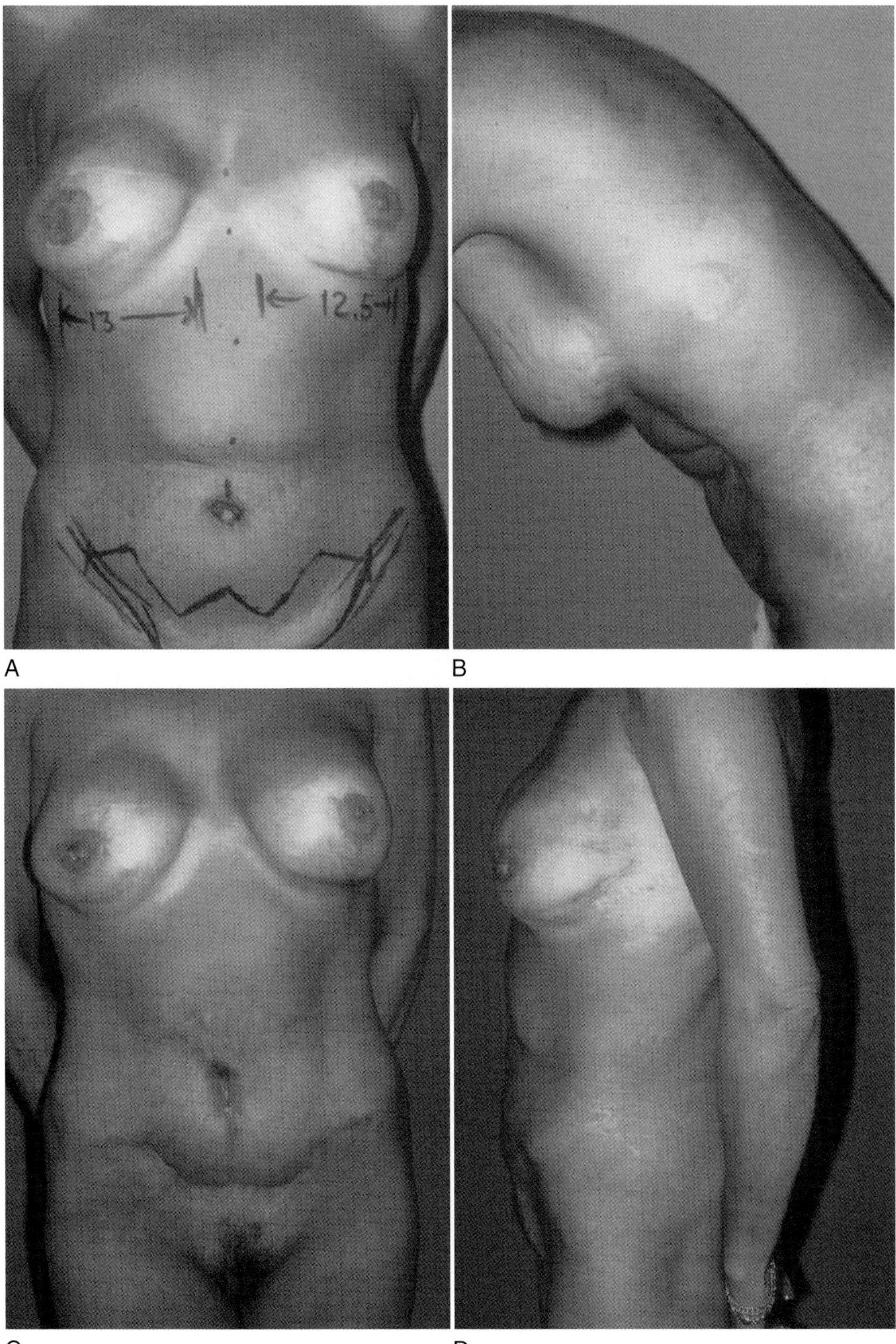

FIGURE 129-7. An example of skin wrinkling illustrated by a 55-year-old woman who desired abdominoplasty. *A* and *B,* Preoperative analysis revealed that she was thin and had "crepe paper" wrinkling of the skin above the umbilicus extending for a distance of 6 cm. She was a smoker, and for that reason the undermining at the first operation was limited to the level of the midabdomen. *C* and *D,* Postoperatively, the wrinkled skin persisted. A second operation was needed to correct the persistent deformities.

Continued

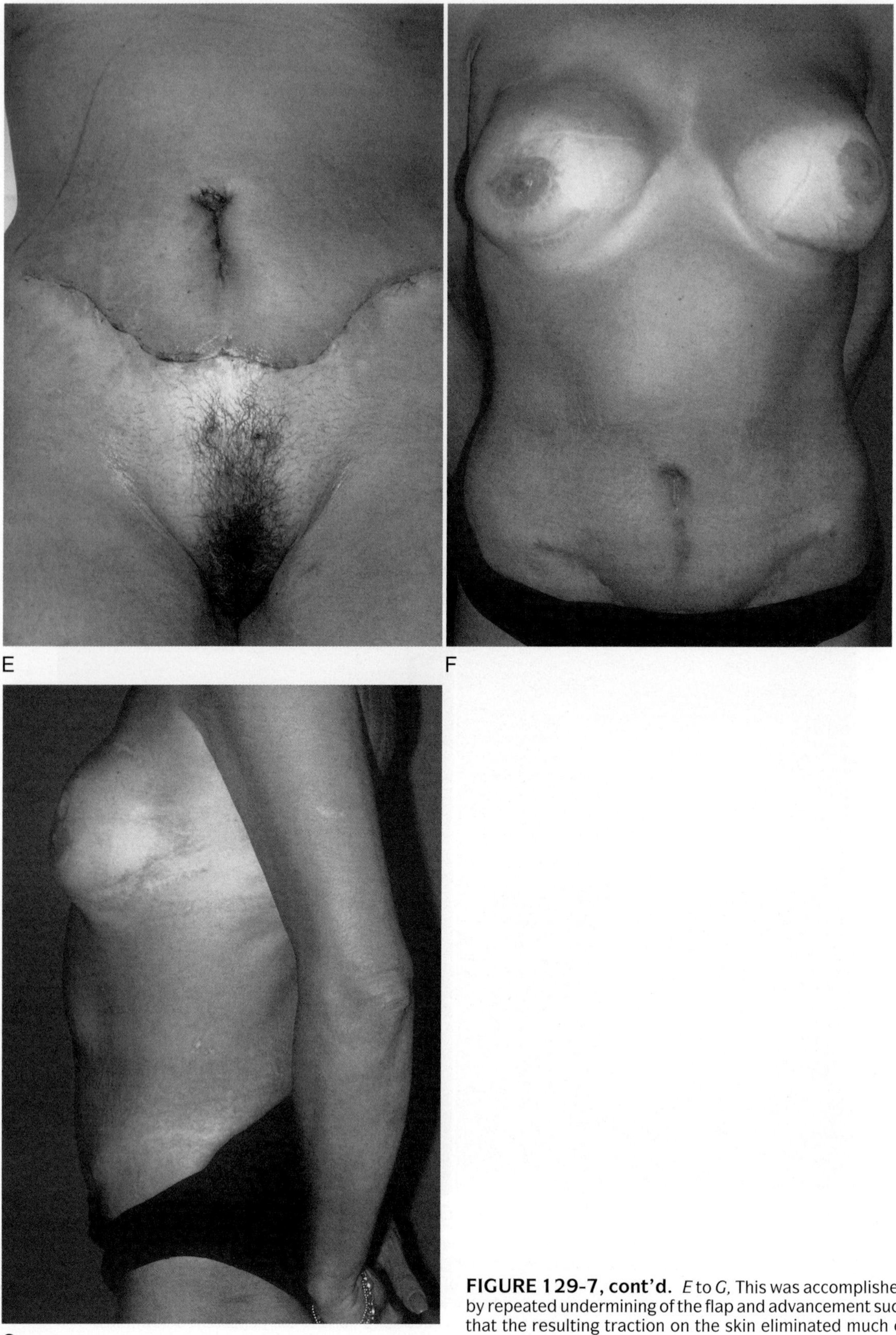

E

F

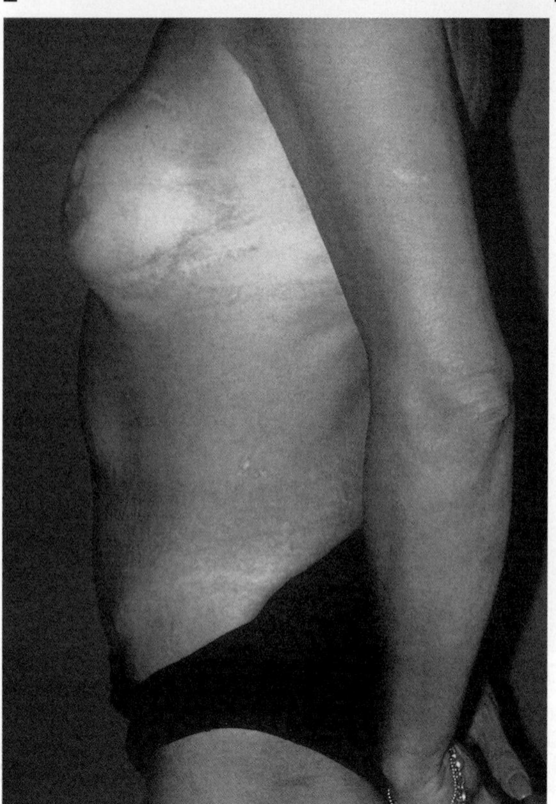

G

FIGURE 129-7, cont'd. *E* to *G*, This was accomplished by repeated undermining of the flap and advancement such that the resulting traction on the skin eliminated much of the previous skin wrinkling.

patients present significant difficulties with any operation that involves skin undermining, advancement, and tightening because this produces "tension" on skin flaps.[18,19] A patient who smokes is instructed to stop completely for at least 4 weeks before surgery and warned that surgery will be postponed if this is not possible. Smoking produces a situation in which there is a decrease in perfusion at the margins of the abdominal flap. With the application of traction on the skin, there is decreased blood flow at the distal edge of the flap and marginal ischemia.

The location and length of previous abdominal scars must also be carefully analyzed.[20] It is of particular importance to note any incision in the upper abdomen, especially those that are oriented horizontally or obliquely. The most common incision encountered is the subcostal incision that was commonly used in the open cholecystectomy procedure. A left upper quadrant oblique incision may have been used for a splenectomy. Any incision in the upper abdominal region will decrease vascular perfusion to some aspect of an advancement flap. This must be taken into account when the skin flap is undermined and tightened. The blood supply to the abdominal wall has been clearly defined by Huger.[21] Such incisions do not contraindicate abdominoplasty. However, the surgeon must carefully analyze conditions and alter the pattern of undermining to maximize flap blood flow.[22] Because the intercostal arterial blood supply becomes important in virtually every abdominoplasty, it is paramount to limit lateral undermining, thereby preserving the maximal amount of blood supply obtained through the intercostal vascular system (Fig. 129-8). Most often, limited or no lateral undermining is required as demonstrated by Lockwood with his procedure of lateral tension abdominoplasty (Fig. 129-9).[15] In summary, although a previous incision does not represent a contraindication to abdominoplasty, the increased risk of skin necrosis below the incision must be pointed out to and discussed with the patient preoperatively.

If skin loss has occurred, it is also critical to support the patient through the difficult time of this unexpected complication. Treatment is almost always conservative in nature. This includes *active* wound management by application of ointments and dress-

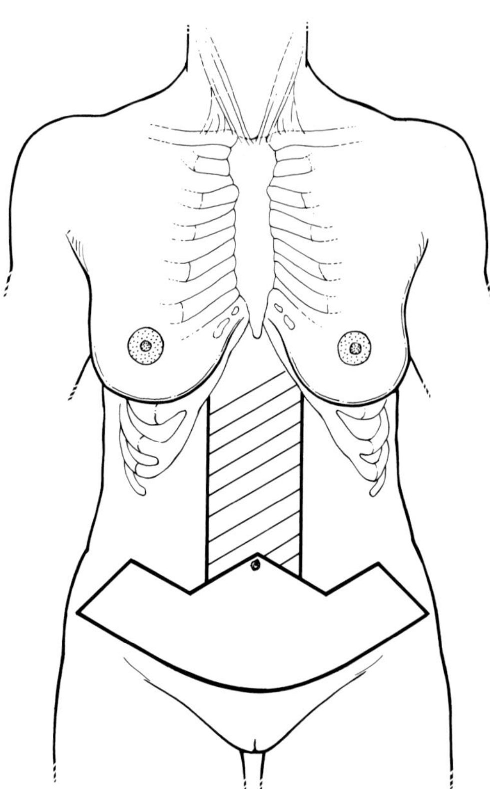

FIGURE 129-9. Modification of Lockwood's technique of lateral tension abdominoplasty.

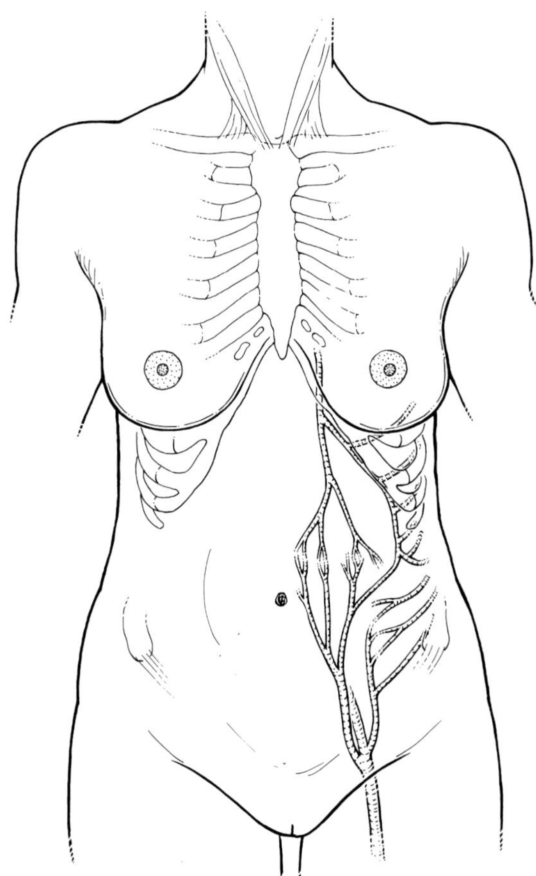

FIGURE 129-8. Blood supply of the abdominal wall. Three systems supply the abdominal wall: the superior epigastric system (zone I), the inferior epigastric system (zone II), and the segmental perforators from intercostal vessels (zone II).

ings (wet to dry with saline). If the problem consists of marginal ischemia with only limited threatened tissue, bacitracin ointment or silver sulfadiazine (Silvadene) cream is applied. It is essential to allow the skin tissues to demarcate. When the process is more severe, conservative débridement can be performed in the office to permit wound healing by epithelialization and contraction. It is usually unwise to repeat undermining and advancement of skin tissues, especially in the subacute phase of wound healing. In certain instances with larger secondary healing areas, the application of negative pressure by use of vacuum sealing can be helpful. This treatment does not necessarily need to be carried out on an inpatient basis; it can also be applied in the outpatient setting. Vacuum sealing can be effective in inducing granulation tissue and shrinking areas of secondary wound healing.[23]

Flap edema and lymphedema of the flap take a minimum of 3 months to resolve substantially. As tissues soften, the possibility for revision of suboptimal contours becomes more realistic and safe, and the results are more predictable. At this time, a limited procedure can most often produce a nice improvement.

"Conservative" therapy is really *active wound therapy*. This includes careful instructions to patients, frequent office visits (several times a week early on), and support for the patients as they heal from this complication.

If a suboptimal contour with a noticeable depression has resulted from tissue loss at the distal margin of the flap, this can be managed with advancement of the superior tissues as a de-epithelialized flap of dermis and subcutaneous adipose tissue, which can markedly improve the contour. It is important to note whether this involves only the skin and superficial aspect of the adipose layer or whether it represents full-thickness flap loss (Fig. 129-10).

SEROMA AND HEMATOMA

Raising a large abdominal flap and advancing it will cause a potential space between the adipose layer of the flap and the abdominal wall. This can lead to a fluid collection, which consists most often of wound fluid (seroma) or, much less frequently, of blood (hematoma). The fluid collection itself is not infectious, but the presence of retained serous or serosanguineous fluid increases the incidence of subcutaneous infection. Furthermore, such a fluid collection prevents apposition of and normal interfascial healing between these two surfaces. There seems to be a higher incidence in patients with a mini-abdominoplasty or limited abdominoplasty when it is combined with extensive liposuction.[2,10]

The diagnosis of such a fluid collection is usually made clinically. If the diagnosis is not clear, ultrasonic examination may be necessary to confirm presence of fluid. Sterile percutaneous aspirations can further characterize the fluid collection and are used to treat it. In general, noticeable fluid collections can be treated successfully by frequent aspirations. After local anesthetic is injected in the skin, the fluid can be aspirated with a large syringe (60 mL) and a larger size needle (18-gauge). The insertion of a drain, either short term or for a few days, may sometimes be necessary. A modified drainage system in the form of a seroma catheter may be used.

In the rare instances when the fluid collection persists, an operative revision is indicated. In a patient with a hematoma, the cavity must be examined for potentially bleeding vessels. A persistent fluid collection, when it is present for an extended period, can lead to the formation of a pseudobursa, and this newly formed lining tissue has to be excised (Fig. 129-11).

For a more rapid closure to be induced, such a wound cavity can be sealed with fibrin glue. In addition, drains should be inserted. In all these procedures, the application of external compression by use of an abdominal binder is helpful in reducing the seroma rate.

The treatment of seromas requires patience from both the patient and the plastic surgeon. It sometimes takes weeks of multiple aspirations for such a cavity to finally be completely resolved.

Scar

Problems related to the scar can present as hypertrophic scar, keloid formation, extensive spreading of the scar, or depression of the scar. In rare instances, the scarring process can result in an unstable or defective scar, which tends to break down. This can result in chronic irritation or infection. This situation is seen most often after delayed primary healing of a large area of skin loss by epithelialization and contraction.

Hypertrophic scars can be treated by repeated intralesional corticoid injections or compression therapy with silicone sheets. Corticoid injections are performed twice in 6 weeks. Care must be taken in limiting the total amount of injected steroid to avoid depressions or color changes in the scar. The preferred substance is triamcinolone acetonide (Kenalog-40) diluted in half with 1% lidocaine (Xylocaine). Injection of no more than 5 mL is recommended per dosage. Persisting hypertrophic areas can be resected; however, the patient should be aware of a potential recurrence.

Many surgeons believe that a careful repair of the superficial fascial system or Scarpa fascial layer done with multiple sutures will limit scar spreading. This concept was proposed by Lockwood.[15,24,25]

Nerve Injury

Injury to the sensory nerves to the skin after abdominoplasty is common. Patients must be told to anticipate

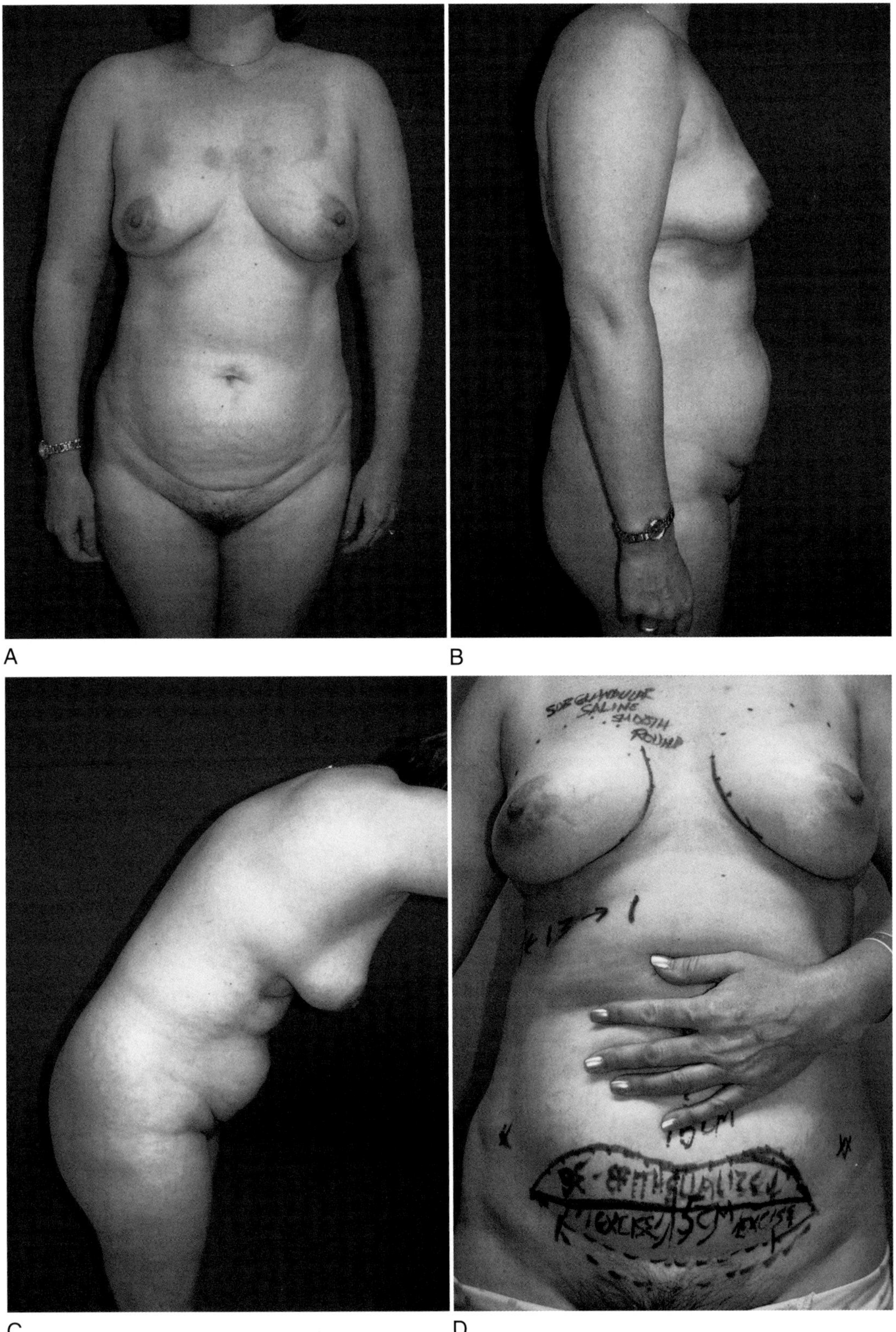

FIGURE 129-10. *A* to *C*, Step-off. *D*, Operative procedure with inferior excision followed by de-epithelialization and advancement. *Continued*

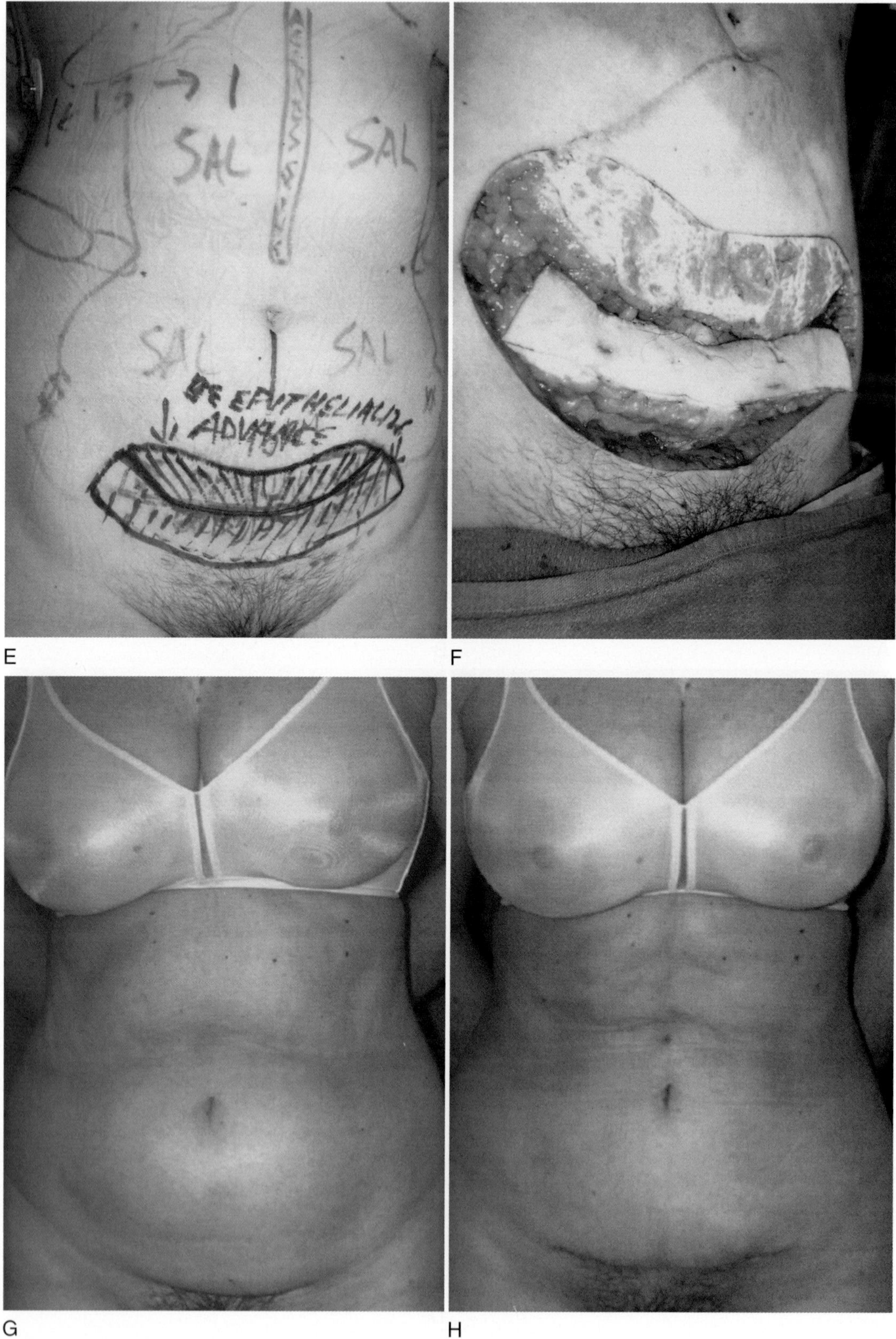

FIGURE 129-10, cont'd. *E* and *F,* Operative procedure with inferior excision followed by de-epithelialization and advancement. *G* and *H,* Second patient.

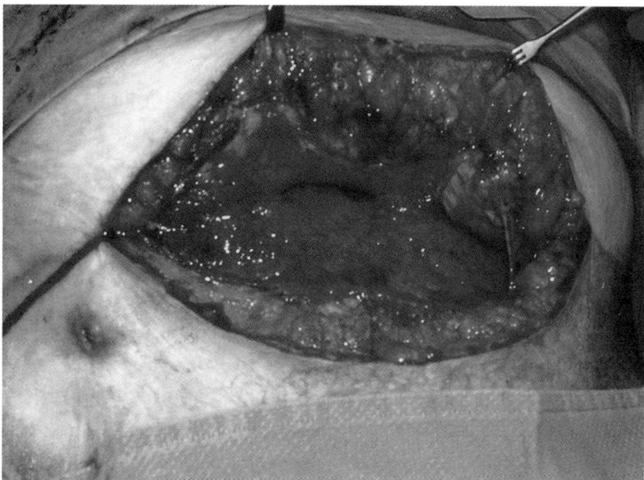

A

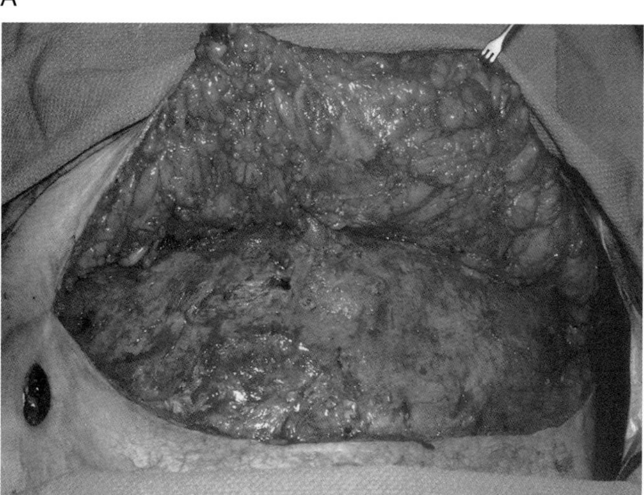

B

FIGURE 129-11. *A* and *B*, Formation of a pseudobursa after a seroma. Preoperative view and postoperative view after resection of the pseudobursa.

decreased or absent feeling in the skin between the umbilicus and the lower incision.

Injuries to major sensory nerves including ilioinguinal, iliohypogastric, and genitofemoral nerves are uncommon, but they can result in pain in the inguinal region.[26] Up to 10% of the patients undergoing abdominoplasty are reported to sustain an injury of the lateral cutaneous nerve of the thigh.[27,28] This occurs when the lateral incision is brought down through the muscle fascia over the anterior superior iliac spine. It is important to sweep the tissue off of the anterior superior iliac spine in the loose layer above the fascia at the anterior superior iliac spine. When the clinical diagnosis is made on the basis of a patient's history and physical examination, a conservative therapeutic approach of injection of local anesthetics can be undertaken. A test blockade of the nerve will reveal the injury and in the same way provide a potential therapy. If the result of test blockade is positive but the pain does not disappear permanently, an operative revision may be indicated.[29] Exact planning of the incision, especially in the lateral portion, is essential to avoid nerve injury.

Flap Contour Deficiency

EDEMA

Edema is seen in virtually every abdominoplasty flap. This is a natural consequence of transecting the lymphatics in the skin with a long horizontal incision. Lymphogenesis and lymph drainage through the scar tissue will occur over time, and the distended appearance of the distal abdominal flap will improve. It is important for the surgeon to avoid any step-off in the contour of the abdominal wound at the time of wound closure. This often requires excision of a significant portion of "subscarpal" adipose tissue or fatty tissue that resides below the superficial fascial system at the time of wound closure. This excess fat is most often present lateral to the midline on either side and is easily excised.

If the patient notices fullness in the lower abdomen and the contour was noted to be satisfactory at surgery, this can be managed with watchful waiting and encouragement. However, if a step-off persists after a period of 6 months, a secondary liposuction can be performed to improve the disharmony of contour. Again, before any surgery is contemplated, it is important to allow tissue equilibrium to occur. This process requires at least 3 months, and postponing surgery for at least 6 months to a year is often helpful. The tincture of time is helpful to both the patient and the surgeon.

EXCESS ADIPOSE TISSUE

Sculpting the fat layer at the time of abdominoplasty must be done only after careful judgment is exercised, again related to the blood supply of the tissues. Contour asymmetries related to excess upper abdominal adipose tissue can be treated most expediently by suction-assisted lipectomy. The patient is marked in the standing position, and areas of excess adipose tissue are directly treated with the aspiration of the adipose tissue at surgery. It is important to use small cannulas, to treat only the deep layer, and to limit the amount of epinephrine in the subcutaneous infiltration fluid to a concentration of 1 to 1,000,000.

LOWER ABDOMINAL STEP-OFF DEFORMITY

A step-off in the lower abdomen can be produced by excess subcutaneous fat in the pubic area. This results anatomically from a thin layer in the supraumbilical area that is brought adjacent to a much thicker adipose layer in the mons pubis. Secondary contouring with liposuction of the mons pubis is a direct way to address this deformity. Advancement of a de-epithelialized distal segment of the abdominal flap can also help correct contour deformities in this area.

An alternative method of addressing a depression in the contour above the pubic hair region is advancement of a de-epithelialized segment of dermis and fat distally after re-elevation of the abdominal flap. This additional soft tissue volume in the subcutaneous adipose layer can dramatically improve step-off deformities in this area. Technically, this is readily done by de-epithelializing and advancing the distal abdominal flap beneath the mons pubis, which is elevated. This gives a natural-appearing, smooth contour to the pubic area. A suction drain is helpful to prevent fluid accumulation in the wound (see Fig. 129-10).

WEIGHT GAIN

The effect of weight gain is difficult to predict because it will affect the entire body contour. Nevertheless, certain areas of the body will gain more weight than others. The preoperative disposition of fat tissue can help predict a potential outcome and contour variations after a substantial weight gain. If there is an increase in the adipose layer accompanying weight gain after abdominoplasty, these areas can in most patients be addressed effectively by liposuction, which can be performed as an outpatient procedure under local anesthesia.

Musculofascial System

RECURRENT LAXITY (INADEQUATE MUSCLE FASCIA PLICATION)

It is not uncommon for patients to notice a "loosening" of a previously "tight" lower abdomen after abdominoplasty. This most often results from a recurrent laxity in the musculature after muscle plication. It is to be expected in many patients, most especially multiparous women with marked protuberance of the lower abdomen. Therefore, it is pointed out to these patients before and immediately after surgery that their contour may in fact undergo a partial relapse of laxity (Fig. 129-12).

The surgeon must carefully study the musculofascial system before surgery and perform appropriate plications, which may include not only vertical but also horizontal plications or even oblique plications. It is important not to "overtighten" patients at the time of surgery because this can be uncomfortable. Nevertheless, the appropriate plication should be undertaken in virtually every patient. In patients with markedly decreased muscle tone and pronounced musculofascial laxity, this most often includes a combination of vertical and horizontal or oblique plication (Fig. 129-13).

Technically, it is important to mark the amount of plication on the musculature with methylene blue before the plication is performed. This will prevent progressive overtightening with the sutures used for plication.

In those patients who develop a recurrent protuberance in the abdomen, it is reasonable to entertain repeated plication of the musculature. This will obviously entail "redoing" this portion of their operation.

In summary, it is common to note a relaxation of the abdominal musculature after abdominoplasty surgery. It is, however, rare to have a patient request retightening of the musculature. It is possible to re-excise and tighten the skin of the lower abdomen in these patients. Therefore, it is necessary to understand the muscle tone of the patient before surgery and to

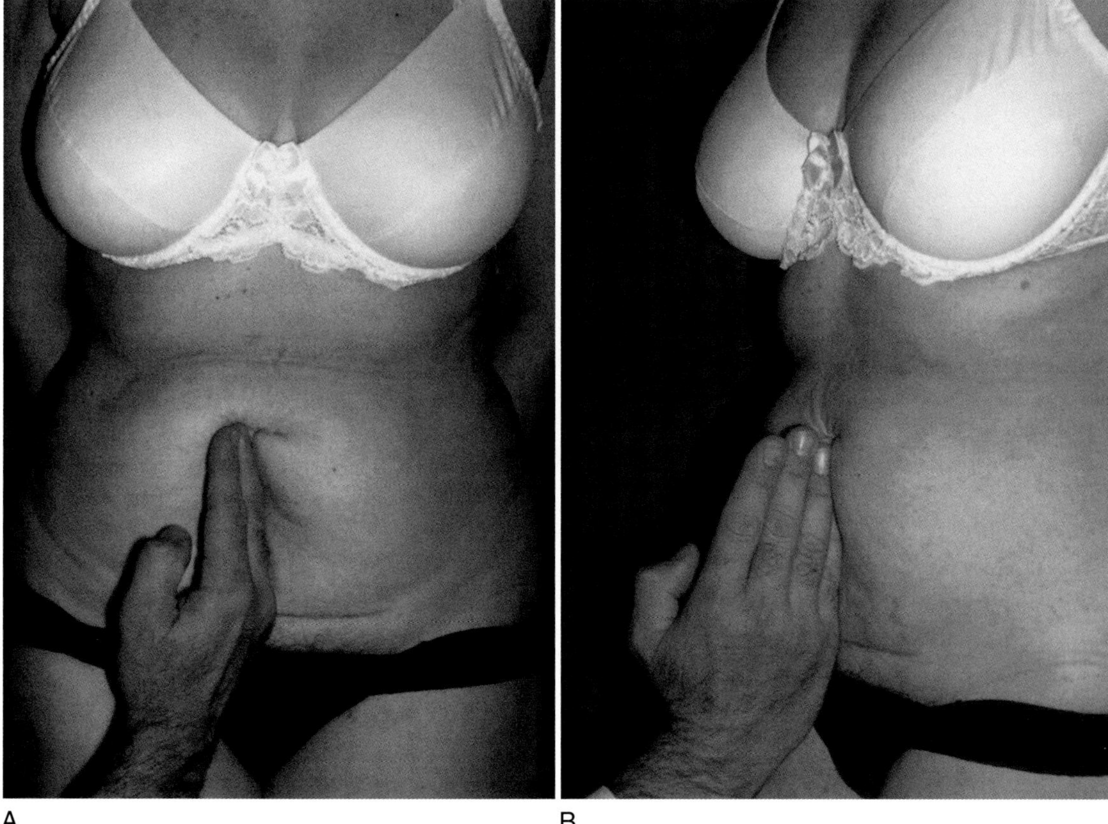

FIGURE 129-12. *A* and *B*, Preoperative evaluation of musculofascial laxity.

have patients watch their weight and exercise in a regular fashion after surgery.

PRONOUNCED RECTUS DIASTASIS WITH VENTRAL HERNIA

In patients in whom muscle plication was not undertaken at the first operation or when this procedure was incomplete, a pronounced bulge with or without ventral hernia can occur. Patients who are multiparous are more predisposed to rectus diastasis with abdominal bulging.[28] These patients frequently have laxity of the entire abdominal wall musculature, and they will most often require aggressive fascial plication in both a vertical and oblique or vertical and horizontal orientation. If a hernia repair is required, the insertion of mesh can be indicated. An increased incidence of inguinal hernias after abdominoplasties has been described.[30]

Umbilicus

ISCHEMIA

Care must be taken at the time of surgery to handle the umbilical tissues carefully, especially in full abdominoplasty operations when the separation of the stalk is performed in a circumferential manner. Although the blood supply emanates from within the umbilicus through remnants of the urachus, it is preferable to leave a small amount of adipose tissue around the umbilicus. This seems to improve the vascularity of the umbilicus and to provide some protection against ischemia.

Nevertheless, umbilical ischemia can occur. It, too, should be managed conservatively; this means the application of dressings and local wound care. Complete healing will most often occur, and the result is usually aesthetically acceptable. The contour of the umbilicus may be somewhat altered by scar contracture, but this can be addressed in a secondary revision. It is unusual to have the umbilicus become eccentric to the degree that the patient is bothered by its appearance. However, should this occur, secondary umbilicoplasty can be performed with a combination of local skin flaps or skin grafts.[31-33]

ECCENTRICITY

In most patients, the natural appearance of the umbilicus is asymmetric. Therefore, a certain asymmetry of approximately 0.5 to 1 cm or less is tolerable.

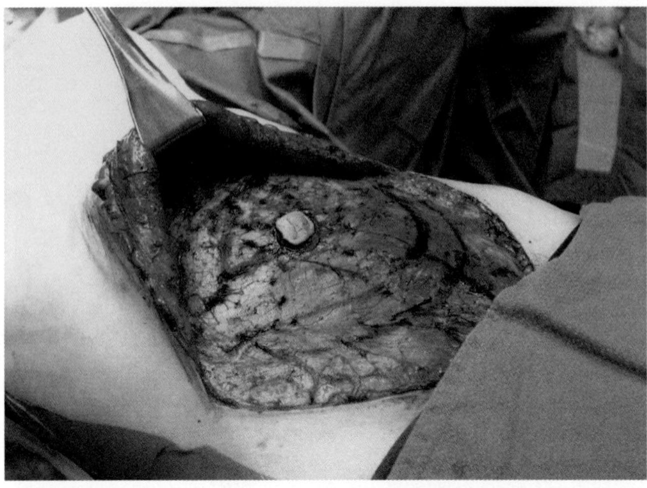

FIGURE 129-13. Combination of vertical and horizontal plication.

If postoperative eccentricity of the umbilicus occurs, additional scars cannot be avoided to move the umbilicus into the correct midline position. In most patients, the necessary changes will be achieved with an extension of the umbilicus that positions it slightly wider and deeper.

If the umbilicus has to be moved over a larger distance, a lateral incision in the shape of a VY-plasty is unavoidable. The lateral incision is localized to the opposite side of the umbilicus migration. If the umbilical pedicle is too long, sutures should be anchored deeply to the fascial layer and used to maintain the desired position (Fig. 129-14).

PREVENTION OF COMPLICATIONS

The key to avoiding certain complications after abdominoplasty is to prevent them. This includes careful planning of the operation, preoperative and postoperative instructions to the patient, and specific precautions undertaken to prevent complications.

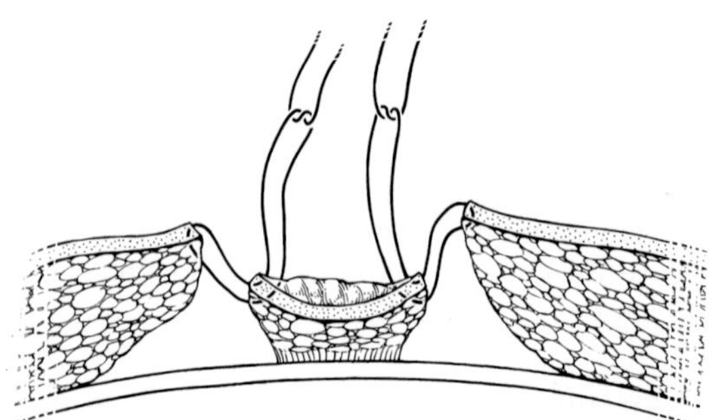

FIGURE 129-14. Reinsertion of the umbilicus. (Modified from Rees TD, LaTrenta GS, eds: Aesthetic Plastic Surgery. Philadelphia, WB Saunders, 1994.)

For prevention of thromboembolism, the use of compression stockings or boots is mandatory. This sequential compression activates the fibrinolytic system. In some situations, subcutaneous heparin may be considered. Obesity is a predisposing factor for thromboembolism. In both abdominoplasty alone and abdominoplasty combined with other procedures, the only risk factor identified in predicting major morbidity, specifically the occurrence of pulmonary embolus, was obesity and not the complexity of the surgical procedure.[34] In those patients with a history of thromboembolic episodes, the decision to proceed with abdominoplasty should be carefully considered and perhaps deferred.

The risk for respiratory decompensation can be minimized by limiting the musculofascial plication in the upper abdomen. A preoperative pulmonary function test is indicated if pulmonary function is compromised. It cannot be emphasized enough that smoking not only is a risk factor for pulmonary problems but also significantly increases the risk of problems related to wound healing.

Because hernia and hernia recurrence are not infrequent problems, a precise preoperative hernia evaluation has to be performed during a careful examination of the patient. If a hernia is diagnosed, a hernia repair at the time of abdominoplasty is indicated. Appropriate bowel preparations should be undertaken before surgery.

The transverse scar may be malpositioned if the laxity of the skin after resection is not appropriately considered. If the suprapubic skin margin is too large, the transverse scar will be moved cranial because of the tension that is applied at the time of wound closure.

Malpositioning of the umbilicus occurs if the harmony of the xiphoid, umbilicus, and pubic area is ignored. It is important to avoid skin overresection, which can result in disharmony. On the other hand, inadequate skin undermining and skin resection can result in a relapse of wrinkled skin.

Excessive skeletonization of the umbilicus should be avoided to prevent ischemia of the umbilicus. For correct and tension-free placement, fixation sutures to the fascia should be used. This technique consistently produces a natural "hooded" appearance of the umbilicus.

A hematoma is usually related to incomplete hemostasis. There is a higher incidence in patients with certain disorders like coagulation defects or in patients receiving anticoagulant therapy. Postoperative hemorrhage can be manifested after a sensation of pressure or pain. Small collections can be managed with serial aspirations; however, large collections require drainage in the operating room.

After a large abdominal flap has been raised, it has to be anticipated that a serous fluid collection will develop. To facilitate sufficient removal and the apposition of the different tissue layers, negative-pressure suction must be instituted. Two drains should usually be placed. The application of fibrin glue, sprayed to seal the wound cavity, can help decrease the risk of seroma development. Furthermore, compression in the form of an abdominal binder should be applied to every patient.

Certain risk factors are associated with impaired wound healing, such as diabetes, hypoproteinemia, obesity, and smoking. These factors must be controlled before surgery. The increased risk of wound healing problems in this setting has to be emphasized to the patient. Local factors involved in impaired wound healing are bleeding, infection, excessive suture material, and technical problems, especially high tension of the wound edges. During suturing, the operating room table should be in a flexed position. This position should be kept postoperatively by placing the patient's leg on a pillow or a knee roll and keeping the bed in a moderately flexed position.

A regimen of perioperative and postoperative antibiotic treatment is carried out and continued for at least 48 hours.

The patient should be restricted from postoperative activities like sports or heavier lifting for at least 4 weeks. This will minimize the chance of hematoma or seroma formation and shorten the period of edema formation.

REFERENCES

1. Cardenas-Camarena L, Gonzales LE: Large-volume liposuction and extensive abdominoplasty: a feasible alternative for improving body shape. Plast Reconstr Surg 1998;102:1698-1707.
2. Matarasso A: Abdominoplasty: a system of classification and treatment for combined abdominoplasty and suction-assisted lipectomy. Aesthetic Plast Surg 1991;15:111-121.
3. Matarasso A: Liposuction as an adjunct to a full abdominoplasty revisited. Plast Reconstr Surg 2000;106:1197-1202.
4. Shestak KC: Marriage abdominoplasty expands the mini-abdominoplasty concept. Plast Reconstr Surg 1999;103:1020-1031.
5. Greminger RF: The mini-abdominoplasty. Plast Reconstr Surg 1987;79:356-365.
6. Dillerud E: Abdominoplasty combined with suction lipectomy: a study of complications, revisions and risk factors in 487 cases. Ann Plast Surg 1990;25:333-338, discussion 339.
7. Floros C, Davis PK: Complications and long-term results following abdominoplasty: a retrospective study. Br J Plast Surg 1991;44:190-194.
8. Grazer FM: Body contouring. Introduction. Clin Plast Surg 1996;23:511-528.
9. Grazer FM, Goldwyn RM: Abdominoplasty assessed by survey, with emphasis on complications. Plast Reconstr Surg 1977;50:513-517.
10. Matarasso A: Abdominal dermolipectomies: early postoperative complications and long-term unfavorable results [discussion]. Plast Reconstr Surg 2000;106:1619-1623.
11. Teimourian B, Rogers WB 3rd: A national survey of complications associated with suction lipectomy: a comparative study. Plast Reconstr Surg 1989;84:628-631.
12. Chaouat M, Levan P, Lalanne B, et al: Abdominal dermolipectomies: early postoperative complications and long-term unfavorable results. Plast Reconstr Surg 2000;106:1614-1618, discussion 1619-1623.
13. Hensel JM, Lehman JA Jr, Tantri MP, et al: An outcome analysis and satisfaction survey of 199 consecutive abdominoplasties. Ann Plast Surg 2001;46:357-363.
14. Fogarty BJ, Khan K, Ashall G, Leonhard AG: Complications of long operations: a prospective study of morbidity associated with prolonged operative time (>6h). Br J Plast Surg 1999;52:33-36.
15. Lockwood T: High-lateral-tension abdominoplasty with superficial fascial system suspension. Plast Reconstr Surg 1995;96:603-615.
16. Kroll SS: Necrosis of abdominoplasty and other secondary flaps after TRAM flap breast reconstruction. Plast Reconstr Surg 1994;94:637-643.
17. Vastine VL, Morgan RF, Williams GS, et al: Wound complications of abdominoplasty in obese patients. Ann Plast Surg 1999;42:34-39.
18. Nolan JM, Jenkins RA, Kurihara K, Schultz RC: The acute effects of cigarette smoke exposure on experimental skin flaps. Plast Reconstr Surg 1985;75:544-549.
19. Rees TD, Liverett DM, Guy CL: The effect of cigarette smoking on skin flap survival in the facelift patient. Plast Reconstr Surg 1984;73:911-915.
20. De Castro CC, Aboudib JH Jr, Salema R, et al: How to deal with abdominoplasty in an abdomen with a scar. Aesthetic Plast Surg 1989;1:67-71.
21. Huger WE Jr: The anatomical rationale for abdominal lipectomy. Ann Surg 1979;45:612-617.
22. Nahai F, Brown GH, Vasconez LO: Blood supply to the abdominal wall as related to planning abdominal incisions. Ann Surg 1976;42:691-695.
23. Fenn CH, Butler PE: Abdominoplasty wound-healing complications: assisted closure using foam suction dressing. Br J Plast Surg 2001;54:348-351.
24. Pollock H, Pollock T: Progressive tension sutures: a technique to reduce local complications in abdominoplasty. Plast Reconstr Surg 2000;105:2583-2586.
25. Shestak KC: Progressive tension sutures: a technique to reduce local complications in abdominoplasty [discussion]. Plast Reconstr Surg 2000;105:2587-2588.
26. Liszka TG, Dellon AL, Manson PN: Iliohypogastric nerve entrapment following abdominoplasty. Plast Reconstr Surg 1994;93:181-184.

27. van Uchelen JH, Werker PM, Kon M: Complications of abdominoplasty in 86 patients. Plast Reconstr Surg 2001;107:1869-1873.
28. al-Qattan MM: Abdominoplasty in multiparous women with severe musculoaponeurotic laxity. Br J Plast Surg 1997;50:450-455.
29. Nahabedian MY, Dellon AL: Outcome of the operative management of nerve injuries in the ilioinguinal region. J Am Coll Surg 1997;184:265-268.
30. Benvenuti D: Increased incidence of inguinal hernias following abdominoplasty [letter]. Plast Reconstr Surg 1999;103:1798.
31. Choudhary S, Tamms KO: Umbilicosculpture: a concept revisited. Br J Plast Surg 1998;51:538-541.
32. Guerrerosantos J, Dicksheet S, Carillo C, Sandoval M: Umbilical reconstruction with secondary abdominoplasty. Ann Plast Surg 1980;5:139-144.
33. Schoeller T, Wechselberger G, Otto A, et al: New technique for scarless umbilical reinsertion in abdominoplasty procedures. Plast Reconstr Surg 1998;102:1720-1723.
34. Hester TR Jr, Baird W, Bostwick J III, et al: Abdominoplasty combined with other major surgical procedures: safe or sorry? Plast Reconstr Surg 1989;83:997-1004.

CHAPTER

130

Secondary Liposuction

MARY K. GINGRASS, MD, FACS ✦ JOHN M. HENSEL, Jr., MD

Liposuction is the most commonly performed aesthetic surgical procedure in the United States, with more than 385,000 patients treated in 2003.[1] With the advent of liposuction for fat removal, there was a shift in body contouring from dermolipectomy, with its sequelae of long, unpredictable scarring, to liposuction, which required only small, inconspicuous scars. Today, liposuction is able to produce dramatic changes in body contour. There is, however, the potential for both major and minor complications. Gargan and Courtiss[2] break down the risks of suction-assisted lipectomy into undesired sequelae and potential complications. Undesired sequelae include surface contour irregularities, hypesthesia, edema, ecchymosis, and skin discoloration. Potential complications include excessive blood loss, hematoma, seroma, infection, thrombosis, fat embolism, and skin necrosis. It is important to address the proper treatment of undesired sequelae of liposuction, in particular contour irregularity, and to provide practitioners with helpful information about prevention and resolution.

CONTOUR IRREGULARITY

Contour irregularity can be defined as an irregular or undesired contour of the body surface that is iatrogenically formed by the aspiration of fat from the subcutaneous tissue. It is the most common permanent undesired sequela of liposuction. A survey of U.S. and Canadian plastic surgeons by Pitman and Teimourian[3] showed that 20.7% of patients undergoing liposuction had unfavorable results as manifested by superficial waviness and asymmetry. Dillerud[4] showed that liposuction performed on more than 2000 healthy patients resulted in undesired results in 10.8% of patients, which consisted mainly of asymmetry, underresection, and skin irregularities. The body sites most at risk for undesirable results were the medial thigh, buttocks, ankle, and face. He also found that proportionally more men (15%) than women (12%) were unhappy with the outcome of their liposuction procedures. Chang[5] reported a series of 175 patients in which 9.7% underwent corrective surgery for post-liposuction contour irregularity. Because of the relatively high incidence of postoperative liposuction contour irregularity, it is important to inform the patient preoperatively of the possible need for secondary procedures.

PHYSICIAN-PATIENT RELATIONSHIP IN SECONDARY LIPOSUCTION

The behavior of patients with unsatisfactory results is unpredictable. They are often angry and disappointed. They want to know why their result is suboptimal and what can be done about it. They are often anxious to have the problem corrected as quickly as possible. It is important that the surgeon give the patient a realistic idea of the expected outcome as well as of the time frame for resolution of the problem. Whatever the situation, an optimistic outlook should be displayed. As long as patients are realistic in their expectations and motivated for successful outcomes, they will usually be happy after the secondary surgery is completed. If the problem cannot be solved completely, honesty with the patient and accurate documentation are paramount for both medicolegal and ethical reasons.

The patient should always be made aware of the possibility of a secondary procedure before the primary procedure. It should be discussed and documented as part of the informed consent. The surgeon's policy of reimbursement for revisionary procedures should also be discussed and documented preoperatively. As an example, patients may not be charged a surgeon's fee for revisionary procedures; however, they may be responsible for anesthesia and facility charges. These issues should be spelled out clearly in the paperwork, which the patient signs preoperatively.

When a surgeon is managing an unfavorable result of another surgeon or colleague, it is advisable *not* to degrade the other surgeon's technique or result. It is best simply to concentrate on the problem at hand and gear the conversation toward what can be done to improve the patient's present condition.

SELECTION OF PATIENTS

Ideally, the best way to "treat" contour irregularity in liposuction is to avoid it. Selection of patients is of utmost importance. The ideal candidate for liposuction is a young healthy patient who has normal body weight and proportion with good skin tone and minimal to moderate localized fat deposits that are unresponsive to diet and exercise. However, in the average plastic surgeon's practice, this type of patient is the exception rather than the rule. Patients of all ages, shapes, and sizes will present for liposuction consultation. The surgeon must determine the type of procedure that is appropriate for each patient on an individual basis.

During the last few years, the indications for liposuction have expanded to include older, more overweight patients. New data suggest that large-volume lipoplasty can produce dramatic weight loss and significant, possibly long-lasting health benefits when it is performed with the strictest criteria for selection of patients.[6] Yet most plastic surgeons remain concerned about the potential risks of large-volume lipoplasty. As more of these patients become candidates for liposuction, the potential for secondary procedures will increase as well. There is little doubt that these patients can benefit from liposuction, but only as long as they understand the limitations of the procedure. They must be made aware that poor skin tone, increased body weight, and musculoaponeurotic weakness increase the risk for contour irregularity and a less than optimal outcome. This type of patient often requires a more extensive procedure for optimal results to be achieved. Liposuction is a body-contouring procedure that results in volume reduction. However, for the average patient, it should not be considered for weight loss.

In most instances, patients want maximal results with minimal surgery. For this reason, it is essential that the surgeon discuss all the surgical options, including risks, benefits, and alternatives for each procedure. The surgeon should give his or her opinion as to which procedure is best, but ultimately the patient must make the decision. If the surgeon thinks that the patient is not a good candidate for liposuction, then the surgeon should turn the patient away. All patients should understand that regardless of the skill of the surgeon, even the optimal candidate under the best of conditions may still require some type of revisionary procedure to optimize the final result.

TYPES OF CONTOUR IRREGULARITY

Chang[5] classifies post-liposuction contour irregularities into major or minor according to the size of the area, difficulty of correction, severity and visual impact of the contour irregularities, and need for dermolipectomy. Contour irregularities generally fall into four categories: undercorrection; overcorrection; failure of skin retraction or abnormal skin retraction; and complex deformities consisting of combinations of undercorrection, overcorrection, and abnormal skin retraction. Illouz[7] beautifully illustrates all of these categories (Figs. 130-1 and 130-2).

If the defect is the result of undercorrection, a simple revision aspiration will correct the defect. If the defect is the result of overcorrection, fat reinjection is the most acceptable method of correction. When the problem is combined (both overcorrection and undercorrection), aspiration and reinjection of fat must be combined to correct the defect. Failure of skin retraction or abnormal skin retraction may require combination procedures or excision of skin.

Undercorrection

Harmonious undercorrection, in which the postoperative result is smooth and proportional but the patient simply desires more removal of fat, is not classified as a contour irregularity and is not part of this discussion. Disproportional undercorrection is one or more residual bulges or an asymmetry wherein one side is undercorrected relative to the other side. Failure to "feather" or taper the transition zone between a suctioned area and a nonsuctioned area can also be an undercorrection problem. The goal in tapering is to remove less and less fat as the periphery of the suctioned area is approached to result in a smooth transition zone. An undercorrected transition zone will leave a residual bulge or a stair-step deformity at the periphery.

Undercorrected areas are treated with further liposuction. In patients with mild or moderate undercorrection, revision can be performed with the administration of local anesthesia, with or without mild

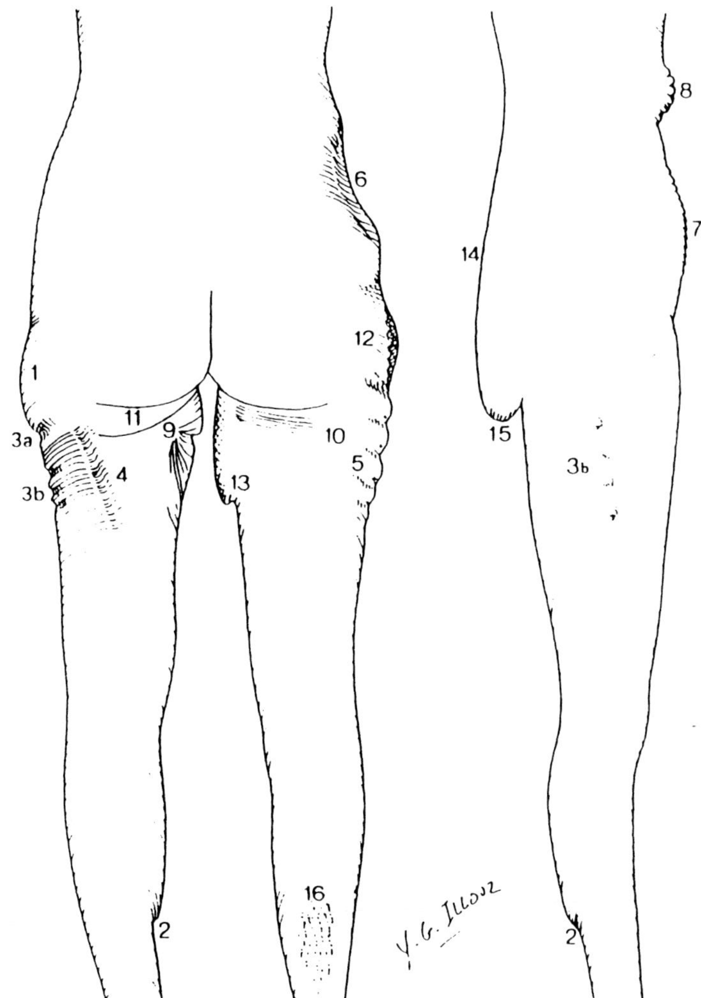

FIGURE 130-1. Schematic representation of the various defects that may result after liposuction: 1, residual bulge; 2, stair-step deformity, frequent in the ankles; 3a, solitary dimple; 3b, multiple dimples, with gaps often seen along the fascia lata; 4, furrow; 5, waves; 6, crater; 7, "French pastry" wrinkling often seen on the abdomen; 8, padded, mattress-like wrinkling resulting from intraclinic seroma formation, almost exclusively seen in the upper abdomen; 9, adhesion to deep, musculoaponeurotic structures that retracts overlying region; 10, "French pastry" wrinkling because of minimal skin excess of a neighboring region after correction of a localized fat deposit; 11, double gluteal fold ("banana"); 12, false bulge because of accordionization of excess skin; 13, ptosis or "sliding" as a result of a neglected seroma; 14, flat buttocks after overcorrection and disregard of the "Bermuda triangle"; 15, gluteal ptosis after liposuction of the inferior segment and overcorrection; 16, residual pigmentation frequently seen in the dependent regions (ankles) and areas where the skin is particularly thin. (From Illouz Y: Body Sculpturing by Lipoplasty. Edinburgh, Churchill Livingstone, 1989:181.)

sedation. Smaller procedures can be done in the office without use of the operating room if proper equipment is available to decrease the cost to the patient. However, the patient's safety and comfort are always of paramount importance in making the decision to use the office or the operating room.

The nature and location of the defect are evaluated with the patient lying down and standing up. Residual bulges, areas of asymmetry, or undercorrected transition zones are carefully marked in the standing position and discussed with the patient so there is a clear understanding of the goals of the revisionary procedure. It is wise to use a different color marking pen for areas of indentation to differentiate them clearly from areas of protuberance (Fig. 130-3). The undercorrected areas are then infiltrated with wetting solution, and secondary liposuction is performed. Feathering or tapering the amount of wetting solution at the periphery of the areas to be treated will help the surgeon establish a smooth transition between suctioned and nonsuctioned areas. As the periphery is approached, the surgeon must make fewer and fewer passes with the cannula or use smaller diameter cannulas.

Overcorrection

Problems of overcorrection result in defects such as dimples, dents, furrows, grooves, and craters. Overcorrection is unfortunately a more difficult problem to correct. When the area of overcorrection can be specifically defined, autologous fat transplantation is the treatment of choice. This technique consists of atraumatic harvesting of fat from the subcutaneous layer. It is then prepared by one of many previously described techniques[8-12] and introduced at a different site for revision of unwanted contour irregularities.[13-15] Simultaneous liposuction around the

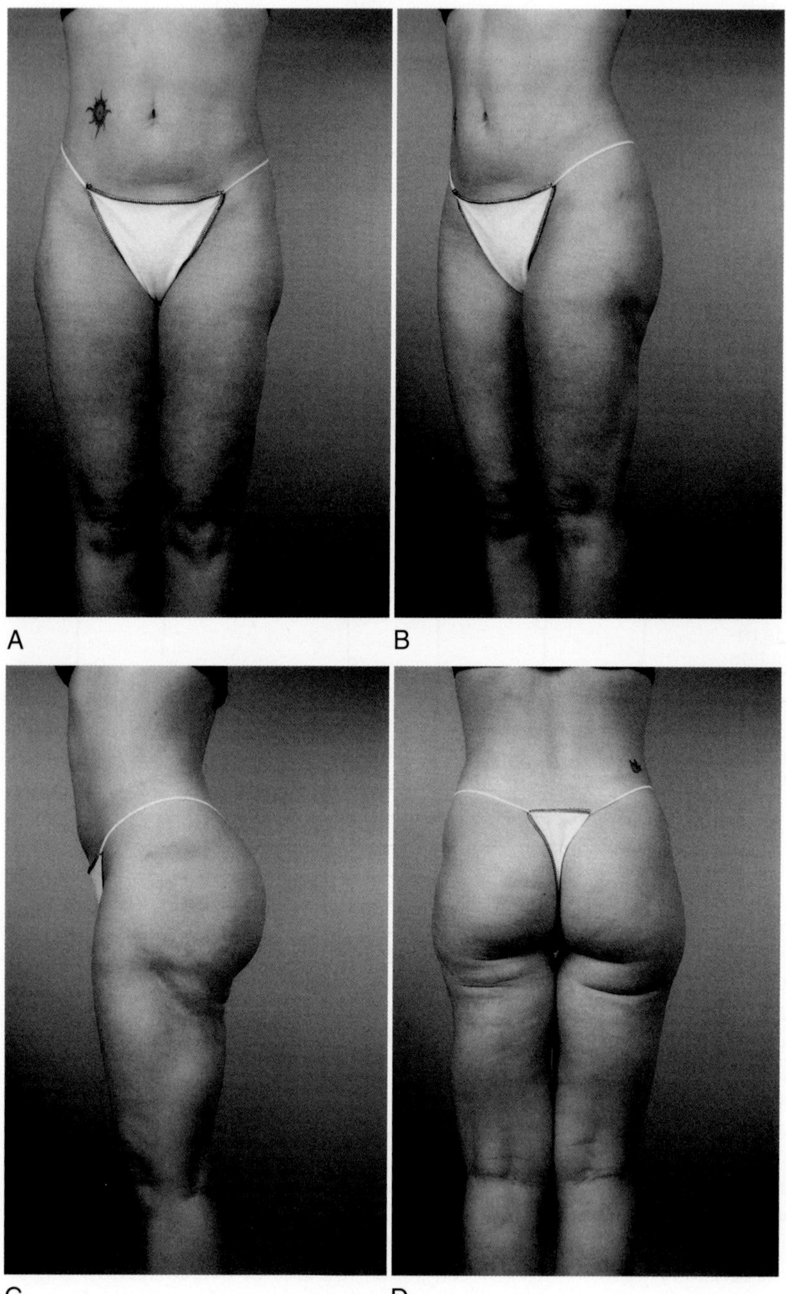

FIGURE 130-2. *A* to *D,* This 32-year-old woman underwent aggressive liposuction of the lateral thighs. She is left with significant contour irregularity of the posterior and lateral thighs. She has furrowing of the left lateral thigh (*B* to *D*) from overcorrection of the deep and superficial fat. The skin in this area is firm, discolored, and adherent to the underlying fascia. The right infragluteal area *(D)* illustrates a banana roll deformity.

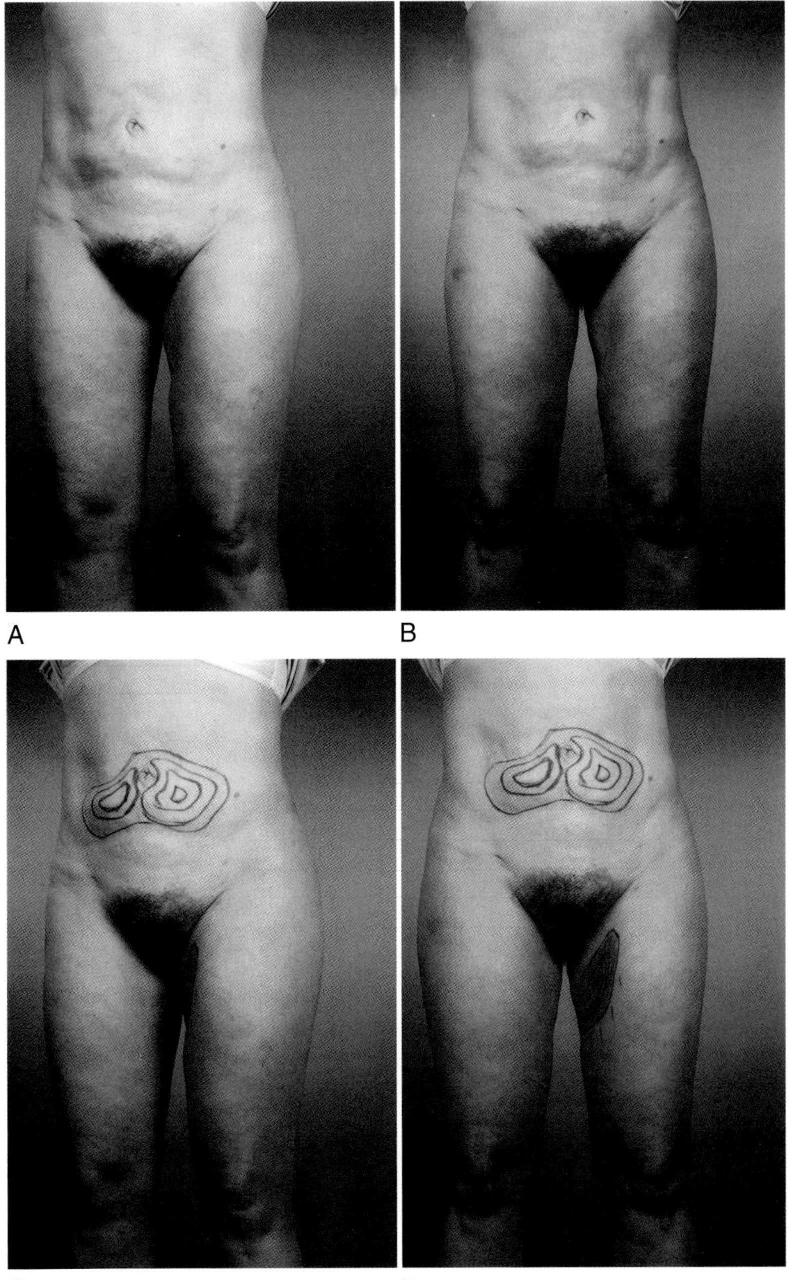

FIGURE 130-3. *A* and *B,* This 44-year-old woman underwent liposuction of the abdomen and thighs. She is left with contour irregularity of the abdomen and a large overcorrection deformity of the left medial thigh. *C* and *D,* She is shown marked for secondary liposuction of the abdomen and autologous fat injection of the left medial thigh. *Continued*

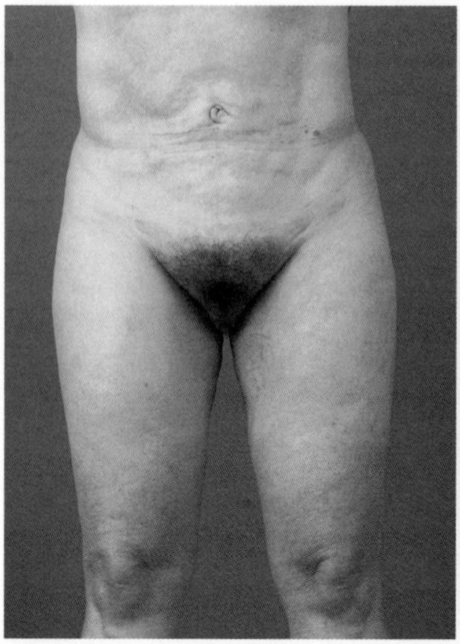
E

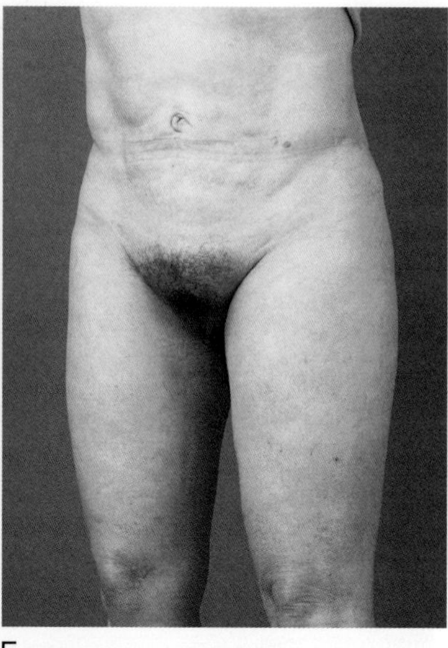
F

FIGURE 130-3, cont'd. *E* and *F*, Patient is shown 1 1/2 years after one session of autologous fat injection to her left medial thigh and revision liposuction of the lower abdomen. She has not elected to have further surgery.

periphery of an area of indentation may also be required to improve the result of the secondary procedure. In this way, it is possible to fill in skin depressions and smooth out soft tissue contour irregularities.

If localized overresection is noted during the primary procedure, immediate fat grafting should be attempted to correct the deformity. The success rate is much better with immediate fat grafting than with delayed grafting because the defect is fresh and there is no scar tissue. However, immediate grafting into a large cavity will produce less than optimal results because the fat grafts must be surrounded by well-vascularized subcutaneous fat to "take." Simply "dumping" nonvascularized fat into a large open cavity will increase the risk of seroma formation, scar tissue, and retractile ligaments if the fat grafts do not become vascularized. Ideally, autologous fat grafts are injected into multiple layers in a systematic fashion so that well-vascularized tissue surrounds each injected "tubule" of fat. For this reason, multiple sessions may be required to fill a particularly deep depression.

Failure of Skin Retraction or Abnormal Skin Retraction

Skin retraction is both the friend and the foe of the liposuction surgeon. Ideally, when an area of protuberance is suctioned, the overlying skin will retract just the right amount to redrape over the suctioned area and leave a smooth appearance. Skin retraction is related to the inherent retractile properties of the skin itself as well as to the underlying fibroconnective tissue lattice that houses the subcutaneous fat. The response of overlying skin to the liposuction procedure itself is also important. Theoretically, skin retraction after superficial liposuction is at least partially related to a "controlled injury" to the undersurface of the skin resulting in scar tissue that contracts.

Simple failure of skin retraction is a problem of poor selection of patients more often than of improper surgical technique. Loose hanging skin after liposuction, no matter how evenly distributed, will be perceived by the patient as an undesired sequela. In rare instances, the postoperative deformity of loose hanging skin may be acceptable to the patient presented with the alternative of excisional surgery. As long as the alternatives and expected results are discussed in detail and carefully documented in the medical record and informed consent, postoperative failure of skin retraction can sometimes be an "acceptable" sequela. It is the authors' opinion that fees for the procedure that were recommended in preference to lipoplasty (abdominoplasty, thigh lift, body lift, or face lift) be discussed and put in writing at the initial consultation because the patient may often come back for this definitive procedure.

Abnormal skin retraction usually results from a combination of overly aggressive liposuction and devascularization of the superficial tissues leading to scar tissue or adhesion formation. Superficial liposuction, when it is performed correctly, can result in predictable postoperative skin retraction.[16,17] If it is performed incorrectly, superficial liposuction can result in severe postoperative contour irregularity. Generally speaking, the superficial fat is the liposuction surgeon's best friend. The goal of liposuction is to remove fat *evenly* from the subcutaneous plane, *leaving* the appropriate amount of residual fat to produce a smooth contour with the surrounding body areas. Uneven removal of fat from any plane, especially the superficial plane, can result in contour irregularity. The superficial plane is the least forgiving for two reasons: it is closest to the surface and therefore most visible, and devascularization or scar tissue involving or extending to the dermis will lead to visible retractile ligaments. Treatment is discussed next.

Complex Deformities

Complex deformities are defined as contour irregularities that involve a combination of undercorrection, overcorrection, and abnormal skin retraction. Complex deformities usually require combined revisionary liposuction, autologous fat transplantation, or skin excision for correction.

When an overcorrection defect is deep and there is scar tissue involving the fascial layer, reinjection of fat often fails because there is no foundation for revascularization of the fat. When localized adhesions complicate the picture, the scar tissue must be released, followed by replacement of the adipose layer by fat grafting. In complex defects, staged or serial grafting may be required. In patients with extensive adhesions, undermining of the skin followed by resection and redraping may be the best option if the patient is willing to accept the required scar. However, this is possible only when there is enough skin laxity to allow excision and when the deformity lies in an area amenable to excision.

Weight fluctuation after liposuction can also affect the problem. With significant weight gain, areas surrounding an overresected and scarred indentation can hypertrophy and magnify the deformity. If there are several episodes of weight gain and loss, skin flaccidity may develop and eventually require resection.

TIMING OF REOPERATIVE SURGERY

Contour irregularity after liposuction can occur even in the best of candidates, under the most ideal conditions, and with the most experienced surgeons. With increasing experience, the incidence of complications decreases. When defects do occur, patients should be made aware of the possibility for improvement. They should be informed that some resolution may occur with time and that any operative intervention should be delayed for at least 6 months to allow all postoperative edema to resolve. When significant scar tissue is involved, it is important that the scar be allowed to mature fully before revisional procedures are attempted. During this period, massage, Endermologie, and external ultrasound can be used as conservative measures in an attempt to improve the problem or to hasten the resolution of edema.

AVOIDANCE OF CONTOUR IRREGULARITY

Avoidance of contour irregularity begins with proper selection of the patient. This should always be addressed in the initial consultation. However, proper selection of patients can be undermined by poor or careless surgical technique. Many changes in technique and equipment have occurred during the years to assist the surgeon in minimizing the problem. The original liposuction cannulas were large and sharp with a single hole. These have largely been replaced by smaller (1.5- to 4.0-mm-diameter), blunt-tipped cannulas with multiple holes. The smaller cannulas are less traumatic and easier to pass through fat, especially in more fibrous areas. Smaller cannulas are more likely to form numerous small tunnels, whereas the larger cannulas may result in cavities. Cavities heal differently than tunnels do and can be responsible for postoperative seromas and abnormal skin retraction. Excessive crisscrossing even with small cannulas can result in cavities.

The tumescent technique was introduced in the late 1980s by Jeffrey Klein.[18-20] Originally described in the dermatology literature as a means of local anesthesia, the infiltration of wetting solution has become standard practice in liposuction surgery. Not only does wetting solution offer the benefits of local anesthesia and decreased blood loss, but it can also assist the surgeon in the avoidance of contour irregularity. Better hemostasis, provided by the epinephrine solution, allows the surgeon adequate time for careful attention to contouring. Even infiltration at multiple levels in the subcutaneous fat, as well as feathering or tapering of the amount of wetting solution at the transition zones between suctioned and nonsuctioned areas, is paramount to avoidance of contour irregularity.

The late 1990s saw the introduction of ultrasound-assisted liposuction, which some authors suggest enhances the surgeon's ability to achieve smooth contour.[21,22] The ultrasound-assisted technique involves a two-step liposuction process. The subcutaneous fat is first subjected to ultrasonic energy by a titanium cannula or probe vibrating at ultrasonic frequency, thereby emulsifying the fat. Any remaining emulsified fat is then evacuated from the subcutaneous space by traditional liposuction cannulas. The suggested improvement comes from the feathering effect with each stroke of the ultrasound-assisted liposuction cannula. The subcutaneous fat is thereby systematically liquefied or destroyed in a smooth fashion rather than by the less efficient methods of traditional lipoaspiration.

No instrument or technique will make up for careless technique or poor surgical judgment. Liposuction requires meticulous technique and constant attention to the final outcome to achieve a harmonious, proportional body contour. Overcorrection can occur quickly, and certain areas of the body are particularly unforgiving. Different areas of the body respond differently to liposuction. The hip rolls and back tend to be relatively forgiving areas and are less susceptible to contour irregularity. This is at least partially so because the overlying skin tends to be thick and the fat tends to be fibrous in nature, therefore having better retractile properties. Fibrous fat has a higher density of fibroconnective tissue within the subcutaneous space, and this tissue lattice is partially responsible for the postoperative skin retraction. The abdomen is somewhat less forgiving in that the skin quality is often compromised by pregnancy and weight fluctuations. The lateral thighs can also be difficult when skin quality is poor and areas of adherence complicate skin redraping. The medial thighs, arms, and face are even less forgiving in that the overlying skin tends to be thin and the fat tends to be loose, with sparse fibroconnective tissue. The anterior thighs and arms, posterior thighs, calves, and ankles are particularly unforgiving in that they are visible when even minor contour irregularities occur. The proximity of the underlying muscle to the skin can lead to accentuation of a deformity with muscle contraction. The lower buttocks have long been considered a taboo area in that loss of support of the overlying skin can cause an unsightly buttocks ptosis. The infragluteal roll should also be approached with extreme caution. Overcorrection, especially in the deep plane, can lead to loss of support and the development of a postoperative banana roll deformity that is extremely difficult to fix, often requiring excisional measures.

SUMMARY

The final result of any liposuction procedure depends on a combination of appropriate fat removal and predictable skin retraction. The surgeon's ability and experience dictate the correct amount of fat aspiration needed to obtain the desired result. In the words of Illouz,[7] "I would insist that this technique is not easy, not simply the suctioning of fat with a cannula, a tube and a pump. Instrumentation alone is not sufficient to make one an expert, let alone an artist. It is the hand as an instrument of the brain that executes the procedure."

REFERENCES

1. American Society for Aesthetic Plastic Surgery: 2003 Statistics on Cosmetic Surgery. Available at: www.surgery.org
2. Gargan TJ, Courtiss EH: The risks of suction lipectomy: their prevention and treatment. Clin Plast Surg 1984;11:457.
3. Pitman GH, Teimourian B: Suction lipectomy: complications and results by survey. Plast Reconstr Surg 1985;76:65.
4. Dillerud E: Suction lipoplasty: a report on complications, undesired results and patient satisfaction based on 3511 procedures. Plast Reconstr Surg 1991;88:239.
5. Chang KN: Surgical correction of postliposuction contour irregularities. Plast Reconstr Surg 1994;94:126.
6. Giese SY, Bulan EJ, Commons GW, et al: Improvements in cardiovascular risk profile with large-volume liposuction: a pilot study. Plast Reconstr Surg 2001;108:510.
7. Illouz YG: Body Sculpturing by Lipoplasty. Edinburgh, Churchill Livingstone, 1989.
8. Coleman SR: Facial recontouring with liposculpture. Clin Plast Surg 1997;24:347.
9. Rubin A, Hoefflin S: Fat purification: survival of the fittest. Plast Reconstr Surg 2002;109:1463.
10. Bartynski J, Marion MS, Wang TD: Histopathologic evaluation of adipose autografts in a rabbit ear model. Otolaryngol Head Neck Surg 1990;102:314.
11. Eppley BL, Smith PG, Sadove AM, Delfino J: Experimental effects of graft, revascularization and consistency on cervicofacial fat transplant survival. J Oral Maxillofac Surg 1990;48:54.
12. Niechajev I, Sevcuk O: Long-term results of fat transplantation: clinical and histologic studies. Plast Reconstr Surg 1994;94:496.
13. Agris J: Autologous fat transplantation: a 3 year study. Am J Cosmet Surg 1987;4:95.
14. Johnson GW: Body contouring by macroinjection of autogenous fat. Am J Cosmet Surg 1987;4:103.
15. Krulig E: Lipoinjection. Am J Cosmet Surg 1987;4:123.
16. Courtiss EH: Suction lipectomy: a retrospective analysis of 100 patients. Plast Reconstr Surg 1984;73:780.
17. Gasparotti M: Superficial liposuction: a new application of the technique for aged and flaccid skin. Aesthetic Plast Surg 1992;16:141.
18. Klein JA: Tumescent technique for regional anesthesia permits lidocaine doses of 35 mg/kg for liposuction. J Dermatol Surg Oncol 1990;16:248.
19. Klein JA: The tumescent technique. Anesthesia and modified liposuction technique. Dermatol Clin 1990;8:425.
20. Klein JA: Tumescent technique for local anesthesia improves safety in large-volume liposuction. Plast Reconstr Surg 1993;91:1085.
21. Rohrich RJ, Raniere J Jr, Kenkel JM, Beran SJ: Operative principles for optimizing results in circumferential body contouring with ultrasound-assisted lipoplasty. Clin Plast Surg 1999;26:305.
22. Gingrass MK: Lipoplasty complications and their prevention. Clin Plast Surg 1999;26:341.

CHAPTER

131

Aesthetic Genital Surgery

GARY J. ALTER, MD

Identity and self-esteem are intimately related to a person's image of his or her genitalia. Self-esteem can be impaired if a person feels inadequate compared with a perceived ideal. A normal man may think his penis is too small, or a woman may consider her genital appearance unsightly. These feelings develop from self-comparisons with pornographic photographs or videos, media attention, or comments from a sexual partner or friend.

Patients' awareness, partially related to increased media coverage, has led to significant demand for aesthetic surgery of the male and female genitalia. New techniques to enhance the appearance of male and female genitalia, based primarily on improved reconstructive pediatric and adult surgical procedures, have been developed. Considerable aesthetic improvement in the genital appearance is now possible. The surgery is challenging and requires strict attention to detail and meticulous technique.

MALE GENITAL COSMETIC SURGERY

Several procedures are now available to enhance or improve the aesthetic appearance of the penis or scrotum. Penile lengthening is performed by release of the suspensory ligament of the penis followed by use of penile weights or stretching devices. Penoscrotal webbing is corrected by one or several Z-plasties. Penile girth is increased by injection of autologous fat or by placement of dermal fat grafts or AlloDerm around the penile circumference. The hidden or buried penis is corrected with a suprapubic lipectomy, possible upper pubic skin resection, and tacking of penopubic and penoscrotal skin. A variety of procedures are performed with differing results because no standardized procedures exist. Many of the complications and deformities result from faulty theoretical or anatomic design, especially if the surgeon is not technically meticulous.

Men are initially resistant to psychiatric evaluation before penile enlargement surgery. Many of the men presenting for penile enlargement have significant self-esteem issues, so refusal to perform the surgery is not unwarranted. The psychological motivations of men with hidden penis, penoscrotal webbing, scrotal enlargement, or true congenital deformities are different from those of men with normal penis size who desire only enlargement, so their care is more rewarding.

Measurements

Schonfeld and Beebe[1] determined that the length of the fully stretched flaccid penis correlates closely with the erect penis. The dorsal length from the junction of the penopubic skin to the tip of the glans in the fully stretched flaccid penis correlated closely to the erect penis. Erect girth or circumference correlated with girth measurements of the flaccid penis according to a more complicated ratio.

Da Ros and Teloken[2] performed artificial erections on 150 white men, measuring penis length from the center of the pubic bone to the tip of the glans and penis circumference at the corona and base. Average penis length was 5.7 inches; 18 were shorter than 4.7 inches and 18 longer than 6.3 inches. Circumference ranged from 3.5 to 5.9 inches (average, 4.7 inches) at the base of the penis and from 3.2 to 5.5 inches (average, 4.4 inches) at the coronal groove.

Wessells et al[3] compared penile length in the flaccid stretched and erect states and also concluded that there is a positive relationship. The average flaccid stretched penile length was 11 cm; the average erect penile length was 12.5 cm. The correlation between stretched length and erect length was $r^2 = .769$. Average flaccid circumference was 10 cm, with an average erect circumference of 12.5 cm; therefore, correlation was not favorable for circumference. They also stated that a thick pubic fat pad decreases visible flaccid penile length but not functional penile length during intercourse.

Aging has an effect on male genitals displayed by descent of the pubic fat pad, possibly causing a hidden penis, and enlargement and lowering of the scrotum with laxity of the fasciae of the scrotum.

Examination

The patient is evaluated both standing and supine to determine variations that change with gravity. While the patient is standing, the penis is checked for concealment due to descent of the pubic fat pad and escutcheon from gravity; supine positioning often eliminates this abnormality. A protuberant abdomen with excess skin and fat may overhang the penis and functionally interfere with sexual intercourse. Release of the suspensory ligament does little to help this patient, who may need an abdominoplasty in addition to a suprapubic lipectomy and skin excision. The amount of suprapubic fat between the pubic symphysis and the skin should be evaluated to determine potential length improvement from suprapubic lipectomy or liposuction. Penis position must be checked to see whether it is partially encircled by the scrotum, and tightness of the suspensory ligament and infrapubic skin is judged by stretching the penis and palpating the infrapubic area. Measurements are taken from the pubic bone and from the skin over the pubis to the tip of the glans on full stretch, with the penis at 90 degrees to the abdomen. Circumference is measured at the base and corona with the penis on full stretch. The underside of the penis is examined for webbing that causes the appearance of a shorter penis. The penis is palpated for Peyronie plaques.

It is important to evaluate function before penile surgery. Urinary and orgasmic function should be normal but are not affected by these procedures. The patient is asked if he has any erectile difficulties or penile curvature. Most men have some minor curvatures, but these are not bothersome and are not an issue. However, if girth surgery is considered, any known or suspected curvature should be photographed. The patient is asked to present photos showing his erect penis from various angles. If the patient is unwilling to present photos, an erection can be obtained by self-stimulation or by intracavernosal injection of prostaglandin E_1. The pharmacologic agent is injected with a 30-gauge needle at the base of the penis transversely into the cavernosal bodies. The dosage is usually 1 mL of 10 μg/mL in the normal man. Photos should be taken of the erection as documentation. The patient is cautioned about the possibility of priapism and the mandatory reversal of the erection if it persists longer than 4 or 5 hours.

Once the diagnosis is made, the possible procedures as well as risks and benefits are discussed with the patient. Penoscrotal webbing and extensive suprapubic fat are not usually presenting complaints, but the physician must describe these abnormalities and possible corrective surgery. Each individual is evaluated to determine the best method to achieve his goals because several procedures are available, depending on the patient's anatomy. He must have a realistic understanding of the design and limitations of the surgery to prevent misconceptions and dissatisfaction. Exaggerated promises lead to the patient's disappointment, depression, and hostility; therefore, honesty, clear communication, and compassion are mandatory for both patient and physician. Because not all malpractice carriers will cover physicians for penile enhancement procedures, verification of coverage is recommended. An extensive consent document helps prevent misunderstanding and provides some protection for the physician.

Anatomy

The suspensory ligament of the penis is a thick, triangular band extending from the linea alba and the upper portion of the symphysis pubis and arcuate ligament to the dorsal midline of the penis.[4] It derives from the outer investing fascia of the abdomen and divides into a sling at the junction of the fixed and mobile portions of the penis. In addition, thickened bands of Scarpa fascia, called the fundiform ligaments, firmly attach to the rectus fascia above the pubic symphysis and extend onto the dorsal and lateral penis, possibly restricting penile excursion.[5]

The skin of the penis is thin and hairless (more distally) and has loose connections with the deeper structures of the penis. No adipose tissue is present under the skin. The superficial or subcutaneous fascia of the penis (dartos fascia) is continuous with the Scarpa and Camper fasciae of the lower abdomen and extends to the corona of the penis. The dartos fascia contains scattered smooth muscle cells. Branches of the superficial external pudendal vessels provide the blood supply to the dartos fascia and skin. The internal pudendal system, which includes the deep dorsal arteries and veins and the cavernosal and urethral vessels, usually communicates with the external pudendal system only at the glans and corona.[6] Because the dartos fascia is highly vascular, it provides an excellent tissue bed for grafts. Buck fascia invests the shaft of the penis deep to the dartos fascia. The deep dorsal vessels and the dorsal nerve travel in the pudendal canal along the ischial ramus and then pass ventrally along the margin of the inferior ramus of the pubis in the deep perineal pouch. The neurovascular bundle pierces the perineal membrane ½ inch from the symphysis pubis and continues under the Buck fascia of the penis. The deep dorsal artery lies between the deep dorsal vein medially and the dorsal nerve of the penis laterally.

Penile Enlargement

PENILE LENGTHENING

Mild length increase by inferior displacement of the penis occurs by release of the suspensory ligament and restricting bands of Scarpa fascia (Fig. 131-1).[7-9] Release of the ligament frees more of the penis to be stretched, thereby allowing a greater gain. Real length gain can be achieved by combining ligament release with the use of special penile weights or stretching devices that act as an external tissue expander.

Technique

The most common incision is a 4-cm transverse pubic incision placed several centimeters above the penopubic junction. Skin advancement onto the proximal dorsal shaft of the penis is rarely necessary unless the patient has a relative deficiency of shaft skin, usually resulting from an overly aggressive circumcision. Nonetheless, many surgeons still advance infrapubic skin onto the penis, theoretically making it longer and giving the appearance of length gain. However, such a gain is disputed. Some physicians use V-Y advancement flaps of various sizes based distally at the penopubic junction or several centimeters proximal to the penopubic junction (see Fig. 131-1).[10,11] However, the base of the penis may develop a hump or appear thicker with hair-bearing skin advanced onto the proximal penile shaft. A large V-Y advancement flap is not recommended because it often produces a deforming dorsal hair-bearing hump at the base of the penis, large dog-ears, and the appearance of penile shortening, especially if there is a relative penoscrotal transposition or a thick suprapubic fat pad.[12-14] Because of compromised blood supply, healing problems at the Y junction often occur. Z-plasties in the pubic region are rarely necessary.

Scarpa fascia is transversely incised to the pubic symphysis.[7-9] The restricting bands of Scarpa fascia and the suspensory ligament are delineated by pulling the penis and by bluntly dissecting on both sides of the midline (Fig. 131-2). While the penis is stretched, the suspensory ligament is cut directly on the periosteum to the inferior border of the pubic bone. No injury will

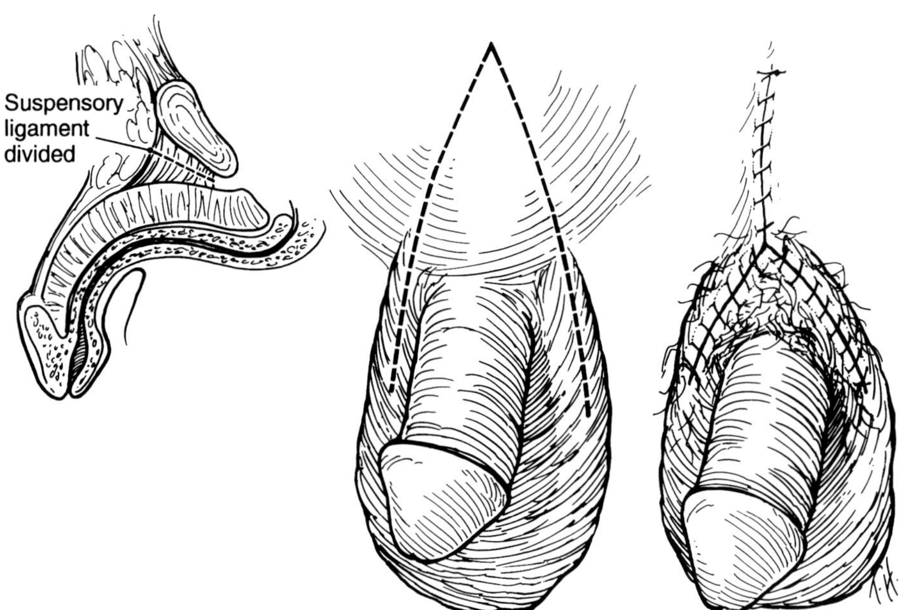

FIGURE 131-1. Method of penile lengthening that often causes penile deformities. The suspensory ligament is released *(left)*. A large V-Y advancement flap is marked *(center)*. The flap is advanced *(right)*, resulting in hair on the proximal shaft of the penis, bilateral dog-ears, and a lower hanging penis.

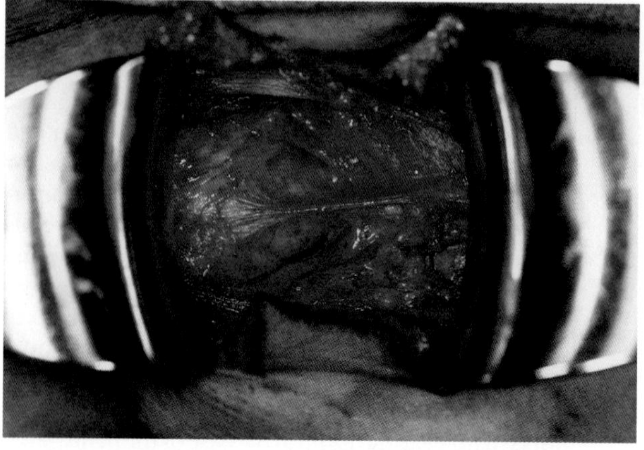

FIGURE 131-2. The suspensory ligament of the penis in the midline and restraining bands of Scarpa fascia bilaterally. The corporal bodies are on the left.

occur to the dorsal neurovascular structures if the ligament is released only 1 cm on each side of the midline. Once this ligament is released, more restraining bands of Scarpa fascia are incised transversely with the penis on stretch. Care must be taken to prevent injury to the spermatic cords.

The release creates a dead space between the corpora and the pubis, which must be filled to prevent reattachment of these structures and possible shortening of the penis. Lipomatous tissue is usually present medial to the spermatic cord.[9] A proximally or distally based fat flap of this fatty tissue is used to fill this space. It is dissected off the cord and divided proximally or distally, leaving an intact random blood supply (Fig. 131-3*A*). This fat flap is then transposed into the dead space and sutured to the periosteum with 000 Vicryl (Fig. 131-3*B*). This vascularized fat is superior to a fat graft in terms of survival and fibrosis. A closed system drain is inserted, and Scarpa fascia is closed vertically. Buried intradermal absorbable sutures are placed, followed by a subcuticular layer of small absorbable or monofilament sutures.

Results

It is difficult to interpret the results of penile lengthening because no standardized measurement technique exists. Dorsal measurements are taken preoperatively and postoperatively from the pubic symphysis and from the suprapubic skin to the tip of the glans penis on full stretch at a 90-degree angle to the abdomen.

Suspensory ligament release alone may occasionally increase flaccid penile length by up to 1 to 2 cm, but often no gain is achieved. Real flaccid and erect length gain can be obtained by use of penile weights or penile stretching devices (Fig. 131-4). Patients can use these devices without undergoing ligament release, but the ligament release frees more of the penis to be expanded, thereby increasing the amount of eventual length gain. The amount of length gain achieved is controversial. A patient should not undergo release of the suspensory ligament unless he is willing to use the weights. Approximately 1 week after surgery, the patient suspends the weights from the end of the penis several times daily for a period of months, stretching

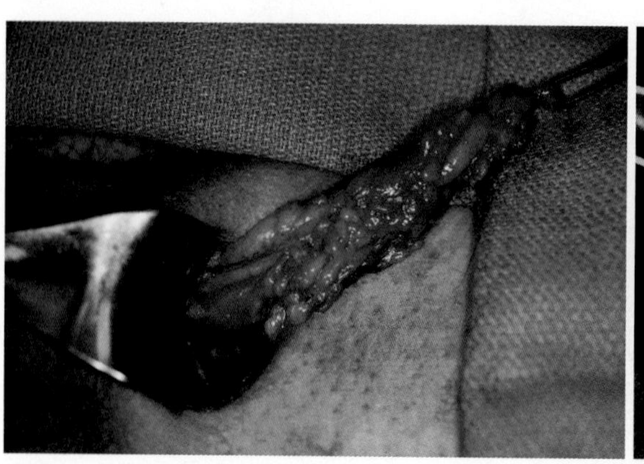

A

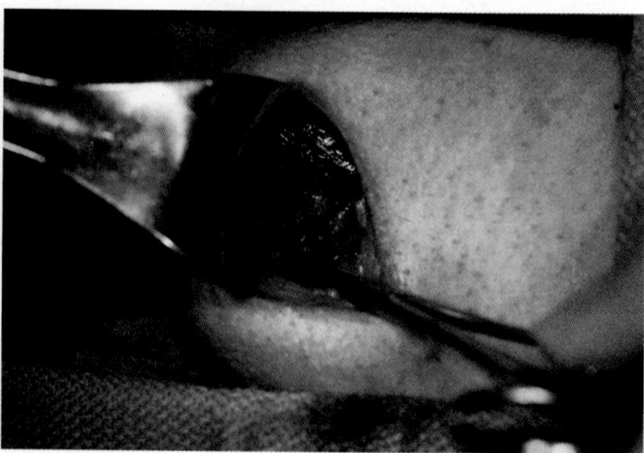

B

FIGURE 131-3. Fat flap used to fill the dead space between the corporal bodies and the pubic symphysis. *A,* Distally based fat flap from the right spermatic cord. *B,* Fat flap transposed.

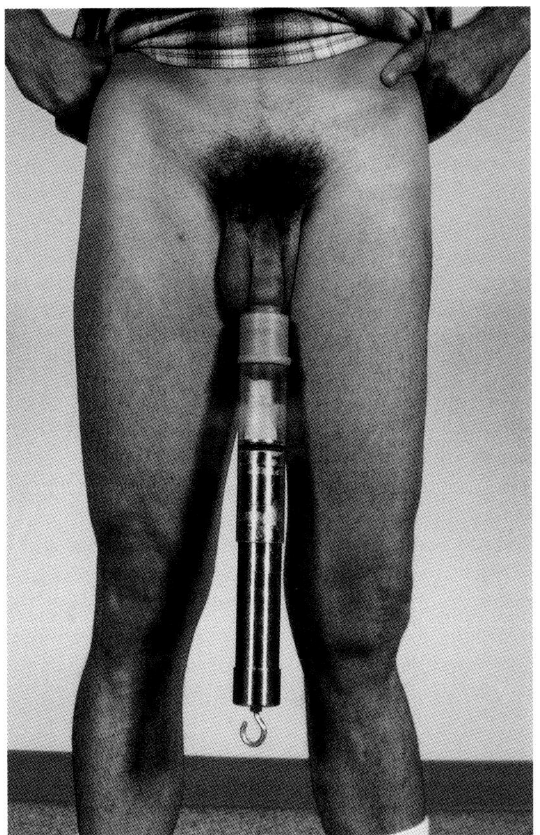

FIGURE 131-4. Patient using penile stretching device known as the MegaTrac.

the corporal bodies. The amount of weight required as well as the duration and frequency of use are still evolving. Other devices are being designed to produce constant penile stretching and traction.

Actual length gains of several inches are uncommon but may occur if a suprapubic lipectomy is also performed on thick subcutaneous tissue. However, anecdotal flaccid as well as erect gains of several inches have been reported by some compulsive weight users. In fact, a 1-inch gain is considered successful even with weights (Fig. 131-5).

GIRTH INCREASE

Techniques to increase penile girth are in a constant state of evolvement and are associated with the largest incidence of complications. The difficulty of achieving girth enhancement is the necessity to create a symmetric and relatively cylindrical phallus. Any graft that may resorb can cause visual or functional deformities. Thus, many techniques have been used with varying success.

Fat Injections

Autologous fat injections are still used by some physicians to increase penile thickness. The fat is injected into the dartos fascia. The fat is movable and gives a somewhat spongy texture to the penis. Less than 50% of injected fat normally survives in other parts of the body.[15-18] Ideally, small amounts of fat are injected in multiple tunnels.[19] Small amounts of total injected fat produce only minimal girth gain but do not have much risk of complications.

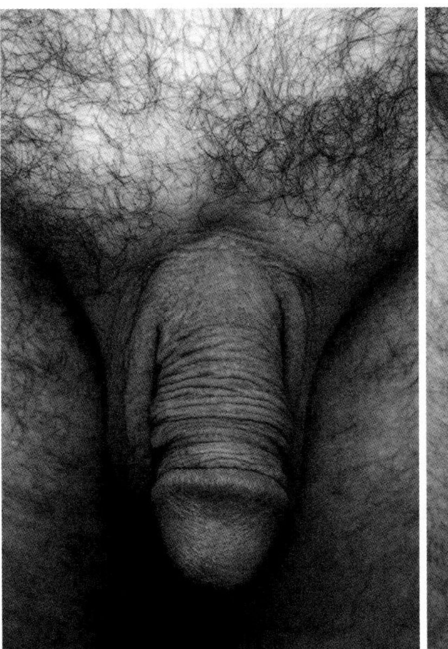

A

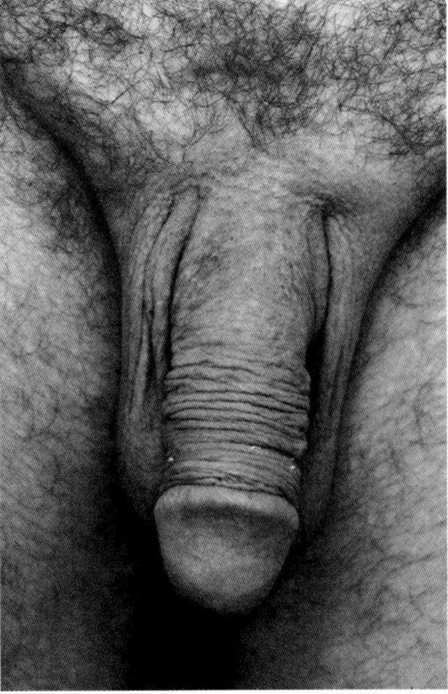

B

FIGURE 131-5. A 59-year-old man before *(A)* and after *(B)* suspensory ligament release. Stretched flaccid length gain of more than $1^1/_2$ inches was achieved after release of the suspensory ligament and use of a stretching device.

Dermal Fat Grafts

Girth enlargement is also performed by inserting dermal fat strips into the dartos fascia or by wrapping dermal fat sheets circumferentially between the dartos and Buck fasciae (Fig. 131-6).[7-9] The strips can be placed through either a partial circumcision incision or a transverse pubic incision. The sheet graft is usually placed through a hemicircumcision incision and wrapped about 80% of the circumference of the penis; the urethra is left uncovered. The grafts are stabilized proximally and sutured distally to prevent migration. Dermal fat grafts have been used successfully in plastic surgery for decades and have higher reliability than autologous fat injections. Dermis "takes" easily and provides support, enabling accurate graft placement. The dermal fat grafts usually take well and provide girth increase. However, difficulties with penile immobilization and the thickness of the grafts increase the risk of poor take and subsequent complications. Circumference is increased 1 to 2 inches with dermal fat graft augmentation (Figs. 131-7 and 131-8). The procedure is far more invasive than fat injections and requires several hours of surgery. Donor site scars from the buttock crease, suprapubic region, or flanks can be unsightly. Nodules and fat resorption are less common with dermal fat grafts than with fat injections. Significant penile edema and induration exist for 6 weeks after surgery, and relatively normal texture returns in 4 to 6 months. Wrapping a sheet of dermal fat grafts rather than inserting strips provides smooth texture with less risk of ridges and displacement.

AlloDerm has recently been used to increase girth (D. Whitehead, personal communication, 2001). AlloDerm is stacked and placed above the Buck fascia in the dartos fascia. The lack of donor site scar is a major advantage over dermal fat grafts.

Simultaneous lengthening and girth enhancement procedures are not performed by some physicians because weight use needs to be delayed several weeks owing to penile swelling and discomfort, which risk premature ligament reattachment. Moreover, the

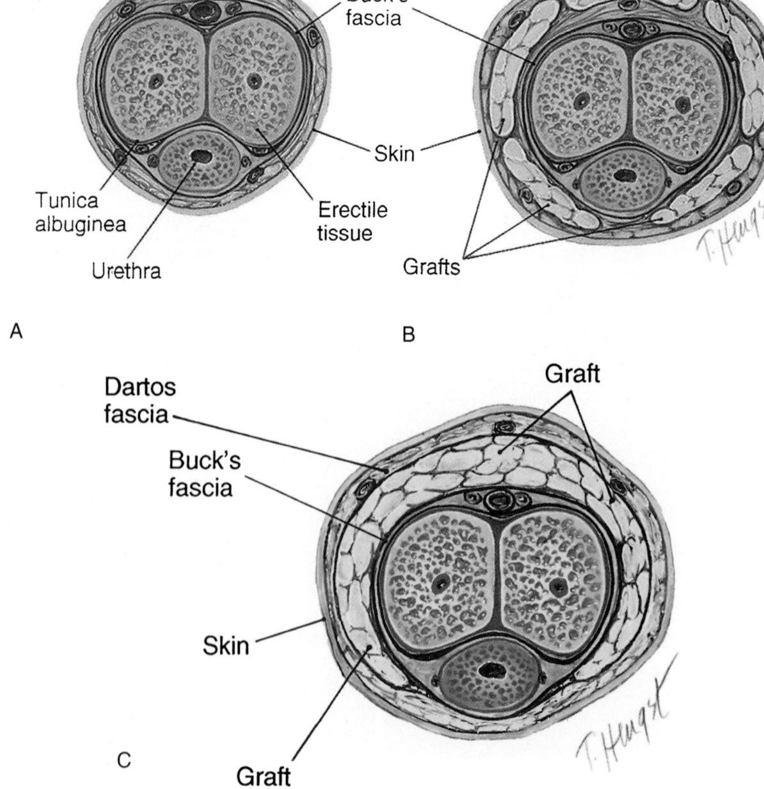

FIGURE 131-6. *A,* Normal penile anatomy. *B,* Dermal fat grafts inserted in the dartos fascia. *C,* Dermal fat graft wrapped circumferentially between the dartos and Buck fasciae.

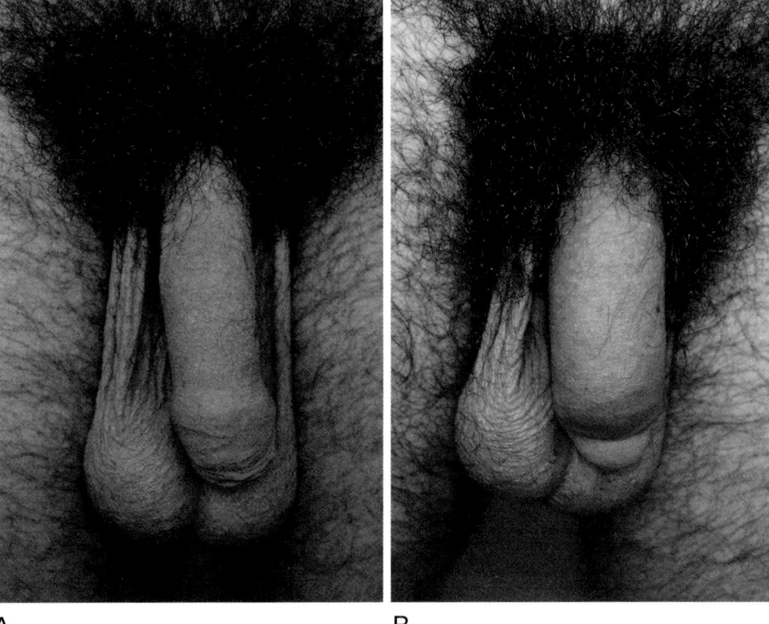

FIGURE 131-7. A 39-year-old patient who underwent dermal fat graft wrap augmentation and conservative circumcision. *A,* Preoperative appearance. *B,* Postoperative appearance. At 5 months, his proximal circumference increased by 1 1/4 inches and distal circumference by 1 1/4 inches.

complication rate increases if both operations are performed simultaneously, resulting in wound problems and decreased graft survival. Once length is achieved, the girth procedure is sometimes performed.

Complications of Penile Enlargement

PENILE LENGTHENING

Complications from release of the suspensory ligament are uncommon. If ligament release is limited to 1 cm on each side of the midline of the symphysis pubis, penile instability will not occur. If the ligament is cut directly on the periosteum of the pubis with the penis on full stretch, dorsal nerve injury will not occur. Decrease in length due to corporal reattachment after ligament release is uncommon if a spermatic cord fat flap is inserted into the space between the corpora and the pubis and if weights are used. If this space is not filled, reattachment of these structures and possible shortening of the penis can occur. If the man is markedly shortened, the attached corporal bodies must be released off the pubic symphysis. Care must be taken because of the potential risk of causing damage to the dorsal neurovascular bundles. A mild decrease in the elevation of the erection can occur with release.

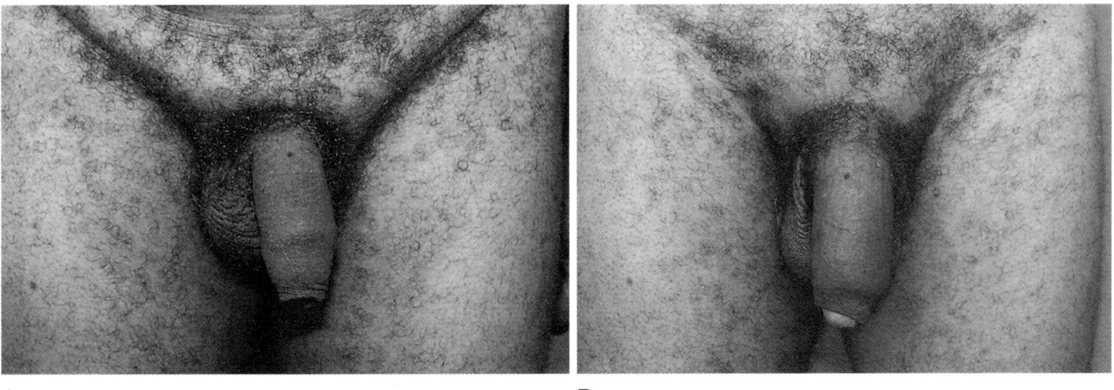

FIGURE 131-8. A 49-year-old who underwent dermal fat graft wrap augmentation, conservative circumcision, and escutcheon elevation (the lower abdominal skin was used as the dermal fat graft donor site). *A,* Preoperative appearance. *B,* Postoperative appearance. At 8 months, the patient gained approximately 1 1/4 inches in proximal circumference and 1 inch in distal circumference. The escutcheon lift gave him a more youthful genital appearance. The dermal fat grafts were obtained from the lower abdomen.

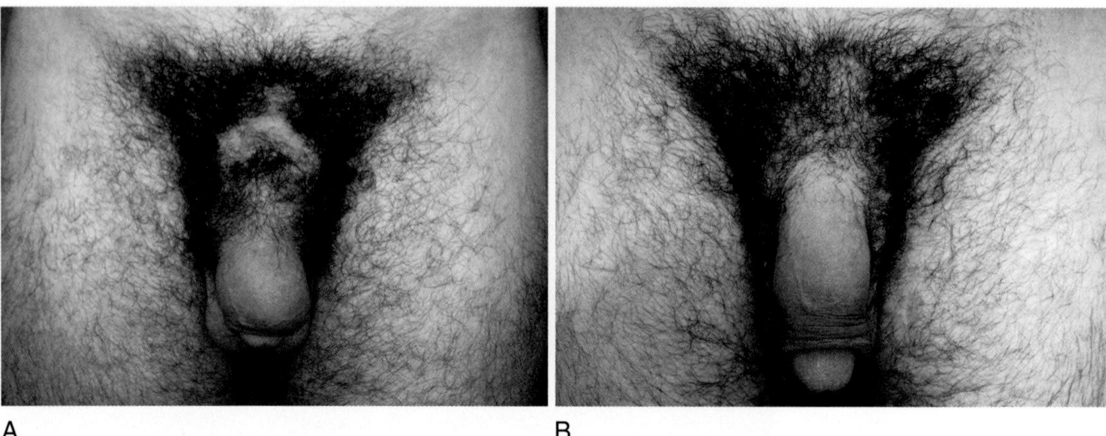

FIGURE 131-9. A 20-year-old who underwent release of the suspensory ligament, a large V-Y advancement flap, and multiple fat injections. *A,* Deformity showing a low-lying penis, hair on the proximal shaft, bilateral dog-ears at the penoscrotal junction, a shorter-appearing penis, wide pubic scars, and a large amount of fat in the shaft. *B,* Reconstruction after complete reversal of V-Y advancement flap resulting in a semicircular incision line, correction of V-Y dog-ears, scar revision, selective removal of fat nodules, and contouring of the left side of the penis.

A large V-Y advancement flap encompasses the entire dorsal penile base and part of the scrotum, partially circumcising and interrupting a significant portion of the proximal penile dartos fascia and skin (see Fig. 131-1). Proximal interruption of the external pudendal vessels and lymphatics diminishes skin and dartos viability.[14] Because these V-Y flaps are distally based, flap viability is compromised by injury to its blood supply. Therefore, flap tip loss, poor wound healing with wound dehiscence, and marked postoperative penile swelling can occur. These wound healing problems predispose to wide, hypertrophic scars, which create hairless suprapubic scars and depressions (Fig. 131-9). The large V-Y flap also advances thick, hair-bearing tissue onto the penis, often creating an unnatural hump at the penile base and the appearance of a low-hanging penis. "Scrotalization" occurs most commonly when there is more suprapubic fat; the thick V-Y flap and suprapubic fat overhang the penis, making it seem shorter and more hidden (Fig. 131-10). Dog-ears at the distal scrotal flap incisions are another common result of the large V-Y advancement flap. Smaller V-Y advancement flaps also predispose to wound and aesthetic complications, but not as severe as with larger flaps (Fig. 131-11).

GIRTH INCREASE

Fat Injections

Lack of take from an inadequate tissue bed, difficulty in penile immobilization, and fat cell trauma result in fat necrosis and resorption.[12-14] Injection of fat into the dartos fascia can cause severe deformities such as curvature or asymmetry due to resorption or migration of fat in the relatively cylindrical penis. Nodules of liquefied necrotic fat or calcified fat develop if injected fat does not survive, deforming the appearance or texture of the penis. Many patients receiving large fat injections (well above 60 mL of fat) will have varying degrees of asymmetry and nodules; with small fat quantities, there is no significant long-term girth gain (Fig. 131-12*A;* see also Figs. 131-9*A* and 131-11).

Large amounts of injected fat occasionally migrate distally during the initial postoperative period, causing unsightly fat deposits at the corona (Fig. 131-12*B*). Distal fat deposits associated with massive swelling of penile skin and a V-Y advancement flap advance the normal shaft skin over the glans. Excision of this "excess

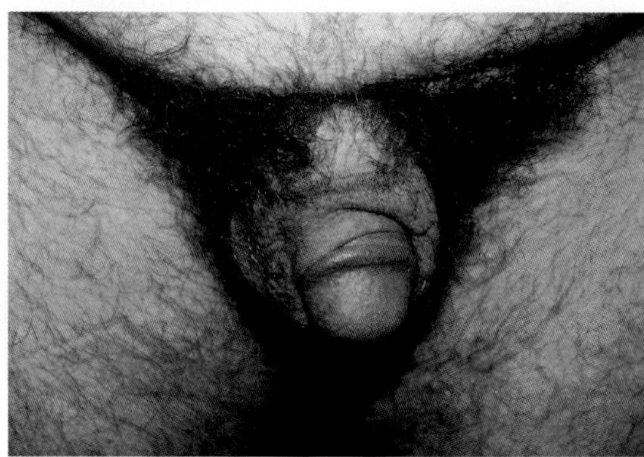

FIGURE 131-10. Scrotalization. The patient started with a short penis that was relatively hidden. The large V-Y advancement flap made his penis appear smaller and surrounded by his scrotum.

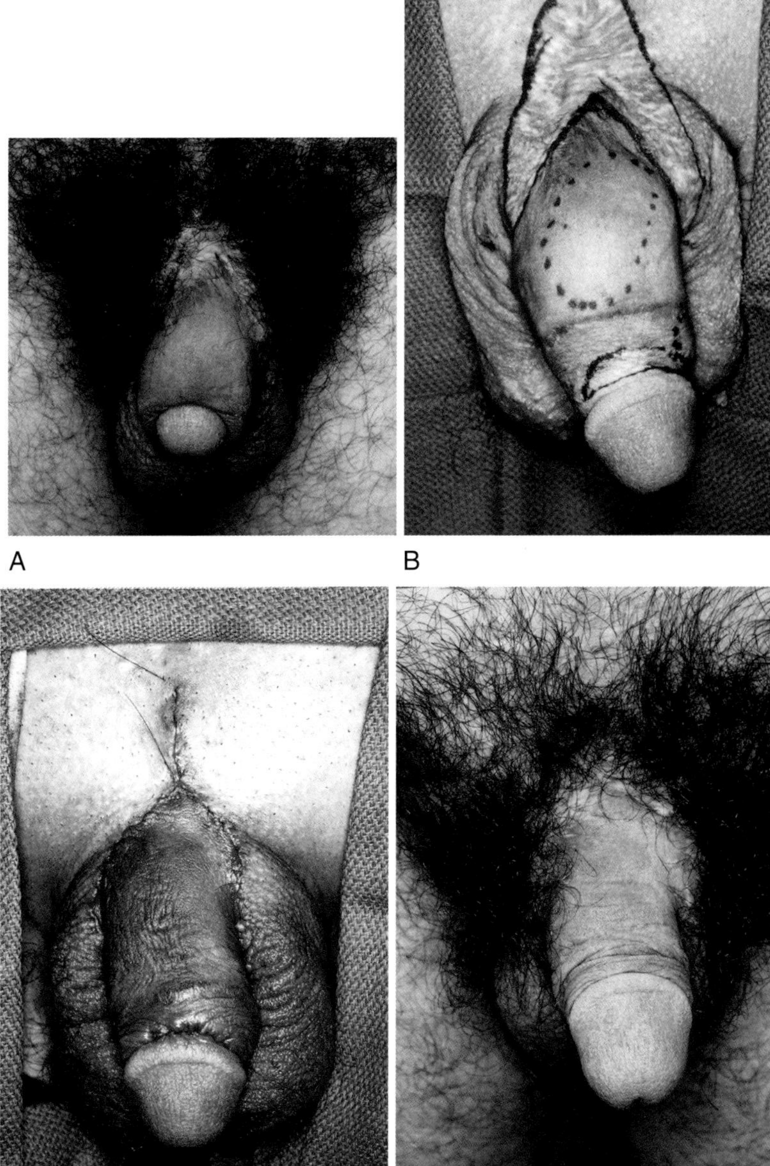

FIGURE 131-11. A 24-year-old who underwent release of the suspensory ligament, a large V-Y advancement flap, and fat injections. *A,* Deformity showing a low-lying penis, hair on the proximal shaft, bilateral dog-ears at the penoscrotal junction, a shorter-appearing penis, wide pubic scars, and fat in the shaft. *B,* Intraoperative markings outlining pubic and distal coronal scars and dorsal fat deposit. *C,* Reconstruction after partial reversal of V-Y advancement flap, correction of V-Y dog-ears, scar revisions, and selective removal of fat. The V-Y flap was aligned and reversed, leaving a Y-shaped scar. Complete reversal of the V-Y flap was not possible because of previous partial loss of a portion of the flap. The dog-ears can be removed by extending the incision along the lateral scrotum or by making lateral darts. *D,* Postoperative appearance at about 9 months. The penis looks normal.

foreskin" shaft skin in patients who have previously been circumcised should not be done. This repeated circumcision frequently leaves inadequate shaft skin if a later reversal of the V-Y advancement flap is desired, thereby limiting the reconstructive options.

Survival of a large volume of injected fat can lead to complaints of inadequate erectile rigidity; the fat overwhelms the firmness of the corporal bodies. If fat injection is combined with a large V-Y flap, difficulty with intercourse can occur by the combination of loose penile skin and a soft penile shaft.

Dermal Fat Grafts

Venous congestion of the surrounding dartos and skin with possible skin injury or necrosis can occur if overly thick dermal fat grafts (more than 1 cm) are inserted, penile skin is overstretched, or an excessively tight dressing is applied. Resorption of a portion of the dermal fat graft can occur with time, but most patients gain stability of the graft. Partial or complete lack of graft viability results in fibrosis and firmness, which can cause penile curvature or shortening due to loss of penile

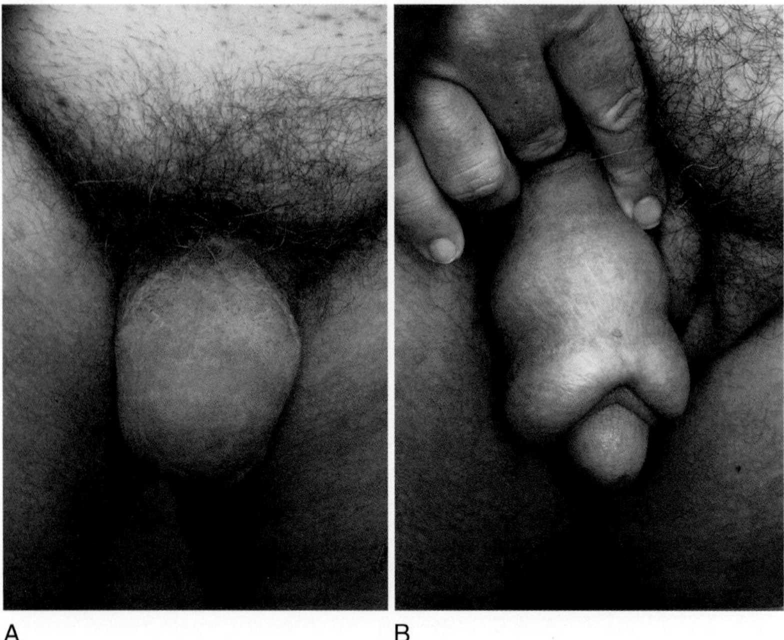

FIGURE 131-12. Patient who underwent V-Y advancement flap with massive fat injections. *A,* The deformed globular penis with massive bulk makes intercourse difficult. *B,* The penile skin is pulled proximally to display the fat deformity at the subcoronal region.

extensibility. The patient may complain of firm areas, curvature, shortening, or penile asymmetry (Fig. 131-13). These complications can be devastating because the patient may become cosmetically and functionally disabled. Therefore, many physicians no longer perform dermal fat graft enlargement. Because grafts can contract with healing, penile weights are used after 1 month to counteract any possible shrinkage or restriction in erections.

Most physicians using AlloDerm claim good survival of the graft with a low complication rate (D. Whitehead, personal communication, 2001). However, complications of AlloDerm erosion, fibrosis, and resorption can occur. Further long-term follow-up will elucidate the success of this graft material.

Reconstruction of Penile Enlargement

Patients may have a combination of penile lengthening with V-Y flaps or fat injections. The patient must prioritize his reconstructive goals because complete correction of all the deformities may not be possible at one operation, if at all.[14] He may want only limited fat removal, partial or no V-Y flap reversal, or minimal scar revisions. Realistic expectations must be emphasized.

The most common repair is partial or complete reversal of the V-Y advancement flap with excision of the wide scars.[13,14] Reversal and scar revision accomplish the following objectives: improvement of the wide or hypertrophic scars, elimination of the suprapubic concavity, and eradication of the unsightly dorsal penile hump and proximal hair-bearing tissue by redraping of the penis with the normal shaft skin and elevation of the penis to its normal position. The V flap is advanced and re-elevated near to its previous location, aligning the hair on the V-Y flap with the pubic hair. Complete V-Y reversal resulting in a semicircular incision is ideal (see Fig. 131-9*B*), but it is often impossible or undesirable. Part of the flap tip may have necrosed after the first procedure or must be excised on this revision to prevent tip flap loss. Complete reversal may also cause penile shortening (either real or illusory) and may restrict an erection, especially if the patient has had multiple circumcisions after fat injections. Partial V-Y reversal results in a Y-shaped scar with a shorter vertical limb (see Fig. 131-11). Patients complaining of suprapubic concavity are usually corrected

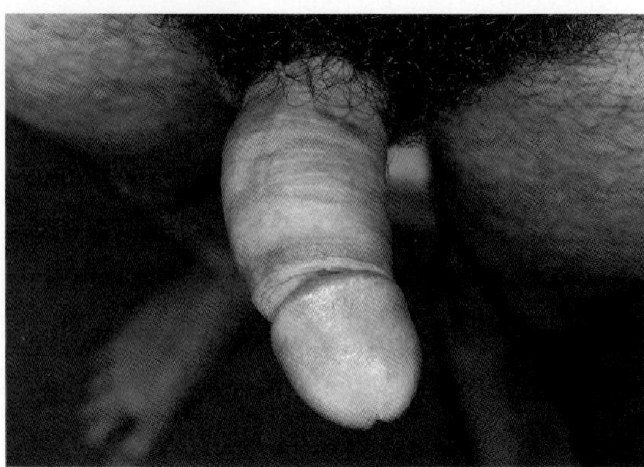

FIGURE 131-13. Patient who underwent circumferential dermal fat graft girth enhancement. He developed partial graft loss with subsequent fibrosis and penile curvature.

by partial or complete reversal of the V-Y flap, excision of scar tissue, mobilization of Scarpa fascia and skin from both sides of the vertical scar, and approximation of the wound.

Reversal of the V-Y flap can cause scrotal dog-ears, which are usually followed along the lateral scrotum. The method of closure and dog-ear excision is determined by judging the tightness of the penile skin, taking care not to restrict an erection. If skin discrepancy or dog-ears are excised by making a circular incision through the skin and dartos fascia at the penile base, prolonged lymphedema or skin loss can occur. Alternatively, the dog-ear is excised from the midportion on the scrotal side of the incision, making a lateral dart instead of following the dog-ear around the penile base.

Excision and scar revision require meticulous skin closure without tension, thus reducing the potential for redevelopment of a hypertrophic scar. A suction drain is used. Despite careful wound closure, minor healing problems often occur at the common junction of the V flap with the vertical closure. In addition, spreading of the scar is common.

Re-release of the suspensory ligament is performed only if the patient complains of penile shortening because the risk of injury to the dorsal neurovascular structures increases. To prevent reattachment of the corporal bodies to the symphysis in a shortened position, a fat flap transposed from spermatic cord lipomatous tissue should be placed between the corpora and the pubis (see earlier).

Most patients with fat injections do not want complete removal of the fat. They usually complain of nodules or penile asymmetry with various concavities or convexities. Removal of fat nodules or penile contouring is performed through limited or complete circumcising incisions, a medial raphe incision, or part of a previous V-Y incision. Shaft incisions are cosmetically unacceptable and unnecessary. Deforming or firm fat deposits are removed first, followed by contouring of the residual fat. Overresection of fat creates unsightly concavities, so contouring is performed by removal of small increments of the deforming fat.

Large diffuse areas of injected fat are usually removed through a circumcision incision, but this may be performed through one side of a previous distal V-Y flap scar. The fat deposits are conservatively removed, preserving as much dartos fascia as possible; overly aggressive removal of dartos may cause skin necrosis, chronic lymphedema, or skin attachment to Buck fascia. Contouring instead of complete fat removal is the goal. Fortunately, few patients want removal of most of the fat because this can lead to prolonged lymphedema and skin attachment to the Buck fascia. Attempts to dissuade them from complete fat removal should be made. The fat is removed through a circumcision or hemicircumcision incision with the necessity of leaving as much dartos fascia as possible attached to the skin, even if it contains some fat. Postoperative closed suction drainage and penile compression dressings are used. Despite all attempts to leave dartos, a high complication rate occurs; lymphedema may persist for up to 6 months, skin attachment may occur, and fibrous attachments from the dorsal corpora to the pubic skin can shorten the penis. These skin and fibrous attachments may necessitate another difficult operation to release this scar tissue and transpose a fat flap to fill the dead space or the area of the skin attachment.

If V-Y flap reversal is performed, simultaneous removal of fat nodules or deforming fat deposits is limited. Removal of large diffuse fat deposits should not be done at the same time as the V-Y reversal; further flap disruption and dartos fascia injury decrease vascularity of the V flap and possibly prolong edema. This fat removal must not be done earlier than 6 months after V-Y flap reversal, allowing time for revascularization of the scarred areas. Fat is removed through a tunnel of several centimeters on one or both sides of the most distal aspect of the V-Y incisions without undermining the V flap or through a limited circumcision incision. One side of the penis must be kept relatively unviolated to ensure adequate lymphatic and blood drainage. Residual deposits are removed through a circumcision, median raphe, or previous distal V-Y incision. However, a proximal medial raphe incision in a patient with a large V-Y flap reversal will injure the remaining untraumatized proximal dartos fascia.

Dermis, dermal fat grafts, and AlloDerm present with a variety of different problems, including penile shortening, curvature, and areas of induration. Removal of the grafts is performed through one or a combination of circumcision, median raphe, and low pubic incisions. An indurated, scarred graft that is not adherent to the Buck fascia can be removed without much difficulty, thereby correcting the deformity. However, the graft may be extensively adherent to the Buck fascia, so extreme care must be used to prevent injury to the dorsal neurovascular structures. Loupe magnification is usually necessary. Removal of the scarred dermal graft may eliminate the deformity, curvature, or penile restriction, but full return of penile length may not occur because of permanent scarring of the skin, dartos, or Buck fascia. As much dartos fascia as possible is left to prevent skin adhesions to Buck fascia. A spermatic cord fat flap or a flap of scrotal dartos fascia is used to fill dead space at the penopubic junction or areas of skin adherence to the Buck fascia to prevent recurrent penile shortening. Closed suction drains are used.

Penoscrotal Web

Scrotal skin extending on the ventral penile shaft causes a more obtuse angle to the penoscrotal junction, thereby obscuring the normal definition to the junction of the

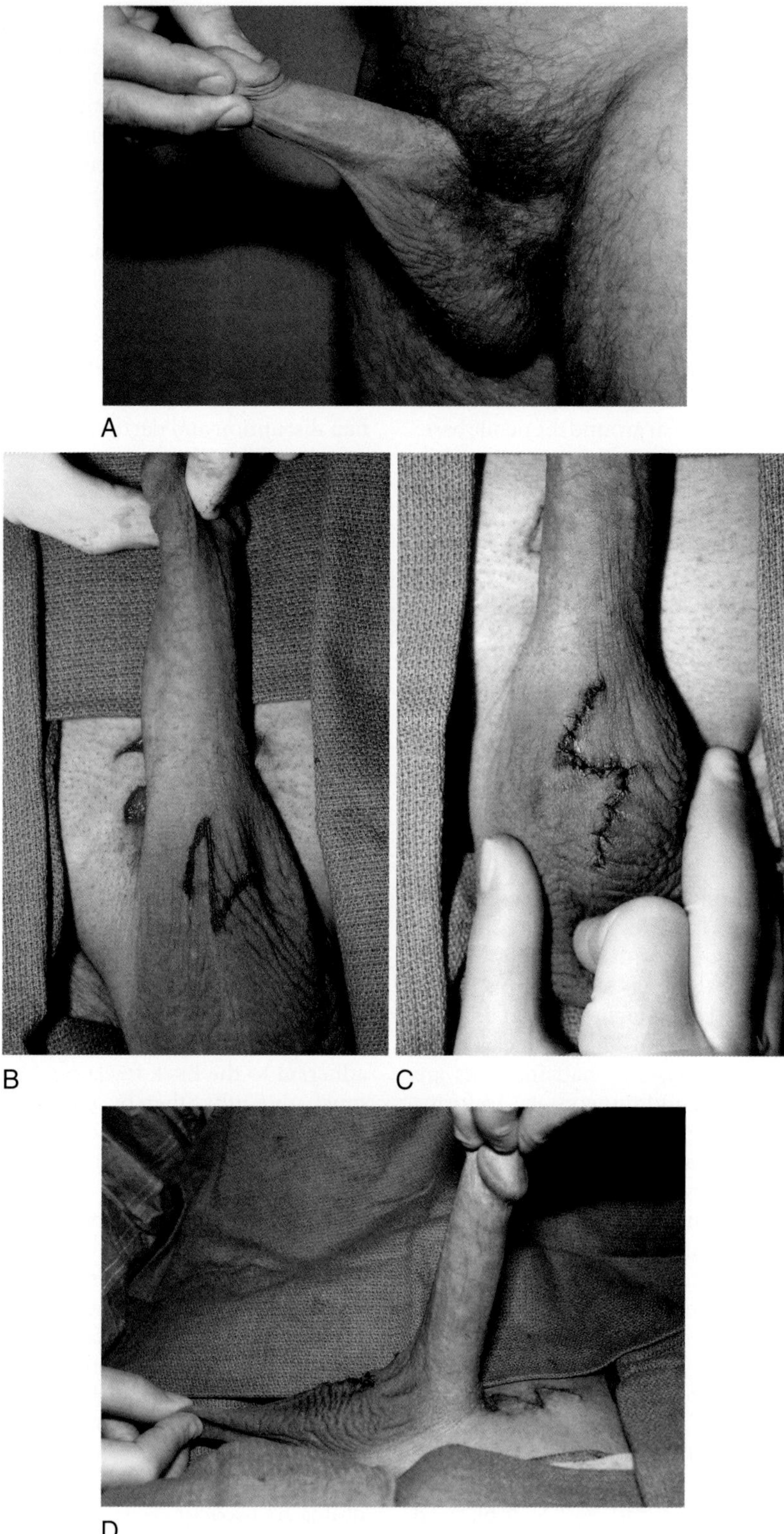

FIGURE 131-14. *A,* Penoscrotal web. *B,* Z-plasty markings at penoscrotal junction. *C,* Closed Z-plasty. *D,* Elimination of web.

scrotum and penis (Fig. 131-14*A*). The penis appears longer if the penoscrotal junction is well defined. The cause of this webbing may be congenital but is more often due to overresection of the ventral penile skin during circumcision.

The web is eliminated by a single or double Z-plasty with the vertical limb centered along the penoscrotal junction (Fig. 131-14).[20] Transposition of the flaps lengthens the shortened web and sharpens the penoscrotal junction, which gives the appearance of more

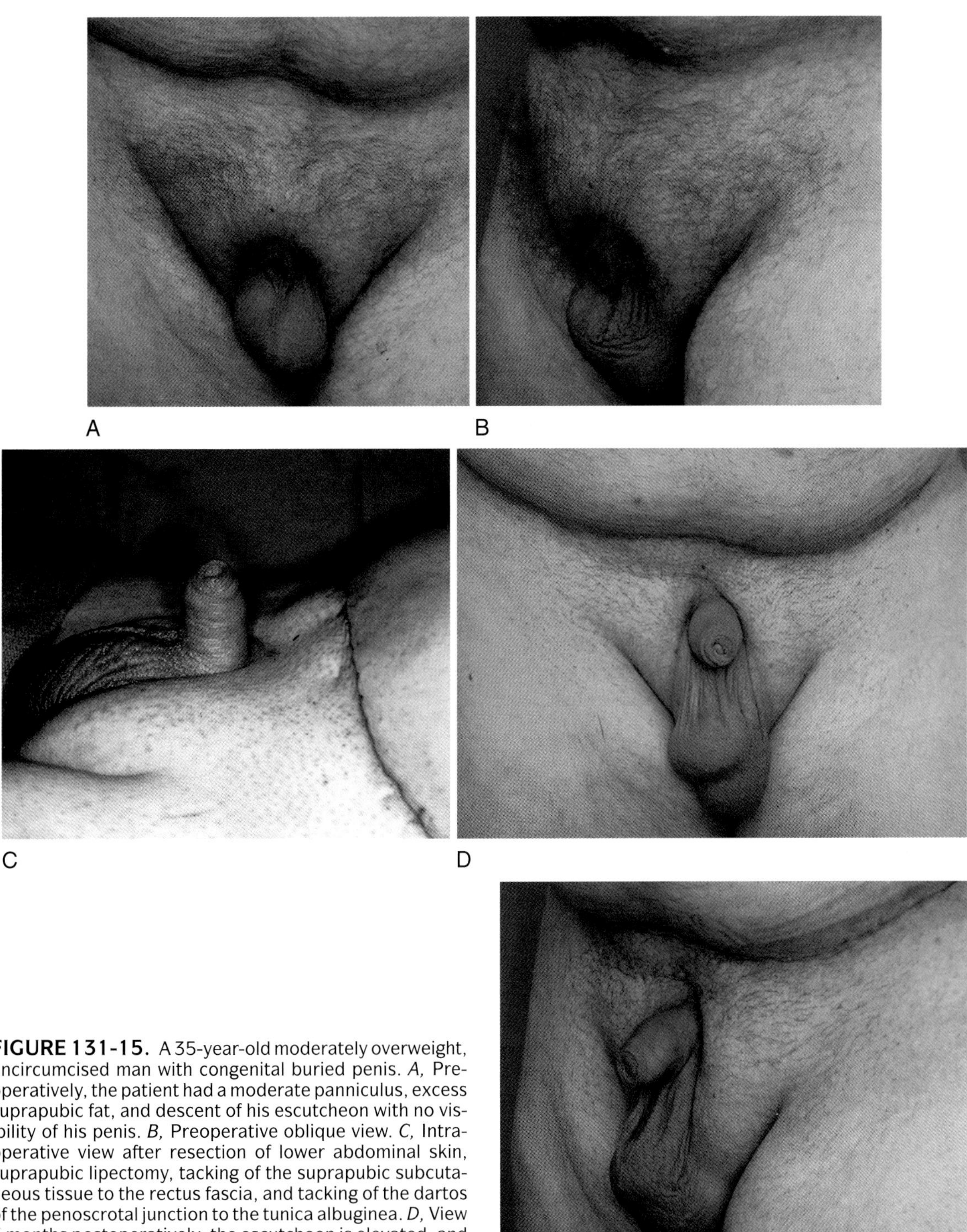

FIGURE 131-15. A 35-year-old moderately overweight, uncircumcised man with congenital buried penis. *A,* Preoperatively, the patient had a moderate panniculus, excess suprapubic fat, and descent of his escutcheon with no visibility of his penis. *B,* Preoperative oblique view. *C,* Intraoperative view after resection of lower abdominal skin, suprapubic lipectomy, tacking of the suprapubic subcutaneous tissue to the rectus fascia, and tacking of the dartos of the penoscrotal junction to the tunica albuginea. *D,* View 3 months postoperatively; the escutcheon is elevated, and the penis is visible. *E,* Oblique view at 3 months postoperatively; the suprapubic concavity was tapered to prevent an abnormal appearance.

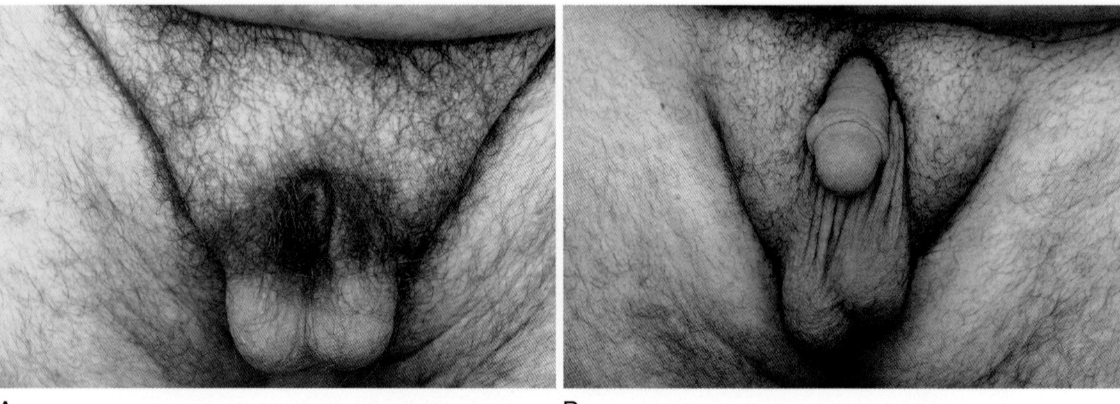

FIGURE 131-16. *A,* A 32-year-old obese, circumcised man with a severe buried penis. *B,* View at 3 months postoperatively revealing a normal-sized penis. Notice that pubic skin and fat were excised, which elevates the penopubic skin.

ventral length. Excision of the web may cause more severe webbing from scar contracture and skin shortage.

Hidden Penis

The terms *hidden, concealed,* and *buried* refer to a penis in which the functional and visual penile length is obscured (Figs. 131-15 and 131-16*A*).[21-37] Penile corporal length may be normal but not visible. Congenital buried penis is uncommon. More often, the penis shaft may be buried below the surface of the prepubic skin by a large suprapubic fat pad, obesity, or pubic skin and fat descent from aging or weight loss. Other causes of concealed penis are overly aggressive circumcision, abdominoplasty with aggressive release of dartos fascia attachments to Scarpa fascia, and penile lengthening by use of an ill-advised large pubic V-Y advancement flap.[34] This section describes the surgical technique to correct the hidden, concealed, or buried adult or pediatric penis that has adequate penile shaft skin. Skin grafts or local flaps for patients with overly resected shaft skin are beyond the scope of this chapter.[37-39]

Surgery is derived from the principles and techniques used to correct the pediatric buried penis.[21-37] These patients usually have inadequate attachments of the Buck fascia to the skin and dartos fascia, so the corporal bodies telescope proximally without the skin and dartos covering.[37] The corporal bodies may bury into the prepubic fat or into the scrotum. Therefore, it is necessary to reattach and stabilize the dartos and skin to the corporal bodies dorsally and ventrally to ensure success.

SURGICAL TECHNIQUE

In these cases, excess fat is conservatively excised and restricting bands of Scarpa fascia are released to increase penile visual and functional length. The suspensory ligament is usually partially released. Moreover, aging causes suprapubic skin and fat to descend, concealing the penis when the patient is standing. Combining fat and skin excision in the aging man provides a more attractive and youthful appearance to the escutcheon while increasing visual and, often, functional penile length (see Figs. 131-15*D* and 131-16*B*). Examination of the patient in the standing position is therefore required for an accurate diagnosis.

Preoperative markings are made with the patient standing to determine the amount of excess skin. A low transverse incision is made in the pubic hair if subcutaneous fat only is removed. If excess skin is excised to raise the escutcheon to give a more youthful appearance to the aging patient, the incision is made above the level of the pubic hair. If the patient is obese, the incision is made in the panniculus fold. Fat is incised to the rectus fascia, and excess fat is excised. A layer of subcutaneous fat is left on the dermal side to prevent a concavity or deformity. Suprapubic fat is contoured to match the abdominal side of the incision and not overly resected, which can result in an unsightly pubic depression. Fat around the spermatic cords and some scrotal fat are removed, but overly aggressive fat removal in the inguinal regions can cause genital lymphedema and injury to the superficial sensory nerves of the genitalia. The buried corporal bodies are seen and freed from the deep subcutaneous tissue. The suspensory ligament is often partially released. To prevent adhesion of the released penis to the pubic symphysis after suspensory ligament release, a fat flap from the lipomatous tissue adjacent to a spermatic cord can be transposed to fill the space (see Fig. 131-3). This flap is proximally or distally based and is sutured to the periosteum of the symphysis.

To prevent the corporal bodies from retracting under the penile skin into the scrotum and pubis, tacking

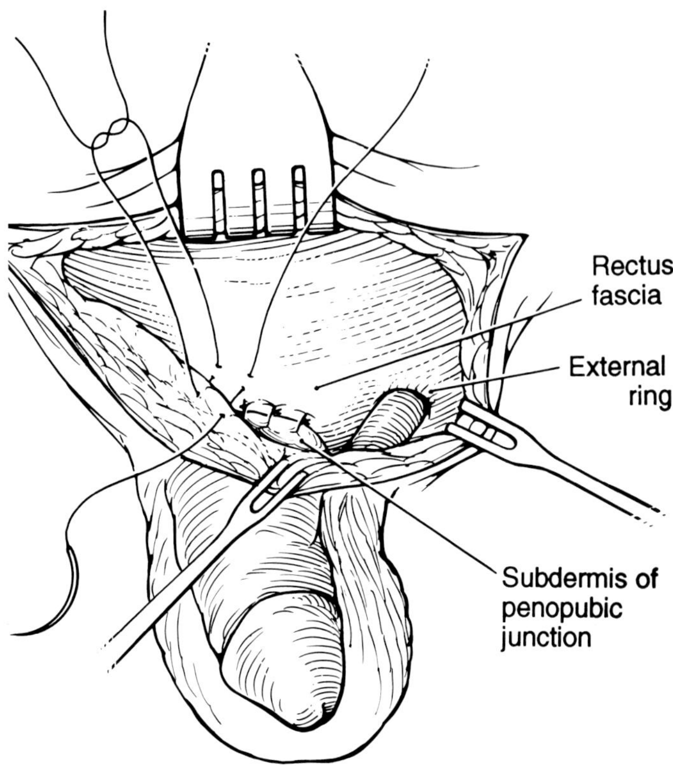

FIGURE 131-17. Technique of tacking the subcutaneous penopubic junction and suprapubic region to the rectus fascia with multiple rows of polyester sutures.

sutures of 0 polyester (Ethibond, Ti-Cron, or Mersilene) are placed in the pubic area (Fig. 131-17). Several rows of sutures are placed from the fibrous fatty tissue at the penopubic junction to the rectus fascia or anterior pubic symphysis. Tacking this fibrofatty tissue of the suprapubic skin to the rectus fascia maintains the upward position of the escutcheon and stabilizes dorsal penile skin to the penis. Rows of sutures are placed medial to the external inguinal rings. Care is taken to prevent dimpling or a deep suprapubic concavity. A closed suction drain is placed, and the wound is closed.

Despite suprapubic tacking, the corpora still tend to retract into the scrotum if the ventral skin is not stabilized.[37] Many of these patients also have penoscrotal webbing. A midline or Z-plasty incision is made at or just inferior to the penoscrotal junction, and dissection is performed through the dartos fascia to the spongiosum and tunica albuginea. Two tacking polyester braided sutures of 2-0 or 3-0 are placed on each side of the urethra at the penoscrotal junction from tunica albuginea to ventral subdermal dartos fascia just inferior to the lateral penoscrotal junction (Fig. 131-18). These sutures maintain the ventral penile skin to the corpora and prevent retraction into fat or scrotum. Care must be taken not to cause excessive skin dimpling from the tacking sutures. The dartos fascia and skin are closed.

At the conclusion of the procedure, the penis should be prominent, and inward pressure on the glans should not allow the penis to bury into the scrotum or abdomen.

Scrotal Enlargement

Men may have stretching and laxity of the scrotum as aging occurs (Fig. 131-19). A large, low-hanging scrotum can cause discomfort or a cosmetic loss of self-esteem. Reduction of the scrotum can be performed in many ways, but the preferred technique maintains its normal sack-like appearance (G. J. Alter, unpublished data, 2001).

The posterior scrotum should be saved because of its superior lymphatic drainage. The markings are made with the patient in the standing position. A superior transverse incision angling up to each pubic region is marked (Fig. 131-19*B* and *C*). The inferior incision is transverse, with an inverted V on the right and left sides of the scrotum to eliminate the dog-ears. This usually results in excision of midscrotal skin and an M-shaped closure, but the closure may be varied to maintain normal scrotal shape (Fig. 131-19*D*). The testicles and tunica vaginalis are not altered. The scrotum tends to stretch after surgery, so resection should allow for this. The skin and underlying dartos fascia are excised. The dartos is reapproximated with 4-0 resorbable sutures, and the skin is closed with a subcuticular resorbable suture. Penrose drains are placed.

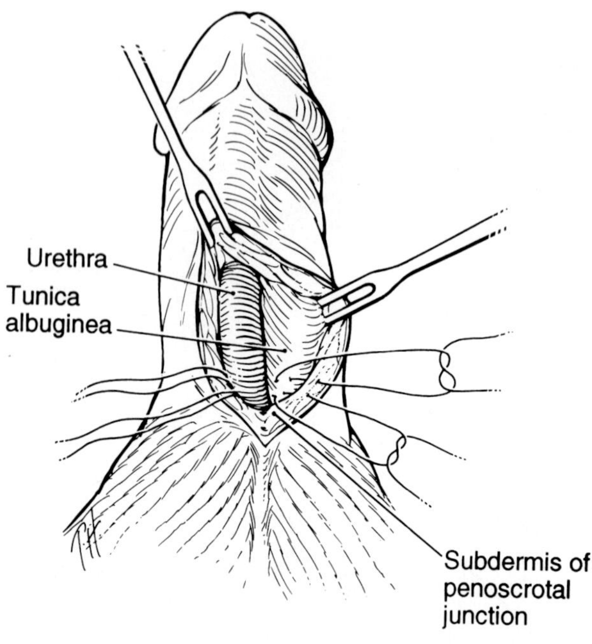

FIGURE 131-18. Technique of bilateral tacking of the subdermal dartos fascia of the penoscrotal junction to the periurethral tunica albuginea.

Significant swelling may occur initially, so meticulous hemostasis is important. Most patients are extremely pleased after the swelling resolves (Fig. 131-19*E*).

FEMALE GENITAL COSMETIC SURGERY

Labia Minora Reduction

The aesthetic genital ideal is derived from cultural influences and each woman's personal concept of beauty. In recent years, women are more aware of their genital appearance because of the popularity of genital shaving or waxing and the proliferation of pornographic photographic material. Therefore, women compare themselves with others and create an aesthetic ideal. Protrusion of the labia minora past the labia majora, especially while standing, is considered aesthetically unacceptable to some women (Figs. 131-20 and 131-21). If the labia minora are enlarged or unequal in size, some women feel deformed or abnormal, resulting in embarrassment or loss of self-esteem.[40,41,48-50] These women frequently refrain from social and sexual situations that may require visualization of their genitals, including wearing tight swimsuits, group showers, or sexual intimacy. They often avoid gynecologic examinations and are too self-conscious to mention their concern to the physician, who frequently dismisses it. Other women complain of discomfort during sexual intercourse or when wearing tight clothing. Massively enlarged labia cause difficulty with hygiene, interfere with sexual intercourse, hamper urinary self-catheterization, and cause chronic inflammation. Labia minora enlargement is congenital in most cases, but some women claim enlargement with age and after childbirth, chronic irritation, or hormone therapy.[42-46]

Reassurance concerning normal variations of the labia may be adequate to allay some women's insecurities, but others seek surgical correction, which achieves improved confidence. Labia minora reduction is indicated in women as young as 15 years when the enlargement severely affects self-esteem. Fear of embarrassment due to one's genitals is a powerful antisocial force.

Most physicians correct protuberant or asymmetric labia minora by excising or amputating the abnormal area and oversewing it.[40-46] Other surgeons have reported W-plasties.[47] The ideal for any cosmetic procedure is to preserve normal anatomy, including the normal labial edge. These procedures are not ideal because the unique contour and color of the labial edge are removed. The removal of medial and lateral de-epithelialized labium eliminates the protrusion, but the total labium remains elongated.[48,49] However, a technique that excises a wedge of the most protuberant labium and reapproximates the edges preserves the normal anatomy of the labial edge.[50]

ANATOMY

The external genitalia have extensive blood supply.[51] It consists of branches from the external superficial pudendal artery, the internal pudendal artery, and frequent contributions from the internal circumflex artery. The external superficial pudendal artery anastomoses with the posterior labial artery, a branch of the internal pudendal artery, in the labia majora. Multiple arterial arches in the labia minora arise from this initial anastomosis, which provides a rich blood supply.

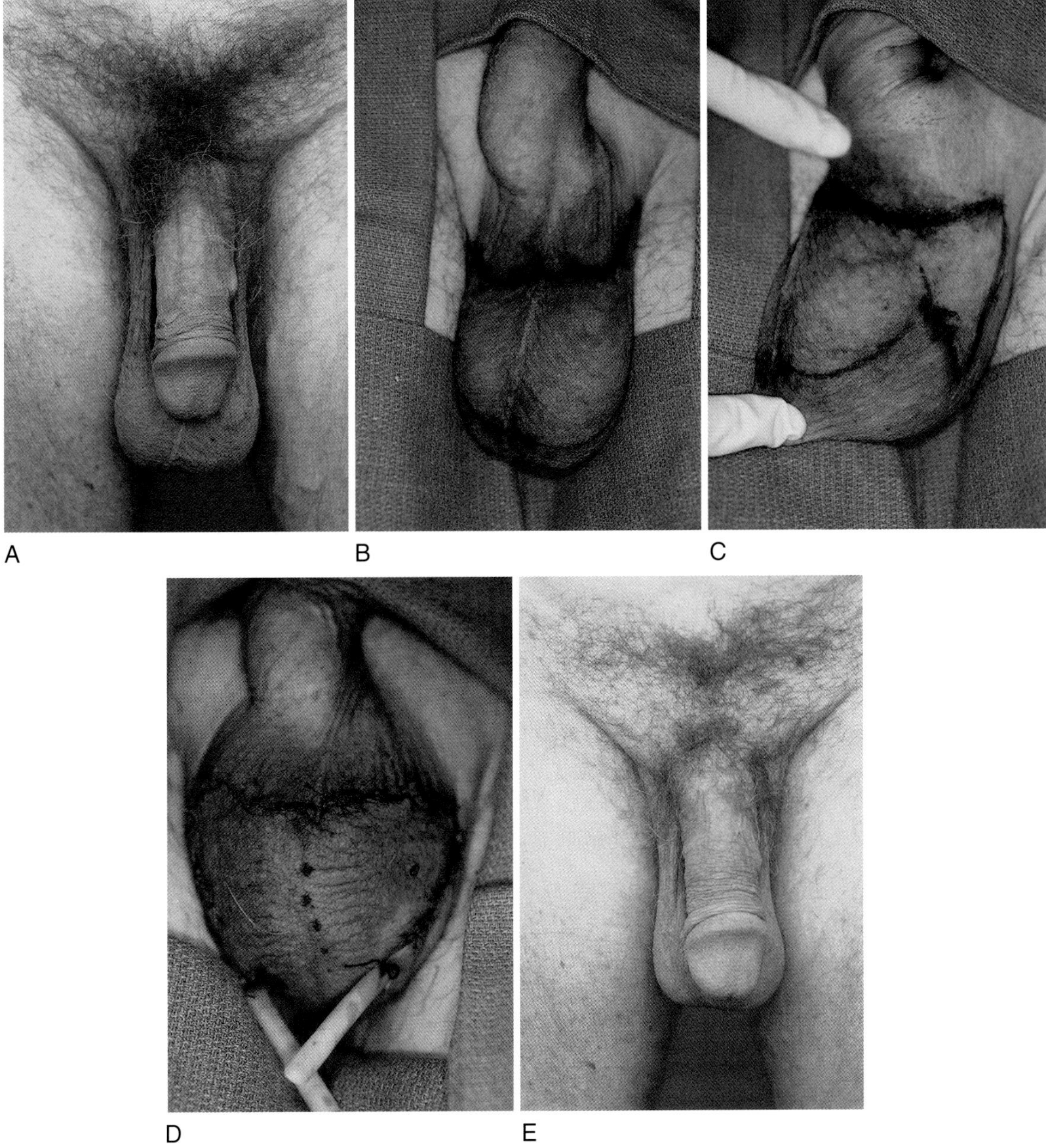

FIGURE 131-19. A 68-year-old man with laxity and descent of his scrotum. *A,* Preoperative appearance. *B,* Markings revealing a superior transverse incision angling toward each pubic region. *C,* The inferior incision is transverse, using an inverted V on the right and left scrotum to eliminate dog-ears. *D,* The resulting closure is M shaped. *E,* Postoperative appearance at 4 months.

TECHNIQUE

The woman is examined preoperatively in the lithotomy position with her head elevated. While using a mirror to visualize her genitalia, she indicates her concerns. The proposed surgical plan is explained and illustrated.

The operation is performed under general or regional anesthesia in the lithotomy position. Labia minora vary greatly in length, thickness, and form. Some women have a prominent labial edge leading to the clitoris, whereas other women have an indistinct edge to the clitoris with the dominant edge leading to the clitoral hood. Asymmetry is common. Therefore, the surgical technique varies according to the anatomy.

The basic reduction is performed by excising a V-shaped wedge of the most protuberant portion of the labium (Fig. 131-20*B*). While the V-shaped excision is marked, several fingers are placed in the vagina, stretching the labia minora to make sure the closure will not cause an overly tight introitus. The

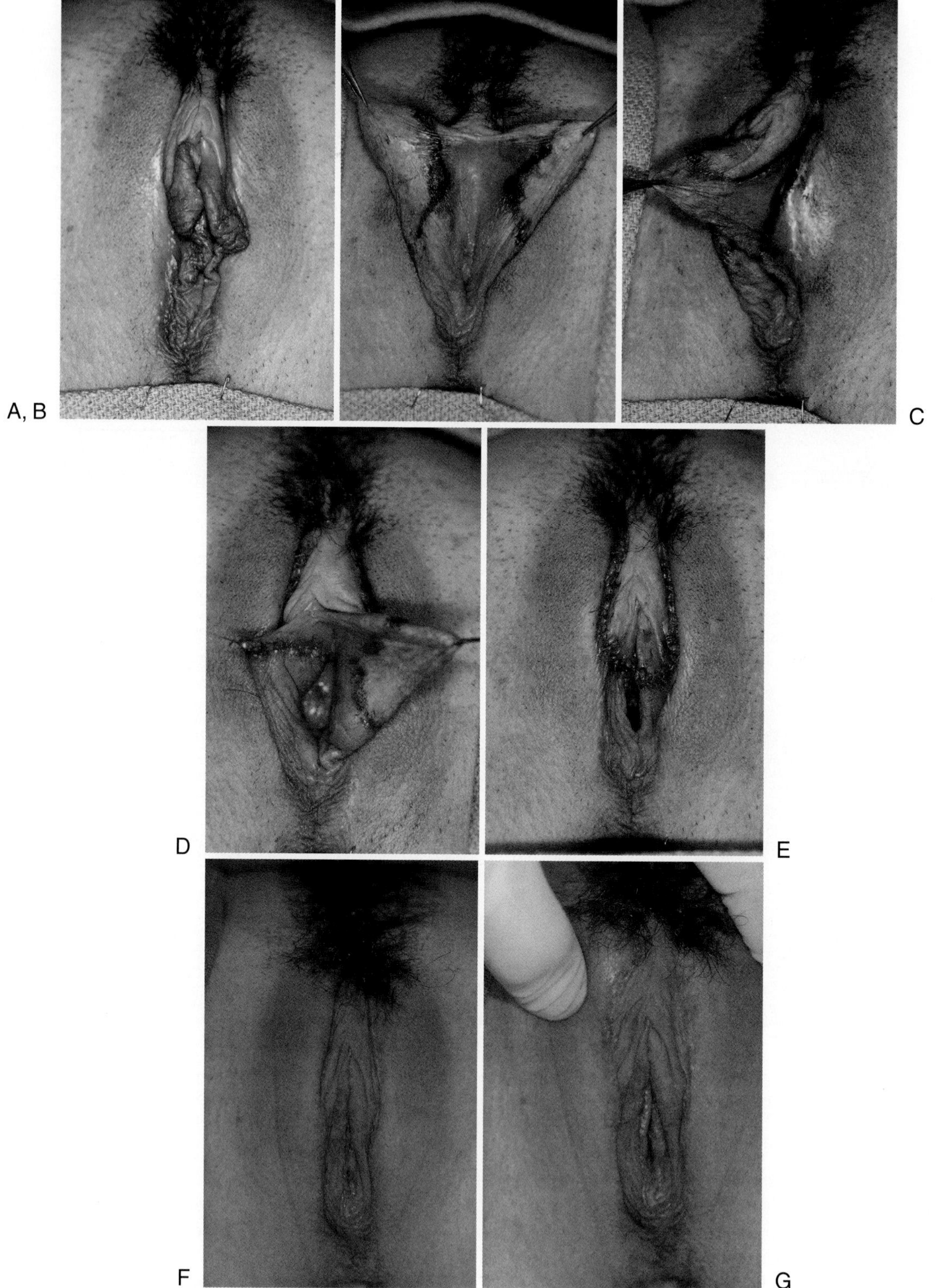

FIGURE 131-20. *A,* Preoperatively, a 24-year-old patient has enlarged labia minora with moderate excess of her clitoral hood. *B,* Preoperative appearance with her labia minora spread open. The markings reveal the protuberant areas to be excised. *C,* The markings showing the lateral labium and lateral clitoral hood, which will be excised. *D,* The right side is completed. *E,* The appearance at the conclusion showing preservation of the normal labial edges. *F,* Postoperative appearance at 4 months. *G,* Postoperative appearance at 4 months with her labia spread open.

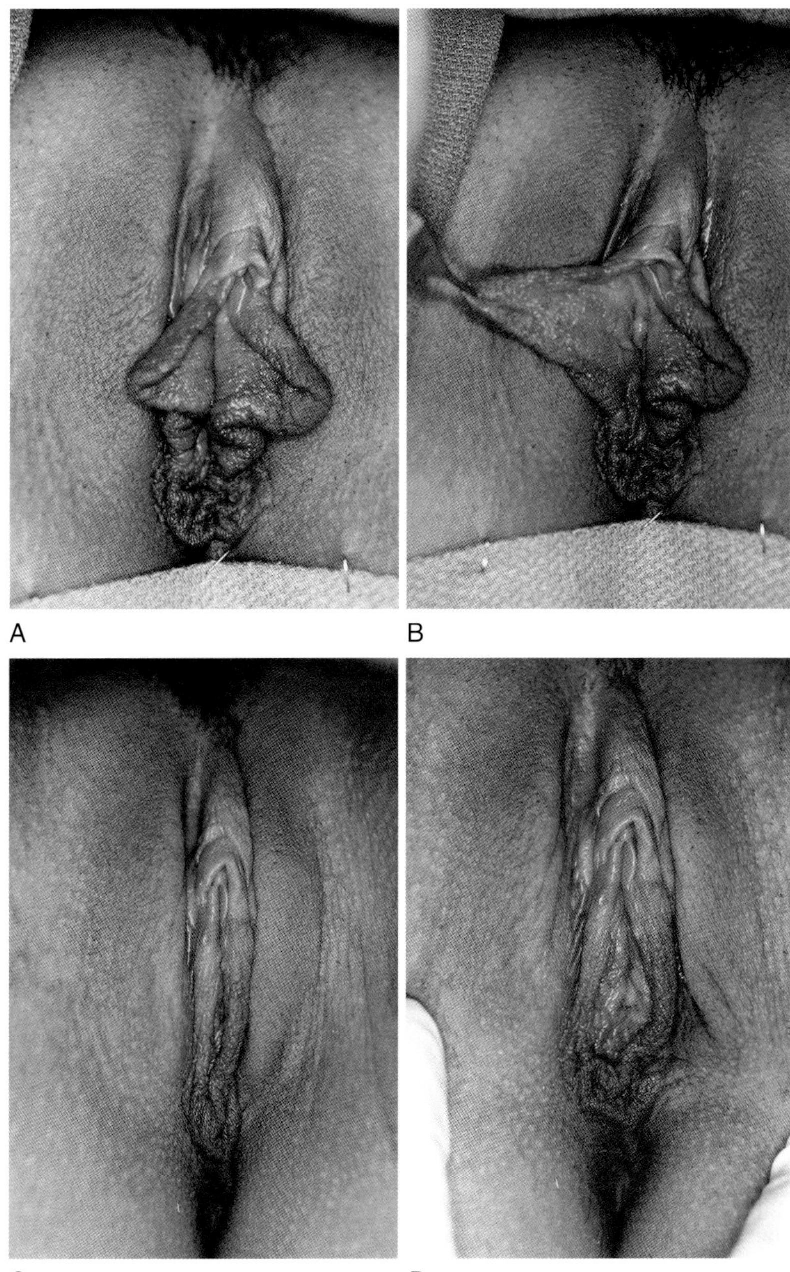

FIGURE 131-21. *A,* Preoperatively, a 29-year-old woman with enlarged labia minora and mild excess of lateral clitoral hood. *B,* Preoperative appearance with her labia minora spread open. *C,* Postoperative appearance at 6 months. *D,* Postoperative appearance at 6 months with her labia spread open.

anterior mark should be a safe distance from the clitoris to prevent interference with sexual sensation. The marks extend medially into the outer vagina and curve laterally into the depression between the labia minora and majora. If the patient has enlargement of the clitoral hood or an extra clitoral hood fold, the lateral resection can be extended to the top of the anterior fourchette to excise the most lateral clitoral hood (G. J. Alter, unpublished data, 2001) (Fig. 131-20*C*).

Conservative infiltration of the labia is performed with lidocaine with epinephrine and bupivacaine after marking to prevent distortion of the anatomy. The smaller labium is corrected first and the second side is matched. The skin and vaginal mucosa are deepithelialized with care to leave as much subcutaneous tissue as possible; a good subcutaneous tissue closure is mandatory to prevent dehiscence of the closure. The anterior and posterior labial edges are reapproximated by first closing the distal subcutaneous tissue with several 6-0 Vicryl sutures (Fig. 131-20*D*). The labial edge is then reapproximated with several 6-0 Vicryl sutures. The internal and external subcutaneous dog-ears are excised. The thicker subcutaneous tissue is closed with interrupted subcutaneous Monocryl sutures, and the medial and lateral labium is closed with interrupted 5-0 Vicryl sutures. The lateral clitoral hood closure is performed by using a subcuticular 5-0 Monocryl with a few interrupted 6-0 Vicryl sutures. Loupe magnification is usually necessary to achieve accurate approximation. The only suture line on the leading edge of the labium is a small transverse line (Fig. 131-20*E*). The remainder of the lateral scar passes along the lateral labium into the fold between the labia majora and minora. If possible, the labia should protrude only slightly past the introitus, but this may not be possible if the labia are massively enlarged.

Antibiotic ointment followed by a vaginal napkin is applied to the surgical site. No vaginal packing or urinary catheterization is necessary. The Vicryl sutures dissolve, but some can be removed if irritation occurs. The patient must wear protective padding and prevent shear forces and trauma for 6 weeks. Sexual intercourse is not allowed during that time.

Patients heal well with normal-appearing labia minora (Fig. 131-20*F* and *G* and Fig. 131-21*C* and *D*). The most common complication is a slight separation of the labial edge closure or a small fistula (Fig. 131-22). Major dehiscence is uncommon. The minor separation or fistula can easily be repaired in 4 to 6 months by combining local anesthetic cream and injections. No patient has complained of loss of sexual sensation, chronic scar discomfort, or interference with intercourse. This technique is a major advance over amputation and closure or techniques requiring long suture lines along the labial edges.

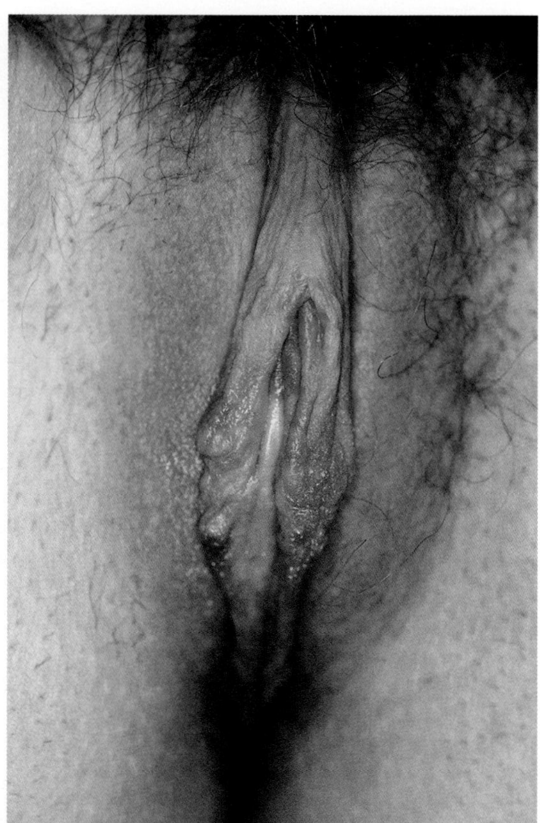

FIGURE 131-22. Minor dehiscence of the right labium. The area was easily repaired under local anesthesia by excision and closure.

Labia Majora

Some women lack fullness of their labia majora or lose fullness with age or childbirth. A combination of lack of labia majora fullness and a prominent clitoris or clitoral hood skin creates a protuberant clitoral region that causes the patient to be self-conscious (G. J. Alter, unpublished data, 2001). The distress of a prominent clitoris has caused some patients to question their sexual identity. In addition, loss of labia majora fullness is a sign of aging, which can cause loss of self-esteem. The fullness can be restored through fat injections by multiple passes of small amounts of fat. If the clitoris appears prominent, injections are concentrated in the anterior labia majora to overlap or hide the clitoris. As in other areas, much of the fat resorbs, but improvement occurs in many, and repeated injections can be performed.

Pubic Descent and Fat Deposits

The pubic region can have large unsightly fat deposits (Fig. 131-23). Many women refrain from wearing tight clothes or swimsuits because of this pubic bulge. Liposuction of this suprapubic fat deposit can improve contour. However, the pubic region can also descend with excess skin, and the bulging frequently extends to the upper labia majora. In such cases, the excess skin and fat must be excised by a transverse lower abdominal incision similar to that for the hidden penis (see previous section) (G. J. Alter, unpublished data, 2001). The large suprapubic and upper labia majora fat deposits are sharply reduced. Care must be taken not to injure the clitoris and not to cause an unsightly concavity. The pubic skin is stabilized to the rectus fascia in a manner also similar to that for the hidden penis (see Fig. 131-20). The dermatolipectomy and elevation of the pubic area cause reversal of the bulging deformity or aged appearance of the external genitalia.

CONCLUSION

During the past decade, innovative techniques have been developed to treat a variety of genital aesthetic deformities. Oftentimes, these procedures enable men and women to overcome psychologically crippling feelings of low self-esteem. Unfortunately, misinformation

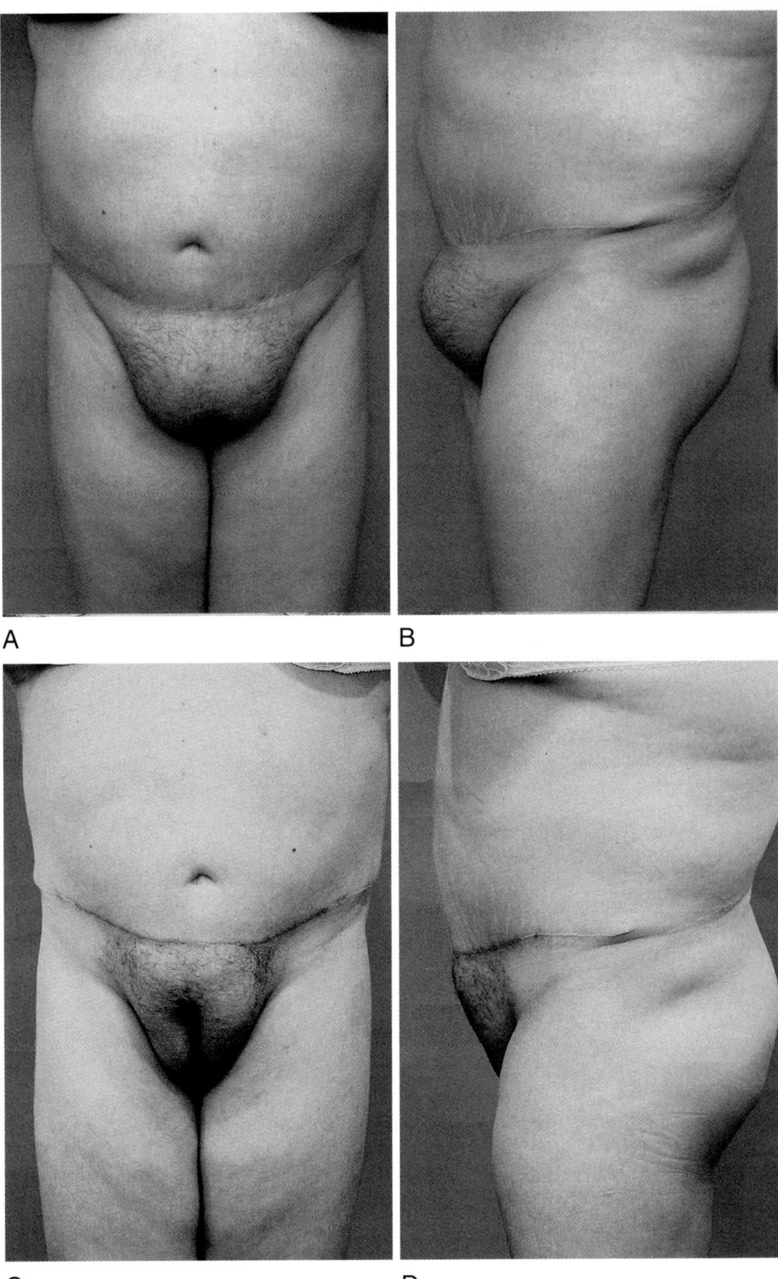

FIGURE 131-23. A 30-year-old woman with large pubic fat pad. She previously underwent abdominoplasty by another physician. *A,* Preoperative frontal view. *B,* Preoperative lateral view. *C,* Postoperative frontal view at 6 months after suprapubic dermatolipectomy and labia majora fat reduction. *D,* Postoperative lateral view at 6 months.

is widespread. For example, patients undergoing penile enlargement procedures often receive overly optimistic promises from some physicians, who are appealing to the insecurities of men while offering guarantees of enlargement with minimal discomfort and absence of complications. Male and female aesthetic genital techniques will continue to evolve with more data and experience. Many patients achieve substantially improved self-esteem, justifying the continued exploration of new and better methods. As more people become aware of the surgical possibilities, these procedures and other new innovations will be more common.

REFERENCES

1. Schonfeld WA, Beebe GW: Normal growth and variation in the male genitalia from birth to maturity. J Urol 1942;48: 759.
2. da Ros C, Teloken C: Caucasian penis: what is normal size? Presented at American Urological Association 89th annual meeting, San Francisco, May 16, 1994.
3. Wessells H, Lue T, McAninch JW: The relationship between penile length in the flaccid and erect states: Guidelines for penile

lengthening. Presented at American Urological Association 90th annual meeting, Las Vegas, April 1995.
4. Basmajian JV, Slonecker CE, eds: Grant's Method of Anatomy, 11th ed. Baltimore, Williams & Wilkins, 1989.
5. Clemente CD, ed: Anatomy of the Human Body by Henry Gray, 30th ed. Philadelphia, Lea & Febiger, 1985.
6. Grossman J, Caldamone A, Khouri R, Kenna DM: Cutaneous blood supply of the penis. Plast Reconstr Surg 1989;83:213.
7. Alter GJ: Augmentation phalloplasty. Urol Clin North Am 1995;22:887.
8. Alter GJ: Penile enhancement. Advances in Urology, vol 9. Chicago, Mosby, 1996:225–254.
9. Alter GJ: Penile enhancement surgery. Techniques Urol 1998;4:70.
10. Long DC: Elongation of the penis [in Chinese]. Zhonghua Zheng Xing Shao Shang Wai Ke Za Zhi 1990;6:17.
11. Roos H, Lissoos I: Penis lengthening. Int J Aesthetic Restorative Surg 1994;2:89.
12. Wessells H, Lue TF, McAninch JW: Complications of penile lengthening and augmentation seen at 1 referral center. J Urol 1996;155:1617.
13. Alter GJ: Re: Complications of penile lengthening and augmentation seen at 1 referral center [letter]. J Urol 1996;156:1784.
14. Alter GJ: Reconstruction of deformities resulting from penile enlargement surgery. J Urol 1997;158:2153.
15. American Society of Plastic and Reconstructive Surgeons: Report on autologous fat transplantation by the ASPRS ad hoc committee on new procedures. Chicago, ASPRS, 1987.
16. Ersek RA: Transplantation of purified autologous fat: a 3-year follow-up is disappointing. Plast Reconstr Surg 1991;87:219.
17. Fredericks S: Discussion: Transplantation of purified autologous fat: a 3-year follow-up is disappointing. Plast Reconstr Surg 1991;87:228.
18. Niechajev I, Sevcuk O: Long-term results of fat transplantation: clinical and histologic studies. Plast Reconstr Surg 1994;94:496.
19. Coleman SR: Structural fat grafting. Aesthetic Surg J 1998;18:386.
20. Vorstman B, Horton CE, Winslow BH: Repair of secondary genital deformities of epispadias/exstrophy. Clin Plast Surg 1988;15:381.
21. Maizels M, Zaontz M, Donovan J, et al: Surgical correction of the buried penis: description of a classification system and a technique to correct this disorder. J Urol 1986;136:268.
22. Crawford BS: Buried penis. Br J Plast Surg 1977;30:96.
23. Devine CJ, Jordan GH, Horton CE: Concealed penis. Soc Pediatr Urol Newslett 1984;115.
24. Horton CE, Vorstman B, Teasley D, Winslow B: Hidden penis release: adjunctive suprapubic lipectomy. Ann Plast Surg 1987;19:131.
25. Alter GJ, Horton CE, Horton CE Jr: Buried penis as a contraindication for circumcision. J Am Coll Surg 1994;178:487.
26. Donahoe PK, Keating MA: Preputial unfurling to correct the buried penis. J Pediatr Surg 1986;21:1055.
27. Boemers TM, DeJong TP: The surgical correction of buried penis: a new technique. J Urol 1995;154:550.
28. Wollin M, Duffy PG, Malone PS, Ransley PG: Buried penis. A novel approach. Br J Urol 1990;65:97.
29. Klauber GT, Sant GR: Disorders of the male external genitalia. In Kelalis PP, King LR, Belman AB: Clinical Pediatric Urology. Philadelphia, WB Saunders, 1985:825–861.
30. Shapiro S: Surgical treatment of the "buried" penis. Urology 1987;30:554.
31. Kubota Y, Ishii N, Watanabe H, et al: Buried penis: a surgical repair. Urol Int 1980;46:61.
32. Shepard GH, Wilson CS, Sallade RL: Webbed penis. Plast Reconstr Surg 1980;66:453.
33. Masih RK, Bresman SA: Webbed penis. J Urol 1974;111:690.
34. Perlmutter AD, Chamberlain JW: Webbed penis without chordee. 1972;107:320.
35. Badhakrishnan J, Reyes HM: Penoplasty for buried penis secondary to "radical" circumcision. J Pediatr Surg 1984;19:629.
36. Adham MN, Teimourian B, Mosca P: Buried penis release in adults with suction lipectomy and abdominoplasty. Plast Reconstr Surg 2000;106:840.
37. Alter GJ, Ehrlich RM: A new technique for correction of the hidden penis in adults and children. J Urol 1999;161:455.
38. Donatucci CF, Ritter EF: Management of the buried penis in adults. J Urol 1998;159:420.
39. Alter GJ, Ehrlich RM: Reconstructive and Plastic Surgery of the External Genitalia. Philadelphia, WB Saunders, 1999.
40. Hodgkinson DJ, Hait G: Aesthetic vaginal labioplasty. Plast Reconstr Surg 1984;74:414.
41. Friedrich EG: Vulvar Disease, 2nd ed. Philadelphia, WB Saunders, 1983.
42. Caparo V: Congenital anomalies. Clin Obstet Gynecol 1971;14:988.
43. Radman HM: Hypertrophy of the labia minora. Obstet Gynecol 1976;48(suppl):78S.
44. Kato K, Kondo A, Gotoh M, et al: Hypertrophy of labia minora in myelodysplastic women. Labioplasty to ease clean intermittent catheterization. Urology 1988;31:294.
45. Gowen RM, Martin VL: Labia minora reduction in an iron-lung disabled woman. Obstet Gynecol 1988;71:488.
46. Chavis WM, LaFerla JJ, Niccolini R: Plastic repair of elongated, hypertrophic labia minora. A case report. J Reprod Med 1989;34:373.
47. Maas SM, Hage JJ: Functional and aesthetic labia minora reduction. Plast Reconstr Surg 2000;105:1453.
48. Choi HY, Kim KT: A new method for aesthetic reduction of labia minora (the deepithelialized reduction labioplasty). Plast Reconstr Surg 2000;105:419.
49. Laub DR: Re: A new method for aesthetic reduction of labia minora (the deepithelialized reduction labioplasty). Plast Reconstr Surg 2000;105:423.
50. Alter GJ: A new technique for aesthetic labia minora reduction. Ann Plast Surg 1998;40:287.
51. Hwang W, Chang T, Sun P, Shung T: Vaginal reconstruction using labia minora flaps in congenital total absence. Ann Plast Surg 1983;18:534.

CHAPTER

132

Reconstruction of the Chest

JAMES KNOETGEN III, MD ✦ CRAIG H. JOHNSON, MD ✦ PHILLIP G. ARNOLD, MD, FACS

HISTORY

The reconstruction of the human chest poses a formidable challenge. Perhaps no other reconstructive challenge to the plastic surgeon is so intertwined with human physiology. The ABCs of airway, breathing, and circulation have a tremendous impact on the management of chest wall extirpation, reconstruction, and eventual function. No other area of reconstructive surgery is so closely tied not only to form and function but also to the mandatory requirements of life itself—a sustained airway exchange, circulatory pressure, and airway patency. For nearly a century, chest wall reconstruction was a challenge that surgeons confronted with varying levels of trepidation as evidenced by Parham's description in 1898 of the surgically formed pneumothorax:

> One of the most startling clinical pictures that the surgeon can ever be called upon to witness. At such a sight the most stout heart will quiver. No wonder the older surgeons discounted such operations. . . . So sudden in my case was the pneumothorax and so striking were the manifestations of profound shock, threatening almost instant disolusion before our eyes, that I resolve to acquaint myself more thoroughly with the dangers of thoracic surgery.[1]

Surgical and medical advances in the early 20th century allowed the evolution of chest reconstruction into its current state. Two of the most significant contributions during this time were the development of positive-pressure ventilation and the ability to control the upper airway, as discussed by Fell[2] and O'Dwyer.[3] The first successful pneumonectomy for carcinoma of the lung was performed in the 1930s by Graham and Singer.[4] Endotracheal ventilation, closed chest drainage, and antibiotics allowed further advances in thoracic resections as well as chest wall reconstruction. Fascia lata grafts were described for closure of chest wall defects,[5] and the resected sternum was reconstructed with rib grafts.

Musculocutaneous flaps made a large contribution to the advancement of chest reconstruction, as they did in other anatomic areas. In 1906, coverage of the anterior chest wall after a radical mastectomy was described by Tansini.[6] In 1950, Campbell[7] described latissimus dorsi transposition for an anterior thoracic defect. But it was really not until the early 1970s that the interest in axially perfused flaps was revived and further delineated.

In the early 20th century, although it may have been technically feasible to remove a tumor, these procedures were not often performed because the defect was not reconstructable with the described techniques of the time. Further major advances occurred during the military conflicts of the 20th century. Patients who presented with a pneumothorax or hemothorax were treated and managed by use of chest tubes, open drainage, and direct visualization of the airway.

ANATOMY AND PHYSIOLOGY

Dual functionality of protection and respiration is addressed in the unique design of the thoracic cage. The framework, or walls, of the thoracic cage simultaneously provides protection for vital organs and a mechanical construct to generate inspiratory force. The framework is formed by the vertebral column posteriorly, the ribs and intercostal spaces on either side, and the sternum and costal cartilages anteriorly.

The ribs have been described as a bucket-handle type of apparatus to allow changes in the size of the pleural space and shape of the thoracic cage on respiratory activity (Fig. 132-1). This action is allowed by the hinging of the ribs posteriorly to the vertebral column and anteriorly to the sternum and costal margin. The rib articulates with the vertebral body of origin as well as with the vertebral body immediately above.

Intercostal spaces occupy the area between each rib. The inferior aspect of each rib has a neurovascular bundle consisting of an intercostal vein, an intercostal artery, and a nerve. Each space contains three muscles: the external intercostal, the internal intercostal, and the transverse thoracic muscles. This musculature corresponds to similar muscle anatomy of the abdominal wall. When the intercostal muscles contract, they all tend to pull the ribs closer together. If the first rib is fixed by contraction of the scalene musculature, intercostal contraction will raise the second through twelfth ribs. If, alternatively, the twelfth rib is fixed by contraction of the quadratus lumborum muscle, the

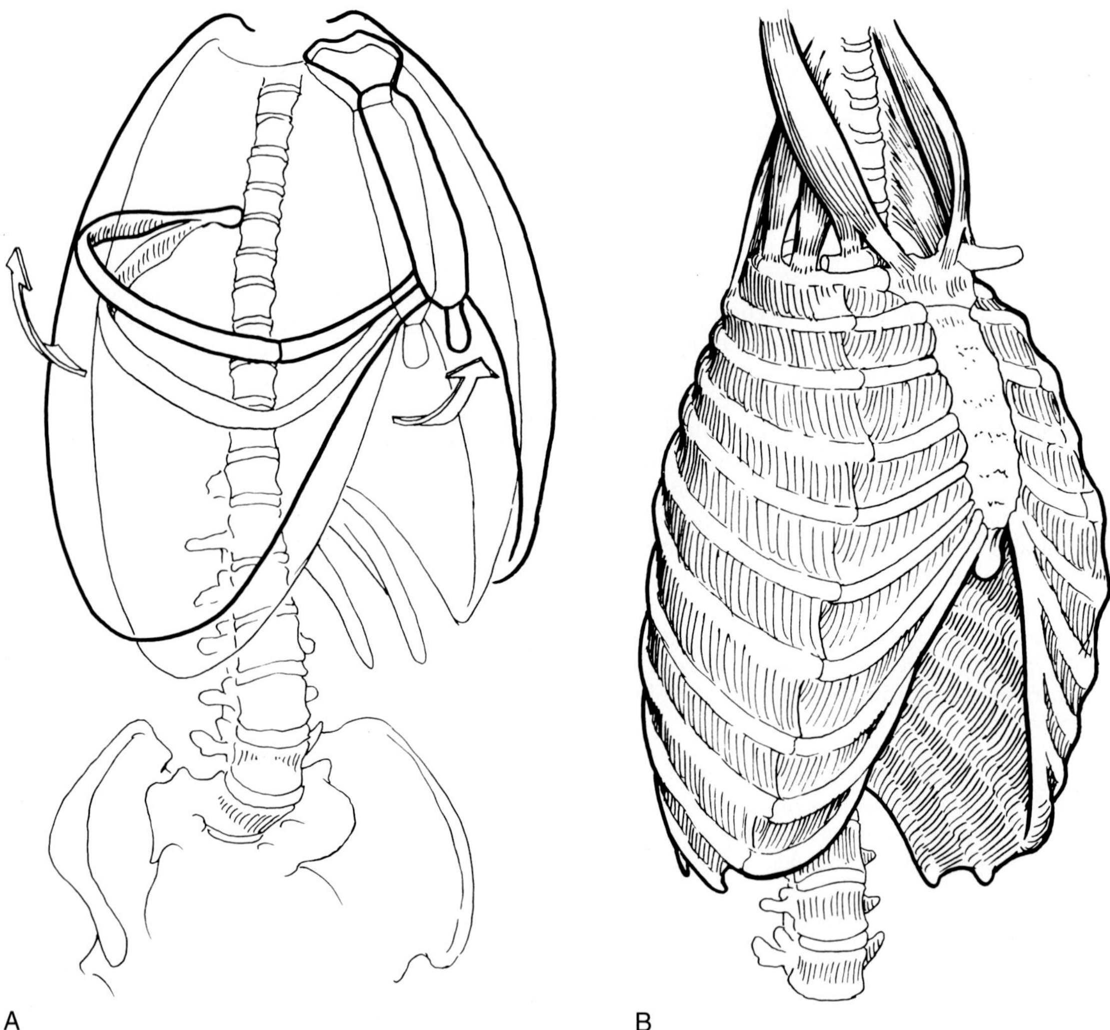

FIGURE 132-1. *A,* Forced inspiration depends on the "bucket-handle" motion of the ribs and the "pump-handle" motion of the sternum. This energy-consuming effort is mediated through the accessory muscles of respiration and occurs when metabolic demand outstrips ventilatory capabilities at rest. Excessive removal of the chest wall in the wrong patient can activate this response and lead to exhaustion. *B,* The accessory muscles of inspiration include the sternocleidomastoids, the scalene muscles, the external intercostals, and the parasternal intercartilaginous muscles. These activate the bucket-handle and pump-handle mechanisms. (From Seyfer A, Graeber G, Wind G, eds: Atlas of Chest Wall Reconstruction. Rockville, MD, Aspen Publications, 1986:28.)

first through eleventh ribs will be lowered. Respiration consists of two phases, inspiration and expiration. Alternating increases and decreases in the thoracic cavity capacity accomplish respiration. By contraction of the diaphragm, the vertical dimensions of the pleural space are increased. The anterior-posterior diameter increases with the pump-handle action of the sternum, and the transverse diameter increases with the bucket-handle mechanism of the anatomy and shape of the ribs. This maneuver is facilitated by the downward sloping of the ribs as they proceed from the vertebral column anteriorly to the sternum.

The sternum consists of three parts: the upper portion (manubrium), the main body, and the inferior portion (xiphoid). The manubrium articulates with the clavicles and the first and upper part of the second costal cartilages on each side. It lies opposite the third and fourth thoracic vertebrae. The body of the sternum articulates with the manubrium by means of a fibrocartilaginous joint. On each side of the body are notches for articulation with the second through seventh costal cartilages.

The diaphragm also helps in respiratory mechanics by serving to elevate the ribs. As the diaphragm contracts and shortens, it eventually contacts the abdominal viscera and uses them as a platform. Further diaphragmatic contraction will then assist with the intercostal elevation of the lower ribs.

It is important to note the movement and changes of the intrathoracic structures during respiration. The root of the lung descends. The tracheal bifurcation may move as many as two vertebral levels inferiorly. The elastic recoil of the lungs and the relaxation of the musculature then allow expiration. Forced expiration is assisted largely by the forceful contraction of the abdominal wall.

In babies and young children, the ribs are nearly horizontal. Therefore, babies and young children have to rely on diaphragmatic action much more than on rib motion to increase their thoracic cavity. By the age of 3 years, the ribs have become more oblique and sloping from posterior to anterior, allowing the development of a more adult-type respiratory pattern.

In discussing defects of the chest, it is helpful to use one of several anatomic classification systems. A commonly accepted and referenced system describes the sternal area as limited to the confines of the sternum; the anterior chest wall is between the sternal border and the anterior axillary line, the lateral chest wall is between the anterior and posterior axillary line, and the posterior chest wall encompasses that area between the posterior axillary line and the vertebral column.

INDICATIONS

The need to reconstruct the chest usually arises out of the management of tumors, trauma, infection (with entry either externally or from an airway problem internally), radiation injury, and congenital anomalies. Each of these indications carries its own subtle nuances with respect to reconstructive strategies.

EVALUATION OF THE PATIENT

In addition to the initial history and physical examination of the patient presenting with a chest wall or thoracic cavity and mediastinal problem, a standard chest radiograph should be obtained. This may help delineate the need for bronchoscopy, including questions involving airway obstruction, bronchopleural fistulas, and esophageal patency. For diagnosis and assessment as well as preoperative planning, it is imperative that the patient have a high-resolution computed tomographic (CT) scan with axial cuts from the neck to the area below the diaphragm.

Numerous studies have documented the importance of a multidisciplinary team approach in working with the patient in need of reconstruction of the chest and the conditions leading up to reconstruction. A multispecialty modality assists in meeting the overall needs of the patient requiring chest reconstruction. In particular, the thoracic surgeon and plastic surgeon should work in concert to deal with the primary problem and help plan the reconstruction. Adjunctive support is also provided by the internal medicine and pulmonology teams, especially in the preoperative and work-up phase, as well as by the critical care and anesthesiology teams working in the operating room and in the immediate postoperative period.

TREATMENT GOALS AND TECHNIQUE SELECTION

The goal of surgical treatment and concurrent reconstruction should be to provide ablation, cure, and treatment of the primary disease process as well as reconstruction to the extent that it allows a return to acceptable respiratory parameters, the control of wounds, and the elimination of the need for respiratory support measures. For patients who require chest wall resection and reconstruction, skeletal reconstruction is often necessary once the defect of the chest wall has reached a significant and consequential size.

Several series have looked at the extent of chest wall reconstruction and tabulated this extent by the number of ribs resected.[8,9] Reconstruction of full-thickness defects of the chest wall remains somewhat controversial. Small defects of skeletal chest components need not be reconstructed, and the defect in general can often be addressed by closure of only soft tissue defects. Structural stability can be provided when necessary by a variety of autogenous tissues, such as fascia lata and rib, or prosthetic materials, such as mesh, metal, and soft tissue patches. There are a variety of different mesh materials available, including polypropylene (Marlex) and polytetrafluoroethylene (Gore-Tex). In general, the adult human thoracic skeleton will tolerate a two-rib resection without the need for autologous or alloplastic support. Once three-rib resections are undertaken, it is a general practice to provide prosthetic support for the chest wall. In one large series,[8] the median number of ribs resected was three, with a range of one to eight.

Traditionally, substantial chest wall defects were reconstructed by a sandwich of polypropylene mesh and methyl methacrylate glue. The sandwich may be constructed and allowed to solidify outside the body on the operating table and then sutured in place, or it may be formed within the defect during reconstruction. When this structure hardens, a rigid shell that adheres to the chest replaces the area of excision.

Methyl methacrylate glue undergoes an endothermic reaction while it is curing. One must be careful to allow partial drying of the glue before it is applied to chest tissue. In addition, the drying and curing process may cause systemic acidosis if the glue is exposed to raw tissue surfaces. For these reasons, in many institutions, polypropylene mesh alone replaced methyl methacrylate sandwiches because of difficulties with methyl methacrylate in the sandwich construction. However, polypropylene mesh alone is more difficult to remove when it is infected and tends to fray and fragment. Therefore, the preferred prosthetic material is 2-mm polytetrafluoroethylene (because the 1-mm sheet is too thin to hold sutures under tension). The 2-mm polytetrafluoroethylene sheet may be stretched tight and maintains the rigidity necessary to reconstruct a stable chest wall. Also, given its nonpermeable state, it allows a watertight and airtight closure for the generation of a negative inspiratory force. In most instances, the placement of the polytetrafluoroethylene patch will then require autogenous soft tissue coverage in the form of either a muscle flap or an omental flap to provide a well-vascularized tissue cover for the mesh. In certain patients, a myocutaneous flap both to cover the mesh and to provide skin coverage may be used.

A standard array of muscle flaps have been delineated during the past 2 decades for use in reconstruction of the chest wall. Before the identification of these axial-based flaps, chest wall reconstruction was a difficult task with many challenges for the surgeon and the patient. Muscle flap selection is largely dependent on the location of the defect around the chest wall. Two of the most commonly used muscle flaps, the latissimus dorsi and the pectoralis major, exist in paired sets in the thoracic cavity and are described as type V musculature (Figs. 132-2 and 132-3). The latissimus dorsi and pectoralis major have a dominant axial perfusion as well as multiple midline segmental perforators that can also fully supply the muscle. These two muscles can be mobilized on either

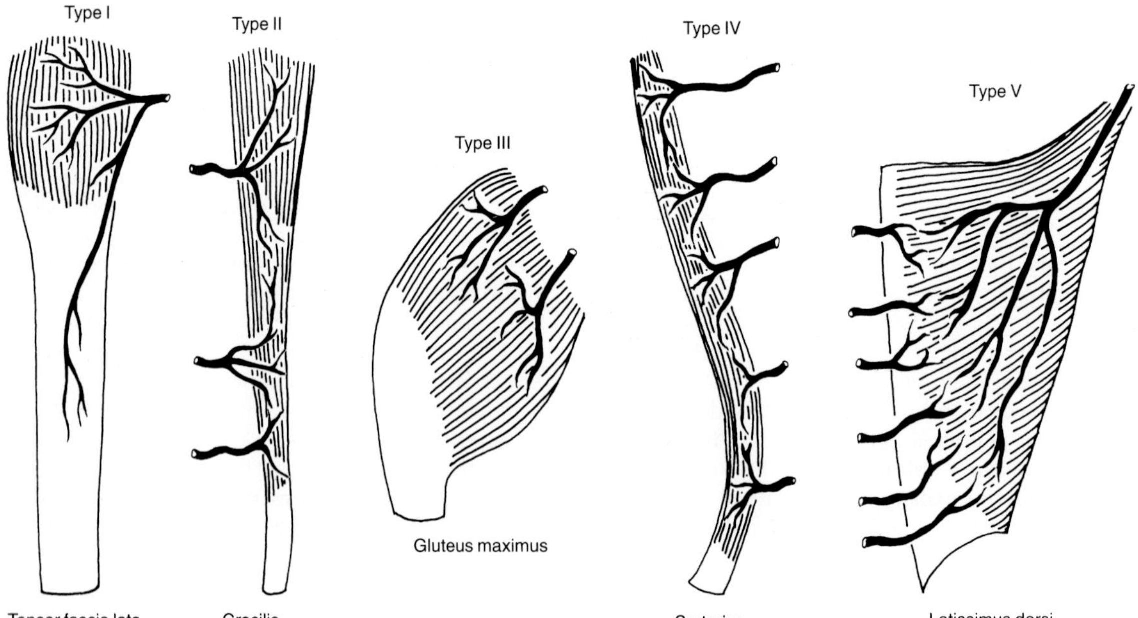

FIGURE 132-2. Mathes-Nahai classification of muscle and musculocutaneous flaps. Patterns of vascular anatomy: type I, one vascular pedicle; type II, dominant pedicle and minor pedicle; type III, two dominant pedicles; type IV, segmental vascular pedicles; type V, one dominant pedicle and secondary segmental pedicles. (From Mathes SJ, Nahai F: Classification of the vascular anatomy of muscles: experimental and clinical correlation. Plast Reconstr Surg 1981;67:177.)

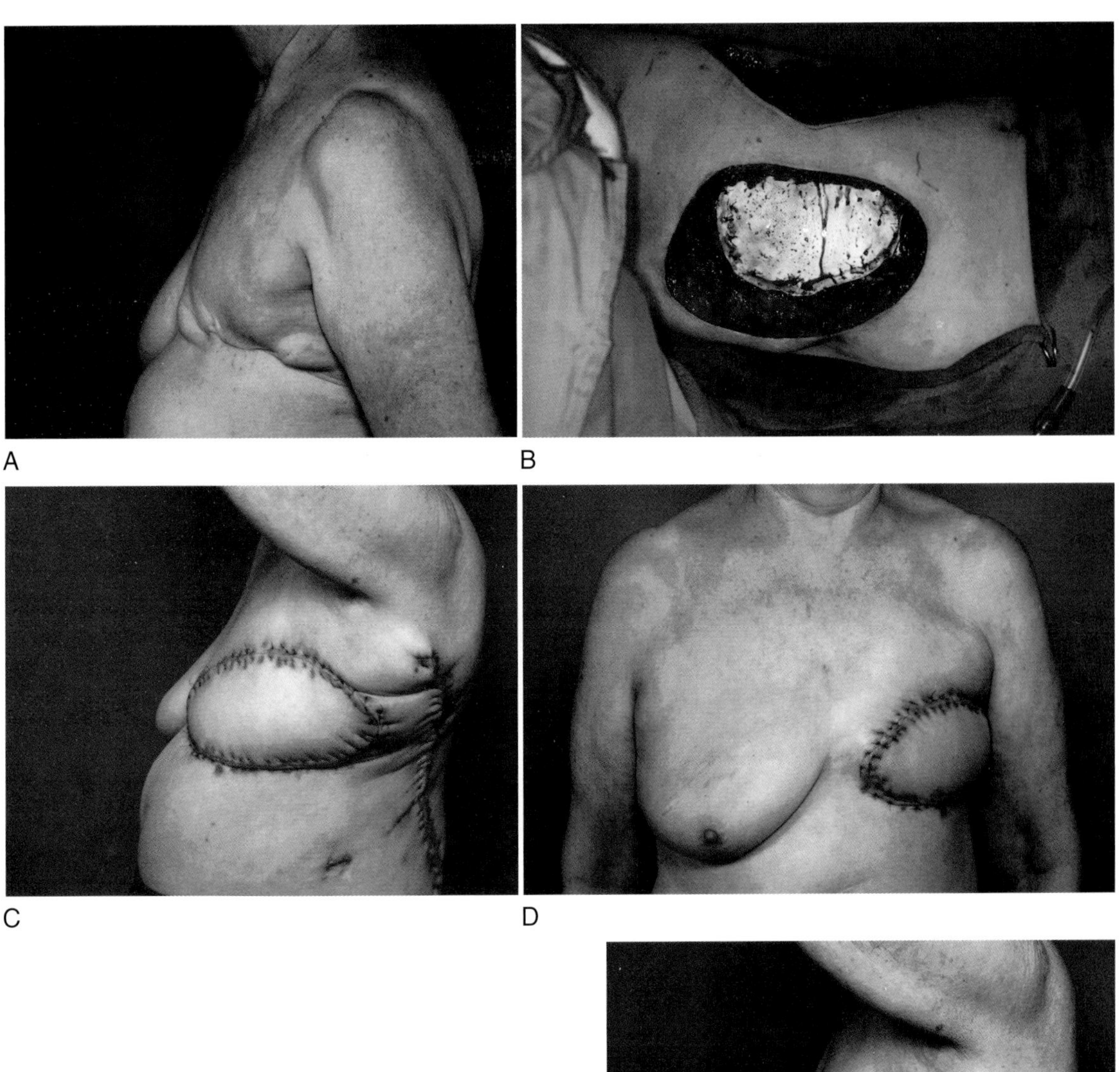

A B C D E

FIGURE 132-3. A 67-year-old with recurrent breast cancer invasive to chest wall. *A,* Preoperative view. *B,* Resection of tumor, chest, and four ribs. Polytetrafluoroethylene (Gore-Tex) mesh is used for reconstruction. *C,* Left latissimus dorsi myocutaneous flap for coverage of mesh reconstruction and chest wall reconstruction. *D,* Postoperative result. *E,* Late postoperative result.

vascular arcade to achieve an arc of rotation sufficient to cover anterior midline and anterolateral chest wall defects (Fig. 132-4).

The pectoralis major muscle can be based on the thoracoacromial vascular leash and easily transposed across the midline for sternal defects or to reach the medial aspect of the opposite side to assist with coverage of anterior chest wall defects on the contralateral side (Fig. 132-5). It can also be based as a turnover flap on the midline perforators, deriving perfusion from internal mammary access (Fig. 132-6).

The latissimus dorsi muscle may be used to reconstruct posterior, posterior midline, posterolateral, and anterior defects (Fig. 132-7). This muscle can be mobilized on its thoracodorsal leash, and it will usually achieve a large arc of motion to reach the lateral aspect

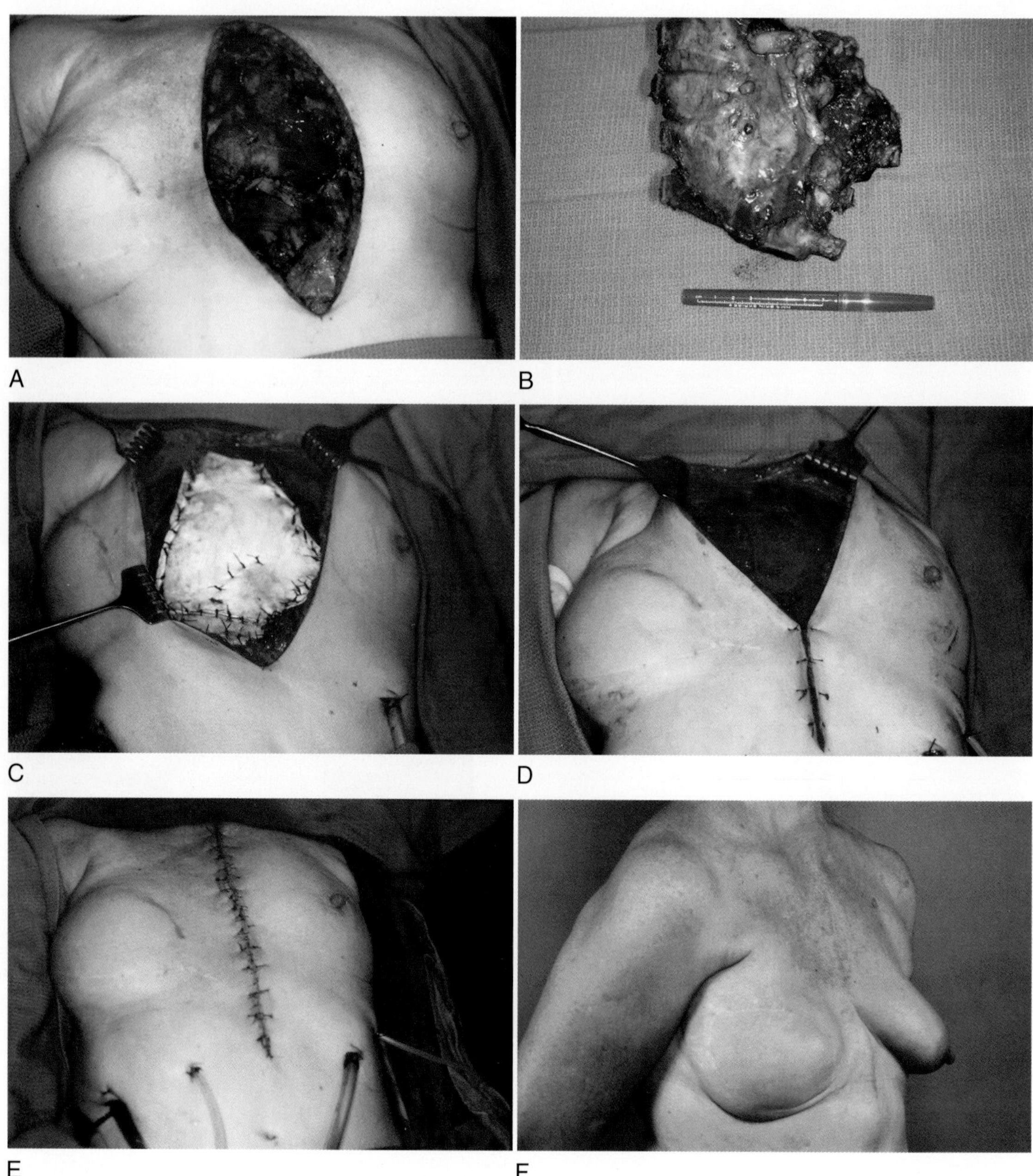

FIGURE 132-4. Sternal resection for radiation-induced sarcoma. *A,* Sternal resection. *B,* Radiation-induced sarcoma. *C,* Polytetrafluoroethylene (Gore-Tex) mesh, 2 mm, used for reconstruction. *D,* Bilateral pectoralis major flaps for mesh coverage and sternal reconstruction. *E,* Wound at closure. *F,* Long-term result.

of the anterior chest wall as well as the true anterior thorax, posterior thorax, and posterior midline. The latissimus can also be based as a turnover flap on the paraspinal and intercostal perforators for reconstruction of the posterior midline or intrathoracic reconstruction of the congenital diaphragm (see the section on congenital defects).

In addition to the latissimus dorsi and pectoralis major, the serratus anterior can be employed alone or in conjunction with the latissimus dorsi muscle for chest reconstruction (Fig. 132-8). Its main perfusion, like that of the latissimus dorsi, comes off the subscapular system and the thoracodorsal leash after it gives rise to the main pedicle to the latissimus dorsi muscle. Donor site morbidity for both the pectoralis major and the latissimus dorsi muscle is minimal from a functional standpoint. Each muscle serves as an adjunctive rotator of the humerus, and the functions of both are largely duplicated by the other primary muscles of the shoulder girdle, such as the rotator cuff. The serratus anterior can be used as a solo muscle flap for lateral chest wall defects, and when it is brought in a combined fashion with the latissimus muscle, it can add further bulk and surface coverage as a combined latissimus dorsi-serratus anterior muscle unit (Fig. 132-9; see also Color Plate 132-1).

Other muscle flap units employed in chest wall reconstruction include the rectus abdominis with or without a myocutaneous vertical or transverse skin component. The rectus abdominis is, however, sometimes precluded by absence of the internal mammary system if the defect has resulted in removal of the portion of the chest wall containing the internal mammary vessel. Likewise, ligation of the internal mammary artery or its procurement for revascularization of coronary arteries precludes its use. External oblique and trapezius muscle and myocutaneous flaps have also been used for chest wall reconstruction. A variety of thoracoepigastric flaps can also be designed for the more inferior portions of the lateral and anterolateral chest wall.

On occasion, one will find a chest wall wound that lacks available local and regional flaps, even if they are used in combination. Free tissue transplantation presents one solution and has been effective.[10] Vein grafting or the use of vein loops may be necessary if suitable recipient vessels are unavailable or damaged by irradiation. Another strategy involves the use of prosthetic material sutured to the chest wall for stability and support with coverage provided by the omentum.

The greater omentum is a versatile organ that has been used by surgeons for a variety of purposes for

Text continued on p. 424

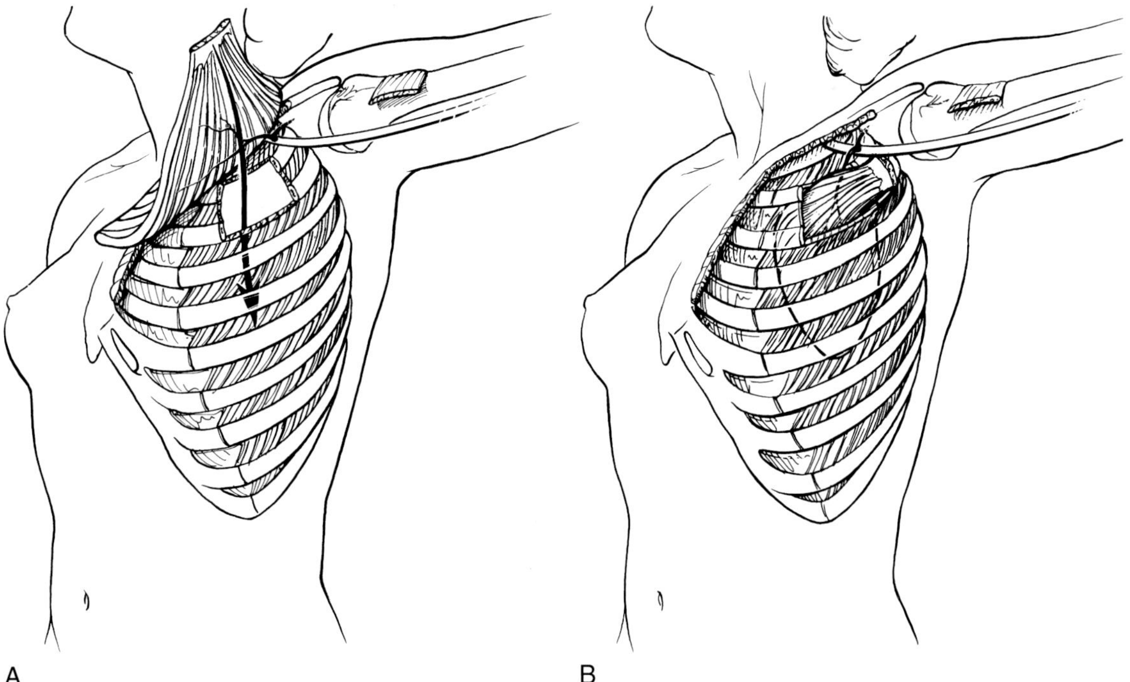

FIGURE 132-5. Pectoralis major flap. An island pectoralis muscle flap based on the dominant thoracoacromial pedicle will provide intrathoracic filling for the upper part of the thoracic cavity. Portions of the second, third, or fourth ribs are resected to allow the island muscle flap to be placed in the chest cavity. *A* and *B*, Arc to intrathoracic cavity.

Continued

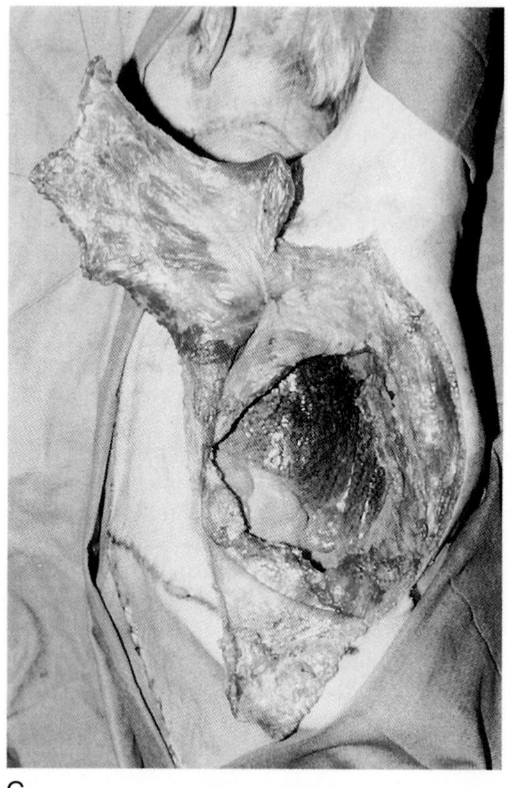

C

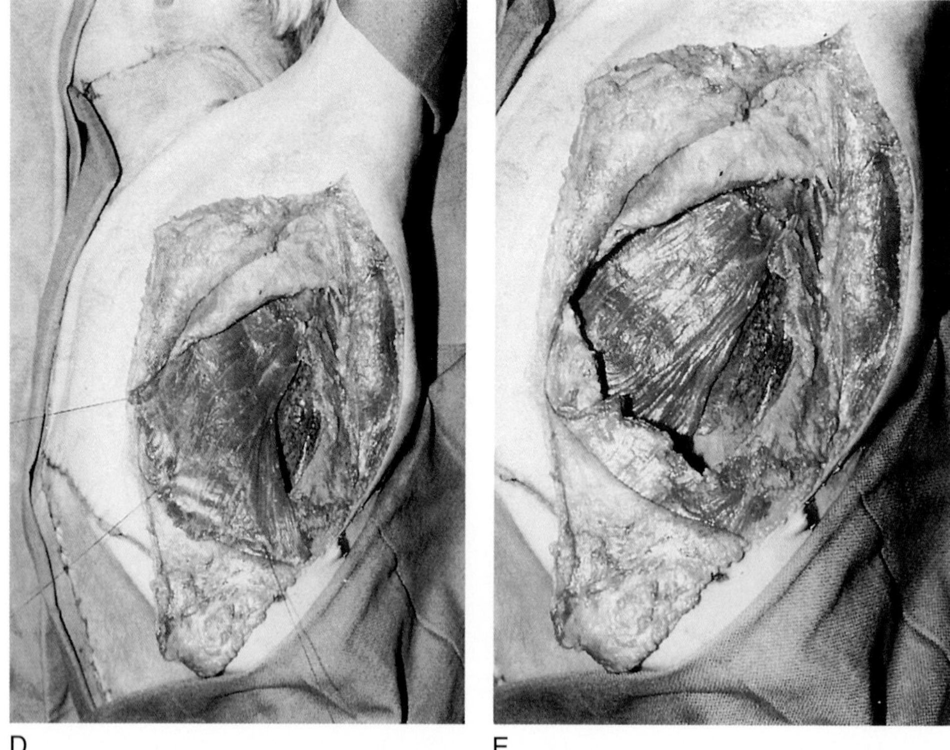

D E

FIGURE 132-5, cont'd. *C,* Elevation of flap. *D,* Coverage of intrathoracic cavity. *E,* Close-up view of flap inset. (From Mathes SJ, Nahai F: Reconstructive Surgery: Principles, Anatomy, and Technique. New York, Churchill Livingstone, 1997:450-451.)

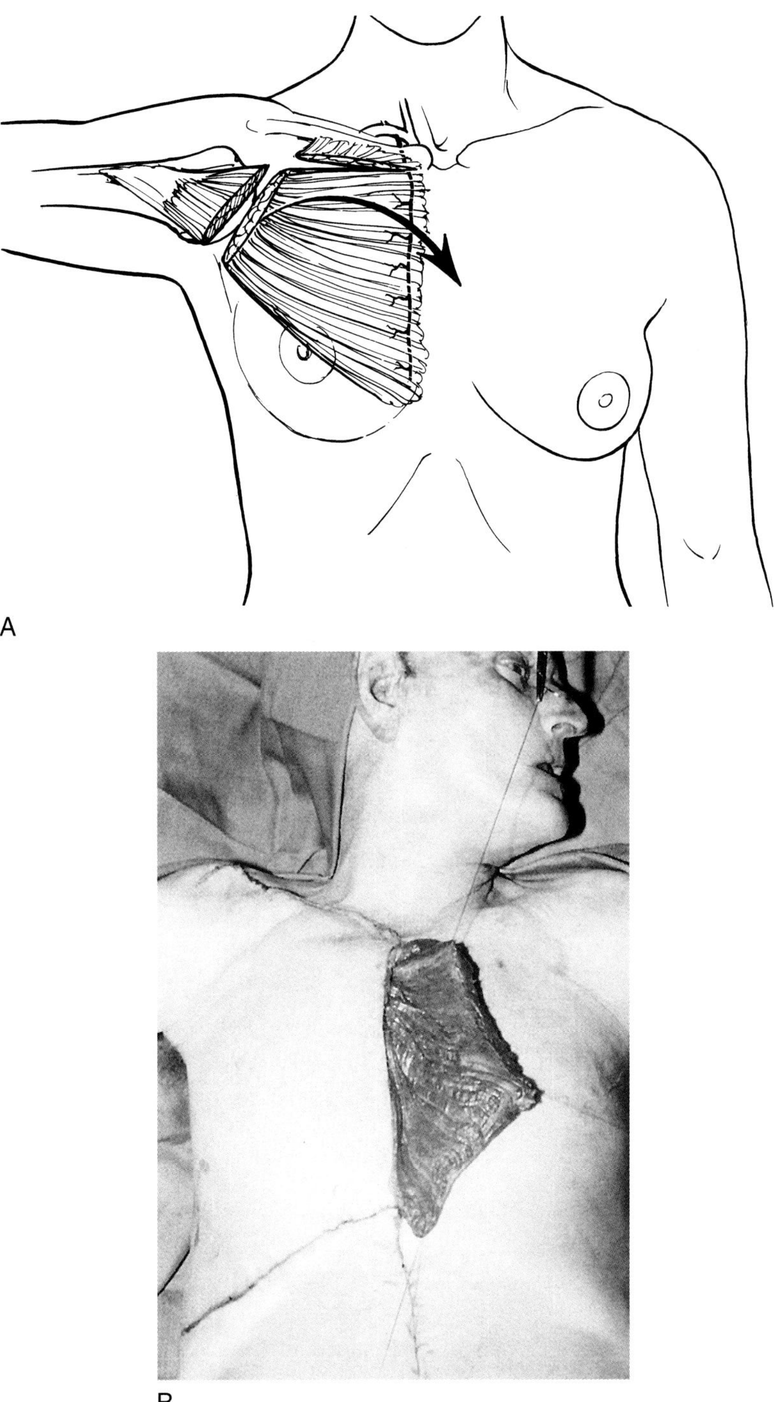

FIGURE 132-6. Pectoralis major turnover flap. The pectoralis major turnover flap is based on the minor segmental pedicles and used predominantly for coverage of the sternum and mediastinum. This modified flap will preserve the anterior axillary fold. *A,* Arc to sternum and anterior mediastinum. *B,* Coverage of anterior mediastinum. (From Mathes SJ, Nahai F: Reconstructive Surgery: Principles, Anatomy, and Technique. New York, Churchill Livingstone, 1997:450-453.)

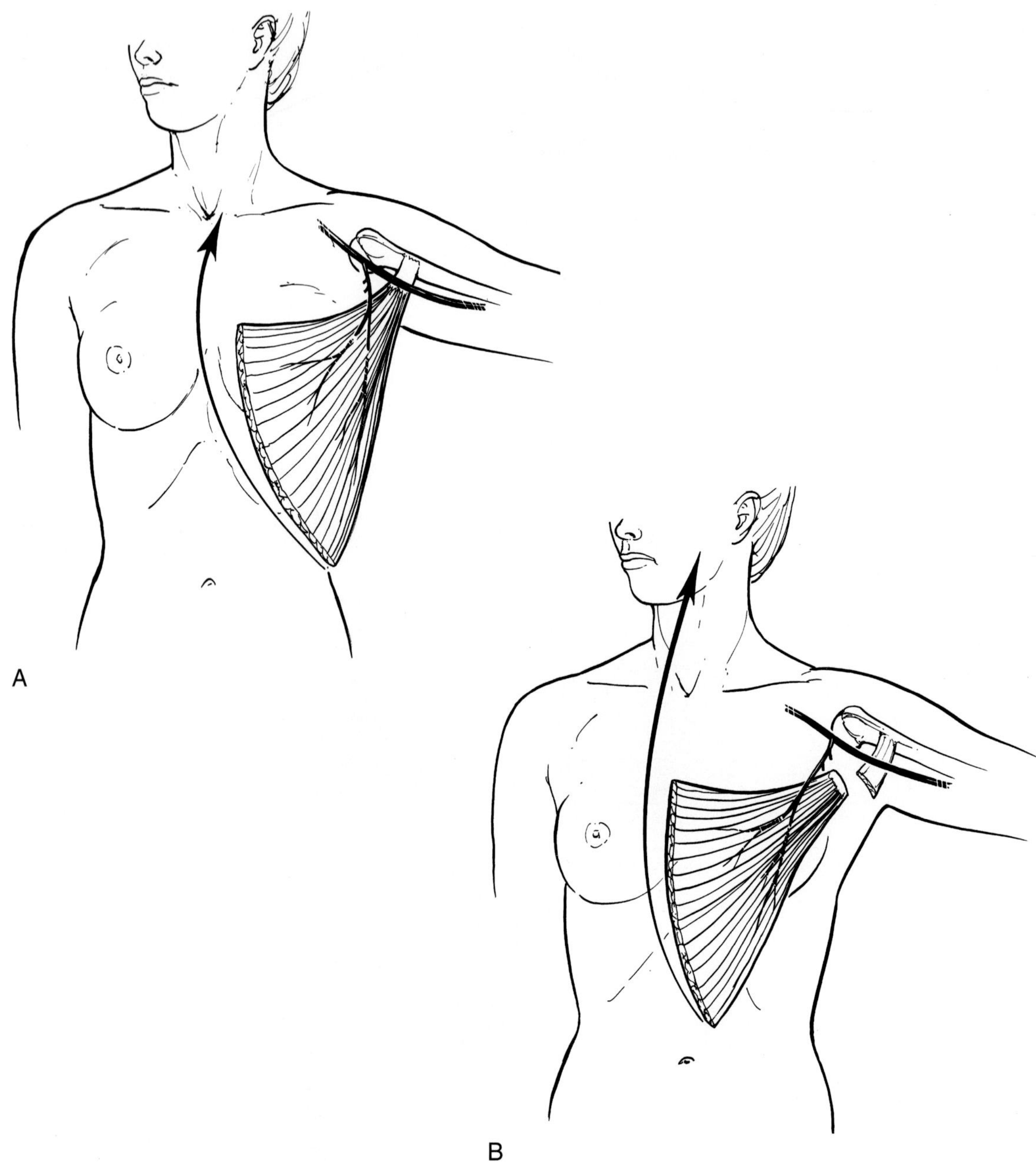

FIGURE 132-7. Latissimus dorsi flap. The point of rotation is located at the posterior axilla where the thoracodorsal pedicle enters the muscle. The muscle then has an anterior and posterior arc of rotation. The anterior arc of the latissimus dorsi flap includes the ipsilateral hemithorax and sternum. The standard arc of rotation is extended approximately 5 to 10 cm by division of the latissimus dorsi fibers of insertion and mobilization of the vascular pedicle (e.g., division of the branch to the serratus anterior muscle). *A,* Arc to anterior thorax with insertion intact. *B,* Arc after release of muscle insertion.

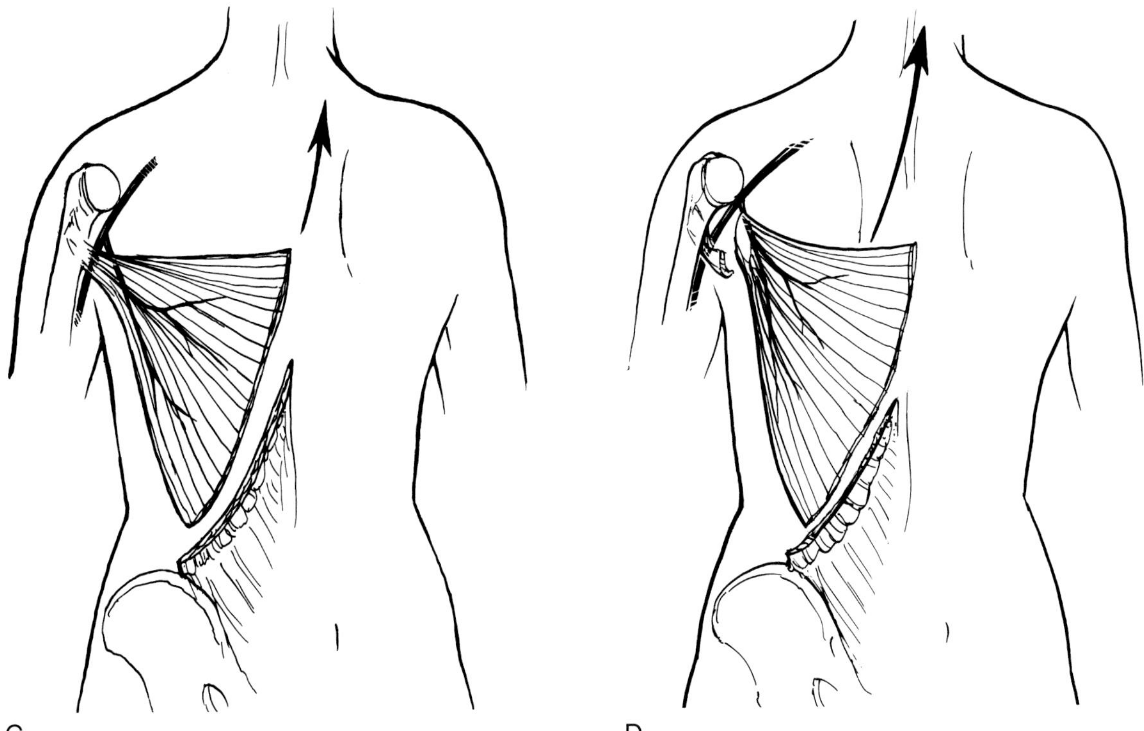

FIGURE 132-7, cont'd. *C,* Arc to posterior thorax with insertion intact. *D,* Arc after release of muscle insertion. (From Mathes SJ, Nahai F: Reconstructive Surgery: Principles, Anatomy, and Technique. New York, Churchill Livingstone, 1997:574, 576.)

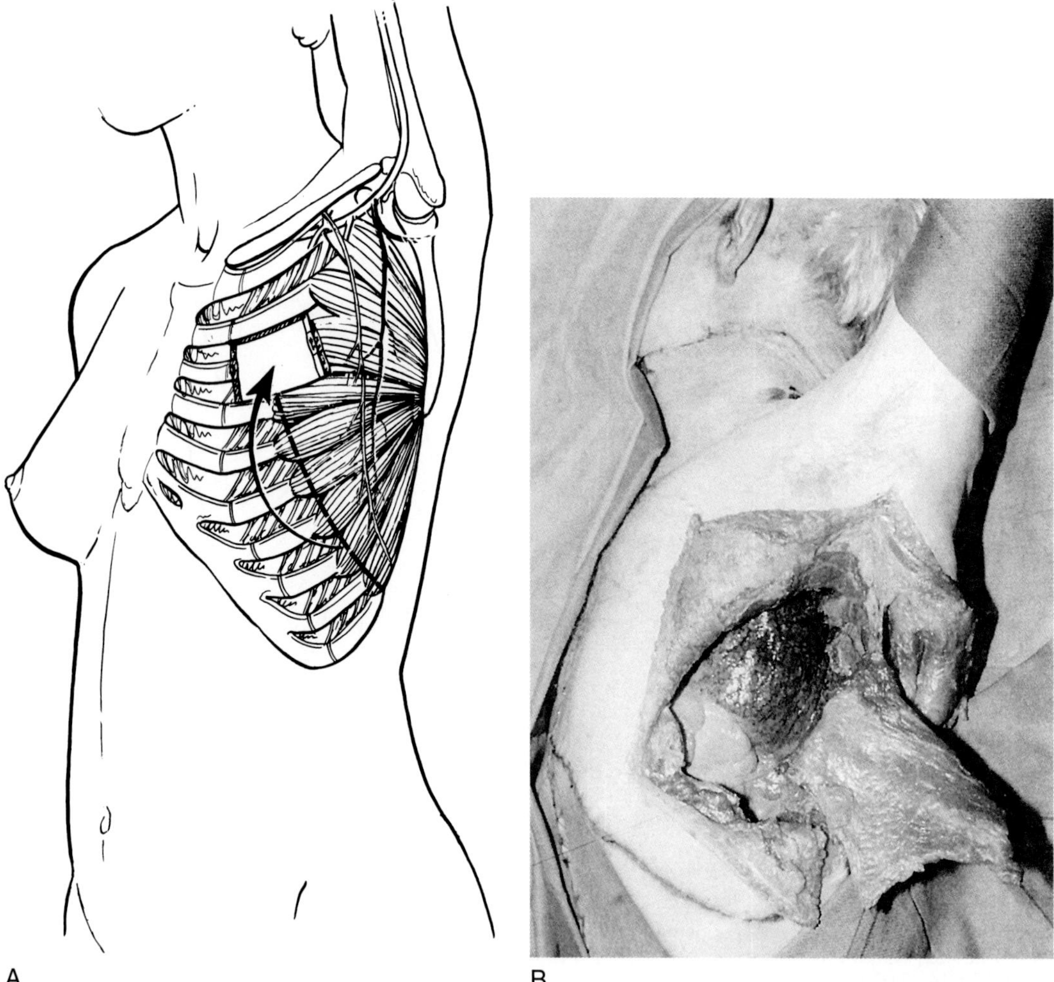

FIGURE 132-8. Serratus anterior flap. Based on its long pedicles in the axilla, the serratus flap has a long arc of rotation that will reach the chest wall, shoulder, axilla, and back. It will also reach the intrathoracic cavity. Division of the thoracodorsal pedicle will increase the anterior arc of rotation. Division of the lateral thoracic pedicle will increase the posterior arc. *A,* Rib resection required for flap arc into thoracic cavity. *B,* Flap inset (lateral chest wall resected to demonstrate intrathoracic position of flap. (From Mathes SJ, Nahai F: Reconstructive Surgery: Principles, Anatomy, and Technique. New York, Churchill Livingstone, 1997:483.)

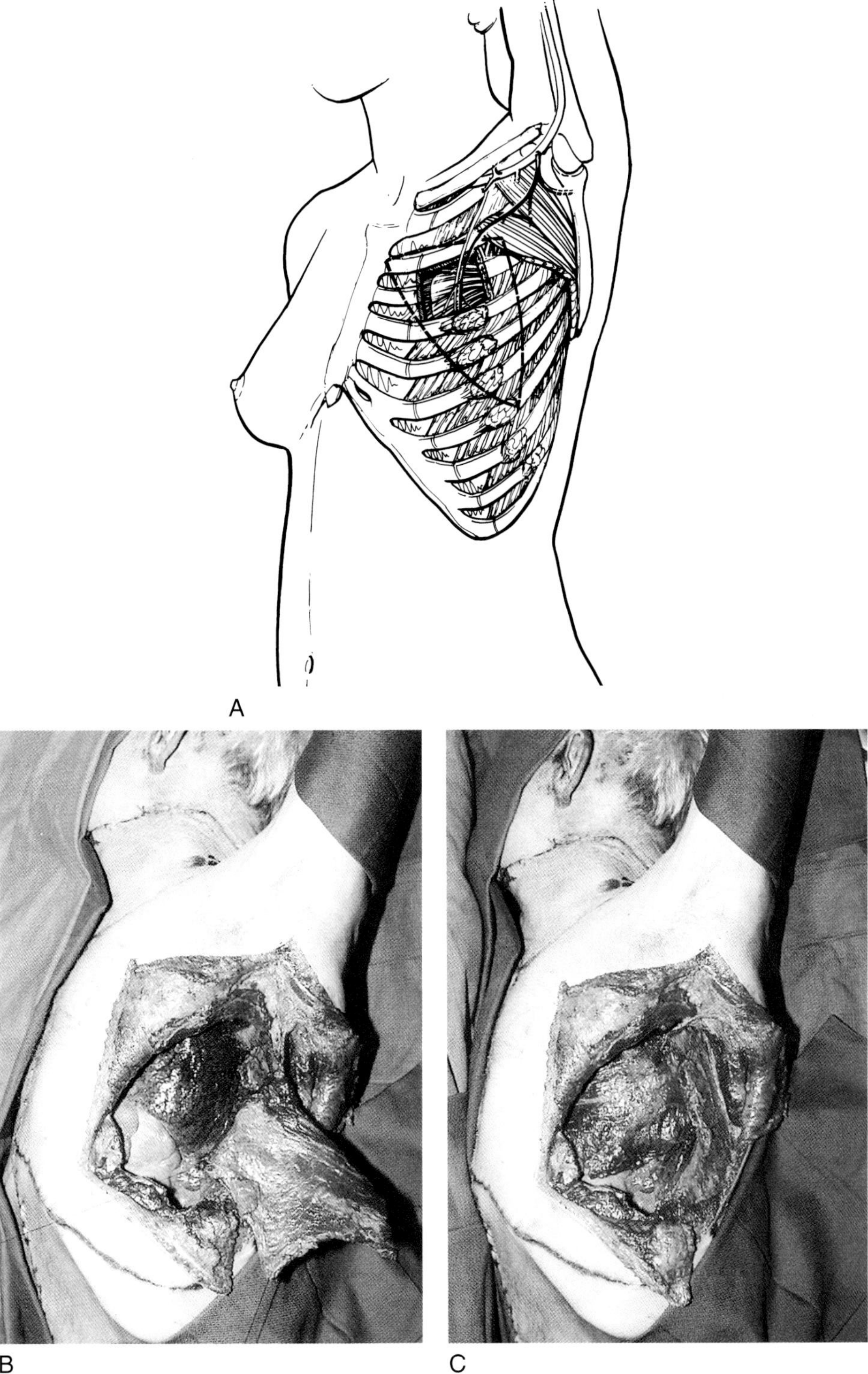

FIGURE 132-9. Latissimus dorsi-serratus anterior muscle coverage (see also Color Plate 132-1). The serratus anterior can be used both as a solo muscle flap for lateral chest wall defects and in combination with the latissimus muscle to add further bulk and surface coverage as a combined latissimus dorsi-serratus anterior muscle unit. *A,* Position of intrathoracic serratus muscle flap *(dotted line). B,* Intrathoracic placement of serratus flap. (Note: resection of lateral chest wall demonstrates flap position.) *C,* Flap inset. (From Mathes SJ, Nahai F: Reconstructive Surgery: Principles, Anatomy, and Technique. New York, Churchill Livingstone, 1997:488-489.)

many years.[11-13] Its large surface area and malleability, the length of both its potential pedicles, the lack of a donor defect, the ease of harvest, and its immunogenic and angiogenic properties[14] make the omentum an excellent option for soft tissue reconstruction of poorly vascularized wound beds. Potential intra-abdominal complications, such as gastric outlet obstruction and gastric, colonic, and splenic injury, increase the risk associated with harvesting of this flap. The omentum can be isolated on either the right or left gastroepiploic artery and brought through a cruciate stab incision in the prosthetic material. It is then spread out and draped over the prosthetic mesh and secured to the lateral skin edges, with skin grafting in approximately 72 hours.

OUTCOMES

Few long-term outcome studies of chest wall resection and reconstruction have been published. However, several publications demonstrate the safety and efficacy of chest wall reconstruction in both the short and long term.[8,9,15-17] Patients requiring chest wall resection and reconstruction generally have life-threatening conditions with significant associated comorbidities; therefore, complications can be expected but are not prohibitive. Despite the risks and potential complications, aggressive chest wall débridement followed by an equally aggressive attempt at reconstruction has yielded acceptable results.

The largest series of chest wall resections and reconstructions in the English literature is by Arnold and Pairolero.[18] Their first paper described their early experience with 100 consecutive patients at the Mayo Clinic in Rochester, Minnesota. They subsequently published a report of 205 patients,[16] followed by a series of 500 consecutive chest wall reconstructions during an 18-year period[9] (Table 132-1). In their series, patients were treated for chest wall tumors, infected median sternotomies, radiation necrosis, and combinations of these pathologic processes. In their series of 500 consecutive patients, the average follow-up was 57 months. The 500 patients underwent an average of 2.3 operations with an average hospitalization of 21 days. In this group, there were 15 perioperative deaths, and 23 patients required tracheostomy. Long-term follow-up revealed 229 late deaths. The deaths were attributed to cancer (147 patients), cardiac causes (49 patients), pulmonary causes (7 patients), and other (26 patients). Excellent results with asymptomatic and healed chest walls were reported in 403 of the 485 patients (83.1%) who were alive 30 days after surgery. The authors concluded that chest wall resection and reconstruction is a safe and durable procedure associated with acceptable long-term survival.

Mansour et al[15] reported a retrospective review of 200 patients during a 25-year period. The group reported a 93% 30-day survival but did not report long-term survival. Seyfer[19] reported an 11-year experience with 295 flaps for chest wall reconstruction. This series reported one death and 13 minor dehiscences. Deschamps et al[8] described 197 patients who underwent chest wall resection and reconstruction with prosthetic material. Soft tissue coverage was achieved with

TABLE 132-1 ✦ INDICATIONS AND MUSCLE REPAIR FOR 500 CONSECUTIVE CHEST WALL RECONSTRUCTIONS

No. of Muscles, by Type	Indication for Reconstruction								
	Tumor	*IMS*	*Irradiation*	*Tumor, Irradiation*	*IMS, Irradiation*	*IMS, Tumor*	*Infection*	*Other*	*Total*
PMM	67	228	4	15	13	0	9	3	339
PMC	8	0	2	5	1	0	0	0	16
LDM	75	2	3	19	0	0	3	2	104
LDC	13	0	12	7	1	0	4	0	37
SAM	0	0	0	2	0	0	0	0	2
SAC	18	0	0	5	0	1	1	0	25
RAM	1	0	3	2	1	0	2	0	9
RAC	2	1	3	0	1	0	1	1	9
EOM	7	0	1	4	0	0	4	0	16
EOC	3	2	7	2	0	0	0	0	14
TRM	2	0	0	1	0	0	0	0	3
TRC	1	0	1	1	0	0	0	0	3
Other	15	1	6	10	0	0	2	0	34
Total	212	234	42	73	17	1	26	6	611

IMS, infected median sternotomy; PMM, pectoralis major muscle; PMC, pectoralis major myocutaneous; LDM, latissimus dorsi muscle; LDC, latissimus dorsi myocutaneous; SAM, serratus anterior muscle; SAC, serratus anterior myocutaneous; RAM, rectus abdominis muscle; RAC, rectus abdominis myocutaneous; EOM, external oblique muscle; EOC, external oblique myocutaneous; TRM, trapezius muscle; TRC, trapezius myocutaneous.

From Arnold PG, Pairolero PC: Chest-wall reconstruction: an account of 500 consecutive patients. Plast Reconstr Surg 1996;98:804-810.

primary wound closure (41.1%), muscle flaps (58.9%), and pedicled omental flaps (1.5%). The authors reported a 4.1% operative mortality rate and 46.2% complication rate. Complications included respiratory compromise (24.4%), seroma (7.1%), wound infection (4.6%), arrhythmia (2.5%), hemorrhage (2.0%), myocardial infarction (1.5%), prolonged air leak (1.0%), and other (3.0%). With a median follow-up of 26 months, 127 patients (70.9%) had a well-healed asymptomatic wound. The authors compared their outcomes of chest wall reconstruction with Prolene mesh and 2-mm polytetrafluoroethylene and found no significant difference between the two. The authors concluded that chest wall resection and reconstruction with prosthetic material yielded satisfactory results in most patients.

TABLE 132-2 ✦ CLASSIFICATION OF INFECTED STERNOTOMY WOUNDS

Classification	No. of Patients
Type I Occurs within first few days Serosanguineous drainage Cellulitis of skin absent Mediastinum soft and pliable Osteomyelitis and costochondritis absent Cultures usually negative	11
Type II Occurs within first few weeks Purulent drainage Cellulitis of skin present Mediastinal suppuration Osteomyelitis frequent, costochondritis rare Cultures positive	84
Type III Occurs months to years later Chronic draining sinus track Cellulitis of skin localized Mediastinitis rare Osteomyelitis, costochondritis, or retained foreign body always present Cultures positive	5
Total	100

From Pairolero PC, Arnold PG: Chest wall tumors. Experience with 100 consecutive patients. J Thorac Cardiovasc Surg 1985;90:367-372.

RECONSTRUCTION OF SPECIFIC DEFECTS

Sternal and Mediastinal Defects

The sternum can be involved with any condition afflicting the chest wall, including primary and metastatic tumors of the sternum. Because of its central and anterior location, the sternum is also a frequent recipient of trauma. Infection can ensue in the sternum as a result of post-sternotomy surgical efforts. As irradiation of breast tumors became popular, the sternum, in association with the anterior chest wall, frequently became involved with osteoradionecrosis. A variety of congenital anomalies can also afflict the sternum.

STERNAL INFECTION

One of the more common issues involving the sternum is sternal infection. Although the advent of the median sternotomy approach afforded the cardiothoracic surgeon unprecedented exposure of the mediastinum, early experiences reported high complication rates. Sternal wound infection leading to sternal wound dehiscence and mediastinitis were not uncommon. Mortality rates in these patients were often as high as 50%. Early treatment modalities for the infected sternal wound were too conservative, employing open drainage, dressing changes, and antibiotic irrigation. Outcomes improved as surgeons became more aggressive in their débridement of infected and nonviable tissue and as the reconstructive armamentarium grew with muscle and omental flaps.

Sternal infection is an uncommon complication of transsternal cardiothoracic surgery. The reported incidence ranges from 0.4% to 5.1%.[20-22] Many papers in the literature have investigated the risk factors for median sternotomy infection and dehiscence. Although some disagreement exists, most authors agree that risk factors include diabetes, female gender, obesity, prolonged postoperative ventilation, parasternal muscle sutures, postoperative dialysis, hypertension, smoking, and use of one or both internal mammary arteries for revascularization.[22-25] Several authors have disputed the claim that use of internal mammary arteries is an independent risk factor.[26,27]

A useful classification system for infected median sternotomy wounds based on the timing of presentation and character of the wound was described by Pairolero and Arnold[17] (Table 132-2). Type I sternal infections occur in the acute phase during postoperative days 1 to 3. They present with serosanguineous drainage, negative wound cultures, no evidence of skin cellulitis, and a soft and pliable mediastinum. This is in contrast to a type II infection, which occurs in the first 2 to 3 weeks of the postoperative period. These infections are marked by purulent drainage, skin cellulitis, positive wound cultures, and mediastinal suppuration and are frequently associated with osteomyelitis. In their series of 100 consecutive patients, 84% of the sternal infections were type II. Type III infections present months to years postoperatively, with a small, chronic draining sinus track. Localized cellulitis is frequently present, and wound cultures are positive. Sternal osteomyelitis, costochondritis, or a retained foreign body is almost universally present. The presence or absence of sternal dehiscence and nonunion must be assessed and noted.

Evaluation and Management of the Patient

The work-up of a patient with a sternal infection problem starts with a chest radiograph and a CT scan of the chest. The CT scan provides valuable information about the union of the primary median sternotomy and the status of the mediastinum, and it shows radiographic evidence of frank mediastinitis. Patients with frank mediastinitis tend to be systemically ill. They may have physiologic parameters consistent with a severe illness, and their hospital course, length of stay, and recovery will be much longer and arduous than for those patients whose infection is exterior to the mediastinum in the subcutaneous soft tissues. The average length of stay for the patients with the type III sternal infection will be 3 weeks, and they will undergo several procedures for débridement until definitive closure is attempted and achieved. A multidisciplinary team approach is best established to care for these patients much in the same way the chest wall is addressed. A general thoracic surgeon plays a critical role in this endeavor. It is widely accepted that adequate débridement is the primary first step in the treatment plan of these sternal infections, especially in those patients with chronic conditions that contain sinus tracks. The initial primary surgeon, who may be the cardiac surgeon who performed a revascularization procedure, may be hesitant to do the aggressive widespread débridement that is often necessary to treat these problems adequately. In support of this, numerous pieces of literature attest to the theory that should the initial attempt at débridement, coverage, and closure fail and infection recur, the usual primary cause is retained sequestrum and inadequate débridement at the first treatment attempt.

Critical care teams play an invaluable role in the care of these patients in the intensive care unit. These patients often require prolonged ventilatory support, and their airway management, ventilatory parameters, and need for possible tracheostomy should be regularly assessed and evaluated. The extent of débridement is critical in treatment of all sternal infections. Those in the acute phase, with serous drainage within the first few days of surgery, can be treated by more conservative measures, and this has some support in the literature.[28] Treatment for patients in the acute phase often involves opening the skin only and instituting wet-to-dry dressing changes. Should the drainage and the wound process be in contact with the sternum, a decision must be made whether to reopen the entire wound or to try to pack the superficial areas of the wound only. Motion at the sternotomy site and frank exposure of the osteotomized ends of the sternum are indications for unwiring of the sternum and multiple washings and irrigations. Identification of healthy, bleeding cortical and cancellous bone on minimal débridement in the operating room is an indication to try to salvage as much of the manubrium, sternum, and xiphoid as possible. However, if the bone looks unhealthy, is soft, or lacks adequate blood supply or any of the costal cartilage is involved, a more aggressive and widespread débridement must be performed. This is especially true if the costal cartilage is exposed and open to the environment.

Numerous muscle flaps have been employed in the treatment of sternal infections. The mainstay of treatment continues to be the pectoralis major muscle (Fig. 132-10). Whereas midline perfusion has been reported by some to provide excellent results, the safest and most reliable technique is transposition of the pectoralis muscle toward the midline on the thoracoacromial vascular leash. An intraoperative assessment is made as to whether the tendinous insertion needs to be released from the humerus. This release can often be done through the midline incision, but if it cannot be done, one should not hesitate to make a counter-incision to safely release the tendinous insertion to allow further transposition. Inferiorly, the pectoralis major can often be maintained in continuity with the upper portion of the rectus sheath. This continuity allows transposition of a bulky muscle unit for obliteration of dead space and coverage of the bone and costal cartilage that has been débrided back to bleeding, healthy tissue.

In patients with chronic sternal infection, repeated serial débridement performed during the course of several days is often required to obtain a stable wound before closure. Although the timing of wound closure has not been successfully measured with any definitive technique, wounds that are closed too soon will result in the recurrence of infection. It is therefore more prudent to leave a wound open "too long" than to close it too soon. In general, a healthy granulation bed with a decrease in serous and fibrinous debris and no evidence of devitalized tissue or foreign body are indications for wound closure. Once the wound surface is nearly covered with a healthy granulation bed, it indicates an intact wound healing mechanism, nutrition suitable for wound healing, and a falling bacterial count. These parameters are indications that the mediastinal wound should accept further soft tissue coverage and closure over drains. In procedures with midline movement of the pectoralis major muscles, the generous use of four drains, two below each muscle unit and two above each muscle unit in the subcutaneous space, is often employed. Their removal is dictated by the amount of output (drainage in the range of 30 to 50 mL) during a 24-hour period.

There are reports in the literature of midline turnover of the pectoralis major muscle based on medial perforating vessels from the internal thoracic artery.[28,29] This muscle flap has drawbacks for two

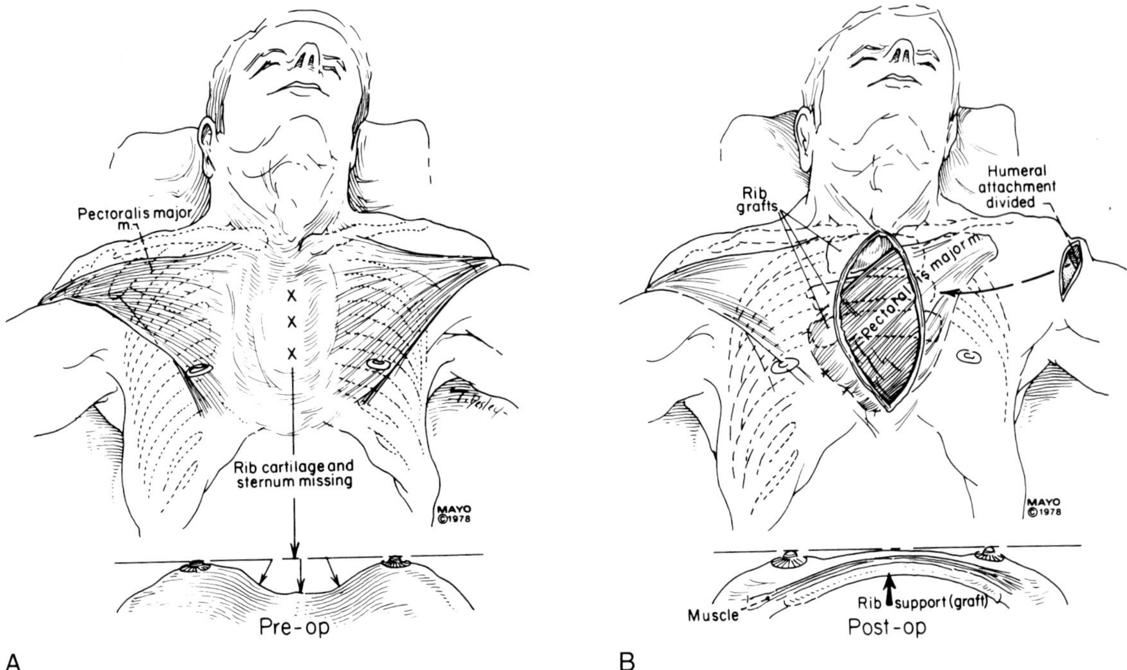

FIGURE 132-10. *A* and *B*, After the humeral insertion is divided, the pectoralis major muscle can be mobilized well across the midline and into the median sternotomy defect. (From Arnold PG, Pairolero PC: Use of pectoralis major muscle flaps to repair defects of anterior chest wall. Plast Reconstr Surg 1979;63:205.)

reasons. First, many patients who present with sternal infection have had their internal mammary arteries used for coronary revascularization, thus making the midline turnover of the pectoralis muscle impossible. Second, patients requiring a second sternotomy for further myocardial revascularization risk injury to the vascular supply to their mediastinal soft tissue coverage. This problem is avoided if the muscles have been transposed to the midline with use of the thoracoacromial vascular leash. One can then reinstitute the previous midline sternal incision. The rectus abdominis has also been reported to be useful as a vertical myocutaneous muscle for sternal infections. Whereas the obvious bulk is advantageous, the rectus abdominis should be a second or third choice based on the previous discussion.

Should the initial attempts with the pectoralis major muscle be unsuccessful, the next step in the reconstructive ladder is often repeated débridement and dressing changes followed by transposition of the omentum. The omentum can be successfully harvested endoscopically, although numerous series continue to report that there is no problem with the upper midline incision with respect to infection, hernia, or other supposed complications.[12] The omentum is usually mobilized on the right gastroepiploic artery (Fig. 132-11). Care must be taken to avoid tethering of the pyloric outlet and formation of a gastric outlet obstruction. The omentum is brought up onto the chest wall, where it can be further unfolded. This maneuver is best performed in the wound bed so the omental flap can be made to fit the defect. Limitations of the greater omental flap include its sometimes limited size, particularly in patients who have undergone previous abdominal surgery, and tethering of the flap by a limited vascular pedicle.

STERNAL TUMORS

Both primary and secondary metastatic tumors arise in the sternum, the manubrium, and the xiphoid. The majority of these tumors are chondrosarcomas. Local control of disease is usually accomplished with a wide local excision of the tumor and 5 cm of normal tissue. This often requires resection of adjacent chest wall. Reconstruction after partial or complete sternectomy is necessary to provide protection of the underlying mediastinal structures and to prevent their herniation. Reconstruction often consists of prosthetic material covered with viable soft tissue (muscle or omentum) and a skin graft.

Intrathoracic Defects and Management of the Pleural Space

Many of the muscles used for reconstruction of the chest wall can also be used for reconstructive endeavors within the thorax. A variety of pathologic processes

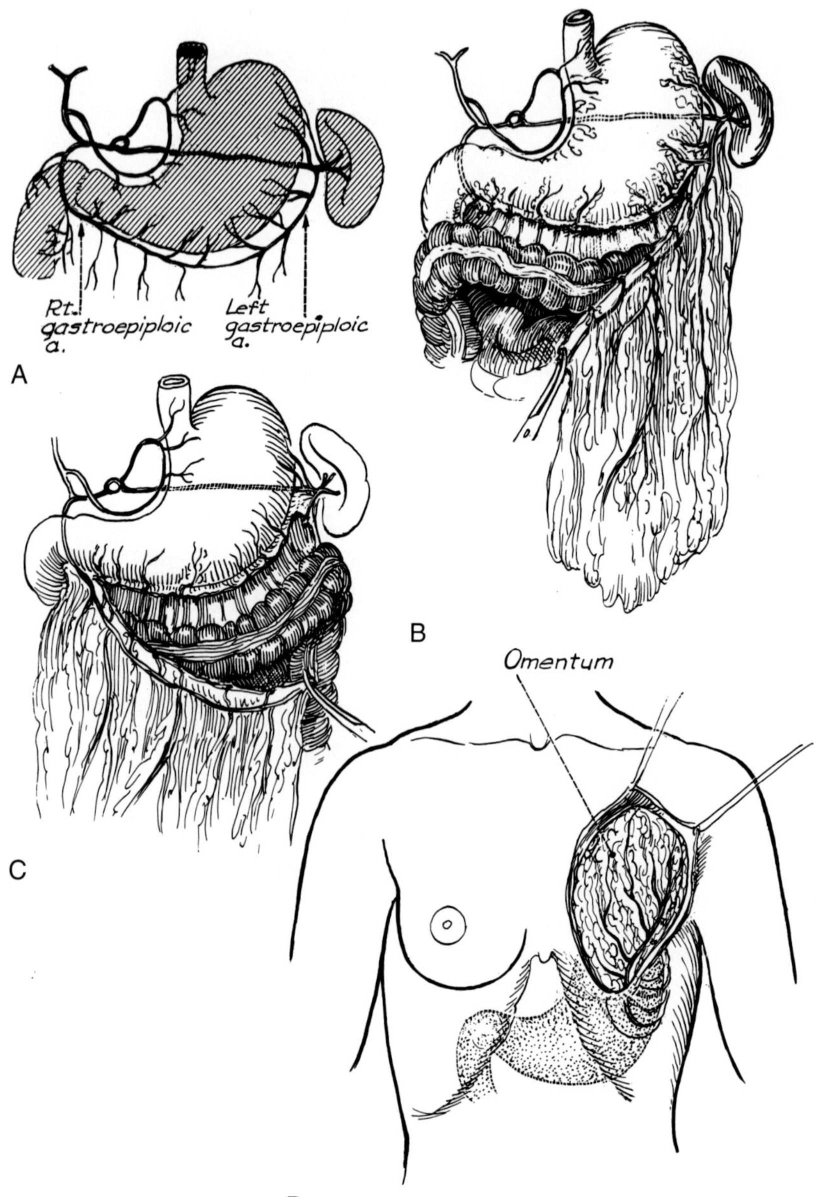

FIGURE 132-11. Closure of a chest wall defect with greater omentum. *A,* Main arterial supply of the greater omentum. *B* and *C,* The greater omentum can be pedicled on the right or left gastroepiploic artery, depending on the site of the defect to be closed. The omental flap is freed from the stomach at the muscularis layer to maintain the integrity of the vascular gastroepiploic arch. *D,* The greater omentum is transferred to the thoracic defect through the superior portion of the abdominal wall incision or through a separate stab wound. A subcutaneous tunnel may be used to pass the omentum to the defect. (After Dupont C, Menard Y: Transposition of the greater omentum for reconstruction of the chest wall. Plast Reconstr Surg 1972;49:263.)

are often treated with intrathoracic muscle flaps (Tables 132-3 and 132-4). The most common indication is a bronchopleural fistula. In the preantibiotic era, bronchopulmonary fistulas were seen as common sequelae of pneumonia. Currently, most bronchopleural fistulas present after pulmonary resection for malignant disease. At particularly high risk are those patients who undergo radiation therapy as an adjunct to their treatment regimen for pulmonary malignant disease and then proceed to completion pneumonectomy. The irradiated bronchial stump is predisposed to dehiscence and subsequent contamination of the pleural space. Reconstructive endeavors useful for the management of this difficult problem can also be used for the management of patients with post-pneumonectomy empyema. The appropriate initial step in treatment of these problems is aggressive wound débridement and control of infection. Débridement and control of infection are followed by the intrathoracic transfer of a well-vascularized muscle to reinforce the closed fistula. This type of management is often adequate for the treatment of the bronchopleural fistula. In patients with empyema, the wound is then treated with frequent dressing changes and irrigation as necessary. Once a clean and granulating wound is established, the wound can be closed after the instil-

TABLE 132-3 ✦ INDICATIONS FOR INTRATHORACIC MUSCLE TRANSPOSITION (MAYO CLINIC, 1977-1987)

Indication	No. of Patients
Infection group (65 patients)	
Bronchopleural fistula	23
Bronchopleural fistula and post-pneumonectomy empyema	17
Esophageal fistula	8
Heart or great vessel perforations	8
Post-pneumonectomy empyema	5
Empyema	2
Tracheal fistula	2
Prophylactic group (22 patients)	
Airway tension	16
Intrathoracic irradiation	6
Total	87

From Arnold PG, Pairolero PC: Intrathoracic muscle flaps: a 10-year experience in the management of life-threatening infections. Plast Reconstr Surg 1989;84:92-98, discussion 99.

lation of an antibiotic solution as described by Clagett.[30,31]

Initial management of an empyema includes complete exposure of the pleural space, meticulous débridement of all nonviable tissue, and vigorous irrigation with jet lavage on a low-pressure setting. Although it is not mandatory, this lavage can be done with any number of antibiotic solutions. Patients often require a prolonged stay in the intensive care unit with ventilatory support, possibly requiring tracheostomy. However, this may not be necessary for the majority of patients who are adequately treated with 1 to 2 weeks of daily dressing changes. Although there are no consistently reliable and objective criteria for establishing when to close the pleural space, there are many helpful indicators. The appearance of a healthy granulation bed in the depths of the pleural cavity in a patient with a resolving leukocytosis suggests a falling bacterial count, an intact wound healing mechanism, and a satisfactory nutritional state. This clinical picture is generally associated with readiness of the pleural space for closure (Fig. 132-12).

During initial surgical débridement, the bronchopleural fistula must be identified, débrided to viable and healthy tissue, and surgically closed. Preoperative CT scanning and bronchoscopy can facilitate its identification and location. In addition, intraoperative bronchoscopy consultation is often useful in identifying the anatomy. Common muscles used for muscle transposition include the serratus anterior muscle based on the subscapular and thoracodorsal leash, the latissimus based on the thoracodorsal axis, and the pectoralis major based on the thoracoacromial perfusion (see Figs. 132-5 to 132-10). Much of the decision as to which muscle to use is based on the placement of the initial thoracotomy incision and the potential division of these chest wall muscles. The placement of a high thoracotomy incision, the routine division of the latissimus submusculature, or the routine division of the serratus anterior musculature can complicate and possibly eliminate the use of one or all local muscle flaps. It should therefore be strongly advocated to all general thoracic and cardiothoracic

TABLE 132-4 ✦ RESULTS ACCORDING TO INDICATION (SERIES OF 87 PATIENTS WITH INTRATHORACIC MUSCLE TRANSPOSITION, MAYO CLINIC, 1977-1987)

Indication	No. of Patients	Result	
		Excellent	*Failure*
Infected group (65 patients)			
Bronchopleural fistula	23	15	8
Bronchopleural fistula and post-pneumonectomy empyema	17	11	6
Esophageal fistula	8	7	1
Heart or great vessel perforations	8	7	1
Post-pneumonectomy empyema	5	3	2
Empyema	2	2	0
Tracheal fistula	2	0	2
Prophylactic group (22 patients)			
Airway tension	16	12	4
Intrathoracic irradiation	6	4	2
Total	87	61	26

From Arnold PG, Pairolero PC: Intrathoracic muscle flaps: a 10-year experience in the management of life-threatening infections. Plast Reconstr Surg 1989;84:92-98, discussion 99.

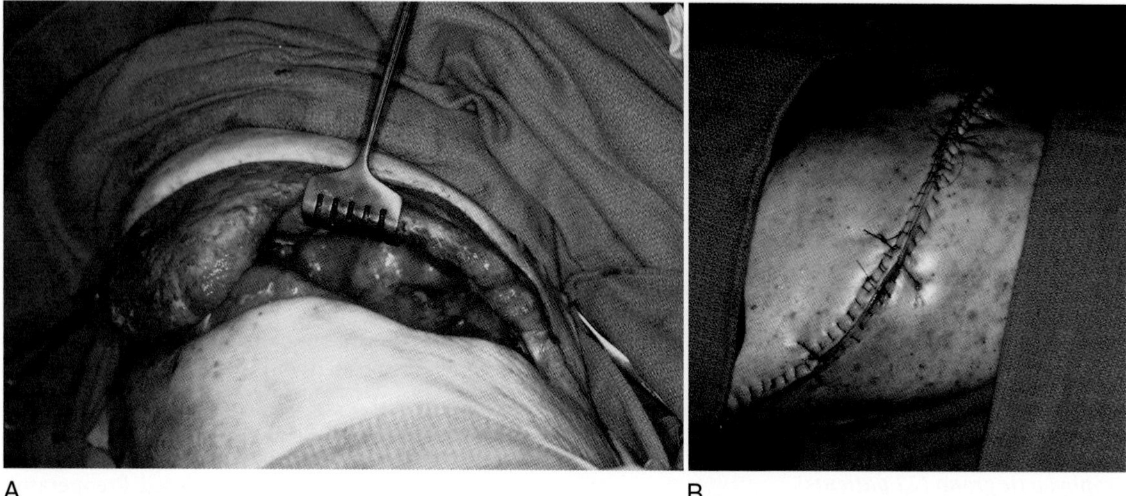

FIGURE 132-12. Coverage of bronchial stump and obliteration of pleural space with antibiotic solution. *A,* Transposed right serratus anterior (below retractor) to cover bronchial stump. *B,* Obliterated pleural space with use of antibiotic solution (based on a formula of 1 liter of normal saline combined with 80 mg of gentamicin, 500 mg of neomycin, and 1 million units of polymyxin B) and closure.

surgeons to place the thoracotomy incision through the resected or unresected bed of the fifth or sixth rib, if possible. Incisions placed higher than this, without strict dissection and preservation of the muscle unit, place these future muscle flaps in jeopardy. If possible, the entire length of the latissimus dorsi and serratus anterior muscles should be preserved.

The most common strategy is the intrathoracic transposition of the serratus anterior muscle, usually delivered through a second thoracotomy by removal of a 7- to 10-cm segment of rib at the second or third interspace. The muscle and vascular pedicle can then be passed through this new thoracotomy incision without tethering or kinking the vascular pedicle. Once it is delivered into the pleural space, the muscle can be sutured over the hilar structures to achieve reinforcement and even a sealed, watertight closure of a vital structure such as the bronchial tree. This healthy tissue will protect the primary suture line from contaminating the pleural space.

Timing of closure is critical, and in general, later rather than immediate coverage in a contaminated situation is probably advantageous for obtaining long-term healing. One can look for signs and conditions to help and guide in the timing of the closure, but no firm objective data on which to base this decision exist. In a large chest wall reconstruction practice, one can be uncertain as to the number of patients who have waited too long to proceed to closure, but clearly those who have been closed too early identify themselves with recurrent infection and wound breakdown.

Once a muscle flap has been used for coverage of the vital structures and reinforced closure, it is then necessary to obliterate the pleural space. Two strategies can be employed. Some advocate complete obliteration of the pleural space with all muscle and muscle bulk, including rotation of the latissimus, pectoralis, and serratus musculature. Whereas successful results may be possible with this strategy, in most human anatomy, there simply is not enough muscle bulk available for rotation and transposition into the normal hemithorax to completely obliterate the space. A second strategy can be employed that obviates the need for multiple muscle transposition into the pleural space. The Clagett procedure[30] has been advocated and used for the past 4 decades. After repeated cleaning and wound inspections have been performed and the pleural space is deemed ready to be closed, an antibiotic solution is used to obliterate the pleural space. The antibiotic solution based on a formula of 1 liter of normal saline combined with 80 mg of gentamicin, 500 mg of neomycin, and 1 million units of polymyxin B can be used; 2 to 3 liters of the antibiotic fluid should be available in the operating room for closure.

Because these wounds have often been left open for an extended time, retraction of the skin and subcutaneous tissue of the chest wall flaps, superiorly and inferiorly, often occurs. These tissues can be mobilized again with fairly extensive undermining to allow tension-free skin and subcutaneous tissue closure. The wounds are then closed from anterior and posterior toward the center of the chest with the patient in the lateral decubitus position. Large, permanent sutures are used for initial support of the wound, followed by fine, meticulous dermal closure to obtain a watertight approximation. One must be certain that all air has been removed from the pleural cavity and obliterated as the space is filled with the antibiotic solution. Should there be any question of remaining air, a cross-table lateral radiograph can be taken on full and complete closure of the wound. Once the wound is completely obliterated with the antibiotic solution, the last few central dermal stitches are placed and closed such that the entire pleural space is now obliterated and the skin edges are reapproximated. Petroleum gauze is applied to the suture line. On postoperative day 4, the large approximating permanent sutures are removed to prevent fistulization of the antibiotic solution through the skin. Past review of a Clagett management type of strategy shows a 75% to 80% long-term wound healing success rate.[32] The long-term successful management of the Clagett procedure in the patient with a lethal combination of irradiation and fungal infection after contamination of the pleural space has yet to be reported.

Should the Clagett procedure fail, it is often worthwhile to make a second attempt after a new series of débridement and dressing changes. A secondary attempt achieves another series of healed wounds in approximately four of five patients, such that long-term healing can be obtained in 90% to 93% of all patients. Should repeated failures of the Clagett thoracoplasty occur or should the patient never achieve a pleural space void of contamination, the final option is an open thoracoplasty with long-term dressing changes. Whereas this is a suboptimal situation and a burden on the patient and family, there are occasions when this is the only treatment option. This situation usually occurs in heavily irradiated patients with multiorganism contamination, including highly resistant strains of bacteria or fungal contamination.

In addition to those patients who may require intrathoracic muscle transposition for management of infectious complications or treatment of a bronchopleural fistula, prophylactic placement of an intrathoracic muscle flap to cover a bronchial stump that is at high risk for disruption and breakdown may be used. Intrathoracic muscle transposition may also be indicated for closure, coverage, or reinforcement of repaired esophageal defects as well as for coverage and reinforcement of aortic and cardiac aneurysmal repair. Likewise, intrathoracic muscle flaps can also reinforce the repairs and prosthetic materials in the reconstruction of great vessels. Muscle flaps may be particularly useful when prosthetic material has to be placed in an infected, contaminated, or irradiated bed.

Congenital Defects

Chest wall reconstruction of congenital problems poses physiologic and anatomic as well as aesthetic considerations (see also Chapter 134). These problems include pectus excavatum, pectus carinatum, Poland syndrome, and sternal clefts anteriorly and myelomeningoceles posteriorly. Like the treatment of adult chest wall deformities, the treatment of congenital problems of the chest wall usually requires a multidisciplinary approach including surgeons from other subspecialties, such as cardiothoracic surgery, pediatric surgery, and neurosurgery.

Congenital clefts of the sternum are rare and are often associated with other thoracic, cardiac, or abdominal anomalies. Ravitch[33,34] described 47 patients with sternal clefts in his review of the literature from 1888 to 1977.[33,34] Few reports have been added since this report. It is suggested that sternal clefts result from a failure of maturation or fusion of the mesenchymal elements of the chest, as should normally occur by the eighth week of fetal life. Sternal clefts are classified as complete or incomplete. The incomplete versions are more common. Sternal clefts can also be classified as total sternal clefts, superior sternal clefts, inferior sternal clefts (including pentalogy of Cantrell), and sternal clefts as part of a total ventral cleft.[35-37]

Sternal clefts should be treated in the neonatal period, usually the first month of life. The relative elasticity of the neonatal chest wall usually allows closure of the clefts with sutures. Concomitant anomalies such as ectopia cordis (complete or partial displacement of the heart outside the thoracic cavity) or pentalogy of Cantrell (inferior sternal cleft, abdominal wall defect, diaphragmatic hernia, aplasia of the diaphragmatic pericardia, and cardiac anomalies) require surgical correction and may require multistage procedures.

Patients who are not treated in the neonatal period and present as children or adults are more difficult to treat. The increasing rigidity of the chest wall makes primary suture closure of the cleft difficult if not impossible. Closure of the cleft in this population of patients may decrease chest wall dimensions, thereby compromising the heart, mediastinal structures, and lungs. Therefore, careful reconstruction of the cleft is required in these patients. A variety of procedures for closure of the adult sternal cleft have been described. Reconstruction has been performed by use of split rib grafts, costal cartilage grafts, autologous tibial periosteum grafts, pectoralis muscle transposition, and a variety of prosthetic materials. Sabiston[38] described a technique using multiple bilateral sliding chondrotomies, which has the advantage of preventing collapse of the chest dimensions. Because patients presenting with this defect are rare and the majority of references in the literature are individual reports, few published outcome data are available.

Occurring as often as once in every 300 births, pectus excavatum is one of the most common congenital anomalies.[39,40] The diagnosis is usually established in infancy, with the deformity becoming more pronounced during the adolescent growth years. It remains stable during adulthood. In pectus excavatum, the superior manubrium, the first and second ribs, and the corresponding costal cartilages are normal. The lower three fourths of the sternum has a symmetric depression, extending laterally to the costochondral junctions. The currently accepted etiology is misdirected overgrowth in the costochondral regions. Although it is usually asymptomatic in childhood, symptoms including exercise intolerance, chest pain, palpitations, wheezing, asthma, and increased frequency of respiratory infections can develop by adolescence. Patients may also present in adulthood with aesthetic concerns.

Reconstruction of pectus excavatum in both the pediatric and adult populations continues to challenge surgeons of many different disciplines. Traditionally, the "gold standard" of care for these patients was the Ravitch procedure,[39] or a modification of this procedure, first described in 1949 (Fig. 132-13). The Ravitch procedure basically includes the resection of involved cartilages subperichondrially and division of the xiphoid to permit elevation of the sternum, followed by a posterior transverse osteotomy superiorly and an anterior transverse osteotomy inferiorly. The sternum is fractured outward, and the osteotomies are stabilized with bone wedges. Internal fixation is performed to maintain the correction. The optimal age at repair by this technique is between 12 and 16 years.

A second strategy includes the use of custom-made prostheses, such as those made of soft silicone rubber. A preoperative moulage can be made of the patient with a plaster of Paris type of material placed directly on the skin, which is prepared with a petroleum jelly layer for easy removal of the hardened moulage. The patient and physician can both apply the plaster of Paris to obtain the correction of the contour deformity that the patient is seeking. A mold is made from the moulage, and the custom-made soft silicone implant is then cast. It is useful to have several strong suture tabs as anchor points placed on the periphery of the prosthetic device. Placement is then usually obtained through a small incision, often located in the xiphisternum region.

In 1998, Nuss[40] reported the first minimally invasive repair of pectus excavatum. This original report included 42 patients during a 10-year experience. This technique has become widely accepted by pediatric and thoracic surgeons with multiple series reported in the world literature. The technique includes thoracoscopic visualization, introduction of a convex metallic bar under the sternum, rotation of the bar to correct the pectus deformity, and insertion of a bar stabilizer. Single bars are usually used, although double bars can be used if necessary. The hardware is removed in approximately 2 years after remodeling has occurred. This is a minimally invasive technique that does not require cartilage incision or resection. Modifications of the technique continue to reduce complications. Nuss reported a series of 303 patients with excellent results in 85% and failure in only 1 patient.[41]

Pectus carinatum is a protrusion deformity of the sternum. This anomaly occurs much less commonly than pectus excavatum and is usually not associated with symptoms or abnormal cardiopulmonary function, except in patients with extreme defects. The usual cause for concern of patients and parents is one of cosmesis. The surgical correction of this deformity uses a technique similar to the Ravitch procedure. A subperichondrial resection is performed, and the sternum is repositioned to form an aesthetically pleasing contour. A substernal metallic strut supports the sternum, and wires maintain the position. In women with milder defects, breast augmentation is occasionally performed as an attempt to mask the chest wall deformity.

Although a constellation of hypoplastic chest wall and upper extremity anomalies were reported more than 150 years ago by Lallemand[42] (1826) and Froriep[43] (1839), it is the anatomist Alfred Poland[44] who has been most credited and recognized for the description, and this condition therefore bears his name. Poland syndrome continues to pose reconstructive challenges to contemporary plastic surgeons. The current theory regarding its etiology is hypoplasia of the subclavian artery or its branches, leading to a spectrum of ipsilateral hypoplastic changes in the chest wall and upper extremity. Presentation is usually in childhood or adolescence for aesthetic concerns, as there is little disability associated with this syndrome.

Absence of the sternocostal head of the pectoralis major muscle is always present, but absence of the entire muscle may also occur in this anomaly. The pectoralis minor muscle is usually absent as well. The latissimus dorsi, external oblique, and serratus anterior muscles may be affected as well. Other structures are affected to varying degrees. The most mild instances of Poland syndrome may be marked only by hypoplasia, elevation, and hypopigmentation of the nipple-areola complex. The nipple may be completely absent (athelia), as may the entire breast (amastia). Varying degrees of hypoplasia of the breast are present in more than a third of female patients, and breast asymmetry may be their presenting complaint. Any parietal component of the chest wall, with the exception of skin and the pleurofascial membrane, may be absent, including costochondral cartilage, sternum, and portions of the second, third, and fourth ribs. The chest wall is usually depressed on one side, caused by hypoplasia of ribs and cartilage. Brachysyndactyly may also occur, with varying degrees of hypoplasia of the musculoskeletal components of the upper extremity, foreshortening of the fingers, and congenital fusion with extension contractures of the interphalangeal joints.

Treatments vary and are directed toward the patient's deformity and concerns. If breast asymmetry

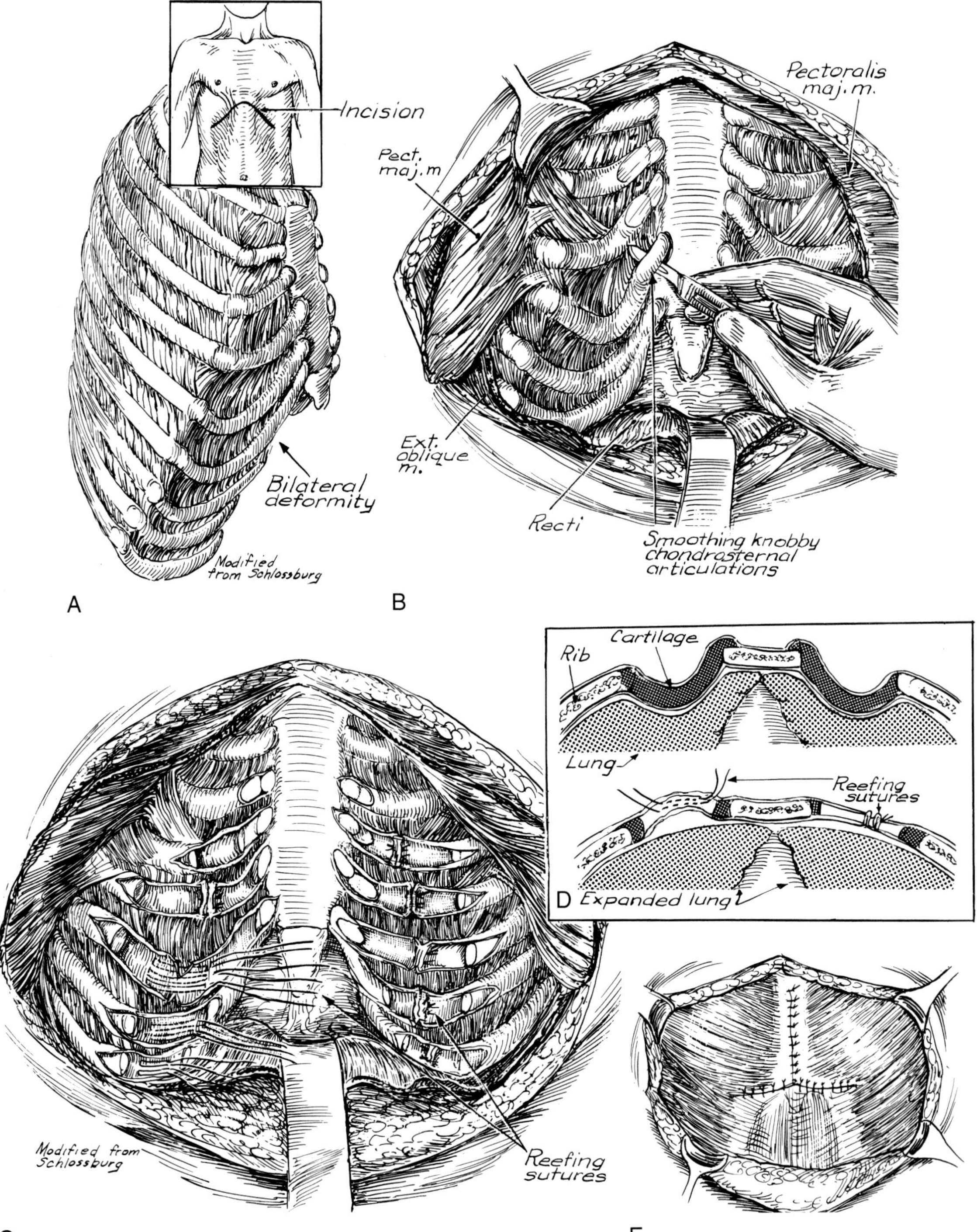

FIGURE 132-13. Ravitch technique for correction of chondrogladiolar type of pectus carinatum. *A* and *B,* A transverse curvilinear incision is used to elevate flaps down to and including the pectoralis muscles. The rectus muscle attachments are divided. Cartilaginous irregularities and knobby projections of the chondrosternal articulations are sharply smoothed out. *C* and *D,* The posteriorly curved, deformed cartilage is resected subperichondrially. The redundant perichondrium is tightened by mattress silk reefing sutures so that the new cartilage will grow in a straight line from the ribs to the sternum. *E,* The pectoralis muscles and recti are reattached to the sternum. (After Ravitch MM: General Thoracic Surgery. Philadelphia, Lea & Febiger, 1972.)

is the only visible manifestation, insertion of a unilateral breast prosthesis or a contralateral breast reduction or mastopexy may be all the required treatment. Concave contours of the chest wall may be corrected with a transaxillary transfer of an ipsilateral pedicled latissimus dorsi muscle flap. The muscle is fixed to the chest wall, and attempts are made to establish an aesthetically pleasing anterior axillary fold. A submuscular breast prosthesis can be added in a female patient. Large contour deformities may not be adequately treated with muscle transfer alone. In these patients, it may be prudent to use a custom-made chest wall prosthesis or alloplastic material to help fill the defect.

More difficult is the treatment of the child with severe aplasia of the chest wall. This can best be accomplished with a two-stage procedure. The first stage addresses repair of the rib defect to protect the underlying thoracic structures. After puberty, a muscle flap transfer can be performed, with an implant in female patients, for formation of a more aesthetically pleasing chest contour.

Myelomeningocele is a congenital disorder that can have devastating consequences if it is not treated adequately. As with other congenital disorders, a multidisciplinary approach is required. The child with myelomeningocele has suffered from an embryologic failure of mesoderm migration, resulting in malformation of the meninges, posterior spine, and overlying skeletal and soft tissues. The meninges and neural elements are contained within the spina bifida cystic herniation. Motor and sensory deficits are the norm, and other potential sequelae include hydrocephalus, paraplegia, incontinence, and sexual dysfunction.

The neurosurgeon must achieve the first treatment goal of closure of the spinal defect and ventricular shunting of cerebrospinal fluid to prevent or correct meningitis, ventriculitis, and hydrocephalus. After the spinal canal and exposed neural elements are securely covered, soft tissue coverage must be ensured by the plastic surgeon. The majority (approximately 75%) of myelomeningocele soft tissue defects can be managed by simple undermining and primary wound closure. Larger defects need more tissue and may require a combination of techniques to ensure a well-healed and stable wound. A variety of techniques and procedures have been described to achieve this goal, including but not limited to skin grafting, cutaneous rotation flaps, double rhomboid Z-plasties, lateral relaxing incisions with bipedicle flap closure, tissue expansion, and a variety of muscle flaps, pedicled and free, alone and in combination. Treatment must be individualized and tailored according to the patient's overall health and the size and character of the soft tissue defect.

Skin grafts do not provide durable cover for the underlying meninges and neural elements and are therefore not often used. Bipedicled musculocutaneous flap closure, when the latissimus dorsi muscles are incorporated, is an attractive and relatively straightforward technique for treatment of these wounds.[45] Mobilization is begun in the midline and is performed in a plane deep to the bilateral latissimus dorsi muscles. This is continued laterally until the wound edges approximate without tension or until the posterior axillary line is reached. If the wound edges still cannot be approximated tension free, a relaxing incision is made in the posterior axillary line. The contralateral posterior axillary line may also be incised, if necessary. This technique is usually adequate to provide enough well-vascularized soft tissue to close almost all myelomeningocele defects with a stable three-layered (muscle, subcutaneous tissue, skin) closure. Alternatively, other authors have suggested a bilateral latissimus dorsi-gluteus maximus musculocutaneous flap without relaxing incisions.[46] This procedure takes advantage of the anastomotic plexus that exists between the skin overlying the gluteus maximus and the latissimus dorsi muscles, without requiring relaxing incisions. The authors reported on a series of 34 patients using a one-stage technique of dural closure and soft tissue coverage with a bilateral latissimus dorsi-gluteus maximus musculocutaneous flap.[47]

Another rare congenital clinical entity that requires surgical reconstruction is agenesis of the diaphragm. Diaphragmatic agenesis is a rare and potentially lethal clinical situation. Reconstruction of the defect with a synthetic patch in the neonatal period is usually adequate for separation of the thoracic and abdominal cavities; however, postoperative early and late complications, such as recurrent hernia, restrictive pulmonary disease, and chest wall deformity, are common after this procedure.

An alternative or additional technique includes reconstruction of the defect with a reversed latissimus dorsi muscle flap based on the intercostal and paraspinous vessels. This procedure is often performed in a staged fashion after failure of a synthetic patch reconstruction. Neuroanastomosis of the phrenic and thoracodorsal nerves potentially allows the neodiaphragm to function in concert with the remnant native diaphragm. Several series have reported growth of the muscle flap with the child, improvement of chest wall deformity and restrictive pulmonary disease, adequate separation of thoracic and abdominal cavities, and lack of paradoxical chest motion.[48-51]

Posterior Midline Chest Wall Defects

Posterior chest wall defects, especially those approximating the midline of the trunk, provide significant surgical challenges. Useful muscle flaps for coverage include the trapezius and the latissimus dorsi. Indications for coverage in this region include trauma, tumor resection, and congenital anomalies such as spina bifida. Traumatic injury and tumor extirpation, especially with the addition of radiation therapy, may preclude the use of muscle flaps for coverage. In patients with inadequate posterior musculature, the rectus abdominis muscle can occasionally be used for coverage of posterior defects. Designed as a transverse rectus abdominis musculocutaneous (TRAM) flap or vertical rectus abdominis musculocutaneous flap, retroperitoneal tunneling or direct transabdominal transfer with tunneling through the retroperitoneum may adequately deliver enough soft tissue to the posterior defect to achieve a stable wound closure.

An alternative to the rectus abdominis muscle flap is the greater omentum (see Fig. 132-11). The omentum has proved to be useful as a salvage procedure for these types of problems. Five patients have been successfully managed by the authors, for the indications of both traumatic injury and tumor extirpation with exposed hardware, with pull-through of the omentum based on the right gastroepiploic artery through a tunnel in the retroperitoneum. Depending on the location of the defect on the back, one can proceed posteriorly through a tunnel and through the back of the chest wall, either above or below the right kidney. Care must be taken to avoid injury to the renal vein, the adrenal vein, and the adrenal gland itself. Once the omentum is passed through, it can be further isolated on its vascular supply and wrapped around exposed hardware (Fig. 132-14; see also Color Plate 132-2). Obviously contaminated open wounds with visible hardware have been successfully managed with this strategy. Once the hardware is wrapped and the defects have been obliterated and filled with the omentum, it is carefully dressed much in the same way that it is managed with sternal wounds and radiation necrosis. After several days of dressing changes, the omentum has usually granulated enough to allow skin grafting.

Problems with this technique have included wound dressing management during the 72 to 96 hours

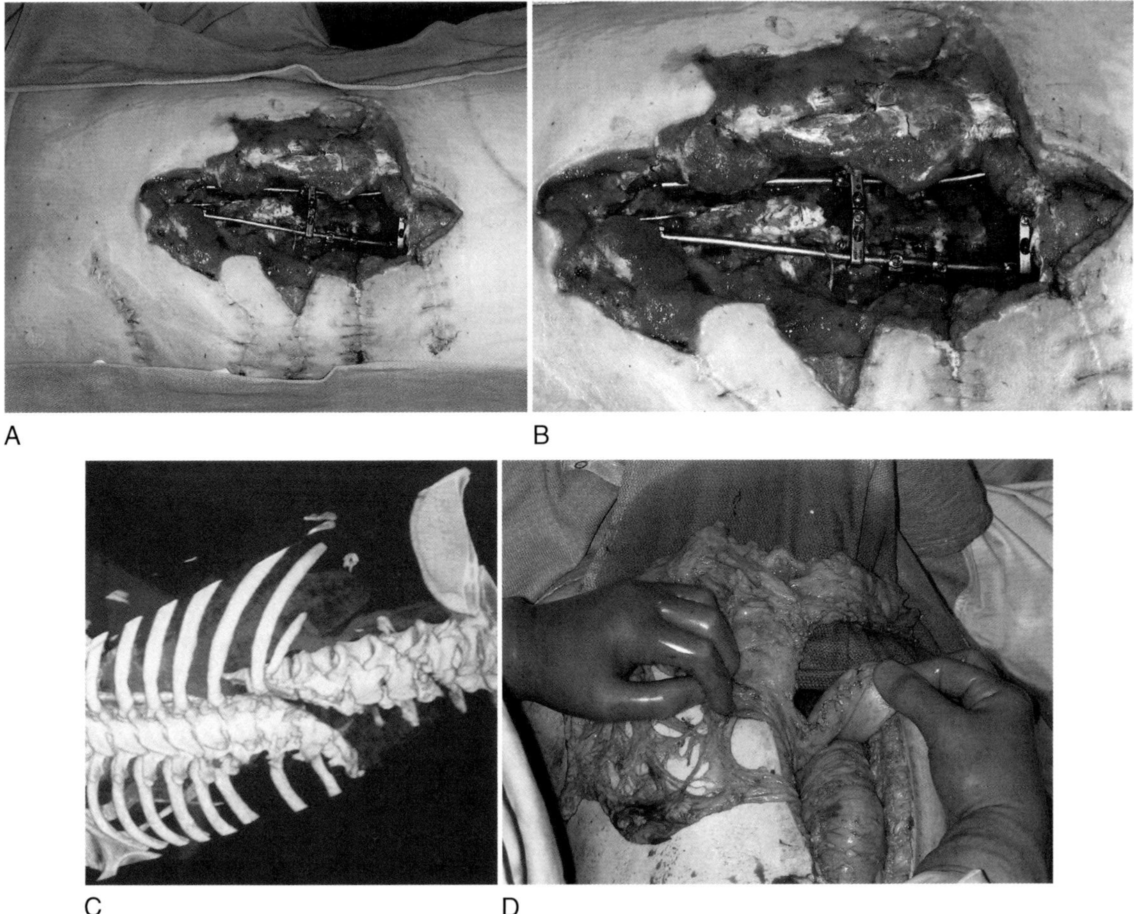

FIGURE 132-14. Coverage of exposed hardware by omental flap (see also Color Plate 132-2). *A*, Exposed Harrington rods after personal watercraft-boat collision. *B*, Close-up view. *C*, CT scan of magnitude of injury. *D*, Omentum harvested on right gastroepiploic artery.

Continued

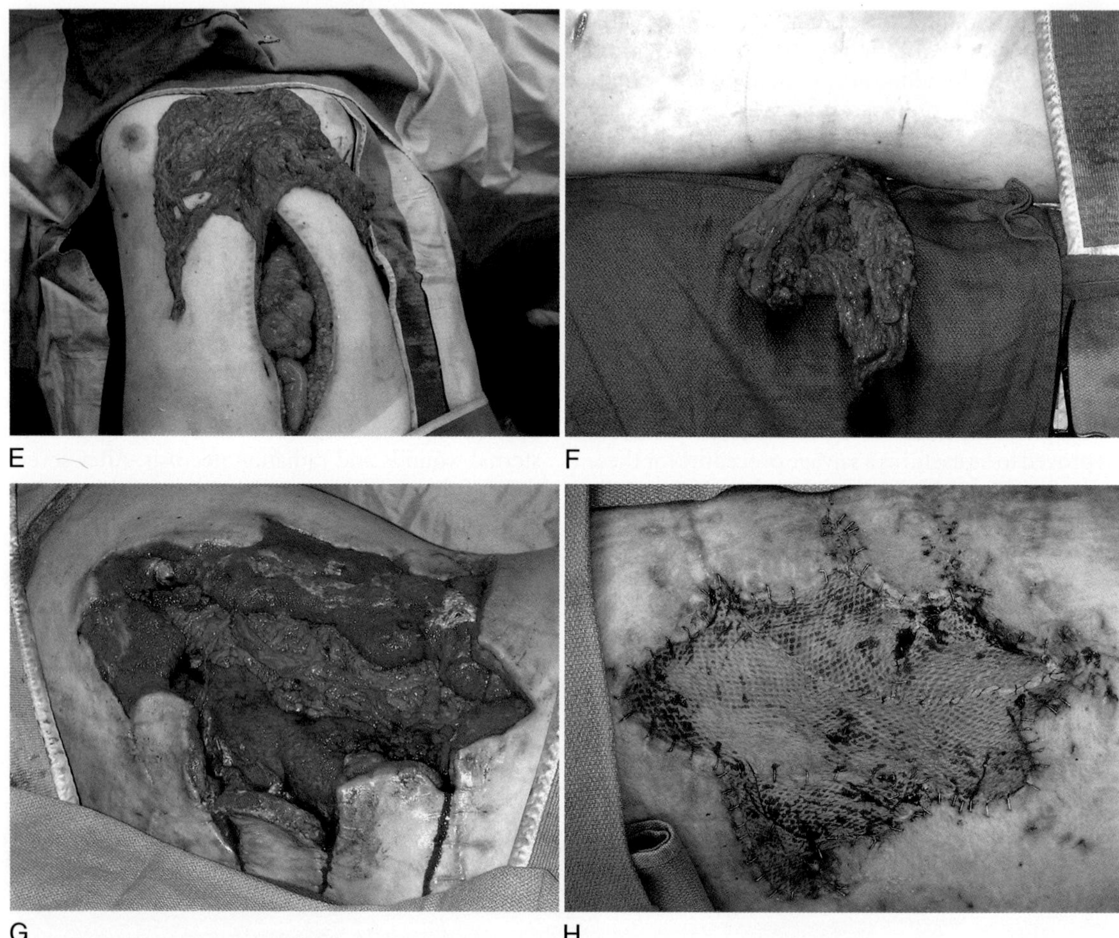

FIGURE 132-14, cont'd. *E,* Omentum fully mobilized. *F,* Omentum is passed through the retroperitoneum over right adrenal gland. *G,* Coverage of hardware with omental flap. *H,* Split-thickness skin graft at 72 hours after procedure.

required for an adequate bed to accept a skin graft. Traditionally, this has been managed with a large, sterile, sticky plastic operating room drape over the entire wound (Fig. 132-15). This drape can be used to cover a saline-soaked gauze sponge that is in contact with the omentum. On the first postoperative day for dressing changes, the sterile drape is cut in the middle, and the dressing is changed to a Nu-Gel type of dressing, which is then changed on a daily basis. The Nu-Gel can provide excellent coverage and maintenance of an environment that allows proliferation of granulation tissue from the omentum. It is also somewhat hydrophilic so that the wound does not become unduly macerated or soggy.

The omentum has been treated with the vacuum-assisted closure (VAC) system to decompress fluid from the often edematous omental flap and help generate a bed of granulation tissue. After the omentum is inset into the wound, it is covered with a sheet of petroleum gauze and the wound VAC with settings of 75 mm Hg intermittent suction. The VAC is changed every 48 hours during the early postoperative period (approximately 5 to 7 days). After this period, a healthy bed of granulation tissue is usually observed on the omentum. This time also allows the surgeon to débride nonviable portions of omentum as necessary and to recontour and reinset the omental flap as needed. A meshed split-thickness skin graft is then applied and covered with a light petroleum dressing and a new VAC sponge for 3 to 5 days at 75 mm Hg of continuous suction. In the authors' limited experience with this technique, we have had success with both the omentum and the skin graft (Fig. 132-16).

SUMMARY

Chest wall reconstruction continues to provide a formidable challenge to the plastic surgeon. Prolonged

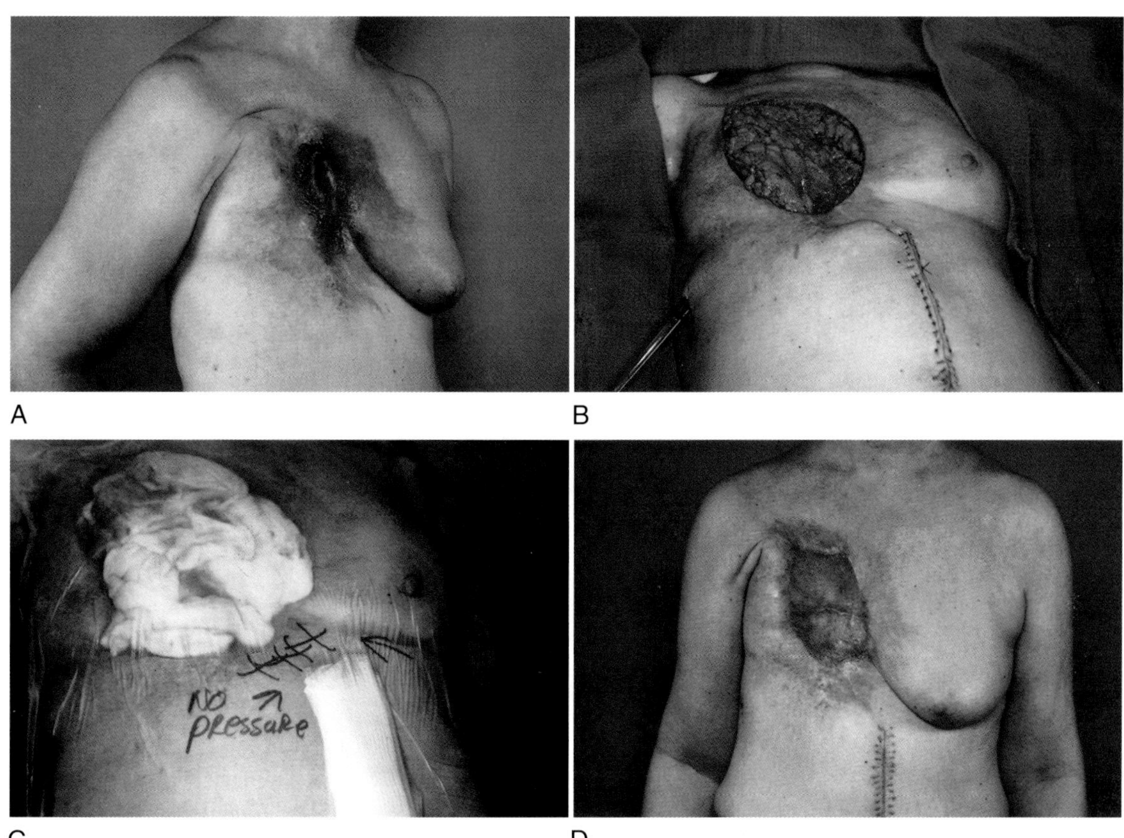

FIGURE 132-15. Omental flap for coverage of anterior chest wall. *A,* Radiation necrosis of right anterior chest wall. *B,* Omental flap transposition. *C,* Dressing of wound should not exert pressure. *D,* Postoperative result.

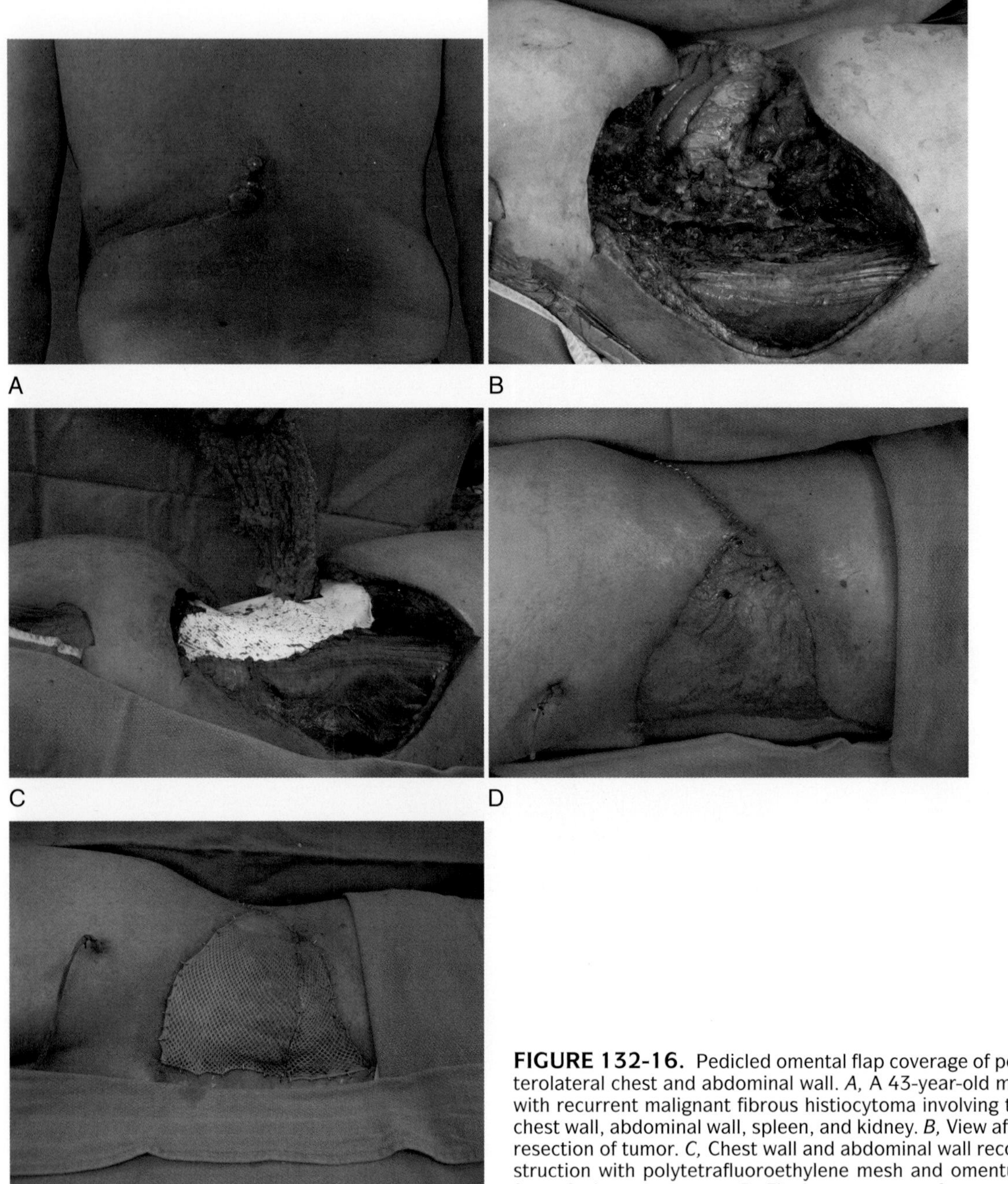

FIGURE 132-16. Pedicled omental flap coverage of posterolateral chest and abdominal wall. *A,* A 43-year-old man with recurrent malignant fibrous histiocytoma involving the chest wall, abdominal wall, spleen, and kidney. *B,* View after resection of tumor. *C,* Chest wall and abdominal wall reconstruction with polytetrafluoroethylene mesh and omentum for soft tissue coverage. *D,* Final appearance of omentum before skin grafting. *E,* Skin-grafted omental flap.

hospitalization of 2 to 3 weeks is often necessary, and patients at centers with large volumes of experience often undergo on average at least two operations before final closure. Multiple reviews, however, have demonstrated that this problem has been successfully treated through the past 2 to 3 decades. Eighty-five percent of patients alive 30 days after operation had a healed asymptomatic chest wall, and most deaths in patients undergoing chest wall reconstruction result from the underlying disease process, usually related to malignant neoplasia.[15]

REFERENCES

1. Parham F: Thoracic resection for tumors growing from the bony wall of the chest. Trans South Surg Gynecol Assoc 1898;11:223.
2. Fell GE: Forced respiration. JAMA 1891;16:325.

3. O'Dwyer J: Fifty cases of croup in private practice treated by intubation of the larynx, with a description of the method and of the dangers incident thereto. Med Rec 1887;32:557.
4. Graham EA, Singer JJ: Successful removal of an entire lung for carcinoma of the bronchus. JAMA 1933;101:1371.
5. Watson WL, James AG: Fascia lata grafts for the chest wall defects. J Thorac Surg 1947;16:399.
6. Tansini I: Sopra il mio nuovo processo di amputazione della mammella. Gazz Med Ital 1906;57:141.
7. Campbell DA: Reconstruction of the anterior thoracic wall. J Thorac Surg 1950;19:456.
8. Deschamps C, et al: Early and long-term results of prosthetic chest wall reconstruction. J Thorac Cardiovasc Surg 1999;117: 588-591, discussion 591-592.
9. Arnold PG, Pairolero PC: Chest-wall reconstruction: an account of 500 consecutive patients. Plast Reconstr Surg 1996;98:804-810.
10. Cordeiro PG, Santamaria E, Hidalgo D: The role of microsurgery in reconstruction of oncologic chest wall defects. Plast Reconstr Surg 2001;108:1924-1930.
11. Jurkiewicz MJ, Arnold PG: The omentum: an account of its use in the reconstruction of the chest wall. Ann Surg 1977;185: 548-554.
12. Hultman CS, et al: Thoracic reconstruction with the omentum: indications, complications, and results. Ann Plast Surg 2001;46:242-249.
13. Arnold PG, Hartrampf CR, Jurkiewicz MJ: One-stage reconstruction of the breast, using the transposed greater omentum. Case report. Plast Reconstr Surg 1976;57:520-522.
14. Zhang QX, et al: Vascular endothelial growth factor is the major angiogenic factor in omentum: mechanism of the omentum-mediated angiogenesis. J Surg Res 1997;67:147-154.
15. Mansour KA, et al: Chest wall resections and reconstruction: a 25-year experience. Ann Thorac Surg 2002;73:1720-1725, discussion 1725-1726.
16. Pairolero PC, Arnold PG: Thoracic wall defects: surgical management of 205 consecutive patients. Mayo Clin Proc 1986; 61:557-563.
17. Pairolero PC, Arnold PG: Chest wall tumors. Experience with 100 consecutive patients. J Thorac Cardiovasc Surg 1985;90: 367-372.
18. Arnold PG, Pairolero PC: Chest wall reconstruction. Experience with 100 consecutive patients. Ann Surg 1984;199:725-732.
19. Seyfer A: Chest wall reconstruction. In Achauer BM, Eriksson E, Guyuron B, et al, eds: Plastic Surgery: Indications, Operations, and Outcomes. St. Louis, Mosby, 2000:547-562.
20. Risk factors for deep sternal wound infection after sternotomy: a prospective, multicenter study. J Thorac Cardiovasc Surg 1996;111:1200-1207.
21. Hugo NE, et al: Single-stage management of 74 consecutive sternal wound complications with pectoralis major myocutaneous advancement flaps. Plast Reconstr Surg 1994;93:1433-1441.
22. Golosow LM, et al: Risk factors for predicting surgical salvage of sternal wound-healing complications. Ann Plast Surg 1999;43:30-35.
23. Stahle E, et al: Sternal wound complications—incidence, microbiology and risk factors. Eur J Cardiothorac Surg 1997;11:1146-1153.
24. McDonald WS, et al: Risk factors for median sternotomy dehiscence in cardiac surgery. South Med J 1989;82:1361-1364.
25. Stahl KD, et al: Association of sternal wound infection with parasternal muscle sutures. J Card Surg 2002;17:498-501.
26. Lytle BW, et al: Perioperative risk of bilateral internal mammary artery grafting: analysis of 500 cases from 1971 to 1984. Circulation 1986;74(pt 2):III37-41.
27. Cosgrove DM, et al: Does bilateral internal mammary artery grafting increase surgical risk? J Thorac Cardiovasc Surg 1988;95:850-856.
28. Nahai F, et al: Primary treatment of the infected sternotomy wound with muscle flaps: a review of 211 consecutive cases. Plast Reconstr Surg 1989;84:434-441.
29. Nahai F, et al: Pectoralis major muscle turnover flaps for closure of the infected sternotomy wound with preservation of form and function. Plast Reconstr Surg 1982;70:471-474.
30. Clagett OT, Geraci JE: A procedure for the management of post-pneumonectomy empyema. J Thorac Cardiovasc Surg 1963; 45:141-145.
31. Stafford EG, Clagett OT: Postpneumonectomy emphema. Neomycin instillation and definitive closure. J Thorac Cardiovasc Surg 1972;63:771-775.
32. Arnold PG, Pairolero PC: Intrathoracic muscle flaps: a 10-year experience in the management of life-threatening infections. Plast Reconstr Surg 1989;84:92-98, discussion 99.
33. Ravitch M: Congenital Deformities of the Chest Wall and Their Operative Correction. Philadelphia, WB Saunders, 1977.
34. Ravitch M: Congenital deformities of the chest wall. In Ravitch M, ed: Pediatric Surgery. Chicago, Year Book, 1977: 406.
35. Morales JM, et al: Ectopia cordis and other midline defects. Ann Thorac Surg 2000;70:111-114.
36. de Campos JR, et al: Repair of congenital sternal cleft in infants and adolescents. Ann Thorac Surg 1998;66:1151-1154.
37. Daum R, Zachariou Z: Total and superior sternal clefts in newborns: a simple technique for surgical correction. J Pediatr Surg 1999;34:408-411.
38. Sabiston D: The surgical management of congenital bifid sternum with partial ectopia cordis. J Thorac Surg 1958;35:118-122.
39. Ravitch M: The operative treatment of pectus excavatum. Ann Surg 1949;129:429-444.
40. Nuss D, et al: A 10-year review of a minimally invasive technique for the correction of pectus excavatum. J Pediatr Surg 1998;33:545-552.
41. Croitoru DP, et al: Experience and modification update for the minimally invasive Nuss technique for pectus excavatum repair in 303 patients. J Pediatr Surg 2002;37:437-445.
42. Lallemand L: Absence de trois cotes simulant un enfoncement accidentel. Ephemerides Medicales de Montpelier 1826;1:144-147.
43. Froriep R: Beobachtung eines Falles von Mangel der Brustdruse. Notizen Gebiete Natur Heilkunde 1839;10:9-14.
44. Poland A: Deficiency of the pectoral muscles. Guys Hosp Rep 1841;6:191-193.
45. Desprez JD, Kiehn CL, Eckstein W: Closure of large meningomyelocele defects by composite skin muscle flaps. Plast Reconstr Surg 1971;47:234-238.
46. Ramasastry SS, Cohen M: Soft tissue closure and plastic surgical aspects of large open myelomeningoceles. Neurosurg Clin North Am 1995;6:279-291.
47. Ramirez OM, et al: A new surgical approach to closure of large lumbosacral meningomyelocele defects. Plast Reconstr Surg 1987;80:799-809.
48. Samarakkody U, Klassen M, Nye B: Reconstruction of congenital agenesis of hemidiaphragm by combined reverse latissimus dorsi and serratus anterior muscle flaps. J Pediatr Surg 2001;36:1637-1640.
49. Lee SL, Poulos ND, Greenholz SK: Staged reconstruction of large congenital diaphragmatic defects with synthetic patch followed by reverse latissimus dorsi muscle. J Pediatr Surg 2002;37:367-370.
50. Whetzel TP, Stokes RB, Greenholz SK, Saunders CJ: Reconstruction of the toddler diaphragm in severe anterolateral congenital diaphragmatic hernia with the reverse latissimus dorsi flap. Ann Plast Surg 1997;39:615-619.
51. Wallace CA, Roden JS: Reverse, innervated latissimus dorsi flap reconstruction of congenital diaphragmatic absence. Plast Reconstr Surg 1995;96:761-769.

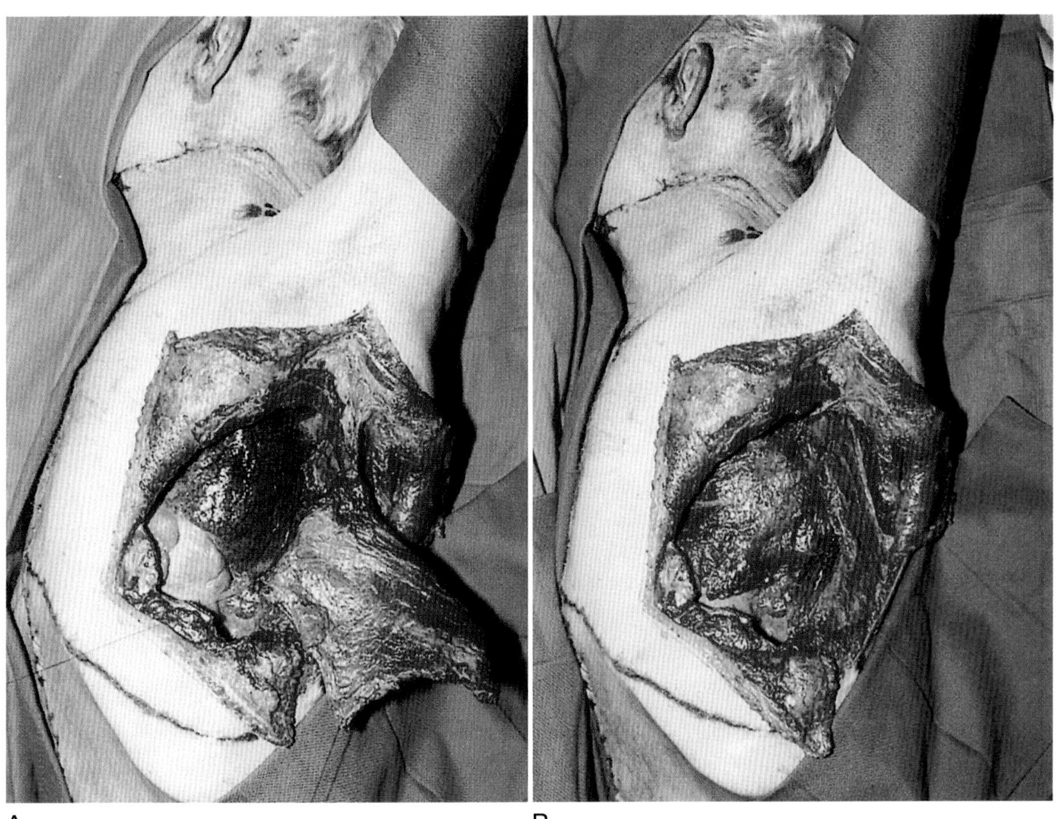

A B

COLOR PLATE 132-1. Latissimus dorsi–serratus anterior muscle coverage. The serratus anterior can be used both as a solo muscle flap for lateral chest wall defects and in combination with the latissimus muscle to add further bulk and surface coverage as a combined latissimus dorsi–serratus anterior muscle unit. *A,* Intrathoracic placement of serratus flap. (Note: resection of lateral chest wall demonstrates flap position.) *B,* Flap inset. (From Mathes SJ, Nahai F: Reconstructive Surgery: Principles, Anatomy, and Technique. New York, Churchill Livingstone, 1997:488-489.)

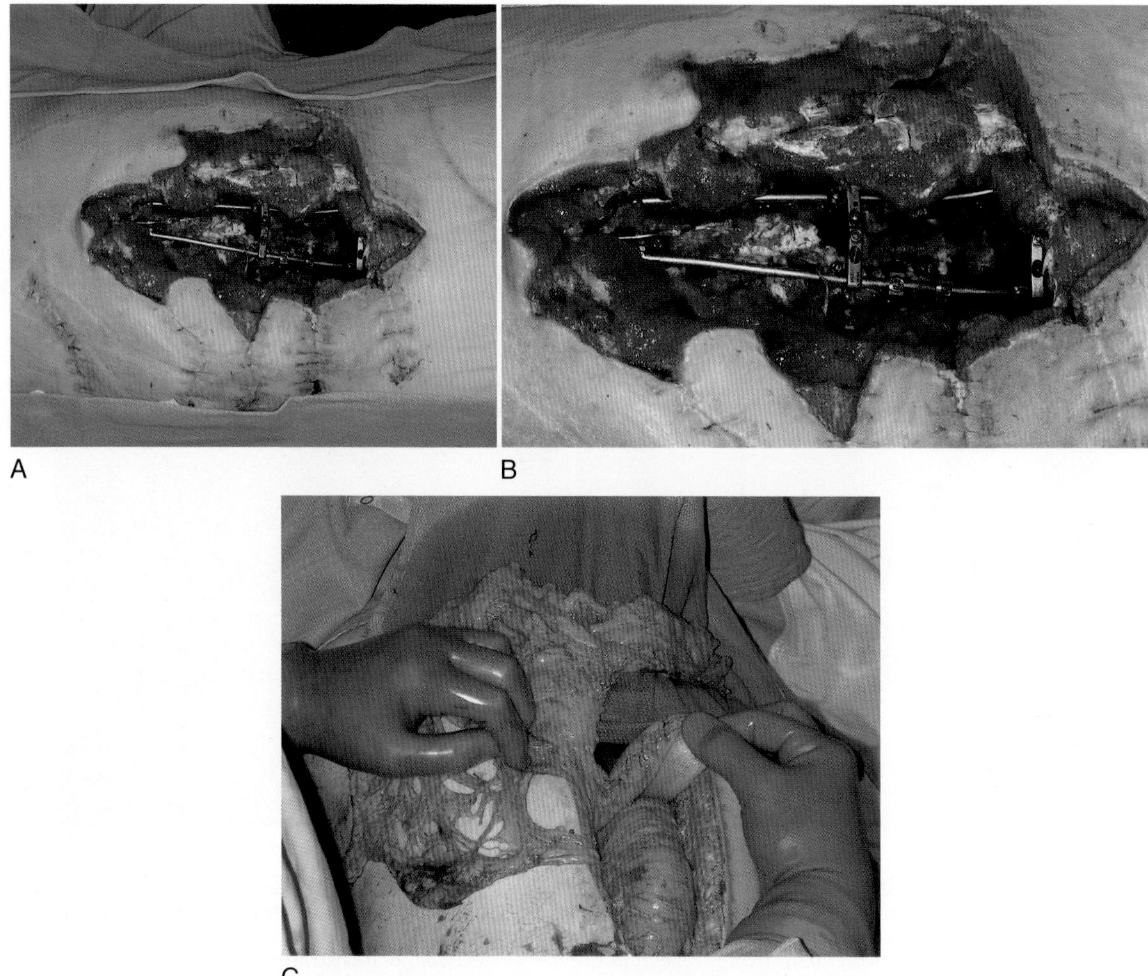

COLOR PLATE 132-2. Coverage of exposed hardware by omental flap. *A,* Exposed Harrington rods after personal watercraft-boat collision. *B,* Close-up view. *C,* Omentum harvested on right gastroepiploic artery.

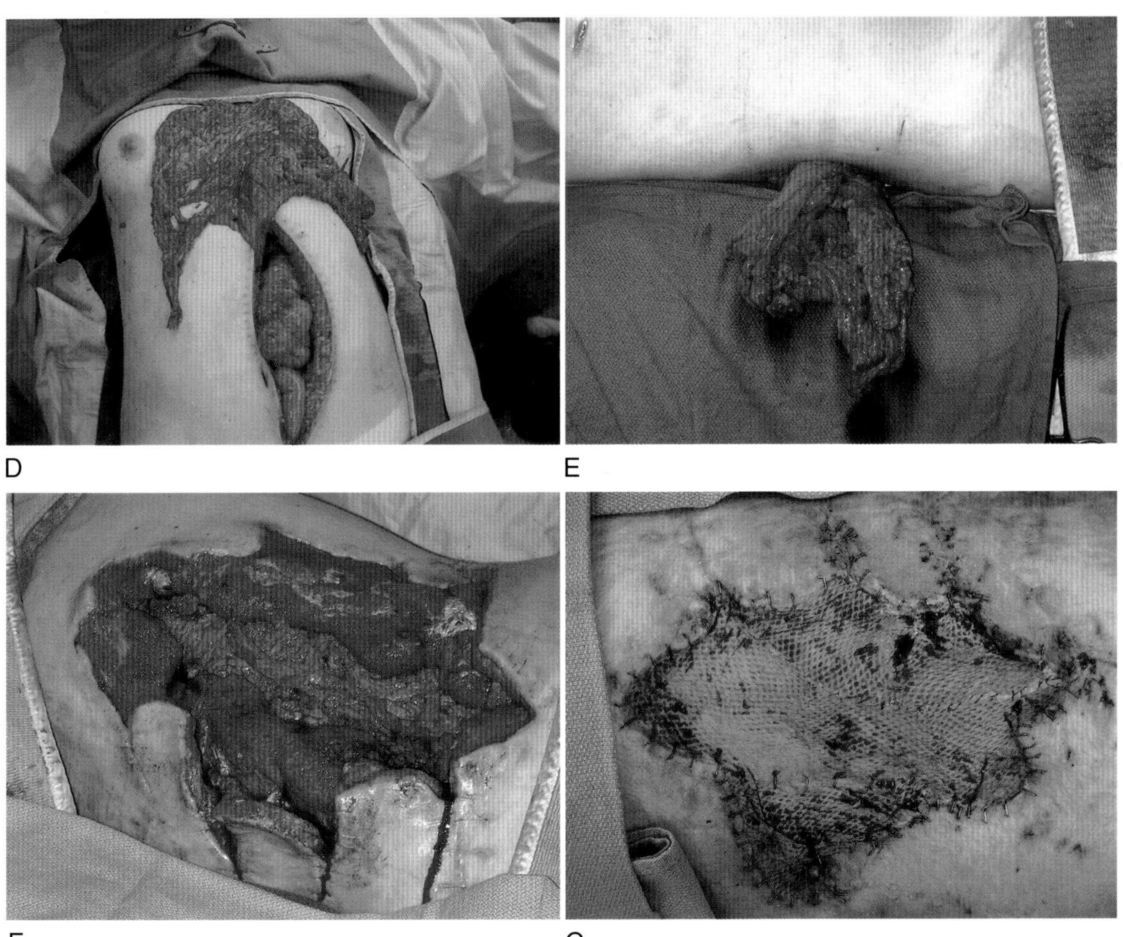

COLOR PLATE 132-2, cont'd. *D,* Omentum fully mobilized. *E,* Omentum is passed through the retroperitoneum over right adrenal gland. *F,* Coverage of hardware with omental flap. *G,* Split-thickness skin graft at 72 hours after procedure.

CHAPTER

133 Reconstruction of the Back

Julius W. Few, MD, FACS ✦ Foad Nahai, MD, FACS

The reconstruction of posterior trunk defects requires a systematic diagnosis and treatment plan. The back is divided into three anatomic areas for reconstruction, the upper, middle, and lower thirds (Fig. 133-1). The upper third extends from the base of the neck to the midscapula; the middle third extends from the midscapula to the waistline, and the lower third from the waist to the sacrococcygeal region. Each area has unique anatomic challenges with preferred local flap options.

Posterior trunk wounds are classified as complex or simple. In a previously reported series, complex wounds have been characterized by one or more of the following: large surface area (>200 cm^2), history of radiation therapy, history of complex infection, exposed hardware, osteodestructive process, spinal instability, and multiple failed attempts at reconstruction.[1]

The underlying pathologic process and systemic condition of the patient are as important as the location of the defect. The patient's past history, especially previous surgical treatment, should be noted. The importance of previous radiation therapy, infection, orthopedic hardware, and status of the spinal column cannot be overstated.

Midline back defects represent the majority of back wounds and serve as the focus for this discussion. However, the following principles can be applied to all back wounds, midline and elsewhere.

RECONSTRUCTION OF NONCOMPLEX BACK WOUNDS

The simplest procedure for effectively closing a back wound should be chosen. Unfortunately, the most effective and reliable technique may involve more effort than a less complex solution, which will only temporize the problem. The reconstructive ladder is a useful guide with certain considerations. Casas and Lewis[2] have shown that it is ideal to obtain two-layered closure for midline back defects. One should consider the use of skin grafting cautiously, with a primary emphasis on closure of donor site defects. A variety of local flaps are available for simple wounds, based on the anatomic location of the given defect. Tissue expansion is of value in the properly selected, motivated patient with a simple defect.

Upper Third

Reconstruction of the upper back requires analysis of the surrounding skin and underlying musculature. The anatomy and reconstructive application of the trapezius (type II circulation), latissimus dorsi (type V circulation), and paraspinous musculature (type IV circulation) are well described.[3] The trapezius is preferred for defects that involve the cephalad portion of the upper third (Fig. 133-2). The latissimus is ideal for the reconstruction of the caudal portion of the upper third (Fig. 133-3). Other local flaps include fasciocutaneous flaps, axial or random based, for smaller, nonmidline simple defects. The use of random flaps with a length-to-width ratio greater than 2:1 may lead to distal wound complications.

Middle Third

The latissimus dorsi, with a type V pattern of circulation, is the ideal source for reconstruction of the middle third (see Fig. 133-3). The musculocutaneous flap based

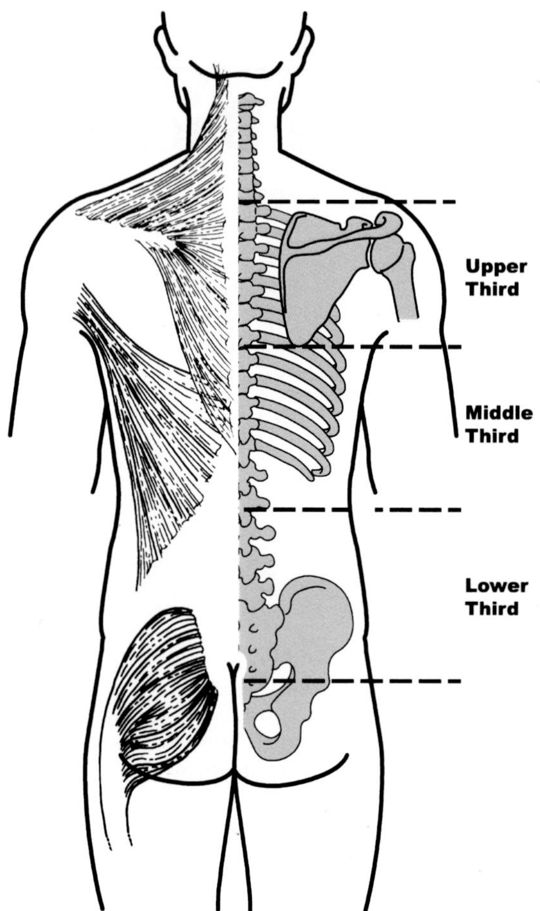

FIGURE 133-1. Anatomic division of the back into upper, lower, and middle thirds.

on the thoracodorsal laterally or the paraspinal perforator medially is a versatile and reliable means of transfer. The use of the musculocutaneous flap has the advantage of providing volume to obliterate a potential dead space in addition to providing skin coverage. The musculocutaneous perforator system is extremely robust and reliable. The latissimus can also be the basis for fasciocutaneous flap circulation in patients in whom dead space obliteration is not required. Tissue expansion may be added for staged reconstruction to minimize the donor site and may be used in patients in whom a skin graft would otherwise be required. For simple defects, tissue expansion or skin grafting is rarely required.

The latissimus is an expendable muscle in patients with intact synergistic shoulder girdle muscles. In patients with contralateral shoulder disease, extreme caution must be exercised to prevent disability. In such patients, segmental transposition of a reversed musculocutaneous flap will preserve function.[3]

Lower Third

In addition to the paraspinous musculature, the lower third is occupied by the latissimus (caudal portion of muscle) and gluteal muscles.[4] The lower third represents a number of unique anatomic challenges that are important in considering reconstruction. The lower third is an area that is exposed to the greatest amount of potential shear stress. In addition, this is an area requiring significant amounts of dynamic motion. In planning flap closure, one must design a flap that is larger than expected to accommodate the local stress.

The gluteus is the first choice for the majority of lower third reconstruction. It has a reliable type III circulation, with significant versatility.[4] The gluteus offers moderate donor site morbidity without significantly impairing ambulation (Fig. 133-4).

The transverse back flap is useful for coverage of the noncomplex wound of the lower third (Fig. 133-5). Transverse back flaps represent a fasciocutaneous flap with type C circulation pattern.[5] This flap can provide a surface of 20 × 7 cm. A preexisting incision at the lower midline is an absolute contraindication to the transverse back flap. The donor site requires skin grafting. The lateral extent of the flap should be limited to the posterior axillary line for optimal distal flap survival. Patients must be kept in a prone position in the early postoperative period to preserve circulation.

RECONSTRUCTION OF COMPLEX BACK WOUNDS

By definition, complex wounds include congenital or acquired defects that have been subject to irradiation, failed attempts at conservative surgical intervention, local infection, spinal instability, or massive secondary wounds. The approach to these patients requires an understanding of the underlying pathologic process and the most likely etiology. The surgical team must then be prepared to stabilize or to reverse local and systemic disease.

Pathophysiologic Considerations

The treatment of complex back wounds is based on the results of experimental work that examined the role of various types of flaps relative to the local environment. Factors considered included response to bacterial inoculation, oxygen and leukocyte delivery, osteomyelitis, vascularity, radiation damage, and prosthetic exposure.

In 1967, Krizek, Robson, and Kho[6] observed that successful delayed wound closure could be obtained with quantitative cultures of less than 10 organisms/g of tissue. Additional studies by Chang and Mathes[7] demonstrated the advantages of muscle versus random

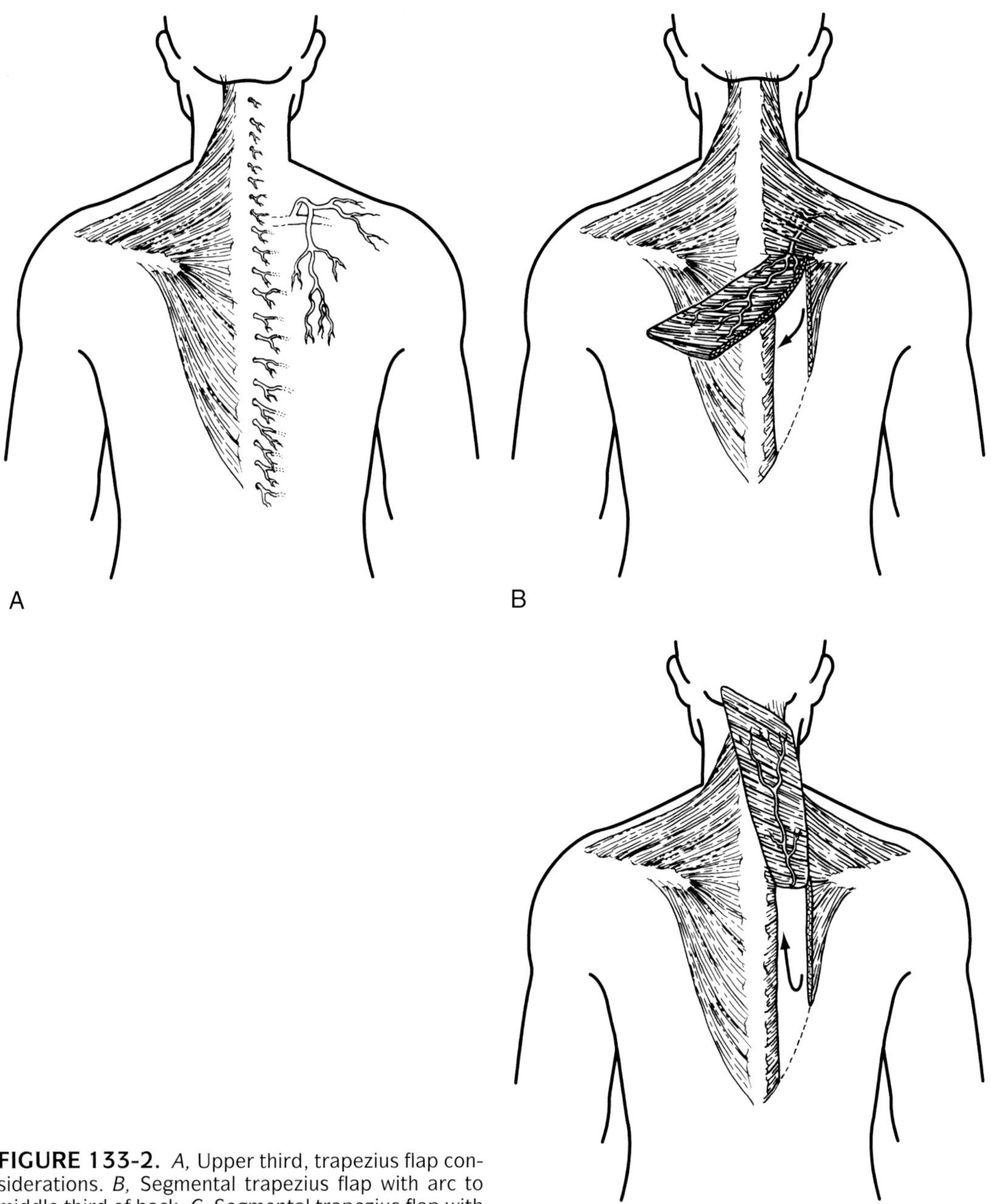

FIGURE 133-2. *A,* Upper third, trapezius flap considerations. *B,* Segmental trapezius flap with arc to middle third of back. *C,* Segmental trapezius flap with arc to upper third of back.

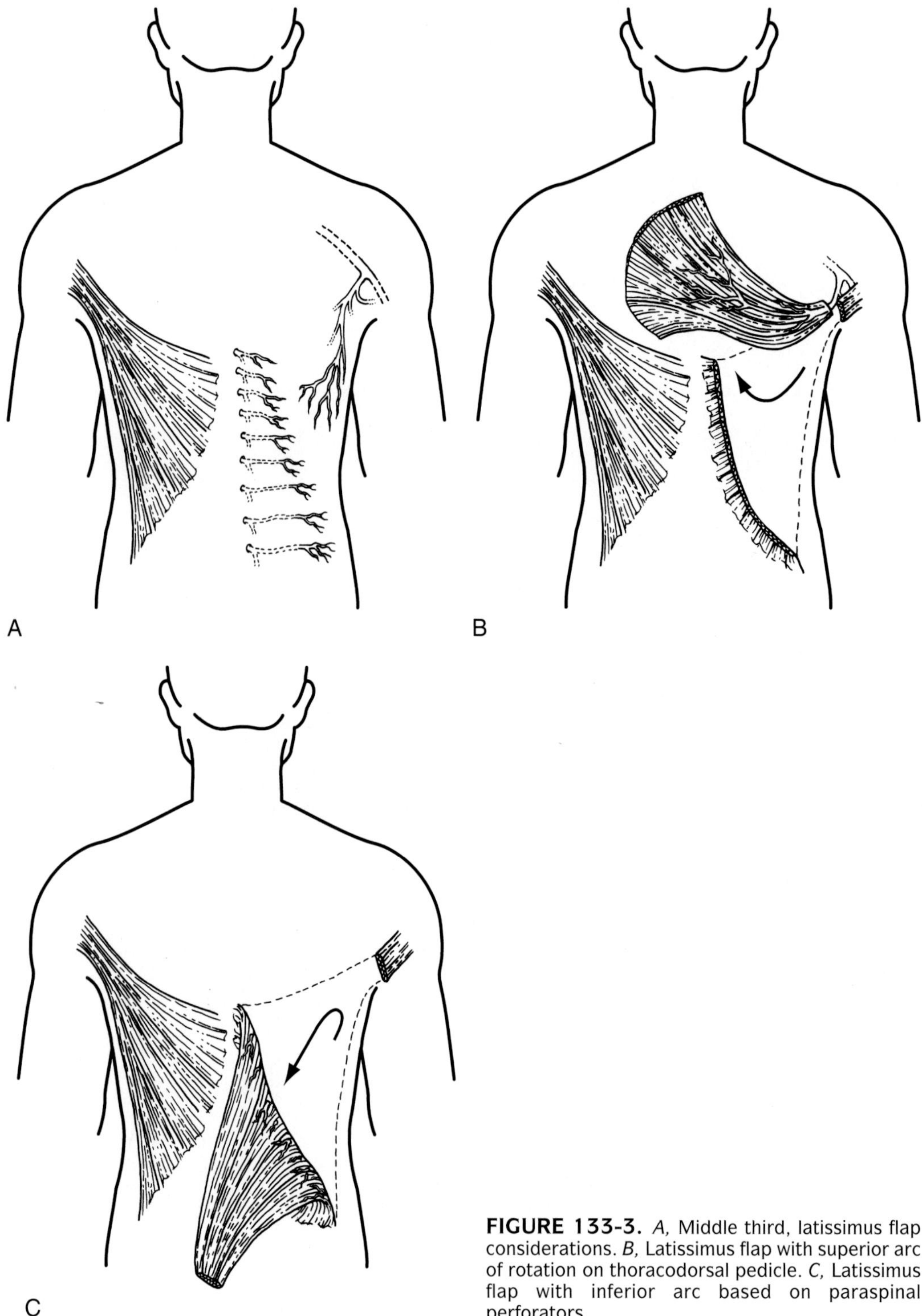

FIGURE 133-3. *A,* Middle third, latissimus flap considerations. *B,* Latissimus flap with superior arc of rotation on thoracodorsal pedicle. *C,* Latissimus flap with inferior arc based on paraspinal perforators.

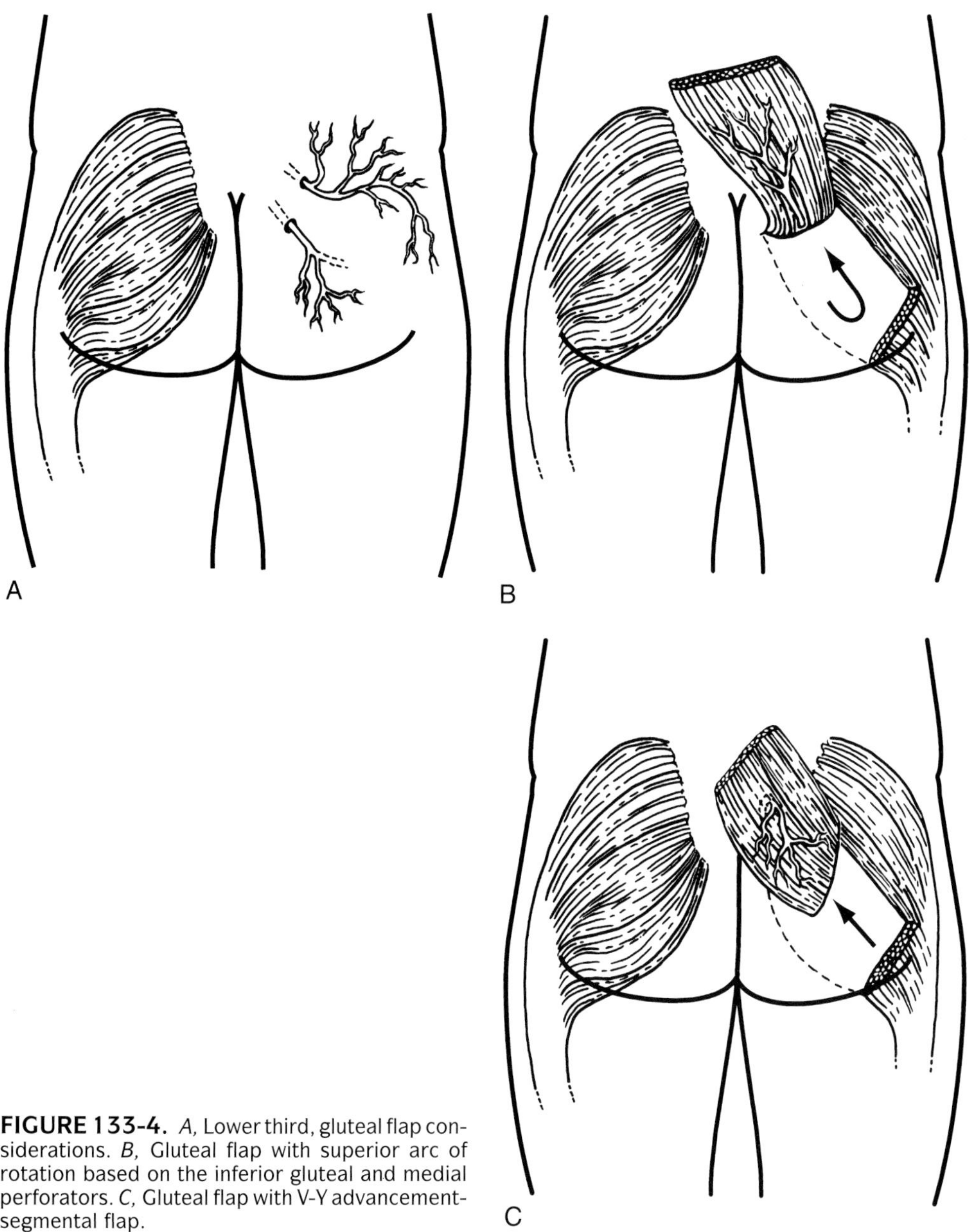

FIGURE 133-4. *A,* Lower third, gluteal flap considerations. *B,* Gluteal flap with superior arc of rotation based on the inferior gluteal and medial perforators. *C,* Gluteal flap with V-Y advancement-segmental flap.

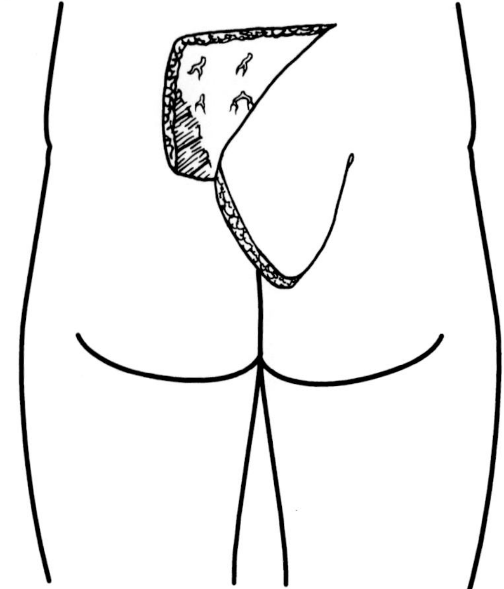

FIGURE 133-5. Transverse back flap.

skin flaps in the control of bacterial inoculation. These animal studies showed relative resistance of musculocutaneous flaps to flap necrosis and propagation of infection compared with random-pattern flaps.

Calderon, Chang, and Mathes[8] examined the bacterial resistance of musculocutaneous flaps versus fasciocutaneous flaps. There was no significant difference in the zone of skin necrosis secondary to infection, but there was a significantly greater bacterial count on deep fluid aspiration from the fasciocutaneous compared with the musculocutaneous flaps.

In studies that more directly identify immunocompetence, random and musculocutaneous flaps also show distinct differences.[9] Leukocyte mobilization and blood flow changes after infection are superior in the musculocutaneous model compared with the random flap model. In addition, oxygen delivery is better with the musculocutaneous flap, leading to improved free radical product and bactericidal function. Fasciocutaneous flaps lie between random and musculocutaneous flaps in their ability to control a hostile wound. A delayed procedure in random flaps appears to improve oxygen delivery when it is performed 15 days before definitive flap elevation.[10] This improvement approaches the delivery of the musculocutaneous flap; however, a delay in the musculocutaneous flap has a minimal effect on oxygen delivery. All flaps have improved oxygen delivery when the inspired oxygen is increased; the most profound effect is seen in the random flap.[11] In the random flap model, increased inspired oxygen leads to decreased flap necrosis secondary to infection. The response to increased inspired oxygen provides the basis for improved outcome with hyperbaric oxygen therapy. In the final analysis, musculocutaneous flaps provide the greatest delivery system for nutrient material.[12] The local and systemic factors can modulate the pathophysiologic process to further complicate the issue.

The pathophysiologic considerations set the stage for appropriate complex back wound reconstruction. In general, all systemic conditions are optimized. This includes control of diabetes, surveillance of cancer, multiorgan function, tobacco use, and overall immune state. Attention is then turned to local factors, such as blood supply, stability of the spine, radiation history, presence of prosthetic material, osteomyelitis or infection, and local tissue availability for reconstruction.

Clinical Considerations

Once the patient's issues have been identified, it is paramount to prepare the wound with aggressive débridement. The wound must be débrided to well-vascularized, relatively healthy tissue. Failure to use a systematic and aggressive intervention plan will result in not only failure of the plan but worsening of the patient's overall condition. The wound is clinically assessed for perfusion in addition to cultures to ensure less than 1×10^5 colony-forming units.

A modified reconstructive ladder is used in this population of patients. Local skin flaps, skin grafting, tissue expansion, and distant skin, alone, are typically not suitable for complex back reconstruction. Musculocutaneous or muscle with skin flap or graft is necessary for the reconstruction of such disease. In addition, it is critical to stabilize the spine rigidly and to correct underlying cerebrospinal disorders. The importance of a multidisciplinary team approach, consisting of surgical oncology, orthopedic surgery, neurosurgery, and plastic surgery, cannot be overstated.

Specific Treatment Options

Musculocutaneous or muscle flaps are preferred to fasciocutaneous flaps for the reconstruction of complex wounds. Muscle flap coverage is especially important for obliteration of dead space. The use of the trapezius is generally most desirable for the upper third of the back.[13] The latissimus offers great versatility in reconstruction of the middle third, based on the standard or distal circulation. Finally, the gluteus maximus is a local solution for the distal third defect.[4] In the situation in which there is minimal dead space and local undisturbed transverse lower back tissue is available, the transverse back flap is a reasonable consideration with the preceding caveats. The use of omentum through the intra-abdominal route or an extended rectus abdominis musculocutaneous flap to reach a

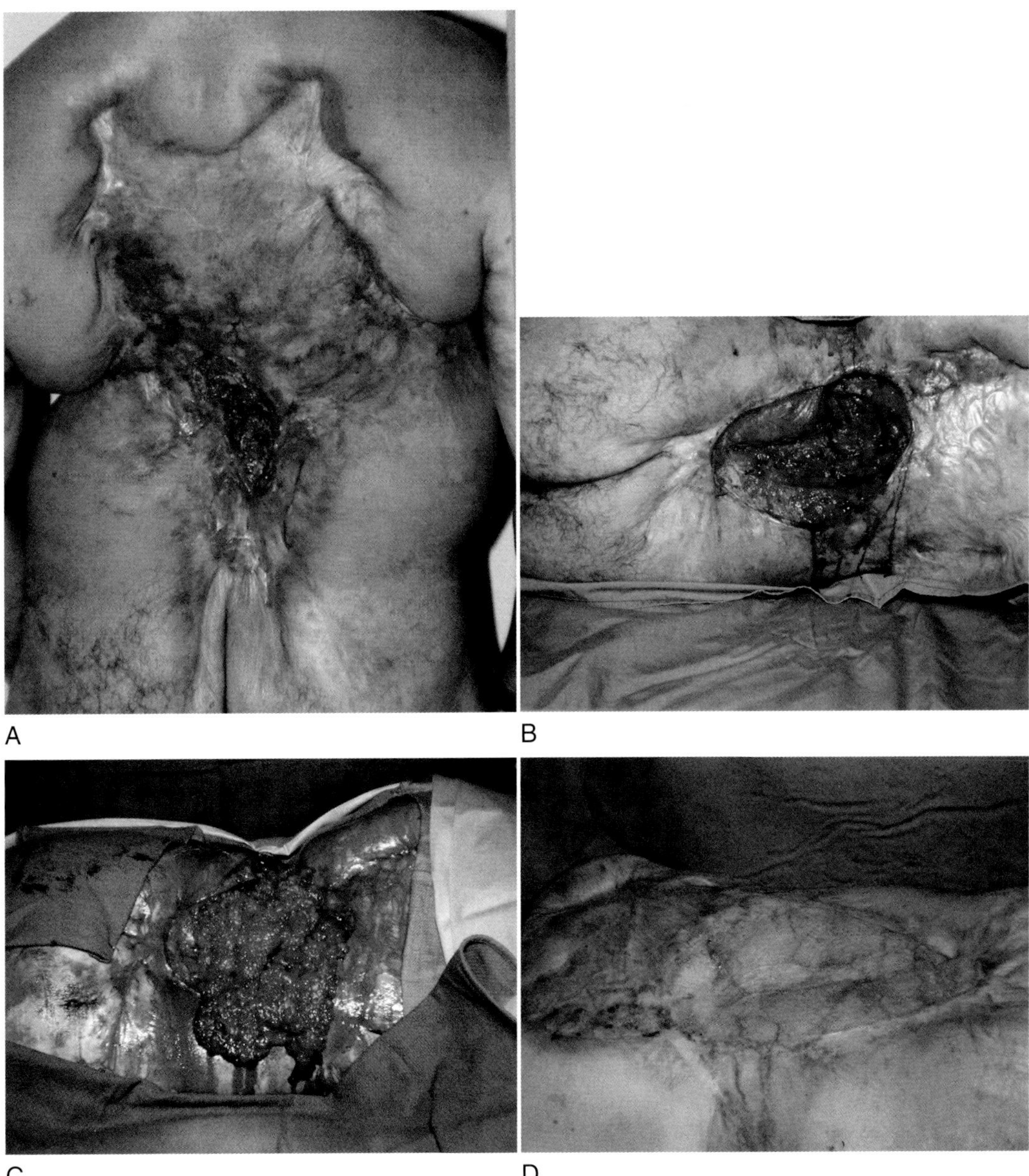

FIGURE 133-6. Reconstruction of Marjolin ulcer of the back with a tunneled omental flap and skin graft. *A,* Preoperative view. The patient has a history of significant burns involving the back, trunk, and extremities. He has a squamous cell carcinoma-Marjolin ulcer in the center of this burn area. All other free flap donor sites are burned. *B,* Defect of the back after resection of Marjolin ulcer. *C,* Reconstruction with omental flap, omentum mobilized and tunneled through into the back. *D,* Final result—stable coverage with omentum and skin graft.

complex defect of the back may also be considered (Fig. 133-6).[14] Free tissue transfer on long vein grafts is reserved for the most severe deformity with inadequate local or distant tissue available.[15]

MYELOMENINGOCELE COVERAGE

Disruption of neural tube closure at 29 days of gestation leads to an open spinal defect known as a meningomyelocele. The neonate born with meningomyelocele has exposure of the spinal canal and neural elements, with associated hydrocephalus. The defect is typically at the thoracolumbar level (spina bifida cystica aperta), allowing soilage risk and cerebrospinal fluid leakage. Kyphosis and other anomalous spine deformities contribute to the pathologic process. The neural plaque is the area of highest risk for cerebrospinal fluid leak.[16-19]

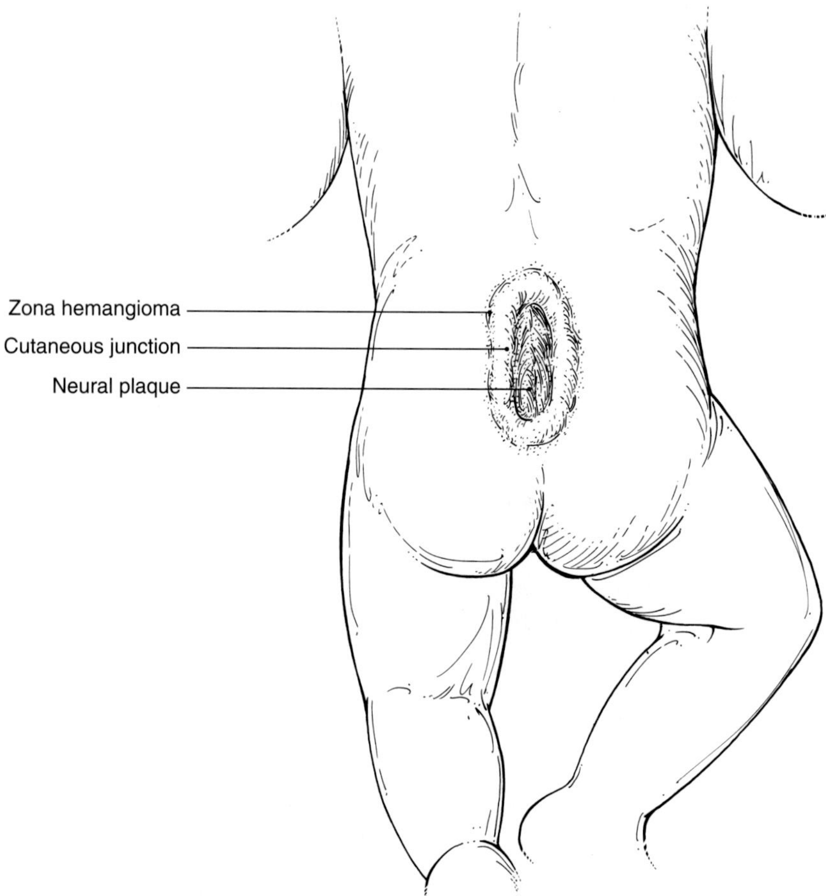

FIGURE 133-7. Thoracolumbar meningomyelocele after split-thickness skin graft cover of the neural plaque. The epithelialized, thin dural sac wall borders the neural plaque and forms the junction with a narrow rim of the dermal hemangioma. Between the neural plaque and its border is the area at greatest risk for cerebrospinal fluid leak.

The infants are typically in a neonatal intensive care unit setting and require neurosurgery for placement of a ventriculoperitoneal shunt. It is of the utmost importance to have a comprehensive multidisciplinary approach to the treatment of these patients.

The initial treatment of such infants involves stabilization of other medical conditions. The placement of a split-thickness skin graft over the central neural plaque provides a temporary biologic shield (Fig. 133-7). The use of the temporary split-thickness skin graft has been popularized by authors such as Laurence, Luce, and Seyfer.[17-19] After the myelomeningocele is temporarily covered, preparations are made for definitive closure of both the neurologic tube and the overlying soft tissue defect. Neurosurgery participates in the reconstruction and closure of the central nervous system followed by plastic surgery closure of the soft tissue defect. Local, random flaps can be used to close small, uncomplicated soft tissue defects. Local musculocutaneous or fasciocutaneous flaps are useful for the larger or more complicated meningomyelocele lesion (Fig. 133-8). Composite advancement of the musculocutaneous gluteus and latissimus flaps has been advocated by Ramasastry and Cohen[16] (Fig. 133-9). Distal or "reversed" musculocutaneous flaps of the latissimus and gluteus are versatile, but skin viability may be less predictable. Doppler assessment is needed to verify the presence of a skin island perforator. Combinations of these techniques can be used to provide the most reliable reconstruction with the least potential morbidity. The goal of reconstruction is to obliterate potential dead space with a reliable tension-free closure.[17,19-24]

RADIATION DEFECTS

Radiation penetrates beneath the dermis to cause damage to blood vessels in addition to the surrounding tissue. Animal studies have shown that a radiation dose of 20 to 30 Gy will lead to permanent hair loss and increased subcutaneous edema with fat and muscle atrophy. There is no significant change in the number of lymphocytes, but rather the ability to phagocytose is decreased. These findings make the use of

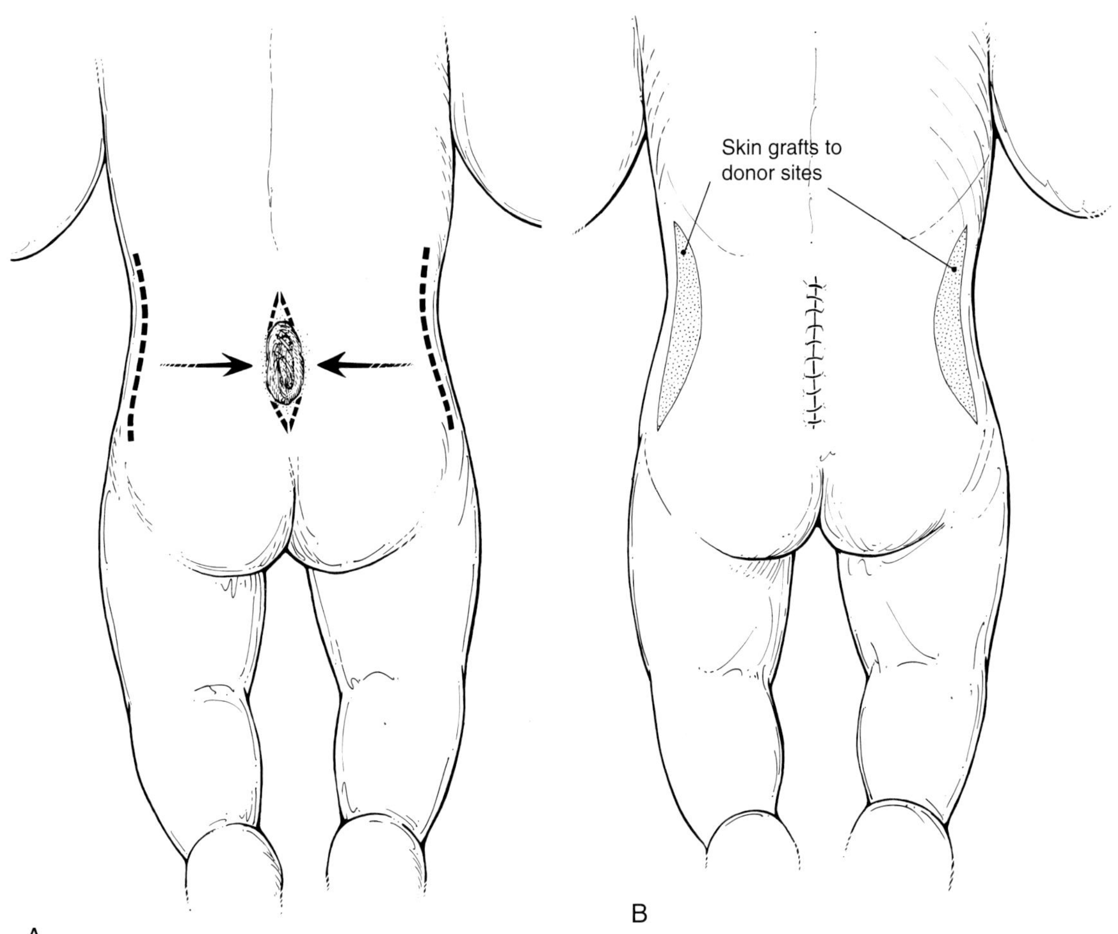

FIGURE 133-8. *A,* Closure of the myelomeningocele can be achieved with bilateral fasciocutaneous or musculocutaneous (latissimus or gluteus) advancement flaps. Relaxing incisions can be used for larger defects to eliminate tension and to divide the insertions of the gluteus or latissimus. *B,* The donor site is closed with a split-thickness skin graft, as needed. The relaxing incisions are rarely required. Small myelomeningocele defects can be closed by a variety of local skin (random) flaps. These techniques should not be used on large or complex myeloceles.

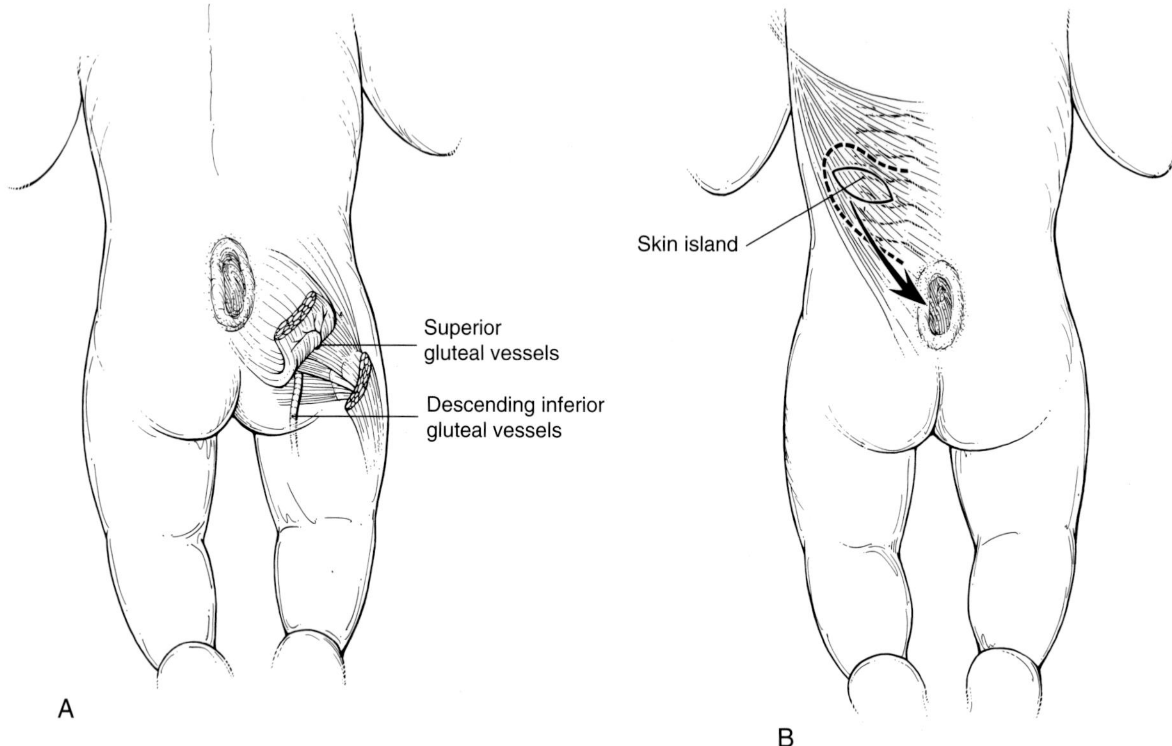

FIGURE 133-9. *A,* Closure of myelomeningocele by use of superiorly based gluteal flap, with or without cutaneous island. The muscle flap alone can be covered with a skin graft. The blood supply to the flap is the superior gluteal system. *B,* Distal latissimus flap, with or without skin paddle, based on paramedian perforators. Doppler assessment should confirm two to four perforators.

irradiated tissue unpredictable.[25] Because skin grafts typically fail, arterial flaps, whether free, regional, musculocutaneous, or fasciocutaneous, are the preferred means of reconstruction. These flaps fill the defect, and their vascularity enhances the local blood flow of the compromised wound bed (Figs. 133-10 and 133-11).

WOUND CLOSURE AFTER ORTHOPEDIC MANIPULATION

The exposure of hardware adds an additional level of complexity to already complex wounds. It is not possible to determine clinically whether an exposed portion of hardware is infected or contaminated.[26] With this uncertainty, the most critical variable is the state of the covering tissue (Figs. 133-12 and 133-13).

There are multiple clinical situations in which closure of a midline defect after orthopedic manipulation is required across multiple zones of the back. A useful tool for this purpose is the paraspinal muscle turnover flap. These muscles are supplied by paramedian perforators coming off the thoracolumbar circulatory system. This tissue provides a reliable muscle system that can be used, in a turnover fashion, to cover the midline posterior spine. The versatility and flexibility of this approach can be increased by incising the muscle fascia proper of the paraspinal muscles. The operating surgeon must be extremely careful to confirm perforator supply to the paraspinal muscles, however, because orthopedic manipulation of this area can result in disruption of the perforator blood vessels, rendering the flap nonviable (Fig. 133-14).

CHRONIC OSTEOMYELITIS

Chronic osteomyelitis is composed of bone devoid of its blood supply and colonized by a wide variety of organisms. Mathes[27] has shown that muscle flap coverage is ideal after wide local débridement of diseased bone.

CONCLUSION

A systematic approach is required in the treatment of posterior trunk defects. The anatomic location and classification of the back wound dictate possible treatment options. The most difficult back defects can be successfully treated with a well-planned, systematic approach.

Text continued on p. 456

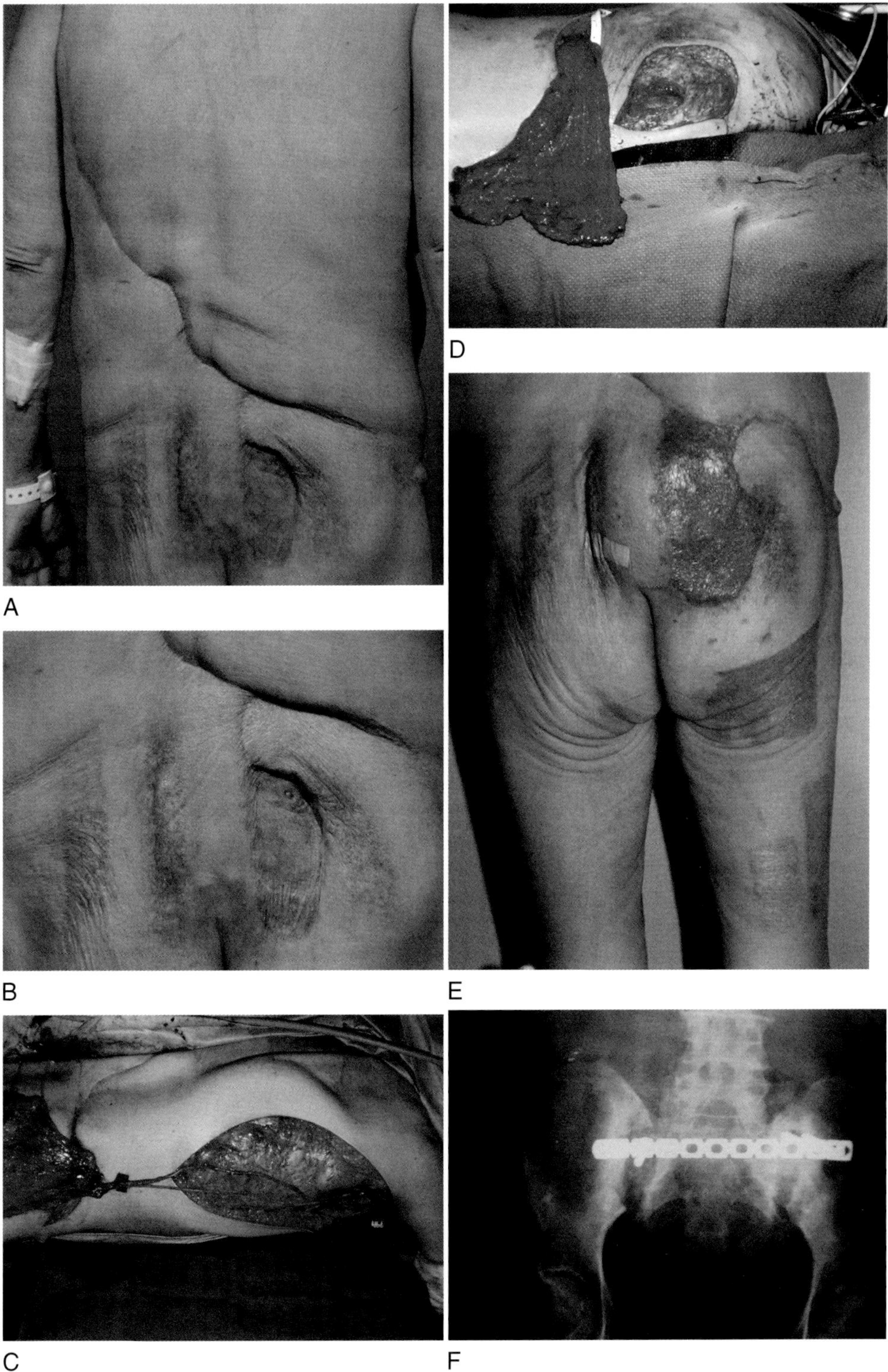

FIGURE 133-10. Reconstruction of osteoradionecrosis of the sacrum with a latissimus dorsi free flap and extensive vein graft. This patient presented with osteoradionecrosis involving the sacroiliac joint. There was a history of gynecologic malignant disease and radiation through the anterior abdominal port. A previous attempt at reconstruction with a free latissimus flap and long vein grafts at another institution had failed. *A* and *B,* Preoperative views. *C,* Intraoperative view demonstrating 25-cm vein grafts sewn into the thoracodorsal vessels proximally and distally. *D,* Viable extended free latissimus dorsi flap and débrided wound. *E,* Stable reconstruction. *F,* Final reconstruction with bone grafting and plating of sacroiliac joint.

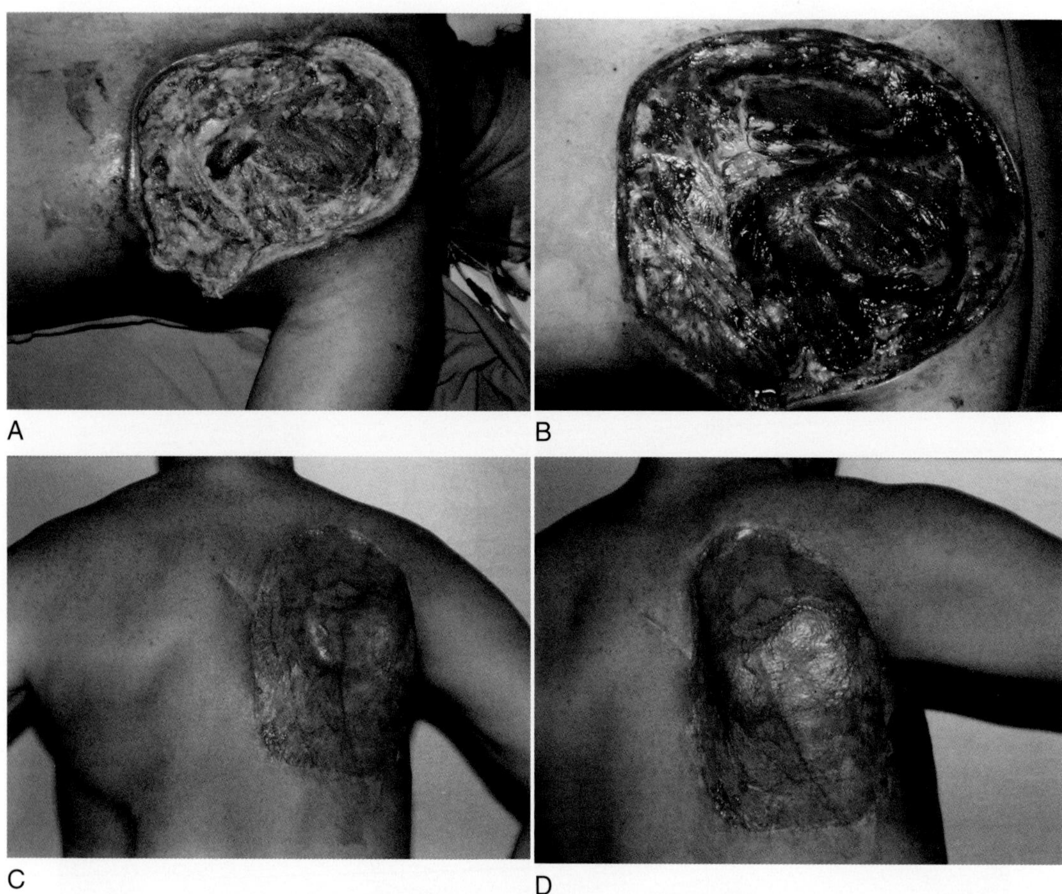

FIGURE 133-11. Reconstruction of upper back radionecrotic defect with free latissimus flap. A young man with fibrosarcoma of the right shoulder who underwent chemotherapy and irradiation resulting in a significant defect is presented. *A,* Defect of right shoulder. *B,* Defect after débridement. *C* and *D,* Reconstruction of radionecrotic ulcer with latissimus free flap from opposite side.

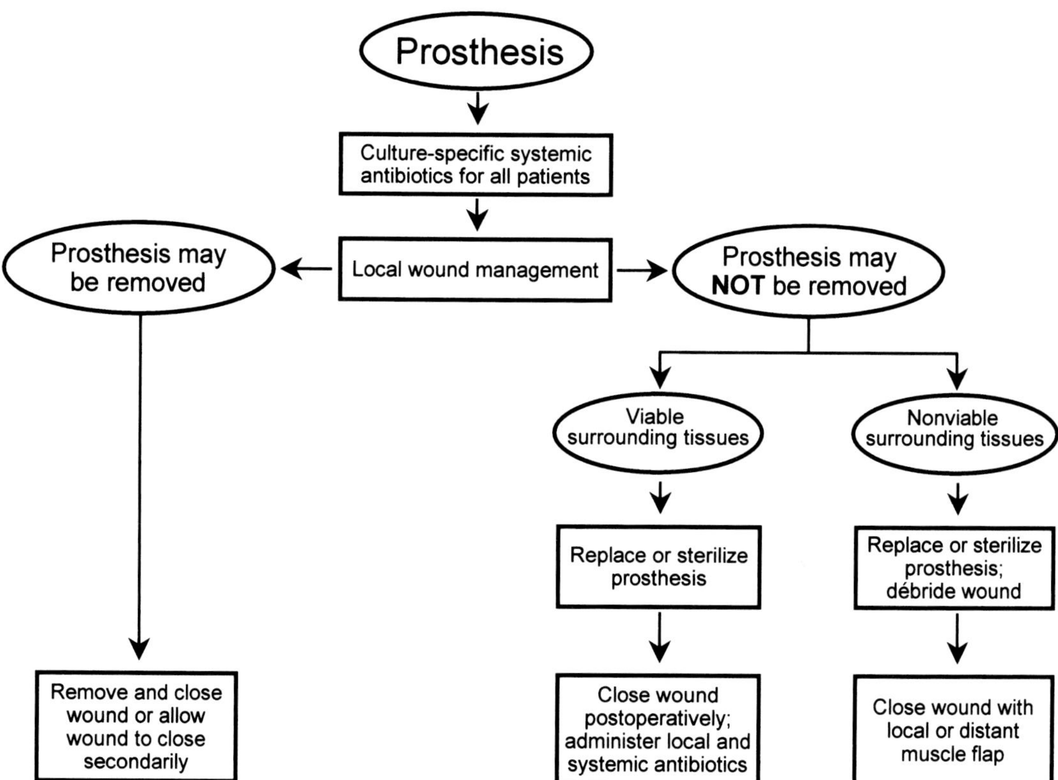

FIGURE 133-12. Management of exposed or infected prosthesis.

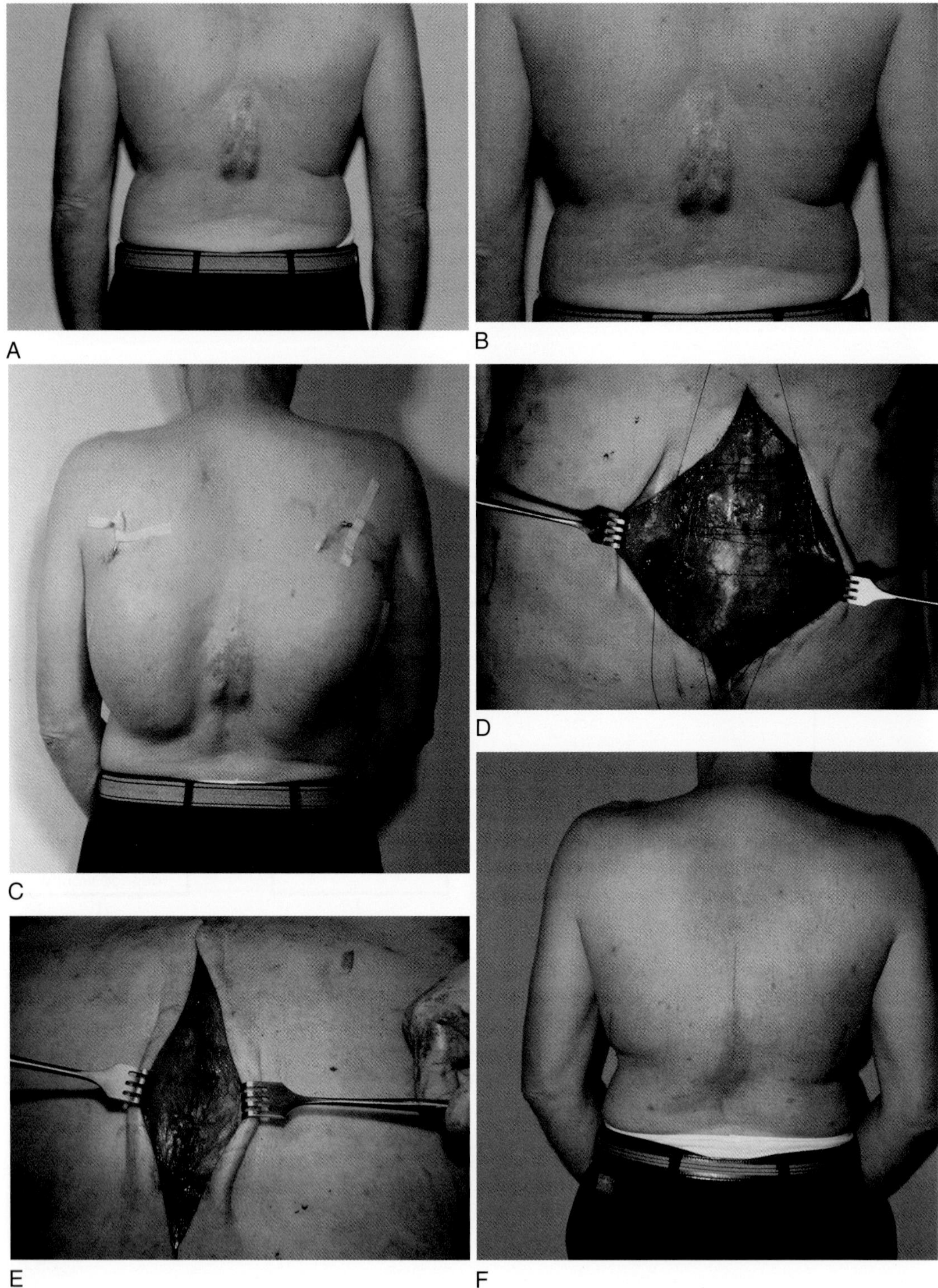

FIGURE 133-13. Staged reconstruction and fusion of back with expanded latissimus dorsi musculocutaneous flaps. A patient with a history of irradiation involving the lower thoracic and upper lumbar vertebrae is presented. He was a candidate for fusion and required stable coverage. *A* and *B*, Preoperative condition. *C*, Expansion of latissimus dorsi musculocutaneous flaps with external ports. Note that access incisions are lateral. *D* and *E*, Intraoperative views after fusion and rod fixation of spine by an orthopedic surgeon. Coverage was achieved by bilateral expanded latissimus dorsi musculocutaneous flaps. *F*, Final result.

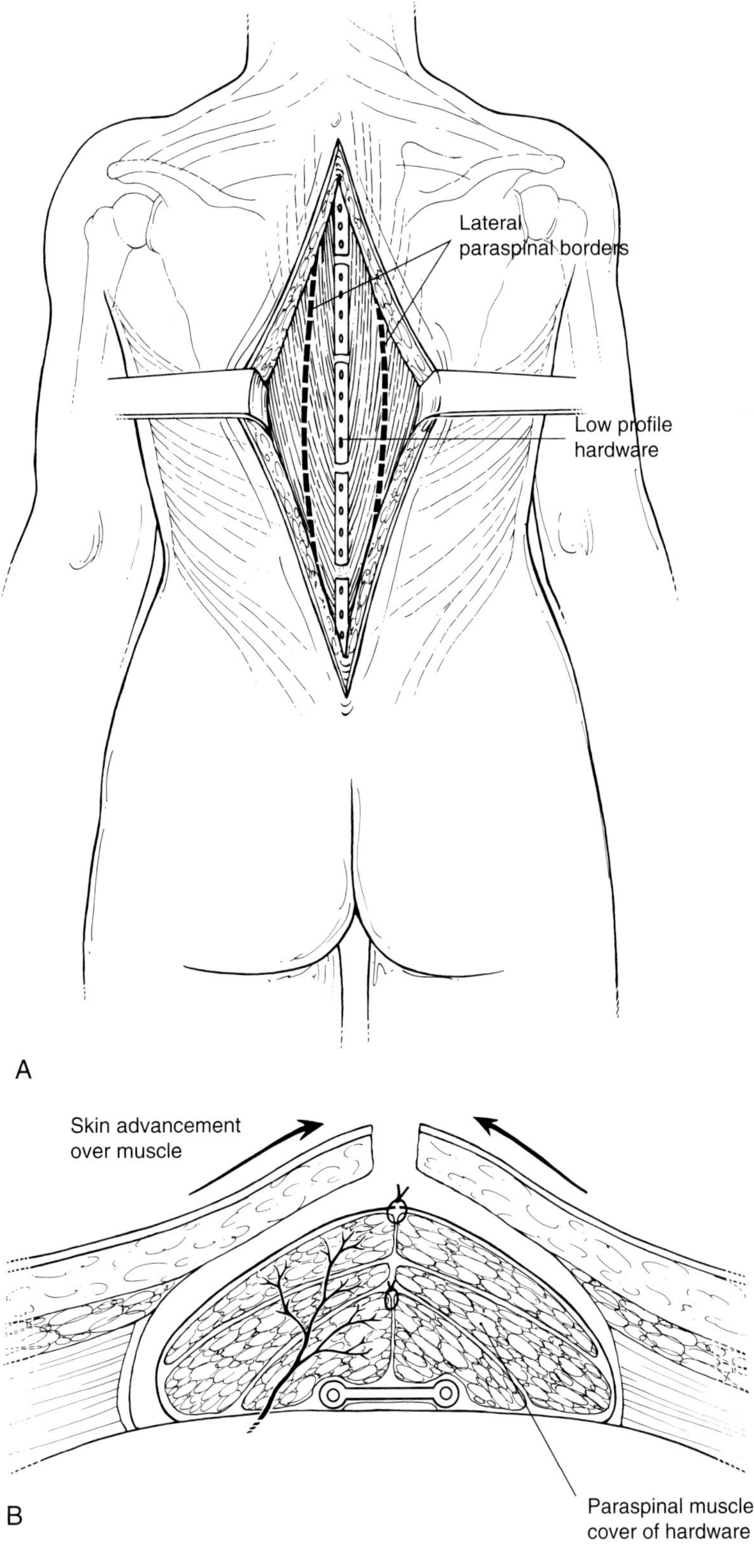

FIGURE 133-14. *A* and *B*, Coverage of spinal (low-profile) hardware with paired paraspinal flaps. The paraspinal flaps are then covered with bilateral skin advancement. Viable perforators must be confirmed before the use of these flaps.

REFERENCES

1. Few J, Marcus J, Lee M, Dumanian G: Treatment of hostile midline back wounds: an extreme approach. Plast Reconstr Surg 1999;105:2448.
2. Casas L, Lewis V: A reliable approach to the closure of large acquired midline defects of the back. Plast Reconstr Surg 1988;84:632.
3. Bostwick JB III, Scheflan M, Nahai F, Jurkiewicz MJ: The "reverse" latissimus dorsi muscle and musculocutaneous flap: anatomical and clinical considerations. Plast Reconstr Surg 1980;65:390.
4. Evans G, Reece G: Lower back reconstruction: an approach to wound closure in the cancer patient. Plast Reconstr Surg 1995;96:635.
5. Hill L, Brown RG, Jurkiewicz MJ: The transverse lumbosacral back flap. Plast Reconstr Surg 1978;62:177.
6. Krizek TJ, Robson MC, Kho E: Bacterial growth and skin graft survival. Surg Forum 1967;18:518.
7. Chang N, Mathes SJ: Comparison of the effect of bacterial inoculation in musculocutaneous and random-pattern flaps. Plast Reconstr Surg 1982;70:1.
8. Calderon W, Chang N, Mathes SJ: Comparison of the effect of bacterial inoculation in musculocutaneous and fasciocutaneous flaps. Plast Reconstr Surg 1986;77:785.
9. Eshima I, Mathes SJ, Paty P: Comparison of the intracellular bacterial killing activity of leukocytes in musculocutaneous and random pattern flaps. Plast Reconstr Surg 1990;86:541.
10. Jonsson K, Hunt TK, Brennan SS, Mathes SJ: Tissue oxygen measurements in delayed skin flaps: a reconsideration of the mechanisms of the delay phenomenon. Plast Reconstr Surg 1988;82:328.
11. Gottrup F, Firmin R, Hunt TK, Mathes SJ: The dynamic properties of tissue oxygen tension in healing flaps. Surgery 1984;95:527.
12. Gottrup F, Orededdon S, Price DC, et al: A comparative study of skin blood flow in musculocutaneous and random pattern flaps. J Surg Res 1984;34:443.
13. Seyfer AE: The lower trapezius flap for recalcitrant wounds of the posterior skull and spine [scalp]. Ann Plast Surg 1988;20:414.
14. Mixter R, Wood W, Dibbell D: Retroperitoneal transposition of rectus abdominis myocutaneous flaps to the perineum and back. Plast Reconstr Surg 1990;85:437.
15. Karanas YL, Yim KK, Johannet P, et al: Use of 20 cm or longer interposition vein grafts in free flap reconstruction of the trunk. Plast Reconstr Surg 1998;101:1262.
16. Ramasastry SS, Cohen M: Soft tissue closure and plastic surgical aspects of large open myelomeningoceles. Neurosurg Clin North Am 1995;6:279.
17. McDonell DE, Seyfer AE: Myelomeningocele. In Cohen M, ed: Mastery of Plastic Surgery. Boston, Little, Brown, 1994:1240.
18. Laurence KM: Effects of early surgery for spina bifida cystica on survival and quality of life. Lancet 1974;1:301.
19. Luce EA, Walsh J: Wound closure of the meningomyelocele defect. Plast Reconstr Surg 1985;75:389.
20. Stevenson TR, Rohrich RJ, Pollock RA, et al: More experience with the "reverse" latissimus dorsi musculocutaneous flap: precise location of blood supply. Plast Reconstr Surg 1984;74:237.
21. Clark DH, Walsh JW, Luce EA: Closure of myeloschisis defects with reverse latissimus dorsi myocutaneous flaps. Neurosurgery 1982;3:423.
22. Mustoe TA, Gifford GH, Lash E: Rapid tissue expansion in the treatment of myelomeningocele. Ann Plast Surg 1988;21:70.
23. Sharrad WJW, Zachary RB, Lorber J, Bruce AM: A controlled trial of immediate and delayed closure of spina bifida cystica. Arch Dis Child 1963;38:18.
24. Ramasastry S, Cohen M, Radhakrishnan J: Congenital back defects. In Bentz ML: Pediatric Plastic Surgery. Stamford, Conn, Appleton & Lange, 1997:763-771.
25. Gabka CJ, Benhaim P, Mathes SJ, et al: An experimental model to determine the effect of irradiated tissue on neutrophil function. Plast Reconstr Surg 1995;96:1676.
26. Lesavoy MA, Dubrow TJ, Wackym PA, Eckardt JJ: Muscle-flap coverage of exposed endoprostheses. Plast Reconstr Surg 1989;83:90.
27. Mathes SJ: The muscle flap for management of osteomyelitis. N Engl J Med 1982;306:294.

CHAPTER

134

Congenital Anomalies of the Chest Wall

STEPHEN J. MATHES, MD ✦ ALAN E. SEYFER, MD ✦ EDWARD P. MIRANDA, MD

Congenital chest wall deformities present unique reconstructive challenges. The expression of the abnormality may be incomplete, and anatomic components are often missing, deformed, or weakened. In addition, there may be associated diagnoses that have an impact on the reconstructive options and timing of the surgery. The patient may initially be seen in adulthood or in the neonatal intensive care unit, and each scenario affects the decision and the timing of any reconstructive effort. Both common and rare congenital anomalies of the chest wall are reviewed, with emphasis on diagnosis and appropriate treatment.

THORAX

Development of the breast and thorax begins at the fourth week of gestation and continues well into adulthood. The complex processes of thoracic and breast development are highlighted by the congenital disorders, each characterized by errors at different stages of development. Many are amenable to surgical therapy (Table 134-1).

Embryology

After approximately 4 weeks of gestation, tissue destined to form the body wall is organized into somites in an axial manner under direction from the notochord. The cell populations of the somites are of mesodermal origin and give rise to osteocytes and chondrocytes—ultimately forming the bony and cartilaginous structures. Superficial to these cells are the myotome and the dermatomal layers, giving rise to the musculature and the deep connective tissues of the skin.[1]

At 5 weeks, the tissues forming the body wall muscles have again divided into two distinct populations, the dorsal epimere and the ventral hypomere. The deep extensors of the back develop from the epimere; the ventrolateral flexors (external intercostals, internal intercostals, and transverse thoracic muscles) develop from the hypomere. The ribs and hypomeric musculature extend ventrally to meet the developing sternal structure.[1]

The sternum is a structure of mesodermal origin that begins development at approximately 6 weeks. At that time, the lateral mesodermal plates move ventrally and medially, giving rise to mesenchymal strips. These strips begin to merge during the seventh week in the craniocaudal direction, generating a cartilaginous manubrium and sternal body and the pectoralis muscles.[2] Fusion is complete by 10 weeks, and ossification of the cartilage begins at 5 to 6 months with the manubrium and progresses caudally.[3] Further ossification of the sternum also occurs bilaterally at four centers where the sternal bands fused. The ossification of the sternum is completed at about 25 years of age. The ribs begin ossification from their angle at 8 weeks of gestation; this slowly progresses until about 16 years of age, at which time multiple centers of ossification form, culminating in complete ossification at about 25 years.[1]

Sternum

In recent years, the medical community has come to appreciate that chest wall deformities can result in clinically significant but surgically correctable derangements. Of all possible chest wall deformities,

TABLE 134-1 ✦ EMBRYOLOGIC CHARACTERIZATION OF CONGENITAL BREAST AND THORACIC DEFORMITIES

Anatomic Site	Disorder
Sternum	Pectus excavatum Pectus carinatum Cleft sternum
Ventral body wall	Ectopia cordis Pentalogy of Cantrell
Thoracic musculature	Poland syndrome
Breast	Supernumerary breasts Congenital absence of the breast Tuberous breast Gynecomastia

the pectus deformities are as common as 1 in 300 live births.[4]

PECTUS EXCAVATUM

Pectus excavatum (Latin *pectus,* breast; *ex,* out of; *cavare,* to hollow out), also referred to as funnel chest, is a disorder morphologically characterized by a depression of the sternum, which is often asymmetric (50%).[5,6] This pectus deformity usually involves the anterior thoracic cage below the sternal angle (of Louis), with depression of the middle (body; gladiolus) and lower (xiphoid) sternum and an incurving of the lower costal cartilages that attach to these segments. The superior portion of the manubrium, the first and second ribs, and the corresponding cartilages are usually spared. Although the affected cartilages are inwardly curved, the ribs lateral to the costochondral junctions are often unaffected. There may also be a component of sternal twisting. The pectoralis major muscles and other chest wall components are usually present in the isolated defect and, other than displacement (with the affected cartilages), are normal.

Pectus excavatum varies significantly in its presentation, ranging from a subtle depression to a major cavity causing displacement of the lungs, the mediastinal organs, and even the spinal column. The most common appearance is a symmetric depression of the inferior two thirds to three fourths of the sternum with extension to the costal cartilages, which along with the xiphoid may be distorted.[6] It frequently presents not only as an aesthetic disturbance but also in association with exercise intolerance, obstructive pulmonary mechanics, asthma, and abnormal cardiac physiology.

Incidence

Pectus excavatum is the most common congenital thoracic deformity that is referred for surgical evaluation. It has a reported incidence of between 1 in 1000 and 8 in 1000 live births,[7,8] with a male-to-female ratio ranging from 3:1[7] to 9:1.[9] Studies have estimated the incidence in females to be 1 in 1500.[10] It occurs most commonly in white individuals.[6]

Etiology

Pectus excavatum was originally hypothesized to be a disorder of overgrowth of the costosternal cartilages[11]; however, this explanation is somewhat unsatisfactory in the modern age of molecular surgery. There seems to be a genetic component to the pathogenesis of pectus excavatum, with 40% of patients reporting a family member with a similar deformity.[6] There has been neither a gene locus nor a definitive mendelian pattern established, however.

The sternum forms independently from bilateral islands of somatic mesoderm in the ventral body wall. At approximately the sixth week, these longitudinal sternal bars fuse in the midline, in a cranial to caudal fashion.[12] Failure to fuse properly can result in ectopia cordis.[13] The ribs form independently of this process from the costal processes of the thoracic vertebrae during the fifth week and grow ventrally with the body wall. As the sternal bars from each side fuse in the midline, they connect on their lateral margins with the advancing rib cartilage.[14] Overgrowth of these lower costal cartilages, forcing the malleable lower sternum inward, is sometimes cited as the embryonic pathway to pectus excavatum.[15,16]

Evaluation

Most patients with pectus excavatum have formation of a defect by the age of 6 years, and mild deformities may be self-limited (Fig. 134-1). More severe anomalies can cause physiologic derangements as well as embarrassment about appearance. The patient, especially in preadolescence, complains to his or her parents after being confronted by situations such as physical education classes and swimming or of apprehension at changing into athletic gear. Such psychosocial implications may be as compelling as the physiologic disorders in prioritizing the indications for repair. In addition to the cosmetic defect, it can be associated with diminished cardiopulmonary function.[17]

The depression of the sternum can significantly reduce the prevertebral space and result in displacement and axial rotation of the heart and great vessels. This has the effect of reducing the volume within the pleural space on one side (and therefore reducing ventilatory capacity), compromising venous return to the heart, and causing cardiorespiratory symptoms (Fig. 134-2). It has long been appreciated that there is an increased association between pectus excavatum, exercise intolerance, and upper respiratory ailments in later childhood.[18]

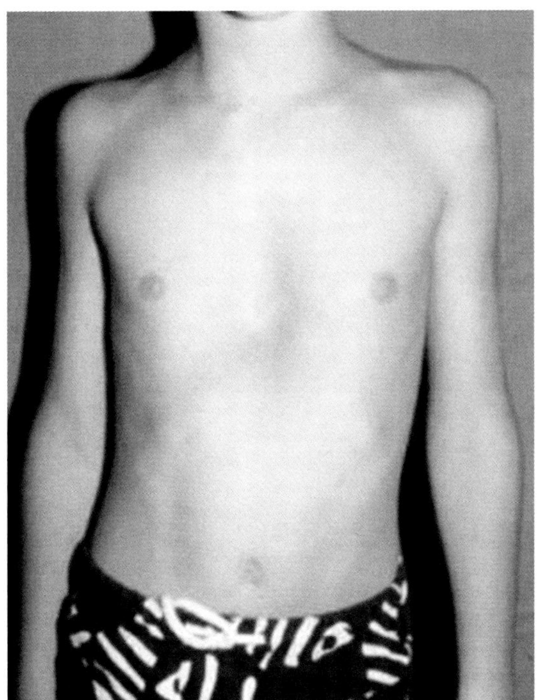

FIGURE 134-1. Pectus excavatum, anterior view of chest. Note central sternal deformity typical of mild symmetric pectus excavatum.

Presentation and Diagnosis

The extent of the structural irregularity and the degree of pectus-related cardiopulmonary dysfunction are critical issues in assessing the anatomic and physiologic severity of the deformity and the indications for repair.[16] Baseline evaluations usually include standard chest radiographs, electrocardiogram, axial computed tomographic (CT) scans, and static or dynamic pulmonary function tests (Fig. 134-3). Coronal and three-dimensional reconstructed CT scans are useful in selected patients. At 6 years of age, the sternovertebral distance less than 5 cm is considered a severe deformity, 5 to 7 cm is moderate, and greater than 7 cm is mild. The ratio of the transverse chest diameter to the anterior-posterior dimension from the anterior border of the spinal column to the deepest part of the sternum is also used as an index of severity. A ratio of greater than 3:2 is considered clinically significant.[16]

Patients with pectus excavatum present with a variety of symptoms. A careful history will often reveal more than simply psychological distress about cosmetic appearance, although in both young children and adults, self-consciousness about appearance is manifested by a reluctance to have their chest exposed. Dyspnea, chest pain, fatigue, and exercise intolerance are often elicited from the patient, although the true significance of these symptoms is controversial. A restrictive pattern of ventilation is often detected with pulmonary function tests. Palpitations are also reported, typically during exertion.[9] Patients often present with other malformations, including scoliosis in 65%.[6] The condition has been reported to progress in certain patients over time (late adolescence to early adulthood) with advancement of the aesthetic deformity or the progression of physiologic derangements, including exercise tolerance.[19]

Because by definition pectus excavatum causes a shortening of the distance between the sternum and the vertebrae, this measurement has been used to radiologically characterize the severity of the disorder. The pectus severity index (PSI, Haller index) is calculated by dividing the internal transverse thoracic diameter by the smallest anterior-posterior distance between the vertebrae and the most depressed portion of the chest wall[20] (Fig. 134-4). The normal value is approximately 2.5 with an upper limit of approximately 3.25. The more severe the deformity, the higher the calculated PSI value. Mean PSI values of 4.8 (ranging from 3.2 to 12.7) have been reported in the literature for patients referred for operative intervention.[21] More severe PSI scores have been observed but are atypical.

Physiology

There has been much debate about the physiologic consequences of pectus excavatum and responses to treatment. Many of the earlier reports contending both for and against a true physiologic syndrome either associated with or caused by its anatomic deformity were anecdotal in nature. More recently, however, several

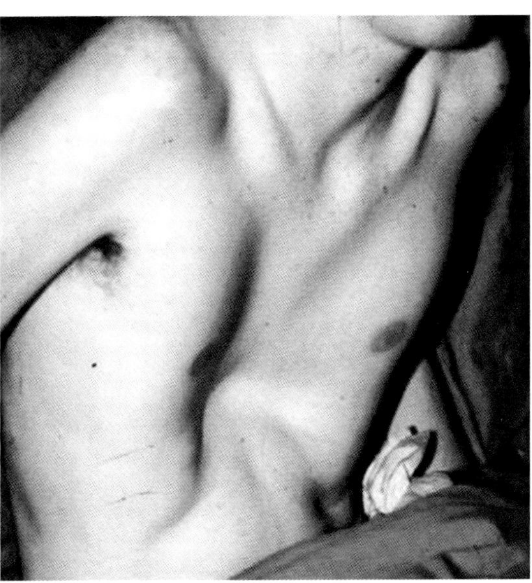

FIGURE 134-2. Pectus excavatum, oblique view of anterior chest. Note severe asymmetric sternal deformity.

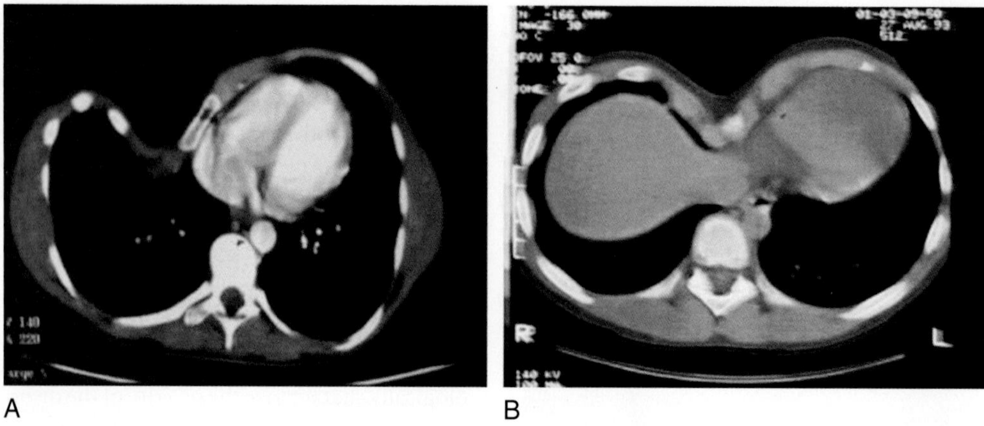

FIGURE 134-3. CT scans of pectus excavatum. *A,* Asymmetric severe deformity. *B,* Symmetric severe deformity.

studies have described the sequelae with more reliable data.

VENTILATORY MECHANICS. In a controlled prospective trial, Quigley et al[22] compared pulmonary function test results before intervention of 36 patients with pectus excavatum (mean age, 16 ± 3 years) and 10 age-matched, healthy control subjects. The patients with pectus excavatum had significantly lower forced vital capacity (81% ± 14% of expected) than the control subjects did (98% ± 9% of expected). The total lung capacity was significantly and inversely correlated with PSI. Of the patients with pectus excavatum, 58% complained of exercise limitations; however, both the test subjects and the control subjects responded similarly to an exercise challenge. Despite these significant data, the mean observed value of 81% is within the normal range, which casts some doubt on the meaningfulness of these data. Furthermore, during exercise testing, there were no differences in pulse oximetry or maximal heart rate.[22]

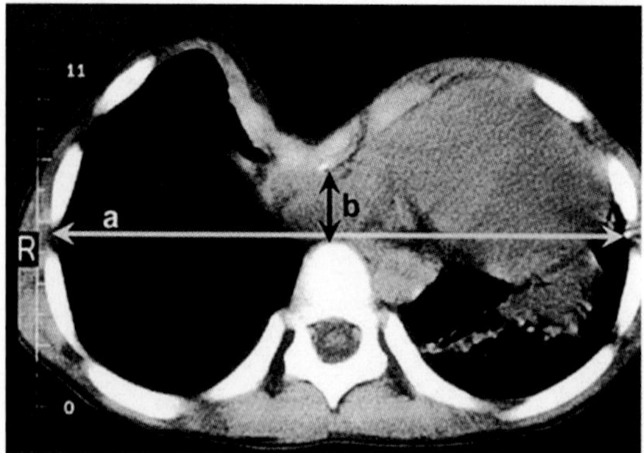

FIGURE 134-4. CT scan used to determine pectus severity index (PSI). The PSI is derived by dividing the internal transverse diameter of the thorax, *a,* by the vertebral-sternal distance at the most depressed portion of the deformity, *b,* by use of a CT scan. (From Malek MH, Fonkalsrud EW, Cooper CB: Ventilatory and cardiovascular responses to exercise in patients with pectus excavatum. Chest 2003;124:870.)

RESPIRATORY PARAMETERS. The common complaint of exercise intolerance among patients with pectus excavatum cannot be adequately explained by the observed restrictive ventilatory pattern or completely discounted by normal pulse oximetry and maximal heart rate (both observed by Quigley[22]). These conflicting findings have prompted a more detailed investigation of respiratory parameters. Malek[9] examined four respiratory tests as more adequate markers of exercise tolerance: maximum oxygen uptake ($\dot{V}O_2max$), the metabolic threshold ($\dot{V}O_2\theta$, the limit above which elevated lactate concentrations are measurable), work efficiency (the rate of change of $\dot{V}O_2$ with respect to work ($\delta\dot{V}O_2/\delta W$), and the time constant for oxygen uptake ($\tau\dot{V}O_2$).[6] In Malek's study,[9] adolescents and adults with pectus excavatum (n = 21) underwent testing for these parameters and standard pulmonary function tests. The pulmonary function test results obtained were consistent with those of the Quigley[22] study and others showing significantly reduced forced vital capacity and forced expiratory volume in 1 second as well as reduced maximum voluntary ventilation (82% of expected) and reduced gas diffusion as measured by the diffusing capacity of the lung for carbon monoxide (84% of expected).[9] Again, although significantly different from the results expected, all mean pulmonary function test results lie in the low end of the accepted normal range. The $\dot{V}O_2max$ in the study patients was observed to be significantly less than predicted (76%), whereas $\dot{V}O_2\theta$, $\delta\dot{V}O_2/\delta W$, and $\tau\dot{V}O_2$ were unchanged. When stratified by PSI, $\dot{V}O_2max$ significantly deteriorates at values worse than 4.0. Subgroup analysis revealed that patients with PSI above 4.0 also have an odds ratio of 8:1 to have a reduced $\dot{V}O_2\theta$ compared with pectus excavatum patients with less severe disease. Although there is uncertainty in the data, it is reasonable to conclude that there is a mild aerobic deficiency in patients with PSI above 4.0 (Table 134-2).[9]

CARDIAC FUNCTION. It has been shown from both radiography and cardiac catheterization studies that patients with pectus excavatum have displacement of the heart.[23,24] However, the same cardiac catheterization study showed that chamber sizes were unchanged.[24] Cardiac output and stroke volume have been shown to be normal at rest; however, cardiac catheterization has documented a diminished ability to augment stroke volume during exercise in an upright position (19% observed versus 51% expected).[25] Malek et al[9] also studied cardiac function by examining $\dot{V}O_2$ divided by heart rate ($\dot{V}O_2/\int c$), which can be used as an estimate of stroke volume, and found a small but significant reduction (86% of expected).[25] Mitral valve prolapse is found incidentally on echocardiography in 15% of patients.[21]

Aesthetic and Psychological Considerations

By far the most consistent complaint of patients with pectus excavatum is the aesthetic deformity caused by the sternal depression. Children have consistently reported dissatisfaction with their appearance without a shirt.[26] A small study of patients aged 12 to 21 years and their parents with PSI ranging from 3.7 to 9.5 who were selected to undergo operative correction of pectus excavatum qualitatively expressed self-consciousness, confidence and self-esteem problems, and limited participation in certain activities where there was a risk for the deformity to be seen (e.g., wearing a tight shirt or swimming).[27]

Classification

A classification system has been proposed by Park et al[28] (Fig. 134-5 and Table 134-3). The primary division is between symmetric (type 1) and asymmetric (type 2) deformities. Symmetric deformities are characterized by co-localization of the center of the depression with the center of the sternum. Asymmetric (type 2) deformities have either a midline sternum with maximal depression lateral to the midline (type 2A) or a median depression but with markedly different slopes on each side of the deformity (type 2B). The most severe deformity has been described as the "Grand Canyon" type, which is a longitudinal depression extending from the lower chest to the clavicle (type 2C).

Operative Treatment

INDICATIONS. Despite the relative uncertainty of abnormal physiology in pectus excavatum, subjective complaints of exercise intolerance, dyspnea, and similar symptoms are relative indications for operation, especially when the symptoms correlate with severe deformity. The risk of progression and documented progression of the deformity are also indications for intervention. Aesthetic concern is always a relative indication for repair.

The optimal age for intervention is not clear and has been the subject of disagreement. It has been argued that asymptomatic young children (2 to 5 years) should

TABLE 134-2 ✦ MEASUREMENTS FOR EXERCISE TOLERANCE IN PATIENTS WITH PECTUS EXCAVATUM

			PSI							
	Overall (n = 21)		*3.0-3.9 (n = 3)*		*4.0-4.9 (n = 9)*		*5.0-5.9 (n = 4)*		*≥6.0 (n = 5)*	
Parameters	*Mean*	*% Ref*	*Mean*	*% Ref*	*Mean*	*% Ref*	*Mean*	*% Ref*	*Mean*	*% Ref*
$\dot{V}O_2$max, L/min	2.14	75	2.57	86	2.04	74	1.44	62	2.63	80
$\dot{V}O_2\theta$, L/min	1.16	41	1.37	47	1.12	41	0.81	37	1.25	38
$\delta\dot{V}O_2\delta W$, mL/min/W	10.6		11.0		10.0		11.2		10.8	
on-$\tau\dot{V}O_2$, s	37.4		34.7		34.7		33.9		39.2	
off-$\tau\dot{V}O_2$, s	41.6		46.5		37.2		45.8		40.1	
∫c rest,*min	84		84		87		92		74	
∫c max,*min	185	98	185	98	177	91	176	91	174	87
$\dot{V}O_2$∫c, mL	12.4	85	13.9	89	11.9	84	9.2	77	14.9	92
RPE, Borg scale[†]	15.4		16.0		16.1		13.5		15.4	

* ∫c rest, ∫c at rest; ∫c max, maximum ∫c.
[†]Scale of 6 to 20 points. RPE, rating of perceived exertion.
From Malek MH, Fonkalsrud EW, Cooper CB: Ventilatory and cardiovascular responses to exercise in patients with pectus excavatum. Chest 2003;124:870.

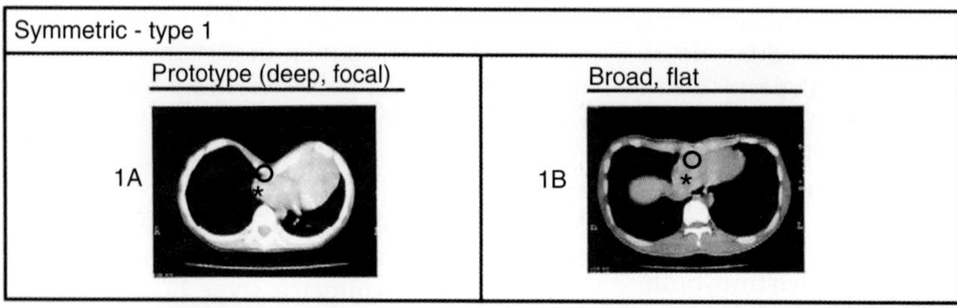

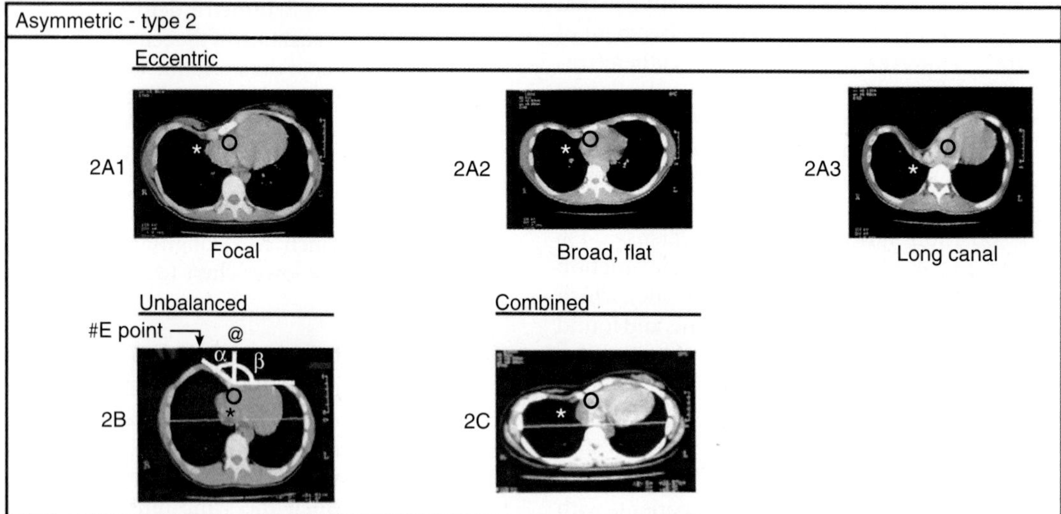

FIGURE 134-5. CT scans illustrate the morphologic types and subtypes of pectus excavatum as defined in the Park classification. The primary division is between symmetric (type 1) and asymmetric (type 2) deformities. See Table 134-3 for details. O, center of the sternum (C point); *, center of the depression (P point); #E point, protruded point of chest wall; @, angles of each chest wall are different ($\alpha < \beta$). (Modified from Park HJ, Lee SY, Lee CS, et al: The Nuss procedure for pectus excavatum: evolution of techniques and early results on 322 patients. Ann Thorac Surg 2004:77:289. Reprinted with permission from The Society of Thoracic Surgeons.)

TABLE 134-3 ✦ CLASSIFICATION OF PECTUS EXCAVATUM BY MORPHOLOGIC TYPES

Morphologic Type and Subtype	Characteristics
Type 1: symmetric	Center of sternum and depression are co-located
Type 1A: prototype (deep, focal)	Typical deep, focal symmetric sternal depression
Type 1B: broad, flat	Broad, flat symmetric sternal depression
Type 2: asymmetric	Center of depression is not located in center of sternum but found laterally to left or right
Type 2A: eccentric	Center of sternum is in midline, but maximal depression is located laterally in cartilage to left or right
1: focal	Deep, focal asymmetric depression
2: broad, flat	Broad, flat asymmetric depression
3: long canal	Extreme form of symmetric depression ("Grand Canyon" type) with deep longitudinal groove from clavicle to lower chest; majority of depression in parasternal cartilage, not sternum
Type 2B: unbalanced	Center of depression is in midline, but one wall of depression is more severely depressed than other; angles formed by each wall and vertical axis are different ($\alpha < \beta$); see Figure 134-5
Type 2C: combined	Combination of types 2A and 2B

Modified from Park HJ, Lee SY, Lee CS, et al: The Nuss procedure for pectus excavatum: evolution of techniques and early results on 322 patients. Ann Thorac Surg 2004;77:289. Reprinted with permission from The Society of Thoracic Surgeons.

undergo operation because of the compliance of the rib cage and ease of operation, but this has been changing with new data for repair in older children and adults.

Timing. The timing of the repair can be an issue. Resectional repairs on young children can limit the growth of the thorax and have been associated with severe chest wall constriction, which is extremely disabling.[29] Thus, resection techniques should probably not be employed in patients younger than 13 years, with optimal repair being delayed until after the age of 16 years. Again, in patients with less severe defects, the procedure is cosmetic, and this must be taken into consideration in subjecting the patient to any procedure. The family and patient are brought into the decision, and the surgeon always has the option of declining and referring the patient to another team if the risk-benefit ratio is not deemed to be acceptable. This problem occurs when the family has unrealistic expectations and refuses to delay the procedure when further sternal development will improve the surgical result.

Treatment Principles. If an operative repair is planned, evaluations by cardiology, pulmonary disease, and anesthesiology specialists are warranted. Their assessments of the risk and safety of the anesthetic and operative procedures have been extremely valuable and may uncover unknown yet critical findings. At this stage, patients may be selected for static and dynamic pulmonary function tests, radionuclide imaging, echocardiography, or ultrasonography. Current data suggest that only patients with a severe pectus excavatum can expect cardiopulmonary improvement after corrective surgery.[30]

The operative options described in the literature for repair of the pectus deformity are numerous. Most described in the first 40 years of pectus excavatum repair have been modifications of the original technique developed by Ravitch[31] in the 1950s, which is still used today. However, in the last 10 years, there has been an explosion in the surgical literature of pectus excavatum repair, initiated by the description by Nuss[10] of a minimally invasive repair of pectus excavatum (Nuss procedure) in 1998.

In patients with *mild* defects that are causing few or no physiologic symptoms, a custom silicone implant may be considered. With such devices, the risk of infection, prolonged seromas, migration, and soft tissue erosion should be taken into account. These complications associated with the implant and the option to reconstruct the chest wall by direct correction of the abnormality serve as indications for resection-osteotomies and anatomic repair as the preferred method of correction.[32] However, in the adult with mild deformity, the custom silicone implant in the male patient or bilateral breast augmentation with mammary prostheses with central custom implant in the female patient can effectively camouflage the deformity (Figs. 134-6 and 134-7).

For more severe defects, both minimally invasive repair and resection techniques have been employed.[33,34] Current studies suggest that both of these approaches provide satisfactory clinical results. In young patients with resilient tissues, the minimally invasive repair is appealing and less traumatic to the tissues. In this procedure, a curved metallic bar is inserted under thoracoscopic control (or after the insertion of a large substernal clamp) through incisions in the anterior axillary line. After substernal positioning, the bar is then inverted to place its convex side ventrally, putting pressure on the deep aspect of the sternum and forcing the sternum anteriorly. Both sides of the bar are then fixed to the sternum or to the lateral chest wall. Although modifications (including the use of surgical steel rather than titanium bars) have allowed higher rates of successful long-term outcome (86.6%),[35] the procedure has had high complication and reoperation rates, prolonged need for pain medication, and lack of efficacy in older teenagers that may limit its applicability.[6,8,35-37]

Ravitch Procedure and Modifications. In the patient whose sternum and cartilages are more mature and less resilient, resection techniques (removal of deformed rib cartilage and sternal repositioning) can be employed. The most widely used resection technique was pioneered by Ravitch[38] (Fig. 134-8). It involves bilateral resection of the deformed costal cartilages and a correctional sternal osteotomy. Although this method requires more operating time than the minimally invasive repair does, it is associated with shorter hospital stays, fewer complications, and decreased use of pain medications[36] (Figs. 134-9 and 134-10). Unfortunately, accurately matched, long-term comparisons of the minimally invasive and resection techniques may not be available for some time.

As pectus excavatum has been hypothesized to be caused by overgrowth of the costal cartilages, Ravitch introduced a procedure that was centered around the resection of costal cartilages.[36] The procedure has been modified numerous times since its original description, with a consistent theme being less extensive resection of the cartilages.[36]

A midline sternal or an inframammary chevron incision with midline extension (if needed) is made with the patient in the supine position. The skin is mobilized laterally, and pectoralis and rectus abdominis flaps are elevated for exposure of the costal cartilages. Small segments of cartilage are resected both medially and laterally, leaving the perichondrial sheaths. The xiphoid-sternal junction is identified and divided. A transverse anterior table osteotomy is made at the

Text continued on p. 469

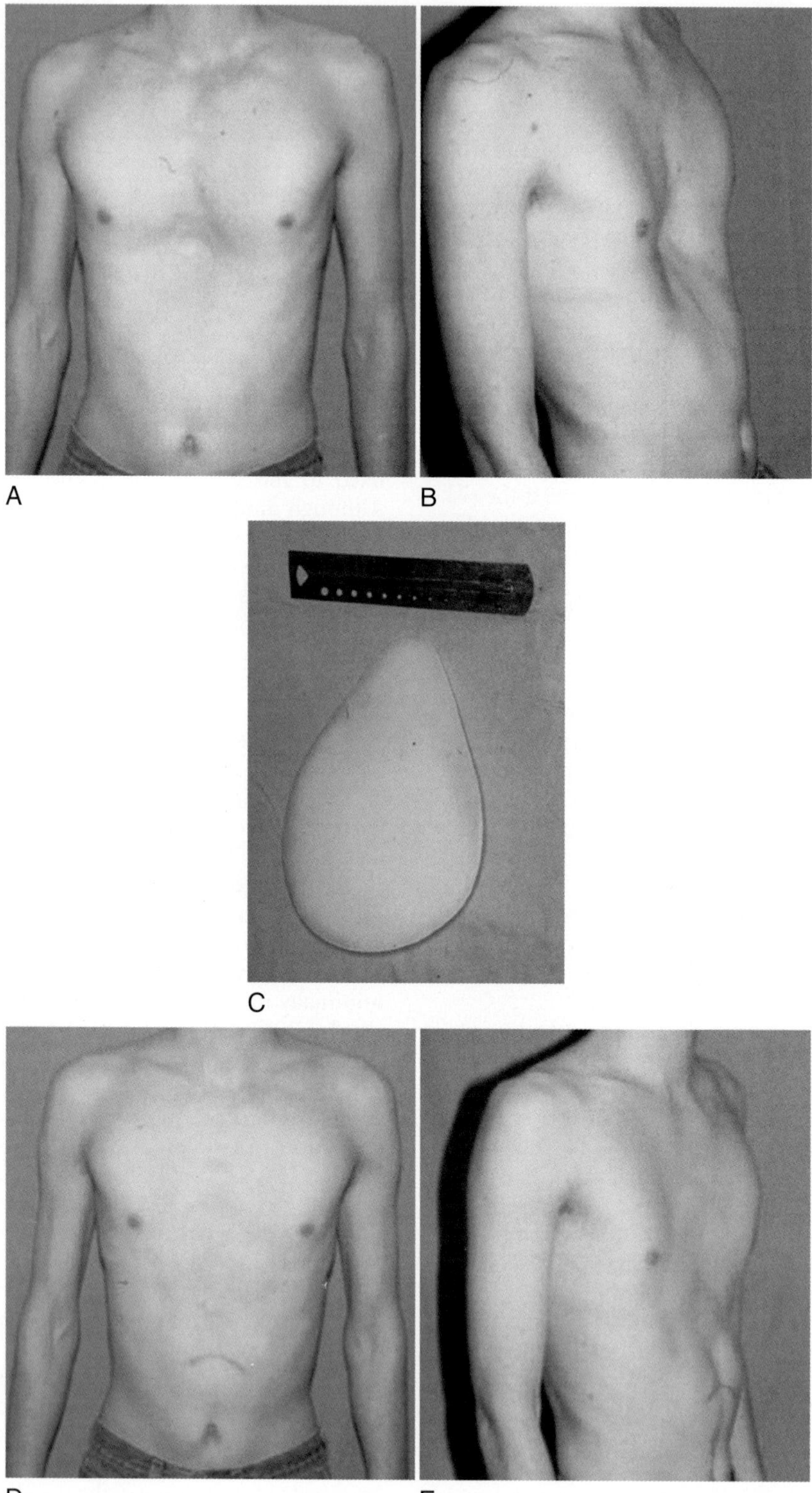

FIGURE 134-6. Use of custom implant to correct adult pectus excavatum. *A,* Anterior view, mild pectus deformity. *B,* Oblique view. Note central concavity. *C,* Custom silicone implant (deep surface of implant). *D,* Anterior postoperative view 6 months after implant insertion. Note transverse epigastric incision for implant insertion. *E,* Oblique view, concave sternal deformity corrected by implant.

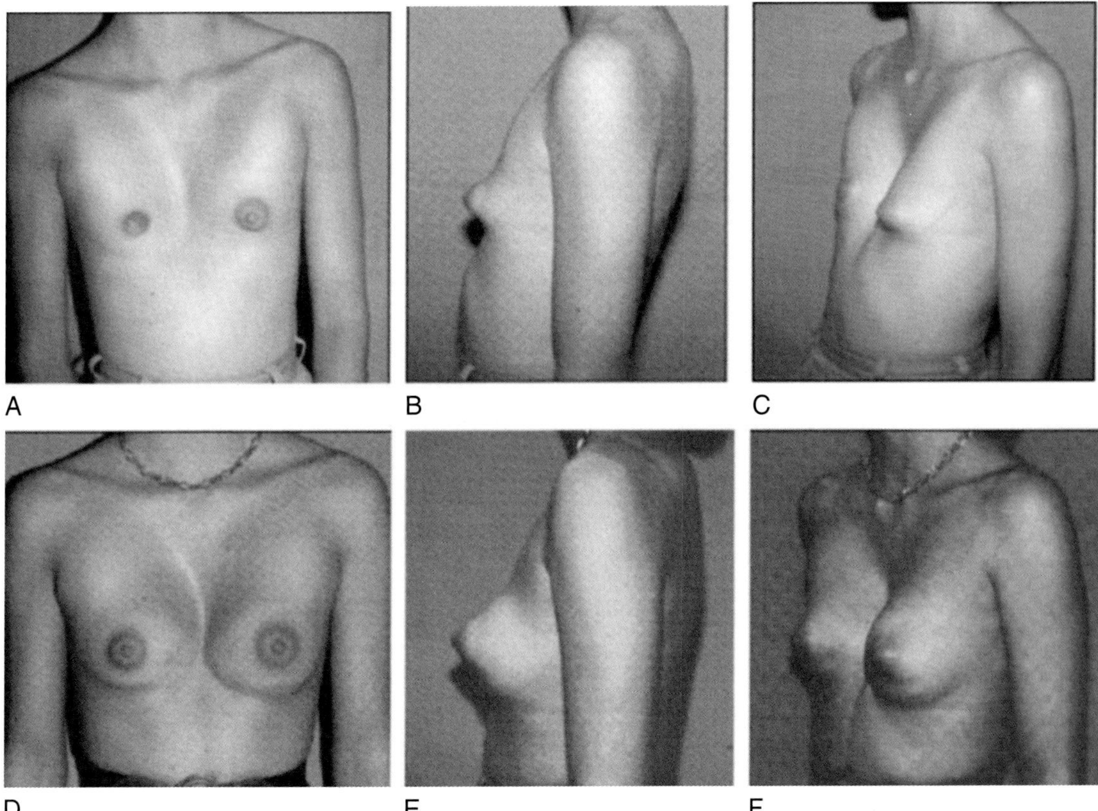

FIGURE 134-7. Pectus excavatum with bilateral tuberous breasts corrected with breast implantation. *A,* Anterior view, mild pectus deformity. *B,* Lateral view, tuberous breast deformity. *C,* Oblique view. Mild pectus deformity/concavity is clearly seen in this view. *D,* Anterior postoperative view at 1 year. Implants have been used to correct the breast deformity. (The patient refused a custom implant for the pectus deformity.) *E,* Postoperative lateral view. *F,* Postoperative oblique view. The pectus concavity is not completely corrected by bilateral breast implants.

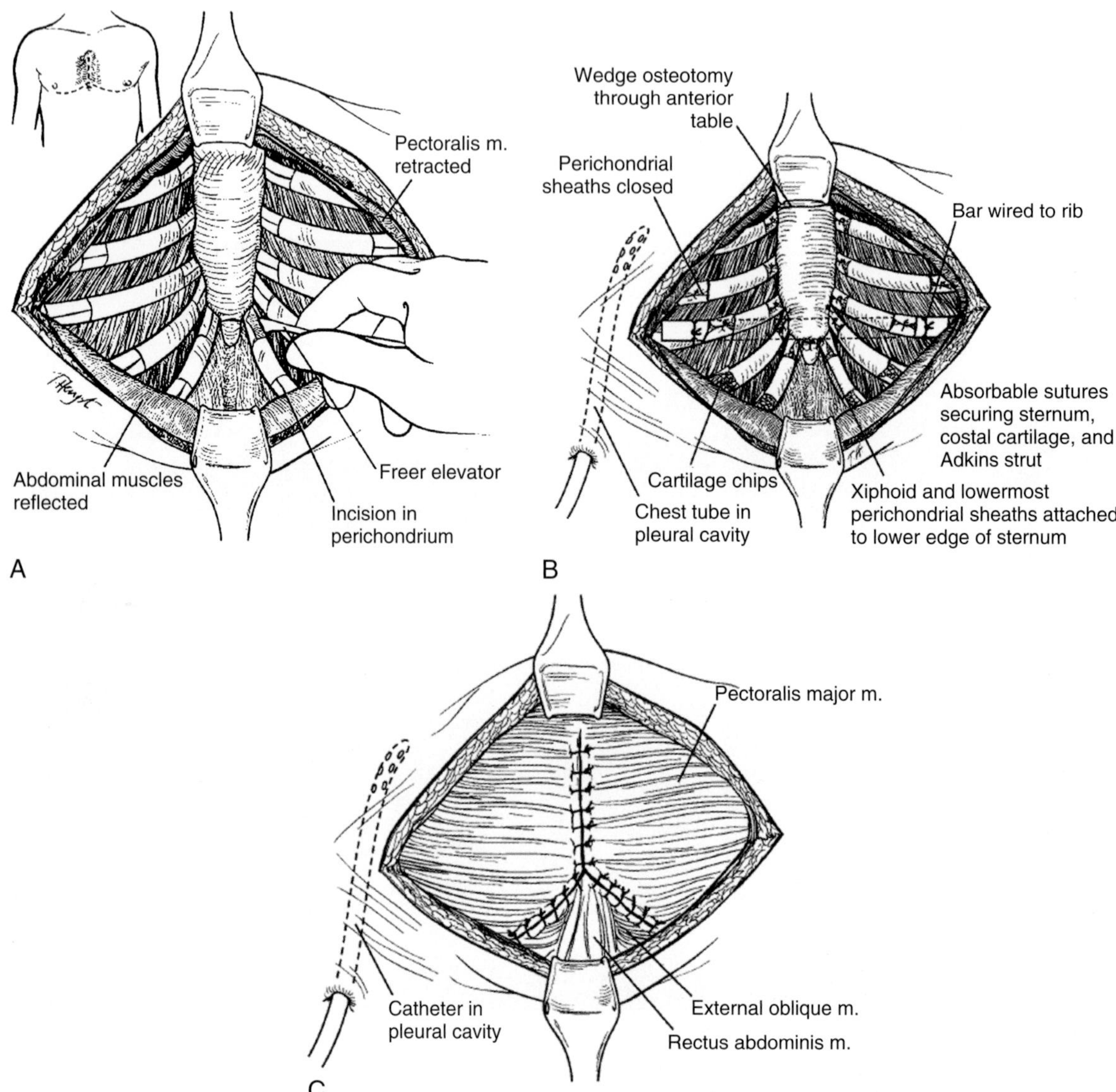

FIGURE 134-8. Pectus excavatum repair, modified Ravitch procedure. *A,* Transverse inframammary incision with upward curvature in the midportion and a small vertical extension superiorly is commonly used. Cutaneous as well as pectoralis and abdominal muscle flaps are elevated to expose the deformed costal cartilages. Incisions are made through the perichondrium on the medial and lateral ends of the deformed cartilages, and short segments of cartilage are removed. *B,* A transverse wedge osteotomy is made across the lower anterior table of the sternum at the desired level. The posterior table of the sternum is fractured but not detached. The lower sternum is elevated to the desired level, and an Adkins strut is placed across the lower anterior chest posterior to the sternum and costal cartilages, with the tip of the strut attached to the anterior surface of a rib on each side with wire. The xiphoid and lowermost perichondrial sheaths are reattached to the sternum. Finely minced fragments of autologous costal cartilage are placed into the open perichondrial sheaths. *C,* A drainage catheter is placed into the right pleural cavity in the majority of patients. The pectoralis muscles are reapproximated over the cartilaginous repair. The abdominal muscles are attached to the pectoralis muscles across the lower anterior chest. (From Fonkalsrud EW: Current management of pectus excavatum. World J Surg 2003;27:502-508.)

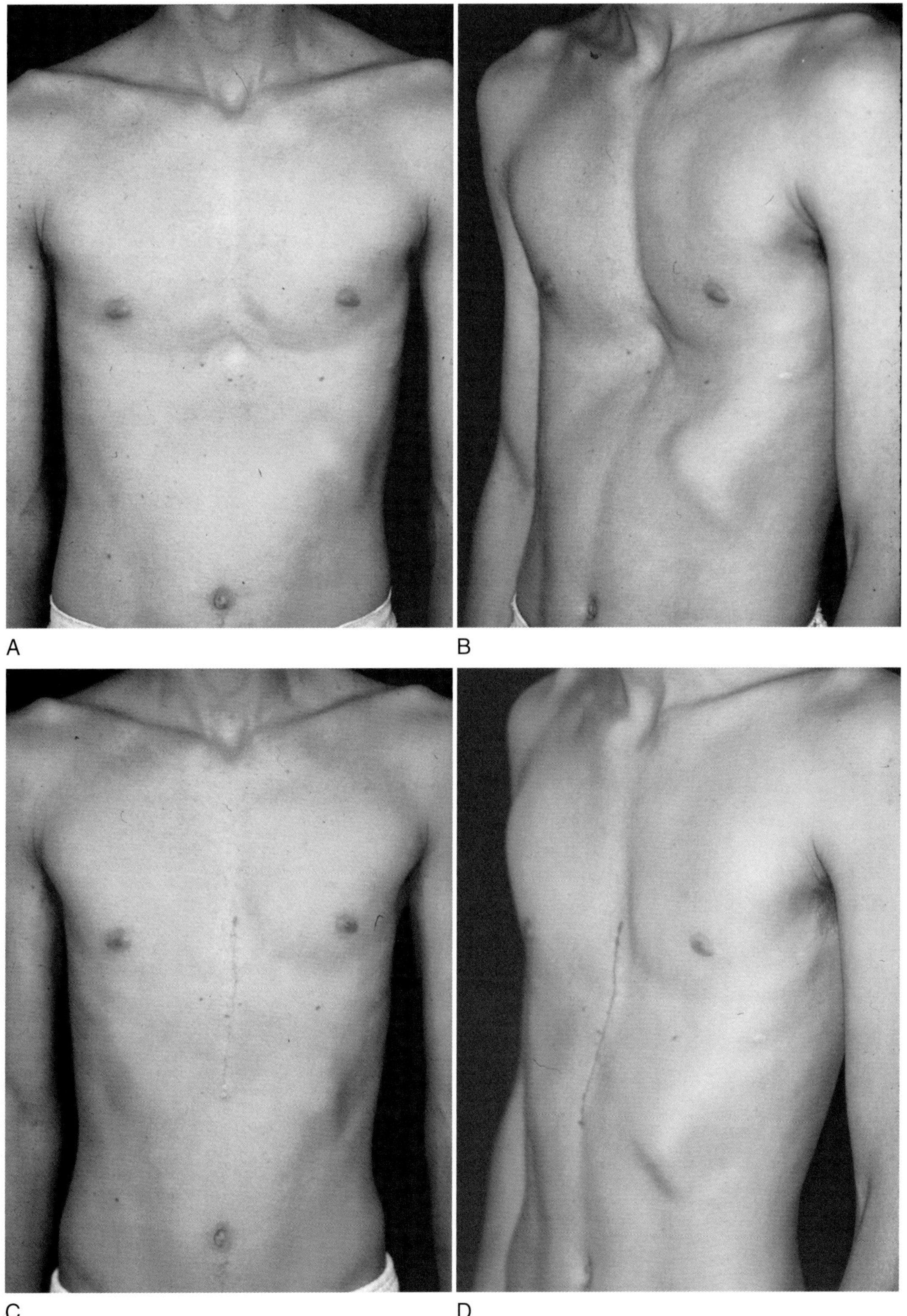

FIGURE 134-9. Pectus excavatum repair, sternum secured with sternal wires. *A,* Anterior view of 18-year-old male patient referred for moderate pectus excavatum. *B,* Oblique view. *C,* Postoperative anterior view. After removal of abnormal cartilage and sternal osteotomies, the sternum was secured with wire sutures. Healing was uneventful; the patient was discharged on the third postoperative day and resumed an active, healthy lifestyle. *D,* Postoperative oblique view.

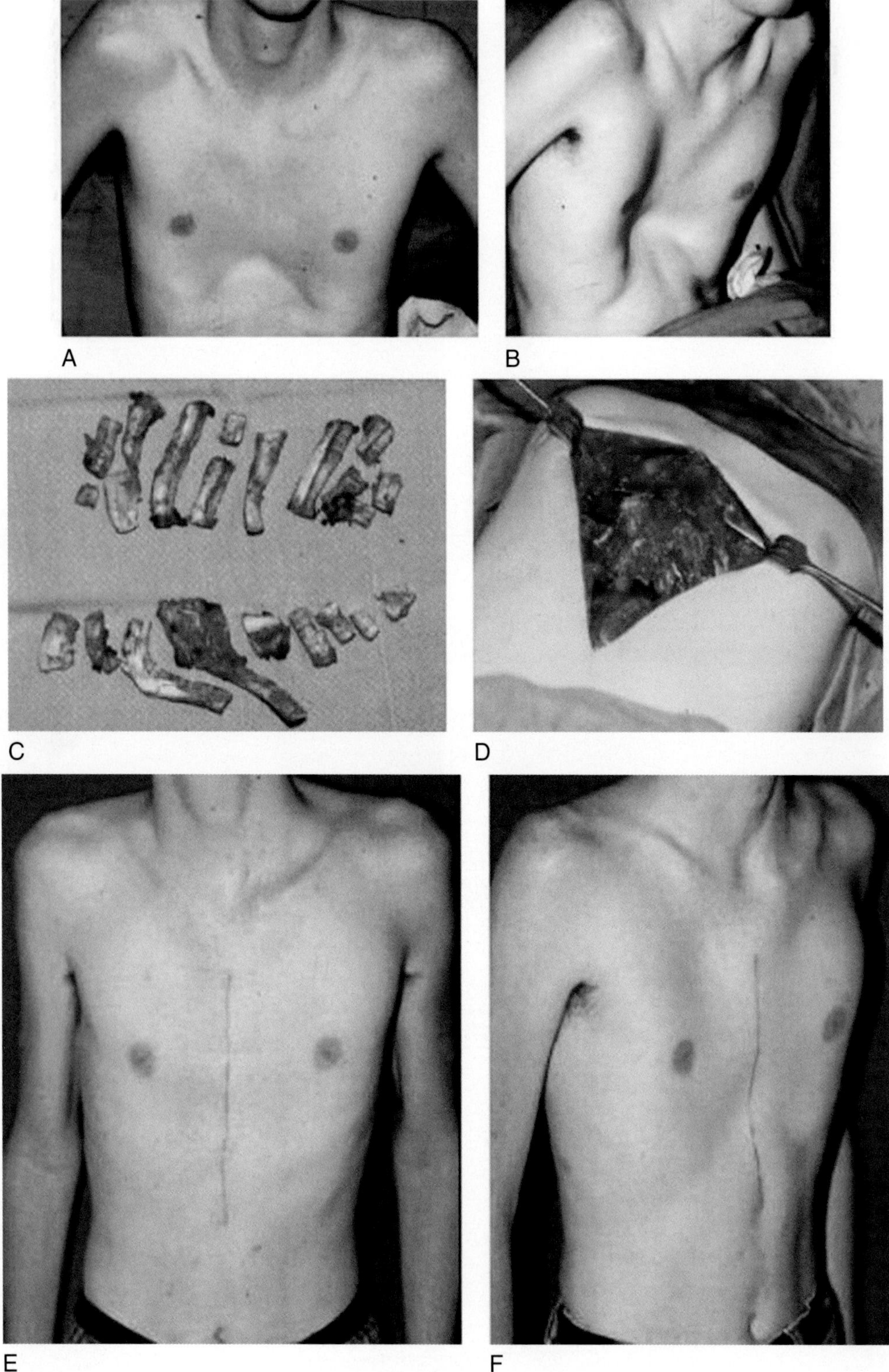

FIGURE 134-10. Pectus excavatum repair, sternum secured with Washington strut. *A,* Anterior view of 17-year-old male patient referred for severe pectus excavatum. *B,* Oblique view. *C,* Rib cartilage (deformed) that was removed. *D,* After osteotomies, the flattened sternum was secured with a Washington strut. *E* and *F,* Postoperative anterior and oblique views. (From Garcia VF, Seyfer AE, Graeber GM: Reconstruction of congenital chest-wall deformities. Surg Clin North Am 1989;69:1103.)

superior margin of the sternal depression after mobilization of the posterior surface of the sternum. The sternum is now elevated, causing a nondisplaced fracture of the posterior sternal table. A small metallic strut can be placed posterior to the sternum and secured to the anterior surface of the ribs laterally where there is normal contour. The xiphoid is reattached to the sternum, and the perichondrial sheaths that were opened are filled with minced autologous cartilage grafts and closed. The pectoralis and rectus abdominis flaps are advanced over the repair and closed. Closed suction drains are placed to eliminate dead space, and tube thoracostomies are used in patients with entrance into the pleural space.[6] The sternal strut is removed at a second procedure approximately 6 months later.

Minimally Invasive Repair: Nuss Procedure. In 1998, Nuss[10] reported a novel, minimally invasive technique for pectus excavatum repair that avoided cartilage resection, osteotomy, and a major anterior chest scar. In addition, the introduction of this procedure has reduced operating time and has stimulated interest in pectus excavatum repair from pediatricians, surgeons, and patients.

The central concept of the Nuss technique is the elevation of the sternum by use of a curved metallic strut (pectus bar) that is inserted laterally (Fig. 134-11). General endotracheal anesthesia is induced, and the patient is placed in the supine position on the operating room table. A 5-mm 30-degree thoracoscope is introduced into the left side of the chest to allow direct observation of the sternum and mediastinal structures. A small incision is made over the fourth intercostal space laterally on each side. Traditionally, a pectus clamp (similar in concept to a vascular tunneling device) was passed under the sternum, exiting through the contralateral incision. Umbilical tape was then attached to the tip of the pectus clamp and drawn through the tunnel by removal of the clamp. A recent modification of the procedure is the "introducer" instrument, which facilitates formation of the substernal tunnel and passage of umbilical tape as well as elevation of the sternum before bar insertion (Fig. 134-12*A*). After passage of the introducer across the mediastinum, the anterior chest wall can be carefully elevated by lifting the introducer on each side of the chest, thus correcting the pectus excavatum before bar insertion. The introducers range from small to extra large with varying degrees of curvature to suit the patient.[35]

The curved (typically U-shaped) pectus bar (Fig. 134-12*B*) is then attached to the umbilical tape and drawn inverted through the tunnel to exit through the opposite wound. By use of rotation or "flipper" instruments (which have largely replaced the vise grips once used) attached to both exposed ends, the bar is

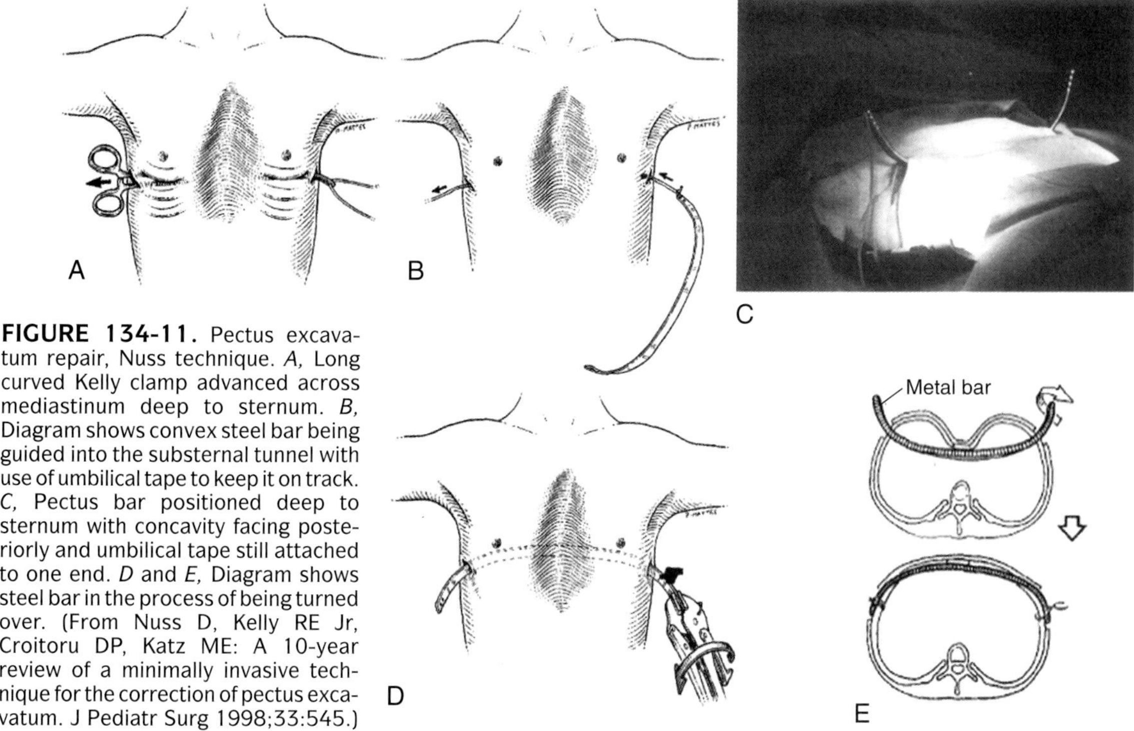

FIGURE 134-11. Pectus excavatum repair, Nuss technique. *A,* Long curved Kelly clamp advanced across mediastinum deep to sternum. *B,* Diagram shows convex steel bar being guided into the substernal tunnel with use of umbilical tape to keep it on track. *C,* Pectus bar positioned deep to sternum with concavity facing posteriorly and umbilical tape still attached to one end. *D* and *E,* Diagram shows steel bar in the process of being turned over. (From Nuss D, Kelly RE Jr, Croitoru DP, Katz ME: A 10-year review of a minimally invasive technique for the correction of pectus excavatum. J Pediatr Surg 1998;33:545.)

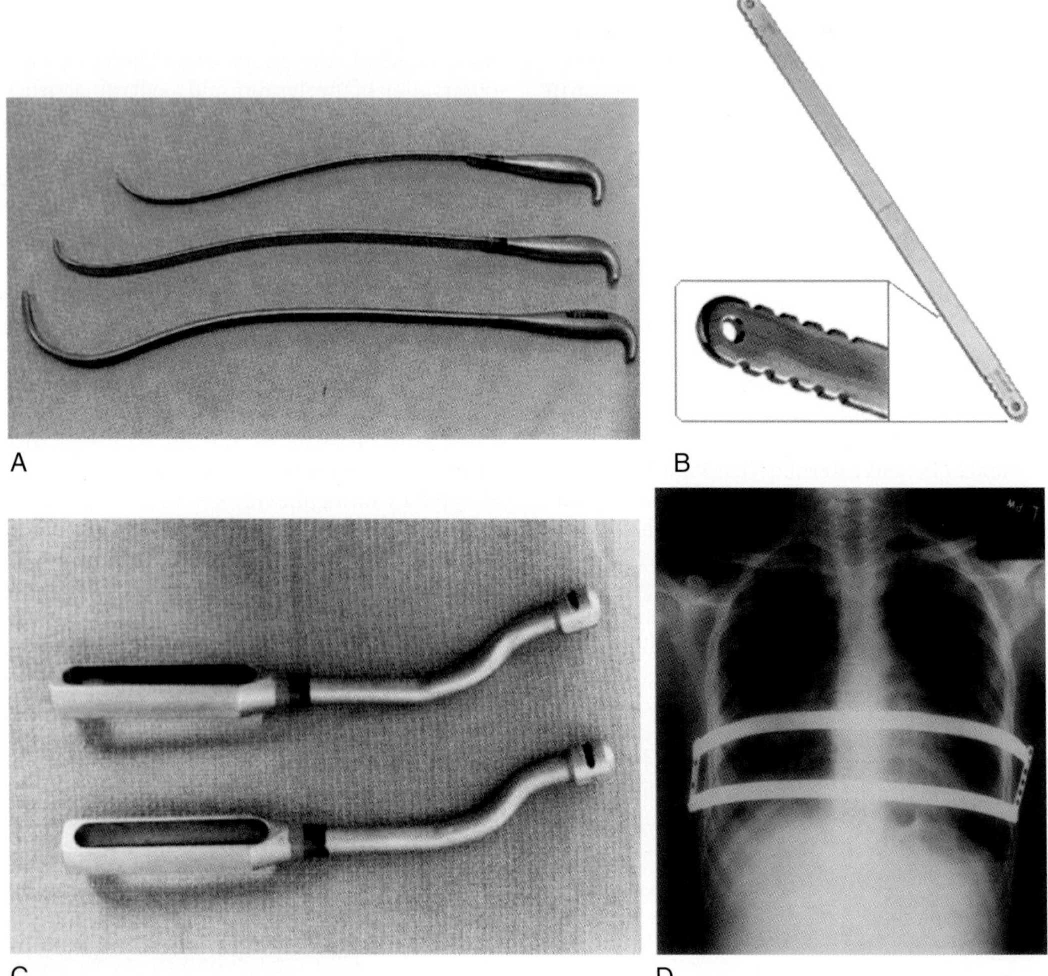

FIGURE 134-12. Instrumentation for Nuss procedure. *A,* Introducer. *B,* Pectus bar. Bar is bent to fit chest size before insertion. *C,* Flipper. *D,* Anterior radiograph demonstrates double pectus bar. (*A* to *C* from Croitoru DP, Kelly RE Jr, Goretsky MJ, et al: Experience and modification update for the minimally invasive Nuss technique for pectus excavatum repair in 303 patients. J Pediatr Surg 2002;37:437. *D* courtesy of Lorenz Surgical, Jacksonville, Fla.)

inverted and elevates the sternum (Fig. 134-12*C*). Additional bars placed cephalad or caudad to the initial bar can occasionally be used to improve the symmetry or extent of the sternal elevation (Fig. 134-12*D*). Once inverted, the bars are secured to the ribs with heavy suture or, in patients with instability, with lateral T supports. The bar remains in place for approximately 2 years, at which time it is removed by opening the original incisions.

REPAIR WITH SILICONE IMPLANTS. The use of custom silicone implants to treat the pectus deformity has the advantage of being a relatively minor procedure. However, it addresses only the cosmetic deformity and none of the potential intrathoracic physiologic disturbances. The risk of progression remains. Consequently, it should be reserved for those who would derive no potential benefit from increasing the intrathoracic volume and those for whom a more invasive operation is too risky. It offers the advantage over the Ravitch procedure of not requiring a midline sternal incision.

Modified Technique for Repair with Custom Silicone Implants. The custom implant is designed from a moulage of the chest taken with the patient in the supine position. The moulage may be made with dental alginate, papier mâché, or plaster compounds from commercially available moulage kits.* CT scans have also been used to assist in forming a model for a custom implant. Scans of the chest are taken with 5-mm cuts from the sternal notch to the xiphoid process; by combination of a composite tracing of the submuscular sternal contour from each section, a

*Specialty Surgical Products, Victor, Montana.

three-dimensional model of the chest may be constructed.[39] The accuracy of the moulage contributes significantly to the fabrication of a custom implant.

When the custom implant, made of a silicone polymer, is received from the manufacturer, the operative procedure is scheduled. The implant is inserted through a small superior transverse epigastric incision. A pocket is dissected superficial to the sternal contour irregularity and the implant is then inserted. The implant made of soft silicone can be modified with a scalpel if it demonstrates excessive projection or the edges are too thick. In general, the implant fits nicely into the defect and does not require a patch on the deep surface or sutures to maintain its appropriate position. After implant placement, the pocket is closed. Drains may be used but require an additional incision and usually are not required. The technique is useful for the young adult or patient with a mild pectus deformity (Fig. 134-13).

RESECTION AND STERNAL FIXATION: MODIFIED TECHNIQUE. The following describes a technique that has been effective for pectus deformities. This technique can be delayed until late adolescence with high satisfaction of patients and families. The procedure is performed under a general anesthetic, and an epidural catheter can be inserted for postoperative pain control. The patient is supine with the arms abducted to 90 degrees, and other appropriate lines and monitoring devices are applied. Although transverse (submammary) incisions have been employed in the past, the central portion of the scar is often hypertrophic and poorly accepted by the patient. Consequently, a short vertical midline incision is used to access the deformity, beginning at the sternal angle (or lower) and ending at the xiphoid. It offers excellent, safe exposure and usually heals with a more favorable scar. The subcutaneous tissues are divided and the pectoralis major muscles liberated from the sternum and costal perichondrium with electrocautery. This effectively exposes the defect, and costal cartilages from ribs two to seven are exposed by incision of the perichondrium over each segment. By use of the Alexander (rib dissector) and the pediatric Y-shaped elevators (strippers), the perichondrium is circumferentially reflected from the cartilage from the sternocostal junction to the costochondral junction on each rib, with care taken to avoid entering the pleura (Fig. 134-14). The deformed cartilage is then removed, leaving a bed of perichondrium for eventual cartilage regrowth. The xiphoid process, often quite deformed, is grasped with a Kocher clamp, and by finger dissection, the sternum is bluntly elevated on its deep aspect from the pleura and the pericardium. A wide malleable retractor is inserted into this space to protect the heart and the great vessels, and the oscillating sternal saw is used to section the sternum. Usually, the anterior table can be cut and the sternum gently "greensticked" forward to provide a nice contour. On occasion, two osteotomies are required to flatten the curved bone.

After the osteotomy, thin orthopedic titanium alloy plates are secured to the sternum with blunt (non–self-tapping) corticocancellous screws. With the malleable retractor in position, appropriate holes are drilled to accept the screws, and depending on the number of osteotomies, one or two thin, flat titanium T-shaped plates are used for sternal fixation. A depth gauge is used to customize the length of the screws. After the final screws are in place, the posterior sternal surface is digitally assessed to ensure that the screws do not protrude against the pericardium. The xiphoid process, if it is badly deformed, is excised. The incision is closed in layers over a soft suction drain. Chest auscultation and a postoperative chest film are performed in the recovery room to assess for an occult pneumothorax.

In a recent series,[40] the average duration of this procedure was between 3 and 4 hours, and the hospital stay ranged from 1 to 3 days. Satisfaction of patients was uniformly high. Although there were no major complications, there was one mild recurrence in a patient who underwent repair at the age of 14 years. No recurrences were observed in patients whose repair was performed at the age of 17 years or later. Follow-up averaged 2.91 years (Fig. 134-15).

Although cartilage removal remains a fairly standard part of the resection, methods of sternal fixation vary and have employed Steinmann pins (Fig. 134-16), silk sutures, metal bars, vascularized rib struts, wires, Marlex mesh, and bioabsorbable mesh.[41-45] Steel and mandibular plates have been used but can be bulky. Thin titanium plates, less bulky than mandibular plates but stronger than miniplates, offer excellent sternal healing and immediate stability, with few complications (Table 134-4). Bioabsorbable plates (see following section, "Bioabsorbable Mesh and Plates") are also effective and do not require removal.[46-49]

Bioabsorbable Mesh and Plates. Successful repair of pectus excavatum has also been reported with use of mesh as well as plates and screws for fixation instead of a retrosternal bar.[43,45,49,50] In 1978, Robicsek[45] reported the use of Marlex mesh for stabilization of the sternum for severe pectus deformity. This technique, although stable, was criticized for establishing a noncompliant chest wall and symptomatic chest wall heaviness.[43] The use of bioabsorbable mesh was introduced as a means to alleviate the rigidity.[43,51] Luzzi[43] reported the results of 28 patients who underwent pectus excavatum repair by the Robicsek technique with use of bioabsorbable polyglactin 910 (Vicryl) for sternal fixation. The mesh was placed retrosternally and secured to the perichondrium, the intercostal muscles, the inferior border of the pectoralis major,

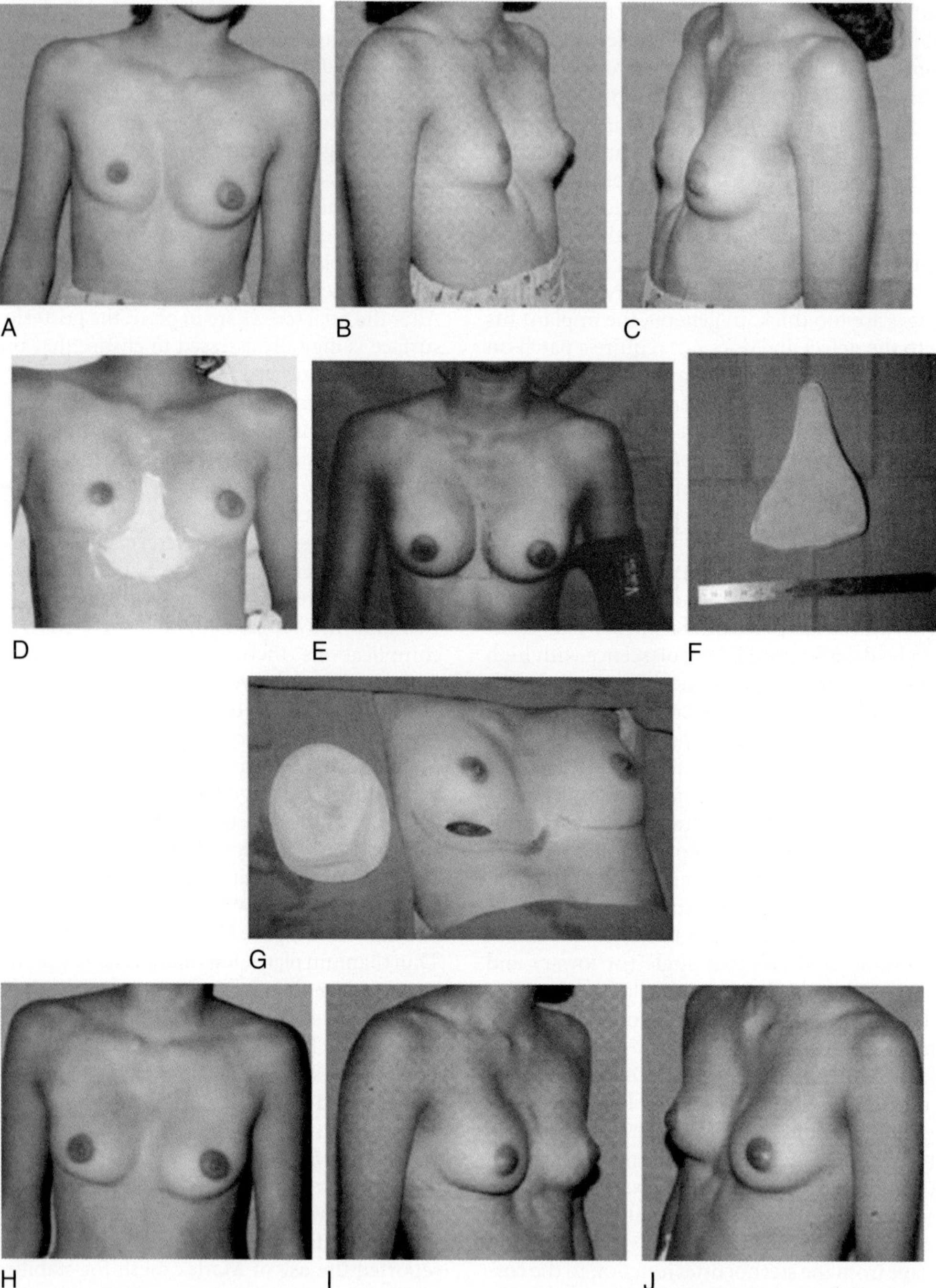

FIGURE 134-13. Pectus excavatum repair, custom implant. *A,* Anterior view of adult patient with pectus excavatum and right constricted breast. *B,* Oblique view of central sternal contour deformity. *C,* Lateral view. Note right inferior breast constriction. *D,* Moulage prepared for design of custom silicone implant for central sternal contour deformity. *E,* Anterior view 3 months after release of inferior breast constriction and insertion of expanders; preoperative second-stage right breast implant and custom sternal implant insertion. *F,* Custom silicone implant for sternal defect. *G,* Anterior intraoperative view, second stage. Both the custom implant for the sternum and the right breast implant have been inserted through a right inframammary incision. *H,* Anterior postoperative view at 1 year of sternal custom implant and right breast augmentation for breast symmetry. *I,* Oblique view. Note correction of sternal defect and constricted hypoplastic right breast. *J,* Oblique view. Note right breast adjustment of inframammary line and inferior breast quadrant parenchyma deficiency.

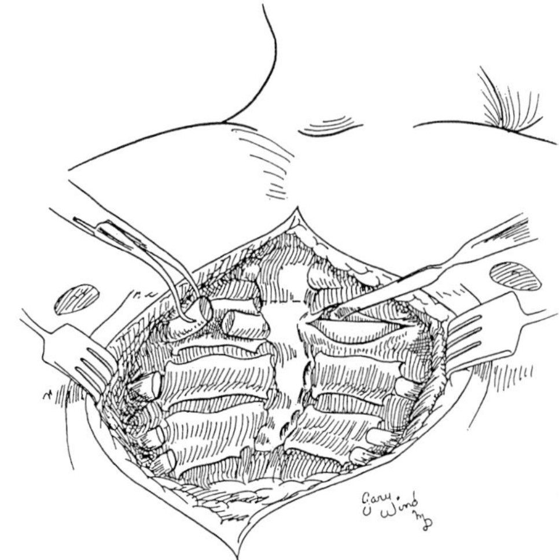

FIGURE 134-14. The deformed cartilage is removed, leaving the perichondrium intact for regeneration of new cartilage. (From Garcia VF, Seyfer AE, Graeber GM: Reconstruction of congenital chest-wall deformities. Surg Clin North Am 1989;69:1103.)

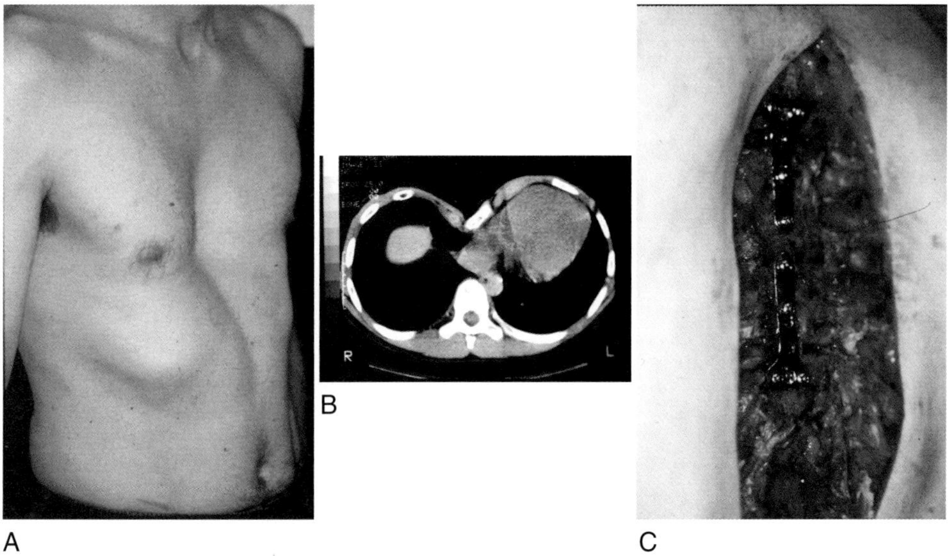

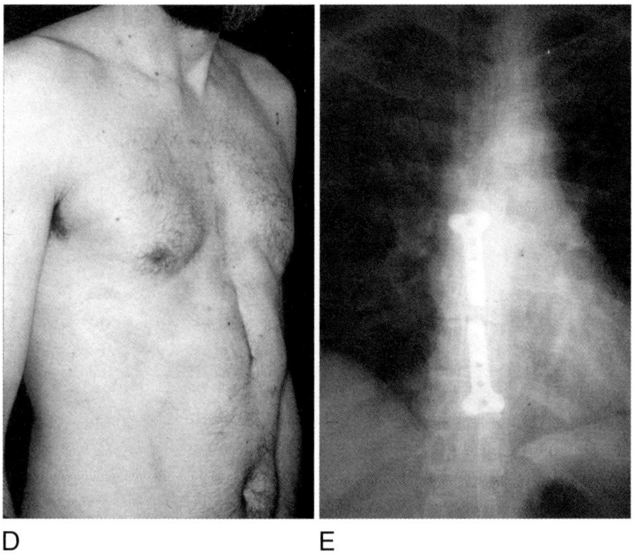

A B C D E

FIGURE 134-15. *A,* A 35-year-old patient in good health who desired repair of his moderate asymptomatic pectus excavatum deformity. *B,* Axial CT scan showed displacement of the cardiac silhouette and mild twisting (dextrorotation) of the sternum. *C,* After resection of deformed cartilage, the two sternal osteotomies were secured with thin titanium alloy plates. *D,* Postoperative appearance. The patient regained his active lifestyle early. *E,* Postoperative chest film.

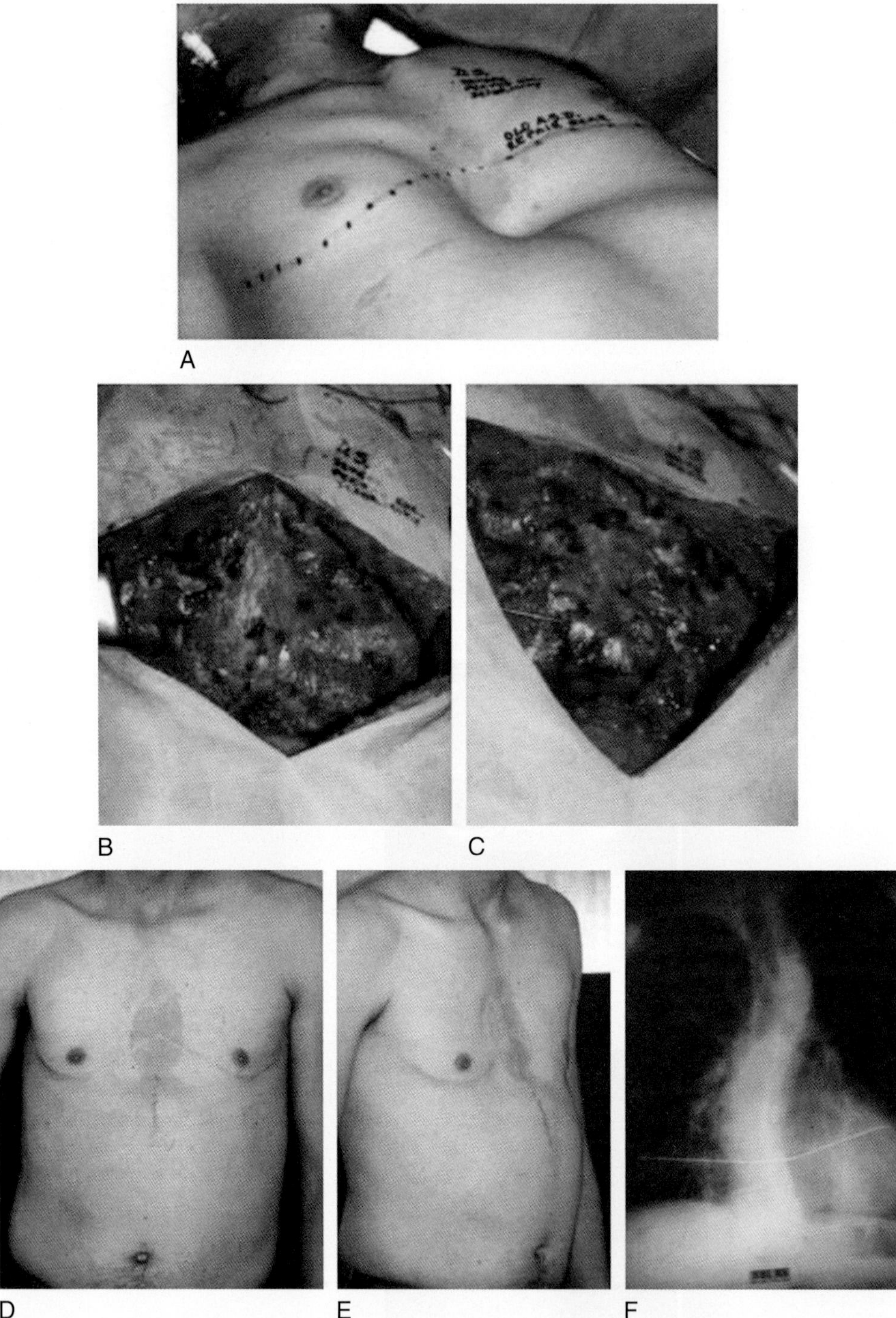

FIGURE 134-16. Pectus excavatum repair, sternum secured with Steinmann pin. *A,* A 31-year-old man with previous repair of an atrial septal defect. *B,* Pericardium was fused to posterior sternal table, making dissection difficult. Deformed cartilage is shown before removal. *C,* After sternal osteotomies, the flattened sternum is secured to the rib bone with a threaded Steinmann pin. *D,* The patient is shown after uneventful healing. *E,* Lateral view. *F,* The patient sustained blunt chest wall trauma 3 years later, breaking the Steinmann pin. Chest radiograph shows the broken pin. It was removed with difficulty because the sternum had healed well.

TABLE 134-4 ✦ NONABSORBABLE STERNAL FIXATION DEVICES

Fixation Device	Long-term Stability	Complications
Retrosternal bar	Removal indicated	Fracture of bar Displacement Internal organ injury
Washington strut	Stable	Palpable hardware
Steinmann (threaded) pin	Stable	Fracture of pin
Steel plate and screws	Stable	Fracture of plate Loosening of screws Internal organ injury
Titanium plate and screws	Stable	Fracture of plate Loosening of screws Internal organ injury

and the cartilaginous stumps. After 2 years of follow-up, results were significant for excellent results in 65% and recurrence in 7% of patients (Table 134-5). All patients were older than 10 years, and no major complications (other than recurrence) were reported. Consistent with other techniques, no significant changes in prospectively acquired pulmonary function test results were noted. Early mobilization was encouraged.[43]

The use of metallic plates and screws for retrosternal support was reported in 1959 by Paltia[50]; however, the presence of metal in the anterior mediastinum still raised concerns about rare but critical complications, including dislodgment leading to cardiac perforation as well as discomfort and the need for removal.[52] Lansman[49] reported a retrospective series of eight patients (mean age, 5.0 years) in whom polylactide plates were placed retrosternally and compared them

TABLE 134-5 ✦ RESULTS OF BIOABSORBABLE MESH FIXATION FOR REPAIR OF PECTUS EXCAVATUM (N = 28)

Result	Polyglactin Mesh (n = 28)	Polylactide Plates (n = 8)
Excellent	18 (65%)	3 (37.5%)
Good	7 (25%)	3 (37.5%)
Fair	1 (3.5)	1 (12.5%)
Poor (recurrence)	2 (7%)	0 (0%)
No evaluation	—	1 (12.5%)

From Lansman S, Serlo W, Linna O, et al: Treatment of pectus excavatum with bioabsorbable polylactide plates: preliminary results. J Pediatr Surg 2002;37:1281-1286.

Reprinted with permission from The Society of Thoracic Surgeons.

with patients with similarly placed metallic plates. Results after a mean of 2.2 years (range, 0.5 to 4.9 years) of follow-up were good but not different from those of the controls. Fracture of the plate requiring reoperation occurred in one patient (12.5%).[49] A brief retrospective series using the modified Ravitch technique in 33 males (14 years and older) with absorbable copolymer (LactoSorb) plates and screws placed anterior to the sternal osteotomy showed no major complications or recurrence after 12 months of follow-up.[53]

Preliminary data indicate that satisfactory results with use of bioabsorbable mesh and plating systems for pectus excavatum repair can be achieved, although good prospective data are lacking. Caution should be exercised in the use of these materials outside of clinical trials until a level of experience with and data on these techniques have been accumulated, allowing accurate comparisons with more traditional methods.

Results

Ravitch Technique. Several good retrospective studies have examined the outcomes for the modified Ravitch technique. Mansour[54] described 68 patients with medical symptoms (mostly adults; mean age, 22 years) and reported excellent results after a mean follow-up of 12 years; 91% reported improvement in symptoms (none worse), and there was only one recurrence. In a patient satisfaction study by Davis[55] with 24 respondents (mean age, approximately 12 years), the median patient satisfaction score was 4 of a possible 5 after a median of 2 years of follow-up. Fonkalsrud[56] reported 75 consecutive reconstructions with substernal strut use; 74 patients responded that the repair was good or excellent at a mean of 8.2 months of follow-up. The mean operating time and length of hospitalization in this high-volume center were 174 minutes and 2.7 days, respectively.

Objective physiologic testing of the Ravitch repair was done in two studies. By radionuclide scanning prospectively of 13 patients before and 6 months after repair, improvement was noted in the left ventricular end-diastolic index and the stroke volume index, suggesting the relief of cardiac compression.[23] However, a prospective study of 15 adolescents with pectus excavatum and 10 age-matched controls who underwent preoperative and postoperative pulmonary function tests and exercise testing revealed no changes in forced vital capacity, but a slight improvement was noted in exercise tolerance and oxygen saturation during exercise after repair. The clinical benefits of the observed response are unclear[22] (Tables 134-6 and 134-7).

Nuss Technique. Several studies, originating from Nuss's institution and elsewhere, confirm the adequacy of minimally invasive repair of pectus excavatum. Nuss retrospectively reported the results of 303 patients. The mean age was 12.4 years (range, 1.75 to 29 years), and

TABLE 134-6 ✦ PREOPERATIVE AND POSTOPERATIVE (8 ± 3 MONTHS) PULMONARY FUNCTION TEST RESULTS

	Pectus Excavatum (n = 15)		Control Subjects (n = 6)	
	Preoperative	*Postoperative*	*Initial*	*Follow-up*
FVC (L)	3.5 ± 1.0	3.7 ± 1.0*	3.3 ± 1.3	3.7 ± 1.6
FVC (% predicted)	81 ± 17	80 ± 16	93 ± 8	97 ± 7
RV (% predicted)	117 ± 33	109 ± 52	101 ± 14	109 ± 42
RV/TLC (%)	27 ± 5	27 ± 9	23 ± 3	23 ± 6

Data are shown only for those subjects who completed both initial and follow-up tests. *$P < .01$: for initial versus follow-up tests.

FVC, forced vital capacity; RV, residual volume; TLC, total lung capacity.

Modified from Quigley PM, Haller JA, Jelus KL, et al: Cardiorespiratory function before and after corrective surgery in pectus excavatum. J Pediatr 1996;128 (pt 1):638.

the mean PSI was 5 (range, 2 to 21). Excellent cosmetic results were achieved in 85%, and only one failure was reported. Two bars were required in 13% of the patients. Bar shifting occurred in 5%, which was improved from the 16% rate when stabilizers were placed.[35] This study was confirmed with equivalent results from a study of 322 patients in Asia with a mean follow-up of 8 years. A broad age range was operated on (1.25 to 49 years, 22% older than 15 years). Successful and relatively easy bar removal after 2 years was demonstrated in 42 patients who achieved the 2-year landmark.[28]

Several studies have evaluated other outcomes of the Nuss technique in children. One small prospective pilot study revealed improved quality of life after repair.[27] A subjective prospective study of 19 children and 22 of their parents with a validated questionnaire revealed improvements after Nuss repair. The children reported subjective improvements in exercise tolerance, shortness of breath, tiredness, and personal satisfaction of their bodies; their parents confirmed these findings and reported fewer instances of frustration, isolation, and self-consciousness in their children.[26] Prospective study of pulmonary function test results before and after the Nuss procedure revealed that at 3 months after operation, there was significant improvement in stroke volume (suggesting relief of cardiac compression) but significant reductions in forced vital capacity and $\dot{V}O_2$max.[57] A different prospective study revealed that at 6 to 12 months after the Nuss repair,

TABLE 134-7 ✦ PREOPERATIVE AND POSTOPERATIVE (8 ± 3 MONTHS) EXERCISE TEST RESULTS

	Pectus Excavatum (n = 15)		Control Subjects (n = 6)	
	Preoperative	*Postoperative*	*Initial*	*Follow-up*
Duration (min)	12 ± 3	13 ± 2*	12 ± 3	12 ± 3
Speed (km/hr)	7 ± 0	8 ± 1*	7 ± 1	7 ± 0
Grade (%)	17 ± 5	19 ± 2†	18 ± 5	18 ± 5
Maximal heart rate (beats/min)	193 ± 11	193 ± 13	193 ± 7	195 ± 12
Respiratory exchange ratio	1.17 ± 0.14	1.31 ± 0.29	1.18 ± 0.06	1.14 ± 0.13
O_2 pulse (mL/beat)	11.5 ± 3.7	12.9 ± 3.6‡	10.8 ± 5.0	11.7 ± 5.5
$\dot{V}E$ (L/min)	88 ± 30	92 ± 30	86 ± 38	86 ± 40
ΔVT (%)	299 ± 80	316 ± 89	240 ± 110	271 ± 111
Maximal $\dot{V}O_2$ (mL/kg/min)	40 ± 8	40 ± 7	39 ± 5	40 ± 7
Anaerobic threshold (mL/kg/min $\dot{V}O_2$)	23 ± 6	23 ± 4	24 ± 4	25 ± 4
Breathing reserve (L/min)	27 ± 20	30 ± 16	19 ± 23	29 ± 15
Maximal $\dot{V}E/\dot{V}O_2$	40 ± 6	44 ± 10	42 ± 8	43 ± 8
Maximal $PETCO_2$ (mm Hg)	42 ± 4	44 ± 3	43 ± 6	44 ± 5
Minimal SaO_2 (%)	96 ± 1	96 ± 2	95 ± 1	96 ± 0

For initial versus follow-up tests: *$P < .02$. †$P < .05$. ‡$P < .005$.

$PETCO_2$, end-tidal PCO_2 tension; $\dot{V}E$, minute ventilation; $\dot{V}O_2$, oxygen consumption; ΔVT, maximal tidal volume divided by the initial VT, expressed as a percentage. $\dot{V}O_2$ and related data were unavailable for one patient with pectus excavatum; heart rate and related data were unavailable for another.

Modified from Quigley PM, Haller JA, Jelus KL, et al: Cardiorespiratory function before and after corrective surgery in pectus excavatum. J Pediatr 1996;128 (pt 1):638.

TABLE 134-8 ✦ COMPLICATIONS OF SURGERY FOR PECTUS EXCAVATUM

	Nuss (n = 273)	Ravitch (n = 251)
Results (n = 76 removed)		
Complications		
Mortality	0	0
Wound seroma	0	12
Pleural effusion	0	13
Pneumonia	3 (0.9%)	12
Pneumothorax	52% (2.7% required treatment)	6
Pericardial effusion, pericarditis	8 (2.4%)	3
Recurrence needing further surgery	6	5 (3 revision)
Protruding cartilage remnants	0	21 (5 revision)
Hypertrophic scar	0	35
Wound infection	7 (2.1%)	Not stated
Bar displacement	29/329 (8.8%)	N/A

From Williams AM, Crabbe DC: Pectus deformities of the anterior chest wall. Paediatr Respir Rev 2003;4:237-242.

no differences in pulmonary function test results (including forced vital capacity) or $\dot{V}O_2$max were observable, suggesting that the decreases in forced vital capacity and $\dot{V}O_2$max reported at 3 months postoperatively were residual effects of the operation.[58]

Complications. Complications in both the Ravitch and the Nuss repairs are relatively low and have been reported in depth (Table 134-8). Several complications require special mention. Early in the Nuss experience, significant injury to the thoracic organs occurred when the bar was passed blindly. The use of a thoracoscope allows direct observation of the intrathoracic organs and has markedly reduced the incidence of major injury.[35] Pericarditis similar to the postpericardiotomy syndrome is a persistent problem occasionally requiring pericardiocentesis. Both the Nuss and the Ravitch techniques have been used to salvage failed attempts of each technique. When implants are used, reoperations are necessary for the usual complications, including infection, rupture, and migration.

Summary

Pectus excavatum is a highly variable disorder presenting with aesthetic and possibly physiologic problems. There are several options for repair (Table 134-9). The Ravitch repair has proved to be a safe and effective technique but is a complex dissection and requires a midline sternotomy scar. The Nuss procedure has been shown to be a successful, minimally invasive alternative to the Ravitch repair with similar results. It is not yet clear whether either repair truly improves the patient's physiology. Both the Nuss and Ravitch repairs can be performed on patients of all ages; however, concealment of the deformity with a custom implant is a reasonable treatment option in asymptomatic adults.

PECTUS CARINATUM

Pectus carinatum (Latin *pectus*, breast, and *carina*, keel) is a disorder morphologically characterized by anterior displacement of the sternum. The entire sternum may protrude, with the most severe protrusion over the middle and lower portions (body and xiphoid) of the sternum. It can also present as a Z-like sagittal shape in which there is a mild depression of the midsternum and a severe protrusion of the lower sternal body and xiphoid. In both variations, the cartilages adjacent to the sternum (particularly rib cartilages two through six) are malformed on both sides. There is significant variation in the presentation of pectus carinatum, ranging from a small protuberance of the midsternum to large anterior displacements of the sternum and costal cartilages.[59]

The skin and subcutaneous fat may be thin over the apex of the deformity and, being draped over the

TABLE 134-9 ✦ PROCEDURES FOR PECTUS EXCAVATUM REPAIR

	Type of Repair		
Variables	*Sternal Resection*	*Sternal Bar*	*Custom Implant*
Age			
Preadolescent		X	
Adolescent	X		
Adult			X
Cardiopulmonary correction	X	X	
Mid-sternotomy scar	X		
Relapse		X	
Contour irregularities	X		X

underlying bone and cartilage, may be subject to more trauma than is usual. In these patients, the prevention of ulceration or injury may be ample indication to ameliorate the defect. As with most pectus problems, the patients usually complain more about the appearance of their chest rather than any functional difficulties.[16,32] These complaints usually surface in adolescence or early adulthood and are similar to those of patients with pectus excavatum.

Incidence

Pectus carinatum is seven times less common than pectus excavatum, making it an unusual but not rare disorder affecting between 1 in 10,000 and 1 in 1000 births. Pectus carinatum has a 6:1 male-to-female ratio.[60]

Etiology

The true cause of pectus carinatum is unknown. Pectus carinatum has been hypothesized to occur secondary to abnormal growth of the cartilage at the costochondral junction. It has a familial predilection as evidenced by observations that approximately 26% of patients with pectus carinatum have relatives with either pectus carinatum or pectus excavatum.[61]

Presentation and Diagnosis

Unlike pectus excavatum, which is generally recognized early in childhood, pectus carinatum is often not diagnosed until adolescence. The patients are generally asymptomatic, although there have been reports of asthmatic and dyspneic symptoms associated with pectus carinatum. Some authors have observed limitations in chest wall motion during ventilation due to the deformity, but this is disputed by some and has not been investigated thoroughly.[62-64] The primary complaint is typically an aesthetic one.

The deformity itself has considerable variation. In general, the mid and lower sternum is protruding. The upper sternum (manubrium) is anteriorly displaced in about 12% of patients, often with concurrent depression of the lower sternum.[65] Severity of the deformity can be characterized by the PSI.

Operative Treatment

The repair of pectus carinatum is similar to that of pectus excavatum. The Ravitch technique and its modifications have been the most common methods studied in the literature. Several retrospective series indicate that excellent results are the norm for this technique.[31,38,66] Fonkalsrud[56] reported a series of 154 patients with pectus carinatum with a mean follow-up of 7.9 years. The mean PSI was 1.76 (range, 1.19 to 1.98), and 136 patients were older than 11 years. In this series, 97% had an excellent result, six required minor revisions, and three had poor outcomes. For the first 94 patients, the standard modified Ravitch approach was used, and for the last 60 patients, a less extensive cartilage resection was performed (Fig. 134-17). In both groups, Adkins struts were placed anterior to the sternum. There was difference observed in the primary outcome (resolution of the pectus carinatum deformity), but the less extensive resections were associated with less pain and shorter hospital stays.

COMPLICATIONS. Complications reported in the group with less extensive resections included seroma (3.3%), pneumothorax (1.7%), persistent mild protrusion of one or two upper or lower cartilages (6.7%), and hypertrophic scarring (6.7%).[56] Similar results have been reported by Davis,[55] who also reported a mean and median patient satisfaction score of 5 of a possible 5.

MODIFIED PECTUS REPAIR TECHNIQUE. The patient is in the same position as for other pectus repairs (supine with the arms abducted and appropriate access lines and monitors applied). A short midline incision is made, and the sternum and ribs are exposed. The deformed cartilage segments are removed as described for pectus excavatum, leaving the perichondrium intact and taking care to protect the underlying heart and vessels. Assessment for sternal osteotomy is then performed; two osteotomies may be needed to reposition the sternum. The bone is secured in its new shape with thin titanium plates or wire sutures. Because the outer table of bone may need trimming for the desired flattening to be obtained, such sutures may offer more flexibility than plates for this defect. In some patients, especially those who have had a previous cardiac operation, the pericardium is extremely adherent to the deep bony table of the sternum. If there is concern about mediastinal adhesions, it may be a safer option to avoid substernal dissection and to remove only a superficial layer of the bone and cartilage to give the chest wall a more normal appearance. Once the protuberant bone and cartilage are removed, the perichondrium is closed and imbricated as deemed necessary to attain a more natural contour, and the incision is closed in layers over a soft suction drain. As with other pectus procedures, the patient is assessed in the recovery room for an occult pneumothorax (Fig. 134-18).

Summary

Pectus carinatum has undergone much less investigation than the related disorder, pectus excavatum. The techniques developed by Ravitch and subsequently modified are successful not only in pectus excavatum but in pectus carinatum as well. As pectus carinatum is generally asymptomatic and unnoticed until early adolescence, repair should be performed in the second decade with the expectation of excellent results as evidenced by retrospective analyses.

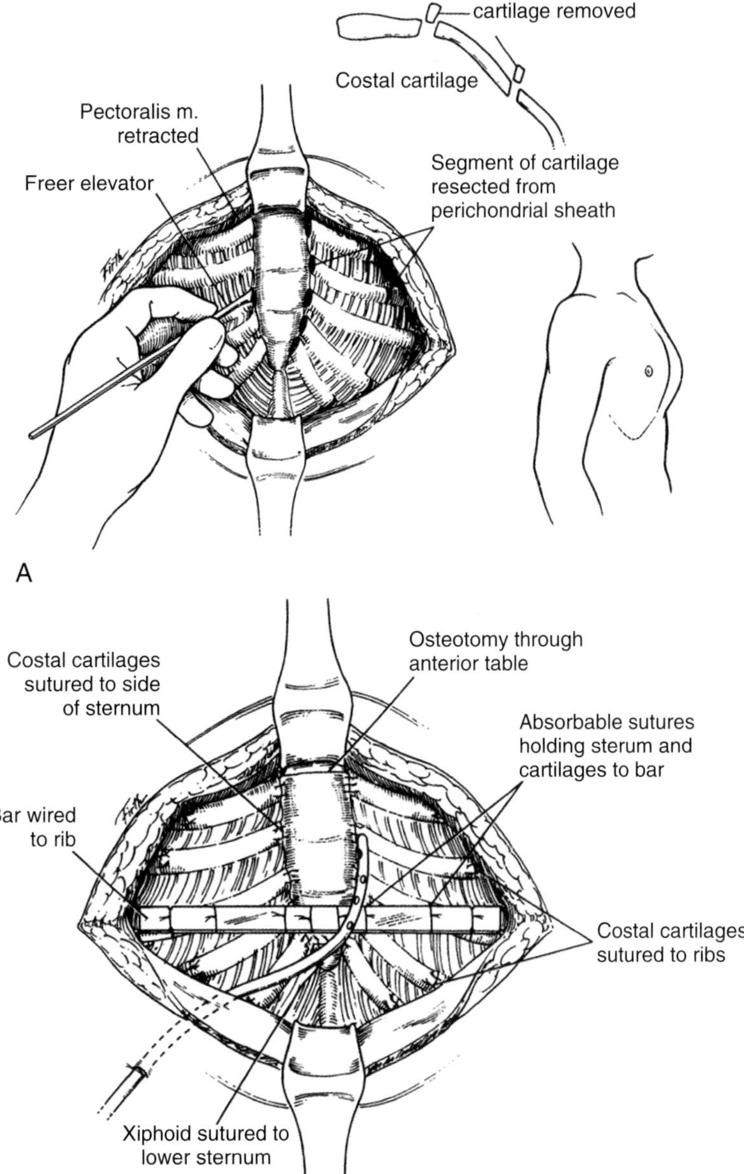

FIGURE 134-17. Modified Ravitch approach for pectus carinatum repair. *A,* A chevron incision is made inferior to the nipples with a midline vertical extension. The pectoralis muscles are reflected laterally over a short distance, and abdominal muscles are reflected inferiorly to expose the deformed cartilages. Incisions through the perichondrium are made on the medial and lateral ends of the deformed cartilages, and short chips of cartilage are removed with a Freer elevator. *B,* The medial ends of the costal cartilages are sutured to the sternum, and the lateral ends are sutured to ribs. The deformed xiphoid is reattached to the sternum. An Adkins strut with mild convex curvature is placed across the lower chest anterior to the sternum and attached to a rib on each side with wire. Large absorbable sutures placed through the anterior table of the sternum and adjacent costal cartilages are attached to the strut. A suction drainage catheter is placed between the cartilage repair and the muscle closure. (From Fonkalsrud EW, Anselmo DM: Less extensive techniques for repair of pectus carinatum: the undertreated chest deformity. J Am Coll Surg 2004;198:898.)

CLEFT STERNUM

Isolated cleft of the sternum is a rare disorder that was first reported in 1740 in "Torres a la Sociéte Royale" and again by Groux in 1858.[3] The first attempt at repair was by Lannelongue in 1888.[1] A successful repair was not reported until Burton[67] published his repair 59 years later (1947).

Incidence

Isolated cleft sternum is very rare, with only about 100 instances being reported in the literature.[68] In one series, isolated cleft sternum occurred in 0.15% of all patients referred for management of chest malformations.[3]

Etiology

Sternal cleft has been hypothesized to result from abnormal or no fusion of the lateral plate mesoderm during the seventh to tenth weeks of gestation.[3] There have been no genetic abnormalities or teratogenic agents identified that cause this malunion.[69] However, a mouse model in which the *HOXB4* gene was mutated yielded cleft sternum in the mouse.[70]

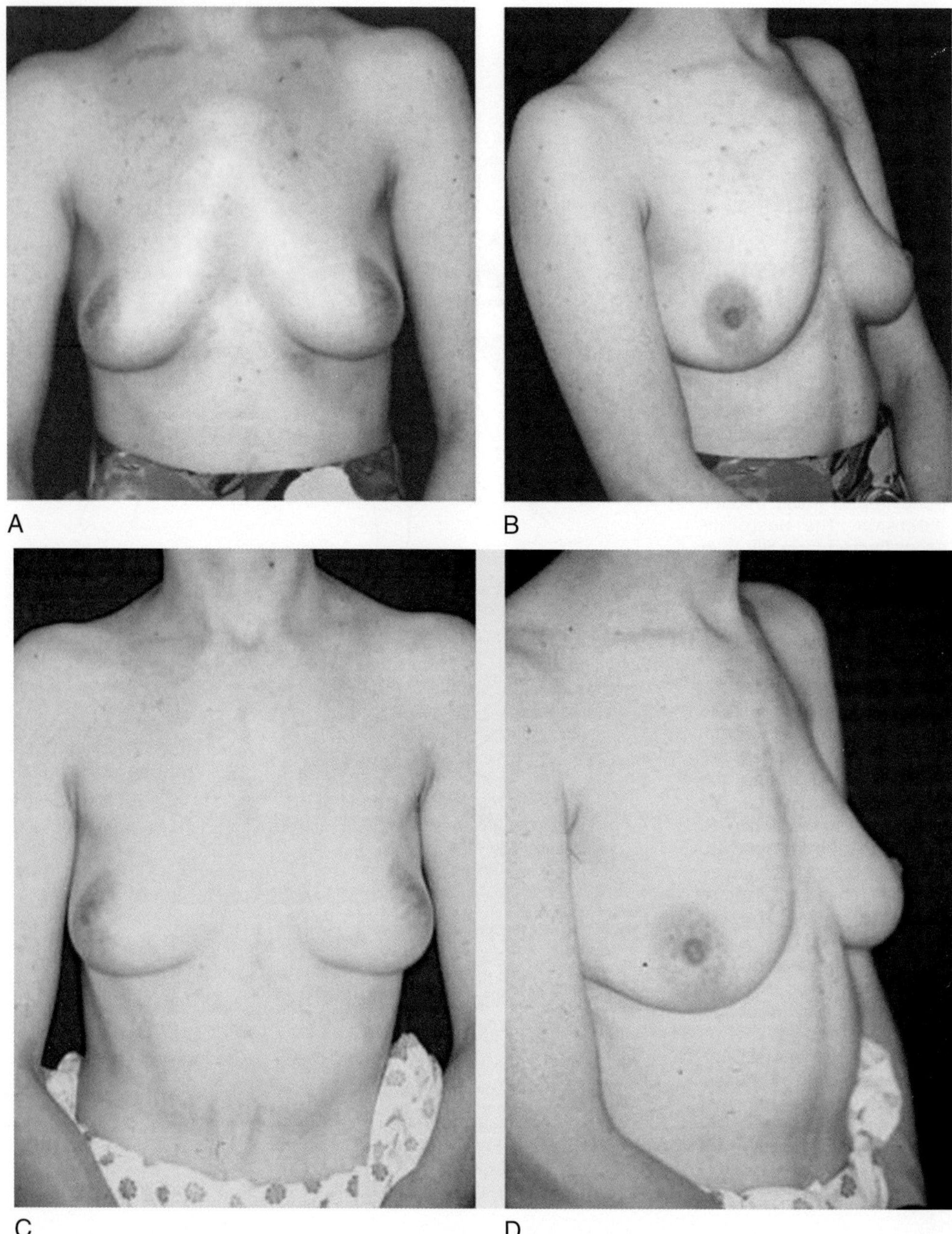

FIGURE 134-18. *A,* Preoperative anterior view of a 28-year-old woman who desired repair of her pectus carinatum deformity. *B,* Preoperative oblique view. The patient was concerned about the cosmetic aspect of the deformity and was in good health. *C,* Postoperative anterior view. After resection of the deformed cartilages, two transverse sternal osteotomies were secured with wire sutures. *D,* Postoperative oblique view. The patient healed uneventfully and was pleased with the result.

Presentation and Diagnosis

Although a sternal cleft can be diagnosed prenatally with ultrasound examination, isolated sternal clefts generally present after birth.[71] The primary observation is great vessel and cardiac motion that is visible through the anterior midline chest because of the malfusion of the sternum, particularly during the Valsalva maneuver. The children are generally otherwise asymptomatic, but dyspnea and recurrent pulmonary infections can occur. The skin and soft tissues are generally intact. Sternal clefts must be differentiated from ectopia cordis because of the profound difference in

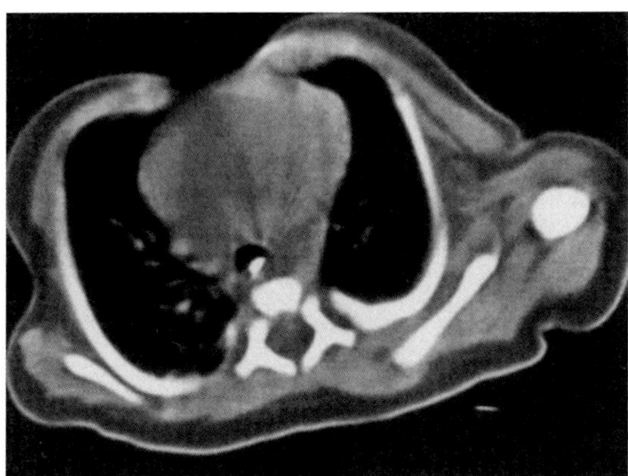

FIGURE 134-19. Cleft sternum. CT scan from 5-day-old infant.

prognosis. Both are generally identified shortly after birth. Sternal clefts are rarely associated with cardiac defects and have excellent long-term survival rates. Conversely, patients with ectopia cordis frequently have cardiac defects and have a much poorer survival.[72] See "Thoracic (True) Ectopia Cordis."

The sternal defect itself is variable, ranging from bifid sternum to complete failure of the sternal fusion (the rarest) (Fig. 134-19). On the basis of the arrangement of the sternal defect, bifid sternums can be either V or U shaped.[68]

Interestingly, sternal clefts are often associated with vascular malformations, particularly in children. In a metareview of the literature, 31 of 73 reviewed reports were associated with hemangiomas. The 31 patients with hemangiomas were almost exclusively female, accounting for the female preponderance observed in the disorder and possibly suggesting a separate cause for this subset of patients with sternal clefts.[73] An additional metareview revealed 9 of 36 patients with defects associated with hemangiomas, 3 with congenital heart defects, and 9 with a connecting midline raphe.[74]

Operative Treatment

Indications. Although sternal clefts are typically asymptomatic at presentation, operative repair is indicated for many. By the nature of the defect, the heart or the great vessels are exposed, risking injury to them from trauma. In addition, sternal repair enables proper excursion of the thoracic cage during ventilation. In the remainder of patients, concern about an aesthetic deformity is the primary motive for repair.[68] Repair typically occurs in infancy when the chest wall is most compliant and a sudden fusion of the sternum is not likely to cause an intolerable compression of the heart.[75]

Technique. The major variables of the sternal cleft repair are the age at time of repair, the extent of the defect, and the technique. Three major categories of repair have been described: primary closure, Ravitch technique, and use of autologous material or prosthetics. Because of the low incidence of this deformity, there have been no prospective studies. However, there have been several studies of these repairs (retrospective reviews and reports) that provide some guidance.

The most solid evidence is found in reports of neonates who underwent primary repair of their defect. Daum[76] reported a retrospective review of six infants with clefts in which the clefts were divided, forming complete clefts that were then closed. The repairs were conducted in the first weeks of life, and all results were good. Domini[68] reported two primary repairs in asymptomatic neonates at 2 and 4 weeks. Excellent results were observed through 15 and 18 months of follow-up.

Data are less definitive for patients later in life. Acastello[3] retrospectively described incomplete superior clefts in eight patients who were stratified by age and technique with 1 to 8 years of follow-up. Primary closure was used in three infants younger than 1 year with results consistent with those of Daum[76] and Domini.[68] The Ravitch procedure was used (to increase chest wall compliance and sternal mobility) for three patients between the ages of 1 and 3 years with similarly excellent results. In two patients older than 3 years, extensive mobilization of all muscles—including the sternocleidomastoid—was performed, followed by a rib homograft that was secured by mesh. One of the patients required major revisions that were accomplished by the Ravitch technique.[3] The successful use of iliac bone grafts combined with bilateral pectoralis major flaps has been reported in adults (Fig. 134-20).[75] A successful repair with bilateral pectoralis major flaps and bilateral fasciocutaneous advancement flaps was performed in an infant.[72]

Sabiston[77] reported the use of sliding chondrotomies in 1958, and they were studied by de Campos[69] in a 1998 retrospective review of eight patients with both complete and incomplete superior clefts ranging in age from 1.5 to 19 years. Sliding chondrotomies were attempted in six patients but achievable only in three. When the chondrotomies would not extend far enough to close the defect in these three patients and one other, the gap was bridged with posterior periosteal flaps from each side of the cleft sternum, which were then sutured together (Fig. 134-21). The gap was filled with two or three chondral grafts, followed by resection of the junction point of the sternal cleft to allow further approximation. All patients whose sliding chondrotomies failed were older (4 to 19 years), contrasted to the young children (1.5 to 2 years) in whom it succeeded. Excellent results were achieved in all patients at a mean of 7.6 years of follow-up.[69]

Summary

Excellent results can be achieved in treatment of isolated sternal clefts of all types regardless of age.

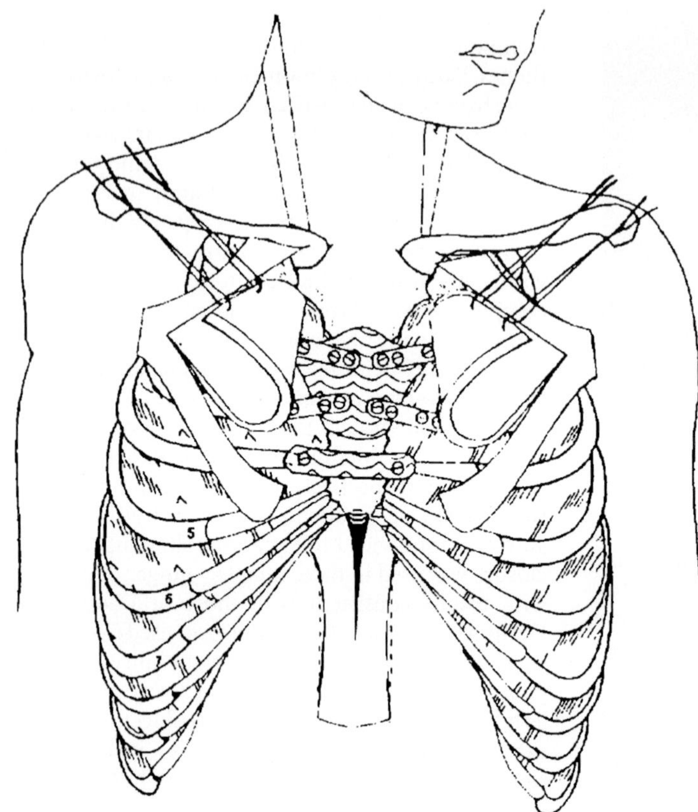

FIGURE 134-20. Cleft sternum. Suri technique with iliac bone grafts and bilateral pectoralis major flaps for adult repair of cleft sternum. (From Suri RK, Sharma RK, Jha NK, Sharma BK: Complete congenital sternal cleft in an adult: repair by autogenous tissues. Ann Thorac Surg 1996;62:573. Reprinted with permission from The Society of Thoracic Surgeons.)

However, the age of the patient dictates the type of procedure to be used (Table 134-10). With advancing age, more invasive procedures are required because of the decreasing compliance of the thoracic cage. Optimally, sternal clefts are identified and repaired during infancy while primary closure of the defect is still possible.

Disorders of Ventral Closure

THORACIC (TRUE) ECTOPIA CORDIS

Thoracic ectopia cordis is a rare disorder characterized by location of the heart outside of the thoracic cage. The incidence has been reported at 5.5 to 8 instances per million births.[78,79] The diagnosis is made

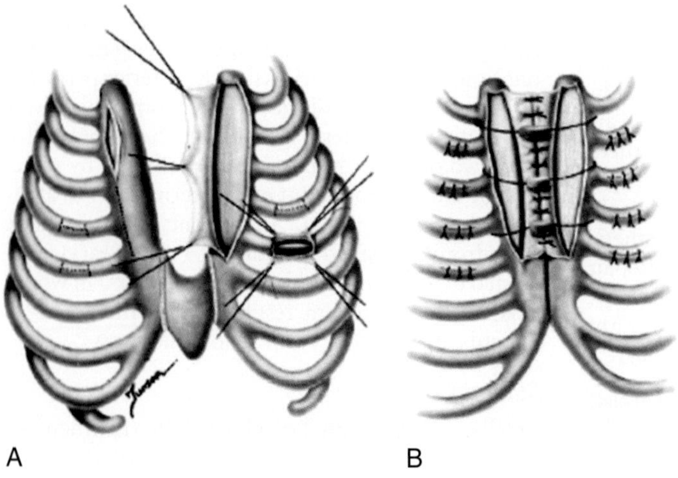

FIGURE 134-21. Cleft sternum, repair of superior sternal cleft with posterior periosteal flaps. *A,* The anterior periosteum is dissected from each sternal bar. Subperichondrial dissection of the ribs is also performed to harvest the chondral grafts. *B,* The periosteal flaps are sutured together to form the posterior wall of the repair, and the cartilaginous junction joining the inferior portion of the bars is resected. The chondral grafts are put in place and secured by sternal wires. (From de Campos JR, Filomeno LT, Fernandez A, et al: Repair of congenital sternal cleft in infants and adolescents. Ann Thorac Surg 1998;66: 1151. Reprinted with permission from The Society of Thoracic Surgeons.)

TABLE 134-10 ✦ SUGGESTED TECHNIQUE FOR STERNAL CLEFT REPAIR STRATIFIED BY AGE

Age of Patient	Operative Technique
0-1 years	Primary closure Bilateral pectoralis major flaps
1-3 years	Ravitch technique Sliding chondrotomies Iliac bone grafts with bilateral pectoralis major flaps
>3 years to adulthood	Posterior periosteal flaps with chondral grafts Ravitch technique Iliac bone grafts with bilateral pectoralis major flaps

either prenatally by ultrasound examination or immediately after birth with the observation of the heart being at least partly out of the chest.[80] Ectopia cordis has a high mortality rate both because there are often associated cardiac anomalies and from the repair itself, which returns the heart to the chest, where it has lost its right of domain.[78,81]

There are five classes of ectopia cordis based on the location of the heart. Cervical and cervicothoracic ectopia cordis are uniformly fatal. Thoracoabdominal ectopia cordis is commonly associated with the pentalogy of Cantrell (see "Pentalogy of Cantrell") and is amenable to operation. Abdominal ectopia cordis with displacement of the heart into the abdomen often needs no intervention for survival.[81] Thoracic (true) ectopia cordis with displacement across the chest wall occurs in about 38% of patients.[82] A concurrent sternal cleft or agenesis is therefore required.[81] There is often no cutaneous covering of the heart (complete thoracic ectopia cordis) or no pericardial sac (Fig. 134-22).[83]

Cardiac defects are present in 80% of patients with complete thoracic ectopia cordis. The most common defects are ventricular septal defects (reported in all patients who have a cardiac anomaly in one series), atrial septal defects (53%), tetralogy of Fallot (20%), and hypoplastic lungs.[83,84] Cardiac defects portend a grave prognosis. In a series of 91 instances of true thoracic ectopia cordis, only one patient with a cardiac defect achieved long-term survival.[82]

The choice of treatment of true ectopia cordis depends initially on whether the ectopia is complete. Incomplete defects can be dealt with less urgently than complete defects, which have a 100% mortality rate when they are left untreated.[85] When soft tissue coverage is present and (most important) intact, it is reasonable to delay repair for optimization of the patient's medical condition and to coincide with the sternal repair and any needed cardiac palliation (e.g., Blalock-Taussig shunt).

There are few data on the optimal treatment of complete defects. Only four successful repairs have been reported in the literature. The immediate priority is to obtain tissue coverage of the heart, which can be done by mobilization of pectoralis or rectus abdominis musculocutaneous flaps. Polytetrafluoroethylene mesh and skin flaps have also been reported to be useful; however, the use of skin flaps must be approached with caution because of the less certain blood supply and the frequent need for vasoconstricting agents for cardiac support.[86] Necrosis of the skin flaps with subsequent severe infection has been reported.[84] The secondary treatment objectives are to return the heart to the thoracic cavity, to repair the sternal defect, and finally to repair or palliate any associated cardiac defects.[83] Four patients with complete ectopia cordis with a successful repair and long-term survival have been described in the literature.[79,84,85] One patient survived to at least 10 years of age.[81] Three others survived repair but died shortly after of other nonrelated causes.[83]

Depending on the severity of the ectopia and the underlying cardiac defects, a staged approach may be optimal. An attempt should be made to return the heart at least partially to the chest at the first operation. After time has allowed the hemodynamics to adjust to the heart within the thoracic cage, palliation or treatment of cardiac defects should be performed.[83] Extracorporeal membrane oxygenation may be helpful.

PENTALOGY OF CANTRELL

The pentalogy of Cantrell is a rare congenital disorder characterized by defects of the lower sternum, anterior diaphragm, parietal pericardium, thora-

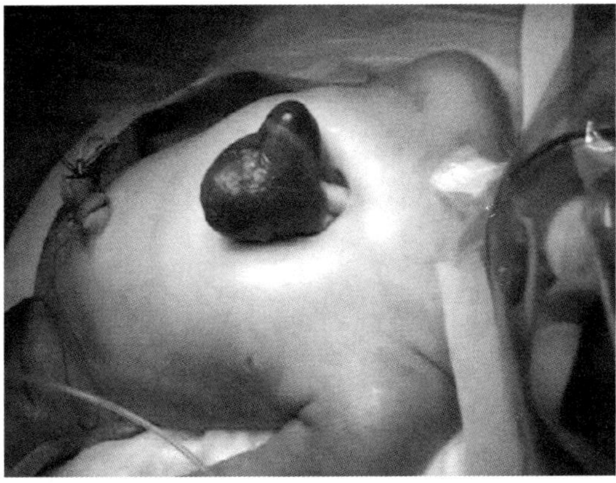

FIGURE 134-22. Thoracic ectopia cordis. (From Alphonso N, Venugopal PS, Deshpande R, Anderson D: Complete thoracic ectopia cordis. Eur J Cardiothorac Surg 2003;23:426.)

coabdominal wall (omphalocele), and heart (including partial herniation).[87] Its incidence has been estimated at approximately 1 in 65,000 live births with a slight (57.5%) male predominance.[88] The cause has been proposed to be an injury or a defect in differentiation of the mesoderm during gestation affecting global midline fusion.[88] The syndrome can be diagnosed by ultrasound examination in utero and has an extremely poor prognosis.[89] If it is not detected in utero, it is generally recognized immediately after birth; however, an instance has been reported of the diagnosis being made in an adult.[88]

Abdominal wall defects occur in 74.5% of patients, sternal defects in 59.4%, and diaphragmatic defects in 56.8%.[88] The repair of the body wall and diaphragmatic defects should be secondary to the repair of symptomatic cardiac anomalies except when a complete thoracoabdominal ectopia cordis is present. As in true ectopia cordis, soft tissue coverage is immediately mandatory. If the cardiac anomalies are minor or asymptomatic, the omphalocele and diaphragmatic hernia can be reduced by the standard methods, and major sternal defects can be closed primarily or by techniques similar to those discussed before.[88] Single-stage repairs have been reported.[84]

Disorders of the Rib Cage

ASPHYXIATING THORACIC DYSTROPHY (JEUNE SYNDROME)

Asphyxiating thoracic dystrophy (ATD) is a rare autosomal recessive congenital disorder described by Jeune[90] in 1954 in which the thoracic cage is elongated and narrow due to abnormal development of the ribs. Additional bone anomalies include an irregular curvature of the clavicles; shortening of the ulnae, radii, tibiae, and fibulae; and a small, irregular pelvis (Fig. 134-23).[91] Other organs that can be affected include the retina, kidney, pancreas, and liver. Polydactyly of hands and feet is often present. A gene locus, *ATD*, mapped to chromosome 15q13 has been identified, although the molecular basis of the disorder is still unkown.[92]

The most common clinical presentation of Jeune syndrome is that of respiratory distress from a restrictive, narrow thoracic cage. The condition of the underlying lungs can range from normal to severely hypoplastic, with associated pulmonary hypertension.[93] ATD is commonly lethal in utero, and those individuals who are born alive generally become ventilator dependent and die within the first year of life.[94] Some patients with ATD without pulmonary failure have been described, and those patients who have survived remain at risk for renal failure and blindness from retinal dystrophy.[95,96]

Steady advancement in pediatric critical care has given surgeons an opportunity to correct the otherwise nearly uniformly fatal ATD. Several methods to provide expansion have been attempted, including rib grafts, bone grafts, and methyl methacrylate implants.[97-99] These provide static expansion of the chest wall that is quickly outgrown, causing recurrence of pulmonary failure.

Two methods have been reported that expand the chest wall and avoid recurrence. Kaddoura[94] reported the implantation of a modified sternal spreader with an accessible ratchet in one neonate that allowed expansion of the thoracic wall over time. After 8 months of

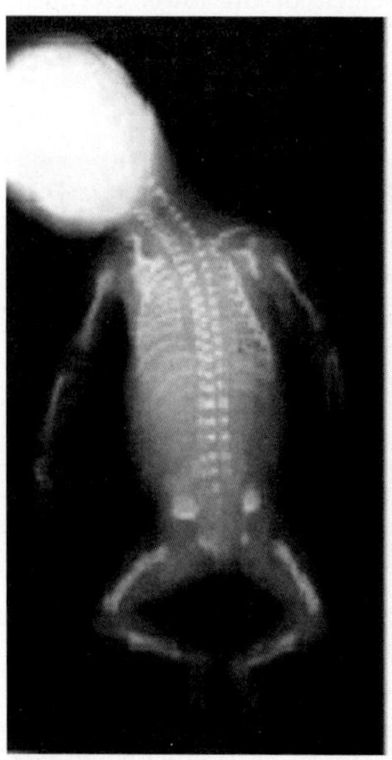
A

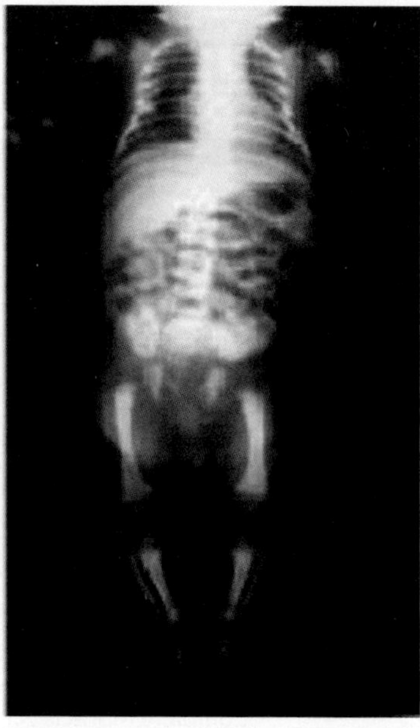
B

FIGURE 134-23. Asphyxiating thoracic dystrophy (Jeune syndrome). Note horizontal ribs, narrow "bell-shaped" thoraces, shortening of lower limbs, and pelvic abnormalities. *A,* Fetus at 30 weeks of gestation. *B,* Infant at 3 months. (From Morgan NV, Bacchelli C, Gissen P, et al: A locus for asphyxiating thoracic dystrophy, ATD, maps to chromosome 15q13. J Med Genet 2003; 40:431-435.)

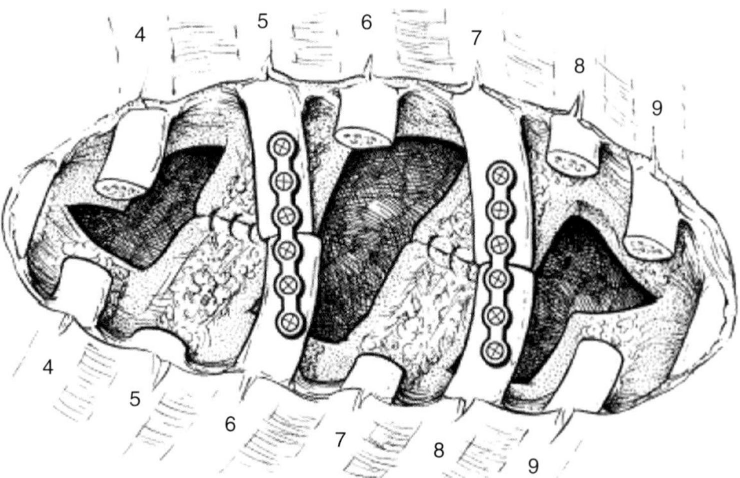

FIGURE 134-24. Lateral thoracic expansion technique. Ribs five through eight are transected on alternate sides and then rigidly fixed with titanium plates end-to-end, resulting in expansion of the thoracic cage. (From Davis JT, Heistein JB, Castile RG, et al: Lateral thoracic expansion for Jeune's syndrome: midterm results. Ann Thorac Surg 2001;72:872. Reprinted with permission from The Society of Thoracic Surgeons.)

follow-up, the patient was ventilator and recurrent pulmonary infection free.

Davis[100] has presented a staged lateral thoracic expansion technique for Jeune syndrome. In this technique, the patient is placed in the lateral position and ribs four through nine are transected on one side; ribs four and nine are transected in the middle, ribs five and seven are transected far anteriorly, and ribs six and eight are transected posteriorly. Ribs five and six are plated end-to-end with a titanium plate, as are ribs seven and eight, expanding the thorax (Fig. 134-24). The contralateral side is expanded 6 months to 1 year later.

Davis[100] reported results for 16 operations in 10 patients. Seven of the patients were children (range, 3 to 17 years), implying a relatively mild presentation of Jeune syndrome in these patients. Three of these patients were ventilator dependent; the remainder had chronic pulmonary problems, including recurrent infections. The other three patients were ventilator-dependent infants younger than 1 year.[100]

Results for the older group were good. Two of the three ventilator-dependent patients achieved the ability to breathe without assistance. The other four patients had global improvements in their functional status as evidenced by decreased cyanosis, increased exercise tolerance, and fewer infections. The infants (who required operations at an earlier age and thus probably had more severe disease) had a much poorer outcome with two postoperative deaths; the third achieved only a 50% decrease in ventilator requirements.[100] With follow-up ranging from about 3 to 9 years, no patient has required reoperation for recurrence except for patients in whom symptomatic plate fracture occurred. It is hypothesized that further expansion (preventing recurrence) may occur from growth at the rib epiphyses, which are uninjured during lateral thoracic expansion. Evidence of bone healing across the plate is present at the plate sites by 3 weeks after operation and continues over time.[55]

Patients with ATD being referred for thoracoplasty will continue to become more frequent as neonatal and pediatric intensive care medicine advances. ATD remains a life-threatening disease; no good solution has been demonstrated for infants with severe disease. For those patients with milder disease who survive infancy, lateral thoracic expansion is the technique that is best supported by the literature, although more data are needed.

Disorders of Thoracic Musculature

POLAND SYNDROME

History

In 1841, Alfred Poland,[101] a London medical student, reported some unusual anatomic findings after a cadaver dissection at Guy's Hospital. The subject of his report, George Elt, had died as a prisoner at the age of 27 years and had been described in life as unable to draw his left arm across his chest. Poland noted that Elt's left torso and upper extremity were underdeveloped and that "the whole of the sternal costal portions of the pectoralis major muscles were deficient . . . the pectoralis minor muscle was wholly absent . . . the serratus magnus muscle was also, for the most part, deficient, its two superior digitations only being present" (Fig. 134-25).[101]

Poland adds that the left hand was shorter than the right, that the digits had a web, and that the middle phalanges were replaced by a ring of bone. Poland was not the first to report findings similar to those that are now referred to as Poland syndrome. However, although Lallemand[102] and Froriep[103] presented patients with similarities, Poland's description was by far the most precise and comprehensive.

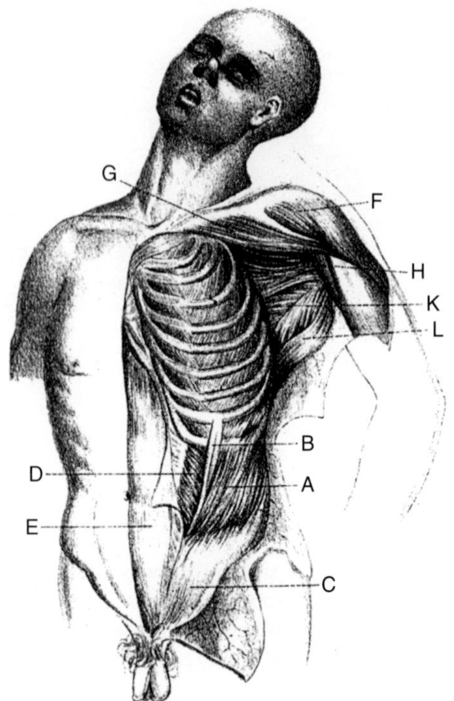

FIGURE 134-25. The illustration from Alfred Poland's original article published in *Guy's Hospital Reports* in 1841 shows the severe form of Poland syndrome. A, External abdominal oblique muscle. B, A slip of the same muscle arising from the eighth rib. C, Tendon of the external oblique muscle. D, Part of the internal oblique muscle, uncovered by the external muscle. E, Sheath of the rectus. F, Deltoid. G, Clavicular portion of the pectoralis major. H, K, and L, Subscapularis, teres major, and latissimus dorsi muscles. (Two origins of the serratus magnus are not shown in the drawing, being concealed by the ribs in this view.) (From Poland A: Deficiency of the pectoral muscles. Guys Hosp Rep 1841;6:191-193.)

Incidence

If Poland syndrome is defined by the unilateral absence or hypoplasia of the thoracic muscles, the incidence ranges from 1 in 7000 to 1 in 100,000 (e.g., male versus female, congenital versus female).[104] Ten percent of these patients also express some of the other features of the disorder, making some estimates of Poland syndrome as infrequent as 1 in 100,000.[104,105] There is a male-to-female ratio of 2:1 to 3:1. Interestingly, in boys, there is a right-side predilection of more than 2:1, but in girls, there is no favored side. Bilateral Poland syndrome has been reported once.[106] In rare familial instances of Poland syndrome, there seems to be neither a favored gender nor a favored side.[104]

Absence of the sternocostal head of the pectoralis major muscle is pathognomonic, but the complex sometimes includes a variety of ipsilateral torso and upper extremity defects. Absence of the anterior portions of ribs two to five as well as loss of the latissimus dorsi, serratus anterior, and anterior abdominal oblique muscles can also occur. The breast tissues can be small or absent and the nipple-areola complex, if present, small and displaced toward the axilla (Fig. 134-26).

Associations have been drawn with renal abnormalities, hemivertebrae, leukemia, and Möbius and Sprengel anomalies. The significance and true occurrence of these associated components are undetermined.

Etiology

The precise mechanism causing Poland syndrome has not been elucidated. Some data suggest that disruption of the early embryonic blood supply in the subclavian or vertebral systems causes the syndrome during the sixth to seventh weeks of gestation.[107] The cause of the disruption has been postulated to be mechanical, focal compression of the vessels.[108] Further evidence is that on the limb, the second, third, and fourth fingers are most severely affected. These digits are the most distal targets of the subclavian artery during the sixth week of gestation.[109] Magnetic resonance angiography of these vessels has been reported to show no abnormalities, indicating that if the vascular hypothesis is true, the vessel injury must be transient.[110] However, alternative theories suggest that injury or developmental failure of the embryonic mesodermal plate during the third and fourth weeks of gestation (which gives rise to the pectoralis muscle) can culminate in Poland syndrome.[111]

Poland syndrome seems to be sporadic in nature (less than 1% risk of a second family member affected).[112] Despite this, 20 patients have been linked to familial transmission, with unaffected parents giving rise to affected children. This mode of transmission is characteristic of a delayed dominant germline mutation.[113]

Presentation and Diagnosis

Although highly variable, Poland syndrome has several common features (Fig. 134-27). The absence of the sternal head of the pectoralis major muscle is constant. The ipsilateral chest wall can suffer from several anomalies, including alopecia of the breast and axilla, lack of subcutaneous tissues, absent pectoralis minor muscle, and absence or distortion of ribs two to four or three to five (reported to be present in 15% of right-sided defects).[104] The chest wall often has a deeply depressed appearance in 11% to 25% of patients.[114-116] Paradoxical motion of the chest wall can be observed in some. Lung herniation through the defect occurs in 8%. The latissimus dorsi, serratus anterior, and external oblique muscles are occasionally absent. Ipsilateral limb anomalies are present in 13% to 56% of patients, including brachysyndactyly (particularly of digits two, three, and four) as well as shortening of the limb, and are highly variable.[104]

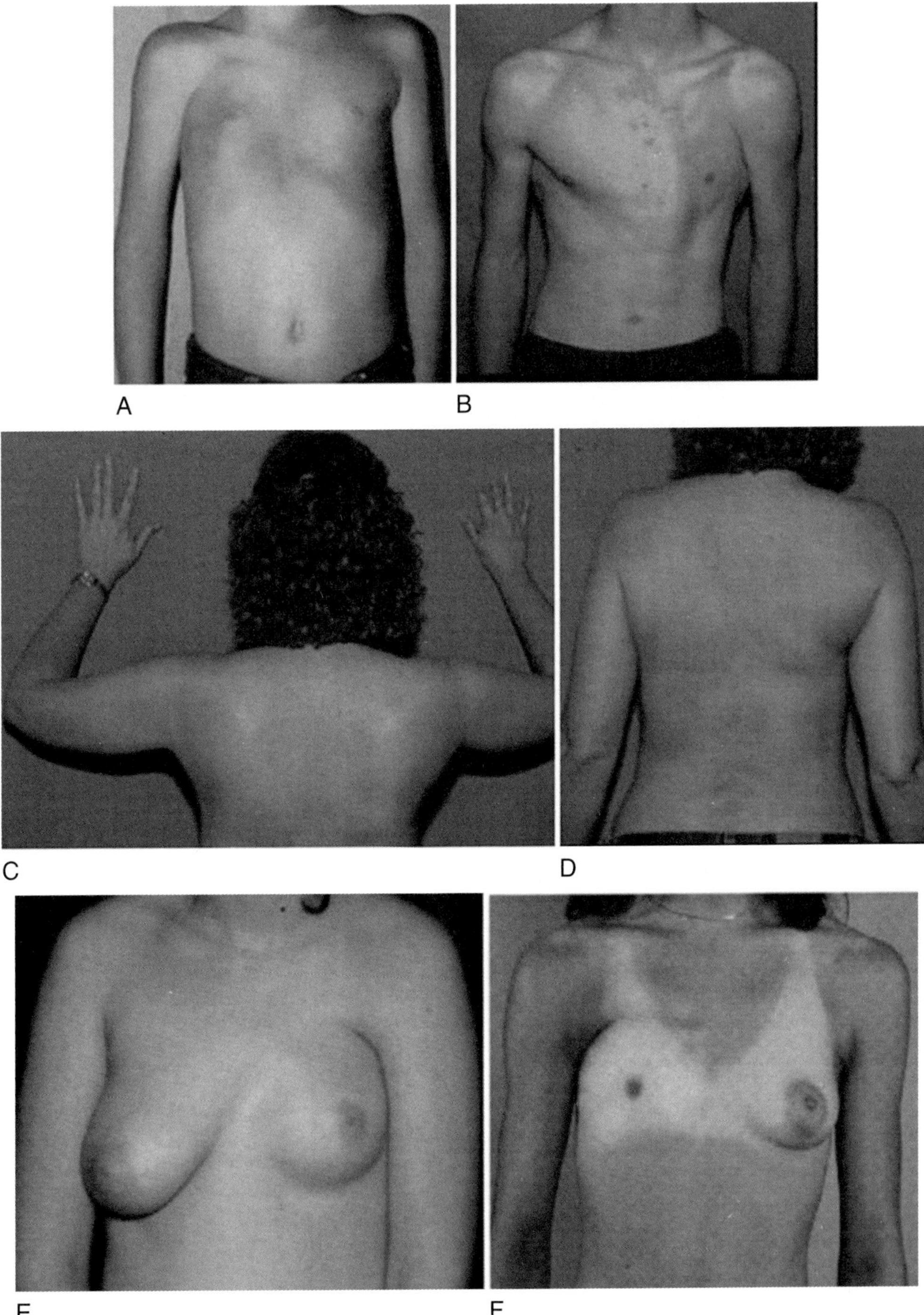

FIGURE 134-26. Poland syndrome. *A*, Preadolescent with absent right pectoralis major muscle. *B*, Adult with absent left pectoralis major muscle and sternal-chest deformity. *C*, Posterior view of patient with Poland syndrome (right side). Note right brachysyndactyly. *D*, Posterior view of Poland syndrome (right side). Note absence of right latissimus dorsi muscle. *E*, Adult with absent left pectoralis major muscle and hypomastia of ipsilateral breast. *F*, Adult with absent right pectoralis major muscle and absence of ipsilateral breast.

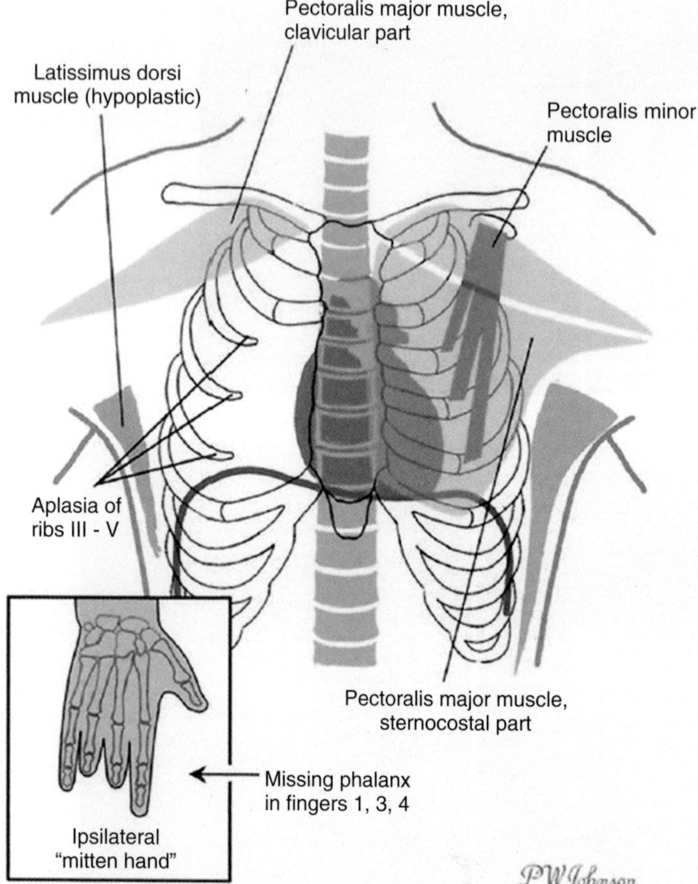

FIGURE 134-27. Schematic representation of features of Poland syndrome. (From Fokin AA, Robicsek F: Poland's syndrome revisited. Ann Thorac Surg 2002;74:2218. Reprinted with permission from The Society of Thoracic Surgeons.)

The breast is affected in one third of patients. Defects range from amastia to simple hypoplasia. The nipple is often either absent or elevated and hypoplastic.[104,115] These features are highly variable in presentation.

The diagnosis can be made on prenatal ultrasound examination but is more often made by visual inspection of the constellation of defects in a severely affected individual.[117] However, many presentations are much more subtle, as evidenced by the fact that Poland syndrome is diagnosed by mammography with a rate of 1 per 19,000 mammograms.[118] The observation of syndactyly should prompt a search for other features of Poland syndrome because the syndrome is present in 10% of all patients with syndactyly.[119]

Evaluation

In the diagnosis of which type of Poland syndrome applies to a particular patient, inspection of the entire torso and both upper extremities is routine. Palpation of the ribs and measurement of the upper extremity (e.g., acromion-olecranon distance) are done. The pectoralis major, serratus anterior, and latissimus dorsi muscles are tested. Standard muscle testing is employed, and each muscle is palpated during the testing to gain an appreciation of its function, volume, and size. Other signs may be apparent. For example, when the serratus anterior is absent, a winged scapula is present. Other muscles, such as the levator scapulae, may be weak or absent. It is important to test and to obtain baseline photographs for both clinical and medicolegal reasons.

A routine chest radiograph can confirm the physical findings, such as the absence of the upper lateral rib segments, smallness of the scapula, or hypoplasia of the hemithorax. Other studies and consultations are performed as dictated by the findings and the age and condition of the patient. The diagnosis and repair of syndactyly are covered in Chapter 204. The syndactyly of Poland syndrome has many variations, as noted before, and is usually the first component to be repaired.

EVALUATION FOR TECHNIQUE SELECTION. In assessment of the deformity, two anatomic variations deserve mention, the simple (mild) form and the complex (severe) form. These differing types require different reconstructive solutions.

The simple form is the most common and is limited to absence of part of the pectoralis major muscle, with variable hypoplasia of other minor components (such as the size of the breast and the size and position of the nipple-areola complex). In the simple form of Poland syndrome, the clavicular head of the pectoralis major muscle is present as a thin triangular bundle that runs along the inferior border of the clavicle. The larger fan-shaped sternocostal head is missing. This deficiency includes its insertion on the humerus, the tendon of which normally spirals so that the anterior fibers become inferior as it approaches the humerus, giving fullness to the anterior axillary fold. Thus, the deficiency causes the anterior axillary fold to be deficient as well, a facet that is noticed by the patient compared with the contralateral (normal) side. Although the ribs and other musculoskeletal components are present and usually normal, the breast tissue may be partially absent and the nipple-areola complex small and displaced toward the axilla. Because the pectoralis minor cannot be seen or reliably tested, the presence of this minor component cannot be confirmed.

The complex (severe) form is characterized by absence of the sternocostal head of the pectoralis major muscle, rib and sternal aberrations, and a relatively severe brachysyndactyly. This is the form that Alfred Poland[101] described, and if one looks closely, one finds that the entire hemithorax and upper extremity components are smaller on the affected side (see Fig. 134-25). In this form, the sternal body can be short and bifid. The cartilage on the affected side may be coalesced into a bar that is rotated and protruding anteriorly. The insertion of the rectus abdominis muscle is abnormally high, having been pulled up by the affected shortening of the affected chest wall. The clavicle is shortened, and the scapula is smaller and may be rotated and higher than on the normal side, as in Sprengel deformity. The cartilages of ribs two through five are missing superolaterally and replaced by a tough pleurofascial membrane that, in younger patients, can be seen to move with respirations. This aspect can be tested by having the patient hold a deep breath while bearing down as with a bowel movement (Valsalva maneuver). The skin, subcutaneous fat, and pleurofascial membrane are noted to bulge outward.

Activities of daily living are rarely limited by either form of Poland syndrome, and the most functionally symptomatic component relates to the syndactyly. Indeed, even with the complex form of the anomaly, most patients in our series indicated that it was the appearance that bothered them the most. One such patient related that his only functional difficulty was in performing pull-ups. His only medical problem was that he broke his arm (humerus) on the affected side while hang-gliding! Thus, providing reassurance to the patient and the patient's family is an important component of the surgeon's mission. Career opportunities are usually not compromised.

The severe form, however, may restrict one from military service (because of inability to pass the physical examination or the physical fitness testing) and certain jobs that require strong upper extremities. With the mild form, there should be no compromise on a functional basis. Indeed, in our series of 63 patients, several patients with the mild form were on active duty in the military and had done well.[40]

The dimensions of upper extremity components are often less on the affected side, but this may not be apparent with the simple form unless one measures the acromion-olecranon and the olecranon-ulnar styloid distances and compares them with the unaffected side. Digital length can also be measured and compared. A simple estimate can be made by having the patient hold the palms together with the digits extended (prayer position). A discrepancy is easy to observe with this maneuver. With the severe form, the upper extremity and chest wall differences are easily noted, and ipsilateral syndactyly (webbed fingers), brachydactyly (short digits), or brachysyndactyly is present (see Chapter 204).

Operative Treatment

Indications. The degree of instability of the chest wall and aesthetic concerns are the two major factors that determine the treatment plan for patients with Poland syndrome. As previously discussed, the thoracic cage provides protection for the underlying organs and aids in both inspiration and expiration. A serious deficiency in either of these functions is an indication for reconstruction of the chest wall.

In both women and men, Poland syndrome can cause an aesthetically unsatisfactory appearance due to hypoplasia or absence of a breast or nipple or the absence of the pectoralis major muscle and the axillary fold.

Timing. Once the decision to operate is made and the planning phase is entered, timing can be an issue. With both forms of this anomaly, the indications for surgical intervention are largely cosmetic because of the asymmetry that exists between the left and right sides of the thorax.[15] Different stages of development have been cited as the optimal time to correct Poland syndrome. Although some think that preadolescent patients are candidates for repair, others believe that reconstructive procedures can be delayed until late adolescence.[36,120] The arguments for waiting include the risk of growth inhibition if operative trauma is conducted too early, the right of the patient to participate in decisions that affect his or her body, and the need for multiple revisions to keep up with breast and chest wall growth. It certainly seems appropriate to gain the patient's concurrence and informed consent before any

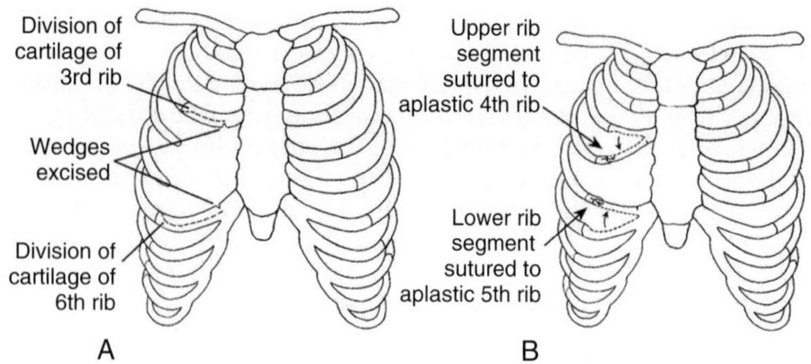

FIGURE 134-28. *A* and *B,* Repair of minor thoracic defects with split rib rotational grafts. (From Fokin AA, Robicsek F: Poland's syndrome revisited. Ann Thorac Surg 2002;74:2218. Reprinted with permission from The Society of Thoracic Surgeons.)

operation, especially one that is cosmetic in nature. Operating before full growth is attained may have certain risks as well. Therefore, waiting until the patient is an adolescent or adult has advantages. If there are cogent psychosocial reasons for performing the operation earlier than in adolescence, it may also be appropriate to gain the concurrence of the family physician. Again, as in pectus deformities, one must not feel pressured by either the patient or the parents to operate. If this is happening, it is reasonable to refer the patient and the family to another team for treatment.

TECHNIQUES. When the chest wall defect is severe, stabilization of the rib cage should be performed promptly after diagnosis. In a series of 27 patients, 20 required an operation for chest wall stabilization. In 14 minor defects, reconstruction was provided either by splitting of an intact rib adjacent to an aplastic one and subsequently fusing the split end to the aplastic one (typically for aplasia of two ribs) (Fig. 134-28) or by separation of abnormally fused ribs. For six patients with severe rib defects, two autologous split rib grafts were harvested and placed across the defect. The remainder of the defect was closed with a Marlex mesh prosthesis (Fig. 134-29). Both techniques are reported to give good results, but mesh closure is reported to appear flattened unless muscle is placed over the defect.[104]

The transposition of autologous muscle over the Poland syndrome defect can provide additional protection and aesthetic contouring of the chest wall in both men and women (Fig. 134-30). Ohmori[121] reported the use of latissimus dorsi flaps to restore the axillary and infraclavicular muscle contour characteristic of an intact pectoralis major muscle. Late atrophy of the flap has been observed, and preservation of the innervation is recommended to minimize the risk of atrophy.[122] The use of customized silicone implants has been reported in male patients with good results; however, malpositioning is reported as a problem.[123-125]

Custom Implant Insertion. If the patient is treated with a custom implant, the newer materials offer flexibility. For fabrication of a custom implant, that is, one that is made for a single patient's unique anatomy, a

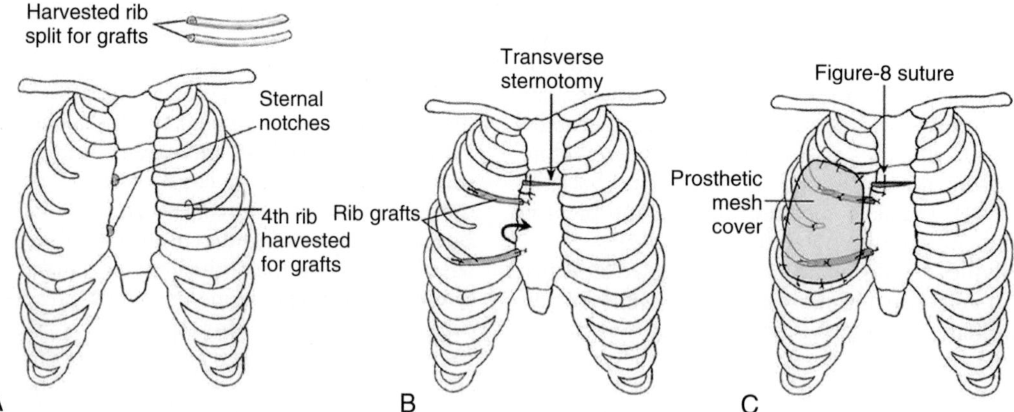

FIGURE 134-29. Stabilization of major chest wall defects with split rib grafts and mesh prosthesis. *A,* Contralateral split ribs are harvested. Notches are made into the sternum to fix the transplanted rib grafts. *B,* Sternal osteotomy performed (if necessary) to rotate sternum into normal position and split rib grafts inset. *C,* Prosthetic mesh is sutured on top of the rib grafts and to the edges of the defect. (From Fokin AA, Robicsek F: Poland's syndrome revisited. Ann Thorac Surg 2002;74:2218. Reprinted with permission from The Society of Thoracic Surgeons.)

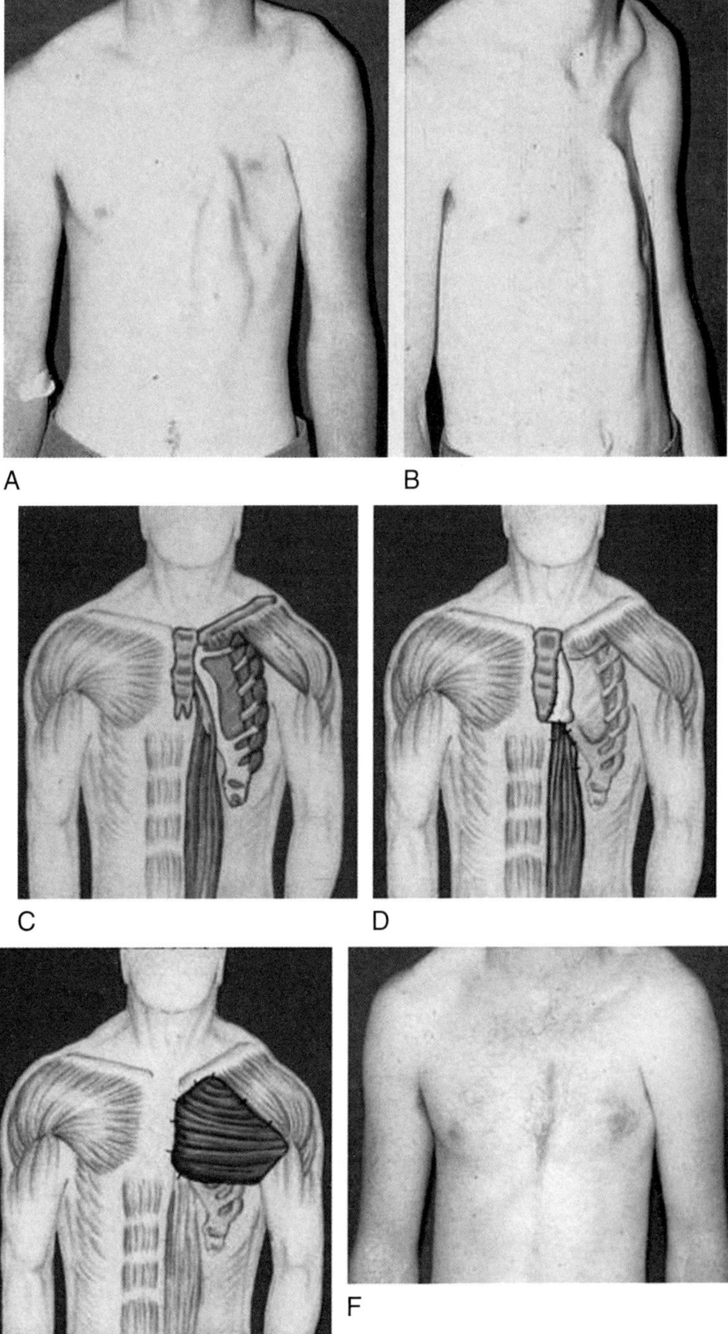

FIGURE 134-30. *A,* Anterior view of a 21-year-old man referred for evaluation and treatment of severe type of Poland anomaly. Affected hemithorax and upper extremity are smaller; in addition to absence of the sternocostal pectoralis major, portions of the anterior upper ribs are missing. The sternum is short, there is a cartilaginous bar protruding from the left sternocostal edge, and the rectus abdominis muscle is inserted abnormally high. Despite this, he was athletic and functioned well. *B,* Oblique view of same patient. Note the protruding cartilage and upper chest wall deficiency. *C,* Schematic diagram of the defect as it was seen at surgery. *D,* Diagram shows the appearance after the first operative stage. The sternal bar and rectus insertion have been repositioned. *E,* Schematic shows the chest wall after the latissimus transfer. *F,* The patient's postoperative appearance after repositioning of the nipple-areola complex. He was able to flex the latissimus muscle and reported that weight training has increased its bulk. (*A, C,* and *F* from Seyfer AE, Icochea R, Graeber GM: Poland's anomaly. Natural history and long-term results of chest wall reconstruction in 33 patients. Ann Surg 1988;208:776.)

mold is fashioned on the patient's chest, as described by the manufacturer's kit. The mold of the patient's chest is then sent to the manufacturer, and a reverse model of the chest wall is fabricated that is unique for that patient and conforms to the specifications submitted by the surgeon (Fig. 134-31). These may specify that the silicone rubber chest wall prosthesis should have the consistency of muscle tissue for a portion of the implant and the consistency of breast tissue for another portion. An alternative approach is the construction of an implant that has two separate chambers. A textured shell superiorly maintains position

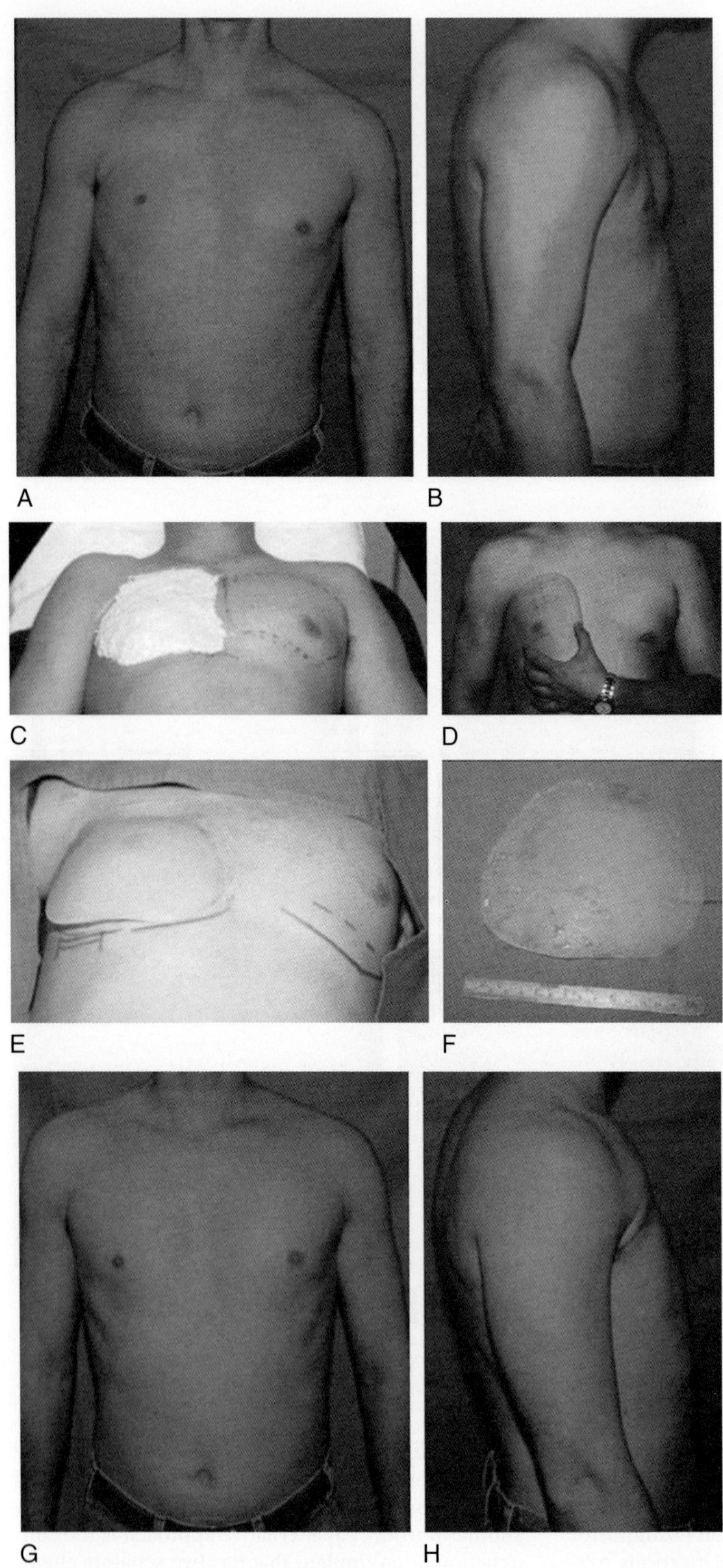

FIGURE 134-31. Poland syndrome, correction with custom implant. *A,* Anterior view, absent sternal pectoralis major muscle. *B,* Lateral view. Note contour deformity with absent pectoralis major muscle. *C,* Moulage for preparation of custom implant. *D,* Mold for custom implant construction. *E,* Intraoperative view. The custom silicone implant is ready for insertion. *F,* Custom implant tailored in operating room as required before final insertion in dissected pocket overlying the sternum. *G,* Anterior postoperative view at 1 year. The silicone custom implant is in place with contour correction. *H,* Lateral view; natural contour on lateral chest provided by implant.

to simulate the missing pectoralis, and a smooth shell inferiorly provides for reconstruction of the breast mound. The implant is sent back to the surgeon and sterilized in preparation for insertion (Fig. 134-32*A*).

For insertion of the implant, the patient is in the supine position with the arms abducted. An incision is entered through the anterolateral chest wall, where the inframammary crease should reside (at approximately the level of the xiphoid and over the lower slips of the serratus anterior). The skin and subcutaneous tissues are dissected free of the ribs over the deep fascia, and a generous pocket is developed in this space (Fig. 134-32*B* and *C*). Because there is no pectoralis major muscle, the dissection plane is on the rib periosteum and the fascia of the serratus anterior muscle. A subserratus pocket offers little to the inferior portion of the pocket, and the muscle slips are usually too friable to dissect without shredding. The custom implant is inserted and secured into position by closing the lateral portions of the pocket (Fig. 134-32*D*). The patient is raised to the sitting position for assessment of symmetry, and any adjustments that are needed are made. If a separate implant for the missing pectoralis is used, a breast implant is inserted to restore adequate breast. Often, a breast reduction, mammary prosthesis, or mastopexy procedure is required on the contralateral side based on preoperative planning with the patient and her family. The incision is closed in layers. The patients may require additional procedures as they grow older and as the body habitus changes on the unaffected side to attain symmetry. For this reason, one may elect to insert an implant with a distant valve that can be adjusted postoperatively until the opposite breast has fully developed.

A custom implant works nicely for the female patient because only the infraclavicular portion of the contour deformity is visible. If the breast is hypoplastic, breast reconstruction with an implant will also be required. However, functional muscle transposition is preferred. At the time of the functional muscle transfer, either a permanent implant or a tissue expander may be inserted to provide breast mound reconstruction if hypomastia is part of the Poland deformity (Fig. 134-33).

In the male patient, the custom implant will simulate the missing pectoralis and improve the contour deformity on the involved hemithorax. However, with motion, the implant does not change and provides a less natural reconstruction than functional muscle transposition does. If the patient is actively involved in bodybuilding, the latissimus muscle will enlarge with physical activity, whereas the implant will not change to correspond to hypertrophy of the opposite pectoralis muscle.

Autogenous Reconstruction. Functional muscle transposition represents the optimal treatment for the absent pectoralis major muscle (Figs. 134-34 to 134-37). An innervated muscle with appropriate origin and insertion will replace the absent pectoralis major muscle and will function to restore missing shoulder abduction. A successful muscle transfer will correct the contour defect, and the transferred innervated muscle has the potential to enlarge if the patient with Poland disease is intent on bodybuilding (Fig. 134-38). Many of the adolescent boys have already begun bodybuilding in an effort to overcome the absent muscle related to the Poland syndrome. The contralateral pectoralis muscle is often already enlarged as a result of exercise.

The other option is autogenous microvascular flap transplantation. The rectus abdominis musculocutaneous flap designed as a perforator flap has been advocated for contour correction. Although rectus muscle function preservation is feasible with the deep inferior epigastric perforator flap design, the resultant correction will not change with physical activity often common in the adolescent or young adult patient and will not replace the absent pectoralis function. Both the latissimus dorsi functional muscle transfer and microvascular composite tissue transplantation do offer advantages over the use of a custom implant because the autogenous tissue, whether muscle or vascularized fascia and subcutaneous tissue, will more naturally restore the contour resulting from the absent pectoralis major muscle. The donor site scar and the more complex operation may influence the patient and family to select the custom implant procedure. Also, with the latissimus transfer from the ipsilateral chest or contralateral microvascular transplantation, the patient will accept loss of latissimus function from the posterior chest in exchange for anterior muscle function. If the custom implant is elected, the patient can later decide to proceed with autogenous reconstruction if there is dissatisfaction with the implant reconstruction.

Latissimus Dorsi Functional Muscle Transposition. If the latissimus dorsi muscle transposition is elected, the physical examination must confirm that the ipsilateral muscle is present. With the patient forcefully pressing the hand into the pelvis, the latissimus muscle contraction is palpable (Fig. 134-39). If the muscle is absent, the opposite muscle may be transplanted by microvascular surgery. The dissection is identical with the exception that the recipient vessels and suitable motor nerve in the axilla must be identified to revascularize the muscle after it is inset into the opposite hemithorax.

The exposure of the latissimus dorsi muscle and the anterior chest wall may be approached in three ways:

1. a posterior transverse or oblique incision for the harvest of the latissimus dorsi muscle and a

Text continued on p. 501

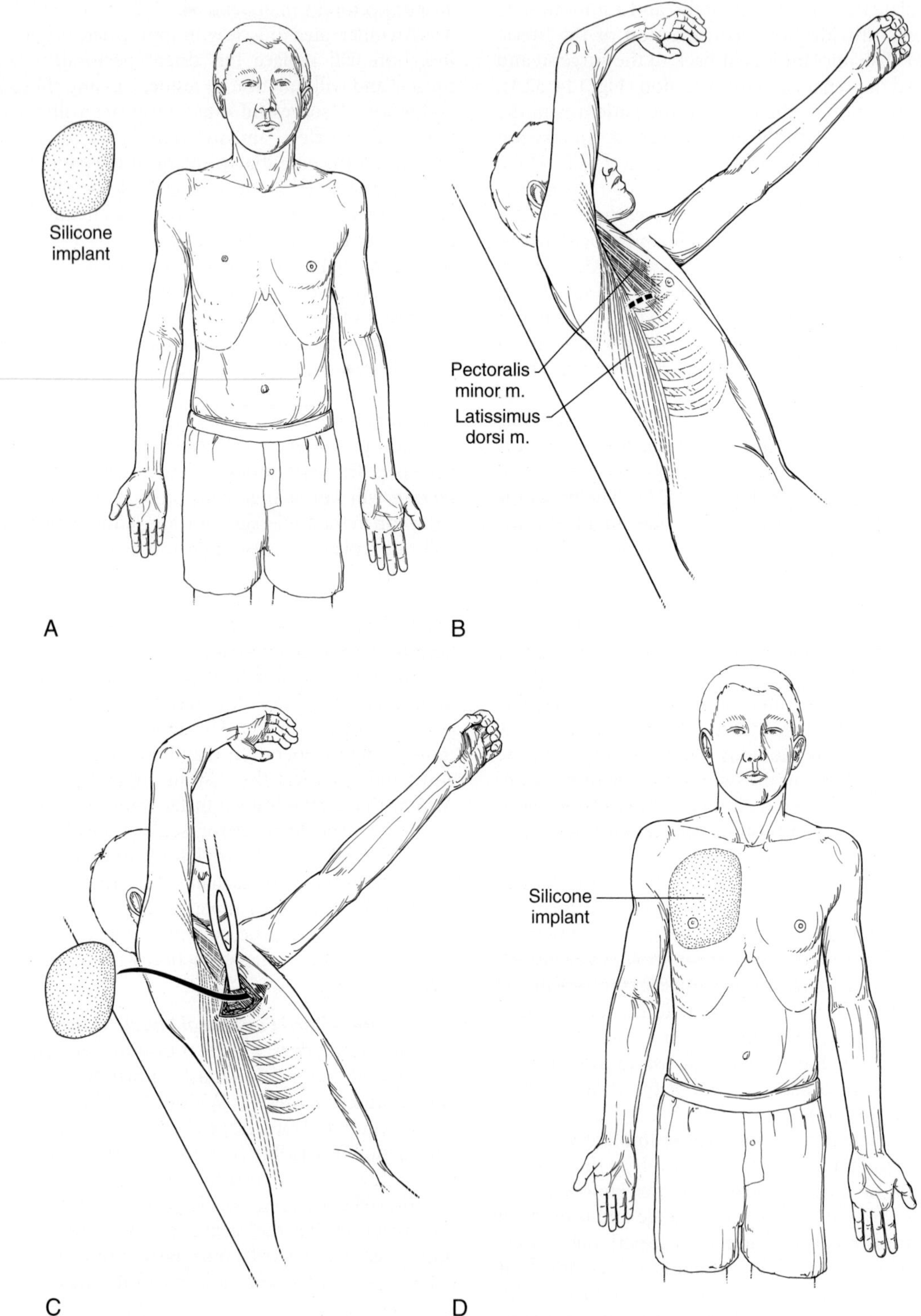

FIGURE 134-32. Poland syndrome, technique for custom silicone implant for pectoralis major contour defect correction. *A,* Absent right pectoralis major muscle custom implant prepared by manufacturer from moulage of defect. *B,* Patient placed in lateral decubitus position. In male patients, exposure for pocket dissection is through a lateral chest wall incision between the anterior and posterior axillary lines. *C,* After pocket dissection between sternum, anterior axillary line, sixth intercostal space, and clavicle, the implant is inserted into position over the pectoralis minor and exposed chest wall. *D,* If the implant is correctly designed and dissection limited to the pectoralis defect, no implant fixation is required.

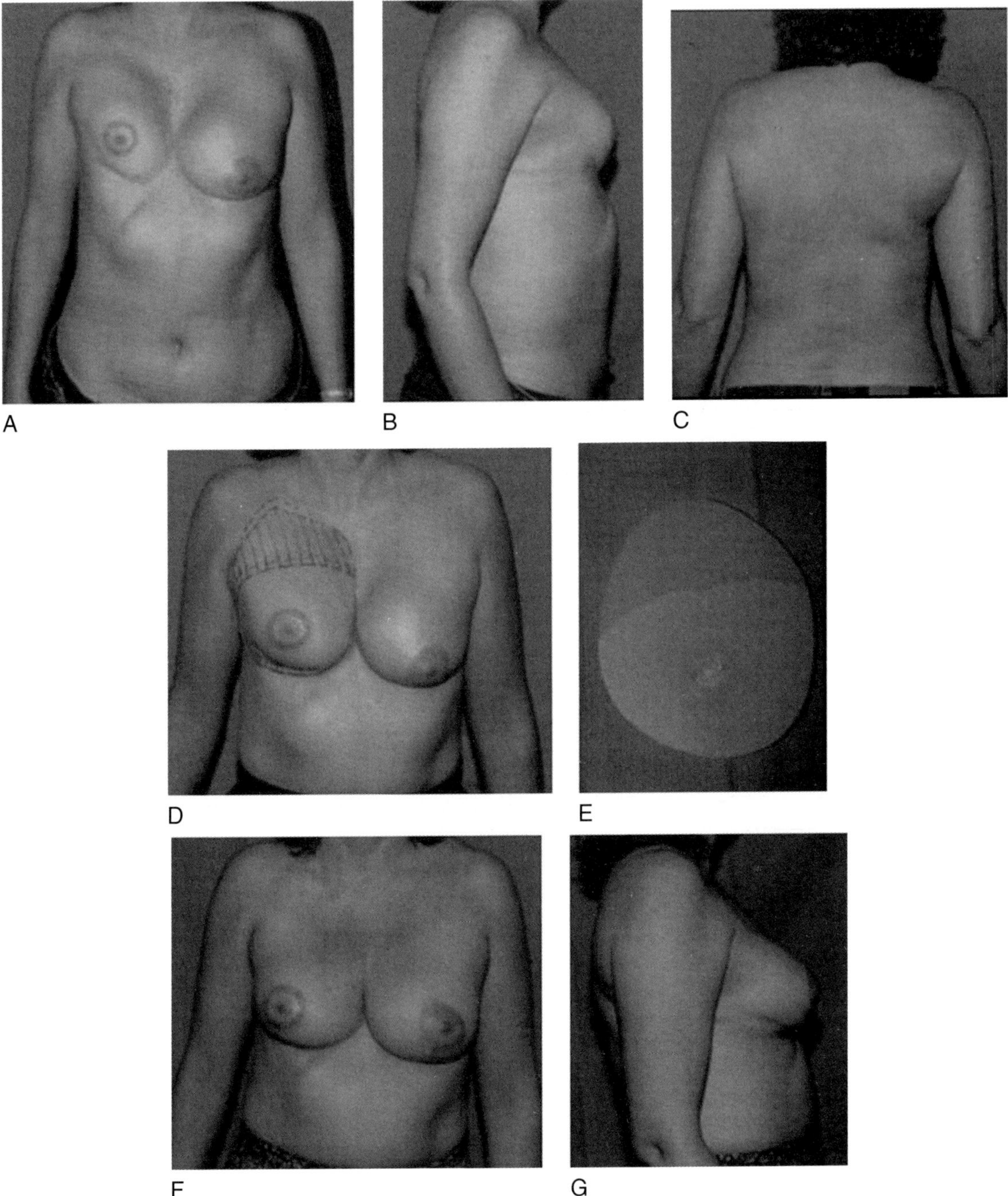

FIGURE 134-33. Poland syndrome, correction with custom implant. *A,* Anterior view. The patient presented with prior breast implant failure for adequate correction of Poland syndrome deformity. *B,* Lateral view. Note position of previously inserted breast implant. *C,* Absent ipsilateral latissimus dorsi muscle. *D,* Anterior postoperative view 3 months after explantation, capsulectomy, and expander insertion; preoperative second-stage custom implant design. *E,* Custom implant with textured implant shell for breast hypomastia and smooth shell for infraclavicular pectoralis major contour defect. *F,* Anterior postoperative view at 1 year with improved breast symmetry and infraclavicular contour correction. *G,* Lateral view. Note adequate breast projection and size with pectoralis major contour provided by custom implant.

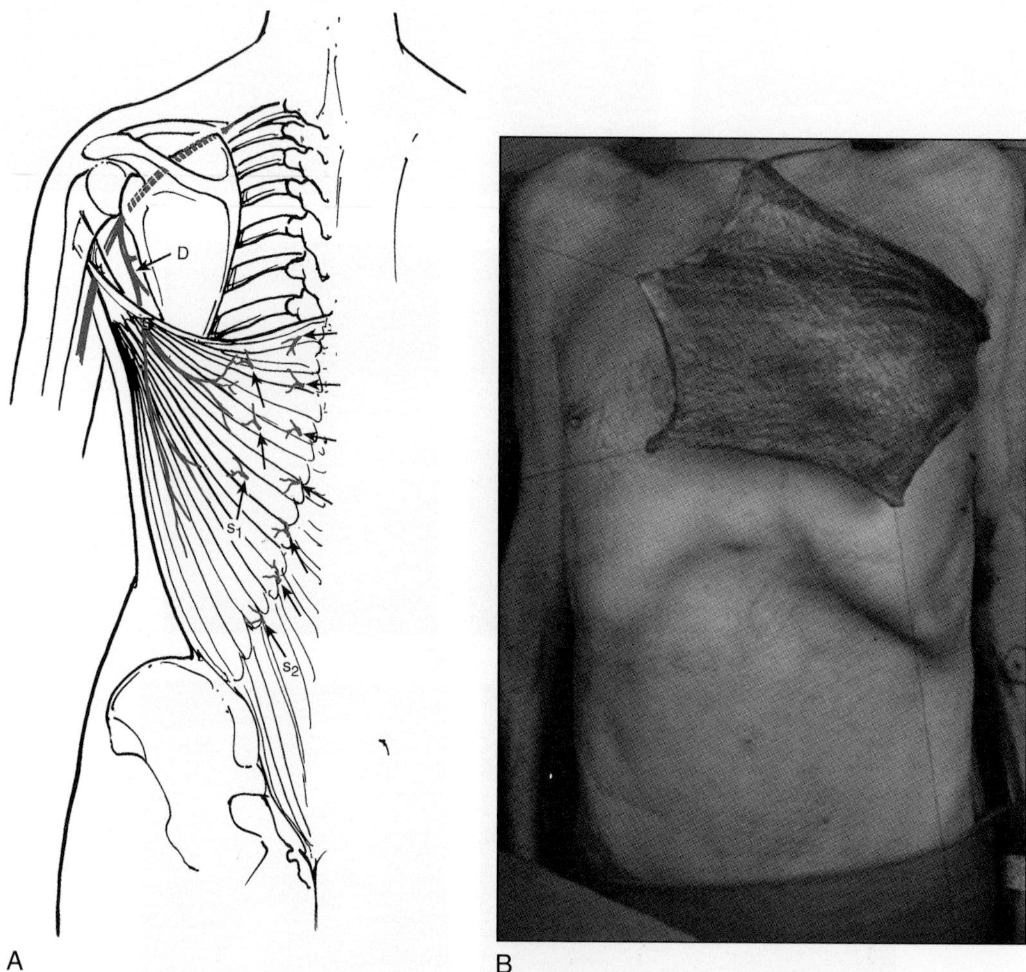

FIGURE 134-34. Anatomy, functional latissimus dorsi muscle transposition. *A,* Vascular anatomy of latissimus dorsi muscle. D, major pedicle—thoracodorsal artery and associated veins. Secondary segmental pedicles: lateral row, branches of posterior intercostal artery and vein (s_1); medial row, branches of lumbar artery and vein (s_2). *B,* Cadaver dissection demonstrates transposition of latissimus dorsi to anterior chest. Note similarity of latissimus dorsi to pectoralis major muscle. (From Mathes SJ, Nahai F: Reconstructive Surgery: Principles, Anatomy, and Technique. New York, Churchill Livingstone, 1997.)

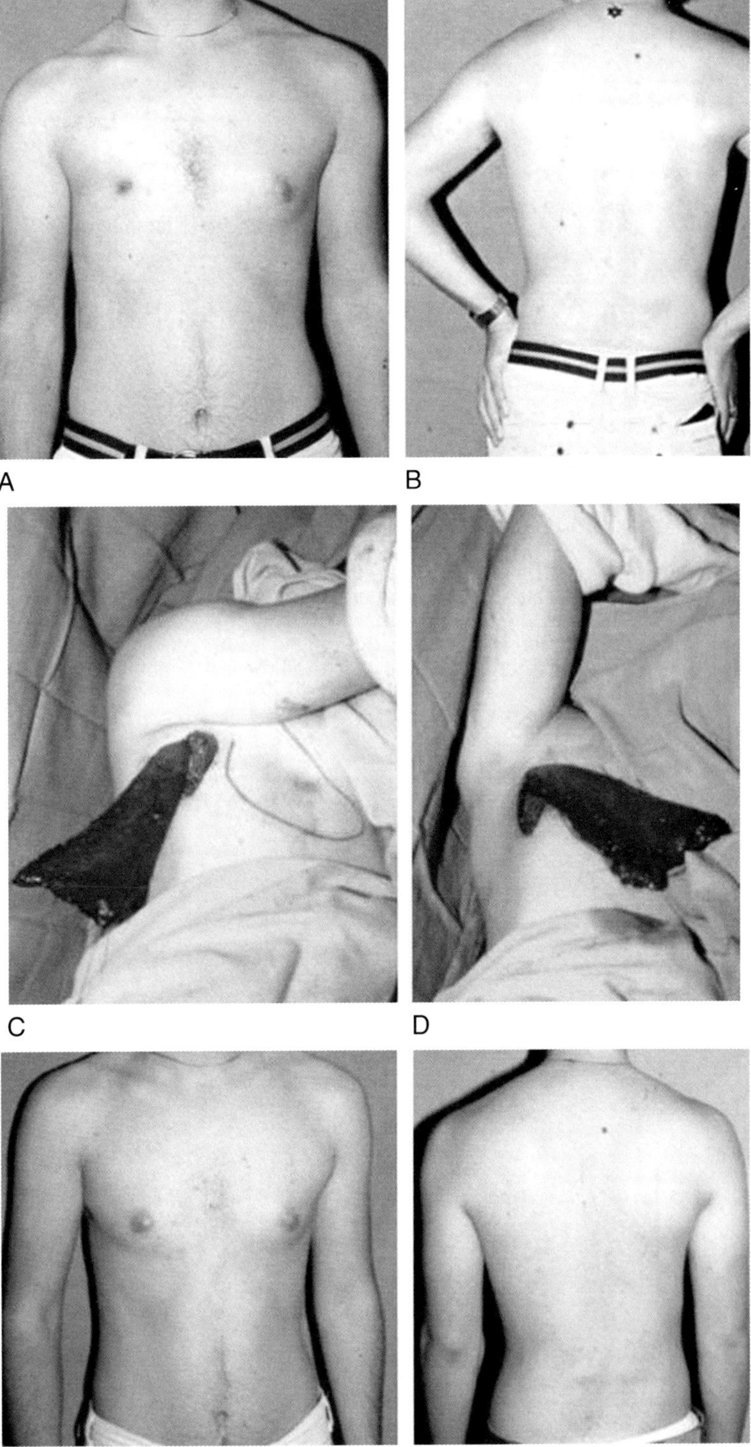

FIGURE 134-35. Latissimus dorsi functional muscle transposition for Poland syndrome. *A,* Anterior view of chest. Note congenital absence of inferior two thirds of pectoralis major muscle. The patient lacks anterior axillary fold and normal right chest projection. *B,* Posterior view, ipsilateral (right) latissimus muscle intact. No hand anomalies were noted. *C,* Intraoperative view, latissimus dorsi muscle detached from origin. *D,* Intraoperative view, arc of rotation of latissimus dorsi muscle. Note that the point of rotation occurs in the axilla to ensure direct alignment of muscle from insertion to new origin on sternum. *E,* Anterior postoperative view 1 year after chest wall reconstruction. *F,* Posterior view. Note normal contour at donor site for latissimus dorsi muscle transposition. (From Mathes SJ, Nahai F: Clinical Atlas of Muscle and Musculocutaneous Flaps. St. Louis, CV Mosby, 1979.)

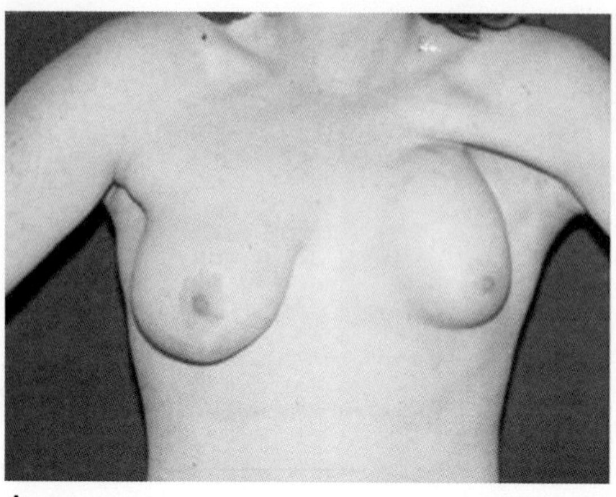

A

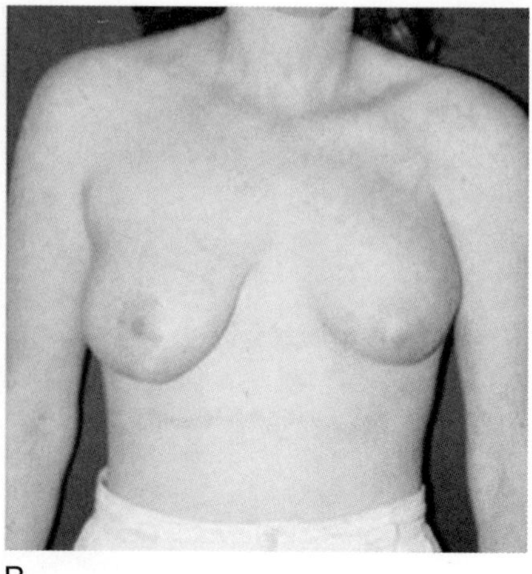

B

FIGURE 134-36. *A,* Preoperative anterior view of 18-year-old female patient referred after an attempt at reconstruction of the mild type of Poland anomaly with a mammary prosthesis alone. The flexing of the clavicular head of the pectoralis major accents the volume that is missing due to absence of the sternocostal head. Unfortunately, the mammary prosthesis does not provide for a natural restoration of the subclavicular hollowing because of the absence of the muscle. *B,* The patient is seen postoperatively after latissimus dorsi muscle transposition and insertion of another mammary prosthesis. This repair provided a more natural result. (*B* from Seyfer AE, Icochea R, Graeber GM: Poland's anomaly. Natural history and long-term results of chest wall reconstruction in 33 patients. Ann Surg 1988;208:776.)

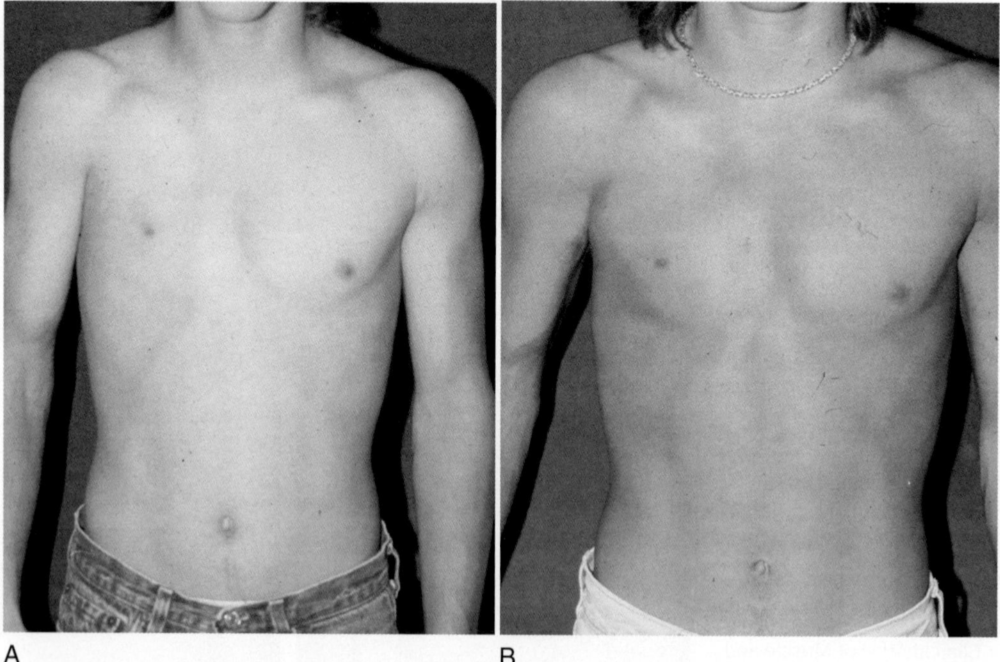

A B

FIGURE 134-37. *A,* Preoperative anterior view of 17-year-old male patient referred for evaluation of Poland anomaly. He was concerned about his appearance and was an accomplished athlete. *B,* The patient is shown after latissimus dorsi muscle transfer. The insertion of the muscle was also moved to improve the axillary fold. (From Seyfer AE, Icochea R, Graeber GM: Poland's anomaly. Natural history and long-term results of chest wall reconstruction in 33 patients. Ann Surg 1988;208:776.)

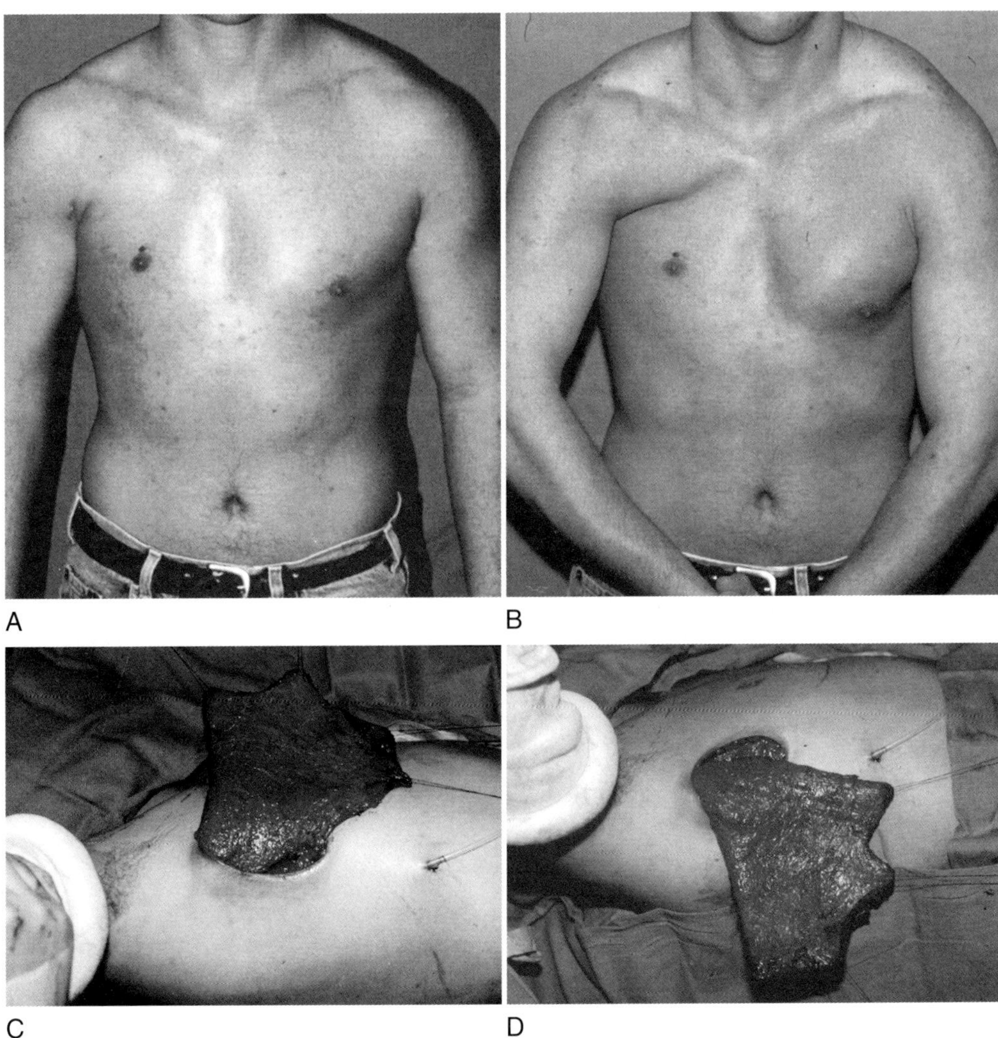

FIGURE 134-38. Latissimus dorsi functional muscle transplantation for Poland syndrome. *A,* Anterior view of chest demonstrates contour defect resulting from absence of sternum head—inferior two thirds of pectoralis major muscle. *B,* Anterior view of chest with forceful contraction of contralateral pectoralis major muscle. The deformity in the right hemithorax is accentuated. *C,* Intraoperative view, dissection of latissimus dorsi muscle performed in lateral decubitus position. After the muscle is released from its origin and ready for transfer to the anterior chest, the patient is rolled to the supine position (beanbag deflated). *D,* Intraoperative view, sutures placed in latissimus dorsi muscle origin and passed through skin to ensure correct anatomic position of new muscle origin at inframammary line and sternal edge.

Continued

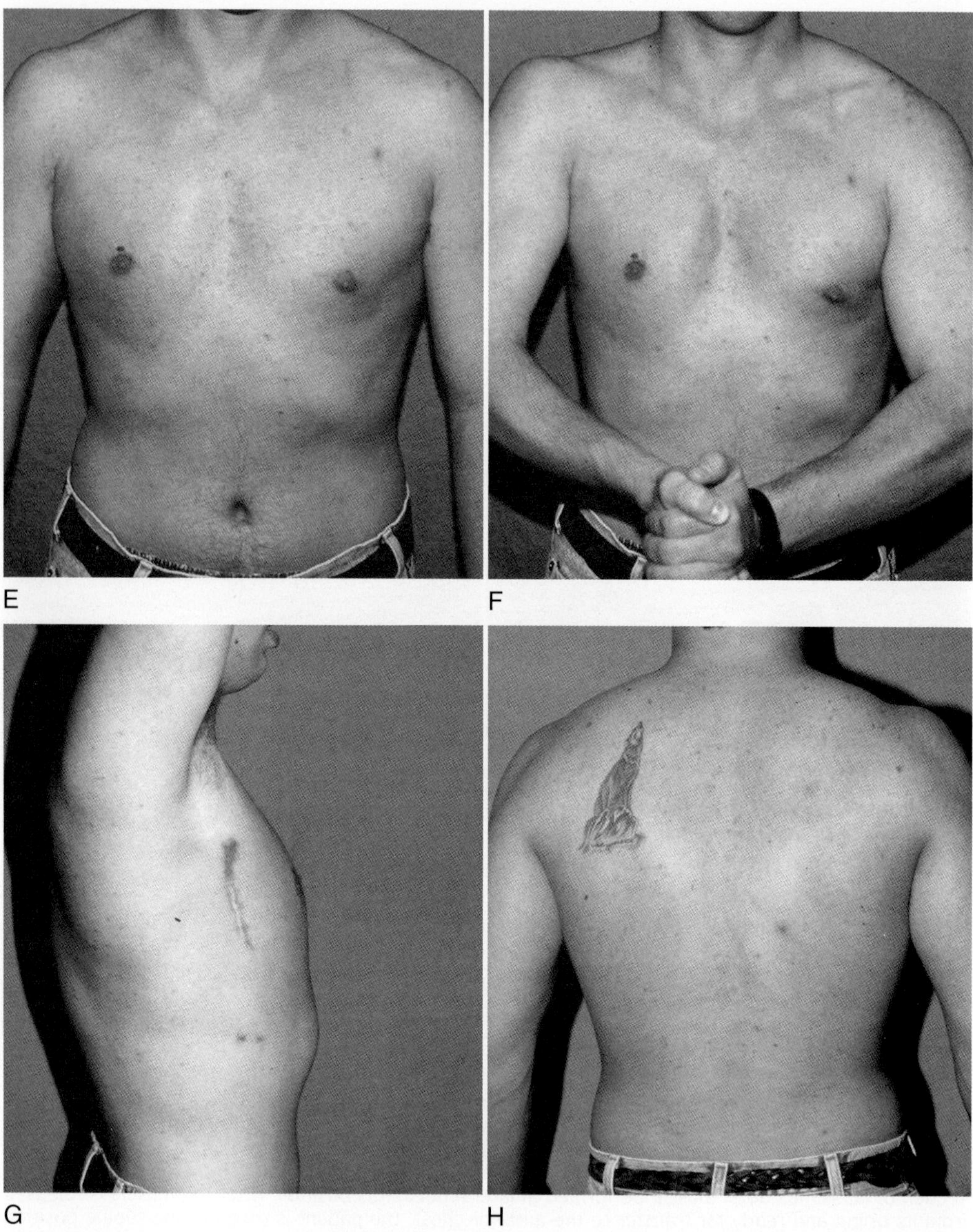

FIGURE 134-38, cont'd. *E,* Anterior postoperative view at 1 year. Latissimus dorsi provides contour correction. *F,* Anterior view with forceful contraction of contralateral pectoralis major muscle; ipsilateral functional latissimus dorsi muscle contraction noted. *G,* Lateral view. The single incision located between the anterior and posterior axillary lines provides adequate exposure for the procedure. The incision is concealed with arm adduction. *H,* Posterior view; minimal contour defect at donor site.

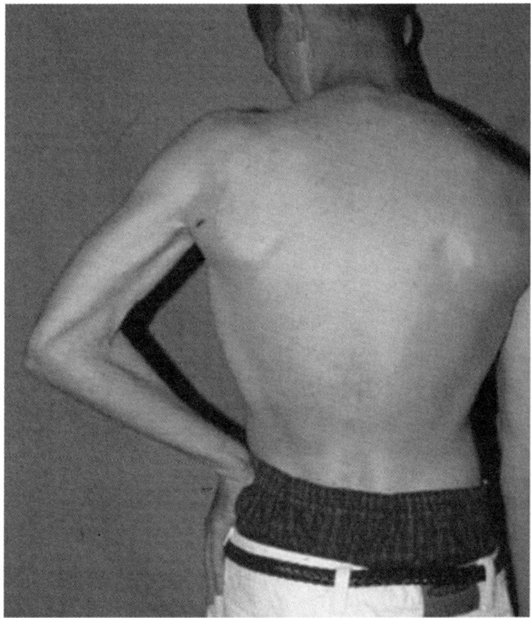

FIGURE 134-39. Preoperative evaluation for latissimus dorsi functional muscle transposition. Forceful adduction of the upper extremity is used to determine whether the latissimus muscle is present in Poland syndrome. Note that the anterior edge of the contracting latissimus dorsi muscle is visible.

separate incision at either the anterior axillary line or the inframammary line for exposure for muscle transfer inset;

2. a vertical or transverse short incision at the midaxillary line, which will provide exposure initially for dissection of the latissimus dorsi muscle and subsequently the dissection over the anterior hemithorax for exposure of the inset site for the muscle transfer; and
3. a lateral chest and posterior chest small incision for endoscopic harvest of the latissimus dorsi muscle and an anterior axillary line or inframammary incision for inset of the muscle.

The exposure through the vertical or lateral short (6 cm) incision at the midaxillary line is preferred because it provides both anterior and posterior chest exposure, and the incision is hidden fairly well beneath the upper extremity. Although the endoscopic harvest is useful, a larger incision is still required to transfer the bulky muscle to the anterior hemithorax and accomplish a careful inset maintaining the appropriate origin-insertion tension to preserve muscle function.

Before surgery, the patient is placed in the sitting position, and the following landmarks are outlined:

- the inframammary line to coincide with the opposite inframammary line;
- the proposed inset of the functional muscle transfer, including the clavicle, the medial sternal edge, and the anterior axillary line;
- the posterior axillary line at the lateral edge of the latissimus muscle (identified while the patient forcefully contracts the muscle against resistance);
- the inferior tip of the scapula, representing the superior posterior edge to the latissimus muscle; and
- the appropriate incision planned for exposure of the latissimus muscle and inset site on the anterior hemithorax.

In the operating room, the patient is placed in the lateral decubitus position, and both the anterior and posterior hemithorax is included in the field of operation (Fig. 134-40*A*). In the male patient or the female patient in whom the breast mound is adequate, the entire operation can be performed in this position. However, in the female patient in whom implant or expander insertion is planned, the patient must be returned to the supine position after donor site closure to position the implant. During this phase of the procedure, the patient is placed in the sitting position to confirm adequate size and position of the implant. If an expander is used, the expander may be placed at the time of the muscle inset, avoiding a shift in position since the patient will be returning to the operating room after expansion is completed for insertion of the permanent implant. A postoperative inflatable implant does require accurate positioning and placement with the patient supine, and confirmation of the patient in the sitting position is recommended.

With the patient supported by an inflatable beanbag, the table is tilted toward the anterior chest to improve exposure of the posterior thorax. The incision preferred is a 6- to 8-cm incision at the midaxillary line. Dissection proceeds posteriorly to identify the lateral latissimus dorsi muscle edge. Once it is visualized, the posterior surface of the muscle is exposed by elevation of the posterior skin and subcutaneous tissue with an electrocautery dissection (Fig. 134-40*B*). Fiberoptic retractors and a surgeon's headlight are required to complete the exposure to the posterior midline of the posterior axilla. The dissection superiorly must expose the latissimus dorsi fibers of insertion into the humerus. After the posterior surface is fully exposed, the deep surface is elevated. This dissection should begin at the axillary tip of the scapula and proceed posteriorly at the free superior edge of the muscle. At the posterior edge of the muscle where its fibers insert into the lumbosacral fascia, the fibers of origin are divided starting superiorly at the lower six thoracic vertebrae and continuing inferior at the sacral vertebrae and the supraspinal ligament. If a single axillary incision is used, it is difficult to coagulate the segmental pedicles (posterior intercostal and lumbar

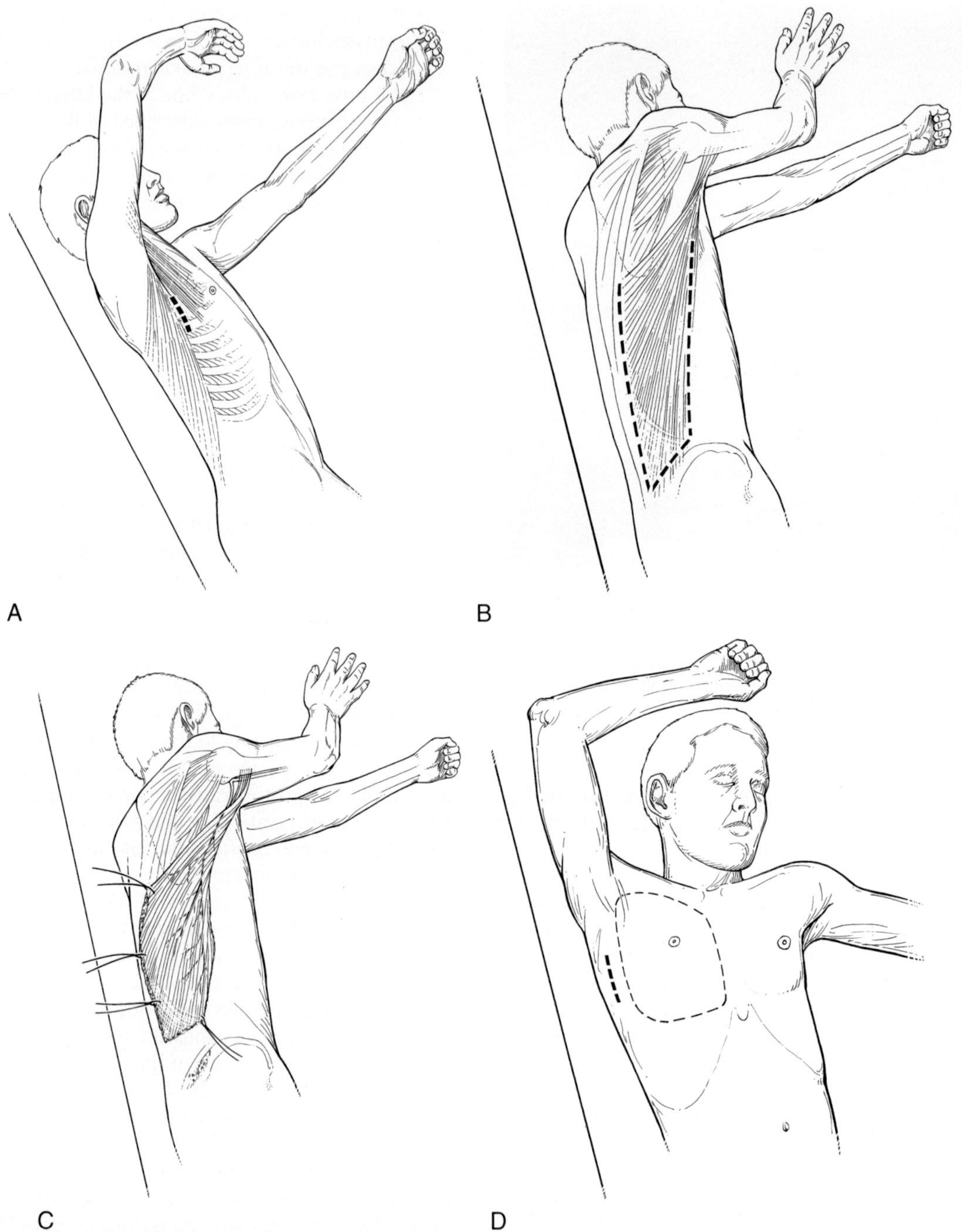

FIGURE 134-40. Operative technique, latissimus dorsi functional muscle transposition. *A,* The lateral decubitus position is used for muscle dissection and inset. An inflatable beanbag provides support on the operating room table and rotation of the patient anterior for back exposure and posterior for anterior chest exposure. *B,* Muscle dissection on the posterior trunk includes release of congenital adhesions to the serratus muscle and division of muscle fibers of origin from thoracolumbar fascia, thoracic and sacral vertebrae, supraspinal ligament, and posterior iliac crest. *C,* Muscle dissection proceeds into the axilla with division of congenital adhesions to teres major muscle and identification of thoracodorsal artery, veins, and nerve. *D,* After latissimus dorsi posterior dissection is completed, the patient is rotated into supine position (deflation of beanbag) for anterior dissection of space for muscle transposition.

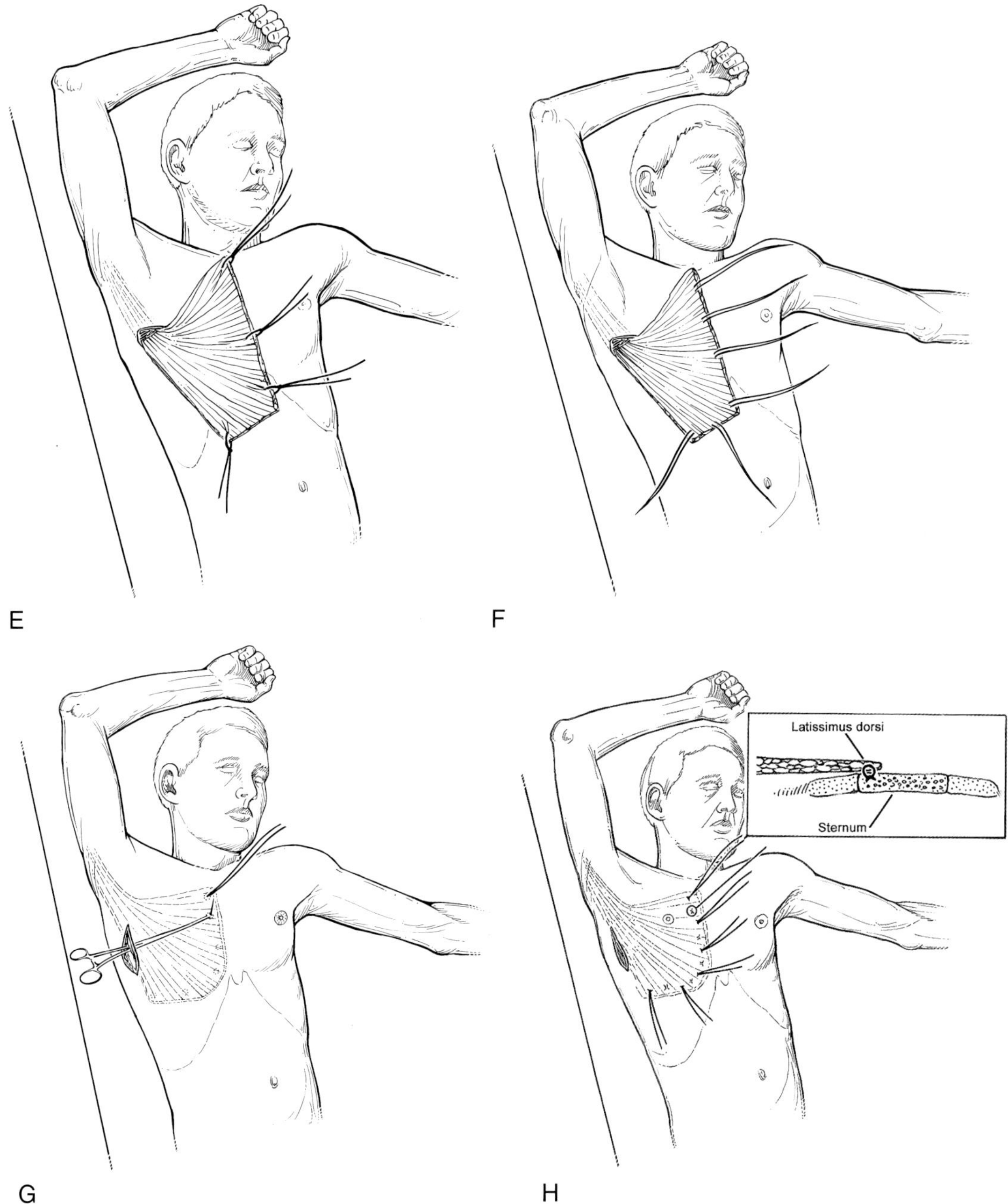

FIGURE 134-40, cont'd. *E,* New latissimus muscle origin is established at inframammary line and along sternal edge. With straight pull of muscle transfer along anterior axillary fold, release of latissimus dorsi muscle insertion is generally not required. *F,* Nonabsorbable sutures passed through muscle origin in horizontal mattress fashion at intervals of 2 to 3 cm. *G,* A Keith needle with both suture ends threaded through the needle eye is passed through the skin slightly medial to the sternal edge and inferior to the inframammary line. *H,* After nonabsorbable sutures are passed through the skin, the position of the muscle origin can be confirmed by pulling the sutures, which advances the muscle into position. Before these sutures passing through the skin are tied, absorbable sutures are placed on the deep surface of muscle origin to the sternal edge and the sixth rib periosteum. *Continued*

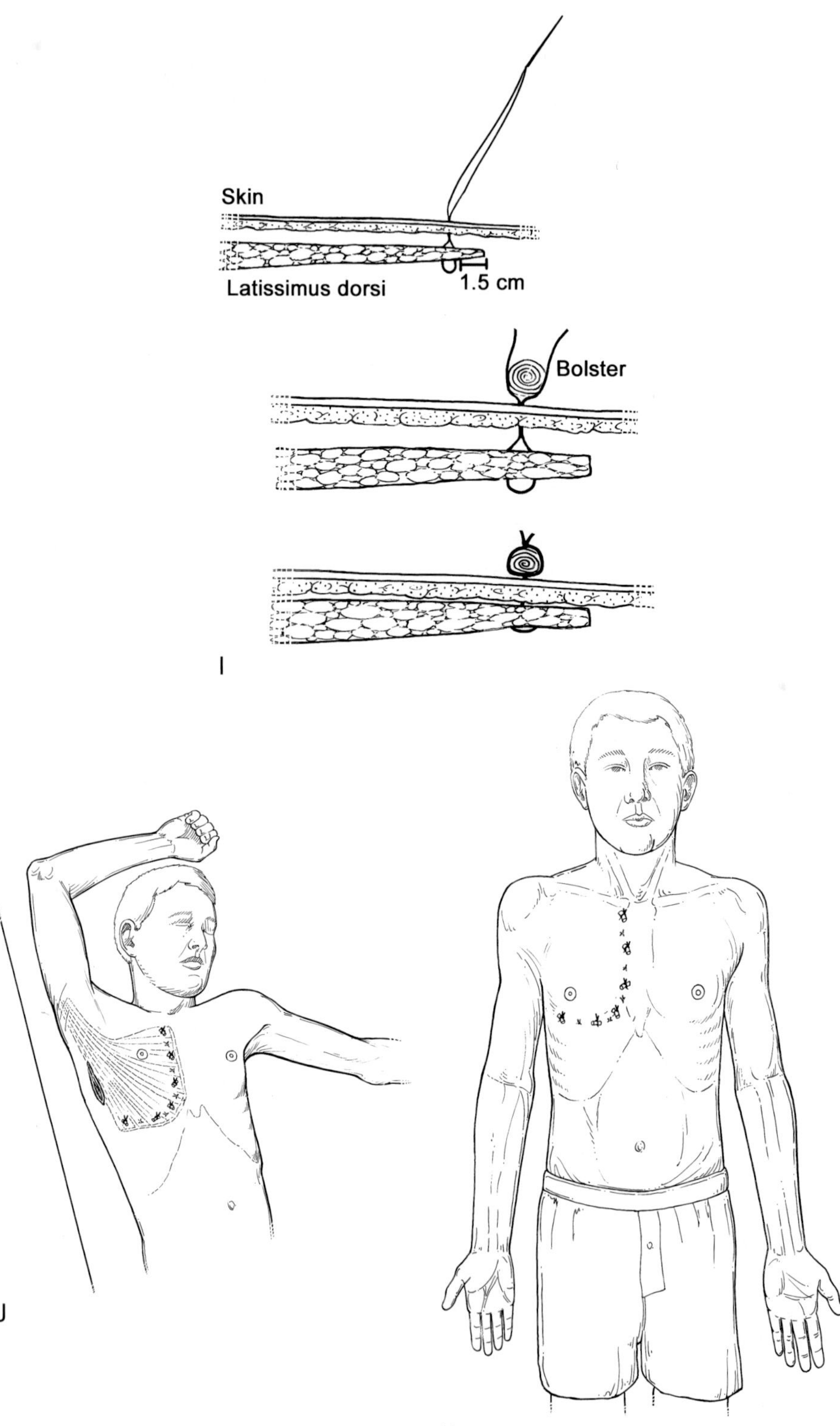

FIGURE 134-40, cont'd. *I,* Close-up of technique to re-establish latissimus dorsi muscle origin. Nonabsorbable sutures are passed through muscle origin and tied over bolster dressing. *J,* Latissimus dorsi muscle origin is established with nonabsorbable bolster sutures through the skin and deep absorbable sutures to sternum and along inframammary line at the sixth rib. *K,* Bolster sutures are removed in 10 to 14 days. Muscle contraction is avoided for 6 weeks.

pedicles) entering the muscle at its posterior origin. If the vessels are difficult to visualize, this area of the dissection is packed with later control of bleeding after the muscle dissection is completed and the muscle transposed toward the anterior chest. If visualization is difficult, a second posterior incision or endoscopic portal may be established. It is important to include the entire muscle in this dissection because it will be transferred as a functional muscle to the anterior chest.

The inferior fibers of origin of the latissimus dorsi into the posterior iliac spine are partially left intact because it is helpful to have muscle stretch while the posterior superior dissection is completed to visualize the point of entry of the thoracodorsal artery, veins, and nerve into the muscle. Because the ipsilateral upper extremity is included in the field of surgery, the assistant abducts the extremity, which allows better exposure into the axilla. Dissection posteriorly and superiorly should extend to the muscle insertion and include division of congenital adhesions posteriorly to the teres major muscle. After the thoracodorsal artery and paired venae comitantes are identified and preserved, the branch to the serratus anterior may be divided as required to allow the arc of rotation into the anterior chest.

The dissection should proceed to the latissimus dorsi fibers of origin into the intertubercular groove of the humerus. The muscle must have a direct line of pull between its insertion and the inset into the anterior chest. Thus, the dissection must establish a space in the superior anterior axilla to connect with the anterior chest. If a direct line of transfer is established, the insertion may be left intact (Fig. 134-41*A*). The insertion may be divided with reattachment to the acromion anterior or passed along the anterior axillary fold and resutured to the humerus (Fig. 134-41*B*). Release of the insertion and its relocation may alter the origin-insertion muscle length and provide a tenotomy effect, which may result in loss of muscle function. If a direct transposition of the muscle is not accomplished by the dissection, reinset of the insertion into the anterior chest may be preferable. The decision regarding relocation of the insertion will depend on the surgeon's preference and familiarity with functional muscle transfer procedures. If the transfer is direct, extending along the anterior axillary fold into the anterior hemithorax, latissimus muscle function is well maintained on the anterior hemithorax without the necessity to relocate the fibers of insertion.

After the dissection of the latissimus muscle is completed, the muscle is removed from the posterior thorax field and rotated onto the surface of the anterior chest (Fig. 134-40*C*). With the muscle removed, it is now easy to establish hemostasis through the single midaxillary incision. A closed suction drain is inserted at this time.

The latissimus dorsi muscle is returned to the posterior chest donor site to proceed with the anterior hemithorax dissection. The table is now tilted toward the posterior chest to improve anterior chest visualization. Through the midaxillary incision or alternative incisions if they are used, the skin of the anterior

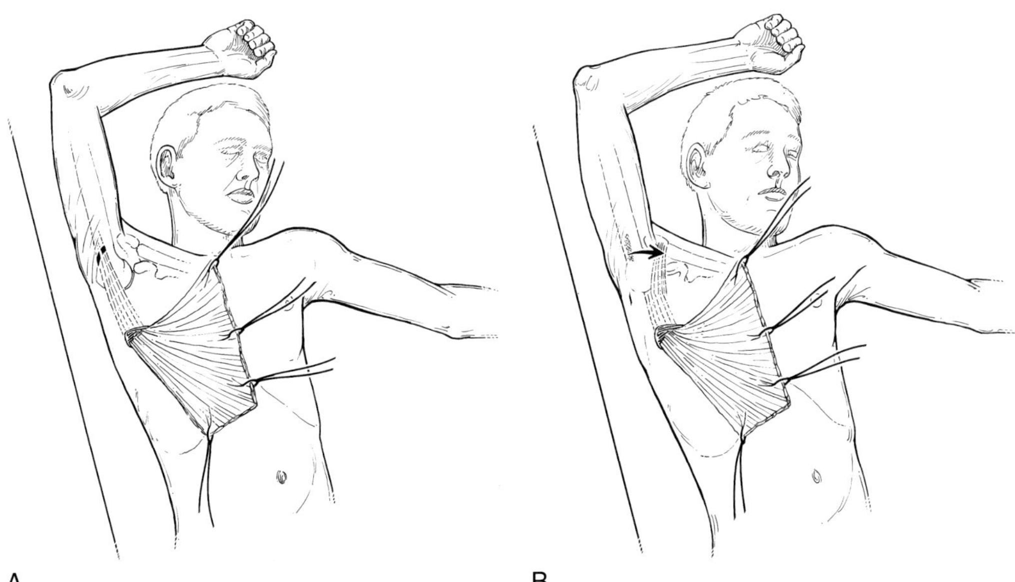

FIGURE 134-41. Latissimus dorsi functional muscle transposition, transfer of insertion. *A,* With pedicle protected, fibers of insertion into intertubercular groove of humerus are divided. *B,* Insertion reattached to acromion or tunneled through anterior axillary fold and reattached to humerus.

chest is elevated, with the dissection plane starting on the superficial fibers of the serratus anterior and proceeding to the anterior ribs, intercostal muscles, and pectoralis minor. The dissection extends from the clavicle superiorly, to 2 cm medial to the medial edge of the sternum, and to the inframammary line as marked before surgery (Fig. 134-40*D*). During the superior dissection, the subclavian vein is not protected by the pectoralis muscle, so the vein must be protected during this part of the dissection. Residual fibrotic fibers of the pectoralis major muscle may be encountered, and these fibers are released because they are nonfunctional and may limit inset of the latissimus dorsi muscle. If the superior aspect of the pectoralis major muscle appears normal and is functional as determined by preoperative evaluation, these fibers are preserved, and the muscle transfer is located inferior to the infraclavicular pectoralis muscle. After the pocket is established, the latissimus dorsi muscle may be transposed to the anterior chest through the anterior superior axillary space in the direction of the anterior axillary fold (Fig. 134-40*E*).

The latissimus muscle is inset so that its fibers are distributed evenly between the superior aspect of inset at the junction of the first rib with the sternum and the sixth intercostal space. The distal muscle may be folded on itself to increase muscle bulk along the sternal edge and to shorten the muscle to ensure appropriate tension between the muscle's origin and new insertion. Techniques for muscle inset vary, but it is helpful to pass a nonabsorbable suture through the muscle edge or folded muscle edge and through the skin by a needle. This techniques ensures adequate distribution of the wide muscle origin along the sternal edge (Fig. 134-40*F* to *H*). Tension on these sutures through the skin will confirm that the muscle is correctly inset in regard to accurate restoration of the origin-insertion length to re-establish natural tension of the muscle. A second row of buried absorbable sutures is now placed to internally establish a new muscle origin along the sternal edge. The sutures passing through the skin are then tied over bolster dressings (Fig. 134-40*I* to *K*).

In the female patient in whom the ipsilateral breast is absent or hypoplastic, a tissue expander may be placed beneath the transposed muscle. If a postoperative inflatable implant is selected (see Chapter 143), the patient should be placed supine with the operative field prepared to allow the patient to be placed in a sitting position. The implant is placed beneath the latissimus muscle and partially inflated, and the position is confirmed to have symmetry with the opposite breast. If contralateral breast surgery is planned, it is preferable to delay this surgery until the site of the latissimus dorsi functional muscle transposition is healed and the expansion process (expander or postoperative inflatable implant) is completed. The anterior hemithorax wound is not usually drained because the posterior donor site has continuity and is drained by a closed suction system.

THE COMPLEX (SEVERE) DEFORMITY. In dealing with the complex (severe) defect, the abnormal sternal and rib contour may be corrected at the initial stage and the latissimus muscle transfer performed at a later stage. However, if the chest wall deformity is repaired with custom implant and not cartilage dissection, implant insertion for sternal deformity and latissimus dorsi functional muscle transposition may be performed simultaneously to avoid a sternal incision (Fig. 134-42).

In the first stage, the patient is supine with the arms abducted. A short midline incision is entered, and the skin and fat are dissected free to expose the defect. The rectus abdominis muscle and its fascia are dissected free from the sternal-rib margins and reflected inferiorly. The sternum is often short and bifid, and a thick bar of abnormal cartilage is present on the affected side. For repair of the contour, the sternal bar of cartilage is sectioned laterally and, like a door on a hinge, turned over to meet the sternal edge, where it is sutured to complete the deficient edge of the sternum. Other pieces of aberrant cartilage are trimmed and either discarded or used as grafts to establish a more natural sternal and chest wall contour. The sternum is now flattened and more natural appearing. The rectus abdominis insertion is mobilized a short distance from its abdominal moorings and reattached to the sternum and chest wall in a more normal position. The incision is closed in layers.

In the second stage, a latissimus muscle transfer is performed as described before. A final third stage can be performed under local anesthetic and is designed to move the nipple-areola complex inferiorly and medially on a local skin flap.

RECONSTRUCTION OF THE BREAST IN POLAND SYNDROME. The optimal timing of the breast or aesthetic chest reconstruction for Poland syndrome is late in the second decade. This operation is usually the second stage of thoracic repair for those with more severe chest wall deformities, but it can occasionally be combined with stabilization of the thoracic cage in patients diagnosed as adults. The delay until the end of adolescence ensures that puberty has passed and that the contralateral chest and breast are fully developed, optimizing the chances of obtaining a symmetric result. Breasts can be augmented with autologous flaps or implants. The latissimus dorsi musculocutaneous flap with an implant can provide adequate projection and satisfactory results.[114] The major disadvantage is the possible loss of arm movement, which may be associated with endoscopic harvest of the latissimus muscle. Only a 6-cm incision in women and a 4-cm

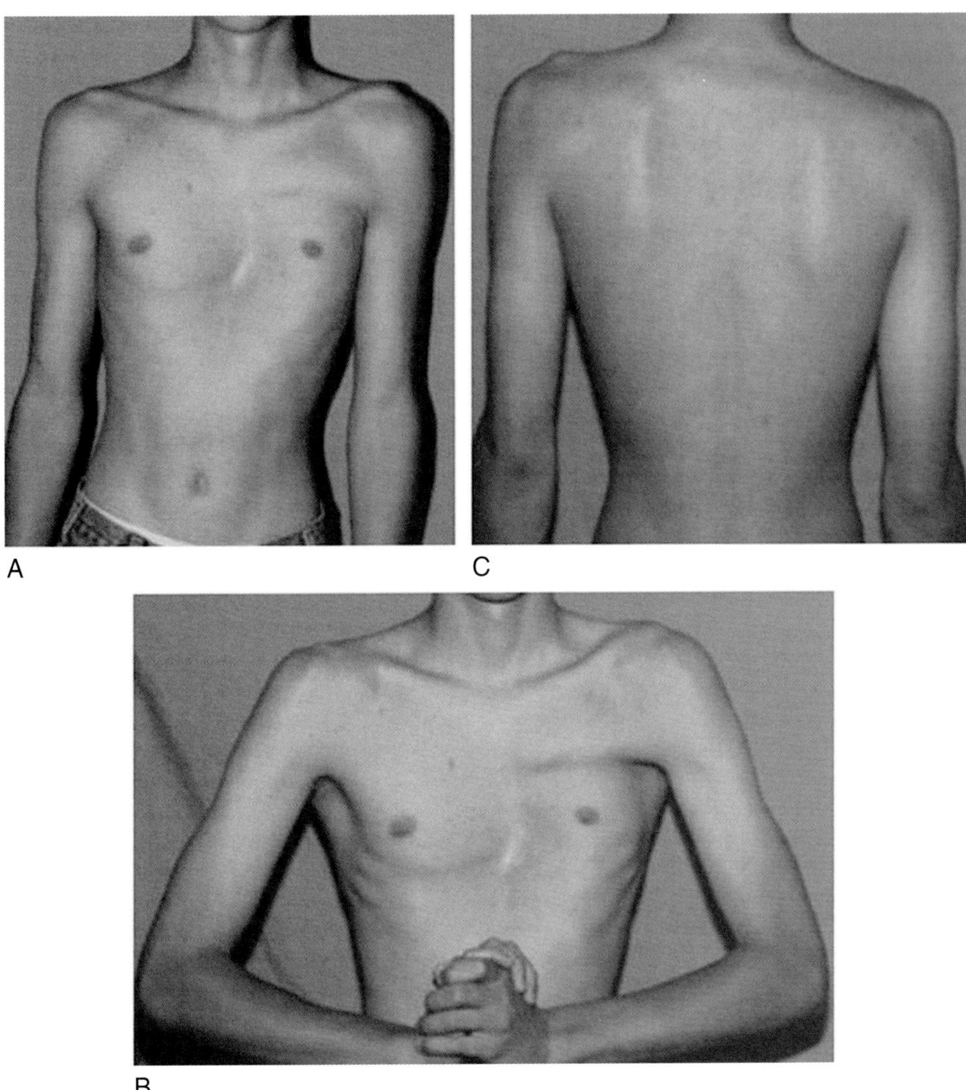

FIGURE 134-42. Latissimus dorsi functional muscle transposition and custom implant for correction of pectus excavatum. *A,* Anterior view of Poland syndrome with pectus excavatum deformity. *B,* Anterior view of forceful upper extremity adduction demonstrates clavicular head of pectoralis major muscle. Inferior two thirds (sternal head) of pectoralis major muscle is absent. *C,* Posterior view of ipsilateral latissimus dorsi muscle available for transplantation. *Continued*

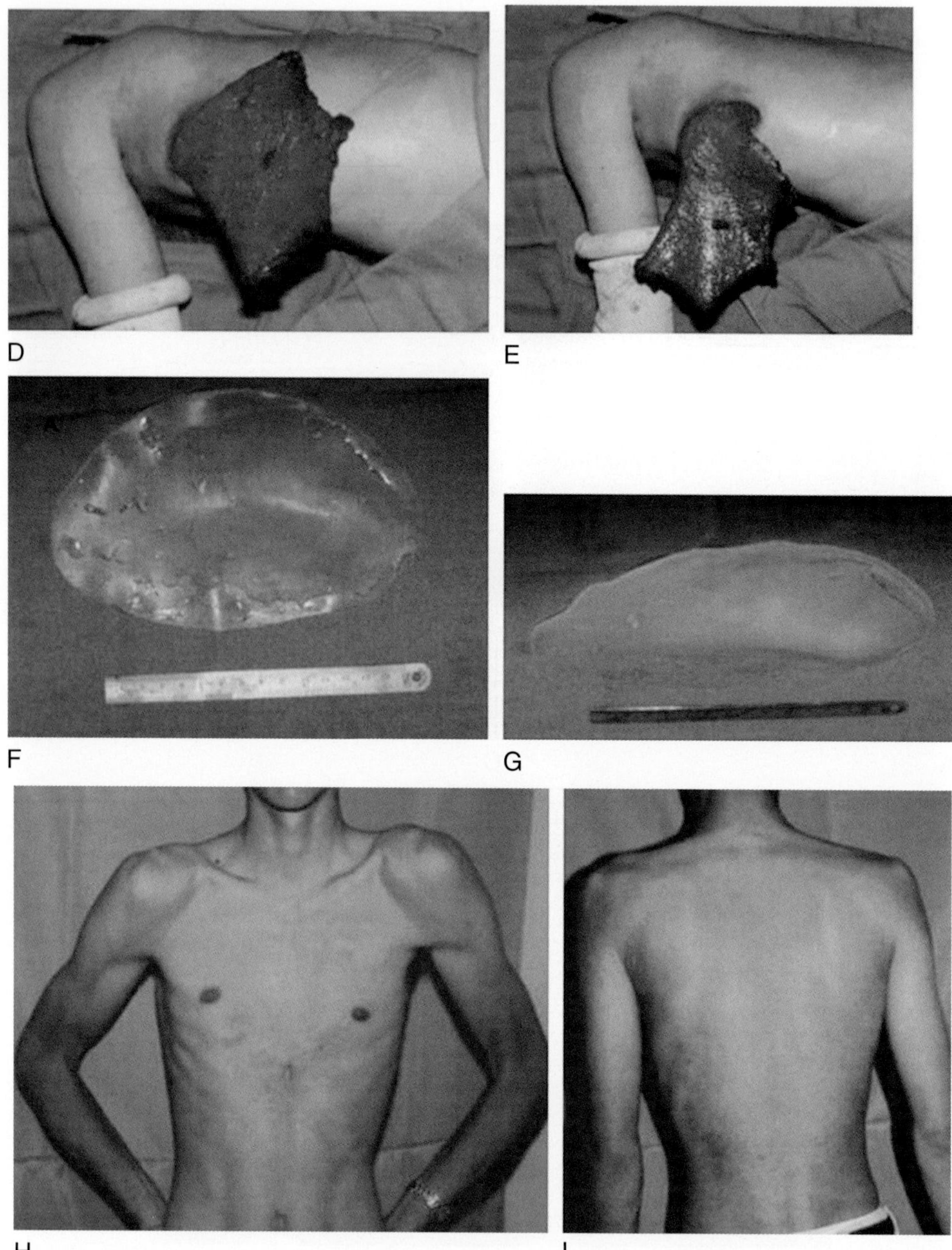

FIGURE 134-42, cont'd. *D,* Intraoperative view of latissimus dorsi muscle fibers of origin divided and muscle flap ready for transposition. *E,* Intraoperative view of latissimus dorsi muscle arc of rotation to anterior chest. *F,* Intraoperative view of anterior surface of custom implant for pectus excavatum correction. *G,* Intraoperative view of posterior convex surface of custom soft silicone implant. *H,* Anterior postoperative view at 1 year of functional transposition of latissimus dorsi muscle and simultaneous pectus excavatum deformity correction. *I,* Posterior view of trunk demonstrates minimal contour deformity at donor site.

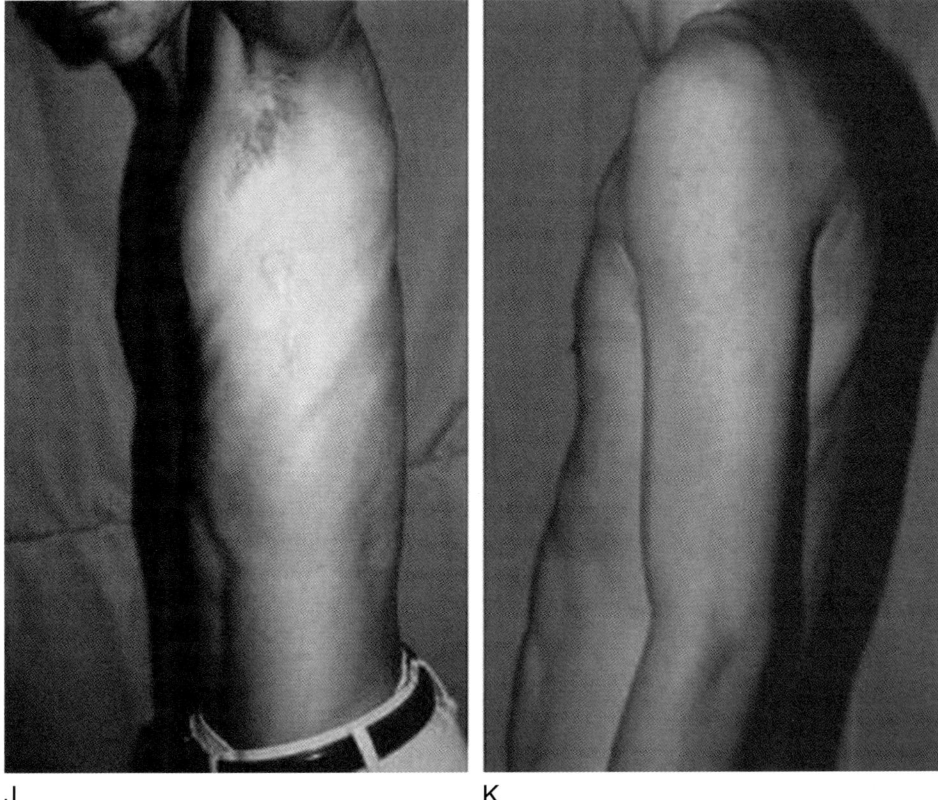

J K

FIGURE 134-42, cont'd. *J,* Lateral view with arm abducted. Healed incision used for operative exposure is visible between anterior and posterior axillary lines. *K,* Lateral view with arm adducted, the scar is concealed.

incision in men was needed to place the permanent implant.[126] Endoscopic harvest has been shown to be effective and to improve satisfaction of patients compared with the open technique.[127]

The use of microvascular free composite tissue transplantation has been reported in a retrospective series of nine patients. Donor sites included the transverse rectus abdominis flap, the contralateral latissimus flap, and superior and inferior gluteal flaps. One flap failed (a superior gluteal flap) because of anomalous venous drainage and was replaced by a second superior gluteal flap. Breast symmetry was established in all patients; however, each patient required 0.4 revisions (ranging from 0 to 2).[128] As the vascular supply to the affected region is uncertain, preoperative ultrasonography or angiography may be helpful in selected patients.[129] As previously noted, the use of free flaps for autogenous contour correction is superb for the breast mound (see Chapter 138) but not as effective in regard to function as ipsilateral latissimus dorsi functional muscle transposition or microvascular functional muscle transplantation of the contralateral latissimus dorsi muscle when the ipsilateral muscle is absent.

Summary

Poland syndrome is a highly variable disorder of the thoracic musculature. The timing and technique of thoracic repair are based on the structures affected and the severity of the disorder. Instability of the chest wall should be corrected promptly with autologous rib grafts and in severe defects with prosthetic mesh. Ultimately, a muscle transfer with or without a prosthesis is needed as a separate stage of reconstruction for those with prior chest wall stabilizations or aesthetic concerns about the appearance of the chest and breast.

BREAST

Embryology

The breast is a tissue that begins to develop from the ectoderm during the fifth week of gestation. The earliest identifiable breast tissue is the mammary ridge, which expands bilaterally from the axillae in a caudad direction to the groin. The ridge undergoes apoptotic regression during the seventh and eighth weeks of gestation, leaving only the primordial breast tissue that exists on the ventral thorax. During weeks 10 to 14, the primordial breast tissue penetrates the underlying mesenchyme. The mesenchymal connective tissue surrounds the breast and ultimately forms a superficial fascia, the outer layer being continuous with Camper fascia and the deeper layer forming the posterior boundary of the breast. These fasciae remain connected to each other by means of a system of interdigitating bundles of connective tissue that exist throughout the mammary tissue and form the suspensory ligaments of Cooper (Fig. 134-43). The outer layer of the superficial fascia envelops the entire breast except directly below the areola. At approximately 20 weeks, canalization occurs.[130] Differentiation of the ectodermal breast tissue continues approximately until birth, at which time development ceases until puberty.[131]

At the time of puberty, the mammary tissue beneath the areola expands, enlarging the areola and ultimately the adjacent skin, and extends radially outward with additional growth toward the ipsilateral axilla, forming the tail of Spence. Growth typically ends at about 16 years of age.[132]

Supernumerary Nipples and Breasts

SUPERNUMERARY NIPPLES (POLYTHELIA)

Supernumerary nipples, or polythelia (*poly,* many, *thelia,* nipple), form along a line from the axilla to the groin that is the remnant of the mammary ridge or milk lines (Figs. 134-44 and 134-45). Remnants of these lines remain after improper regression of the mammary ridge at approximately 3 months of gestation; these may give rise to accessory nipples.[133] Polythelia is relatively common and is observable at birth with an incidence of 0.2% to 2.5%. The lowest frequency has been reported in white Europeans (0.2%); in black American and Jewish newborns, frequencies of 1.6% and 2.5% have been reported, respectively.[134-137] Reasons for these differences are controversial, but studies with higher rates may reflect the use of more thorough examination techniques.[133] The most common site is inferior to the normal breast but superior to the lower abdominal-inguinal regions; in approximately 50% of patients, it is bilateral.[138,139] Sites outside of the milk lines have been described, including the scapula, posterior thigh, head, and neck.[140]

Whereas polythelia rarely causes more than an aesthetic concern to the patient, an accessory nipple or rudimentary nipple-areola complex can both respond in a physiologic manner and suffer the same diseases as normal breast tissue.[141] Supernumerary nipples have also been associated with several other congenital deformities, including occult urogenital and vertebral malformations, as well as cardiac arrhythmias and renal cell carcinoma (Table 134-11).[142] However, much of the data has been derived from reports and retrospective studies. When the renal system was examined by ultrasound in a controlled prospective study, no significant differences in the rate of anomalies were detected between children with polythelia (3.74%, n = 496) and controls (3.17%, n = 410).[143] Study of children with recurrent urinary tract infections also revealed no differences in the prevalence of polythelia between those with radiographically demonstrable urogenital anomalies and those without.[144]

Polythelia has also been associated with testicular cancer. Two relatively small studies suggest an elevated risk. In the Health and Nutrition Examination Study,[145] polythelia was present in 27 of 7004 (0.4%) white males studied; based on a comparison with the overall male cohort, a relative risk for development of testicular cancer (in the context of polythelia) was found to be 31.8 (95% confidence interval, 13.9 to 72.6). Goedert et al[145] studied 299 males with an incidence of polythelia of 2.7%. In these patients, a relative risk of testicular cancer of 4.5 (95% confidence interval, 1.6 to 12.4) was calculated. It is reasonable to conclude from these reports that male patients with supernumerary nipples have an increased risk for testicular tumors, but the actual relative risk remains uncertain because of the relatively low incidence of both diseases.

The treatment of choice for supernumerary nipples is simple excision, although care must be taken first to exclude a breast mass. In addition, alternative diagnoses including malignant melanoma must be considered. In men, a testicular examination is warranted—particularly for those with a history of an undescended testis. As for the urinary system, it has been suggested that an investigation for anomalies be reserved for symptomatic patients.[140]

TABLE 134-11 ✦ POLYTHELIA AND POSSIBLY ASSOCIATED CONDITIONS

Urinary Tract Abnormalities	Cardiac Abnormalities	Miscellaneous Abnormalities
Renal agenesis	Cardiac conduction disturbances, especially left bundle branch block	Pyloric stenosis
Renal cell carcinoma	Hypertension	Epilepsy
Obstructive disease	Congenital heart anomalies	Ear abnormalities
Supernumerary kidney(s)		Arthrogryposis multiplex congenita

From Pellegrini JR, Wagner RF Jr: Polythelia and associated conditions. Am Fam Physician 1983;28:129-132.

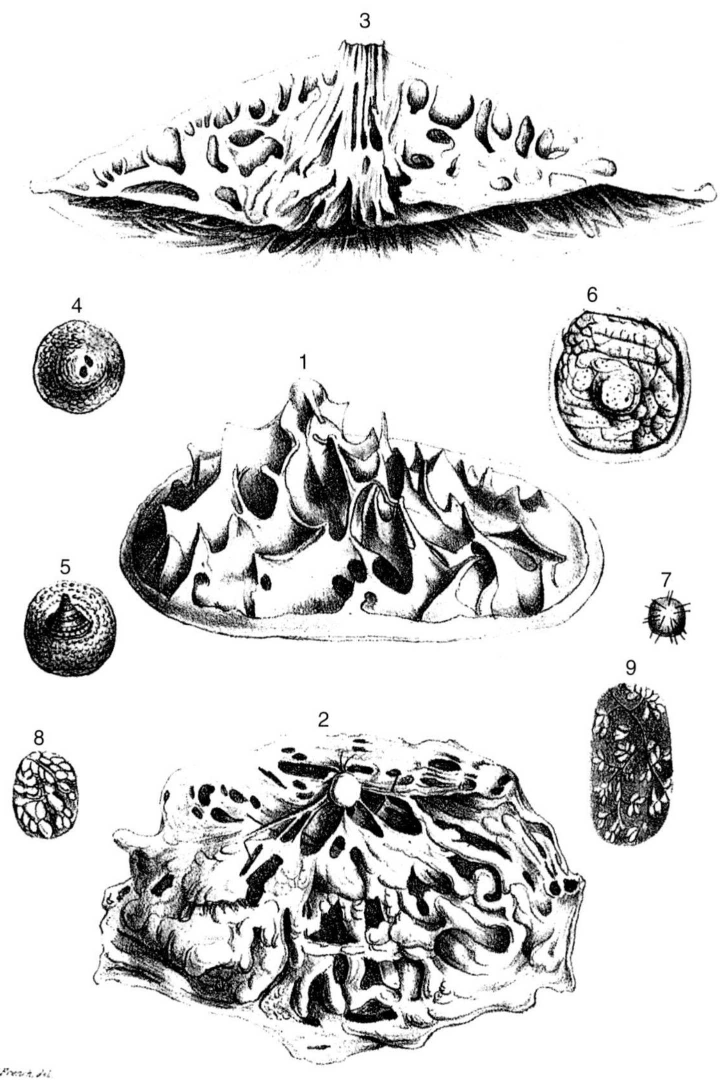

FIGURE 134-43. Illustration from *Anatomy and Diseases of the Breast* by Sir Astley Cooper published in 1845. Ligamenta suspensoria and sections. 1, A preparation made to show the ligamenta suspensoria supporting the folds of the breast to the inner side of the skin. The nipple is seen in the center, a portion of skin in the circumference, and the folds of the breast are sustained by the ligamenta suspensoria, which are continued to the skin; but their connection with it is here cut off. Thus the surface of the breast is greatly increased, while its diameter remains the same. 2, A view of the gland dissected and unravelled, to show the ducts over bristles, the lobuli, and the glandules. 3, A section of the mammary gland through the nipple, showing the ducts over a bristle, unravelled, and proceeding to the posterior part of the gland. The ligamenta suspensoria may be seen passing from the anterior surface of the gland to the skin, supporting the folds or processes of the former, and leaving considerable cavities between them, in which the fat is contained in its proper membrane. The fascia may be observed passing to each extremity of the gland, and dividing into two portions; the anterior proceeding upon the surface of the gland to form the ligamenta suspensoria; the posterior behind the gland, sending processes between which a smaller quantity of fat is contained; and both these layers assist in producing the fibrous tissue of the gland. It also sends processes of fascia backwards, to join the aponeurosis of the pectoral muscle, forming the line from one extremity of the gland to the other. The section, therefore, clearly shows the various cords by means of which the breast is slung and sustained. 4, Shows the depressions of the nipple, in which the orifices of the lactiferous tubes are placed. 5, A dried preparation of the nipple and areola; showing the papillae of each: those of the nipple taken in this mode of preparing them in a rather spiral direction, and those of the areola arranged in circles. 6, The nipple and areola, after being placed in alcohol, by which they have been somewhat constrained. The nipple is placed near the center, and the orifices of the lactiferous tubes are seen in it. Numerous orifices are also visible around it, placed in the tubercles of the areola. These orifices are from one to five, and sometimes more in number. 7, Sixteen bristles in the orifices of the lactiferous tubes. 8, Shows some of the larger glandules of the breast. 9, Exhibit some of the smaller, with ducts unravelled. (From Cooper A: Anatomy and Diseases of the Breast. Philadelphia, Lea & Blanchard, 1845.)

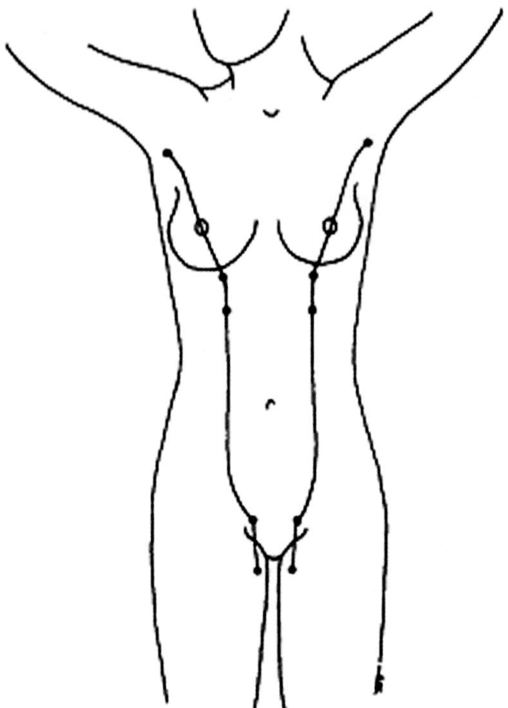

FIGURE 134-44. The mammary ridges or milk lines along which ectopic breast tissue tends to form. Bullets represent common locations of supernumerary nipples. (From Bland KI, Romwell LJ: Congenital and acquired disturbances of breast development and growth. In Bland KI, Copeland EM III, eds: The Breast: Comprehensive Management of Benign and Malignant Disorders, 3rd ed. Philadelphia, Elsevier, 2004:200.)

SUPERNUMERARY BREASTS (POLYMASTIA)

Whereas polythelia is simply an accessory nipple, a supernumerary breast (polymastia: *poly,* many, *mastia,* breast) implies the development of ectopic breast parenchyma with or without the presence of a nipple. Typically, supernumerary breasts develop from residual mammary ridge tissue after hormonal stimulation. The presentation can vary widely, with all combinations of breast tissue and elements of the nipple-areola complex. The overall incidence has been estimated at 0.1% to 1.0%.[146,147] The most common site noted for ectopic breast tissue is the axilla, but there is some doubt as to whether the axillary breast is truly polymastia or whether the extra axillary tissue simply represents hypertrophy of the tail of Spence (Fig. 134-46).[148,149] Other sites are generally along the milk lines and on the vulva.[150]

Ectopic breasts must be evaluated for the same diseases as in normal breasts. Fibroadenomas, fibrocystic breast disease, and other benign diseases have been described in ectopic breast tissue.[151] Adenocarcinoma and cystosarcoma phyllodes tumors have been reported, making the evaluation of the supernumerary breast for malignant neoplasia essential.[141,152] The differential diagnosis includes lipoma, lymphadenopathy, other soft tissue tumors, vascular lesions, and abscess.

The presence of ectopic breast tissue, particularly if it is extra-axillary, poses concerns similar to those for other anomalies in patients with polythelia.[133] Familial polymastia has been reported and has an association with abnormalities of chromosomes 3 and 8.[147,153] Renal anomalies have been documented in 8 of 20 children identified in a longitudinal study to have supernumerary breasts.[135] Associations have also been drawn between renal malignant neoplasms and polymastia.[145]

The treatment of polymastia is generally elliptical excision. If the primary complaint is mastodynia during pregnancy or lactation, an expectant approach is reasonable because it is likely that the pain will resolve. The evaluation of breast masses in ectopic tissue should follow the same procedures as for the normal breast. The management of breast cancer in an ectopic location is less clear. A retrospective review of 90 patients with carcinoma in ectopic locations (71%

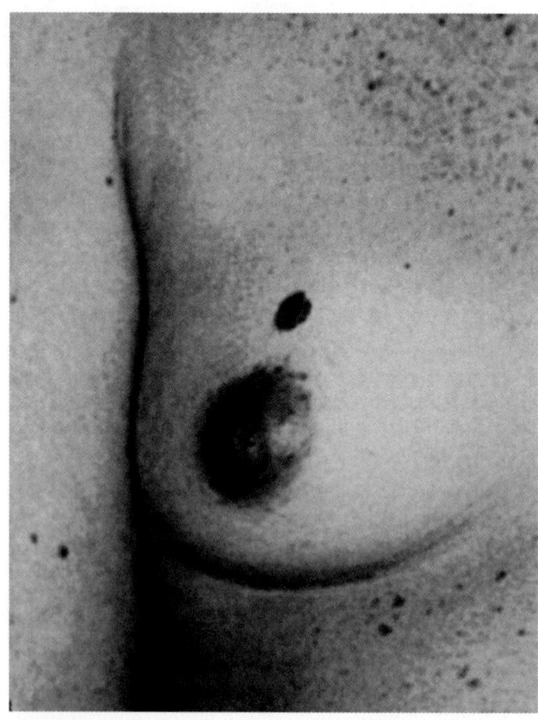

FIGURE 134-45. Supernumerary nipple and areola complex (rudimentary) in upper right breast of a 22-year-old woman. (From Bland KI, Romwell LJ: Congenital and acquired disturbances of breast development and growth. In Bland KI, Copeland EM III, eds: The Breast: Comprehensive Management of Benign and Malignant Disorders, 3rd ed. Philadelphia, Elsevier, 2004:214.)

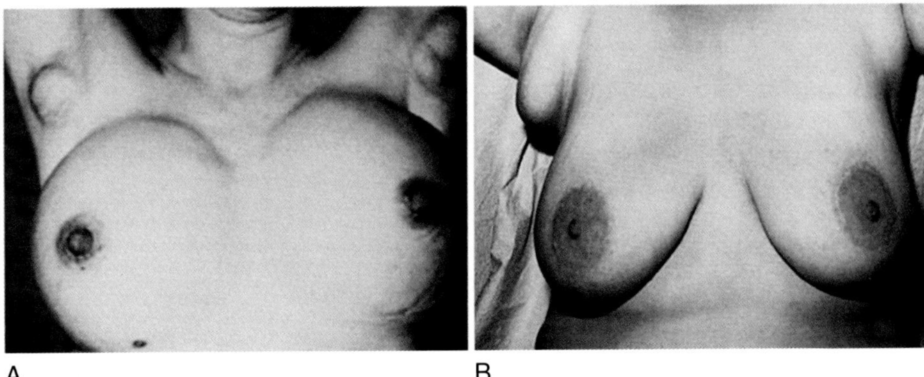

FIGURE 134-46. *A* and *B*, Supernumerary breasts presenting as accessory (ectopic) breast tissue bilaterally in the axilla. In *A*, the right supernumerary inframammary nipple presents in the mammary milk line. (*A* from Greer KE: Accessory axillary breast tissue. Arch Dermatol 1974;109:88. Copyright 1974, American Medical Association. *B* courtesy of Dr. Michael M. Meguid, SUNY Health Sciences Center, Syracuse, NY. Taken from Bland KI, Romwell LJ: Congenital and acquired disturbances of breast development and growth. In Bland KI, Copeland EM III, eds: The Breast: Comprehensive Management of Benign and Malignant Disorders, 3rd ed. Philadelphia, Elsevier, 2004:217.)

in the axilla) demonstrated no differences in survival between wide local excision and modified radical mastectomy.[154] In the age of selective sentinel lymphadenectomy, this uncertainty may lessen as lymphoscintigraphy combined with selective sentinel lymphadenectomy can identify sentinel lymph nodal metastasis even in atypical basins, improving staging and treatment recommendations.[155]

SUMMARY

Supernumerary nipples and breasts are relatively common congenital anomalies with a generally benign course. Accessory breast tissues are subject to the diseases that affect the normal breast and must be treated accordingly. Furthermore, evidence exists that links polythelia and polymastia with other congenital anomalies and malignant neoplasms, particularly of the urogenital system.

Anomalous Breast Development

The tuberous breast deformity was first described by Rees and Aston[156] in 1976 and was named for its similarity to a tuber root. Subsequently, there has been some confusion in the literature with the introduction of several other named syndromes, including "snoopy breast," "tubular breast," "herniated areolar complex," "lower-pole hypoplasia," and "narrow-based breast," all of which are similar to or incorrectly equated with tuberous breast disorder.[156-162] All of these variations in anomalous breast development have common characteristics but are incorrectly equated with tuberous breast as originally described. As a result of the variations of the anomalies in breast development, the diagnostic criteria for tuberous breast in many publications have been extended to include all of the deformities observed in breast shape. Asymmetry of the breast is common; as many as 88% of women presenting for augmentation mammaplasty have some degree of asymmetry, and 29% have base constriction.[163] The patient who presents with tuberous breast syndrome as originally noted to have herniated breast tissue through the areola and constricted base must be identified.

TUBEROUS BREAST

The tuberous breast is a developmental disorder of the breast in which the fundamental anatomic feature is a herniation of breast tissue through a constricting fascial ring beneath the areola.[164] A narrow mammary base, elevation of the inframammary fold, and relative hypoplasia of one or more quadrants are also variable features of the disorder.[157,165] The tuberous breast can be distinguished from the *tubular* breast. Both can have breast base constriction, but only the tuberous breast has herniation of breast tissue through the areola, causing its enlargement (Figs. 134-47 and 134-48).[164]

Incidence

Tuberous breast is a rare disorder, and there have been no adequate estimations of its incidence or prevalence.[166] It is generally sporadic with little risk of occurrence in relatives.[167]

Etiology

The proposed cause of the tuberous breast is the presence of a ring of fascia that constricts the radial outgrowth of the breast tissue in one or more directions, causing herniation of breast tissue through

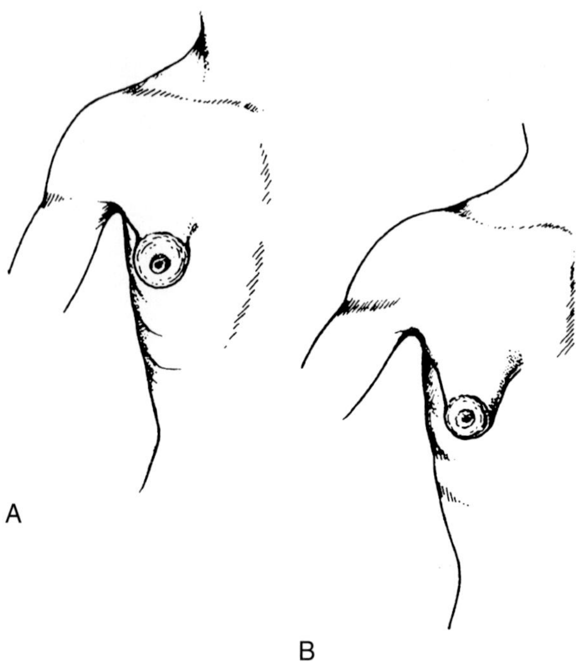

FIGURE 134-47. *A,* Tuberous breast. Base diameters are reduced both vertically and horizontally, and mega-areola is evident. *B,* Tubular breast. Only the vertical diameter is reduced, and no mega-areola is present. (From Panettiere P, Del Gaudio GA, Marchetti L, et al: The tuberous breast syndrome. Aesthetic Plast Surg 2000;24:445.)

the natural hiatus in the outer layer of the superficial fascia just posterior to the nipple-areola complex (Fig. 134-49).[166,168]

It has been proposed that this constricting ring is a thickened ring of the superficial fascia (most commonly, growth is restricted inferiorly, with a short and high inframammary line causing a tuberous appearance with ptosis). In many instances, but not all, the mammary tissue herniates through the hiatus in the fascia located directly deep to the areola.[165] The tuberous deformity ranges from a small tissue deficiency of the lower medial quadrant to constriction in 360 degrees with all existing breast tissue herniated through the areolar fascial hiatus.[168] There is little information on the underlying cause of the ring. No genetic mutation or noxious stimulus during gestation has been attributed to the development of tuberous breasts.[166]

Presentation and Diagnosis

Tuberous breast disorder characteristically does not present until at least 12 or 13 years of age; referral for surgical care typically occurs in the mid teens or earlier. The patient's complaint is an aesthetic one, but the psychological ramifications can be severe.[169] Often, the patient initially seeks augmentation mammaplasty and then discovers the existence of her deformity.[170] Approximately 89% (73% to 100%) of patients have bilateral defects, and 70% of patients with bilateral defects have an asymmetry of more than 100 g.[157,166,168,171,172] Although hypoplasia of one or more quadrants is a prominent feature of the disorder, only 27% of tuberous breasts are deficient in overall volume; 28% are reported to be hypertrophic.[157]

Classification

Several classification schemes for tuberous breast have been proposed. The system described by von Heimburg[165] and subsequently modified has become the most commonly used.[157]

The von Heimburg classification is divided into four categories (Table 134-12) based on the degree of hypoplasia and the size of the skin envelope. It has been argued that von Heimburg's type II and type III breasts are really the same because the amount of skin envelope is simply dependent on the size of the glandular tissue itself.[157,170]

The degrees of the disorder have been reduced to three classes solely based on the degree of hypoplasia of the base of the breast (Fig. 134-50). Type I is the least severe and is characterized by hypoplasia of the lower medial quadrant; type II breasts are hypoplastic in both lower quadrants, and the areola points downward; type III breasts have hypoplasia in all four quadrants.[157] In a series of 37 patients, most breasts (54%) that were operated on were type I, and 81% of patients had at least one type I breast.

Operative Treatment

Anomalous breast development presents with variations in abnormal anatomy, resulting in multiple surgical techniques described for correction of the tuberous breast deformity. The tuberous breast with herniation of breast tissue through a constriction fascial

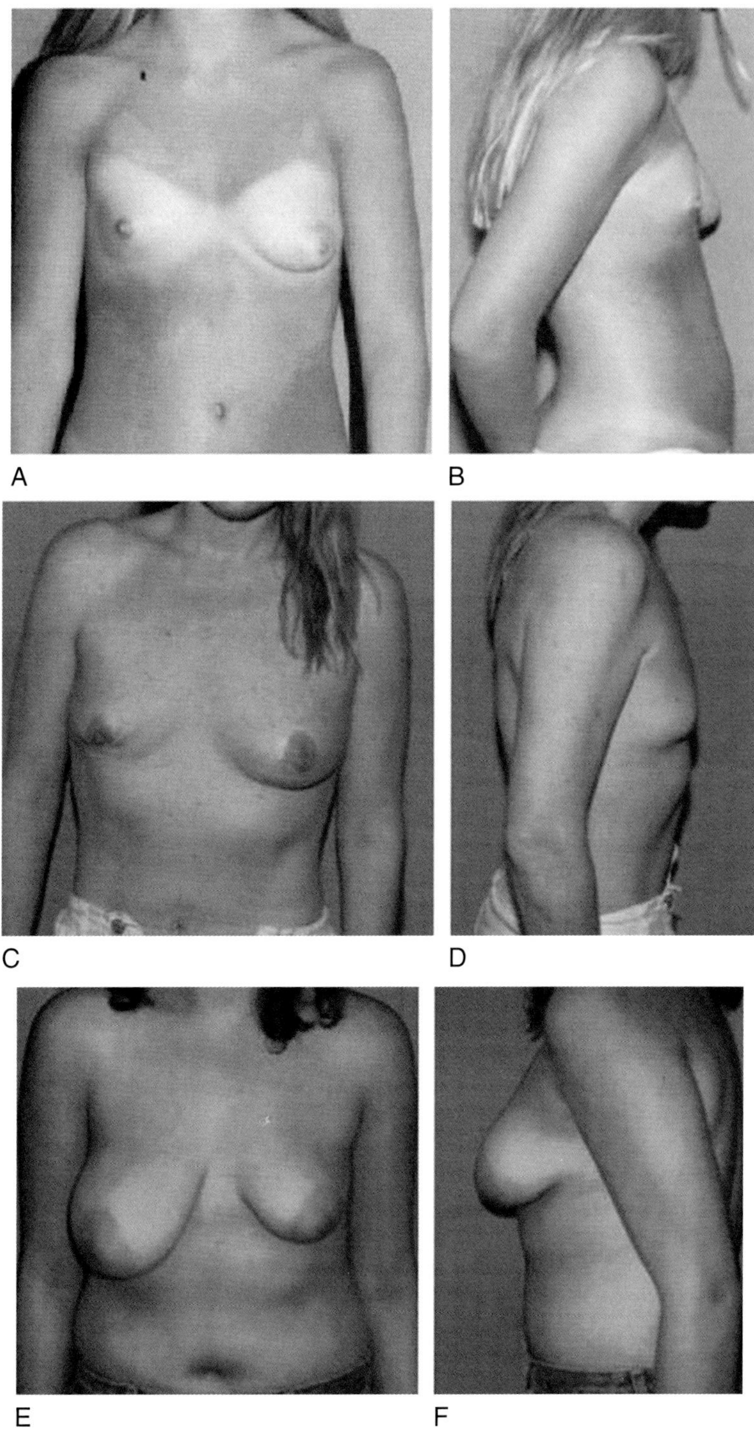

FIGURE 134-48. Breast developmental anomalies, constricted hypoplastic breast. *A,* Anterior view of asymmetry with right breast hypomastia and inframammary constriction; left breast, mild ptosis. *B,* Lateral view. *C,* Anterior view of asymmetry with constricted breast. *D,* Lateral view. Note malpositioned inframammary line. *E,* Anterior view, asymmetry with left constricted breast and right breast ptosis. *F,* Lateral view of constricted breast.

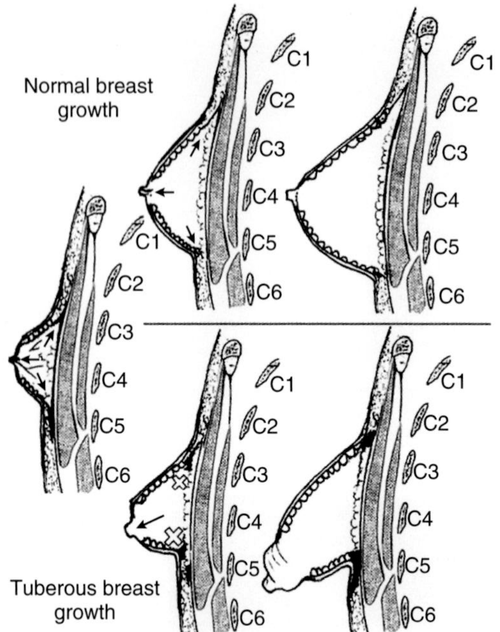

FIGURE 134-49. *Top,* Normal breast development with forward and peripheral expansion. *Bottom,* Development of a tuberous breast, with limited peripheral expansion and exaggerated forward expansion. (From Grolleau JL, Lanfrey E, Lavigne B, et al: Breast base anomalies: treatment strategy for tuberous breasts, minor deformities, and asymmetry. Plast Reconstr Surg 1999;104:2040.)

ring may be approached through a periareolar incision, allowing areola reduction and release of the constricting ring. Undermining of the periareola incision allows tissue rearrangement for correction of breast shape and inferior breast position.[157]

Because the anomalous breast development may also include a narrow base with superior displacement of the inframammary line, the inframammary approach is another effective way to release the constricting bands and adjust the inferior position of the breast. The use of a tissue expander is also helpful in correction of the skin envelope deficiency in the inferior breast mound. Correction of volume deficiency

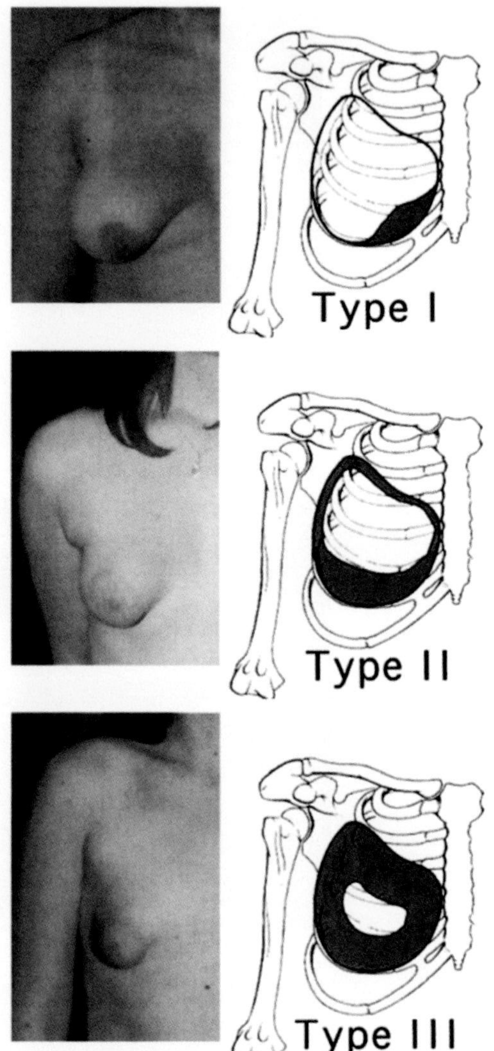

FIGURE 134-50. Classification system for breast base anomalies. Type I breasts have hypoplasia of the lower medial quadrant. Type II breasts have hypoplasia of both lower quadrants. Type III breasts have hypoplasia of all four quadrants. (From Grolleau JL, Lanfrey E, Lavigne B, et al: Breast base anomalies: treatment strategy for tuberous breasts, minor deformities, and asymmetry. Plast Reconstr Surg 1999;104:2040.)

TABLE 134-12 ✦ VON HEIMBURG'S TUBEROUS BREAST CLASSIFICATION

Class	Anatomic Features
von Heimburg class I	Hypoplasia of lower medial quadrant
von Heimburg class II	Hypoplasia of both lower quadrants with adequate areolar skin
von Heimburg class III	Hypoplasia of both lower quadrants with limited areolar skin
von Heimburg class IV	Hypoplasia of all quadrants

From von Heimburg D, et al: The tuberous breast deformity: classification and treatment. Br J Plast Surg 1996;49:339-345.
Reprinted with permission from The British Association of Plastic Surgeons.

may be accomplished with rearrangement of breast parenchyma with internal breast flaps, a permanent implant, or a combination of techniques. Technique selection must consider the anatomic variations in the anomalous breast development to achieve an adequate correction of the deformity.

MAILLARD Z-PLASTY. The inferior Z-plasty introduced by Maillard[173] in 1986 for reduction mammaplasty has been adapted for the tuberous breast. The Z-plasty technique primarily adds tissue to the inferior pole of the breast, where type I and type II deformities are hypoplastic. A circumareolar and a triangular infra-areolar de-epithelialization is performed (Fig. 134-51*A* and *B*). The inferior portion of the breast is extensively mobilized in the subcutaneous plane, and dissection is extended inferiorly to the inframammary fold, which can be adjusted at this time. Dissection in extended around the lower edge of the breast tissue to the posterior surface of the breast. The areola is moved superiorly, and the inferior portion of the breast is reshaped by overlapping the elevated inferior skin flaps in the fashion of a Z-plasty (Fig. 134-51*G*).[173]

SUPERIOR PEDICLE MAMMAPLASTY WITH A LATERAL DERMOGLANDULAR FLAP. The superior pedicle mammaplasty with a lateral dermoglandular flap technique recontours the breast by elevating the nipple-areola complex and provides contour to the lower pole (and the deficient lower medial quadrant in particular) with a laterally based flap. After a keyhole incision and de-epithelialization (including the excess areola), the breast is mobilized laterally from the anterior chest wall. A lateral triangular dermoglandular flap is preserved. The breast is mobilized medially in the same plane, and the flap is then transposed to the medial breast, deep to the existing breast tissue, augmenting the hypoplastic area. The flap is secured to the deep fascia, resulting in an L-shaped scar (Fig. 134-52). When the tissue is inadequate to compensate for the medial deficiency, as in a type II or type III breast, the scar takes on the shape of an S and is less aesthetically pleasing.[156] Consequently, data from Grolleau et al[157] suggest that this technique is ideal for type I deformities.

RIBEIRO TECHNIQUE. Ribeiro's technique[174] is a circumareolar method combined with an inferior pedicle to allow shaping of the inferior pole of the tuberous breast (Fig. 134-53*A* to *H*). After the induction of general anesthesia, the patient is placed in a semisitting position. The breast is marked with the outline of the desired areola, and the remaining extra areola is de-epithelialized. An inferior flap is made by dividing the lower pole of the breast from the upper pole and nipple-areola complex. This disrupts the constricting fascial ring. The flap is mobilized medially and laterally while the intercostal perforating vessels are preserved. The medial and lateral projections are divided, further disrupting the fascial constriction. The inferior flap is then folded over itself to give inferior pole projection and a normal appearance (Fig. 134-53*I* and *J*).[174] Other modifications of this technique have been described, including one by Mandrekas et al[168]; rather than division of the lateral and medial projections, the inferior flap is divided in the middle and then folded over to enhance the inferior projection. Mandrekas et al[168] reported correction of the deformity and satisfaction of patients with this method in 11 of 11 patients with primarily bilateral type II deformities. Complete symmetry was achieved in 9 of the 11 patients, all 9 of whom had type II deformities. Symmetry was made no worse in the remaining two patients, each of whom had mispaired deformities (types III/II and types I/II).

Ribeiro reported that this technique is optimal for the reconstruction of small breasts and typically never used implants for augmentation. This observation has been confirmed to be true for type II and type III tuberous breasts by Grolleau et al[157] in a small, highly selective series. Choupina et al[166] have reported the successful use of this technique combined with implant placement for type III breasts.

IMPLANT RECONSTRUCTION. The use of implants in treatment of the tuberous breast is common. Implants are used for hypoplastic breasts, to balance significant asymmetry with the contralateral breast, and when a larger breast size is desired. Breast implants, however, will not always correct the parenchyma tissue imbalance and the skin envelope deficiency in the inferior breast mound. It has been observed that the placement of an implant behind the breast parenchyma as sole treatment may accentuate the appearance of the deformity.[175] It has been noted that for type II tuberous breasts, placement of an implant generates the appearance of a second inframammary fold. However, with correction of the inframammary line position and release of the constricting ring and shortened ligaments, implants may be used simultaneously with a satisfactory result (Fig. 134-54). If symmetry is not satisfactory in the operating room, insertion of a tissue expander is recommended.

Puckett Technique. In patients with a moderate to severe tuberous breast deformity, breast hypoplasia is often present. If a patient desires reconstruction with an implant, the technique described by Puckett[162] may be used. The initial steps are similar to the Ribeiro technique, including de-epithelialization and inferior dissection. The breast is then dissected from the chest wall in a superior direction. After half of the breast has been mobilized, an inferior breast flap based from just deep to the nipple-areola complex is elevated (Fig.

Text continued on p. 522

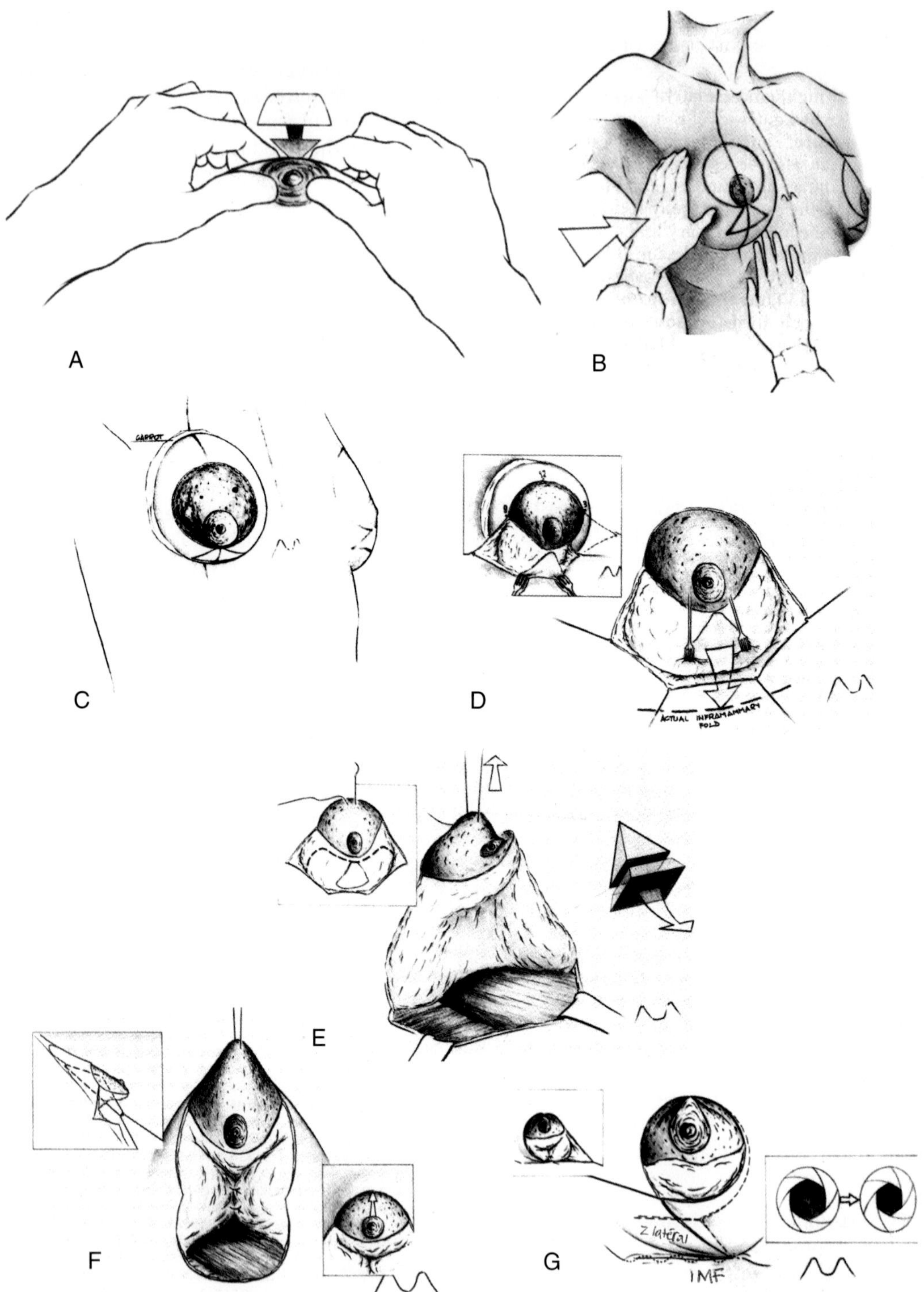
A
B
C
D
ACTUAL INFRAMAMMARY FOLD
E
F
G
Z lateral
IMF

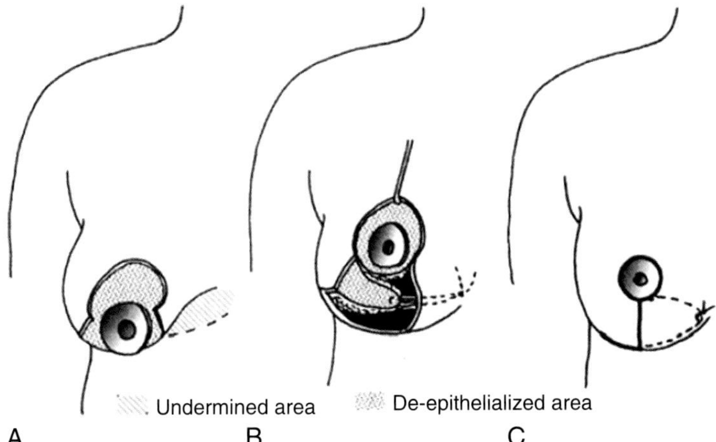

FIGURE 134-52. Superior pedicle mammaplasty with a lateral dermoglandular flap for tuberous breast. *A,* Incisions and areas of de-epithelialization. *B,* Design of lateral-based dermoglandular flap. *C,* Closure. Note dermoglandular flap with corrected medial lower quadrant contour defect. (From Grolleau JL, Lanfrey E, Lavigne B, et al: Breast base anomalies: treatment strategy for tuberous breasts, minor deformities, and asymmetry. Plast Reconstr Surg 1999;104:2040.)

FIGURE 134-51. The Maillard Z-plasty, preoperative markings. *A,* Periareolar de-epithelialization in the vertical axis is estimated by pinching the skin. *B,* Preoperative markings illustrate the planned incisions and areas for de-epithelialization. *C,* A tourniquet is applied to the base of the breast to facilitate the de-epithelialization. *D,* A wide subcutaneous dissection is performed at the deepest level of the ligaments of Cooper as far as the 3- and 9-o'clock positions. By pulling upward on two clamps fixed to the isosceles triangle, the dissection is extended to the inframammary fold, which is widely undermined. Beginning with an initial purely subcutaneous approach, the retromammary space is finally completely dissected. *E,* Glandular resection is carried out at the base of the mammary cone, converting the large pyramid into a small one. *F,* Placement of a single suture between the gland just above the areola and pectoralis fascia in the infraclavicular region produces a fullness in the upper quadrant. *G,* After elevation of the nipple-areola complex, the elevated skin flaps are interlocked as a standard Z-plasty. First, the lateral triangle is sutured into the new inframammary fold, followed by the medial flap, which is gently advanced and rotated to diminish the tension around the areola (like the diaphragm of a camera). (From Maillard GF: A Z-mammaplasty with minimal scarring. Plast Reconstr Surg 1986;77:66.)

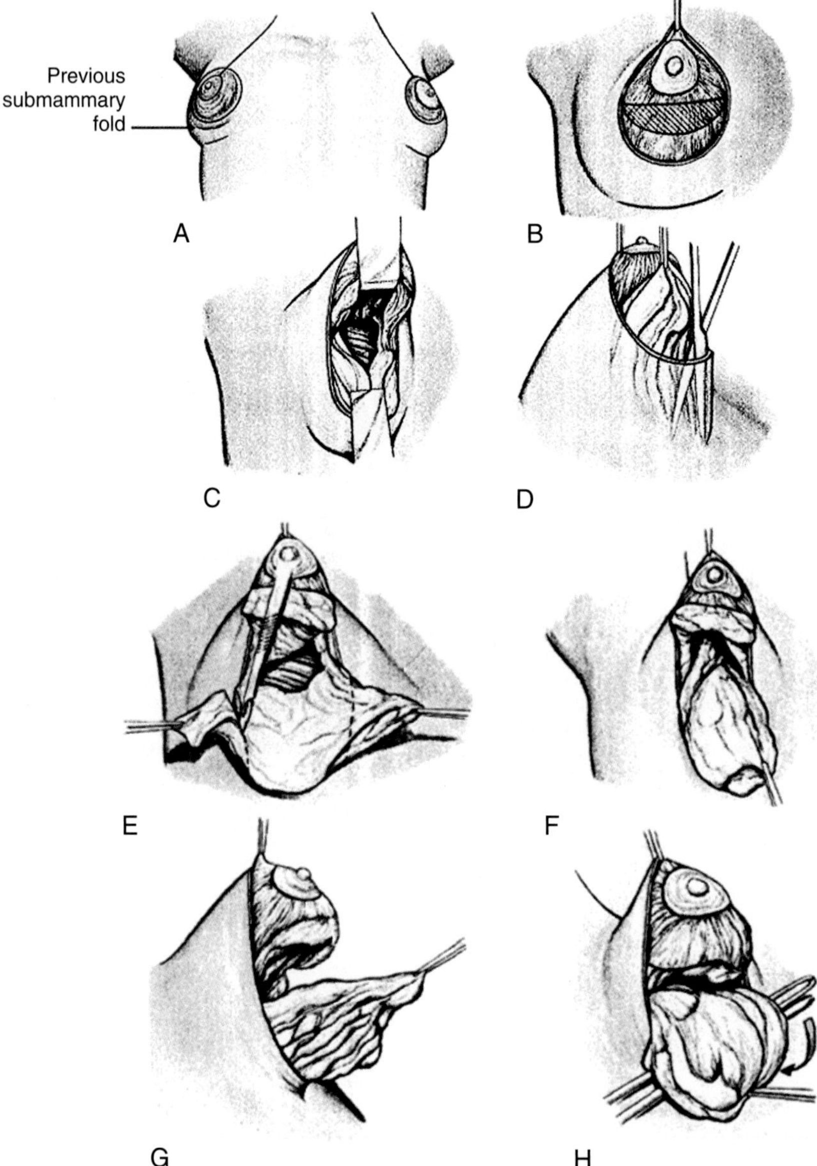

FIGURE 134-53. *A,* Preoperative markings with areas of de-epithelialization. *B,* Division of inferior breast tissue into superior pedicle with nipple-areola and inferior breast contour correction. *C,* Dissection to pectoralis major muscle. *D,* Subcutaneous dissection to new inframammary line. *E,* Division of lateral and medial edges of inferior flap. *F,* Completion of inferior pedicle elevation. *G,* Flap is ready for inset. *H,* Completion of inferior pedicle elevation.

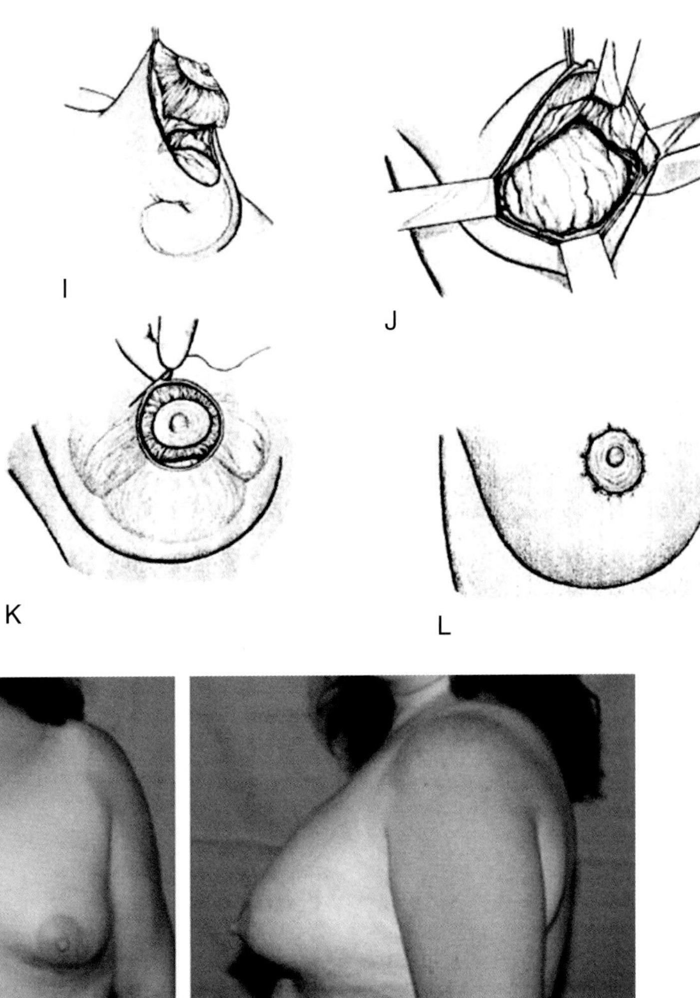

FIGURE 134-53, cont'd. *I,* Folding of inferior pedicle for autoaugmentation of inferior quadrants of tubular breast. *J,* Flap inset into pectoralis major fascia. *K,* Pursestring suture around nipple-areola. *L,* Interrupted areola-cutaneous sutures. (From Ribeiro L, Canzi W, Buss A, Accorsi A Jr: Tuberous breast: a new approach. Plast Reconstr Surg 1998;101:42.)

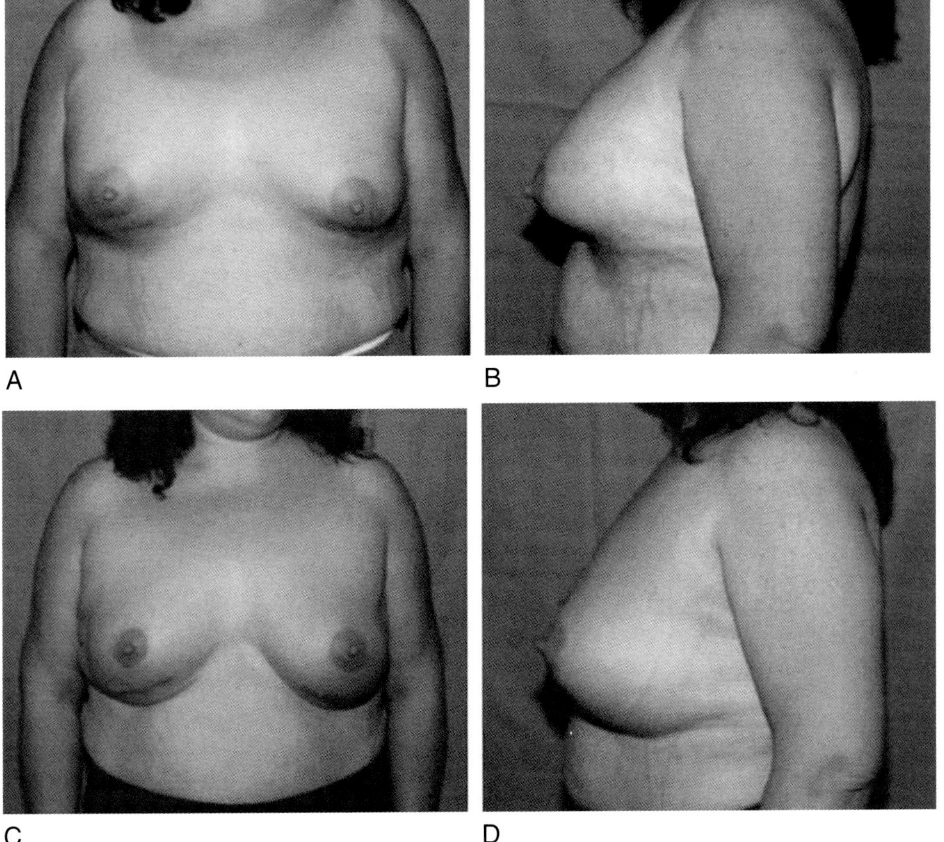

FIGURE 134-54. Breast asymmetry with constricted breast, correction with constricting band release and implants. *A,* Anterior view of breast asymmetry and left constricted breast (type II). *B,* Lateral view. Note constricted and elevated left inframammary line. *C,* Anterior postoperative view 1 year after bilateral breast augmentation and release of constriction of left inframammary region. *D,* Lateral view.

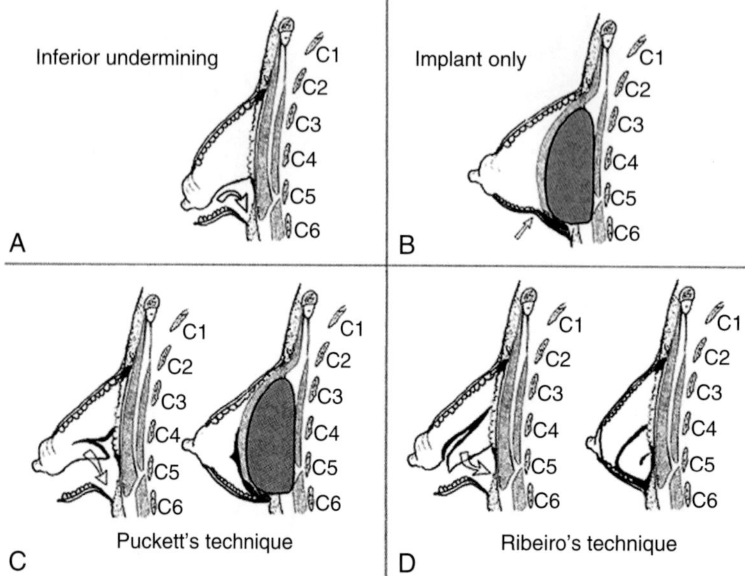

FIGURE 134-55. Reconstruction of breast hypoplasia (types II and III) and constriction of inferior breast quadrants. *A,* Inferior undermining of site of constriction. *B,* Implant-alone correction of inferior quadrant hypomastia and constriction bands. Note possible contour irregularity at prior abnormal inframammary line. *C,* Puckett and Concannon's technique using superiorly based parenchymal flap for inferior quadrant contour correction. *D,* Ribeiro's technique using inferior pedicle for inferior quadrant contour correction. (From Grolleau JL, Lanfrey E, Lavigne B, et al: Breast base anomalies: treatment strategy for tuberous breasts, minor deformities, and asymmetry. Plast Reconstr Surg 1999;104:2040.)

134-55). A submuscular implant is placed and the breast is unfurled inferiorly over the implant, transferring tissue bulk to the inferior pole.

Tissue Expansion. Tissue expansion has been reported as a means of augmenting the hypoplastic tuberous breast, but it will also expand the deficient skin envelope and the abnormal fascial band after release of the fascial constricting ring. Scheepers and Quaba[176] described four patients in whom tissue expansion during 2 to 3 months was used to successfully repair type II and type III breasts in which there was an inframammary skin deficiency with an elevated inframammary fold. However, many investigators do not agree with the theory that a relative skin deficiency is associated with an elevated inframammary crease but instead believe that inhibition of inferior radial growth causes an apparent elevation of the inframammary fold without true skin deficiency.[168] Tissue expansion does mitigate the "double bubble" characteristic of repairs using only an implant but may not completely correct the crease at the former abnormal inframammary line, especially if the release of the fascial bands is not accomplished at the time of the expander insertion (Fig. 134-56). The use of tissue expanders early in breast development with expansion to maintain symmetry with a larger contralateral breast may be useful in patients with unilateral tuberous breast if tissue rearrangement is planned at the time of the permanent implant placement and if the diagnosis is clear at an early stage (Figs. 134-57 and 134-58).

Expander-Implant with Release of Constricting Fascia. With an inframammary incision, it is possible to release the constricting fascial ring and to re-establish the appropriate location of the inframammary line with inferior dissection. An expander is then inserted, with the superior portion of the expander in a subpectoral position and the inferior fibers of the pectoralis major released from the sternum between the fourth and sixth intercostal space and along the sixth intercostal space. The expander is located with the inferior shell at the new inframammary line. The expander is partially inflated to confirm release of all constricting bands. The expander is inflated during the next 3 to 6 months. If the opposite breast is still developing, the expander can be left in place until the opposite breast is fully developed. At the second stage, the inframammary incision is used to replace the expander with a permanent implant. If the areola is too large, the areola is reduced to match the contralateral side. Also, if the opposite breast has congenital ptosis, a mastopexy is performed simultaneously (Fig. 134-59).

Summary

Despite the relative paucity of outcomes data for surgical correction of the tuberous breast, several generalizations can be made (Table 134-13). The presence of a tuberous deformity does not always imply an overall hypoplasia of the breast. The use of an implant with or without tissue expansion requires release of constricting bands and additional tissue rearrangement depending on extent of the deformity. Finally, selection of the technique of reconstruction should be based on degree of severity of the disorder.

CONGENITAL ABSENCE OF THE BREAST

The absence of one or both breasts is an extremely rare disorder. It occurs either as an isolated deformity

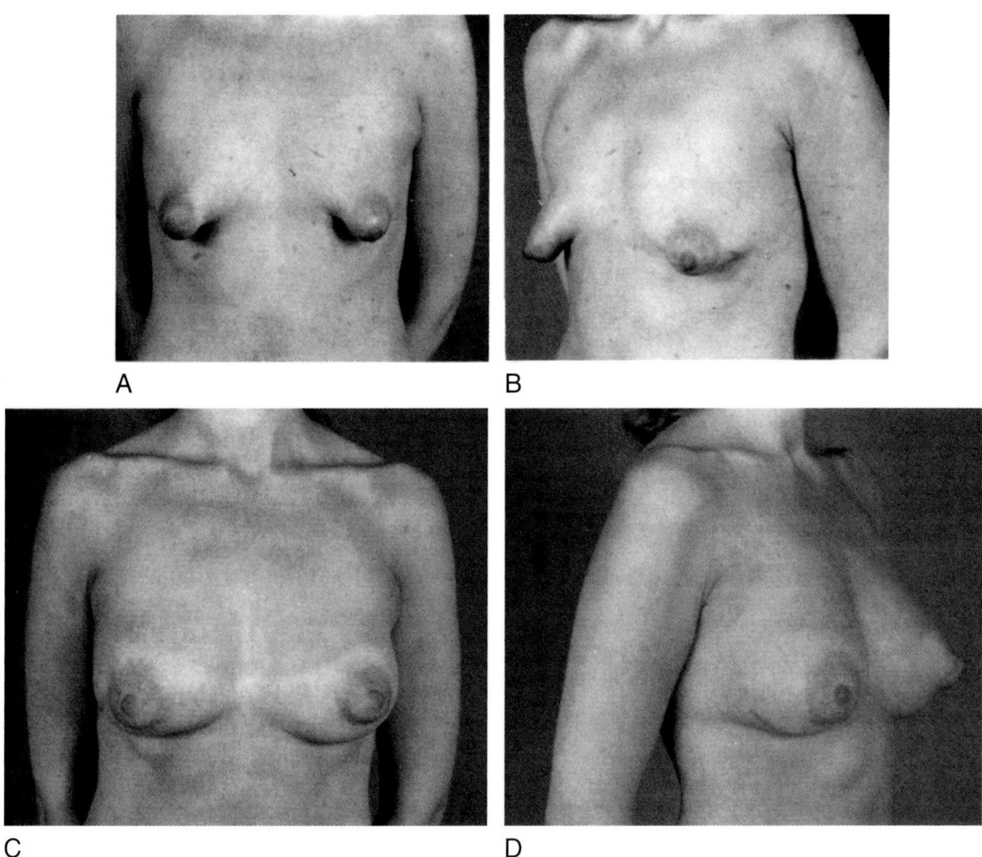

FIGURE 134-56. Reconstruction of the tuberous breast with release of constriction bands and expansion-implant sequence. *A,* Anterior view of tuberous breasts. *B,* Oblique view. *C,* Anterior postoperative view after reconstruction. *D,* Oblique view. (From Scheepers JH, Quaba AA: Tissue expansion in the treatment of tubular breast deformity. Br J Plast Surg 1992;45[7]:529.)

TABLE 134-13 ✦ SUGGESTED TECHNIQUES BASED ON TUBEROUS BREAST CLASSIFICATION

Tuberous Class	Recommended Techniques
Type I	Maillard Z-plasty Superior pedicle mammaplasty with lateral dermoglandular flap Release constricting bands with expander-implant
Type II	Ribeiro technique (if no need for augmentation) Puckett technique (if concurrent augmentation is desired) Release constricting bands with expander-implant
Type III	Puckett technique (if concurrent augmentation is desired) Ribeiro technique (if no need for augmentation) Release constricting bands with expander-implant

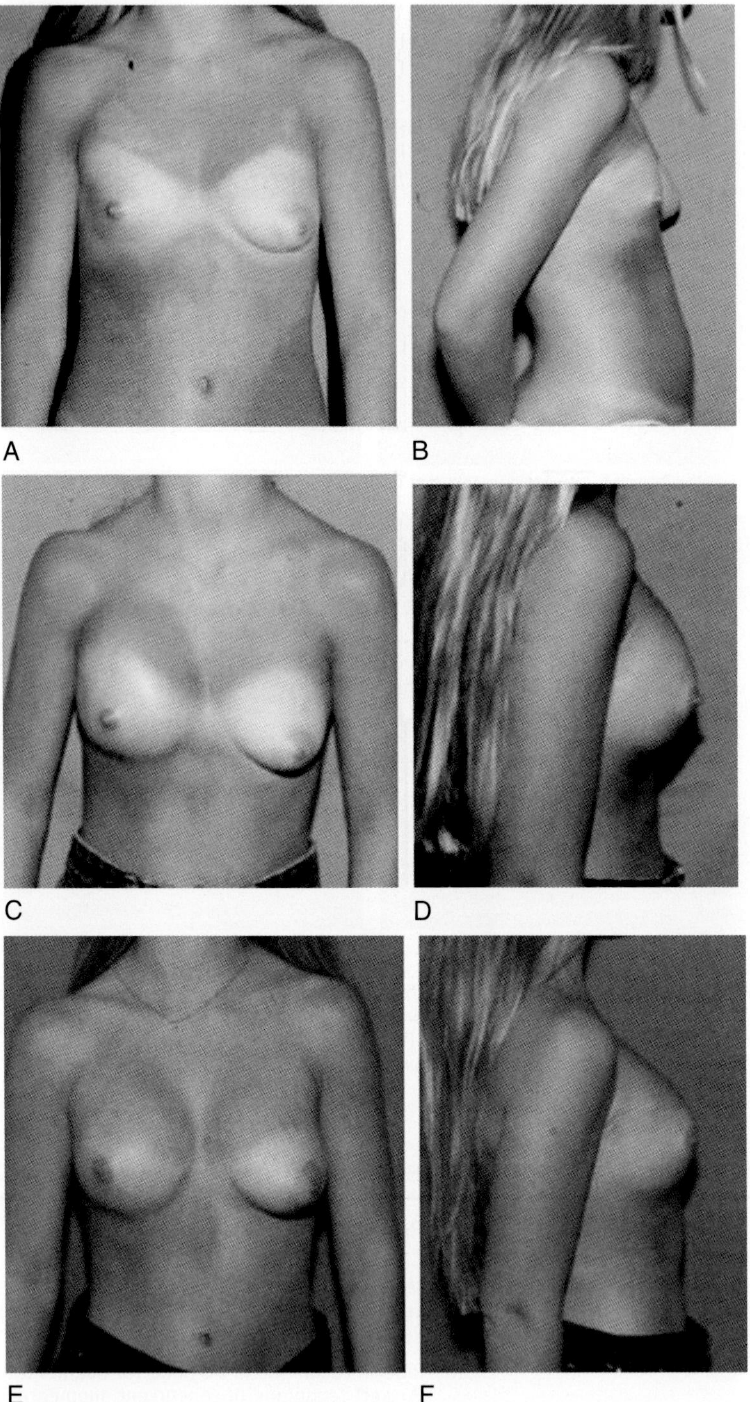

FIGURE 134-57. Reconstruction of congenital breast hypomastia with release of constriction of inframammary lower quadrants. *A,* Anterior view of constriction of right inframammary region with breast hypomastia. *B,* Lateral view. *C,* Anterior postoperative view 3 months after release of constricting bands and insertion of tissue expander. *D,* Lateral view. Note new inframammary line. *E,* Anterior postoperative view 1 year after expander-implant sequence. *F,* Lateral view. Note corrected position of inframammary line and normal distance between areola-cutaneous junction and inframammary line corrected by constriction release and expansion.

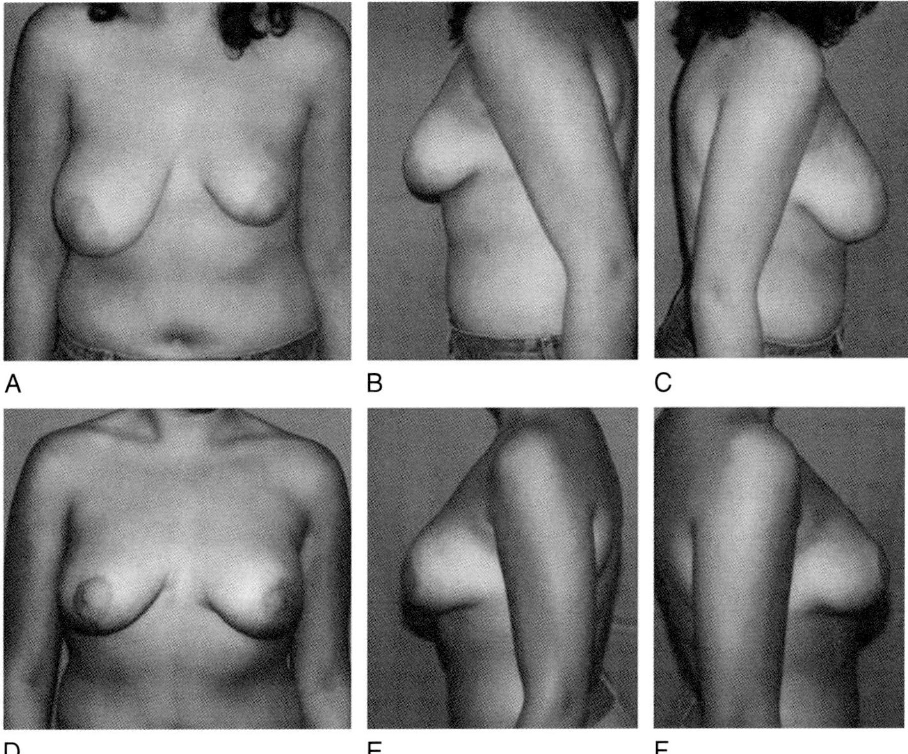

FIGURE 134-58. Reconstruction of breast asymmetry with constricted breast (type II) and ptosis with constricting band release and expander-implant sequence. *A,* Anterior view of left constricted breast and right breast ptosis. *B,* Lateral view of malpositioned inframammary line with constricted lower quadrants of breast. *C,* Lateral view of congenital breast ptosis. *D,* Anterior postoperative view 1 year after expander-implant sequence. *E,* Lateral view of repositioned inframammary line and expanded inferior quadrants of breast with subsequent implant insertion. *F,* Lateral view of postoperative mastopexy.

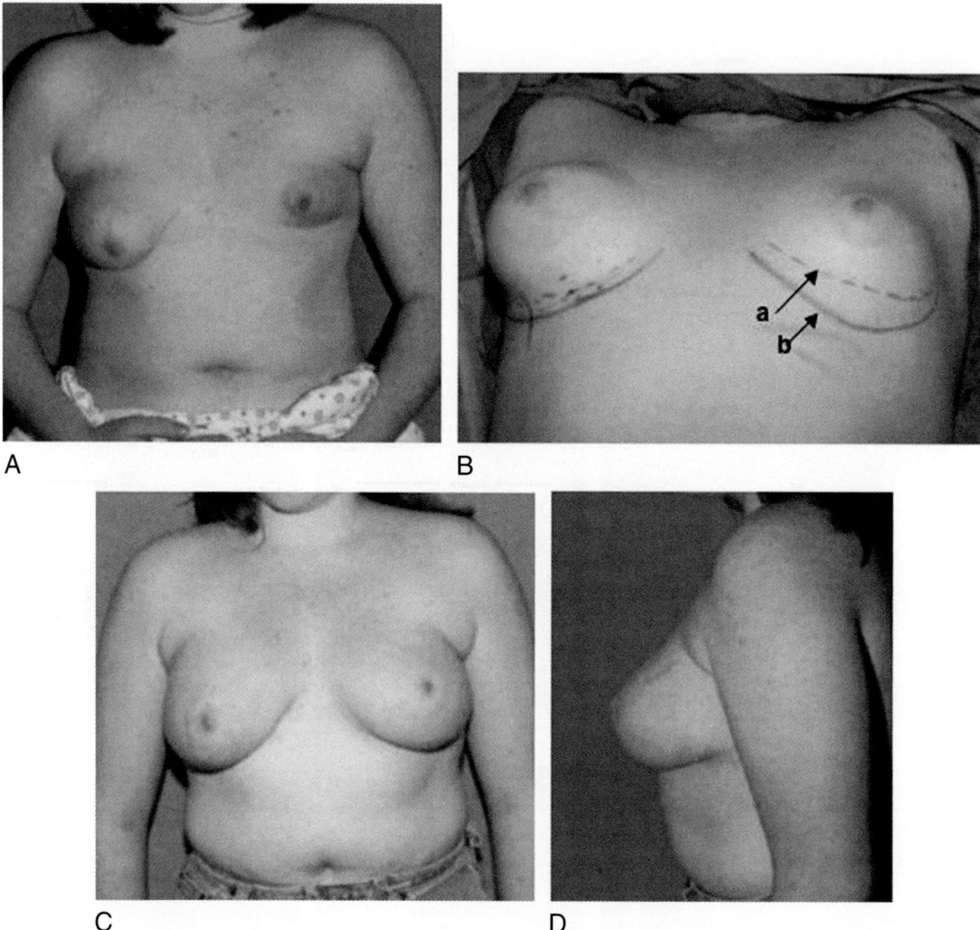

FIGURE 134-59. Reconstruction of bilateral breast asymmetry with bilateral hypomastia and constricted breasts with constricting band release and expander-implant sequence. *A,* Anterior view of left breast with hypomastia and lower quadrant constriction (type II) and right breast constricted inframammary line (type I). *B,* Intraoperative view; *a* denotes current abnormal inframammary line; *b* denotes planned new inframammary line after release of constricting bands. *C,* Anterior postoperative view 1 year after left breast expander-implant sequence and right breast augmentation. *D,* Lateral view demonstrates corrected inframammary line and inferior areola-cutaneous-inframammary line distance.

or in conjunction with several developmental syndromes, including the Ullrich-Turner syndrome (agenesis of breast and left nipple, pectoralis major muscle, and hair follicles of the breast), the AREDYLD syndrome (bilateral amastia, ectodermal dysplasia, lipoatrophy, and diabetes mellitus), and the autosomal dominant syndrome of ureteral triplication-bilateral amastia, pectus excavatum, umbilical hernia, patent ductus arteriosus, low-set ears, palpebral ptosis, hypertelorism, cubitus valgus, and syndactyly.[177] Variations of these disorders have different degrees of athelia (absent nipple), amazia (absent mammary gland), and amastia (absent mammae).[178]

Isolated absence of the breast was first reported by Froriep[103] in 1839. If unilateral, it is most likely to occur in patients with the diagnosis of Poland syndrome, but other variants have been reported. Bilateral absence is rare, although 16 patients were described in 1965, 62.5% of whom had no other identifiable anomaly.[179]

Familial inheritance in either an autosomal dominant or undefined mendelian pattern, affecting both sexes, was also observed in both isolated and syndromic bilateral absences.[130,179] No genetic locus has been identified for nonsyndromic (isolated, familial or otherwise) absences of the breasts. Sporadic reports of possible teratogens exist in the literature, but no definitive data exist.[180]

Construction of breasts for isolated congenital absence is not well documented in the literature. Techniques using either autologous tissue (e.g., transverse rectus abdominis myocutaneous [TRAM] flap, latissimus dorsi flap; see Chapter 138) or expansion and subsequent implant placement are reasonable options. Lin et al[178] reported on reconstruction of a patient by use of a TRAM flap with excellent results.

GYNECOMASTIA

Gynecomastia ("woman breast") is the development of breast tissue in men. It possesses a complex physiology with both congenital and acquired features.

Incidence

Gynecomastia has a relatively high incidence of 32% to 40%.[181-183] Studies have shown the incidence to be as high as 65% in adolescents.[184] Gynecomastia is bilateral in 25% to 75% of patients.[185,186]

Etiology

The traditional view of the cause of gynecomastia is that abnormal male breast development stems from elevated estrogen levels (absolute or relative), decreased androgen levels, or insensitivity to androgens, possibly due to receptor insensitivity. The mechanisms causing gynecomastia can be divided into two classes, congenital and acquired. The varied causes of gynecomastia are numerous and beyond the scope of this discussion. Despite the advances in understanding the mechanisms causing gynecomastia, idiopathic causes remain the most frequent diagnosis (25%).[185]

Congenital causes of gynecomastia can be further classified as physiologic or pathologic. Physiologic congenital gynecomastia occurs in the neonatal, adolescent, or elderly phases of life. Exposure to high maternal estrogen concentrations in utero leads to the development of breast tissue in neonates. This process resolves within a few weeks of birth as the estrogen levels return to normal.[187] During puberty, the estradiol-to-testosterone ratio is elevated in some boys, leading to gynecomastia in up to 65% of patients. The clinical syndrome can be subtle and may go unnoticed unless it is detected by physical examination. Most instances resolve by the end of puberty.[185] In the elderly, peripheral conversion of testosterone to estrogen by aromatase remains intact in the peripheral fat even as systemic production declines, causing elevation of the estrogen-to-testosterone ratio and inducing breast development.[185]

Pathologic congenital gynecomastia is caused by genetic or embryologic disorders that exhibit as either hypogonadism or hyperestrogenism (Table 134-14). Klinefelter syndrome (karyotype 47 XXY) requires special mention. Unlike in studies of gynecomastia in general, in which no additional risk of breast cancer has been observed, patients with Klinefelter syndrome have been estimated to have up to a 60-fold increased risk of breast cancer. Whereas male breast cancer accounts for only approximately 1% of breast cancer patients, the incidence of breast cancer in patients with Klinefelter syndrome has been estimated between 1 in 400 and 1 in 1000.[188] Evaluation of patients with Klinefelter syndrome must have an adequate consideration of their elevated breast cancer risk.

Acquired gynecomastia can be subdivided into pathologic and pharmacologic causes. Pathologic causes can be primarily endocrine, metabolic, or neoplastic (Table 134-15).[189] Gynecomastia is caused by numerous drugs that directly or indirectly alter estrogen or testosterone concentrations (Table 134-16).

TABLE 134-14 ✦ CONGENITAL GYNECOMASTIA: SELECTED CAUSES

Physiologic	
Neonatal	
Pubertal	
Senile	
Pathologic	
Hypogonadal	Androgen resistance Enzymatic defect of testosterone synthesis Congenital anorchism Klinefelter syndrome
Hyperestrogenic	True hermaphroditism Congenital adrenal hyperplasia Elevated peripheral aromatase

TABLE 134-15 ✦ ACQUIRED GYNECOMASTIA: SELECTED CAUSES

Metabolic	Renal failure Hepatic failure Starvation Alcoholism
Endocrine	Acquired hypogonadism Thyrotoxicosis Pituitary failure
Neoplastic	Adrenal tumors Testicular tumors HCG-producing tumors Bronchogenic carcinoma Pituitary tumors
Miscellaneous	Chest wall trauma Spinal cord injury Psychological stress HIV infection Herpes zoster infection
Drug induced	
Idiopathic	

HCG, human chorionic gonadotropin; HIV, human immunodeficiency virus.

From Glass AR: Gynecomastia. Endocrinol Metab Clin North Am 1994;23:825.

TABLE 134-16 ✦ DRUG-INDUCED GYNECOMASTIA

Drug classes associated with gynecomastia

Estrogens
Gonadotropins
Androgens (aromatizable)
Antiandrogens (cyproterone, flutamide)
Cancer chemotherapy agents (especially alkylating agents)
Calcium channel blockers (verapamil, nifedipine, diltiazem)
Angiotensin-converting enzyme inhibitors (captopril, enalapril)
Antihypertensives (methyldopa, reserpine)
Digitalis preparations
Dopamine blockers (phenothiazines, metoclopramide, domperidone)
Central nervous system agents (tricyclics, diazepam, phenytoin, diethylpropion)
Drugs of abuse (marijuana, heroin, methadone, amphetamines)
Antituberculous agents (isoniazid, ethionamide, thiacetazone)

Individual drugs commonly associated with gynecomastia

Cimetidine
Spironolactone
Ketoconazole

Miscellaneous drugs related to gynecomastia

Amiodarone
Auranofin
Clomiphene
Etretinate
Metronidazole
Omeprazole
Penicillamine
Sulindac
Theophylline

From Glass AR: Gynecomastia. Endocrinol Metab Clin North Am 1994;23:825.

Histologic Analysis

Three histologic patterns have been described in breast tissue explanted from men with gynecomastia: florid, intermediate, and fibrous. The florid pattern has increased cellularity in the stroma with budding ducts. Fibrous gynecomastia has little or no ductal proliferation but dense fibrosis in the stroma. The intermediate class has features of both.[185] No increased frequency of breast cancer has been observed except in Klinefelter syndrome.[185] A progression from florid to fibrous generally takes place during 1 year.[190]

Presentation and Diagnosis

Gynecomastia generally presents as an aesthetic complaint. A careful history and physical examination are mandatory, with special attention directed toward the endocrine system, genital system, and signs of malignant neoplasia. Drug use, both prescribed and illegal, should be reviewed. If hypogonadism is suspected, karyotype analysis should be performed to test for Klinefelter syndrome because treatment may be different. Biopsy should be performed for unilateral gynecomastia in the context of Klinefelter syndrome. Further diagnostic action needs to be taken only if the history or physical examination suggests an underlying pathologic cause.

Examination of the breasts should be detailed and needs to exclude nodules or discharge. The presence of a nodule requires evaluation. An enlargement of 0.5 cm has been used as a standard for diagnosis.[191] Standard parameters of the male breast and nipple-areola complex have been reported and can be used as a reference for comparison. The average diameter of the nipple-areola complex is 2.8 cm, and it lies approximately 20 cm from the sternal notch.[192] The length of time that the gynecomastia has been present should also be evaluated because beyond 12 months, the breast usually becomes irreversibly fibrotic.[189]

Simon[193] proposed a classification system as an aid to directing therapy in 1973. The classification is divided on the basis of size into three overall grades, which are further subdivided by the presence or absence of skin excess (Table 134-17).

Although gynecomastia presenting to the general practitioner, pediatrician, or even pediatric endocrinologist—particularly in the adolescent—might not routinely provoke routine laboratory testing, the clinical spectrum of disease presenting to the surgeon potentially is significantly different.[194] The primary reason for this is that the self-limited causes have generally been excluded (i.e., the offending drug has been removed or puberty has ended). In a cohort study evaluating the risk of malignant transformation with gynecomastia in 446 men, each of whom had received an operation for the treatment of gynecomastia, there was no overall increase in the incidence of malignant tumors. However, there was a significant increase in risk for testicular tumors (standardized incidence ratio [SIR] = 5.8; 95% confidence interval, 1.2-17.0) and nonmelanoma skin cancer (SIR = 3.2; 95% confidence

TABLE 134-17 ✦ SIMON CLASSIFICATION OF GYNECOMASTIA

Grade	Enlargement	Skin Excess
I	Small	Absent
IIA	Moderate	Absent
IIB	Moderate	Present
III	Large	Present

interval, 1.7-5.5). There may also be a predilection for unilateral gynecomastia.[194]

Subgroup analysis suggested that the increased incidence for testicular cancer was primarily in those younger than 50 years at the time of diagnosis (for those younger than 50 years, SIR = 6.7; for those 50 years and older, SIR = 0.0).[194] This has been confirmed in an additional retrospective study of 175 men presenting to a breast surgery clinic for breast enlargement, in which 4 of 127 men diagnosed with gynecomastia had testicular tumors at presentation.[195] Three of the four had a palpable testicular mass; all four had tumor visible on ultrasound examination. A fifth was diagnosed with a testicular tumor 9 months after evaluation for gynecomastia. Of these five patients, the mean age was 39.4 years (range, 31 to 61 years); two had an elevated alpha-fetoprotein concentration, and one had elevated β-human chorionic gonadotropin. Two other patients (without tumors) had an elevated alpha-fetoprotein concentration (false-positive), and five had elevated prolactin levels (one was ultimately diagnosed with a microadenoma of the pituitary).[195]

For nonmelanoma skin cancer, the increased incidence occurred in patients older than 50 years, regardless of the age at diagnosis, and at least 10 years after operation for gynecomastia (making skin cancer education at the time of diagnosis more important than screening).[194]

At the time of presentation to the surgeon, testicular examination is reasonable in all patients and should be considered mandatory in postpubertal men younger than 50 years. Routine screening for endocrine markers (alpha-fetoprotein, β-human chorionic gonadotropin) is more controversial because of the presence of false-positives; however, it is reasonable in the high-risk age group.[195] Abnormal laboratory results or a palpable testicular mass should be followed up with an ultrasound examination. For patients with small testicles but with other signs of more advanced puberty, karyotyping should be considered to rule out Klinefelter syndrome.[196] Adolescent boys with marked (>4 cm in diameter) gynecomastia should be referred to an endocrinologist; 12% have been reported to have a major endocrine disorder, and most if not all have other major medical problems.[197] Education about skin cancer prevention and detection should always be provided.

Treatment

The treatment of gynecomastia is in evolution. Originally, gynecomastia was treated exclusively by limited intra-areolar incision mastectomy, but the operative treatment options have progressed to include suction-assisted lipectomy (SAL) and ultrasound-assisted liposuction (UAL). These techniques have been used alone or in combination with standard excision. Further elucidation of the pathogenesis of gynecomastia has led to attempts at medical therapies, with limited success.

Nonoperative Treatment. Expectant management is appropriate in certain patients, particularly in neonatal and pubertal gynecomastia. Neonatal gynecomastia generally resolves in a matter of weeks; pubertal gynecomastia resolves within about 2 years as evidenced by a rate of 7.7% at the age of 17 years (compared with 65% at the peak of puberty).[191]

For many etiologies, treatment of the underlying cause may resolve the gynecomastia. This spontaneous resolution is particularly true of drug-induced gynecomastia. The caveat to this treatment plan is that most breasts progress to severe fibrosis, so that after 1 year, the only option is surgical. The exception is pubertal gynecomastia, which can resolve during 2 years or more.[190]

Operative Treatment. Surgical resection of gynecomastia remains the mainstay of treatment. Several options are available to the surgeon, including traditional excision and SAL or a combination of both. Traditional excision can be performed through three different incisions: semicircular at the inferior areola-cutaneous junction; transverse or hemitransverse areola, dividing the nipple-areola complex in half; and inframammary (for mastectomy) (Figs. 134-60 and 134-61). Initial considerations include the size of the breast, the presence of excess skin, and the degree of ptosis (if any). The classification scheme presented by Simon has worked well as an aid for deciding among treatment modalities.

Grade I breasts often have just a small protuberance of fibrous breast tissue below the areola. These can be treated by simple excision through a small periareolar or transverse incision. Colombo-Benkmann et al[198] treated 31 grade I breasts through the small periareolar incision with no recurrences or hypesthesias. Additional excess skin was present after resection in 7% of patients. Nipple retraction was present in 29% of patients; hence, care must be taken not to overresect the subareolar region.

SAL and UAL have been used in the treatment of grade I gynecomastia generally as an adjunct to excision (Figs. 134-62 and 134-63; see also Fig. 134-60*D*). Wiesman et al[199] reported 116 grade I breasts and used SAL in conjunction with excision in 27% and SAL alone in 3.5%. Approximately 10% of patients required revisions across all techniques. No patients required skin resection. Grade I breasts generally have a high amount of fibrous glandular tissue, making at least a partial excision necessary. UAL has been advocated as a method able to remove even dense fibrous tissue and to minimize complications and overresection. UAL has been used as the only modality of treatment in one series of 18 grade I breasts without need for

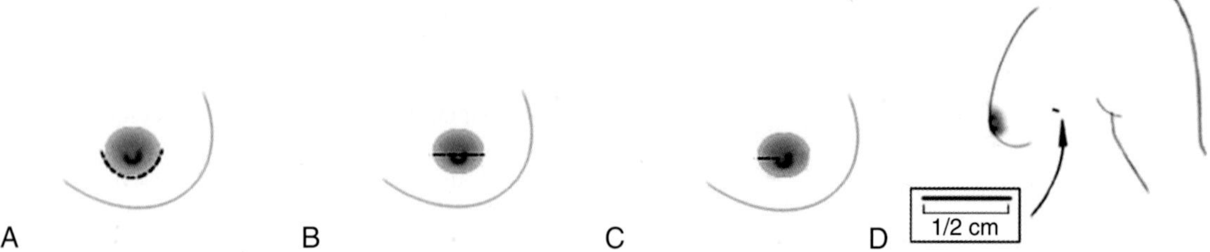

FIGURE 134-60. Gynecomastia incisions. *A,* Inferior semicircular areola incision. *B,* Transverse transareolar incision. *C,* Radial or hemitransverse areola incision. *D,* Lateral incision for suction-assisted lipectomy.

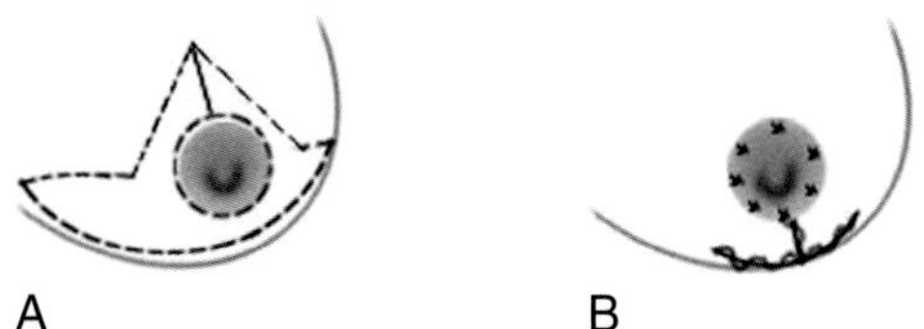

FIGURE 134-61. *A* and *B,* Illustration of incision for gynecomastia correction with skin and tissue resection and nipple-areola grafts.

reoperation.[187] However, photographs reveal residual gynecomastia, suggesting that UAL alone may not be adequate for fibrous tissue.[200]

Grade II breasts are larger than grade I breasts and are associated with a broader and often a fatter chest. On occasion, there is excess skin. Colombo-Benkmann et al[198] treated 67 grade II breasts with excision alone and were able to use a semicircular periareolar incision in most (94%) and extended the incision in 6%. They observed recurrences in 8%, hypesthesia in 25%,

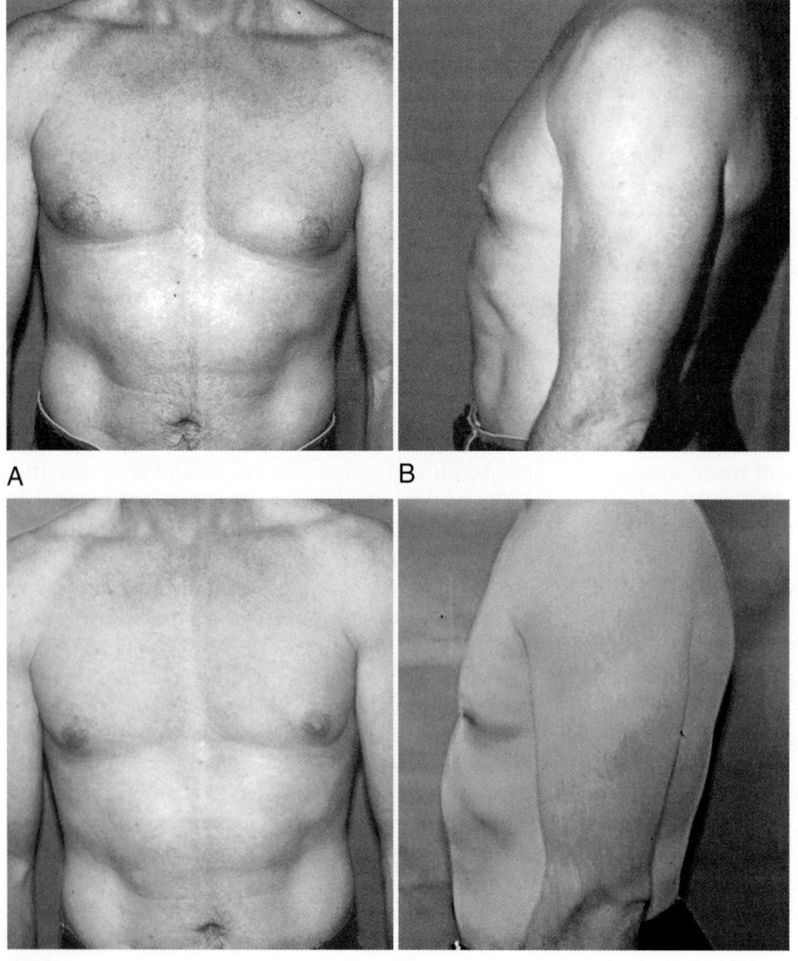

FIGURE 134-62. Gynecomastia corrected with suction-assisted lipectomy. *A,* Anterior view of gynecomastia (grade I). *B,* Lateral view. *C,* Anterior postoperative view 1 year after suction-assisted lipectomy for removal of breast tissue. *D,* Lateral view.

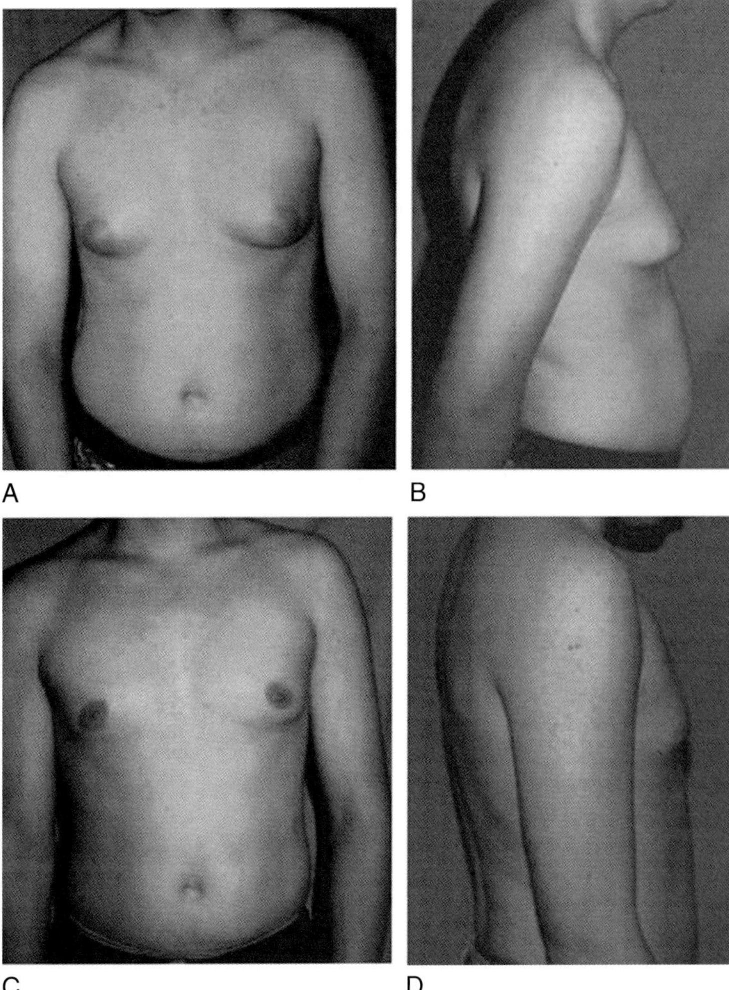

FIGURE 134-63. Gynecomastia corrected with suction-assisted lipectomy. *A,* Anterior preoperative view of gynecomastia (grade I). *B,* Lateral view. *C,* Anterior postoperative view 1 year after suction-assisted lipectomy for removal of breast tissue. *D,* Lateral view.

redundant skin in 5%, and nipple retraction from over-resection in 38%.

Wiesman et al[199] treated 138 grade II breasts and selected the technique by observation of the breast. Excision alone was used in 32.6%, excision and SAL in 56.5%, and SAL alone in 8.7%. Skin resection was required in only 2.2% of patients. Seromas and hematomas were present in 13%, and revisions were needed in 14.5% of patients. Rohrich et al[187] reported UAL of 24 patients with no need for revision; however, the concerns of residual glandular tissue causing persistent projection of the breast remain.[200] Rosenberg[201] reported good results of SAL alone in a series of 10 patients with primarily fatty breasts without dense glandular tissue. Courtiss[202] reported similar results. SAL has also been useful in tapering the resection margins in broadly based breasts to prevent a "saucer deformity" in combination with excision. From these data, it is reasonable to conclude that the addition of SAL or UAL in selected patients may improve aesthetic outcome and maintain low complication rates. SAL will usually provide satisfactory treatment for the larger breast without ptosis and without excessive fibrosis. No specific advantage is noted with use of UAL, but both forms of suction lipectomy are effective either alone or in conjunction with subareola direct excision (Fig. 134-64).

The treatment of grade III gynecomastia remains controversial. The large size and presence of excess skin make a good aesthetic outcome difficult to achieve. A broad spectrum of procedures have been advocated for high-grade gynecomastia, including total mastectomy with free nipple grafting (Fig. 134-65) and modified reduction mammaplasty with a dermal pedicle for breasts with ptosis.[203,204] Wiesman et al[199] treated 69 grade III breasts and resected skin with or without SAL in 61%; no patients were treated with SAL alone. Of the patients who did not require skin resection, only 30% required reoperation for residual laxity after 6 to 9 months of follow-up, suggesting that

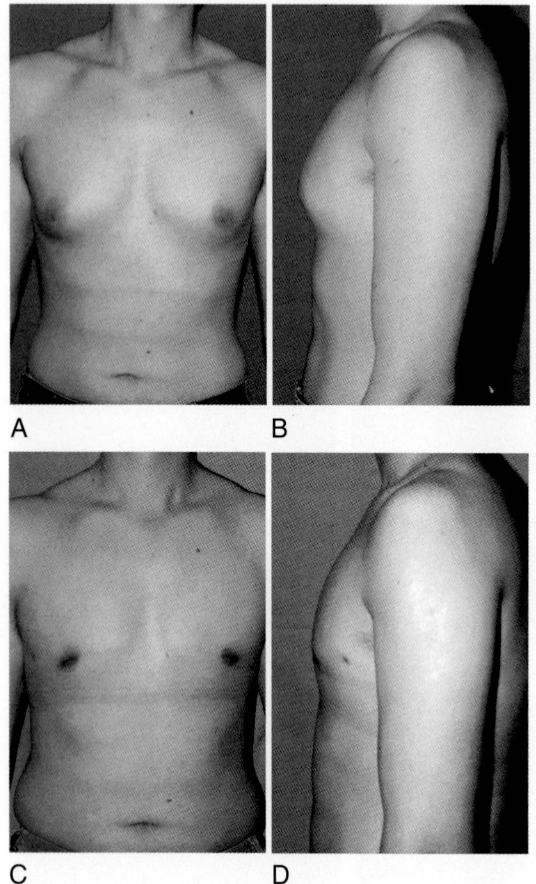

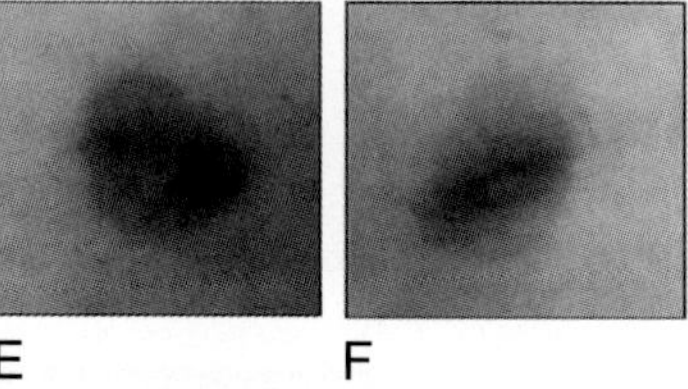

FIGURE 134-64. Gynecomastia corrected with direct excision and suction-assisted lipectomy. *A,* Anterior view of gynecomastia (grade II). *B,* Lateral view. *C,* Anterior postoperative view 1 year after transverse areola incision for direct excision of subareola breast tissue and suction-assisted lipectomy. *D,* Lateral view. *E* and *F,* Close-up view of left (*E*) and right (*F*) nipple-areola incision sites. Note minimal scarring at healed incision sites.

in selected patients, a large skin resection scar can be avoided if skin resection is delayed until a second procedure in 6 to 9 months. When all grades and all techniques are evaluated, there is no significant increase in complication rates observed over increasing grade, but performance of a skin resection significantly increases the complication rate from 14% to 40% (independent of grade). Furthermore, the revision rate for patients who had a skin excision at the initial operation was 38% (no different from those who did not have a revision), so skin resection at the initial operation does not necessarily reduce the number of operations that an individual needs.

The use of UAL alone for the treatment of grade III gynecomastia in 19 patients was reported. However, revisions were required 6 to 9 months afterward for 42% of patients because of excess skin laxity, particularly in patients with grade II or grade III ptosis. The interesting result is that despite significant preoperative skin laxity, it appears to resolve in more than 50% of the patients. This finding is consistent with that of Wiesman et al,[199] but long-term follow-up is needed.

Summary

Gynecomastia is a common disorder with many complex causes. A thorough history and physical examination are needed for accurate diagnosis and management. Grade I and grade II gynecomastia with firm glandular tissue are best treated with excision. Combination with SAL is likely to give better body contouring. For fatty low-grade breasts without significant glandular tissue, SAL or UAL alone may be the best treatment option. Grade III gynecomastia remains controversial. If ptosis is not severe, suction lipectomy is effective, and some shrinkage of the skin envelope will occur. Repeating SAL in approximately 3 months may provide adequate contour in patients with grade III gynecomastia without excessive ptosis. If ptosis is severe, skin reduction in combination with subcutaneous mastectomy with nipple grafting is effective treatment. Although the patient will have an inframammary incision, the functional and psychological sequelae of a grade III breast with ptosis will be relieved. With this approach, secondary procedures are rarely required.

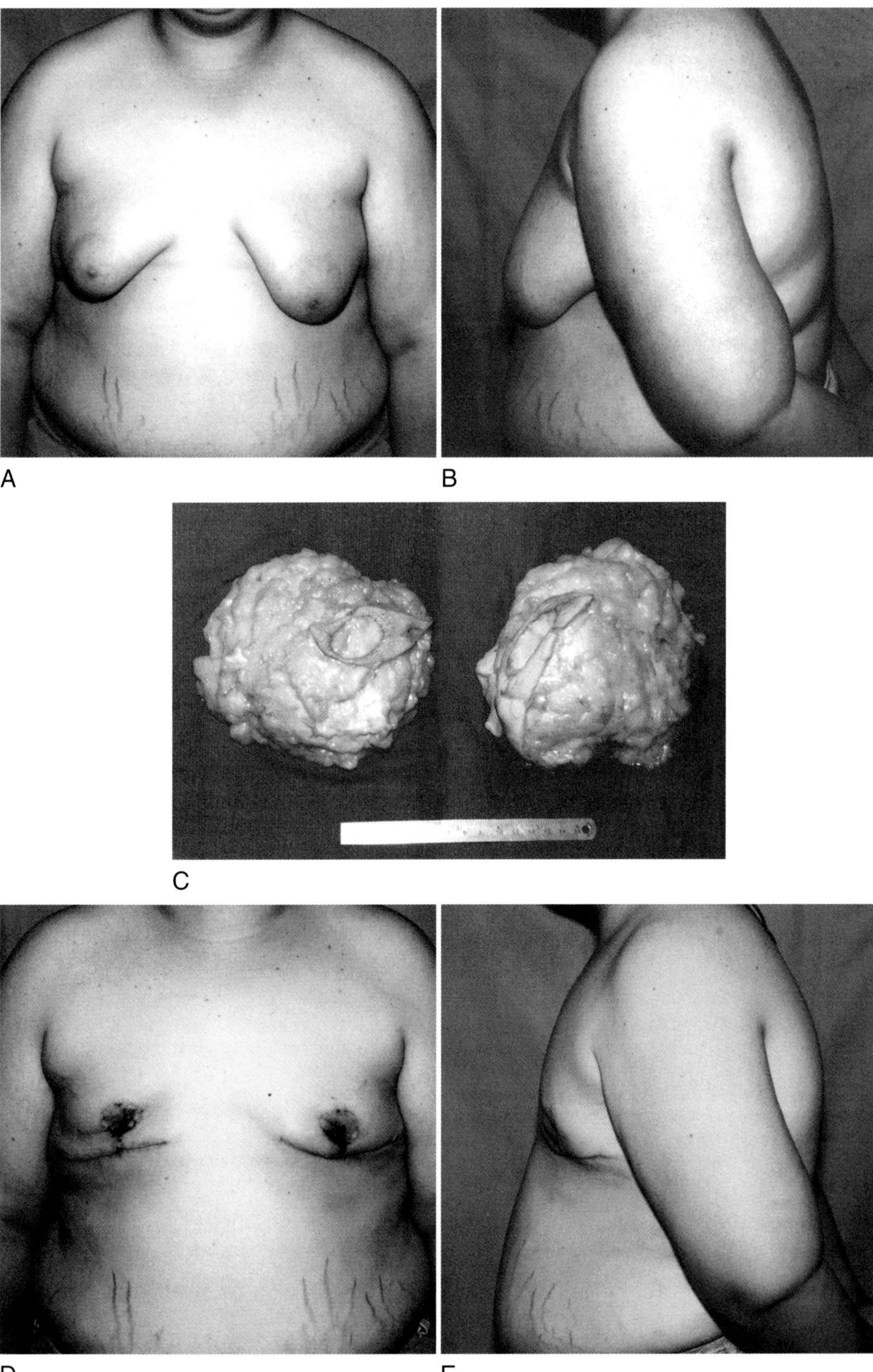

FIGURE 134-65. Correction of gynecomastia (grade III) with skin and tissue resection and bilateral nipple full-thickness grafts. *A,* Anterior view of bilateral severe gynecomastia with ptosis. *B,* Lateral view. *C,* Intraoperative view of specimen with nipple-areola removed for reinsertion as free full-thickness graft. *D,* Postoperative anterior view at 3 months of bilateral subcutaneous mastectomy with skin resection and free nipple-areola grafts. *E,* Lateral view. (From Hamilton S, Gault D: The tuberous male breast. Br J Plast Surg 2003;56:295. Reprinted with permission from The British Association of Plastic Surgeons.)

REFERENCES

1. Netscher DT, Peterson R: Normal and abnormal development of the extremities and trunk. Clin Plast Surg 1990;17:13-21.
2. Williams PL: Gray's Anatomy: The Anatomical Basis of Medicine and Surgery, 38th ed. New York, Churchill Livingstone, 1995.
3. Acastello E, Majluf R, Garrido P, et al: Sternal cleft: a surgical opportunity. J Pediatr Surg 2003;38:178-183.
4. Ravitch MM: Congenital Deformities of the Chest Wall and Their Operative Correction. Philadelphia, WB Saunders, 1977.
5. Morshuis WJ, Mulder H, Wapperom G, et al: Pectus excavatum. A clinical study with long-term postoperative follow-up. Eur J Cardiothorac Surg 1992;6:318-328, discussion 328-329.
6. Fonkalsrud EW: Current management of pectus excavatum. World J Surg 2003;27:502-508.
7. Saxena AK, Schaarschmidt K, Schleef J, et al: Surgical correction of pectus excavatum: the Munster experience. Langenbecks Arch Surg 1999;384:187-193.
8. Molik KA, Engum SA, Rescorla FJ, et al: Pectus excavatum repair: experience with standard and minimal invasive techniques. J Pediatr Surg 2001;36:324-328.
9. Malek MH, Fonkalsrud EW, Cooper CB: Ventilatory and cardiovascular responses to exercise in patients with pectus excavatum. Chest 2003;124:870.
10. Nuss D, Kelly RE Jr, Croitoru DP, Katz ME: A 10-year review of a minimally invasive technique for the correction of pectus excavatum. J Pediatr Surg 1998;33:545.
11. Robicsek F: Surgical treatment of pectus excavatum. Chest Surg Clin North Am 2000;10:277-296.
12. Moore KL: The Developing Human: Clinically Oriented Embryology, 3d ed. Philadelphia, WB Saunders, 1982:351.
13. Sadler TW: Langman's Medical Embryology, 7th ed. Baltimore, Williams & Wilkins, 1995:174.
14. Larsen WJ: Human Embryology. New York, Churchill Livingstone, 1993:71.
15. Ochsner A, DeBakey M: Chone-chondrosternon: report of a case and review of the literature. J Thorac Surg 1939;8:469.
16. Garcia VF, Seyfer AE, Graeber GM: Reconstruction of congenital chest-wall deformities. Surg Clin North Am 1989; 69:1103-1118.
17. Morshuis W, Folgering H, Barentsz J, et al: Pulmonary function before surgery for pectus excavatum and at long-term follow-up. Chest 1994;105:1646-1652.
18. Brodkin SH: Pectus excavatum: surgical indications and time of operation. Pediatrics 1953;11:582.
19. Shamberger RC: Cardiopulmonary effects of anterior chest wall deformities. Chest Surg Clin North Am 2000;10:245.
20. Haller JA Jr, Kramer SS, Lietman SA: Use of CT scans in selection of patients for pectus excavatum surgery: a preliminary report. J Pediatr Surg 1987;22:904.
21. Fonkalsrud EW, DeUgarte D, Choi E: Repair of pectus excavatum and carinatum deformities in 116 adults. Ann Surg 2002;236:304.
22. Quigley PM, Haller JA, Jelus KL, et al: Cardiorespiratory function before and after corrective surgery in pectus excavatum. J Pediatr 1996;128(pt 1):638.
23. Peterson RJ, Young WG Jr, Godwin JD, et al: Noninvasive assessment of exercise cardiac function before and after pectus excavatum repair. J Thorac Cardiovasc Surg 1985;90:251-260.
24. Garusi GF, Dettorre A: Angiocardiographic patterns in funnel-chest. Cardiologia 1964;45:313-330.
25. Bevegard S: Postural circulatory changes at rest and during exercise in patients with funnel chest, with special reference to factors affecting the stroke volume. Acta Med Scand 1962;171:695-713.
26. Lawson ML, Cash TF, Akers R, et al: A pilot study of the impact of surgical repair on disease-specific quality of life among patients with pectus excavatum. J Pediatr Surg 2003;38:916.
27. Roberts J, Hayashi A, Anderson JO, et al: Quality of life of patients who have undergone the Nuss procedure for pectus excavatum: preliminary findings. J Pediatr Surg 2003;38:779.
28. Park HJ, Lee SY, Lee CS, et al: The Nuss procedure for pectus excavatum: evolution of techniques and early results on 322 patients. Ann Thorac Surg 2004;77:289.
29. Haller JA Jr, Colombani PM, Humphries CT, et al: Chest wall constriction after too extensive and too early operations for pectus excavatum. Ann Thorac Surg 1996;61:1618-1624, discussion 1625.
30. Kowalewski J, Barcikowski S, Brocki M: Cardiorespiratory function before and after operation for pectus excavatum: medium-term results. Eur J Cardiothorac Surg 1998;13:275-279.
31. Ravitch MM: The operative treatment of pectus excavatum. J S C Med Assoc 1955;51:244-249.
32. Seyfer AE, Graeber GM, Wind GL: Atlas of Chest Wall Reconstruction. Rockville, Md, Aspen Press, 1986:234.
33. Nuss D, Kelly RE, Croitoru DP, Katz ME: A 10-year review of a minimally invasive technique for the correction of pectus excavatum. J Pediatric Surg 1988;33:545-552.
34. Hebra A: Minimally invasive pectus surgery. Chest Surg Clin North Am 2000;10:329-339.
35. Croitoru DP, Kelly RE Jr, Goretsky MJ, et al: Experience and modification update for the minimally invasive Nuss technique for pectus excavatum repair in 303 patients. J Pediatr Surg 2002;37:437-445.
36. Fonkalsrud EW, Beanes S, Hebra A, et al: Comparison of minimally invasive and modified Ravitch pectus excavatum repair. J Pediatr Surg 2002;37:413-417.
37. Coln D, Gunning T, Ramsay M, et al: Early experience with the Nuss minimally invasive correction of pectus excavatum in adults. World J Surg 2002;26:1217-1221. Epub 2002 Sep 06.
38. Ravitch MM: The operative treatment of pectus excavatum. Ann Surg 1949;129:429-444.
39. Johnson PE: Refining silicone implant correction of pectus excavatum through computed tomography. Plast Reconstr Surg 1996;97:445.
40. Seyfer AE: in progress.
41. Carachi R, Audry G, Ranke A, et al: Collagen-coated Vicryl mesh: a new bioprosthesis in pediatric surgical practice. J Pediatr Surg 1995;30:1302.
42. Nakanishi Y, Nakajima T, Sakakibara A, Nishiyama T: A vascularized rib strut technique for funnel chest correction. Br J Plast Surg 1992;45:364-366.
43. Luzzi L, Voltolini L, Zacharias J, et al: Ten year experience of bioabsorbable mesh support in pectus excavatum repair. Br J Plast Surg 2004;57:733-740.
44. Gilbert JC, Zwiren GT: Repair of pectus excavatum using a substernal metal strut within a Marlex envelope. South Med J 1989;82:1240.
45. Robicsek F: Marlex mesh support for the correction of very severe and recurrent pectus excavatum. Ann Thorac Surg 1978;26:80.
46. Bentz ML, Futrell JW: Improved chest wall fixation for correction of pectus excavatum. Br J Plast Surg 1992;45: 367-370.
47. Gotzen L, Dragojevic D: Funnel chest correction by use of AO implants and instruments. Thorac Cardiovasc Surg 1979;27:61-64.
48. De Agustin-Asensio JC, Banuelos C, Vazques JJ: Titanium miniplates for the surgical correction of pectus excavatum. J Am Coll Surg 1999;188:455-458.
49. Lansman S, Serlo W, Linna O, et al: Treatment of pectus excavatum with bioabsorbable polylactide plates: preliminary results. J Pediatr Surg 2002;37:1281-1286.
50. Paltia V, Parkkulainen KV, Sulamaa M, Wallgren GR: Operative technique in funnel chest; experience in 81 cases. Acta Chir Scand 1959;116:90-98.

51. Brooks JP, Tripp HF: Bioabsorbable weave technique for repair of pectus excavatum. J Thorac Cardiovasc Surg 2000;119:176-178.
52. Pircova A, Sekarski-Hunkeler N, Jeanrenaud X, et al: Cardiac perforation after surgical repair of pectus excavatum. J Pediatr Surg 1995;30:1506-1508.
53. Gurkok S, Genc O, Dakak M, Balkanli K: The use of absorbable material in correction of pectus deformities. Eur J Cardiothorac Surg 2001;19:711-712.
54. Mansour KA, Thourani VH, Odessey EA, et al: Thirty-year experience with repair of pectus deformities in adults. Ann Thorac Surg 2003;76:391-395, discussion 395.
55. Davis JT, Weinstein S: Repair of the pectus deformity: results of the Ravitch approach in the current era. Ann Thorac Surg 2004;78:421-426.
56. Fonkalsrud EW, Anselmo DM: Less extensive techniques for repair of pectus carinatum: the undertreated chest deformity. J Am Coll Surg 2004;198:898-905.
57. Sigalet DL, Montgomery M, Harder J: Cardiopulmonary effects of closed repair of pectus excavatum. J Pediatr Surg 2003;38:380-385, discussion 380-385.
58. Borowitz D, Cerny F, Zallen G, et al: Pulmonary function and exercise response in patients with pectus excavatum after Nuss repair. J Pediatr Surg 2003;38:544-547.
59. Fonkalsrud EW: Pectus carinatum: the undertreated chest malformation. Asian J Surg 2003;26:189-192.
60. Shamberger RC, Welch KJ: Surgical correction of pectus carinatum. J Pediatr Surg 1987;22:48.
61. Shamberger RC: Congenital chest wall deformities. Curr Probl Surg 1996;33:469-542.
62. Robicsek F, Cook JW, Daugherty HK, Selle JG: Pectus carinatum. Coll Works Cardiopulm Dis 1979;22:65-78.
63. Picard LR, Tepas JJ, Shermeta DW, Haller JA Jr: Pectus carinatum: results of surgical therapy. J Pediatr Surg 1979;14:228.
64. Cahill JL, Lees GM, Robertson HT: A summary of preoperative and postoperative cardiorespiratory performance in patients undergoing pectus excavatum and carinatum repair. J Pediatr Surg 1984;19:430-433.
65. Fonkalsrud EW, Beanes S: Surgical management of pectus carinatum: 30 years' experience. World J Surg 2001;25:898-903.
66. Ravitch MM: Congenital Deformities of the Chest Wall and Their Operative Correction. Philadelphia, WB Saunders, 1958.
67. Burton JF: Method of correction of ectopic cordis: two cases. Arch Surg 1947;54:79-81.
68. Domini M, Cupaioli M, Rossi F, et al: Bifid sternum: neonatal surgical treatment. Ann Thorac Surg 2000;69:267-269.
69. de Campos JR, Filomeno LT, Fernandez A, et al: Repair of congenital sternal cleft in infants and adolescents. Ann Thorac Surg 1998;66:1151-1154.
70. Ramirez-Solis R, Zheng H, Whiting J, et al: Hoxb-4 (Hox-2.6) mutant mice show homeotic transformation of a cervical vertebra and defects in the closure of the sternal rudiments. Cell 1993;73:279-294.
71. Rose NC, Coleman BG, Wallace D, et al: Prenatal diagnosis of a chest wall hamartoma and sternal cleft. Ultrasound Obstet Gynecol 1996;7:453-455.
72. Snyder BJ, Robbins RC, Ramos D: Primary repair of complete sternal cleft with pectoralis major muscle flaps. Ann Thorac Surg 1996;61:983-984.
73. Gorlin RJ, Kantaputra P, Aughton DJ, Mulliken JB: Marked female predilection in some syndromes associated with facial hemangiomas. Am J Med Genet 1994;52:130-135.
74. Shalak L, Kaddoura I, Obeid M, et al: Complete cleft sternum and congenital heart disease: review of the literature. Pediatr Int 2002;44:314-316.
75. Suri RK, Sharma RK, Jha NK, Sharma BK: Complete congenital sternal cleft in an adult: repair by autogenous tissues. Ann Thorac Surg 1996;62:573.
76. Daum R, Zachariou Z: Total and superior sternal clefts in newborns: a simple technique for surgical correction. J Pediatr Surg 1999;34:408-411.
77. Sabiston DC Jr: The surgical management of congenital bifid sternum with partial ectopia cordis. J Thorac Surg 1958;35:118-122.
78. Khoury MJ, Cordero JF, Rasmussen S: Ectopia cordis, midline defects and chromosome abnormalities: an epidemiologic perspective. Am J Med Genet 1988;30:811-817.
79. Dobell AR, Williams HB, Long RW: Staged repair of ectopia cordis. J Pediatr Surg 1982;17:353-358.
80. Tongsong T, Wanapirak C, Sirivatanapa P, Wongtrangan S: Prenatal sonographic diagnosis of ectopia cordis. J Clin Ultrasound 1999;27:440-445.
81. Ley EJ, Roth JJ, Kim KA, et al: Successful repair of ectopia cordis using alloplastic materials: 10-year follow-up. Plast Reconstr Surg 2004;114:1519-1522.
82. Morello M, Quaini E, Nenov G, Pome G: Extrathoracic ectopia cordis. Case report. J Cardiovasc Surg (Torino) 1994;35:511-515.
83. Alphonso N, Venugopal PS, Deshpande R, Anderson D: Complete thoracic ectopia cordis. Eur J Cardiothorac Surg 2003;23:426-428.
84. Morales JM, Patel SG, Duff JA, et al: Ectopia cordis and other midline defects. Ann Thorac Surg 2000;70:111-114.
85. Hornberger LK, Colan SD, Lock JE, et al: Outcome of patients with ectopia cordis and significant intracardiac defects. Circulation 1996;94:II32-II37.
86. Amato JJ, Zelen J, Talwalkar NG: Single-stage repair of thoracic ectopia cordis. Ann Thorac Surg 1995;59:518-520.
87. Cantrell JR, Haller JA, Ravitch MM: A syndrome of congenital defects involving the abdominal wall, sternum, diaphragm, pericardium, and heart. Surg Gynecol Obstet 1958;107:602-614.
88. Falcao JL, Falcao SN, Sawicki WC, et al: Cantrell syndrome. Case report of an adult. Arq Bras Cardiol 2000;75:323-328.
89. Ghidini A, Sirtori M, Romero R, Hobbins JC: Prenatal diagnosis of pentalogy of Cantrell. J Ultrasound Med 1988;7:567-572.
90. Jeune M, Carron R, Beraud C, Loaec Y: Polychondrodystrophie avec blocage thoracique d'évolution fatale. Pediatrie 1954;9:390-392.
91. Turkel SB, Diehl EJ, Richmond JA: Necropsy findings in neonatal asphyxiating thoracic dystrophy. J Med Genet 1985;22:112-118.
92. Morgan NV, Bacchelli C, Gissen P, et al: A locus for asphyxiating thoracic dystrophy, ATD, maps to chromosome 15q13. J Med Genet 2003;40:431-435.
93. Williams AJ, Vawter G, Reid LM: Lung structure in asphyxiating thoracic dystrophy. Arch Pathol Lab Med 1984;108:658-661.
94. Kaddoura IL, Obeid MY, Mroueh SM, Nasser AA: Dynamic thoracoplasty for asphyxiating thoracic dystrophy. Ann Thorac Surg 2001;72:1755-1758.
95. Kozlowski K, Masel J: Asphyxiating thoracic dystrophy without respiratory disease: report of two cases of the latent form. Pediatr Radiol 1976;5:30-33.
96. Shah KJ: Renal lesion in Jeune's syndrome. Br J Radiol 1980;53:432-436.
97. Barnes ND, Hull D, Milner AD, Waterston DJ: Chest reconstruction in thoracic dystrophy. Arch Dis Child 1971;46:833-837.
98. Aronson DC, Van Nierop JC, Taminau A, Vos A: Homologous bone graft for expansion thoracoplasty in Jeune's asphyxiating thoracic dystrophy. J Pediatr Surg 1999;34:500-503.
99. Todd DW, Tinguely SJ, Norberg WJ: A thoracic expansion technique for Jeune's asphyxiating thoracic dystrophy. J Pediatr Surg 1986;21:161-163.

100. Davis JT, Heistein JB, Castile RG, et al: Lateral thoracic expansion for Jeune's syndrome: midterm results. Ann Thorac Surg 2001;72:872.
101. Poland A: Deficiency of the pectoral muscles. Guys Hosp Rep 1841;6:191-193.
102. Lallemand LM: Ephemerides Medicales de Montpellier 1826;1:144-147.
103. Froriep R: Beobachtung eines Falles von Mangel der Brustdrüse. Notizen Gebiete Natur Heilkunde 1839;10:9-14.
104. Fokin AA, Robicsek F: Poland's syndrome revisited. Ann Thorac Surg 2002;74:2218.
105. Pearl M, Chow TF, Friedman E: Poland's syndrome. Radiology 1971;101:619-623.
106. Karnak I, Tanyel FC, Tuncbilek E, et al: Bilateral Poland anomaly. Am J Med Genet 1998;75:505-507.
107. Fraser FC, Ronen GM, O'Leary E: Pectoralis major defect and Poland sequence in second cousins: extension of the Poland sequence spectrum. Am J Med Genet 1989;33:468-470.
108. Cobben JM, Robinson PH, van Essen AJ, et al: Poland anomaly in mother and daughter. Am J Med Genet 1989;33:519-521.
109. Bouvet JP, Leveque D, Bernetieres F, Gros JJ: Vascular origin of Poland syndrome? A comparative rheographic study of the vascularization of the arms in eight patients. Eur J Pediatr 1978;128:17-26.
110. Mentzel HJ, Seidel J, Sauner D, et al: Radiological aspects of the Poland syndrome and implications for treatment: a case study and review. Eur J Pediatr 2002;161:455-459.
111. Bamforth JS, Fabian C, Machin G, Honore L: Poland anomaly with limb body wall disruption defect: case report and review. Am J Med Genet 1992;43:780-784.
112. Gorlin R: J Risk of recurrence in usually nongenetic malformation syndromes. Birth Defects Orig Artic Ser 1979;15:181-188.
113. David TJ: Familial Poland anomaly. J Med Genet 1982;19:293-296.
114. Shamberger RC, Welch KJ, Upton J 3rd: Surgical treatment of thoracic deformity in Poland's syndrome. J Pediatr Surg 1989;24:760-765, discussion 766.
115. Walker JC Jr, Meijer R, Aranda D: Syndactylism with deformity of the pectoralis muscle. Poland's syndrome. J Pediatr Surg 1969;4:569-572.
116. Mace JW, Kaplan JM, Schanberger JE, Gotlin RW: Poland's syndrome. Report of seven cases and review of the literature. Clin Pediatr (Phila) 1972;11:98-102.
117. Paladini D, D'Armiento MR, Martinelli P: Prenatal ultrasound diagnosis of Poland syndrome. Obstet Gynecol 2004;104:1156-1159.
118. Perez-Aznar JM, Urbano J, Garcia Laborda E, et al: Breast and pectoralis muscle hypoplasia. A mild degree of Poland's syndrome. Acta Radiol 1996;37:759-762.
119. Al-Qattan MM: Classification of hand anomalies in Poland's syndrome. Br J Plast Surg 2001;54:132-136.
120. Schaarschmidt K, Kolberg-Schwerdt A, Dimitrov G, Straubeta J: Submuscular bar, multiple pericostal bar fixation, bilateral thoracoscopy: a modified Nuss repair in adolescents. J Pediatr Surg 2002;37:1276-1280.
121. Ohmori K, Takada H: Correction of Poland's pectoralis major muscle anomaly with latissimus dorsi musculocutaneous flaps. Plast Reconstr Surg 1980;65:400-404.
122. Marks MW, Iacobucci J: Reconstruction of congenital chest wall deformities using solid silicone onlay prostheses. Chest Surg Clin North Am 2000;10:341-355.
123. Avci G, Misirlioglu A, Eker G, Akoz T: Mild degree of Poland's syndrome reconstruction with customized silicone prosthesis. Aesthetic Plast Surg 2003;27:112-115.
124. Gatti JE: Poland's deformity reconstructions with a customized, extrasoft silicone prosthesis. Ann Plast Surg 1997;39:122-130.
125. Seyfer AE, Icochea R, Graeber GM: Poland's anomaly. Natural history and long-term results of chest wall reconstruction in 33 patients. Ann Surg 1988;208:776.
126. Borschel GH, Izenberg PH, Cederna PS: Endoscopically assisted reconstruction of male and female Poland syndrome. Plast Reconstr Surg 2002;109:1536-1543.
127. Lin CH, Levin LS: Free flap expansion using balloon-assisted endoscopic technique. Microsurgery 1996;7:330-336.
128. Longaker MT, Glat PM, Colen LB, Siebert JW: Reconstruction of breast asymmetry in Poland's chest-wall deformity using microvascular free flaps. Plast Reconstr Surg 1997;99:429-436.
129. Beer GM, Kompatscher P, Hergan K: Poland's syndrome and vascular malformations. Br J Plast Surg 1996;49:482-484.
130. Nelson MM, Cooper CK: Congenital defects of the breast—an autosomal dominant trait. S Afr Med J 1982;61:434-436.
131. Osbourne M: Breast development and anatomy. In Harris J, ed: Breast Diseases. Philadelphia, JB Lippincott, 1991:1-13.
132. Moore KL: The integumentary system. In Moore KL: The Developing Human: Clinically Oriented Embryology, 4th ed. Philadelphia, WB Saunders, 1988:426-428.
133. Bland KI, Copeland : The Breast: Comprehensive Management of Benign and Malignant Disorders, 3rd ed. Philadelphia, Elsevier, 2004:212-215.
134. Mehes K: Association of supernumerary nipples with other anomalies. J Pediatr 1983;102:161.
135. Mehes K, et al: Supernumerary nipples and urologic malignancies. Cancer Genet Cytogenet 1987;24:185.
136. Rahbar F: Clinical significance of supernumerary nipples in black neonates. Clin Pediatr 1982;21:46.
137. Mimouni F, et al: Occurrence of supernumerary nipples in newborns. Am J Dis Child 1983;137:952.
138. Moore JA, Schosser RH: Becker's melanosis and hypoplasia of the breast and pectoralis major muscle. Pediatr Dermatol 1985;3:34.
139. Abramson DJ: Bilateral intra-areolar polythelia. Arch Surg 1975;110:1255.
140. Velanovich V: Ectopic breast tissue, supernumerary breasts, and supernumerary nipples. South Med J 1995;88:903.
141. Cheong JH, Lee BC, Lee KS: Carcinoma of the axillary breast. Yonsei Med J 1999;40:290-293.
142. Pellegrini JR, Wagner RF Jr: Polythelia and associated conditions. Am Fam Physician 1983;28:129-132.
143. Jojart G, Seres E: Supernumerary nipples and renal anomalies. Int Urol Nephrol 1994;26:141.
144. Grotto I, Browner-Elhanan K, Mimouni D, et al: Occurrence of supernumerary nipples in children with kidney and urinary tract malformations. Pediatr Dermatol 2001;18:291-294.
145. Goedert JJ, McKeen EA, Javadpour N, et al: Polythelia and testicular cancer. Ann Intern Med 1984;101:646-647.
146. Chung CS, Myrianthopoulos NC: Factors affecting risks of congenital malformations. I. Analysis of epidemiologic factors in congenital malformations. Report from the Collaborative Perinatal Project. Birth Defects Orig Artic Ser 1975;11:1.
147. Orti E, Qazi QH: Polymastia. In Bergasma D, ed: Birth Defects Compendium. New York, Alan R. Liss, 1979.
148. John C: Über akzessorische Milchdrüsen und Warzen, insbesondere über milchdrüsemähnliche Bildungen in der Achselhöhle. Arch Gynakol 1925;126:689.
149. Jeffcoate TN: Principles of Gynecology. London, Butterworth, 1967.
150. Garcia JJ, Verkauf BS, Hochberg CJ, Ingram JM: Aberrant breast tissue of the vulva. A case report and review of the literature. Obstet Gynecol 1978;52:225-228.
151. DeCholnoky T: Accessory breast tissue in the axilla. N Y State J Med 1951;51:2245.
152. Saleh HA, Klein LH: Cystosarcoma phyllodes arising synchronously in right breast and bilateral axillary ectopic breast tissue. Arch Pathol Lab Med 1990;114:624-626.

153. DeGrouchy J, Turleau C: Clinical Atlas of Human Chromosomes. New York, John Wiley & Sons, 1977.
154. Evans DM, Guyton DP: Carcinoma of the axillary breast. J Surg Oncol 1995;59:190.
155. Thorne AL, Jackson A, Yiangou C: The use of sentinel node biopsy in the treatment of cancer of an accessory breast. Breast 2003;12:153-155.
156. Rees TD, Aston SJ: The tuberous breast. Clin Plast Surg 1976;3:339-347.
157. Grolleau JL, Lanfrey E, Lavigne B, et al: Breast base anomalies: treatment strategy for tuberous breasts, minor deformities, and asymmetry. Plast Reconstr Surg 1999;104:2040-2048.
158. Williams G, Hoffman S: Mammoplasty for tubular breasts. Aesthetic Plast Surg 1981;5:51-56.
159. Bass CB: Herniated areolar complex. Ann Plast Surg 1978;1:402-406.
160. Gruber RP, Jones HW Jr: The "donut" mastopexy: indications and complications. Plast Reconstr Surg 1980;65:34.
161. Brink RR: Evaluating breast parenchymal maldistribution with regard to mastopexy and augmentation mammaplasty. Plast Reconstr Surg 1990;86:715-719, discussion 720-721.
162. Puckett CL, Concannon MJ: Augmenting the narrow-based breast: the unfurling technique to prevent the double-bubble deformity. Aesthetic Plast Surg 1990;14:15.
163. Rohrich RJ, Hartley W, Brown S: Incidence of breast and chest wall asymmetry in breast augmentation: a retrospective analysis of 100 patients. Plast Reconstr Surg 2003;111:1513-1519, discussion 1520-1523.
164. Panettiere P, Del Gaudio GA, Marchetti L, et al: The tuberous breast syndrome. Aesthetic Plast Surg 2000;24:445.
165. von Heimburg D, et al: The tuberous breast deformity: classification and treatment. Br J Plast Surg 1996;49:339-345.
166. Choupina M, Malheiro E, Pinho C, et al: Tuberous breast: a surgical challenge. Aesthetic Plast Surg 2002;26:50.
167. Parano E, Falsaperla R, Pavone V, et al: Intrafamilial phenotypic heterogeneity of the Poland complex: a case report. Neuropediatrics 1995;26:217-219.
168. Mandrekas AD, Zambacos GJ, Anastasopoulos A, et al: Aesthetic reconstruction of the tuberous breast deformity. Plast Reconstr Surg 2003;112:1099.
169. Muti E: Personal approach to surgical correction of the extremely hypoplastic tuberous breast. Aesthetic Plast Surg 1996;20:385.
170. Dinner MI, Dowden RV: The tubular/tuberous breast syndrome. Ann Plast Surg 1987;19:414-420.
171. Meara JG, Kolker A, Bartlett G, et al: Tuberous breast deformity: principles and practice. Ann Plast Surg 2000;45:607.
172. Pardo A, Watier E, Georgieu N, et al: Tuberous breast syndrome. Report on a series of 22 operated patients. Ann Chir Plast Esthet 1999;44:583.
173. Maillard GF: A Z-mammaplasty with minimal scarring. Plast Reconstr Surg 1986;77:66-76.
174. Ribeiro L, Canzi W, Buss A, Accorsi A Jr: Tuberous breast: a new approach. Plast Reconstr Surg 1998;101:42.
175. Atiyeh BS, Hashim HA, El-Douaihy Y, Kayle DI: Perinipple round-block technique for correction of tuberous/tubular breast deformity. Aesthetic Plast Surg 1998;22:284.
176. Scheepers JH, Quaba AA: Tissue expansion in the treatment of tubular breast deformity. Br J Plast Surg 1992;45:529.
177. Martinez-Chequer JC, Carranza-Lira S, Lopez-Silva JD, et al: Congenital absence of the breasts: a case report. Am J Obstet Gynecol 2004;191:372-374.
178. Lin KY, Nguyen DB, Williams RM: Complete breast absence revisited. Plast Reconstr Surg 2000;106:98-101.
179. Trier WC: Complete breast absence. Case report and review of the literature. Plast Reconstr Surg 1965;36:431-439.
180. Greenberg F, Elder FF, Ledbetter DH: Neonatal diagnosis of Prader-Willi syndrome and its implications. Am J Med Genet 1987;28:845-856.
181. Carlson HE: Gynecomastia. N Engl J Med 1980;303:795.
182. Nuttall FQ: Gynecomastia as a physical finding in normal men. J Clin Endocrinol Metab 1979;48:338.
183. Williams MJ: Gynecomastia: its incidence, recognition and host characterization in 447 autopsy cases. Am J Med 1963;34:103.
184. Nydick M, Bustos J, Dale JH, Rawson RW: Gynecomastia in adolescent boys. JAMA 1961;178:449.
185. Cohen IK, Pozez AL, McKeown JE: Gynecomastia. In Courtiss EH, ed: Male Aesthetic Surgery. St. Louis, Mosby, 1991.
186. Neuman JF: Evaluation and treatment of gynecomastia. Am Fam Physician 1997;55:1835.
187. Rohrich RJ, Ha RY, Kenkel JM, Adams WP Jr: Classification and management of gynecomastia: defining the role of ultrasound-assisted liposuction. Plast Reconstr Surg 2003;111:909-923, discussion 924-925.
188. Jackson AW, Muldal S, Ockey CH, O'Connor PJ: Carcinoma of male breast in association with the Klinefelter syndrome. Br Med J 1965;1:223.
189. Bannayan GA, Hajdu SI: Gynecomastia: clinicopathologic study of 351 cases. Am J Clin Pathol 1972;57:431.
190. Hands LJ, Greenall MJ: Gynaecomastia. Br J Surg 1991;78:907-911.
191. McGrath MH: Gynecomastia. In Jurkiewicz MJ, Mathes SJ, Krizek TJ, Ariyan S, eds: Plastic Surgery: Principles and Practice. St. Louis, Mosby, 1990:1119.
192. Beckenstein MS, Windle BH, Stroup RT: Anatomical parameters for nipple position and areolar diameter in males. Ann Plast Surg 1996;36:33.
193. Simon BE, Hoffman S, Kahn S: Classification and surgical correction of gynecomastia. Plast Reconstr Surg 1973;51:48.
194. Olsson H, Bladstrom A, Alm P: Male gynecomastia and risk for malignant tumours—a cohort study. BMC Cancer 2002;2:26.
195. Daniels IR, Layer GT: Testicular tumours presenting as gynaecomastia. Eur J Surg Oncol 2003;29:437-439.
196. Bertrand J: Pediatric Endocrinology. Baltimore, Williams & Wilkins, 1993.
197. Sher ES, Migeon CJ, Berkovitz GD: Evaluation of boys with marked breast development at puberty. Clin Pediatr (Phila) 1998;37:367-371.
198. Colombo-Benkmann M, Buse B, Stern J, Herfarth C: Indications for and results of surgical therapy for male gynecomastia. Am J Surg 1999;178:60.
199. Wiesman IM, Lehman JA Jr, Parker MG, et al: Gynecomastia: an outcome analysis. Ann Plast Surg 2004;53:97-101.
200. Strasser EJ: Ultrasound aspiration for gynecomastia. Plast Reconstr Surg 2003;112:1967-1968.
201. Rosenberg GJ: Gynecomastia: suction lipectomy as a contemporary solution. Plast Reconstr Surg 1987;80:379.
202. Courtiss EH: Gynecomastia: analysis of 159 patients and current recommendations for treatment. Plast Reconstr Surg 1987;79:740.
203. Murphy TP, Ehrlichman RJ, Seckel BR: Nipple placement in simple mastectomy with free nipple grafting for severe gynecomastia. Plast Reconstr Surg 1994;94:818.
204. Ward CM, Khalid K: Surgical treatment of grade III gynaecomastia. Ann R Coll Surg Engl 1989;71:226-228.

CHAPTER

135

Breast Reduction

GLYN JONES, MD

DEFINITION

Breast reduction can be defined as surgical reduction of breast volume to achieve a smaller, aesthetically shaped breast mound with concomitant relief of the potential symptoms of mammary hypertrophy. In addition, there is some evidence to suggest that breast reduction may reduce the individual risk of breast cancer.

HISTORY OF BREAST REDUCTION TECHNIQUES

Reduction surgery for gynecomastia was described as early as the 6th century AD. Schaller described a breast amputation mammaplasty in the 19th century, and Dieffenbach[1] performed lower pole reduction through an inframammary scar in 1848. One of the earliest accounts of a reproducible breast reduction technique hails from the end of the 19th century, when Pousson[2] described a superior wedge resection of the upper pole of the breast to both lift and reduce the breast. Sporadic reports of breast reduction procedures with discontinuous resections of up to 1400 g through an inframammary approach were described by authors such as Morestin and Guinard,[3] but it was Morestin who used a nipple transposition technique for the first time. It was not until the 1920s that more reliable operations began to appear. Transverse amputation of the lower pole of the breast with free nipple grafting was advocated by Thorek[4] in 1922 and is still used today in selected patients, albeit now with the incorporation of Wise's inverted T scar. Aubert[5] published his approach in 1923, emphasizing the importance of leaving the skin attached to the gland to minimize vascular complications. In 1925, Passot[6] described a nipple transposition into a buttonhole incision higher on the breast mound (Fig. 135-1). Schwarzmann[7] suggested maintaining the nipple on a superomedial dermal pedicle in 1930 (Fig. 135-2). This revolutionary concept led to the evolution of the wide array of reduction techniques currently employed that base the nipple on a dermoglandular pedicle, with the location of the pedicle determining where glandular resection occurs. Biesenberger[8] was the first to develop a

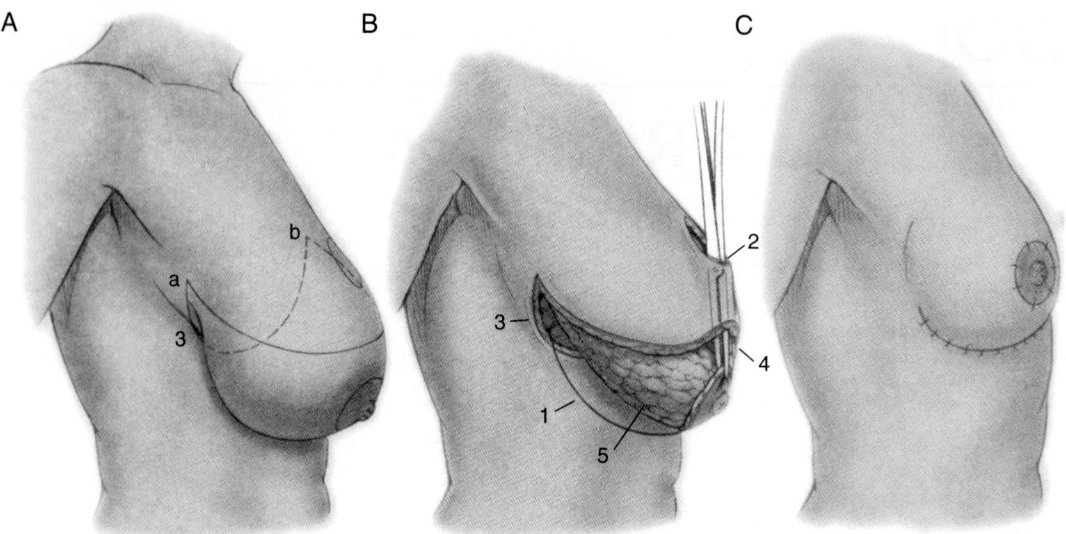

FIGURE 135-1. *A* to *C*, Passot technique of nipple transposition. (From Lickstein LH, Shestak KC: The conceptual evolution of modern reduction mammaplasty. Operative Techniques Plast Reconstr Surg 1999;6:88.)

reproducible parenchymal pedicle-based technique with an inverted T scar and a "cut as you go" pattern to achieve skin resection (Fig. 135-3). The procedure relied heavily on wide subcutaneous undermining with folding of the breast pedicle. Although reproducible, the technique carried a high complication rate in terms of skin and nipple necrosis. It persisted as a dominant reduction technique into the 1950s but was ultimately abandoned in favor of the more reliable pedicled techniques described later. Planning of the skin excision remained an inexact science, and Aufricht[9] commented on the importance of skin brassiere shaping in his publication in 1949. Bames[10] had already begun to note the importance of preoperative breast marking and together with the work of Penn[11] in South Africa provided the impetus for Wise to develop his concept of a measured keyhole pattern in 1956, which has become the mainstay of modern skin resection designs.

Schwarzmann's concepts were extended by Strombeck,[12] who devised a horizontal dermoglandular bipedicled flap to maintain nipple viability (Fig. 135-4). Skoog[13] also published a technique for superolateral dermoglandular support of the nipple. Strombeck's technique was combined with Wise's keyhole skin excision pattern, which together became a widely accepted and reliable method of breast reduction in the 1960s.[14] In 1972, McKissock[15] modified this approach by developing the concept of a vertical bipedicled flap, which is still popular with some surgeons today (Fig. 135-5). McKissock's pedicle was very thin and folded easily but did not carry as much vascularity as the modern techniques can afford. Pitanguy[16] and Weiner[17] had both popularized superior pedicle techniques in the 1960s, incorporating Wise's keyhole skin resection pattern (Fig. 135-6). The mid to late 1970s saw a number of surgeons (Courtiss, Georgiade, Goldwyn, Ribiero, Robbins) working on the refinement of an inferior dermoglandular pedicle with a broad base to improve vascularity and sensation[18-21] (Fig. 135-7). The resulting techniques, including Hester's modification,[22] the central mound technique, have become the "gold standard" procedures against which others are measured (Fig. 135-8). These operations incorporate the Wise-pattern skin resection. They are reliable, reproducible, and appropriate for a wide variety of breast sizes and shapes. Long experience with these reduction procedures gradually led to the realization that "bottoming out" of the breast with time seemed an inevitable consequence with an often unpleasant scaphoid appearance to the upper pole of the breast and lengthening of the inferior vertical scar (Fig. 135-9). Orlando and Guthrie[23] popularized the superomedial pedicle in an effort to reduce bottoming out (Figs. 135-10 and 135-11). They reasoned that maintaining volume in the upper pole would lessen the impact of gravitational descent. Concerns about the descent of inferior pedicles and the possibility of scar hypertrophy in long inferior horizontal scars led a number of surgeons in Europe and South America to explore short-scar techniques based on superior pedicles. Foremost among these were Lassus, Lejour, Marchac, Peixoto, Goes, and Benelli, to name but a few.[24-31] This movement has spread to North America, and several techniques, such as Hammond's SPAIR (short-scar periareolar inferior pedicle reduction) mammaplasty[32] and Hall-Findlay's modification

Text continued on p. 550

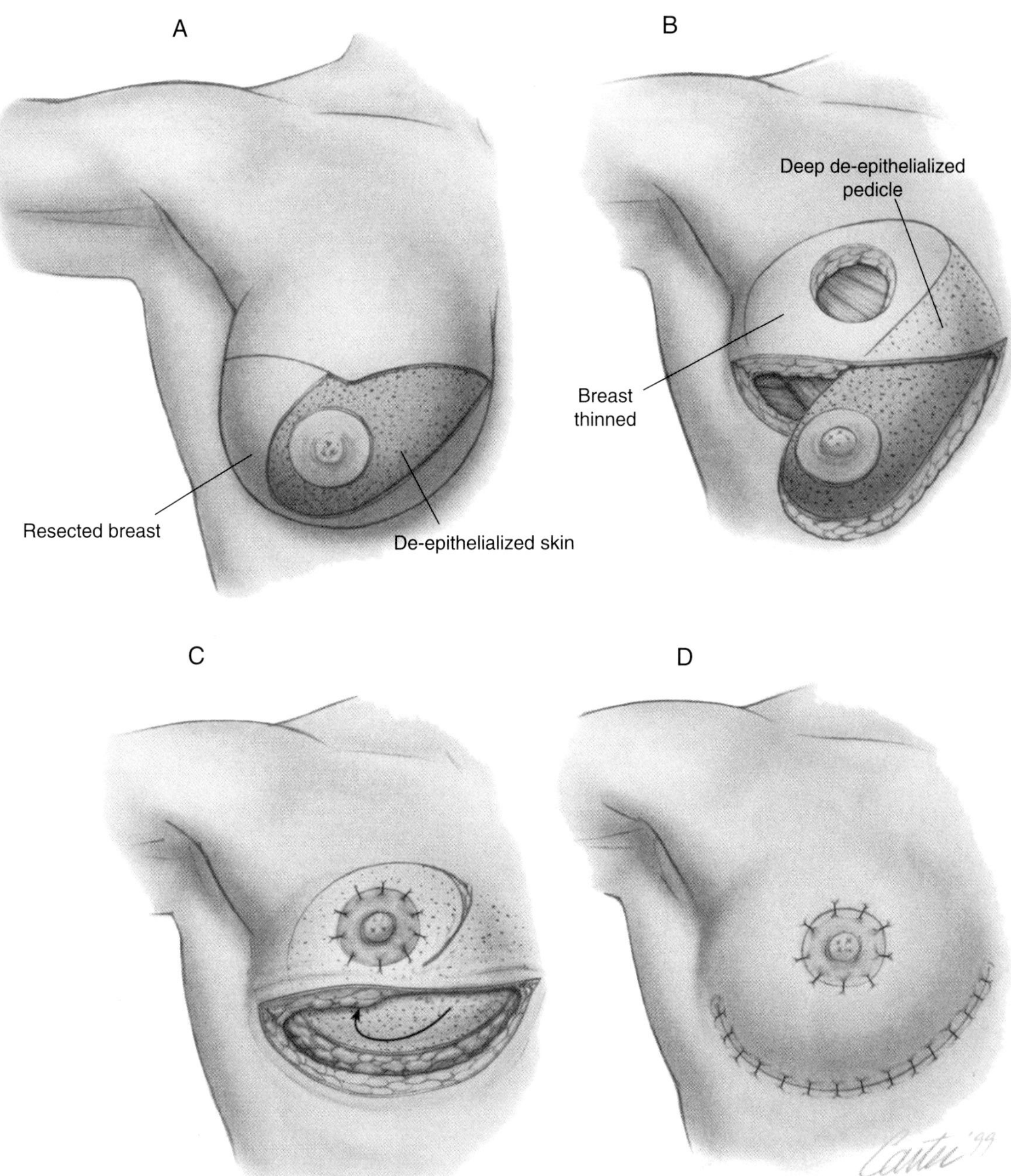

FIGURE 135-2. *A* to *D,* Schwarzmann reduction with superomedial dermoglandular pedicle. (From Lickstein LH, Shestak KC: The conceptual evolution of modern reduction mammaplasty. Operative Techniques Plast Reconstr Surg 1999;6:88.)

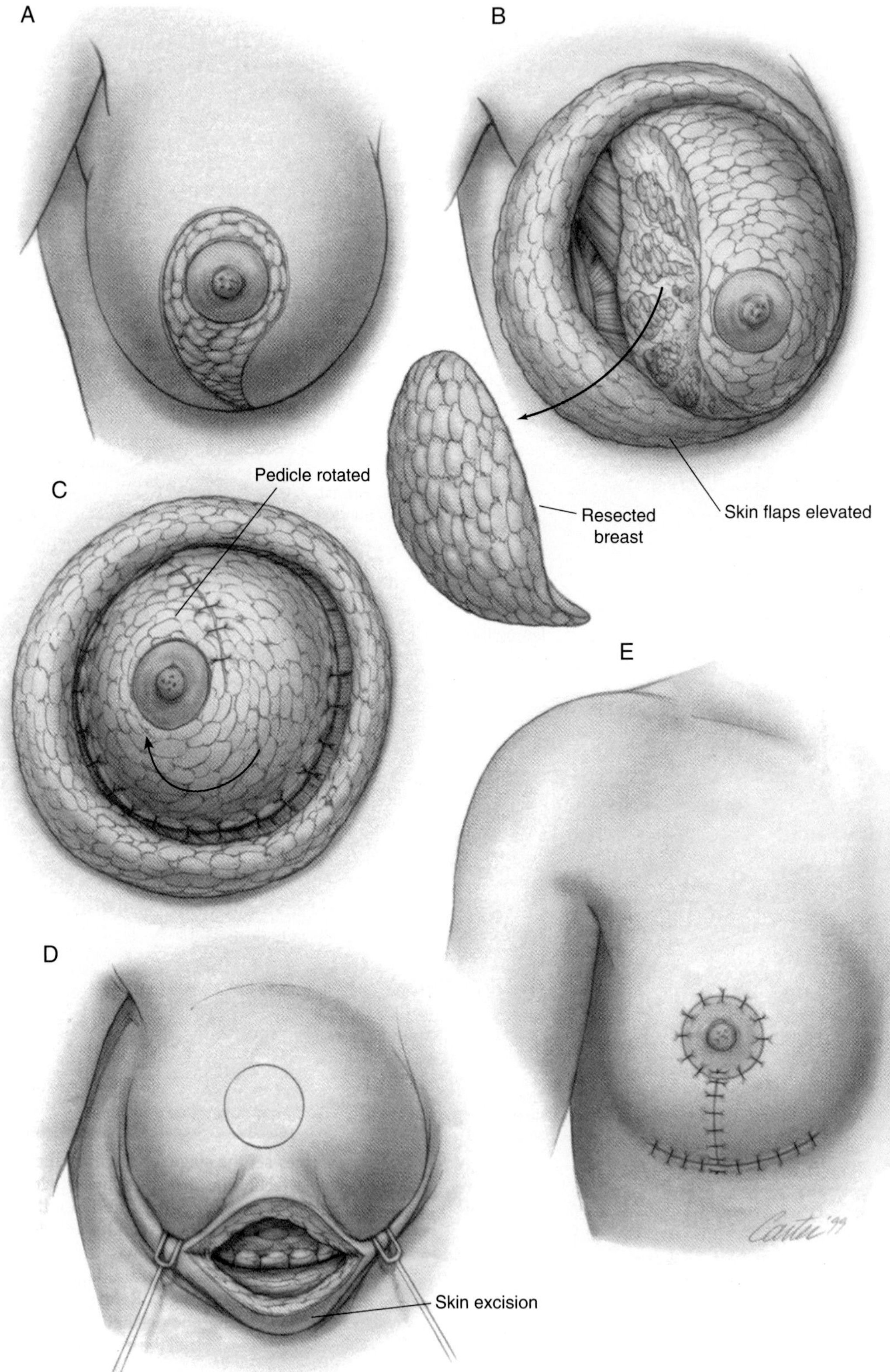

FIGURE 135-3. *A* to *E*, Biesenberger reduction—degloving the breast with inverted T closure. (From Lickstein LH, Shestak KC: The conceptual evolution of modern reduction mammaplasty. Operative Techniques Plast Reconstr Surg 1999;6:88.)

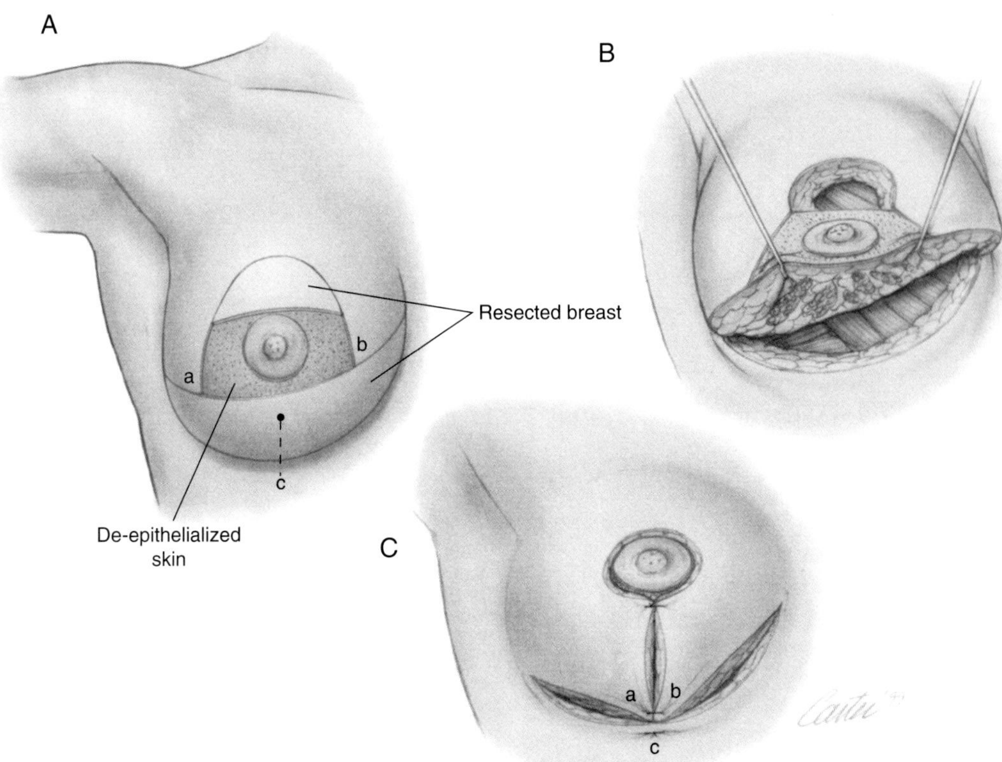

FIGURE 135-4. *A* to *C*, Strombeck horizontal bipedicle technique. (From Lickstein LH, Shestak KC: The conceptual evolution of modern reduction mammaplasty. Operative Techniques Plast Reconstr Surg 1999;6:88.)

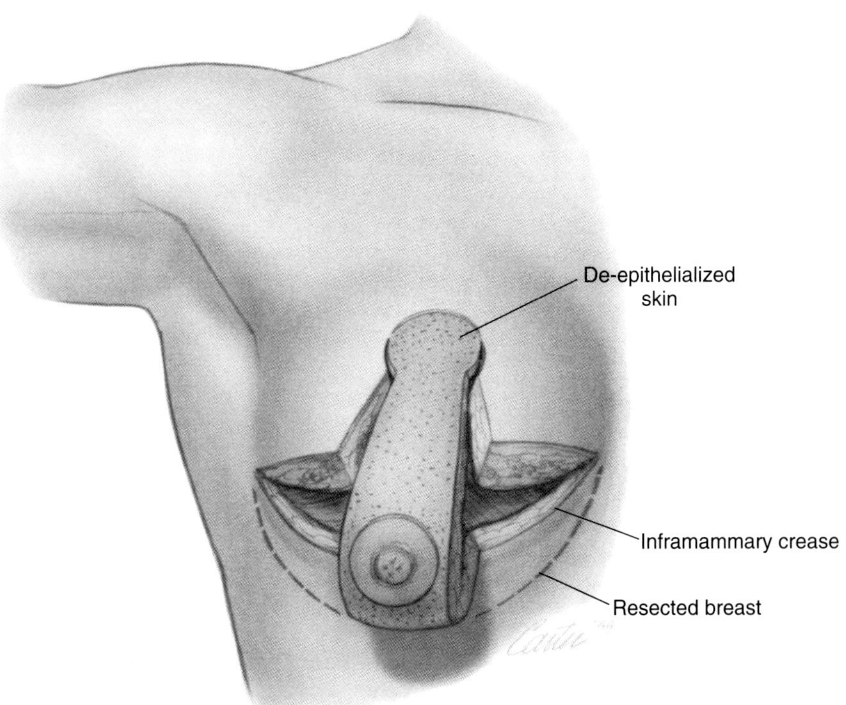

FIGURE 135-5. McKissock vertical bipedicled dermoglandular flap with Wise-pattern skin excision. (From Lickstein LH, Shestak KC: The conceptual evolution of modern reduction mammaplasty. Operative Techniques Plast Reconstr Surg 1999;6:88.)

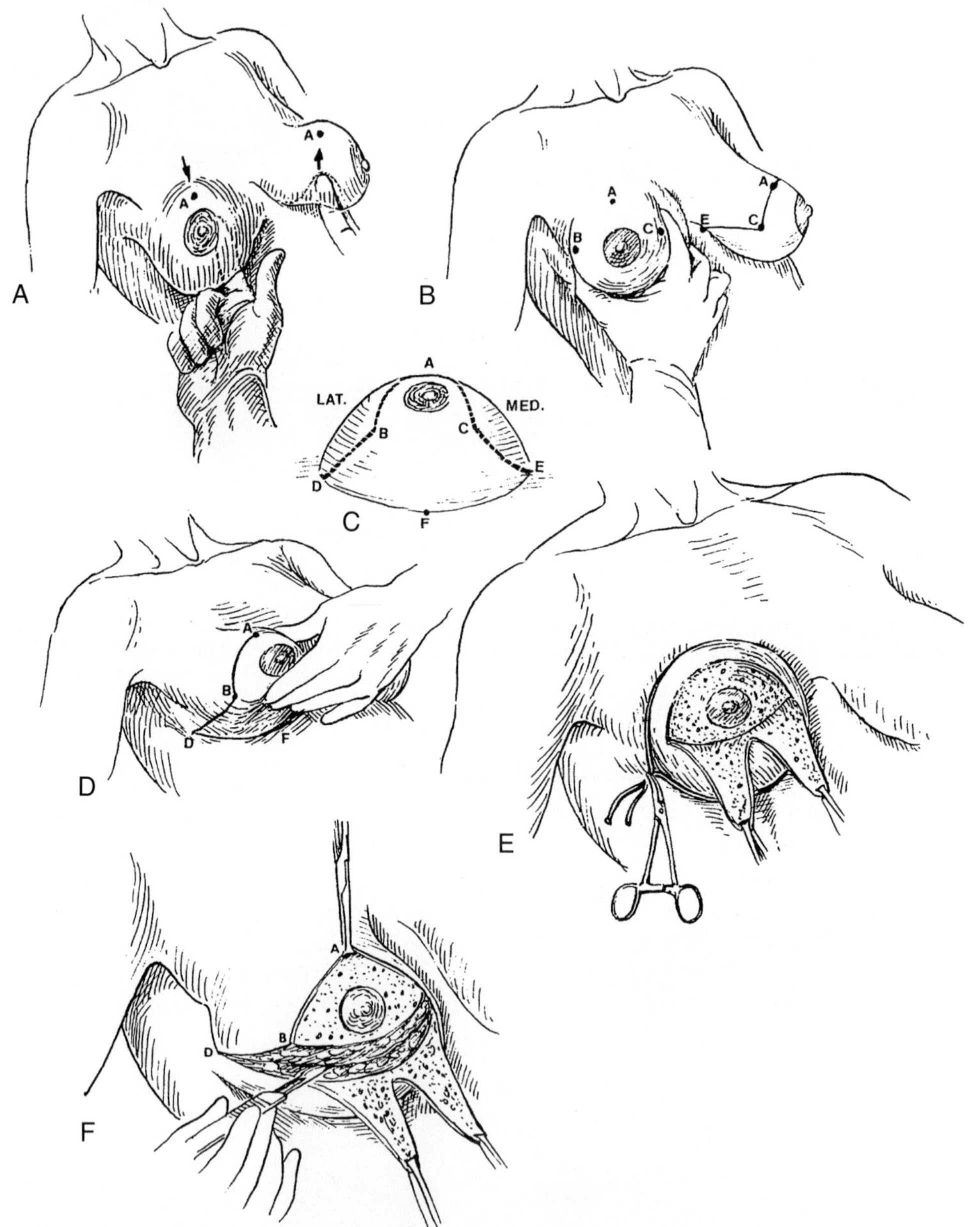

FIGURE 135-6. *A* to *N*, Pitanguy reduction with inferior resection and superior pedicle. (From Aston JJ, Rees TD: Breast reduction and mastopexy. In Rees TD: Aesthetic Plastic Surgery. Philadelphia, WB Saunders, 1980:930.)

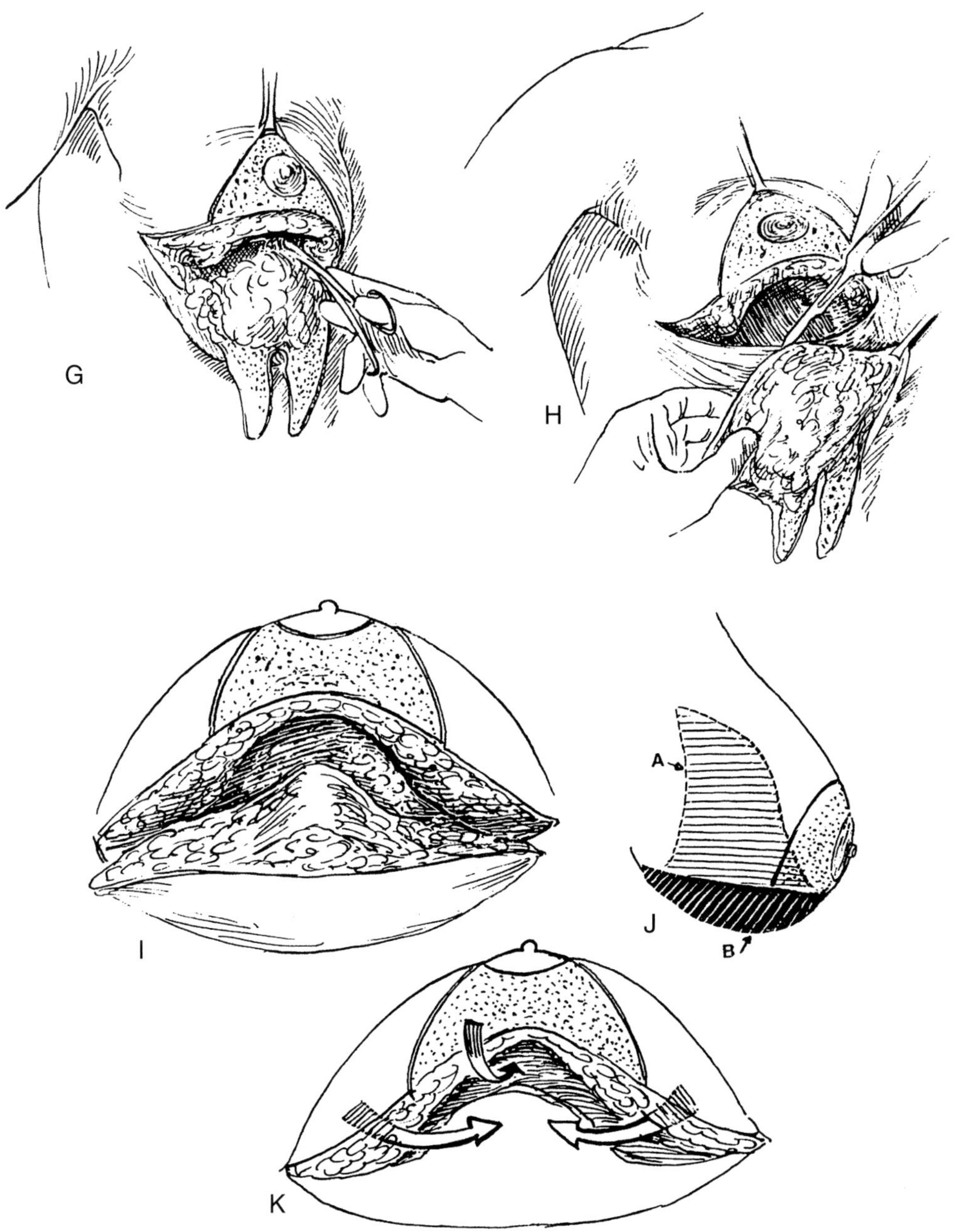

FIGURE 135-6, cont'd.

Continued

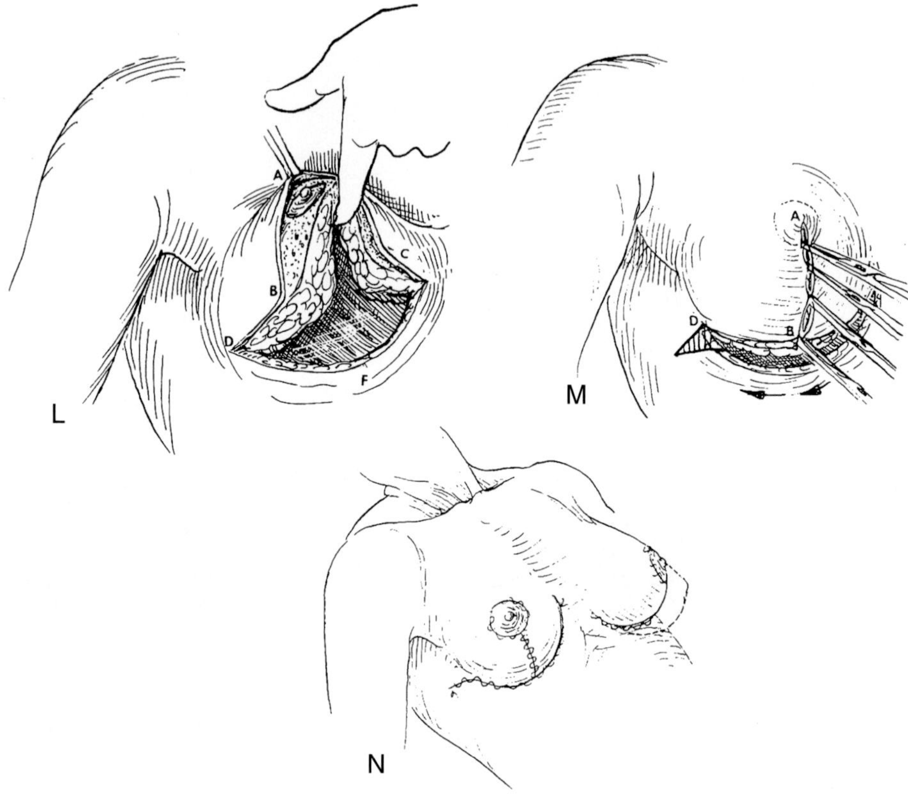

FIGURE 135-6, cont'd.

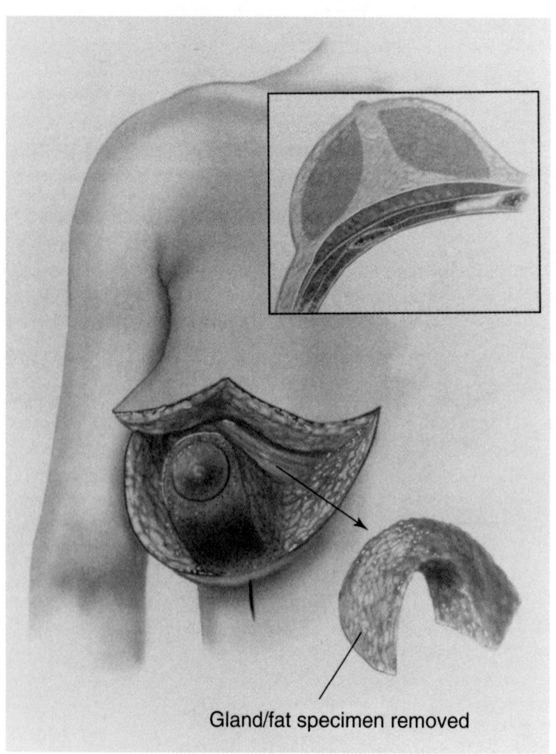

FIGURE 135-7. Inferior pedicle technique with Wise-pattern skin excision.

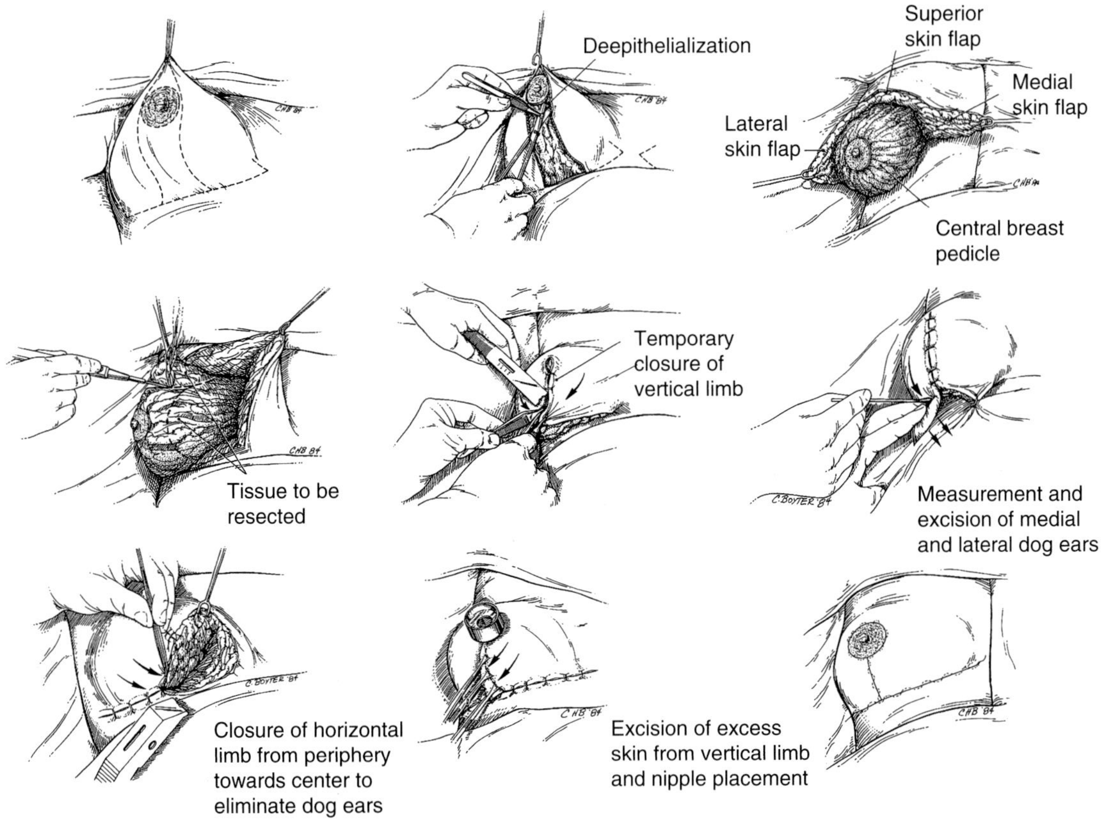

Deepithelialization

Superior skin flap

Medial skin flap

Lateral skin flap

Central breast pedicle

Temporary closure of vertical limb

Tissue to be resected

Measurement and excision of medial and lateral dog ears

Closure of horizontal limb from periphery towards center to eliminate dog ears

Excision of excess skin from vertical limb and nipple placement

FIGURE 135-8. Central mound technique popularized by Hester. (From Hester TR Jr, Bostwick J III, Miller L: Breast reduction utilizing the maximally vascularized central pedicle. Plast Reconstr Surg 1985;76:890.)

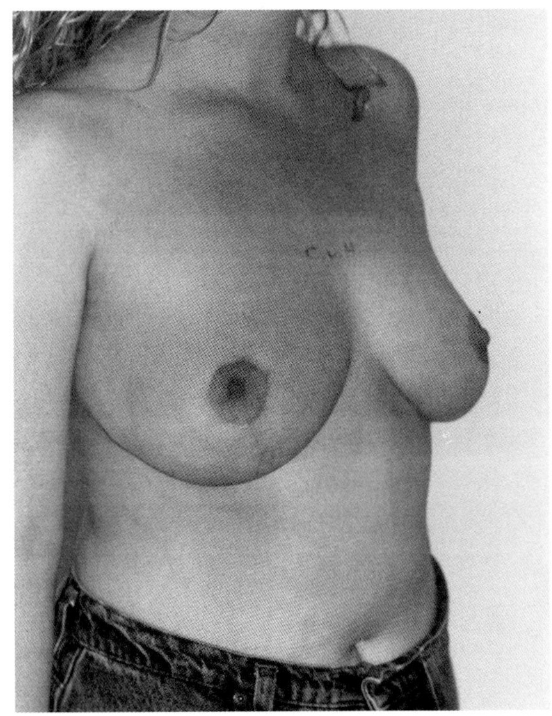

FIGURE 135-9. One-year postoperative view of a young woman after inferior pedicle reduction of 500 g per side demonstrating bottoming out with loss of upper pole fullness.

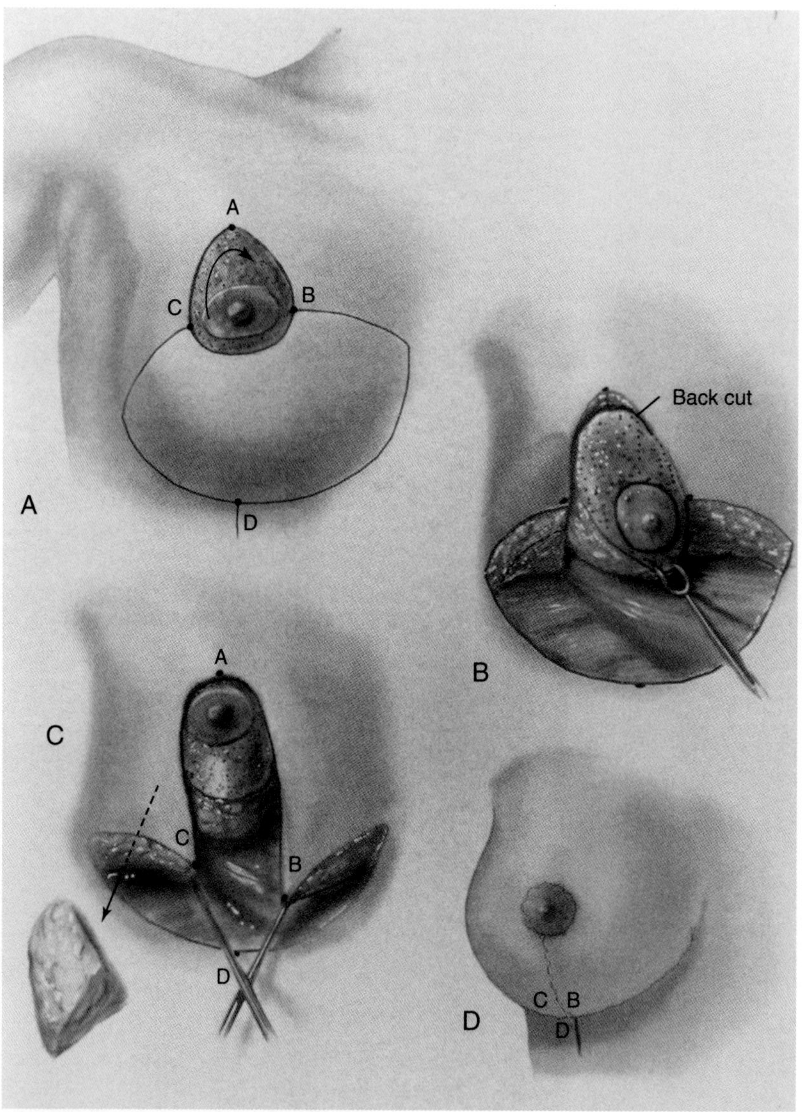

FIGURE 135-10. *A* to *D*, Superomedial pedicle with Wise-pattern skin closure.

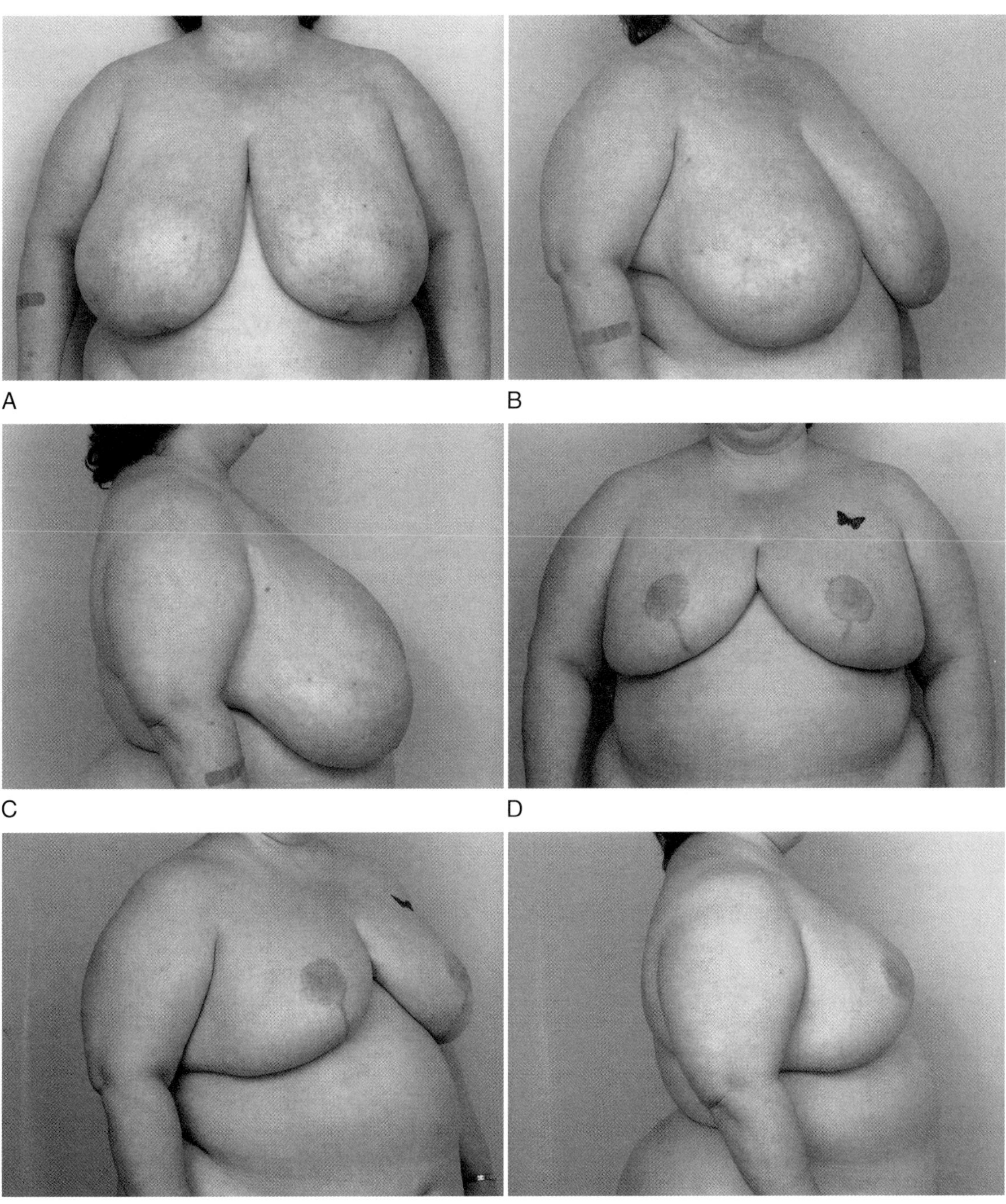

FIGURE 135-11. Preoperative views of patient for superomedial reduction through a Wise-pattern skin excision: *A,* anterior view; *B,* oblique view; *C,* lateral view. Postoperative views at 1 year after resection of 1800 g per side: *D,* anterior view; *E,* oblique view; *F,* lateral view.

TABLE 135-1 ✦ MAJOR ADVANCES IN MODERN BREAST REDUCTION TECHNIQUES

Horizontal bipedicle (Strombeck, 1960)
Superior pedicle (Pitanguy, Weiner, 1962)
Superolateral pedicle (Skoog, 1963)
Vertical bipedicle (McKissock, 1972)
Inferior pedicle (Courtiss, Goldwyn, Ribiero, Robbins, Georgiade, 1975-1977)
Superomedial pedicle (Orlando, 1975)
Central mound (Biesenberger, 1928; Hester, 1985)

Historically, skin excision in these techniques has been based on the Wise-pattern keyhole design. Vertical and short-scar techniques include the following:
Vertical scar (Lassus, Lejour, Hammond SPAIR, Hall-Findlay, 1970-1999; see Figs. 135-17, 135-18, and 135-26)
Vertical scar with short inframammary scar (Marchac, Peixoto, 1980-1982; see Fig. 135-21)
B or J scar reduction (Regnault, Chiari, 1970-1974; see Fig. 135-22)
Periareolar reduction (Benelli, Sampao-Goes, 1990-1996; see Figs. 135-24 and 135-25)

of the Lejour procedure,[33] have emerged. Key to most of these procedures have been the elimination or drastic shortening of any horizontal scars and an emphasis on some form of superior or superomedial pedicle (with the exception of Hammond's SPAIR technique, which uses a modified inferior pedicle). The techniques have proved immensely useful and are gaining in popularity, although the learning curves are steep. They have helped reduce the tendency to severe bottoming out and produce a rounded projectile breast that patients value. The reduction in horizontal scar length or, better still, its complete elimination has been particularly useful in patients prone to hypertrophic scarring (Table 135-1).

Renewed interest is being shown in the horizontal scar techniques as popularized by Passot[6] (see Fig. 135-1). Although there are some pleasing results with this technique, breast flattening may be a problem. In addition, hypertrophic scarring most commonly complicates the horizontal scar component in Wise-pattern reductions, and it seems unfortunate to emphasize this scar once more.

When reviewing these techniques, the reader should be cognizant that it is not how much tissue is taken but what is left behind that will determine outcome. Second, it is not the skin brassiere that molds final breast shape; rather, it is the parenchyma beneath that is crucial to permanence and projection of the reduced breast.

BREAST EMBRYOLOGY

The breast arises from the linear ectodermal ridge or mammary ridge, which extends from the axilla to the groin.[34] This so-called milk line appears at the sixth week of fetal development and may give rise to varying degrees of breast and nipple development at any point along its length if the natural involution of the majority of the mammary ridge does not take place. By the 16th week in utero, the ectodermal ridge has penetrated into the underlying mesoderm and sends approximately 20 ingrowths radially into the developing breast. Each ectodermal bud deepens in its growth pattern and ultimately canalizes into the lactiferous ducts of the established breast. By 28 weeks, the acini develop around the terminal tips of the lactiferous system; the ducts concentrate superficially into a pit in the skin of the embryonic chest wall. Mesodermal proliferation in the area gives rise to the circular and longitudinal smooth muscle fibers of the nipple-areola complex. The areola is of ectodermal origin and contains apocrine glands, enlarged versions of which become Montgomery tubercles. The mature breast contains approximately 20 lobules, each with a primary ductal drainage system. There is overlap between the drainage systems, however, and the lobes cannot be readily identified clinically as distinct anatomic units. Support for the breast comes from both the skin envelope and the fibrous suspensory ligaments of Astley Cooper that anchor the breast to the pectoralis major fascia.

BREAST ANATOMY

The base of the breast overlies the pectoralis major muscle between the second and sixth ribs in the nonptotic state. The gland is anchored to the pectoralis major fascia by the suspensory ligaments first described by Astley Cooper[35] in 1840. The lower pole of the breast is fuller than the upper pole. The tail of Spence extends obliquely up into the medial wall of the axilla. The breast overlies the pectoralis major muscle as well as the uppermost portion of the rectus abdominis muscle inferomedially. The nipple lies above the inframammary crease and is usually level with the fourth rib and just lateral to the midclavicular line. The average nipple to sternal notch measurement in a youthful, well-developed breast is 21 to 22 cm; an equilateral triangle formed between the nipples and sternal notch measures an average of 21 cm per side. This figure is remarkably consistent, considering the enormous variety of shapes seen in the female breast. Ptosis tends to increase both the notch to nipple length and the inframammary fold to nipple distance. The second to sixth intercostal nerves supply breast innervation. Lateral innervation is predominantly from the anterior rami of the lateral cutaneous branches of the third through sixth intercostal nerves. Medial innervation arises from the anterior cutaneous branches of the second through sixth intercostal nerves. Nerve supply to the nipple is from the third, fourth, and fifth anterior and lateral cutaneous nerves.[36] Courtiss and Goldwyn[37] have labeled the fourth intercostal nerve the most important nipple innervator. Whereas this has almost become dogma in plastic surgical teaching, Sarhadi[38] has demonstrated that the lateral cutaneous branches of the third through fifth intercostal nerves and the anterior cutaneous branches of the second through fifth intercostal nerves all contribute to nipple supply. This is probably the explanation for the fact that a remarkably high number of patients retain nipple sensitivity after reduction despite enormous variations in technique and pedicle location. Sarhadi traced the lateral cutaneous branch of the fourth intercostal nerve into the nipple and described two branches. The superficial branch passes up through superficial parenchyma; the deep branch passes inferolaterally on the pectoralis major fascia before coursing up into the areola. This fact might give one pause in considering techniques that rely heavily on inferolateral resection of the gland.

Blood supply to the breast is from multiple sources, including the internal mammary perforators (most notably the second to fifth perforators), the thoracoacromial vessels, the vessels to serratus anterior, the lateral thoracic vessels, and the terminal branches of the third to eighth intercostal vessels.[22] The superomedial perforator supply from the internal mammary vessels is particularly robust and accounts for some 60% of the total breast blood supply. The lateral thoracic supply contributes about 30% of total breast vascularity.[39] There is, however, some degree of variation in dominance of breast blood supply. Maliniac[40] has proposed that one should attempt to preserve as much vascularity as possible during breast reduction.

PHYSIOLOGY OF THE NORMAL BREAST

The breast undergoes three major cycles of development. The initial phase occurs between birth and puberty, during which time there is a gradual increase in breast stroma and glandular tissue. The breast ducts elongate and canalize in preparation for milk storage in later life. Numerous hormonal influences come to bear on the developing breast, including estrogen, progesterone, prolactin, insulin, thyroxine, and growth hormone. The pituitary-based release factors follicle-stimulating hormone and luteinizing hormone trigger the release of estrogen and progesterone, which stimulate breast development at puberty and during pregnancy. Progesterone strongly affects the terminal glandular component; prolactin triggers the differentiation of alveolar epithelial cells into milk-producing cells.[41,42]

During the menstrual cycle, breast size and consistency vary. In the resting phase, the ducts are lined with a bilaminar layer of cuboidal cells; the terminal ductal alveoli have a single cuboidal cell lining. The major draining ducts are lined with pseudostratified columnar epithelium. Stromal tissue increases in density as the periphery of the breast is approached. There are a high number of fibroblasts, plasma cells, lymphocytes, mast cells, and histiocytes in the unstimulated breast.

In the proliferative phase of the menstrual cycle, estrogen rises between days 3 and 7. Intraductal epithelial proliferation occurs, producing two or three layers of polygonal B cells that almost obscure the lumen of the ducts. Stromal density increases, as do the numbers of fibroblasts and plasma cells.

During the second week or luteal phase, progesterone release from the stimulated follicles results in further epithelial proliferation. Myoepithelial cells in the basal layer become more prominent, and B cells increase in number. Columnar A cells with a high RNA content become visible. Inflammatory cells are less obvious.

During the secretory phase of the third week, estrogen, progesterone, and prolactin influence the breast. Steroid hormones trigger lipid droplet formation in the alveoli, and this, combined with water retention, is responsible for the 15% to 30% increase in breast volume premenstrually. The increase in water retention within the stroma appears to be related to an estrogen-induced histamine release affecting the stromal microcirculation. Prolactin stimulates an increase in ribosomes and RNA content within luminal epithelial cells; the stroma becomes less dense with edema and venous congestion. This can become a major source of discomfort.

The final withdrawal phase of the cycle is associated with decline of estrogen and progesterone. While luminal secretions are transiently retained, the stroma reverts to its more densely compacted nonedematous state.

Menopause is characterized by a decline in estrogen associated with a rise in progesterone. Glandular involution occurs with partial regression of glandular epithelium and decreased vascularity and cellularity of the stroma. After menopause, fat infiltration into the breast occurs with increased elasticity and reduced vascularity. Lymphocytic infiltration around the ductal remnants may occur.

Breast enlargement is usually complete by the late teens but may continue into early adulthood. It may be associated with physical abnormalities including hypertrophy, gigantomastia, asymmetry, and ptosis. Excessive weight gain may contribute to massive breast enlargement. Whereas some women experience breast atrophy after menopause, others develop significant secondary breast enlargement with fatty infiltration of the breast. Excessive breast growth may precipitate functional symptoms that cause the patient discomfort and embarrassment.

Mammary hypertrophy appears to be related to abnormal end-organ responsiveness to estrogens.[43-45]

Jabs[46] has shown that women with hypertrophy have a normal number of estrogen receptors and usually have normal estrogen levels, suggestive of end-organ hypersensitivity. The breast stroma increases (both fat and fibrous elements) while the glandular component remains fairly low. Eliasen[47] has shown that benign ductal hyperplasia is a common component of hypertrophied breasts, but there does not seem to be an increased cancer risk in these patients unless obesity is associated as a risk factor. Juvenile hypertrophy manifests in late childhood or early adolescence and was first described as early as 1670 by Durston.[48] Gigantomastia is defined as a breast size requiring a resection of at least 1800 g per side. It usually starts in early adolescence and is independent of body weight. Patients are highly symptomatic and require radical surgery because spontaneous involution is rare. Ongoing breast development after reduction is a risk and may necessitate further surgery at a later age. Unilateral enlargement should be carefully evaluated to exclude giant fibroadenoma, cystosarcoma phyllodes, virginal hamartoma, virginal hypertrophy, hematoma, and of course the rare but occasional breast cancer in adolescence. Attempts to suppress breast development with hormone manipulation have been ineffective. Baker[49] has shown tamoxifen to have a positive effect in some young girls with virginal hypertrophy, but the adverse effects of long-term tamoxifen therapy, especially in a young patient, preclude its safe use.

EVALUATION OF BREAST ENLARGEMENT

History

In taking a history of patients with mammary hypertrophy, there are several important areas of investigation (Table 135-2). In younger patients, psychological issues and personal embarrassment are key elements in the patient's decision to seek surgery. It is common to see these women walk into the office wearing loose-fitting clothing; their body posture reflects a desire to hide the true size of the breasts by hunching and rounding of the shoulders or stooping. Older women tend to complain more about the physical symptoms of mammary hypertrophy, and backache is often a more prominent complaint. Older women may also complain about the difficulties inherent in achieving adequate mammograms, and compression pain may be significant. If women are married or have partners, the attitude of a significant other toward the patient's large breasts should also be tactfully ascertained. Some spouses are extremely hostile to the concept of reduction surgery; they can be reassured that the procedure will be performed in such a way as to leave the patient with a breast size and shape still in proportion to the woman's body habitus. Active women may also complain about their inability to exercise without discomfort, and sports bras may be inadequate to provide the support necessary for effective participation in a physically active lifestyle.

TABLE 135-2 ✦ PATIENT'S HISTORY—IMPORTANT AREAS OF INVESTIGATION

Evaluate the symptoms of hypertrophy, including upper thoracic backache, grooving of the shoulders by bra straps, breast pain, rashes beneath or between the breasts during summer months, and psychological factors such as embarrassment and anxiety.
Review breast cancer risk factors (personal and familial).
Discuss scarring tendencies.
Review the history of any bleeding disorders, diabetes, or collagen vascular disease.
Discuss smoking history.
Review general medical background.

Physical Examination

Physical examination should be thorough and include a competent general examination as well as a local breast examination. The patient's height and weight are attained together with an evaluation of the patient's general body habitus. Full physical examination should be performed at the initial assessment and should incorporate psychological assessment of the patient's demeanor and expectations.

Local breast examination is performed to exclude masses, and any suspicious lesion should be fully evaluated with appropriate investigations before surgery. It is advisable to obtain preoperative mammograms in all patients older than 35 years. The axillae and supraclavicular fossae are palpated for lymphadenopathy. Breast skin is evaluated for striae and scars, and patients should be warned that striae might be more visible postoperatively after stretching of the breast skin envelope with reduction surgery. Assessment of breast scars is important because they may transgress pedicle designs and compromise flap blood supply, especially if they have been recently incurred. The nipple-areola complex is assessed for size, shape, and sensitivity. In general, the larger the breast, the more likely a patient is to start experiencing reduction in sensitivity preoperatively, possibly owing to the effects of extreme traction on cutaneous nerves by the weight of the breast. Although a generalization, it is also true that the more radical the reduction, the more likely a patient is to suffer long-term postoperative numbness of the nipples. The surgeon should evaluate asymmetry and bring this to the patient's attention; any postoperative asymmetry will become a focus of attention, and patients may also question why differing amounts of tissue were removed from each breast if they happen to read an operative report related to a breast asymmetry procedure.

It is crucial to measure the nipple to sternal notch, nipple to inframammary fold, and internipple distances. Not only does this give the surgeon an opportunity to measure subtle differences in breast size and shape, but it also allows one to assess the technique to be used for reduction. Sternal notch to nipple distance usually lies between 19 and 22 cm in the "ideal" breast and may be anywhere from 25 to 50 cm or more in patients with very large breasts. The longer the nipple to notch measurement, the less likely a patient is to be a candidate for a superiorly based pedicle reduction. Similarly, if the inframammary fold to nipple distance is excessively long, this may preclude the use of an inferior pedicle technique. Vertical short-scar techniques such as that described by Lassus are preferred and may be performed comfortably if the nipple to notch measurement is less than 38 cm. If the inframammary fold to nipple distance is more than 22 cm, there may be difficulty with inferior pedicle or central mound techniques. With nipple to notch distances of more than 40 cm, one should seriously consider lower pole breast amputation through a Wise skin pattern with either free nipple grafting or preferably immediate nipple reconstruction with subsequent tattoo of the areola.

Specific Investigations

Mammography should be performed preoperatively in all patients with risk factors and in any patient older than 35 years. High-resolution digital mammography is making inroads into the field, but its availability is still limited. Ultrasound evaluation should be performed if lesions may be cystic and amenable to aspiration for cytology. Magnetic resonance imaging is still finding its true place in the evaluation of the breast. Although its role is clearly preeminent in evaluation of implant rupture, its role in breast cancer is limited to the high-risk breast with lesions that are difficult to clarify by conventional techniques. Investigations for associated musculoskeletal symptoms should also be conducted. It is also recommended that all minors requesting breast reduction undergo psychological evaluation and counseling.

TREATMENT PLANNING

Indications for Surgery

There are both minor and major indications for surgery (Table 135-3). In addition to these indications, breast cancer management has established a novel reason for therapeutic breast reduction. The ongoing move toward breast conservation internationally has led to difficulties when radiation oncologists are faced with providing adequate dosages to the entire gland in women with mammary hypertrophy. The high dosages required to achieve adequate treatment of a large breast parenchymal volume may predispose the patient to greater risks of fat necrosis and fibrosis in the long term. Lumpectomy followed by a therapeutic or "oncoplastic" reduction as described by Audretsch[50] and Clough[51] has made breast conservation feasible in patients who would otherwise not have been good candidates for this treatment modality. Aside from this aspect of cancer management, there are also data to suggest that reduction surgery in the benign breast may reduce the incidence of breast cancer development at a later stage in the patient's life.[52]

TABLE 135-3 ✦ MAJOR AND MINOR INDICATIONS FOR BREAST REDUCTION SURGERY

Major Indications
Very large breasts
Shoulder pain
Cervical and upper thoracic backache
Severe embarrassment, physically or sexually
Recurrent intertrigo
Minor Indications
Inability to exercise due to breast discomfort
Difficulty with breathing during exercise
Difficulty finding clothing to fit
Grooving and hyperpigmentation of shoulder strap areas

Although symptoms of mammary hypertrophy can be divided into local, musculoskeletal, and dermatologic, the spectrum of complaints progresses as breast size increases. Mammary hypertrophy is typically associated with heaviness, discomfort, and a dragging sensation in the breasts. The large breast mass lying in front of the body's normal center of gravity may establish a tendency to exaggeration of the natural thoracic lordosis. Cervical and upper thoracic backaches are almost ubiquitous complaints among women suffering from mammary hypertrophy.[53] This in turn leads to a need for the muscles bracing the shoulder girdle to work excessively at keeping the patient's shoulders back, resulting in hypertrophy, particularly true in the trapezius muscles. These muscles bulge unattractively above the patient's shoulders while the downward traction of bra straps may form grooves in the distal insertion of the trapezius to the acromion. Prolonged friction within these grooves produces hyperpigmentation in the bra strap lines. The pendulous nature of most massive breasts may cause problems with personal hygiene; in the summer months, trapped moisture and body heat provide an excellent milieu in which fungal infections can take root. Patients often mention a need for the use of antifungal and steroid creams to reduce these heat-induced and fungal rashes. Staphylococcal superinfection of these inframammary rashes can result in impetigo. Body odor may become offensive in some patients.

The larger the breast, the more difficult it becomes to exercise or to find clothes that fit. The patient's embarrassment in front of family and friends can lead to significant psychological effects including unwillingness to be seen naked by a spouse. The inability to exercise may potentiate a preexisting tendency to obesity and result in further deterioration in breast size. As the breasts enlarge, the ease of finding a bra of appropriate size becomes increasingly difficult, and patients resort to buying expensive custom bras or, more commonly, attempt to force their oversized breasts into bras several sizes too large for their chest circumference as these bras tend to incorporate bigger cup sizes. Large breasts out of proportion to the lower body also have an impact on the patient's ability to purchase clothing that fits both the upper and lower halves of the body comfortably. Frequently, the chest size dictates purchase of larger tops with smaller skirt or pants sizes and precludes patients from wearing dresses.

The overall impact of mammary hypertrophy on a patient's daily life becomes highly significant. It is particularly distressing for younger girls and women, especially when they think that they are the object of unwanted stares and derision. Kerrigan[54,55] has been responsible for evaluating the impact of breast hypertrophy on women's health in several well-designed prospective studies. In her initial study, she identified the impact of macromastia as being as significant as that of serious health conditions like moderate angina and kidney transplants. In a subsequent study, Kerrigan demonstrated that patients with hypertrophy experienced a significant negative impact on their health, whether or not they sought treatment for macromastia. Of particular note was the finding that the symptoms associated with hypertrophy were more important than the actual breast volume, a finding corroborated by Netscher.[56] Netscher also found that symptoms are independent of the patient's age and weight. In another landmark study by Kerrigan's group, a surgical treatment group was matched with two control groups, one with D cup breasts and another with breasts smaller than a D cup, both of which groups did not receive surgery.[57] The nonoperative group with large breasts failed to achieve symptomatic relief despite conservative measures. By contrast, the surgical group with hypertrophy had a decrease in back-centered pain from 50% preoperatively to less than 10% postoperatively. Preoperatively, all patients had scored poorly in tests measuring quality of life and mental and physical parameters. Postoperatively, the study group's scores were above the national average scores in all areas tested.

Mammary hypertrophy has a significant impact on women's lives, and reduction surgery offers real medical and psychological benefits to these patients. Insurance companies need to understand these outcome studies as they seek to limit access of patients to surgery.[58-65]

Selection of Technique

The specific technique one should use for a given patient depends on several factors, including breast size, estimated resection volume, breast shape, and the more elusive concept of experience (Table 135-4). Breast hypertrophy may be divided into mild, moderate, major, and gigantic. These are represented by resections of less than 200 g, 200 to 500 g, 500 to 1500 g, and more than 1500 g per side.

EVALUATION OF BREAST SIZE AND ESTIMATION OF RESECTION VOLUMES

Technique selection is based on the surgeon's preference and breast size and shape. Chest wall and breast diameters also factor into this decision. Patients should have their bra strap circumference measured in inches at the level of the strap, just beneath the inframammary crease, as well as under the arms. The breast

TABLE 135-4 ✦ OPERATIVE TECHNIQUES IN BREAST REDUCTION

Early horizontal and combined scar techniques
- Passot procedure (see Fig. 135-1)
- Schwarzmann medial dermoglandular pedicle (see Fig. 135-2)
- Biesenberger technique (see Fig. 135-3)

Wise-pattern approaches
- Inferior pedicle technique (see Fig. 135-7)
- Pitanguy technique (see Fig. 135-6)
- Strombeck horizontal pedicle technique (see Fig. 135-4)
- McKissock technique (see Fig. 135-5)
- Lateral pedicle technique
- Superomedial pedicle technique (see Fig. 135-10)
- Central mound technique (see Fig. 135-8)
- Breast amputation and free nipple graft, Wise pattern (see Fig. 135-27)

Short-scar techniques
- Lassus-Lejour technique (see Fig. 135-17)
- Hall-Findlay technique (see Fig. 135-18)
- Marchac short-scar technique (see Fig. 135-21)
- Regnault B technique (see Fig. 135-22)
- L reduction (see Fig. 135-23)
- Benelli round block technique (see Fig. 135-24)
- Goes periareolar approach (see Fig. 135-25)
- Hammond SPAIR approach (see Fig. 135-26)

Liposuction-assisted reduction (Courtiss and Matarasso) (see Fig. 135-13)

circumference at the nipple can then be measured with the breasts in a bra (Fig. 135-12). For every inch above the strap size, cup size increases by a factor of 1. For example, a woman with a 34-inch strap size and a 36-inch breast circumference has a 34B cup bra; if her breast measurement is 38 inches, she has a 34D cup bra. In terms of breast volume per cup size, various formulas have been described. One suggested concept is as follows: for a bra strap size of 32 to 34 inches, each cup size represents 100 g; 36 to 38 inches, 200 g; 40 to 42 inches, 300 g; 44 to 46 inches, 400 g. Theoretically, a patient with a 40DD bra wishing to have a C cup final result would require a resection of at least 300 × 2 or 600 g per side. In practice, this figure is often greater, and these formulas should be used only as a rough guide. The goal of surgery is to form a mature, slightly

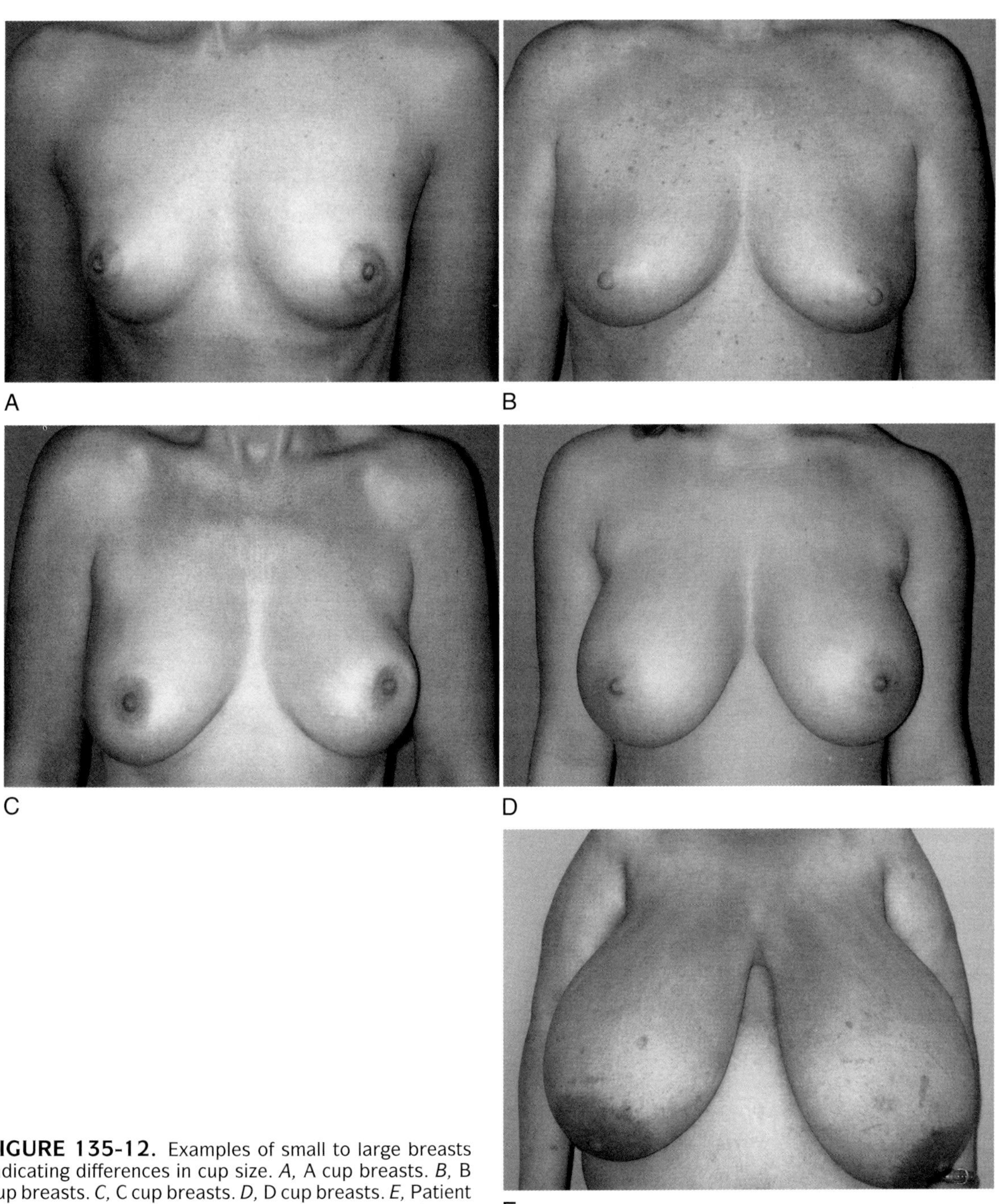

FIGURE 135-12. Examples of small to large breasts indicating differences in cup size. *A,* A cup breasts. *B,* B cup breasts. *C,* C cup breasts. *D,* D cup breasts. *E,* Patient with large asymmetric breasts who wears a J cup bra.

pendulous breast in proportion to the patient's overall body habitus. Several authors have cautioned against offering a patient a virginal-looking breast.[9,11,66] Technically, this goal is rarely feasible.

DETERMINING NIPPLE LOCATION AND SIZE

Penn[11] demonstrated that the nipple lies 21 cm from the sternal notch and midsternal point and forms an equilateral triangle with the other nipple and the notch. The average nipple to inframammary fold distance in his study was about 7 cm. Heavier projectile breasts often require a longer nipple to inframammary fold distance. This is often seen in vertical reductions, where this distance may settle at 8 to 12 cm yet appear entirely normal to the examining eye and provide a pleasing aesthetic effect. Pitanguy[16] recommended use of the midhumeral point plus 2 or 3 cm for determining the new nipple level. Nipple diameter is often grossly dilated in patients with huge breasts and areolar reduction is an integral part of breast reduction surgery. The average areola diameter is 38 to 45 mm.

SMALL TO MODERATE REDUCTIONS (150-500 g per side)

Vertical scar techniques are particularly suited to these reductions with minimal risk of skin redundancy at the inframammary fold.[24-27,32,33] Periareolar techniques, such as the Benelli and Goes procedures, can be valuable, but attention must be paid to careful breast shaping to avoid flattening of the breast mound, and permanent pursestring sutures should be placed to avoid spreading of the areolar diameter in the long term.[30,31]

For minor resections, almost any technique will suffice, but the short-scar procedures are particularly helpful because an unnecessary horizontal scar is avoided on a breast that could easily be handled with a vertical or periareolar reduction. The same indications for vertical reductions apply to moderate resections of less than 500 g per side.

MAJOR REDUCTIONS (500-1500 g per side)

For reductions in excess of 500 g per side, the periareolar procedures are generally not appropriate. One should select either a vertical technique, such as the Lassus-Lejour, Hall-Findlay, or SPAIR operation, or a standard Wise-pattern technique, such as the inferior or central pedicle or a superomedial pedicle approach.[14-22] Again, it is preferable to use short-scar vertical reductions for these patients. Results are predictable and complications are few if the procedure is well executed. These operations produce well-rounded breasts with excellent projection and much less tendency to bottom out with time. Scars are minimized.

MASSIVE REDUCTIONS (>1500 g per side)

When it comes to resections of more than 1500 g per side, many of the same principles described for major reductions apply; but once resections approach 1800 to 2000 g per side, one should consider breast amputation rather than relying on a pedicle to maintain a nipple's viability. If the inframammary fold to nipple distance is less than 22 cm in such patients, a central mound reduction is still reliable and safe. Its use can be extended if the patient is not too ptotic because the pedicle length may still be within acceptable limits even in the presence of a massive breast. When the breasts are much larger, it is often difficult to achieve a small enough pedicle to give adequate reduction volume while still keeping the nipple vascularized. One also runs into the difficulty of trying to produce a pleasing shape in these huge reductions when dealing with the presence of a large pedicle.

Breast amputation is preferable for patients with gigantomastia.[67,68] The real dilemma with this procedure is the morbidity associated with free nipple grafts in patients of color. Although scattered melanocyte loss in white patients may not be that noticeable, it can be significant for black patients, who develop a piebald appearance to the grafted nipple in some circumstances. Even with good graft thinning and an apparently excellent take, it is surprising how many of these women may develop hypopigmentation of their nipple grafts. Tattooing of color into the depigmented areas is almost universally useless because the color tends toward a dull gray rather than dark brown. A reasonable solution is to perform total nipple-areola reconstruction, which, although radical, provides an extremely pleasing shape and appearance to the breast.

TECHNIQUE SELECTION AND PREOPERATIVE BREAST SHAPE

Patients with large axillary fat rolls benefit from suction lipectomy of the axillary area. Patients having liposuction should be warned that lateral suction may prove to be the most painful part of the procedure postoperatively. True accessory breast tissue is best dealt with by direct resection, including skin, leaving a linear scar at the anterior axillary fold.

Patients with a broad breast are well served by the Lassus-Lejour and vertical Arie-Pitanguy techniques,[16,69] which narrow the base of the breast more effectively than the standard Wise-pattern techniques, which may flatten the breast unattractively.[70] The SPAIR procedure is effective in shaping the broad breast by virtue of the internal shaping sutures integral to this technique.

Narrow-chested women also benefit from the narrowing achieved with the Lassus-Lejour type of reductions. With experience in vertical reduction, the Wise pattern is less frequently used in small to moderate breast reductions.

Patients having periareolar procedures should be warned that the anteroposterior projection of the breast may be flattened and the pursestring closure may stretch out with time unless a permanent suture such as Gore-Tex is inserted.

Additional Preoperative and Perioperative Considerations

Several issues should be clarified before proceeding with reduction surgery. The use of prophylactic antibiotics, the possibility of transfusion, the use of drains, the place of local anesthetic infiltration, and the use of tumescent infiltration should be addressed in planning the operative procedure.

PROPHYLACTIC ANTIBIOTICS

Antibiotic prophylaxis in elective breast surgery has been widely practiced for decades. Perioperative antibiotic therapy in the form of an intravenous dose of medication with induction followed by one or two doses postoperatively seems a reasonable course of action. Perioperative dosing is certainly recognized as being efficacious in other areas of surgery. The use of longer term therapy is less clearly established.

Several studies have produced conflicting reports in the plastic surgical literature. Platt et al[71] described 2587 patients who underwent breast surgery ranging from benign lumpectomies to reductions and mastectomies. Their conclusion was that antibiotic prophylaxis significantly reduced sepsis rates. In a much smaller study, Serletti[72] prospectively evaluated two groups of breast reduction patients; one group received prophylactic antibiotics and the other did not. Antibiotic prophylaxis made no difference to infection rates, whereas risk factors such as obesity and large reduction volumes did affect wound healing rates and infection.

Antibiotic prophylaxis is recommended for all implant procedures as well as for most major breast operations, such as TRAM flaps and reductions.

AUTOLOGOUS BLOOD TRANSFUSION

Autologous transfusion is almost certainly unnecessary. Numerous techniques exist to reduce blood loss during reduction surgery. The use of tumescent infiltration with epinephrine-containing wetting solution has had a major impact on reducing blood loss during breast reduction, allowing the surgeon to use scalpel dissection for quick and relatively bloodless resection. Clugston[73] evaluated the use of autologous blood transfusion in reduction mammaplasty and found no benefit in terms of postoperative hemoglobin level, length of stay, and cost.

DRAINS

The use of drains has been a surgical dictum in breast reduction surgery for decades. A study failed to show any major benefit to the routine use of drains after breast reduction.[74] They add to the patient's discomfort and will not prevent hematoma formation. Meticulous attention to securing hemostasis is more important in achieving a reduction in hematoma rates than is the use of drains.

TUMESCENT INFILTRATION OF EPINEPHRINE-CONTAINING SOLUTIONS

The use of wetting solutions containing epinephrine has made a major difference to both the safety and efficacy of liposuction.[75] Blood loss has been dramatically reduced as a direct consequence of this use. It would seem logical to apply the same technology to other procedures, including breast reduction. As mentioned before, transfusion has been used after breast reduction because the procedure can be bloody. Whereas electrocautery makes a substantial difference to blood loss, it does slow the procedure, and it works poorly in a saturated environment. Tumescent infiltration of a wetting solution along planned resection lines forms a relatively bloodless track along which scalpel dissection may be used with minimal blood loss. It allows quick and easy dissection with little staining of the field by blood, and when bleeding does occur, the bleeding point is readily identified and treated with electrocautery. It does not appear to interfere with pedicle viability, but infiltration directly into the pedicle is generally avoided. The solution should also contain local anesthetic solution as a means of providing some degree of local intraoperative analgesia. Epinephrine is typically infiltrated at a concentration of 1:1,000,000 when wetting solutions are used.

HOSPITALIZATION—IS IT NECESSARY?

Several studies have documented a safe experience with outpatient breast reduction surgery. Davies[76] and Short[77] have both reported safe, cost-effective outcomes with outpatient reductions. One of the largest studies to date has been reported by Buenaventura et al.[77a] They described a series of 338 patients undergoing breast reduction, 286 of whom (84.6%) were treated as outpatients. The remaining 52 (15.4%) were treated as inpatients and were older on average by 8 years, often requiring larger volume resections (1896 g versus 1486 g). They reported a high degree of satisfaction of patients with outpatient care, and up to $2500 was saved per patient. It is clear from these studies that outpatient management is both feasible and safe. It is probably still wise to admit patients undergoing larger reduction and older women with potentially serious medical histories. When admission is required, 23-hour observation is usually all that is necessary.

MAMMOGRAPHY AND BREAST REDUCTION

Mammography, an essential tool in breast screening, may be compromised by the effects of postsurgical scarring. In an effort to evaluate the radiologic changes induced in the breast after reduction mammaplasty, Danikas et al[78] reviewed the mammograms of 113 patients operated on during a 7-year period. Surgeons involved in the study had used either the vertical bipedicle McKissock technique or the inferior pedicle approach. There were no significant differences on the basis of technique. Reduction surgery resulted in parenchymal redistribution (90%) and elevation of the nipple (84.9%) secondary to glandular pseudoptosis. Calcification was seen in 25% and oil cysts in 19%, both due to fat necrosis. Retroareolar fibrosis was seen in 20%. Areolar thickening was present in 5.3% and skin thickening was found in 1.7% compared with the nonsurgical control group.

OPERATIVE TECHNIQUES

(see Table 135-4)

Liposuction-Assisted Reduction

Liposuction reduction was proposed originally by Grazer[79] and subsequently by Teimourian[80] in 1985. Teimourian recommended suction lipectomy as an adjunct to excisional reduction; Matarasso and Courtiss[81] proposed suction alone as a means for reducing breast volume without excision in selected patients, publishing a series of nine patients in 1991 (Fig. 135-13). Selection criteria included patients with elastic skin and predominantly fatty breasts with nipples in a normal nonptotic position. Early reports represented suction volumes of less than 500 mL per side, but Courtiss[82] later reported suction volumes of up to 835 mL per side. Breast edema lasted for up to a year but eventually settled, and nipple-areola diameters decreased with time while nipple levels rose slightly. Complications were absent in his small initial series, and patients were satisfied with the lack of extensive breast scars. Breast size is not dramatically changed, but for the patient wishing conservative reduction and who is afraid of scarring or who suffers from keloids, it may be a reasonable option. Gray has reported suction volumes up to 2250 mL in a series of 45 patients without complications. Skin retraction was satisfactory, and ptosis responded well. Matarasso continues to advocate its use but advises increasing tumescent infiltration levels to 1.5 mL per milliliter of aspirate instead of a 1:1 ratio. He advocates undercorrection of postmenopausal women but suggests reducing younger premenopausal women to their desired size.

One of the primary initial concerns with suction was the possibility of inducing fat necrosis, leading to intramammary calcification. A 2-year follow-up of Courtiss' original patients has failed to demonstrate any traumatic calcification. This observation has been corroborated by Lejour,[83] who performed extensive whole breast liposuction in her series of vertical reductions without evidence of traumatic calcification. She did not advocate use of liposuction alone except for the older woman desiring a conservative reduction without extensive scars or a major operation. Greater concern has been voiced about the use of ultrasound-assisted liposuction in the breast. Calcification has not been seen as a cause for concern after either suction modality. The role of ultrasonic energy in inducing malignant change remains unclear, although this is probably more theoretical than practical. At this time, ultrasound-assisted liposuction is not strongly advised if breast suction alone is planned. A more significant concern is that of obtaining tissue for pathologic examination after liposuction. This should be discussed carefully with the patient and a full breast examination should be performed preoperatively, including mammography as indicated. At this time, most surgeons tend to relegate suction to male patients with gynecomastia or use it as an adjunct to conventional reduction techniques for spot reduction.

Wise-Pattern Marking Design and Techniques

The Wise skin pattern remains the most commonly used design for pedicled breast reduction techniques today.[14] Skin marking is done preoperatively with the patient in the erect position.

The nipple location is marked with the weight taken off the breast to prevent unsightly elevation of the areola above the edge of the bra postoperatively as the lightened breast rides up on the chest wall. This deformity is almost impossible to correct without producing unsightly scars on the upper pole of the breast. Nipple height is placed opposite the inframammary fold, 19 to 23 cm from the suprasternal notch (depending on the patient's height) or 1 to 2 cm below the midhumeral point (Pitanguy point).

If a Wise pattern is used, the vertical limbs should be designed to leave a final postoperative length of 4.5 to 5 cm from the inframammary fold to the edge of the areola because the inframammary scar will lengthen with time in most of these patients as the breast bottoms out. Horizontal limbs should "steal" up onto the breast mound medially and laterally to remain within the final postoperative breast crease. The wider the angle of the Wise pattern apex, the greater

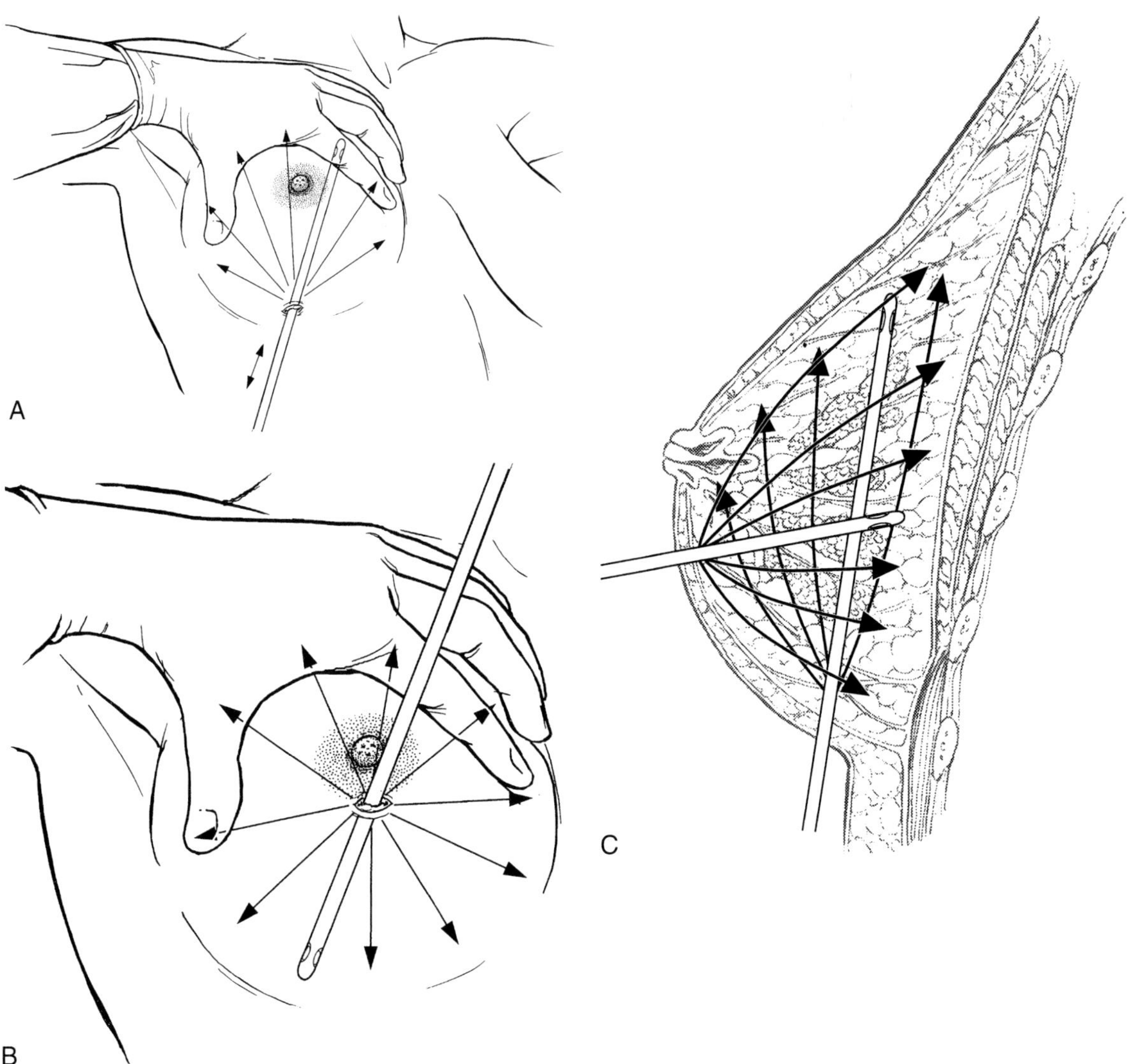

FIGURE 135-13. *A* to *C*, Suction reduction technique. (From Matarasso A: Breast reduction by suction mammaplasty. Operative Techniques Plast Reconstr Surg 1999;6:136.)

the theoretical projection of the resulting breast mound. It is wise to err on the side of leaving redundant skin with a more acute angle that can be trimmed at the end of the procedure because tension at the confluence of the skin flaps may lead to necrosis in wide-angle closures (Fig. 135-14).

INFERIOR PEDICLE TECHNIQUE

The basis of this operation is preservation of nipple-areola viability on an inferiorly based dermal-parenchymal pedicle.[17-21] Because a relatively large amount of breast tissue is left beneath the nipple, breast-feeding is potentially more likely than it is with some of the other techniques. Retention of lateral and medial mesenteries running out onto the chest wall also preserves vascularity and may result in higher levels of nipple sensory preservation. Mandrekas et al[84] reported a series of 371 patients with use of this technique of "mesenteric preservation." The overall complication rate was only 11.4%. Nipple insensitivity was recorded in only 1.3% of patients, and of those patients who became pregnant subsequent to reduction, 72% were able to breast-feed. In terms of design features, Georgiade[19] advised a length-to-breadth ratio of 3:1 for the inferior pedicle, particularly in very large patients. This ratio for pedicle dimension was challenged by Ariyan,[85] who believes that larger pedicles may compromise vascularity by establishing venous congestion. Certainly, the larger the pedicle, the greater the difficulty one has in achieving a satisfactory reduction. The most limiting factor in deciding whether to

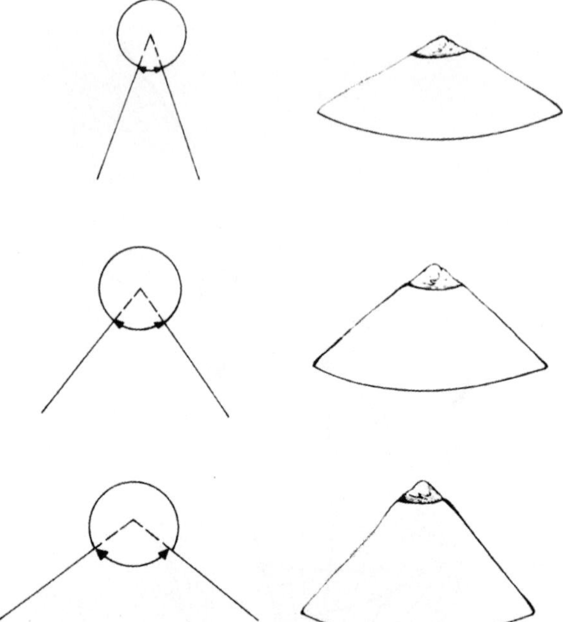

FIGURE 135-14. The wider the keyhole pattern is opened, the greater the coning effect when the medial and lateral flaps are brought together. (From Gradinger G: Reduction mammaplasty with free nipple-areola graft. Operative Techniques Plast Reconstr Surg 1999;6:141.)

use this technique is related to the length from the nipple to inframammary fold. As this length begins to exceed 20 cm, the width of the pedicle required to safely support the nipple becomes a rate-limiting step in achieving an effective reduction. If the pedicle is narrowed, the length-to-breadth ratio may easily become 5 or 6:1; nipple blood flow becomes tenuous, and the pedicle may be at risk for fat necrosis. The ensuing calcification may have longer term implications for mammographic follow-up of these patients. In terms of Wise-pattern design, Courtiss and Goldwyn[18] suggest rotating the keyhole more laterally to preserve lateral intercostal innervation from the fourth and fifth intercostal nerves.

The patient is marked in the erect position; the weight is taken off the breast slightly to allow more accurate assessment of final nipple level. Failure to perform this maneuver may lead to postreduction elevation of the nipple above the intended position as the lighter breast rides up the chest wall. The apex of the keyhole is marked as the top of the areola diameter, allowing 42 to 45 mm for areola diameter plus another 45 mm for the vertical breast scar to the inframammary crease; the total length of the preoperative vertical limb from the upper pole of the new areola position is then 9 cm. Crepeau and Klein[86] have confirmed these measurements, including the postoperative lengthening that inevitably takes place. The midaxis of the breast is marked to provide accurate positioning of the inverted T closure. The nipple-areola diameter is cut at 42 to 45 mm, and the inferior pedicle is de-epithelialized. This is performed with a No. 10 blade with the skin under tension.

The procedure can be continued in one of two directions at this point. Some surgeons elect to incise and shape the breast flaps, leaving 1 to 2 cm of breast tissue on the undersurface of the flaps. This dissection gradually thickens down to the chest wall. The pedicle can then be carved and fitted up beneath the skin flaps. Lateral and medial mesenteries are left gently shelving onto the chest wall to preserve blood and nerve supply. Care should be taken in carving the pedicle that the nipple-areola complex is not pulled away from the chest wall during dissection; this maneuver can result in excessive thinning of the base of the pedicle with a reduction in blood flow to the nipple. Another approach is to carve the pedicle first and then shape the surrounding skin flaps. This allows more leeway in skin flap shaping and more of a "tailor-tack" approach to shaping and reducing skin tension. The pedicle can be gently pressed against the chest wall during its dissection, ensuring that the lateral and medial mesenteries taper gently onto the pectoralis major fascia. The redundant tissue to be resected is removed en bloc as a single horseshoe excision. Care should be taken to debulk the inferolateral and inferomedial portions of the breast to prevent the "boxy breast deformity" so often seen when surgeons first start performing inferior pedicle reductions. Additional liposuction of the breast tail and lateral chest wall fold may further reduce fullness in this area and improve breast shape. Tacking of the pedicle to the pectoral fascia is one of the methods used to attempt to maintain breast fullness in the upper pole. It can cause distortion and should be used judiciously, and there are no convincing data that it prevents bottoming out in the long term.

Closure is then undertaken, making sure that skin tension is stolen in from lateral to medial, leaving as tension free a closure as possible at the T juncture inferiorly. There is little doubt that most instances of T junction necrosis arise from too much tension being exerted on the tips of the skin flaps during closure. These flap tips should be lying loosely together without any tension before the final subcuticular suture is inserted. The incision lines are taped with SteriStrips, and loose dry dressings are applied. Circumferential dressings are unnecessary and cumbersome. The use of drains has not been shown to reduce hematomas or seromas in breast reduction surgery, and many surgeons have abandoned their use. Postoperative care involves supporting the breasts in a soft bra for 4 weeks and the use of scar taping with occlusive tape, or scar massage is encouraged. In patients with a tendency to hypertrophy, early application of silicone gel strips or cream may reduce scar complications (Figs. 135-15 and 135-16).

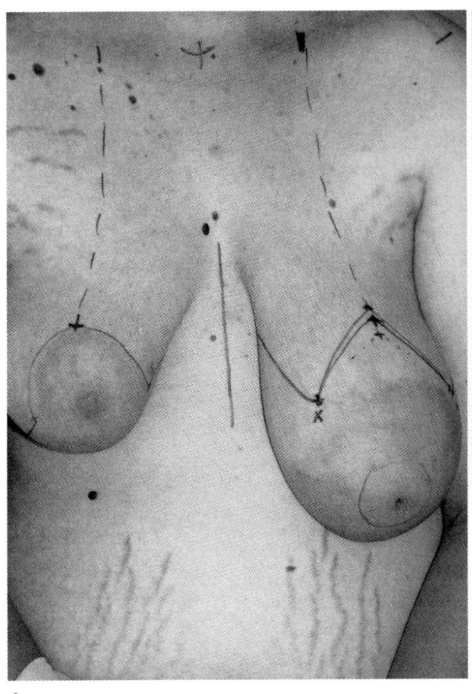

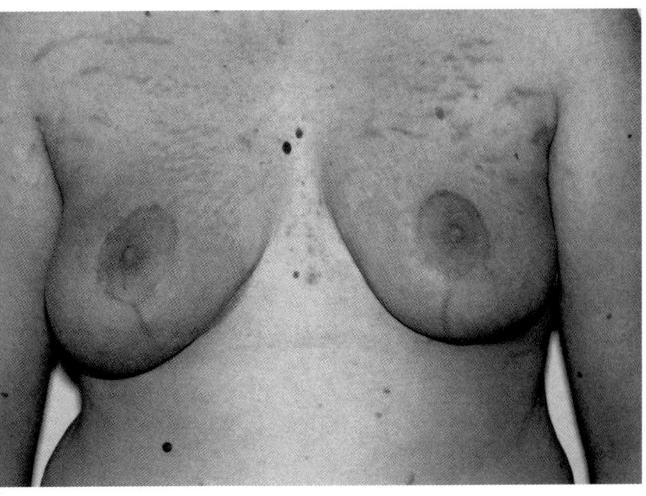

FIGURE 135-15. *A,* Preoperative view of young adult with breast asymmetry and grade III ptosis. *B,* Left inferior pedicle reduction of 650 g and right mastopexy by Wise-pattern technique, 1 year after surgery.

SUPERIOR PEDICLE TECHNIQUE

The superiorly based dermal flap nipple transposition was described by Weiner[17] in 1973. In 1992, Robbins and Hoffman[87] described their experience with a superior dermoglandular flap extending down to the chest wall. Nipple necrosis developed in 1.4% of 193 patients; blistering occurred in another 4.3%. Nipple sensation appeared good. They recommended the procedure for patients having resections of up to 1200 g. Abramo[88] reported similarly good experience with a superior pedicle with few complications. Arie[69] and Pitanguy[16] described superiorly based techniques in 1957 and 1967, respectively (see Fig. 135-6). In a review by Matarasso and Pitanguy[89] in 1996, the degree of breast volume resection and ptosis correction determined whether a vertical or inverted T scar was used for closure. These techniques are reliable and reproducible, but the superior pedicle is difficult to rotate on itself in patients with densely glandular breast tissue, which feels stiff and unyielding. Such patients are better served by inferior pedicle, medial pedicle, and central mound procedures.

STROMBECK HORIZONTAL BIPEDICLE TECHNIQUE

In 1960, Strombeck[12] described the horizontal bipedicle techniques for breast reduction, using Schwarzmann's concept of nipple preservation on a dermal flap[7] (see Fig. 135-4). Strombeck took this a step further by incorporating a bipedicled attachment, thereby bolstering nipple blood supply. He also advised against dissecting skin from the breast parenchyma and incorporated the Wise pattern into the basic design. The procedure was widely used, but surgeons experienced difficulty with rotating the horizontal pedicle into its new inset, and lack of nipple sensitivity was a major problem. The technique was almost entirely abandoned with the advent of the McKissock and other pedicled techniques relying on dermoglandular flaps.

McKISSOCK VERTICAL BIPEDICLE TECHNIQUE

McKissock[15] described the vertical bipedicle technique in 1972 (see Fig. 135-5). Unlike Strombeck's operation, this technique relied on a dermoglandular pedicle inferiorly and superiorly, thinning to a dermal-only component just above the nipple. Many surgeons modified this technique to maintain the dermoglandular flap throughout its length. The flap was folded on itself at inset. The procedure proved reliable in patients with nipple to notch lengths of up to 40 cm and provided better nipple sensation than the Strombeck procedure. It is still used by some surgeons today.

LATERAL PEDICLE TECHNIQUE

Whereas Skoog[13] is credited with promoting a lateral dermal pedicle for nipple support, it was Nicolle[90] who incorporated the parenchyma to form a lateral dermoglandular flap. Because the lateral flaps tend to rely on the less dominant lateral vascular supplies for the nipple, nipple necrosis is a more significant issue. As

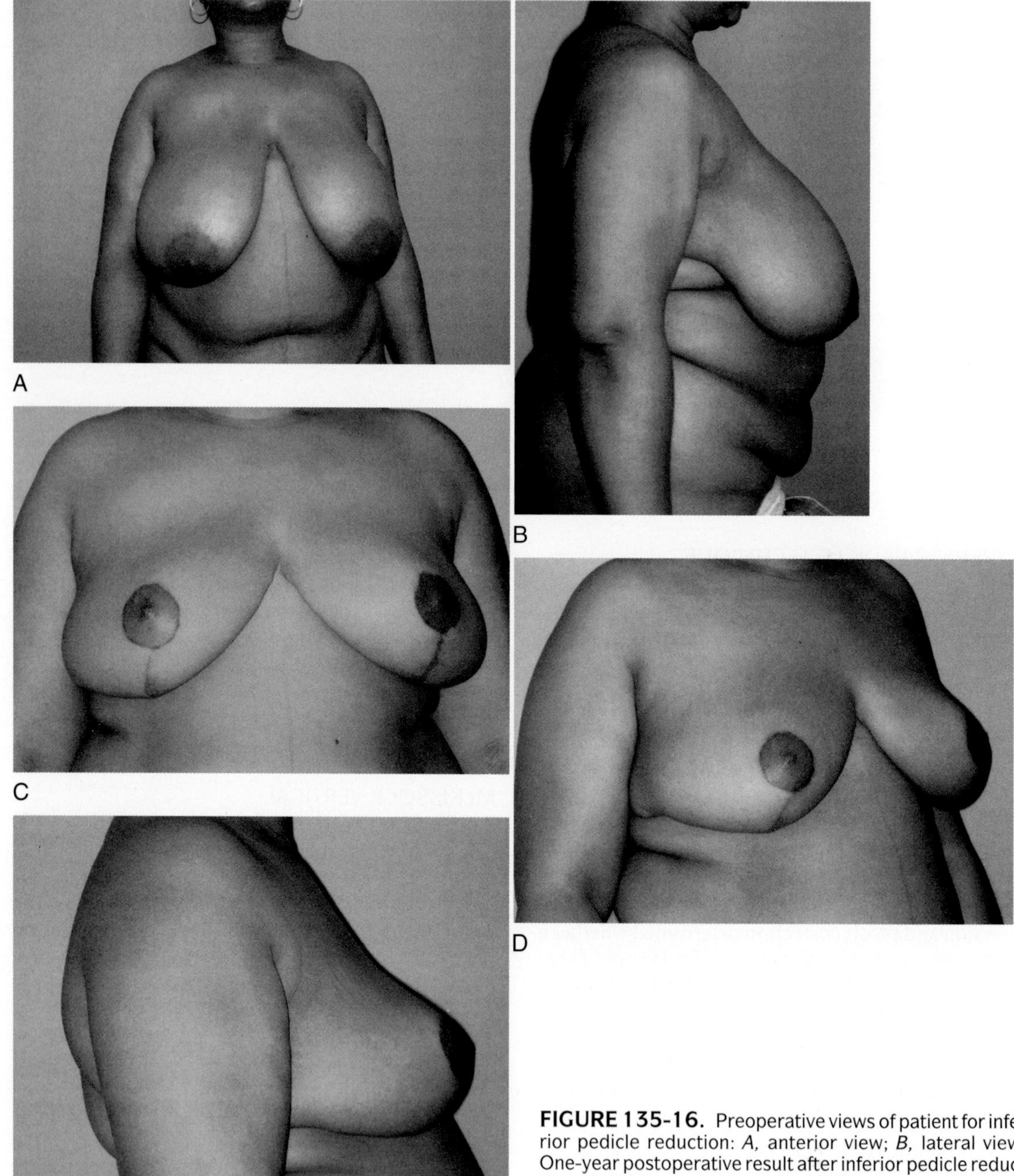

FIGURE 135-16. Preoperative views of patient for inferior pedicle reduction: *A*, anterior view; *B*, lateral view. One-year postoperative result after inferior pedicle reduction of 1500 g per side through Wise-pattern skin excision: *C*, anterior view; *D*, oblique view; *E*, lateral view.

a consequence, Botta and Rifai[91] advised against transposing the nipple more than 15 cm on a lateral dermoglandular flap. These techniques are not popular in the United States but are still used in certain areas of Europe and Scandinavia.

MEDIAL PEDICLE TECHNIQUE

A purely medial pedicle reduction was reported by Nahabedian.[92] In a small series of 45 patients, 44 patients had satisfactory outcomes; nipple sensitivity was achieved in 98% of the patients. One patient was converted to free nipple graft because of vascular compromise of the pedicle. As with all medial pedicle techniques, adequate volume resection remains the key concern, but flap rotation into the areola inset is usually easier than with vertical or superior pedicles. One of the key advantages to basing a pedicle medially is that it incorporates a substantial vascular inflow from the internal mammary perforators, particularly those arising from the second and third interspaces.

CENTRAL MOUND MODIFICATION OF THE INFERIOR PEDICLE TECHNIQUE

All of the procedures described have been based on the use of a dermoglandular pedicle to support nipple viability. The basis for a dermal strip is that it may preserve the subdermal plexus more reliably than if the dermis were to be stripped away. Biesenberger[93] was the first surgeon to incorporate this concept, followed by Climo and Alexander[94] in 1980. Other surgeons to capitalize on this idea included Lexer-Kraske,[95] Penn,[11] Arie,[69] and Pitanguy.[16] The Dufourmentel-Mouly procedure[96]—another popular parenchymal Kraske,[95] Penn,[11] Arie,[69] and Pitanguy technique widely practiced in Europe—involves a lateral wedge resection with the nipple based on a superomedial parenchymal pedicle. Regnault's B technique was popular in Canada.[97]

The central mound approach described by Hester[22] in 1985 relies on the nipple's being carried on a central block of breast tissue without incorporation of an inferior de-epithelialized strip of dermis (see Fig. 135-8). The pedicle is thus completely glandular. A conical or mound shape is carved with a gentle taper onto the chest wall all around the central nipple-areola complex. Skin flap shaping is similar to that described before with the exception that Hester effectively uses tailor-tacking to assess the skin resection to be performed. The more rounded central pedicle may provide a better shape for the new breast compared with the standard inferior pedicle. This is not unlike the original Biesenberger technique in terms of use of a central parenchymal block of tissue; but unlike in the Biesenberger approach, there is no rotation of the pedicle, and a layer of parenchyma is left attached to the surrounding skin flaps as in all of the other modern approaches to breast reduction. Hester achieves pleasing conical breast shapes at the time of surgery. Bottoming out is still a problem with these central parenchymal procedures, and some surgeons have implied that the lack of an inferior dermal support may predispose these patients to more parenchymal descent with time.

Short-Scar Techniques

PRINCIPLES

Disillusionment with the procedures based on the Wise pattern resulted from the problems of bottoming out and scar aesthetics in the long term. While surgeons in the United States focused on pedicle variations within the confines of the Wise pattern, their European and South American counterparts began aggressively exploring short-scar alternatives (Table 135-5).

These procedures have evolved progressively and are rapidly gaining acceptance in the United States and other parts of the world. Although initially thought to be suitable for small to moderate reductions in young women with elastic skin, many procedures are now finding utility in larger reductions in older women.

VERTICAL MAMMAPLASTY

Lassus[24,25] pioneered the use of a vertical scar technique in 1964 and has developed a 40-year experience with this approach. He emphasized the use of a superior pedicle, inferior pyramidal glandular resection, no skin undermining, and closure with a vertical scar only. He does not use breast liposuction at all, nor does he use suspensory suturing of the breast to the pectoralis major fascia. He also maintains skin attachments to the underlying breast parenchyma. In 1996, he published a 30-year experience with the technique in 710 patients.[98] He reported no nipple necroses, provided that the nipple was not transposed more than 9 cm vertically. The results were stable in the long term, and conical projection was maintained well. Twenty hypertrophic scars developed, four of which were severe. This is no worse than the reports from T-shaped scarring, and it at least eliminated the potential for more extensive scarring underneath the breast. Lassus did not report nipple sensitivity. He subsequently updated the series in 1999, and long-term aesthetic results were excellent.[99]

TABLE 135-5 ✦ SHORT-SCAR ALTERNATIVES TO THE WISE PATTERN

Vertical mammaplasty
Vertical mammaplasty with short horizontal scars
L-shaped scar techniques
Periareolar techniques
Inframammary scar technique

Lejour[26,27] modified Lassus' technique and brought it to wider acceptance in this country. Her modifications included skin undermining adjacent to the vertical parenchymal pillar edges, suture suspension of the pedicle to the pectoralis major fascia, total breast liposuction, and tumescent fluid infiltration into the breast gland (Fig. 135-17). Lejour[100] reviewed the data of 250 patients and reported them in 1999. Shape retention was excellent; delayed wound healing at the base of the breast was the most common complication at 5.4%, followed by seroma formation at 5%. Lejour was wary of performing the procedure for reductions in excess of 1200 g per side. Complication rates for vertical reductions appear similar to those for inferior pedicle techniques overall as reported by others.[101-104] Deconinck et al[105] evaluated their results in 243 vertical reductions with an average resection of 905 g per side and found low complication rates, rapid operating times, and high satisfaction of patients and surgeons. Satisfaction of patients and surgeons was also found to be higher for vertical mammaplasties as opposed to Wise-pattern techniques in a study by Godwin.[106] Nipple sensitivity has been evaluated by Greuse[107] and found to be comparable to that of other techniques, with larger breasts taking longer to recover than smaller reductions. The learning curve is steep, and most surgeons focus on their concerns about inferior dog-ear formation.[108] This problem and its prevention are addressed in the technical description in the following section.

Hall-Findlay[33] reported a variation on the vertical scar theme by use of a medial pedicle with inferolateral resection of the gland. The average resection reported in her initial series of 400 breasts was 525 g. Like Lassus, she does not use suspensory or purse-string suturing, and liposuction is targeted to certain areas and not the breast as a whole. She pioneered the technique in an effort to shorten the learning curve associated with mastery of the vertical techniques. The technique is particularly effective in small to moderate reductions, but larger resections may cause flattening or blunting of the inferolateral quadrant of the breast, and care should be taken in reshaping the breast in larger patients (Fig. 135-18). Like the Lassus and Lejour procedures, the Hall-Findlay approach forms a conical, well-supported breast that tends to maintain its shape better in the long term with less of a tendency to bottom out.

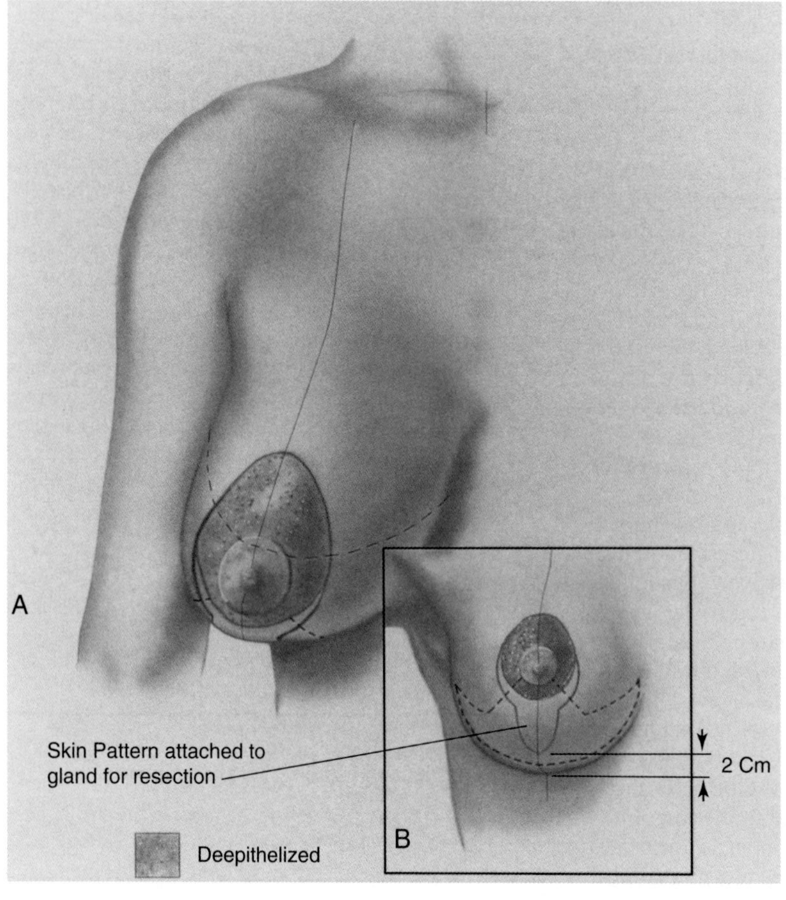

FIGURE 135-17. *A* to *F*, Vertical reduction as proposed by Lassus and Lejour.

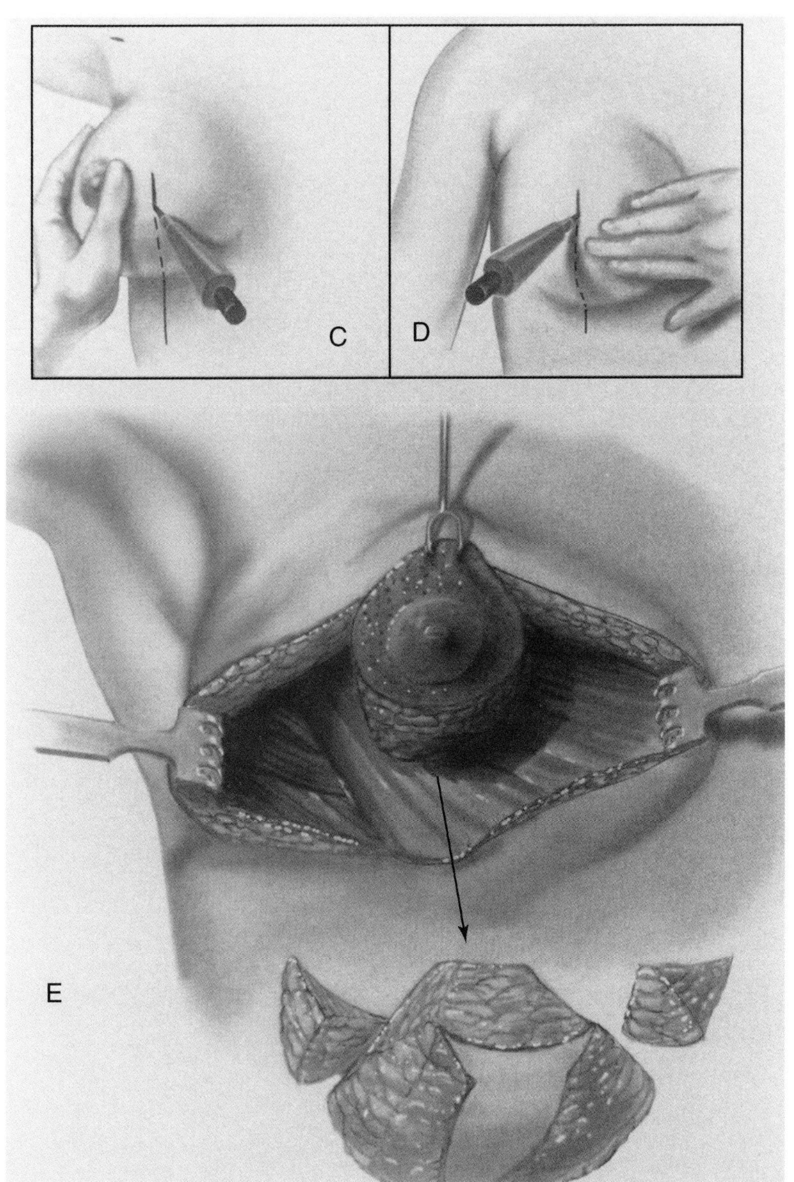

FIGURE 135-17, cont'd. *Continued*

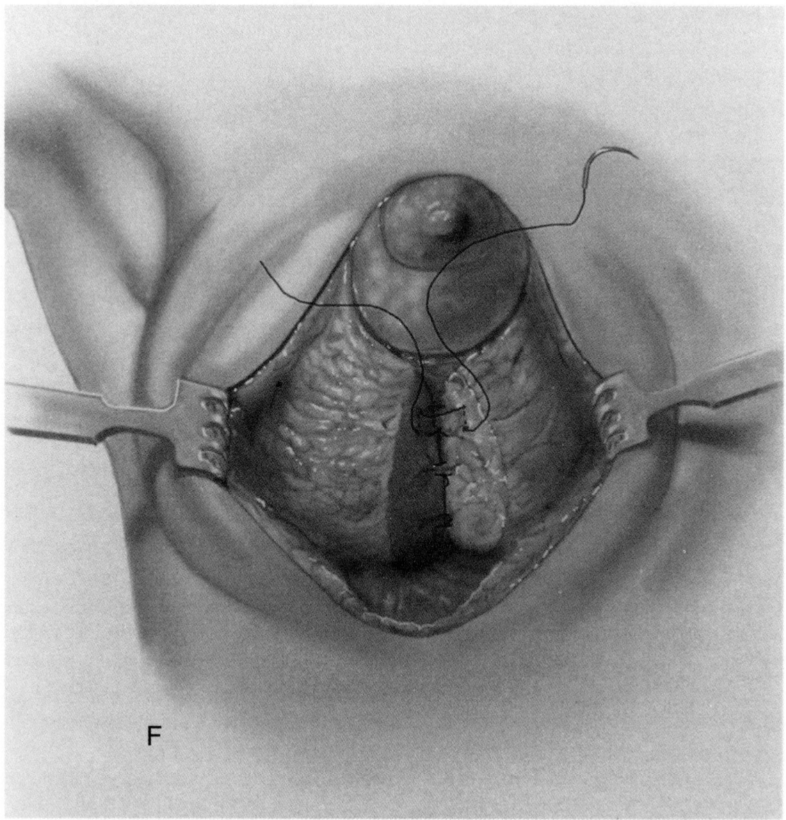

FIGURE 135-17, cont'd.

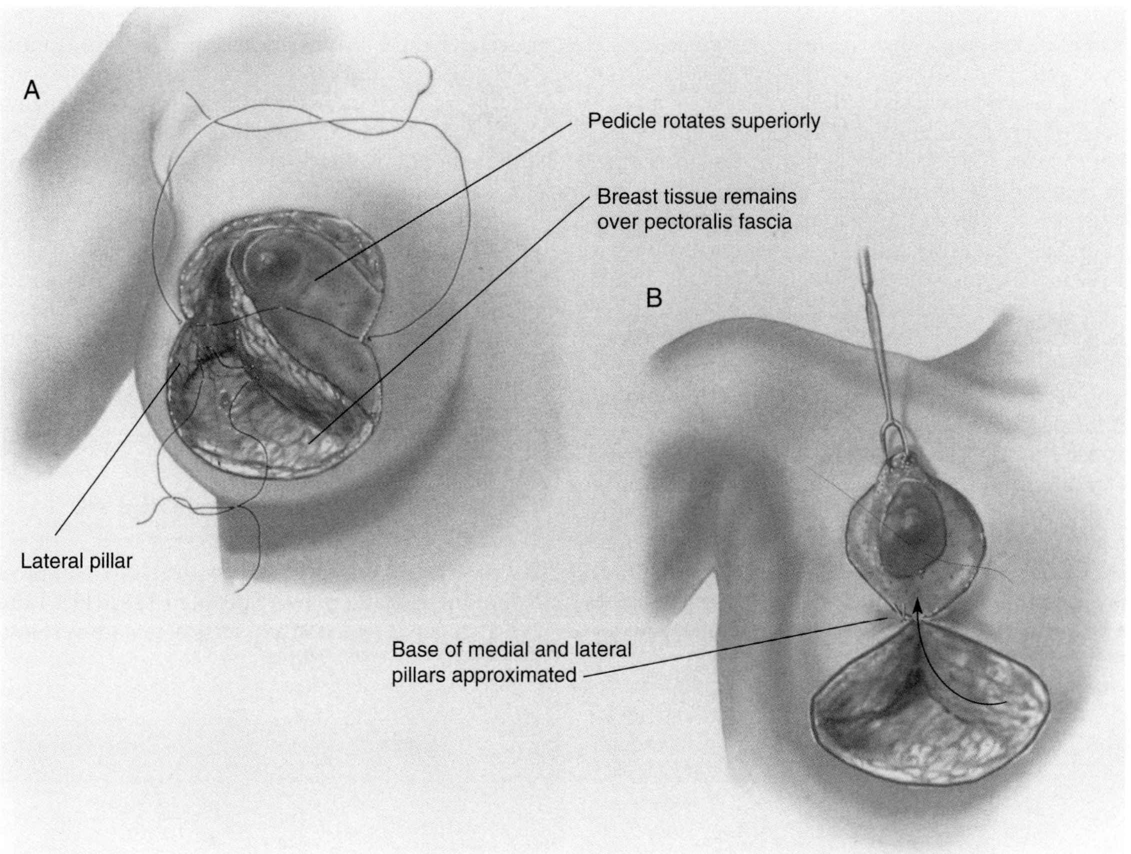

FIGURE 135-18. *A* and *B*, Hall-Findlay vertical reduction with superomedial pedicle.

LASSUS-LEJOUR TECHNIQUE (see Fig. 135-17)

Marking is performed in the erect position, and the weight of the breast is supported when the nipple to areola distance is measured.[17-19] A perpendicular is dropped from the midclavicular line through the natural nipple. The sternal notch to areola distance is measured typically at 22 to 23 cm. The areola inset is inscribed as an open circle, and it is preferable to use the mosque or onion dome shape suggested by Lejour. The midaxis of the breast is marked at the inframammary crease. The breast is pushed laterally, and a perpendicular is dropped from the appropriate point on the circumference of the areola inset circle to a point 3 cm above the midpoint of the breast crease. The breast is pushed medially, and the same maneuver is performed laterally. When the breast is relaxed once more, these two lines assume the appearance of splayed out limbs radiating from the areola inset. The two ends are joined by a gentle U-shaped curve about 2 cm above the inframammary crease. The superior pedicle is drawn in with a progressively wider base as the pedicle meets the circumference of the areola inset.

The breast is then infiltrated with tumescent fluid with use of an infusion system. Fluid is infiltrated only along the resection lines and into the inframammary crease and tail of the breast. Liposuction of the breast tail is performed together with some suctioning of the inframammary area to assist with reducing dog-ear formation. Liposuction of the tail of the breast is usually the most uncomfortable part of the procedure postoperatively and may cause some bruising. The areolar diameter is cut at 42 mm, and the superior pedicle is de-epithelialized (the technique can be adapted to suit a medial or lateral pedicle as well). The medial and lateral breast pillar incisions are made with a No. 10 blade; the tumescent fluid provides effective enough hemostasis for almost all of the breast shaping to be done with knife rather than cautery dissection. This technique provides for quick and easy shaping of the gland. Dissection is taken down to the chest wall in a beveled manner to form a central pyramid-like resection excavated beneath the pedicle. The two pillar incisions communicate around the inferior edge of the nipple-areola complex. The incision at this point is made only 1 cm deep; the tip of the areola is grasped with an Allis clamp, and the breast is allowed to fall under its own weight. The pedicle is then carved from 1 cm at its tip, gently shelving to a thicker base at the chest wall. This maneuver completes the apex of the central resection, which comes away as a pyramidal block of breast tissue. Medial and lateral inframammary wedge resections are performed at the crease immediately subdermally. This resection reduces the tendency to dog-ear formation. The entire inframammary skin crease should be evacuated of breast tissue to the dermis and down to the chest wall for this reason. A superomedial pedicle could be used rather than a true vertical pedicle. The medial approach does allow easier transposition into the areola inset and may cause less nipple ischemia because there is less folding of the pedicle to take place.

After the resections are completed, the medial and lateral pillars are approximated with deep Vicryl sutures to help with glandular shaping. The pedicle is gently infolded into the center of the breast and inset. The author does not use the pedicle suspension sutures advocated by Lejour, and suctioning of the entire gland is not recommended because it may precipitate necrosis if it is carried out aggressively. At the end of the procedure, there is some puckering of the skin around the nipple inset and along the vertical limb of the scar, but this usually flattens out within 4 to 6 weeks. Breast shape is conical with marked projection and settles within about 6 weeks. The shape is well maintained, and bottoming out is much less of a problem than it is with inferior pedicled reductions (Figs. 135-19 and 135-20). Patients are encouraged to tape all scars for 2 months regardless of technique; underwire bras can be used as soon as the patient is comfortable. Use of underwiring helps compress the inferior dog-ear onto the chest wall, allowing early adhesion of the skin to the chest. This compression may be another useful aid in dog-ear reduction.

VERTICAL REDUCTION INCORPORATING A SHORT HORIZONTAL SCAR

Marchac[28] published his results with a short-scar procedure in 1982 and in more detail in 1988 (Fig. 135-21). The central resection and vertical closure were not

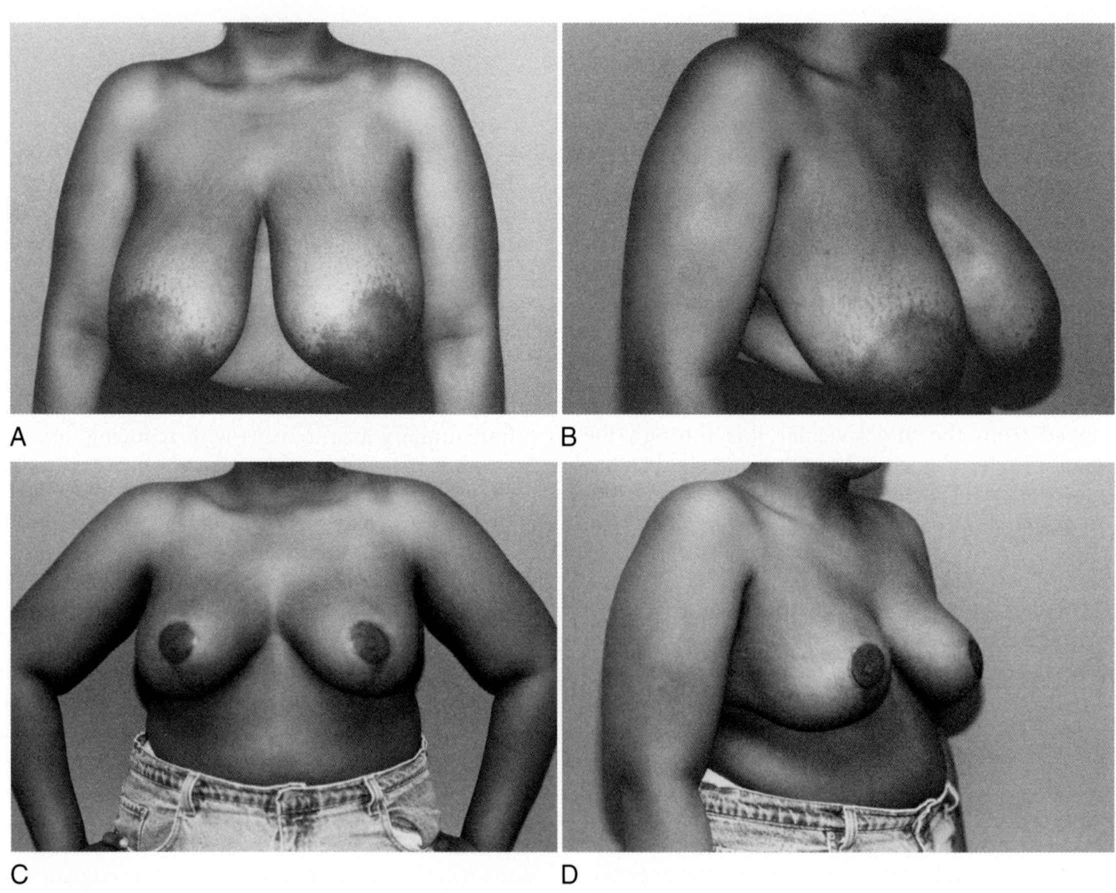

FIGURE 135-19. Preoperative views of patient for whom a vertical reduction is planned: *A*, anterior view; *B*, oblique view. One-year postoperative result after vertical reduction of 1200 g per side illustrates the well-rounded shape of the breast: *C*, anterior view; *D*, oblique view.

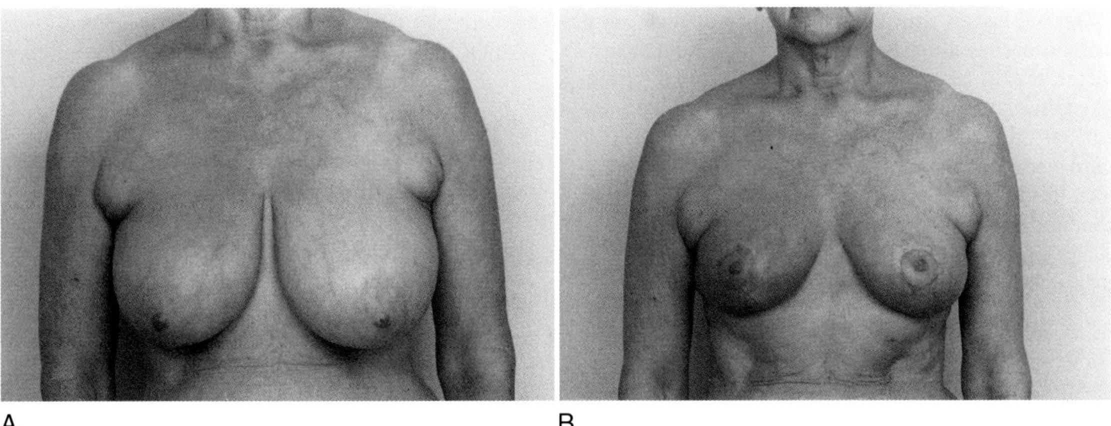

FIGURE 135-20. *A,* Preoperative view of a 55-year-old woman for whom a vertical reduction is planned. *B,* One-year postoperative view of same patient showing the result of a 500-g vertical reduction.

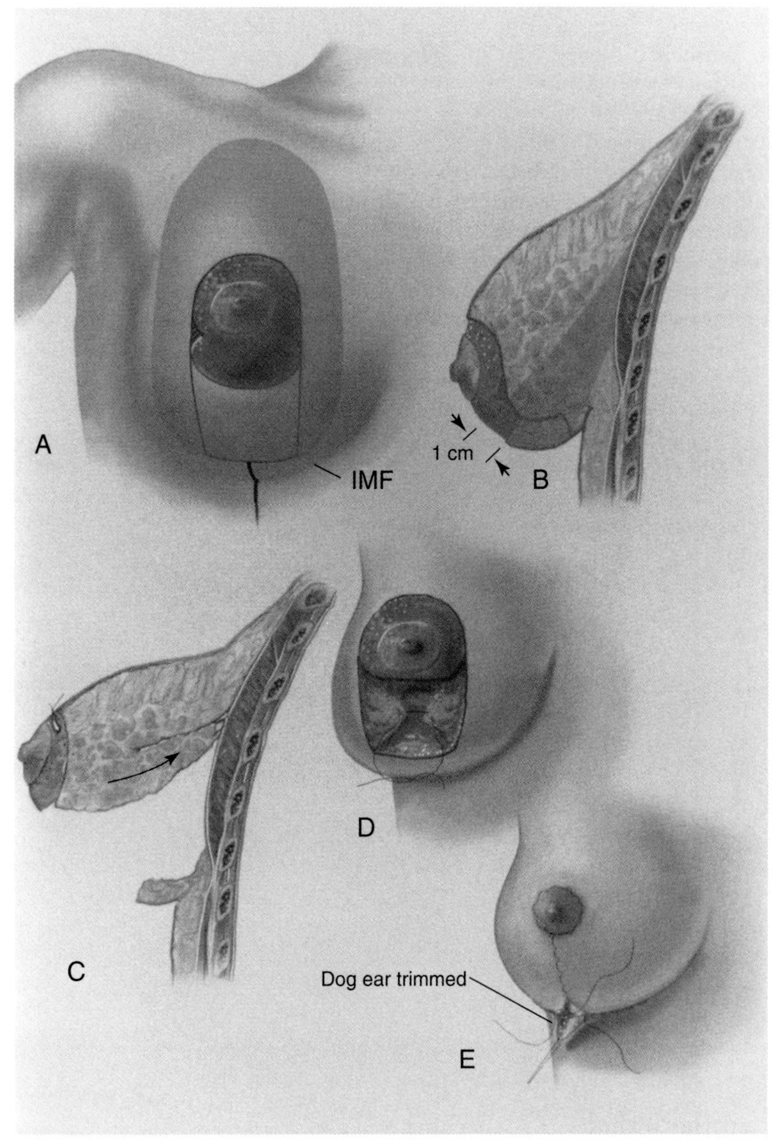

FIGURE 135-21. *A* to *E,* Marchac short-scar technique with a short horizontal component to the scar to deal with inferior dog-ears. IMF, inframammary fold.

unlike the Lassus procedure in some respects, but a horizontal component was an integral part of the preoperative skin resection design. Shin and Lee[109] published their small experience of the "short submammary scar" or SSS technique similar to that of Lassus but again incorporating a preplanned horizontal skin resection. Results were good, but resection volumes were small to moderate, the largest being 750 g per side.

L-SHAPED SCAR REDUCTION

Regnault[97] reported her B technique mammaplasty in 1974, a procedure that eliminated the medial component of the horizontal scar (Fig. 135-22). A similar procedure was described by Bozola.[110] The nipple is preserved on a superomedial dermoglandular pedicle, with good shapes being achieved from the inferolateral glandular resection, but the scar sometimes encroaches on the upper abdominal wall below the bra strap line. Skin tailoring has to be carefully judged to maintain a higher scar. The resection bears great similarity to the glandular resection advocated in the Hall-Findlay technique, which has largely superseded these procedures. In 1994, Born[111] published his experience with a modified L scar technique (Fig. 135-23). His procedure uses a medial triangular flap interdigitating with a lateral rectangular flap. In a series of 275 patients with an average reduction volume of 775 g per side, complications were few and cosmetic results appear excellent. Similarly positive results have been reported by Chiari[112] with his variant of the L scar reduction.

HORIZONTAL SCAR REDUCTION

Passot[6] was the first surgeon to describe a horizontal scar reduction by an inferior horizontal wedge resection with transposition of the nipple into a buttonhole incision higher up on the breast mound (see Fig. 135-1). Variations on this theme have been devised by Yousif,[113] basing the nipple on a central or inferior pedicle, and Savaci,[114] using a central mound approach. Problems with potential skin viability and puckering at the inframammary crease remain minor concerns, and these techniques have not seen much widespread acceptance. Flattening of the breast mound with time tends to be an inherent problem because of the lack of vectors pulling the medial and lateral quadrants of the breast centrally.

PERIAREOLAR REDUCTION

In an effort to minimize scarring still further, some surgeons have explored the use of periareolar techniques. Bennelli[31] described the "round block" technique in 1990 (Fig. 135-24). The skin excess is taken up in a pursestring manner around the areola, and puckering tends to settle with time. Although there is a high degree of satisfaction of patients when it is possible to use this technique, the drawback to these

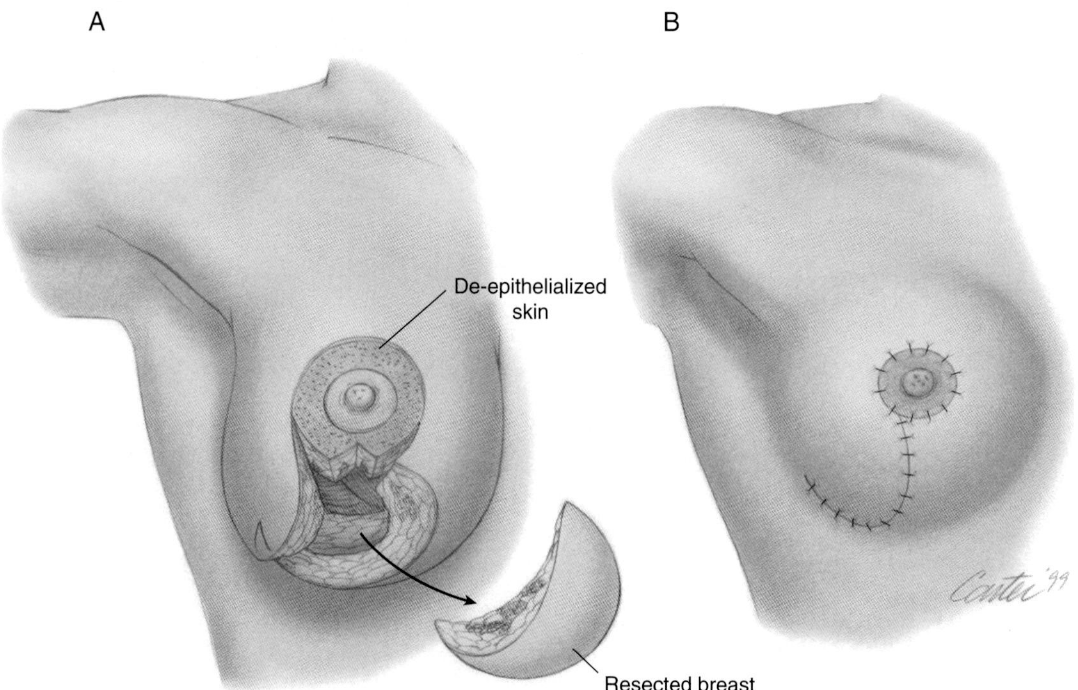

FIGURE 135-22. *A* and *B*, Regnault B technique. (From Lickstein LH, Shestak KC: The conceptual evolution of modern reduction mammaplasty. Operative Techniques Plast Reconstr Surg 1999;6:88.)

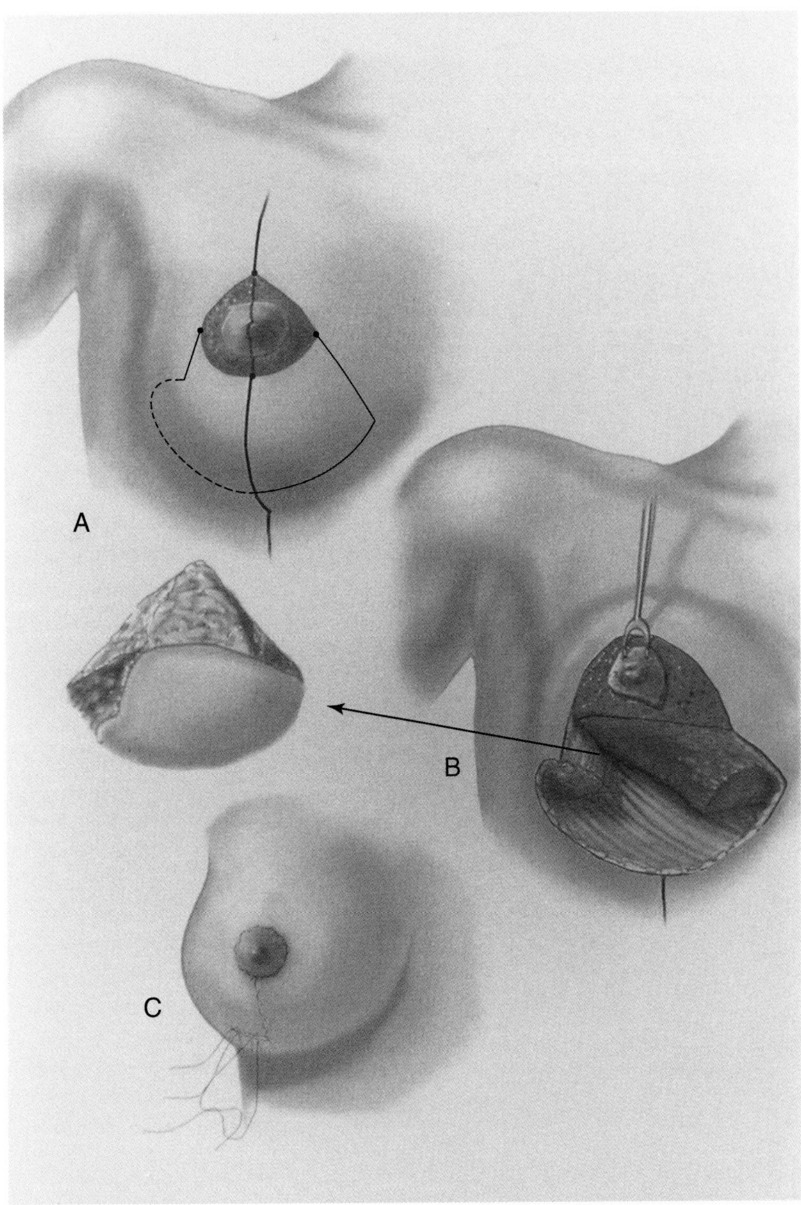

FIGURE 135-23. *A* to *C*, L reduction.

procedures is the tendency to flatten the breast in the anteroposterior dimension, resulting in a "pancake" look to the breast. There is also a considerable tendency for the areolae to widen with time. This problem has led Hammond[32] to use a Gore-Tex pursestring suture in an effort to control areola widening. Felicio[115] reported his experience with 380 patients having small to moderate reductions and found the complication rates to be similar to those of other procedures. He did not think that it was of value in larger reductions.

Goes[30] has been a major proponent of the periareolar mammaplasty, which he terms the double skin technique. He reported his 7-year experience with 254 patients in 1996. The concept involves elevation of fairly thin skin flaps and removal of a superior horizontal wedge with a vertical upper pole wedge, which is then closed to cone the breast (Fig. 135-25). The exposed central pedicle is then supported with a Vicryl mesh cone to provide further support and shaping of the mound. This allows less skin resection in an effort to reduce the flattening mentioned earlier and has not had deleterious effects on breast imaging as the mesh is resorbed. The procedure is not advocated for breast resections of more than 500 g per side. Goes is currently exploring the use of more permanent internal mesh in an effort to improve long-term results.

Hammond[32] described the SPAIR technique in 1999 in an effort to provide a simpler inferior pedicle-based vertical approach to reduction surgery (Fig. 135-26). At that time, 98 patients were described with average

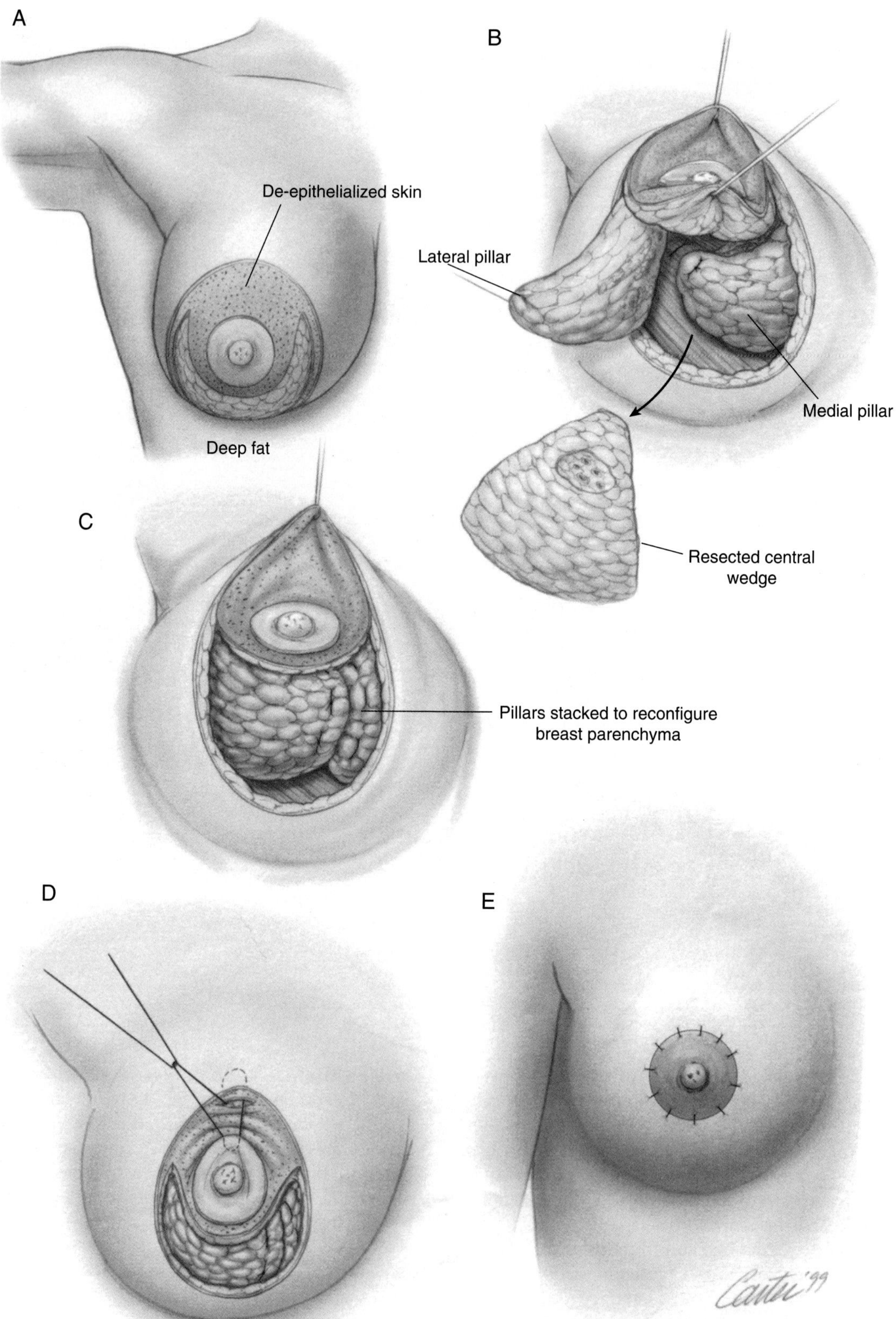

FIGURE 135-24. *A* to *E*, Benelli round block procedure. (From Lickstein LH, Shestak KC: The conceptual evolution of modern reduction mammaplasty. Operative Techniques Plast Reconstr Surg 1999;6:88.)

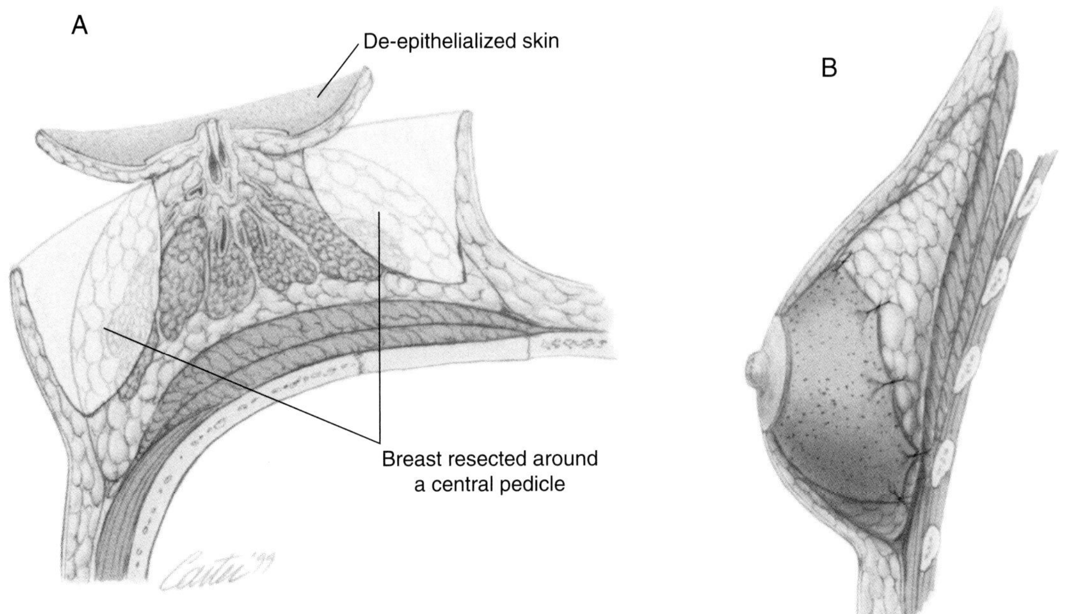

FIGURE 135-25. *A* and *B*, Goes procedure. (From Lickstein LH, Shestak KC: The conceptual evolution of modern reduction mammaplasty. Operative Techniques Plast Reconstr Surg 1999;6:88.)

A B

C D

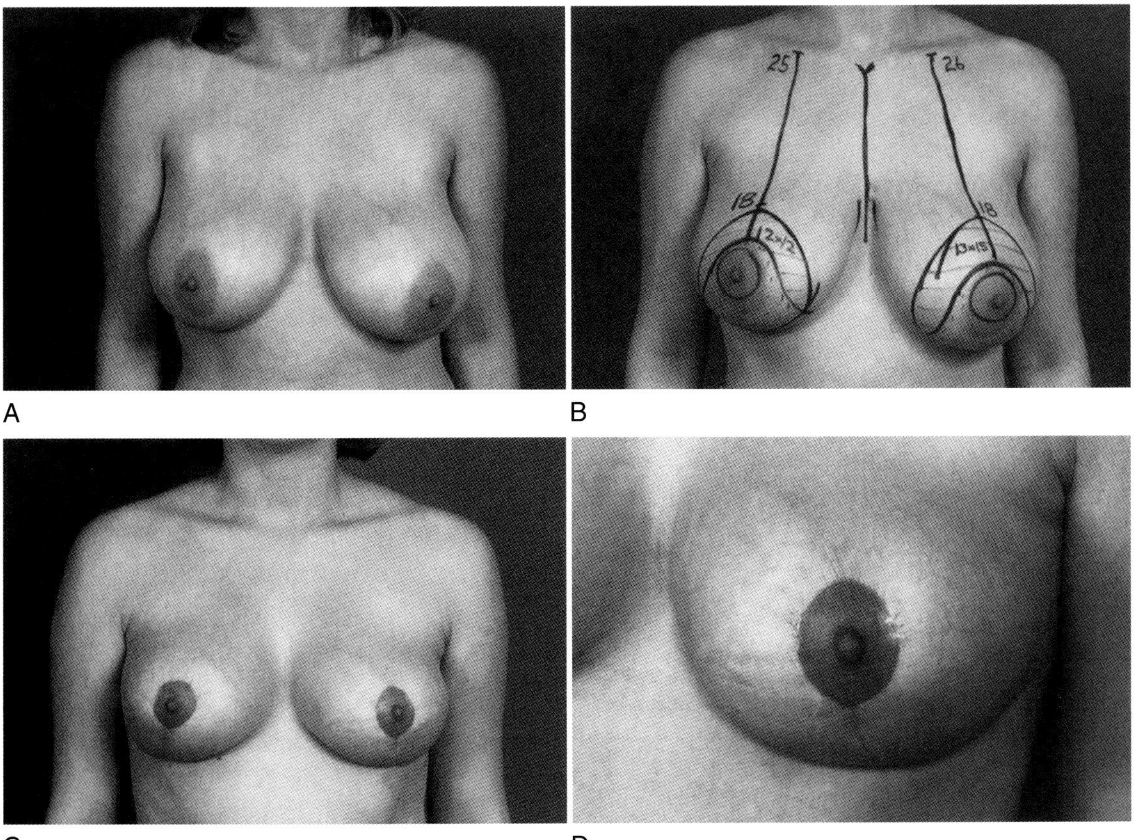

FIGURE 135-26. *A* to *D*, Hammond's SPAIR technique. (From Lickstein LH, Shestak KC: The conceptual evolution of modern reduction mammaplasty. Operative Techniques Plast Reconstr Surg 1999;6:88.)

follow-up of almost 8 months. The nipple is based on a modified inferior dermoglandular pedicle that is tethered to the chest wall superiorly with anchoring sutures. The skin resection is primarily vertical in nature, but Hammond does not hesitate to curve it laterally into a J-shaped scar if redundancy is a major problem. The issue of areolar dilatation is tackled by insertion of a Gore-Tex pursestring suture into the periareolar dermis approximately 5 to 10 mm outside the skin edge to avoid palpability or erosion of the Gore-Tex suture or its knot. Hammond shows excellent results and claims that pedicle suspension eliminates bottoming out. Whereas this has been debated, his results are pleasing and complications are few. Neophytes should start using this procedure with mastopexies before applying this technique to smaller reductions.

REDUCING THE MASSIVE BREAST

Attempts at reducing massive breasts by maintaining the nipple on a dermoglandular pedicle are often hampered by the excessive bulk of the pedicle required to achieve nipple viability. Fat necrosis may occur in the dermal breast flap with resultant difficulty in mammographic screening. Lower pole breast amputation with free nipple grafting as proposed by Thorek[67] has become a mainstay of treatment in this population of patients.[68] The procedure has also gained acceptance in patients who require breast reduction but suffer from significant medical comorbidities that might preclude use of conventional pedicled techniques. Lower pole breast amputation is quick and provides a projectile breast if central tissue is preserved to augment the closure. The thinned nipple graft is applied to a central de-epithelialized disk on the dome of the breast mound (Fig. 135-27). Oneal et al[116] reviewed the procedure in 11 such patients with comorbidities and found it to be safe and effective with a high degree of satisfaction of patients (Fig. 135-28).

One of the most common problems associated with breast amputation is that of resecting breast tissue with exactly the same pattern as that of the skin. If this is performed, there is a tendency to have too little tissue centrally to establish projection, resulting in a flattened breast. This is particularly true of patients with severe ptosis in whom the majority of breast volume resides in the lower pole, which is then resected. This leaves inadequate volume on the upper pole skin flaps with resulting poor projection after closure. By leaving a bridge of breast tissue on the pectoralis major fascia between the vertical limbs of the Wise pattern and by beveling the resection from above downward to the inframammary crease, the surgeon is able to leave a central mound of breast tissue to aid in shaping the new mound and to provide fullness to the central breast (Fig. 135-29). This simple precaution provides excellent shapes after breast amputation and nipple grafting. Casas[117] described incising longer 7-cm vertical limbs to the Wise pattern; the inferior vertical redundancy is infolded under the breast as de-epithelialized flaps to improve projection if necessary. Koger[118] reported use of a de-epithelialized inferiorly based pyramid of breast tissue that is tacked up into the central breast to augment the area of deficient volume.

Despite these apparent solutions to the volume problem, nipple graft depigmentation remains a major source of concern, particularly in patients of color. Darkly pigmented nipples may have piebald depigmentation, with pink areas developing within normal dark areas. The melanocyte population appears particularly sensitive to hypoxia, and even in the face of apparently successful graft take, depigmentation may ensue (Fig. 135-30). Tattooing has been a universally poor salvage for these patients because the color takes on a grayish hue rather than dark brown. Overgrafting dark split-thickness skin grafts onto fresh dermabrasion of these areas can be effective. A seemingly more radical but highly effective technique is to perform breast amputation with immediate nipple reconstruction by use of redundant breast skin at the apex of the Wise-pattern vertical limbs. This technique is frequently used for massive reductions, followed by areola tattooing similar to that performed with conventional nipple reconstruction after mastectomy. The technique produces a projectile, reasonably sensate nipple, and tattoo dye uptake into the normal breast skin around the nipple is excellent and even. Four-year follow-up of these patients indicates that nipple projection remains good. Satisfaction of patients has been extremely high.

PROBLEM AREAS IN BREAST REDUCTION

Secondary Breast Reduction

All surgeons ultimately face the problem of dealing with patients who have had reductions years before and now require another procedure. Indications for repeated reduction include breast volume increase due to ongoing hypertrophy or weight gain, poor shape or asymmetry from the initial procedure, and recurrent symptoms. Whenever possible, the same pedicle used originally should be used again. Hudson[119] has shown that in a series of 16 patients undergoing repeated reduction, transection of the original pedicle occurred in 3 patients, resulting in nipple necrosis in 2 patients. Losee[120] described 10 patients undergoing secondary reductions, 3 of whom had transection of their pedicles; 2 of the 3 patients had delayed healing that ultimately settled in response to conservative dressing care. It is advisable to use the previous pedicle if at all possible to minimize complications.

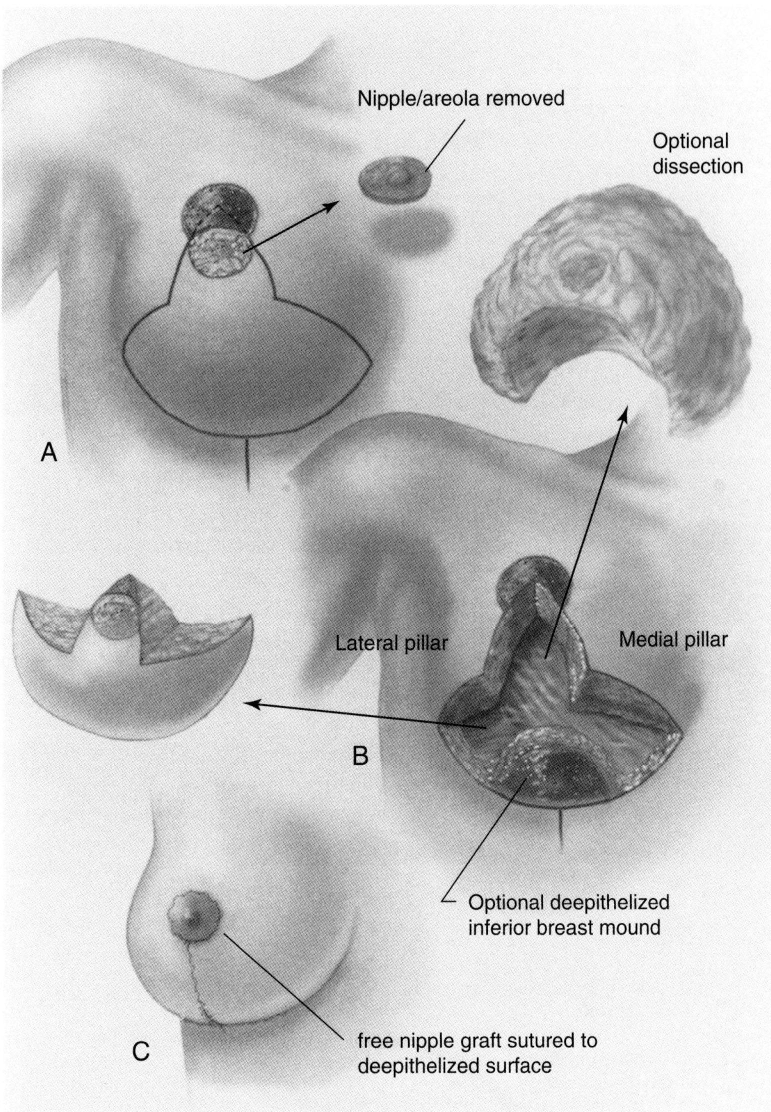

FIGURE 135-27. *A* to *C*, Breast amputation and free nipple grafting by use of the Wise pattern.

Breast Reduction and Prior Irradiation Injury

With the increased use of breast conservation therapy for breast cancer, plastic surgeons are seeing an increase in the number of patients requiring reduction in the face of prior irradiation of the breast. Spear[121] has reviewed this in three such patients and found no increase in complication rates but advocates use of wider, shorter pedicles with no undermining whatsoever. Handel[122] reported a postirradiation reduction in which the nipple was transplanted as a free nipple graft with satisfactory aesthetic outcome. If reduction is required, at least 6 months should pass between completion of radiotherapy and reduction surgery. It is reasonable to ask radiation therapists to reduce the daily fraction from 2 cGy to 1.8 cGy to minimize the daily insult to the breast tissues. It is far preferable, however, to perform reduction before radiation therapy as an integral part of the treatment plan. Oncoplastic surgery as advocated by Audretsch[50] and Clough[51] provides an opportunity to remove the malignant mass, to reduce breast volume, and to improve breast shape, and it provides a more acceptable breast volume for the radiation oncologist to treat. This approach eliminates the adverse effects of irradiation on breast vasculature before surgery and allows the reconstructive surgeon to operate in a field without scars from previous surgery or adverse effects from radiation therapy.

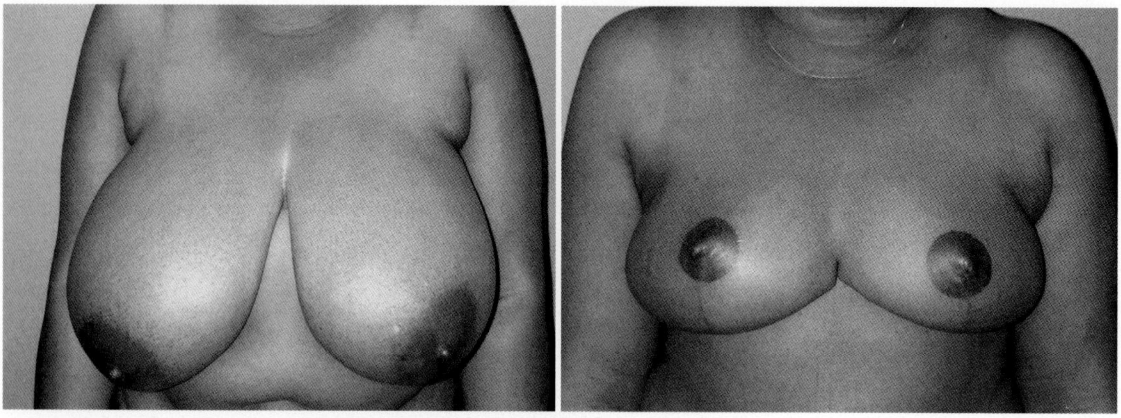

A B 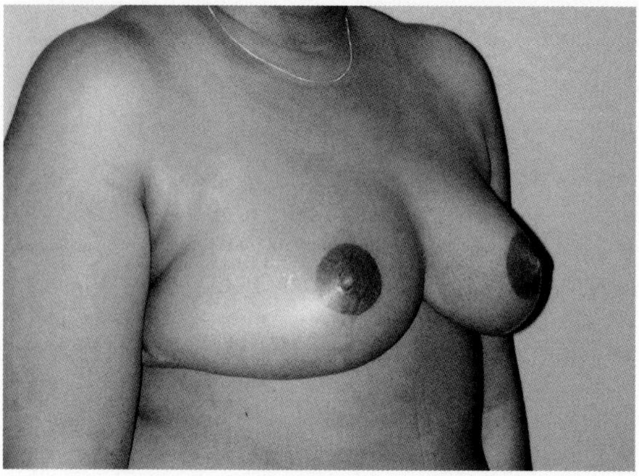 C

FIGURE 135-28. *A,* Preoperative view of patient with gigantomastia. Nipple to notch measurements: 42 cm (right), 44 cm (left); inframammary fold to nipple distances: 23 cm (right), 25 cm (left). *B,* Anterior postoperative view 9 months after lower pole breast amputation (2500 g on right side, 2900 g on left side) and immediate nipple reconstruction with areolar tattooing shows uniform color and nipple projection. *C,* Oblique view demonstrates nipple projection.

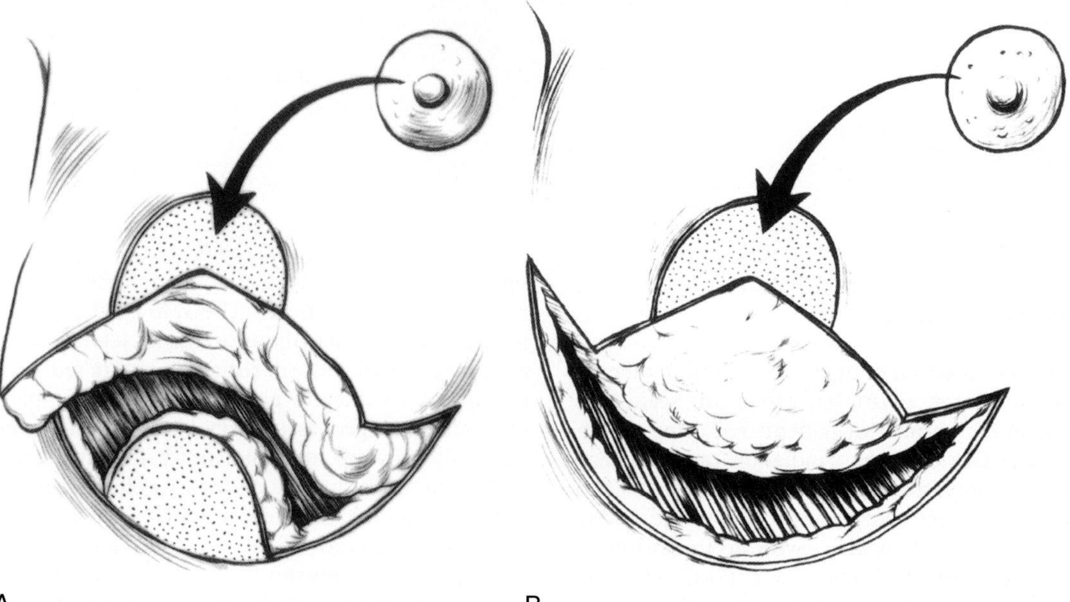

FIGURE 135-29. Two variations in the approach to improvement of projection in free nipple grafting. *A,* Beveled parenchymal resection. *B,* Lower retained mound. (From Gradinger G: Reduction mammaplasty with free nipple-areola graft. Operative Techniques Plast Reconstr Surg 1999:6:145.)

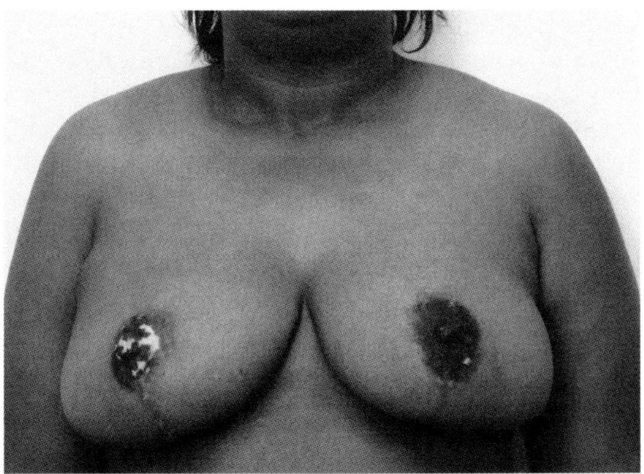

FIGURE 135-30. Six-month postoperative view of a patient who had unilateral areolar hypopigmentation after free nipple grafting despite apparently successful graft.

Adolescent Breast Reduction for Juvenile Hypertrophy

Juvenile hypertrophy may cause significant symptoms in adolescent girls, who ultimately require reductions in their early teens at a time when the breast may still be growing. This presents a significant dilemma for the surgeon. If symptoms are severe enough to warrant reduction at an early age, one simply has to warn the patient and her family that further breast growth is a probability and the operation may need to be repeated in the future. When juvenile hypertrophy leads to gigantomastia, the decision is relatively simple; but in the older adolescent who presents with symptomatic large breasts, the decision-making process becomes more difficult. At the core of this problem lies the issue of the patient's ability to accept the real consequences of reduction when she may be emotionally and psychologically immature to handle these sequelae. How does a 16- or 17-year-old handle scarring and diminished nipple sensitivity or reduced ability to breast-feed when she may be facing courtship and marriage in a few years?

Several studies have been conducted in the hope of answering these pressing concerns. Evans and McMahan reported survey results in 15 and 48 women, respectively, who had reductions at an average age of 17.5 years. Average follow-up ranged from 42 to 70 months. In McMahan's study,[123] 94% of patients were comfortable enough with their surgery to recommend it to others. Their most common complaint was scarring in 60% and diminished nipple sensitivity in 35%. Pain relief was reported in more than 80% of respondents. One patient required reoperation for further breast growth. In Evans' study,[124] similar satisfaction was noted. Both authors concluded that adolescent breast reduction for intractable symptoms is both safe and psychologically beneficial. It is still prudent to suggest waiting until breast growth has been stable for at least 1 year as opposed to the 2 years suggested previously.

OUTCOME STUDIES

One of the problems with trying to deliver comparable outcome studies in breast reduction is the wide variety of techniques used in the treatment of hypertrophy. Variables such as age, weight, symptoms, and body habitus add further complexity to the equation. It is clear that breast symptoms are independent of body weight, and the patient's relief is usually not achieved by weight reduction alone. The following studies summarize some of the most pertinent outcomes generated to date.

In a study of 406 patients undergoing reduction by inferior pedicle with occasional Strombeck procedures, Davis[102] found an overall complication rate of 53%. Diminished nipple sensation was found in 25%, wound healing problems occurred in 19%, and infection requiring antibiotic therapy was present in 12%. Loss of nipple-areola skin occurred in 6%, and secondary reduction was required in 5%. Satisfaction of patients was high in 83%, but patients were dissatisfied with scars (18%), breast size too large (9%), breast size too small (9%), contour asymmetry (8%), and poor aesthetic outcome (8%).

Few studies have been performed to compare techniques. Woods[125] evaluated complications after Maliniac, Skoog, Dufourmentel-Mouly, and McKissock procedures; of these, the McKissock procedure had the lowest complication rate. Comparing the McKissock and inferior pedicle reductions, Hughes[126] demonstrated similar results with increasing satisfaction of the patient and acceptance with time.

Blomquist[127] evaluated 49 women after reduction and found improvement in all quality of life parameters measured except sleep patterns. The obese population benefited just as much as their nonobese counterparts did, an important observation for third-party payers to note. Miller[128] found a 93% reduction in symptoms after reduction in 133 patients with a 62% improvement in activity levels after surgery. The improvements in outcome did not correlate with breast volume resection, but there was an inverse relationship between preoperative breast size and activity levels, a finding corroborated by Sood et al.[129] In Sood's study, pulmonary function was significantly improved in all patients undergoing reduction for symptomatic macromastia as measured both subjectively and objectively. He also found no correlation between the volume of resection and improvement in symptom complex. Dabbah[59] described 185 postreduction patients averaging more than 800 g per side. He found 97% improvement in back, shoulder, and neck pain; 59% of patients were completely asymptomatic. In this study, fat necrosis and infection occurred in 22%, nipple necrosis developed in 4%, and excess scarring occurred in 4% of patients. Of the 185 patients questioned, 95% were happy with their results. Gonzalez[60] conducted an interesting study involving 33 reduction patients, and the same survey was given to 40 volunteers of similar age, height, and weight but with small breasts. In this study, reduction surgery reduced backache and shoulder and neck pain in all patients and totally eliminated it in 25%. Symptomatic improvement was independent of height-to-weight ratios, again calling into question the benefits of attempting to lose weight as an effective conservative intervention in this population of patients.

Operating on patients for breast pain has always been a difficult issue for plastic surgeons. Patients with mammary hypertrophy often complain of breast pain, but how does this respond to surgery? In answer to this question, Wallace[130] surveyed 282 women who presented with breast pain after surgery, including 49 women who had breast reductions. The breast reduction patients had the lowest incidence of postoperative pain at only 22%. Much of this pain was probably neurogenic in origin because it tended to improve steadily with time. With regard to a woman's primary motivation for reduction, Schnur[131] found that 78% desired symptomatic relief, 5% were motivated by cosmetic reasons, and 17% had a mixed motive. Whereas these are all powerful arguments in favor of insurance coverage for breast reduction, third-party carriers still place arbitrary weight restrictions on the planned resection before they will consider covering the procedure. Typically, this number is 500 g per side. This is reasonable for some women, but short women may be highly symptomatic with much smaller breasts than their taller counterparts are. Seitchik[132] has suggested that different resection weights should be applied to different patient weights: 400 g for a body weight of less than 60 kg; 700 g for 61 to 70 kg; and 1000 g for more than 80 kg. Although these numbers may seem reasonable, they are not supported by the data currently available. They do not take into account the fact that reduction patients benefit from surgery based on breast size and symptoms with little or no correlation with body weight.

COMPLICATIONS

Hematomas and Seromas

Hematomas are rare, with an incidence of less than 1%.[103,111] They typically occur within the first 12 hours after surgery and are usually unilateral. Hematomas manifest with increasing pain, swelling, and bruising of the affected side and may be associated with evidence of vascular impairment to a previously viable nipple or skin envelope secondary to tension-induced ischemia. Bleeding intercostal perforators are the most common source. Treatment involves surgical evacuation and sealing of the bleeding point. Drains have not been shown to be of any real value in reducing hematoma rates, and their use is not recommended.[74] Seromas are also rare, with an incidence between 1% and 5%. Aspiration is usually adequate to deal with the problem, but ultrasound-guided aspiration with insertion of a seroma drain may be required in difficult procedures.

Infection

Infection in the form of cellulitis requiring antibiotics or abscess formation is fortunately rare, with an incidence of 1%. Cellulitis is treated with antibiotics. Abscesses require open drainage and are usually a consequence of infection within an undiagnosed hematoma. Davis[102] reported a 12% incidence of cellulitis requiring antibiotic therapy, a figure that seems high. Dabbah[59] reported a 22% incidence of infection and fat necrosis. Perioperative antibiotic therapy may be helpful in maintaining lower infection rates, as may saline lavage of the reduction site before closure.

Skin Necrosis

Skin necrosis is often tension related in Wise-pattern reductions and is virtually absent in vertical techniques. In Wise-pattern closures, tension at the inverted T closure compromises blood flow to the tips of the skin flaps, and necrosis follows. It is crucial to redistribute tension from lateral to medial in these closures, thereby ensuring that the flap tips are under no tension whatsoever. It is also important to avoid undermining the tips of these flaps in an effort to maintain good vascularity to the tissues.

The incidence of necrosis after breast reduction is unclear and is obviously related to surgical expertise, technique, and procedure. Skin necrosis and wound healing complications occur more frequently than does invasive infection. Davis[102] reported a 19% incidence of wound healing problems related to skin viability underneath the breast. Lejour[100] noted a 5.4% incidence of delayed healing at the inframammary crease associated with vertical reductions, and wound healing problems were directly proportional to the preoperative breast size and quantity of fat within the breast. Minimizing the size of the inferior dog-ear deformity and paying careful attention to meticulous vertical incision coaptation are crucial to improved wound healing at this site.

Fat Necrosis

Fat necrosis is also rare but more common with long central or inferior pedicles in huge breasts. Folding of a long superior pedicle may also precipitate fat necrosis. Sutures incorporating large portions of breast fat may induce patchy fat necrosis beneath suture lines. The incidence of fat necrosis is grossly underreported because it may exist without obvious palpable lesions that are, however, visible on mammography. Dabbah[59] noted a 22% rate of clinically palpable fat necrosis and infection. Fat necrosis may cause the patient anxiety about cancer. Its appearance on mammography is fairly typical with densely whorled calcification rather than the finely stippled calcification of carcinoma.[78] Fine-needle aspiration can provide accurate tissue diagnosis where uncertainty exists.

Nipple Loss

Nipple loss is uncommon, but it is reported in association with smoking. Long pedicles or a thick pedicle folded in vertical technique may also predispose to nipple loss from inadequate vascular perfusion. It is more common in massive pedicled reductions. Davis[102] reported a 6% incidence in inferior pedicled and bipedicled McKissock techniques; Dabbah[59] noted a 4% rate. With vertical reduction, blistering occurred in 3% with no nipple losses. Nipple blistering is more likely than true full-thickness necrosis. If blistering occurs, it should be allowed to heal secondarily, but patients should be warned that depigmentation of the areola may result. If frank necrosis occurs, it should also be allowed to heal before nipple reconstruction is performed.

Laser Doppler flowmetry may be used to evaluate perfusion to nipples that appear to be marginal, particularly in black patients with very dark areolae. Roth[133] determined perfusion rates in patients without complications (average perfusion, 4.8 mL/min per 100 g), in those with blistering (1.4 mL/min per 100 g), and in those with frank necrosis (0.8 mL/min per 100 g), demonstrating significant quantitative differences in flow. Perbeck[134] has shown enormous reserves in nipple blood flow even once the pedicle is cut, and deepithelialization actually increased blood flow to the nipple above resting preoperative values. In another study by Scheufler,[135] near-infrared reflection spectroscopy measurement of blood flow to the skin and areola of post-breast reduction patients found a good correlation between decreased tissue oxygenation and poor surgical outcome. Because instrument calibration and standardization are still widely disparate between manufacturers, the routine use of such devices for assessment of cutaneous blood flow is unlikely in the near future.

Nipple Numbness

Nipple numbness is common in most techniques to some degree; the tendency is for feeling to return with time, but it may never return to normal levels. Courtiss and Goldwyn[37] and Slezak and Dellon[136] have observed that many women with large breasts do not have much tactile sensation in their nipples preoperatively, and this should be discussed with the patient preoperatively. On the basis of our understanding of nipple nerve supply, central pedicles are probably more likely to preserve sensation than are upper pole pedicles, but the multiplicity of innervation sources tends to maintain some degree of sensitivity in most patients.

Several studies have attempted to quantify nipple sensitivity postoperatively. Gonzalez[137] reported a 9% loss of sensation in central and inferior pedicle techniques but made the observation that if less than 440 g of tissue is resected per side, nipple sensation is usually preserved. On occasion, patients may develop hyperesthetic nipples, but this usually resolves spontaneously. Some patients report an improvement in nipple sensation after reduction, and this may reflect a reduction in traction on nerves after reduction of breast mass. This observation has been corroborated by Temple and Hurst,[138] who noted improved sensation in 43 of 45 patients undergoing inferior pedicle reduction, with loss of sensation in only 2 patients. Free nipple grafting may be associated with return of sensation in a significant number of patients. Townsend reported his data of 45 patients with free nipple grafts, and 82% noted some degree of sensory return to light touch. A comparison by Hamdi[139] of superior pedicle reduction with inferior pedicle reduction yielded interesting results. Patients with superior pedicles had better initial breast skin sensitivity, whereas patients with inferior pedicles had better nipple sensation. By 6 months, both groups had similar sensation without any patients reporting total insensibility, but 50% of the patients had less sensation than preoperative levels.

Critics have often suggested that vertical mammaplasties may fare more poorly in terms of recovering sensation. Greuse[107] reviewed 80 vertical mammaplasties with Lejour's technique. Patients were evaluated on the basis of the volume of resection and nipple to notch measurement. Group 1 had less than 500 g resected per side with nipple to notch measurements of less than 29 cm; group 2 had more than 500 g resected per side with nipple to notch measurements of more than 29 cm. Group 1 patients experienced an initial decline in sensation with progressive return to normal. Group 2 patients had recovery of pressure sensation, but vibration and temperature sensitivities were still diminished at 1 year. Patients did not complain of nipple numbness in this series. Loss of sensation appears to worry surgeons more than it does patients, but careful preoperative counseling is essential to prevent the patient's misunderstanding about this condition.

Hypertrophic Scars

Hypertrophic scars usually occur with the most medial or lateral ends of the horizontal limb of a Wise-pattern scar. Reducing tension and postoperative taping or topical silicone application may be of value. Steroid injections are also helpful in more recalcitrant scars.

One of the most common causes of litigation after breast reduction is unsatisfactory scarring. Vertical techniques may reduce this complication, but even these procedures carry their share of problems. Lassus described 20 patients with unsatisfactory scars in his series of 710 patients, 4 of them categorized as "serious." Davis reported an 18% incidence of poor scarring with a Wise-pattern approach. Excess scarring continues to be the major source of breast reduction-based litigation in the United States at the time of writing.

Asymmetry

Asymmetry should be avoided at all costs by intraoperative evaluation of breast size and shape after reduction and loose tailor-tacking of the breast with temporary staples. It is not what is removed but rather what is left behind that really matters in reduction surgery. Flap thickness should be palpated carefully, and resection lines should be meticulously drawn and compared for symmetry with the patient in the erect position preoperatively. Davis reported an 8% incidence of asymmetry. Failure to achieve symmetry is a fairly common cause of litigation after reduction surgery. Prevention of this complication is essential because reoperation may be required if asymmetry occurs after reduction.

Inadequate Reduction or Overresection

Inadequate reduction tends to be more of a problem for the neophyte than for experienced surgeons. It can be a problem with vertical techniques when this approach is first learned. The estimation of resection volumes mentioned earlier should give the surgeon a rough guide of how much tissue to resect for any given breast size.

Overresection is especially risky in patients with grade III ptosis with empty upper poles in whom inferior glandular resection is done. It is a serious enough problem to warrant some women's requesting postreduction breast augmentation if overresection has been radical. Great caution should be exercised in dealing with very ptotic breasts or patients who have undergone massive weight loss. The problem is even more serious in performing breast amputation techniques through a Wise-pattern keyhole in massive breasts with severe ptosis. The problem can be avoided by beveling the resection inferiorly to conserve more lower pole tissue, which can be folded into the new breast when flap closure is performed. When reductions are performed in obese patients, care should be taken to leave the breasts a little larger than usual to maintain normal body proportions. If the patient undergoes weight loss or has a gastric bypass, subsequent weight loss from the breasts may leave them looking too small and disproportionate.

"Boxy" Breast Deformity

A result of "boxy" breast deformity is due to inadequate inferolateral-inferomedial resections, particularly prevalent when an inferior pedicle technique is used. Failure to empty the medial and lateral inframammary quadrants causes fullness in these areas, contributing to the appearance of lower pole squareness.

Intramammary Scarring

Intramammary scarring visible on mammography is rarely a major clinical problem. Fat necrosis calcification has a typical whorled appearance on mammography; its incidence was quoted as 25% in a study by Danikas,[78] who evaluated inferior pedicle and vertical bipedicle reductions.

Recurrent Enlargement

Recurrent enlargement is secondary to massive weight gain or ongoing virginal hypertrophy. Patients with virginal hypertrophy must be warned that their breasts are still growing and may need a secondary reduction. It is probably wise to wait until breast growth has been static for at least 1 year before proceeding with reduction in young girls unless symptoms are incapacitating or ulceration is imminent. Secondary reduction (discussed earlier) is definitely more risky than primary reduction and should incorporate use of the original pedicle whenever possible.

Inability to Breast-feed

An inability to breast-feed is a significant issue for many young women seeking breast reduction. Many women with large breasts tend to be poor breast-feeders, but this is a generalization. They should be warned that although some women are able to breast-feed after reduction, many cannot; and of those who can, few are able to nourish their children entirely from breast-feeding.

In a study of the Pitanguy technique, Aboudib[140] found that of 11 patients who became pregnant after reduction, 9 (91%) were able to lactate and to breast-feed successfully. In another study, Marshall[141] followed up 30 women who breast-fed after reduction mammaplasty. At discharge from the hospital, 93% were successfully breast-feeding; but by 3 months post partum, only 27% were still breast-feeding, and almost all required supplementary formula feedings. Sandsmark[142] observed a cohort of 292 patients, 49 of whom attempted to breast-feed after delivery. Of 49 patients, 32 (65%) were able to breast-feed, but all of them required supplemental feeding to provide adequate nutrition for their infants. Similar findings were borne out by Souto et al,[143] who found that few mothers were able to maintain adequate levels of breast milk production after reduction. Harris[144] followed up 20 of 68 women who had inferior pedicle reductions and found that of those women who lactated, 35% nursed for at least 2 months, 45% persisted for only 2 weeks, and the remainder did not even attempt to breast-feed. In yet another study, Brzozowski[145] found that of 78 women who bore children after inferior pedicle reductions, 52.6% became engorged and did not attempt to breast-feed; only 19% breast-fed successfully without requiring formula supplementation. Putting all of these data together, it is clear that although breast-feeding is technically possible after a wide variety of reduction techniques, successful breast-feeding is rarely achieved without supplemental formula feedings.

Cancer and Breast Reduction

There are potentially serious medicolegal implications when breast cancer is found at the time of breast reduction. Breast reduction does not cause cancer; in fact, because of the resection of a significant amount of breast tissue, the risk of breast cancer has been shown to be slightly reduced. It is still imperative, however, that patients continue to perform breast self-examination and have regular mammograms at the appropriate age. In a study by Tang,[146] patients diagnosed with breast cancer at the time of breast reduction were shown to have earlier stage lesions with a higher incidence of node-negative lesions. Their 5-year survival was also higher at 88% as opposed to a 77% survival for matched controls in the general population. Similarly, Brinton[52] found that patients who previously had breast reductions and then developed breast carcinoma experienced lower risk than that of unreduced patients.

Inadequate Mastopexy Result

An inadequate mastopexy effect is due to inadequate skin resection to shape the gland or may result from breast suction. Suction lipectomy of the breast has been described by Courtiss. It is appropriate only for smaller reductions and relies heavily on adequate skin retraction to shape the gland. It is not useful in severely ptotic breasts.

Dog-ears

Dog-ears occur laterally and medially in Wise-pattern reductions and inferiorly with vertical reductions. Minor revisions under local anesthesia in the office operating room will usually provide adequate correction if these dog-ears have not settled spontaneously within 6 months of the original reduction. In obese patients, dog-ears may extend onto the posterior chest because of the large amount of axillary fullness so prevalent in this population of patients. These patients may need more extensive revisions under general anesthesia with both excisional and suction contouring of the lateral chest and back.

CONCLUSION

Breast reduction is an established, highly successful surgical technique aimed at reducing both the size of the large female breast and the complications associated with mammary hypertrophy. Satisfaction of patients is high, and the results are reasonably predictable. The advent of scar reduction techniques has added significantly to the success of these procedures and has, to some extent, enhanced long-term retention of breast projection. Outcome studies are increasingly demonstrating the value of these procedures in terms of their positive impact on patients' physical and psychological well-being. Their incorporation into oncologic breast surgery has enabled breast conservation to be offered more safely to women with larger breasts.

REFERENCES

1. Dieffenbach JF: Die Operative Chirurgie, vol 2. Leipzig, Brockhaus, 1848:370.
2. Pousson M, Michel X: Sur un cas de mastopexie. J Med Bordeaux 1897;27:495.
3. Guinard M: Comment on: Rapport de l'ablation esthetique des tumeurs du sein, par M.H. Morestin. Bull Mem Soc Chir (Paris) 1903;29:568.
4. Thorek M: Possibilities in the recognition of the human form. N Y Med J 1922;116:572.
5. Aubert V: Hypertrophie mammaire de la puberte: resection partielle restauratrice. Arch Franco-Belg Chir 1923;3:284.
6. Passot R: La correction esthetique du prolapsus mammaire par le procede de la transposition du mamelon. Presse Med 1925;33:317.
7. Schwarzmann E: Die Technik der Mammaplastik. Chirurg 1930;2:932.
8. Biesenberger H: Eine neue Methode der Mammaplastik. Zentrabl Chir 1928;55:2383.
9. Aufricht G: Mammaplasty for pendulous breasts. Empiric and geometric planning. Plast Reconstr Surg 1949;4:13.
10. Bames HO: Reduction of massive breast hypertrophy. Plast Reconstr Surg 1948;3:560.
11. Penn J: Breast reduction. Br J Plast Surg 1955;7:357.
12. Strombeck JO: Mammaplasty: report of a new techniques based on the two pedicle procedure. Br J Plast Surg 1960; 13:79.
13. Skoog TA: A technique of breast reduction, transposition of the nipple on a cutaneous vascular pedicle. Acta Chir Scand 1963;126:453.
14. Wise RJ: A preliminary report on a method of planning the mammaplasty. Plast Reconstr Surg 1956;17:367.
15. McKissock PK: Reduction mammaplasty with vertical dermal flap. Plast Reconstr Surg 1972;49:245.

16. Pitanguy I: Surgical correction of breast hypertrophy. Br J Plast Surg 1967;20:78.
17. Weiner DL, Aiache AE, Silver L, Tittiranonda T: A single dermal pedicle for nipple transposition in subcutaneous mastectomy, reduction mammaplasty, or mastopexy. Plast Reconstr Surg 1973;51:115.
18. Courtiss E, Goldwyn RM: Reduction mammaplasty by the inferior pedicle technique. Plast Reconstr Surg 1977;59:500.
19. Georgiade NG, Serafin D, Morris R, et al: Reduction mammaplasty utilizing an inferior pedicle nipple-areolar flap. Ann Plast Surg 1979;3:211.
20. Ribiero L: A new technique for reduction mammaplasty. Plast Reconstr Surg 1975;55:330.
21. Robbins TH: A reduction mammaplasty with the areola-nipple based on an inferior dermal pedicle. Plast Reconstr Surg 1977;59:64.
22. Hester TR Jr, Bostwick J III, Miller L: Breast reduction utilizing the maximally vascularized central pedicle. Plast Reconstr Surg 1985;76:890.
23. Orlando JC, Guthrie RH Jr: The superomedial pedicle for nipple transposition. Br J Plast Surg 1975;28:42.
24. Lassus C: A technique for breast reduction. Int Surg 1970;53:69.
25. Lassus C: Breast reduction: evolution of a technique—a single vertical scar. Aesthetic Plast Surg 1987;11:107.
26. Lejour M, Abboud M: Vertical mammaplasty without inframammary scar and with breast liposuction. Perspect Plast Surg 1990;4:67.
27. Lejour M: Vertical mammaplasty and liposuction of the breast. Plast Reconstr Surg 1994;94:100.
28. Marchac D, de Olarte G: Reduction mammaplasty and correction of ptosis with a short inframammary scar. Plast Reconstr Surg 1982;69:45.
29. Peixoto G: Reduction mammaplasty: a personal technique. Plast Reconstr Surg 1980;65:217.
30. Goes JCS: Periareolar mammaplasty: double skin technique with application of polyglactine or mixed mesh. Plast Reconstr Surg 1996;97:959.
31. Benelli L: A new periareolar mammaplasty: round block technique. Aesthetic Plast Surg 1990;14:93.
32. Hammond DC: Short scar periareolar inferior pedicle reduction (SPAIR) mammaplasty. Plast Reconstr Surg 1999; 103:890.
33. Hall-Findlay EJ: A simplified vertical reduction mammaplasty; shortening the learning curve. Plast Reconstr Surg 1999;104: 748.
34. Gray SW, Skandalakis JE: Embryology for Surgeons. Philadelphia, WB Saunders, 1972:405.
35. Cooper AP: On the Anatomy of the Breast, vol 2. London, Longmans, 1840:1-89.
36. Craig RDP, Sykes PA: Nipple sensitivity following reduction mammaplasty. Br J Plast Surg 1970;23:165.
37. Courtiss EH, Goldwyn RM: Breast sensation before and after plastic surgery. Plast Reconstr Surg 1976;58:1.
38. Sarhadi NS, Dunn JS, Lee FD, Soutar DS: An anatomical study of the nerve supply of the breast, including the nipple and areola. Br J Plast Surg 1996;49:156.
39. Palmer JH, Taylor GI: The vascular territories of the anterior chest wall. Br J Plast Surg 1986;39:287.
40. Maliniac JW: Arterial supply of the breast. Arch Surg 1943;47:329.
41. Hollinshead WH: Anatomy for Surgeons, vol 2. New York, Harper & Row, 1971:17.
42. Russo J, Hu YF, Silva ID, Russo IH: Cancer risk related to mammary gland structure and development. Microsc Res Tech 2001;52:204.
43. Pang S: Premature thelarche and premature adrenarche. Pediatr Ann 1981;10:29.
44. Ilicki A, Prager Lewin R, Kauli R, et al: Premature thelarche—natural history and sex hormone secretion in 68 girls. Acta Paediatr Scand 1984;73:756.
45. Root AW, Shulman DI: Isosexual precocity. Current concepts and recent advances. Fertil Steril 1986;45:749.
46. Jabs AD, Frantz AG, Smith-Vaniz A, Hugo NE: Mammary hypertrophy is not associated with increased estrogen receptors. Plast Reconstr Surg 1990;86:64.
47. Eliasen CA, Cranor ML, Rosen PP: Atypical duct hyperplasia of the breast in young females. Am J Pathol 1992;16:246.
48. Durston W: Concerning a very sudden and excessive swelling of a woman's breast. Philosoph Trans R Soc Lond 1670;4:1047.
49. Baker SB, Burkey BA, Thornton P, LaRossa D: Juvenile gigantomastia: presentation of four cases and review of the literature. Ann Plast Surg 2001;46:517.
50. Audretsch WP, Rezai M, Kolotas C, et al: Tumor specific immediate reconstruction in breast cancer patients. Perspect Plast Surg 1998;11:71.
51. Clough KB, Nos C, Calmon RJ, et al: Conservative treatment of breast cancers by mammaplasty and irradiation: a new approach to lower quadrant tumors. Plast Reconstr Surg 1995;96:363.
52. Brinton LA, Persson I, Boice D Jr, et al: Breast cancer risk in relation to amount of tissue removed during breast reduction operations in Sweden. Cancer 2001;91:478.
53. Letterman G, Schurter M: The effects of mammary hypertrophy on the skeletal system. Ann Plast Surg 1980;5:425.
54. Kerrigan CL, Collins ED, Kneeland TS, et al: Measuring health state preferences in women with breast hypertrophy. Plast Reconstr Surg 2000;106:280.
55. Kerrigan CL, Collins ED, Striplin D, et al: The health burden of breast hypertrophy. Plast Reconstr Surg 2001;108:1591.
56. Netscher DT, Meade RA, Goodman CM, et al: Physical and psychological symptoms among 88 volunteer subjects compared with patients seeking plastic surgery procedures to the breast. Plast Reconstr Surg 2000;105:2366.
57. Collins ED, Kerrigan CL, Kim M, et al: The effectiveness of surgical and nonsurgical interventions in relieving the symptoms of macromastia. Plast Reconstr Surg 2002;109:1556.
58. Boschert MT, Barone CM, Puckett CL: Outcome analysis of reduction mammaplasty. Plast Reconstr Surg 1996;98:451.
59. Dabbah A, Lehman JA Jr, Parker MG, et al: Reduction mammaplasty: an outcome analysis. Ann Plast Surg 1995; 35:337.
60. Gonzalez F, Walton RL, Shafer B, et al: Reduction mammaplasty improves symptoms of macromastia. Plast Reconstr Surg 1993;91:1270.
61. Klassen A, Fitzpatrick R, Jenkinson C, Goodacre T: Should breast reduction surgery be rationed? A comparison of the health status of patients before and after treatment: postal questionnaire. BMJ 1996;313:454.
62. Klassen A, Fitzpatrick R, Jenkinson C, Goodacre T: Patients' health related quality of life before and after aesthetic surgery. Br J Plast Surg 1996;49:433.
63. Maxwell-Davis G, Ringler SL, Short K, et al: Reduction mammaplasty: long term efficacy, morbidity and patient satisfaction. Plast Reconstr Surg 1995;96:1106.
64. Miller AP, Zacher JB, Berggren RB, et al: Breast reduction for symptomatic macromastia: can objective predictors for operative success be identified? Plast Reconstr Surg 1995;95:77.
65. Raispis T, Zehring RD, Downey DL: Long-term functional results after reduction mammaplasty. Ann Plast Surg 1995; 34:113.
66. Berry EP: Geometric planning in reduction mammaplasty. Plast Reconstr Surg 1968;42:232.
67. Thorek M: Plastic reconstruction of the breast and free transplantation of the nipple. J Int Coll Surg 1946;9:194.
68. Gradinger GP: Breast reduction with free nipple graft technique. In Spear SL, ed: Surgery of the Breast: Principles and Art. Philadelphia, Lippincott-Raven, 1998:807-821.
69. Arie G: Una nueva tecnica de mastoplastia. Rev Iber Latino Am Cir Plast 1957;3:28.

70. Mathes SJ, Nahai F, Hester TR: Avoiding the flat breast in reduction mammaplasty. Plast Reconstr Surg 1980;66:63.
71. Platt R, Zucker JR, Zaleznik DF, et al: Perioperative antibiotic prophylaxis and wound infection following breast surgery. J Antimicrob Chemother 1993;31(suppl B):43.
72. Serletti JM, Davenport MS, Herrera HR, Caldwell EH: Efficacy of antibiotic prophylaxis in reduction mammaplasty. Ann Plast Surg 1994;33:476.
73. Clugston PA, Fitzpatrick DG, Kester DA, et al: Autologous blood use in reduction mammaplasty. Is it justified? Plast Reconstr Surg 1995;95:824.
74. Arrowsmith J, Eltigani E, Krarup K, Varma S: An audit of breast reduction without drains. Br J Plast Surg 1999;52:586.
75. Bell MSG: The use of epinephrine in breast reduction [comment]. Plast Reconstr Surg 2003;112:693.
76. Davies BW, Lewis RD, Pennington GA: Reduction mammaplasty: a comparison of outpatient and inpatient procedures. Aesthetic Plast Surg 1996;20:77.
77. Short KK, Ringler SL, Bengston BP et al: Reduction mammaplasty: a safe and effective outpatient procedure. Aesthetic Plast Surg 1996;20:513.
77a. Buenaventura S, Severinac R, Mullis W, et al: Outpatient reduction mammaplasty: a review of 338 consecutive cases. Ann Plast Surg 1996;36:162.
78. Danikas D, Theodorou SJ, Kokkalis G, et al: Mammographic findings following reduction mammaplasty. Aesthetic Plast Surg 2001;25:283.
79. Grazer FM: Suction-Assisted Lipectomy. Its Indications, Contraindications and Complications. Chicago, Year Book, 1984. Advances in Plastic and Reconstructive Surgery, vol 51.
80. Teimourian B, Massac E Jr, Wiegering CE: Reduction suction mammaplasty and suction lipectomy as an adjunct to breast surgery. Aesthetic Plast Surg 1985;9:97.
81. Matarasso A, Courtiss EH: Suction mammaplasty: the use of suction lipectomy to reduce large breasts. Plast Reconstr Surg 1991;87:709.
82. Courtiss EH: Reduction mammaplasty by suction alone. Plast Reconstr Surg 1993;92:1276.
83. Lejour M: Discussion of "Reduction mammaplasty by suction alone" by E.H. Courtiss. Plast Reconstr Surg 1993;92:1286.
84. Mandrekas AD, Zambacos GJ, Anastopoulos A, Hapsas DA: Reduction mammaplasty with the inferior pedicle technique: early and late complications in 371 patients. Br J Plast Surg 1996;49:442.
85. Ariyan S: Reduction mammaplasty with the nipple-areola carried on a single, narrow inferior pedicle. Ann Plast Surg 1980;5:167.
86. Crepeau R, Klein H: Reduction mammaplasty with inferiorly based glandular pedicle flap. Ann Plast Surg 1982;9:463.
87. Robbins LB, Hoffman DK: The superior dermoglandular pedicle approach to breast reduction. Ann Plast Surg 1992;29:211.
88. Abramo AC: Pattern of reduction mammaplasty that uses a superior vertical dermal pedicle. Aesthetic Plast Surg 1991;15:265.
89. Matarasso A, Pitanguy I: The keel resection/Pitanguy reduction mammaplasty. Operative Techniques Plast Reconstr Surg 1996;3:156.
90. Nicolle F: Improved standards in reduction mammaplasty and mastopexy. Plast Reconstr Surg 1982;69:453.
91. Botta SA, Rifai R: Personal refinements in the single pedicle Skoog technique for reduction mammaplasty. Aesthetic Plast Surg 1991;15:257.
92. Nahabedian MY, McGibbon BM, Manson PN: Medial pedicle reduction mammaplasty for severe mammary hypertrophy. Plast Reconstr Surg 2000;105:896.
93. Biesenberger H: Deformitaten und kosmetische Operationen der weiblichen Brust. Vienna, W Maudrich, 1931.
94. Climo MS, Alexander JE: Intercostothelial circulation: nipple survival in reduction mammaplasty in the absence of a dermal pedicle. Ann Plast Surg 1980;4:128.
95. Kraske H: Operative treatment of hypertrophied mamma. Munch Med Wochenschr 1923;70:672.
96. Dufourmentel C, Mouly R: Plastie mammaire par la methode oblique. Ann Chir Plast 1961;6:45.
97. Regnault P: Reduction mammaplasty by the "B" technique. Plast Reconstr Surg 1974;53:19.
98. Lassus C: A 30 year experience with vertical mammaplasty. Plast Reconstr Surg 1996;97:373.
99. Lassus C: Update on vertical mammaplasty. Plast Reconstr Surg 1999;104:2289.
100. Lejour M: Vertical mammaplasty: early complications after 250 personal consecutive cases. Plast Reconstr Surg 1999;104:764.
101. Pickford MA, Boorman JG: Early experience with the Lejour vertical scar reduction mammaplasty technique. Br J Plast Surg 1993;46:516.
102. Davis GM, Ringler SL, Short K, et al: Reduction mammaplasty: long-term efficacy, morbidity and patient satisfaction. Plast Reconstr Surg 1995;96:1106.
103. Tapia A, Blanch A, Salvador J, et al: Evolution of the vertical Lejour's mastoplasty technique. Aesthetic Plast Surg 1996;20:377.
104. Asplund OA, Davies DM: Vertical scar breast reduction with medial flap or glandular transposition of the nipple-areola. Br J Plast Surg 1996;49:507.
105. Deconinck C, de Greef C, Walravens C, Calteux N: Report of 243 vertical mammaplasties for very large, heavy breasts and/or severe ptosis. Analysis of the result and technical. Ann Chir Plast Esthet 2002;47:623.
106. Godwin Y, Wood SH, O'Neill TJ: A comparison of the patient and surgeon opinion on the long-term aesthetic outcome of reduction mammaplasty. Br J Plast Surg 1998;51:444.
107. Greuse M, Hamdi M, De Mey A: Breast sensitivity after vertical mammaplasty. Plast Reconstr Surg 2001;107:970.
108. Berthe JV, Massaut J, Greuse M, et al: The vertical mammaplasty: a reappraisal of the techniques and its complications. Plast Reconstr Surg 2003;111:2192.
109. Shin KS, Lee HK: Reduction mammaplasty with the short submammary scar (S-S-S) technique. Aesthetic Plast Surg 1992;16:109.
110. Bozola AR: Breast reduction with short L scar. Plast Reconstr Surg 1990;85:728.
111. Born G: The "L" reduction mammaplasty. Ann Plast Surg 1994;32:383.
112. Chiari A Jr: The L short-scar mammaplasty. 12 years later. Plast Reconstr Surg 2001;108:489.
113. Yousif NJ, Larson DL, Sanger JR, Matloub HS: Elimination of the vertical scar in reduction mammaplasty. Plast Reconstr Surg 1992;89:459.
114. Savaci N: Reduction mammaplasty by the central pedicle avoiding a vertical scar. Aesthetic Plast Surg 1996;20:171.
115. Felicio Y: Periareolar reduction mammaplasty. Plast Reconstr Surg 1991;88:789.
116. Oneal RM: Reduction mammaplasty with free nipple transplantation: indications and refinements. Ann Plast Surg 1991;26:117.
117. Casas LA, Byun MY, Depoli PA: Maximizing breast projection after free-nipple-graft reduction mammaplasty. Plast Reconstr Surg 2001;107:955.
118. Koger KE, Sunde D, Press BHJ, Hovey LM: Reduction mammaplasty for gigantomastia using inferiorly based pedicle with free nipple transplantation. Ann Plast Surg 1994;33:561.
119. Hudson DA, Skoll PJ: Repeat reduction mammaplasty. Plast Reconstr Surg 1999;104:401.
120. Losee JE, Caldwell EH, Serletti JM: Secondary reduction mammaplasty. Is using a different pedicle safe? Plast Reconstr Surg 2000;106:1004.
121. Spear SL, Burke JB, Forman D, et al: Experience with reduction mammaplasty following breast conservation surgery and radiation therapy. Plast Reconstr Surg 1998;102:1913.

122. Handel N, Lewinsky B, Waisman JR: Reduction mammaplasty following radiation therapy for breast cancer. Plast Reconstr Surg 1992;85:953.
123. McMahan JD, Wolfe JA, Cromer BA, Ruberg RL: Lasting success in teenage reduction mammaplasty. Ann Plast Surg 1995; 35:227.
124. Evans GRD, Ryan JJ: Reduction mammaplasty for the teenage patient: a critical analysis. Aesthetic Plast Surg 1994;18:291.
125. Woods JE, Borkowski JJ, Masson JK, Irons GB: Experience with and comparison of methods of reduction mammaplasty. Mayo Clin Proc 1978;53:487.
126. Hughes LA, Mahoney JL: Patient satisfaction with reduction mammaplasty: an early survey. Aesthetic Plast Surg 1993; 17:345.
127. Blomquist L, Eriksson A, Brandberg Y: Reduction mammaplasty provides long-term improvement in health status and quality of life. Plast Reconstr Surg 2000;106:991.
128. Miller AP, Zacher JB, Berggren RB, et al: Breast reduction for symptomatic macromastia: can objective predictors for operative success be identified? Plast Reconstr Surg 1995;95:77.
129. Sood R, Mount D, Coleman J III, et al: Effects of reduction mammaplasty on pulmonary function and symptoms of macromastia. Plast Reconstr Surg 2003;111:688.
130. Wallace MS, Wallace AM, Lee J, Dobke MK: Pain after breast surgery: a survey of 282 women. Pain 1996;66:195.
131. Schnur PL, Hoehn JG, Ilstrup DM, et al: Reduction mammaplasty: cosmetic or reconstructive procedure? [comment]. Ann Plast Surg 1991;27:232.
132. Seitchik MW: Reduction mammaplasty: criteria for insurance coverage. Plast Reconstr Surg 1995;95:1029.
133. Roth AC, Zook EG, Brown R, Zamboni WA: Nipple-areolar perfusion and reduction mammaplasty: correlation of laser Doppler readings with surgical complications. Plast Reconstr Surg 1996;97:381.
134. Perbeck L, Proano E, Maatanen H: Skin circulation in the nipple after reduction mammaplasty with a bipedicle vertical dermal flap. Scand J Plast Reconstr Surg Hand Surg 1991;25:41.
135. Scheufler O, Andresen R: Tissue oxygenation and perfusion in inferior pedicle reduction mammaplasty by near-infrared reflection spectroscopy and color-coded duplex sonography. Plast Reconstr Surg 2003;111:1131.
136. Slezak S, Dellon AL: Quantitation of sensibility in gigantomastia and alteration following reduction mammaplasty. Plast Reconstr Surg 1993;91:1265.
137. Gonzalez F, Brown FE, Gold ME, et al: Preoperative and postoperative nipple sensibility in patients undergoing reduction mammaplasty. Plast Reconstr Surg 1993;92:809.
138. Temple CLF, Hurst LN: Reduction mammaplasty improves breast sensibility. Plast Reconstr Surg 1999;104:72.
139. Hamdi M, Greuse M, De Mey A, Webster MHC: A prospective quantitative comparison of breast sensation after superior and inferior pedicle mammaplasty. Br J Plast Surg 2001;54:43.
140. Aboudib JH, de Castro CC, Coelho RS, Cupello AM: Analysis of late results in post-pregnancy mammaplasty. Ann Plast Surg 1991;26:111.
141. Marshall DR, Callan PP, Nicholson W: Breastfeeding after reduction mammaplasty. Br J Plast Surg 1994;47:167.
142. Sandsmark M, Amland PF, Abyholm F, Traaholt L: Reduction mammaplasty: a comparative study of the Orlando and Robbins methods in 292 patients. Scand J Plast Reconstr Surg Hand Surg 1992;26:203.
143. Souto GC, Giugliani ER, Giugliani C, Schneider MA: The impact of breast reduction surgery on breast feeding performance. J Hum Lact 2003;19:43.
144. Harris L, Morris SF, Freiberg A: Is breast feeding possible after reduction mammaplasty? Plast Reconstr Surg 1992; 89:836.
145. Brzozowski D, Niessen M, Evans HB, Hurst LN: Breast feeding after inferior pedicle reduction mammaplasty. Plast Reconstr Surg 2000;105:530.
146. Tang C, Brown M, Levine R, et al: Breast cancer found at the time of breast reduction. Plast Reconstr Surg 1999;103: 1682.

CHAPTER

136

Vertical Reduction: Techniques

KRISTIN BOEHM, MD ✦ FOAD NAHAI, MD, FACS

Breast reduction techniques have evolved through multiple adaptations and variations since their inception in the early 1900s. Early techniques, such as that of Biesenberger,[1] involved complete dissection of the skin from the underlying breast tissue; Pitanguy,[2] Strombeck,[3] and Skoog[4,5] introduced pedicle techniques, leaving breast parenchyma attached to the skin. In particular, those procedures based on the inferior pedicle proved technically easier in the hands of most surgeons and led to a certain popularity of the inferior pedicle technique that persists even today.[6,7] Whereas all of these techniques were successful in the treatment of mammary hypertrophy and its associated symptoms, they relied on the inverted T incision and resultant conspicuous scar. Recognizing the need to improve on length and quality of these scars, surgeons have recently focused on the development of reduction mammaplasty techniques that eliminate the transverse incision and improve the aesthetic result of the reduced breast.

In 1969, Lassus[8] revived the vertical reduction technique originated by Dartigues[9] and later modified it to effectively establish a vertical scar that did not cross the inframammary fold.[10-12] Marchac[13,14] and Marconi and Cavina[15] made further modifications, but it was Lejour[16,17] who most notably popularized the technique that led to its widespread acceptance in Europe and South America. On the other hand, North American surgeons have been reluctant to adopt vertical reduction techniques, most likely because of the associated steep learning curve, the familiarity with inferior pedicle techniques, and a certain discomfort with the superior pedicle and early postoperative appearance of the breasts. However, as the technique has continued to evolve and superior results are consistently reproduced, enthusiasm for the procedure has grown and sparked increased interest in learning the details of the vertical approach. As experience with vertical reduction continues to increase, improved results and fewer complications should lead to a high satisfaction rate among both surgeons and patients.

SELECTION OF PATIENTS

Standard breast reduction operations are effective in reducing breast size and alleviating the associated symptoms of macromastia. The vertical mammaplasty is no exception and as such is applicable to all women deemed appropriate candidates for reduction surgery. There is, however, a subset of patients who seem to yield consistently superior results and are ideally suited for vertical reduction. Patients in this category include young women with normal skin elasticity and moderate breast hypertrophy. In these patients, the optimal aesthetic result is obtained after only a few postoperative weeks once the breasts have settled and skin puckering around the incision has flattened. In older patients with less elastic skin, it may take longer for the wrinkles along the vertical scar to become flat and unnoticeable. In addition, in those patients whose breasts are primarily composed of fat as opposed to glandular tissue, the pillars that are dissected are inevitably weak, and the sutures used to approximate these pillars and to shape the breast will have little substance to hold. Consequently, the breast shape may become distorted over time as the breast tissue tends to pull away from the midline and widen the scars in the process.

Some controversy has centered on the size limitations of the vertical mammaplasty and its applicability to large-volume breast reductions. In her series of 250 patients, Lejour noted a higher rate of wound healing complications in patients with larger, fatty breasts and concluded that techniques other than the vertical mammaplasty should be considered in patients with a resection of more than 1000 g per breast.[18] In contrast, Nahai and Lacotte have both performed 2000-g reductions without increased incidence of complications or areolar loss.[19] Others who have applied short-scar techniques to large-breasted individuals have reported abundant inferior pole skin with only limited postoperative shrinkage and consequently also limit the technique to resections of less than 1000 g per breast. However, it remains unclear and a source of speculation whether the inelastic, stretched breast skin failed to shrink or the mere size of the breasts led to suboptimal results.

Although it may seem that the vertical reduction is of limited utility in large-volume reductions, it is more likely that these patients with severe hypertrophy are simply more likely to encounter complications, including delayed healing and seroma formation, regardless of the technique used. Given the learning curve associated with any new procedure, it is reasonable to initially select patients with normal skin elasticity and smaller reductions in using the vertical reduction early on to develop a certain familiarity with the nuances of the procedure.

MARKINGS

With the patient in an upright position, the midline of the chest is drawn from the suprasternal notch down onto the abdomen. A second line is drawn from the midclavicular point to the nipple. The inframammary fold is also marked; this is particularly important because this mark denotes the lower limit of skin and breast dissection during the procedure. The vertical axis of the breast is then marked 10 to 14 cm from the abdominal midline below the level of the inframammary crease. The absolute distance from the midline will vary according to the width of the chest and position of the breasts.

To mark the new nipple position, an index finger is placed in the inframammary crease and a mark then made on the forward projection of the index finger onto the anterior surface of the breast (Fig. 136-1). This mark should be made along the line that was previously drawn from the midclavicle to the nipple. This new nipple site is usually 10 to 14 cm from the midline and 18 to 22 cm from the sternal notch. These distances can be compared between the sides and adjusted to achieve optimal symmetry postoperatively.

The lateral and medial markings are determined next. For the medial line, the breast is pushed laterally and a line is made projecting the previously made vertical axis onto the breast. Similarly, the lateral line is drawn by pushing the breast medially and continuing the vertical axis located below the inframammary crease onto the breast (Fig. 136-2). The greater the force used to push the breast laterally and medially, the further apart these two lines will be from each other and the larger the volume of reduction.

The upper and lower limits of skin excision are now marked. For the lower mark, a curved line is made connecting the lower ends of the medial and lateral

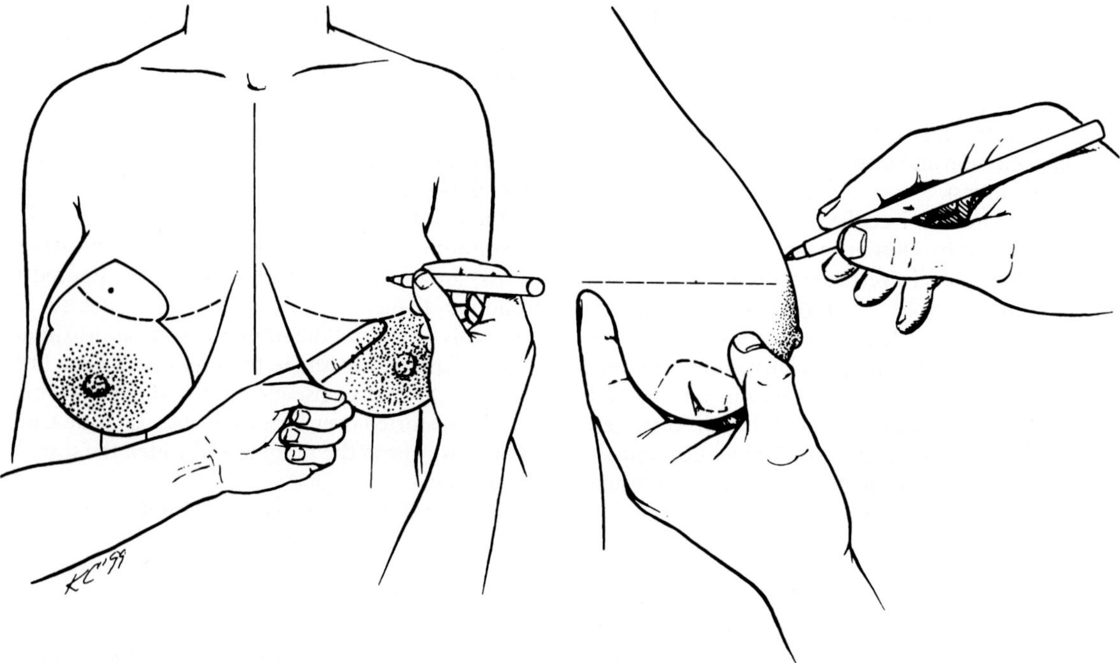

FIGURE 136-1. Marking the new nipple position by transposing the level of the inframammary crease anteriorly onto the breast.

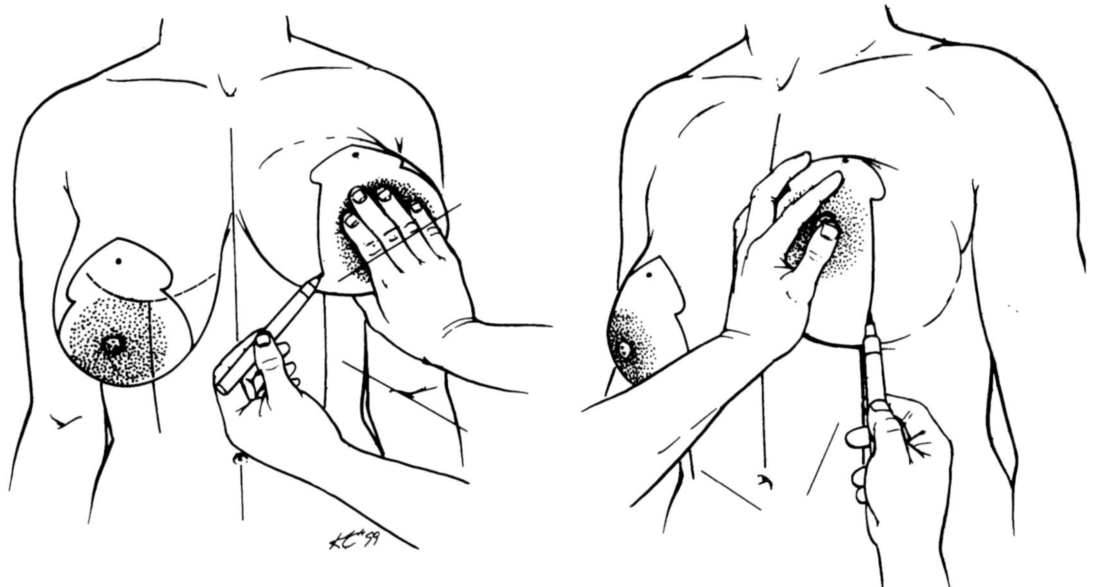

FIGURE 136-2. Determining the medial and lateral markings by pushing the breast laterally and medially, respectively.

lines, somewhere between 4 and 6 cm above the existing inframammary fold. This marking should be placed higher in larger breast reductions. A lower line made too close to the existent inframammary crease will result in a scar extending onto the upper abdomen.

The upper limit will ultimately represent the superior margin of the areola and is usually 2 cm above the future nipple. The shape of this periareolar marking is dependent on the size of the breast. For moderate to large reductions, an ellipse is constructed such that the lower half meets the medial and lateral breast markings. For smaller reductions, more of a dome shape is made at the most superior aspect in an effort to reduce tension in this upper aspect (Fig. 136-3). Last, a 40- to 42-cm-diameter circle is drawn around the existing nipple without stretching the breast skin or areola.

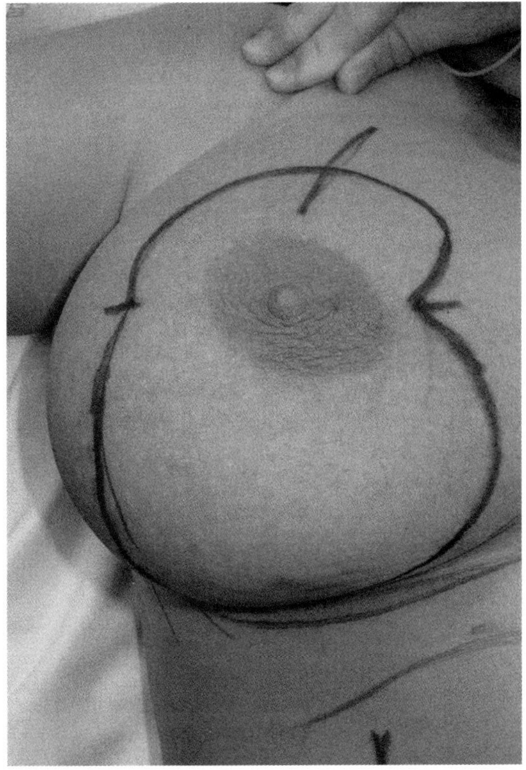

FIGURE 136-3. Photograph showing final markings including the curved lines connecting the medial and lateral marks. These curved lines represent superior and inferior limits of skin excision.

SURGICAL TECHNIQUE

With the patient supine on the operating table and general anesthesia established, the arms are extended 70 to 90 degrees and secured in anticipation of sitting the patient up during the procedure; 0.5% lidocaine with 1:200,000 epinephrine is infiltrated between the lower markings, sparing the area around the nipple. The base of the breast is constricted with a mammostat, and the area around the areola is deepithelialized within the markings and down 3 to 4 cm beneath the areola (Fig. 136-4). The use of the mammostat not only facilitates holding of the breast

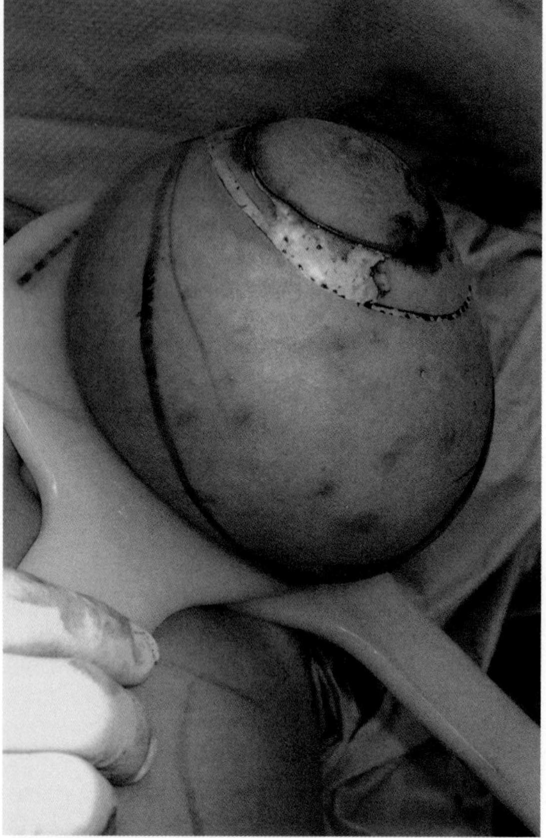

FIGURE 136-4. Intraoperative photograph demonstrating use of mammostat. Periareolar de-epithelialization is performed to 3 to 4 cm below the areola.

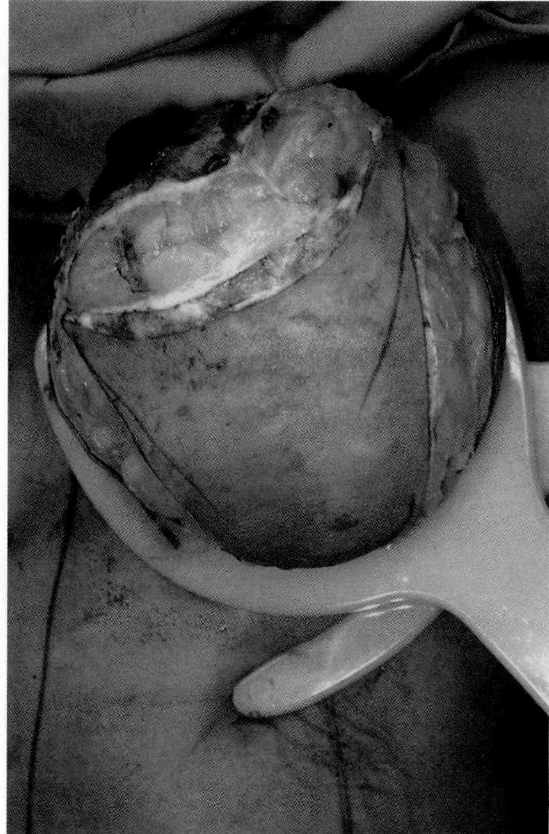

FIGURE 136-5. Full-thickness incisions through skin markings into underlying breast parenchyma.

tissue during de-epithelialization but also reduces blood loss.

Incisions are then made through the medial, inferior, and lateral markings (Fig. 136-5). The skin is elevated from the lower breast as a thin 1.0- to 1.5-cm flap extending from the lower incision to the inframammary crease (Fig. 136-6). At the level of the inframammary fold, the scalpel is repositioned such that breast and fatty tissue are excised perpendicular to the chest wall. At this point, the whole lower breast tissue is now entirely free of overlying skin.

For the medial dissection to be performed, the breast is pulled laterally so that the medial breast markings are in continuity with the vertical axis of the breast marked on the upper abdomen. The medial incision is made through breast tissue down to pectoralis fascia. This is repeated for the lateral incision, with care taken to pull the breast medially such that the lateral mark is in line with the vertical axis (Fig. 136-7). With inferior, medial, and lateral incisions now made through the gland, the central and lower bulk of the breast can be elevated off the chest wall. The most inferior aspect of the breast tissue at the level of the

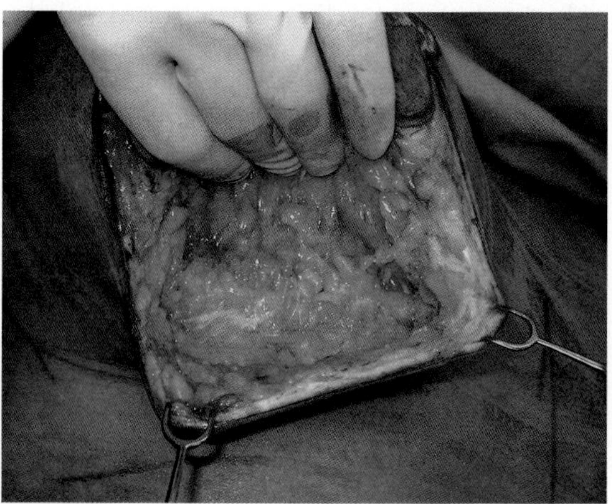

FIGURE 136-6. Skin elevation along the inferior pole of the breast. A flap 1.0- to 1.5-cm thick should be raised to the level of the inframammary crease.

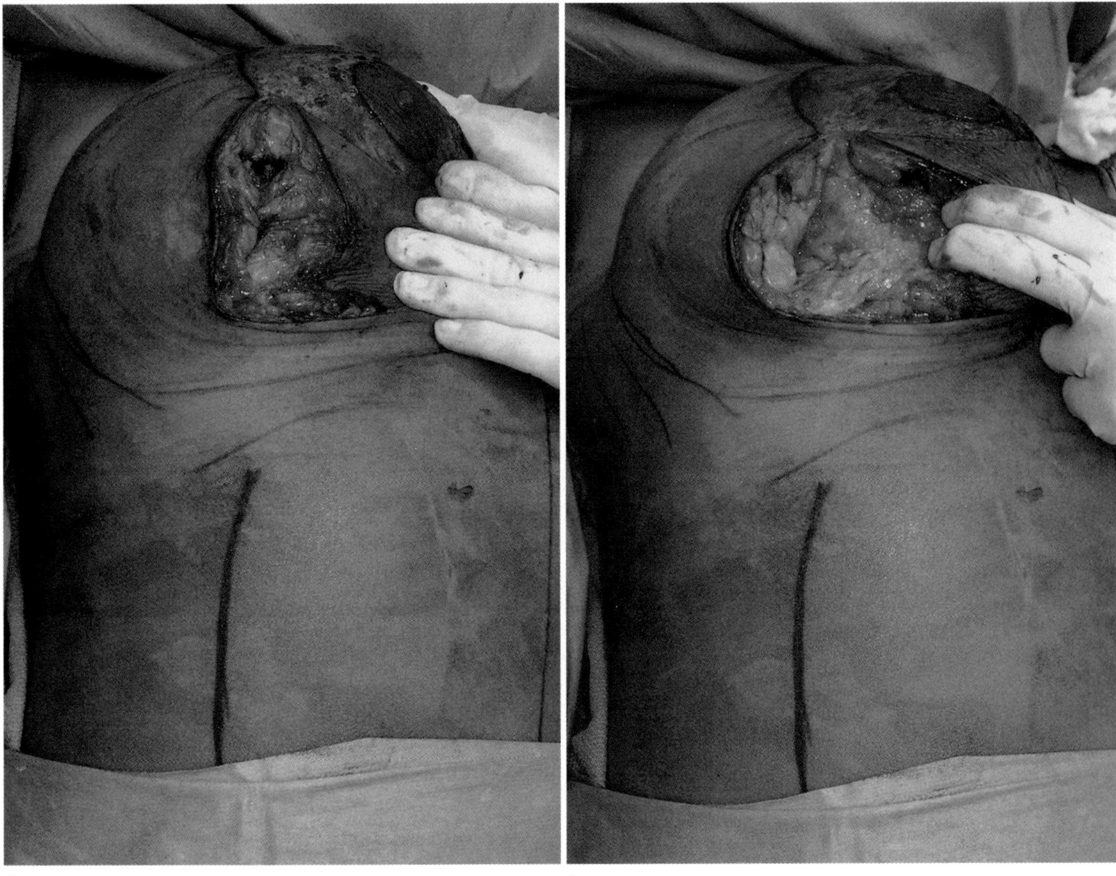

FIGURE 136-7. *A,* To define the lateral extent of resection, the breast is pulled medially such that the preoperative lateral mark is in line with the vertical axis of the breast. *B,* Dissection proceeds through breast tissue down to the level of the pectoralis fascia.

inframammary fold is dissected off the pectoralis in an upward direction (Fig. 136-8). This dissection is continued up to the level of the new nipple. In this manner, a portion of the breast has been adequately mobilized and prepared for resection (Fig. 136-9).

An incision is then made along the lower border of de-epithelialized tissue, below the areolar margin. A superiorly based flap encircling the nipple-areola complex is then elevated in a cephalad fashion. Once elevated, the parenchymal tissue medial to, lateral to, and below the areola can be excised en bloc (Fig. 136-10). In the patients with large breasts, additional tissue must be sharply excised from behind the areolar pedicle. The longer the dermal pedicle, the thinner it should be to facilitate nipple inset. After this central wedge excision, medial and lateral pillars are left (Fig. 136-11).

For closure, the nipple-areola complex is temporarily inset into its new position, and a 7-mm Blake drain is placed over the pectoralis fascia and brought out through the skin. The drain not only will evacuate any residual fluid but also serves to obliterate the dead space beneath the lower breast skin. The remaining medial and lateral pillars of breast tissue are brought together and sutured in two layers with 2-0 and 3-0 Vicryl (Fig. 136-12). If any size discrepancies exist between the breasts or further size reduction is desired, the sutures can be removed and additional tissue excised from the pillars or behind the areola. For definitive closure, the pillars are once again secured to each other with two layers of Vicryl, and the nipple is inset with interrupted Vicryl and intracuticular Monocryl. The lower end of the vertical scar is closed as a pursestring, and the remainder of the incision is closed with a Monocryl intracuticular suture pulled tight to gather the skin in a short vertical scar (Fig. 136-13). The skin margins along the vertical limb are not elevated from the underlying breast tissue to minimize tissue ischemia and to prevent flap loss.

At the end of the procedure, SteriStrips are placed over the incisions and around the nipple-areola complex. The patient is placed in a surgical bra, which

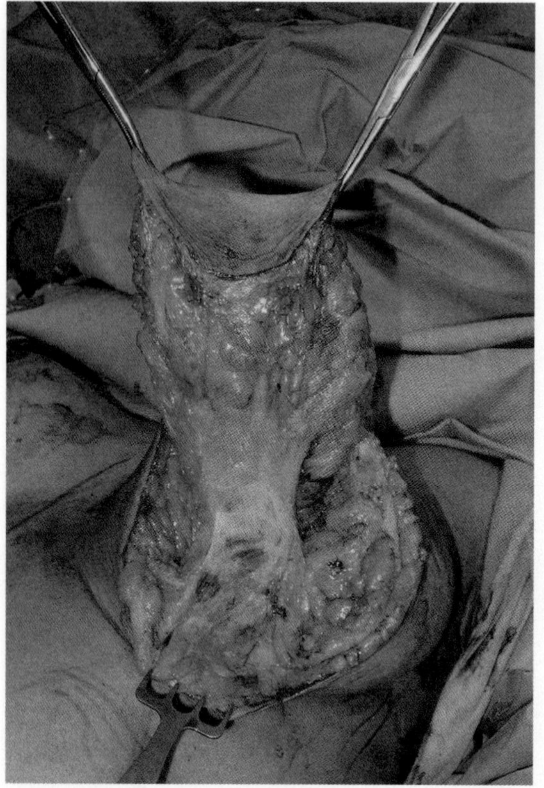

FIGURE 136-8. Elevating breast tissue in a cephalad direction at the level of the pectoralis fascia.

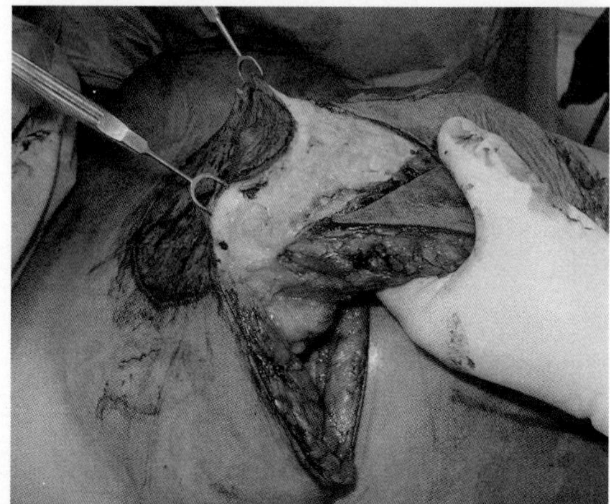

FIGURE 136-9. Breast tissue dissection is carried up to the level of the nipple-areola complex.

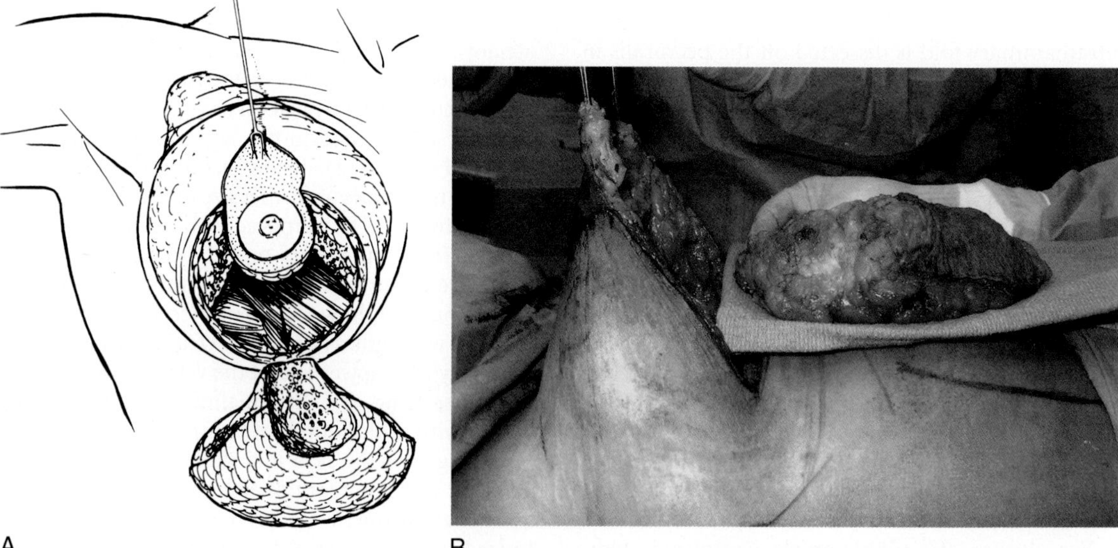

FIGURE 136-10. *A,* Schematic demonstrating tissue below, medial to, and lateral to the areola included in resection. For additional volume reduction, retroareolar tissue can also be removed. *B,* Intraoperative photograph showing en bloc removal of specimen.

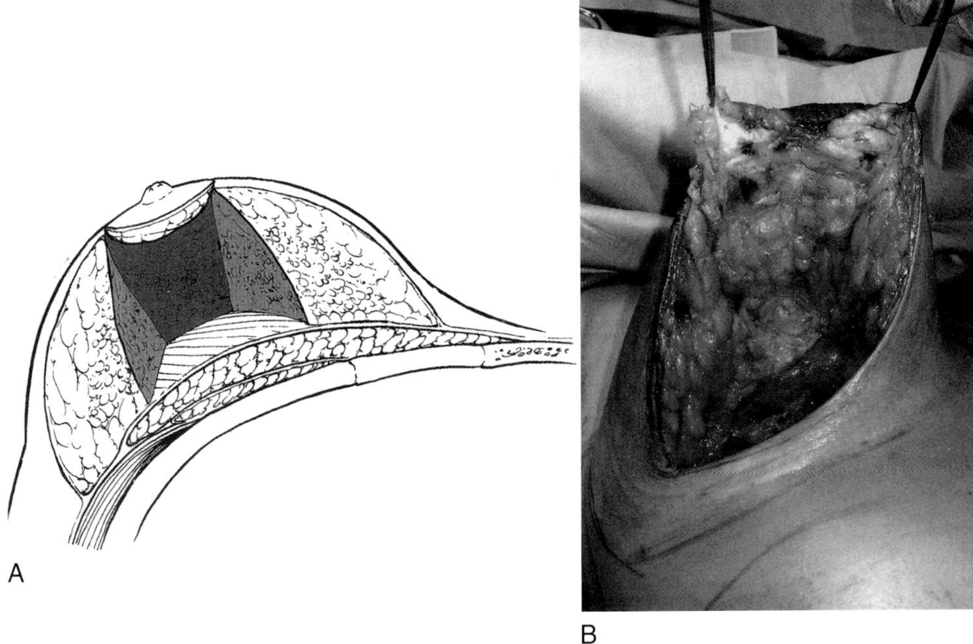

FIGURE 136-11. *A* and *B*, Illustration and photograph showing medial and lateral pillars that will eventually be reapproximated to re-establish breast projection.

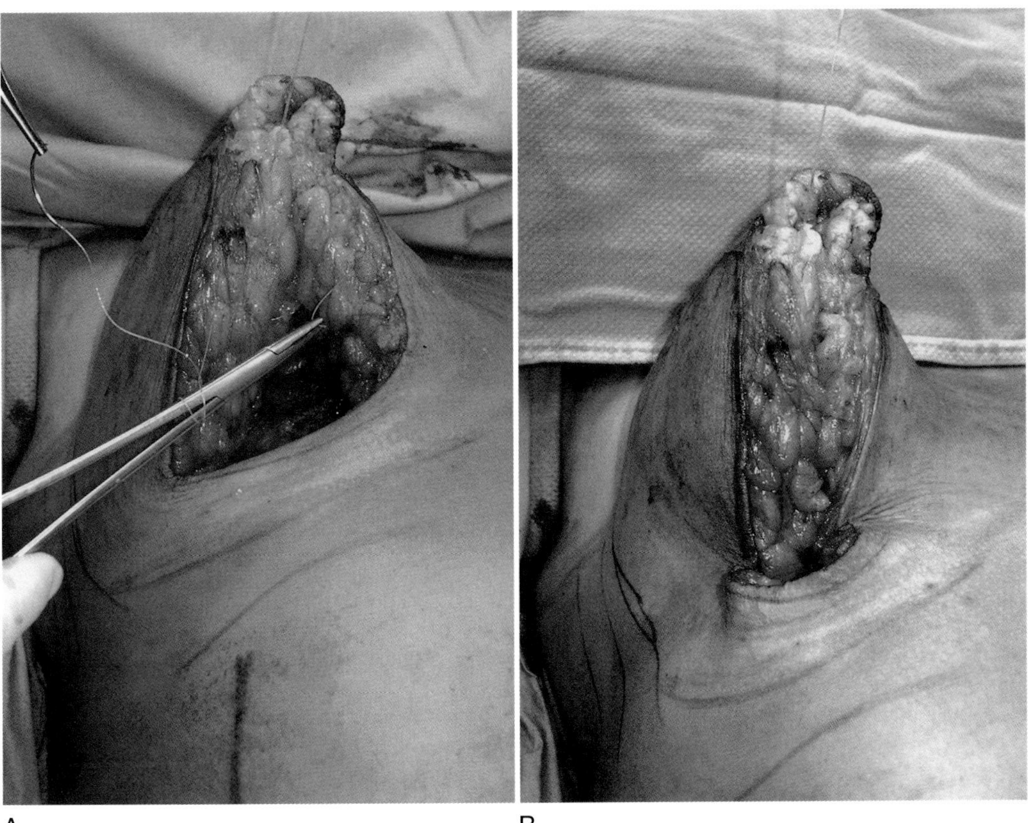

FIGURE 136-12. *A* and *B*, Suturing together of medial and lateral breast pillars. Note how this maneuver narrows the breast base diameter and contributes to breast projection.

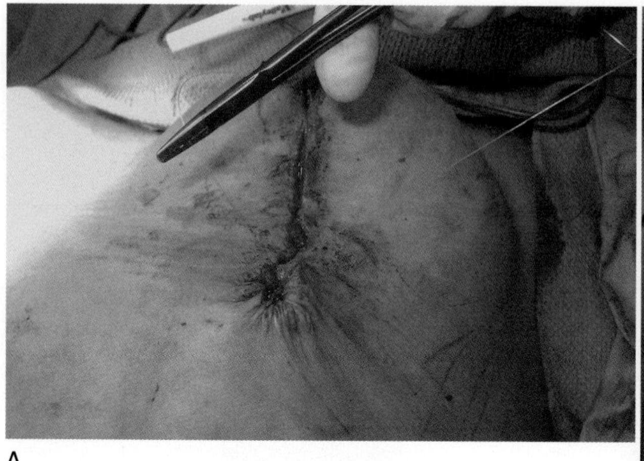

A

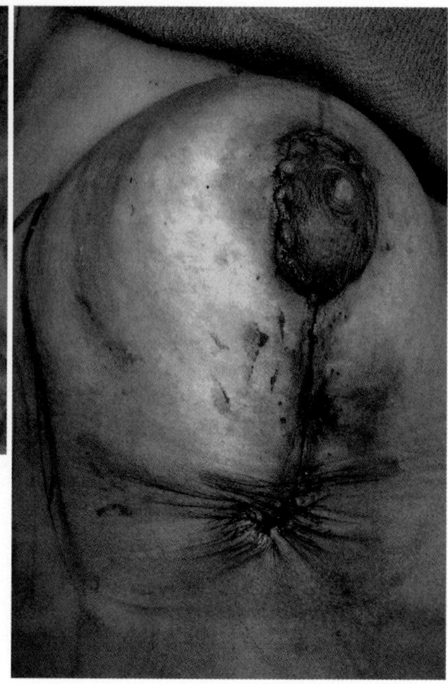

B

FIGURE 136-13. *A*, Pursestring closure along lower end of vertical scar. The puckering will tend to smoothen over time. *B*, Final on-table appearance of breast at completion of the procedure.

she is to wear continuously for 3 weeks. Drains are removed at 24 hours postoperatively.

TECHNIQUE MODIFICATIONS

The technique discussed in the preceding section relies on concepts introduced by Lejour and Lassus, including a vertical scar with a superior pedicle and suturing of the lateral and medial pillars to maintain breast shape and to prevent postoperative ptosis. Over the years, other surgeons have introduced their individual modifications of the vertical scar technique, often in response to technical difficulties related to the superior pedicle. Published reports of these techniques also suggest that consistent and excellent results can be achieved with these design variations.

In 1999, Hall-Findlay[20] published her experience with a modified vertical reduction in 400 patients. Her technique relies on a medial or lateral pedicle as opposed to a superior pedicle. She reports that this facilitates insetting of the nipple-areola complex and ensures circulation to the nipple because the pedicle is shorter. Her preoperative markings include placement of the nipple at the level of the inframammary crease. Medial and lateral vertical limbs are drawn and joined above the level of the inframammary fold. A mosque dome design is used around the areola.

The medial pedicle is designed with a 6- to 8-cm base and a 1-cm cuff left around the areola (Fig. 136-14). Once it is de-epithelialized, the pedicle is incised as a dermoglandular pedicle. With the need for any pedicle undermining averted, a robust blood supply to the nipple-areola complex is ensured. The skin and breast tissue located laterally are excised. The remaining medial pedicle can easily be rotated into position and brought out in the area designed for the areola. Once again, suturing of the medial and lateral glandular pillars will narrow the breast base diameter and give a conical shape to the breast.

In her series, Hall-Findlay[20] found her technique applicable to reductions of both small and large volume. Specific advantages include the ease of insetting the short medial pedicle and preservation of vascularity and sensation to the nipple-areola complex because of a thicker dermoglandular pedicle. By elimination of wide skin undermining, the theoretical risk of postoperative wound healing problems is minimized. In addition, reliance on a superomedial pedicle should minimize the risk of postoperative pseudoptosis and actually facilitate raising of the inframammary crease.[21]

The short-scar periareolar inferior pedicle reduction (SPAIR) mammaplasty popularized by Hammond[22] uses an inferior pedicle with which most surgeons are already familiar but successfully eliminates the horizontal component of the scar. This technique relies on an 8-cm inferiorly based pedicle that is centered about the breast meridian. No undermining of the pedicle is performed. Breast flaps are developed medially, superiorly, and laterally, and the tissue between these flaps and the chest wall is removed. The inferior pedicle can now fit into this defect, and it is

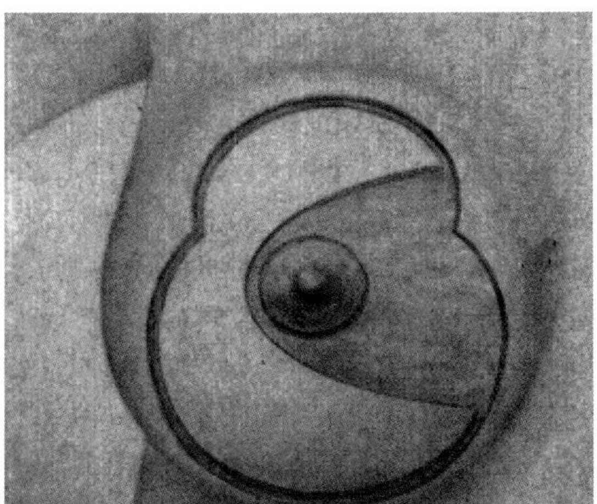

FIGURE 136-14. The de-epithelialized medial pedicle as described by Hall-Findlay.

held in place by sutures to the pectoralis fascia that in addition restore upper pole volume. A Gore-Tex suture is used to pursestring the areolar defect, and redundant skin along the inferior limb is gathered but never beyond the inframammary crease. Because of the inferior pedicle, this method does not produce the exaggerated flat inferior pole, and there is less reliance on postoperative settling for ultimate results. This technique has been successfully applied to breasts of all sizes with good long-term maintenance of shape and projection. Compared with other vertical scar techniques, the SPAIR does not rely on the sometimes unpredictable postoperative settling to shape the breast mound. Control over final breast shape is more appropriately in the hands of the surgeon at the time of the operation. As with the Hall-Findlay technique, difficulty of insetting a superiorly based nipple-areola complex is avoided with minimal risk of vascular compromise to the nipple-areola complex.

The technique of Beer et al[23] relies on a central mound breast excision, but all preoperative markings and subsequent resections are based on precise geometric measurements, thereby making the procedure easily reproducible. A periareolar skin resection is also included to produce a round breast shape.

RESULTS

Traditional reduction mammaplasty techniques using an anchor-shaped incision often result in lengthy and poor-quality scars along the inframammary crease. Vertical reduction techniques not only reduce scarring but, in addition, incorporate internal parenchymal sutures that improve overall breast shape and projection. By elimination of the reliance on a skin brassiere, the breast shape is preserved over time, and the risk of postoperative "bottoming out" as is often seen in Wise-pattern reductions is minimized. Maintenance of breast shape as long as 20 years postoperatively has been demonstrated.[24]

Despite hesitation by some to use the vertical scar technique in large-volume reductions, it has proved applicable to a range of size reductions (Figs. 136-15 to 136-18). Both Nahai and Lacotte have reported safely performing vertical scar reductions in patients with reductions of more than 2000 g.[19] Not unexpectedly, body mass index and breast volume contribute to postoperative results and complication rates. As cited by Korchin,[25] Tapia et al,[26] and Berthe et al,[27] a certain percentage of these patients may require minor revision, particularly those undergoing large-volume reduction. It is precisely this same group of patients who benefit from elimination of the lengthy inframammary scar, particularly that subset susceptible to hypertrophic or keloid scar formation. Specifically in one prospective, randomized study comparing outcomes of inferior pedicle versus vertical scar reductions, the vertical mammaplasty cohort ranked their scar quality and overall aesthetic results significantly higher than did their Wise-pattern counterparts.[25]

In addition to shape and scar, preservation of nipple-areola sensitivity is of primary importance to patients undergoing breast procedures. Using Semmes-Weinstein pressure threshold testing, Gonzalez et al[28] reported that nipple-areola sensitivity was retained in 96% of breasts after reduction of 550 g or less and in 85% of breasts after reduction of 550 g or more. The technique for reduction was either a central pedicle or an inferior pedicle. Many have criticized the vertical scar reduction with a superior pedicle because of the risk of sensory damage secondary to disruption of the lateral fibers of the fourth intercostal nerve. However, anatomic studies have demonstrated that medial and lateral branches of the second through sixth intercostal contribute to nipple sensation.[29] Subjective data obtained by Hall-Findlay[21] from follow-up questionnaires of patients with vertical scar showed that 85% had sensation close to preoperative levels, regardless of superior, lateral, or medial pedicle. More objective data have been reported by Hamdi et al[30] in a study that compared sensation after superior and inferior pedicle mammaplasties. They concluded that by the sixth postoperative month, the mean value of nipple-areola pressure sensation was comparable between these two subsets of patients. Mofid et al[31] further validated this by using even more sophisticated computer-assisted neurosensory testing to compare nipple sensation after inferior and medial pedicle reduction techniques. In comparison of medial and inferior pedicle techniques, there were no significant differences in postoperative sensory outcomes of patients. Additional studies have corroborated the lack of statistically significant variation in postoperative nipple-areola sensation in patients undergoing

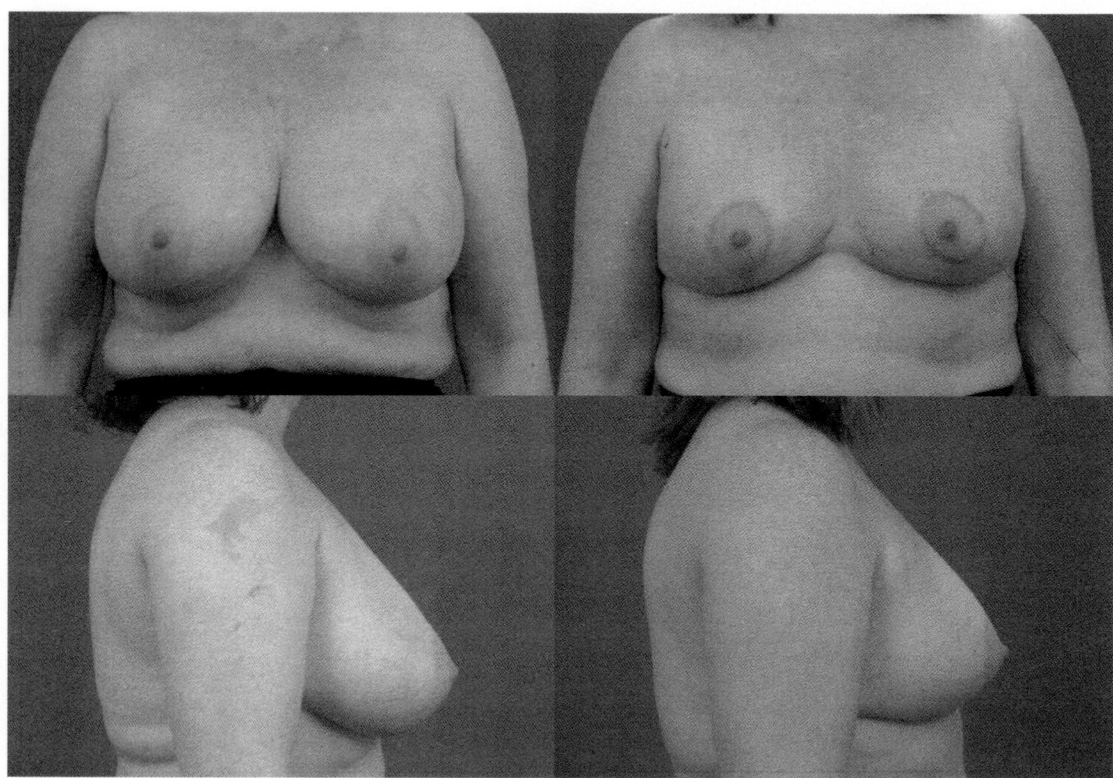

FIGURE 136-15. Preoperative and postoperative results in a small reduction; 388 g was resected from the right breast and 432 g from the left.

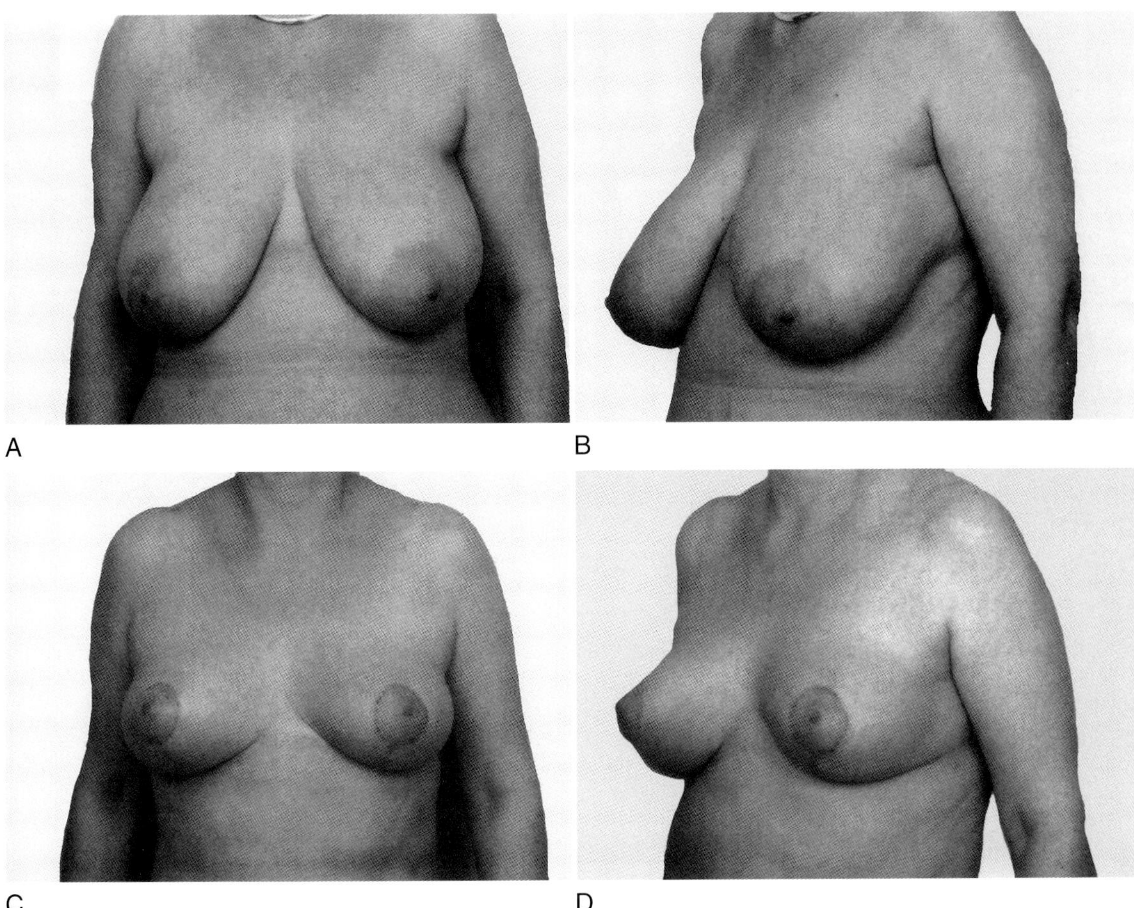

FIGURE 136-16. *A* and *B*, Preoperative photographs in a moderate-sized reduction. *C* and *D*, Postoperative results after 500-g reduction on each side.

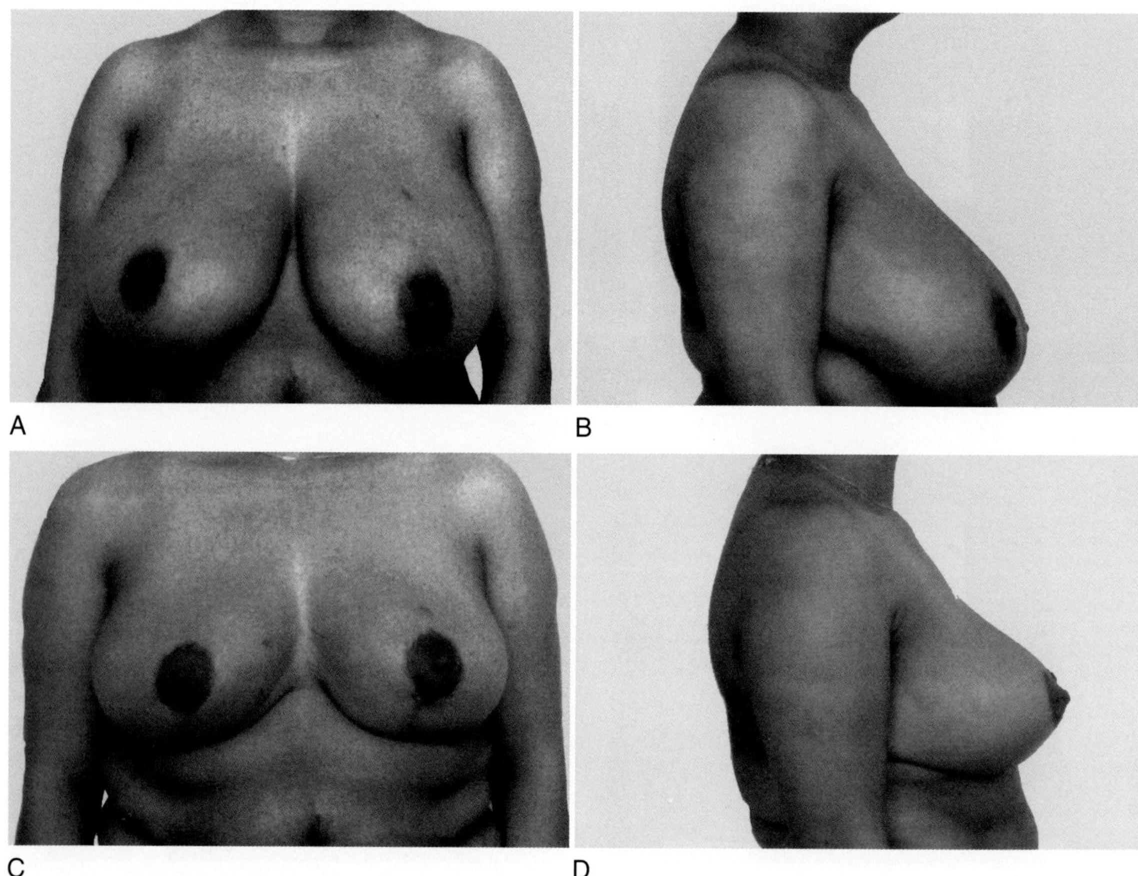

FIGURE 136-17. *A* and *B*, Preoperative views of patient undergoing vertical reduction. *C* and *D*, Postoperative views after 800-g reduction on each side.

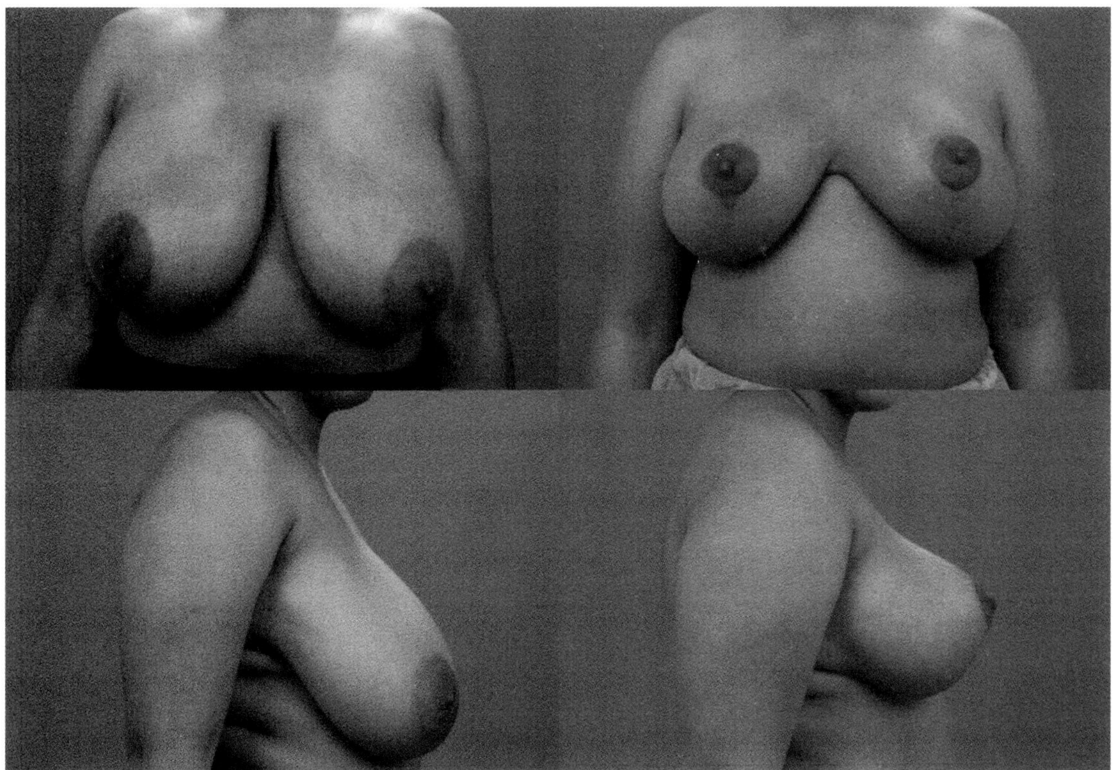

FIGURE 136-18. Preoperative and postoperative results in a large-volume reduction; 951 g was resected from the right breast and 1037 g from the left.

traditional Wise-pattern reductions versus vertical scar reductions.[25] Because a portion of both medial and lateral parenchyma is preserved with all the various vertical scar techniques along with dermoglandular tissue around the areola, the potential for retained postoperative sensation exists.

Retained nipple-areola sensitivity should theoretically contribute to the ability to lactate after vertical reduction. From an anatomic standpoint, postoperative lactation would also necessitate intact connections between the lactiferous ducts and nipple. Depending on the amount of desired volume reduction, retroareolar breast tissue can be left in the form of a dermoglandular pedicle in the course of vertical reduction. Preservation of this tissue should therefore confer some success in postoperative breast-feeding and not inherently represent a shortcoming of the technique.

COMPLICATIONS

One of the most comprehensive evaluations of early postoperative complications was published by Lejour[18] in 1999. In her series, there were five types of early complications: seroma (5% incidence), hematoma (1.2% incidence), infection (0.004% incidence), partial areola necrosis (0.004% incidence), and delayed healing (5.4% incidence). The more minor of these complications were treated conservatively, including aspiration of seromas and administration of antibiotics for infection, without compromise of final results. In patients with areolar loss and wound dehiscence, healing ultimately occurred with dressing changes during the course of weeks to months but often resulted in thicker, wider scars. Unlike the technique described in this text, Lejour relied on liposuction and wide undermining to shape the breast, both of which may have compromised tissue viability and predisposed to necrosis. The techniques reported by Lassus and Nahai, which do not include a large amount of liposuction or skin undermining, seem to have fewer problems with postoperative seroma, skin slough, or glandular necrosis.[24] Additional reviews of the vertical technique have cited a significant decrease in the occurrence of minor complications such as seroma and wound dehiscence when the technique was modified to decrease skin undermining and to eliminate liposuction.[27]

Delayed complications tend to be somewhat more serious in nature and often necessitate surgical revision for their correction. The most common complication in this category is related to excess scarring. When scar revisions were added to other complications in one study,[25] the vertical scar technique had a 19% complication rate compared with 8% in a Wise-pattern cohort. Because redundant skin is not resected along the inferior pole, settling and softening of the scar in this region require a prolonged time. If such settling does not occur, residual wrinkles can persist along the vertical limb and compromise appearance. Whereas scar massage, compression, and triamcinolone (Kenalog) injections may help fade or soften the scar, it is rare that a widened scar will spontaneously shrink into a fine line. In these situations, scar revision or addition of a short horizontal scar can be performed under local anesthesia with overall improvement in scar color and quality. Not unexpectedly, patients undergoing large-volume reduction with more skin redundancy are at higher risk for requiring a second procedure for scar revision. Although admittedly the higher rate of scar revision does raise economic issues, Lassus[24] concluded that it is far better to revise a wide but shorter scar than to resort at the onset to lengthy horizontal scars, which can never ultimately be removed.

Despite careful surgical planning that places the inferior limb of the vertical incision well above the inframammary fold, the vertical scar may on occasion extend onto the upper abdomen, where it is easily conspicuous. The likelihood of the scar's lengthening over time is actually less than with other more conventional reduction methods that rely on skin-only techniques and allow the breast parenchyma to exert pressure and deformational forces on the overlying skin. Once again, larger breasted patients with excess skin are at greater risk for a lengthy scar. In those patients, the lower extent of the vertical scar should be placed well above the preexisting inframammary fold to prevent extension of the scar onto the abdomen.[19] In those situations in which scar length does pose a problem, a minor secondary procedure is all that is needed to correct this deformity. After several months of postoperative descent of the breast, a horizontal crescent of skin and scar can be excised at the lower pole and the scar relocated more superiorly in the inframammary fold. Once again, the resultant horizontal scar is much shorter than that typically associated with the inverted T incision.

An often-cited aesthetic shortcoming of the vertical reduction technique is a nipple-areola complex situated too high on the breast. In addition, asymmetries of the nipples may become apparent as the breast settles. In this situation, the short inframammary fold excision can once again remove excess skin and reposition the nipple-areola complex in a lower and more natural position. Differential skin excisions can correct asymmetries between the sides. In an effort to avoid this complication, it is important during the initial surgery to remove all excess breast tissue in the lower pole and adequately tighten the medial and lateral pillars to form a flat lower breast and full superior breast. In this way, the potential for any residual lower pole tissue to persist and give a bottoming out appearance is eliminated. Others have found success by intraoperative placement of the nipple-areola complex 1.0 to 1.5 cm below the anterior projection of the inframammary crease and use of a pursestring to accommodate any residual excess skin along the upper pole.[32] This modification may prove particularly beneficial in those patients with very large, ptotic breasts who may be subject to more settling of the breast in the postoperative period.

Finally, although the initial appearance of the breast is somewhat unusual with a flat inferior pole and exaggerated superior pole fullness, postoperative settling allows the breast to assume a more natural shape. Because this eventual result depends on factors such as gravity and skin elasticity, the final shape of the breast is to a certain extent out of the surgeon's control, and the possibility of a poor result or noticeable asymmetries is perhaps greater than with some of the more traditional techniques. The frequency of this problem should appreciably decrease as each individual surgeon gains familiarity with the technique and can more appropriately predict the role of the aforementioned postoperative changes. In those instances in which volume and shape issues continue to be a problem, the vertical incision can be opened under local anesthesia or monitored anesthesia care and either additional volume resected or the pillar sutures tightened or loosened, depending on the desired effect.

CONCLUSION

As experience with the vertical mammaplasty has grown and appropriate modifications have been made, it appears that the technique has been able to fulfill the basic goals of breast reduction surgery while improving on aesthetic shape and minimizing scar.

Sheer volume can be removed by any number of methods, but the vertical mammaplasty does so in such a way that the projection of the breast is increased and a pleasing shape ultimately obtained. The suturing of the medial and lateral pillars effectively controls this breast reshaping without reliance on a skin brassiere to mold the breast. Lejour's experience with more than 250 patients in 10 years has shown the durability of this technique over time.[33] Her results ranging from 1 to 3 years postoperatively clearly demonstrate the stability of the breast shape over time and its resistance to recurrent ptosis and flattening. Lassus[24] has similarly achieved long-lasting results documenting impressive results 9 to 23 years postoperatively.

Clearly, then, the vertical reduction mammaplasty has proved to be effective both in solving the functional problems of macromastia and in establishing an aesthetically pleasing breast with superior pole fullness and minimal scars.

REFERENCES

1. Biesenberger H: Eine neue Methode der Mammaplastik. Zentralbl Chir 1928;55:2382.
2. Pitanguy I: Surgical correction of breast hypertrophy. Br J Plast Surg 1967;20:78-85.
3. Strombeck JO: Mammaplasty: report of a new technique based on the two-pedicle procedure. Br J Plast Surg 1960;13:79-90.
4. Skoog T: A technique of breast reduction; transposition of the nipple on a cutaneous vascular pedicle. Acta Chir Scand 1963;126:453-465.
5. Skoog T: Plastic Surgery: New Methods and Refinements. Stockholm, Almqvist and Wiksell, 1974.
6. Robbins TH: A reduction mammaplasty with the areola-nipple based on an inferior pedicle. Plast Reconstr Surg 1977;59:64-67.
7. Georgiade NG, Serafin D, Morris R, Georgiade G: Reduction mammaplasty utilizing an inferior pedicle nipple-areolar flap. Ann Plast Surg 1979;3:211-218.
8. Lassus C: Possibilities et limites de la chirurgie plastique de la silhouette feminine. L'Hopital 1969;801:575.
9. Dartigues L: Traitement chirurgical du prolapsus mammaire. Arch Franc Belg Chir 1925;28:313.
10. Lassus C: New refinements in vertical mammaplasty. Chir Plast 1981;6:81.
11. Lassus C: Breast reduction: evolution of a technique. A single vertical scar. Aesthetic Plast Surg 1987;11:107-112.
12. Lassus C: A 30-year experience with vertical mammaplasty. Plast Reconstr Surg 1996;97:373-380.
13. Marchac D, De Olarte G: Reduction mammaplasty and correction of ptosis with a short inframammary scar. Plast Reconstr Surg 1982;69:45-55.
14. Marchac D, Sagher U: Mammaplasty with a short horizontal scar. Evaluation and results after 9 years. Clin Plast Surg 1988;15:627-639.
15. Marconi F, Cavina C: Reduction mammaplasty and correction of ptosis: a personal technique. Plast Reconstr Surg 1993;9:1046-1056.
16. Lejour M, Abboud M, DeClety A, et al: Reduction des cicatrices de plastie mammaire de l'ancre courte a la verticale. Ann Chir Plast Esthet 1990;35:369-379.
17. Lejour M: Vertical Mammaplasty and Liposuction. St. Louis, Quality Medical Publishing, 1994.
18. Lejour M: Vertical mammaplasty: early complications after 250 personal consecutive cases. Plast Reconstr Surg 1999;104:764-770.
19. Nahai F: Discussion on update on vertical mammaplasty. Plast Reconstr Surg 1999;104:2299-2302.
20. Hall-Findlay E: A simplified vertical reduction mammaplasty: shortening the learning curve. Plast Reconstr Surg 1999;104:748-759.
21. Hall-Findlay E: Pedicles in vertical breast reduction and mastopexy. Clin Plast Surg 2002;29:379-391.
22. Hammond D: Short scar periareolar inferior pedicle reduction (SPAIR) mammaplasty. Plast Reconstr Surg 1999;103:890-901.
23. Beer GM, Morgenthaler W, Spicher I, Meyer VE: Modifications in vertical scar breast reduction. Br J Plast Surg 2001;54:341-347.
24. Lassus C: Update on vertical mammaplasty. Plast Reconstr Surg 1999;104:2289-2304.
25. Korchin L, Cruz-Korchin N: Vertical versus Wise pattern breast reduction: patient satisfaction, revision rates and complications. Plast Reconstr Surg 2003;112:1573-1581.
26. Tapia A, Blanch A, Salvador J, et al: Evolution of the vertical scar in Lejour's mastoplasty technique. Aesthetic Plast Surg 1996;20:377-384.
27. Berthe JV, Massaut J, Greuse M, et al: The vertical mammaplasty: a reappraisal of the technique and its complications. Plast Reconstr Surg 2003;111:2192-2199.
28. Gonzalez F, Brown F, Gold M, et al: Preoperative and postoperative nipple-areola sensibility in patients undergoing reduction mammaplasty. Plast Reconstr Surg 1993;92:809-818.
29. Schlenz I, Kuzbari R, Gruber H, Holle J: The sensitivity of the nipple-areola complex: an anatomic study. Plast Reconstr Surg 2000;105:905-909.
30. Hamdi M, Greuse M, DeMey A, Webster MH: A prospective quantitative comparison of breast sensation after superior and inferior pedicle mammaplasty. Br J Plast Surg 2001;54:39-42.
31. Mofid M, Dellon AL, Elias J, Nahabedian M: Quantitation of breast sensibility following reduction mammaplasty: a comparison of inferior and medial pedicle techniques. Plast Reconstr Surg 2002;109:2283-2288.
32. Vogt P, Muhlberger T, Torres A, et al: Method for intraoperative positioning of the nipple-areola complex in vertical scar reduction mammaplasty. Plast Reconstr Surg 2000;105:2096-2099.
33. Lejour M: Vertical mammaplasty: update and appraisal of late results. Plast Reconstr Surg 1999;104:771-781.

CHAPTER

137

Inferior Pedicle Reduction: Techniques

STEPHEN J. MATHES, MD ✦ WESLEY SCHOOLER, MD

Reduction mammaplasty is designed to accomplish the following goals: to reduce breast weight and size to improve the patient's comfort and to relieve stress on the trunk and neck musculoskeletal system; to establish a normal relationship between breast size and chest and body dimensions to improve the patient's body image; to allow physical activities without limitations resulting from excess breast size, redundancy, and weight; to reduce breast size for improvement of breast surveillance through self-examination and mammography; and to eliminate breast contact with the abdomen for prevention of intertriginous skin irritation and infection. For these goals to be accomplished, any surgical technique must encompass three components: excision of excess breast tissue, reduction of size of the skin envelope, and relocation of the nipple-areola complex. The procedure should be designed to accomplish these goals with the following critical considerations: safety, reliability, avoidance of skin or breast avascular necrosis, nipple-areola survival, minimization of scars, and maintenance or restoration of breast symmetry. The evolution of techniques has appropriately focused on these considerations. Initially, the focus was placed on techniques to remove breast tissue and to reduce the skin envelope to match the new breast size. The next phase of surgical procedures focused on the process of shifting the nipple-areola complex without loss of its circulation and innervation. With identification of the vascularity of the breast and effective ways to move the nipple-areola to an appropriate position on the new breast mound, the emphasis has shifted to development of methods to minimize scars while accomplishing the goals of reduction mammaplasty. During the past 30 years, the inferior pedicle technique has been widely used for breast reduction because of its ability to accomplish a safe and effective breast reduction.[1] Details of reduction mammaplasty are reviewed, including anatomic basis, technique, modifications, limitations, and results.

The techniques introduced for reduction mammaplasty have focused on removal of excess breast tissue while blood supply to the nipple-areola is maintained. The nipple-areola has been located on a pedicle of dermis and underlying layer of breast tissue to capture blood supply for later transposition of the nipple-areola to an appropriate position on the reduced breast mound. Historically, the pedicle has been based on all quadrants of the breast. Aufricht[2] described the inferior pedicle. Skoog[3] and Weiner[4] used a superior pedicle, and Strombeck[5] and McKissock[6] developed the bipedicle technique to ensure survival of the nipple-areola.

In general, breast resection is performed with an effort to preserve the origin of the blood supply to the base of the pedicle. The vascular anatomy is reviewed to explain the anatomic basis for survival of the nipple-areola regardless of the direction selected for the base of the nipple-areola flap. The skin closure after the mobilization of the nipple-areola pedicle and breast parenchyma resection is generally based on the Wise pattern[7] (Fig. 137-1), which consists of diverging limbs

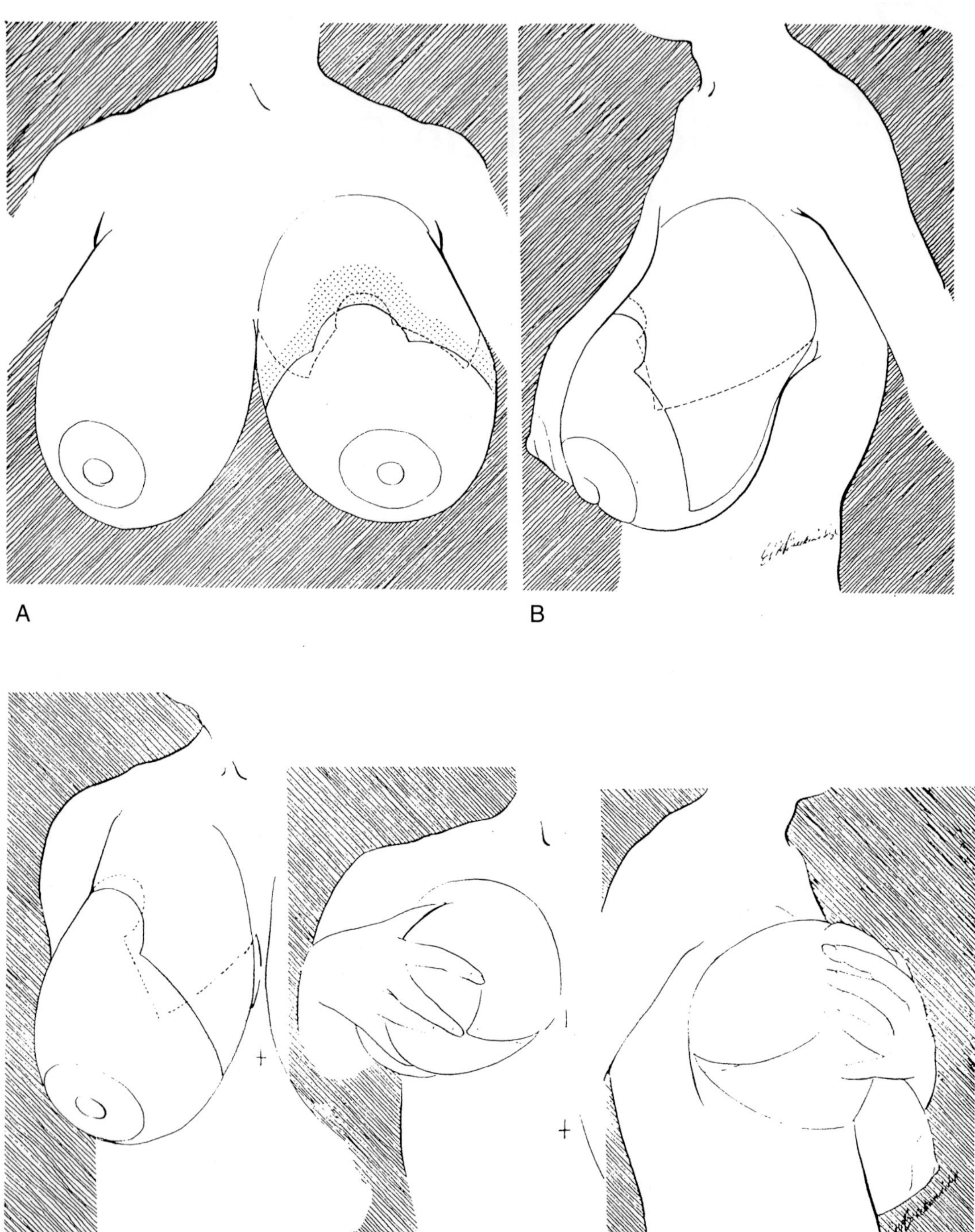

FIGURE 137-1. *A* to *C*, Pattern of skin resection in reduction mammaplasty. In *A*, the stippling represents the extent of undermining of the skin flaps. *D* and *E*, Modification of original marking to broaden and shorten the skin flaps and to shorten the submammary incision. (From Wise RJ: A preliminary report on a method of planning the mammaplasty. Plast Reconstr Surg 1956;17:367.)

starting at the selected site for the future location of the nipple-areola and extending 5 to 6 cm. The remainder of the skin resection extends medial and lateral from the inferior central limbs as a lazy S configuration to resect redundant skin and breast parenchyma and to ensure a conical shape to the breast skin envelope. A keyhole is frequently designed at the superior apex of the Wise pattern that represents the site for later inset of the nipple-areola. Modifications are reviewed and include design without the keyhole skin resection and selection of the nipple-areola site after completion of the skin and breast parenchyma resection. Furthermore, the medial and lateral skin resection can be delayed until the central mound is established. The variations in technique for breast reduction include design on the pedicle for transposition of the nipple-areola, skin resection pattern, areas of breast parenchyma resection, and potential shifting of the preserved breast parenchyma to improve breast mound shape and projection.

HISTORICAL PERSPECTIVES

The modern era of breast reduction began in 1972 when McKissock[8] changed the orientation of the pedicle to support the nipple-areola from horizontal to vertical with the description of the vertical dermal flap (Fig. 137-2). This technique allowed safety in transposition of the nipple-areola and simultaneous effective resection of breast tissue, maintaining a natural breast shape by use of the "coning principle."

Ribeiro[9] introduced a dermal-lipoglandular flap based on the inferior aspect of the breast mound and used this tissue to "autoaugment" the breast after superior, medial, and lateral breast tissue resection (Fig. 137-3). Courtiss and Goldwyn[10] identified the mammaplasty technique in which the inferior pedicle contains the nipple-areola and the closure is accomplished by conversion of the keyhole incision into an inverted T incision (Fig. 137-4). The safety and reliability of this approach using the inferior pedicle technique was confirmed by Reich.[11] Robbins[12] also confirmed the maintenance of nipple-areola sensation with the inferior pedicle technique. Georgiade[13] further perfected the technique by decreasing the width of the inferior pedicle to 6 to 9 cm, emphasizing the importance of maintaining attachments to the pectoral fascia and demonstrating the reliability with pedicle lengths up to 28 cm (Fig. 137-5).

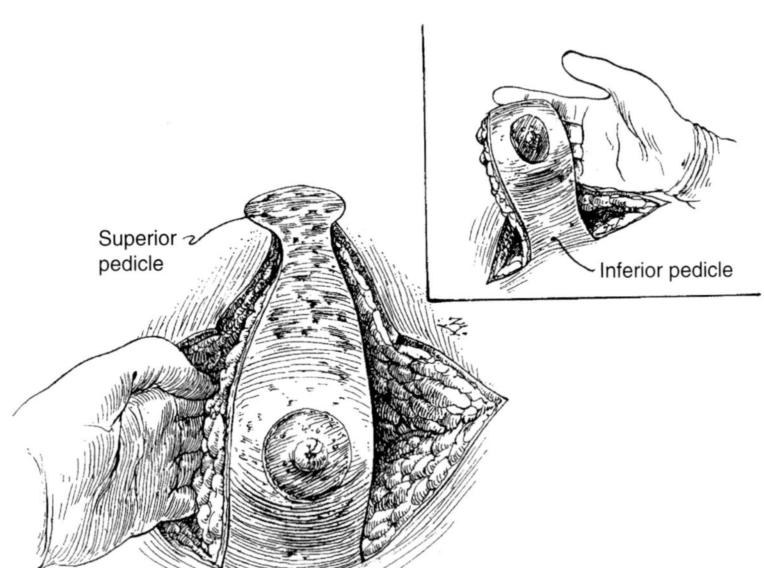

FIGURE 137-2. Development of vertical bipedicle flap to support nipple-areola circulation and to allow resection of excess breast parenchyma. (From McKissock PK: Reduction mammaplasty with a vertical dermal flap. Plast Reconstr Surg 1972;49:245.)

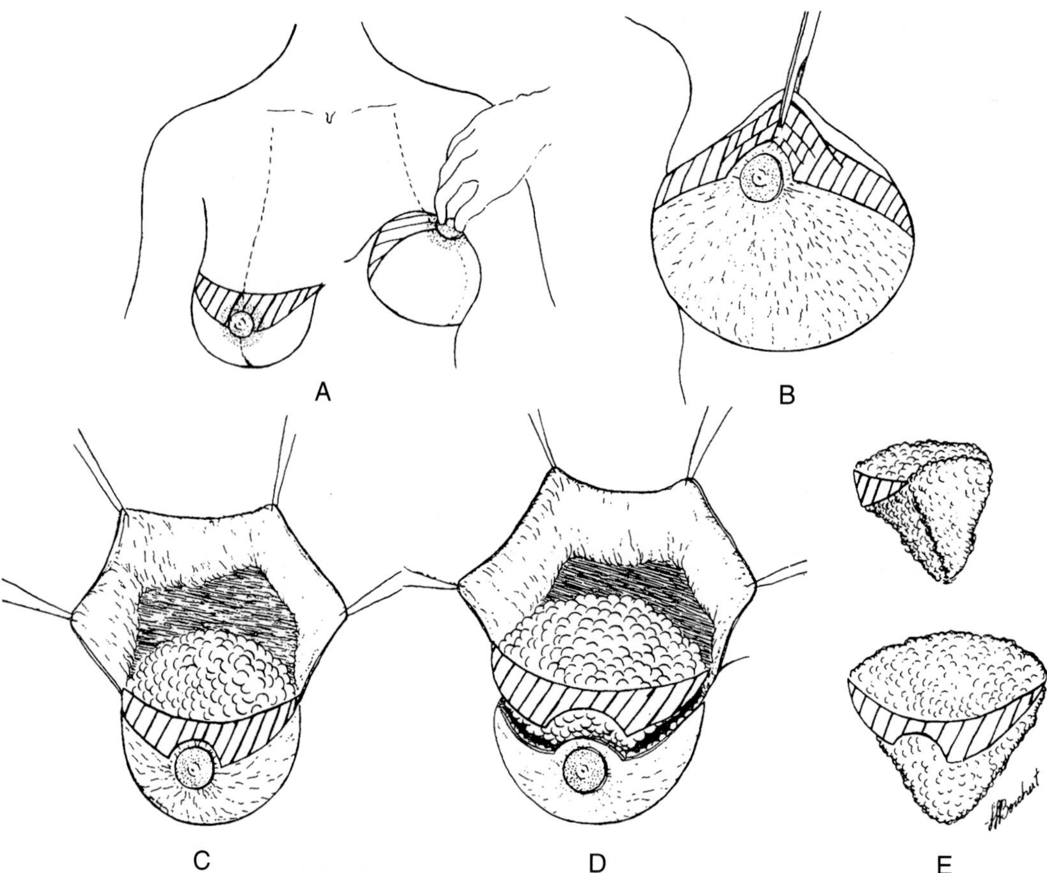

FIGURE 137-3. Development of inferior pedicle to support nipple-areola circulation and to allow resection of excess breast parenchyma. *A,* The superior and middle incision lines are shown on the right breast, and the inferior incision line is shown on the left breast. *B,* Dotted area is the "de-epithelialized" area. *C,* The superior skin flap has been raised. (Note the area of pectoral fascia exposed above.) *D* and *E,* Resection of mammary tissue and a crescent of attached skin. (From Ribeiro L: A new technique for reduction mammaplasty. Plast Reconstr Surg 1975;55:330.)

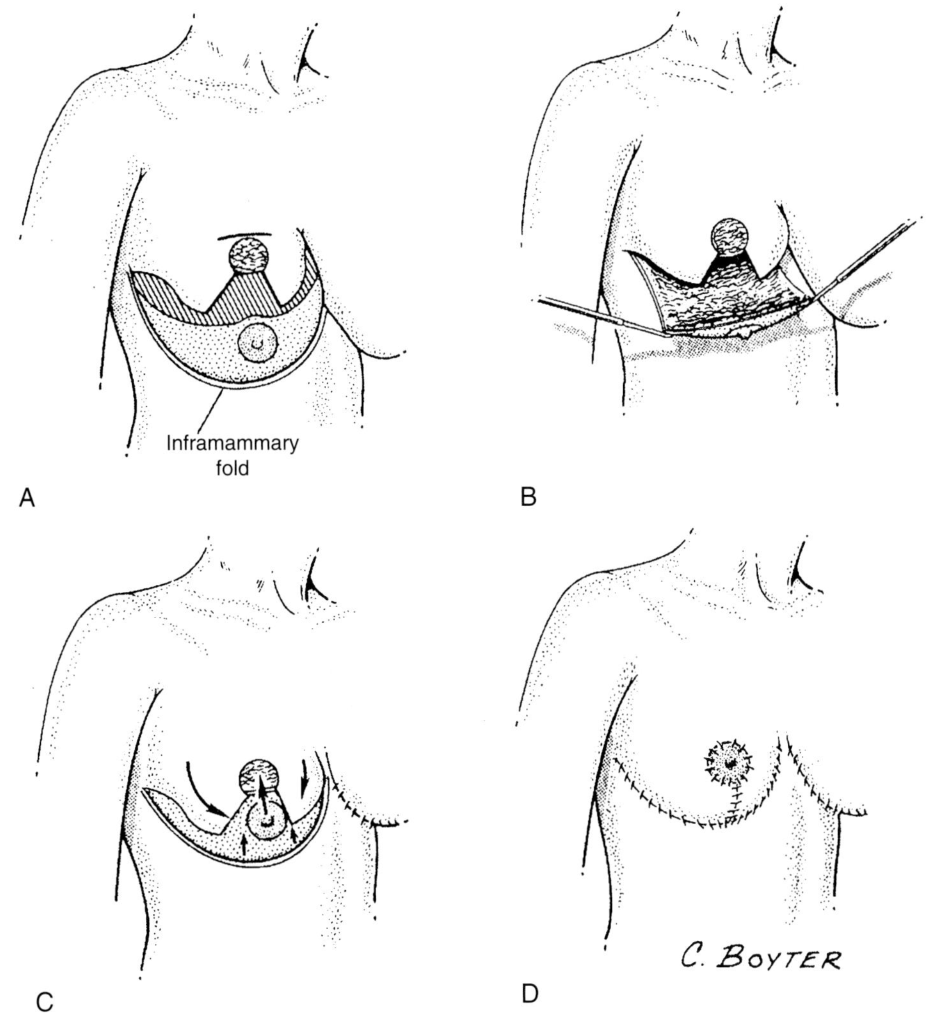

FIGURE 137-4. Development of keyhole design in association with inferior pedicle for breast reduction. *A,* First, the keyhole and the future medial and lateral skin flaps are marked. Next, the broad inferior pedicle is marked (with its inferior margin 1 cm above the entire length of the inframammary fold) and a split skin graft is removed from its surface (stippled area). *B,* The inferior pedicle, the width of the breast and 2 to 4 cm high, is dissected down through the breast to the pectoral muscle. Only the skin is removed from the circular areolar site in the keyhole. After this, one can remove as much of the breast as necessary above the inferior pedicle and between the limbs of the keyhole. *C,* The nipple and areola, on their inferior pedicle, are brought up and fastened on the circular part of the keyhole. The medial and lateral skin flaps are approximated beneath the areola. *D,* The closure. (From Courtiss EH, Goldwyn RM: Reduction mammaplasty by the inferior pedicle technique. Plast Reconstr Surg 1977;59:500.)

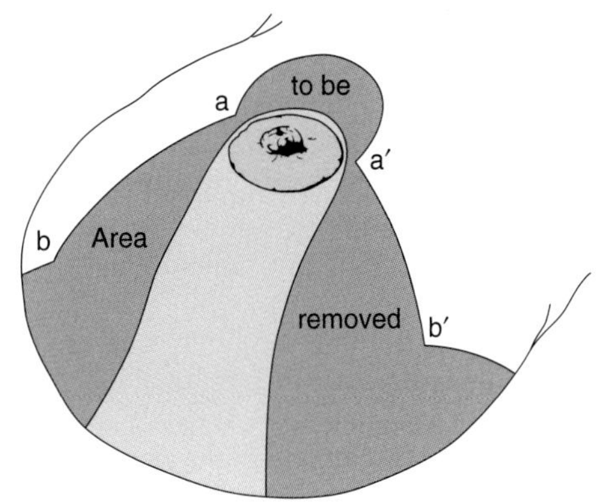

FIGURE 137-5. Modification of inferior pedicle with decreased width while reliable nipple-areola circulation is maintained. The areas of breast and skin excision are shown. Note the narrow cuff of dermis (1 to 2 cm) around the areola. The width at the base of the dermal pedicle will vary from 6 to 9 cm. (From Georgiade NG, Serafin D, Morris R, Georgiade GS: Reduction mammaplasty utilizing an inferior pedicle nipple-areola flap. Ann Plast Surg 1979;3:211.)

BREAST CIRCULATION

A knowledge of breast circulation is essential for planning safe reduction mammaplasty. Sources of blood supply for the breast include the medial perforating branches of the internal mammary. The lateral chest wall pedicle is the lateral thoracic artery, which provides circulation for the lateral aspect of the breast mound. The breast is located over the pectoralis major muscle. The major pedicle for this muscle is the thoracoacromial artery. The breast receives numerous musculocutaneous perforating vessels from the underlying pectoralis major muscle. The intercostal branches are not directly a source of circulation with the exception of the inferior lateral breast. All these arteries are accompanied by paired veins (Fig. 137-6; see also Color Plate 137-1).

The design of the bipedicle approach for relocation of the nipple-areola position by McKissock[6] incorporated the segmental pedicles from both the intermammary and lateral thoracic artery for the superior pedicle and the musculocutaneous branches from the thoracoacromial artery and the inferior segmental branches of the internal mammary artery and communications via the intercostal arteries. Division of this bipedicled, de-epithelialized flap is accomplished without impairment of the nipple-areola circulation, allowing use of either the superior or inferior-based

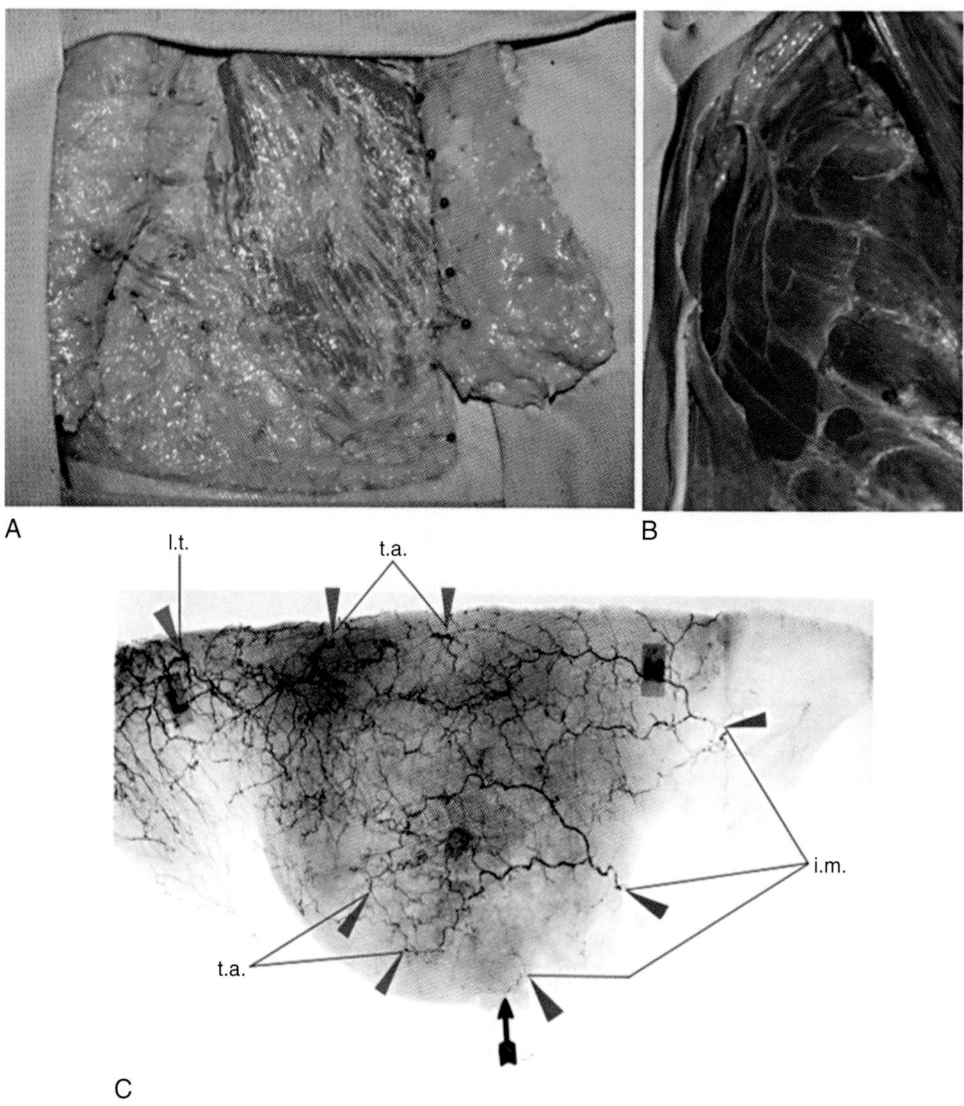

FIGURE 137-6. Vascular anatomy of the breast (see also Color Plate 137-1). *A,* Anterior hemithorax. Beads on left side designate branches of the lateral thoracic artery entering the lateral breast, and the beads on the right designate site of segmental branches of the internal mammary artery into the medial breast. *B,* Selective latex injection of lateral thoracic artery. *C,* Selective barium latex injection into internal mammary (i.m.), lateral thoracic (l.t.), and thoracoacromial (t.a.) arteries demonstrates contribution to breast circulation.

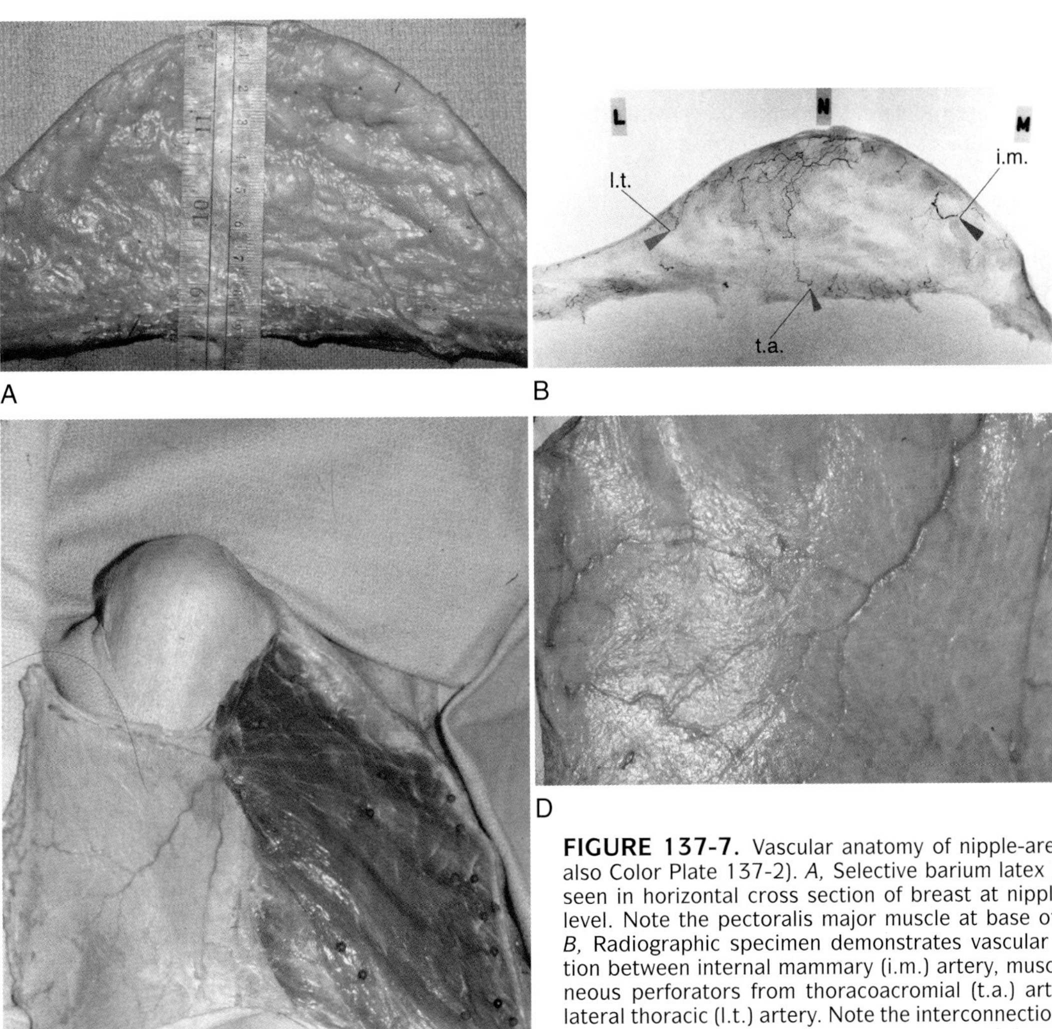

FIGURE 137-7. Vascular anatomy of nipple-areola (see also Color Plate 137-2). *A,* Selective barium latex injection seen in horizontal cross section of breast at nipple-areola level. Note the pectoralis major muscle at base of breast. *B,* Radiographic specimen demonstrates vascular connection between internal mammary (i.m.) artery, musculocutaneous perforators from thoracoacromial (t.a.) artery, and lateral thoracic (l.t.) artery. Note the interconnections of the three vascular systems at the nipple-areola. *C,* Latex vascular injection of breast and hemithorax. Chest skin is divided at sternal edge and reflected laterally to visualize deep surface of breast region. Note the segmental branches of the internal mammary artery and lateral branches of the lateral thoracic artery. *D,* Close-up of deep surface of breast at nipple-areola site. Note the arterial-arterial direct anastomosis between branches of internal mammary artery and lateral thoracic artery.

flap to carry the nipple-areola to a new location on the breast mound (Fig. 137-7; see also Color Plate 137-2). The classic approach for the inferior pedicle leaves the nipple-areola attached to the inferior dermal breast flap for autoaugmentation of the breast envelope after reduction and allows safe transposition of the nipple-areola to the apex of the new breast mound (Color Plate 137-3*A* to *C*). The versatility of the location for the dermal flap for vascular support of the nipple-areola is based on the direct communication of the vascular network between the terminal branches of the lateral thoracic, the internal mammary, and the musculocutaneous branches of the thoracoacromial arteries and associated veins (Color Plate 137-3*C* to *E*).

INDICATIONS

Symptomatic macromastia is the primary indication for reduction mammaplasty. Both physical and psychological symptoms from macromastia can adversely affect a woman's quality of life. Common musculoskeletal complaints include neck, breast, shoulder, and upper and lower back pain. Physical features of women with macromastia include hunched or rounded shoulders due to scapula rotation forward, kyphosis, and chronic skin indentation of the shoulders and back due to brassiere pressure.[14] Chronic skin problems include striations of the upper breast and intertrigo at the inframammary crease due to maceration, which can lead to chronic fungal infections and recurrent mastitis.

Psychological effects of macromastia are often most apparent in adolescent patients and include poor perception of body image and poor self-esteem, which may ultimately contribute to depression. Women with macromastia limit participation in physical fitness activities and most modify their wardrobe to wear clothing that is comfortable, accommodates increased chest wall girth, and is not revealing. These deviations from normal compared with peers can lead to poor self-esteem. Limitations in physical fitness can contribute to generalized obesity.

SELECTION OF THE PATIENT

Patients requesting breast reduction can be divided into three categories on the basis of an estimate of the amount of breast tissue required to restore breast size compatible with body physique. The range of reduction is based on preoperative breast size and includes moderate reduction (<800 g), large reduction (800 to 2500 g), and gigantomastia reduction (>2500 g). Reduction of the very large breast requires special techniques and considerations because of potential complications (Fig. 137-8). If this patient is

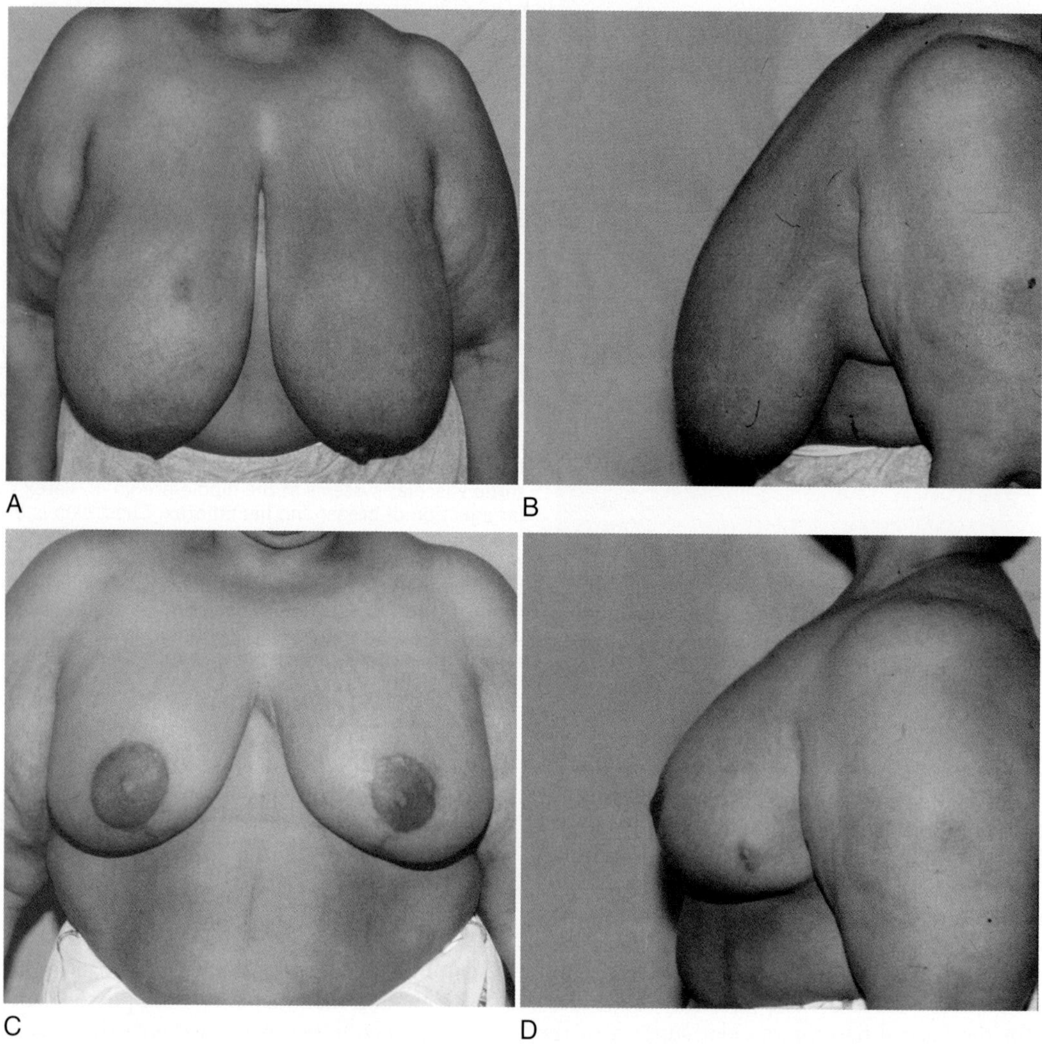

FIGURE 137-8. Gigantomastia reduction with inferior pedicle technique. *A,* Preoperative anterior view. *B,* Preoperative lateral view. *C,* Postoperative anterior view 1 year after reduction. *D,* Postoperative lateral view 1 year after reduction.

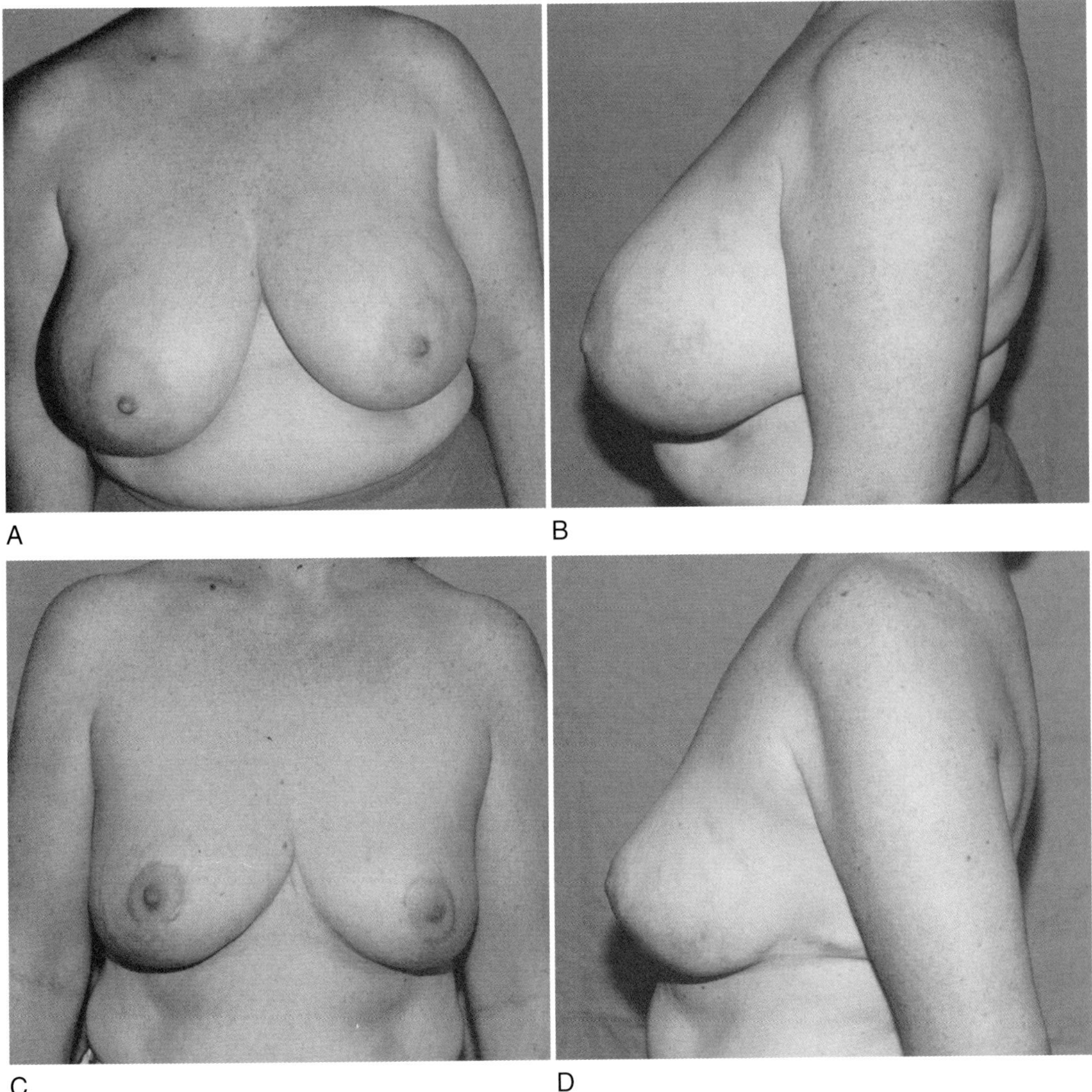

FIGURE 137-9. Large reduction with inferior pedicle technique. *A*, Preoperative anterior view. *B*, Preoperative lateral view. *C*, Postoperative anterior view 1 year after reduction. *D*, Postoperative lateral view 1 year after reduction.

obese, reduction may not be appropriate until weight loss is accomplished. Many patients cannot lose weight and still are anxious to undergo a reduction mammaplasty. Selection of the patient in this category therefore requires careful discussion of the increased morbidity associated with reduction mammaplasty and options for bariatric surgery preceding reduction mammaplasty. The inferior pedicle technique in the very large breast is still useful as a mechanism to autoaugment the breast mound after completion of reduction, but the pedicle may be too long to adequately support circulation for the nipple-areola. Even if the long inferior pedicle will support the nipple-areola, the long length of the pedicle may incorporate excessive breast tissue when it is transposed to the appropriate position for the nipple-areola in relationship to the breast mound and result in an inadequate reduction. For the very large breast reduction, the nipple-areola is grafted with the length of the inferior pedicle adjusted solely for the purpose of the re-established projecting conical breast mound (autoaugmentation).

The large breast reduction will require removal of 800 to 2500 g of breast tissue (Fig. 137-9). The medium-sized breast is appropriate for the inferior pedicle technique. The shape and projection of the breast can be enhanced by use of the inferior pedicle after breast resection is performed. Furthermore, with

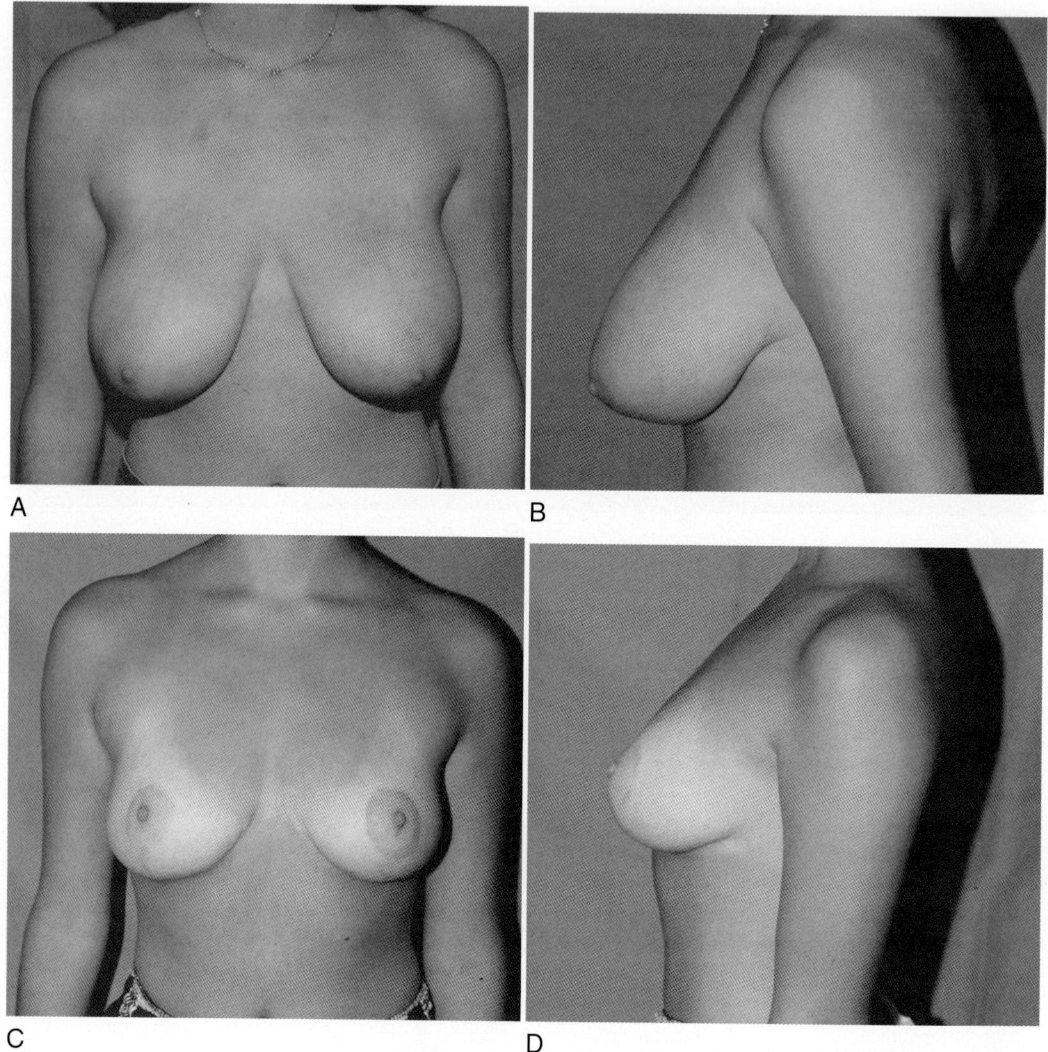

FIGURE 137-10. Moderate reduction with inferior pedicle technique. *A,* Preoperative anterior view. *B,* Preoperative lateral view. *C,* Postoperative anterior view 1 year after reduction. *D,* Postoperative lateral view 1 year after reduction.

a 6- to 8-cm width on the inferior pedicle and a length up to 21 cm, the nipple-areola will have adequate perfusion. The bulk of the pedicle after it is rotated into position will not be so excessive to impair skin closure or to require the presence of excess breast tissue in the inferior aspect of the new breast mound.

The moderate breast reduction usually has a major component of breast ptosis (Fig. 137-10). In this patient, the reduction is minimal and primarily relates to resection of medial and lateral tissue with preservation of most central breast tissue. The inferior pedicle is primarily used to accomplish transposition of the nipple-areola to an appropriate position in association with breast skin envelope resection to correct the ptosis and loss of support for the breast.

The age of patients requesting reduction varies greatly. In the very young patient (younger than 18 years), the family must be part of the consultation process, and their support is essential for a decision to proceed with a reduction mammaplasty. If there is concern about mental stability of the adolescent patient or if the procedure is requested to improve athletic performance, psychiatric consultation is required before the parents and the surgeon agree to proceed with the reduction mammaplasty. The young professional and middle-aged patients who have suffered with heavy breasts are usually capable of making a reasonable informed decision in regard to reduction mammaplasty. However, the patient who insists on a postoperative reduction breast size below the normal size for her height and weight may not have appropriate indications for reduction mammaplasty.

Patients with concurrent illness may have increased risk of complications. Patients with cardiopulmonary insufficiency and collagen diseases may have wound healing and circulatory complications. If the breast is in the intermediate to large category, a reduction mammaplasty may improve quality of life. These patients need explicit information about complications especially related to wound healing.

Tobacco use is an absolute contraindication to reduction mammaplasty. If the patient will stop smoking for a minimum of 6 weeks, the risk of skin loss and fat necrosis appears reduced, allowing the surgeon to proceed with the inferior pedicle technique. If there is question about reliability concerning cessation of tobacco use, the patient should not be selected as a surgical candidate for reduction mammaplasty, or a preoperative nicotine test is indicated to verify abstinence from smoking. A simple, accurate, and inexpensive test for nicotine content in urine was approved by the Food and Drug Administration in 1996.[15] Disposable NicCheck* test strips are inserted into a urine sample and will change color according to the nicotine content in a patient's urine. This test has been reported as accurate and reliable,[15] and it may be useful in determining those patients who will not be candidates for reduction mammaplasty because of continued tobacco use.

A patient's risk for breast cancer should be reviewed before selection for reduction mammaplasty. Although the procedure will not change future risk for cancer, the patient should be aware of the risk factors. A mammogram for patients older than 30 years should be available for review within 6 months of the date of reduction mammaplasty. Any abnormalities identified should undergo appropriate evaluation before proceeding with reduction mammaplasty. If the patient is identified as high risk for breast cancer related to hereditary predisposition (see Chapter 138) or if the breast has evidence of atypia from prior biopsies, a prophylactic mastectomy with immediate reconstruction should be considered.

The patient's concerns about aesthetics and function of the breast after reduction mammaplasty may affect suitability for the procedure and technique selected. The inferior pedicle technique with nipple-areola transposition usually incorporates the nipple and areola sensory innervation. However, the patient who is concerned about maintenance of sensation must accept the potential decrease in sensation. Fortunately, this technique is usually effective in maintaining satisfactory sensation compatible with preoperative status. Gonzalez[14] found that 90.5% of patients who underwent inferior pedicle reduction mammaplasty retained nipple-areola sensation. A wide inferior pedicle with less inferior lateral dissection may be effective in avoiding sensory changes when this aspect of the surgery is of major importance for the patient.

The amount and duration of breast and musculoskeletal pain, extent of preoperative disability, and exercise intolerance related to the large breasts should be noted. The patient must be prepared to return to normal activities in a reasonable interval after reduction mammaplasty.[16] Posture abnormalities should be noted. If there are excess musculoskeletal symptoms or posture abnormalities, an orthopedic consultation should be obtained before proceeding with reduction mammaplasty.

The physical examination should document breast size, degree of ptosis, and breast asymmetry. The patient should be fully informed about risk of persistent asymmetry and changes in breast size related to diet, particularly since weight loss may occur after the reduction mammaplasty is completed.

The younger patient who may subsequently become pregnant should be informed about potential inability to breast-feed after reduction mammaplasty. The inferior pedicle technique does maintain ductal connections with preserved inferior breast parenchyma. In addition, preservation of postoperative nipple sensitivity allows breast milk let-down and expression.[17] Many patients who have undergone inferior pedicle reduction mammaplasty have successfully breast-fed their babies, but the ability to nurse may be adversely affected by all reduction techniques. The most important factors necessary for breast-feeding after reduction mammaplasty are appropriate preservation of breast lobules and lactiferous ducts (breast tissue) to allow milk production and expression, respectively,[17] and encouragement from medical professionals to breast-feed postoperatively.[18]

Transposition of the nipple-areola and reduction of the skin envelope will require external visible breast mound scars. The inferior pedicle technique generally requires an inverted T scar with a vertical component between the inframammary line and the inferior border of the areola. A transverse component will be present along the inframammary line, often extending between the lateral sternal line and the anterior axillary line. A scar surrounds the areola in its new position. The patient may have interest in the vertical mammaplasty technique that eliminates the horizontal scar on the inframammary line (see Chapter 136). The technique should be presented to the patient and its advantages and disadvantages reviewed. If the patient requests a vertical reduction, the surgeon who does not use this approach should review the inferior pedicle technique but help the patient seek consulta-

*Dynagen, Inc., Cambridge, Massachusetts.

TABLE 137-1 ✦ COMPARISON OF INFERIOR PEDICLE VERSUS VERTICAL REDUCTION MAMMAPLASTY

		Predictable Results*		Optimal Nipple-Areola Position†		Preservation of Shape†		Scars	
	Technical Ease	*Early Experience*	*Late Experience*	*Early*	*Late*	*Early*	*Late*	*Acceptable*	*Risk of Hypertrophy*
Inferior pedicle									
Moderate (<800 g)	++++	+++	++++	+++	++	++++	+++	++	Yes
Large (800-2500 g)	+++	+++	+++	+++	++	+++	++	+++	Yes
Gigantomastia (>2500 g)	++	++	+++	+++	++	+++	++	++	Yes
Vertical pedicle									
Moderate (<800 g)	++++	++	++++	++	+++	++	++++	+++	No
Large (800-2500 g)	+	+	++	+	+	+	++	++	No
Gigantomastia (>2500 g)	Not generally recommended for gigantomastia.								

Excellent, ++++; good, +++; fair, ++; acceptable, +.
*Early experience, <15 procedures; late experience, >15 procedures.
†Follow-up for critique of results: early, <6 months; late, >6 months.

tion for a second opinion regarding suitability for alternative techniques to accomplish a reduction mammaplasty (Table 137-1).

PREOPERATIVE PREPARATION AND MARKING

For large breast and gigantomastia reductions, a 1-unit autotransfusion is usually obtained before surgery. Photographs are taken to document the size, shape, and symmetry of the breasts. The patient is generally scheduled for one night of hospitalization. If the patient uses tobacco, confirmation of abstinence for 6 weeks should be confirmed by interview of the patient or by laboratory or urine testing immediately before surgery.

In the preoperative area, the patient is placed in the sitting position to locate the site of the nipple-areola placement. The inframammary line is located as well as the midline of each breast. Areas of lipodystrophy that may be present in the lateral chest and axillary region are outlined. The markings begin with the inframammary line from the sternal edge to the midaxillary line (Fig. 137-11*A*). A mark is made at the center of the manubrium to designate the midline of the sternum. A second mark is made at the midclavicle. From this mark, a line is drawn inferiorly to bisect the nipple-areola and extends to the previously marked inframammary line (Fig. 137-11*B*). This line will designate the midline of the breast and determine the vertical position of the nipple-areola on the reduced breast. The horizontal position of the nipple-areola is now determined. There are three methods that may be used to plan this position:

1. By placing the finger at the previously marked inframammary line, one can project through the breast parenchyma to the future site of the nipple-areola (Fig. 137-11*B* and *C*).
2. A line is drawn from the sternal notch to the previously drawn midline of the breast (the midclavicular line) at the site selected for the new position of the nipple-areola. This distance will vary with the height of the patient and breast size, but it usually ranges from 20 to 25 cm (Fig. 137-11*D*).[13]
3. The nipple-areola is usually located at the same level on the horizontal axis of the midpoint of the upper arm (Fig. 137-11*E*).

All three measurements are used to confirm optimal position for the nipple-areola. After the new site of the nipple-areola is located, the diverging limbs extend inferior to this point for a distance of 5 to 6 cm. These limbs represent the vertical skin closure of the reduced breast mound extending from the nipple-areola to the inframammary line. If a keyhole is designed, the areola circumference should be planned at 4 to 5 cm. A McKissock keyhole pattern device (Padgett Instruments) may be used to design both the keyhole and the limbs representing the vertical closure. The angle of divergence of the limbs should not be excessive or excess tension will result at the closure site at the junction of the inframammary line and the vertical line extending from the inferior areola to the midline of

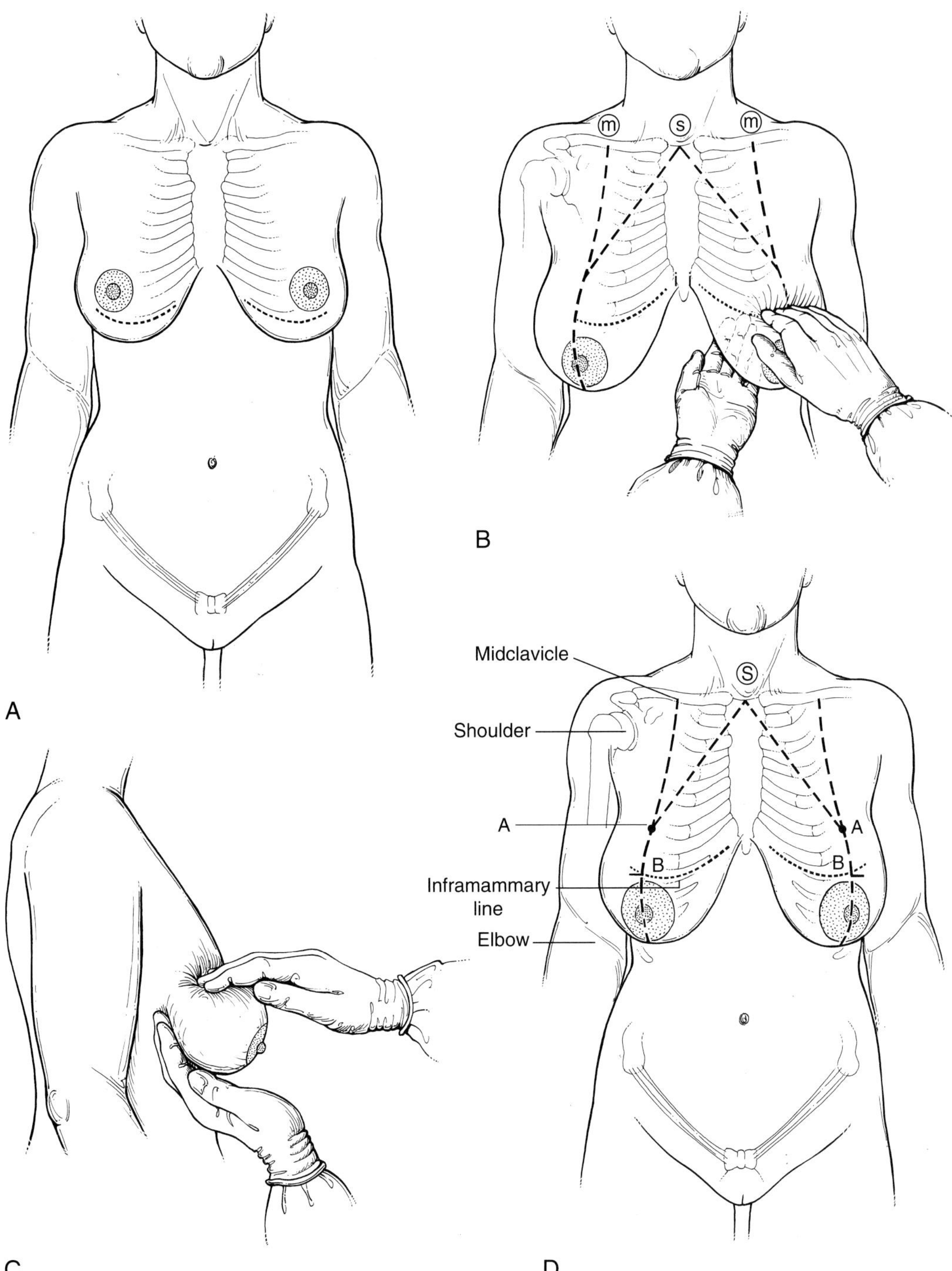

FIGURE 137-11. Preoperative markings for inferior pedicle technique. *A,* Inframammary line. *B,* Location of nipple-areola placement site. Midclavicular line represents axis for nipple-areola site. New nipple site coincides with inframammary line. m, midclavicular line; s, sternal notch-nipple-areola site; i, inframammary line. *C,* Determination of nipple-areola site after reduction. *D,* Sternal-nipple distance ranges from 20 to 25 cm, depending on the patient's height and postoperative reduction breast size. Planned nipple-areola site (A) is determined by the inframammary line as well as by the distance from the sternal notch and mid-upper arm.

Continued

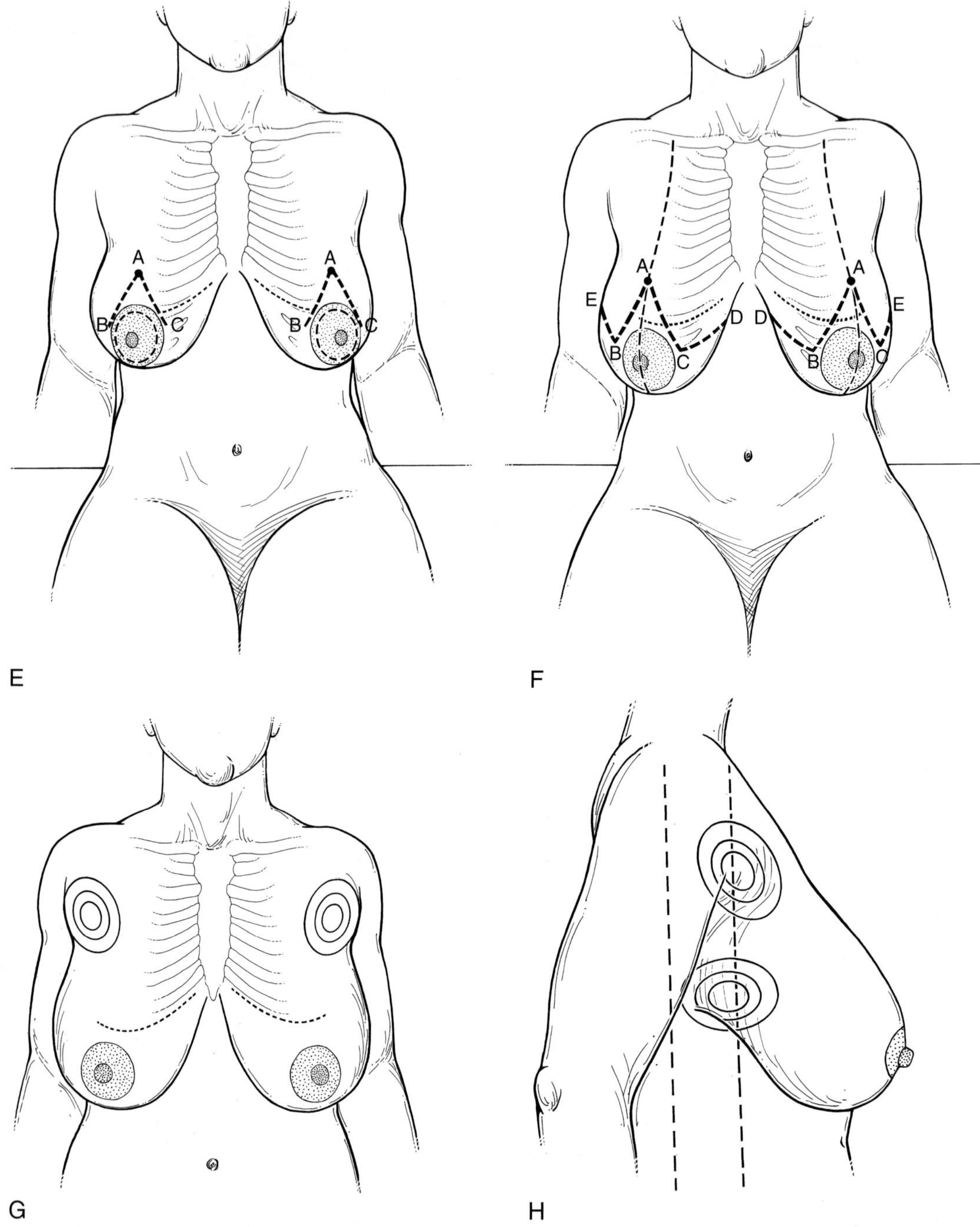

FIGURE 137-11, cont'd. *E,* Lines A-B and A-C represent vertical closure site after reduction. The length of A-B and A-C ranges from 5 to 8 cm, with an average of 6 cm. B-C distance should not exceed 7 to 8 cm. Areola size is reduced to correspond with breast mound reduction. *F,* Lines C-D and B-E represent areas of skin and breast resection to restore conical shape to the breast mound. C-D and B-E generally have a lazy S shape. Markings serve as guidelines and may be altered after central breast resection and closure are completed. A, selected site for nipple-areola transposition. *G,* Areas of lipodystrophy at superior anterior lateral chest are marked for liposuction. *H,* Areas of lipodystrophy are outlined on the lateral chest. Liposuction in larger breasts and gigantomastia reductions should be located between the anterior axillary and midaxillary lines to avoid lateral contour irregularity after breast reduction.

the breast at the inframammary line. The distance between the vertical limbs should not exceed 6 to 7 cm (Fig. 137-11*E*). Excess tension as a result of too wide an angle of divergence will apply pressure to the underlying inferior pedicle and distort the inferior shape of the new breast mound. Excessive tension at the inverted T closure may also increase the risk of avascular skin necrosis. The inferior pedicle may be designed in the preoperative area, or the design can be completed after the patient is under anesthesia and prepared and draped for surgery (Fig. 137-11*F*).

If the patient has areas of lipodystrophy in the superior lateral chest and the mid to lateral chest, these areas of excess contour may be improved by liposuction. Liposuction, particularly in the area of the lateral chest, will assist in closure of the lateral aspect of the breast and enable the surgeon to shorten the lateral aspect of the inframammary line closure without a contour irregularity due to excess tissue at the end of the incision. With the patient in the sitting position, a topographic map of areas of planned liposuction should be outlined (Fig. 137-11*G* and *H*).

INTRAOPERATIVE POSITIONING AND MARKING

The patient is placed supine with the arm abducted at 90 degrees and pronated, with care taken to provide padding particularly in the elbow and wrist regions. Because the patient will be seated intraoperatively, it is important to test the operating room table mechanism to confirm that the patient is properly positioned for elevation into the 70- to 90-degree sitting position. Also, wraps around the upper and lower arm should be checked to confirm that the upper extremity position is maintained while the patient is elevated. It is helpful to place the patient in an upright position to confirm symmetry of breast parenchyma resection, adequate resection of skin and breast in the medial and lateral areas, and nipple-areola position if the site is not predetermined by a keyhole design before surgery. It is essential to avoid hyperabduction of the upper extremity throughout the duration of the reduction mammaplasty. Patients who suffer preoperative upper extremity or shoulder disabilities may require only a 45-degree abduction of the upper extremities during the procedure.

OPERATIVE PROCEDURE

The design of the inferior pedicle is centered on the midline of the breast (midclavicular line), with a width of 8 cm. The width may be shorter (6 cm) in a small reduction or wider for a large reduction (10 cm) if the patient has risk factors that may affect pedicle circulation (prior radiation therapy, collagen disease, obesity, tobacco use) (Fig. 137-12*A*). Also, in the patient with great concern about a possible decrease in nipple-areola sensation, the lateral aspect may be extended to ensure that dissection for pedicle elevation will incorporate the fourth to sixth intercostal nerves. When the inframammary line is drawn with the patient sitting in the preoperative area, the weight of the breast may pull skin inferiorly. After the reduction, the pull will be less, so it appears helpful to arbitrarily move the inframammary line 1 cm superiorly to adjust for the effect of the reduction mammaplasty. The size of the areola is generally excessive in the macromastia patient. The size is reduced to 3 to 4 cm, depending on the surgeon's and patient's preference, and marked with a cookie cutter or circular device to plan the new areola dimensions.

After completion of all markings, the incisions are marked with the scalpel so that they are not washed away during the process of de-epithelialization of the inferior pedicle. De-epithelialization is accomplished by use of the knife or scissors, preserving the underlying dermis (Fig. 137-12*B*). Preservation of the dermis avoids injury to the underlying subdermal plexus and provides a layer of tissue to help support the inferior pedicle. Excess areola is resected, with preservation of the central areola and nipple based on the intraoperative design. If liposuction is planned, tumescent fluid is injected through a small incision at the inferior lateral edge of the inferior pedicle. After the tumescent fluid is delivered, appropriately sized cannulas are used to remove designated areas of lipodystrophy. Liposuction is not used to reduce fatty tissue within the breast parenchyma since this tissue will be resected under direct visualization.

The inferior pedicle is now elevated (Fig. 137-12*C*). The inferior breast tissue is included with the inferior pedicle, which is elevated to the pectoral fascia. After the pedicle is elevated, it is reflected inferiorly and covered with a moist dressing. The remainder of the breast parenchyma is elevated from the pectoralis major muscle and adjacent serratus anterior muscle extending from the sternal edge to the anterior axillary line. The breast tissue with the overlying skin is elevated superiorly to the clavicle. The breast tissue above the inferior pedicle, including the keyhole area if this area has been designated, is resected along with excess breast tissue included with the superior flap. In general, a 1.5- to 2.0-cm layer of subcutaneous tissue and breast parenchyma is left intact with the superior preserved skin envelope. When the flap is pulled inferiorly to the inframammary line, the thickness of the superior flap should be similar for both breasts and resemble a breast requiring augmentation to restore volume and projection. The inferior pedicle will shortly be used to autoaugment the breasts (Fig. 137-12*D* to *F*).

Bilateral inferior pedicles are elevated and examined. Excess breast tissue is resected with care while

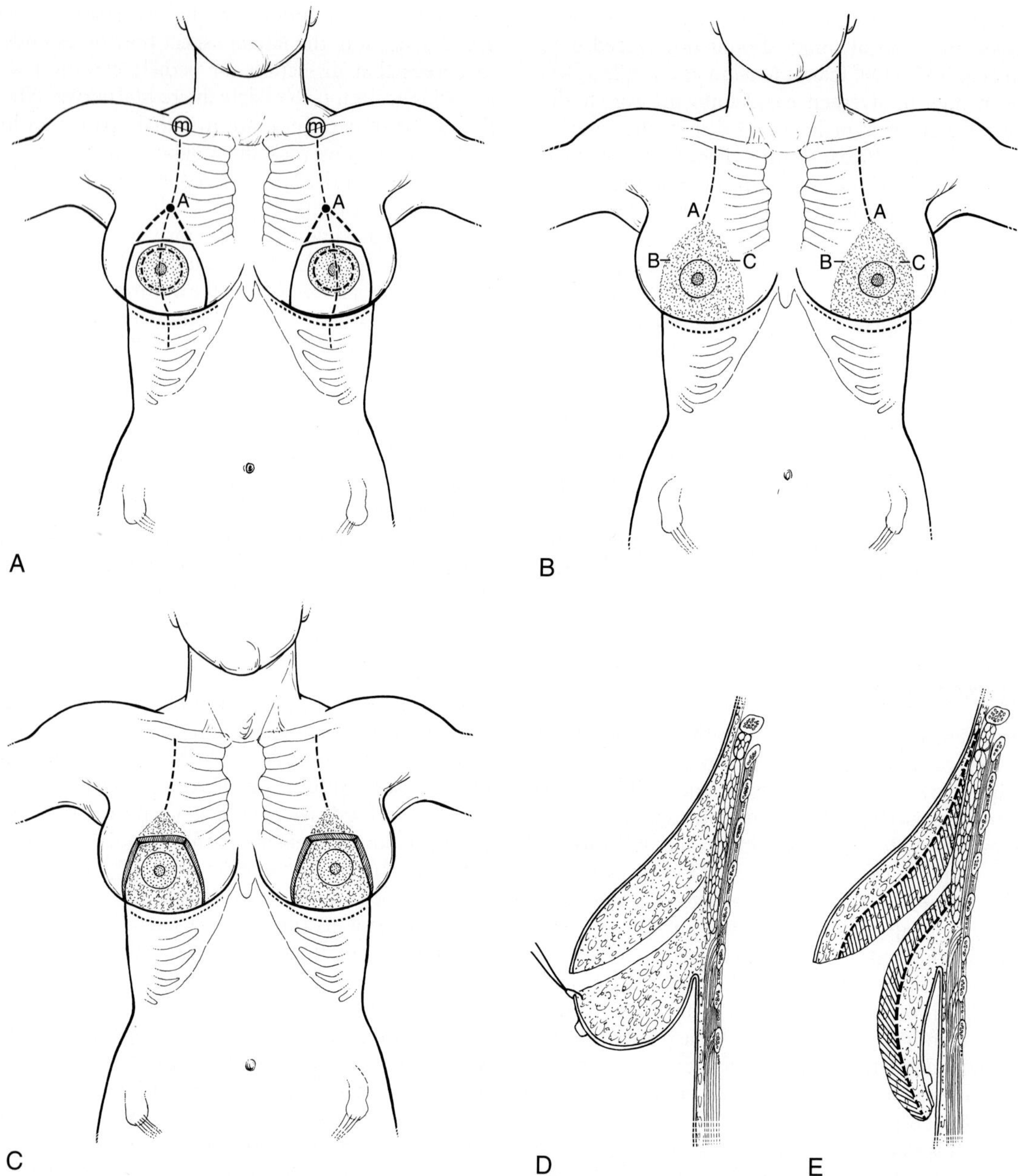

FIGURE 137-12. Operative technique: inferior pedicle reduction. *A,* Inferior pedicle is centered on the midclavicular line with dimension of 6 to 10 cm. The areola is reduced to 3.5 to 4.5 cm. m, midclavicular line; A, selected site for nipple-areola transposition. *B,* Inferior pedicle and skin between limbs of Wise pattern (A-B, A-C) are de-epithelialized. *C,* Incisions are made to elevate inferior pedicle. *D,* Inferior pedicle is elevated to pectoralis muscle, and superior breast is elevated to clavicle superiorly, sternum medially, and anterior axillary line laterally. *E,* Breast tissue is resected from the deep surface of the superior breast mound and from inferior pedicle. (See crosshatched areas indicating site of breast parenchyma reduction.)

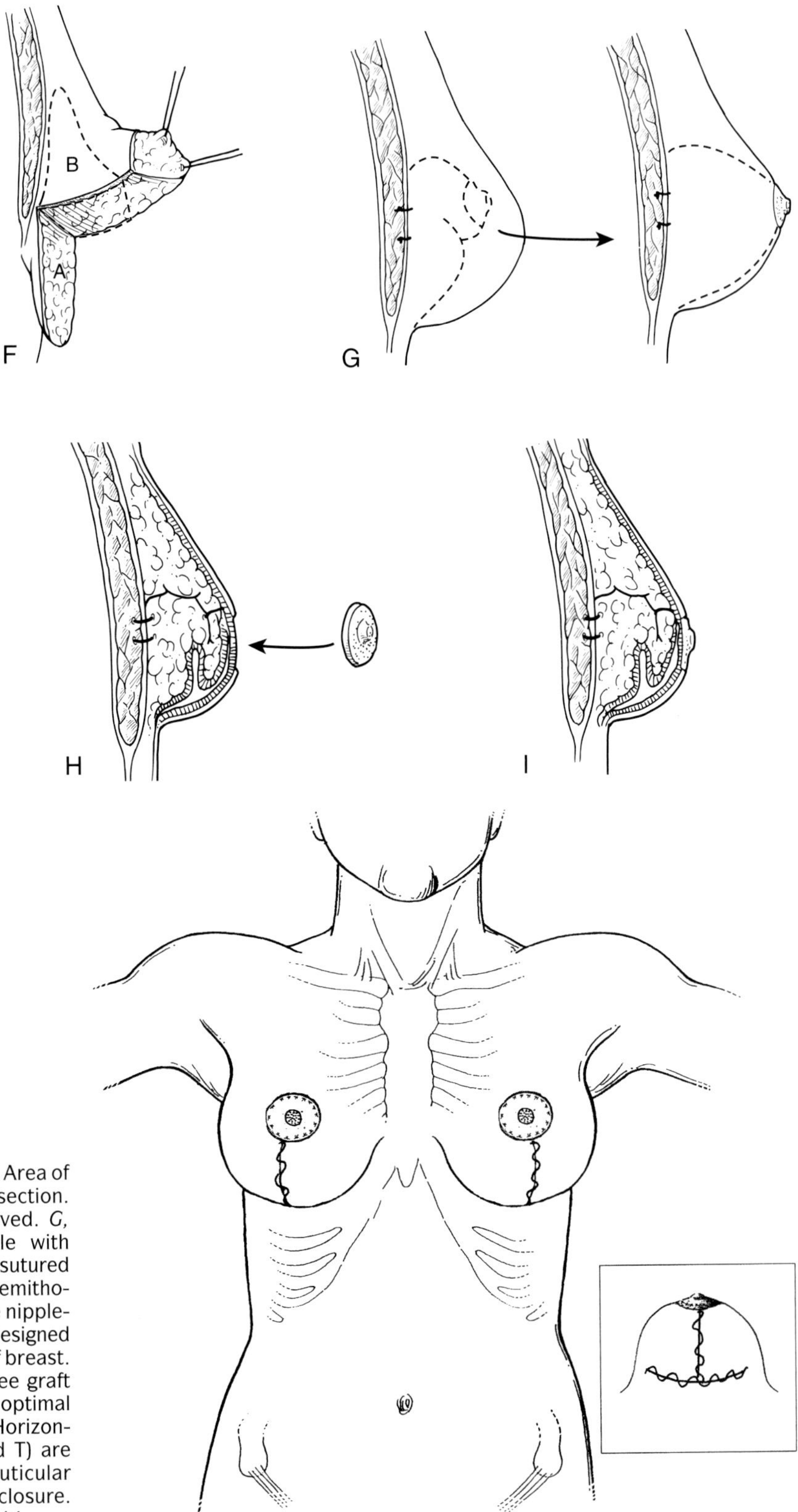

FIGURE 137-12, cont'd. *F,* Area of central breast parenchyma resection. B, breast resection; A, preserved. *G,* Dermal breast inferior pedicle with nipple-areola. Inferior pedicle is sutured in centralized position on each hemithorax. *H,* Inferior pedicle with free nipple-areola grafts. Inferior pedicle is designed to provide autoaugmentation of breast. *I,* Nipple-areola is placed as free graft after completion of reduction in optimal position on breast mound. *J,* Horizontal and vertical limbs (inverted T) are closed with running subcuticular sutures. *Inset* shows inverted T closure. Nipple-areola site is sutured with vertical mattress sutures.

preserving the base of the flap where the vascular pedicles from the perforating branches of the thoracoacromial artery and associated veins and the internal mammary artery and veins enter the pedicle. Also, the inferior pedicles can be placed on the chest and briefly covered by the superior preserved skin envelope to visualize the size of the breast. The weight of the resected tissue is monitored, and this process is continued until the reduction appears adequate and weights are compatible. The visualized size and projection of the preserved breast tissue in association with the inferior pedicle are more important in determining extent of parenchymal resection than are measured weights because the majority of breasts have asymmetry and the remaining tissue is more important than the tissue removed for correction of asymmetry.

The inferior pedicles, which contain the nipple-areola and the preserved breast tissue, are now ready for placement on the central aspect of each hemithorax. The pedicles are sutured to the chest wall with absorbable sutures to align each inferior pedicle in a central position along the midclavicular line. One suture is usually placed for the medial and lateral aspect of the inferior pedicle. The medial suture is located at the fourth interspace between the deep surface of the midpedicle and the pectoralis major muscle, and the lateral suture is placed at the same level through the lateral edge of the pectoralis major. The distal half of the pedicle should remain mobile so the pedicle will easily transpose the nipple-areola on its superficial surface to the appropriately selected site on the breast mound after skin closure of the envelope (Fig. 137-12*G*).

After the inferior pedicle is attached to the chest wall, the vertical limbs of the superior flaps are approximated to the inframammary line at the midclavicular line. If the keyhole incision has been incorporated into the reduction design, the nipple-areola may be sutured to the keyhole area in several strategic areas. If the nipple-areola position is not yet declared, the vertical closure is completed over the inferior pedicle with plans to later determine the site of the nipple-areola.

The medial and lateral skin and associated breast tissue may be resected on the basis of preoperative markings. A preferred method is to sit the patient on the operating room table and resect the medial and lateral redundant breast tissue with the central mound already established. Although the skin resection generally corresponds to the preoperatively designed lazy S incisions, the resection of medial and lateral skin and associated breast parenchyma is accomplished while visualizing the central pedicle and central inverted T closure with the chest in an upright position. This allows the surgeon to precisely resect tissue with the goal of symmetry and optimal projection.

After completion of the resection of the excess breast parenchyma and associated skin and subcutaneous tissue, the vertical and horizontal inframammary incision is closed by direct approximation with buried dermal and subcuticular sutures. With the patient still in the sitting position, the position of the nipple-areola is selected if it is not predetermined by a keyhole incision. The distance from the inframammary line to the future site of the inferior aspect of the areola should range from 4 to 5 cm. These sites are marked, and the patient is examined from the end of the operating room table. When symmetry is achieved in both breasts (and nipple-areola positioning appears symmetric), the nipple-areola sites are selected and the patient is returned to the supine position. The skin is resected, including underlying subcutaneous tissues. The nipple-areola is retrieved and sutured into position with half vertical mattress interrupted sutures with the knots oriented on the areola to avoid possible suture marks on the skin adjacent to the new areola-cutaneous junction (Figs. 137-12*H* to *J* and 137-13).

Intraoperative Assessment of Nipple-Areola Circulation

If circulation of the nipple-areola appears compromised or borderline compromised after closure of the breast mound and inset of the nipple-areola, intravenous administration of fluorescein is indicated. After a test dose to confirm no allergies to this medication, 2 g of fluorescein are given to the patient. After a 15-minute interval, Wood's lamp is used to deliver ultraviolet light to the nipple-areola. A yellow-green fluorescence to the nipple-areola confirms an intact dermal circulation (Color Plate 137-4). A dark blue appearance indicates inadequate dermal perfusion and represents an indication to evaluate potential problems with the circulation of the inferior pedicle. If there is excessive tension at the inverted T closure, reduction in size of the inferior pedicle may restore circulation to the pedicle and the nipple-areola. If there is no evidence of constriction at the base of

FIGURE 137-13. Moderate reduction with inferior pedicle technique. *A*, Preoperative anterior view. *B*, Preoperative lateral view. *C*, Intraoperative view of 10-cm inferior pedicle de-epithelialization. *D*, Intraoperative view of left inferior pedicle elevated off chest. Right inferior pedicle is sutured in centralized position on right hemithorax. *E*, Pedicles are reflected inferiorly. Note superior, medial, and lateral breast parenchyma reduction. *F*, Pedicles inset for autoaugmentation. The final nipple-areola site is selected after reduction is completed. *G*, Postoperative anterior view 1 year after reduction. *H*, Postoperative lateral view 1 year after reduction.

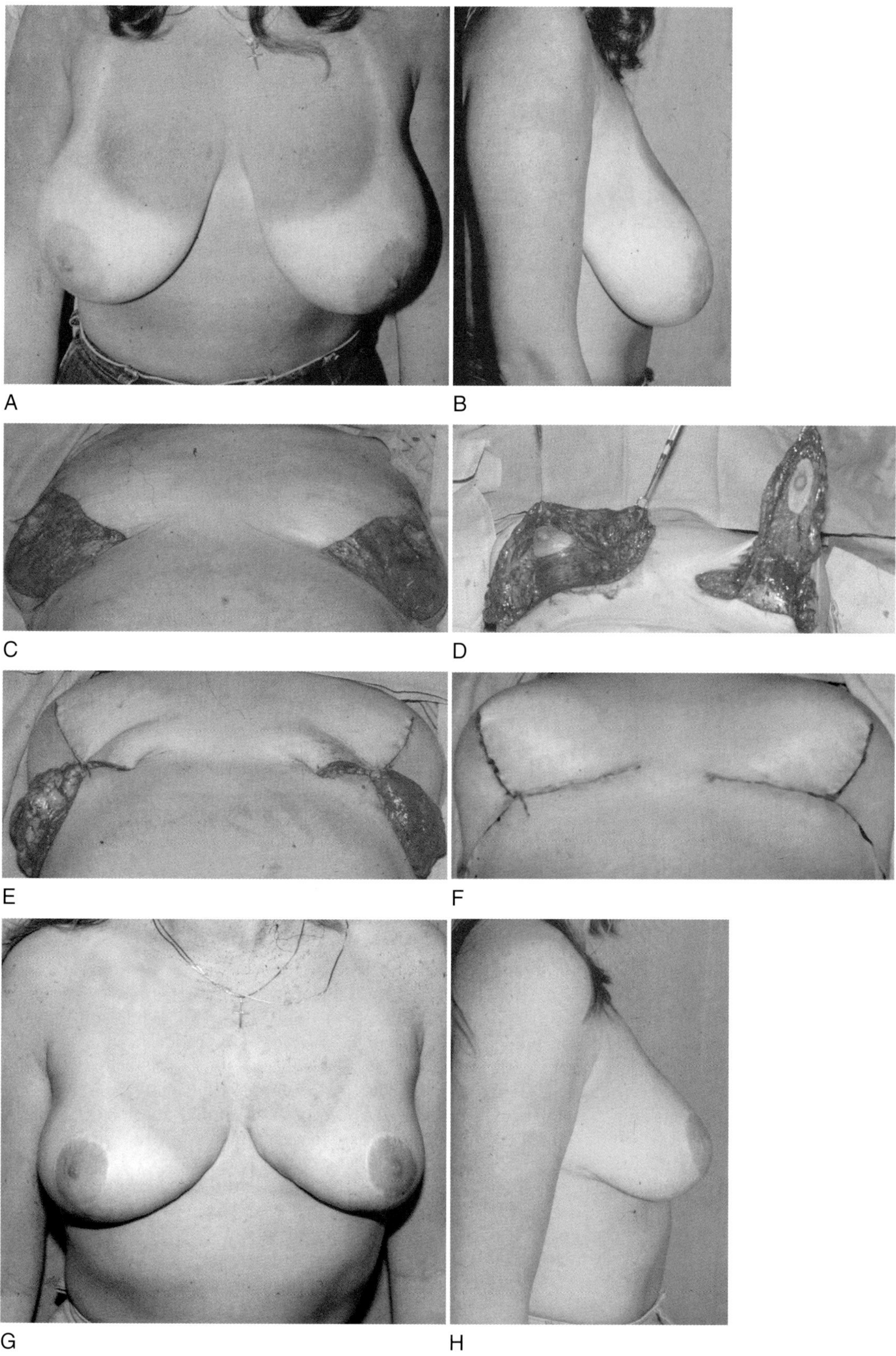
A
B
C
D
E
F
G
H

the inferior-based dermal breast flap and no hematoma or hypotension, it is advisable to remove the nipple-areola from the inferior pedicle and place the nipple-areola as a free nipple-areola graft (see following section, "Inferior Pedicle with Nipple-Areola Grafts").

MODIFICATIONS IN OPERATIVE TECHNIQUE

Inferior Pedicle with Nipple-Areola Grafts

One method of preserving nipple viability and decreasing the chance of abnormal pigmentation has been free nipple grafting after amputation of the nipple-areola complex. This technique was originally introduced by Adams[19] in 1944. Indications for this procedure include patients with gigantomastia, high-risk surgical candidates (i.e., elderly and patients with chronic severe illness), and patients with previous operative scars or who require a resection of breast tissue in the region of the inferior pedicle.[20] The technique is performed by removal of the nipple-areola complex as a full-thickness unit, thinning of the graft with scissors, de-epithelialization of the recipient site of the new areola location, and suturing the graft in place.[21] Traditionally, free nipple grafting was thought to ensure a viable nipple at the expense of nipple sensation and erectile function[22]; however, the literature has not supported this conclusion. Nipple erectile function has been shown to return in 70% of patients after free nipple grafting.[23] Sensation with free nipple grafting has been comparable to sensation changes after pedicle techniques such as the McKissock reduction.[24] One study comparing nipple sensation after free nipple grafting versus the inferior pedicle technique showed improved sensation in the majority of patients in both groups, although pressure thresholds were much lower in the inferior pedicle group.[25] Free nipple grafting should be considered in patients with gigantomastia and when intraoperative compromise of nipple vascularity is evident.

The inferior pedicle technique for breast reduction may not provide adequate perfusion for the very large breast because of excess pedicle length (>25 cm). However, the inferior pedicle is still useful to provide autoaugmentation to achieve optimal breast size and projection with safety in survival of preserved breast tissue. This technique is described as inferior pedicle with nipple-areola grafts. Intraoperative appearance may require urgent evaluation of the circulation of the inferior pedicle and the nipple-areola. If circulation appears inadequate, free nipple-areola grafts are indicated.

If the breasts are very large (>2500 g), the nipple-areola may require removal and replacement as a graft. The decision to use the nipple-areola as a free graft may be made in the preoperative planning session, or this decision may be delayed until the inferior pedicle is elevated. If the nipple-areola circulation appears inadequate after the inferior pedicle is elevated, or if the length of the pedicle necessary to include the nipple-areola results in excessive breast tissue to provide the extent of reduction planned, the surgeon has the option of removing the nipple-areola from the inferior pedicle and replacing the nipple-areola as a full-thickness graft. If the decision is delayed until after the inferior pedicle is elevated, resection of the dermis in the area of the keyhole or the area planned for the site of the nipple-areola is delayed until assessment of nipple-areola circulation. In all these situations, the inferior pedicle is still useful for autoaugmentation of the breast mound after resection of the superior, medial, and lateral excess breast parenchyma and reduction of the breast tissue included with the inferior pedicle until appropriate reduction of the breast mound is achieved. The retained portion of the pedicle usually measures approximately 15 to 20 cm in length from the flap base at the inframammary line (Fig. 137-14; see also Fig. 137-12*H* and *I*).

If free nipple-areola grafts are planned, the patient is placed in the sitting position after the inferior pedicle is inset and the vertical and horizontal inframammary incisions are closed. After the appropriate location is determined, the nipple-areola grafts, which have all subcutaneous tissue removed, are sutured in place with half vertical mattress sutures. These sutures are left long and tied over a cotton bolster dressing.

Reduction Mammaplasty After Lumpectomy and Radiation Therapy

With the increasing frequency of lumpectomy and radiation therapy, there are patients who have macromastia with ptosis who request bilateral reduction. Although ptosis is less on the lumpectomy-irradiated side because of the late effect of the radiation therapy, the patients may request bilateral reduction. Unless the lumpectomy was located inferior to the nipple-areola, it is possible to perform an inferior pedicle with safety if the base of the inferior pedicle is extended to 10 cm and the undermining superiorly is minimized. The contralateral breast reduction is modified slightly to maintain symmetry. The patient is informed of increased risk for complications, including loss of nipple-areola, skin envelope necrosis particularly at the junction of the inverted T incision, and fat necrosis. If wound healing complications are severe, the patient may require use of a

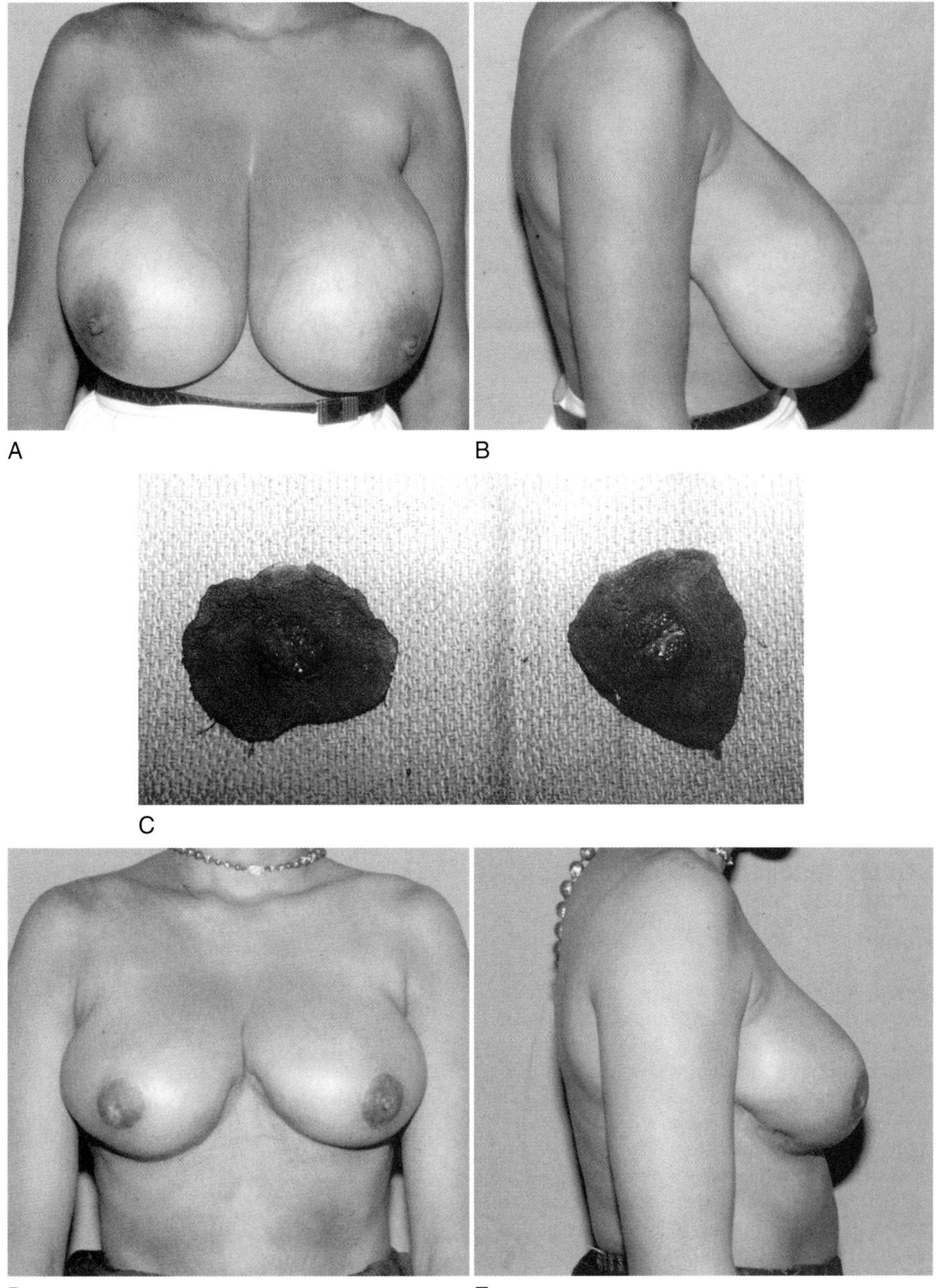

FIGURE 137-14. Large reduction with inferior pedicle technique and nipple-areola grafts. *A,* Preoperative anterior view demonstrating gigantomastia. *B,* Preoperative lateral view. *C,* Pedicle used to autograft breast after reduction. Note nipple-areola grafts. *D,* Postoperative anterior view 1 year after reduction. *E,* Postoperative lateral view 1 year after reduction. Note adequate projection and size provided by inferior pedicle.

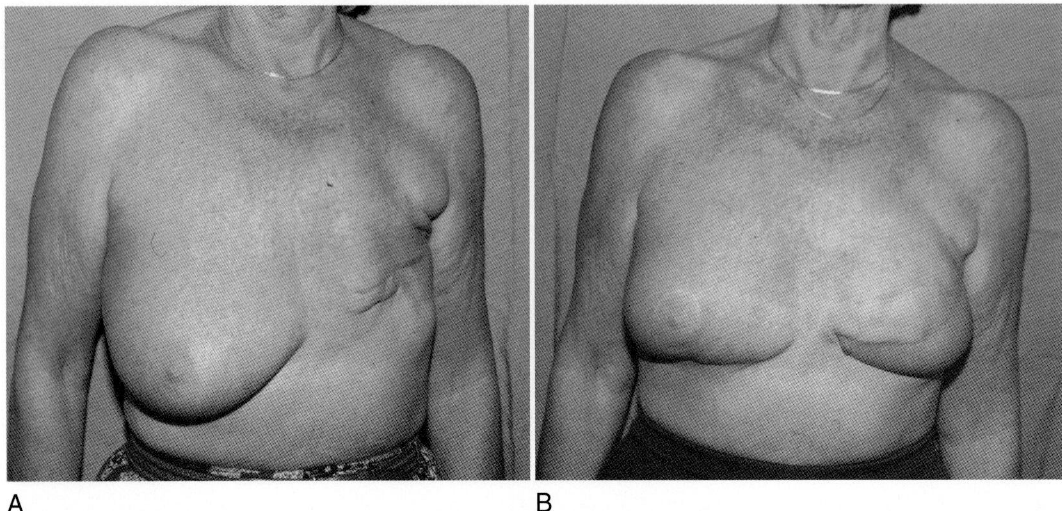

A B

FIGURE 137-15. Inferior pedicle technique in postlumpectomy patient who underwent breast radiation therapy and a left modified radical mastectomy. *A,* Preoperative view. *B,* Postoperative view 9 years after right inferior pedicle reduction and left latissimus dorsi-implant breast reconstruction.

distant flap (e.g., latissimus dorsi musculocutaneous flap). Fortunately, wound healing problems and loss of nipple-areola and skin envelope in selected patients presenting for bilateral reduction are rare (Fig. 137-15).

Secondary Reduction Mammaplasty

In the patient who develops recurrent macromastia and ptosis after reduction mammaplasty, inferior pedicle reduction mammaplasty may be repeated. The inferior pedicle can be redesigned and can include the nipple-areola. The surgeon must be certain that the preceding reduction procedure was accomplished by use of an inferior pedicle. It is not likely that the nipple-areola will have adequate perfusion if it was previously based on a superior or medial pedicle. Furthermore, the breast parenchymal resection may have included the inferior central breast between the fourth and sixth intercostal space, eliminating the normal vascular connections that allow safe elevation of the inferior pedicle.

Malposition of the Nipple-Areola After Inferior Pedicle Reduction

The nipple-areola should never be placed too high on the breast mound after inferior pedicle technique for reduction. In general, the inferior areola-cutaneous junction should be located in the range of 4 to 5 cm superior to the inframammary line. With time, the fullness in the inferior quadrant of the reduced breast will increase (Figs. 137-16 to 137-18),[26] although this process does not impair the quality of the result because it is a normal process in the aging breast and occurs slowly in the reduced breast. However, if the nipple-areola starts in an abnormally superior position, the maturation of the reduced breast will accentuate the deformity. Many patients are extremely displeased with the result because the nipple-areola may be slightly visible over the superior edge of the bra or bathing garment.

COMPLICATIONS

Early complications related to the inferior pedicle technique include hematoma, excessive bleeding, nipple or pedicle necrosis, skin flap necrosis, and wound dehiscence. A retrospective review by Mandrekas et al[27] of 371 patients who had breast reductions by the inferior pedicle technique showed an overall complication rate of 11.4%, with an equal number of early and late complications. Wound dehiscence was the most common early complication (4.6%), which occurred at the inferior T junction (Tables 137-2 and 137-3).

Other retrospective studies using patient surveys, various techniques, and a wide range of breast tissue

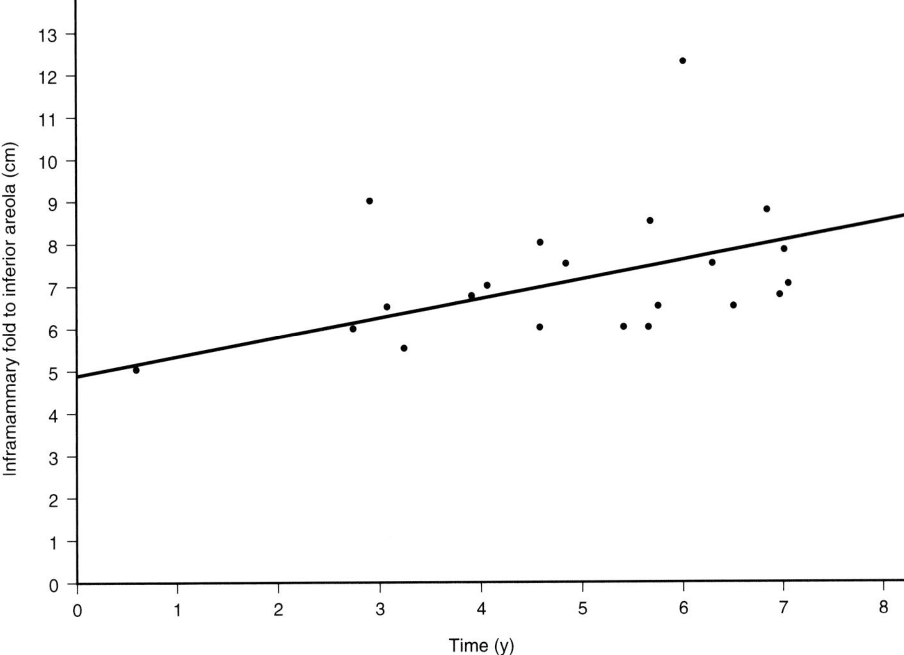

FIGURE 137-16. Graph of the distance from the inframammary fold to inferior border of the areola (cm) versus duration (years) from operation to follow-up. (From Reus WF, Mathes SJ: Preservation of projection after reduction mammaplasty: long-term follow-up of the inferior pedicle technique. Plast Reconstr Surg 1988;82:644.)

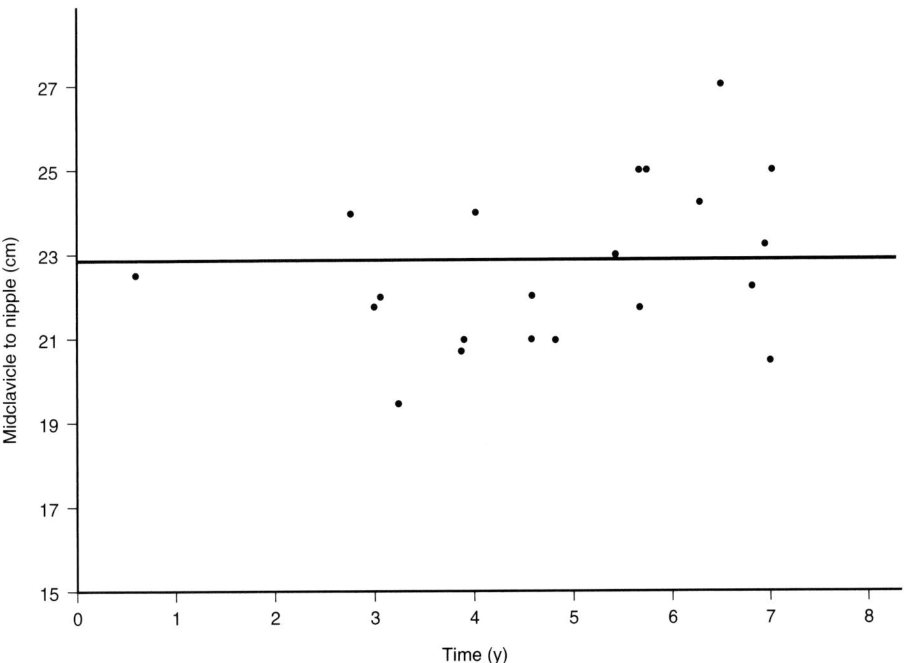

FIGURE 137-17. Graph of the distance from midclavicle to nipple (cm) versus duration (years) from operation to follow-up. (From Reus WF, Mathes SJ: Preservation of projection after reduction mammaplasty: long-term follow-up of the inferior pedicle technique. Plast Reconstr Surg 1988;82:644.)

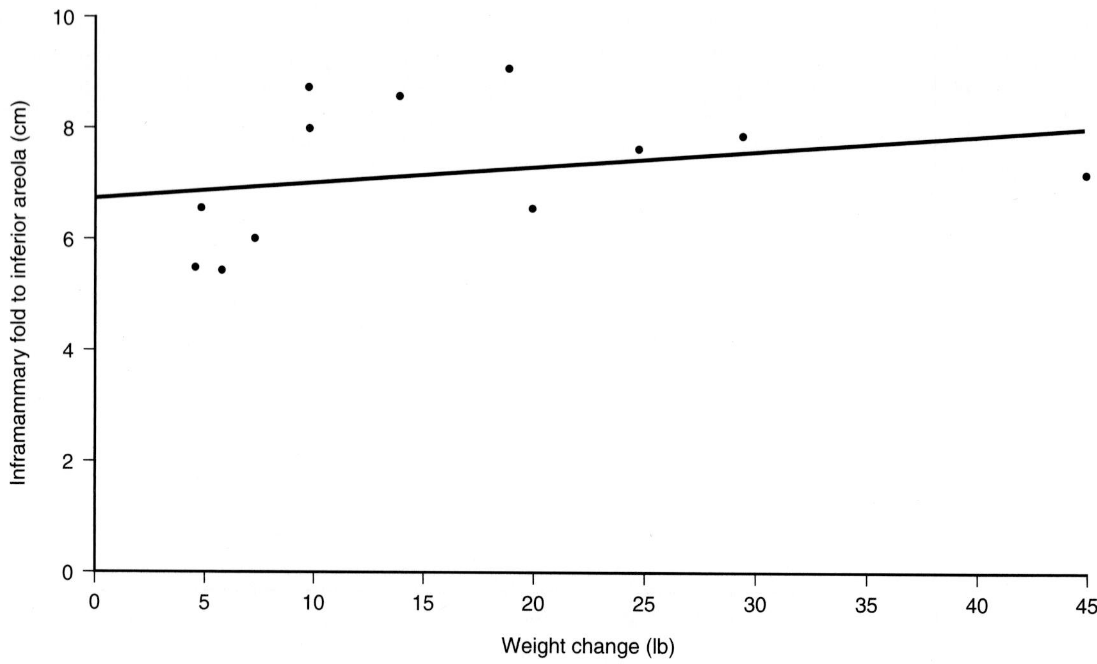

FIGURE 137-18. Graph of the distance from inframammary fold to inferior border of the areola (cm) versus change in body weight (pounds) from time of operation to follow-up. (From Reus WF, Mathes SJ: Preservation of projection after reduction mammaplasty: long-term follow-up of the inferior pedicle technique. Plast Reconstr Surg 1988;82:644.)

TABLE 137-2 ✦ COMPLICATIONS FROM INFERIOR PEDICLE BREAST REDUCTION

Study	Author	Wound Dehiscence (%)	Areolar Necrosis (%)	Infection (%)	Seroma (%)	Hematoma (%)
1	Cruz-Korchin[29]	4	1	1	1	1
2	Mandrekas[27]	4.6	0.8	0	0	0.3
3	Erdogan[34]	2	2	0	0	2
4	Davis[30]	19	6	12	NA	NA

TABLE 137-3 ✦ COMPARISON OF OUTCOMES OF INFERIOR PEDICLE TECHNIQUE BREAST REDUCTION

Study	Author	No. of Patients	Size of Reduction*	Revision Rate (%)	Complication Rate (%)	Satisfaction Rate (%)
1	Cruz-Korchin[29]	105	Mild (553 g)	0	8	8/10 (10-point scale)
2	Mandrekas[27]	371	Mild (870 g)	3	11.4	NA
3	Erdogan[34]	52	Moderate (1100 g)	NA	13	NA
4	Davis[30]	345	Moderate (676 g)	10	50	NA

*Mild, <600 g per breast; moderate, 600-1200 g per breast; massive, >1200 g; gigantomastia, >2500 g.

resected had much higher complication rates. A study by Dabbah et al[28] showed an overall complication rate of 50% with a mean of 855 g of breast tissue removed and fat necrosis or infection as the most common complication at 22%. Other complications included hematoma (2%), wound dehiscence (10%), loss of nipple-areola tissue (4%), and seroma (1%). Complications occurred much more frequently when more than 1000 g of breast tissue was resected. A randomized prospective study by Cruz-Korchin and Korchin[29] comparing the inferior pedicle technique and the vertical pedicle technique showed no difference between the two techniques with an overall complication rate of 8%, with wound dehiscence being most common (4%) and 1% rates for infections, seromas, alveolar necrosis, and hematomas.

Long-term complications from the inferior pedicle technique include fat necrosis, loss of nipple sensation, hypertrophic scarring, and breast asymmetry requiring secondary surgery.[27] Unacceptable scarring, particularly of the inverted T, has ranged from 4%[28] to 18%,[30] whereas fat necrosis has been documented less frequently. Occult carcinoma was present in 0.16% of specimens in a survey of 2576 patients.[31] A study of breast reduction specimens in 182 patients revealed proliferative changes in 10%, including proliferation without atypia (5%), proliferation with atypia (3%), sclerosing adenosis (2%), papillomatosis (0.5%), and lobular carcinoma in situ (0.5%).[32] The loss of lactation ability has also been a known side effect of reduction mammaplasty, with 30% of patients being unable to produce adequate milk for breast-feeding.[27]

Loss of sensation of the nipple-areola complex, which has been attributed to injury of the fourth to sixth intercostal nerves, has been a concern with reduction mammaplasty. The degree of sensation loss has been more difficult to quantify in patients with macromastia and patients who have undergone reduction mammaplasty. Breast sensation was found to be diminished in patients with gigantomastia when thresholds for vibration and pressure were assessed by a vibrometer and Semmes-Weinstein monofilaments, and there was a range of changes with reduction mammaplasty, even including some patients with improved sensation after free nipple grafting.[24] Another study using a pressure-specified sensory device to compare light touch in 41 patients who underwent reduction by the medial pedicle technique and 31 patients who underwent reduction by the inferior pedicle technique showed preservation of sensation in 86% in the medial pedicle group and 92% in the inferior pedicle group, although the average resection weight was 1490 g in the medial pedicle group and 720 g in the inferior pedicle group.[33] Several studies have suggested that reduced sensation of the nipple-areola complex is more likely to occur after larger volume reductions (>1000 g).[14]

Loss of viability of the nipple-areola complex after reduction mammaplasty with partial or total necrosis has an incidence of 0.8% to 2%; it has been attributed to large resections[33] (>1500 g) and pedicle lengths traditionally longer than 15 cm,[8] although reductions have been performed safely with pedicles as long as 38 cm.[34] Laser Doppler flowmetry measurements of preoperative and postoperative nipple-areola blood flow showed a decrease to 79% of preoperative values with an average resection of 283 g of tissue per breast.[35] Other risk factors for nipple-areola necrosis also include age older than 30 years and obesity.[33]

LONG-TERM RESULTS

One of the criticisms of the inferior pedicle technique is the progressive "bottoming out" of the breast over time with inferior migration of the breast parenchyma, an increasing inframammary fold to nipple distance at a rate of 0.44 cm per year, and the superior migration of the nipple-areola complex.[26] Proposed techniques to reduce this effect include lower placement of the nipple-areola complex[35,36] and shaping the breast by securing the pedicle to the chest wall with sutures to decrease tension on the skin envelope (Figs. 137-19 to 137-21).[37,38]

Outcome studies of the satisfaction of patients and relief of symptoms including back and neck pain have been supportive of reduction mammaplasty. A study by Schnur et al[39] showed a patient satisfaction rate of 88%, with 94% of 324 patients who thought that the operation was successful. Another study by Chao et al[16] demonstrated a patient satisfaction rate of 96% with relief of chronic neck and back pain, less intertrigo, and improved posture.

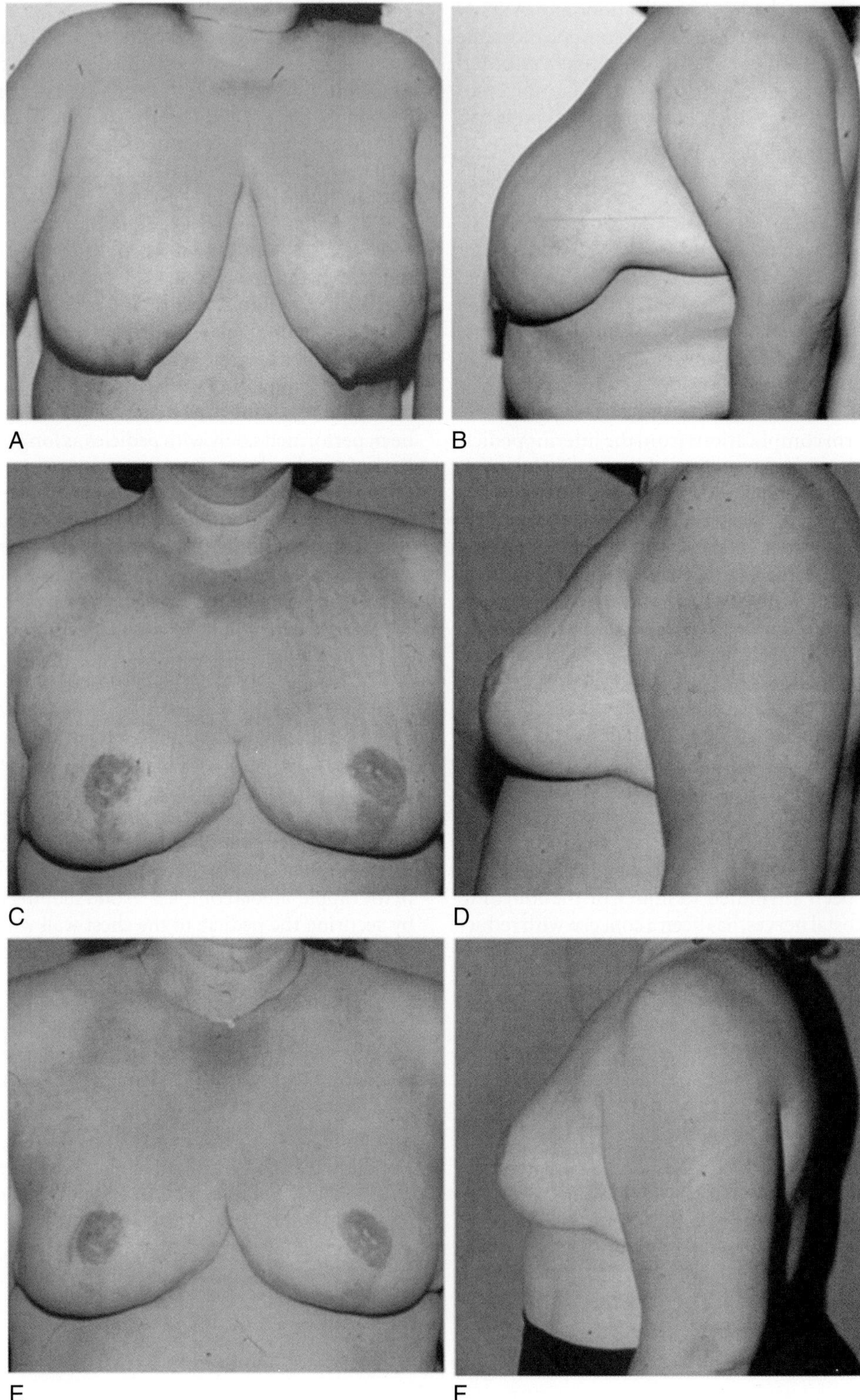

FIGURE 137-19. Long-term follow-up of large reduction with inferior pedicle technique. *A,* Preoperative anterior view. *B,* Preoperative lateral view. *C,* Postoperative anterior view 2 years after reduction. *D,* Postoperative lateral view 2 years after reduction. *E,* Postoperative anterior view 7 years after reduction. *F,* Postoperative lateral view 7 years after reduction.

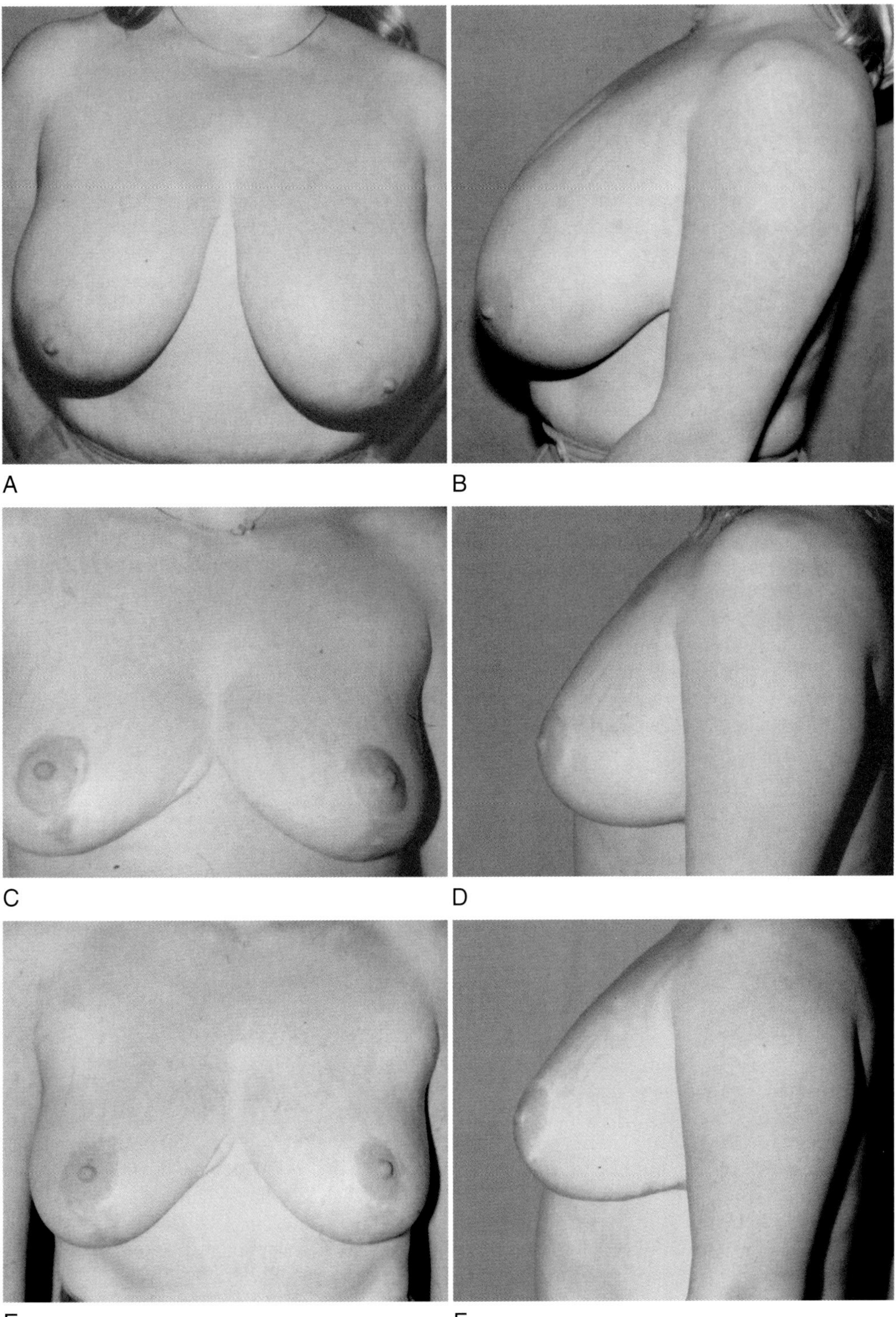

FIGURE 137-20. Long-term follow-up of large reduction with inferior pedicle technique. *A,* Preoperative anterior view. *B,* Preoperative lateral view. *C,* Postoperative anterior view 2 years after reduction. *D,* Postoperative lateral view 2 years after reduction. *E,* Postoperative anterior view 4 years after reduction. *F,* Postoperative lateral view 4 years after reduction.

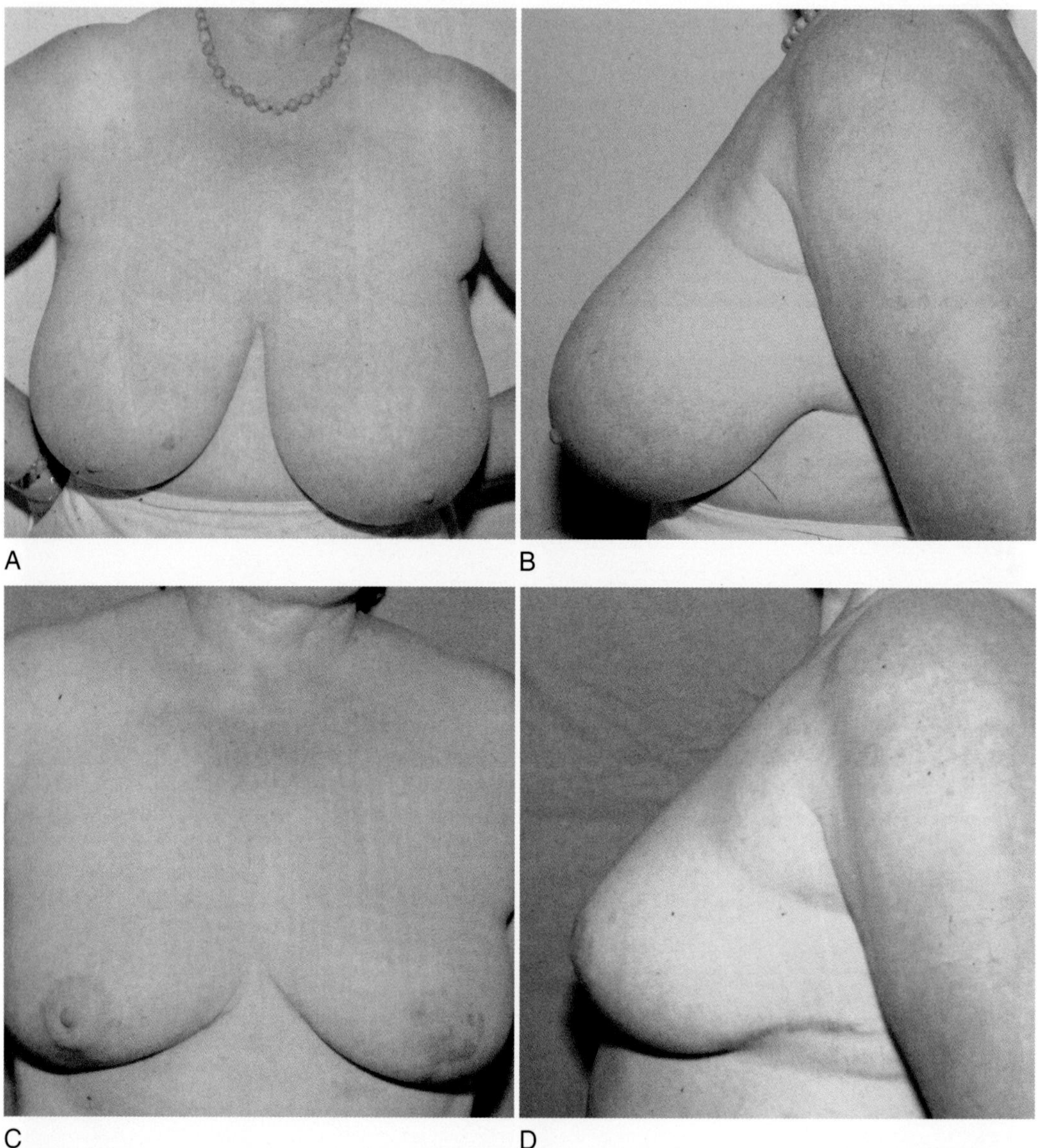

FIGURE 137-21. Long-term follow-up of gigantomastia reduction by inferior pedicle technique with free nipple-areola grafts. *A,* Preoperative anterior view. *B,* Preoperative lateral view. *C,* Postoperative anterior view 1 year after reduction. *D,* Postoperative lateral view 1 year after reduction.

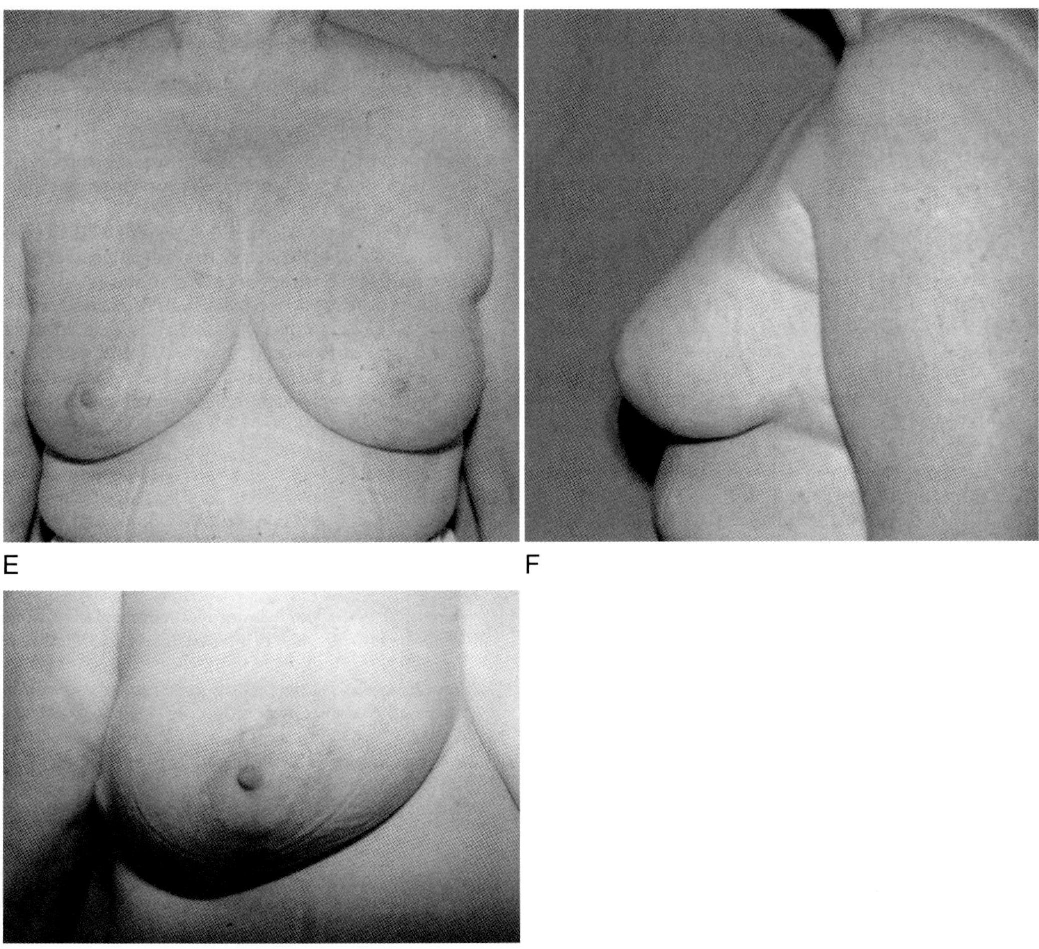

FIGURE 137-21, cont'd. *E,* Postoperative anterior view 8 years after reduction. *F,* Postoperative lateral view 8 years after reduction. *G,* Nipple demonstrates retained projection after nipple-areola grafts.

REFERENCES

1. Ribeiro LA, Accorsi A, Buss A, Marcal-Pessoa M: Creation and evolution of 30 years of the inferior pedicle in reduction mammaplasties. Plast Reconstr Surg 2002;110:960.
2. Aufricht G: Mammaplasty for pendulous breasts. Plast Reconstr Surg 1949;4:13.
3. Skoog T: A technique of breast reduction: transposition of the nipple on a cutaneous vascular pedicle. Acta Chir Scand 1963;126:453.
4. Weiner DL, Aiache AE, Silver L, Tittiranonda T: A single dermal pedicle for transposition of the nipple on a cutaneous vascular pedicle. Acta Chir Scand 1963;126:453.
5. Strombeck JO: Mammaplasty—report of a new technique based on the two pedicle procedure. Br J Plast Surg 1960; 13:79.
6. McKissock PK: Reduction mammaplasty by the vertical bipedicle flap technique. Rationale and results. Clin Plast Surg 1976;3:309.
7. Wise RJ: A preliminary report on a method of planning the mammaplasty. Plast Reconstr Surg 1956;17:367.
8. McKissock PK: Reduction mammaplasty with a vertical dermal flap. Plast Reconstr Surg 1972;49:245.
9. Ribeiro LA: A new technique for reduction mammaplasty. Plast Reconstr Surg 1975;55:330.
10. Courtiss EH, Goldwyn RM: Reduction mammaplasty by the inferior pedicle technique: an alternative to free nipple and areola grafting for severe macromastia or extreme ptosis. Plast Reconstr Surg 1977;59:500.
11. Reich J: The advantages of a lower central breast segment in reduction mammaplasty. Br J Plast Surg 1983;36:196.
12. Robbins TH: A reduction mammaplasty with the areola-nipple based on an inferior dermal pedicle. Plast Reconstr Surg 1977;59:64.
13. Georgiade NG, Serafin D, Morris R, Georgiade GS: Reduction mammaplasty utilizing an inferior pedicle nipple-areola flap. Ann Plast Surg 1979;3:211.
14. Gonzalez F, Brown FE, Gold ME, et al: Preoperative and postoperative nipple-areola sensibility in patients undergoing reduction mammaplasty. Plast Reconstr Surg 1993;92:809.
15. Leichow SJ, Merikas EP, Cook G, et al: An evaluation of NicCheck I: a dipstick method for analyzing nicotine and its metabolites. Addict Behav 1999;24:145.

16. Chao JD, Memmel HC, Redding JF, et al: Reduction mammaplasty is a functional operation, improving quality of life in symptomatic women: a prospective, single-center breast reduction outcome study. Plast Reconstr Surg 2002;110:1644.
17. Edwards EA: Surgical anatomy of the breast. In Goldwyn RM, ed: Plastic and Reconstructive Surgery of the Breast. Boston, Little, Brown, 1976:37.
18. Brzozowski D, Niessen M, Evans HB, Hurst LN: Breast-feeding after inferior pedicle reduction mammaplasty. Plast Reconstr Surg 2000;105:530.
19. Adams WM: Free transplantation of the nipples and areolae. Surgery 1944;5:186.
20. O'Neal RM, Goldstein JA, Rohrich R, et al: Reduction mammoplasty with free-nipple transplantation: indications and technical refinements. Ann Plast Surg 1991;26:117.
21. Gradinger GP: Reduction mammoplasty utilizing nipple-areola transplantation. Clin Plast Surg 1988;19:1641.
22. Hoopes JE, Jabaley ME: Reduction mammaplasty: amputation and augmentation. Plast Reconstr Surg 1969;44:441.
23. Townsend PLG: Nipple sensation following breast reduction and free nipple transplantation. Br J Plast Surg 1974;27:308.
24. Slezak S, Dellon AL: Quantitation of sensibility in gigantomastia and alteration following reduction mammaplasty. Plast Reconstr Surg 1993;91:1265.
25. Ahmed OA, Kolhe PS: Comparison of nipple and areolar sensation after breast reduction by free nipple graft and inferior pedicle techniques. Br J Plast Surg 2000;53:126.
26. Reus WF, Mathes SJ: Preservation of projection after reduction mammaplasty: long-term follow-up of the inferior pedicle technique. Plast Reconstr Surg 1988;82:644.
27. Mandrekas AD, Zambacos GJ, Anastasopoulos A, Hapsas DA: Reduction mammaplasty with the inferior pedicle technique: early and late complications in 371 patients. Br J Plast Surg 1996;49:442.
28. Dabbah A, Lehman JA Jr, Parker MG, et al: Reduction mammaplasty: an outcome analysis. Ann Plast Surg 1995; 35:337.
29. Cruz-Korchin N, Korchin L: Vertical versus Wise pattern breast reduction: patient satisfaction, revision rates, and complications. Plast Reconstr Surg 2003;112:1573.
30. Davis GM., Ringler SL, Short K, et al: Reduction mammaplasty: long-term efficacy, morbidity, and patient satisfaction. Plast Reconstr Surg 1995;96:1106.
31. Jansen DA, Murphy M, Kind GM, Sands K: Breast cancer in reduction mammoplasty: case reports and a survey of plastic surgeons. Plast Reconstr Surg 1998;101:361.
32. Blansfield JA, Kukora JS, Goldhahn RT Jr, Buinewicz BR: Suspicious findings in reduction mammaplasty specimens: review of 182 consecutive patients. Ann Plast Surg. 2004;52:126.
33. Nahabedian MY, Mofid MM: Viability and sensation of the nipple-areolar complex after reduction mammaplasty. Ann Plast Surg 2002;49:24.
34. Erdogan B, Ayhan M, Deren O, Tuncel A: Importance of pedicle length in inferior pedicle technique and long-term outcome of areola-to-fold distance. Aesthetic Plast Surg 2002;26:436.
35. Tracy CA, Pool R, Gellis M, Vasileff W. Blood flow of the areola and breast skin flaps during reduction mammaplasty as measured by laser Doppler flowmetry. Ann Plast Surg 1992; 28:160.
36. Marchac D, de Olarte G: Reduction mammaplasty and correction of ptosis with a short inframammary scar. Plast Reconstr Surg 1982;69:45.
37. Crepeau R, Klein HW: Reduction mammaplasty with inferiorly based glandular pedicle flap. Ann Plast Surg 1982;9:463.
38. Mathes SJ, Nahai F, Hester TR: Avoiding the flat breast in reduction mammaplasty. Plast Reconstr Surg 1980;66:63.
39. Schnur PL, Schnur DP, Petty PM, et al: Reduction mammaplasty: an outcome study. Plast Reconstr Surg 1977;100:875.

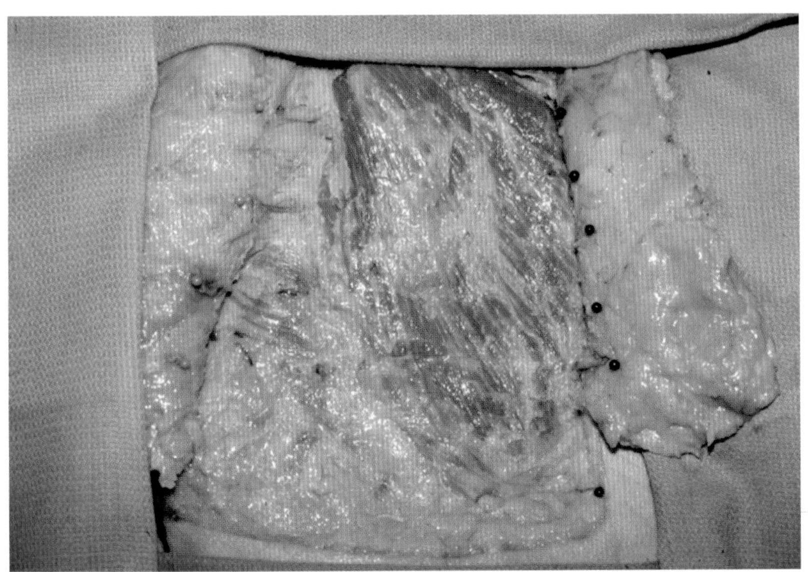

A

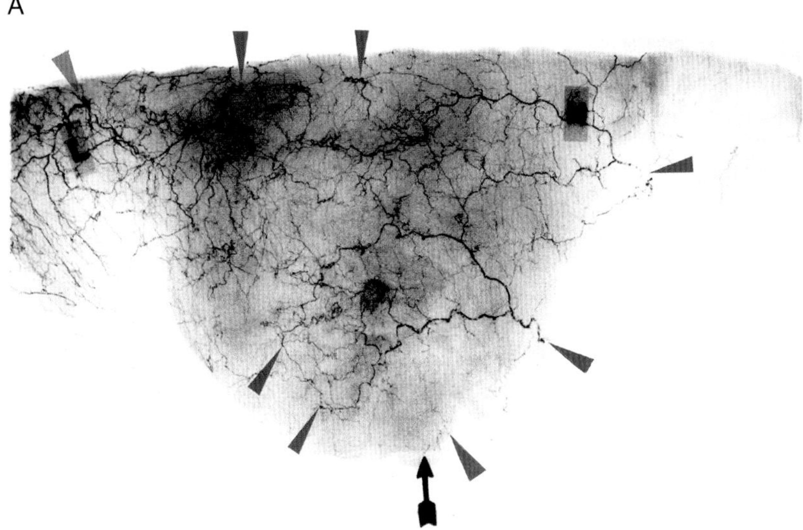

B

COLOR PLATE 137-1. Vascular anatomy of the breast. *A,* Anterior hemithorax. Purple beads on left designate branches of the lateral thoracic artery entering the lateral breast, and the black beads on the right designate site of segmental branches of the internal mammary artery into the medial breast. *B,* Selective barium latex injection into internal mammary (*blue arrows*), lateral thoracic (*green arrow*), and thoracoacromial (*red arrows*) arteries demonstrates contribution to breast circulation.

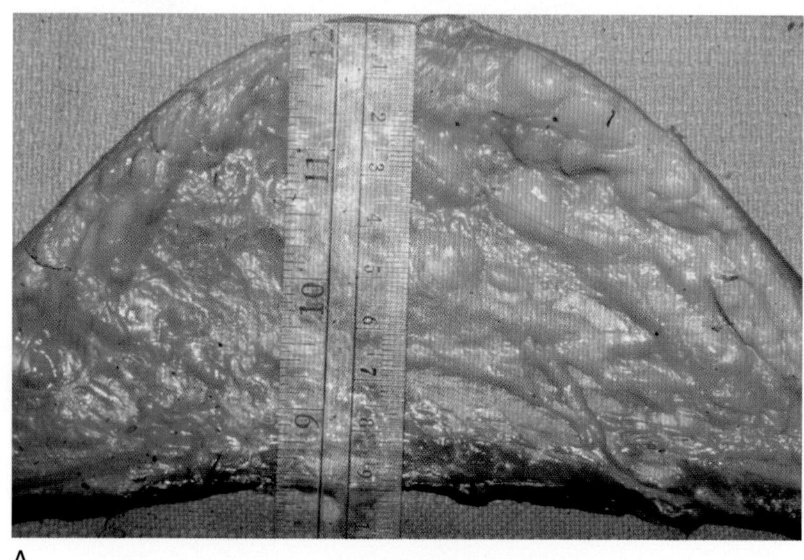

A

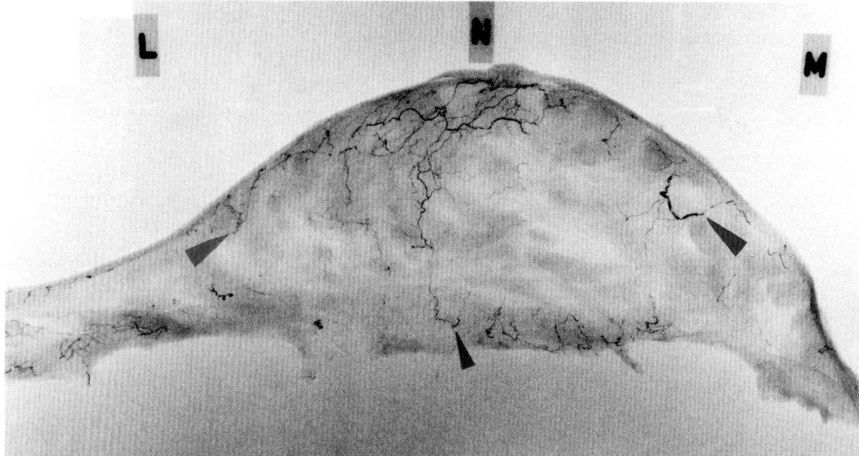

B

COLOR PLATE 137-2. Vascular anatomy of nipple-areola. *A,* Selective barium latex injection seen in horizontal cross section of breast at nipple-areola level. Note the pectoralis major muscle at base of breast. *B,* Radiographic specimen demonstrates vascular connection between internal mammary (*blue arrow*) artery, musculocutaneous perforators from thoracoacromial (*red arrow*) artery, and lateral thoracic (*green arrow*) artery. Note the interconnections of the three vascular systems at the nipple-areola. *Continued*

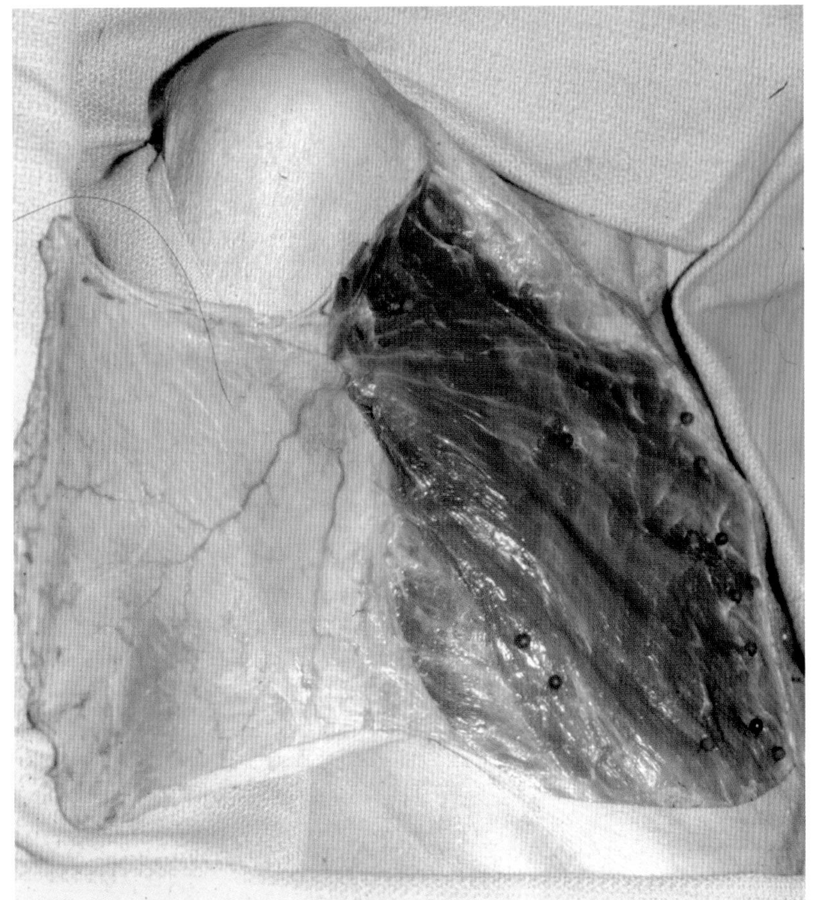

C

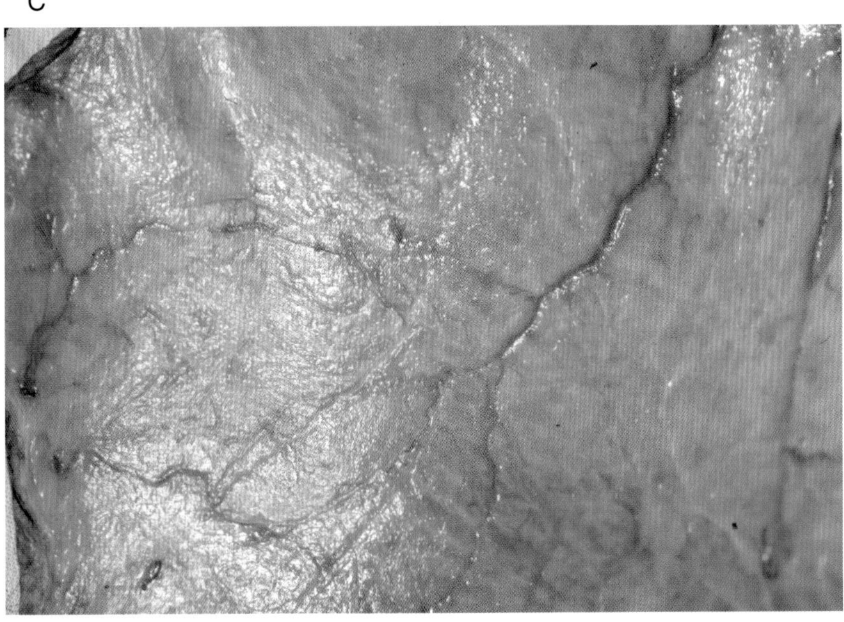

D

COLOR PLATE 137-2, cont'd. *C,* Latex vascular injection of breast and hemithorax. Chest skin is divided at sternal edge and reflected laterally to visualize deep surface of breast region. Note the segmental branches of the internal mammary artery and lateral branches of the lateral thoracic artery. *D,* Close-up of deep surface of breast at nipple-areola site. Note the arterial-arterial direct anastomosis between branches of internal mammary artery and lateral thoracic artery.

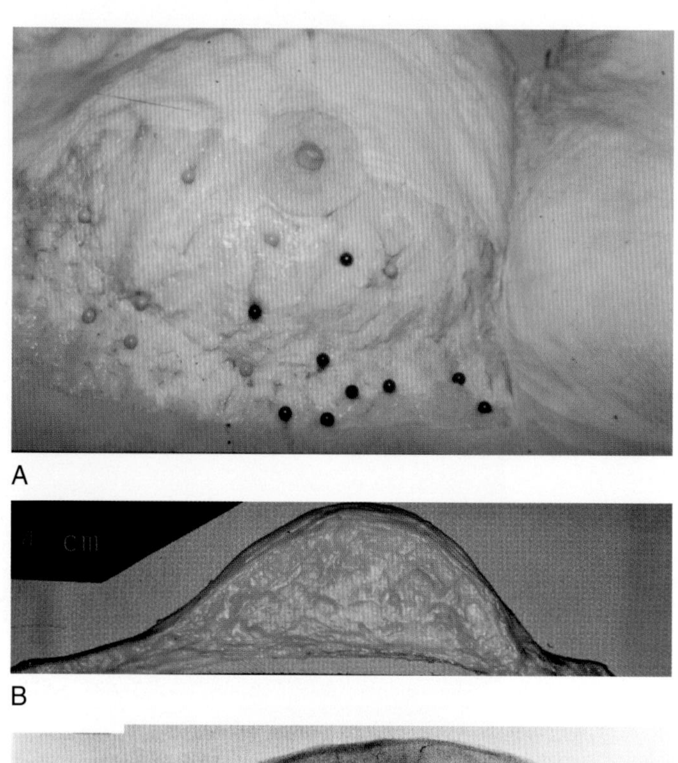

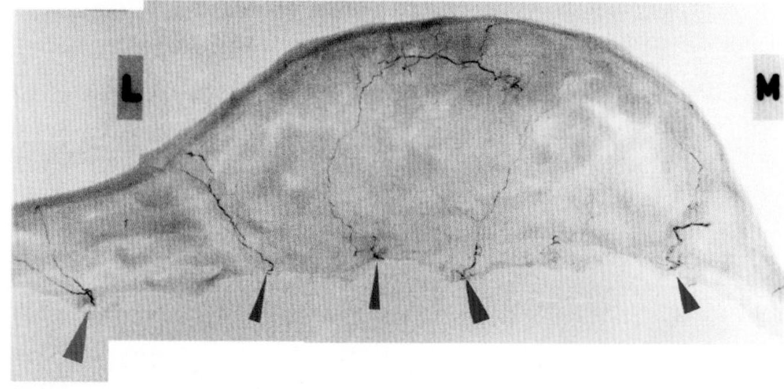

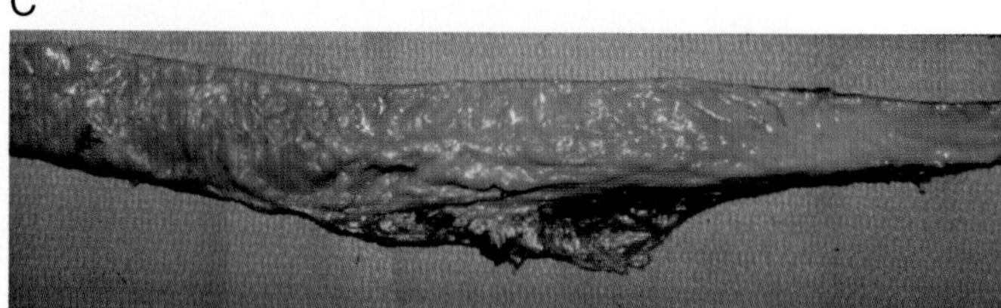

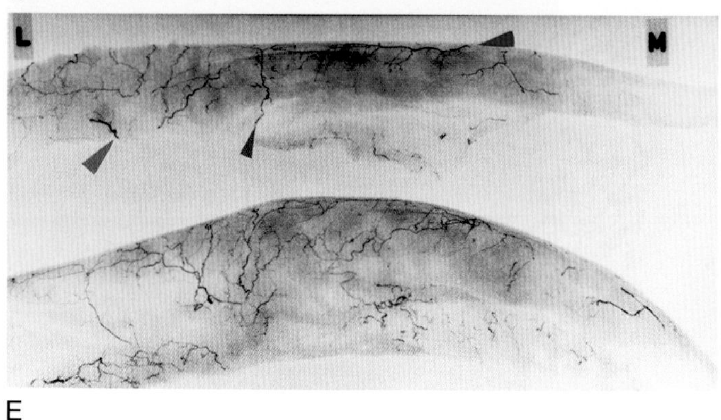

COLOR PLATE 137-3. Circulation of inferior pedicle. *A,* Selective ink-injected breast specimen: green, lateral thoracic artery; red, internal mammary artery. Black beads denote sites of vascular communication via internal mammary artery. Purple beads denote sites of vascular communication via lateral thoracic artery. *B,* Horizontal cross section 4 cm inferior to nipple-areola. *C,* Radiograph of a horizontal cross section 4 cm inferior to nipple-areola. Note vascular connection to breast parenchyma via thoracoacromial artery (*red arrows*) and internal mammary artery (*blue arrows*). The lateral thoracic (*green arrow*) vascular connections may be seen in the lateral breast beyond the dimensions of the inferior pedicle. *D,* Horizontal cross section of breast 6 cm inferior to nipple-areola. Note the pectoralis major muscle at base of specimen. *E,* Radiograph of a horizontal cross section of breast 6 cm inferior to nipple-areola.

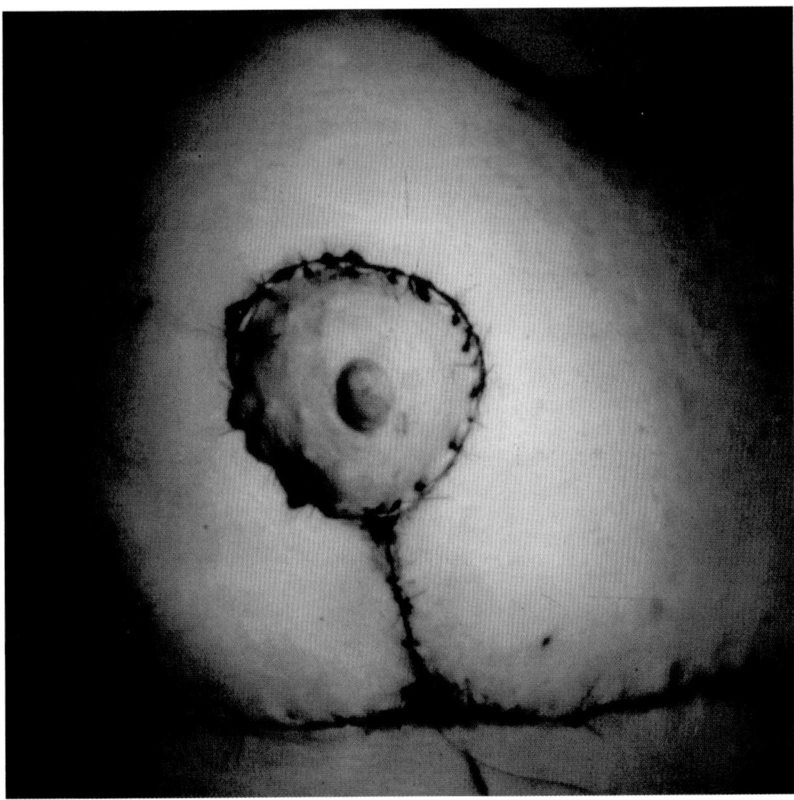

COLOR PLATE 137-4. Fluorescein evaluation of nipple-areola circulation: intravenous administration of 2 g of fluorescein after inset of nipple-areola based on inferior pedicle. Ultraviolet light (Wood's lamp) demonstrates yellow fluorescence indicating viable nipple-areola.

CHAPTER

138

Breast Cancer: Diagnosis, Therapy, and Postmastectomy Reconstruction

STEPHEN J. MATHES, MD ✦ JULIE LANG, MD

A large component of many general surgical and breast specialty practices is the diagnosis and treatment of breast cancer. On occasion, a patient will present to the plastic surgeon with breast complaints as well; thus, knowledge of the current diagnostic and therapeutic approaches is essential. The expertise of a plastic surgeon may be called on in planning of a screening or diagnostic program for a previously augmented patient. Because the breast is an important organ for a woman's body image, many patients opt for reconstruction after mastectomy for breast cancer. The diagnosis and treatment of breast cancer have become a multidisciplinary practice. With growing numbers of patients seeking plastic surgical consultation for recommendations for reconstructive options, plastic surgeons are an important part of the multidisciplinary care of the patient with breast cancer.

INCIDENCE

In the United States, breast cancer is the most common noncutaneous cancer among women. The lifetime incidence of breast cancer for American women is approximately 8%. In 2001, approximately 192,000 new patients were diagnosed with invasive breast cancer, and approximately 47,100 additional patients were diagnosed with in situ breast cancer. There were approximately 40,200 deaths attributable to breast cancer in the year 2001; only lung cancer is responsible for more cancer-related deaths. Male breast cancer represents 1% of all breast cancers, with approximately 1500 new diagnoses and 400 deaths in 2001.[1]

Independent risk factors for breast cancer (Table 138-1) include early age at menarche, late menopause, first full-term pregnancy after the age of 30 years, history of premenopausal breast cancer for a patient's mother and sister (i.e., two or more first-degree relatives with a diagnosis of breast cancer at an early age), and personal history of breast cancer or of benign proliferative disease.[2] The *BRCA1* and *BRCA2* mutations occur in less than 1% of women. These inherited mutations account for 5% to 10% of breast cancers; thus, the majority of occurrences are sporadic. Whereas the incidence of breast cancer has been rising during the last 2 decades, the mortality rates have remained stable since the 1950s. Much of the increased incidence is attributable to improved screening with physical examination and mammography, although screening alone does not appear to fully explain the increased incidence.[2]

TABLE 138-1 ✦ FACTORS THAT INCREASE THE RELATIVE RISK FOR BREAST CANCER IN WOMEN[293,294]

Relative Risk*	Factor
Relative risk > 4.0	Certain inherited genetic mutations for breast cancer Two or more first-degree relatives with breast cancer diagnosed at an early age Personal history of breast cancer Age 65+ vs. <65 years (although risk increases across all ages until the age of 80 years)
Relative risk 2.1-4.0	One first-degree relative with breast cancer Nodular densities on mammogram (>75% of breast volume) Atypical hyperplasia High-dose ionizing radiation to the chest Ovaries surgically removed <40 years
Relative risk 1.1-2.0	High socioeconomic status Urban residence Northern U.S. residence Early menarche (<12 years) Late menopause (≥55 years) Late age at first full-term pregnancy (≥30 years) Never breast-fed a child Postmenopausal obesity Recent oral contraceptive use Tall Personal history of cancer of the endometrium, ovary, or colon Jewish heritage

*Relative risk is defined as a measure of how much a particular risk factor influences the probability of a specified outcome, such as the diagnosis of breast cancer. A relative risk of 2 associated with a risk factor means that persons with that risk factor have a 2-fold increased risk of having a specified outcome compared with persons without that risk factor.

DIAGNOSIS

The benign and malignant conditions of the breast may be subdivided into two diagnostic categories: (1) conditions that present as symptomatic breast disease with clinical signs and symptoms and (2) asymptomatic disease detected by screening mammography.[3] Diagnostic strategies for symptomatic breast disease include clinical breast examination, breast imaging (mammography, ultrasonography, or magnetic resonance imaging), and tissue diagnosis (fine-needle aspiration biopsy, core needle biopsy, or surgical excisional biopsy). Asymptomatic disease by definition is not detectable by any physical signs or symptoms; rather, it is brought to the clinician's attention by an abnormal screening mammogram.

Diagnostic Modalities

CLINICAL BREAST EXAMINATION

Despite numerous advances in breast imaging, the clinical breast examination remains of utmost importance in the assessment of the breast and its associated lymph node basins. Like physical examination of all other regions of the body, the clinical breast examination consists of visual inspection followed by physical examination of four key elements: (1) breast parenchyma, (2) nipple-areola complex, (3) skin envelope, and (4) ipsilateral axillary and supraclavicular lymph node basins. The clinical breast examination is a routine part of annual breast screening by primary care physicians as well as an integral part of the breast surgeon's assessment of a patient. For early breast cancer detection, the American Cancer Society (*www.cancer.org*) recommends that between the ages of 20 and 39 years, women should have a clinical breast examination by a health professional every 3 years; after the age of 40 years, they should have a clinical breast examination every year. Beginning around 20 years of age, all women should be informed of the benefits of breast self-examination and instructed in proper technique; however, in 2004, for the first time, the American Cancer Society has made the breast self-examination an optional part of screening because it has not been shown to have an impact on mortality.

DIAGNOSTIC IMAGING MODALITIES

Mammography

Mammography is a widely used, highly effective screening modality. The typical views include a mediolateral oblique view and a craniocaudal view. Supplemental views may be required to better investigate specific diagnostic problems. For example, rotated or exaggerated craniocaudal views visualize either more lateral or more medial than standard views.[4] With

TABLE 138-2 ✦ BI-RADS CLASSIFICATION[295]

BI-RADS* Category	Interpretation
0	Assessment incomplete; needs additional imaging evaluation
1	Negative; routine mammogram in 1 year recommended
2	Benign finding; routine mammogram in 1 year recommended
3	Probably benign finding; short-interval follow-up suggested (6 months)
4	Suspicious abnormality; biopsy should be considered
5	Highly suggestive of malignancy; appropriate action should be taken

*Breast Imaging Reporting and Data System developed by the American College of Radiology.

questionable lesions, specific magnified views are obtained to better delineate the area of interest.

A study correlated the mammographic appearance and pathologic results of 543 nonpalpable breast tumors.[5] The majority of masses (95%), masses with calcifications (68%), and architectural distortions (79%) were due to invasive cancers. The majority of isolated calcifications without masses (68%) were due to ductal carcinoma in situ. In addition, microcalcifications may develop in the conservatively treated breast, posing additional diagnostic challenges.[6]

The BI-RADS (Breast Imaging Reporting and Data System) classification is the most commonly used reporting system for mammography. These standardized criteria (Table 138-2) provide a means of radiographically risk-stratifying lesions such that the significance of the mammogram is clear to all clinicians. In this classification, BI-RADS 4 (suggestive of malignant disease) or BI-RADS 5 (highly suggestive) should always prompt biopsy for tissue diagnosis of a mammographic abnormality (Fig. 138-1).

The more frequent use of mammography for screening purposes has resulted in increased recommendations for breast biopsies for clinically occult lesions. As a result of screening mammography, many breast cancers may now be detected at an earlier stage; it is estimated that implementation of regular mammography for women older than 50 years can reduce breast cancer mortality by 20% to 30% for this population.[7] The only screening modality available for the detection of nonpalpable breast cancer is mammography, but less than 50% of women older than 50 years undergo annual screening mammography.[8] Even if 100% of patients complied with screening mammography and if mammograms had 100% diagnostic accuracy, 13% of breast cancers would still be mammographically occult—detectable only when they became clinically palpable.[6] Screening mammography has been shown to have a sensitivity of 68% to 92%[9] and a specificity of 95%[10]; in one study, Yankaskas et al[9] found a 29% rate of false-negative findings that were detectable by other radiologists blinded to whether the patient had a diagnosis of cancer.

Nonpalpable lesions account for 17.5% to 58% of diagnosed breast cancers in published series. Palpable breast cancers have a significantly worse 8-year survival rate than do nonpalpable cancers (87% versus 95%). Skinner et al[11] have shown that palpable tumors have a less diffuse growth pattern, higher metastatic potential, higher proliferative activity, more nuclear abnormalities, and worse prognosis. Palpable cancers have a higher probability of being node positive than nonpalpable cancers do.[12] From Skinner's data, independent of primary tumor size, palpable cancers are twice as likely as nonpalpable cancers to spread to axillary lymph nodes. This tendency toward metastasis corresponds to a worse prognosis for these patients.

The National Cancer Institute recommends annual mammography beginning at the age of 40 years for women at normal risk for breast cancer. Although most physicians agree with this practice guideline, a small but vocal group of epidemiologists, physicians, and other advocates challenge this recommendation. An article called "Search and Destroy: Why mammograms are not the answer" in *The New Republic* criticized mammographic screening programs, claiming that early detection merely "picks up many times more cancers that would never have become symptomatic during the patient's lifetime or that could have been treated just as easily had they not been detected until the woman could feel the lump herself."[13] This article argues that mammography has done nothing to reduce the overall death rate from breast cancer while incurring high financial costs to society. As is true in most sensationalist journalism, this article is simply not well grounded in medical facts. As previously discussed, there is a definite survival advantage for patients with nonpalpable (small) breast cancers over those with palpable disease. The potential for breast-conserving surgery rather than mastectomy also diminishes with increasing mass size because of the likelihood of a final operative result with acceptable symmetry. Several studies have concluded that mammographic screening is an effective tool in reducing breast cancer mortality.[14-16] These studies demonstrated a 30% to 50% reduction in 5-year mortality for patients undergoing screening mammography.

Ultrasonography

Breast ultrasonography is widely used to differentiate solid from cystic breast masses. Other indications include evaluation of palpable masses in young women

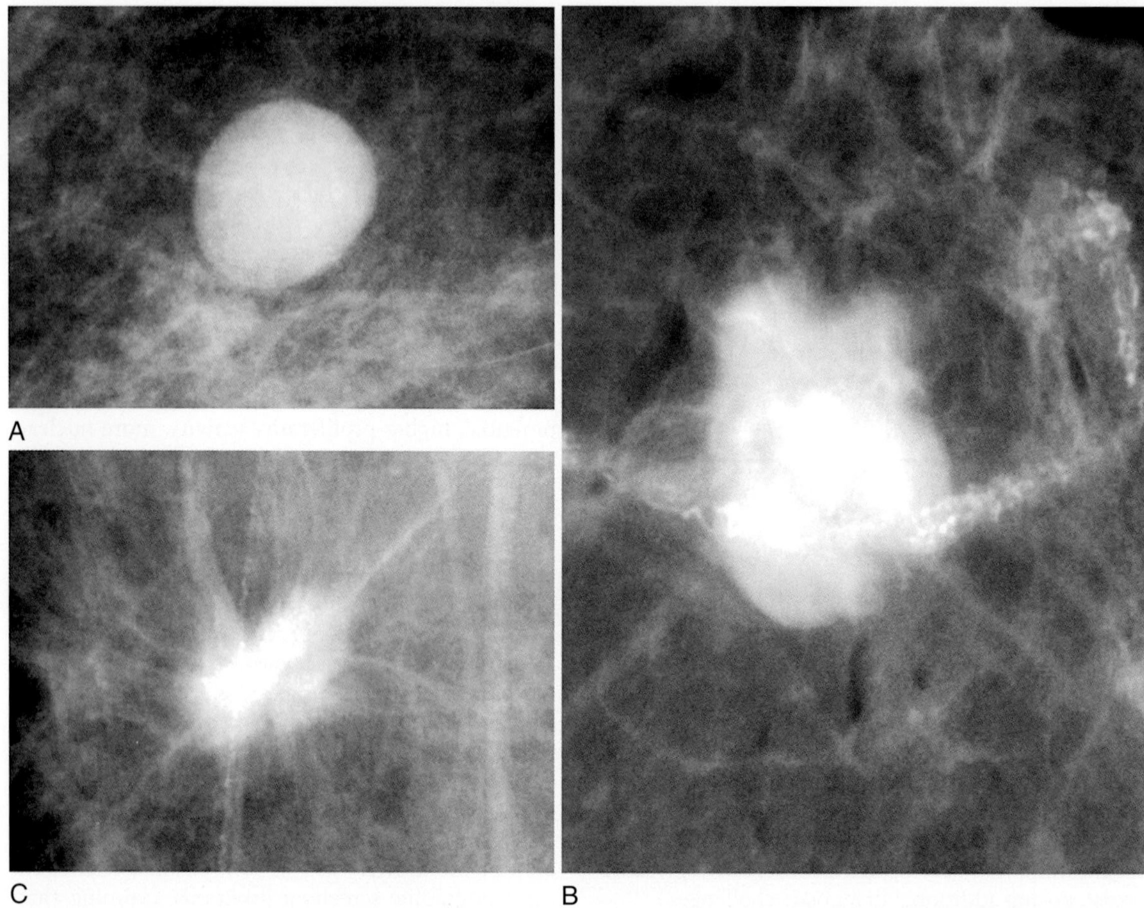

FIGURE 138-1. *A,* BI-RADS 3 mammogram, probably a benign lesion. *B,* BI-RADS 4 mammogram, suspicious abnormality. *C,* BI-RADS 5 mammogram, highly suggestive of malignant disease. (Images courtesy of Edward Sickles, MD, UCSF Department of Radiology.)

with radiographically dense breasts, evaluation of masses incompletely characterized by mammography, guidance for biopsy or evacuation of cysts, and evaluation in the patient who has undergone augmentation mammaplasty.[17] It is the imaging modality of choice for pregnant woman or during lactation because of the low potential for irradiation. Many breast surgeons use focused breast ultrasonography as an extension of the physical examination. A focused breast ultrasound examination looking specifically at a suspicious area of breast tissue for solid or cystic lesions may be performed in the office. Whereas whole-breast or focused breast ultrasound examinations are highly useful for these specific indications, unacceptably high false-negative and false-positive rates make whole-breast ultrasonography a poor general screening tool for breast cancer for large populations (Table 138-3).[18]

Several ultrasonographic criteria help differentiate malignant from benign lesions. The most specific signs are the presence of spiculations, a taller than wide shape, multiple projections from a nodule within ducts coursing away from the nipple, and the presence of calcifications.[19] Other malignant sonographic criteria include angular margins, a markedly hypoechoic lesion, posterior shadowing, and a heterogeneous internal structure.[20] Stavros et al[21] stated that a solid nodule may be classified as benign if two of the following patterns are noted without any malignant characteristics by ultrasonography: (1) homogeneous hyperechogenicity, (2) thin echogenic pseudocapsule

TABLE 138-3 ✦ INDICATIONS FOR FOCUSED BREAST ULTRASONOGRAPHY

Determination of solid vs. cystic breast mass
Evaluation of palpable masses in young women with radiodense breasts
Evaluation of masses incompletely characterized by mammography
Guidance for image-directed biopsy or evacuation of cysts
Evaluation of patients who have undergone augmentation mammaplasty

pattern, and (3) ellipsoid shape with fewer than four macrolobulations.

Magnetic Resonance Imaging

In recent years, contrast-enhanced magnetic resonance imaging (MRI) has been used for the evaluation of the breast for cancer. One study has compared the accuracy of MRI to mammography and ultrasonography in the detection of tumor size and multifocality in 61 women who underwent mastectomy for breast carcinoma.[22] The index tumor was missed by mammography 10% of the time, by ultrasonography 15% of the time, and by MRI 2% of the time. Tumor size was underestimated by mammography and ultrasonography 14% and 18% of the time, respectively. MRI showed no significant difference in size compared with that found on final pathologic diagnosis. In this study, mammography detected 31% of additional invasive lesions, ultrasonography found 38%, and MRI showed 100%.

MRI has been shown to be significantly more accurate than mammography in the characterization of infiltrating lobular carcinoma (Fig. 138-2).[23] MRI is also useful in the management of patients with axillary node metastases and unknown primary malignant neoplasm.[24] MRI is often a helpful addition to the work-up of the breast cancer patient with locally advanced disease to better define the extent of tumor invasion. For select patients, MRI has been found to be useful in the preoperative evaluation of breast cancer, and future practice will probably tend to use it increasingly. The main disadvantages are cost (which precludes widespread use as a screening modality) and limited availability compared with mammography or ultrasonography. Discomfort of the patient is also a consideration because the examination is difficult for claustrophobic patients and may require prone positioning. In addition, although some centers may have MRI available, many as yet do not have MRI-directed biopsy protocols. When a lesion is only identified on MRI, it is helpful to have the ability to perform MRI-directed biopsy. As standardized MRI-directed biopsy protocols develop, many of these lesions not well visualized by mammography or ultrasonography may be amenable to MRI-directed biopsy.

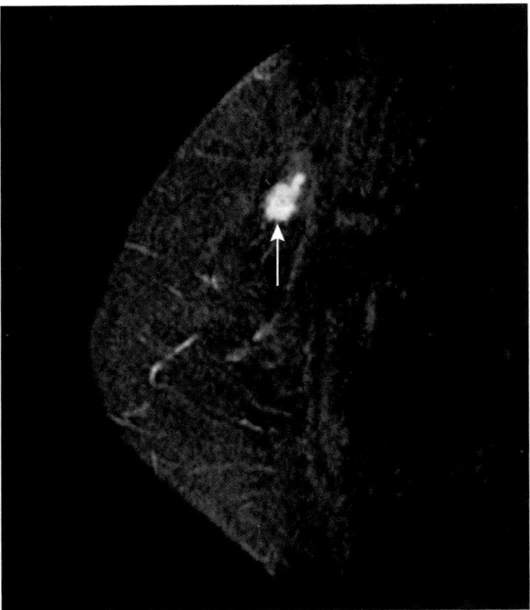

FIGURE 138-2. A mass *(arrow)* was identified by MRI examination that was not seen on ultrasound examination. MRI-guided localization of the region was performed, and pathologic examination yielded infiltrating lobular carcinoma. (From Morris EA: Breast cancer imaging with MRI. Radiol Clin North Am 2002;40:443.)

Although MRI is now widely used as a technique for the imaging of silicone breast implants, mammography is still the preferred initial imaging modality of choice.[25] High field strength MRI emphasizes signals from silicone, water, or fat; therefore, it is the technique of choice in imaging breasts to rule out implant rupture (Fig. 138-3).

Diagnostic Imaging in Patients with Breast Implants

As breast implants are widely used for both reconstructive and augmentative purposes, the efficacy of breast cancer screening with mammography is important for this population of patients. An implant is radiopaque on mammography and obscures some breast tissue, which in theory might reduce visualization of breast tumors. With submuscular placement of the implant, special mammographic techniques and additional surveillance views of the augmented breast tissue through mammography can be effective (Figs. 138-4 and 138-5).[26] Furthermore, specialized mammography techniques for the examination have been described to improve breast tissue visualization by displacement of the implant.[26] If the implant is not freely mobile, a straight lateral view is obtained to adequately visualize the tissue posterior to the implant. The estimated proportion of breast tissue that is obscured from mammographic examination ranges in the literature from 25% to 80%.[27]

Screening mammography is more difficult in a patient with implants. Women who have implants should have their mammograms performed at a certified mammography center and should inform the personnel of their implants. Several studies have examined the possible association of augmentation mammaplasty with delayed detection of breast cancer. The difficulty with single-center studies of this topic is that thus far, most studies reported in the literature have been small, retrospective cohort studies. Cahan et al[28] reported a retrospective analysis of patients diagnosed with a new primary breast cancer. Twenty-two

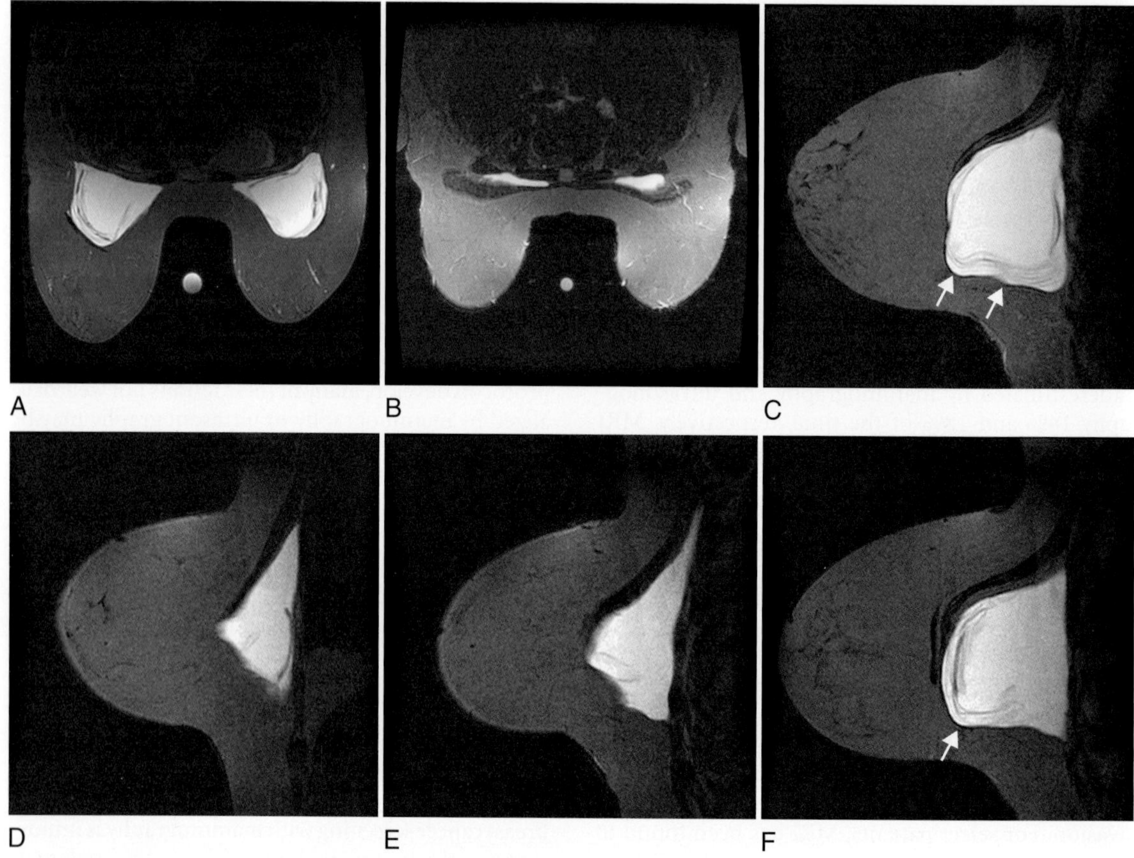

FIGURE 138-3. *A* to *F*, MRI of ruptured implants. Note "linguini sign" (*arrows*).

women who underwent prior implant augmentation mammaplasty (group A) were compared with 611 nonaugmented women (group B). The study patients were also compared with the Surveillance, Epidemiology, and End Results (SEER) data group (group C). No significant difference was found between groups A and B in mean tumor size. There was no significant difference between groups A, B, or C in incidence of axillary nodal involvement. They concluded that nonpalpable invasive and in situ breast cancer can be detected in augmented patients by mammography. Stage at presentation for the augmented patients was no different from that for the nonaugmented patients.

Concern about the potential delay in breast cancer diagnosis in the augmented breast was also addressed by Holmich et al[29] in 2003 in a study of 2955 women who received cosmetic breast implants in Denmark during the period 1973-1997. The authors found that women with breast implants on average were diagnosed with breast cancer at the same stage as were control subjects. There was no significant difference in overall survival between the two groups after an average of 6.4 years of follow-up.

In an outcome study by Miglioretti et al,[30] a matched prospective cohort of 137 women with augmentation and 685 women without augmentation diagnosed with breast cancer was compared with a retrospective review of 10,533 women with augmentation and 974,915 women without augmentation and without breast cancer from seven mammographic centers; the study was designed to determine mammographic accuracy and cancer characteristics in these four groups. Among symptomatic women, both sensitivity and specificity were lower for women with augmentation compared with women without augmentation, but differences were not significant. Tumors were of similar stage, size, estrogen receptor status, and nodal status, but they tended to be lower grade for women with breast augmentation than for those without. The study concluded that breast augmentation decreases the sensitivity of screening mammography among asymptomatic women but does not increase the false-positive rate. Despite the lower accuracy of mammography in women with augmentation, the prognostic characteristics of tumors are not influenced by augmentation.

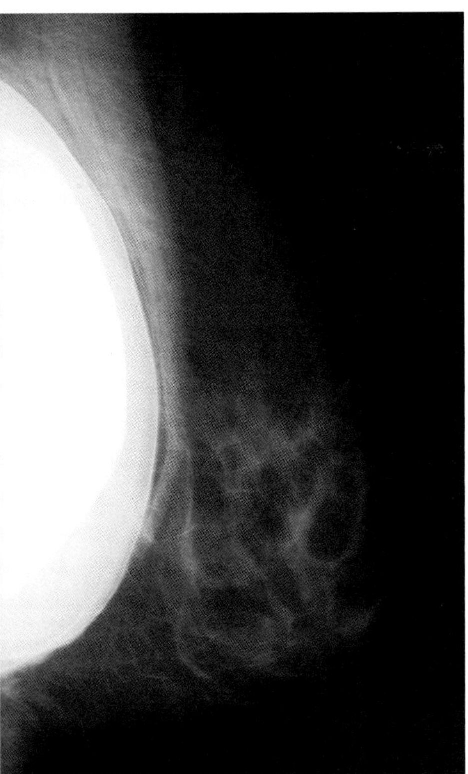

FIGURE 138-4. Mammography with implants (implant: two-lumen retropectoral).

Diagnostic Imaging of Breast Implant Complications

Imaging studies have increasingly been used to evaluate the complications of breast implants, such as rupture, silicone extravasation, gel bleed, polyurethane breakdown, and peri-implant fluid collections.[31] The use of multiple imaging modalities has been helpful in providing an overview of the status of the breast implant. Implant rupture may be classified as either intracapsular or extracapsular, depending on whether the silicone has migrated out of the fibrous capsule.

Mammography is excellent for detecting extracapsular rupture but often fails to detect intracapsular rupture because the fibrous capsule maintains the normal shape of the ruptured implant. Mammographic signs of implant rupture include a contour abnormality or bulge and the migration of silicone away from the site of the implant. Ruptured or injected silicone can obscure breast cancer, hindering detection on routine screening.

The sonographic appearance of saline implants is similar to that of silicone implants. The most useful sonographic sign of a ruptured implant is the step-ladder sign, echogenic lines corresponding to the ruptured elastomer shell that has retracted from the fibrous capsule.[32] The sonographic finding of free silicone is the most specific sign for implant rupture.

MRI provides an excellent representation of the anatomy of the breast, implant, axilla, and chest wall. The silicone shell is of lower signal than the silicone used as prosthetic filler material because of greater cross-linking of methyl groups. The MRI sign of an internal linear focus of decreased intensity within the implant (the linguini sign) is often found, representing the collapsed outer shell.[33]

A study comparing the radiographic evaluation of symptomatic patients with silicone breast implants to rule out rupture with results at explantation operation found mammography to have a sensitivity of 11% with a specificity of 89%, ultrasonography to have a sensitivity of 70% with a specificity of 92%, and MRI to have a sensitivity of 81% with a specificity of 92%.[34]

Factors Associated with Delay of Cancer Diagnosis

Not all breast cancers are detectable clinically by either physical examination or mammography. The most common cause of malpractice litigation in the United States is failure to diagnose a breast cancer. The average age of the litigant is currently 39 years, which suggests that breast cancer in younger women is more difficult to detect.[35]

Although more widespread use of mammography has increased the detection of early breast cancers, a study reported that the physician's delay in the diagnosis of breast cancer is common.[36] In a study of 454 breast cancer patients, 9% (42 patients) experienced delay of diagnosis for a median of 9 months. In this study, delay is defined as "physical action that completed an episode of care without diagnosing cancer of which there was a sign." The most frequent cause of delay in making the diagnosis of breast cancer is the physician's inappropriately reassuring the patient that a mass is benign without biopsy (Table 138-4). For women younger than 50 years, the most common chief

TABLE 138-4 ✦ REASONS FOR DELAY OF DIAGNOSIS FOR 42 (9%) OF 454 BREAST CANCERS[36]

Reason*	Number (%)
Inappropriate reassurance by physician that lump is benign without biopsy	21 (50)
Mammographer failed to notice new mass or suspicious calcifications	14 (33)
Misread pathology report	4 (9)
Poorly performed fine-needle aspiration by physician without formal training in the technique	5 (12)

*Both misread mammograms and inappropriate reassurance by a physician without biopsy occurred for 2 patients and are counted in both categories.

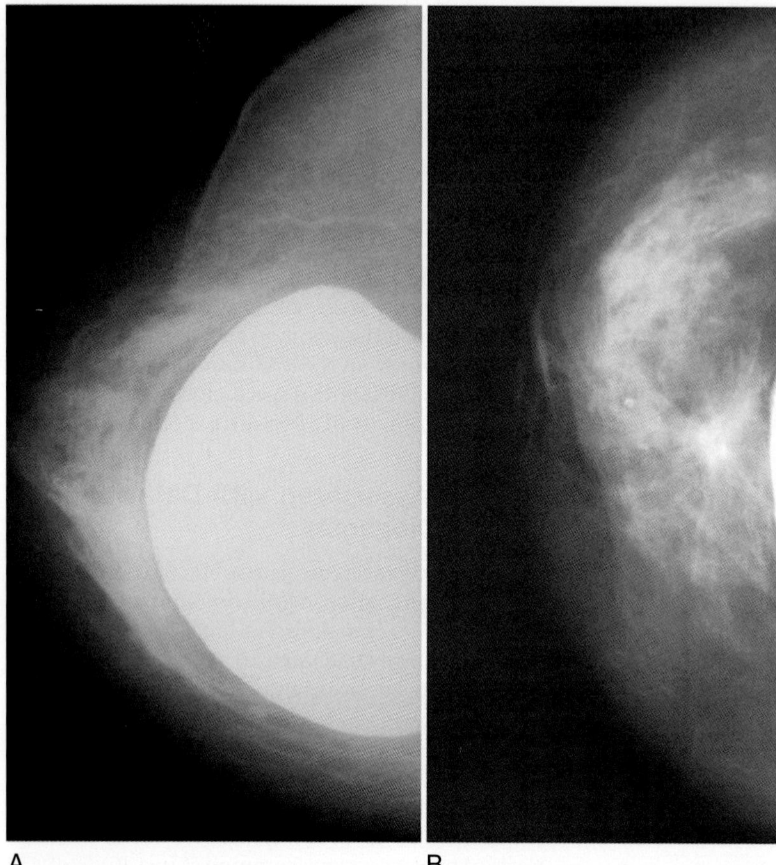

FIGURE 138-5. Displacement of a patient's implant (Eklund maneuver) is required at the time of mammography for optimal screening. *A*, Normal mammogram without implant displacement. *B*, After displacement of the patient's implant, a malignant neoplasm is detectable.

complaint was a mass; for women older than 50 years, the most common chief complaint was an abnormal mammogram (the investigators found that women with normal mammograms were 10 times more likely to have delay of diagnosis, regardless of whether a mass was present). In this study, misinterpretation of mammograms resulted in a delay of diagnosis for 7% of the patients. For those patients who presented with a chief complaint of finding a lump in the breast on self-examination, 32% who had normal mammograms had a delay in diagnosis, but only 4% of these same patients who had suggestive mammograms had a delay in diagnosis. On the basis of these findings, Goodson suggested the following recommendations to reduce delay by physicians:

- Focus the clinical breast examination on the presence or absence of a mass, without interpretation of what it might be.
- Expect tissue sampling for all palpable breast masses.
- Recommend tissue sampling of all palpable masses, even if the mammogram shows no signs of cancer.
- Verify that physicians doing fine-needle aspirations have specific training in the procedure.
- Re-evaluate patients after a short interval if a tentative decision is made that an area identified by a patient falls within the narrowly defined rules of predictable variations of breast structure.

As Goodson's study suggests, a tissue diagnosis is the standard of care for the work-up of a palpable breast mass. For women younger than 30 years who present with a breast mass that remains throughout the menstrual cycle, ultrasonography should be used to determine whether it is a solid or cystic mass. If it appears to be a simple cyst, needle aspiration of the cyst cavity should be performed; if this produces a resolution of the mass by ultrasonography and palpation, the risk of cancer is minimal. If the mass persists or if the aspiration was not consistent with cystic fluid, biopsy should be considered. All complex cysts should prompt biopsy (preferably core biopsy) because a neoplasm could be located in the cyst wall.

Histologic Diagnostic Modalities

The majority of lesions for which women undergo breast biopsy prove to be benign. In addition, many women must undergo multiple biopsies over the course of their lifetime. The most widely used techniques for breast biopsy are fine-needle aspiration, core needle biopsy, and excisional biopsy. Most tumors are now diagnosed without the use of excisional biopsy; minimally invasive diagnostic approaches are advantageous in terms of minimal scar, decreased anatomic deformity permitting improved mammographic surveillance (minimal or no scarring on subsequent mammograms), decreased pain, and significantly decreased cost while diagnostic accuracy is maintained. In addition, translational research is being performed on the utility of the analysis of ductal fluid by the techniques of ductal lavage and nipple discharge analysis. The diagnosis of cancer is thus generally known preoperatively, facilitating appropriate planning and counseling about treatment options.

IMAGE-GUIDED CORE BIOPSY

Image-guided core biopsy is performed by either stereotactic x-ray or ultrasound guidance. The technique of stereotactic biopsy involves use of a specially equipped mammography unit to calculate the three-dimensional position of a lesion in real time. Two stereotactic systems are widely available; one may be an add-on to normal upright mammography equipment, whereas the other requires specially designed prone equipment, used separately from the normal mammography suite. The add-on unit is typically less costly and provides the ability to sample lesions close to the chest wall that cannot be reached with the prone table.[4] The advantage of the dedicated stereotactic table is that the patient is positioned prone and cannot see the biopsy procedure; thus, there is less likelihood of the patient's movement. Digital images are taken and processed by the computer, which calculates the position of the lesion in three-dimensional space. Although many surgeons can accommodate ultrasound-guided biopsies in the office, stereotaxis is more involved in equipment requirements and thus generally is performed in a radiology suite, by either a surgeon or radiologist.

Ultrasound guidance is increasingly being incorporated into surgical practice in the care of breast disease. It is less costly than stereotaxis and can frequently be performed in the surgeon's office. Ultrasonography provides excellent guidance for core biopsy, fine-needle aspiration, and drainage of cysts.

FINE-NEEDLE ASPIRATION

Fine-needle aspiration (FNA) is performed under guidance by palpation, ultrasonography, or stereotactic mammography. The examiner places a 20- to 23-gauge needle into the lesion. On aspiration with a syringe, material is sampled for cytopathologic examination. Numerous multidirectional passes through the area increase the likelihood of successful sampling, particularly in small lesions.[37] The cellular material is placed on slides for review by an experienced cytopathologist. The procedure is rapidly accomplished, is well tolerated, and is cost-effective.

The National Cancer Institute recommends reporting cytologic results according to five categories: unsatisfactory, benign, indeterminate/atypical, suspicious/probably malignant, and malignant (Color Plate 138-1).[38] FNA does not provide enough tissue architecture for the diagnosis of invasive carcinoma to be made. With experience in use of needle aspiration, FNA has a reported false-negative rate of 2%, similar to that of intraoperative frozen sections. When atypia is found on FNA, 61% ultimately proves to actually be malignant disease.[39] Therefore, findings of atypia should result in surgical excision. The biggest pitfall to use of FNA is the problem of sampling error; false-negative rates of 2% to 22% have been reported in the literature.[40] FNA provides cytologic diagnoses that must be closely correlated with clinical and imaging findings to improve sensitivity of diagnosis (the so-called triple test of clinical, radiographic, and pathologic findings). One of the main disadvantages of FNA is the close follow-up required in equivocal patients, and noncompliance may be an issue. The high false-negative rate often makes it unclear how to manage a patient with a negative result. In Pijnappel's series,[41] a benign initial FNA result required an additional invasive procedure for 58% of the patients (needle-localized breast biopsy or core biopsy) to verify nonmalignant disease because false-negative results were often suspected by clinicians.

Ljung et al[42] reviewed the diagnostic accuracy of FNA in two groups of physicians based on prior experience with FNA: formally trained physicians (at least 150 FNA biopsies during fellowship training or the equivalent, currently performing at least 100 FNAs per year; 729 FNA biopsies total) and physicians without formal training (median of 2 FNA biopsies per year, range of 1 to 43 FNA biopsies; 314 FNA biopsies total). They found that formally trained physicians missed 2% of patients, whereas physicians without formal training missed 25%. Of the patients with benign lesions seen by formally trained physicians, 8% went on to surgery, whereas 30% of those examined by physicians without formal training in FNA required surgery. Formal training clearly improves the diagnostic accuracy of FNA for evaluation of breast tissue.

CORE NEEDLE BIOPSY

Core needle biopsy involves use of an automated biopsy gun with a 14- to 18-gauge needle attached to the end. The needle is positioned by either stereotactic or sonographic guidance. When the spring-loaded biopsy gun is fired, the needle advances into the lesion and takes a core of tissue (Fig. 138-6). Four passes through the lesion are required to optimize sensitivity and to

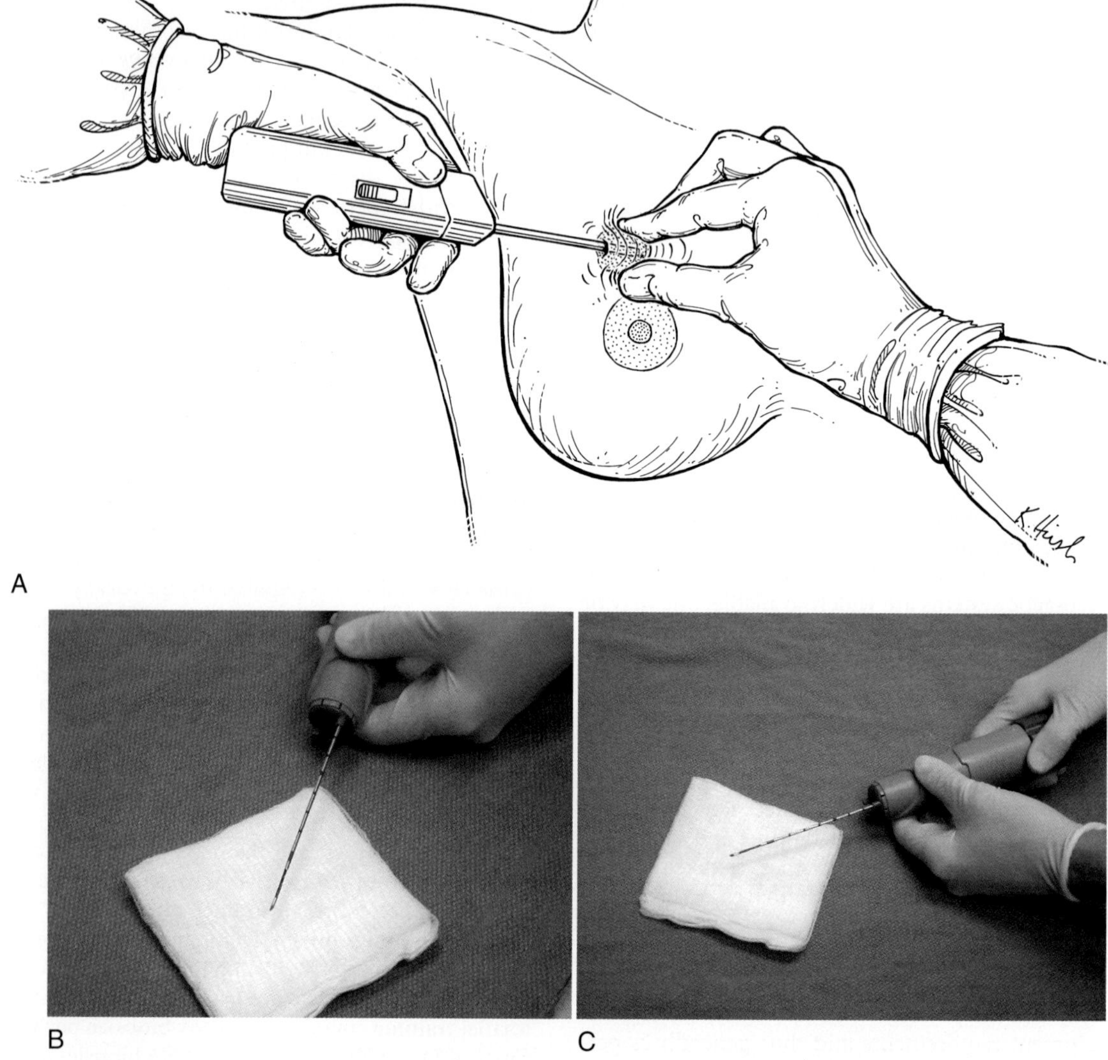

FIGURE 138-6. *A,* Technique of core biopsy. *B* and *C,* Biopsy needle with core of tissue.

determine histologic grade with accuracy.[43] The diagnostic sensitivity of core needle biopsy with two or more passes is 95% (as later confirmed by excisional biopsy for verification); with four or more passes, the histologic grade of the tumor could be accurately determined with 74% accuracy, after which point results began to plateau with further passes.

One difficulty of core needle biopsy is that the technique provides a monodirectional sampling of the target lesion; if multiple passes are to be undertaken, this potentially involves reinsertion of the needle multiple times. This problem is overcome by use of vacuum-assisted instrumentation. These systems use a vacuum to aspirate tissue into a chamber, where it is sampled. Examples of these instruments are the Mammotome,* the ABBI,† and the SiteSelect‡ system. The Mammotome system uses a 3-mm skin puncture to accommodate an 11-gauge instrument that is positioned in the lesion under image guidance; the core biopsy specimen is obtained by suction and rotation of the instrument repeatedly to a different area of the lesion until a sufficient number of biopsy samples are taken. The ABBI device uses a 1- to 2.5-cm skin incision to accommodate a cannula (10, 15, or 20 mm in diameter) that is positioned under image guidance. With suction assistance, high-speed oscillating knives

*Ethicon Endo-Surgery, Cincinnati, Ohio.
†United States Surgical, Norwalk, Conn.
‡Imagyn Surgical, Irvine, Calif.

pull a cylinder of tissue into a chamber outside the breast. The advantage of these techniques is that multiple passes are accomplished by rotating the needle sequentially rather than by reinsertion; thus, only one needle stick is required. The SiteSelect uses image guidance to completely excise small lesions through a 1.5-cm skin incision; this technique is an excisional biopsy variant of a traditional core biopsy.[44] Accuracy of the vacuum-assisted breast biopsy approaches 100% in one series.[45] Further studies of the diagnostic accuracy of each of these vacuum-assisted modalities would certainly be beneficial because initial results have been encouraging.

Core biopsy specimens are preserved in formalin for pathologic analysis. The advantages over FNA include accurate diagnosis of specific benign or malignant histologic features, decreased likelihood of sampling error secondary to much larger tissue specimens, and an en bloc core specimen rather than a cytologic specimen (Color Plate 138-2). Thus, the subsequent pathologic analysis will allow determination of invasive versus noninvasive disease and histologic grade (although there is a discrepancy of 25% between core biopsy grade and grade of surgical tumor specimen). Although histologic grade cannot be determined by FNA, nuclear grade may be determined by both FNA and core biopsy. In most instances, a core biopsy specimen can provide enough tissue to analyze estrogen receptor status and the presence of the HER-2/neu oncoprotein, neither of which is provided by an FNA specimen. Overexpression of the HER-2/neu antigen, which occurs in 30% of breast cancer patients, is associated with poorer prognosis and less likelihood of response to conventional chemotherapy.[46]

Contraindications to stereotactic- or ultrasound-guided core biopsy include mammographic presence of a radial scar (a complex sclerosing lesion that simulates carcinoma mammographically and on physical examination; these lesions are in fact associated with carcinoma anywhere within the lesion, thus predisposing to sampling error); lesions not well visualized in the imaging suite; patients who cannot tolerate lying prone for 30 minutes; and patients with small breasts that compress to less than 2 cm. Those patients with a radial scar (Color Plate 138-2*A*) should undergo excisional biopsy. In any of the other situations, patients should undergo ultrasound-guided core biopsy if the lesion can be well visualized, stereotactic biopsy if visualization is not possible by ultrasound guidance, or needle-localized excisional biopsy if the lesion cannot be visualized by either of these means.[47] The presence of an implant is a relative contraindication to core needle biopsy by either technique.

The advantage of core biopsy over excisional biopsy is that the diagnosis is made preoperatively and thus only one operation (lumpectomy or mastectomy) is required for definitive treatment of the breast cancer. This technique is highly accurate, less invasive than excisional biopsy, and considerably less expensive. The downside potentially is that since core biopsy is an incisional biopsy technique, tumor could theoretically be seeded across the biopsy site and into the skin. Tumor seeding of core biopsy sites has been reported.[48] Not all biopsy sites are located in the optimal position for lumpectomy incisions; therefore, the surgeon must decide for each patient whether to excise the biopsy site. Routine lumpectomy does not involve resection of skin at the site of a core breast biopsy. King et al[47] performed a retrospective analysis of 211 patients treated by breast-conserving therapy; 132 were diagnosed by image-guided core needle biopsy and 79 by wire-localized excisional breast biopsy. They found a local recurrence rate of 3% for patients diagnosed by image-guided core needle biopsy and 2.5% for patients diagnosed by wire-localized excisional breast biopsy. These results compared favorably between the two techniques. They argued that most patients select breast-conserving therapy to improve cosmetic results; thus, they advocated use of postoperative radiation therapy to achieve local control of any residual disease remaining as a result of the core needle biopsy. Chao et al[49] disagree, instead recommending excision of the biopsy track when definitive surgical resection of the tumor is performed. The stereotactic site is excised in continuity with the operative specimen. When this is not possible, an additional incision may have to be made to excise the skin entry site and also the needle track (Table 138-5).[49]

TABLE 138-5 ✦ ANALYSIS OF DIAGNOSTIC PROCEDURES FOR BREAST BIOPSY

Procedure	Sensitivity	Specificity	Cost	Feasibility for Office Procedure
Fine-needle aspiration	+	+++	$	+++*
Core biopsy	++	+++	$$	++*
Needle-localized excisional biopsy	+++	+++	$$$	+

*Feasible for office use only if no image guidance is required or if the lesion is visible on portable office-based ultrasonography.

Sensitivity is defined as the probability that the test result will be positive in someone with the disease. Specificity is defined as the probability that the test result will be negative in someone who does not have the disease.

Morrow[7] raised several concerns in regard to the replacement of excisional biopsy with core biopsy. She cited diagnostic inaccuracy for patients with mammographically detectable microcalcifications (frequently ductal carcinoma in situ) rather than mass lesions with this technique. She also reported misdiagnosis by core biopsy of the histologic finding of atypical hyperplasia when excisional biopsy specimens ultimately showed ductal carcinoma in situ or infiltrating carcinoma. These concerns emphasize the necessity of tailoring the diagnostic techniques and follow-up techniques that the clinician selects to the specific patient's clinical data.

NEEDLE-LOCALIZED EXCISIONAL BIOPSY

Indications for needle-localized excisional breast biopsy include any nonpalpable abnormality visualized on mammography that is BI-RADS 3, 4, or 5 (see Table 138-2).[50] The technique of needle-localized excisional biopsy is being used less frequently for the purpose of obtaining a tissue diagnosis in centers with stereotactic- or ultrasound-guided breast biopsy. In these centers, its use is typically reserved for assisting the surgeon in locating a nonpalpable lesion for lumpectomy. With the increasing use of percutaneous image-guided biopsy, specialized indications have evolved to include[51] disagreement between the mammographic or clinical impression and histologic findings of percutaneous biopsy, atypical ductal hyperplasia on percutaneous biopsy,[52] and radial scar on mammography or percutaneous biopsy.[53,54] When percutaneous biopsy is nondiagnostic for nonpalpable radiographic lesions, a needle-localized breast biopsy is recommended.

Needle-localized breast biopsy is performed by placing a 20-gauge Kopans needle advanced to the site of the mammographic lesion by ultrasound or stereotactic guidance. A hook wire is threaded into the needle and deployed within the site of the abnormality. Two orthogonal mammographic views are taken to ensure proper placement of the wire within the lesion. The radiologist positions the needle and wire to achieve the shortest distance from the skin to the lesion such that no extraneous tissue is excised. The surgeon performs an excisional biopsy through a 2- to 5-cm skin incision, guided by the position of the wire. Care is taken not to transect the wire and to achieve 1-cm margins circumferentially.

OPEN EXCISIONAL BIOPSY

Excisional biopsy may be performed without needle localization for palpable masses (e.g., if FNA or core needle biopsy results are negative but the clinician suspects potential sampling error). The surgical incision is carefully chosen so that it may be incorporated by a mastectomy incision in the event that definitive resection is necessary. Excisional biopsy must always be approached as if it is a biopsy for a cancer. The specimen is carefully marked for orientation to assist the pathologist in determination of margins. The false-negative rates of excisional biopsies range from 1% to 5% in most series.[3]

With the advent of image-guided biopsies, most patients can be diagnosed preoperatively without a surgical excisional biopsy, sparing them an anxiety-producing trip to the operating room to procure a diagnosis. If sufficient tissue is resected with negative margins at the time of an excisional biopsy for invasive disease or ductal carcinoma in situ, this procedure is essentially equivalent to a lumpectomy—in this instance, both diagnostic and therapeutic. If the patient and surgeon agree on a breast-conserving surgical approach, the excisional biopsy with negative 1-cm margins may constitute the definitive resection of the tumor, necessitating consultation with a radiation oncologist to arrange radiation therapy. However, for those patients who are scheduled to undergo a mastectomy on the basis of the results of their excisional biopsy, this biopsy technique results in one additional operation. Percutaneous biopsy before operation offers the patient the psychological advantage of time to prepare for the cancer surgery and to consider what extirpative and reconstructive options would best suit her.

Aesthetic considerations should be an important part of the operative plan for the patient with benign breast disease. When possible, an areolar-cutaneous incision may be chosen to minimize scar formation. This incision is preferred for young patients with fibroadenomas.

Experimental Modalities

DUCTAL LAVAGE AND NIPPLE DISCHARGE ANALYSIS

Spontaneous nipple discharge is found in only 10% of breast cancer patients; malignant cells are not always present and are more common if the tumor lies in a major duct. Whereas sensitivity is low, specificity of cytologic analysis of nipple discharge for breast carcinoma is close to 100%.[55] Studies indicate that breast carcinoma tends to occur in a segmental fashion within a particular ductal system rather than throughout the entire breast.[56] Ductal lavage is an experimental technique that uses a microcatheter inserted into the ductal system through the nipple surface orifices (Color Plate 138-3). The physician irrigates the duct with saline to wash out cells for cytologic examination.[57] Preliminary studies indicate that it may be useful for the early detection of intraductal breast carcinomas.[58] Approximately 78% of patients undergoing ductal lavage produced samples that had an adequate number of cells for diagnostic purposes; the mean number of epithelial cells yielded was 13,500 (an adequate number of cells for diagnostic purposes in ductal lavage is defined as 10 epithelial cells per specimen).[59] This technique could benefit the general population for the purposes of screening and risk assessment; healthy individuals are not likely to subject themselves to invasive screening tests, but if such an assay could be developed with excellent levels of comfort, many patients would be compliant with screening. Klein et al[60] performed a pilot study of a noninvasive technique of nipple aspiration. They were able to obtain nipple aspiration fluid from 80% of the women participating in the study and stated that patients reported a minimal level of discomfort. There were no serious adverse effects. They explored the feasibility of obtaining DNA and proteins for molecular investigation from these specimens and had good results. Ductal lavage is still in the experimental stages, although many groups are currently performing clinical trials.

Morrow et al[59] suggest the following guidelines for the implementation and management of ductal lavage. This procedure should be used in asymptomatic women with normal breast examination findings because it is intended as a method of risk assessment only. It is important for the surgeon performing the procedure to communicate directly with the cytopathologist when findings of atypia are made so that the degree of atypia, cellularity, and quality of the specimen are confirmed. If the specimen is deemed inadequate, lavage should be repeated. An adequate lavage specimen that shows atypia should lead the clinician to confirm that the findings on breast examination and mammography are normal, and the patient should be counseled on her increased risk for breast cancer (with emphasis on close follow-up). With a suspicious finding on ductal lavage, the next evaluation should be ductography or ductoscopy. If these studies detect abnormalities, core or needle-localized biopsy should be directed by these studies to the abnormal focus. If the findings on ductography or ductoscopy are normal, breast MRI should be obtained next, followed by biopsy if any abnormal densities are localized. If the breast MRI is normal, Morrow recommends repeated clinical breast examination in 3 months, repeated ductoscopy or ductography in 3 months, unilateral mammography in 6 months, and consideration of tamoxifen prophylaxis.

STAGING

The American Joint Committee on Cancer TNM (tumor, nodes, metastasis) breast cancer staging system is the "common language" for clinicians to describe clinical situations and to assess treatment outcomes. This system is best suited to cancers that spread according to an orderly halstedian manner, but it does not work as well when it is applied to small tumors that spread directly by hematogenous pathways early in their course, not necessarily invading lymph nodes (Tables 138-6 and 138-7).[61]

MANAGEMENT

Surgical Treatment Modalities

Surgical management of breast cancer involves four major aspects: the breast parenchyma, the skin envelope, the nipple-areola complex, and the lymph nodes. There has been a trend toward a more conservative approach to the surgical extirpation of breast cancer. For more than a century, the primary treatment of breast cancer was the Halsted radical mastectomy. This procedure was quite disfiguring and left the patient with increased morbidity postoperatively. The resection of the pectoralis muscles and the complete axillary nodal basin (levels I, II, and III) along with the mastectomy specimen taken with a wide skin margin frequently necessitated skin graft coverage for closure. It is now clear that such radical surgery is often not necessary for the treatment of breast cancer. The treatment preference is now modified radical mastectomy (resection of all visible breast tissue with the axillary nodal basin en bloc). Current surgical management of early breast cancer (stage I and stage II) focuses on providing the patient with information about the options of breast-conserving therapy versus mastectomy.

There are currently two approaches to breast cancer extirpation: (1) removal of the tumor with a 1- to 2-cm margin of surrounding tissue and (2) removal of all breast tissue. This second approach is variable on the basis of the approach to the skin envelope. The contributing factors to this decision include indications for resection of the skin envelope in continuity with the breast parenchyma and indications for resection of the nipple-areola complex. The evolution of breast cancer surgical care is based on collaboration between breast surgical oncologists, medical and radiation oncologists, radiologists, pathologists, and plastic surgeons. Both diagnostic and therapeutic modalities are progressing toward minimally invasive techniques. Breast-conserving therapy has proved to be oncologically sound for stage I and stage II breast cancers[62] and results in minimal scar and less physical and psychological trauma to the patient. Lumpectomy with axillary dissection and radiation therapy has been shown to be equivalent to modified radical mastectomy for overall survival.

In the United States, modified radical mastectomy remains the most common procedure for the treatment of stage I and stage II breast cancer. Approximately 20% of women who would be good candidates for breast conservation therapy elect instead to undergo modified radical mastectomy, suggesting that

TABLE 138-6 ✦ AMERICAN JOINT COMMITTEE ON CANCER TNM STAGING SYSTEM FOR BREAST CANCER[296]

TNM Staging

Primary Tumor (T)

Definitions for classifying the primary tumor (T) are the same for clinical and for pathologic classification. If the measurement is made by the physical examination, the examiner uses the major headings (T1, T2, or T3). If other measurements, such as mammographic or pathologic measurements, are used, the subsets of T1 can be used. Tumors should be measured to the nearest 0.1-cm increment.

TX	Primary tumor cannot be assessed
T0	No evidence of primary tumor
Tis	Carcinoma in situ
Tis (DCIS)	Ductal carcinoma in situ
Tis (LCIS)	Lobular carcinoma in situ
Tis (Paget)	Paget disease of the nipple with no tumor
	Note: Paget disease associated with a tumor is classified according to the size of the tumor.
T1	Tumor 2 cm or less in greatest dimension
T1mic	Microinvasion 0.1 cm or less in greatest dimension
T1a	Tumor more than 0.1 cm but not more than 0.5 cm in greatest dimension
T1b	Tumor more than 0.5 cm but not more than 1 cm in greatest dimension
T1c	Tumor more than 1 cm but not more than 2 cm in greatest dimension
T2	Tumor more than 2 cm but not more than 5 cm in greatest dimension
T3	Tumor more than 5 cm in greatest dimension
T4	Tumor of any size with direct extension to (a) chest wall or (b) skin, only as described below
T4a	Extension to chest wall, not including pectoralis muscle
T4b	Edema (including peau d'orange) or ulceration of the skin of the breast or satellite skin nodules confined to the same breast
T4c	Both T4a and T4b
T4d	Inflammatory carcinoma

Regional Lymph Nodes (N)

Clinical

NX	Regional lymph nodes cannot be assessed (e.g., previously removed)
N0	No regional lymph node metastasis
N1	Metastasis to movable ipsilateral axillary lymph node(s)
N2	Metastases in ipsilateral axillary lymph nodes fixed to one another (matted) or in clinically apparent ipsilateral internal mammary nodes in the absence of clinically evident axillary lymph node metastasis
N2a	Metastases in ipsilateral axillary lymph nodes fixed to one another (matted) or to other structures
N2b	Metastases only in clinically apparent ipsilateral internal mammary nodes and in the absence of clinically evident axillary lymph node metastasis
N3	Metastasis in ipsilateral infraclavicular lymph node(s), with or without axillary lymph node involvement, or in clinically apparent ipsilateral internal mammary lymph node(s) and in the presence of clinically evident axillary lymph node metastasis; or metastasis in ipsilateral supraclavicular lymph node(s), with or without axillary or internal mammary lymph node involvement
N3a	Metastasis in ipsilateral infraclavicular lymph node(s)
N3b	Metastasis in ipsilateral internal mammary lymph node(s) and axillary lymph node(s)
N3c	Metastasis in ipsilateral supraclavicular lymph node(s)

Pathologic (pN)

pNX	Regional lymph nodes cannot be assessed (e.g., previously removed or not removed for pathologic study)
pN0	No regional lymph node metastasis histologically and no additional examination for isolated tumor cells (ITCs)
	Note: ITCs are defined as single tumor cells or small cell clusters not greater than 0.2 mm that are usually detected only by immunohistochemical (IHC) or molecular methods but may be verified on hematoxylin and eosin stains. ITCs do not usually show evidence of malignant activity (e.g., proliferation or stromal reaction).
pN0(i–)	No regional lymph node metastasis histologically, negative IHC
pN0(i+)	No regional lymph node metastasis histologically, positive IHC, no IHC cluster greater than 0.2 mm
pN0(mol–)	No regional lymph node metastasis histologically, negative molecular findings (RT-PCR)

TABLE 138-6 ✦ AMERICAN JOINT COMMITTEE ON CANCER TNM STAGING SYSTEM FOR BREAST CANCER[296]—cont'd

pN0(mol+)	No regional lymph node metastasis histologically, positive molecular findings (RT-PCR)
pN1	Metastasis in 1 to 3 axillary lymph nodes, or in internal mammary nodes with microscopic disease detected by sentinel lymph node dissection, but not clinically apparent
pN1mi	Micrometastasis (greater than 0.2 mm, none greater than 2.0 mm)
pN1a	Metastasis in 1 to 3 axillary lymph nodes
pN1b	Metastasis in internal mammary nodes with microscopic disease detected by sentinel lymph node dissection, but not clinically apparent
pN1c	Metastasis in 1 to 3 axillary lymph nodes and in internal mammary nodes with microscopic disease detected by sentinel lymph node dissection, but not clinically apparent (If associated with more than 3 positive axillary lymph nodes, the internal mammary nodes are classified as pN3b to reflect increased tumor burden.)
pN2	Metastasis in 4 to 9 axillary lymph nodes or in clinically apparent internal mammary lymph nodes in the absence of axillary lymph node metastasis
pN2a	Metastasis in 4 to 9 axillary lymph nodes (at least one tumor deposit greater than 2.0 mm)
pN2b	Metastasis in clinically apparent internal mammary lymph nodes in the absence of axillary lymph node metastasis
pN3	Metastasis in 10 or more axillary lymph nodes, in infraclavicular lymph nodes, or in clinically apparent ipsilateral internal mammary lymph nodes in the presence of 1 or more positive axillary lymph nodes; or in more than 3 axillary lymph nodes with clinically negative microscopic metastasis in internal mammary lymph nodes; or in ipsilateral supraclavicular lymph nodes
pN3a	Metastasis in 10 or more axillary lymph nodes (at least one tumor deposit greater than 2.0 mm), or metastasis to the infraclavicular lymph nodes
pN3b	Metastasis in clinically apparent ipsilateral internal mammary lymph nodes in the presence of 1 or more positive axillary lymph nodes; or in more than 3 axillary lymph nodes and in internal mammary lymph nodes with microscopic disease detected by sentinel lymph node dissection, but not clinically apparent
pN3c	Metastasis in ipsilateral supraclavicular lymph nodes

Distant Metastasis (M)

MX	Distant metastasis cannot be assessed
M0	No distant metastasis
M1	Distant metastasis

Stage Grouping

Stage 0	Tis	N0	M0
Stage I	T1	N0	M0
Stage IIA	T0	N1	M0
	T1	N1	M0
	T2	N0	M0
Stage IIB	T2	N1	M0
	T3	N0	M0
Stage IIIA	T0	N2	M0
	T1	N2	M0
	T2	N2	M0
	T3	N1	M0
	T3	N2	M0
Stage IIIB	T4	N0	M0
	T4	N1	M0
	T4	N2	M0
Stage IIIC	Any T	N3	M0
Stage IV	Any T	Any N	M1

Note: Stage designation may be changed if postsurgical imaging studies show distant metastases, provided that the studies are carried out within 4 months of diagnosis in the absence of disease progression and provided that the patient has not received neoadjuvant therapy.

TABLE 138-7 ✦ BREAST CANCER SURVIVAL BY STAGE[218]

Stage	5-Year Relative Survival Rate
0	100%
I	98%
IIA	88%
IIB	76%
IIIA	56%
IIIB	49%
IV	16%

TABLE 138-8 ✦ CONTRAINDICATIONS TO BREAST-CONSERVING THERAPY[64]

First or second trimester of pregnancy (due to need for radiation therapy)
History of prior therapeutic irradiation to the breast region
Multiple primary tumors in separate quadrants of the breast (multicentricity)
Extensive indeterminate or malignant-appearing calcifications throughout the breast

breast-conserving therapy is still underused in the general community.[63] Both patients and their surgeons frequently elect mastectomy as opposed to breast conservation to avoid the risk of late local recurrence, a new primary tumor, or distortion of the breast's shape or size and position. Four absolute contraindications to breast-conserving therapy were developed at a multidisciplinary meeting including representatives from the American College of Surgeons, the American College of Radiology, the College of American Pathologists, and the Society of Surgical Oncology in 1992 (Table 138-8).[64] Relative contraindications include a large tumor-to-breast ratio that precludes acceptable aesthetic results and collagen vascular disease. Prophylactic mastectomy for high-risk individuals is another example of a medical indication for mastectomy. Despite strong evidence in support of breast-conserving therapy, Morrow et al[65] found in an analysis of 16,643 patients with stage I and stage II breast cancer nationwide that only 42.6% actually received breast-conserving surgery. Although breast conservation is sound on the basis of oncologic principles, may patients will elect mastectomy to avoid the risk of local recurrence and the necessary surveillance of the remaining breast tissue. In patients with smaller breasts and ptotic breasts, a lumpectomy procedure and subsequent radiation therapy may distort the breast shape and accentuate asymmetry. Reconstructive breast surgery can provide an immediate or delayed restoration of the breast, which now allows the patient to select mastectomy and avoid these potential undesirable aspects of breast conservation surgery (Table 138-9).

Because the purpose of breast conservation is to preserve a breast with intact sensation and a reasonable symmetry with the opposite breast, the con-

TABLE 138-9 ✦ COMPARISON OF TYPES OF BREAST SURGERY AND EXTENT OF RESECTION

	Radical Mastectomy	Modified Radical Mastectomy	Simple Mastectomy	Breast-Conserving Surgery	Skin-Sparing Mastectomy
Breast tissue	Completely resected	Completely resected	Completely resected	Tumor plus margins resected	Completely resected
Skin envelope	Resected	Resected	Partially preserved	Preserved	Preserved
Nipple-areola complex	Resected	Resected	Resected	Preserved	Resected*
Axilla	Complete dissection en bloc	Complete dissection en bloc	Spared	Sentinel node dissection before axillary lymph node dissection	Sentinel node dissection before axillary lymph node dissection
Pectoralis major	Resected	Spared	Spared	Spared	Spared
Reconstruction	Skin graft or local flap required for defect coverage Delayed	Possible† Immediate or delayed	Possible† Immediate or delayed	Not required‡	Immediate*

*The epidermal component of the nipple-areola may be preserved in selected patients.
†Based on the surgeon's and patient's considerations.
‡Late distortion of breast due to loss of breast parenchyma and radiation effects may require reconstructive procedures.

tralateral breast must also be considered in the decision-making process. Certain patients, on the basis of an increased risk for breast cancer, may elect contralateral prophylactic mastectomy. If the opposite breast has an undesirable shape, has excess skin, or is malpositioned, contralateral breast procedures may be elected for symmetry and aesthetic considerations. Finally, in breast conservation procedures, there is an increasing interest in reconstruction of the breast defects resulting from lumpectomy and radiation therapy.

LUMPECTOMY

Lumpectomies along with irradiation have been shown to be roughly equivalent to mastectomies for long-term survival. Multiple randomized studies with follow-up periods from 6 to 13 years found no difference in overall or distant disease-free survival between these two therapies.[66-68] The resection specimen is sent for an ex vivo radiograph to ascertain whether the calcifications in question were removed. Postoperatively, the patient receives a mammogram before radiation therapy to be certain that all suspicious calcifications were removed.

Recommendations Regarding Breast Conservation Techniques

In one of the more decisive position statements on the roles of mastectomy versus lumpectomy, the Canadian Steering Committee on Clinical Practice Guidelines for the Care and Treatment of Breast Cancer[69] made the following recommendations:

1. For patients with stage I or stage II disease, breast-conserving therapy is recommended in the absence of specific reasons for selecting mastectomy.
2. Mastectomy should be considered if
   - factors that tend to increase the risk of local recurrence are present, such as extensive malignant-type calcifications on mammography, multiple primary tumors (multicentricity is an absolute contraindication), and failure to obtain negative margins;
   - the patient is unable to lay flat or abduct the arm, precluding the use of radiation therapy;
   - there are any absolute contraindications, such as pregnancy or previous radiation therapy to the breast tissue;
   - there are relative contraindications, such as lupus or scleroderma;
   - the tumor-to-breast ratio is large, such that the lumpectomy itself would be disfiguring; and
   - the patient has a strong preference for mastectomy.
3. Breast-conserving surgery is not contraindicated by a centrally located tumor, axillary lymph node involvement, or breast implants.
4. The surgeon must make a full and fair assessment of the risk and benefits of lumpectomy versus mastectomy to the patient.
5. Every open biopsy, even with the slightest suspicion for breast cancer, should in effect be a lumpectomy—resecting the mass with wide local excision of tumor along with a cuff of normal breast tissue (by palpation and visualization).
6. All tumor-involved margins should undergo re-excision.
7. The primary tumor and axillary dissections should be performed by separate incisions, except when the tumor is close to the axilla anatomically.
8. Drains and sutures should not be used in the breast parenchyma for lumpectomy.

Breast-conserving surgery may at times be appropriate for stage III disease that was down-staged with neoadjuvant chemotherapy, but it should never be offered for stage IV tumors or inflammatory breast cancer.[70]

A multivariate analysis of predictive factors for local recurrence in a large cohort of patients (2006) found that between lumpectomy and mastectomy patients, the most significant variable predictive of local recurrence was young age.[71] In this study, patients younger than 40 years had a fivefold increased risk of a recurrent breast cancer after breast-conserving surgery compared with patients older than 60 years. This effect was not noted in patients undergoing mastectomy.

Technique

The diagnosis is confirmed by core biopsy preoperatively, and the patient is re-examined before the operation is commenced. The lesion is marked while the patient is awake to facilitate location of the tumor in the operating room. The patient is placed in the supine position with the arm abducted to 90 degrees; the shoulder is internally rotated. In general, incisions should be made in an arcuate fashion parallel to the areolar margin. The exception is the rare patient with a mass in the "keyhole area" in the inferior portion of the breast (Fig. 138-7).[72] The rationale for use of a radial incision in this area is that adequate nipple projection will be preserved if a lumpectomy is performed through this incision, whereas with an arcuate incision, the nipple may be distorted inferiorly. Excision and radiation therapy combine to cause additive tissue loss; therefore, it is necessary to take great care in choosing the most advantageous incision. Some surgeons advocate excising any preoperative biopsy site with an elliptical skin incision, although this is not routine practice at most centers because the decision

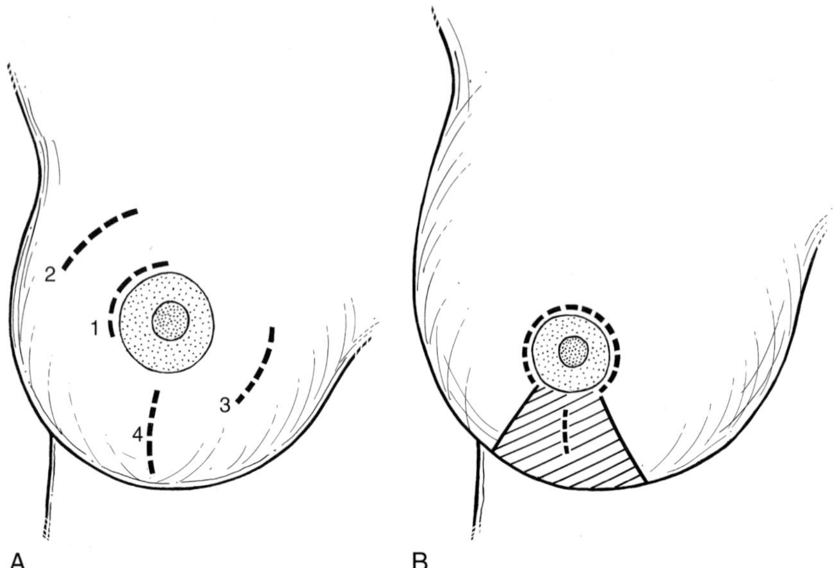

FIGURE 138-7. Lumpectomy incisions. *A,* The proper incision for a lumpectomy is generally curvilinear except for the "keyhole" area inferior to the nipple-areola complex. *B,* In the shaded area (keyhole area) shown inferior to the nipple-areola complex, lesions should be approached through a vertical incision.

to use lumpectomy implies that radiation therapy will occur.

After the incision is made, the skin is grasped with tissue forceps and electrocautery is used to dissect circumferentially around the tumor, taking 2-cm margins. The dissection will often continue to the pectoralis fascia for the deep margin, although for small, superficial tumors, this depth of resection may not be necessary. If the tumor is within 2 cm of the skin, an ellipse of skin should be resected to ensure that 2-cm margins have been obtained circumferentially. The tumor is oriented with marking sutures. If there is any doubt about obtaining negative margins, the lumpectomy cavity is re-excised. These re-excision specimens are sent separately from the main specimen for pathologic evaluation. Close attention is given to achieving adequate hemostasis with electrocautery. The skin incision is closed with a subcuticular absorbable suture and Steri-Strips.

SEGMENTAL RESECTION (QUADRANTECTOMY)

Before adequate evidence existed to support the performance of lumpectomies with radiation therapy, studies from Milan demonstrated that quadrantectomy with axillary dissection and radiation therapy is equivalent to the Halsted radical mastectomy in overall survival. Quadrantectomy is defined as an ample radical resection of the tumor along with the entire surrounding breast quadrant but conserving the remainder of the breast parenchyma.[73] Veronesi et al[74,75] published the Milan experience with quadrantectomy plus axillary dissection and radiation therapy in 1977 and 1981, demonstrating that this treatment is equivalent to the Halsted mastectomy in regard to local recurrence and overall survival rates.

In this technique, the incision incorporates any previous biopsy sites, generally in an elliptical fashion. The dissection proceeds by resection of a generous cone of normal breast tissue surrounding the tumor, continuing posteriorly to expose the pectoralis fascia. As originally described, if the tumor is close to the pectoralis major muscle, superficial muscle tissue is resected to achieve 2-cm margins.[73] This procedure achieves better aesthetic results with lesions in the upper-outer quadrant than it does for other areas, particularly for central or lower quadrant lesions. Whereas breast-conserving therapy is well within the standard of care for routine practice now, as recently as 2 decades ago it was not. Quadrantectomy has an important historical significance as a precursor to lumpectomy but has little role in modern breast surgery because it is unnecessarily disfiguring with no added benefit.

MASTECTOMY: TERMINOLOGY AND TECHNIQUES

The mastectomy procedure has evolved from the Halsted radical mastectomy, a procedure that involved a wide excision of all breast tissue, all overlying skin, and the pectoralis major muscle and a full en bloc dissection of level I, II, and III nodes. Because of the increased morbidity incurred without any demonstrated benefit in terms of local recurrence, radical mastectomies are rarely performed today. Several other types of mastectomy procedures are available to the breast surgeon. The most commonly performed mastectomy is the modified radical mastectomy, which removes all breast tissue including the nipple-areola complex, an ellipse of skin overlying the nipple-areola complex, and the axillary nodes en bloc. A skin-sparing mastectomy resects all breast tissue through a circumareolar incision but preserves the skin envelope, thus facilitating immediate reconstruction. The status of the axillary nodes may be determined by a sentinel lymph node dissection that is performed at the beginning of the extirpative procedure. A simple mastectomy involves the resection of all breast tissue and the nipple-areola complex (similar to a modified radical mastectomy) but does not include axillary lymphadenectomy. Total mastectomy implies that the surgeon resects all breast tissue, usually preserving the skin envelope. Because the term *mastectomy* implies complete removal of breast parenchyma, the term *total mastectomy* is not necessary. A subcutaneous mastectomy involves the use of a noncentral incision (such as an inframammary or axillary approach) to perform a mastectomy, thereby preserving the skin, skin envelope, and cutaneous portion of the nipple-areola complex. Again, all mastectomies involve a subcutaneous dissection where the skin envelope is preserved, so this term, like total mastectomy, is not helpful for the analysis of outcomes.

Breast tissue is distributed widely over the anterolateral chest and axilla. Haagensen[76] pointed out that breast parenchyma protrudes into the underlying pectoral muscles, extends along Cooper ligaments to the skin, may cross the midline, and laterally may reach the apex of the axilla. Temple et al[77] showed that breast tissue extends high into the axilla and is adherent to the pectoralis fascia. It is thus doubtful that any type of mastectomy can completely resect all breast tissue.[78]

Simple Mastectomy

Simple mastectomy is a total mastectomy without axillary node or sentinel node dissection. It involves resection of breast tissue, skin, and the nipple-areola complex through a wide elliptical skin incision with primary closure or reconstruction. The pectoral muscles and their fascia remain intact. The mastectomy is classified as simple mastectomy in contradistinction to modified radical mastectomy. However, the term *mastectomy* would suffice as the surgeon may designate whether sentinel node biopsy is performed with the mastectomy.

There are three other groups of patients for whom the risk of axillary nodal disease is so low that axillary lymph node dissection and sentinel node dissection can routinely be avoided: (1) patients with extensive ductal carcinoma in situ that cannot be managed with breast-conserving therapy because of multifocal disease, (2) patients with pure tubular carcinoma, and (3) patients with microinvasive carcinoma (these patients would typically be good candidates for breast-conserving therapy). Microinvasive carcinoma of the breast is defined in the TNM staging classification as "the extension of cancer cells beyond the basement membrane and into the adjacent tissue with no focus more than 0.1 cm in greatest dimension."[79] Patients with microinvasive carcinoma of the breast have a less than 10% rate of axillary nodal metastases; therefore, studies support therapy with local treatment alone because the cure rate approaches 100%.[80]

Most surgeons elect to perform sentinel node biopsy to document nodal status at the time of simple mastectomy for cancer. Simple mastectomy has the oncologic advantage of resection of all skin tissue as well as the nipple-areola complex, leaving no possibility of residual breast tissue behind from these sites; it is therefore considered the standard in terms of risk of local recurrence for ductal carcinoma in situ, for optimal prophylactic mastectomy, and for the treatment of recurrent disease previously managed with lumpectomy. This procedure may be performed alone or with a sentinel node dissection. If the sentinel node dissection is positive for malignant disease, formal axillary node dissection is performed. In this situation, the procedure is classified as a modified radical mastectomy rather than a simple mastectomy.

Total Mastectomy

Total mastectomy is a somewhat vague term usually referring to a simple mastectomy procedure with skin envelope preservation. Procedures designed to remove breast tissue in patients with increased risk for breast cancer or with chronic breast pain associated with fibrocystic disease were termed subcutaneous mastectomy. Because many of these patients had incomplete breast tissue removal often associated with breast implant insertion, the term *total mastectomy* was introduced to indicate a technique in which all breast tissue is removed; this term is itself a misnomer because many studies have shown that no mastectomy completely removes all breast tissue. The classic study that affirms this concept was performed by Goldman and Goldwyn[81] (Table 138-10); they performed subcutaneous mastectomies on six female cadavers with biopsy of all borders of the resection. They found residual breast tissue in each retroareolar area and in nearly all of the peripheral margin biopsy specimens. No study has been reported looking objectively at the percentage of residual breast tissue in simple or modified radical mastectomies, but many studies estimate that 90% to 95% of breast tissue is removed with these procedures (Fig. 138-8).[82]

TABLE 138-10 ✦ SITES OF REMNANT BREAST TISSUE AFTER SUBCUTANEOUS MASTECTOMY OF SIX CADAVERS

	Cadavers (6 total)
Subareolar remnant breast tissue	6
Unilateral remnant breast tissue (other than subareolar)	2
Bilateral remnant breast tissue (other than subareolar)	3
No remnant breast tissue (other than subareolar)	1

Modified from Goldman LD, Goldwyn RM: Some anatomical considerations of subcutaneous mastectomy. Plast Reconstr Surg 1977;51:501-505.

Subcutaneous Mastectomy

Subcutaneous mastectomy is another term for mastectomy. The term initially designated procedures designed to remove breast tissue prophylactically for patients with increased risk for later development of breast cancer and patients in whom surveillance is difficult because of size and shape of the breast. Unfortunately, because the incision is remote to breast tissue (inframammary or axillary incision), this procedure will often not allow complete removal of breast parenchyma. However, if it is performed as a prophylactic procedure in a patient with high risk for future development of breast carcinoma or as a mastectomy technique for documented stage I disease, it may be an effective surgical approach. Studies in the last decade have shown that subcutaneous mastectomy for stage I and stage II breast cancer has local recurrence rates similar to those of simple mastectomy.[83] The subcutaneous mastectomy technique may be performed with either an inframammary or axillary incision. Both incisions permit access to the axilla for clearance of level I and II lymph nodes. Flaps are elevated at approximately 5-mm-thick skin flaps (or by visualization that all breast tissue is dissected off fatty tissue or skin). The flap is raised from the incision to the sternal border medially, superiorly to the clavicle, and inferiorly to the inframammary crease. The surgeon attempts to perform a complete mastectomy through this incision, but unlike in the simple mastectomy, all the skin and the nipple-areola complex are left intact (Fig. 138-9).

Numerous indications for unilateral or bilateral subcutaneous mastectomy have been described.[84,85] Indications for the procedure include fibrocystic disease with multiple biopsies that result in extensive scarring; proliferative epithelial changes in postmenopausal patients (not receiving exogenous hormones); lobular carcinoma in situ or lobular neoplasm[86]; premalignant disease proven by one or more biopsies in which epithelial proliferation, atypical ductal or lobular hyperplasia, cellular atypia, or florid papillomatosis is the predominant finding; family history of bilateral

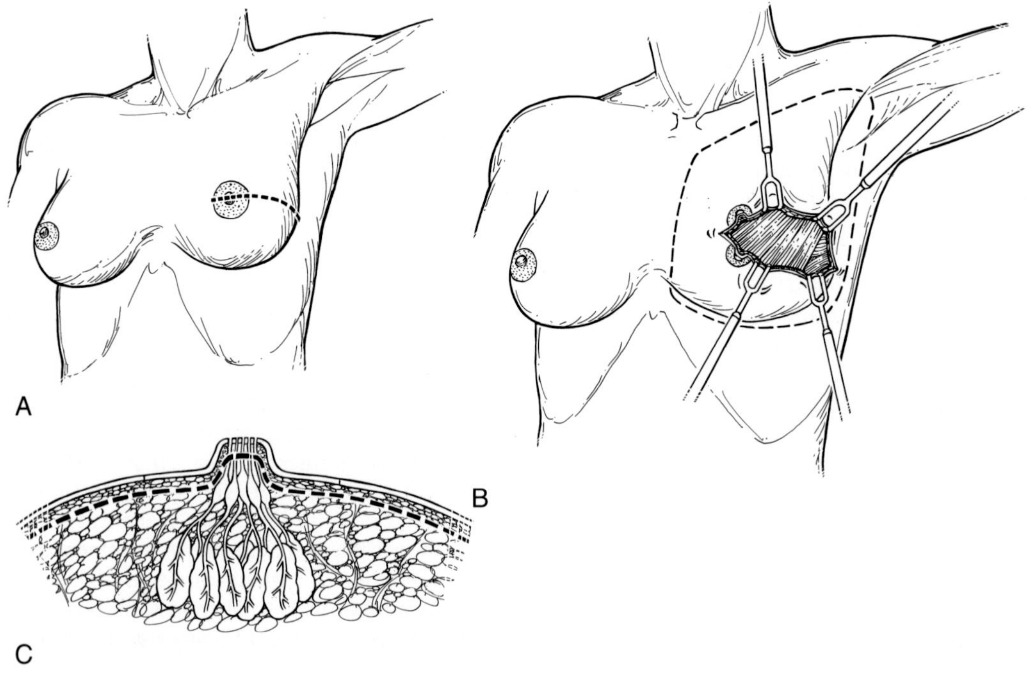

FIGURE 138-8. *A* to *C,* Total mastectomy with a central incision.

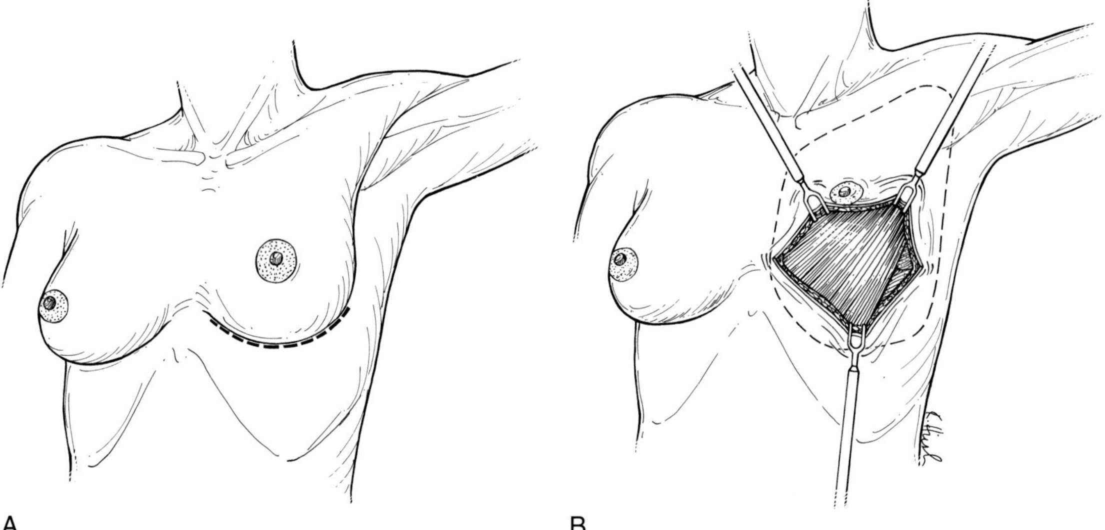

FIGURE 138-9. Subcutaneous mastectomy. *A,* Incision placement. *B,* The extent of resection is indicated with a dashed line.

premenopausal breast cancer or other strong genetic predisposition; chronic mastitis with recurrent infections refractory to conservative treatment; selected patients with mastodynia refractory to treatment; parenchymal loss or scarring resulting from trauma, infection, or previous biopsies; proven malignant disease in one breast and a suspicious mammogram of the other; large benign breast tumors; cancer phobia associated with a realistic risk of breast cancer; and silicone mastopathy from silicone injections.[87]

Whereas some centers support use of the subcutaneous mastectomy for primary breast cancer or ductal carcinoma in situ, in general, it is not recommended for these indications. It is extremely difficult to perform an adequate cancer operation through a remote breast incision (inframammary or axillary incision). The incision needs to be centrally located to adequately visualize the thickness of skin flaps and to ensure that the mastectomy plane is equivalent to a modified radical mastectomy. In addition, the breast flap below the nipple-areola complex is subject to ischemia because of partial devascularization. The nipple-areola complex is preserved with this procedure, increasing the likelihood of residual breast tissue and the risk for later cancer development. Historically, many patients who underwent a subcutaneous mastectomy did not have an adequate resection for these reasons. There is a certain negative connotation associated with this procedure from the many reports of incomplete resections. Obviously, all mastectomies are subcutaneous in regard to technique. Because subcutaneous mastectomy implies an incision distant from the nipple-areola complex, it is probably not an adequate approach to prophylactic mastectomy.

Cheung et al[88] reported similar rates of local recurrence between subcutaneous mastectomy (16%) and simple mastectomy (14%) for invasive cancer in their series; this study included only patients who underwent either of these operations without postoperative irradiation. This study included 134 patients who underwent subcutaneous mastectomy without irradiation. They noted that in those patients with local recurrence, four of five were located in the nipple. On the basis of this finding, they adjusted their practice so that those subcutaneous mastectomy patients in whom the nipple was noted to be microscopically involved and those with poor histologic grade, nodal involvement, or lymphovascular invasion were given prophylactic flap irradiation or radiation treatment directed at the nipple, as appropriate. They argue that subcutaneous mastectomy is less expensive and quicker to perform than reconstructive flap procedures such as transverse rectus abdominis musculocutaneous (TRAM) or latissimus dorsi flaps. They favored prosthetic implant placement after subcutaneous mastectomy. However, this may result in increased scarring and significant risk of implant complications if radiation therapy is used. Their postoperative complications included skin flap or areola necrosis, wound infection, hematoma formation, and capsule formation.

Al-Ghazal et al[89] reported a series of 101 patients who had subcutaneous mastectomy with implant reconstruction for treatment of primary breast cancer. They found the following factors to be associated with improved result with this technique: submuscular insertion of the implant, lateral incision approach, and immediate insertion of the prosthesis. They find that subcutaneous mastectomy with immediate reconstruction as a one-stage procedure is safe and gives a better aesthetic result and higher satisfaction of patients than a two-stage procedure does, in agreement with Ward and Edwards.[90] They noted that the major criticisms of this technique are early local recurrence and capsular contracture.[91,92]

Sufi et al[93] reported a small series of patients who underwent subcutaneous mastectomy with immediate reconstruction with a latissimus dorsi flap plus a tissue expander. They reported using a lazy S vertical incision in the midaxillary line to perform the mastectomy, axillary dissection, and elevation of an ipsilateral latissimus dorsi flap. All breast tissue is removed from the back of the nipple, leaving only the skin. They contend that reconstruction with a component of autologous tissue provides superior cosmetic results compared with implants alone.[93,94]

Although use of autologous tissue when possible is mainstream practice today for breast reconstruction, the idea of nipple preservation is not—it is a highly controversial topic. Subcutaneous mastectomy is well accepted by some centers on the basis of these data; however, others are reluctant to offer this procedure on the basis of existing data because of concerns of potential involvement of the nipple-areola complex. Because subcutaneous mastectomy implies an incision distant from the nipple-areola complex, this approach may imply inadequate management of the nipple-areola complex. An approach directly involving the nipple-areola complex may be more effective in removal of breast parenchyma.

Total Mastectomy Versus Subcutaneous Mastectomy

Both terms as techniques for breast removal have different connotations based on indications and extent of breast tissue removal. Total mastectomy is essentially a simple mastectomy with skin envelope preservation. The incision includes nipple or nipple-areola complex removal, with care taken to remove all ductal tissue. Subcutaneous mastectomy implies removal of all breast tissue, but this term is generally used in conjunction with an inframammary or axillary incision with preservation of the nipple and areola. Peripheral incisions with preservation of the nipple-areola complex generally leave breast tissue directly beneath the nipple-areola complex. This technique may allow development of a new primary cancer in the retained breast tissue.

Some centers use a rigorous approach to breast tissue extirpation including the subareolar region and report excellent long-term follow-up documenting no cancer development in high-risk patients. In general, the term *skin-sparing mastectomy* is preferred to describe prophylactic mastectomy in which the skin envelope is preserved and the areola may be preserved.

Skin-Sparing Mastectomy

For women who will require mastectomy as the surgical management of their breast cancer, skin-sparing mastectomy with immediate reconstruction is an excellent choice for complete breast parenchyma resection and acceptable breast mound provided by an implant or flap. This procedure preserves as much of the patient's breast skin as possible—the breast parenchyma, nipple-areola contents, and at times axillary contents are removed through a circumareolar incision (sentinel lymph node dissection may be performed through a separate incision first if it is indicated). Any existing biopsy scar may be resected along with the main specimen. By preserving the inframammary fold and native skin envelope, the plastic surgeon can reconstruct a breast that is an excellent match to the contralateral breast in size, color, and shape.[95]

The operation for skin-sparing mastectomy is technically more difficult than traditional mastectomy because of decreased exposure secondary to a smaller incision. Five types of incisions are described: periareolar incision, tennis-racket incision (periareolar with a lateral extension for better access to the axilla), reduction mammaplasty incision (periareolar with extension inferiorly), modified elliptical incision encircling the areola, and periareolar incision with medial and lateral extensions.[96] Many surgeons have been trending toward use of the periareolar incision as they become more familiar with technical aspects of the procedure.[97,98] This approach is technically more challenging than others unless the areola is wide relative to the breast size.

The surgical team of general and plastic surgeons mark the skin preoperatively. If the tumor is superficial, the incision is carefully planned to remove any breast skin required to obtain a negative margin (particularly any tumor within 1 cm of breast skin)—this point is imperative (Figs. 138-10 to 138-12). If the tumor is

FIGURE 138-10. Skin-sparing mastectomy. *A*, Incision placement for skin-preserving mastectomy with sentinel node dissection. Note that the surgeon has elected not to excise the previous core biopsy site in this example. *B*, Extent of resection. Although the incision is circumareolar, the surgeon attempts to perform the same extent of resection as would be accomplished with a simple mastectomy. *C*, Wider periareolar incision secondary to tumor in retroareolar location. With a retroareolar tumor, the surgical oncologist may attempt a skin-preserving mastectomy with a wider extent of resection *(D)*. *E*, Skin-preserving mastectomy with excision of biopsy site. The dashed line indicates a tennis-racket incision for resection of previous excisional biopsy site and extent of resection *(F)*.

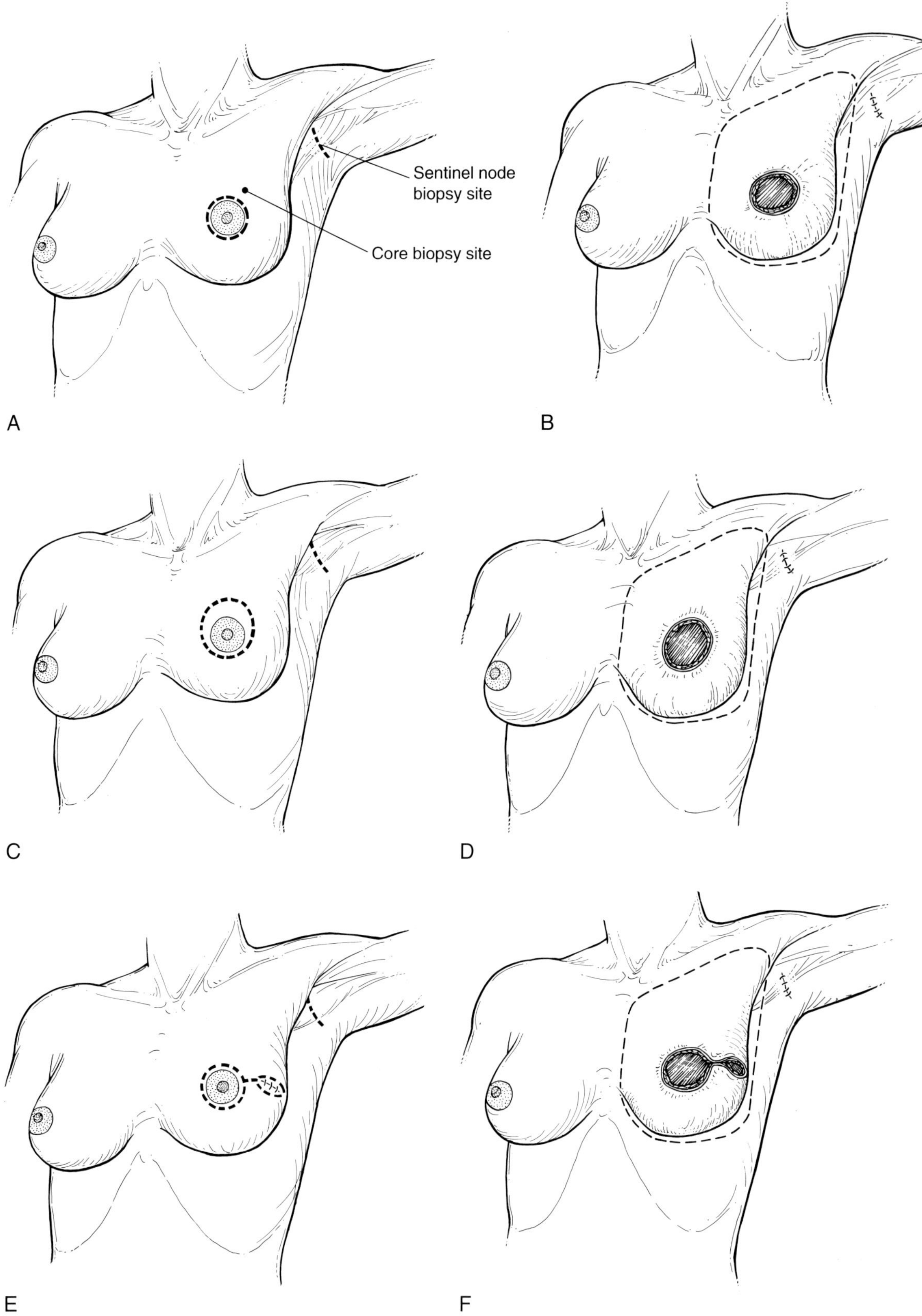
Sentinel node
biopsy site
Core biopsy site
A
B
C
D
E
F

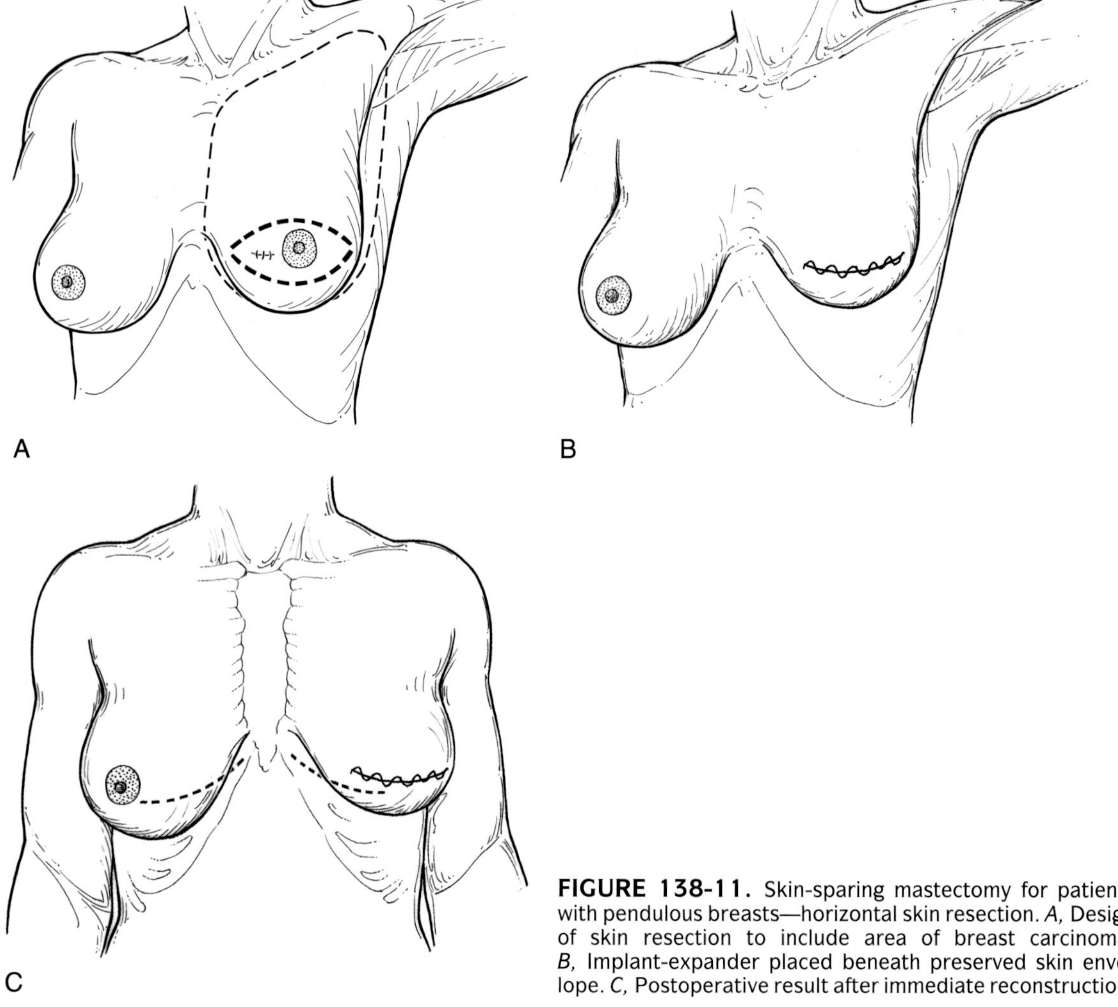

FIGURE 138-11. Skin-sparing mastectomy for patients with pendulous breasts—horizontal skin resection. *A,* Design of skin resection to include area of breast carcinoma. *B,* Implant-expander placed beneath preserved skin envelope. *C,* Postoperative result after immediate reconstruction.

deep within the breast, no additional skin is resected. Singletary et al[95] recommend excision of previous biopsy incisions with 1-cm margins. By use of electrocautery, the skin flap is elevated circumareolarly with the assistance of fine-tipped skin hooks for skin retraction. It is unnecessary and undesirable to make unusually thin skin flaps because no improvement in the rate of local recurrence is gained; very thin skin flaps often result in flap necrosis and poor cosmetic outcome. The flaps are dissected and the breast is resected en bloc off the pectoralis major muscle, leaving its fascia intact.

If desired, an axillary nodal dissection or sentinel node dissection may be performed. It has been shown that axillary nodal dissections yield equivalent results when they are performed in conjunction with either skin-sparing mastectomy or modified radical mastectomy.[99] Sentinel node dissection may be performed immediately before skin-sparing mastectomy through a separate incision in the axilla in the standard fashion (see "Sentinel Lymph Node Biopsy").

Several studies have shown that skin-sparing mastectomy has an acceptable rate of local recurrence compared with traditional mastectomy. Local recurrence is defined as biopsy-proven carcinoma in the skin flaps, muscle flaps, or flaps incorporated into the breast reconstruction procedure. Kroll et al[100] studied 154 patients with stage I or stage II breast cancer; 114 had skin-sparing mastectomies and 40 had non–skin-sparing mastectomies. The local recurrence rate in the skin-sparing mastectomy cohort was 7.0%; in the conventional mastectomy group, it was 7.5%. Simmons et al[99] studied 231 patients treated with mastectomy; 77 had skin-sparing mastectomy and 154 had non–skin-sparing mastectomy. They found local recurrence rates of 5.6% for skin-sparing mastectomy and 3.9% for non–skin-sparing mastectomy. Carlson et al[101] found a local recurrence rate of 4.8% in 187 patients

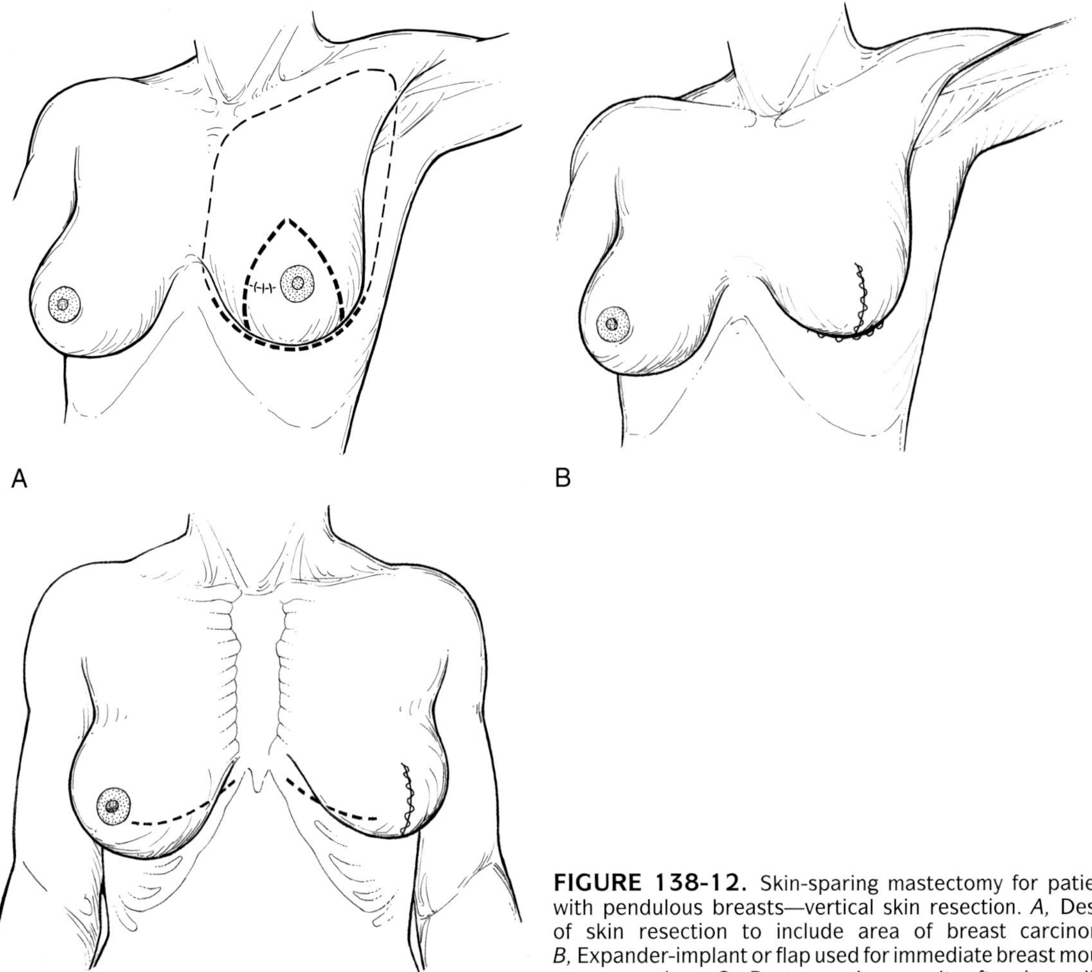

FIGURE 138-12. Skin-sparing mastectomy for patients with pendulous breasts—vertical skin resection. *A,* Design of skin resection to include area of breast carcinoma. *B,* Expander-implant or flap used for immediate breast mound reconstruction. *C,* Postoperative result after immediate closure with inverted T to re-establish breast envelope.

with skin-sparing mastectomy and a rate of 9.5% for non–skin-sparing mastectomy. Newman et al[102] reported one of the largest series in the current literature addressing the incidence of local recurrence for skin-sparing mastectomy. They found a local recurrence rate of 6.2% for 437 skin-sparing mastectomies; for their non–skin-sparing mastectomies, their rate was 7.4%. Based on these series and others, the local recurrence rates for skin-sparing mastectomy and modified radical mastectomy are equivalent (Table 138-11).

Slavin et al[97] studied 32 consecutive skin-sparing mastectomy patients; an incision was made with a 5-mm border margin of skin circumareolar for each operation. Multiple biopsy specimens of the remaining skin edges were obtained by excision of strips measuring roughly 1 cm in length by 3 to 4 mm in width; this skin represents tissue that would have been excised if a traditional modified radical mastectomy had been performed. Each of the 114 biopsy specimens was assessed histologically, and no specimens revealed evidence of any breast ducts in the dermis.

The skin of the chest wall is the most frequent site of local recurrence after skin-sparing mastectomy. Slavin et al[97] argued that local recurrence should be viewed as representing a matter of aggressive tumor biology more than failed operative technique. Standard practice is resection of skin to achieve negative 1- to 2-cm margins but otherwise no resection of additional skin unless for the purpose of clear margins.

Local recurrence has been found to be an independent variable in prediction of survival after skin-sparing mastectomy. In the study by Newman[102] referred to before, 14 of 23 skin-sparing mastectomy patients with local recurrence were alive and free of disease at a median follow-up of 26 months. Of 23 patients, 7 died of metastatic disease at a median interval of 18 months postoperatively. Two were alive with persistent but stable distant disease and one patient was alive with stable local disease but no evidence of

TABLE 138-11 ✦ LOCAL AND SYSTEMIC RECURRENCE RATES AFTER SKIN-SPARING MASTECTOMY

Summary of studies of local recurrence (LR) data for skin-sparing mastectomy (SSM) compared with non–skin-sparing mastectomy (non-SSM) for invasive cancer

First Author	*No. of SSM*	*No. of non-SSM*	*LR for SSM (%)*	*LR for non-SSM (%)*	*Mean Follow-up (years)*
Kroll[100]	114	40	7.0	7.5	6
Simmons[99]	77	154	3.9	3.25	5
Carlson[101]	327	188	4.8	9.5	3.4

Summary of studies of local and systemic recurrence after SSM

First Author	*No. of SSM*	*LR for SSM (%)*	*Systemic Recurrence (%) after LR with SSM*	*Mean Follow-up (months)*
Newman[102]	437	6.2	39	50
Carlson[107]	565	5.5	77.4	78.1
Medina-Franco[103]	176	4.5	75	73

distant disease at a median follow-up of 26 months. Most of the skin-sparing mastectomy patients in this series who had recurrence were managed with a multidisciplinary approach of local control by limited surgical resection, radiotherapy, and systemic therapy. Simmons et al[99] also examined the local and distant recurrence rates of skin-sparing mastectomies by comparing these patients with a matched-stage cohort who underwent non–skin-sparing mastectomy. They found the 5-year survival rate for skin-sparing mastectomy patients with local recurrences to be 95.29%; for non–skin-sparing mastectomy patients with local recurrence, the 5-year survival rate was 95.18%. The distant recurrence rates for skin-sparing mastectomy and conventional mastectomy were equivalent in this study at 3.9% (3 of 77 patients and 6 of 154 patients, respectively). In another series, patients had a 5-year survival rate of 90% when no local recurrence developed, but the 5-year survival rate dropped to 50% in patients with local recurrence, suggesting the close link between local recurrence and systemic disease.[103] Historically, patients undergoing conventional mastectomy who manifest local recurrence have a 30% to 60% rate of synchronous metastatic disease, with a corresponding overall survival of 18% to 42% at 5 years.[104-106] As stated by Carlson[107] in an editorial reviewing the data on local recurrence after skin-sparing mastectomy, longer follow-up periods and additional studies are required for any firm conclusions to be made on prognosis after local recurrence in skin-sparing mastectomy patients.

There is limited evidence on what stages of breast cancer are appropriate to undergo skin-sparing mastectomy. In a commentary by Danforth[108] of a study by Rivadeneira et al,[109] the authors noted that 45% of the study patients had stage 0 or stage I breast cancer; there were no local or regional recurrences with either skin-sparing or non–skin-sparing mastectomies. Danforth suggested that these patients appear to be the best candidates for skin-sparing mastectomy. The local recurrence rate for patients assigned to stage II was 11.5% (3 of 26); for patients assigned to stage III, it was 25%[108] with skin-sparing mastectomy (not very many patients with stage III disease were included in this study). Kroll[100] generally excluded patients with stage III or stage IV disease from undergoing skin-sparing mastectomy.

Skin-sparing mastectomy has been used in patients with locally advanced breast cancers (stage IIB and stage III).[110] In this population, because of the frequent need for neoadjuvant or adjuvant therapy, special concerns arise. These issues involve risk of delaying postoperative chemotherapy or radiation therapy because of surgical recovery from skin-sparing mastectomy or reconstruction, poor wound healing, and thus poor cosmetic result overall secondary to chemotherapy or radiation therapy. Foster et al[110] reported a series of 25 patients with locally advanced breast cancer (stage IIB and stage III) who underwent skin-sparing mastectomy with reconstruction.[110] In addition to their surgical procedure, the patients in this study received the following therapies: 52% neoadjuvant chemotherapy, 92% postoperative chemotherapy, and 48% postoperative radiation therapy. The local recurrence rate in this series was 4% at an average of 4 years of follow-up. Few centers have studied the use of skin-sparing mastectomy for locally advanced disease. This initial report is favorable and suggests that further investigation is warranted. More data will be necessary to better determine the safety of skin-sparing mastectomy for this population; however, initial results with autologous reconstruction appear to be promising for this population.

Prophylactic Mastectomy

The most common indications for prophylactic mastectomy include women with a known genetic predisposition for breast cancer and those with a unilateral breast cancer desiring contralateral prophylactic mastectomy. The Society of Surgical Oncology[111] established a position statement describing indications for consideration of prophylactic mastectomy (Table 138-12).

Genetic testing for susceptibility to breast cancer should include screening for *BRCA1, BRCA2,* Cowden disease, Li-Fraumeni syndrome, and ataxia-telangiectasia.[112] As advances in genetic testing have made it possible to identify patients with a genetic predisposition to breast cancer (most commonly *BRCA1* or *BRCA2*), more patients are now undergoing these tests and seeking recommendations from clinicians concerning the preventive measures available. Breast oncologists, general surgeons, and plastic surgeons will increasingly be asked about the data supporting prophylactic mastectomy as use of genetic testing increases.

Five percent to 10% of breast cancer results from an inheritable genetic mutation. Patients with *BRCA1* or *BRCA2* mutations have a 40% to 85% lifetime risk for breast cancer. In addition, age at diagnosis of the *BRCA* mutation is an important factor to consider. Schrag et al[113] performed mathematical analyses of the benefits of prophylactic mastectomy for patients with *BRCA* mutations. They found that a 30-year-old woman with a *BRCA* mutation who undergoes prophylactic mastectomy could expect an additional survival of 2.9 to 5.3 years; a 60-year-old woman with a *BRCA* mutation undergoing prophylactic mastectomy would gain negligible benefit. Those *BRCA* mutation carriers who reach 60 years of age without developing a breast cancer have a favorable risk profile; by this age, other comorbidities compete for cause of death, and thus there is less benefit to prophylactic mastectomy for these patients.

TABLE 138-12 ✦ SOCIETY OF SURGICAL ONCOLOGY POSITION STATEMENT ON INDICATIONS FOR CONSIDERATION OF PROPHYLACTIC MASTECTOMY[111]

Women with no prior history of breast cancer
Atypical hyperplasia
Family history of premenopausal bilateral breast cancer
Women with unilateral breast cancer (contralateral breast)
Diffuse microcalcifications
Lobular carcinoma in situ
Large breast, difficult to evaluate
History of lobular carcinoma in situ followed by unilateral breast cancer
History of atypical hyperplasia
Primary family history
Age at diagnosis <40 years

Verhoog et al[114] studied the risk of contralateral breast cancer in 164 patients with a proven *BRCA1* mutation and a primary breast cancer. They studied age at diagnosis of the first breast cancer in relation to risk for development of a contralateral breast cancer during a 10-year period of follow-up. Of the 124 *BRCA1* patients who were younger than 50 years at initial diagnosis of breast cancer, 40% developed a contralateral breast cancer, in contrast to 12% of the 40 patients older than 50 years at initial diagnosis of breast cancer.

In the current era of breast-conserving surgery, some patients and surgeons have had difficulty accepting prophylactic mastectomy because it is a more radical procedure performed on those without cancer than what is often being offered to patients with early-stage breast cancer (lumpectomy and radiation therapy). However, the multifocal predisposition for cancer development within the breast parenchyma does not allow preservation of breast tissue as is now possible with isolated invasive cancer in specific segments of the breast. There are historical precedents for prophylactic surgery for those with hereditary predispositions for cancer. Prophylactic resections are the standard of care for conditions such as familial adenomatous polyposis (prophylactic colectomy) and multiple endocrine neoplasia type 2 (prophylactic thyroidectomy).[82] As the use of genetic testing for *BRCA1* and *BRCA2* genes increases, there will be increased interest on the part of patients and clinicians alike for prophylactic mastectomy.

Three types of mastectomies are currently being performed prophylactically. The term *prophylactic mastectomy* itself has no descriptive value regarding the skin envelope. A total (simple) mastectomy excises the nipple-areola complex, all visible breast tissue, and an ellipse of skin such that primary closure may still be accomplished. A subcutaneous mastectomy resects all visible breast tissue through an inframammary or axillary incision, leaving the nipple-areola complex and skin intact. A skin-sparing mastectomy removes all visible breast tissue through a transverse incision bisecting the nipple-areola complex or a circumareolar incision with preservation of only the cutaneous component of the nipple-areola complex (Fig. 138-13). Although historically the subcutaneous mastectomy was frequently used for prophylaxis, most surgeons currently do not favor attempting to excise all breast tissue through an inframammary or axillary

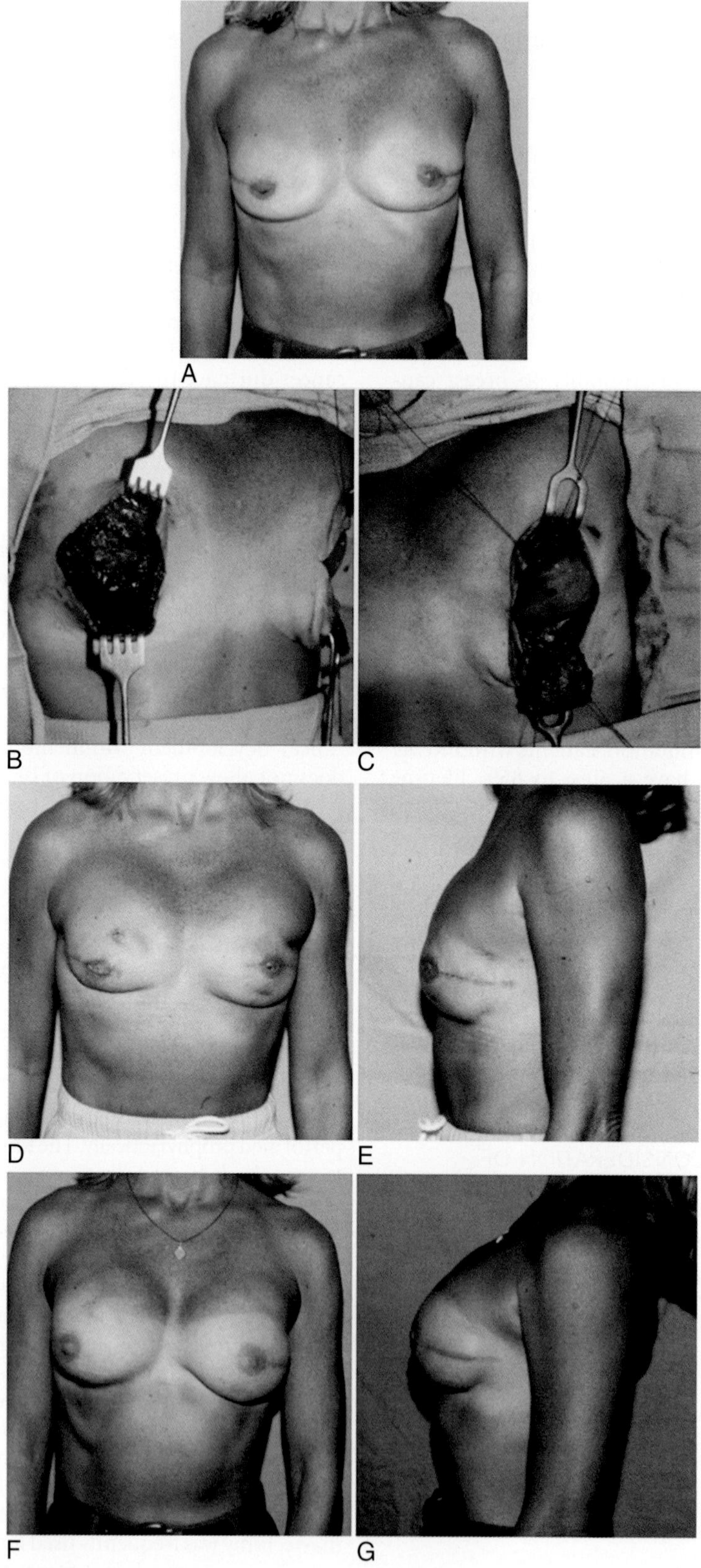

FIGURE 138-13. See *legend on opposite page.*

incision because it is extremely difficult to perform a mastectomy properly through a noncentral incision (as was previously discussed in the section on subcutaneous mastectomies; see "Simple Mastectomy," "Subcutaneous Mastectomy," and "Skin-Sparing Mastectomy" for a more detailed discussion of these techniques). No mastectomy is likely to completely eradicate all breast tissue; therefore, consideration must be given to how to perform the best possible mastectomy by the selected approach.

Hartmann et al[115] reported the Mayo Clinic experience with bilateral prophylactic mastectomies between 1960 and 1993. They found that 1065 women had undergone bilateral prophylactic mastectomies, and of these, 639 women had a family history of breast cancer. Subcutaneous mastectomies were performed for 90% of the patients; they describe their procedure as removal of 90% or more of the breast tissue with residual tissue left immediately under the nipple and areola, where it is easily palpable. Of these patients, 94% then had immediate breast reconstruction. This study represents one of the largest reported experiences with subcutaneous mastectomies for prophylaxis. They compared the incidence of breast cancer development in the high-risk population of the study patients with the incidence of breast cancer development in their sisters (who did not undergo prophylaxis) and found that prophylactic mastectomy resulted in a 90% reduction in incidence of breast cancer for those at high risk on the basis of family history.

Another consideration is elective synchronous contralateral prophylactic mastectomy at the time of ipsilateral mastectomy for a primary breast cancer. Gershenwald et al[116] reviewed the M.D. Anderson experience with synchronous elective contralateral mastectomy. They concluded that for a carefully chosen population of a young age, with anticipated difficulties in following clinical or mammographic surveillance, and with an increased lifetime risk (based on family history) for development of a second primary breast cancer, elective contralateral mastectomy is indicated. This procedure should be offered only if the primary tumor is resected with curative intent—that is, no evidence of distant disease is noted.

FIGURE 138-13. *A*, Postoperative anterior view of prior partial bilateral mastectomy for silicone mastitis (the patient has previously undergone non-medical grade liquid silicone injections). *B*, Right mastectomy defect. The expander is in place beneath the pectoralis muscle superiorly. The inferior segmental rectus flap is elevated for expander coverage. *C*, Left pectoralis major muscle with inferior segmental rectus–external oblique flap provides expander-implant coverage. *D*, Postoperative anterior view after bilateral prophylactic mastectomy. Subpectoral and regional rectus flaps and expanders are in place. *E*, Lateral postoperative view. *F*, Anterior postoperative view at 1 year with permanent saline implants in place. *G*, Lateral postoperative view.

Modified Radical Mastectomy

Modified radical mastectomy is the most common treatment of stage I and stage II breast cancer, despite the increasing use of breast-conserving therapy.[117,118] Patients with stage III disease are usually treated with neoadjuvant therapy before modified radical mastectomy. In general, patients with stage IV disease require palliative mastectomy to control tumor growth on the chest wall, but treatment is directed toward systemic therapy.

In an analysis of predictive factors for local recurrence in 1289 patients treated with mastectomy, moderate or high histologic grade (II or III) and extensive axillary node involvement (10 nodes or more) were found to be statistically significant factors.[71]

Modified radical mastectomy removes the breast tissue, the nipple-areola complex, and the ipsilateral axillary lymph nodes en bloc. The pectoralis major fascia is left intact to facilitate implant reconstruction. Variations of the procedure, such as removal of the pectoralis minor muscle, division of the pectoralis minor tendon for better axillary exposure, and resection of the fascia of the pectoralis major, are not required.[119] Tumor located adjacent to the pectoralis muscle with possible muscle involvement may warrant muscle resection.

The incision is marked as an ellipse to include the nipple-areola complex, any previous biopsy site, and any excess breast skin (Fig. 138-14). Care should be taken to avoid extension of the incision medial to the sternum or lateral to the breast mound because this will produce dog-ears.[119] Skin edges are elevated with skin hooks while skin flaps are dissected with electrocautery. A plane between the subcutaneous fat and breast parenchyma is defined; the surgeon palpates frequently to ensure that the breast tissue is being adequately dissected without forming a "buttonhole" through the skin. The dissection proceeds superiorly to the level of the clavicle, medially to the level of the sternum, inferiorly to the superior aspect of the rectus sheath, and laterally to the latissimus dorsi muscle. The breast is dissected free of the pectoralis fascia but left attached at the lateral edge to provide countertraction during axillary dissection. The technique of axillary dissection as part of the modified radical mastectomy procedure is identical to the technique when axillary dissection is performed as a separate procedure and is discussed later. The wound is irrigated, and hemostasis is carefully obtained. A closed suction drain is placed in the mastectomy cavity and brought out through a separate stab incision. If no immediate reconstruction is planned, deep dermal interrupted 3-0 absorbable

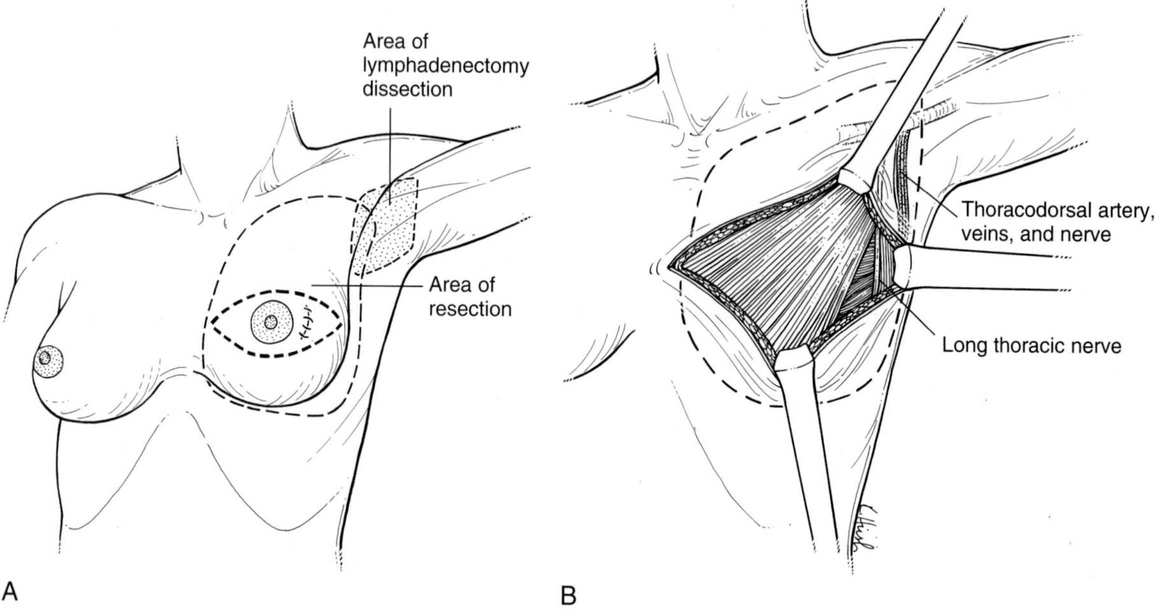

FIGURE 138-14. Modified radical mastectomy. *A,* Incision placement. *B,* Extent of resection.

sutures are placed to reapproximate the wound followed by a running subcuticular 4-0 absorbable suture. Patients generally remain in the hospital overnight unless they prefer otherwise and are medically able to be discharged the same day. The next day, the dressings are removed and the patient receives instructions in caring for the drain. Instructions for arm exercises are provided before discharge. The drain is removed in the office when the output is less than 30 mL per day. To ensure adequate wound healing, chemotherapy or radiotherapy commences at least 2 weeks after surgery.

Radical Mastectomy

The Halsted procedure, which is now used infrequently and not recommended, is the most common type of radical mastectomy. This procedure involves making a large oblique elliptical incision that extends to the axillary fossa. The pectoralis major and minor muscles are completely removed along with the breast specimen. A complete axillary lymphadenectomy (levels I, II, and III) is performed as well.

Fisher et al[120] published the 25-year follow-up of the National Surgical Adjuvant Breast and Bowel Project (NSABP). This prospective, randomized study compared the 25-year outcomes for 1765 women who were treated for primary breast cancer. Of the patients with clinically negative axillary nodes, one third underwent a Halsted radical mastectomy, one third underwent total mastectomy without axillary dissection but with regional radiation therapy, and one third underwent total mastectomy alone without any axillary treatment. Of the patients with clinically positive axillary nodes, half underwent radical mastectomy and the other half underwent total mastectomy and regional axillary radiation therapy. Hazard ratio is defined as the odds that an adverse outcome will occur; hazard ratios less than 1 indicate that the treatment reduced the odds of the adverse outcome being studied, whereas hazard ratios greater than 1 indicate that the treatment failed to reduce the odds of the adverse outcome. Among patients with clinically negative nodes, the hazard ratio for death among those treated with total mastectomy plus axillary radiation therapy was 1.08 compared with those treated with radical mastectomy—essentially equivalent. The hazard ratio for node-negative women who underwent total mastectomy without radiation therapy was

1.03 compared with those treated with radical mastectomy, again equivalent results. Among those patients with clinically positive nodes, the hazard ratio for death among those who underwent total mastectomy and radiation therapy was 1.06 compared with radical mastectomy. This large study with long-term follow-up failed to show any significant survival benefit to removal of occult positive nodes. They estimated that because of the randomization process, 40% of those patients who underwent total mastectomy had positive nodes that were not removed at the time of the initial surgery. This study also emphasizes the importance of long-term follow-up for determination of breast cancer prognosis; 25% of recurrences and 50% of contralateral breast carcinomas were diagnosed 5 years after mastectomy.

PRESERVATION OF THE NIPPLE-AREOLA COMPLEX

The literature is quite divided on the issue of whether the nipple-areola complex may ever safely be spared in a mastectomy. Fisher et al[121] published the NSABP Protocol B-06, which randomized women with tumors smaller than 4 cm in diameter (regardless of nodal status) to one of three treatment arms: mastectomy, lumpectomy alone, or lumpectomy with radiation therapy. No survival advantage was found for any of the treatment groups after 12 years of follow-up. Jensen[122] used this study to argue that since the nipple-areola complex was spared in two thirds of the patients in this study and no survival difference was found between treatment groups, it is safe to spare the nipple-areola complex when surgical margins are clear.

Laronga et al[123] retrospectively looked at 286 mastectomy specimens from patients who had skin-sparing mastectomies. Occult tumor involving the nipple-areola complex was found in 5.6%. They cited multiple older studies that found the risk of occult nipple-areola complex involvement to be increased with increasing proximity of the primary to the nipple-areola complex, tumor larger than 2 cm, poorly differentiated histologic features, and positive axillary lymph nodes.[124-126] On the basis of these findings, they contend that women who have small, solitary tumors on the periphery of the breast with no detectable metastatic lymph nodes are good candidates for skin-sparing mastectomy with nipple-areola preservation.[123]

Simmons et al[127] published a study in which the mastectomy specimens of 217 patients were retrospectively analyzed to look for frequency of malignant nipple or areola involvement. Specimens were sectioned at 3-mm intervals across the nipple and by tangential sectioning of the remaining nipple-areola tissue. The overall frequency of nipple involvement was 10.6%. Those patients with tumors smaller than 2 cm, peripheral tumors, and two or fewer positive nodes had an incidence of 6.7% nipple involvement. They concluded that nipple preservation is not a reasonable option for mastectomy patients.

Cense et al[128] reviewed the literature on the frequency and predictive factors of nipple involvement. They concluded that the risk is lowest in patients with tumor smaller than 2 cm (T1) and at a distance of 2.5 cm or more from the nipple-areola complex. These patients would benefit the most from breast-conserving therapy. They propose that for this set of patients who choose mastectomy when they are offered breast-conserving therapy, the surgeon could offer a nipple-sparing procedure with immediate reconstruction. They noted that if a woman chooses mastectomy because she is at high risk for a recurrence or second primary due to a genetic predisposition, a nipple-sparing mastectomy may not be the wisest choice of procedure as it leaves more residual breast tissue behind than other procedures do. There have been numerous reports of breast cancer in residual tissue after subcutaneous mastectomy performed for prophylaxis.[115,129,130] More studies will be necessary to safely delineate whether it is ever safe to spare the nipple-areola complex in the surgical management of invasive breast cancer. Until there is further evidence regarding the safety of nipple-sparing procedures, these operations are not recommended for breast cancers outside of clinical studies. Procedures designed to preserve the nipple-areola complex (such as subcutaneous mastectomy) should be offered to patients who are at high risk for breast cancer but without an actual current diagnosis of breast cancer. If it is more than 2 cm distant from the primary tumor, the nipple-areola complex epidermis may technically be preserved after all ducts have been excised. Preservation of the epidermal components of the nipple-areola complex requires precise removal of all ductal tissue. Resultant wound contracture generally reduces nipple projection, and nipple loss is possible due to vascular insufficiency; however, areola survival is fairly constant if the incision is in proximity to the nipple-areola complex.

SENTINEL LYMPH NODE BIOPSY

The single most important predictor of survival in patients with breast cancer is the histologic status of the axillary lymph nodes.[131] Most breast cancers are currently detected in stage I or stage II; as breast cancer surgical management of the primary tumor has evolved to more conservative procedures, so too has the management of the axillary nodes of the breast cancer patient. Sentinel lymph node (SLN) dissection is a minimally invasive alternative to a formal axillary node dissection that has the potential to spare 70% to 80% of patients a more extensive axillary dissection because only 30% of breast cancers today have

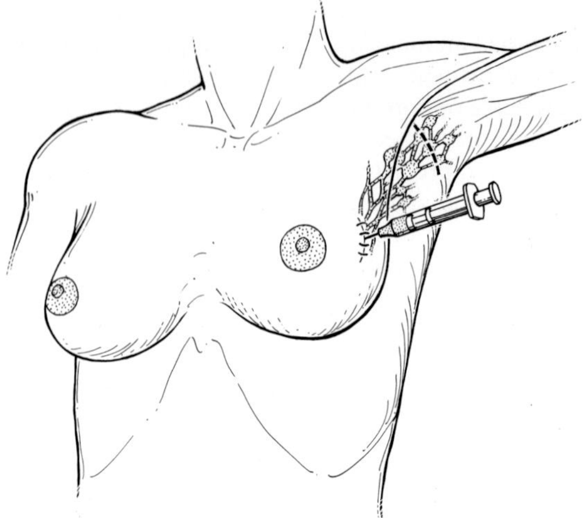

FIGURE 138-15. Sentinel lymph node procedure consisting of intraoperative injection of vital blue dye and/or radioactive sulfur colloid for mapping of lymphatics.

axillary metastases on presentation.[132] The SLN is defined as the node or nodes that most directly drain the tumor bed, and this node should be positive histologically first if any axillary metastasis has occurred. If the SLN is found to be negative on pathologic evaluation with hematoxylin and eosin staining, no further axillary dissection is required; if it is found to be positive for cancer cells, an axillary node dissection is indicated.

The procedure involves an intradermal injection of a vital blue dye (1% Lymphazurin) or radioactive sulfur colloid to localize the first lymph node that drains the tumor (Fig. 138-15). This approach was introduced for breast cancer surgery in the mid-1990s and has been successfully used to locate the first node or collection of nodes from which metastasis from breast cancer spreads. This node is most often an axillary lymph node (usually in the central area of level I), but it may also be found at level II (behind the pectoralis minor muscle), at level III (medial to the pectoralis minor), interpectorally (Rotter node), supraclavicularly, or in the internal mammary chain.[133] Most centers do not perform biopsy of the internal mammary chain, although there is no clear consensus on this issue. Positive internal mammary nodes could be detected only by intraparenchymal injection of radioisotope (as opposed to intradermal injection).

The advantage of this technique is that the critical prognostic status of the axillary lymph nodes is obtained to make oncologic decisions without incurring the morbidity associated with an axillary nodal dissection. The degree of postoperative pain, lymphedema, paresthesias, infection, and restriction of arm range of motion are much decreased with sentinel node dissection as opposed to axillary node dissection.

Specific contraindications to sentinel node dissection are few and include palpable axillary nodes, other nodes already confirmed to be positive by FNA cytology, and previous axillary surgical procedures.[134] Neoadjuvant chemotherapy for locally advanced breast cancer is not an absolute contraindication; however, sentinel lymphadenectomy in this setting has been shown not to be reliable for inflammatory breast cancer.[135] In the setting of neoadjuvant chemotherapy, the main problems with SLN dissection are that fibrosis of lymphatics secondary to chemotherapy may mask or alter the lymphatic drainage pattern and that locally advanced disease requiring chemotherapy is more likely to have positive lymphatic vessels and nodes, which could be so choked with tumor that normal lymphatic drainage could be altered.[136] Thus, until this issue is definitively answered, all patients undergoing SLN dissection after neoadjuvant chemotherapy should undergo formal axillary lymph node dissection. Since neoadjuvant chemotherapy is being used with increased frequency, many surgeons are interested in being able to offer SLN dissection to these patients, particularly patients who have no clinical evidence of nodal disease at presentation. A large, multicenter, randomized study, the NSABP B-27, found that SLN biopsy after neoadjuvant chemotherapy performs equivalently to SLN biopsy after systemic therapy.[137] Several small, single-institution studies have reported widely discordant results with SLN biopsy in the setting of neoadjuvant chemotherapy.[138] The potential role of SLN biopsy in the setting of neoadjuvant chemotherapy remains a controversy in the management of patients with locally advanced breast cancer.

The pathologic and histologic techniques are critical to the outcomes of sentinel node dissection. Some centers use intraoperative frozen sections or intraoperative touch preparations, moving to immediate axillary dissection if these techniques detect cancer cells in the sentinel lymph nodes. Most breast surgeons currently do not rely on these techniques, however, because the false-negative rates are high and even if the nodes are later found to have isolated tumor cells (which is defined as a focus of lymph node metastases less than 0.2 mm in diameter), the axillary nodes are not considered to be positive and are staged as pN0(i+).[139] In contrast, according to the sixth edition of the *American Joint Committee on Cancer Staging Manual,* micrometastatic disease (defined as a focus of carcinoma less than 2 mm in diameter) is classified as pN1(mi).[61] The sensitivity of intraoperative frozen section of sentinel lymph nodes for T1 breast cancer is 40%; for T2 breast cancer, it is 76%.[140] The sensitivity for macrometastatic disease (>2 mm) is 83% to 92%, whereas the sensitivity for micrometastatic disease (<2 mm) is 17% to 78% (although micrometastatic disease detectable only by immunohistochemistry is missed on intraoperative frozen section analysis).[140,141] The benefit for intraoperative frozen section analysis thus clearly increases with larger tumor size. Intraoperative touch preparations (imprint cytologic examination) were found to have a sensitivity of 87% and a specificity of 100% for a series of 74 SLN dissections[142]; further studies will be necessary to determine the sensitivity for a larger population of patients. Currently, the standard remains awaiting the final hematoxylin and eosin staining results of the sentinel lymph nodes, although practice patterns do vary somewhat, depending on the local availability and reliability of these types of intraoperative pathologic studies. Micrometastases have been detected by techniques such as immunohistochemistry and reverse transcription–polymerase chain reaction; however, it is thought that these tests are overly sensitive and thus should not be routinely used unless hematoxylin and eosin staining results are equivocal.[143]

Hill et al[144] reported on the lessons learned from 500 patients who underwent SLN biopsies at a single center. A planned axillary lymph node dissection was performed for 104 patients; the first 60 SLN biopsies were each followed by an axillary node dissection. Thereafter, surgeons who were inexperienced with SLN biopsy continued to perform axillary node dissection after SLN biopsy. They found that the SLN was successfully identified by blue dye in 80%, by isotope in 85%, and by a combination of both in 93%. Success in locating the SLN did not correlate with the route of administration of the isotope, tumor size, location, multicentricity, lymphovascular invasion, or a previous surgical biopsy. Abnormal lymphoscintigraphy was significantly associated with successfully finding the SLN. The overall false-negative rate of SLN biopsy was found to be 10.6% based on histologic examination of the completion axillary lymph node specimens. The majority of these false-negative results were early in each surgeon's experience with the SLN procedure, suggesting that there is a learning curve associated with the procedure. The authors noted that although this false-negative rate of 10.6% seems higher than that reported in most studies, most series in the literature report their false-negative rates using the total number of patients rather than calculating it as the number of false-negative SLN dissections/number of planned axillary lymph node dissections with positive nodal disease.

False-negatives are the most important problem of the technique of SLN dissection. Some rate of false-negative results will be inherent to the procedure due to arborization of lymphatics, tumor obstruction of lymphatic pathways, errors in radioactive colloid or blue dye injection, or errors in histologic sampling.[145]

Studies support the implementation of SLN dissection by demonstrating few problems with axillary recurrences after a negative SLN dissection without any further axillary dissection.[146] Two large multicenter trials are studying the utility of axillary node dissection. The NSABP-32 study randomizes patients with breast cancer and negative SLN dissection to axillary lymph node dissection or no axillary lymph node dissection. The American College of Surgeons Z11 trial randomizes patients with SLNs that are positive for tumor to either axillary lymph node dissection or no axillary lymph node dissection. These large trials should help determine what the role of SLN dissection should be and if it is safe to abandon axillary lymph node dissection as a routine procedure.

The SLN dissection technique may be performed with vital blue dye or radioactive sulfur colloid. The radiocolloid is injected in the nuclear medicine department, and the results of the lymphoscintigram are communicated to the surgeon preoperatively to facilitate location of the SLN. The blue dye is injected by the surgeon in the operating room; several techniques for the injection have been described. The most frequently used are peritumoral, intratumoral, subcutaneous, subdermal, and subareolar. Studies now suggest that the intradermal route may identify more clearly the rich lymphatic network of the skin and provide a lesser degree of scatter than peritumoral injection.[147] Approximately 5 mL of dye is injected; some surgeons prefer to perform the operation with radiocolloid only because anaphylactic reactions to vital blue dye have been described. After approximately 5 minutes to allow the dye to reach the axilla, the skin incision is made obliquely beginning near the anterior axillary line and about 1 cm inferior to the hair-bearing portion of the axilla.[148] The subcutaneous tissues are dissected with electrocautery; the sentinel lymph nodes are always found deep to the claviculopectoral fascia. The patient's arm may be raised to help bring the deeper axillary contents toward the incision. Blue lymphatics are followed, guiding the surgeon to the sentinel lymph nodes. Once these nodes with dye are identified, they are excised by ligation of the lymphatics with suture to avoid obscuring the field with blue dye, and the specimens are passed off the field. The afferent lymphatics are traced proximally toward the breast, searching for any additional sentinel lymph nodes. When radiocolloid is administered, the gamma probe is used to locate "hot" radioactive areas. Sentinel nodes are removed until the radioactive counts in the basin return to background levels. With the use of radiotracer and lymphoscintigraphy, the success rate for harvesting of SLNs has been shown to be 95%.[149] With the blue dye technique, a similar success rate of 96% has been shown. A consensus conference on the use of SLN dissection recommends that surgeons new to the technique use both the blue dye and radiotracer methods to optimize their rates of successful SLN dissections.[133]

Sentinel node biopsy was developed for use in conjunction with the rise in prevalence of breast-conserving surgery. Because of the enormous potential to reduce morbidity by avoidance of an axillary node dissection, many surgeons have also adopted the use of SLN dissection along with simple mastectomy. A consensus conference on the use of SLN biopsy supported this technique, concluding that SLN biopsy works well in patients undergoing mastectomy.[133] The main concern with combining these two procedures is that unlike SLN dissection at the time of lumpectomy, SLN dissection with mastectomy results in more technical difficulty if a second operation for a completion axillary dissection is required when the final histopathologic diagnosis of the sentinel nodes is made. Difficulties associated with delayed axillary lymph node dissection are particularly true if an immediate reconstruction was performed and reoperation for axillary clearance is necessary. The thoracodorsal vessels are often used for recipient vessels for a free TRAM flap or as a vascular pedicle for a latissimus dorsi musculocutaneous flap. These vessels could be compromised during a reoperative axillary procedure; use of the internal mammary artery and vein as the receptor vessels for microvascular flap transplantation minimizes the risk of vascular damage on reoperation for patients undergoing mastectomy and SLN dissection who may potentially require axillary lymph node dissection subsequently.[150]

AXILLARY LYMPH NODE DISSECTION

The technique of axillary lymph node dissection is the same regardless of whether the procedure is performed at the time of a modified radical mastectomy or through a separate incision for patients undergoing breast-conserving surgery.[151] When it is performed as part of a modified radical mastectomy, the mastectomy incision is designed as an ellipse encompassing the nipple-areola complex and any previous biopsy site. Skin flaps are elevated superiorly to the level of the clavicle, medially to the level of the sternum, and inferiorly to the level of the rectus sheath. Dissection then continues laterally until the anterior border of the latissimus dorsi muscle is identified. Beginning inferiorly, the breast is resected off the pectoral muscles but left attached at the axilla so that an en bloc resection of the breast tissue and axillary contents may be accomplished.

The axilla may be divided into three levels anatomically on the basis of the relationship of the node in question to the pectoralis minor muscle. The goal of the operation is to completely remove all level I, II, and III lymph nodes (Fig. 138-16). Level I nodes are located lateral to the pectoralis minor muscle. Level II nodes are found posterior to the pectoralis minor muscle and are termed Rotter nodes. Level III nodes are located medial to the pectoralis minor muscle. Some surgeons now perform a modified version of the axillary node dissection, leaving the level III nodes in situ unless there are palpable nodal metastases. This method may reduce the risk of postoperative lymphedema.[152]

The breast is next retracted medially, and dissection proceeds superiorly along the anterior border of the latissimus dorsi muscle until the axillary vein is

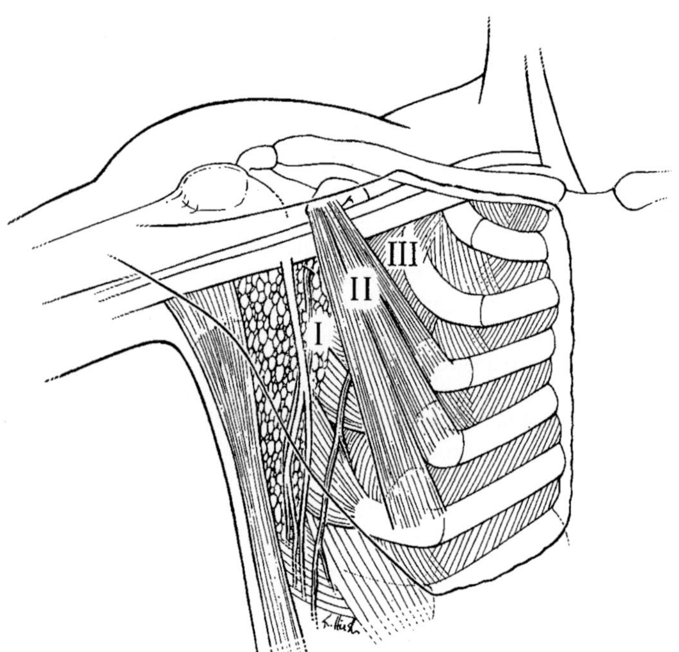

FIGURE 138-16. Levels of dissection for axillary lymph nodes. The anatomy of nodal levels is defined by the pectoralis minor muscle: level I is lateral to the pectoralis minor, level II is posterior to the pectoralis minor, and level III is medial to the pectoralis minor.

identified. It is crucial to always be aware of the location and course of the axillary vein in performing an axillary node dissection; all dissection should occur inferior to this landmark (preferably by about 1 cm inferior to the vein) to ensure its preservation. By staying 1 cm below the vein, many small lymphatics are preserved. Small branches of the axillary vein may be ligated with absorbable ties.

A peanut sponge is used to gently sweep downward along the fatty tissue and lymph nodes anterior and inferior to the axillary vein. The intercostobrachial nerve traverses the axilla, running directly through axillary fat. This position makes this nerve difficult to preserve, but great care should be taken to attempt its preservation because transection results in an annoying anesthesia of the inner aspect of the upper arm. The subscapular artery and vein are next identified and preserved. The thoracodorsal nerve, which supplies innervation to the latissimus dorsi muscle, is next carefully identified and preserved. The long thoracic nerve is found against the chest wall, where it supplies innervation to the serratus anterior muscle. It is carefully identified and preserved; inadvertent injury to the long thoracic nerve results in a winged scapula deformity. The medial pectoral nerve is found crossing the axilla around the lateral edge of the pectoralis major muscle. Damage to this nerve will result in atrophy of the lateral pectoralis major muscle.

Most level I nodes will remain readily attached to the specimen. On full mobilization of the resection specimen, the axillary lymph node dissection is completed from superolateral to inferomedial, and the main specimen is passed off the table. Level II and level III nodes are located by dissecting with the index finger adjacent to the costoclavicular ligament at the thoracic inlet and gently palpating for nodes in level III. The line of dissection remains inferior to the axillary vein. Level II nodes are identified posterior to the pectoralis minor. The axillary vein and medial pectoral nerve are preserved and protected when the pectoralis minor is retracted. The axillary vein and the thoracodorsal, long, thoracic, and medial pectoral nerves are again visualized to confirm that no injury has occurred.

For patients undergoing axillary lymph node dissection with breast conservation, the lumpectomy is performed first, with instruments changed before the axillary lymph node dissection is begun. An oblique incision is made along the posterior border of the pectoralis major in the anterior axilla, usually near the anterior axillary line. The incision is anterior to the hair-bearing area of the axilla and is usually well hidden when the patient is standing. Dissection continues with electrocautery until the axillary fat is encountered. The axillary vein is next identified. An assistant retracts the pectoralis major and minor muscles medially and superiorly, providing access to the axilla. The dissection then proceeds as described before, with identification of each structure.

After wound irrigation, two closed suction drains are placed through the inferior lateral chest wall for mastectomy patients, with one lying in the anterior chest wall and the other positioned in the axilla. For patients treated with breast conservation, a single closed suction drain is placed in the axilla. Axillary node dissection specimens typically consist of 15 to 20 lymph nodes within the specimen.

The patient records the daily drain output, and the drains are removed in the office when each drains less than 30 mL per day. Range-of-motion exercises commence at least 2 weeks after surgery but not before the drains are removed. Normal arm movement (particularly of the shoulder) is encouraged in the early postoperative period.

Morbidity is associated with the procedure, including lymphedema (5% to 25%), seroma, hematoma, paresthesias, wound infection, and decreased shoulder range of motion. Postmastectomy pain syndrome has been shown to be associated with axillary node dissection; it is thought to be related to surgical nerve injury. The use of sentinel lymph node dissection has been shown to reduce the incidence of postmastectomy pain syndrome.[153]

Multidisciplinary Breast Cancer Management

Whereas surgery is the primary treatment of breast cancer, for patients with stage III or stage IV disease, chemotherapy and radiation therapy are highly effective at decreasing the tumor burden and in some instances may allow delayed resection if the breast tumor responds to treatment. Chemotherapy or radiation therapy given before surgery is referred to as neoadjuvant therapy. The philosophy of this approach is to attempt to kill local tumor cells at the primary to make the lesion operable as well as to eradicate micrometastatic disease foci. In addition, the hormonal milieu plays a role in carcinogenesis. Tamoxifen treatment may help control and palliate these patients as well. Many centers are currently studying outcomes after neoadjuvant therapy and surgical resection; these studies will help guide future treatment decisions.

Locally advanced breast cancer includes stage III and some stage IV disease. These cancers are characterized by primary tumors larger than 5 cm, bulky or matted lymph nodes, inflammatory carcinoma, and isolated ipsilateral supraclavicular lymph nodes as the only site of metastasis.[154] Locally advanced breast cancer represents approximately 10% of breast cancer presentations in the United States. In underserved populations in the United States, this rate increases to 20%. In developing countries, the rate is greater than 50%.[155] These patients are at a very high risk for micrometastatic disease, which can circulate undetected and ultimately progress to grossly metastatic disease, organ dysfunction, and death.

The goals of treatment of locally advanced breast cancer are therefore to obtain and to maintain (1) local control by surgery or radiation therapy, or both, and (2) control of systemic disease with chemotherapy or hormonal therapy, or both. The 5-year survival rates have been reported to be 36% to 80% for locally advanced breast cancer.[156-158] These patients are at high postoperative risk for complications including skin breakdown, tissue necrosis, bleeding, pain, and infection. The use of chemotherapy or radiation therapy in the preoperative or postoperative setting affects the patient's ability to heal her wound. Plastic surgery consultation is often required for reconstruction to provide flap coverage; skin graft will generally not provide stable coverage because of the prior radiation therapy. As multidisciplinary treatment has clearly been shown to benefit the patient with locally advanced breast cancer, it is crucial for all involved specialists (breast surgeon, diagnostic radiologists, pathologists, medical oncologists, and radiation oncologists) to work closely together and to tailor multimodality therapy on the basis of the patient's available data. Breast tumor boards are highly effective venues for the discussion of patients with locally advanced breast cancer. This disease underscores the necessity for a team-based approach to breast cancer care.

Patients with metastatic disease must be identified before surgery is performed. The supraclavicular nodes, bone, lung, liver, and brain are the most prevalent sites of distant metastatic disease. A history of bone or abdominal pain, weight loss, or neurologic changes requires special work-up for metastatic disease. Physical examination of the supraclavicular nodes and liver may be able to detect metastatic disease by finding adenopathy or a mass. Liver function tests may suggest liver metastasis and should be followed by a computed tomographic (CT) scan of the abdomen or a right upper quadrant ultrasound examination to look at the liver if the test results are elevated.[159] Bone metastasis may be identified by elevated alkaline phosphatase and calcium levels. Chest radiographs are unlikely to detect lung metastasis, and if suspicion is high for metastatic disease, CT scans of the chest and abdomen should be obtained. Bone scans are indicated for patients with suggestive symptoms or an elevated alkaline phosphatase level.[160] Neither CT scans nor bone scans should be routinely obtained, but they are indicated if the patient demonstrates signs and symptoms compatible with distant metastatic disease.

NEOADJUVANT RADIATION THERAPY

Some T2 or T3 breast cancers are unsuitable for breast-conserving surgery initially because of tumor-to-breast volume ratio. Calitchi et al[161] studied the long-term outcome of neoadjuvant radiation therapy for this population. Seventy-five patients with noninflammatory, nonmetastatic T2 and T3 breast cancers underwent radiotherapy followed by breast-conserving surgery; 47% ultimately relapsed, with a median time to relapse of 13 years; 27 patients subsequently showed evidence of systemic disease. Nine local recurrences (12%) were treated by re-excision in one patient and mastectomy in the remaining eight. The overall and disease-free survival in this series is similar to that of conservative treatment for T2 and T3 breast cancer. Darai et al[162] performed a similar study of neoadjuvant radiotherapy for patients with T2 breast cancers before lumpectomy; they reported a local recurrence rate of 13% and a disease-free survival rate of 70% at 5 years.

Further investigation of the use of neoadjuvant radiation therapy is required, but these initial studies look promising for the prospect of reducing tumor burden sufficiently to be able to offer breast-conserving surgery to patients with T2-3 tumors. Unfortunately, neoadjuvant radiation therapy combined with later conservative surgery may distort breast shape and increase risk of complication for later mastectomy or reconstruction. As systemic chemotherapy has improved markedly during the last decade, most centers focus their neoadjuvant therapies on neoadjuvant chemotherapy rather than on radiation therapy. Neoadjuvant chemotherapy offers the potential to reduce tumor volume so that breast-conserving surgery may be offered, and it provides preliminary systemic therapy.

NEOADJUVANT CHEMOTHERAPY

Neoadjuvant chemotherapy has become the standard of care for locally advanced breast cancers (T3, T4, or N2 [fixed axillary] or N3 [ipsilateral internal mammary lymph nodes]), and it is increasingly being used in patients with otherwise operable stage I and stage II disease with large tumor-to-breast ratios to achieve successful breast conservation.[163] The M.D. Anderson experience with neoadjuvant chemotherapy for stage II and stage III breast cancers found excellent response rates, permitting breast-conserving therapy for local control (Table 138-13).[164]

Although attempts to use neoadjuvant chemotherapy have been made for 20 years, few multi-institution randomized trials exist. The largest existing study is the NSABP B-18 trial.[165] In this study, 1523 women with palpable, operable breast cancers (T1-3, N0-1, M0) were randomized to receive four cycles of doxorubicin and cyclophosphamide (AC) either before or after surgery. Whereas the overall clinical response rate after chemotherapy was high (80% showed a partial response or a complete clinical

TABLE 138-13 ✦ CLASSIFICATION OF RESPONSE TO THERAPY (COMPARED WITH PRETREATMENT SIZE)[164]

Complete response	No measurable tumor
Partial response	Reduction in tumor size ≥50%
Minor response	Reduction in tumor size ≥25% and <50%
No change	<25% decrease or increase in tumor size
Progressive disease	>25% increase in tumor size

response), the 5-year disease-free survival rates were the same (67.3% versus 66.7%), as were the overall survival rates (80% versus 79.6%). The main advantage of this therapy appeared to be that patients who received neoadjuvant chemotherapy had a higher rate of lumpectomy than did the standard postoperatively treated patients (67% versus 60%). Multiple single-institution studies of various chemotherapy regimens have been reported, with no consensus on the optimal neoadjuvant regimen.[166,167] Many centers have recently been interested in the neoadjuvant use of docetaxel. Docetaxel is a highly active cytotoxic agent shown to have marked activity in the setting of primary chemotherapy for metastatic disease and for anthracycline-resistant disease.[168] Additional multi-institution, prospective, randomized studies will be required to better define the future role of neoadjuvant chemotherapy.

POSTOPERATIVE RADIATION THERAPY

The four most common indications for radiation therapy for breast cancer are (1) ductal carcinoma in situ, (2) early-stage (stage I-II) disease treated by lumpectomy, (3) locally advanced breast cancer, as postmastectomy therapy (for the high-risk patient and patients with chest wall recurrences), and (4) involved surgical margins.[169,170] The management of ductal carcinoma in situ with radiation therapy is more controversial than the other indications for radiotherapy. This treatment is discussed later in the section on management of ductal carcinoma in situ (see "Ductal Carcinoma In Situ" under "Management of Breast Carcinoma In Situ").

Tumor size does not influence the rate of local recurrence when a complete excision with negative margins is performed and the patient receives radiation therapy.[171] When patients are treated with lumpectomy alone without irradiation, the local failure risk correlates significantly with larger tumor size. Studies have looked at how patients with early invasive breast cancer with negative nodal status have done after wide excision alone without radiotherapy; at 56 months of median follow-up, 16% of patients experienced locally recurrent disease.[172] The National Surgical Adjuvant Breast and Bowel Project trial found that with lumpectomy alone without radiation therapy, the local recurrence rate was 40% at 8 years of follow-up, whereas those patients treated with lumpectomy and radiation therapy had a local recurrence rate of less than 10%.[121]

Certain patients have a higher risk for failure of local control, such as patients whose breast cancer histologically is found to have an extensive intraductal component. An extensive intraductal component is defined as an in situ component of 25% or more of the primary infiltrating carcinoma and in situ carcinoma present in the surrounding normal breast tissue.[173] The Joint Center for Radiation Therapy at Harvard reported that breast cancer patients whose tumors had an extensive intraductal component treated with resection and irradiation had a 7.6% risk for local recurrence; patients without an extensive intraductal component had only a 3.1% risk for local recurrence.[174]

After breast-conserving surgical excision of the primary tumor and either sentinel lymph node dissection or axillary lymph node dissection, radiation is delivered to the entire affected breast for a total of 4500 to 5000 cGy during 5 weeks of treatment. A boost of 1000 to 1600 cGy is delivered to the lumpectomy site frequently, although this is not yet of proven benefit. Tangentially oriented photon fields are implemented to reduce exposure to the heart and lungs; the patient is carefully repositioned in exactly the same manner each treatment, sometimes with wedges for support. For complex studies (complex tangents and internal mammary chain fields), CT scan images are used to plan the three-dimensional treatment plan. With current radiation therapy protocols, dosimetry studies have shown no decreased effect of radiation in the setting of existing implants (either preexisting from augmentation or placed at the time of breast reconstruction for cancer).[175]

The role of irradiation for positive axillary lymph nodes is not clearly defined presently. Patients whose nodes are histologically negative or who have one to three positive nodes have not been proved to benefit significantly by the addition of regional axillary irradiation.[121] The American College of Surgeons Oncology Group is currently conducting a prospective, randomized trial (Z11) of patients clinically staged to T1-2, N0, M0 who have a positive sentinel node. This study compares sentinel node–positive patients treated with breast-conserving surgery and radiation therapy who have either completion axillary nodal dissection or no further axillary therapy. This study will be informative as to whether completion axillary dissection actually benefits patients with positive sentinel nodes or if radiation therapy after sentinel node dissection is appropriate local treatment without the necessity of completion axillary nodal dissection.

Routine use of axillary radiation therapy is typically reserved for patients with four or more positive axillary nodes. It has been shown that there is no added benefit to irradiation of the axilla if a thorough axillary node dissection has been performed, even if it demonstrates multiple positive nodes with extracapsular extension. Extracapsular involvement of the node, therefore, does not influence prognosis independently; rather, the total number of involved axillary nodes is the significant determinant of risk.[176] Irradiation may be used for patients whose axillary dissection was incomplete; however, level I nodes are almost always already included in the breast fields.

The optimal sequence of breast-conserving surgery, chemotherapy, and radiation therapy for early-stage, node–positive breast cancer patients is not known.[177] Slotman[178] reported that delay of radiation therapy for more than 7 weeks after lumpectomy results in an increased local recurrence rate. However, for those patients with positive nodes and negative surgical margins, it is now clearly advantageous to begin systemic chemotherapy before radiation therapy.[179] Radiation therapy for patients who had lumpectomy typically consists of four or more positive lymph nodes after an adequate axillary dissection.[180]

Another controversy in breast cancer treatment is the issue of postmastectomy irradiation. It is generally accepted that patients with a high risk for local recurrence (four or more positive nodes, primary tumor of 5 cm or larger, or pectoralis fascia involvement) should have postmastectomy radiation therapy.[181] Radiation therapy for these patients typically includes the chest wall as well as comprehensive nodal therapy, including the internal mammary lymph nodes. The locoregional recurrence rate is decreased in this population from 20% to 30% to less than 10% with postmastectomy radiation therapy. It is generally accepted that for patients with low risk for local recurrence (5% to 10%), postmastectomy radiation therapy is not beneficial because morbidities related to the radiation therapy do not merit the small benefit gained in terms of local control. The controversy exists for the patients with intermediate levels of risk (10% to 25% risk for local recurrence), such as patients with one to three positive nodes. Several clinical trials are in progress to evaluate this issue and help resolve this controversy.

Radiation Therapy and Implant or Flap Reconstruction

Radiation therapy is known to significantly impair wound healing by inhibition of fibroblasts and microvascular occlusion. For the reconstructive surgeon, the status of the treatment plan regarding potential radiation therapy for a patient is particularly important so that the most appropriate procedure is chosen to achieve the optimal reconstructive result.

TABLE 138-14 ✦ MODIFIED BAKER CLASSIFICATION OF CAPSULAR CONTRACTURE AFTER BREAST RECONSTRUCTION[297]

Grade	Description
IA	Soft
IB	Soft but implant visible
II	Implant with mild firmness
III	Implant with moderate firmness
IV	Excessively firm and symptomatic breast

Studies have shown that previously irradiated patients undergoing expander placement prior to implants had a very high complication rate (with up to 20% developing Baker III or IV capsular contracture and up to 60% having either a complication or an unfavorable result) (Table 138-14).[182] Changes in the skin secondary to irradiation resulted in poor outcomes when expansion was attempted compared with the nonirradiated study population.[183] Krueger et al[184] studied 81 patients who underwent mastectomy and expander-implant reconstruction; 19 of these patients also underwent radiation therapy. Complications occurred in 68% of the irradiated patients compared with 31% of the patients who did not receive radiation therapy. With the use of tissue expanders and implants in the setting of an irradiated field, there is a higher rate of infection, extrusion, and inadequate results due to poor breast envelope expansion and subsequent capsular contracture.

Radiation therapy after immediate breast reconstruction with implants is associated with a markedly increased risk for capsular contracture. Vandeweyer et al[185] found that in their series, 100% of the patients who underwent immediate reconstruction with implants followed by radiation treatment developed either a grade III or grade IV capsular contracture. Whereas many of the earlier studies on implant reconstruction in the setting of radiation therapy concur in their high complication rates, these studies are problematic for several reasons. Most of the studies are small, especially when patients are stratified according to whether radiation therapy occurred before or subsequent to implant reconstruction (Table 138-15). There is also the issue of whether the expander was replaced with a permanent implant before the radiation treatment. Different subsets of patients also received different radiation therapy, depending on the institution and the time of the study.

Cordeiro et al[186] addressed these concerns by conducting a relatively large study of patients (n = 81) who were treated in the identical fashion with tissue

TABLE 138-15 ✦ COMPARISON OF COMPLICATIONS ASSOCIATED WITH IMPLANT RECONSTRUCTION FROM RADIATION THERAPY

		No. with Radiation Therapy			% Grade 3 and Grade 4 Capsular Contracture (grade 3/grade 4)		
Author (Year)	**No. of Patients**	*After Immediate Expander and Implant Reconstruction Fully Completed*	*Before Any Implant Reconstruction*	*After Expansion, Before Permanent Implant*	*Nonirradiated Control Patients*	*Irradiated Implant-Reconstructed Patients*	**% Any Complication (irradiated implants/ nonirradiated implants)**
Cordeiro[186] (2004)	81	81	0	0	9.3/1.3	33.8/5.9	68/40
Spear[271] (2000)	40	5	9	19	0	32.5	52.5/10
Vandeweyer[185] (2000)	6	6	0	0	3.3/0	66/33	100/19.4
Krueger[184] (2001)	19	9	3	0	10	26	68/31
Forman[182] (1998)	10	0	10	0	Not reported	20	60/not reported

expander placement at the time of mastectomy, tissue expansion during postoperative chemotherapy, exchange of the tissue expander for a permanent implant 4 weeks after the completion of chemotherapy, and chest wall irradiation 4 weeks after placement of the permanent implant device. Although this study noted higher rates of Baker grade III and grade IV capsular contracture in the irradiated population (33.8% and 5.9%, respectively) than in the nonirradiated population (9.3% and 1.3%), they found that overall complication rates were high in both the irradiated and nonirradiated groups (68% and 40%). Despite these high complication rates for each group, 80% of the irradiated group and 88% of the nonirradiated group demonstrated good to excellent aesthetic results. This study provides compelling evidence that tissue expander–implant reconstruction is an acceptable choice even when it is followed by postoperative radiation therapy. Further large studies carefully designed to keep treatment arms constant are necessary.

A history of chest irradiation does not have a prohibitive impact on musculocutaneous flap reconstruction, as nonirradiated, well-vascularized tissues are brought into the defect. In the largest reported series, Williams et al[187] studied 118 patients with breast cancer who underwent radiation therapy followed by a TRAM flap compared with 572 patients matched for age, smoking, obesity, and hypertension with no radiation therapy before similar reconstruction. A significantly increased complication rate was noted only for fat necrosis (17.6% in the irradiated group versus 10.1% for the nonirradiated group) (Table 138-16). TRAM flaps are therefore an excellent reconstructive choice in this population with excellent flap survival and an overall good symmetric result.

Immediate reconstruction with a flap for autogenous reconstruction followed by radiation therapy may adversely affect the quality of the breast mound. Although the patient benefits from a single procedure that accomplishes both mastectomy and flap reconstruction, the flap may exhibit increased fat necrosis and scar contracture.

Plastic surgeons debate the merits of immediate flap reconstruction or delay in flap reconstruction pending completion of radiotherapy. With the necessity of immediate flaps for skin-sparing mastectomy and the effectiveness of radiation oncologists to minimize skin and underlying soft tissue damage, it is currently the consensus that the advantages of immediate reconstruction with postoperative radiation therapy outweigh the disadvantages of skin contraction in skin-sparing mastectomy when no breast mound is present during radiation therapy.

When modified mastectomy is performed, adequate skin envelope will require flap skin. Therefore, delay in reconstruction until radiation therapy is completed may actually improve the quality of the reconstruction and avoid complications. Immediate reconstruction may warrant flap use preceding radiation therapy after modified radical mastectomy.

POSTOPERATIVE ADJUVANT CHEMOTHERAPY

It is now recognized that systemic chemotherapy treats occult micrometastatic disease; the difficulty lies in recognizing which patients would benefit from undergoing adjuvant chemotherapy versus which may be considered cured by local therapy alone. The best established prognostic factors for invasive breast cancer are lymph node status and tumor diameter. When nodal involvement is considered, the risk groups include node

TABLE 138-16 ✦ COMPLICATIONS AFTER TRAM RECONSTRUCTION IN THE SETTING OF RADIATION THERAPY

	Group 1	Group 2	Group 3
First Author (Year)	*No. of TRAM→XRT*	*No. of XRT→TRAM*	*No. of Unirradiated TRAM*
Williams[298] (1997)	19	108	57
Tran[299] (2001)	32	70	0

% Complications (by Group 1/2/3)

First Author (Year)	*Infection*	*Fat Necrosis*	*Contracture-Fibrosis*	*Flap Loss, Partial*	*Flap Loss, Total*
Williams[298] (1997)	5.3/6.6/2.8	15.8/17.6/10	10/0/0	NA/2.8/NA	0/0/0
Tran[299] (2001)	NA/NA/—	43.8/8.6/—	75/0/—	0/7.1/—	0/1.4/—

XRT, radiation therapy.

negative, 1 to 3 involved nodes, 4 to 9 involved nodes, and 10 or more involved nodes.[188] Some clinicians use these different nodal risk groups to make therapeutic decisions; others simply distinguish between the presence or absence of nodal involvement.

The second most important factor affecting prognosis is tumor diameter, particularly for women with node-negative disease. One group that has generally not been treated with systemic therapy is women with node-negative breast cancer of less than 1 cm in diameter. Rosen et al[191] reported that the risk for recurrence in this population older than 20 years is 13%.[189] In addition, patients with tumors of tubular, medullary, or colloid histology up to 3 cm in diameter have a better prognosis than do patients with ductal or lobular carcinoma.[190,191]

Another factor to be considered in planning for systemic therapy is the estrogen and progesterone receptor status because tamoxifen should be offered to all estrogen receptor–positive patients.[192] HER-2/neu, a transmembrane tyrosine kinase receptor, is the biomarker with the greatest prevalence in breast cancer (overexpressed in 30% of patients).[193] HER-2/neu amplification or overexpression is associated with a poorer prognosis in node–positive women; some studies have found relative methotrexate resistance and a requirement for higher doses of doxorubicin to treat these patients.[194] Trastuzumab, a recombinant monoclonal antibody against HER2, has been approved by the Food and Drug Administration (FDA) for patients with advanced metastatic breast cancer whose tumors overexpress HER2.[195]

At the Sixth International Conference on Adjuvant Therapy of Primary Breast Cancer at St. Gallen, Switzerland, in 1998, a panel of experts proposed recommendations and guidelines for the use of adjuvant chemotherapy for patients with primary breast cancer.[196] According to this consensus conference, patients with axillary node metastases should be considered for adjuvant chemotherapy regardless of age, menopausal status, or hormone receptor status.[197] It has been demonstrated that regimens containing an anthracycline (doxorubicin or epirubicin) provide better results than cyclophosphamide, methotrexate, and 5-fluorouracil (CMF).[198] One of the most commonly used regimens in the United States today is doxorubicin-cyclophosphamide (AC). Preliminary data indicate that a survival benefit exists for the addition of paclitaxel to the AC regimen[199]; further studies of this are ongoing. For lower risk patients, CMF is a commonly used regimen. A Cochrane Database review noted that polychemotherapy (either anthracycline based with AC or non–anthracycline based with CMF) produces a 7% to 11% improvement in absolute 10-year survival for women younger than 50 years with early breast cancer.[200] It also reported that women aged 50 to 69 years gained a 2% to 3% survival benefit at 10 years. Most oncologists favor AC over CMF and are encouraged by the early trials of taxane-based therapy.[201,202]

According to the St. Gallen consensus conference, node-negative premenopausal women with moderately or poorly differentiated invasive tumors greater than 1 cm in diameter and negative hormonal receptors should undergo adjuvant chemotherapy.[197] Node-negative patients with a low risk for recurrence should not receive adjuvant chemotherapy; this includes patients older than 35 years with tumors less than 1 cm in diameter, estrogen receptor– or progesterone receptor–positive status, and well-differentiated grade. Other patients who may not require chemotherapy are patients with pure mucinous, tubular, papillary, or adenocystic carcinoma if the tumor is less than 3 cm. Medical contraindications to chemotherapy include severe cardiovascular, hepatic, or renal disease; concurrent terminal illness; severe bone marrow deficiency; severe immunodeficiency; and mental illness.

ENDOCRINE THERAPY

Treatment with tamoxifen for patients with estrogen receptor–positive tumors has been shown to be effective as adjuvant therapy. In a study of the effects of 5 years of tamoxifen therapy, the odds of recurrence for node–negative women were reduced by 14.9% and mortality was reduced by 5.6%; for node–positive women, the odds of recurrence were reduced by 15.2% and mortality was reduced by 10.9%.[203] All estrogen receptor–positive breast cancer patients should be considered for tamoxifen therapy. Prevention studies have shown that 5 years of tamoxifen reduced the risk for invasive breast cancer by 49% for a cohort of 6681 patients compared with 6707 control subjects; this study included patients aged 60 years or older, patients aged 35 to 59 years with a 5-year predicted risk for breast cancer of at least 1.66%, and patients with lobular carcinoma in situ.[204]

Whereas tamoxifen has long been the mainstay of endocrine therapy for breast cancer, its side effect profile makes it nonoptimal therapy for many patients. It has been associated with increased incidence of endometrial cancer and thromboembolism. Many patients also suffer side effects including hot flashes, nausea, and other complaints. Tamoxifen acts as both an estrogen agonist and antagonist, which may result in incomplete blockage of the estrogen receptor and contribute to its adverse effects. Other agents, such as raloxifene, a selective estrogen receptor modulator like tamoxifen that has antiestrogenic effects on breast tissue, have been approved for use in endocrine therapy. Cummings et al[205] found that among postmenopausal women with osteoporosis, raloxifene for 3 years reduced the risk of breast cancer by 76%.

There is currently much interest in the efficacy of aromatase inhibitors such as letrozole and anastrozole. Aromatase inhibitors are effective against estrogen receptor–positive breast cancers and have a lower risk of thromboembolism than tamoxifen does. They are approved as first-line endocrine therapy for postmenopausal women with hormone receptor–positive metastatic breast cancer. Several major ongoing clinical trials are comparing the efficacy of aromatase inhibitors in terms of response rate and long-term survival with tamoxifen.[206,207] Some of these studies are investigating the role of aromatase inhibitors and selective estrogen receptor modulators as neoadjuvant therapy as well as the potential additive effects of these drugs.

MANAGEMENT OF BREAST CARCINOMA IN SITU

Ductal Carcinoma In Situ

Ductal carcinoma in situ (DCIS) is diagnosed much more commonly than in previous years because of the widespread use of screening mammography. In some centers, 25% of the breast cancers diagnosed are DCIS.[208] Although DCIS is molecularly not distinguishable from invasive carcinoma by looking at gains and losses of genes over the entire set of chromosomes (comparative genomic hybridization), by evaluation of specific base pair abnormalities, by analysis of genetic expression (microarrays), or by studies of particular molecular markers,[209] DCIS clearly is a separate and important disease entity. It is a nonobligate precursor lesion to an invasive cancer, with risk of progression depending on a combination of factors, including histologic grade, lesion size, and margin status.[210] Approximately 90% of DCIS is diagnosed by mammography; microcalcifications are the most common mammographic evidence of DCIS.[210]

Whereas DCIS was traditionally classified on the basis of architectural patterns (comedo, micropapillary, solid, cribriform, and papillary), these are now recognized to be of limited value in prognosis. The histologic grade of DCIS has replaced the pattern as the most predictive guide to clinical behavior and treatment. The most reproducible classification scheme appears to be the Van Nuys system[211] (Table 138-17). One to three points are given for each of three different prognostic indicators of local breast recurrence (size, margins, and pathologic classification). Under this system, DCIS can be divided into three groups. Group 1 (low grade) manifests low- or intermediate-grade nuclei and no necrosis. Group 2 (intermediate grade) includes tumors with low- or intermediate-grade nuclei and comedo necrosis. Group 3 (high grade) consists of tumors with high-grade nuclei regardless of the presence or absence of necrosis.

Other pathologic factors, such as tumor size and margin width, are important but problematic; because DCIS is rarely palpable and often indistinguishable from surrounding tissue, both tumor size and margins must be determined by the pathologist by microscopic sectioning. Because most recurrent DCIS is probably simply incompletely resected initial disease, establishing that negative margins are achieved is crucial. If any calcifications remain postoperatively, plans must be made to re-excise the lumpectomy cavity or to convert to a mastectomy if it is not possible to achieve negative margins with a reasonable effort at breast-conserving therapy.

It is important not to overtreat or undertreat DCIS; patients with this diagnosis should be advised of their overall excellent prognosis (Table 138-18). If a hypothetical 100 patients were diagnosed with DCIS and had margin-negative surgery (lumpectomy) and postoperative radiation therapy, at least 80 patients would enjoy long-term local control.[212] Twenty patients would have local recurrences, with 10 being DCIS and 10 being invasive. Those with recurrent DCIS could achieve a nearly 100% cure rate with a completion mastectomy. The 10 patients with invasive disease would have a 75% 5-year survival rate with a completion modified radical mastectomy.[212]

Treatment options for DCIS include mastectomy and breast-conserving therapy with or without irradiation. A consensus conference held in Philadelphia in 1999 concluded that the goal of treatment for DCIS should be breast conservation.[213] Although there have been several single-institution reports, no clinical trial has reliably and reproducibly identified a population of patients who may safely undergo breast-conserving therapy without radiation therapy for DCIS. As for invasive disease, mastectomy is indicated if multicentric disease is noted or if diffuse, malignant-appearing microcalcifications that are DCIS are found

TABLE 138-17 ✦ VAN NUYS PROGNOSTIC INDEX[152]

Score	1 point	2 points	3 points
Size	<15 mm	15-40 mm	>40 mm
Margins	>10 mm	1-9 mm	<1 mm
Pathologic classification	Non-high grade without necrosis	Non-high grade with necrosis	High grade with or without necrosis

TABLE 138-18 ✦ MANAGEMENT ALGORITHM FOR DCIS BASED ON THE VAN NUYS PROGNOSTIC INDEX (VNPI) AT THE BREAST HEALTH CENTER, WOMEN AND INFANTS HOSPITAL, PROVIDENCE, RHODE ISLAND[213]

VNPI 3 or 4	Primary cancer	Excision to 1-cm surgical margins
	Axillary dissection	None
	Adjuvant radiation therapy	None
VNPI 5, 6, or 7	Primary cancer	Excision or re-excision to 1-cm surgical margins, if possible
	Axillary dissection	None
	Adjuvant radiation therapy	Selection between observation and radiation therapy, depending on excision margins; if 1-cm margin or negative re-excision, no radiation therapy
VNPI 8 or 9	Primary cancer	Mastectomy
	Axillary dissection	None or sentinel biopsy only
	Adjuvant radiation therapy	None after mastectomy

throughout the breast. The risk/benefit analysis of breast-conserving surgery versus mastectomy must be thoroughly discussed with the patient. There is no indication for sentinel node dissection or axillary node dissection because the risk of nodal metastasis is less than 1%. Sentinel lymph node dissection should be considered, however, for all patients undergoing mastectomy for DCIS because once mastectomy is performed, it will be impossible to do a sentinel node dissection. Patients undergoing mastectomy for a preoperative diagnosis of multifocal or diffuse DCIS may be harboring occult invasive disease that will be diagnosed on the final surgical pathologic examination. It is thus advantageous to perform sentinel lymph node dissection before mastectomy for DCIS.[214]

Lobular Carcinoma In Situ

Foote and Stewart[215] provided the first description of a lesion they termed lobular carcinoma in situ (LCIS). The key features they described were as follows: the lesion is a microscopic diagnosis—it cannot be identified clinically or by gross pathologic examination; the lesion is multicentric, often throughout the breast; and the invasive carcinomas that subsequently develop may be infiltrating lobular or infiltrating ductal in type. It is now clear that the lesion of LCIS itself does not represent an obligate precursor lesion to invasive cancer but rather represents a marker of an increased risk for breast cancer in both breasts.[216] A review of 6287 biopsies performed because of abnormal mammograms revealed that LCIS was present in 2.3% of patients.[217] Most studies agree that LCIS is associated with a relative risk for the development of breast cancer that is 7 to 10 times higher than that of control subjects.[218]

Because the risk for development of cancer is equal in bilateral breasts (LCIS itself is not the immediate precursor of invasive carcinoma), local excisional surgeries are not indicated. The only operative intervention that may be beneficial is bilateral mastectomy. Mastectomy is a difficult decision for a patient. If the annual risk of 1% for the development of breast cancer is not acceptable, the patient may elect prophylactic surgery. Most patients prefer to undergo a lifetime of careful screening rather than to undergo bilateral prophylactic mastectomies. This is acceptable because 75% of patients with LCIS will never develop invasive breast cancer.[219]

POSTMASTECTOMY BREAST RECONSTRUCTION

General Considerations

Concurrent with the evolution in breast cancer surgical treatment toward minimally invasive approaches, those patients who do undergo mastectomy have increasingly expressed an interest in pursuing breast reconstruction. Any breast cancer patient with no evidence of local or systemic disease who is medically fit to undergo a reconstructive breast procedure may be considered a potential candidate. In certain instances, women with systemic metastatic disease may be considered for breast reconstruction on the basis of personal issues and with support of their oncologist. Today, an estimated 15% of mastectomy patients undergo breast reconstruction in the United States according to a study that evaluated the incidence of reconstruction of 10,406 mastectomy-treated patients reported to the SEER registry in 1998.[220] An earlier study found that between 1985 and 1990, 3.4% of mastectomy patients had immediate or early delayed reconstruction; between 1994 and 1995, 8.3% of these patients had reconstruction.[221] Whereas mastectomy patients may be undergoing breast reconstruction more frequently than in the past, in a recent survey, more than one third of referring physicians (general surgeons, medical oncologists, and primary care physicians) and 90% of plastic surgeons believed that eligible patients were not being offered referrals for reconstruction because of inadequate knowledge of the referring physician on this subject.[222] The likelihood of referral for breast reconstruction is directly related to the patient's age, with age older than 49 years decreasing the likelihood of referral to a plastic surgeon. August et al[223] demonstrated that the full array of breast reconstructive options are safe in older women (older than 65 years) by comparing the rates of complications and reoperations in patients stratified by age, autogenous or implant reconstruction, and immediate or delayed reconstruction.

Breast reconstruction has been shown to improve a woman's self-image after mastectomy.[224] The main objective of breast reconstruction is to improve the quality of life of the breast cancer patient. Therefore, a treatment plan must be defined that is acceptable to both the patient and the plastic surgeon. In counseling patients on their options, it must be emphasized that no single reconstructive procedure is right for everyone. Reconstruction must be individualized to reflect the patient's general health condition, the type of mastectomy performed, the extent of the disease process, and the goal of symmetry with the contralateral breast.

There has been a trend in recent years toward immediate reconstruction because of both the improved overall result with this technique[225] and the demonstration that immediate reconstruction is psychologically beneficial to patients.[226,227] Another benefit is that breast reconstruction is also technically accomplished more readily at the time of mastectomy for several reasons.[228] The skin envelope is more pliable, and the native inframammary fold is easier to delineate in this setting. Because of the superior results of immediate reconstructive procedures, fewer revisions and contralateral symmetry procedures are necessary.[229] Immediate breast reconstruction has been shown to be significantly less costly than delayed reconstruction,[230] to require less total operating time, and to result in shorter total length of hospitalization.[231] Immediate breast reconstruction does not delay the likelihood of detection of recurrent invasive cancer[232]; the oncologic safety of breast reconstruction is well established by several studies.[233-235] For these reasons, immediate breast reconstruction is considered the standard of care, with many breast centers offering this option at the time of mastectomy. It is important to consider, however, the potentially higher rate of complications in immediate reconstruction; risks must be considered to be the additive risk of the mastectomy plus the reconstruction.[236]

Goals of Reconstruction

There are four major objectives in breast reconstructive surgery. The first is a natural-appearing breast mound with adequate volume for projection and size.[237] The second goal is the optimal reconstruction of the skin envelope. In skin-sparing mastectomies, the skin envelope may be intact. When no skin is resected (i.e., prophylactic mastectomy), the breast mound must be contoured to provide an inframammary fold and an anterior axillary line. In patients with an inadequate skin envelope, a decision must be made as to the replacement of skin through the use of expansion or with a regional or distant flap. The third objective is symmetry. If necessary, a procedure is performed on the contralateral breast to achieve symmetric projection and size or shape. The final objective is the reconstruction of a nipple-areola complex that matches the opposite side in color and projection. In immediate reconstruction in skin-sparing mastectomy, the resected nipple-areola or extended incision requires additional coverage for continuity of the skin envelope and a platform for nipple-areola reconstruction (Table 138-19).

TABLE 138-19 ✦ GOALS OF RECONSTRUCTION

Volume (size and projection)
Envelope (shape and position)
Symmetry with contralateral breast
Nipple-areola complex

Technique Selection

Two major factors have influenced choices available for breast reconstruction: type of mastectomy and technical advances in breast reconstruction. As noted in the discussion of breast cancer treatment, the extent of the resection has been reduced from the radical mastectomy with loss of an extensive portion of the skin envelope and the underlying pectoralis major muscle (Fig. 138-17) to the now-common simple mastectomy with sentinel lymph node dissection or axillary lymph node dissection. In many instances, skin-sparing techniques minimize the skin deficiency and corresponding complexity of techniques needed to restore the breast. Techniques available now fall into two main categories: use of local existing skin envelope within which to restore the breast mound and use of tissue from regional or distant sites to provide additional skin envelope or to provide for the breast mound (Fig. 138-18).

The first clinical experience with tissue expansion was described in 1957 when Neumann[238] related the use of a rubber balloon placed subcutaneously in the postauricular region. After gradual expansion during a 2-month period, sufficient skin was present for coverage of a traumatic defect of a patient's ear. Despite this evidence of the feasibility of tissue expansion,

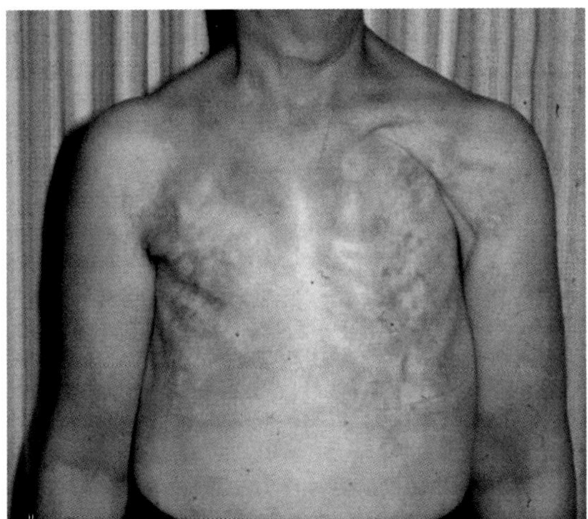

A

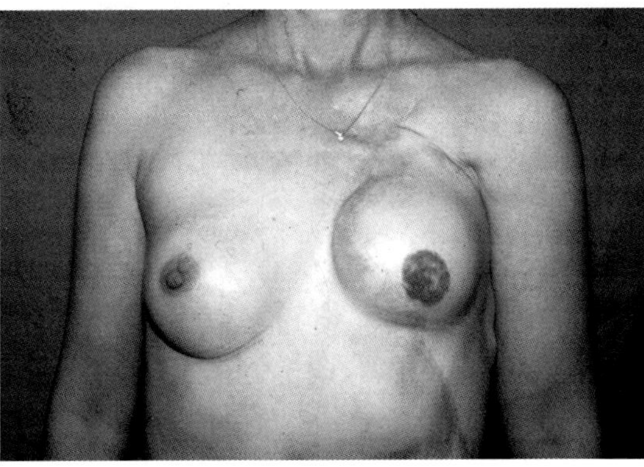

B

FIGURE 138-17. Radical mastectomy. *A*, Anterior view of patient with bilateral mastectomy (left radical mastectomy and right modified radical mastectomy). Note absence of pectoralis muscle on the left with infraclavicular contour defect and skin grafts for wound closure. *B*, Reconstruction with implant following left radical mastectomy. Despite local flaps, the skin envelope is inadequate, and there is no correction of infraclavicular contour defect.

major interest in tissue expansion did not occur for another 20 years. Working independently, Radovan[239] and Austad[240] both developed silicone tissue expanders and published their findings in 1982. Radovan performed his first tissue expansion in 1976. Austad developed a self-inflating silicone prosthesis and investigated the histologic effects of tissue expansion. Subsequent to this early work, tissue expansion has been investigated thoroughly and gained widespread acceptance on the basis of its proven safety and efficacy.

The tissue expander, as originally described, allows stretching of the remaining skin envelope to cover the nonautogenous breast implant to provide a mound and to complete the first two goals of reconstruction: a breast mound with projection and an adequate skin envelope. In some instances, an adequate skin envelope allows direct use of an implant that is fully inflated or has a distant valve for gradual filling with later removal of the distant port after satisfactory implant volume is achieved. Specific approaches not requiring flap replacement of the missing skin envelope and using a synthetic implant (gel- or saline-filled silicone implants) to provide the substance of the mound are described to illustrate specific indications and techniques.

The regional or distant flap offers more options for the reconstructive surgeon in terms of an additional immediate source of well-vascularized skin and soft tissues (see Fig. 138-18). When the skin defect is too extensive to allow immediate insertion of a permanent implant or temporary expander, the flap provides additional skin to restore a normal or nearly normal skin envelope and to cover the implant, or the required volume of vascularized soft tissue to restore the required breast volume, to satisfy both reconstructive goals of volume (projection) and adequate skin envelope.

With the advances in flap design and the ability to transplant tissue by microsurgical technique (composite tissue transplantation), there are a number of regional and distant tissue sources available to the patient who elects or is advised to use additional tissue to complete breast reconstruction. Specific approaches requiring regional and distant flaps are described to illustrate specific indications and techniques.

Although the major influence on the method selected for breast reconstruction is extent of the mastectomy, timing of the reconstruction and the status of the opposite breast have considerable influence on the choice of reconstructive method. The reconstruction will be either immediate (at the time of the mastectomy) or delayed (usually after chemotherapy and radiation therapy are completed or a time selected by the patient). The extent of the mastectomy may require flap use for defect closure or limit the use of an expander-implant. Also, one of the goals of the reconstructive process is to establish a breast that has symmetry with the opposite breast. If the opposite breast is large or pendulous, expansion of the skin envelope after mastectomy may not be adequate to establish symmetry. However, in many instances, the patient does not want to match the opposite breast and instead wants the opposite breast size or shape altered. If the surgeon knows that the opposite breast will be altered, the options available for the breast reconstruction will increase because the skin envelope at the site of reconstruction does not have to fully match the opposite side. Procedures selected for the opposite breast may include augmentation, mastopexy, and reduction mammaplasty. There is also increasing interest in prophylactic mastectomy, which then requires simultaneous or sequential mastectomy and reconstructive procedures for the contralateral breast to achieve symmetry.

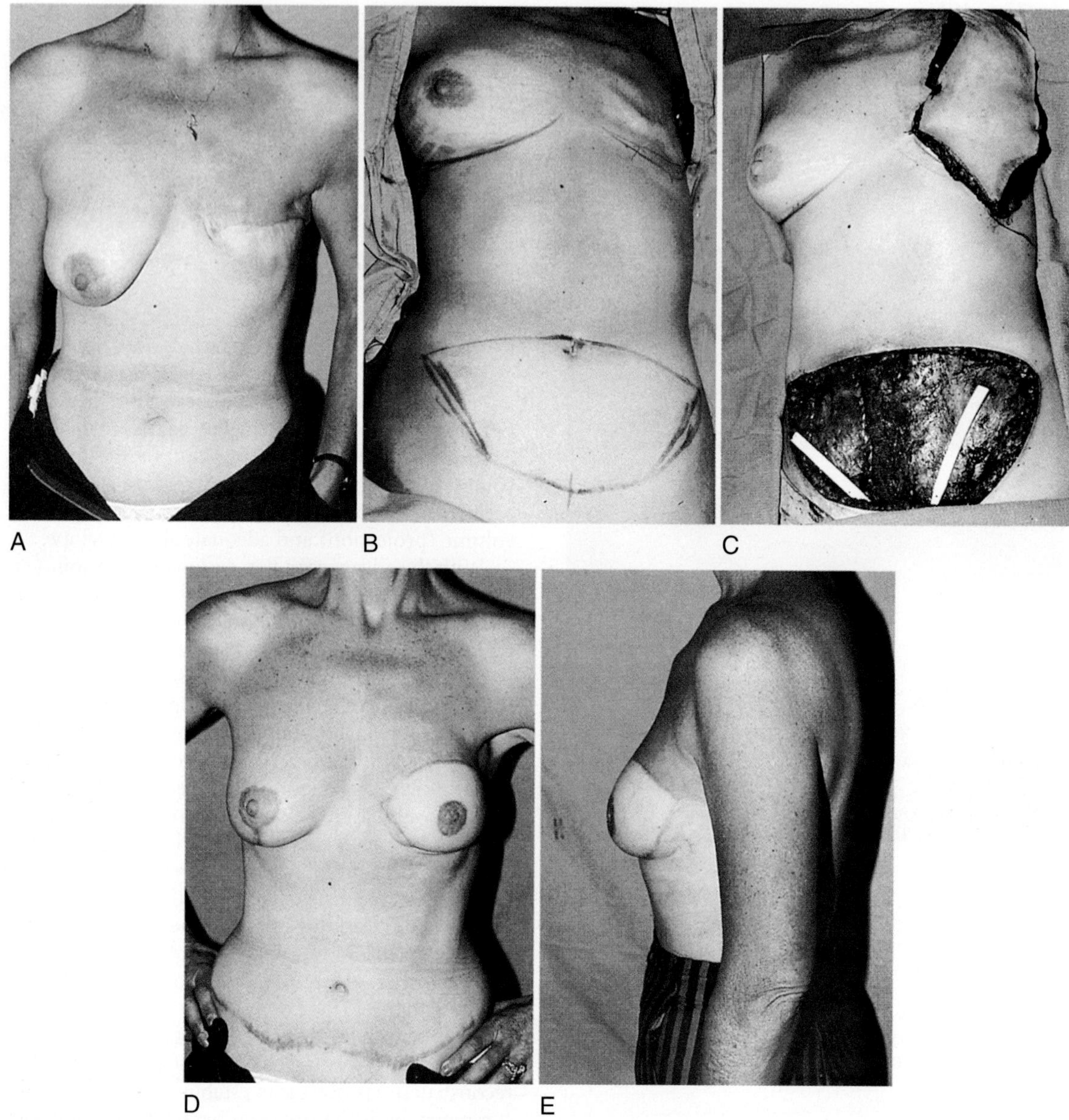

FIGURE 138-18. *A,* Left modified radical mastectomy defect. *B,* Design of contralateral TRAM flap based on superior epigastric artery and associated venae comitantes for autogenous breast reconstruction. *C,* Flap transposed 90 degrees to contralateral chest wall defect to provide soft tissue and skin for breast reconstruction. The abdominal fascial defect is reconstructed with Prolene mesh. *D* and *E,* Postoperative view at 1 year demonstrates results of single-stage breast reconstruction with direct closure of donor defect and adequate autogenous tissue to achieve breast mound projection. (From Mathes SJ, Nahai F: Reconstructive Surgery: Principles, Anatomy, and Technique. New York, Churchill Livingstone, 1997:113.)

Expander-Implant Reconstruction

Breast reconstruction may be accomplished with immediate or delayed insertion of an implant alone when sufficient soft tissues exist to permit coverage of a permanent prosthesis placed subpectorally with tension-free skin closure. In general, this option of permanent implant placement without prior expansion is appropriate only for patients in whom the skin envelope is preserved, that is, patients treated by skin-sparing mastectomy or subcutaneous mastectomy.

For most patients who choose implant reconstruction, it will be necessary to undergo a two-stage expander/implant sequence. The design of the expander has changed since its inception. Advances in design include port location (distant to the actual implant or incorporated into the wall of the expander), shape of the expander (round to rectangular), wall

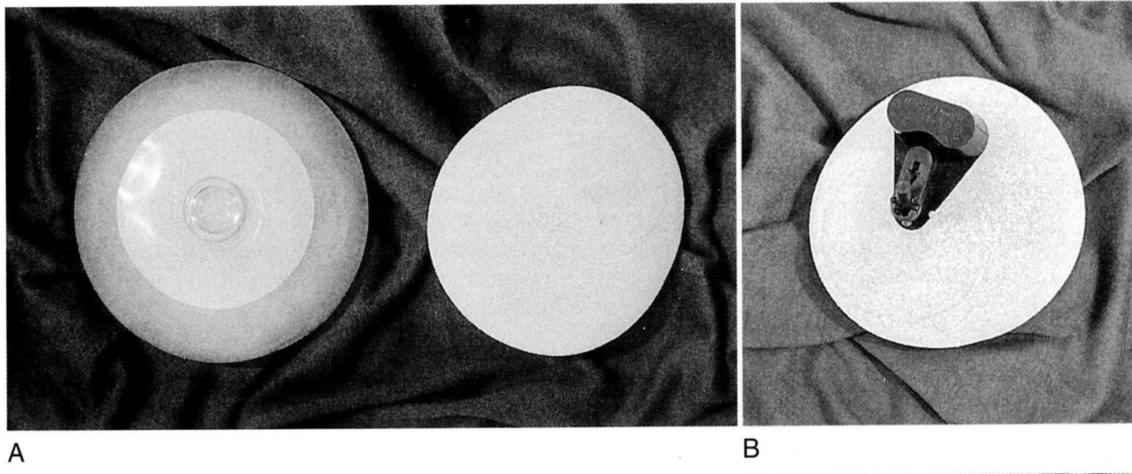

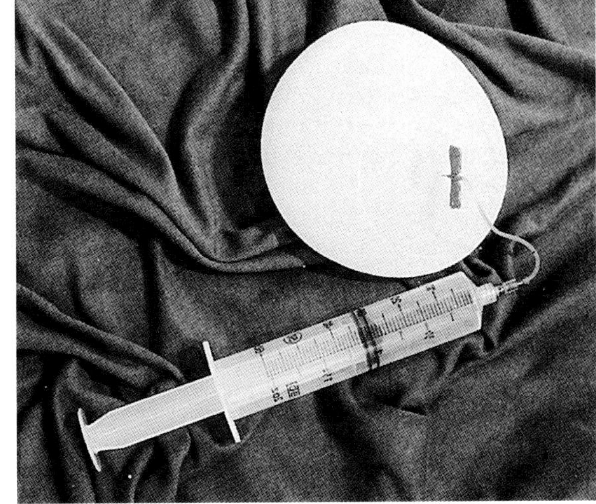

FIGURE 138-19. Round expanders with integral port for breast reconstruction. *A,* Mentor 700 mL *(left)* and McGhan 400 mL *(right)*. *B,* McGhan style 133 implant: magnetic detector for location of port. *C,* Insertion of 23-gauge needle for saline injection (magnetic metallic backing prevents needle puncture of expander wall). (From Mathes SJ, Nahai F: Reconstructive Surgery: Principles, Anatomy, and Technique. New York, Churchill Livingstone, 1997:60.)

composition (smooth and textured), and duration of the device (temporary and permanent); the permanent implant has a distant port allowing removal of the port while the implant is maintained when appropriate volume is established (Fig. 138-19).

Despite advances in design, the use of implants alone and the expander/implant sequence for immediate or delayed reconstruction has declined, and there has been an increase in the use of local and distant flaps for breast reconstruction. This trend in less frequent use of implant/expanders is in part due to the silicone implant controversy. In 1992, the FDA withdrew the use of gel-filled silicone breast implants, allowing use of only saline-filled silicone wall implants unless the surgeon is included in an approved clinical trial. In a study by Alderman et al[220] of 1607 reconstructed patients in 1998, the ratio of total autogenous reconstructions (autogenous reconstructions plus autogenous with implant) to the number of implants alone was 2:1. The Alderman study concurs with a study by Trabulsy and Mathes[241] of 455 postmastectomy reconstructions that occurred in three chronologic study groups: group I, 1979-1983; group II, 1984-1987; and group III, 1988-1991. This study found a significant decrease over time in the use of implants alone and also with latissimus dorsi flap with implant. Use of the TRAM flap, which gives the patient an autogenous wound reconstruction, increased markedly over the study period.

BREAST IMPLANT SAFETY

Because many mastectomy patients prefer the simplicity of an implant for breast reconstruction, and many breast reconstruction patients undergo augmentation or mastopexy augmentation of the contralateral breast for symmetry, a review of the current status of the implant in regard to safety is appropriate. Breast implants were introduced in the United States in the 1960s and were widely available for breast augmentation and breast reconstruction until 1992.

At that time, it was estimated that approximately 1 million women in the United States had received breast implants for augmentation or reconstruction. In 1992, the FDA limited the use of silicone gel–filled implants[242] to patients undergoing silicone gel implant replacement and postmastectomy patients undergoing reconstruction performed by surgeons approved for clinical trials of the silicone implant. Saline implants were approved for both augmentation and reconstruction. On the basis of the clinical trial results and implant review at FDA hearings, an FDA advisory committee recommended approval of one manufacturer's silicone gel–filled breast implants in 2003.[243] The agency responded with additional research requirements for companies applying to market their breast implants in the United States.[244] Silicone gel–filled breast implants continue to be available under FDA-approved clinical studies. Saline-filled breast implants made by two manufacturers were approved for marketing in the United States in 2000.[245]

Patients may have many questions associated with the long-term effects of silicone breast implants for breast augmentation or reconstruction, including the following: Are breast implants associated with difficulty in screening? Do patients who undergo reconstruction with implants have an increased rate of breast cancer recurrence or a decreased length of survival? Are there links between breast implants and systemic disease, particularly connective tissue disorders? These are key questions for women considering surgery with breast implants and their physicians.

Screening in Patients with Breast Implants

The Eklund maneuver facilitates the optimization of mammography for patients with implants (see "Diagnostic Imaging in Patients with Breast Implants"), but not all women with implants will necessarily have access to mammographers familiar with imaging of the augmented breast.

Young et al[246] reported a study in 1993 evaluating the relative radiolucencies of five breast implant filler materials: silicone gel, saline, breast tissue equivalent, peanut oil (triglycerides), and polyvinylpyrrolidone (Bio-Oncotic gel). Peanut oil demonstrated the highest clarity of imaging, required the least radiation exposure, and was found to be four times more radiolucent than saline or polyvinylpyrrolidone; peanut oil was 45 times more radiolucent than silicone gel. Whereas peanut oil implants were available only for a brief period under clinical trials, it is important to consider the benefits of more radiolucent prosthetic filler materials in future implant design. As noted in the section on diagnostic imaging in patients with implants, cancer diagnosis is not delayed in augmented versus control patients. Mammography, despite limitations from the presence of an implant, is effective in screening for breast cancer.

Breast Implants and Breast Cancer Risk

The lifetime incidence of breast cancer in the American female population is approximately 8%, and it follows that a corresponding percentage of the patients who received implant placement will go on to develop breast cancer. Birdsell et al[247] in 1993 studied the stage of breast cancer at time of detection and survival rates for 41 women who developed breast cancer after cosmetic implant placement and compared how these women fared versus women without implants who were diagnosed with breast cancer. They found no significant difference in the stage at diagnosis between the two populations, and in fact, for unclear reasons, the tumors of the women with breast implants were smaller at the time the diagnosis was made. Earlier, in 1985, Georgiade et al[248] compared 101 women who underwent implant reconstruction after mastectomy for breast cancer with 377 women with breast cancer who did not have implants. They looked at risk of recurrence or death and found no significant difference in relapse-free survival between the implant and control group patients when adjustments were made for nuclear grade, nodal status, age, and histologic grade. Hoshaw et al[249] performed a meta-analysis looking at the same questions posed by the Birdsell and Georgiade studies. Numerous other studies corroborated their results.[28,250,251] Bryant et al[252] looked at whether breast implants placed for cosmetic surgery imparted any additional risk for breast cancer in a study population. They found that the patients who had breast augmentation had the same incidence of breast cancer as that of the general population during the period in which their cohort was observed. Another study compared two subgroups of breast cancer patients who underwent either implant or autogenous reconstruction with matched-stage control breast cancer patients who did not undergo reconstruction.[253] They found no significant difference in length of survival or local recurrence between either subgroup of reconstructed patients and the control patients.

Deapen et al[27] in 2000 reported a large retrospective cohort study of 3182 patients who had cosmetic breast augmentation. Breast cancer incidence from their cohort was compared with population-based cancer registry reports from Los Angeles County and with the SEER database. Only 37 patients of their cohort developed an invasive or in situ breast cancer. The stage at presentation and 5-year survival of these patients were similar to those predicted by the SEER database survival rates.

Each individual study that addressed the question of whether breast implant patients experience a delay in diagnosis and consequent decrease in survival is limited by the small number of patients who were diagnosed with breast cancer, making a statistically significant conclusion difficult to achieve, even in very large cohort studies. Taken together, these studies concur that augmented patients have equivalent outcomes in terms of breast cancer incidence, stage at diagnosis, and overall survival compared with nonaugmented patients.

Silicone Breast Implants and Risk for Connective Tissue Disorders

Whereas early studies,[254] anecdotal reports, and legal claims filed against silicone implant manufacturers suggested a linkage between silicone breast implants and connective tissue disorders (particularly scleroderma), subsequent epidemiologic studies did not show any significant difference in the prevalence of connective tissue disorders in women with and without silicone breast implants.[255,256] A comprehensive meta-analysis of 20 studies of silicone gel-filled breast implants by Janowsky et al[257] published in 2000 found that breast implants contribute no detectable influence on the number of women in whom connective tissue disorders develop. The definitive study on the safety of breast implants—the government-funded Institute of Medicine study,[258] published in 2000—reviewed more than 1000 research reports and concluded that silicone gel implants do not increase the risk for autoimmune diseases or cancer. The study by Kjoller et al[259] of Danish women with implants also supported the same conclusions.

From a public health perspective, elimination of silicone implants from the market would likely not have an impact on the incidence of connective tissue diseases such as rheumatoid arthritis, systemic lupus erythematosus, scleroderma or systemic sclerosis, and Sjögren syndrome. Connective tissue disorders appear to be no more common in women with silicone breast implants than in women without implants.

Although questions about the long-term safety of silicone breast implants have been answered by the many studies conducted during the past decade, non–life-threatening localized problems that may occur in the area of the breast implant remain the primary concern. The FDA's updated data requirements for implant manufacturers call for additional data on mechanical testing, implant rupture, clinical information, and product labeling to address issues that remain.[260]

INDICATIONS

In general, implant reconstruction alone is considered only in patients whose contralateral breast is small, and thus a symmetric breast mound may be established by this technique. Unfortunately, the initial wound healing milieu surrounding the site of implant insertion (immediate reconstruction) or dissection of preserved skin envelope with scar release (delayed reconstruction) risks implant exposure and increased scar around the implant, resulting in capsular contracture and lack of natural breast ptosis (Table 138-20).

The advantages of permanent implant reconstruction are decreased operative time, no requirement for a second procedure, technical ease of the procedure, no additional scars, good color match, and no donor site morbidity as is inherent to flap reconstruction.

The expander has allowed more consistent results and decreased complications (such as severe capsular contracture or implant exposure) when the existing skin envelope after mastectomy is used without additional flap tissue. The expander is generally used as a temporary device to prepare the skin envelope for the permanent implant. Because the implant does not have to be filled to the final desired volume for breast size at the time of initial insertion, there is less concern about pressure and subsequent impaired circulation in the remaining overlying skin (Table 138-21).

IMPLANT SELECTION

Implant selection will vary with the surgeon's preference and experience, and there is no specific implant that provides superior results. Implant categories include shape (round or biodimensional), fill (silicone liquid, cohesive silicone gel, or saline), and surface variation (smooth or textured). Several choices of implant type exist. Round and dome-shaped implants are commonly used, one potential disadvantage being excessive upper pole fullness. Biodimensional implants attempt to avoid this problem by forming an implant

TABLE 138-20 ✦ INDICATIONS FOR AND CONTRAINDICATIONS TO IMPLANT BREAST RECONSTRUCTION

Indications	Contraindications
Skin envelope adequate for implant use	Unstable circulation in existing skin envelope (relative)
Contralateral breast surgery is planned for symmetry (augmentation, mastopexy, or reduction mammaplasty)	Opposite ptotic or large breast that patient wishes to preserve and match with reconstructed breast mound (relative)
Distant donor site unacceptable to patient or surgical risk unacceptable	Planned postoperative radiation therapy
	Implant unacceptable to patient
	Current smoker (relative contraindication)

TABLE 138-21 ✦ INDICATIONS FOR AND CONTRAINDICATIONS TO IMPLANT-EXPANDER RECONSTRUCTION

Immediate	Delayed
Indications	*Indications*
Skin envelope adequate for coverage of expander	Skin envelope adequate for coverage of expander
Contralateral breast small without ptosis or minimal ptosis	Revision of contralateral breast planned for symmetry with reconstructed breast mound (augmentation, reduction mammaplasty, or mastopexy)
Surgery of contralateral breast planned for symmetry with reconstructed breast mound (augmentation, reduction mammaplasty, or mastopexy)	Distant donor site unacceptable to patient or surgical risk unacceptable
Distant donor site unacceptable to patient or surgical risk unacceptable	
Contraindications	*Contraindications*
Skin envelope circulation impaired without adequate local muscle or fascial flaps available for expander coverage	Unstable skin envelope secondary to surgical scars or radiation injury
Opposite large or ptotic breast and patient wishes reconstructed mound to match existing opposite breast	Implant unacceptable to patient
Chest wall radiation therapy planned (relative contraindication)	Opposite large or ptotic breast and patient wishes reconstructed mound to match existing opposite breast
Current smoker (relative contraindication)	Current smoker (relative contraindication)
Implant unacceptable to patient	

with a nonround, more anatomic shape. Silicone gel–filled breast implants are once again available for use if the surgeon participates in clinical trials of implant safety and complications.[262,263] Although silicone breast implants are not yet approved for unrestricted use for breast augmentation and reconstruction, current studies support the safety of the silicone gel[249,264] (see Chapter 143). Given the concern about the safety of silicone gel–filled implants in the last decade, some reconstructive surgeons began using saline-filled implants with good results and have continued using the saline implants. The texture of the implant is another consideration. Implants with textured surfaces promote tissue adherence, theoretically reducing the likelihood of implant migration or capsular contracture.

TECHNIQUE (IMPLANT)

Implant insertion for breast reconstruction is generally used for immediate reconstruction where a small implant is required for breast mound symmetry with the contralateral breast, or in delayed reconstruction if the patient has an adequate skin envelope (Fig. 138-20). If the required volume of implant is large (more than 400 mL), the implant size may result in excessive pressure on the preserved skin envelope and may make muscle coverage of the implant (if it is planned at implant site insertion) difficult. The Becker implant has a distant port that allows only partial implant expansion on an immediate basis with delay completion of implant filling with saline and provides an alternative approach to immediate implant insertion. Although it is not a two-stage procedure, later removal of the distant port is likely to be necessary.

TECHNIQUE (EXPANDER/IMPLANT)

The process of expansion counteracts the early tendency for wound contracture, particularly in immediate reconstruction, where the entire deep surface of the skin envelope has been injured by breast tissue resection. Unless a permanent expander-implant device is used, the expander-implant technique requires a staged procedure generally involving two operations: expander insertion, which avoids two reconstructive procedures if it is done at the time of mastectomy; and removal of the expander and insertion of the permanent implant. In general, the two-stage expander-implant is selected because the combination expander-implant is not as well designed for both expansion and permanent breast implant.

The expander is inserted beneath the pectoralis major muscle (Fig. 138-21). Many surgeons do not obtain complete muscle coverage, preferring to allow the inferior part of the expander to lie at the inferior

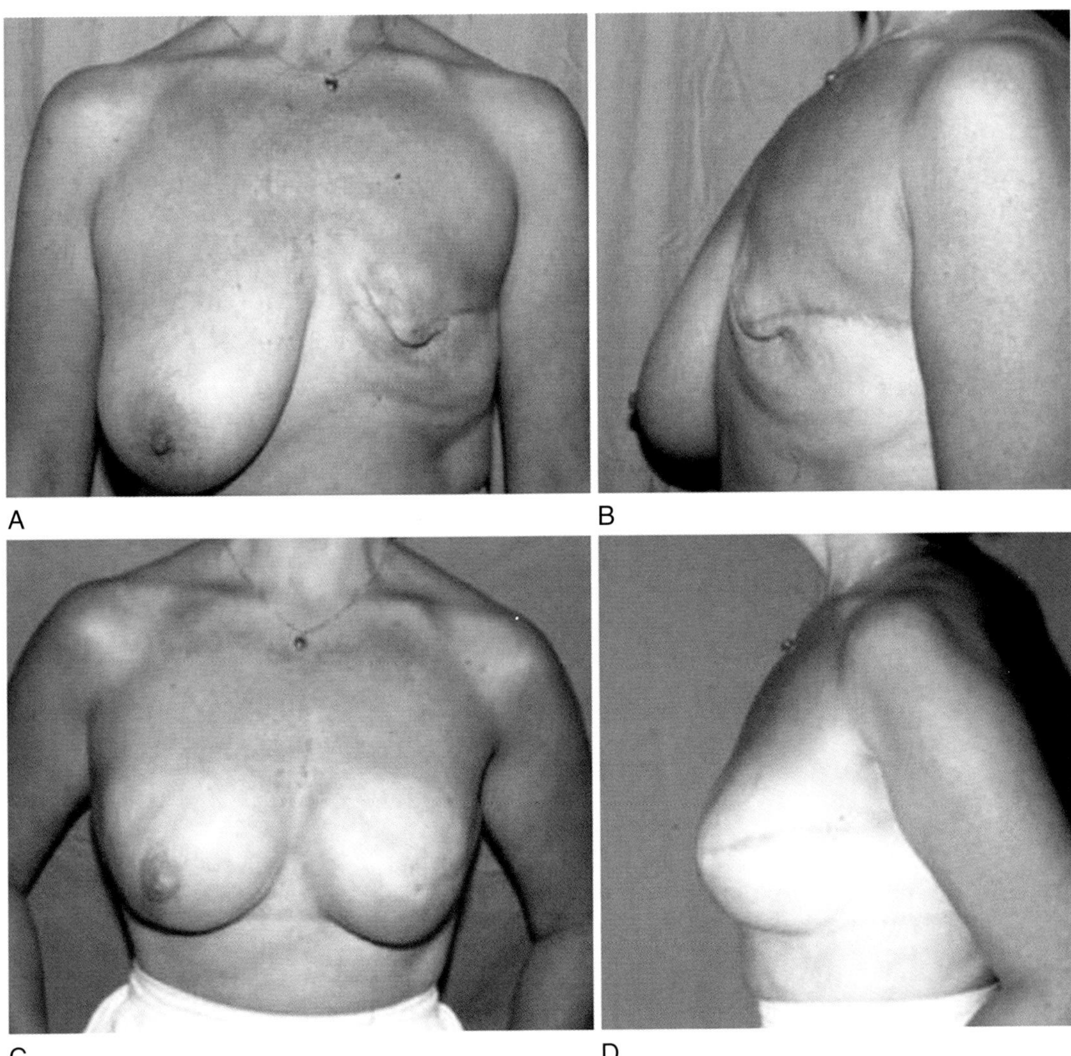

FIGURE 138-20. Implant reconstruction of postoperative left modified radical mastectomy. *A,* Skin envelope adequate for single-stage reconstruction with implant. *B,* Lateral view of mastectomy defect. *C,* Postoperative view 1 year after single-stage breast reconstruction with implant. The contralateral breast underwent reduction mammaplasty for symmetry. *D,* Postoperative lateral view demonstrates adequate projection and definition of inframammary line.

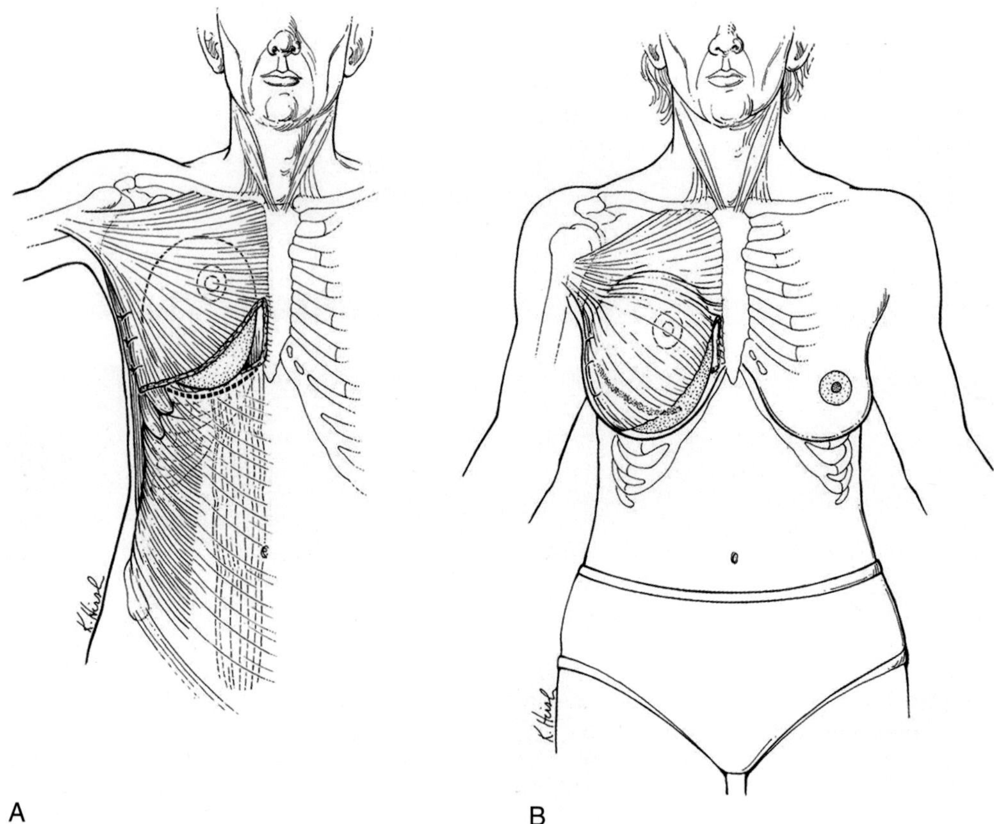

FIGURE 138-21. Expander in position *(A)* and filled *(B)*.

mammary line with the lower third directly beneath the preserved skin envelope, where maximal projection during the expansion process is most desired. In the immediate reconstruction, there is greater risk of skin loss and implant exposure. When overlying skin circulation appears impaired, complete submuscular expander placement is desirable. Complete expander-implant coverage requires a combination of the pectoralis major and either the serratus anterior muscle or segmental rectus abdominis–external oblique flaps (see Chapter 143). In 2 to 3 weeks, the patient is ready for saline injections to begin the expansion process. The goal is generally overexpansion of the skin envelope (20% larger than planned permanent breast implant volume). This process usually requires saline injections weekly or every 2 to 3 weeks (approximately 50 to 100 mL per visit). When adequate expansion is complete, generally in 3 months, the patient is returned to the operating room for permanent implant insertion (see Fig. 138-21). If alteration of the opposite breast is planned, this procedure is usually performed simultaneously. If the opposite breast is undergoing this procedure for symmetry, performing the second-stage reconstructive procedure and the contralateral breast modification allows intraoperative decisions to ensure optimal symmetry. The time interval between expander insertion and permanent implant placement may vary on the basis of the surgeon's recommendations and the patient's preference. Delay of more than 3 months does not seem to alter outcome, although after 6 months of expander placement, there is often increased capsular contracture around the expander. Decreasing the interval between procedures (less than 2 to 3 months) may not allow time for adequate expansion and for the completion of the wound healing process associated with the mastectomy, particularly after immediate reconstruction. If the patient is receiving chemotherapy or radiation therapy, the second stage is generally delayed until these therapeutic treatments are complete. As previously noted, radiation therapy represents a relative contraindication for an expander because damage to the skin envelope decreases the skin envelope volume and elicits capsular contracture when the permanent implant is inserted.

Many groups have reported their experience with staged expander-implant reconstruction.[265,266] Anatomic expanders may provide a more naturally shaped breast reconstruction result as they preferentially expand the lower pole.[267] Spear et al[265] find staged implant reconstruction with serial expansion to give superior results to one-stage implant alone procedures. Gui et al[268] reported on immediate breast reconstruction with biodimensional anatomic permanent expander implants. They found that this one-stage procedure with shaped implants gave good results. The implant was filled with saline intraoperatively after placement and closure of the submuscular and subcutaneous pockets. Final implant filling was performed in the outpatient setting.

Although implant reconstruction often provides a satisfactory result, there is general agreement that autologous reconstruction produces a more natural breast reconstruction. It is important to tailor the reconstructive plan to the patient's needs; some patients are clearly medically unsuitable for the additional morbidity incurred by undergoing flap reconstruction. In addition, some patients simply will not want to undergo TRAM flap reconstruction, the current standard of care. Only one group of patients should be particularly cautioned to avoid implant reconstruction—patients who will undergo radiation treatment. It has been clearly demonstrated that radiation therapy results in an increased incidence of capsular contracture. Several groups have reported increased rates of capsular contracture (30% to 45%) after postmastectomy radiation therapy in the setting of implant reconstruction.[269,270] Spear et al[271] found in their series that 47.5% of irradiated breasts with saline implants ultimately required conversion to flap reconstruction because of problems with the appearance of the implants. The expander-implant technique requires minimal hospital and recuperative time and is appealing to the active patient who cannot or is unwilling to miss work or personal obligations. Many patients are able to return to work or exercise programs within 7 to 10 days after each procedure—expander insertion and the later permanent implant insertion (Figs. 138-22 and 138-23).

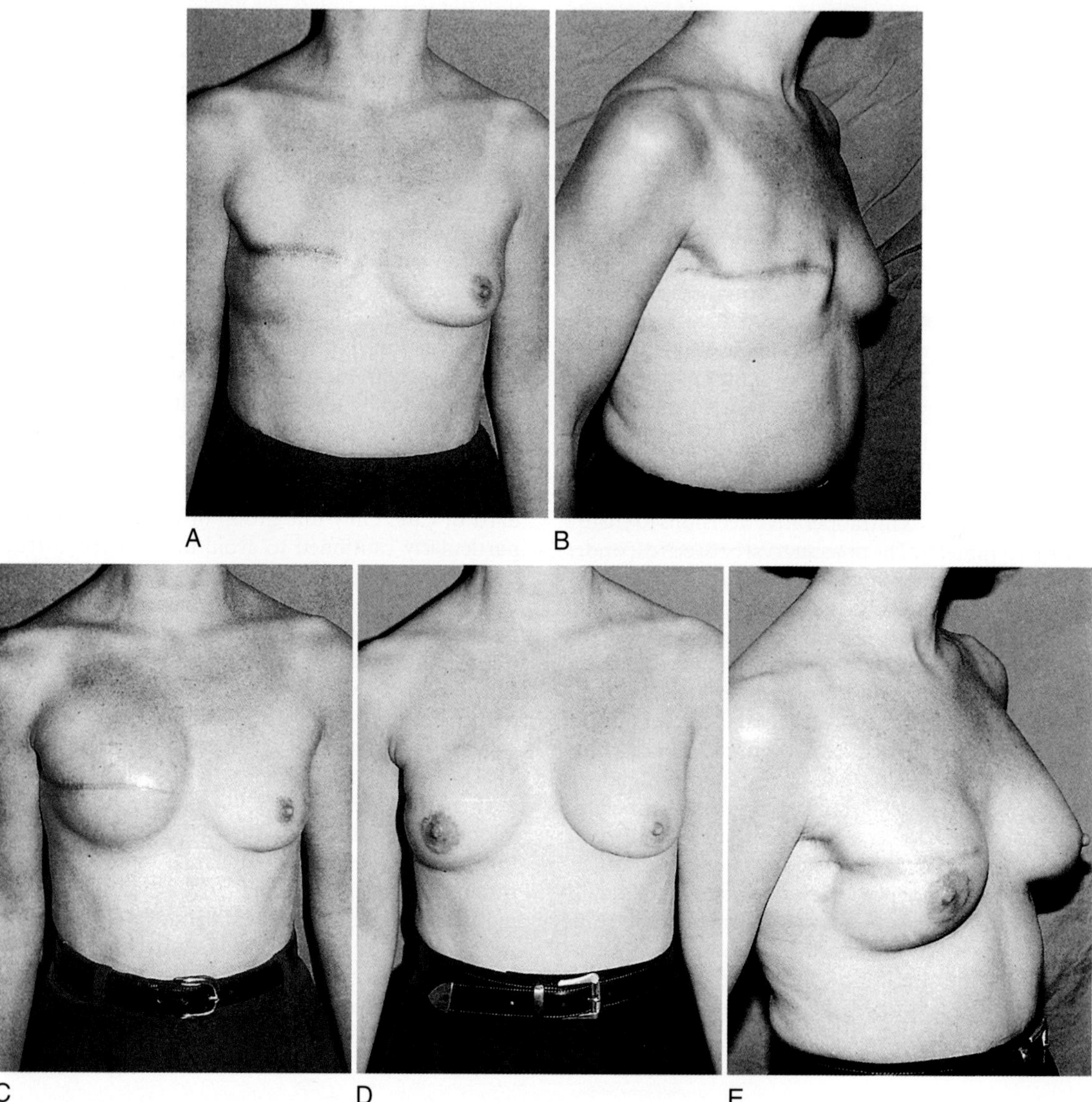

FIGURE 138-22. Tissue expansion for breast reconstruction. *A* and *B,* Modified radical mastectomy defect with stable chest wall skin. *C,* Postoperative view at 3 months shows the well-defined inframammary line with skin expansion centered between the third and sixth intercostal spaces. *D* and *E,* Views at 1 year after second-stage expander removal and permanent implant insertion. The expanded skin provides an adequate envelope for the silicone wall saline-filled permanent implant. (From Mathes SJ, Nahai F: Reconstructive Surgery: Principles, Anatomy, and Technique. New York, Churchill Livingstone, 1997:72.)

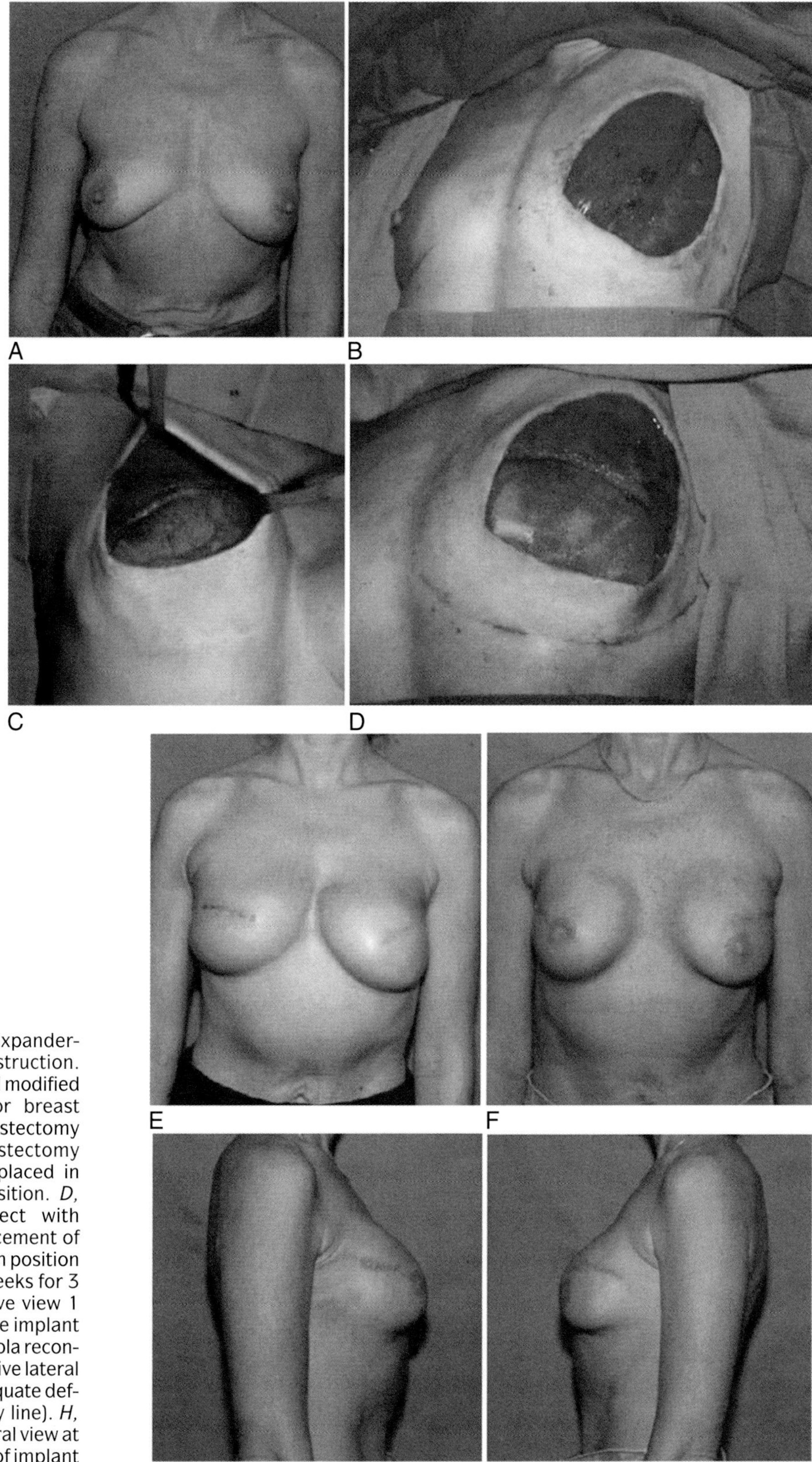

FIGURE 138-23. Expander-implant breast reconstruction. *A,* Preoperative bilateral modified radical mastectomy for breast carcinoma. *B,* Left mastectomy defect. *C,* Right mastectomy defect with expander placed in partial subpectoral position. *D,* Left mastectomy defect with partial subpectoral placement of expander. *E,* Expander in position with inflation every 3 weeks for 3 months. *F,* Postoperative view 1 year after bilateral saline implant insertion and nipple-areola reconstruction. *G,* Postoperative lateral view at 1 year (note adequate definition of inframammary line). *H,* Postoperative right lateral view at 1 year, superior aspect of implant in subpectoral position.

Transposition Flap Reconstruction

When the silicone implant was introduced in 1964 by Cronin and Gerow,[272] most patients underwent a radical mastectomy with resultant loss of a majority of the skin envelope (many patients required skin grafts for wound closure at the time of mastectomy) and the pectoralis major muscle. As a result, use of the implant alone provided an unnatural breast mound, so the implant could not be used for reconstruction without first providing flap coverage. Flap coverage was accomplished by abdominal cutaneous-fasciocutaneous flaps (e.g., thoracoepigastric flap) followed by staged implant insertion; see the later section entitled "Thoracoepigastric (Transverse Abdominal) Flap." The infraclavicular hollow, due to absence of the pectoralis major, was not corrected because of lack of soft tissue availability. The other option for breast reconstruction was the tubed pedicle flap (Fig. 138-24). Although it was a multistaged procedure,[272,273] it did provide adequate soft tissue and skin to allow autogenous reconstruction.

In the 1970s, anatomic research on muscle flaps revisited the latissimus musculocutaneous flap originally used by Tansini[274,275] for immediate coverage of a mastectomy defect in 1896. This technique provided the patient with cutaneous coverage of the defect as well as functional muscle to replace the absent pectoralis major muscle (Fig. 138-25). Unfortunately, this technique was lost for many years until it was rediscovered and used in the late 1970s, and this technique continues to be widely used for breast reconstruction, chest wall coverage, and head and neck reconstruction.[274] The reintroduction of the latissimus dorsi musculocutaneous flap provided a safe and reliable method to accomplish a satisfactory breast reconstruction for the large population of women with unsightly and difficult chest deformity after radical mastectomy. Despite the trend away from the aggressive radical mastectomy to the more conservative modified radical mastectomy and, in many patients, the skin-sparing mastectomy, the latissimus muscle flap is frequently used to provide implant coverage, the latissimus dorsi musculocutaneous flap for complex defect reconstruction (i.e., large skin envelope deficiency with impaired circulation due to radiotherapy) and secondary reconstruction. It often represents the only available method for patients with unavailable regional and distant flap donor sites. Furthermore, the flap can be designed in certain individuals to include adequate soft tissue to provide an autogenous reconstruction (no implant device is used to restore breast mound volume).

In the late l970s, plastic surgeons began the search for other sources of regional flap tissue suitable for breast reconstruction. Mathes[276] identified the rectus abdominis musculocutaneous flap and successfully used the vertical skin island for inferior anterior chest wall reconstruction (Fig. 138-26). Subsequently, Hartrampf[277] envisioned a transverse skin island using the redundant skin and soft tissue between the umbilicus and the pubis. He successfully transferred the rectus abdominis musculocutaneous flap with the transverse skin (TRAM) island for autogenous single-stage breast reconstruction. The skin of this flap was incorporated into the remaining postmastectomy envelope, and the underlying fatty tissue and muscle provided the required breast mound volume and projection. The donor site closure was transversely located above the pubic hair line, and with loss of the abdominal panniculus, the multiparous woman was provided with improved abdominal contour similar to the resultant appearance after abdominoplasty. This method of breast reconstruction is now commonly used for autogenous reconstruction, particularly after skin-sparing mastectomy. This method also works well for the postmastectomy patient and for patients in whom implant or other techniques have failed.

With the identification of the pedicles for flaps that may provide both skin and soft tissue applicable for breast reconstruction, microvascular composite tissue transplantation soon was applied to the field of breast reconstruction. The initial interest in transplantation of the TRAM flap based on its inferior pedicle, the deep inferior epigastric artery and paired venae comitantes, gained great acceptance for autogenous breast reconstruction. When the TRAM flap was unavailable, the superior or inferior half of the gluteus maximus musculocutaneous flap based on the superior or inferior gluteal artery and associated venae comitantes was transplanted to suitable receptor vessels in proximity to the mastectomy defect. The donor site closure did alter buttock symmetry, but this autogenous tissue provided a reasonable source of flap for breast reconstruction. Because perforator vessels that pass between the muscle's superficial surface to the overlying skin may be dissected independently of the muscle and eventually traced to their origin from the major muscle pedicle, it has become attractive to use this perforator flap for transplantation to the mastectomy defect to provide breast reconstruction. This dissection preserves continuity of the donor muscle and avoids potential weakness at the donor site. Perforator flaps have been based on the deep inferior epigastric vascular pedicle and the superior and inferior gluteal vascular pedicle. These two donor sites, based on perforator vessel dissection, preserve muscle function of the rectus abdominis or gluteus maximus.

As the quest for other donor sites has increased during the past 2 decades, successful transplantation of other tissues has provided breast mound

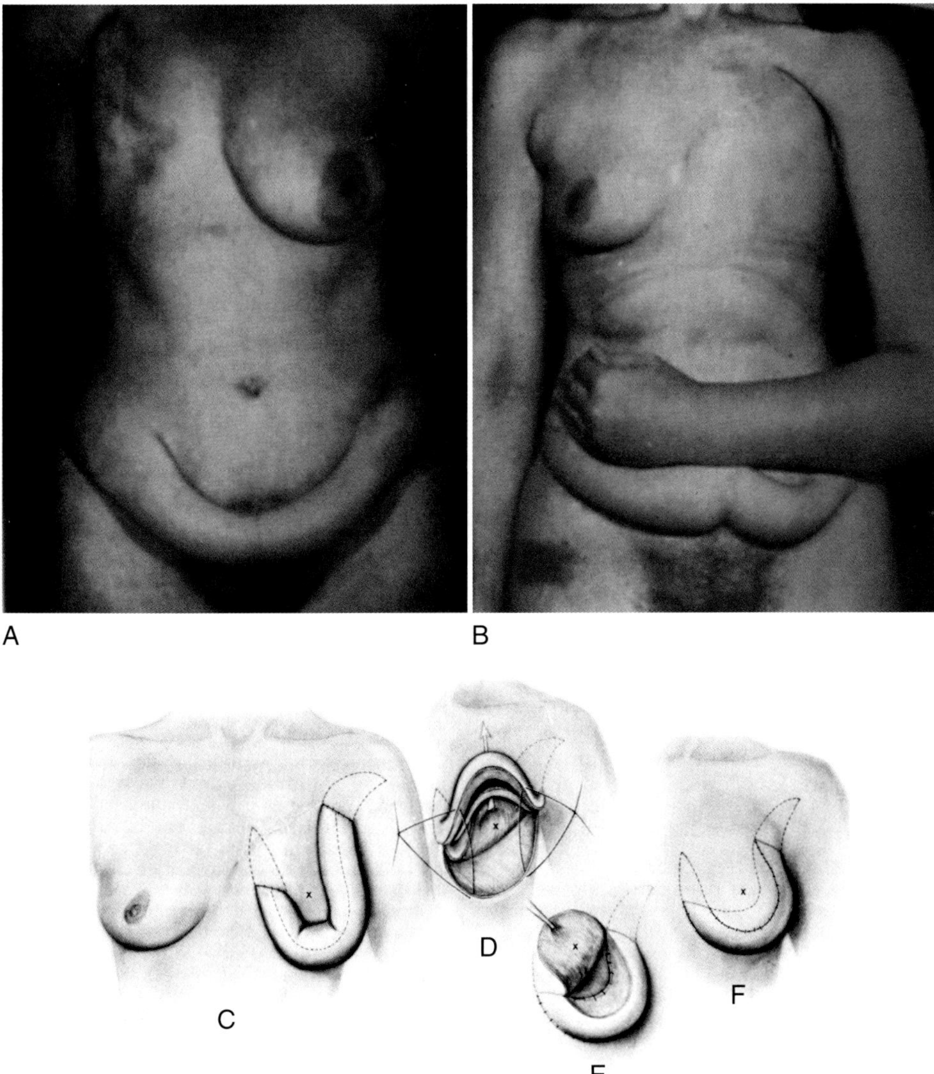

FIGURE 138-24. Breast reconstruction by tubed pedicle flap. The initial stage of the procedure is the design of the tubed pedicle flap, and the second stage is inset of the tubed pedicle flap to restore the breast mound. *A,* Design of an abdominal tube flap for breast reconstruction. After an abdominal lipectomy, a tube is formed from the excess tissue for later inset into the breast mound. *B,* Design of abdominal tube for breast reconstruction by use of an arm carrier. After an abdominal lipectomy, a tube is formed from the excess skin and tissue for later inset into the breast defect. A small wrist attachment is made just to the right of the old midline scar in the flap, as the flap is swung on its pedicle for breast mound reconstruction. *C,* The broken line on the tube indicates its seam; the broken lines extending above the two pedicles indicate the areas in which they are implanted. *D,* The seam of the tubed abdominal flap has been opened, and the chest flap X has been elevated after a chest incision has been made in the inframammary line from one pedicle of the tubed flap to the other. The lower margin of the partially opened tubed flap will be sutured to the lower edge of the inframammary incision. *E,* The upper half of the surface of the tubed flap has been denuded where the chest flap will cover it, and its upper edge has been sutured up in place. *F,* The overlapping chest flap has been sutured down on the tubed flap. After healing, the soft tissue mound will be ready for a breast implant (if necessary) and for free nipple and areola grafts. (*C* to *F* from Millard DR Jr: Breast reconstruction after a radical mastectomy. Plast Reconstr Surg 1976;58:283-291.)

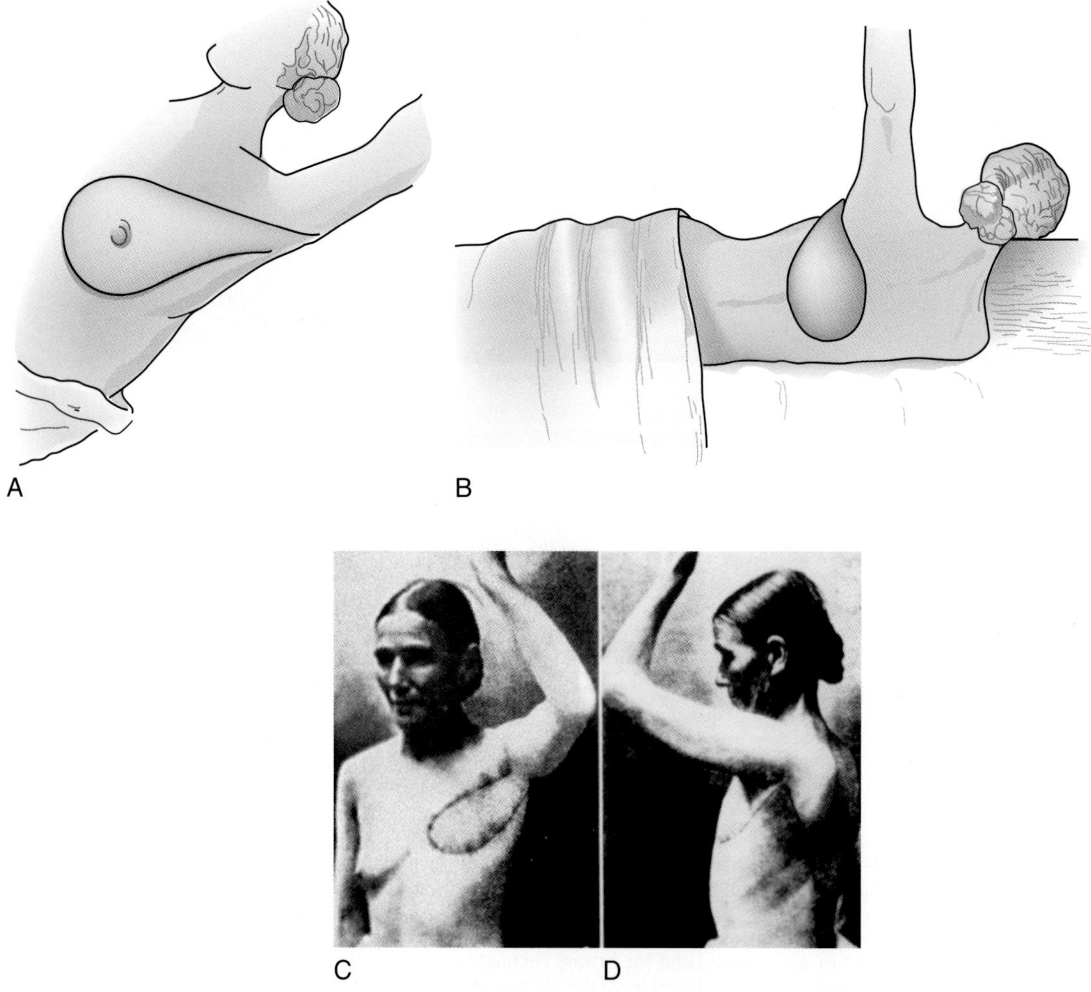

FIGURE 138-25. Breast reconstruction by Tansini latissimus dorsi musculocutaneous flap. *A,* The area of skin to be excised with the mastectomy. *B,* The design of the posterior musculocutaneous flap for defect coverage. *C,* One of Tansini's patients; result after radical mastectomy with latissimus dorsi musculocutaneous flap coverage. *D,* Primary closure of donor site. (*A* and *B* redrawn from Tansini I: Nuovo processo per l'amputazione della mammella per cancre. Riforma Med 1896;12:3. From Maxwell GP: Iginio Tansini and the origin of the latissimus dorsi musculocutaneous flap. Plast Reconstr Surg 1980;65:686-692. *C* and *D* from Purpura F: Tansini method for cure of cancer of the breast. Lancet 1908;1:634.)

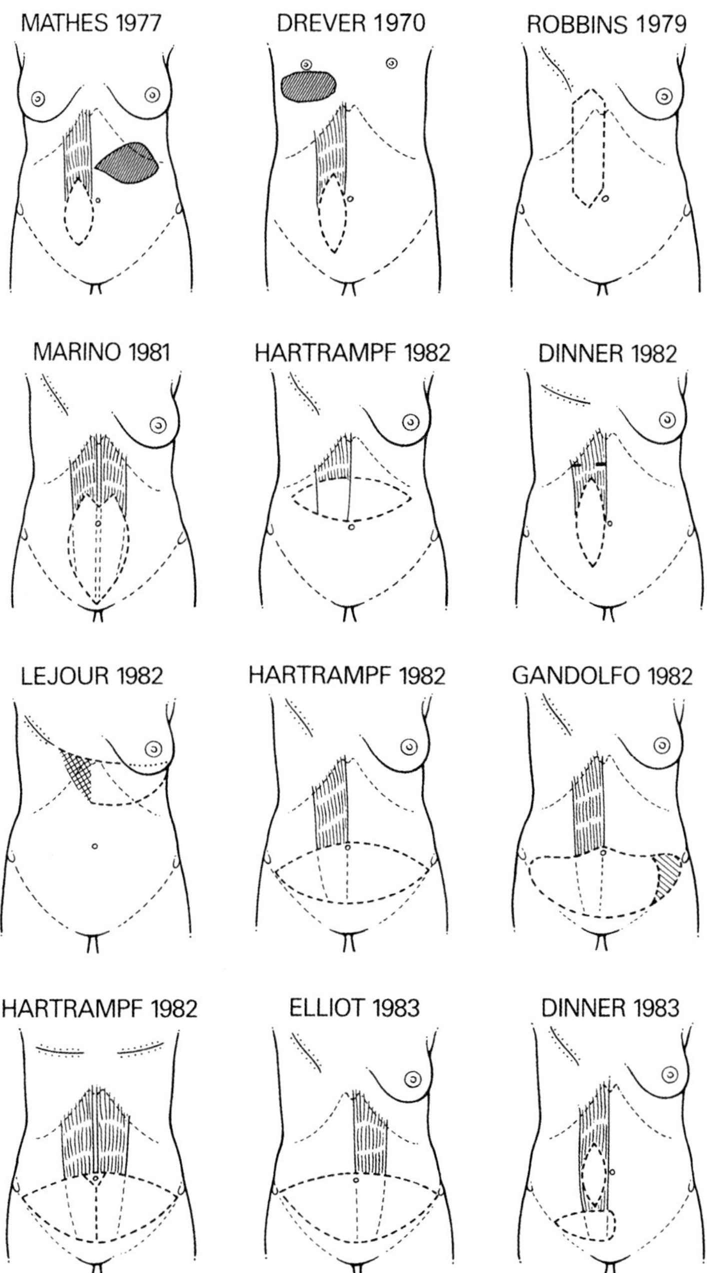

FIGURE 138-26. Evolution of skin territory designs for superiorly based rectus abdominis musculocutaneous flaps. (From Cormack GC, Lamberty BG: The Arterial Anatomy of Skin Flaps. Edinburgh, Churchill Livingstone, 1986.)

autogenous reconstruction. Examples include the superficial epigastric artery and venae comitantes (lower abdomen), the deep branch of the circumflex iliac artery and venae comitantes (deep groin or Rubens flap), the medial and lateral femoral circumflex descending artery and venae comitantes (medial and lateral thigh flap), and the medial femoral circumflex artery and venae comitantes (gracilis). With the exception of the gracilis musculocutaneous flap, all of the fasciocutaneous flaps are generally based on septocutaneous vessels. Each has both skin and soft tissue capable of providing autogenous breast reconstruction. Because pedicle location may vary and donor site closure scar is more obvious, the rectus abdominis musculocutaneous flap based on its inferior deep pedicle and the modified design based solely on the perforator vessels and their connection with the deep inferior epigastric are the most common methods involving microvascular transplantation (free flap method). Each category of flap used solely for skin envelope correction or for both skin envelope and breast mound size and projection is discussed in regard to indications, technique, and outcome (Table 138-22).

LATISSIMUS DORSI MUSCULOCUTANEOUS FLAP

The latissimus dorsi musculocutaneous flap is useful for breast reconstruction in patients without sufficient redundant abdominal skin necessary for donor site closure for a TRAM flap. In nulliparous thin patients, the TRAM flap may provide necessary skin for the skin envelope reconstruction but not adequate soft tissue for autogenous breast mound reconstruction. In this group of patients, use of the TRAM flap would still require implant for the breast mound. Since the patient has a preexisting youthful contour to her abdomen, the latissimus musculocutaneous flap with implant is a more acceptable donor site and provides an equivalent result. It is also useful for patients who require a flap for the skin envelope but have abdominal incisions in which the rectus muscle was divided and is not available for use as a superiorly based transposition flap for breast mound reconstruction. Most patients who are candidates for the latissimus dorsi flap will also be candidates for the TRAM flap. However, certain patients may want to avoid abdominal incisions, preferring instead the back donor sites that can easily be hidden within the bra line. In general, the donor site incision is long (approximately 20 cm) in the subscapular area. Endoscopic muscle harvest has been reported with good results, thereby minimizing incisions,[278] but most patients require both muscle and the overlying skin island for satisfactory reconstruction.

Most patients who receive latissimus dorsi flap reconstruction will require an implant for a breast mound of sufficient size. It is possible to include subcutaneous tissue adjacent to the skin island, and in selected patients, an autogenous reconstruction can be accomplished (Table 138-23).

The major vascular pedicle of this flap is the thoracodorsal artery, a branch of the subscapular artery (Fig. 138-27). It is important to ascertain patency of this artery before operation by verifying the innervation of the muscle by assessing for isometric contraction since the artery and nerve course in close proximity. Loss of muscle innervation may indicate associated injury to the thoracodorsal artery and vein. Although muscle bulk is atrophic in a denervated muscle, the vascular communications to the muscle belly and skin are still intact; thus, a denervated flap may be used if other reconstructive options are not available.[276] Even if the thoracodorsal artery has been ligated during mastectomy or axillary dissection, the latissimus dorsi flap may still be used, based on communicating vessels between the serratus anterior with arterial reversal of flow into the thoracodorsal pedicle and the latissimus dorsi.

Preoperative Markings and Preparation

In immediate reconstruction, the extent of skin resection is confirmed with the responsible oncologic breast surgeon. The posterior skin island, based on the planned mastectomy dissection, is marked

TABLE 138-22 ✦ COMPARISON OF IMMEDIATE TRANSPOSITION FLAPS BY TYPE[237,241,286,300-303]

	Latissimus Dorsi	TRAM (Unipedicled)	TRAM (Bipedicled)
Potential for coverage	Excellent	Excellent	Excellent
Potential for mound	Implant required	Good	Good
Mean operative time (hours)	3.8	5.5	6.6
Hospitalization (days)	4	4	7.6
Complications (% by type)	38.8	23.6	26.9
Seroma	2-3	1.4	5
Partial flap loss	7	5	13
Donor site hernia	N/A	5.9	2

TABLE 138-23 ✦ INDICATIONS FOR AND CONTRAINDICATIONS TO LATISSIMUS DORSI FLAP RECONSTRUCTION

Indications	Contraindications
Inadequate skin envelope, other flap sources not available	Prior lateral thoracotomy with division of the latissimus muscle
Skin-sparing mastectomy: skin island for nipple-areola defect or muscle implant coverage desirable	Prior division of thoracodorsal artery and venae comitantes (relative contraindication if branches via serratus anterior muscle to latissimus dorsi intact)
Autologous reconstruction requested, TRAM or other donor site unavailable	Plans for adjuvant radiation therapy after reconstruction (relative contraindication)
Secondary breast reconstruction, flap required	Prior irradiation to ipsilateral posterior superior trunk
Reconstruction of quadrantectomy segmental defect from breast-conserving surgery	Competitive athletic endeavors requiring use of latissimus dorsi muscle (relative contraindication)
Reconstruction of Poland syndrome with breast agenesis	Current smoker (relative contraindication)

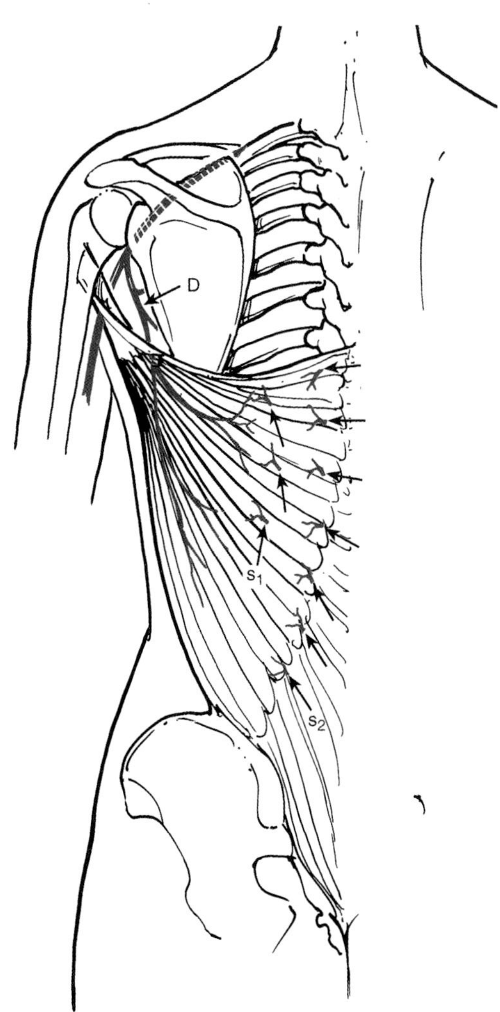

FIGURE 138-27. Vascular anatomy of latissimus dorsi muscle. Dominant pedicle: thoracodorsal artery (D). Secondary segmental pedicles: lateral row, branches of posterior intercostal artery and vein (s_1); medial row, branches of lumbar artery and vein (s_2). (From Mathes SJ, Nahai F: Reconstructive Surgery: Principles, Anatomy, and Technique. New York, Churchill Livingstone, 1997:566.)

preoperatively. In delayed reconstruction, planning of the skin island should be based on the existing mastectomy defect and the orientation of scars on the anterior chest. A skin island of approximately 8 by 25 cm is selected. In most instances, the widest skin island that will allow primary closure is chosen. Preoperative markings are placed with the patient in a sitting position in the preoperative area. On the posterior trunk, the tip of the axilla and posterior iliac spine are also marked for later orientation of the skin island and muscle flap elevation (Figs. 138-28 to 138-30).

Attention is then turned to the anterior chest. For immediate reconstruction, confirmation of the extent of mastectomy resection is obtained from the oncologic breast surgeon. If skin-sparing mastectomy is planned, optional extensions of the periareolar incision should be considered for patients with pendulous breasts to design the skin envelope and to avoid skin loss due to devascularization (see Figs. 138-11 and 138-12). In some instances, the periareolar incision includes an extension to the primary tumor biopsy site. The inframammary line is also marked bilaterally for use at the time of flap inset.

In delayed reconstruction, the surgeon has the option to enter the skin envelope through the mastectomy scar or at the level of the inframammary line (Fig. 138-31). In the latissimus dorsi flap, the original mastectomy scar is generally retained, and the initial incision for flap inset is made approximately 2 cm superior to the projected location of the inframammary line as determined by the contralateral inframammary line (the skin will retract inferiorly when this incision is made because of scar contracture, and the ultimate inframammary line will be symmetric with the contralateral breast).

If simultaneous contralateral breast surgery is planned, marking of the opposite breast will also be required at this time. Many surgeons elect to delay symmetry procedures until the final position of the reconstructed breast mound is achieved. If there is any doubt

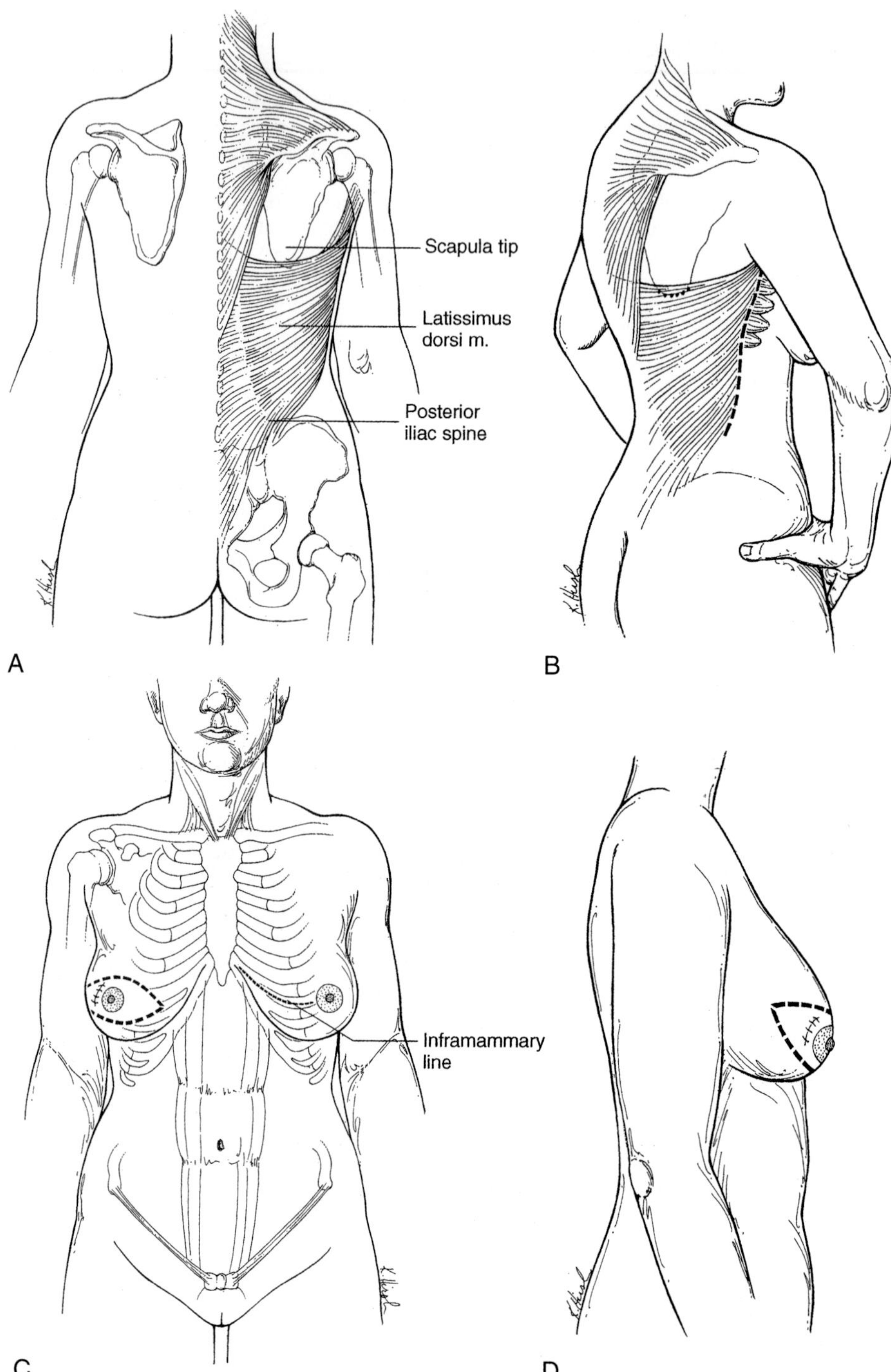

FIGURE 138-28. Latissimus dorsi musculocutaneous flap for breast reconstruction. *A,* Surface landmarks. *B,* Contraction of muscle allows surgeon to palpate anterior edge of muscle. *C,* Anterior chest markings for immediate reconstruction should be discussed with the oncologic surgeon. In some instances, the periareolar incision includes an extension to the primary tumor biopsy site. The inframammary line is also marked bilaterally for use at the time of flap inset. *D,* Lateral view of anterior chest markings.

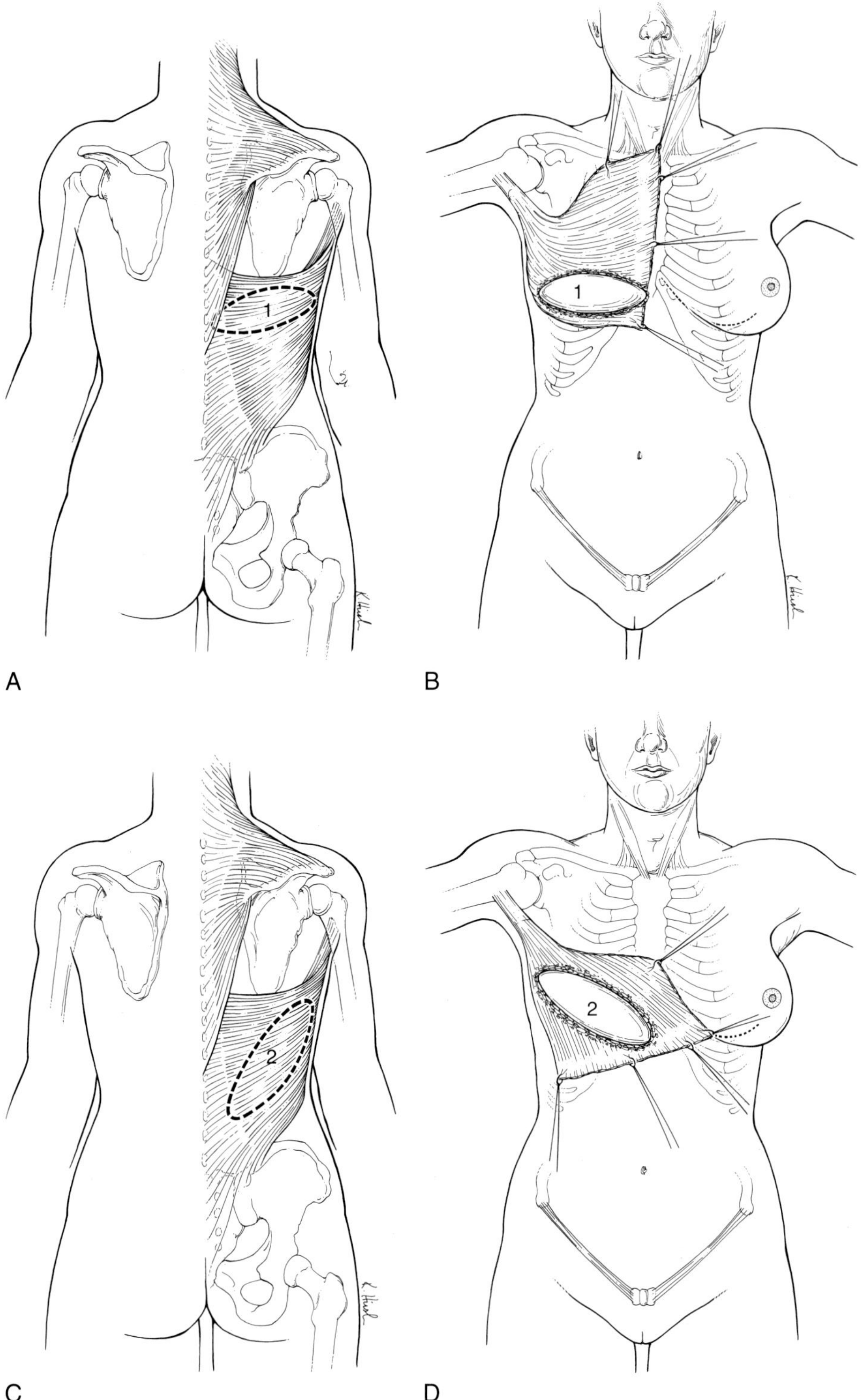

FIGURE 138-29. *A,* Design of skin island: superior. Donor site closure will fall beneath bra strap. *B,* After transposition to anterior chest, skin island will be located inferiorly with majority of muscle located superiorly. *C,* Design of skin island: oblique. The skin island is located medial to the muscle with the superior end directed toward the axilla. *D,* After transposition to anterior chest, skin island will be adjacent to inframammary line with muscle available both superior and inferior to skin island. *Continued*

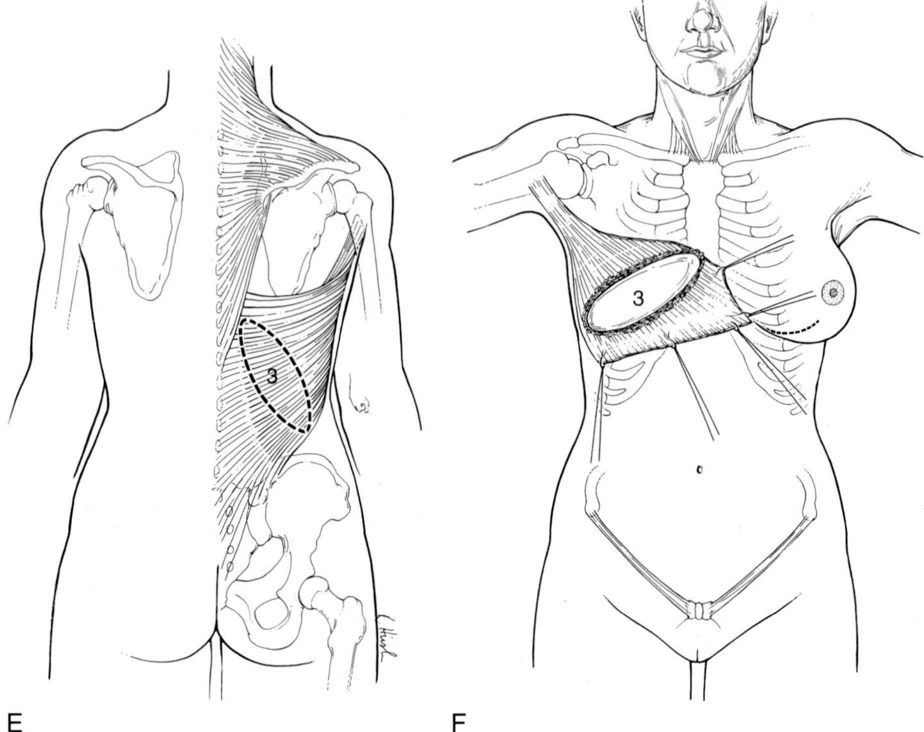

FIGURE 138-29, cont'd. Design of skin island: oblique. *E,* The skin island is located medial to the inferior muscle with tip directed posterior midline. Flap donor site closure is along normal skin lines. The island design allows the most subcutaneous tissue desirable for autogenous reconstruction. *F,* After flap transposition, skin island is adjacent to medial or inferior hemithorax muscle. Muscle is available to both superior and inferior skin island.

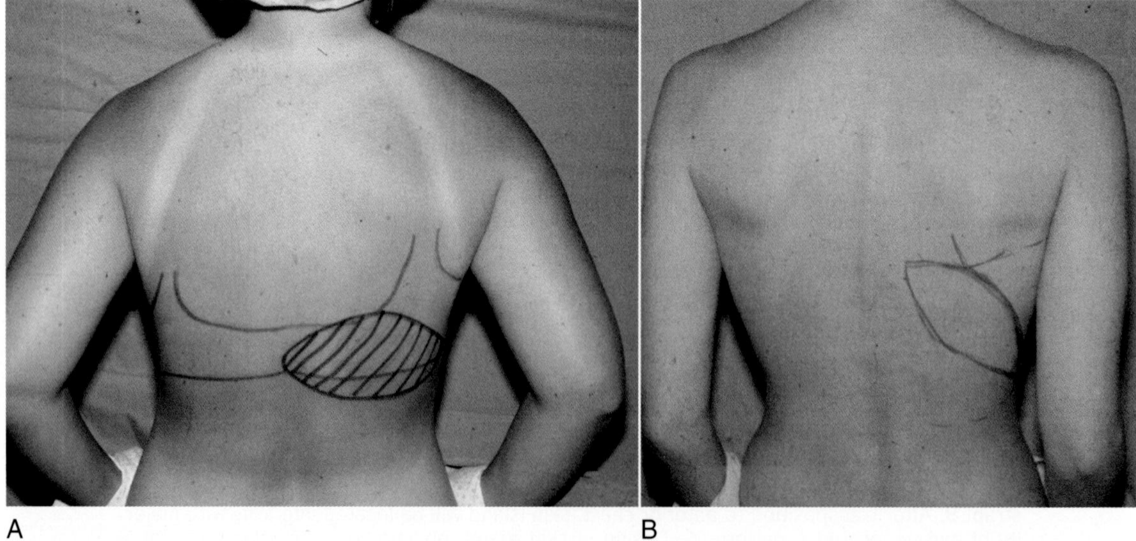

FIGURE 138-30. *A,* Transverse design of skin island allows the donor site closure to fall beneath the bra. The proximity of incision to axilla provides exposure for the axillary dissection. *B,* Oblique design provides latissimus muscle both above and below the skin island for implant coverage.

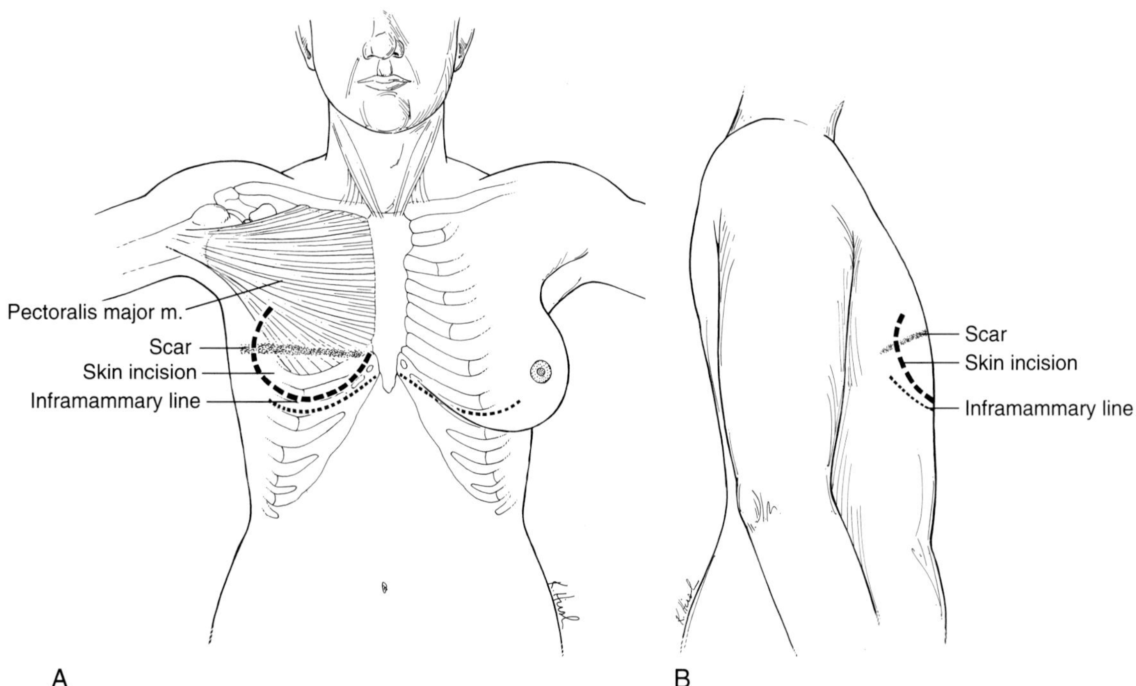

FIGURE 138-31. Latissimus dorsi musculocutaneous flap for delayed breast reconstruction. *A*, Preoperative markings. Inframammary line marking is based on opposite side. Incision with subsequent scar release is 1 to 2 cm superior to inframammary line and crosses mastectomy scar to ensure release of potential scar contracture. *B*, Planned incision to release scar extends through lateral aspect of mastectomy scar.

as to the reliability of the latissimus flap inset or if the patient is unsure of desired size or shape at either the reconstruction site or the opposite breast, it is preferable to delay the contralateral breast surgery until a suitable interval of follow-up (6 weeks to 3 months).

When the patient is taken to the operating room, she is initially placed in the lateral decubitus position to allow latissimus flap elevation and simultaneous preparation of the flap recipient site at the mastectomy defect. At the completion of this phase of the procedure, the flap will be ready for final inset at the mastectomy defect, and the donor site will be closed. After donor site closure is achieved, the patient is then prepared again and draped in the supine position with arms extended. With the patient in this position, the surgeon can accurately complete flap inset and select the appropriate implant size for breast mound reconstruction.

Technique

The procedure starts with the patient in the lateral decubitus position (for bilateral latissimus musculocutaneous flaps, the patient is placed prone to allow simultaneous elevation of both flaps). The skin island is redrawn, and its position and size are confirmed (Fig. 138-32*A*). The initial incision is made inferior to the skin island to locate the muscle. The incision is beveled away from the edge of the skin island to preserve musculocutaneous perforating vessels (Fig. 138-32*B*). If a thin atrophic muscle is encountered, it indicates a denervated muscle, and the surgeon should be cautious during the superior skin island incision and superficial muscle identification. Injury to the muscle by inadvertent muscle incision may result in loss of the skin island. After the superior and inferior incisions around the skin island are completed, the skin is elevated off the superficial surface of the muscle inferiorly to the posterior iliac spine and superiorly into the axilla. With the assistant holding the arm abducted (flexed position), it is possible to expose the muscle within the axilla to its insertion in the humerus. After the entire superficial surface of the muscle is exposed, the muscle origin along the vertebral column at the lumbosacral fascia is released by sharp dissection with both a knife and electrocautery (Fig. 138-32*C*). The anterior edge of the muscle is identified and separated from the underlying serratus anterior muscle (Fig. 138-32*D*). The inferior origin of the muscle is divided and the muscle is elevated from posterior to anterior, with care to separate the deep surface of the latissimus from the underlying serratus anterior muscle (Fig. 138-32*E*). Now that the entire origin is released, the deep surface of the muscle is exposed toward the axilla (Fig. 138-32*F*). The crossing branch to the serratus anterior from the thoracodorsal pedicle is preserved. If the thoracodorsal artery and paired venae comitantes are already divided or injured during the axillary dissection, the flap may be based on retrograde flow through the serratus anterior and vein branches.

As dissection progresses into the axilla, the posterior muscle is separated from the teres major and scapula. Small communicating vessels will need division and cauterization. On the deep surface of the muscle within the superior axilla, the major pedicle, the thoracodorsal artery and vein, is identified and preserved. The muscle is dissected to the level of its insertion into the humerus. The thoracodorsal nerve is identified and preserved (Fig. 138-32*G*). Some surgeons advocate division of the insertion; however, this maneuver is not recommended because it allows direct tension on the pedicle after the flap is transposed to the anterior chest. Some surgeons advocate denervation of the muscle by selective division of the thoracodorsal nerve within the axilla. In general, the nerve is preserved because atrophy of the muscle is avoided, particularly when the muscle bulk is desirable for breast mound reconstruction. The anterior axilla is divided to prepare a tunnel between the posterior donor site dissection and the mastectomy wound. For delayed reconstruction, an incision is made at the preselected site on the mastectomy defect and the tunnel completed. The latissimus dorsi musculocutaneous flap is now transposed to the anterior chest, and the donor site is closed directly (Fig. 138-32*H*). Two suction drains are placed in the donor site space and exit through a small incision along the midaxillary line.

The patient is now reprepared and draped in the supine position with arms extended, and the inset phase of the procedure is started. In delayed unilateral reconstruction, the flap has already been transposed to the anterior chest and placed in the defect between the inframammary incision and the existing breast envelope (for delayed bilateral latissimus dorsi reconstruction, flaps remain in the axillae until the anterior chest incisions are made for bilateral flap inset) (Fig. 138-33*A*). For immediate latissimus dorsi reconstruction, the flap is inset directly into the defect formed by the skin resection or, in skin-sparing mastectomy, placed beneath the preserved skin envelope.

A pocket is then established beneath the pectoralis major muscle for implant placement (Fig. 138-33*B* and *C*). The inferior fibers of the pectoralis major originate at the sixth intercostal space. The muscle origins along the sternal edge between the fourth and sixth intercostal space are released to avoid excessive pressure on the implant due to muscle tightness. A sizer implant approximately the size of the contralateral breast is placed beneath the latissimus musculocutaneous flap (inferior) and the pectoralis major–preserved skin envelope (superior) (Fig. 138-33*D*).

The patient is then raised to a sitting position. After appropriate inflation of the sizer implant, the inframammary incision is extended at the medial and lateral aspects of the anterior hemithorax (across the existing transverse mastectomy scar in delayed reconstruction) to release the skin envelope. As the skin envelope is released, the skin island of the latissimus flap will gradually extend inferiorly, demonstrating mild ptosis (Fig. 138-33*E* and *F*).

When satisfactory mound size, projection, and ptosis are established, the patient is returned to a supine position and an implant of appropriate size is selected. The implant will be covered by both the existing pectoralis major muscle and the latissimus dorsi muscle. The inferior edge of the latissimus, now located superior to the skin island on the anterior chest, may remain unattached, or it can be sutured to the inferior edge of the pectoralis major muscle. The skin island will extend along the inframammary line and form the inferior portion of the skin envelope (Fig. 138-33*G* to *I*). Severely scarred or devascularized skin between the neo–inframammary line and the transverse mastectomy scar is excised and replaced by the skin island of the latissimus dorsi flap.

For radical mastectomy reconstruction, the skin island on the posterior trunk is designed as far inferior as possible so that after flap transposition to the anterior chest, the muscle now superior to the skin

Text continued on p. 704

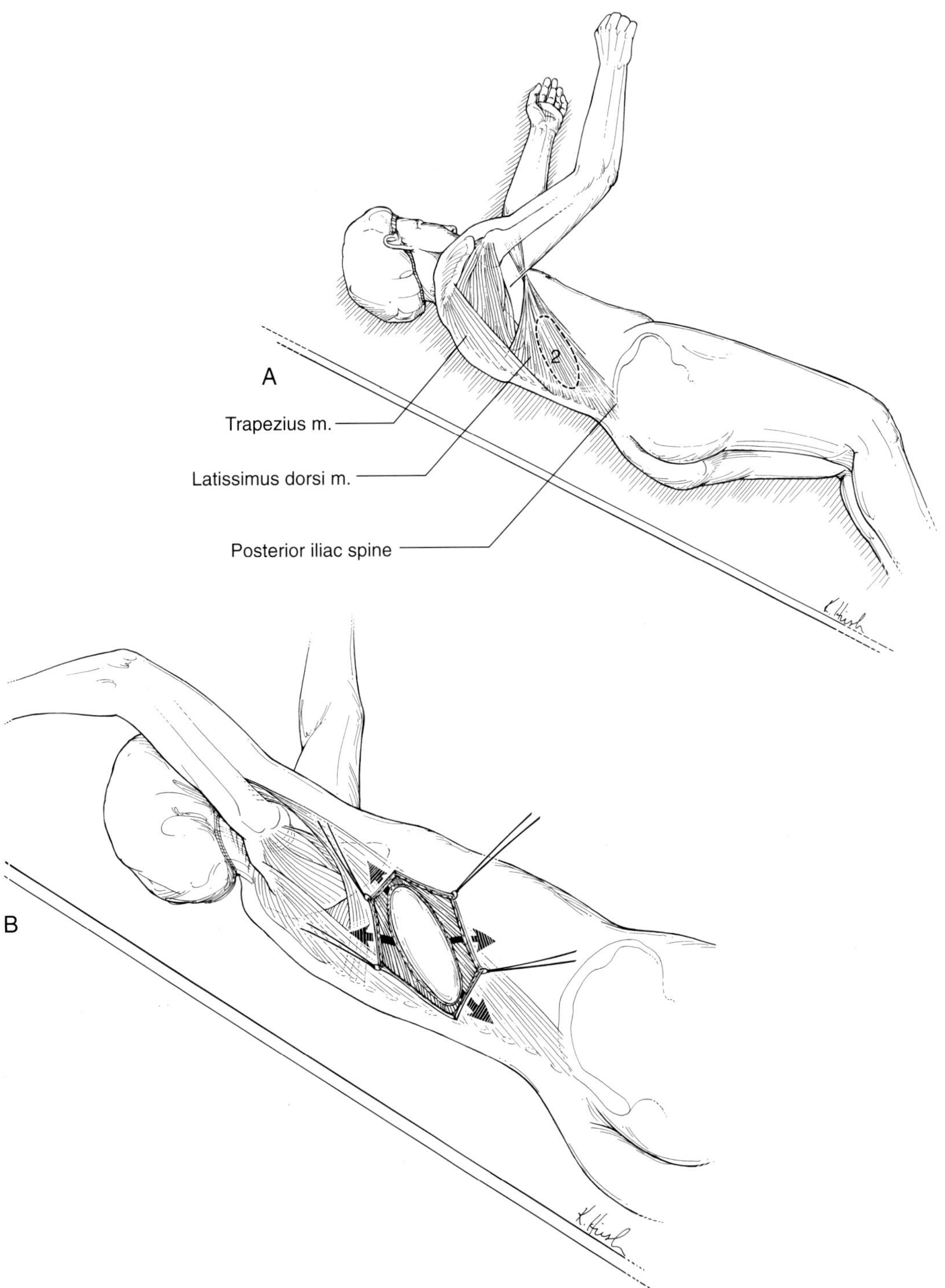

FIGURE 138-32. Technique for latissimus dorsi musculocutaneous flap. *A,* Patient positioned in lateral decubitus position. Posterior chest (flap donor site) and anterior chest (breast mound reconstruction site) are included in the operative field. *B,* Incision around skin island allows dissection to expose anterior surface of latissimus dorsi muscle.

Continued

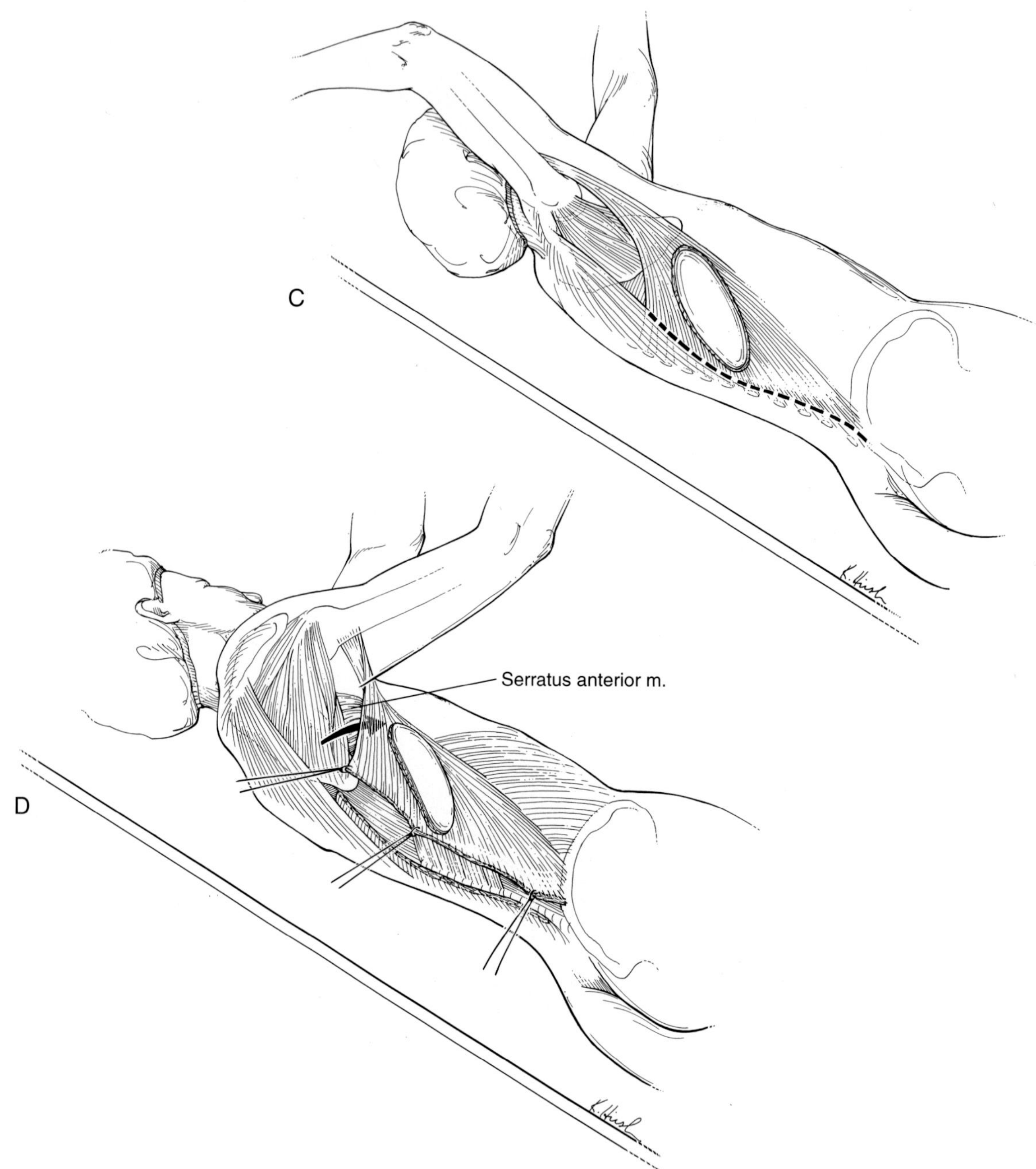

FIGURE 138-32, cont'd. *C,* Latissimus dorsi fibers of origin from lumbosacral fascia and vertebrae are divided. *D,* Deep surface of muscle is exposed. Care is taken to avoid flap dissection deep to the serratus anterior muscle. The latissimus muscles are separated from the underlying serratus anterior, with dissection starting posterior where the muscle plane is easily identified.

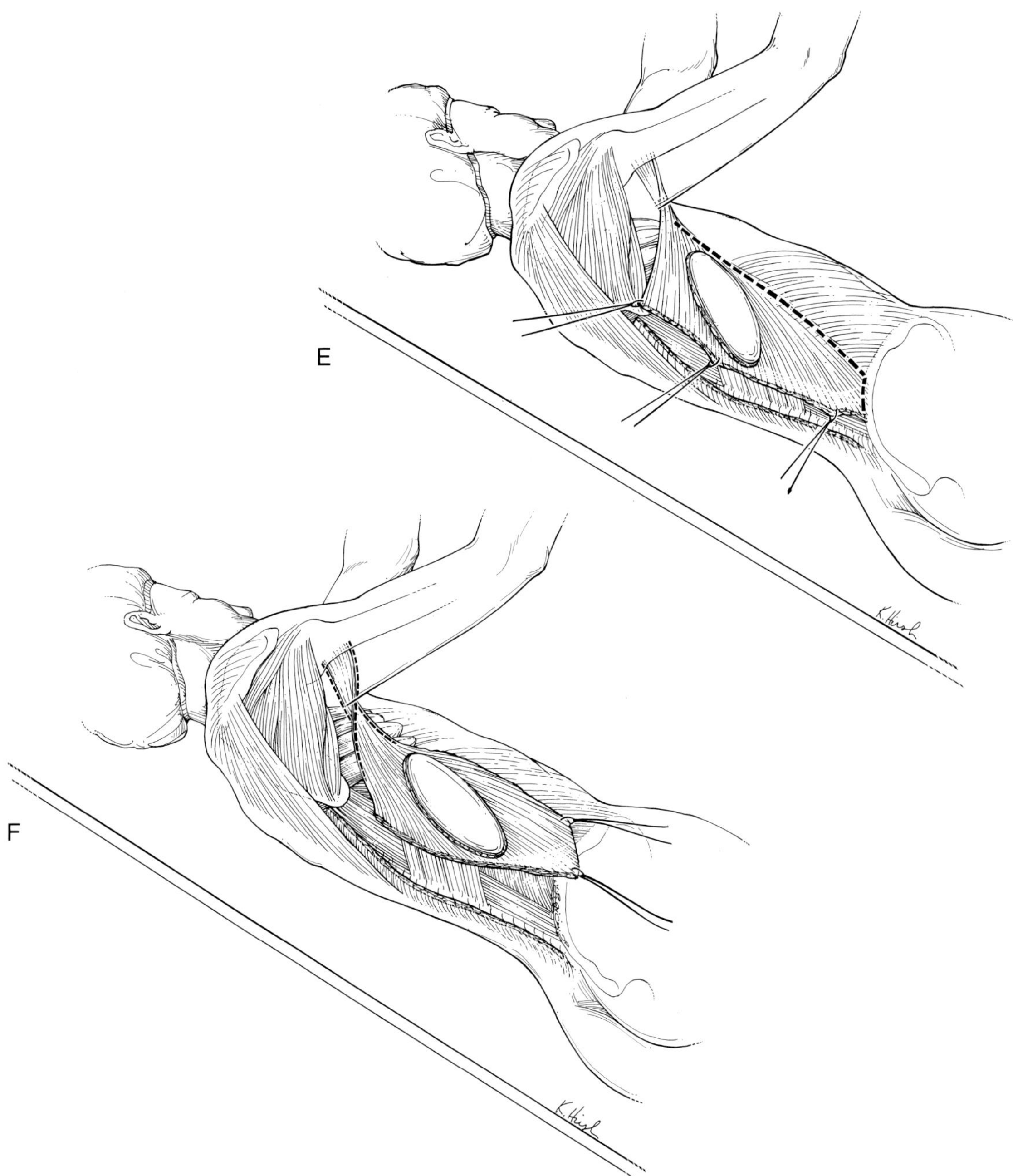

FIGURE 138-32, cont'd. *E,* Final mobilization of the latissimus dorsi muscle is separation from congenital adhesions with adjacent musculature at the anterior axillary line. *F,* Proximal dissection toward latissimus dorsi insertion required for identification and preservation of the thoracodorsal artery, veins, and nerve. A lighted retractor allows visualization of the pedicle while dissection is performed to muscle insertion. *Continued*

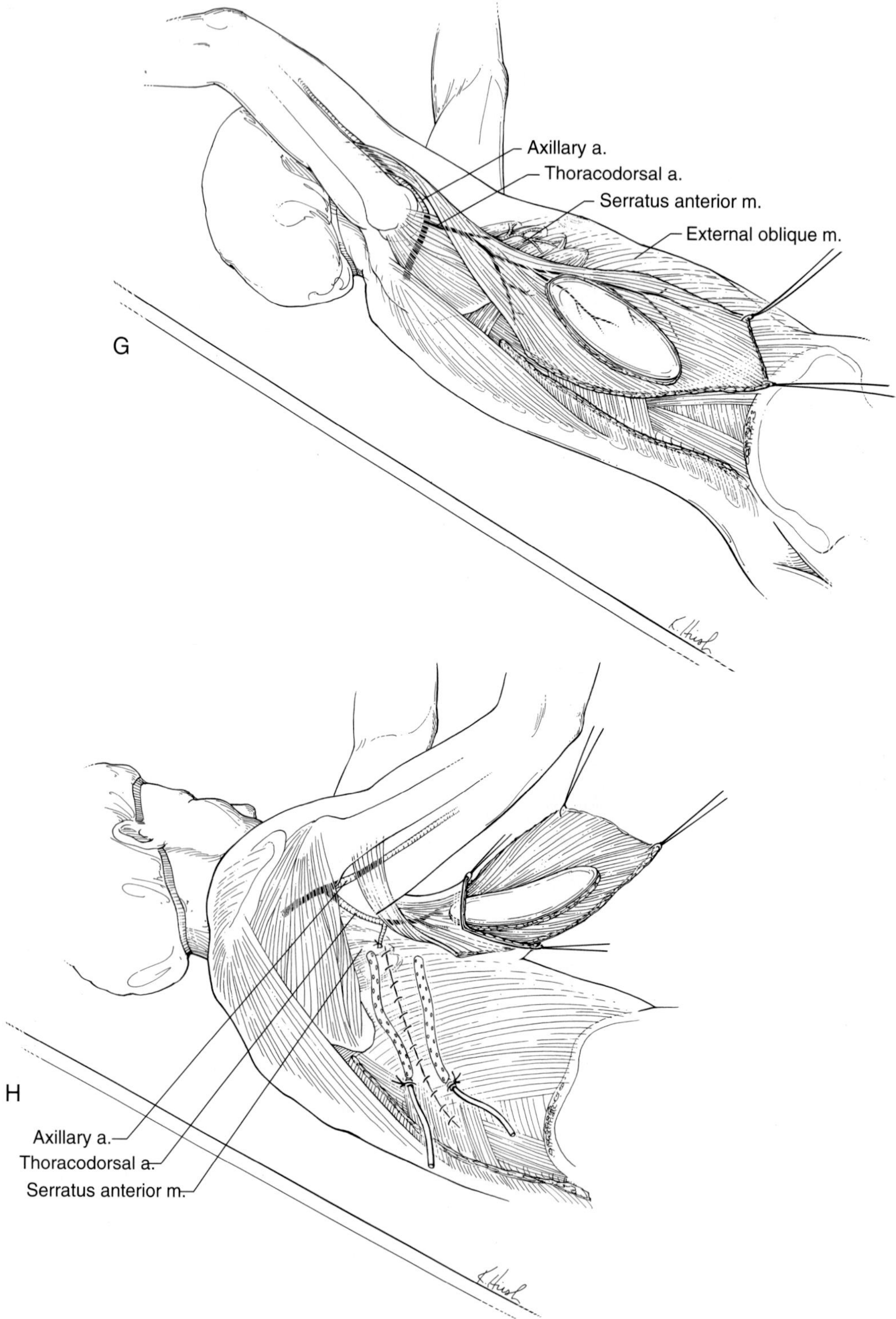

FIGURE 138-32, cont'd. *G,* Complete elevation of the latissimus dorsi muscle with skin island. Thoracodorsal branch to serratus can generally be left intact. *H,* Incision is made adjacent to inframammary line, and remaining skin envelope and pectoralis muscle are elevated together. A tunnel is made in the superior axilla, and the flap is transposed to the anterior chest. The donor site is closed, and the patient is ready for repositioning in the supine position for flap inset.

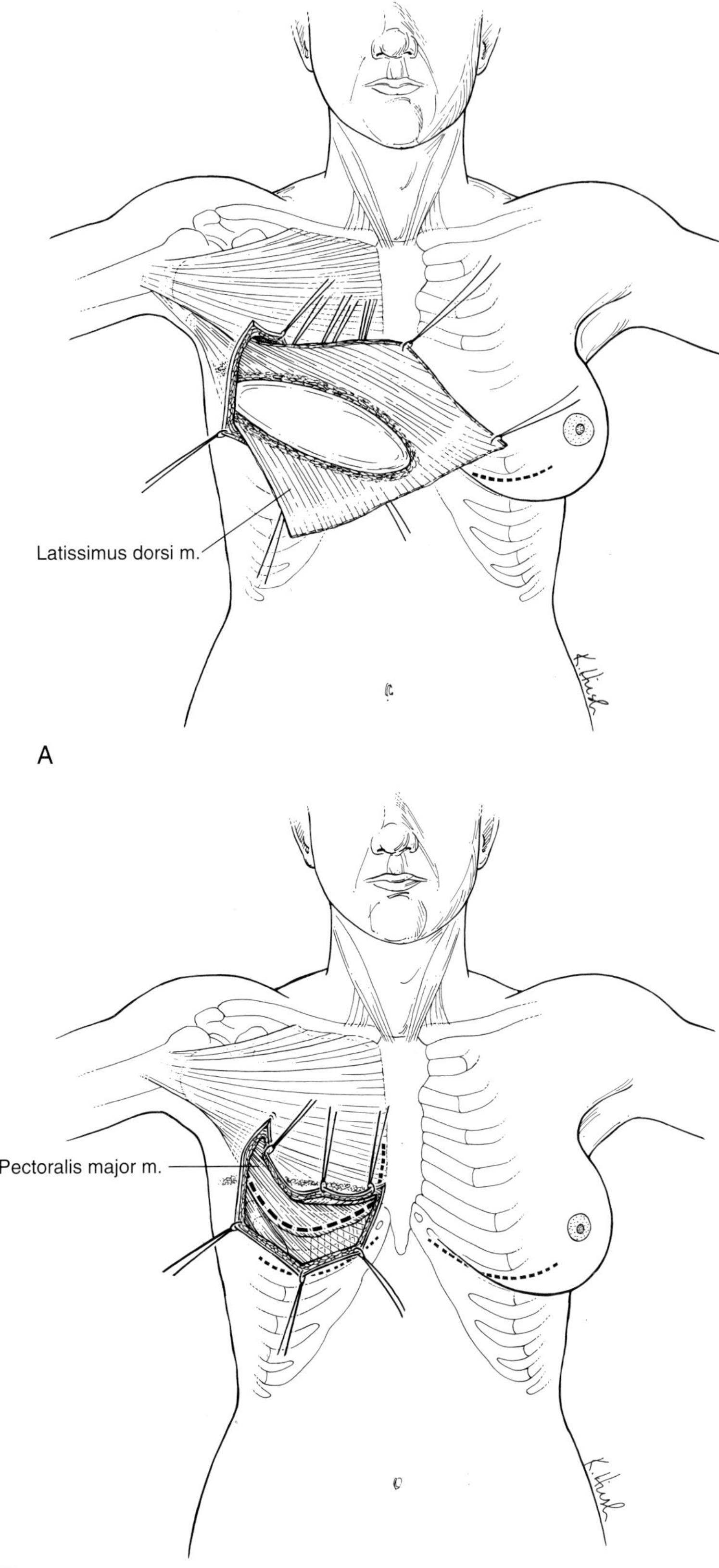

FIGURE 138-33. Latissimus dorsi musculocutaneous flap inset for delayed breast reconstruction. *A,* Patient is reprepared and draped in supine position. Flap is placed in axilla while recipient site is prepared. *B,* Inset of latissimus dorsi musculocutaneous flap for delayed breast reconstruction. Skin envelope is elevated with underlying pectoralis major muscle. Care is required to preserve vascular connection between skin envelope and pectoralis muscle. If the pectoralis muscle is absent (radical mastectomy), skin is elevated from ribs and costal muscles.

Continued

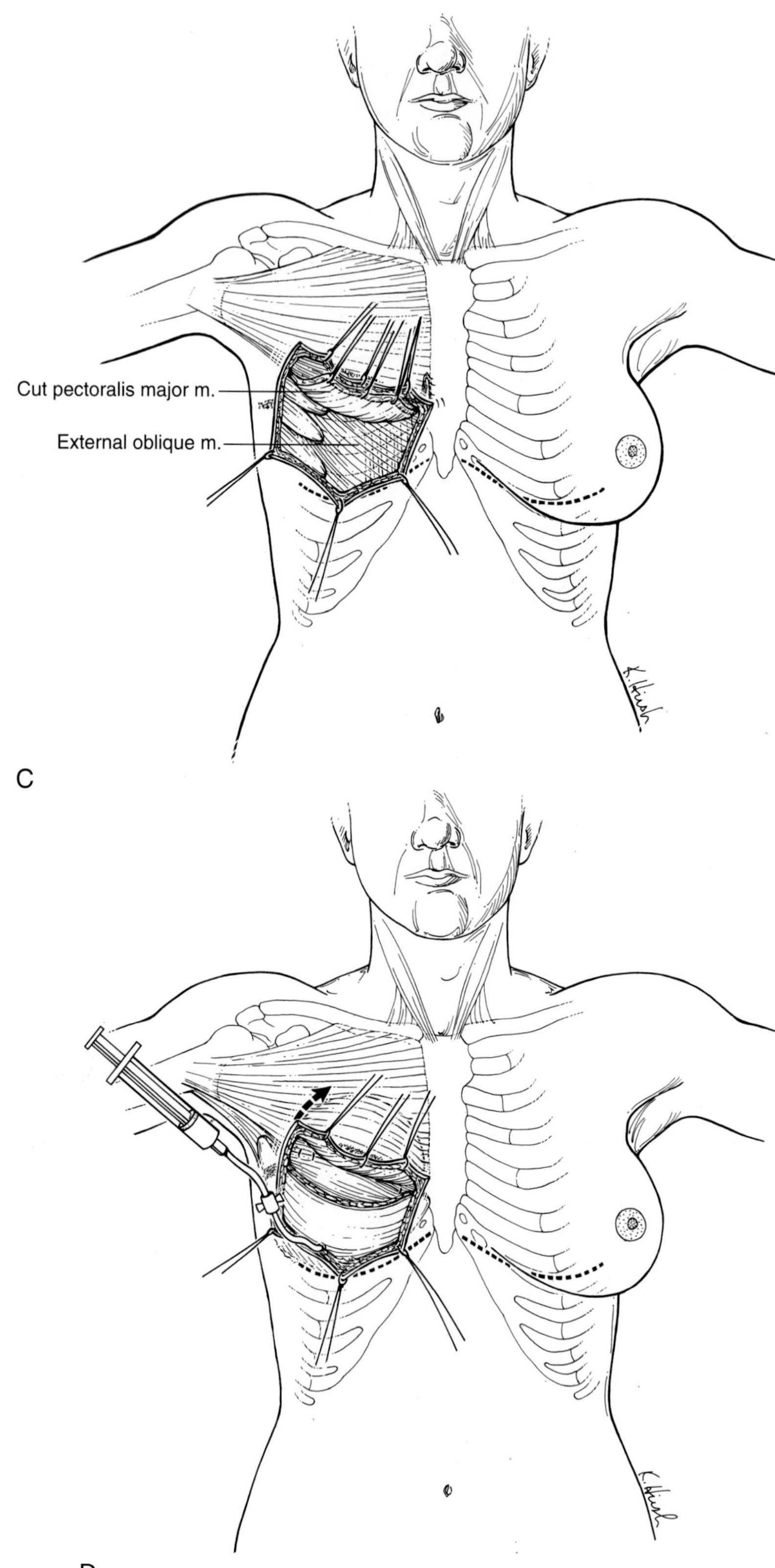

FIGURE 138-33, cont'd. *C,* Pocket is formed between pectoralis major muscle and chest wall. Pectoralis major fibers of origin are divided along the inframammary line and at sternal edge between fourth and sixth intercostal spaces. *D,* Latissimus dorsi skin island is placed over defect. The patient is placed in the sitting position for final inset of the flap and selection of appropriately sized implant. Implant sizer is beneath latissimus muscle inferiorly and pectoralis major muscle superiorly.

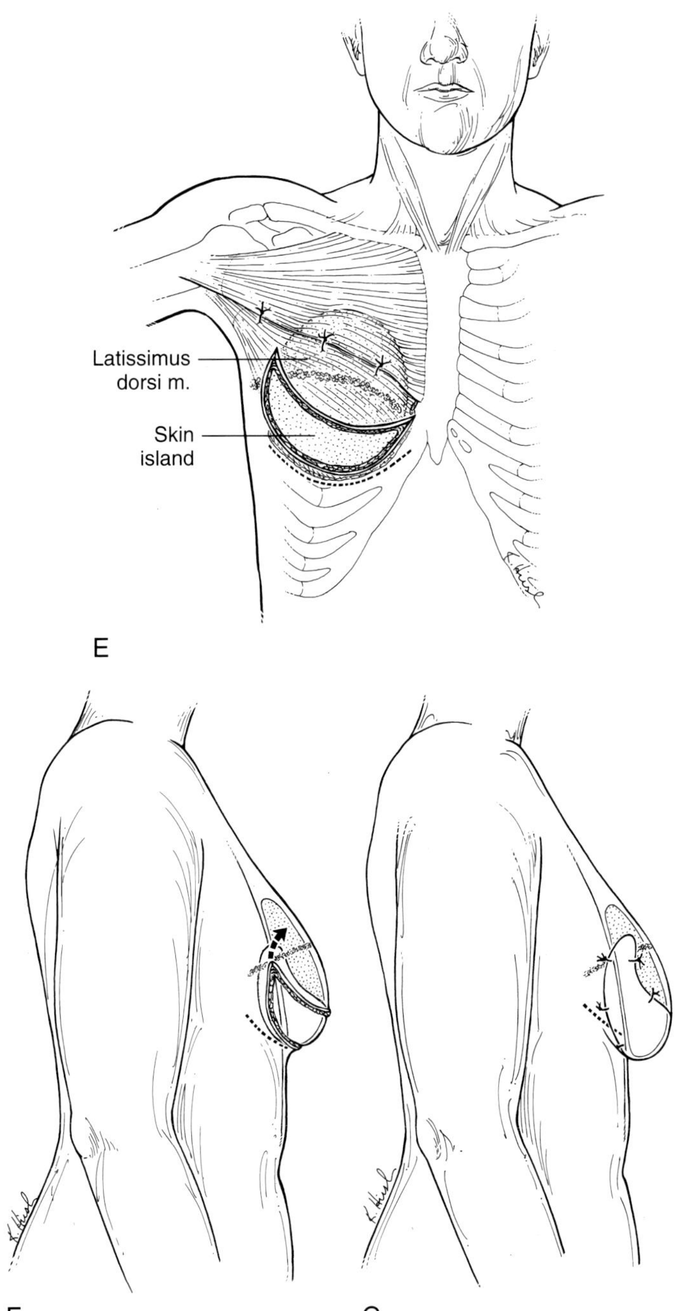

FIGURE 138-33, cont'd. *E,* Lateral mastectomy scar is released and skin island inset to provide inferior skin envelope. The permanent implant is selected on the basis of the sizer and placed in a pocket beneath the pectoralis and latissimus dorsi muscles. *F,* Release of lateral mastectomy scar will allow skin envelope to drape and demonstrate slight ptosis. *G,* After release of mastectomy scar laterally, skin island is inset. The distal skin envelope below the mastectomy scar is resected if adequate skin envelope is provided by latissimus skin island. *Continued*

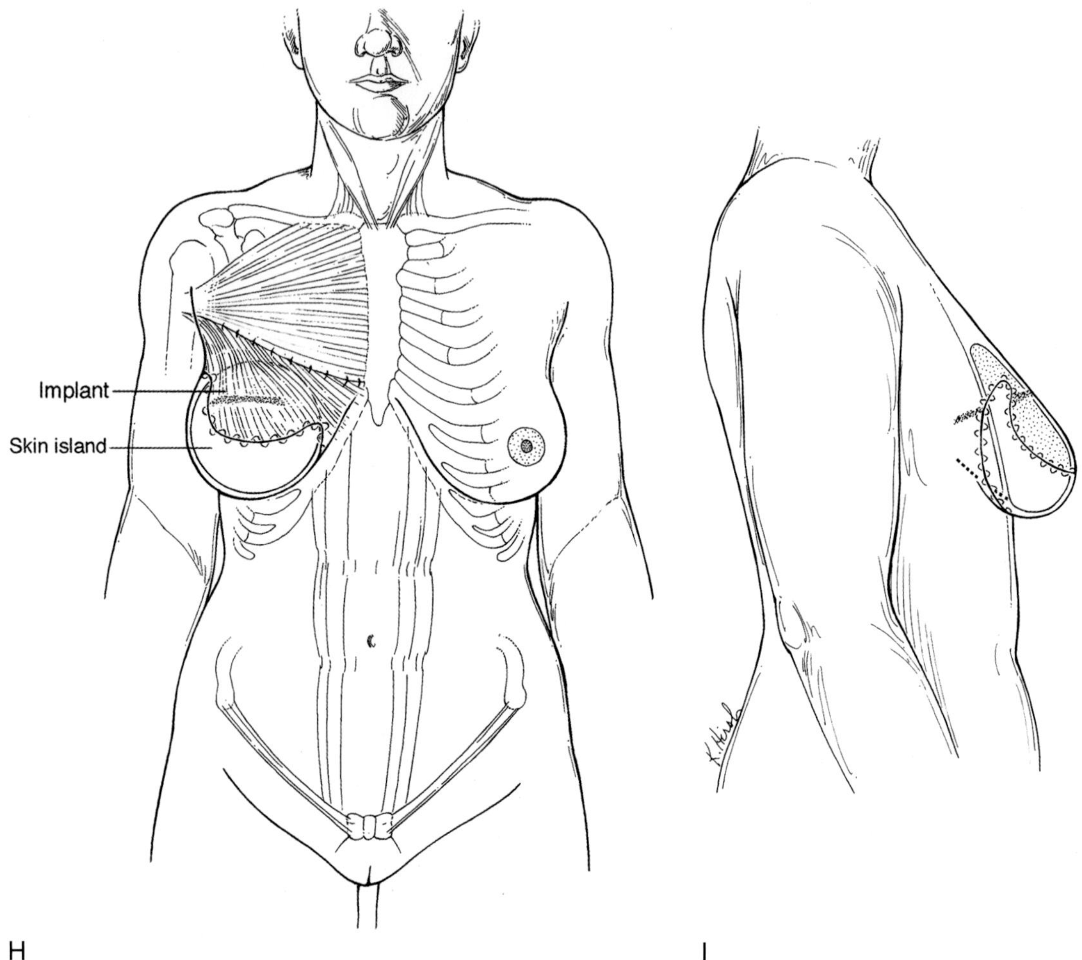

FIGURE 138-33, cont'd. *H,* Permanent implant is positioned behind latissimus and pectoralis muscles. Superior edge of latissimus muscle is loosely sutured to edge of pectoralis muscle. *I,* Permanent implant size should be selected on the basis of symmetry to contralateral breast. If the skin envelope appears inadequate despite addition of latissimus dorsi skin island, a tissue expander should be selected with plans to expand the region.

island will reach the clavicle to replace the resected pectoralis major muscle.

In immediate skin-sparing mastectomy reconstruction, the flap is placed within the preserved skin envelope. The nipple-areola has generally been resected. The portion of the skin island in position under the limited skin defect is marked. The flap is then brought through the nipple-areola onto the chest wall (note: the central defect at the nipple-areola site is generally stretched during mastectomy to allow exposure for the mastectomy and the skin island for de-epithelialization), and the portion of the skin island to be buried beneath the existing skin envelope is de-epithelialized (Fig. 138-34). An implant of appropriate size is chosen (based on sizer inset and inflation as described previously) and inserted through the nipple-areola defect beneath the inferior edge of the pectoralis major muscle. The flap is then reinserted through the nipple-areola defect, and the preserved skin island is inset into the skin envelope defect and sutured in place.

The surgeon may elect to add another drain to the anterior chest, but it is generally not required. If the skin envelope is still tight despite the addition of the skin island provided by the latissimus flap (due to prior irradiation or in secondary breast reconstruction), an expander may be inserted instead of the permanent implant. After a period of inflation of the expander, the patient is taken back to the operating room, and the expander is exchanged for a permanent implant (Figs. 138-35 to 138-40).

Complications for the latissimus dorsi musculocutaneous flap include donor site seroma, hematoma, capsular contracture, fat necrosis, implant displacement, implant rupture, wound infection, partial or total flap loss, muscle weakness as a result of the latissimus dorsi donor site, and asymmetry. Results with

Text continued on p. 712

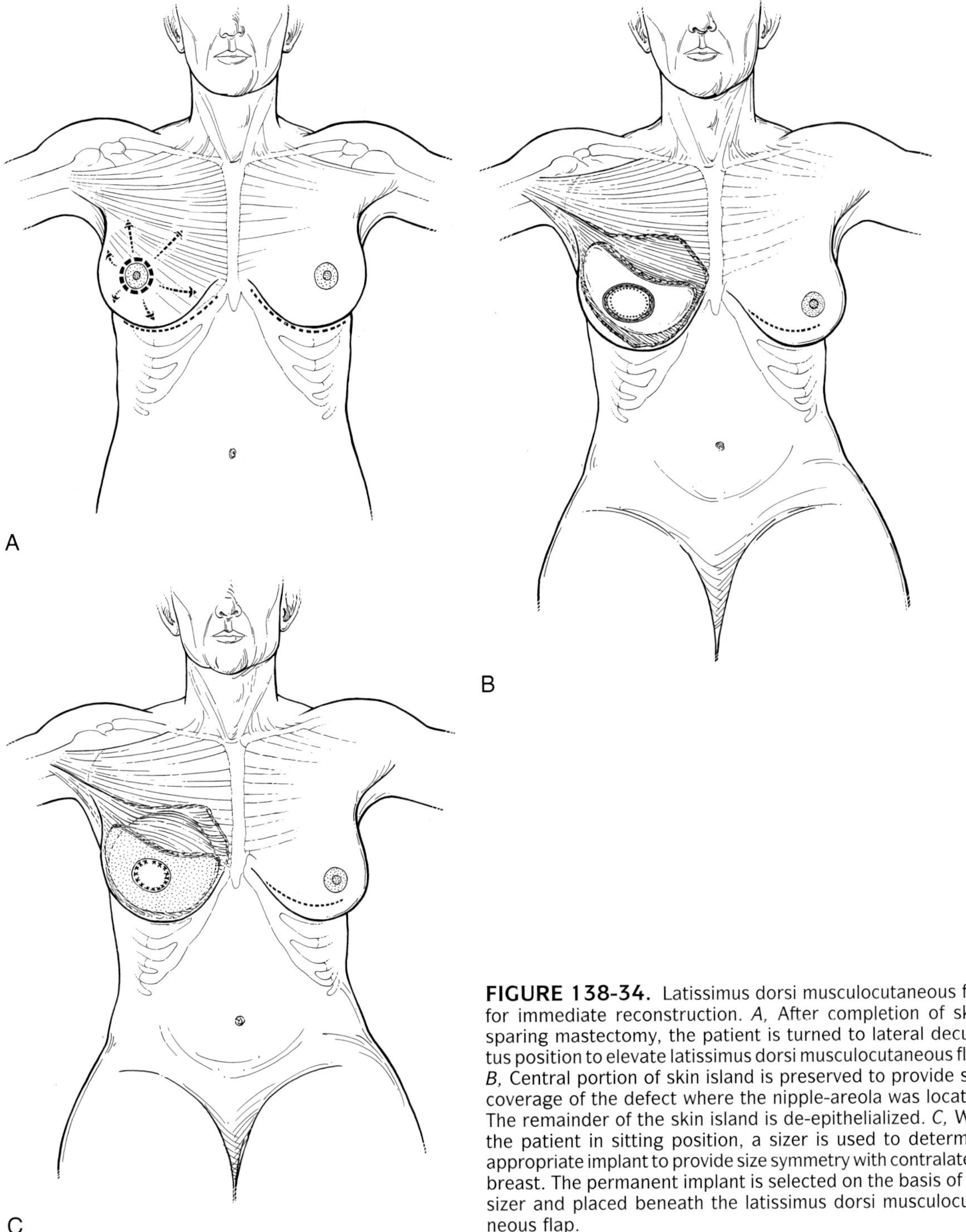

FIGURE 138-34. Latissimus dorsi musculocutaneous flap for immediate reconstruction. *A,* After completion of skin-sparing mastectomy, the patient is turned to lateral decubitus position to elevate latissimus dorsi musculocutaneous flap. *B,* Central portion of skin island is preserved to provide skin coverage of the defect where the nipple-areola was located. The remainder of the skin island is de-epithelialized. *C,* With the patient in sitting position, a sizer is used to determine appropriate implant to provide size symmetry with contralateral breast. The permanent implant is selected on the basis of the sizer and placed beneath the latissimus dorsi musculocutaneous flap.

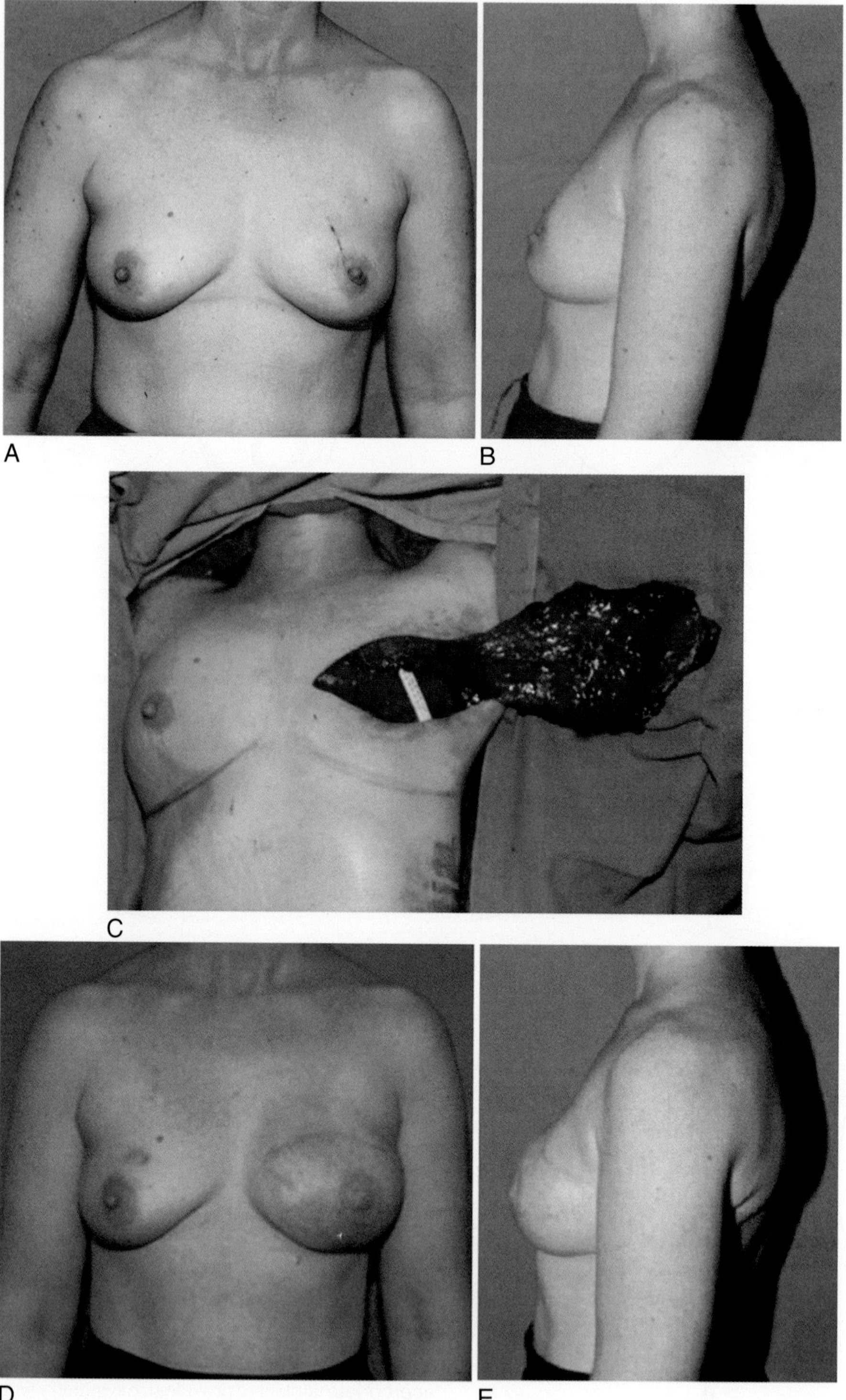

FIGURE 138-35. Latissimus dorsi musculocutaneous flap with implant for immediate breast reconstruction. *A,* Preoperative anterior view; left invasive breast carcinoma. *B,* Preoperative lateral view. *C,* Mastectomy defect; left latissimus dorsi musculocutaneous flap transposed into defect. *D,* Postoperative view 1 $^{1}/_{2}$ years after immediate reconstruction including nipple-areola. The skin island provides adequate restoration of the breast skin envelope. *E,* Postoperative lateral view demonstrates adequate projection and volume provided by implant and flap.

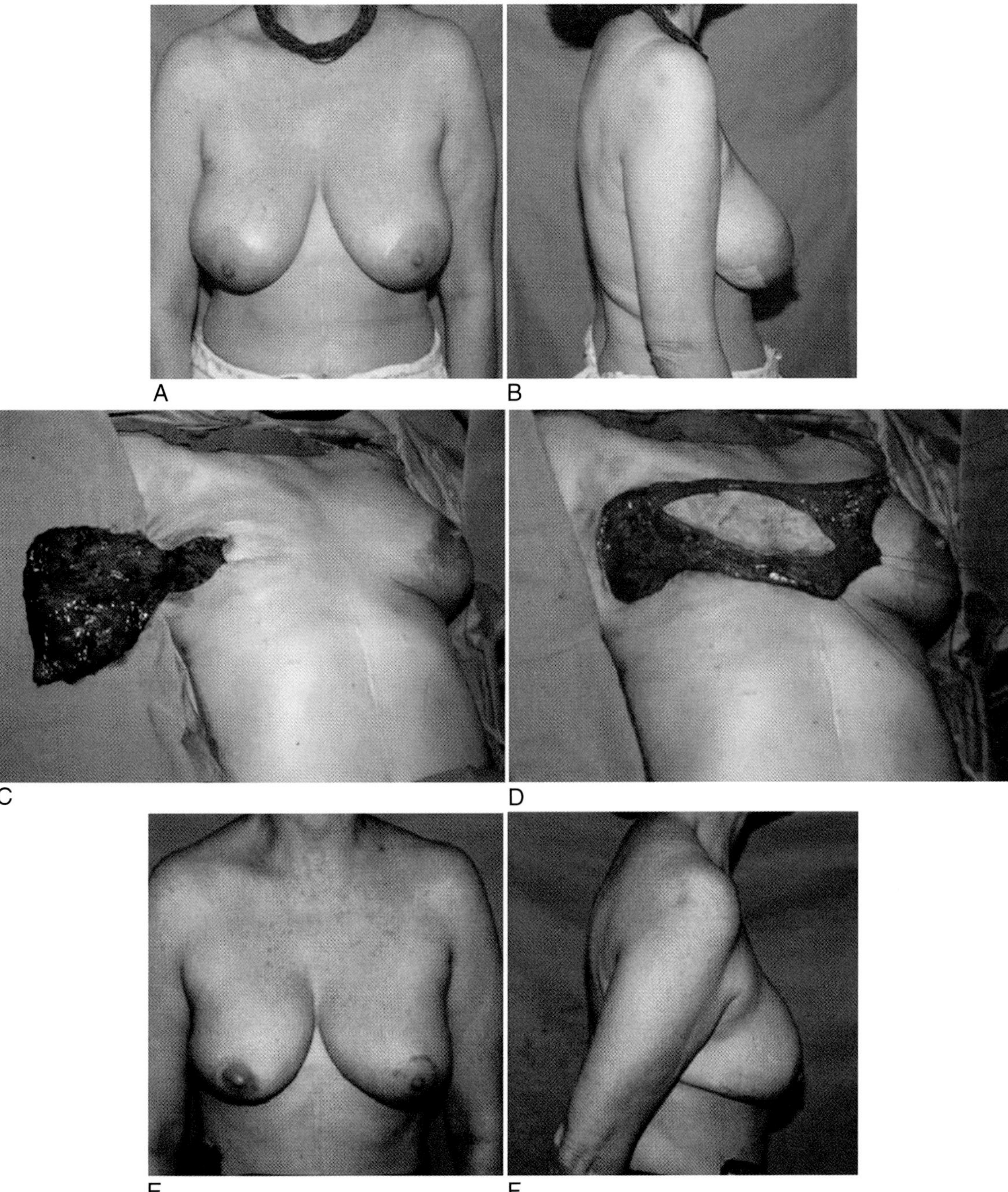

FIGURE 138-36. Latissimus dorsi musculocutaneous flap for immediate right breast reconstruction with implant. *A,* Preoperative right skin-sparing mastectomy. The patient desires reconstruction to match the contralateral ptotic breast. *B,* Preoperative lateral view. Bandage covers biopsy site for tumor. *C,* Right mastectomy defect (areola preserved); right latissimus dorsi musculocutaneous flap transposed into defect. *D,* Flap will provide muscle coverage of implant. Skin island will be used to restore normal right breast skin envelope. *E,* Postoperative view at 1 year. Flap provides adequate skin envelope to allow restoration of breast shape and projection. Nipple reconstruction is completed. *F,* Lateral view demonstrates reconstructed breast mound, exhibiting adequate ptosis to match opposite breast.

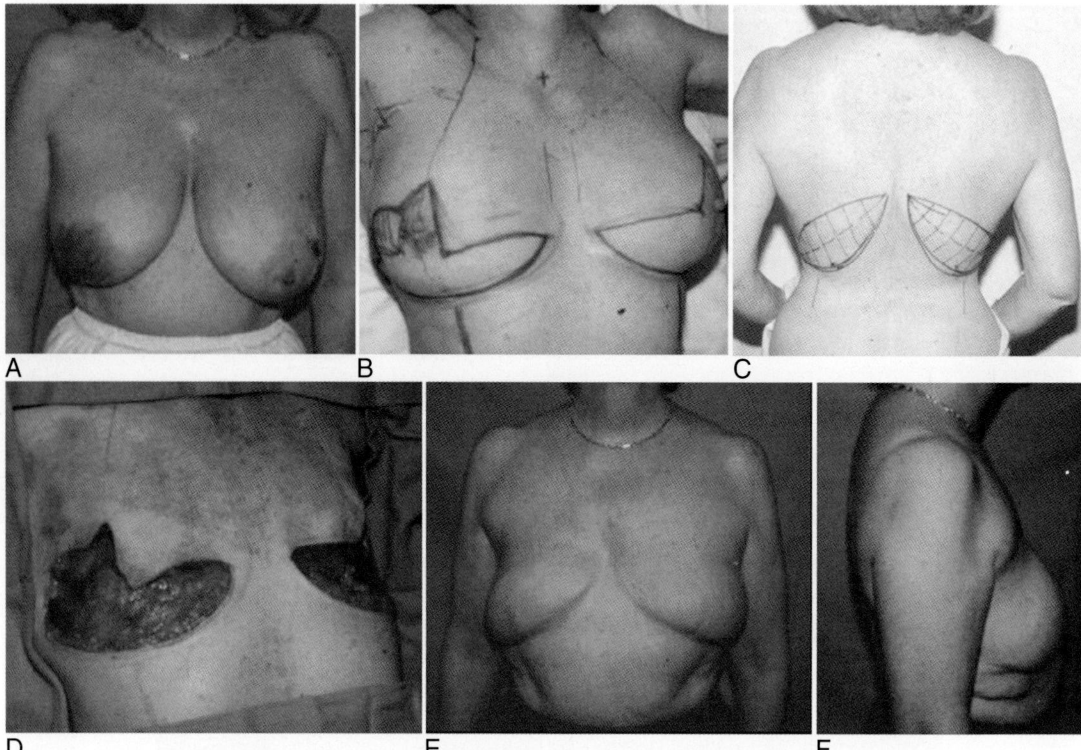

FIGURE 138-37. Bilateral latissimus dorsi musculocutaneous flaps for immediate breast reconstruction. *A,* Preoperative view of patient with bilateral breast cancer. The patient desires bilateral autogenous breast reconstruction. Abdominal donor sites are not available. *B,* Mastectomy incisions designed to provide adequate mastectomy margins and breast envelope reductions. *C,* Bilateral latissimus dorsi musculocutaneous flaps planned. Note oblique skin island selected in areas of greatest adipose tissue in skin territory of latissimus dorsi muscle. *D,* Bilateral mastectomy defects. *E,* Postoperative anterior view at 1 year. Flaps provide adequate soft tissue (skin islands de-epithelialized) for autogenous reconstruction. *F,* Lateral view demonstrates adequate projection and natural breast ptosis.

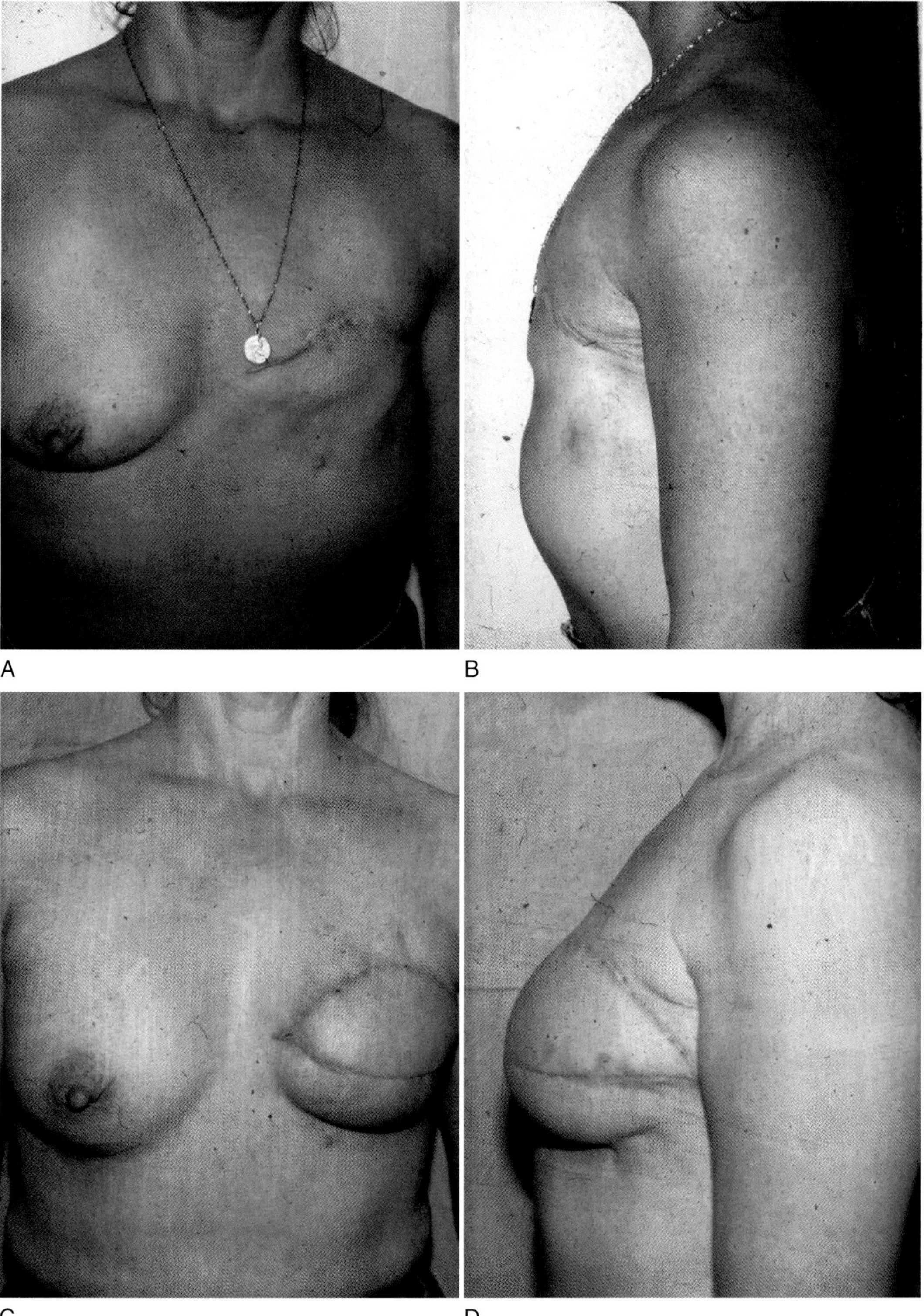

FIGURE 138-38. Latissimus dorsi musculocutaneous flap for delayed breast reconstruction (unnatural appearance with skin island inset in old mastectomy scar). *A,* Preoperative anterior view of mastectomy defect. *B,* Postoperative lateral view after mastectomy. *C,* Postoperative anterior view 6 months after breast reconstruction. Inset of skin island at existing scar restores skin envelope but allows visibility of skin island. *D,* Postoperative lateral view after reconstruction. Skin island site is visible on breast mound.

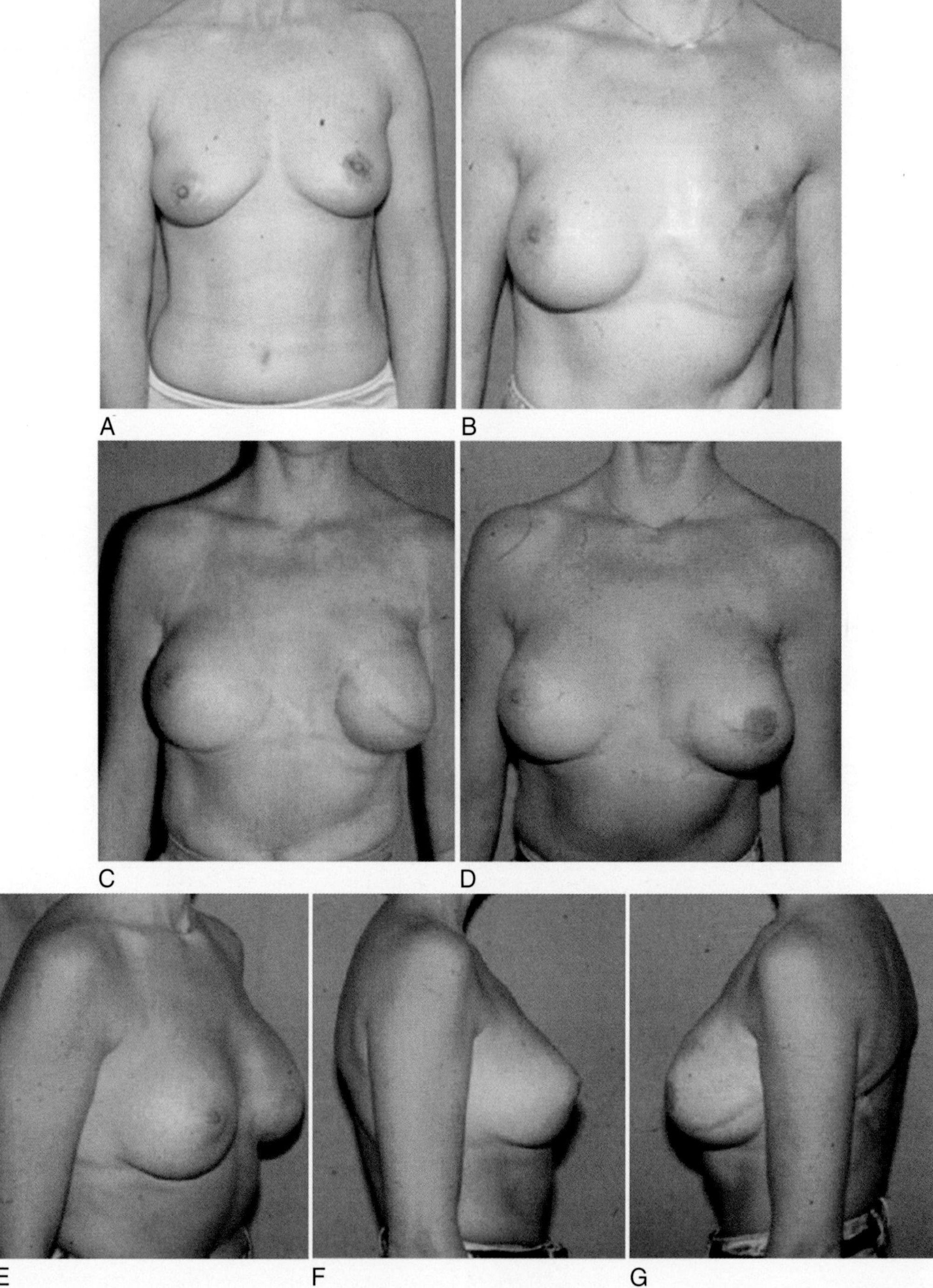

FIGURE 138-39. Latissimus dorsi musculocutaneous flaps for delayed breast reconstruction (flap hidden with inset in inframammary line and lateral release of mastectomy scar with flap). *A,* The patient has undergone bilateral breast augmentation; preoperative for mastectomy of left breast for invasive breast cancer. *B,* Left modified radical mastectomy defect. *C,* Postoperative view at 3 months of left latissimus dorsi musculocutaneous flap with implant for breast mound reconstruction. The skin island is not placed within the mastectomy scar but inset in inferior skin envelope. *D,* Postoperative view at 1 year demonstrates adequate breast projection and volume to match contralateral augmented breast. *E,* Oblique view demonstrates adequate restoration of inframammary line and reasonable breast projection. *F,* Lateral view of augmented right breast. *G,* Lateral view of reconstructed left breast.

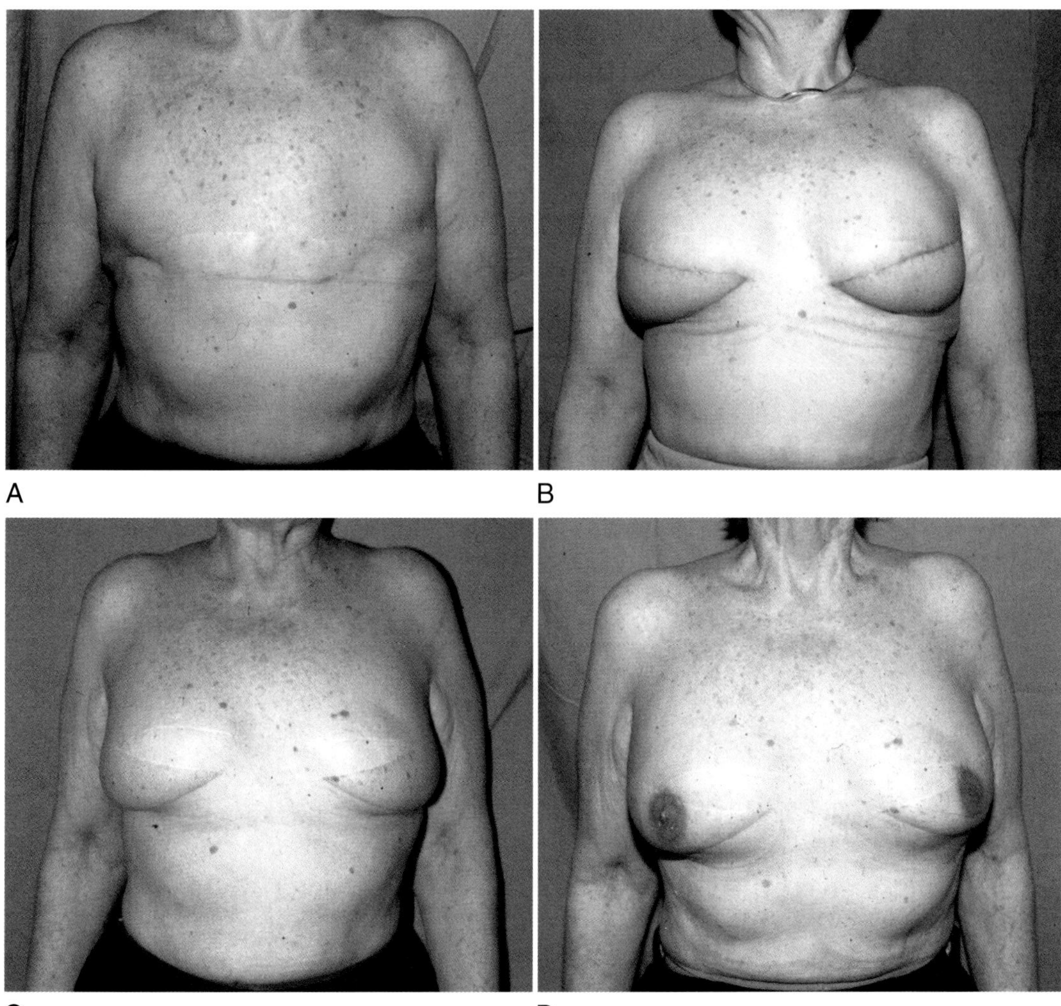

FIGURE 138-40. Bilateral latissimus dorsi flaps for delayed breast reconstruction. *A,* Preoperative anterior view of patient after bilateral modified radical mastectomies. *B,* Skin island is inset between mastectomy scar and inframammary line. Implants provide mound volume and projection. *C,* Postoperative view at 6 months. Skin islands are less visible when they are located over the inferior breast mound. *D,* Anterior view 1 year after bilateral flaps plus implants and nipple-areola reconstruction. Latissimus dorsi flap provides adequate restoration of skin island.

latissimus dorsi myocutaneous flap are generally very good. Most problems with this form of reconstruction are related to the implant rather than to the autogenous flap used to re-establish a normal skin envelope and provide implant coverage.

TRANSVERSE RECTUS ABDOMINIS MUSCULOCUTANEOUS (TRAM) TRANSPOSITION FLAP

Interest in the rectus abdominis flap centered on its dual blood supply (type III) with its skin territory based on the vertical orientation of the muscle (Fig. 138-41). The flap was initially used for inferior anterior chest wall reconstruction[276] based on its superior pedicle, the superior epigastric artery and associated veins. Later, the rectus abdominis musculocutaneous flap was based inferiorly on its inferior pedicle, the deep inferior epigastric artery and associated veins.[276] In each instance, the skin island was designed vertically over the primary territory of the rectus muscle. In 1981, Hartrampf et al[277] envisioned the flap's incorporating a transverse skin island located on the inferior abdominal wall, allowing a transverse donor site closure. This modification of the musculocutaneous flap would allow use of the redundant abdominal wall skin and subcutaneous tissue for breast reconstruction and provide a donor site closure scar located on the inferior trunk similar to an abdominoplasty scar. This approach was readily incorporated into breast reconstruction since the transverse skin island between the umbilicus and the pubic region provided both skin for envelope deficiency and the required soft tissue to re-establish a breast mound (generally without the need for implant) and an acceptable donor site scar. With the concern for silicone implant safety in the early 1990s, the flap provides a method to use autogenous tissues for complete breast reconstruction. For these reasons, the TRAM flap soon became the first choice for breast reconstruction

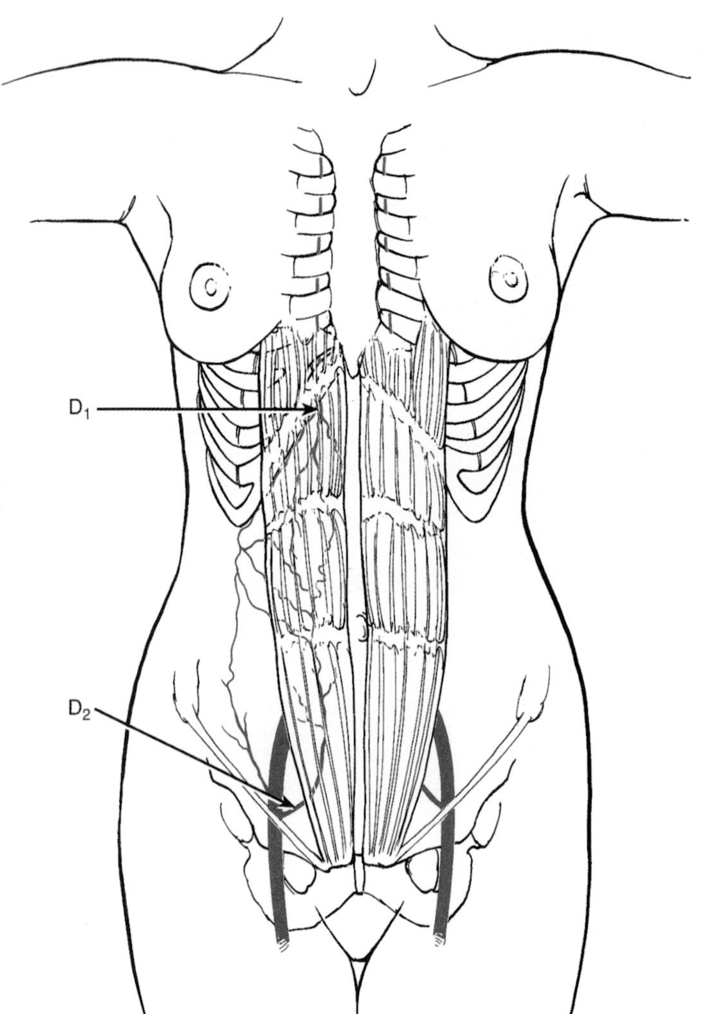

FIGURE 138-41. Rectus abdominis flap. Dominant pedicles: superior epigastric artery (D_1) and inferior epigastric artery (D_2). (From Mathes SJ, Nahai F: Reconstructive Surgery: Principles, Anatomy, and Technique. New York, Churchill Livingstone, 1997:1044.)

(Figs. 138-42 to 138-44). Later, as interest developed in skin-sparing mastectomy, where use of tissue expanders could be followed by insertion of saline implants without the concerns associated with the gel-filled silicone implant, the use of expanders either with pectoralis major coverage or in association with the latissimus dorsi muscle or musculocutaneous flaps was frequently selected, avoiding the use of the TRAM flap. Also, there remains concern about loss of rectus muscle function (either single or bilateral) as a consequence of use of the TRAM flap for breast reconstruction.

With interest in microvascular transplantation of the rectus abdominis musculocutaneous flap for breast reconstruction, a modification in the flap harvest techniques has been identified in which selected perforator branches of the deep inferior epigastric artery and associated venae comitantes are identified and dissected from the adjacent rectus muscle, thus preserving integrity of the majority of the inferior third of the rectus muscle (perforator flap) (see Fig. 138-75). There is ongoing debate as to the advantages of the microvascular transplantation of the TRAM flap or the perforator modification in regard to improvement in the quality of the breast mound reconstruction and the abdominal wall function at the donor site since the perforator dissection allows maintenance of the continuity of the rectus muscle. At present, both quality of the breast mound reconstruction (especially skin or subcutaneous tissue loss or fat necrosis) and problems at the donor site (especially hernia or abdominal weakness) are related to the experience of the surgeon and not necessarily inherent to the specific technique used.

The standard transposition technique using either the ipsilateral or contralateral rectus muscle with the transverse skin island has proved reliable in regard to flap survival, quality of breast mound reconstruction, and avoidance of donor site problems. This approach still remains the first choice for breast reconstruction when the skin envelope is inadequate and a flap is necessary or when autogenous reconstruction is requested by the patient.[241]

Primary indications for use of the transposition TRAM flap for breast reconstruction are the necessity of a flap due to inadequate skin envelope and a request by the patient for autogenous reconstruction (eliminating the need for a breast prosthesis). Although other flap sources are available and reliable (e.g., the latissimus dorsi musculocutaneous flap), the donor site allows use of redundant inferior abdominal wall tissue (often excessive in the multiparous patient), and the donor site scar is less obvious on the inferior trunk compared with other sites. The concept of an autogenous breast reconstruction is appealing to patients because it eliminates concern of implant failure or adverse reaction to a foreign body. In addition, the autogenous breast will age much like the contralateral breast, unlike the breast mound dependent on an implant for size and projection.

The rectus abdominis musculocutaneous flap does require a fairly extensive dissection compared with expander-implant reconstruction or even the latissimus dorsi musculocutaneous flap. The patient must accept the possibility of a longer hospitalization (average, 5 days) and a period of limited physical activity due to donor site closure of the important fascial layers of the inferior abdomen (6 weeks). Although the flap is reliable based on its type III circulation via the superior epigastric artery and associated venae comitantes,[277] the procedure is complex and stressful for the patient with medical problems.[183] Medical disabilities, obesity, diabetes, cigarette addiction, or adjuvant chemoradiation may represent relative contraindications to use of this technique for breast reconstruction.[279-281] Although the donor site represents one of the positive features for TRAM flap selection, there is risk of donor site morbidity due to weakness or hernia from use of one or both rectus muscles for the flap design and the incision through the rectus sheath, especially inferior to the arcuate line where abdominal hernia or weakness is possible. Fortunately, with care in abdominal closure of the fascial layers, the incidence of incisional hernia in the inferior abdomen remains low (7% to 9%) (Table 138-24).[236,282,283]

With the shift of the skin island from vertical as originally described[276] to transverse,[277] the donor site location improved, but the inclusion of a donor area containing the most subcutaneous tissue (panniculus) available for breast mound reconstruction was far more significant. The transverse skin island extends in the vertical direction between the umbilicus (or 1 to 3 cm superior to the umbilicus) and the pubic hair line (or 1 to 5 cm superior, depending on laxity of abdominal panniculus) and transversely between the anterior iliac spines. The skin island of the flap has been divided into zones based on the reliability of its circulation and survival (Fig. 138-45). Zone 1 is located directly over the muscle and represents its primary cutaneous territory. Directly across the midline of the abdomen is zone 2, which extends from the midline of the abdomen to the lateral edge of the contralateral muscle. Zone 2 of the skin island has proved reliable because of the circulation provided by the subdermal and deeper vascular communications of musculocutaneous perforating vessels from the rectus muscle beneath zone 1. However, the two more lateral zones—zone 3, the portion of the skin island lateral to the primary rectus muscle, and zone 4, the portion of the skin island most distant from the primary flap territory (zone 1) located between the lateral edge of the contralateral rectus sheath and

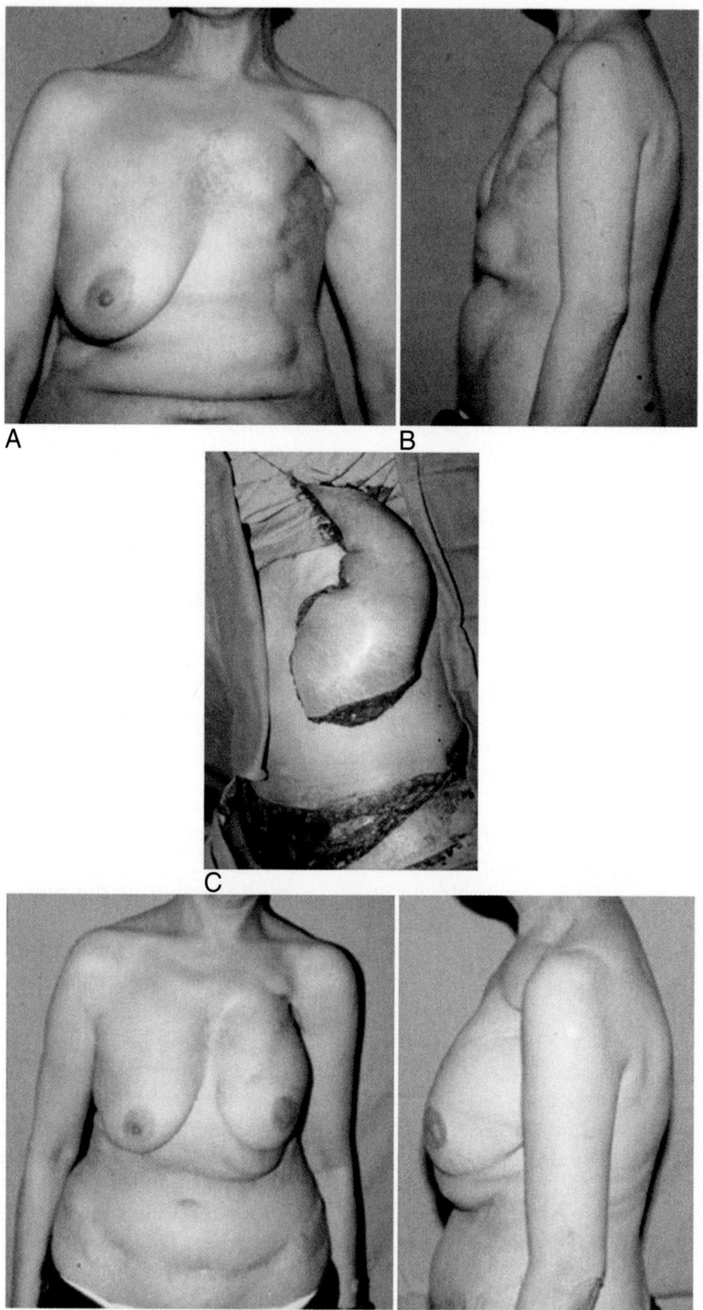

FIGURE 138-42. TRAM flap for delayed left mastectomy reconstruction. *A,* Anterior view of left radical mastectomy defect. *B,* Lateral view of left mastectomy defect. *C,* Transposition of contralateral TRAM flap to provide left autogenous reconstruction. *D,* Postoperative view at 2 years demonstrates autogenous breast mound provided by contralateral TRAM flap. *E,* Lateral view demonstrates correction of contour deformity due to loss of pectoralis major muscle.

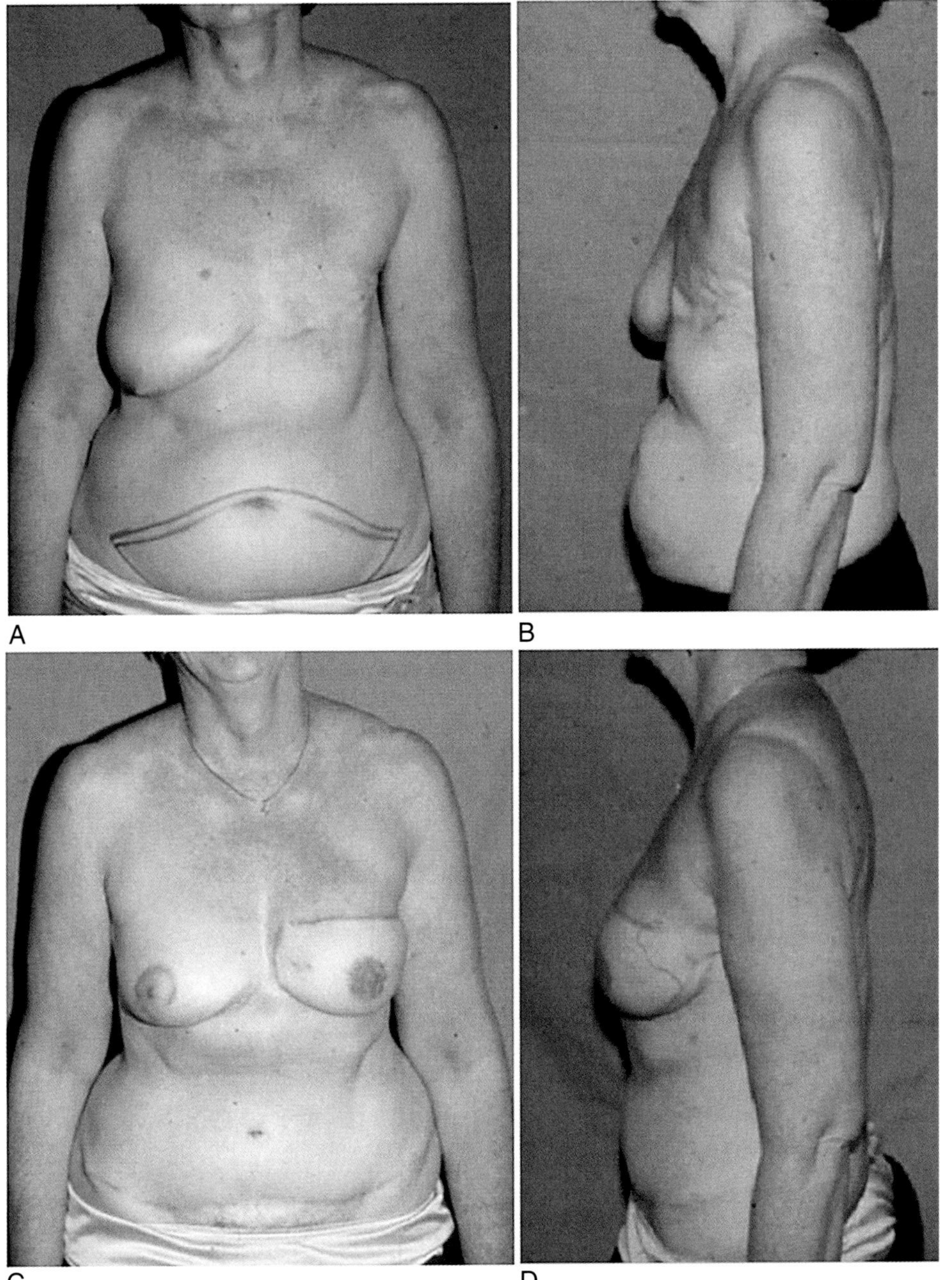

FIGURE 138-43. TRAM flap for delayed left breast reconstruction. *A,* Postoperative left modified radical mastectomy. The TRAM skin island is outlined for autogenous reconstruction. *B,* Preoperative lateral view. Abdominal panniculus will be transposed as TRAM flap for autogenous reconstruction. *C,* Postoperative view at 1 year of left breast reconstruction with contralateral TRAM flap. Nipple-areola reconstruction is completed. The breast mound demonstrates adequate size for symmetry with the opposite breast. *D,* Postoperative lateral view. TRAM autogenous reconstruction demonstrates adequate mound projection. Donor site contour is improved after panniculectomy.

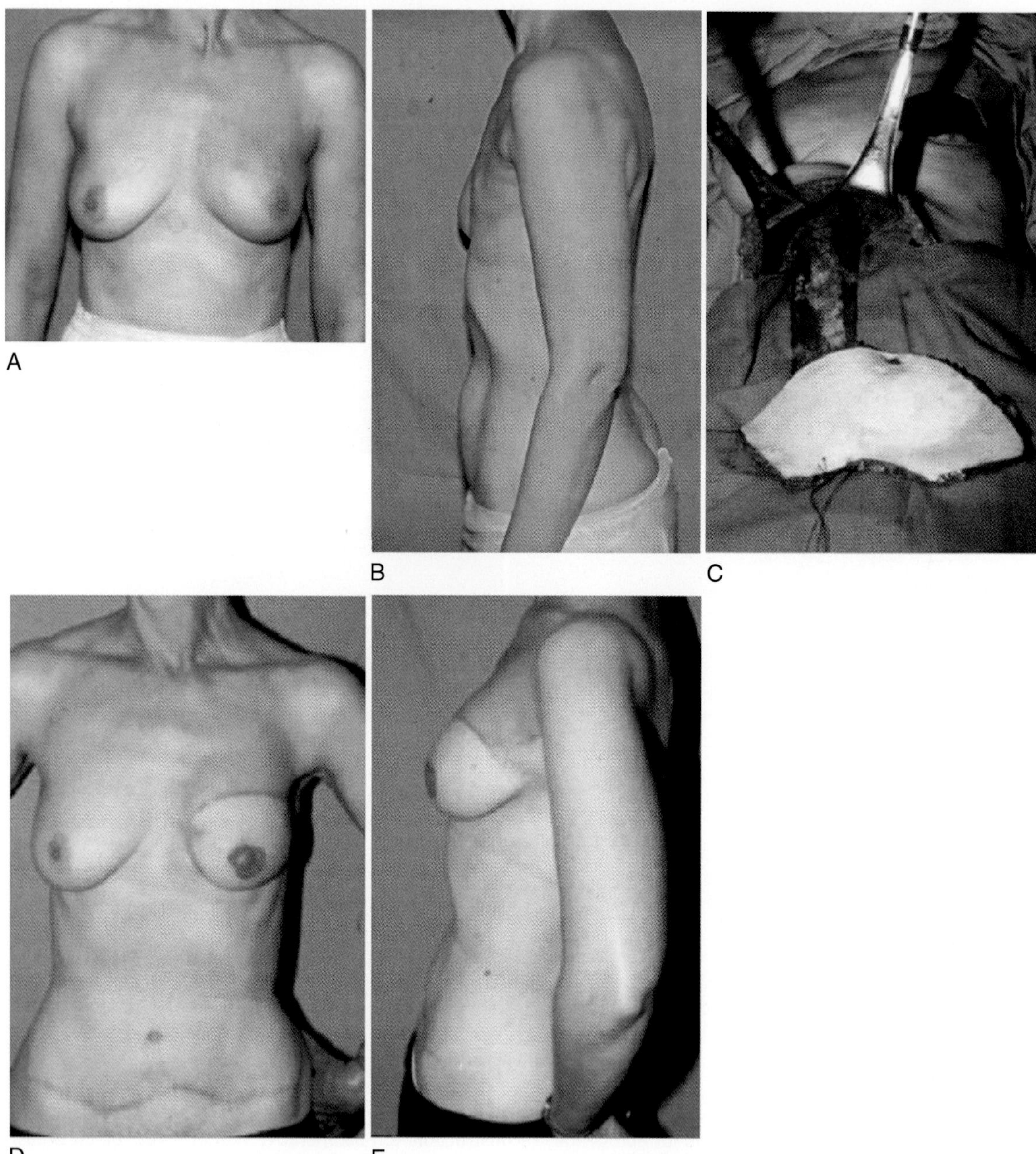

FIGURE 138-44. Rectus abdominis musculocutaneous flaps for delayed breast reconstruction. *A,* Preoperative anterior view of left mastectomy for invasive breast carcinoma. *B,* Postoperative lateral view after left mastectomy; preoperative for breast reconstruction. *C,* Right TRAM flap ready for transposition to left chest defect. *D,* Postoperative view at 2 years of left autogenous breast reconstruction with TRAM flap and later nipple-areola reconstruction. *E,* Postoperative lateral view demonstrates adequate mound projection and definition of inframammary line.

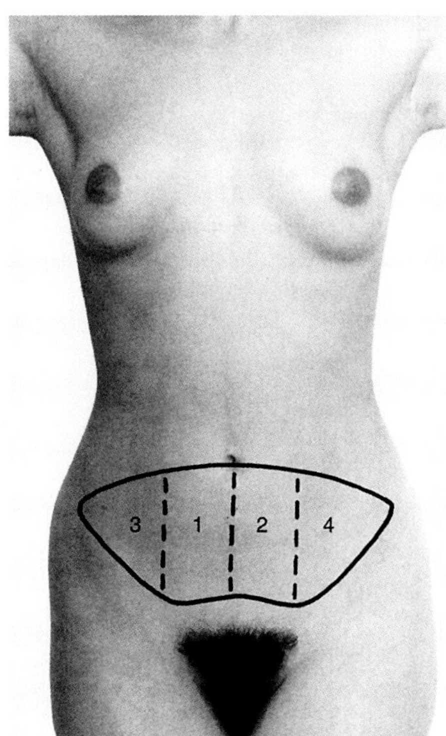

FIGURE 138-45. Rectus abdominis musculocutaneous flap; transverse inferior skin island design (extended skin island). Note zones 1 to 4 designate relationship of skin island to rectus muscle flap. (From Mathes SJ, Nahai F: Reconstructive Surgery: Principles, Anatomy, and Technique. New York, Churchill Livingstone, 1997:1053.)

the iliac crest—are less reliable in regard to circulation based on one rectus abdominis muscle. In general, most of zone 4 and certainly the lateral aspect of zone 3 are discarded because of inadequate perfusion. In the obese patient or patients with collagen or vascular disease, efforts are under analysis to improve flap circulation especially to zones 1 and 2 of the skin island. Two methods advocated are shifting the skin island to the midabdomen, where there are more perforating vessels from the underlying superior epigastric pedicle, and providing a flap delay.

The ability to improve skin and muscle survival of a musculocutaneous flap by strategic delay was initially demonstrated by Mathes and Nahai[284,285] and has subsequently been applied clinically for the superior-based rectus abdominis musculocutaneous flap. Although different approaches are used, the concept primarily involves strategic division of the inferior pedicle to the rectus muscle, the deep inferior epigastric artery and venae comitantes, at varying intervals before flap elevation for the reconstructive procedure. The vessel ligation is typically performed 2 to 3 weeks before flap elevation; however, reports have shown that as little as 3 days may be sufficient.[286] Variations include incisions at the planned design of the skin island, division of ipsilateral or bilateral superficial epigastric artery and venae comitantes, division of the contralateral deep inferior epigastric artery and venae comitantes, and preliminary partial elevation of zones 3 and 4. Although delay is effective in improving skin island circulation,[287-289] the TRAM flap is most often elevated as a single-stage procedure and can be effectively used in most abdomens including the mildly obese patient. If delay is required, other flap options should be considered, including vertical design of the skin island and alternative flaps (e.g., the latissimus dorsi musculocutaneous flap) (Fig. 138-46).

Efforts to improve the reliability of the TRAM skin island have also focused on the vascular pedicle. As a type III muscle flap, its dual blood supply extends from the costal margin via the superior epigastric artery and the pelvis via the deep inferior epigastric artery. Both pedicles have accompanying venae comitantes that provide muscle venous drainage. The entire muscle and primary skin territory will reliably survive transposition on either pedicle. However, with the inferior transverse skin island based superiorly for the TRAM

TABLE 138-24 ✦ DELAYED UNIPEDICLED TRAM FLAP COMPLICATIONS

Author	No. of Patients	Delay (mean)	Interval Technique	Partial Flap Loss (%)	Total Flap Loss (%)	Hernia (%)
Erdmann[304]	76	13.9 days	Bilateral deep inferior epigastric artery and vein ligated	6.6	0	6.6
Rickard[288]	15	14 days	Bilateral deep and superficial inferior epigastric artery and vein ligated	0	0	7
Scheufler[305]	40	3.6 months	Embolization of bilateral deep inferior epigastric arteries (87%), unilateral artery (13%)	7.5	0	10
Restifo[306]	15	7 days	Deep and superficial inferior epigastric artery and vein ligated	13	0	0

flap, there is venous insufficiency visible in the nonprimary territories of the skin island due to required reversal of flow for venous drainage via the pedicle most distant from the skin island. Fortunately, in most circumstances, zone 1 and zone 2 will survive—hence the established reliability of the TRAM transposition flap for breast reconstruction. However, partial areas of flap necrosis occur with a variable frequency of 5% to 15%.[236,283] Efforts to improve skin island circulation have also focused on use of the deep inferior epigastric pedicle as the basis of flap circulation or to augment circulation in addition to the superior pedicle. The microvascular transplantation of the TRAM flap based on the deep inferior epigastric artery and associated venae comitantes places the skin island close to its normal circulation and eliminates the reversal of venous flow observed in the superior-based pedicle (see "Microvascular Composite Tissue Transplantation"). However, the microvascular transplantation of the TRAM flap requires restoration of blood

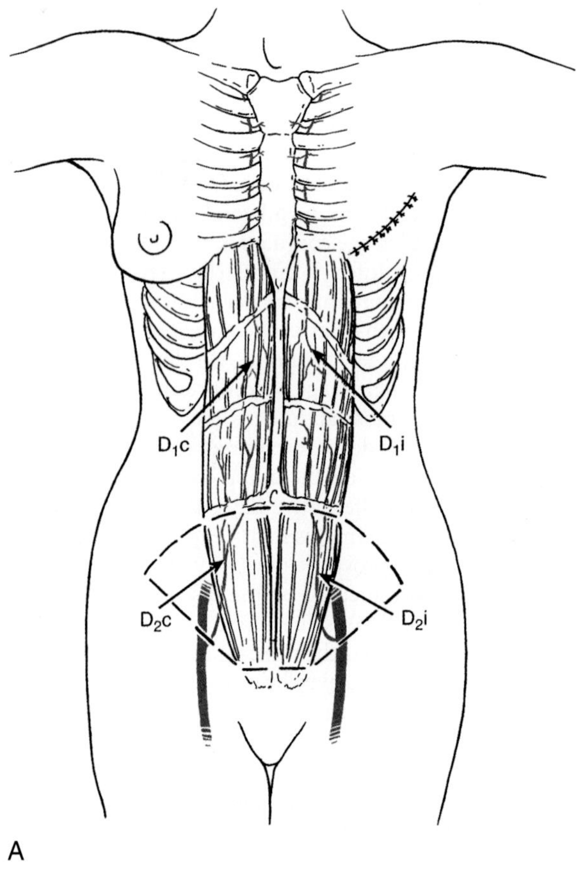

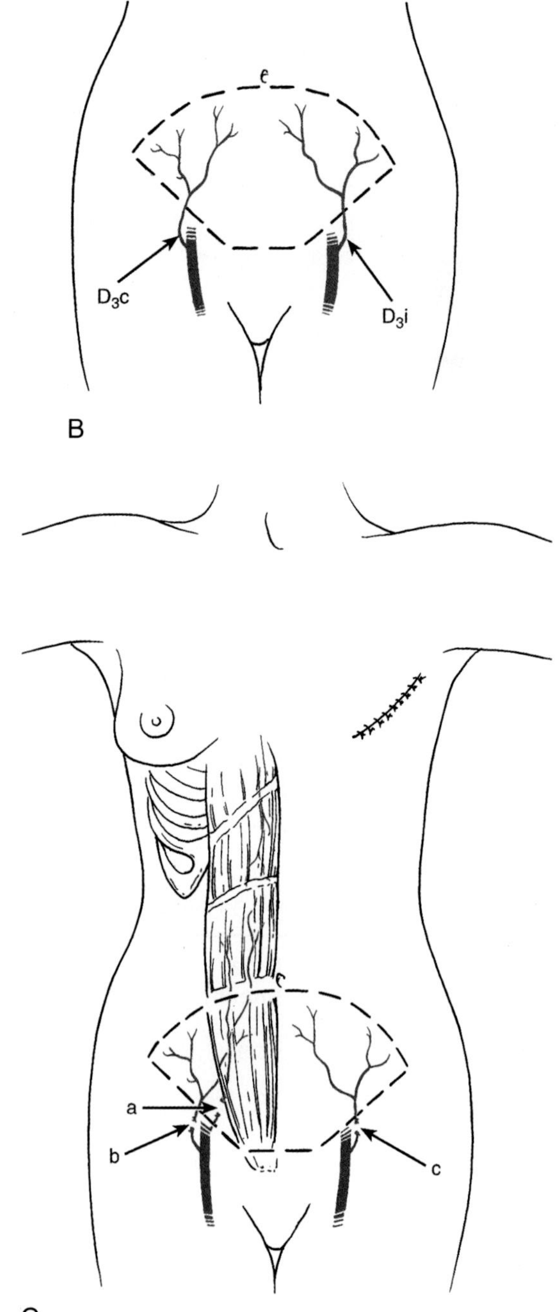

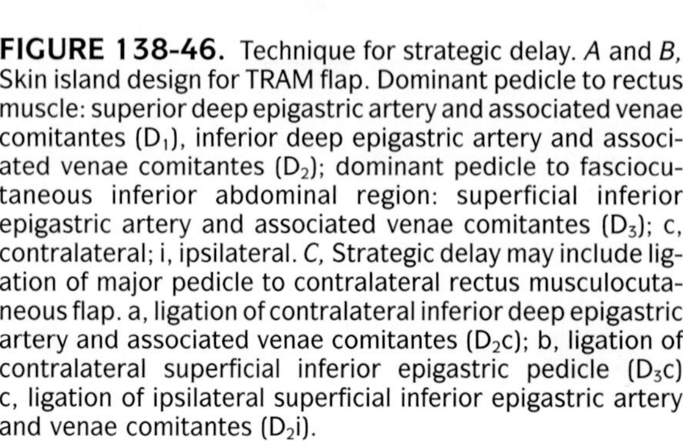
FIGURE 138-46. Technique for strategic delay. *A* and *B*, Skin island design for TRAM flap. Dominant pedicle to rectus muscle: superior deep epigastric artery and associated venae comitantes (D_1), inferior deep epigastric artery and associated venae comitantes (D_2); dominant pedicle to fasciocutaneous inferior abdominal region: superficial inferior epigastric artery and associated venae comitantes (D_3); c, contralateral; i, ipsilateral. *C,* Strategic delay may include ligation of major pedicle to contralateral rectus musculocutaneous flap. a, ligation of contralateral inferior deep epigastric artery and associated venae comitantes (D_2c); b, ligation of contralateral superficial inferior epigastric pedicle (D_3c) c, ligation of ipsilateral superficial inferior epigastric artery and venae comitantes (D_2i).

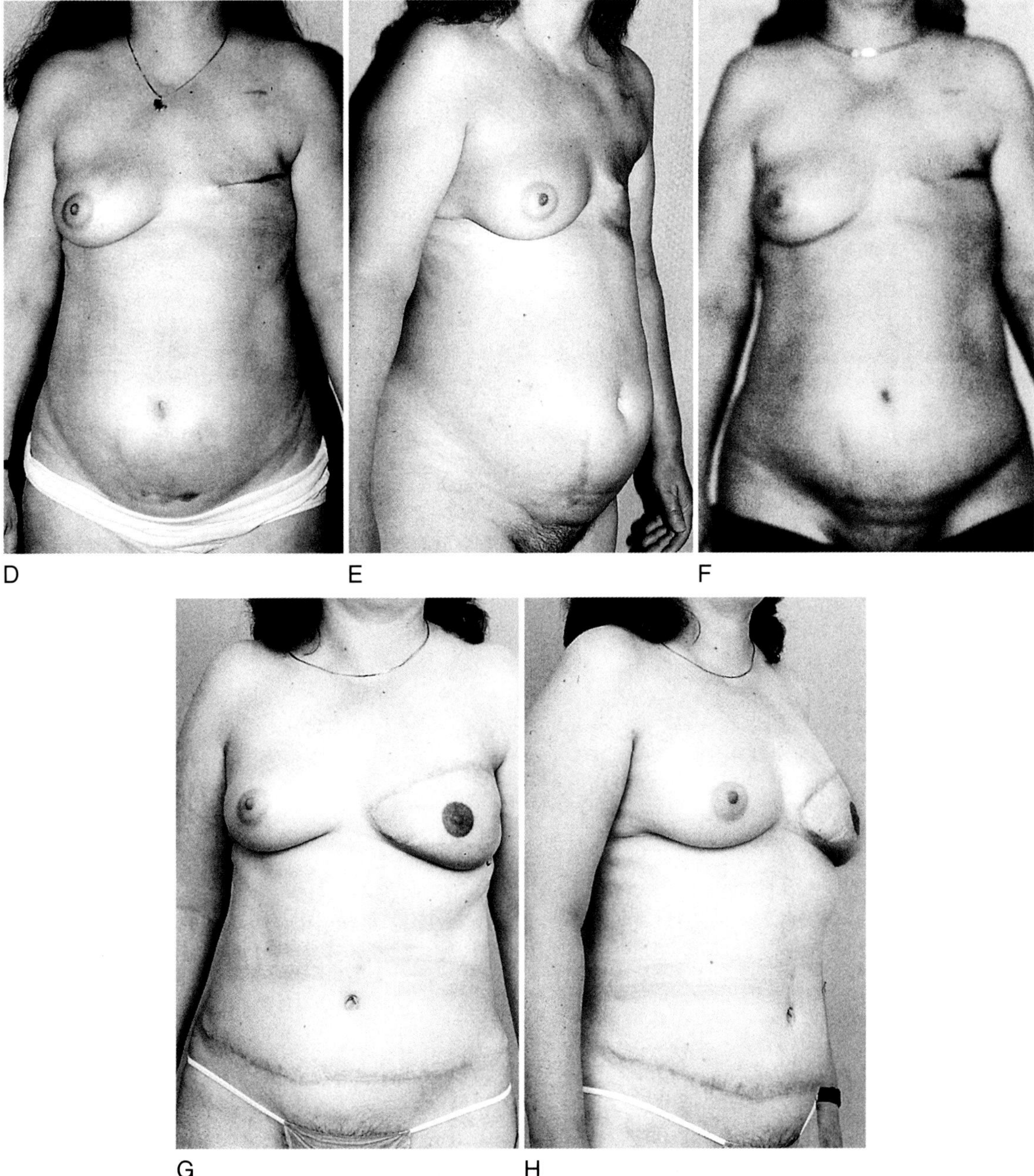

FIGURE 138-46, cont'd. *D* and *E,* Preoperative views of 45-year-old obese woman with right paramedian scar and lower transverse abdominal scar who underwent radiation therapy after mastectomy. A unipedicled delayed TRAM flap breast reconstruction was planned in this high-risk patient. *F,* Three weeks after strategic delay. Both superficial inferior epigastric vessels and the left deep inferior epigastric vessels were divided through the existing lower transverse abdominal scar. *G* and *H,* Final result at 2 years. (From Mathes SJ, Nahai F: Reconstructive Surgery: Principles, Anatomy, and Technique. New York, Churchill Livingstone, 1997:102-104.)

flow by microvascular anastomosis into suitable receptor vessels in proximity to the mastectomy defect with the risk of complete flap loss if the anastomosis should fail. An alternative approach is the transposition of the TRAM flap based on the superior epigastric pedicle with an additional anastomosis of the deep inferior epigastric artery, vein, or both to suitable receptor vessels, usually within the axilla. This technique has been termed supercharging the flap, and although it is rarely used in clinical practice, it serves as a salvage step if the flap seems to have arterial or venous insufficiency at the time of inset. Most surgeons preserve length on the deep inferior epigastric pedicle before division and ligation during the flap harvest process. If needed, the pedicle will reach the axilla, where receptor vessels are available to supplement either arterial input or venous output or both.

The use of a bipedicled rectus abdominis musculocutaneous flap will also improve skin island circulation and converts the TRAM skin zones into zone 1 between the lateral edges of both rectus muscles and the remaining lateral aspects of the flap into zone 2. Bipedicled TRAM flaps are especially useful in bilateral breast reconstruction; in reconstruction requiring complete use of the skin island; with radical mastectomy, where part of the skin island will be used to fill the contour defect resulting from resection of the pectoralis major muscle; and for autogenous reconstruction when the contralateral breast is large and extra volume is needed with the flap for symmetry (Fig. 138-47). When bilateral TRAM flaps are used for bilateral reconstruction, the flaps are elevated as two independent flaps with the transverse skin island divided at the midline of the abdomen incorporating zone 1 and zone 3 for each flap. If it is used for one side, the surgeon may elect to leave the skin island intact with the two underlying muscles or to divide the skin island in the midline and elevate two independent flaps that can be stacked or shifted independently on the reconstructive site to achieve symmetry with the opposite breast.

Technique Selection

If the TRAM transposition flap is selected for ipsilateral breast reconstruction, the flap design must take the opposite breast into consideration. If the patient requests matching for a large or ptotic breast, the size of the panniculus will determine whether a unilateral or bilateral TRAM flap is required. Most patients elect to undergo reduction or mastopexy either simultaneously or subsequently, so bilateral TRAM flaps for modified radical or skin-sparing mastectomy are rarely required. However, if the defect is extensive (radical mastectomy with absence of pectoralis major) or the remaining skin envelope severely damaged (e.g., prior radiation therapy), bilateral TRAM flaps should be considered. When bilateral mastectomy reconstruction is planned, bipedicled TRAM flaps with two hemitransverse skin islands should be considered unless one side represents a prophylactic mastectomy and the patient prefers to maintain one rectus muscle intact. In this instance, the TRAM flap will be used for the more extensive defect, and the contralateral side may be reconstructed by the expander-implant method.

The surgeon must also decide on which muscle to base the skin island for the unilateral TRAM flap. Either the ipsilateral or contralateral flap is effective and equally reliable for breast reconstruction. Many surgeons have used both sides with equal efficiency and quality of results. Proponents of the contralateral TRAM flap note that the arc of rotation is close to the xiphoid and does not require disruption of the inframammary line. The flap rotates only 90 to 180 degrees, resulting in less twisting of the muscle below the skin island. The proponents of the ipsilateral TRAM flap note ease of arc of rotation through the medial inframammary line and the ability to flip the reversed flap back so the cutaneous portion of the flap aligns with the retained breast skin. If inset is achieved with an adequate tunnel and without tension, both ipsilateral and contralateral flaps provide safe and quality results.

Preoperative Markings and Preparation

Preoperative markings are completed immediately before surgery. Two areas require careful markings: the TRAM skin island dimension and location on the inferior abdomen and the intended site of inset of the TRAM flap at the mastectomy defect. If immediate reconstruction is planned, the extent of skin resection can be planned with the oncologic breast surgeon since this will represent the inset site for the exposed portion of the TRAM skin island. In general, the skin island is designed to include the entire lower abdominal panniculus to allow a youthful abdominal donor site with defect closure (similar to abdominoplasty approach). When there is not excessive lower abdominal skin and subcutaneous tissue (nulliparous patient) or in the obese patient, skin marking must take into consideration the potential difficulty in donor site closure with increased width of the skin island (Figs. 138-48 and 138-49).

ABDOMINAL MARKING. The skin island is located between the umbilicus and the pubic hair line extending between the anterior iliac spines. In general, the superior skin island is located 1 to 3 cm superior to the umbilicus. If the distance between the xiphoid and pubis is short, the skin island is placed slightly more inferiorly on the abdomen to ensure an adequate arc of rotation to the chest wall. The inferior mark will extend immediately superior to the pubic hair line

Text continued on p. 725

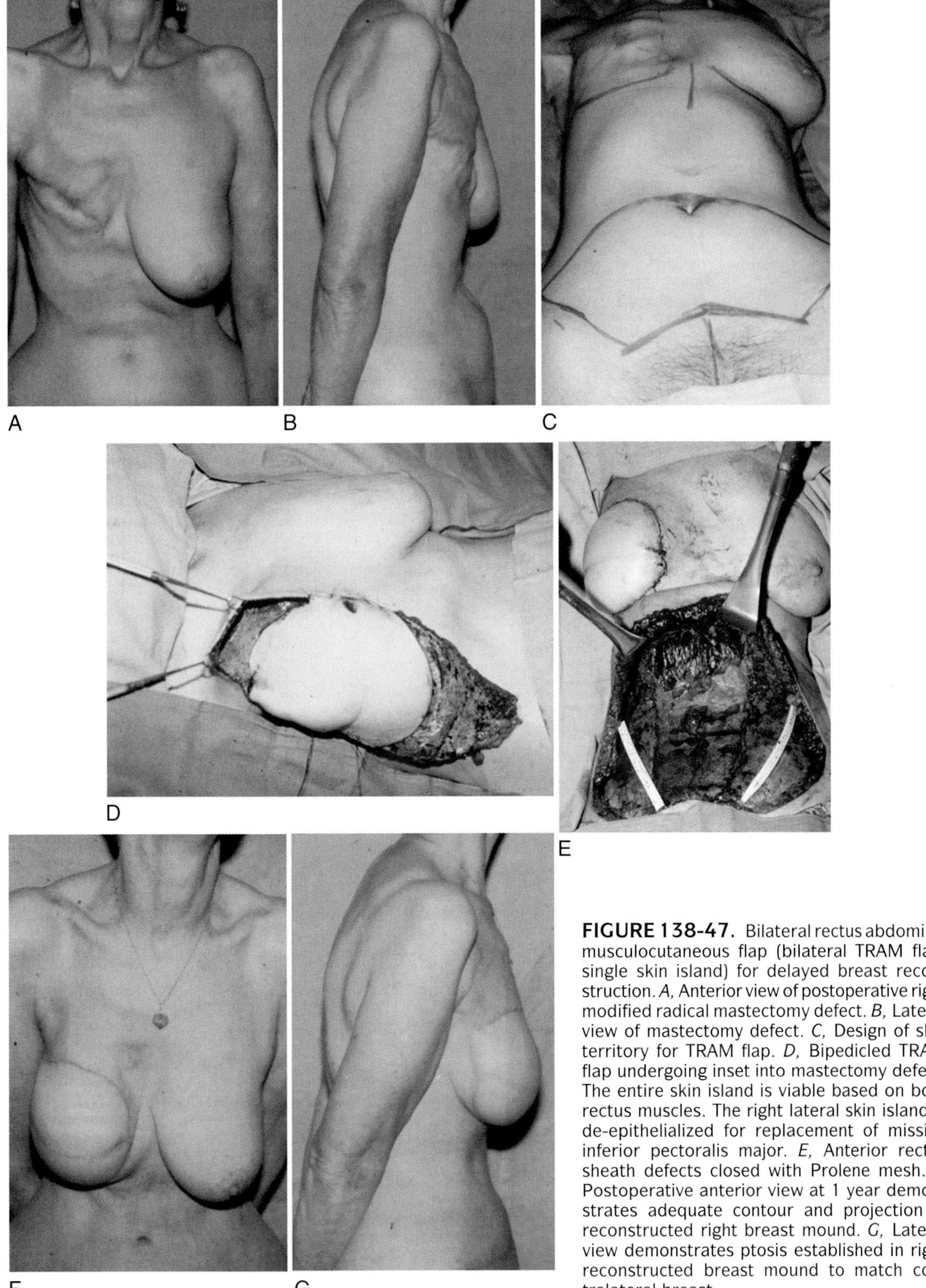

FIGURE 138-47. Bilateral rectus abdominis musculocutaneous flap (bilateral TRAM flap, single skin island) for delayed breast reconstruction. *A,* Anterior view of postoperative right modified radical mastectomy defect. *B,* Lateral view of mastectomy defect. *C,* Design of skin territory for TRAM flap. *D,* Bipedicled TRAM flap undergoing inset into mastectomy defect. The entire skin island is viable based on both rectus muscles. The right lateral skin island is de-epithelialized for replacement of missing inferior pectoralis major. *E,* Anterior rectus sheath defects closed with Prolene mesh. *F,* Postoperative anterior view at 1 year demonstrates adequate contour and projection in reconstructed right breast mound. *G,* Lateral view demonstrates ptosis established in right reconstructed breast mound to match contralateral breast.

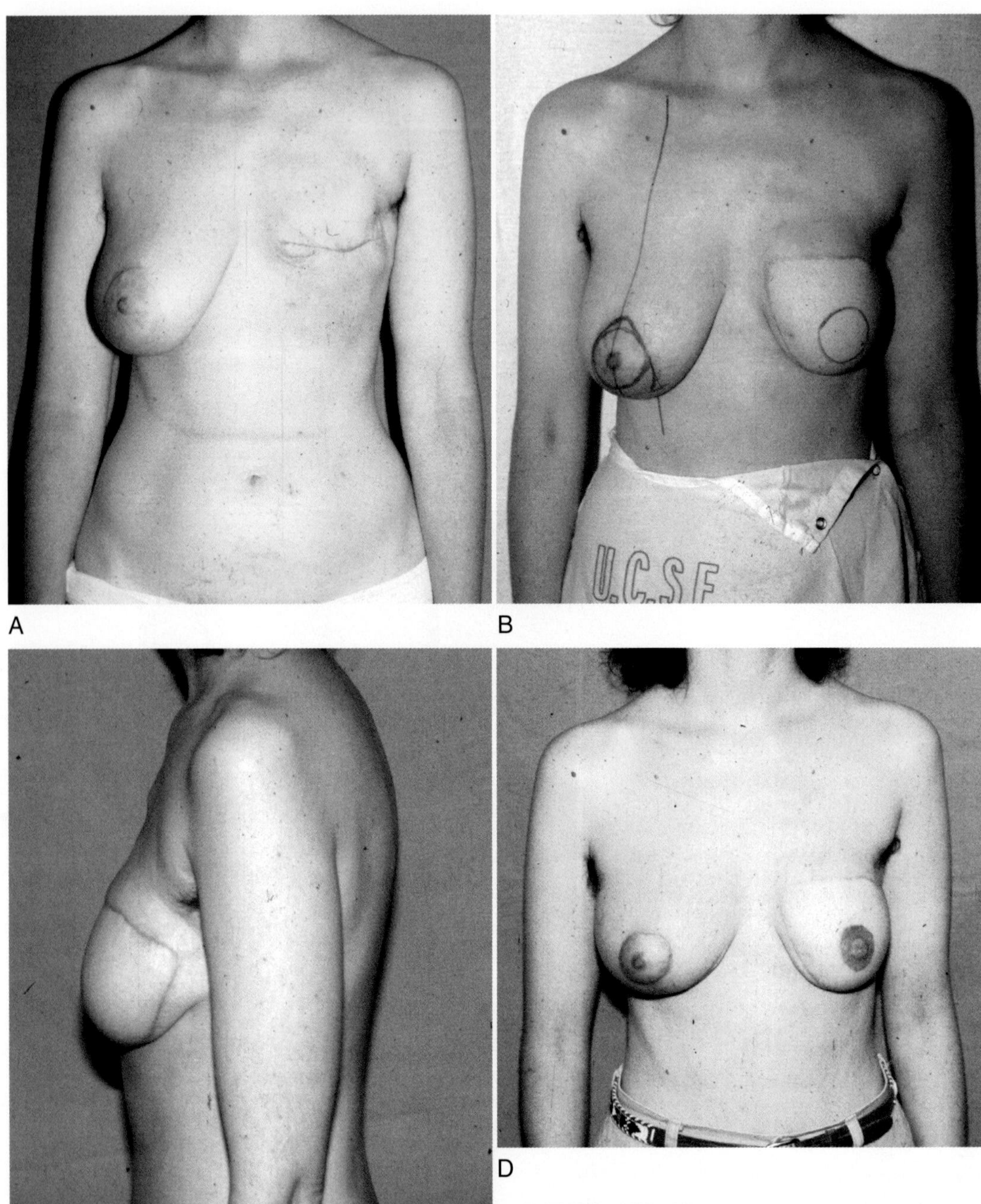

FIGURE 138-48. TRAM flap for delayed breast reconstruction. *A,* Postoperative view of left modified radical mastectomy. Nulliparous patient requests autogenous reconstruction. *B,* Postoperative view 6 months after left breast TRAM flap reconstruction; markings for left nipple reconstruction and right mastopexy. *C,* Postoperative lateral view demonstrates adequate mound projection after TRAM flap reconstruction. *D,* Postoperative view at 1 year of left breast TRAM flap reconstruction and right mastopexy for symmetry.

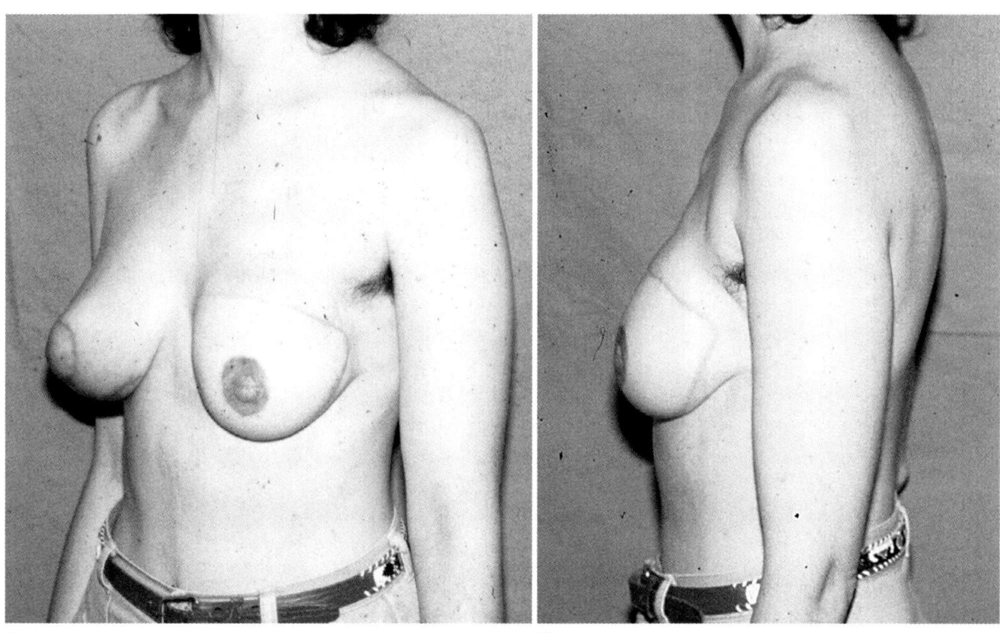

FIGURE 138-48, cont'd. *E,* Postoperative oblique view. *F,* Postoperative lateral view after nipple-areola reconstruction.

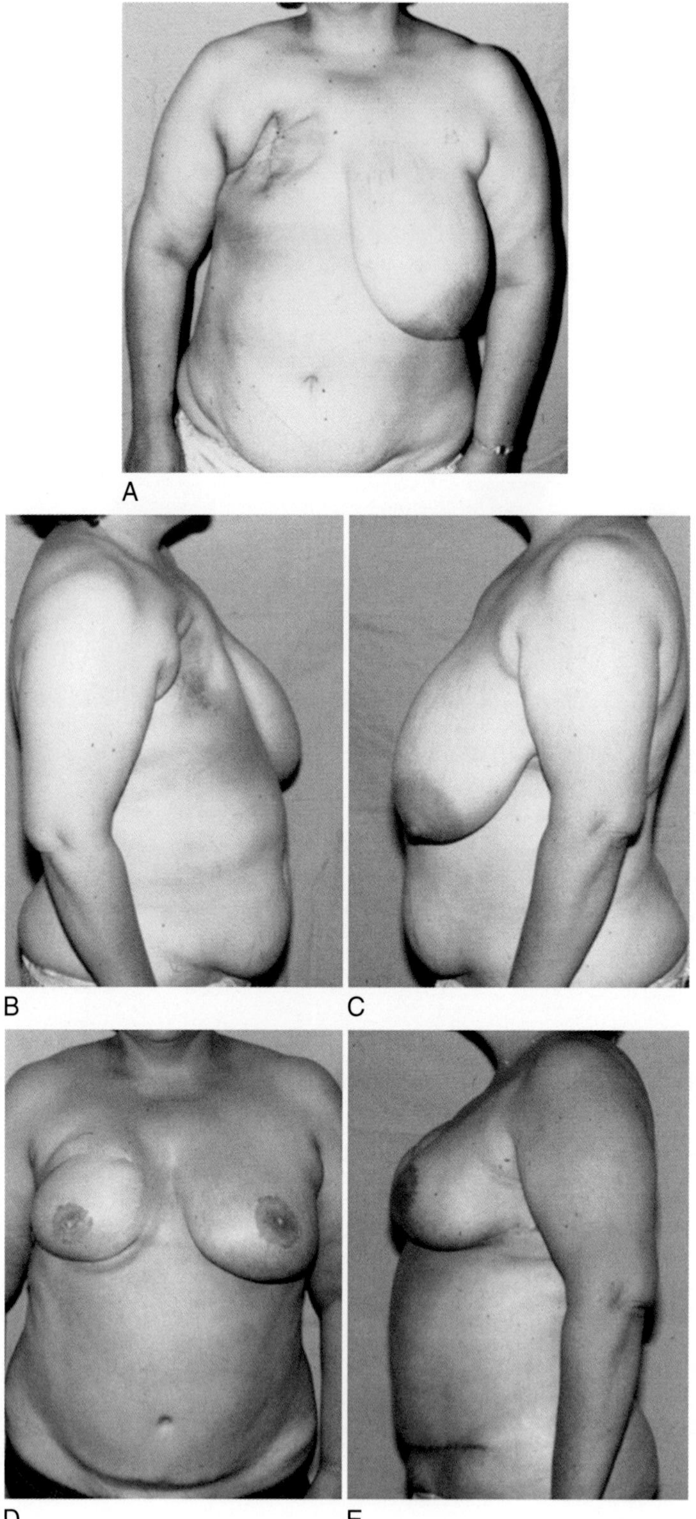

FIGURE 138-49. TRAM flap for delayed breast reconstruction. *A,* Anterior postoperative view of modified radical mastectomy. *B,* Lateral view of mastectomy defect. Note panniculus available as donor site for autogenous breast reconstruction. *C,* Lateral preoperative view of left breast macromastia. *D,* Postoperative view at 1 year of right breast reconstruction by contralateral TRAM flap. *E,* Postoperative view of left reduction mammaplasty for symmetry.

(Fig. 138-50*A*). If the patient has a prior transverse cesarean scar, this scar is selected as the inferior margin of the skin island. During surgery, the inferior margin of the skin island may be moved superiorly if direct closure as measured with retraction of the superior abdominal flap over the skin island with the patient's body flexed on the operating room table appears difficult or too tight.

CHEST MARKING. In immediate reconstruction, the extent of skin resection is confirmed with the responsible oncologic breast surgeon. If skin-sparing mastectomy is planned, optional lateral transverse extension of the periareolar incision is considered. In some instances, the periareolar incision includes an extension to the primary tumor biopsy site. The inframammary line is also marked bilaterally for use at the time of flap inset. In delayed reconstruction, the surgeon has the option to enter the skin envelope through the mastectomy scar or at the level of the inframammary line. In general, it is preferable to enter the mastectomy defect through an incision that is 2 to 3 cm superior to the level of the contralateral inframammary line since the skin will be pulled inferiorly after abdominal wall closure. With flap inset, the mastectomy scar and the intervening skin between the mastectomy scar and the inframammary scar will be excised and replaced by the TRAM skin island.

If simultaneous contralateral breast surgery is planned, the breast marking will also be required at this time. Many surgeons elect to delay the symmetry procedures, awaiting the final position of the reconstructed breast mound before performing surgery on the opposite breast. With experience, the TRAM flap inset will provide a predicable result that will allow simultaneous contralateral breast procedures for symmetry. When there is doubt about the reliability of the flap inset or in patients unsure of desired size or shape at either the reconstruction site or the opposite breast, it is preferable to delay the contralateral breast surgery until a suitable interval of follow-up (6 weeks to 3 months).

Text continued on p. 730

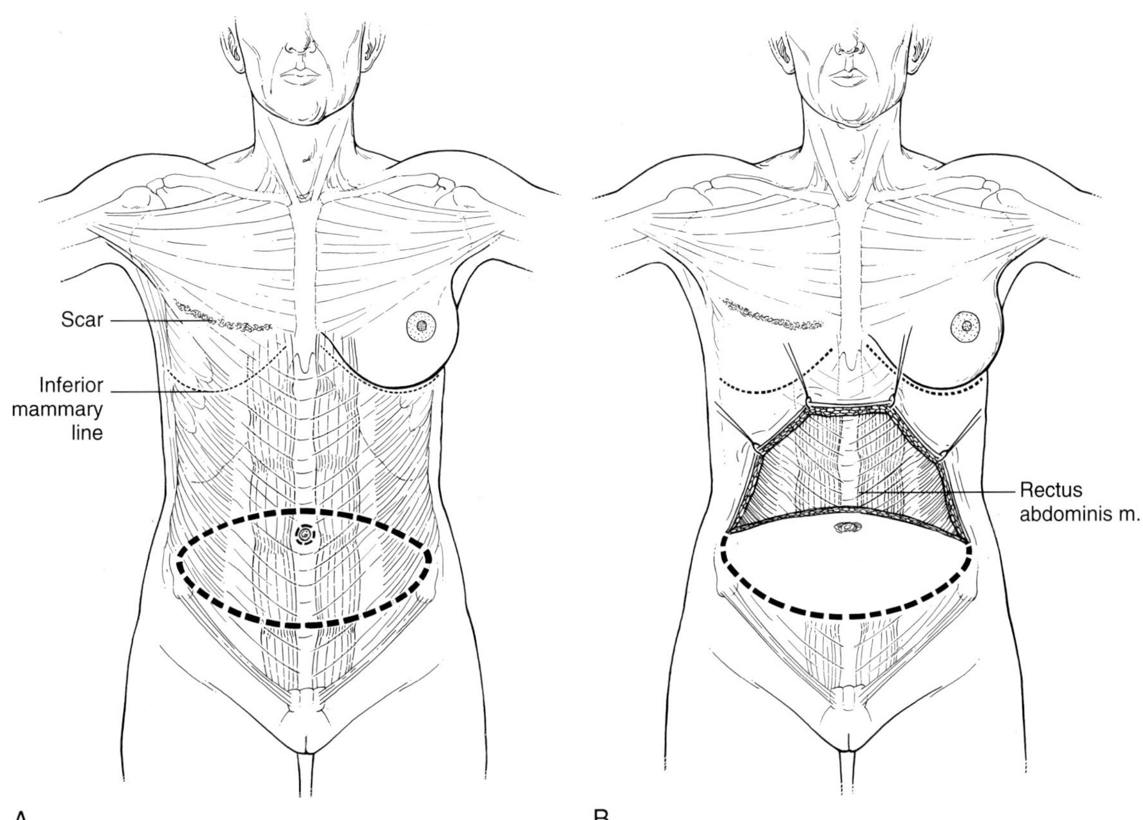

FIGURE 138-50. Technique of elevation: TRAM flap. *A,* Skin island located between anterior iliac spines and between umbilicus and pubis. *B,* Superior abdominal flap elevated to costal margin and inferior sternum. *Continued*

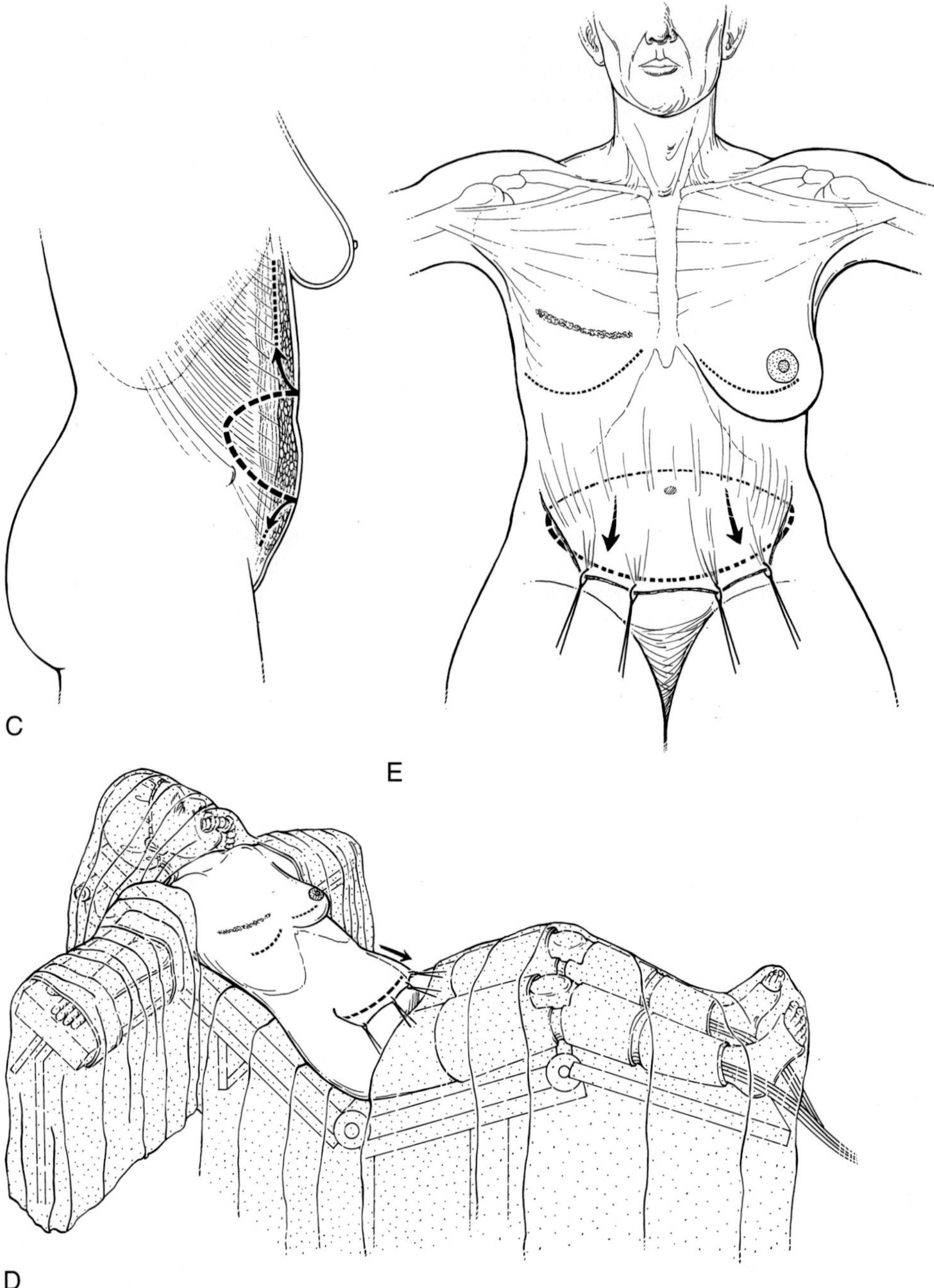

FIGURE 138-50, cont'd. *C,* Plane of dissection flap to Scarpa layer and superficial to rectus sheath and external oblique fascia. *D,* After superior flap is elevated, the patient is flexed and the superior flap is advanced over the designed skin island to ensure that direct donor site closure is possible based on width of designed skin island (TRAM). *E,* Confirmation of adequate superior flap for direct donor site closure.

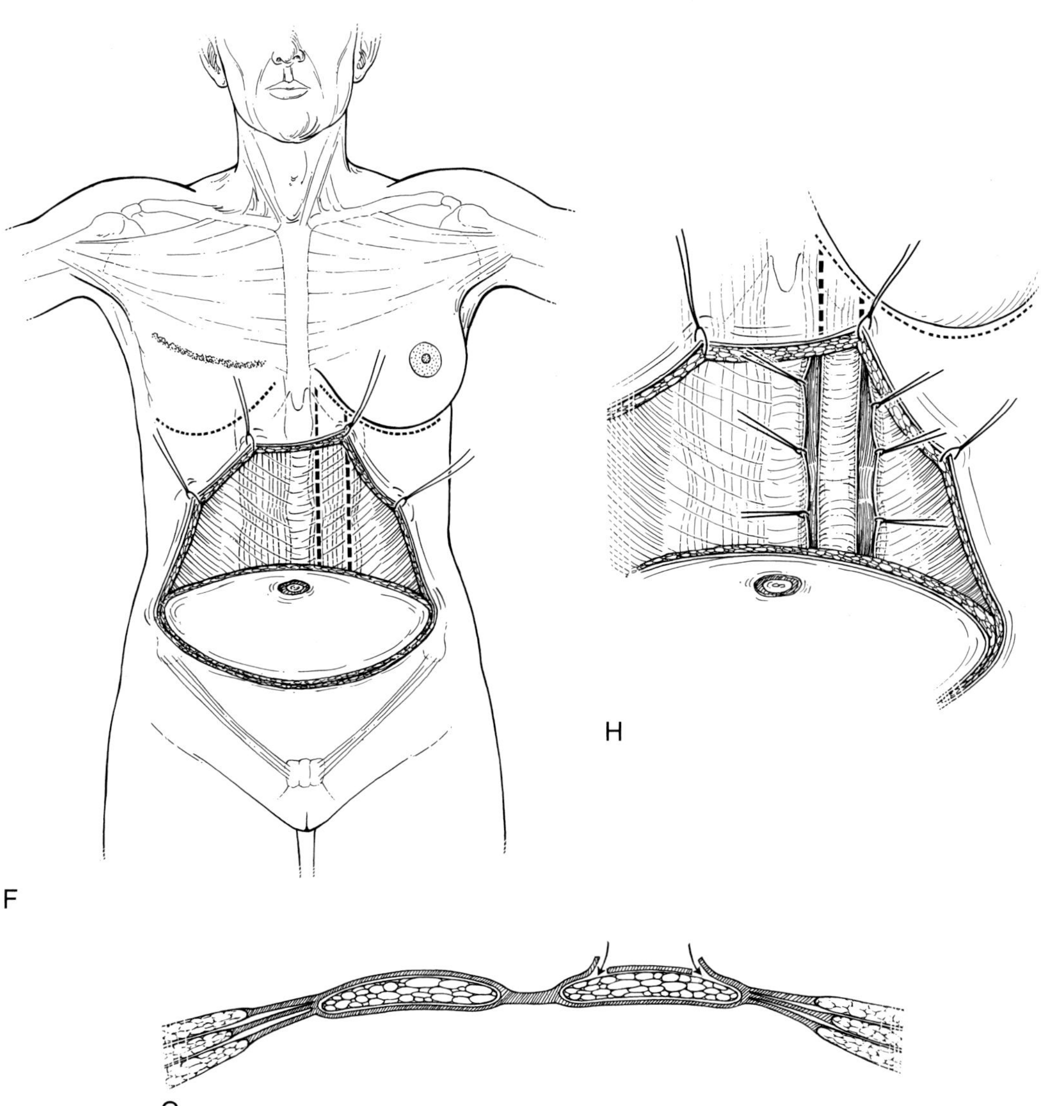

FIGURE 138-50, cont'd. *F,* Parallel incisions are made over the rectus sheath, each approximately 2 cm from the edge of the sheath. Central anterior rectus sheath will be included with rectus muscle. *G,* Cross section demonstrates plane of dissection to separate muscle edges from medial and lateral rectus sheath. *H,* Preservation of medial and lateral anterior sheath will allow defect anterior sheath closure in most patients.

Continued

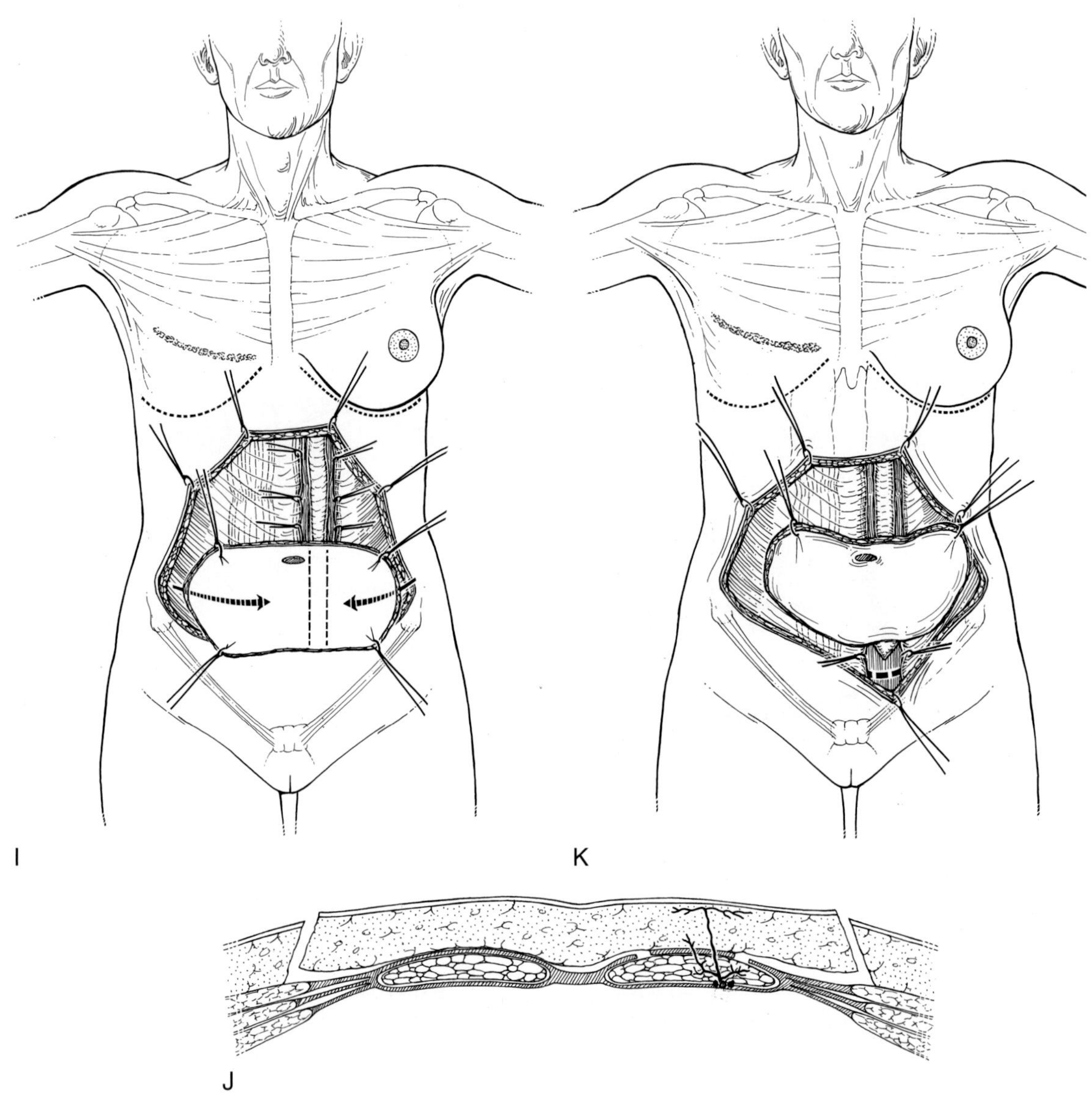

FIGURE 138-50, cont'd. *I,* Contralateral skin island (zone 2 and zone 4) elevated from external oblique and anterior sheath. The location of the divided musculocutaneous perforators from the opposite rectus muscle is noted because the pattern may be repeated on the flap side. Ipsilateral flap (zone 3) is elevated. Both sides are elevated from medial and lateral 2 cm from the anterior rectus sheath or until significant perforators (1 mm in diameter) are encountered. Large perforators are preserved. *J,* Cross section of inferior abdomen demonstrates plane of dissection and preservation of rectus sheath fascial edge for later donor site closure. *K,* Anterior sheath is divided, and sutures approximate medial and lateral rectus muscle edge to edge of central rectus sheath and deep surface of flap. These sutures will prevent inadvertent disruption of musculocutaneous perforating vessels. The rectus muscle distal to the superior margin of the skin island is divided.

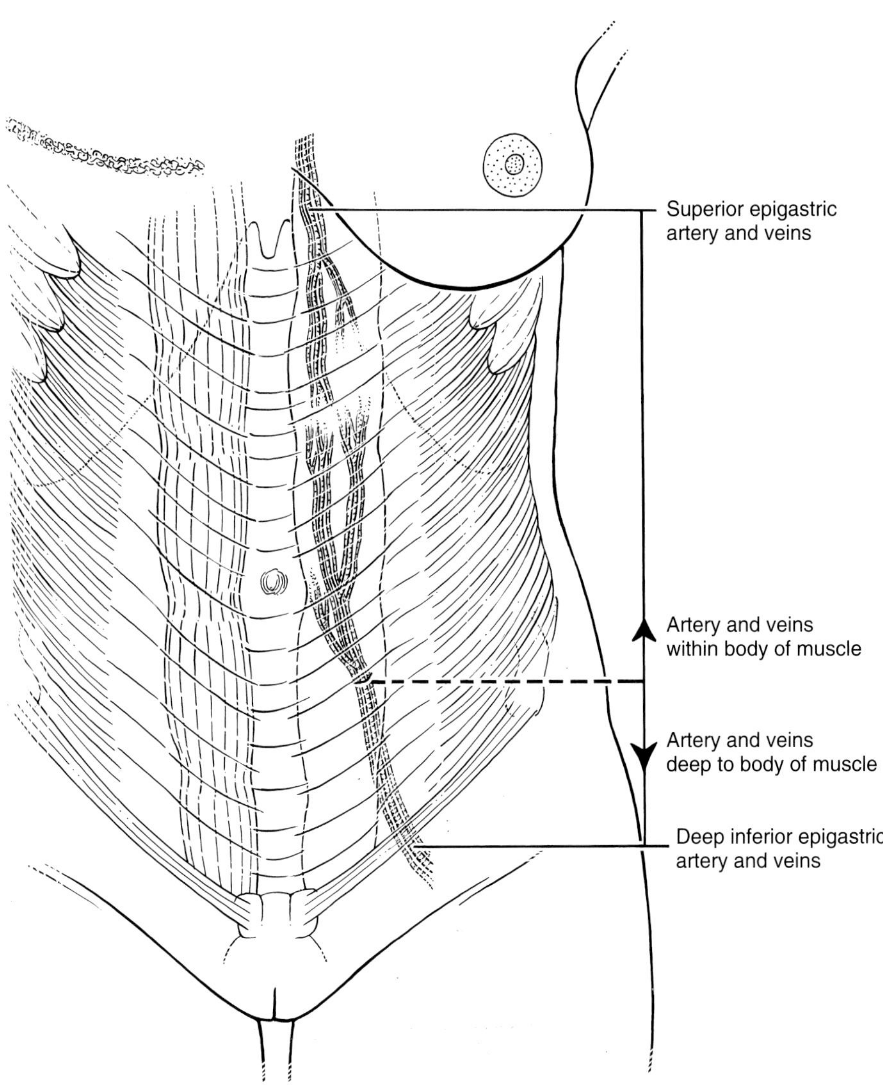

FIGURE 138-50, cont'd. *L,* Vascular anatomy of superior and inferior deep epigastric artery and venae comitantes below skin island. The rectus muscle is divided without injury to the deep inferior epigastric pedicle. *Continued*

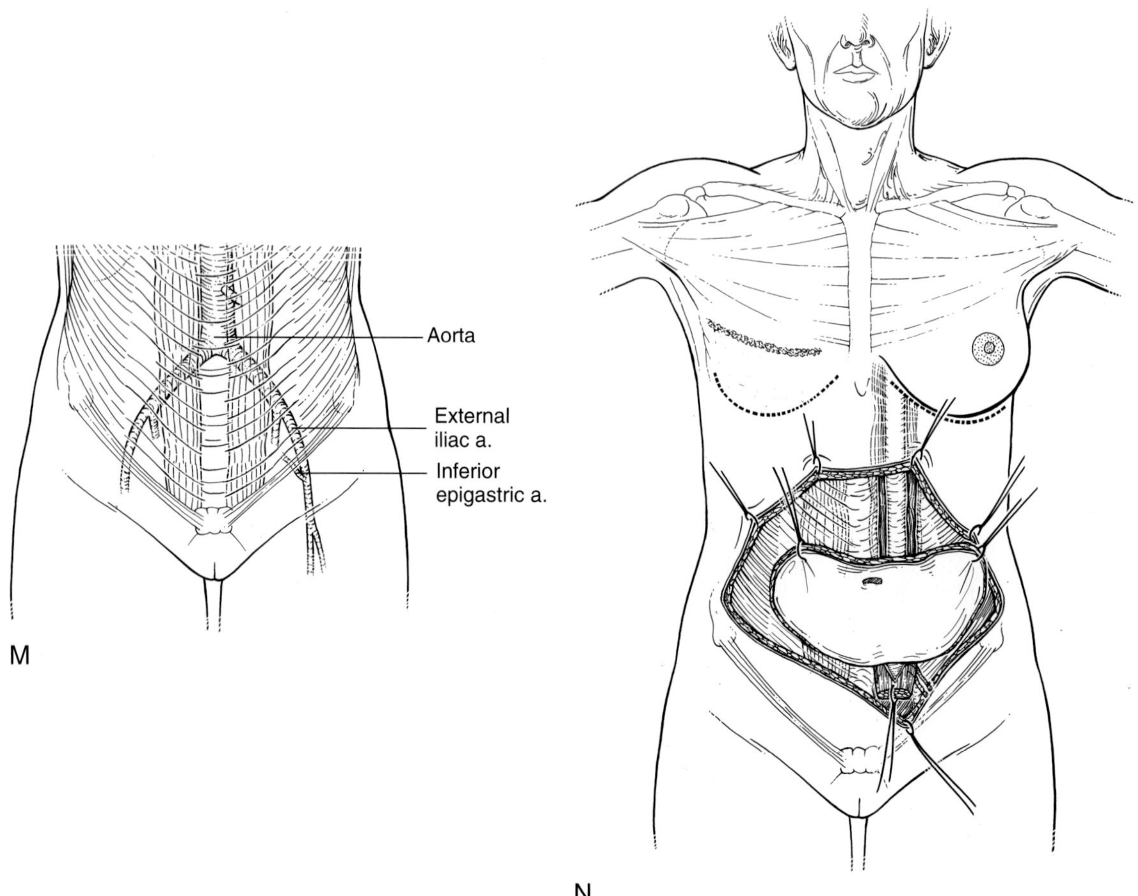

FIGURE 138-50, cont'd. *M,* The deep inferior epigastric pedicle and associated areas are dissected to the pelvis to provide length. It is divided and ligated with the pedicle available as donor flap vessels in the event that proximal pedicle flap perfusion appears inadequate. *N,* Flap is elevated from posterior sheath, and minor pedicles and motor nerves are divided and ligated to level of costal margin. The flap is returned to the donor site and covered with moist warm dressing while the recipient site at the mastectomy defect is prepared for flap inset.

If the decision is made to use the TRAM flap for breast reconstruction, initial preparation includes certain optional steps that many reconstruction breast surgeons find advisable. If the patient notes recent weight gain during chemoradiation treatments, a weight loss program before reconstruction may be advisable, especially if the patient plans to return to her normal weight after breast cancer treatment is completed. In the immediate reconstruction patient, this option will not be available, but in this group of patients, recent weight gain is less common. Donation of one or two units of blood for autotransfusion should be considered. In delayed reconstruction, use of transfusion is less likely, but in immediate reconstruction, two surgeons are involved and blood loss may be more extensive than predicted. Avoidance of abdominal distention may help with donor site closure and avoid ileus after surgery. For this reason, restricted diet of liquids may be helpful for the 48 hours before surgery, and laxative and enema may be used the night before surgery. Anesthesia consultation is useful in regard to possible epidural catheter placement for pain relief postoperatively. Patients who are concerned about muscle strength changes after surgery may benefit from a bodybuilding protocol at a health club emphasizing abdominal strength before surgery if time permits. Patients who are fit before surgery generally will not have difficulty returning to preoperative physical activities.[290] Similarly, patients who are less active and not inclined to sports will not be impaired in their postsurgery activities but may be slower to resume physical activities.

Technique

The TRAM flap may be based on a single rectus muscle (frequently called unipedicled TRAM flap) or on bilateral rectus muscles (bipedicled TRAM flap). There are differences in technique in the areas of flap elevation,

TABLE 138-25 ✦ INDICATIONS FOR AND CONTRAINDICATIONS TO PEDICLED TRAM FLAP RECONSTRUCTION

Indications

Unipedicled TRAM Flap	*Bipedicled TRAM Flap (single skin island)*	*Bipedicled TRAM Flap (two hemitransverse skin islands)*
Skin-sparing mastectomy, autogenous reconstruction Inadequate or damaged skin envelope Contralateral large or ptotic breast, patient requests match with reconstructed breast mound Autogenous reconstruction, patient and surgeon select abdominal donor site	Inadequate skin envelope, absent pectoralis muscle (status post radical mastectomy) Extensive skin envelope defect or postmastectomy damaged skin envelope Unilateral autogenous, reconstruction minimal redundant skin or fat at abdominal donor site Planned large mound reconstruction with avoidance of potential for fat necrosis	Bilateral mastectomy, inadequate or damaged skin envelopes Bilateral mastectomy, autogenous reconstruction Inadequate skin envelope, absent pectoralis major muscle (status post radical mastectomy) Unilateral reconstruction with prior midline incision and planned use of entire lower abdominal panniculus for mound reconstruction Unilateral autogenous reconstruction, minimal redundant skin or fat at abdominal donor site Planned large mound reconstruction with avoidance of potential for fat necrosis

Contraindications

Prior subcostal incision or prior ligation of or injury to pedicle(s)
Prior abdominoplasty
Prior lower abdominoplasty lipoplasty (relative contraindication)
Morbid obesity (relative, depending on body mass index)
Smoker (relative contraindication)
Medical comorbidities (relative contraindication)
Competitive athletic endeavors requiring use of rectus abdominis muscle (relative contraindication)

arc of rotation, and final flap inset, depending on the patient's defect (unilateral or bilateral), use of the unipedicled or bipedicled TRAM flap, and use of a single skin island or two hemi-skin islands. These modifications in technique are specified in the following discussion (Table 138-25).

Endotracheal inhalation anesthesia is used, frequently simultaneously with epidural regional anesthesia; the epidural is used after surgery for pain relief. Nitrous oxide inhalational gas is not used to avoid intestinal distention that may adversely affect later donor site closure. Antiembolism stockings and sequential compression devices are applied before induction of general anesthesia. A Foley catheter is inserted to monitor urine output. The preparation includes both anterior chest and entire abdomen. The patient is positioned on the operating room table so that she may be placed in sitting position for flap inset and abdominal closure. The upper extremities are padded to avoid compression and wrapped to arm boards in 90 degrees of abduction so that they will remain in position while the patient is in the sitting position. The lower extremities are placed in antiembolism sequential compression devices to avoid venous pooling during the lengthy procedure.

Flap Elevation. For immediate reconstruction, the flap may be elevated while the general surgeon is completing the mastectomy, or the plastic surgeon may await completion of the mastectomy. For delayed reconstruction, the procedure starts with elevation of the TRAM flap. An incision around the umbilicus allows release of the umbilical stalk to the midline fascia (Fig. 138-50*B*). The superior skin island incision is completed with a bevel of subcutaneous tissue superior to the skin incision to capture as many perforating vessels as possible and to add fatty tissue to the flap for the breast mound reconstruction. The superior abdominal skin and subcutaneous tissue are elevated from the abdominal fascia from the superior skin island incision to superior to the costal margin and to the sternum in the midline (Fig. 138-50*C*). The flap extends laterally to the anterior axillary line. After the abdominal flap elevation is completed, the patient is flexed into a partial sitting position and the superior-based abdominal flap is advanced toward the pubis. If the flap covers the marked inferior incision for the TRAM skin island without tension, closure of the donor site is readily accomplished after TRAM flap transposition (Fig. 138-50*D* and *E*). If closure appears unlikely without tension, the width of the flap is reduced so that closure will be possible.

The patient is returned to the supine position, and the inferior skin island incision is made to the underlying fascia. Unless flap bulk may not be adequate, the inferior incision is not beveled away from the skin island. With gentle retraction of the superior flap, the exposed anterior sheath of the flap is visualized. Incisions are made through the anterior sheath superior to the skin island to expose the rectus muscle (Fig. 138-50*F* and *G*). A central strip of anterior rectus sheath may be left over the muscle with two parallel incisions located approximately 2 cm lateral to the medial edge of the sheath and 2 cm medial to the lateral edge of the sheath (Fig. 138-50*H*). The central portion of the anterior sheath is included with the flap. The exposed muscle is dissected from the medial and lateral edge of the sheath (Fig. 138-50*I*). At the tendinous inscriptions, the muscle is adherent to the medial and lateral sheath, so this portion of the dissection is performed with care to avoid disruption of the continuity of the muscle. If the surgeon elects to preserve the medial or lateral portion of the rectus muscle to provide a function-preserving technique, a Doppler probe is used to locate the course of the superior epigastric artery within the muscle. Rather than separation of the muscle from the edge of the rectus sheath, the muscle is divided along the line lateral, medial, or at both edges, avoiding injury to the pedicle branches in the central portion of the rectus muscle. This technique places the flap circulation at risk, and the function-preserving aspect of this maneuver is questionable; the central portion of the muscle may be denervated because the segmental innervation from the intercostal motor branches enters the lateral posterior muscle. Although this technique is advocated by some experienced surgeons, the majority of TRAM transposition flaps include the entire width of the muscle and rely on the remaining abdominal wall muscles with fascial reconstruction to maintain normal abdominal function.

The skin island is now elevated from the external oblique fascia on the side of the rectus muscle flap and from the external oblique, opposite rectus sheath, and midline fascia on the opposite side of the abdomen (Fig. 138-50*J* and *K*). When the medial and lateral edge of the rectus sheath is reached, the skin island is carefully elevated an additional 1 to 2 cm medial to the lateral edge of the rectus sheath and a similar distance lateral to the medial edge of the sheath. If a large perforator is encountered, it is carefully preserved, although the perforators are usually located over the central portion of the muscle (Figs. 138-50*L* and *M* and Fig. 138-51). Parallel incisions are made through the rectus sheath, exposing the underlying rectus muscle. To avoid inadvertent disruption of the perforating musculocutaneous branches, the surgeon may elect to place sutures between the medial and lateral edge of the muscle and the edge of the divided rectus sheath and the overlying deep surface of the skin island. These segmental sutures are placed approximately every 3 to 5 cm during the process of dividing the rectus sheath beneath the skin island, starting at the superior edge of the skin island and progressing inferior to the inferior edge of the skin island. This suture technique is optional but serves the purpose of holding the muscle, rectus sheath, and deep surface of the skin island together during the process of flap elevation. These sutures may be left in place after flap transposition or removed, depending on the surgeon's preference.

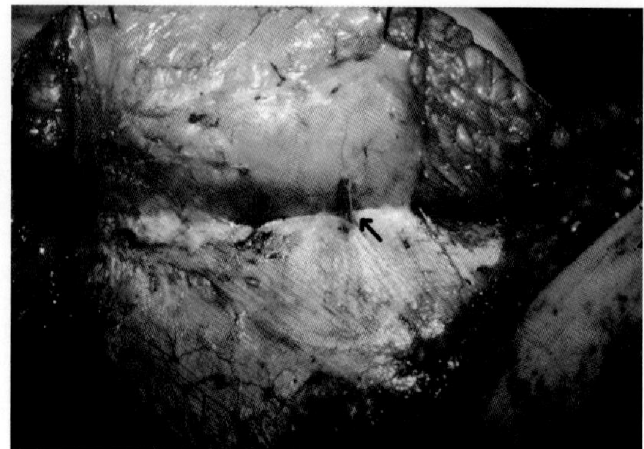

FIGURE 138-51. Perforating vessels: rectus abdominis musculocutaneous (TRAM) flap. During skin island elevation, at zone 1, lateral perforating vessels are preserved. Dissection allows preservation of 1.5 to 2 cm of lateral anterior rectus sheath for later donor site closure. Close-up lateral view of TRAM perforator vessels. For deep inferior epigastric pedicle flap dissection, the perforator is dissected through rectus muscle to origin from deep inferior epigastric artery and venae comitantes.

The rectus muscle is identified inferior to the skin island and elevated from the posterior sheath. The posterior sheath is thin at this level below the arcuate line (semicircular line of Douglas), so the surgeon must use care not to inadvertently enter the peritoneal cavity. Also, the deep inferior epigastric artery and associated venae comitantes are located lateral to the muscle within the posterior sheath. This pedicle should not be inadvertently included with the rectus muscle but left on the posterior sheath to be subsequently individually divided. The rectus muscle is divided between the inferior aspect of the skin island and the pubis (Fig. 138-50*N*). If the function-preserving technique is used, only the central or medial two thirds of the muscle is divided with preservation of the deep inferior epigastric pedicle into the preserved lateral rectus muscle. If the muscle is completely divided, the deep inferior epigastric artery and the paired venae comitantes are now identified and dissected to the pelvis, where they are divided and ligated. It is a common practice to preserve as much length as possible before division so that the pedicle could be used to revascularize the flap through microvascular anastomosis with suitable receptor vessels on the chest wall if the superior epigastric pedicle proves to be inadequate to support the flap. Fortunately, this so-called supercharging of the flap by this additional anastomosis is rarely if ever needed, but preservation of the deep inferior pedicle length is not difficult and is always then available if needed.

The rectus muscle including the skin island is now elevated from the posterior rectus sheath starting at the lower abdomen up to the costal margin. If the entire muscle is included in the flap, the lateral segmental minor vascular connections and intercostal motor nerves are divided and ligated with sutures or hemoclips. At the level of the costal margin, the superior motor branch is located and divided because complete denervation of the rectus muscle is desirable to allow muscle atrophy that will decrease muscle bulk within the tunnel, allowing the muscle to pass from the donor site onto the chest wall.

For the bipedicled flap with a single skin island, the release of the midline fascia and medial edges of the rectus sheaths is more difficult than in the unipedicle technique just described (Fig. 138-52*A*). The superior and inferior midlines of the flap are gently elevated, and a tunnel is made with sharp dissection between the subcutaneous tissue and the midline fascia (Fig. 138-52*B*). The lateral aspects of the skin island are elevated off the external oblique fascia. As noted for the unipedicled flap, the lateral rectus sheath is incised and the muscle elevated from the posterior sheath. With the surgeon now approaching the medial aspect of the rectus sheath from posterior to the rectus muscle, it is possible to release the medial edge of the sheath without disruption of the perforating vessels to the skin island from the rectus muscle. At the level of the medial edge of the rectus sheath for the exposed rectus muscle, the anterior sheath is incised 1 to 2 cm lateral to the medial edge of the anterior sheath (Fig. 138-52*C* and *D*).

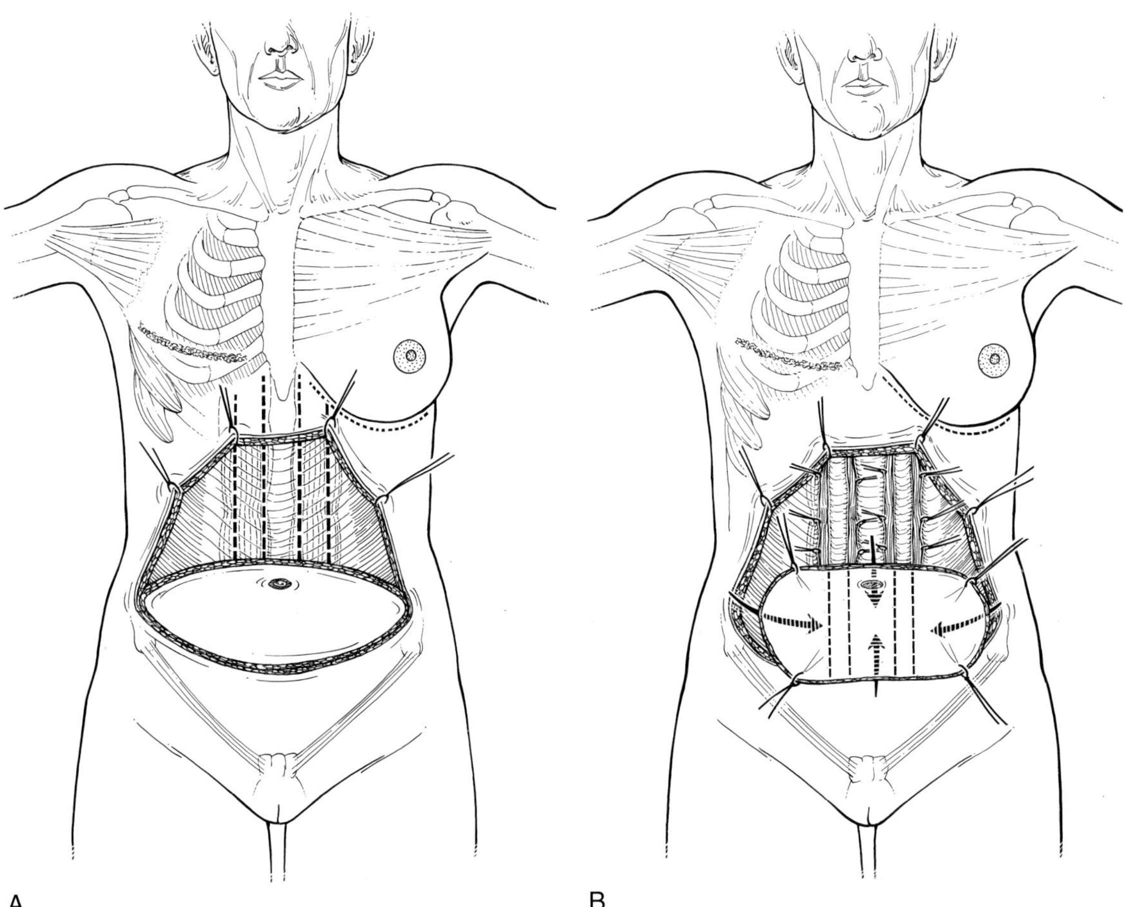

FIGURE 138-52. Bilateral rectus abdominis musculocutaneous flap with single skin island (bipedicled TRAM flap). *A,* Initial dissection is similar to single TRAM flap. Note parallel incisions at anterior edges for both muscles. *B,* Skin island (zone 2) is elevated bilaterally from external oblique to lateral edge of rectus sheath. The medial portion of the skin island requires dissection between the muscles, primarily from the midline fascia. *Continued*

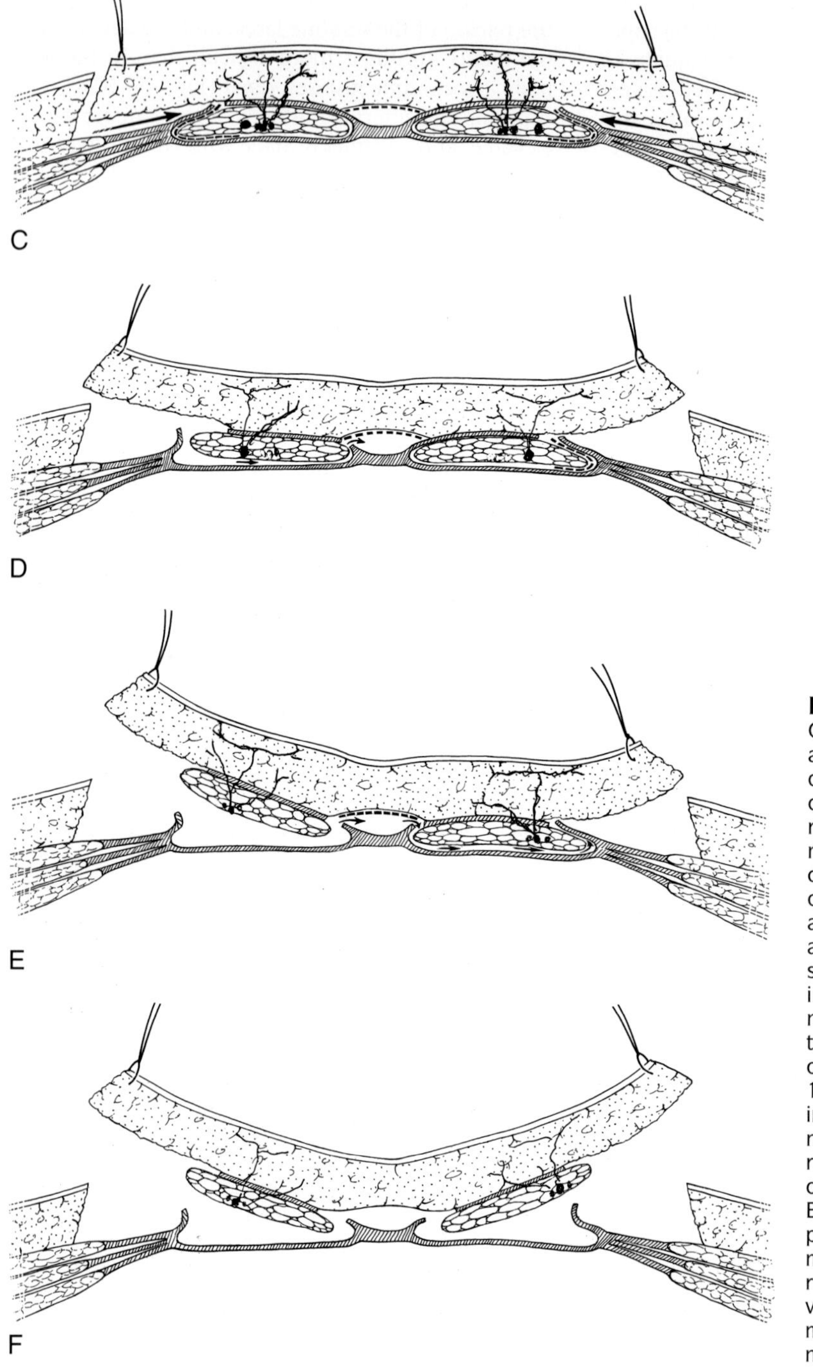

FIGURE 138-52, cont'd. *C,* Cross section of medial inferior abdominal wall demonstrates initial dissection of flap from external oblique fascia and lateral edge of rectus sheath. *D,* Cross section of medial inferior abdominal wall demonstrates technique to elevate one muscle from posterior sheath and enter through medial edge of anterior rectus sheath into midline space. *E,* Cross section of medial inferior abdominal wall. With one muscle fully elevated, it is possible to dissect the medial rectus sheath on the opposite rectus to preserve 1 to 2 cm of medial sheath. After incision of the sheath, the opposite muscle is elevated from the posterior rectus sheath. *F,* Cross section of medial inferior abdominal wall. Both muscles are elevated with intact posterior sheath and preserved medial and lateral edges of each rectus sheath. Both muscles are elevated from posterior sheath to costal margin. Bipedicled TRAM flap is needed for inset.

At this point, one rectus muscle is fully elevated and safely connected to the overlying skin island. With release of one rectus muscle from its rectus sheath, the tunnel made at the level of the midline fascia is entered and will provide exposure to the opposite medial rectus sheath. The exposure of the medial edge of the rectus sheath of the second muscle will enable TRAM flap elevation after release of the anterior rectus sheath 1 to 2 cm lateral to the medial edge (Fig. 138-52*E* and *F*). When two hemi–skin islands are required for reconstruction of either a unilateral or bilateral defect, the elevation technique is the same, except that the transverse skin island is divided at the level of the midline fascia, with each hemi–skin island based on its underlying rectus muscle (Fig. 138-53).

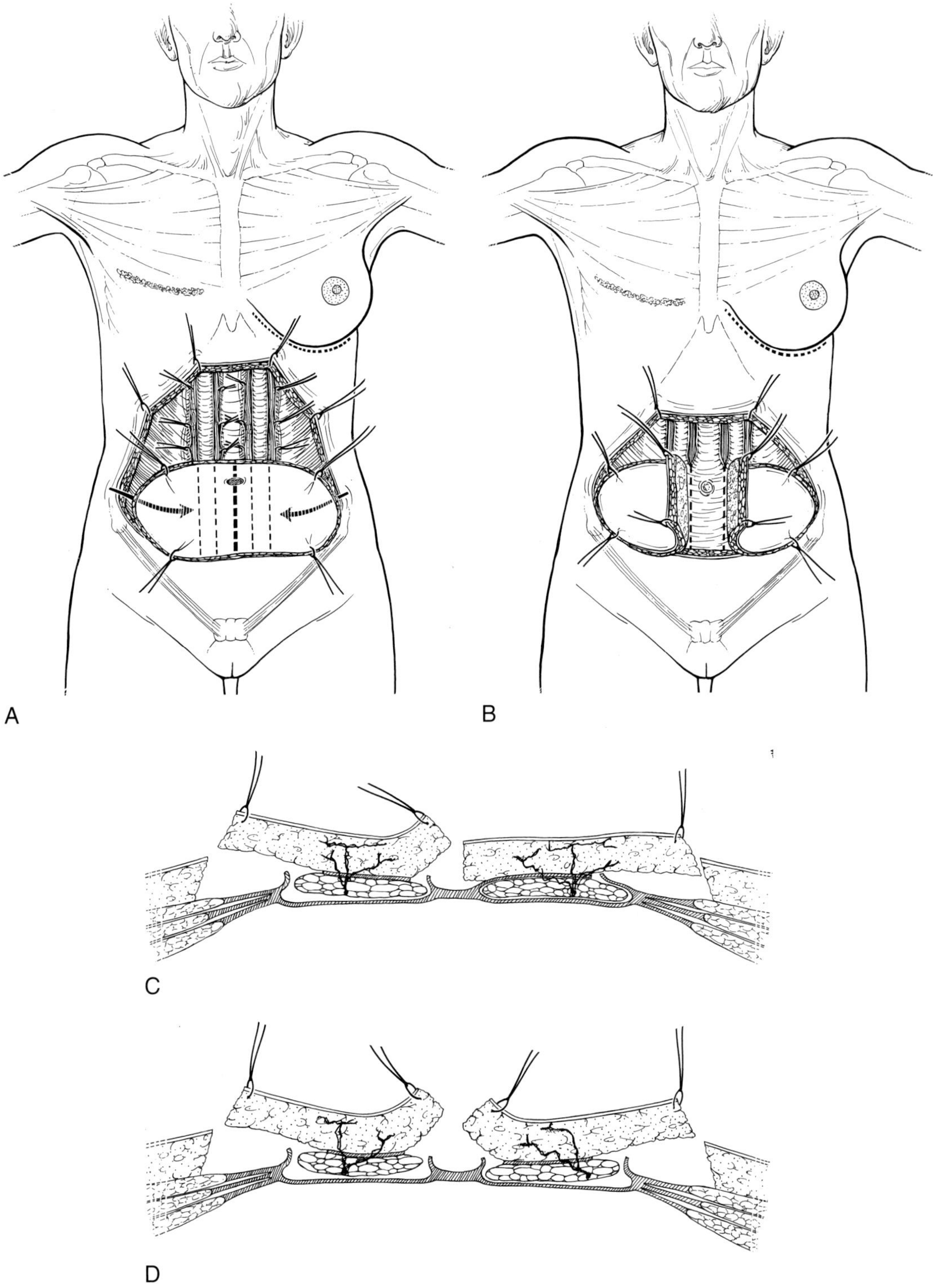

FIGURE 138-53. Technique of elevation: bilateral rectus abdominis musculocutaneous flap with hemitransverse skin islands (bilateral TRAM flaps). *A,* Skin island is divided at midline. Lateral aspect of each hemitransverse skin island is elevated from external oblique to lateral edge of rectus sheath. *B,* Medial edges of hemitransverse skin islands are elevated from midline fascia and medial edges of rectus sheath. *C,* Cross section of medial inferior abdominal wall. Midline incision provides exposure to elevate each hemitransverse skin island to expose medial edge of rectus sheath. *D,* Cross section of medial inferior abdominal wall. Both rectus muscles are divided inferior to the skin island, and the rectus muscles are elevated from posterior sheath to costal margin. Bilateral TRAM flaps are ready for inset.

The completely elevated flap is placed in the donor site and covered with moist dressing while the chest wall tunnel and recipient site are prepared.

CHEST WALL PREPARATION AND FLAP TRANSPOSITION. In immediate reconstruction, the mastectomy should have been completed and the plastic surgeon must prepare a tunnel between the mastectomy defect and the abdominal wall dissection space. The tunnel is generally located between the sternum and the medial third to the inferior mammary line. The dissection is located immediately superficial to the pectoralis muscle fibers of origin between the fourth and sixth intercostal spaces, progressing superficial to the superior rectus muscle fibers of origin to the costal margin. Resection of subcutaneous tissue superficial to the tunnel beneath the overlying skin reduces the contour fullness sometimes visible where the rectus muscle traverses the tunnel onto the chest wall. The tunnel size should be twice the width of the rectus muscle to ensure that there will not be constriction of the muscle within the tunnel. If a skin-sparing mastectomy has been performed, only the nipple-areola defect will require cutaneous coverage. The flap is transposed through the tunnel into the mastectomy defect (Fig. 138-54*A*). The cutaneous defect is marked on the skin island, and the flap is returned to the abdominal donor site where the remaining skin is de-epithelialized (Fig. 138-54*B* to *D*). If the defect at the mastectomy site is large enough to bring the skin island through the defect, de-epithelialization of the skin island may be completed on the chest wall, eliminating the necessity of returning the flap to the abdomen.

For delayed reconstruction, more preparation is required at the mastectomy site before the TRAM flap is transposed to the chest wall. The surgeon has the option of incising the mastectomy scar or using an incision below the mastectomy scar at the predicted site of the new inframammary line. The advantage of the incision at the new inframammary line is that the

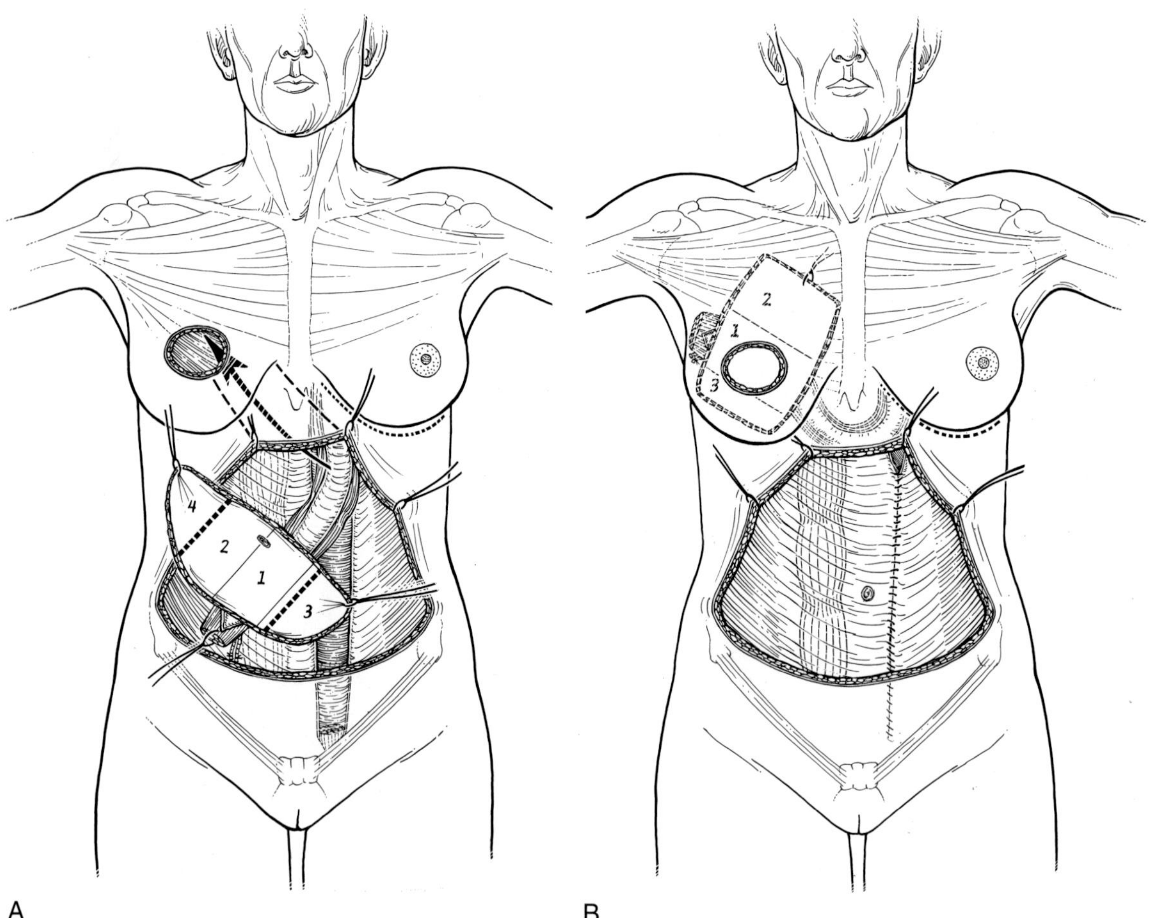

FIGURE 138-54. TRAM flap for immediate breast reconstruction. *A*, Defect after skin-sparing mastectomy. Contralateral TRAM flap is passed through tunnel into mastectomy defect. *B*, With flap in place beneath preserved skin envelope, abdominal fascia is closed directly with running permanent sutures. Zone 4 is resected, and zone 1 will be placed at nipple-areola defect.

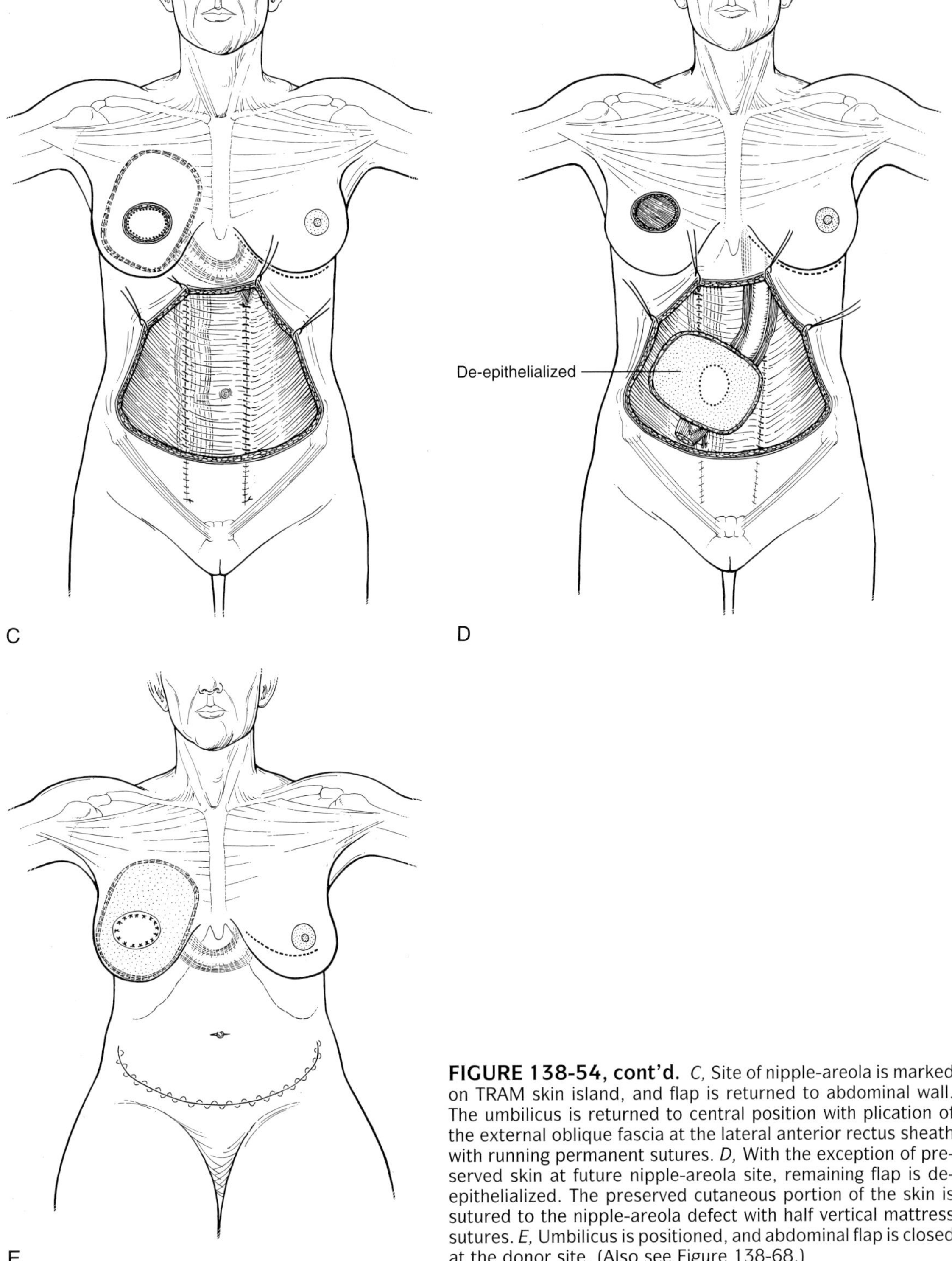

FIGURE 138-54, cont'd. *C,* Site of nipple-areola is marked on TRAM skin island, and flap is returned to abdominal wall. The umbilicus is returned to central position with plication of the external oblique fascia at the lateral anterior rectus sheath with running permanent sutures. *D,* With the exception of preserved skin at future nipple-areola site, remaining flap is de-epithelialized. The preserved cutaneous portion of the skin is sutured to the nipple-areola defect with half vertical mattress sutures. *E,* Umbilicus is positioned, and abdominal flap is closed at the donor site. (Also see Figure 138-68.)

inferior edge of flap inset will coincide with the inframammary line and avoid visualization of the inferior flap inset scar. Regardless of the initial incision used, the mastectomy skin flaps are elevated to the clavicle superiorly, the sternum medially, the anterior axillary line laterally, and the inferior mammary line inferiorly if the initial incision is not made at this level. For a radical mastectomy defect, this dissection is performed over the ribs and intercostal muscles and the pectoralis minor muscle. For a modified radical mastectomy, the surgeon has the option of performing the dissection superficial or deep to the pectoralis major muscle. If the skin island of the TRAM flap is well vascularized, the dissection superficial to the pectoralis muscle allows easier manipulation of the flap for mound reconstruction because the flap will not be compressed by the pectoralis major muscle in the subpectoral position. However, dissection superficial to the pectoralis may result in devascularization of the skin envelope in proximity to the mastectomy incision, particularly if the chest wall has been irradiated. This skin is best removed because there will be adequate skin from zone 1 and zone 2 of the flap to provide a generous new breast skin envelope. After the mastectomy site dissection is completed, a tunnel is made and the flap transposed to the chest wall in a manner similar to that described for immediate reconstruction (Fig. 138-55).

The arc of rotation will be different if the muscle flap is ipsilateral or contralateral to the mastectomy defect. The ipsilateral TRAM flap will generally rotate 180 degrees, or the flap may be turned upside down through the tunnel with the skin island then rotated a second time on the chest wall to bring the skin island facing the skin of the preserved breast envelope at the mastectomy defect. If the opposite (contralateral) TRAM flap is used, the flap will also rotate 180 degrees across the midline and through the tunnel, or the flap may be turned over the costal margin with the skin island facing posterior and then the skin island direction reversed on the chest wall. In general, zone 4 is excised before the flap is transposed to the chest wall. All or part of zone 3 may be resected before the flap is transposed through the tunnel or the unreliable portions of the flap may be resected on the chest wall. Removal of zone 4 and the distal part of zone 3 before flap transposition to the chest wall allows more gentle passage of the flap onto the chest wall through the tunnel.

For the bipedicled TRAM flap (single skin island), the entire skin island is retained and included with the underlying muscles for transposition to the chest wall. (The zones of the skin island include only zone 1 and zone 2 for each muscle.) The flap is rotated 180 degrees through the tunnel onto the mastectomy defect (Fig. 138-56).

For the bipedicled TRAM flaps with separate hemitransverse skin islands, each flap will have a separate arc of rotation to the same hemithorax if it is used for single breast reconstruction or for bilateral reconstruction (Fig. 138-57). When both flaps are used for a unilateral reconstruction, each flap will have a 180-degree arc of rotation through the same tunnel to the mastectomy defect (Fig. 138-57*A*). The tunnel size must ensure no constriction on the two rectus muscles. When bipedicled TRAM flaps with hemi–skin islands are used for bilateral breast reconstruction, most surgeons elect to use the ipsilateral flap for each side, requiring a clockwise rotation for the left side and counterclockwise for the right side (Fig. 138-57*B*). It is also possible to cross the flaps across the epigastric sternal area with each flap's arc of rotation to the opposite mastectomy site. Although both methods of rotation for bilateral reconstruction are safe, increased tunnel bulk may result at the level where the muscle bellies of the two flaps cross immediately inferior to the sternum in the superior epigastrium.

If zone 2 is unavailable for use in the breast mound reconstruction, or if a patient is very thin without a significant panniculus in the lower abdomen, adequate breast mound volume may not be provided by the TRAM flap. Under these circumstances, other flaps should be considered; however, there will be circumstances when the TRAM flap is selected, but because of limitations noted or when zones 1 and 2 are needed to provide a stable skin envelope, implant use beneath the flap may be necessary to provide symmetry with the contralateral breast. For these patients, either an expander or saline implant with a distant port is recommended. The implant-expander is placed beneath the flap and not immediately inflated to avoid pressure on the overlying TRAM flap. After surgery, the implant can be inflated to appropriate dimensions, and the port may be removed or the expander replaced with a permanent saline implant (Fig. 138-58).

Donor Site Closure. The surgeon may return to the abdomen for donor site closure before final flap inset or work with a second surgeon who can close the abdomen simultaneously. Because restoration of abdominal fascial continuity is of great importance, it is helpful for the surgical team to concentrate on abdominal wall closure before final flap inset is completed. The key to abdominal closure is repair of the anterior sheath defect by restoration of the continuity of the midline fascia and preserved cuff of medial rectus sheath with the preserved cuff of lateral sheath and the external and internal oblique fascia. Below the arcuate line, the internal oblique fascia often retracts laterally; if it is not reattached to the anterior sheath reconstruction, abdominal hernia or weakness will result. If adequate fascia is present, direct suture approximation will be adequate for fascial repair (Fig. 138-59). If the fascia cannot be approximated without

Text continued on p. 746

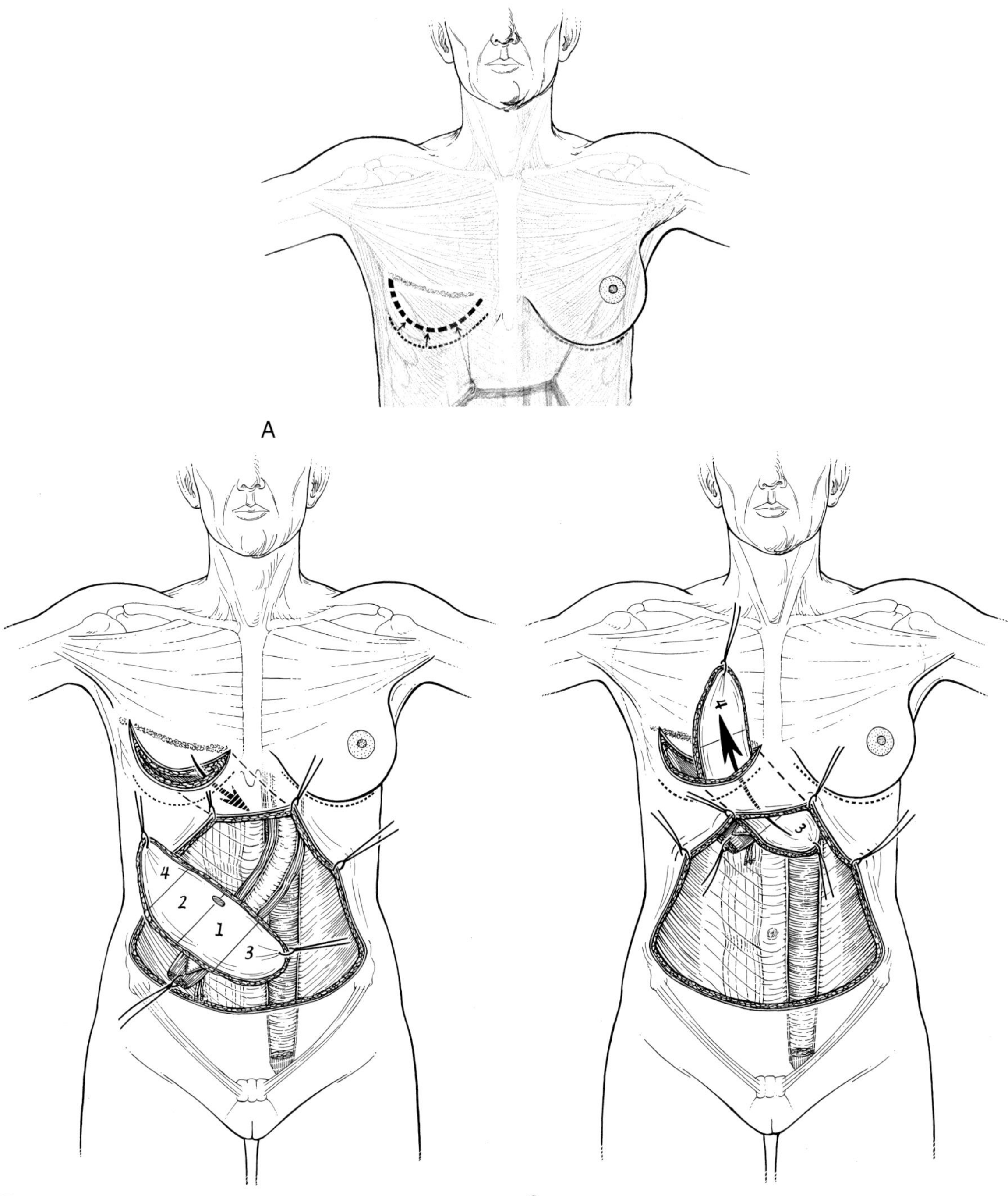

FIGURE 138-55. TRAM flap inset for breast reconstruction. *A,* Initial incision is made 1 to 2 cm superior to inframammary line *(dashed line)* and prepared for flap inset. *B,* Skin envelope is elevated superficial to pectoralis major muscle. A tunnel is made between the mastectomy defect and the abdominal dissection space. The inframammary incision extends through the lateral aspect of the mastectomy scar. *C,* TRAM flap is transposed through tunnel into mastectomy defect. The flap is placed in the defect and covered with moist dressing. Abdominal fascial repair is accomplished before flap inset is completed.

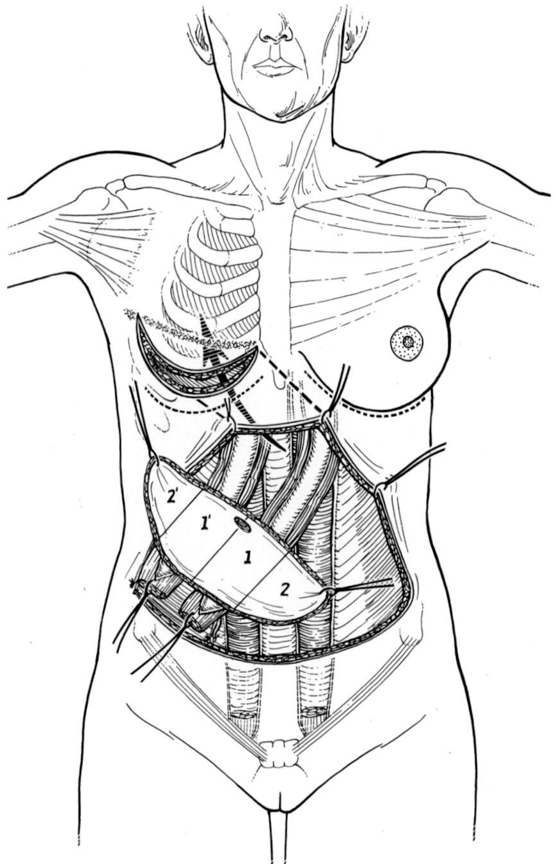

FIGURE 138-56. Bilateral TRAM flaps (single skin island, bipedicled) for delayed breast reconstruction. The arc of rotation to the mastectomy defect is through the tunnel.

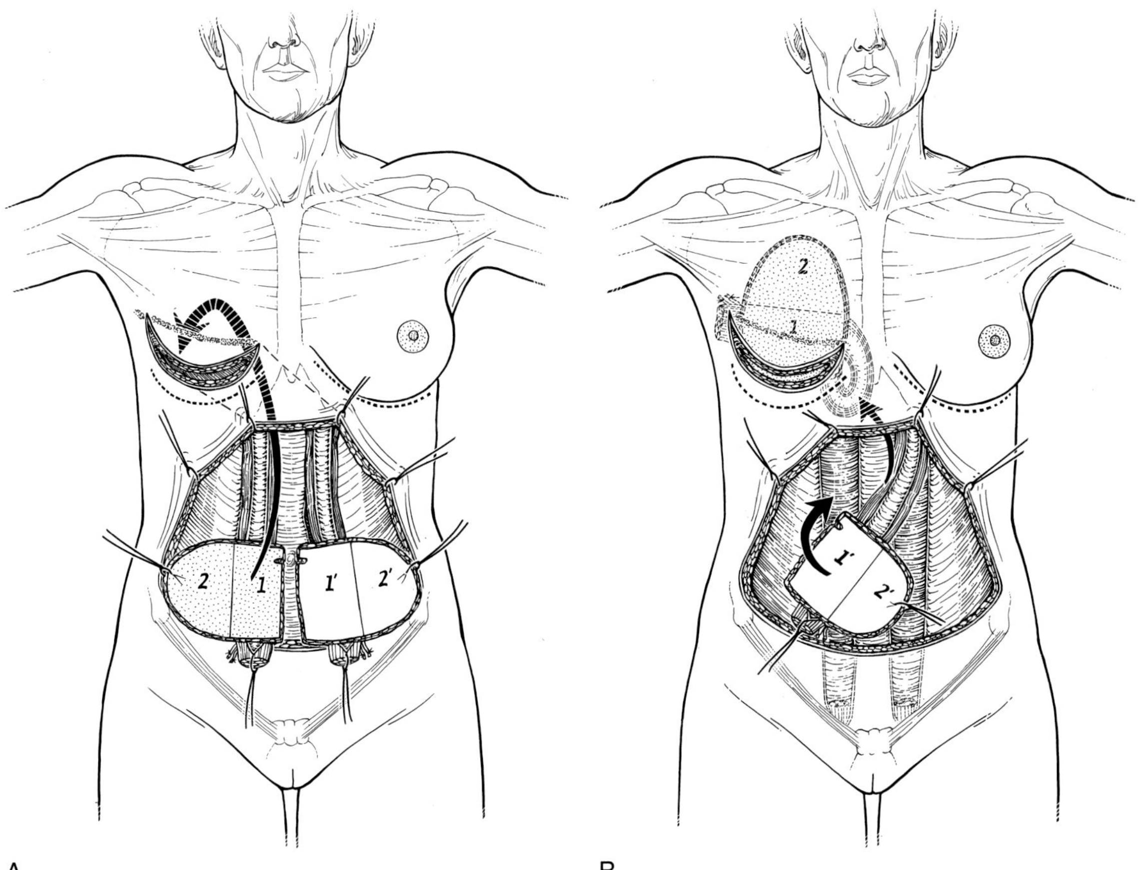

FIGURE 138-57. Bilateral TRAM flaps (two separate flaps with hemitransverse skin island). *A,* Arc of rotation for ipsilateral flap. *B,* Arc of rotation for contralateral flap. Stacked flaps can improve projection and size of the reconstructed breast mound.

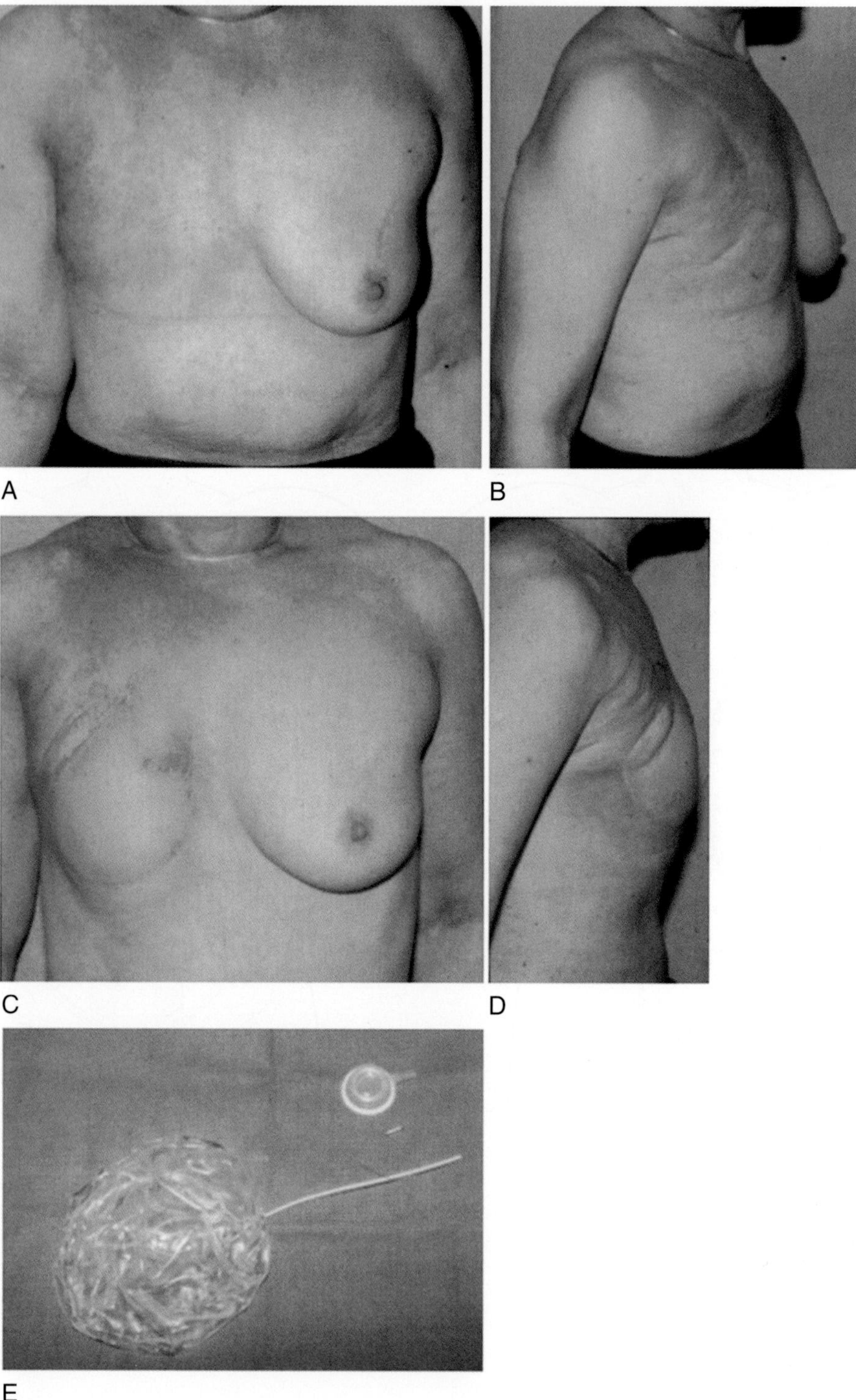

FIGURE 138-58. TRAM flap for delayed right breast reconstruction. *A,* Preoperative anterior view of modified radical mastectomy defect with postoperative radiation therapy. *B,* Lateral preoperative oblique view demonstrates scar contracture on right hemithorax. *C,* Postoperative view at 3 months of transposition of contralateral TRAM flap with immediate insertion of inflatable saline implant. Zone 2 is not available because of abdominal scar. *D,* Postoperative lateral view 3 months after contralateral TRAM flap. *E,* Saline inflatable implant placed beneath TRAM flap inset site.

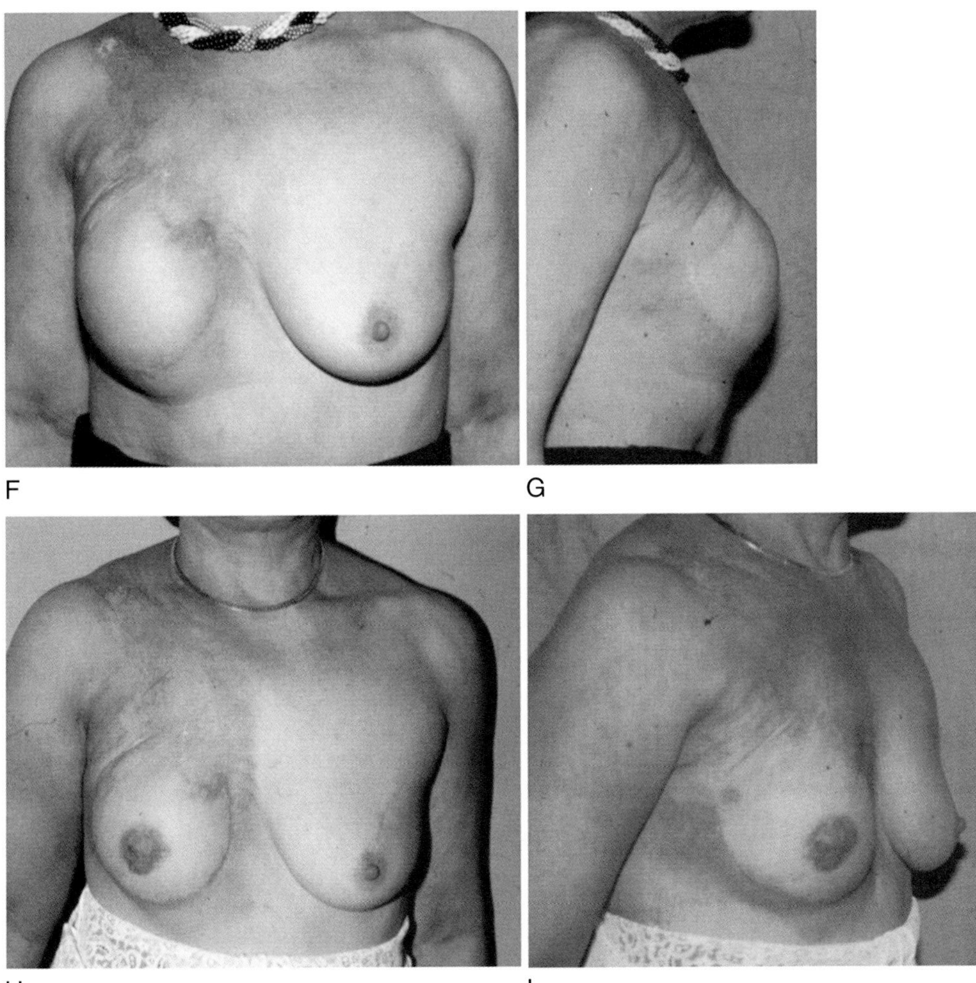

FIGURE 138-58, cont'd. *F,* Postoperative anterior view at 6 months. Saline implant inflation is in progress. *G,* Postoperative lateral view at 6 months. Breast volume is improved with inflation of saline implant. *H,* Postoperative anterior view at 1 year of combined TRAM flap and implant providing adequate mound size and symmetry in radiation-damaged chest. *I,* Postoperative oblique view. Mound projection is adequate. Nipple-areola reconstruction is completed.

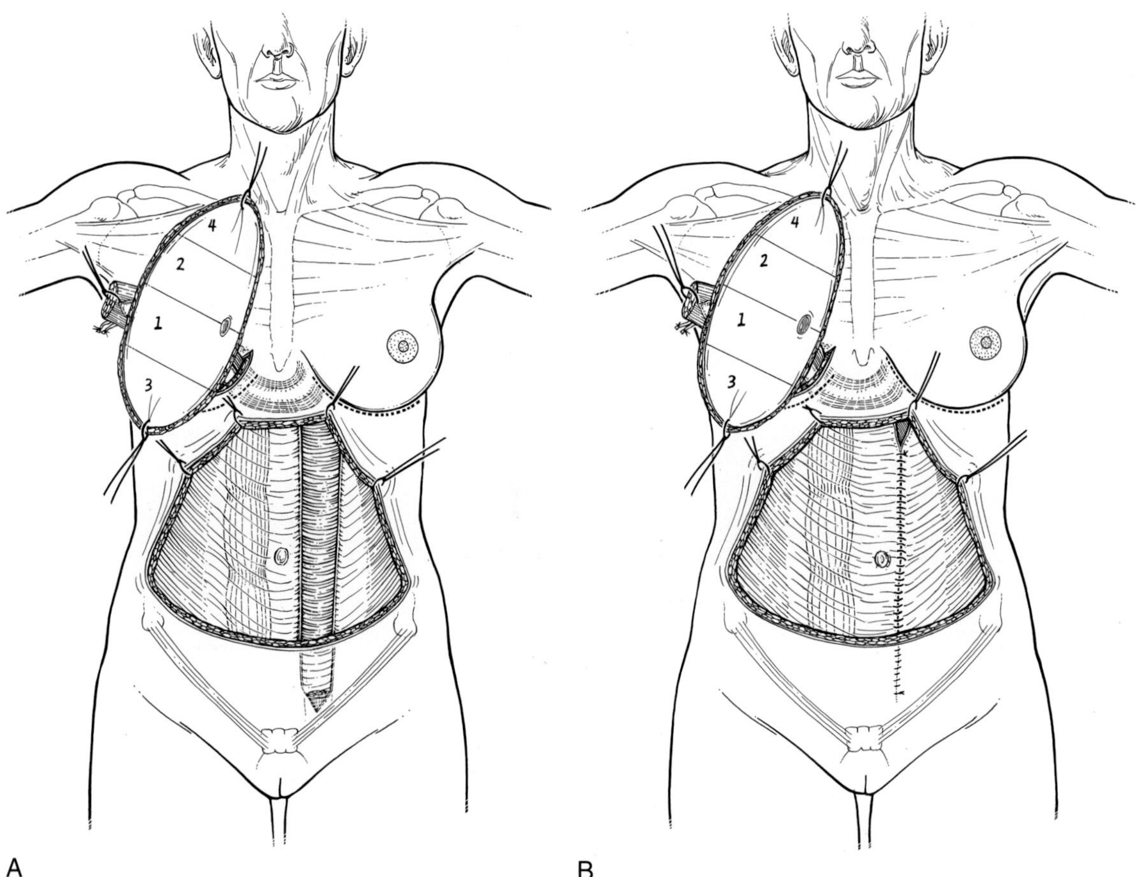

FIGURE 138-59. Unilateral TRAM flap. Donor site: abdominal fascial closure. *A,* After flap is transposed onto chest defect, abdominal fascial closure is completed. *B,* In nonobese patients, direct closure of fascial edges can usually be accomplished with running permanent sutures.

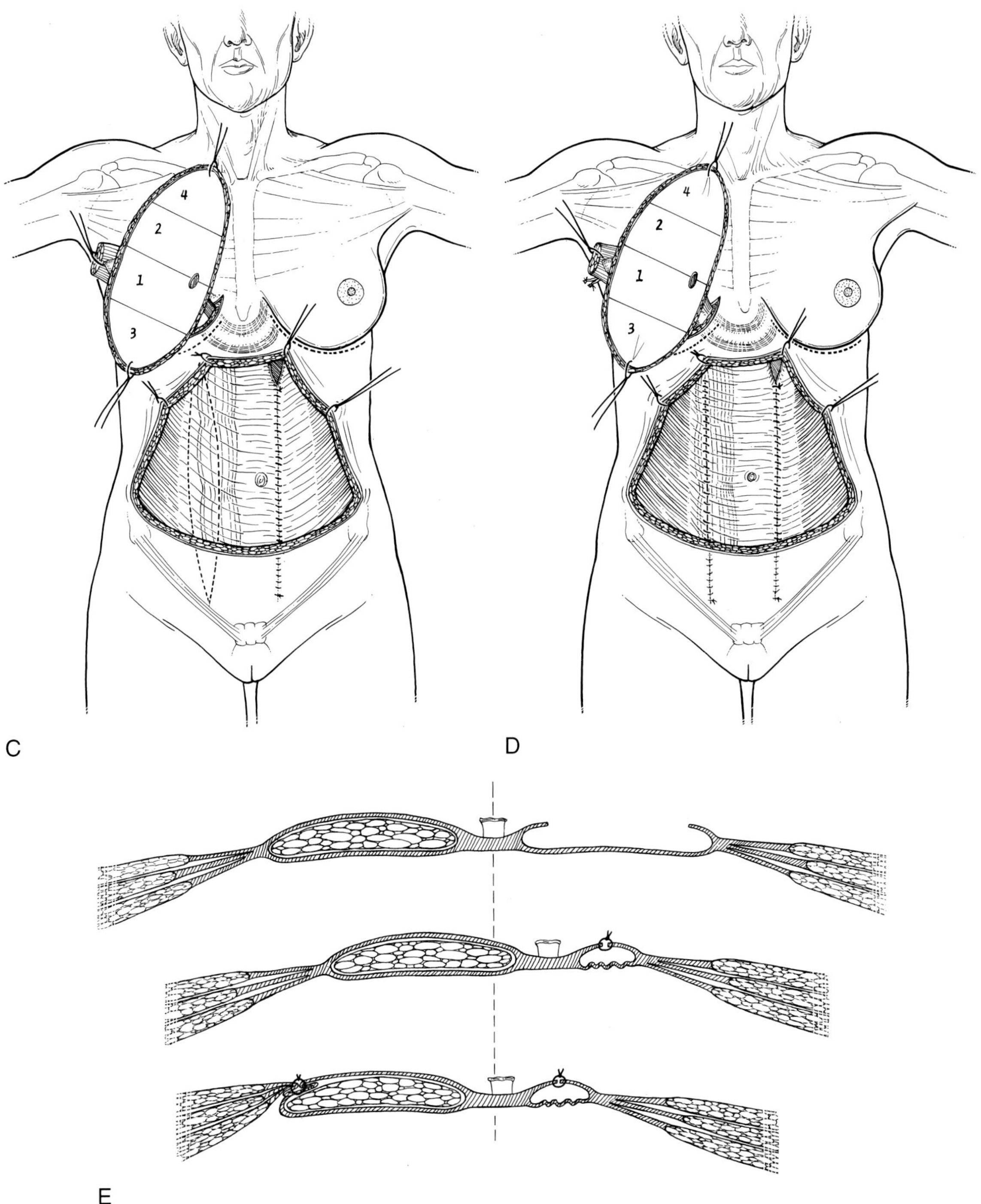

FIGURE 138-59, cont'd. *C,* Plication of fascia on opposite side of abdominal wall will maintain umbilicus in midline position. Note outline of planned plication between external oblique fascia and lateral rectus sheath. *D,* Donor site plication accomplished with running permanent sutures. *E,* Cross section of medial inferior abdominal wall. Medial and lateral edges of preserved anterior sheath are approximated with running sutures. Suture closure and plication of lateral fascia shift umbilicus to appropriate site on the flap and will maintain umbilicus in midline.

tension (excessive tension is evidenced by tearing of the fascia as sutures are applied), synthetic mesh as interposition graft is indicated. Use of a synthetic mesh patch has been advocated to reinforce the closure (Fig. 138-60). Although the patch is helpful, if tension-free closure of the fascia is not accomplished, the patch may not prevent late hernia formation. The interposition mesh is sutured between the midline fascia and preserved cuff of medial anterior sheath and the lateral cuff of anterior rectus sheath and external and internal oblique fascial layers. The mesh width should be equivalent to the excised portion of the rectus sheath

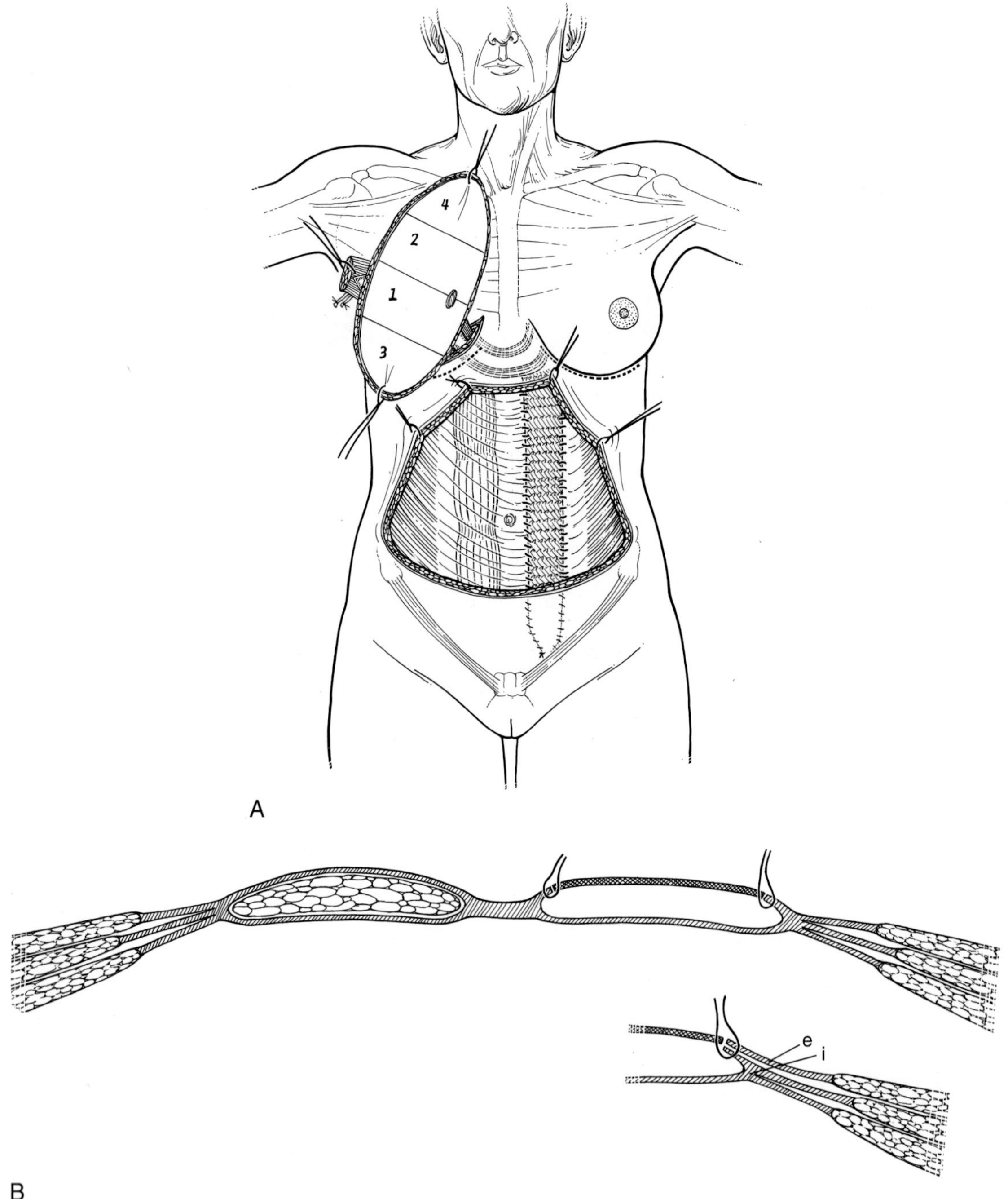

FIGURE 138-60. Donor site: abdominal fascial closure. *A,* If fascia tears or cannot be approximated directly, permanent Prolene mesh is used as interpositional graft to replace missing anterior rectus sheath. *B,* Cross section of medial abdomen. Mesh is sutured to preserved lateral and medial edges of anterior sheath. A running permanent suture is used. Note that the internal oblique layer may separate from the external oblique. Both layers must be included in the lateral mesh suture line. e, external oblique fascia; i, internal oblique fascia.

(anterior sheath included with the TRAM flap) to restore appropriate abdominal girth. With direct suture closure or use of interpositional mesh, as the closure approaches the costal margin, compression of the rectus muscle as it exits the superior rectus sheath and enters the tunnel for its transposition to the mastectomy defect must be avoided.

Direct suture closure will shift the umbilicus toward the donor side of the abdomen. Many surgeons elect to plicate the external oblique fascia to the lateral rectus sheath on the contralateral side of the abdomen to relocate the umbilicus to a central position and also to maintain balance at the site of abdominal wall closure (see Fig. 138-59*C*).

Fascial closure techniques after bipedicled TRAM flap elevation may be more complex than those for the unipedicled TRAM flap. The extent of difficulty will depend on the strength and laxity of the abdominal fascial layers. If 1 to 2 cm of anterior fascia is preserved on the medial and lateral edge of each rectus sheath and the patient has normal body weight, usually both anterior sheath closures are possible with direct suture techniques. The actual suture closure technique varies among surgeons and includes a single running suture, double running closure, and interrupted sutures (Fig. 138-61).

A synthetic mesh patch is often used to reinforce the closure. If extensive tension is observed after the rectus sheath is closed, as frequently indicated by suture tearing fascia on the opposite side during closure, interposition mesh is recommended. Techniques for mesh insertion vary. The mesh must, however, provide continuity between the lateral sheath remnants including both external and internal oblique fascial layers and the midline fascia. The mesh must be inserted with adequate tension to restore normal preexisting abdominal girth, or protrusion of the abdomen will be observed (Fig. 138-62). The most reliable technique for Prolene mesh use consists of initially suturing the mesh to one lateral side, with suture of the mesh to the lateral sheath including the medial aspect of the external and internal oblique fascia. The mesh is next sutured to the medial edge of the rectus sheath, including the lateral aspect of the midline fascia. The third

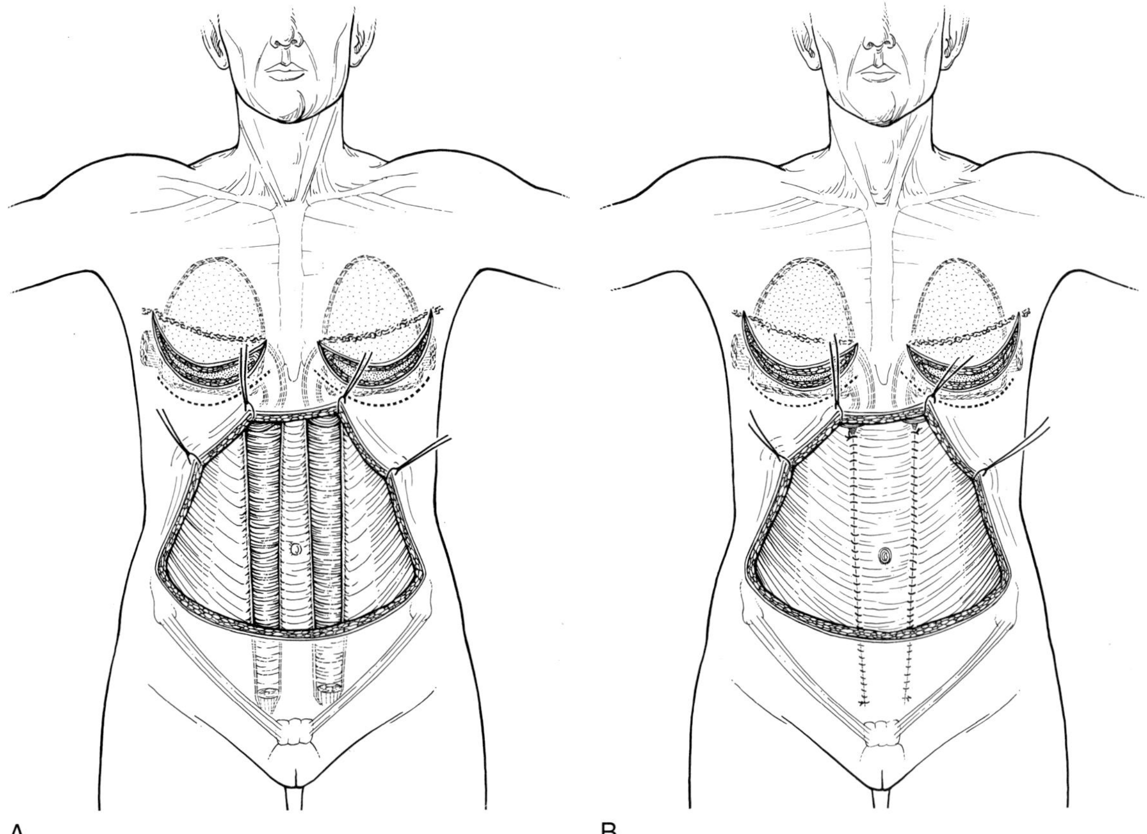

FIGURE 138-61. Bilateral TRAM flap. Donor site: abdominal fascial closure. *A,* In the younger patient without obesity and when medial and lateral edges of both anterior rectus sheaths are preserved, the fascial continuity can be restored with two running permanent sutures. *B,* Closure of the lateral anterior rectus sheath defects with parallel running sutures.

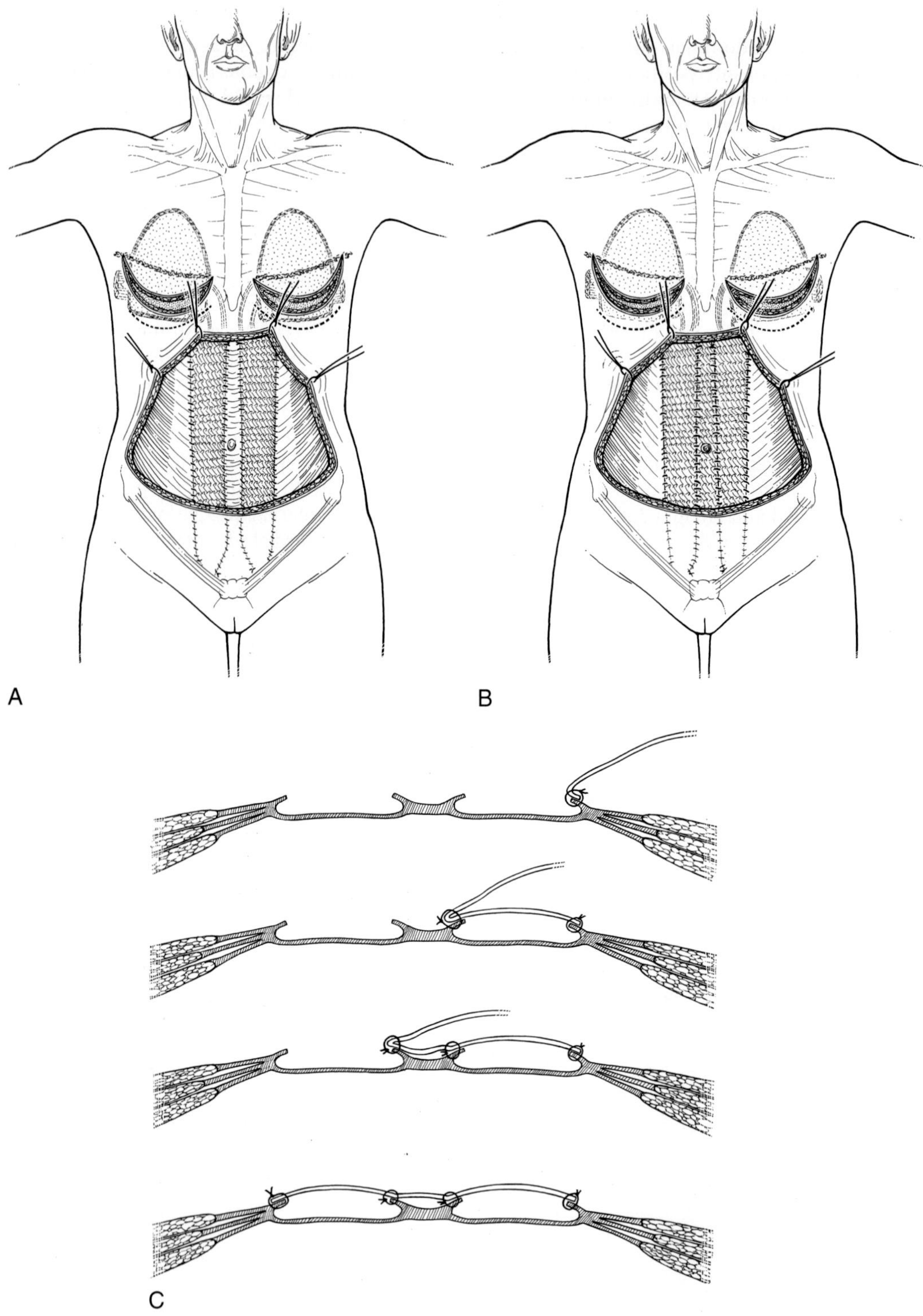

FIGURE 138-62. Bilateral TRAM flap. Donor site: fascial defect closure. *A,* If fascia tears or will not approximate, interpositional Prolene mesh is used for fascial reconstruction. Two separate sheets of mesh can be used, one for each anterior sheath fascial defect. *B,* A simple piece of Prolene mesh may be used with four suture lines: lateral sheath, medial sheath, opposite medial sheath, and lateral sheath. A small incision is made through the mesh spanning the midline fascia to release the umbilicus for later skin approximation. *C,* Cross section of medial inferior abdominal wall; technique for use of single piece of mesh to replace anterior rectus sheath fascial defects. Each suture line is consecutively applied starting laterally and then medially. Fascial approximation is kept tight to improve abdominal contour and function.

suture line occurs on the opposite medial sheath and lateral aspect of the midline fascia. Finally, the fourth suture line represents the inset of the mesh at the medial remnants of the contralateral lateral sheath, including the medial attachments of the internal and external oblique fascia. The mesh is kept tight where it is used to replace each missing anterior sheath. At the costal margin, compression of the rectus muscle is avoided at the level of the muscle entry into the tunnel for its transposition to the chest wall. Since the mesh is in continuity across the abdominal wall, a small incision is made over the midline portion of the mesh at the location of the umbilicus so the umbilicus may be pulled through the mesh for subsequent passage through the abdominal advancement flap after cutaneous donor site closure.

On completion of fascial closure, the surgeon may return to the chest wall for final inset of the TRAM flap to restore the breast mound. Since the patient is returned to the sitting or flexed position, it is possible simultaneously to inset the TRAM flap and to advance the superior-based abdominal advancement flap for donor site closure (Fig. 138-63). Drains are placed in the abdominal closure site. Excess subcutaneous tissue deep to Scarpa fascia may be excised to match the fatty layer adjacent to the pubic and lateral inferior abdominal wall.

The defect is closed temporarily by staples to approximate neoumbilical positioning. A fiberoptic retractor is used to visualize the umbilicus position beneath the abdominal flap. A needle is then passed through the abdominal flap to mark the appropriate position for the umbilical inset site (Fig. 138-64*A*). With completion of the abdominal flap closure of the donor defect of the TRAM skin island, a transverse or vertical ellipse of skin is resected at the selected neoumbilical site. The umbilicus is retrieved and sutured to the skin edge (Fig. 138-64*B* and *C*). A number of modifications have been proposed for the umbilical suture technique and include fascial

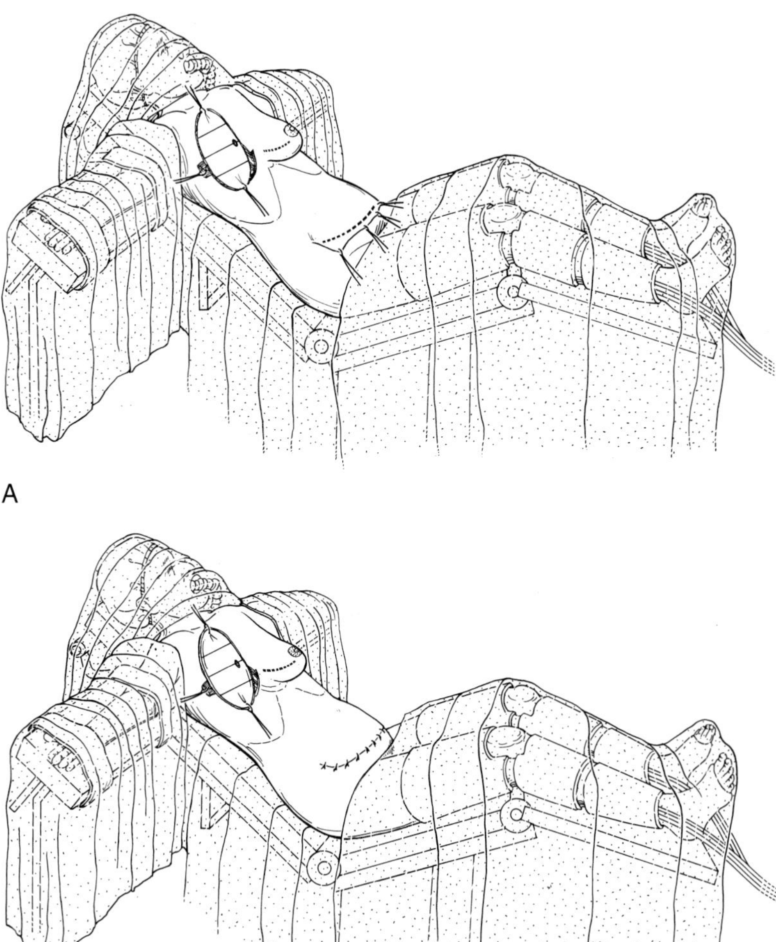

FIGURE 138-63. Abdominal flap closure. *A,* The patient is placed in sitting position. Superior-based abdominal flap is advanced to inferior edge of TRAM donor site defect. *B,* The abdomen is initially closed with large interrupted sutures to balance the closure and to trim dog-ears. These sutures are then replaced with buried absorbable sutures followed by subcutaneous closure.

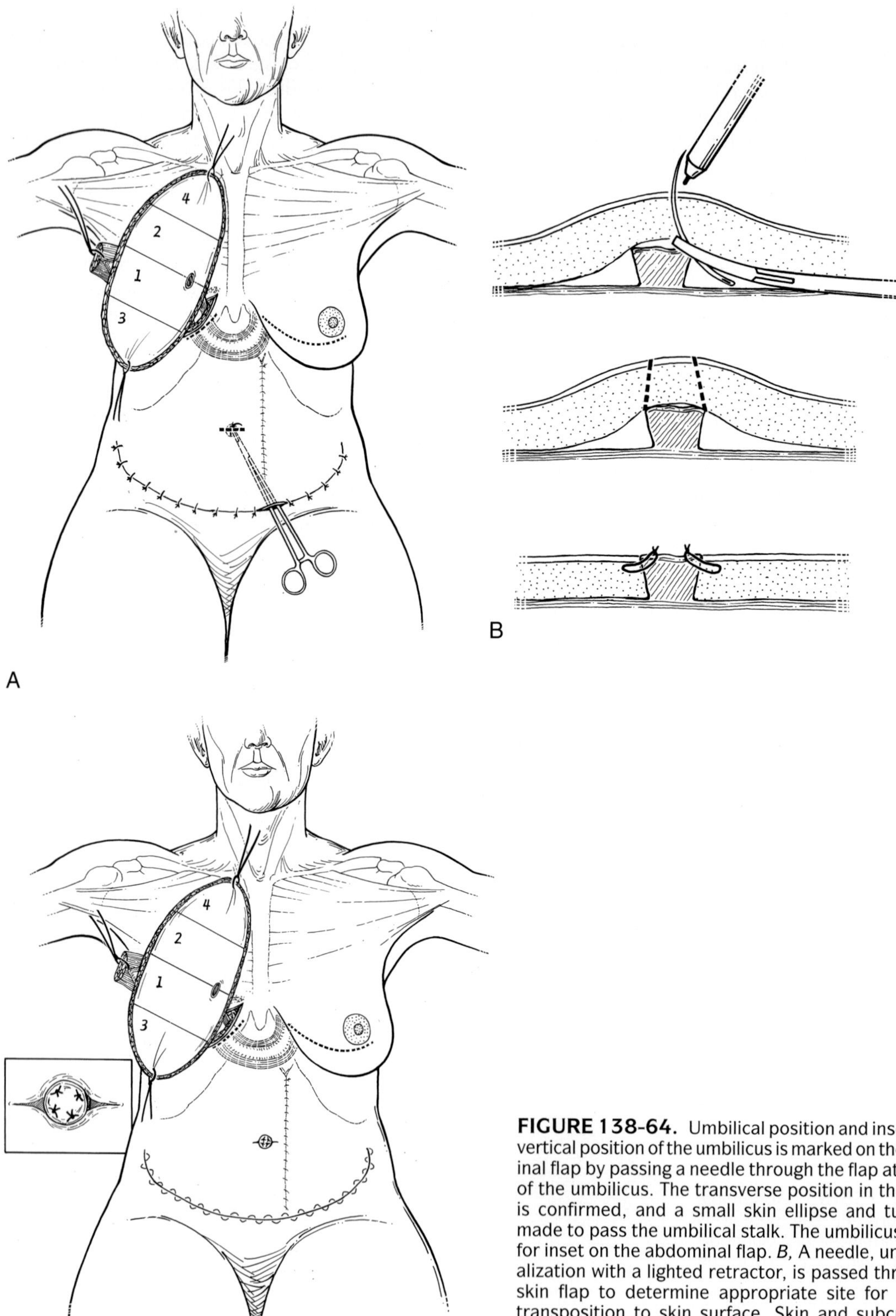

FIGURE 138-64. Umbilical position and inset. *A,* The vertical position of the umbilicus is marked on the abdominal flap by passing a needle through the flap at the level of the umbilicus. The transverse position in the midline is confirmed, and a small skin ellipse and tunnel are made to pass the umbilical stalk. The umbilicus is ready for inset on the abdominal flap. *B,* A needle, under visualization with a lighted retractor, is passed through the skin flap to determine appropriate site for umbilical transposition to skin surface. Skin and subcutaneous tissue are resected. The umbilicus is sutured to the skin edge with half vertical mattress sutures. *C,* Completion of umbilical placement suture. Abdominal flap closure is accomplished with running subcuticular sutures.

attachment of the umbilical deep surface to improve the appearance. The umbilical modifications are discussed in more detail in the abdominoplasty chapters (Fig. 138-65).

Final Flap Inset. The method chosen for final inset of the TRAM flap at the mastectomy defect site will depend on the surgeon's preference in regard to technique and the type of defect. Each surgeon will perform the flap inset differently for each patient, depending on the extent of the skin envelope deficiency, the extent of hemithorax scarring (particularly after irradiation changes), and the requirements to match a contralateral breast, especially if no contralateral breast surgery is planned.

In immediate reconstruction, especially after skin preservation mastectomy, the preserved portion of the skin island is generally located in zone 1. If skin-sparing mastectomy has been performed, only the nipple-areola defect will require cutaneous coverage (Fig. 138-66). The remainder of the de-epithelialized flap is positioned to simulate the resected breast tissue. Suture of the flap is minimal because the preserved skin envelope and the fixation of the flap at the areola site will provide appropriate contour and projection. The inset for the delayed reconstruction is more complex, depending on the status of the skin envelope at the mastectomy site and plans for the opposite breast.

There are three potential positions for the skin island on the chest wall. In the first position, the envelope is oriented vertically or obliquely with zone 1 at the region of the inframammary line and zone 2 at the midbreast. Zone 3 may be either rotated laterally toward the anterior inferior axilla or tucked beneath zone 1 to provide more projection for the breast mound. With this position of the skin island, there is more central flap bulk and the zone 2 portion of the flap extends superiorly toward the clavicle (Fig. 138-67).

The second position of the skin island is a transverse orientation with the flap rotated approximately 270 degrees, with zone 1 placed laterally and zone 2 placed medially for the contralateral flap. The ipsilateral flap has the opposite orientation with the entire skin island located inferior to the midsternal region. Zone 3 is generally excised, although it can be tucked beneath zone 1 to provide more breast projection if necessary.

The third position of the skin island is also transverse. The turnover rotation is most commonly used for the ipsilateral flap. With this transposition, the inferior portion of the flap stays inferior (at the inferior mammary line), unlike the ipsilateral or contralateral 270-degree arc of rotation. Regardless of the arc of rotation, it is helpful to keep zone 1 in the area of skin envelope replacement, although the medial portion of zone 2 is also safe skin to preserve for the new skin envelope (Fig. 138-68).

TABLE 138-26 ✦ COMPLICATIONS OF PEDICLED UNILATERAL TRAM FLAP BREAST RECONSTRUCTION (IMMEDIATE AND DELAYED)[236,283]

Complication	Percentage of Patients*
Partial flap loss	5.0-16.2
Fat necrosis	10.6
Abdominal hernia	7.8-8.8
Pulmonary embolism, deep venous thrombosis	0.7
Pneumonia	0.7
Wound infection	5.0-11.7
Wound dehiscence	5.6
Hematoma	1.3
Lymphedema	5.6
Any complication	23.7-31

*Range of percentage of patients with complications as reported in the literature.

After the inferior breast mound is established with the flap, a decision may be safely made regarding the extent of scarred residual skin envelope and mastectomy scar that should be resected to improve breast mound appearance and shape. In general, in the delayed reconstruction, it is advantageous to resect the unstable central skin between the inframammary line and the mastectomy scar. The mastectomy scar is not expansile and will impede breast mound projection; hence, its resection will allow better breast mound shape and projection. With the inframammary line inset completed and with vertical or oblique orientation of the skin island, it is possible to slide the skin island inferiorly to establish ptosis in the reconstructed breast mound. Once the desired ptosis is achieved, a suction drain may be placed in the axillary area, followed by closure of the recipient site (Fig. 138-69).

After inset of the skin island is complete, with the patient in the sitting position, the flap is carefully examined to ensure adequate cutaneous circulation. If there is evidence of arterial insufficiency or increasing venous insufficiency (there is often slight venous insufficiency immediately after flap elevation that gradually improves when the flap is transposed to the chest wall), sutures should be released to prevent flap compression and the skin island adjusted in regard to its inset. A light noncompressive dressing is applied. The patient is maintained in semisitting position to avoid excessive tension on the abdominal advancement flap (Table 138-26).

For the bipedicled TRAM flap with a single skin island, the entire skin island will be available for use in mastectomy defect reconstruction. The position of

Text continued on p. 758

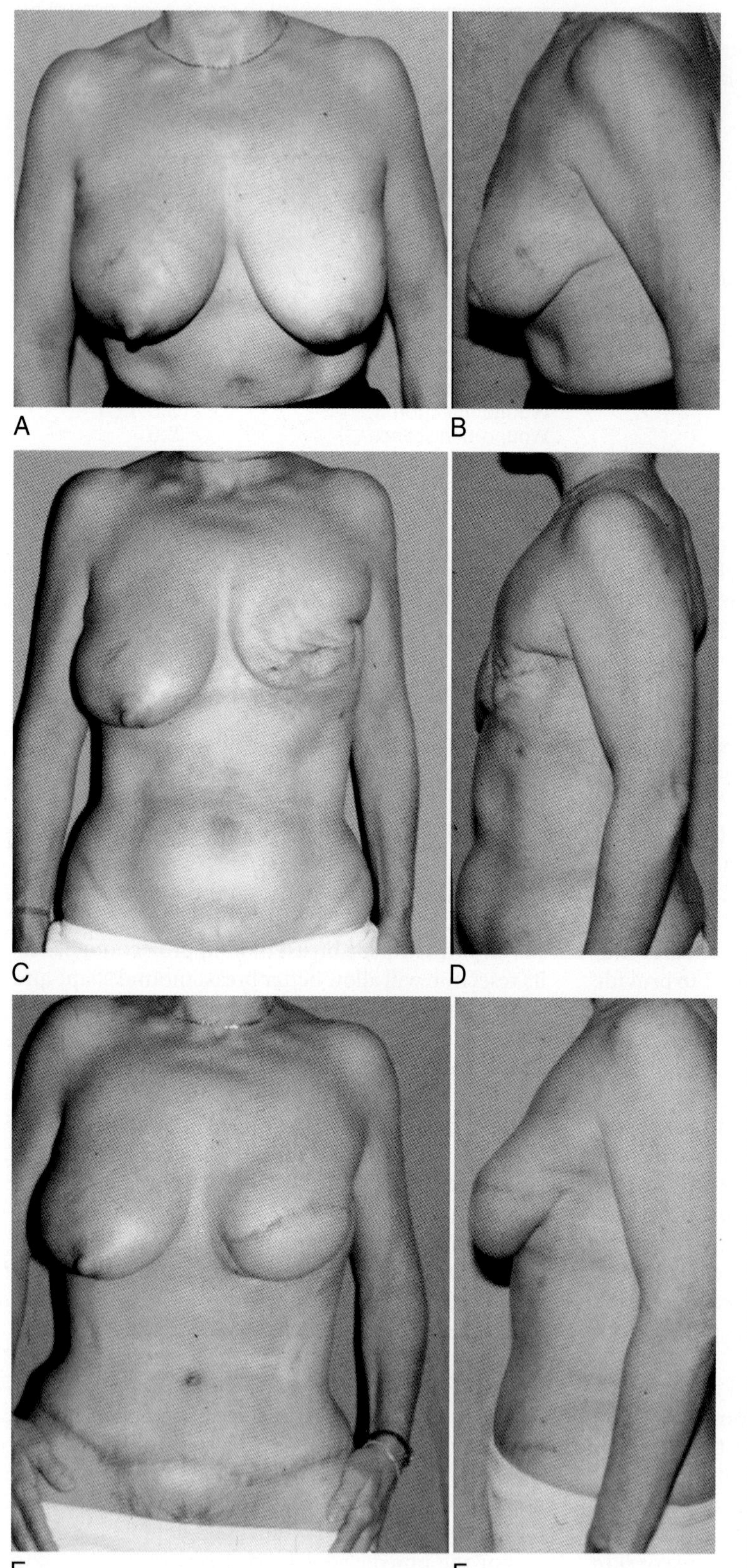

FIGURE 138-65. TRAM flap for delayed left breast reconstruction. Improved abdominal contour after donor site closure. *A,* Preoperative anterior view. The patient has undergone left lumpectomy and radiation therapy; preoperative view of left modified radical mastectomy for invasive breast cancer. *B,* Preoperative lateral view, left breast. *C,* Postoperative left modified radical mastectomy. The patient requests autogenous reconstruction. *D,* Lateral view of left modified radical mastectomy. Redundant abdominal tissue is available at donor site of inferior abdomen. *E,* Postoperative view at 1 year of left breast TRAM reconstruction. Adequate symmetry is achieved with the opposite breast. Abdominal closure provides improved contour. The umbilicus is centralized after direct closure of right rectus donor site with plication sutures between left rectus sheath and exterior oblique fascia. *F,* Lateral view. TRAM skin island provides natural ptosis to match contralateral breast. Abdominal contour is improved with no physical limitations.

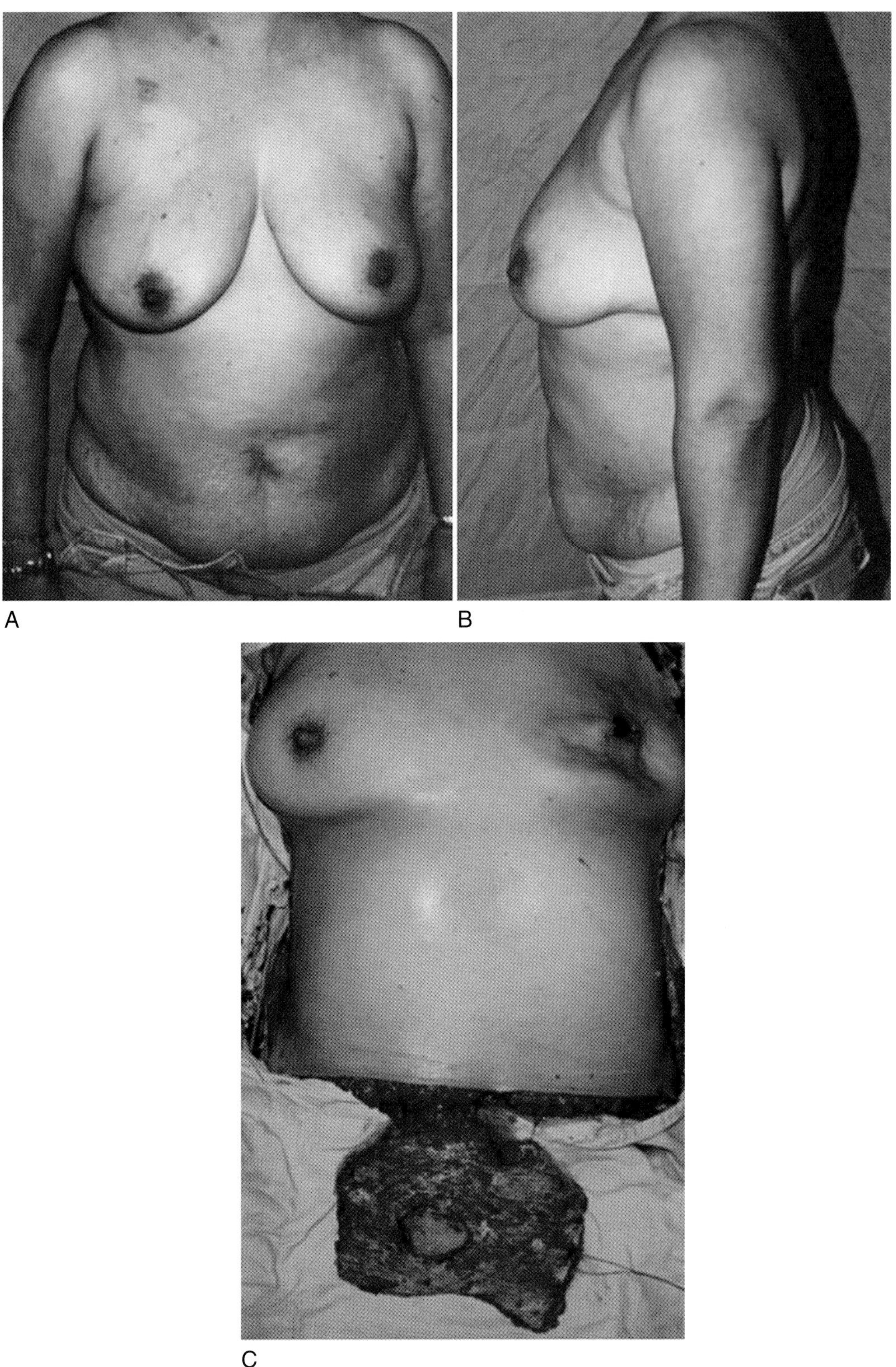

FIGURE 138-66. Immediate skin-sparing TRAM flap. *A,* Anterior preoperative view. *B,* Preoperative lateral view. *C,* Intraoperative view of skin island design for skin-sparing TRAM flap. TRAM flap is partially elevated. Note left skin-sparing mastectomy with skin envelope prepared for inset of TRAM flap.

Continued

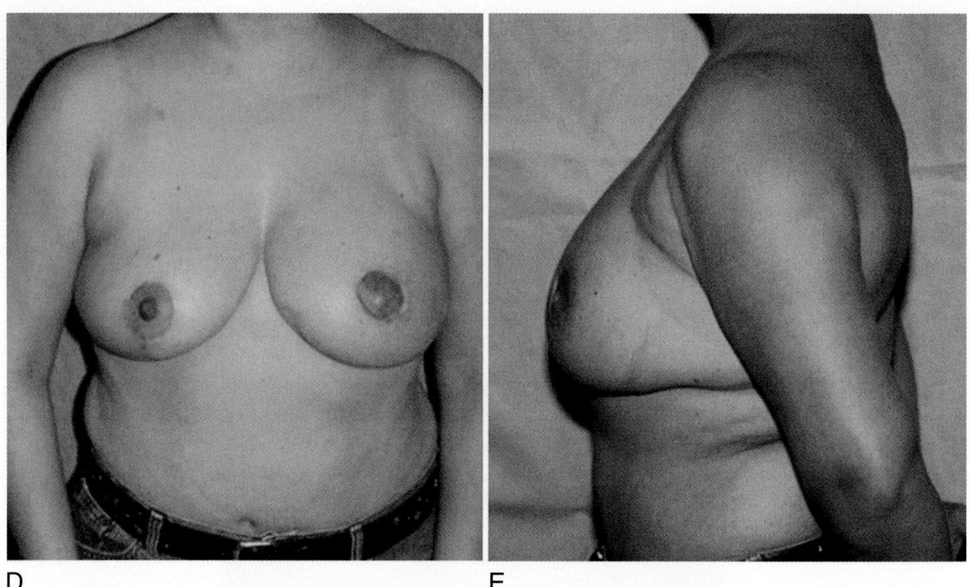

FIGURE 138-66, cont'd. *D,* Postoperative anterior view. *E,* Postoperative lateral view. (Also see Figure 138-55.)

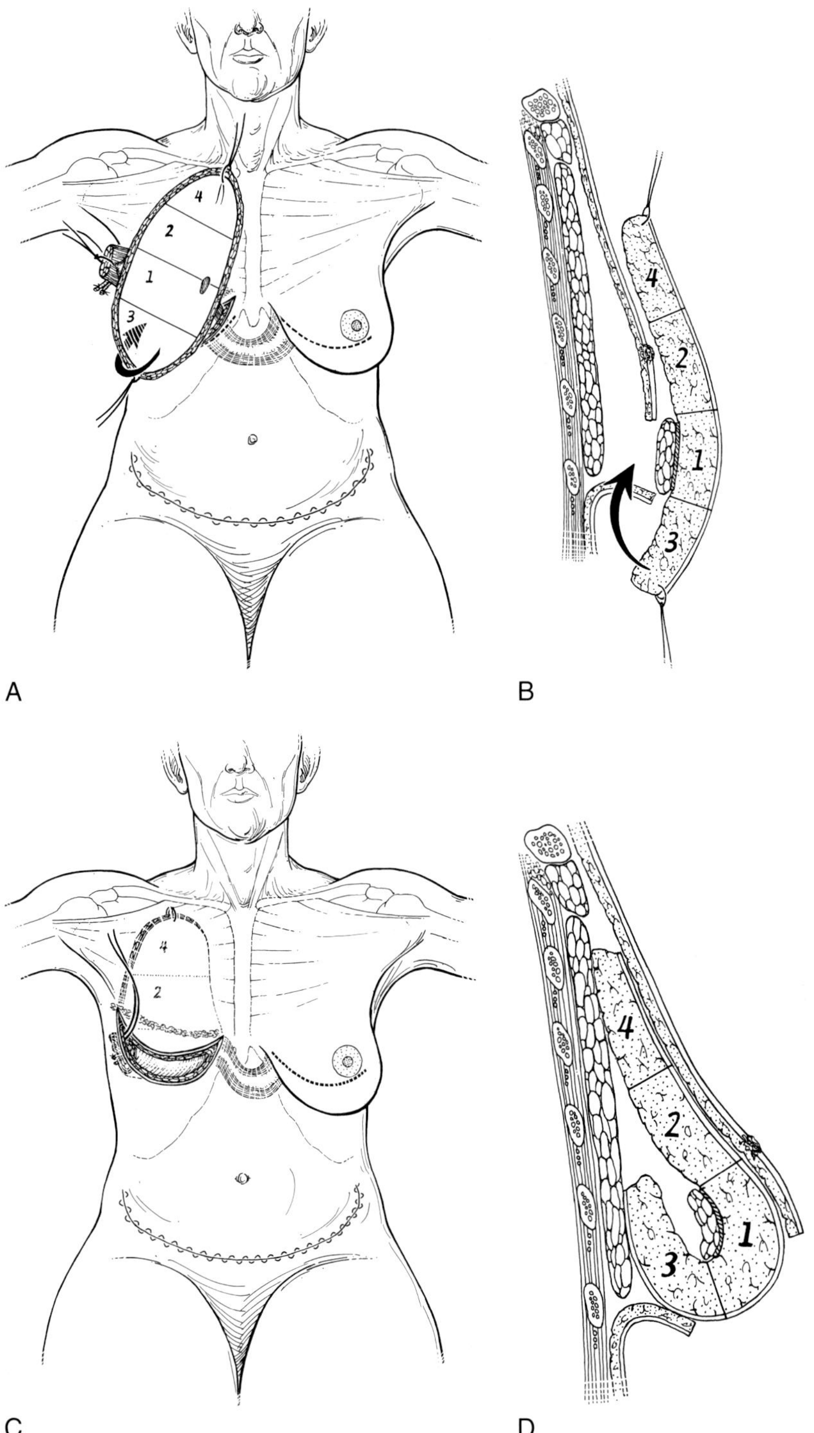

FIGURE 138-67. Flap inset: contralateral TRAM flap. *A,* Zone 1 will be located in area of skin envelope replacement. Zone 4 will be discarded. Zone 2 and zone 3 will be de-epithelialized, with zone 3 folded beneath zone 1 to increase projection. Zone 2 will provide upper breast contour corrections. *B,* Cross section of contralateral flap during inset. Zone 1 and part of zone 2 will provide cutaneous coverage to improve skin envelope. Remaining zone 2 and zone 3 will be used for contour and projection. *C,* The skin envelope between mastectomy scar and inframammary line will be resected and replaced by skin island zone 1 and zone 2. Zone 2 can be lowered toward the inframammary line to increase ptosis. *D,* Cross section of flap during inset. Zone 4 will be discarded. Zone 3 is stacked behind muscle to increase projection.

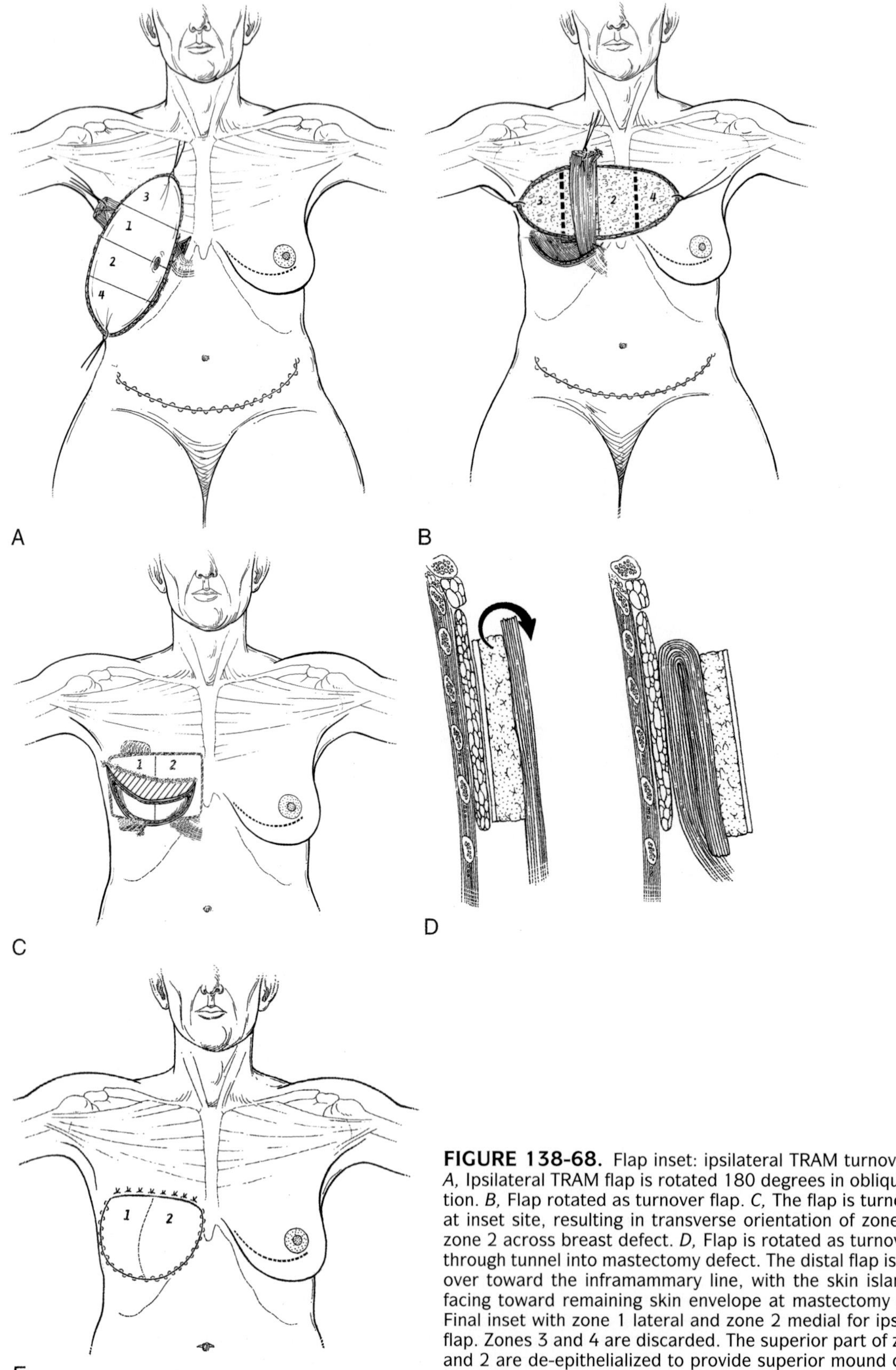

FIGURE 138-68. Flap inset: ipsilateral TRAM turnover flap. *A,* Ipsilateral TRAM flap is rotated 180 degrees in oblique position. *B,* Flap rotated as turnover flap. *C,* The flap is turned over at inset site, resulting in transverse orientation of zone 1 and zone 2 across breast defect. *D,* Flap is rotated as turnover flap through tunnel into mastectomy defect. The distal flap is turned over toward the inframammary line, with the skin island now facing toward remaining skin envelope at mastectomy site. *E,* Final inset with zone 1 lateral and zone 2 medial for ipsilateral flap. Zones 3 and 4 are discarded. The superior part of zones 1 and 2 are de-epithelialized to provide superior mound contour beneath preserved skin envelope.

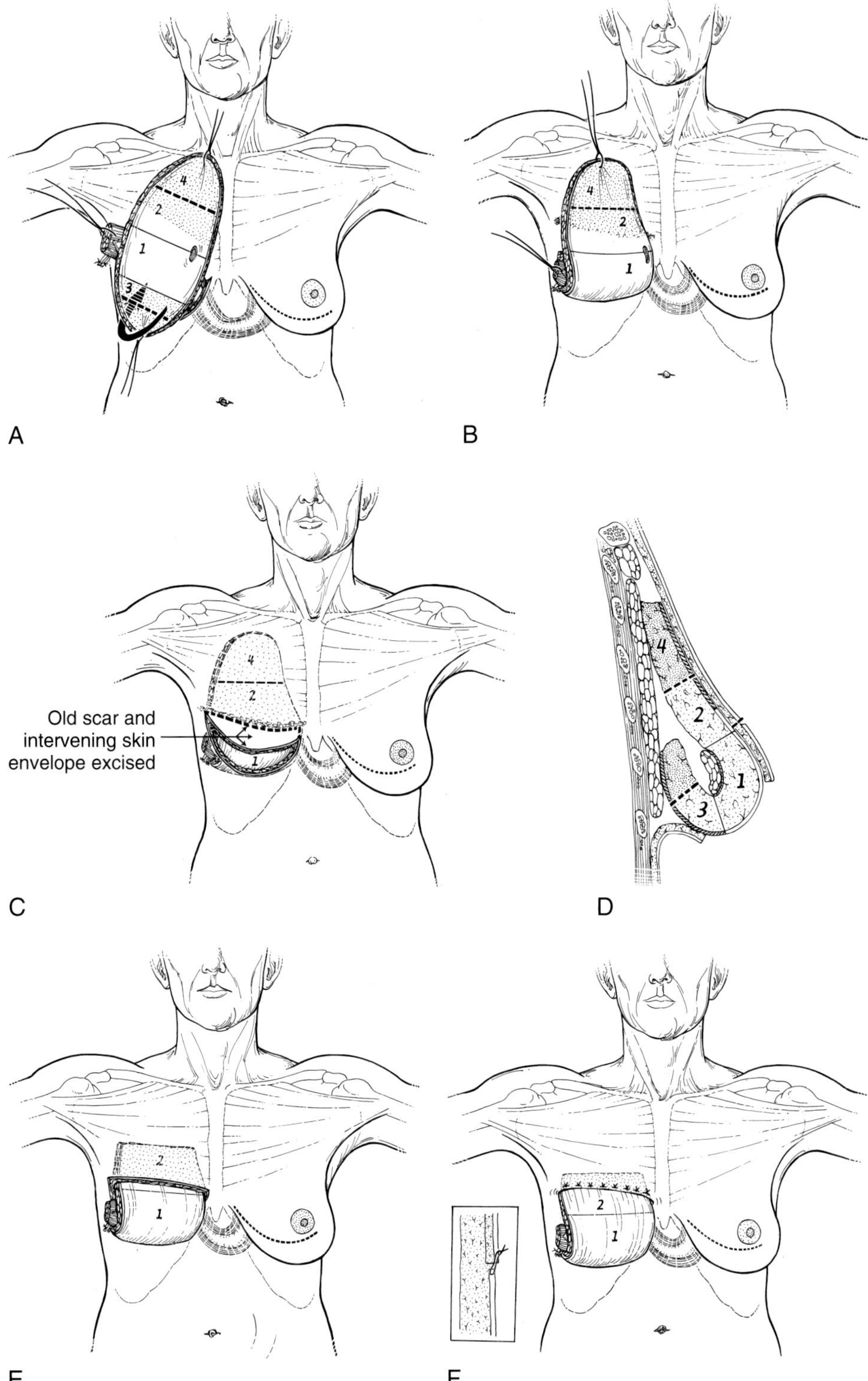

FIGURE 138-69. Flap inset: contralateral TRAM flap. *A,* With a 270-degree arc of rotation, skin island has oblique position at mastectomy site. *B,* Zone 4 is discarded. Zone 3 is rotated laterally to provide contour improvement based on shape of opposite breast. *C,* Old scar and skin envelope between scar and inframammary line are excised. *D,* All of zone 4 and distal part of zone 3 are excised. Skin envelope between mastectomy scar and inframammary region is resected and replaced with zone 1. *E,* TRAM flap ready for final inset. *F,* Junction of retained skin envelope and skin of TRAM approximated with half vertical mattress sutures. Remaining flap is inset with buried absorbable and subcutaneous sutures.

Continued

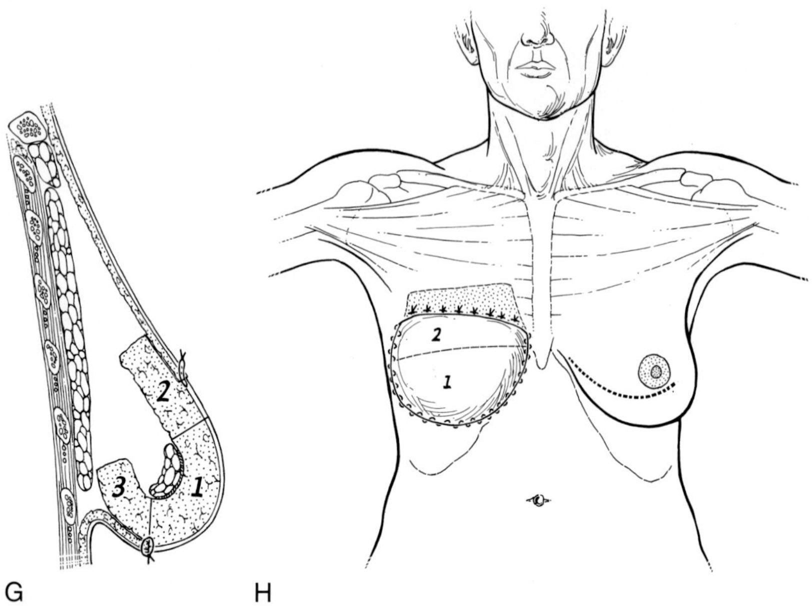

FIGURE 138-69, cont'd. *G,* Cross section demonstrates final position of TRAM flaps. *H,* Flap inset completed.

the flap will be either vertical or transverse. If the flap is vertical, the ipsilateral rectus muscle's zone 2 portion of the skin island is positioned at the infraclavicular region and the contralateral rectus muscle's zone 2 is located below the inframammary region (Fig. 138-70). In general, zone 2 of the contralateral muscle will be folded under the remaining flap to augment size and projection. Zone 2 of the ipsilateral muscle will be used to simulate the missing pectoralis major muscle for radical mastectomy or to allow inferior migration of the entire flap to provide more ptosis for the breast mound. If the flap is placed transversely on the chest wall, both zones 2 will be used for fullness both medial and lateral to the central mound.

For bilateral TRAM flaps with two separate hemitransverse skin islands, the two flaps are usually stacked to improve projection in a unilateral reconstruction. The advantage of this flap design (as opposed to the single skin island) is the ability to move the two flaps independently (Fig. 138-71). The disadvantages of two hemi–skin islands are the loss of skin island continuity for replacement of the missing skin envelope; difficulty in maintaining position of the tissues used for infraclavicular filling of areas of absent soft tissue or pectoralis muscle; and separation of the arterial and venous systems, which may increase the likelihood of venous insufficiency.

When bilateral TRAM flaps with separated hemitransverse skin islands are transposed simultaneously for bilateral breast reconstruction, each flap may be transposed to the ipsilateral hemithorax or the flaps may cross to the contralateral sides (Fig. 138-72). If each flap is transposed to the ipsilateral side, the left flap is rotated clockwise 270 degrees so that zone 1 is located at the inframammary region. The right flap is rotated counterclockwise to a similar position at the right inframammary region. Zone 2 is directed toward the superior aspect of each hemithorax. Each flap may also be transposed to assume a transverse position, with zone 1 medial and zone 2 lateral. A third alternative arc of rotation involves rotating the flap as a turnover flap. In the hemithorax, the skin territory will be facing toward the chest wall. The hemitransverse skin island is flipped over so that the inferior portion of the skin island is now located at the inframammary region with zone 1 medial and zone 2 lateral with a transverse orientation.

With crossing flaps, each flap is rotated 270 degrees so that the hemitransverse skin island assumes a vertical orientation with zone 1 located at the medial inframammary region. With each arc of rotation, the zone 1 portion of the skin island should be located so that this portion of the skin island is used to replace the missing skin envelope. The remainder of the flap is de-epithelialized and used to provide breast mound replacement. As noted, there is great versatility in the positioning of skin islands after bilateral breast reconstruction. In general, the skin island with a rectus muscle carrier is positioned to avoid vascular compromise and to fit the defect and provide optimal breast mound size and projection.

Postoperative Management

After surgery, standard postoperative care is required with the appropriate emphasis on early ambulation and respiratory care. The Foley catheter is generally removed the first postoperative day. A temporary ileus

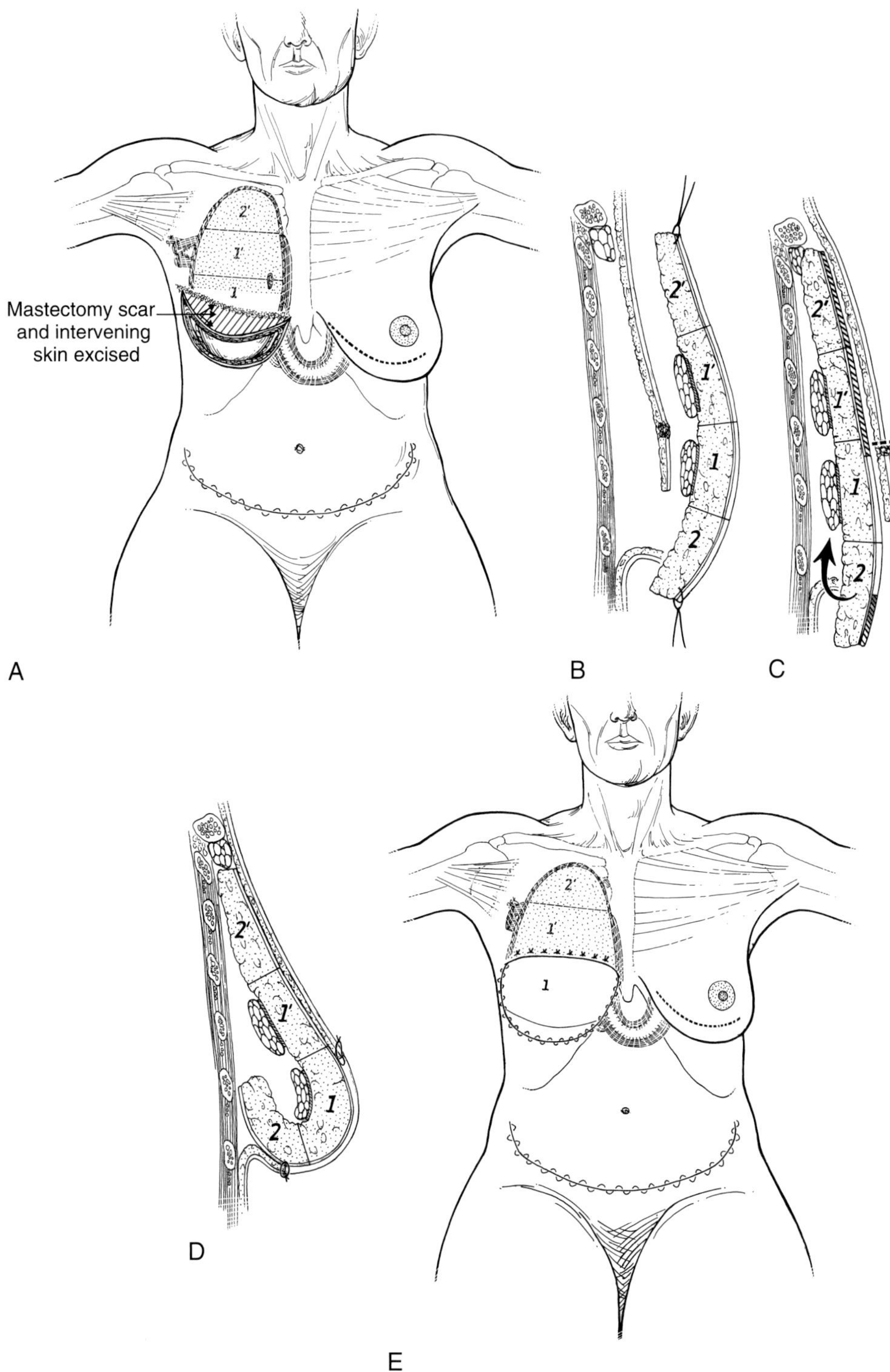

FIGURE 138-70. Flap inset: bilateral TRAM flap with single skin island (bipedicled). *A,* Skin island is positioned with ipsilateral rectus for zones 1′ and 2′ and contralateral rectus muscle for zones 1 and 2. *B,* Cross section of bilateral TRAM flap positioned on chest with zones 2′ and 1′ based on ipsilateral muscle and zones 1 and 2 on contralateral muscle. *C,* Skin envelope between mastectomy scar and inframammary region will be excised with use of zone 1 for inferior skin envelope. Zone 3 will be folded beneath zone 1 to provide breast mound projection. All areas of buried skin island will be de-epithelialized. *D,* Final appearance of inset of bilateral TRAM flap. *E,* Final appearance of inset for bilateral TRAM flap with one skin island for breast reconstruction.

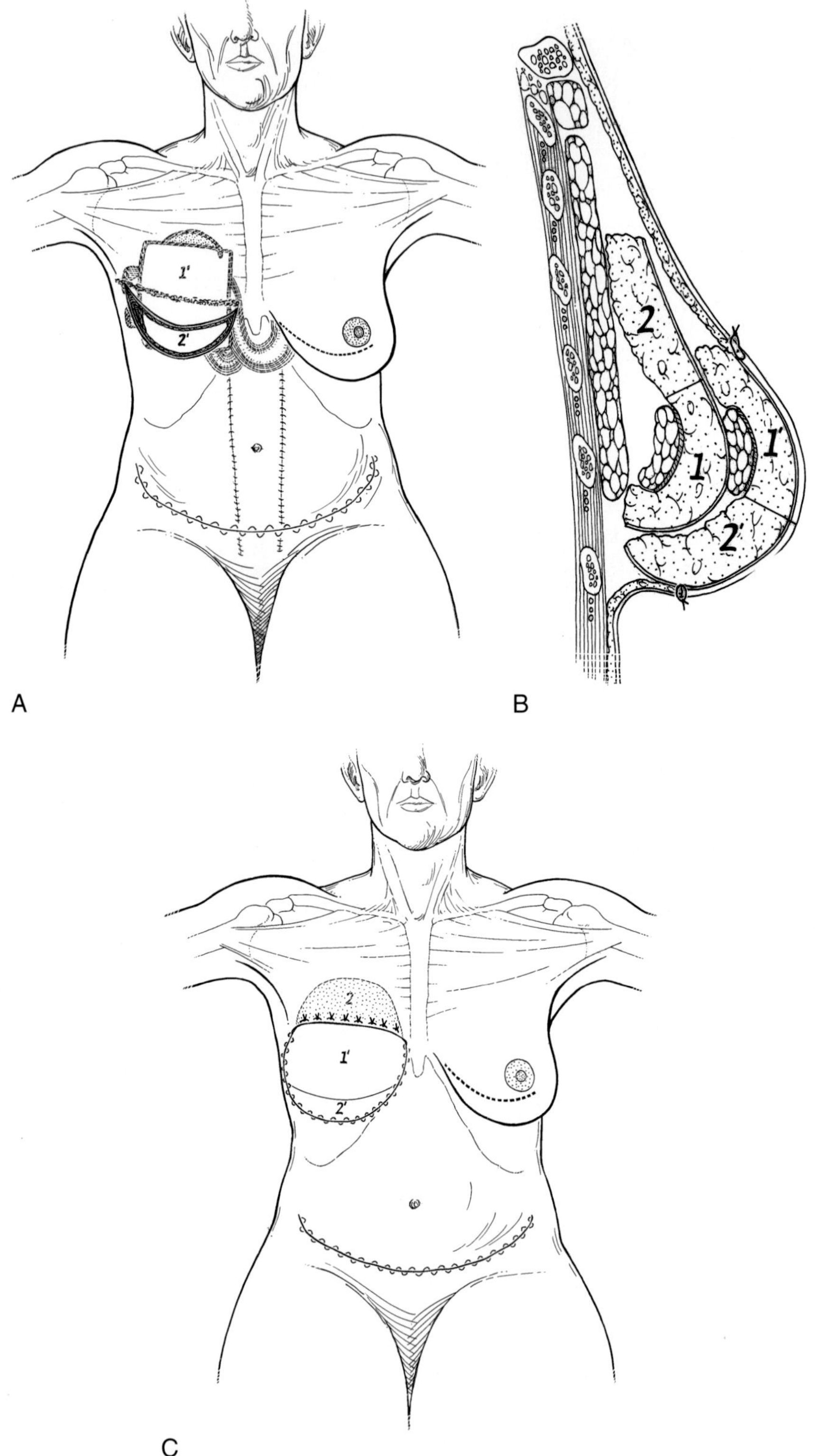

FIGURE 138-71. Flap inset: bilateral TRAM flap with hemitransverse skin islands for breast reconstruction. *A,* The flaps are stacked with the contralateral flap on the surface of the reconstructed breast mound (zones 2′ and 1′). *B,* Ipsilateral TRAM skin island buried and skin de-epithelialized (zones 2 and 1). Contralateral TRAM skin island used to provide skin envelope coverage (zones 1′ and 2′). *C,* Final appearance after bilateral TRAM flap inset. Two independent flaps can be used to provide appropriate contour and may be stacked to improve projection.

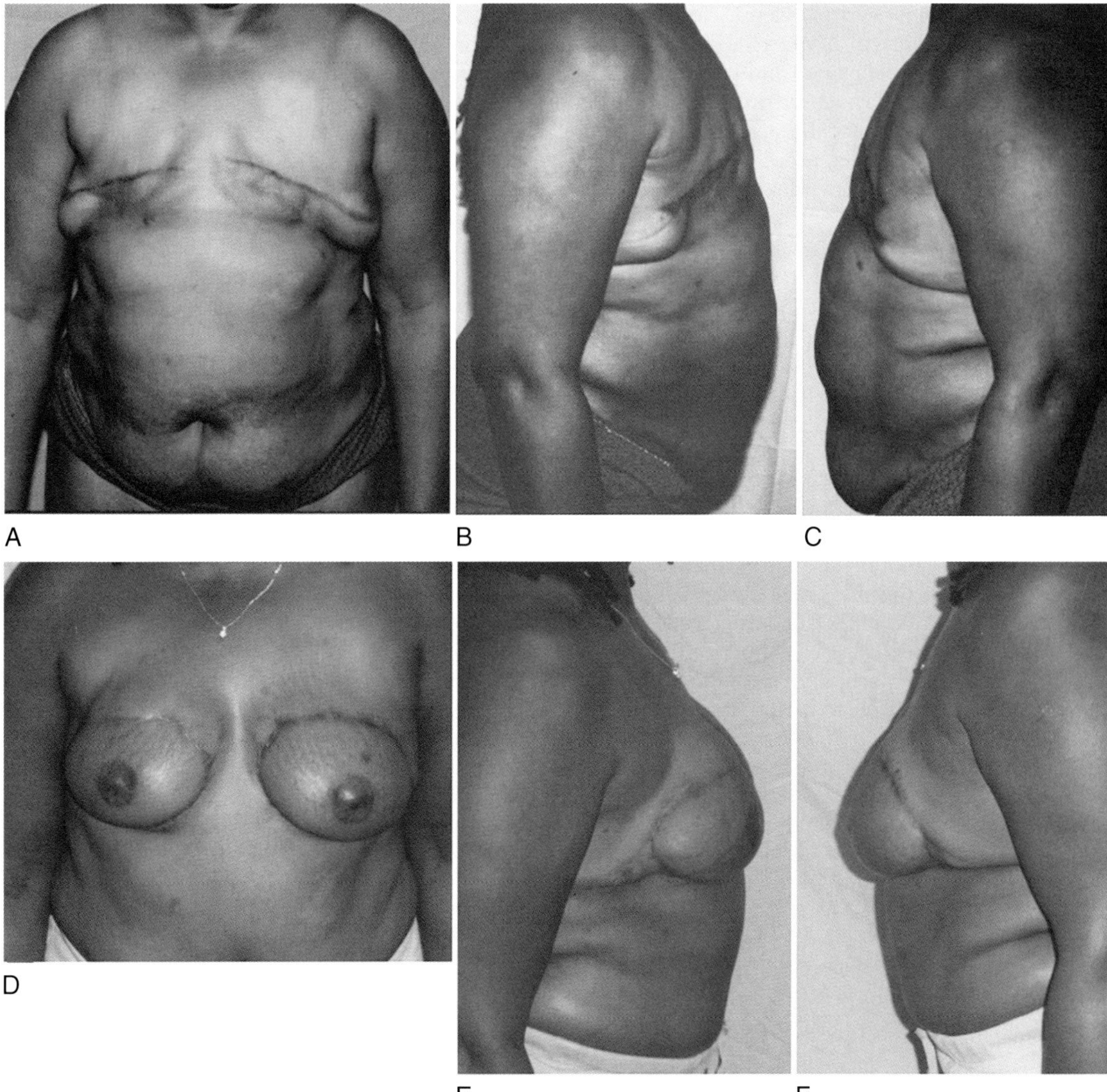

FIGURE 138-72. Bilateral TRAM flap for delayed breast reconstruction. *A,* Preoperative anterior view of patient after bilateral mastectomy. *B* and *C,* Preoperative lateral views. *D,* Postoperative view 1 year after bilateral TRAM flap with use of both pedicles. Two hemitransverse skin islands provide adequate breast mound projection. *E* and *F,* Postoperative lateral views.

is possible and more commonly observed in the patient with epidural regional anesthesia for pain relief. Usually, the patient is ready for discharge by the fifth postoperative day. The patient is usually discharged with drains in place, which are subsequently removed between postoperative days 7 and 10 when serous drainage has stopped. The patient's physical activities are usually restricted for 6 weeks postoperatively to allow healing of the abdominal wall donor site.

Microvascular Composite Tissue Transplantation

Microvascular composite tissue transplantation or the free flap allows use of distant tissue for defect reconstruction. Requirements for use of a free flap include availability of a source of tissue with a reliable pedicle, suitable receptor vessels in proximity to the site of planned tissue transplantation, and a microvascular team and required equipment capable of performing microsurgery with safety and reliability. For breast reconstruction, microvascular composite tissue transplantation offers several possible advantages when a flap is required for restoration of the breast skin envelope or for soft tissue for autogenous reconstruction: a suitable flap source when transposition flaps are unavailable or contraindicated; a flap with potential for improved tissue perfusion due to improved flap design compared with standard transposition flap design; a distant donor site more acceptable to the patient; and the ability to preserve muscle continuity with use of a perforator flap in which the muscle pedicle is dissected to include single or multiple perforating vessels to the skin territory of the musculocutaneous flap without incorporation of the actual muscle in the flap (perforator flap). This approach in harvest of the free flap offers the potential of muscle function preservation. Because the free flap depends on the microvascular anastomosis between the flap pedicle and the receptor vessel for survival, there is always the risk of vascular complications at the anastomosis site with subsequent flap loss (Fig. 138-73).

Sources of tissue suitable for microvascular transplantation include the inferior abdominal skin and subcutaneous tissue, generally based on the deep inferior epigastric artery and associated veins or the superficial inferior epigastric artery and associated vein. The second option for suitable autogenous tissue is located overlying the gluteus maximus muscle and is based on either the superior or inferior gluteal artery and associated veins. These tissues are usually transplanted with a segment of underlying muscle (e.g., rectus abdominis muscle or superior or inferior half of gluteus maximus muscle) to capture the musculocutaneous perforators to the skin territory of the muscle flaps. In an effort to preserve muscle function, flap design is evolving to eliminate muscle excision by elevation of the lower abdomen based on the superficial inferior epigastric artery and associated vein or use of a perforator flap based on the major pedicle to the rectus abdominis or gluteus maximus muscle.

Flap design as a perforator flap requires splitting the muscle at the site of the perforating vessels to use the pedicle connected to the perforator to the overlying skin territory while preserving muscle continuity. Both the TRAM flap and the gluteus maximus muscle flap, or perforator modification of the flaps, have acceptable donor sites as initially appreciated in their use as standard transposition flaps. When these donor sites are not available, any established free flap donor site can be selected. Another donor site used as an alternative option is the deep circumflex iliac fasciocutaneous flap[291] (termed the Rubens flap because the skin island includes the skin and soft tissue located at the lateral trunk flank region, where there is often adequate volume of subcutaneous tissue to provide tissue for autogenous breast reconstruction). The lateral thigh fasciocutaneous and gracilis musculocutaneous flaps have less desirable donor site locations but can be considered potential flap donor sites, particularly when a flap is required for breast reconstruction and other more standard flaps are unavailable. The TRAM free flap and its modification as a perforator flap and the gluteus maximus as standard and perforator flap are reviewed in regard to indications and technique for breast reconstruction.

The indications for a free flap for breast reconstruction are similar to those for a standard transposition flap, including the necessity for restoration of the skin envelope and a patient's request for autogenous tissue for mound replacement. The results comparing standard flaps and free flaps for breast reconstruction are similar and primarily relate to the experience of the surgical team with the technique. Many centers rely on standard TRAM transposition for autogenous reconstruction and have excellent results. Community plastic surgeons may not wish to undertake the complexity of the microvascular procedure and may provide results comparable to those of centers that rely largely on microvascular techniques for autogenous breast reconstruction.

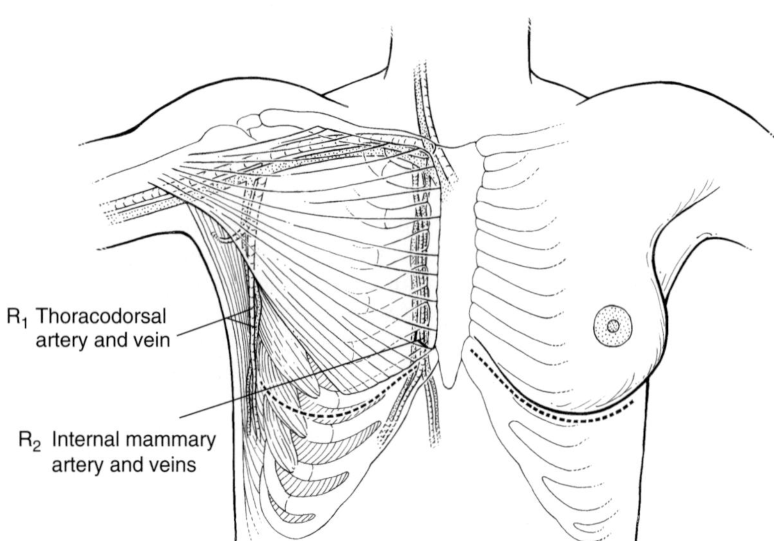

FIGURE 138-73. Receptor vessels available for microvascular composite tissue transplantation for breast reconstruction. Thoracodorsal artery and venae comitantes or internal mammary artery and venae comitantes are available as reliable receptor vessels. Visualization of internal mammary vessels requires resection of one or two costal cartilages (generally third and fourth).

TABLE 138-27 ✦ INDICATIONS FOR AND CONTRAINDICATIONS TO MICROVASCULAR COMPOSITE TISSUE TRANSPLANTATION

Indications	Contraindications
Inadequate skin envelope, other flap sources not available or not selected by patient	Donor site pedicle unavailable
Autogenous reconstruction, patient's or surgeon's preference	Receptor site vessels unavailable
Muscle function-preserving technique, patient's or surgeon's preference	Lack of microvascular support systems

The use of the perforator flap offers the option of muscle function preservation that is an advantage to this technique for flap harvest. Fortunately, the use of the muscle in standard transposition techniques is not associated with loss of abdominal function for the athletic patient if the donor closure is properly performed. Risk of hernia is reduced in the perforator flap with muscle integrity preservation, but since the anterior sheath is partially removed, risk of hernia or weakness is not totally eliminated. In standard flap design, particularly with the TRAM flap, the pedicle is distant from the incorporated skin island, increasing risk of venous insufficiency in the portion of the flap distant from the muscle (zones 3 and 4 of the TRAM skin island), with resultant risk of partial flap loss or fat necrosis. The free flap design allows more precise design of the skin island close to the pedicle (deep inferior epigastric artery and venae comitantes), point of entrance into the muscle, and its subsequent vascular connections (musculocutaneous perforating vessels) into the overlying skin territory. When muscle is incorporated with the skin island in this free flap design, more perforating vessels are incorporated into the skin island. There is improved flap circulation and reduced risk of venous insufficiency and subsequent fat necrosis. With the design of the free flap as a perforator flap, there may be reduced vascular communication between the pedicle and the overlying skin island, introducing more risk of late fat necrosis. In general, composite tissue transplantation is now frequently used for breast reconstruction with excellent safety and outcomes. In certain patients, it represents the only option available for satisfactory breast reconstruction (Table 138-27).[292]

DONOR FLAP SELECTION

When the surgeon and patient elect to undertake breast reconstruction with microvascular flap transplantation, the options for flap selection are increased by the availability of distant flap sites (Table 138-28). The two most commonly used donor sites are the lower abdomen and the buttock. The lower abdomen offers skin and subcutaneous fat that can be moved to the chest as a transposition flap (see previous discussion of pedicled TRAM flap) or may be transplanted based on the deep inferior epigastric artery and associated veins or the superficial inferior epigastric artery and vein. Because the skin island for the flap is based immediately adjacent to the pedicle, there is more direct arterial and venous perfusion via the inferior pedicle than is observed when the superior pedicle (superior epigastric artery and associated venae comitantes) is selected as the flap pedicle. Although the skin island and associated lower abdominal tissue will survive on either pedicle, advocates of the deep inferior epigastric pedicle (DIEP) as the vascular basis of the TRAM flap think that zones 2 and 3 are better perfused with less fat necrosis despite preservation of the borderline flap areas for the breast reconstruction. Since there is concern about division of the rectus muscle, only a segment of the muscle is harvested with the standard DIEP-TRAM flap. With identification of the central muscle perforators, the medial and lateral thirds of the muscle may be preserved, maintaining continuity of the rectus muscle. With careful identification of a single large perforator or two or three smaller perforators, the muscle may be split to allow release of the deep inferior epigastric pedicle through the muscle during the harvest. With the perforator flap, the entire continuity of the rectus muscle is preserved. (A small segment of the muscle may be denervated lateral to the muscle split.) This approach is attractive to the athletic young patient who wishes to preserve rectus muscle if possible. With the perforator dissection, the advantage of using the DIEP flap in terms of skin island perfusion is lost because the number of perforators may be diminished without use of the distal segment of the rectus muscle as part of the flap. In general, the DIEP-TRAM flap with muscle preservation or the DIEP perforator flap is used as the donor flap. Thus, either part or all of the muscle continuity is maintained.

For immediate reconstruction, when an axillary node dissection is performed, the thoracodorsal artery and veins are generally selected as the recipient vessels for flap revascularization. Because sentinel lymph node dissection frequently eliminates the need for axillary node dissection, the plastic surgeon must dissect the axilla to locate the thoracodorsal pedicle or may frequently use the internal mammary artery and veins as the receptor vessels. For immediate reconstruction

TABLE 138-28 ✦ DONOR FLAP SELECTION

Pedicle Name	Length/ Diameter	Skin Territory (cm)	Function Preservation	Position for Harvest	Fat Necrosis Risk	Dissection Complexity	Hernia Risk
DIEP-TRAM (segmental)	5 cm/2.5 mm	25 × 6	Possible	Supine	+	+	++
DIEP, perforator (art. + vc)	5 cm/2.5 mm	25 × 6	Yes	Supine	++	++	+
SIEP (art. + vc)	4-6 cm/1-1.5 mm	20 × 15	Yes	Supine	+	+++	N/A
SGAP, superior gluteus (segmental) (art. + vc)	3 cm/2.5 mm	24 × 12	Yes	Lateral decubitus or prone	+	+++	N/A
SGAP, perforator (art. + vc)	3 cm/2.5 mm	24 × 12	Yes	Lateral decubitus or prone	+	+++	N/A
IGAP, inferior gluteus (segmental) (art. + vc)	3 cm/2.5 mm	24 × 12	Yes	Lateral decubitus or prone	+	+++	N/A
IGAP, perforator (art. + vc)	3 cm/2.5 mm	24 × 12	Yes	Lateral decubitus or prone	+	+++	N/A
DCIA (art. + vc)	6-8 cm/2-2.5 mm	12 × 6	N/A	Lateral decubitus	++	+++	N/A

(art. + vc), artery and venae comitantes.
Risk: +++, high; ++, moderate; +, low; N/A, not applicable.

TABLE 138-29 ✦ COMPLICATIONS OF FREE UNILATERAL TRAM FLAP BREAST RECONSTRUCTION[236,307,308]

Complication	Percentage of Patients*
Partial flap loss	1.1-14.9
Total flap loss	1.5-2
Fat necrosis	16
Anastomotic thrombosis	4.7-6.0
Delayed wound healing	7-11
Abdominal hernia	2.8-11.9
Pulmonary embolism, deep venous thrombosis	0.5
Wound infection	2.3-17.9
Wound dehiscence	1.5
Hematoma	2.3
Lymphedema	4.5
Back pain	6.0
Any complication	37-60

*Range of percentage of patients with complications as reported in the literature.

after mastectomy and sentinel lymph node biopsy, it is preferable to use the internal mammary artery and vein to avoid axillary dissection. If the patient should require a delayed axillary dissection after pathologic evaluation of sentinel lymph node specimens, the dissection would not be adjacent to the flap pedicle. In some instances, removal of the third or fourth costal cartilages allows better visualization of the receptor vessels. With increasing interest in perforator flaps, some surgeons are now using the medial chest perforator vessels that emerge through the pectoralis major muscle as the receptor vessels and not dissecting posterior to the level of the internal mammary artery and vein (Tables 138-29 and 138-30).

For both immediate and delayed breast reconstruction using the TRAM flap, the patient is positioned supine for the entire procedure. The flap is outlined as described for the standard TRAM transposition flap. Vein grafts may rarely be required if suitable receptor vessels are not readily located, so the leg is also prepared and draped in the event that vein graft harvest is required. If an upper extremity vein graft is preferred, it should be taken on the extremity opposite the mastectomy site (Fig. 138-74).

TRAM FLAPS BASED ON THE DEEP INFERIOR EPIGASTRIC ARTERY AND VEINS (DIEP)

Segmental TRAM Flap

The technique for elevation of the rectus musculocutaneous flap for microvascular transplantation is similar to that for standard flap elevation. During the initial dissection, the superficial epigastric artery and vein, when encountered, are preserved. This pedicle, which is adequate for microanastomosis in only 15% to 30% of patients, may be considered for the flap pedicle or preserved on the contralateral side of the flap pedicle (DIEP) to enhance circulation by second microanastomosis if necessary. After the musculocutaneous flap is elevated from the posterior rectus sheath, the inferior epigastric artery and associated venae comitantes are identified and dissected inferiorly to their origin from the external iliac artery and vein. In general, the paired venae comitantes will form a single vein before entering the external iliac vein. At this point, the pedicle is ready for transection, and flap elevation is completed.

Segmental elevation of the inferior lateral rectus muscle with an overlying skin island is an alternative technique for rectus abdominis musculocutaneous flap elevation. A Doppler probe is used to locate paraumbilical musculocutaneous perforating vessels over the lateral half of the middle third of the rectus muscle. Only the segment of muscle containing perforating vessels is included with the skin island based on the inferior epigastric artery and associated venae comitantes. The medial third or lateral third of the muscle is left intact to maintain the continuity of the entire muscle between the costal margin and pubis for function preservation.

The lateral and medial thirds of the muscle are arbitrarily divided after identification and preservation of the central musculocutaneous perforating vessels to the overlying skin island, or the perforating vessels are fully dissected in the muscle to their junction with the lateral branch of the inferior epigastric artery and associated venae comitantes. This latter approach ensures inclusion of the dominant lateral branch of the vascular pedicle and allows inclusion of minimal rectus muscle fibers with the flap (Fig. 138-75).

TABLE 138-30 ✦ COMPLICATIONS OF DIEP FLAP[309-311]

Complication	Percentage of Patients*
Partial flap loss	7
Total flap loss	2-5
Fat necrosis	6-10
Anastomotic thrombosis	10
Abdominal hernia	0
Wound infection	3
Hematoma	2
Scar hypertrophy	2
Axillary seroma	1

*Range of percentage of patients with complications as reported in the literature.

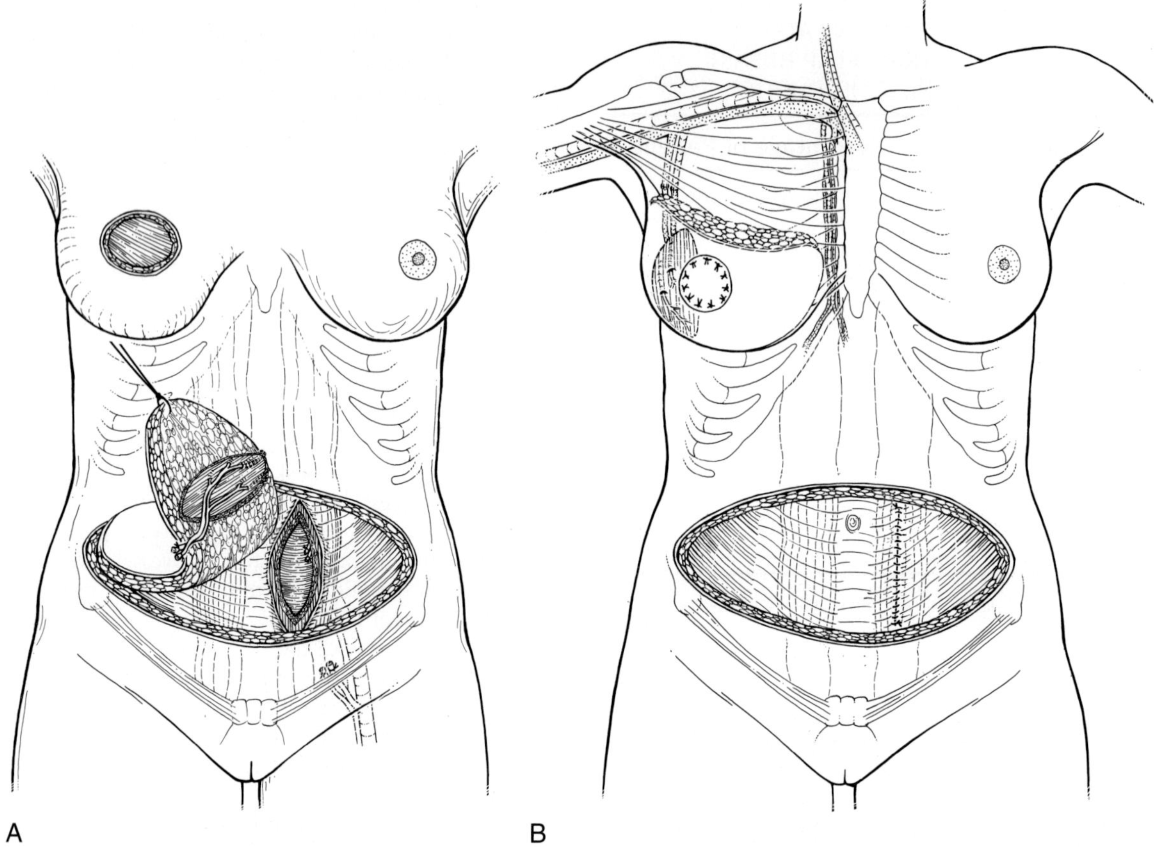

FIGURE 138-74. Microvascular transplantation of DIEP-segmental rectus. *A,* Central small segment of muscle that contains three perforating vessels dissected in continuity with deep inferior epigastric artery and venae comitantes. If a single perforator is 1.5 to 3 mm, it can be dissected through rectus muscle to DIEP, and excision of segment of muscle can be avoided. If perforators are small, a strip of rectus muscle will allow inclusion of several perforating vessels connected to DIEP. *B,* Flap inset using zones 1 and 2. Microanastomosis is between DIEP artery and veins and thoracodorsal artery and vein.

Perforator Flap

A smaller lower abdominal flap may be elevated precisely on a single large musculocutaneous perforator vessel from the inferior epigastric artery and associated venae comitantes. A Doppler probe is used to locate musculocutaneous pedicles from the rectus muscles with the planned skin island inferior to the umbilicus. The skin island is incised and elevated to the site where the perforator enters the skin island. The anterior rectus sheath is incised, and the perforator is dissected from its intermuscular course to its origin from the inferior epigastric artery and venae comitantes. If the perforator is small (<1.5 mm), it may be necessary to dissect several perforators in the medial or lateral row and include a small segment of muscle to ensure adequate flap perfusion. Proximal dissection of the deep inferior epigastric pedicle is performed as required for pedicle length. Although this technique requires splitting of the rectus muscle a short distance for dissection of the perforator through its intermuscular course, a segment of muscle is generally not included with the flap, and function of the muscle is preserved.

SUPERFICIAL INFERIOR EPIGASTRIC ARTERY (SIEA) FASCIOCUTANEOUS FLAP

In selected patients, the superficial inferior epigastric artery (SIEA) fasciocutaneous flap may be used for autogenous breast reconstruction by microvascular transplantation based on the superficial epigastric artery and venae comitantes or a separate superficial vein. In general, the lower abdominal donor site is planned for transplantation based on the DIEP. However, during the initial dissection of the skin territory, the surgeon may elect to identify the superficial inferior epigastric artery and vein during the dissection of the inferior aspect of the skin island. These vessels are not consistent and may not always be present. The venous drainage is via the venae comitantes with the SIEA or through the superficial

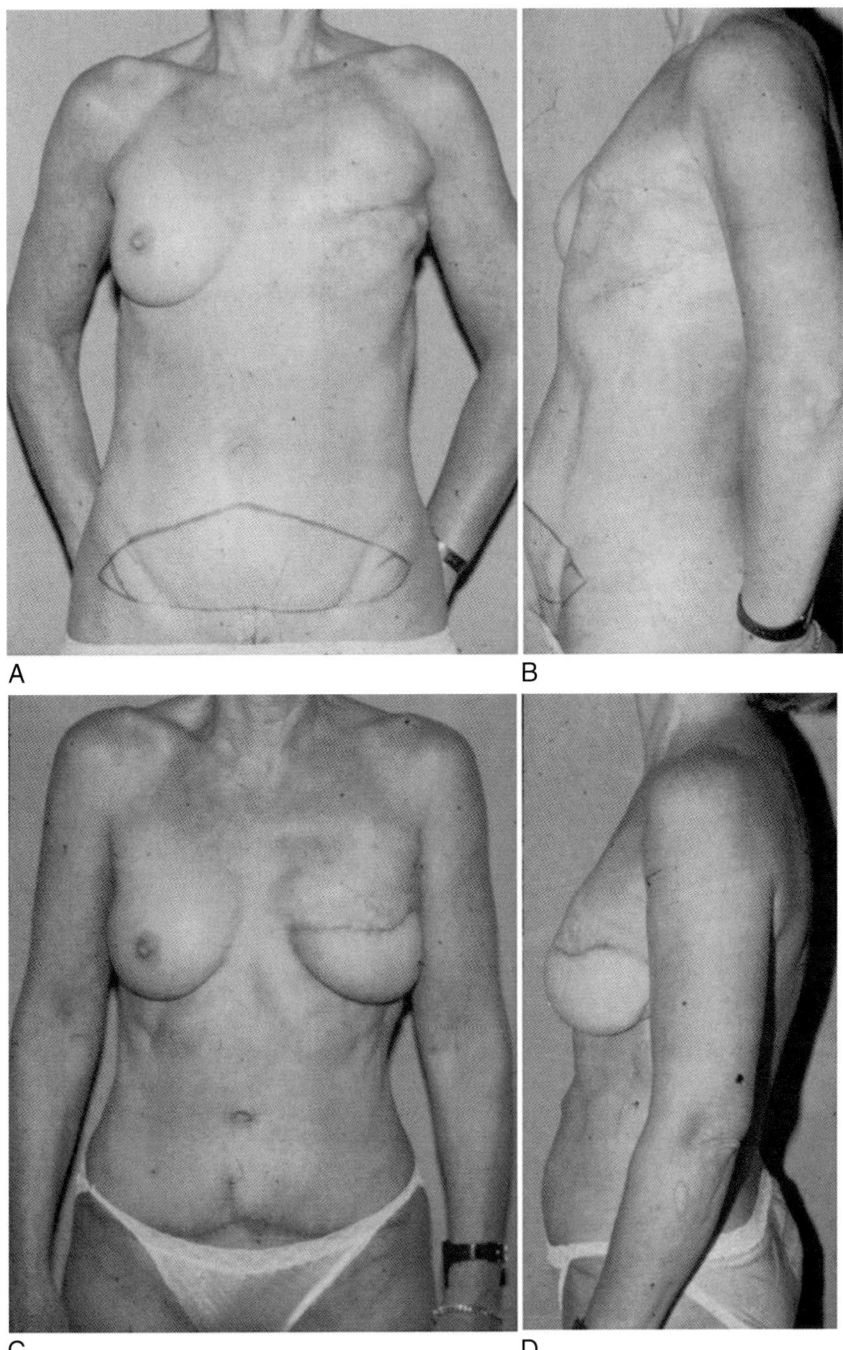

FIGURE 138-75. Microvascular transplantation of rectus abdominis musculocutaneous flap (TRAM-segmental rectus muscle) for delayed breast reconstruction. *A,* Anterior view of left mastectomy defect. The patient requests autogenous reconstruction. Markings for left segmental-TRAM free flap. *B,* Lateral view demonstrates mastectomy defect and TRAM free flap donor site. *C,* Postoperative view at 6 months demonstrates breast mound with adequate size for symmetry. TRAM flap receptor vessels—thoracic dorsal artery and vein. *D,* Postoperative view demonstrates adequate breast mound projection provided by free TRAM flap.

inferior epigastric vein, which is a large, superficially located, vertically oriented vein draining the lower abdomen. This vein is more superficially located than the SIEA. The SIEA originates from the anterior surface of the femoral artery 4 to 5 cm below the inguinal ligament. In up to 48% of patients, it may arise from a common trunk with the superficial circumflex artery. It courses vertically upward, crossing the inguinal ligament at a point halfway between the anterior superior iliac spine and the pubis. It courses deep to Scarpa fascia (Fig. 138-76).[284,285]

The skin island is limited to zone 1 and medial portion of zone 2 of the territory of the rectus abdominis musculocutaneous flap. If the skin island is designed for the DIEP, the inferior incision between the pubis and the anterior iliac spine will be used to locate the superficial inferior epigastric artery and vein. After the initial incision, the dissection is continued

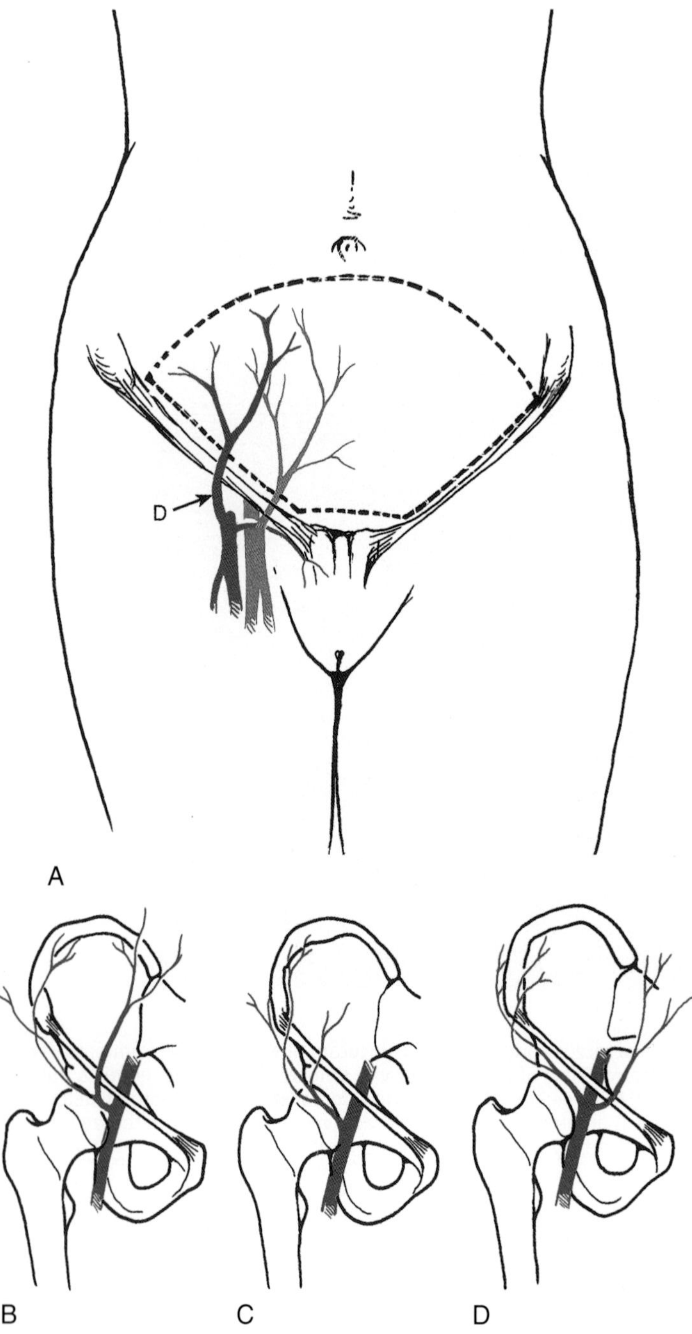

FIGURE 138-76. SIEA flap and variations of superficial circumflex iliac artery and superficial inferior epigastric artery. *A,* Dominant pedicle: superficial epigastric artery (D). *B,* Common origin (48%). *C,* Large superficial circumflex iliac artery without superficial inferior epigastric artery (10% to 15%). *D,* Separate origins (42% to 47%). (From Mathes SJ, Nahai F: Reconstructive Surgery: Principles, Anatomy, and Technique. New York, Churchill Livingstone, 1997:1096.)

through the subcutaneous tissue to Scarpa fascia. The superficial inferior epigastric vein lies superficial within this layer and is encountered during this part of the dissection. It is identified and preserved. Dissection then continues deep to Scarpa fascia. Loupe magnification is recommended for this dissection. Deep to Scarpa fascia, the SIEA is identified coursing vertically. It measures approximately 1 mm in diameter at this level. If the superficial inferior epigastric artery and vein are selected for the flap pedicle, extension of pedicle length will be required for adequate flap inset in proximity to recipient vessels on the chest wall (usually either the internal mammary artery and veins or large perforators from the internal mammary vessels). Dissection of the vascular pedicle toward its femoral artery origin will significantly increase the length of the arterial pedicle. The superficial inferior epigastric vein is traced to the saphenous or femoral vein to increase its venous pedicle length.

If the superficial inferior epigastric perforator and vein are inadequate in size or absent on one side of the midline, contralateral dissection may provide adequate pedicle to base the inferior abdominal tissue as a fasciocutaneous flap. In the event that the superficial inferior epigastric perforator and vein are inadequate as donor flap pedicles for microvascular transplantation, it is preferable to continue the dissection for the DIEP. As noted earlier in this chapter, the DIEP has greater pedicle length and diameter and is well established as a reliable and consistent donor vessel for transplantation of the inferior abdominal skin territory for autogenous breast reconstruction.

SUPERIOR AND INFERIOR GLUTEUS MAXIMUS MUSCULOCUTANEOUS FLAPS (SGAP AND IGAP)

An excellent donor site for composite tissue for breast reconstruction is located in the posterior inferior trunk incorporating the skin territory of the gluteus maximus muscle. Although the inferior abdomen is generally the first choice for tissue for transplantation to the breast, this donor site may not be available or practical because of prior surgery in the inferior abdomen (e.g., prior abdominoplasty, suction lipectomy, or laparotomy) or inadequate adipose tissue for autogenous reconstruction. In some instances, the patient may desire to avoid lower abdominal donor site scars in favor of use of the buttock as a donor site. Initially, the surgeon selected either the superior or the inferior half of the muscle with associated skin island as the flap for transplantation to the mastectomy site. The superior segmental muscle with overlying skin island is based on the superior gluteal artery and venae comitantes. The inferior segmental muscle with overlying skin island is based on the inferior gluteal artery and venae comitantes. Because only half or a segment of half of the muscle is incorporated in the flap, gluteus maximus muscle function is preserved. Muscle function preservation is extremely important for the ambulatory patient. Loss of gluteus maximus muscle function may lead to hip instability (Tables 138-31 and 138-32).

More recently, the concept of the perforator flap is used in which the musculocutaneous perforator is dissected through the muscle to its origin from the muscle pedicle, allowing preservation of all or the majority of the muscle. Dissection of the perforator allows development of a longer flap pedicle, which is helpful for the gluteus maximus flap modification as the inferior and superior gluteal pedicles are short and difficult to dissect to increase pedicle length to their points of origin adjacent to the lateral edge of the sacrum.

The superior gluteal segmental musculocutaneous flap (SGAP) and its perforator modification and the inferior gluteal segmental musculocutaneous flap (IGAP) and its perforator modification are fairly similar in design and approach. The superior half of

TABLE 138-31 ✦ INDICATIONS FOR AND CONTRAINDICATIONS TO SGAP OR IGAP RECONSTRUCTION[312]

Indications	Contraindications
Previous abdominoplasty or failed TRAM flap	Donor site pedicle unavailable
Lack of available superior and inferior epigastric vessels (previous abdominal scars)	Receptor site vessels unavailable
Second breast after previous TRAM flap	Lack of microvascular support systems
Inadequate abdominal fat for TRAM flap (extremely thin patients)	Patient medically unable to tolerate length of the procedure or recovery
	No suitable perforator vessels available

TABLE 138-32 ✦ COMPLICATIONS OF SGAP RECONSTRUCTION[313]

Complication	Percentage of Patients*
Total flap necrosis	5
Fat necrosis	5
Wound dehiscence (buttock)	10
Gluteal seroma	35
Gluteal depressions	20
Scar hypertrophy	5

*Range of percentage of patients with complications as reported in the literature.

the muscle is slightly easier to dissect, and the approach to the pedicle superior to the piriformis muscle is fairly direct. The thickness of the fatty layer is less, so the bulk of the flap for autogenous reconstruction will be less. The donor site is slightly more visible located in the midbuttock. The inferior half of the muscle is more difficult to dissect, and the approach to the inferior gluteal artery and associated vein is slightly more difficult. In addition, the pedicle has proximity to the sciatic nerve. The fatty layer is thicker and more suitable for breast reconstruction. The donor site is better concealed in the gluteal crease. If the entire inferior half of the muscle is removed, there is concern due to loss of soft tissue overlying the sciatic nerve. However, use of the segmental muscle or perforator flap has eliminated this disadvantage. Unfortunately, the flap dissection requires the lateral decubitus or prone position, so the patient's position must be altered for both immediate and delayed breast reconstruction.

The technique for microvascular transplantation generally involves elevation of a musculocutaneous flap based on either the superior or inferior gluteal pedicle. The initial technique is similar to elevation of the standard superior or inferior gluteus maximus musculocutaneous flap. Because the gluteus is rarely if ever transplanted as a functional muscle, an effort is made to remove only a small segment or no gluteus maximus muscle (perforator flap) with the overlying skin island. For this reason, the skin island is designed at either the superior or inferior edge of the muscle.

Technique

SGAP FLAP. For the SGAP flap, the skin island is centered over a line connecting the posterior iliac spine and the superior edge of the posterior sacrum. The skin island is incised to expose the superficial surface of the underlying gluteus maximus muscle. If a segment of the superior half of the muscle is included with the flap, the muscle fibers of insertion are divided 2 to 3 cm distal to the skin island. Dissection deep to the muscle now allows identification of the superior gluteal artery and vein. With the superior gluteal pedicle under visualization, the muscle is now split to the sacral edge.

Superior fibers of the muscle origin are divided immediately medial to the point of entrance of the vascular pedicle into muscle. The superior gluteal artery and vein are then dissected beneath the sacral edge superior to the piriformis muscle until adequate pedicle length is achieved.

An alternative approach (perforator flap) to elevation of a superior skin island involves identification of the point of entry of the musculocutaneous perforators into the designed skin island. This is accomplished by elevation of the lateral edge of the skin island until major perforating vessels are encountered as dissection proceeds toward the sacral edge. These musculocutaneous perforating vessels entering the skin island are then dissected through the medial superior gluteus maximus muscle until the superior gluteal artery and vein are identified. By splitting of the superior fibers of the gluteus maximus muscle, incorporation of the superior half of the gluteus maximus muscle in this musculocutaneous flap can be avoided. Elevation of the remainder of the pedicle beneath the sacrum is similar to that described for the standard superior gluteus maximus musculocutaneous flap.

IGAP FLAP. For the IGAP flap, the inferior skin island is centered over the gluteal crease lateral to the ischium. The initial incision through the skin island exposes the inferior fibers of the gluteus maximus muscle at the superior edge of the skin island and the fascia of the posterior thigh at the inferior edge of the skin island. The posterior thigh fascia is incised, permitting identification of the descending branch of the inferior gluteal artery and associated venae comitantes and the posterior femoral cutaneous nerve. Dissection proceeds superiorly beneath the deep fascia and the inferior half of the gluteus maximus muscle. With use of fiberoptic lighted retractors, the descending branch of the inferior gluteal artery and vein can be followed to its junction with the inferior gluteal artery and vein. A small segment of the inferior half of the gluteus maximus muscle is generally included with the flap so that the muscle branches of the flap's vascular pedicle will not have to be divided. However, the posterior femoral cutaneous nerve can be separated from the vascular pedicle and transection of this sensory nerve avoided during flap elevation. Proximal dissection of the inferior gluteal artery and veins immediately inferior to the piriformis muscle will increase pedicle length. Care is necessary to avoid injury to the sciatic nerve inferiorly and the inferior gluteal nerve immediately superior to the vascular pedicle.

As noted with the SGAP, it is possible to elevate the lateral edge of the designed skin island from the underlying inferior half of the gluteus maximus muscle. When perforators are encountered, the skin island is based on a large musculocutaneous perforator. The perforator is dissected through the muscle to its junction with the inferior gluteal artery and its associated veins. A portion of the muscle is split adjacent to the selected musculocutaneous perforator vessels for visualization of the intramuscular and posterior muscular dissection. Once the junction of the perforator vessels and the inferior gluteal vessel is identified, the remainder of the skin island is elevated from the superficial surface of the muscle. If several large perforating vessels are encountered, these perforators may be incorporated into the flap design. Each perforating vessel may be dissected independently, or a small segment of muscle may be included in the flap design. After the skin island is completely mobilized with its vascular attachments to the pedicle, the inferior gluteal artery and veins may be dissected beneath the sacral lateral edge to preserve adequate pedicle length.

Both the superior and inferior gluteal musculocutaneous flaps and the perforator modification represent function-preserving techniques. After the flaps are fully dissected and adequate pedicle length is achieved, the pedicle is divided beneath the sacrum and the flaps are set aside on the operating room table with a cool dressing. The donor site is drained with closed suction drainage, and the donor site is closed directly. The patient is returned to the supine position, and the microvascular revascularization of the flap is started. If the recipient vessels are not yet prepared, it is possible to prepare the recipient vessels while the patient is still in the lateral decubitus position. With this approach, the flap pedicle is not divided, maintaining flap circulation until the surgeon is ready to reposition the patient and begin flap revascularization and flap inset. Flap inset is similar to that described for the TRAM flap and its DIEP modification.

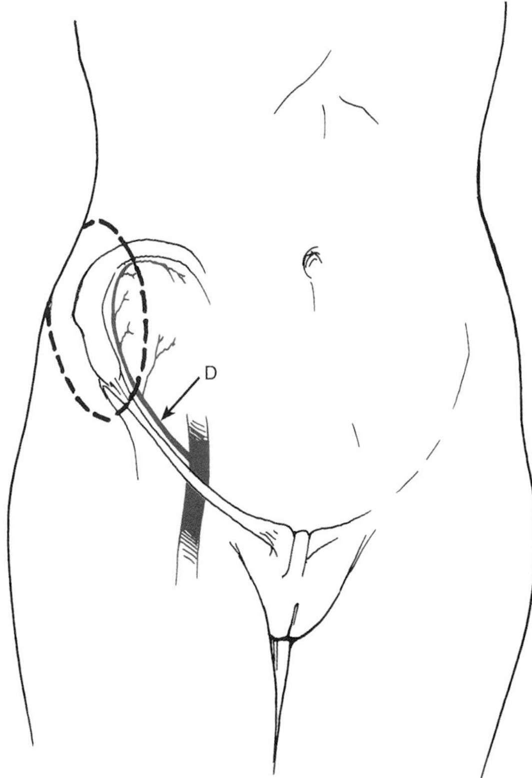

FIGURE 138-77. Vascular anatomy: deep circumflex iliac artery flap (DCIA flap, Rubens flap). (From Mathes SJ, Nahai F: Reconstructive Surgery: Principles, Anatomy, and Technique. New York, Churchill Livingstone, 1997:967.)

DEEP CIRCUMFLEX ILIAC ARTERY FLAP (DCIA FLAP, RUBENS FLAP)

An alternative donor site for composite tissue for breast reconstruction is the lateral inferior trunk immediately superior to the anterior iliac spine extending to the posterior iliac spine. In this region, the patient may have adequate subcutaneous tissue for design of a flap for autogenous breast reconstruction. In general, this flap, based on the deep circumflex iliac artery and its associated veins, is a more difficult flap to elevate, and donor site closure is less well disguised than with the rectus and gluteus maximus modified flaps for microvascular transplantation. For this reason, it is selected as an alternative donor site when the inferior abdomen and the gluteal region are unavailable or already used for prior breast reconstruction (Fig. 138-77).

Technique

The skin island is designed to incorporate the maximum volume of lower lateral abdominal and flank fat. It can extend well beyond the iliac crest onto the lower back. The initial groin incision is made, and the deep circumflex artery and associated venae comitantes are located. The pedicle is initially identified at its origin from the external iliac artery. The external oblique aponeurosis is divided, and the round ligament of the uterus or spermatic cord is retracted medially and upward to expose the DCIA and associated venae comitantes. At this stage, a cuff of internal oblique and transverse muscle may be included with the pedicle. The skin island incision is then completed, and the upper half of the island is dissected off the external oblique down to within 5 to 6 cm of the iliac crest. Here the upper half of the dissection extends through muscle, including the external oblique, internal oblique, and transverse muscles. This compound musculocutaneous flap contains perforating vessels into the overlying skin. These perforators are preserved, and muscle is dissected to the iliac crest below the course of the DCIA pedicle. The lower half is then elevated off the tensor fascia lata and gluteus medius to the lower border of the iliac crest and over the crest and down along the periosteum of the inner surface of the crest. Perforating osseous branches of the DCIA are divided during this part of the dissection. Laterally, the skin and fat beyond the iliac crest are elevated as a fasciocutaneous extension. The dissection is deep to the fascia up to the level of the iliac crest and then deep to the muscles as previously described. Final muscle flap elevation is completed by dissecting the muscles and pedicle off the inner surface of the iliac crest. The flap now based on the DCIA pedicle is ready for transplantation to the chest for coverage and breast reconstruction. Donor site closure requires approximation of the internal oblique, external oblique, and transverse muscles to the iliac crest (Fig. 138-78).

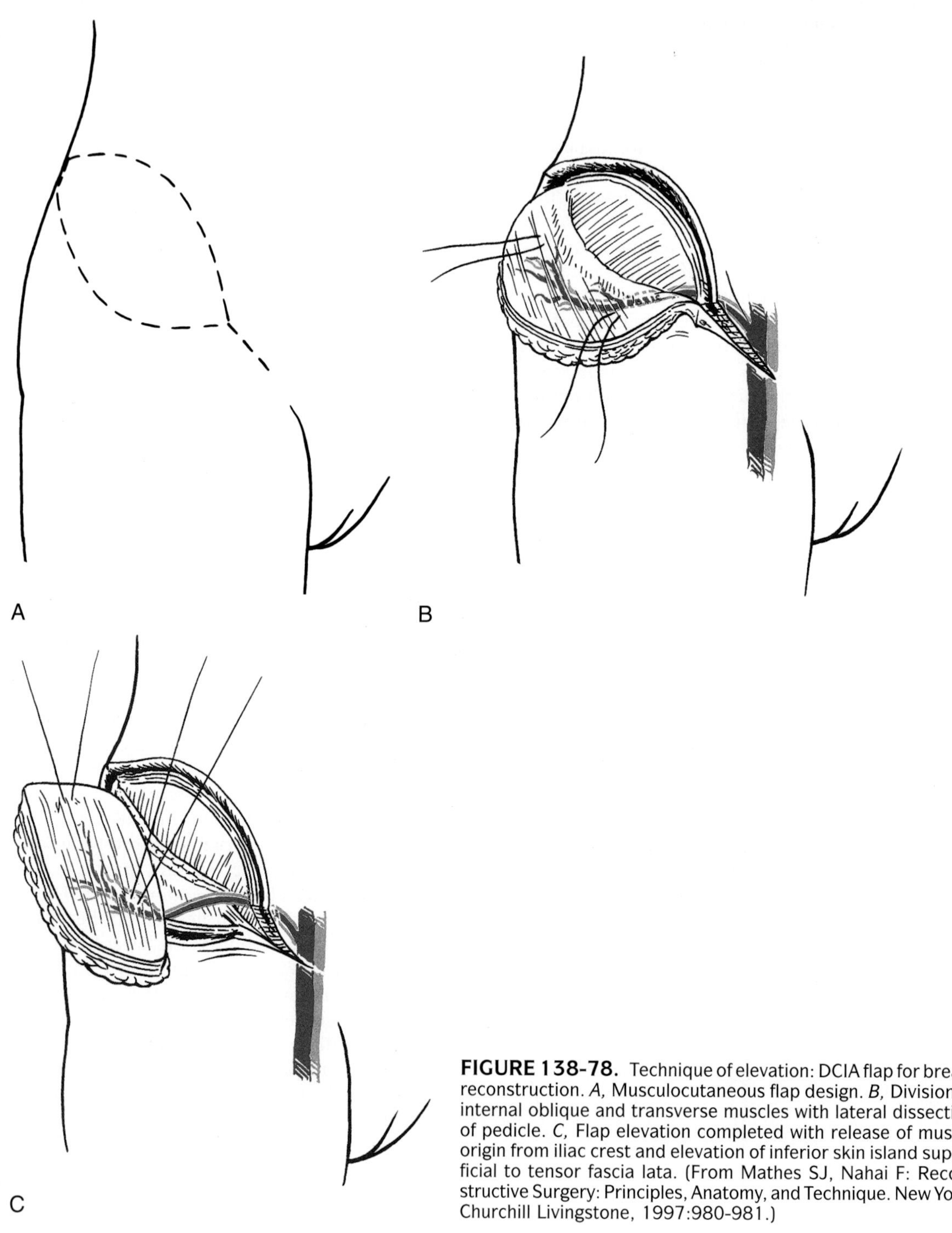

FIGURE 138-78. Technique of elevation: DCIA flap for breast reconstruction. *A,* Musculocutaneous flap design. *B,* Division of internal oblique and transverse muscles with lateral dissection of pedicle. *C,* Flap elevation completed with release of muscle origin from iliac crest and elevation of inferior skin island superficial to tensor fascia lata. (From Mathes SJ, Nahai F: Reconstructive Surgery: Principles, Anatomy, and Technique. New York, Churchill Livingstone, 1997:980-981.)

Complex Mastectomy Defect: Coverage and Delayed Reconstruction

Patients who present with inflammatory breast carcinoma or advanced invasive cancer may require a palliative mastectomy with both preoperative and postoperative chemotherapy and postoperative radiation therapy. The plastic surgeon may need to provide coverage because the large chest wall defect may not be suitable for skin graft coverage. Some of these patients may respond to chemotherapy and radiation therapy and eventually may be suitable candidates for breast reconstruction. Options for coverage of the large mastectomy defect include the thoracoepigastric flap, the latissimus dorsi musculocutaneous flap, and the rectus abdominis musculocutaneous flap with either a vertical or transverse (TRAM) skin island (Fig. 138-79). The thoracoepigastric flap (transverse abdominal flap) is a regional fasciocutaneous flap that will cover a large mastectomy defect with direct donor site closure. Located beneath the mastectomy site, this flap is available to the plastic surgeon if it is required, without altering the patient's position after the extensive mastectomy is completed. This type of mastectomy is generally classified as radical mastectomy because the invasive tumor usually has infiltrated into the pectoralis major muscle, requiring excision of both total breast parenchyma and underlying pectoralis major muscle. The use of the thoracoepigastric flap still preserves the territory of the rectus abdominis musculocutaneous flap and the latissimus dorsi musculocutaneous flap for future coverage if further tumor resection is required or if the patient has good treatment response and becomes a candidate for breast reconstruction. See the following section, "Thoracoepigastric (Transverse Abdominal) Flap."

If the patient is obese, it is preferable to use the rectus abdominis musculocutaneous flap with a vertical skin island. If the patient has an extensive defect from the tumor resection that extends across the sternum, the thoracoepigastric flap may not provide adequate coverage because of inadequate arc of rotation to central anterior chest defects. With a mastectomy defect that extends beyond the ipsilateral sternal edges medially and the anterior axillary line laterally, it is preferable to use the bilateral rectus abdominis musculocutaneous flap with a transverse skin island (bilateral TRAM flap) (Fig. 138-80). If the extensive defect extends into the axilla or midaxillary line laterally and to the sternal edge medially, a combined thoracoepigastric flap plus the latissimus dorsi musculocutaneous flap will provide adequate coverage. Previous sections describe the latissimus dorsi and the rectus abdominis musculocutaneous flaps in regard to design and technique of elevation.

THORACOEPIGASTRIC (TRANSVERSE ABDOMINAL) FLAP

The territory of the thoracoepigastric flap extends from the central abdomen to the lateral trunk. The midline of the abdomen denotes the flap base. The flap is located between the xiphoid process and midpoint between the xiphoid and umbilicus. The flap extends laterally to a point between the anterior axillary line and the midaxillary line. The flap has a width of 7 to 8 cm and extends from the midline to the anterior axillary line. The flap may be extended to the midaxillary line, although the extended flap may demonstrate inadequate circulation. The flap length ranges from 15 to 25 cm. The flap base is centered over the superior rectus musculocutaneous perforating vessels and vascular communications with the subcostal arteries and associated venae comitantes.

The flap is elevated with the patient in the supine position. It is helpful to place a beanbag or towels to

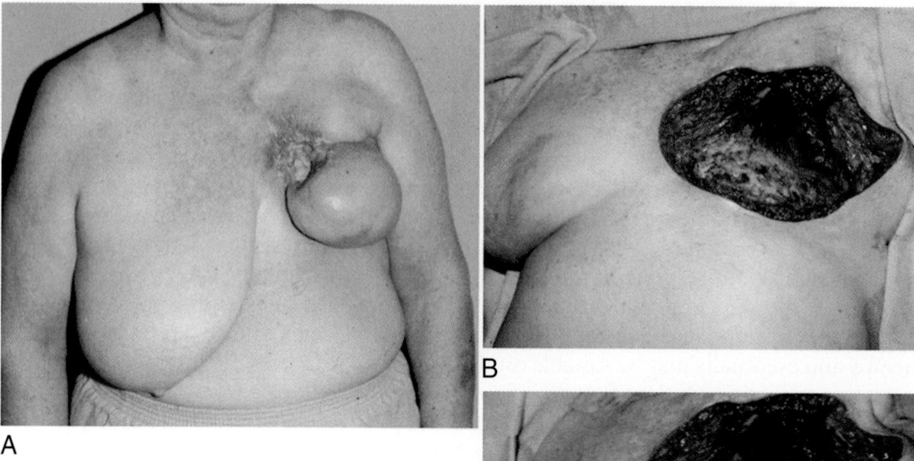

FIGURE 138-79. Complex mastectomy defect. *A,* Postoperative anterior view of lumpectomy and radiation therapy of left breast. The patient had recurrent breast cancer. *B,* Postoperative anterior view of completion of mastectomy. *C,* Design of contralateral rectus abdominis musculocutaneous flap for mastectomy defect coverage. Vertical skin island is selected because of obesity at TRAM donor site. *D,* Postoperative view 6 months after immediate chest coverage with rectus abdominis musculocutaneous flap. *E,* Postoperative lateral view. Flap provides stable coverage.

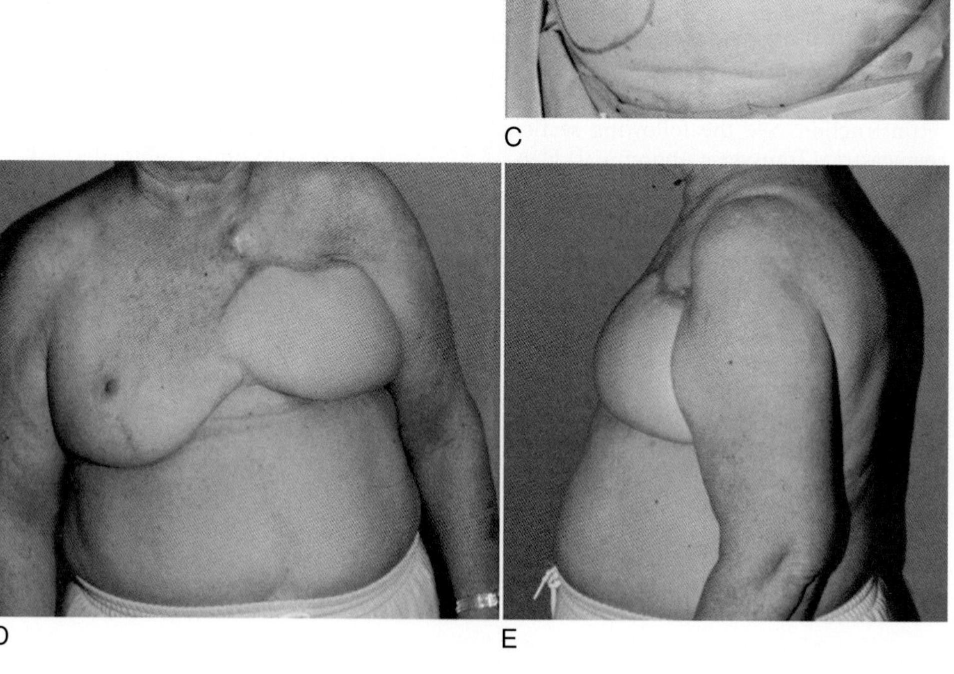

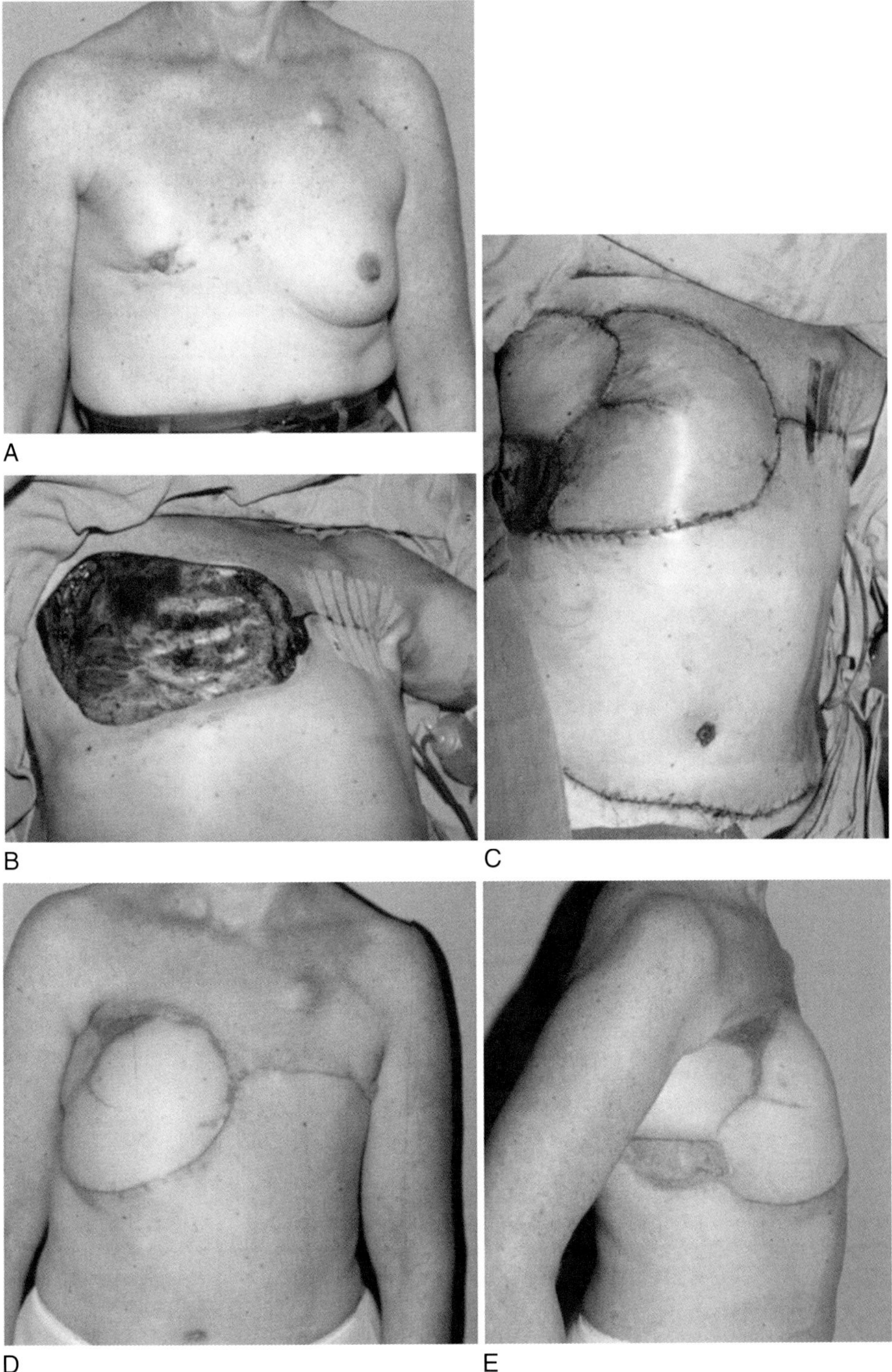

FIGURE 138-80. Complex mastectomy defect: bilateral rectus abdominis musculocutaneous flap with single skin island (TRAM) and ipsilateral latissimus dorsi musculocutaneous flap. *A,* Anterior view of advanced right breast carcinoma and left invasive breast carcinoma. *B,* Anterior view of palliative right mastectomy and left modified radical mastectomy. Right chest wall defect extends from left sternal edge to right medial axillary line. *C,* Immediate postoperative view of chest wall coverage with bilateral TRAM flap (single skin island and right latissimus dorsi musculocutaneous flap). *D,* Postoperative anterior view 3 months after bilateral TRAM flap and latissimus dorsi musculocutaneous flap. *E,* Postoperative lateral view demonstrates stable coverage for complex defect.

elevate the lateral posterior chest wall if the flap is extended to the midaxillary line. The ipsilateral arm is prepared in the field and covered with a stockinette. This allows arm movement to assist in donor site closure (Fig. 138-81).

The superior incision extends to the midpoint of the ipsilateral rectus abdominis muscle. The inferior incision is parallel to the superior incision extending to the midline of the abdomen. The skin outlines of the flap are incised to the level of the serratus anterior muscle laterally and external oblique fascia over the superior abdomen. The flap is then elevated by sharp dissection immediately superficial to the external oblique fascia. The flap is elevated to the lateral edge of the rectus sheath, and the inferior incision extends to the rectus sheath and midline fascia. Further dissection medial to the lateral edge of the rectus sheath is performed as required for adequate flap rotation, with care taken to avoid division of musculocutaneous perforating vessels over the central area of the rectus sheath. A back-cut may be required on the inferior incision to expedite flap rotation.

The flap cannot be extended beyond its initial design as a fasciocutaneous flap. However, it can be converted to a superiorly or inferiorly based rectus abdominis musculocutaneous flap. If the epigastric flap is converted to a superiorly based rectus abdominis musculocutaneous flap with a transverse skin island, the skin island will be too close to the muscle point of rotation at the costal margin, which is not an ideal flap design for a wide arc of rotation.

The flap is rotated 45 to 90 degrees in a superior direction for mastectomy site coverage. It is directly inset into the defect without use of a tunnel. A two-layered closure is performed incorporating the fascial and cutaneous layers of the flap.

Donor site closure is key to successful use of this flap. The skin of the anterior abdominal wall below the defect is undermined as required, advanced superiorly, and approximated to the superior edge of the donor site defect with heavy buried absorbable sutures (2-0 polyglycolic sutures). This maneuver relieves tension on the flap base and allows its advancement onto the chest wall. Direct donor site closure assists flap rotation and avoids a contour defect at the donor site (Fig. 138-82).

Most of these patients will not be candidates for breast reconstruction owing to problems with metastatic disease. However, the inflammatory breast cancer patients may have excellent response to chemotherapy and radiation therapy. If this type of patient wishes reconstruction, the plastic surgeon and the breast oncologist will have to review planned treatment protocols to be certain that efforts at reconstruction will not delay cancer treatment recommendations. In those patients approved by the breast cancer team including the plastic surgeon and surgical oncologist, planning for reconstruction is started. If the flap providing coverage is stable, it may be used to cover a tissue expander. If expansion is successful, a permanent implant can be inserted after a minimum of 3 months of tissue expansion (Fig. 138-83).

If the flap is not stable or is too tight for expansion, it is preferable to use a distant flap for autogenous reconstruction or with tissue expander with options to later provide a permanent implant. Because the patient has probably undergone an axillary lymph node dissection and received axillary radiation therapy, the latissimus may not be available as a safe flap. The rectus abdominis musculocutaneous flap (TRAM flap) represents the best option under these circumstances. The contralateral flap is used if standard transposition is planned because the ipsilateral internal mammary artery space would probably have been in the field of radiation therapy (Table 138-33).

TABLE 138-33 ✦ FLAP CHOICES FOR SPECIFIC DEFECT LOCATIONS

Flap	Defect		
	Central breast defect (between sternal edge and anterior axillary line)	Medial defect extension (between anterior axillary line and across sternum)	Lateral defect extension (between sternal edge and midaxillary line)
Thoracoepigastric flap	X		
TRAM flap (bilateral)		X	
Latissimus dorsi musculocutaneous flap			X
Combined		X	X

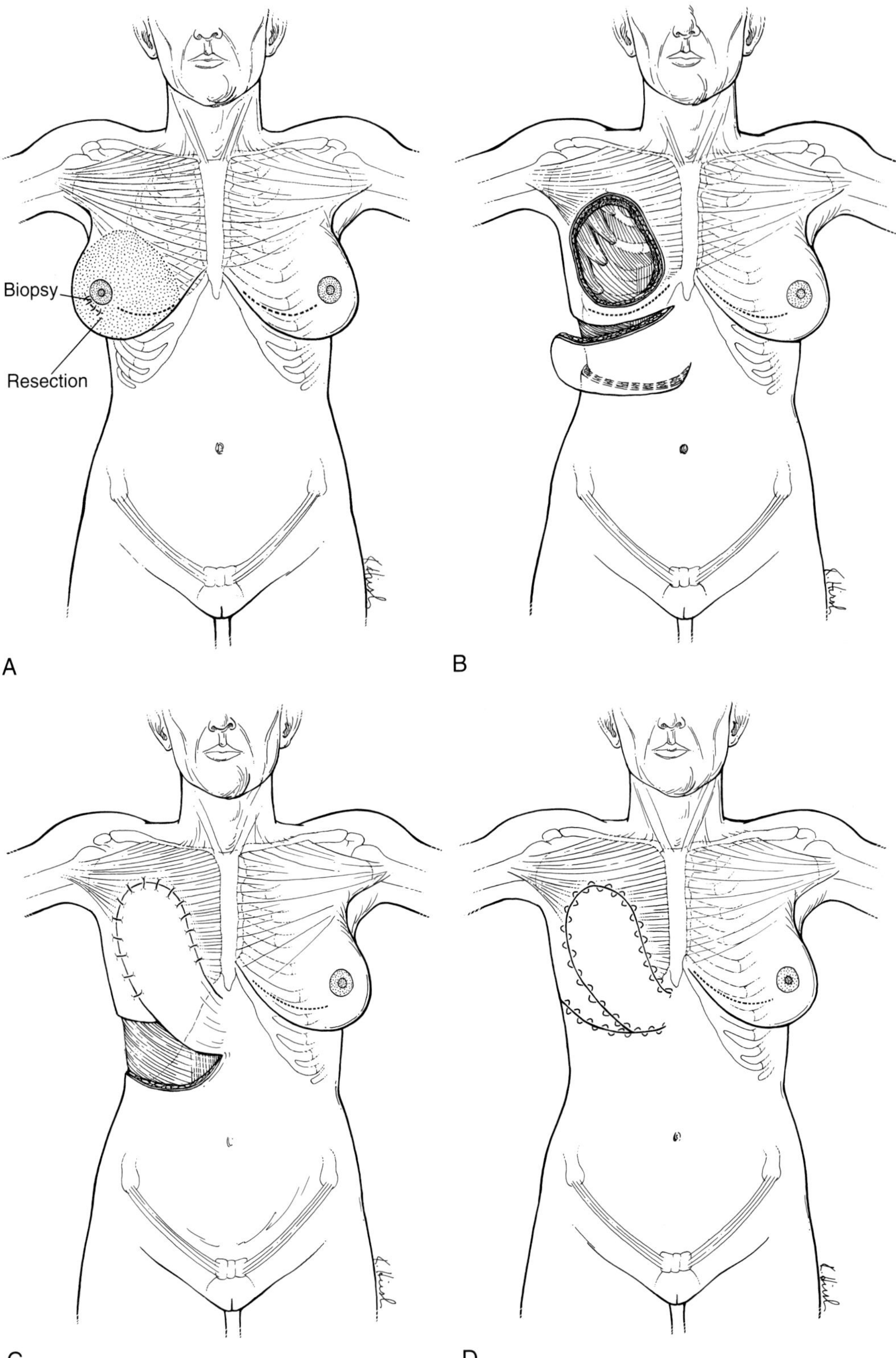

FIGURE 138-81. Thoracoepigastric (transverse abdominal) flap for coverage of complex mastectomy defects for advanced breast carcinoma. *A,* Stippled areas will be removed, including all breast tissue. *B,* Design of thoracoepigastric flap. Flap may extend to the midaxillary line. *C,* Flap inset into complex mastectomy defect. *D,* Abdominal flap advanced for donor site closure. (Also see Figure 138-81.)

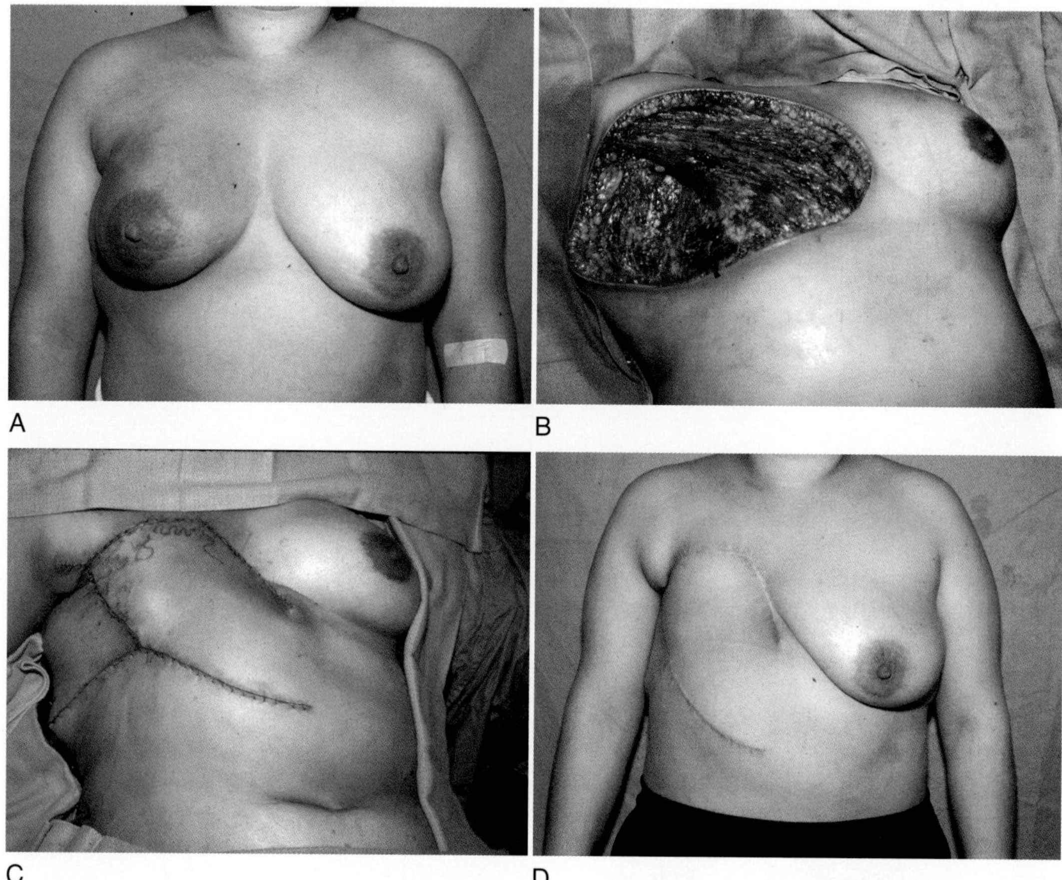

FIGURE 138-82. Complex mastectomy defect coverage: thoracoepigastric fasciocutaneous flap. *A,* Postoperative right lumpectomy and radiation therapy for recurrent right breast carcinoma. *B,* Mastectomy defect extends from sternum to anterior axillary line. *C,* Thoracoepigastric flap inset for defect coverage. *D,* Postoperative view at 6 months demonstrates stable coverage. (Also see Figure 138-83.)

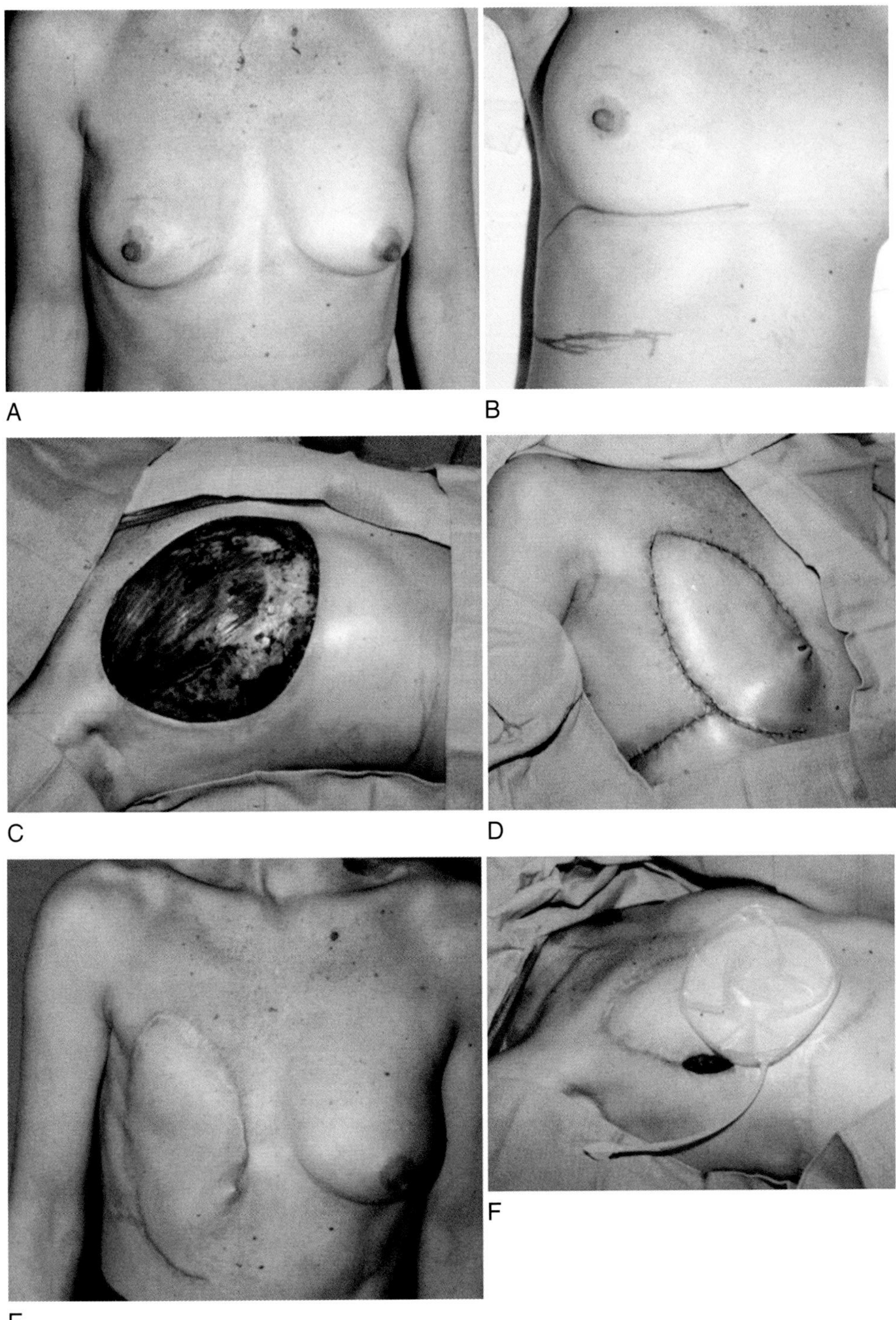

FIGURE 138-83. Complex mastectomy defect with flap coverage. *A,* Anterior view of right breast inflammatory carcinoma after neoadjuvant radiation therapy and chemotherapy. *B,* Preoperative design of thoracoepigastric flap for coverage of mastectomy defect. *C,* Intraoperative lateral view of complex mastectomy defect. *D,* Closure of defect with thoracoepigastric flap. *E,* Postoperative anterior view. Thoracoepigastric flap provided stable coverage of right breast defect. The patient demonstrates no recurrent or metastatic disease. *F,* Expander insertion for breast mound reconstruction to match contralateral breast. *Continued*

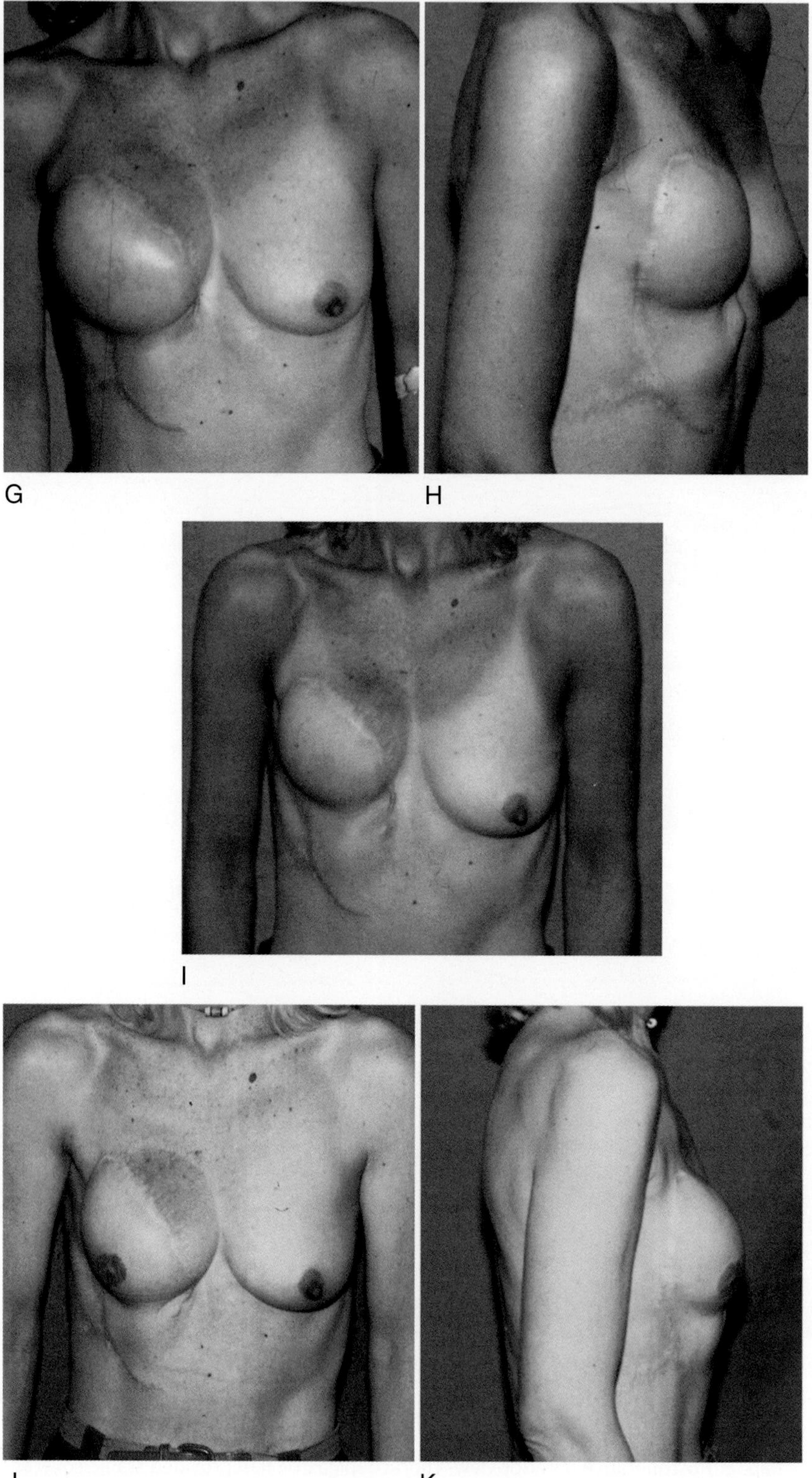

FIGURE 138-83, cont'd. *G* and *H,* Expansion in progress. *I,* Anterior view of completion of expander process at 3 months. *J,* Postoperative anterior view after permanent implant placement and nipple-areola complex reconstruction. *K,* Postoperative lateral view demonstrates adequate breast mound projection.

SUMMARY

Trends in Breast Cancer Management

Current trends in breast cancer management include improved diagnostic modalities; accurate noninvasive and minimally invasive histologic diagnostic modalities; predictors now available to define populations at high risk for breast cancer; advances in breast conservation techniques for treatment of invasive breast cancer; and advances in mastectomy techniques, including sentinel node biopsy and skin-sparing mastectomy. These advances allow earlier diagnosis and encourage women to seek consultation for breast surveillance and treatment if high-risk breast parenchymal changes or invasive breast cancers are detected. Multidisciplinary breast cancer management allows coordination of treatment modalities, including neoadjuvant radiation therapy and chemotherapy, endocrine therapy, and surgical therapy, to ensure optimal chance for cure and long-term palliation for local recurrence or systemic breast cancer. This chapter addresses these areas in the management of the breast cancer patient to inform the plastic surgeon of the rationale for diagnostic and therapeutic procedures and the effect these evolving procedures will have on outcome for the patient with breast cancer. With a thorough knowledge of these aspects of breast cancer management, the plastic surgeon will be able to advise the woman at risk or under treatment for breast cancer about the options for reconstruction with emphasis on timing, coordination of treatment efforts with the surgical oncologist, techniques, and quality of results.

Questions now facing the plastic surgeon in consultation with the patient include the following:

- What is the role of prophylactic mastectomy for the medium-risk patient, such as the patient with no genetic predisposition for breast cancer who develops breast cancer and now worries about the contralateral breast?
- With stage I breast cancer, will the patient decide on breast conservation techniques or skin-sparing mastectomy?
- When there is a chance that postoperative radiation therapy will be required, will reconstruction be immediate or delayed?
- When the skin envelope is largely preserved, does the patient desire expander-implant or autogenous reconstruction with a flap?
- Is the slightly increased risk of flap loss in microvascular composite tissue transplantation compared with standard flap transposition worth the potential benefits of muscle preservation at the donor site?
- If additional skin envelope is required, which is better, the TRAM or the latissimus dorsi?
- When there is breast deformity after lumpectomy and radiation therapy, is it better to elect completion mastectomy with reconstruction or to use flaps to correct the deformity, preserving the remaining breast tissue?
- If microvascular techniques are planned, should standard muscle flap with pedicle or perforator flap be selected?

Many of these questions and others that surface during the patient's consultation with the plastic surgeon have no one answer. The appropriate advice relates to the patient's tumor status, body configuration, physical status, and requirements; the surgeon's experience and skills; and above all, the patient's expectations. This chapter provides an overview of all reconstructive techniques and common indications for their use. Subsequent chapters will further address all reconstructive options with emphasis on indications, contraindications, techniques, advances, and outcomes.

Selection of Techniques for Breast Reconstruction

Recommendation for reconstructive techniques can be based on timing of the reconstruction, skills and outcomes of the surgical oncologist, mastectomy technique selected, plans and timing for adjuvant treatment, physical status and age of the patient, skills and outcomes of the plastic surgeon, contralateral breast status, and expectations of the patient. All these variables will influence the safety and quality of the reconstruction and need to be considered in advising the patient about the choices for reconstruction and recommendations by the plastic surgeon. Working as part of a team in breast care will certainly help answer these questions. The surgical oncologist and plastic surgeon can coordinate their evaluation and decision in regard to diagnosis, treatment, and reconstruction when appropriate.

TIMING OF RECONSTRUCTION

For immediate reconstruction, both expander-implant and flap use are appropriate, depending on extent of skin resection, expertise of the plastic surgeon, and expectations of the patient. If skin preservation mastectomy or modified radical mastectomy is planned, the expander-implant option is available. The postoperative recovery is quick, allowing the patient's rapid return to preexisting lifestyle activities. If the surgical oncologist's outcomes have increased risk for skin loss in a preserved skin envelope, it may be preferable to use an autogenous flap for breast reconstruction. If the patient desires autogenous reconstruction, the rectus abdominis musculocutaneous flap (TRAM), as either a transposition flap or a free flap (DIEA or TRAM–segmental rectus), should be considered.

MASTECTOMY TECHNIQUE

For skin-sparing mastectomy, the surgeon may select either expander-implant or autogenous reconstruction with TRAM or free flap (DIEA or TRAM–segmental rectus). If a patient has prior irradiation (recurrence after lumpectomy and irradiation), the use of an expander-implant is high risk for exposure and failure. Either flap transposition or transplantation should be selected. For an extensive defect, the surgeon should consider wound closure and delayed reconstruction because this type of patient usually has a larger tumor and will require adjuvant treatment. If primary closure is not feasible, the patient is a candidate for TRAM, latissimus dorsi, or thoracoepigastric flap.

PLANS AND TIMING FOR ADJUVANT TREATMENT

If the patient is scheduled for radiation therapy after mastectomy, there is an increased risk of local complications for both implant-expander and flap. Unfortunately, the decision for radiation therapy is often not made until the pathologist's final report becomes available. If the mastectomy site will require irradiation and an expander-implant is selected, this type of reconstruction must have an expander in place before the radiation therapy is started. When the radiation therapy is completed, the plastic surgeon can replace the expander with a permanent implant. Local problems including capsular contracture will be increased and future revisions may become necessary. If a flap is selected, most patients now will by preference want the flap in place after the mastectomy is completed. However, delay in reconstruction when a flap is planned will avoid increased risk of fat necrosis and shrinkage with postponement until radiation therapy is completed. Many patients in this category are unsure of reconstruction because their initial focus is breast cancer survival. In these patients, delay in reconstruction allows family to concentrate on optimal breast cancer treatment. When treatment of the cancer is completed, the patient and family can begin to plan breast reconstruction.

CONTRALATERAL BREAST

Many options are available to the breast cancer patient related to the opposite breast. If the patient is at high risk for bilateral breast cancer because of the tumor's pathologic characteristics, family history, or genetic predisposition, a prophylactic mastectomy may be advisable. With the bilateral surgery planned, the reconstructive surgery options will change. This type of patient may prefer an expander-implant to avoid bilateral flaps. With skin-sparing mastectomy and emphasis on autogenous reconstruction, selection of the patient may dictate bilateral TRAM transposition flaps or bilateral microvascular composite tissue transplantation (DIEA or TRAM–segmental rectus). If the patient has a large or pendulous opposite breast, symmetry is unlikely if an expander-implant is selected. However, if the patient desires reduction or mastopexy for the contralateral breast, symmetry can be achieved with the simpler technique of an expander-implant on the mastectomy side. If the patient wants the opposite breast matched, the optimal choice will be either latissimus dorsi musculocutaneous flap with implant or autogenous reconstruction with TRAM or DIEA flap.

PLASTIC SURGEON'S SKILLS AND EXPERIENCE

Many patients have made up their minds as to what technique they expect for breast reconstruction. The plastic surgeon should describe all techniques to every patient and then report which techniques would most likely fulfill the patient's expectations and accomplish the reconstruction with minimal risk and optimal outcome in regard to quality of result. If the technique proposed by the patient is not performed by the plastic surgeon, the patient should be referred to an appropriate colleague or center. If equal or superior results can be accomplished by alternative techniques, the patient should receive this information. It is possible that the patient may prefer the surgeon and not pursue the preconceived idea of the best technique for reconstruction.

EXPECTATION

The patient should express her goals for breast reconstruction in regard to timing, complexity of technique, contralateral breast symmetry, work and family schedules, and physical activities. Many patients are unwilling to miss work or family obligations and seek breast reconstruction with minimal potential morbidity. With the expander-implant option, the patient can be home quickly and return to normal routine earlier than when a flap is used. Other patients are committed to the most natural reconstruction with use of autogenous tissue and will accept a more complex technique to reach this goal. This patient is likely to prefer the TRAM flap or microvascular transplantation of the segmental TRAM or the DIEP flap. Certain patients are committed to special activities or sports for which certain muscles are important. For instance, the patient may be reluctant to have the latissimus dorsi or rectus muscle used as a flap. Fortunately, many studies have documented no loss of function when these muscles are used because of synergistic activity of adjacent musculature. Nevertheless, multiple options are now available for breast reconstruction, so the plastic surgeon may offer options that should satisfy most realistic expectations of patients.

The goal of breast reconstruction is restoration of form and function with safety. Fortunately, the plastic surgeon has local, regional, and distant options to accomplish breast reconstruction. The future will include continued efforts to improve both the expander and permanent implant design. With the identification of regional and distant flaps, breast reconstruction may be accomplished without an implant as an autogenous reconstruction, or the flap may be used to restore the skin envelope in combination with an implant to provide symmetry with the opposite breast. Modifications in mastectomy technique including skin-sparing techniques allow the plastic surgeon to concentrate on breast mound size and projection to minimize the deformity related to mastectomy. Now the reconstructed breast mound with intact original skin envelope may be preferable to scarring associated with breast-conserving mastectomy. The process of detection and treatment of breast cancer is evolving with continual improvements in diagnosis, treatment, and reconstruction.

REFERENCES

1. American Cancer Society: Breast Cancer Facts and Figures 2001-2002. American Cancer Society Department of Epidemiology and Surveillance Research, 2002.
2. Racial/Ethnic Patterns of Breast Cancer in the United States. National Cancer Institute Web publication, 2002.
3. Kern K: Diagnostic options in symptomatic breast disease. In Cameron JL: Current Surgical Therapy, 7th ed. St Louis, Mosby, 2001:678-686.
4. Grainger RG, Allison DJ: Grainger and Allison's Diagnostic Radiology: A Textbook of Medical Imaging, 4th ed. New York, Churchill Livingstone, 2001.
5. Gajdos S, et al: Mammographic appearance of nonpalpable breast cancer reflects pathologic characteristics. Ann Surg 2002;235:246-251.
6. Giess CS, et al: Comparison of rate of development and rate of change for benign and malignant breast calcifications at the lumpectomy bed. AJR Am J Roentgenol 2000;175:789-793.
7. Morrow M: When can stereotactic core biopsy replace excisional biopsy? A clinical perspective. Breast Cancer Res Treat 1995;36:1-9.
8. Cady B, et al: The new era in breast cancer. Invasion, size, and nodal involvement dramatically decreasing as a result of mammographic screening. Arch Surg 1996;131:301-308.
9. Yankaskas BC, et al: Reassessment of breast cancers missed during routine screening mammography: a community-based study. AJR Am J Roentgenol 2001;177:535-541.
10. Baker LH, et al: Breast Cancer Detection Demonstration Project: five-year summary report. CA Cancer J Clin 1982;32:194-225.
11. Skinner KA, et al: Palpable breast cancers are inherently different from nonpalpable breast cancers. Ann Surg Oncol 2001;8:705-710.
12. Tafra L, et al: Nonpalpable versus palpable invasive breast tumors treated with breast-conserving surgical management. Am Surg 1996;62:395-399.
13. Brownlee S: Search and destroy: Why mammograms are not the answer. The New Republic Online, April 2002.
14. Nystrom L, et al: Breast cancer screening with mammography. Overview of the Swedish randomized trials. Lancet 1993;341:973-978.
15. Tabar L, et al: Beyond randomized controlled trials: organized mammographic screening substantially reduces breast carcinoma mortality. Cancer 2001;91:1724-1731.
16. Wojcik BE, et al: Effects of screening mammography on the comparative survival rates of African American, white, and Hispanic beneficiaries of a comprehensive health care system. Breast J 2003;9:175-183.
17. Flobbe K: The role of ultrasonography as an adjunct to mammography in the detection of breast cancer: a systemic review. Eur J Cancer 2002;38:1044-1050.
18. Kopans DB: Breast-cancer screening with ultrasonography. Lancet 1999;354:2096-2097.
19. Tardivon AA: Imaging and management of nonpalpable lesions of the breast. Eur J Radiol 2002;42:2-9.
20. Syllabus of the American College of Surgeons: Skills-Oriented Postgraduate Course in Breast Ultrasound, April 12-15, 2003:52.
21. Stavros AT, et al: Solid breast nodules: use of sonography to distinguish between benign and malignant lesions. Radiology 1995;196:123-134.
22. Boetes C: Breast tumors: comparative accuracy of MR imaging relative to mammography and US for demonstrating extent. Radiology 1995;197:33-42.
23. Rodenko GN, et al: MR imaging in the management before surgery of lobular carcinoma of the breast: correlation with pathology. AJR Am J Roentgenol 1996;167:1415-1419.
24. Orel SG, et al: Breast MR imaging in patients with axillary node metastases and unknown primary malignancy. Radiology 1999;212:543-549.
25. Azavedo E, et al: Imaging breasts with silicone implants. Eur Radiol 1999;9:349-355.
26. Eklund GW, et al: Improved imaging of the augmented breast. AJR Am J Roentgenol 1988;151:469.
27. Deapen D, et al: Breast cancer stage at diagnosis and survival among patients with prior breast implants. Plast Reconstr Surg 2000;105:535-540.
28. Cahan A, et al: Breast cancer after breast augmentation with silicone implants. Ann Surg Oncol 1995;2:121-125.
29. Holmich LR, et al: State of breast cancer at diagnosis among women with cosmetic breast implants. Br J Cancer 2003;88:832.
30. Miglioretti DL, Rutter CM, Geller BM, et al: Effect of breast augmentation on the accuracy of mammography and cancer characteristics. JAMA 2004;291:442.
31. O'Toole M, Caskey CI: Imaging spectrum of breast implant complications: mammography, ultrasound, and magnetic resonance imaging. Semin Ultrasound CT MR 2000;21:351-361.
32. DeBruhl ND: Sonographic evaluation of silicone breast implants. Radiology 1993;189:95.
33. Gorczyca DP, et al: Silicone breast implants in vivo: MR imaging. Radiology 1992;185:407-410.

34. Ahn CY, et al: Comparative silicone breast implant evaluation using mammography, sonography, and magnetic resonance imaging: experience with 59 implants. Plast Reconstr Surg 1994;94:620-627.
35. Esserman LJ: Imaging, diagnosis, and biopsy of breast lesions. The UCSF Postgraduate Course in General Surgery, 2002:441-444.
36. Goodson WH, et al: Causes of physician delay in the diagnosis of breast cancer. Arch Intern Med 2002;162:1343-1348.
37. Meunier M, et al: Fine needle aspiration cytology versus percutaneous biopsy of nonpalpable breast lesions. Eur J Radiol 2002;42:10-16.
38. The uniform approach to breast fine needle aspiration biopsy. The final version. Breast J 1997;3:148-168.
39. Mitnick JS, et al: The clinical significance of cytologic atypia in stereotactic fine needle aspiration biopsies of mammogram-detected breast lesions. Radiology 1996;198:319-322.
40. Collaco LM, et al: Value of fine needle aspiration in the diagnosis of breast lesions. Acta Cytol 1999;43:587-592.
41. Pijnappel RM, et al: Diagnostic strategies in non-palpable breast lesions. Eur J Cancer 2002;38:550-555.
42. Ljung BM: Diagnostic accuracy of fine-needle aspiration biopsy is determined by physician training in sampling technique. Cancer 2001;93:263-268.
43. McIlhenny C: Optimum number of core biopsies for accurate assessment of histological grade in breast cancer. Br J Surg 2002;89:84-85.
44. Corn CC: SiteSelect: minimally invasive excision of breast lesions. Breast J 2001;7:427-429.
45. Simon JR, et al: Accuracy and complication rates of US-guided vacuum-assisted core breast biopsy: initial results. Radiology 2000;215:694-697.
46. Burton A: FISHy decisions in breast cancer treatment choice. Lancet Oncol 2001;2:654.
47. King TA, et al: Biopsy technique has no impact on local recurrence after breast-conserving therapy. Breast J 2001;7:19-24.
48. Youngson BJ, et al: Displacement of carcinomatous epithelium in surgical breast specimens following stereotaxic core biopsy. Am J Clin Pathol 1995;103:598-602.
49. Chao C, et al: Local recurrence of breast cancer in the stereotactic core needle biopsy site: case reports and review of the literature. Breast J 2001;7:124-127.
50. Yim JH, et al: Mammographically detected breast cancer. Benefits of stereotactic core versus wire localization biopsy. Ann Surg 1996;223:688-697, discussion 697-700.
51. Mroz CT: Needlewire localized excisional breast biopsy. Operative Techniques Gen Surg 2000;2:96-103.
52. Brem RF, et al: Atypical ductal hyperplasia: histologic underestimation of carcinoma in tissue harvested from impalpable breast lesions using 11-gauge stereotactically guided directional vacuum-assisted biopsy. AJR Am J Roentgenol 1999;172:1405-1407.
53. Jacobs TW, et al: Radial scars in benign breast-biopsy specimens and the risk of breast cancer. N Engl J Med 1999;340:430-436.
54. Frouge C, et al: Mammographic lesions suggestive of radial scars: microscopic findings in 40 cases. Radiology 1995;195:623-625.
55. Sakorafa GH: Nipple discharge: current diagnostic and therapeutic approaches. Cancer Treat Rev 2001;27:275-282.
56. Johnson JE, et al: Recurrent mammary carcinoma after local excision: a segmental problem. Cancer 1995;75:1612-1618.
57. Singletary SE: New approaches to surgery for breast cancer. Endocr Relat Cancer 2001;8:265-286.
58. Dooley WC, et al: Detection of premalignant and malignant breast cells by ductal lavage. Obstet Gynecol 2001;97(suppl 1):S2.
59. Morrow M, et al: Evaluation and management of the woman with an abnormal ductal lavage. J Am Coll Surg 2002;94:648-656.
60. Klein P, et al: Biomarker assays in nipple aspiration fluid. Breast J 2001;6:378-387.
61. Benson JR, et al: The TNM staging system and breast cancer. Lancet Oncol 2003;4:56-57.
62. Fisher B, et al: Eight-year results of a randomized clinical trial comparing total mastectomy and lumpectomy with or without irradiation in the treatment of breast cancer. N Engl J Med 1989;320:822-828.
63. Staradub VL, et al: Modified radical mastectomy. Operative Techniques Gen Surg 2000;2:118-126.
64. Winchester DP, et al: Standards for breast-conservation treatment. CA Cancer J Clin 1992;42:134-176.
65. Morrow M, et al: Factors predicting the use of breast-conserving therapy in stage I and II breast carcinoma. J Clin Oncol 2001;19:2254-2262.
66. Veronesi U, et al: Breast conservation is the treatment of choice in small breast cancer: long-term results of a randomized trial. Eur J Can 1990;26:668-670.
67. Sarrazin D, et al: Ten-year results of a randomized trial comparing a conservative treatment to mastectomy in early breast cancer. Radiother Oncol 1989;14:177-184.
68. Jacobson JA, et al: Ten-year results of a comparison of conservation with mastectomy in the treatment of stage I and II breast cancer. N Engl J Med 1995;332:907-911.
69. The Steering Committee on Clinical Practice Guidelines for the Care and Treatment of Breast Cancer: Mastectomy or lumpectomy? The choice of operation for clinical stages I and II breast cancer. CMAJ 1998;158(suppl):S15-S21.
70. Doughty JC: Lumpectomy for malignant disease. Operative Techniques Gen Surg 2000;2:127-131.
71. Arriagada R, et al: Predictive factors for local recurrence in 2006 patients with surgically resected small breast cancer. Ann Oncol 2002;13:1404-1413.
72. Cox CE, et al: Breast biopsy for benign disease. Operative Techniques Gen Surg 2000;2:86-95.
73. Veronesi U, et al: Quadrantectomy for malignant disease. Operative Techniques Gen Surg 2000;2:132-136.
74. Veronesi U, et al: Conservative treatment of breast cancer. Cancer 1977;39:2822-2826.
75. Veronesi U, et al: Comparing radical mastectomy with quadrantectomy, axillary dissection, and radiotherapy in patients with small cancers of the breast. N Engl J Med 1981;305:6-11.
76. Haagensen CD: Diseases of the Breast, 2nd ed. Philadelphia, WB Saunders, 1971:16-17.
77. Temple WJ, et al: Technical considerations for prophylactic mastectomy in patients at high risk for breast cancer. Am J Surg 1991;161:413-415.
78. Yugueros P, et al: Current concepts and techniques in subcutaneous mastectomy. Operative Techniques Gen Surg 2000;2:110-117.
79. Hermanek P, et al: TNM Atlas: Illustrated Guide to the TNM/pTNM Classification of Malignant Tumors, 4th ed. Berlin, Springer-Verlag, 1997:201-212.
80. Hoda RS, et al: Microinvasive carcinoma of the breast—a commonly misdiagnosed entity. Arch Pathol Lab Med 2001;125:1259-1260.
81. Goldman LD, Goldwyn RM: Some anatomical considerations of subcutaneous mastectomy. Plast Reconstr Surg 1977;51:501-505.
82. Eisen A, et al: Prophylactic surgery in women with a hereditary predisposition to breast and ovarian cancer. J Clin Oncol 2000;18:1980-1995.
83. Palmer BV, et al: Subcutaneous mastectomy with immediate reconstruction as treatment for early breast cancer. Br J Surg 1992;79:1309-1311.

84. Georgiade N, et al: Subcutaneous mastectomy: an evolution of concept and technique. Ann Plast Surg 1982;8:8-19.
85. Jarrett JR, et al: Aesthetic refinements in prophylactic subcutaneous mastectomy with submuscular reconstruction. Plast Reconstr Surg 1982;69:624-631.
86. Woods JE: Detailed technique of subcutaneous mastectomy with and without mastopexy. Ann Plast Surg 1987;18:51-61.
87. Chen TH: Silicone injection granulomas of the breast: treatment by subcutaneous mastectomy and immediate subpectoral breast implant. Br J Plast Surg 1995;48:71-76.
88. Cheung KL, et al: Subcutaneous mastectomy for primary breast cancer and ductal carcinoma in situ. Eur J Surg Oncol 1997; 23:343-347.
89. Al-Ghazal SK, et al: Subcutaneous mastectomy with implant reconstruction: cosmetic outcome and patient satisfaction. Eur J Surg Oncol 2000;26:137-141.
90. Ward DC, Edwards MH: Early results of subcutaneous mastectomy with immediate silicone prosthetic implant for carcinoma of the breast. Br J Surg 1983;70:651-653.
91. Capozzi A: Long-term complication of polyurethane-covered breast implants. Plast Reconstr Surg 1987;88:458-461.
92. Holzgreve W, Beller FK: Surgical complications and follow-up evaluation of 163 patients with subcutaneous mastectomy. Aesthetic Plast Surg 1987;11:45-48.
93. Sufi PA: Envelope mastectomy with immediate reconstruction (EMIR). Eur J Surg Oncol 2000;26:367-370.
94. Baker RR: The management of breast cancer with immediate or delayed reconstruction. Adv Surg 1992;25:51-64.
95. Singletary SE, et al: Skin-sparing mastectomy with immediate breast reconstruction. Operative Techniques Gen Surg 2000;2:137-151.
96. Simmons RM: Skin-sparing mastectomies. Am J Surg 2000; 180:290-293.
97. Slavin SA, et al: Skin-sparing mastectomy and immediate reconstruction: oncologic risks and aesthetic results in patients with early-stage breast cancer. Plast Reconstr Surg 1998;102: 49-62.
98. Toth BA, et al: Modified skin incision for mastectomy: the need for plastic surgical input in preoperative planning. Plast Reconstr Surg 1991;87:1048-1053.
99. Simmons RM, et al: Local and distant recurrence rates in skin-sparing mastectomies compared with non–skin-sparing mastectomies. Ann Surg Oncol 1999;6:676-681.
100. Kroll SS, et al: Local recurrence risk after skin-sparing and conventional mastectomy: a 6-year follow-up. Plast Reconstr Surg 1999;104:421-425.
101. Carlson GW, et al: Skin-sparing mastectomy, oncologic and reconstructive considerations. Ann Surg 1998;225:570-578.
102. Newman LA, et al: Presentation, treatment, and outcome of local recurrence after skin-sparing mastectomy and immediate breast reconstruction. Ann Surg Oncol 1998;5: 620-626.
103. Medina-Franco H, et al: Factors associated with local recurrence after skin-sparing mastectomy and immediate breast reconstruction for invasive breast cancer. Ann Surg 2002;6:814-819.
104. Gilliland MD, et al: The implications of local recurrence of breast cancer as the first site of therapeutic failure. Ann Surg 1983;197:284-287.
105. Willner J, et al: Locoregional recurrence of breast cancer following mastectomy: always a fatal event? Results of a univariate and multivariate analysis. Int J Radiat Oncol Biol Phys 1997;37:853-863.
106. Andry G, et al: Locoregional recurrences after 649 modified radical mastectomies: incidence and significance. Eur J Surg Oncol 1989;15:476-485.
107. Carlson GW: Local recurrence after skin-sparing mastectomy: a manifestation of tumor biology or surgical conservatism? Ann Surg Oncol 1998;5:571-572.
108. Danforth DN: Comments on skin-sparing mastectomy and immediate breast reconstruction: a critical analysis of local recurrence. Cancer J 2000;6:285-286.
109. Rivadeneira DE, et al: Skin-sparing mastectomy with immediate breast reconstruction: a critical analysis of local recurrence. Cancer J 2000;6:331-335.
110. Foster RD, et al: Skin-sparing mastectomy and immediate breast reconstruction: a prospective cohort study for the treatment of advanced stages of breast carcinoma. Ann Surg Oncol 2002;9:462-466.
111. Society of Surgical Oncology: SSO develops position statement on prophylactic mastectomy. SSO News Summer 1993; 1:10.
112. Anderson BO: Prophylactic surgery to reduce breast cancer risk: a brief literature review. Breast J 2001;7:321-330.
113. Schrag D, et al: Decision analysis—effects of prophylactic mastectomy and oophorectomy on life expectancy among women with BRCA1 or BRCA2 mutations. N Engl J Med 1997; 336:1465-1571.
114. Verhoog LC, et al: Contralateral breast cancer risk is influenced by the age at onset in BRCA1-associated breast cancer. Br J Cancer 2000;83:384-386.
115. Hartmann LC, et al: Efficacy of bilateral prophylactic mastectomy in women with a family history of breast cancer. N Engl J Med 1999;340:77-83.
116. Gershenwald JE, et al: Synchronous elective contralateral mastectomy and immediate bilateral breast reconstruction in women with early-stage breast cancer. Ann Surg Oncol 1998;5:529-538.
117. Morrow M, et al: Factors responsible for the under-utilization of breast-conserving therapy. Proc Am Soc Clin Oncol 1998;17:98a.
118. Guadagnoli E, et al: Use of breast-conserving surgery for treatment of stage I and stage II breast cancer. J Clin Oncol 1998;16:101-106.
119. Staradub VL, et al: Modified radical mastectomy. Operative Techniques Gen Surg 2000;2:118-126.
120. Fisher B, et al: Twenty-five year follow-up of a randomized trial comparing radical mastectomy, total mastectomy, and total mastectomy followed by irradiation. N Engl J Med 2002; 347:567-574.
121. Fisher B, et al: Reanalysis and results after 12 years of follow-up in a randomized clinical trial comparing total mastectomy with lumpectomy with or without irradiation in the treatment of breast cancer. N Engl J Med 1995;333:1456.
122. Jensen J: When can the nipple-areola complex safely be spared during mastectomy? Plast Reconstr Surg 2002;109:805-807.
123. Laronga C, et al: The incidence of occult nipple-areola complex involvement in breast cancer patients receiving a skin-sparing mastectomy. Ann Surg Oncol 1999;6:609-613.
124. Lagios MD, et al: A guide to the frequency of nipple involvement in breast cancer. A study of 149 consecutive mastectomies using a serial subgross and correlated radiographic technique. Am J Surg 1979;138:135-142.
125. Santini D, et al: Neoplastic involvement of nipple-areolar complex in invasive breast cancer. Am J Surg 1989;158:399-403.
126. Morimoto T, et al: Involvement of nipple and areola in early breast cancer. Cancer 1985;55:2459-2463.
127. Simmons RM, et al: Analysis of nipple/areolar involvement with mastectomy: can the areola be preserved? Ann Surg Oncol 2002;9:165-168.
128. Cense HA, et al: Nipple-sparing mastectomy in breast cancer: a viable option? Eur J Surg Oncol 2001;27:521-526.
129. Eldar S, et al: Cancer of the breast after prophylactic subcutaneous mastectomy. Am J Surg 1984;148:692-693.
130. Willemsen HW, et al: Breast carcinoma in residual breast tissue after prophylactic bilateral subcutaneous mastectomy. Eur J Surg Oncol 1998;24:331-332.

131. Rosen PP, et al: A long-term follow-up study of survival in stage I (T1N0M0) and stage II (T1N1M0) breast carcinoma. J Clin Oncol 1989;7:355-366.
132. Leong SP, et al: Multidisciplinary approach to selective sentinel lymph node mapping in breast cancer. Breast Cancer 2000;7:105-113.
133. Schwartz GF, et al: Proceedings of the consensus conference on the role of sentinel lymph node biopsy in carcinoma of the breast, April 19-22, 2001, Philadelphia, PA, USA. Breast J 2002;8:126-138.
134. Cady B: Consensus on sentinel node biopsy. Breast J 2002;8:123-125.
135. Stearns V, et al: Sentinel lymphadenectomy after neoadjuvant chemotherapy for breast cancer may reliably represent the axilla except for inflammatory breast cancer. Ann Surg Oncol 2002;9:235-242.
136. Nason K, et al: Increased false negative sentinel node biopsy rates after preoperative chemotherapy for invasive breast carcinoma. Cancer 2000;89:2187-2194.
137. Mamounas E, et al: Accuracy of sentinel node biopsy after neoadjuvant chemotherapy in breast cancer: updated results from the NSABP B-27 [abstract]. Proc Am Soc Clin Oncol 2002;21:36a.
138. Mamounas E: Sentinel lymph node biopsy after neoadjuvant systemic therapy. Surg Clin North Am 2003;83:931-942.
139. Singletary SE, et al: Classification of isolated tumor cells: clarification of the 6th edition of the American Joint Committee on Cancer Staging Manual. Cancer 2003;98: 2740-2741.
140. Weiser MR, et al: Is routine intraoperative frozen-section examination of sentinel lymph nodes in breast cancer worthwhile? Ann Surg Oncol 2000;7:651-655.
141. Menes TS, et al: Touch preparation or frozen section for intraoperative detection of sentinel lymph node metastases from breast cancer. Ann Surg Oncol 2003;10:1166-1170.
142. Van Diest PJ, et al: Reliability of intraoperative frozen section and imprint cytological investigation of sentinel lymph nodes in breast cancer. Histopathology 1999;35:14-18.
143. Noguchi M: Sentinel lymph node biopsy and breast cancer. Br J Surg 2002;89:21-34.
144. Hill AD, et al: Lessons learned from 500 cases of lymphatic mapping for breast cancer. Ann Surg 1999;229:528-535.
145. Nano MT: Clinical impact of false-negative sentinel node biopsy in primary breast cancer. Br J Surg 2002;89:1430-1434.
146. Giuliano AE, et al: Prospective observational study of sentinel lymphadenectomy without further axillary dissection in patients with sentinel node-negative breast cancer. J Clin Oncol 2000;18:2553-2559.
147. Motomura K, et al: Intradermal radioisotope injection is superior to subdermal injection for the identification of the sentinel node in breast cancer patients. J Surg Oncol 2003;82:91-96, discussion 96-97.
148. Haigh PI, et al: Intraoperative lymphatic mapping and sentinel lymphadenectomy for breast cancer. Operative Techniques Gen Surg 2000;2:161-165.
149. Giuliano AE: Mapping a pathway for axillary staging; a personal perspective on the current status of sentinel lymph node dissection for breast cancer. Arch Surg 1999;134:195-199.
150. Kronowitz SJ, et al: Implications of axillary sentinel lymph node biopsy in immediate autologous breast reconstruction. Plast Reconstr Surg 2002;109:1888-1896.
151. Martin JK: Axillary dissection. Operative Techniques Gen Surg 2000;2:152-160.
152. Chung MA, et al: Breast cancer: surgical therapy. In Cameron JL, ed: Current Surgical Therapy, 7th ed. St Louis, Mosby, 2001:702-709.
153. Miguel R, et al: The effect of sentinel node selective axillary lymphadenectomy on the incidence of postmastectomy pain syndrome. Cancer Control 2001;8:427-429.
154. Carlson RW, et al: Multidisciplinary management of locally advanced breast cancer. Breast J 1999;5:303-307.
155. Seidman H, et al: Survival experience in the Breast Cancer Demonstration Project. CA Cancer J Clin 1987;37:258-290.
156. Valagussa P, et al: T3b-T4 breast cancer: factors affecting results in combined modality treatment. Clin Exp Metastasis 1983;1:191-202.
157. Jacquillat C, et al: Results of a conservative treatment combining induction (neoadjuvant) and consolidation chemotherapy, hormonotherapy, and external and interstitial irradiation in 98 patients with locally advanced breast cancer (IIIA-IIIB). Cancer 1988;61:1977-1982.
158. Touboul E, et al: Possibility of conservative local treatment after combined chemotherapy and preoperative irradiation for locally advanced noninflammatory breast cancer. Int J Radiat Oncol Biol Phys 1996;34:1019-1028.
159. Shuster TD: Multidisciplinary care for patients with breast cancer. Surg Clin North Am 2000;80:505-533.
160. Baker RR, et al: An evaluation of bone scans as screening procedures for occult metastases in primary breast cancer. Ann Surg 1977;186:363-368.
161. Calitchi E, et al: Long-term results of neoadjuvant radiation therapy for breast cancer. Int J Cancer 2001;96:253-259.
162. Darai E, et al: Conservative surgery after radiotherapy with preoperative doses in the treatment of breast cancer. Presse Med 1991;20:2144-2148.
163. Wolff AC, et al: Preoperative therapy in breast cancer: lessons from the treatment of locally advanced disease. Oncologist 2002;7:239-245.
164. Singletary SE: Neoadjuvant chemotherapy in the treatment of stage II and III breast cancer. Am J Surg 2001;182:341-346.
165. Fisher B, et al: Effect of preoperative chemotherapy on the outcome of women with operable breast cancer. J Clin Oncol 1998;16:2672-2685.
166. Merajver SD, et al: Breast conservation and prolonged chemotherapy for locally advanced breast cancer: the University of Michigan experience. J Clin Oncol 1997;15:2873-2881.
167. Eltahir A, et al: Treatment of large and locally advanced breast cancers using neoadjuvant chemotherapy. Am J Surg 1998; 175:127-132.
168. Amat S, et al: Neoadjuvant docetaxel for operable breast cancer induces a high pathological response and breast-conservation rate. Br J Cancer 2003;88:1339-1345.
169. Taghian AG, et al: The role of radiation therapy for primary breast cancer. Surg Clin North Am 1999;79:1091-1109.
170. Fowble B: Postmastectomy radiation: then and now. Oncology 1997;11:213-240.
171. Cuzick J, et al: Cause-specific mortality in long-term survivors of breast cancer who participated in trials of radiotherapy. J Clin Oncol 1994;12:447-453.
172. Schnitt SJ, et al: A prospective study of conservative surgery alone in the treatment of selected patients with stage I breast cancer. Cancer 1996;77:1094-1100.
173. Schnitt SJ: Updated results on the influence of pathologic features on treatment outcomes in stage I and II breast cancer treated by primary radiation therapy. Int J Radiat Oncol Biol Phys 1985;11(suppl I):104-105.
174. Galper S, et al: Factors associated with regional nodal failure in patients with early stage breast cancer with 0-3 positive axillary nodes following tangential irradiation alone. Int J Radiat Oncol Biol Phys 1999;45:1157-1166.
175. Victor SJ, et al: Treatment outcome with radiation therapy after breast augmentation or reconstruction in patients with primary breast carcinoma. Cancer 1998;82:1303-1309.
176. Donegan W, et al: Implications of extracapsular nodal metastasis for treatment and prognosis of breast cancer. Cancer 1993;72:778-782.
177. Ruo Redda MG, et al: Timing of radiotherapy in breast cancer conserving treatment. Cancer Treat Rev 2002;28:5-10.

178. Slotman BJ, et al: Importance of timing of radiotherapy in breast conserving treatment for early stage breast cancer. Radiother Oncol 1994;30:206-212.
179. Gage I: Radiation therapy and breast cancer. Curr Opin Oncol 1997;9:527-531.
180. Halverson KJ: Regional nodal management and patterns of failure following conservative surgery and radiation therapy for early-stage breast carcinoma. J Clin Oncol 1991;9:988-996.
181. Ryu JK: Radiotherapy for breast cancer: today and tomorrow. Cancer Biother Radiopharm 2002;17:255-266.
182. Forman DL, et al: Breast reconstruction in previously irradiated patients using tissue expanders and implants: a potentially unfavorable result. Ann Plast Surg 1998;40: 360-364.
183. Lin KY, et al: An outcome study of breast reconstruction: presurgical identification of risk factors for complications. Ann Surg Oncol 2001;8:586-591.
184. Krueger EA, et al: Complications and patient satisfaction following expander/implant breast reconstruction with and without radiotherapy. Int J Radiat Oncol Biol Phys 2001;49:713-721.
185. Vandeweyer E, et al: Radiation therapy after immediate breast reconstruction with implants. Plast Reconstr Surg 2000;106:56-58.
186. Cordeiro PG, et al: Irradiation after immediate tissue expander/implant breast reconstruction: outcomes, complications, aesthetic results, and satisfaction among 156 patients. Plast Reconstr Surg 2004;113:877-881.
187. Williams JK, et al: TRAM flap breast reconstruction after radiation therapy. Ann Surg 1995;221:756-766.
188. Munster PN, et al: Adjuvant therapy for resectable breast cancer. Hematol Oncol Clin North Am 1999;13:391-413.
189. Rosen PP, et al: Factors influencing prognosis in node-negative breast carcinoma: analysis of 767 T1N0M0/T2N0M0 patients with long-term follow-up. J Clin Oncol 1993;11:2090.
190. Fisher ER, et al: Medullary cancer of the breast revisited. Breast Cancer Res Treat 1990;16:215.
191. Rosen PP: Lobular carcinoma in situ: recent clinicopathologic studies at Memorial Hospital. Pathol Res Pract 1980;166:430.
192. Early Breast Cancer Trialists' Group: Systemic treatment of early breast cancer by hormonal, cytotoxic, or immune therapy. 133 randomised trials involving 31,000 recurrences and 24,000 deaths among 75,000 women. Lancet 1992;339:71-85.
193. Ross JS: The HER-2/neu gene and protein in breast cancer 2003: biomarker and target of therapy. Oncologist 2003;8:307-325.
194. Muss HB, et al: c-erbB-2 expression and response to adjuvant therapy in women with node–positive early breast cancer. N Engl J Med 1994;330:1260.
195. Park JW, et al: Biological therapy of breast cancer. BioDrugs 2000;14:221-246.
196. Esteva FJ, et al: Adjuvant systemic therapy for primary breast cancer. Surg Clin North Am 1999;79:1075-1090.
197. Goldhirsch A, et al: Meeting highlights: International Consensus Panel on the Treatment of Primary Breast Cancer. J Natl Cancer Inst 1998;90:1601-1608.
198. Early Breast Cancer Trialists' Collaborative Group: Polychemotherapy for early breast cancer: an overview of the randomised trials. Lancet 1998;352:930-942.
199. Mamounas EP, et al: NSABP Protocol B-27. Preoperative doxorubicin plus cyclophosphamide followed by preoperative or postoperative docetaxel. Oncology (Huntingt) 1997;11:37-40.
200. Early Breast Cancer Trialists' Collaborative Group: Multi-agent chemotherapy for early breast cancer. Cochrane Database Syst Rev 2002;1:CD000487.
201. Coleman RE: Current and future status of adjuvant therapy for breast cancer. Cancer Suppl 2003;97:880-886.
202. Singletary SE: Systemic treatment after sentinel lymph node biopsy in breast cancer: who, what, and why? J Am Coll Surg 2001;192:220-230.
203. Early Breast Cancer Trialists' Group: Tamoxifen for early breast cancer: an overview of the randomised trials. Lancet 1998;351:1451.
204. Fisher B, et al: Tamoxifen for prevention of breast cancer: report of the National Surgical Adjuvant Breast and Bowel Project P-1 Study. J Natl Cancer Inst 1998;90:1371-1388.
205. Cummings SR, et al: The effect of raloxifene on risk of breast cancer in postmenopausal women. JAMA 1999;281: 2189-2196.
206. Goss PE: Emerging role of aromatase inhibitors in the adjuvant setting. Am J Clin Oncol 2003;26:S27-33.
207. Dixon JM: Neoadjuvant tamoxifen and aromatase inhibitors: comparisons and clinical outcomes. J Steroid Biochem Mol Biol 2003;86:295-299.
208. Miller NA, et al: In situ duct carcinoma of the breast: clinical and histopathologic factors and association with recurrent carcinoma. Breast J 2001;7:292-302.
209. Hwang ES, et al: Management of ductal carcinoma in situ. Surg Clin North Am 1999;79:1007-1022.
210. Winchester DP, et al: The diagnosis and management of ductal carcinoma in-situ of the breast. CA Cancer J Clin 2000;50:184-200.
211. Silverstein MJ, et al: A prognostic index for ductal carcinoma in situ of the breast. Cancer 1996;77:2267-2274.
212. Winchester DP, et al: Standards for diagnosis and management of ductal carcinoma in situ (DCIS) of the breast. CA Cancer J Clin 1998;48:108-128.
213. Schwartz GF, et al: The current treatment of ductal carcinoma in situ. Breast J 2001;7:308-310.
214. Intra M, et al: Axillary sentinel lymph node biopsy in patients with pure ductal carcinoma in situ of the breast. Arch Surg 2003;138:309-313.
215. Foote FW, Stewart FW: Lobular carcinoma in situ: a rare form of mammary carcinoma. Am J Pathol 1941;17:491-499.
216. Schnitt SJ, et al: Lobular carcinoma in situ: current concepts and controversies. Semin Diagn Pathol 1999;16:209-223.
217. Frykberg ER, et al: In situ breast carcinoma. Adv Surg 1993;26:29-72.
218. American Cancer Society: Cancer reference information. Available at: www.cancer.org.
219. Goldschmidt RA, et al: Lobular carcinoma in situ of the breast. Semin Surg Oncol 1996;12:314-320.
220. Alderman A, et al: The national utilization of immediate and early delayed breast reconstruction and the effect of sociodemographic factors. Plast Reconstr Surg 2003;111:695-702.
221. Morrow M, et al: Factors influencing the use of breast reconstruction postmastectomy: a National Cancer Database study. J Am Coll Surg 2001;192:1-8.
222. Wanzel K, et al: Reconstructive breast surgery: referring physician knowledge and learning needs. Plast Reconstr Surg 2002;110:1441-1450.
223. August D, et al: Breast reconstruction in older women. Surgery 1994;115:663-668.
224. Pusic A, et al: Surgical options for early-stage breast cancer: factors associated with patient choice and postoperative quality of life. Plast Reconstr Surg 1999;104:1325-1333.
225. Georgiade G, et al: Rationale for immediate reconstruction of the breast following modified radical mastectomy. Ann Plast Surg 1982;8:20-28.
226. Schain WS, et al: The sooner the better: a study of psychological factors in women undergoing immediate versus delayed breast reconstruction. Am J Psychiatry 1985;142:40-46.
227. Wellisch D, et al: Psychosocial correlates of immediate versus delayed reconstruction of the breast. Plast Reconstr Surg 1985;76:713-718.
228. Bostwick J, et al: Reconstruction of the breast. Surg Oncol Clin North Am 1997;6:71-89.
229. Elliott L, et al: Breast reconstruction: progress in the past decade. World J Surg 1990;14:763-775.

230. Elkowitz A: Various methods of breast reconstruction after mastectomy: an economic comparison. Plast Reconstr Surg 1993;92:77-83.
231. Khoo A, et al: A comparison of resource costs of immediate and delayed breast reconstruction. Plast Reconstr Surg 1998;101:964-968.
232. Langstein H, et al: Breast cancer recurrence after immediate reconstruction: patterns and significance. Plast Reconstr Surg 2003;111:712-720.
233. Slavin S, et al: Recurrent breast cancer following immediate reconstruction with myocutaneous flaps. Plast Reconstr Surg 1994;93:1191.
234. Noone RB, et al: Recurrence of breast carcinoma following immediate reconstruction. Plast Reconstr Surg 1994;93:96-106.
235. Johnson C, et al: Oncological aspects of immediate breast reconstruction following mastectomy for malignancy. Arch Surg 1989;124:819.
236. Alderman A: Complications in postmastectomy breast reconstruction: two-year results of the Michigan Breast Reconstruction Outcome Study. Plast Reconstr Surg 2002;109: 2265-2274.
237. Oliva A, et al: Techniques of breast reconstruction. Probl Gen Surg 1989;6:564-584.
238. Neumann CG: The expansion of an area of skin by progressive distention of a subcutaneous balloon. Plast Reconstr Surg 1957;19:124.
239. Radovan C: Breast reconstruction after mastectomy using the temporary expander. Plast Reconstr Surg 1982;69:195-208.
240. Austad ED, Rose GL: A self-inflating tissue expander. Plast Reconstr Surg 1982;70:588-594.
241. Trabulsy PP, Anthony JP, Mathes SJ: Changing trends in postmastectomy breast reconstruction: a 13-year experience. Plast Reconstr Surg 1994;93:1418-1427.
242. Breast implants available only under controlled clinical studies. U.S. Food and Drug Administration, April 16, 1991. Available at: http://www.fda.gov/bbs/topics/NEWS/NEW00273.html. Accessed June 28, 2004.
243. Summary from the General and Plastic Surgery Devices Panel meeting, October 14 and 15, 2003. U.S. Food and Drug Administration. Available at: http://www.fda.gov/cdrh/panel/summary/gpsd101403.html. Accessed June 28, 2004.
244. Saline, silicone gel, and alternative breast implants—draft guidance for industry and staff. U.S. Food and Drug Administration, January 8, 2004. Available at: http://www.fda.gov/cdrh/ode/guidance/1239.html. Accessed June 28, 2004.
245. Two firms get FDA approval to continue marketing saline-filled breast implants. U.S. Food and Drug Administration, May 10, 2000. Available at: http://www.fda.gov/bbs/topics/NEWS/NEW00727.html. Accessed June 28, 2004.
246. Young V, et al: The relative radiolucencies of breast implant filler materials. Plast Reconstr Surg 1993;91:1066-1072.
247. Birdsell DC, et al: Breast cancer diagnosis and survival in women with and without breast implants. Plast Reconstr Surg 1993;92:795.
248. Georgiade GS, et al: Long-term clinical outcome of immediate reconstruction after mastectomy. Plast Reconstr Surg 1985;76:415.
249. Hoshaw SJ, et al: Breast-implants and cancer: causation, delayed detection, and survival. Plast Reconstr Surg 2001;107:1393-1408.
250. Joseph E, et al: Survival from breast carcinoma after augmentation mammoplasty. Proceedings of the 67th annual scientific meeting of the American Society of Plastic and Reconstructive Surgeons, the Plastic Surgery Educational Foundation, and the American Society of Maxillofacial Surgeons, Boston, Mass, October 3-7, 1998.
251. Petit JY: Does long-term exposure to gel-filled silicone implants increase the risk of relapse after breast cancer? Tumori 1998;84:525.
252. Bryant H, et al: Breast implants and breast cancer—reanalysis of a linkage study. N Engl J Med 1995;332:1535-1539.
253. Duskova M, et al: Breast reconstruction as an integral part of breast carcinoma therapy (a self-present final report of a research project IGA MZ CR). Acta Chir Plast 2001;43:42-53.
254. Varga J: Systemic sclerosis after augmentation mammoplasty with silicone implants. Ann Intern Med 1989;111:377-383.
255. Edworthy S, et al: A clinical study of the relationship between silicone breast implants and connective tissue disease. J Rheumatol 1998;25:254-260.
256. Holmich LR, et al: Self-reported diseases and symptoms by rupture status among unselected Danish women with cosmetic silicone breast implants. Plast Reconstr Surg 2003;111:723-732.
257. Janowsky EC, et al: Meta-analyses of the relation between silicone breast implants and the risk of connective-tissue diseases. N Engl J Med 2000;342:781-790.
258. Committee on the Safety of Silicone Breast Implants, Institute of Medicine: Safety of Silicone Breast Implants. Washington, DC, National Academy Press, 2000.
259. Kjoller K: Connective tissue disease and other rheumatic conditions following cosmetic breast implantation in Denmark. Arch Intern Med 2001;161:973.
260. Saline, silicone gel, and alternative breast implants—draft guidance for industry and staff. U.S. Food and Drug Administration, January 8, 2004. Available at: http://www.fda.gov/cdrh/ode/guidance/1239.html. Accessed June 28, 2004.
261. Gabriel S, et al: Complications leading to surgery after breast implantation. N Engl J Med 1997;336:677-682.
262. Collis N: Ten-year review of a prospective randomized controlled trial of textured versus smooth subglandular silicone gel breast implants. Plast Reconstr Surg 2000;106:786-791.
263. Muzaffar A: The silicone gel-filled breast implant controversy: an update. Plast Reconstr Surg 2001;109:742-748.
264. Janowsky EC, et al: Meta-analyses of the relation between silicone breast implants and the risk of connective-tissue diseases. N Engl J Med 2000;342:781-790.
265. Spear S, et al: Immediate breast reconstruction in two stages using textured integrated-valve tissue expanders and breast implants: a retrospective review of 171 consecutive breast reconstructions from 1989-1996. Plast Reconstr Surg 1998; 101:53.
266. Slavin S: Sixty consecutive breast reconstructions with the inflatable expander: a critical appraisal. Plast Reconstr Surg 1990;86:910.
267. Spear S, et al: Breast reconstruction with implants and expanders. Plast Reconstr Surg 2001;107:177-188.
268. Gui G, et al: Immediate breast reconstruction using biodimensional anatomical permanent expander implants: a prospective analysis of outcome and patient satisfaction. Plast Reconstr Surg 2003;111:125-138.
269. Evans G: Reconstruction and the radiated breast: is there a role for implants? Plast Reconstr Surg 1994;96:1111-1115.
270. Kraemer O, et al: Breast reconstruction and tissue expansion in irradiated versus not irradiated women after mastectomy. Scand J Plast Reconstr Surg Hand Surg 1996;30:201-206.
271. Spear S, et al: Staged breast reconstruction with saline-filled implants in the irradiated breast: recent trends and therapeutic implications. Plast Reconstr Surg 2000;105:930-942.
272. Cronin TD, et al: Augmentation mammoplasty: a new "natural feel" prosthesis. Transactions of the Third International Congress of Plastic and Reconstructive Surgeons. Amsterdam, Excerpta Medica, 1964.
273. Millard DR Jr: Breast reconstruction after a radical mastectomy. Plast Reconstr Surg 1976;58:283-291.

274. Maxwell GP: Iginio Tansini and the origin of the latissimus dorsi musculocutaneous flap. Plast Reconstr Surg 1980;65:686-692.
275. Tansini I: Nuovo processo per l'amputazione della mammella per cancre. Riforma Med 1896;12:3.
276. Mathes SJ, Bostwick J 3rd: A rectus abdominis myocutaneous flap to reconstruct abdominal wall defects. Br J Plast Surg 1977;30:282-283.
277. Hartrampf CR, Scheflan M, Black PW: Breast reconstruction with a transverse abdominal island flap. Plast Reconstr Surg 1982;69:216-225.
278. Pomel C: Endoscopic muscular latissimus dorsi flap harvesting for immediate breast reconstruction after skin sparing mastectomy. Eur J Surg Oncol 2003;29:127-131.
279. Lipa JE, Youssef AA, Kuerer HM, et al: Breast reconstruction in older women: advantages of autogenous tissue. Plast Reconstr Surg 2003;111:1110-1121.
280. Larson DL, Yousif NJ, Sinha RK, et al: A comparison of pedicled and free TRAM flaps for breast reconstruction in a single institution. Plast Reconstr Surg 1999;104:674-680.
281. Chang DW, et al: Effect of obesity on flap and donor site complications in free-transverse rectus abdominis myocutaneous flap breast reconstruction. Plast Reconstr Surg 2000;105:1640.
282. Mizgala CL, Hartrampf CR Jr, Bennett GK: Assessment of the abdominal wall after pedicled TRAM flap surgery: 5- to 7-year follow-up of 150 consecutive patients. Plast Reconstr Surg 1994;93:988-1002, discussion 1003-1004.
283. Watterson P, et al: TRAM flap anatomy correlated with a 10-year clinical experience with 556 patients. Plast Reconstr Surg 1995;95:1185-1193.
284. Mathes SJ, Nahai F: Clinical Atlas of Muscle and Musculocutaneous Flaps. St Louis, Mosby, 1979.
285. Mathes SJ, Nahai F: Muscle flap transposition with function preservation: technical and clinical considerations. Plast Reconstr Surg 1980;66:242-249.
286. Malata CM, et al: Immediate breast reconstruction after mastectomy. Br J Surg 2000;87:1455-1472.
287. Codner MA, Bostwick J 3rd: The delayed TRAM flap. Clin Plast Surg 1998;25:183-189.
288. Rickard RF, Hudson DA: Influence of vascular delay on abdominal wall complications in unipedicled TRAM flap breast reconstruction. Ann Plast Surg 2003;50:138-142.
289. Ribuffo D: A hemodynamic approach to clinical results in the TRAM flap after selective delay. Plast Reconstr Surg1997;99:1706-1714.
290. Simon AM, Bouwense CL, McMillan S, et al: Comparison of unipedicled and bipedicled TRAM flap breast reconstructions: assessment of physical function and patient satisfaction. Plast Reconstr Surg 2004;113:136-140.
291. Hartrampf CR Jr, Noel RT, Drazan L, et al: Ruben's fat pad for breast reconstruction: a peri-iliac soft-tissue free flap. Plast Reconstr Surg 1994;93:402-407.
292. Serletti J, et al: Microvascular reconstruction of the breast. Semin Surg Oncol 2000;19:264-271.
293. Hulka BS, Stark AT: Breast cancer: cause and prevention. Lancet 1995;197:33.
294. Kelsey JL, Horn-Ross PL: Breast cancer: magnitude of the problem and descriptive epidemiology. Epidemiol Rev 1993;15:7.
295. Liberman L, Menell JH: Breast imaging reporting and data system (BI-RADS). Radiol Clin North Am 2002;40:409.
296. Abeloff MD, Armitage JO, Niederhuber JE, et al: Clinical Oncology, 3rd ed. Philadelphia, Elsevier, 2004:2394.
297. Spear SL, Baker JL Jr: Classification of capsular contracture after prosthetic breast reconstruction. Plast Reconstr Surg 1995;96:1119.
298. Williams JK, et al: The effects of radiation treatment after TRAM flap breast reconstruction. Plast Reconstr Surg 1997;100:1153-1160.
299. Tran NV, et al: Comparison of immediate and delayed free TRAM flap breast reconstruction in patients receiving post-mastectomy radiation therapy. Plast Reconstr Surg 2001;108:78-82.
300. Baldwin BJ: Bilateral breast reconstruction: conventional versus free TRAM. Plast Reconstr Surg 1994;93:1410-1416.
301. Shestak KC: Breast reconstruction with a pedicled TRAM flap. Clin Plast Surg 1998;25:167-182.
302. Carlson GW, et al: Results of immediate breast reconstruction after skin-sparing mastectomy. Ann Plast Surg 2001;46:222-228.
303. Paige KT, et al: A comparison of morbidity from bilateral, unipedicled and unilateral, unipedicled TRAM flap breast reconstructions. Plast Reconstr Surg 1998;101:1819-1827.
304. Erdmann D, et al: Delay in unipedicled TRAM flap reconstruction of the breast: a review of 76 consecutive cases. Plast Reconstr Surg 2002;110:762-767.
305. Scheufler O: Clinical results of TRAM flap delay by selective embolization of the deep inferior epigastric arteries. Plast Reconstr Surg 2000;105:1320-1329.
306. Restifo RJ, et al: Timing, magnitude, and utility of surgical delay in the TRAM flap: II. clinical studies. Plast Reconstr Surg 1997;99:1217-1223.
307. DeBono R: Immediate versus delayed free TRAM breast reconstruction: an analysis of perioperative factors and complications. Br J Plast Surg 2002;55:111-116.
308. Grotting J: Immediate breast reconstruction using the free TRAM flap. Clin Plast Surg 1994;21:207-221.
309. Nahabedian M, et al: Breast reconstruction with the free TRAM or DIEP flap: patient selection, choice of flap, and outcome. Plast Reconstr Surg 2002;110:466-475.
310. Blondeel P, et al: One hundred free DIEP flap breast reconstructions: a personal experience. Br J Plast Surg 1999;52:104-111.
311. Nahabedian M, et al: Contour abnormalities of the abdomen after breast reconstruction with abdominal flaps: the role of muscle preservation. Plast Reconstr Surg 2002;109:91-101.
312. Shaw WW: Superior gluteal free flap breast reconstruction. Clin Plast Surg 1998;25:267-282.
313. Blondeel PN: The sensate free superior gluteal artery perforator (S-GAP) flap: a valuable alternative in autologous breast reconstruction. Br J Plast Surg 1999;52:185-193.

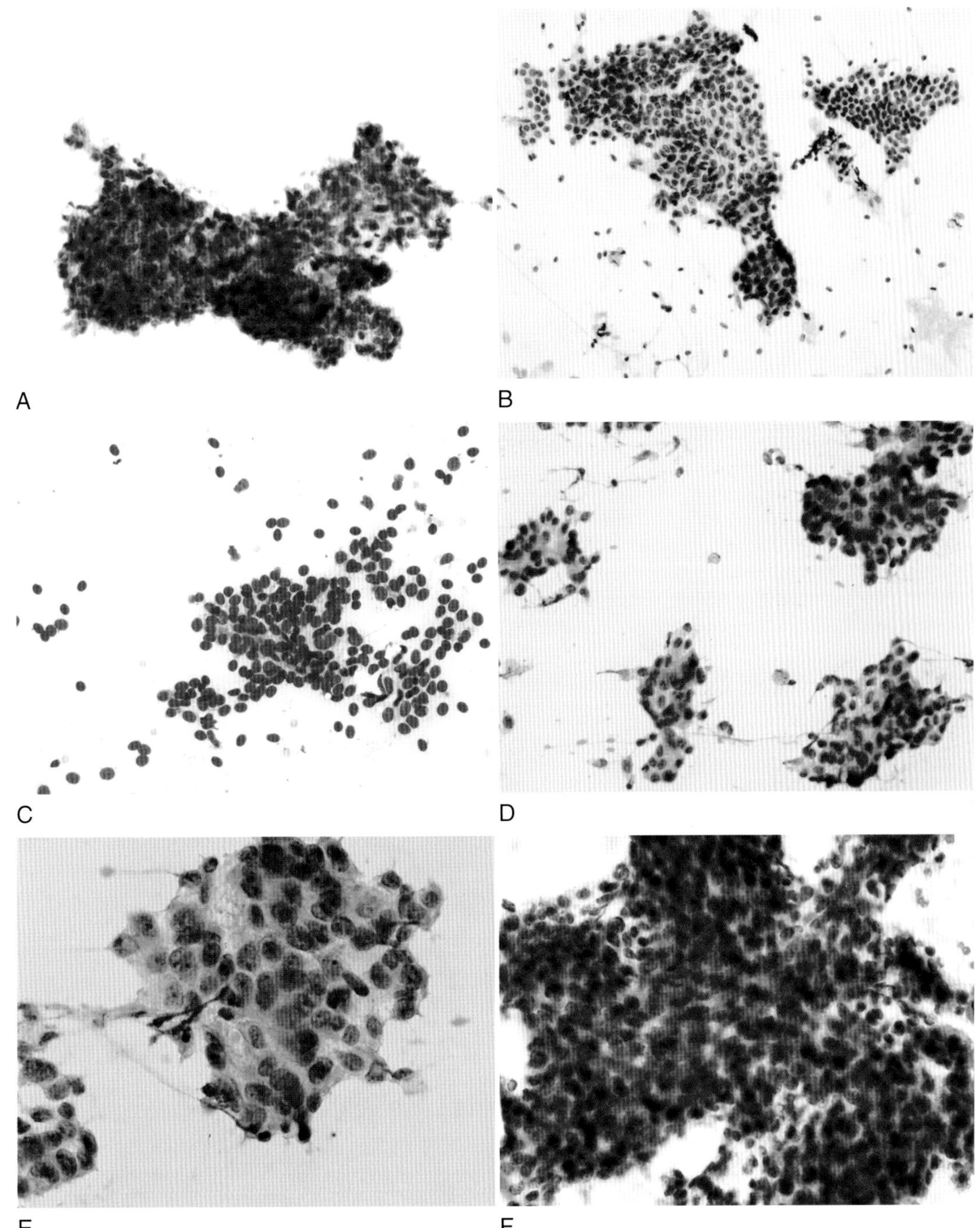

COLOR PLATE 138-1. Fine-needle aspiration biopsy. *A,* Breast, atypical. Slightly enlarged epithelial cells are seen in a cohesive cluster. The arrangement is multilayered and irregular, causing this sample to be considered atypical and triggering further work-up (usually open biopsy). *B,* Fibrocystic change. Two clusters of unremarkable breast epithelium are seen in well-organized clusters including small, oval, dark-staining nuclei of myoepithelial cells. Single bare benign nuclei are seen in the background. (Papanicolaou stain; magnification ×200.) *C,* Benign epithelium; loosely organized, small benign breast epithelial cells including myoepithelial cells. (May-Grunewald-Giemsa stain; original magnification ×200.) *D,* High-grade breast cancer (×400); irregularly arranged, enlarged malignant breast epithelial cells. The chromatin pattern in the nuclei is coarse, and nucleoli are present. The nuclei vary significantly in size and shape. Myoepithelial cells are absent. (Papanicolaou stain; original magnification ×400.) *E,* High-grade breast cancer (×200); irregularly arranged, enlarged malignant cells in several clusters. Focally gland-like arrangements are present. Myoepithelial cells are absent. (Papanicolaou stain; original magnification ×200.) *F,* Low-grade breast cancer; mildly enlarged, hyperchromatic epithelial cells in a multilayered, irregularly arranged cluster. Myoepithelial cells are absent. (Papanicolaou stain; original magnification ×400.)

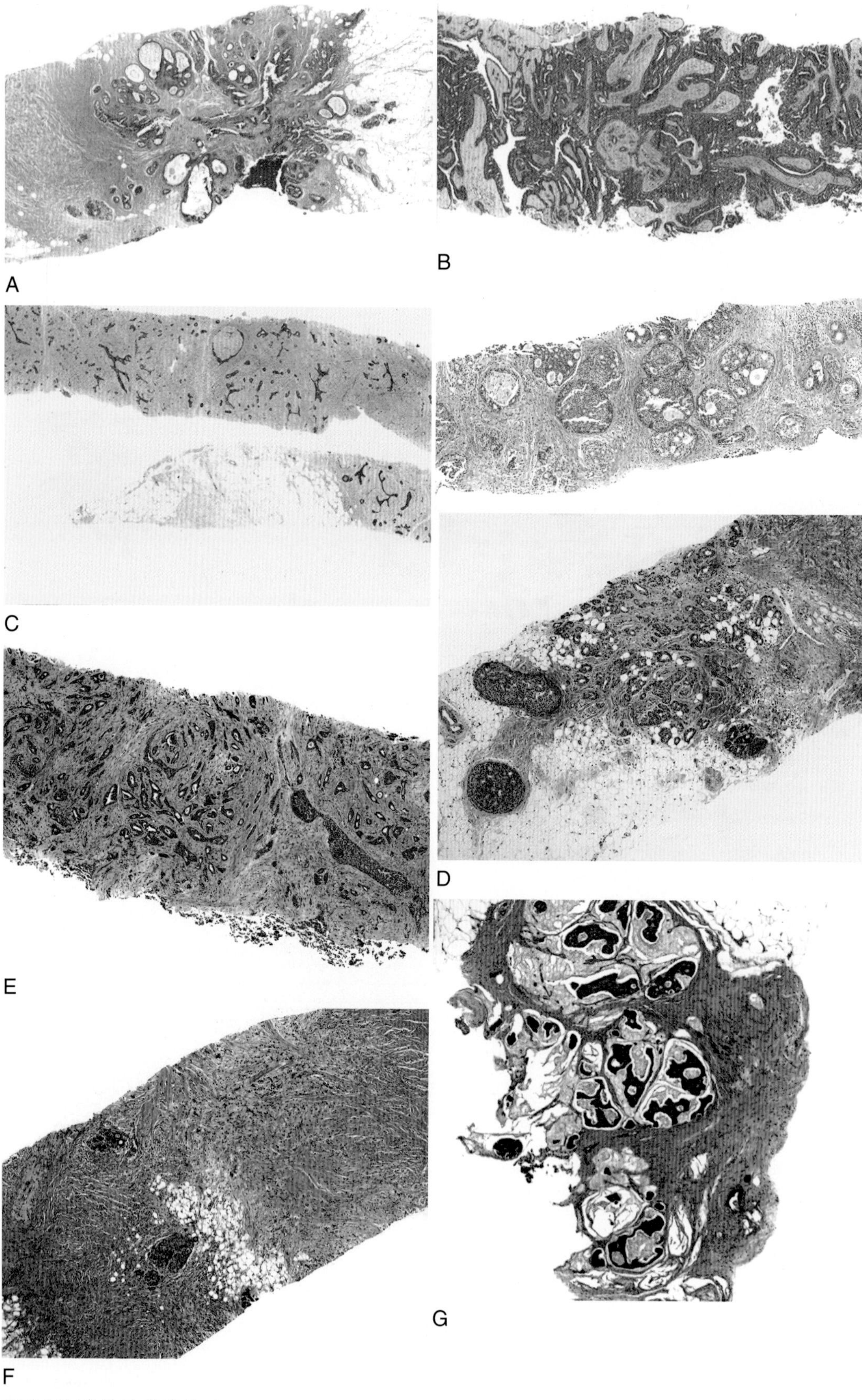

COLOR PLATE 138-2. *See opposite page.*

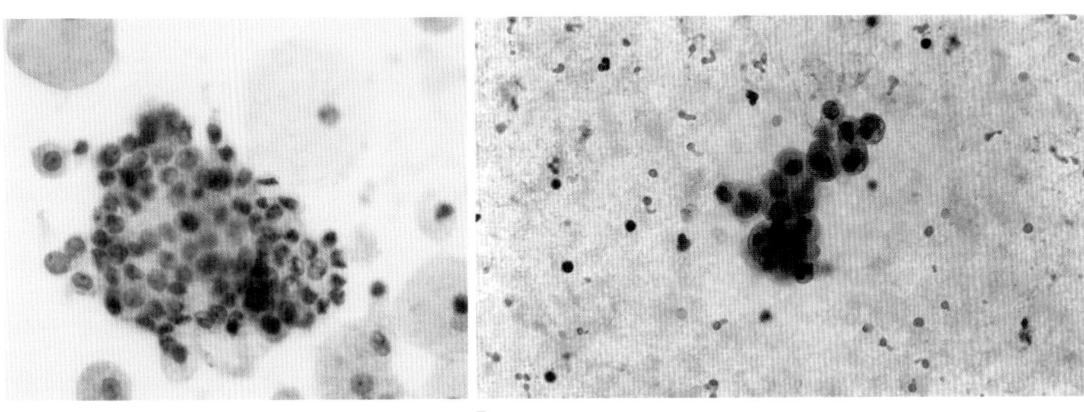

COLOR PLATE 138-3. Cytologic findings by ductal lavage. *A,* Benign specimen; well-organized clusters of bland epithelial cells including small, dark-staining myoepithelial cells. Several single histiocytes are seen surrounding the epithelial cells. (Papanicolaou stain; original magnification ×400.) *B,* Marked atypia; cluster of slightly enlarged, hyperchromatic epithelial cells. There is significant variability in both size and shape of the nuclei. The arrangements are somewhat irregular, and myoepithelial cells are not present. Scattered lymphocytes and erythrocytes are seen in the background. (Papanicolaou stain; magnification ×400.) (Images courtesy of Britt-Marie Ljeung, MD, UCSF Department of Pathology.)

COLOR PLATE 138-2. Histologic specimens obtained by core biopsy. *A,* Radial scar with fibrotic tissue. Patients with this finding should undergo an excisional biopsy to rule out carcinoma. *B,* Small duct breast papilloma. Typical histologic view of a core biopsy specimen of a small duct breast papilloma. Normal two-cell epithelium lines demonstrate a fibrovascular core. Frond-like projections are also present. *C,* Fibroadenoma. The fibrous capsule demarcates the fibroadenoma tumor from the surrounding breast tissue. As the name implies, both fibrous and glandular structures are neoplastic. *D,* Ductal carcinoma in situ (DCIS). Most patients with DCIS manifest a mixture of patterns. Comedonecrosis is characterized by sheets of neoplastic cells with central necrosis. This necrosis often calcifies and may be detectable on mammography. In cribriform DCIS, intraepithelial spaces are regular in morphologic appearance. *E,* Infiltrating ductal carcinoma. Note the abundant dense, fibrous stroma that gives the tumor a hard consistency. *F,* Invasive lobular carcinoma. Typical histologic appearance of lobular carcinoma showing parallel arrays of single cells in a fibrous stroma. This type of tumor constitutes approximately 10% of breast cancers. *G,* Mucinous breast carcinoma. Mucinous carcinomas are invasive carcinomas characterized by mucin production. They are usually well-circumscribed masses. (Images courtesy of Yunn-Yi Chen, MD, and Alfred Au, MD, UCSF Department of Pathology.)

CHAPTER

139

Reconstruction of the Nipple-Areola Complex

STEPHEN J. MATHES, MD ✦ CRISTIANE M. UENO, MD

The nipple-areola complex (NAC) is routinely excised as part of the skin envelope resection during mastectomy, especially if the tumor is close to it.[1] The nipple and areola are usually resected and included with the mastectomy specimen with skin-sparing mastectomy.

The nipple contains ductal tissue and may contain cancer cells (Fig. 139-1). However, the areola is a skin appendage, and it does not require resection unless the surgeon thinks that resection is necessary to obtain adequate skin margins on the basis of established criteria to avoid potential local recurrence (see Chapter 138). When prophylactic mastectomy is performed, the areola may be preserved with a transverse incision through its center with a short lateral extension for exposure and excision of the breast parenchyma. In prophylactic mastectomy and in selected mastectomies for breast cancer, the cutaneous portion of the nipple may also be preserved if the surgeon carefully removes all ductal tissue from the nipple. The nipple will lose some projection, but it can be preserved with this approach without increased risk of local recurrence. Because the process of mastectomy and reconstruction represents a team approach, both the surgical oncologist and the plastic surgeon should jointly discuss the planned skin resection and advisability of areola or NAC preservation. For most patients presenting with invasive carcinoma, the surgical oncologist will elect to remove the central skin envelope including the NAC. The multiple approaches to nipple-areola reconstruction offer an excellent opportunity to provide a patient with optimal breast reconstruction, including the NAC and adjacent skin.

Postmastectomy patients also suffer a distortion of the body image that may result in negative psychological consequences. Replacement of the breast restores the self-image that may be lost as a consequence of mastectomy. With successful restoration of a breast mound, many patients desire a nipple-areola to complete reconstruction of the breast and achieve symmetry.

Reconstruction of the breast mound has consistently improved with multiple techniques that are selected on the basis of the extent of the defect and the patient's and surgeon's preferences. Nipple-areola reconstruction has also made significant strides in regard to multiple surgical options. Since 1944, when Adams[2] described the reconstruction of the NAC with the nipple-areola graft,[2] the techniques for NAC reconstruction have improved with grafts of a variety of donor areas[2-13] and local flaps.[14-25] The most popular techniques include the skate flap[20] and the star flap.[23] With improved techniques, nipple-areola reconstruction has become more popular in the past 2 decades as many patients consider the idea of a reconstructed breast without the NAC undesirable.[1,26-28]

ANATOMY

The NAC is ideally located at the most prominent point of the breast or above the level of the projected inframammary crease. Average projection of the nipple is 5 mm.

The areola projects slightly and has an average diameter of 35 to 45 mm. The areola texture can be smooth or rough at the location of the Montgomery tubercles. There is a wide variation in color, shape, size, and projection of the NAC as a result of race, the aging process, hormonal changes (pregnancy and menopause), and variation in weight (Fig. 139-2).

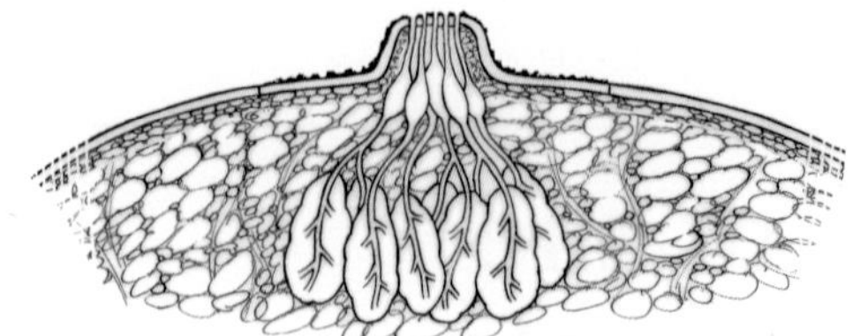

FIGURE 139-1. Cross section of the breast demonstrating nipple surface, skin, subcutaneous tissue, lactiferous ducts, and segmental and subsegmental ducts.

TABLE 139-1 ✦ GOALS OF NIPPLE-AREOLA RECONSTRUCTION

Position
Symmetry
Color
Size
Projection
Sensitivity

GOALS OF NIPPLE-AREOLA RECONSTRUCTION

Position of the nipple-areola reconstruction is usually determined by the shape of the reconstructed breast mound. However, in skin-sparing mastectomy when a flap is used to fill the cutaneous defect at the former nipple-areola site, this area of the flap is usually used for the future nipple-areola location. Optimal symmetry is usually difficult to achieve because of the differences in shape and size between the reconstructed and the contralateral breast. Symmetry is often best achieved in a delayed procedure, allowing wound maturation within the reconstructed breast mound before determination of location and choice of technique. Color, size, and projection relate both to the nipple and to the areola. There are now many well-described techniques that can be selected to best achieve nipple and areola dimensions and surface characteristics to match the contralateral nipple-areola or to provide an acceptable reconstruction in bilateral mastectomy reconstructions. Restoration of sensation does occur in regard to protective sensation through both the retained breast skin envelope and flaps when they are used for skin envelope replacement. Reinnervation of flaps by coaptation of sensory nerves to the flap with recipient nerves in proximity to the hemithorax is currently done in selected patients. Within 6 months after the breast mound reconstruction, patients often note gradual restoration of sensation in the breast mound. Future techniques, it is hoped, will reliably achieve this goal of restoration of nipple-areola sensation (Table 139-1).

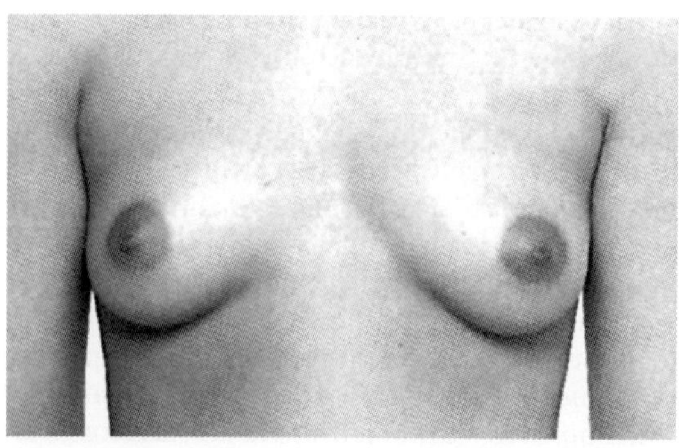

A

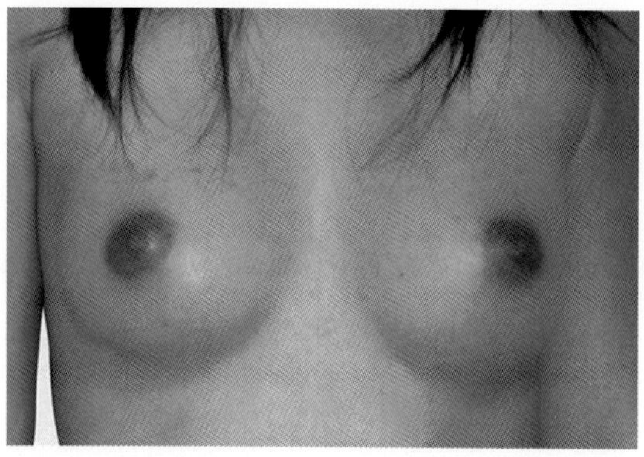

B

FIGURE 139-2. Normal nipple-areola color seen in white patient *(A)* and Asian patient *(B)*.

RECONSTRUCTIVE OPTIONS AND TIMING

In general, nipple-areola reconstruction is delayed pending breast mound and skin envelope reconstruction.[1,26,27] Even if the areola is preserved, postmastectomy reconstruction of the breast may shift the areola position compared with the opposite breast. The altered shape of the reconstructed breast may require repositioning of the NAC to establish symmetry. The exception to the delayed nipple reconstruction is the patient undergoing the skin-preserving mastectomy and immediate reconstruction of the breast mound with a transposition or microvascular transplanted flap. Because the only part of the flap skin preserved is the portion for inset into the former site of the nipple-areola, this flap skin may undergo a simultaneous technique for nipple reconstruction. If the flap has volume equivalent to the opposite breast or modification of the opposite breast is planned (e.g., reduction mammaplasty or mastopexy), the nipple should have an appropriate position for symmetry with the opposite breast. Even in this situation, delay in nipple-areola reconstruction may be preferable in the event that the reconstructed breast mound is subsequently altered for symmetry or excessive or inadequate size is observed in the postoperative period. Nipple reconstruction should be performed as a final stage, after adjustments to the flap and contralateral breast. It is usually performed 2 to 3 months after the final breast shape is achieved. If subsequent surgical procedures are planned for the opposite breast for symmetry with the reconstructed breast, it is preferable to delay nipple reconstruction until the opposite breast surgery is performed. Because the nipple reconstruction is performed electively under local anesthesia, a delay is preferable until the patient can decide her preference for NAC location and nipple projection.

Although the majority of patients choose to have the NAC reconstructed, some postmastectomy patients elect not to undergo the procedure. If an adequate breast mound is established with symmetry with the opposite breast, the patient may believe that adequate balance and body image issues are resolved and not wish to pursue further surgical procedures. There is no time limit on nipple-areola reconstruction, so the patient may decide to forgo the procedure or wait until she is comfortable with her breast reconstruction and past anxiety regarding recurrence of her breast cancer.

POSITIONING

When the patient has agreed to proceed with nipple-areola reconstruction, the patient and the plastic surgeon must determine the optimal position. If the patient has undergone a skin-preserving procedure, it is preferable to use the prior nipple-areola site if a flap has been used to fill this space, restoring the preoperative dimensions of the skin envelope. If the skin island extends beyond the limits of the former site of the nipple-areola area, the surgeon and the patient will plan together to determine the optimal position for symmetry and breast mound appearance. In bilateral mastectomy, simultaneous nipple reconstruction is performed, and planning will therefore include placement of both nipple-areola sites.[1,26,27]

Two approaches for planning the nipple-areola site include

1. providing the patient with a nipple-areola prosthesis to wear for a short period to determine her preferred position and,
2. in the preoperative room, taking measurements with the patient in the sitting position, arms at sides; measurements are taken of the chest to determine nipple-areola distances from inframammary line, sternal notch, midclavicular line, and midline adjacent to the fourth intercostal space.

On the basis of these measurements on the contralateral and reconstructed breast mound, placement of the drawing of the areola on the breast mound at the location that most closely matches the opposite nipple-areola site or, if the reconstruction is bilateral, that matches the preexisting nipple-areola location is determined (Fig. 139-3*A*). After completion of one or both techniques to determine location, a Polaroid or digital photograph is taken and shown to the patient and accompanying family (Fig. 139-3*B*). If the patient and the plastic surgeon jointly approve the selected position documented by the photograph, the patient is ready for the nipple or simultaneous nipple-areola reconstruction. Because both breasts may not be identical, particularly in comparing a reconstructed breast mound with a normal breast or in comparing bilateral reconstructed breast mounds by different techniques, it may be difficult to determine the optimal nipple-areola position. Sometimes alterations in these measurements have to be made to ascertain the best position of the NAC, and a difference between the measurements and the visual impression has to be accepted. The final location is marked after an agreement between the surgeon and the patient on the ideal position. In bilateral reconstruction, the process is the same, and the location of the new NAC will be chosen by the measurements and review of photographs of the selected site with the patient and her family.

TECHNIQUES

Although most techniques will give a satisfactory result in nipple-areola reconstruction, the choice of the technique must be individualized. The individual scars should be taken into consideration for the donor area and nipple reconstruction. Moreover, the vasculature of the flap must be adequate to accept the reconstruction, diminishing the risks of complications. Donor site morbidity is another factor that must be considered.

The nipple and areola may be reconstructed simultaneously, or the nipple reconstruction may be completed first and later followed by areola reconstruction. Presently, the nipple is most often reconstructed by a variety of local flap designs. After healing of the nipple is confirmed, the entire nipple and the areola are tattooed for appropriate pigmentation. If the nipple and areola are reconstructed simultaneously, the approach usually involves local flaps to provide the nipple mound in conjunction with a skin graft for areola reconstruction.

Nipple Reconstruction

SKIN GRAFTS

Use of a skin graft for reconstruction of the nipple was first described in 1944 by Adams,[2] who performed a transplantation of the nipple and areola. Concerns about the inability to sustain projection or to acquire

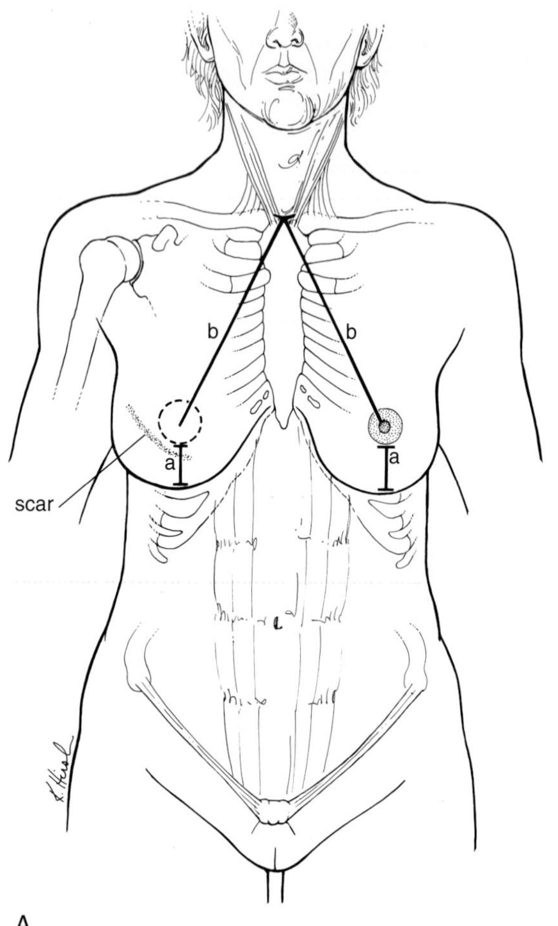

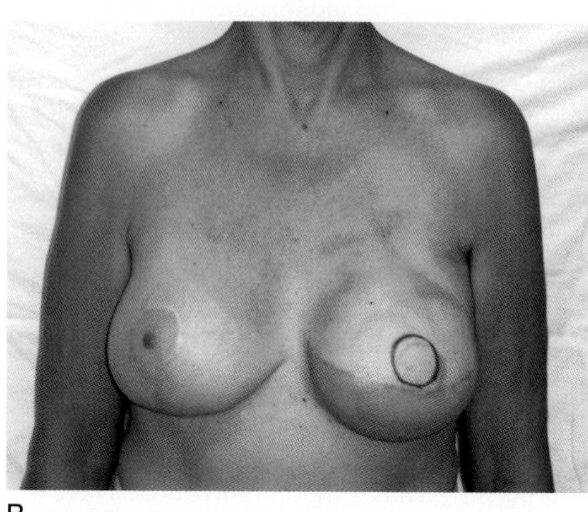

FIGURE 139-3. Nipple-areola position. *A,* Measurements useful in location of nipple-areola include sternal notch to nipple distance based on contralateral nipple (b) and inframammary line to inferior areola (a), cutaneous distance based on contralateral nipple. *B,* Preoperative picture of patient showing planned location of nipple-areola complex.

an exact color match have motivated others to develop additional nipple-areola reconstructive options. In 1972, Millard[6] introduced the idea of a split graft from the contralateral side. Brent and Bostwick,[9] in 1977, proposed the use of auricular tissues and cartilage to project the nipple. In 1981, Klatsky and Manson[12] reported the use of a toe pulp graft for nipple projection. Continued improvements in skin graft techniques offer the surgeon a variety of techniques and donor sites to achieve optimal results in individual patients (Table 139-2).

If a skin graft is planned for the nipple, a full-thickness graft from the opposite nipple may be considered.[6] If the opposite nipple has excess projection as observed by the patient (usually a projection of more than 5 mm), a full-thickness graft from the opposite nipple may be suitable. A graft from the contralateral nipple will slightly reduce its projection and simultaneously provide ideal skin for grafting of the opposite nipple. Most patients are not candidates for nipple-sharing reconstruction, and many patients fear donor site morbidity, including diminished projection of the donor site, risks of diminishing the sensitivity, and transfer of potentially malignant ductal tissue.[1,26,27]

When the opposite nipple is absent or lacks projection or the procedure is undesirable to the patient, grafting, flaps, and tattoo are the primary reconstructive choices. Full-thickness skin grafts may be selected close to the perineum,[10] generally adjacent to the posterior aspect of the labia majora. In this location, the grafts will have adequate pigmentation and will not often require intradermal tattoo. However, because this donor site is painful for the patient during the healing process, other donor sites may be preferable. Skin grafts taken from the groin or from redundant skin adjacent to the breast mound reconstruction will provide excellent coverage but are likely to require later intradermal tattoo.[26]

LOCAL FLAPS

Reliable local flap techniques[14-25] have been described that provide a nipple with reasonable projection. For this reason, most patients now undergo local flaps for nipple reconstruction followed by intradermal tattoo

TABLE 139-2 ✦ HISTORY OF NIPPLE-AREOLA RECONSTRUCTION

Type of Reconstruction	Year	Author	Technique
Skin grafts	1944	Adams[2]	Autologous nipple-areola graft
	1946	Thorek[50]	Autologous nipple-areola graft
	1949	Adams[3]	Labia minora graft
	1972	Millard[6]	Nipple-sharing reconstruction
	1977	Brent and Bostwick[9]	Reconstruction with auricular tissue
	1978	Muruci et al[11]	Mucous membrane free graft
	1979	Dubin[51]	Two-stage procedure (areola graft followed by nipple from a central graft with device for mechanical traction)
	1981	Klatsky and Manson[12]	Toe pulp free graft
Tattoo-dermabrasion	1975	Rees[8]	Intradermal tattoo
	1981	Cohen[13]	Dermabrasion to form nipple-areola in African Americans
Flaps	1933	Berson[52]	Three partial-thickness skin flaps for nipple
	1952	Di Pirro[52]	Modification of Berson technique (using four triangles)
	1970	Di Pirro[4]	V-Y technique
	1972	Snyder[5]	V-Y advancement technique with modified design
	1978	Muruci et al[11]	Full-thickness turnover flap (from denuded areolar bed, covered with a mucous membrane graft)
	1982	Serafin and Georgiade[14]	Two-stage technique
	1983	Little et al[15]	Quadrapod flap (one-stage reconstruction)
	1984	Hartrampf and Culbertson[17]	Dermal fat flap
	1984	Chang[16]	T flap
	1986	Cohen et al[19]	Pinwheel flap
	1987	Little[20]	Skate flap
	1987	Kroll[22]	Double opposing tab flap
	1988	Cronin et al[21]	S flap
	1991	Anton, Eskenazi, and Hartrampf [23]	Star flap
	1993	Hugo et al[24]	Double opposing pennant flap
	1993	Eskenazi[25]	Modified star flap
	1993	Hallock[54]	H flap
	1994	Jones and Bostwick[57]	C-V flap
	1995	Zhang et al[53]	Beta flap
	1996	Eng[39]	Bell flap
	1997	Ramakrishnan[55]	Twin flap
	1999	Kroll[56]	Wraparound flap
	2000	Horn et al[58]	Box nipple flap
Combined: flap and nipple prosthesis	1990	Hallock[41]	Flap and polyurethane nipple prosthesis
Combined: flap and autologous grafts	1997	Tanabe-Yanaga et al[59]	Dermal fat flap and rolled auricular cartilage graft
	2003	Bernard and Beran[42]	Fat graft
Combined: flap and autologous cartilage grafts	2003	Guerra et al[44]	Arrow flap and costal cartilage
	2003	Wei et al[43]	Modified top hat flap and costal cartilage
Combined: flap and artificial bone	2003	Yanaga[36]	Dermal fat flap and artificial bone
Ectoprosthesis	1992	Ullmann et al[40]	Nipple-areola reconstruction with a custom-made silicone ectoprosthesis

after the nipple flaps have healed.[29-32] There are numerous flaps and modifications that are effective in establishing the NAC. Each technique offers advantages, but there are also disadvantages related to donor site vascularity and quality of tissue (flaps versus preserved breast skin envelope), maintenance of nipple mound size and projection, and potential complications. Five flaps are discussed, including the dermal fat flap (which may include immediate areola reconstruction), skate flap, star flap, bell flap, and double opposing tab flap.

In most techniques (with the exception of the double opposing tab flap), the key to success is designing the flap base away from the mastectomy incision. The flap should have adequate dimensions to provide adequate height for the nipple mound. In patients who have undergone breast reconstruction by a flap, the local flap for nipple-areola reconstruction will be based, when it is feasible, on site selection on the surface of the flap where healthy full-thickness tissue will be available for nipple reconstruction. In the patient who has undergone reconstruction by immediate implant or expander-implant, the skin envelope is thin and the resultant flaps are more likely to atrophy and to lose projection over time. In this group, subsequent contralateral full-thickness nipple graft or a cartilage graft may be helpful in providing secondary augmentation of the nipple.

Dermal Fat Flap

The dermal fat flap was first described by Hartrampf and Culbertson[17] in 1984, and it is known to provide a sustained result in terms of nipple projection.[33,34] However, there is an associated decrease in projection over time as determined by the gradual absorption of the central-wedge fat associated with the maturation of scar tissue. In addition, this technique is not always a reliable reconstructive option for patients with implants because tension on the skin plane associated with a thin fat layer causes loss of projection and risk of wound dehiscence.[1] In spite of these disadvantages, a skin graft used to cover the flap can provide an adequate color match and texture.[27]

MODIFIED DERMAL FLAP TECHNIQUE WITH IMMEDIATE GRAFTING. If dermal fat flaps are selected to establish the nipple mound with immediate full-thickness skin grafts to provide coverage of the nipple mound and areola donor site, the site for nipple reconstruction is selected and de-epithelialized (Fig. 139-4). Three centrally based dermal flaps are designed, usually at 12-, 3-, and 9-o'clock positions. The flaps may be altered in position to avoid the mastectomy incision. The flaps are based on the center of the designed areola and taper at the periphery of the areola. Each of the three dermal flaps is elevated to include a thin layer of subcutaneous tissue (3 to 5 mm). One should not undermine the central base of the three flaps. The three flaps are rotated to the midpoint of the nipple site and sutured together. The deep surface of each flap is exposed on the reconstructed nipple mound. The donor sites for the flaps are left open for graft coverage.

A full-thickness skin graft is harvested from a pigmented site in the perineum, generally between the posterior labia and rectum.[10,11] Groin skin is more convenient, but it may require tattoo because of inadequate pigmentation. In patients with pigmented skin with very darkly pigmented areola, labial skin may be harvested to match a very dark opposite areola. The ellipse of skin is designed to include a central piece of skin to match and cover the entire areola. The ends of the ellipse will represent skin used for the nipple coverage and allow direct linear closure of the full-thickness donor site. After the graft is defatted, the peripheral segments of the skin graft are sutured to the nipple mound. The larger central graft is sutured to the areola site with the sutures left long to fix a bolster dressing over the nipple-areola grafted site. A small hole is cut in the center of the areola graft, allowing the nipple (now covered with the graft) to project through the opening. The entire nipple-areola site is covered with cotton bolster dressing. This dressing is usually removed in 3 to 5 days (Fig. 139-5).

Skate Flap

The skate flap, first described by Little[20] in 1987 (Fig. 139-6), is considered by many to be the optimal procedure for nipple projection to match a contralateral nipple that is more than 5 mm in height. According to Cederna et al,[35] the skate flap can provide a reasonable projection even after long-term follow-up. The main disadvantage consists of distortion in the areola associated with the closure of the radial-positioned defect of the donor site.[1] However, the closure can be modified and corrected subsequently at the time of areola reconstruction.[36]

MODIFIED SKATE FLAP TECHNIQUE. The skate flap is a reliable technique for reconstruction of a nipple (Figs. 139-7 and 139-8).[20] After the appropriate site for the nipple-areola is determined, the diameter of the nipple is established on the basis of the opposite areola; if bilateral nipple-areola reconstruction is planned, the diameter is 3.5 to 4.5 cm. A line extending across the width of the areola is drawn to establish the base of the skate flap. The base is oriented away from the mastectomy scar, and it can be oriented either transversely or vertically, with the flap oriented perpendicular to the base and extending within the planned areola site. In general, the base is oriented transversely and located either inferior or superior to the midaxis of the areola. The middle third of the base line represents the actual base of the flap and is usually 1.5 cm in width. The outer thirds of this line represent the "wings" of the skate flap (approximately 1 cm in length) and will become the flaps that form the bottom half of the nipple. A semicircular line is now drawn between the ends of the base line previously established. The height of the semicircular line is generally 1.5 cm from the midpoint of the base line, but it may be altered, depending on the desired height of the reconstructed nipple. The entire flap should be designed within the planned site of the areola to avoid visible scars outside the area of the subsequent pigmented areola.

The initial incision extends along the base and around the hemicircle, preserving only the skin bridge at the middle third of the base line. The two wings are then elevated to include the dermis and a thin layer

Text continued on p. 807

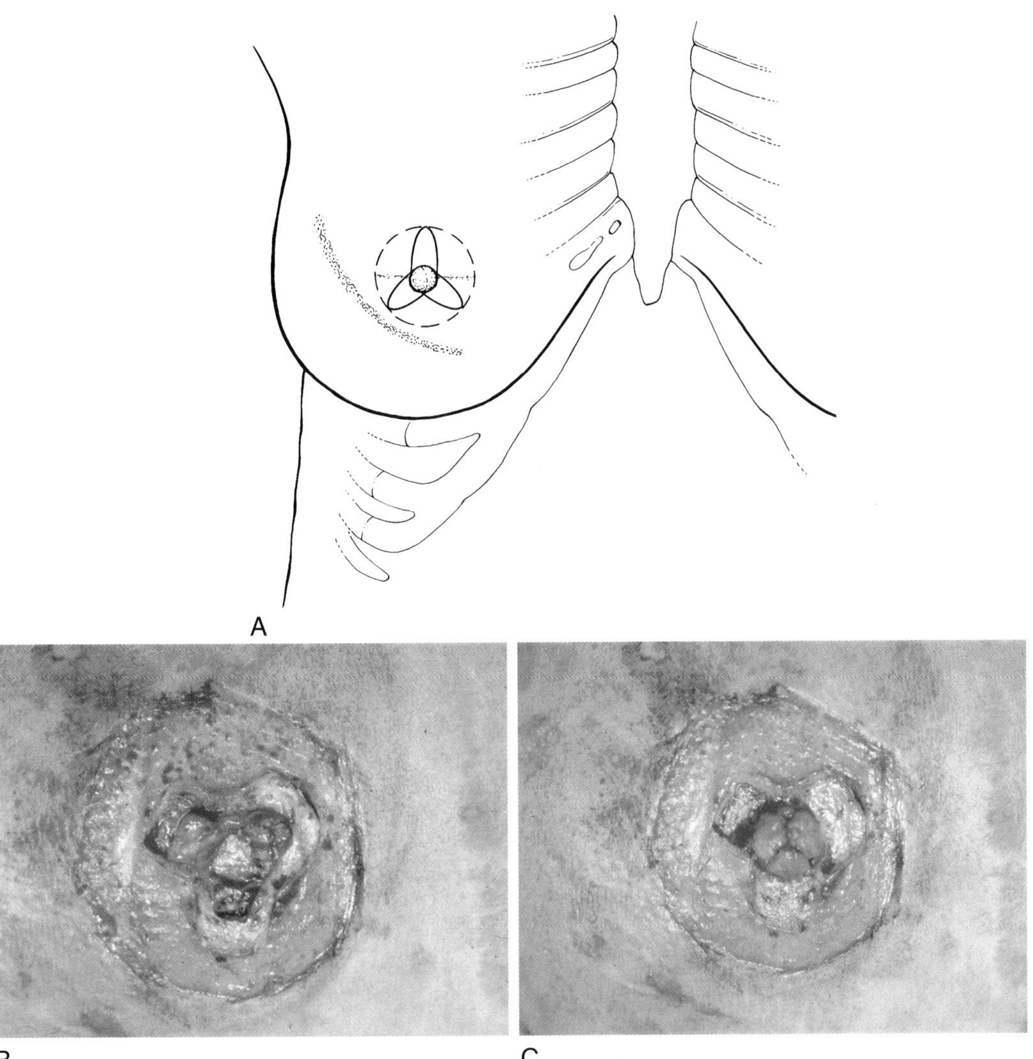

FIGURE 139-4. Dermal full-thickness skin graft areola reconstruction. *A,* Preoperative drawing of three dermal flaps after nipple-areola site is de-epithelialized. *B,* Dermal flap elevated, based centrally. Each flap includes a thin layer of subcutaneous tissue. *C,* Three dermal flaps rotated 90 degrees to center of planned nipple site and sutured together with buried absorbable sutures. *Continued*

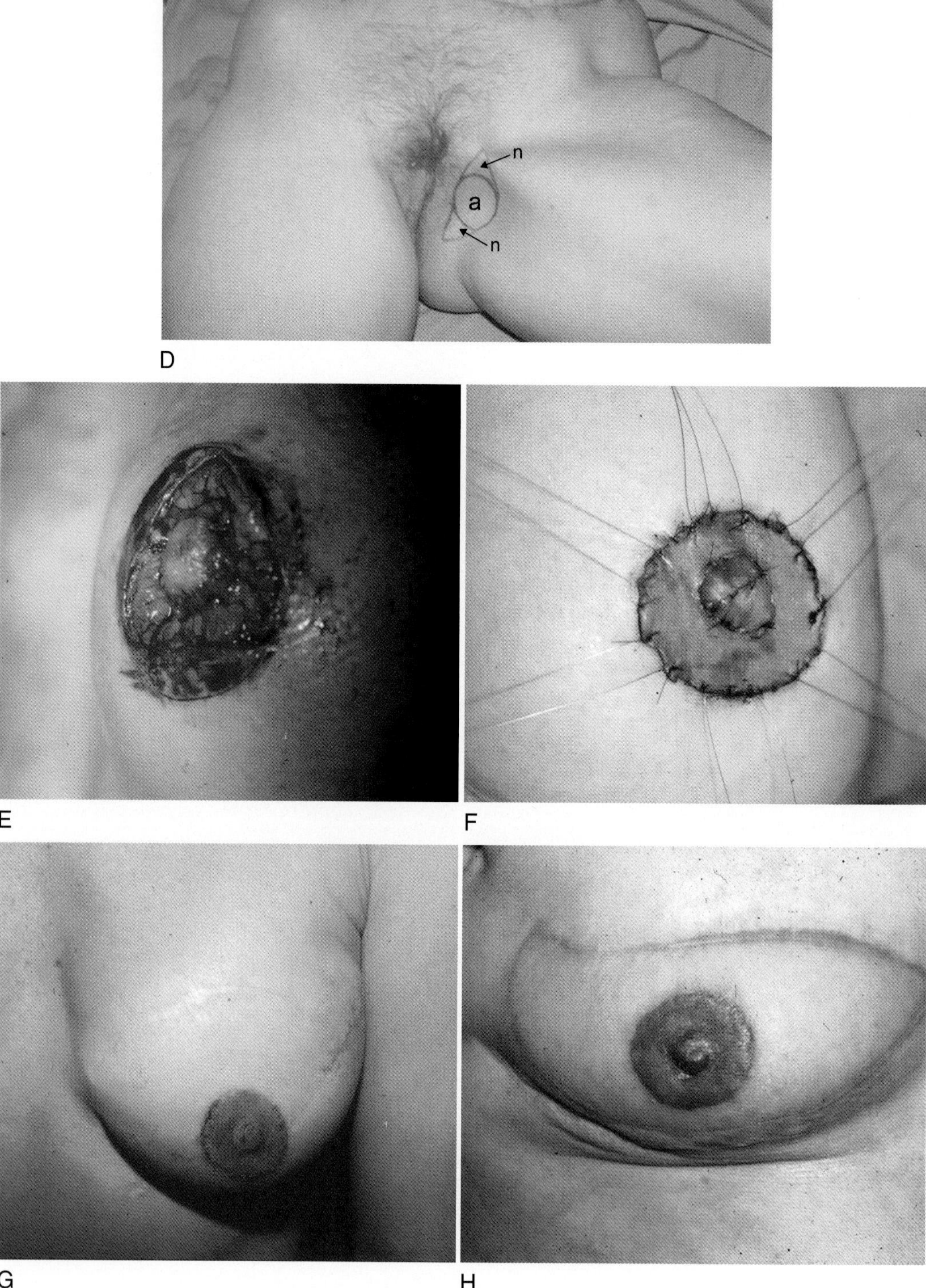

FIGURE 139-4, cont'd. *D,* Full-thickness skin graft. The donor site is located in the pigmented area adjacent to the perineum. Center ellipse for areola (a) and distal parts of graft for nipple mound (n) are depicted. *E,* Lateral view demonstrates suture of the full-thickness skin graft for nipple mound coverage. *F,* Full-thickness skin graft placed to cover areola ("a" area from *D*). Small central cut in graft allows position of nipple mound through graft. Sutures are left long for tie-over bolster dressing. *G,* Anterior view of early postoperative single-stage nipple-areola reconstruction. *H,* Anterior postoperative view of another dermal flap (full-thickness skin graft) nipple-areola reconstruction at 1 year.

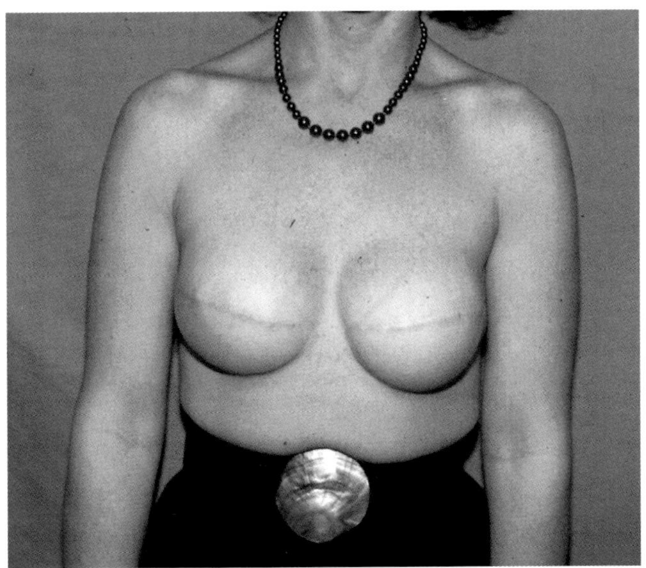

A

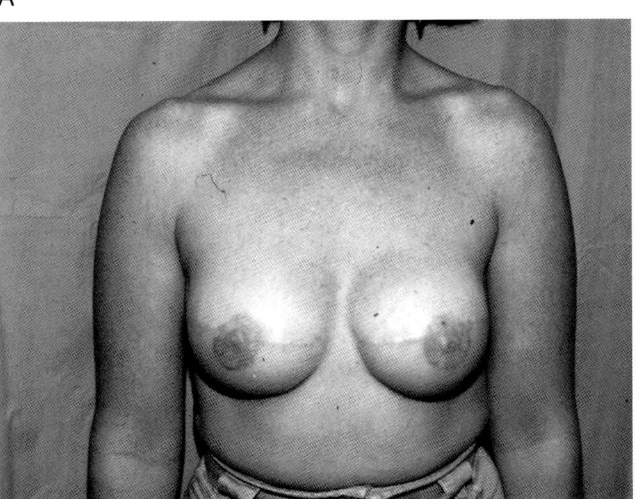

B

FIGURE 139-5. Dermal flap full-thickness skin graft nipple-areola reconstruction. *A,* Anterior postoperative view of bilateral expander-implant reconstruction. *B,* Anterior postoperative view of bilateral single-stage nipple-areola reconstruction at 1 year.

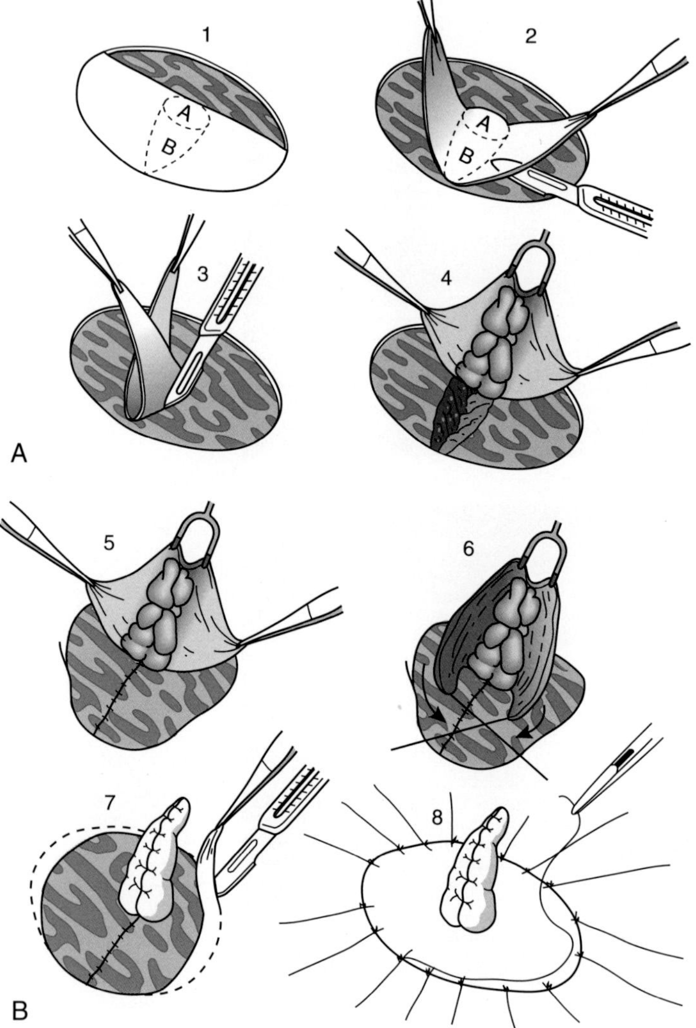

FIGURE 139-6. Nipple reconstruction by the skate flap. *A:* 1, area beyond tangent to nipple disk A denuded; lines from 3- and 9-o'clock of nipple disk to 6-o'clock of areolar pattern outline body of skate; 2, wings of skate elevated deep split-thickness up to body; 3, dissection changes from horizontal to vertical as dermis and fat are cut through to form composite body; 4, body dissected centrally and elevated; deep trough remains in dermal bed. *B:* 5, areolar bed closed; areolar pattern distorts; 6, wings of skate brought around body to each other; 7, completed nipple cone; areolar pattern revised; 8, areolar doughnut graft added. (From Little JW: Nipple-areolar reconstruction. Adv Plast Surg 1987;3:43.)

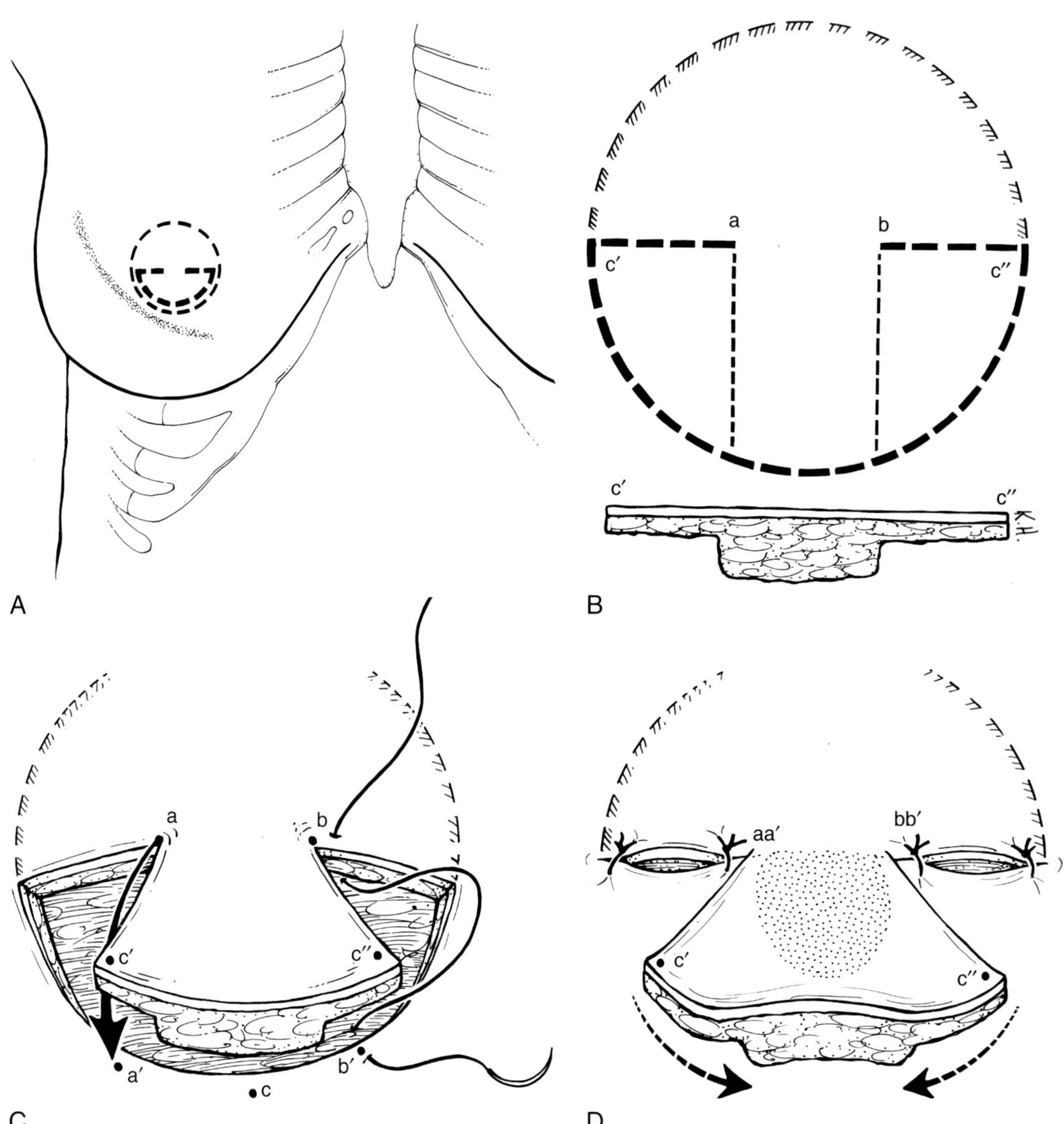

FIGURE 139-7. *A,* Design of skate flap. Base is directed away from the preexisting mastectomy scar. *B,* Markings for skate flap located within future site of areola with diameter of 4 to 4.5 cm (distance based on contralateral areola). Wings (c′, c″) will include less subcutaneous fat than the central (c) base of the flap. *C,* After skate flap is elevated, wings of donor site are closed. *D,* Wings rotated 90 degrees to approximate with midline of central flap of donor site.

Continued

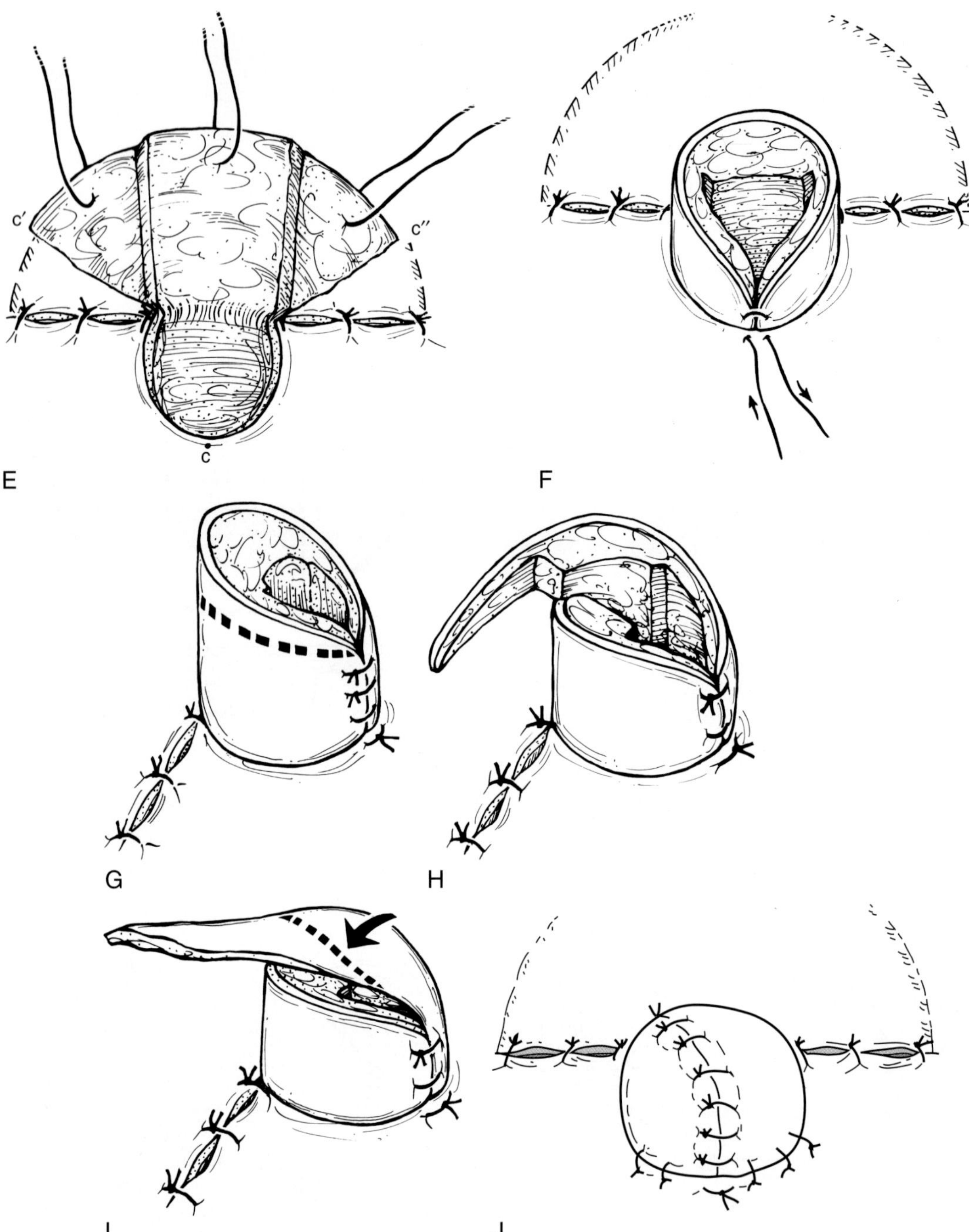

FIGURE 139-7, cont'd. *E,* Deep surface of skate flap demonstrates flap base and subcutaneous tissue included with flap. *F,* Horizontal mattress suture used to approximate flap wings to midline of central flap donor site. *G,* Base of nipple formed by approximation of wings of skate flap. The tip of the flap is excised to form a flat nipple tip. *H,* One wing of the skate flap is folded to form tip of nipple mound. *I,* Redundant skin resected. Height of nipple can be determined to match opposite nipple. *J,* Closure of donor site and nipple mound, and nipple base completed.

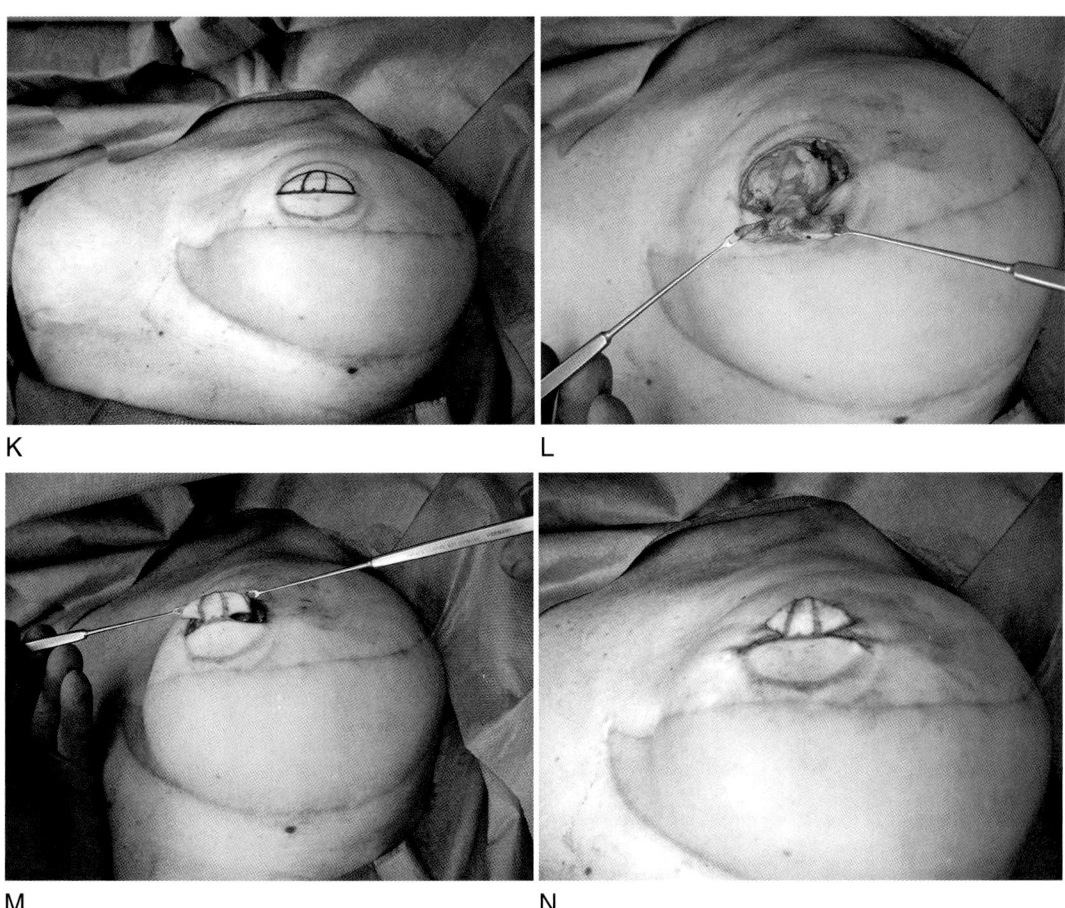

FIGURE 139-7, cont'd. *K* to *Q,* Intraoperative photographs of patient undergoing unilateral modified skate flap. *Continued*

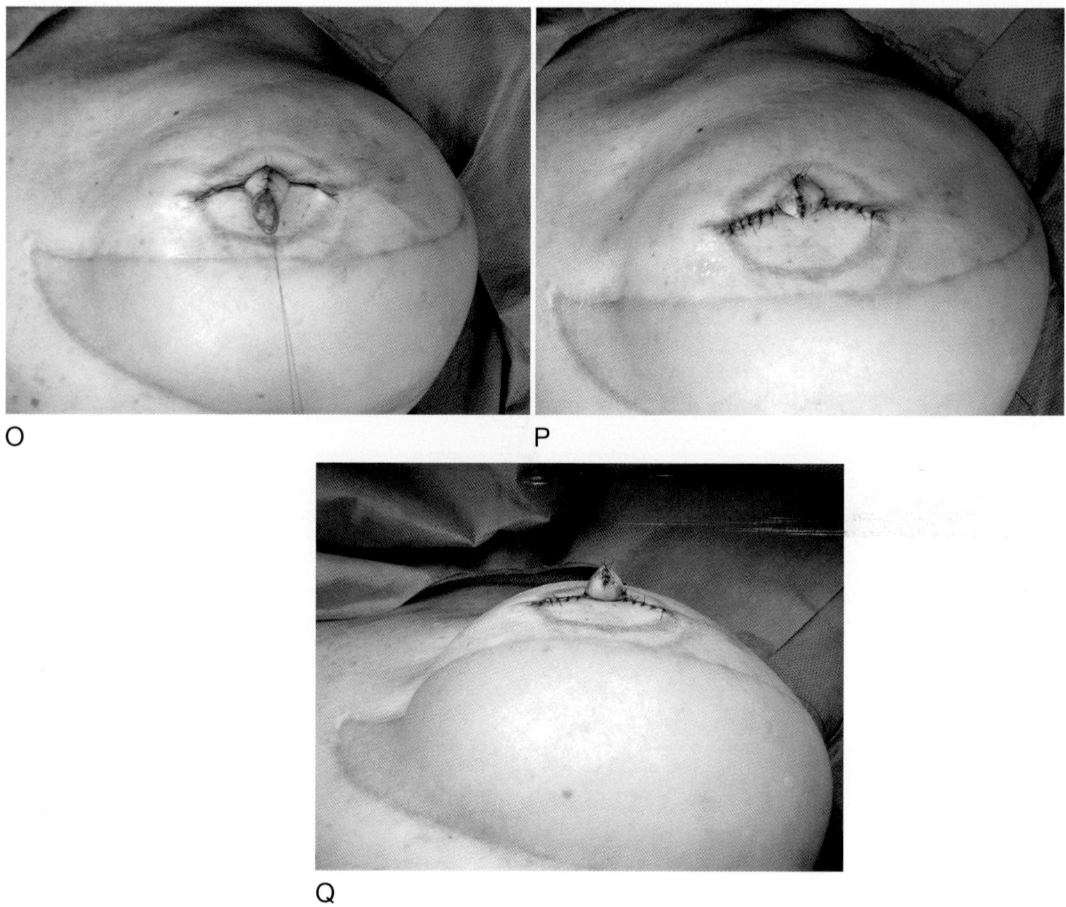

FIGURE 139-7, cont'd.

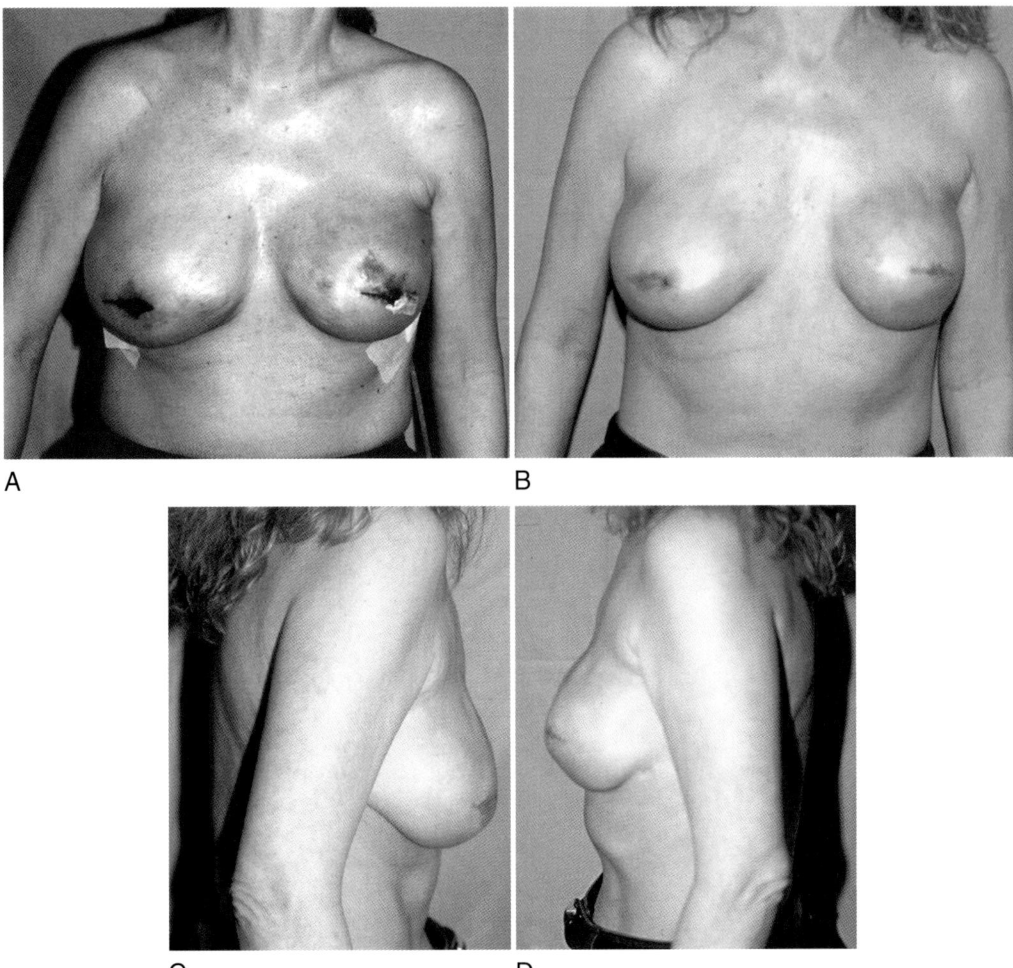

FIGURE 139-8. *A,* Anterior view, immediate postoperative bilateral mastectomy and bilateral latissimus dorsi musculocutaneous flap with implants. *B,* Anterior postoperative view 3 months after bilateral reconstruction by latissimus dorsi musculocutaneous flaps and implants for immediate reconstruction. *C* and *D,* Lateral postoperative views at 3 months.

Continued

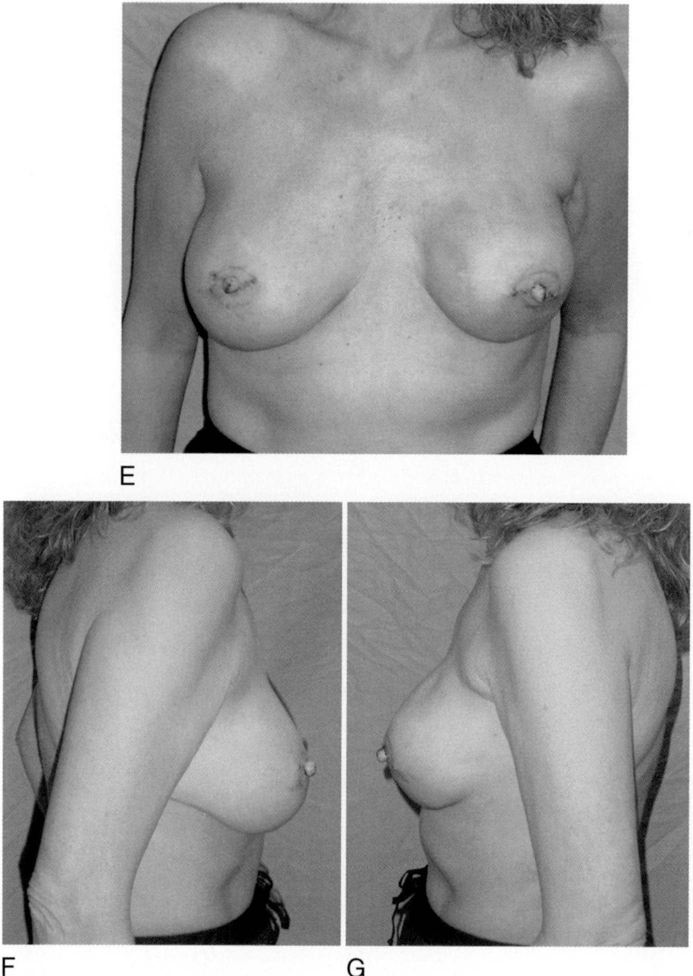

FIGURE 139-8, cont'd. *E,* Anterior postoperative view 6 weeks after bilateral modified skate flaps for nipple reconstruction. *F* and *G,* Lateral views demonstrate skate flap projection.

of subcutaneous fat (approximately 4 mm of fat beneath the dermis). The central pedicle is elevated to include a thicker layer of fat (5 to 8 mm), and care is required to not undermine the base of the flap. When the skate flap is designed on flap skin, less fat is required because dermis is thicker (especially on the latissimus dorsi skin island). When the skate flap is designed on a preserved breast skin envelope, the dermis is often thin, so fat down to the capsule (if there is underlying implant reconstruction) is elevated with the pedicle to ensure adequate bulk to the nipple. The two wings of the flap are now rotated 90 degrees to a position opposite the midpoint of the flap base. The distal tips of these flaps are sutured together to the midpoint of the hemicircle. The two donor sites for the wings are closed directly. The wings are then approximated to form a nipple tube. The end of the tube will require dog-ear modification to establish a flat plane as opposed to a pointed tip of the nipple. The bases of the wings are sutured to complete the nipple reconstruction.

Star Flap

The star flap, first described by Anton, Eskenazi, and Hartrampf[23] in 1991, is performed in those patients in whom the projection of the opposite nipple is around 5 mm (Figs. 139-9 and 139-10). It is a relatively simple technique for establishing a new nipple by use of scar tissue.[1] The projection limitation is a result of the limited wing length of the star flap,[34,37] which is associated with the loss in projection over time.[23] Even though this limitation can be an issue in use of the star flap, in a comparison study by Shestak et al,[38] there was no difference in loss of projection in the long-term follow-up between the skate flap and the star flap.

After the correct adjustment of the new nipple position, a star pattern with three wings is drawn. It can be superiorly or inferiorly based (depending on the position of the mastectomy scar). The lengths of the two lateral wings vary according to the size of the opposite nipple. The lateral wings and the distal portion of the central wing are carefully elevated in the subcutaneous fat plane to maintain the dermal and subdermal base blood supply. Once the star edges are raised, the remaining donor area is approximated with interrupted sutures, avoiding the constriction of the flap's base. The wings are then sutured together. One lateral wing is sutured along the nipple base, and at the endpoint of this suture, the opposing lateral wing begins to be sutured. The distal portion of the central wing will be the top of the nipple.

Bell Flap

The bell flap, described by Eng[39] in 1996 (Fig. 139-11), is most often applied in patients who have a contralateral nipple with less than 5 mm of projection. As it is elevated and folded on itself, the maximum projection of the flap will be half of its length. The flap closure is accomplished by placing a pursestring suture, which helps in establishing projection of the areola and provides primary closure of the donor site.[26,39] However, in a study performed by Shestak et al[38] analyzing the bell flap, skate flap, and star flap, the bell flap provided less long-term projection.

The bell flap is based on Japanese origami and is formed from a bell-shaped model. The halo area has to be 15% to 20% larger in diameter than the size desired for the opposite nipple, and the wide area of the bell is placed at the 6-o'clock position. The pedicle is based in the central area of the halo. The bell-shaped flap is elevated in the subcutaneous fat plane and wrapped like an inverted box. The residual cut edges are advanced and sutured together, forming the shape of a cone. The resultant nipple (inverted box) is settled above this cone, completing the nipple reconstruction. Even though the cone may sometimes assume an inverted form as a result of the forces applied by the coning process, the nipple complex is everted after a pursestring closure that runs along the outer skin circle.

Double Opposing Tab Flap

The double opposing tab flap was devised by Kroll[22] in the late 1980s. It is similar to the bell flap technique, consisting of an S-shaped pattern that gives it a cylindrical shape (Fig. 139-12). Like the skate flap, it is composed of lateral appendages (like wings) containing skin and subcutaneous fat. An incision is made (through the existing scar if the patient has one) to allow these lateral appendages to fold and form the edges of the nipple. These edges are then brought into opposition by key sutures to support one another (Fig. 139-12*C*). The final nipple shape tends to be oval (Fig. 139-12*C*). The width of the flap ranges from 18 to 22 mm. As the flap gets wider, the nipple becomes more oval. The bottom of the flap has a sawtooth design to facilitate the interdigitating closure. As in the skate flap technique, the donor site area is covered with a skin graft.

Flaps Incorporating Autogenous or Alloplastic Materials for Nipple Projection

Because nipple projection can be difficult to achieve and to maintain, several techniques using autogenous and alloplastic materials have been developed to achieve this goal.[27] If local tissue cannot provide adequate nipple projection or if there is gradual loss of projection after the nipple flap has healed, implants may be used to reinforce or to re-establish nipple projection.

ECTOPROSTHESIS. A custom-made ectoprosthesis is designed by the impression of a breast mold (as a cast copy of a real breast). The ectoprosthesis is made of silicone and is colored with pigments that match

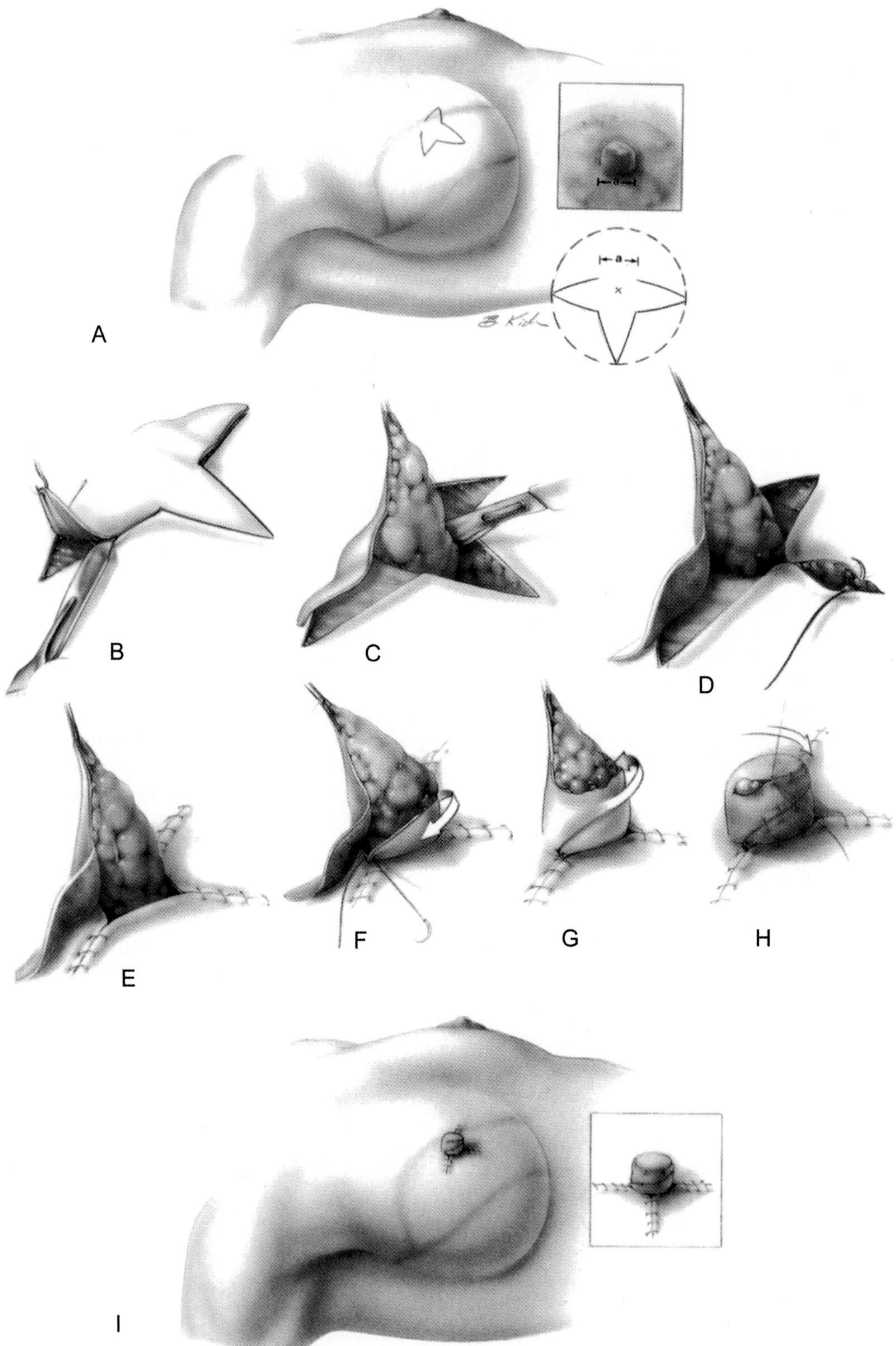

FIGURE 139-9. *A* to *I*, Planning, elevation, assembly, and donor site closure of the star flap. (From Anton M, Eskenazi LB, Hartrampf CR: Nipple reconstruction with local flaps: star and wrap flaps. Perspect Plast Surg 1991;5:67.)

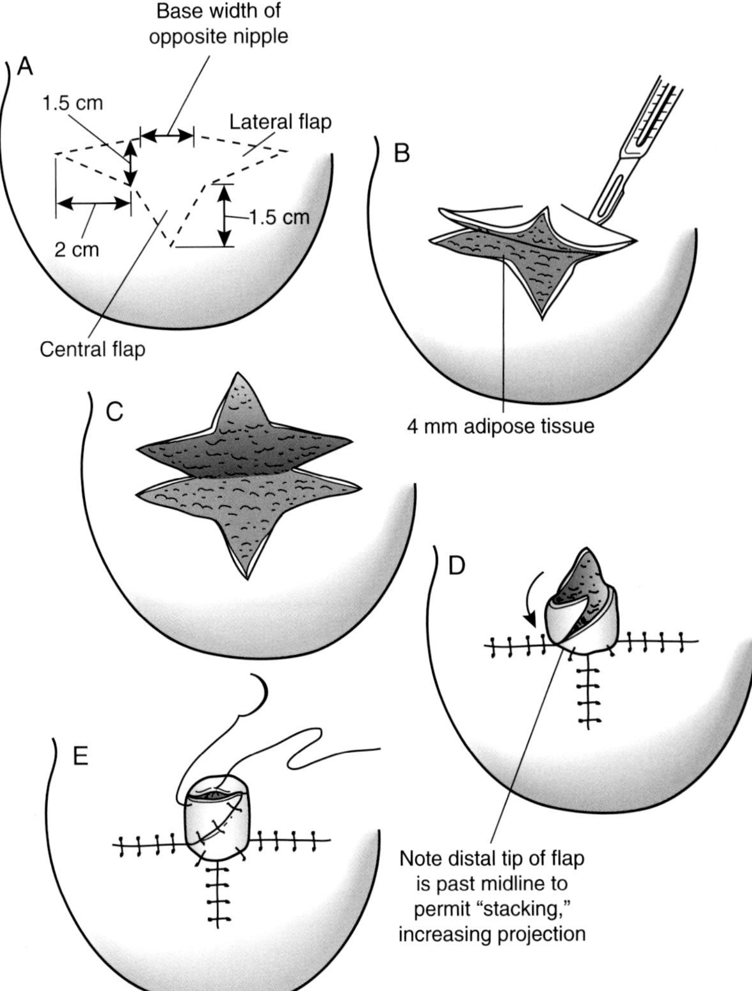

FIGURE 139-10. *A* to *E,* Planning, elevation, assembly, and donor site closure of the modified star flap. (From Shestak KC, Gabriel A, Landecker A, et al: Assessment of long-term projection: a comparison of three techniques. Plast Reconstr Surg 2002;110:780.)

the opposite nipple. Ullmann et al[40] relate the use of this artificial nipple that is glued to the patient's body. The results presented with a high rate of satisfaction by the patients and no adverse effects related to the glue or the prosthesis material.

ALLOPLASTIC MATERIALS. Alloplastic materials have been described to optimize nipple projection. Hallock[41] performed a study with a polyurethane-coated silicone gel implant in patients for 1 year without loss of projection or complications. At present, autogenous tissues are preferred for nipple projection when it is required.

AUTOGENOUS TISSUES. Autogenous tissue as a combined material to improve projection has been extensively described (Table 139-3). Brent and Bostwick[9] introduced the use of auricular tissue in 1977. Bernard and Beran[42] have been studying the applications of autogenous fat graft from the umbilicus area to acquire projection of the nipple. Although the study results demonstrated adequate projection and bulk within the nipple, the fat graft procedure needed to be repeated at least two times.

The most common techniques use costal cartilage combined with a local flap to improve the nipple projection. Yamamoto et al[37] described a combined technique using the star flap and a costal cartilage graft. The authors presented an excellent long-term projection result and the advantage of no donor site morbidity because the cartilage is extracted at the time of breast reconstruction and maintained in a tissue bank until the nipple reconstruction. This technique may provide a definitive advantage for Asian patients who present with a prominent nipple and a small areola surface, as advocated by Wei et al.[43] This technique can maintain the height and width equal to the opposite nipple in this population of patients. Guerra et al[44] described use of the costal cartilage graft with a follow-up of more than 7 years and reported that nipple projection was stable and reliable. There was, however, an

TABLE 139-3 ✦ AUTOGENOUS TISSUES FOR NIPPLE PROJECTION

Types	Dimension	Donor Site	Complications: Donor Site	Complications: Receptor Site	Resorption
Auricular cartilage[59]	1 × 2 cm	Auricular concha	Additional scar	2 partial necrosis	Bilobed flap: 5.4% of patients had partial resorption Trilobed flap: 61% of patients had partial resorption
Fat graft[42]	1-2 mL	Paraumbilical region	None	Requires repeat procedures (usually 2 steps)	~50% of patients have loss of projection with only one procedure
Banked cartilage[43]	1 cm in length × 0.6 cm in diameter	Third costal cartilage	None (no distortion/no thorax discomfort)	None	Final height > 1 cm (no resorption)
Conserved cartilage (under skin)[44]	1.5 cm in length × 0.1-0.15 cm in diameter	Third costal cartilage	None (no distortion/no thorax discomfort)	4% exposure	Projection stable: 20% of patients had revision
Artificial bone (Ceratite)[36]	~1 × 2 cm—shaped to size that does not cause tension on dermal fat flap	—	—	5% partial flap necrosis, 5% exposure	Projection stable

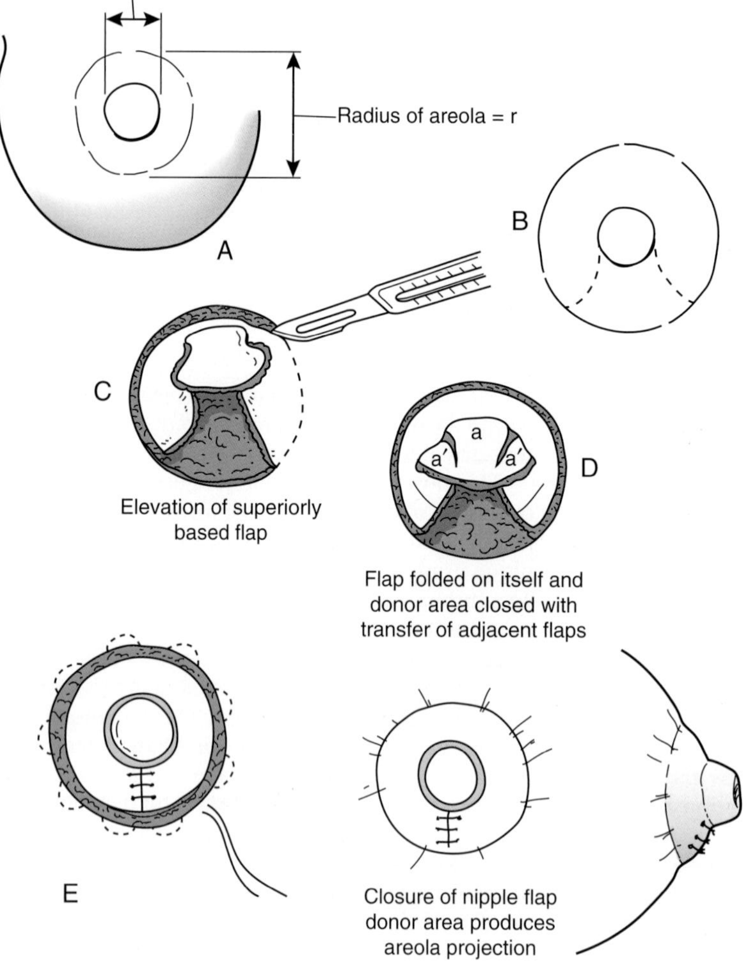

FIGURE 139-11. *A* to *E,* Planning, elevation, assembly, and donor site closure of the bell flap. (From Shestak KC, Gabriel A, Landecker A, et al: Assessment of long-term projection: a comparison of three techniques. Plast Reconstr Surg 2002;110:780.)

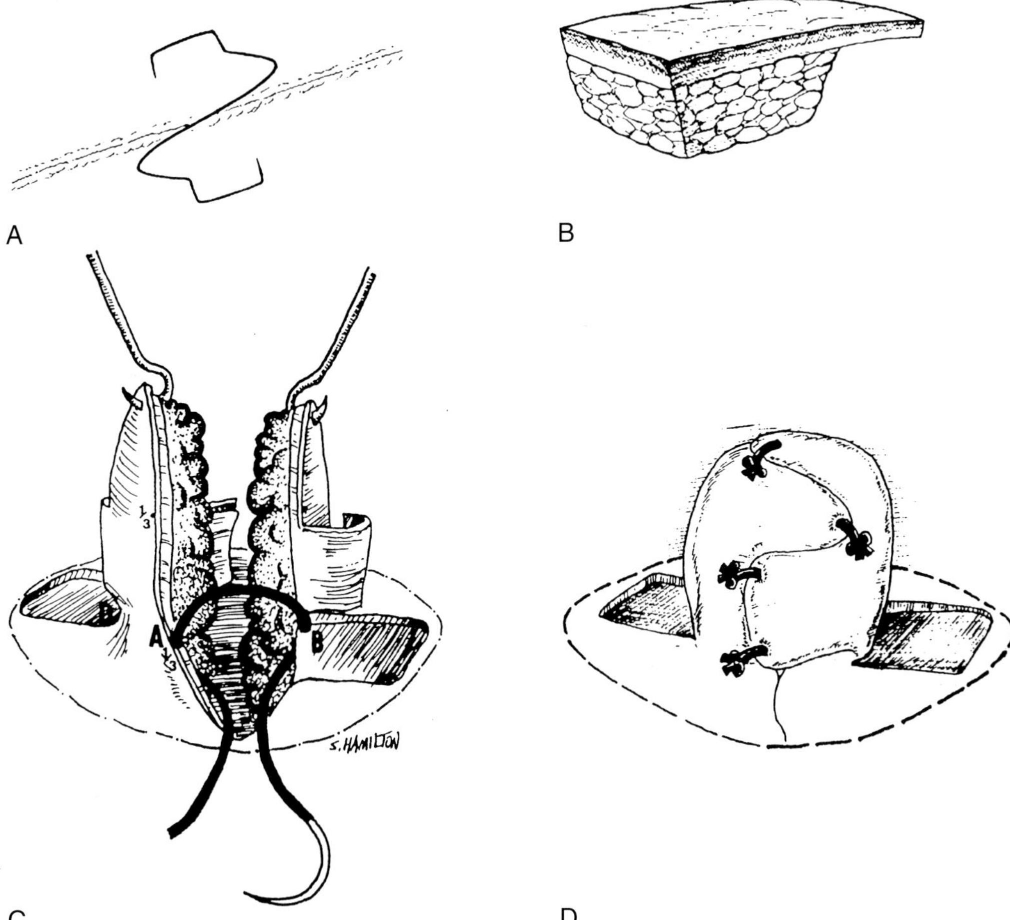

FIGURE 139-12. *A,* Diagram of double opposing tab flaps showing correct orientation to underlying scar (if present). *B,* Cross section of one flap showing relationship of tab to the dermal fat portion. *C,* The key suture that will bring the flaps into opposition and determine the amount of projection. *D,* The completed nipple. (From Kroll SS, Hamilton S: Nipple reconstruction with the double-opposing-tab flap. Plast Reconstr Surg 1989;84:523.)

incidence of 4% cartilage graft loss due to exposure of the cartilage and ischemia of the nipple flap.

Yanaga[36] reported the use of artificial bone with an average nipple height of 80.5% of the measurement of the opposite side. Support at the center of the dermal base confers stability to the bone, which is not depressed, maintaining the circulation.

When there is adequate flap tissue on which to design a local flap, an autogenous or alloplastic implant to enhance nipple projection is generally not necessary. However, use of an alloplastic implant or autogenous tissue as a salvage procedure after failure of a conventional technique for nipple reconstruction may be appropriate.

Postoperative Management

After nipple reconstruction, an ointment is placed over the nipple, and 2 × 2 gauze squares, with central holes the size of the diameter of the new nipple, are placed over the breast in layers. The dressing is taped to the breast skin and should remain in place for 5 to 7 days.

The dressing is removed in a subsequent visit in approximately 5 to 7 days, and the sutures are also removed. A new dressing is applied that is left in place for approximately 7 days. The tattoo is usually delayed for 4 to 6 weeks, and pressure to the nipple reconstruction site is avoided. With techniques that involve the use of a graft, the bolster dressing is removed in 3 to 5 days.

Complications

The most common complication is loss of projection. Projection usually decreases in the first 6 months. In general, it follows partial or complete failure of the reconstruction, which may be due to an error in timing of reconstruction or choice of technique (Fig. 139-13).[28,34]

Intraoperative planning and execution are critical steps in achieving optimal results. Complications such as epidermolysis, partial or complete necrosis, and open wounds are problems associated with ischemia of the flap, separation of the tissues as a result of shearing forces during the manipulation of the tissues, or an error in planning the amount of soft tissue necessary to maintain the vascularization of the flaps (Fig. 139-14).[1,26,27]

Infection is not a common complication, and it is most often associated with use of synthetic material to perform the nipple reconstruction.[27,34] Avoidance of direct pressure over the nipple for approximately 3 weeks and adherence to the postoperative regimen are also crucial for optimal results.[26,34]

Areola Reconstruction

Areola reconstruction can usually be performed by skin grafting or tattooing, approximately 2 to 3 months after the nipple reconstruction (Table 139-4).[1,8,26,27,29,30-32] The major advantage of a skin graft is the resultant irregular surface, which resembles the normal areola with Montgomery tubercles. Therefore, grafting followed by tattoo may provide a more natural appearance and the possibility of a sensory reinnervation with the graft by neurotization of the flap by the edges of normal tissue.

TABLE 139-4 ✦ GOALS OF AREOLA RECONSTRUCTION

Size
Pigmentation
Texture
Sensitivity

Areola reconstruction may be performed as a single-stage procedure at the time of nipple reconstruction or may be delayed until nipple reconstruction is completed. Correct positioning of the site has been emphasized. When dermal flaps are used for the nipple, skin grafting for cutaneous coverage is required. When flaps are used for the nipple, the surgeon has the option of immediate versus delayed skin grafting or tattoo of the NAC. If grafting of the areola is planned, immediate grafting at the time of nipple reconstruction is preferable.

The goals of size and pigmentation can be achieved with grafts, tattoos, or a combination of these techniques. Texture is best achieved with grafts because they provide a more natural, irregular surface. Sensory

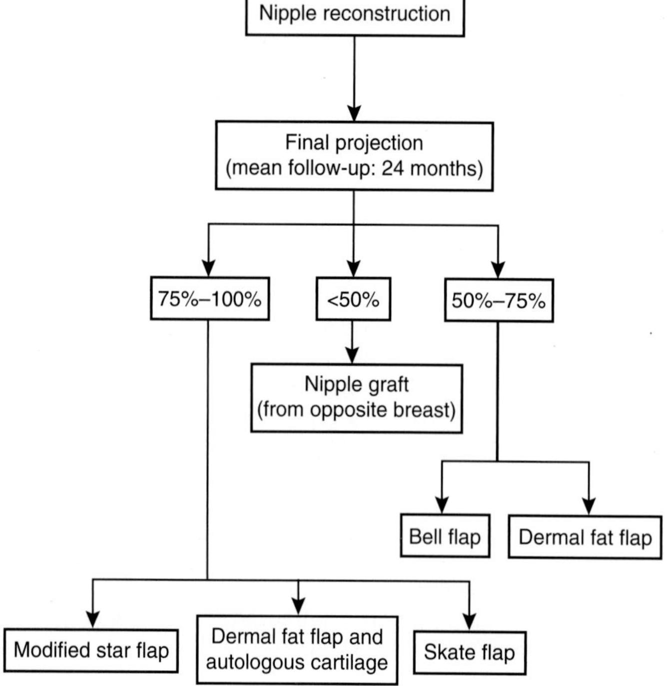

FIGURE 139-13. Comparison of final nipple projection (mean follow-up, 24 months) of nipple grafts and various local flaps. (Data from references 33, 35, 38, 43, 47.)

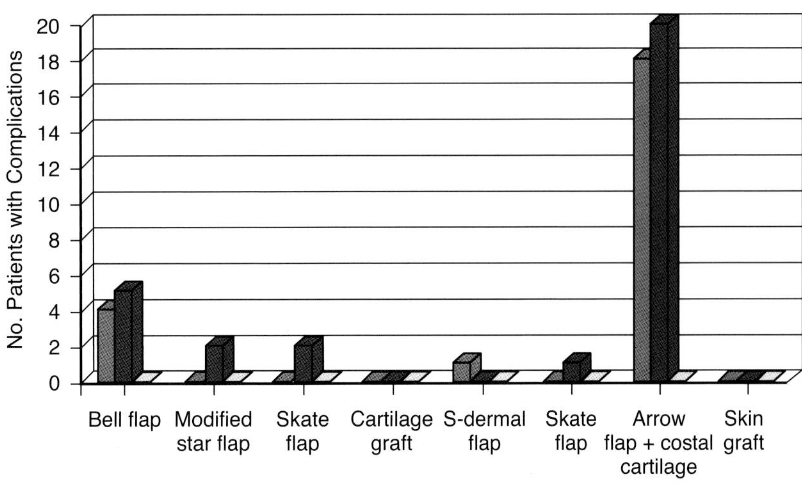

FIGURE 139-14. Comparison of complications of nipple grafts and various local flaps. (Data from references 33, 35, 38, 43, 44, 47.)

results are independent of the nipple-areola reconstruction and related to skin envelope preservation at the time of mastectomy and postoperative neurotization of flaps when they are used. Edsander-Nord et al[45] reported the return of sensation in breast flaps with and without nerve repair. The authors evaluated breast reconstructions with the deep inferior epigastric artery perforator (DIEP) flap reconstruction with (DIEP+) and without (DIEP–) nerve repair and transverse rectus abdominis musculocutaneous (TRAM) flap reconstruction without (TRAM–) nerve repair. The results presented were as follows: 30% of DIEP+, 8% of DIEP–, and 4% of TRAM– patients reported having erogenous sensation in the reconstructed breast.

Cooter et al[46] obtained data from 55 breast reconstruction patients to evaluate the degree of satisfaction with the breast reconstruction. Patients reported a 90% satisfaction rate with the appearance of the breast with a bra compared with a 52% satisfaction rate with the NAC color (skin graft and tattoo).

Cohen et al[28] evaluated 110 patients who underwent breast reconstruction with TRAM flap (59%), latissimus dorsi flap (19%), expander followed by an implant (9%), implant reconstruction (4%), and other (9%) and who subsequently underwent nipple reconstruction with star flap (35%), nipple sharing (10%), keyhole flap (9%), skate flap (9%), S flap (8%), full-thickness skin graft (6%), and other (23%). Of the patients studied, 12% refused nipple reconstruction. Patients reported an 81% satisfaction rate with the breast mound reconstruction compared with a 64% satisfaction rate with the nipple reconstruction. The decreased level of satisfaction with the NAC reconstruction was related to the longer time interval between the reconstruction of the breast and completion of the reconstructive process with the NAC (mean of 39 months). In a distribution of all factors analyzed by the patients, dissatisfaction was related to lack of projection, color, shape, size, texture, and position. Despite these data, 91% of patients confirmed that they would undergo a breast reconstruction again under the same circumstances.

Cheng et al[47] reported a study of 25 Chinese women who underwent nipple reconstruction with an S-dermal fat flap followed by intradermal tattoo. The authors collected a score based on a questionnaire that revealed the following results: the highest score was given to color followed by symmetry, size, and projection. Eighty-six percent of the patients were satisfied with the reconstruction, and all would recommend the NAC reconstruction to other women.

SKIN GRAFTS

The advantage of the skin graft for the areola is the slight wrinkling that occurs, unlike the smooth appearance of the tattoo directly placed on the breast mound skin. Full-thickness skin grafts for areola reconstruction can be harvested from the opposite areola (when patients undergo reduction or mastopexy and the opposite areola is wide), which may offer the best color match.[2,5,10] The skin graft may also be selected from a pigmented area (e.g., perineum, labia, and groin), where there will be adequate pigment for both the nipple and areola. If adequate pigment is not achieved—because of selection of a skin graft donor site where skin is not pigmented (skin graft donor site may come from skin resected at the breast mound reconstruction site during revision and may not contain increased pigmentation compared with the reconstructed breast mound) or if the nipple flaps include skin envelope surface—a second procedure to tattoo the nipple or the skin grafts will be required after healing of the nipple and areola graft is confirmed.

TATTOO

The reconstruction may also be accomplished with tattooing, described by Rees[8] in 1975, which has largely replaced skin grafting techniques,[30-32,48] avoiding donor site morbidity related to the harvest of the full-thickness skin graft. Although an exact color match is not always available and the tattoo tends to fade with time, avoidance of the donor site morbidity associated with graft harvest makes tattooing the preferred choice for many surgeons.

Tattooing has the advantage of providing a reasonable coloration of the areola and nipple from a wide choice of pigments, and an easy secondary revision may be performed. Furthermore, there is no donor site morbidity, and few complications are associated with the tattooing procedure. However, the pigments and tattooing are in a nonregulatory status by the Food and Drug Administration.[30,31] The base powder of some pigments consists of soluble inorganic salts of metal as iron oxides (for brown pigments); however, several colors have been changed to a highly stable inorganic metal (e.g., titanium) to decrease skin sensitivity.[31,49] Sterilization of materials and instruments, such as needles and containers, is mandatory.[31,32,48,49]

The initial tattoo must be darker than the desired final color because the result will fade with time. This phenomenon is related to the quantity of blood that is resorbed during the procedure associated with the ingestion of the pigments by the macrophages.[31]

The position of the areola is determined by the patient and the surgeon before the tattooing procedure (see section entitled "Positioning") (Fig. 139-15). The procedure is performed with the patient supine. A topical anesthetic is used to anesthetize the area of areola placement. In general, however, the procedure may be tolerated without local anesthesia. By selecting between the wide variations in pigments ranging from dark brown to pink to yellow, the surgeon can enhance the visual analysis of the areola and the gradations of color observed in the opposite areola or in the preoperative pictures of the patients undergoing bilateral nipple-areola reconstruction. The pigments are mixed by the surgeon, and the shade is tested on normal skin and compared with the opposite areola.

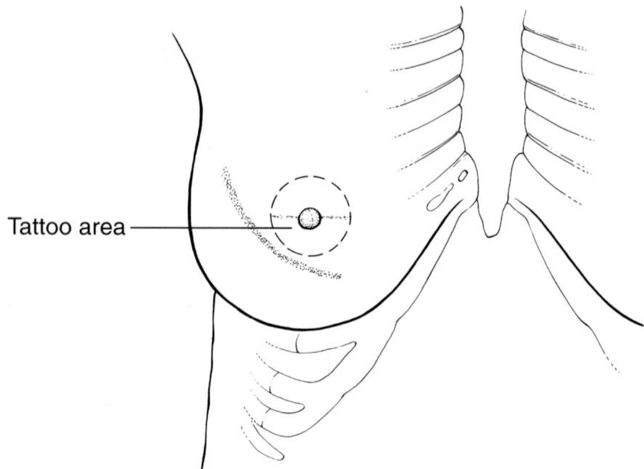

FIGURE 139-15. Nipple-areola tattoo. The nipple reconstruction site determines center of areola. The dimension of the areola is matched with the contralateral areola.

It is preferable to begin in the peripheral area and work toward the central area (Color Plate 139-1).

Some patients may present with a redness after the procedure associated with an edema and an itching sensation that remains for a few hours.[31] Fading of the pigments is common; however, fading may be revised with touch-ups in approximately 3 months (Figs. 139-16 and 139-17).

POSTOPERATIVE MANAGEMENT

Skin Grafts

The skin graft site is covered immediately either with a bolster dressing to compress the full-thickness graft to the donor site or with gauze, avoiding motion at the recipient site. The areola dressing should compress the graft to prevent shearing forces. After the initial dressing is removed, an ointment should be applied to the graft area to provide a moist environment and comfort for the patient. The dressing must remain intact and is removed in the subsequent visit (5 to 7 days) for evaluation. A new dressing is then applied, and the stitches are removed in 1 week.

Tattoo

After the tattoo procedure, there will be an excess of pigment deposited over the tattoo, which can be removed with moist gauze. Bacitracin or petroleum jelly is applied to the area, and it is covered with gauze. The gauze coverage should be removed in 3 to 5 days and the area evaluated. As a result of the punctures required for tattooing, discrete bleeding will give rise to crusts that separate in a few days.

SUMMARY

A wide variety of techniques have been introduced for reconstruction of the NAC. Each technique has

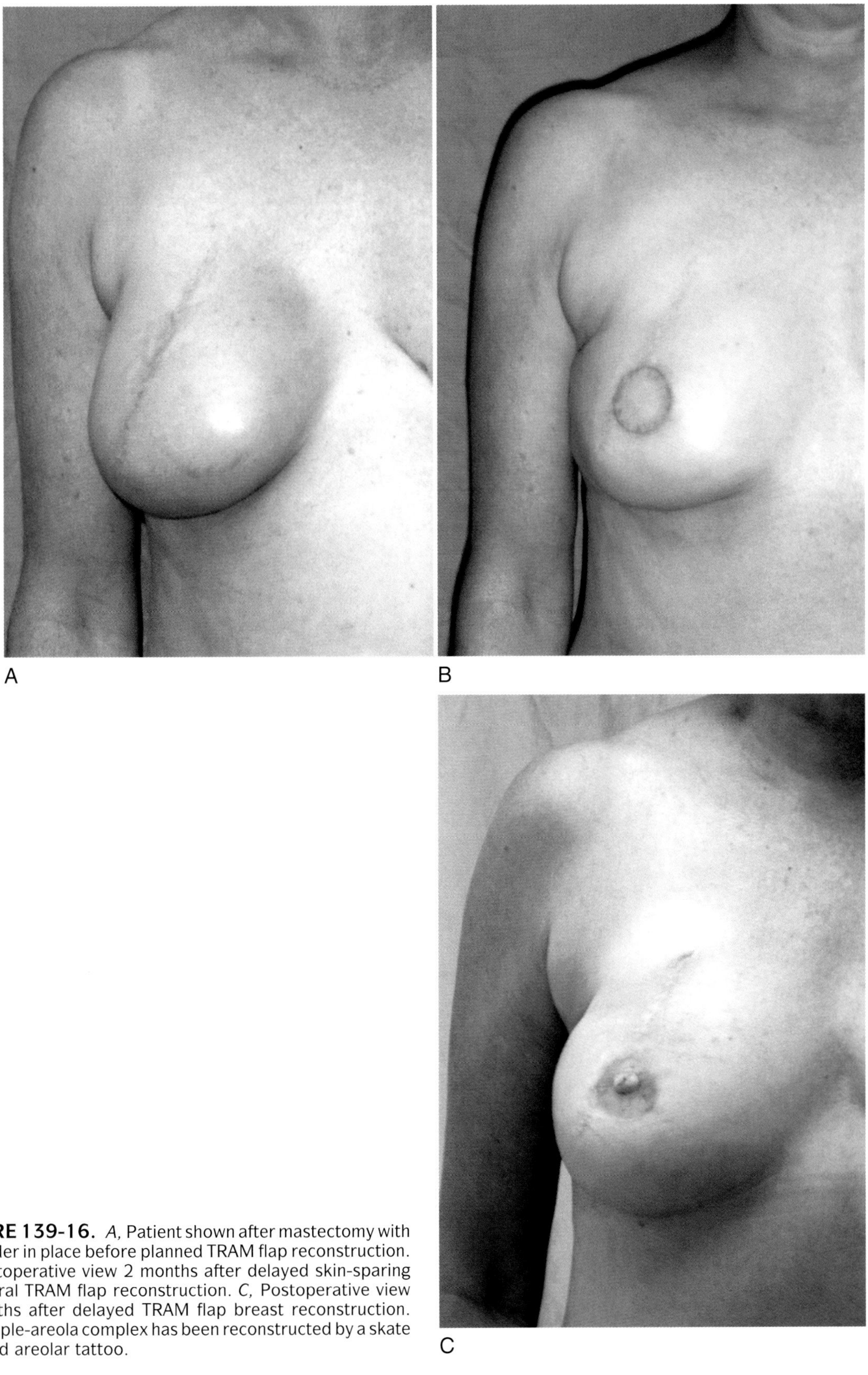

A

B

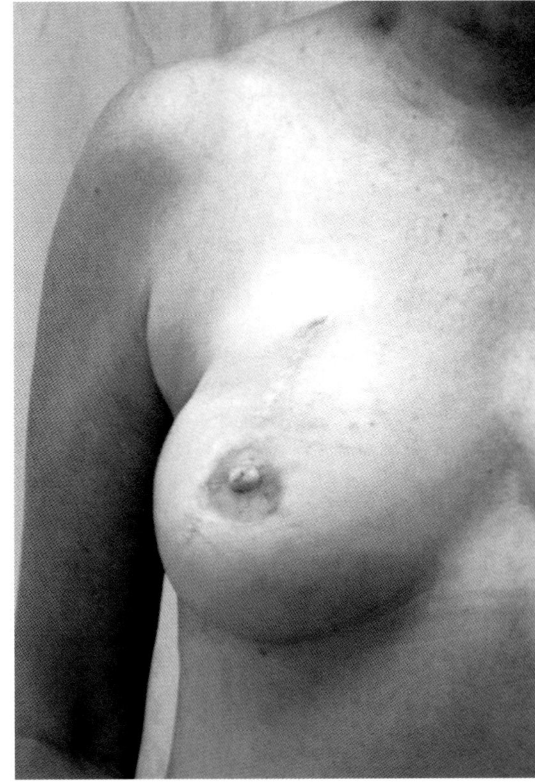

C

FIGURE 139-16. *A,* Patient shown after mastectomy with expander in place before planned TRAM flap reconstruction. *B,* Postoperative view 2 months after delayed skin-sparing unilateral TRAM flap reconstruction. *C,* Postoperative view 6 months after delayed TRAM flap breast reconstruction. The nipple-areola complex has been reconstructed by a skate flap and areolar tattoo.

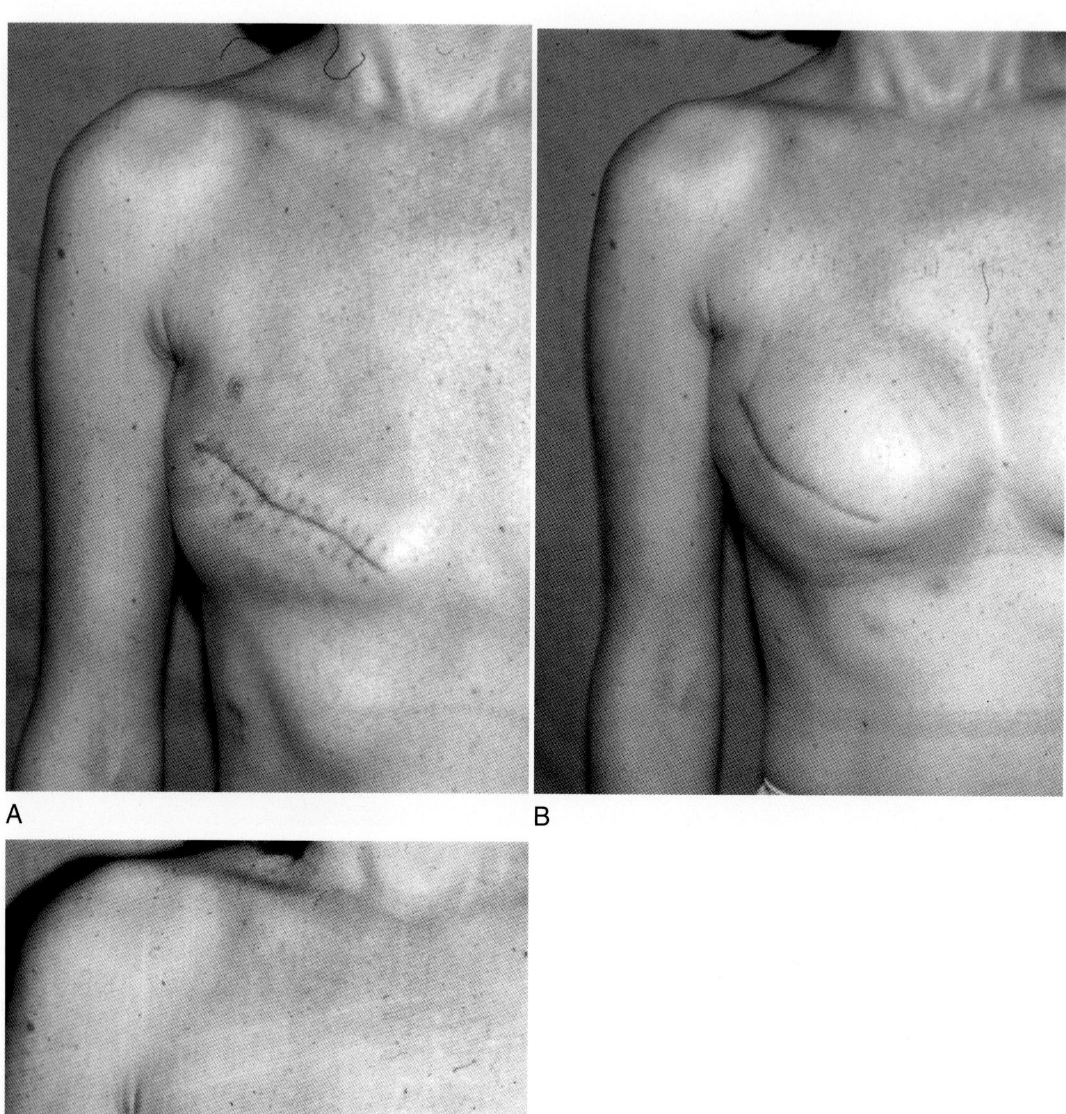

FIGURE 139-17. *A,* Patient is seen after unilateral mastectomy. *B,* Postoperative view demonstrating stable implant-expander breast reconstruction. *C,* Postoperative view after nipple-areola reconstruction.

advantages and disadvantages in regard to fulfilling the goals of nipple-areola reconstruction.

Postmastectomy reconstruction patients can be subdivided into three groups in regard to nipple-areola reconstruction: (1) patients who have no interest in further surgery, (2) patients who have unstable central mound skin or present with irradiation injury to the central breast mound, and (3) patients with a stable skin envelope or flap at the central breast mound. For the first group, selected patients may have interest in an external silicone ectoprosthesis. For the second group, a delayed reconstruction of the NAC should be planned. A cartilage graft may be helpful if a local flap is not possible or will provide inadequate projection. In group three, immediate or delayed nipple-areola reconstruction is safe and should provide an acceptable result.

As to technique, there are many local flaps available for nipple reconstruction, and the surgeon will develop preferences for those techniques that provide reliable and predictable results. Both skin grafts and tattoo are excellent choices for nipple-areola pigmentation. In general, nipple-areola reconstruction represents a final, positive step in a sometimes difficult process from diagnosis to treatment and reconstruction for breast cancer.

REFERENCES

1. Bohmert H, von Hesler FW: Techniques of reconstruction of nipple-areolar complex. In Bohmert H, ed: Breast Cancer: Conservative and Reconstructive Surgery. New York, Thieme, 1989:356.
2. Adams WM: Free transplantation of the nipples and areola. Surgery 1944;15:186.
3. Adams WM: Labial transplant for correction of loss of the nipple. Plast Reconstr Surg 1949;4:295.
4. Di Pirro ME: Reconstruction of the nipple and areola after a burn. Plast Reconstr Surg 1970;46:299.
5. Snyder CC, et al: Surgery of the areola-nipple complex. Symposium on Aesthetic Surgery of the Face, Eyelid, and Breast. St. Louis, Mosby, 1972:192.
6. Millard DR: Nipple and areola reconstruction by split-skin graft from the normal side. Plast Reconstr Surg 1972;50: 350.
7. Bunchman HH 2nd, Larson DL, Huang TT, Lewis SR: Areola and nipple reconstruction in burned breast: "double bubble" technique. Plast Reconstr Surg 1974;54:531.
8. Rees TD: Reconstruction of the breast areola by intradermal tattoo and transfer. Plast Reconstr Surg 1975;55:620.
9. Brent B, Bostwick J: Nipple-areola reconstruction with auricular tissues. Plast Reconstr Surg 1977;60:353.
10. Broadbent TR, Woolf RM, Metz PS: Restoring the mammary areola by a skin graft from the upper inner thigh. Br J Plast Surg 1977;30:220.
11. Muruci DJ, Dantas JJ, Noguerira LR: Reconstruction of the nipple-areola complex. Plast Reconstr Surg 1978;61:558.
12. Klatsky SA, Manson PN: Toe pulp free grafts in nipple reconstruction. Plast Reconstr Surg 1981;68:245.
13. Cohen IK: Reconstruction of the nipple-areola by dermabrasion in a black patient. Plast Reconstr Surg 1981;67:231.
14. Serafin D, Georgiade M: Nipple-areola reconstruction postmastectomy. Ann Plast Surg 1982;8:29.
15. Little JW, Munasifi T, McCulloch DT: One-stage reconstruction of a projecting nipple: the quadrapod flap. Plast Reconstr Surg 1983;71:126.
16. Chang WHJ: Nipple reconstruction with a T flap. Plast Reconstr Surg 1984;73:140.
17. Hartrampf C, Culbertson J: A dermal-fat flap for nipple reconstruction. Plast Reconstr Surg 1984;73:982.
18. Thomas SV, Gillis MB, Pool R: Nipple reconstruction with a new local tissue flap. Plast Reconstr Surg 1996;97:1053.
19. Cohen IK, Ward JA, Chandrasekhar B: The pinwheel flap nipple and barrier areola graft reconstruction. Plast Reconstr Surg 1986;77:995.
20. Little JW: Nipple-areolar reconstruction. Adv Plast Surg 1987;3:43.
21. Cronin ED, Humphreys DH, Ruiz-Razura A: Nipple reconstruction: the S-flap. Plast Reconstr Surg 1988;81:783.
22. Kroll SS: Nipple reconstruction with the double-opposing-tab flap. Plast Surg Forum 1987;10:219.
23. Anton M, Eskenazi L, Hartrampf CR: Nipple reconstruction with local flaps: star and wrap flaps. Perspect Plast Surg 1991;5:67.
24. Hugo NE, Sultan MR, Hardy SP: Nipple-areola reconstruction with intradermal tattoo and double opposing pennant flaps. Ann Plast Surg 1993;30:510.
25. Eskenazi L: A one-stage nipple reconstruction with the "modified star" flap and immediate tattoo: a review of 100 cases. Plast Reconstr Surg 1993;92:671.
26. Hartrampf CR: Nipple-areola reconstruction. In Hartrampf CR, ed: Breast Reconstruction with Living Tissue. Norfolk, Va, Hampton Press, 1991:327-345.
27. Lemperle G, Nievergelt J: Nipple-areola reconstruction. In Lemperle G, Nievergelt J: Plastic and Reconstructive Breast Surgery—An Atlas. Berlin, Springer-Verlag, 1991:141.
28. Cohen BE, et al: Nipple-areola reconstruction: satisfaction and clinical determinants. Plast Reconstr Surg 2002;110:457.
29. Spear SL, Convit R, Little JW III: Intradermal tattoo as an adjuvant to nipple-areola reconstruction. Plast Reconstr Surg 1989;83:907.
30. Spear SL, Little JW, Convit R: Intradermal tattoo as an adjunct to nipple-areola reconstruction. Plast Reconstr Surg 1989;83:907.
31. Spear SL, Arias J: Long-term experience with nipple-areola tattooing. Plast Reconstr Surg 1995;35:232.
32. Bhatty MA, Berry RB: Nipple-areola reconstruction by tattooing and nipple sharing. Br J Plast Surg 1997;50:331.
33. Kargul G, et al: Reconstruction of the breast areola complex. Comparison of different techniques. Handchir Mikrochir Plast Chir 2001;33:133.
34. Few JW, Marcus JR, Casas LA: Long-term predictable nipple projection following reconstruction. Plast Reconstr Surg 1999;104:1321.
35. Cederna P, et al: Modified technique for nipple-areolar reconstruction: a case series. Plast Reconstr Surg 2003;112:1274.
36. Yanaga H: Nipple-areola reconstruction with a dermal fat flap: technical improvement from rolled auricular cartilage to artificial bone. Plast Reconstr Surg 2003;112:1863.
37. Yamamoto Y, et al: Two innovations of the star flap technique for nipple reconstruction. Br J Plast Surg 2001;54:723.
38. Shestak KC, Gabriel A, Landecker A, et al: Assessment of long-term projection: a comparison of three techniques. Plast Reconstr Surg 2002;110:780.
39. Eng JS: Bell flap nipple reconstruction: a new wrinkle. Ann Plast Surg 1996;36:485.
40. Ullmann Y, Pelled LJ, Laufer D, Blumenfeld L: Nipple-areola reconstruction with a custom-made silicone ectoprosthesis. Ann Plast Surg 1992;28:485.
41. Hallock GG: Polyurethane nipple prosthesis. Ann Plast Surg 1990;24:80.
42. Bernard RW, Beran SJ: Autologous fat graft in nipple reconstruction. Plast Reconstr Surg 2003;112:964.

43. Wei FC, et al: Nipple reconstruction in Asian female using banked cartilage graft and modified top hat flap. Br J Plast Surg 2003;56:692.
44. Guerra AB, Khoobehi K, Metzinger SE, Allen RJ: New technique for nipple-areola reconstruction: arrow flap and rib cartilage graft for long-lasting nipple projection. Ann Plast Surg 2003;50:31.
45. Edsander-Nord A, Wickman M, Hansson P: Somatosensory status after pedicled or free TRAM flap surgery: a retrospective study. Plast Reconstr Surg 1999;104:1642.
46. Cooter RD, Dean NR, Neild T, et al: Fading of nipple-areolar reconstruction: the last hurdle in breast reconstruction? Br J Plast Surg 2002; 55:574.
47. Cheng MS, Ho CM, Cheung WY, et al: Nipple-areola reconstruction in autologous breast reconstruction. Chinese patients' perspective. Ann Plast Surg 2004;53:328.
48. Fourie le R, Bruce-Chwatt A: Professional tattooing: alternative method to nipple reconstruction. Br J Plast Surg 2004;57:693.
49. Masser MR, Di Meo L, Hobby JA: Tattooing in reconstruction of the nipple and areola: a new method. Plast Reconstr Surg 1989;84:677.
50. Thorek M: Plastic reconstruction of the breast and free transplantation of the nipple. J Int Coll Surg 1946;9:194.
51. Dubin DB: A new simplified method for nipple reconstruction. Presented at the Annual Meeting of the American Society of Plastic and Reconstructive Surgeons, New Orleans, 1980.
52. Gruber RP: Nipple-areola reconstruction: a review of techniques. Clin Plast Surg 1979;6:71.
53. Zhang Z, Xia Z, Li D: One-stage reconstruction of nipple-areola: the beta flap [in Chinese]. Zhonghua Zheng Xing Shao Shang Wai Ke Za Zhi 1995;11:241.
54. Hallock GG, Altobelli JA: Cylindrical nipple reconstruction using an H flap. Ann Plast Surg 1993;30:23.
55. Ramakrishnan VV, Mohan D, Krishna A: Twin flap technique for nipple reconstruction. Ann Plast Surg 1997;39:241.
56. Kroll SS: Integrated breast mound reduction and nipple reconstruction with the wraparound flap. Plast Reconstr Surg 1999;104:687.
57. Jones G, Bostwick J III: Nipple-areolar reconstruction. Operative Techniques Plast Reconstr Surg 1994;1:35.
58. Horn MA, Cimino V, Angelats J: Modified autogenous latissimus breast reconstruction and the box top nipple. Plast Reconstr Surg 2000;106:763.
59. Tanabe-Yanaga H, Tai Y, Kiyokawa YT, Yamauchi T: Nipple-areola reconstruction with a dermal-fat flap and rolled auricular cartilage. Plast Reconstr Surg 1997;100:431.

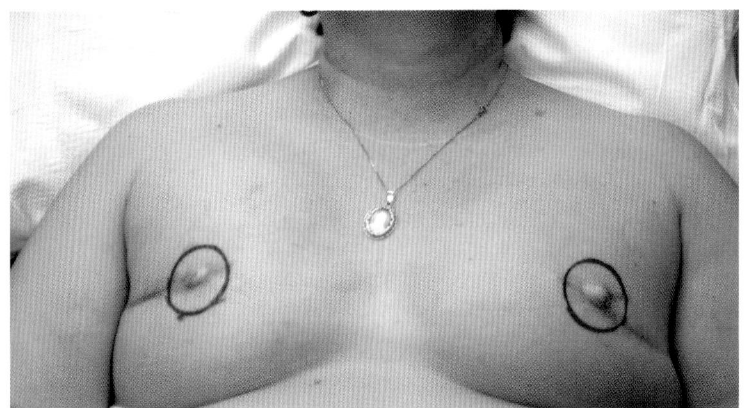

A

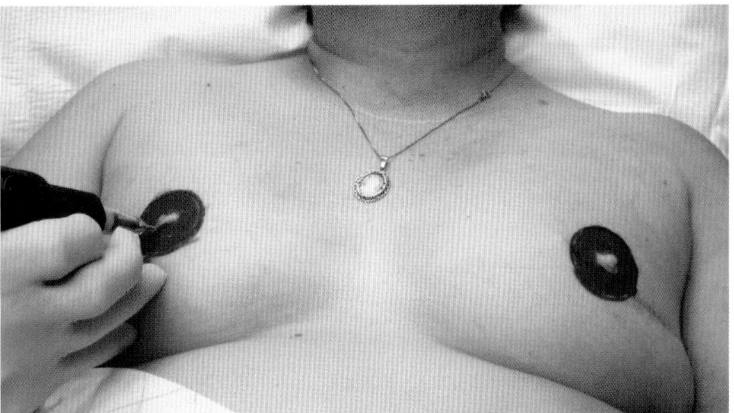

B

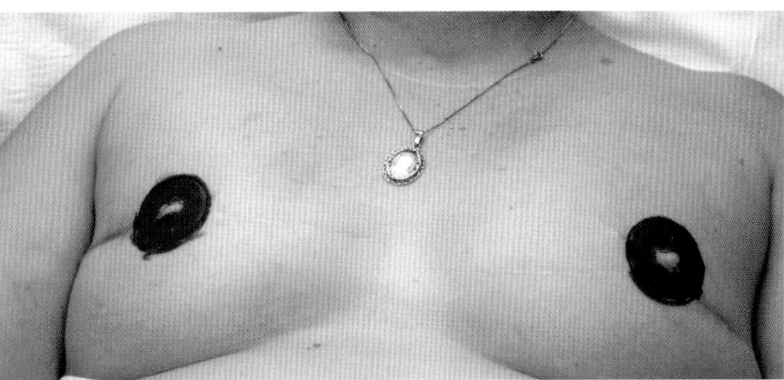

C

COLOR PLATE 139-1. Nipple-areola intradermal tattoo. The patient is seen 3 months after expander-implant reconstruction for bilateral mastectomy and 6 weeks after skate flap nipple reconstruction. *A,* Preoperative outline of areola. *B* and *C,* Brown pigments placed on areola (if unilateral nipple-areola reconstruction is performed, pigments that match the contralateral side would be selected) and pushed into dermis by electric hand set. *Continued*

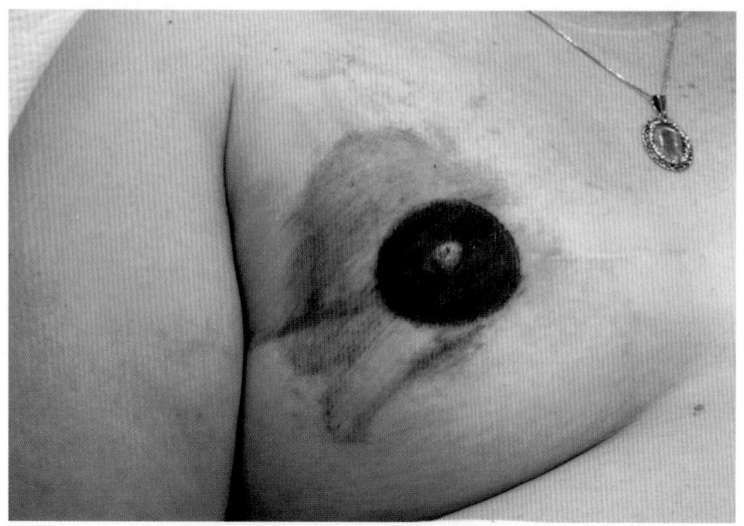

D

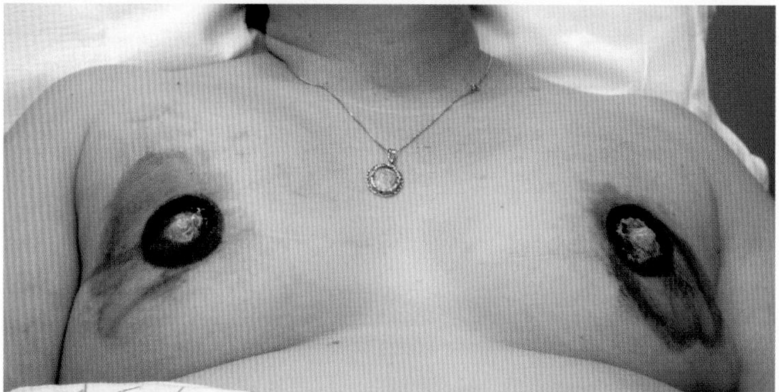

E

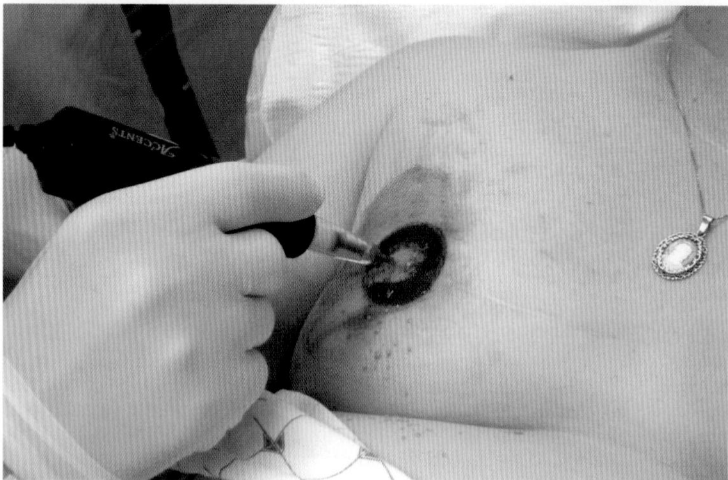

F

COLOR PLATE 139-1, cont'd. *D,* Brown pigments injected into dermis. *E,* Rose pigments selected for nipple. *F,* Pigments injected into dermis of skate flap.

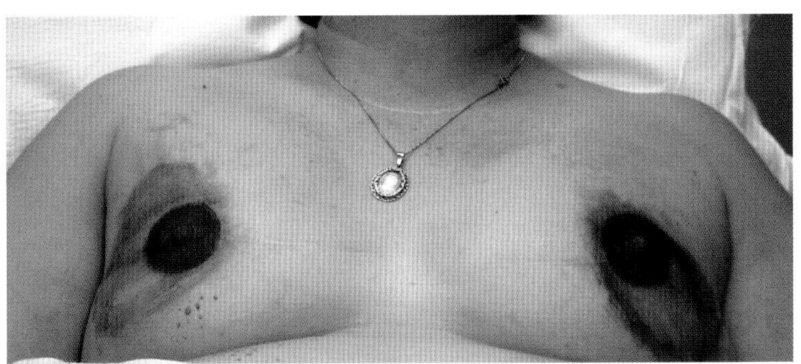

G

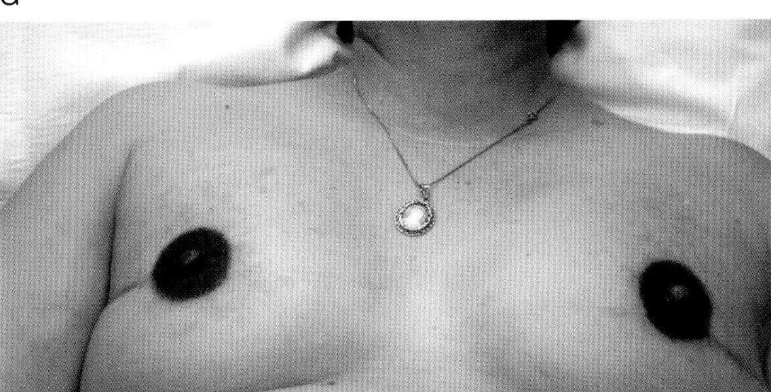

H

COLOR PLATE 139-1, cont'd. *G,* Darker brown pigment placed at base of nipple to accentuate height of nipple. *H,* Tattoo for bilateral nipple-areola completed.

CHAPTER

140

Immediate Postmastectomy Reconstruction: Latissimus Flap Techniques

SCOTT L. SPEAR, MD ✦ AMER A. SABA, MD

The latissimus dorsi muscle flap was originally described by Tansini[1,2] in 1906 for use as an axial musculocutaneous flap to cover mastectomy defects. This technique of mastectomy wound management became popular in Europe for some time but eventually fell from favor. In 1977, Schneider[3] described the anatomy of the flap and outlined its use for reconstruction of the breast. The technique of the skin island over the muscle was popularized by Bostwick[4] in 1978. This allowed the possible replacement of skin deficiencies and reconstruction of the radical mastectomy defects. McCraw[5] defined the vascular territory of the latissimus dorsi musculocutaneous flap, and Maxwell[6] concluded that the flap could be raised successfully even when the thoracodorsal arterial trunk is ligated, to be sustained presumptively by secondary perfusion.[7] This secondary source of circulation to the flap was later shown to be the serratus collateral branch.[8] The description of the transverse rectus abdominis musculocutaneous (TRAM) flap by Hartrampf[9] in 1979 and the ability to reconstruct the breast completely with autogenous tissue resulted in decline of the use of the latissimus dorsi muscle flap. Today, with the advancements in techniques and the tremendous improvements in the aesthetic results of breast reconstruction, the latissimus dorsi muscle flap with its versatility is undergoing resurgence in popularity as different applications are being developed. It is commonly used in immediate breast reconstruction to replace skin, to add tissue to reduce the size of the breast implant needed, and to provide more cushion and cover to establish a more natural breast contour. New approaches now allow additional fat and subcutaneous tissue to be harvested over the latissimus dorsi muscle, making purely autologous latissimus dorsi flap breast reconstruction possible for certain candidates. Partial breast reconstruction is also possible after quadrantectomy or lumpectomy by use of this flap with specific designs. Thus, the latissimus dorsi flap is now frequently used as a primary method of immediate reconstruction as well as a supplement to other techniques.

ANATOMY

The latissimus dorsi muscle is a large, flat, triangular muscle measuring approximately 25 by 35 cm and covering the posterior inferior half of the trunk. The major part of its outer surface is subcutaneous. Its superomedial fibers are deep to the trapezius muscle. The remainder of the muscle is superficial to the serratus anterior and posterior muscles, a portion of the external oblique muscle, and the erector spinae.

The muscle originates from the iliac crest, the posterior layer of the thoracolumbar fascia, the lower six thoracic spines, and the lower third to fourth ribs laterally, where it is closely associated with some origins of the external oblique muscle. As the muscle passes toward the axilla, near the tip of the scapula, it converges in a spiral fashion and joins with fibers of the teres major to form the posterior axillary fold. The latissimus dorsi insertion is through a 3-cm-broad tendon attached to the intertubercular groove of the humerus.

At the level of the tenth to eleventh rib, there is a firm, thick aponeurotic attachment between the serratus anterior and the latissimus. These aponeurotic attachments correspond to the lower border of the serratus anterior; they must be divided during latissimus dorsi flap elevation to prevent inadvertent elevation of the serratus anterior muscle along with the latissimus dorsi flap.

The pattern of circulation of the latissimus dorsi muscle is type V according to the Mathes and Nahai classification.[10,11] The dominant pedicle is composed of the thoracodorsal artery, two veins, and the thoracodorsal nerve. The length of the thoracodorsal artery is 8 cm with a diameter of 2.5 mm. This vessel's relatively large diameter, predictability, and minimal anatomic variation along with the large musculocutaneous unit it supplies make the latissimus dorsi flap a highly reliable donor site as a transposition or free flap for breast reconstruction.

The thoracodorsal artery, along with the circumflex scapular artery, is a branch of the subscapular artery arising from the axillary artery. The thoracodorsal artery gives off a branch to the serratus muscle shortly after entering the underside of the latissimus muscle in the posterior axilla 10 cm inferior to the muscle insertion into the humerus (Fig. 140-1). Understanding of the anatomy in this area is important. In patients with previous axillary dissection, when the thoracodorsal pedicle has been divided, a reversal of flow through the serratus branch can provide adequate blood flow to the flap, allowing the use of the latissimus dorsi muscle as a transposition flap based on its dominant vascular pedicle.[8] Once it is in the muscle, the vascular pedicle bifurcates into a large lateral branch and a smaller transverse branch. These branches arborize within the muscle to produce extensive intramuscular collateralization.[12-14] A precise knowledge of the internal vascular anatomy of the muscle makes it

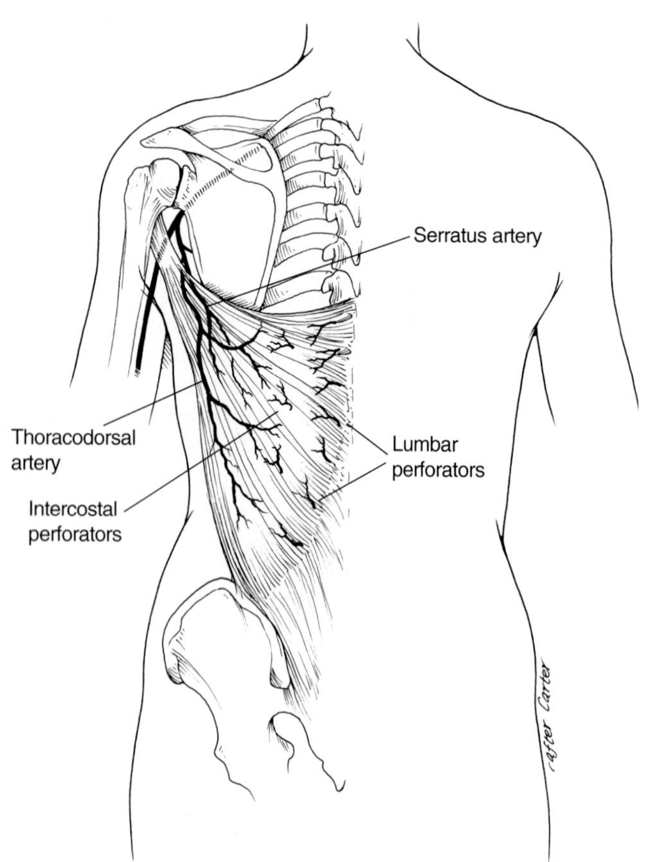

FIGURE 140-1. The blood supply to the latissimus dorsi muscle.

possible to split it for use as a double flap or to preserve half of the muscle to maintain function.

Secondary segmental pedicles enter the underside of the muscle through the lateral perforators row off the posterior intercostal arteries 5 cm from the posterior midline and through the medial perforators row off the lumbar artery adjacent to the site of muscle origin. These perforators allow the use of the latissimus dorsi as a foldover flap to cover midback defects.[15,16]

Numerous musculocutaneous perforators extend from this rich intramuscular vascular network into the overlying skin and subcutaneous tissue, allowing skin islands to be safely designed anywhere within the margin of the muscle. The largest perforators branch from the lateral branch of the thoracodorsal artery, making safest the skin island located in a lateral vertical orientation.[12-14]

The latissimus dorsi muscle adducts, extends, and rotates the humerus medially. It also assists in securing the tip of the scapula against the posterior chest wall. It is an expendable muscle because function is preserved by the remaining synergistic shoulder girdle muscles. Transposition of this muscle anteriorly has been shown to be well tolerated by patients and results in only a minimal functional deficit,[17,18] although dynamic weakness in shoulder extension and adduction may occur.[19]

PREOPERATIVE ASSESSMENT AND APPROPRIATE CONSULTATION

A preoperative consultation should gather detailed information about the patient's medical history, the state of local tissues, the condition of the breast, the possible donor sites, and the patient's wishes.

In patients who will undergo immediate breast reconstruction, the planning requires an estimate of how much skin and breast tissue will be removed. Particular attention is given to the amount of skin and subcutaneous tissue obtainable in the dorsal region. A good indication is given by pinching the lateral dorsal pad to estimate the thickness of the adipose layer. It is vital to compare the mass available with that which will be needed to achieve a suitable breast size.

It is also important preoperatively to assess the function of the latissimus dorsi muscle. Denervated and nonfunctional muscle after an axillary dissection increases the risk of damaged thoracodorsal vessels or inadequate circulation. In this instance, the latissimus dorsi must then be elevated on an intact serratus collateral pedicle. Functioning muscle is most often a favorable sign for the integrity of the pedicle; however, it does not guarantee intact thoracodorsal vessels.

Arteriography is not ordinarily thought to be necessary to obtain information about the status of the thoracodorsal artery when there is good muscle function. The flap's nearly perfect reliability when the serratus collateral is preserved makes arteriography and electromyography virtually unnecessary.

INDICATIONS

The decision to select the latissimus flap reconstruction must take into account the patient's motivations, the anatomy of the breast as well as of the back, the nature of underlying breast disease, and the competency of the surgical team.

The latissimus dorsi is helpful for breast reconstruction after a skin-sparing mastectomy when a breast prosthesis is part of the plan. The latissimus dorsi skin can be used to replace the missing skin at the site of the nipple-areola, and the muscle can be used to provide improved soft tissue coverage of the breast implant or expander. Placement of a tissue expander under the latissimus muscle allows postoperative adjustment of breast volume and ultimately better symmetry with the opposite breast. Use of the autogenous latissimus dorsi alone without a prosthesis does not allow as much range in the size of the reconstructed breast. In either instance, it is difficult to assess the final volume of the reconstructed breast at the initial setting because of swelling and settling of the breast in the postoperative course.

Primary reconstruction can still be accomplished without an implant, especially for women with a small to medium-sized breast (Fig. 140-2).[20] An extended latissimus dorsi musculocutaneous flap without an implant could even be used for a larger breast, especially in patients with at least 2 cm of pinch thickness of back fat (Fig. 140-3).[21-25] The texture of the breast

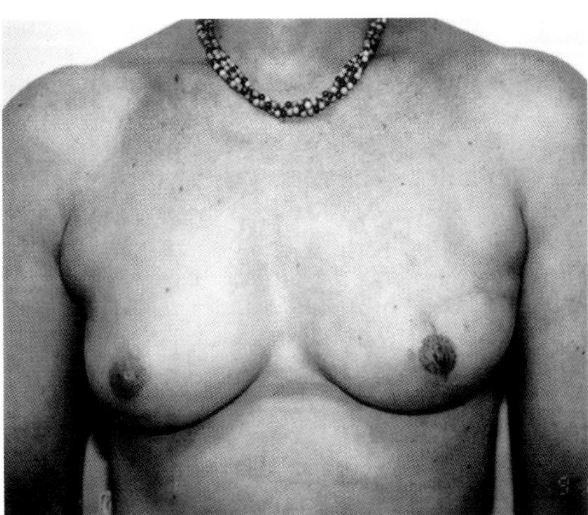

FIGURE 140-2. Postoperative result for a woman with medium-sized breasts who had a left mastectomy for breast cancer and immediate reconstruction by the autogenous latissimus dorsi flap with the boomerang design. (Courtesy of Dr. Richard W. Dabb.)

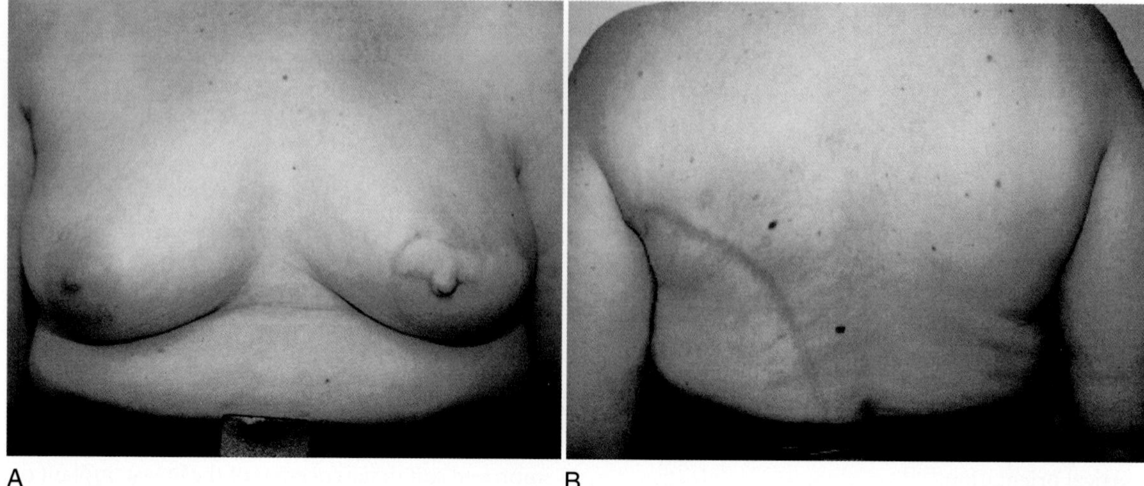

FIGURE 140-3. *A,* Postoperative result for a woman with large breasts who had a left mastectomy for breast cancer and immediate reconstruction by the autogenous latissimus dorsi flap with the boomerang design. The flap design provided adequate volume and projection to achieve good symmetry with the contralateral breast. *B,* Appearance of the back postoperatively, showing an acceptable donor site scar. (*A* and *B* courtesy of Dr. Richard W. Dabb.)

and the absence of an implant are major advantages of the purely autogenous breast reconstruction.[26]

Finally, the latissimus dorsi flap is particularly useful for reconstruction of partial mastectomy or lumpectomy deformities. In such patients, in whom irradiation is certain to aggravate the lumpectomy deformity, the latissimus flap can replace some or all of the missing tissue and thus mitigate the eventual damage.

SPECIFIC INDICATIONS

Patients Who Are Not Candidates for a TRAM Flap

Some women who need supplementary autologous tissue for a satisfactory breast reconstruction or who wish to have purely autogenous breast reconstruction may not be candidates for the TRAM flap (Fig. 140-4).[27] This includes women who have had a previous abdominoplasty or TRAM flap, and it may also include women with insufficient abdominal skin or fat. Women who smoke, have diabetes, or are obese may be considered to be too high risk to undergo a TRAM flap. Some women may choose not to undergo on operation as extensive and lengthy as a TRAM flap, particularly in light of the time required for recuperation.

When a TRAM flap is not available or advisable, the latissimus flap becomes an obvious option. Aside from being an alternative when a TRAM flap is not the right choice, the latissimus flap has certain attributes and advantages that may make it a better choice. The latissimus flap includes a large well-vascularized flat muscle that may be better suited for dealing with poorly vascularized defects or for covering an implant. In patients with small defects, particularly laterally, the latissimus may be the best choice.

Previous Irradiation During Breast Conservative Therapy

The skin flaps of a previously irradiated breast are unreliable from a circulatory point of view and inelastic from a tissue expansion perspective. The addition of a latissimus musculocutaneous flap at the time of immediate postmastectomy reconstruction makes the operation safer and improves the odds that the ultimate result will be satisfactory (Fig. 140-5).[28]

Partial Mastectomy Defects

In women in whom a lumpectomy would establish an undesirable defect, the latissimus flap can replace or make up for the missing tissue (Fig. 140-6).[29]

Excessively Thin or Unreliable Skin Flaps over an Implant

The latissimus dorsi flap can provide additional skin cover and soft tissue padding to properly cover an implant or expander.[30,31]

After a Previous Mastopexy or Reduction

The skin flaps in these patients may be unreliable. A skin-sparing mastectomy approach to these patients makes them good candidates for the latissimus flap

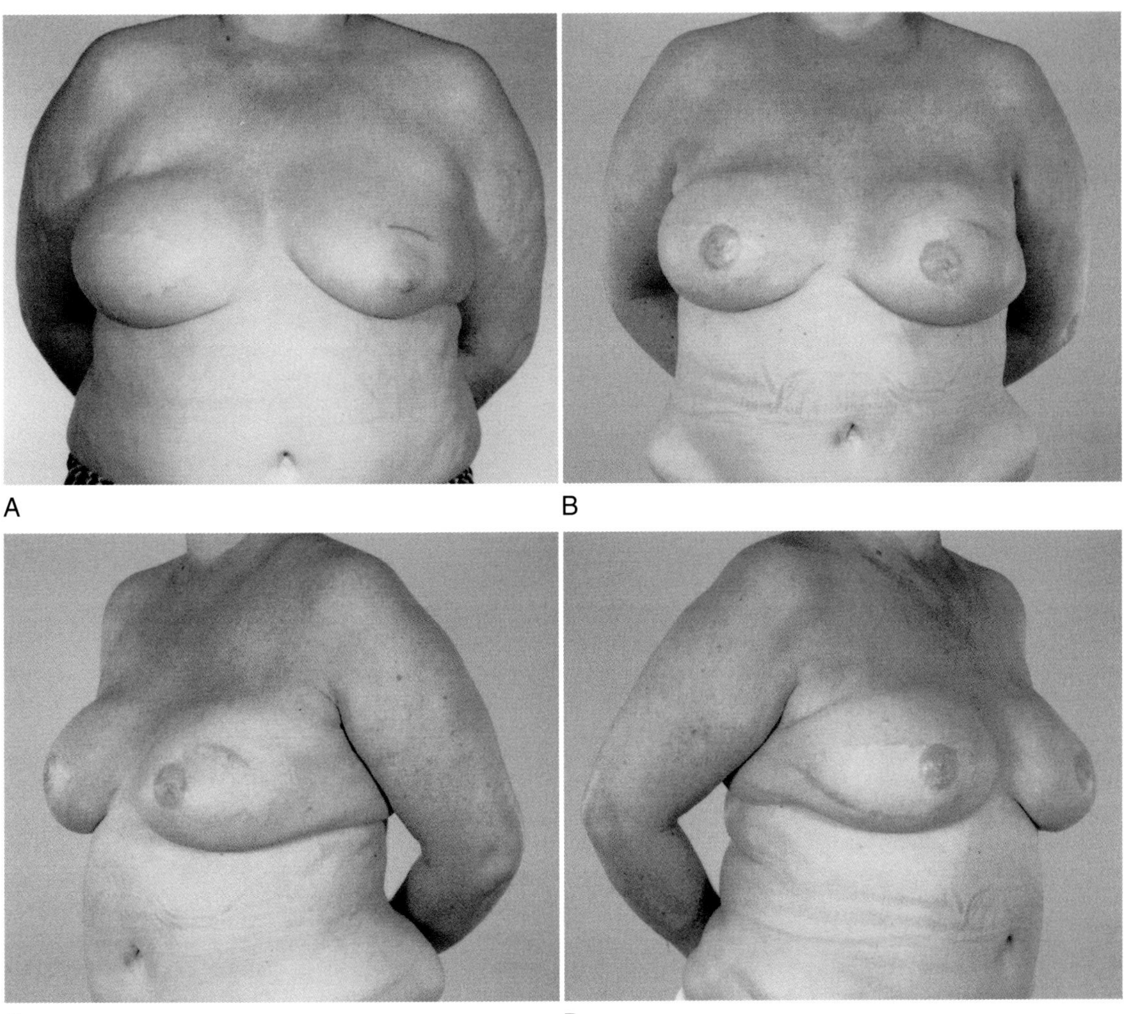

FIGURE 140-4. *A,* Preoperative appearance of a patient with cancer of the left breast. The patient has a history of right mastectomy and TRAM flap reconstruction. *B* to *D,* Postoperative result with excellent symmetry after a left mastectomy and immediate reconstruction with latissimus dorsi flap and a prosthesis.

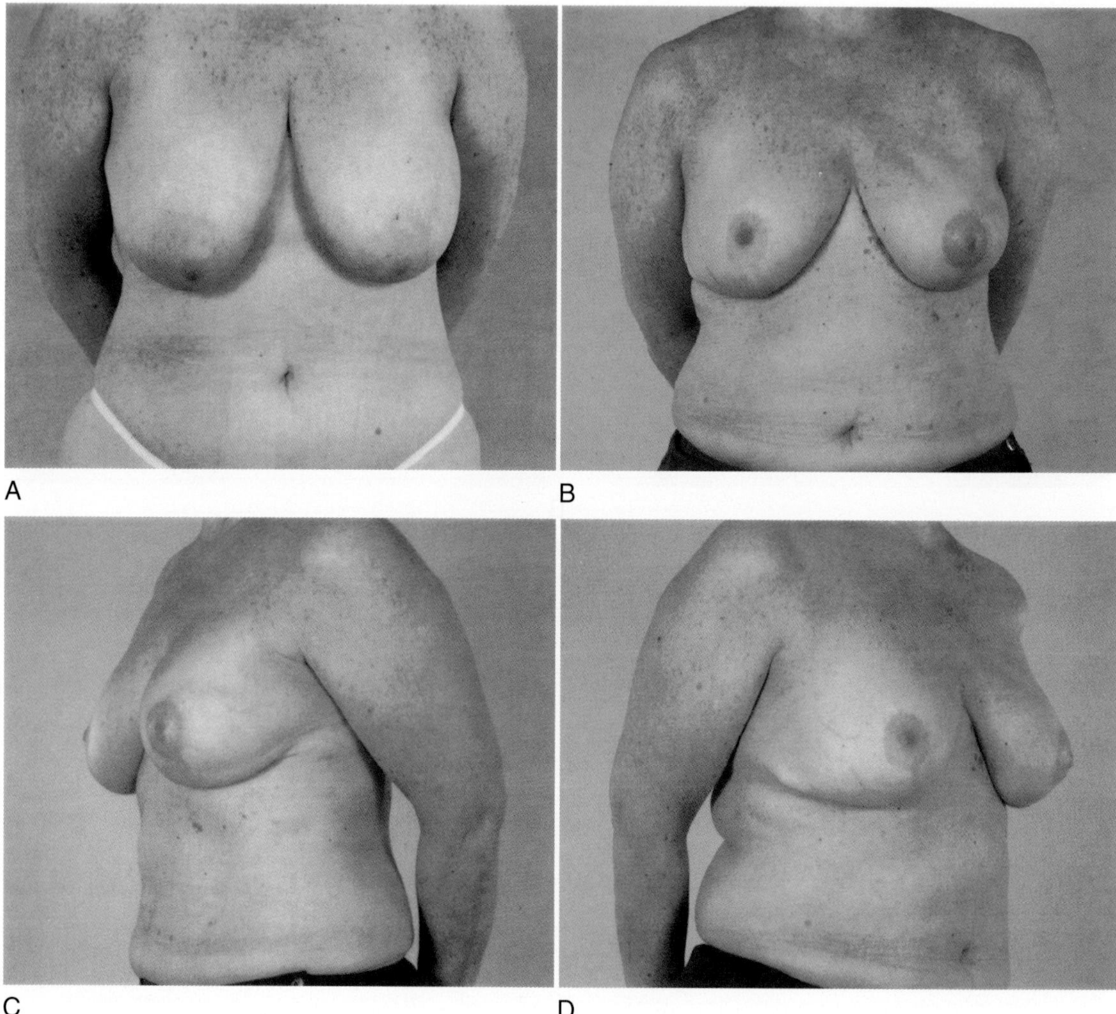

FIGURE 140-5. *A,* Preoperative appearance of a 52-year-old woman who had left lumpectomy and radiation treatment for breast cancer. *B* to *D,* After a recurrence of cancer in the left breast 11 years later, she underwent a left mastectomy and immediate reconstruction with latissimus dorsi flap and a prosthesis as well as a reduction mastopexy of the right breast for better symmetry.

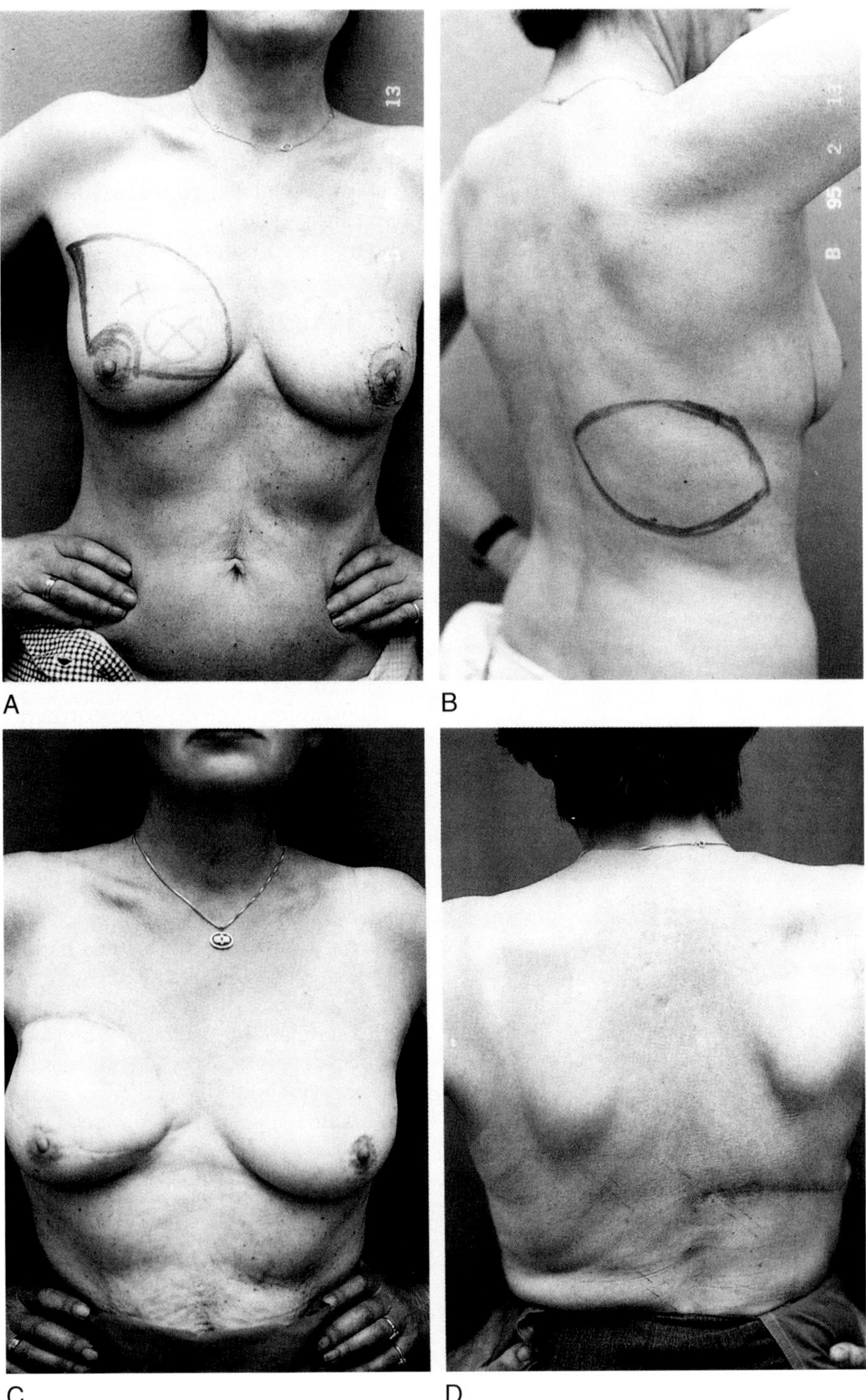

FIGURE 140-6. *A* and *B,* Before surgery. Front and donor site views illustrate direct access to the former tumor bed; partial mastectomy includes overlying irradiated skin. *C* and *D,* After surgery; result of skin and volume reconstruction after irradiation. Scar of donor site disappears over time. The natural breast shape is maintained. (From Spear SS: Surgery of the Breast: Principles and Art. Philadelphia, Lippincott-Raven, 1998:182.)

over a prosthesis to provide safe cover if flap necrosis should develop.

Augmented Breasts

Women who have had breast augmentation previously may select a skin-sparing mastectomy with a latissimus flap over their breast prosthesis to have the greatest likelihood of symmetry and an attractive result from their reconstruction.[32]

Large Ptotic Breasts

Reconstruction of a large or ptotic breast is complicated by the long flaps generated by the mastectomy as well as by the frequent need to plan the mastectomy with breast reduction patterns and techniques. The use of the latissimus flap in these patients provides safer cover over the implant and facilitates the use of reduction design patterns to allow the reconstruction to more closely simulate the opposite breast.

Prophylactic Mastectomy

For some women, particularly younger women undergoing prophylactic mastectomy, the ultimate cosmetic results can be important. The latissimus flap can be used in these women to maximize the aesthetic results, including retention of the nipple as a skin graft (Fig. 140-7).

Surgeon's Preference

Finally, because of the inherent advantages in adding a latissimus flap to a prosthetic reconstruction, some surgeons simply prefer the addition of a flap to many if not most of their implant reconstructions.

CONTRAINDICATIONS

The main contraindication to use of the latissimus dorsi flap is a previous posterolateral thoracotomy in which the latissimus muscle had been divided. This makes the dorsal donor site unavailable for ipsilateral breast reconstruction. A relative contraindication is an atrophic latissimus dorsi muscle after division of the thoracodorsal nerve during an axillary dissection. The volume of the latissimus dorsi muscle is decreased by denervation atrophy. This may not provide enough tissue to permit breast reconstruction or to achieve symmetry, especially in planning total autogenous reconstruction. Moreover, the risk of damaged thoracodorsal vessels is increased in a nonfunctioning latissimus muscle, necessitating an intact serratus collateral pedicle to elevate the flap.

Finally, the use of the latissimus flap electively with skin-sparing mastectomy before radiation therapy is probably unwise. The immediate use of the latissimus dorsi muscle would result in the needless irradiation of the flap and the likely corresponding damage to it. In such circumstances, it is a safer and more predictable strategy to postpone the latissimus flap reconstruction until after the mastectomy and subsequent radiation therapy.[33] Skin-sparing mastectomy with a latissimus flap thus should be reserved for patients unlikely to undergo postmastectomy adjuvant radiation therapy.

TECHNIQUES

One advantage of the immediate reconstruction is that the plastic surgeon and general surgeon can work together to preserve important landmarks, such as the inframammary fold and the native unaffected breast skin envelope, which define the unique shape of a woman's breast. This preservation allows the reconstructed breast to assume a more natural and symmetric shape once the volume is restored. The quantity of skin excised during mastectomy dictates the skin requirement for breast restoration. Knowing the exact skin requirement and replacing it facilitate the reconstruction.

In planning immediate reconstruction with a latissimus flap, surgical planning and marking should be done in an unhurried fashion with appropriate consideration given to how the plan to use the latissimus flap may affect the method of the mastectomy itself. In virtually all patients with invasive breast cancer, in most patients with in situ cancer, and in many prophylactic mastectomies, the nipple-areola will need to be excised. When the latissimus flap is planned, the nipple-areola can be removed as the aesthetic unit of a circle, rather than as an ellipse as is typically done with a standard mastectomy. When a biopsy has been performed previously or the tumor is close to the skin, that skin too should be marked for excision. This additional skin to be removed may be excised as a separate ellipse or as a piece contiguous to the areola, thus requiring a larger patch for its replacement. An axillary incision, when it is considered, is usually done through a separate incision, which should be closed primarily. After the likely skin requirement resulting from the mastectomy has been determined, consideration can be given to planning of the latissimus flap itself. Some thought should also be given to how much muscle may be needed as well as where it may be needed and in what relationship to the skin island.

The preoperative planning and markings are done with the patient in the upright position. The planned skin excision, midline, and inframammary folds are marked first. Before designing the flap itself, examine the patient's back and mark the lateral margin of the latissimus dorsi muscle along the posterior axillary line down to the posterior iliac crest by supporting the patient's abducted arm and palpating the muscle

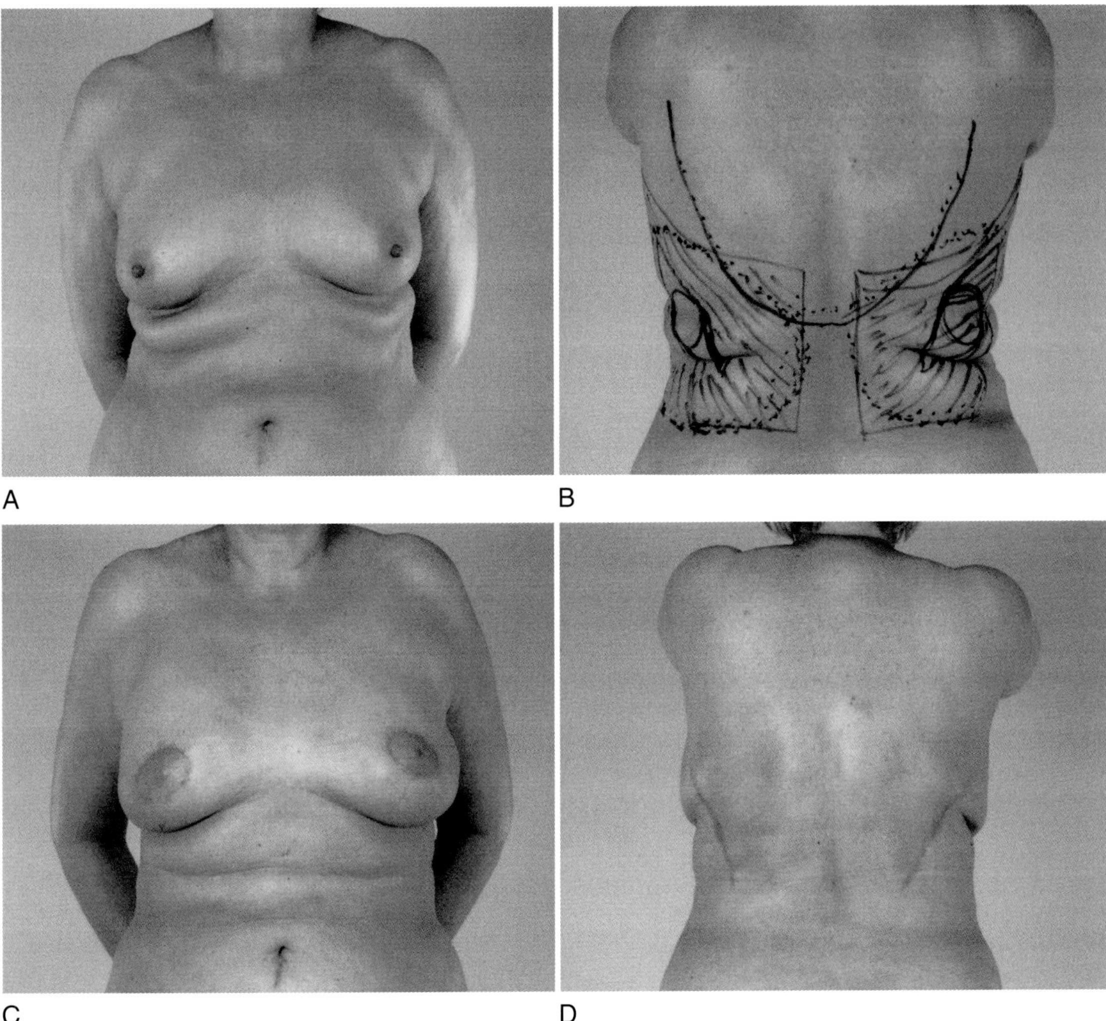

FIGURE 140-7. *A,* Preoperative appearance of a 52-year-old woman with a strong family history of breast cancer who is *BRCA1* positive. The patient desired to have bilateral prophylactic mastectomy and immediate reconstruction. *B,* Preoperative markings in preparation for elevation of bilateral latissimus dorsi muscles with discrete small skin islands designed obliquely in a natural skin line along the lower midback. *C,* Postoperative view after bilateral mastectomy and immediate breast reconstruction with latissimus dorsi flap and prosthesis as well as free nipple grafts for ultimate aesthetic results. *D,* Favorable postoperative donor site scars that will be well hidden in a dress with a "low-cut" back.

laterally as the patient pushes downward. The superior margin of the flap is identified by locating the tip of the scapula, with the patient's arms at the sides, and drawing a line across this landmark up into the axilla over the top of the posterior axillary fold. The posterior or medial margin is represented for all practical purposes by the posterior midline. The inferior margin is marked at the posterior iliac crest.

The planning of the skin pattern is variable, depending on the circumstances of the mastectomy.[34] It may be a discrete small island when reconstruction is planned with an implant after a skin-sparing mastectomy (Fig. 140-8). Alternatively, it may require all the available excess back skin and fat when a total autogenous latissimus breast reconstruction is attempted (Fig. 140-9). The skin island is designed laterally, obliquely in a natural skin line along the lower midback, or transversely where the scar can be hidden within the confines of the bra straps. The donor site back scars should be designed with the patient's preference for the location of the scar taken into consideration. Ironically, even though the latissimus flap may be designed to replace the circular aesthetic unit of the areola, the skin pattern of the latissimus flap itself is ultimately closed always as an ellipse, thus leaving a linear scar at the donor site.

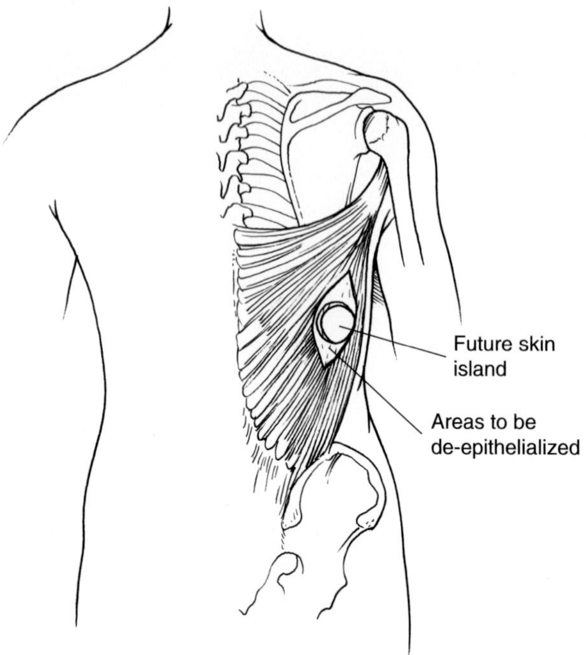

FIGURE 140-8. Common placement of the skin island in planning of latissimus dorsi flap reconstruction with a prosthesis.

After the mastectomy is performed by the general surgeon, latissimus flap elevation is performed in the lateral decubitus position (Fig. 140-10). To begin with, the skin island is incised. When an autologous latissimus dorsi flap reconstruction without an implant is planned, dissection is carried out just beneath the superficial fascia, leaving the deep fat attached to the surface of the muscle (Fig. 140-11). The fascia superficialis is a useful guide for this procedure because it ensures that a consistent thickness of fat is kept on the cutaneous flaps, thus helping avoid any secondary dorsal irregularities or, worse, flap loss. The fat left attached to the surface of the muscle is well vascularized by the perforators coming from the muscle itself. The entire surface of the muscle to be used is exposed in this same plane. The dissection then proceeds laterally to identify the lateral border of the latissimus dorsi muscle. The latissimus dorsi muscle is separated from the serratus anterior, and the flap is elevated along its lateral edge. The lumbosacral fascia is divided at the level of the posterior axillary line, then the latissimus fibers of origin are separated from the

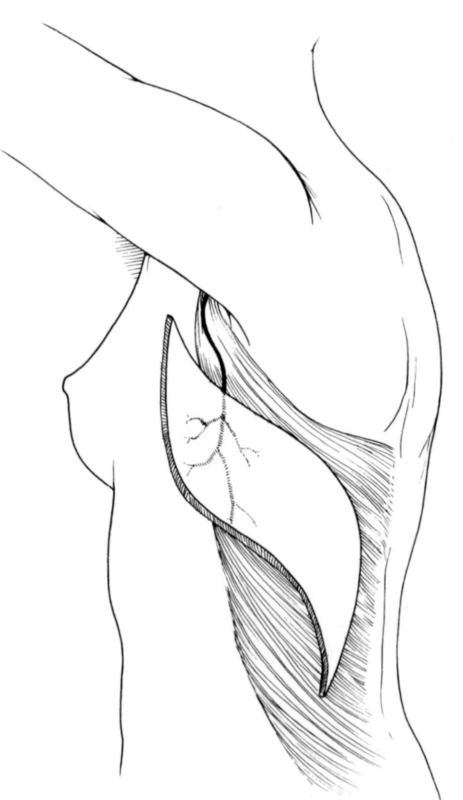

FIGURE 140-9. When total autogenous latissimus breast reconstruction is planned, the skin island is designed to include all available excess back skin and fat.

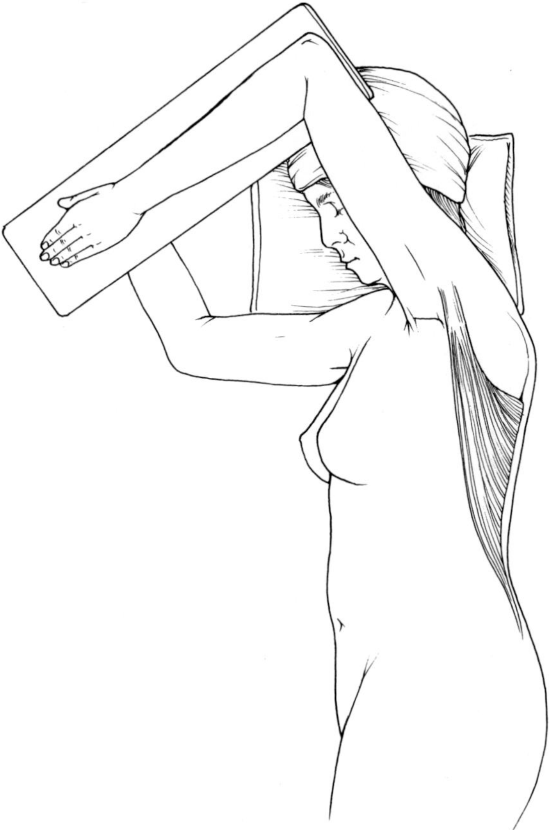

FIGURE 140-10. The patient is positioned in the lateral decubitus position for latissimus flap elevation. This allows easy access to the entire muscle and its insertion.

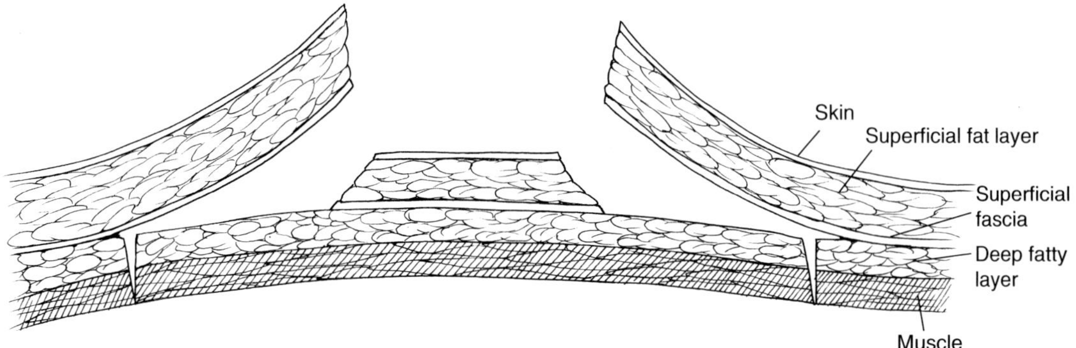

FIGURE 140-11. In the autogenous latissimus flap, the deep fat is left attached to the muscle as the dissection is carried out just beneath the fascia superficialis. This ensures adequate volume for reconstruction and preservation of the dorsal skin flaps.

paraspinous muscle fascia. Care must be taken to avoid incising through the paraspinous fascia because this makes identification of the proper plane of dissection difficult. The remaining fibers of origin are divided medially from the vertebral column. In dividing these fascial attachments, large intercostal perforating vessels should be carefully controlled to prevent bleeding and postoperative hematoma formation. Superomedially, the covering fibers of the trapezius muscle are identified and elevated away from the underlying latissimus muscle. After the superior border of the latissimus is identified, dissection is carried out laterally toward the axilla, separating away the fibers of the teres major muscle that diffuse with those of the latissimus. The entire muscle flap is then elevated toward the axilla (Fig. 140-12*A*). The thoracodorsal artery and vein are identified at the point of entrance into muscle. The serratus branch is easily identified and may be left intact, especially if the patient had axillary dissection in which the thoracodorsal artery may have been injured. The additional blood inflow through the serratus branch may be critical. It is desirable in most patients to divide the latissimus dorsi muscle near its insertion at its attachment to the humerus. Release of the insertions helps avoid the displeasing bulge in the low axilla that is sometimes seen when the insertion is left intact.[35] Care must be taken during this step to preserve the thoracodorsal vessels. The flap is then transferred to the mastectomy defect through a subcutaneous tunnel high in the axilla to further prevent an unnatural lateral bulge and to fill the axilla (Fig. 140-12*B*). Suturing of the muscle at the anterior axillary line should be performed to prevent lateral migration of the flap and implant and to protect the pedicle from tension.

The back incision is first temporarily stapled closed over a suction drainage tube. When fibrin glue is used, several transverse lines of approximation are then marked with a pen, and the staples are removed. Fibrin sealant adhesive, in appropriate concentrations, may be used to encourage the adherence of the superficial skin flaps to the underlying deep tissues. The fibrin sealant is sprayed, and the patient is then stapled again as previously marked. The spray is applied in less than 60 seconds so that the fibrin does not set up before the closure has occurred. Pressure is then maintained on the skin flap for 4 or 5 minutes to promote a good fibrin bond. The donor site is then closed over the previously inserted suction drain in layers including 2-0 polydioxanone to the fascia superficialis followed by interrupted and running intradermal 3-0 Monocryl to the dermis.

The patient is then placed in a supine position for insetting of the flap. The placement of the flap depends on the particular circumstances of the reconstruction. For immediate reconstruction after a modified radical mastectomy, the skin paddle is positioned at the site of the skin excision. After a skin-sparing mastectomy in which only the areola is excised, only an areolar size disk of back skin over the latissimus is preserved; the rest of the dorsal cutaneous paddle is de-epithelialized. In prophylactic skin-sparing mastectomy, the nipple-areola may be preserved as a full-thickness skin graft and sutured back in place on top of the de-epithelialized latissimus skin island.

When reconstruction is planned with use of the latissimus flap over an expander, it is easier and quicker to leave the pectoralis major muscle intact and to place the expander between the latissimus and pectoralis major muscles (Fig. 140-13). The latissimus muscle is inset just beneath the upper mastectomy skin flap. This position helps achieve some soft tissue filling of the upper pole of the reconstructed breast. The latissimus dorsi muscle is sutured medially and inferiorly to the underlying muscle and fascia in such a way as to help establish those borders of the breast. Superiorly, marionette half-mattress sutures are used between the overlying breast skin and the edge of the latissimus muscle to help cover the entire mastectomy defect with the latissimus muscle. Not tying these sutures provides access for placement of the expander. The expander is

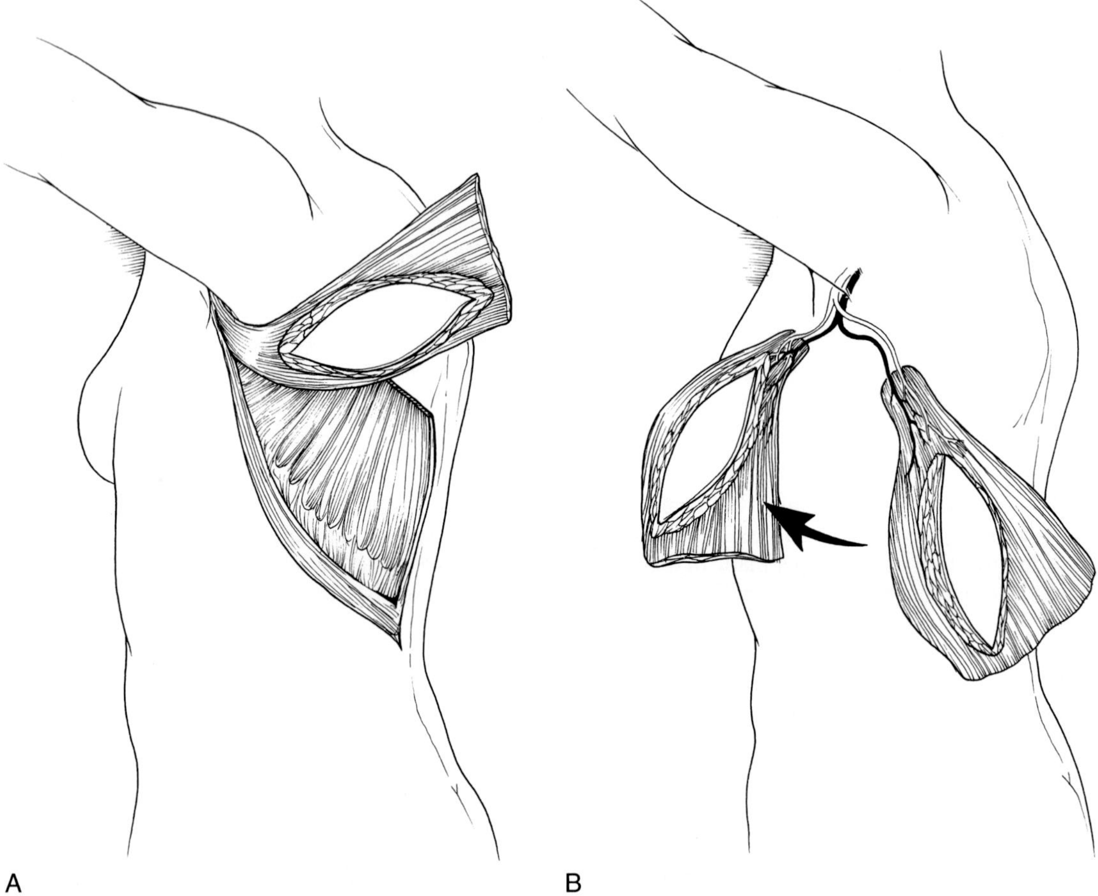

FIGURE 140-12. *A,* Elevation of the latissimus dorsi musculocutaneous flap and the underlying anatomy. *B,* After division of the muscle insertion, the latissimus flap is transposed anteriorly to the mastectomy defect through a subcutaneous tunnel high in the axilla.

inserted from above and may be filled with several hundred milliliters of saline because there is generally no tightness to the sublatissimus pocket. Postoperatively, the tissue expander is further inflated until the desired volume is achieved, starting 2 weeks postoperatively or once the wound is healed. The second stage of the reconstruction is typically performed after 4 to 8 months, allowing adequate healing and settling of the soft tissue. An implant of appropriate size and shape is then inserted through the previous incision after the expander is removed. Symmetry can be improved by correction of any soft tissue or contour deformity as well as by correction of the inframammary fold. The nipple and areola are usually reconstructed at the same procedure.

When reconstruction is planned with use of the total autogenous latissimus dorsi flap, the cutaneous paddle is molded in the form of an asymmetric U (Fig. 140-14). The curved base of the U gives the apex of the breast. The distal part of the muscle and its underlying fat are folded under this breast cone to increase the volume and the projection of the breast. Various moldings can be tried until one arrives at a satisfactory shape for the rebuilt breast. This procedure of molding is crucial to the final quality of the result, and one must understand how to achieve the different arrangements necessary for a good morphologic result.

The extended latissimus dorsi flap can provide 300 to 400 mL or more of soft tissue volume for breast reconstruction. Postoperative muscle atrophy of 20% to 25% should be taken into consideration during the insetting and sizing of the flap. Some surgeons think that the intact thoracodorsal nerve may help preserve maximum volume of the flap in the long term and therefore advocate not dividing the thoracodorsal nerve when the flap is used in this fashion. They also argue that because the latissimus dorsi muscle is fixed to the chest wall in a relaxed manner, little contraction is noticed in the flap postoperatively when the nerve is left intact. On the other hand, when the muscle is used over an expander, postoperative voluntary muscle

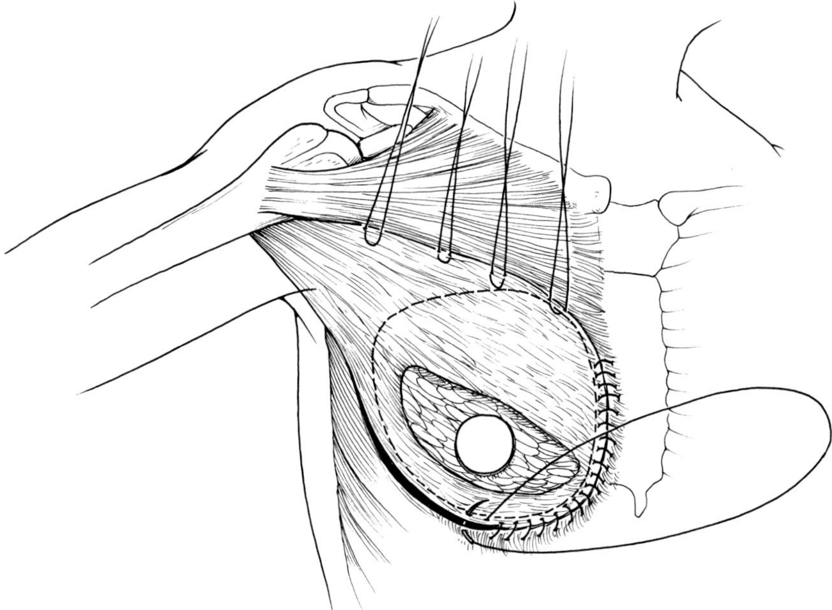

FIGURE 140-13. When immediate latissimus flap reconstruction is planned with a prosthesis for skin-sparing mastectomy, the skin pattern is designed as a discrete small island. After transposition of the flap, the expander is placed between the latissimus and pectoralis major muscles.

contraction can be significant when the thoracodorsal nerve is left intact.

COMPLICATIONS

Flap Necrosis

The latissimus dorsi flap is a hardy flap that has an excellent and reliable circulation. There is a minimal risk of flap necrosis even in smokers and diabetics. Significant flap necrosis is unusual and nearly always associated with injury to the vascular pedicle. The pedicle can be injured either directly during the dissection around the pedicle or indirectly by twisting or thrombosis from tension on the pedicle by the weight of the flap, especially if the flap is not properly secured to the chest wall.

Partial flap necrosis has been noted in up to 7% of patients but is more common when an extended flap has been elevated.[36] On the other hand, necrosis of the mastectomy skin flaps is a more common complication.

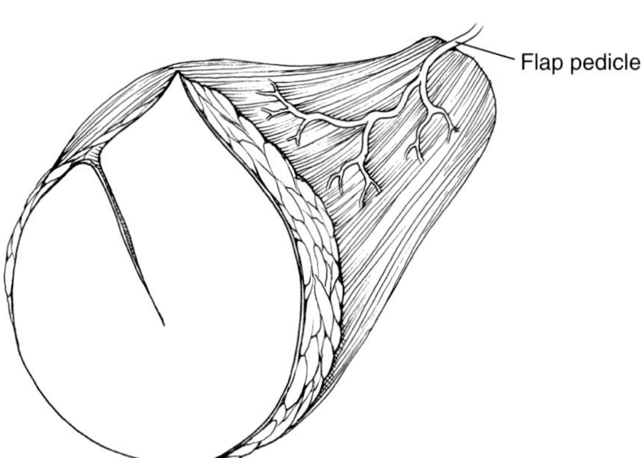

FIGURE 140-14. For total autogenous latissimus reconstruction, the flap is folded into a cone shape to increase the volume and projection of the reconstructed breast.

Donor Site Morbidity

By far the most common complication is seroma at the back donor site.[37] The rate of dorsal seroma may be increased when an extended flap is performed.[38,39]

Dorsal skin flap necrosis also occurs, especially with large skin paddles, resulting in excessive tension on the back closure. Dissection in too superficial a plane in trying to leave subcutaneous fat on the flap also puts the skin flaps at greater risk. Other possible donor site problems are loss of shoulder mobility, shoulder weakness, winging of the scapula, and dorsal hernia.[40]

Prosthesis-Related Complications

A complication related to the use of prosthetic devices in conjunction with the latissimus flap is migration of the expander or implant through the axilla and into the back.[41] This should be avoidable by secure suturing of the latissimus muscle to the lateral chest wall. Other implant-related complications include capsular contracture,[42,43] device failure, periprosthetic infection, and device extrusion. Fortunately, the incidence of all of these is fairly low.

FUTURE CONSIDERATIONS AND UNSOLVED PROBLEMS

Breast reconstruction for the purpose of improving quality of life of patients with breast cancer has become more widespread. However, reports in the literature have described thermal injuries to reconstructed breasts caused by heating pads, sun exposure, and hair dryers.[44-46] Division of various sensory nerves including the sensory nerve in the reconstructed breast flap and the subsequent sensory changes can lead to such burn injuries.

Although the spontaneous recovery of sensation in breast reconstruction with musculocutaneous flaps without sensory neurorrhaphy has been reported in the literature,[47] such sensory recovery is rare. The predictable recovery of sensibility would be highly desirable. A sensate flap could be achieved by neurorrhaphy between the lateral cutaneous branch of the dorsal primary divisions of the seventh thoracic nerve and the lateral cutaneous branch of the fourth intercostal nerve.[48]

Although the aesthetic results of breast reconstruction have monopolized the attention of plastic surgeons for some time, bringing sensibility to the reconstructed breast constitutes the next challenge.

CONCLUSION

Breast reconstruction and conservation have become an integral part of breast cancer treatment, and more and more patients are benefiting from an immediate reconstruction after skin-sparing mastectomy.

The latissimus dorsi musculocutaneous flap continues to play an important role in such immediate breast reconstruction. This flap is reliable, and its elevation is technically straightforward. Outstanding results can be obtained over and above those obtained with tissue expanders and implants alone. Complications are few and results are predictable, especially in appropriately selected patients.

It is frequently combined with tissue expansion or an implant to enhance symmetry and to reduce capsular contracture. It is useful for supplementing other techniques, for filling in contour deformities after breast conservation surgery, and for autogenous tissue reconstruction for women who have excess lateral back tissue. The extended latissimus dorsi flap is a reliable method for totally autologous breast reconstruction and can be considered a primary choice for breast reconstruction, particularly in women who otherwise are at high risk for a TRAM flap or an implant procedure.

REFERENCES

1. Maxwell GP: Iginio Tansini and the origin of the latissimus dorsi musculocutaneous flap. Plast Reconstr Surg 1980;65:686.
2. Lassen M, Krag C, Nielsen IM: The latissimus dorsi flap: an overview. Scand J Plast Surg 1985;19:41.
3. Schneider WJ, Hill HL, Brown RG: Latissimus dorsi myocutaneous flap for breast reconstruction. Br J Plast Surg 1977;30:277.
4. Bostwick J, Vasconez LO, Jurkiewicz MJ: Breast reconstruction after a radical mastectomy. Plast Reconstr Surg 1978;61:682.
5. McCraw JB, Dibbell DG, Carraway JH: Clinical definition of independent myocutaneous vascular territories. Plast Reconstr Surg 1977;60:341.
6. Maxwell GP, McGibbon BM, Hoopes JE: Vascular considerations in the use of a latissimus dorsi myocutaneous flap after a mastectomy with an axillary dissection. Plast Reconstr Surg 1979;64:771.
7. Levine RA, DeFelice CA: Possible explanation of successful latissimus dorsi flap without the thoracodorsal artery [letter]. Plast Reconstr Surg 1980;65:532.
8. Fisher J, Bostwick J III, Powell RW: Latissimus dorsi blood supply after thoracodorsal vessel division: the serratus collateral. Plast Reconstr Surg 1983;73:502.
9. Hartrampf CR, Scheflan M, Black PW: Breast reconstruction with a transverse abdominal island flap. Plast Reconstr Surg 1982;69:216.
10. Mathes SJ, Nahai F: Classification of the vascular anatomy of muscles: experimental and clinical correlation. Plast Reconstr Surg 1981;67:177.
11. Mathes SJ, Nahai F: Latissimus dorsi flap. In Mathes SJ, Nahai F, eds: Reconstructive Surgery: Principles, Anatomy, and Technique, vol I. New York, Churchill Livingstone, 1997:565.
12. Bartlett SP, May JW Jr, Yaremchuk MJ: The latissimus dorsi muscle: a fresh cadaver study of the primary neurovascular pedicle. Plast Reconstr Surg 1981;67:631.
13. Tobin GR, Schusterman M, Peterson GH, et al: The intramuscular anatomy of the latissimus dorsi muscle: the basis for splitting the flap. Plast Reconstr Surg 1981;67:631.
14. Rowsell AR, Eisenberg N, Davies DM, et al: The anatomy of the thoracodorsal artery within the latissimus dorsi muscle. Br J Plast Surg 1986;39:206.
15. Bostwick J III, Scheflan M, Nahai F, et al: The reverse latissimus dorsi muscle and musculocutaneous flap: anatomical and clinical considerations. Plast Reconstr Surg 1980;65:395.
16. Stevenson TR, Rohrich RJ, Pollock RA, et al: More experience with the reverse latissimus dorsi musculocutaneous flap: precise location of blood supply. Plast Reconstr Surg 1984;74:237.
17. Laitung JKG, Peck F: Shoulder function following the loss of the latissimus dorsi muscle. Br J Plast Surg 1985;38:375.
18. Russell RC, Pribaz J, Zook EG, et al: Functional evaluation of latissimus dorsi donor site. Plast Reconstr Surg 1986;78:336.
19. Fraulin FOG, Louie G, Zorrilla L, et al: Functional evaluation of the shoulder following latissimus dorsi muscle transfer. Ann Plast Surg 1995;35:349.
20. Papp C, Wechselberger G, Schoeller T: Autologous breast reconstruction after breast-conserving cancer surgery. Plast Reconstr Surg 1998;102:1932.
21. Papp C, Zanon E, McCraw J: Breast volume replacement using the de-epithelialized latissimus dorsi myocutaneous flap. Eur J Plast Surg 1988;11:120.
22. McCraw JB, Papp C, Edwards A, McMellin A: The autogenous latissimus breast reconstruction. Clin Plast Surg 1994;21:279.
23. Germann G, Steinau H-U: Breast reconstruction with the extended latissimus dorsi flap. Plast Reconstr Surg 1996;97:519.

24. Papp C, McCraw JB: Autogenous latissimus breast reconstruction. Clin Plast Surg 1998;25:261.
25. Baumholtz MA, Al-Shunnar BM, Dabb RW: Boomerang flap reconstruction for the breast. Ann Plast Surg 2002;49:44.
26. Delay E, Gounot N, Bouillot A: Autologous latissimus breast reconstruction: a 3 year clinical experience with 100 patients. Plast Reconstr Surg 1998;102:1461.
27. Chang DW, Kroll SS, Dackiw A, et al: Reconstructive management of contralateral breast cancer in patients who previously underwent unilateral breast reconstruction. Plast Reconstr Surg 2001;108:352.
28. Salmon RJ, Razaboni R, Soussaline M: The use of the latissimus dorsi musculocutaneous flap following recurrence of cancer in irradiated breasts. Br J Plast Surg 1988;41:41.
29. Clough KB, Kroll SS, Audretsch W: An approach to the repair of partial mastectomy defects. Plast Reconstr Surg 1999;104:409.
30. Lejour M, Alemanno P, De Mey A, et al: Analysis of fifty-six breast reconstructions using the latissimus dorsi flap. Ann Chir Plast Esthet 1985;30:7.
31. Pendergrast WJ, Bostwick JB III, Jurkiewicz MJ: The subcutaneous mastectomy cripple: surgical rehabilitation with the latissimus dorsi flap. Plast Reconstr Surg 1980;66:554.
32. Spear SL, Slack C, Howard MA: Postmastectomy reconstruction of the previously augmented breast: diagnosis, staging, methodology, and outcome. Plast Reconstr Surg 2001;107:1167.
33. Spear SL, Onyewu C: Staged breast reconstruction with saline-filled implants in the irradiated breast: recent trends and therapeutic implications. Plast Reconstr Surg 2000;105:930.
34. Millard DR Jr: Variations in the design of the latissimus dorsi flap in breast reconstruction. Ann Plast Surg 1981;7:269.
35. Greber B, Krause A, Reimer T, et al: Breast reconstruction with latissimus dorsi flap: improved aesthetic results after transection of its humeral insertion. Plast Reconstr Surg 1999;103:1876.
36. Hokin JAB, Silfverskiold KL: Breast reconstruction without an implant: results and complications using an extended latissimus dorsi flap. Plast Reconstr Surg 1987;79:58.
37. Menke H, Erkens M, Olbrisch RR: Evolving concepts in breast reconstruction with latissimus dorsi flaps: results and follow-up of 121 consecutive patients. Ann Plast Surg 2001;47:107.
38. Clough KB, Louis-Sylvestre C, Fitoussi A, et al: Donor site sequelae after autologous breast reconstruction with an extended latissimus dorsi flap. Plast Reconstr Surg 2002;109:1904.
39. Chang DW, Youssef A, Cha S, et al: Autologous breast reconstruction with the extended latissimus dorsi flap. Plast Reconstr Surg 2002;110:751.
40. Mickel TJ, Barton FE Jr, Rohrich RJ, et al: Management and prevention of lumbar herniation following a latissimus dorsi flap. Plast Reconstr Surg 1999;103:1473.
41. De Mey A, Lejour M, Declety A, et al: Late results and current indications of latissimus dorsi breast reconstructions. Br J Plast Surg 1991;44:1.
42. Smith BK, Cohen BE, Biggs TM, et al: Simultaneous bilateral breast reconstruction using latissimus dorsi myocutaneous flaps: a retrospective review of an institutional experience. Plast Reconstr Surg 2001;108:1174.
43. Peltoniemi H, Asko-Seljavaara S, Harma M, et al: Latissimus dorsi breast reconstruction. Long term results and return of sensibility. Scand J Plast Reconstr Surg Hand Surg 1993;27:127.
44. Maxwell GP, Tornambe R: Second and third degree burns as a complication in breast reconstruction. Ann Plast Surg 1989;22:386
45. Lejour M: Burn of a reconstructed breast. Plast Reconstr Surg 1996;97:1306.
46. Alexandrides IJ, Shestak KC, Noone RB: Thermal injuries following TRAM flap breast reconstruction. Ann Plast Surg 1997;38:335.
47. Delay E, Jorquera F, Lucas R, et al: Sensitivity of breasts reconstructed with the autologous latissimus dorsi flap. Plast Reconstr Surg 2000;106:302.
48. Yano K, Hosokawa K, Takagi S, et al: Breast reconstruction using the sensate latissimus dorsi musculocutaneous flap. Plast Reconstr Surg 2002;109:1897.

CHAPTER

141

Immediate Postmastectomy Reconstruction: TRAM Flap Transposition Techniques

SCOTT L. SPEAR, MD ✦ JASON C. GANZ, MD

HISTORY

The transverse rectus abdominis musculocutaneous flap, or TRAM flap, was first widely introduced for reconstruction of the breast by Hartrampf in 1982.[1] In his landmark paper, Hartrampf described a procedure in which tissues that would normally be discarded during an abdominal lipectomy were instead transferred to a mastectomy defect based on the proximal rectus abdominis muscle and the superior epigastric vessels contained within it. The skin and subcutaneous tissue of the abdomen were left in continuity with the anterior rectus sheath and its perforators from the deep epigastric vascular system, on which the flap relied.[1] At the time of its introduction, the TRAM flap provided an attractive alternative to implant reconstruction and to the other options for autogenous breast reconstruction that either did not provide enough soft tissue (e.g., the latissimus dorsi myocutaneous flap) or involved multiple stages to be completed (e.g., the tubed abdominal flaps). Since its introduction, the TRAM flap has undergone countless refinements and modifications; today, it is widely considered the most reliable and attractive option for breast reconstruction.

GOALS

The goal in breast reconstruction is the formation of a breast that has a natural contour and feel, has reasonable symmetry to the contralateral breast, and is in harmony with the patient's anatomy and needs. In evaluating the options for breast reconstruction, there are several factors to be considered. These include the size of the opposite breast, the plans for altering the opposite breast, the nature of the mastectomy defect, the pathologic stage of the breast cancer, the likelihood of postmastectomy irradiation, the general health of the patient, the availability of donor tissue, the lifestyle of the patient, and finally the patient's goals and expectations. With all of these considerations, the reconstructive surgeon has a wide variety of options from which to choose, including prosthetic techniques, autologous techniques, and combined autologous tissue and implant techniques. In addition, a number of matching procedures are available for the contralateral breast to help with symmetry.[2]

At present, it is generally agreed that the best method of breast reconstruction is autologous tissue. Among the available variations of autologous tissue, the TRAM flap alone is the best alternative. This is not to say that the TRAM flap is best in every situation and in every patient; rather, on average, TRAM flaps generally produce superior results. The decision whether to reconstruct with a TRAM flap and what type of TRAM flap to use can be complex. In addition to the patient's motivations, it is important to take into account the anatomy of the breast and abdomen, the nature of the underlying breast disease, and the competency of the surgical team. The best candidates are those patients in whom the transposition of abdominal tissue will leave the abdominal donor site in an improved state compared with its preoperative condition. Thus, an abdomen with excess skin and fat as well as a lax muscle wall is a preferable donor site compared with the trim abdomen and firm abdominal wall of the nulliparous woman. The patient with a larger breast is also a better candidate for a TRAM flap than is the patient with a small breast that might be more easily reconstructed with some other simpler and less invasive technique.

Patients with early-stage breast cancer, particularly those who will not require radiation therapy, can often be corrected with a smaller operation and may not need a TRAM flap. On the other hand, patients with previous irradiation after lumpectomy or those who have undergone postmastectomy irradiation are likely to be better treated later with a TRAM flap to allow replacement of as much irradiated tissue as possible.

Whereas many articles in the literature attest to the benefits of the TRAM flap, not all patients obtain good results with TRAM flaps, and there are certainly some patients who have suffered significant abdominal donor site complications. Therefore, it is advisable not to underestimate the morbidity of the abdominal donor site, particularly in inexperienced hands.

Although it might seem that the TRAM flap is a single operation, in reality it represents a number of different operations wrapped in one. Included under the title of TRAM flap are single-pedicled TRAM flaps, double-pedicled TRAM flaps, bilateral TRAM flaps for bilateral breast reconstruction, single- or double-pedicled TRAM flaps with a preliminary delay of the inferior epigastric artery, free TRAM flaps (either unilateral or bilateral), deep inferior epigastric artery perforator flap (either unilateral or bilateral), and any of these varieties of TRAM flap with a prosthesis beneath for added volume. In addition to these variations, several types of TRAM flap have been described that are even more complicated in their design but infrequently used. This presentation focuses on the use of the pedicled TRAM flap for breast reconstruction.

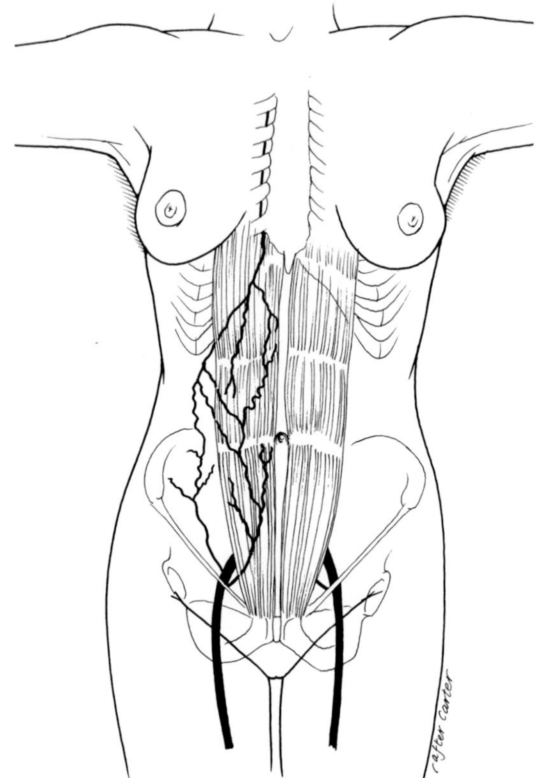

FIGURE 141-1. Vascular anatomy of the deep epigastric system.

ANATOMY

The TRAM flap is based on the circulation to the anterior abdominal wall that derives from perforating vessels through the rectus abdominis muscle and the deep epigastric system (Fig. 141-1). These perforating vessels are supplied primarily as branches from the deep inferior epigastric artery but can also be supplied by the adjacent territory of the superior epigastric artery. The anatomy of the perforating vessels is somewhat variable and may be predominantly along the lateral third of the muscle, in the central third of the muscle, or even in the medial third. The concept of the epigastric artery as the pedicle source was originally described by Mathes.[3] The vascular anatomy of the epigastric arteries as they relate to the TRAM flap was described by Moon and Taylor.[4] They described three basic arterial schemata. In a type I pattern, a single intramuscular vessel extends from the superior epigastric artery to the deep inferior epigastric artery. The majority of patients in their study exhibited a type II system, in which the inferior epigastric artery branches into two vessels at the arcuate line and communicates with the superior epigastric through anastomosing choke vessels. Patients with a type III pattern exhibited three branches of the inferior epigastric artery at the arcuate line. These patients, on average, showed an even greater number of anastomoses with the superior epigastric artery. Only 2% of patients showed symmetry between their rectus muscles; most showed different vascular patterns on each side. The epigastric vessels send perforators through the rectus muscle that cross the anterior rectus sheath in two rows, one medial and one lateral. The rectus abdominis muscle is a type III muscle as described by Mathes[3] and has, in addition to the superior and inferior epigastric vessels, circulation from branches of the 8th, 9th, 10th, 11th, and 12th intercostal vessels. These vessels enter the rectus muscle after anastomosis with the superior and deep inferior epigastric vessels posterior to the muscle. They penetrate the posterior rectus sheath just medial to the linea semilunaris. The rectus abdominis muscles also derive their motor innervation from the intercostal nerves T8 through T12.

The primary blood supply to the lower rectus muscle is from the deep inferior epigastric artery. Hence, the blood supply with use of the inferior epigastric artery for the free TRAM flap or perforator flap is substantially richer than the blood supply available from the superior epigastric artery.[5]

The circulation from either rectus muscle across the lower abdomen is divided into four zones (Fig. 141-2). Zone I is the zone immediately overlying the rectus muscle. Zone II is described as a zone immediately across the midline. Zone III is the ipsilateral zone just lateral to the rectus muscle border, and zone IV is the contralateral zone lateral to the contralateral rectus border. The circulation is best in zone I, somewhat variable in zones II and III, and usually poor in zone IV, particularly with a pedicled TRAM flap. In each of these zones, the blood supply is improved to some degree by use of the perforator flap, free flap, or pedicled flap after a delay procedure.

The rectus abdominis muscle is covered on its superficial surface by the anterior rectus sheath, which is composed of the external oblique fascia throughout its length, the entire internal oblique fascia below the arcuate line, and part of the internal oblique fascia above the arcuate line (Fig. 141-3). The anterior rectus sheath contains tendinous inscriptions, which are adherences of the anterior sheath to the underlying rectus muscle. The average patient has three tendinous inscriptions on each side, the first at the level of the costal margin, the second halfway between the costal margin and the umbilicus, and the third at the level of the umbilicus.[6] On its posterior surface, the rectus muscle lies on top of the posterior rectus sheath, which is composed of the internal oblique fascia above the arcuate line; but it is thinned out at the level

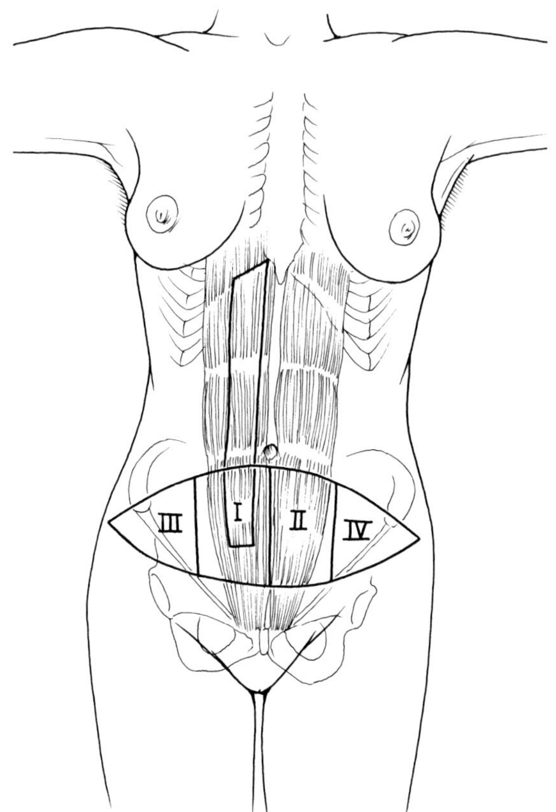

FIGURE 141-2. Circulatory zones of the TRAM flap.

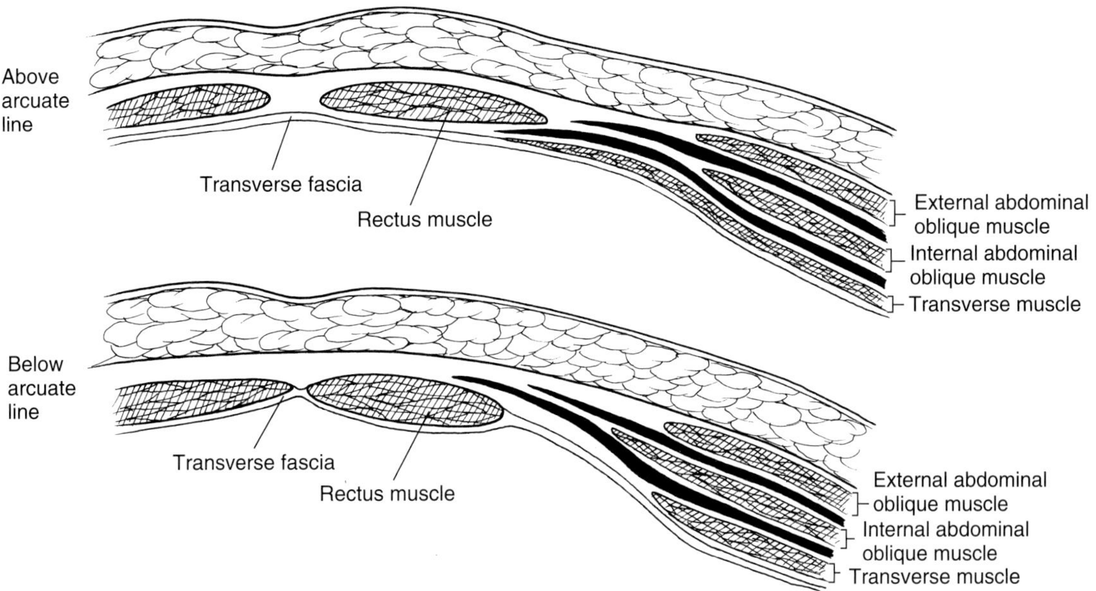

FIGURE 141-3. Anatomy of the rectus sheath above and below the arcuate line.

of the arcuate line down to the pubic ramus because of the lack of internal oblique fascia, which now courses within the anterior rectus sheath. In younger patients, the muscles tend to be fairly narrow and lie adjacent to the midline on either side. In older patients, particularly in patients who are overweight or who have had multiple pregnancies, the muscles tend to be less thick, widened, and often separated at the midline by thinning of the abdominal wall fascia termed a diastasis of the rectus abdominis muscles. Anatomic variations in the size, strength, and width of the rectus abdominis muscle are important to bear in mind when the operation is planned and executed. Likewise, variations in the strength of the abdominal wall fascia, particularly the linea alba, are important to note before the dissection of the muscle.

Generally speaking, sophisticated diagnostic studies are not required in planning breast reconstruction with the TRAM flap. Although angiography of the abdominal wall circulation or the thoracic circulation might be informative in terms of planning TRAM flaps or free TRAM flaps when surgery has previously been performed close to major vascular pedicles, in general, these procedures are not undertaken because of their limited usefulness. Some surgeons employ Doppler or laser color Doppler studies to better define the location of the perforators when either free or TRAM flaps are planned, but this is not thought to be necessary by most surgeons. The most important diagnostic study when a TRAM flap is planned is careful assessment of the soft tissues of the chest, breast, and abdomen. A preoperative plan that provides adequate amounts of skin and soft tissue to reconstruct the breast is critical. Once the required amount of soft tissue is known, the second critical step is to be certain that the blood supply to move that tissue will also be provided. This diagnostic study is essentially a good physical examination, and it should be performed before final decisions are made in planning a TRAM flap.

The treatment goal of TRAM flap breast reconstruction is the reconstruction of a beautiful, natural, and comfortable breast. At the same time, an equally important goal is to leave the abdominal donor site undamaged and if possible improved as a result of the operation. Thus, it is recommended that the TRAM flap be thought of as an abdominoplasty in which the tissues are not discarded but rather used to reconstruct a breast. This concept requires the TRAM flap donor site to correspond to an abdominoplasty plan, and the repair of the abdominal wall, skin, fat, and superficial fascia should be accomplished with aesthetic standards. It is unfortunate that the insurance industry does not appreciate the complexity and time required to execute these procedures; nevertheless, this should be the goal.

There is some variability from surgeon to surgeon in the selection of the many TRAM flaps available, but there are some overriding principles. It has become clear during the last 2 decades that some factors significantly increase the risk for complications to both the TRAM flap and the donor site. These are obesity, smoking, diabetes, hypertension, collagen vascular disease, and other significant systemic illnesses (such as pulmonary, renal, or cardiac disease). So, in terms of circulation, the single-pedicled TRAM flap has its best application in patients who do not have any of these risk factors and who have enough tissue in the lower abdomen for reconstruction of the breast to the desired size and shape. Generally speaking, approximately 50% of the lower abdominal tissue typically removed in an abdominoplasty will be available in most patients without risk factors to provide tissue for breast reconstruction. Patients who have risk factors or who need more tissue than 50% of the lower abdomen need a TRAM flap with more robust circulation. This moves them into the category of patients who would benefit from a free TRAM flap, a TRAM flap with a preliminary delay procedure of the deep inferior epigastric vessels, or a double-pedicled TRAM flap.[7,8] There is also the option of performing a single-pedicled TRAM flap with the addition of a prosthesis in patients who have no risk factors but who need more volume than the TRAM flap alone will provide. The deep inferior epigastric artery perforator (DIEP) flap is a free flap based on one, two, or more perforator vessels, but it does not carry the whole, most, or in some instances any of the lower rectus abdominis muscle. This procedure provides an enhanced circulation compared with a single-pedicled TRAM flap, but it is most likely not as hearty or as simple to harvest as a free TRAM flap, which carries all the perforators and a corresponding segment of the rectus abdominis muscle.[9]

At present, it is likely that the majority of TRAM flaps done in North America are single-pedicled procedures. This fact reflects the reliability of the procedure, the simplicity of the technique, and the facility of performing this operation in most hospitals. The free TRAM flap and DIEP flap offer the exciting possibility of breast reconstruction with the use of less muscle and with a better blood supply, but at the risk of a higher frequency of total flap loss and with the requirement of a greater commitment of time and resources to perform the operation.[10,11] Thus, the free flap and DIEP flap are most commonly performed in a small number of centers around the United States where the commitment has been made to perform these operations literally at any cost. This section is limited to pedicled TRAM flap options.

TECHNIQUE

In the truest sense of the word, technique in TRAM flap reconstruction of the breast begins with the planning stage. In immediate breast reconstruction, the planning requires an estimate of how much skin and breast tissue will be removed. An abdominoplasty pattern is then drawn on the abdomen to incorporate the amount of skin and fat that can be removed. Design of the flap is based on a French-cut bikini pattern so the final scar will be oblique upward, following the same line as a thong from groin to iliac crest (Fig. 141-4). Once the abdominoplasty pattern has been drawn, the requisite amount of skin is drawn on the abdomen overlying one or the other pedicle. The ipsilateral flap is preferred, with the flap based on the same side as the mastectomy. After it is determined how much skin and fat will be required, a final decision must be made whether to do a single-pedicled, double-pedicled, or free flap. It is to be hoped the decision was made correctly at an earlier moment during the consultation so the plan does not have to be changed at this point.

Regardless of the initial plan, allowances must be made for possible surprises at the time of surgery. For that reason, a final decision in terms of skin planning should be left until after the mastectomy is complete and the mastectomy flaps can be re-examined to make sure additional abdominal skin is not required. When possible, it is preferable to de-epithelialize appropriate portions of the flap while it still sits on the abdomen because this facilitates the de-epithelialization process. The umbilicus is dissected out, leaving a modest amount of fat along the stalk to ensure its blood supply. The upper abdominal skin and subcutaneous fat are undermined off the fascia up to the costal margins, and a tunnel is made into the mastectomy defect along the meridian of the breast. On average, this tunnel should accommodate four of the surgeon's fingers, although this may vary on the basis of flap volume. The patient is then sat upright in the operating room to make certain that the upper abdominal flap can be closed to the planned inferior incision. Once this has been demonstrated, the inferior incision is made, and the TRAM flap is then elevated, bringing the contralateral side to the midline in the single-pedicled TRAM flap and on the ipsilateral side to the lateral border of the anterior rectus sheath.

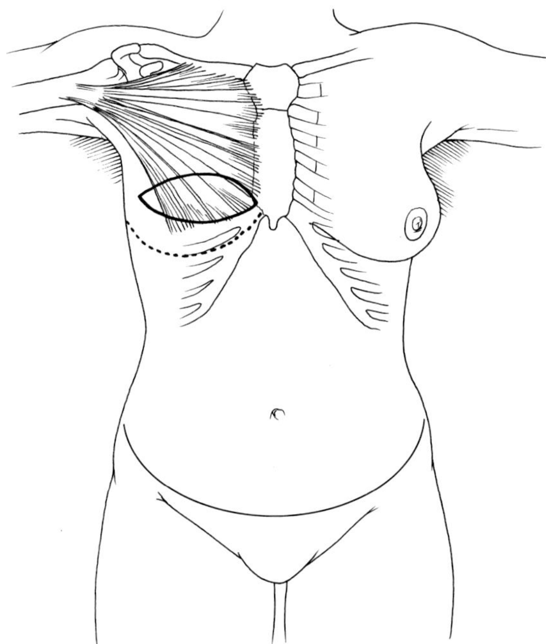

FIGURE 141-4. The final lines of closure of the TRAM flap are designed to mimic an abdominoplasty incision.

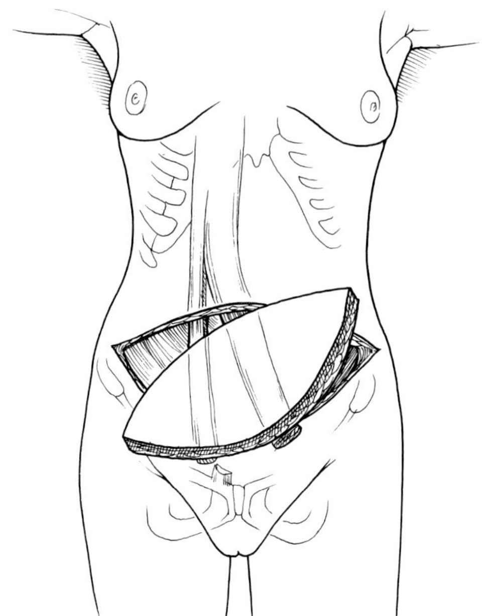

FIGURE 141-5. The rectus muscle is split longitudinally, including only the muscle that carries the medial and lateral perforator rows in the TRAM flap.

The flap is then carefully dissected off the anterior abdominal wall fascia until perforators are encountered both medially and laterally. A muscle-splitting technique is preferred (Fig. 141-5), in which only the amount of rectus muscle necessary to carry both medial and lateral rows of perforators is included in the flap. Generally speaking, the medial perforator row is approximately 5 to 10 mm off the medial border of the anterior rectus sheath, and the lateral perforator row is usually 3.5 to 4 cm lateral to the medial perforators and 1 or 2 cm medial to the lateral muscle edge. Thus, in the muscle-splitting technique, the fascial incisions extend from 1 cm lateral to the medial border of the anterior rectus sheath to 3.5 to 4 cm lateral. The strip of fascia therefore tends to be approximately 3.5 to 4 cm in width and extends from the costal margin down to just below the arcuate line. Inferiorly, the lines are brought together at a tapered point, much as when an ellipse of skin is excised (Fig. 141-6). After the fascia

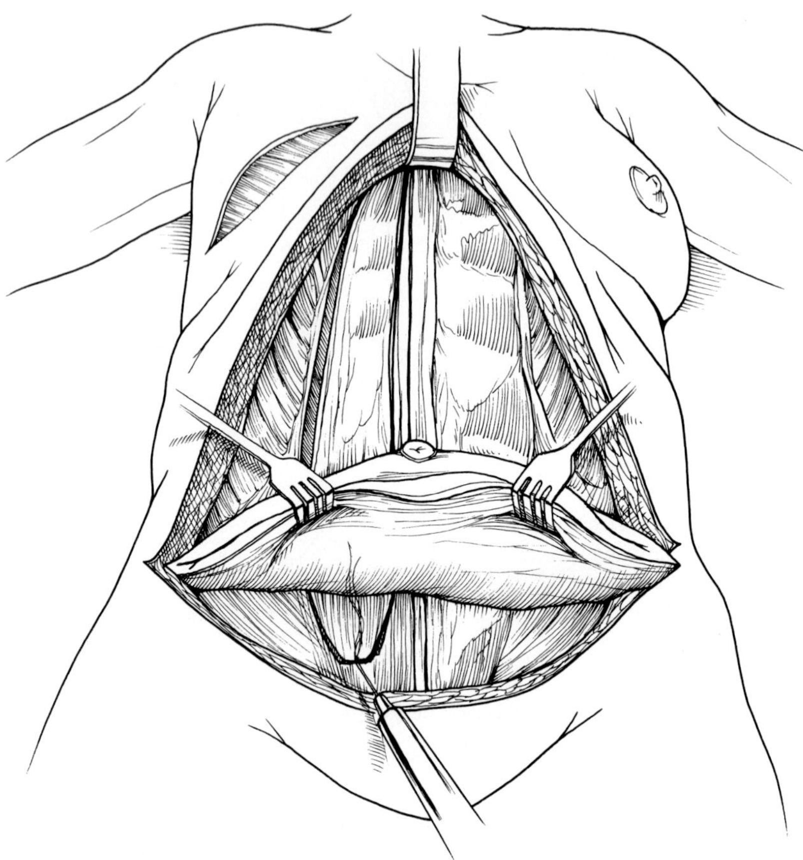

FIGURE 141-6. The anterior rectus sheath fascia is incised inferiorly in a wedge-shaped fashion.

has been incised laterally, the muscle is separated in the direction of its fibers three or four fingerbreadths above the pubic tubercle, identifying the site where the inferior epigastric vessels traverse the muscle at that point. The vessels are then dissected more widely and ligated with sutures as well as clipped. When possible, a length of inferior epigastric artery is left dangling from the flap itself for the rare instance in which a vascular anastomosis might be required later (Fig. 141-7). The muscle is then split from an inferior to superior direction, being careful not to move obliquely medially across its blood supply. If anything, the dissection should be carried in an upward and somewhat lateral direction just to be sure the blood supply is left intact. It is also a good idea to be sure the inferior epigastric vessels enter the segment of muscle one is going to use, which may be more lateral than expected. Medially, the muscle is separated from the anterior and posterior rectus sheaths near the midline. The muscle is transected with cautery or ligatures below the arcuate line and below the lowest perforator that is included in the flap. In transection of the muscle, care is taken not to reinjure the inferior epigastric vessels that have already been transected. The flap is ultimately mobilized relatively easily off the rectus sheath with use of hemoclips to ligate the intercostal perforators going up toward the costal border and including the eighth intercostal nerve and vessels (Fig. 141-8). The muscle is transected approximately 80% across above the costal margin so there is less of a bulge of muscle as it traverses the costal margin. A small amount of muscle and fascia is left intact to reduce the tension on the vessels. The TRAM flap that will form the new breast is then brought into the mastectomy defect through the meridian tunnel and left on the chest.

The abdominal wall is closed in one of several ways. In most patients, the sheath is closed primarily in layers beginning with a figure-of-eight 2-0 polydioxanone (PDS) suture followed by a running looped 0 Prolene suture. This closure goes down to the pubic tubercle and up to the costal margin, leaving approximately only a 1- or 2-cm aperture around the muscle flap pedicle base. The contralateral side is plicated with a 2-0 PDS suture in a running horizontal mattress pattern followed by an over-and-over stitch. If there is undue tension, rather than closing the donor site sheath primarily, mesh (Prolene or other synthetic materials such as AlloDerm) may be sutured to the midline or even across the midline to help stabilize the donor site. In these patients, it is important that

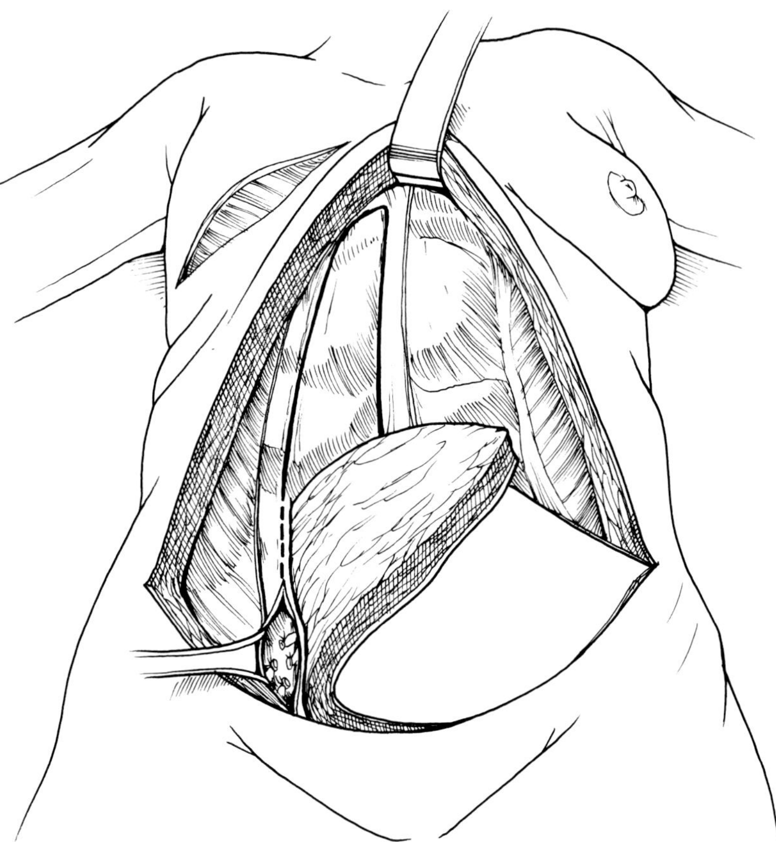

FIGURE 141-7. The deep inferior epigastric vessels are identified laterally and ligated.

the posterior sheath be closed to the anterior sheath to prevent a hernia through the weak fascia below the arcuate line.

The skin of the umbilicus is tacked down to the fascia with suture material, either 3-0 Vicryl or 3-0 Monocryl suture, leaving the needles attached until they can be brought through a new umbilical aperture at a later point in the operation (Fig. 141-9). The abdominal skin flap is then defatted deep to Scarpa fascia along its most distal 3 to 5 cm. This line of definition is clear laterally and less distinct centrally. The patient is then sat upright, and the incision is temporarily stapled in place. The site for the new umbilicus is marked, and an incision is made there in the form of a small and narrow upside-down U or horseshoe. The umbilical tacking sutures that were previously placed are then brought through that aperture after conservative defatting of the tissues surrounding that hole. At this point, fibrin tissue glue is used in appropriate concentrations to assist the fixation of the superficial and deep tissues. After placement of drains, the tissue glue is sprayed and the patient is stapled again as previously marked. This needs to be done in less than 60 seconds so the glue does not set up before the closure has occurred. Pressure is maintained on the skin flap for 4 to 5 minutes to encourage a good bond between the superficial and deep tissues. The donor site incision is closed in layers including interrupted 2-0 PDS to Scarpa fascia followed by interrupted and running intradermal 3-0 Monocryl to the dermis. The umbilicus is stabilized with the four tacking sutures that were previously placed; the dermis is now tacked from the abdominal skin to the dermis of the umbilicus and then down to the abdominal wall fascia. Fine sutures of 5-0 Monocryl, either as small skin stitches or as dermal stitches, are used to further close the umbilicus.

With the abdomen closed, the TRAM flap is rotated as appropriate, anywhere from 90 to 180 degrees. It is tacked in place and further shaped and de-epithelialized. It is helpful to remove some of the fat deep to Scarpa fascia even on the TRAM flap to reduce the potential amount of fat necrosis. This maneuver can be done with the TRAM flap still on the abdomen before it is brought through the tunnel. The inframammary fold may be further defined by sutures between the mastectomy skin flaps and the chest wall as well as by sutures between the TRAM flap and the pectoralis fascia. The TRAM flap is finally shaped and further de-epithelialized as required. Marionette

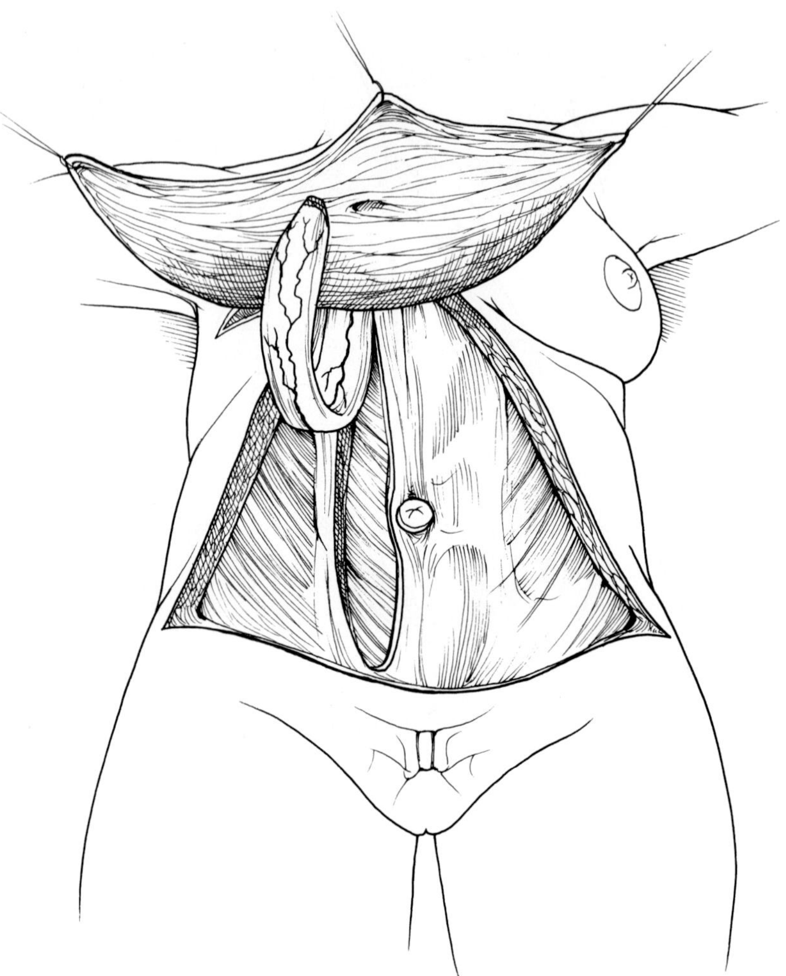

FIGURE 141-8. After the rectus muscle is divided inferiorly, the remaining muscle is split longitudinally and elevated off the posterior rectus sheath.

sutures may be used to help suspend the TRAM flap laterally, medially, and superiorly. Alternatively, the TRAM flap can be sutured directly to the overlying skin or the underlying fascia. It is particularly important to prevent the flap from migrating inferiorly or laterally, which it is prone to do.

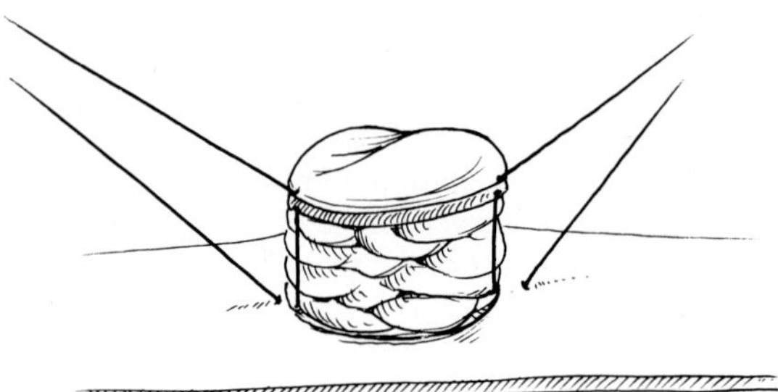

FIGURE 141-9. Sutures are placed from the umbilical stalk to the abdominal wall. These sutures are later passed through the umbilical incision and used to fix the umbilicus to the skin.

The skin of the TRAM flap is sutured in place much like the abdominal donor site with interrupted and running sutures of intradermal Monocryl. Both the abdomen and TRAM flap reconstruction sites are drained with large drains, which are typically left in place for at least 7 days if not significantly longer.

The procedure for harvesting a double-pedicled TRAM flap has many similarities to the single-pedicled procedure. When both muscles are used as bilateral flaps, it is preferable to preserve the lateral muscle by the muscle-splitting technique. Preoperative markings are made as previously described. After the mastectomy is performed, the recipient defect is evaluated, and the operative plan is confirmed, de-epithelialization of the appropriate portions of the flap may be performed while the flap remains in situ. The umbilicus is incised, and the superior incision is made down to the level of the abdominal wall fascia. The superior skin flap is dissected to the level of the costal margin, and the subcutaneous tunnel to the mastectomy defect is formed. The patient is then flexed, and the ability to close the abdominal defect is ascertained. At this point, the table is flattened and the inferior incision is made. The flap is elevated from the external oblique fascia bilaterally to the lateral aspect of the rectus sheath. The flap is then further elevated until the lateral row of perforators is identified on each side. Fascial incisions are planned as before, allowing a 3.5- to 4-cm fascial strip, with approximately 1 cm of anterior rectus sheath fascia remaining medially over each muscle. The muscle is split as previously described, and the inferior epigastric vessels are dissected free and ligated. The muscle splitting is then completed, and the rectus is transected as necessary at its inferior aspect. The muscle is elevated off the posterior rectus sheath and rotated into the defect.

Careful closure of the bipedicled TRAM defect is of particular importance; this defect is considerably larger than the unilateral defect, and simple primary fascial closure is not always possible. Synthetic fascial replacement with Prolene or Gore-Tex mesh may be used to attain closure of the rectus sheath. Autologous tissue is preferred to close the rectus sheath whenever possible. Attempts are first made to close the fascial defects with interrupted figure-of-eight sutures, alternating from one side to the other to distribute tension evenly. If this cannot be accomplished without tearing or excessive tightness, external oblique flaps may be used.[12] Relaxing incisions are first made through the external oblique fascia, parallel to the external oblique fibers and approximately 1 cm medial to the anterosuperior iliac spine. This incision is continued cranially and caudally, extending to the inguinal ligament inferiorly and over the external oblique muscle belly superiorly. The rectus sheath defect is then closed as before, often with a mesh overlay for additional support. The remainder of the abdominal closure and flap inset are performed as in the single-pedicled TRAM flap.

There are seemingly as many options in TRAM flap harvest as there are surgeons performing it. In the patient whose volume needs for reconstruction outstretch the amount of abdominal tissue available, an implant may be placed beneath the TRAM flap; alternatively, the TRAM flap may be "stacked."[13] A double-pedicled TRAM flap is harvested and then split vertically through the midline, as for a bilateral reconstruction. The ipsilateral flap is completely de-epithelialized and placed deep to the contralateral flap after delivery into the defect. This technique is particularly useful for patients who have considerable breast projection without significant ptosis (Figs. 141-10 to 141-12).

COMPLICATIONS

Serious complications resulting from TRAM flap operations are fortunately rare. These are more often than not due to underlying disease. A careful history and physical examination should be performed with referral to the appropriate specialists for clearance before surgery. Patients with breast cancer are at considerable risk for deep venous thrombosis, and the appropriate prophylaxis should be undertaken before, during, and after surgery.

More common complications of TRAM flap reconstruction can be subdivided into flap complications and donor site morbidity. Flap complications may consist of total or partial flap necrosis or, more commonly, fat necrosis. Proper preoperative planning should avoid most of these problems, ensuring that a plan is chosen that will provide adequate blood supply to the tissue needed. If a large amount of tissue is needed, a bipedicled technique, surgical delay, or even free tissue transfer should be considered to minimize fat necrosis and flap loss. Fat necrosis may be completely asymptomatic, or it may present as a firm, calcified mass or with drainage of turbid fluid through the incision. Treatment may range from simple observation to direct partial or total excision at the time of any revision surgery. Flap necrosis can result from several causes. Undue tension or torsion on the pedicle as it rotates into the defect can cause venous congestion or even arterial insufficiency. Care should be taken at the time of surgery to ensure that the pedicle is lying comfortably and without tension on its route into the mastectomy defect. In addition, the flap should be carefully examined after delivery into the defect to evaluate for any congestion or ischemia. Congested regions may be excised before inset. Should a flap appear threatened in the immediate postoperative period, simple steps may be taken to minimize pressure on the pedicle. Any binding dressings about the abdomen should be loosened or removed. A binder over the lower abdomen is desirable, making certain it does not encroach on the pedicle by carefully marking on the patient's abdomen where the pedicle lies. Sutures may be released in the area of ischemia to relieve tension. If necrosis should occur, small necrotic regions may often be débrided at the bedside or in the office; the wound is resutured primarily or left to heal secondarily. Larger areas of necrosis most often need to be débrided in the operating room, where the defect can then be closed primarily. Total flap loss is more common in free tissue transfer and is a rare complication of pedicled TRAM flaps.[14]

Abdominal wall complications may include hernia or abdominal wall laxity, seroma, skin flap necrosis, or wound dehiscence. Hernia is a relatively uncommon complication of TRAM flap surgery if a careful fascial closure is undertaken.[15] More often, patients will complain of abdominal weakness. Hartrampf et al performed a retrospective review of 150 patients who underwent unipedicled or bipedicled TRAM flap operations 5 to 7 years previously. Although no hernias were present, 60% of patients with bipedicled

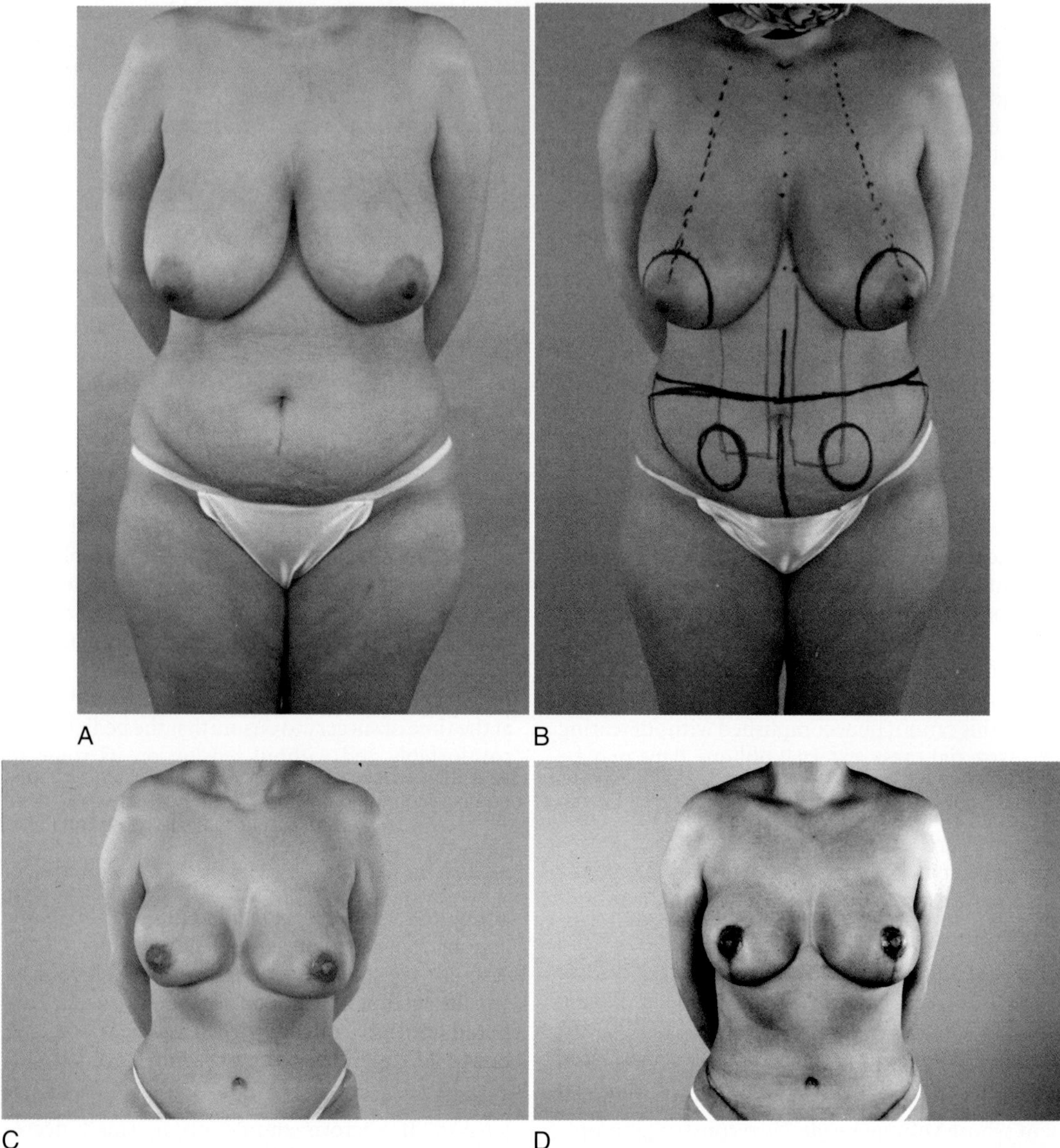

FIGURE 141-10. This 41-year-old patient underwent a bilateral TRAM delay procedure, followed by bilateral prophylactic mastectomy and immediate bilateral TRAM reconstruction. The nipple-areola complex was removed at the time of mastectomy and reattached as a composite graft after reconstruction. *A,* Preoperative frontal view. *B,* Markings for bilateral TRAM reconstruction. *C,* Initial postoperative frontal view. *D,* Final postoperative frontal view after bilateral TRAM reconstruction.

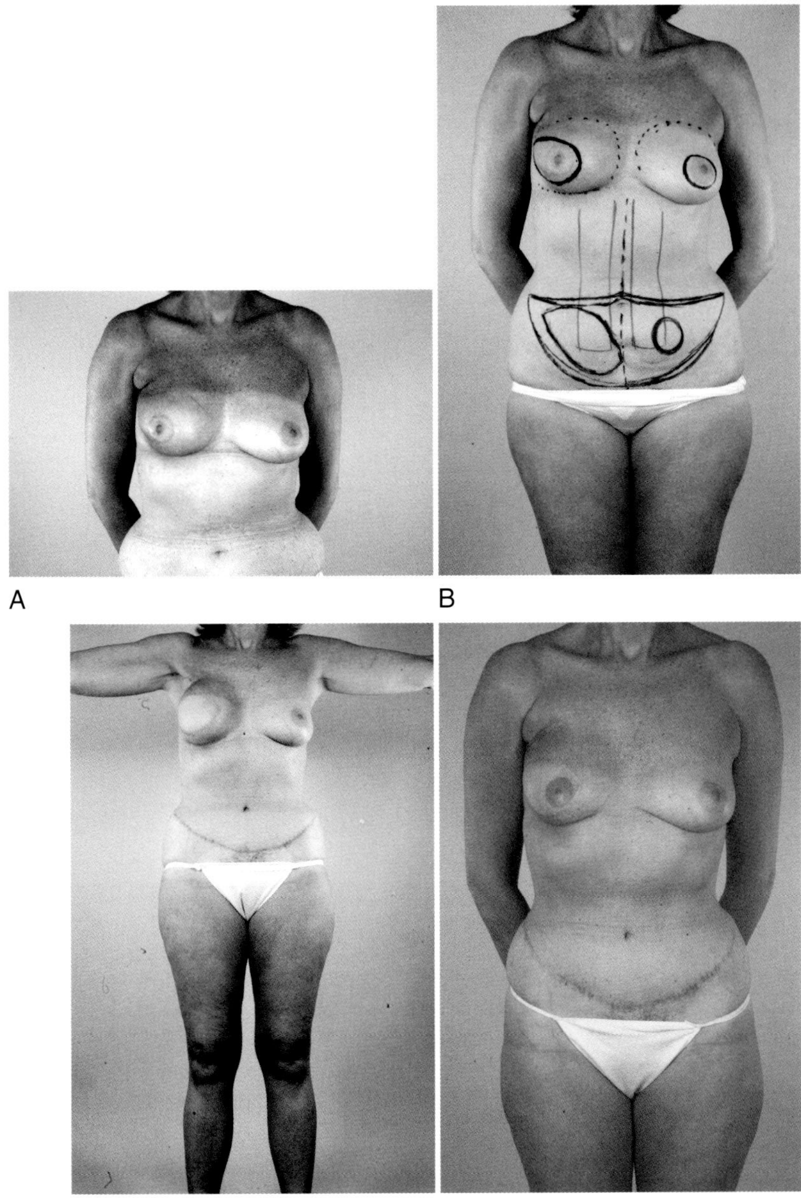

FIGURE 141-11. This 55-year-old patient underwent a lumpectomy and axillary dissection, followed by chemotherapy and radiation therapy. After a local recurrence, she underwent a mastectomy with immediate single-pedicled TRAM reconstruction. *A,* Preoperative frontal view. *B,* Markings for a single-pedicled TRAM flap. The left breast was initially marked for a prophylactic mastectomy; however, the patient decided not to undergo this portion of the procedure on the day of surgery. *C,* Initial postoperative result. *D,* Final postoperative result after nipple reconstruction and tattooing.

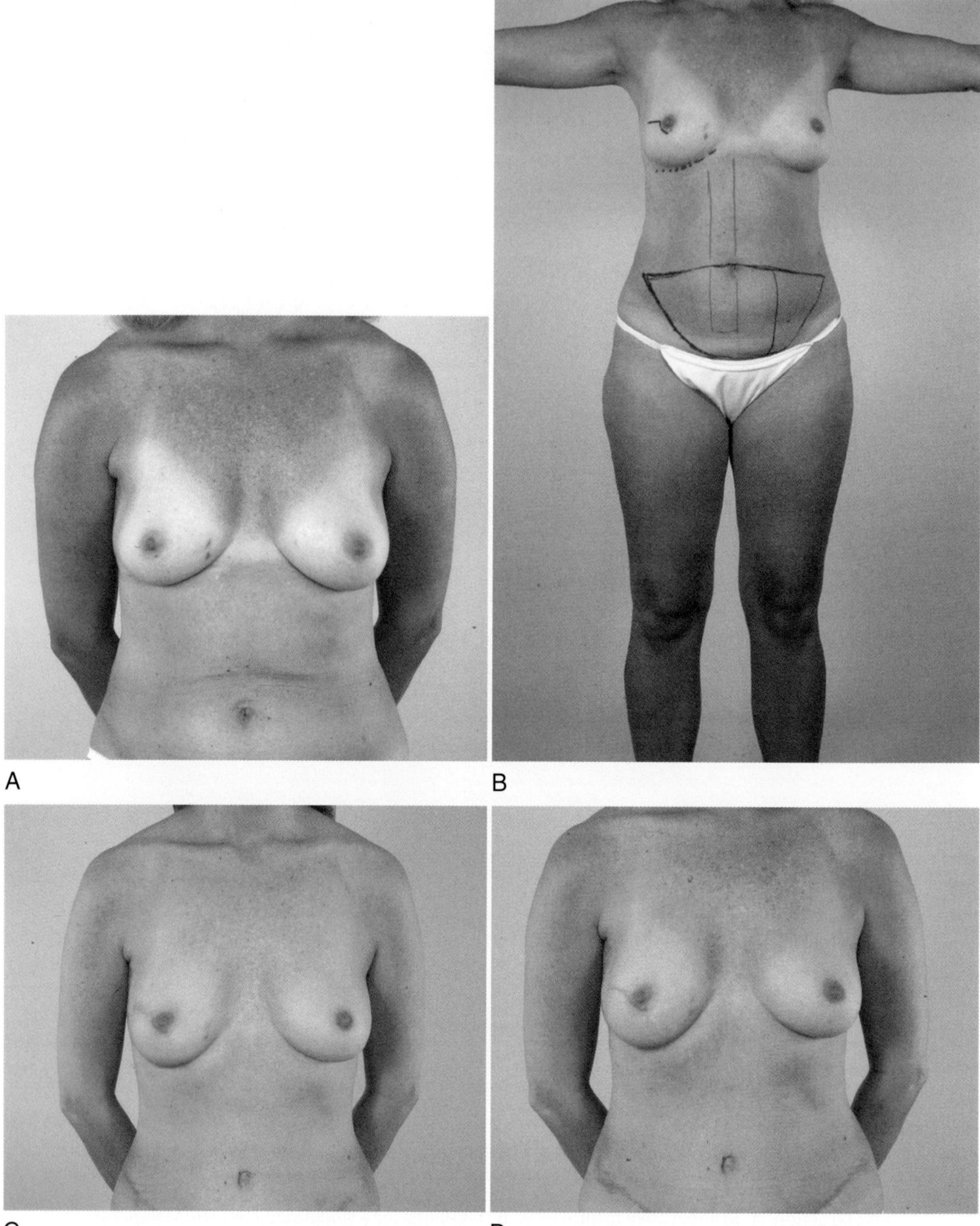

FIGURE 141-12. This 46-year-old patient with multicentric ductal carcinoma in situ underwent a nipple-sparing mastectomy with immediate single-pedicled TRAM reconstruction. *A*, Preoperative frontal view. *B*, Initial postoperative result. *C*, Immediate postoperative result. *D*, Final postoperative frontal view.

flaps and 35% of patients with unipedicled flaps admitted to some abdominal weakness, and 35% and 16%, respectively, mentioned decreased exercise ability. Patients should be educated about this possibility before undergoing surgery.

CONCLUSIONS

The TRAM flap can give appropriately selected patients a dual benefit—it can provide an aesthetically superior breast reconstruction, in both appearance and feel, while simultaneously giving patients the benefit of an abdominoplasty. It is important that the appropriate type of TRAM flap be chosen for each individual patient. Careful selection of patients and preoperative planning can improve the likelihood of a satisfying operation for both patient and surgeon.

REFERENCES

1. Hartrampf CR, Scheflan M, Black PW: Breast reconstruction with a transverse abdominal island flap. Plast Reconstr Surg 1982;69:216-224.
2. Spear SL: Surgery of the Breast: Principles and Art. Philadelphia, Lippincott-Raven, 1997.
3. Mathes SJ: A rectus abdominis myocutaneous flap to reconstruct abdominal wall defects. Br J Plast Surg 1977;30:282-283.
4. Moon HK, Taylor GI: The vascular anatomy of rectus abdominis musculocutaneous flaps based on the deep superior epigastric system. Plast Reconstr Surg 1988;82:815-831.
5. Mathes SJ, Logan SE: The use of a rectus abdominis myocutaneous flap to reconstruct a groin defect. Br J Plast Surg 1984; 37:351-353.
6. Codner MA, Bostwick J: The delayed TRAM flap. Clin Plast Surg 1998;25:183-189.
7. Kroll SS, Baldwin B: A comparison of outcomes using three different methods of breast reconstruction. Plast Reconstr Surg 1992;90:455-462.
8. Allen RJ, Treece P: Deep inferior epigastric perforator flap for breast reconstruction. Ann Plast Surg 1994;32:32-38.
9. Baldwin BJ, Schusterman MA, Miller MJ, et al: Bilateral breast reconstruction: conventional versus free TRAM. Plast Reconstr Surg 1994;93:1410-1416.
10. Grotting JC, Urist MM, Maddox WA, Vasconez LO: Conventional TRAM flap versus free microsurgical TRAM flap for immediate breast reconstruction. Plast Reconstr Surg 1989;83:828-841.
11. Spear SL, Walker RK: The external oblique flap for reconstruction of the rectus sheath. Plast Reconstr Surg 1992;90: 608-613.
12. Spear SL, Walker RK, Stefan MM: The stacked transverse rectus abdominis musculocutaneous flap revisited in breast reconstruction. Ann Plast Surg 1994;32:565-571.
13. Watterson PA, Bostwick J, Hester TR, et al: TRAM flap anatomy correlated with a 10-year clinical experience with 556 patients. Plast Reconstr Surg 1995;95:1185-1194.
14. Paige KT, Bostwick J, Bried JT, Jones G: A comparison of morbidity from bilateral, unipedicled and unilateral, unipedicled TRAM flap breast reconstructions. Plast Reconstr Surg 1998;101:1819-1827.
15. Mizgala CL, Hartrampf CR, Bennett GK: Assessment of the abdominal wall after pedicled TRAM flap surgery: 5- to 7-year follow-up of 150 consecutive patients. Plast Reconstr Surg 1994;93:988-1002.

CHAPTER

142

Postmastectomy Reconstruction: Free TRAM Flap Techniques

JAMES C. GROTTING, MD ✦ MICHAEL S. BECKENSTEIN, MD ✦ STEPHEN M. CHEN, MD

The evolution of microsurgical principles and their application to breast reconstruction led to the development of the free TRAM flap.[1-3] Whereas the overall philosophy for choosing a TRAM flap for reconstruction of a breast is the same for the free TRAM flap, the use of the dominant pedicle and less abdominal wall morbidity provide several advantages over the pedicled TRAM flap.[4-6] The rationale for use of the free TRAM flap is discussed, as are the indications, operative technique, perioperative care, complications, secondary operations, and unsolved problems.

RATIONALE FOR USE OF THE FREE TRAM FLAP

The same qualities that make the TRAM flap the "gold standard" for autogenous tissue breast reconstruction are applicable to the free TRAM flap. However, several additional advantages are available with the free TRAM flap. The dominant pedicle (deep inferior epigastric vessels) is employed, which yields a higher perfusion pressure and better flow within the flap (Fig. 142-1).[4,5,7] This property diminishes the frequency of fat necrosis compared with risk-matched pedicled procedures.[3,8,9] Various shaping maneuvers can be used with this flap that yield arguably superior aesthetic results.[1,2,8-11] The flap can be safely folded on itself to establish more ptosis or to increase projection. These maneuvers cannot be safely performed on the pedicled TRAM flap. Less rectus muscle is required with free TRAM flap elevation, resulting in a lower incidence of abdominal wall weakness and hernia formation.[4,8,12,13] The lesser abdominal wall insult results in a more expedient recovery and less hospitalization compared with the pedicled TRAM flap.[2-4,8,13,14]

The deep inferior epigastric artery perforator flap was developed to eradicate abdominal wall morbidity by dissection of the chosen perforators from the investing abdominal wall fascia. The dissection continues to incorporate the major, intramuscular branches and finally the deep inferior epigastric vessels. Because no muscle or fascia is incorporated into the flap, no hernias or weaknesses should develop.[8,15,16] The perforator flap concept is compelling because it essentially nullifies the incidence of hernia formation; however, there is debate as to whether a large amount of tissue can be safely transferred with this method.[8] The muscle-sparing technique, for free TRAM flap harvest, allows large volumes of abdominal adipose tissue to be safely transferred with an acceptably low incidence of abdominal wall hernia formation.[4,8,14,17] Incorporation of a small cuff of muscle and fascia saves operative time and minimizes potential injury to the perforators. These

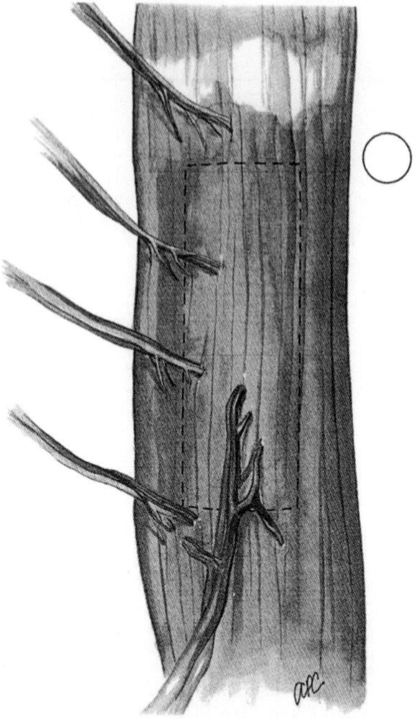

FIGURE 142-1. The rectus abdominis muscle seen from its deep surface. The inferior epigastric artery and its accompanying vein usually enter at approximately the level of the semicircular line in the middle third of the muscle. The artery usually sends a branch caudally to supply the inferior portion of the rectus abdominis muscle. The intercostal neurovascular bundles enter obliquely at intervals, with the main trunk of the nerve penetrating the central third of the muscle. However, small twigs of the nerve may occasionally be seen piercing the lateral third of the muscle. These branches can be preserved, thereby leaving a strip of innervated muscle in situ with the free TRAM flap technique. The medial strip remains vascularized but denervated. It may regain function by neurotization. (From Grotting JC, Oslin BD: Free TRAM flap breast reconstruction. In Spear SL, ed: Surgery of the Breast: Principles and Art. Philadelphia, Lippincott-Raven, 1998:555.)

benefits outweigh the low risk of abdominal wall weakness.

The major disadvantage of the free TRAM flap is the potential for complete flap loss. For the conventional TRAM flap, this is a negligible concern.[4,8,18] The rate of total flap loss for the free TRAM flap is less than 1%, which is low enough to be offset by the added benefits attainable.[2,4,8,7] Microsurgical skills and proficiency are required to perform free TRAM flap breast reconstruction, which should be developed in current plastic surgery training programs. Microsurgical breast reconstruction can be performed expediently, safely, economically, and with consistent results.[4,19] These factors make the free TRAM flap an attractive option for autogenous tissue breast reconstruction and justify its frequent use.

INDICATIONS AND CONTRAINDICATIONS

Any patient who is a candidate for a pedicled TRAM flap can undergo a free TRAM flap reconstruction with a few exceptions.[18,20] This method is precluded in patients who have had both deep inferior epigastric pedicles divided from surgery or trauma and in those with midline incisions requiring zone II and most of zone IV regions. In these patients, a double-pedicled TRAM flap or other more complex microsurgical maneuvers might be considered.

The indications for the free TRAM flap are extended to include some absolute and relative contraindications for the pedicled TRAM flap.[18,20] Patients with a smoking history can undergo free TRAM flap breast reconstruction because the higher flow vessels (pedicle) are more resistant to the deleterious effects of carbon monoxide and other noxious agents in cigarette smoke compared with a conventional TRAM flap pedicle. Smoking, however, should be stopped in the perioperative period. Patients with diabetes are better suited for free TRAM flap breast reconstruction. Obese patients tend to have more flap and donor site complications because the adipose tissue and skin are poorly perfused by the perforators.[4,8,21] This results in higher incidences of fat necrosis and abdominal or flap skin ischemia. The enhanced perfusion of the free TRAM flap diminishes fat necrosis in these patients. Less undermining of the abdominal wall flap is required than for the conventional TRAM flap because there is no need for the tunnel connecting the abdomen with the mammary pocket. This preserves more of the zone II and zone III blood supply to the abdominal wall, which diminishes the potential for tissue ischemia.[8,21]

Patients who require a large volume of tissue to reconstruct the breast are better suited for the free TRAM flap. Larger volumes of tissue survive with the enhanced perfusion pressure of the free TRAM flap with a lower incidence of fat necrosis. Delay procedures or a double-pedicled TRAM flap would be necessary to safely transfer a similar volume of tissue. This requires additional surgery and entails more abdominal wall morbidity.

A subcostal incision with transection of the rectus muscle divides the superior epigastric vessels, negating use of a pedicled TRAM flap on the affected side. A free TRAM flap, however, can be used on the side of a subcostal incision. This is especially relevant when a right subcostal incision is present and a contralateral TRAM flap is required to reconstruct the left breast.

PREOPERATIVE CONSIDERATIONS

Initial Assessment

The surgeon must carefully evaluate the patient to determine whether she is a candidate for free TRAM flap breast reconstruction. A careful history and physical examination are essential in this determination. The medical and surgical history will provide insight into conditions that might preclude elective reconstruction. Various medications that induce vasospasm or bleeding should be identified and adjusted after consultation with the prescribing physician. A history of cigarette smoking is important, and smoking should be ceased a minimum of 2 weeks preoperatively and for 1 month postoperatively. Previous surgeries and the location of incisions also influence operative decision-making and planning. A consultation with the oncologist is warranted to determine whether a mastectomy is prudent on the contralateral side or whether perioperative radiation therapy or chemotherapy is required.

A careful physical examination includes evaluation of both breasts to determine the flap volume requirement. Asymmetries in size, shape, volume, inframammary fold position, and nipple-areola differences should be noted and demonstrated to the patient. The potential for alteration of the contralateral breast with reduction, mastopexy, or augmentation should also be assessed. With these factors in mind, an assessment of the abdominal wall adipose distribution is made. The surgeon must determine whether there is enough tissue that can safely be shaped into a flap. The presence and location of scars should be noted and factored into the decision process. Pfannenstiel, midline, and paramedian scars demand attention and careful, thoughtful flap design. These factors should help determine whether a free TRAM flap reconstruction is feasible.

If the free TRAM flap option is viable, the procedure should be explained to the patient in detail with all risks, benefits, and alternatives. It is the patient who ultimately makes the decision. The patient's expectations and the surgeon's abilities must be carefully discussed to establish a realistic scenario for the patient. Finally, an informed consent must be obtained. Preoperative photographs are essential in making final preoperative plans; essential details not noted in the physical examination are often readily visible in photographs. Communication with the oncologic surgeon is important to coordinate the surgery and to plan the mastectomy incisions. Routine preoperative laboratory studies, a chest radiograph, and an electrocardiogram are obtained. Donation of two units of autologous or directed blood should be encouraged for bilateral reconstruction if there is enough intervening time. For unilateral reconstruction, we no longer require blood donation.

Flap Design

The shape and volume distribution requirements of the reconstructed breast determine the flap design. A breast that is more ptotic with lower pole fullness and less projection can be formed with an ipsilateral flap that is rotated 90 degrees, with the umbilicus positioned inferomedially. The base width of the breast corresponds to the vertical "height" of the flap as marked on the abdomen. The inferior portion of the flap can be folded beneath itself to establish more projection. A full, conical breast with good projection requires a contralateral flap that is rotated 180 degrees with the umbilicus placed at the 6-o'clock position. The base width of the breast corresponds to the width of the flap before elevation. The flap can be oriented more obliquely if the anterior axillary fold needs to be defined. These designs are based on use of axillary recipient vessels. For internal mammary anastomosis, the same concepts are applied but the opposite pedicle is used. Ipsilateral flaps are usually employed in bilateral reconstruction (Fig. 142-2).

To simulate the flap and to determine whether there is enough abdominal tissue, the dimensions of the breast are transcribed onto the abdomen according to the chosen orientation. The surgeon then places two hands on the breast to be removed to obtain a "sense" of volume. This maneuver is repeated on the abdominal area designated for the flap. With the estimate of breast volume kept in mind, a determination as to the adequacy of abdominal tissue is made. Closure of the abdominal wound must be performed without undue tension and is dependent on the skin requirement of the new breast. In the multiparous patient, laxity and an excess of the abdominal wall tissues facilitate wound closure after flap harvest. Nulliparous patients and those with more resilient tissue present more of a challenge. Closure potential must be verified in all patients by pinching the skin of the designated flap, approximating the closure. If it is excessively tight, after factoring in some tension release after skin undermining, adjustments must be made. The skin-sparing mastectomy has decreased the requirement for donor skin. Beveling the flap incisions allows the incorporation of the needed adipose tissue with less skin excision, thereby facilitating closure.

Recipient Vessels

It is preferable to use the thoracodorsal vessels as the recipient site. These vessels are of sufficient caliber and length for anastomosis to the donor vessels (Fig. 142-3).[8,10,11,22-24] In immediate reconstruction, these vessels are readily dissected and often visible in the axillary bed after axillary node dissection. If there is no axillary dissection, these vessels are easily accessible through the modified radical mastectomy wound or through a separate axillary incision if a periareolar approach is used.[4,8] If these vessels are not sufficient on exploration, the circumflex scapular or more proximal vessels can be used. On occasion, unnamed

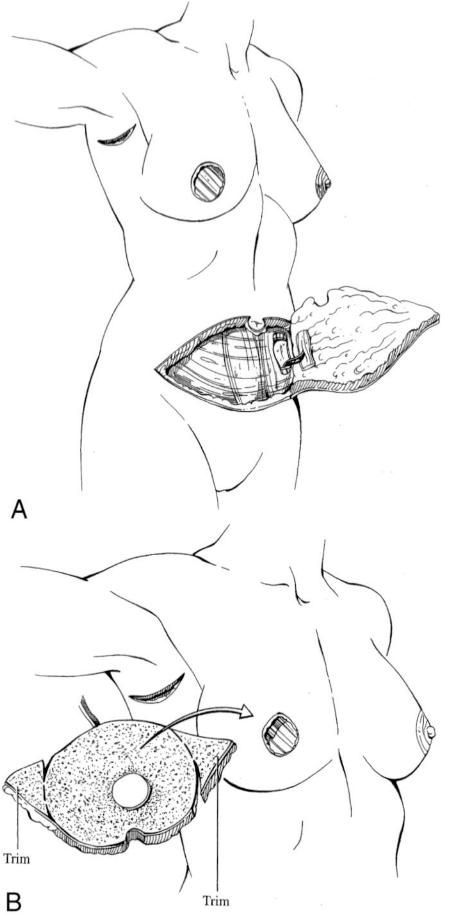

FIGURE 142-2. *A,* Schematic representation of flap design. The flap is based on the deep inferior epigastric artery and vein. The authors' preferred method is to spare a strip of rectus muscle both laterally and medially, basing the flap on both the medial and lateral row of rectus abdominis perforators. *B,* For a more mature-looking breast, the flap is oriented transversely with the umbilicus at the 6-o'clock position. This rotates the inferior epigastric artery and vein 180 degrees to lie close to the preferred recipient vessels, the thoracodorsal artery and vein. (From Grotting JC, Oslin BD: Free TRAM flap breast reconstruction. In Spear SL, ed: Surgery of the Breast: Principles and Art. Philadelphia, Lippincott-Raven, 1998:555.)

vessels of sufficient caliber can be used. In delayed reconstruction, there is the possibility that the thoracodorsal or other potential vessels were ligated or damaged. The original operative report might be helpful to determine whether this occurred. If there is a question as to the status of these vessels, noninvasive Doppler studies can be obtained to make this determination.

An initial exploration of these vessels can be performed before flap design to determine recipient vessel adequacy. If the axilla was previously irradiated, these vessels may not be suitable. However, with extensive scar release and adventiciectomy around the vessels, these vessels might still be used, provided that good inflow and outflow are demonstrable. Many times, clipping a large proximal arterial branch will greatly improve inflow by preventing a "steal phenomenon." If the axillary vessels are not sufficient or there is any doubt, the internal mammary vessels should be used. The flap orientation may have to be altered to form the desired breast shape. If either is available, it is recommended that the recipient vessels be found to be satisfactory before the flap pedicle is chosen.

OPERATIVE TECHNIQUE

Preoperative Marking

The patient is marked in the standing position. For a skin-sparing mastectomy, a periareolar incision is marked with a margin of approximately 0.5 cm from the areola. If the biopsy site must be re-excised, it is marked with an ellipse. If there is a narrow bridge of skin between the areola and biopsy site, the intervening portion is excised to minimize potential skin loss. A small incision is marked in the axilla for the anastomosis. This is oriented in a natural crease just at the lower border of the axillary hair. If a modified radical mastectomy is planned, the appropriate ellipse encompassing the nipple-areola complex is designed. The oncologic surgeon should be included in the planning of these incisions.

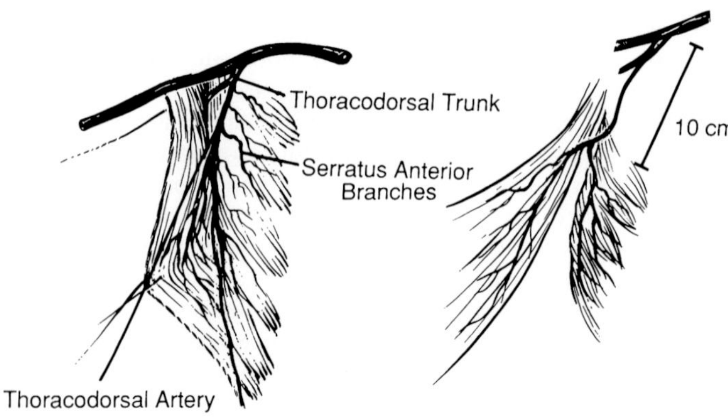

FIGURE 142-3. The most convenient vessels for microvascular anastomosis are the thoracodorsal artery (approximately 10 cm long) and vein. The vessels can be safely divided for end-to-end anastomosis, which facilitates positioning of the flap without tension on the pedicle. (From Bostwick J III: Breast reconstruction. In McCarthy JG, ed: Plastic Surgery. Philadelphia, WB Saunders, 1990:3897.)

The midline is marked from the sternal notch through the xiphoid, umbilicus, and pubis. The flap is marked in the hypogastric region, which should contain dimensions of the desired flap as well as an additional portion to facilitate symmetric closure of the defect. The lowest edge of the flap should border, when possible, an existing Pfannenstiel scar. Flap design varies according to flap dimensions, body habitus, adipose distribution, and scar location. The conventional elliptical pattern in heavier patients and an aesthetic abdominoplasty ("handlebar") pattern in the more slender patient are advocated (Fig. 142-4).[20,25]

Positioning of the Patient

Operating room setup and positioning of the patient are essential to facilitate the procedure. The anesthesia equipment is placed at the patient's feet with the head toward the center of the room. This allows two teams to work simultaneously, unencumbered, minimizing cross-contamination. The flap can be elevated simultaneously with the mastectomy. Contralateral breast alteration may be performed by a third team member at this time. The abdominal wall defect can be repaired and closed along with the anastomosis.

The patient is centered on the bed with the shoulders squared, arms abducted 90 degrees, elbows slightly flexed, and thumbs oriented upward. All pressure points are padded, and pneumatic sequential compression is used. Before induction of anesthesia, verify that the patient's head is lying comfortably on a neurosurgical headrest to prevent postoperative neck discomfort. The intravenous tubing and endotracheal tubes are secured along the side of the table to keep them away from the operative field. Foam padding is placed over the patient's face, with the nose exposed, for protection against the assistant's arm pressure

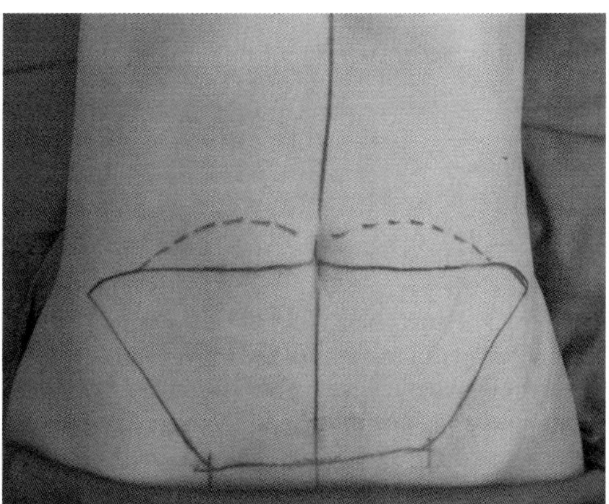

FIGURE 142-4. The patient is marked preoperatively (in the standing position) with a "handlebar" flap design. The markings can be modified according to the amount of excess tissue, just as in aesthetic abdominoplasty.

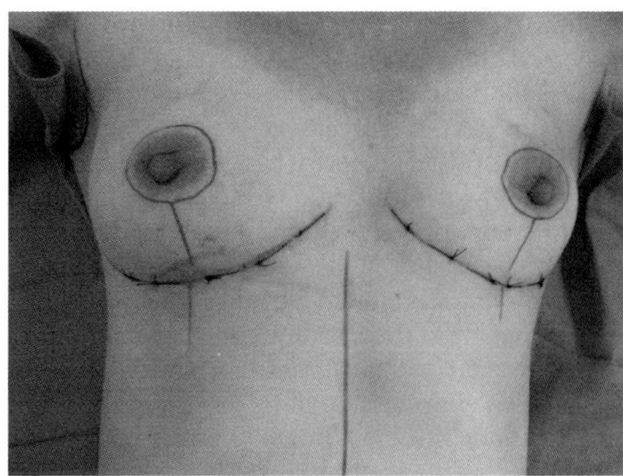

FIGURE 142-5. A skin-sparing mastectomy is marked along with a separate incision for the axillary dissection and anastomosis. The silk sutures to delineate the inframammary fold are in place. Only the periareolar incision is required for breasts of this size and shape.

during the microsurgical portion. The microscope can readily be brought into the field from the center of the room along with a video monitor to enable the entire surgical team to view the anastomotic portion of the procedure. Before preparation of the skin, silk sutures are placed along the inframammary fold to delineate and preserve it during the mastectomy. These sutures are carefully placed through the skin and into the pectoralis-rectus fascia (Fig. 142-5). The patient is then prepared and draped in the usual manner. Heparin (5000 units) is administered subcutaneously, on call to the operating room, as an attempt to reduce the incidence of pulmonary emboli. Eighteen-inch, 2-0 silk sutures are placed in the sternal notch, xiphoid region, and midline of the pubis. They are used for triangulation to verify symmetry and the true midline.

Anesthesia Requirements

The operating room should be warm so that the patient's core temperature remains above 36°C. The patient should be adequately hydrated to maintain blood pressure and urine output. The minimum amount of intravenous fluid to accomplish this is used; if additional fluid is needed, colloid is preferred. Hydration of the patient minimizes "relative" hemodilution and the third-space mobilization that occurs around the third postoperative day. Nitrous oxide is avoided to minimize bowel distention, which may compromise abdominal wall closure. The anesthesia team is provided with a written protocol addressing these requirements and room setup.

Flap Dissection

The umbilicus is then circumscribed; two single skin hooks are placed at the 12-o'clock and 6-o'clock positions. A No. 15 scalpel is used to incise the periumbilical skin. With the aid of a double hook placed on the abdominal skin, Metzenbaum scissors are used to dissect the umbilical stalk, circumferentially, away from the flap and down to the fascia. The cephalic skin incisions are made, and the electrocautery is used to dissect the adipose tissue down to the rectus fascia. If more adipose tissue is needed as compared with skin, this dissection is beveled away from the flap. The angle is determined by the amount of fat needed. When the fascia is reached, the abdominal flap is elevated in the suprafascial plane. This dissection is confined to the borders of the rectus musculature and proceeds to the costal margins. This dissection is not as extensive as for a pedicled TRAM flap because no tunnel is required. The inferior incision is made, and electrocautery is used to dissect down to the fascia.

It is best to commence flap elevation from zone IV of the flap because the surgeon may obtain insight as to the location of the desired perforators on the opposite side. The medial row of perforators is then divided on the opposite side, making sure the midline is crossed. The flap is then elevated off the fascia, laterally to medially, past the edge of the rectus muscle, until a row of lateral perforators of sufficient caliber is encountered (Fig. 142-6*A* and *B*).[3,5,20] Suprafascial dissection from caudal to cephalad continues to the most inferior perforator (Fig. 142-6*C*). Adjacent to the lateral perforators, the fascia is incised longitudinally down below the most inferior perforator (Fig. 142-6*D*).

The inferior portion of the flap is elevated up to the largest of the inferior perforators approximately at the level of the arcuate line. A dotted line is marked. At this point, a transverse fascial incision is made delineating the lower border of the muscle to be harvested (Fig. 142-6*E*). If needed, an incision can be extended from above the caudal line to facilitate dissection of the deep inferior epigastric vessels.

From this point, the longitudinal incision is obliquely extended an additional 4 cm inferiorly to facilitate vessel dissection. Allis clamps are placed on the lateral edge of the incised fascia above the transverse cut (Fig. 142-6*F* and *G*).

The lateral edge of the rectus muscle is then dissected free, exposing the deep inferior epigastric vessels. The twelfth intercostal vessels are divided to provide access to these vessels. A finger is inserted to bluntly dissect the muscle and pedicle from the posterior sheath. With sharp and blunt dissection, the vascular pedicle is dissected from the overlying muscle at the caudal edge of the flap, which should allow two fingers to be placed in this space to protect the vessels during muscle harvest (Fig. 142-6*H* and *I*).

The lateral muscle is split to the cephalic border of the flap by first placing a right-angled clamp through the muscle's underside, between the lateral edge of the muscle and the perforators, with extreme care to protect the pedicle (Fig. 142-6*J* and *K*). Electrocautery, with diminished power settings, is used to incise the muscle at this point to establish a space that will accommodate a finger. The finger is placed facing cephalad and is used to protect the pedicle as the muscle is split (Fig. 142-6*L* and *M*).

Once this is completed, the inferior border of the flap is divided, again with one finger placed between the vessels and the muscle. The muscle is divided below the inserted finger, which ensures the safety of the pedicle (Fig. 142-6*N* and *O*). The medial border of the flap is dissected in a similar manner, ensuring that a finger protects the pedicle at all times. The cephalic border of the rectus muscle, including the superior epigastric branches, is left intact until an intact deep inferior epigastric pedicle and adequate recipient inflow are verified. This preserves the option for a pedicled TRAM flap if needed (Fig. 142-6*P*).

The deep inferior epigastric vessels are then dissected free with the aid of a lighted fiberoptic retractor. Deaver retractors are placed on the caudal muscle in addition to a cephalically placed malleable retractor pushing down toward the pelvic floor (Fig. 142-7).

Careful dissection toward the iliac vessels is performed until an adequate pedicle length is attained. Bipolar cautery and vascular clips are used to divide the various branches. Once adequate recipient vessel inflow is verified, the rectus muscle is transected at the superior margin of the flap with electrocautery. This maneuver is followed by pedicle division between medium vascular clips (Fig. 142-8). The flap is then transferred to the chest, where it is held for several seconds to allow the vessels to "dangle" and assume their natural orientation, preventing torsion. Several staples are placed to secure the flap to the chest skin.

Vascular Anastomosis

Before division of the vascular pedicle of the flap, the recipient vessels are dissected and prepared for anastomosis. It is preferable to use the thoracodorsal vessels and divide them proximal to the serratus branch. This preserves retrograde flow to the latissimus dorsi muscle, keeping it available as a salvage option. The artery is divided to assess inflow visually before the division of the cephalic portion of the rectus muscle. Exposure is obtained with an Adson-Beckman retractor to retract the lateral skin and latissimus muscle. A Deaver retractor is placed at the cephalic skin and secured with a towel clip to the foam over the patient's

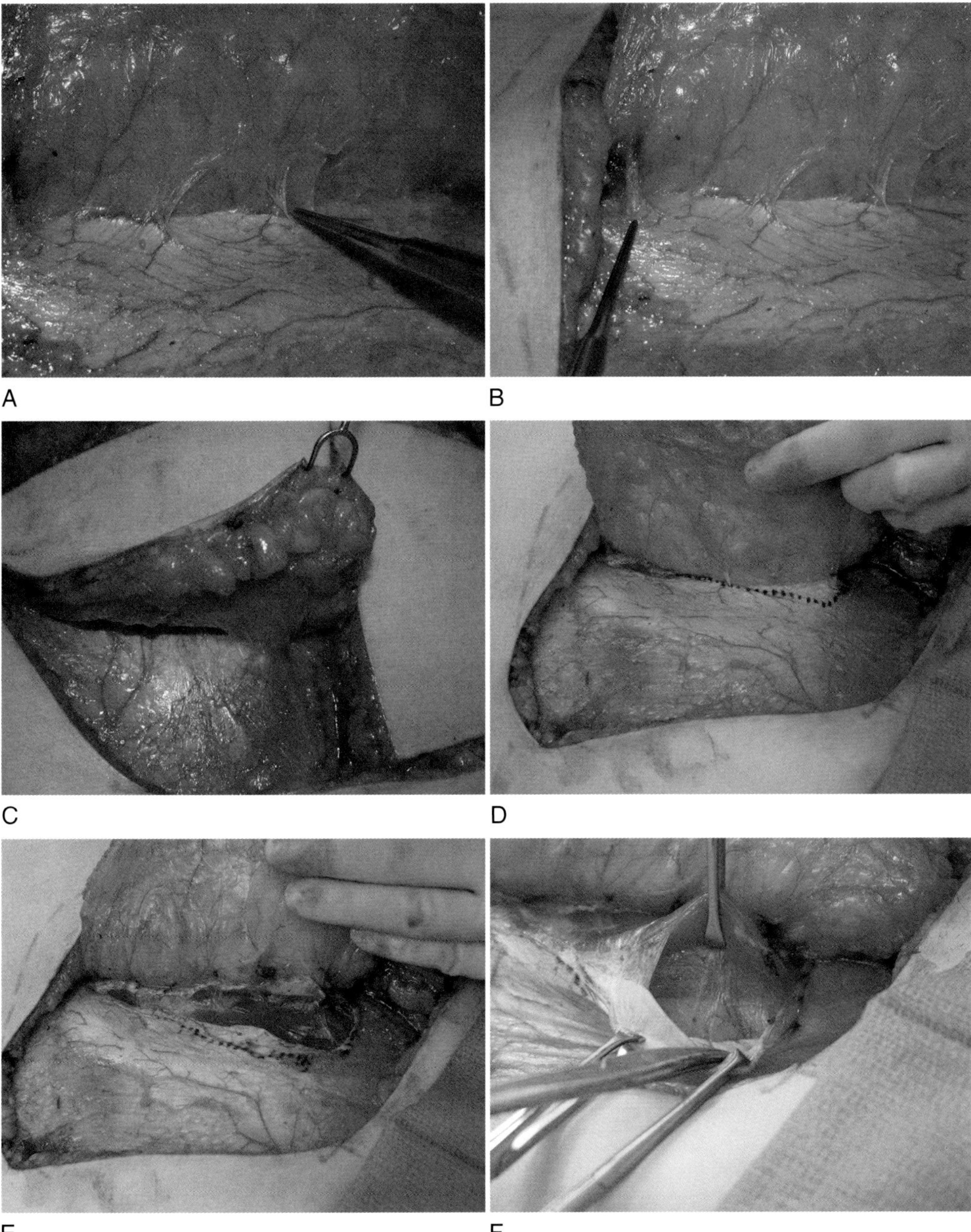

FIGURE 142-6. *A,* Flap dissection from lateral to medial until a lateral row of perforators is encountered. *B,* Forceps pointing to largest lateral perforator at the cephalad portion of the flap. *C,* Suprafascial dissection from caudal to cephalad until the most inferior perforator is encountered. *D* and *E,* Line of fascial incision lateral to the lateral row of perforators and transverse below the most inferior perforator. Note that the incision is medial to the dotted line because perforators were located more medially; thus, more fascia could be preserved for wound closure. *F,* Exposure of the lateral edge of the rectus muscle demonstrates the twelfth intercostal vessels, which serve as a landmark for the deeper and more medial deep inferior epigastric pedicle.

Continued

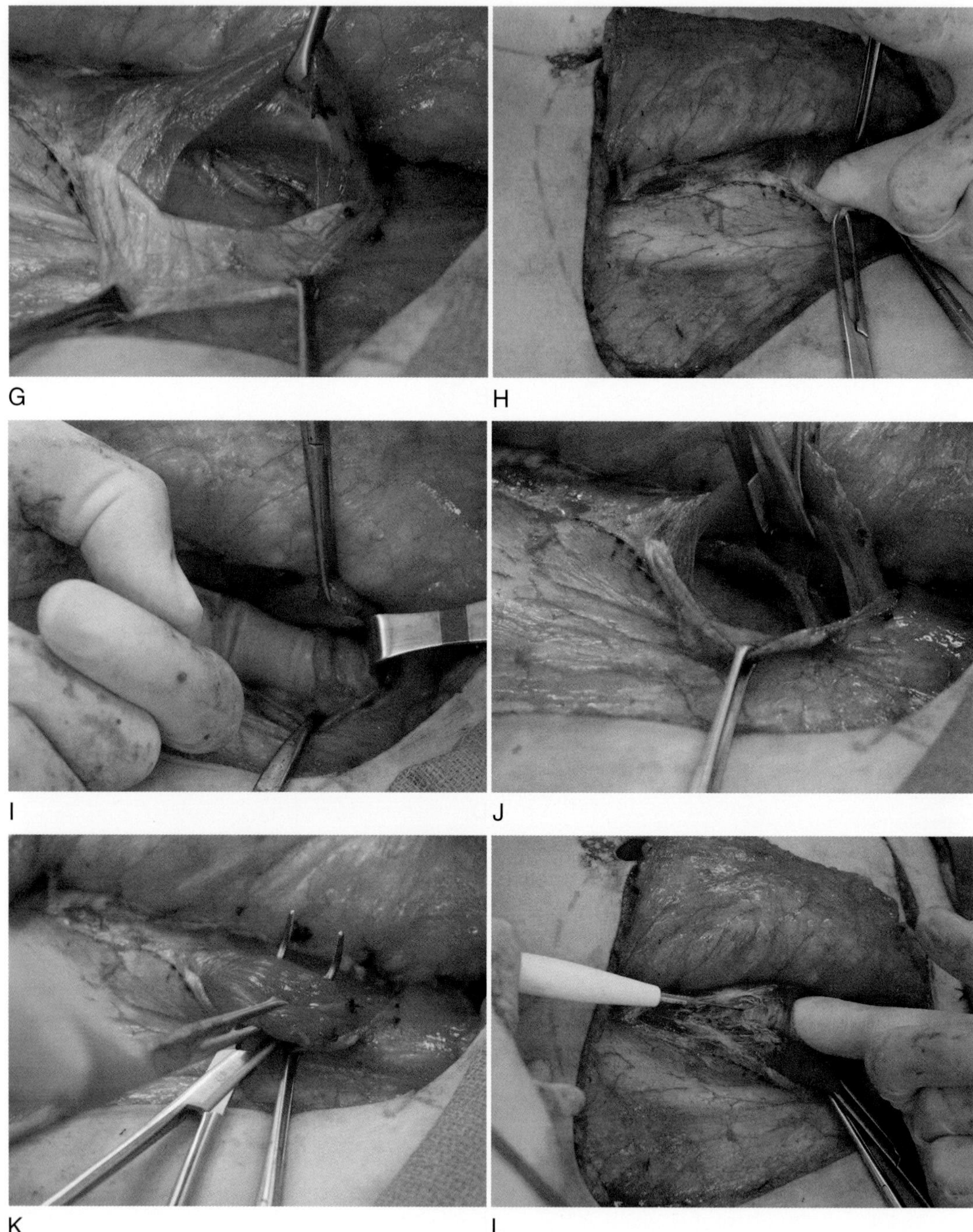

FIGURE 142-6, cont'd. *G,* Deep inferior epigastric vessels. *H,* Finger is used to bluntly dissect muscle and pedicle from the areolar attachments to the posterior sheath. *I,* Deep inferior epigastric vessels identified before splitting of the muscle. *J* and *K,* The right-angled clamp is placed through the muscle under direct vision to protect the deep inferior epigastric vessels. *L,* Electrocautery dissection dividing the lateral edge of the rectus with the finger present to protect the deep inferior epigastric vessels.

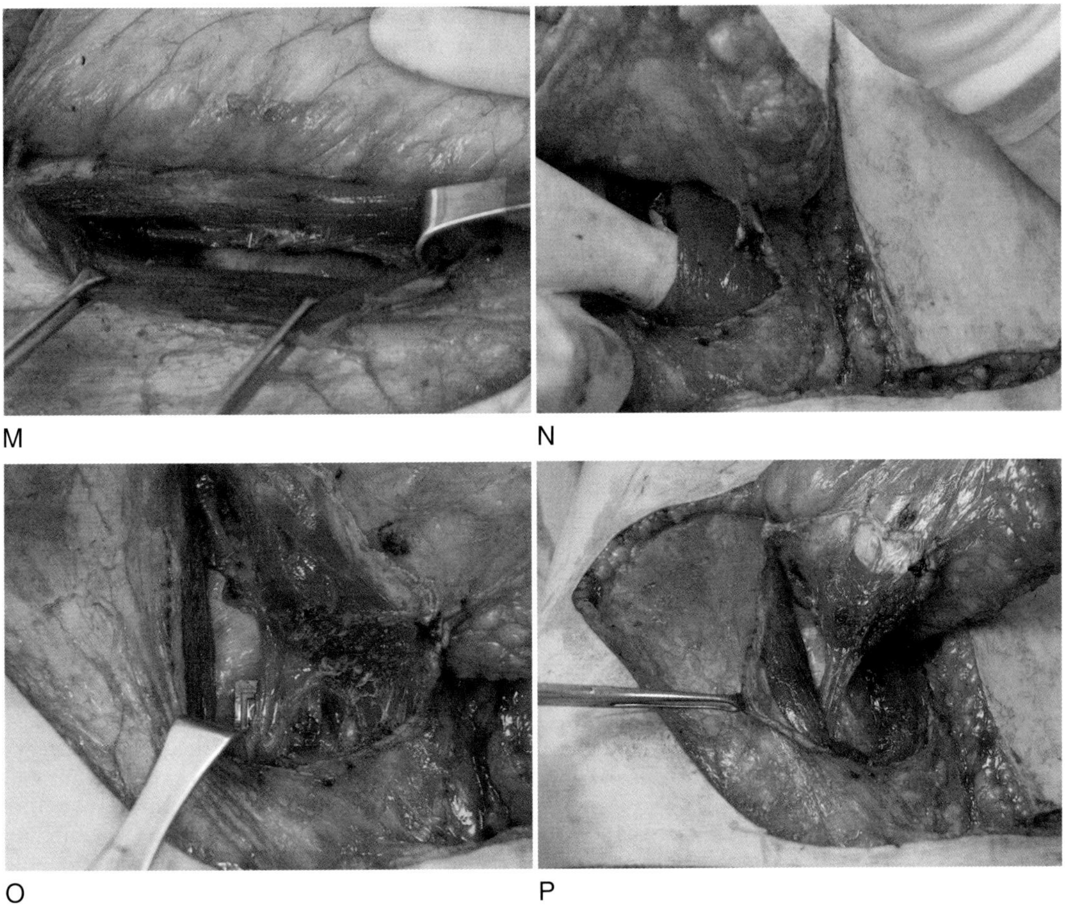

M N

O P

FIGURE 142-6, cont'd. *M,* Completed dissection of the lateral rectus from the deep inferior epigastric vessels. *N,* Division of the transverse portion of the rectus muscle below the level of the most inferior perforator. The finger is protecting the deep inferior epigastric pedicle. *O,* Completion of the transverse section of the rectus muscle. Note the deep inferior epigastric pedicle. *P,* Completed dissection of the muscle. The deep inferior epigastric vessels have not been sectioned yet.

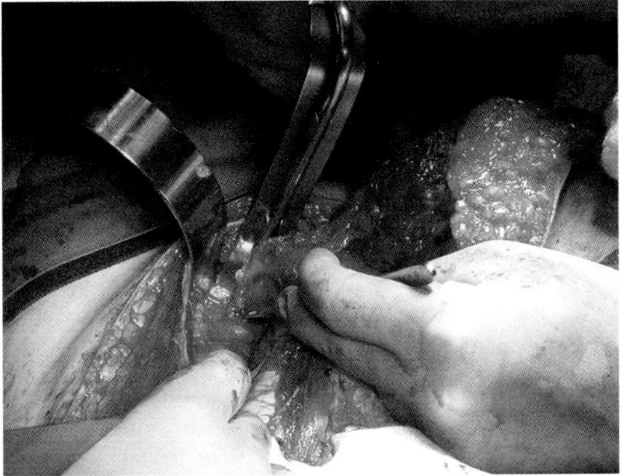

FIGURE 142-7. The dissection of the donor vessels is facilitated by use of fiberoptic, Deaver, and malleable retractors.

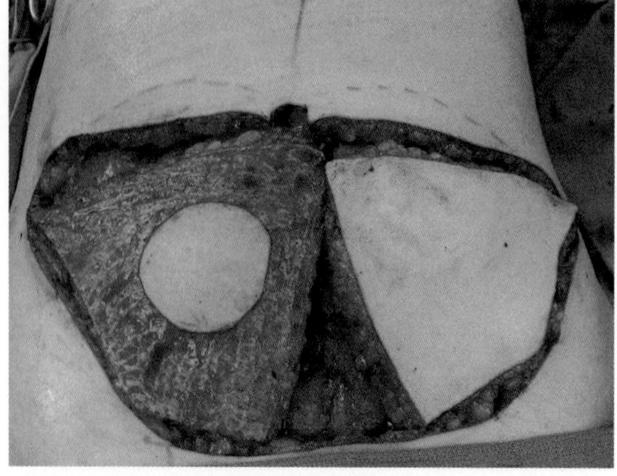

A

B

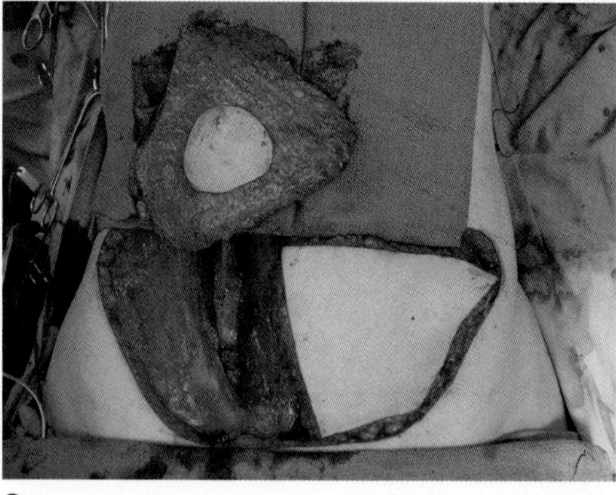

C

FIGURE 142-8. *A,* Flap dissection just before division of deep inferior epigastrics for transfer to the chest. Each hemiflap will be rotated 90 degrees, and the skin island will be situated within the periareolar defect from the skin-sparing mastectomy. *B,* Division of the deep inferior epigastric pedicle. *C,* Approximate in situ position of the TRAM flap (90-degree clockwise rotation) on transfer to the mastectomy defect.

head by use of a lap pad looped through the retractor handle (Fig. 142-9).

The donor vessels are placed through the mastectomy incision and brought in proximity to the recipient vessels. If periareolar and axillary incisions are used, the donor vessels must be brought through a tunnel connecting these sites (Fig. 142-10). The microscope can readily be brought into the field from the center of the room along with a video monitor to enable the entire surgical team to view the anastomotic portion. An end-to-end anastomosis is performed with standardized microsurgical techniques by suturing of the artery and use of a coupling device for the vein (Fig. 142-11). Verification of adequate flow is made by release of the venous clamps first, followed by the arterial clamps.

Flap Insetting and Shaping

The flap is first secured to the chest wall by suturing the segment of rectus muscle to the pectoralis muscle centrally with 2-0 Vicryl sutures, taking care not to compress the pedicle. The distal zones of the flap are trimmed as needed, and the dermis of the flap is sutured along the inframammary fold. A suture is placed at the lateral extent of the inframammary fold and along the base of the fold, ending at the medial border of the fold. Similar sutures are also placed along the cephalic border of the flap for exaggerated upper pole fullness. The flap should be placed slightly higher and medial because it will descend laterally and inferiorly as the tissues mature (Fig. 142-12).

Additional trimming of the flap to obtain the desired shape is performed. If a contralateral breast adjustment is necessary, it is performed before these maneuvers. To increase projection, the lower, central portion of the flap can be plicated; an apex, upward wedge of skin is marked, this portion is de-epithelialized, and the skin is sutured, resulting in a linear closure. The wedge must not be too wide because excessive tension can compromise the blood flow across this portion of the flap, leading to ischemia. A portion of the flap can be de-epithelialized and folded under itself to enhance projection or lateral fullness.

The patient is placed in the sitting position, the mammary skin is stapled to the flap, and symmetry is verified. The skin island is marked and incised, and the remainder of the flap is de-epithelialized and sutured to the mammary skin. The dermis is divided down to the fat at the edge of the skin island to avoid a thickness discrepancy at the final closure. Closed suction drains are placed in the axilla and along the sternal border. For the skin-sparing method, a purse-string suture is not recommended because it may compromise mammary skin perfusion (Fig. 142-13). The flap skin island can be varied in size to ensure a tension-free closure. If there is excess mammary skin,

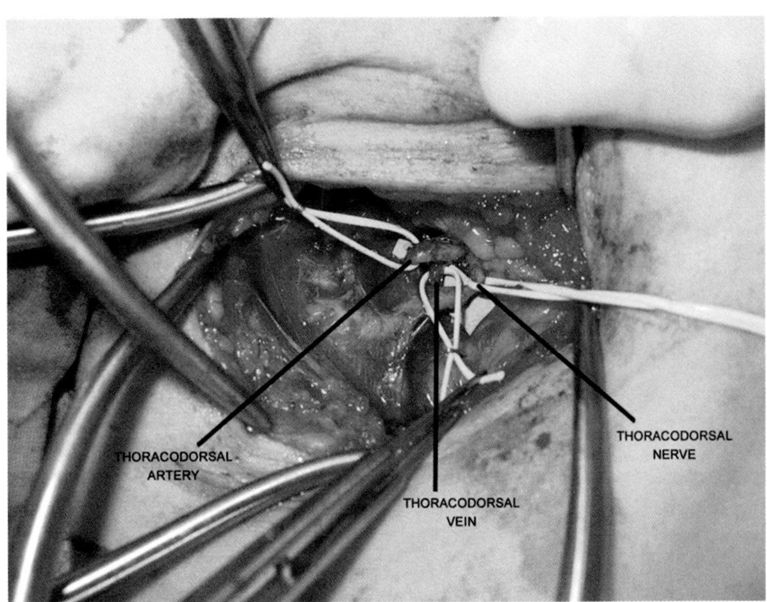

FIGURE 142-9. Axillary dissection to identify the thoracodorsal artery (left, superior), vein (center), and nerve (right).

it can be excised by de-epithelialization of a vertical wedge of mammary skin in the inferior pole that is similar to a mastopexy. The skin should not be completely transected, to preserve dermal plexus circulation. Approximation of the edges will simulate the vertical limb of a reduction or mastopexy while increasing projection. If a contralateral reduction or mastopexy is needed, this maneuver helps establish symmetry (Fig. 142-14).

Abdominal Wall Repair and Closure

The abdominal wall defect is repaired by first reapproximating the lowest portion of the defect, where the fascial incision extends below the caudal border of the flap; 2-0 Prolene sutures are used to close this defect in a pants-over-vest manner. Next, the entire defect is repaired with a running, double-stranded, 0 nylon suture. The repair commences at the costal margin and is run toward the pubis. Care is taken to incorporate both internal and external oblique layers in the closure. Failure to reapproximate the internal oblique layer is one of the causes of subsequent hernias and weakness.[4,18]

In unilateral procedures, the contralateral side is plicated in a similar manner. The sutures are placed at the junction of the external oblique muscle and the rectus fascia. This helps equalize tension on the abdominal wall and moves the umbilicus back toward the midline. A midline plication from the xiphoid process to the umbilicus is usually helpful to further equalize tension and to prevent epigastric bulges. Closure in bilateral procedures is similar to that in unilateral procedures. If the fascia cannot be approximated without undue tension, onlay, synthetic mesh reinforcement should be used. By employment of this muscle-sparing method, the use of synthetic mesh has dramatically decreased.[4]

With the patient in the sitting position, the wound is temporarily closed with staples. The position of the neoumbilicus is marked by palpation of its position through the abdominal skin. Closed suction drains are placed through separate incisions, and the wound is closed in layers. The neoumbilicus is formed by excision of a curvilinear ellipse of skin and sharp removal of a full-thickness "core" of fat until the umbilical stalk is exposed. The umbilical skin is sutured to the abdominal skin with interrupted, half-buried, 4-0 nylon

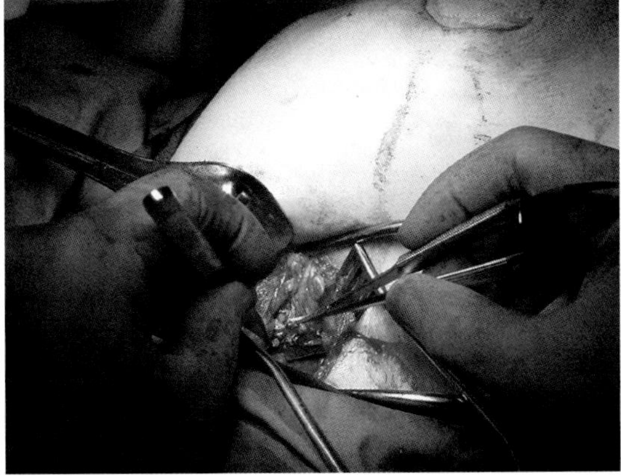

FIGURE 142-10. Anastomosis through axillary approach. Exposure is provided with a Deaver retractor, which is anchored to the foam padding over the patient's head, and two Adson-Beckman retractors.

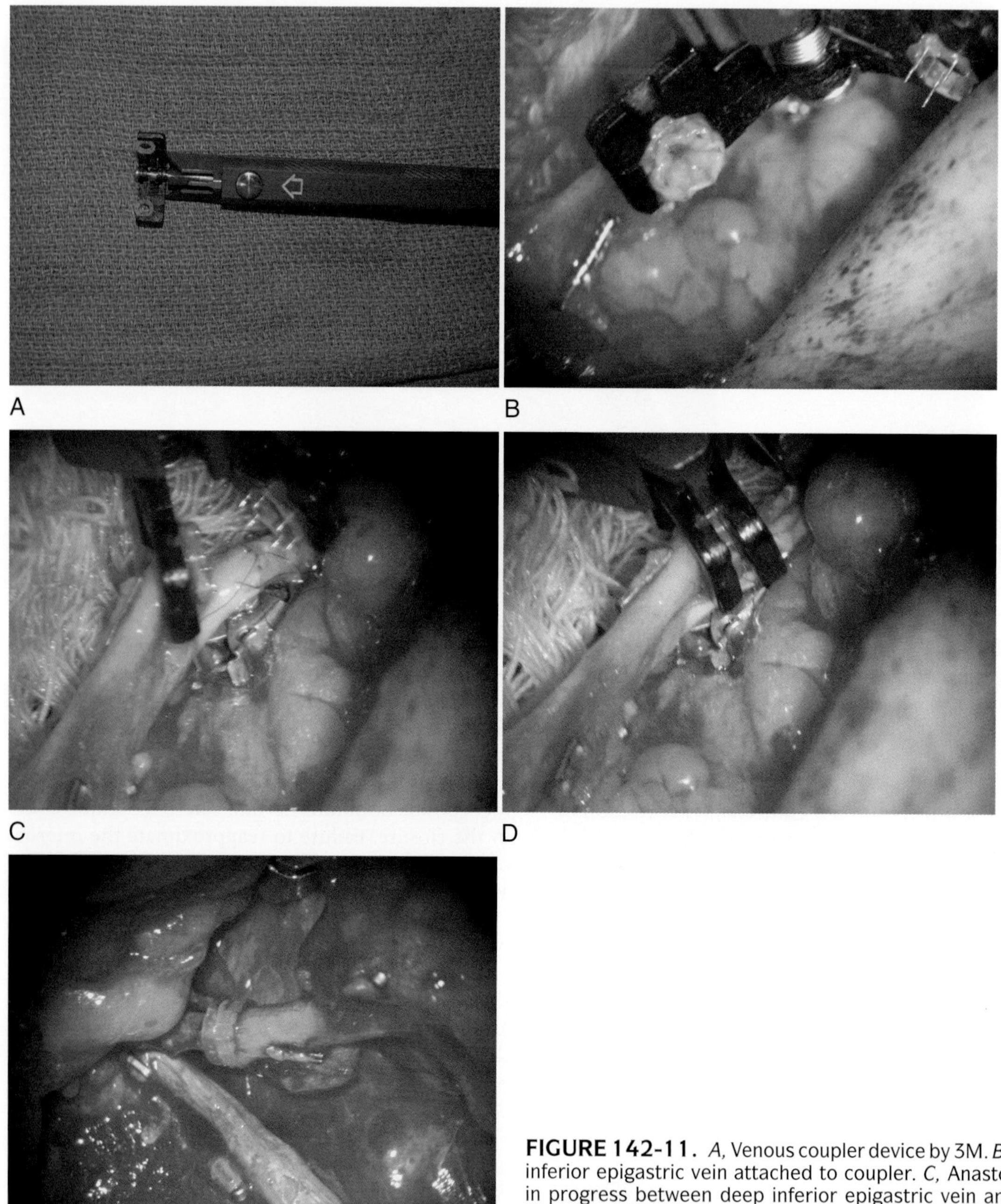

FIGURE 142-11. *A,* Venous coupler device by 3M. *B,* Deep inferior epigastric vein attached to coupler. *C,* Anastomosis in progress between deep inferior epigastric vein and thoracodorsal vein. Note completed arterial anastomosis in background. *D,* Venous anastomosis is almost complete. *E,* Completed venous anastomosis.

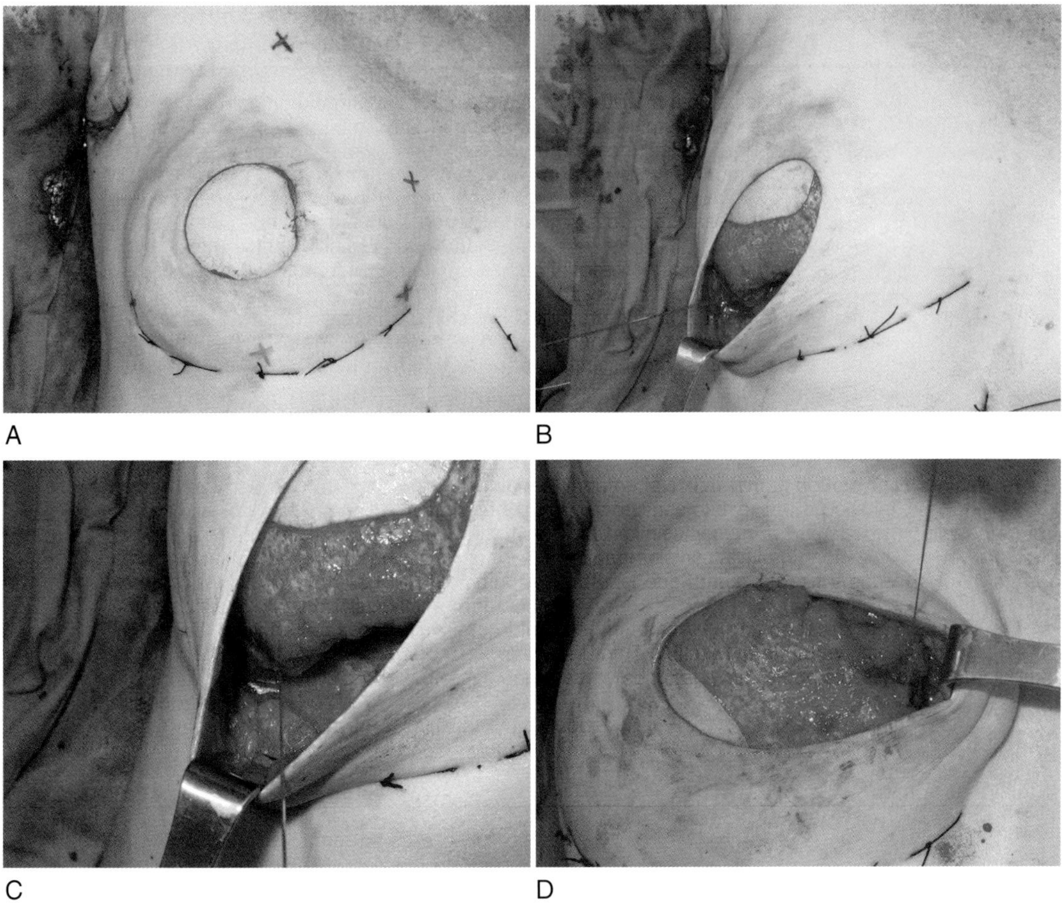

A B

C D

FIGURE 142-12. *A,* Sites of fixation for the inset of the TRAM flap onto the chest wall. *B,* The first and most important step for flap inset is suturing of the rectus segment to the pectoralis to prevent inadvertent traction injury to the pedicle. *C,* The triangular hemiflap (in bilateral reconstruction) must be sutured into a projecting shape. This is accomplished by "gathering" the flap from lateral to medial. *D,* Fixation of the dermis to the chest wall.

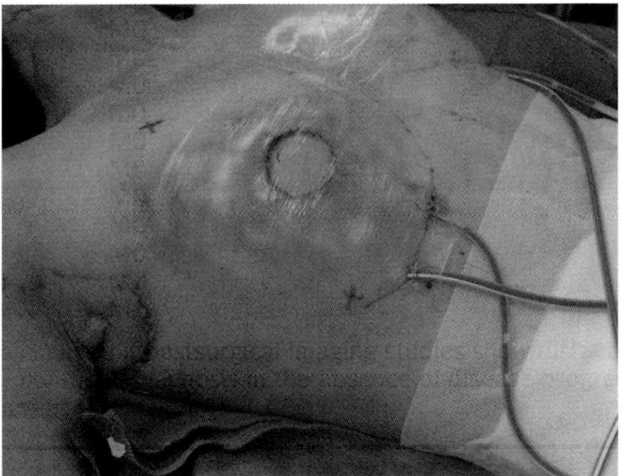

FIGURE 142-13. Postoperative dressing demonstrates placement of two drains in each breast. The lateral drain is for the axilla; the medial drain is for the sternal border. Venous blood in the medial drain could be an early sign of a venous outflow problem.

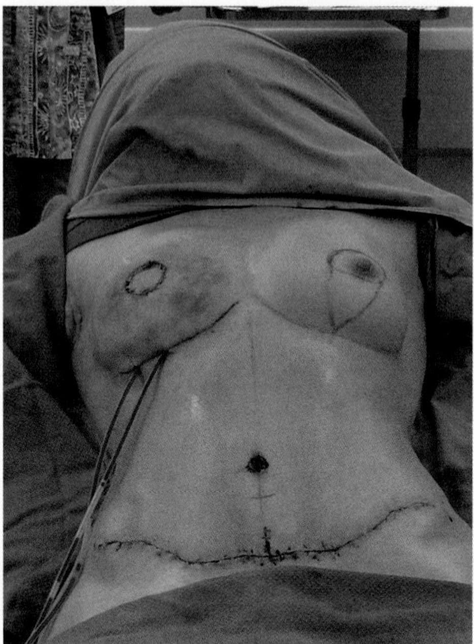

FIGURE 142-14. The completed reconstruction. The mammary skin was cyanotic with capillary refill approaching 2 seconds. This improved in the immediate postoperative period, and no skin loss occurred. The left breast was marked for a mastopexy; however, because the flap's shape and volume were close to those of the left breast, it was decided to forgo the mastopexy. If necessary, it can be performed at the second stage.

mattress sutures. The abdominal closure can be completed as the microsurgical portion is being performed. The patient can be flexed at the waist and placed in the Trendelenburg position, which facilitates both abdominal wall closure and anastomosis.[4,5,8]

A large sheet of clear, adhesive dressing (Tegaderm) is placed on the reconstructed breast. Gauze dressings are placed over the abdominal wound.

Postoperative Care and Flap Monitoring

The patient is transferred to the recovery room, where monitoring commences. Classic clinical signs, a conventional Doppler probe, and a transcutaneous laser Doppler probe are used to monitor and assess flap perfusion. The small flap skin island provides an adequate surface for assessment of flap perfusion. The laser probe is placed on the cutaneous portion of the flap, and the alarm is set at 50% of the initial, stabilized baseline value. The patients may recuperate on a regular surgical floor rather than using an intensive care bed. Nurses are trained to monitor the flaps and perform hourly assessments. Strong indications of venous congestion or arterial insufficiency warrant urgent re-exploration to salvage a potentially failing flap.[26,27] Waiting or employing other diagnostic measures prolongs ischemic time and allows further thrombosis or irreversible reperfusion injury to progress. The vessels are explored, and any necessary revisions in the anastomosis are made. The patient is always made aware of this potential complication during the informed consent process.

A written protocol for the postoperative course has been established to ensure consistency in care of patients (Fig. 142-15). The room is kept above 75°F. Patients sit in a chair on the first postoperative day and ambulate by the third day. They are discharged on the fourth or fifth postoperative day and are seen in the office at weekly intervals for the first month. One baby aspirin and a caffeine-free diet are prescribed for 2 months. The patient should be carefully instructed not to abduct the arm of the reconstructed breast above the level of the shoulder for 10 days. This minimizes the potential for avulsion of the anastomosis.[27] Beginning at 10 days, the patient performs "creep up the wall" exercises several times daily, with her fingertips to the side and forward with the elbow straight.

Secondary or Revisional Surgery

The second stage usually consists of additional shaping of the flap and a nipple reconstruction. This is performed 3 to 6 months after the initial reconstruction. If a patient is to undergo adjuvant chemotherapy, this stage is delayed until the treatments are completed and the patient's blood cell counts normalize. Because the mammary skin envelope is preserved in immediate reconstruction with the periareolar approach, there is seldom a need to excise flap skin to attain symmetry with the contralateral breast. The difference is usually volumetric. A delayed reconstruction may require skin excision. Conventional suction-assisted lipectomy is usually all that is required to recontour and diminish flap bulk. When larger amounts of fat need to be excised, the native mammary skin flaps may have to be elevated with performance of tangential excision.[21,27] If there is any significant fat necrosis, it is excised at this time. The resulting defect may need secondary reconstruction with an implant or an additional flap. The latissimus flap is an available option, *provided that the serratus branch was preserved at the initial surgery.*

At the time of secondary revisions, the nipple is reconstructed, preferably with a modified fishtail flap (Fig. 142-16).[27] The fishtail flap is usually raised from the TRAM flap skin island, but the mammary skin may also serve as donor tissue. If a significant alteration of the flap is required, it may be prudent to delay nipple reconstruction to avoid malposition of the nipple. Areolar tattooing completes the entire reconstructive

PHY0260

SURG #74 - STANDING ORDERS -
POST-OP ORDERS FOR FREE TRAM FLAP
BREAST RECONSTRUCTION
DR. JAMES GROTTING
EFFECTIVE 1/97
PAGE 1 OF 2

DATE:

1. Recovery Room to floor s/p free TRAM Flap breast reconstruction.
2. Patient stable, vital signs q 4 hours, I&O q shift.
3. Flap checks q 1 hour x 24 hours, q 2 hours x 48 hours, then q 4 hours for color, turgor, warmth, capillary refill, A and V doppler signals*, record laser doppler flow value*.
4. Activity: bedrest in modified Fowler position, OOB to chair in a.m., adjust bed to patient comfort on day 2.
5. Room comfortable, 72 - 75 degrees, warm blanket over reconstructed breasts.
6. Diet: Ice chips only for first night, clear liquids post-op day 1, may advance to caffeine-free regular diet starting post-op day 3.
7. IVF: D51/4NS + 20meq KCL at 125cc per hour.
8. Meds:
   Ancef 1 gram IV q 8 hours.
   PCA per anesthesia pain service.
   Tylenol 650mg po q 6 hours prn for temperature $\geq$ 101.5 or pain.
   Toradol 10mg IV q 6 hours.
   Benadryl 25mg po q 6 hours prn itching.
   Restoril 15 - 30 mg HS prn insomnia.
   ECASA 325mg po QD beginning post-op day 3.
   Phenergan 25mg I.M. q 4 - 6 hours prn nausea and vomiting, if no relief Zofran 4 mg IV q 6 hours prn.
9. Full length SCD hose x 72 hours.
10. Labs: HCT in Recovery Room.
    HCT in a.m.
11. J-P drains to bulb suction, empty and record q shift - record 24 hours totals for each drain.
12. Notify MD or SA for unstable vitals, change in flap appearance, UOP less than 200cc / 8 hours, excessive J-P output.

CONTINUED

A

FIGURE 142-15. *A* and *B*, Routine postoperative orders for free TRAM flap patients. *Continued*

PHY0260
SURG #74 - STANDING ORDERS -
POST-OP ORDERS FOR FREE TRAM FLAP
BREAST RECONSTRUCTION
DR. JAMES GROTTING
EFFECTIVE 1/97
PAGE 2 OF 2

DATE:

13. O2 - 2 liters per nasal cannula x 48 hours.

14. Laser doppler setup at bedside (SA will set alarms)*.

15. Patient may shower post-op day 4.

* Omit for conventional TRAM flap.

ALL FURTHER ORDERS TO BE WRITTEN ON STANDARD PHYSICIAN'S ORDER SHEET.

St. Vincent's Hospital ~ Birmingham, Alabama

B

FIGURE 142-15, cont'd.

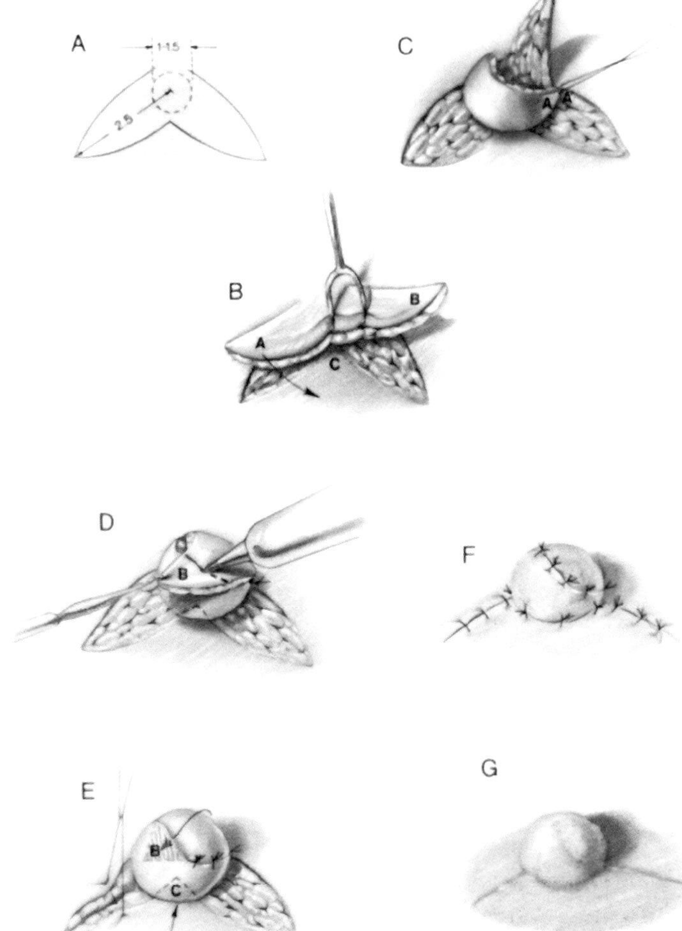

FIGURE 142-16. *A* to *G*, Modified fishtail flap nipple reconstruction. (From Grotting JC: Reoperation following free flap breast reconstruction. In Grotting JC: Reoperative Aesthetic and Reconstructive Plastic Surgery. St. Louis, Quality Medical Publishing, 1995:1093.)

process 6 to 8 weeks after the nipple is reconstructed (Figs. 142-17 to 142-22).

The abdomen might benefit from revision surgery, especially in contour. An epigastric fullness often persists as a result of the repositioning of the adipose tissue. Lateral dog-ears may be present in the lower abdomen after flap harvest. Suction-assisted lipectomy readily recontours these areas and can be performed during the second stage.

COMPLICATIONS

Complications can be categorized into early and delayed events. Hematoma, seroma, infection, anastomotic failure, flap loss, and skin necrosis are usually manifested in the early postoperative period. Deep venous thrombosis and pulmonary embolism are other early complications. Fat necrosis, abdominal wall weakness, and hernias are more common complications arising later in the postoperative course.

In the authors' series of 355 free TRAM flaps, the incidence of complete flap loss was 0.8%, with a 1.6% incidence of partial flap loss, necessitating débridement and additional reconstruction.[8] Depending on the magnitude of the partial flap loss, reconstruction can be performed with implants or other flaps. The latissimus flap is an excellent option, but if there is doubt about the pedicle's integrity, other free flaps may have to be used. The Rubens and gluteal flaps are good alternatives.

Significant fat necrosis requiring excision occurred in 1.9%, and minor fat necrosis was noted in 4.5% of flaps, which were untreated.[8] Fat necrosis is manifested as focal areas of hard tissue, distinct from the adipose tissue. It has distinct characteristics on a mammogram that make it distinguishable from tumor recurrences. If there is ever doubt, these areas should be examined by biopsy or excised. Smaller foci, if they are not suspicious, can be observed.

Text continued on p. 872

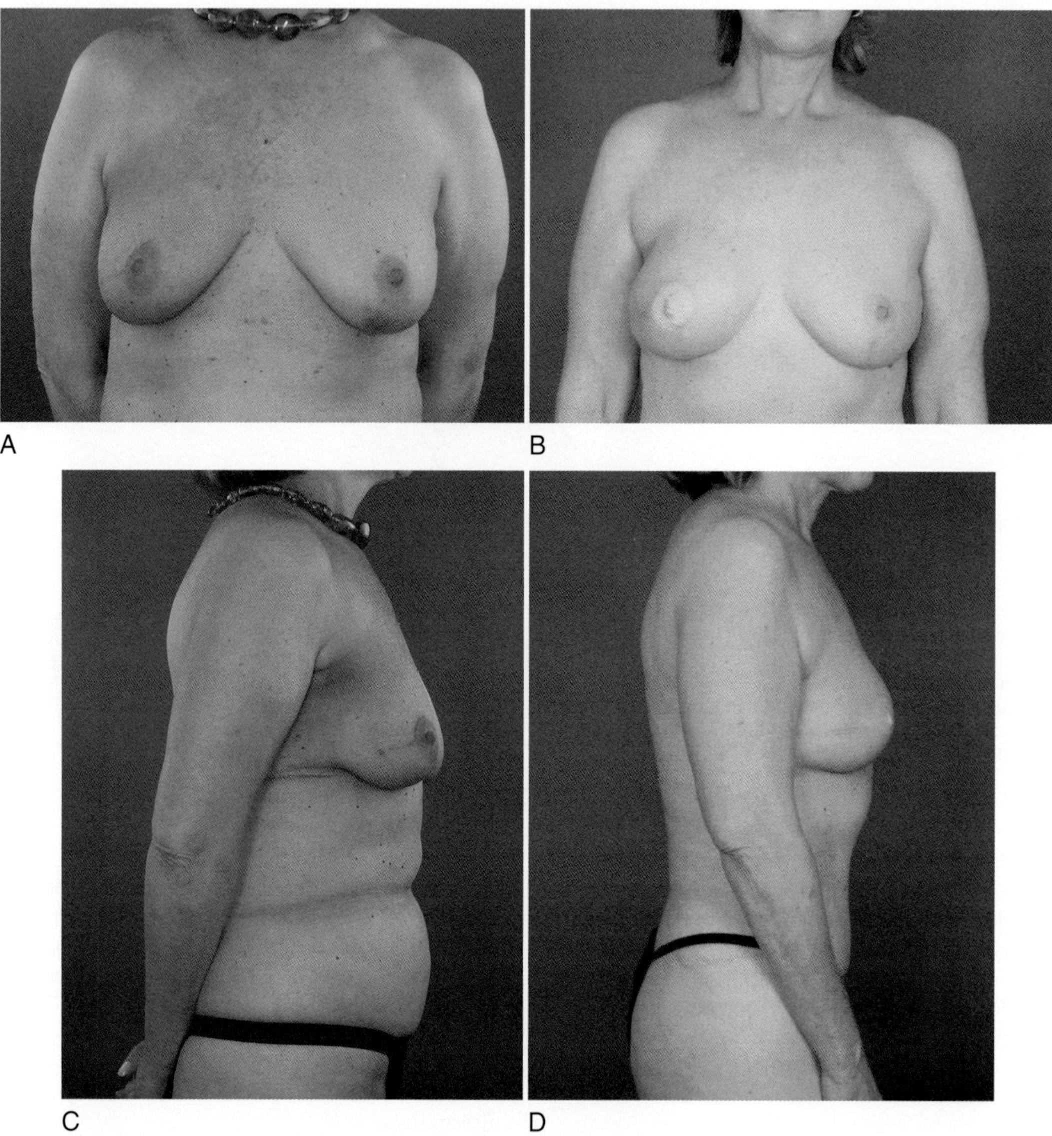

FIGURE 142-17. Unilateral immediate breast reconstruction in a 56-year-old white woman. Preoperative radiation therapy was followed by modified radical mastectomy with immediate breast reconstruction by the right free TRAM flap and mastopexy of the left breast. *A* and *C,* Preoperative views. *B* and *D,* Postoperative views.

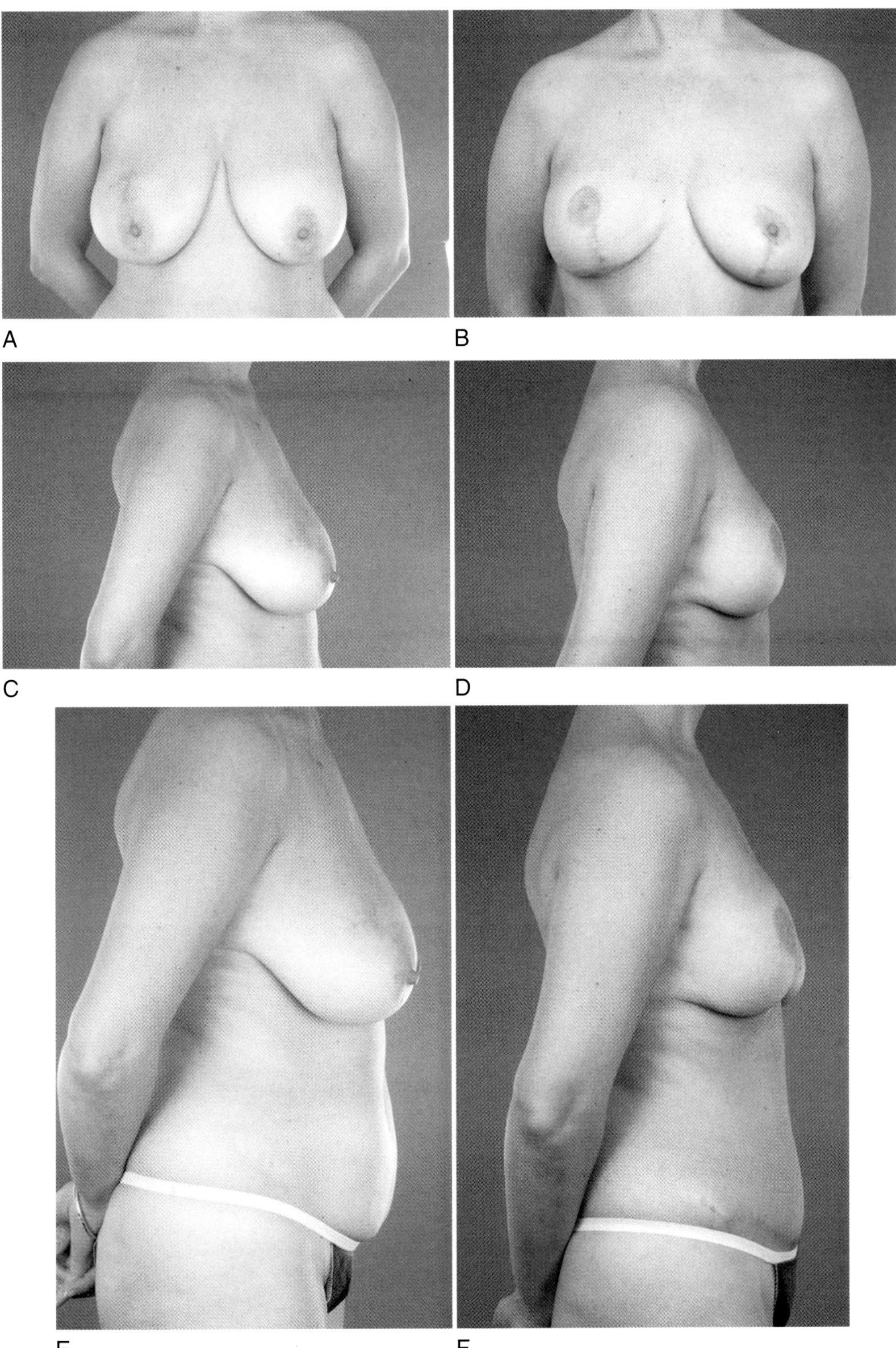

FIGURE 142-18. Unilateral immediate breast reconstruction in a 44-year-old white woman after right mastectomy. Immediate reconstruction was performed by the right free TRAM flap with a left breast reduction. *A, C,* and *E,* Preoperative views. *B, D,* and *F,* Postoperative views at 1 year.

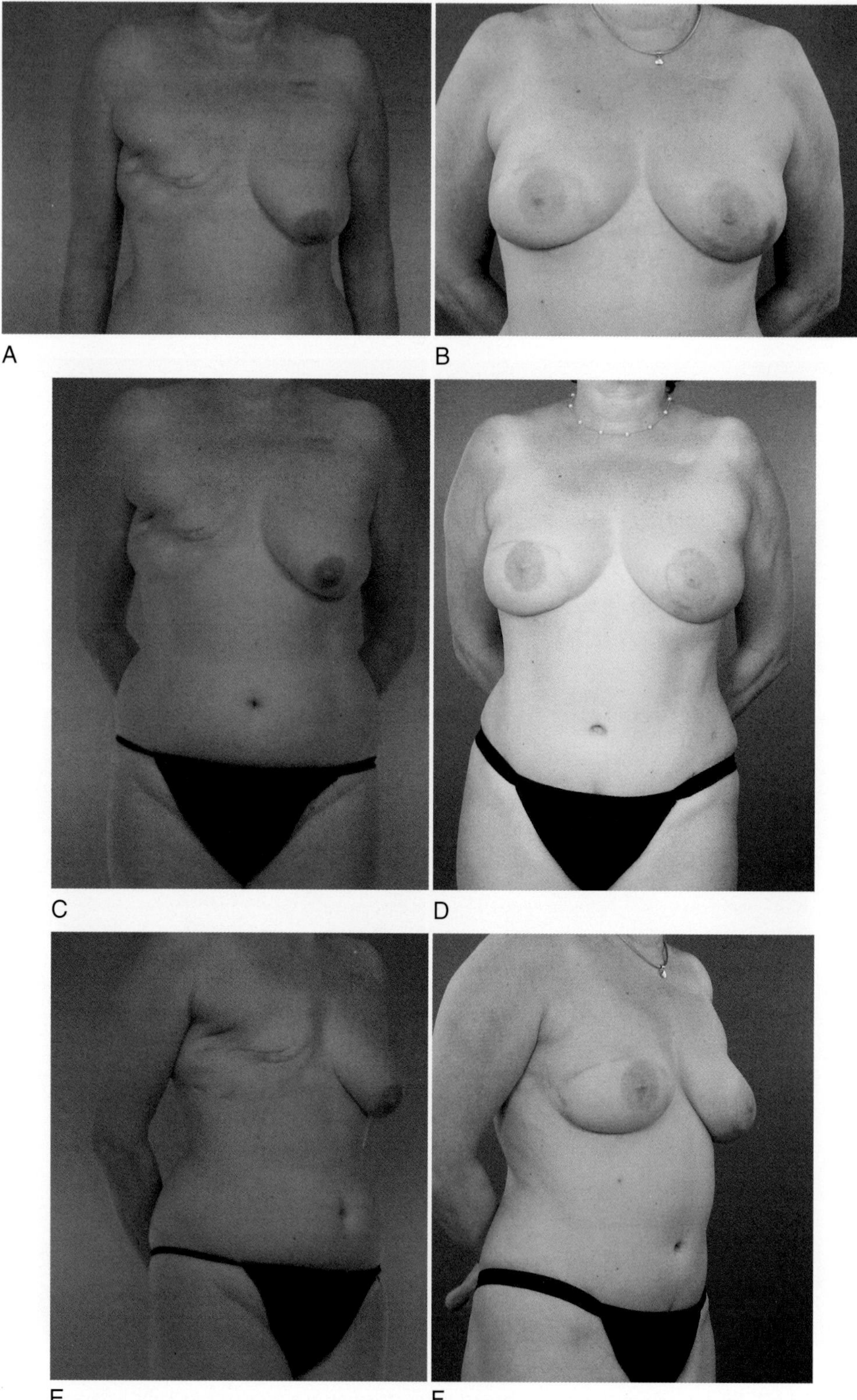

FIGURE 142-19. Unilateral delayed reconstruction in a 50-year-old white woman after right modified mastectomy and postoperative chemotherapy. Reconstruction was performed 9 months later by the right free TRAM flap and a left mastopexy. *A, C,* and *E,* Preoperative views. *B, D,* and *F,* Postoperative views at 18 months.

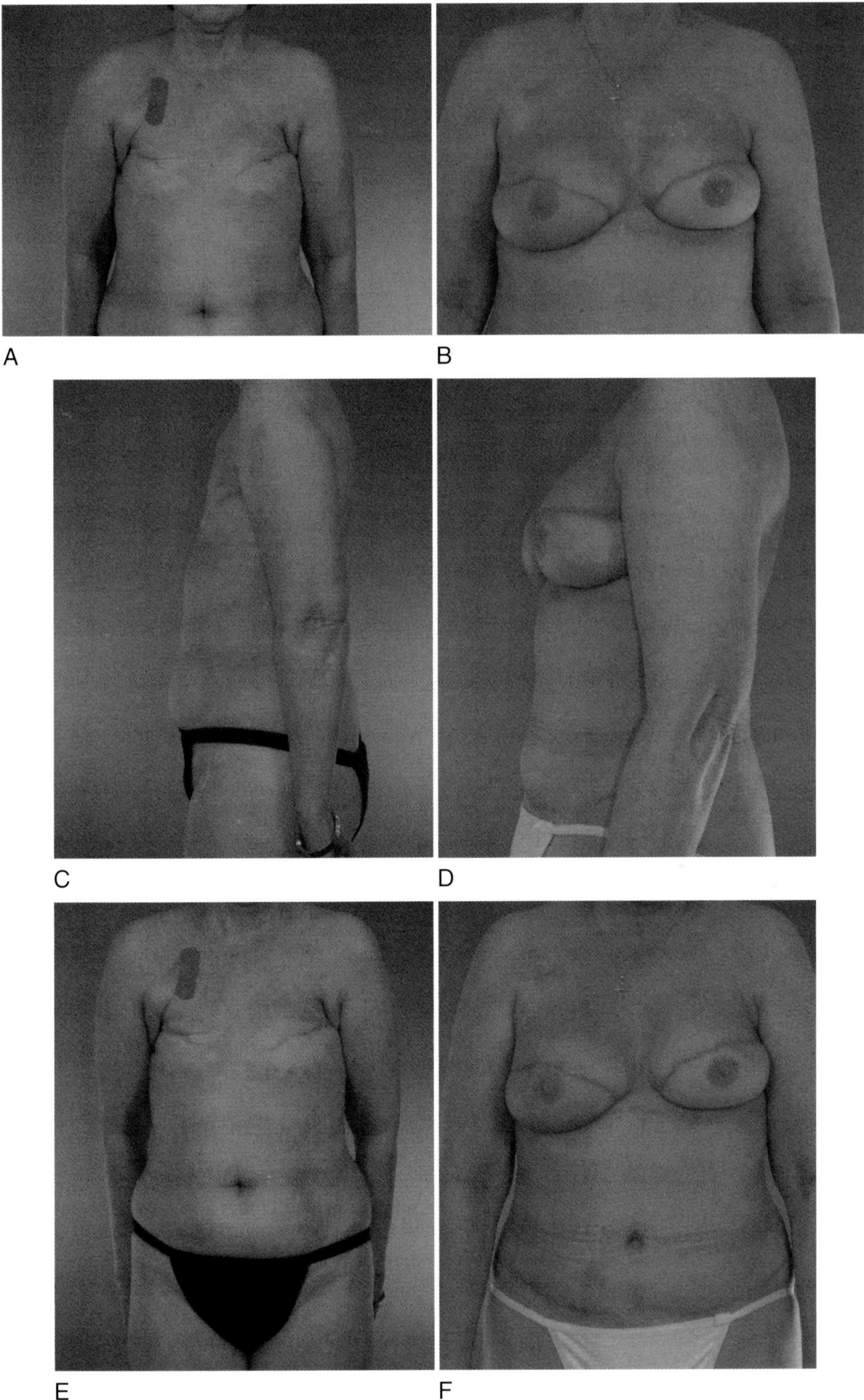

FIGURE 142-20. Bilateral delayed reconstruction in a 58-year-old white woman after right simple mastectomy and left modified radical mastectomy, chemotherapy, and radiation therapy. One year later, she underwent bilateral free TRAM flap reconstruction. *A, C,* and *E,* Preoperative views. *B, D,* and *F,* Postoperative views at 6 months.

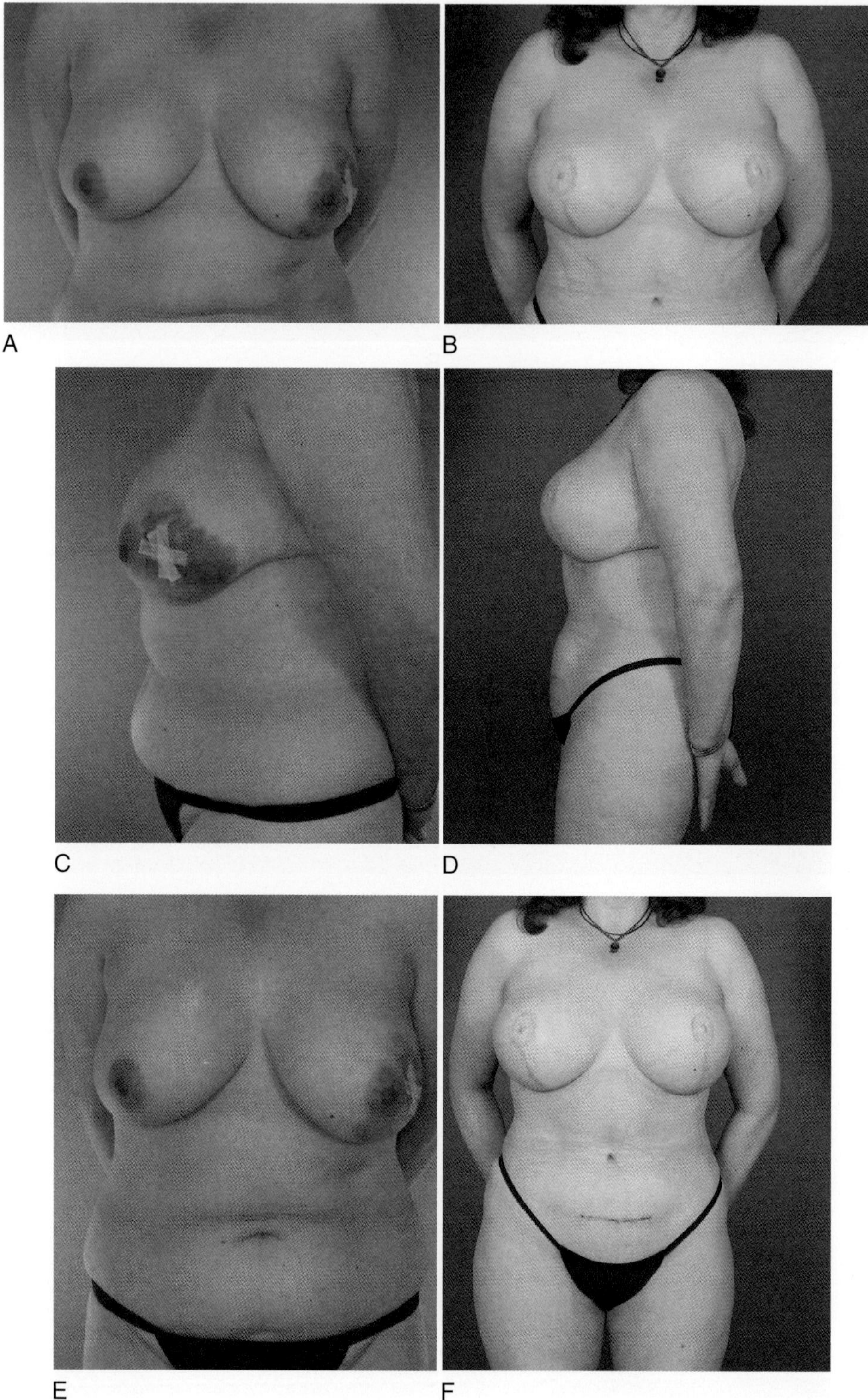

FIGURE 142-21. Bilateral immediate reconstruction in a 52-year-old white woman with augmentation by silicone implants. She underwent bilateral mastectomies for breast cancer and immediate reconstruction with bilateral free TRAM flaps. *A, C,* and *E,* Preoperative views. *B, D,* and *F,* Postoperative views at $2^{1}/_{2}$ years.

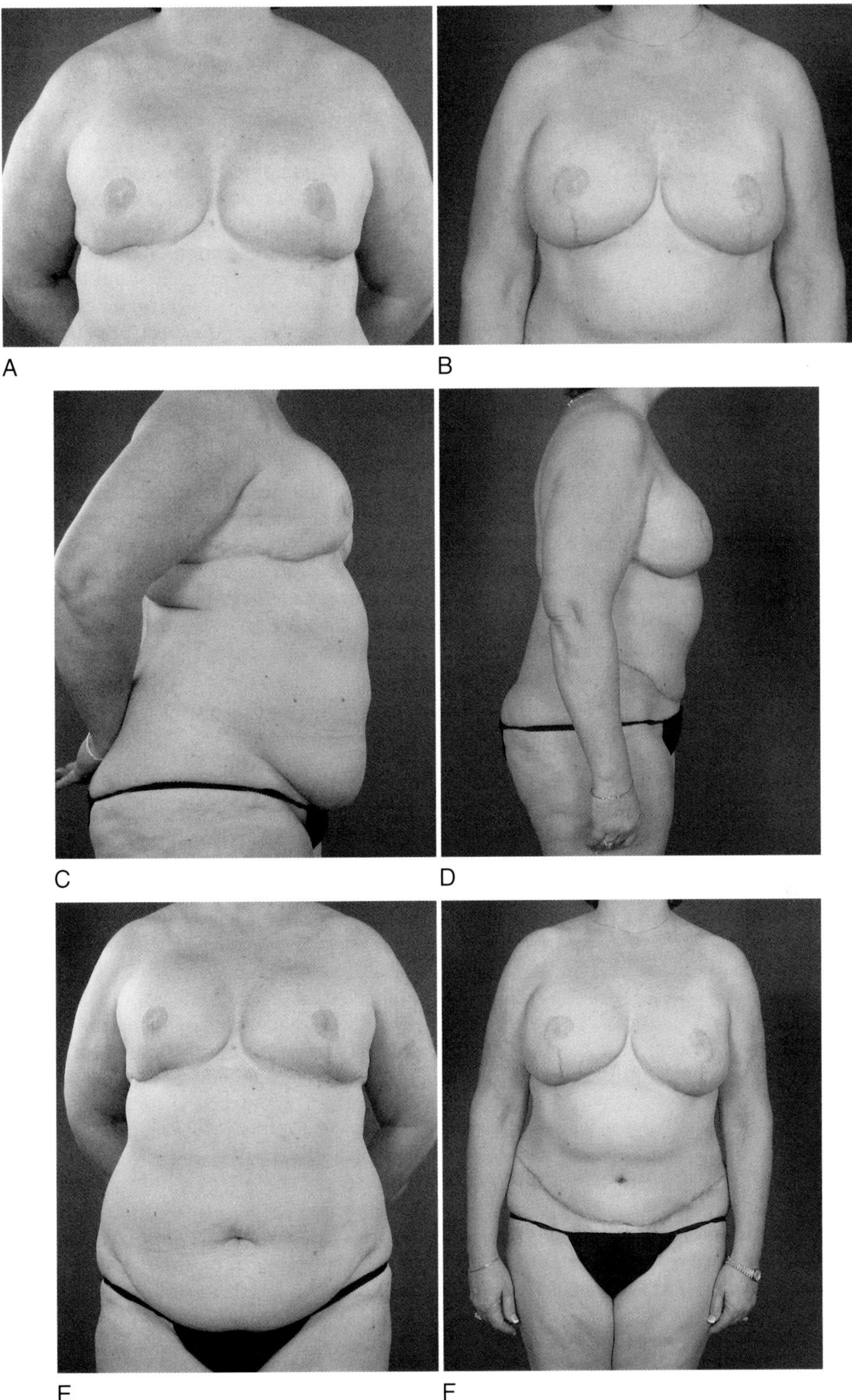

FIGURE 142-22. Salvage of implant reconstruction. A 48-year-old white woman presented with painful breasts from capsular contracture after bilateral subcutaneous mastectomies and immediate reconstruction with expanders and implants for severe fibrocystic disease. She underwent explantation of the implants with bilateral free TRAM flap reconstruction. *A, C,* and *E,* Preoperative views. *B, D,* and *F,* Postoperative views at 3 months.

Arterial thrombosis occurred in 0.84% of flaps, and venous thrombosis manifested in 3.1%. The overall re-exploration rate, in the authors' series, was 4.8%.[8] This is comparable to other series.[3] All but two of the flaps were explored within 48 hours from the initial reconstruction, and all were salvaged. If arterial or venous compromise is suspected, re-exploration is mandatory because any delay diminishes the chance of successful flap salvage. Among all free flaps, re-exploration within 6 hours of transplantation has an 84% salvage rate, whereas this rate diminishes to 58% when re-exploration is performed between 6 and 24 hours.[26]

A total of 9 hematomas developed in the 355 flaps, 7 in the TRAM flaps and 2 in the abdominal wound.[8] Hematomas, especially in TRAM flaps, should be evacuated because they can compromise the anastomosis. There were five instances of seromas requiring drainage in the authors' series.[8] It is preferable to aspirate the fluid initially and use a compression garment. If the fluid reaccumulates, a drain is placed in a dependent region. An old drain site can drain the lower abdomen, and access through the umbilicus can drain the epigastric area.

Infection is rare and is often just a cellulitis that is readily treated with antibiotics. Purulent infections require drainage, débridement, dressing changes, and culture-specific antibiotic regimen. Skin necrosis, if it is minor, can be managed conservatively, allowing the eschar to separate and the wound to heal by secondary intention. More extensive skin necrosis may warrant débridement and possible coverage with skin grafting or flap advancement. Large wounds can also be allowed to heal secondarily. Later revisions may be necessary. In the authors' series, the overall incidence of skin necrosis was 4.2%, 2.8% mammary skin loss and 1.4% abdominal skin loss.[8] Umbilical slough can often be treated conservatively with débridement and dressing changes. An acceptable neoumbilicus usually results; however, if an unacceptable result is obtained, an umbilicus can be established with local flaps.[27]

Deep venous thrombosis and pulmonary embolism are serious complications that must be diagnosed and treated early. It is recommended that 5000 units of heparin be injected subcutaneously on call to the operating room as well as sequential compression devices that are worn until the third day after surgery. Intravenous heparin is frequently administered during the microsurgical portion to diminish platelet aggregation in the recipient vessels. Aspirin and ketorolac are used postoperatively, which might help further propagation of any existing thrombi. Despite adequate prophylaxis, a deep venous thrombosis can still develop. Any signs of calf tenderness, swelling, Homans sign, or discomfort should raise suspicion, and noninvasive studies are ordered. If deep venous thrombosis is diagnosed, anticoagulation is commenced. Dyspnea, pleuritic chest pain, fever, and tachycardia can be signs of pulmonary embolism. Again, if there is a suspicion, a ventilation-perfusion scan should be obtained with treatment rendered urgently. One patient in the authors' series died of a saddle embolus despite emergency pulmonary thrombectomy.[8]

Hernias are manifested later in the postoperative course, and presentation varies from frank bulges to symptoms of vague abdominal discomfort. Patients with pain in the abdomen should be carefully examined for areas of weakness of hernias. Having the patient strain, flex at the waist, or perform sit-ups can aid in the diagnosis. Areas of asymptomatic weakness can be managed expectantly, but hernias should be repaired. Herniorrhaphy requires opening of the donor site incision and elevation of the skin flap to expose the hernia. Repair might entail dissection to the costal margins. The sac should be excised, fascial edges identified, and primary closure attempted. If a secure closure is not feasible, reinforcement with synthetic mesh should be employed with either an inlay or an onlay method. The hernia rate in the authors' series was 4.8% (n = 17); 2.8% of patients (n = 10) required herniorraphy.[8]

THE FUTURE

Breast reconstruction with the free TRAM flap has evolved to where an aesthetically pleasing breast can be consistently formed. However, there are some details that would refine this method and elevate the level of attainable results. A varying degree of sensation returns to the new breast a year or more after reconstruction. If better sensory function can be incorporated into the breast, it would be noted as a significant improvement. Despite the increased ability to shape the free TRAM flap, compared with the pedicled TRAM flap, sufficient projection often remains elusive. An innovative method or perhaps a new flap that increases projection would dramatically enhance the level of results currently obtainable. Another aspect that requires improvement is areolar projection and sensation. The development of a sensate flap providing sensation to this region has been proposed, but the associated morbidity may not justify the result.[28] There is always room for improvement, and it should be encouraged rather than merely accepting the status quo.

REFERENCES

1. Friedman RJ, Argenta LC, Anderson R: Deep inferior epigastric free flap for breast reconstruction after radical mastectomy. Plast Reconstr Surg 1985;76:455.
2. Feller AM, Biemer E, Steinau HU: The free TRAM flap. In Strauch B, Vasconez L, Hall-Findlay EJ, eds: Grabb's Encyclopedia of Flaps. Boston, Little, Brown, 1990:1326.

3. Grotting JC, Urist M, Maddox WA, Vasconez LO: Conventional TRAM flap versus free microsurgical TRAM flap for immediate breast reconstruction. Plast Reconstr Surg 1989;83:828.
4. Grotting JC, Beckenstein MS, Arkoulakis NS: The art and science of autologous breast reconstruction. Breast J 2003;9:350.
5. Grotting JC: The free abdominoplasty flap for immediate breast reconstruction. Ann Plast Surg 1991;27:351.
6. Kroll SS, Schusterman MA, Reece GP, et al: Abdominal wall strength, bulging and hernia after TRAM flap breast reconstruction. Plast Reconstr Surg 1995;96:616.
7. Elliott LF: Free TRAM flap. Operative Techniques Plast Reconstr Surg 1994;1:39.
8. Beckenstein M, Grotting JC: Breast reconstruction with free tissue transfer. Plast Reconstr Surg 2001;108:1345.
9. Baldwin BJ, Schusterman MA, Miller M, et al: Bilateral breast reconstruction: conventional versus free TRAM. Plast Reconstr Surg 1994;93:1410.
10. Grotting JC: Immediate breast reconstruction using the free TRAM flap. Clin Plast Surg 1994;21:2.
11. Grotting JC: Breast reconstruction with free tissue transfer. In Cohen M: Mastery of Plastic and Reconstructive Surgery, vol 2. Boston, Little, Brown, 1994:1304.
12. Schusterman MA: The free TRAM flap. Clin Plast Surg 1998;2:191.
13. Feller AM: Free TRAM. Clin Plast Surg 1994;21:223.
14. Arnez ZM, Bajec J, Barsdley AF, et al: Experience with 50 free TRAM flap breast reconstructions. Plast Reconstr Surg 1991;87:470.
15. Allen RJ, Treece P: Deep inferior epigastric perforator flap for breast reconstruction. Ann Plast Surg 1994;32:32.
16. Allen RJ: Perforator flaps in breast reconstruction. In Spear SL, ed: Surgery of the Breast: Principles and Art. Philadelphia, Lippincott-Raven, 1998.
17. Nahabedian MY, Tsangaris T, Momen B: Breast reconstruction with the DIEP flap or the muscle-sparing (MS-2) free TRAM flap: is there a difference? Plast Reconstr Surg 2005;115(2):436.
18. Hartrampf CR, Bennett GK: Autogenous tissue reconstruction in the mastectomy patient: a critical review of 300 patients. Ann Surg 1987;205:508.
19. Kroll SS, Evans GR, Reece GP, et al: Comparison of resource costs of free and conventional TRAM flap breast reconstruction. Plast Reconstr Surg 1996;98:74.
20. Hartrampf CR, Black PB, Scheflan M: Breast reconstruction with a transverse rectus abdominal island flap. Plast Reconstr Surg 1982;69:216.
21. Bostwick J III: Finishing touches after breast reconstruction with pedicled flaps. In Grotting JC: Reoperative Aesthetic and Reconstructive Plastic Surgery. St. Louis, Quality Medical Publishing, 1995:1053.
22. Laritieri AL, Mitranoff M, Rimareix F, et al: Use of circumflex scapular vessels as a recipient pedicle for autologous breast reconstruction: a report of 40 consecutive cases. Plast Reconstr Surg 1999;104:2049.
23. Kroll SS, Baldwin B: A comparison of outcomes using three different methods of breast reconstruction. Plast Reconstr Surg 1993;75:455.
24. Dupin CL, Allen RJ, Glass CA, et al: The internal mammary artery and vein as a recipient site for free flap breast reconstruction: a report of 110 consecutive cases. Plast Reconstr Surg 1996;98:685.
25. Bared R, Kept EM, Toss Neo F: Abdominoplasty. Plast Reconstr Surg 1974;54:161.
26. Olivia A, Bunke HJ: Failed and failing free flaps. In Grotting JC: Reoperative Aesthetic and Reconstructive Plastic Surgery. St. Louis, Quality Medical Publishing, 1995:155.
27. Grotting JC: Reoperation following free flap breast reconstruction. In Grotting JC: Reoperative Aesthetic and Reconstructive Plastic Surgery. St. Louis, Quality Medical Publishing, 1995:1093.
28. Hartrampf CR: Reconstruction of a sensate nipple-areolar complex with a costal neuromuscular island flap. Unpublished data.

CHAPTER

143

Postmastectomy Reconstruction: Expander-Implant Techniques

STEPHEN J. MATHES, MD ✦ MARGA MASSEY, MD

Factors including type of mastectomy, timing of reconstruction, tissue expansion, and implant design have made expander-implant techniques an important method for breast reconstruction. Tissue expansion was first reported by Neumann[1] in 1957 for coverage of a subauricular defect. Although Neumann's report appeared in *Plastic and Reconstructive Surgery* and demonstrated the feasibility of the procedure, major interest in tissue expansion did not occur for another 20 years. Working independently, Radovan[2] and Austad[3] developed silicone tissue expanders and published their findings in 1982. Radovan[2] performed his first tissue expansion in 1976. Austad[3] developed a self-inflating silicone prosthesis and investigated the histologic effects of tissue expansion. Subsequent to this early work, tissue expansion has been investigated thoroughly and gained widespread acceptance on the basis of its proven safety and efficacy.

The silicone implant was initially incorporated into breast reconstruction as a device to provide a safe and stable breast mound. At the time of its inception, the radical mastectomy and modified radical mastectomy were routinely used to extirpate breast cancer. The implant could rarely be used under the preserved skin envelope because of existing scar tissue and inadequate and often unstable skin coverage at the mastectomy site. Therefore, the implant was used in conjunction with a flap for coverage. With the evolution of mastectomy techniques and diagnosis of breast cancer at an earlier stage, more conservative approaches to mastectomy, including skin-preserving and skin-sparing mastectomy, have been used. As skin envelope preservation became possible, the use of an implant without a flap was a safe option for breast reconstruction.

With increasing recognition of the value of immediate reconstruction for the mastectomy patient, the option of expander-implant became more practical for incorporation into techniques for reconstruction. With the development of the concept of tissue expansion, a deflated implant can be inserted beneath the mastectomy skin that will not adversely affect mastectomy skin survival. The expander can subsequently undergo inflation both to stretch the dimensions of the retained skin envelope and to avoid wound contraction during the process of wound maturation after the mastectomy. With improvement in the design of tissue expanders, the port is now incorporated into the surface of the implant, eliminating the dissection distant to the mastectomy site to place the valve for later expander inflation. With the use of a textured expander, the expander will not migrate away from the area of greatest skin tightness (usually the inferior half of the preserved breast skin envelope) and will maintain a well-defined inframammary line despite the mastectomy dissection. These innovations have made the expander-implant for breast reconstruction a reliable technique to restore form at the site of mastectomy.

The process of reconstruction with use of an expander-implant is generally a two-stage procedure. The first stage is insertion of the expander either at the time of mastectomy or delayed until the patient is referred or presents for reconstruction. If the first stage is not performed at the time of the mastectomy, it is preferable to delay reconstruction a minimum of 3 months and until adjuvant treatments are completed. Two factors may allow this technique to be used in a single-stage procedure for immediate reconstruction:

1. Development of implants with a distant removable port. The implant may be inflated, and when inflation is completed, the port and tubing may be removed through a small incision at the port site. The port is designed for removal without loss of saline within the inflated implant.
2. With total skin-sparing techniques now available for select patients with early-stage breast cancer, it is possible to insert the permanent implant at the time of mastectomy.

Three factors may allow use of this technique for a single-stage delayed expander-implant reconstruction:

1. Incorporation of local tissue to improve dimension of the skin envelope may allow immediate permanent insertion.
2. When a large breast undergoes mastectomy, preservation of the majority of the skin envelope may allow late permanent implant insertion, especially if the patient elects to undergo mastopexy-reduction of the contralateral breast (Fig. 143-1).
3. Use of an adjustable permanent implant-expander with a distant removal port. When the expansion process is completed, the implant can be reduced to normal size and the distant port removed.

The advantages of the expander-implant technique for breast reconstruction include the following:

- Minimal morbidity.
- Reduced operative time. Although there are usually two procedures, each is short in the range of 1 to 1.5 hours and requires only one night in the hospital. The second stage may be performed on an outpatient basis according to the preference of the patient and the surgeon.
- No donor site morbidity, unlike in flap procedures, when the patient will have an additional scar at the flap harvest site.
- If the patient becomes dissatisfied with the result, all preexisting flaps are still available, and the expander-implant maintains the breast space if the flap is later incorporated into a secondary reconstruction (Figs. 143-2 and 143-3).

The disadvantages related to expander-implant use include the following:

- Complications inherent to implant use, including implant deflation or malfunction, capsular contracture, and fear of adverse interactions between the patient's immune system and the device (see data on implant use in Chapter 138).
- Exposure and infection. The implant is generally located beneath thin cutaneous coverage. Exposure may result in infection that will not generally respond to antibiotics, requiring implant removal.
- Contour irregularities visible on skin surface due to underlying implant. Again, because the implant is gradually encapsulated with scar, the adhesions of the scar to the implant and skin may result in unnatural appearance.
- The implant will not behave like normal vascularized tissue. It will remain cooler than adjacent body parts when ambient temperature is low, and the reconstructed breast will not develop natural ptosis with advancing age because of scar attachment between implant and chest wall and overlying skin envelope as opposed to the contralateral breast.

Certain criteria are required before a patient represents an appropriate candidate for implant-expander reconstruction. The patient must have an adequate skin envelope to support the expander-implant. If the skin has poor vascularity from circulatory injury during the mastectomy (immediate reconstruction), the implant must have muscle coverage. In delayed reconstruction, irradiated skin represents a relative contraindication to the expander-implant because implant exposure may occur and the skin envelope will usually not respond to the expansion process. If the patient is a smoker or is being treated for scleroderma, use of an expander-implant is a relative contraindication. Cessation of smoking for 6 weeks may be acceptable to proceed with the expander-implant, although skin circulation may still be adversely affected. The patient must be aware of limitations of the expander-implant technique in regard to sym-

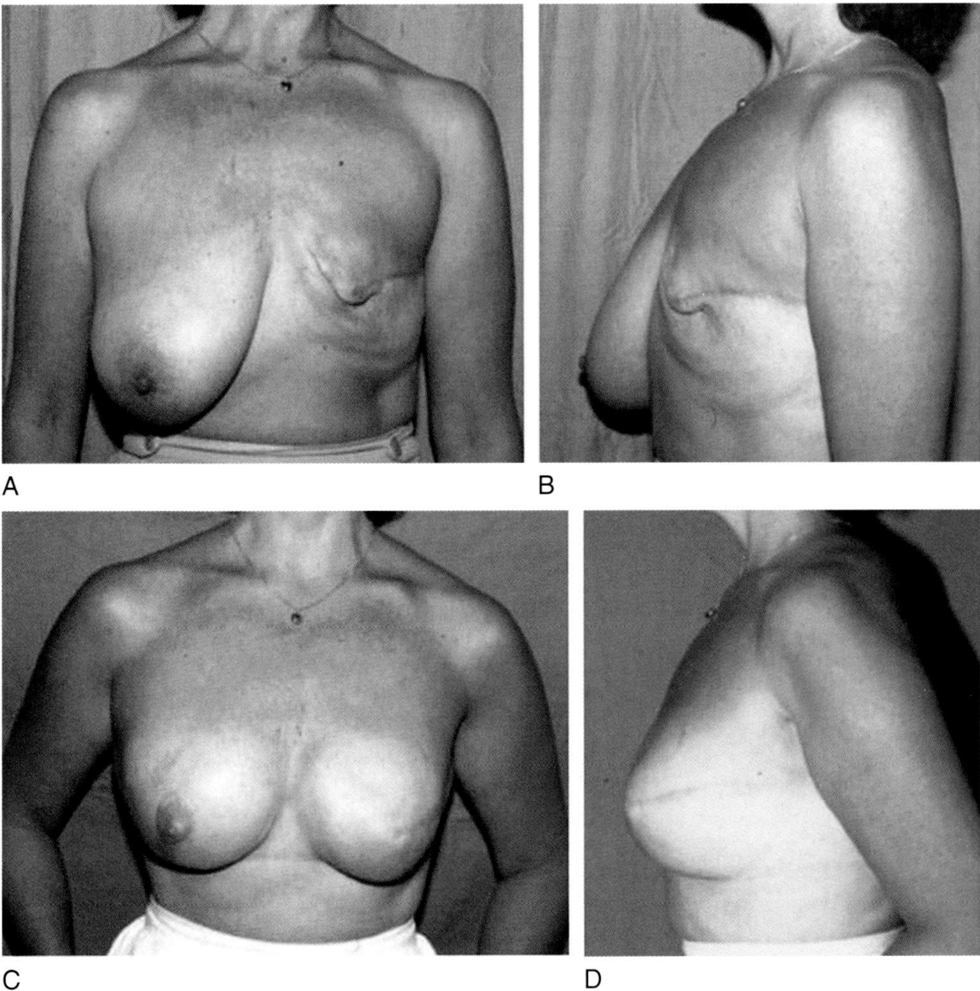

FIGURE 143-1. Delayed implant reconstruction. *A,* Postoperative anterior view of left modified radical mastectomy. Note that the mastectomy skin envelope has redundant skin. *B,* Lateral view of mastectomy defect. *C,* Postoperative anterior view 1 year after left breast reconstruction with single-stage implant insertion and contralateral mastopexy. *D,* Postoperative lateral view 1 year after left breast and nipple-areola reconstruction.

metry. If the opposite breast is ptotic or large, it is unlikely that the expansion process will be able to provide a result that will match the opposite breast. The patient must agree to delayed surgery of the opposite breast to establish symmetry with the reconstructed breast mound (reduction mammaplasty or mastopexy). If the contralateral breast is very small (A cup), the expansion process will be effective, but when a very small implant is inserted, capsular contracture may impair the final result. In general, this type of patient will agree to an augmentation of the opposite side to allow symmetry and a slightly larger implant to maintain the expanded skin envelope on the mastectomy side.

The patient must be well informed about all options for breast reconstruction. In general, autogenous breast reconstruction will provide a more natural breast but will require more complex surgery and additional donor site scars. In immediate reconstruction with skin-sparing mastectomy, the addition of the latissimus dorsi musculocutaneous flap will preserve the space for the nipple-areola with use of the skin island and provide excellent implant coverage. The transverse rectus abdominis musculocutaneous (TRAM) transposition flap, the deep inferior epigastric pedicle (DIEP)–segmental TRAM flap, or the DIEP perforator flap microvascular transplantation will provide skin for the nipple-areola defect and autogenous tissue to replace the resected breast tissue. Finally, the patient must be willing to accept the use of a permanent prosthesis. At present, both the silicone gel– and saline-filled implants are approved by the Food

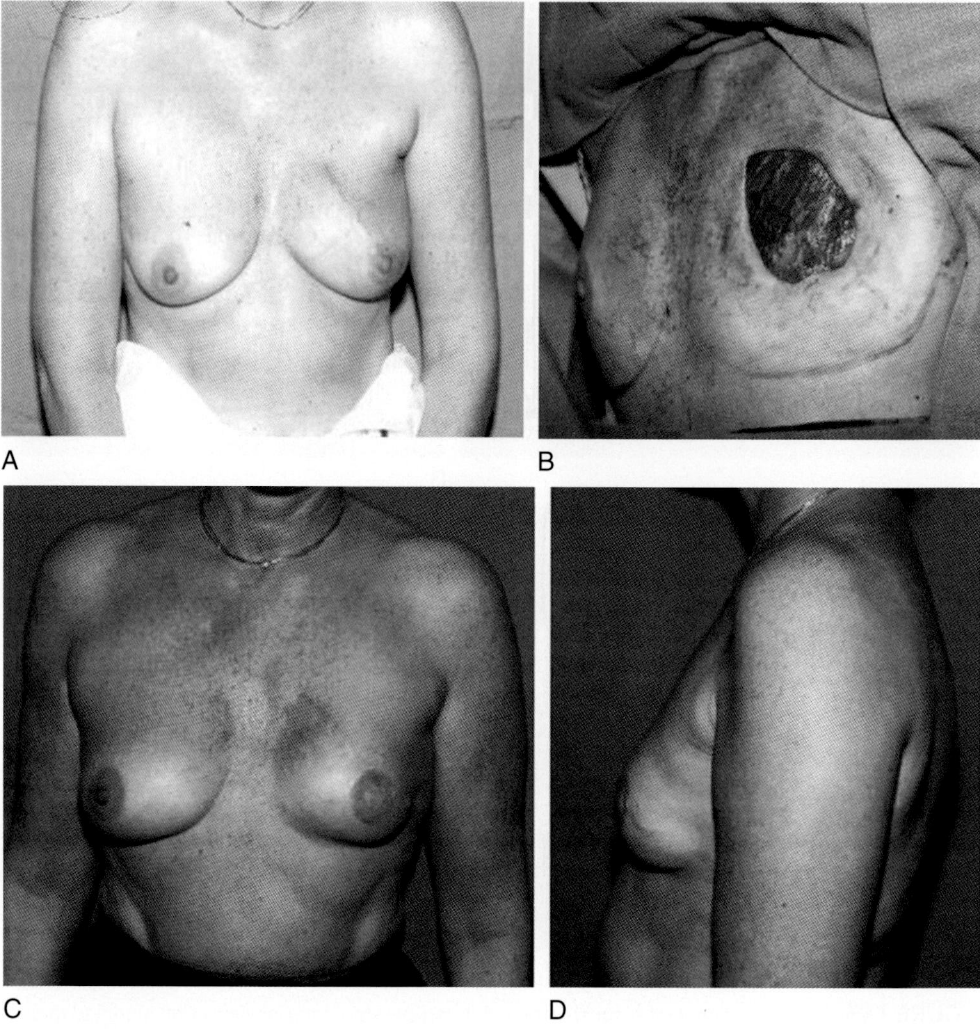

FIGURE 143-2. Immediate expander-implant reconstruction. *A,* Anterior view of left stage I breast cancer. *B,* Modified radical mastectomy defect. Note preserved inframammary line. *C,* Postoperative anterior view at 1 year after left breast reconstruction and right mastopexy with augmentation. *D,* Postoperative lateral view at 1 year. Note definition of inframammary line.

and Drug Administration (FDA) for breast reconstruction. However, as of 1992, the FDA required that silicone gel–filled implants be limited only to women participating in scientific protocols. The patient must agree to participate in an approved adjunct clinical study to be eligible for use of silicone gel implants.[4]

The technique for expander-implant use generally requires two stages. Each stage is discussed in regard to marking, position, dissection, closure, dressing, and postoperative care. Special considerations, including single-stage expander-implant reconstruction, techniques for expander-implant muscle coverage, alternative approaches for expander-implant use in patients with an inadequate skin envelope, and outcomes, are also reviewed.

STAGE 1

Markings

For immediate reconstruction, mark the inframammary line with the patient in the upright position (Fig. 143-4*A*). Mark the tumor site and plan the extent of skin resection with a general surgeon. If the breast is large or ptotic, skin envelope reduction may be necessary at the time of the mastectomy. Incorporate the tumor and skin resection in the plan for skin envelope reduction. Mark prior incisions for biopsy or other procedures, and incorporate these scars into the plan for skin resection or skin envelope reduction. The incision for sentinel node biopsy or axillary dissection is generally separate from the mastectomy incision. If the general surgeon plans to extend the incision from

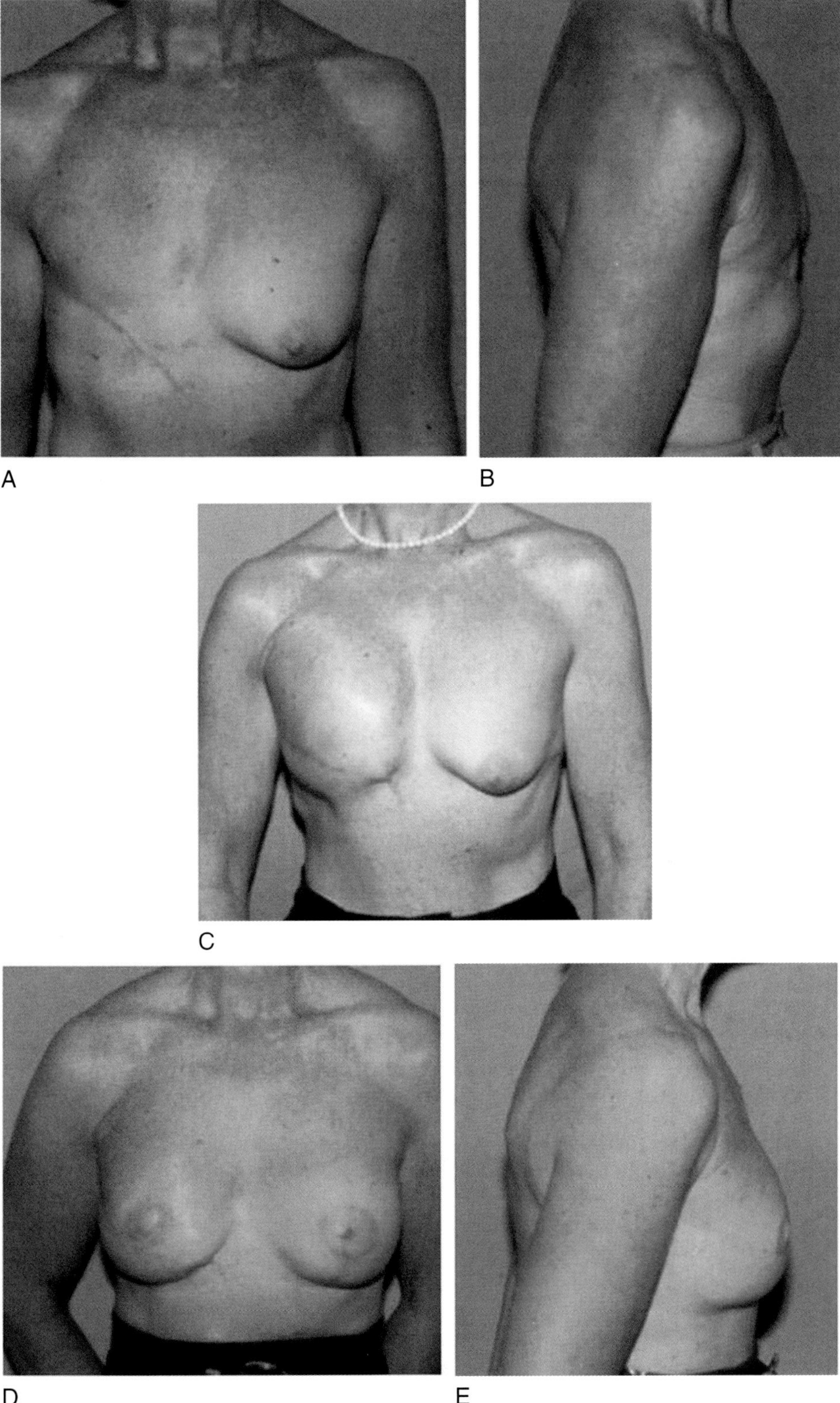

FIGURE 143-3. Delayed expander-implant reconstruction. *A,* Anterior view of right modified radical mastectomy defect. *B,* Lateral view of mastectomy defect. *C,* Postoperative anterior view, stage 1: expander in place. *D,* Postoperative anterior view at 1 year, stage 2: permanent implant in place. *E,* Postoperative lateral view at 1 year.

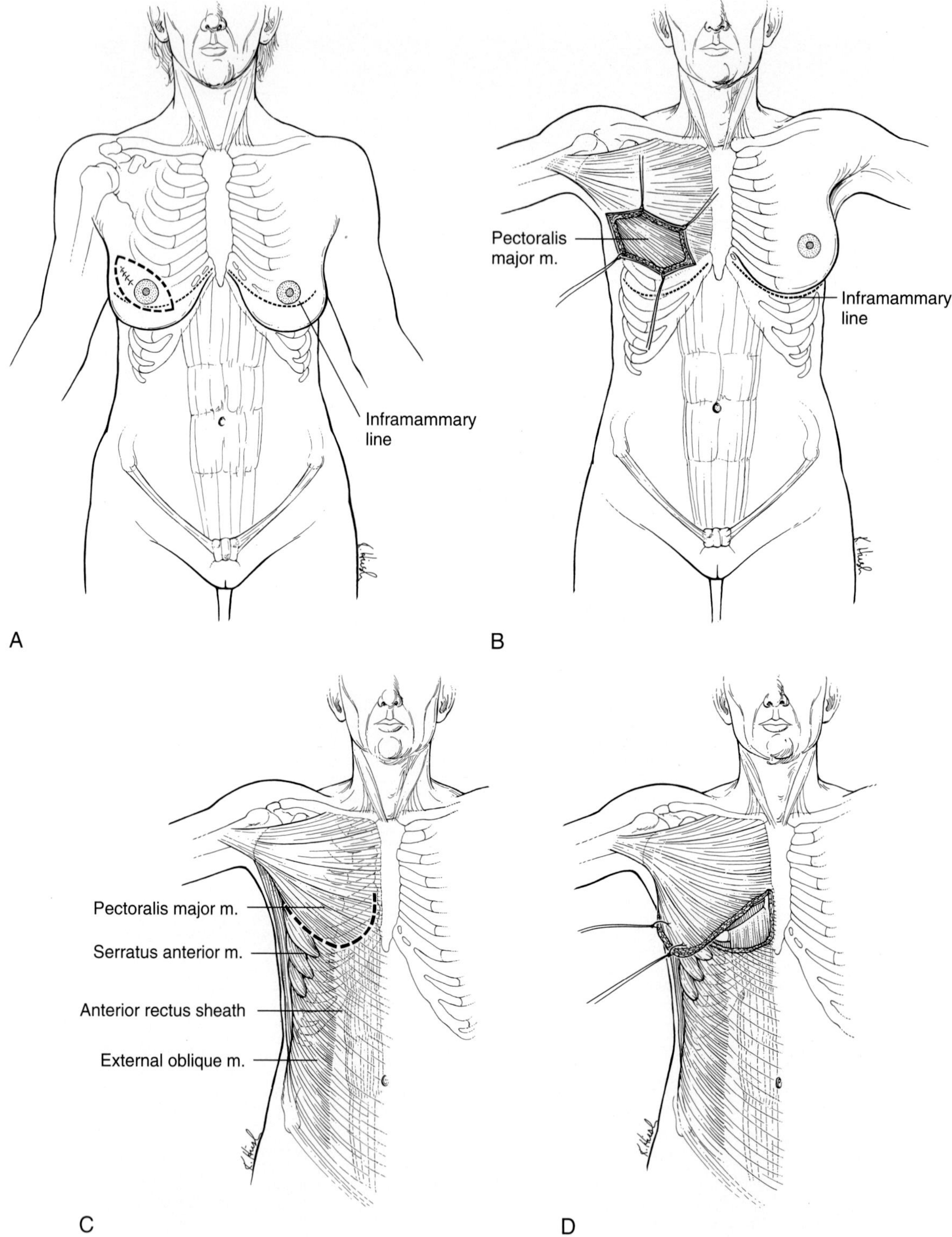

FIGURE 143-4. Stage 1, expander-implant reconstruction. *A,* Markings. Determine inframammary line at time of mastectomy or, in delayed reconstruction, on the basis of the opposite inframammary position. *B,* Expose superficial surface of pectoralis major muscle. *C,* Release pectoralis major muscle from origin at inframammary line or sixth intercostal space and along sternum from fourth to sixth intercostal spaces. *D,* After subpectoral space is prepared for expander insertion, rotate pectoralis major muscle laterally to anterior axillary line.

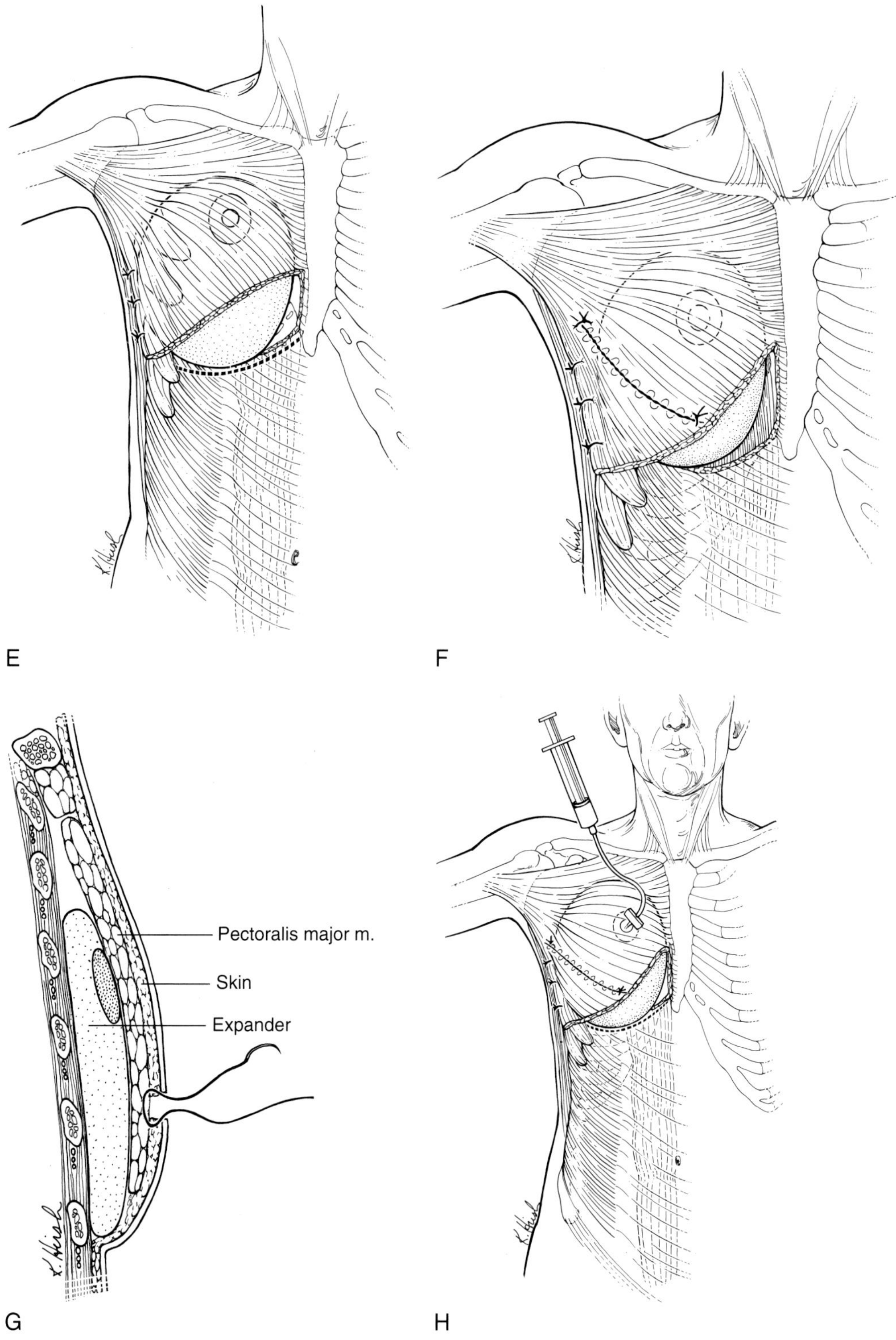

FIGURE 143-4, cont'd. *E,* Place expander beneath pectoralis major muscle flap with inferior edge of expander located at inframammary line. Suture lateral edge of pectoralis major flap at anterior axillary line. *F,* Expander is generally inflated with 50 to 100 mL of saline before insertion. A closed suction drain is generally inserted through the lateral chest wall incision. Note that total muscle coverage is not provided by this technique. The inferior central skin envelope is directly over the expander. If skin viability is questionable, do not release inferior pectoralis muscle or add rectus abdominis-external oblique segmental flap. *G,* Lateral view demonstrates position of expander with relationship to inframammary line. *H,* Expander port patency is checked after skin closure to ensure that the port is accessible and patent.

the mastectomy skin resection into the axilla, incorporate this incision into the plans for the skin envelope procedure. Although the final decision for the extent and location of the mastectomy skin resection should be made by the oncologic surgeon, consider the following options:

1. Preserve the areola if the tumor is remote from the nipple-areola complex in normal or small nonptotic breasts.
2. Avoid extending an incision into the infraclavicular, sternal, and inframammary regions (tumor location may necessitate extension of the incision into these areas).
3. A separate axillary incision may be preferable to arbitrary extension of the mastectomy incision into the axilla for sentinel node biopsy or axillary dissection. If the axillary dissection is in continuity with the mastectomy wound, it is important to drain both the axilla and the mastectomy site with separate closed suction drains. The axillary dissection closed drainage system will usually remain in place longer to avoid seroma formation.

The inframammary line is defined by a marking, and the contralateral breast is similarly marked to serve as a reminder of this important anatomic landmark. Dissection below the inframammary line at the time of mastectomy should be avoided. Preservation of skin and soft tissue continuity below the inframammary line will allow preservation of this anatomic landmark during the first stage of breast reconstruction.

For delayed reconstruction, position of the inframammary line should be based on the contralateral breast or chest wall anatomy (approximately the sixth intercostal space) for bilateral staged breast reconstruction with an expander followed by permanent implants. Mark the mastectomy incision and plan the location of the incision to perform expander insertion (in general, a 4-cm incision at the lateral aspect of the mastectomy scar).

Position

A supine position with the arm extended is the preferred position for the patient. If the general surgeon prefers a special position in regard to elevation of the hemithorax or fixation of the ipsilateral arm over the patient (attached to the ether screen), repositioning is not required for expander insertion. If skin envelope reduction is planned, repositioning of the patient with arms extended may be required (Fig. 143-4*B*).

Dissection

For immediate reconstruction, the plastic surgeon is generally called to the operating room for expander insertion after completion of the mastectomy. Expander placement is preferred in a subpectoral position after release of the pectoralis major muscle fibers from its origin along the costal margin and from the sternum between the fourth and sixth intercostal spaces. The muscle is then transposed laterally to define the lateral edge of the breast mound reconstruction and still provide coverage of the expander from the clavicle to the level of the mastectomy incision, usually occurring in the midbreast (lateral transposition of the partially released pectoralis major muscle also avoids later migration of the expander into the area of the axillary dissection or lateral chest wall) (Fig. 143-4*C* and *D*). At the subpectoral elevation of the pectoralis major to the level of the clavicle superiorly, sternum medially, and anterior axillary line laterally and release of its origin as noted, the expander is placed on the exposed chest wall and over the preserved pectoralis minor muscle (Fig. 143-4*E*). Size and type of expander are based on the plastic surgeon's preference. As noted in the review of available expanders (see "Expander Selection"), expander diameter should match the space between the sternal edge and the anterior axillary line in the mastectomy defect. A textured expander will generally not migrate and will preserve the inframammary line (Fig. 143-4*F* to *H*).

If the oncologic surgeon will avoid dissection inferior to the defined inframammary line (see "Markings"), the expander will enhance the inframammary fold during the expansion process. If dissection extends below the inframammary line, the inferior edge of the expander may be placed at the true inframammary line and will generally maintain this position, particularly if a textured expander is used, allowing restoration of the inframammary fold during the expansion. The plastic surgeon may prefer to expand below the inframammary line in an effort to incorporate abdominal skin into the breast envelope. Suture restoration of the inframammary line will then become necessary at the second stage when the expander is removed and the permanent implant is inserted. When possible, use of the inferior expander edge at the true inframammary line is preferred because expansion efforts are better directed toward the inferior breast envelope rather than the abdominal skin.

If skin viability is in question between the mastectomy incision and the inframammary line, the surgeon has four options:

1. Delay expander insertion and simply close the mastectomy incision. A delayed reconstruction will then be required after healing of the mastectomy site is achieved. All patients scheduled for first-stage expander insertion should be made aware of the possibility that expander insertion will not be performed if skin damage appears extensive after the mastectomy procedure.

2. Place the expander in the complete submuscular (subpectoral) position. This technique is avoided because an expander is less efficient when it is located completely beneath the intact pectoralis major muscle. Because its fibers of origin have not been released, the expander tends to provide expansion of only the superior muscle fibers and the overlying skin.
3. Achieve total muscle coverage of the expander. Complete submuscular coverage is accomplished by splitting the lateral aspect of the pectoralis major muscle at the fourth or fifth intercostal space and dissecting the pocket for the expander by elevation of the pectoralis major from sternum to anterior axillary line and from clavicle to sixth intercostal space, including release of the fibers of pectoralis origin at the inframammary line. The dissection laterally proceeds beneath the lateral edge of the serratus anterior muscle to ensure complete muscle coverage of the implant. After expander insertion, the split fibers of the pectoralis major are reapproximated (Fig. 143-5).
4. Switch to a distant or regional flap to provide muscle coverage of the inferior aspect of the exposed expander with the release and transposition of the limited pectoralis major muscle flap. This flap may be muscle alone (latissimus dorsi or segmental rectus abdominis), or it may provide immediate skin and soft tissue replacement (latissimus dorsi musculocutaneous flap or rectus abdominis musculocutaneous flap). In the skin-sparing technique, staging the expander-implant technique without a distant flap defeats the purpose of preservation of all the skin envelope with the exception of the nipple-areola. The distant or regional flaps (latissimus dorsi musculocutaneous flap or rectus abdominis musculocutaneous flap) will provide skin to replace the nipple-areola and for coverage of the implant (latissimus dorsi muscle) or immediate mound reconstruction (rectus abdominis musculocutaneous flap).

Expander Selection

Expander selection is based on the surgeon's preference and experience, the planned reconstructive method (e.g., delayed or immediate), the irradiation requirements, and the patient's anatomic requirements (e.g., residual skin envelope dimensions, post-expansion volume requirements to achieve desired cup size or to match contralateral breast) (Table 143-1). The most commonly used expanders have an incorporated saline injection port. Incorporation of the injection port is preferable because additional dissection for port placement is not required. During saline inflation, the port is located by direct palpation or with a magnetic finder. In addition, most expanders are now anatomically "shaped" to permit greater expansion of the inferior half of the device. This design provides greater expansion of the skin immediately superior to the inframammary line and minimizes the deformity of the upper chest observed during expansion with a round device. Increasing the inferior volume of the skin envelope will provide a natural contour with appropriate ptosis after permanent implant placement.[5] The majority of expanders used for breast reconstruction have a textured surface to allow capsular ingrowth into the device to inhibit migration during the expansion process and to decrease capsular contracture, allowing the expansion process to have a direct effect on the overlying skin.

TABLE 143-1 ✦ EXPANDER SELECTION CRITERIA

	Full height	Moderate height	Low height (inferior pole expansion)	Immediate skin-sparing mastectomy	Immediate modified radical mastectomy	Immediate postoperative radiation planned	Delayed (tight envelope)	Delayed (loose envelope)
133 FV (INAMED)	X			X	X	X		X
133 MV (INAMED)		X		X	X	X		X
133 LV (INAMED)			X				X	
6100 (Mentor)			X				X	
6200 (Mentor))		X		X	X	X		X
6300 (Mentor)	X			X	X	X		X

For unilateral procedures, the size of the tissue expander is determined by measuring the base width and height of the contralateral breast with an additional allowance for overinflation of one third of breast volume to provide an adequate skin envelope for final implant insertion. For bilateral procedures, the size of the tissue expander should be based on the patient's skin envelope and the desired postoperative breast size.

For patients undergoing immediate breast reconstruction after a skin-sparing or modified radical mastectomy, the volume of the skin envelope most often permits placement of a full- or moderate-height expander. In some patients, the skin envelope volume may permit placement of a permanent implant;

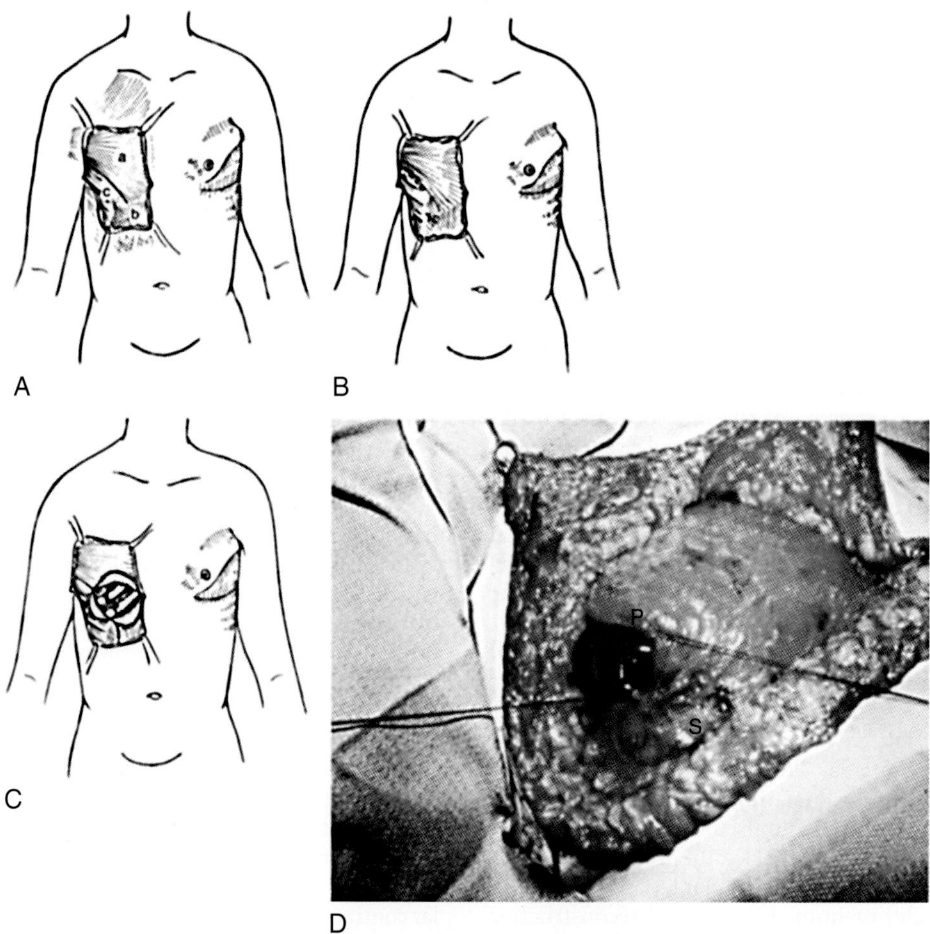

FIGURE 143-5. *A,* Expander-implant coverage provided by pectoralis major (a), rectus abdominis (b), and serratus anterior (c) muscles. *B,* Serratus anterior and pectoralis muscle fibers split near axilla for exposure of submuscular space. *C* and *D,* Submuscular pocket elevated. Fibers of origin of pectoralis major from fifth and sixth ribs are divided. P, pectoralis major; S, serratus anterior.

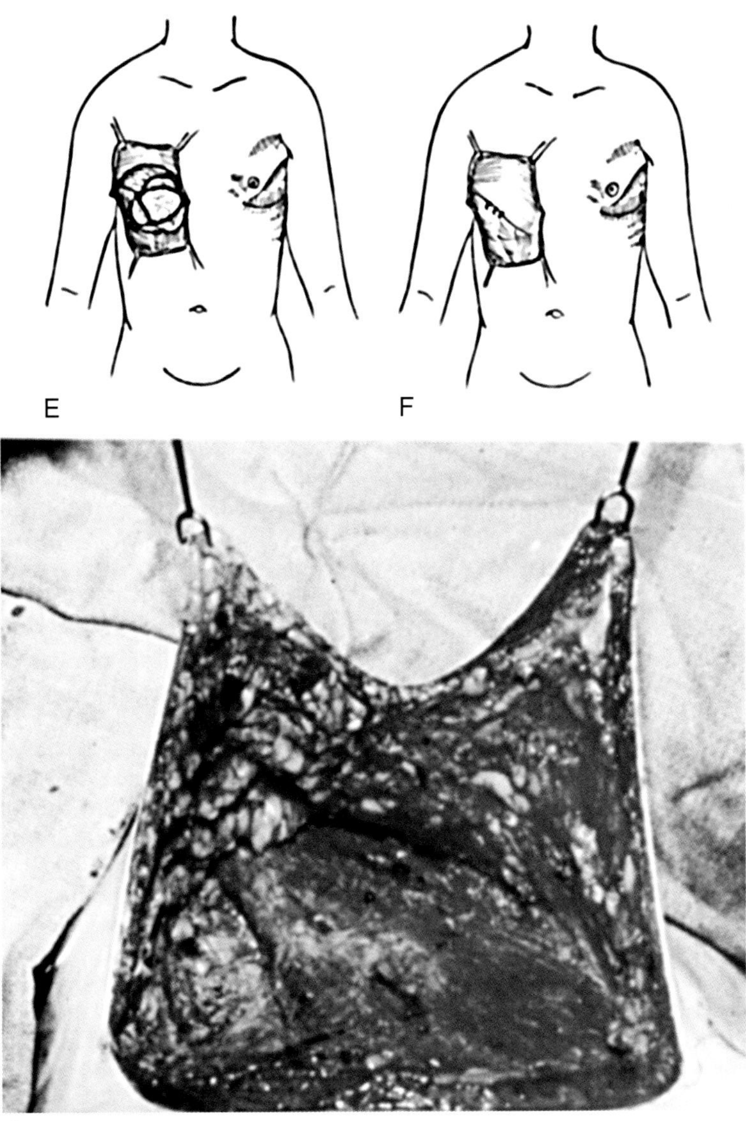

FIGURE 143-5, cont'd. *E,* Expander or implant is inserted beneath muscles with adequate pocket to ensure normal breast position. *F* and *G,* Muscle closed over implant and preserved breast skin closed directly. (From Mathes SJ, Nahai F: A systematic approach to flap selection. In Mathes SJ, Nahai F, eds: Clinical Applications for Muscle and Musculocutaneous Flaps. St. Louis, CV Mosby, 1982:285.)

however, this approach is not recommended unless the skin envelope circulation appears intact and the volume required to match the opposite breast is not excessive (see "Single-Stage Expander-Implant Reconstruction"). Postoperative mastectomy patients undergoing delayed reconstructive procedures may also be candidates for full- or moderate-height expanders if they have an adequate residual skin envelope. For patients undergoing delayed reconstruction with a tight skin envelope, a low-height expander may be used to provide limited upper pole and maximum lower pole expansion for appropriate contour and ptosis after placement of a permanent implant. A reduced amount of upper pole expansion with a greater degree of lower pole expansion will seat the permanent implant lower within the implant pocket, requiring less revision of the inframammary fold at the second stage of reconstruction. Late postoperative mastectomy patients who have undergone prior radiation therapy are generally not candidates for expander-implant reconstruction because implant exposure may occur, and the skin envelope is not usually responsive to the expansion process. Furthermore, as a result of the effect of irradiation on the chest wall and the resistance of the skin envelope to the process of expansion, the chest wall may become depressed by the posterior pressure of the expander.

Round tissue expanders are not commonly used for breast reconstruction; however, some patients may be candidates for these types of devices. For example, a patient with implants from an elective augmentation procedure undergoing skin-sparing mastectomy with planned irradiation may be best served with a round implant to preserve the skin envelope for subsequent delayed reconstruction with a permanent round implant. These types of expanders have either a textured or smooth wall and an incorporated saline injection port or a remote port connected by a closed tube system. Placement of the distant port requires a tunnel between the port site and the expander for the connecting tube. The remote port is placed just below the skin surface and is identified by palpation for saline inflation. An incorporated port is preferred as it does not require additional dissection, and the patient is not inconvenienced by the palpable port site.

The following discussion contains specific product information for expander devices that are currently available to assist in determining the optimal choice for the patient's reconstructive needs.

ANATOMIC-SHAPED EXPANDERS

Traditional expander-based breast reconstruction has evolved by use of anatomic or shaped tissue expanders with a focus on expansion of skin in the lower pole of the reconstructed breast. This approach is evidenced by the development of a broad selection of tissue expanders with device design characteristics that address not only projection of the area of tissue expansion but also the transverse dimension of expansion relative to the final volume of the reconstructed breast mound. Specific devices have even been developed that provide a distinct lack of expansion of tissue above the meridian of the anticipated breast mound in an attempt to provide a more natural appearance of the final reconstruction and to limit the amount of additional surgery at the level of the inframammary fold during the second stage.

INAMED Aesthetics Breast Reconstruction Tissue Expanders

INAMED Aesthetics (Santa Barbara, Calif) has developed a unique line of shaped BioDIMENSIONAL tissue expanders for use in the first stage of traditional expander-based breast reconstruction. These expanders, designated the 133 V series, all have integrated infusion ports that are anterior in location and easily identified in the clinic by the Magna-Site device. Each is engineered with a patented BIOSPAN textured surface that has been specifically developed for rapid tissue expansion with secure tissue adherence and integration. These devices have been designed to produce a distinct inframammary fold that requires minimal adjustment and an implant pocket that is soft and acceptable for any type of final implant, whether it is saline or silicone filled.

INAMED Style 133 FV Tissue Expander: Full Height. The INAMED Style 133 FV tissue expander is a full-height device designed to provide traditional upper pole expansion in a variable projection profile. Expander volumes from 300 to 850 mL are provided in devices with a transverse base width of 11 to 16 cm. Maximum projection at the lower pole ranges from 5.0 to 6.8 cm (Table 143-2 and Fig. 143-6).

TABLE 143-2 ✦ INAMED STYLE 133 FV TISSUE EXPANDER: FULL HEIGHT

Style	Catalog No.	Fill Volume (mL)	Width (cm)	Height (cm)	Projection (cm)
133 FV	67-133FV11	300	11	11.5	5
133 FV	67-133FV12	400	12	12.5	5.3
133 FV	67-133FV13	500	13	13.5	5.7
133 FV	67-133FV14	600	14	14.5	6.2
133 FV	67-133FV15	750	15	15.5	6.7
133 FV	67-133FV16	850	16	16.5	6.8

Shape: BioDIMENSIONAL; profile: full height; surface: BIOSPAN; port style: Magna-Site.

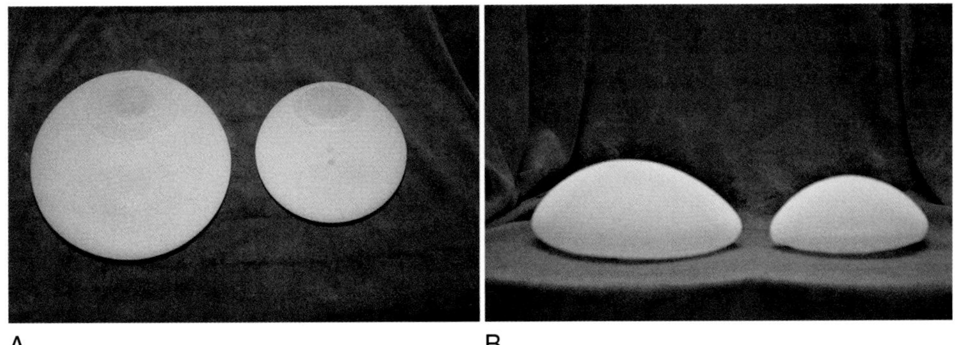

A B

FIGURE 143-6. INAMED Style 133 FV tissue expander: full height. *A,* Anterior view. *B,* Lateral view.

INAMED STYLE 133 MV TISSUE EXPANDER: MODERATE HEIGHT. The INAMED Style 133 MV tissue expander is a moderate-height device designed to provide less upper pole expansion in a variable projection profile. Expander volumes from 250 to 700 mL are provided in devices with a transverse base width of 11 to 16 cm, reflecting a reduced volume per transverse dimension provided by the Style 133 FV series. Maximum projection at the lower pole is only minimally affected by the reduction of volume relative to the transverse dimension and ranges from 4.9 to 6.6 cm (Table 143-3 and Fig. 143-7).

TABLE 143-3 ✦ INAMED STYLE 133 MV TISSUE EXPANDER: MODERATE HEIGHT

Style	Catalog No.	Fill Volume (mL)	Width (cm)	Height (cm)	Projection (cm)
133 MV	67-133MV11	250	11	10	4.9
133 MV	67-133MV12	300	12	11	5.2
133 MV	67-133MV13	400	13	12	5.6
133 MV	67-133MV14	500	14	13	6
133 MV	67-133MV15	600	15	14	6.3
133 MV	67-133MV16	700	16	15	6.6

Shape: BioDIMENSIONAL; profile: moderate height; surface: BIOSPAN; port style: Magna-Site.

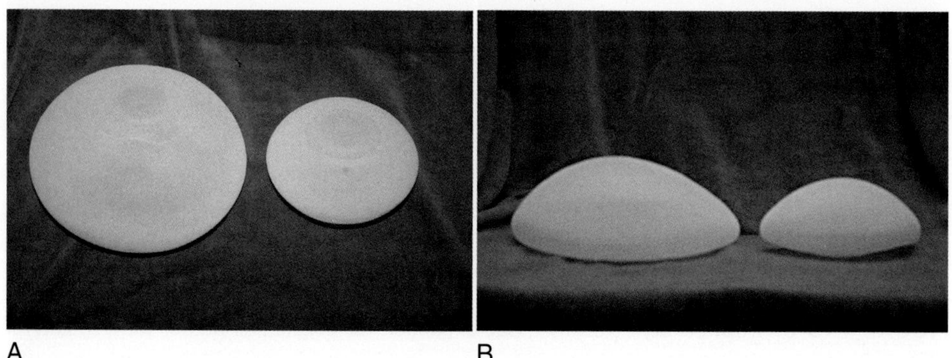

A B

FIGURE 143-7. INAMED Style 133 MV tissue expander: moderate height. *A,* Anterior view. *B,* Lateral view.

INAMED STYLE 133 LV TISSUE EXPANDER: LOW HEIGHT. The INAMED Style 133 LV tissue expander is a low-height device that employs a "semi-lunar" shape to provide a maximum centralized lower pole projection during the expansion process. Specifically, this device has an "intra-arc" height or height of the expander in the longitudinal dimension ranging from 7.0 to 9.5 cm relative to expander volumes of 150 to 500 mL with transverse base dimensions of 11 to 16 cm. The reduction in expander volume relative to the base diameter of the Style 133 FV and Style 133 MV series reflects the lack of expansion of the upper pole of the reconstructed breast mound. This device has gained recent popularity given its association with less superior implant migration. However, if a tissue expander is being used as a bridge to autologous tissue reconstruction in the patient requiring radiation therapy, this would be a less pleasing device to choose for interim cosmesis. Higher profile devices from the Style 133 FV and Style 133 MV series would be more appropriate for such patients requiring irradiation and a secondary autologous reconstructive procedure 6 to 9 months after the completion of radiation therapy (Table 143-4 and Fig. 143-8).

TABLE 143-4 ✦ INAMED STYLE 133 LV TISSUE EXPANDER: LOW HEIGHT

Style	Catalog No.	Fill Volume (mL)	Width (cm)	Height (cm)	Projection (cm)	Width Tip to Base (cm)
133 LV	67-133LV11	150	11	7	4.7	7.6
133 LV	67-133LV12	200	12	7.5	5.3	8.4
133 LV	67-133LV13	300	13	8	5.7	9.1
133 LV	67-133LV14	350	14	8.5	6	9.7
133 LV	67-133LV15	400	15	9	6.3	10.5
133 LV	67-133LV16	500	16	9.5	6.3	11.3

Shape: BioDIMENSIONAL; profile: low height; surface: BIOSPAN; port style: Magna-Site.

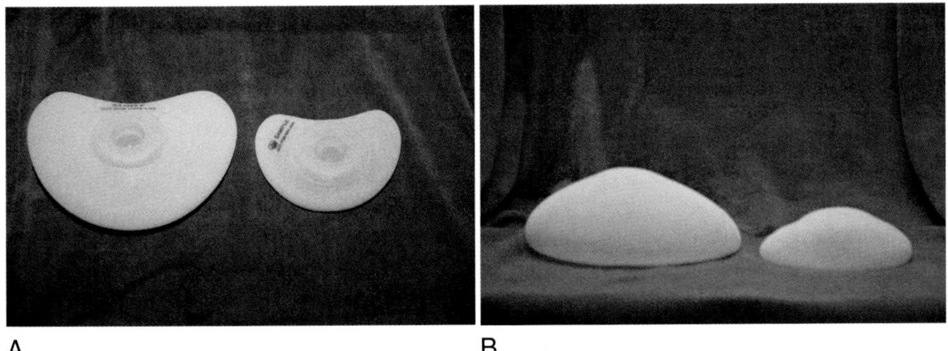

A B

FIGURE 143-8. INAMED Style 133 LV tissue expander: low height. *A,* Anterior view. *B,* Lateral view.

Mentor Corporation Breast Reconstruction Tissue Expanders

Mentor Corporation (Santa Barbara, Calif) has developed a line of shaped Contour Profile tissue expanders for use in the first stage of traditional two-stage breast reconstruction. These expanders all have integrated infusion ports that are anterior in location and easily identified in the clinic by an included magnetic finding device. Each is engineered with a patented Siltex textured surface to prevent expander migration or rotation.

Mentor Style 6100 Tissue Expander: Low Height. Mentor Style 6100 tissue expanders are low-height, shaped devices offering tissue expansion to obtain breast mound volumes of 250 to 750 mL based on a range of base transverse dimensions of 11.4 to 16.5 cm. Device heights in the 6100 series range from 8.1 cm with 6.1 cm of projection in the 250-mL expander to 11.9 cm with 8.1 cm of projection in the 750-mL expander. Minimal upper pole expansion is provided with the use of this device. The upper border of this device is transverse in its orientation and does not assume a crescent shape as is seen in the INAMED Style 133 LV device. Mentor Style 6100 devices provide a larger volume range (250 to 750 mL) relative to the INAMED 133 LV series (150 to 500 mL). However, the INAMED 133 LV series can provide a lower pole projection tissue expander for patients requiring an expander with volume requirements of 150 mL and 200 mL, which is not available in the Mentor Style 6100 series. Caution is again warranted for use of this device as a bridge to autologous tissue reconstruction in the patient requiring irradiation. The appearance of this low-height device is less projecting for the time after the completion of radiation therapy. Patients may be more pleased with a device with a more generous height simulating the contralateral breast (Table 143-5 and Fig. 143-9).

TABLE 143-5 ✦ MENTOR STYLE 6100 TISSUE EXPANDER: LOW HEIGHT

Style	Catalog No.	Fill Volume (mL)	Width (cm)	Height (cm)	Projection (cm)	Width Tip to Base (cm)
6100	354-6111	250	11.4	8.1	6.1	NA
6100	354-6112	350	12.7	9.4	6.5	NA
6100	354-6113	450	14	10.2	7.1	NA
6100	354-6114	550	15	10.9	7.4	NA
6100	354-6115	650	15.7	11.2	7.9	NA
6100	354-6116	750	16.5	11.9	8.1	NA

Shape: contour profile; profile: low height; surface: Siltex; port style: integrated.

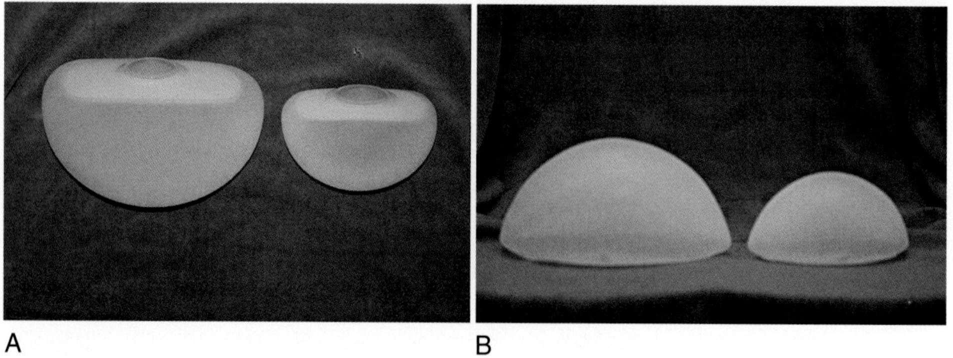

A B

FIGURE 143-9. Mentor Style 6100 tissue expander: low height. *A*, Anterior view. *B*, Lateral view.

MENTOR STYLE 6200 TISSUE EXPANDER: MEDIUM HEIGHT. Mentor Style 6200 tissue expanders are medium-height, shaped devices offering tissue expansion to obtain volumes of 350 to 800 mL based on a range of base transverse dimensions of 11.7 to 15.6 cm. Distinctly, the 6200 series has a shorter base diameter-to-volume ratio relative to the Mentor 6100 series. The medium-height design of this series provides expansion of the upper pole of the reconstruction site with expanders with a height of 10 cm for the 350-mL expander to 15.6 cm for the 800-mL expander. Projection for this device ranges from 6.6 to 8.0 cm, which is relatively concordant with the 6100 series. Reduction in the transverse dimension with extension of the height of individual devices results in the maintenance of projection for a selected volume (Table 143-6 and Fig. 143-10).

TABLE 143-6 ✦ MENTOR STYLE 6200 TISSUE EXPANDER: MEDIUM HEIGHT

Style	Catalog No.	Fill Volume (mL)	Width (cm)	Height (cm)	Projection (cm)	Width Tip to Base (cm)
6200	354-6212	350	11.7	10	6.6	NA
6200	354-6213	450	12.7	10.8	7	NA
6200	354-6214	550	13.5	11.7	7.4	NA
6200	354-6215	650	14.6	12.6	7.6	NA
6200	354-6216	800	15.6	13.3	8	NA

Shape: contour profile; profile: medium height; surface: Siltex; port style: integrated.

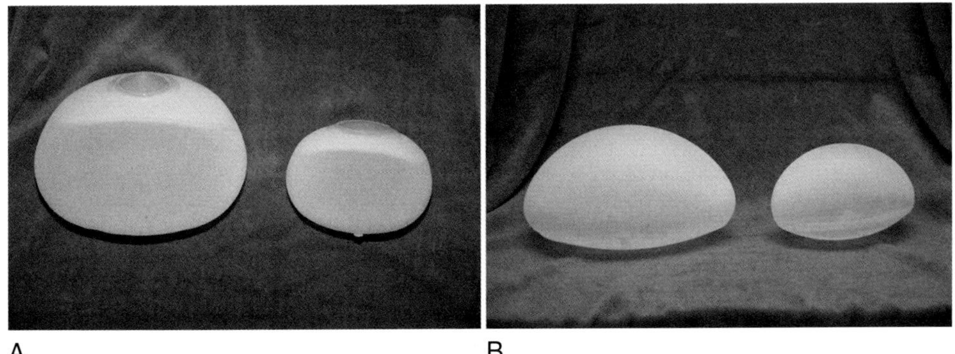

FIGURE 143-10. Mentor Style 6200 tissue expander: medium height. *A*, Anterior view. *B*, Lateral view.

MENTOR STYLE 6300 TISSUE EXPANDER: TALL HEIGHT. Mentor Style 6300 tissue expanders are tall-height, shaped devices offering tissue expansion to obtain volumes of 250 to 850 mL based on a range of base transverse dimensions of 10.1 to 15.4 cm. The 6300 series alters base diameter relative to height with an additional reduction in projection for a given volume. For patients with significant projection relative to volume, one would be better served with the 6200 series with the sacrifice of height of the expander in the first stage of the reconstruction (Table 143-7 and Fig. 143-11).

TABLE 143-7 ✦ MENTOR STYLE 6300 TISSUE EXPANDER: TALL HEIGHT

Style	Catalog No.	Fill Volume (mL)	Width (cm)	Height (cm)	Projection (cm)	Width Tip to Base (cm)
6300	354-6311	250	10.1	10.7	5.6	NA
6300	354-6312	350	11.3	11.8	6	NA
6300	354-6313	450	12.3	12.9	6.5	NA
6300	354-6314	550	13.2	13.8	6.9	NA
6300	354-6315	650	14	14	7.3	NA
6300	354-6316	750	14.6	14.6	7.6	NA
6300	354-6317	850	15.4	15.4	7.9	NA

Shape: contour profile; profile: tall height; surface: Siltex; port style: integrated.

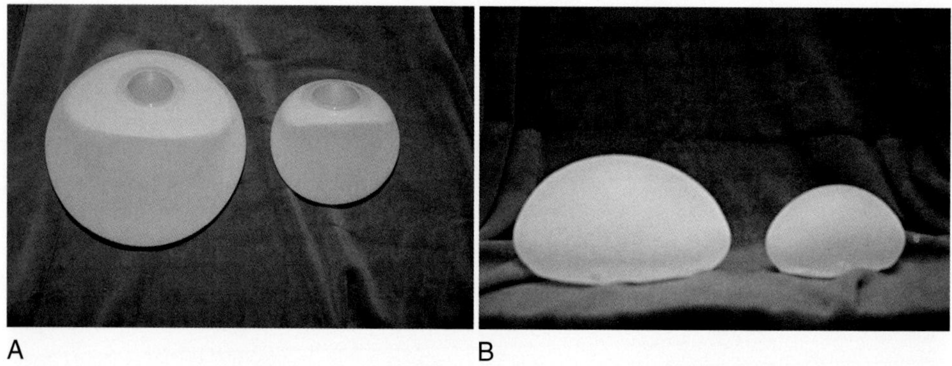

FIGURE 143-11. Mentor Style 6300 tissue expander: tall height. *A,* Anterior view. *B,* Lateral view.

DISSECTION

In summary, dissection includes the following steps:

1. Release the pectoralis major muscle from the sixth intercostal space and the medial origin from the fourth through the sixth intercostal spaces (Color Plate 143-1; see also Fig. 143-4*C* and *D*).
2. Insert expander. Confirm that the inferior margin of the expander is located at the premarked inframammary line. Place the expander beneath the pectoralis major muscle between the clavicle and the fourth intercostal space with muscle coverage extending laterally to the anterior axillary line (see Fig. 143-4*F* and *G*). Suture the lateral edge of the mobilized pectoralis major muscle to the anterior axillary line.
3. Insert two drains (10-mm JP drains are preferred). These will provide drainage of axillary dissection or sentinel node biopsy and drainage of the subpectoral space. Exit the drains either within the axillary skin or lateral to the site of the inframammary fold along the bra line at the lateral chest wall region.
4. Close the mastectomy incision if possible. Incorporate the inferior edge of the pectoralis major muscle in the skin closure to provide muscle curvature in the event of partial skin loss at the incision site. Another technique to ensure coverage of the implant in proximity to the incision is use of a suture passed through the edge of the pectoralis muscle. With advancement of the pectoralis muscle flap, these sutures are passed through the skin by a Keith needle and tied over bolster dressings. This technique will maintain the position of the muscle for implant coverage during the early postoperative period.
5. Inflate the expander through the skin and add an additional 50 to 100 mL, depending on skin laxity of remaining envelope and circulation status. This maneuver confirms appropriate positioning of the expander port and patency with a 23-gauge needle or butterfly insertion (see Fig. 143-4*H*).

Additional steps of the dissection phase of staged expander-implant insertion are as follows:

1. If skin appears unstable (inadequate circulation) between the fourth and the sixth intercostal spaces, a segmental rectus muscle flap for additional implant coverage should be considered (see technique description for segmental rectus flap). As noted, alternative options if skin circulation is in question include complete local muscle coverage of the expander-implant or use of a distant flap for immediate reconstruction, including the latissimus dorsi and rectus abdominis muscle or musculocutaneous flaps (see Chapter 138).
2. In patients with breast ptosis or hypertrophy, skin envelope reduction should be incorporated in the mastectomy site closure. Skin envelope reduction will avoid skin loss and improve eventual contour of the reconstructed breast mound.

Closure

The dermal layer is closed with 4-0 absorbable sutures that incorporate the anterior surface of the inferior pectoralis major muscle with skin closure. Subcuticular skin closure is then completed with breast fluffs and a supportive dressing.

Postoperative Care

Broad-spectrum antibiotic coverage, started intraoperatively, should be given intravenously at the time of the mastectomy and continued for 5 to 7 days in an oral form. Drains should stay in place for 7 to 10 days (they can be removed as early as day 5 if drainage is below 30 mL per 24 hours). Oral antibiotics may be continued until drains are removed.

Expansion Process

The first inflation of the expander at 2 to 3 weeks is usually 60 to 100 mL of saline, followed by expansion every 3 to 4 weeks for 3 months. If the patient is receiving chemotherapy during the expansion process, it may be helpful to expand the patients 1 week before each of their cycles of chemotherapy, depending on the time intervals used by the oncologist. This regimen will expand the breast mound for approximately a 20% to 30% greater volume than the opposite breast or planned volume of bilateral reconstruction or alteration of the contralateral breast to accomplish breast enlargement (augmentation), uplift (mastopexy), or reduction (Fig. 143-12).

The expansion process is not started until 2 to 3 weeks after expander insertion to allow complete healing of the insertion site. There are two approaches to expansion: (1) injection of saline solution to a maximal endpoint, when discomfort or blanching of the skin territory is observed, and subsequent deflation until skin capillary refill or discomfort has resolved; and (2) injection of 10% to 20% of the total volume of expander capacity at each visit without attempting to inject the maximal volume tolerated by the patient and flap circulation. The theoretical advantage of the first approach is faster expansion and rupture of scar tissue. The expansion device can be inflated to several times its design volume without risk of rupture. In general, the expander is inflated to the maximal

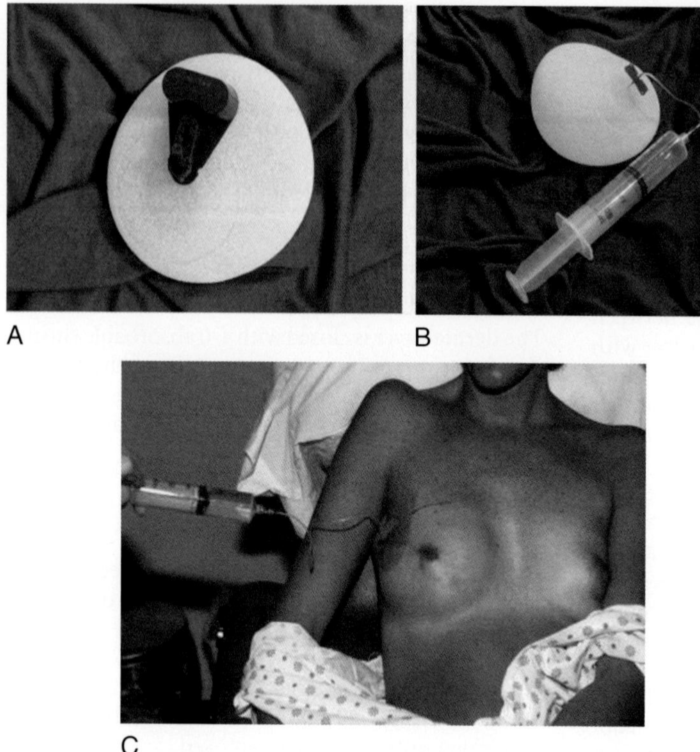

FIGURE 143-12. *A,* Location of expander port with magnetic device or by direct palpation. *B,* Small-caliper needle (23-gauge) is inserted into port to instill saline. *C,* Expander inflation. The patient is placed in a comfortable position to accomplish inflation of the expander.

volume tolerated during a specific time interval of 2 to 3 months. Expanders used for breast reconstruction are frequently left in place for longer intervals to accommodate the patient's schedule or to allow completion of cytotoxic or adjuvant chemotherapy. The patient returns to the office for expansion every 2 to 4 weeks, depending on the schedules of the patient and the surgeon.

The incorporated or distant port is located and prepared with antiseptic solution (povidone-iodine preferred). A 23-gauge needle is attached to an intravenous connector with three-way stopcock. The needle is passed into the valve, and withdrawal of saline will confirm needle location within the port. The first expansion generally consists of 50 to 100 mL of saline, and a 100-mL volume is subsequently injected at each visit.

Complications

ERYTHEMA AND CELLULITIS. Erythema frequently represents response of the skin to dissection and will resolve spontaneously. If erythema is associated with symptoms of infection (malaise, fever, or an increase in drainage through the suction catheters), intravenous antibiotic therapy either on an inpatient basis or by a home care service should be provided. Failure of cellulitis to resolve indicates peri-implant infection. Expander removal is required with repeat of stage 1 in 3 to 6 months.

PERSISTENT SEROUS DRAINAGE THROUGH SUCTION CATHETER. After 10 days, wound contamination at the drain exit site becomes a real risk. Drain removal and aspiration of fluid lateral to the anterior axillary line are feasible because implant migration lateral to the anterior axillary line is avoided by the pectoralis major muscle flap. If serous accumulation is extensive, reoperation with culture of the expanders, irrigation of the space, and insertion of new drains are appropriate.

PARTIAL OR COMPLETE SKIN NECROSIS. If partial or complete skin necrosis at the suture line is observed, muscle coverage of the expander in this region is generally provided by the pectoralis major muscle or a segmental rectus muscle flap. For small areas of necrosis, the use of topical antibiotics and local wound care are generally adequate. The expansion process is delayed pending healing of areas of partial or complete skin loss. If there is concern about impending expander exposure, options include (1) excision of the area of skin necrosis and advancement of the remaining envelope for closure and implant closure and implant coverage, (2) use of a distant flap, and (3) expander removal with plans for delayed reconstruction.

In general, if the skin necrosis is extensive, expander removal with a plan for delayed reconstruction is preferred. If the implant-expander is exposed with periimplant purulent drainage, expander removal is also recommended. With implant removal, culture-specific antibiotic therapy on an outpatient basis will resolve the infection. Expander-implant reinsertion can be scheduled after a minimum of 3 to 6 months, depending on the status of the overlying skin envelope.

EXPANDER FAILURE OR MALFUNCTION. Expander failure or malfunction may occur if the expander will not retain saline injections because of loss of expander wall integrity. In this instance, expander replacement as an operative procedure is required. The position of the expander port should be confirmed both at the time of the expander insertion (intraoperative position) and immediately before inflation of the expander (outpatient facility). Position of the expander port may be determined by a combination of palpation and use of an appropriate port locater based on the manufacturer's recommendations.

If the expander or a distant port has been placed upside down or rotated during the postoperative period, the position must be altered to allow inflation with saline. If attempts to manipulate the expander or port fail, the patient will require intraoperative relocation of the device to allow sequential inflation. This problem can usually be avoided if the port location and access are confirmed after wound closure while the patient is still under anesthesia.

STAGE 2

The final injection for expander inflation generally occurs 3 to 4 weeks before the planned second-stage procedure. During this time, patients should consider implant size. Frequently, size is determined by the contralateral breast. If, however, contralateral breast adjustments are planned, in general, permanent implant size will be approximately 50% to 75% of the end-volume within the expander. Obviously, volume adjustments can be made according to the patient's preference (Fig. 143-13).

If the patient is scheduled to receive radiation therapy, there are two approaches to the timing of the expansion and permanent implant insertion. The radiation therapy may be delayed until the expander-implant sequence is completed (delay of radiation therapy), or the radiation therapy can be completed during the expansion process with a delay of insertion of the permanent implant until radiation therapy is completed. (If an adjustable implant is used, the final volume may be adjusted after radiation therapy is completed with removal of the distant port.)

Markings

Determine the location of the inframammary line with the patient upright. Any adjustment required in the inframammary position should be planned at this time in consultation with the patient.

At this time, markings for the contralateral breast are required if adjustments are planned:

1. Augmentation. Mark the inframammary line and the incision planned for the augmentation (see Chapters 118 and 119).
2. Mastopexy-reduction. Mark the skin envelope and plan the incision and location for the nipple-areola (see Chapter 120).

Mark the incision for entry into the expander space and exposure for implant exchange. It is preferable to use the lateral aspect of the mastectomy incision to minimize the required area for later scar maturation (Fig. 143-13*C*).

Position

A supine position with the arms extended is the preferred position. The arms are secured so the patient may be placed in a sitting position to check selected implant position, size, projection, and symmetry.

Dissection

An incision is made lateral to the mastectomy scar at the expander site, followed by an incision through the capsule with removal of the expander. Release the residual scar or adjust the implant pocket according to preoperative markings. If the expander has been placed at the true inframammary line position, minimal adjustments of the inframammary fold will be required. If, however, the expander has been placed below the inframammary line, pocket closure at the planned inframammary line will require placement of sutures between the anterior capsule surface and the opposed side of the inframammary line. In general, a 3-0 or 2-0 suture is used for this purpose. Frequent placement of the patient in a sitting position will confirm accurate positioning of the inframammary line. Also, redundant expander skin below the planned inframammary line is advanced superiorly to incorporate the skin into the breast envelope.

Implant selection is based on the surgeon's preference and experience in regard to implant type and shape. Implant volume is based on discussions with the patient about preferred breast size, appearance during expander inflation, skin envelope limitations, and, in unilateral reconstruction, matching of the contralateral breast (see following section, "Contralateral Breast Adjustment"). A sizer is used before permanent implant placement. The sizer is placed within the pocket and inflated with

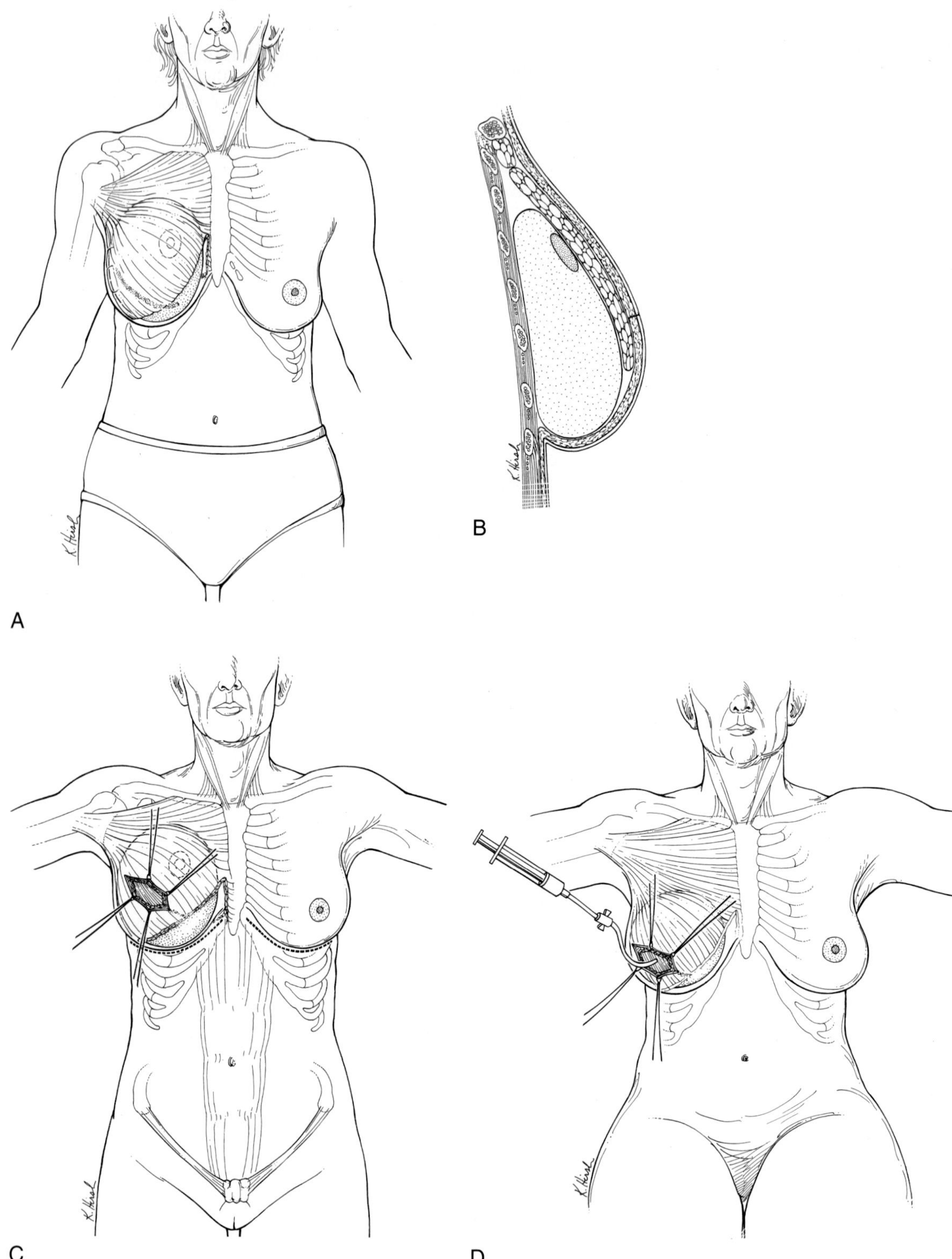

FIGURE 143-13. Stage 2, expander-implant reconstruction. *A,* Expansion process completed with breast mound approximately 25% larger than anticipated permanent implant. *B,* Lateral view, with proper placement and without muscle fiber restriction. Increased expansion will occur at the inferior half of the skin envelope. *C,* Lateral incision through mastectomy scar allows deflation of expander and its removal. Capsulotomy or pocket adjustment can be accomplished, if required. *D,* Sizer is inserted. The patient is placed in sitting position, and volume is determined for selection of permanent implant.

the patient in a sitting position to confirm optimal shape, position, and volume (Fig. 143-13*D*). If unilateral breast reconstruction is performed without surgery to the opposite breast, symmetry should be achieved at this time. If augmentation, mastopexy, mastopexy-augmentation, or reduction is planned for the contralateral breast, one should proceed with the opposite breast surgery after the desired size is achieved with the sizer on the side of the reconstruction. If bilateral breast reconstruction is performed, the opposite dissection (see preceding steps) should be completed and the symmetry confirmed. The permanent breast implant is placed in the subpectoral position.

Implant Selection

Selection of the permanent implant is based on shape, silicone wall characteristics (smooth versus textured), and volume. The type and shape of the implant are generally based on the surgeon's preference and experience. Implant volume is determined according to the preoperative discussion with the patient about the desired size of the reconstructed breast mound, the preoperative and postoperative size of the contralateral breast, and the appearance of the expanded skin envelope. In general, permanent implant size will be approximately 50% to 75% of the end-volume within the expander; however, precise implant volume is determined intraoperatively by use of a sizer inflated to the desired volume before placement of the permanent implant. After implant insertion, the skin envelope may also be adjusted for optimal ptosis and contour.

Permanent implants may have a smooth or textured silicone shell and are either saline or silicone gel filled. As of 1992, the FDA limited the use of silicone gel-filled breast implants in the United States to specific patients, including those undergoing reconstructive procedures for breast cancer who agree to participate in approved clinical trials.

The complications associated with expander-implants (see "Complications") should be thoroughly explained to the patient before expander placement. Patients can also be provided the Internet Web site addresses for INAMED, Mentor, and the American Society of Plastic Surgeons, where an extensive amount of educational information for patients is available for their review concerning implant options and potential complications.

ANATOMIC-SHAPED SALINE-FILLED IMPLANTS

INAMED Aesthetics Anatomic-Shaped Saline-Filled Breast Implants

INAMED Aesthetics offers three distinct BioDIMENSIONAL-compatible, shaped, saline-filled breast implant series for the second stage of implant-based breast reconstruction. All three series of implants are protected by the patented BIOCELL textured surface specifically to reduce capsular contracture and to prevent postoperative malpositioning.

INAMED STYLE 163 SALINE-FILLED BREAST IMPLANTS: FULL HEIGHT. INAMED Style 163 saline-filled, shaped, textured breast implants are offered for a volume as low as 360 mL to 820 mL with associated base diameters of 12 to 15.5 cm and projection of 4.9 to 6.1 cm. The height of this implant is 12.8 cm for the 360- to 380-mL device. The height of the 780- to 820-mL device is 16.5 cm, making this line of saline-filled implants compatible with all three of the INAMED 133 V series tissue expanders. One must note that the upper portion of the implant pocket will have to be designed at the second stage when the INAMED 133 LV (low height) series or the Mentor Style 6100 (low height) series tissue expanders are used. Note that this breast implant has a posterior fill valve diaphragm that is distinct from the INAMED Style 363LF and 468 series (Table 143-8 and Fig. 143-14).

TABLE 143-8 ✦ INAMED STYLE 163 SALINE-FILLED BREAST IMPLANTS: FULL HEIGHT

Style	Catalog No.	Fill Volume (mL)	Width (cm)	Height (cm)	Projection (cm)
163	27-163361	360-380	12	12.8	4.9
163	27-163441	440-460	12.8	13.6	5.2
163	27-163531	530-555	13.5	14.6	5.5
163	27-163656	655-690	14.6	15.6	5.8
163	27-163781	780-820	15.5	16.5	6.1

Shape: BioDIMENSIONAL; height: low; profile (projection): full; surface: BIOCELL; diaphragm valve: posterior.

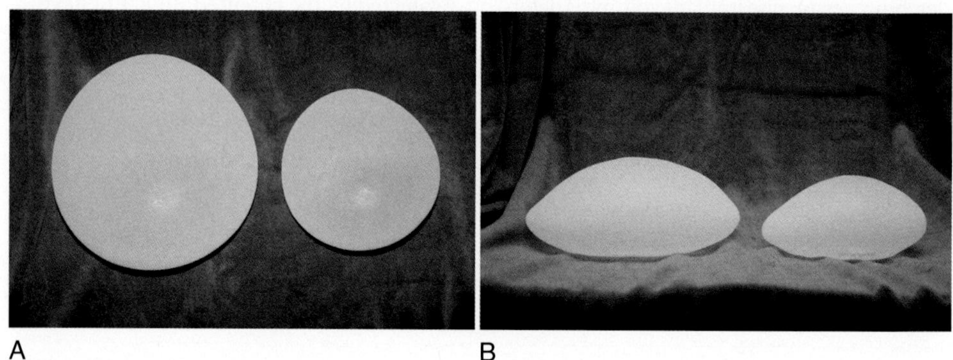

A B

FIGURE 143-14. INAMED Style 163 saline-filled breast implant: full height. *A,* Anterior view. *B,* Lateral view.

INAMED STYLE 363LF SALINE-FILLED BREAST IMPLANTS: LOW HEIGHT. INAMED Style 363LF saline-filled, shaped, textured breast implants are low-height BioDIMENSIONAL-compatible implants. They were specifically designed for use with INAMED Style 133 LV and 133 MV tissue expanders. Volumes from 170 to 180 mL (base diameter, 10. 4 cm; height, 8.6 cm; and projection, 4.2 cm) to a maximum of 690 to 720 mL (base diameter, 15.8 cm; height, 13.4 cm; and projection, 6.8 cm) are available with an anterior fill diaphragm (Table 143-9 and Fig. 143-15).

TABLE 143-9 ✦ INAMED STYLE 363LF SALINE-FILLED BREAST IMPLANTS: LOW HEIGHT

Style	Catalog No.	Fill Volume (mL)	Width (cm)	Height (cm)	Projection (cm)
363LF	27-363104LF	170-180	10.4	8.6	4.2
363LF	27-363108LF	200-210	10.8	9	4.5
363LF	27-363112LF	230-240	11.2	9.4	4.7
363LF	27-363118LF	260-275	11.8	9.8	4.9
363LF	27-363122LF	300-315	12.2	10.2	5.1
363LF	27-363126LF	330-350	12.6	10.6	5.3
363LF	27-363130LF	370-390	13	11	5.5
363LF	27-363136LF	410-430	13.6	11.4	5.6
363LF	27-363140LF	450-475	14	11.8	5.8
363LF	27-363144LF	510-535	14.4	12.2	6.1
363LF	27-363150LF	560-585	15	12.6	6.2
363LF	27-363154LF	620-645	15.4	13	6.5
363LF	27-363158LF	690-720	15.8	13.4	6.8

Shape: BioDIMENSIONAL; height: low; profile (projection): full; surface: BIOCELL; diaphragm valve: anterior.

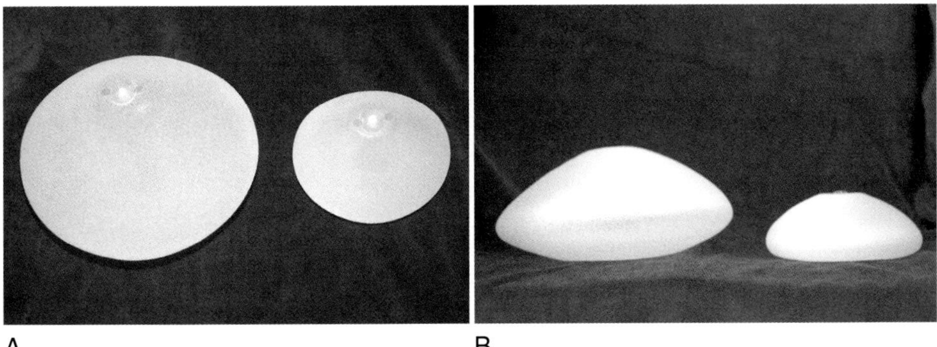

A B

FIGURE 143-15. INAMED Style 363LF saline-filled breast implant: low height. *A,* Anterior view. *B,* Lateral view.

INAMED STYLE 468 SALINE-FILLED BREAST IMPLANTS: FULL HEIGHT. INAMED Style 468 saline-filled, shaped, textured breast implants are full-height BioDIMENSIONAL-compatible implants. They were specifically designed for use with INAMED Style 133 HV tissue expanders but may easily be adapted to the INAMED Style 133 MV and 133 LV series with appropriate adjustment of the upper pole pocket at the second operative intervention. These implants are offered in volumes from 195 to 650 mL in 10 distinct implant sizes. They present with an anterior fill diaphragm valve (Table 143-10 and Fig. 143-16).

TABLE 143-10 ✦ INAMED STYLE 468 SALINE-FILLED BREAST IMPLANTS: FULL HEIGHT

Style	Catalog No.	Fill Volume (mL)	Width (cm)	Height (cm)	Projection (cm)
468	27-468196	195-205	10	10.5	4
468	27-468231	230-240	10.5	11	4.2
468	27-468271	270-285	11	11.5	4.3
468	27-468301	300-315	11.5	12	4.6
468	27-468351	350-370	12	12.5	4.8
468	27-468381	380-400	12.5	13	4.9
468	27-468451	450-475	13	13.5	5.3
468	27-468496	495-520	13.5	14	5.5
468	27-468561	560-590	14	14.5	5.7
468	27-468621	620-650	14.5	15	5.9

Shape: BioDIMENSIONAL; profile (projection): low; surface: BIOCELL; diaphragm valve: anterior.

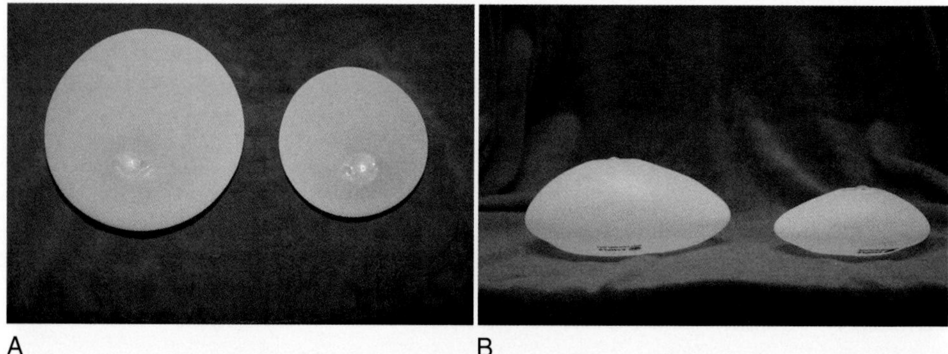

A B

FIGURE 143-16. INAMED Style 468 saline-filled breast implant: full height. *A,* Anterior view. *B,* Lateral view.

Mentor Corporation Anatomic-Shaped Saline-Filled Breast Implants

Mentor Corporation offers two distinct series of Contour Profile-compatible, shaped, saline-filled breast implants for the second stage of implant-based breast reconstruction. Both series of implants are protected by the Siltex textured surface and are produced with anterior fill diaphragm valves.

MENTOR STYLE 2900 SALINE-FILLED BREAST IMPLANTS: MODERATE PROJECTION PROFILE. Mentor Style 2900 saline-filled, shaped, textured breast implants were designed for use with Mentor Contour Profile tissue expanders. Specifically, these implants are of a moderate projection profile design. Implants with volumes from 175 to 200 mL and 525 to 575 mL are available in six distinct implant sizes. Base diameters range from 10.2 to 14.9 cm with heights from 8.5 to 12.5 cm and projection of 4.3 to 5.6 cm (Table 143-11 and Fig. 143-17).

TABLE 143-11 ✦ MENTOR STYLE 2900 SALINE-FILLED BREAST IMPLANTS: MODERATE PROJECTION PROFILE

Style	Catalog No.	Fill Volume (mL)	Width (cm)	Height (cm)	Projection (cm)
2900	354-2910	175 + 25	10.2	8.5	4.3
2900	354-2911	225 + 25	11.2	9.4	4.5
2900	354-2912	275 + 25	12.2	10.3	4.5
2900	354-2913	350 + 50	13.1	11	4.7
2900	354-2914	425 + 50	13.8	11.6	5.2
2900	354-2915	525 + 50	14.9	12.5	5.6

Shape: contour profile; profile (projection): moderate; surface: Siltex; diaphragm valve: anterior.

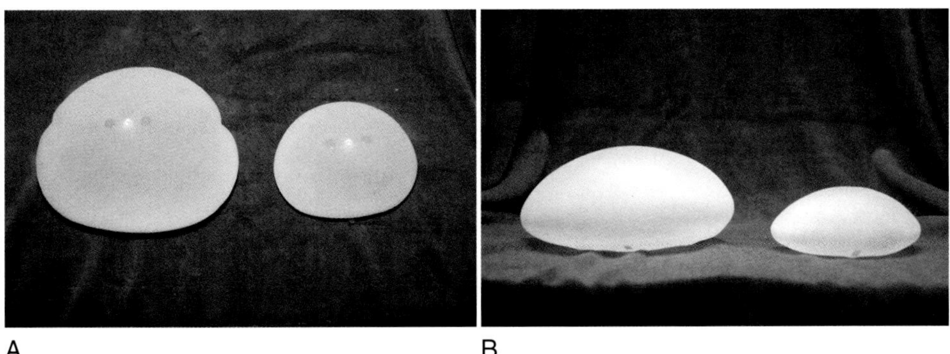

A B

FIGURE 143-17. Mentor Style 2900 saline-filled breast implant: moderate projection profile. *A,* Anterior view. *B,* Lateral view.

MENTOR STYLE 2700 SALINE-FILLED BREAST IMPLANTS: HIGH PROJECTION PROFILE. Mentor Style 2700 saline-filled, shaped, textured breast implants were designed for use with the Mentor Contour Profile tissue expanders. This series of implants differs from the 2900 series in that base diameter dimensions are foreshortened in exchange for augmented projection parameters. For example, the 2900 series 350-mL implant with a base diameter of 13.1 cm has 4.7 cm of projection relative to the 2700 series implant with the same volume, which has a base diameter of 12.3 cm and a projection of 5.3 cm. Height of the 2700 series implant also contributes to increased projection (11 cm versus 10.5 cm for a 350-mL fill volume) (Table 143-12 and Fig. 143-18).

TABLE 143-12 ✦ MENTOR STYLE 2700 SALINE-FILLED BREAST IMPLANTS: HIGH PROJECTION PROFILE

Style	Catalog No.	Fill Volume (mL)	Width (cm)	Height (cm)	Projection (cm)
2700	354-2711	275 + 25	11.5	9.5	5.1
2700	354-2712	350 + 50	12.3	10.5	5.3
2700	354-2713	450 + 50	13.2	11	6.1
2700	354-2714	550 + 50	14	11.9	6.4
2700	354-2715	650 + 75	15	12.7	6.6

Shape: contour profile; profile (projection): high; surface: Siltex; diaphragm valve: anterior.

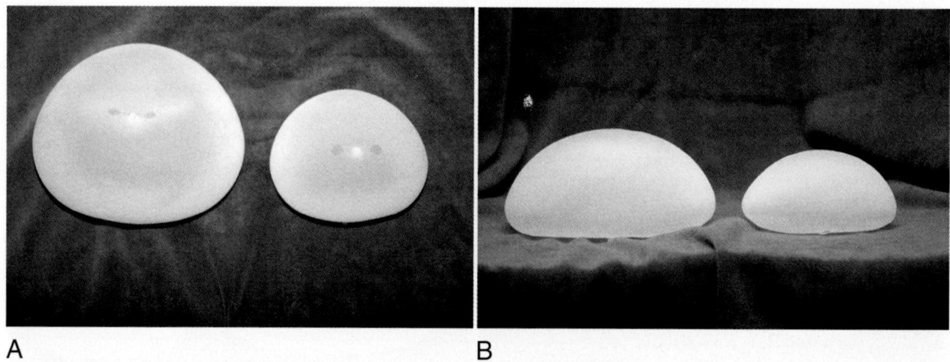

A B

FIGURE 143-18. Mentor Style 2700 saline-filled breast implant: high projection profile. *A,* Anterior view. *B,* Lateral view.

ROUND SALINE-FILLED BREAST IMPLANTS

INAMED Aesthetics Round Saline-Filled Breast Implants

INAMED offers four distinct styles of round saline-filled breast implants. Three of the styles offered are smooth walled and distinctly are not textured. Style 168 is offered with BIOCELL texturing to prevent capsular contracture. The styles differ with regard to their projection profile (low, moderate, and high). Implant base diameter and height parameters are diminished to provide increased projection. Implants with minimum and maximum volume recommendations and final base diameter and projection dimensions are provided by the manufacturer. Overfilling to more than the maximum volume is not recommended. All styles are offered with anterior fill diaphragm valves.

INAMED STYLE 68LP SALINE-FILLED BREAST IMPLANTS: LOW PROJECTION PROFILE. INAMED Style 68LP breast implants are low-projection profile, smooth-walled, round, saline-filled prostheses that can be used for second-stage breast reconstruction. Volumes from 125 to 700 mL are offered in 19 distinct implant sizes. A minimum diameter of 9.3 cm with an associated 3.2 cm projection is provided by the 125- to 145-mL volume implant. The largest implant of this style is 680 to 700 mL with a base diameter of 16.1 cm and an associated projection of 4.7 cm (Table 143-13 and Fig. 143-19).

TABLE 143-13 ✦ INAMED STYLE 68LP SALINE-FILLED BREAST IMPLANTS: LOW PROJECTION PROFILE

		Dimensions at Minimum Volume		Dimensions at Maximum Volume	
Style	**Fill Volume (mL)**	*Diameter (cm)*	*Projection (cm)*	*Diameter (cm)*	*Projection (cm)*
68LP	125-145	9.5	2.6	9.3	3.2
68LP	150-170	10	2.7	9.9	3.2
68LP	175-195	10.6	2.8	10.4	3.3
68LP	200-220	11	3	10.9	3.4
68LP	225-245	11.4	3.1	11.3	3.4
68LP	250-270	11.9	3.2	11.7	3.5
68LP	275-295	12.2	3.3	12.1	3.6
68LP	300-320	12.5	3.4	12.4	3.7
68LP	325-345	12.9	3.5	12.7	3.8
68LP	350-370	13.3	3.6	13.2	3.8
68LP	400-420	13.5	3.8	13.4	4.2
68LP	420-440	13.9	3.9	13.8	4.1
68LP	440-460	14.2	3.9	14.1	4.1
68LP	480-500	14.5	4	14.4	4.3
68LP	535-545	14.8	4.2	14.7	4.5
68LP	550-570	15.1	4.3	15	4.5
68LP	600-620	15.4	4.4	15.3	4.6
68LP	640-660	15.8	4.5	15.7	4.7
68LP	680-700	16.2	4.5	16.1	4.7

Shape: round; profile (projection): low; surface: smooth; diaphragm valve: anterior.

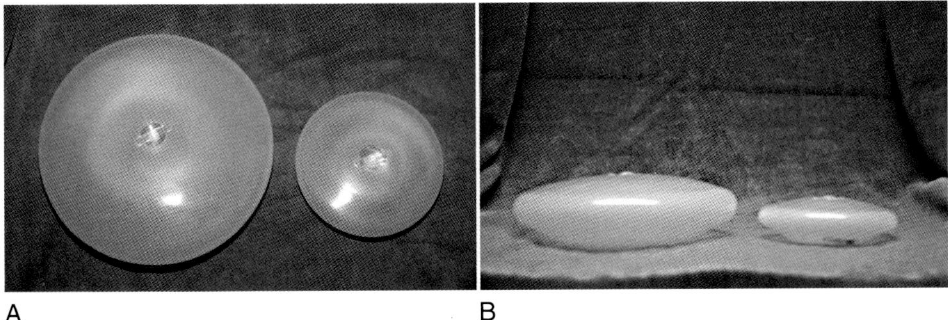

FIGURE 143-19. INAMED Style 68LP saline-filled breast implant: low projection profile. *A,* Anterior view. *B,* Lateral view.

INAMED STYLE 68MP SALINE-FILLED BREAST IMPLANTS: MODERATE PROJECTION PROFILE. INAMED Style 68MP breast implants are moderate-projection profile, smooth-walled, round, saline-filled prostheses that can be used for second-stage breast reconstruction. Volumes from 120 to 850 mL are offered in 20 distinct implant sizes. The smallest of this style of implant (120 to 150 mL) has a base diameter of 9 cm and an associated projection of 3 cm as reported by the manufacturer. Whether this reflects dimensions of the 120-mL fill volume (minimum recommended fill volume) or a 150-mL fill volume (maximum recommended fill volume) is not defined by INAMED. Comparison of the Style 68LP 700-mL fill volume implant with a projection of 4.7 cm with the Style 68MP 700-mL fill volume implant with projection of 5.3 cm illustrates this concept of differential projection profiles (Table 143-14 and Fig. 143-20).

TABLE 143-14 ✦ INAMED STYLE 68MP SALINE-FILLED BREAST IMPLANTS: MODERATE PROJECTION PROFILE

Style	Catalog No.	Fill Volume (mL)	Diameter (cm)	Projection (cm)
68MP	25-68121	120-150	9	3
68MP	25-68151	150-180	9.6	3.3
68MP	25-68181	180-210	10.2	3.4
68MP	25-68211	210-240	10.6	3.7
68MP	25-68241	240-270	11	3.8
68MP	25-68271	270-300	11.6	3.9
68MP	25-68301	300-330	11.9	4.1
68MP	25-68331	330-360	12.3	4.2
68MP	25-68361	360-390	12.7	4.2
68MP	25-68391	390-420	13	4.5
68MP	25-68421	420-450	13.4	4.5
68MP	25-68451	450-480	13.7	4.6
68MP	25-68481	480-510	14.1	4.6
68MP	25-68511	510-540	14.4	4.6
68MP	25-68551	550-600	14.6	4.9
68MP	25-68601	600-650	15	5
68MP	25-68651	650-700	15.2	5.3
68MP	25-68701	700-750	15.6	5.4
68MP	25-68751	750-800	15.9	5.6
68MP	25-68801	800-850	16.4	5.6

Shape: round; profile (projection): moderate; surface: smooth; diaphragm valve: anterior.

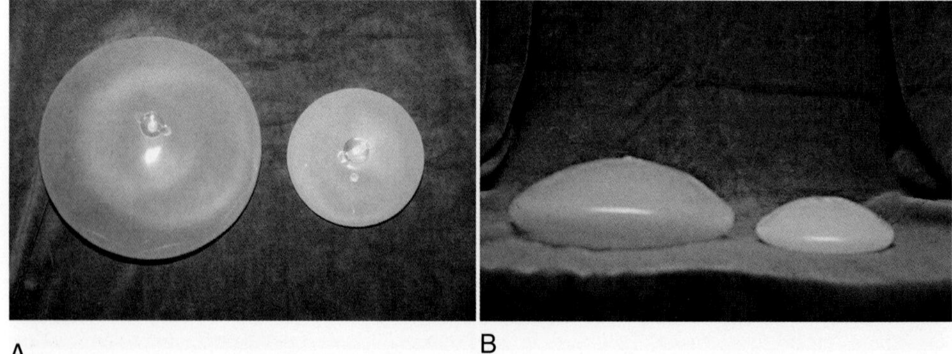

A B

FIGURE 143-20. INAMED Style 68MP saline-filled breast implant: moderate projection profile. *A*, Anterior view. *B*, Lateral view.

INAMED STYLE 68HP BREAST IMPLANTS: HIGH PROJECTION PROFILE. INAMED Style 68HP breast implants are high-projection profile, smooth-walled, round, saline-filled prostheses that can be used for second-stage breast reconstruction. Volumes from 160 to 850 mL are offered in 16 distinct implant sizes. The smallest of this style implant is 160 to 175 mL with a minimum fill base diameter of 9 cm and projection of 3.9 cm and a maximum fill base diameter of 8.8 cm and projection of 4.3 cm. The largest implant of this style is 800 to 850 mL with a minimum fill base diameter of 15 cm and projection of 6.7 cm and a maximum fill base diameter of 14.7 cm and projection of 7.2 cm. This implant offers the most significant projection-to-volume ratio commercially available by INAMED Aesthetics (Table 143-15 and Fig. 143-21).

TABLE 143-15 ✦ INAMED STYLE 68HP SALINE-FILLED BREAST IMPLANTS: HIGH PROJECTION PROFILE

			Dimensions at Minimum Volume		Dimensions at Maximum Volume	
Style	**Catalog No.**	**Fill Volume (mL)**	*Diameter (cm)*	*Projection (cm)*	*Diameter (cm)*	*Projection (cm)*
68HP	25-68160HP	160-175	9	3.9	8.8	4.3
68HP	25-68200HP	200-220	9.6	4.2	9.5	4.6
68HP	25-68240HP	240-260	10.2	4.4	10	5
68HP	25-68280HP	280-300	10.6	4.7	10.5	5.2
68HP	25-68320HP	320-340	11.1	4.9	11	5.3
68HP	25-68350HP	350-380	11.6	4.9	11.4	5.5
68HP	25-68400HP	400-430	11.9	5	11.7	5.9
68HP	25-68425HP	425-455	12.3	5.3	12.1	5.9
68HP	25-68465HP	465-505	12.6	5.6	12.5	6.1
68HP	25-68500HP	500-540	13	5.7	12.8	6.3
68HP	25-68550HP	550-590	13.3	5.8	13.1	6.4
68HP	25-68600HP	600-640	13.7	6	13.5	6.6
68HP	25-68650HP	650-700	14	6.1	13.8	6.9
68HP	25-68700HP	700-750	14.4	6.2	14.1	7.1
68HP	25-68750HP	750-800	14.6	6.5	14.4	7.2
68HP	25-68800HP	800-850	15	6.7	14.7	7.2

Shape: round; profile (projection): high; surface: smooth; diaphragm valve: anterior.

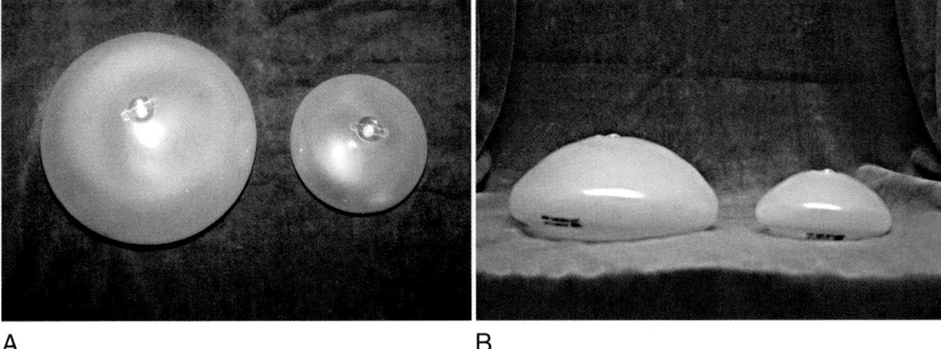

A B

FIGURE 143-21. INAMED Style 68HP saline-filled breast implant: high projection profile. *A,* Anterior view. *B,* Lateral view.

INAMED Style 168 Breast Implants: Moderate Projection Profile. INAMED Style 168 breast implants are moderate-projection profile, BIOCELL textured surface-walled, round, saline-filled prostheses that can be used for second-stage breast reconstruction. Volumes from 120 to 850 mL are offered in 20 distinct implant sizes as are offered in the INAMED Style 68MP profile, exactly. INAMED Style 168 is a textured form of the INAMED Style 68MP series (Table 143-16 and Fig. 143-22).

TABLE 143-16 ✦ INAMED STYLE 168 SALINE-FILLED BREAST IMPLANTS: MODERATE PROJECTION PROFILE

Style	Catalog No.	Fill Volume (mL)	Diameter (cm)	Projection (cm)
168	27-168121	120-150	9	3
168	27-168151	150-180	9.6	3.3
168	27-168181	180-210	10.2	3.4
168	27-168211	210-240	10.6	3.7
168	27-168241	240-270	11.1	3.8
168	27-168271	270-300	11.6	3.9
168	27-168301	300-330	11.9	4.1
168	27-168331	330-360	12.3	4.2
168	27-168361	360-390	12.7	4.2
168	27-168391	390-420	13	4.5
168	27-168421	420-450	13.4	4.5
168	27-168451	450-480	13.7	4.6
168	27-168481	480-510	14.1	4.6
168	27-168511	510-540	14.4	4.6
168	27-168551	550-600	14.6	4.9
168	27-168601	600-650	15	5
168	27-168651	650-700	15.2	5.3
168	27-168701	700-750	15.6	5.4
168	27-168751	750-800	15.9	5.6
168	27-168801	800-850	16.4	5.6

Shape: round; profile (projection): moderate; surface: moderate; diaphragm valve: anterior.

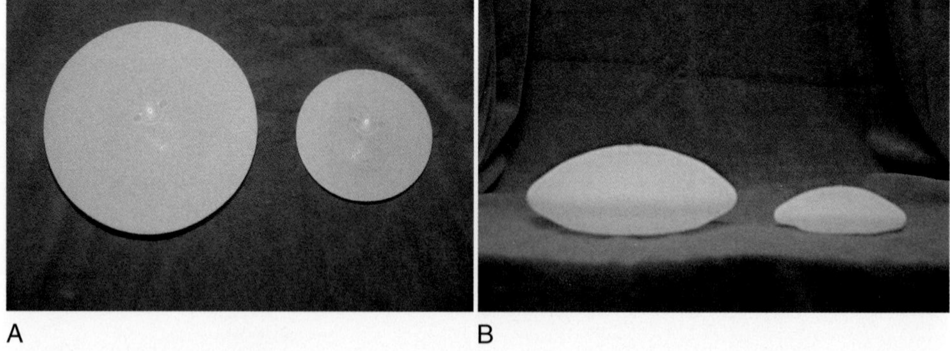

A B

FIGURE 143-22. INAMED Style 168 saline-filled breast implant: moderate projection profile. *A,* Anterior view. *B,* Lateral view.

Mentor Corporation Round Saline-Filled Breast Implants

Mentor Corporation offers three styles of round saline-filled breast implants. Two styles are smooth walled, with either a moderate or high projection profile. The characteristics of the high-projection profile smooth-walled model and the moderate-projection textured model are described here. The moderate-projection profile smooth-walled model, Mentor Style 1600, is also available. Mentor Corporation may be contacted for further details.

MENTOR STYLE 3000 SALINE-FILLED BREAST IMPLANTS: HIGH PROJECTION PROFILE. Mentor Style 3000 breast implants are high-projection profile, smooth-walled, round, saline-filled prostheses that can be used for second-stage breast reconstruction. Volumes from 170 to 750 mL are offered in 15 distinct implant sizes. Comparison of the Mentor Style 3000 (500 to 600 mL) filled to 500 mL with the INAMED Style 68HP (500 to 540 mL) filled to 500 mL indicates base diameters of 12.8 cm versus 13.0 cm and projections of 5.6 cm versus 5.7 cm. As a generality, the Mentor Style 3000 has a larger fill range (30 to 80 mL) than the INAMED 68HP (15 to 50 mL) from the smallest to the largest implant (170 versus 160 mL, 750 versus 850 mL), which may reflect a difference in the appearance of the implant at lower filling volumes. It is suggested that one might elect to preferentially use Mentor Style 1600 breast implants at the higher fill volumes to prevent rippling and contour irregularities. Overfilling of this implant is not recommended (Table 143-17 and Fig. 143-23).

TABLE 143-17 ✦ MENTOR STYLE 3000 SALINE-FILLED BREAST IMPLANTS: HIGH PROJECTION PROFILE

			Dimensions at Minimum Volume		Dimensions at Maximum Volume	
Style	**Catalog No.**	**Fill Volume (mL)**	*Diameter (cm)*	*Projection (cm)*	*Diameter (cm)*	*Projection (cm)*
3000	350-3170	170-200	9	4	8.8	4.9
3000	350-3190	190-225	9.3	4.1	9.1	5.1
3000	350-3210	210-250	9.6	4.2	9.5	5.3
3000	350-3230	230-275	10	4.3	9.8	5.5
3000	350-3250	250-300	10.2	4.5	10	5.6
3000	350-3270	270-325	10.4	4.6	10.2	5.8
3000	350-3290	290-350	10.8	4.7	10.5	5.9
3000	350-3310	310-375	11	4.8	10.7	6
3000	350-3330	330-400	11.3	4.8	11	6.2
3000	350-3380	380-450	11.7	5.2	11.4	6.4
3000	350-3420	420-500	12	5.4	11.7	6.7
3000	350-3460	460-550	12.4	5.5	12.1	6.9
3000	350-3500	500-600	12.8	5.6	12.4	7.1
3000	350-3560	560-675	13.4	5.7	13.1	7.3
3000	350-3630	630-750	13.8	5.9	13.4	7.4

Shape: round; profile (projection): high; surface: smooth; diaphragm valve: anterior.

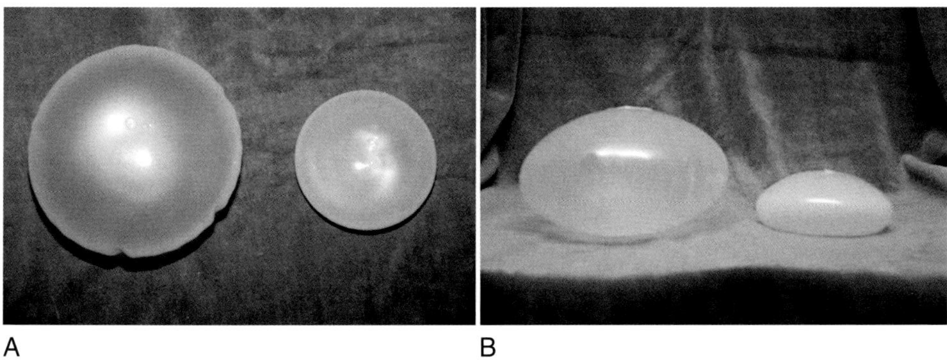

A B

FIGURE 143-23. Mentor Style 3000 saline-filled breast implant: high projection profile. *A,* Anterior view. *B,* Lateral view.

MENTOR STYLE 2600 SALINE-FILLED BREAST IMPLANTS: MODERATE PROJECTION PROFILE. Mentor Style 2600 breast implants are moderate-projection profile, Siltex textured, round, saline-filled breast implants that can be used for second-stage breast reconstruction. Volumes from 125 to 525 mL are offered in 13 distinct implant sizes. Nominal and maximum fill implant dimensions are not provided by the manufacturer. Comparison of the Mentor Style 2600 implant size 375 to 425 mL with the INAMED Style 168 implant size 390 to 420 mL relates base diameters of 13.6 cm versus 13 cm and projections of 4 cm versus 4.5 cm. Note that these comparisons may be compromised on the basis of the 50-mL fill range reported for the Mentor implant (Table 143-18 and Fig. 143-24).

TABLE 143-18 ✦ MENTOR STYLE 2600 SALINE-FILLED BREAST IMPLANTS: MODERATE PROJECTION PROFILE

Style	Catalog No.	Fill Volume (mL)	Diameter (cm)	Projection (cm)
2600	354-2610	125 + 25	9.5	3
2600	354-2615	150 + 25	10	3.1
2600	354-2620	175 + 25	10.6	3.3
2600	354-2625	200 + 25	11	3.4
2600	354-2630	225 + 25	11.5	3.5
2600	354-2635	250 + 25	11.9	3.6
2600	354-2640	275 + 25	12.3	3.7
2600	354-2645	300 + 25	12.6	3.7
2600	354-2650	325 + 50	13	3.8
2600	354-2655	350 + 50	13.3	3.9
2600	354-2660	375 + 50	13.6	4
2600	354-2670	425 + 50	14.2	4.1
2600	354-2680	475 + 50	14.8	4.2

Shape: round; profile (projection): moderate; surface: Siltex; diaphragm valve: anterior.

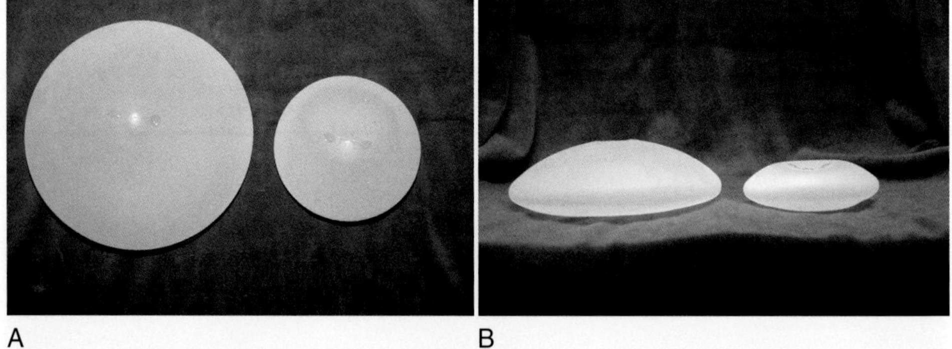

A B

FIGURE 143-24. Mentor Style 2600 saline-filled breast implant: moderate projection profile. *A,* Anterior view. *B,* Lateral view.

ANATOMIC-SHAPED SILICONE-FILLED BREAST IMPLANTS

INAMED Aesthetics is currently the only manufacturer to offer an anatomic or shaped silicone-filled breast implant for breast reconstruction. This implant is INAMED Style 153 and is compatible with the BioDIMENSIONAL system Style 133 V of INAMED tissue expanders. It is BIOCELL textured and is released with a low-diffusion shell that features a barrier coat between two layers of silicone elastomer (Intrashiel barrier). It is described as full height and full projection, which can be translated to full height and high-projection profile as these terms have previously been used in the text. Silicone-filled breast implants are available in the United States only by participation in restricted clinical trials. Contact INAMED for additional eligibility information for participation by physicians and patients (Table 143-19 and Fig. 143-25).

TABLE 143-19 ✦ INAMED STYLE 153 (SILICONE-FILLED) BREAST IMPLANTS: FULL HEIGHT AND FULL PROJECTION PROFILE

Style	Catalog No.	Shape	Fill Volume (mL)	Width (cm)	Height (cm)	Projection (cm)
153	27-153361	BioDIMENSIONAL	360	12.3	13.1	4.5
153	27-153451	BioDIMENSIONAL	450	13.1	14.1	4.9
153	27-153541	BioDIMENSIONAL	540	13.9	14.9	5.2
153	27-153631	BioDIMENSIONAL	630	14.6	15.7	5.5
153	27-153721	BioDIMENSIONAL	720	15.9	16.9	5.6

Height: full; projection: full; surface: BIOCELL; shell characteristics: Intrashiel barrier.

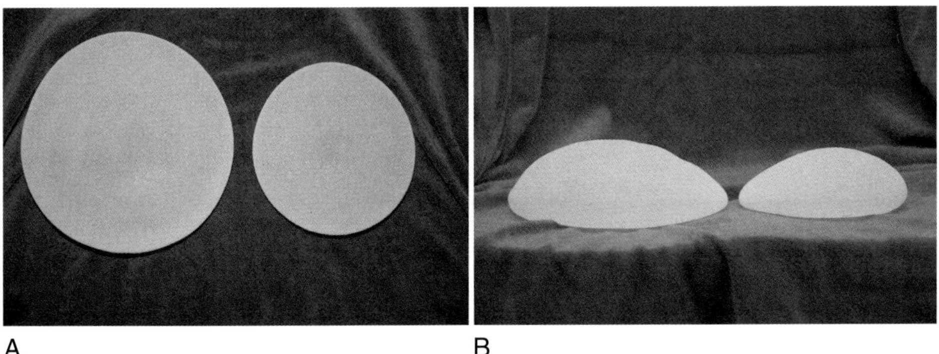

A B

FIGURE 143-25. INAMED Style 153 silicone-filled, anatomic-shaped breast implant: full height and high projection profile. *A,* Anterior view. *B,* Lateral view.

ROUND SILICONE-FILLED BREAST IMPLANTS

INAMED Aesthetics Round Silicone-Filled Breast Implants

INAMED Aesthetics offers a wide selection of round silicone-filled breast implants for use in two-stage breast reconstruction given participation by patients and physicians in appropriate clinical trials. Four styles of smooth-walled implants and two styles of textured implants are available in a wide selection of sizes for optimal and precise implant-based breast reconstructions.

INAMED Style 10 Silicone-Filled Breast Implants: Moderate Projection Profile. INAMED Style 10 breast implants are smooth shell implants with a moderate projection profile. Implant volumes range from 120 to 800 mL in 20 distinct implant sizes. Base diameters range from 9.4 to 17.2 cm with projection ranges from 2.5 to 4.9 cm (Table 143-20 and Fig. 143-26).

TABLE 143-20 ✦ INAMED STYLE 10 SILICONE-FILLED BREAST IMPLANTS: MODERATE PROJECTION PROFILE

Style	Catalog No.	Fill Volume (mL)	Diameter (cm)	Projection (cm)
10	24-10120	120	9.4	2.5
10	24-10150	150	10.1	2.7
10	24-10180	180	10.7	2.9
10	24-10210	210	11.2	3
10	24-10240	240	11.7	3.2
10	24-10270	270	12.2	3.3
10	24-10300	300	12.6	3.5
10	24-10330	330	13	3.6
10	24-10360	360	13.4	3.7
10	24-10390	390	13.6	3.8
10	24-10420	420	14	3.8
10	24-10450	450	14.4	3.9
10	24-10480	480	14.8	3.9
10	24-10510	510	15.1	4
10	24-10550	550	15.4	4
10	24-10600	600	15.8	4.3
10	24-10650	650	16	4.5
10	24-10700	700	16.4	4.6
10	24-10750	750	16.8	4.8
10	24-10800	800	17.2	4.9

Shape: round; profile (projection): moderate; surface: smooth; shell characteristics: Intrashiel barrier.

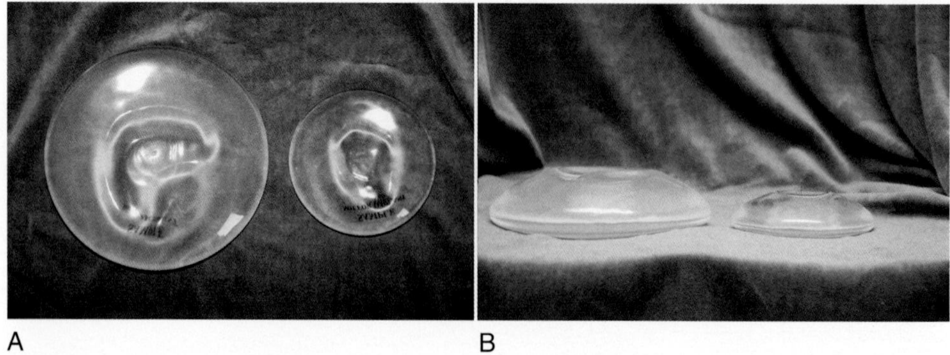

FIGURE 143-26. INAMED Style 10 silicone-filled breast implant: moderate projection profile. *A*, Anterior view. *B*, Lateral view.

INAMED STYLE 20 SILICONE-FILLED BREAST IMPLANTS: HIGH PROJECTION PROFLE. INAMED Style 20 silicone-filled breast implants are smooth shell implants with a full (high) projection profile. Implant volumes range from 120 to 800 mL in 23 distinct implant sizes. Base diameters range from 9.0 to 15.3 cm with projection ranges from 2.7 to 6.1 cm. Transition to the full (high) projection profile again reflects loss of base diameter and height for increased projection (Table 143-21 and Fig. 143-27).

TABLE 143-21 ✦ INAMED STYLE 20 SILICONE-FILLED BREAST IMPLANTS: FULL PROJECTION PROFILE

Style	Catalog No.	Fill Volume (mL)	Diameter (cm)	Projection (cm)
20	24-20120	120	9	2.7
20	24-20140	140	9.1	3.3
20	24-20160	160	9.4	3.5
20	24-20180	180	9.6	3.8
20	24-20200	200	9.7	4
20	24-20230	230	10	4.2
20	24-20260	260	10.4	4.3
20	24-20280	280	10.6	4.5
20	24-20300	300	10.9	4.5
20	24-20325	325	11.2	4.6
20	24-20350	350	11.4	4.9
20	24-20375	375	11.7	4.9
20	24-20400	400	11.9	5
20	24-20425	435	12	5.2
20	24-20450	450	12.4	5.2
20	24-20475	475	12.6	5.5
20	24-20500	500	13	5.2
20	24-20550	550	13.5	5.6
20	24-20600	600	13.8	5.7
20	24-20650	650	14.2	5.9
20	24-20700	700	14.5	6.2
20	24-20750	750	15	6
20	24-20800	800	15.3	6.1

Shape: round; profile (projection): full; surface: smooth; shell characteristics: Intrashiel barrier.

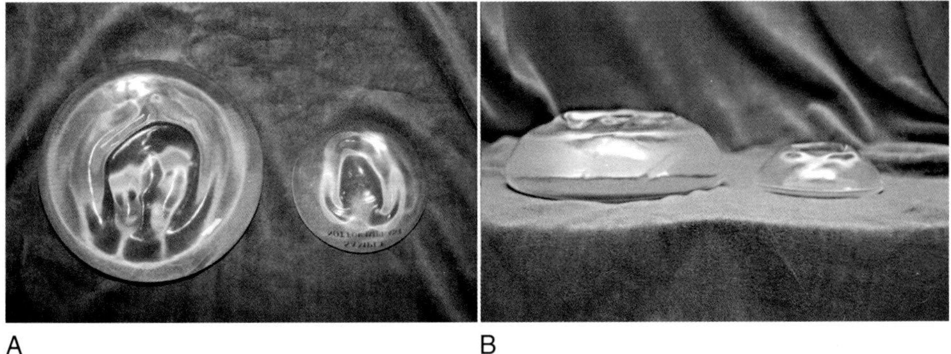

A B

FIGURE 143-27. INAMED Style 20 silicone-filled breast implant: high projection profile. *A*, Anterior view. *B*, Lateral view.

INAMED STYLE 40 SILICONE-FILLED BREAST IMPLANTS: MODERATE PROJECTION PROFILE. INAMED Style 40 silicone-filled breast implants are smooth shell implants with a standard (moderate) projection profile. Implant volumes range from 80 to 560 mL in 19 distinct implant sizes. Base diameters range from 8.8 to 14.7 cm with projection ranges from 1.7 to 4.6 cm (Table 143-22 and Fig. 143-28).

TABLE 143-22 ✦ INAMED STYLE 40 SILICONE-FILLED BREAST IMPLANTS: MODERATE PROJECTION PROFILE

Style	Catalog No.	Fill Volume (mL)	Diameter (cm)	Projection (cm)
40	25-40081	80	8.8	1.7
40	25-40101	100	8.9	2.2
40	25-40121	120	9.1	2.5
40	25-40141	140	9.4	2.7
40	25-40161	160	9.7	3.1
40	25-40181	180	10	3.3
40	25-40201	200	10.2	3.5
40	25-40221	220	10.5	3.6
40	25-40241	240	10.9	3.7
40	25-40261	260	11.2	3.8
40	25-40281	280	11.4	3.8
40	25-40301	300	11.7	3.9
40	25-40321	320	12	3.9
40	25-40341	340	12.3	4
40	25-40361	360	12.5	4.1
40	25-40401	400	12.7	4.2
40	25-40461	460	13.8	4.2
40	25-40501	500	14.2	4.3
40	25-40561	560	14.7	4.6

Shape: round; profile (projection): moderate; surface: smooth; shell characteristics: Intrashiel barrier.

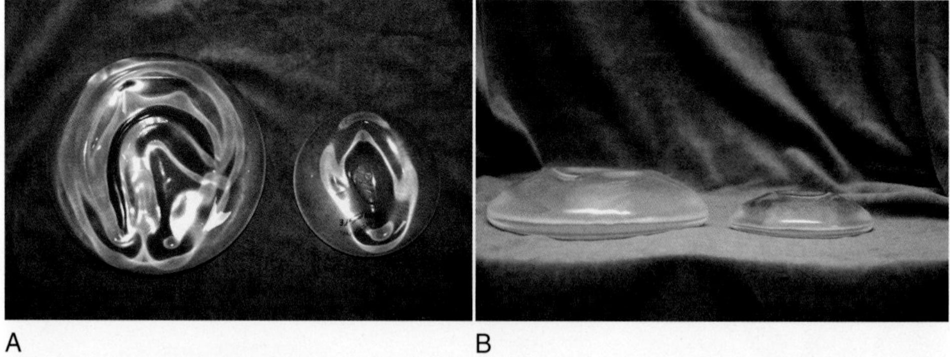

A B

FIGURE 143-28. INAMED Style 40 silicone-filled breast implant: moderate projection profile. *A*, Anterior view. *B*, Lateral view.

INAMED STYLE 45 SILICONE-FILLED BREAST IMPLANTS: HIGH "UPPER PORTION" PROJECTION PROFILE. INAMED Style 45 silicone-filled breast implants are smooth shell implants with a high "upper portion" breast projection. Implant volumes range from 120 to 800 mL in 15 distinct implant sizes. Base diameters range from 7.4 to 14.2 cm with projection ranges from 3.6 to 6.7 cm (Table 143-23 and Fig. 143-29).

TABLE 143-23 ✦ INAMED STYLE 45 SILICONE-FILLED BREAST IMPLANTS: HIGH "UPPER PORTION" PROJECTION PROFILE

Style	Catalog No.	Fill Volume (mL)	Diameter (cm)	Projection (cm)
45	25-45121	120	7.4	3.6
45	25-45161	160	8.2	3.8
45	25-45201	200	9	4.1
45	25-45241	240	9.6	4.3
45	25-45281	280	10	4.6
45	25-45321	320	10.4	4.8
45	25-45361	360	10.8	5.1
45	25-45401	400	11.2	5.1
45	25-45461	460	11.4	5.9
45	25-45501	500	11.9	5.7
45	25-45551	550	12.4	6
45	25-45601	600	12.8	6.1
45	25-45651	650	13.2	6.2
45	25-45701	700	13.5	6.4
45	25-45801	800	14.2	6.7

Shape: round; profile (projection): full; surface: smooth; shell characteristics: Intrashiel barrier.

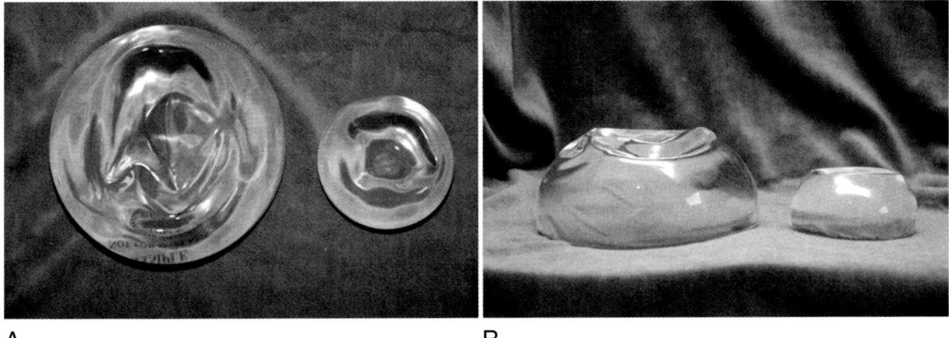

A B

FIGURE 143-29. INAMED Style 45 silicone-filled breast implant: high "upper portion" projection profile. *A*, Anterior view. *B*, Lateral view.

INAMED STYLE 110 SILICONE-FILLED BREAST IMPLANTS: MODERATE PROJECTION PROFILE. INAMED Style 110 silicone-filled breast implants are textured shell implants with a moderate projection profile. Implant volumes range from 90 to 510 mL in 15 distinct implant sizes. Base diameters range from 8.7 to 15.5 cm with projection ranges from 2.0 to 3.4 cm (Table 143-24 and Fig. 143-30).

TABLE 143-24 ✦ INAMED STYLE 110 SILICONE-FILLED BREAST IMPLANTS: MODERATE PROJECTION PROFILE

Style	Catalog No.	Fill Volume (mL)	Diameter (cm)	Projection (cm)
110	27-110091	90	8.7	2
110	27-110121	120	9	2.4
110	27-110151	150	9.7	2.5
110	27-110181	180	10.3	2.7
110	27-110211	210	11.1	2.8
110	27-110241	240	11.7	2.9
110	27-110271	270	12.3	3
110	27-110301	300	12.6	3.1
110	27-110331	330	12.8	3.1
110	27-110361	360	13.5	3.2
110	27-110391	390	13.7	3.2
110	27-110421	420	13.9	3.3
110	27-110451	450	14.3	3.3
110	27-110481	480	15.1	3.3
110	27-110511	510	15.5	3.4

Shape: round; profile (projection): moderate; surface: BIOCELL; shell characteristics: Intrashiel barrier.

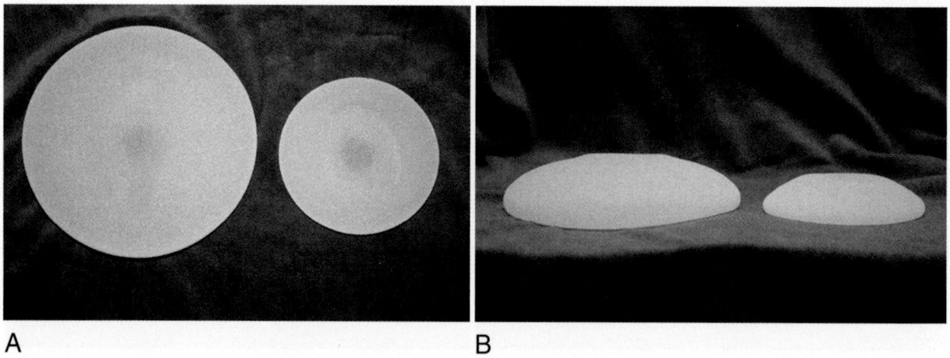

FIGURE 143-30. INAMED Style 110 silicone-filled breast implant: moderate projection profile. *A*, Anterior view. *B*, Lateral view.

INAMED STYLE 120 SILICONE-FILLED BREAST IMPLANTS: HIGH PROJECTION PROFILE. INAMED Style 120 silicone-filled breast implants are textured shell implants with a high projection profile. Implant volumes range from 180 to 650 mL in 11 distinct implant sizes. Base diameters range from 9.4 to 15.5 cm with projection ranges from 3.3 to 5.0 cm (Table 143-25 and Fig. 143-31).

TABLE 143-25 ✦ INAMED STYLE 120 (SILICONE-FILLED) BREAST IMPLANTS: HIGH PROJECTION PROFILE

Style	Catalog No.	Fill Volume (mL)	Diameter (cm)	Projection (cm)
120	27-120181	180	9.4	3.3
120	27-120221	220	9.9	3.7
120	27-120261	260	10.6	4
120	27-120301	300	11	4.2
120	27-120341	340	11.5	4.3
120	27-120401	400	12.1	4
120	27-120441	440	12.7	4.6
120	27-120501	500	13.5	4.7
120	27-120551	550	13.9	4.8
120	27-120601	600	14.5	4.9
120	27-120651	650	15.5	5

Shape: round; profile (projection): high; surface: BIOCELL; shell characteristics: Intrashiel barrier.

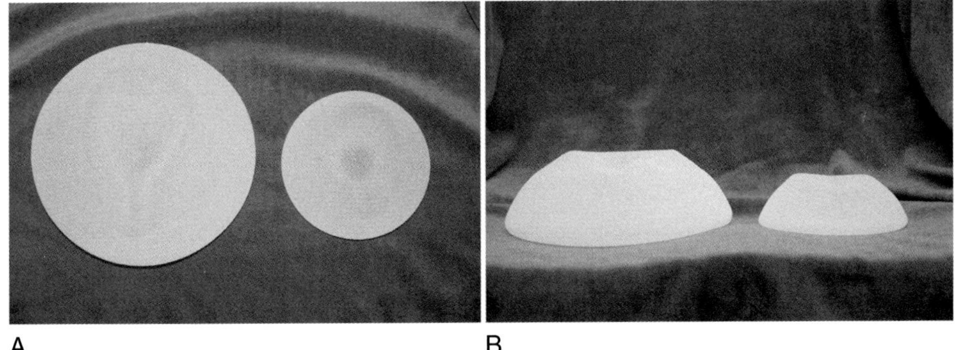

FIGURE 143-31. INAMED Style 120 silicone-filled breast implant: high projection profile. *A*, Anterior view. *B*, Lateral view.

Mentor Corporation Round Silicone-Filled Breast Implants

MENTOR STYLE 350 SILICONE-FILLED BREAST IMPLANTS: MODERATE PROJECTION PROFILE. Mentor Style 350-Moderate Projection Profile series of silicone breast implants are smooth shell implants with a moderate projection profile. Implant volumes range from 100 to 800 mL in 19 distinct implant sizes. Base diameters range from 9.3 to 18.2 cm with projection ranges from 2.1 to 4.1 cm (Table 143-26 and Fig. 143-32).

TABLE 143-26 ✦ MENTOR STYLE 350 (SILICONE-FILLED) BREAST IMPLANTS: MODERATE PROJECTION PROFILE

Style	Catalog No.	Fill Volume (mL)	Diameter (cm)	Projection (cm)
350	350-7100BC	100	9.3	2.1
350	350-7125BC	125	10	2.2
350	350-7150BC	150	10.3	2.3
350	350-7175BC	175	11.2	2.4
350	350-7200BC	200	11.7	2.5
350	350-7225BC	225	12.2	2.6
350	350-7250BC	250	12.3	2.8
350	350-7275BC	275	13.2	2.9
350	350-7300BC	300	13.5	3
350	350-7325BC	325	13.9	3
350	350-7350BC	350	14.2	3.1
350	350-7375BC	375	14.4	3.2
350	350-7400BC	400	14.5	3.2
350	350-7450BC	450	14.9	3.4
350	350-7500BC	500	15.2	3.6
350	350-7550BC	550	15.9	3.6
350	350-7600BC	600	16.5	3.7
350	350-7700BC	700	17.4	3.9
350	350-7800BC	800	18.2	4.1

Shape: round; profile (projection): moderate; surface: smooth.

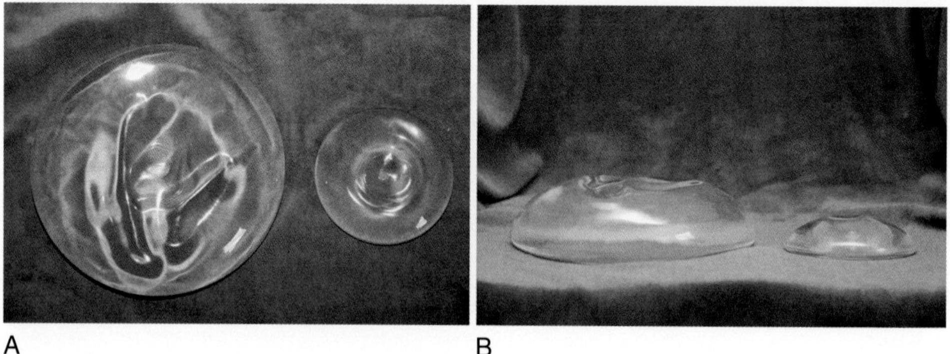

FIGURE 143-32. Mentor Style 350 silicone-filled breast implant: moderate projection profile. *A*, Anterior view. *B*, Lateral view.

MENTOR STYLE 350 SILICONE-FILLED BREAST IMPLANTS: MODERATE *PLUS* PROJECTION PROFILE. Mentor Style 350-Moderate *Plus* Projection Profile series of silicone breast implants are smooth shell implants with a "moderate plus" projection profile. Implant volumes range from 100 to 800 mL in 19 distinct implant sizes. Base diameters range from 8.2 to 16.5 cm with projection ranges from 2.7 to 5.1 cm. Base diameter and projection comparisons within the Mentor styles are much easier to ascertain because of the 19 constant implant volumes sizes (Table 143-27 and Fig. 143-33).

TABLE 143-27 ✦ MENTOR STYLE 350 (SILICONE-FILLED) BREAST IMPLANTS: MODERATE *PLUS* PROJECTION PROFILE

Style	Catalog No.	Fill Volume (mL)	Diameter (cm)	Projection (cm)
350	350-1001BC	100	8.2	2.7
350	350-1251BC	125	8.9	2.8
350	350-1501BC	150	9.5	2.9
350	350-1751BC	175	10	3.1
350	350-2001BC	200	10.5	3.2
350	350-2251BC	225	10.9	3.3
350	350-2501BC	250	11.3	3.4
350	350-2751BC	275	11.7	3.5
350	350-3001BC	300	12	3.6
350	350-3251BC	325	12.3	3.8
350	350-3501BC	350	12.5	3.9
350	350-3751BC	375	12.8	4
350	350-4001BC	400	13.1	4
350	350-4501BC	450	13.6	4.2
350	350-5001BC	500	14.1	4.3
350	350-5501BC	550	14.6	4.5
350	350-6001BC	600	15	4.6
350	350-7001BC	700	15.8	4.9
350	350-8001BC	800	16.5	5.1

Shape: round; profile (projection): moderate *plus*; surface: smooth.

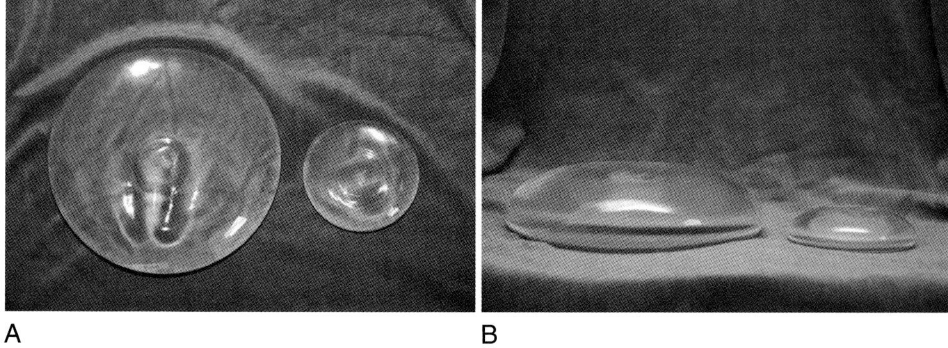

A B

FIGURE 143-33. Mentor Style 350 silicone-filled breast implant: moderate *plus* projection profile. *A,* Anterior view. *B,* Lateral view.

Mentor Style 350 Silicone-Filled Breast Implants: High Projection Profile. Mentor Style 350-High Projection Profile series of silicone breast implants are smooth shell implants with a high projection profile. Implant volumes range from 125 to 800 mL in 20 distinct implant sizes. Base diameters range from 8.3 to 15.5 cm with projection ranges from 3.5 to 6.0 cm. Progression from moderate to moderate plus to high projection profile reflects diminution of the base diameter and height with proportional increase in the projection profile (Table 143-28 and Fig. 143-34).

TABLE 143-28 ✦ MENTOR STYLE 350 (SILICONE-FILLED) BREAST IMPLANTS: HIGH PROJECTION PROFILE

Style	Catalog No.	Fill Volume (mL)	Diameter (cm)	Projection (cm)
350	350-1254BC	125	8.3	3.5
350	350-1504BC	150	8.8	3.7
350	350-1754BC	175	9.3	3.9
350	350-2004BC	200	9.7	4
350	350-2254BC	225	10.1	4.2
350	350-2504BC	250	10.5	4.3
350	350-2754BC	275	10	4.4
350	350-3004BC	300	11.1	4.5
350	350-3254BC	325	11.4	4.6
350	350-3504BC	350	11.7	4.8
350	350-3754BC	375	12	4.8
350	350-4004BC	400	12.2	5
350	350-4254BC	425	12.5	5
350	350-4504BC	450	12.8	5.1
350	350-5004BC	500	13.2	5.3
350	350-5504BC	550	13.6	5.5
350	350-6004BC	600	14	5.6
350	350-6504BC	650	14.4	5.7
350	350-7004BC	700	14.8	5.8
350	350-8004BC	800	15.5	6

Shape: round; profile (projection): high; surface: smooth.

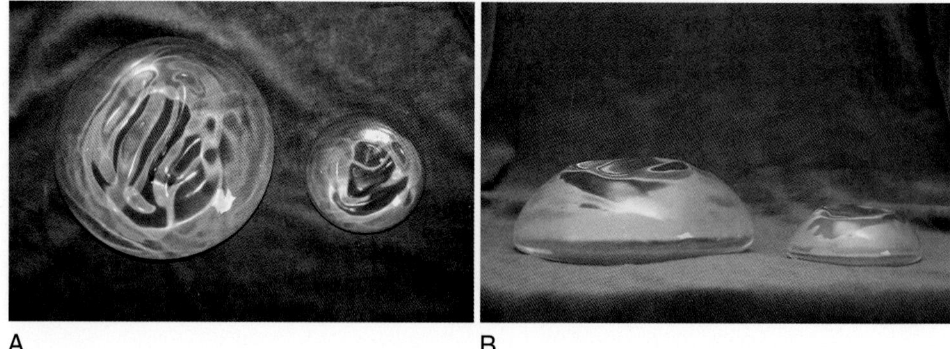

A B

FIGURE 143-34. Mentor Style 350 silicone-filled breast implant: high projection profile. *A,* Anterior view. *B,* Lateral view.

Mentor Style 354 Silicone-Filled Breast Implants: Moderate Projection Profile. Mentor Style 354-Moderate Projection Profile series of silicone breast implants are textured shell implants with a moderate projection profile. Implant volumes range from 100 to 800 mL in 19 distinct implant sizes. Base diameters range from 8.8 to 17.2 cm with projection ranges from 2.5 to 4.6 cm (Table 143-29 and Fig. 143-35).

TABLE 143-29 ✦ MENTOR STYLE 354 (SILICONE-FILLED) BREAST IMPLANTS: MODERATE PROJECTION PROFILE

Style	Catalog No.	Fill Volume (mL)	Diameter (cm)	Projection (cm)
354	354-1007	100	8.8	2.5
354	354-1257	125	9.3	2.8
354	354-1507	150	10.2	2.7
354	354-1757	175	10.7	2.8
354	354-2007	200	11.2	2.8
354	354-2257	225	11.4	3
354	354-2507	250	11.5	3.3
354	354-2757	275	12.4	3.4
354	354-3007	300	12.6	3.5
354	354-3257	325	12.9	3.6
354	354-3507	350	13.4	3.7
354	354-3757	375	13.4	3.8
354	354-4007	400	13.5	3.9
354	354-4507	450	13.9	4.1
354	354-5007	500	14.2	4.3
354	354-5507	550	14.8	4.4
354	354-6007	600	15.4	4.5
354	354-7007	700	16.8	4.3
354	354-8007	800	17.2	4.6

Shape: round; profile (projection): moderate; surface: Siltex.

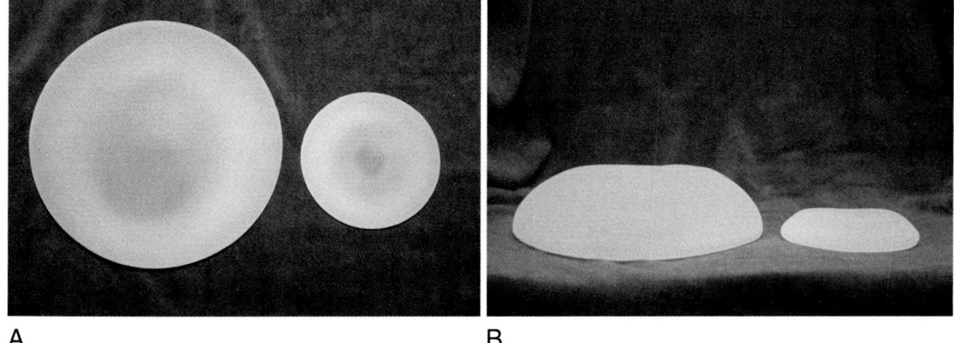

A B

FIGURE 143-35. Mentor Style 354 silicone-filled breast implant: moderate projection profile. *A,* Anterior view. *B,* Lateral view.

Mentor Style 354 Silicone-Filled Breast Implants: Moderate *Plus* Projection Profile. Mentor Style 354-Moderate *Plus* Projection Profile series of silicone breast implants are textured shell implants with a moderate plus projection profile. Implant volumes range from 100 to 800 mL in 19 distinct implant sizes. Base diameters range from 8.1 to 16.6 cm with projection ranges from 2.7 to 5.0 cm (Table 143-30 and Fig. 143-36).

TABLE 143-30 ✦ MENTOR STYLE 354 (SILICONE-FILLED) BREAST IMPLANTS: MODERATE *PLUS* PROJECTION PROFILE

Style	Catalog No.	Fill Volume (mL)	Diameter (cm)	Projection (cm)
354	354-1001	100	8.1	2.7
354	354-1251	125	8.8	2.9
354	354-1501	150	9.4	3
354	354-1751	175	10	3.2
354	354-2001	200	10.5	3.3
354	354-2251	225	10.9	3.5
354	354-2501	250	11.3	3.6
354	354-2751	275	11.7	3.7
354	354-3001	300	12	3.7
354	354-3251	325	12.3	3.8
354	354-3501	350	12.6	3.8
354	354-3751	375	12.9	3.9
354	354-4001	400	13.2	4
354	354-4501	450	13.7	4.1
354	354-5001	500	14.1	4.2
354	354-5501	550	14.4	4.4
354	354-6001	600	14.7	4.5
354	354-7001	700	15.7	4.8
354	354-8001	800	16.6	5

Shape: round; profile (projection): moderate *plus*; surface: Siltex.

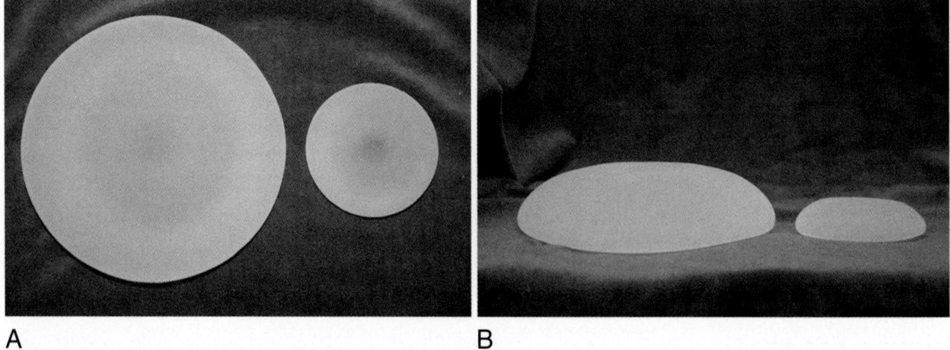

A B

FIGURE 143-36. Mentor Style 354 silicone-filled breast implant: moderate *plus* projection profile. *A,* Anterior view. *B,* Lateral view.

MENTOR STYLE 354 SILICONE-FILLED BREAST IMPLANTS: HIGH PROJECTION PROFILE. Mentor Style 354-High Projection Profile series of silicone breast implants are textured shell implants with a high projection profile. Implant volumes range from 125 to 800 mL in 20 distinct implant sizes. Base diameters range from 8.4 to 15.4 cm with projection ranges from 3.6 to 6.3 cm (Table 143-31 and Fig. 143-37).

TABLE 143-31 ✦ MENTOR STYLE 354 (SILICONE-FILLED) BREAST IMPLANTS: HIGH PROJECTION PROFILE

Style	Catalog No.	Fill Volume (mL)	Diameter (cm)	Projection (cm)
354	354-4125	125	8.4	3.6
354	354-4150	150	8.9	3.8
354	354-4175	175	9.4	4
354	354-4200	200	9.9	4.1
354	354-4225	225	10.2	4.3
354	354-4250	250	10.5	4.5
354	354-4275	275	10.9	4.6
354	354-4300	300	11.1	4.7
354	354-4325	325	11.5	4.8
354	354-4350	350	11.7	4.9
354	354-4375	375	12	5
354	354-4400	400	12.3	5.1
354	354-4425	425	12.5	5.2
354	354-4450	450	12.7	5.2
354	354-4500	500	13.2	5.4
354	354-4550	550	13.5	5.6
354	354-4600	600	14	5.7
354	354-4650	650	14.3	5.8
354	354-4700	700	14.7	6
354	354-4800	800	15.4	6.3

Shape: round; profile (projection): high; surface: Siltex.

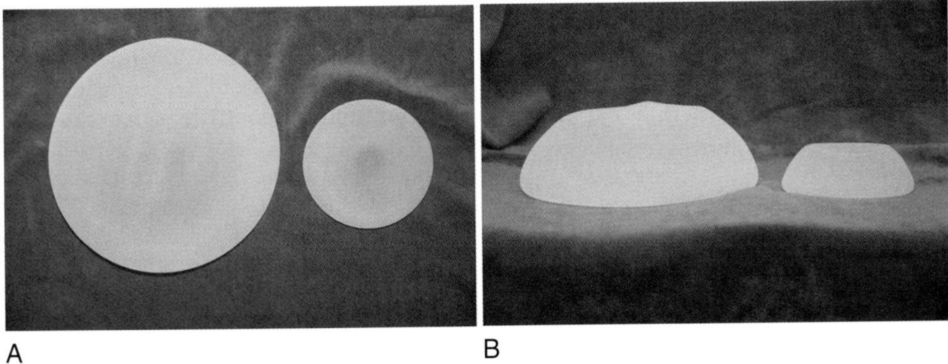

A B

FIGURE 143-37. Mentor Style 354 silicone-filled breast implant: high projection profile. *A*, Anterior view. *B*, Lateral view.

Contralateral Breast Adjustment

The order of the procedure generally consists of completion of second-stage reconstruction at least to the point of sizer insertion followed by contralateral breast adjustment to include augmentation, mastopexy, mastopexy-augmentation, or reduction. Adjustment of the implant pocket, including the inframammary line in the medial or lateral extension, may be necessary to match the contralateral breast as closely as possible. The implant pocket adjustment is accomplished by inspection of the reconstructed mound position and the shape and size of the implant in place with the patient in a sitting position.

Pocket Adjustment

Pocket adjustment may require use of internal sutures. Buried sutures are placed to adjust the pocket, particularly if the expander was located below the inframammary line. The smooth expander tended to migrate superiorly during the inflation process, so the expander was placed purposely below the inframammary line to ensure that the inferior preserved skin envelope was expanded. Routinely, the inframammary line was adjusted superiorly at the time of permanent implant insertion. Now, with the availability of textured expanders, this expander will remain at the inframammary line and effectively expand the lower half of the breast envelope without migration superiorly during the inflation process. With careful placement of the expander at the initial insertion, internal pocket adjustment is less commonly required.

Closure

Closures are generally limited to an absorbable layer in the dermis followed by a subcuticular suture or closure with a topical skin adhesive. Contralateral breast closure is accomplished in a similar manner on the basis of the procedures required to establish breast symmetry. Drains should be inserted through separate stab incisions in the axillary region if extensive capsulectomy, capsulotomy, or inframammary line adjustments are required.

Postoperative Care

Dressings should be removed by the second or third day with either soft bra (without underwire) or braless tank top support. The patient should resume normal activity within 5 days. Sporting activities can be resumed within 2 weeks if no inframammary line adjustment is required or within 6 weeks if suture repair of the inframammary line is required.

SINGLE-STAGE EXPANDER-IMPLANT RECONSTRUCTION

In immediate reconstruction after mastectomy for invasive stage I breast cancer or prophylactic mastectomy, the safer approach for a single-stage procedure at present is the use of an expander or implant with a remote port. This device initially serves as an expander that is then later reduced to a selected saline volume implant followed by removal of the connecting tubing and valve through an incision over the port. Although the combined implant-expander with the remote port is used effectively in breast reconstruction, the implant may lack features beneficial to expansion (textured surface and convenience and comfort of incorporated valve) or features that may be desirable to adjust at a second procedure (size, shape). Not all changes that occur with expansion are predictable, and the opportunity to perform a second procedure with an expander-implant allows modification of the implant pocket to provide optimal form for the reconstructed breast mound.

When skin-sparing mastectomy is performed with either resection of the nipple or preservation of the cutaneous portion of the nipple, it is possible to place the permanent expander-implant in a submuscular position and to provide an excellent result in one stage. However, long-term results are not yet available, and there is a risk of increased local complications, including capsular contracture, because the implant will be surrounded in the environment of wound healing as a result of the mastectomy.

In delayed reconstruction, a single-stage procedure may be accomplished by direct implant placement in selected patients with a redundant skin envelope preserved at the time of mastectomy. In most patients, the concept of expansion and implant insertion as separate procedures offers the advantage of an improved skin envelope in regard to dimensions, circulation, and wound healing environment compared with immediate implant insertion. The patient must be informed of potential risks of implant exposure and the possibility of inadequate skin to provide slight ptosis at the inferior half of the breast mound. When the skin is tight, it is possible to advance abdominal skin to the sixth intercostal space (see section entitled "Abdominal Advancement Flap" under "Inadequate Skin Envelope: Alternative Approaches"). This maneuver allows use of the existing inferior chest wall skin as part of the inferior skin envelope. This technique is similar to recruitment of skin accomplished over the time interval of expansion, but by immediate advancement of the skin flap, it is possible to use the increased breast mound skin as a part of the skin envelope. Immediate placement of a permanent expander-implant may then allow adequate breast mound reconstruction in a single stage.

Adjustable, Permanent Expander-Implant

In 1984, Hilton Becker[6] designed the first adjustable, permanent implant-expander with a detachable reservoir to allow the device to be left in place as a permanent implant. In 1992, about 14% of reconstructions with implants were estimated to be permanent expander-implants.[7]

The original Becker-type design of expander-implant has a silicone gel-filled outer lumen (25% or 50% overall volume) that surrounds an expandable saline inner lumen. The newer Mentor Spectrum implant is saline filled and more widely used because of the FDA restrictions placed on silicone gel-filled implants in 1992.[4] Improvements made as a result of early experience include a textured surface (to mitigate both capsular contracture and implant migration) and the availability of anatomically shaped devices.

The obvious advantages of the adjustable, permanent expander-implant include the single-stage procedure, no additional scars on the breast mound (there will be a scar at the site of port removal), good color match, and ability to adjust the size of the implant postoperatively. The use of Mentor Spectrum postoperatively adjustable implants in patients requesting an increase in breast volume is distinctive. Patients with smaller breasts can undergo skin-sparing mastectomy with immediate Mentor Spectrum implant placement with nominal saline fill volumes. Postoperatively, they then undergo serial expansion to achieve an "augmented" reconstruction. Addition of a latissimus dorsi musculocutaneous flap to this approach provides a small skin island to fill the areola defect. With preservation of the complete skin envelope and the addition of latissimus muscle coverage of the implant, a breast mound can be established with the adjustable implant without limitations resulting from closure of the areola excision site.

A disadvantage of a single-stage implant-based reconstruction is the inability to adjust the breast (and contralateral breast) aesthetically at a second procedure. Immediate reconstruction with the permanent implant-expander is also a relative contraindication in patients requiring postoperative radiotherapy. However, it is a novel bridge to autologous reconstruction for patients with a need for radiation therapy. Such patients can undergo an immediate one-stage, implant-based reconstruction with no delay to the initiation to chemotherapy and no delay to radiation therapy. They benefit from a subcutaneous prosthesis in the 6 to 9 months after irradiation while they are waiting for a final autologous reconstruction. Some patients even elect to maintain an implant-based reconstruction in an irradiated field and delay their intended autologous reconstructions until a later date if at all. However, increased complications have also been noted for patients undergoing delayed reconstruction procedures with permanent expander-implants.[8] Disadvantages are also related to the increased complications, such as capsular contracture, rupture, hematoma, wound infection, wound seroma, extrusion of implant, migration of implant, leakage of implant, chronic pain, skin or fat necrosis, and wound dehiscence.[8-13]

Gui et al[12] reported on immediate breast reconstruction with biodimensional anatomic permanent expander-implants. They found that this one-stage procedure with anatomically shaped implants gave good results. The implant was filled to 50% with saline intraoperatively after placement and closure of the submuscular and subcutaneous pockets. Final implant filling was usually achieved in one or two outpatient visits, as opposed to the multiple visits most often reported. Although no information about capsule formation was reported because of the short-term follow-up of patients, early complication rates were moderate to low, including infection (5.2%), hematoma (1.6%), seroma (0%), skin necrosis (3%), implant loss or extrusion (3.9%), and deflation (0%). The results of a questionnaire, to which 96 of the 107 patients studied responded, indicated that 88% of patients were satisfied with their reconstructive outcome.

Camilleri et al[13] described 111 consecutive women with reconstruction by the Mentor Becker (reverse double-lumen, gel outside, textured surface) permanent expander-implant with an average follow-up of 1 year. Early complications encountered were more typical of expanders, such as wound dehiscence (8%), filling port failure (6%), infection and removal (5%), skin flap necrosis, expander exposure (5%), and pain on expansion (20%). The capsular contracture rate was reported at 9% at 1 year. This lower rate of contracture than in previous studies (e.g., 15.8% and 28% for immediate and delayed reconstructions, respectively, as reported by Mandrekas et al[8]) is attributed to the textured surface of the implants as well as to overfilling of the device. Despite the reported complications, 89% of women expressed satisfaction during follow-up to the plastic surgeon.

With the popularity of the skin-sparing mastectomy, when immediate single-stage reconstruction is planned with use of a permanent adjustable implant, the closure of the defect at the site of the resection of the nipple-areola complex is difficult to accomplish without some distortion of the preserved skin envelope. Direct closure usually requires extension of the incision laterally to avoid unnatural appearance of the retained skin in proximity to the areola defect closure. An innovation reported by Toth[14] consists of insertion of an adjustable permanent implant in a subpectoral position followed by a pursestring closure at the areola defect (Fig. 143-38). This approach avoids

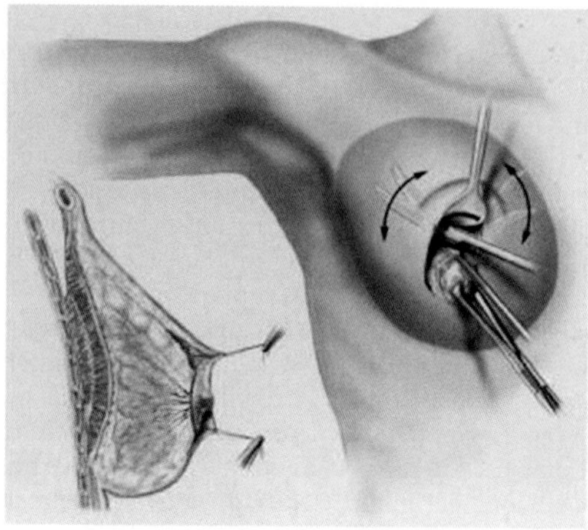

A

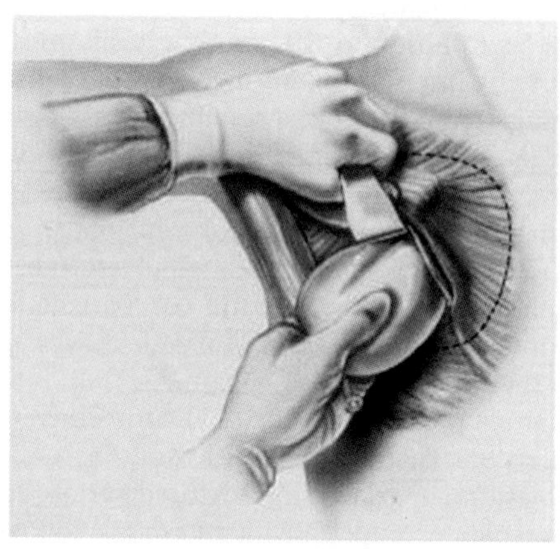

B

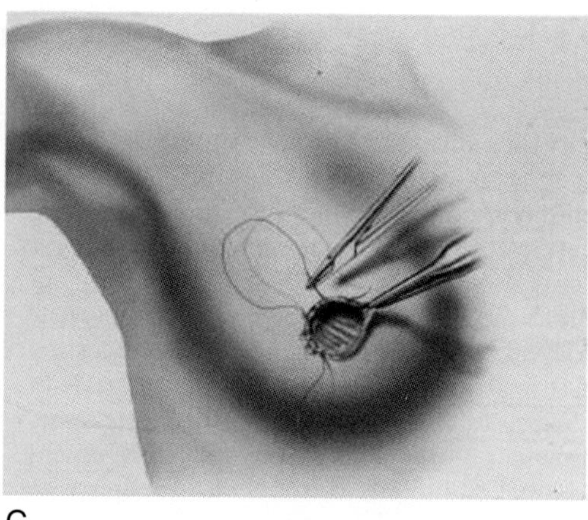

C

FIGURE 143-38. *A,* The planning of skin-sparing mastectomy with immediate pursestring reconstruction involves collaboration with the patient's general surgeon in choosing a favorable biopsy site, preferably with a circumareolar incision. As shown in the surgical diagram, the nipple-areola complex and biopsy site are always included in the specimen. Skin flaps are first elevated circumferentially above the breast tissue. Discontinuous axillary and inframammary incisions may be added for additional exposure. *B,* A small tissue expander is placed completely within a submuscular pocket formed beneath the pectoralis major and serratus muscles. This is facilitated by adduction of the patient's arms on the operating table. *C,* The pursestring skin closure is completed with a 2-0 monofilament absorbable suture. (From Toth BA, Daane SP: Purse-string mastectomy with immediate prosthetic reconstruction: an improved skin-sparing technique for small breasts. Plast Reconstr Surg 2003;111:2333.)

a scar extending beyond the site of the later areola reconstruction. It appears to be an excellent approach for smaller breast reconstruction and for providing temporary maintenance of the skin envelope if the patient must undergo postoperative irradiation with later possible autogenous reconstruction (Fig. 143-39).

The following discussion contains product information for adjustable, permanent expander-implants that are currently available in the United States.

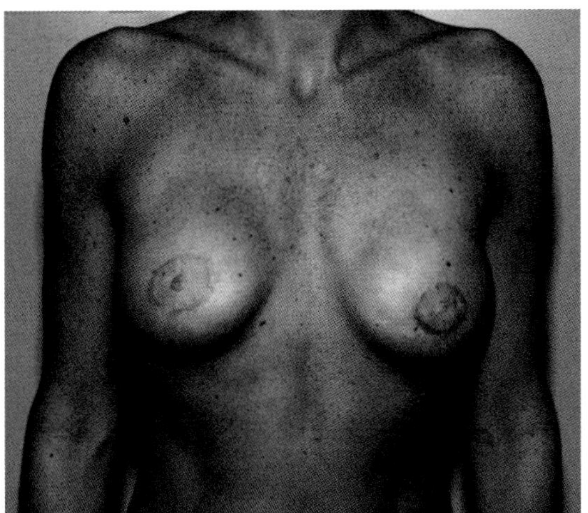

FIGURE 143-39. Postoperative view of a 31-year-old patient after bilateral circumareolar mastectomy, followed by submuscular tissue expander placement and purse-string closure. The final reconstruction was assessed 6 months after nipple-areola reconstruction. Preservation and projection of breast shape are observed. (From Toth BA, Daane SP: Purse-string mastectomy with immediate prosthetic reconstruction: an improved skin-sparing technique for small breasts. Plast Reconstr Surg 2003;111: 2333.)

MENTOR CORPORATION SPECTRUM ADJUSTABLE BREAST IMPLANTS

Mentor Corporation offers three distinct styles of an exclusive postoperatively adjustable saline-filled breast implant known as the Spectrum implant. The Spectrum implant is designed as a permanent breast implant with a remote fill port for volume adjustments up to 6 months after its insertion. The fill port can be removed under a local anesthetic in an office-based procedure once an appropriate breast reconstruction volume is attained. It has a distinct role in immediate implant-based, single-stage breast reconstruction in the setting of a skin-sparing mastectomy. The initial volume of the implant can be reduced to alleviate undue pressure on the skin-sparing mastectomy skin flaps. Serial "expansion" can then be performed in the office and the remote port later removed through a separate incision, therefore eliminating the need for a formal second-stage operative procedure whereby a tissue expander must be removed and replaced with a permanent breast implant.

Mentor Spectrum Style 1400 Adjustable Breast Implants

Mentor Spectrum Style 1400 breast implants are smooth shell, round, saline-filled devices designed to allow postoperative adjustability of reconstruction site implant volumes. Implant volumes from 125 to 690 mL are available in 10 distinct implants. Base diameters range from 9.3 to 14.2 cm with projection of 3.2 to 6 cm (Table 143-32 and Fig. 143-40).

TABLE 143-32 ✦ MENTOR SPECTRUM STYLE 1400 BREAST IMPLANTS (SMOOTH SHELL)

			Minimum Fill			Maximum Fill		
Style	**Catalog No.**	**Temporary Minimum Volume (mL)**	*Final Volume (mL)*	*Diameter (cm)*	*Projection (cm)*	*Final Volume (mL)*	*Diameter (cm)*	*Projection (cm)*
1400	350-1410	105	125	9.4	2.7	150	9.3	3.2
1400	350-1420	150	175	10.3	3.1	210	10.2	3.8
1400	350-1430	190	225	10.8	3.5	270	10.9	4.3
1400	350-1440	230	275	11.6	3.8	330	11.5	4.6
1400	350-1450	275	325	12.4	4	390	12.1	4.9
1400	350-1460	320	375	13.5	4.1	450	13	4.9
1400	350-1470	360	425	14	4.2	510	13.7	4.8
1400	350-1480	405	475	14.3	4.4	570	13.8	5.4
1400	350-1485	450	525	15	4.4	630	14.4	5.6
1400	350-1490	490	575	14.7	4.8	690	14.2	6

Shape: round; surface: smooth.

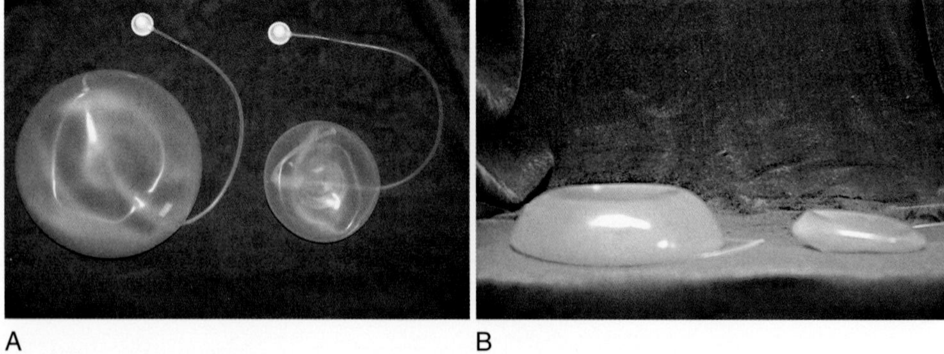

FIGURE 143-40. Mentor Spectrum Style 1400 adjustable breast implant. *A,* Anterior view. *B,* Lateral view.

Mentor Spectrum Style 2400 Adjustable Breast Implants

Mentor Spectrum Style 2400 breast implants are Siltex textured, round, saline-filled devices designed to allow postoperative adjustability of breast reconstruction site implant volumes. Implant volumes from 150 to 570 mL are available in eight distinct implants. Base diameters range from 9.2 to 15.2 cm with a projection range of 3.5 to 5.7 cm (Table 143-33 and Fig. 143-41).

TABLE 143-33 ✦ MENTOR SPECTRUM STYLE 2400 BREAST IMPLANTS (TEXTURED SHELL)

			Minimum Fill			Maximum Fill		
Style	Catalog No.	Temporary Minimum Volume (mL)	*Final Volume (mL)*	*Diameter (cm)*	*Projection (cm)*	*Final Volume (mL)*	*Diameter (cm)*	*Projection (cm)*
2400	354-2410M	105	125	9.4	3	150	9.2	3.5
2400	354-2420M	150	175	10.5	3.1	210	10.4	3.9
2400	354-2430M	190	225	11.3	3.3	270	11.1	4.2
2400	354-2440M	235	275	12	3.6	330	11.4	4.4
2400	354-2450M	275	325	12.9	3.7	390	12.6	4.5
2400	354-2460M	320	375	13.4	3.9	450	13.1	4.8
2400	354-2470M	360	425	14	4.2	510	13.6	5
2400	354-2480M	400	475	14.5	4.5	570	15.2	5.7

Shape: round; surface: smooth.

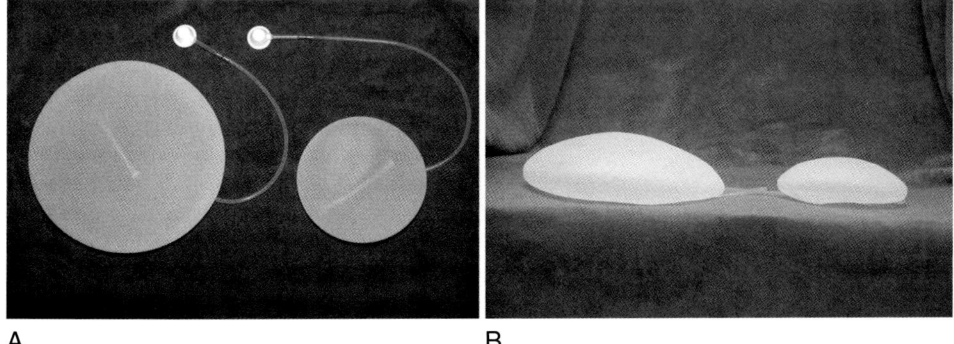

A B

FIGURE 143-41. Mentor Spectrum Style 2400 adjustable breast implant. *A,* Anterior view. *B,* Lateral view.

Mentor Spectrum Style 2500 Adjustable Breast Implants

Mentor Spectrum Style 2500 breast implants are Siltex textured, shaped, saline-filled devices designed to allow postoperative adjustability of breast reconstruction site implant volumes. Implant volumes from 330 to 780 mL are available in five distinct implants. Base diameters range from 9.4 to 12.5 cm with a projection range of 6.3 to 8.2 cm (Table 143-34 and Fig. 143-42).

TABLE 143-34 ✦ MENTOR SPECTRUM STYLE 2500 BREAST IMPLANTS (TEXTURED SHELL)

			Minimum Fill			Maximum Fill		
Style	**Catalog No.**	**Temporary Minimum Volume (mL)**	*Final Volume (mL)*	*Diameter (cm)*	*Projection (cm)*	*Final Volume (mL)*	*Diameter (cm)*	*Projection (cm)*
2500	354-2511	275	11.5	9.5	5.1	330	9.4	6.3
2500	354-2512	350	12.3	10.5	5.3	420	10.1	6.9
2500	354-2513	450	13.2	11	6.1	540	11	7.5
2500	354-2514	550	14	11.9	6.4	660	11.9	7.9
2500	354-2515	650	15	12.7	6.6	780	12.5	8.2

Shape: contour profile; surface: Siltex.

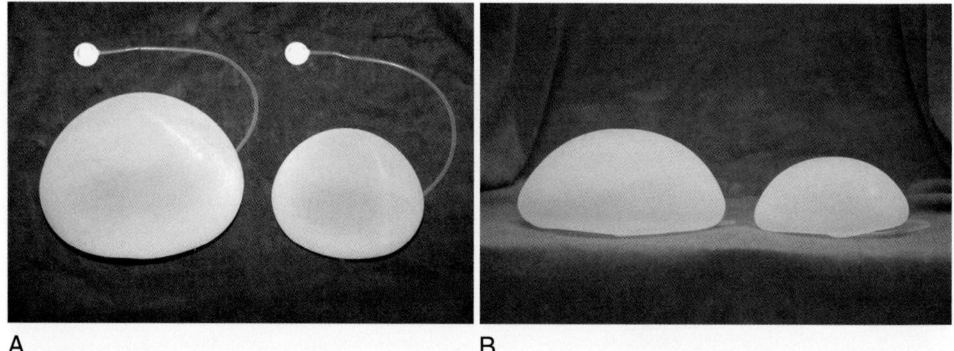

A B

FIGURE 143-42. Mentor Spectrum Style 2500 adjustable breast implant. *A,* Anterior view. *B,* Lateral view.

MENTOR BECKER ADJUSTABLE BREAST IMPLANTS

Mentor Corporation offers a distinctive outer silicone-filled and inner saline-filled postoperatively adjustable Becker expander-mammary implant. Four unique styles are offered to include a 25% outer silicone shell versus an outer 50% silicone shell. The 25% versus the 50% silicone outer shell is calculated on the basis of the anticipated final implant volume. Both the 25% and the 50% Becker expander-implant are available in a smooth shell and in a Siltex textured shell. All styles of the Becker expander-implant are round in their configuration.

Mentor Becker Style 25-350 Adjustable Breast Implants

The Mentor Becker Style 25-350 is a smooth shell, round, 25% by volume outer shell silicone-filled, 75% by volume inner shell saline-filled permanent breast implant with a remote infusion port. Final implant volumes range from 150 to 800 mL in 10 distinct implant sizes. Recommended overexpansion volumes are provided by the manufacturer. Final base diameters of 10.1 to 16.5 cm are associated with a projection range of 3.1 to 5.4 cm (Table 143-35 and Fig. 143-43).

TABLE 143-35 ✦ MENTOR BECKER STYLE 25-350 BREAST IMPLANTS (SMOOTH SHELL)

				Temporary Overexpansion Volumes					
Style	**Catalog No.**	**Size (mL)**	**Gel Volume (mL)**	*Maximum Saline (mL)*	*Total Gel-Saline (mL)*	**Total Saline (mL)**	**Total Gel-Saline (mL)**	**Diameter (cm)**	**Projection (cm)**
25	350-0150	150	40	185	225	85-150	125-190	10.1	3.1
25	350-0200	200	50	250	300	125-200	175-250	10.9	3.3
25	350-0250	250	60	315	375	165-255	225-315	11.4	3.7
25	350-0300	300	75	375	450	200-300	275-375	12.5	3.8
25	350-0350	350	90	435	525	235-350	325-440	13.2	3.9
25	350-0400	400	100	500	600	275-400	375-500	13.5	4.2
25	350-0500	500	125	625	750	350-500	475-625	13.9	4.9
25	350-0600	600	150	750	900	425-600	575-750	14.9	4.9
25	350-0700	700	175	875	1050	500-700	675-875	16.2	5
25	350-0800	800	200	1000	1200	575-800	775-1000	16.5	5.4

% Silicone gel outer lumen: 25; % saline inner lumen: 75; shape: round; surface: smooth; port style: remote.

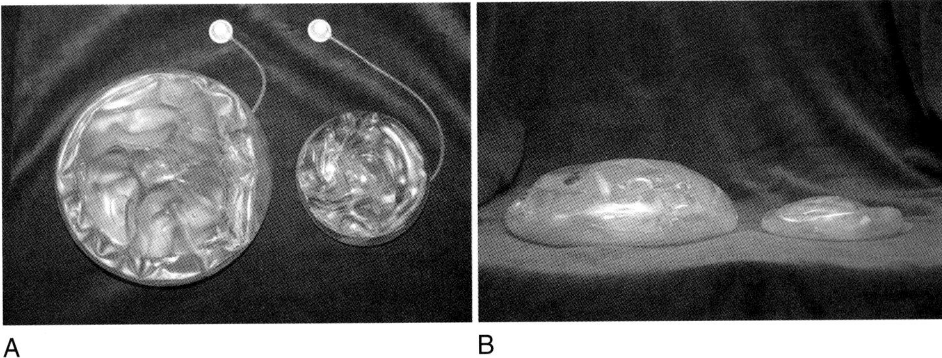

A B

FIGURE 143-43. Mentor Becker Style 25-350 adjustable breast implant. *A,* Anterior view. *B,* Lateral view.

Mentor Becker Style 50-350 Adjustable Breast Implants

The Mentor Becker Style 50-350 is a smooth shell, round, 50% by volume outer shell silicone-filled, 50% by volume inner shell saline-filled permanent breast implant with a remote infusion port. Final implant volumes range from 300 to 700 mL in five distinct implant sizes. Recommended overexpansion volumes are provided by the manufacturer. Final base diameters of 12.7 to 16.1 cm are associated with a projection range of 3.8 to 5.1 cm (Table 143-36 and Fig. 143-44).

TABLE 143-36 ✦ MENTOR BECKER STYLE 50-350 BREAST IMPLANTS (SMOOTH SHELL)

Style	Catalog No.	Size (mL)	Gel Volume (mL)	Total Saline (mL)	Total Gel-Saline (mL)	Diameter (cm)	Projection (cm)
50	350-1515	300	150	150-200	300-350	12.7	3.8
50	350-2020	400	200	200-300	400-500	13.6	4.1
50	350-2525	500	250	250-350	500-600	13.8	5
50	350-3030	600	300	300-425	600-725	15.1	5
50	350-3535	700	350	350-500	700-850	16.1	5.1

% Silicone gel outer lumen: 50; % saline inner lumen: 50; shape: round; surface: smooth; port style: remote.

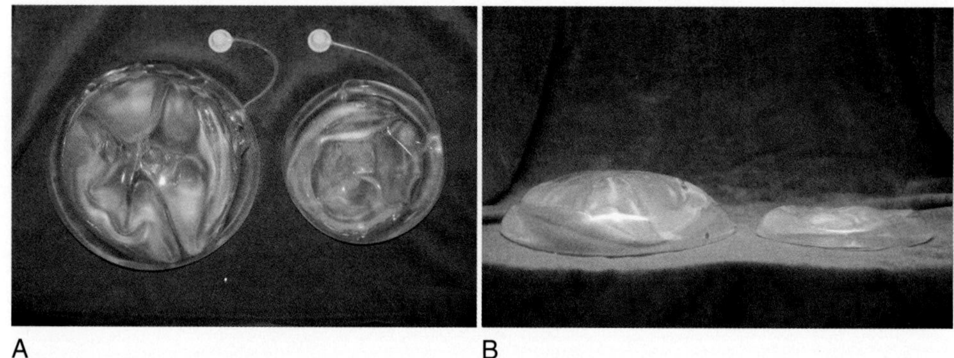

A B

FIGURE 143-44. Mentor Becker Style 50-350 adjustable breast implant. *A,* Anterior view. *B,* Lateral view.

Mentor Becker Style 25-354 Adjustable Breast Implants

The Mentor Becker Style 25-354 is a Siltex textured, round, 25% by volume outer shell silicone-filled, 75% by volume inner shell saline-filled permanent breast implant with a remote infusion port. Final implant volumes range from 150 to 800 mL in 10 distinct implant sizes. Recommended overexpansion volumes are provided by the manufacturer. Final base diameters of 10.7 to 17.2 cm are associated with a projection range of 2.4 to 4.6 cm (Table 143-37 and Fig. 143-45).

TABLE 143-37 ✦ MENTOR BECKER STYLE 25-354 BREAST IMPLANTS (TEXTURED SHELL)

				Temporary Overexpansion Volumes					
Style	**Catalog No.**	**Size (mL)**	**Gel Volume (mL)**	*Maximum Saline (mL)*	*Total Gel-Saline (mL)*	**Total Saline (mL)**	**Total Gel-Saline (mL)**	**Diameter (cm)**	**Projection (cm)**
25	354-1500	150	40	185	225	85-150	125-190	10.7	2.4
25	354-2000	200	50	250	300	125-200	175-250	11.6	2.7
25	354-2500	250	60	315	375	165-255	225-315	12.1	3
25	354-3000	300	75	375	450	200-300	275-375	12.9	3
25	354-3500	350	90	435	525	235-350	325-440	14.1	3
25	354-4000	400	100	500	600	275-400	375-500	13.9	3.4
25	354-5000	500	125	625	750	350-500	475-625	14.7	3.7
25	354-6000	600	150	750	900	425-600	575-750	15.6	4.2
25	354-7000	700	175	875	1050	500-700	675-875	16.8	4.3
25	354-8000	800	200	1000	1200	575-800	775-1000	17.2	4.6

% Silicone gel outer lumen: 25; % saline inner lumen: 75; shape: round; surface: Siltex; port style: remote.

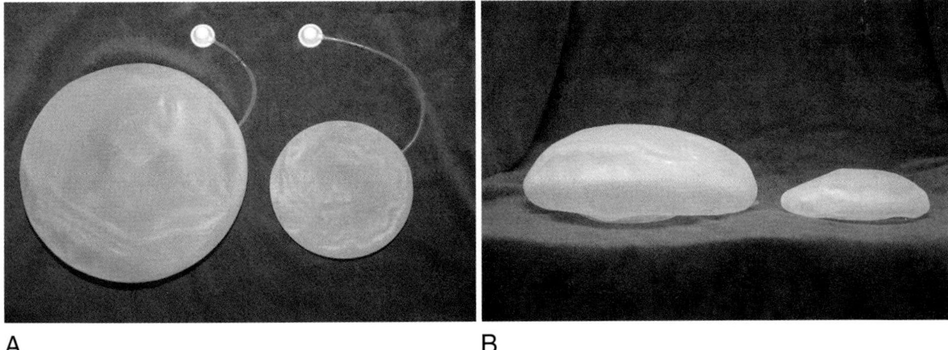

A B

FIGURE 143-45. Mentor Becker Style 25-354 adjustable breast implant. *A,* Anterior view. *B,* Lateral view.

Mentor Becker Style 50-354 Adjustable Breast Implants

The Mentor Becker Style 50-354 is a Siltex textured, round, 50% by volume outer shell silicone-filled, 50% by volume inner shell saline-filled permanent breast implant with a remote infusion port. Final implant volumes range from 300 to 700 mL in five distinct implant sizes. Recommended overexpansion volumes are provided by the manufacturer. Final base diameters of 12.9 to 16.0 cm are associated with a projection range of 3.0 to 5.0 cm (Table 143-38 and Fig. 143-46).

TABLE 143-38 ✦ MENTOR BECKER STYLE 50-354 BREAST IMPLANTS (TEXTURED SHELL)

Style	Catalog No.	Size (mL)	Gel Volume (mL)	Total Saline (mL)	Total Gel-Saline (mL)	Diameter (cm)	Projection (cm)
50	354-1515	300	150	150-200	300-350	12.9	3
50	354-2020	400	200	200-300	400-500	13.9	3.4
50	354-2525	500	250	250-350	500-600	14.7	3.7
50	354-3030	600	300	300-425	600-725	15.6	4.2
50	354-3535	700	350	350-500	700-850	16	5

% Silicone gel outer lumen: 50; % saline inner lumen: 50; shape: round; surface: Siltex; port style: remote.

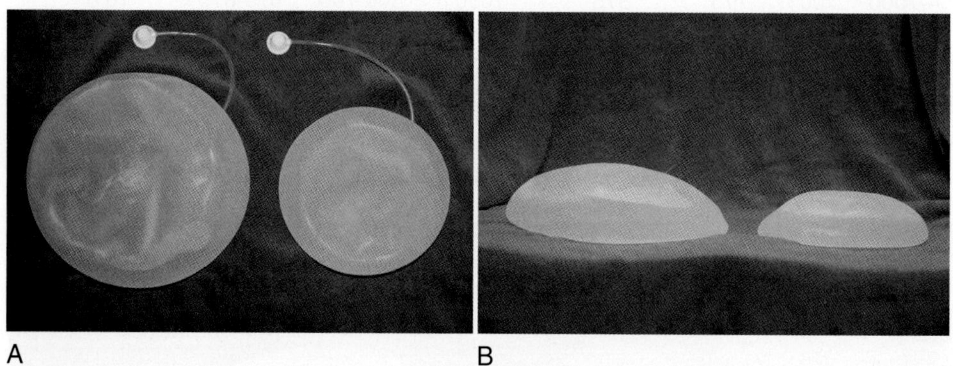

A B

FIGURE 143-46. Mentor Becker Style 50-354 adjustable breast implant. *A,* Anterior view. *B,* Lateral view.

EXPANDER-IMPLANT MUSCLE COVERAGE

Muscle coverage of the expander is desirable to avoid potential implant exposure if skin envelope necrosis or wound separation should occur. Also, implant coverage of the superior half of the reconstructed breast mound avoids direct contact with and adherence of the implant to the skin envelope, which may be visible when the patient is sitting or standing. Placement of the expander-implant in the subpectoral position is recommended. However, it is helpful to release the pectoralis major muscle origin from the inframammary line and from the fourth to the sixth intercostal spaces. The distal muscle is then transposed laterally to maintain the implant in a central position and avoid migration into the area of the lateral chest wall and axillary dissection. Without muscle coverage over the inferior third of the expander, improved expansion of the inferior preserved breast envelope is expected (Fig. 143-47).

When skin viability is questionable in the inferior aspect of the skin envelope, failure to have muscle coverage of the expander may result in eventual expander exposure and necessity for its removal. Although complete coverage by the pectoralis major and serratus anterior muscles can be achieved, these muscles with origin intact may impair the expansion process.

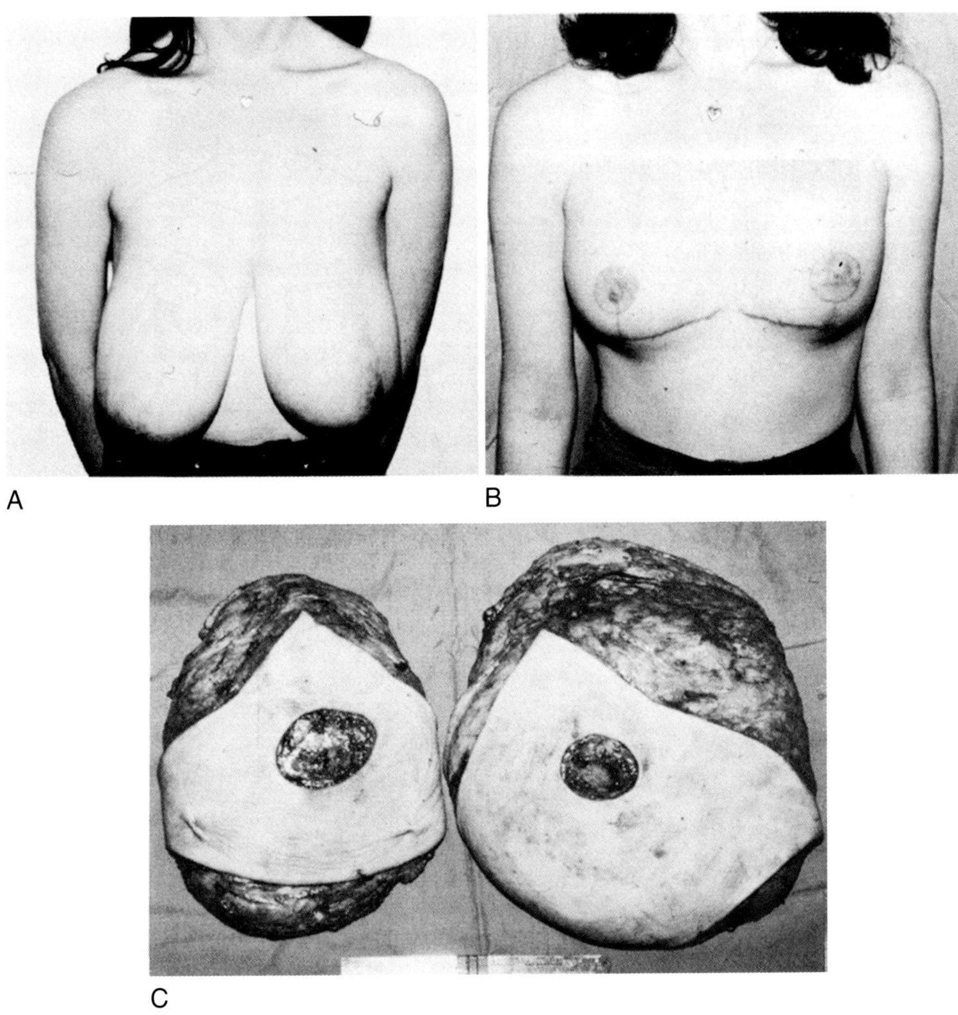

FIGURE 143-47. Expander-implant muscle coverage. *A,* Bilateral macromastia. Breast growth is controlled only by estrogen antagonists. *B,* Postoperative view of bilateral immediate breast reconstruction, 6 months after subcutaneous mastectomy with nipple-areola grafts incorporating placement of silicone implants beneath pectoralis major, serratus anterior, and anterior rectus sheath. *C,* Specimens from bilateral subcutaneous mastectomies. (From Mathes SJ, Nahai F: A systematic approach to flap selection. In Mathes SJ, Nahai F, eds: Clinical Applications for Muscle and Musculocutaneous Flaps. St. Louis, CV Mosby, 1982:285.)

Segmental Rectus–External Oblique Flap

If the skin viability of the inferior preserved skin envelope is in question, it is possible to obtain complete central inferior expander coverage and still avoid tight coverage by the segmental rectus flap over the inferior aspect of the expander (Fig. 143-48*A* and *B*). The abdominal skin is elevated from the inframammary line to the costal margin. The rectus muscle is divided at the costal margin and elevated as a segmental flap to the sixth intercostal space (Fig. 143-48*C* and Color Plate 143-2*A*). The lateral fascial fibers of the external oblique are also included with the segmental rectus flap. This flap does not divide the superior epigastric artery and associated veins because the muscle is divided at the costal margin. Although proximal fibers of rectus abdominis muscle insertion from the fifth, sixth, and seventh ribs are divided, the inscriptiones tendineae are preserved below the costal margin, preserving muscle function. The segmental flap is based on branches of the sixth intercostal artery and associated veins. The segmental flap is rotated 180 degrees and approximated to the inferior fibers of the previously released pectoralis major (Fig. 143-48*D* to *G* and Color Plate 143-2*B*). The pectoralis major combined with this segmental flap will protect the expander if skin necrosis should occur but will not limit the effect of the expander on the preserved inferior breast envelope (Figs. 143-49 and 143-50).

INADEQUATE SKIN ENVELOPE: ALTERNATIVE APPROACHES

In immediate reconstruction, the process of expansion is effective even when the mastectomy has not included an extensive portion of the skin envelope. Fortunately, the trend is preservation of the majority of the skin envelope in dealing with breast cancer resection. In delayed reconstruction, the process of wound contraction is not avoided by simultaneous expansion, so shrinkage of the retained skin envelope may be observed, particularly if a large segment of the skin envelope has been resected. If the surgeon is concerned that tissue expansion of the preserved skin envelope will not be adequate for breast mound reconstruction, it is possible to incorporate abdominal skin or the skin of an alternative flap (e.g., a latissimus dorsi musculocutaneous flap) into the skin envelope to establish an adequate breast envelope for reconstruction.

Several techniques may be used to incorporate additional skin into the breast mound. Placement of the expander below the inframammary line may be used to expand the skin in proximity to the costal margin. After the expansion is completed, internal suture of the expanded skin envelope can elevate the inferior anterior chest wall skin above the established inframammary line. This skin will now become part of the inferior breast mound coverage, providing a more natural contour to the reconstructed breast mound. An abdominal advancement flap may be used to establish the new inframammary line with the skin above the flap incorporated into the inferior aspect of the breast mound. This approach can be used as a single-stage technique for delayed reconstruction or be preceded by staged expansion. Because a transverse incision below the planned inframammary line is required, this approach is not suitable for immediate reconstruction as there will be a second, more superior incision used for the mastectomy.

At present, the most common solution for patients with an inadequate breast envelope is reconstruction with an autologous flap. A flap is generally used for immediate or delayed reconstruction to avoid the two-stage procedure required with an expander (with the exception of the expander-implant with the distant removable port). However, there are specific instances in both immediate and delayed breast reconstruction when a flap is required but the use of a tissue expander in conjunction with a flap will benefit the reconstructive process.

Text continued on p. 939

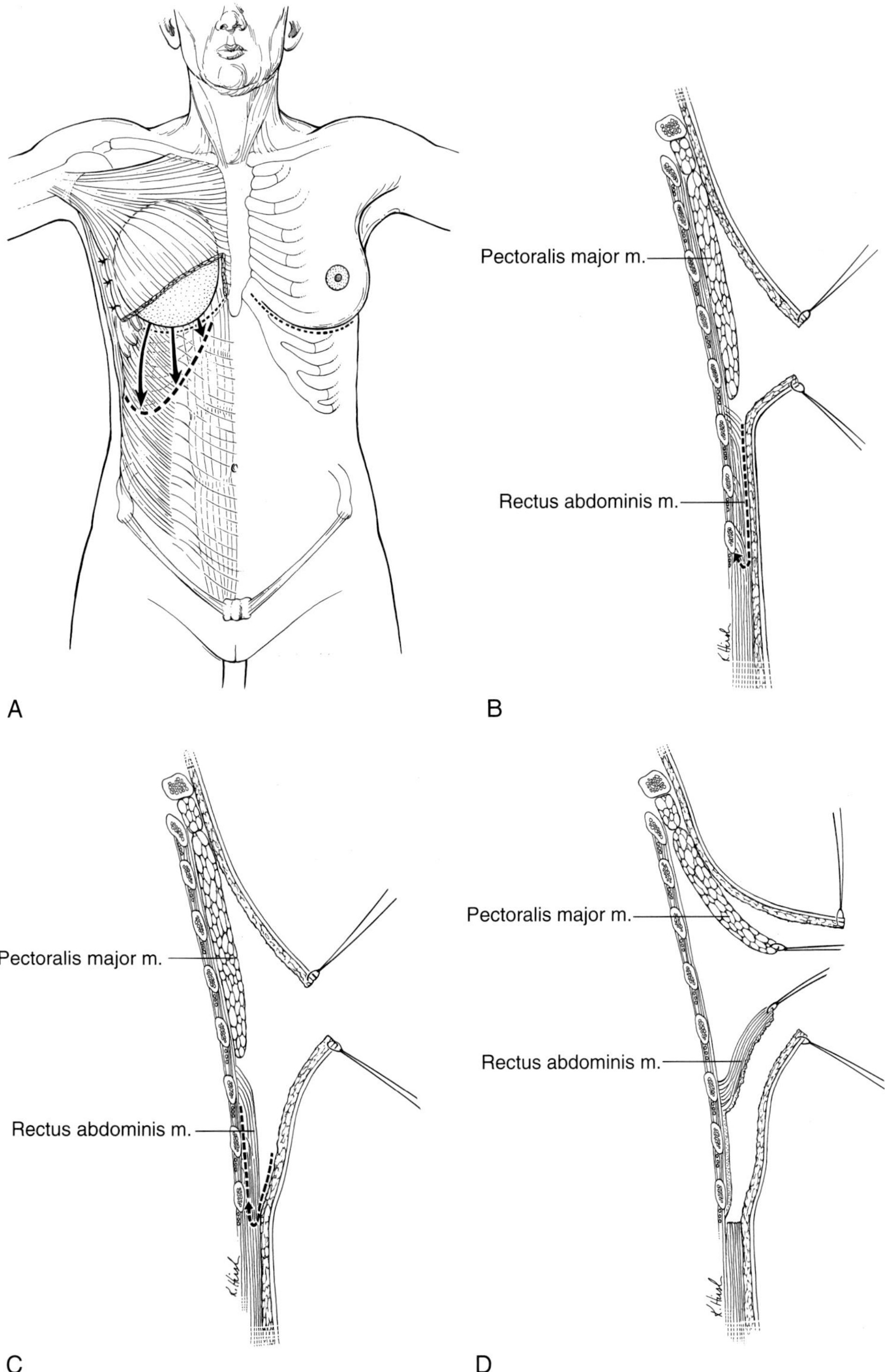

FIGURE 143-48. Segmental rectus abdominis–external oblique flap. *A,* Subcutaneous dissection from inframammary line to costal margin to expose segmental muscle flap. *B,* Lateral view demonstrates dissection plane to expose thoracic portion of rectus abdominis muscle insertion and superior external oblique muscle and fascia. *C,* At costal margin, rectus muscle is transected (superior to entry of superior epigastric pedicle into muscle), and lateral external oblique fibers are divided. Muscle is elevated superiorly to sixth intercostal space. *D,* Segmental muscle flap elevated to inferior aspect of sixth rib where pedicle to segmental flap is located. *Continued*

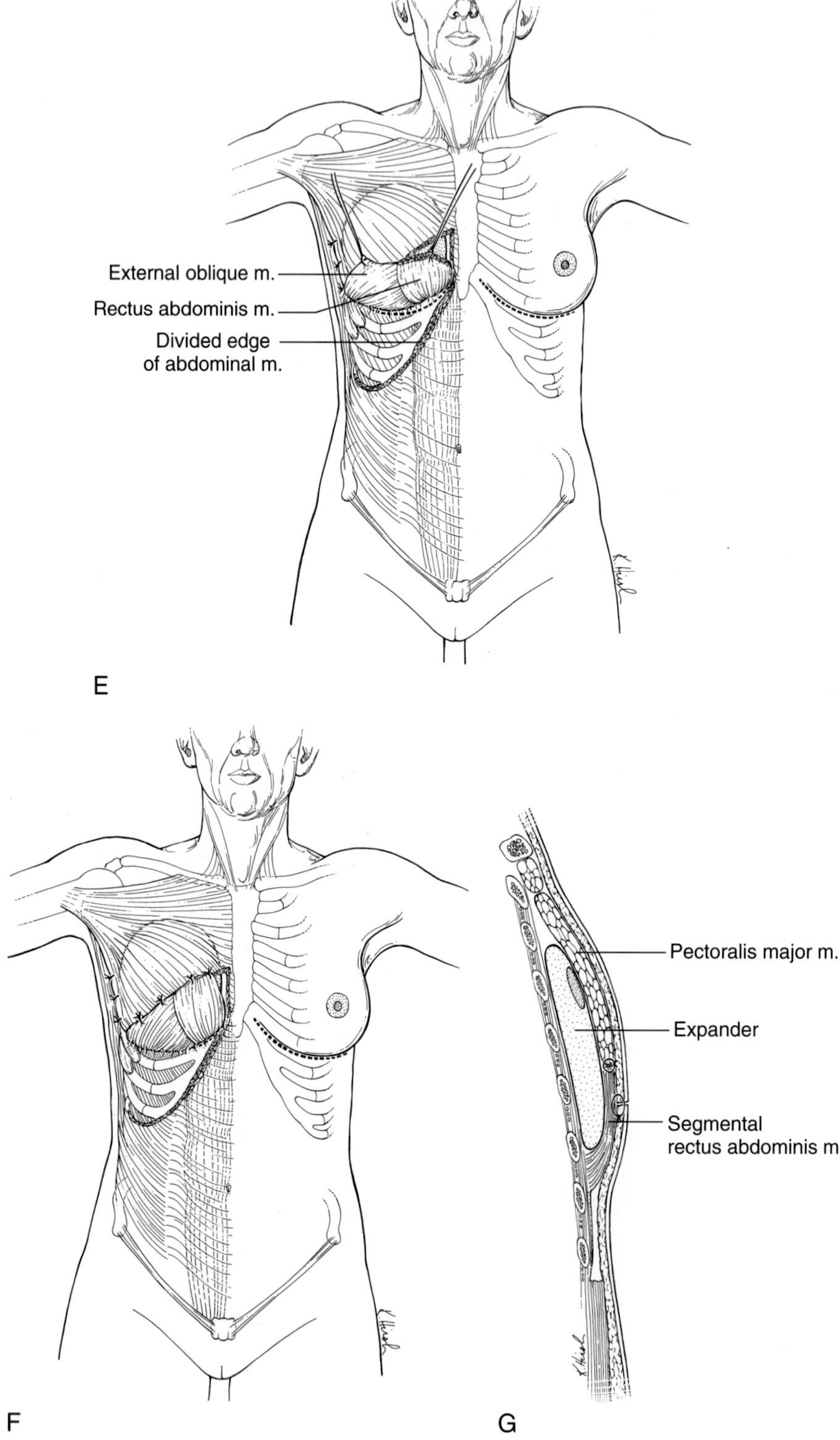

FIGURE 143-48, cont'd. *E* and *F,* Segmental flap is sutured to edge of pectoralis major muscle flap, providing coverage over central inferior expander-implant without restricting expansion process by tight muscle coverage. *G,* Lateral view. The inframammary line is preserved by the muscle arc of rotation at the sixth intercostal space.

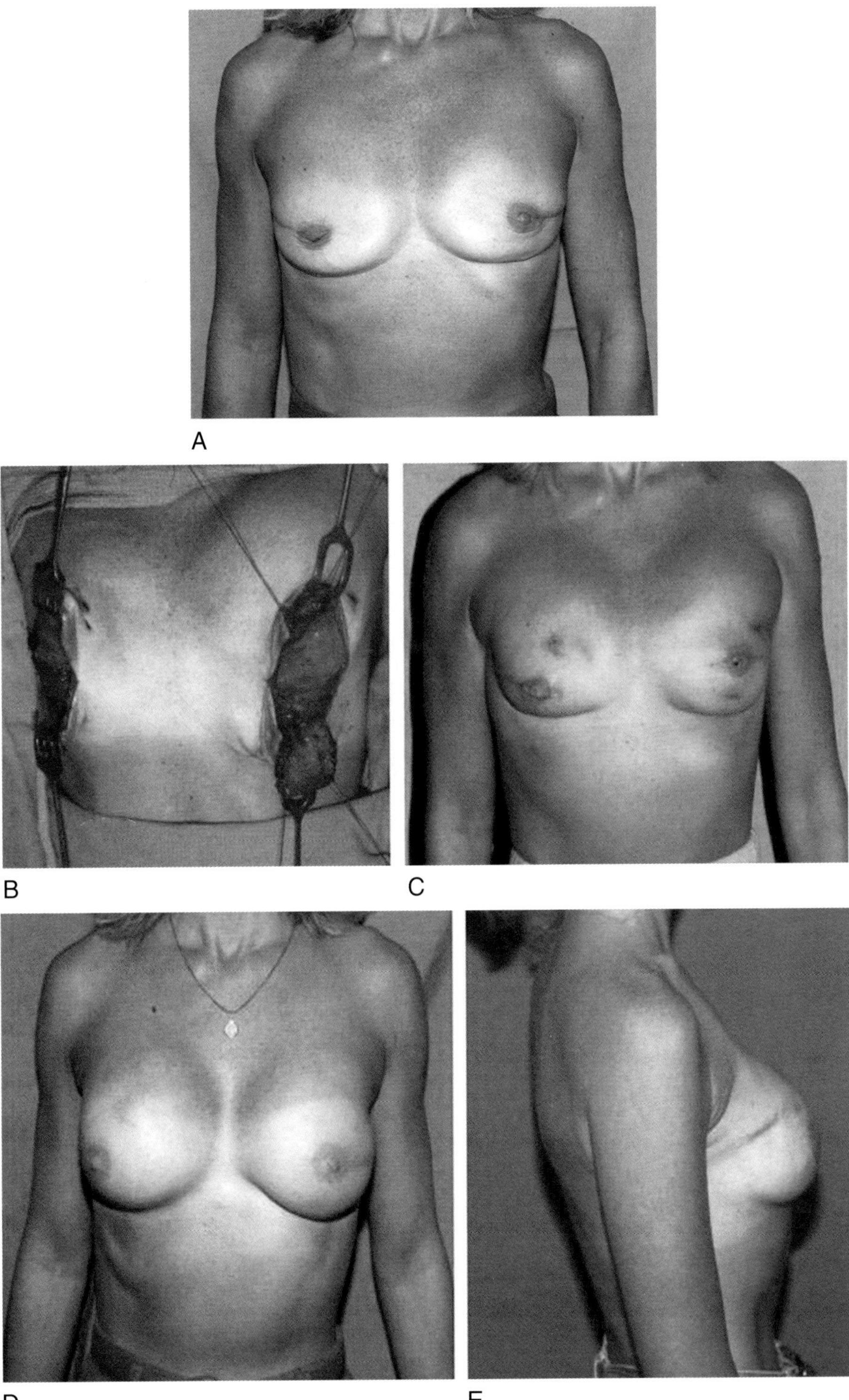

FIGURE 143-49. Immediate expander-implant reconstruction: expander coverage with segmental rectus abdominis–external oblique flap. *A,* Silicone mastitis after non–medical grade silicone breast injections. *B,* Bilateral subcutaneous mastectomy with bilateral segmental flaps elevated for inferior expander coverage. *C,* Postoperative stage 1, expanders in place. Skin envelope survival is noted despite subdermal dissection to remove free silicone. *D,* Postoperative view at 1 year, stage 2: bilateral reconstruction with permanent saline implant. *E,* Postoperative stage 2 lateral view at 1 year.

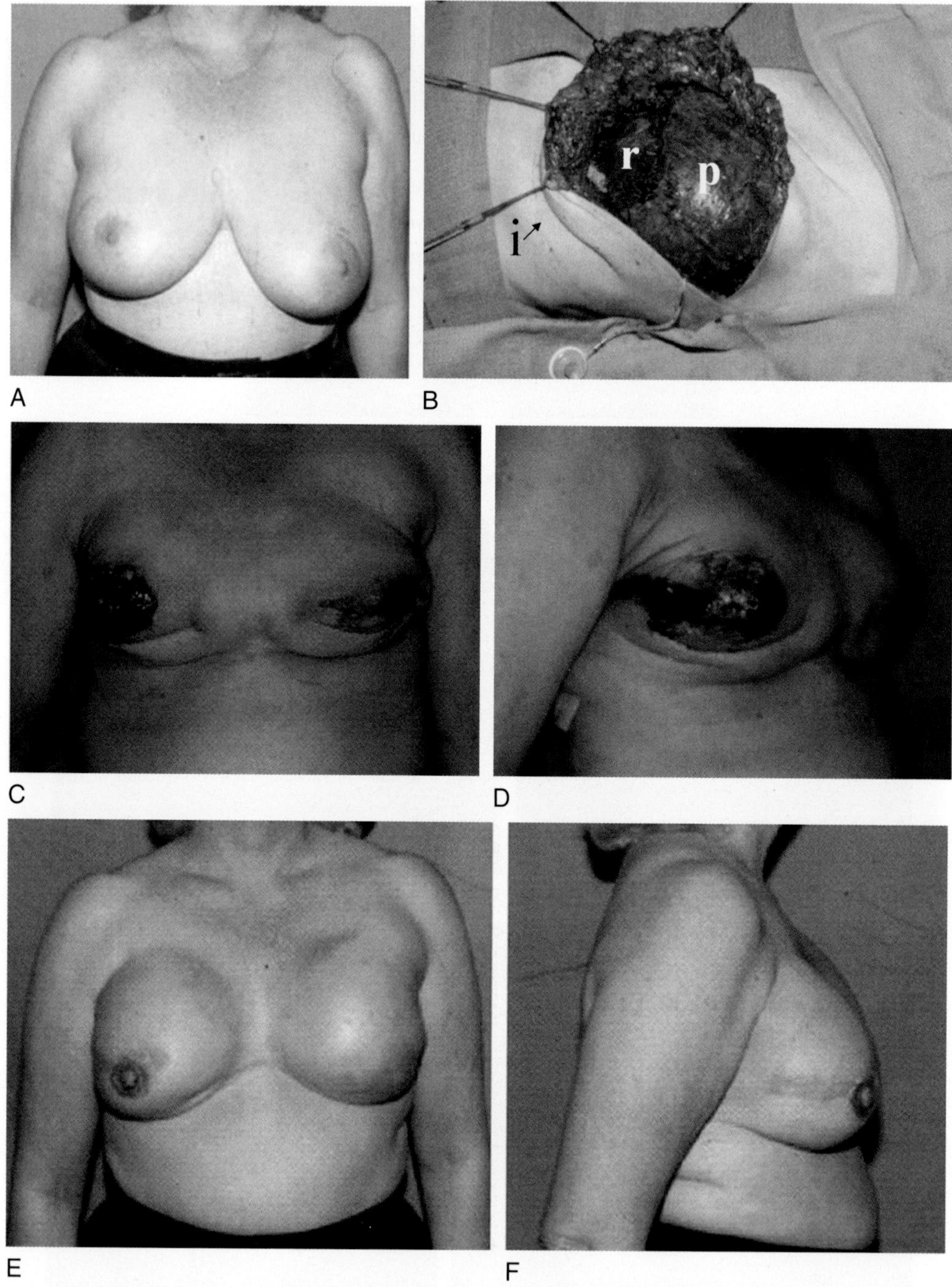

FIGURE 143-50. Immediate expander-implant reconstruction with segmental rectus–external oblique flap. *A,* Preoperative anterior view of right stage I breast cancer and left atypia on biopsy. *B,* Stage 1, expander coverage with pectoralis major flap (p) superiorly and laterally and segmental rectus flap (r) inferiorly; i, inframammary line. *C,* Postoperative stage 1 anterior view at 3 weeks. There is bilateral partial skin necrosis. The wounds were treated with silver sulfadiazine (Silvadene). Expanders have complete muscle coverage. *D,* Postoperative lateral view at 3 weeks. *E,* Postoperative stage 2 anterior view at 6 months. After healing of areas of skin necrosis, the expansion process was completed and permanent implants were inserted. *F,* Postoperative stage 2 lateral view at 6 months.

Expansion Below Anticipated Inframammary Line

The technique of expansion below the inframammary line was often used with the smooth-walled expander because the expander often migrated toward the clavicle, where there is less resistance during the expansion process. By starting inferior to the anticipated inframammary line, the inferior chest wall skin is the center of expansion, providing a more natural skin envelope to cover the permanent implant in the second stage of expander-implant reconstruction. With the textured expander, the expander can be placed exactly at the inframammary line, with the expansion process centered over the inferior aspect of the breast mound because this implant is less likely to migrate superiorly to the area of least resistance. Tissue adhesions to the textured surface hold the implant in place. However, if the surgeon requires the skin below the inframammary line to be incorporated into the breast coverage, the expander can effectively be placed below the inframammary line and this additional expanded skin used for the breast mound (Fig. 143-51*A* to *D*).

At the second stage, internal plication of the expanded skin at the inframammary line will provide more skin for the inferior breast mound, with natural ptosis of the reconstructed breast mound (Fig. 143-51*E* and *F*). Internal plication with sutures can be applied through the mastectomy incision, avoiding further breast mound scars. After the inferior expanded skin is plicated superiorly, the sizer is inserted with the patient in a sitting position. Standing at the foot of the operating room table, the surgeon can determine when sufficient plication of the inferior skin has provided additional skin for the inferior aspect of the reconstructed breast mound and the correct location of the inframammary line for symmetry with the contralateral breast or appropriate position if bilateral reconstruction is required. Additional sutures are applied or removed until the breast mound has a natural appearance and bilateral breast symmetry has been accomplished. When the surgeon is satisfied with the position of the inframammary line and the size of the permanent implant determined by use of the sizer, the permanent breast implant is inserted, completing the second-stage breast reconstruction (Figs. 143-51*G* to *I* and 143-52).

Text continued on p. 944

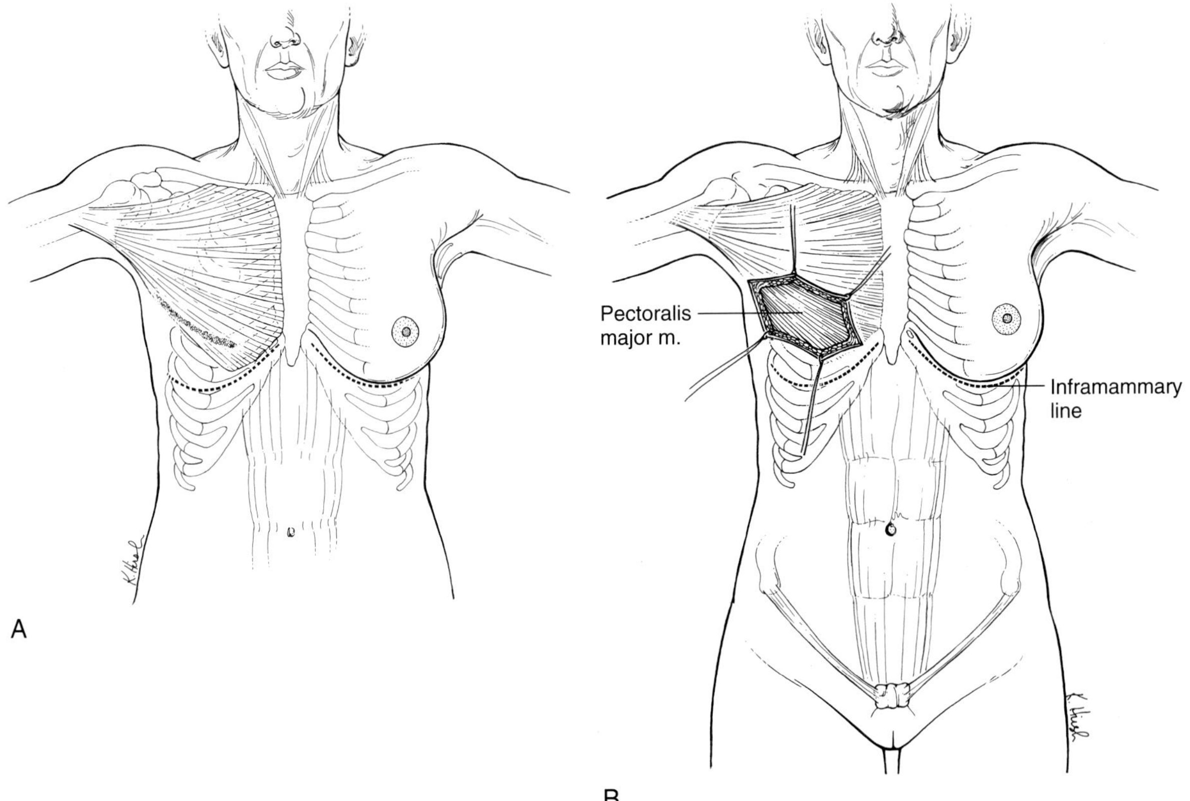

FIGURE 143-51. Expansion below anticipated inframammary line. *A,* Delayed reconstruction: dissection for expander-implant extends below defined inframammary line to inferior chest wall space. *B,* Dissection through mastectomy scar. *Continued*

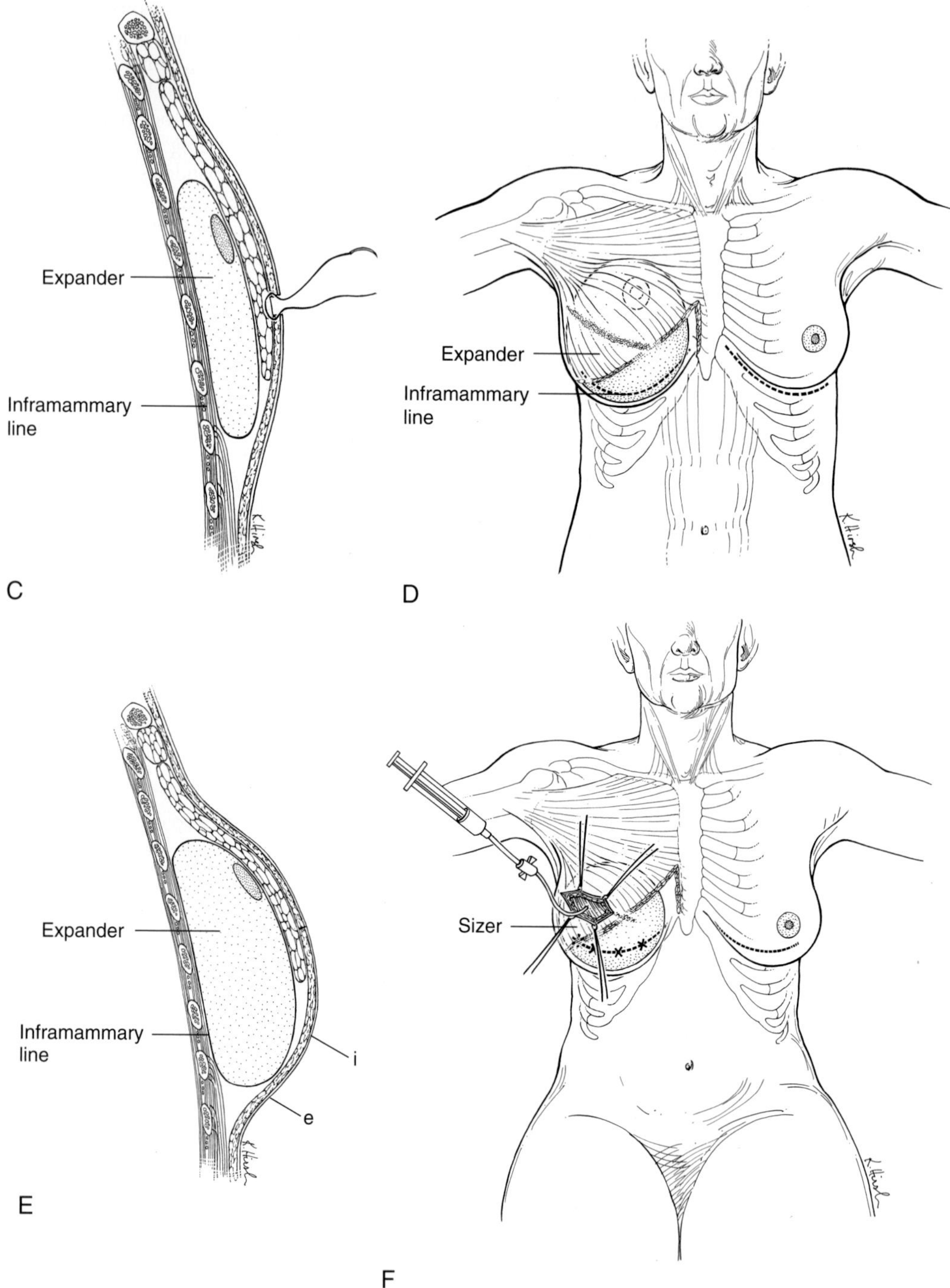

FIGURE 143-51, cont'd. *C,* Lateral view. The expander is placed in a subpectoral position with release of inferior (sixth intercostal space) pectoralis major muscle origin. Note that expander space extends inferior to defined inframammary line to inferior chest wall skin. *D,* Stage 1: expansion incorporates inferior chest wall flap into breast skin envelope. *E,* Stage 1, lateral view. Note that expander increases dimension of inferior skin envelope. i, inframammary line; e, expanded skin envelope inferior to i. *F,* Stage 2: sizer is placed beneath expander skin envelope. With the patient in a sitting position, the skin envelope is plicated.

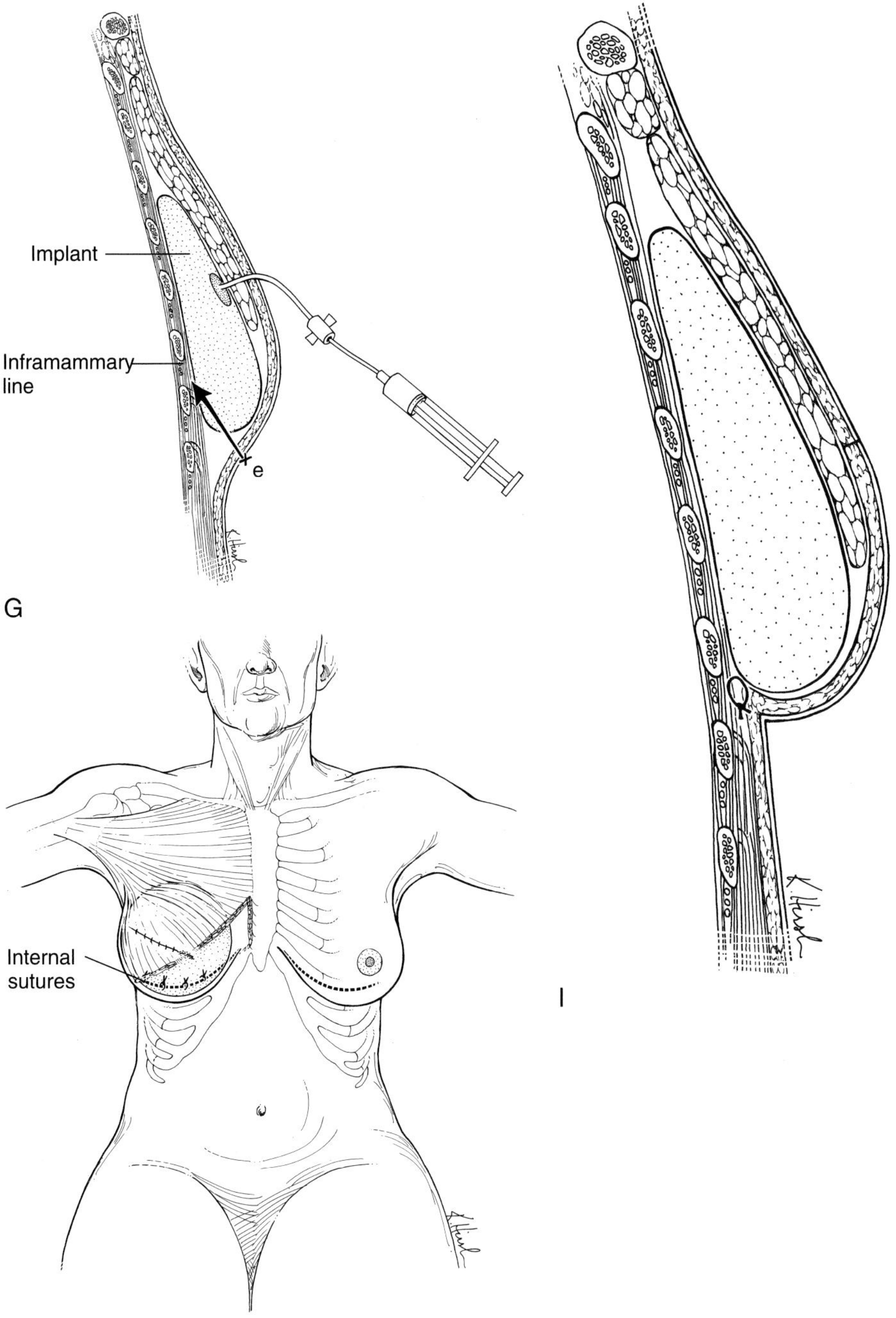

FIGURE 143-51, cont'd. *G,* Stage 2, lateral view. Expanded skin originally below the inframammary line is incorporated into inferior breast skin envelope. The inframammary line is established by plication of expanded skin (e) to the chest wall with internal sutures. *H,* Stage 2: with position of inframammary line defined, implant size is determined by sizer. The permanent implant is inserted, and the mastectomy defect is closed. *I,* Stage 2: lateral view at completion of expander-implant reconstruction. Note suture plication of new inframammary line.

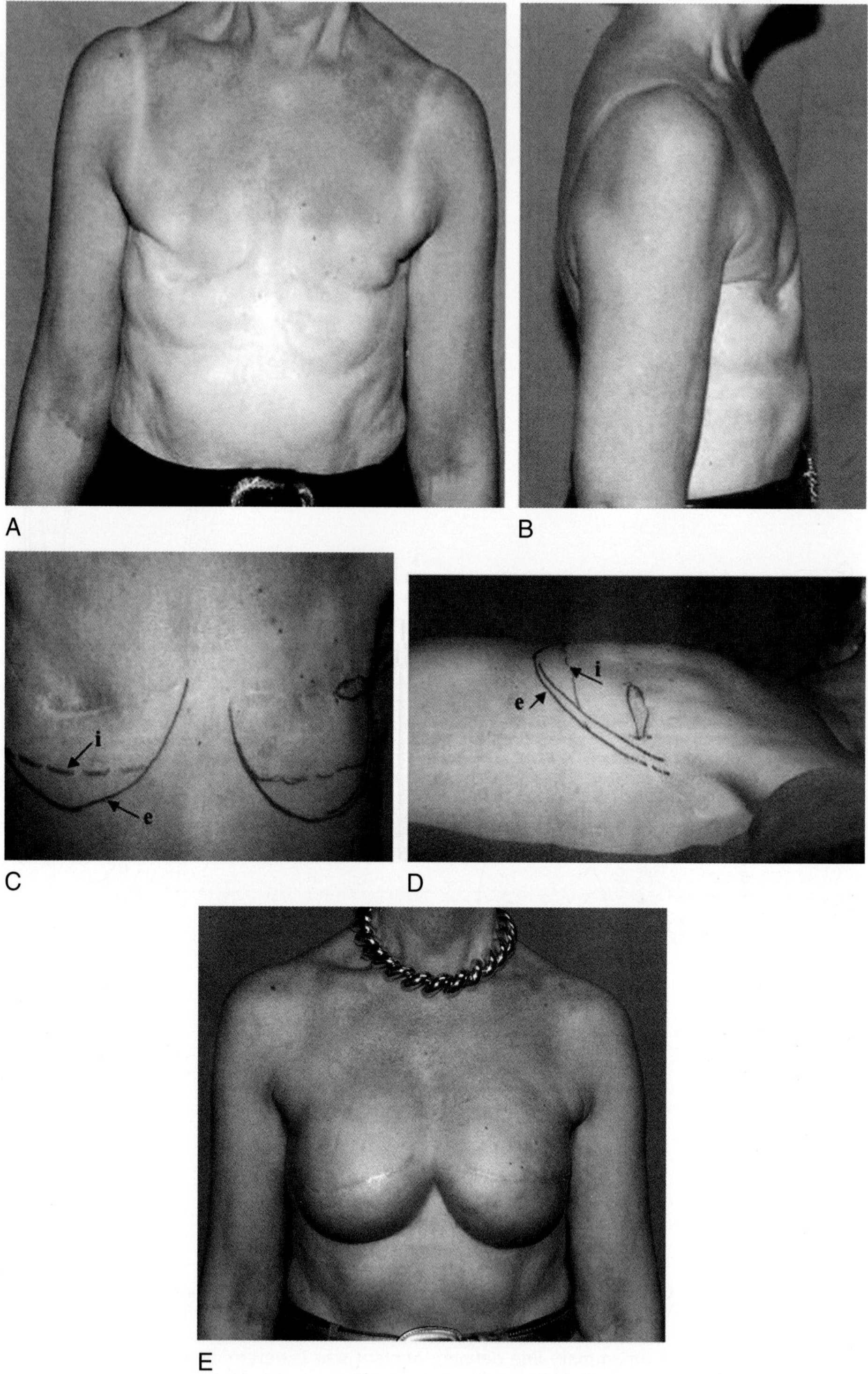

FIGURE 143-52. Delayed expander-implant reconstruction with expansion below the inframammary line. *A,* Anterior postoperative view after bilateral mastectomy. Note tight skin envelopes. *B,* Lateral view of right mastectomy defect. *C,* Anterior preoperative view, stage 1. Expander will be placed below inframammary line (i) to expand inferior chest wall skin (e). *D,* Lateral preoperative stage 1 view demonstrates extension of zone of expansion from inframammary line (i) to inferior anterior chest skin above costal margin (e). *E,* Postoperative anterior view, stage 1: expanders in place.

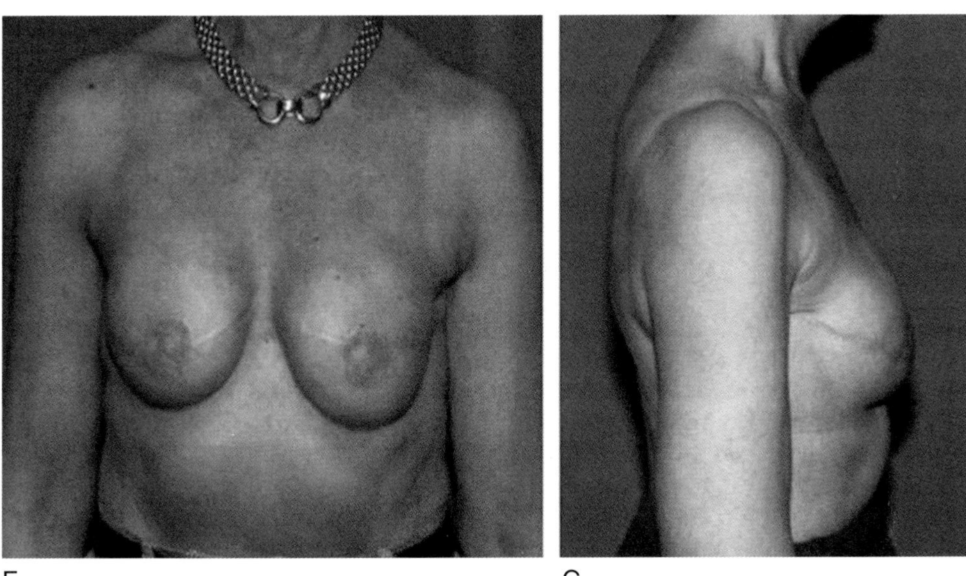

F G

FIGURE 143-52, cont'd. *F,* Postoperative anterior view, stage 2, at 1 year: internal advancement and plication of skin allowing improved skin envelope. *G,* Lateral postoperative view, stage 2. Note well-defined inframammary line.

Abdominal Advancement Flap

The abdominal advancement flap technique was developed before the tissue expander was used to establish a suitable skin envelope for implant breast reconstruction. It is not commonly required if staged breast reconstruction is selected with an expander-implant.[15,16] However, it is useful when a single-stage delayed reconstruction is selected or when secondary breast reconstruction is performed (Fig. 143-53).[17,18]

The inframammary line is marked at the site of reconstruction. A second line is then drawn inferior to the anticipated marked inframammary line. The second line will represent the incision site and the leading edge of the abdominal advancement flap (Fig. 143-53*A*). This line is usually marked 1 to 2 cm below the inframammary line. This advancement flap will move the inferior line to the inframammary line. The superior skin envelope will be sutured to the flap edge, forming the new inframammary line. The skin between the original and the new inframammary line is now located on the inferior aspect of the breast mound skin envelope. The advancement flap is elevated superficial to the anterior rectus sheath and the external oblique fascia laterally. The flap is usually elevated either to the costal margin or further inferiorly to the level of the umbilicus, depending of how much flap is required to establish an adequate skin envelope. The distal 3 to 5 mm of the advancement flap is de-epithelialized to allow inset of the inferior aspect of the skin envelope into the advancement flap that has been sutured to the chest wall at the inframammary line. If the dissection for the advancement flap extends into the upper quadrant of the abdomen, the donor site is generally drained with closed suction catheters (10-mm JP drains are preferred). After the inframammary line is inset, the sizer is placed beneath the skin envelope and the patient is placed in the sitting position to confirm correct position of the inframammary line and implant size.

When the surgeon is satisfied with implant position and size, the temporary sutures are removed. The permanent implant is placed, followed by a two-layer closure at the inframammary line (Figs. 143-54 to 143-56).

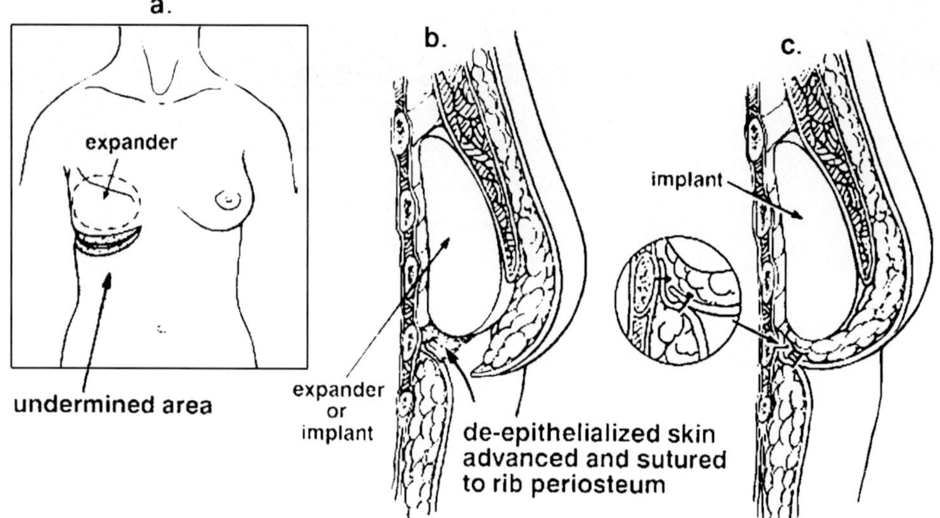

FIGURE 143-53. Lower thoracic advancement flap. *A,* Inset demonstrates anterior view of expander-implant in place and area to be undermined. *B,* Lateral view of expander-implant in place. *C,* De-epithelialized skin is advanced and sutured to rib periosteum. (From Oliva A, Mathes SJ: Technique of breast reconstruction. Prob Gen Surg 1989;6:564.)

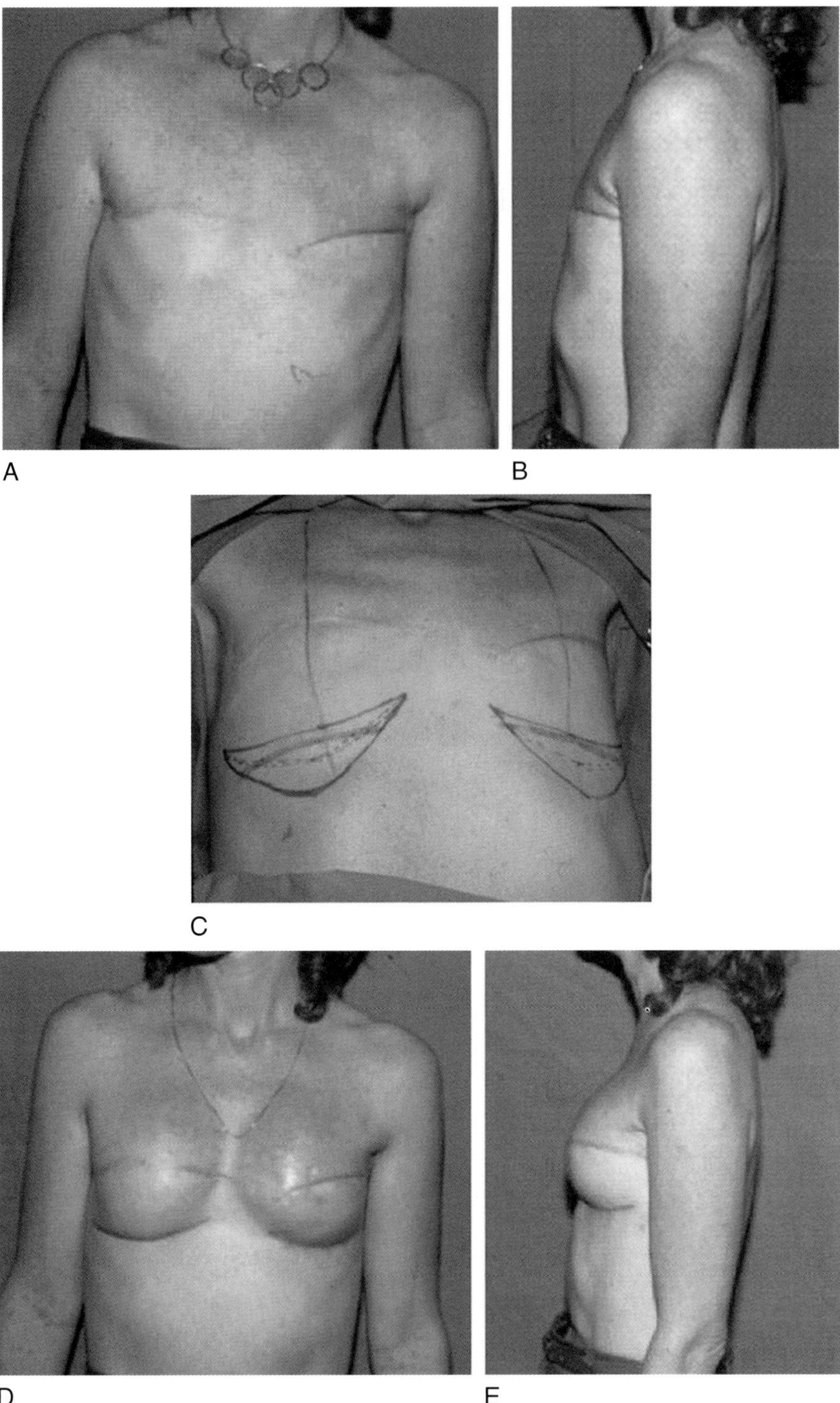

FIGURE 143-54. Delayed implant reconstruction with abdominal advancement flap. *A,* Anterior view of bilateral mastectomy defect. *B,* Left lateral view of mastectomy defect. *C,* Preoperative markings for abdominal advancement flap. Distal abdominal advancement flap will be advanced to inframammary line. Intervening skin (crosshatched) will be incorporated into inferior breast skin envelope. *D,* Postoperative anterior view at 6 months of abdominal advancement flap, which allowed single-stage implant reconstruction. *E,* Postoperative lateral view at 6 months. The inframammary line is defined at suture closure of the distal abdominal advancement flap and inferior breast skin envelope.

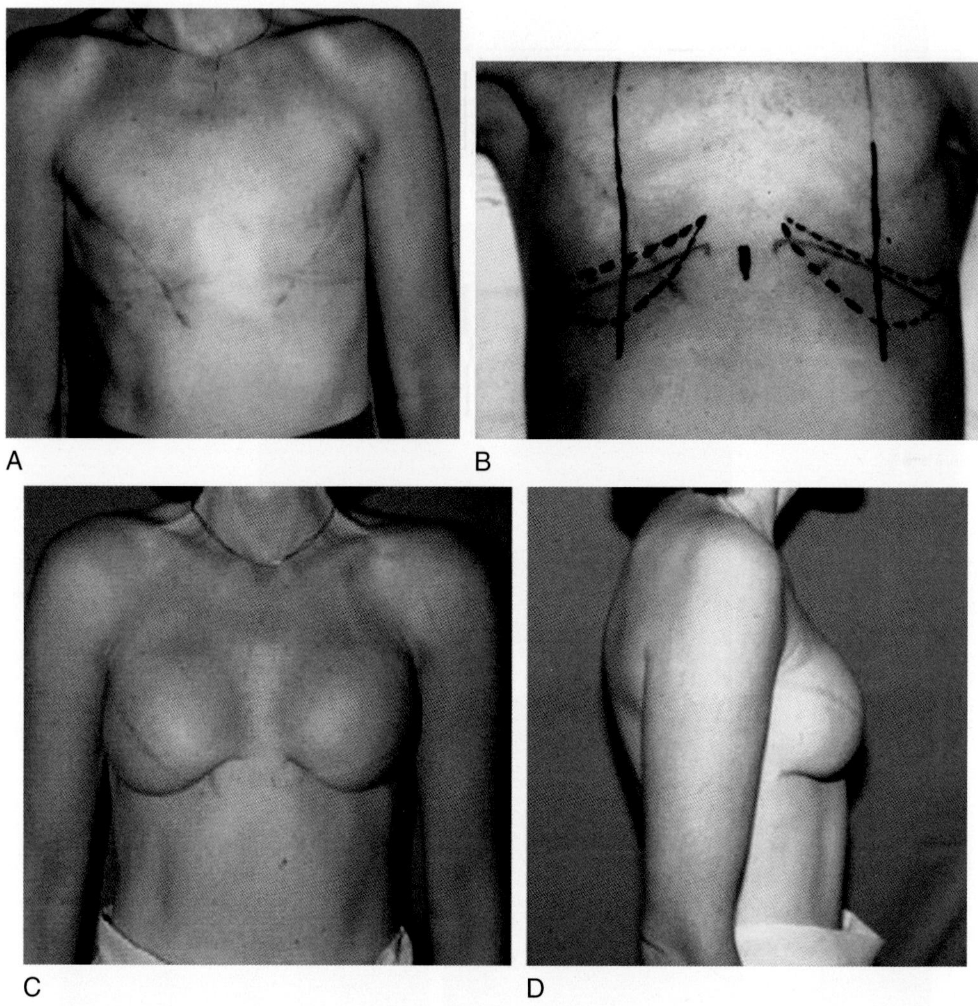

FIGURE 143-55. Delayed implant reconstruction with abdominal advancement flap. *A,* Preoperative anterior view. *B,* Preoperative markings for abdominal advancement flap. *C,* Postoperative anterior view 1 year after bilateral reconstruction. *D,* Postoperative lateral view at 1 year.

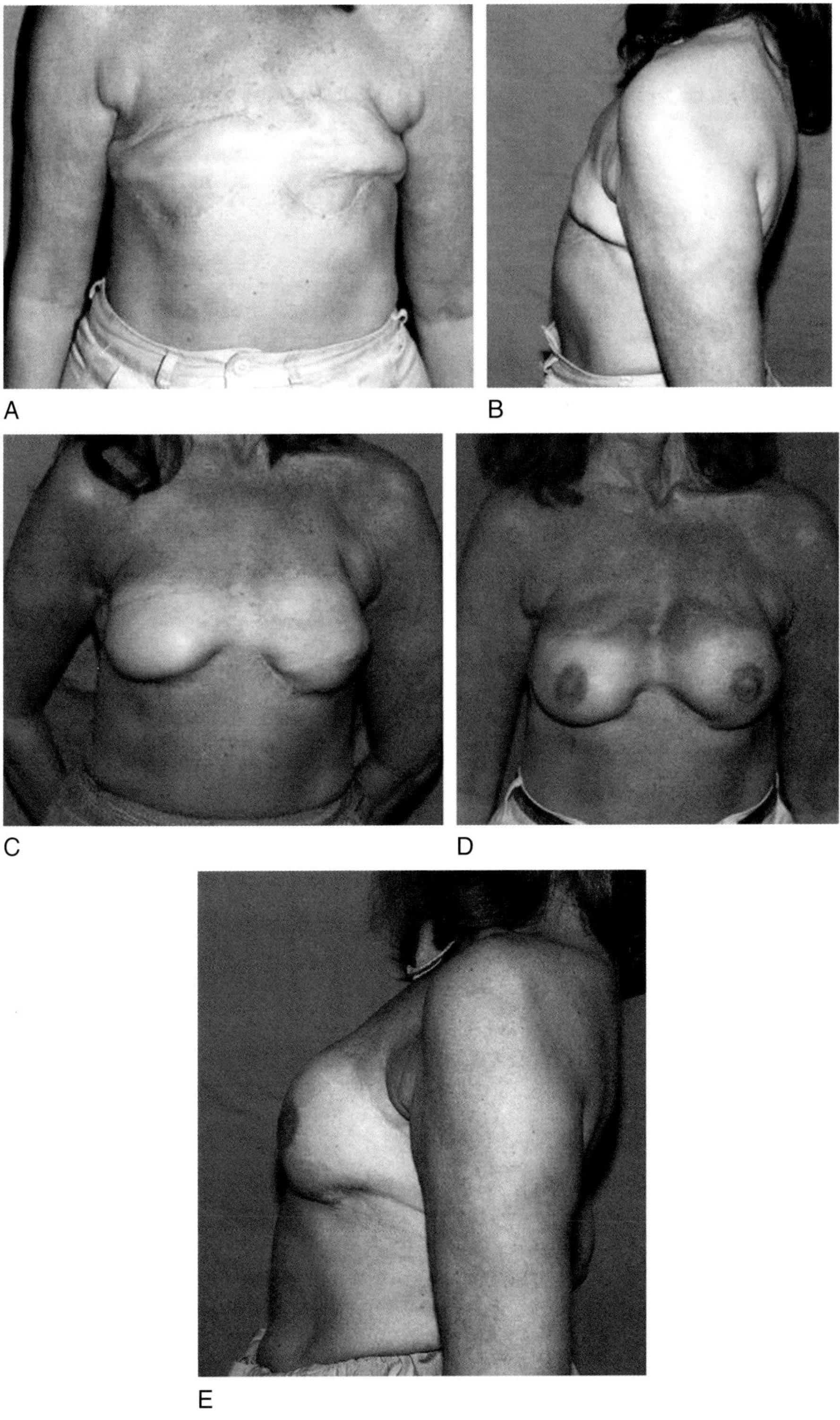

FIGURE 143-56. Delayed expander-implant reconstruction: abdominal advancement flap. *A*, Anterior view of postoperative bilateral mastectomy and failed prior reconstruction attempt with tight chest wall skin envelope. *B*, Lateral view of mastectomy defect. *C*, Postoperative anterior view at 3 months: abdominal advancement flap with implant reconstruction. *D*, Postoperative anterior view at 1 year: bilateral reconstruction. Abdominal advancement flap allows incorporation of inframammary skin into inferior breast skin envelope *E*, Postoperative lateral view at 1 year. Site of inset of abdominal flap defines inframammary line.

Total Skin-Sparing Mastectomy

The skin-sparing approach is now a well-accepted technique in regard to tumor management and for skin envelope preservation for reconstruction. The concept of nipple-areola sparing was originally introduced by Parry et al[19] in 1977. Anatomic evaluations of the areola reveal a combination of sebaceous, sweat, and areolar glands.[20] As a skin appendage, these glands should not have breast parenchymal tumors, with the exception of the areolar glands, which may be identical to the extralobular ducts in breast parenchyma.[21] For this reason, Simmons et al[22] performed pathologic analysis of 217 mastectomy specimens in search of tumor involvement of the areola. Of these specimens, there was only a 1% occurrence of malignant involvement of the areola and 10% involvement of the nipple. The nipple does contain ductal tissue that may harbor tumor cells with varying reports of tumor involvement (5% to 58% tumor involvement of the nipple-areola complex).[23] If the mastectomy incision is in proximity to the nipple, it is possible to remove all ductal tissue and confirm margins with frozen section but preserve the cutaneous portion of the nipple. This approach has been used with success with both areola-sparing and nipple-areola (total skin-sparing) approaches, with use of similar criteria for preservation of the areola or entire nipple-areola complex (Table 143-39).[24-26] With appropriate selection of patients, including prophylactic mastectomy and stage I (<3.5 cm), peripheral tumors or tumors not in proximity to the nipple-areola complex (>2 cm), and confirmation of no tumor involvement with frozen section analysis, local recurrence rates have not been increased above skin-sparing mastectomy data.[25] However, nipple-areola ischemic necrosis or wound contraction in the preserved nipple epidermis may result in loss of the nipple height or unacceptable distortion of the nipple appearance. Furthermore, with skin loss, there is risk of implant exposure and loss of the reconstruction. If an autogenous reconstruction is performed, loss of the nipple presents less risk in regard to eventual outcome. Use of the flap skin island in replacement of the nipple-areola in skin-sparing mastectomy may provide a better vascularized base for subsequent nipple-areola reconstruction (see Chapter 139).

In the series by Crowe et al[24] of 54 attempted nipple-sparing mastectomies, 6 were noted to have neoplastic involvement on frozen section analysis. The remaining 44 patients underwent nipple preservation with 6% partial loss of the nipple. In the series by Simmons et al[26] with 2-year follow-up, 17 areola-sparing mastectomies were performed in 12 patients (prophylaxis, n = 10; ductal carcinoma in situ, n = 4; <2 cm peripheral infiltrating cancer, n = 3); no local recurrence was noted. Gerber et al[25] reported an analysis of 286 patients with indications for modified radical mastectomy with tumor margins greater than 2 cm for the nipple. Of these patients, 112 underwent skin-sparing mastectomy and 134 underwent modified radical mastectomy. Intraoperative frozen section analysis was used to determine whether the nipple-areola complex could be preserved. In this group of skin-sparing mastectomy, the nipple-areola complex was preserved in 61 patients (54.5%) and resected in 51 patients (45.5%). Indications for resection of the nipple-areola were based on frozen section findings, including extensive intraductal component (defined as more than 25% of tumor cells in ducts), tumor growth closer than 2 cm from the nipple, and suspicious cells in the base of the nipple. With a mean follow-

TABLE 143-39 ✦ SELECTION CRITERIA FOR AREOLA- AND NIPPLE-SPARING MASTECTOMY

Study	n (ASM or NSM)	Inclusion Criteria
Gerber et al[25]	61 (NSM)	Age <75 years BMI range 21–35 kg/m^2 Absence of skin involvement Noncentral tumor Radiographic distance of at least 2 cm between the NAC and tumor Intraoperative frozen section of breast parenchyma free of tumor cells closer than 2 cm to the NAC
Crowe et al[24]	48 (NSM)	Non–centrally located tumors Tumor <3.5 cm in size Frozen section analysis of nipple core free of malignancy
Simmons et al[26]	17 (ASM)	Non–centrally located tumors Tumors <4 cm in size In patients with multifocal DCIS with microinvasion, negative touch-prep cytology to the posterior portion of the areola

ASM, areola-sparing mastectomy; NSM, nipple-sparing mastectomy; BMI, body mass index; NAC, nipple-areola complex; DCIS, ductal carcinoma in situ.
From Simmons RM, Hollenbeck ST, Latrenta GS: Two-year follow-up of areola-sparing mastectomy with immediate reconstruction. Am J Surg 2004;188:403.

TABLE 143-40 ✦ FOLLOW-UP DATA COMPARING SKIN-SPARING MASTECTOMY (SSM) WITH AND WITHOUT NIPPLE-AREOLA COMPLEX (NAC) CONSERVATION AND MODIFIED RADICAL MASTECTOMY (MRM)

	SSM with NAC Conservation (n = 61)	SSM without NAC Conservation (n = 51)	MRM (n = 134)	P
Local recurrences	3 (5%)	3 (6%)	11 (8%)	.666
Distant metastases	14 (23%)	10 (20%)	28 (21%)	.906
Death	9 (15%)	5 (10%)	17 (13%)	.733
Procedures performed on the opposite breast to achieve symmetry	8 (13%)	8 (16%)	9 (7%)	n.d.
NAC reconstruction	—	33 (65%)	17 (13%)	.733
Secondary breast reconstruction	—	—	11 (8%)	n.d.
Would today decide for SSM	—	—	12 (9%)	n.d.

n.d., not done.

From Gerber B, Krause A, Reimer T, et al: Skin-sparing mastectomy with conservation of the nipple-areola complex and autologous reconstruction is an oncologically safe procedure. Ann Surg 2003;238:120.

up of 59 months, local recurrence occurred in six patients (5.4%) in the skin-sparing mastectomy group (one recurrence in nipple preservation; after resection, the patient was reported tumor free with 52-month follow-up). Local recurrence developed in 11 patients (8.2%) in the modified radical mastectomy group (Table 143-40).[25] The aesthetic results were analyzed as superior in the skin-preserving mastectomy group and were reported to be significantly better in the patients in the skin-sparing mastectomy group with nipple preservation.

For areola preservation, the incision may extend directly through the areola with an incision around the nipple so that the nipple is included in the mastectomy specimen. Other incisions may be used distant to the areola with a separate incision around the nipple so that it is included with the mastectomy specimen (Fig. 143-57). For prophylactic mastectomy, the transverse incision extending from the medial areola-cutaneous margin through the areola and then extending laterally beyond the lateral areola toward the anterior axillary line provides excellent exposure and preserves circulation to the superior- and inferior-based flaps. For nipple preservation, the transverse nipple-areola incision (Fig. 143-58) allows excellent exposure to the ductal system for direct inspection of the nipple. Furthermore, if additional exposure is required, the incision may be extended laterally toward the anterior axillary line with preservation of circulation to the split nipple-areola complex. A separate areola-cutaneous incision may be used, but the areola between the nipple and the incision may be more likely to have loss of subdermal vascular connections (Fig. 143-59).

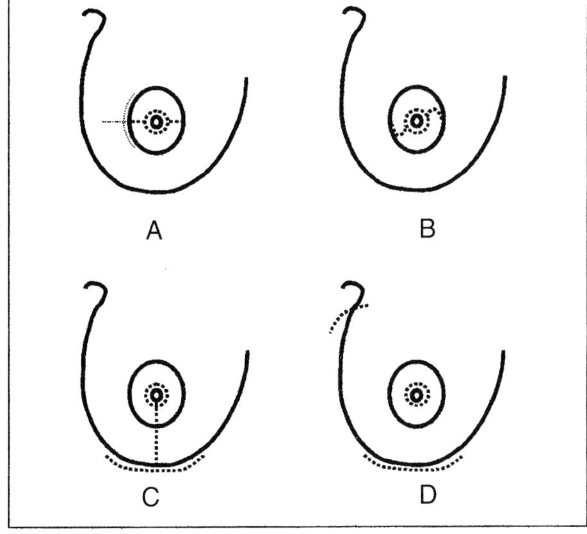

FIGURE 143-57. Schematic representation of incisions used for areola-sparing mastectomy (small dotted line indicates line of incision). *A,* Linear intra-areolar incision with extra-areolar extension shaped as either a "tennis racquet" or a T. *B,* S-shaped intra-areolar incision. *C,* Inverted T inframammary crease incision. *D,* Triple incision (inframammary crease, perinipple, and axillary). (From Simmons RM, Hollenbeck ST, Latrenta GS: Areola-sparing mastectomy with immediate breast reconstruction. Ann Plast Surg 2003; 51:547.)

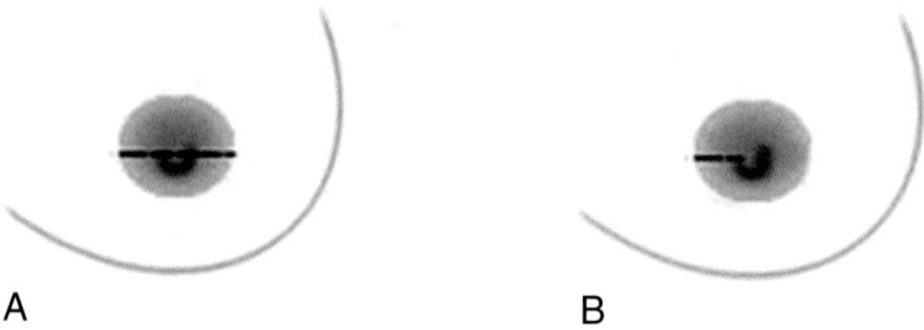

FIGURE 143-58. *A,* Transverse nipple-areola incision. *B,* Hemitransverse nipple-areola incision.

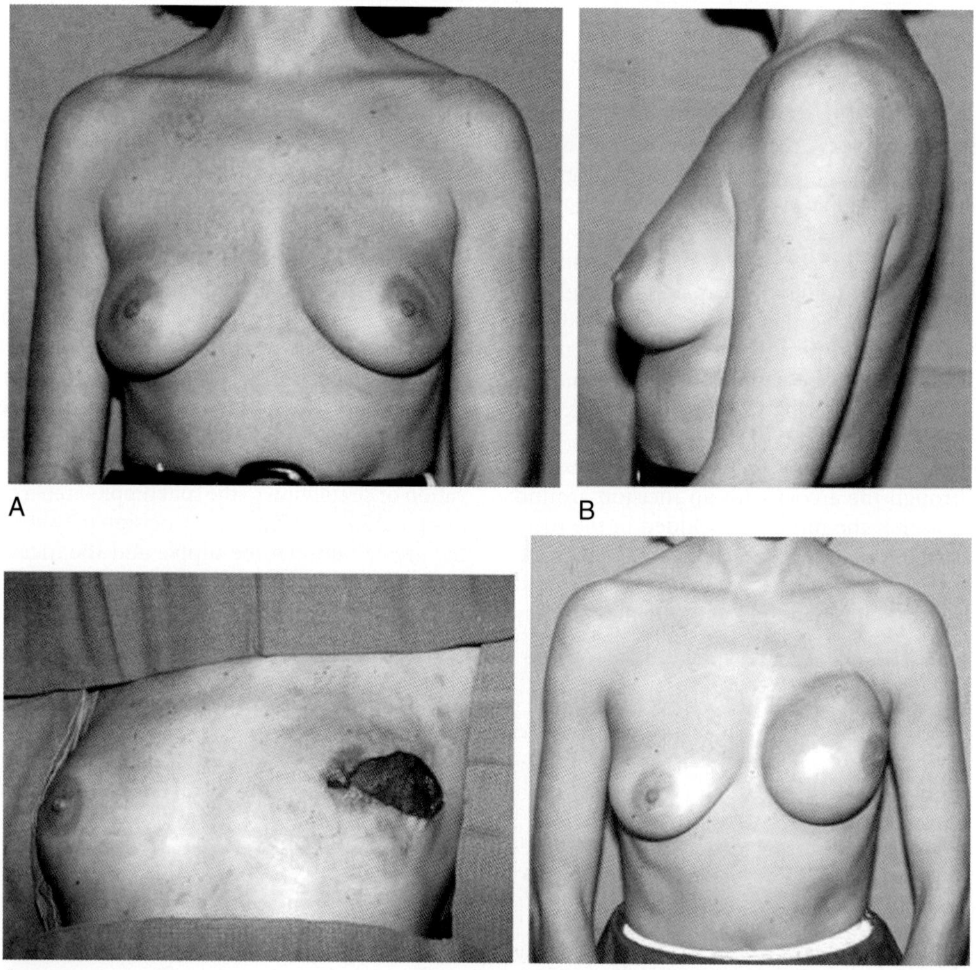

A
B
C
D

FIGURE 143-59. *A,* Anterior view of left invasive breast cancer (stage I). *B,* Lateral view. *C,* Mastectomy incision transects nipple-areola and extends to anterior axillary line. Nipple and areola-cutaneous portion are preserved with dissection of nipple ductal tissue through the incision. *D,* Anterior view of completion of tissue expansion 3 months after mastectomy.

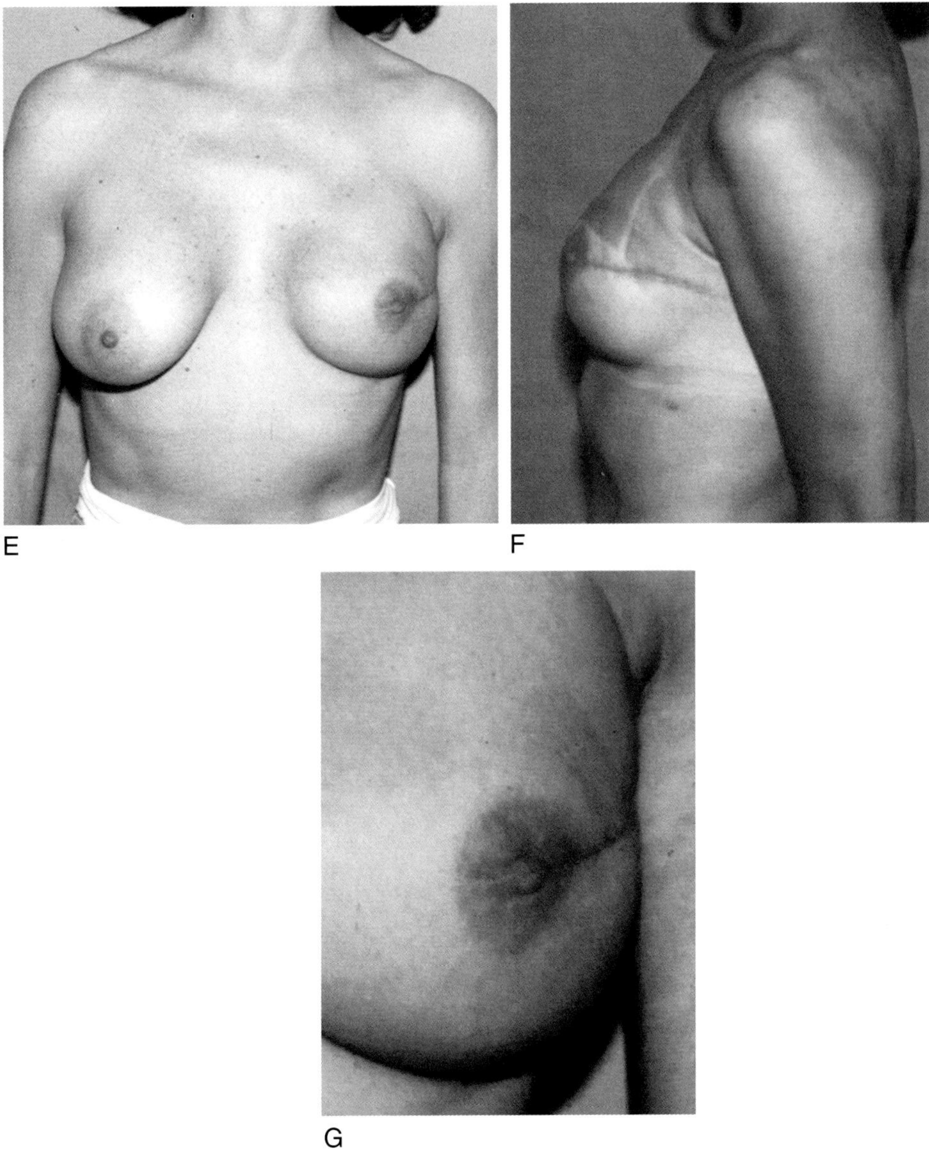

FIGURE 143-59, cont'd. *E,* Anterior view 1 year after insertion of permanent implant to complete breast reconstruction. Note adequate mound with slight loss of breast ptosis and preserved nipple-areola. *F,* Lateral view. *G,* Close-up anterior and lateral view of preserved cutaneous portion of nipple-areola.

Expander-Implant Use in Association with Flaps

A flap is often used for breast reconstruction to avoid a staged procedure, which is required when an expander is used. However, there are instances in which an expander used in association with a flap will enhance or even enable the reconstructive process. The tissue expander may be used in the following ways in conjunction with immediate or delayed flap use: to preserve a suitable breast envelope for staged incorporation of a flap; to allow observation of the preserved skin envelope before use of a flap; to expand the remaining skin envelope after a flap has been inset; and to expand the skin envelope in preparation for later flap insertion.

BREAST ENVELOPE PRESERVATION FOR STAGED FLAP RECONSTRUCTION

When use of a flap is anticipated for immediate breast reconstruction, there may be concern about tumor margins or requirements for radiation therapy based on pathologic examination of the permanent specimen. Temporary use of an expander allows preservation of the skin envelope, particularly after skin-sparing mastectomy. If radiation therapy is required, flap reconstruction can be delayed until after therapy is completed to avoid damage to an autogenous flap. During the process of radiation therapy, the expander will preserve the skin envelope and reduce the requirement for skin replacement at the second-stage reconstruction.

There is still an ongoing discussion of the value of immediate flap reconstruction with irradiation of the flap versus delay in the flap until the radiation therapy is completed (see Chapter 138) (Fig. 143-60).

OBSERVATION OF THE PRESERVED SKIN ENVELOPE

After skin-sparing mastectomy, there is always a risk of skin loss due to devascularization of the skin flaps. If there is doubt about the status of the skin envelope, an expander is a safe way to observe the skin envelope to make a final decision as to timing and dimensions of a delayed flap procedure for breast reconstruction. An expander may also be used in immediate reconstruction to observe the viability of the skin envelope.

When an immediate flap is used after skin-sparing mastectomy, the cutaneous portion of the flap is tailored to precisely fit the area of skin resected during the mastectomy. If adequate skin envelope circulation is impaired, this skin may be resected and a larger cutaneous portion of the flap inset to preserve the required dimensions of skin envelope to provide an adequate breast mound reconstruction. However, it may be difficult to accurately predict skin envelope survival because of ecchymosis of the preserved skin envelope. Even with the use of fluorescein, it may be difficult to accurately determine which portion of the preserved skin envelope will survive and which portion should be resected. The use of the expander will allow observation of the skin envelope in the early postoperative period. In most instances, within 7 to 10 days, an accurate assessment of the skin envelope is possible, allowing precise design of the flap for breast reconstruction. If the plastic surgeon works closely with the oncologic surgeon, the survival of the skin envelope may be predicted accurately, allowing immediate use of the flap and avoiding a staged procedure when the expander is initially inserted to observe skin envelope survival.

EXPANSION OF SKIN ENVELOPE AFTER FLAP RECONSTRUCTION

In delayed reconstruction or secondary reconstruction, there may be extensive damage to the preserved skin envelope, or the flap may have inadequate dimension to fully restore the required skin envelope. Simultaneous placement of an expander beneath the remaining skin envelope and flap will allow later expansion of the skin envelope after the flap is healed. At a later stage, a permanent implant may be placed beneath the expanded skin envelope. This approach is more commonly used in the latissimus dorsi musculocutaneous flap, in which the skin island dimension is more limited than in the TRAM flap; however, if zone 2 is unavailable for use in the breast mound reconstruction, or if a patient is very thin without a significant panniculus in the lower abdomen, adequate breast mound volume may not be provided by the TRAM flap (Figs. 143-61 and 143-62).

The required implant size may put undesirable pressure on the flap and impair its circulation. The expander is inflated after the flap is healed to prepare a space for later permanent implant insertion. The latissimus flap usually requires simultaneous insertion of the permanent implant at the time of inset. However, insertion of an expander may help avoid excess scar development beneath the flap during the early healing process, allowing later insertion of the permanent implant after the expansion process is completed.

EXPANSION OF THE SKIN ENVELOPE FOR FLAP INSERTION

In immediate or delayed reconstruction, preliminary skin expansion of the retained skin envelope will prepare the space for staged autogenous flap breast reconstruction. With this approach, the flap can primarily be used for the breast mound, and minimal skin island will be required for the breast envelope. In

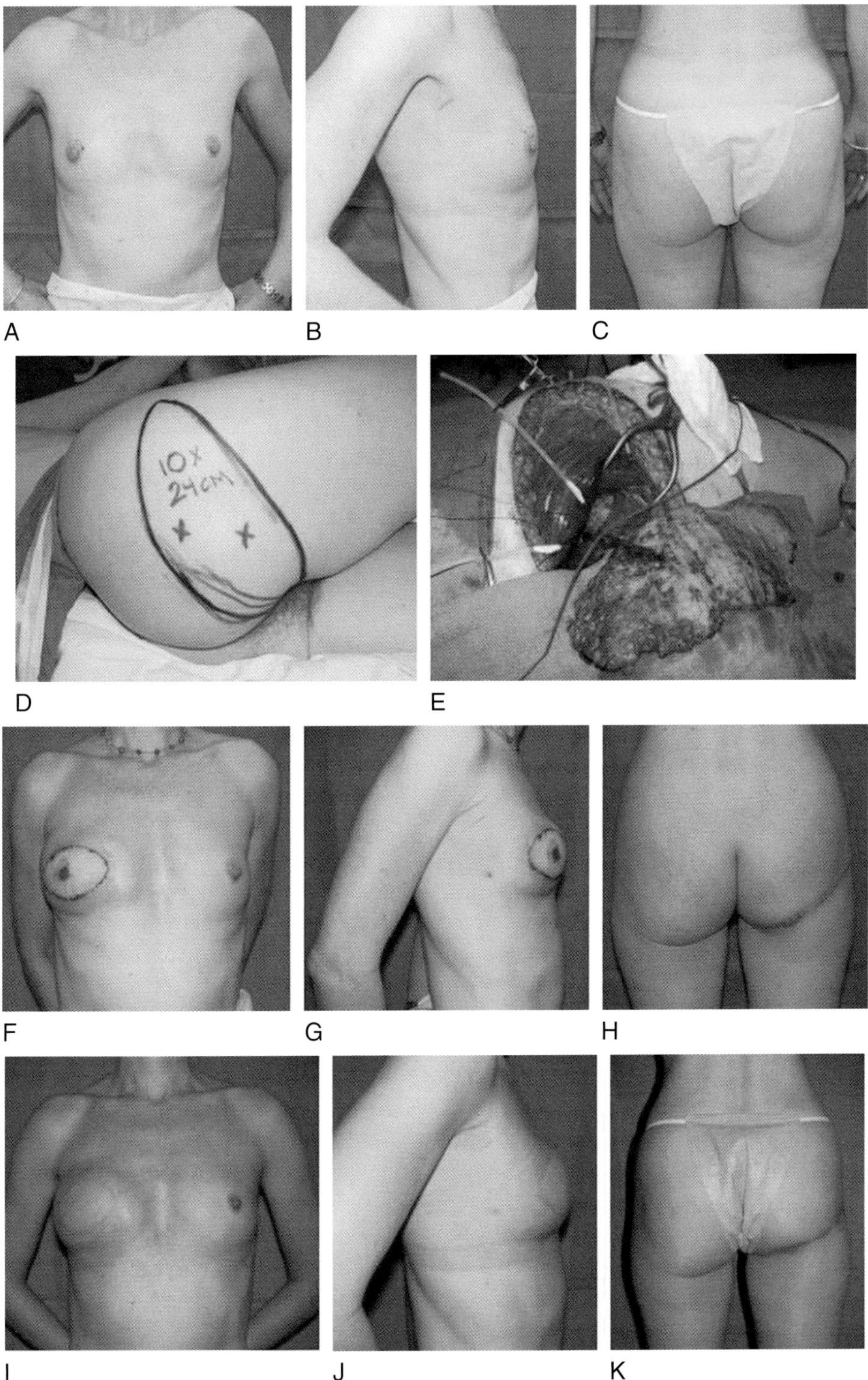

FIGURE 143-60. Expander reconstruction with staged inferior gluteal artery perforator (IGAP) flap. *A,* Preoperative anterior view of patient with stage I breast cancer. *B,* Preoperative lateral view. *C,* Preoperative posterior view of potential gluteal donor site. *D,* IGAP flap design. *E,* IGAP flap dissection and elevation. *F,* Day 21, postoperative anterior view after expander and staged IGAP flap reconstruction. *G,* Day 28, postoperative lateral view. *H,* Day 28, postoperative posterior view showing donor site and "in the crease" closure. *I,* Postoperative anterior view at 2 months. *J,* Postoperative lateral view at 2 months. *K,* Postoperative posterior view at 2 months showing donor site.

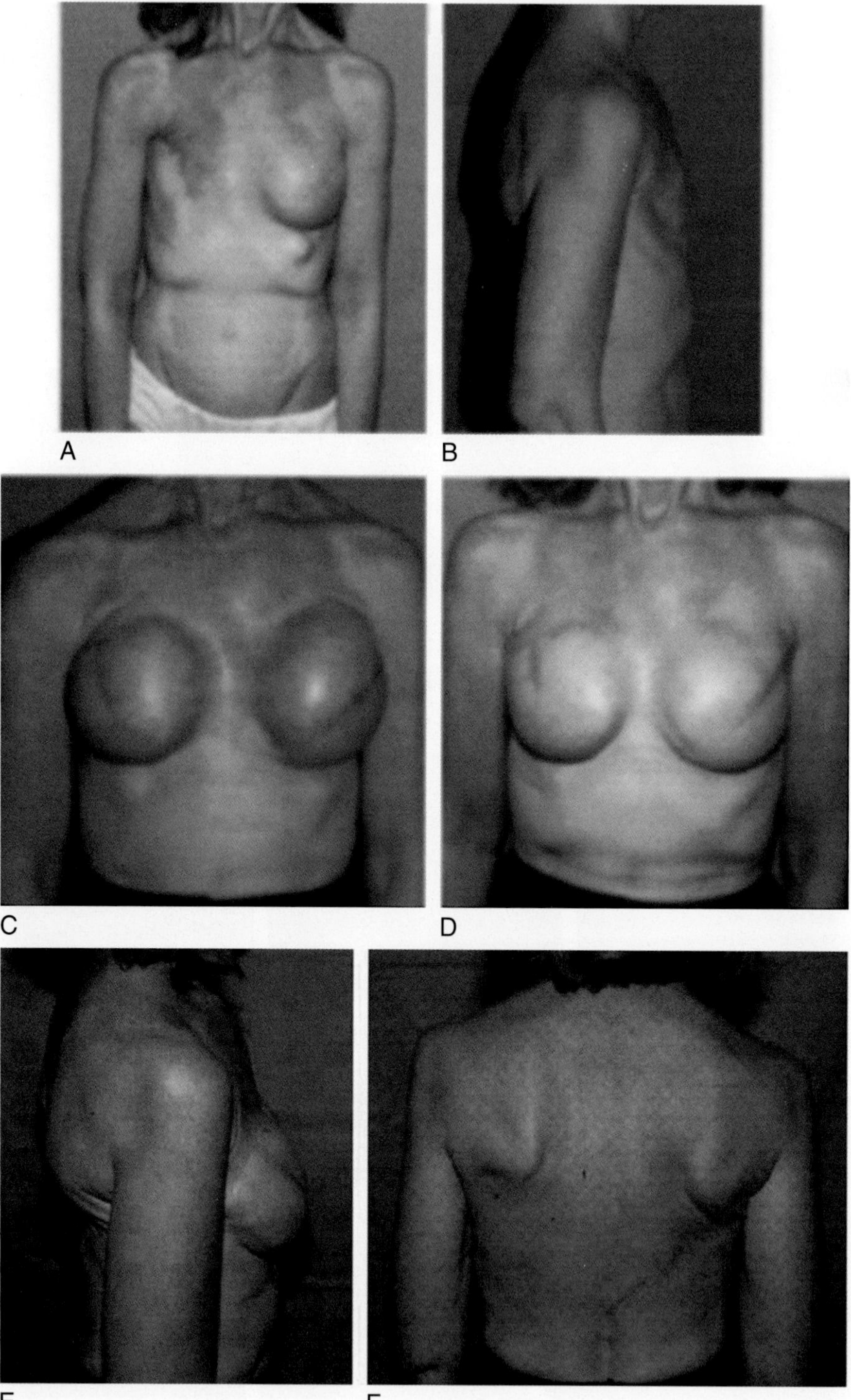

FIGURE 143-61. Expansion of skin envelope after flap inset. *A,* Anterior view of right modified radical mastectomy defect with irradiation and attempted reconstruction of left breast (expander in place for 1 year). *B,* Lateral view, mastectomy and radiation defect. *C,* Postoperative view of bilateral expander inflation and latissimus dorsi musculocutaneous flap reconstruction on the right. *D,* Postoperative anterior view at 1 year after permanent saline implant placement after a latissimus dorsi musculocutaneous flap on the right side and bilateral staged expansion and removal. *E,* Postoperative lateral view at 1 year. *F,* Postoperative view at 1 year of posterior donor site for latissimus dorsi musculocutaneous flap.

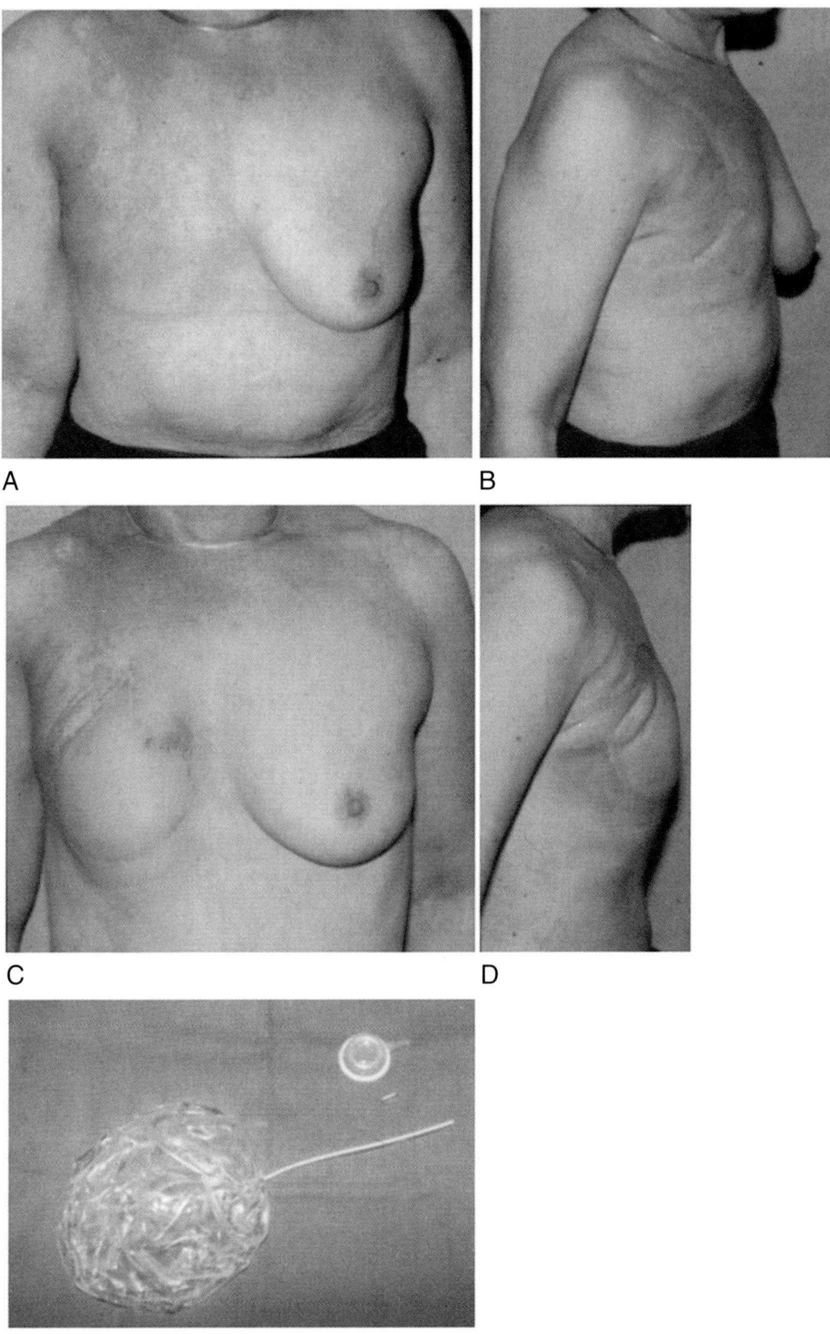

FIGURE 143-62. TRAM flap for delayed right breast reconstruction with adjustable implant for breast mound volume improvement. *A,* Preoperative anterior view of modified radical mastectomy defect with postoperative radiation therapy. *B,* Lateral preoperative oblique view demonstrates scar contracture on right hemithorax. *C,* Postoperative view at 3 months of transposition of contralateral TRAM flap with immediate insertion of inflatable saline implant. Zone 2 was not available because of abdominal scar. *D,* Postoperative lateral view 3 months after contralateral TRAM flap.

Continued

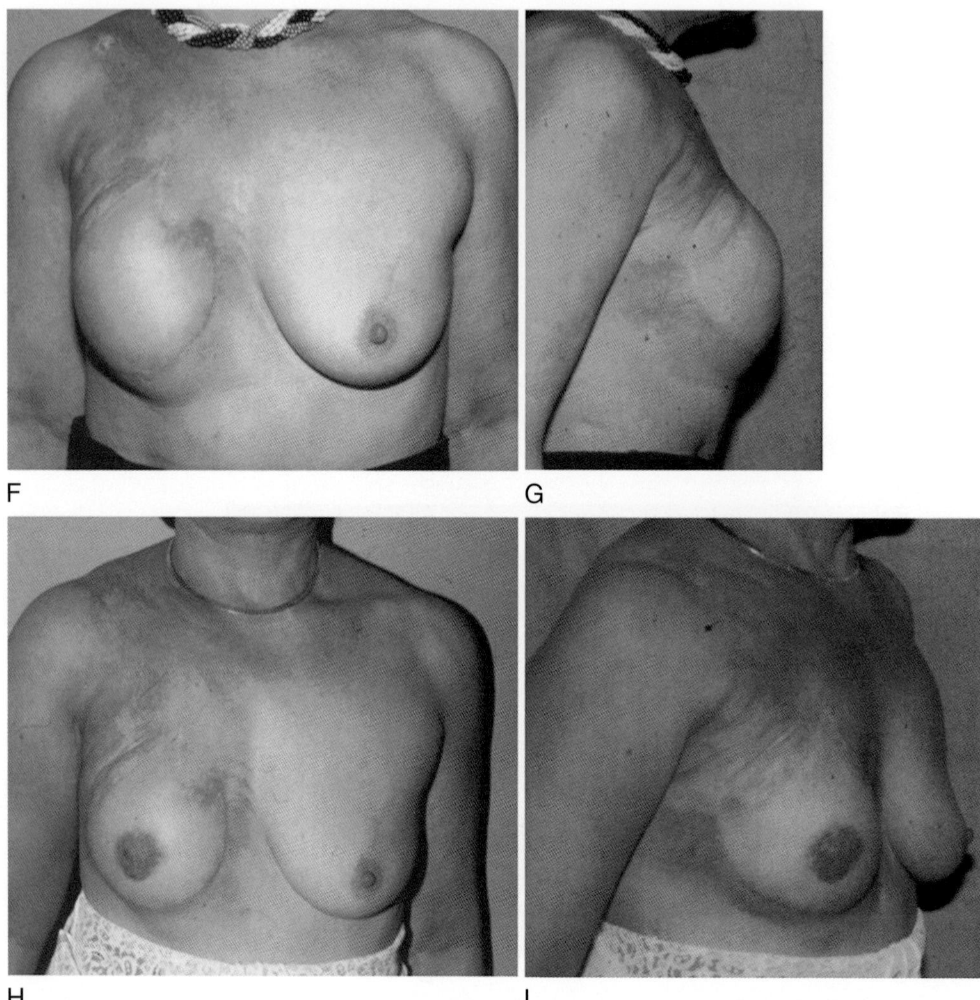

FIGURE 143-62, cont'd. *E,* Saline inflatable implant placed beneath TRAM flap inset site. *F,* Postoperative anterior view at 6 months. Saline implant inflation is in progress. *G,* Postoperative lateral view at 6 months. Breast volume is improved with inflation of the saline implant. *H,* Postoperative anterior view at 1 year of combined TRAM flap and implant providing adequate mound size and symmetry in radiation-damaged chest. *I,* Postoperative oblique view demonstrating adequate mound projection. Nipple-areola reconstruction is completed.

selected patients, the first stage of expansion will allow the patient to decide whether to proceed with second-stage implant insertion or with flap use for autogenous reconstruction. In delayed reconstruction, depending on the extent of the original mastectomy resection, donor site skin available, and preference of the patient for aesthetic outcome, the skin envelope may not be sufficient to restore the breast mound with an appropriate autologous flap. For these patients, expanders may be used to increase the volume of the skin envelope to enable delayed placement of a permanent, autologous flap (Fig. 143-63).

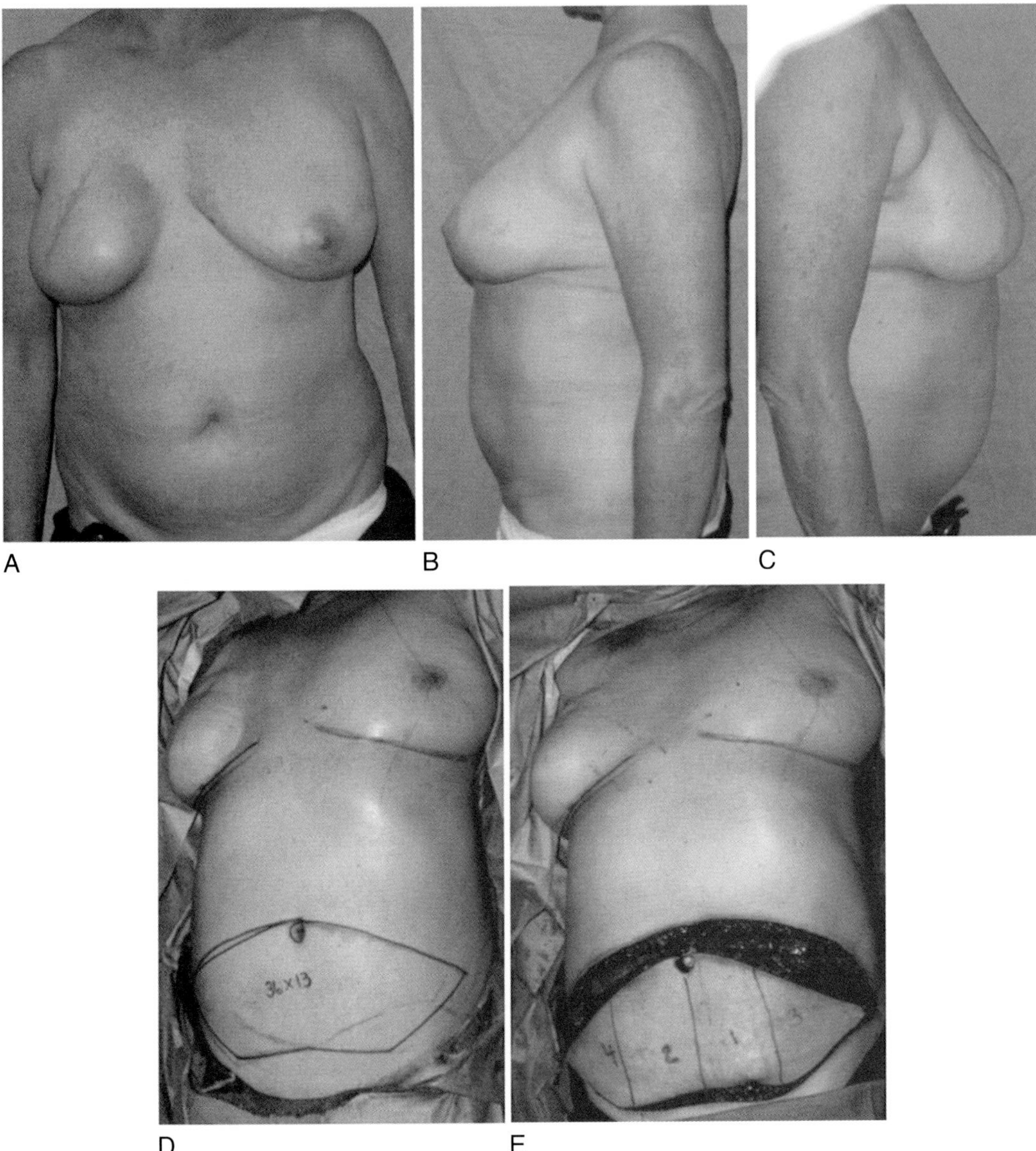

FIGURE 143-63. Expansion of skin envelope for delayed flap insertion with use of expanders to provide adequate skin envelope. *A,* Anterior preoperative view after unilateral skin-sparing mastectomy. The patient is seen with the expander in place in preparation for TRAM flap placement. *B* and *C,* Preoperative lateral views. *D,* Intraoperative view of skin island design for skin-sparing TRAM flap. *E,* TRAM flap is partially elevated.

Continued

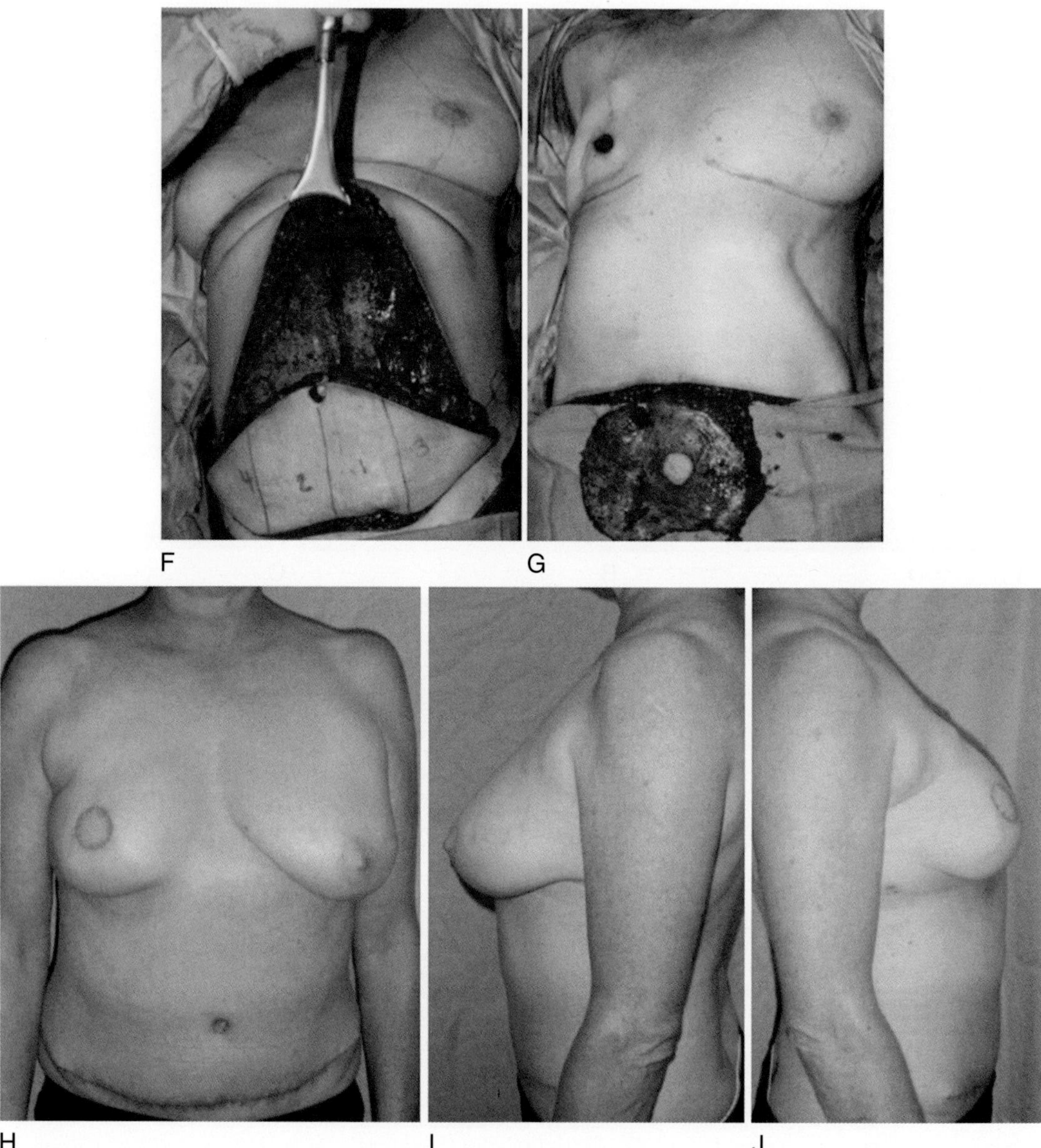

FIGURE 143-63, cont'd. *F,* Flap pedicle release for rotation and inset into defect. The flap will be rotated for temporary placement within the skin envelope. The area of skin necessary for nipple-areola reconstruction will be preserved on the skin island. The remainder of the skin island will be de-epithelialized, and the excess tissue will be trimmed. *G,* The skin envelope has been prepared. The flap has been de-epithelialized and trimmed and is ready for final inset into the defect. *H,* Anterior postoperative view at 3 months demonstrating nipple-areola site designed intraoperatively. *I* and *J,* Postoperative lateral views at 3 months.

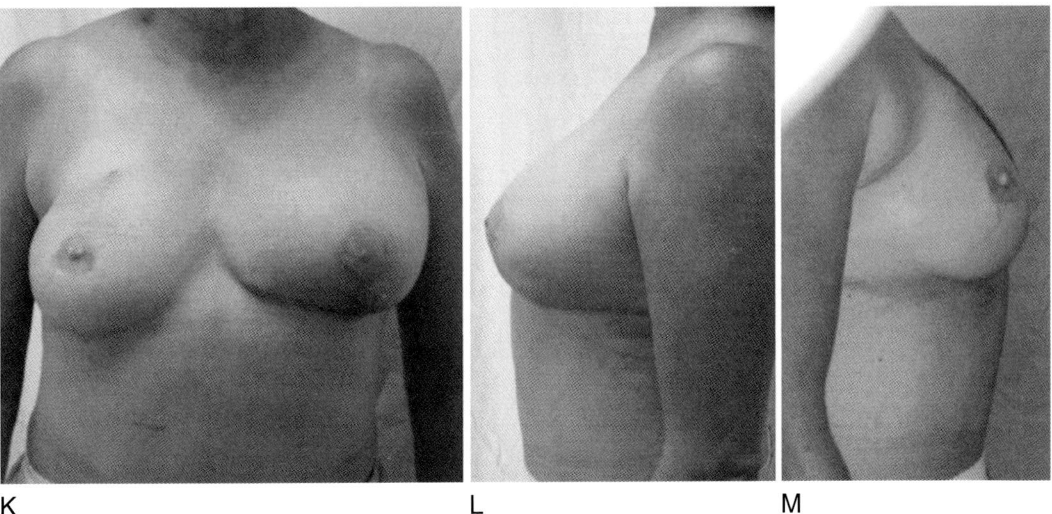

FIGURE 143-63, cont'd. *K,* Postoperative view 8 months after skin-sparing TRAM flap and nipple-areola reconstruction demonstrating adequate breast mound projection and ptosis. *L* and *M,* Lateral postoperative views at 8 months.

OUTCOMES

In a study comparing three consecutive study groups, there was no significant difference in major and minor complication rates between autogenous and nonautogenous reconstruction[27] (Fig. 143-64). Similarly, in the Michigan Breast Reconstruction Outcome Study,[28] total complication rates between the expander-implant reconstructive groups and the combined TRAM flap groups showed no significant difference (Table 143-41). When the operative time is compared, the total time for expander-implant procedures remains much less than for flap procedures, but the average number of procedures is greater (Table 143-42).[27] Thus, the patient's choice, the status of the mastectomy site, and the status of the contralateral breast will determine which procedure offers the best outcome for the individual patient. Because of decreased technique complexity, no additional donor site scar and potential complications, and shorter recovery time, many patients will select nonautogenous expander-implant reconstruction.

The choice in breast reconstruction primarily centers on nonautogenous versus autogenous. Nonautogenous reconstruction encompasses a wide range of techniques, including implant alone, postoperative adjustable implant, staged expander-implant, and flaps incorporating an implant for breast mound volume (e.g., latissimus dorsi muscle, TRAM, abdominal advancement). Similarly, there is a wide variety of autogenous reconstruction techniques, including pedicled TRAM flap, free TRAM flap, perforator flaps, and latissimus dorsi musculocutaneous flaps. It is therefore difficult to compare outcome results because each surgeon and breast care center emphasize different procedures on the basis of experience and confidence with specific techniques. Implant-expander techniques are widely used throughout the world, providing safe and reliable breast reconstruction. The Michigan Breast Reconstruction Outcome Study[28] demonstrated greater aesthetic and general satisfaction of patients undergoing reconstruction by pedicled and free TRAM flaps compared with patients undergoing expander-implant reconstruction. However, pedicled or free TRAM flap

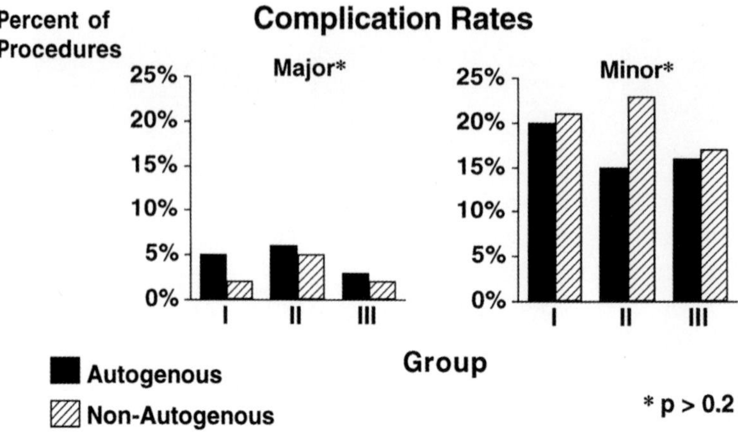

FIGURE 143-64. Comparison of major and minor complication rates between nonautogenous and autogenous methods of breast reconstruction for three consecutive study groups. (From Trabulsy PP, Anthony JP, Mathes SJ: Changing trends in postmastectomy breast reconstruction: a 13-year experience. Plast Reconstr Surg 1994;93:1418-1427.)

procedures are more complex and require longer hospitalization and outpatient recovery time. Post-reconstruction satisfaction rates vary for expander-implants, but in most studies, they range from 78%[29] to 61%.[30] Clough[31] noted a decline in aesthetic satisfaction from an initial rate of 86% at 2 years to 54% at 5 years after implant reconstruction. The linear decrease in satisfaction is multifactorial but may be a result of long-term complications, such as capsular contracture and asymmetric contralateral ptosis.

TABLE 143-41 ✦ FREQUENCY OF COMPLICATIONS BY TYPE OF RECONSTRUCTION

	Implants		Pedicle TRAM Flaps		Free TRAM Flaps	
Complication	*No.*	*%*	*No.*	*%*	*No.*	*%*
Back pain	1	1.3	4	2.2	4	6.0
Hernia/abdominal wall laxity	—		14	7.8	8	11.9
Lymphedema	3	3.8	10	5.6	3	4.5
Capsular contracture	12	15.2	—		—	
Implant shift	1	1.3	—		—	
Wound dehiscence	3	3.8	10	5.6	1	1.5
Partial flap loss (fat necrosis)	5	6.3	29	16.2	10	14.9
Total flap loss	0		2	1.1	1	1.5
Anastomotic thrombosis	—		—		4	6.0
Implant failure	3	3.8	—		—	
Infection	28	35.4	21	11.7	12	17.9
Clostridium difficile colitis	0		1	0.5	0	
Hematoma/seroma of the breast	4	5.1	7	3.9	6	9.0
Hematoma/seroma of the abdomen	—		7	3.9	3	4.5
Abdominal wall necrosis	—		3	1.7	0	
Cardiac/pulmonary complications	1	1.3	6	3.4	6	9.0

From Wilkins EG, Cederna PS, Lowery JC, et al: Prospective analysis of psychosocial outcomes in breast reconstruction: one-year postoperative results from the Michigan Breast Reconstruction Outcome Study. Plast Reconstr Surg 2000;106:1014.

TABLE 143-42 ✦ AVERAGE OPERATIVE TIME FOR EACH TECHNIQUE AND AVERAGE NUMBER OF PROCEDURES FOR FINAL RESULT

	Average Operative Time by Technique	Average No. of Procedures* on Reconstructed Breast by Technique
Implant, n = 82	1.2 h	1.8
Staged tissue expander-implant, n = 142	3.2 h	2.4
Latissimus dorsi implant, n = 107	3.8 h	1.7
TRAM flap, n = 106	5.5 h	1.2
Free flap, n = 12	9.0 h	1.2

*Does not include nipple-areola reconstruction.

Note: Operative techniques have improved with experience, and time required for free flaps has been reduced by 3 hours on average.

From Trabulsy PP, Anthony JP, Mathes SJ: Changing trends in postmastectomy breast reconstruction: a 13-year experience. Plast Reconstr Surg 1994;93:1418-1427.

COMPLICATIONS

Complications occur in the perioperative period, early (3 to 6 weeks), and late. Studies investigating complications common to expander-implant reconstruction show great variability in reported rates (Table 143-43).[12] Perioperative complications include hematoma, seroma, and infection. Hematoma requires reoperation and ranges from 0% to 5.8%. Seroma is usually avoided with a closed suction system, but if it is extensive, it may require open drainage. Infection rates range from 0% to 15%. Antibiotic therapy for early cellulites may be effective. Perioperative antibiotics in immediate reconstruction are recommended.

Early complications usually involve skin envelope necrosis, infection, and expander-implant malfunction. Skin envelope necrosis may occur in the range of 0% to 21%.[12] A rate exceeding 10% may represent a relative contraindication to immediate reconstruction, particularly in skin-sparing mastectomy. Usually, a small segment of skin at the incision site may be vulnerable to ischemic necrosis. With muscle coverage of the expander-implant, local wound care, and topical antibiotics, healing should occur without jeopardy to the implant. When skin necrosis is more extensive, unless the implant is well covered with muscle, implant exposure may occur, and subsequent removal may become necessary. When infection occurs in the implant space, implant removal is necessary with delayed secondary reconstruction after wound healing and scar maturation are achieved. Tenderness, late seroma development, low-grade fever, and leukocytosis usually indicate implant space infection.

Malfunction of the expander-implant in the early postoperative period should be rare. Proper placement of the expander and confirmation of port patency after skin closure during the operative procedure should avoid problems. Confirmation with devices to locate the port during early expansion will avoid inadvertent puncture of the expander. If malfunction occurs in the early postoperative period, re-exploration is required with replacement of the nonfunctional expander-implant.

Late complications related to expander-implant reconstruction extend throughout the life of the patient. Delayed implant deflations and rupture represent the greatest concern for the patient. Deflation and rupture rates are difficult to determine because the design of both saline- and gel-filled implants is constantly changing. The risk, however, does increase with implant age. A minimum of 15% of modern implants can be expected to rupture between the third

TABLE 143-43 ✦ SUMMARY OF COMPLICATIONS AFTER IMPLANT BREAST RECONSTRUCTIVE SURGERY

Reference	n	Reconstruction Details	Infection (%)	Hematoma (%)	Seroma Around Implant (%)	Native Skin Necrosis (%)	Implant Loss or Extrusion (%)	Difficulty in Expansion (%)	Valve Failure (%)	Deflation (%)
Mansel et al[40] (1986)	12	I, immediate	7.9	0	0	0	16.7	0	0	0
Schuster et al[41] (1990)	38	LD + I, immediate	8.3	0	0	2.6	23.7	0	0	0
	56	E/I, silicone, immediate	5.4	3.6	7.1	12.5	7.1	0	0	0
Mandrekas et al[8] (1995)	44	Becker, immediate and delayed	2.3	0	0	2.3	0	0	2.3	0
Hunter-Smith and Laurie[42] (1995)	54	Becker, immediate and delayed	3.7	0	1.9	3.7	1.9	0	1.9	1.9
McGeorge et al[43] (1996)	19	E/I, saline, immediate and delayed	5.3	0	5.3	5.3	0	0	0	0
Ramon et al[44] (1997)	52	E/I, silicone, delayed	9.6	5.8	0	1.9	5.8	11.5	3.8	3.8
Spear and Majidian[45] (1998)	171	E/I, saline, immediate	3.5	1.2	0	5.3	10.5	0	0	4.0
Slavin et al[46] (1998)	51	LD + I, saline, immediate	2.0	0	0	21.6	3.9	0	0	0
Al-Ghazal and Blamey[47] (2000)	101	I, silicone, Becker, immediate and delayed	0	0	0	8.9	10-13	0	0	0
Peyser et al[48] (2000)	71	LD + Becker or McGhan 150, immediate	4.2	1.4	0	9.9	0	0	1.4	0
Berry et al[49] (1998)	100	Becker, immediate	15	0	0	4	14	0	1	0
Gui[12] (2003)	129	McGhan 150, immediate	6.2	1.6	0	3	3.9	0	0	0

E/I, tissue expander replaced by implant; saline, saline implant; I, implant alone; silicone, silicone implant; Becker, Becker permanent expander-implant; McGhan 150, McGhan style 150 permanent expander-implant; LD, latissimus dorsi flap.

From Gui GP, Tan SM, Faliakou EC, et al: Immediate breast reconstruction using biodimensional anatomical permanent expander implants: a prospective analysis of outcome and patient satisfaction. Plast Reconstr Surg 2003;111:125.

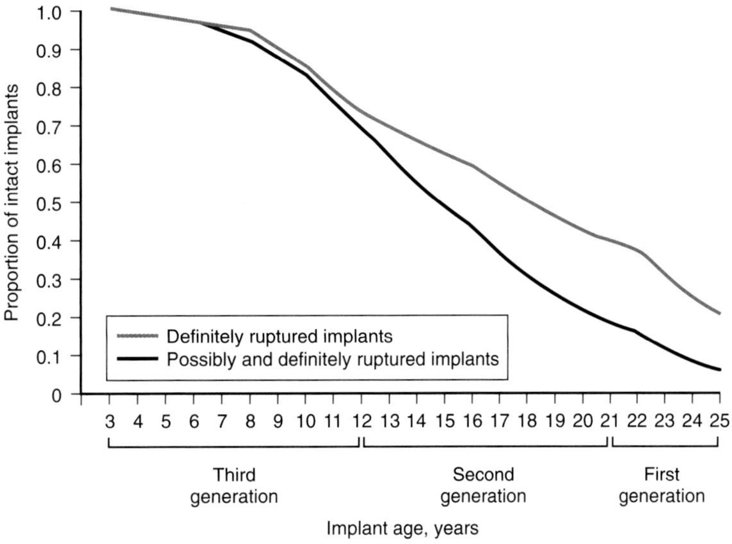

FIGURE 143-65. Cumulative rupture-free implant survival. First-generation implant used from 1974-1978 (constructed with thick silicone walls); second-generation implant used from 1979-1987 (softer, thin-walled implants); third-generation implants used from 1988-present (barrier-coated, low-bleed implants). For third-generation implants intact at 3 years: rupture-free survival of 98% at 5 years and 83% to 85% at 10 years. (From Holmich LR, Friis S, Fryzek JP, et al: Incidence of silicone breast implant rupture. Arch Surg 2003; 138:801-806.)

and tenth years after implantation. This observation is based on a study of 271 women who had received breast implants at least 3 years before their evaluation by sequential magnetic resonance imaging (Fig. 143-65).[32] Long-term saline implant deflation rates are reported in the 5% to 6% range.[33] The diagnosis of saline implant failure is easily made because of implant deflation and loss of breast volume. Exploration and implant exchange are required. With the silicone gel implant, it is difficult to diagnose implant rupture. The breast size and shape will not necessarily change because the silicone remains in the breast pocket, and a mammogram will not always detect implant rupture. Magnetic resonance imaging can help confirm diagnosis of a ruptured silicone gel implant with a reported sensitivity for detection of implant rupture of 86.7% with a specificity of 88.5%.[34]

The Baker classification continues to be the most common rating system for capsular contracture (Table 143-44).[35] Capsular contracture occurs at a variable rate ranging from 1% to 38%. The capsular contracture rate is similar after reconstruction with either saline or silicone gel implants and appears to be in the 16% to 30% range (Baker III/IV) based on implant studies reported at FDA hearings for the major implant manufacturers.* The most common reason for reoperation in the expander-implant patient is for correction of capsular contracture or implant shell failure with rupture or leak. Wrinkling is another long-term problem observed with implants and may be observed in the range of 20% to 25% of patients.* Submuscular positioning of the implant will avoid adherence of the skin envelope to the implant and resultant distortion of the skin overlying the implant. The use of a textured implant shell may prevent symptomatic capsular contracture but seems to increase the rate of wrinkling due to adhesions of the skin envelope to the implant shell.

Since 1980, there has been concern about the possible association between silicone gel implants and autoimmune diseases (see Chapter 138). In the Institute of Medicine study of Safety of Silicone Implants report, it was noted that there is no plausible evidence of a novel autoimmune disease because of silicone gel implants.[36] Similar observations reviewed by large meta-analyses have concluded that there is no association between implants and autoimmune diseases (e.g., rheumatoid arthritis, systemic lupus erythematosus, scleroderma).

Several clinical studies have been conducted by both INAMED and Mentor to determine the most common complications as well as the benefits of their implants. INAMED conducted several clinical studies to test its saline-filled breast implants, including the Large

TABLE 143-44 ✦ BAKER CLASSIFICATION OF CAPSULAR CONTRACTURE

Grade	Description
I	Soft
II	Less soft, but implant not visible
III	Moderate firmness, implant can be palpated or distortion can be seen
IV	Very firm, hard, tender, painful, and cold

From Baker JL Jr: Classification of spherical contractures. Paper presented at the Aesthetic Breast Symposium, Scottsdale, Arizona, 1975.

*http://www.fda.gov/cdrh/breastimplants.

Simple Trial (LST), the 1995 Reconstruction Study (R95) (and augmentation cohort, A95), and the Post Approval Survey Study.[37,38] The LST was designed to determine the 1-year rates of capsular contracture, infection, implant leakage or deflation, and implant replacement or removal. There were 2333 patients enrolled for augmentation, 225 for reconstruction, and 317 for revision (replacement of existing implants). Of these enrolled patients, 62% returned for their 1-year follow-up visit. The R95 and A95 studies were designed to assess all complications as well as the patient's satisfaction, body image, body esteem, and self-concept during the initial 5 years after breast reconstruction. Patients were observed annually, and data through 3 years (with partial 4-year data) were presented to the FDA for premarket device approval. The most common complications reported were asymmetry and capsular contracture (Table 143-45). During the 5 years reviewed by the study, there were 70 devices removed in 62 patients. Of these 70 devices, 49 were replaced and 21 were not. The most common reason for implant removal through 5 years was capsular contracture (31% of the 70 implants removed) (Table 143-46).

After premarket approval, INAMED transitioned data collection to a post-approval study. The Post Approval Survey Study (PASS) was designed to collect long-term safety data from patients 6 to 10 years after implant placement. The patients receive surveys each year. The PASS data are shown for both the R95 (reconstructive) cohorts. The data presented through 7 years include earlier data shown in the tables with new information added (Tables 143-47 and 143-48). Of the patients who provided satisfaction scores at 7 years after implant placement, 88% indicated that they were satisfied with their implants.

Mentor also conducted clinical testing of its saline-filled breast implants in two major studies, the Large Simple Trial (LST) and the Saline Prospective Study (SPS). The LST was designed to determine the 1-year rates of capsular contracture, infection, deflation, and implant removal. There were 2066 augmentation patients, 104 reconstruction patients, and 215 revision patients enrolled. Of these enrolled patients, 47% returned for their 1-year visit. The SPS was designed as a 3-year study to assess all complications with breast implants as well as the patient's satisfaction, body image, and self-concept. Patients were observed annually, and data for the following 3 years were collected. The SPS enrolled 1264 augmentation patients and 428 reconstruction patients. Of these, 76% of augmentation patients and 78% of reconstruction patients

TABLE 143-45 ✦ COMPLICATIONS REPORTED FOR RECONSTRUCTION PATIENTS (INAMED R95 STUDY)[37]

	N = 237 Patients	
Complications	*3-Year Complication Rate*† *(%)*	*5-Year Complication Rate (%)*
Additional operation (reoperation)	39	45
Asymmetry*	33	39
Capsular contracture	25	36
Implant replacement or removal for any reason	23	28
Wrinkling*	23	25
Implant palpability or visibility*	20	27
Breast pain*	15	18
Loss of nipple sensation*	12	18
Implant malposition*	12	17
Irritation or inflammation*	7	7
Leakage or deflation	6	8
Intense skin sensation*	6	6
Scarring complications	6	6
Infection	5	6
Capsule calcification*	5	5
Seroma	4	4
Skin or tissue necrosis	4	4
Delayed wound healing*	3	3
Implant extrusion	3	3
Rash	3	3
Hematoma	1	1

*These complications were assessed with severity ratings. Only the rates for moderate, severe, and very severe (excludes mild and very mild ratings) are shown in this table.

†As reported in original premarket approval submission.

TABLE 143-46 ✦ PRIMARY REASON FOR IMPLANT REMOVAL IN RECONSTRUCTION PATIENTS (INAMED R95 STUDY)[37]

Primary Reason for Implant Removal	Through 4 Years* (%) (N = 62 Implants Removed)	Through 5 Years (%) (N = 70 Implants Removed)
Capsular contracture III/IV	26	31
Patient choice	23	21
Leakage or deflation†	16	17
Infection	10	10
Implant extrusion	6	6
Implant malposition	6	4
Other‡	3	4
Wrinkling	3	3
Asymmetry	3	1
Recurrent breast cancer	3	1
Total	100	100

*As reported in original premarket approval submission with additional data clarification.
†Includes removals where the reason for removal was unknown.
‡Through 4 years, other reasons were abnormality of computed tomographic scan at mastectomy site and poor tissue expansion due to irradiation. Through 5 years, other reasons were abnormality of computed tomographic scan at mastectomy site, poor tissue expansion due to irradiation, and second-stage breast reconstruction.

TABLE 143-47 ✦ COMPLICATIONS (INAMED PASS STUDY)[37]

Complication	7-Year Complication Rate (%) (N = 237 Patients)
Reoperation	49
Capsular contracture	43
Implant removal	31
Breast pain	26
Implant deflation	12

TABLE 143-48 ✦ PRIMARY REASON FOR IMPLANT REMOVAL (INAMED PASS STUDY)[37]

Primary Reason for Implant Removal	Through 7 Years (%) (N = 81 Implants Removed)
Implant deflation	25
Capsular contracture	25
Patient choice	24
Infection	9
Implant extrusion	5
Other*	5
Implant malposition	4
Wrinkling	3
Asymmetry	3
Total	100

*Other reasons as reported by the physician were recurrent carcinoma (n = 1), abnormality on computed tomographic scan at mastectomy site (n = 1), poor tissue expansion due to irradiation (n = 1), and second-stage breast reconstruction (n = 1).

returned for their 3-year visit. The 3-year complication rates for reconstruction patients (including all levels of severity, mild to severe) were reported (Table 143-49). The rates reflect the number of reconstructive patients who experienced the listed complications at least once within the first 3 years after implantation. Some complications occurred more than once for some patients. Approximately 40% of reconstruction patients had an additional operation within the first 3 years of implantation. The most common com-

TABLE 143-49 ✦ COMPLICATION RATES FOR RECONSTRUCTION PATIENTS (MENTOR SPS STUDY)[38]

Reconstruction Complications	3-Year Complication Rate (%) (N = 416 Patients)
Additional operation (reoperation)	40
Loss of nipple sensation	35
Capsular contracture III/IV or grade unknown	30
Asymmetry	28
Implant removal	27
Wrinkling	20
Breast pain	17
Infection	9
Leakage or deflation	9
Irritation or inflammation	8
Delayed wound healing	6
Seroma	6
Scarring	5
Extrusion	2
Necrosis	2
Hematoma	1
Position change	1

TABLE 143-50 ✦ REASONS FOR IMPLANT REMOVAL IN RECONSTRUCTION PATIENTS (MENTOR SPS STUDY)[38]

Main Reason for Reconstruction Implant Removal Through 3 Years*	% (N = 116 Implants Removed)
Capsular contracture	30
Infection	24
Leakage or deflation	22
Patient request for size or style change	6
Necrosis or extrusion	5
Asymmetry	4
Breast pain	3
Delayed wound healing	2
Cosmetic revision	1
Wrinkling	1
Breast cancer	1
Total	100

*Corrections to some rates reported at 3 years. Total number of implants removed did not change.

plication, loss of nipple sensation, was reported by 35% of patients within the first 3 years following reconstruction. There were 116 implants removed in 97 reconstruction patients during the 3 years reported in the SPS study (Table 143-50). Of the 116 implants removed among reconstruction patients, 60% were replaced. The most common reasons for implant removal were correction of capsular contracture (30%) and infection (24%).

After product approval, Mentor switched data collection to a post-approval study. The post-approval study is designed to collect data from patients through the 10-year post-implantation period by use of a questionnaire mailed to patients each year. To date, data have been collected from patients through the 7-year post-implantation period. The post-approval data include earlier data collected for the SPS study with current information added (Tables 143-51 and 143-52).

TABLE 143-51 ✦ COMPLICATIONS IN RECONSTRUCTION PATIENTS (MENTOR POST-APPROVAL STUDY)[38]

Reconstruction Complications	5-Year Complication Rate (%) by Patient (N = 416)	7-Year Complication Rate (%) by Patient (N = 416)
Reoperation	43	50
Implant removal	30	39
Capsular contracture III/IV or unknown	29	49
Implant deflation	18	27
Breast pain	16	29

SUMMARY

Breast reconstruction with the expander-implant, if it is selected properly, provides an excellent form at the site of mastectomy and is a safe procedure. Selection requirements have been reviewed and include an

TABLE 143-52 ✦ PRIMARY REASON FOR IMPLANT REMOVAL IN RECONSTRUCTION PATIENTS (MENTOR POST-APPROVAL STUDY)[38]

Main Reason for Removal	5 Years (%) (N = 135 Implants Removed)	7 Years (%) (N = 180 Implants Removed)
Capsular contracture	29	29
Leakage or deflation	25	28
Infection	21	16
Patient request for size or shape change	8	9
Necrosis or extrusion	5	4
Asymmetry	4	4
Breast pain	3	2
Breast mass or cancer	1	2
Delayed wound healing	1	1
Wrinkling	1	1
Cosmetic revision	1	1
Contralateral replacement	0	2
Position change	0	1
Hypertrophic scarring	0	1
Irritation or inflammation	0	1

adequate and stable skin envelope as well as an opposite breast that is not extremely ptotic or large (or which the patient desires to have revised with augmentation, mastopexy, mastopexy-augmentation, or reduction mammaplasty). Finally, the patient must be comfortable with an implant that is either a silicone shell, saline-filled implant or a silicone shell, gel-filled implant. If the expander is used to prepare the skin envelope for the permanent implant, a two-stage procedure is required. With early diagnosis and skin-preserving techniques, single-stage implant insertion at the time of mastectomy may be available to selected patients. Both the single-stage implant insertion and the two-stage expander-implant sequence are fairly simple procedures that require only a 1-day hospitalization, and the recovery period is fairly short with minimal disability. Most patients may begin limited activities within 2 weeks and generally return to work in 3 weeks. Most patients are pleased with the result, particularly the patient who is well informed about the procedure and its limitations (Figs. 143-66 and 143-67).

Special techniques have been described, including expansion below the inframammary line and use of the abdominal advancement flap. Both modifications of the expander-implant technique will enhance the inferior portion of the skin envelope and may be helpful when the skin is heavily scarred at the mastectomy site in delayed reconstruction. The additional skin incorporated into the breast skin envelope may improve the coverage of the permanent implant and

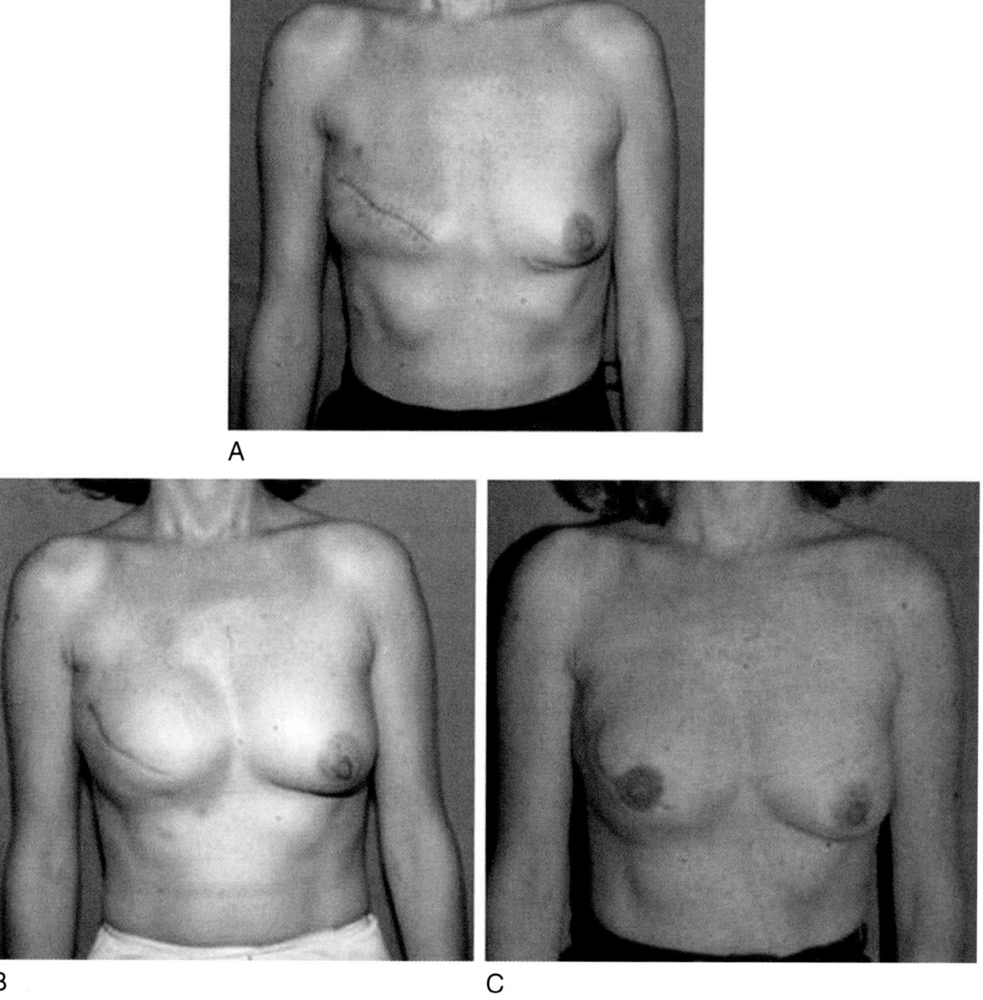

FIGURE 143-66. Delayed expander-implant reconstruction. *A,* Postoperative anterior view of right modified radical mastectomy. *B,* Postoperative anterior view, stage 1: expander in place. *C,* Postoperative anterior view, stage 2, 1 year after implant placement and nipple-areola reconstruction.

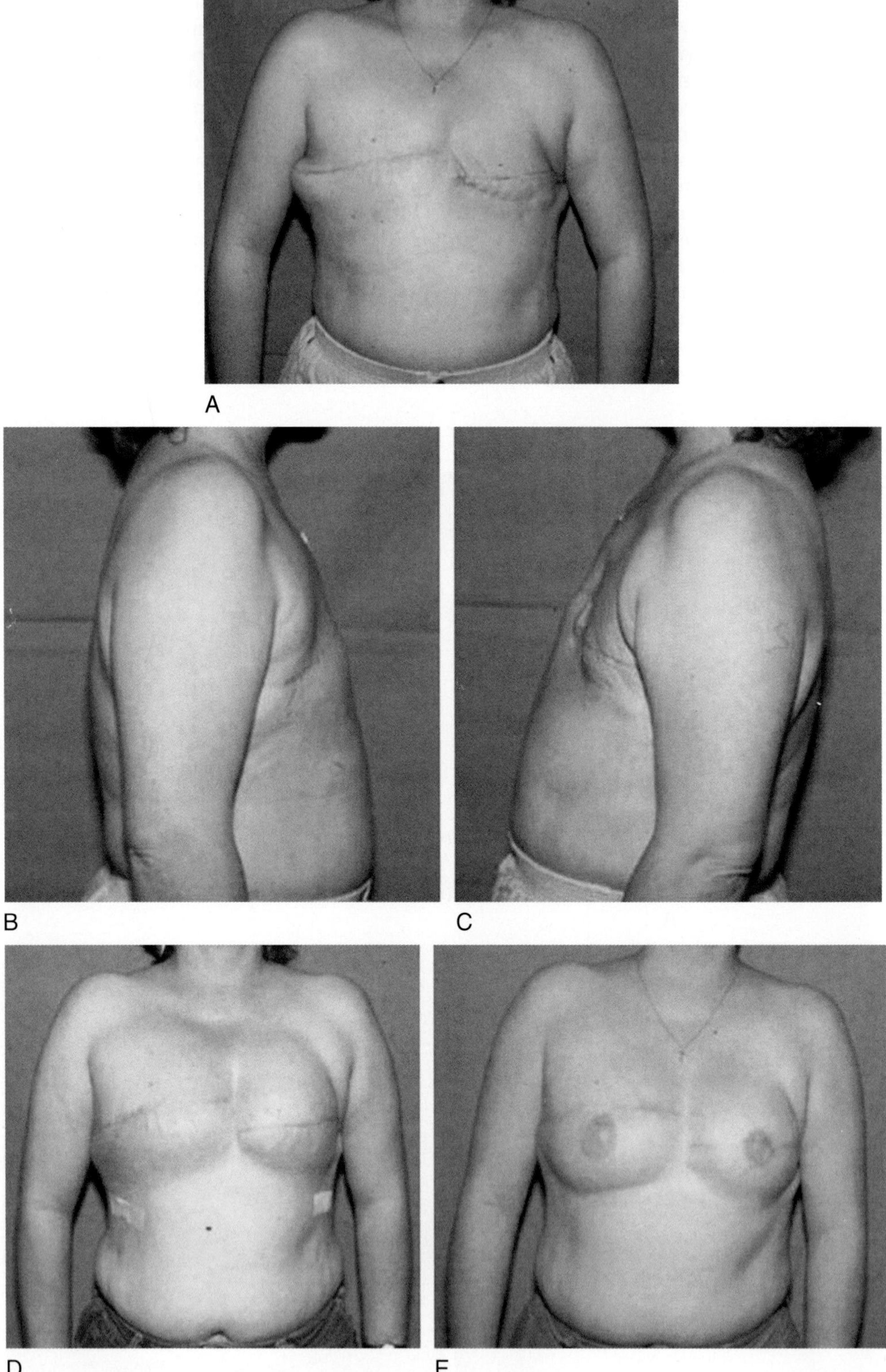

FIGURE 143-67. Delayed expander-implant reconstruction. *A,* Postoperative view of bilateral modified mastectomy. *B,* Right lateral view of mastectomy defect. *C,* Left lateral view of mastectomy defect. *D,* Postoperative anterior view, stage 1: expander in place. *E,* Postoperative anterior view, stage 2, 1 year after bilateral reconstruction and nipple-areola reconstruction.

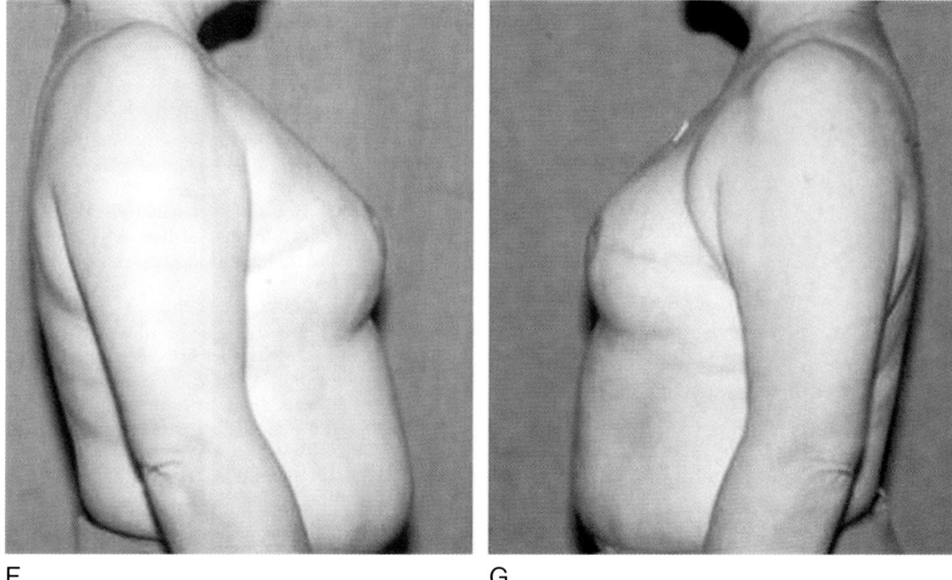

F G

FIGURE 143-67, cont'd. *F,* Postoperative right lateral view at 1 year. *G,* Postoperative left lateral view at 1 year.

provide a more natural contour for the breast reconstruction.

The addition of a well-vascularized flap will provide either an autogenous reconstruction (TRAM flap or selected perforator flaps) or an adequate skin envelope for immediate permanent implant insertion. Indications for expander use in conjunction with a flap have been described. The expander will provide a safe space for later implant insertion or use of autogenous technique after radiation therapy is completed. Finally, the expander may improve the skin envelope when the flap does not fully restore the skin envelope to a desirable dimension to allow appropriately sized permanent implant insertion.

Designs of expanders and permanent implants that are currently available have been provided. Extensive efforts are currently under way to improve the safety and effectiveness of implants. Innovative forms of biopolymer technology are being applied to the development of breast implants. In the mid-1990s, cohesive gel implants were introduced outside of the United States. The dense silicone polymer-filled implants are anatomically shaped, retain their shape against gravity and external forces, and are not susceptible to wrinkling as seen in silicone gel- or saline-filled implants (Fig. 143-68). In addition, if a cohesive gel implant ruptures, it maintains both its shape and integrity (Fig. 143-69). European experience indicates that capsular contracture seems to occur less often with cohesive gel implants; however, because these implants are relatively new, long-term studies of capsular contracture rates are not available. The largest published study to date reported that cohesive gel implants showed an overall capsular contracture rate of less than 5%. The majority of these contractures were minor in nature, with only 4 of 600 patients having a severe (Baker IV) contracture.[39] Some speculate that the lowered capsular contracture rate may be due to the increased firmness of the implant, which inhibits the body from contracting around it. The firmness of

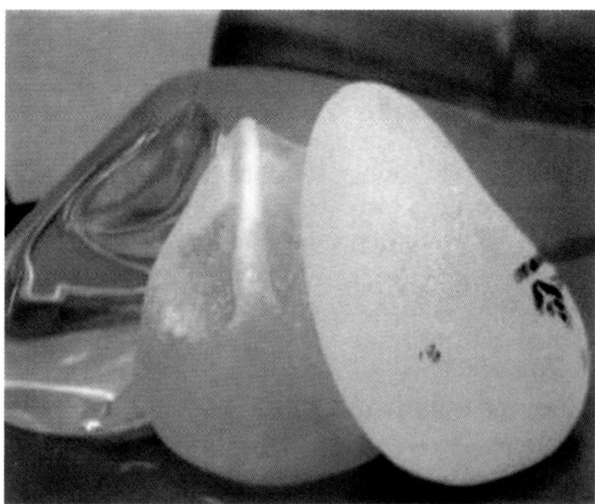

FIGURE 143-68. A silicone gel, saline, and cohesive gel implant *(right)* are stacked together to demonstrate how only the cohesive gel implant maintains its shape against gravity, devoid of wrinkles. (From Drever JM: Cohesive gel implants for breast augmentation. Aesthetic Surg J 2003;23:405.)

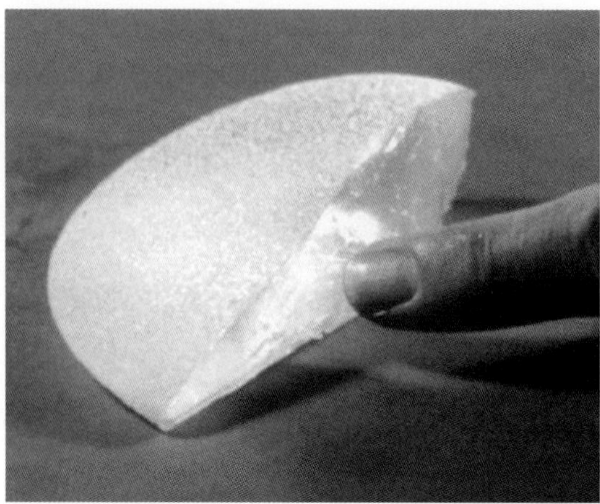

FIGURE 143-69. Cohesive gel implant divided in half to expose the gel. Note the textured surface, consistency of the cohesive gel, and how the gel retains its shape. (From Drever JM: Cohesive gel implants for breast augmentation. Aesthetic Surg J 2003;23:405.)

the implant may also become a problem if the implant should shift its position beneath the breast envelope with resultant loss of optimal projection and contour. Studies with careful follow-up are necessary before any conclusions can be drawn in regard to complications with this device.

Other new concepts in implant development are currently being studied outside of the United States. Another unique implant currently under development is a silicone-polyurethane copolymer with extended biostability (e.g., Elast-Eon breast implant by AorTech Biomaterials, Victoria, Australia). This implant has been designed in response to the FDA guidance documents of 2003 addressing silicone implant leakage and rupture. Development of this implant has been focused on biostability with an increase in device tear strength, tensile strength, abrasion resistance, and fatigue performance and improved barrier properties. In addition, development is focused not only on the outer shell of the implant and the cohesive properties of the implant fill copolymer but also on the potential of offering an in situ polymerization gel that can be introduced into empty implants. Although implant design represents the direction of most of the commercial endeavors to eliminate concerns about implants, the future direction of breast replacement may ultimately rely on tissue engineering to provide patients with autogenous reconstruction without the need of a flap, thereby replacing the use of an implant for breast reconstruction.

Currently, the expander-implant is an appropriate approach for many patients who desire reconstruction after mastectomy. When it is selected properly, the expander-implant represents a useful technique for breast reconstruction.

REFERENCES

1. Neumann CG: The expansion of an area of skin by progressive distention of a subcutaneous balloon. Plast Reconstr Surg 1957;19:124.
2. Radovan C: Breast reconstruction after mastectomy using the temporary expander. Plast Reconstr Surg 1982;69:195.
3. Austad ED, Rose GL: A self-inflating tissue expander. Plast Reconstr Surg 1982;70:588.
4. U.S. Congress House of Representatives: The FDA's Regulation of Silicone Breast Implants. A staff report prepared by the Human Resources and Intergovernmental Relations Subcommittee of the Committee on Government Operations. Washington, DC, U.S. Government Printing Office, 1992.
5. Hammond DC, Perry LC, Maxwell GP, Fisher J: Morphologic analysis of tissue expander shape using a biochemical model. Plast Reconstr Surg 1993;92:255.
6. Becker H: Breast reconstruction using an inflatable breast implant with detachable reservoir. Plast Reconstr Surg 1984;73:678.
7. Zones JS: The political and social context of silicone breast implant use in the United States. J Long Term Eff Med Implants 1992;1:225.
8. Mandrekas AD, Zambacos GJ, Katsanton PN: Immediate and delayed breast reconstruction with permanent tissue expanders. Br J Plast Surg 1995;48:572.
9. Spear SL, Onyewu C: Staged breast reconstruction with saline-filled implants in the irradiated breast: recent trends and therapeutic implications. Plast Reconstr Surg 2000;105: 930.
10. Maxwell GP, Falcone PA: Eighty-four consecutive breast reconstructions using a textured silicone tissue expander. Plast Reconstr Surg 1992;89:1022.
11. Cederna PS, Yates WR, Chang P, et al: Postmastectomy reconstruction: comparative analysis of the psychosocial, functional, and cosmetic effects of transverse rectus abdominis musculocutaneous flap versus breast implant reconstruction. Ann Plast Surg 1995;35:458.
12. Gui GP, Tan SM, Faliakou EC, et al: Immediate breast reconstruction using biodimensional anatomical permanent expander implants: a prospective analysis of outcome and patient satisfaction. Plast Reconstr Surg 2003;111:125.
13. Camilleri IG, Malata CM, Stavrianos S, McLean NR: A review of 120 Becker permanent tissue expanders in reconstruction of the breast. Br J Plast Surg 1996;49:346.
14. Toth BA, Daane SP: Purse-string mastectomy with immediate prosthetic reconstruction: an improved skin-sparing technique for small breasts. Plast Reconstr Surg 2003;111:2333.
15. Tai Y, Hasegawa H: A transverse abdominal flap for reconstruction after radical operations for recurrent breast cancer. Plast Reconstr Surg 1974;53:52.
16. Brown RG, Vasconez LO, Jurkiewicz MJ: Transverse abdominal flap and the deep epigastric arcade. Plast Reconstr Surg 1975;55:416.
17. Pennisi VR: Making a definite inframammary fold under a reconstructed breast. Plast Reconstr Surg 1977;60:523-525.
18. Ryan JJ: A lower thoracic advancement flap in breast reconstruction after mastectomy. Plast Reconstr Surg 1982;70:153-160.
19. Parry RG, Cochran TC Jr, Wolfort FG: When is there nipple involvement in carcinoma of the breast? Plast Reconstr Surg 1977;59:535.
20. Giacometti L, Montagna W: The nipple and areola of the human female breast. Anat Rec 1962;144:191.
21. Schnitt SJ, Goldwyn RM, Slavin SA: Mammary ducts in the areola: implications for patients undergoing reconstructive surgery of the breast. Plast Reconstr Surg 1993;92:1290.
22. Simmons RM, Hollenbeck ST, Latrenta GS: Areola-sparing mastectomy with immediate breast reconstruction. Ann Plast Surg 2003;51:547.

23. Cense HA, Rutgers EJ, Lopes Carkoza M, et al: Nipple-sparing mastectomy in breast cancer—a viable option. Eur J Surg Oncol 2001;27:521.
24. Crowe JP Jr, Kim JA, Yetman R, et al: Nipple-sparing mastectomy: technique and results of 54 procedures. Arch Surg 2004;139:148.
25. Gerber B, Krause A, Reimer T, et al: Skin-sparing mastectomy with conservation of the nipple-areola complex and autologous reconstruction is an oncologically safe procedure. Ann Surg 2003;238:120.
26. Simmons RM, Hollenbeck ST, Latrenta GS: Two-year follow-up of areola-sparing mastectomy with immediate reconstruction. Am J Surg 2004;188:403.
27. Trabulsy PP, Anthony JP, Mathes SJ: Changing trends in post-mastectomy breast reconstruction: a 13-year experience. Plast Reconstr Surg 1994;93:1418-1427.
28. Wilkins EG, Cederna PS, Lowery JC, et al: Prospective analysis of psychosocial outcomes in breast reconstruction: one-year postoperative results from the Michigan Breast Reconstruction Outcome Study. Plast Reconstr Surg 2000;106:1014.
29. Racano C, Fania PL, Motta GB, et al: Immediate and delayed two-stage post-mastectomy breast reconstruction with implants. Our experience of general surgeons. Minerva Chir 2002;57:135-149.
30. Alderman AK, Wilkins EG, Lowery JC, et al: Determinants of patient satisfaction in postmastectomy breast reconstruction. Plast Reconstr Surg 2000;106:769.
31. Clough KB, O'Donoghue JM, Fitoussi AD, et al: Prospective evaluation of late cosmetic results following breast reconstruction: I. Implant reconstruction. Plast Reconstr Surg 2001;107:1702.
32. Holmich LR, Friis S, Fryzek JP, et al: Incidence of silicone breast implant rupture. Arch Surg 2003;138:801-806.
33. Gutowski KA, Mesna GT, Cunningham BL: Saline-filled breast implants: a Plastic Surgery Educational Foundation Multicenter Outcomes Study. Plast Reconstr Surg 1997;100:1019.
34. Herborn CU, Marincek B, Erfmann D, et al: Breast augmentation and reconstructive surgery: MR imaging of implant rupture and malignancy. Eur Radiol 2002;12:2198.
35. Baker JL Jr: Classification of spherical contractures. Paper presented at the Aesthetic Breast Symposium, Scottsdale, Arizona, 1975.
36. Bondurant S, et al: Safety of Silicone Breast Implants. Washington, DC, National Academy Press, 2000.
37. Making an Informed Decision [patient brochure]. Santa Barbara, Calif, INAMED Aesthetics, January 2005.
38. Saline-Filled Breast Implant Surgery: Making an Informed Decision. Santa Barbara, Calif, Mentor Corporation, January 2004.
39. Heden P, Jernbeck J, Hober M: Breast augmentation with anatomical cohesive gel implants: the world's largest current experience. Clin Plast Surg 2001;28:531.
40. Mansel RE, Horgan K, Webster DJ, et al: Cosmetic results of immediate breast reconstruction post-mastectomy: a follow-up study. Br J Surg 1986;73:813.
41. Schuster RH, Rotter S, Boonn W, Efron G: The use of tissue expanders in immediate breast reconstruction following mastectomy for cancer. Br J Plast Surg 1990;43:413.
42. Hunter-Smith DJ, Laurie SW: Breast reconstruction using permanent tissue expanders. Aust N Z J Surg 1995;65:492.
43. McGeorge DD, Mahdi S, Tsekouras A: Breast reconstruction with anatomical expanders and implants: our early experience. Br J Plast Surg 1996;49:352.
44. Ramon Y, Ullmann Y, Moscona R, et al: Aesthetic results and patient satisfaction with immediate breast reconstruction using tissue expansion: a follow-up study. Plast Reconstr Surg 1997;99:686.
45. Spear SL, Majidian A: Immediate breast reconstruction in two stages using textured, integrated-valve tissue expanders and breast implants: a retrospective review of 171 consecutive breast reconstructions from 1989 to 1996. Plast Reconstr Surg 1998;101:53.
46. Slavin SA, Schnitt SJ, Duda RB, et al: Skin-sparing mastectomy and immediate reconstruction: oncologic risks and aesthetic results in patients with early-stage breast cancer. Plast Reconstr Surg 1998;102:49.
47. Al-Ghazal SK, Blamey RW: Subcutaneous mastectomy with implant reconstruction: cosmetic outcome and patient satisfaction. Eur J Surg Oncol 2000;26:137.
48. Peyser PM, Abel JA, Straker VF, et al: Ultra-conservative skin-sparing "keyhole" mastectomy and immediate breast and areola reconstruction. Ann R Coll Surg Engl 2000;82:227.
49. Berry MG, al-Mufti RA, Jenkinson AD, et al: An audit of outcome including patient satisfaction with immediate breast reconstruction performed by breast surgeons. Ann R Coll Surg Engl 1998;80:173.

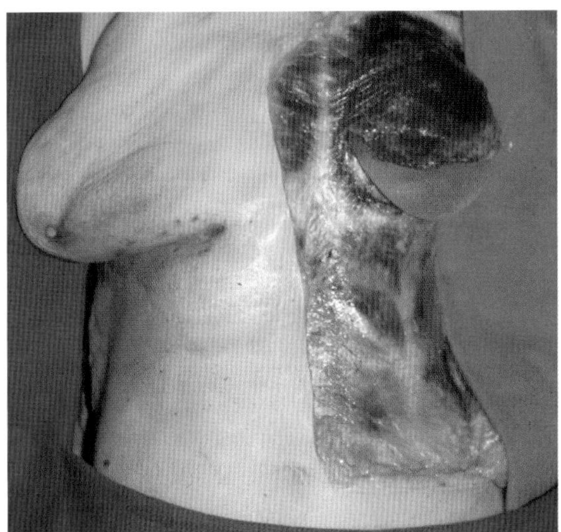

COLOR PLATE 143-1. Expander-implant reconstruction, stage 1. Anatomic dissection demonstrates release of pectoralis major origin from sixth intercostal space inferiorly and from fourth to sixth intercostal spaces medially. Pectoral muscle fibers will not restrain implant projection over the inferior breast mound.

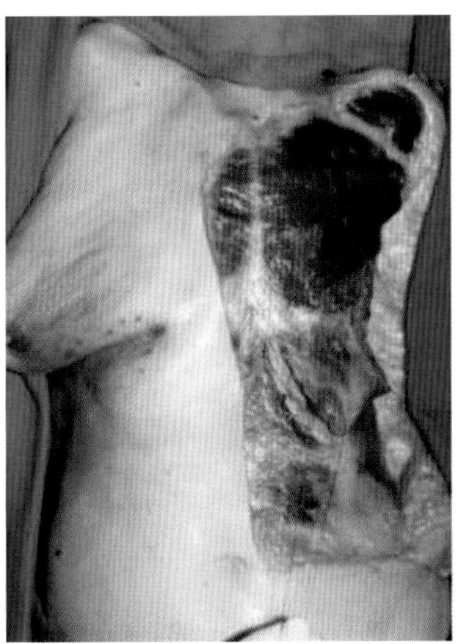

A

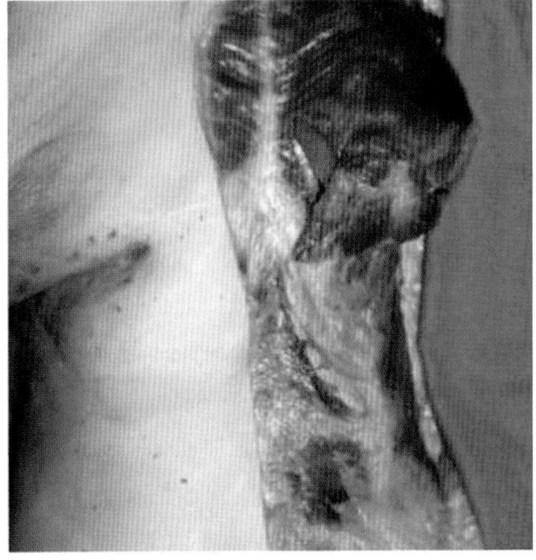

B

COLOR PLATE 143-2. Segmental rectus abdominis-external oblique flap. *A,* Cadaver dissection demonstrates rectus elevation at costal margin. *B,* Segmental rectus flap rotated at the sixth intercostal space and sutured to inferior pectoralis flap to provide implant coverage.

CHAPTER

144

Delayed Postmastectomy Reconstruction: TRAM Transposition Techniques

GLYN JONES, MD

The surgical management of breast reconstruction has undergone a gradual evolution with the promotion of autologous techniques.[1] Before their development, breast reconstruction focused on the formation of a breast mound by use of round gel or saline implants placed beneath a tight skin envelope. The associated distortion and frequency of capsular contracture did little to encourage reconstructive surgeons and may have contributed significantly to the thrust to achieve control of breast cancer by breast conservation techniques coupled with radiation therapy. The development of the transverse rectus abdominis myocutaneous (TRAM) flap for breast reconstruction revolutionized breast reconstruction and enabled surgeons to rebuild the breast entirely from autologous tissue. A successful TRAM flap reconstruction is soft, warm, and well integrated into a patient's psyche, given that she does not have to deal with the artificial feel of an implant-based reconstruction.

Skin-sparing mastectomy has been another landmark advance in breast reconstruction, heralding a new era in achieving the goal of a natural reconstructed breast. It is oncologically safe and does not compromise the mastectomy.[2-4] Combined with TRAM flap reconstruction, skin-sparing mastectomy offers exciting possibilities for both patient and surgeon, with the potential for increasing the patient's acceptance of mastectomy as an alternative to lumpectomy and radiation therapy for breast cancer.

Whereas many patients undergoing mastectomy at this time have the option of immediate reconstruction with skin-sparing mastectomy, many patients still present for delayed reconstruction. This may be due to a failure on the part of the oncologic surgeon to offer this approach to the patient, or immediate reconstruction may have been deliberately withheld because of the need for postoperative administration of radiation therapy. There are also those patients who are uncomfortable with the magnitude of combined surgery and therefore elect to separate their mastectomy and reconstructive procedures.

INDICATIONS

Breast reconstruction may be delayed for a variety of reasons (Table 144-1). Delayed reconstruction carries

TABLE 144-1 ✦ INDICATIONS FOR DELAYED BREAST RECONSTRUCTION

Patient's preference
Oncologic surgeon's preference
Patient will undergo postoperative radiation therapy
Patient is not fit enough medically to undergo reconstruction
Patient is not psychologically ready for reconstruction
Doubt about the viability of mastectomy skin flaps

with it a series of implications that may affect patient outcomes both positively and negatively. By delaying reconstruction, a patient is forced to live with her mastectomy defect for a variable period. Living with a mastectomy allows the patient to experience life without a breast and to see if she is able to adapt to and use a simple bra prosthesis. Many patients find life without a breast unacceptable, particularly when breast cancer strikes at a younger age. Having experienced life with a mastectomy deformity, many patients undergoing subsequent reconstruction are more accepting of their reconstructive outcomes. In addition, delay affords the mastectomy flaps time to settle, and any problems with delayed wound healing or necrosis can be resolved. Scars soften with time and edema resolves. It also affords an opportunity for patients with more advanced tumors to undergo radiation therapy without any direct negative effect on the autologous reconstruction. On the negative side, delay mandates another operative procedure with the additional cost of a separate hospital stay, anesthesia, and surgical expenses. It also requires the surgeon to operate in a scarred, often irradiated bed with loss of tissue compliance and elasticity.

HISTORY

In 1976, Millard[5] described a tubed lower abdominal pedicled flap as a source of tissue for reconstruction of the radical mastectomy defect. The flap was inset onto the chest through the wrist, achieving a remarkable autologous tissue reconstruction for the time. Following Mathes' initial description of the vascular anatomy and use of the rectus abdominis musculocutaneous flap for abdominal wall reconstruction,[6] Robbins[7] described a vertical rectus abdominis flap for breast reconstruction in 1979. Working independently, Drever, Dinner, and Sakai refined variations on the use of vertical rectus abdominis myocutaneous flaps for breast reconstruction.[8-11] It was Carl Hartrampf and his colleagues who took the bold step of changing the skin island orientation to a transverse one, making a more sizeable volume of tissue available for breast reconstruction with a more cosmetically acceptable donor site.[12-15] Scheflan's dissections at Emory University confirmed the dominant inferior epigastric arterial supply to the lower abdominal skin and fat. Blood supply was most robust directly over the muscle belly where perforators were most abundant, whereas the periphery of the flap appeared to rely on the superficial epigastric and circumflex iliac terminal branches. Milloy had already evaluated the blood supply within the rectus muscles in 1960, and these findings together with Scheflan's work were confirmed in the anatomic studies of Taylor, Moon, and Palmer with their publication of the angiosome concept, an extension of Michel Salmon's pioneering studies.[16-18] From these early beginnings, the TRAM flap was destined to become the "gold standard" procedure for breast reconstruction, with free flap options developing as refinements of the original pedicled technique. The following discussion focuses on the most popular and widely used procedure, the pedicled TRAM flap and its variations.

VASCULAR BASIS

The tissue of the lower abdomen and periumbilical area is supplied by perforators arising from five sources (Table 144-2). Of these five sources, only the first is used in raising a pedicled TRAM flap, although the eighth intercostal vessels can be incorporated into the pedicle to augment blood supply if necessary. It is clear, however, that the primary blood supply of the lower abdominal wall skin and fat is from the deep inferior epigastric system.[15-18] The vessels from both epigastric systems penetrate the rectus muscles on their deep surfaces and travel as single or duplicated vessels up and down the flap to communicate in the periumbilical region.[18-20] In addition, several vascular patterns are noted within the rectus muscles (Table 144-3).

On the basis of these observations, Moon and Taylor postulated three major variations in skin island design: the upper abdominal, midabdominal, and lower abdominal flaps. Injection studies suggested decreasing density of musculocutaneous perforating vessels to the lower skin paddle compared with the mid and upper skin islands. This finding was corroborated by

TABLE 144-2 ✦ PERFORATORS ARISING FROM FIVE SOURCES THAT SUPPLY LOWER ABDOMEN

Superior epigastric vessels arising from the termination of the internal mammary axis supplemented by costal margin intercostal vessels
Deep inferior epigastric vessels
Superficial inferior epigastric vessels
Intercostal segmental vessels
Terminal branches of the superficial and deep circumflex iliac vessels

TABLE 144-3 ✦ TRAM FLAP VASCULAR PATTERNS*

Type I (29%)	Single superior and inferior arterial supply
Type II (57%)	Double-branched system from each source artery
Type III (14%)	Triple-branched system from each vessel

*Bilateral vascular symmetry was noted in only 2% of patients.
From Moon HK, Taylor GI: The vascular anatomy of rectus abdominis musculocutaneous flaps based on the deep superior epigastric system. Plast Reconstr Surg 1988;82:815.

Harris.[21] The net result of these studies in a clinical context is that it is important to center the flap on the periumbilical perforators for maximal capture of available blood supply.

Only 40% to 50% of patients have macroscopic communications between the two systems; up to 60% of patients have choke vessels of a microscopic caliber.[17,22] The superior vessels pass into the substance of the muscle at or above the costal margin and run down within the muscle toward the umbilicus. The inferior supply enters the posterolateral aspect of the muscle below the arcuate line and runs up to anastomose with the superior vessels in the periumbilical area. It provides a more robust circulation to the flap and is accompanied by two large venae comitantes that drain into the iliac circulation.[15,20] These venae comitantes are larger than the superior veins, which partially explains the improved venous drainage associated with the free TRAM flap. The periumbilical anastomosis has a bidirectional venous outflow confirmed by Taylor. When a pedicled TRAM flap is raised, distal venous flow has to reverse and follow the drainage pattern of the superior veins, overcoming the venous valves within the choke system described by Taylor.[17,18] Arterial perforators arise from both systems and run in two roughly parallel sets on either side of the linea alba. The lateral row lies 2 to 3 cm within the lateral border of the rectus sheath; the medial row lies 1 to 2 cm from the linea alba.[18] In the region of the medial portion of the arcuate line, the deep system sends a peritoneal perforator toward the umbilicus, which needs separate ligation or cauterization.

The fascia overlying the rectus muscles is densely adherent to the muscle at the tendinous inscriptions. During flap elevation, a gently tapering cuff of this fascia is left on the muscle with its apex toward the costal margin. This facilitates maintaining the integrity of the muscle, thereby reducing the risk of injury to the pedicle, and it aids in relieving tension during closure.[23] A muscle-sparing technique can be used to leave some muscle laterally or medially to assist in maintaining abdominal wall strength. Whether this muscle strip remains innervated or vascularized is debatable; the intercostal nerves and vessels penetrate the posterior aspect of the rectus muscle at the junction of the mid and lateral thirds of the muscle and not in the lateral third. Any lateral segment is probably devoid of neurovascular input.[24,25] Harris[21] demonstrated an 80% reduction in intraoperative blood flow when the medial and lateral thirds of the rectus muscle are clamped to simulate muscle-sparing harvest. Given this observation, it is probably unwise to incorporate muscle-sparing surgery into TRAM flap harvest.

The vascular zones of the unipedicled flap (and free TRAM flap) are divided into four areas (Table 144-4). These zones have functional significance from a vascular standpoint. Zone I is unquestionably the most reliable portion of the flap, followed by the medial portion of zone III. The end of zone III becomes increasingly unreliable as one moves toward the tip of the flap, and it is wise to discard it in most patients. The medial portion of zone II is also usually reliable, but the lateral part is less predictable, followed by zone IV, which is rarely useful even in many free flaps. Zone IV should be discarded as a matter of routine. Taylor documented the anatomic theory behind these maneuvers in his discussion of the angiosome concept.[17] It is his belief that a single adjacent vascular territory could be captured relatively reliably, but more than one angiosome capture becomes increasingly unpredictable, particularly once the midline is crossed. This is borne out in practice. These observations led Taylor to popularize the concept of TRAM flap delay in an effort to bolster the blood flow to the flap before elevation.

Anatomic and Physiologic Basis of Vascular Delay

Vascular delay is not a new concept, and its efficacy was well documented during the era of tubed pedicled flaps for general reconstruction.[26] Its effectiveness in musculocutaneous flaps has been demonstrated in studies by Mathes and Nahai.[27] Moon and Taylor[18] recommended surgical delay of the TRAM flap 1 week before definitive elevation. The procedure focused on ligation of the superficial and deep inferior epigastric

TABLE 144-4 ✦ UNIPEDICLED TRAM FLAP VASCULAR ZONES

Zone I overlies the muscle pedicle
Zone II lies across the midline, immediately adjacent to zone I
Zone III lies lateral to zone I on the ipsilateral side
Zone IV lies lateral to zone II on the contralateral side from the pedicle

TABLE 144-5 ✦ INDICATIONS FOR TRAM FLAP VASCULAR DELAY

Higher risk patients—obesity, smoking, prior irradiation
Patients with multiple abdominal scars
Alternative for plastic surgeons not comfortable with microsurgical reconstruction

systems in an outpatient setting. Although it was timed for a week before flap elevation and breast reconstruction, Taylor believed the delay phenomenon to have reached an effective peak at 72 hours after surgery rather than during the classic 10-day window suggested historically in the literature.[26] There is little doubt that the procedure is effective. Codner[28] demonstrated a dramatic, statistically significant rise in vascular inflow to the pedicle after delay, with increased arterial pressure and greater perfusion pressures in the delayed pedicles. This was corroborated by Restifo[29] and Ribuffo.[30] Restifo demonstrated a flow in the superior epigastric vessels similar to that of the inferior system once delay had been performed. Like Taylor, he was able to demonstrate no benefit to waiting longer than 1 week after delay before formal flap elevation. Ribuffo[30] used color Doppler studies to demonstrate increased caliber of and flow within the superior epigastric system after vascular delay (Table 144-5).

Experience with minimal incision approaches to delay has not been as reliable in the author's practice as a more formal extensive delay. Taylor advises a complete lower abdominal incision with undermining of the tips of the flap (zones III and IV), with care being taken to ensure division of the superficial inferior epigastric arterial and venous systems as well as of the deep inferior system.[18] Vascular compromise of the TRAM flap is all too often related to venous congestion rather than to arterial inadequacy, and the superficial venous system contributes significantly to the venous drainage of the TRAM skin island. Its division at delay promotes flap reliance on the cephalad venous outflow. Delay is rarely performed because it is preferable to proceed to a free flap when the surgeon is willing to use microvascular transplantation based on the deep inferior epigastric artery and associated venae comitantes as an alternative approach. For the non-microsurgeon, however, delay remains a potentially useful tool in reducing the risk of pedicled procedures.

ANATOMIC CONSIDERATIONS

The rectus sheath is an essential element to success with this procedure.[23,31,32] Laterally, the rectus sheath consists of two fascial components derived from the external and internal oblique muscles. These blend into a confluent anterior sheet that fuses at the linea alba with the contralateral sheath. It is imperative that both lateral components be incorporated into the fascial closure when the donor defect is closed if hernias or bulges are to be prevented.[23,33] The technical considerations pertinent to this closure are discussed in the operative technique section to follow.

Nerve supply to the muscle is segmental and must be divided when the flap is raised. It is essential to denervate the eighth intercostal nerve at the costal margin. This maneuver causes the muscle to atrophy, which prevents muscle bulging at the costal margin tunnel when the patient is in a sitting position.

SKIN-SPARING MASTECTOMY IN BREAST RECONSTRUCTION: TECHNICAL CONSIDERATIONS

Pedicled and free TRAM flaps are frequently used in conjunction with skin-sparing mastectomy in the form of immediate reconstruction. Increasing numbers of surgeons are performing skin-sparing mastectomies even when delayed reconstruction is planned, and it is appropriate that a short discussion of this important procedure be included. Skin-sparing mastectomy involves removal of the breast through the nipple-areola complex excision site, with axillary dissection performed through the same incision or through an additional skin crease incision in the axillary floor. This leaves behind the patient's natural skin brassiere together with a defined inframammary fold to help form the newly reconstructed breast.[2] Whereas this is most valuable in immediate reconstruction, it does offer maintenance of the inframammary crease for delayed reconstruction. The original breast shape may be more readily matched as a consequence.[34]

The traditional mastectomy wound leaves a large skin defect, making access to the chest wall, axilla, and TRAM flap tunnel communicating with the abdominal dissection simple. When skin-sparing mastectomy is performed, the excision usually incorporates a periareolar biopsy site if biopsy has been performed, and axillary dissection is done either through the nipple-areola complex wound or through a separate axillary incision.[3] On occasion, a high lateral biopsy site may be excised separate from the nipple-areola complex area. If the biopsy site wound is close to the axilla, axillary clearance or sentinel node biopsy may be performed through this incision. The closer an excised skin biopsy site is to the excised nipple-areola disk, the greater the risk of skin bridge necrosis. Skin incisions for the procedure have been suggested by Carlson,[3] Toth,[35] and Skoll,[36] all of whom emphasize the risks of the Wise-pattern approach for ptotic patients. Carlson has emphasized the critical importance of handling skin flaps gently to minimize the risks of skin necrosis. Retractors with "toe-in" tips to their blades may easily damage the delicate subdermal capillary network during dissection of the mastectomy skin flaps, resulting in extensive areas of necrosis. Prolonged traction with a retractor blade in one area may induce localized areas of skin necrosis. Every attempt should be made to preserve the inframammary fold because Carlson has shown that this does not compromise the oncologic safety of the procedure and greatly enhances the ultimate appearance of the reconstruction.[37]

Whereas skin-sparing mastectomy may be used without immediate reconstruction, the retention of the additional breast skin does little to ease the reconstructive surgeon's task when delayed reconstruction is finally performed. This is particularly true of irradiated patients. Data published by Kronowitz[38] have supported the contention that skin mastectomy flaps may be held out to size by an immediately placed expander that can be inflated and maintained during radiation therapy if reconstruction is to be delayed. The expander can be removed subsequently and replaced with a TRAM flap. This approach has been given the label of "immediate-delayed" reconstruction. It does allow the surgeon to take advantage of skin-sparing mastectomy in the face of delayed reconstruction, although the author has generally found this irradiated skin envelope to be of poor quality in the long term because it retracts and becomes fibrotic to some extent, necessitating its excision. By contrast, the expansion does allow the upper pole to remain stretched out, thereby preventing the constriction band effect produced by nonexpanded mastectomy scars. It may still be preferable to undertake true delayed reconstruction when radiation therapy is planned.

IMPACT OF PREVIOUS INCISIONS, BODY HABITUS, AND IRRADIATION

Previous mastectomy with or without radiation therapy poses a number of significant concerns for the reconstructive surgeon. Incision placement on the chest wall may be high (Fig. 144-1) or low (Fig. 144-2), horizontal or oblique, and it may extend from the midline anteriorly to the midaxilla or posterior axillary line. If radiation has been applied, pigmentation may further compromise the skin color and consistency. In delayed reconstruction, it is generally preferred to disregard the previous mastectomy scar in deciding where to place the TRAM flap. Essentially, the flap must be placed where it will give the optimum breast shape irrespective of the location of previous scars. One should try to resect the old scar to prevent a patchwork appearance to the reconstructed chest wall, but this is not always possible. The emphasis should be on correct positioning of the reconstruction in relation to the inframammary crease level. Failure to position the flap correctly will result in only poor aesthetic outcomes. Of particular significance in delayed reconstruction is the problem of dealing with linear mastectomy scar contracture when the old scar is incorporated into the reconstruction. When the old scar is opened out to receive the TRAM flap, the upper skin flap tends to act as a restraining band across the upper pole of the TRAM flap, forming a transverse groove at the juncture of the TRAM flap with the chest wall. A transverse groove is most easily addressed by performing a lateral Z-plasty superolaterally in the region of the anterior axillary fold, immediately releasing this band-like effect. This should be planned as part of the reconstruction and discussed with the patient preoperatively. When it is possible to incorporate the old mastectomy scar into the reconstruction, the scar should be excised and submitted for pathologic examination to exclude any evidence of local recurrence. The lower mastectomy skin flap is usually of poor quality with adhesion to the chest wall and may be puckered, rendering it unusable (Fig. 144-3). This skin is resected and replaced by TRAM flap skin wherever possible.

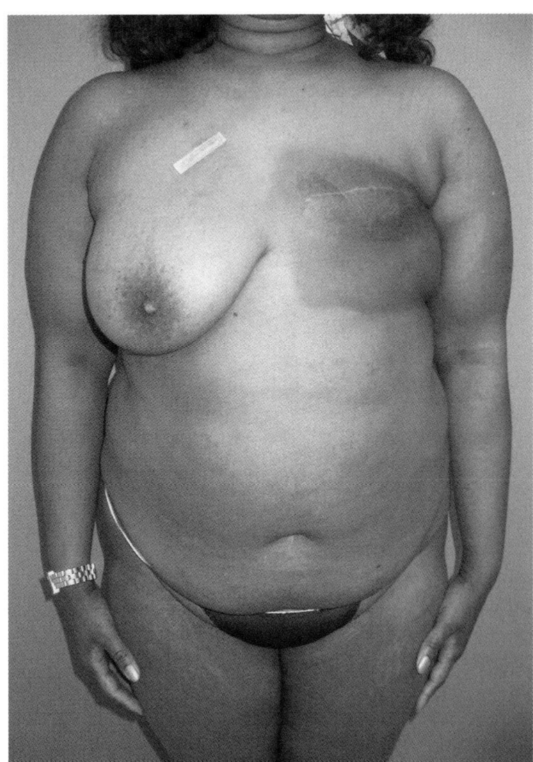

FIGURE 144-1. Obese patient with irradiated mastectomy site and high mastectomy scar.

Body habitus has a significant impact on decision-making in both immediate and delayed TRAM flap reconstruction. In the delayed setting, obesity may

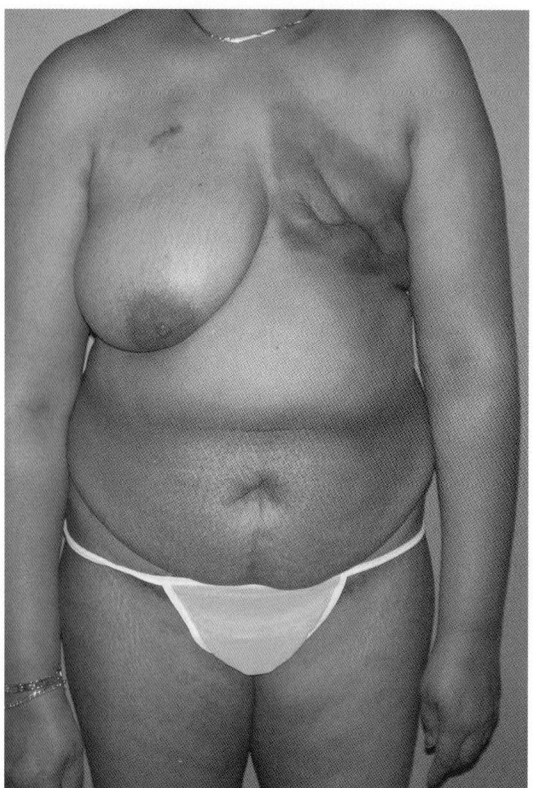

FIGURE 144-2. Obese patient with low mastectomy scar, radiation changes, and severe cutaneous puckering.

contribute to a hollowed out appearance to the mastectomy site where thinned skin flaps are adherent to the pectoralis major muscle; at the periphery of the mastectomy, fat builds up progressively to the thickness of the normal surrounding tissue (see Fig. 144-2). This crater-like deformity may absorb a significant volume of the flap before any external projection can be achieved, and one needs to take this additional volume requirement into account in planning the flap design. The length and breadth of the chest wall also affect flap design and orientation. Patients with a long chest dimension require more vertical or oblique flap positioning. If they also have a wide transverse breast diameter, the width of TRAM flap harvested will have to be correspondingly generous. Failure to provide enough upper pole fill will result in unattractive hollowing of the infraclavicular area, and this is difficult to correct later. Similarly, inadequate transverse volume will produce a narrow, constricted-looking breast. Patients with broad breasts and short vertical chest height tend to require a more transverse flap orientation, but care must again be exercised in an effort to maintain good upper pole fill. This is particularly true of the anterior axillary fold area, where residual post-mastectomy hollowing detracts from what may otherwise be an excellent TRAM flap reconstruction. The ability to place some of the tail of the flap into this area should also enter preoperative planning concerning the dimensions of the flap.

Radiation therapy administered after mastectomy alters the color, texture, and consistency of the residual chest wall skin. It is typically rendered less pliable, edematous, less well vascularized, and somewhat darker by ionizing radiation. It also results in potential damage to the internal mammary vessels feeding the pedicled TRAM flap. Studies of internal mammary caliber after radiation therapy have not demonstrated significant flow reduction in these vessels, and yet many studies have found increased rates of fat necrosis in TRAM flaps elevated on previously irradiated internal mammary vessels. If a pedicled flap is to be used, the flap should either be based on the contralateral nonirradiated side or be planned as a bipedicled procedure. If a unipedicled flap is planned, the incorporation of vascular delay 1 week before flap elevation is another alternative that dramatically improves vascular inflow. Alternatively, a free TRAM flap is an excellent choice. The use of the immediate-delayed approach has been advocated as a means of preserving the breast skin envelope of a skin-sparing mastectomy through the course of radiation therapy. Although this is certainly feasible, the author's experience with this approach has been less than gratifying. Shrinkage and pigmentation changes in the irradiated skin envelope appear all too common, and the quality of the reconstruction appears to deteriorate with time. The one major benefit to this approach is that the ability to design a more natural slope to the upper pole of the breast may be enhanced.

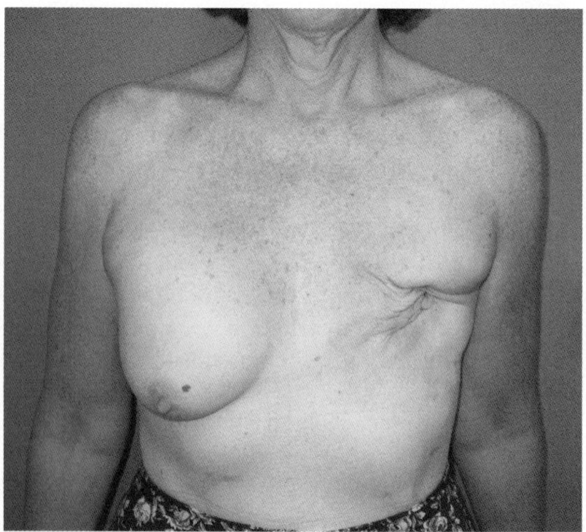

FIGURE 144-3. Central mastectomy scar with severe skin puckering that necessitated resection of lower pole skin at the time of reconstruction.

SELECTION OF PATIENT AND TECHNIQUE

TRAM flap breast reconstruction is a significant surgical undertaking for both patient and surgeon. The first prerequisite for this procedure is a patient willing to undergo what the operation demands—major surgery, a prolonged hospital stay, and a 4- to 8-week recovery period before the patient begins to feel that life is returning to some degree of normalcy. The second major requirement is an available donor site. The patient should have a thorough history taken, including an evaluation of comorbidities such as gastroesophageal reflux, abdominal bloating and irritable bowel syndrome, lumbar spine problems, smoking history, and cardiovascular risk factors. Diabetes mellitus does not appear to pose unusually high additional risk to flap perfusion,[33] although Hartrampf[12] has assigned it a significant value. Collagen vascular disease is a potential problem, although the procedure may be performed safely in patients with systemic lupus erythematosus and mild rheumatoid arthritis. Scleroderma would present more of a risk if anterior chest tightness is present because this could compromise abdominal skin closure. Prior abdominoplasty and abdominal liposuction represent contraindications to the procedure in theory, although the procedure has been successfully performed by the author in a patient with complete abdominal wall undermining 20 years previously as well as in patients with conservative liposuction. Preoperative Doppler ultrasound evaluation of perforators can be extremely helpful in evaluating the potential reliability of the skin island under these circumstances. A full clinical examination should be performed noting body habitus and weight. The abdomen should be examined for old scars, particularly right upper quadrant cholecystectomy scars or vertical midline incisions.[39] Pfannenstiel incisions are not regarded as a risk factor for this operation. Laparoscopic incisions are rarely a problem, but port sites may injure the vessels within the rectus muscle in the upper abdomen, and Doppler evaluation is recommended. It is probably unwise to operate within 6 weeks after laparoscopic surgery. A final factor in flap selection is that of the patient's occupation and lifestyle. Active, young individuals are better served by a free TRAM or perforator flap, and patients engaged in musical careers occasionally express concerns about the impact of muscle loss on their ability to sing. The loss of muscle, however, does not appear to be a significant issue in practice (Figs. 144-4 and 144-5).

Hartrampf[12] attempted to assign risk scores to patients to determine their eligibility for TRAM flap reconstruction. Risk factors included smoking, obesity, psychological instability, autoimmune disease and diabetes mellitus, severe systemic disease, and inexperience of the surgeon. In this rating system, two risk factors or a score below 5 represented a patient with borderline risk, whereas patients with three or more risk factors or a score above 5 were not considered candidates for surgery.[12] Diabetes did not correlate well with complications, but obesity, smoking, abdominal scars, and prior radiation therapy are indications for potential problems with flap circulation.[32,33]

TECHNIQUE

Preoperative Preparation

Some surgeons institute a full bowel preparation before TRAM flap surgery. Others prescribe a low-residue

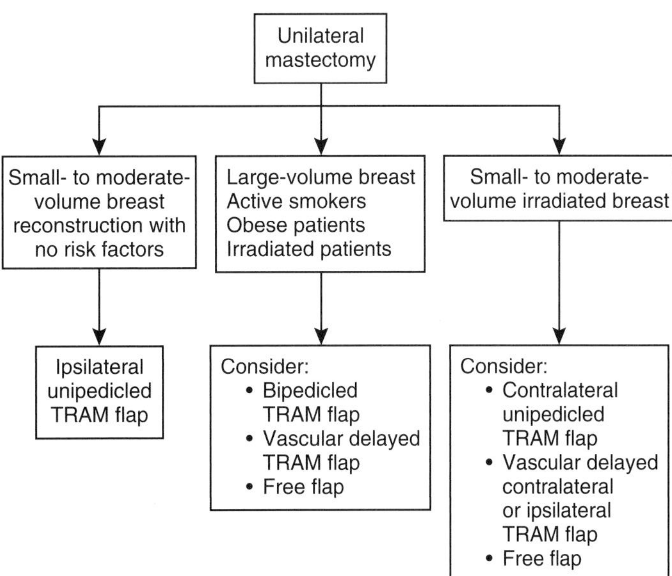

FIGURE 144-4. Delayed breast reconstruction: algorithm for choosing pedicled technique in patients with unilateral mastectomies.

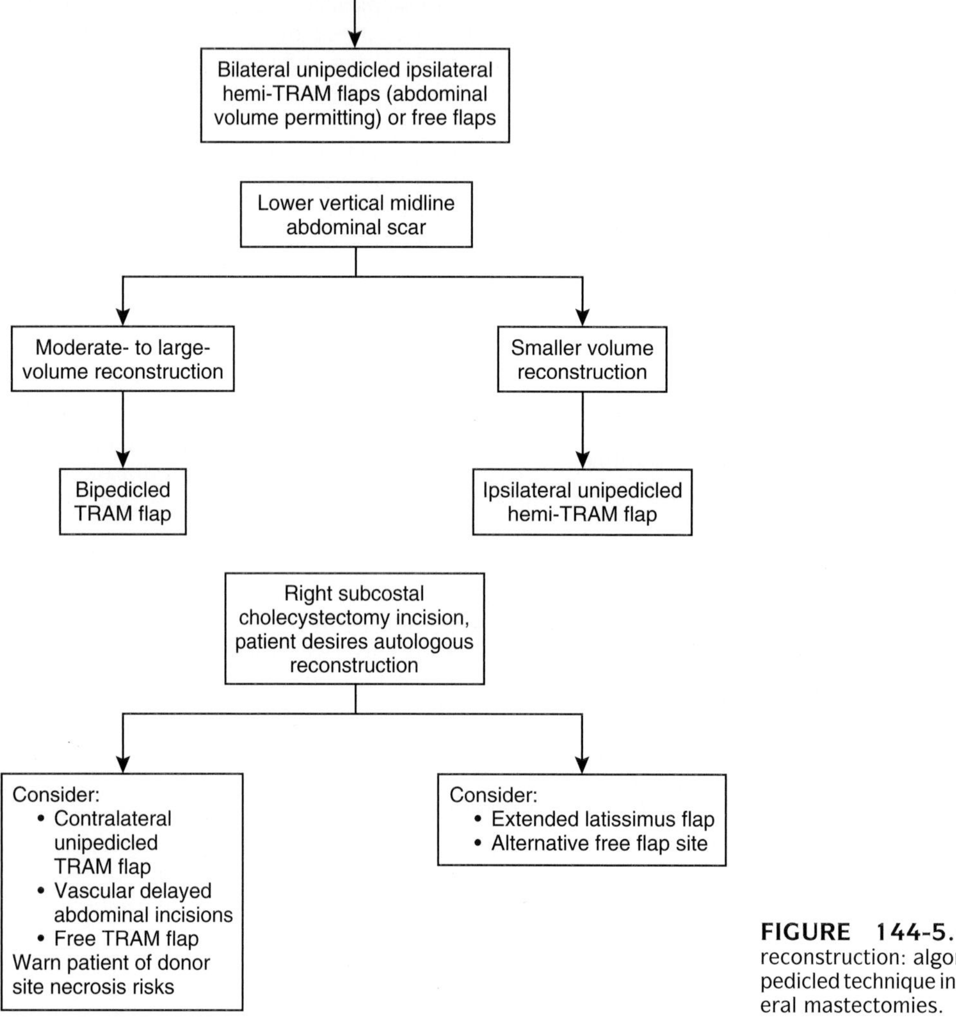

FIGURE 144-5. Delayed breast reconstruction: algorithm for choosing pedicled technique in patients with bilateral mastectomies.

diet for 24 to 48 hours before surgery to limit potential discomfort during the mild, transient ileus that often follows the abdominal wall closure.

Anesthetic Requirements

Patients are kept warm and well hydrated to provide a vasodilated, bounding circulation.[12] Urine output should be high throughout the procedure. Nitrous oxide administration can cause small bowel distention, resulting in potential difficulties with abdominal wall closure. It is recommended that all nitrous oxide inhalation be discontinued from the end of the mastectomy. Intraoperative body warming blankets are used routinely, as are leg compression stockings. The use of prophylactic heparin therapy or low-molecular-weight heparin does not appear to dramatically increase the risk of hematomas, and the use of intravenous ketorolac for postoperative pain has not been shown to increase hematoma rates.[40,41] The reported incidence of deep venous thrombosis complicated by pulmonary embolism is just under 1%; the incidence of fatal pulmonary embolism is approximately 0.1%.[32,33]

Operative Positioning

Patients are placed on the operating table in the supine position with the arms abducted to 80 to 90 degrees; further abduction may cause transient palsy to the lower trunk of the brachial plexus. Care should be taken to pad all pressure points, with particular attention being paid to elbows and heels. Patients should be on an operating table that can be flexed to the fully erect position to allow accuracy in flap shaping and to facilitate abdominal wound closure. Intraoperative patient warming devices are used routinely.

Ipsilateral Versus Contralateral Unipedicled TRAM Flap

The controversy over the use of ipsilateral versus contralateral unipedicled flaps continues. The author was trained to perform the contralateral procedure but has switched to the ipsilateral procedure wherever possible for several reasons. The ipsilateral transfer is associated with a much less obtrusive pedicle bulge in the long term, in part because the pedicle twist is less bulky owing to a direct 180-degree transposition over the costal margin when the ipsilateral transfer is performed; any rotation within the mastectomy site occurs above the inframammary crease as a consequence. By contrast, the contralateral flap begins its pedicle and flap rotation within the tunnel before reaching the breast, resulting in a more deforming bulge. Inframammary crease definition is far more crisp with the ipsilateral procedures, whereas the contralateral procedure causes more blunting of the medial inframammary fold, resulting in a visually disturbing lack of definition that is difficult to correct, even with subcutaneous suction up to the dermis. Flap perfusion appears better with less venous congestion in the ipsilateral procedure.

Unipedicled Operative Procedure

The upper abdominal incision is made first, and the upper abdominal skin flap is elevated over the costal margins laterally and to the xiphoid centrally. The patient is flexed to assess the adequacy of closure to the inferior incision line. The inferior incision may need to be elevated slightly to avoid tension at the donor site closure. Tight closure can seriously compromise blood flow to the skin edges, causing skin necrosis, particularly in the area between the umbilicus and pubis. The risk of skin necrosis is greater in obese patients. Preexisting Pfannenstiel incisions are routinely ignored because they do not have an impact on the survival of suprapubic skin and do not affect TRAM flap viability negatively. The distal incision is then made, and TRAM flap elevation is undertaken from lateral to medial, identifying the lateral row of perforators and the lateral border of the rectus abdominis muscle. The decision as to the side on which to base the flap depends on abdominal anatomy and the surgeon's preference. A conventional open cholecystectomy scar mandates a left-sided unipedicled flap. In the unscarred abdomen, either side may be used (Fig. 144-6), and it is generally based on the surgeon's preference. Ipsilateral transfer is beneficial in terms of reduction of initial intermammary bulging; definition of the ipsilateral inframammary crease tends to be excellent, pedicle tension is reduced, and flap positioning tends to be easier. Vascular supply to the flap appears better with ipsilateral transfer.[42] Ipsilateral transfer has become the author's preference wherever possible for these reasons. The contralateral pedicle tends to cause more medial inframammary crease bulging and somewhat limits the ease of flap positioning in terms of more lateral motion.

Radiation treatment of the affected breast necessitates either a contralateral unipedicled flap (with or

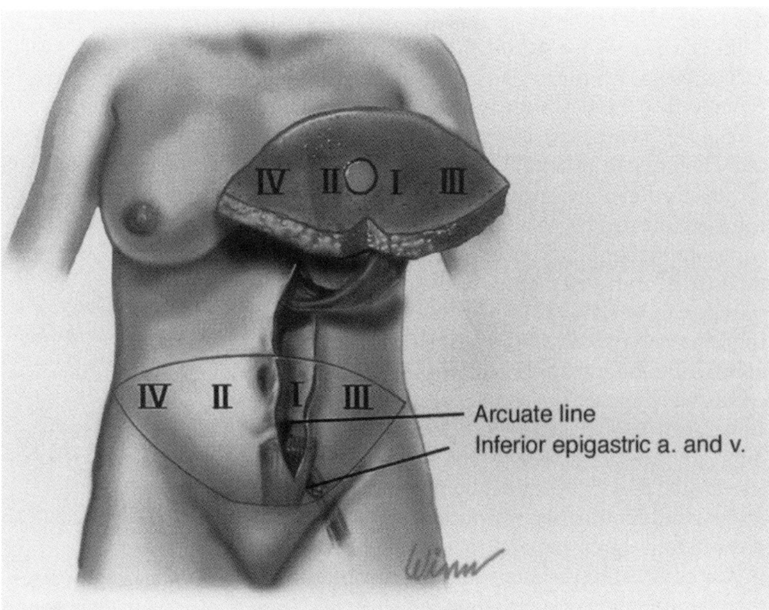

FIGURE 144-6. Ipsilateral unipedicled TRAM flap with 180-degree flap rotation.

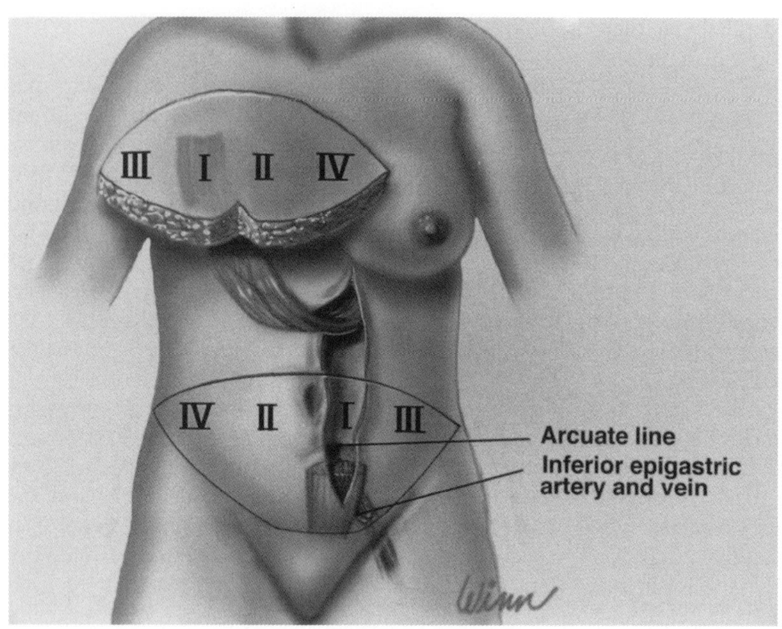

FIGURE 144-7. Contralateral unipedicled TRAM flap with 180-degree flap rotation.

without surgical delay) or preferably a bipedicled or free TRAM flap. The ipsilateral irradiated pedicle may be unreliable and has shown a higher fibrosis rate and slightly increased fat necrosis rate in patients with preoperative radiation treatment of the internal mammary supply.[43] A contralateral pedicle is useful in these patients but tends to cause some degree of blunting of the medial inframammary fold and softens the depth of the intermammary space (Fig. 144-7).

A surgical delay performed 5 to 7 days previously significantly improves TRAM flap blood supply, and this should be considered for the pedicled procedures if a large breast is to be fashioned.[26-28,44,45] If vascular delay is performed, it should include an incision right across the lower inferior end of the TRAM flap with elevation of the flap tips as described by Taylor.[26,46] The rectus fascia is incised as a long ellipse to facilitate closure and maintenance of muscle integrity at the inscriptions and is freed from the underlying rectus muscle. Care must be taken not to penetrate the muscle while the tendinous inscriptions are separated from the medial and lateral edges of the rectus sheath. The muscle can be elevated in its entirety or by a muscle-sparing technique (Fig. 144-8). Muscle sparing involves identifying the intramuscular course of the superior epigastric vessels with a Doppler probe and then leaving a lateral strip of muscle some 2 cm in diameter. Theoretically, this preserved strip of muscle leaves muscle innervated and vascularized by the intercostal vessels and nerves for further abdominal wall competence postoperatively. In practice, however, the intercostal supply penetrates the rectus muscle in its middle third, thereby leaving no innervation and probably little if any blood supply to the lateral muscle strip. A medial strip of muscle may also be left, but its functional value is also questionable. As noted earlier, Harris[21] demonstrated an 80% reduction in pedicled blood flow by clamping the medial and lateral thirds of the rectus muscle intraoperatively. Data on the diminishing size and strength of residual upper rectus muscle left after

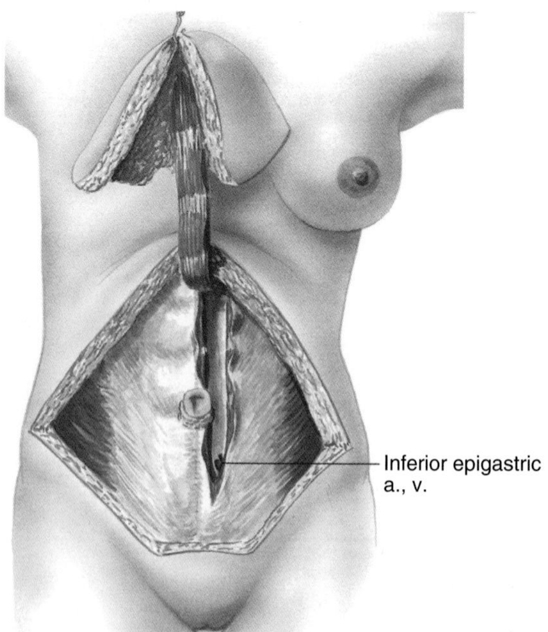

FIGURE 144-8. Muscle-sparing unipedicled TRAM flap as described by Hartrampf.

free TRAM flap harvest further call into question the validity of performing muscle-sparing procedures.[25] However, the additional muscle left behind may facilitate closure with less fascial tearing and may provide some further fibrosis to buttress the abdominal wall in the long term.

The rectus muscle is divided distally, and the deep inferior epigastric vessels are ligated with Ligaclips. These vessels should be dissected out with the flap because they may be needed for conversion to a free flap in the event of vascular compromise of a pedicled flap.

Flap elevation is based on the superior epigastric supply. Care should be taken to divide the eighth intercostal nerve as it enters the muscle near the costal margin. This essential maneuver facilitates muscle atrophy, reducing epigastric bulk in the long term, and eliminates the need for muscle sparing as a means of reducing pedicle bulk at the costal margin. A wide subcutaneous tunnel is made between the abdominal dissection and the mastectomy site, allowing passage of the pedicle without compression. When a contralateral pedicle is used, it is tunneled adjacent to the medial border of the normal breast. Ipsilateral flaps are passed straight up through the inframammary fold of the mastectomy site. If venous congestion occurs, repositioning may be helpful. In addition, one may remove the Ligaclip on the deep inferior epigastric vein stump and allow it to bleed for several minutes for venous decompression. Flap congestion should gradually decrease as venous flow in the flap adjusts to the new flap location and drainage direction. Alternatively, Hartrampf's "mechanical leech" drainage system may be inserted into the deep inferior vascular system to aid in venous decompression.[47] This involves inserting a pediatric feeding tube or venous cannula into the deep inferior epigastric vein and using this as a decompression valve that can be opened periodically to bleed the flap of congested, poorly oxygenated venous blood under pressure. It mandates that the surgeon harvest a usable stump of deep inferior epigastric vein at the time of TRAM flap harvest. The catheter can be flushed with dilute heparin solution to maintain its patency for a period of 2 or 3 days as needed.

Abdominal closure should be carefully undertaken because poor closure dramatically increases the risk of hernia formation. It is essential to incorporate both the internal and external oblique aponeuroses into the sheath closure.[48] If fraying of the fascia occurs, it can be darned with a suture weave or covered with an onlay of Prolene mesh or AlloDerm. Bucky and May[49] have reported the routine incorporation of mesh into all TRAM flap abdominal closures with excellent success; of 65 patients treated, 1 patient developed a mesh infection and 1 patient developed a hernia. The author minimizes the risks of fascial fraying by using a double mattress figure-of-eight closure in patients with high abdominal tension. To limit the use of foreign material, mesh closure should be limited. Once abdominal fascial closure has been securely achieved, the upper abdominal skin flap is redraped over suction drains and closed. An umbilicoplasty is then performed, preferably by use of the Avelar technique. This technique provides a naturally hooded umbilicus and gives the impression of a slightly Rubenesque natural contour to the lower abdomen. Appearance is further enhanced by a high lateral tension abdominoplasty skin design for the TRAM flap, producing a closure with less tension at the midline suprapubic region that is characteristic of the standard elliptical design to establish maximal tension at the midline. TRAM flap shaping follows, and technical caveats are discussed later in this chapter.

Careful attention should be paid to designing the lateral inframammary fold with quilting sutures to prevent loss of definition at this site. This maneuver should be performed with the patient in the erect position to evaluate the effect of gravity on the final shape of the reconstruction. Additional sutures can be placed at the inferolateral edge of the flap to infold the bottom of the flap for a rounder final breast shape as well as additional projection. With skin-sparing mastectomies, most of the flap is de-epithelialized, leaving only a disk of TRAM skin to resurface the skin deficit at the nipple-areola excision site. In conventional mastectomy skin excisions, a significant area of TRAM skin is required externally to reconstruct the skin deficit. It is preferable to delay adjustments on the contralateral breast to a later procedure after complete healing at the site of reconstruction (Figs. 144-9 to 144-11).

Bipedicled TRAM Flap

Indications for a bipedicled TRAM flap often represent indications for free TRAM flap transplantation for many surgeons (Table 144-6). Bipedicled flaps are robust and probably have a better blood supply than free TRAM flaps because of the conversion of zones II and IV to additional zones I and III, respectively. They allow more reliable survival of a greater proportion of the flap at the expense of greater abdominal donor site muscle loss. Whereas this affects the patient's abdominal strength in the short term, longer term function appears eminently compatible with

TABLE 144-6 ✦ INDICATIONS FOR BIPEDICLED TRAM FLAP

Large-volume reconstruction
Patients with midline abdominal incisions
Smokers
Obesity
Patients with radiation injury to one pedicle

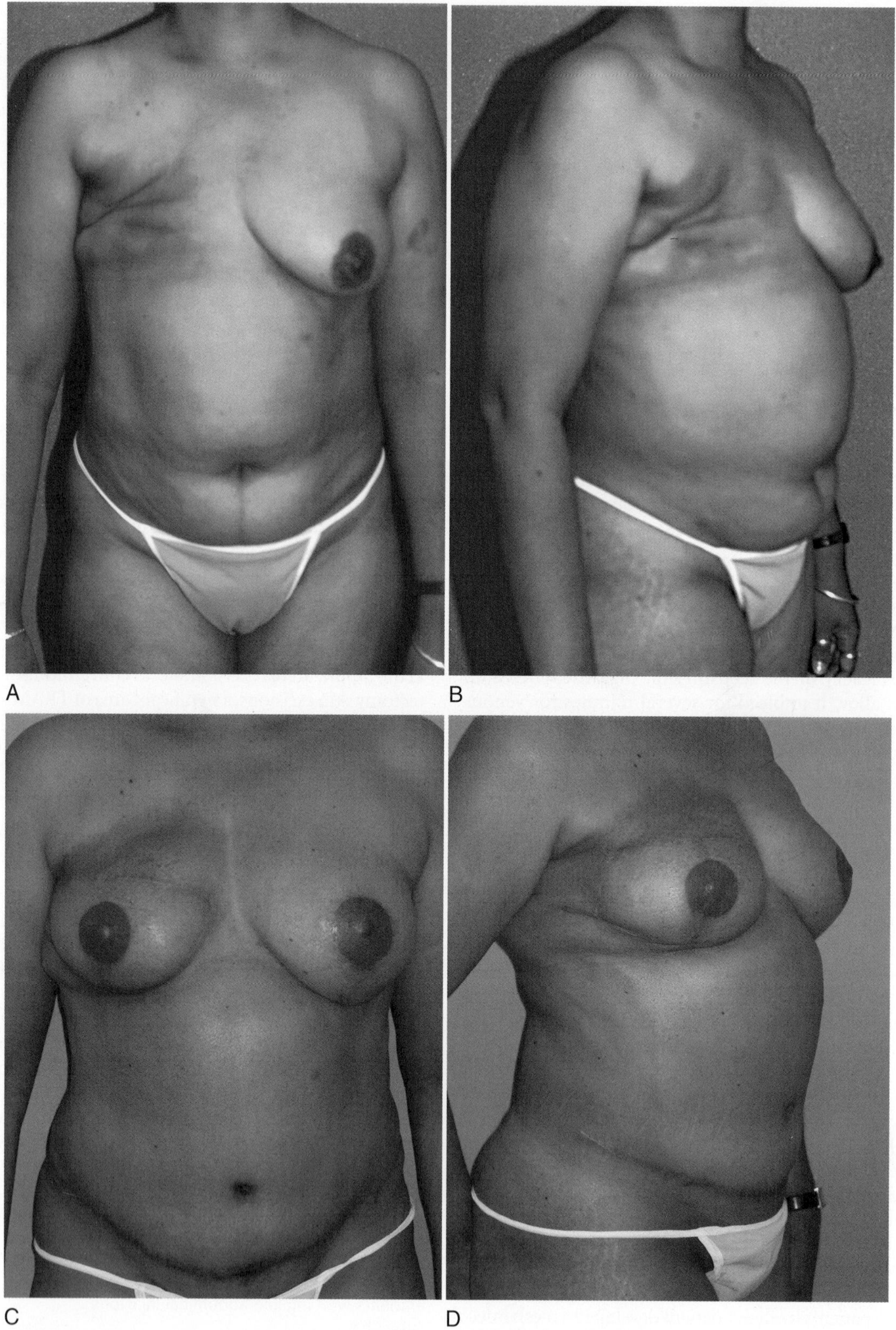

FIGURE 144-9. *A,* A 45-year-old woman with right mastectomy and postoperative irradiation, left breast ptosis. *B,* Oblique view. *C,* Anteroposterior view after left contralateral unipedicled TRAM flap. *D,* Oblique view.

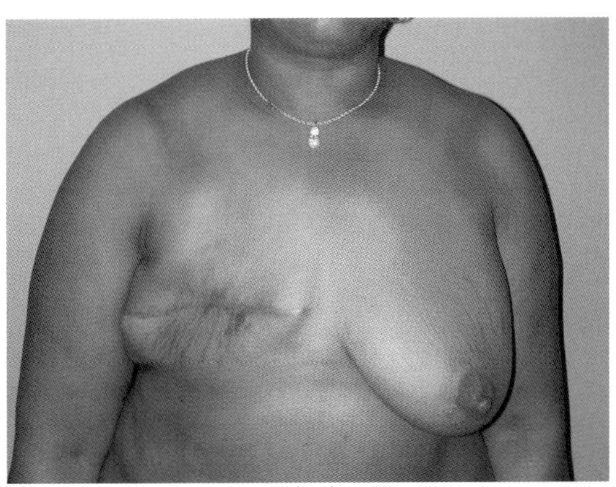

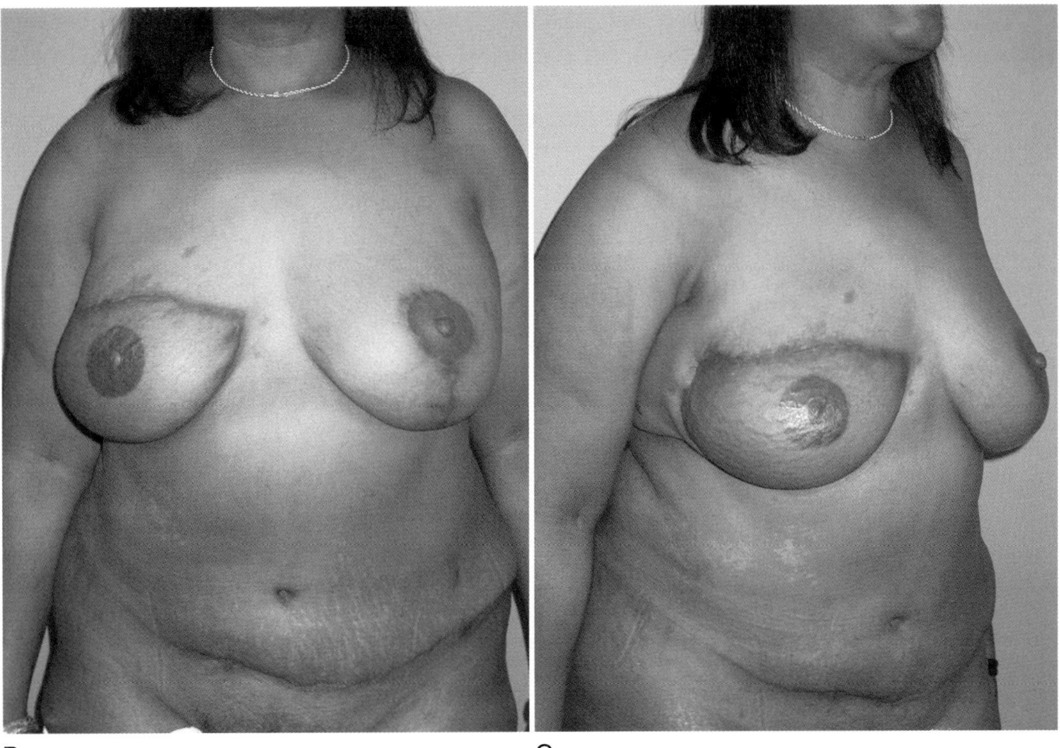

FIGURE 144-10. *A,* Preoperative view after right mastectomy; no irradiation. *B,* Postoperative result with ipsilateral unipedicled TRAM flap and C-V flap nipple reconstruction and tattoo, anteroposterior view. *C,* Oblique view.

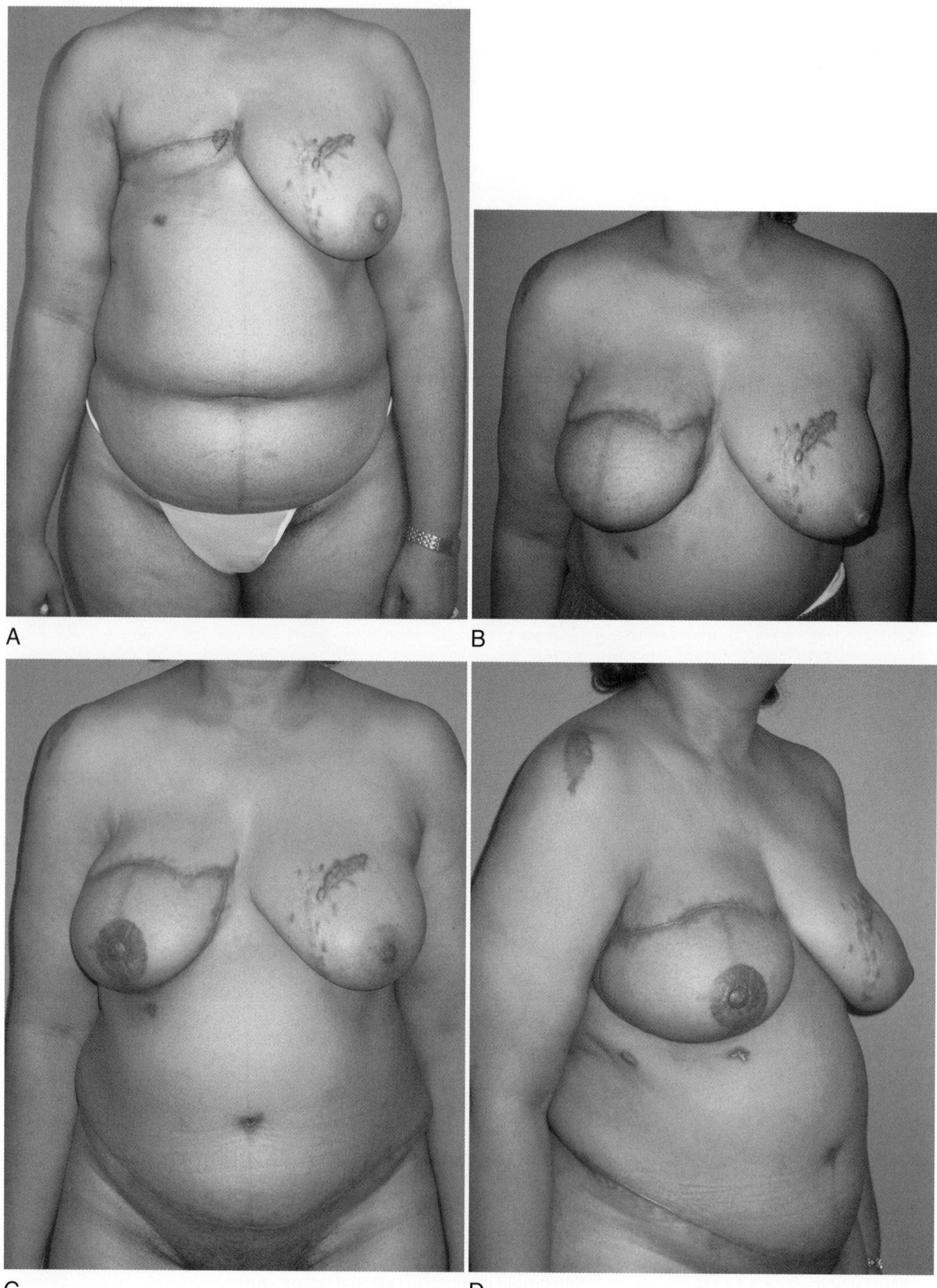

FIGURE 144-11. *A,* Preoperative anteroposterior view of a 50-year-old woman with right mastectomy, left breast ptosis, and keloid formation. The patient specifically desired TRAM flap reconstruction despite the potential for further keloid formation. *B,* Early postoperative result after ipsilateral unipedicled TRAM flap, anteroposterior view. *C,* Final result at 1 year with nipple reconstruction in place, anteroposterior view. *D,* Oblique view.

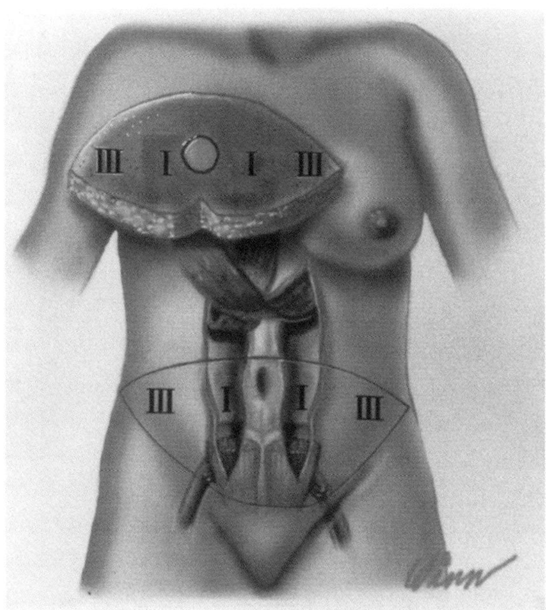

FIGURE 144-12. Bipedicled TRAM flap procedure.

activities of daily living. There are also fewer flap complications, and the procedure enables the non-microsurgeon to safely perform TRAM flap breast reconstruction in higher risk patients.[32]

Preoperative preparation and positioning are similar to those outlined for the unipedicled procedure. Initial flap elevation is identical in that both sides of the flap are dissected to the lateral perforators. Medial dissection differs in that a tunnel must be fashioned down the linea alba between the two pedicles (Fig. 144-12). This leaves a fascial strip on either side of the linea for fascial closure. As two pedicles have to pass up onto the chest wall, a more generous tunnel has to be fashioned, causing more initial bulging, and the patient should be informed of this preoperatively.

Once the flap is elevated, it is passed onto the chest, with care taken to prevent compression of the pedicles within the tunnel. If fascial tearing occurs during abdominal closure, precautions similar to those described for the unipedicled procedure are taken. Mesh closure is rarely required but should be used without hesitation if fascial closure is tenuous in any way. Abdominal wall strength is almost certainly more compromised compared with the unipedicled procedure,[50,51] and it should be performed with caution in the younger patient. Problems with backache, early satiety, and constipation may bother some patients. In young women, a free TRAM flap is safer than a bipedicled flap in terms of abdominal morbidity, but this has never been clearly proved. In the Emory review of bipedicled flap results, flap complications and abdominal wall complications were no worse than with unipedicled flaps, and flap blood supply was predictably better given the dual blood supply.[32] The author's large experience with bilateral and bipedicled flaps has confirmed initial experience with this procedure as safe and reliable with remarkably few complications considering the higher risk patients in whom it is performed. The abdominal strength objections voiced by some surgeons do not appear to be as significant as initially thought, and patients cope remarkably well with activities of daily living. Whereas it is true that strength is diminished significantly initially, particularly with respect to patients' ability to perform sit-ups, abdominal wall function improves with time, and a remarkable number of patients have little or no negative impact on activities of daily living. Hernia rates are not significantly higher with this procedure compared with unipedicled TRAM flaps. These issues are discussed at greater length in the outcomes section. It is an excellent option for the non-microsurgeon who performs large numbers of breast reconstructions in higher risk patients (Fig. 144-13).

Bipedicled TRAM Flap with Two Skin Islands

Bilateral reconstruction with two pedicled TRAM flaps follows an operative sequence identical to that described for the bipedicled procedure, the exception being that the skin island is split down the midline during the initial dissection, forming two flaps of equal size (Figs. 144-14 to 144-16). The flaps are transposed to the chest wall through ipsilateral tunnels to prevent possible compression and kinking through a common central tunnel. Flap rotation on the chest wall is typically 90 degrees. Abdominal closure is identical to that for the bipedicled TRAM flap.

Whereas bilateral bipedicled TRAM flaps are most commonly used in bilateral reconstructions, they have also been used successfully in unilateral reconstruction as stacked flaps to increase projection. A single-pedicle flap in a slim woman with a thin pannus will result in a relatively small volume flap because zone IV and part of zone III will usually be discarded. By use of two hemi-TRAM flaps, the entire pannus volume may be incorporated successfully into the reconstruction, with the deeper placed flap providing additional central volume for projection. In such circumstances, it would be reasonable to split the flap slightly off-center, using the larger side superficially to provide as much skin surface as possible while reserving the slightly smaller flap for deep fill.

Intraoperative Volume and Scar Assessment

During immediate reconstruction, the mastectomy specimen can be weighed off the surgical field. The

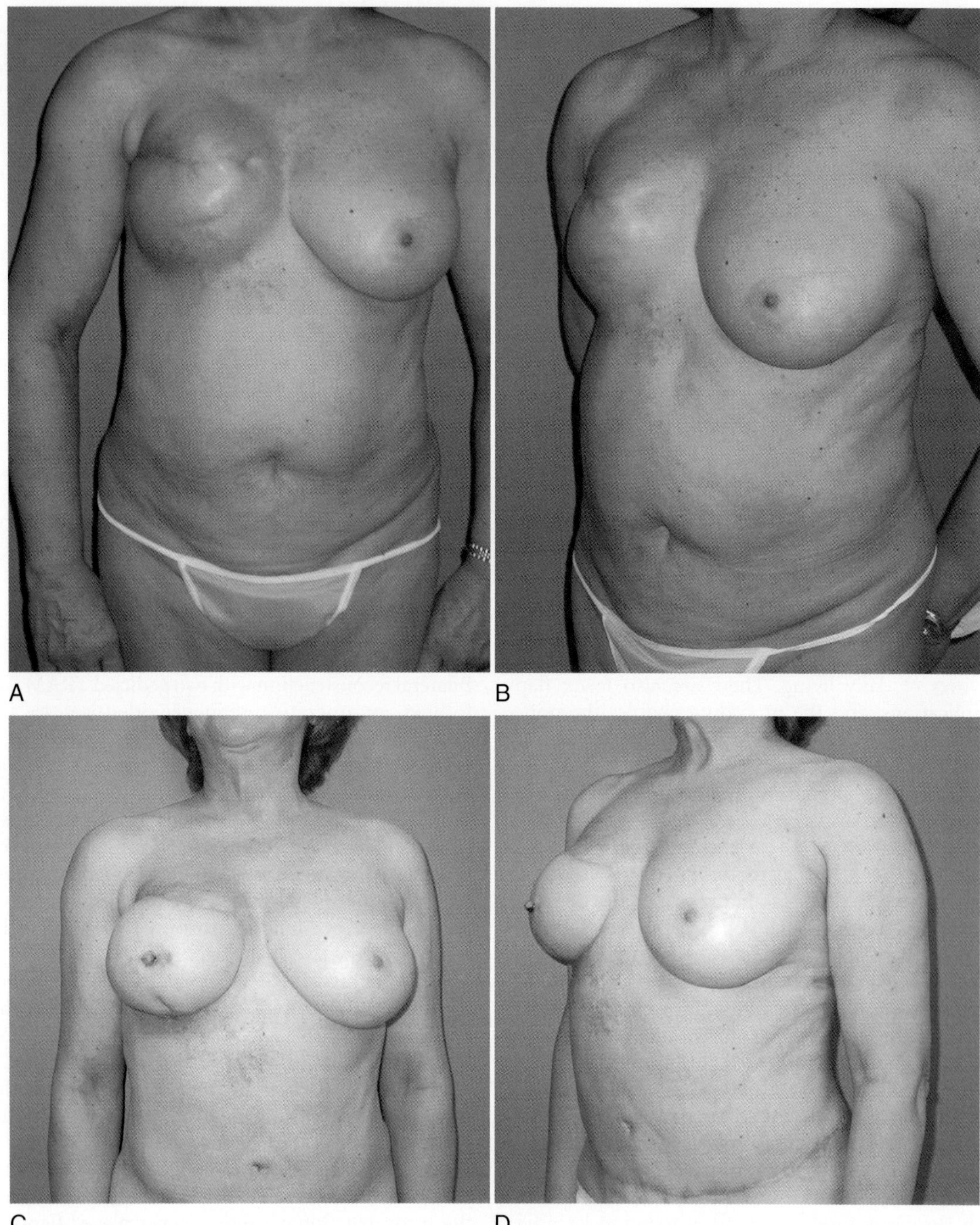

FIGURE 144-13. *A,* A 52-year-old woman after right mastectomy with immediate expander-implant reconstruction performed 3 years previously, anteroposterior view. She presented with pain, tightness, and persistent discomfort associated with grade III capsular contracture. *B,* Oblique view. *C,* Early postoperative result showing delayed bipedicled TRAM flap breast reconstruction after explantation with resection of the lower pole breast skin and subsequent nipple reconstruction before tattoo, anteroposterior view. The patient had complete resolution of her chest wall discomfort. *D,* Oblique view.

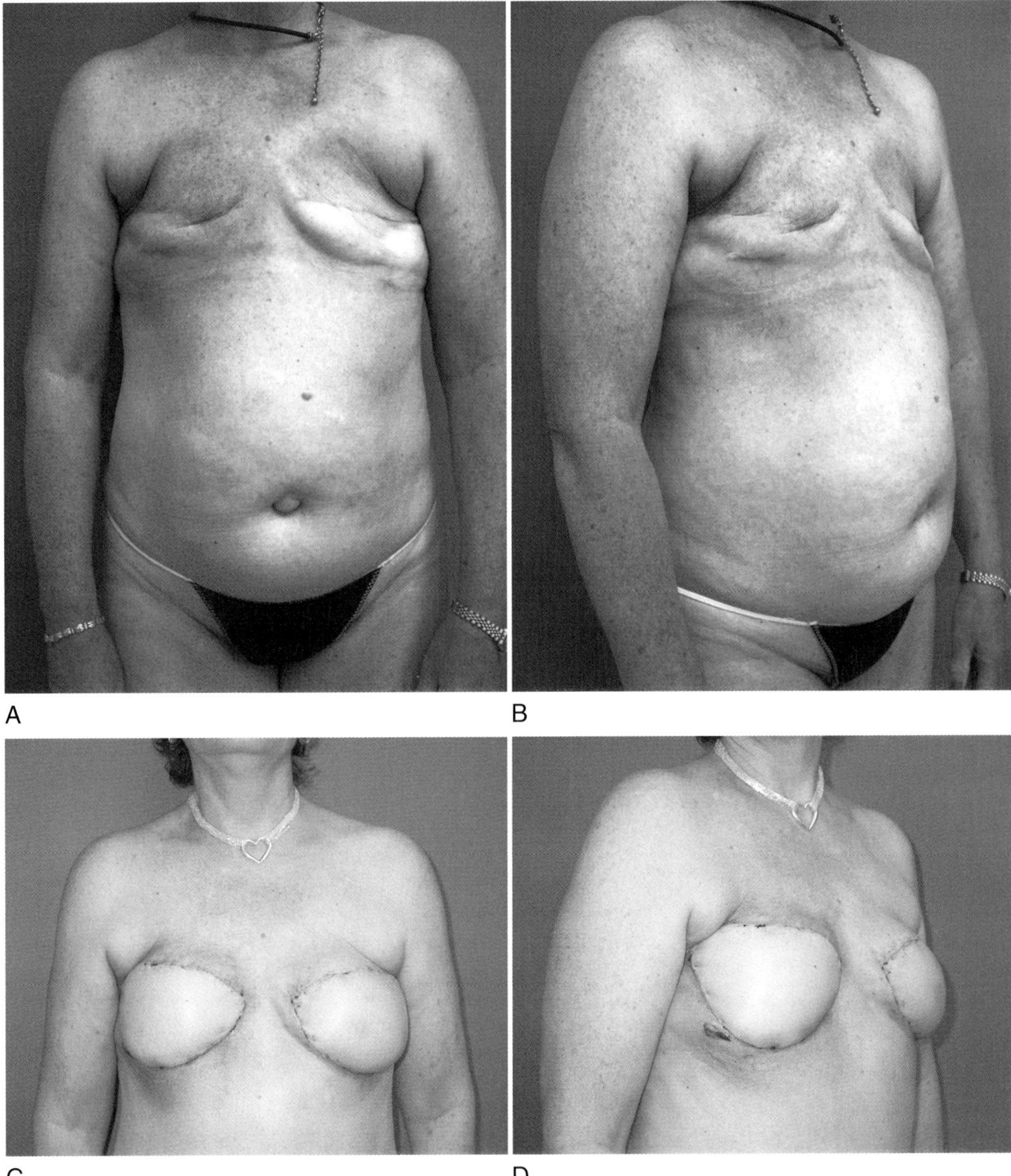

FIGURE 144-14. *A,* Patient 1 year after bilateral mastectomies for breast cancer with irradiated right chest wall. The patient is relatively slim and a nonsmoker. *B,* Oblique view. *C,* Early postoperative result after bilateral ipsilateral pedicled TRAM flaps, anteroposterior view. *D,* Oblique view.

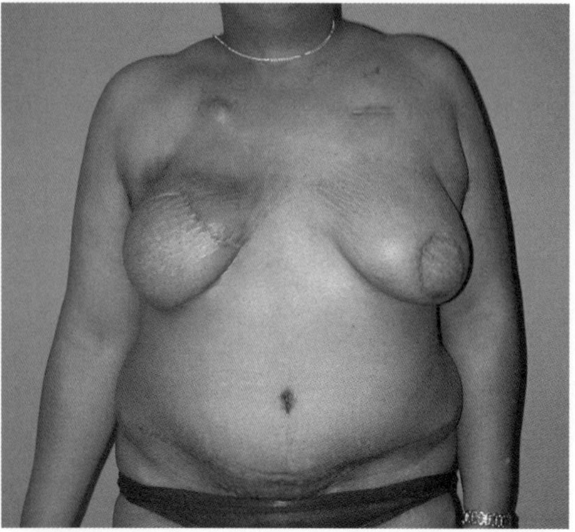

FIGURE 144-15. Early postoperative view after right mastectomy without reconstruction in a 57-year-old woman who developed left breast cancer. She underwent a left skin-sparing mastectomy and immediate left unipedicled hemi-TRAM flap reconstruction, with effectively a delayed right breast reconstruction by the right hemi-TRAM flap. Oblique orientation of the flaps was used in an effort to fill her upper pole hollowing after her initial right mastectomy. Symmetry is reasonable and nipple reconstruction is pending.

problem becomes how to determine the volume of the TRAM flap available to achieve a match for the contralateral breast. Wagner[51] devised a formula to calculate flap volume (V):

$$L \times W \times T \times 0.81 = V$$

where L, W, and T represent the length, width, and thickness of the TRAM flap. Hudson[52] has suggested the use of a simple hanging balance gas sterilized for intraoperative measurement of flap weight rather than volume. Volumetric assessment by hand is a simple but crude and somewhat inaccurate alternative.

The previous mastectomy scar, whether irradiated or not, poses significant technical problems. If it is incised and used as the inset for the TRAM flap, its tight horizontal contraction tends to act as a band across the upper pole of the reconstruction, forming a linear groove. If this occurs, the scar should be excised completely, and a lateral modified Z-plasty should be performed to soften the contour of the inset (Fig. 144-17). The procedure is more of an oblique back-cut than a true Z-plasty is, allowing a tongue of the TRAM flap skin island to angle up toward the axilla. The acute angles of the skin flaps are usually trimmed to blunt the contours. This breaks the contracture band and allows a more natural juncture between the

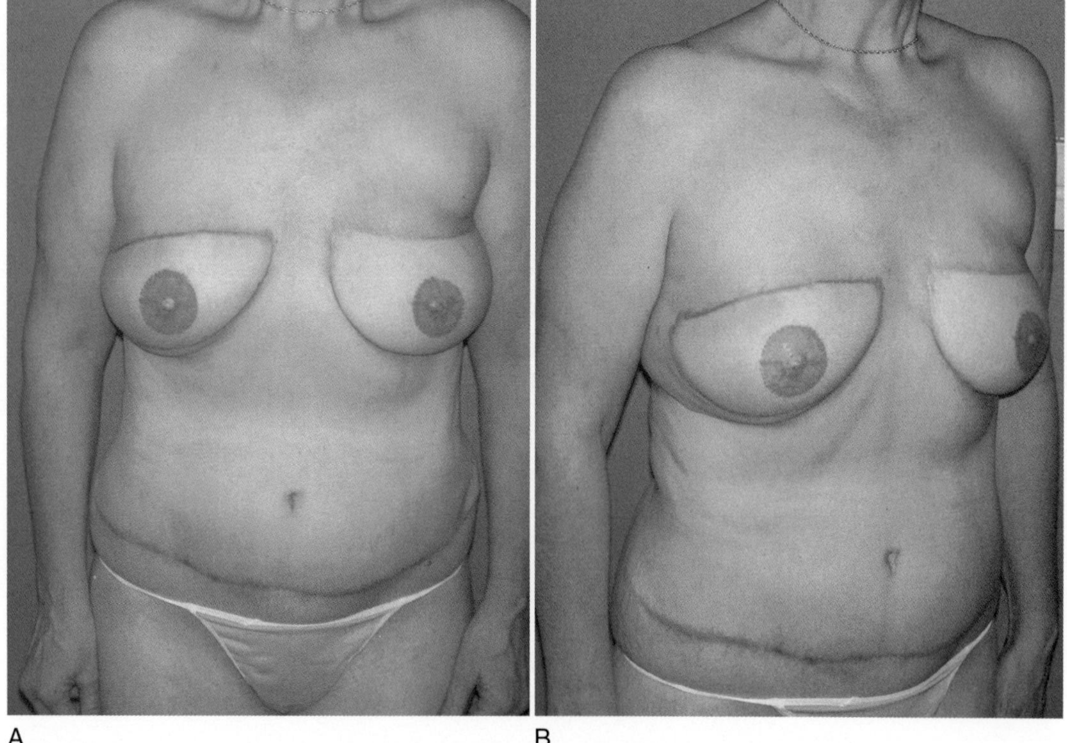

FIGURE 144-16. *A,* Bilateral delayed pedicled ipsilateral TRAM flap reconstruction in a slim patient with a long chest wall dimension demonstrating the need for a long oblique inset to the TRAM flaps. *B,* Oblique view.

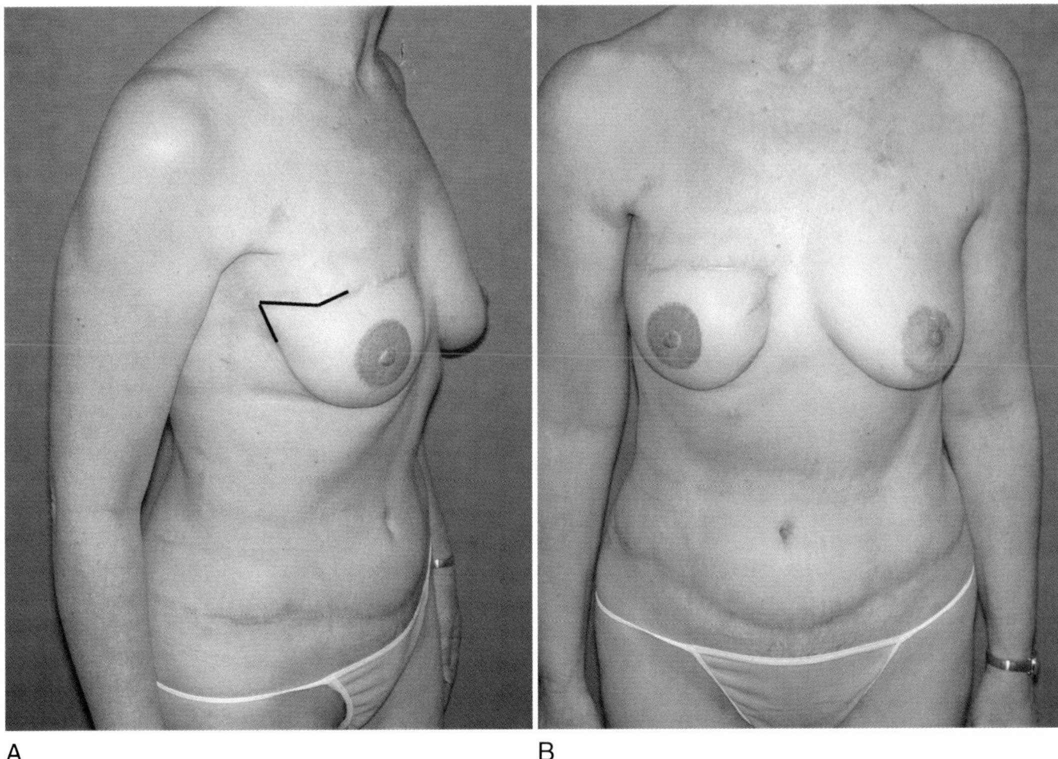

FIGURE 144-17. *A,* Right unipedicled TRAM flap inset showing oblique back-cut toward the axilla outlined in black. A wedge of TRAM flap skin is shown sliced into the back-cut. *B,* Anteroposterior view.

mastectomy flap and TRAM flap. Another alternative is to ignore the mastectomy scar completely, particularly if it is situated high on the chest wall, and place the TRAM flap exactly where it needs to be irrespective of the location of other breast scars. High mastectomy scars do not need to expand as much as more inferior scars do, and horizontal tightness may not be as much of an issue in these patients. Regardless of where the flap is ultimately placed, the inferior mastectomy skin flap should be completely excised down to the inframammary crease. This maneuver allows the TRAM flap skin island to form the lower pole of the breast and the new inframammary fold, and it also reduces the tendency of the breast to look like a "patchwork quilt" of differing skin colors and textures. This is particularly important when the chest wall has been irradiated. The lower mastectomy flap almost never expands sufficiently to accommodate the bulk of the TRAM flap anyway, and there seems little if any benefit to preserving it intact.

Flap Shaping and Positioning

The tip of zone III and almost all of zone IV should be discarded unless their blood supply appears unusually good. Flap orientation is critical to obtaining a natural shape and good symmetry. Whereas secondary shaping is always feasible and often necessary,[53] time spent shaping the flap at the initial operation is well spent, and it is possible to achieve excellent shape and symmetry at this first stage when adjustments are made most easily.[34,54-56] The most common orientations of the flap are transverse with a 180-degree rotation (Fig. 144-18) and oblique with a 120-degree or 80-degree rotation (see Fig. 144-17). In general, it is preferable to place as much bulk laterally and inferiorly to provide maximal projection and natural breast shape. This positioning allows less superior bulk, a desirable feature permitting optimal feathering of the TRAM flap's bulk into the space between the mastectomy skin flap and underlying pectoral muscle. The flap should be neatly anchored into this space to prevent unsightly step-offs, bulges, or hollows resulting from poor positioning. In addition, the edges of the flap should be beveled to further accentuate a gentle transition onto the chest wall. The 180-degree rotation allows the surgeon to take advantage of the well-vascularized, bulky fat in the periumbilical and infraumbilical areas, and this orientation is particularly useful for the patient with a broad-based breast. Closure of the umbilical donor site as a wedge cones the flap to produce more central, inferior projection

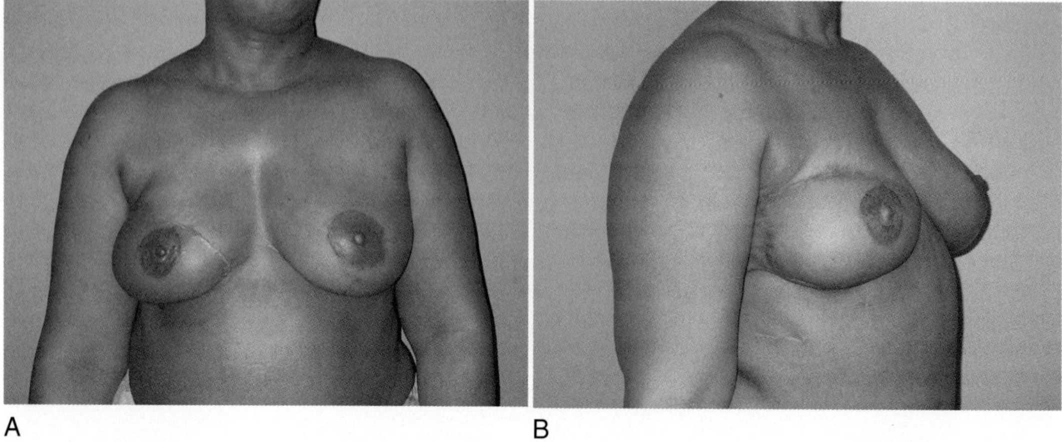

FIGURE 144-18. *A,* Anteroposterior view of completed right unipedicled ipsilateral TRAM flap reconstruction in a patient with a broad transverse chest diameter showing transverse flap orientation; contralateral left breast vertical reduction for symmetry. *B,* Oblique view.

mimicking the shape of the mature, slightly ptotic breast. The more coning required, the greater the degree of suturing needed to achieve this goal. If the 180-degree rotation is used, this positioning usually places the nipple-areola skin disk immediately above the umbilical wedge closure (with the flap on the chest wall), again taking advantage of the central fat bulk for projection of the nipple at the summit of the breast. It also provides a more gradual tapering of flap thickness toward the periphery of the breast superiorly and medially as the TRAM shelves off onto the pectoral muscle. If lateral fullness is required, zone III can be folded beneath zone I, but this should only be done once the lateral breast crease has been established and the flap has been secured to the chest wall in an appropriate position. It is preferable not to fold these flaps because this may increase fat necrosis. TRAM flap patients may complain of lateral displacement of the flap, causing abutment of the breast against the inner aspect of the arm. This lateral displacement can best be prevented by firmly anchoring the flap medially and superiorly with suture fixation at the time of tissue transfer.

Oblique flap rotation is used for those patients with narrower breasts or in the rare patient in whom a 180-degree rotation causes persistent venous congestion. Vertical orientation is used in patients with a narrow breast and long, thin chest wall or in patients with significant ptosis who do not wish to have a contralateral mastopexy. As rotation approaches 90 degrees with the umbilicus medially, medial bulk tends to become difficult to eradicate, and the inferolateral area tends to become deficient of fullness. This is due to the tapering of fat thickness that occurs naturally as one moves from zone I toward the tip of zone III.

TRAM flap folding is a contentious issue. The lower pole can be filled by folding zone III under zone I to project the summit of the breast; rotation through approximately 120 to 130 degrees allows folding of zone III beneath zone I if it is needed for lateral breast fullness, and the tail of zone III may be lifted into the anterior axillary fold to fill this area as needed. The main problem encountered with folding in this position is that the folded free edge of the flap may produce a visible line or step-off in the inferior contour, and it may be technically impossible in patients with stiff abdominal fat. Careful tapering of the folded zone III edge may blunt this effect successfully. Congestion of the folded zone is a potential problem with flap necrosis and increased areas of fat necrosis. On occasion, this degree of rotation may result in difficulties with venous congestion when pedicled flaps are used. Whether pedicled or free flaps are used, it is preferable to rely more on careful TRAM flap positioning than on folding to achieve projection, as the folded zone may experience vascular compromise distal to the fold.

The flap is tacked into position with key staples initially, and the patient is placed into a sitting position on the operating table to assess shape and symmetry. Once the flap size, shape, and position have been determined, the patient can be returned to a supine position. Any areas requiring burial beneath existing mastectomy skin flaps superiorly can be de-epithelialized with large scissors; the flap is then tacked to the pectoralis major muscle with suspensory sutures of Vicryl or PDS. Some surgeons prefer nonabsorbable sutures for this purpose in an effort to minimize the potential for inferolateral drift of the flap in the early postoperative period. The flap is then sewn into its recipient skin margin after incorporation of the superolateral Z-plasty alluded to earlier. Running subcuticular suturing is used throughout, and a drain is routinely placed to the bed of the reconstruction.

Donor Site Closure

Donor site closure is critical to the successful completion of TRAM flap breast reconstruction. A few words on donor closure are pertinent.

Sheath closure should always incorporate both the internal and external oblique fascial layers to limit the risk of hernia formation. A deep layer of either running or interrupted No. 1 Prolene suture followed by a second layer of running No. 1 PDS suture is commonly used. Closure with double figure-of-eight No. 1 Prolene interrupted sutures provides an extremely powerful closure with a built-in pulley-like mechanism to reduce fascial tearing as the fascia is closed. This suture layer is reinforced with a running No. 1 PDS layer secondarily. Contralateral vertical sheath plication may be performed to centralize the umbilicus in unilateral pedicled flaps; this additional step is obviously unnecessary in bipedicled or bilateral flaps. However, in the author's experience, contralateral plication seems to do relatively little to centralize the umbilicus in practice while simultaneously increasing intra-abdominal tension unnecessarily. Horizontal plication inferiorly can be performed to add further tightening in select patients, but this is almost never necessary or possible. The skin pannus is defatted around the umbilicus inset, which the author prefers to reconstruct by the Avelar umbilicoplasty.[57] This provides a naturally hooded umbilicus and gives the impression of a slightly Rubenesque natural contour to the lower abdomen. Appearance is further enhanced by a high lateral tension abdominoplasty skin design (Lockwood abdominoplasty design) for the TRAM flap, producing a closure with less tension at the midline suprapubic region that is characteristic of the standard elliptical design to establish maximal tension at the midline. Mesh is not recommended unless there is extensive tearing of weak fascial components during closure. If mesh is required, onlay of the mesh is preferable to use of inlay techniques, although Bucky[49] describes excellent results with extensive inlay achieving attractive abdominal contouring.

Nipple Reconstruction

It is preferable to wait 6 to 8 weeks before performing nipple reconstruction. A waiting period of 6 to 8 weeks allows resolution of flap edema, and gravitational pull will allow some settling of the flap for more accurate assessment of nipple placement. A C-V flap is used for nipple reconstruction, which forms a nipple some 50% longer than required as atrophy will cause further slight loss of projection with time. In an effort to maintain nipple projection in TRAM flap reconstructions, it is preferable to place the reconstructed nipple's free edge on a shelf of de-epithelialized adjacent TRAM flap skin to prevent the nipple from falling back into the donor site. This technique often gives improved long-term projection in the author's experience. Tattooing is usually performed 8 weeks later to minimize the effect of tattoo-induced traumatic atrophy of the nipple (see Figs. 144-10 and 144-11). Immediate nipple reconstruction has been advocated by some and is certainly more cost-effective than staged procedures.[58] The difficulty with this approach is that settling of the TRAM flap may result in an incorrectly placed nipple reconstruction. A traditional skate flap with surrounding skin graft unquestionably provides the best long-term projection in the author's opinion, but its mandatory requirement for a skin graft detracts from its value to some extent.[59] Tattooing is still required for the areolar graft in these patients, but the results are usually excellent.

Secondary Shaping and Contralateral Breast Surgery

Secondary shaping is usually not necessary if careful attention was paid to flap shaping and symmetry at the initial operation. Where possible, it is preferable to match the reconstruction to the contralateral breast unless this breast is in need of reduction or mastopexy at the patient's request. If secondary shaping is necessary, it is preferable to perform it at the time of nipple reconstruction.[53] Careful contouring with 3- to 4-mm cannulas will help define blunted inframammary folds or lateral breast creases and effectively reduces minor contour defects produced by overfilling with excess flap bulk. If a flap is too low or too lateral, it is preferable to separate it from the surrounding skin envelope and attempt to relocate it into its appropriate position with anchoring stay sutures placed between the flap's deep surface and the pectoralis major fascia. The need for this maneuver can almost be eliminated by careful intraoperative positioning, taking particular care to avoid upper pole hollowing. Contralateral reduction, mastopexy, or augmentation will be necessary in some patients and can be performed either at the initial operation or subsequently at the time of nipple reconstruction.

COMPLICATIONS AND OUTCOMES

The major complications of delayed TRAM flap reconstruction include scarring, skin and fat necrosis, flap loss, hernia formation, deep venous thrombosis, asymmetry, abdominal tightness, early satiety, and the psychosexual and acceptance issues surrounding any breast reconstruction.

Skin and Fat Necrosis

Skin and fat necrosis is a relatively common occurrence in any TRAM flap reconstruction, whether it is free or pedicled. The problem in unraveling the data available is that observers differ in the estimate of "clinically significant" fat necrosis. In the author's series at Emory Clinic, a definition of 10% or more of the flap surface containing palpable firmness was used. This yielded a "significant fat necrosis" rate of 10.6%.[33] In this series, risk factors associated with fat necrosis included prior irradiation ($P < .001$), abdominal scarring ($P < .01$), and obesity ($P < .02$). Among patients with unipedicled TRAM flaps, two or more risk factors pushed the fat necrosis rate up to 24.7% compared with 8.3% in patients without risk factors ($P < .002$). Interestingly, patients with multiple risk factors undergoing bipedicled flaps did not have an increased risk for fat necrosis, suggesting that the bipedicled procedure eliminated the impact of the risk factors by boosting flap blood supply. Paige's review[32] of bipedicled TRAM flap reconstructions demonstrated no increased risk of fat necrosis or flap loss among bilateral patients. The risk factors identified were identical to those identified in an earlier study published by Watterson.[33] Bilateral procedures showed a slight increase in general complications such as atelectasis. Abdominal complications were not increased significantly. In a study from M.D. Anderson Cancer Center, Kroll[60] compared clinical and radiologic evidence of fat necrosis between 49 free and 67 pedicled TRAM flaps. The size of the lesions was not clear, but all lesions were visible mammographically. Predictably, free TRAM flaps demonstrated an 8.2% incidence of detectable fat necrosis compared with 26.9% in pedicled TRAM flaps ($P < .01$). Interestingly, fat necrosis was more common in obese patients and smokers, but this did not attain statistical significance. Elliott et al[61] confirmed similar findings for their series of patients, but in all of these studies, measurement of the amount of fat necrosis has been subjective to a considerable degree.

Radiation treatment negatively affects TRAM flaps, causing both fibrosis and fat necrosis. In a 1995 study, Williams[43] reported the Emory experience with radiation therapy administered either before or after TRAM flap reconstruction. Nineteen patients received radiation therapy after pedicled TRAM flap surgery, 108 received radiation therapy before reconstruction, and 572 patients underwent breast reconstruction without radiotherapy. Mean follow-up was 47 months. Fibrosis within the reconstruction was found in 31.6% of irradiated TRAM flaps but not in patients who received preoperative therapy. Fat necrosis was similar in both irradiated groups at 17.6% versus 10% in the nonirradiated patients. Obesity further compounded fat necrosis rates when it was coupled with radiation therapy. Rogers[62] found a similar trend when free deep inferior epigastric perforator (DIEP) flaps were exposed to postoperative irradiation. By contrast, Zimmerman[63] described 21 patients with free TRAM flap reconstruction and claimed little negative impact in the majority of patients. The question of whether it is worthwhile to perform a microsurgical turbocharged anastomosis to reduce fat necrosis has been addressed in a small series of patients by El-Mrakby et al.[64] Turbocharged pedicled flaps had almost twice the rate of fat necrosis of free flaps, although the fact that these patients required turbocharging suggests an inevitable sample bias. Their conclusion is that free flaps are superior to turbocharged pedicled flaps. The use of turbocharging by anastomosis of the deep inferior epigastric vessels to the thoracodorsal vessels seems to incorporate the worst of both pedicled and microsurgical worlds. It is, however, reasonable to perform a venous anastomosis in an effort to improve venous outflow because this is the most common cause of flap failure.

Abdominal Wall Strength and Contour

There has long been contention about the impact of pedicled versus free TRAM flaps on abdominal wall function. It seems intuitive that a free flap would have far less impact than pedicled flaps on abdominal wall function, with bipedicled flaps demonstrating the worst outcome. In practice, this is not strictly true, particularly when activities of daily living are evaluated by the patients themselves. It appears that there is considerable recruitment of adjacent muscle groups to achieve strength, and this tends to improve with time. Furthermore, it appears that even with free flap harvest, the residual rectus muscle tends to atrophy significantly, and hernia rates are not that much less than with pedicled flaps.

Hartrampf[12] reported a 1.5% hernia rate in 351 unipedicled TRAM flap reconstructions. The Emory group reported a hernia rate of 8.8%, a figure strongly skewed by one surgeon's use of small inlay mesh repairs; this figure has since been reduced to approximately 3.9%.[32,33] This is similar to the data presented by Petit[65,66] from Milan, who reported 251 TRAM flap reconstructions with a hernia rate averaging 7%, now reduced to 2%. Paige's review of the Emory experience with 257 bilateral versus unilateral pedicled reconstructions during a 7-year period revealed no significant difference between the two groups in terms of abdominal morbidity. In a review of 268 patients who had undergone either free TRAM or conventional pedicled TRAM flap reconstructions at least 6 months before, Kroll found similar hernia rates whether unipedicled or bilateral flaps were harvested (3.8% versus 2.6%, not statistically significant). Patients with single-pedicle free TRAM flaps were more likely to perform sit-ups than were patients with conventional unipedicled flaps, who in turn were more likely to be able to do sit-ups than were patients with bilateral free or bipedicled flaps. His conclusion was that the abdominal hernia or bulge rate is relatively independent of the type of TRAM flap used and the number of muscle pedicles harvested.

By contrast, measured abdominal strength was affected by these factors as far out as 6 months postoperatively. Nahabedian[67] evaluated 108 women with free TRAM flaps, 37 women with pedicled flaps, and 10 women with DIEP flaps. Lower abdominal contour defects were far more common after bilateral free TRAM flaps than with DIEP flaps. Blondeel[68,69] found that free TRAM flaps had a far more negative impact on abdominal strength than did free DIEP flaps, but even free DIEP flaps may cause some degree of abdominal weakness.[70] Suominen[24,25,71] has performed several studies to accurately measure abdominal strength and function up to 12 months postoperatively. In a magnetic resonance imaging study of the residual rectus muscles left after free and pedicled flaps, the donor rectus muscle on the free flap side had atrophied by at least 25% compared with the nonsurgical side, and fatty degeneration was significantly higher in the donor muscle. No hernias were detected in either group.[25] In another study by the same author, long-term follow-up (mean, 23 months) of the pedicled and free TRAM flap groups was performed. By this time, there were no significant differences in abdominal flexion-extension strengths between the groups.[24] Edsander-Nord[72] performed a prospective study of 19 free versus 23 pedicled TRAM flap patients, assessing strength at 3, 6, and 12 months postoperatively. Apart from an initial transient decrease in strength that was worse in pedicled than in free flap patients, the strength differences resolved almost entirely by 12 months. What is interesting is that free TRAM flap patients experienced a greater incidence of lower abdominal bulging (82%) than did their pedicled counterparts (48%).

In a meta-analysis of previously published data, Reece and Kroll[31] attempted to collate the evidence concerning abdominal wall morbidity after TRAM flap reconstruction. The data are interesting, but firm conclusions are difficult to arrive at given the widely disparate data collected. In conclusion, there is no doubt that the more muscle harvested, the greater the initial impact on abdominal strength. However, as time progresses, pedicled and free TRAM flap patients develop similar functional outcomes with little impact on the activities of daily living. Abdominal bulge and hernia rates appear to be independent of the type of flap harvested and may relate to the care with which repair has been undertaken as well as the quality of the fascia to be repaired. The exact mechanism for these observed differences has yet to be explained satisfactorily.

Partial Flap Loss

Whereas complete flap loss is extremely rare in pedicled TRAM flap reconstruction (2 of 350 unipedicled and 0 of 39 bipedicled TRAM flaps in Hartrampf's series[12]), partial flap loss is more common. Hartrampf reported an 8.5% incidence in his series; Kroll[73] reported an incidence of 15.4% in slim patients that increased to 41.7% in obese patients. Elliott[61] reported a 10% incidence in a series of 128 patients who underwent unipedicled TRAM flaps, and Trabulsy et al[1] noted an incidence of 6% partial flap loss and 4% complete flap loss in their series of 99 patients. By comparison, Chang,[74] reporting on more than 700 free TRAM flap breast reconstructions, found total flap loss in 5.1% and partial flap loss in 6.2%. This pushes total flap necrosis-related complications to above 11% in a center of excellence. These figures should be borne in mind when occasional microsurgeons are tempted to embark on complex free flap procedures in higher risk patients. It may also explain why many surgeons who are comfortable with microsurgery are reluctant to convert to performing free TRAM flaps routinely in their practices, given the time and cost restraints of these complex procedures.

Factors Influencing Outcome

OBESITY

The most comprehensive study to date detailing the impact of obesity on human flap viability is that presented by Chang et al.[74] In this study, free TRAM flap results were evaluated on the basis of the patient's body mass. Normal weight patients (n = 442) had no total flap losses and a 1.6% partial flap necrosis rate. Overweight patients (n = 212) experienced 1.9% total flap loss with a 1.4% partial flap necrosis rate. By contrast, 64 obese patients had a 3.2% total flap necrosis rate and a 3.2% partial flap necrosis rate. Fat necrosis rates were 6.1% in normal patients, 9% in the overweight group, and 7.8% in the obese category. Abdominal bulges were 3 times more common in overweight patients compared with normal, and seromas were 10 times more common in obese patients. In the Emory University study of 556 patients, obesity correlated with both fat necrosis and general complications at the $P < 0.02$ level.[33]

SMOKING

Watterson's study[33] demonstrated a significant correlation between smoking and general complications ($P < .002$), but interestingly, smoking did not correlate strongly with fat necrosis. Hartrampf[12] accorded heavy smoking a moderate risk in his scoring system for TRAM flap patient selection criteria. Chang[74] found a significant risk for both the reconstruction and the donor site in smokers compared with nonsmokers, with those having more than a 10 pack-year history faring worse than those with shorter histories. Former smokers and nonsmokers had similar complication rates. In another study, Padubidri[75] found overall complications to be greater in smokers at 39.4% versus 25% in ex-smokers and nonsmokers.

RADIATION THERAPY

Until recently, adjunctive radiation therapy has been reserved for those patients with more advanced breast cancers and more than three positive axillary lymph nodes. The publication of two papers, one from Denmark and the other from Canada, initiated a major swing toward adjunctive radiation treatment of patients with early breast cancer in an effort to improve survival.[76,77] Although the trend has not been strongly supported by the Consensus Conference on Breast Disease, more patients than ever before are being advised to have adjunctive radiation therapy. The result has been that more and more patients with TRAM flap reconstructions are now facing postoperative radiotherapy and the consequences of radiation's impact on the flap. Add to this the dramatic impact of skin-sparing mastectomy on breast reconstruction and one can see what a dilemma the reconstructive surgeon now faces. Should the patient who faces radiotherapy in her future proceed with mastectomy first and then have delayed reconstruction, or should we go ahead with a skin-sparing mastectomy with all of its benefits, reconstruct the breast with a TRAM flap, and then proceed to radiation therapy, accepting its negative consequences? This dilemma is the subject of constant debate at national and international meetings. Surgeons who frequently perform TRAM flaps are aware of radiation's impact on these flaps, whether they are pedicled or free. TRAM flaps tolerate irradiation better than expander-implant reconstructions do and with fewer complications.[78] Williams[79] reviewed the Emory experience with radiation treatment and found it to increase fibrosis as well as fat necrosis, depending on the timing of treatment in relation to surgery. Flap loss was not increased, a finding corroborated by Kroll's review[80] of 428 flaps (of 1384 free flaps total) transferred to previously irradiated beds. It was Kroll's belief that radiation treatment significantly affected the feel and shape of TRAM flaps when it was administered after reconstruction as evidenced by Williams' data. His conclusion was that patients in whom postmastectomy radiotherapy is likely should complete their radiation treatment and then proceed to TRAM flap reconstruction, forgoing the benefits of skin-sparing mastectomy and immediate reconstruction. In this manner, the final reconstruction may be spared the deleterious effects of radiation injury in the long term even though there is a greater likelihood that such patients may need free or bipedicled TRAM flap procedures. There is certainly merit in this argument given the possible prospect of fibrosis, distortion, and fat necrosis that may supervene in an irradiated TRAM flap.

The impact of radiation treatment should be considered when a surgeon is deciding whether to perform a free or pedicled TRAM flap in an irradiated, postmastectomy reconstruction. It is certainly safe to advocate free TRAM flap reconstruction in the face of prior irradiation, but it does mandate a high degree of microsurgical expertise with a 95% to 98% flap success rate if this is to be routinely offered to patients. The use of either a bipedicled flap or a contralateral unipedicled flap in patients with no other risk factors is a perfectly reasonable approach. However, when a free flap is planned, one is performing a microvascular anastomosis in an irradiated field, and the vessels may be scarred and fragile. This is particularly true of the internal mammary veins, which may be fragile even when they have not previously been irradiated. It is the author's practice to plan for a free TRAM flap in patients with multiple risk factors in addition to radiation treatment. At the time of reconstruction, the axilla or internal mammary vessels are explored first in an effort to determine suitability for anastomosis. If these vessels are usable, a free TRAM flap is performed. If the recipient vessels are poor, a bipedicled procedure is performed. The patient is made aware of this reconstructive decision-making process before surgery.

Pregnancy After Pedicled TRAM Flaps

Despite the loss of muscle function after pedicled TRAM flap harvest, it is still possible for patients to conceive and carry a pregnancy to term as well as to achieve normal vaginal delivery.[81] Johnson[82] described the successful vaginal delivery of monozygotic twins after bilateral pedicled TRAM flap reconstruction, indicating that patients can be reassured that their abdomens will in all likelihood perform satisfactorily even under the considerable stress of twin pregnancy. Parodi[83] cautions against patients becoming pregnant within 12 months after TRAM flap surgery, reporting a single instance of a woman becoming pregnant at 4 months postoperatively and developing a hernia. She delivered vaginally at term.

Patient Satisfaction Outcomes

The emotional outcome after breast reconstruction is difficult to predict and highly individual.[84] Numerous factors may influence the aesthetic outcome.[85] In a study of 125 women diagnosed with breast cancer, Keith[86] found that 49.6% of his respondents desired breast reconstruction if it was available. Younger women and more depressed women tended to favor reconstruction more than older patients did. In this study, marital status, tumor size, extrovertism, neuroticism, and tough-mindedness did not independently predict the desire for reconstruction. Of those women requesting reconstruction, 63% were concerned that reconstruction might mask recurrence, but 94% thought that it would greatly benefit their self-esteem. Age does not appear to be a significant risk factor for pedicled TRAM flap use as evidenced by a study of 84 patients aged 65 years or older.[87]

In a small study of women's acceptance of the procedure, Nissen[88] found that although women were generally highly satisfied with their reconstruction, their greatest anxiety remained the fear of recurrence as well as a desire to be as informed as possible about complications and recovery. This was reinforced in a study by Tykka,[89] who found that most women were highly satisfied with their TRAM flap reconstructions, all of which in this study had been performed to replace inconvenient bra prostheses. The patients were particularly pleased with the autologous nature of the reconstructions but had been surprised by the extent of the surgery and length of the recovery process.

It appears that patients are more accepting of the quality of their reconstruction than are their surgeons as evidenced by a study of 20 patients whose level of satisfaction was much higher than that of their surgeons.[90] In another study of 60 inner-city women undergoing breast reconstruction, demographic analysis failed to show any differences in education, economic status, or insurance status of women undergoing reconstruction. In this study, reconstructed women had a higher satisfaction with their sex lives and body image than did non-reconstructed women.[91] Women without reconstructions tended to feel more embarrassed naked in front of a spouse and had lower partner satisfaction with their bodies. Although these trends are culled from relatively small populations of patients, it is apparent that breast reconstruction can be an immensely satisfying procedure for many patients and can have a positive impact on a patient's daily life and convenience.

CONCLUSION

Pedicled TRAM flap breast reconstruction remains the first choice for autologous reconstruction and is readily learned by any competent surgeon. It provides excellent contour and softness in most patients, and abdominal complications are few. Given the potential for free flap failure and the added cost involved in additional operating time for microsurgical procedures,[92] pedicled TRAM flaps remain the most cost-effective method of autologous breast reconstruction in most surgeons' hands.[92] Although TRAM flap reconstruction is a major operative procedure, it provides both patient and surgeon with a unique tool to achieve a natural, soft, warm, well-integrated reconstruction after mastectomy.

The decision to delay breast reconstruction should be made before mastectomy, if possible. If a patient has a large tumor, palpable axillary lymph nodes, or an inflammatory lesion, it can almost be guaranteed that radiation treatment will be a part of her future therapeutic program. Given the negative impact of radiation treatment on any reconstruction including TRAM flaps (pedicled or free), it is preferable to delay the reconstruction. If the patient is opposed to the magnitude of immediate reconstruction or has grossly unrealistic expectations about what reconstruction can offer, it is often preferable to defer reconstruction to a later time when the patient's expectations may have been tempered by the reality of life without a breast. Many such patients are grateful for this opportunity and are much more realistic about what they are undertaking when delayed breast reconstruction is finally chosen. From the reconstructive surgeon's perspective, delay may allow more flexibility with scheduling without the need to adjust operating schedules to match those of the oncologic surgeon.

REFERENCES

1. Trabulsy PP, Anthony JP, Mathes SJ: Changing trends in postmastectomy breast reconstruction: a 13 year experience. Plast Reconstr Surg 1994;93:1418.
2. Carlson GW, Grossl M, Lewis MM: Preservation of the inframammary fold: what are we leaving behind? Plast Reconstr Surg 1996;98:447.
3. Carlson GW: Skin sparing mastectomy: anatomic and technical considerations. Am Surg 1996;62:151.
4. Bostwick J 3rd, Carlson GW: Reconstruction of the breast. Surg Oncol Clin North Am 1997;6:71.
5. Millard DR Jr: Breast reconstruction after a radical mastectomy. Plast Reconstr Surg 1976;58:283.
6. Mathes SJ, Bostwick J 3rd: A rectus abdominis myocutaneous flap to reconstruct abdominal wall defects. Br J Plast Surg 1977;30:282.
7. Robbins TH: Rectus abdominis myocutaneous flap for breast reconstruction. Aust N Z J Surg 1979;49:527.
8. Drever JM: Total breast reconstruction with either of two abdominal flaps. Plast Reconstr Surg 1977;59:185.
9. Dinner MI, Labandter HP, Dowden RV: The role of the rectus abdominis myocutaneous flap in breast reconstruction. Plast Reconstr Surg 1982;69:209.
10. Dinner MI, Dowden RV, Scheflan M: Refinements in the use of the transverse abdominal island flap for postmastectomy reconstruction. Ann Plast Surg 1983;11:362.
11. Sakai S, Takahashi H, Tanabe H: The extended vertical rectus abdominis myocutaneous flap for breast reconstruction. Plast Reconstr Surg 1989;83:1061, discussion 1068.
12. Hartrampf CR Jr: The transverse abdominal island flap for breast reconstruction. A 7-year experience. Clin Plast Surg 1988;15:703.
13. Hartrampf CR Jr, Bennett GK: Autogenous tissue reconstruction in the mastectomy patient. A critical review of 300 patients. Ann Surg 1987;205:508.

14. Scheflan M, Hartrampf CR, Black PW: Breast reconstruction with a transverse abdominal island flap. Plast Reconstr Surg 1982;69:908.
15. Scheflan M, Dinner MI: The transverse abdominal island flap: part I. Indications, contraindications, results, and complications. Ann Plast Surg 1983;10:24.
16. Milloy FJ, Anson BJ, McAfee DK: The rectus abdominis muscle and the epigastric arteries. Surg Gynecol Obstet 1960;110:293.
17. Taylor GI, Palmer JH: The vascular territories (angiosomes) of the body: experimental study and clinical applications. Br J Plast Surg 1987;40:113.
18. Moon HK, Taylor GI: The vascular anatomy of rectus abdominis musculocutaneous flaps based on the deep superior epigastric system. Plast Reconstr Surg 1988;82:815.
19. Taylor GI, Corlett RJ, Boyd JB: The versatile deep inferior epigastric (inferior rectus abdominis) flap. Br J Plast Surg 1984;37:330.
20. Watterson PA, Taylor GI, Crock JG: The venous territories of muscles: anatomical study and clinical implications. Br J Plast Surg 1988;41:569.
21. Harris NR, Webb MS II, May JW Jr: Intraoperative physiologic blood flow studies in the TRAM flap. Plast Reconstr Surg 1992;90:553, discussion 559.
22. Miller LB, Bostwick J 3rd, Hartrampf CR Jr, et al: The superiorly based rectus abdominis flap: predicting and enhancing its blood supply based on an anatomic and clinical study. Plast Reconstr Surg 1988;81:713.
23. Dinner MI, Dowden RV: The value of the anterior rectus sheath in the transverse abdominal island flap. Plast Reconstr Surg 1983;72:724.
24. Suominen S, Asko-Seljavaara S, von Smitten K: Sequelae in the abdominal wall after pedicled or free TRAM flap surgery. Ann Plast Surg 1996;36:629.
25. Suominen S, Tervahartiala P, von Smitten K, Asko-Seljavaara S: Magnetic resonance imaging of the TRAM flap donor site. Ann Plast Surg 1997;38:23.
26. Dhar SC, Taylor GI: The delay phenomenon: the story unfolds. Plast Reconstr Surg 1999;104:2079.
27. Mathes SJ, Nahai F: Classification of the vascular anatomy of muscles: experimental and clinical correlation. Plast Reconstr Surg 1981;67:177.
28. Codner MA, Bostwick J 3rd, Nahai F, et al: TRAM flap vascular delay for high-risk breast reconstruction. Plast Reconstr Surg 1995;96:1615.
29. Restifo RJ, Syed SA, Ward BA, et al: Surgical delay in TRAM flap breast reconstruction: a comparison of 7- and 14-day delay periods. Ann Plast Surg 1997;38:330, discussion 333.
30. Ribuffo D, Muratori L, Antoniadou K, et al: A hemodynamic approach to clinical results in the TRAM flap after selective delay. Plast Reconstr Surg 1997;99:1706.
31. Reece GP, Kroll SS: Abdominal wall complications. Prevention and treatment. Clin Plast Surg 1998;25:235.
32. Paige KT, Bostwick J 3rd, Bried JT, Jones G: A comparison of morbidity from bilateral, unipedicled and unilateral, unipedicled TRAM flap breast reconstructions. Plast Reconstr Surg 1998;101:1819.
33. Watterson PA, Bostwick J 3rd, Hester TR Jr, et al: TRAM flap anatomy correlated with a 10-year clinical experience with 556 patients. Plast Reconstr Surg 1995;95:1185.
34. Slavin SA, Schnitt SJ, Duda RB, et al: Skin-sparing mastectomy and immediate reconstruction: oncologic risks and aesthetic results in patients with early-stage breast cancer. Plast Reconstr Surg 1998;102:49.
35. Toth BA, Forley BG, Calabria R: Retrospective study of the skin-sparing mastectomy in breast reconstruction. Plast Reconstr Surg 1999;104:77.
36. Skoll PJ, Hudson DA: Skin-sparing mastectomy using a modified Wise pattern. Plast Reconstr Surg 2002;110:214.
37. Carlson GW, Bostwick J 3rd, Styblo TM, et al: Skin-sparing mastectomy. Oncologic and reconstructive considerations. Ann Surg 1997;225:570, discussion 575.
38. Kronowitz SJ, Hunt KK, Kuerer HM, et al: Delayed-immediate breast reconstruction. Plast Reconstr Surg 2004;113:1617.
39. Losken A, Carlson GW, Jones GE, et al: Importance of right subcostal incisions in patients undergoing TRAM flap breast reconstruction. Ann Plast Surg 2002;49:115.
40. Kroll SS, Miller MJ, Reece GP, et al: Anticoagulants and hematomas in free flap surgery. Plast Reconstr Surg 1995;96:643.
41. Sharma S, Chang DW, Koutz C, et al: Incidence of hematoma associated with ketorolac after TRAM flap breast reconstruction. Plast Reconstr Surg 2001;107:352.
42. Clugston PA, Gingrass MK, Azurin D, et al: Ipsilateral pedicled TRAM flaps: the safer alternative? Plast Reconstr Surg 2000;105:77.
43. Williams JK, Bostwick J 3rd, Bried JT, et al: TRAM flap breast reconstruction after radiation treatment. Ann Surg 1995;221:756, discussion 764.
44. Morris SF, Taylor GI: The time sequence of the delay phenomenon: when is a surgical delay effective? An experimental study. Plast Reconstr Surg 1995;95:526.
45. Hudson DA: The surgically delayed unipedicled TRAM flap for breast reconstruction. Ann Plast Surg 1996;36:238, discussion 242.
46. Taylor GI, Corlett RJ, Caddy CM, Zelt RG: An anatomic review of the delay phenomenon: II. Clinical applications. Plast Reconstr Surg 1992;89:408, discussion 417.
47. Hartrampf CR Jr, Drazan L, Noel RT: A mechanical leech for transverse rectus abdominis musculocutaneous flaps. Ann Plast Surg 1993;31:103.
48. Kroll SS, Schusterman MA, Mistry D: The internal oblique repair of abdominal bulges secondary to TRAM flap breast reconstruction. Plast Reconstr Surg 1995;96:100.
49. Bucky LP, May JW Jr: Synthetic mesh. Its use in abdominal wall reconstruction after the TRAM. Clin Plast Surg 1994;21:273.
50. Evans GR, Schusterman MA, Kroll SS, et al: Reconstruction and the radiated breast: is there a role for implants? Plast Reconstr Surg 1995;96:1111, discussion 1116.
51. Wagner DS, Michelow BJ, Hartrampf CR Jr: Double-pedicle TRAM flap for unilateral breast reconstruction. Plast Reconstr Surg 1991;88:987.
52. Lazarus D, Hudson DA: A simple method for determining the weight of the TRAM flap intraoperatively at the time of breast reconstruction. Plast Reconstr Surg 2001;107:818.
53. Maxwell GP, Andochick SE: Secondary shaping of the TRAM flap. Clin Plast Surg 1994;21:247.
54. Kroll SS, Coffey JA Jr, Winn RJ, Schusterman MA: A comparison of factors affecting aesthetic outcomes of TRAM flap breast reconstructions. Plast Reconstr Surg 1995;96:860.
55. Carlson GW, Losken A, Moore B, et al: Results of immediate breast reconstruction after skin-sparing mastectomy. Ann Plast Surg 2001;46:222.
56. Restifo RJ: The "aesthetic subunit" principle in late TRAM flap breast reconstruction. Ann Plast Surg 1999;42:235.
57. Avelar J: Fat suction versus abdominoplasty. Aesthetic Plast Surg 1985;9:265.
58. Hudson DA, Skoll PJ: Single-stage, autologous breast restoration. Plast Reconstr Surg 2001;108:1163, discussion 1172.
59. Jones GW: Nipple-areola reconstruction. Operative Techniques Plast Surg 1993;1:35.
60. Kroll SS, Gherardini G, Martin JE, et al: Fat necrosis in free and pedicled TRAM flaps. Plast Reconstr Surg 1998;102:1502.
61. Elliott LF, Eskenazi L, Beegle PH Jr, et al: Immediate TRAM flap breast reconstruction: 128 consecutive cases. Plast Reconstr Surg 1993;92:217.
62. Rogers NE, Allen RJ: Radiation effects on breast reconstruction with the deep inferior epigastric perforator flap. Plast Reconstr Surg 2002;109:1919, discussion 1925.

63. Zimmerman RP, Mark RJ, Kim AI, et al: Radiation tolerance of transverse rectus abdominis myocutaneous-free flaps used in immediate breast reconstruction. Am J Clin Oncol 1998;21:381.
64. El-Mrakby HH, Milner RH, McLean NR: Supercharged pedicled TRAM flap in breast reconstruction: is it a worthwhile procedure. Ann Plast Surg 2002;49:252.
65. Petit JY, Rietjens M: Complications and abdominal wall sequelae in pedicle TRAM breast reconstruction [in French]. Ann Chir Plast Esthet 1997;42:131.
66. Petit JY, Rietjens M, Garusi C, et al: Abdominal complications and sequelae after breast reconstruction with pedicled TRAM flap: is there still an indication for pedicled TRAM in the year 2003? Plast Reconstr Surg 2003;112:1063.
67. Nahabedian MY, Dooley W, Singh N, Manson PN: Contour abnormalities of the abdomen after breast reconstruction with abdominal flaps: the role of muscle preservation. Plast Reconstr Surg 2002;109:91.
68. Blondeel N, Vanderstraeten GG, Monstrey SJ, et al: The donor site morbidity of free DIEP flaps and free TRAM flaps for breast reconstruction. Br J Plast Surg 1997;50:322.
69. Blondeel N, Boeckx WD, Vanderstraeten GG, et al: The fate of the oblique abdominal muscles after free TRAM flap surgery. Br J Plast Surg 1997;50:315.
70. Futter CM, Webster MH, Hagen S, Mitchell SL: A retrospective comparison of abdominal muscle strength following breast reconstruction with a free TRAM or DIEP flap. Br J Plast Surg 2000;53:578.
71. Suominen S, Asko-Seljavaara S, Kinnunen J, et al: Abdominal wall competence after free transverse rectus abdominis musculocutaneous flap harvest: a prospective study. Ann Plast Surg 1997;39:229.
72. Edsander-Nord A, Jurell G, Wickman M: Donor-site morbidity after pedicled or free TRAM flap surgery: a prospective and objective study. Plast Reconstr Surg 1998;102:1508.
73. Kroll SS, Netscher DT: Complications of TRAM flap breast reconstruction in obese patients. Plast Reconstr Surg 1989;84:886.
74. Chang DW, Wang B, Robb GL, et al: Effect of obesity on flap and donor-site complications in free transverse rectus abdominis myocutaneous flap breast reconstruction. Plast Reconstr Surg 2000;105:1640.
75. Padubidri AN, Yetman R, Browne E, et al: Complications of postmastectomy breast reconstructions in smokers, ex-smokers, and nonsmokers. Plast Reconstr Surg 2001;107:342, discussion 350.
76. Overgaard M, Hansen PS, Overgaard J, et al: Postoperative radiotherapy in high-risk premenopausal women with breast cancer who receive adjuvant chemotherapy. Danish Breast Cancer Cooperative Group 82b Trial. N Engl J Med 1997;337:949.
77. Ragaz J, Jackson SM, Le N, et al: Adjuvant radiotherapy and chemotherapy in node-positive premenopausal women with breast cancer. N Engl J Med 1997;337:956.
78. Chawla AK, Kachnic LA, Taghian AG, et al: Radiotherapy and breast reconstruction: complications and cosmesis with TRAM versus tissue expander/implant. Int J Radiat Oncol Biol Phys 2002;54:520.
79. Williams JK, Carlson GW, Bostwick J 3rd, et al: The effects of radiation treatment after TRAM flap breast reconstruction. Plast Reconstr Surg 1997;100:1153.
80. Kroll SS, Robb GL, Reece GP, et al: Does prior irradiation increase the risk of total or partial free-flap loss? J Reconstr Microsurg 1998;14:263.
81. Chen L, Hartrampf CR, Bennett GK: Successful pregnancies following TRAM flap surgery. Plast Reconstr Surg 1993;91:69.
82. Johnson RM, Barney LM, King JC: Vaginal delivery of monozygotic twins after bilateral pedicle TRAM breast reconstruction. Plast Reconstr Surg 2002;109:1653.
83. Parodi PC, Osti M, Longhi P, et al: Pregnancy and TRAM-flap breast reconstruction after mastectomy: a case report. Scand J Plast Reconstr Surg Hand Surg 2001;35:211.
84. Boughton B: Emotional outcome after breast surgery is highly individual. J Natl Cancer Inst 2000;92:1375.
85. Caffee HH: A comparison of factors affecting aesthetic outcomes of TRAM flap breast reconstructions. Plast Reconstr Surg 1996;98:182.
86. Keith DJ, Walker MB, Walker LG, et al: Women who wish breast reconstruction: characteristics, fears, and hopes. Plast Reconstr Surg 2003;111:1051, discussion 1057.
87. Lipa JE, Youssef AA, Kuerer HM, et al: Breast reconstruction in older women: advantages of autogenous tissue. Plast Reconstr Surg 2003;111:1110.
88. Nissen MJ, Swenson KK, Kind EA: Quality of life after postmastectomy breast reconstruction. Oncol Nurs Forum Online 2002;29:547.
89. Tykka E, Asko-Seljavaara S, Hietanen H: Patient satisfaction with delayed breast reconstruction: a prospective study. Ann Plast Surg 2002;49:258.
90. Veiga DF, Neto MS, Garcia EB, et al: Evaluations of the aesthetic results and patient satisfaction with the late pedicled TRAM flap breast reconstruction. Ann Plast Surg 2002; 48:515.
91. Zweifler M, Rodriguez E, Reilly J, et al: Breast reconstruction among inner city women with breast carcinoma. Ann Plast Surg 2001;47:53.
92. Kroll SS, Evans GR, Reece GP, et al: Comparison of resource costs of free and conventional TRAM flap breast reconstruction. Plast Reconstr Surg 1996;98:74.

CHAPTER

145

Delayed Postmastectomy Reconstruction: Free TRAM Techniques

STEPHEN S. KROLL, MD†

WHY THE FREE TRAM FLAP?

Breast reconstruction with autologous tissue can be performed successfully both with the free transverse rectus abdominis myocutaneous (TRAM) flap[1-3] and with the conventional, pedicled TRAM flap.[4,5] Neither technique is perfect. Each has advantages and disadvantages. The best choice for any individual patient will depend on her anatomy, the nature of the defect, the availability of recipient vessels, and the size of the desired breast as well as the abilities of the surgeon and the facilities that are available. At the author's institution, however, the free TRAM flap is generally preferred for most patients.[6,7]

The advantages of the free TRAM flap over the pedicled TRAM flap are a better blood supply and reduced donor site morbidity. The blood supply is better because the deep inferior epigastric vessels that supply the flap are closer to the flap than are the superior epigastric vessels that supply the pedicled TRAM flap.[8] They are also larger vessels, capable of delivering more blood to the flap. More of the TRAM flap is therefore available for reconstruction of the breast mound, and the risk of partial flap loss or fat necrosis is reduced.

Donor site morbidity is reduced because only a small piece of the rectus abdominis muscle needs to be sacrificed in elevation and transfer of the flap. There is therefore less postoperative pain. Moreover, the abdominal wall is weakened less than after a conventional TRAM flap. Patients recover more quickly, and the recovery is more complete. Most patients (93% of the author's patients) who have had a bilateral free TRAM flap, for example, can perform sit-ups after recovery, whereas only 27% of patients who have had bilateral pedicled TRAM flaps can do them.[9]

Free TRAM flaps do have certain disadvantages. Training in microsurgery is required, and so are well-maintained microsurgical instruments. A good-quality operating microscope is usually necessary, although there are some surgeons who prefer to perform the anastomosis with loupes. A well-trained assistant is almost essential, and the surgery is more complex than that of the conventional, pedicled flap.

The main disadvantage of the free TRAM flap is the risk of total flap loss if the vascular anastomosis is not successful. Even in the most experienced hands, success is not 100%. Failure rates as low as 1% or 2% are not rare,[10] but patients must understand that success is not guaranteed. Even so, the free TRAM flap is preferred by many surgeons because it provides a better overall chance to achieve an aesthetically successful

†Deceased.

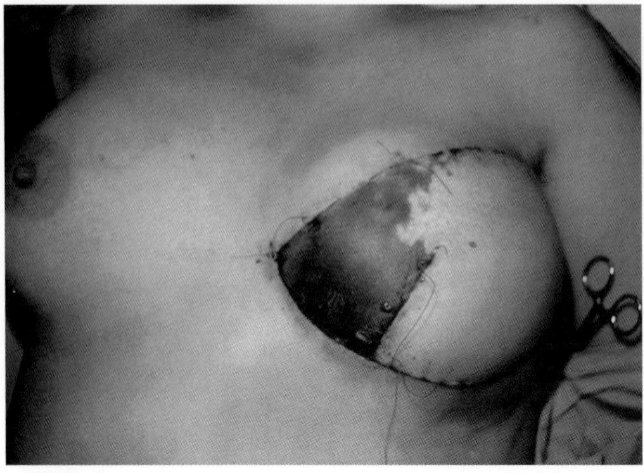

FIGURE 145-1. Partial flap loss in a conventional, pedicled TRAM flap. Approximately 30% of the flap was lost. This will obviously affect the final outcome. (From Kroll SS: Breast Reconstruction with Autologous Tissue: Art and Artistry. New York, Springer-Verlag, 1999.)

result. Whereas the risk of total flap loss is higher with use of the free TRAM flap, the risk of partial flap loss is much lower (Table 145-1) and the amount of necrotic tissue lost in partial flap losses is usually smaller. Because these partial (but sometimes major) flap losses in pedicled TRAM flaps can lead to complete failure to achieve a reconstructed breast (Fig. 145-1), the overall chances of success are better when the free TRAM flap is used.[11] Moreover, the quality of the result is usually better as well (Fig. 145-2).

TYPES OF FREE TRAM FLAP

The free TRAM flap includes several variations on the basic theme of transferring the tissue on the deep inferior epigastric blood supply. The simplest version is the flap that harvests the entire width of the rectus abdominis muscle and fascia. This is the easiest to perform but gives up many of the advantages of the free TRAM flap by maximizing donor site morbidity. Because it is not necessary to sacrifice the full width of the muscle, many surgeons prefer to split it. It is preferable to preserve at least some of the muscle and to sacrifice as little of the fascia as possible. This can be accomplished in almost every case by use of a muscle-sparing free TRAM flap (Fig. 145-3). With less fascia width harvested, there is usually less postoperative pain and a faster recovery.[12] In almost all cases, enough blood supply is maintained to make an adequate breast mound with the flap.

If the surgeon wants to reduce donor site morbidity as much as possible, a deep inferior epigastric perforator (DIEP) flap can be used.[13,14] In the DIEP flap (Fig. 145-4), no muscle or fascia is sacrificed so that there is almost no tension on the fascial repair, and postoperative pain is dramatically reduced. One to three perforators are dissected through the muscle, which must be split and therefore sustains some damage but remains in situ. Patients recover much more quickly from this operation and have stronger abdomens once recovery has been completed. Because only a few perforators are kept intact, however, the blood supply is less robust than that of the standard free TRAM flap.[15] To avoid an increased incidence of partial flap loss and fat necrosis, some care in selection of patients must be exercised.

One other modification of the free TRAM flap is the fascia-sparing free TRAM flap.[16] This is similar to the DIEP flap in that virtually no fascia is removed from the abdominal wall, but it is like the standard free TRAM flap in that perforators from both the medial and lateral rows are maintained (Fig. 145-5). This is an option that can be selected when survival of most of the flap will be required to achieve an adequate breast but there are no really large single perforators in either the medial or lateral row. The fascia-sparing free TRAM flap causes more morbidity than does the DIEP flap, however, because although all of the fascia is preserved in situ, the muscle is not.

TABLE 145-1 ✦ FLAP LOSS AND FAT NECROSIS AFTER TRAM FLAPS

Flap Type	n	Total Loss	Partial Loss	Fat Necrosis
Free TRAM	655	0.9%	1.4%	5.0%
Conventional TRAM	412	0.5%	10.3%	20.3%

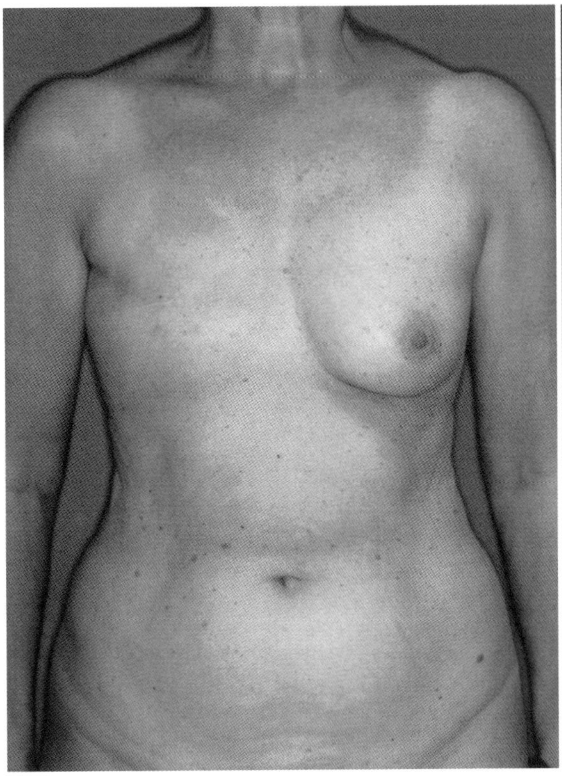

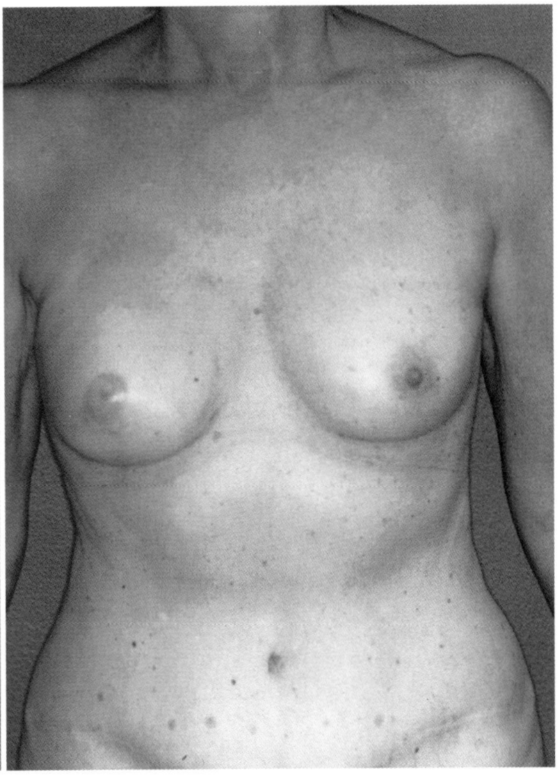

A B

FIGURE 145-2. *A,* Patient after right modified radical mastectomy. *B,* After delayed reconstruction with a free TRAM flap.

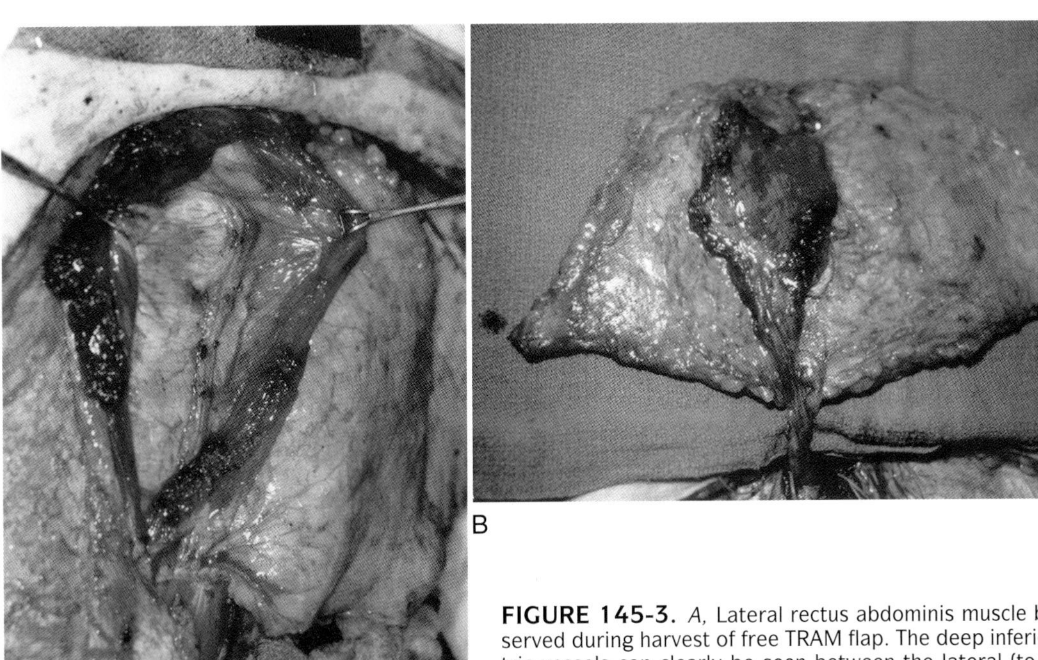

A B

FIGURE 145-3. *A,* Lateral rectus abdominis muscle being preserved during harvest of free TRAM flap. The deep inferior epigastric vessels can clearly be seen between the lateral (to the right) and medial (to the left) muscle. *B,* Posterior surface of free TRAM flap. Only part of the width of the rectus muscle has been harvested.

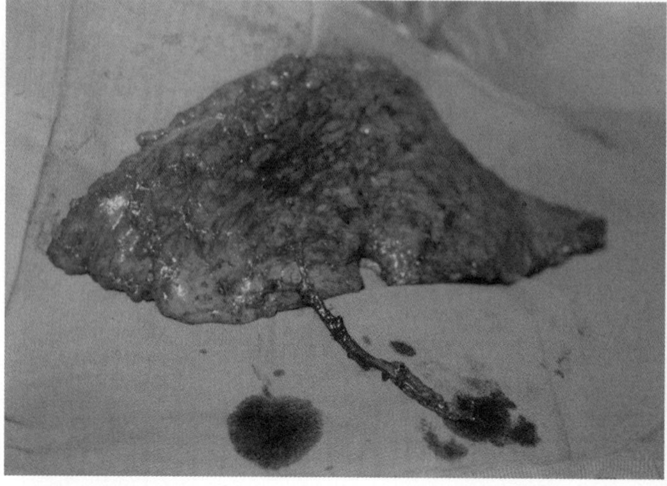

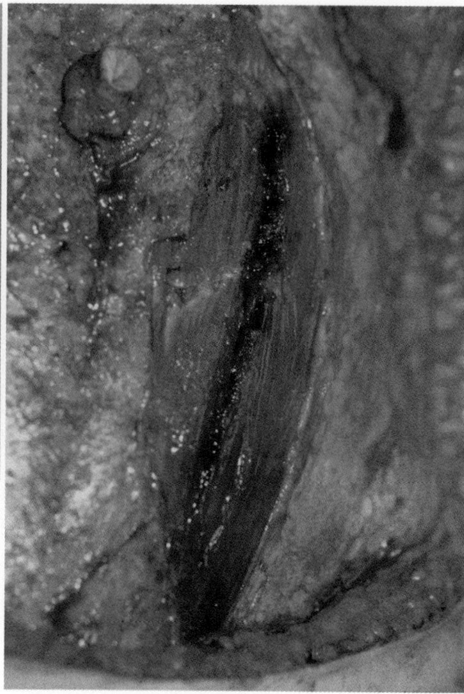

FIGURE 145-4. *A,* DIEP flap, which contains no muscle. *B,* DIEP flap donor site.

CHOICE OF RECIPIENT VESSELS

When *immediate* breast reconstruction with free flaps is performed, the thoracodorsal vessels are usually chosen as recipients because they are exposed during the axillary dissection that usually accompanies the mastectomy and therefore are readily available. In *delayed* reconstruction, however, there is no real advantage to use of the thoracodorsal vessels. If they are available, the internal mammary vessels are usually preferable (Fig. 145-6).[17,18] They are closer to the breast, they are usually not scarred from previous surgery, and the artery is less likely to be affected by vascular spasm. Moreover, the arms of the patient can be placed at her side so that they do not interfere with the positioning of the surgeons. Most surgeons who perform many delayed breast reconstructions therefore prefer to use the internal mammary vessels rather than the thoracodorsal ones, provided they are available and are of suitable size.

The main disadvantage of the internal mammary vessels is the inconsistent size of the vein (the artery is almost always adequate). Especially on the left side, the internal mammary vein can be small. Removal of the third rather than the fourth costal cartilage is helpful for access, but even in the third interspace, the vein may sometimes be less than 2 mm in diameter. If the donor vein is a large one, the anastomosis can be a problem.

To minimize the impact of this anatomic variability, the use of preoperative color ultrasound Doppler (duplex) scanning can be helpful.[19] With this test, the surgeon can determine whether adequate internal mammary vessels are present and which rib should be removed for maximum ease of anastomosis. An adequate vein is usually present. If not, the surgeon can select the thoracodorsal vessels as recipients instead, thereby avoiding a difficult anastomosis.

DESIGNING AND PLANNING

The first step in shaping of the reconstructed breast is proper planning of the pocket in which the flap will be placed. To do this, the midline is marked along with the outline of the opposite, normal breast. The mirror image of that outline is then marked on the side to be reconstructed (Fig. 145-7).

If bilateral delayed reconstruction is necessary, there is no opposite breast to use as a template. The surgeon can then use the position of the patient's brassiere to mark the position of the breasts. Outlines similar to those discussed in the preceding paragraph are then drawn on each side (see Fig. 145-7).

The free TRAM flap is then designed symmetrically on the abdomen. The tips of the flap should be placed in a natural concavity, if one is present, to minimize the dog-ear. The upper border of the flap is usually

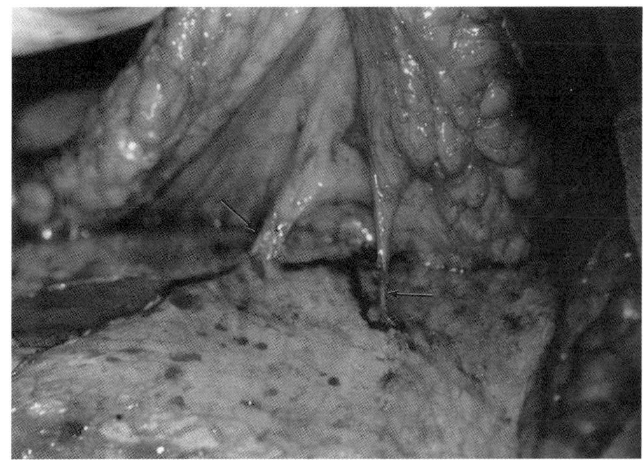
A

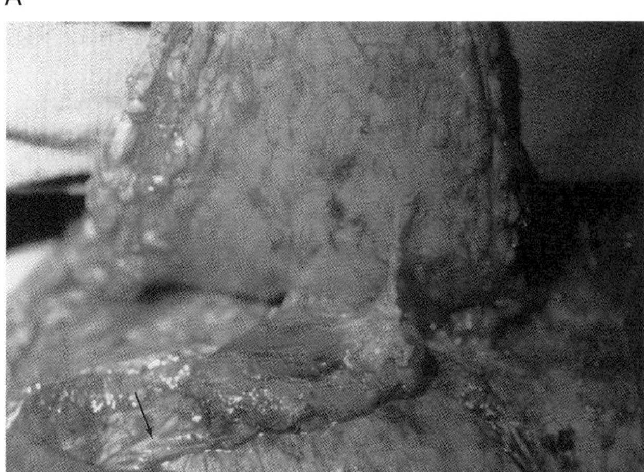
B

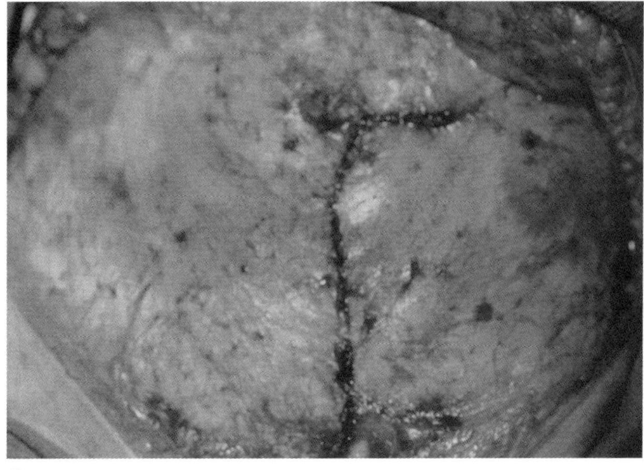
C

FIGURE 145-5. *A,* Two perforators *(arrows),* one lateral and the other medial, are visibly isolated as the remaining flap has been separated from the rectus abdominis sheath. The flap midline is to the left, and the vertical portion of the fascial incision has been started. *B,* After elevation, the flap contains two medial perforators and one prominent lateral one. Each perforator is surrounded by a small button of fascia. The deep inferior epigastric pedicle is clearly visible *(arrow)*. *C,* The closed donor site does not displace the umbilicus or form fascial dog-ears because essentially no fascia has been removed.

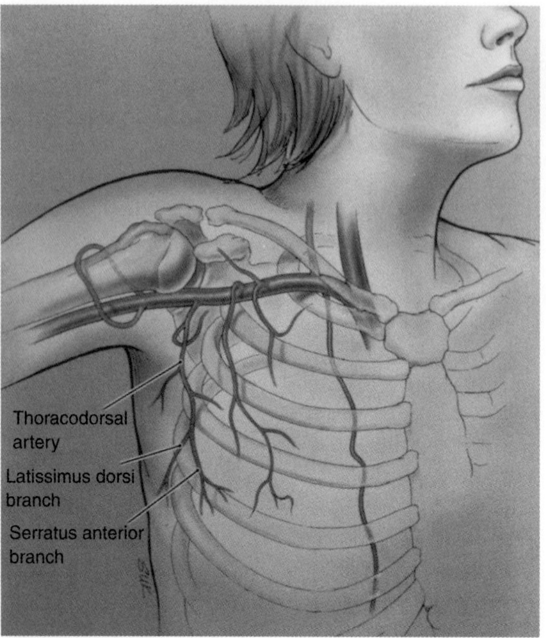

FIGURE 145-6. Anatomy of internal mammary and of thoracodorsal vessels. (From Kroll SS: Breast Reconstruction with Autologous Tissue: Art and Artistry. New York, Springer-Verlag, 1999.)

placed 1 or 2 cm above the umbilicus, although some surgeons prefer to place it at the umbilicus. The lower border is usually at the point where the thickness of the subcutaneous flap decreases, just at or above the pubic hairline. It is usually possible to estimate the amount of flap width that can be harvested by having the patient bend forward to flex her waist.

Design of the DIEP flap is identical to that of the free TRAM flap except that the surgeon should not expect to be able to use as much of the flap as is available when a free TRAM flap is used (Fig. 145-8). In most instances, tissue from any part of zone IV (the part of the flap farthest across the midline from the pedicle) is not reliable.

DISSECTING THE POCKET AND EXPOSING THE RECIPIENT VESSELS

The surgery begins with opening of the old mastectomy incision and dissection of the pocket into which the flap will be inserted. The pocket dissection is completed superiorly, but inferiorly it is usually best to leave dissection of the lowest 1 or 2 cm of the pocket until later. That way, closure of the abdominal donor site will not drag the lower border of the breast down lower than the surgeon had intended.

For exposure of the internal mammary vessels, the pectoralis muscle is usually split over the third costal cartilage. The attachment of the rib to the sternum is exposed. Near the junction between the cartilage and bone of the rib, lateral to the internal mammary vessels, the periosteum is incised and partially removed. With Langenbeck, Freer, and Joseph periosteal elevators, the periosteum is freed circumferentially from the cartilage. A Doyen (pigtail) elevator is then used to separate the periosteum medially from the undersurface of the rib.

The cartilage is then incised laterally and removed as far medially as possible. If the deep layer of the periosteum is still intact, it is then incised laterally. With loupe magnification (4.5× is preferred), the internal mammary vessels are exposed. Bipolar electrocautery is essential to achieve hemostasis without damaging the main vessels. Clips can be used away from the planned anastomotic site but should be avoided close to the vessel ends because they interfere with performance of the anastomosis.

Dissection of the vessels all the way from the second to the fourth rib increases effective pedicle length and makes the anastomosis easier. This extra dissection does, however, increase operative time.

If the thoracodorsal vessels will be used, they should be approached through the scar tissue from below so that if they are injured during identification, the more proximal portion can still be used for the anastomosis. The vessels should be dissected from the serratus branch to as close to the axillary vessels as possible without dividing the circumflex scapular branches. This allows the pedicle to rotate anteriorly so that the anastomosis need not be performed deep in a hole and so that the effective pedicle length of the flap is increased.

FLAP ELEVATION AND TRANSFER

Free TRAM Flap

When a free TRAM flap is performed, the abdominoplasty flap is elevated up toward the xiphoid, then stapled up out of the way so that free access to the TRAM flap is obtained. The TRAM flap is elevated off the deep abdominal fascia from lateral to medial until perforating vessels are seen entering the flap from the rectus abdominis sheath (Fig. 145-9). A vertical incision is then made in the fascia, approximately 5 mm lateral to the perforators. The fascia is dissected laterally to expose part of the rectus abdominis muscle.

The muscle is then split with a hemostat (Fig. 145-10), and the deep inferior epigastric vessels are identified. These are dissected inferiorly all the way to their origin at the external iliac vessels. The dissection can be performed by extending the muscle split or, alternatively, by dissecting around the muscle laterally. This dissection all the way to the origin of the vessels maximizes pedicle length and increases the

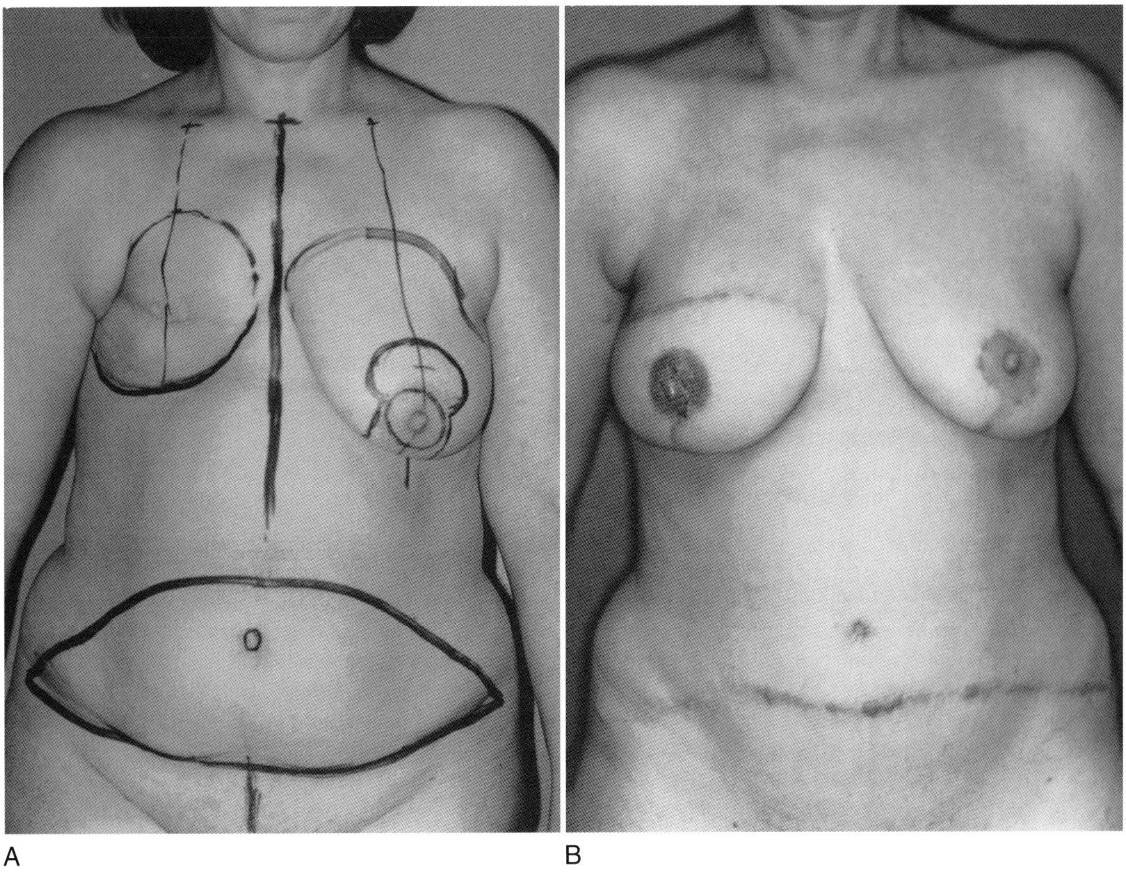

A B

FIGURE 145-7. *A,* Plan for delayed reconstruction of the right breast, with design of TRAM flap on abdomen. *B,* Early result. The scars are prominent, but breast shape and symmetry are reasonably good.

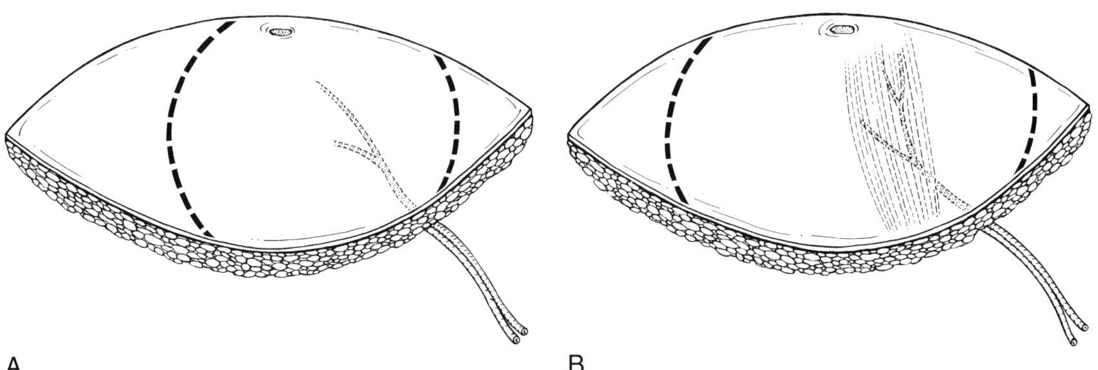

A B

FIGURE 145-8. *A,* Estimated tissue viability when a DIEP flap is used. *B,* Estimated tissue viability when a free TRAM flap is used.

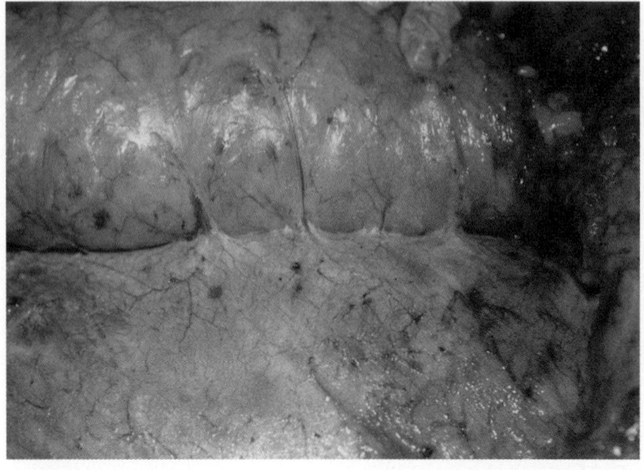

FIGURE 145-9. The lateral row of perforators found when the TRAM flap is elevated off the deep abdominal fascia.

caliber of the vessels at the site of the anastomosis. The anastomosis is thereby made easier, and the reach of the flap, which is critical when the thoracodorsal vessels are used, is increased. The dissection is facilitated by extending the fascial incision sufficiently inferiorly that retraction is easy (Fig. 145-11). By using two retractors and a sponge on a stick, the surgeon can see clearly what he or she is doing, and the risk of errors is minimized (Fig. 145-12).

All muscle lateral to the muscle split is preserved in situ. Medially, muscle should be preserved only if there are no large perforators close to the medial border of the muscle. Any muscle that is preserved medially is completely denervated, so it makes no sense to jeopardize flap survival to preserve it. If there are no large perforators close to the border, however, a medial strip of muscle can be preserved.

Once the flap pedicle has been dissected, the flap is freed from the contralateral side and its viability assessed. It is then allowed to perfuse in situ while the recipient vessels are divided and prepared for the anastomosis.

DIEP Flap

When making the incision for the lower border of the DIEP flap, the surgeon should look carefully for the superficial inferior epigastric vein. If this vein is of unusually large caliber (>2.5 mm), the surgeon should dissect it inferiorly for several centimeters and preserve it. The presence of a large superficial vein may be an indication that the usual venous drainage of the flap may be inadequate. In that case, the surgeon will have to either drain the flap by use of the superficial inferior epigastric vein (this will require vein grafting) or convert the operation into a standard free TRAM flap.

Otherwise, the beginning of the DIEP flap dissection is identical to that of the free TRAM flap until after the lateral row of perforators has been identified. The perforators are isolated under loupe magnification so they can be carefully examined (Fig. 145-13). Two or three of the largest perforators are examined closely to see if they contain a vein at least 1 mm in diameter and have a palpable pulse. If at least one perforator meets this criterion, a DIEP flap is usually possible. Care should be taken that what appears to be a large lateral perforator is not really just small vessels accompanied by a large sensory nerve.

The fascia is then opened widely with vertical incisions above and below the chosen perforator. The fascia is dissected laterally, and the muscle is exposed. The perforator is separated from the medial fascia and a vessel loop placed around it. Lifting the muscle on either side of the perforator with fine-toothed forceps (by both surgeon and assistant) helps facilitate separation of the perforator from the surrounding muscle. Loupe magnification (3.5 to 6.0) is essential.

Small side branches should be coagulated with bipolar electrocautery. Even the tiniest of branches must be carefully cauterized to avoid bleeding and vascular spasm. Larger ones can be ligated with small clips or silk ties. Careful hemostasis must be maintained at all times. The dissection is meticulous and cannot be rushed. This slow, careful dissection is continued until the perforator joins the deep inferior epigastric vessels deep to the muscle. Vessel loop retraction is useful, and much of the muscle dissection can be done with the bipolar forceps. Extreme care must be taken to avoid inadvertent traction on the perforators, which are delicate and fragile until they reach the deep inferior epigastric vessels.

If a second perforator is included, it is dissected through the muscle in an identical fashion until it, too, joins either the deep inferior epigastric vessels or the first perforator. Motor nerves (Fig. 145-14) are dissected away from the perforators and preserved, if possible. If the motor nerve runs between two perforators,

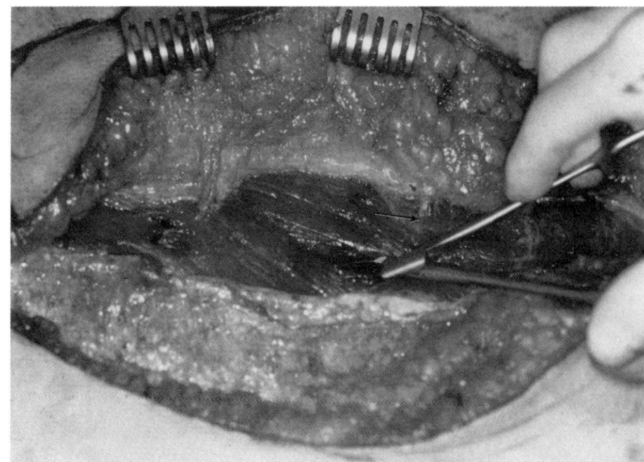

A

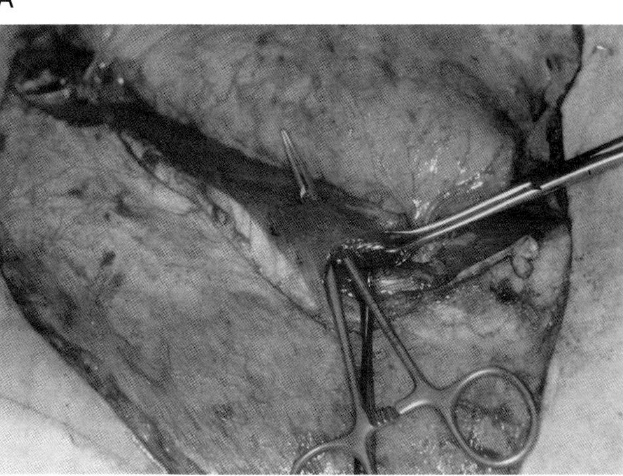

B

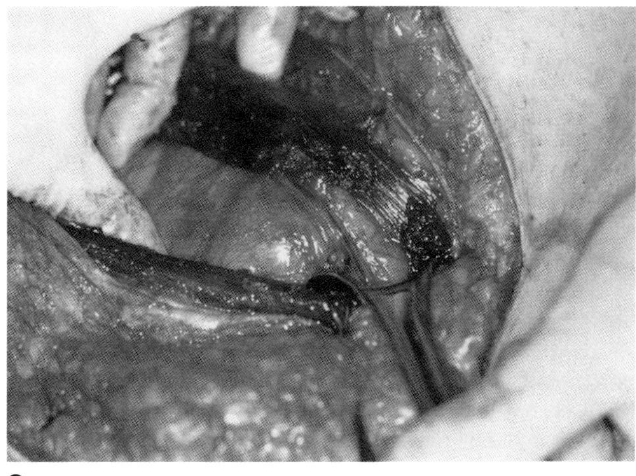

C

FIGURE 145-10. *A,* The muscle is split carefully with a hemostat just lateral to one of the perforators *(arrow)*. Care is taken to avoid injury to the underlying deep inferior epigastric vessels. *B,* The dissection is continued superiorly, dividing muscle fibers if necessary to stay lateral to the perforators. *C,* After the muscle is split, the pedicle can clearly be seen entering the muscle from beneath the retractor.

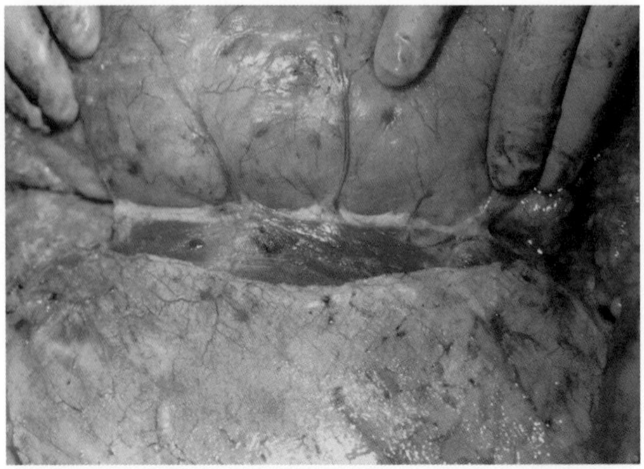

A

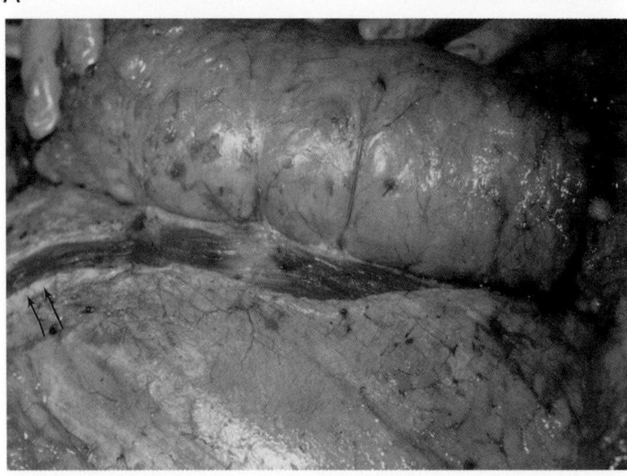

B

FIGURE 145-11. *A,* The fascia is incised just lateral to the lateral row of perforators. *B,* Extending this fascial incision inferiorly *(arrows)* improves exposure without adding visible scar or increasing the risk of hernia.

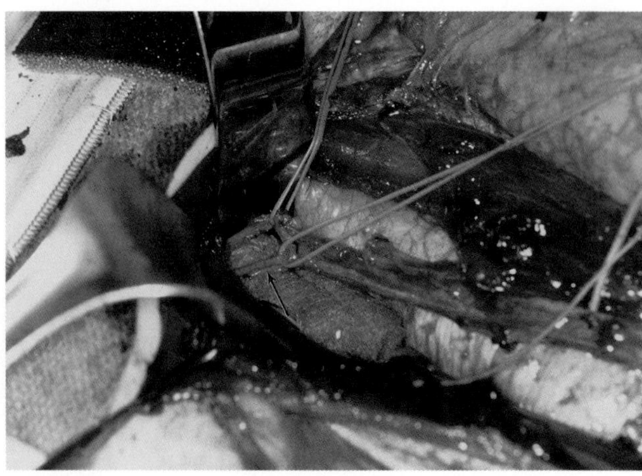

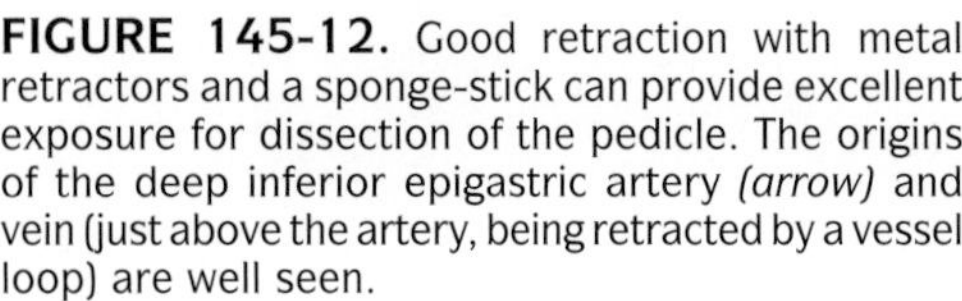

FIGURE 145-12. Good retraction with metal retractors and a sponge-stick can provide excellent exposure for dissection of the pedicle. The origins of the deep inferior epigastric artery *(arrow)* and vein (just above the artery, being retracted by a vessel loop) are well seen.

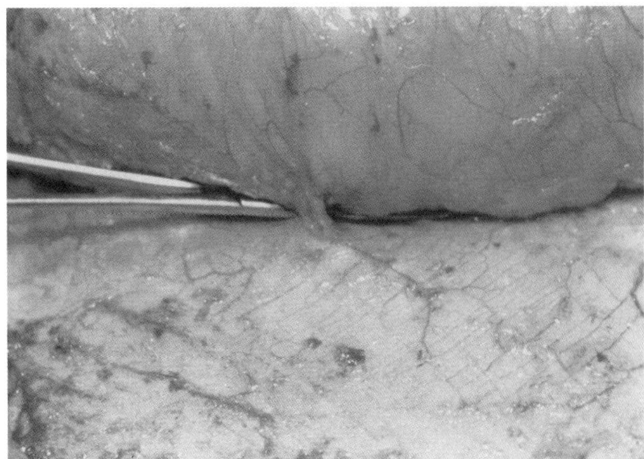

FIGURE 145-13. Large lateral perforator that is suitable for use in a DIEP flap.

it must be divided. If the divided motor nerve is of significant size, however, it can be repaired after the flap has been harvested.

A separate dissection around the lateral edge of the muscle is required inferiorly to locate and dissect the most inferior part of the deep inferior epigastric pedicle. Some surgeons omit this part of the dissection because a long pedicle is not really required for anastomosis to the internal mammary vessels. For any reconstruction using the thoracodorsal vessels as recipients, however, the longer pedicle is essential. Even when the internal mammary vessels are used, the longer pedicle is preferred to make the anastomosis technically easier and to allow the flap to be positioned more freely when the breast is shaped.

Once the pedicle has been successfully dissected (Fig. 145-15), the contralateral side can be elevated and its perforators ligated. The opposite side is preserved until the last step so that if the pedicle is injured during the dissection, the operation can still be completed successfully with use of the deep inferior epigastric vessels on the other side. The flap is then stapled into a stable position and allowed to perfuse while final preparation of the recipient vessels is completed.

Flap Transfer

The recipient vessels are clamped with nontraumatizing microvascular clamps, then ligated distally. The vessel ends are prepared for an end-to-end anastomosis by removal of any excess adventitia. The microscope is positioned and checked to be sure that it is functioning properly.

The flap is then harvested; the stumps of the deep inferior epigastric vessels are ligated with 2-0 silk. It can be useful to mark the top surface of the vein with a pen before the vessel is divided to help orient the vein during the anastomosis and to avoid twisting it. The vessels are then divided, and the flap is transferred to the chest. The pedicle may be allowed to dangle freely, both to drain excess blood and to allow any twisting to correct itself.

The venous anastomosis is usually performed first. The vein is carefully oriented to avoid twisting and

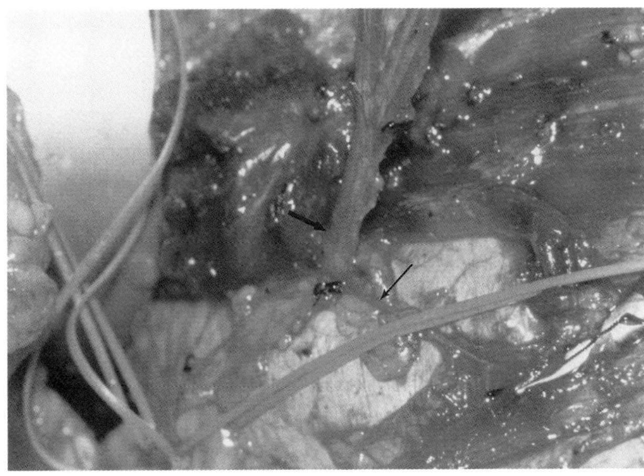

FIGURE 145-14. The motor nerve *(thin arrow)* crosses superficial and inferior to the perforator *(thick arrow)*. It can be separated from the vessels without injuring them by careful, mostly blunt dissection.

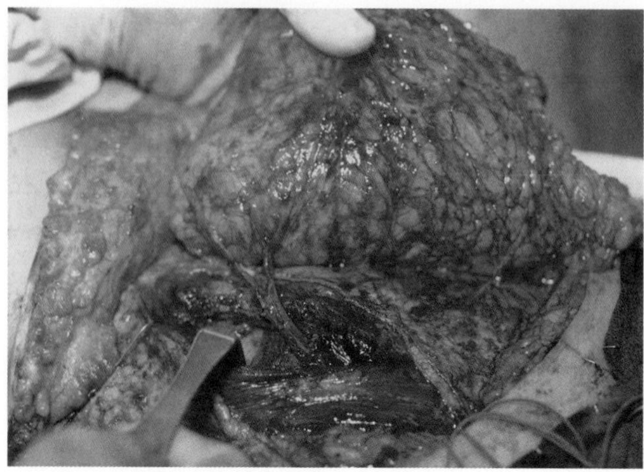

FIGURE 145-15. The flap after dissection of the pedicle. The muscle has been split but not removed.

then placed in a double-approximating clamp. The anastomosis can be done with 8-0, 9-0, or even 10-0 nylon; either running or interrupted sutures are used according to the preference of the surgeon. The clamps are then released, and the venous anastomosis is allowed to perfuse while the arterial anastomosis is performed. For the arterial anastomosis, suture choice and technique are again determined by the surgeon's preference and are probably unimportant. What is important is avoidance of tension on the anastomosis caused by inadequate pedicle length, avoidance of twists, and avoidance of large size mismatches by appropriate choice of donor and recipient vessels.

Once the anastomosis has been completed and the clamps have been released, it should be inspected carefully. Small leaks will usually stop spontaneously, but larger ones often require an extra suture. Spasm in the artery should be corrected by application of papaverine 2% topical solution and by careful, selective removal of adventitia. The surgeon should take special care not to overlook small side branches that have not been tied off. If these are not adequately controlled, they can cause persistent spasm that can lead to loss of a flap or, alternatively, result in a hematoma when the spasm is released.

After the anastomosis has been completed, the flap must be stabilized so that inadvertent tension on the pedicle is avoided. For free TRAM flaps, this can be accomplished by suturing the rectus abdominis fascia to the pectoralis fascia or muscle of the chest wall. For DIEP flaps, there is no such fascia, so the flap is stabilized by placing multiple sutures between the fat at the medial edge of the flap and the medial edge of the breast pocket.

The mastectomy skin flaps can also be stapled to or over the flap to provide additional (although temporary) stabilization. Extreme care should be taken to make sure that the flap does not fall off the chest, an event that could result in either disruption of the anastomosis or avulsion of the perforators of the flap.

CLOSURE OF THE DONOR SITE

Once the flap has been stabilized and is being adequately perfused, attention can be turned to the fascial donor site. The first step in avoiding problems in donor site closure is to avoid removal of too much fascia in the first place. If this has been done, the closure will be under minimal tension and can be accomplished without resorting to mesh reinforcement even if the reconstruction is bilateral. The fascial closure is performed with a running, heavy-gauge monofilament suture (such as No. 1 polypropylene). All knots are buried so they are not palpable, and the inferior oblique (deeper) layer must be included in every stitch (Fig. 145-16). If there are fascial dog-ears above or below the fascial defect, they should be corrected by plicating sutures that extend the full height of the abdominal wall.

If the umbilicus has been displaced by closure of a unilateral fascial defect, it is tacked over to the midline with a 3-0 polyglactic acid suture. If this is not sufficient, plication of the contralateral fascia with sutures will help restore abdominal symmetry but will increase both tension on the closure and postoperative pain. If the sutures are tending to pull through the fascia either because the fascia is weak or because the wound tension is high, reinforcement with synthetic (polypropylene) mesh should be considered. This is accomplished by placing an overlay of mesh on the repair, then suturing it into place with polyglactic acid sutures around the periphery.

At least one suction wound drain should be inserted and a new opening made in the abdominoplasty flap for the umbilicus. Additional undermining of the abdominoplasty flap is performed as necessary, but the lateral perforators to the abdominal skin should

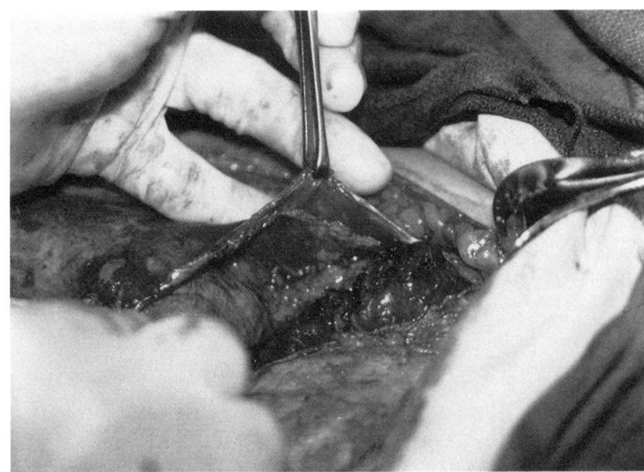

FIGURE 145-16. Abdominal wall closure. The internal oblique fascia can be seen retracting from the external oblique fascia (held in the Allis clamp). It is essential to include this internal oblique fascia on either side of the repair.

be preserved so that the risk of abdominoplasty flap necrosis is minimized.

Closure of the abdominoplasty flap is performed in layers with 2-0 polyglactic acid sutures for Scarpa fascia and 3-0 sutures of the same material for the dermis. The skin is closed with 3-0 polypropylene (or similar) running subcuticular suture. Care should be taken to excise any dog-ears at this time; it is far easier to do this in the operating room than it will be later in the clinic under local anesthesia.

FLAP INSET

Breast shaping in delayed reconstruction consists of three basic steps: formation of the breast pocket, replacement of the missing breast skin, and replacement of the missing breast volume. The accuracy of these steps and the surgeon's success in carrying them out determine the aesthetic quality of the result. In delayed reconstruction, formation of the breast pocket is performed by dissection according to the design that was made preoperatively (a mirror image of the opposite, normal breast). Once the abdominoplasty flap has been closed, the surgeon can complete the dissection of the pocket down to the desired level of the inframammary fold. The sheet of scar tissue that is present beneath the inferior mastectomy flap is released so the skin can expand to its original dimensions. If it will not expand, a vertical incision is made in the mastectomy flap down to the level of the inframammary fold (Fig. 145-17). This will allow the lower panel of the breast skin brassiere to separate, forming a V-shaped defect. The TRAM flap skin fills that defect, restoring lower pole fullness and restoring breast shape.

The horizontal mastectomy incision is allowed to separate vertically, and this defect is also filled by TRAM flap skin (Fig. 145-18). The flap is then trimmed of excess fatty tissue until the volume matches that of the opposite breast.

If the flap is sufficiently wide, the infraclavicular hollow is corrected by suturing the superior edge of the flap to whatever remnants of the breast tissue are present superiorly or to the chest wall if there is nothing else. The flap is thinned superiorly to blend it into the remaining chest wall. The patient is placed in the sitting position so that ptosis and breast symmetry can be evaluated (Fig. 145-19) before final shaping is completed. The mastectomy flaps are then evaluated for viability, and all buried TRAM flap skin is de-epithelialized. A grooved suction drain is inserted, with care taken not to obstruct the pedicle with the drain. The wounds are then closed in layers, usually with 3-0 polyglactic acid sutures for the dermis and 3-0

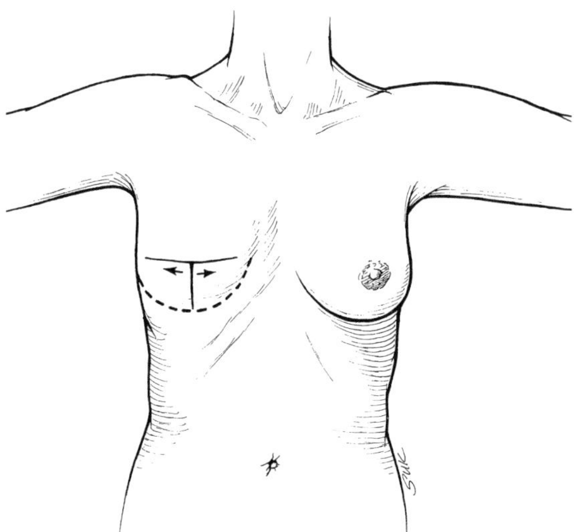

FIGURE 145-17. Vertical incision in lower mastectomy flap to expand skin envelope in the lower pole of the breast. (From Kroll SS: Breast Reconstruction with Autologous Tissue: Art and Artistry. New York, Springer-Verlag, 1999.)

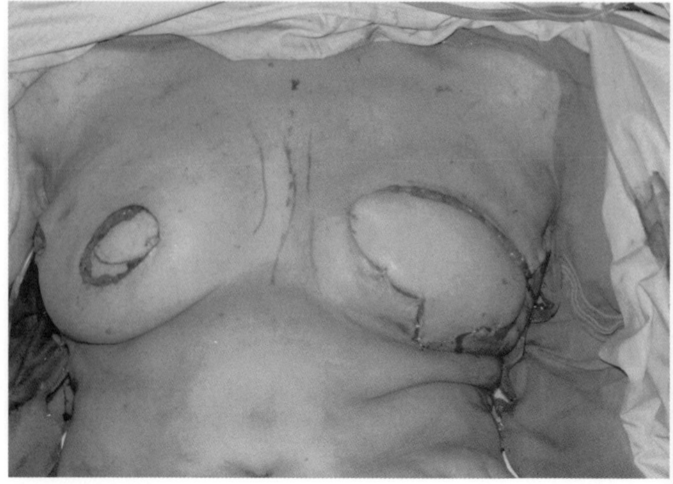

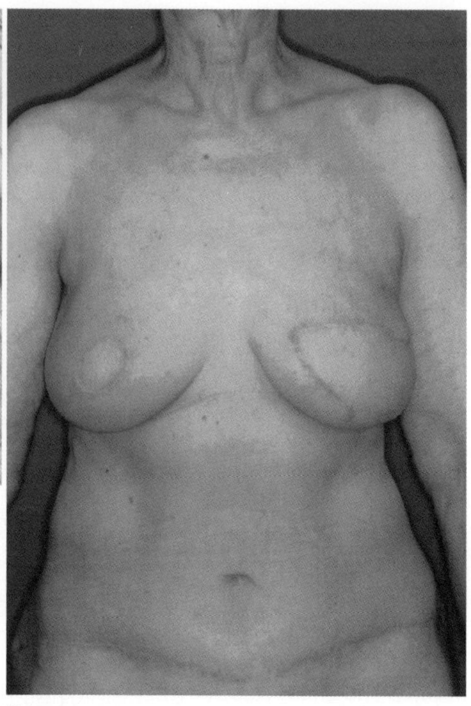

FIGURE 145-18. *A,* The left breast defect made by reopening the mastectomy incision and by making a vertical incision is filled with TRAM flap skin. *B,* The resulting left delayed breast reconstruction matches the shape of the immediate breast reconstruction on the right quite well. (From Kroll SS: Breast Reconstruction with Autologous Tissue: Art and Artistry. New York, Springer-Verlag, 1999.)

polypropylene running subcuticular sutures for the skin.

POSTOPERATIVE CARE

In delayed reconstruction, enough TRAM flap skin is exposed that it is not usually difficult to find a Doppler signal that can be monitored with a hand-held pencil Doppler probe. The site of the signal is marked with a small blue polypropylene suture, and the flap is checked every hour around the clock for 3 days. The nurses check the flap for color, temperature, capillary refill, and presence of the Doppler signal. Any significant change should be reported to the surgeon. If pedicle obstruction is suspected, immediate return to the operating room is required to ensure that the pedicle is patent. If the pedicle is obstructed, attempts to correct the problem will fail unless they are made soon after the obstruction has occurred. It is therefore better to err on the side of caution and return to the operating room if there is any real question about the viability of the flap.

Pain control is usually accomplished with intravenous narcotics (morphine, meperidine [Demerol], or hydromorphone [Dilaudid]) administered by a patient-controlled analgesia pump. This allows the patient to receive a baseline dose of morphine (usually 1 mg/hr) and to obtain additional medication, within limits set by the surgeon (0.5 to 1.0 mg every 15 minutes is typical), at the push of a button. Patients are advised to take only that medication which is necessary for pain relief to avoid the accompanying nausea and constipation that are caused by the narcotics. Intravenous administration of ketorolac (Toradol), 30 mg every 8 hours, can reduce the need for narcotics and does not appear to increase the risk of hematoma.[20] The patient-controlled analgesia pump is discontinued when the patient thinks that it is no longer needed.

In patients in whom the abdominal closure has been tight, insertion of a nasogastric tube may be indicated to prevent gastric dilatation and respiratory distress. The tube can be removed in the morning of the first postoperative day, provided nausea is not present.

Patients are encouraged to get out of bed on the first postoperative day, if possible. This helps prevent atelectasis, reduces postoperative fever, aids bowel function, and helps prevent thrombophlebitis. When patients first stand upright, however, they must be careful not to straighten themselves too rapidly or they will have pain in the donor site. The vertical tightening of the abdomen will force them to walk in a bent-over position for several days, which may cause temporary back pain. In most instances, however, patients will be able to stand up straight within a week

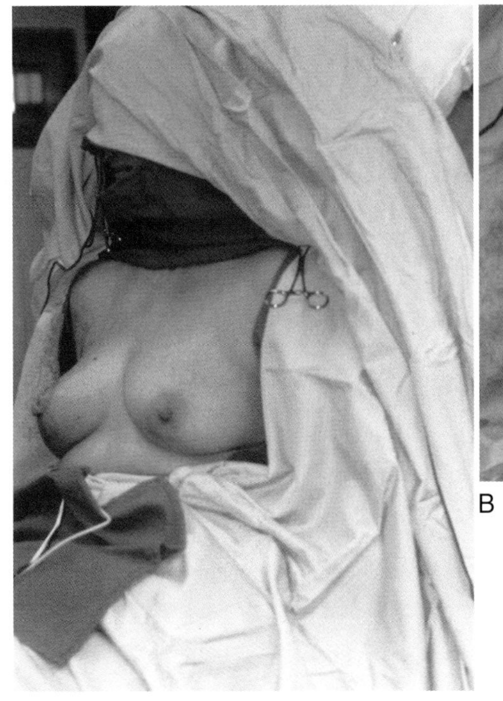

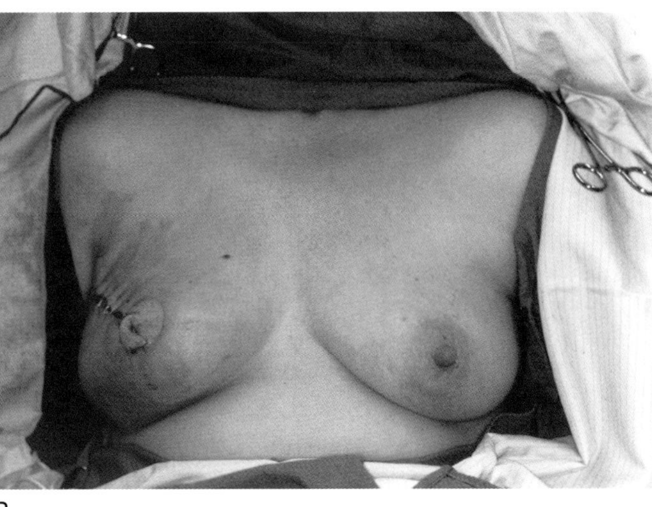

FIGURE 145-19. *A,* In this breast reconstruction revision, the patient is placed in the near-sitting position so that ptosis and symmetry can be evaluated. *B,* Note that the shoulders are exposed so that the surgeon can tell if the patient is leaning off to one side. (From Kroll SS: Breast Reconstruction with Autologous Tissue: Art and Artistry. New York, Springer-Verlag, 1999.)

if they have had children or 2 weeks if they have never been pregnant.

All patients will have some fever on the second and third postoperative days. Effective treatment of this usually consists of adequate fluid intake and ambulation. Surgeons should not ignore other potential causes of the fever, but extensive work-ups that include blood cultures are usually unnecessary.

Patients with large, heavy reconstructed breasts are advised to wear a brassiere that prevents the breast from drooping when the patient stands upright. This helps avoid the tension on the pedicle that unrestricted ptosis could cause, a situation that could easily lead to pedicle thrombosis and flap loss. This breast support is usually continued for 30 days. In cases in which the thoracodorsal vessels have been used as recipients, patients are advised to avoid abducting their arms more than 90 degrees to avoid possible stretching of the pedicle.

Patients usually leave the hospital when flap monitoring has been completed and when they are comfortable taking oral analgesics. For patients with DIEP flaps, 4 days in the hospital are usually sufficient. For free TRAM flap patients, 5 or 6 days may be required. In most cases, one or more drains will remain in place and will have to be cared for at home by the patient. Patients are instructed to empty the drains once per day and to measure the output. Once the daily output has been less than 25 mL for 2 consecutive days, the drains can be removed. Removing the drains earlier risks development of a seroma, which may require insertion of a new drain.

REVISIONS

Although surgeons usually try to achieve symmetry in the first operation, this effort is rarely completely successful. In most cases, at least one revision procedure will be necessary to match the opposite breast. Fortunately, most of these operations can be performed as outpatient procedures under local anesthesia. Useful tools for breast mound revisions include liposuction, direct tissue excision, V to Y island flaps, and breast reduction techniques.[21]

For small changes in breast volume, liposuction can often be useful. Preliminary injection of the breast with saline containing epinephrine 1:1,000,000 helps reduce blood loss and bruising. In some patients, the fat comes out readily, and liposuction is all that is required to achieve the desired modification. In other patients, however, the liposuction is less effective. The surgeon should therefore always be prepared to reopen the old scars and excise tissue directly.

In some patients, there will be an excess of tissue in one part of the breast (usually laterally) while there is a deficiency in another part of the breast. In that case, simple excision is not adequate to correct the problem. This problem can often be helped with a V to Y island flap (Fig. 145-20). Although new

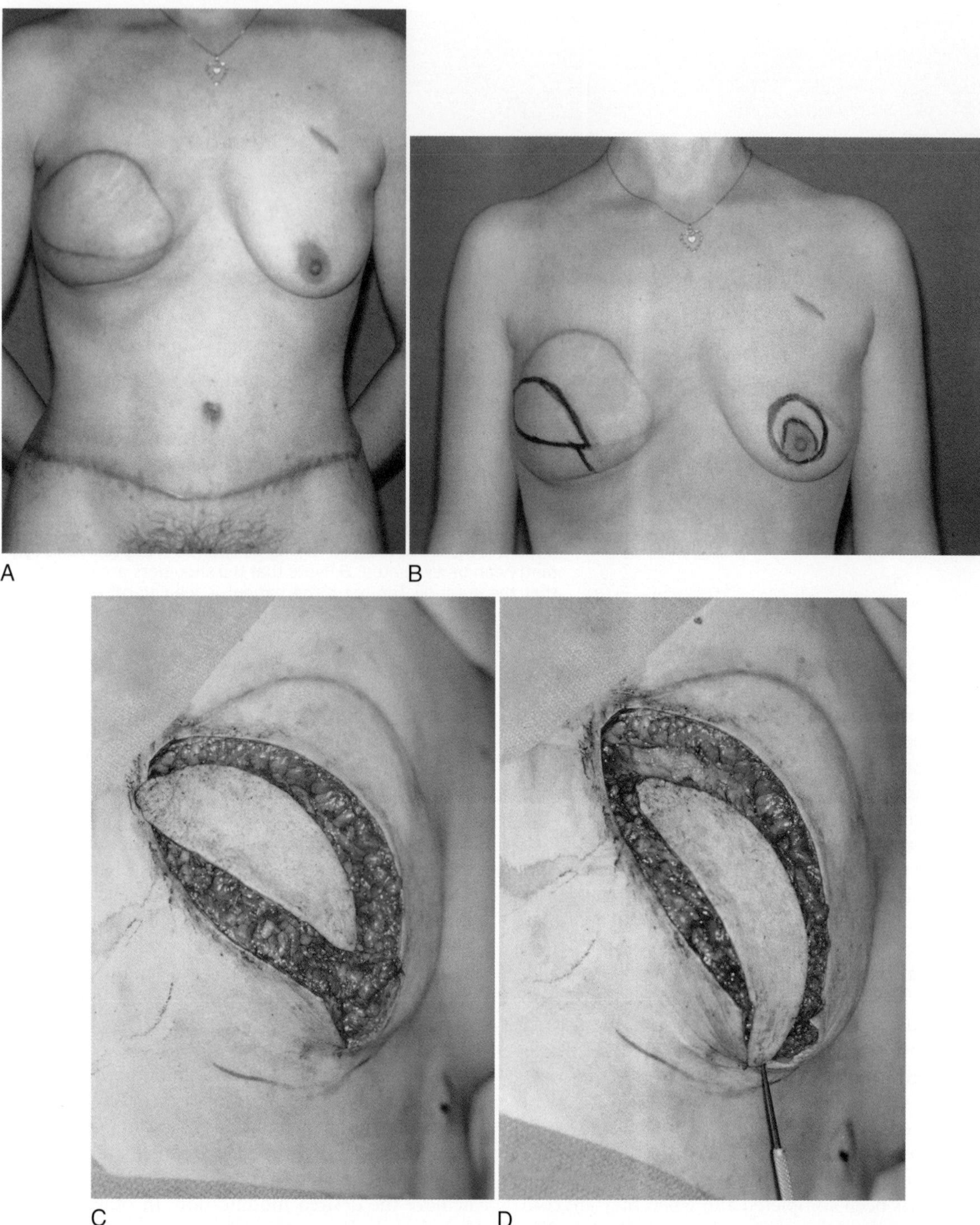

FIGURE 145-20. *A*, Patient with excess fullness in the upper outer quadrant of a breast mound reconstructed with a free TRAM flap. There is insufficient tissue in the lower pole. *B*, Design for V to Y island advancement flap and for opposite concentric mastopexy. *C*, The flap is elevated on a subcutaneous pedicle. *D*, The flap is advanced inferiorly and medially.

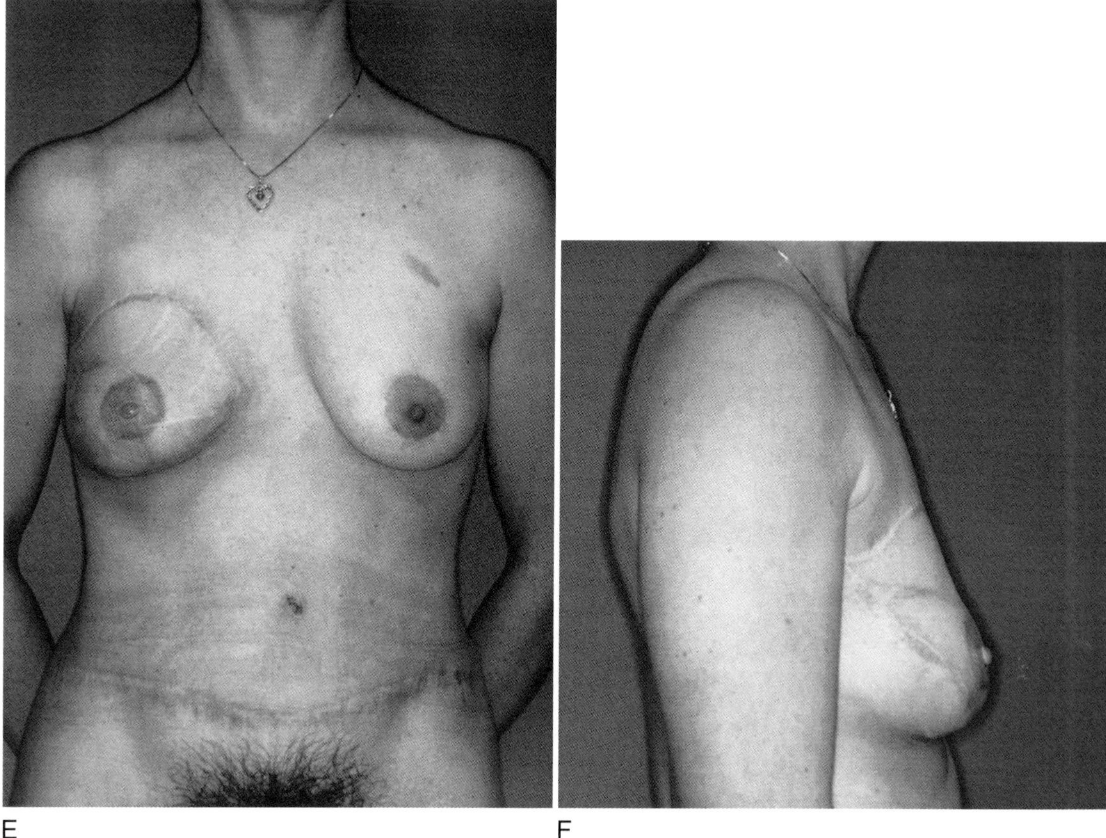

E F

FIGURE 145-20, cont'd. *E* and *F,* Same patient, after healing and nipple reconstruction. (From Kroll SS: Breast Reconstruction with Autologous Tissue: Art and Artistry. New York, Springer-Verlag, 1999.)

scars may be required, the breast shape is changed significantly and the quality of the result therefore improved.

In some patients who have a reconstructed breast mound that is larger than the opposite, normal breast, the projection as well as the symmetry of the breast can be improved by adapting breast reduction techniques to the breast revision. In one version of this approach, the old scars are ignored and a triangle of tissue is removed from the lower pole of the breast (Fig. 145-21). Medial and lateral breast flaps are designed and dissected off the chest wall for a distance of several centimeters above the inframammary fold. The flaps are mobilized toward the breast meridian and closed in an inverted T or J pattern. Some of the excess skin that would otherwise be discarded is preserved as a rectangular "wraparound" flap that can be used for reconstruction of the nipple. The result is a smaller breast with better projection and a nipple that does not depend on taking tissue away from the breast mound for its existence.

OPPOSITE BREAST SURGERY FOR SYMMETRY

If the opposite breast is very large or very ptotic, reduction mammaplasty or mastopexy is usually indicated. Although it is often possible to provide a large or ptotic breast with a free TRAM flap, it is not usually a good idea. Large, heavy flaps can produce severe tension on the flap pedicle when the patient stands upright unless the breast is carefully supported. This tension can easily cause thrombosis and flap loss. The risk of failure is therefore lessened by reducing or lifting the opposite breast and reconstructing a smaller, lighter breast mound to match.

Although the opposite breast reduction or mastopexy can be deferred until a later time, it is usually best performed at the same time as the breast mound reconstruction. In that way, subsequent revisions are easier and can often be done under local anesthesia. Moreover, the surgeon avoids the temptation to make a larger or more ptotic breast than is really safe. In

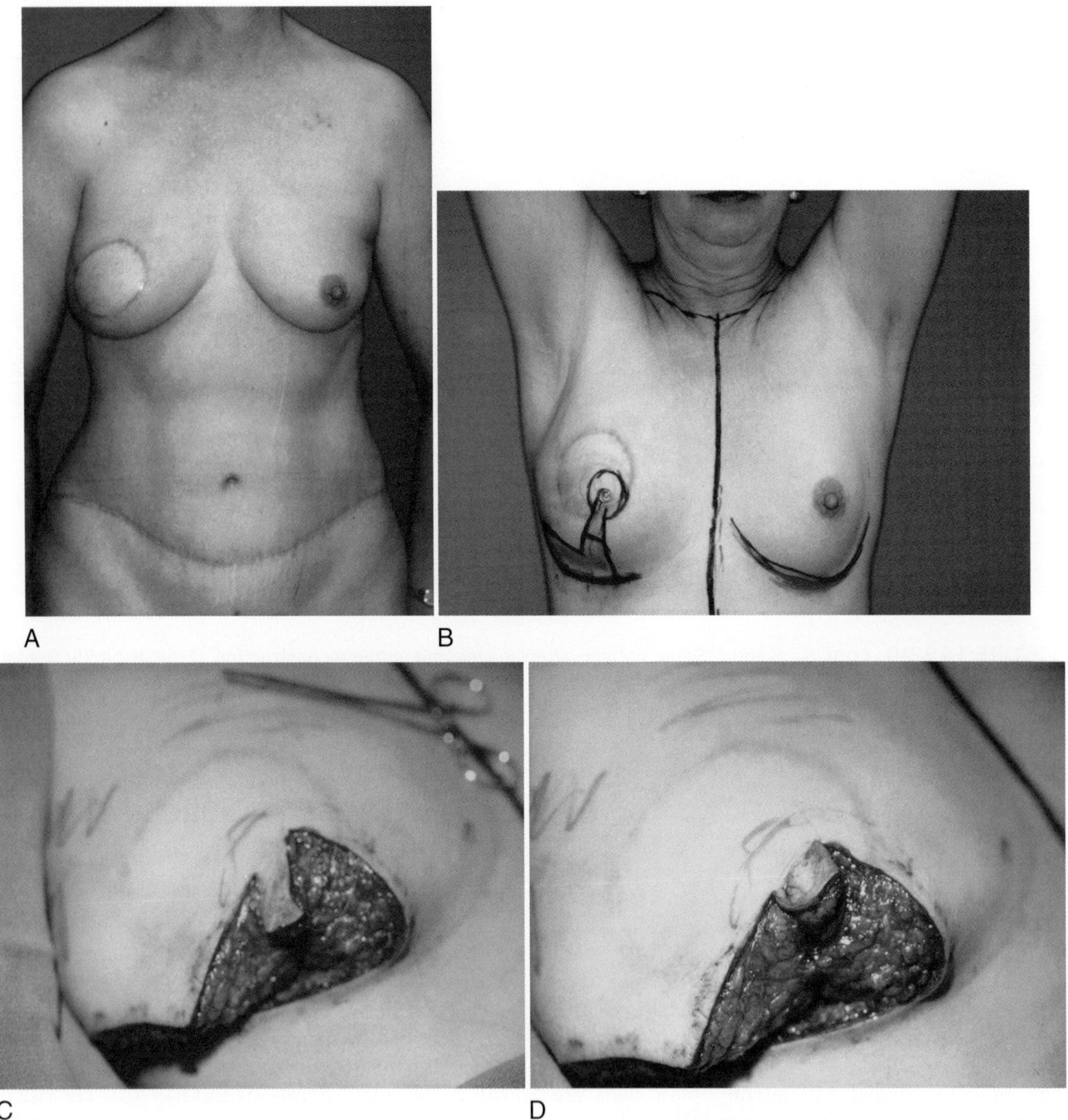

FIGURE 145-21. *A,* Patient after immediate right breast reconstruction with a free TRAM flap. The mound is slightly too large. *B,* Plan for reduction of the reconstructed mound with a J-shaped pattern. *C,* A small rectangular "wraparound" flap has been made out of tissue that would normally have been discarded during the breast reduction. *D,* The tip of the wraparound flap is sutured to its medial base to form a projecting nipple.

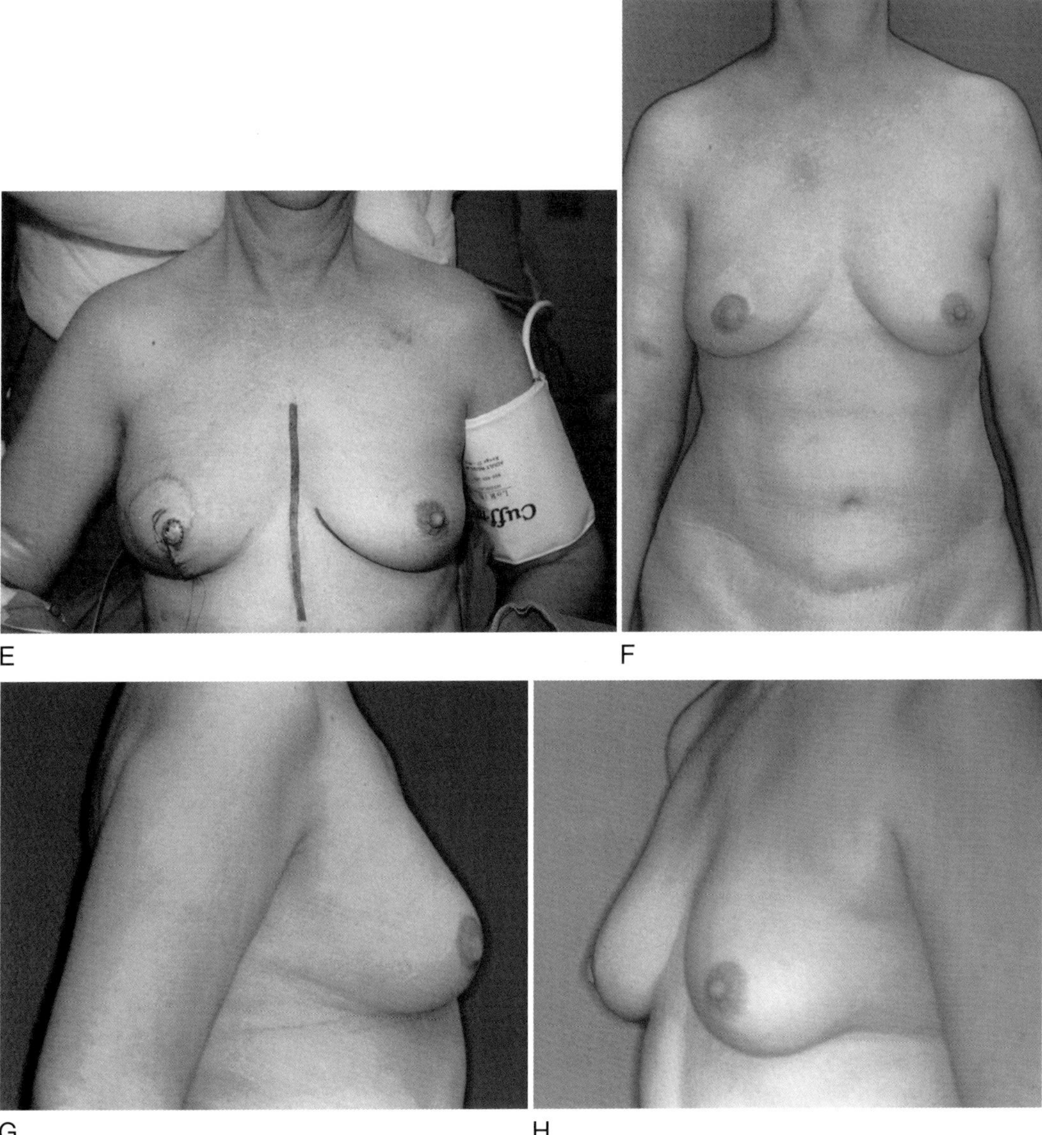

E F G H

FIGURE 145-21, cont'd. *E,* The immediate result shows improved breast symmetry and projection. *F* to *H,* One year later, symmetry and projection have been well maintained. The nipple was achieved without taking any tissue away from the breast mound. (From Kroll SS: Integrated breast mound reduction and nipple reconstruction with the wraparound flap. Plast Reconstr Surg 1999;104:687-693.)

borderline cases, the patient can be prepared for a breast reduction or mastopexy, with the surgeon making the final decision about proceeding with the opposite breast surgery in the operating room.

NIPPLE RECONSTRUCTION

As in real estate, the single most important determinant of success in any nipple reconstruction is its location. If the nipple is in the wrong position on the breast mound, it will detract from the illusion of a restored breast rather than add to it. It is better to have no nipple than to have one in the wrong location.

Most modern nipple reconstruction techniques use local tissue harvested from the breast mound. In most cases, these local flaps flatten the mound around the nipple slightly. This distortion usually is not noticeable in larger breasts but can be significant in small ones. It is to avoid this flattening that the combination of breast mound reduction and nipple reconstruction with the wraparound flap is sometimes indicated.

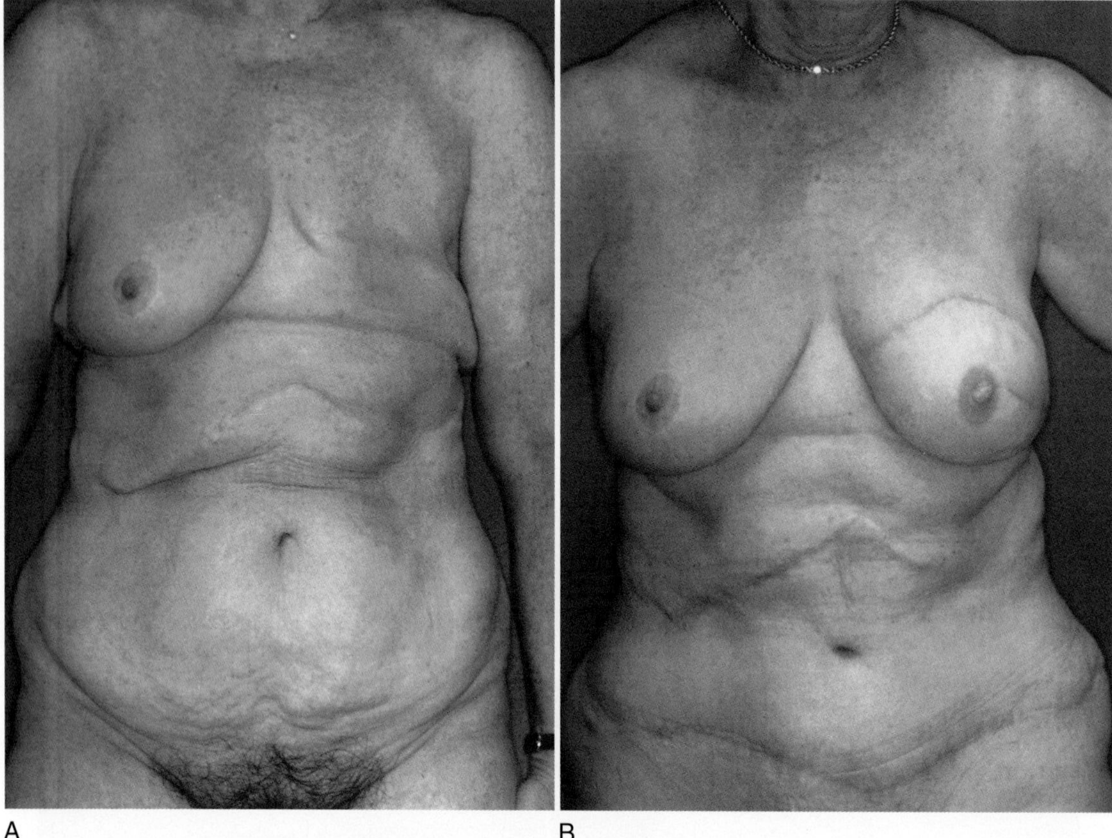

FIGURE 145-22. *A,* Patient after modified radical mastectomy. She also has a scar from a splenectomy. *B,* Result of delayed reconstruction with a DIEP flap. Despite the scars, the overall improvement is considerable.

The areola is established with tattooing. The tattoo process is simple and relatively painless, and it can be done in the office or clinic by a physician's assistant or a nurse. In some cases, better color symmetry can be achieved by also tattooing the opposite side, if the patient will permit it.

Delayed breast reconstruction can provide excellent results in properly selected patients. The aesthetic outcomes may not be as consistently good as those of immediate reconstruction after skin-sparing mastectomy but are still well worth the effort (Fig. 145-22). Patients with more severe defects or with irradiation injury to the surrounding skin will have poorer aesthetic results and should be made aware of this so they will have appropriately reduced expectations. Free TRAM flaps provide the best aesthetic results in most cases. Patients usually appreciate delayed reconstruction very much, perhaps more so than patients who have had immediate reconstructions. Having lived with the deformity of an unreconstructed mastectomy, they are highly motivated and are usually grateful for any improvement that delayed reconstruction is able to provide. When it is properly performed, that improvement can be considerable.

REFERENCES

1. Holmstrom H: The free abdominoplasty flap and its use in breast reconstruction. Scand J Plast Reconstr Surg 1979;13:423-427.
2. Grotting JC, Urist MM, Maddox WA, Vasconez LO: Conventional TRAM flap versus free microsurgical TRAM flap for immediate breast reconstruction. Plast Reconstr Surg 1989;83:842-844.
3. Grotting JC: Immediate breast reconstruction using the free TRAM flap. Clin Plast Surg 1994;21:207-221.
4. Hartrampf CR Jr, Scheflan M, Black PW: Breast reconstruction with a transverse abdominal island flap. Plast Reconstr Surg 1982;69:216-224.
5. Hartrampf CR Jr, Bennett GK: Autogenous tissue reconstruction in the mastectomy patient: a critical review of 300 patients. Ann Surg 1987;205:508-518.
6. Schusterman MA, Kroll SS, Weldon ME: Immediate breast reconstruction: why the free TRAM over the conventional TRAM flap? Plast Reconstr Surg 1992;90:255-262.
7. Baldwin BJ, Schusterman MA, Miller MJ, et al: Bilateral breast reconstruction: conventional vs free TRAM. Plast Reconstr Surg 1994;93:1410-1416.

8. Boyd JB, Taylor GI, Corlett R: The vascular territories of the superior epigastric and the deep inferior epigastric systems. Plast Reconstr Surg 1984;73:1-14.
9. Kroll SS, Schusterman MA, Reece GP, et al: Abdominal wall strength, bulging, and hernia after TRAM flap breast reconstruction. Plast Reconstr Surg 1995;96:616-619.
10. Kroll SS, Schusterman MA, Reece GP, et al: Choice of flap and incidence of free flap success. Plast Reconstr Surg 1996;98: 459-463.
11. Kroll SS, Reece GP, Miller MJ, et al: Comparison of cost for DIEP and free TRAM flap breast reconstructions. Plast Reconstr Surg 2001;107:1413-1416, discussion 1417-1418.
12. Kroll SS, Sharma S, Koutz C, et al: Postoperative morphine requirements of free TRAM and DIEP flaps. Plast Reconstr Surg 2001;107:338-341.
13. Allen RJ, Treece P: Deep inferior epigastric perforator flap for breast reconstruction. Ann Plast Surg 1994;32:32-38.
14. Blondeel PN: One hundred free DIEP flap breast reconstructions: a personal experience. Br J Plast Surg 1999;52:104-111.
15. Kroll SS: Fat necrosis in free TRAM and DIEP flaps. Plast Reconstr Surg 2000;106:576-583.
16. Kroll SS: Breast Reconstruction with Autologous Tissue: Art and Artistry. New York, Springer-Verlag, 1999.
17. Dupin CL, Allen RJ, Glass CA, Bunch R: The internal mammary artery and vein as a recipient site for free-flap breast reconstruction: a report of 110 consecutive cases. Plast Reconstr Surg 1996;98:685-689.
18. Ninkovic M, Anderl H, Hefel A, et al: Internal mammary vessels: a reliable recipient system for free flaps in breast reconstruction. Br J Plast Surg 1995;48:533-539.
19. Ninkovic M, Schwabegger A, Anderl H: Internal mammary vessels as a recipient site. Clin Plast Surg 1998;25:213-222.
20. Sharma S, Chang DW, Koutz C, et al: Incidence of hematoma associated with ketorolac after TRAM flap breast reconstruction. Plast Reconstr Surg 2001;107:352-355.
21. Kroll SS: Integrated breast mound reduction and nipple reconstruction with the wraparound flap. Plast Reconstr Surg 1999;104:687-693.

CHAPTER

146

Delayed Postmastectomy Reconstruction: Latissimus Flap Techniques

SCOTT L. SPEAR, MD ✦ CHRISTOPHER L. HESS, MD

HISTORY

The latissimus dorsi musculocutaneous flap was originally described in 1906 by Tansini to cover mastectomy defects.[1] Although it was popular for a short time, it gradually fell out of favor until 1976, when Olivari[2] redescribed the flap. In 1977, McCraw[3] defined the flap's vascular territory; Schneider[4] described the anatomy of the flap and its use in breast reconstruction. Bostwick[5] subsequently popularized the technique of a skin island over the muscle, allowing the replacement of the skin defect as well as the entire radical mastectomy defect. In 1978, Maxwell[6,7] successfully used the latissimus as a free flap and speculated that the latissimus flap had collateral circulation that would allow it to be raised despite ligation of the thoracodorsal vessels. This collateral circulation was later shown to be the serratus branch of the thoracodorsal artery.[8] With the introduction of the transverse rectus abdominis myocutaneous (TRAM) flap in 1982 by Hartrampf et al[9] and the ability to reconstruct the breast with only autologous tissue, the use of the latissimus in breast reconstruction declined. To extend the utility of the latissimus, Hokin[10] modified the flap's design by elevating a significant amount of subcutaneous fat. This relocation allowed the latissimus to be used for total autologous reconstruction in small to moderate-sized breasts. Today, with the wide variety of options for breast reconstruction, the versatility of the latissimus flap has led to its use in multiple applications in both immediate and delayed breast reconstruction.

As the diagnosis and treatment of breast cancer continue to change, so must the strategies for breast reconstruction. Whereas immediate breast reconstruction became more and more accepted during the last 2 decades of the 20th century, trends have recently moved back toward delayed reconstruction.[11,12] There remain some significant advantages to immediate reconstruction, including the plastic surgeon's help in design of the pattern of skin excision. When the skin defect can be limited to the areola, this allows a reconstruction with no visible scar on the breast. Scars are limited to the areolar skin island, where a small portion of flap skin is transposed to replace the areola. Immediate reconstruction has other benefits to the patient, including psychological as well as those of economies of time, money, and discomfort.

Nevertheless, there are advantages to delayed reconstruction too. Most notably, the final pathologic process will be known and all or most of the cancer treatment will have been completed, including the mastectomy, chemotherapy, and radiation therapy. In the context of delayed reconstruction, the breast skin, chest wall muscles, and soft tissues will be healed, and any resulting defects or problems should be apparent. The risk of infection, hematoma, and, most important, mastectomy flap necrosis should also be less.

INDICATIONS

Poor Candidates for TRAM Flap Reconstruction

When autologous reconstruction is appropriate, the TRAM flap has traditionally been considered the first choice. For various reasons, however, not all patients are good candidates for TRAM flap reconstruction. Although absolute contraindications are limited to previous abdominoplasty and prior use of the TRAM flap (Fig. 146-1), the list of relative contraindications is more extensive. Alternative forms of reconstruction are more likely to be suitable for patients who have either very thin or very obese abdomens; with cigarette smoking; with significant underlying systemic diseases, such as diabetes mellitus and collagen vascular disease; with previous abdominal surgeries, such as an open cholecystectomy or those by the "chevron" or "clamshell" approaches; with prior radiation therapy to the abdominal region; and for highly athletic women.[13,14] Although a free TRAM flap may be applicable in some of these situations, the extended latissimus or standard latissimus with prosthesis is an excellent alternative and avoids the complexity of microsurgical tissue transfer.

HISTORY OF RADIATION THERAPY

If the consultation takes place after radiation therapy, it is important to determine the indications for the radiation, the dose and site of the radiation, and most important, the quality of the remaining tissues. The presence of radiation damage is significant because reconstructions in irradiated tissues, regardless of the method, always lead to a diminished result and a higher rate of complications. Large doses of radiation, as high as 10,000 cGy, typically leave the tissues feeling inelastic, tight, and thickened. This is especially troublesome when the radiation is given during the reconstruction when a tissue expander is already in place. In any case, reconstruction with an implant alone may not be possible and may result in significant complications or, at the very least, a disappointing result. Reconstruction with the help of autologous tissue may be critical because it brings well-vascularized tissue to the ischemic chest wall. The pedicled latissimus flap provides a moderately sized skin island as well as a large amount of well-vascularized muscle (Fig. 146-2). It is a hardy flap that can be used despite irradiation to the axilla.[15]

LARGE CONTRALATERAL OR PTOTIC BREAST

Generally speaking, as the breast gets larger or more ptotic, it becomes more difficult to reconstruct the breast with an implant alone. There is frequently a need for a larger prosthesis associated with longer and frequently thinner skin flaps. A common solution is to reduce or to lift (mastopexy) the opposite side, thus allowing the reconstruction of a smaller or less ptotic breast. However, for a number of reasons, either aesthetic or personal, the decision may be made to reconstruct the breast to a large size or with a significant amount of ptosis. The latissimus musculocutaneous flap allows greater support of the implant by virtue of the muscle. It can also augment the soft tissue cover by interposing the latissimus muscle and perhaps some of its overlying fat between the native breast skin and chest wall muscles. Finally, the availability of a significant skin island (up to 10×30 cm) provides the possibility of true breast ptosis and the placement of an implant substantially larger than otherwise would be possible (Fig. 146-3).

THIN MASTECTOMY SKIN FLAPS

With thicker mastectomy skin flaps, it is easier to obtain an aesthetically pleasing result. For a number of reasons, however, the skin flaps may be thin: the patient is thin, the mastectomy was aggressive, or there were complications at the time of mastectomy or radiation therapy. Whatever the reason, thin skin flaps can lead to several problems. A lack of tissue over an implant increases both its palpability and visibility and can lead to an unnatural appearance. This is particularly troublesome when there is significant capsular contracture; despite full muscle coverage over the prosthesis, this can occur even when the mastectomy flaps are thin. The latissimus flap not only increases the amount of tissue between the breast skin flaps and the prosthesis but also provides well-vascularized muscle that can reduce the amount of capsular contracture (Fig. 146-4).

CONTRAINDICATIONS

Absolute Contraindications

Absolute contraindications for use of the latissimus dorsi myocutaneous flap for breast reconstruction include prior division of the muscle, as would follow a posterolateral thoracotomy, and congenital absence or significant hypoplasia of the muscle.[16]

Relative Contraindications

Prior division of the thoracodorsal artery and vein may occur in the course of axillary dissection during the modified radical mastectomy. This does not necessarily negate the use of the latissimus for breast reconstruction. Several authors have studied the vascularity of this muscle and have determined that the latissimus flap can survive by reverse flow from the serratus anterior branch of the thoracodorsal pedicle.[17-19] Previous

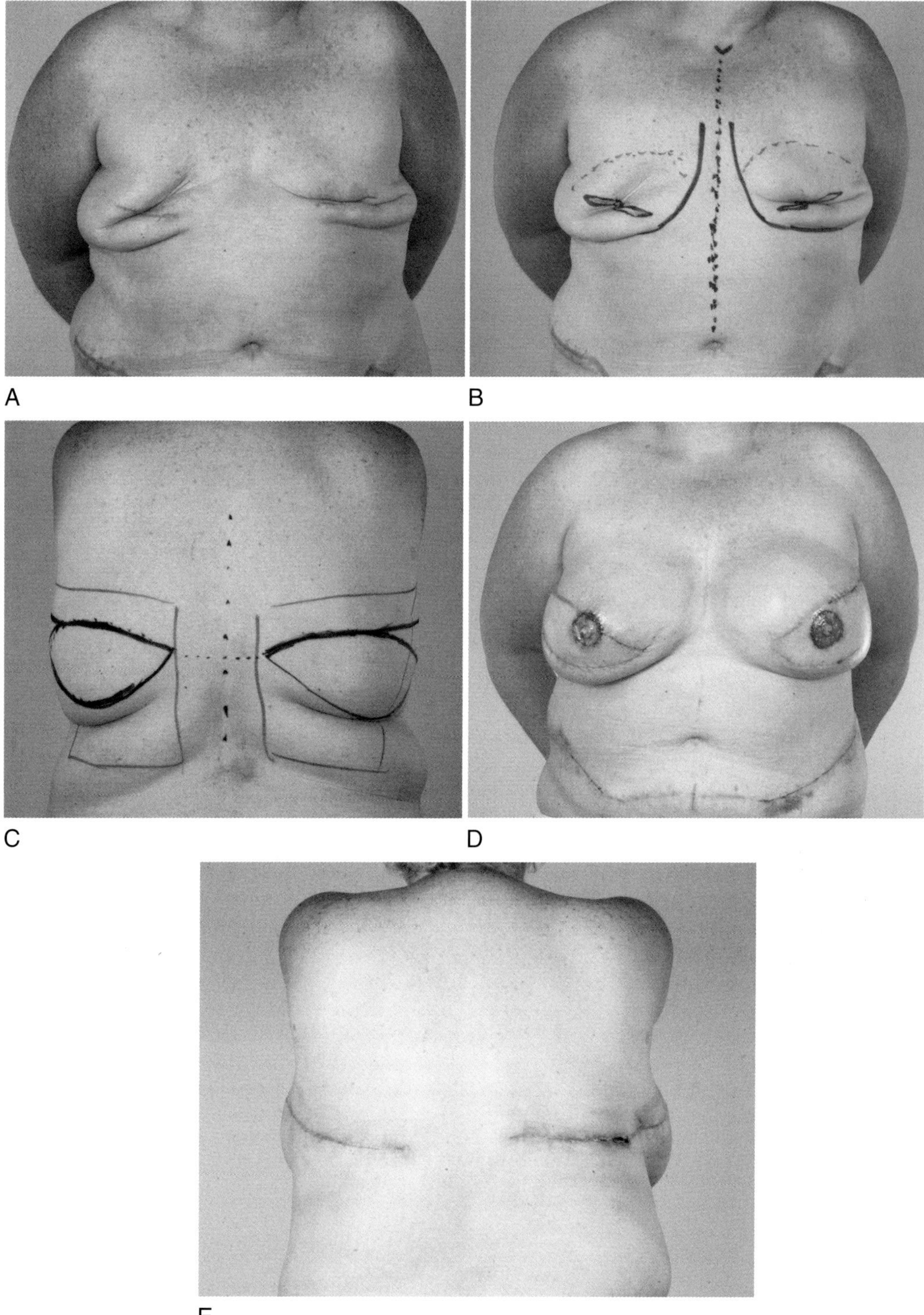

FIGURE 146-1. *A,* Preoperative appearance of a 43-year-old patient who presented to us after a failed bilateral TRAM flap breast reconstruction. *B,* Preoperative markings of the chest wall indicate the previous incisions, inframammary folds, and superior extent of planned dissection. *C,* Preoperative markings of the back illustrate the large skin islands needed to cover the proposed implants. This placement of the skin islands takes advantage of the excess fat over the patient's flanks. *D* and *E,* Early postoperative result demonstrating good bilateral symmetry, lower pole fullness, and donor site scars that will be hidden beneath a brassiere.

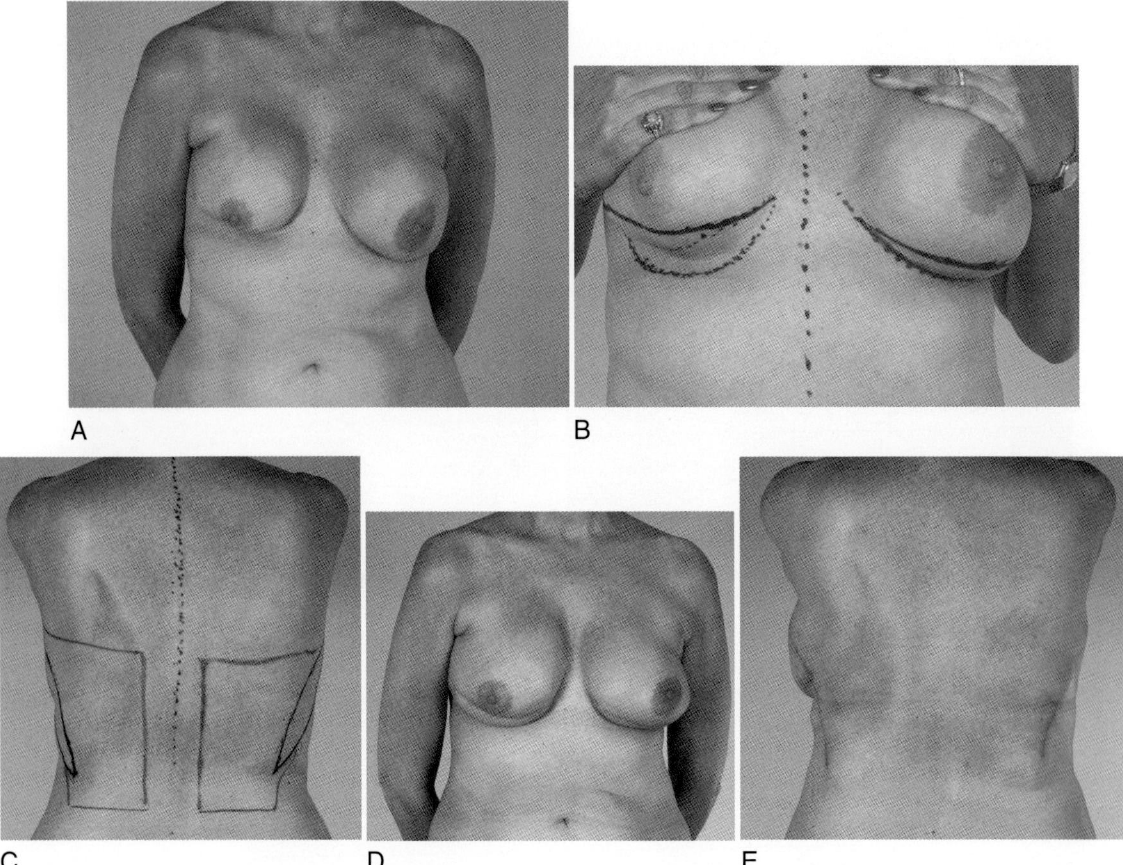

FIGURE 146-2. *A,* Preoperative appearance of a 58-year-old patient after bilateral lumpectomies and radiation therapy demonstrating significant postirradiation breast deformities. The latissimus flap skin islands will be used to replace a portion of the irradiated mastectomy skin flaps in the lower poles. *B,* Preoperative markings of the chest wall indicate the site of latissimus island placement. *C,* Posterior preoperative markings demonstrate the extent of muscle elevation and the placement of skin islands along the lateral border of the muscles. *D* and *E,* Postoperative result demonstrating good symmetry and correction of the breast deformities and favorable posterior scars that will be well hidden in a dress with a "low-cut" back.

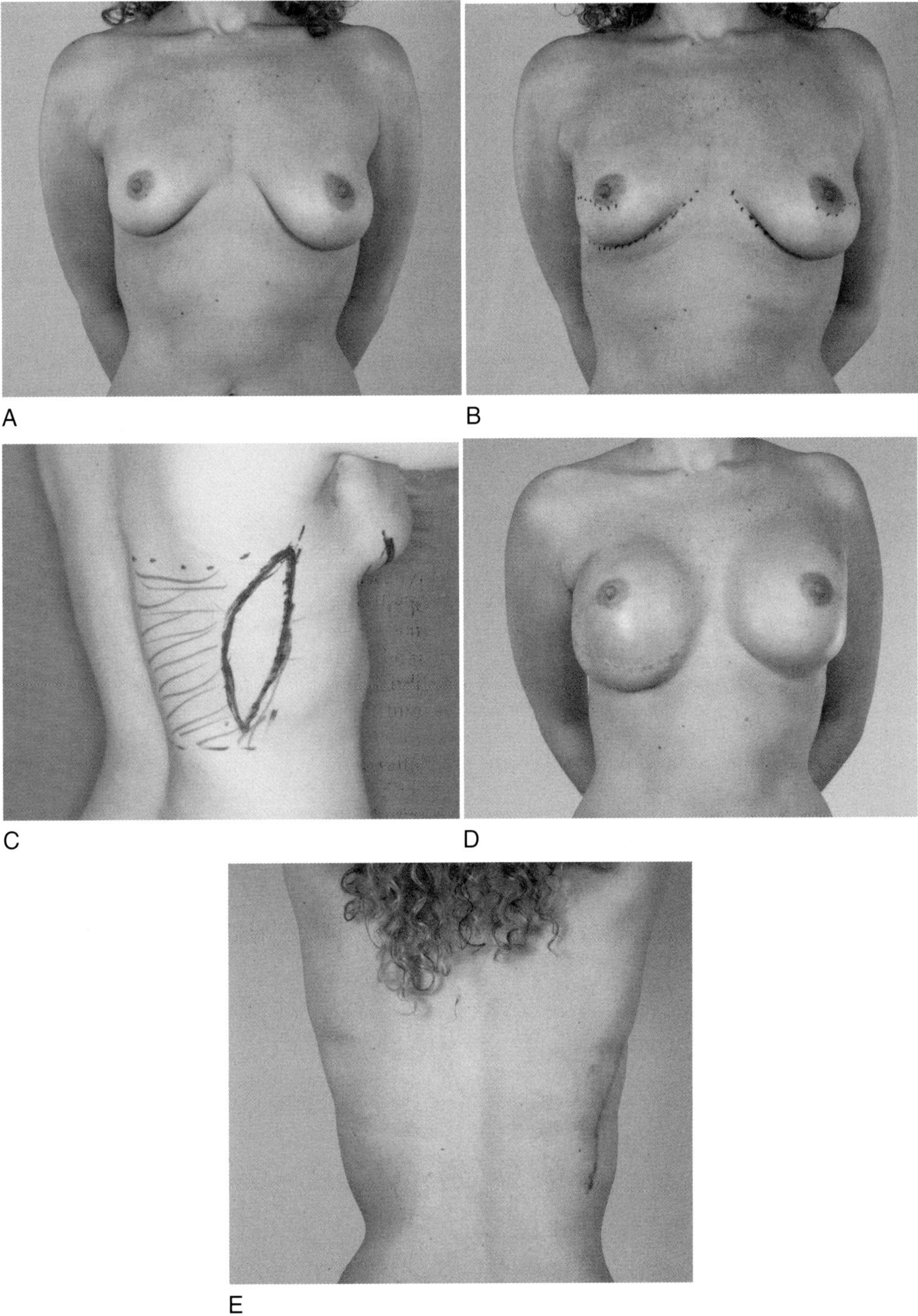

FIGURE 146-3. *A,* The appearance of a 34-year-old patient after a right lumpectomy and radiation therapy. Subsequent testing indicated that the patient was positive for the *BRCA* gene, and she elected to undergo bilateral subcutaneous mastectomies. The patient desired breast size enhancement as part of her reconstruction. *B,* Preoperative markings before subcutaneous mastectomies and immediate placement of tissue expanders demonstrate the proposed incisions. *C,* Posterior preoperative markings for the latissimus myocutaneous flap at the time of the second stage of the procedure. *D,* The final result after a right delayed latissimus flap reconstruction, removal of the tissue expanders, and bilateral placement of 440-mL silicone gel implants. *E,* An acceptable posterior scar.

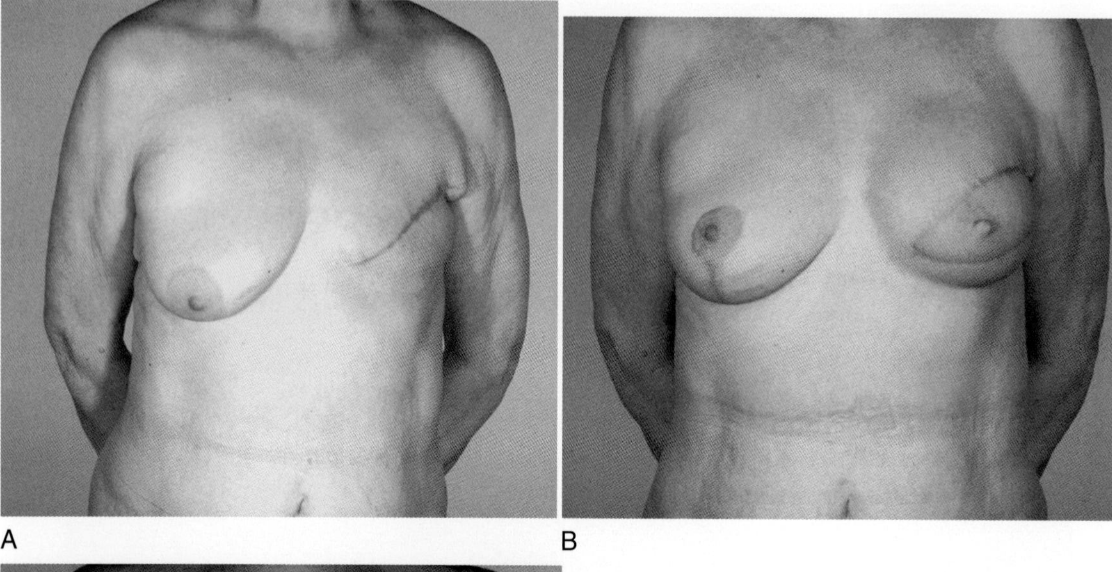

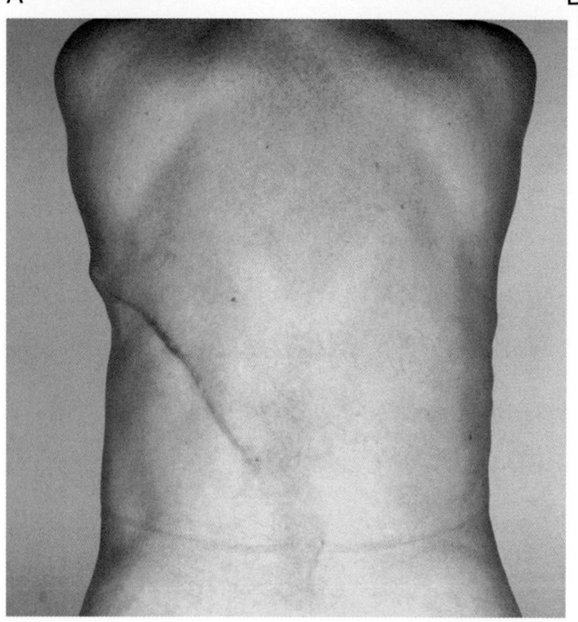

FIGURE 146-4. *A,* The preoperative appearance of a 67-year-old patient with thin-skinned, ptotic breasts after a left modified radical mastectomy. *B* and *C,* The final result after a left latissimus flap with a 370-mL saline-filled implant and a right reduction mammaplasty.

division of the thoracodorsal nerve leaves a thin, atrophic muscle that is somewhat less helpful for coverage of a prosthesis. Preexisting shoulder weakness due to congenital or acquired musculoskeletal disorders requires evaluation by a physiatrist to determine if removing the function of the latissimus will worsen the existing problem. Depending on the nature of the disorder, it would probably be best just to avoid use of the latissimus. Finally, in rare cases, prior aggressive radiation to the axilla and ipsilateral posterolateral trunk could damage the region of the pedicle or leave a fibrotic, atrophic, poorly vascularized muscle that could either prevent an attempt at reconstruction or leave insufficient tissue for the reconstructive purpose.

ANATOMY

The latissimus dorsi muscle, from the Latin meaning "widest of the back," is a large, flat muscle that covers the inferior half of the posterior trunk (Fig. 146-5). It is largely subcutaneous except at its insertion and at its superomedial origin, where it is covered by the trapezius muscle. The remainder of the muscle is superficial to the deep muscles of the back and a portion of the serratus anterior muscle. Although it

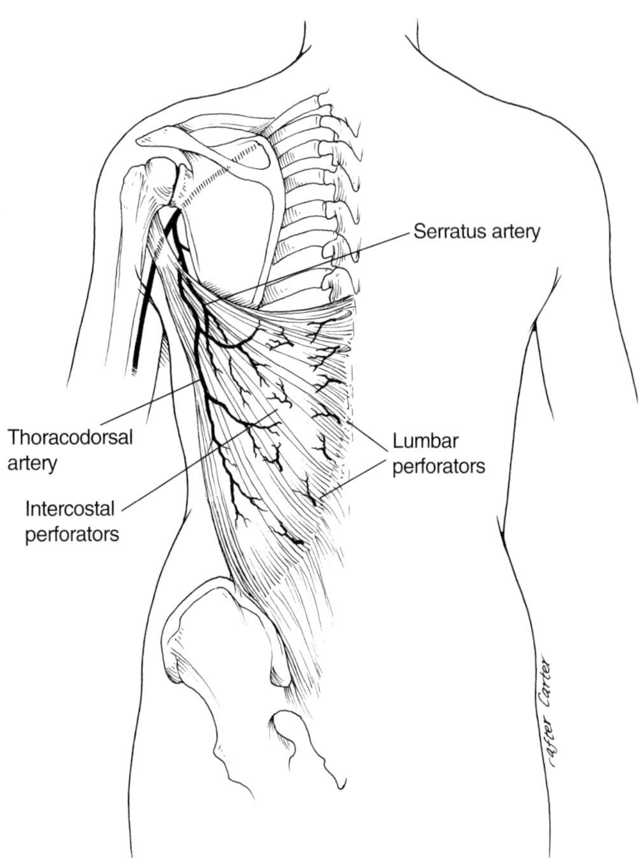

FIGURE 146-5. The latissimus dorsi muscle and its blood supply.

is broad, measuring up to 25 × 35 cm, it is relatively thin, measuring only 1 cm at its origin and 2 to 2.5 cm at its insertion.[15]

The muscle arises from the lower six thoracic vertebrae, sacral vertebrae, and posterior iliac crest as a continuum of the posterior layer of the thoracolumbar fascia. Small muscle slips that arise near origins of the external oblique muscle on the lowest three or four ribs join the muscle as it passes obliquely toward the axilla. The superior edge of the muscle emerges from beneath the trapezius as it crosses the tip of the scapula. As it passes the tip of the scapula, it becomes closely associated with the teres major muscle. The latissimus rotates laterally and anteriorly around the teres major, adding somewhat to the contour of the posterior axillary fold. It then inserts into the inferior aspect of the intertubercular groove of the humerus by a 3-cm tendon.

At the posterolateral aspect of the tenth and eleventh ribs, there are thick fascial attachments between the latissimus and the serratus anterior muscles.[15] These attachments are contiguous with the lower border of the serratus anterior. Failure to divide these attachments during elevation of the latissimus can lead to elevation of the serratus muscle.

According to the Mathes and Nahai classification,[20] the pattern of circulation of the latissimus dorsi muscle consists of a single dominant pedicle and multiple segmental pedicles and is therefore designated type V (see Fig. 146-5). The dominant pedicle is composed of the thoracodorsal artery, two accompanying venae comitantes, and the thoracodorsal nerve. The length of the thoracodorsal artery, from its bifurcation with the circumflex scapular artery, is approximately 8.7 cm; its diameter is typically 1.5 to 3 mm.[15,21] The relatively large diameter of the thoracodorsal artery, its predictability and minimal anatomic variations, and the large musculocutaneous unit it supplies make the latissimus dorsi flap highly reliable for breast reconstruction as a pedicled or free flap.

The subscapular artery arises from the third part of the axillary artery and immediately divides into the circumflex scapular and thoracodorsal arteries. The thoracodorsal artery courses through the posterior axilla before entering the undersurface of the latissimus dorsi muscle 10 to 12 cm below the axillary artery and 2.5 to 3 cm inside the lateral edge of the muscle.[15] Shortly before entering the latissimus muscle, the thoracodorsal artery gives off one to three branches to the serratus anterior muscle.[19] On entering the muscle, the thoracodorsal artery divides into a larger lateral branch that courses parallel to the lateral border of the muscle and a smaller medial branch paralleling the upper border of the muscle.[22,23] Secondary vessels arborize from these deep primary vessels and gradually become superficial within the muscle.[24]

The secondary blood supply to the latissimus muscle consists of segmental pedicles that arise along the medial part of the muscle in two parallel rows. The lateral row consists of four to six perforators that arise from the posterior intercostal vessels. These small vessels pierce the muscle 5 cm lateral to the posterior midline.[25] The medial row consists of four to six perforators that arise from the lumbar artery and pierce the lumbar fascia just lateral to the lumbar vertebrae.[20]

Numerous musculocutaneous perforators extend from the rich intramuscular vascular network into the overlying skin and subcutaneous tissue, allowing skin islands to be safely designed anywhere within the margins of the muscle. Perforators from the medial intramuscular branch allow a skin island to be extended 4 to 6 cm beyond the superior edge of the muscle.[26] The largest perforators arise from the lateral intramuscular branch, making the location of the safest skin island in a vertical orientation up to 2 to 3 cm beyond the lateral edge of the muscle.[14,26]

A thorough understanding of the blood supply of the latissimus dorsi musculocutaneous flap allows the full use of this donor tissue for breast reconstruction. There is great versatility in orientation of skin islands transversely, obliquely, or vertically. The bifurcated intramuscular vessels make it possible to split the muscle for use as a double flap or to preserve half of the muscle to maintain function.[21,23] But, as stated previously, the latissimus dorsi musculocutaneous flap is not solely dependent on a patent thoracodorsal vessel. Fisher and Bostwick's study[19] demonstrated that after division of the thoracodorsal vessels, a reversal of flow through the serratus branch provides approximately the same amount of blood flow to the flap as the thoracodorsal vessel does. In fact, this reverse flow is virtually the same as the primary thoracodorsal flow after 30 days.[19] This reversal in pedicle perfusion allows the latissimus dorsi muscle to be used as a transposition flap despite axillary dissection with division of the thoracodorsal pedicle.

The latissimus dorsi muscle assists in adduction, extension, and medial rotation of the humerus. It also holds the inferior tip of the scapula against the chest wall and somewhat helps in elevating and stabilizing the pelvis. It is an expendable muscle because the remaining synergistic shoulder girdle muscles preserve function. Transposition of this muscle anteriorly has been shown to be well tolerated by patients and results in only a minimal functional deficit, although dynamic weakness in shoulder extension and torque may occur.[27-30]

Diagnostic studies are typically of limited value when the latissimus flap is used for breast reconstruction. However, should there be concerns about the patency of the thoracodorsal pedicle, arteriography of the axillary vessels could provide the answer. Unfortunately, this subjects the patient to an invasive procedure and the risks associated with contrast media. As an acceptable alternative, magnetic resonance angiography could provide adequate visualization of the vessels while avoiding the inherent risks of an invasive procedure.[31] Alternatively, pedicle integrity can be evaluated at the time of reconstruction by initiating flap elevation within the axilla. If it is determined that the thoracodorsal pedicle is patent or, if it is ligated, that the serratus branch is intact, flap elevation can continue. The use of fluorescein has been advocated in the immediate setting to help establish skin flap vascularity.[32] In delayed reconstruction, this is unnecessary because any compromised skin will have declared itself previously.

TECHNIQUE

Marking the Donor Site

With the patient in the sitting or standing position, the anatomic landmarks for the latissimus dorsi are drawn with a marking pen. Landmarks include the "tip" of the scapula, anterior edge of the muscle (drawn on a line from the anterior margin of the posterior border of the axilla to the posterior iliac spine; it is accentuated with contraction), posterior iliac spine, and posterior midline (vertebral column).

The most important determinant in the design of the skin island is where on the breast it is to be placed. With this in mind, one must also take into account the following variables:

- The necessary amount of skin to replace portions of or to add to the breast skin envelope

The length of the skin island is limited only by the margins of the latissimus muscle. However, direct closure of the back wound, when widths exceed 7 to 8 cm, may be possible only with increased skin laxity, prior skin expansion, or skin grafting.[21]

- Position of the skin in relation to the muscle after transposition to the anterior chest wall

A superior transverse or superior oblique skin island allows placement of the skin island, after transposition, to the inferior pole of the reconstructed breast mound. The bulk of the muscle is located in the superior anterior chest for implant coverage or for replacement of deficient or transected pectoralis major muscle.

- The location of the donor site scar on the posterior trunk

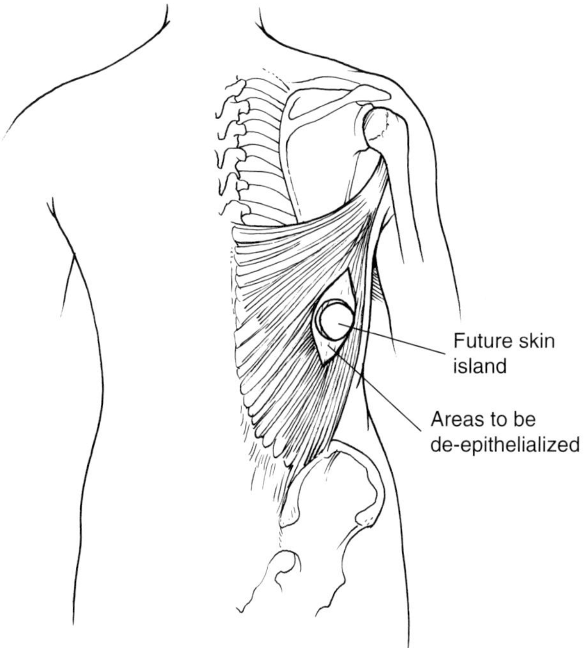

FIGURE 146-6. Typical placement of the skin island for delayed reconstruction.

A superior transverse skin island will allow closure beneath the bra line. An oblique incision across the inferior aspect of the muscle with the superior end at the medial posterior trunk will allow a donor site scar along the lines of least tension and keep the incision on the inferior posterior trunk. Unfortunately, this incision leaves an unacceptably conspicuous scar.

An oblique skin island design along the lateral margin of the muscle with the superior aspect of the skin island located in the direction of the axilla keeps the scar within an inferolateral position. This position is the most favorable because it is not easily seen in a dress with a "low-cut" back (Fig. 146-6). Although this skin island can be elevated up to 3 cm lateral to the lateral border of muscle, design of the skin island 4 to 5 cm medial to the lateral border is preferred.[15] This leaves an inconspicuous scar and provides 4 to 5 cm of muscle superior to the skin island when it is transposed to the chest wall. The other advantage to this skin island placement is the greater arc of rotation and thus transposition to the most inferomedial position of the breast.

Marking the Reconstruction Site on the Anterior Chest Wall

Marking of the anterior chest wall should begin with the inframammary fold of the contralateral breast, the midsternal line, and the mastectomy scar. These are used to determine the appropriate position of the mastectomy site inframammary line. If the patient has undergone previous bilateral mastectomies, the inframammary fold can often still be visualized in the sixth intercostal space. If this location is not appropriate for the new construction, the new fold can be determined intraoperatively.

The radical mastectomy has long since fallen out of favor. However, the rare patient may have an absent pectoralis major muscle. In this case, the planned position of the latissimus muscle may be outlined to simulate the position of the contralateral pectoralis major muscle.

Positioning of the Patient

The patient is initially placed in the lateral decubitus position for the flap elevation to be performed (Fig. 146-7). A beanbag is generally placed under the patient to provide support for the trunk and helps avoid injury to the contralateral brachial plexus. The ipsilateral arm is included in the operative field, covered with a stockinette and supported on an elevated arm

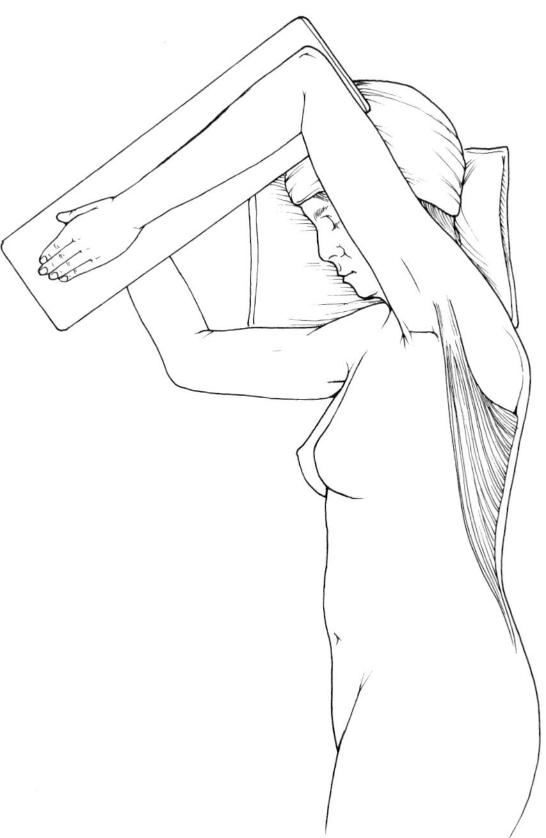

FIGURE 146-7. Placement of the patient in the lateral decubitus position allows easy access to the entire muscle, including its insertion.

board. After flap elevation is completed and the flap is transposed to the axillary tunnel, the donor site is closed in layers including the superficial fascia and dermis. The patient is then placed in the supine position for completion of the procedure. Proper positioning on the operating table is essential; the patient should be elevated to the sitting position to confirm breast mound position during the second stage of flap inset.

Dissection for Standard Flap Elevation

The skin island is initially incised to just below the fascia superficialis. On the medial border, the incision is carried to the muscle in a slightly oblique manner to include 1 to 2 cm of deep fat adjacent to the skin island (Fig. 146-8). Once the muscle is reached, the entire superomedial skin flap is elevated, exposing the latissimus muscle. On the lateral border, the incision may continue in a much more gradual direction so that the deep fat may be included to the edge of the muscle. The preservation of subcutaneous tissue on the muscle will provide for thicker tissue over the prosthesis and greater lower pole fullness. The remainder of the skin flaps are then elevated. The latissimus muscle is separated from the serratus anterior starting at the inferolateral edge and continuing superiorly along the lateral edge. Dissection continues medially as the lumbosacral fascia is divided at the level of the posterior axillary line, and the latissimus fibers of origin are separated from the paraspinous muscle fascia. Care must be taken to avoid incising through the paraspinous fascia; this makes identification of the proper plane of dissection difficult. The remaining fibers of origin are divided medially from the vertebral column as the flap is raised in an inferior to superior direction. When these fascial attachments are divided, large intercostal perforating vessels should be carefully controlled to prevent bleeding and postoperative hematoma formation. As the flap elevation proceeds superomedially, the covering fibers of the trapezius muscle are identified and elevated away from the underlying latissimus muscle. After the superior border of the latissimus is identified, dissection is carried out laterally toward the axilla, separating the fibers of the teres major muscle that coalesce with those of the latissimus. The entire muscle flap is then elevated toward the axilla. The thoracodorsal artery and vein are then identified at their point of entry into muscle. The serratus branch is easily identified and may be left intact, especially if the patient has had an axillary dissection and the thoracodorsal artery may have been injured. In this case, the serratus branch inflow may be the sole pedicle. It is desirable in most cases to divide the latissimus dorsi muscle near its insertion at its attachment to the humerus (Fig. 146-9). This helps avoid the displeasing bulge in the low axilla that is sometimes seen when the insertion is left intact. Of course, care must be taken during this step to preserve the thoracodorsal vessels. The flap is then placed in a subcutaneous tunnel high in the axilla. A high tunnel will help prevent an unnatural bulge lateral to the breast and will fill the axilla.

While the patient is still in the lateral decubitus position, the back incision is first temporarily closed with staples over a suction drainage tube. When fibrin glue is used, several transverse lines of approximation are then marked on the skin with a pen, and the staples are removed. Fibrin sealant adhesive, in appropriate concentrations, may be used to encourage the adherence of the superficial skin flaps to the underlying deep tissues. The fibrin sealant is sprayed, and the patient is then stapled again as previously marked. This closure needs to be completed in less than 60 seconds so that the fibrin does not set up before the closure has occurred. Pressure is then maintained on the skin flap for 4 to 5 minutes to promote a good fibrin bond. The donor site is then closed over a suction drain in layers: 2–0 polydioxanone to the fascia superficialis; followed by interrupted, deep intradermal 3–0 Monocryl; and finished with a running, superficial intradermal 3–0 Monocryl. The patient is then placed in the supine position for the flap to be inset.

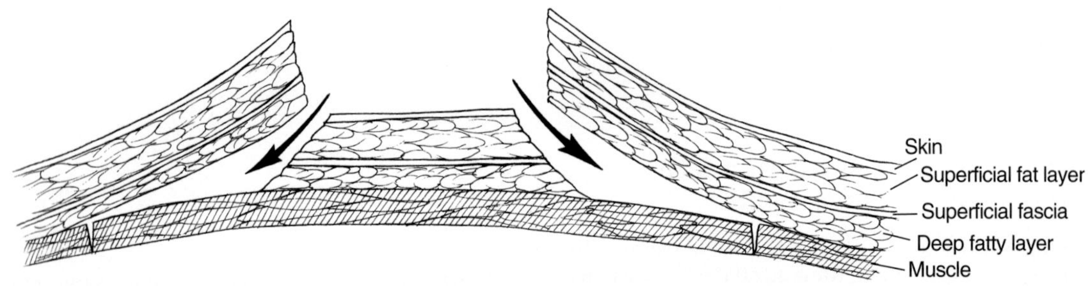

FIGURE 146-8. In the standard latissimus flap, 1 to 2 cm of deep fat adjacent to the skin paddle is included with the flap as the incision continues obliquely in the plane between the deep fat and the muscle.

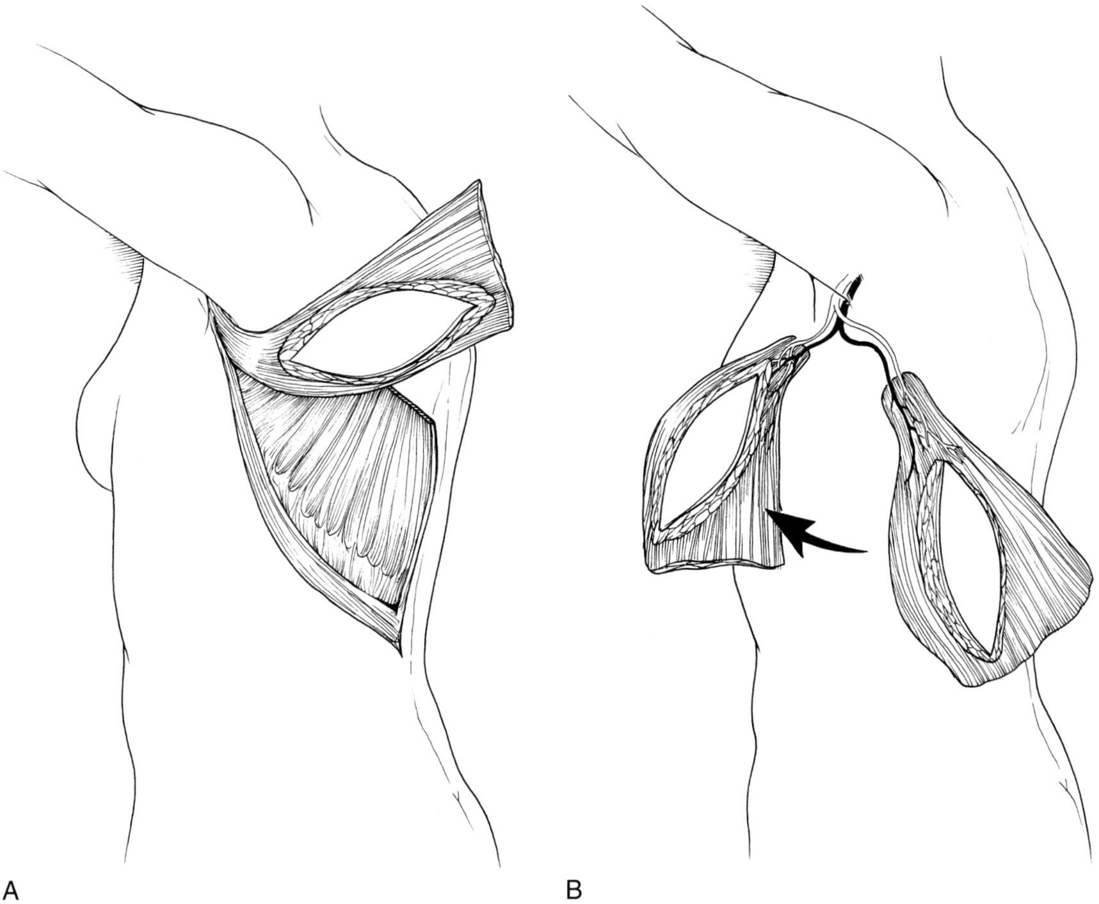

A B

FIGURE 146-9. *A,* Elevation of the flap and the underlying anatomy. *B,* After division of the muscle insertion, the latissimus flap is transposed to the anterior chest wall through a subcutaneous tunnel high in the axilla.

For delayed reconstruction, the latissimus flap is used both for inferior pole fullness and to cover an expander or implant. In most cases, an incision is made at or just above the predetermined inframammary fold along a line from the lateral sternal border to the anterior axillary line (Fig. 146-10). The superior chest wall skin flap is elevated, usually in the subcutaneous plane, and the latissimus flap is brought through the tunnel and into the defect. Suturing of the muscle at or near the anterior axillary line should be performed to prevent lateral migration of the flap and implant and to protect the pedicle from tension. The best projection is achieved when the pectoralis major muscle is left intact and the expander or prosthesis is placed between the latissimus and pectoralis major muscles. The latissimus dorsi muscle is sutured medially and inferiorly to the underlying muscle and fascia in such a way as to help form those borders of the breast. Superiorly, three to five marionette, half-mattress 3–0 Prolene sutures are placed between the overlying breast skin and the edge of the latissimus muscle to help cover the entire mastectomy defect with the latissimus

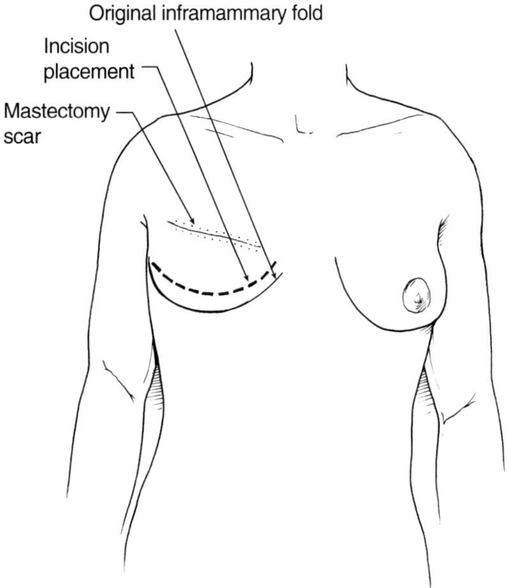

FIGURE 146-10. The chest wall incision is placed approximately 1 cm superior to the original inframammary fold.

muscle. These sutures are tagged with hemostats, thus allowing access to place the expander or prosthesis. The expander or prosthesis is inserted from above and may be filled with several hundred milliliters of saline because there is generally no tightness to the sublatissimus pocket (Fig. 146-11). Finally, the skin paddle is closed to the surrounding breast skin, over a drain, in two dermal layers (Fig. 146-12). Starting 2 to 3 weeks postoperatively, the tissue expander is further inflated, as needed, until the desired volume is achieved.

The second stage of the reconstruction is typically performed after 4 to 8 months. This allows adequate healing and settling of the soft tissue. An implant of appropriate size and shape is then inserted through the previous incision after the expander is removed. Symmetry can be improved by correction of any soft tissue or contour deformities as well as by correction of the inframammary fold. The nipple and areola are usually reconstructed at the same procedure.

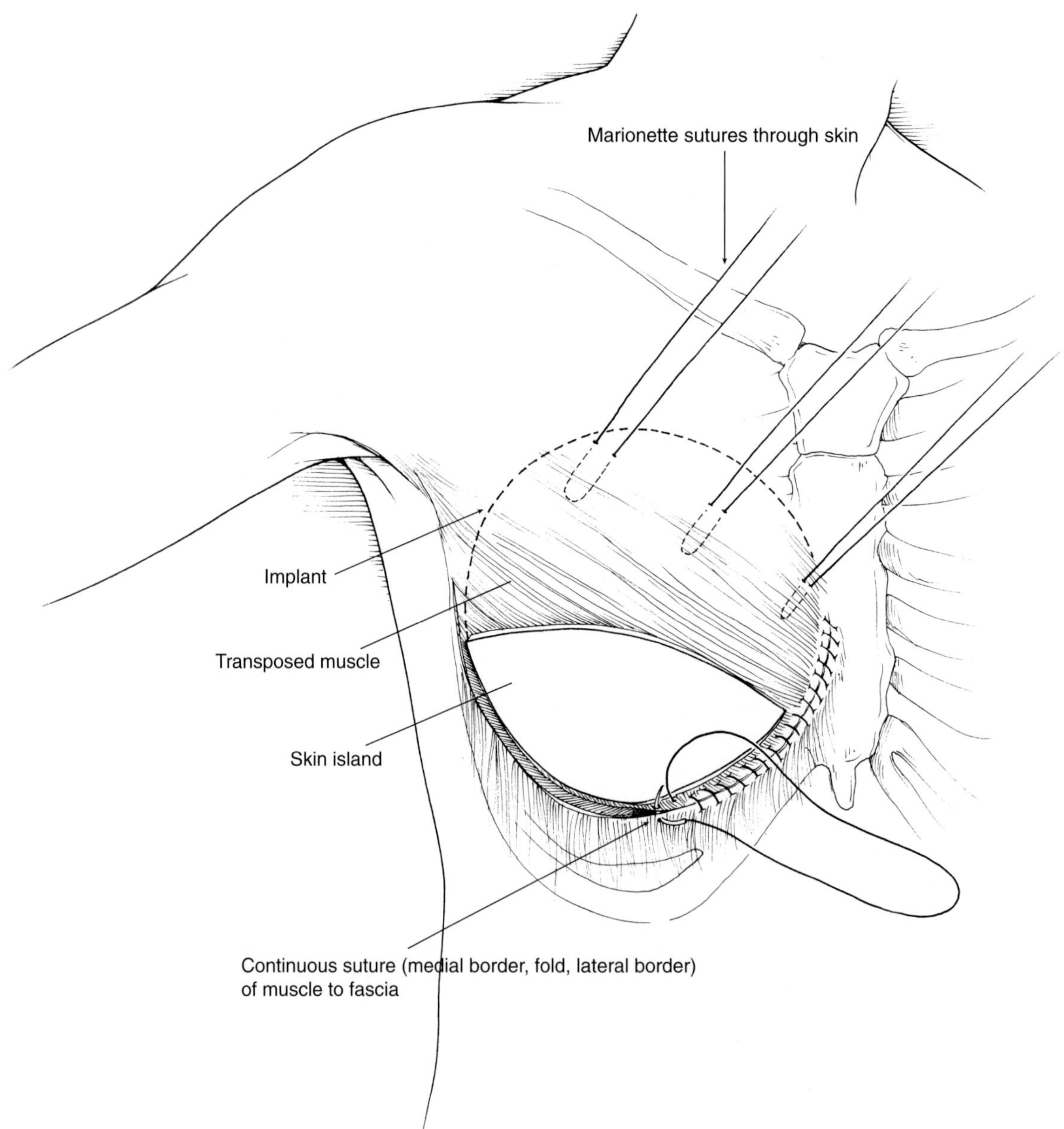

FIGURE 146-11. After transposition, the latissimus muscle is sutured to the deep fascia from the 3-o'clock to 9-o'clock positions. Superiorly, three to five marionette, half-mattress 3–0 Prolene sutures are placed between the overlying breast skin and the edge of the latissimus muscle. The device is placed between the latissimus and pectoralis major muscles, and the marionette sutures are tightened to elevate the latissimus muscle over the device.

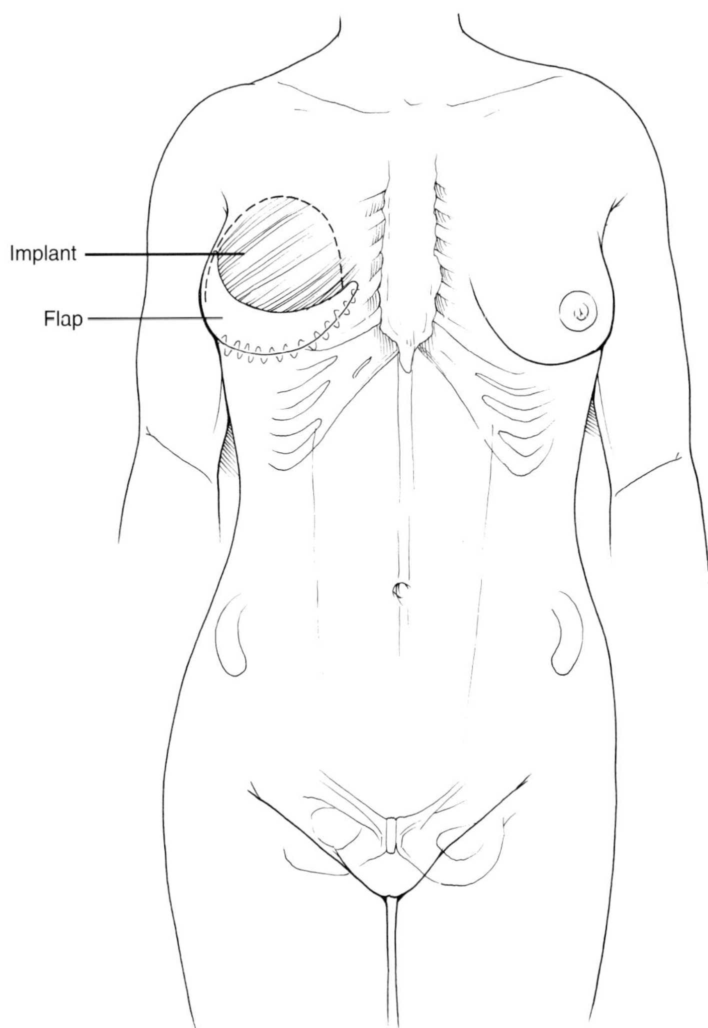

FIGURE 146-12. The latissimus flap in place covering the implant.

Dissection for Extended Latissimus

When total autologous reconstruction with the latissimus flap is planned, the extended latissimus dorsi flap can provide 300 to 400 mL or more of soft tissue volume for breast reconstruction.[33] To begin with, the cutaneous paddle is designed such that it can be molded in the form of an asymmetric U (Fig. 146-13).[34] The curved base of the U gives the apex of the breast. Although the standard description of the extended latissimus flap is of dissection in a plane above the fascia superficialis, it is preferable to raise the flap in a plane just beneath the superficial fascia, leaving the deep fat attached to the surface of the muscle (Fig. 146-14).[35] The fascia superficialis is a useful guide for this procedure because it ensures that a consistent thickness of fat is kept on the cutaneous flaps, thus helping avoid any secondary dorsal irregularities or, worse, flap loss. The fascia superficialis also provides another strength layer to the back closure. The fatty tissue left attached to the surface of the muscle is well vascularized by the perforators coming from the muscle itself. The entire surface of the muscle to be used is exposed in this same plane. Reports of postoperative muscle atrophy of 20% to 25% should be taken into consideration during the insetting and sizing of the flap.[35] After transposition to the chest wall, the distal part of the muscle and its underlying fat are folded under this breast cone to increase the volume and the projection of the breast (Fig. 146-15). Various forms can be tried until one arrives at a satisfactory shape for the rebuilt breast. This procedure of molding is crucial to the final quality of the result, and one must understand how to achieve the different arrangements necessary to obtain a good morphologic result.

Some surgeons think that the intact thoracodorsal nerve may help preserve maximum volume of the flap

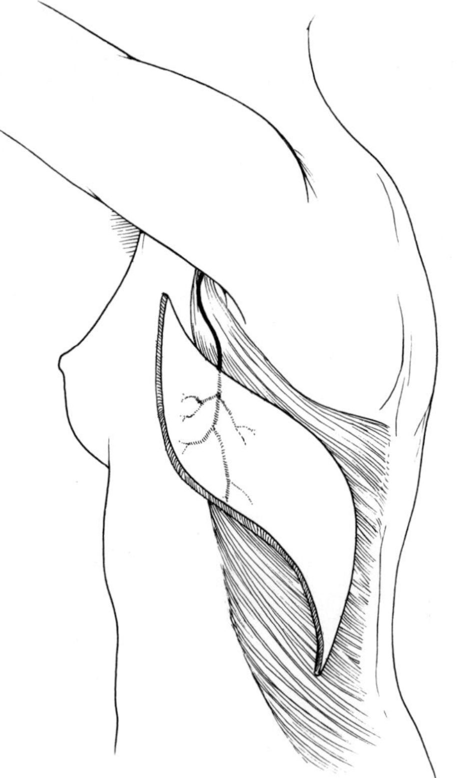

FIGURE 146-13. Flap design for the extended latissimus myocutaneous flap.

in the long term and therefore advocate not dividing the thoracodorsal nerve when the flap is used in this fashion.[36] They also argue that because the latissimus dorsi muscle is fixed to the chest wall in a relaxed manner, little contraction is noticed in the flap postoperatively when the nerve is left intact. On the other hand, with use of the muscle over an expander, postoperative voluntary muscle contraction can be significant when the thoracodorsal nerve is left intact.

COMPLICATIONS

The complications associated with delayed latissimus breast reconstruction are similar to those with immediate reconstruction. These complications are primarily attributed to the donor site and the prosthesis. By far the most common complication is formation of a seroma at the donor site.[37,38] This results because the mobility of the shoulder girdle prevents the elevated back tissue from adhering to the underlying parascapular tissue. The risk of seroma formation is increased when an extended flap is performed.[30,39] The greater amount of tissue removed not only leaves a greater space but also decreases the amount of available tissue for fluid resorption.

Although it is uncommon, dorsal skin flap necrosis can occur, especially with large skin paddles, from excessive tension of the back closure.[40] Dissection in a plane too superficial, in trying to leave subcutaneous fat on the flap, also puts the skin flaps at greater risk. Other possible donor site problems include decreased shoulder mobility, shoulder weakness, winging of the scapula, and dorsal hernia.[41,42]

Complications related to the use of prosthetic devices in conjunction with the latissimus flap include migration of the expander or implant through the axilla and into the back.[43] This problem is avoided by secure suturing of the latissimus muscle to the lateral chest wall.[44] Other implant-related complications include capsular contracture, device failure, periprosthetic infection, and device extrusion.[43] Fortunately, the incidence of all of these is fairly low, especially when the implant is placed between the pectoralis and latissimus muscles.

The latissimus dorsi flap is a hardy flap that has an excellent and reliable circulation. Significant flap necrosis is unusual and is nearly always associated with either recognized or unrecognized injury to the vascular pedicle. Pedicle injury can be either direct, from dissection around the pedicle, or indirect, due to twisting or thrombosis from tension on the pedicle.[39]

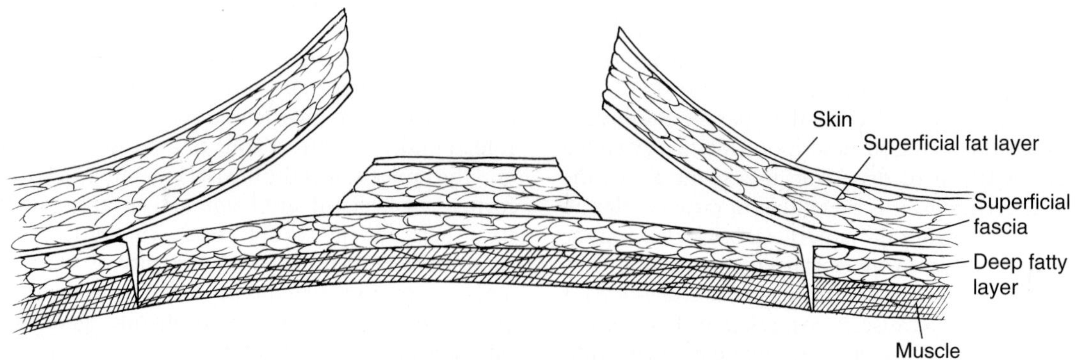

FIGURE 146-14. The plane of dissection for the extended latissimus flap proceeds just deep to the fascia superficialis, leaving the deep fat attached to the flap.

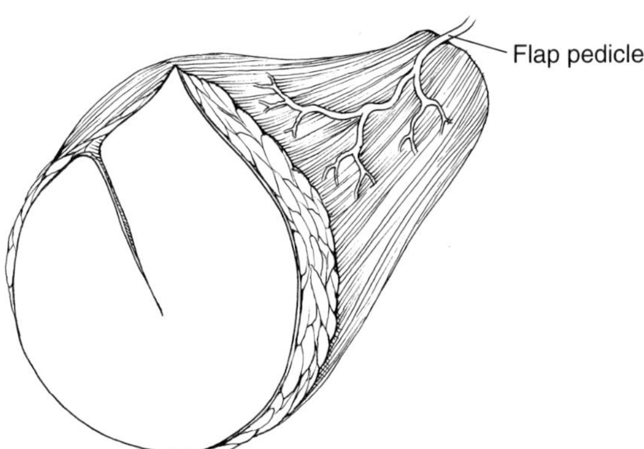

FIGURE 146-15. After transposition to the chest wall, the distal part of the flap is folded into a cone shape to increase the volume and projection of the reconstructed breast.

Tension can be avoided by properly securing the flap to the chest wall. On the other hand, partial flap necrosis has been noted in 3% to 5% of cases but is more common when an extended latissimus flap has been elevated.[37,39]

REFERENCES

1. Maxwell GP: Iginio Tansini and the origin of the latissimus dorsi musculocutaneous flap. Plast Reconstr Surg 1980;65:686.
2. Olivari N: The latissimus flap. Br J Plast Surg 1976;29:126.
3. McCraw JB, Dibbell DG, Carraway JH: Clinical definition of independent myocutaneous vascular territories. Plast Reconstr Surg 1977;60:341.
4. Schneider WJ, Hill HL, Brown RG: Latissimus dorsi myocutaneous flap for breast reconstruction. Br J Plast Surg 1977;30:277.
5. Bostwick J, Vasconez LO, Jurkiewicz MJ: Breast reconstruction after a radical mastectomy. Plast Reconstr Surg 1978;61:682.
6. Maxwell GP, Steuber K, Hoopes JE: A free latissimus dorsi myocutaneous flap. Plast Reconstr Surg 1978;62:462.
7. Maxwell GP, McGibbon BM, Hoopes JE: Vascular considerations in the use of a latissimus dorsi myocutaneous flap after a mastectomy with an axillary dissection. Plast Reconstr Surg 1979;64:771.
8. Fisher J, Bostwick J, Powell RW: Latissimus dorsi blood supply after thoracodorsal vessel division: the serratus collateral. Plast Reconstr Surg 1983;72:502.
9. Hartrampf CR, Scheflan M, Black PW: Breast reconstruction with a transverse abdominal island flap. Plast Reconstr Surg 1982;69:216.
10. Hokin JAB: Mastectomy reconstruction without a prosthetic implant. Plast Reconstr Surg 1983;72:810.
11. Trabulsy PP, Anthony JP, Mathes SJ: Changing trends in postmastectomy breast reconstruction: a 13-year experience. Plast Reconstr Surg 1994;93:1418.
12. Losken A, Carlson GW, Bostwick J III, et al: Trends in unilateral breast reconstruction and management of the contralateral breast: the Emory experience. Plast Reconstr Surg 2002;110:89.
13. Hartrampf CR Jr, Bennett GK: Autogenous tissue reconstruction in the mastectomy patient. A critical review of 300 patients. Ann Surg 1987;205:508.
14. Watterson PA, Bostwick J, Hester TR, et al: TRAM flap anatomy correlated with a 10-year clinical experience in 556 patients. Plast Reconstr Surg 1995;95:1185.
15. Bostwick J III: Reconstruction with latissimus dorsi flap. In Bostwick J III, ed: Aesthetic and Reconstructive Breast Surgery. St. Louis, CV Mosby, 1983:379.
16. Cochran JH Jr, Pauly TJ, Edstrom LE, et al: Hypoplasia of the latissimus dorsi muscle complicating breast reconstruction in Poland's syndrome. Ann Plast Surg 1981;6:402.
17. Maxwell GP, McGibbon BM, Hoopes JE: Vascular considerations in the use of a latissimus dorsi myocutaneous flap after a mastectomy with an axillary dissection. Plast Reconstr Surg 1979;64:771.
18. Bostwick J III, Scheflan M, Nahai F, et al: The "reverse" latissimus dorsi muscle and musculocutaneous flap: anatomical and clinical considerations. Plast Reconstr Surg 1980;65:395.
19. Fisher J, Bostwick J, Powell RW: Latissimus dorsi blood supply after thoracodorsal vessel division: the serratus collateral. Plast Reconstr Surg 1983;72:502.
20. Mathes SJ, Nahai F: Latissimus dorsi flap. In Mathes SJ, Nahai F, eds: Reconstructive Surgery: Principles, Anatomy, and Technique, vol I. New York, Churchill Livingstone, 1997:565.
21. Schusterman MA, Tobin GT, Peterson GH, et al: Intramuscular neurovascular anatomy of the latissimus dorsi: the basis for splitting the flap. Surg Forum 1980;31:559.
22. Bartlett S, May JW, Yaremchuk MJ: The latissimus dorsi muscle: a fresh cadaver study of the primary neurovascular pedicle. Plast Reconstr Surg 1981;67:631.
23. Obin GR, Schusterman M, Peterson GH, et al: The intramuscular neurovascular anatomy of the latissimus dorsi muscle: the basis for splitting the flap. Plast Reconstr Surg 1981;67:637.
24. Rowsell AR, Eisenberg N, Davies DM, et al: The anatomy of the thoracodorsal artery within the latissimus dorsi muscle. Br J Plast Surg 1986;39:206.
25. Stevenson TR, Rohrich RJ, Pollock RA, et al: More experience with the "reverse" latissimus dorsi musculocutaneous flap: precise location of blood supply. Plast Reconstr Surg 1984;74:237.
26. Watson JS, Craig P, Orton CI: The free latissimus dorsi myocutaneous flap. Plast Reconstr Surg 1979;64:299.
27. Salmi A, Tuominen R, Tukiainen E, et al: Morbidity of donor and recipient sites after free flap surgery. A prospective study. Scand J Plast Reconstr Surg Hand Surg 1995;29:337.
28. Fraulin FO, Louie G, Zorrilla L, et al: Functional evaluation of the shoulder following latissimus dorsi muscle transfer. Ann Plast Surg 1995;35:349.
29. Brumback RJ, McBride MS, Ortolani NC: Functional evaluation of the shoulder after transfer of the vascularized latissimus dorsi muscle. J Bone Joint Surg Am 1992;74:377.
30. Cough KB, Louis-Sylvestre C, Fitoussi A, et al: Donor site sequelae after autologous breast reconstruction with an extended latissimus dorsi flap. Plast Reconstr Surg 2002;109:104.
31. Krinsky G, Rofsky NM: MR angiography of the aortic arch vessels and upper extremities. Magn Reson Imaging Clin North Am 1998;6:269.
32. Singer R, Lewis CM, Franklin JD, et al: Fluorescein test for prediction of flap viability during breast reconstruction. Plast Reconstr Surg 1978;61:371.
33. Hokin JAB, Silfverskiold KL: Breast reconstruction without an implant: results and complications using an extended latissimus dorsi flap. Plast Reconstr Surg 1987;79:58.
34. Baumholtz MA, Al-Shunnar BM, Dabb RW: Boomerang flap reconstruction for the breast. Ann Plast Surg 2002;49:44.
35. Germann G, Steinau HU: Breast reconstruction with the extended latissimus dorsi flap. Plast Reconstr Surg 1996;97:519.
36. Lee JW, Chang TW: Extended latissimus dorsi musculocutaneous flap for breast reconstruction: experience in Oriental patients. Br J Plast Surg 1999;52:365.
37. Moore TS, Farrell LD: Latissimus dorsi myocutaneous flap for breast reconstruction: long-term results. Plast Reconstr Surg 1992;89:666.

38. Lejour M, Jabri M, Deraemaecker R: Analysis of long-term results of 326 breast reconstructions. Clin Plast Surg 1988;15:689.
39. Chang DW, Youssef A, Cha S, et al: Autologous breast reconstruction with the extended latissimus dorsi flap. Plast Reconstr Surg 2002;110:751.
40. Delay E, Gounot N, Bouillot A, et al: Autologous latissimus breast reconstruction: a 3-year clinical experience with 100 patients. Plast Reconstr Surg 1998;102:1461.
41. Russell RC, Pribaz J, Zook EG, et al: Functional evaluation of latissimus dorsi donor site. Plast Reconstr Surg 1986;78:336.
42. Mickel TJ, Barton FE, Rohrich RJ, et al: Management and prevention of lumbar herniation following a latissimus dorsi flap. Plast Reconstr Surg 1999;103:1473.
43. Smith BK, Cohen BE, Biggs TM, et al: Simultaneous bilateral breast reconstruction using latissimus dorsi myocutaneous flaps: a retrospective review of an institutional experience. Plast Reconstr Surg 2001;108:1174.
44. Hammond DC, Fisher J: Latissimus dorsi musculocutaneous flap breast reconstruction. In Spear SL, ed: Surgery of the Breast: Principles and Art. Philadelphia, Lippincott-Raven, 1998:447.

CHAPTER

147

Perforator Flaps for Breast Reconstruction

PETER C. NELIGAN, MB, BCh, FRCS(I), FRCSC, FACS
✦ STEVEN F. MORRIS, MD, MSc, FRCSC

The current state of the art in breast reconstruction has reached a level of sophistication that allows predictability in terms of the reconstruction as well as in donor morbidity. Autologous breast reconstruction has evolved parallel to our increasing understanding of soft tissue anatomy and blood flow patterns. The introduction of musculocutaneous flaps in the 1970s saw the development of new techniques in breast reconstruction that were not only more reliable than methods previously available but also more predictable in terms of the ultimate result that we could offer our patients. The latissimus dorsi flap, originally described as early as 1896,[1-3] is widely used, and the transverse rectus abdominis musculocutaneous flap[4-8] plays a pivotal role in our armamentarium. Perforator flaps are evolving as a further option in this area of reconstruction. This has resulted from the pioneering work of Koshima,[9-13] Kroll,[14] Zhou,[15] Itoh,[16] Blondeel,[17] Allen,[18] and others.

Musculocutaneous perforator flaps represent an evolution in the sophistication of flap surgery. It has been shown that careful dissection of the musculocutaneous perforator vessels obviates the need for a passive muscle carrier or underlying fascial plexus.[10,19] Selective harvesting of the skin above the underlying muscle reduces donor site morbidity.[20] When only skin and subcutaneous fat are needed for the reconstruction, it seems logical to preserve the integrity of the underlying muscle. The importance of musculocutaneous perforators to the circulation and viability of skin flaps has been understood for decades. In fact, the design of the cutaneous paddle of musculocutaneous flaps is based on the usual location of these perforators. In flap surgery, muscle and fascia have traditionally been elevated with the skin to ensure that these perforators are protected. As a consequence, the donor defect often results in both functional loss and a poor aesthetic outcome. Koshima and Soeda[10] and Kroll and Rosenfield[14] in the late 1980s introduced a new type of surgical flap based exclusively on these perforator arteries. They showed that preservation of the small arteries perforating the underlying muscle allowed exclusion of the passive muscle carrier and preservation of that underlying muscle. These flaps were therefore composed solely of skin and subcutaneous fat. Kroll and Rosenfield[14] suggested that perforator flaps combine the reliable blood supply of musculocutaneous flaps with the reduced donor site morbidity of a skin flap.

ADVANTAGES OF MUSCULOCUTANEOUS PERFORATOR FLAPS

The primary advantage of the perforator flap technique is that it is muscle sparing. For example, research by Angrigiani et al[21] showed that incorporating the latissimus dorsi muscle does not increase the maximal size of the skin island in the latissimus dorsi flap. However, a correlation has been shown to exist between the size of the skin island and the diameter of the cutaneous perforator.[21]

Many studies have compared the functional[20,22,23] and aesthetic[24,25] postoperative effects of the deep inferior epigastric perforator (DIEP) flap and transverse rectus abdominis musculocutaneous (TRAM) flap procedures. In a series of 50 women and 32 nonsurgical control subjects, Futter et al[26] showed that the TRAM flap group had significantly more weakness in abdominal and back extensor muscles. Patients undergoing the DIEP flap procedure are reported to have decreased postoperative pain compared with TRAM flap patients.[27]

DISADVANTAGES OF MUSCULOCUTANEOUS PERFORATOR FLAPS

Elevation of perforator flaps requires meticulous dissection of the musculocutaneous perforators through the underlying muscle. This places greater technical demands on the surgeon and increases operating time. The dissection of small perforating vessels through the muscle is often difficult and tedious. However, Kaplan and Allen[28] report that operating time decreases by 2 hours for the DIEP flap versus the TRAM flap procedure. Personal experience has shown that an initial increased operating time decreases with increasing familiarity with the procedure.

The unpredictable variability of the perforator vessels is another disadvantage of perforator flaps.[29] Technologic advances continue to make preoperative planning of surgical flaps easier. Doppler ultrasonography is used routinely by many surgeons to locate the perforator arteries before surgery.[30] Other techniques include magnetic resonance imaging,[31] thermography,[32,33] and color flow duplex scanning.[34]

NOMENCLATURE

The literature has become somewhat confusing and conflicting in the area of flap description. Flaps have been categorized according to anatomic location (anterolateral thigh flap),[15] arterial supply (superior gluteal artery perforator),[35] or muscle of origin (gastrocnemius perforator flap).[29] Similarly, flaps have been described according to tissue composition as musculocutaneous, septocutaneous, fasciocutaneous, and so on. We have proposed a standardized method for describing perforator flaps based on vascular supply. In this system, the artery of origin describes all perforator flaps. Therefore, the deep inferior epigastric artery perforator flap, currently known as the DIEP flap, is designated the DIEAP flap; the lateral circumflex femoral artery perforator flap becomes the LCFAP flap.[36] This nomenclature has been adopted for the remainder of this chapter.

DEEP INFERIOR EPIGASTRIC ARTERY PERFORATOR FLAP

Many authors have described the anatomy and clinical uses of the deep inferior epigastric artery perforator (DIEAP) flap.[10,16-18,20,22,23,37-45] The DIEAP flap is based on musculocutaneous perforators from the deep inferior epigastric branch of the external iliac artery. The DIEAP flap has become popular for breast reconstruction[17,18,20,22] and is particularly indicated in physically active patients as well as in patients who are expecting to have children because of complete preservation of the rectus abdominis muscle (Table 147-1).[46]

Anatomy

SURFACE MARKINGS

The surface markings for the DIEAP flap are similar to those for the TRAM flap. We know that there is a concentration of perforators in the periumbilical area, and the majority of larger caliber perforators are found here (Fig. 147-1). Because of the differences in the relationship of the skin paddle of perforator flaps to the underlying muscle, we are not necessarily constrained by the relationship of the skin to the underlying muscle. The skin paddle can theoretically be arranged in any direction around a given perforator. For breast reconstruction, however, the standard TRAM skin paddle is used. This provides optimal donor site scar placement.

VASCULAR ANATOMY

Anatomic studies of the deep inferior epigastric system indicate that the artery originates as a single branch, courses along the inferior surface of the rectus abdominis muscle, and is accompanied by two venae comitantes.[16,47,48] The deep inferior epigastric artery usually divides into a medial and lateral branch at the level of the middle third of the muscle (see Fig. 147-1).[48] The lateral branch is the preferred dominant vascular pedicle for elevation of the DIEAP flap because

TABLE 147-1 ✦ DIEAP FLAP

Advantages
Skin territory same as for TRAM flap
Allows two-team approach to harvest
Muscle sparing
Long pedicle
Disadvantages
Learning curve
Requires microvascular expertise
Increased operating time

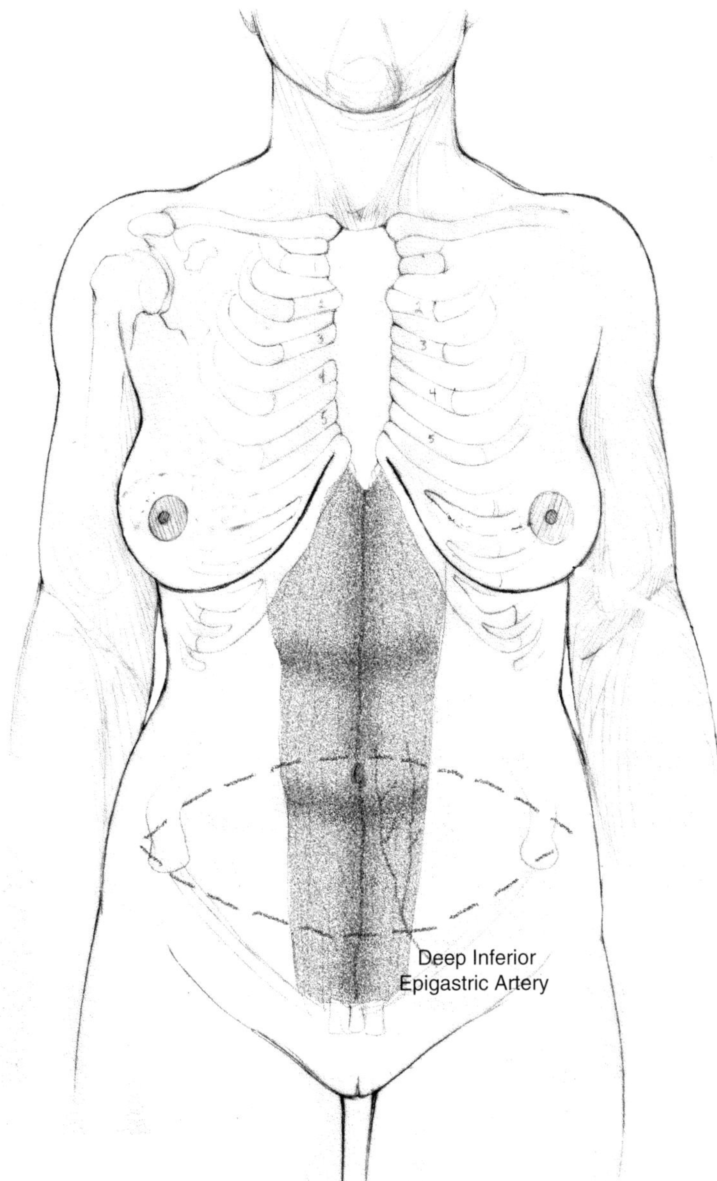

FIGURE 147-1. Illustration of rectus abdominis muscle showing anatomy of deep inferior epigastric vessel system and placement of skin paddle for the DIEAP flap.

of facilitated dissection and muscle preservation.[16] However, dissection is directed by the size of the perforators, and the largest perforator is sometimes found in the medial row, arising from the medial branch of the deep inferior epigastric artery. Although studies of the deep inferior epigastric artery have shown its anatomic variability,[16,48,49] preoperative evaluation of the vascular anatomy has helped identify major perforators and thus reduce the risk associated with intraoperative visualization.[50]

The DIEAP flap territory is similar to that of the TRAM flap.[46] An average pedicle length and diameter of 10 cm and 3.6 mm, respectively, have been reported.[51] In a series of 20 cadavers, El-Mrakby and Milner[48] determined the average number of perforators larger than 0.5 mm and within a 4-cm radius of the umbilicus to be approximately five per side. Survival has been reported of oval skin paddles measuring 20 × 29 cm[18] and 34 × 16 cm[17] based on a single perforator artery from the deep inferior epigastric system.

Surgical Technique

The skin markings are similar to those for a TRAM flap (see Fig. 147-1). Doppler examination of the perforators is performed once preparation and draping are complete. The position of the perforators is marked on both sides of the abdomen. This is a safe flap to raise because one can use a stepwise method in choosing perforators as well as in eliminating them. The skin paddle is outlined in exactly the same way as in a TRAM flap. One feature that is striking is the asymmetry of the perforators from one side to the other. There is a difference in the harvest technique of unilateral versus bilateral DIEAP flaps.

UNILATERAL DIEAP FLAP

The perforators are identified by Doppler signal and marked. The flap borders are incised. The incision cuts through skin and subcutaneous fat down to the deep fascia. Dissection then proceeds from lateral to medial at the suprafascial level. As the lateral margin of the rectus sheath is approached, care is taken to identify the lateral row of perforators. Small vessels can be seen within the fat of the flap as dissection proceeds, and these converge toward the vessel of origin. Once this is seen, dissection proceeds with caution. The appearance of the perforators at this stage often resembles an oak tree (Fig. 147-2). Several features give clues to the size of the perforator. One is the actual size of the branches and whether pulsation can be seen within them. A useful indicator is the size of the fascial opening through which the perforator emerges from the muscle. In general, larger openings are associated with large perforators, although sometimes this may not be apparent if the vessel is in spasm. Some very small perforators will be encountered and these can be eliminated, keeping only the larger ones. In the situation in which at least one of the lateral perforators is large, one can begin dissection by incising the fascia. If the fascial opening is large, this is straightforward. If the fascial opening is small and closely adherent to the perforator, it can be incised lateral to the perforator, with preservation of a cuff of fascia around the perforator at this level. The course of the perforator within the muscle is variable. In general, the perforator is seen to be much larger once the fascia is incised. Then it either goes straight through the muscle to the underlying branch of the deep inferior epigastric artery or runs a more oblique course through the muscle, which makes for a more tedious dissection. On occasion, a perforator will be seen to course along the surface of the muscle directly under the fascia for a variable distance before entering the muscle. In this situation, care must be taken not to damage the perforator as one incises the fascia. It is important to clip or coagulate the muscle branches arising from the perforator. Once the larger deeper vessel is reached, dissection proceeds until sufficient caliber and length are achieved. This will often require dissection back to the deep inferior epigastric artery itself. On occasion, one can divide the pedicle more distally and often preserve one of the main branches of the deep inferior epigastric artery. There may be more than one suitable perforator. When this occurs, size is the determining factor. The largest perforator is the one to choose. If there are two or more suitable perforators, check to see if they are in line and arising from the same vessel. It may be possible to preserve both perforators without sacrificing muscle (Fig. 147-3). However, as multiple perforators are preserved, the segmental motor nerves need to be cut as they cross over the pedicle.

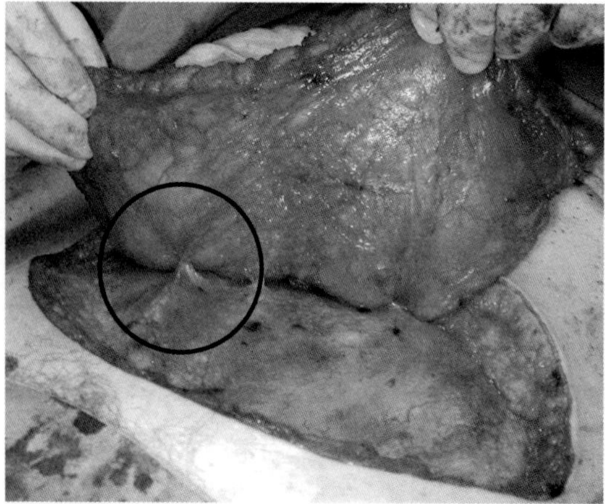

FIGURE 147-2. Deep inferior epigastric artery perforator identified by "oak tree" appearance of vessels traversing the subcutaneous fat *(circled)*.

All of the lateral perforators will occasionally be small. In this case, one may need to select the medial perforators. Once all the lateral perforators are identified and the smaller ones eliminated, dissection proceeds around the superior and inferior borders of the flap. In general, the medial paraumbilical perforators can be identified in this way. Careful dissection between the lateral perforators will reveal the medial row. Once again, size determines the choice of perforator. If all perforators are small, one may need to consider converting to a TRAM flap by incorporating several perforators with a small cuff of muscle.

BILATERAL DIEAP FLAP

Dissection of the bilateral DIEAP flap is easier than dissection of the unilateral flap because the perforators can be approached from both lateral and medial directions. The lateral approach is as already described. The medial approach involves making a midline incision (which has to be done in any event) and dissecting from medial to lateral. Again, size determines the perforator that is most suitable, and the rest of the dissection is as already described.

Defect Closure

Regardless of whether one is dealing with a unilateral or bilateral DIEAP flap, closure of the abdominal wall

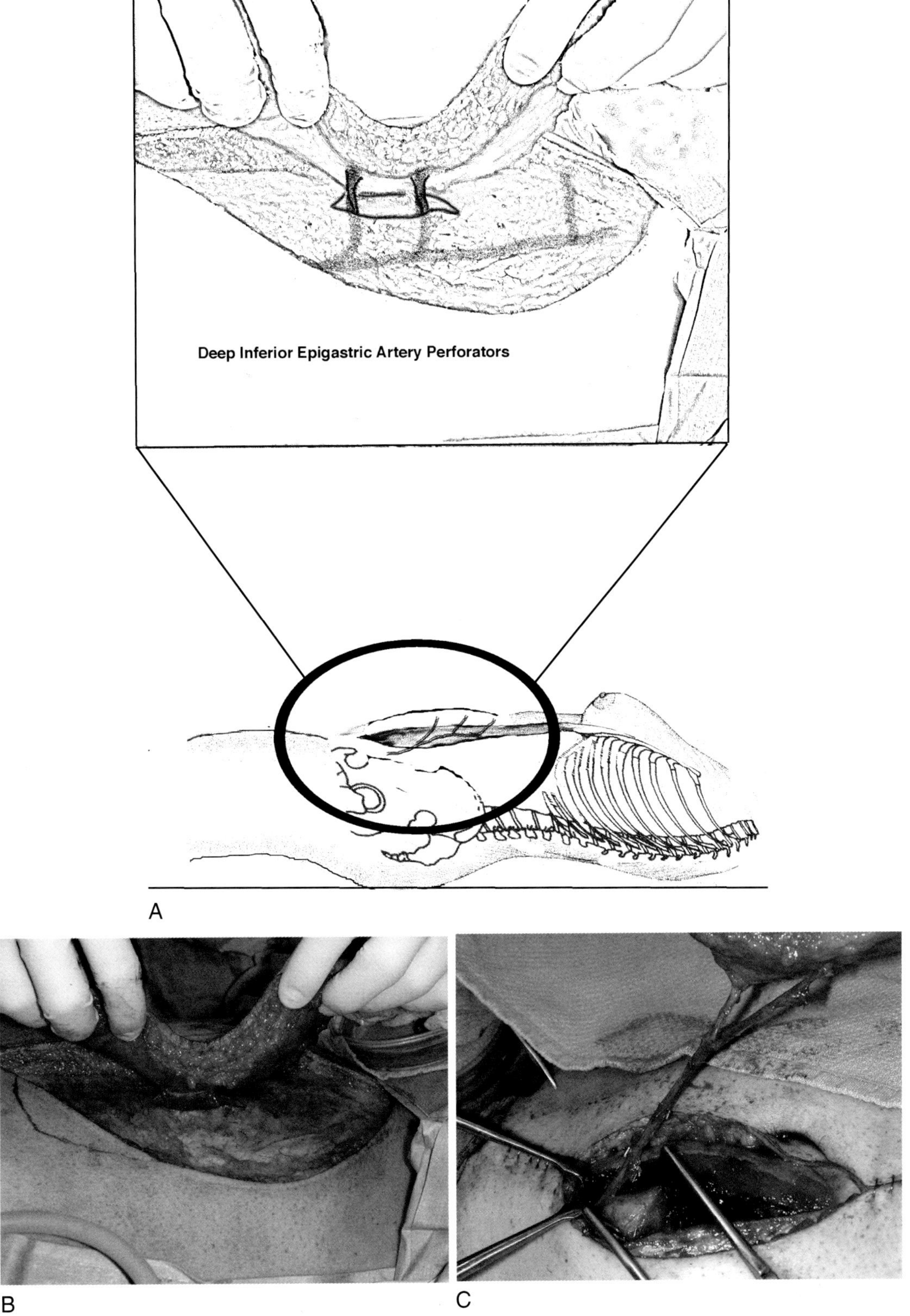

FIGURE 147-3. *A,* Illustration of deep inferior epigastric vessel system with flap being raised incorporating two perforators. *B,* DIEAP flap being raised on two perforators. These perforators arise from the same underlying vessel. *C,* Complete pedicle dissection of the same flap. Note the length of pedicle available.

defect is simple. First, muscle is split along its fibers, not cut. For this reason, muscle repair is not necessary. Again, the fascia is incised, not excised, so that simple repair is all that is required. There is no need for centralization of the umbilicus or plication of the contralateral side as is sometimes the case with TRAM flap defect repair.

Avoiding Complications

Two important factors must be considered in use of these flaps to maximize the safety of the procedure. The first is venous drainage, and the second is the harvest technique. Contraindications to the DIEAP flap are patient specific. Patients who are active smokers, require more than 70% of the usual TRAM flap skin paddle, or have insufficiently small perforators (specifically veins) are not good candidates for the DIEAP flap procedure.[40] According to Kroll,[40] insufficient vascular supply to a DIEAP flap is defined as lack of at least one perforator containing a palpable pulse and a vein with a diameter of at least 1 mm. Also, the presence of an unusually large superficial inferior epigastric vein is a potential indicator of the presence of small veins in the flap system.[23] In this situation, it is advisable to preserve several centimeters of the vein in case it is needed for auxiliary flap drainage.[23] Alternatively, one may elect to convert to a TRAM flap to incorporate the maximum number of perforators.

The stepwise approach to harvest of these flaps makes them a safe option. In unilateral cases, a suitable perforator can be identified and dissected on one side before the perforators on the other side are even disturbed. This is particularly reassuring during the surgeon's early experience with this technique for flap elevation. If the perforator is damaged during dissection, the flap can simply be converted to a contralateral TRAM flap.

SUPERIOR GLUTEAL ARTERY PERFORATOR FLAP

Of the many perforator-based flaps introduced in the last several years, the superior gluteal artery perforator (SGAP) flap is a particularly useful one and has been well described.[35,52-57] Its success can be attributed to the highly vascularized skin of the gluteal region as described by Salmon[58,59] The SGAP skin paddle is on the upper buttock, and as with all perforator flaps, the axis of the skin paddle can be placed in multiple directions (Fig. 147-4). The perforators are identified by Doppler signal preoperatively,[50] and the skin paddle is planned on the basis of their position. This flap can also be used as a pedicled flap for reconstructions, such as for sacral and trochanteric pressure ulcers.[14,35,53] Whereas the lower abdomen is currently the preferred donor site for autologous breast reconstruction, the SGAP has been recognized as an alternative for the DIEAP procedure when the lower abdomen is not suitable because of insufficient tissue or extensive scarring.[18,54,55] The SGAP flap has also been described as a sensate flap based on the second and third lumbar nerves.[57]

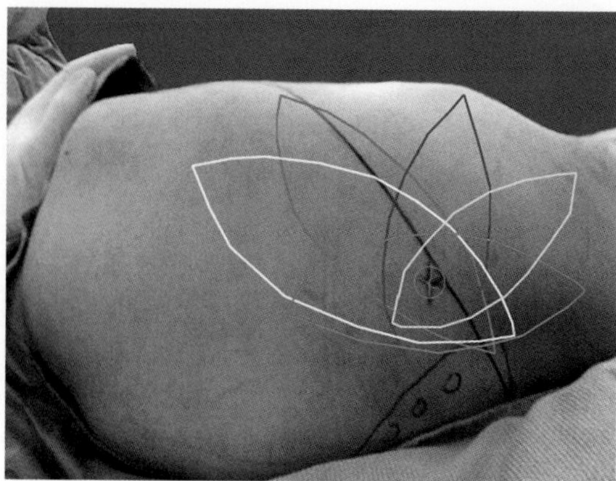

FIGURE 147-4. Potential axes for skin paddle harvest based on the pedicle of an SGAP flap by Doppler signal.

This flap has many advantages over the superior gluteal musculocutaneous flap and has, to a large extent, replaced that flap. Dissection of the musculocutaneous flap is difficult because of the short length of pedicle as well as its deep location. Both of these factors make visualization difficult. With the SGAP flap, pedicle length is significantly greater, and although the dissection is not easy, it is very much easier than dissection of the musculocutaneous pedicle (Table 147-2).

Anatomy

SURFACE MARKINGS

The perforators supplying this flap are fairly constant. A line (A-B) is drawn from the posterior superior iliac spine to the coccyx (Fig. 147-5). A second line (C-D) is drawn at right angles to the midpoint of line A-B and extends to the tip of the greater trochanter. The line A-D joins the posterior superior iliac spine with the tip of the greater trochanter. Line A-D marks the axis of the gluteus maximus muscle, and the proximal third of this line marks the location of the superior gluteal artery as it exits the greater sciatic notch. The piriformis muscle is marked by line C-D. The perforators will be found above the piriformis and lateral to the superior gluteal artery. Two or three perforators can generally be identified by Doppler examination, and the design of the skin paddle can be based on their position. For breast reconstruction, the axis of the skin paddle is positioned superiorly (Fig. 147-6). In this

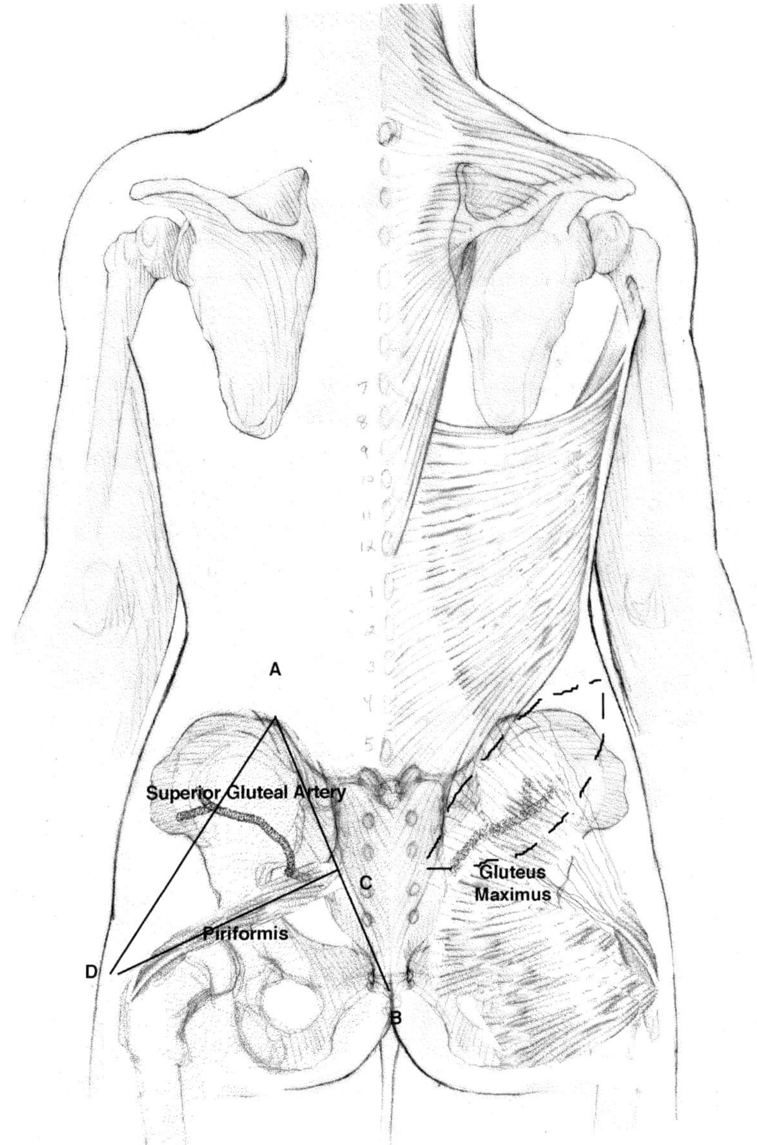

FIGURE 147-5. Illustration of anatomy of superior gluteal artery system showing relationship to piriformis. Surface markings and skin paddle placement are also shown. Line A-B joins the posterior superior iliac spine with the coccyx. Line C-D is at right angles to the midpoint of this line and runs to the greater trochanter. It marks the position of the piriformis muscle. Line A-D joins the posterior superior iliac spine with the greater trochanter. The superior gluteal artery is found along the proximal third of this line.

TABLE 147-2 ✦ SGAP FLAP

Advantages
Generous bulk
Excellent donor defect
Minimal donor morbidity
Disadvantages
Tedious dissection
Vessels occasionally small
Patient requires repositioning for flap harvest and inset
Flap contouring difficult because of globular nature of fat

way, the donor scars can be hidden under the patient's regular clothing. Placement of the axis of the flap in this direction also minimizes the lift on the buttock crease so that even a large flap can be harvested without producing a significant asymmetry of the buttock creases (Fig. 147-7).

VASCULAR ANATOMY

The SGAP flap is based on the superior gluteal artery perforator system. Large-diameter perforators supplying the gluteal skin account for the size of the cutaneous territory of a single musculocutaneous perforator.[53] Twenty to 25 musculocutaneous perforators from the superior and inferior gluteal arteries,

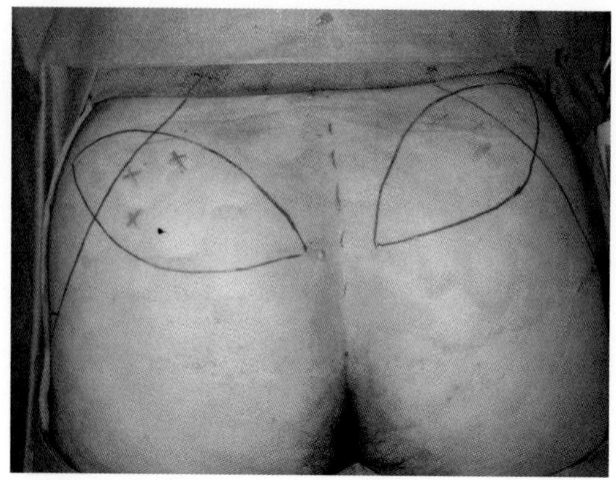

FIGURE 147-6. Bilateral SGAP flaps marked for harvest. Note superior orientation of skin paddle that facilitates hiding of the scar and minimizes lift on the buttock crease.

branches of the internal iliac artery, are responsible for the vascular supply to the integument overlying the gluteus maximus muscle.[53,55] There are predominantly three major musculocutaneous perforators from the superior gluteal artery supplying the superolateral region of the buttock; the inferior gluteal artery supplies the inferolateral and inferomedial areas.[55] Other anatomic studies have verified the consistency of the number and size of superior gluteal artery perforators. The average length of the major perforators is 8 cm, and their average diameter is 1.0 to 1.5 mm. The average diameter of the source artery is 3.5 mm.[52,53,55] Similar to the deep inferior epigastric artery, the superior gluteal artery is accompanied by two venae comitantes averaging between 2 and 4 mm in diameter.[55] The skin paddle of the SGAP flap is smaller than that of the DIEAP flap, averaging 8 to 12 cm × 22 to 32 cm.[55]

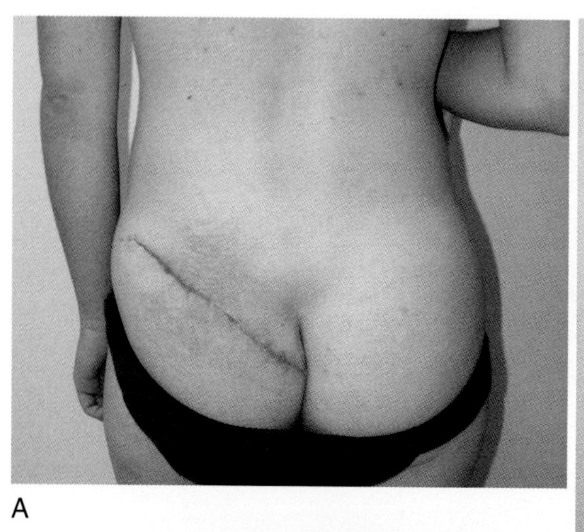

A

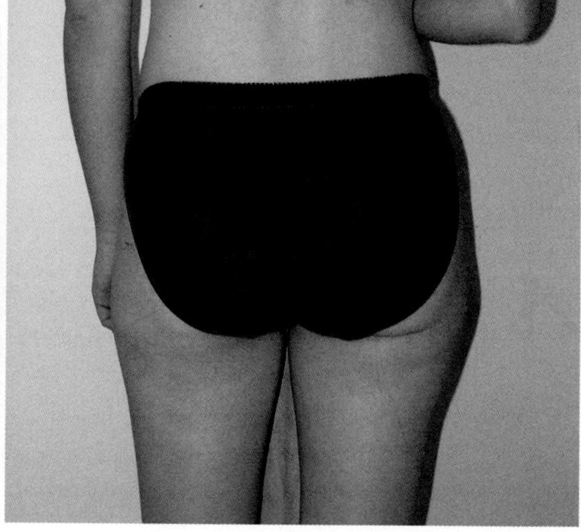

B

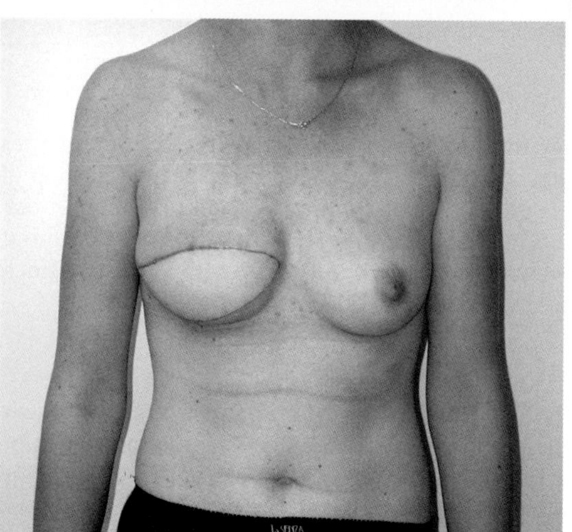

C

FIGURE 147-7. *A,* SGAP donor scar in early postoperative period. *B,* Donor scar hidden under patient's clothing; note minimal lift to buttock crease. *C,* SGAP flap used to reconstruct right breast. Delayed reconstruction after previous modified radical mastectomy.

Although the lower abdomen is currently the preferred donor site for autogenous breast reconstruction,[18,57] the SGAP flap has been recognized as an alternative for the DIEAP procedure when the lower abdomen is not suitable because of insufficient tissue or extensive scarring.[55] The SGAP flap has also been described as a sensate flap based on the second and third lumbar nerves.[57]

Surgical Technique

This flap can be harvested with the patient in either the lateral decubitus or prone position. The lateral decubitus position allows simultaneous approaches to donor and recipient areas and is useful if the thoracodorsal vessels are being used. However, the prone position is preferred despite the need to reposition the patient for inset. In the prone position, dissection is facilitated because the surgeon is looking directly down on the perforators. This is particularly important in dissection around and within the fat pad lateral to the sacrum where numerous venous branches can be encountered. In the lateral decubitus position, one does not have as direct a view of this part of the dissection.

Dissection begins laterally and superiorly (Fig. 147-8). Even in thin patients, the amount of subcutaneous fat is surprising. Above the superior border of the gluteus maximus, there is a deep fat pad that is easily identified because the consistency of the fat is different from that of the subcutaneous fat. This fat pad is above the superior border of the muscle. The gluteus minimus can be identified laterally. It is distinguished by the fact that its fibers run more vertically than those of the gluteus maximus. Once the fat pad is reached, the superior border of the gluteus maximus is easily identified. Dissection now proceeds with caution until the perforators are sequentially identified. The fascia overlying the gluteus maximus is thin and far less discrete than the rectus fascia. Dissection generally proceeds deep to the fascia. Two or three perforators are usually identified. Once they are seen, the largest is selected for continuing dissection. If two or even three perforators are adjacent and can be incorporated into the pedicle without extensively dividing the muscle, this is advantageous. Usually, however, a single perforator is chosen. This can clearly be seen to perforate the muscle. The muscle is easily split along the line of its fibers to facilitate continued dissection (Fig. 147-9). The use of dura hooks as retractors greatly facilitates these dissections. They hold the muscle out of the way and do not interfere with the surgeon's field of vision. They can easily be repositioned by the surgeon and are superior to surgical assistants in terms of maintaining retraction. This frees the assistant to help with vessel clipping and hemostasis. The dissection proceeds slowly initially, with care taken to divide the numerous muscle branches. The course of the perforator through the muscle is variable. The vessel sometimes goes straight down through the muscle and then runs along its undersurface. At other times, the vessel runs a more oblique course through the muscle. Regardless of the course of the vessel, at its proximal end, it runs into a consistent parasacral fat pad. The caliber of the artery and venae comitantes is variable at this level. If the caliber and length are sufficient, dissection can be completed at this level and the vessels divided. If further length or greater caliber is needed, dissection needs to proceed through this fat pad. Dissection needs to proceed only as far as is needed to obtain adequate pedicle length and caliber. Once the fat pad is entered, numerous venous branches are encountered, and each of these must be ligated. At this level, the caliber of the vessels is much larger. Once flap harvest is complete, donor site closure is easily accomplished.

Defect Closure

The gluteal fascia is not nearly as defined a structure as the rectus fascia, and repair of this structure is not necessary. As with the DIEAP defect repair, the muscle fibers have been split, not cut, so no repair is necessary.

Avoiding Complications

Careful identification of the Doppler signals before the beginning of dissection is important. Nevertheless, these should be taken only as indicators of where the perforators are likely to be and are not a substitute for careful dissection. In patients with significant cellulite in the buttock area, the amount of subcutaneous fat is excessive. In these situations, the perforators can be difficult to find and extremely small, and the flap circulation may be compromised. Cellulite is recognized by the presence of multiple dermal indentations on the skin surface. This has been described as the "cottage cheese" appearance. This should be sought during preoperative evaluation. One author (P.C.N.) has abandoned dissection in two such cases and now considers cellulite a contraindication to use of the SGAP flap. Because the dissection is intramuscular, there is little risk to the motor nerve. The piriformis muscle can be seen at the caudal portion of the dissection during dissection of the main trunk of the superior gluteal artery.

FLAP TRANSFER

Decisions about receptor vessels are essential for successful flap transplantation by microsurgery for breast reconstruction (Table 147-3). The internal mammary artery and associated veins are the preferred receptor vessels for flap revascularization. There are several reasons for this choice. The internal mammary artery and vein are easily dissected from behind the second,

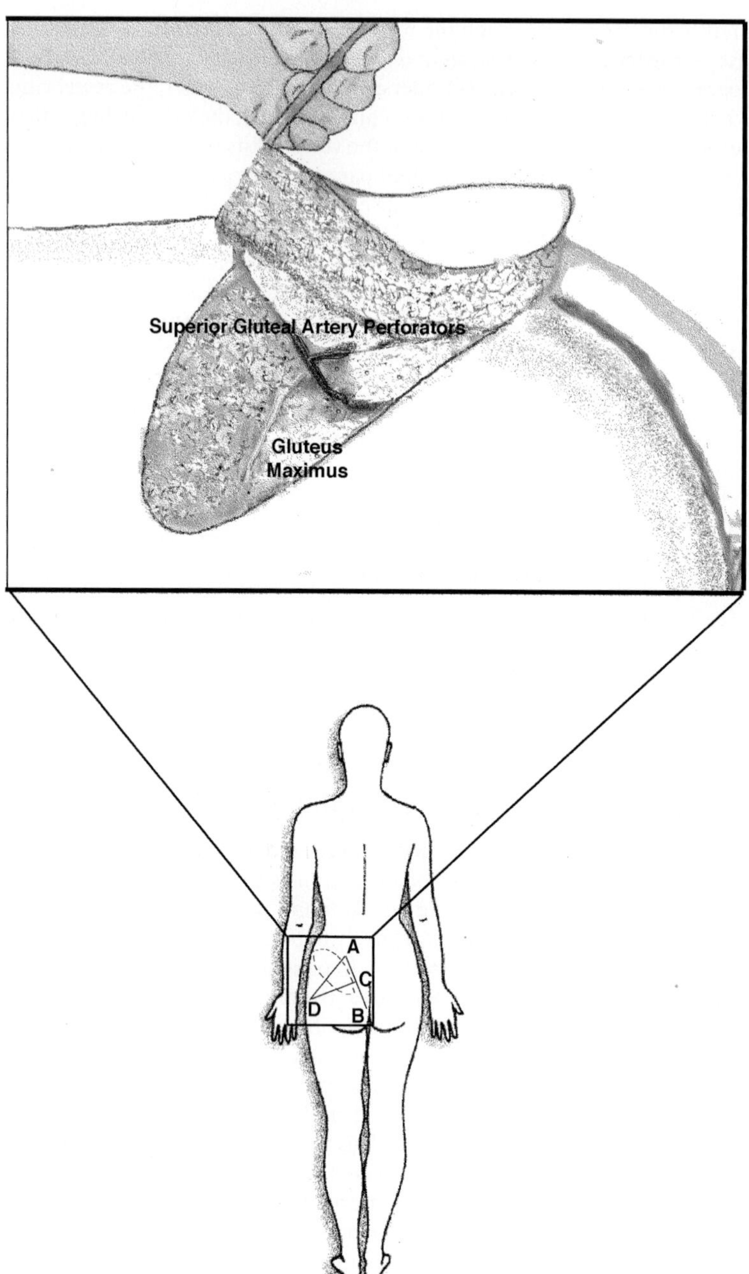

FIGURE 147-8. Illustration of surface markings and skin paddle placement of SGAP flap. Perforators are shown entering the deep surface of the flap as they emerge from the gluteus maximus muscle.

TABLE 147-3 ✦ FEATURES OF RECIPIENT VESSEL OPTIONS IN BREAST RECONSTRUCTION

Recipient Vessels	Artery Diameter	Vein Diameter	Ease of Anastomosis	Ease of Dissection
Internal mammary	1.5-3.0 mm	2-4 mm	+++	++
Subscapular, thoracodorsal	1.5-3.0 mm	1.5-3.0 mm	+	+++

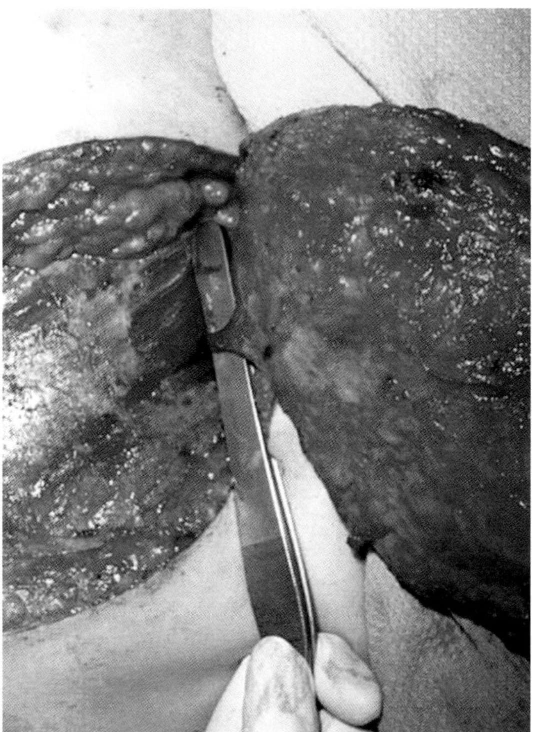

FIGURE 147-9. Superior gluteal artery perforator emerging between muscle fibers.

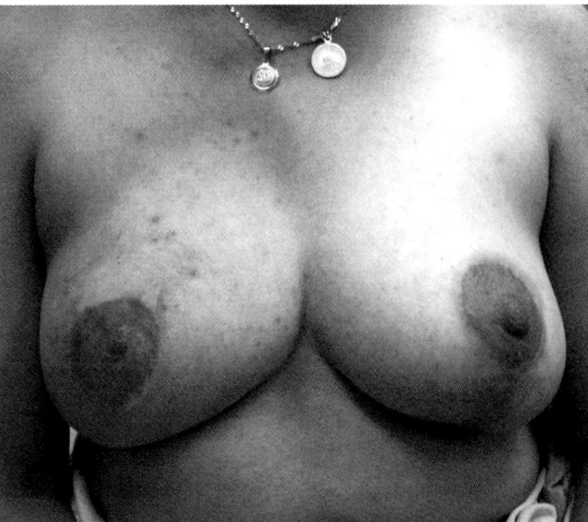

FIGURE 147-10. Postoperative photograph of patient 2 years after right skin-sparing mastectomy with immediate DIEAP flap reconstruction. The patient has also had a right nipple reconstruction with fishtail flap and tattoo as well as a left breast reduction.

third, or fourth costal cartilage. In cases of delayed reconstruction, they are not encased in scar tissue as can sometimes happen with the subscapular system. In immediate reconstructions, there is an increasing use of sentinel node biopsy. In our series, four patients have required axillary node dissection 1 to 2 weeks subsequent to the mastectomy and reconstruction. Not having a pedicle in the axilla has made this a safer procedure. Furthermore, anastomosis to the internal mammary system is technically easier because the vessels are so easily accessible, and positioning of the flap on the chest for anastomosis is easy. The only disadvantage of using these vessels is that the surgeon needs to become accustomed to chest movement during respiration. The anesthesiologist can frequently alter respiratory patterns during the microvascular anastomoses to facilitate this. The authors' current choice is to use the internal mammary vessels for all reconstructions if possible. However, when the internal mammary vessels are unsuitable (such as occasionally after irradiation of the internal mammary nodes), the subscapular system is used. Most frequently, the thoracodorsal artery is the recipient vessel in these cases.

SUMMARY

Perforator flaps have opened a new chapter in the field of breast reconstruction. The DIEAP flap is the first choice and for most patients is an excellent alternative to the traditional rectus abdominis musculocutaneous transposition flap or the free TRAM flap. There is a learning curve in dissecting this flap, but the sequential nature of perforator selection makes it safe. The SGAP flap is an excellent alternative for patients who are not candidates for the DIEAP flap for whatever reason. It is preferred to the superior gluteal musculocutaneous flap, which is more bulky and difficult to dissect, and leaves an acceptable donor site (Table 147-4 and Figs. 147-10 to 147-12).

TABLE 147-4 ✦ COMPARISON OF TRAM FLAPS WITH PERFORATOR FLAP OPTIONS

Flap	Flap Size	Pedicle Length	Pedicle Diameter	Difficulty in Dissection	Position of Patient
DIEAP	Zones I-III	8-15 cm	2-3.6 mm	+++	Supine
Free TRAM	Zones I-IV	6-8 cm	2-3.6 mm	++	Supine
Pedicled TRAM	Zones I-III	NA	NA	+	Supine
SGAP	10 × 22 cm	6-8 cm	1-3.5 mm	++++	Prone or lateral

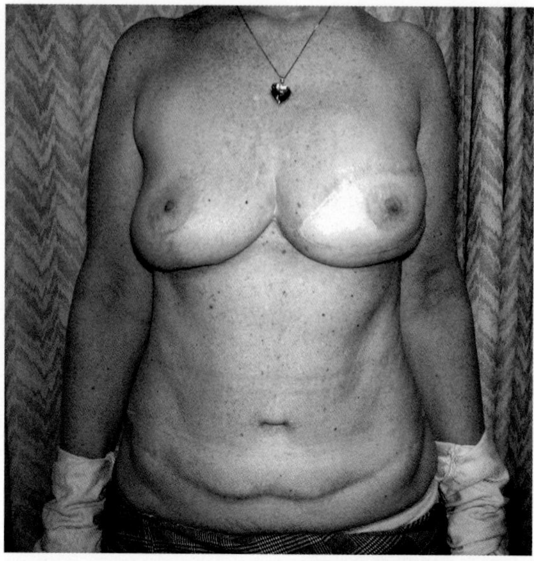

FIGURE 147-11. Postoperative photograph of patient 2 years after left delayed breast reconstruction with DIEAP flap. The patient has also had left nipple reconstruction with fishtail flap and tattoo as well as a right breast reduction.

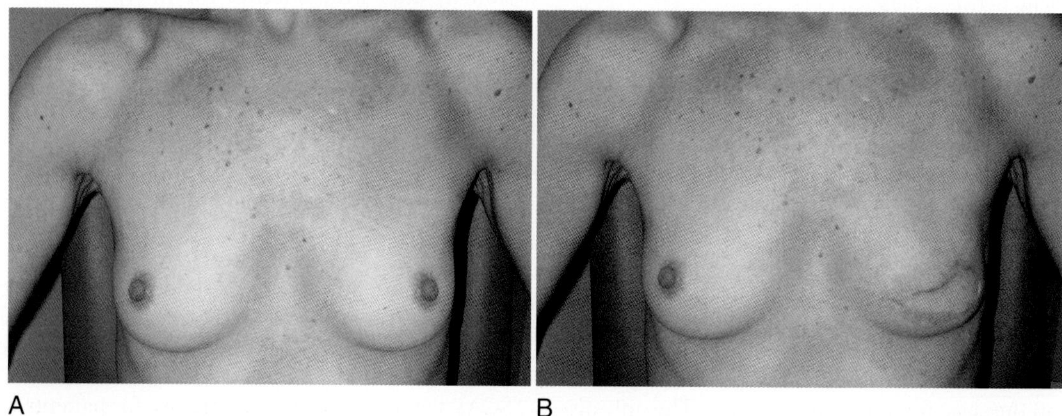

A B

FIGURE 147-12. *A,* Preoperative photograph of patient with carcinoma of the left breast. *B,* Postoperative photograph of the same patient. She had a skin-sparing mastectomy with excision of some medial skin, which was thought to be at risk because of the proximity of the underlying tumor. The patient declined nipple reconstruction.

REFERENCES

1. Schneider WJ, Hill HL Jr, Brown RG: Latissimus dorsi myocutaneous flap for breast reconstruction. Br J Plast Surg 1977; 30:277-281.
2. Bostwick J 3rd, Vasconez LO, Jurkiewicz MJ: Breast reconstruction after a radical mastectomy. Plast Reconstr Surg 1978;61:682-693.
3. Bostwick J 3rd, Scheflan M: The latissimus dorsi musculocutaneous flap: a one-stage breast reconstruction. Clin Plast Surg 1980;7:71-78.
4. Scheflan M, Dinner MI: The transverse abdominal island flap: part I. Indications, contraindications, results, and complications. Ann Plast Surg 1983;10:24-35.
5. Scheflan M, Dinner MI: The transverse abdominal island flap: part II. Surgical technique. Ann Plast Surg 1983;10:120-129.
6. Hartrampf CR, Scheflan M, Black PW: Breast reconstruction with a transverse abdominal island flap. Plast Reconstr Surg 1982;69:216-225.
7. Drever JM, Hodson-Walker NJ: Immediate breast reconstruction after mastectomy using a rectus abdominis myodermal flap without an implant. Can J Surg 1982;25:429-431.

8. Drever JM: The lower abdominal transverse rectus abdominis myocutaneous flap for breast reconstruction. Ann Plast Surg 1983;10:179-185.
9. Koshima I, Soeda S, Yamasaki M, Kyou J: The free or pedicled anteromedial thigh flap. Ann Plast Surg 1988;21:480-485.
10. Koshima I, Soeda S: Inferior epigastric artery skin flaps without rectus abdominis muscle. Br J Plast Surg 1989;42:645-648.
11. Koshima I, Moriguchi T, Fukuda H, et al: Free, thinned, paraumbilical perforator-based flaps. J Reconstr Microsurg 1991;7:313-316.
12. Koshima I, Moriguchi T, Soeda S, et al: Free thin paraumbilical perforator-based flaps. Ann Plast Surg 1992;29:12-17.
13. Koshima I, Moriguchi T, Ohta S, et al: The vasculature and clinical application of the posterior tibial perforator-based flap. Plast Reconstr Surg 1992;90:643-649.
14. Kroll SS, Rosenfield L: Perforator-based flaps for low posterior midline defects. Plast Reconstr Surg 1988;81:561-566.
15. Zhou G, Qiao Q, Chen GY, et al: Clinical experience and surgical anatomy of 32 free anterolateral thigh flap transplantations. Br J Plast Surg 1991;44:91-96.
16. Itoh Y, Arai K: The deep inferior epigastric artery free skin flap: anatomic study and clinical application. Plast Reconstr Surg 1993;91:853-863, discussion 864.
17. Blondeel PN, Boeckx WD: Refinements in free flap breast reconstruction: the free bilateral deep inferior epigastric perforator flap anastomosed to the internal mammary artery. Br J Plast Surg 1994;47:495-501.
18. Allen RJ, Treece P: Deep inferior epigastric perforator flap for breast reconstruction. Ann Plast Surg 1994;32:32-38.
19. Koshima I, Soeda S: Inferior epigastric artery skin flaps without rectus abdominis muscle. Br J Plast Surg 1989;42:645-648.
20. Blondeel N, Vanderstraeten GG, Monstrey SJ, et al: The donor site morbidity of free DIEP flaps and free TRAM flaps for breast reconstruction. Br J Plast Surg 1997;50:322-330.
21. Angrigiani C, Grilli D, Siebert J: Latissimus dorsi musculocutaneous flap without muscle. Plast Reconstr Surg 1995; 96:1608-1614.
22. Hamdi M, Weiler-Mithoff EM, Webster MH: Deep inferior epigastric perforator flap in breast reconstruction: experience with the first 50 flaps. Plast Reconstr Surg 1999;103:86-95.
23. Blondeel PN: One hundred free DIEP flap breast reconstructions: a personal experience. Br J Plast Surg 1999;52:104-111.
24. Nahabedian MY, Dooley W, Singh N, Manson PN: Contour abnormalities of the abdomen after breast reconstruction with abdominal flaps: the role of muscle preservation. Plast Reconstr Surg 2002;109:91-101.
25. Nahabedian MY, Manson PN: Contour abnormalities of the abdomen after transverse rectus abdominis muscle flap breast reconstruction: a multifactorial analysis. Plast Reconstr Surg 2002;109:81-87, discussion 88-90.
26. Futter CM, Webster MH, Hagen S, Mitchell SL: A retrospective comparison of abdominal muscle strength following breast reconstruction with a free TRAM or DIEP flap. Br J Plast Surg 2000;53:578-583.
27. Kroll SS, Sharma S, Koutz C, et al: Postoperative morphine requirements of free TRAM and DIEP flaps. Plast Reconstr Surg 2001;107:338-341.
28. Kaplan JL, Allen RJ: Cost-based comparison between perforator flaps and TRAM flaps for breast reconstruction. Plast Reconstr Surg 2000;105:943-948.
29. Hallock GG: Anatomic basis of the gastrocnemius perforator-based flap. Ann Plast Surg 2001;47:517-522.
30. Taylor GI, Doyle M, McCarten G: The Doppler probe for planning flaps: anatomical study and clinical applications. Br J Plast Surg 1990;43:1-16.
31. Ahn CY, Narayanan K, Shaw WW: In vivo anatomic study of cutaneous perforators in free flaps using magnetic resonance imaging. J Reconstr Microsurg 1994;10:157-163.
32. Zetterman E, Salmi A, Suominen S, et al: Effect of cooling and warming on thermographic imaging of the perforating vessels of the abdomen. Eur J Plast Surg 1999;22:58-61.
33. Chijiwa T, Arai K, Miyazaki N, et al: Making of a facial perforator map by thermography. Ann Plast Surg 2000;44:596-600.
34. Rand RP, Cramer MM, Strandness DE Jr: Color-flow duplex scanning in the preoperative assessment of TRAM flap perforators: a report of 32 consecutive patients. Plast Reconstr Surg 1994;93:453-459.
35. Verpaele AM, Blondeel PN, Van Landuyt K, et al: The superior gluteal artery perforator flap: an additional tool in the treatment of sacral pressure sores. Br J Plast Surg 1999;52:385-391.
36. Geddes CR, Morris SF, Neligan PC: Perforator flaps: evolution, classification and applications. Ann Plast Surg 2003;50:90-99.
37. Feller AM, Galla TJ: The deep inferior epigastric artery perforator flap. Clin Plast Surg 1998;25:197-206.
38. Kostakoglu N, Kecik A: Deep inferior epigastric artery (DIEA) skin flap: clinical experience of 15 cases. Br J Plast Surg 1998; 51:25-31.
39. Spauwen PHM, Deutman HC, Kauer JMG: The area of transposition of the pedicled deep inferior epigastric perforator flap: an anatomical study. Eur J Plast Surg 1999;22: 234-236.
40. Kroll SS: Fat necrosis in free transverse rectus abdominis myocutaneous and deep inferior epigastric perforator flaps. Plast Reconstr Surg 2000;106:576-583.
41. Guzzetti T, Thione A: Successful breast reconstruction with a perforator to deep inferior epigastric perforator flap. Ann Plast Surg 2001;46:641-643.
42. Keller A: The deep inferior epigastric perforator free flap for breast reconstruction. Ann Plast Surg 2001;46:474-479, discussion 479-480.
43. Keller A: Fat necrosis in free rectus abdominis and deep inferior epigastric perforator flaps. Plast Reconstr Surg 2001;107:1611-1612.
44. Rickard R: TRAM and DIEP flap zones. Br J Plast Surg 2001;54:272-273.
45. Yap LH, Whiten SC, Forster A, Stevenson JH: The anatomical and neurophysiological basis of the sensate free TRAM and DIEP flaps. Br J Plast Surg 2002;55:35-45.
46. Koshima I, Inagawa K, Urushibara K, et al: Deep inferior epigastric perforator dermal-fat or adiposal flap for correction of craniofacial contour deformities. Plast Reconstr Surg 2000;106:10-15.
47. Boyd JB, Taylor GI, Corlett R: The vascular territories of the superior epigastric and the deep inferior epigastric systems. Plast Reconstr Surg 1984;73:1-16.
48. El-Mrakby HH, Milner RH: The vascular anatomy of the lower anterior abdominal wall: a microdissection study on the deep inferior epigastric vessels and the perforator branches. Plast Reconstr Surg 2002;109:539-543, discussion 544-547.
49. Taylor GI, Palmer JH: The vascular territories (angiosomes) of the body: experimental study and clinical applications. Br J Plast Surg 1987;40:113-141.
50. Blondeel PN, Beyens G, Verhaeghe R, et al: Doppler flowmetry in the planning of perforator flaps. Br J Plast Surg 1998;51:202-209.
51. Heitmann C, Felmerer G, Durmus C, et al: Anatomical features of perforator blood vessels in the deep inferior epigastric perforator flap. Br J Plast Surg 2000;53:205-208.
52. Allen R, Guarda H, Wall F, et al: Free flap breast reconstruction: the LSU experience (1984-1996). J La State Med Soc 1997;149: 388-392.
53. Koshima I, Moriguchi T, Soeda S, et al: The gluteal perforator-based flap for repair of sacral pressure sores. Plast Reconstr Surg 1993;91:678-683.

54. Allen RJ, Tucker C Jr: Superior gluteal artery perforator free flap for breast reconstruction. Plast Reconstr Surg 1995;95:1207-1212.
55. Allen RJ: The superior gluteal artery perforator flap. Clin Plast Surg 1998;25:293-302.
56. Ao M, Mae O, Namba Y, Asagoe K: Perforator-based flap for coverage of lumbosacral defects. Plast Reconstr Surg 1998;101:987-991.
57. Blondeel PN: The sensate free superior gluteal artery perforator (S-GAP) flap: a valuable alternative in autologous breast reconstruction. Br J Plast Surg 1999;52:185-193.
58. Salmon M: Arteres de la peau. Paris, Masson et Cie, 1936.
59. Salmon M: Arteries of the Skin. Taylor G, ed. London, Churchill Livingstone, 1988.

CHAPTER

148

Postmastectomy Reconstruction: Alternative Free Flaps

L. FRANKLYN ELLIOTT, MD, FACS ✦ PATTI BERGEY, PA-C

Breast cancer continues to be a disturbingly common problem in the United States. Despite earlier diagnosis by increasingly sophisticated detection techniques, a number of patients still must choose mastectomy for treatment of breast cancer for reasons that are familiar to everyone. Therefore, successful techniques in breast reconstruction are extremely important to women. Fortunately, these methods have expanded during the past 2 decades and offer an array of choices to the reconstructive plastic surgeon and to the patient.

Autogenous tissue techniques remain the method of choice in terms of naturalness and long-term result. However, there are patients who prefer to use breast implants for postmastectomy reconstruction to avoid incisions in other areas and to have a faster recovery from the initial operation. Unfortunately, breast implants for reconstruction often require second and third operations to achieve a satisfactory result to the patient and almost never match the naturalness that is achieved with autogenous tissue techniques in the long term.

The transverse rectus abdominis myocutaneous (TRAM) flap is the first choice for autogenous tissue breast reconstruction after mastectomy. However, there are a number of clinical settings wherein autogenous tissue reconstruction is desired but the TRAM flap is not the best choice. An obvious clinical example is the patient with either a previous TRAM flap or an abdominoplasty. Whereas success has been claimed in performance of a secondary TRAM flap or TRAM flap after previous abdominoplasty, this is not recommended. First, there is usually not enough tissue left to construct a second breast. Second, either of these operations has transected all the perforators of the abdominal wall, making a second TRAM flap unreliable in terms of tissue perfusion and survival.

Another clinical setting for avoiding the TRAM flap is the markedly obese patient. Several studies have been published to attest to the higher incidence of complications associated with morbid obesity and TRAM flap use.[1,2] These should be heeded. Furthermore, in the markedly obese patient, there is usually adequate fat deposition in the area of the latissimus. This allows an autogenous latissimus breast reconstruction to form a large breast, with generally lower operative morbidity (Fig. 148-1). Morbid obesity is only one of the significant risk factors in performing a TRAM flap. Other risks include smoking history, diabetes, vasculitis, and scars on the abdomen. Whereas some of these factors militate against the performance of free flap transfer, scars on the abdomen in association with other risk factors might deter the surgeon from use of the TRAM flap specifically.

A final consideration is the body habitus of the patient. Some patients are particularly lacking in fat deposition in the TRAM flap distribution but do have adequate fat deposition in other locations (Fig. 148-2). This type of patient was the initial stimulus for the development of free tissue transfers from the hip and lateral thigh locations. The patients must be willing to accept a scar, but the concern about a scar is often decreased when they understand that the unwanted fullness can be aesthetically improved.

For these reasons, alternative free flaps are indicated for breast reconstruction in those patients desiring autogenous tissue breast reconstruction. The most successful sites for free tissue transfer have been the gluteal free flap, the Rubens free flap (deep circumflex

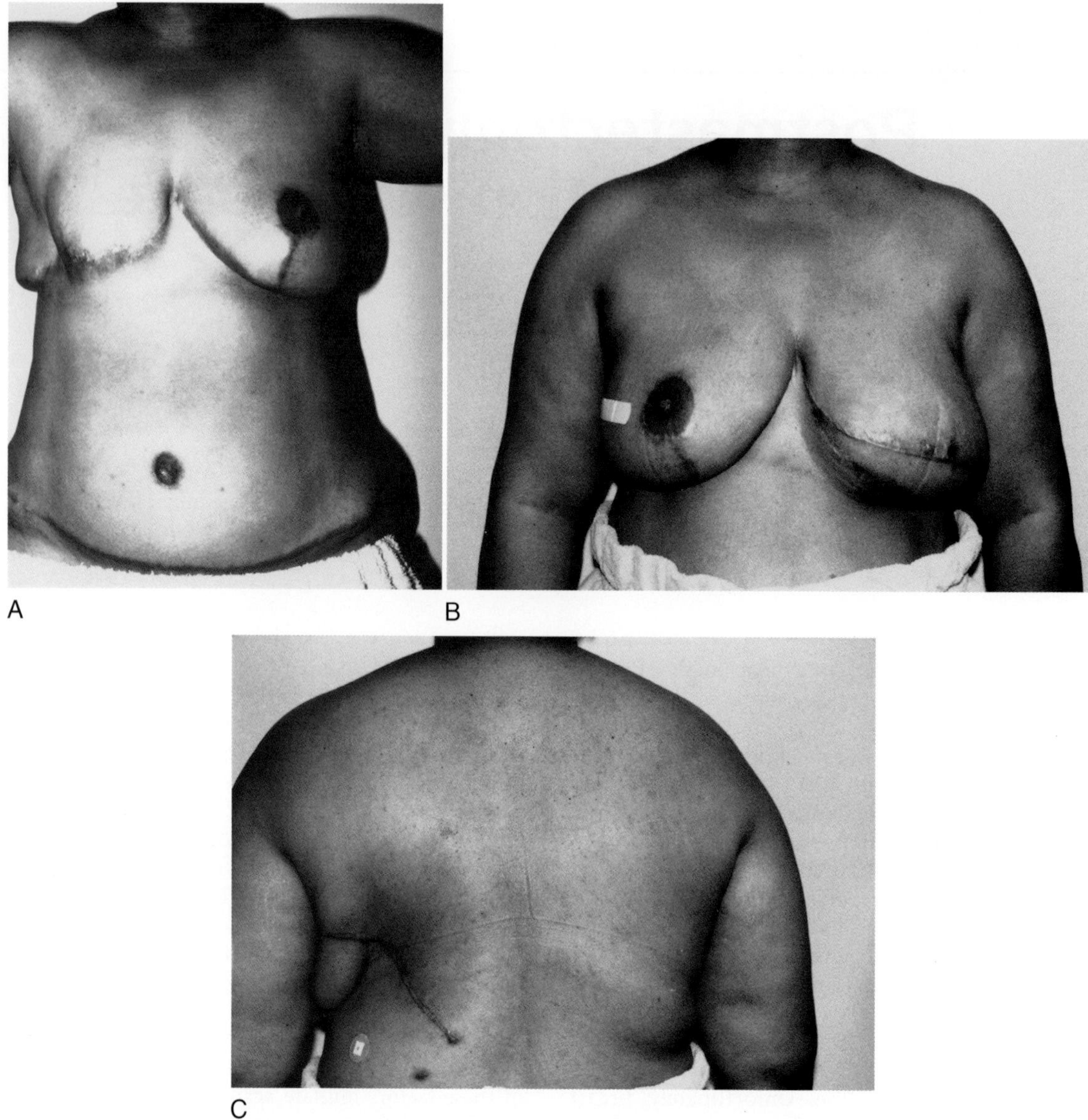

FIGURE 148-1. A 42-year-old patient after unsuccessful right free TRAM flap and left mastopexy. *A,* Frontal view. *B,* One year after secondary reconstruction of the left breast with autogenous latissimus myocutaneous flap. *C,* Donor site 1 year postoperatively.

iliac artery), and the lateral transverse thigh flap (LTTF).

Any of these flaps can be used in either the immediate or the delayed situation. However, in general, the skin islands are not as extensive for any of these flaps as they are for TRAM flaps. For this reason, the use of these flaps in the delayed situation must be carefully evaluated with regard to the amount of skin needed to achieve an aesthetically pleasing breast reconstruction. This is usually not a problem with immediate reconstruction by skin-sparing technique.

The indications for alternative free flaps for breast reconstruction can be the same in either the immediate or the delayed setting. There is really no difference in preoperative preparation in either setting. Blood transfusions are rarely needed, and patients are not routinely required to set aside autologous blood before their operation. This is true even in the performance of simultaneous bilateral reconstructions. However, as mentioned, skin needs must be carefully assessed because skin islands are much more limited with these alternative sites than in the TRAM flap site.

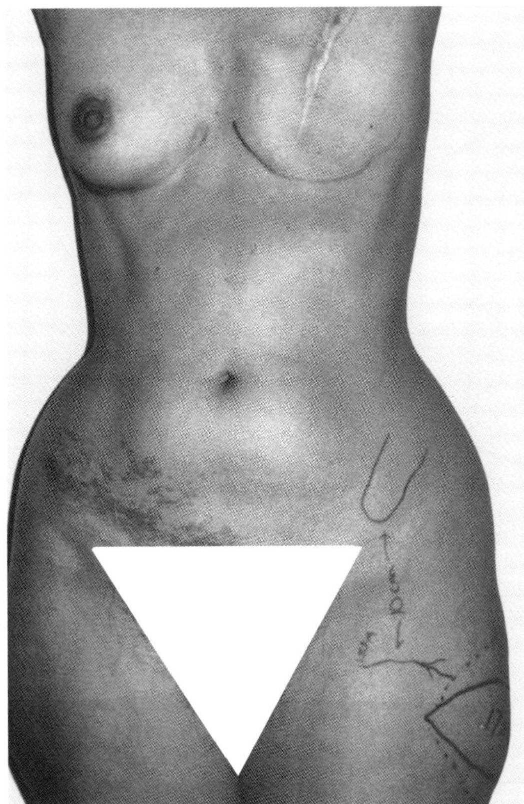

FIGURE 148-2. A 39-year-old patient for breast reconstruction demonstrating little or no TRAM tissue but adequate tissue in the locations of the Rubens and lateral transverse thigh flaps.

The preferred vascular recipient sites are dictated by previous operations and by the type of flap being used for transfer. In almost all delayed situations, use of the internal mammary vessels is preferred. It is best to avoid prolonged dissection in the axilla to isolate the thoracodorsal vessels. These vessels can be encased in considerable scar and, because of this, may lack the length one would anticipate in the immediate, unscarred situation. Thus, because of scarring and difficulty in dissection, the internal mammary vessels are preferred if the axilla has been previously dissected.

Furthermore, the flaps have characteristics that dictate the use of one vascular pedicle over the other. For instance, the gluteal perforator flap is normally characterized by a pedicle of 3 to 4 cm. However, the vessels are usually located centrally under the flap, and the artery is normally of the small caliber of 1 to 2 mm. Because of the location of the perforator and its size, use of the internal mammary vessels is preferred when a shorter length is required to reach the vessels and an end-to-side anastomosis to the internal mammary artery obviates concerns about size discrepancy. On the other hand, both the Rubens flap and the LTTF have longer pedicles of 6 to 8 cm located peripherally on the flap (Fig. 148-3). These vessels easily reach the axilla and permit a versatile placement of the flap onto the chest wall for breast shaping. In the immediate setting, the thoracodorsal vessels are preferred for both the Rubens flap and the LTTF because, in general, they are freshly dissected and readily available. However, in the delayed situation or one in which the pedicle length may not be adequate, we do not hesitate to use the internal mammary vessels.

The technique for dissection of the thoracodorsal vessels is well known. For exposure of the internal mammary vessels, the cartilaginous portion of the third or fourth rib is resected at its junction with the sternum. Only one rib segment is usually removed after dissection off the perichondrium. The vessels are then readily found just deep to the posterior perichondrium but superficial to the pleura.

Monitoring of these flaps can be a problem if no skin island is left for observation. For this reason, even

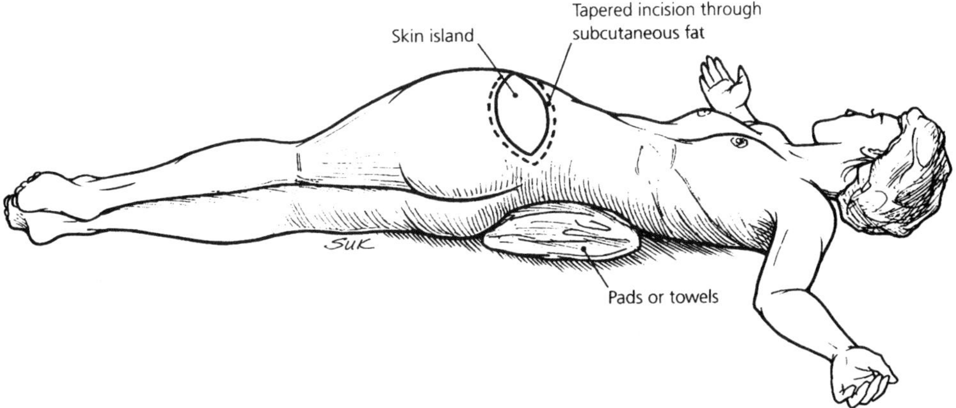

FIGURE 148-3. Illustration of operative positioning for harvest of Rubens flap. (From Kroll SS: The Rubens fat pad free flap. In Kroll SS: Breast Reconstruction with Autologous Tissue. Art and Artistry. New York, Springer-Verlag, 2000:201.)

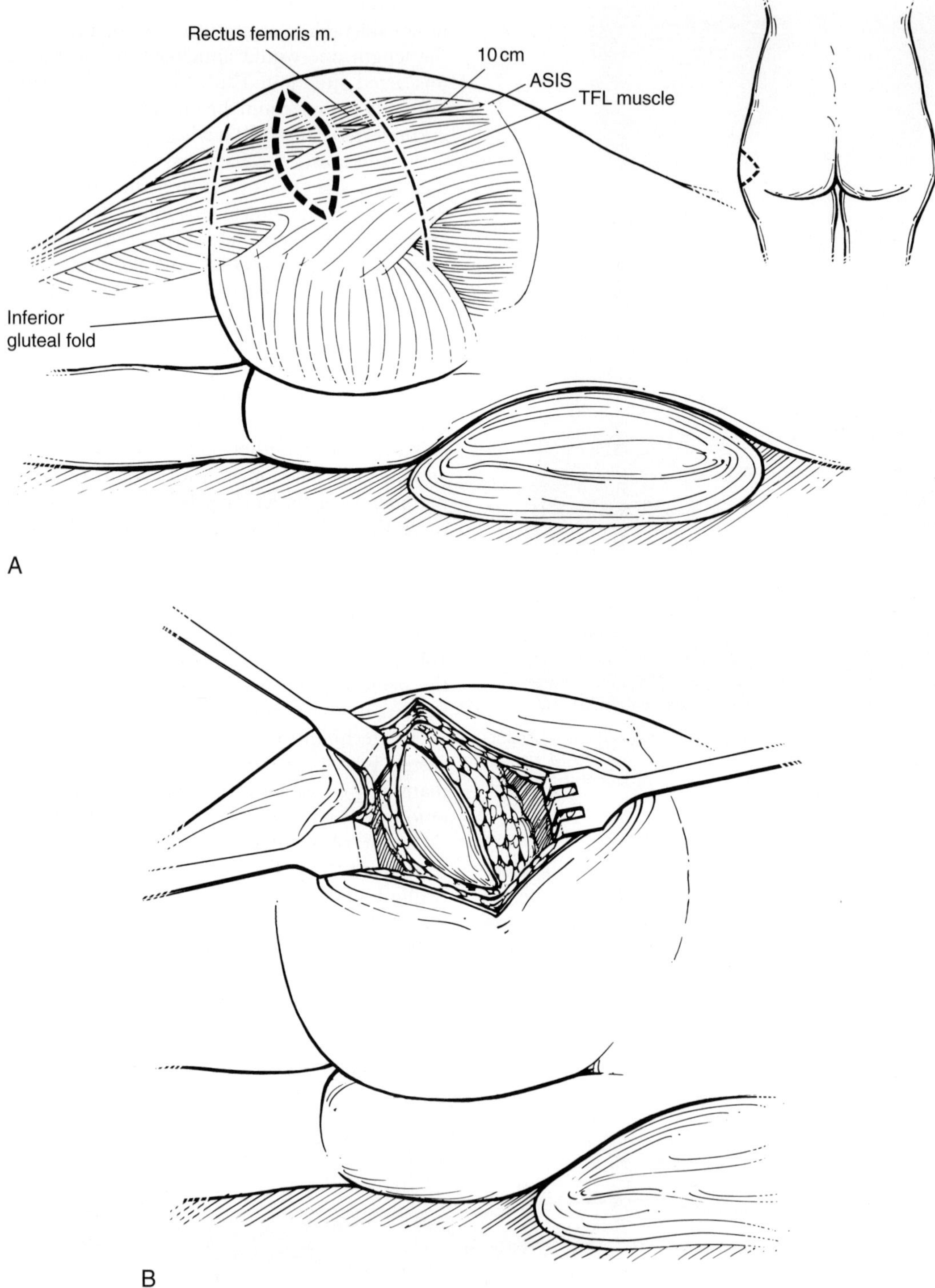

FIGURE 148-4. *A,* Illustration of positioning for harvest of LTTF flap. *B,* Illustration of right LTTF dissection. ASIS, anterior superior iliac spine; TFL, tensor fascia lata.

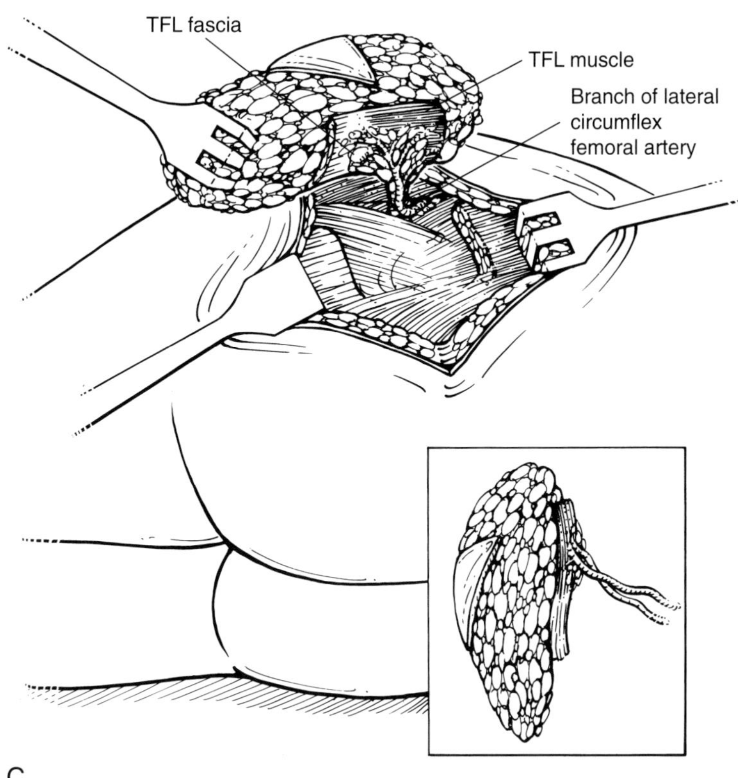

FIGURE 148-4, cont'd. *C,* Illustration of elevated LTTF flap. Inset demonstrates peripheral location of long vascular pedicle of dissected flap. Note division superiorly of TFL muscle and inferiorly of TFL fascia.

in the setting of adequate or excess native skin of the chest wall, a small skin island is always left for monitoring. Monitoring is done by the physician or a trained team of nurses who look for color, temperature, and palpable differences in the flap. Another handy device is the cutaneous Doppler probe. This probe can be applied directly to the skin island, and a perforator can often be detected and thus checked periodically. If the thoracodorsal vessels are used, the laser Doppler probe supplied by the vascular laboratory can be used to document patency of both the artery and the vein. Any changes are treated immediately with return to the operating room for exploration.

FLAP TECHNIQUES

Lateral Transverse Thigh Flap

The LTTF idea was first suggested by Carl R. Hartrampf, Jr. It was then investigated in cadaver injections to determine fat and cutaneous distribution of the blood flow through the lateral circumflex femoral artery. A postulate that blood flow through the lateral circumflex femoral artery would immediately perfuse the "saddlebag" tissues was confirmed. It was well known that this vessel perfused the tensor fasciae latae (TFL) muscle, the vastus lateralis through its descending branch, and fat and skin islands over these muscles. The variation for the LTTF was use of a transverse fat and skin island instead of a vertical one down the thigh.[3,4] The lateral circumflex femoral artery arises off either the common femoral or profundus femoral artery and travels laterally deep to the rectus femoris muscle, providing branches to it as well as subsequent descending branches to the vastus lateralis and branches to the TFL muscle. There are also direct perforators to the skin, but these are relatively small. Most of the branches to the fat overlying the greater trochanter and in the area of maximum projection of the upper lateral thigh come through the TFL muscle as perforators. Fat can be harvested posteriorly to the lateral gluteal region, inferiorly some 5 cm inferior to the greater trochanter, superiorly toward the iliac crest, and anteriorly to the lateral border of the rectus femoris (Fig. 148-4). The surgical technique involves placement of the patient with the side being operated on slightly elevated on a beanbag (see Fig. 148-4). Before positioning, the point of maximum projection is marked on the lateral thigh; the flap borders are marked peripherally out from this point to harvest adequate fat for the proposed breast size. The location of the lateral circumflex femoral vessels can reliably be predicted 10 cm caudad to the anterior superior iliac spine. A line between that level and the inferior gluteal fold is drawn, generally defining the incision line. A skin island of 5 to 7 cm in vertical height with a varying length, depending on the chest needs, is designed along this line. The chest area is first prepared by recreating the breast dimensions and isolating the chosen vascular pedicle.

The flap is then dissected by incising the skin island and dissecting away from this skin island in a beveled manner to shape the flap as it is elevated (see Fig. 148-4*B*). One encounters the TFL muscle superiorly and the TFL fascia inferiorly. The dissection can then be brought up posteriorly, transecting the muscle superiorly and the fascia inferiorly. Further elevation of the flap reveals the entry of the lateral circumflex femoral artery into the posterior TFL muscle. Once this is identified, dissection continues just lateral to the rectus femoris muscle so that the vessels are isolated. Side branches are ligated and divided, and the pedicle is dissected as far under the rectus femoris muscle as length is needed for vascular anastomosis. The flap is then divided and transferred.

Possible pitfalls in the elevation of this flap include harvesting of too little fat, not keeping enough fat or skin over the TFL muscle to ensure adequate perforators, and not dissecting adequate length on the lateral circumflex femoral vessels. All of these can be avoided by careful planning and certainly are reduced by experience.

The donor site is generally closed after the flap has been revascularized. Time should be spent in quilting the closure with deep sutures to obliterate the dead space. This helps alleviate persistent and sometimes massive seromas in the donor site. Quilting does cause more of a significant deformity apparent at the time of operation and initially thereafter in the postoperative period. However, this depression can be treated successfully at the time of nipple-areola reconstruction by a revision with a pants-over-vest secondary closure along with liposuction, both cephalad and caudad to the operative site.

Long-term evaluation of this flap indicates a more projecting fat structure than that of the usual TRAM flap. There has been essentially no disability secondary to the harvesting of the TFL muscle, and few if any pain syndromes are associated with this flap harvest. Shaping of the breast is simple, and it tends to have slightly more projection than that of the TRAM flap if it is used on the opposite side (Fig. 148-5).

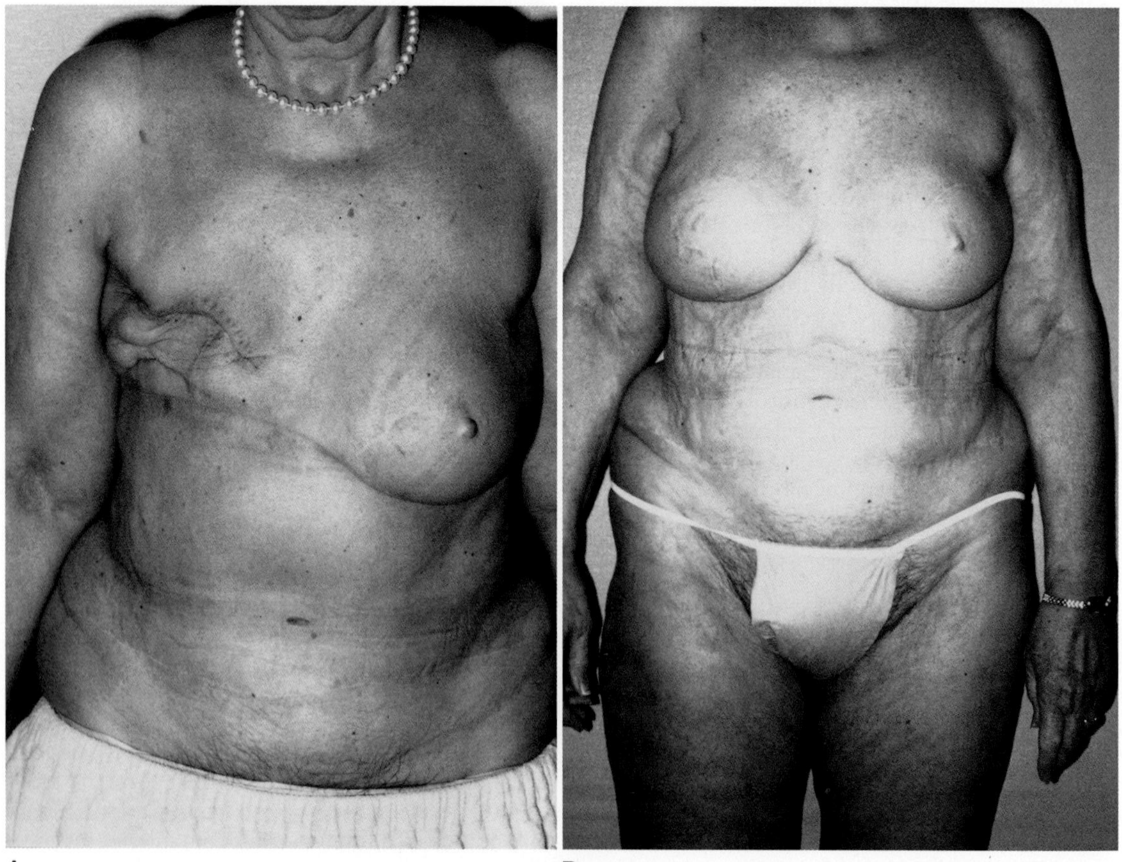

FIGURE 148-5. *A,* Two years after reconstruction of the left breast with pedicled TRAM flap and two months after right mastectomy. *B,* One year after right LTTF and 3 years after left pedicled TRAM flap. Note comparable projection of the two flaps and donor deformity on right lateral thigh.

Rubens Flap

The Rubens flap is the iliac crest flap popularized by Ian Taylor[5] but without the bone. This flap is based on the deep circumflex iliac vessels.[6] The vessels are usually isolated first by a dissection similar to that of a hernia repair. Once the vessels are isolated, elevation of the flap follows, including periosteum of the iliac crest.

The surgical technique involves first marking the patient in a standing position, outlining the fat that one proposes to take in view of the desired breast size. The incision usually extends from just lateral to the midline out to the posterior axillary line. The skin island is located just above the iliac crest, usually at the area of maximum prominence of fat in the hip region (Fig. 148-6). A TRAM flap or abdominoplasty has often been performed previously so that the medial part of this incision is in an old scar. The authors have not found that either of these operations prevents the successful performance of a Rubens flap by interrupting perforators to the skin and fat.

The patient is placed on the table with the hips slightly elevated on a beanbag (see Fig. 148-4). The chest is prepared as described before with exposure of the vascular pedicle. Once the pedicle has been chosen and is found to be appropriate, attention is turned to the abdomen, where the medial portion of the incision is made, extending to the anterior superior iliac spine. Dissection through the external oblique, internal oblique, and transversalis is necessary to reveal the deep inferior epigastric vessels. Preperitoneal fat is retracted superiorly, and the deep circumflex iliac vessels can be found arising from near the origin of the deep inferior epigastric vessels. A sterile Doppler probe may be of some use in locating these vessels in the more obese patient. The vessels travel laterally toward the anterior superior iliac spine, and one must begin to harvest fat and skin at this point because this is where the perforators begin. These perforators penetrate through the external oblique, internal oblique, and transversalis muscles, so a segment of these muscles must be included in the elevation of the flap (Fig. 148-7).

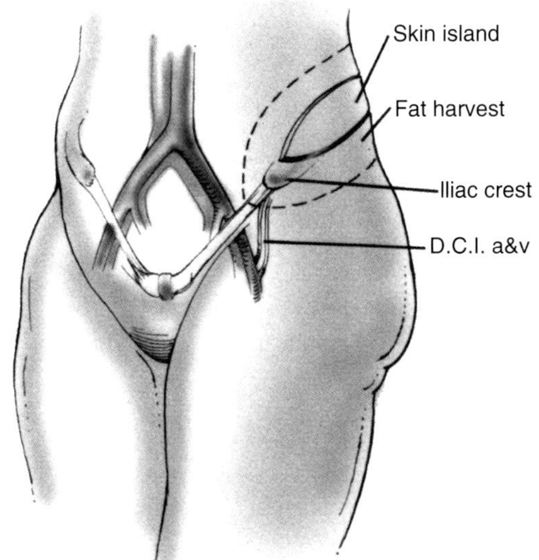

FIGURE 148-6. Illustration of Rubens flap demonstrating location of skin island and incision sites. DCI, deep circumflex iliac.

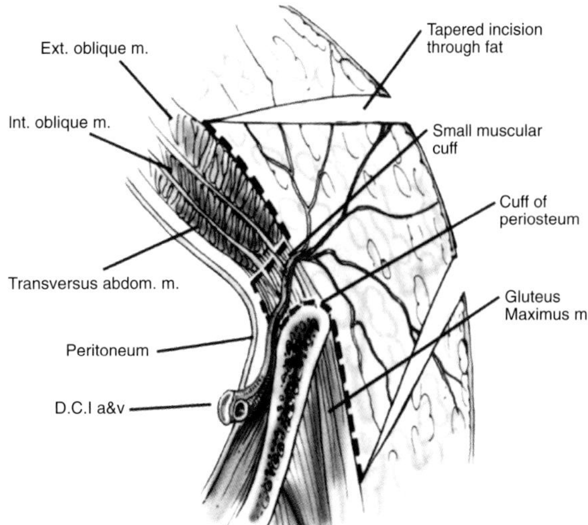

FIGURE 148-7. Illustration of details of Rubens free flap dissection. Dotted line demonstrates lines of flap dissection, incision through oblique musculature, and elevation over the iliac crest. DCI, deep circumflex iliac.

The skin island is incised and the amount of fat to be included in the flap defined by beveling out over the flap inferiorly, posteriorly, and superiorly. Inferiorly, the fat is elevated up to the iliac crest, and the periosteum is incised on its inferior border. Posteriorly, the flap is elevated to the posterior superior iliac spine; superiorly, the fat is developed down to within 2 cm of the iliac crest, exposing the external oblique muscle. All three layers of muscle are incised from the anterior superior iliac spine posteriorly some 5 to 6 cm toward the posterior superior iliac spine. The continuation of the deep circumflex iliac vessels is found just cephalad to the iliac crest. It can be tracked and identified with the intraoperative Doppler probe. Once incisions through these muscles have been completed, the flap is elevated off the iliac crest in a subperiosteal plane beginning on the inferior border. The flap is now completely freed up as an island and its transfer can be completed.

The muscle closure of the donor site must first be completed. Closure of the donor site is relatively tedious, but if it is left until after the flap has been vascularized, it will lead to retraction of the abdominal muscles and a more difficult closure. To avoid subsequent abdominal calamities, a secure closure of the three layers of muscle down to the iliac crest is imperative. Drill holes with K-wires are used to suture the internal oblique and transversalis muscles to the iliac crest with 0 polypropylene sutures. This is accomplished by use of mattress sutures in an interrupted manner. It is generally not possible to suture the muscles to the soft tissue of the iliac crest as this has been elevated with the flap. Once closure is completed to the iliac crest and continued to the midline, as in a hernia repair, the external oblique can be closed over this in a second layer. This closure generally does not require drill holes into the iliac crest because the external oblique can be sutured to soft tissue caudad to the iliac crest. Drains are then placed, and the skin is closed routinely.

The flap is then revascularized and the breast shaped.

Pitfalls in the elevation and transfer of this flap can include dissection too close to the deep circumflex iliac vessels in the superior position; inadequate dissection of the deep circumflex iliac vessels to their origin, leading to diminutive lumens; and inadequate harvesting of fat for flap volume. There is a fine line in terms of how much of the three abdominal muscles is harvested between ease of closure of the abdominal wall and adequate vascularity of the flap itself. The further one narrows the amount of muscle harvested, the easier the closure will be but the more one limits possible perforators to the flap itself. The appropriate width of harvested muscle seems to be 2 cm, but this must be done by transecting the muscle above the iliac crest before the periosteum is freed from the crest; reversing this order releases the muscle from the crest and accordions the whole muscle segment, thereby increasing the chance of injury to the vessels. Adequate fat harvest comes with proper planning and experience. The vessels must be dissected to their origin because it is only at the origin that both the artery and vein are of appropriate size to facilitate subsequent end-to-end anastomosis. Specifically, the artery is usually 2 to 3 mm and the vein can be 3 to 4 mm. This is generally true only if the vessels are followed completely to their origin.

The trim patient may have more trouble with the donor site because coverage of the denuded iliac crest is not as thick. These are probably not the best patients for whom to choose the Rubens flap, and another choice is preferred. Otherwise, if the muscles are repaired securely, problems with Rubens flap donor sites are few. In fact, when the Rubens flap is performed bilaterally, donor sites can leave the patient with improved contour in the hip region compared with preoperatively, without any postoperative revisions (Fig. 148-8).

Long-term evaluation of the Rubens flap suggests that its fat is similar to that of the TRAM flap with slightly less projection but certainly a soft result. These evaluations do hold up with time, similar to the result with the TRAM flap (Fig. 148-9).

Gluteal Flap

The gluteal free flap, as it is performed today, has two dominant characteristics. First, it is a perforator flap. Second, it is based on perforators of the superior gluteal vessels. Originally described by Allen and Tucker[7] and referred to as the superior gluteal artery perforator free flap, it will often yield excellent results. The inferior gluteal pedicle is not recommended because it flattens the inferior buttock unnaturally, involves dissection around or near the sciatic nerve, and results in a scar on which the patient must sit. The use of the superior gluteal pedicle actually results in a buttock lift, avoids dissection near the sciatic nerve, and places the scar higher on the buttock, thus allowing the patient to sit without difficulty. The perforator technique is essential to achieving a longer pedicle, a more appropriately sized pedicle, and essentially no muscle morbidity.

The flap is outlined in the superior buttock region, again with skin and fat elements designed according to what is needed on the chest (Fig. 148-10). Preoperative Doppler evaluation may be used for location and assessment of the size of the perforators. However, the authors have not found this to be of significant accuracy and prefer to locate the largest perforators intraoperatively during the dissection.

The flap can be dissected with the patient in the lateral position, but more commonly, the patient is placed totally prone after the chest has been dissected and the vessels have been located and prepared. The prone position gives the best exposure circumferentially around the flap as it is elevated and is easiest for the surgeon. This is important because the perforator dissection can be somewhat tedious.

The flap is dissected by first incising the skin island and then beveling out peripherally to harvest adequate fat. Once the gluteus muscle is encountered peripherally around the flap, the flap can be elevated from lateral to medial. One should begin looking for perforators approximately 4 cm lateral to the lateral sacral border. Dissection is performed with either a knife or micro-bipolar cautery. Two or three choices can usually be found, and the larger is selected. The perforator is dissected down between the muscle fibers for 2 to 3 cm before a decision is made as to the optimal perforator. Two or more perforators can be chosen, but this adds to the complexity and length of the technique and does not seem necessary as far as flap perfusion is concerned. The perforator is dissected completely through the muscle with use of loupe magnification. It can be dissected further toward the foramen to increase the size of the artery or vein. The vein is usually 4 mm at this point and can easily be

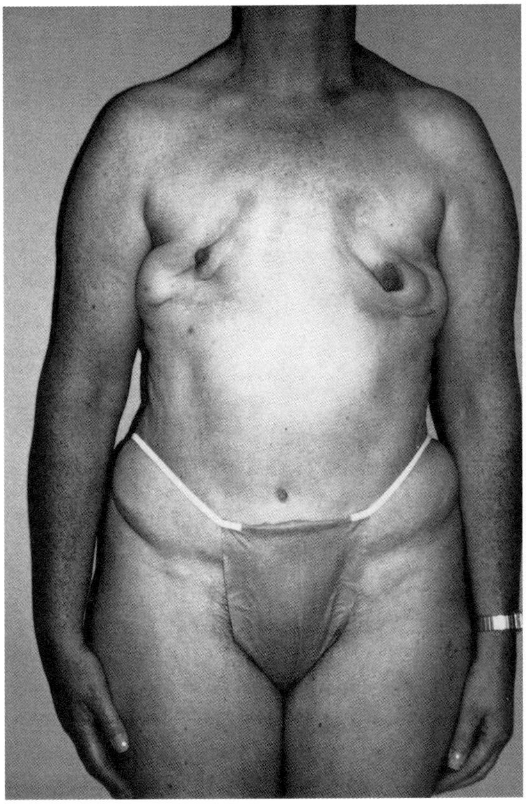

A

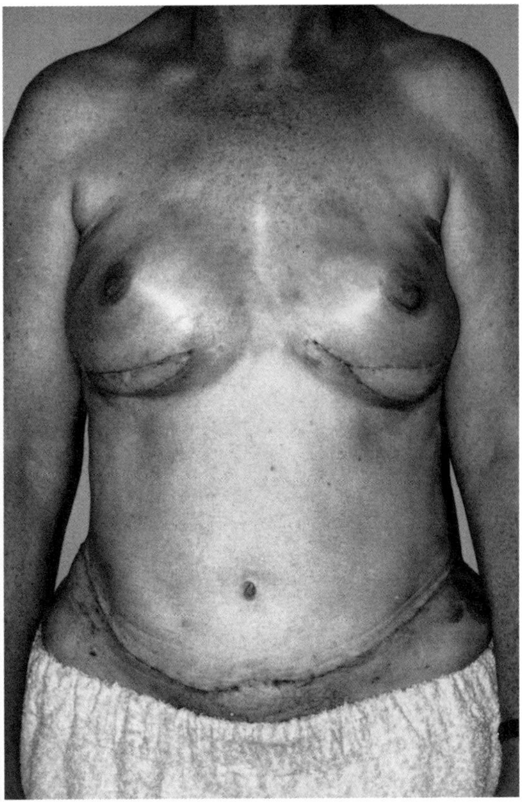

B

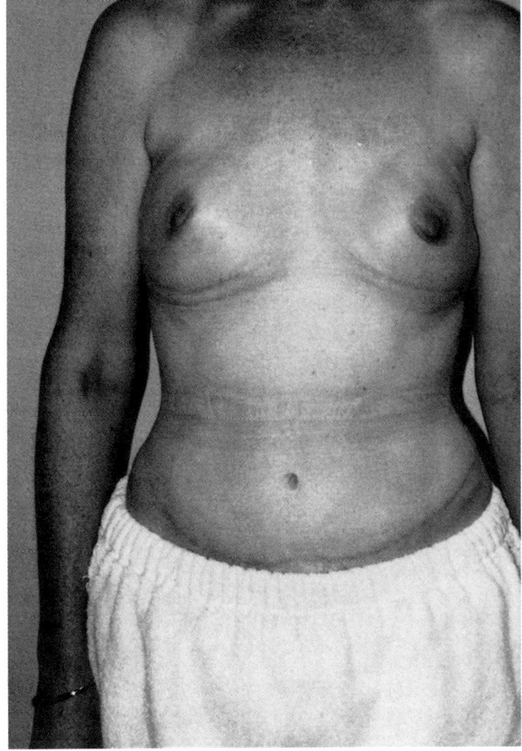

C

FIGURE 148-8. A 41-year-old patient after bilateral prophylactic mastectomies, unsuccessful reconstruction attempted with bilateral implants, and subsequent implant removal. *A,* Preoperative view. *B,* Three months after bilateral Rubens flap reconstruction. Note improved contour. *C,* Two years after bilateral Rubens reconstruction. Note continued improved waist contour.

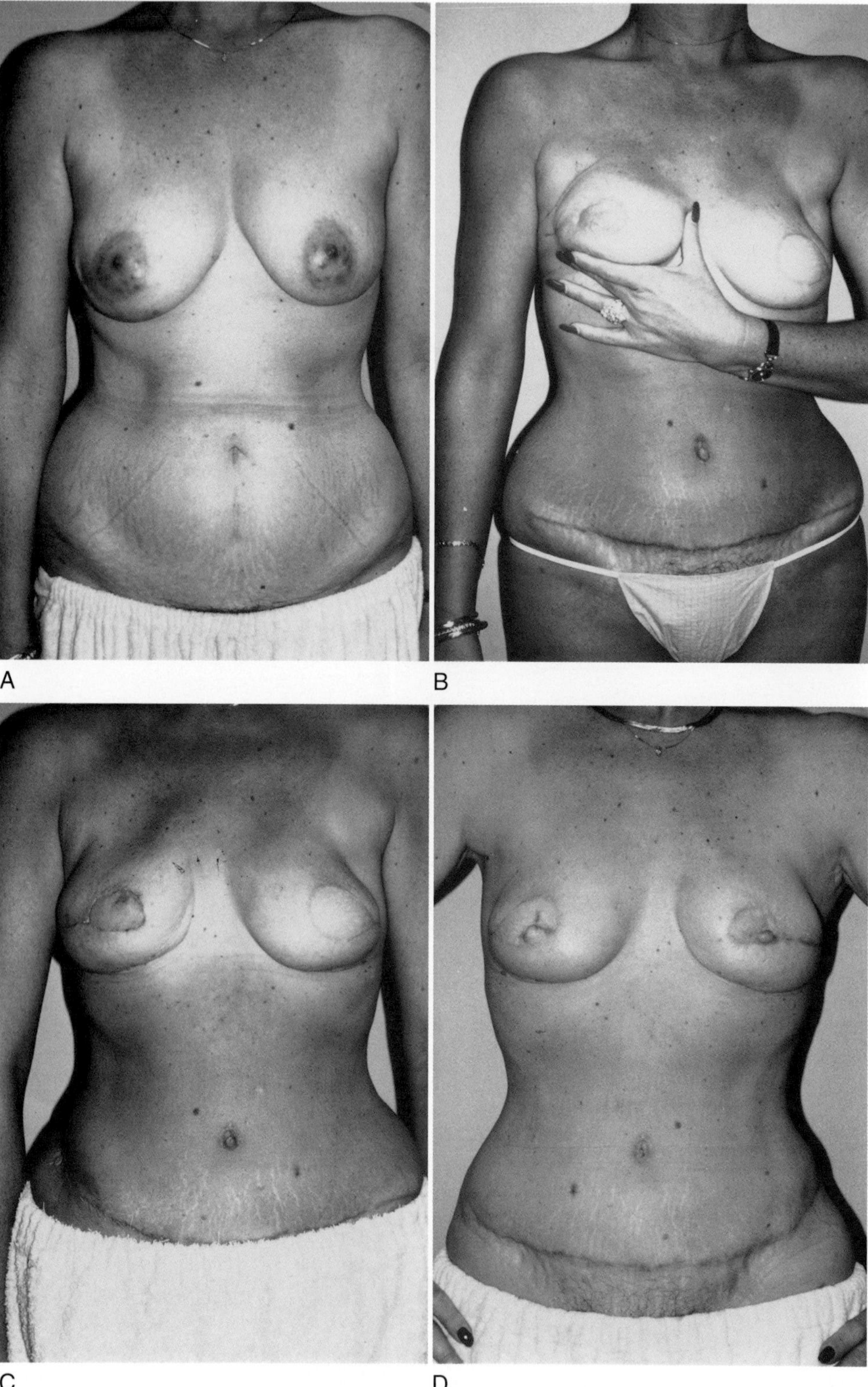

FIGURE 148-9. A 48-year-old patient for bilateral mastectomy and bilateral pedicled TRAM flap reconstruction. *A,* Preoperative view. *B,* Postoperative view at 8 months with diffuse fat necrosis and firmness of right breast reconstruction. *C,* Two months after removal of right TRAM flap and secondary reconstruction with right Rubens flap. *D,* Seven months after right Rubens reconstruction and balancing procedure on left hip.

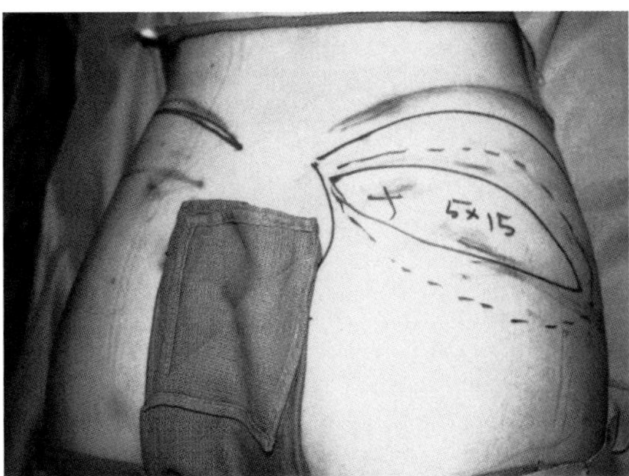

FIGURE 148-10. Design of right free gluteal perforator flap. Solid lines indicate skin island; dotted lines indicate fat harvest.

anastomosed to the internal mammary vein. The artery is small, about 1 mm. It will enlarge if it is dissected further, but this becomes increasingly difficult.

When bilateral gluteal transfer is performed, which is usually done simultaneously, the flaps are not divided until both are elevated. At that time, both are divided, the donor sites are closed rapidly, the patient is repositioned in a supine position, and the flaps are alternately revascularized.

If there is more than a 1.5 to 1.0 size discrepancy between the internal mammary artery and the gluteal perforator artery, an end-to-side anastomosis is performed. This usually involves a 1.0- to 1.5-mm perforator gluteal artery and can be somewhat challenging. It is preferable to use 10–0 nylon for this anastomosis. The veins are usually of matching size and generally are 3 mm or more.

There are many possible pitfalls. Each step of the operation in itself is not difficult, but putting them all together without error requires intense concentration. This is one of the more difficult free flaps to perform. Patience is required to identify and to isolate the proper perforator in dissection of the fat off the gluteus muscle. Dissection of the perforator down to its origin requires microcautery of several branches. Bleeding at the base of the gluteus muscle can be difficult to control and may cause damage to the perforator itself. Finally, anastomosis to the internal mammary vessels does not usually allow a second try. This is a free flap that continues to require microsurgical technique akin to that of a finger replantation.

The closure of the donor site is straightforward. It is usual that a depression is left in the superior gluteal region. However, this does resolve some on its own but is readily treated by a pants-over-vest secondary revision, which gives a buttock lift and is usually appreciated by the patient. Bilateral cases have good buttock symmetry, but in the instance of unilateral harvest, liposuction of the opposite buttock with or without skin removal is indicated (Fig. 148-11).

Long-term evaluation of the gluteal flap reveals that the fat projection is similar to that of the LTTF. It is a more cohesive flap than the Rubens or the TRAM flap. Shaping requires little maneuvering other than to place the flap on the chest wall and to close the skin.

COMPARISON OF FLAP TECHNIQUES

All three flaps have a place in treatment of patients who desire autogenous tissue breast reconstruction in whom the TRAM flap is not the best or first choice. The LTTF should probably be limited to those patients who have a significant and bothersome accumulation of fat in the lateral thigh. The scar is the most visible of the three; thus, the price the patient must pay for the LTTF harvest is compensated for only if the contour is significantly improved. The vascularity is good, however, and the technical performance of the flap is probably the most straightforward of the three. Donor site closure is easy and flap projection is good.

The Rubens flap is usually chosen if the patient's fat accumulation is dominant in the hip area. This is often the case in patients who have had previous abdominoplasty or a TRAM flap because the abdomen has been tightened but the hip area is often left untreated. As mentioned, harvest for bilateral Rubens flaps can often lead to an improved contour of the waist, truly appreciated by the patient. The flap harvest, however, is more difficult than for the LTTF, and the donor site closure is by far the most difficult of all. The vessels are reliable, long, and usually of adequate caliber. Projection and volume are good, although probably not as good as with the other two flaps. The skin island can probably be the largest of the three choices but still not the size of a TRAM flap skin island. The lateral femoral cutaneous nerve of the thigh does run directly through the harvest site and is always divided in the harvesting of this flap. However, morbidity from this nerve division is rarely noted.

Patients almost always have adequate fat in the gluteal site. This factor and the location of the scar are its most attractive elements. When there is simply not adequate fat in other locations, the gluteal flap will almost always suffice. The donor site is associated with virtually no morbidity except for the contour deformity, which can readily be treated. Indeed, patients have been discharged from the hospital in several instances at 2 or 3 days postoperatively. Lying supine is associated with some pain for a week or so, but sitting is not a problem.

The pedicle makes the gluteal operation difficult. The use of the perforator technique, however, has lengthened the pedicle by dissection of the perforator through the muscle without any muscle attached to it.

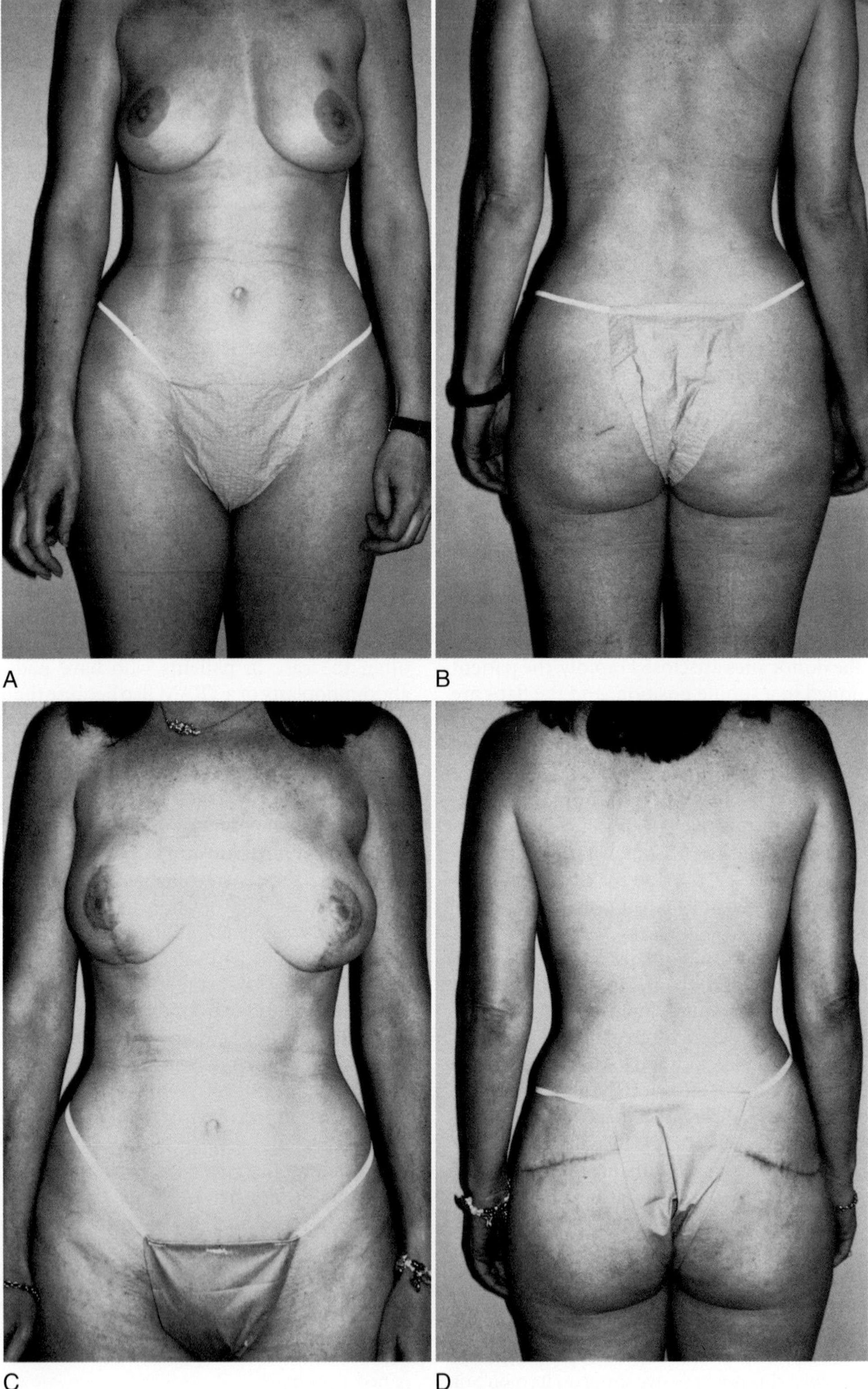

FIGURE 148-11. A 36-year-old patient with premalignant mastopathy for bilateral mastectomy and bilateral immediate reconstruction with free gluteal perforator flaps. *A,* Preoperative frontal view. Note scant abdominal tissue. *B,* Preoperative view of donor sites. *C,* Two months after bilateral free gluteal perforator breast reconstruction, frontal view. *D,* Donor sites at 3 months postoperatively.

This creates a 3- to 4-cm pedicle just by tracing the perforator through the muscle. However, the artery is still small, and to get a larger artery, one must continue down deep to the muscle, where dissection is extremely tedious. If an artery of adequate size can be obtained, end-to-end anastomosis can be performed with the internal mammary artery, converting the operation into a simpler procedure. The fat itself is similar to that of the LTTF and gives excellent projection, which is probably better than with either the Rubens or the TRAM flap.

SUMMARY

Microsurgeons are fortunate to have additional free flap choices for breast reconstruction after mastectomy in those patients who prefer autogenous tissue reconstruction. The TRAM flap remains the first choice, but it cannot be used in a growing number of instances. Each flap truly has its individual indications. Thus, the microsurgeon should be familiar with each of these. Depending on the patient's habitus, one flap may be significantly preferred to the others in each clinical situation. Cadaver dissection of these flaps is a good idea to provide familiarity with the dissection before the clinical application. Obviously, a high level of microvascular capability is required, particularly in the gluteal free flap. Thus, it is probable that these flaps should be applied in a relatively limited number of sites by those who will take the time to familiarize themselves with the anatomy and who maintain a high level of microsurgical expertise and experience.

REFERENCES

1. Kroll SS, Netscher DT: Complications of TRAM flap breast reconstruction in obese patients. Plast Reconstr Surg 1989;84:886-892.
2. Chang DW, Wang B, Robb GL, et al: Effect of obesity on flap and donor site complications in free transverse rectus abdominis myocutaneous flap breast reconstruction. Plast Reconstr Surg 2000;105:1640-1648.
3. Elliott LF: The lateral transverse thigh free flap for autologous tissue breast reconstruction. Perspect Plast Surg 1989;3:80.
4. Elliott LF, Beegle PH, Hartrampf CR: The lateral transverse thigh free flap: an alternative for autogenous tissue breast reconstruction. Plast Reconstr Surg 1990;85:169-178.
5. Taylor GI, Townsend P, Corlett RT: The superiority of the deep circumflex iliac vessels as the supply for free groin flaps. Plast Reconstr Surg 1979;64:745-749.
6. Hartrampf CR, Noel RT, Drozan L, et al: Rubens' fat pad for breast reconstruction: a peri-iliac soft-tissue free flap. Plast Reconstr Surg 1994;93:402-407.
7. Allen RJ, Tucker C Jr: Superior gluteal artery perforator free flap for breast reconstruction. Plast Reconstr Surg 1995;95:1207.

CHAPTER

149

Secondary Reconstructive Surgery: Mastopexy and Reduction

DAVINDER J. SINGH, MD ✦ R. BARRETT NOONE, MD, FACS

Reduction mammaplasty, one of the most common operations in plastic surgery, has produced excellent aesthetic and physical benefits for patients. Numerous studies have reported the overall satisfaction of patients after reduction mammaplasty.[1,2] Despite the improvement and evolution in techniques for this surgery, secondary surgery may be indicated infrequently to correct unfavorable results and complications such as size discrepancies, nipple asymmetry, fat necrosis, and hypertrophic scarring.[3-7]

In addition, the breast will often undergo changes after the initial surgery that are related to weight gain or alterations associated with pregnancy, menopause, and medications, resulting in an unsatisfactory condition for the patient. A small percentage of these patients may present for repeated reduction mammaplasty. Secondary surgery may also be needed for management of breast neoplasms after reduction mammaplasty and treatment of ptosis several years after a breast reduction.

Regardless of the indication for surgery, a second operation is generally psychologically distressing to the patient and may be a financial burden because third-party insurance coverage is a problem. Consequently, the surgeon is faced with the challenges not only of correcting the deformity but also of guiding the patient through a delicate situation.

MANAGEMENT OF THE PATIENT

Psychology and Patient-Physician Rapport

Although most women who undergo reduction mammaplasty are pleased with the results, those who experience complications or secondary hyperplasia can be difficult to manage.[8] The surgeon or a psychiatrist or psychologist should address the psychological aspects of the change in body image, the recurrence of symptoms, and the patient's guilt if weight gain is the cause of an unfavorable result. On occasion, a successful result may be interpreted differently by the patient and the surgeon.

Some patients may experience hostility toward the surgeon because of the physical, emotional, and economic burden the secondary surgery places on them.

Some surgeons may have difficulty managing these patients because of a lack of training or experience and should consult a psychiatrist or psychologist.

The surgeon should also be cognizant of the influence on the patient of third parties such as spouses, family members, and friends and include them in the discussions if the patient so desires. Most important, the patient must be prepared for the psychological sequelae of secondary surgery and for the potential for another complication or unfavorable result.

Medicolegal Considerations

Patients presenting for secondary surgery for rehypertrophy or complications pose medicolegal dilemmas. They may be involved in litigation with the original surgeon and may have heightened, unrealistic expectations from their second surgeon. Eleven percent of plastic surgeons who responded to a questionnaire stated that a dissatisfied patient had sued them at least once after a reduction mammaplasty.[8-10]

To establish realistic expectations and to avoid litigation, it is imperative to obtain informed consent from the patient after explaining the potential results, risks, and complications of secondary surgery. This consent is an opportunity for the surgeon to develop a rapport with the patient as well. Surgeons should include a caveat for the possibility of surgical revision in their initial consents for primary reduction mammaplasty. This early explanation of possible problems enables most patients to cope better with a complication if it occurs.

Once the surgeon and patient have established a rapport and informed consent has been given, the surgeon should obtain the patient's permission for communication with the previous surgeon and for records of operations and preoperative photographs to help obtain optimal results. Photographs before secondary surgery are essential for planning and for medicolegal documentation.

TREATMENT OF UNFAVORABLE RESULTS AND COMPLICATIONS

Scars

The scarring from reduction mammaplasty remains an aesthetic problem, and many different surgical techniques have evolved to minimize the scars.[11,12] Most patients are accepting of the scars; however, hypertrophic scars are displeasing to both the patient and the surgeon and are the most common cause of litigation after reduction mammaplasty (Fig. 149-1).

Preoperative education is key in preparing the patient for wound healing difficulties and possible hypertrophic scarring. A thorough history of previous operations and wound healing should be obtained, and all measures to prevent hypertrophic scarring should be taken. Some causes are infection, suture extrusion, tension on closure, and skin necrosis with healing by second intention. Hypertrophic scars are most commonly located in the inframammary fold and laterally.

Many hypertrophic scars will improve with time and need no treatment. However, symptomatic scars (i.e., pruritic, tender, painful) necessitate intralesional steroid injections (Fig. 149-2). The recommended dose of triamcinolone (40 mg/mL) is spaced at 6-week intervals for two or three cycles. The patient should be aware of the potential for skin discoloration, atrophy, or skin depression with these injections. If intralesional injection of steroids fails and the patient is still disturbed by the scarring 1 year after surgery, surgical revision may be attempted. Surgery is not always successful and may result in further hypertrophy. Compression and massage can help reduce the extent of the recurrence. Silicone gel sheeting has been described as a treatment for scar hypertrophy.

Widened scars may result from flap necrosis secondary to skin tension. The most common location for this is the T junction between the medial and lateral flaps and along the vertical limb. Skin edge necrosis should be allowed to heal by second intention. Although the scar may be widened, revision is rarely needed because the scar is asymptomatic and hidden beneath the ptotic breast.

A frequent postoperative complaint, especially with larger reductions, is the manifestation of dog-ears both medially and laterally when a discrepancy exists between the lengths of the superior and inferior flaps. These dog-ears are often seen laterally, and every attempt should be made to eliminate them at the initial surgery by closing from the end of the wound toward the middle (Fig. 149-3). Some rippling or pleating may result but is inconspicuous and will resolve in a few months. If a dog-ear is unavoidable, it should be observed and allowed to mature for 9 to 12 months before revision.

Fat Necrosis

Fat necrosis is seen more commonly in obese patients undergoing reduction mammaplasty and usually occurs at the end of the pedicle, with or without skin or nipple loss.[8] It may present early postoperatively with the patient experiencing elevated temperatures and localized induration and tenderness. Most areas of fat necrosis spontaneously resolve in a few months but may also present with drainage of yellowish, fatty fluid, often through the vertical limb incision.

If a mass is symptomatic or persists beyond a few months, an imaging study should be performed with subsequent needle or excisional biopsy. The patient

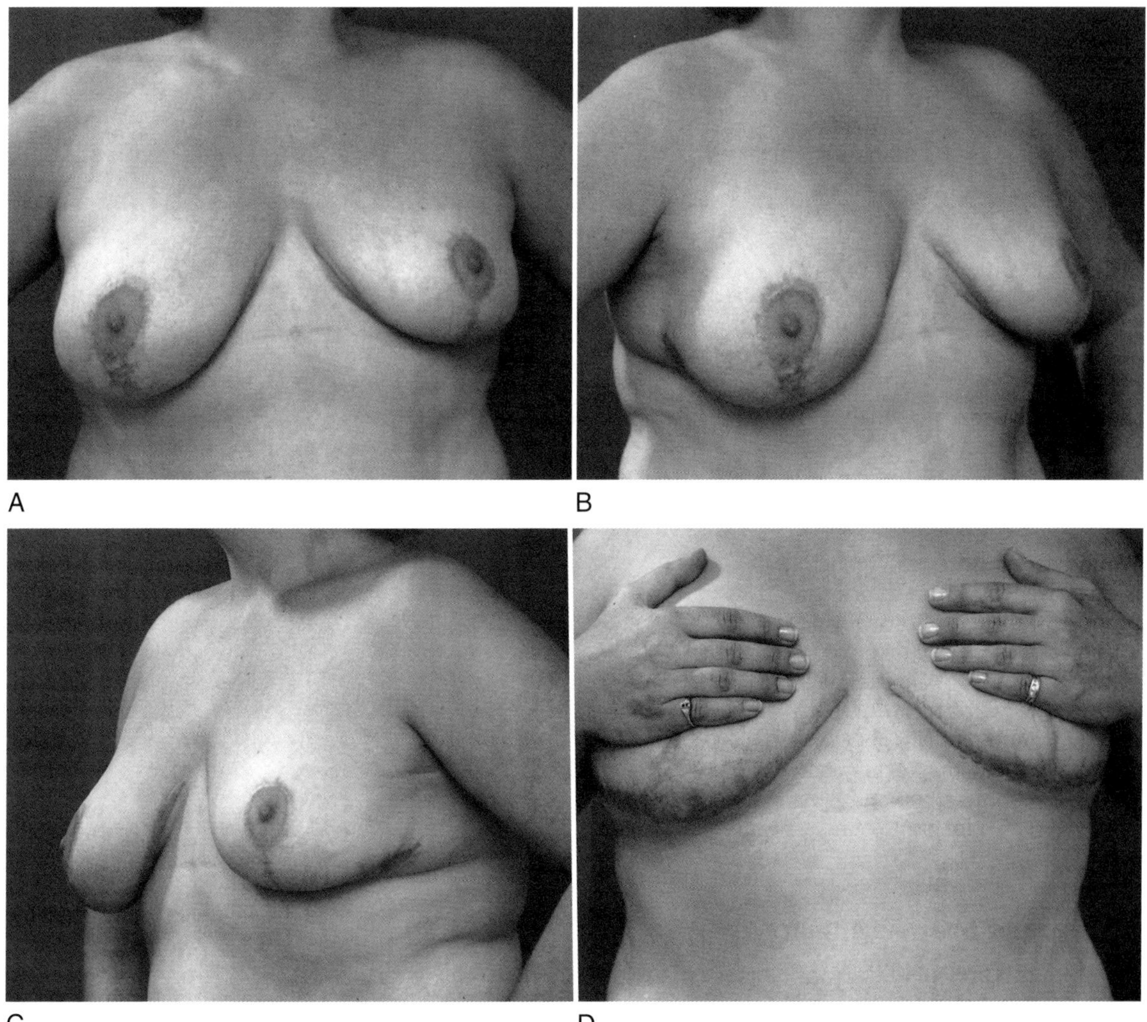

FIGURE 149-1. *A* to *C*, A 32-year-old woman 7 months after bilateral breast reduction. She complained of asymmetry secondary to underreduction of the right breast and hypertrophic scars. *D*, Reduction mammaplasty of the right breast was repeated 18 months after initial surgery.

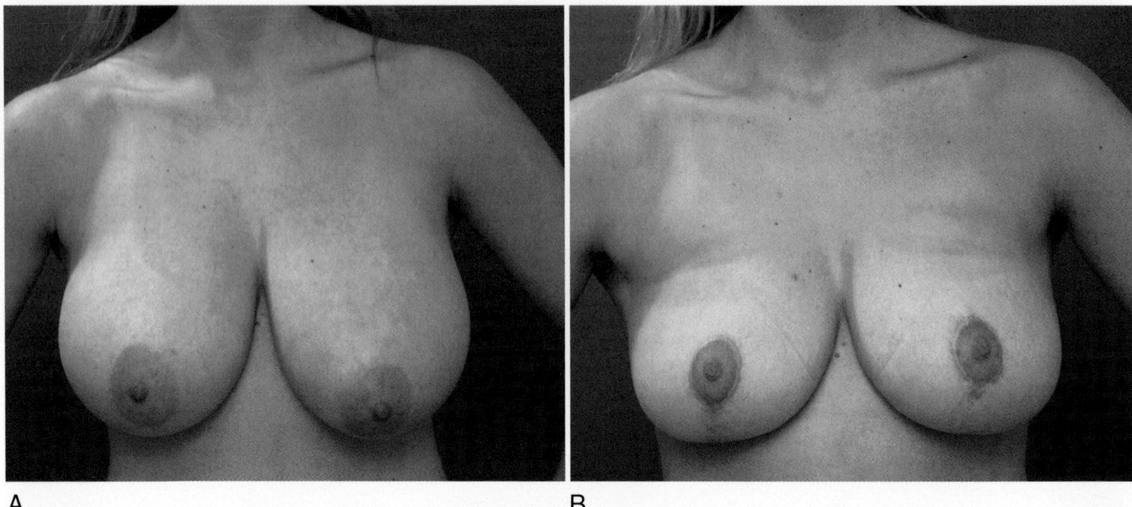

FIGURE 149-2. *A,* An 18-year-old woman with macromastia who underwent reduction mammaplasty. *B,* Resultant hypertrophic scars. She received triamcinolone injections.

should be advised of potential mammographic changes secondary to fat necrosis.

Wound Dehiscence

Wound dehiscence is not frequently seen unless there is excessive tension on the closure or vascular compromise of the flaps. It usually occurs at the T of the inframammary fold or in the vertical limb. Most small areas will heal with limited débridement and local wound care with wet-to-dry dressings or a topical antibiotic ointment (Fig. 149-4). If necrosis is extensive, the patient may experience chronic pain and discomfort from granulation tissue, and revisional surgery with skin grafting may be needed (Color Plate 149-1).

Breast and Scar Asymmetry

Many patients present initially with breast and nipple asymmetry, but some are unaware of it. This should be addressed with the patient during preoperative evaluation because the asymmetry may have an impact on postoperative results. Significant skin flap discrepancies between the breasts result in varying scar length. Also, delayed ptosis may develop differentially on the larger breast that was reduced.

Reoperation for symmetry problems should be delayed for 18 to 24 months because the breasts and scars undergo changes postoperatively with the healing process. Secondary procedures to treat breast asymmetry sometimes require operations on both breasts. More often, though, reduction of the larger of the breasts and reshaping of the skin envelope are adequate for achieving symmetry. When an asymmetric breast is initially treated, the nipple should be set slightly lower on the side to be revised rather than to match the normal side. This allows the nipple elevation that occurs as the skin flaps heal and contract.[5]

If the nipple locations are symmetric and the skin flaps and scars are asymmetric, correction can be performed without disturbing the nipple-areola complex. This can be accomplished by either skin resection or de-epithelialization and inversion of the dermal pedicle if size adjustment is indicated. Liposuction alone may be adequate in improving size asymmetry and can frequently be done as an outpatient procedure.

Overreduction

Overreduction is a difficult problem that generally occurs in three different situations. The first is the older woman with marked ptosis, in which most of the breast tissue is well below the inframammary fold.[8] In these patients, it is helpful to develop an inferior pedicle that is ample to provide upper pole fullness with the patient in a sitting position.

Overreduction may also be seen in situations in which the surgeon promises the patient a certain "cup size" or attempts to meet the weight requirements of resected tissue for insurance coverage (Fig. 149-5). On the initial consultation, a breast size should not be guaranteed.[10] The patient should be assured that her desires are understood.

Breast reduction in the adolescent may lead to hyperplasia a few years after surgery, even in the absence of pregnancy and lactation. This may be disconcerting

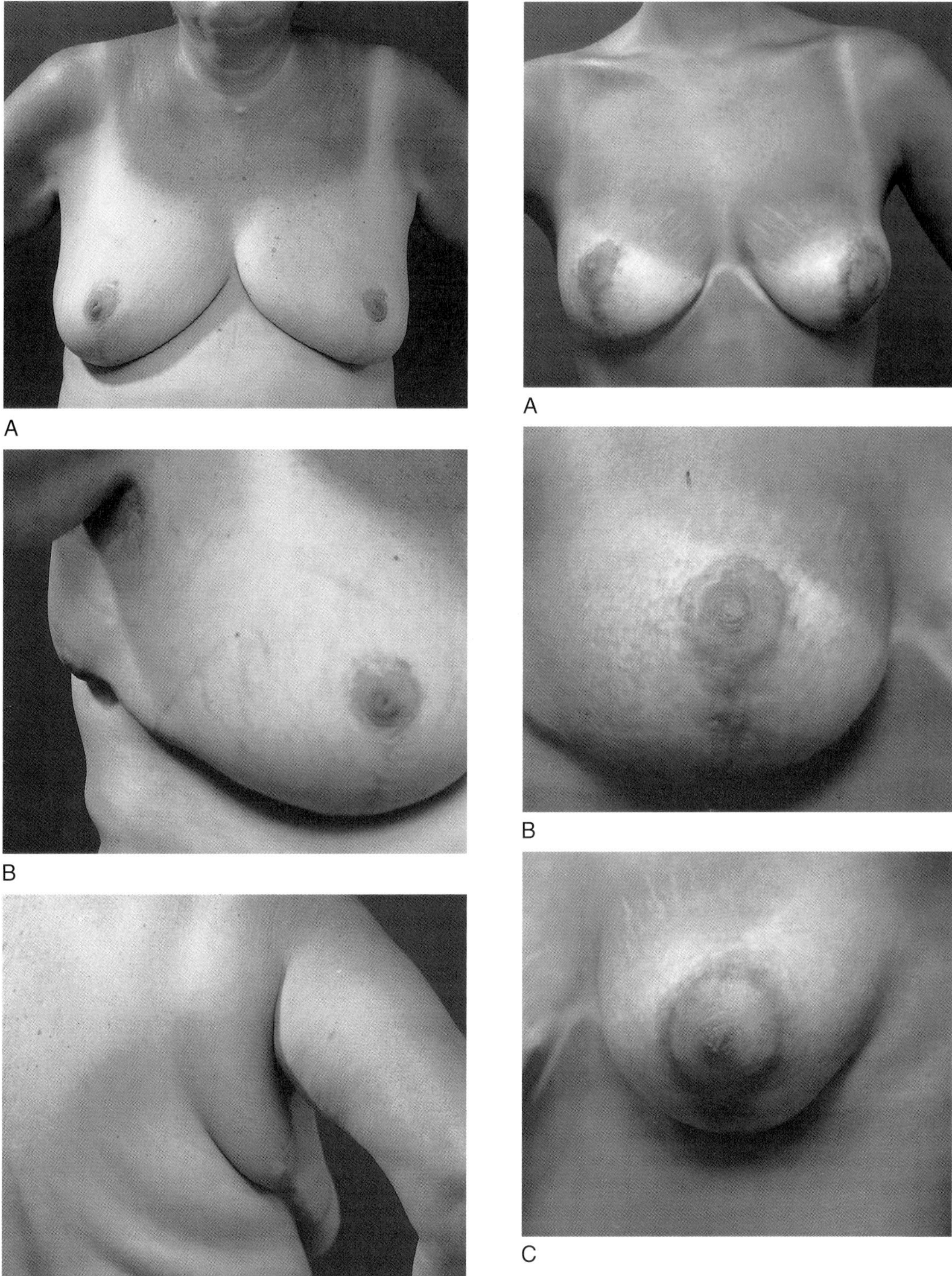

FIGURE 149-3. *A,* A 45-year-old woman 12 months after bilateral reduction mammaplasty. *B* and *C,* Patient presented with a complaint of dog-ears laterally.

FIGURE 149-4. *A* to *C,* An 18-year-old woman evaluated 3 months after bilateral reduction mammaplasty. She presented with a complaint of scars resulting from delayed healing secondary to wound dehiscence of the vertical component. The patient was advised to allow maturation of scars for 6 to 12 months before revision.

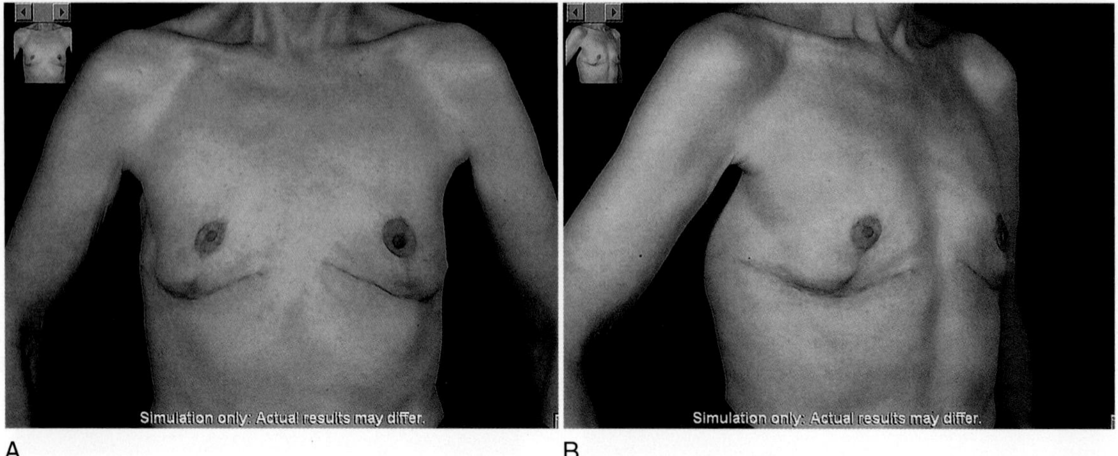

FIGURE 149-5. *A* and *B*, A 49-year-old woman 5 months after reduction mammaplasty. Photographs illustrate overreduction. The patient underwent reconstruction 7 months later with silicone gel mammary prostheses.

to the young patient, who may then wish to have augmentation.

In general, underreduction is much easier to treat than overreduction, which can be addressed only by augmentation. Delaying secondary surgery for 9 to 12 months is appropriate. The psychological and medicolegal implications of secondary surgery with augmentation should be well understood by the surgeon. The patient should understand the problems and complications of breast implants before embarking on the surgery.[8]

The patient may have a more pleasing result with augmentation and mastopexy, and this should be emphasized to the patient. Augmentation may be performed in either the submammary or submuscular position, depending on nipple-areola location and ptosis. If the postreduction patient who becomes hypoplastic demonstrates mammary ptosis, it is best to augment in the submammary plane. Techniques and implant selection are essentially the same in the postreduction patient and in the de novo breast augmentation patient.

Underreduction

Inadequate reduction is a troublesome issue for the patient and consequently the surgeon (see Fig. 149-1). Even though the surgeon may be satisfied with the overall result, he or she will need to address the issue with a patient who is psychologically difficult and perceives her initial complaint of macromastia to persist. She carries with her the body image of macromastia and may be unrealistic in her expectations.[13]

The patient notes most issues of inadequate reduction in the early postoperative period. Immediate revision should be avoided because the breast will undergo changes in size as the swelling resolves and the wounds heal during the first 6 to 12 months. Only then can an assessment be made about final breast size. Most surgeons delay secondary reduction for 18 to 24 months if the patient presents to the same surgeon. They generally employ the same surgical technique as in the first surgery (Fig. 149-6).

Techniques for inadequate reduction are essentially the same as for treatment of rehypertrophy. Debate as to the appropriate technique during secondary surgery has arisen and is discussed later with treatment of rehypertrophy.[14-16]

Nipple-Areola Problems

RECONSTRUCTION AFTER NIPPLE NECROSIS

Nipple necrosis is a devastating complication for the patient and should be discussed as a possibility in the informed consent (Fig. 149-7). Several preventive methods have been described for avoidance and treatment of nipple ischemia. This chapter addresses the secondary treatment of established nipple necrosis.

When necrosis is apparent and systemic antibiotics have been administered, surgical judgment should be employed for débridement of the nipple or pedicle (Fig. 149-8). Often, only partial nipple loss will occur, and débridement is limited to the nonviable areas. Depending on the extent of tissue necrosis, the patient may require serial débridement and local wound care with 25% Dakin solution three times a day on an outpatient basis. Once adequate tissue débridement has been achieved, the wound is allowed to heal by second intention.

Reassurance of the patient is essential during this process of wound healing and maturation. Discussion

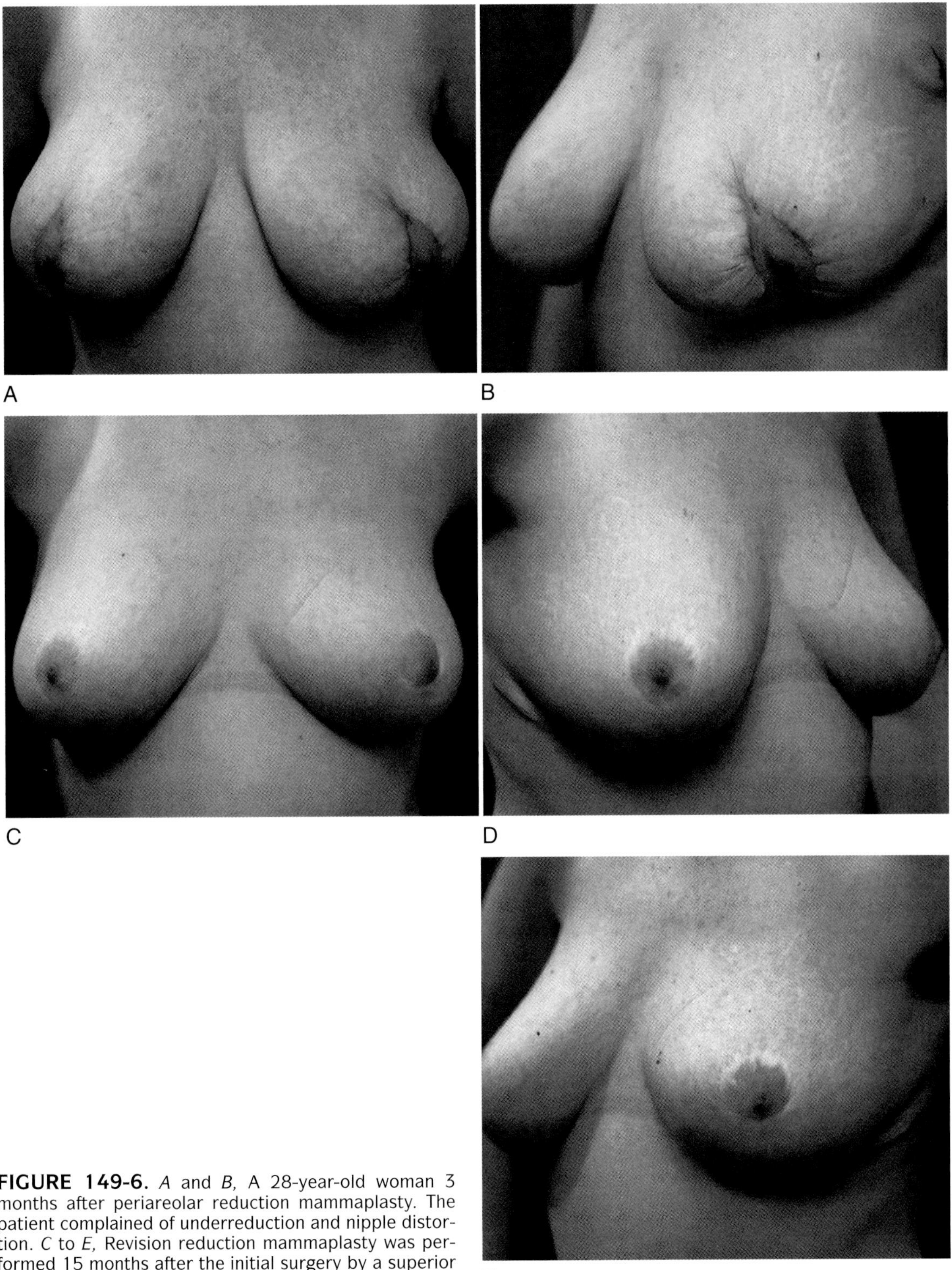

FIGURE 149-6. *A* and *B*, A 28-year-old woman 3 months after periareolar reduction mammaplasty. The patient complained of underreduction and nipple distortion. *C* to *E*, Revision reduction mammaplasty was performed 15 months after the initial surgery by a superior pedicle technique.

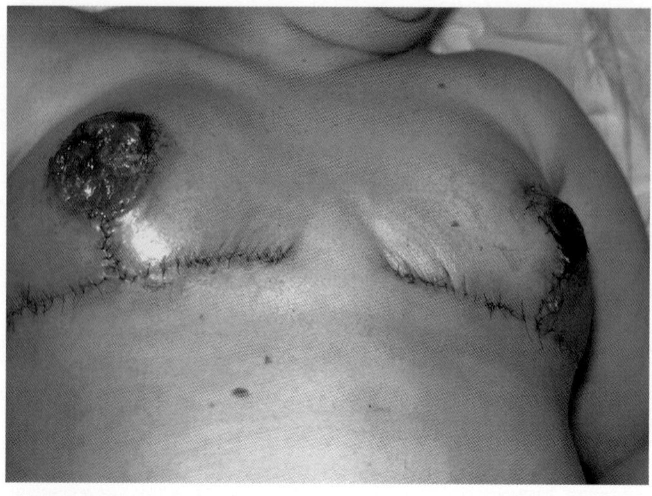

FIGURE 149-7. A 32-year-old woman with bilateral nipple-areola complex necrosis after reduction mammaplasty.

of the surgeon's experience with nipple-areola reconstruction in the breast cancer patient may be appropriate in explaining the options to the patient. Tattooing is often difficult in the chronically scarred tissue, and skin grafting for the areola is more effective. In general, nipple reconstruction after necrosis is delayed for a year after complete healing of the wound.

CORRECTION OF TOO HIGH OR LOW NIPPLE

One of the most common and unfortunate errors in preoperative planning is placement of the proposed nipple-areola complex in a position resulting in a nipple that is too high (Fig. 149-9). The surgeon may notice this in the early postoperative period, but it becomes a more significant problem to the surgeon and the patient later as the tissue in the lower pole of the breast relaxes. This results in a stretching of the skin, which increases the distance between the nipple and inframammary fold. This distance is generally set at 5 cm with the standard patterns and with time stretches into a stable distance of 7 cm. However, in some patients, it is difficult to predict the behavior of the soft tissue, and the final distance is too great. If preoperative planning does not take into account this phenomenon of "bottoming out" and the nipple is placed too high originally, the final result is aesthetically disturbing. Nipples may ride above a bra line or bathing wear and can be irritated by clothing.

Placement of the nipple too high can be avoided by the preoperative marking of the inframammary fold transposed onto the anterior surface of the breast. Obstetric calipers can be used to measure the suprasternal notch to inframammary fold distance, and this can be translated to the anterior breast.

Correction of the nipple placed too high requires repositioning of the nipple at a lower level, with a resultant scar at the present site of the nipple. Lowering can usually be performed with the original pedicle, but it

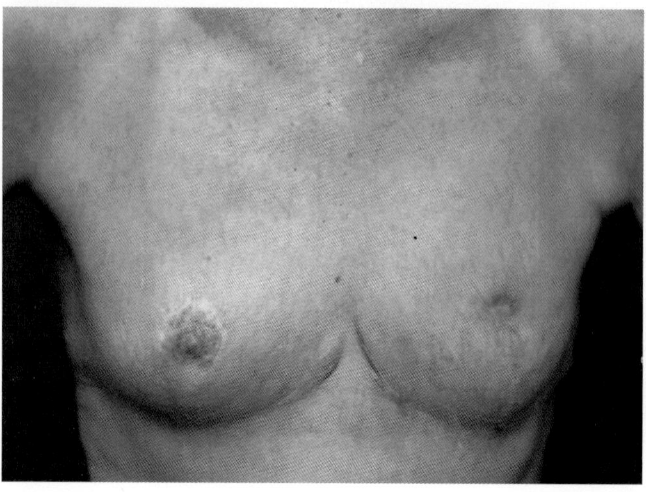

FIGURE 149-8. A 56-year-old woman with history of reduction mammaplasty at age 26 years. The records of her initial surgery were unavailable. She experienced rehypertrophy after weight gain and underwent a second reduction by the inferior pedicle technique. She had postoperative nipple necrosis primarily on the left side. This photograph illustrates the result after débridement and wound care for 9 months. Reconstruction was performed 1 year after secondary reduction with direct nipple revision and full-thickness skin grafts.

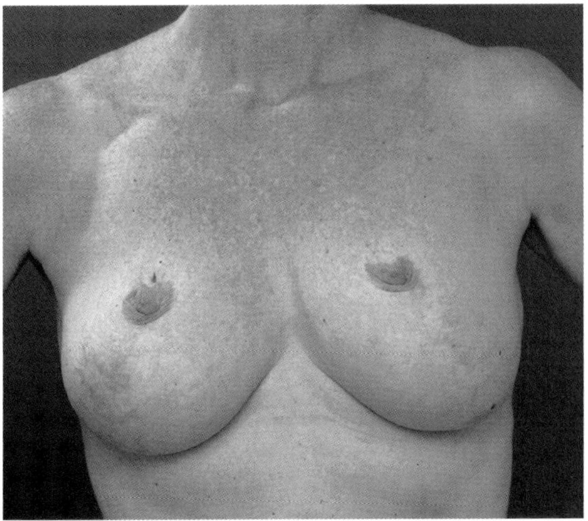

A

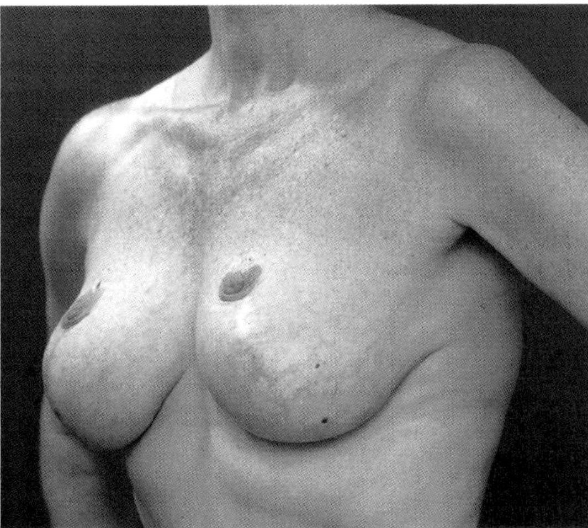

B

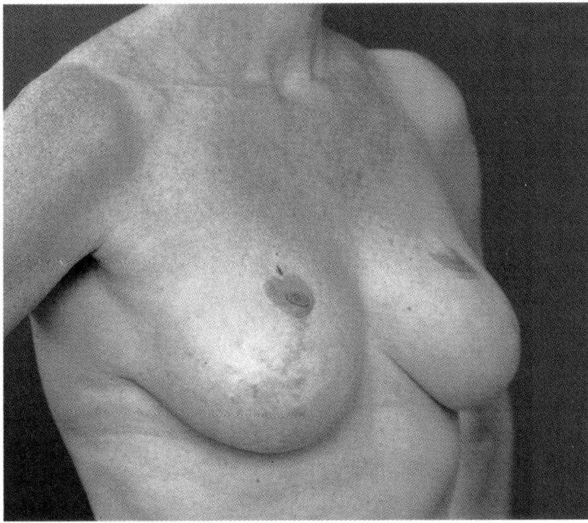

C

FIGURE 149-9. *A* to *C*, A 48-year-old woman after reduction mammaplasty at age 37 years. She complained that the nipple-areola complex was too high and medial. The patient was advised to have transfer of the nipple as a free graft; however, she did not undergo revision.

can also be done as a full-thickness graft. The donor scar from the nipple should be directed obliquely toward the axilla rather than vertically or medially to hide the scar under clothing.[3,5]

If the nipple position is adequate but the distance from the nipple to the inframammary fold is long, some improvement can be obtained by excision of an ellipse of inframammary fold skin. This is essentially a mastopexy on the lower pole of the breast without moving the nipple.

Nipple placement too low may occur because of preoperative misplanning or because of glandular ptosis and nipple ptosis relative to the inframammary fold. This is a relatively easy problem to correct by marking the new nipple position at the inframammary fold and elevating it on a dermal pedicle.

CORRECTION OF NIPPLE CONVERGENCE OR DIVERGENCE

The patient's nipples may have developed eccentrically, either medial or lateral to the line from the midclavicle to the inframammary fold, resulting in natural divergence or convergence. Unless this is recognized and corrected during reduction mammaplasty, there may be accentuated nipple asymmetry (Fig. 149-10; see also Fig. 149-9). These nuances of nipple position may escape the patient and should be discussed preoperatively.

In general, nipple divergence or convergence should be corrected at the time of the original reduction mammaplasty by placing the new nipple on the vertical line from the midclavicle to the inframammary fold. If this is not accomplished intraoperatively, an eccentrically placed nipple will result either unilaterally or bilaterally and be displeasing.

Correction of convergence or divergence can be performed by simple crescent-shaped skin excision on the appropriate side of the nipple if the movement needed is minimal. If greater movement of the nipple is necessary, medial or lateral incisions may be required to preserve the nipple on a dermal pedicle for repositioning. Salema[6] advocated the inferior curved pedicle technique to correct the convergent nipple.

RESIDUAL AREOLA

Residual areola along the vertical limb is unavoidable in certain patients if tension on the skin closure is to be circumvented. This becomes an issue in patients with large areolas with diameters in the range of 6 to 8 cm and when the distance to the new nipple location is short (Fig. 149-11). Patients should be advised of this preoperatively. When the preoperative pattern is placed, the vertical limbs of the pattern may encompass portions of the pigmented areola, and with closure of the limbs, the residual areola appears on either side of the scar of the vertical limb. It is more prudent to leave the residual areola initially instead of excising all

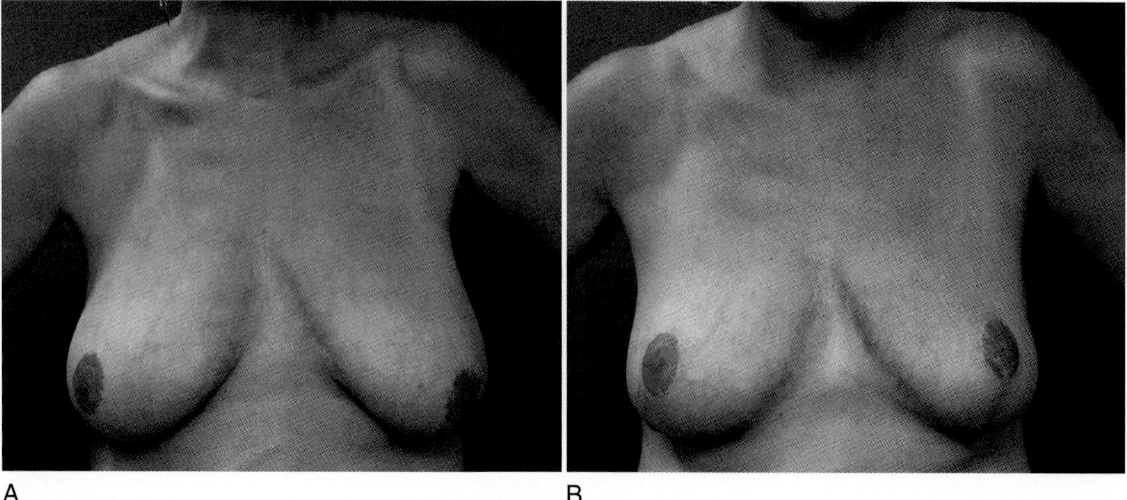

FIGURE 149-10. *A*, A 36-year-old woman with nipple asymmetry. *B*, The patient seen after revision.

of it and establishing a closure of the vertical limb that has too much tension.

Correction of this problem can be performed 9 to 12 months later when the wounds have matured and the skin envelope has loosened. Revision involves an elliptical excision of the vertical limb and direct closure.

IRREGULAR PIGMENTATION

In the severely hypertrophied and ptotic breast, free nipple grafts are occasionally used during reduction mammaplasty. Irregular pigmentation or hypopigmentation may result, especially in black patients. This is explained preoperatively when it is anticipated that a free nipple graft is needed. Patients usually accept the pigment changes, but some may desire correction.

It is best to advise the patient to wait for at least a year after initial surgery because areas of hypopigmentation often improve with time. If no significant improvement is seen within this time frame, intradermal tattoo techniques are effective in restoring pigment to the nipple-areola complex. If the hypopigmented area is small, excision and primary closure can be performed.

NIPPLE-AREOLA CONTOUR IRREGULARITIES

Contour irregularities of the nipple-areola complex may be accentuated by or result from reduction

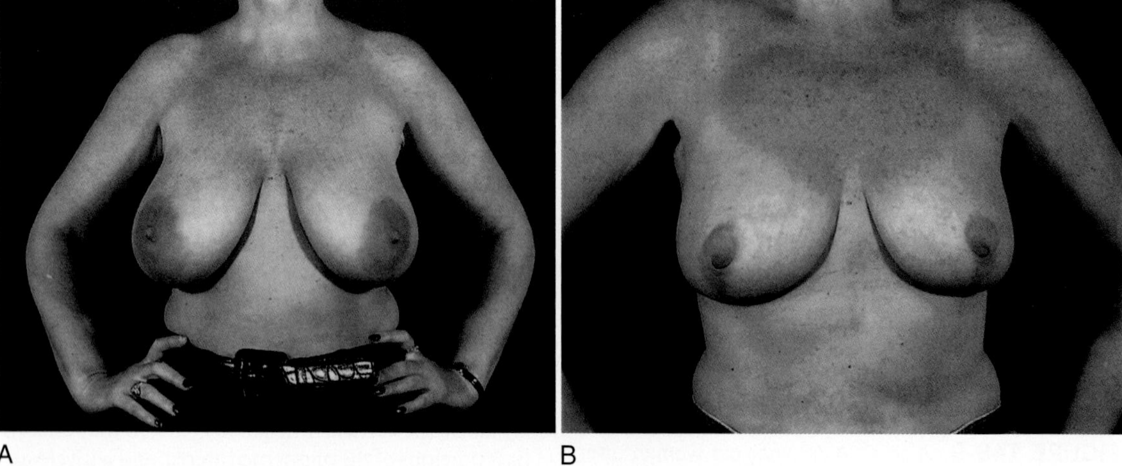

FIGURE 149-11. *A*, A 32-year-old woman with large areolas seen preoperatively. *B*, The patient underwent reduction mammaplasty with resultant residual areola along vertical incision.

mammaplasty. These include nipple inversion or protrusion and areola border irregularities secondary to malalignment of the nipple-areola complex within the keyhole.

Patients should be informed that preexisting inverted nipples will remain so after reduction mammaplasty unless they are corrected. On occasion, nipple inversion is a result of the reduction, more often with the vertical pedicle technique of McKissock and the horizontal pedicle technique of Strömbeck.

Some surgeons attempt correction at the time of primary reduction; however, others think that the blood supply to the nipple-areola complex may be compromised and therefore delay correction. This involves an incision at the junction of the nipple and areola, providing exposure for complete division of the ducts. Dermal flaps of areola can be interposed between the retracted ducts and the nipple to maintain projection and prevent recurrence.[17]

Because preexisting nipple protrusion can become even more pronounced on a smaller breast, the nipple may be reduced at the time of the initial surgery. Nipple vascularity remains a concern, however, with the simultaneous reduction of the breast and the nipple.

After reduction mammaplasty, excessive protrusion of the nipple may occur if the areola diameter is too large for the keyhole that was originally planned. With time, this may correct itself; but if it persists, revision is necessary with a delay of 9 to 10 months for optimal healing. A border of skin around the areola is usually de-epithelialized, and the areola rim is excised. The remaining areola is then stretched to fit the defect, resulting in a less protuberant appearance.

Irregular borders can be corrected, especially when redundant areola is present in one part but not in the other part of the areola. Excision of a border with de-epithelialization of the skin edge or resection of redundant areola can be performed. Contour deformities are more common when the superior dermal pedicle is used instead of the inferior pedicle because of inattention to adequate release of the dermal attachments of the pedicle. Correction may entail only excision at the inferior portion to correct the contour.

Epidermal Cysts

Epidermal cysts in the reduced breast may result from remnants of epithelium left behind because of inadequate de-epithelialization of the pedicle. These cysts can be diagnosed by physical examination, mammography, or ultrasonography and treated by aspiration with possible recurrence. There is also potential for infection if the cyst persists. Definitive treatment is excision, and it may be necessary if the cyst becomes symptomatic or is of concern to the patient or physician.

LATE REGROWTH

Endocrinology and Physiology

The breast is an endocrine organ whose development and behavior are regulated by the neuroendocrine mechanisms that regulate the reproductive system. Mammary growth is affected by various factors in addition to hormones, including mesenchyme, genetics, diet, and environment.

As puberty approaches, there are increasing hormones released by the hypothalamus, pituitary, ovaries, and adrenal glands, and the mammary gland begins a new growth phase. Overall, the major influence on breast development is estrogen; however, the coordinated action of many hormones, including estrogen, prolactin, progesterone, insulin, growth hormone, cortisol, and thyroxine, is necessary.

The cyclic changes in the breast noted during menstruation are caused by rising estrogen levels in the first 2 weeks followed by elevated progesterone in the second half of the cycle. Progesterone and prolactin have been implicated in the discomfort of the premenstrual breasts.

Etiology

IDIOPATHIC HYPERPLASIA

The etiology of breast hypertrophy and gigantomastia is poorly understood. Adolescent breast development should be considered complete before the primary reduction mammaplasty is performed. Some surgeons advocate waiting for 1 year at the end of adolescence to ensure stability of breast size. However, if physical and psychological symptoms become intolerable to the patient who has massive hypertrophy, earlier reduction mammaplasty can be considered. The patient should be advised that secondary reduction might become necessary if rehypertrophy occurs, and even secondary surgery may not be a permanent reduction.

WEIGHT GAIN

Weight gain remains a common cause of rehypertrophy after primary reduction mammaplasty (Fig. 149-12). The psychosocial ramifications of this are not always clearly understood by the patient but should be addressed by the surgeon. The patient may be advised to lose weight before planning secondary surgery. However, many patients with significant rehypertrophy find it difficult to exercise to lose the weight. For these patients, secondary reduction should be considered.

PREGNANCY AND LACTATION

During pregnancy and lactation, estrogen and prolactin levels are elevated and result in changes in breast tissue,

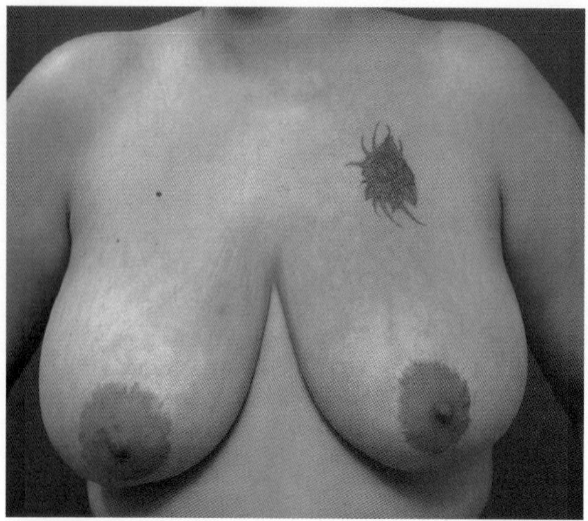

FIGURE 149-12. A 35-year-old woman with history of reduction at age 16 years who presented with rehypertrophy associated with weight gain during the past 3 years. The previous operation was a McKissock vertical mammaplasty. The secondary reduction was performed by inferior pedicle technique with good results. (Postoperative photographs are unavailable.)

including augmentation of milk ducts, hypertrophy of connective tissue, increased fat deposition, and retention of water. The areola skin glands become more prominent, and the nipples often enlarge and become more erect.

These changes take place even in the reduced breasts, which may then rehypertrophy during pregnancy and persist in this state post partum. Most patients and surgeons prefer to delay secondary reduction until completion of the childbearing years.

MENOPAUSE

Between the ages of 35 and 45 years, decreasing estrogen levels preceding menopause cause the glandular epithelium to disappear gradually and the alveoli and lobules to shrink, leading to replacement by fat and fibrous matrix. Regrowth in the menopausal breast, including that which has been previously reduced, is commonly related to generalized weight gain in the postmenopausal woman (Fig. 149-13).

Secondary surgery may be indicated in the postmenopausal patient with rehypertrophy because of symptoms worsened by the aging musculoskeletal system. Suction-assisted lipectomy can be a major adjuvant in postmenopausal secondary breast reduction given the degree of fatty replacement in the breast. After reduction, those women who experience more of an involution of their breast tissue during menopause may desire secondary mastopexy, which can be combined with other procedures such as abdominoplasty or suction-assisted lipectomy.

Treatment of Rehypertrophy

Secondary surgery for rehypertrophy should be delayed until the inciting event is clarified and the appropriate time has passed to allow a stable breast size.

SURGICAL TECHNIQUES

The surgical techniques used for secondary reduction are essentially the same as those for primary reduction mammaplasty (see Chapter 120). Classical teaching emphasizes the importance of using the same technique employed in the primary reduction mammaplasty for the secondary reduction to avoid vascular compromise and nipple or breast tissue necrosis[14] (Fig. 149-14; see also Fig. 149-12). The surgeon should make every effort to determine the original technique (i.e., inferior versus superior versus vertical pedicle). If operative records are not available, a free nipple graft is perhaps the safest technique to preserve nipple viability. Lejour[15] has used vertical mammaplasty as the secondary technique after varying techniques in the primary surgery.

A study published by Losee et al[16] challenges this classical teaching and describes 10 patients, 7 of whom underwent secondary reduction by a technique different from that used in the primary surgery. An average of 4 years separated the reductions of similar technique, whereas an average of 15 years separated the reductions of differing technique. Of this group of 10 patients, 3 experienced self-limited complications; 1 of the 3 patients who underwent the same technique of secondary reduction had minor wound healing problems; 2 of the 7 patients who underwent secondary reduction by a different technique experienced delayed wound healing. No patients in either group suffered significant skin, pedicle, or nipple-areola complex compromise. Although the patients in this study experienced no significant nipple-areola complex or breast tissue necrosis, the results are based on a small series of patients, and the surgeon should use his or her judgment in planning secondary surgery.

Suction Mammaplasty

Suction lipectomy is frequently a good adjunctive technique for secondary reduction mammaplasty.[18] Suction mammaplasty in the already-reduced breast involves suctioning in two planes, the deep plane in the central portion of the breast for overall reduction and the superficial plane in the immediate subcutaneous tissue to promote skin contraction.

Suction lipectomy is also useful for improving the contour of the chest in areas surrounding the breast, especially the anterior and posterior axillary folds and the lateral thorax in patients who have rehypertrophy with weight gain.

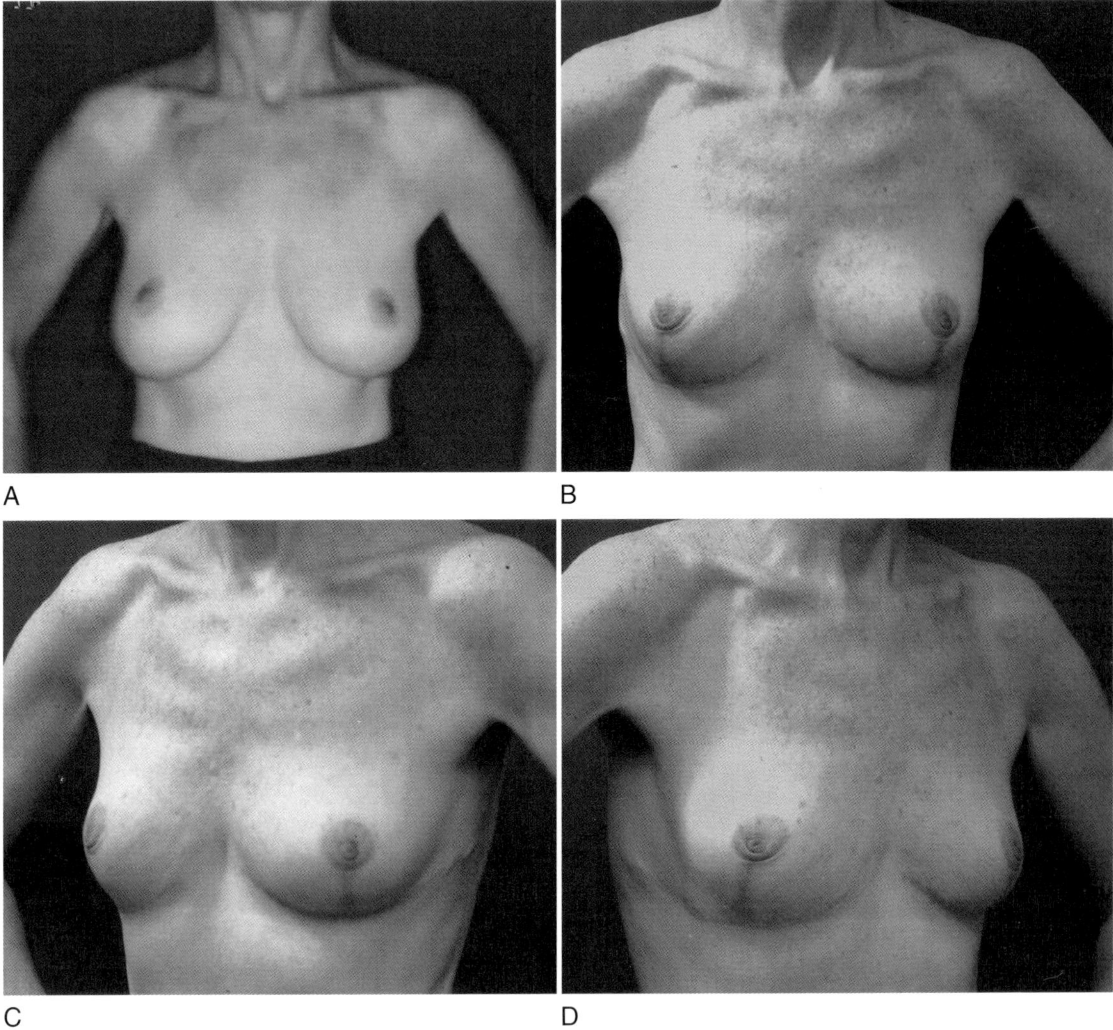

FIGURE 149-13. *A,* A 46-year-old woman after reduction mammaplasty by superior pedicle technique at age 30 years. She experienced rehypertrophy with menopause. *B* to *D,* Reduction mammaplasty was repeated with use of the same technique.

SECONDARY TREATMENT OF PTOSIS

Glandular Ptosis

Glandular ptosis recurs after mastopexy when the nipple position remains constant and the skin undergoes relaxation beneath the nipple, producing a more ptotic position and increased distance from the nipple to the inframammary fold.

Nipple position should be unchanged in the secondary treatment of glandular ptosis. By use of old scars, secondary dermal mastopexy with inversion of the dermis after de-epithelialization produces more fullness in the breast and nipple projection.

Nipple Ptosis

Secondary correction of nipple ptosis is performed by techniques similar to those used to correct a nipple that is too low. Elevation of the nipple can be performed by crescent excision of skin above the nipple or by re-establishing the dermal pedicle.

Ptosis After Implant Removal

Implant removal often results in mammary ptosis or skin laxity in the superior pole of the breast. Conventional mastopexy techniques can be used for correction in patients with large implants, who are then left with significant ptosis, or in those patients with hypoplastic breasts. If the implant is in the

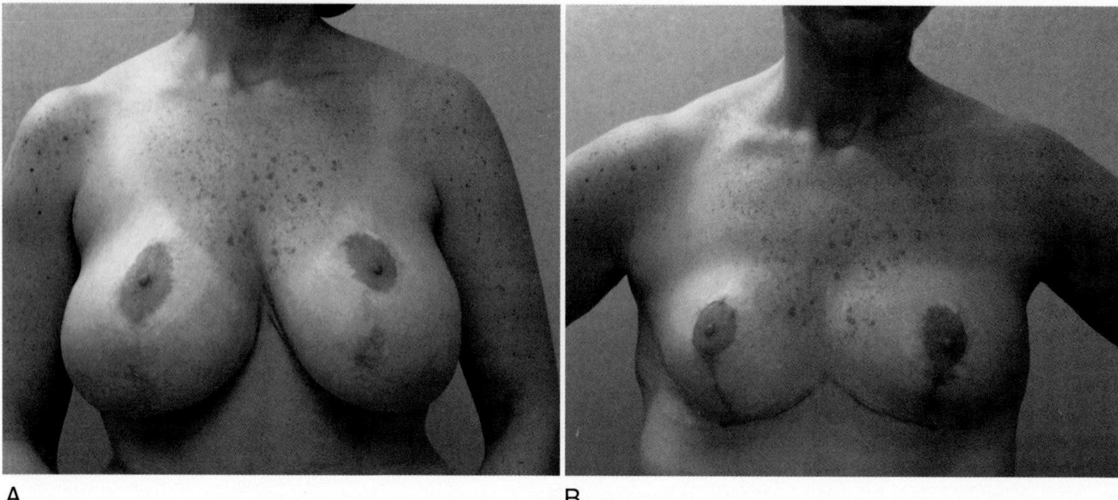

FIGURE 149-14. *A,* A 39-year-old woman with reduction mammaplasty at age 14 years by a superior pedicle technique who presented with rehypertrophy after pregnancy. *B,* The patient is shown after a secondary reduction in which the position of the left nipple was unchanged and a right areola reduction with repositioning was performed.

submammary position, it may be better to delay treatment of mammary ptosis. The use of a dermal pedicle for mastopexy as a second-stage operation after explantation helps prevent vascular compromise of the nipple-areola complex.

At times, the degree of ptosis after implant removal is unpredictable, especially in the younger patient, who may experience significant skin contraction. Some surgeons may opt to delay mastopexy in these patients.

Ptosis with Implant Replacement

Those patients who wish to have implant replacement and simultaneous correction of mammary ptosis may do so by the same techniques used in the original augmentation mammaplasty.

MAMMOGRAPHIC CHANGES AFTER REDUCTION MAMMAPLASTY

Baseline mammograms are obtained for all patients older than 30 years who are undergoing reduction mammaplasty. The postoperative baseline mammogram is acquired 1 year after surgery. Regular mammographic studies after that are determined by the recommendations of the American College of Radiology (*http://www.acr.org*), generally after the age of 40 years on an annual basis.

Reduction mammaplasty results in mammographic changes. Thickening of the skin of the areola and periareola contour changes can be seen. Other postoperative findings include distorted architecture of the breast, fibrosis in the retroareola region, and areas of fat necrosis.[19]

Fat necrosis can be visualized on mammography as well-circumscribed round or oval regions of decreased or increased density with or without calcifications, mimicking cancer. Brown[19] reported a series of patients who underwent mammograms after reduction mammaplasty. He found fat necrosis in 10% of mammograms and asymmetric densities in approximately 50% of mammograms, suggesting varying degrees of scarring. He also reported calcifications in 40% of reduction mammaplasty patients after 2 years. These calcifications are typically coarser than the typical malignant calcifications.

Mammographic changes improve over time. For example, asymmetric densities decrease by 50% after 2 years and then remain stable on serial mammography. Calcifications, on the other hand, increase over time. In the first postoperative year, there is a 3% incidence, which then increases to 20% in the second year and to 40% in the third year.[19] Suspicious calcifications should be treated with biopsy. However, benign calcification, such as that seen after reduction, can be observed with serial mammograms.

MANAGEMENT OF BREAST NEOPLASMS AFTER REDUCTION MAMMAPLASTY

Breast Cancer

Malignant breast lesions may be diagnosed at the time of reduction mammaplasty or at a later time. On occasion, a palpable mass is found at the time of reduction surgery, and pathologic examination demonstrates malignant change. Rarely, the resected breast tissue sent for pathologic evaluation returns with a diagnosis of malignant neoplasia. Occult cancer detected at the time of reduction mammaplasty is particularly traumatic to the patient. Some patients have suspicious mammographic or physical findings in the years subsequent to a reduction mammaplasty and undergo biopsy that reveals a malignant neoplasm.

Regardless of the time of diagnosis, treatment of breast cancer must be decided independently of the technique of reduction mammaplasty. This treatment may require lumpectomy and axillary node dissection or mastectomy with subsequent irradiation or chemotherapy. The patient and her oncologic surgeon should deal with the decisions regarding treatment of breast cancer.

If a mastectomy is performed, the reduction mammaplasty scars may be used with reconstruction by transverse rectus abdominis myocutaneous flap or submuscular implants.

Benign Disease

Benign breast disease such as fibrocystic or fibroadenomatous disease can occur in the postreduction mammaplasty patient. The symptoms of fibrocystic disease may be improved after reduction because large amounts of cyst-containing breast tissue are removed. The disease can persist and may require further treatment, such as aspiration or excision of the cysts. Attention should be given to the dermal pedicles used during the original reduction when benign disease is removed. In most circumstances, surgery for benign disease can be performed through the reduction mammaplasty scars.

COMPLICATIONS OF SECONDARY MASTOPEXY AND REDUCTION

Complications that may occur after secondary reduction and mastopexy are essentially the same as those after primary reduction. There may be a higher incidence of fat and nipple necrosis, depending on the surgical technique used.

REFERENCES

1. Schnur P: Reduction mammaplasty: an outcome analysis. Plast Reconstr Surg 1997;100:875.
2. Serletti J: Long-term patient satisfaction following reduction mammaplasty. Ann Plast Surg 1999;28:363.
3. Elsahy N: Correction of abnormally high nipples after reduction mammaplasty. Aesthetic Plast Surg 1990;14:21.
4. Herman S, Hoffman S, Kahn S: Revisional surgery after reduction mammaplasty. Plast Reconstr Surg 1975;55:422.
5. Millard DR Jr, Mullin WR, Lesavoy MA: Secondary correction of the too-high areola and nipple after a mammaplasty. Plast Reconstr Surg 1976;58:568.
6. Salema R, Aboudib JH, de Castro CC: Convergent nipple-areola complexes corrected by inferior curved pedicle technique. Ann Plast Surg 1987;19:555.
7. Hoffman S: Recurrent deformities following reduction mammaplasty and correction of breast asymmetry. Plast Reconstr Surg 1986;78:55.
8. Hoffman S: Complications of reduction mammaplasty. In Noone RB, ed: Plastic and Reconstructive Surgery of the Breast. Philadelphia, BC Decker, 1991:285-296.
9. Hoffman S: Reduction mammaplasty: a medicolegal hazard? Aesthetic Plast Surg 1987;11:113.
10. Hoffman S: Medicolegal aspects of reduction mammaplasty. In Goldwyn R, ed: Reduction Mammaplasty. Boston, Little, Brown, 1989:60.
11. Lejour M: Vertical mammaplasty: update and appraisal of late results. Plast Reconstr Surg 1999;104:771.
12. Lejour M: Vertical mammaplasty: early complications after 250 personal consecutive cases. Plast Reconstr Surg 1999;104:764.
13. Sarwer DB, Bartlett SP, Bucky L, et al: Bigger is not always better: body image dissatisfaction in breast reduction and breast augmentation patients. Plast Reconstr Surg 1998;101:1956.
14. Hudson DA, Skoll PJ: Repeat reduction mammaplasty. Plast Reconstr Surg 1999;104:401.
15. Lejour M: Vertical mammaplasty as secondary surgery after other techniques. Aesthetic Plast Surg 1997;21:403.
16. Losee JE, Caldwell EH, Serletti JM: Secondary reduction mammaplasty: is using a different pedicle safe? Plast Reconstr Surg 2000;106:1004.
17. Teimourian B, Adham MN: Simple technique for correction of inverted nipple. Plast Reconstr Surg 1980;65:504.
18. Gray LN: Liposuction breast reduction. Aesthetic Plast Surg 1998;22:159.
19. Brown RE, Sargent SK, Cohen SR, Morain WD: Mammographic changes following reduction mammaplasty. Plast Reconstr Surg 1987;80:691.

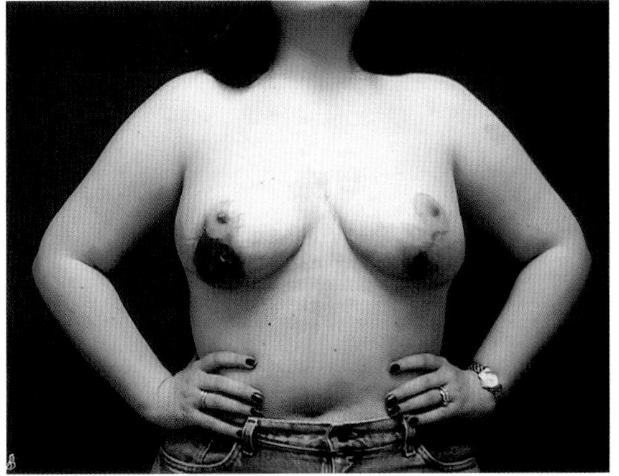

A

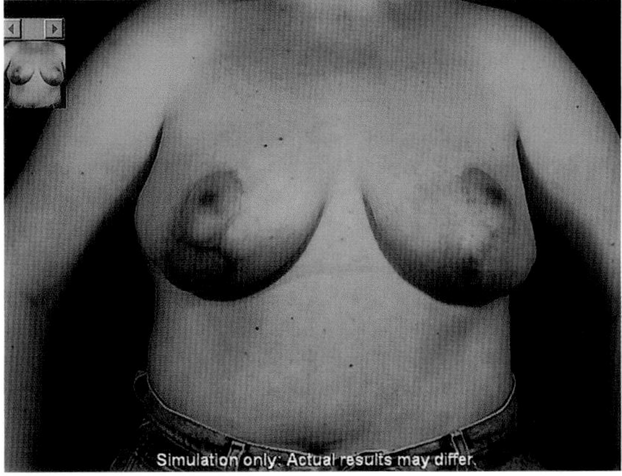

B

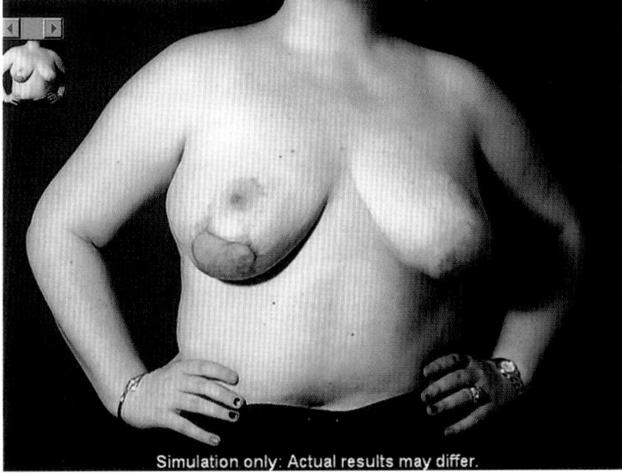

C

COLOR PLATE 149-1. *A,* A 28-year-old woman with significant skin necrosis on the right breast after bilateral reduction mammaplasty. *B,* The wound after skin grafting. *C,* Six-month follow-up.

CHAPTER

150

Secondary Breast Reconstruction

STEPHEN J. MATHES, MD ✦ LEE ALKUREISHI, MD

> *It is important to have an open mind and to rethink the treatment strategy. . . . If the situation calls for a change in strategy and if the surgeon is flexible enough to pursue a new course, the reward will often be a vastly improved result and a satisfied patient.*
>
> —*Kroll and Freeman*[1]

Secondary breast reconstruction is defined as a procedure or procedures performed after the initial reconstructive procedure for the purpose of correcting a complication of the initial procedure or to improve the aesthetics of the breast reconstruction in a dissatisfied patient. The initial procedure may be a single operation (single-stage reconstruction) or staged procedures in which an expander-implant sequence is used or a second-stage implant insertion is planned beneath a previously inset flap to complete the reconstruction. Secondary procedures are not considered contralateral procedures planned for symmetry with the reconstructed breast mound. However, a surgical procedure performed after the planned reconstructive sequence is complete is classified as a secondary procedure. Risk factors that contribute to problems leading to indications for secondary breast reconstruction are presented. Evaluation of the dissatisfied patient requires decisions regarding diagnosis of the problem, selection of the technique to correct the acquired deformity, review of the status of the contralateral breast, and timing of secondary procedures. Finally, each common complication resulting in indications for secondary reconstruction is reviewed in regard to prevalence, etiology, diagnosis, and treatment.

Complications and *reconstructive failures* are terms commonly used to imply the need for secondary procedures. The large number of techniques available for reconstruction correlates with the large number of potential complications that may occur during the initial reconstructive sequence. Although many series discuss complications of breast reconstruction, it is difficult to compare series. The breast reconstruction population is a heterogeneous one, with differences arising in the type of mastectomy, the type of reconstruction, the timing (immediate versus delayed), the patient's characteristics and concurrent risk factors, and finally the surgeon's skills and familiarity with techniques. Furthermore, within each technique, there are a multitude of factors that may affect the outcome.

Malyon et al[2] described a series of 164 patients who underwent reconstruction by implant alone, implant with autogenous tissue, pedicled flap, or free transfer; 62% of the reconstructions were immediate and 38% were delayed. The mean follow-up was 10 months (range, 2 to 19 months). Complication rates were provided for each type of reconstruction, and complications were divided into categories on the basis of severity and necessity for reoperation (secondary reconstruction). In this series of patients, 14 patients (8.5%) suffered complete loss of the reconstruction; 34 patients (21%) required reoperation for moderate complications; and 25 patients (15%) requested secondary reconstructive procedures. The total reoperation rate in this series was 44.9%, with 29% of the secondary procedures performed to correct complications of the previous surgery. The highest rate of secondary reconstruction was associated with implant-only reconstructions, with 21 of 50 patients undergoing two or more procedures before nipple reconstruction. Deep inferior epigastric perforator (DIEP) flap and latissimus dorsi flap secondary reconstructive rates were 17 of 47 (36%) and 8 of 50 (16%), respectively.

Each technique used in the primary reconstruction has specific complications that may result in the necessity for secondary reconstruction. The technique selected affects both the complication incidence and the type of complication encountered. The patient should be carefully informed about these potential complications and subsequent procedures that may be required to correct potential problems, which may impair the quality of the reconstruction. The technique selected by the patient may be less complex, such as implant compared with flap, but it may exhibit increased rates of complications. Conversely, the flap technique may provide the needed tissues to avoid local complications but introduces the potential for donor site complications. All techniques may completely fail their primary purpose of breast mound reconstruction with implant loss or flap failure. With implant loss, the surgeon still has all flap options, whereas with flap loss, the implant-alone option is generally no longer possible and secondary flap options may be limited. The implications of complications, particularly reconstructive failure as related to future secondary procedures, should be discussed with the patient and family.

CHOICE OF PRIMARY BREAST RECONSTRUCTION TECHNIQUE AND OUTCOMES

Expander-Implant

Implants are primarily used either beneath the preserved skin envelope after mastectomy or in association with the latissimus dorsi musculocutaneous flap. In the majority of mastectomies, the expander-implant sequence is used to allow preparation of the preserved skin envelope to receive the permanent implant. This discussion of the implant complications that may lead to secondary procedures focuses on problems with implants, which include expanders, adjustable permanent implants, and permanent implants after the expander-implant staged procedures.

The major complications associated with implants are exposure, infection, and capsular contracture. Exposure usually results from skin envelope necrosis without adequate muscle coverage of the implant. Infection occurs usually as a consequence of exposure but may be related to infected seroma or bacterial contamination of the operative site from breast tissue or skin. Once a peri-implant infection is established, it is generally advisable to remove the implant to allow healing with delay of the secondary procedure for 3 to 6 months. Capsular contracture is a long-term risk that may adversely affect the quality of the reconstruction.

The expander is a prosthetic device that is safe in its use as a temporary prosthetic device pending its replacement with a permanent implant. Clinical studies have reported the rate of complications for implants, and selected studies are reviewed. Unfortunately, the specific implant models are always changing, so it is difficult to predict relevance of data for current patients. Also, follow-up in these patients is often difficult because of the tendency for patients to relocate away from the site of their original surgery. The implant manufacturers are obligated to record data for device approval from the Federal Drug Administration based on clinical trials. These data have better follow-up rates and are helpful for predicting potential complications (see Tables 150-24 to 150-32).[3-6]

Gui et al[7] have published a summary table (Table 150-1) that reviews implant complications from 11 clinical studies between 1986 and 2000. Secondary reconstructive procedures may follow any of these complications. The complications that most likely may lead to a major failure of the reconstruction or unsatisfactory result in regard to projection, size, and symmetry include skin necrosis (0% to 21.6%), implant loss or extrusion (0% to 23.7%), and infection (0% to 15%).

In a retrospective study of Heyer-Schulte Style 1800 implants involving 167 implants (64 for reconstruction), 50 patients (64.9%) had further surgery after the initial implant placement. Reasons for reoperation included open capsulotomy (41% of 83 reoperations), deflation (38.6%), infection (7.2%), and "other" (13.2%).[8] In a similar study[9] of 157 patients (165 breasts) with immediate reconstruction with implants or expanders, an 18% prosthesis loss was noted (22% gel prosthesis and 15% expander). Risk factors cited for gel implant loss included lack of complete muscle coverage, smoking, implant size larger

TABLE 150-1 ✦ SUMMARY OF IMPLANT COMPLICATIONS

Reference	n	Reconstruction Details	Infections (%)	Hematoma (%)	Seroma Around Implant (%)	Native Skin Neurosis (%)	Implant Loss or Extrusion (%)	Difficulty in Expansion (%)	Valve Failure (%)	Deflation (%)
Mansel et al[146] (1986)	12	I, immediate	7.9	0	0	0	16.7	0	0	0
	38	LD + I, immediate	8.3	0	0	2.6	23.7	0	0	0
Schuster et al[147] (1990)	56	E/I, silicone, immediate	5.4	3.6	7.1	12.5	7.1	0	0	0
Mandrekas et al[148] (1995)	44	Becker, immediate and delayed	2.3	0	0	2.3	0	0	2.3	0
Hunter-Smith and Laurie[149] (1995)	54	Becker, immediate and delayed	3.7	0	1.9	3.7	1.9	0	1.9	1.9
McGeorge et al[150] (1996)	19	E/I, saline, immediate and delayed	5.3	0	5.3	5.3	0	0	0	0
Ramon et al[23] (1997)	52	E/I, silicone, delayed	9.6	5.8	0	1.9	5.8	11.5	3.8	3.8
Spear and Majidian[32] (1998)	171	E/I, saline, immediate	3.5	1.2	0	5.3	10.5	0	0	4.0
Slavin et al[151] (1998)	51	LD + I, saline, immediate	2.0	0	0	21.6	3.9	0	0	0
Al-Ghazal and Blamey[152] (2000)	101	I, silicone, Becker, immediate and delayed	0	0	0	8.9	10-13	0	0	0
Peyser et al[153] (2000)	71	LD + Becker or McGhan 150, immediate	4.2	1.4	0	9.9	0	0	1.4	0
Berry et al[39] (1998)	100	Becker, immediate	15	0	0	4	14	0	1	0
Gui[7] (2003)	129	McGhan 150, immediate	6.2	1.6	0	3	3.9	0	0	0

E/I, tissue expander replaced by implant; saline, saline implant; I, implant alone; silicone, silicone implant; Becker, Becker permanent expander-implant; McGhan 150, McGhan Style 150 permanent expander-implant; LD, latissimus dorsi flap.

From Gui GP, Tan SM, Faliakou EC, et al: Immediate breast reconstruction using biodimensional anatomical permanent expander implants: a prospective analysis of outcome and patient satisfaction. Plast Reconstr Surg 2003;111:125.

than 400 mL, and age ($P < .05$). Risk factors for the expander group included detachment of the pectoralis major and lack of muscle coverage. The expander takes pressure off the preserved skin envelope and allows later insertion of an implant required to fulfill the patient's expectations of breast size and symmetry.

Flap

The latissimus dorsi and transverse rectus abdominis musculocutaneous (TRAM) flaps are well-established techniques for breast reconstruction. Unlike an expander-implant, the flap provides well-vascularized tissue to add to the preserved skin envelope after mastectomy. With the flap, both muscle and skin island are now available to improve the dimensions of the skin envelope (both latissimus dorsi and TRAM flaps), to provide muscle coverage of the implant if it is used (latissimus dorsi flap), and to provide autogenous tissue for a new breast volume (primarily TRAM flap). With microsurgical transplantation, the perforator flaps (including the deep inferior epigastric perforator flap, superficial inferior epigastric perforator flap, superior gluteal artery perforator flap, and inferior gluteal artery perforator flap) can also provide both skin for the breast envelope and autogenous tissue for the mound.

The initial steps of flap elevation require preservation of an intact vascular pedicle or flap–receptor vessel anastomosis to avoid the major complication of flap loss. Once the flap is successfully placed at the mastectomy site, the method of and expertise in flap inset will determine the quality of the reconstruction. Failure to achieve adequate inset will necessitate secondary reconstructive procedures. In Hartrampf's review[10] of 300 patients undergoing TRAM flap for reconstruction, 42% of the reconstructed mounds required revision. Breast complications encountered included total flap loss (1 patient, 0.3%), partial flap loss (18 patients, 6%), fat necrosis (21 patients, 7%), breast infection (2 patients, 0.6%), breast hematoma (8 patients, 2.6%), and mastectomy skin flap loss (2 patients, 0.6%). Total complication incidence (including donor site) was 49 of 300 patients (16.3%).

Outcomes

The decision about which reconstructive technique to use in breast surgery is an important variable affecting the possible need for secondary reconstruction. Unfortunately, most of the published data regarding reconstruction techniques and their associated outcomes is applicable only to the particular subset of the population examined in that series and thus cannot be extrapolated to make general conclusions. There are relatively fewer series that examine the outcomes of all or multiple types of reconstruction in a large population of patients, and even fewer are prospective in design.

As such, it is best to acknowledge and understand some of the generally accepted principles involved in breast reconstruction technique. These include the following points:

1. The complication (and revision) rate after prosthetic reconstruction is generally higher than that of autologous reconstruction.[11]
2. The lower revision rate for autologous operations may be attributed to
   - lower overall and major complication rates with autologous techniques[12,13];
   - superior aesthetic outcome with autologous techniques[14]; and
   - longer lasting acceptable results with autologous reconstruction.[15,16]

In a review of 325 postmastectomy breast reconstructions[12] (105 expander-implants, 47 latissimus dorsi flaps, 173 TRAM flaps), failure of the procedure was defined as use of a different technique to rescue the reconstruction, implant removal, or postoperative rating of photographs in the category of poor or failed to complete because of complications. The 21% failure rate for tissue expander-implant reconstructions was significantly higher than that for latissimus dorsi reconstructions (9%) and TRAM flap reconstructions (3%) ($P = .0001$). The causes of expander-implant failure were listed as capsular contracture, implant exposure, and infection. Average overall grade for the TRAM flap was significantly higher than for the other techniques ($P = .0001$), although this difference was reduced if only patients who completed nipple-areola reconstruction were considered ($P = .09$). This difference may be explained by the higher risk of failure in the expander-implant group. In conclusion, the authors noted that scarring was less in the expander-implant group, breast shape and ptosis were better achieved in the TRAM flap and latissimus dorsi flap groups, and outcomes were better with immediate reconstruction, most likely because of the preservation of uninvolved breast skin.

In an analysis of 55 expander-implant patients compared with 74 TRAM flap reconstructions,[17] higher complication rates and decreased satisfaction rates were observed in the expander-implant patients. The number of revisions required was reported as 117 in the 55 expander-implant patients and 78 in the 74 TRAM flap patients. The most important factor in satisfaction of patients was noted to be symmetry after the reconstruction. Similarly, in a study comparing prosthetic (n = 19) and autologous (n = 43) immediate breast reconstructions, the postoperative results were analyzed for complication rates and risk factors. The use of a prosthetic reconstruction was found in this series to be associated with more major wound complications ($P < .05$) compared with autologous techniques.[13]

In a review by Alderman et al[18] of 326 patients undergoing breast reconstruction with an expander-implant (79), pedicled TRAM flap (179), and free TRAM flap (67) for 2 years of follow-up, 223 of 326 (68.4%) patients were free of major complications, 77 (23.6%) had one major complication, and 26 (8%) had two or three major complications. The number of patients requiring reoperation was thus 103 of 326 (31.6%). Total complication rates between the expander-implant sequence and combined TRAM groups showed no significant differences, and the same pattern was seen for major complications. In a similar study comparing outcomes in pedicled TRAM flap, free TRAM flap, and expander-implant groups,[19] major complications occurred at a rate of 26 of 123 (21.2%) in all patients, 15 of 70 (21.4%) for pedicled TRAM flaps, 0 of 14 (0%) for free TRAM flaps, and 11 of 39 (23.1%) for expander-implants. The authors demonstrated a significant risk for major complications associated with body mass index ($P = .06$) and smoking history ($P = .03$) for both prosthetic and autologous reconstructions. After chi-square analysis, an increased risk of major complications after previous radiation therapy was noted in the expander-implant group ($P = .05$) but not in the TRAM flap group. This study illustrates the importance of strict selection of the patient and technique in planning primary and secondary reconstructions.

INDICATIONS FOR AND TIMING OF SECONDARY BREAST RECONSTRUCTION

The classification of complications of breast reconstruction has been approached in a wide variety of ways. Malyon[2] divides the severity of complications into five groups that allow analysis of necessity for secondary reconstructive procedures (Table 150-2). The most important aspect of this classification is that it permits the distinction to be made between those complications requiring further surgery (severe or moderate) and those that do not (mild); clearly, it is important to distinguish between these two groups of complications because the treatment differs greatly.

Concentrating on those complications that do require secondary intervention, it is equally important to distinguish between technique failure, necessitating urgent intervention, and "procedural" complications that may be treated electively. The timing of the secondary reconstruction is key to the types of procedures undertaken (Table 150-3). The patients expressing dissatisfaction and requesting secondary reconstruction are placed in a separate group. The severity of complications, if any, may have little bearing on the patient's perceived need for further surgery, and multiple factors must be taken into consideration in planning secondary surgery, the most important of which is the patient's expectation. These secondary reconstructions are classified as unsatisfactory results.

TABLE 150-2 ✦ CLASSIFICATION OF COMPLICATIONS

Severity	Description
None	No record of any adverse event
Mild	Adverse event not requiring any surgical intervention
Moderate	Adverse event requiring surgical intervention
Severe	Complete loss of reconstruction
Patient request	Patient requests surgical adjustment of reconstruction or opposite breast

From Malyon AD, Husein M, Weiler-Mithoff EM: How many procedures to make a breast? Br J Plast Surg 2001;54:227-231.

Technique Failure

The technique failure group requires immediate intervention either to salvage the procedure or to treat progressive complications. Acute failure presents differently according to the technique. Indications for urgent surgical intervention after breast reconstruction are listed in Table 150-4.

Procedural Complications

Procedural complications requiring surgery are problems that result in loss or impairment of the reconstruction but do not necessarily require urgent surgery. These complications are inherent to the procedure and may occur despite careful precautions; they usually do not occur during the initial postoperative period (Table 150-5).

TABLE 150-3 ✦ CLASSIFICATION OF BREAST RECONSTRUCTION COMPLICATIONS ACCORDING TO TIMING AND SEVERITY

Problem	Description
Technique failure	Complication necessitating urgent intervention
Procedural complication	Requires surgery but may be treated electively
Unsatisfactory results	Patient expresses dissatisfaction with outcome of reconstruction

TABLE 150-4 ✦ TECHNIQUE FAILURE: BREAST RECONSTRUCTION

Technique	Defect
Expander-implant	Skin envelope necrosis Exposure Infection Expander malfunction (port failure) Deflation or rupture Enlarging hematoma
Transposition flap	Vascular compromise (arterial or venous insufficiency) Flap necrosis Dehiscence of flap inset Enlarging hematoma
Microvascular flap transplantation	Vascular compromise (arterial or venous insufficiency) Flap necrosis due to anastomotic failure Dehiscence of flap inset Enlarging hematoma

Unsatisfactory Result

The indication for secondary reconstruction related to dissatisfaction with the outcome may be a result of technical errors in the reconstruction, postoperative complications inherent to the technique, lack of symmetry with the contralateral breast, or unfulfilled expectations of the patient. Many of the procedural complications can lead to late dissatisfaction, and there is considerable overlap between these two categories.

TABLE 150-5 ✦ PROCEDURAL COMPLICATIONS: BREAST RECONSTRUCTION

Technique	Defect
Expander-implant	Expander-implant malfunction Implant deflation Chronic seroma Implant malposition (implant shift into donor site or axilla) Deflation or rupture
Transposition flap	Partial flap loss (related to inadequate vascularity or inappropriate flap design) Malposition of underlying implant (implant shift into donor site or axilla) Deflation of underlying implant Chronic seroma
Microvascular flap transplantation	Partial flap loss (related to inadequate vascularity or inappropriate flap design) Chronic seroma

TABLE 150-6 ✦ UNSATISFACTORY RESULT: BREAST RECONSTRUCTION

Technique	Defect
Expander-implant	Capsular contracture Malposition of breast mound Inadequate symmetry with contralateral breast (size, position, ptosis) Scar Implant appearance (palpable edge or wrinkling) Loss of acceptance of prosthetic device (requested explantation) Implant loss (sequela of technique failure) Implant failure (deflation or rupture)
Transposition flap	Malposition Inadequate symmetry with contralateral breast (size, position, ptosis) Scar Fat necrosis Flap loss (sequela of technique failure)
Microvascular flap transplantation	Malposition Inadequate symmetry with contralateral breast (size, position, ptosis) Scar Fat necrosis Flap loss (sequela of technique failure)

However, dissatisfaction need not arise from the development of complications. The decision to proceed with a secondary reconstructive procedure requires careful evaluation of the cause of the unsatisfactory result, development of a plan to correct the problem, and mutual understanding of the projected outcome between the surgeon and the patient. Problems resulting in indications for secondary procedures can be common to the process of breast reconstruction or unique to the technique selected (Table 150-6).

INCIDENCE OF SECONDARY BREAST RECONSTRUCTION PROCEDURES

In a retrospective review of 888 patients who underwent unilateral (n = 738) or bilateral (n = 150) breast reconstructions with a mean follow-up of 28.5 months, Losken et al[20] reported that the mean number of secondary reconstructions required was 3.99 for unilateral reconstructions and 5.54 for bilateral reconstructions. The following variables were associated with increased risk for secondary reconstructions: delayed reconstruction ($P < .001$), radiotherapy ($P = .032$), and development of any complication ($P < .001$). The number of secondary reconstructions also increased with the number of risk factors, including smoking, diabetes, obesity, hypertension, and radiation therapy.

Nahabedian et al[21] described 382 patients who underwent autologous (n = 217 patients, 277 breasts) or implant (n = 117 patients, 154 breasts) reconstruction with regard to the need for secondary reconstruction to improve symmetry. This study, with mean follow-up of 21 months, found that final volume symmetry and contour symmetry were more often achieved with autologous reconstructions than with implant reconstructions (84% versus 75% for volume symmetry, 78% versus 60% for contour symmetry). Despite these findings, secondary reconstructions were more often performed in autologous reconstructions (59% versus 39%).

The types of ipsilateral secondary reconstructions carried out in this study included skin or fat excision (95%), implant exchange (3%), and implant augmentation (2%). Contralateral breast procedures included reduction mammaplasty (46%), mastopexy (43%), and augmentation (11%). The authors noted that ipsilateral procedures were far more common than contralateral procedures for symmetry (42% versus 10.5%).

Analysis of patients who undergo secondary breast reconstruction will provide information about prevalence of the problem requiring revision and direct efforts to avoid complications that result in technique failure, procedural complications, and dissatisfaction. In preliminary results (S. J. Mathes and L. Alkureishi, unpublished data, 2005), 85 patients (116 breasts) required ipsilateral secondary breast reconstruction between January 1, 1996, and November 1, 2003. Mean follow-up was 9.8 years (range, 1 to 39 years), and an average of 2.2 secondary reconstructions were required per breast (range, 1 to 10). The majority of secondary reconstructions were performed during the 15-month period after the primary reconstruction. More than 80% of secondary reconstructions performed after 2 years were for patients who underwent primary reconstruction with implant.

The most frequent indications for secondary reconstruction were related to dissatisfaction with the aesthetic outcome; asymmetry was cited in 45.5% of all secondary reconstructions, unacceptable scarring in 29.3%, and contour deformities in 24%. Capsular contracture was also commonly seen (26.3%). By comparison, technique failures necessitating urgent intervention were rare; implant failure occurred in 19 patients (11%), vascular supply problems in 18 (11%, all but one of which were partial flap or fat necrosis), problems with the skin envelope in 18 (11%), and infection in 7 (4%) (Table 150-7) (S. J. Mathes and L. Alkureishi, unpublished data, 2005).

TABLE 150-7 ✦ RELATIVE FREQUENCIES OF EACH INDICATION FOR SECONDARY RECONSTRUCTION

Indication	Type	All Operations (n = 167)
Asymmetry (ipsilateral)	Dissatisfaction	76 (45.5%)
Unacceptable scars	Dissatisfaction	49 (29.3%)
Capsular contracture	Dissatisfaction	44 (26.3%)
Contour defects	Procedural	40 (24.0%)
Implant failure	Procedural	19 (11.4%)
Skin envelope problems		18 (10.8%)
Mastectomy skin necrosis	Technique failure	7 (4.2%)
Extrusion	Technique failure	6 (3.6%)
Inadequate skin envelope	Dissatisfaction	2 (1.2%)
Unstable skin	Technique failure	3 (1.8%)
Vascular supply problems		18 (10.8%)
Total flap loss	Technique failure	0
Partial flap loss	Technique failure	4 (2.4%)
Fat necrosis	Procedural	14 (8.4%)
Absent breast mound	Technique failure	14 (8.4%)
Nipple-related problems	Procedural	8 (4.8%)
Infection		7 (4.2%)
Periprosthetic	Technique failure	2 (1.2%)
Other infection	Procedural	5 (3%)
Silicone concerns	Dissatisfaction	4 (2.4%)
Early postoperative complications	Technique failure	3 (1.8%)
Other	Procedural	5 (3.0%)

S.J. Mathes and L. Alkureishi, unpublished data, 2005.

TABLE 150-8 ✦ CLASSIFICATION OF SECONDARY DEFORMITIES

Envelope
Mound
Position
Scar
Symmetry

The secondary reconstruction techniques employed reflected the relative frequencies of the indications: symmetry-related procedures were carried out in 54% of all secondary procedures, correction of capsular contracture in 44%, implant exchange in 40%, and scar revision in 38%. In general, patients presented with multiple indications for secondary reconstruction, and multiple techniques were often used during one operation.

CLASSIFICATION OF BREAST DEFORMITIES AFTER RECONSTRUCTION

In an effort to focus on the component parts of the failure of breast reconstruction, it is helpful to organize the evaluation of the breast into the following areas: envelope, mound, position, scar, and symmetry. As noted in the review of the incidence of secondary surgery, there is a great deal of overlap in the indications for secondary reconstructive procedures (technique failure, procedural complications, and unsatisfactory result). Although there is often one major area of deficiency in the reconstruction, there may be multiple areas in which improvements are required to provide a result satisfying to the patient presenting for secondary breast reconstruction. By focusing on each area of the failed reconstruction, including problems related to envelope, mound, position, and scar, the surgeon can formulate a reconstruction plan that will address each area. Symmetry is included as a separate entity in this classification because the reconstructed breast must ultimately have an appearance similar to the contralateral breast in its unaltered form or after contralateral procedures. The reconstructed breast may satisfy the criteria of excellent envelope, mound, position, and scar but still must have symmetry with the opposite breast (see Chapter 138). Additional areas that may require surgery after breast reconstruction, the nipple-areola complex and flap donor sites, are also included (Table 150-8).

Envelope

The envelope should provide adequate coverage of the implant or autogenous tissue for the mound. Inadequate envelope most commonly presents with inadequate inferior breast mound ptosis compared with the contralateral breast. Acute failure of the envelope results from skin necrosis or flap loss. Failure of the envelope in the expander-implant sequence usually results in loss of the implant. Partial flap failure may distort the breast mound and prevent symmetry with the opposite breast. Complete flap failure may prevent direct closure of the mastectomy wound or distort the mastectomy site.

Excess skin envelope rarely occurs with expander-implant reconstruction but may result with flap inset. Excess flap inset into the preserved mastectomy skin envelope may result in excess ptosis or distortion of the breast mound.

Specific problems related to the envelope include partial flap loss, complete flap loss, deficiency, and excess (Table 150-9).

Mound

The breast mound is formed by a permanent implant, flap tissue, or combination of flap and implant. With implant use, the most common problem is capsular contracture. Capsular contracture will distort the appearance of the breast (Baker III/IV) and frequently causes local discomfort for the patient. Fat necrosis in the autogenous reconstruction causes firmness in the breast mound and often results in apprehension for the patient and oncologist, who are concerned about local tumor recurrence. Visibility of the implant through the skin envelope may be due to the edge of the silicone shell or wrinkling from adherence of the implant wall to the overlying skin envelope. Inadequate size of the mound is a frequent problem for the patient and a source of requests for secondary reconstruction. With both implant and autogenous recon-

TABLE 150-9 ✦ ETIOLOGY OF ENVELOPE DEFORMITY

Envelope	Technique Failure	Procedural	Dissatisfaction
Partial flap loss		X	
Complete flap loss	X		
Deficiency			X
Excess			X

TABLE 150-10 ✦ ETIOLOGY OF MOUND DEFORMITY

Mound	Technique Failure	Procedural	Dissatisfaction
Implant extrusion	X		
Infection	X		
Implant failure		X	
Capsular contracture		X	
Skin wrinkling		X	
Implant palpability		X	
Fat necrosis		X	
Contour			X
Explantation			X

struction, the mound may be too small or too large compared with the opposite breast. Projection of the mound is another aspect of the result after reconstruction that may be inadequate compared with the opposite breast or fall short of the patient's expectations of the result. Finally, fullness in the infraclavicular region is often less than in the contralateral breast. This deficiency of tissue in the superior aspect of the breast mound occurs with expander-implant, flap, and combination reconstruction. Often, the efforts directed to mound reconstruction do not have the ability to provide both mound and infraclavicular fullness.

Both after mastectomy and later after reconstruction, many patients are bothered by fullness and scars in the axilla and lateral chest resulting in contour irregularities. Particularly after axillary dissection, there is often prominence of skin laxity in the lateral chest. Many patients are satisfied with the reconstruction but concerned about excess skin in the lateral chest, resulting in requests for secondary procedures. The problem of contour fullness in the tunnel for transposition flaps may also detract from the reconstruction result.

Specific problems related to the mound include implant extrusion, infection, implant failure, capsular contracture, skin wrinkling, implant palpability, fat necrosis, contour deficiency, and explantation (Table 150-10).

Position

The key to the position on the reconstructed breast is the inframammary line. If the reconstructed mound is too low or too high in relation to the inframammary line, adequate symmetry will not be established; in bilateral reconstruction, the position will not be correct for clothes and appropriate fullness at the superior aspect of the breast mound. If the mound is located below the inframammary line, there will not be adequate fullness in the infraclavicular and superior aspect of the breast mound. If the mound is located above the inframammary line, the breast mound will have excess fullness in the superior chest. Finally, the breast mound may be placed too close to the sternum or too lateral in relation to the hemithorax with the mound located lateral to the midclavicular line. Inappropriate position of the breast mound can be disturbing to the patient and generally requires a secondary reconstructive procedure.

Specific problems related to position include placement and inframammary line (Table 150-11).

Scar

The scar may become a problem in distorting the breast mound shape or may be inherently thick and detract from the overall result. In delayed reconstruction, the plastic surgeon must deal with the presenting mastectomy scar. For the expander-implant sequence, the lateral aspect of the scar can be used to accomplish the reconstructive procedures. Scar medial and superior to the level of the nipple-areola should be avoided. Fortunately, in immediate reconstruction, the plastic surgeon may interact with the surgical oncologist in mastectomy scar location and design. Many scar and color mismatch concerns are unavoidable but fortunately improve with time, and secondary procedures should be delayed for at least a year after the primary reconstruction.

TABLE 150-11 ✦ ETIOLOGY OF POSITION DEFORMITY

Position	Technique Failure	Procedural	Dissatisfaction
Placement		X	
Inframammary line			X

TABLE 150-12 ✦ ETIOLOGY OF SCAR DEFORMITY

Scar	Technique Failure	Procedural	Dissatisfaction
Position		X	
Hypertrophic		X	

Specific problems related to scar include scar malposition and hypertrophic scar (Table 150-12).

Symmetry

Deficiency with envelope, mound, position, and scar affects the quality of the breast reconstruction. Because the breast is a paired organ, the reconstructed breast must resemble the opposite breast, or in the event of bilateral reconstruction, the breasts must resemble each other.

Although the breast may meet qualifications as an adequate reconstruction, the patient will likely express dissatisfaction if symmetry is not established by the reconstruction. If the preoperative plan includes later modification of the opposite breast to meet the patient's desire for correction of abnormalities of the opposite breast (e.g., reduction mammaplasty, mastopexy, augmentation), this opposite procedure is not considered secondary surgery. However, if the patient wishes to match the existing breast or to change the shape of the opposite breast but symmetry is not established, further procedures on the site of reconstruction to provide symmetry are classified as secondary reconstructive procedures. Often, acceptable symmetry cannot be achieved, particularly when different methods are used in bilateral staged reconstruction. As part of the informed consent, the patient and concerned family must understand the goals of the procedure and the limitation in achieving symmetry.

Specific problems related to symmetry include position and mound (Table 150-13).

Additional Deformities

NIPPLE-AREOLA

Nipple-areola reconstruction, when it is requested by patients, may also require secondary procedures because of malposition, loss of the nipple, failure of the nipple to provide adequate form and projection, failure of adequate pigmentation, or a combination of these problems.

DONOR SITE

Donor site problems are reviewed in the individual chapters on techniques for the various flaps, including TRAM, latissimus dorsi, and perforator flaps.

MANAGEMENT OF BREAST DEFORMITIES AFTER RECONSTRUCTION

Whereas problems that follow breast reconstruction can be divided into the separate categories of envelope, mound, position, scar, and symmetry, dissatisfaction with the reconstruction is often multifactorial, and several problems may coexist. The following discussion of problems focuses on the individual problem, but the secondary surgery may have to address several problems simultaneously to provide a successful secondary reconstruction. Similarly, the patient may present with several minor concerns regarding the outcome of her reconstruction, none of which would individually be considered an indication for secondary intervention. However, multiple small problems may combine to become a significantly poorer aesthetic outcome. The best example of this type of problem is "unacceptable scarring"; scar revisions are frequently carried out in conjunction with other, more extensive, secondary procedures.

The decision to reoperate must be realistic in regard to the chance of improving the reconstruction. In consultation with the patient requesting immediate or delayed reconstruction, the expectations of the patient can be accurately ascertained and realistic goals can be established with the patient and family in regard to the likely outcome. If the outcome is fulfilled by the

TABLE 150-13 ✦ ETIOLOGY OF SYMMETRY DEFORMITY

Symmetry	Technique Failure	Procedural	Dissatisfaction
Position			X
Mound			X

surgery with no overt problems, secondary surgery may not be advisable.

Each procedure has shortcomings concerning the reconstructed breast (e.g., expander-implant) or the donor site (flap). Patients should be aware of the possible deficiencies in the outcome for each procedure and the limitations of secondary reconstructive procedures should they become necessary. When the dissatisfied patient arrives from another plastic surgeon requesting further efforts to improve the reconstruction, it is difficult to ascertain the expectations regarding the initial procedure and future secondary procedures. The patient must be well informed as to the problems objectively identified during the evaluation and the potential benefits and limitations of secondary surgery. Patients who underwent prophylactic mastectomy (subcutaneous mastectomy) often expected larger and more natural breast shape and contour because they do not have invasive breast cancer and are electively undergoing bilateral mastectomy. This group of patients may be disappointed with their reconstruction, and secondary procedures often may not improve their acceptance of the result despite the protection against increased risk of subsequent development of breast cancer. Gutowski[22] noted that patients were more likely to be dissatisfied after prophylactic mastectomy compared with patients undergoing augmentation or breast reconstruction for cancer ($P = .0005$).

Envelope

MASTECTOMY SKIN LOSS

Envelope problems may be a direct consequence of the loss of preserved skin at the mastectomy site (Fig. 150-1).[3,7,15,17,18,23-39] If the expander or permanent adjustable implant has been used, muscle coverage will generally allow salvage of the implant while the wound is treated with frequent dressing changes and topical antibiotics. If the skin loss with the expander-implant is extensive, the plastic surgeon has two options: removal of implant, wound closure, and delayed secondary procedure or immediate flap to replace lost skin envelope and to avoid loss of the implant (Table 150-14). In general, implant removal is preferred because the patient may not be able to make an appropriate decision about a flap under the duress of mastectomy for cancer and subsequent immediate secondary procedure. If the flap has minor skin loss, conservative therapy is again appropriate. The eschar will eventually separate and wound healing by the contracture process will occur, with complete wound closure. Because a flap has been used, the skin envelope will remain adequate in most circumstances. If major flap loss is observed, flap débridement will be required, followed by delayed wound closure with use of either local tissue or skin grafts. After adjuvant cancer treatment is completed, if it is required, and wound maturation is observed (3 to 6 months), secondary reconstruction can be planned (Figs. 150-2 to 150-4).

When skin envelope necrosis occurs with skin-sparing mastectomy with an underlying immediate flap, the exposed surface of the flap is well vascularized and will accept skin grafts (Tables 150-15 and 150-16). Some centers have proposed inset of the flap without de-epithelialization of the flap beyond the excised nipple-areola complex; the patient returns to the operating room in several days for excision of any nonviable preserved breast skin, and the underlying flap skin is used to fill this unexpected defect, with the

Text continued on p. 1101

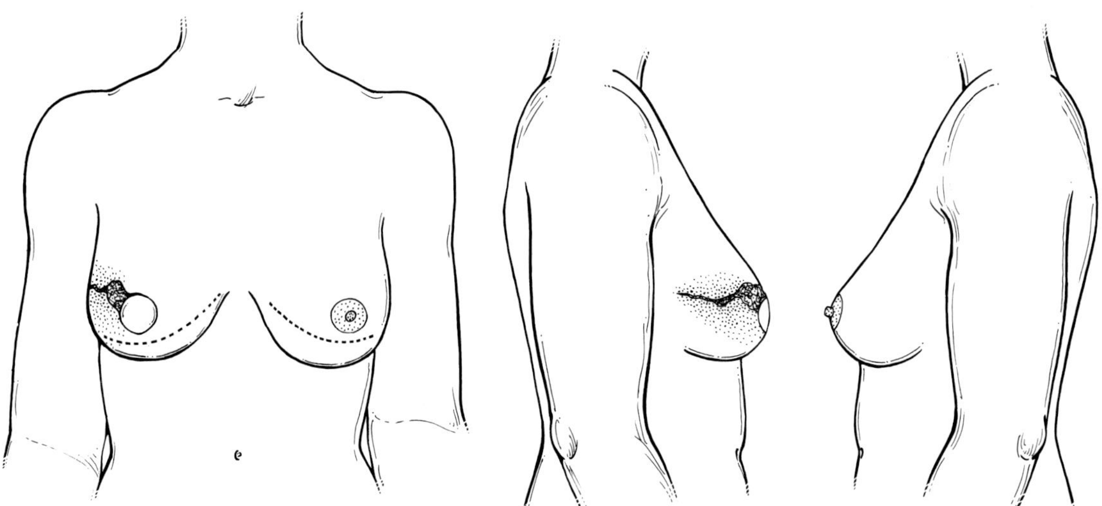

FIGURE 150-1. Mastectomy skin loss: skin-sparing envelope necrosis.

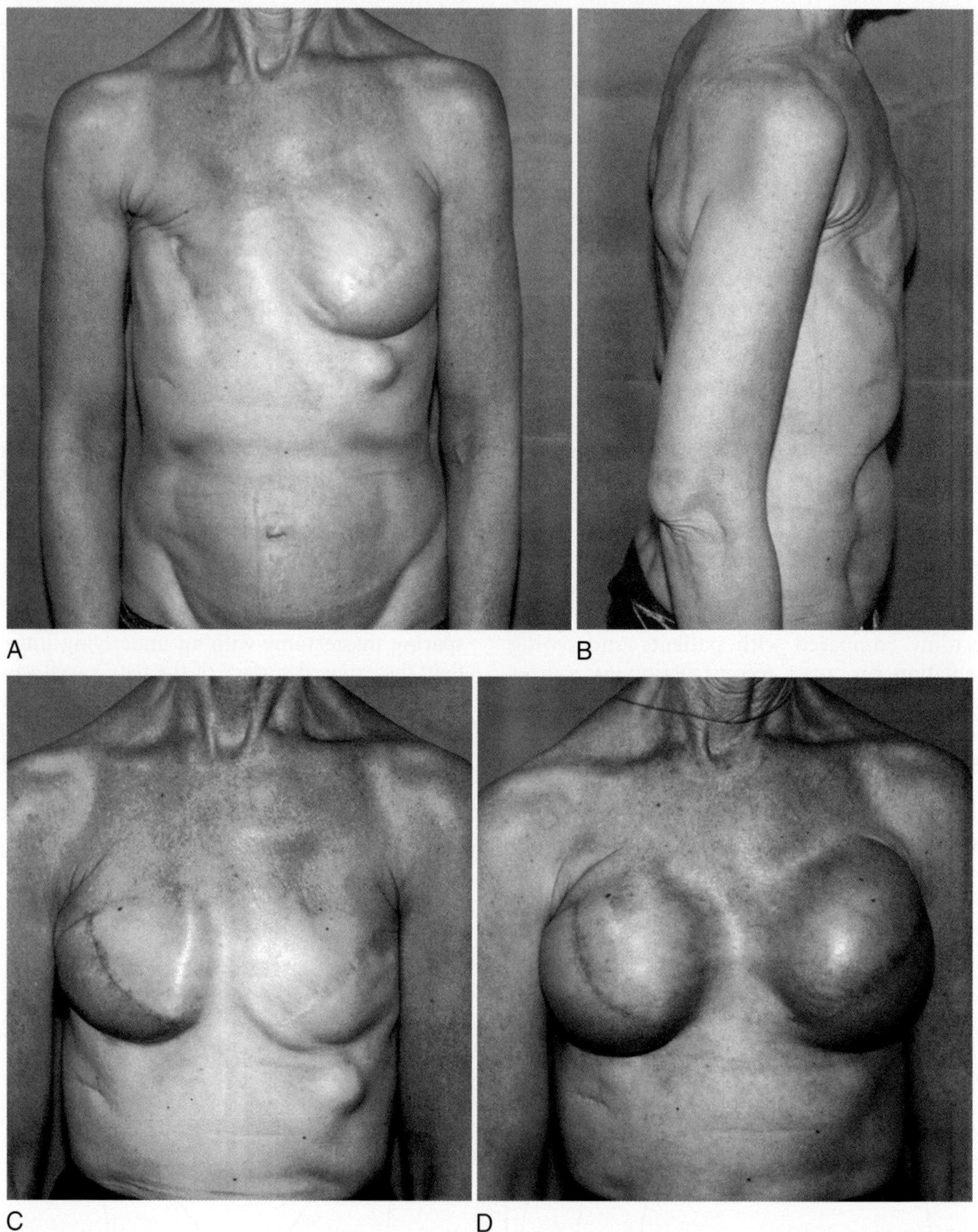

FIGURE 150-2. Mastectomy skin loss *(right)* and implant failure *(left)*. *A,* Anterior view of patient presenting with loss of coverage of right implant with implant removal; left prophylactic mastectomy with expander in place. *B,* Lateral view of inadequate remaining skin envelope for breast mound reconstruction. *C,* Anterior postoperative view of staged secondary reconstruction with right flap (latissimus dorsi musculocutaneous transposition flap) and tissue expander. *D,* Postoperative anterior view of left staged secondary breast reconstruction with capsulectomy and insertion of new expander. The expanders are inflated during 3 months.

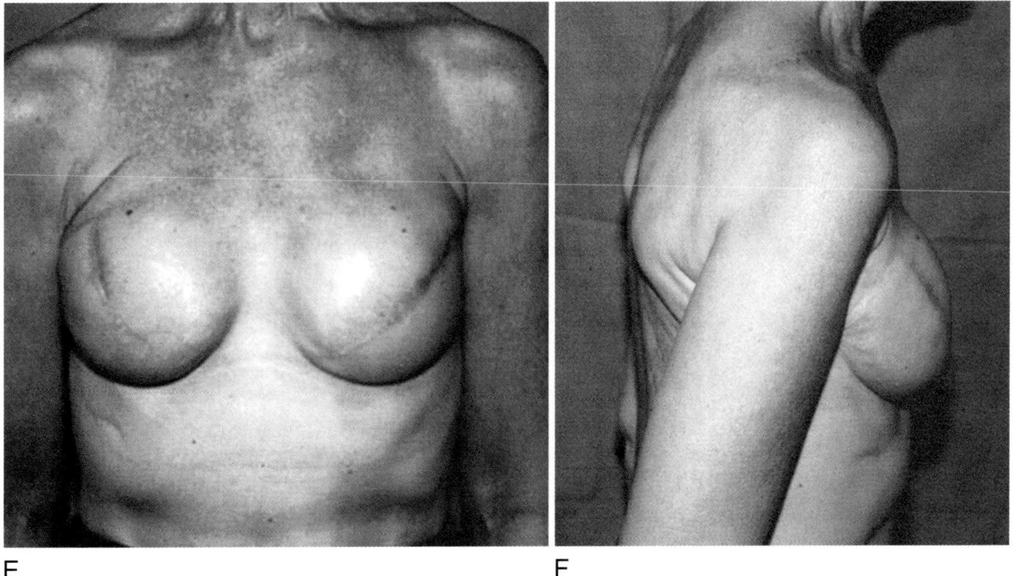

E F

FIGURE 150-2, cont'd. *E,* Anterior postoperative view of completed bilateral secondary reconstruction. *F,* Lateral view. Note that the flap provides an adequate skin envelope for the permanent implant.

TABLE 150-14 ✦ SURGICAL OPTIONS FOR CORRECTION OF MASTECTOMY SKIN LOSS

Problem	Surgical Options
Mastectomy skin flap necrosis	Conservative: wound care (if small) Irrigation and débridement ± explantation Delayed primary closure Skin graft or with skin island flap

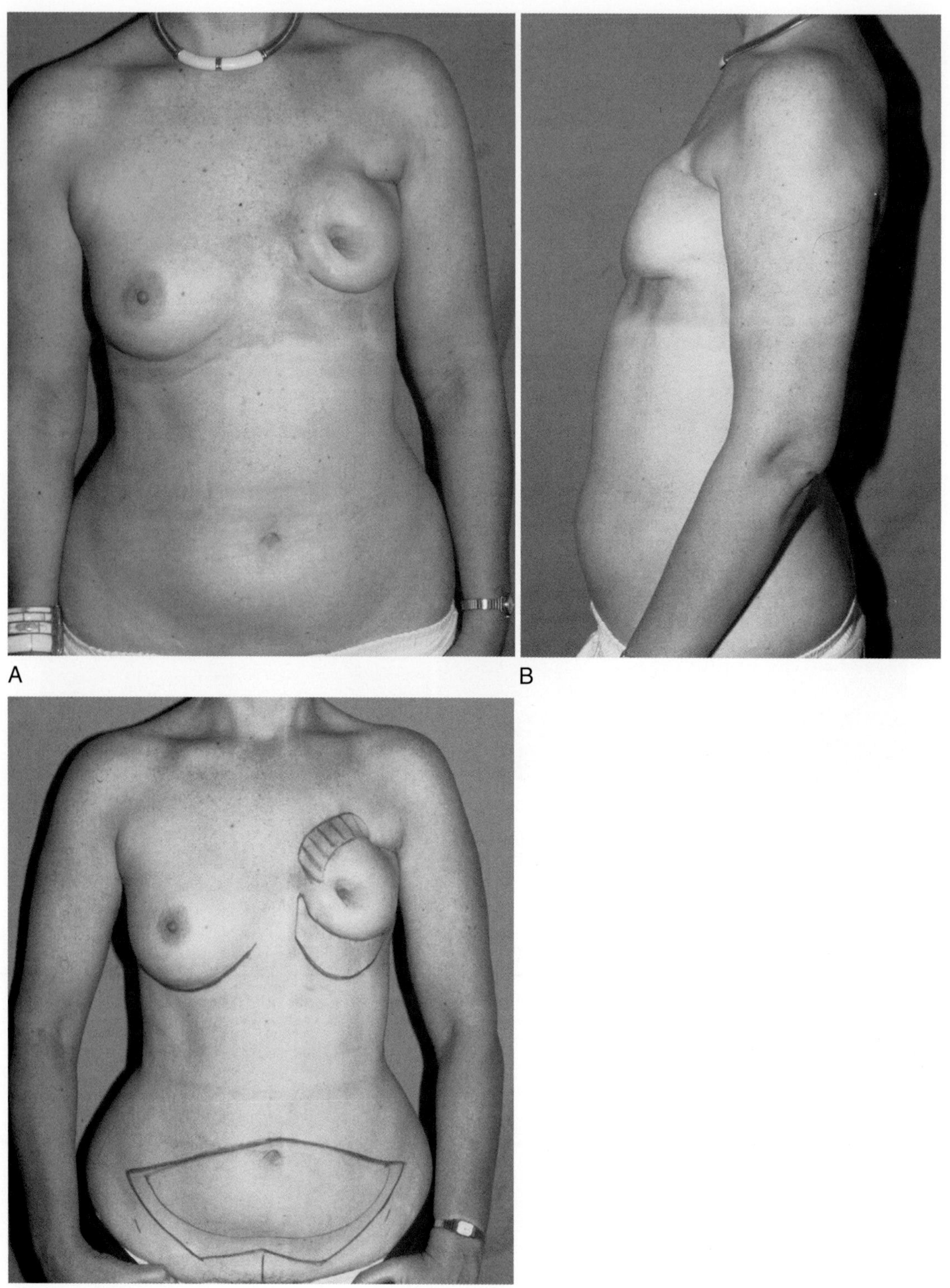

FIGURE 150-3. Mastectomy skin loss. *A,* Anterior view of patient presenting with loss of skin envelope after delayed breast reconstruction. *B,* Lateral view. Note inadequate skin envelope. *C,* Anterior view: design of rectus abdominis musculocutaneous flap with marking for left inframammary line.

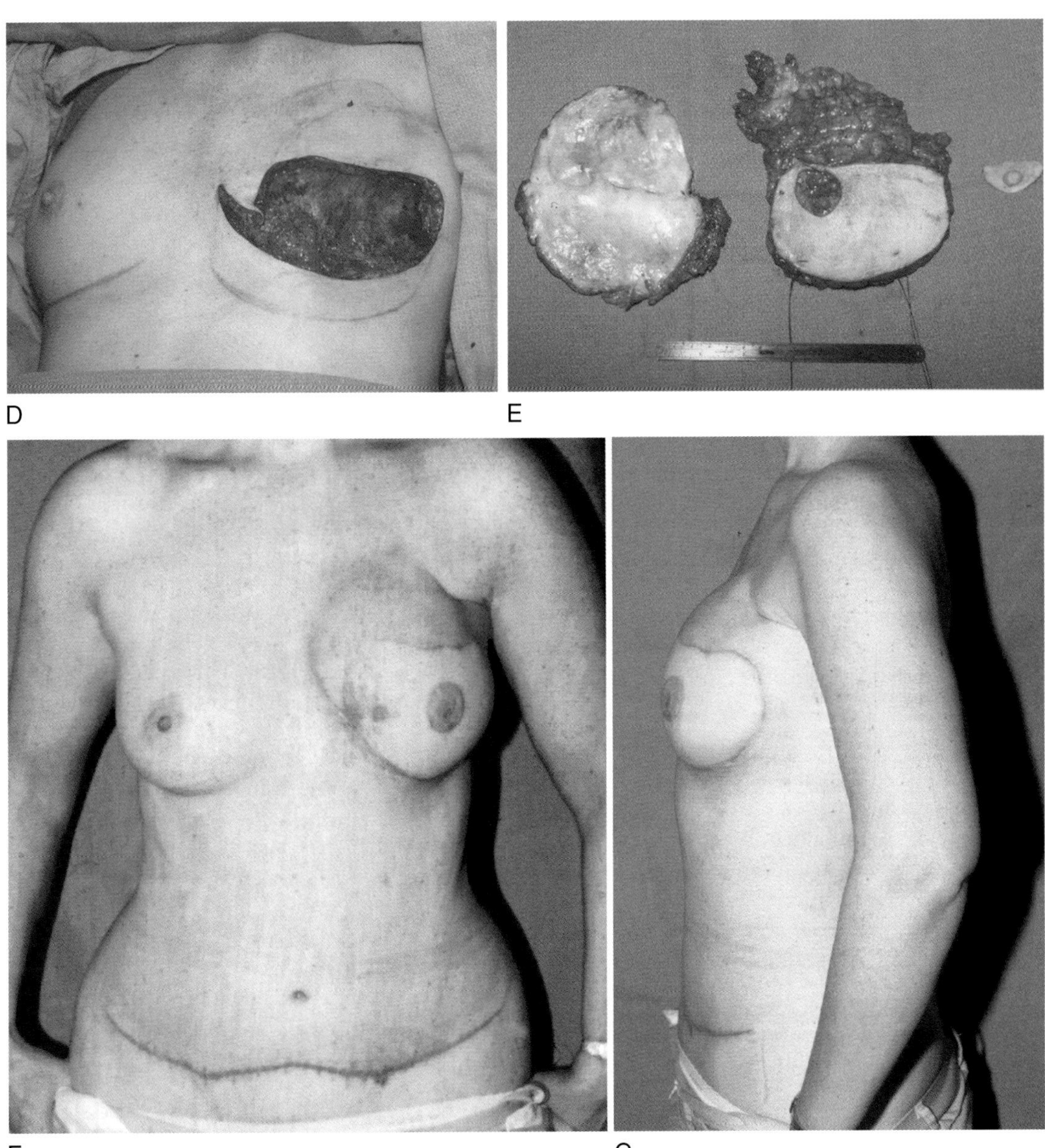

FIGURE 150-3, cont'd. *D,* Intraoperative view of unstable and scarred skin envelope resected. Note that the site for the inframammary line is elevated over the preoperatively determined site because of anticipated lowering of the inframammary line after abdominal donor site closure. *E,* Intraoperative view of specimen. Note explantation with total capsulectomy and unstable preserved mastectomy skin envelope. *F,* Anterior view of postoperative secondary breast reconstruction with capsulectomy, explantation, and TRAM flap for autogenous reconstruction. *G,* Lateral view. Note repositioned inframammary line and adequate skin envelope provided by TRAM skin island and autogenous mound.

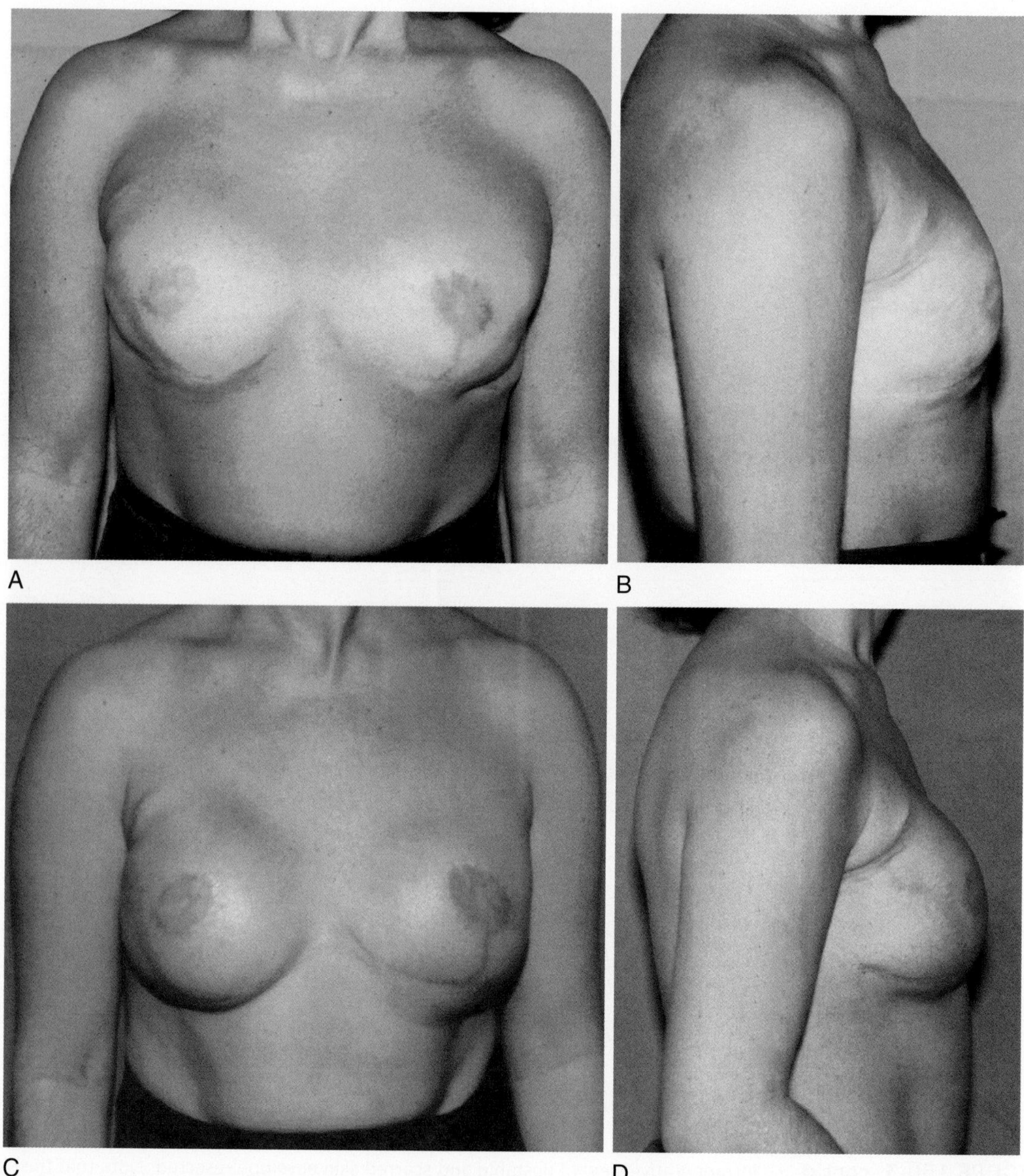

FIGURE 150-4. Mastectomy skin loss. *A,* Anterior view of patient presenting with right breast failed implant reconstruction due to partial mastectomy skin loss. *B,* Lateral view. Because of inadequate skin envelope, the mound lacks inferior fullness. *C,* Postoperative anterior view after single-stage secondary procedures including implant exchange, flap (latissimus dorsi musculocutaneous transposition flap), and capsulectomy. *D,* Lateral view. Note inferior fullness possible with replacement of inadequate envelope.

TABLE 150-15 ✦ RATES OF SKIN NECROSIS, WOUND DEHISCENCE, AND EXTRUSION ASSOCIATED WITH IMPLANTS

Author, Year	N	Technique	Necrosis	Dehiscence	Extrusion	Risk Factors Described	Effect on Incidence
Alderman,[18] 2002	326	E/I or TRAM flap	6.3%	3.8%	—	IBR, DBR	IBR ↑ major complications ($P = .005$)
Ramon,[23] 1997	52	Immediate E/I	1.9%	—	5.8%	None described	—
Crespo,[24] 1994	115	E/I or implant	2.6%			None described	—
Gabriel,[25] 1997	1454 breasts	Augmentation or reconstruction	0.8% of all	0.3% of all	1%	Surgical indication (augmentation, reconstruction)	Higher total complication rate with reconstruction ($P < .005$)
Clough,[15] 2001	360 implants	49.7% saline, 35.6% Becker, 7.2% E/I, 7.5% silicone	5.5%	—	—	—	—
Pusic,[26] 2003	370 breasts	Rapid E/I (<7 weeks)	—	—	0.3%	None described	—
Disa,[27] 1999	770	90% immediate	0.25%	—	0.25%	Concomitant medical illness, prior irradiation	No effect on risk of premature expander removal
O'Brien,[28] 1993	113	83% E/I, 17% autologous	5%	—	2%	None described	—
Furey,[29] 1994	120 breasts	E/I or implant	10% (4.2% required reoperation)	—	0.8%	Chemotherapy	Necrosis → reoperation: 8.3% vs. 2.4%, P value not given
Slavin,[30] 1998	51	SSM, IBR with LD flap + implant	21.6% (may include LD flap)	—	3.9%	None described	—
Schuster,[31] 1988	56 breasts	Immediate E/I	12.5%	—	7.1%	None described	—

Continued

TABLE 150-15 ✦ RATES OF SKIN NECROSIS, WOUND DEHISCENCE, AND EXTRUSION ASSOCIATED WITH IMPLANTS—cont'd

Author, Year	N	Technique	Necrosis	Dehiscence	Extrusion	Risk Factors Described	Effect on Incidence
Spear,[32] 1998	171	E/I (8% with flap), immediate	5.3%	—	10.5%	None described	—
Noone,[33] 1985	185	Implant, 3% E/I (all immediate)	15% (0% loss)	—	4% (2% → loss)	None described	—
Gui,[7] 2003	129	Immediate McGhan 150 ± LD flap	3%	—	3.9% (4.4% for implant, 3.3% for LD flap + implant)	None described	—
Contant,[34] 2000	100	Immediate implant	5% → implant loss	—	—	Radiotherapy	↑ Risk of prosthesis loss ($P < .05$)
Gutowski,[22] 1997	504	Saline implants (6.2% reconstruction)	2.2% "wound complication"	0.3%	—	None specific to skin problems	—
Miller,[35] 1991	83	64% IBR, 36% DBR E/I or implant	"Skin slough" (7.2%)	—	—	Timing (IBR, DBR)	7.2% vs. 0%, $P = .07$
Cooper,[36] 1984	82	Implant ± LD flap	—	—	17%	None described	—
Camilleri,[37] 1996	120 breasts	Becker expander (+LD flap in 30%)	5% "skin breakdown"	—	—	Radiotherapy, smoking	Both ↑ risk of skin problems ($P = .05$)
Pennisi,[38] 1990	115	Polyurethane implants after subcutaneous mastectomy	6.1% → loss		See text—figures combined	None described	—
Berry,[39] 1998	100	Immediate Becker	4%	—	14%	None described	—
McCraw,[17] 1987	55	E/I	9.1% → loss	—	See text	None described	—
Mentor SPS[3]	416	Saline implants, 3-year follow-up	2%	6% "delayed wound healing"	2%	—	—

DBR, delayed breast reconstruction; E/I, expander-implant; IBR, immediate breast reconstruction; LD flap, latissimus dorsi flap; SSM, skin-sparing mastectomy; TRAM flap, transverse rectus abdominis musculocutaneous flap.

TABLE 150-16 ✦ UNSTABLE SKIN, MASTECTOMY SKIN FLAP NECROSIS, AND DEHISCENCE INCIDENCE AFTER AUTOLOGOUS RECONSTRUCTION

Author, Year	N	Technique	Unstable Skin	Mastectomy Skin Flap Necrosis	Dehiscence	Risk Factors
Hartrampf,[10] 1987	383 breasts	Pedicled TRAM flap reconstruction	—	2 (0.6%)	—	Smoking history (58× more likely, $P = .001$) Radiation: no effect
Menke,[40] 2001	121	LD flap ± implant	—	—	3.3%—no reoperations	—
Roy,[41] 1998	111	LD flap + implant (95%)	—	3% "skin loss"	RT	Not significant
Clough,[16] 2001	171	TRAM flap (unipedicled, bipedicled, supercharged, free)	—	—	2.9% "delayed healing"	—
Chang,[43] 2002	75	Extended LD flap without implant	—	17.3%	—	Age, breast size ↑ risk of any breast complications
Chang,[44] 2000	936	Free TRAM flap	—	Smokers, 18.9%; ex-smokers, 10%; nonsmokers 9%	—	Smoking ↑ risk of mastectomy skin flap necrosis (18.9% vs. 9%, $P = .005$)
Tran,[45] 2001	102	Immediate or delayed free TRAM flap	—	5.7% of DBR, 9.4% of IBR	—	IBR then RT vs. RT then DBR
Crespo,[24] 1994	216	TRAM flap (n = 101), tissue expander–implant, or implant	—	3% of TRAM flap group	—	—
Paige,[46] 1998	257	Unilateral unipedicled/ bilateral unipedicled TRAM flap	"Full-thickness skin loss," 8.2%			Laterality NS Obesity, smoking, and prior RT all significant for any complication

DBR, delayed breast reconstruction; IBR, immediate breast reconstruction; LD flap, latissimus dorsi flap; RT, radiation therapy; TRAM flap, transverse rectus abdominis musculocutaneous flap.

remainder of the buried skin island de-epithelialized for the final flap inset. This approach is effective but defeats the advantage of immediate reconstruction as a single-stage procedure. In high-risk patients (smokers, obesity, and connective tissue disease) in whom risk of skin loss is greater, this approach may have some merit. However, these patients may not be good candidates for skin-preserving mastectomy and simultaneous flap use for mound reconstruction. If skin loss is routinely observed in skin-sparing mastectomy, resection of ecchymotic skin or skin without fluorescence (fluorescein injection) may be warranted rather than a second-look procedure.

Delayed skin envelope problems are less dramatic but a frequent cause of dissatisfaction of patients. After expander-implant use, the patient may not have natural ptosis or adequate fullness in the inferior aspect of the breast to match the contralateral breast. Contralateral mastopexy or reduction mammaplasty is a common solution to this problem and should be discussed before the reconstruction. However, if the patient refuses contralateral breast surgery and the opposite breast is mildly ptotic, the expander-implant technique should be avoided. If it has been used and the patient is dissatisfied, a flap inset will increase the dimensions of the skin envelope and allow moderate ptosis to be established, providing symmetry with the opposite breast.

FLAP LOSS

Partial and total flap losses, in the form of skin and subcutaneous tissue necrosis, are ischemic complica-

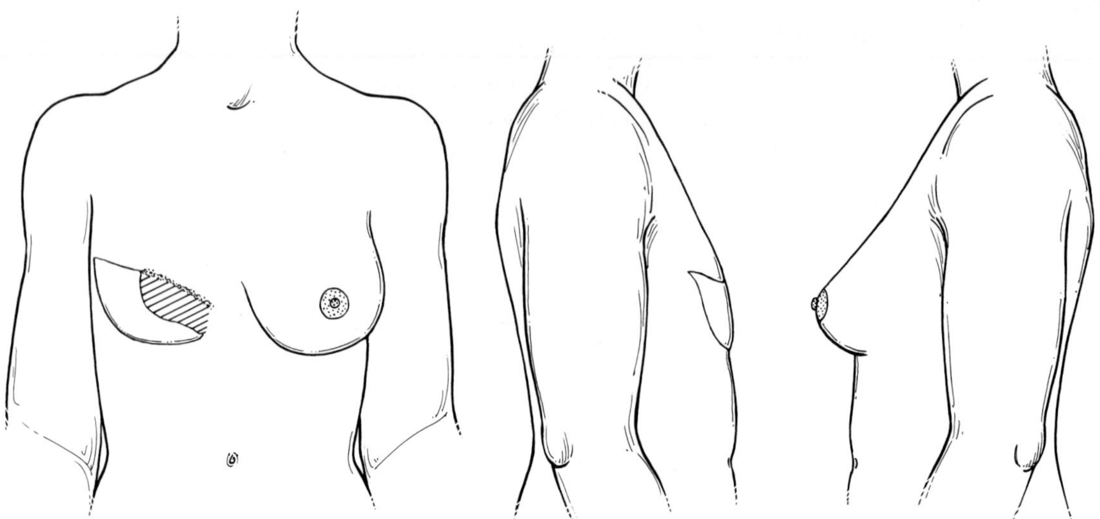

FIGURE 150-5. Partial flap loss.

tions resulting from vascular insufficiency (Fig. 150-5).[10,11,16,24,40-53] They may follow reconstruction with any autologous tissue. The incidence of partial or complete flap loss varies with flap selection and surgeon experience with use of the selected flap.[40-42] The rectus abdominis musculocutaneous flap is generally used to solve two reconstructive requirements: skin envelope deficiency and autogenous volume to establish a breast mound (Table 150-17). Partial or complete skin necrosis will result in both envelope and mound problems but is addressed under the category of envelope. Ischemic necrosis of subcutaneous tissue may have an intact cutaneous portion of the composite flap but will affect the quality of the reconstruction. Fat necrosis is discussed later as a mound problem.

With the increasing frequency of transplantation of the TRAM flap, the incidence of partial flap loss has decreased. Flap loss after microvascular transplantation of the TRAM or perforator (DIEP) flap usually occurs early in the postoperative period (within 4 to 5 days) and may be the result of anastomotic flaws, side-branch injury, vessel spasm, pedicle kinking or compression, hematoma, or tight wound closure.[44] It may also result from venous outflow problems. Depending on perforator vessel anatomy, skin island loss may occur despite successful flap revascularization (Fig. 150-6 and Table 150-18).

Partial loss of the latissimus dorsi musculocutaneous flap ranges from 1.7% to 5.3%; total flap loss is rare, occurring in 0% to 0.3%.[40-43] The TRAM transposition flap has a greater risk of partial flap loss, depending on the design of the skin island.[42,48] Use of the primary territory of the flap, limited to zones 1 and 2, should be safe, but extending the territory to include zones 3 and 4 will increase the risk of partial flap loss. Partial flap loss has a wide reported range from 6% to 10.6%.[11,12,49] Total flap loss of the transposition TRAM flap ranges from 0.3% to 3.9% (Fig. 150-7 and Table 150-19).[44-49]

The wide variation in reported rates of partial and total flap necrosis may be in part explained by a lack of standard definitions for these terms. The line between a large partial flap loss and total flap loss is indistinct, and at the other end of the scale, some authors report partial flap loss only if the extent of necrosis is greater than a set threshold, which can vary between studies.

Kroll,[49] in his review of 302 reconstructions with TRAM flap (n = 162), latissimus dorsi flap (n = 45), and tissue expansion (n = 95), reported on incidence and treatment of flap necrosis. Flap necrosis was most common in the TRAM group (26%), followed by tissue expansion (13%) and latissimus dorsi (11%). The flap necrosis was not always so extensive as to require

TABLE 150-17 ✦ SURGICAL OPTIONS AFTER DEVELOPMENT OF FLAP LOSS

Problem	Surgical Options
Partial or total flap loss	Early re-exploration to prevent further flap loss Conservative: wound care (if small partial) Revision: flap reinset (if remaining volume allows) Irrigation and débridement + closure Conversion to another flap

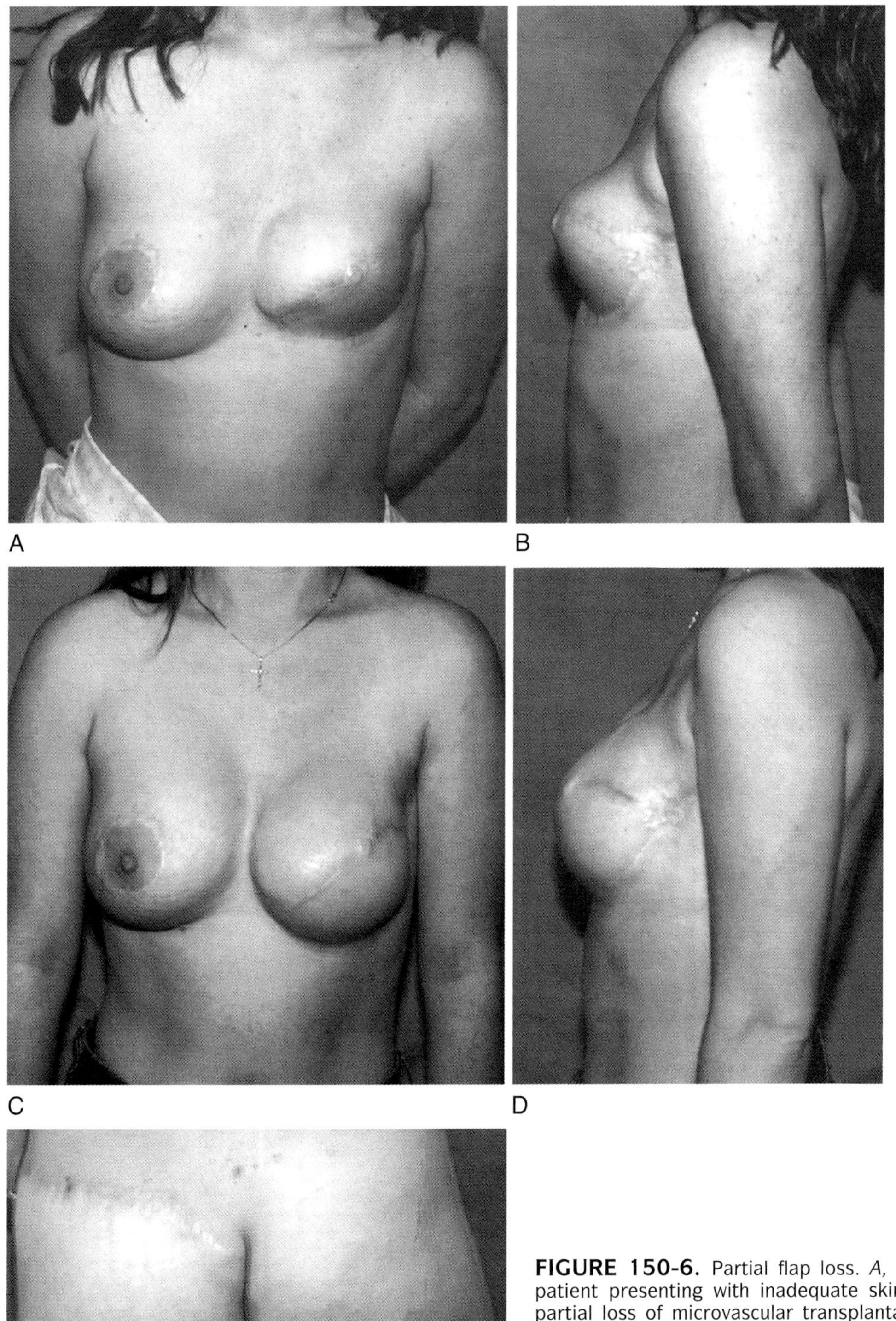

FIGURE 150-6. Partial flap loss. *A,* Anterior view of patient presenting with inadequate skin envelope after partial loss of microvascular transplantation of superior gluteus maximus musculocutaneous flap. *B,* Lateral view. Note inadequate skin envelope for breast mound reconstruction. *C,* Anterior postoperative view of secondary breast reconstruction with latissimus dorsi musculocutaneous transposition flap with permanent implant. *D,* Lateral view. Flap provides adequate skin envelope for implant coverage and inferior breast mound fullness. *E,* Posterior trunk. Note donor site scar for failed gluteus maximus free flap.

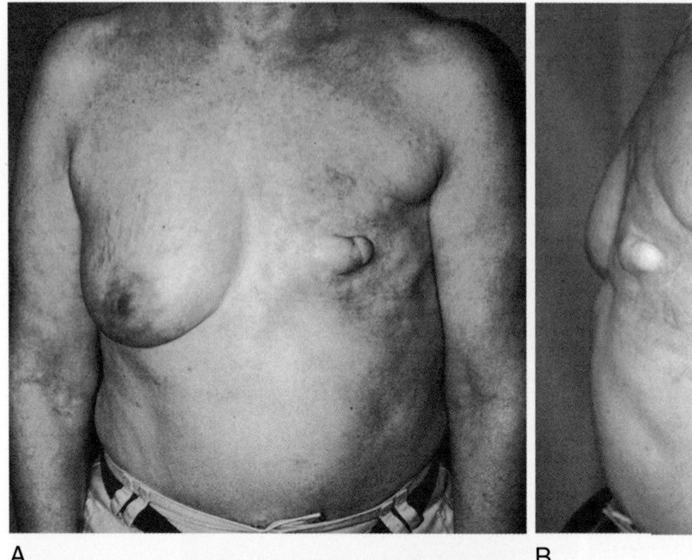

A

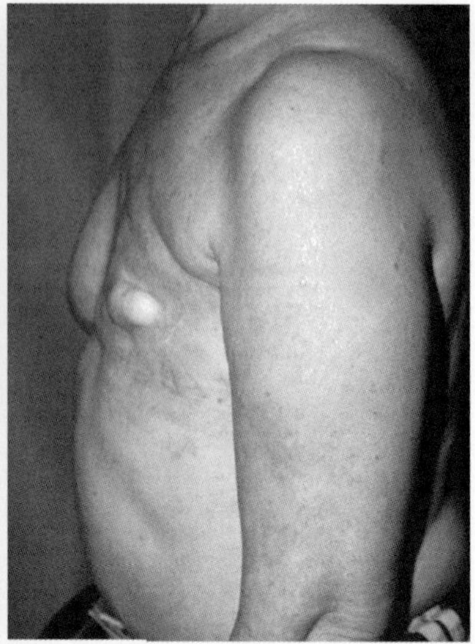

B

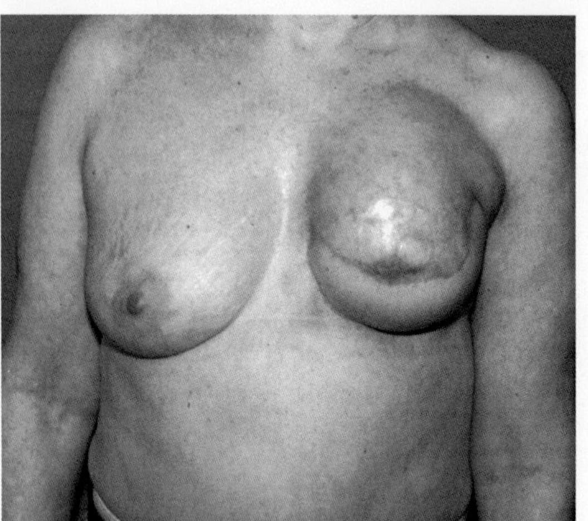

C

FIGURE 150-7. Complete flap loss. *A,* Anterior view of patient presenting with complete loss of TRAM flap. *B,* Lateral view. Note inadequate skin envelope for breast mound reconstruction. *C,* Anterior postoperative view of staged reconstruction with latissimus dorsi musculocutaneous transposition flap and expander (inflated during 3 months). *D,* Anterior postoperative view after insertion of permanent implant. *E,* Lateral view. The flap provides an adequate skin envelope for the permanent implant.

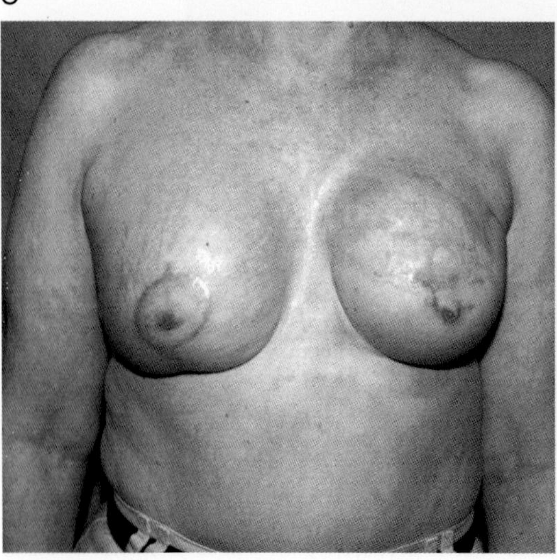

D

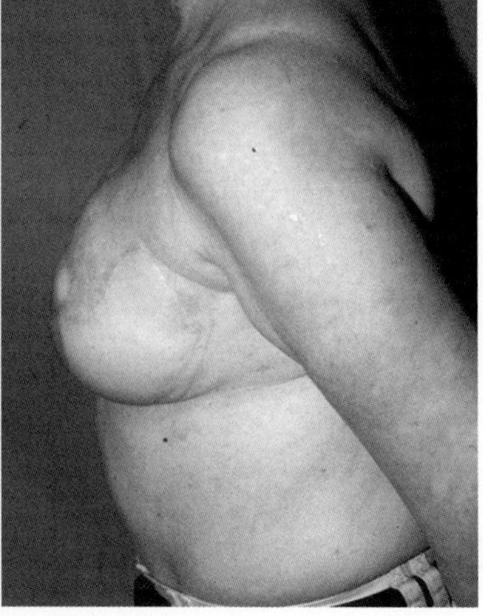

E

TABLE 150-18 ✦ COMPLICATION RATES OF AUTOGENOUS AND NONAUTOGENOUS METHODS*

	Group I 1979-1983		Group II 1984-1987		Group III 1988-1991	
	Major	*Minor*	*Major*	*Minor*	*Major*	*Minor*
Nonautogenous	n = 133		n = 93		n = 111	
Implants	2 (5%)	9 (22.5%)	2 (8%)	3 (12%)	1 (6%)	3 (18%)
Tissue expansion	0 (0%)	3 (75%)	2 (4%)	15 (28%)	1 (1%)	14 (17%)
Latissimus dorsi with implant	1 (1%)	15 (18%)	1 (8%)	3 (25%)	0 (0%)	2 (17%)
Abdominal advance with implant	0 (0%)	2 (33%)	0 (0%)	1 (33%)	0 (0%)	0 (0%)
Total	3 (2%)	29 (21%)	5 (5%)	22 (23%)	2 (2%)	19 (17%)
Autogenous	n = 20		n = 33		n = 65	
TRAM	1 (5%)	4 (20%)	2 (6%)	5 (15%)	1 (2%)	8 (15%)
Free flap	0		0		1 (1%)	3 (25%)
Total	1 (5%)	4 (20%)	2 (6%)	5 (15%)	2 (3%)	11 (17%)

*No. (%) of complications, major and minor (n = 455). $P > .20$ between each pair of study groups.

From Trabulsy PP, Anthony JP, Mathes SJ: Changing trends in postmastectomy breast reconstruction: a 13-year experience. Plast Reconstr Surg 1994;93:1418-1427.

further surgery (10.6% of the 302 reconstructions required surgical revision for management of flap necrosis). The revision rates were reported as follows, according to technique: TRAM flap, 12%; tissue expanders, 13%; and latissimus dorsi flap, 2%. Surgical revision consisted of early aggressive débridement and repeated primary closure. Conversion to a TRAM flap was required in one tissue expansion patient.

When complete flap loss occurs, débridement and closure of the mastectomy defect are required. Immediate use of an alternative flap is also an option. When a transposition flap fails, it may be wise to achieve a healed wound and to plan a delayed secondary reconstruction. If a free flap fails, the patient usually has undergone an urgent technique for flap salvage by exploration of the anastomosis. If the recipient vessels are a source of the difficulty in revascularization of the flap, delay in the secondary flap procedure may be wise while the patient recovers from the initial reconstruction and urgent salvage procedures.

For partial flap loss, the options include conservative management consisting of both topical and parenteral antibiotics and delay in débridement until the area of necrosis forms an eschar and eschar separation occurs. Kroll,[49] in his review of partial flap loss, discusses the relative merits of conservative versus aggressive treatment with the following conclusions: conservative treatment involves little or no débridement, facilitating maximum preservation of tissue; conservative treatment leads to prolonged healing and increased scarring; and aggressive treatment sacrifices some potentially viable tissue but usually results in early healing and less scarring.

In the latissimus dorsi musculocutaneous flap with underlying implant, there is concern about implant infection or exposure. Unless the portion of the skin island necrosis is very small, early débridement and closure are indicated.

In the TRAM transposition flap, the demarcation between a small area of flap necrosis and ischemia may be difficult to determine in the early postoperative phase. Conservative wound care is recommended until eschar separation occurs, and then minimal débridement will be required. However, if the area of necrosis is large, wound sepsis occurs, or there is potential for implant contamination or exposure, early débridement and wound closure are indicated.

If excision is necessary, it should be carried out early (day 2 to 7) before infection can be established. All necrotic skin and discolored fat should be débrided, which can result in volume loss. If excision is required in an aesthetically critical portion of the flap, the flap may require repositioning. Radical débridement may be necessary for subtotal necrosis.

EXCESS

After flap use, the skin island may be excessive, allowing excess ptosis or too large inset of the flap skin island in the skin-sparing nipple-areola defect. The surgeon is often reluctant to excise scarred preserved skin envelope at the time of inset of a flap for delayed breast reconstruction. The excess native skin along with the addition of flap skin may result in excess breast ptosis compared with the contralateral breast. The secondary procedure will include resection of

TABLE 150-19 ✦ PARTIAL AND TOTAL FLAP LOSS AND SELECTED RISK FACTORS FOR AUTOLOGOUS RECONSTRUCTION

Author, Year	N	Technique	Partial or Total Flap Loss Incidence	Risk Factors Described	Effect on Incidence
Hartrampf,[10] 1987	383 breasts	Pedicled TRAM flap reconstruction	Partial, 6% Total, 0.3%	Smoking, RT	Smoking ↑ risk, RT no effect
Menke,[40] 2001	121	LD flap ± implant	Partial, 1.7% Total, 0%	—	—
Roy,[41] 1998	111	LD flap + implant (95%)	4% "skin and fat loss"	RT	Not significant
Clough,[16] 2001	171	TRAM flap (unipedicled, bipedicled, supercharged, free)	Total, 1.2% Partial, 10.6%	—	—
Kroll,[48] 2000	310	Free TRAM flap (279), DIEP flap (31)	Partial: free TRAM flap, 2.2%; unselected DIEP flap, 37.5%; selected DIEP flap, 8.7% (see text)	Free TRAM flap vs. unselected DIEP flap; smoking	Unselected DIEP flap ↑ risk Smoking NS (see fat necrosis section)
Chang,[43] 2002	75	Extended LD flap without implant	Partial, 5.3% Total, 0%	Age, breast size	Both ↑ risk of any flap complication
Kroll,[49] 1991	302 breasts	TRAM flap, LD flap, E/I	Any: 19.5% (includes mastectomy flap necrosis); 10.6% required revision	—	—
Kroll,[50] 1994	284	TRAM flap, LD flap	"Major flap loss" requiring surgery: 3.9%; any degree of flap loss: 27%	TRAM flap vs. LD flap; RT	RT associated with ↑ risk of any breast complication ($P = .03$) Irradiated LD flaps have more complications than irradiated TRAM flaps (small sample, NS)
Moran,[51] 2001	221	Free, pedicled TRAM flap	Total flap loss, 3% (all pedicled) Partial flap loss, 11% (all pedicled) Figures are all for obese patients	Free vs. pedicled TRAM flap, obesity	Total or partial flap loss more common in pedicled TRAM flap than in free TRAM flap Obesity ↑ any complication in free TRAM flap (14% vs. 0%, $P = .008$) but not pedicled
Chang,[44] 2000	936	Free TRAM flap	Total, 0.9% Partial, 1.4%	Smoking	No significant difference
Williams,[52] 1997	699	Pedicled TRAM flap	"Full-thickness skin loss": no RT, 0.1%; prior RT, 2.8%; RT to TRAM flap, 5.3%	Preoperative and postoperative TRAM flap irradiation	Preoperative vs. postoperative, not significant RT vs. no RT, marginal for any complication ($P = .072$)
Tran,[45] 2001	102	Immediate or delayed free TRAM flap	Partial, 7.1% Total, 1.4% Numbers are for DBR; no flap loss seen in 32 IBR patients	IBR then RT vs. RT then DBR	No significant difference
Crespo,[24] 1994	216	TRAM flap (n = 101), E/I, or implant	3% of TRAM flap group	—	—
Banic,[53] 1995	111	Free TRAM flap	Partial, 7.2% (1.8% minor, 5.4% major) Total, 5.4%	RT, chemotherapy, smoking	None significant

DBR, delayed breast reconstruction; DIEP flap, deep inferior epigastric perforator flap; E/I, expander-implant; IBR, immediate breast reconstruction; LD flap, latissimus dorsi flap; RT, radiation therapy; TRAM flap, transverse rectus abdominis musculocutaneous flap.

excess flap or native preserved skin envelope to provide appropriate dimensions for the breast skin envelope. If the excess skin is scarred from the mastectomy, the area of skin is preferentially excised with the flap edge advanced for closure. If the preserved skin envelope is normal in appearance, it is usually preferable to resect the excess flap skin island to tailor the final skin envelope (Fig. 150-8 and Table 150-20).

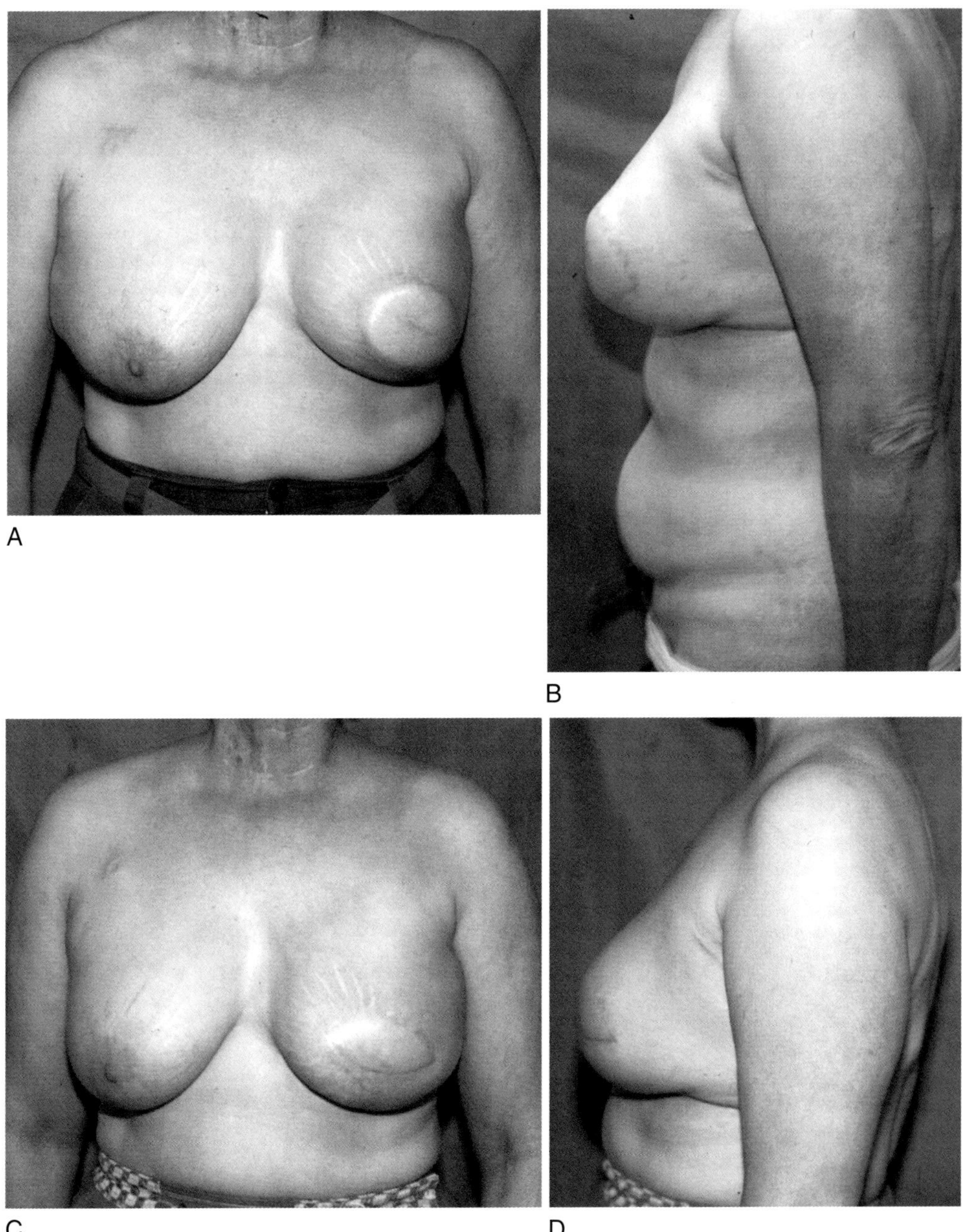

FIGURE 150-8. Excess envelope. *A*, Anterior postoperative view of patient immediately after reconstruction with TRAM flap for skin-sparing mastectomy. Skin island dimensions are excessive at nipple-areola defect. *B*, Lateral view after autogenous reconstruction with TRAM flap. *C*, Anterior postoperative view of secondary reconstruction with reduction of skin island to establish natural contour of breast mound. *D*, Lateral view with appropriately sized skin envelope.

TABLE 150-20 ✦ SURGICAL OPTIONS FOR CORRECTION OF SKIN ENVELOPE EXCESS

Problem	Surgical Options
Skin envelope excess	No treatment Revision: liposuction (select cases) Revision: resection of excess tissue (flap or native skin)

TABLE 150-21 ✦ SURGICAL OPTIONS FOR CORRECTION OF SKIN ENVELOPE DEFICIENCY

Problem	Surgical Options
Skin envelope deficiency	Tissue expansion Revision: reinset of existing flap Addition of flap to existing reconstruction Conversion to flap technique

DEFICIENCY

When the technique selected fails to provide adequate skin envelope, the breast mound is not likely to fulfill the requirements of a natural breast appropriate for the patient's age and will lack symmetry with the opposite breast (Fig. 150-9). This problem occurs most commonly when the implant is inserted in skin-sparing mastectomy and adequate envelope is not available for the implant size selected or tissue expansion fails to provide an adequate envelope and inferior quadrant breast fullness (Table 150-21). When radiation therapy follows immediate breast reconstruction, there may be some shrinkage of the envelope, which will result in a deficiency of the envelope with corresponding loss of desired breast appearance.

With flap use for the breast envelope, design and inset errors may result in inadequate envelope. Particularly in delayed reconstruction, the skin island incorporated in the flap design must account for the loss of skin envelope at the mastectomy site and subsequent wound contraction, particularly if the mastectomy site has undergone radiation treatment.

When the envelope is inadequate, a secondary procedure is usually required. Either tissue expansion or a flap will be required to re-establish an adequate envelope. Most commonly, a flap will be required, especially if tissue expansion has already been attempted in the initial reconstructive procedure (Figs. 150-10 and 150-11).

INFECTION

Infection involving the skin envelope may represent cellulitis resulting from bacterial exposure during the mastectomy and reconstruction. However, it may represent a more serious problem reflecting peri-implant infection or infection involving the deep surface of the flap. With autogenous reconstruction, cellulitis usually responds quickly to antibiotic therapy unless there is flap ischemia. With immediate reconstruction with an expander-implant, cellulitis is more difficult to treat successfully because the preserved skin

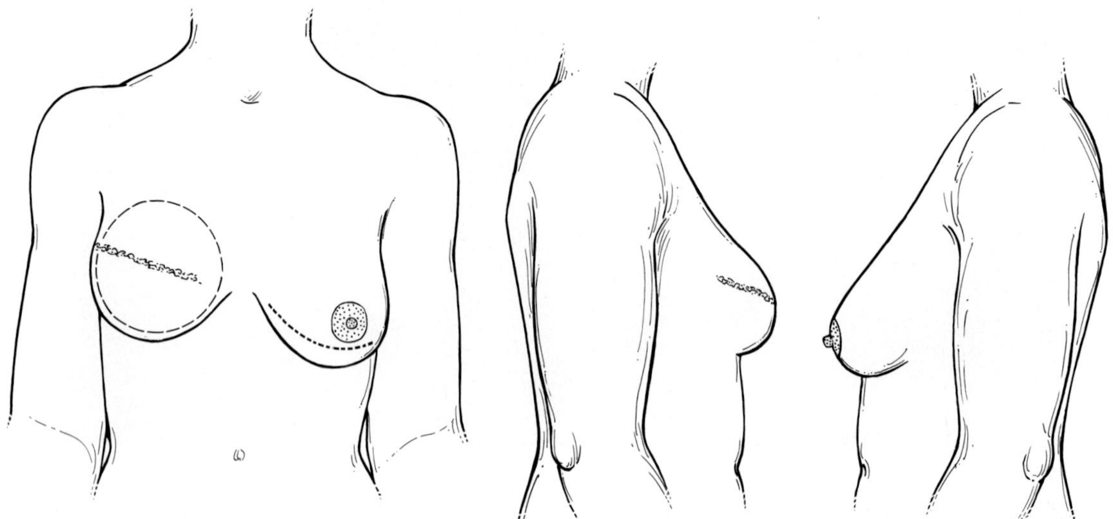

FIGURE 150-9. Skin envelope deficiency. The implant reconstruction has inadequate fullness in the inferior reconstructed mound (lack of natural breast ptosis).

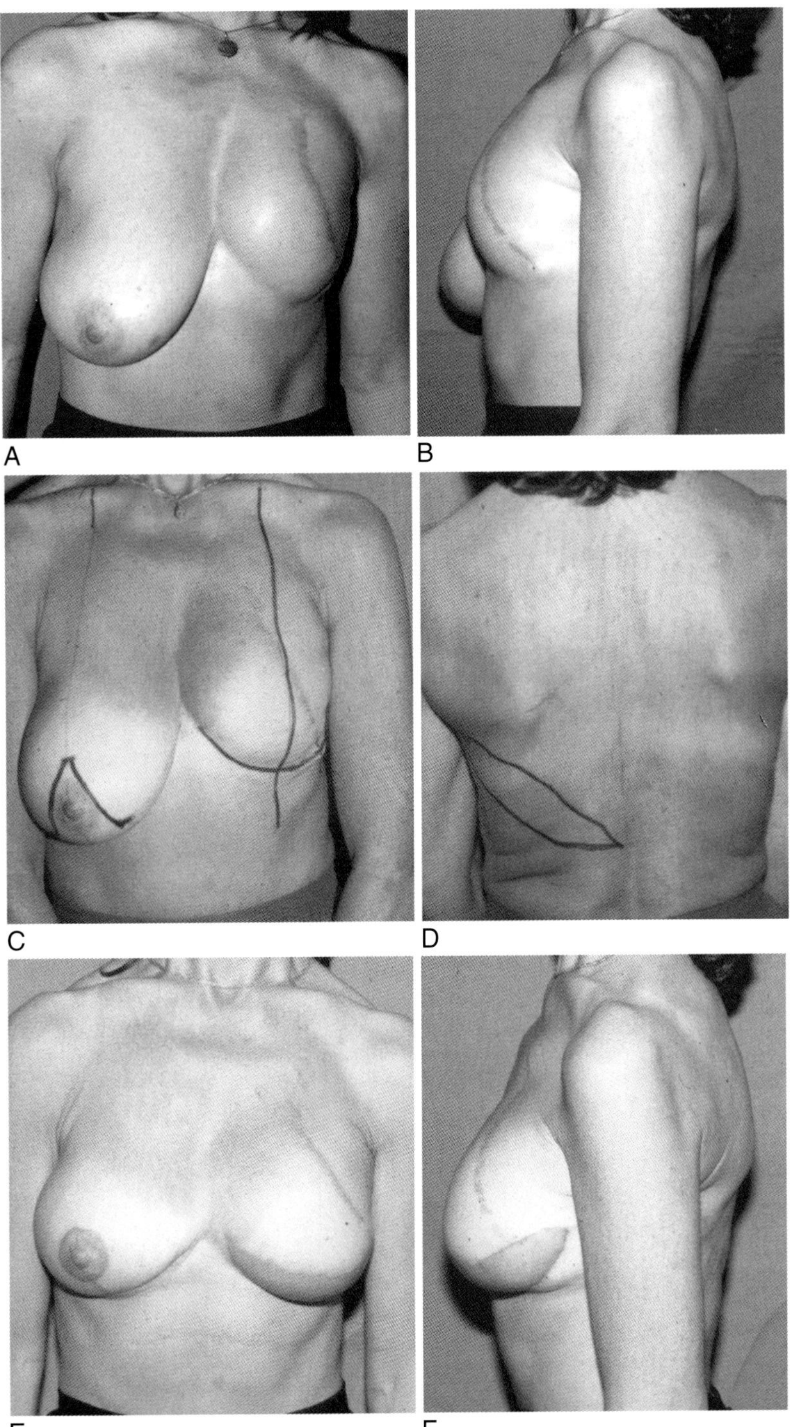

FIGURE 150-10. Deficiency of the skin envelope. *A,* Anterior view: postoperative delayed reconstruction with expander-implant sequence. *B,* Lateral view. Note inadequate skin envelope despite tissue expansion to provide fullness in inferior quadrants of breast mound. *C,* Anterior preoperative view for secondary reconstruction. The plan also included mastopexy for the contralateral breast. *D,* Posterior trunk. Note design of skin island for latissimus dorsi musculocutaneous transposition flap. *E,* Anterior postoperative view after secondary reconstruction with capsulectomy, implant exchange, and latissimus dorsi musculocutaneous flap. *F,* Lateral view. Note that the flap provides adequate skin envelope for coverage of the implant and natural inferior breast fullness.

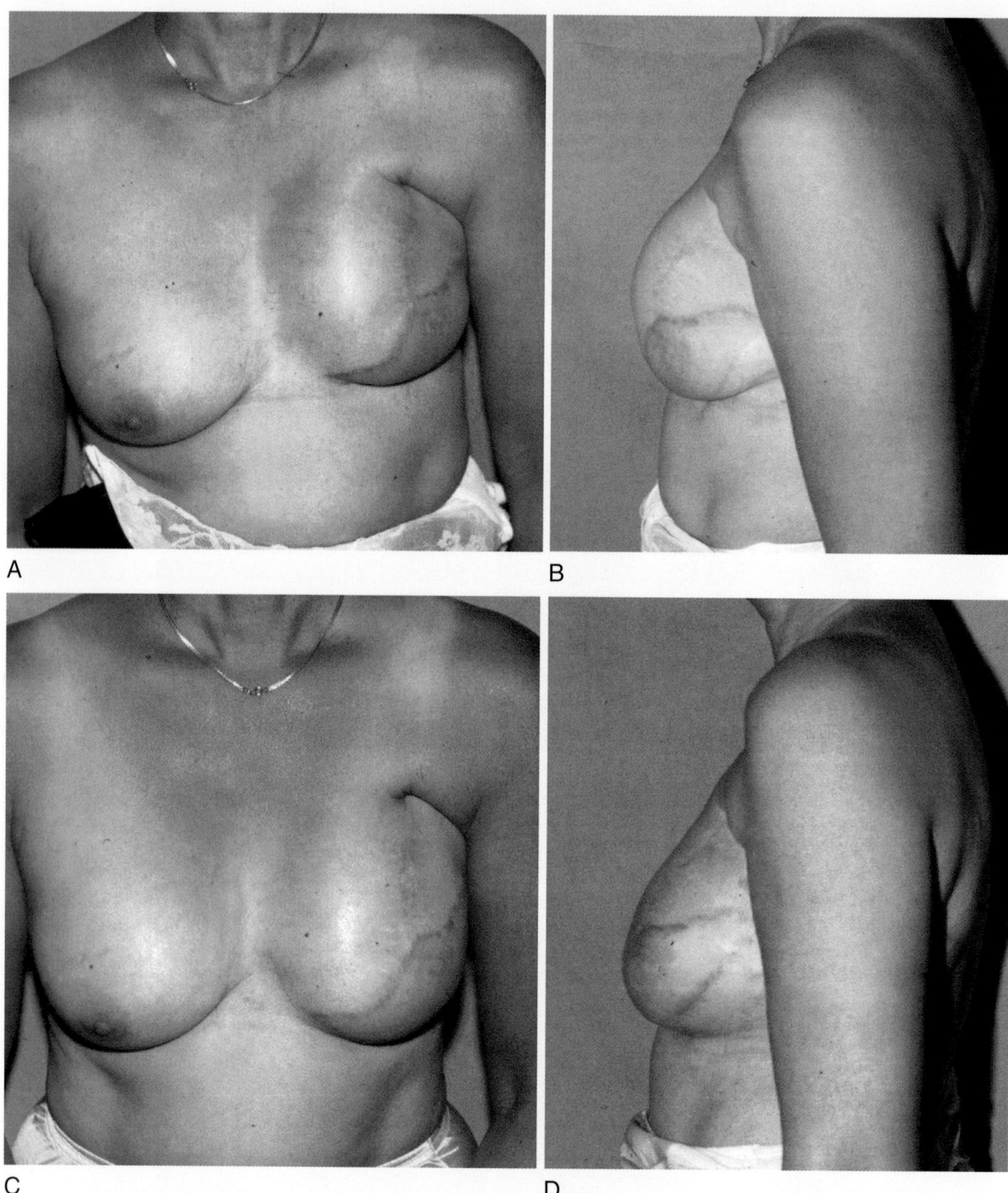

FIGURE 150-11. Skin envelope deficiency. *A,* Anterior view of patient presenting with delayed implant reconstruction after mastectomy. *B,* Lateral view. Note inadequate skin envelope to provide fullness to inferior quadrants of breast mound. *C,* Anterior view after secondary reconstruction with latissimus dorsi musculocutaneous transposition flap with capsulectomy and implant exchange. *D,* Lateral view. Note that the flap provides adequate skin envelope for coverage of the implant and natural inferior breast fullness.

envelope is ischemic from the mastectomy. When cellulitis is observed in the preserved skin envelope with implant reconstruction, a short course of parenteral antibiotics is recommended. If there is no response to the antibiotic course, there is likely contamination and resultant infection in the implant space. The management of this problem relates to the breast mound and is covered in the next section dealing with problems related to the mound.

Mound

Failure of the mound to have a normal breast contour, to provide symmetry with the contralateral breast, or both is a common cause of dissatisfaction of patients. Mound problems are different for expander-implant and flap autogenous reconstructions. The mound in the expander-implant sequence is dependent on an implant, which unfortunately is a source of difficulty because of implant infection, implant loss, capsular contracture, and implant malfunction including deflation and wrinkling. The autogenous mound composed of flap tissue may not have adequate projection or shape if it is inset improperly. Fat necrosis is a frequent complication when the flap dimensions exceed the safe area of the skin territory of the flap (e.g., zones 3 and 4 of the TRAM flap, small perforators in the DIEP flap, or inclusion of distal skin island near the posterior midline of the trunk in the latissimus dorsi musculocutaneous flap). The discussion of mound complications is divided into implant and flap with the understanding that in many instances, the two sources of mound reconstruction are combined.

CAPSULAR CONTRACTURE

The most common problem requiring secondary reconstruction in the implant patient is capsular contracture (Fig. 150-12 and Table 150-22).[3-6,54-60] Significant contracture can lead to problems with malposition of the breast mound, distortion of the breast shape, firmness, implant failure, and pain, and it may lead to secondary surgical procedures when the extent of contracture causes the patient to be dissatisfied with the result. The incidence of symptomatic capsular contracture is high. In a multicenter retrospective review[22] of 504 patients (995 implants for augmentation [93.7%] and reconstruction [6.3%]), the overall percentage of patients who had significant contracture or who had a previous capsulotomy was reported to be 20.4% with a mean follow-up of 6 years (range, 4 to 13 years). The authors suggested that this high rate may be explained by the inclusion of the patient's own evaluations within these figures. The reoperation rate in this study was reported to be 20.6%. The incidence of capsular contracture is variable, and in review of clinical studies, the incidence varies from 5% to 35% (Table 150-23).[3-6,54-60]

TABLE 150-22 ✦ SURGICAL OPTIONS FOR CORRECTION OF CAPSULAR CONTRACTURE

Problem	Surgical Options
Capsular contracture	No treatment (Baker grade I or II) Partial capsulectomy (Baker grade III) Total capsulectomy (Baker grade IV, implant rupture, or capsular calcification) Explantation Explantation with secondary reconstruction (implant exchange, expander-implant sequence, autogenous reconstruction with flap)

The variability in results depends to a large extent on the follow-up of the study patients. The best follow-up rates are available in the reported clinical trials by the implant manufacturers in preparation for prosthesis approval by the Federal Drug Administration. The results of the INAMED (formerly McGhan) R95 study[5] and the longer follow-up Post Approval Survey Study[6] provide data as to the problems observed with implants and the reoperation rates in attempting to correct these observed problems (Tables 150-24 to 150-26). INAMED conducted several clinical studies to test its saline-filled breast implants, including the Large Simple Trial (LST), the 1995 Reconstruction Study (R95) (and augmentation cohort, A95), and the Post Approval Survey Study.[5,6] The LST was designed to determine the 1-year rates of capsular contracture, infection, implant leakage or deflation, and implant replacement or removal. There were 2333 patients enrolled for augmentation, 225 for reconstruction, and 317 for revision (replacement of existing implants). Of these enrolled patients, 62% returned for their 1-year follow-up visit. The R95 and A95 studies were designed to assess all complications as well as the patient's satisfaction, body image, body esteem, and self-concept during the initial 5 years after breast reconstruction. Patients were observed annually, and data through 3 years (with partial 4-year data) were presented to the Federal Drug Administration in 2003 for premarket device approval. The most common complications reported were asymmetry and capsular contracture. During the 5 years reviewed by the study, there were 70 implants removed in 62 patients. Of these 70 implants, 49 were replaced and 21 were not. The most common reason for implant removal through 5 years was capsular contracture (31% of the 70 implants removed)[6] (see Table 143-46).

After premarket approval, INAMED transitioned data collection to a post-approval study. The Post Approval Survey Study (PASS) was designed to collect long-term safety data from patients 6 to 10 years after

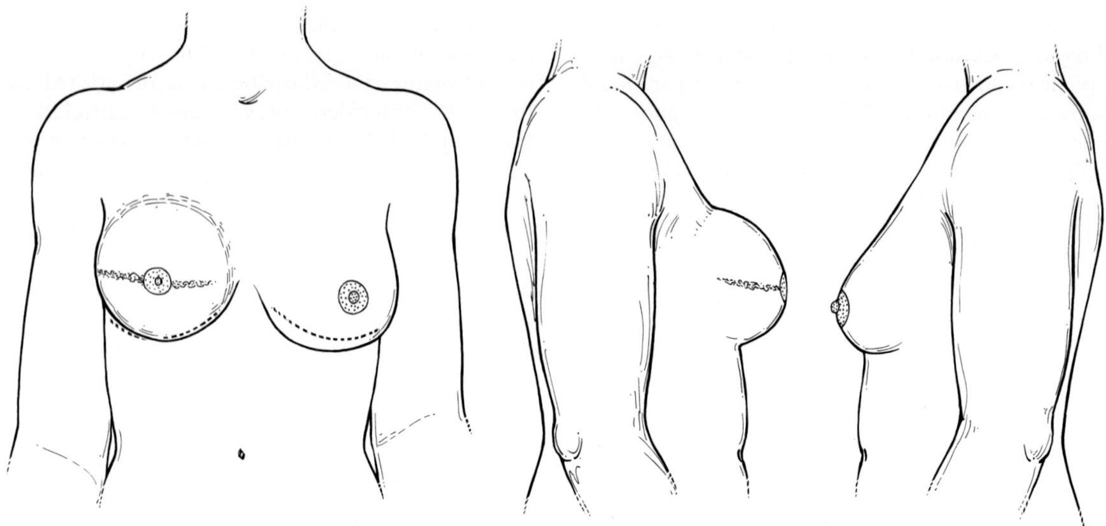

FIGURE 150-12. Capsular contracture.

TABLE 150-23 ✦ INCIDENCE OF CAPSULAR CONTRACTURE

Author, Year	N	Technique	Contracture Incidence	Risk Factors Described	Effect on Incidence
Cunningham,[54] 2000	882 breasts	6.1% reconstruction with saline implant	20.4%*	Implant model, submammary position, implant size	All ↑ risk of contracture (see text)
Gutowski,[22] 1997	995 implants	6.3% reconstruction with saline implant	20.4%*	Several	
Worseg,[8] 1995	167 implants	38% reconstruction with 1800 inflatable	7.8% contracture, 35% previous capsulotomy	Placement, hematoma	Placement: no effect Hematoma ↑ risk of contracture
Handel,[55] 1995	1655 implants	16.9% reconstruction	14% of all patients	Filler, surface texture, placement	See text
Asplund,[56] 1984	72 breasts	Silicone or saline reconstruction	36%	Filler (silicone vs. saline)	Silicone 55% vs. saline 20% ($P = .006$)
Woods,[57] 1980	53	Subcutaneous mastectomy with submuscular reconstruction	5%	—	—
Wickman,[58] 1997	49	Permanent textured expander	8%	Timing (immediate vs. delayed)	Immediate ↑ risk (11% vs. 0%)
Thuesen,[59] 1995	20	Delayed unilateral reconstruction	45% felt "harder than desired," 2% capsulotomy	Smooth vs. textured	No significant difference
Dickson,[60] 1987	92 breasts	E/I (13 immediate, 62 delayed)	8.7%	Radiation	↑ Risk of any complication
Mentor SPS[3]	416 patients	Saline implants, 3-year follow-up	30%	—	—
McGhan R95[5]	237 patients	Saline implants, 3-year and 5-year follow-up	25% 3-year, 36% 5-year	—	—

E/I, expander-implant sequence.
*Not all reported contractures will have been reoperated on.

TABLE 150-24 ✦ REASONS FOR REOPERATION FOR RECONSTRUCTION PATIENTS (INAMED R95 STUDY)[5]

Reasons for Reoperation	4 Years (%) (N = 117 Reoperations)	5 Years (%) (N = 125 Reoperations)
Capsular contracture	27	27
Asymmetry	21	20
Patient choice	11	10
Implant malposition	10	9
Scarring	9	8
Lump, mass, or cyst	8	8
Implant deflation	8	9
Infection	7	7
Tissue or skin necrosis	5	5
Hematoma or seroma	5	5
Breast pain	5	5
Implant extrusion	4	4
Add or remove saline	4	3
Wrinkling	3	4
Implant palpability	2	2
Delayed wound healing	2	2
Unsatisfactory nipple result	<1	<1
Skin lesion or cyst	<1	2
Total*	131	130

*Total is greater than 100% because some reoperations were performed for multiple reasons.

TABLE 150-25 ✦ ADDITIONAL SURGICAL PROCEDURES PERFORMED FOR RECONSTRUCTIVE PATIENTS (INAMED R95 STUDY)[5]

	N = 237 Patients	
Type of Surgical Procedures	*Through 4 Years* (%) (N= 151 Surgical Procedures)*	*Through 5 Years (%) (N= 159 Surgical Procedures)*
Implant removal with replacement†	30	31
Scar revision or wound repair	19	19
Capsule procedure	12	8
Implant removal without replacement	11	13
Add or remove saline	6	6
Removal of excess fluid	5	4
Biopsy or lump removal	5	4
Reposition implant	4	4
Skin-related procedure	4	4
Nipple-related procedures (unplanned)	2	2
Other procedures‡	2	2
Removal of skin lesion or cyst	1	2
Total	100	100

*As reported in original premarket approval submission with additional data clarification.
†Some removals were replaced with an INAMED implant; others were replaced with a non-INAMED implant.
‡Through 4 years, other procedures were liposuction, placement of a stacked implant. Through 5 years, other procedures were liposuction, placement of a stacked implant.

TABLE 150-26 ✦ COMPLICATION RATES AFTER IMPLANT REPLACEMENT (INAMED R95 STUDY)[5]

Complication After Replacement of Reconstruction Implant	2-Year Complication Rate* (%) (N = 40 Implants)	3-Year Complication Rate* (%) (N = 40 Implants)
Capsule contracture III/IV	33	34
Removal or replacement	26	27
Leakage or deflation	5	10
Infection	7	3

*As reported in original premarket approval submission with correction to capsular contracture rate.

implant placement (Tables 150-27 to 150-29). The patients receive surveys each year. The data presented through 7 years include earlier data shown in the tables with new information added.

Similarly, Mentor has also provided data with long-term follow-up related to complications after use of an implant requiring reconstruction. Mentor conducted two major studies, the Large Simple Trial (LST) and the Saline Prospective Study (SPS).[3,4] The LST was designed to determine the 1-year rates of capsular contracture, infection, deflation, and implant removal. There were 2066 augmentation patients, 104 reconstruction patients, and 215 revision patients enrolled. Of these enrolled patients, 47% returned for their 1-year visit. The SPS was designed as a 3-year study to assess all complications with saline breast implants as well as the patient's satisfaction, body image, and self-concept. Patients were observed annually, and data for

TABLE 150-27 ✦ COMPLICATION RATES FOR RECONSTRUCTIVE PATIENTS (INAMED PASS STUDY)[6]

Complication	7-Year Complication Rate (%) (N = 237 Patients)
Reoperation	49
Capsular contracture	43
Implant removal	31
Breast pain	26
Implant deflation	12

TABLE 150-28 ✦ REASONS FOR REOPERATION IN RECONSTRUCTIVE PATIENTS (INAMED PASS STUDY)[6]

Reasons for Reoperation	7-Year (%) (N = 138 Reoperations)
Capsular contracture	25
Asymmetry	18
Implant deflation	12
Patient choice	12
Implant malposition	9
Lump, mass, or cyst	9
Scarring	8
Infection	7
Breast pain	4
Hematoma or seroma	4
Tissue or skin necrosis	4
Implant extrusion	4
Wrinkling	4
Add or remove saline	4
Implant palpability	2
Delayed wound healing	1
Skin lesion or cyst	1
Unsatisfactory nipple result	1
Cancer	<1
Ptosis	<1

*Total is greater than 100% because some reoperations were performed for multiple reasons.

the following 3 years were collected (Tables 150-30 and 150-31). The SPS enrolled 1264 augmentation patients and 428 reconstruction patients. Of these, 76% of augmentation patients and 78% of reconstruction patients returned for their 3-year visit. The 3-year complication rates for reconstruction patients (including all levels of severity, mild to severe) were reported.

After product approval, Mentor switched data collection to a post-approval study. The post-approval study is designed to collect data from patients through the 10-year post-implantation period by use of a questionnaire mailed to patients each year. To date, data

TABLE 150-29 ✦ PRIMARY REASON FOR IMPLANT REMOVAL IN RECONSTRUCTIVE PATIENTS (INAMED PASS STUDY)[6]

Primary Reason for Implant Removal	Through 7 Years (%) (N = 81 Implants Removed)
Implant deflation	25
Capsular contracture	25
Patient choice	24
Infection	9
Implant extrusion	5
Other*	5
Implant malposition	4
Wrinkling	3
Asymmetry	3
Total	100

*Other reasons as reported by the physician were recurrent carcinoma (n = 1), abnormality on computed tomographic scan at mastectomy site (n = 1), poor tissue expansion due to irradiation (n = 1), and second-stage breast reconstruction (n = 1).

TABLE 150-30 ✦ ADDITIONAL SURGICAL PROCEDURES PERFORMED FOR RECONSTRUCTIVE PATIENTS (MENTOR SPS STUDY)[3]

Type of Additional Surgical Treatment	% (N = 353 Procedures)
Capsule related	28
Implant removal with replacement	19
Scar or wound revision	13
Implant removal without replacement	11
Nipple related (unplanned)	8
Saline adjustment	7
Reposition implant	6
Biopsy or cyst removal	<1
Breast reduction or mastectomy	<1
Mastopexy	<1
Total	100

TABLE 150-31 ✦ REASONS FOR IMPLANT REMOVAL FOR RECONSTRUCTION PATIENTS (MENTOR SPS STUDY)[3]

Main Reason for Reconstruction Implant Removal Through 3 Years*	% (N = 116 Implants Removed)
Capsular contracture	30
Infection	24
Leakage or deflation	22
Patient request for size or style change	6
Necrosis or extrusion	5
Asymmetry	4
Breast pain	3
Delayed wound healing	2
Cosmetic revision	1
Wrinkling	1
Breast cancer	1
Total	100

*Corrections to some rates reported at 3 years. Total number of implants removed did not change.

TABLE 150-32 ✦ PRIMARY REASON FOR IMPLANT REMOVAL IN RECONSTRUCTION PATIENTS (MENTOR POST-APPROVAL STUDY)[4]

Main Reason for Removal	5 Years (%) (N = 135 Implants Removed)	7 Years (%) (N = 180 Implants Removed)
Capsular contracture	29	29
Leakage or deflation	25	28
Infection	21	16
Patient request for size or shape change	8	9
Necrosis or extrusion	5	4
Asymmetry	4	4
Breast pain	3	2
Breast mass or cancer	1	2
Delayed wound healing	1	1
Wrinkling	1	1
Cosmetic revision	1	1
Contralateral replacement	0	2
Position change	0	1
Hypertrophic scarring	0	1
Irritation or inflammation	0	1

have been collected from patients through the 7-year post-implantation period. The post-approval data include earlier data collected for the SPS study with current information added.[4] At 5 years and at 7 years, the primary reason for implant removal was capsular contracture (29%) (Table 150-32).

The Baker[61] classification provides data based on appearance of the breast and firmness (Table 150-33). When the breast exhibits a Baker III/IV level, which indicates a firm reconstructed breast with or without an unacceptable aesthetic outcome, the patient will generally request a secondary procedure to restore the mound appearance and a more natural softness.

Tschopp[62] described 92 women who were evaluated for long-term results of latissimus dorsi flap reconstruction. With a minimum follow-up of 6 years, capsular contracture was noted with the implant beneath the latissimus flap (Table 150-34). A Baker grade of III or IV is generally accepted as an indication for intervention, and the authors reported that "70% [of patients] needed no further intervention." This figure corresponds to the number of patients who had grade I (13%) or grade II (57%) contracture. It follows that 30% of patients did require some form of intervention, although the author goes on to say that "only the severe capsular formations (Baker IV) needed capsulotomy (4% of women) and replacement of the prosthesis because the women were unhappy

TABLE 150-33 ✦ BAKER CLASSIFICATION OF CAPSULAR CONTRACTURE AFTER PROSTHETIC BREAST RECONSTRUCTION

Grade	Description
Ia	Absolutely natural, cannot tell breast was reconstructed
Ib	Soft, but the implant is detectable by physical examination or inspection because of mastectomy
II	Mildly firm reconstructed breast with an implant that may be visible and detectable by physical examination
III	Moderately firm reconstructed breast; the implant is readily detectable, but the result may still be acceptable
IV	Severe capsular contracture with an unacceptable aesthetic outcome or significant patient symptoms requiring surgical intervention

From Spear SL, Baker JL Jr: Classification of capsular contracture after prosthetic breast reconstruction. Plast Reconstr Surg 1995;96:1119-1123, discussion 1124.

TABLE 150-34 ✦ TSCHOPP[62] STUDY: INCIDENCE OF CAPSULAR CONTRACTURE WITH MINIMUM FOLLOW-UP OF SIX YEARS

Baker I	13%
Baker II	57%
Baker III	26%
Baker IV	4%

Data from Tschopp H: Evaluation of long-term results in breast reconstruction using the latissimus dorsi flap. Ann Plast Surg 1991;26:328-340.

with the results." The type of "intervention" carried out on the 26% of patients who had a grade III contracture is not stated.

Capsular contracture may represent the only reason for secondary reconstruction or may be associated with problems related to skin envelope, position, and scar (see Table 150-22). When capsular contracture is an isolated problem, subtotal capsulectomy and implant exchange will provide an acceptable result. If there is evidence of a silicone gel implant shell failure or calcification within the capsule, a total capsulectomy is performed with implant exchange. If the patient demands autogenous reconstruction, the standard rectus abdominis transposition flap (TRAM flap) or a perforator flap transplanted by microvascular technique offers the best technique for secondary reconstruction (Figs. 150-13 to 150-15).

Effect of Surface Texturing

Surface texturing has been shown to lower capsular contracture rates compared with smooth-walled implants. The reasons for this are not entirely clear, but it has been suggested that the irregular surface texture leads to disordered deposition of collagen fibrils, producing a thinner, more pliable capsule that is less likely to contract.[63]

However, it has been suggested that the benefit of the textured surface on capsular contracture may be only a short-term effect, with textured and smooth implants exhibiting similar long-term contracture incidence.[55] The authors of this study stated that only polyurethane-covered implants, which are no longer available, confer a long-term advantage over smooth implants ($P < .0001$).

Effect of Filler Material

As noted from the data provided by INAMED and Mentor, capsular contracture rates were high after long-term follow-up regardless of shell and contents (saline versus silicone gel). With low-bleed implants now routinely used, the rates are probably similar. However, in the prospective trial from Asplund et al[56] involving the random allocation of silicone-filled implants (n = 35) or saline-filled implants (n = 37), significant (grade III/IV) capsular contracture was seen more commonly in the silicone implant group than in the saline implant group (55% versus 20%; $P < .006$), and satisfaction of patients with regard to breast consistency was significantly higher in the saline group ($P = .03$). The same population of patients was evaluated by Gylbert et al[64] in 1990, 6 years later. Capsular contracture was observed in 50% of the gel implant group and 16% of the saline group. These results are similar to those seen 6 years earlier, which seems counterintuitive because the incidence of capsular contracture generally increases with time.[55]

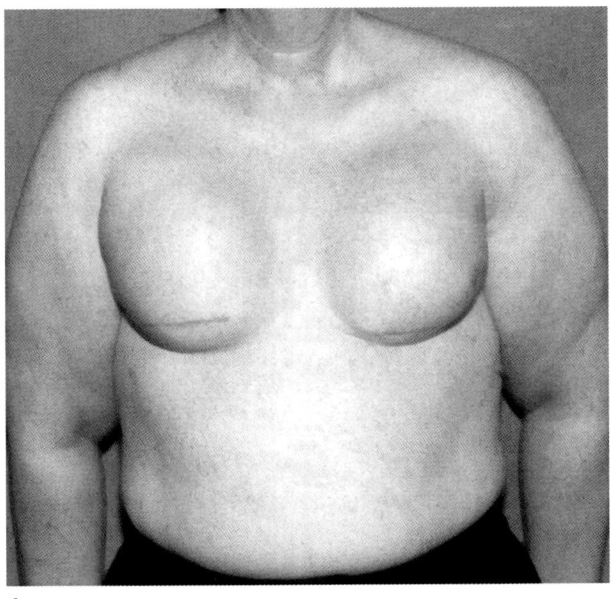
A

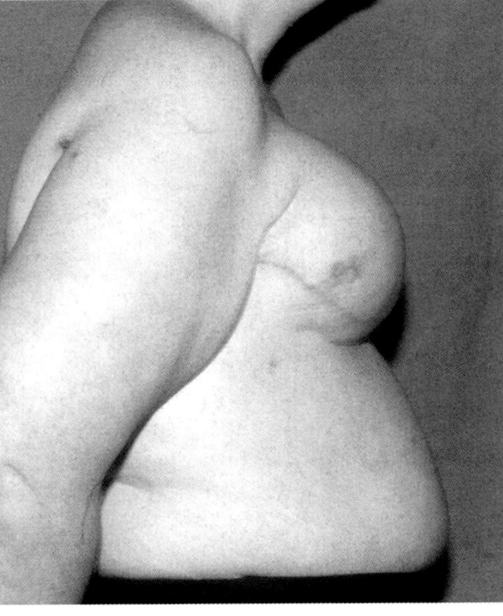
B

FIGURE 150-13. Capsular contracture. *A,* Anterior view of patient after bilateral mastectomy and implant reconstruction. *B,* Lateral view. Note adequate skin envelope, with Baker grade III-IV capsular contracture.

Continued

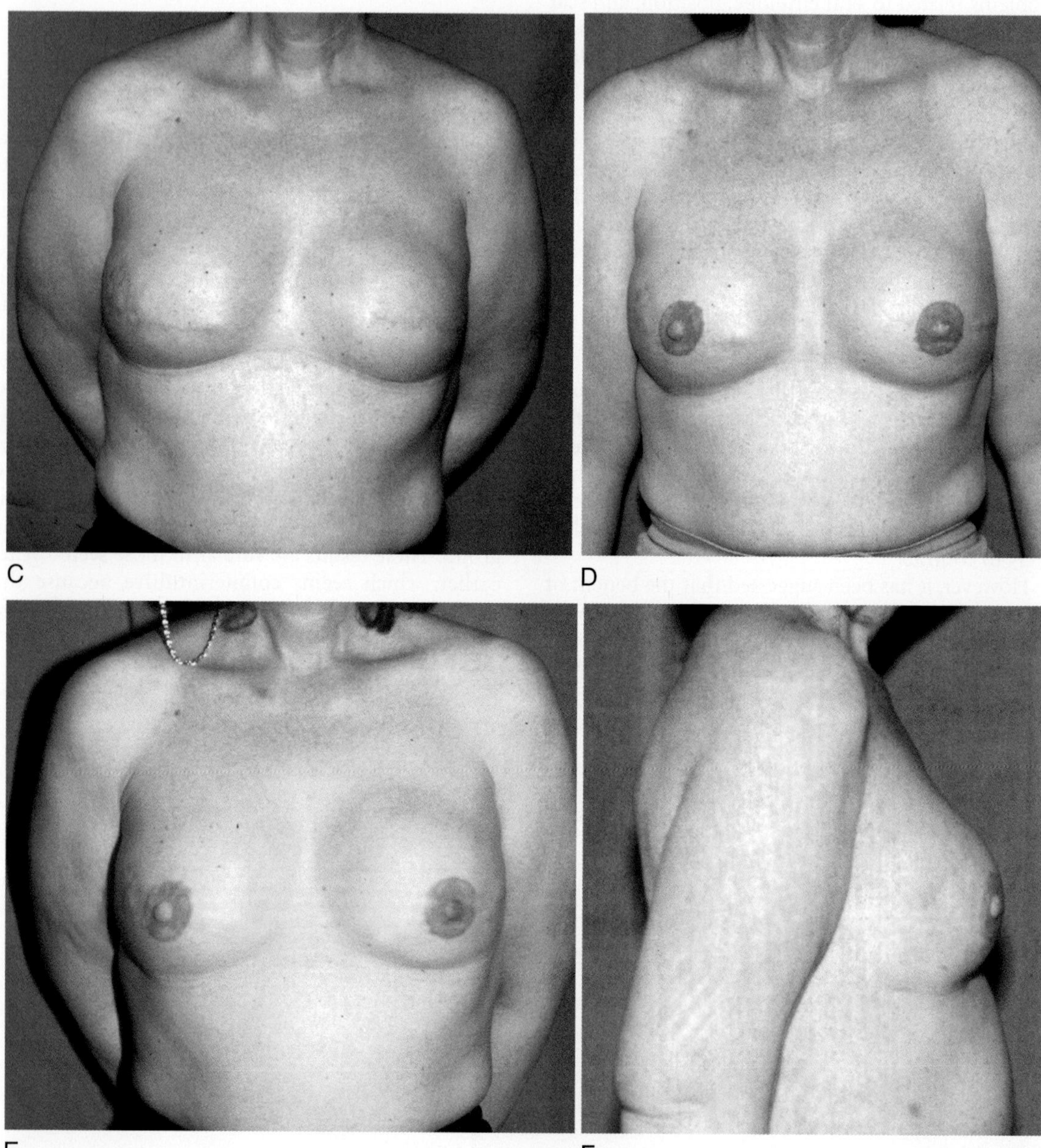

FIGURE 150-13, cont'd. *C,* Postoperative anterior view after bilateral secondary breast reconstruction with capsulectomy and implant exchange. *D,* Anterior view 6 months after bilateral nipple-areola reconstruction. *E,* Postoperative view 2 years after bilateral secondary breast reconstruction. *F,* Lateral view. Note adequate skin envelope with improved breast position and fullness after capsulectomy.

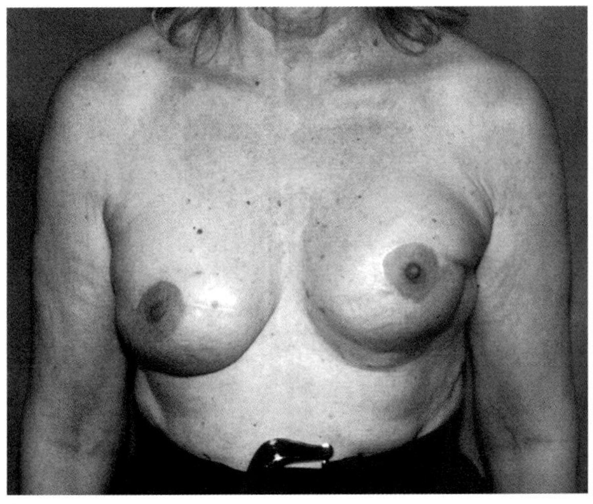

A

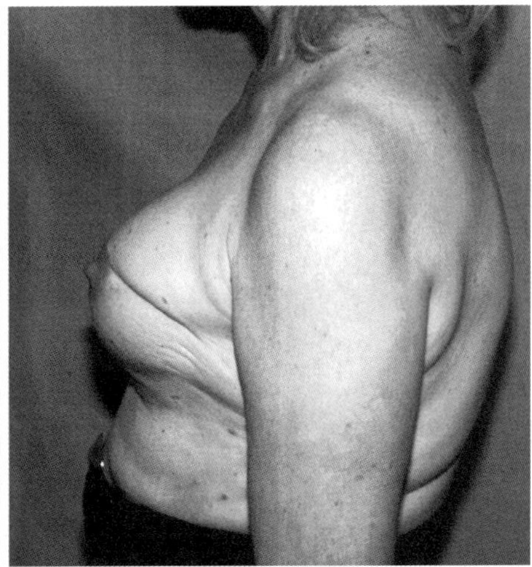

B

FIGURE 150-14. Capsular contracture. *A,* Anterior view of patient after bilateral prophylactic mastectomies with left capsular contracture and inadequate mound contour. *B,* Lateral view. Note adequate skin envelope, with Baker grade III capsular contracture and inadequate fullness in inferior quadrants of breast mounds. *C,* Postoperative anterior view after staged secondary reconstruction with implant removal, capsulectomy, and expander insertion (expanders inflated during 3-month interval). *D,* Anterior postoperative view after expander removal and permanent implant insertion. *E,* Lateral view. Note that capsulectomy and expansion with permanent implant insertion have provided adequate implant coverage and natural fullness in inferior breast mound.

C

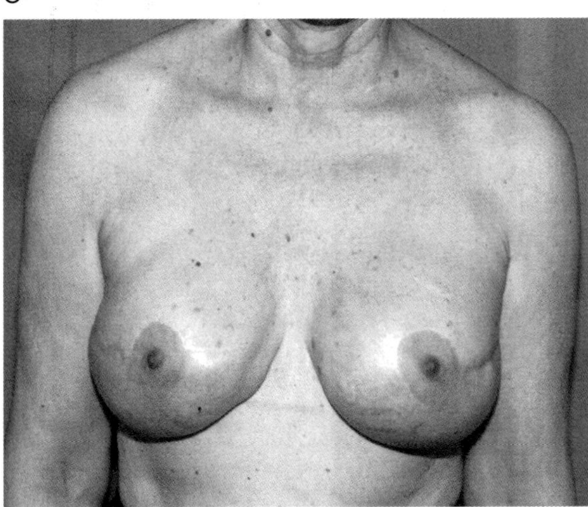

D

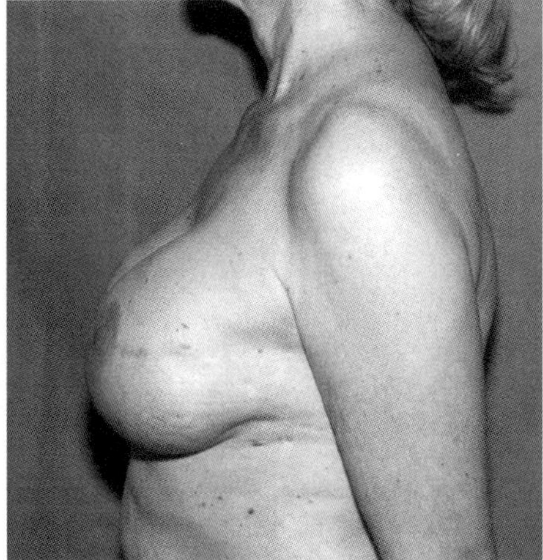

E

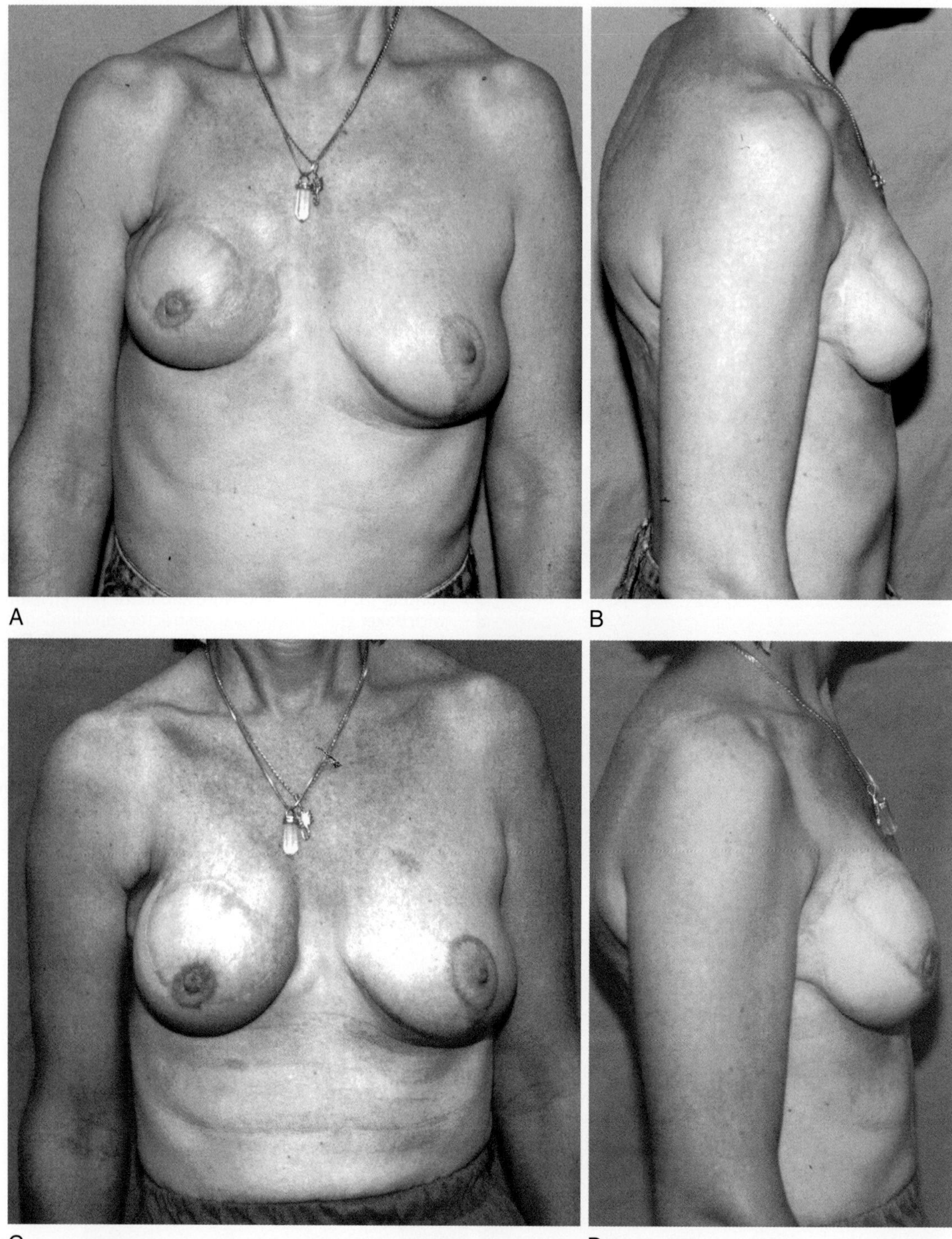

FIGURE 150-15. Capsular contracture. *A,* Anterior view of patient with latissimus dorsi musculocutaneous transposition flap and permanent implant for delayed breast reconstruction. The patient has malposition of the implant due to Baker grade IV capsular contracture. *B,* Lateral view. Note superior migration of implant despite adequate skin envelope. *C,* Postoperative anterior view of secondary reconstruction with capsulectomy and implant exchange. The implant is now correctly placed to fill the inferior skin envelope and to provide natural inferior fullness in the breast mound. *D,* Lateral view. Note improvement in implant position.

SKIN WRINKLING AND IMPLANT PALPABILITY

A breast mound reconstructed with a prosthesis will never feel like a "normal" breast; this is inherent in the technique and is usually accepted by most patients. The same is true for augmented breasts, although the presence of normal breast tissue overlying the implant can help minimize implant palpability. This breast tissue is not available after mastectomy, and as a result, the implant used for reconstruction may be more palpable. Placement of the implant in a submuscular position can help with this problem and may also help reduce the likelihood of capsular contracture (see preceding section).

Skin wrinkling is a problem that tends to occur more often with inflatable saline-filled implants and is related to the formation of folds or creases in the implant silicone elastomer shell. These folds are transmitted through the overlying tissues and are manifested as visible or palpable "wrinkles" in the skin of the reconstructed breast mound. A mild degree of wrinkling is often accepted by the patient and requires no treatment; however, this varies between patients, and some may find any degree of skin wrinkling unacceptable. As noted in the review of outcome studies conducted by the implant manufacturers, wrinkling is frequently observed. Mentor's SPS study[3] reported that 20% of 416 saline reconstruction patients with skin wrinkling related problems at 3-year follow-up. INAMED's R95 trial[5] reported a skin wrinkling incidence of 23% and 25% at 3- and 5-year follow-up in a series of 237 patients. Implant palpability was reported at 20% and 27%, respectively.

In the thin patient with an implant, skin wrinkling and implant palpability may not be completely avoidable, and discussion of this potential problem should be part of the informed consent. With a submuscular position, this problem may be decreased but not completely avoided. The lower part of the implant may not have muscle coverage to allow maximal projection in this area, and wrinkling or the implant's edge may become visible. The fill volume of the implant may also have a relationship with formation of rippling or wrinkles. The development of creases in the implant shell is thought to be related to the fill volume of inflatable saline implants; implants "underfilled" (filled to a volume below the recommended range) are more likely to develop folds. When the patient stands upright, the saline solution falls to the lower pole of the implant, leaving the upper pole relatively empty. The wall of the upper pole, no longer held open by the fluid in the lumen, can then fold on itself, causing creases in the shell that may become permanent over time.

This phenomenon is observed less commonly in breasts reconstructed with silicone gel prostheses, and this is thought to be due to the increased viscosity of the gel. Asplund[56] noted a 3% incidence of palpable skin wrinkling for silicone gel implants versus 14% for saline (not significant) based on reporting by patients. In the 6-year follow-up[64] of this same population of patients, the incidence of palpable wrinkles as measured by the surgeon differed significantly between the two groups ($P = .019$). Implant palpability reported by patients in this study was 15% for silicone implants versus 26% for saline implants, although this was not statistically significant. Handel[55] also demonstrated increased incidence of skin wrinkling with saline-filled implants (7.2%) compared with silicone gel implants (2.1%).

When the patient requests secondary surgery for correction of wrinkling or implant palpability, the most effective solution is to switch to an autogenous reconstruction or to use a latissimus dorsi muscle flap over the area of implant visibility (Table 150-35). Unfortunately, this approach requires a major flap procedure and may not be desirable to most patients. Implant exchange to smooth shell saline or gel filled may offer some improvement. Massiha[65] described the use of either local capsular flaps or fat grafts to provide tissue between the implant and the skin envelope and reported success with this technique. However, introduction of fat grafts may damage the implant and also result in microcalcifications, which may cause concern for recurrence or new primary cancer if mammography is used for surveillance. Currently, there is interest in placement of AlloDerm as a graft between the implant and the skin envelope. If wrinkling is not too extensive and other aspects of the reconstruction related to skin envelope, position, and scar are acceptable to the patient, further surgery may not be advisable.

IMPLANT EXTRUSION

Implant extrusion will obviously affect the mound, so it is a problem that requires secondary mound reconstruction. It results from mastectomy skin or flap loss.

TABLE 150-35 ✦ SURGICAL OPTIONS FOR CORRECTION OF SKIN WRINKLING OR IMPLANT PALPABILITY

Problem	Surgical Options
Skin wrinkling or implant palpability	No treatment (dependent on severity and patient's expectations) Implant exchange (size or fill volume adjustment) Addition of flap tissue (e.g., latissimus dorsi) Conversion to flap reconstruction Dermal grafts (AlloDerm)

Therefore, the appropriate discussion of this problem is presented under "Envelope," with review of data related to both skin envelope and flap complications. Also, infection may predispose a patient to skin necrosis; the problem of infection is reviewed under both "Mound" and "Envelope."

IMPLANT FAILURE

If there is failure of the implant due to rupture or leak, the mound will lose both volume and projection. As a result, the patient will present for secondary surgical procedures to restore the breast mound. With the saline-filled implant, the diagnosis is readily apparent because there is immediate or gradual shrinkage of the implant. With the gel-filled implant, the diagnosis is not easily established because despite shell failure, the silicone gel usually remains within the surrounding capsule and maintains breast volume. In augmentation patients, a leak is usually suspected on the basis of mammography and confirmed by a magnetic resonance imaging scan. In the reconstruction patient, mammography is not routinely applied to the site of reconstruction because all breast tissue has been removed in the prior mastectomy. In general, the patient presents with concern about the gel-filled implants or dissatisfaction with the reconstruction and a request for implant removal and an alternative technique of reconstruction (Table 150-36).

TABLE 150-36 ✦ SURGICAL OPTIONS AFTER IMPLANT FAILURE

Problem	Surgical Options
Implant failure: saline implants	Explantation Capsulotomy or capsulectomy with implant replacement Autologous reconstruction with flap
Implant failure: silicone gel implants	No treatment Explantation Capsulotomy or capsulectomy with implant replacement Autologous reconstruction with flap

Cunningham et al[54] reviewed the incidence of saline implant deflation and found that it varies from 2% to 76% between studies. The authors stated that these previous studies tend to represent "only a single clinical practice experience, multiple manufacturing generations, and/or significantly varying clinical settings," and therefore the conclusions drawn from these studies are limited (Table 150-37).

TABLE 150-37 ✦ INCIDENCE OF SALINE IMPLANT FAILURE

Author, Year	N	Technique	Failure Incidence	Risk Factors Described	Effect on Incidence
Gylbert,[64] 1990	72 breasts	Reconstruction with silicone or saline	16% saline 0% silicone	Filler material	Saline ↑ risk of failure
McGhan R95[5]	237	Reconstruction with saline implants	6% of implants 5% of patients	—	—
Mentor SPS[3]	428	Reconstruction with saline implants	7% of implants 9% of patients	—	—
Gutowski,[22] 1997	995 implants for augmentation and reconstruction	6.3% reconstruction with saline implants	5.5% total failure 4.7% "spontaneous"	Fill volume, model, intraluminal antibiotics/ steroids	All significant (see text)
Cunningham,[54] 2000	450 patients, augmentation and reconstruction	6.1% reconstruction with saline implants	8.3% (5.8% excluding Surgitek)	Model, size	Surgitek ↑ risk Size > 450 mL ↑ risk
Worseg,[8] 1995	167 implants	Augmentation or reconstruction with inflatable implants	23.9%	Open or closed capsulotomy	Both ↑ risk Open, $P = .012$ Closed, $P = .038$
Alderman,[18] 2002	326	Reconstruction with expander-implant or TRAM flap	3.8%	Timing (immediate vs. delayed)	↑ Risk of total and major complications
Gabriel,[25] 1997	749	Augmentation (71%) or reconstruction (29%) with implants	5.7%	Indication for surgery, age at implantation	Both ↑ risk of any complication (see text)
Camilleri,[37] 1996	120	Reconstruction with Becker prosthesis	6% fill port failure 1.6% rupture	—	—

TABLE 150-38 ✦ COMPLICATION RATES FOR RECONSTRUCTION PATIENTS (INAMED R95 STUDY)[5]

	N = 237 Patients	
Complications	*3-Year Complication Rate*[†] *(%)*	*5-Year Complication Rate (%)*
Additional operation (reoperation)	39	45
Asymmetry*	33	39
Capsular contracture	25	36
Implant replacement or removal for any reason	23	28
Wrinkling*	23	25
Implant palpability or visibility*	20	27
Breast pain*	15	18
Loss of nipple sensation*	12	18
Implant malposition*	12	17
Irritation or inflammation*	7	7
Leakage or deflation	6	8
Intense skin sensation*	6	6
Scarring complications	6	6
Infection	5	6
Capsule calcification*	5	5
Seroma	4	4
Skin or tissue necrosis	4	4
Delayed wound healing*	3	3
Implant extrusion	3	3
Rash	3	3
Hematoma	1	1

*These complications were assessed with severity ratings. Only the rates for moderate, severe, or very severe (excludes mild and very mild ratings) are shown in this table.

[†]As reported in original premarket approval submission.

Both INAMED and Mentor provided data to the FDA in 2003 based on prospective clinical trials of saline implants. In the R95 (INAMED) study,[5] 237 patients with saline-filled implants were studied for reconstruction, with a 71% 3-year follow-up. The 3-year risk for deflation was reported at 6%; at 5 years, it was reported at 8% (Table 150-38). Similarly, in the SPS prospective trial (Mentor),[3] 1264 augmentation and 428 reconstructive patients were entered, with 3-year follow-up in 68% of reconstructive patients. The 3-year risk for deflation in this group is 9% of patients and 7% of implants (Table 150-39).

In general, diagnosis of failure with saline implants tends to be technically easier because deflation with these types of implants is usually complete. Failure of silicone implants, on the other hand, including silicone bleeds, pinhole defects, and frank rupture, tends to be more difficult to identify because the silicone may be contained within the capsule and the breast retains its shape.[66,67] Therefore, diagnosis relies on the various imaging modalities available. Magnetic resonance imaging, ultrasonography, and mammography have been employed in the detection of implant failure. The success and accuracy of these techniques are variable. Magnetic resonance imaging and ultrasonography offer promising diagnostic potential in detecting failure. However, the literature reviewing

TABLE 150-39 ✦ COMPLICATION RATES FOR RECONSTRUCTION PATIENTS (MENTOR SPS STUDY)[3]

Reconstruction Complications	**3-Year Complication Rate (%) (N = 416 patients)**
Additional operation (reoperation)	40
Loss of nipple sensation	35
Capsular contracture III/IV or grade unknown	30
Asymmetry	28
Implant removal	27
Wrinkling	20
Breast pain	17
Infection	9
Leakage or deflation	9
Irritation or inflammation	8
Delayed wound healing	6
Seroma	6
Scarring	5
Extrusion	2
Necrosis	2
Hematoma	1
Position change	1

rupture detection sensitivity and specificity for these modalities is lacking, and as such, explantation surgery remains the "gold standard" for detection.[68]

Many clinical studies have attempted to define the rupture or leak rate of silicone gel implants.[66-69] However, the majority of these reports include or are restricted to breast augmentation patients. In INAMED's reported safety outcomes for the Core study[70] in 2003 regarding McGhan BIOCELL textured and smooth silicone-filled breast implants (3-year cumulative first occurrence), a rupture rate of 6.3% by patient (N = 221) and 4.2% by implant (N = 361) was noted. The true rupture rate is still difficult to confirm because diagnosis of silent rupture cannot be made without routine magnetic resonance imaging and confirmation of possible rupture or leak of implants by secondary surgery. Also, the product shell and silicone gel are under constant modification to improve the product. Long-term follow-up studies generally do not reflect the implant currently used in augmentation and reconstruction procedures. As with other complications, there are various options with regard to implant failure treatment (see Table 150-36).

Many patients dissatisfied with their reconstruction because of concern about silicone gel implant failure do not wish to have a gel implant replacement. In these patients, a secondary procedure with a saline implant replacement will provide a satisfactory result. Most patients with a deflated saline implant will accept implant replacement. In the saline implant failure, the implant pocket has generally contracted because of loss of space with the saline absorption. The secondary reconstructive procedure will require a subtotal capsulectomy to restore the shape and projection of the former implant. In long-term deflation or in patients who have received prior irradiation, it may be necessary to recommend a flap to provide an adequate skin envelope or use of a tissue expander (see "Envelope") (Fig. 150-16).

IMPLANT-RELATED INFECTION

Infections of the reconstructed breast may be superficial, involving only the skin and subcutaneous fat, or they may be deeper (periprosthetic infection). Superficial infections usually resolve with antibiotic therapy, whereas periprosthetic infections almost always require operative intervention (Table 150-40). Although most studies do distinguish between superficial and deep infections, some combine the two under the general term of "infection" (Fig. 150-17).

The timing of infection is an important consideration. In general, most infections occurring in conjunction with the initial breast reconstruction procedure represent technique failure and require immediate attention for treatment of the infection in an effort to preserve the reconstructed breast mound. However, late infection may also occur, representing a procedural complication. Nahabedian and Galdino[71] suggest that the majority of complications occur *after* the initial postoperative period, which implies that bacterial contamination at the time of insertion may not be the only route of entry for infecting organisms.

TABLE 150-40 ✦ SURGICAL OPTIONS FOR IMPLANT-RELATED INFECTION

Problem	Surgical Options
Infection (skin)	Parenteral antibiotics + wound care
Infection (periprosthetic)	Explantation without immediate replacement Delayed secondary reconstruction: implant or flap Salvage procedure may be possible (see text)

The route of entry for microbes is also described as an important consideration and differs between early and late infections. Early postoperative infections are thought to be due to the introduction of bacteria at the time of operation, and their incidence can be reduced through meticulous aseptic technique.[72,73] Later infections are caused by microbial entry through other routes, including saline instillation, diffusion through the implant shell, and nosocomial by bacteremia. There are also conflicting reports of microbial growth within saline-filled implants. Becker and Hartman[74] and more recently Brown et al[75] have failed to show significant growth of any organisms from samples of saline from implants and expanders up to 23 years old. Chen et al[76] reported mixed results, with good growth of *Serratia* but poor growth of *Staphylococcus aureus* and *Staphylococcus epidermidis.* Young et al[77] conducted an experimental in vitro and in vivo animal study and determined that *S. epidermidis, Escherichia coli, Enterobacter cloacae, Klebsiella pneumoniae, Pseudomonas aeruginosa, Aspergillus fumigatus,* and *Paecilomyces variotii* could survive in the lumen of a saline-filled implant for up to 6 months (the endpoint of the study). Importantly, both the Chen study and the Young study used in vivo control implants, in which no organisms were inoculated. These controls remained sterile at the end of both study periods. Brown et al[75] concluded that although saline implants appear to be capable of supporting microbial growth, their sterile condition is maintained unless they are inoculated with organisms (e.g., during placement or filling).

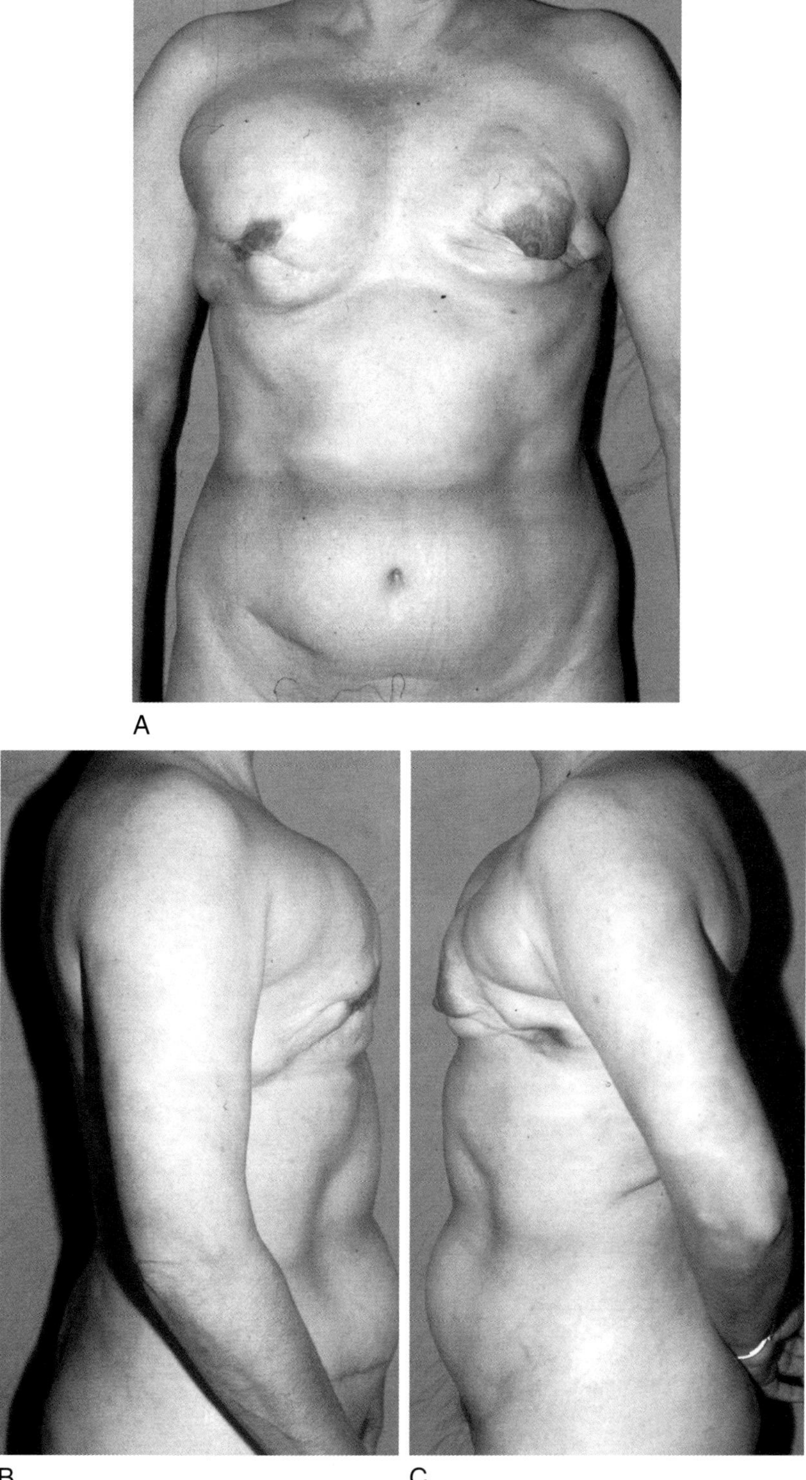

FIGURE 150-16. Implant failure. *A*, Anterior view of patient presenting with bilateral expanders placed for immediate reconstruction for bilateral prophylactic mastectomy. The expanders have failed to provide adequate envelope expansion. *B* and *C*, Lateral views. Note wound contraction occurring in the preserved skin envelope (*C*).

Continued

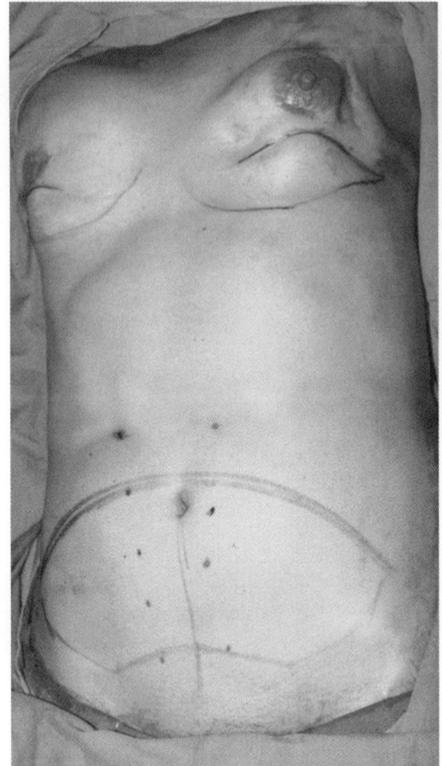

D

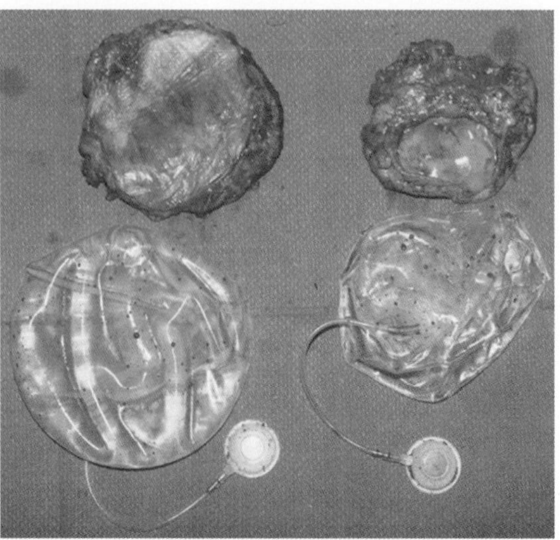

E

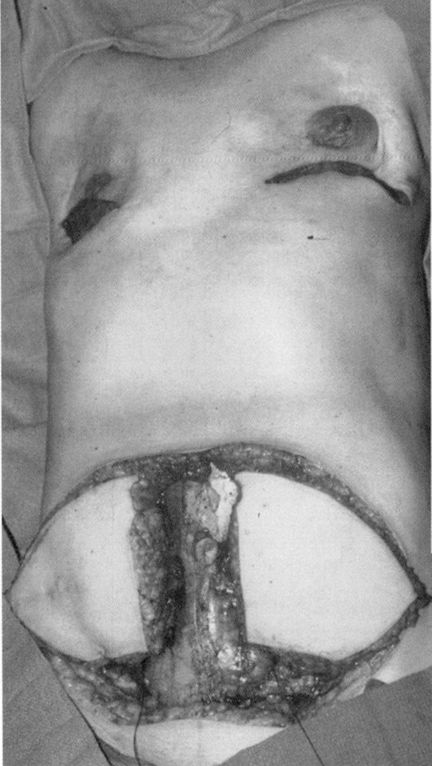

F

FIGURE 150-16, cont'd. *D,* Anterior view: preoperative design of bilateral rectus abdominis musculocutaneous flaps. *E,* Intraoperative view: capsulectomy specimen and explantation of failed expanders. *F,* Intraoperative anterior view. Note bilateral rectus abdominis musculocutaneous flaps ready for transposition to sites of bilateral completion mastectomies.

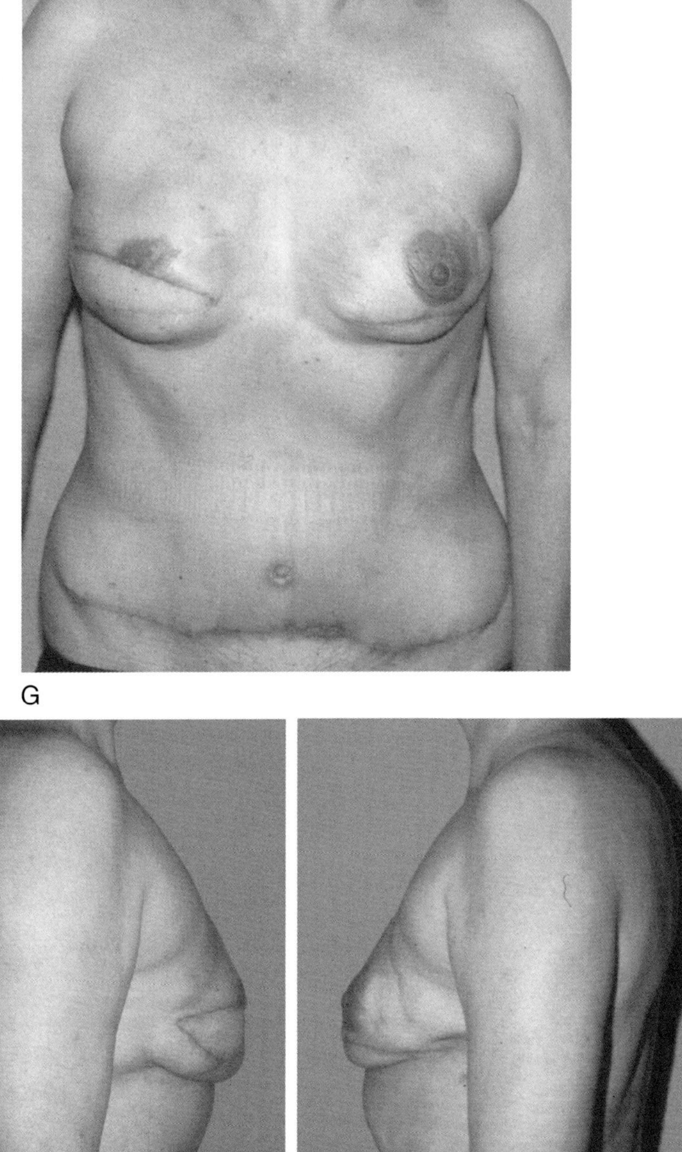

G

H I

FIGURE 150-16, cont'd. *G,* Postoperative anterior view of secondary reconstruction by autogenous breast reconstruction with bilateral TRAM flaps. *H* and *I*, Lateral views. *Continued*

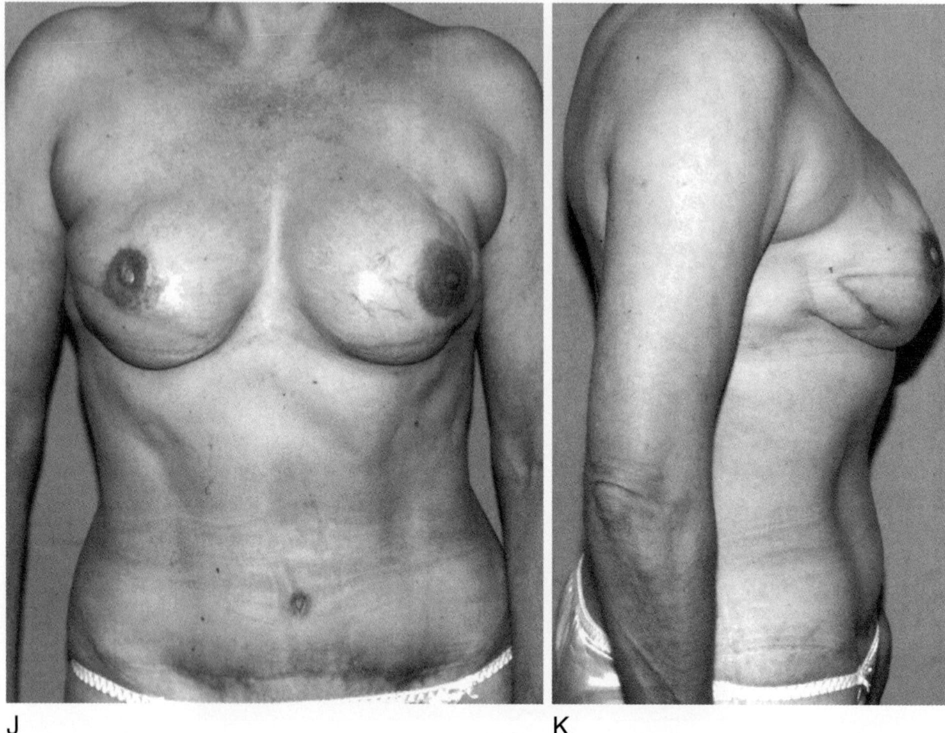

FIGURE 150-16, cont'd. *J,* Anterior postoperative view after secondary reconstruction with permanent implant insertion. The patient desired increased mound projection (contour problem). *K,* Lateral view. Note adequate coverage of implant with TRAM flap and improved breast contour.

Nahabedian and Galdino[71] reviewed 130 patients with 168 implants used in expander-implant breast reconstruction to determine the effects of various factors on the incidence of periprosthetic infection, including chemotherapy, radiotherapy, axillary lymph node dissection, tumor stage, tobacco use, laterality, and diabetes. All expanders were anatomic textured with integrated port. A musculocutaneous flap was used in 15% of the patients. Mean follow-up was 29 months with a range of 12 to 47 months. Infection rate was 7.7% (10 of 130 patients), and implant infection rate was 6% (10 of the 168 implants). Explantation due to the infection was performed an average of 116 days after insertion (eight expanders and one permanent implant). The infection was noted after the initial postoperative period in 90% of the patients. Cultured bacteria included *Staphylococcus aureus* (seven) and *Serratia marcescens* (one). Although only radiotherapy was statistically associated with the infections, other factors were thought to be associated with increased risk for infection, including chemotherapy, axillary node dissection, and tumor stage.

Evaluation of 23 clinical series* reveals a wide range (0.2% to 35%) of reported infection rates (Table 150-41). The INAMED R95 study[5] of 237 patients demonstrates a 5% 3-year rate and a 6% 5-year rate (see Table 150-38). The Mentor SPS study[3] of 416 patients shows a 9% infection rate at 3 years (see Table 150-39).

Periprosthetic infections are defined as a purulent fluid collection around the prosthesis. This definition does not include patients with wound infection or cellulitis who are usually successfully treated with antibiotics. When a periprosthetic infection occurs without implant exposure, parenteral antibiotic therapy should immediately be instituted. If resolution of symptoms

*References 3, 5, 7, 15, 17, 18, 22, 23, 27-30, 32, 33, 35, 37, 55, 78-83.

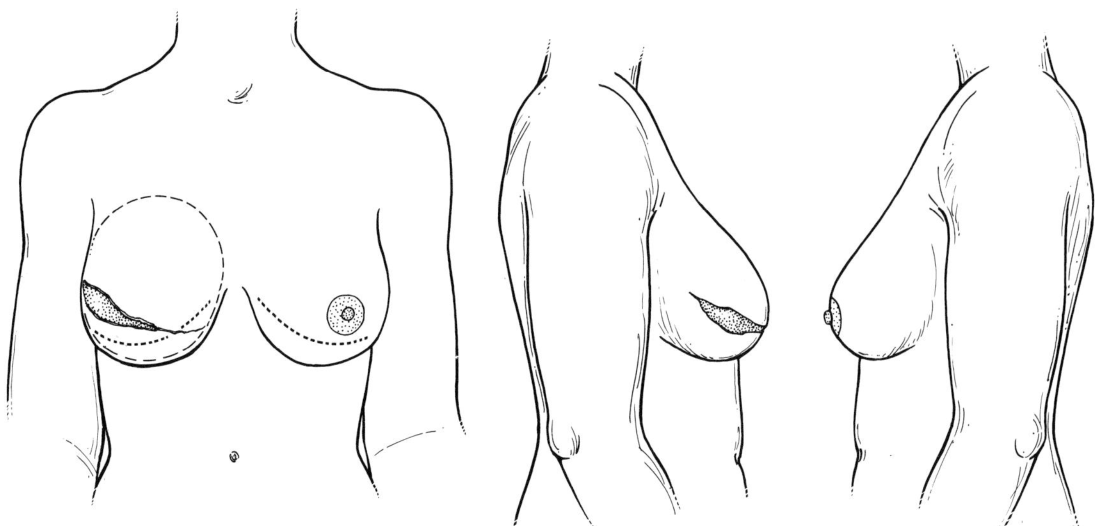

FIGURE 150-17. Implant-related infection: implant exposure with infection.

does not occur within 3 to 7 days, the patient requires exploration and implant removal or one attempt at a salvage procedure including implant removal, débridement of the implant pocket, implant exchange, closed suction drainage, and 7 to 10 days of culture-specific antibiotics. If infection recurs, the implant is removed and delayed secondary reconstruction planned for 3 to 6 months (Figs. 150-18 and 150-19).

Yii and Khoo[84] have provided a retrospective review of 17 patients in which a protocol for salvage of infected expander prostheses in breast reconstruction was evaluated. This protocol, which was applied to 14 of the 17 patients (the remaining three patients elected to have implants removed), included the following technique: (1) admit patient; (2) swab wound or discharge fluid and submit for culture and sensitivity study; (3) commence intravenous antibiotics; (4) salvage procedure. The salvage procedure consisted of opening the capsule and draining fluid, which is sent for culture and sensitivity study. The implant is removed, and the cavity is scrubbed with povidone-iodine with a brush before irrigation with half-strength hydrogen peroxide, then saline. At this point, the authors state that good clinical judgment is required to determine whether salvage is feasible on the basis of severity, the patient's wishes, and vascularity of the recipient bed. Circumferential and radial capsulotomies are then performed, and a new implant is placed into the prepared pocket before closure. Continuous irrigation with normal saline is continued for 12 hours, with intermittent antibiotic instillation through the drains for up to 5 days. The patient should be given intravenous antibiotics for 5 to 7 days, and expansion should be delayed for 3 to 4 weeks.

Of the 17 patients with periprosthetic infections studied by Yii and Khoo,[84] 3 patients did not undergo the salvage procedure and had their prostheses removed. Of the 14 patients remaining, 9 patients had successful salvage surgery (64%). Five patients did not have a successful outcome of salvage surgery. Four of these five patients had infection caused by coagulase-negative staphylococci. The *S. aureus* rate was significantly higher in the failure group ($P = .023$). Two of the five patients in the failure group and five of the nine patients in the successful group had preceding radiotherapy. There was no difference in outcome whether or not the patients had received previous radiotherapy ($P = .50$).

Flap infection is rarely a direct cause for secondary reconstructive procedures. However, infection is generally defined when the patient is started on antibiotic therapy in the postoperative period. In general, flap infections present as cellulitis and respond rapidly to parenteral antibiotics. The rate of reported infections in flaps ranges from 0.6% to 10%, with slightly higher rates when the mastectomy site has been irradiated (Table 150-42).[10,16,24,40,41,43,48,51,52,85-88] In combined autologous and implant reconstructions, if the implant space becomes infected, the infected implant will require management as previously described for implant reconstruction. Fortunately, the well-vascularized coverage by the flap protects the implant, so implant removal due to periprosthetic infection in association with a flap is uncommon.

TABLE 150-41 ✦ INCIDENCE OF IMPLANT-RELATED INFECTION

Author, Year	N	Technique	Incidence of Infection	Risk Factors Evaluated	Effect on Incidence	Organisms Found
Krueger,[78] 2001	81	E/I	23.5%	Radiotherapy	37% vs. 19%, $P = .13$	—
Kraemer,[79] 1996	146	E/I	3.4%	Radiotherapy	2% vs. 3%, NS	—
Yule,[80] 1996	46	Immediate E/I	10.9%	Chemotherapy	13% vs. 9%, $P > .1$	—
Contant,[81] 2000	100	Immediate E/I	5% → loss	Radiotherapy	↑ Risk of prosthesis loss	—
Handel,[55] 1995	1665 breasts	Augmentation or reconstruction	4.3% of reconstructed	Filler material, surface texture, timing	No effect	—
Furey,[29] 1994	124 breasts	E/I or implant	5.8%	Chemotherapy	11.1% vs. 3.6%, significance not given	—
Armstrong,[82] 1989	49 breasts	E/I or implant	24% (18% loss)	IBR + use of expander	Immediate + expander 53% infection vs. 24% overall	Coagulase-negative staphylococcus
Brand,[83] 1993	54,661	Augmentation or reconstruction	0.3%-0.6% for reconstruction	Surface texture, placement, smoking, obesity, diabetes, others	NS (skin atrophy or scarring, additional surgery, pregnancy or lactation, exercise, and trauma significant)	*S. aureus, S. epidermidis,* streptococcus A and B, enterobacteria, *Klebsiella, Pseudomonas,* mycobacteria
Clough,[15] 2001	360 breasts	49.7% saline, 35.6% Becker, 7.2% E/I, 7.5% silicone	1.9%	None described	—	—
O'Brien,[28] 1993	113	E/I 83%, 17% autologous	5.7% loss due to infection	None described	—	—
Slavin,[30] 1998	51	SSM, IBR with LD flap + implant	2%	Not described	—	—

Ramon,[23] 1997	52	Immediate E/I	2%	None described	—	—
Gutowski,[22] 1997	504	Saline implants (6.2% reconstruction)	0.2% "wound infection"	None specific to infection risk	—	—
Miller,[35] 1991	83	64% IBR, 36% DBR E/I or implant	6%	Timing (IBR, DBR)	8.2% vs. 2.6%, $P = .47$	—
Alderman,[18] 2002	326	E/I or TRAM flap	35.4 (E/I)*	IBR, DBR	IBR = ↑ major complications ($P = .005$)	—
Noone,[33] 1985	185	Implant, 3% E/I (all immediate)	0% loss due to infection alone (2% loss with hematoma + infection)	—	—	—
Disa,[27] 1999	770	E/I, 90% immediate	1% removal of infected expander	Not described	—	*S. aureus*, *Enterobacter*
Spear,[32] 1998	171	E/I (8% with flap), immediate	1.2%	None described	—	—
Gui,[7] 2003	129 breasts	Immediate McGhan 150 ± LD flap	6.2% (7.4% for implant, 4.9% for LD flap + implant)*	None described	—	—
Camilleri,[37] 1996[†]	120 breasts	Becker expander (+LD flap in 30%)	5% "pocket sepsis"	Radiotherapy, smoking	Both ↑ risk of skin problems, $P = .05$	—
McCraw,[17] 1987	55	E/I	5.5%*	None described	—	—
Mentor SPS[3]	416	Saline implants, 3-year follow-up	9%	—	—	—
McGhan R95[5]	237 patients	Saline implants, 3- and 5-year follow-up	5% (3-year), 6% (5-year)	—	—	—

Not all of the papers distinguish between superficial infections and periprosthetic infections requiring removal. DBR, delayed breast reconstruction; E/I, expander-implant sequence; IBR, immediate breast reconstruction; LD flap, latissimus dorsi flap; SSM, skin-sparing mastectomy; TRAM flap, transverse rectus abdominis musculocutaneous flap.

*This figure is for all infections, not just those leading to reoperation.

[†]In the study of Camilleri et al, 98% of patients received prophylactic flucloxacillin and pocket irrigation with povidone-iodine at the time of expander insertion.

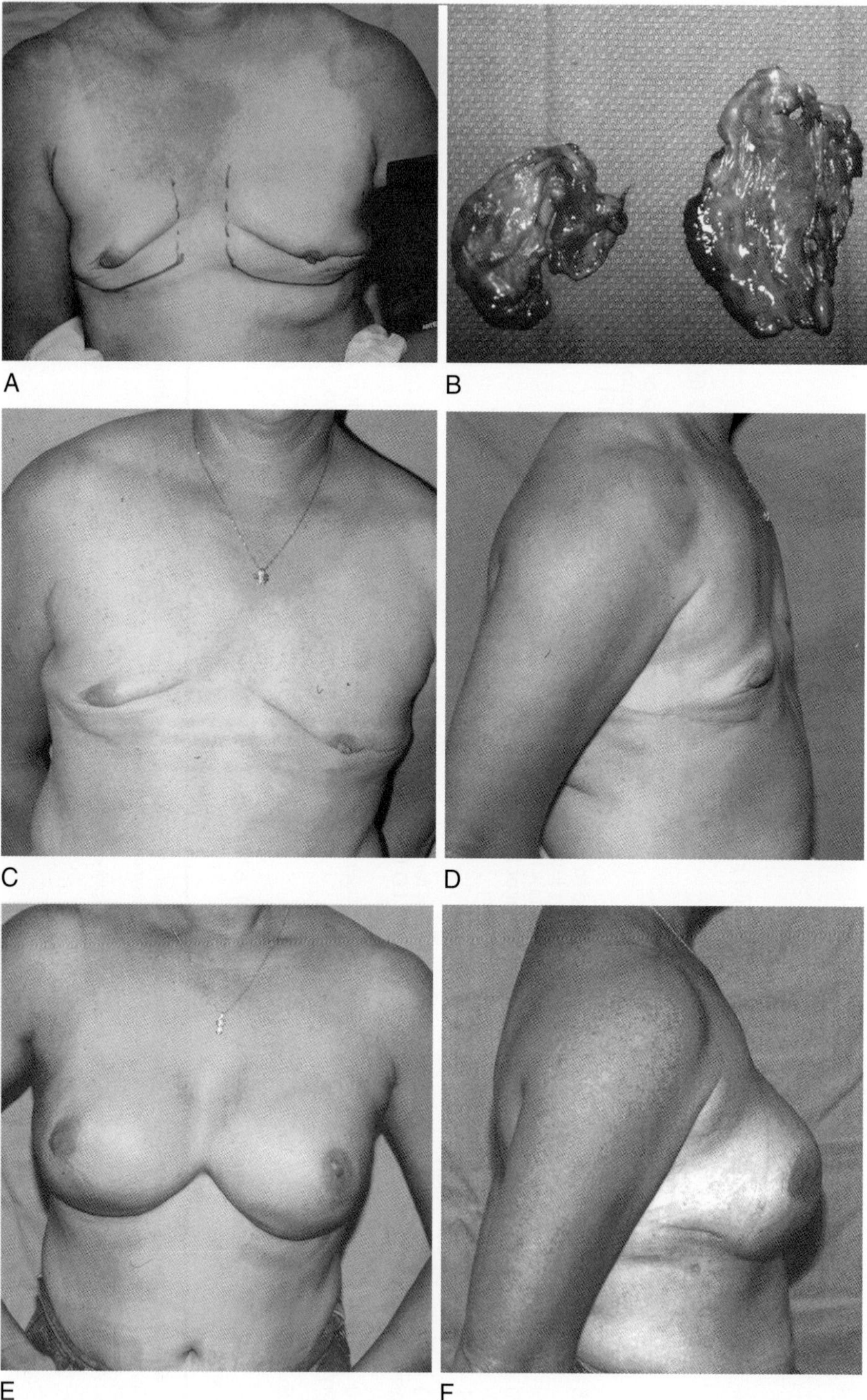

FIGURE 150-18. Implant infection. *A*, Anterior view of patient after bilateral immediate reconstruction of subcutaneous mastectomy with bilateral implant removal for infection. *B*, Intraoperative view: bilateral infected capsular space resected (total capsule resection). *C*, Postoperative anterior view 3 months after capsulectomy and 7-day culture-specific parenteral antibiotic therapy. *D*, Lateral view. The breast envelope is now supple without residual infection. Note adequate skin envelope available for secondary reconstruction. *E*, Postoperative anterior view at 1 year of bilateral secondary reconstruction with permanent implant insertion. Perioperative antibiotic coverage was provided on the basis of prior culture results. *F*, Lateral view. Note that the envelope provides adequate coverage of the implant and allows natural fullness in inferior breast mound.

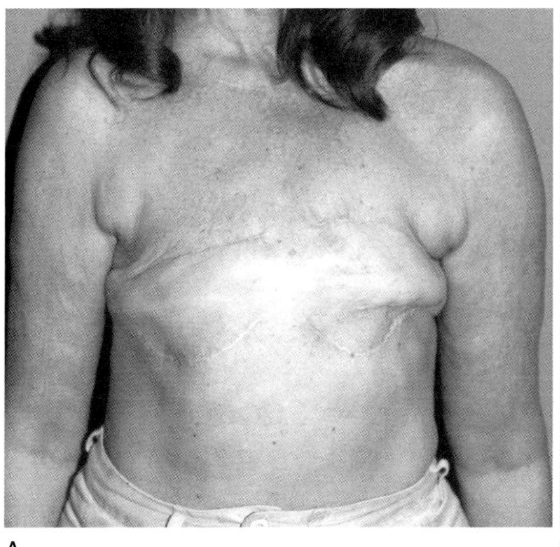
A

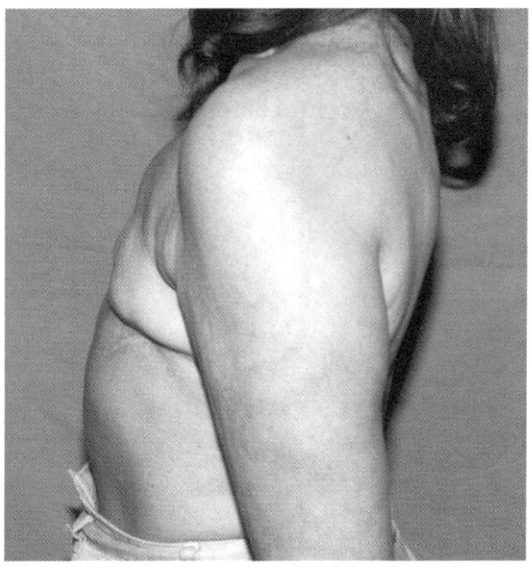
B

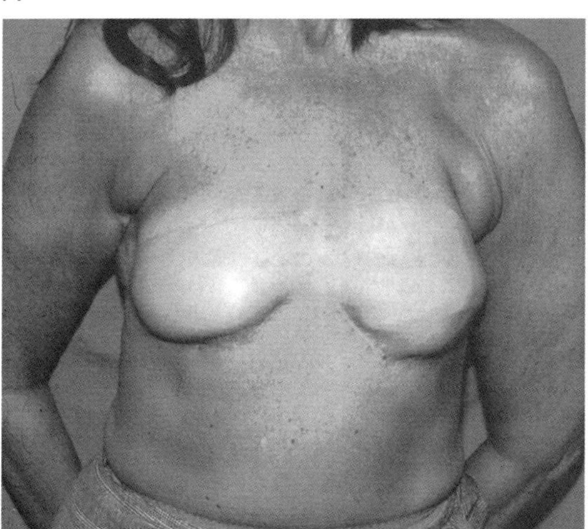
C

FIGURE 150-19. Implant infection. *A,* Anterior view of patient presenting after left modified radical mastectomy and right prophylactic mastectomy. Both implants were removed because of peri-implant infection. Note that adequate skin envelope is still available for expansion-implant sequence. *B,* Lateral view. *C,* Anterior view. The expanders are inserted with total capsulectomy, and antibiotic coverage is provided during the initial postoperative period. *D,* Anterior postoperative view 1 year after bilateral secondary breast reconstruction with expander-implant sequence. *E,* Lateral view. Note adequate envelope for implant coverage.

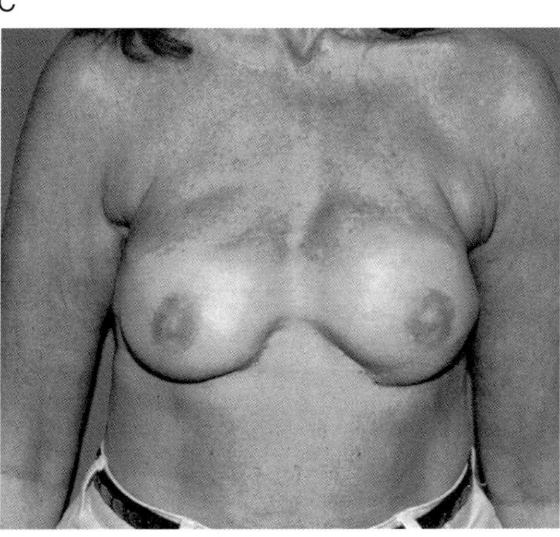
D

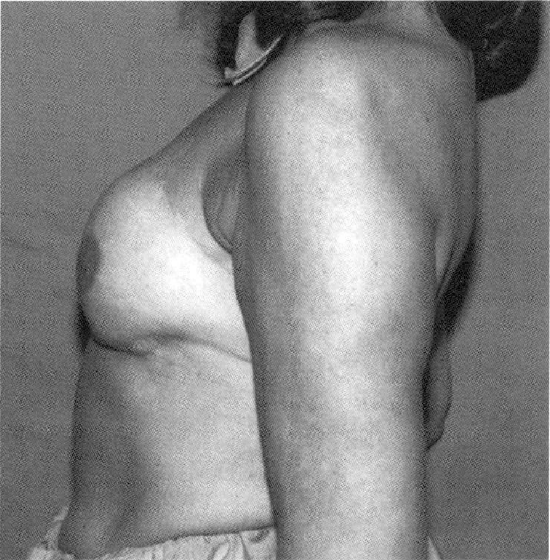
E

TABLE 150-42 ✦ INCIDENCE OF INFECTION AFTER FLAP BREAST RECONSTRUCTION

Author, Year	N	Technique	Infection Incidence	Risk Factors Described	Effect on Incidence
Hartrampf,[10] 1987	383 breasts	Pedicled TRAM flap reconstruction	2 (0.6%)	Relative: smoking, RT	Specific effect on infection not stated
Menke,[40] 2001	121	LD flap ± implant	2%	—	—
Roy,[41] 1998	111	LD flap + implant (95%)	8%	RT	No effect
Clough,[16] 2001	171	TRAM flap (unipedicled, bipedicled, supercharged, free)	Not described	—	—
Scevola,[85] 2002	768 breasts	TRAM or DIEP flap	1.8%	Number of drains	Not significant ($P = .1$)
Chang,[43] 2002	75	Extended LD flap without implant	5.3%	Age, breast size	Both ↑ risk of any flap complication (see text for details)
Moran,[51] 2001	221	Free or pedicled TRAM flap	7.9% (obese patients)	Obesity, free vs. pedicled TRAM flap	Obesity ↑ complications in free TRAM flap ($P = .008$) but not pedicled
Chang,[44] 2000	936	Free TRAM flap	1.8%	Smoking	No significant difference
Williams,[52] 1997	699	Pedicled TRAM flap	No RT, 2.8% RT → TRAM flap, 6.6% TRAM flap → RT, 5.3%	Preoperative and postoperative TRAM flap irradiation	Preoperative vs. postoperative, not significant RT vs. no RT, marginal for any complication ($P = .072$)
Crespo,[24] 1994	216	TRAM flap (n = 101), E/I, or implant	3% of TRAM flap group	—	—
Paige,[46] 1998	257	Unilateral unipedicled/ bilateral unipedicled TRAM flap	3.5% requiring wound intervention, IV antibiotics, or readmission	Unilateral vs. bilateral (all unipedicled), obesity, smoking, diabetes, hypertension	Laterality NS Obesity, smoking, diabetes, and hypertension all significant
Erdmann,[86] 2002	76 breasts	TRAM flap with vascular delay	2.6%	Smoking, obesity, RT, chemotherapy	Smoking, obesity significant for any flap complication
Schusterman,[87] 1992	68 breasts	Pedicled TRAM or free TRAM flap	8% of pedicled, 10% of free TRAM flaps	Free vs. pedicled TRAM flap	Not significant
Serletti,[88] 1997	125 breasts	Pedicled TRAM or free TRAM flap	8% of pedicled, 7% of free TRAM flaps	Free vs. pedicled	Not significant

DIEP flap, deep inferior epigastric perforator flap; E/I, expander-implant; LD flap, latissimus dorsi flap; RT, radiation therapy; TRAM flap, transverse rectus abdominis musculocutaneous flap.

FAT NECROSIS

Fat necrosis is another manifestation of ischemic tissue necrosis, similar to partial or total flap necrosis. However, with fat necrosis, the subcutaneous tissue is affected in the absence of skin necrosis. It therefore presents as an area of firmness in the reconstructed breast, usually within the 3-month postoperative period. It may be confused with recurrence of tumor on clinical examination, and biopsy of suspicious lesions should be performed.[10,89,90]

TABLE 150-43 ✦ SURGICAL OPTIONS FOR MANAGEMENT OF FAT NECROSIS

Problem	Surgical Options
Fat necrosis: circumscribed area of firmness	No treatment Resection If extensive: resection and implant insertion

Kroll[89] defines fat necrosis as "the formation of a small firm area (or areas) of scar tissue in the periphery of a flap caused by ischemic necrosis of subcutaneous fat in the absence of necrosis of overlying flap skin." In the study by Kroll[89] in which 110 patients (116 reconstructions) were evaluated for fat necrosis, pedicled TRAM flaps (n = 67) were found to have a higher incidence of fat necrosis than free TRAM flaps (n = 49) as detected clinically (26.9% versus 8.2%; P = .0113) and mammographically (13.4% versus 2%; P = .031). Risk factors described were smoking and obesity. Both smokers and obese patients had increased incidence of fat necrosis, but the rate of fat necrosis for these groups was not statistically significant.

The incidence of fat necrosis is variable according to clinical studies,* but the range is 7% to 37% for TRAM transposition flaps, 0% to 10% for microvascular transplantation of TRAM flaps, and as high as 62.5% in perforator (DIEP) flaps (see Table 150-45). In the first eight DIEP flaps, the authors found a high incidence of partial flap necrosis (37.5%) and fat necrosis (62.5%). In another study by Kroll,[49] selection of patients for a DIEP flap was limited to anatomic findings at flap dissection of one large perforator (palpable pulse) and vein (>1 mm) and reconstructions in which only 70% of the flap was required. With use of these selection criteria, the authors found a considerably lower incidence of partial flap necrosis (8.7%) and fat necrosis (17.4%) in 23 DIEP flaps. These incidences were marginally higher than those seen in the TRAM flap group (partial flap loss, 2.2%; fat necrosis, 12.9%). Overall partial flap necrosis incidence was reported to be 16.1% (TRAM and DIEP flaps), whereas overall fat necrosis was reported as 29%.

Because it is a clinical diagnosis based on flap palpation, the incidence will vary by the definition of a thickened area and the thoroughness of the examination. Keller[90] compared data with those of Kroll et al[89] and suggested that the significantly lower incidence of fat necrosis in DIEP flaps (6.8%) may be explained by inclusion of areas of fat necrosis less than 2 cm in size by Kroll et al, whereas Keller does not consider these significant.

The incidence of fat necrosis requiring a secondary reconstructive procedure is difficult to ascertain from the literature. However, an area of fat necrosis may be of concern to the patient and oncologist as suggestive of recurrent tumor and may require resection (Table 150-43). Also, it is common to remove areas of fat necrosis in the distal part of zone 3 if this part of the pedicled TRAM transposition flap is retained at the time of flap inset. Although this portion of the flap may survive without fat necrosis, it may be preserved in the superior aspect of the reconstructed breast mound, and if fat necrosis occurs, resection of this part of the flap may be required as a secondary procedure.

CONTOUR DEFECTS

The contour of the reconstructed breast mound should resemble the normal characteristics of the breast for the patient's age. The mound should have greater fullness in the inferior quadrants and a defined sternal and anterior axillary edge. There should be a tapered fullness at the superior aspect of the breast. The breast tissue normally extends to the infraclavicular and axillary regions, so ideally this area of the breast mound is replaced at reconstruction because the mastectomy has excised this area of breast tissue superior to the actual breast mound. The goals of reconstruction must provide for the breast mound and if possible should correct infraclavicular hollowness (Table 150-44).

In implant-expander reconstruction, there is great diversity of permanent saline- and gel-filled implants from which to choose. These implants and their specifications and design characteristics are identified in Chapter 143. Although the implants vary in base

TABLE 150-44 ✦ SURGICAL OPTIONS FOR MANAGEMENT OF INADEQUATE CONTOUR

Problem	Surgical Options
Contour	No treatment Revision: reinset of tissue flap or turnover flap Revision: resection of excess tissue Liposuction Implant exchange for anatomic implant Flap (latissimus dorsi muscle)

*References 10, 16, 40, 43-45, 47, 51-53, 86, 87, 89, 91, 92.

TABLE 150-45 ✦ INCIDENCE OF FAT NECROSIS

Author, Year	N	Technique	Fat Necrosis Incidence	Risk Factors Described	Effect on Incidence
Hartrampf,[10] 1987	383 breasts	Pedicled TRAM flap reconstruction	7%	Smoking, RT (relative)	Not specifically stated for fat necrosis
Menke,[40] 2001	121	LD flap ± implant	1.7%	—	—
Clough,[16] 2001	171	TRAM flap (unipedicled, bipedicled, supercharged, free)	13.5%	—	—
Kroll,[89] 1998	110	Pedicled or free TRAM flap	Pedicled, 37.3% Free, 10.2%	Pedicled vs. free, smoking, obesity	Pedicled ↑ risk Smoking, obesity NS
Kroll,[48] 2000	310	Free TRAM flap (279), DIEP flap (31)	Free TRAM flap, 12.9%; unselected DIEP flap, 62.5%; selected DIEP flap, 17.4% (see text)	Free TRAM flap vs. unselected DIEP flap; smoking	Unselected DIEP flap ↑ risk of fat necrosis Smoking NS (see text)
Jewell,[91] 1999	50	Free or pedicled TRAM flap	All severities, 34% Extent >5 cm in 22% (30% of pedicled, 10% of free; $P < .05$)	Obesity, smoking, cup size	Obesity ↑ risk, $P < .009$ Smoking and cup size, not significant
Moran,[51] 2001	221	Free or pedicled TRAM flap	9.6% (10% of free, 8% of pedicled)—all patients obese	Free vs. pedicled TRAM flap, obesity	Obesity ↑ complications in free TRAM flap ($P = .008$) but not pedicled Free vs. pedicled: not significant for fat necrosis
Chang,[44] 2000	936	Free TRAM flap	5.9%	Smoking	No significant difference
Williams,[52] 1997	699	Pedicled TRAM flap	Preoperative RT, 17.6% Post-TRAM flap RT, 15.8% No RT, <1%	Preoperative and postoperative TRAM flap irradiation	Prior irradiation ↑ incidence of fat necrosis ($P = .032$)
Tran,[45] 2001	102	Immediate or delayed free TRAM flap	8.6% of DBR 43.8% of IBR ($P = .000$)	IBR then RT vs. RT then DBR	IBR vs. DBR (all irradiated) IBR leads to ↑ late complications, including fat necrosis
Banic,[53] 1995	111	Free TRAM flap	9% (4.5% minor, 4.5% major)	RT, chemotherapy, smoking	None significant
Paige,[46] 1998	257	Unilateral unipedicled/ bilateral unipedicled TRAM flap	At least 10% of the flap: 11.3%	Unilateral vs. bilateral (all unipedicled), obesity	Laterality NS Obesity significant
Nahabedian,[92] 2002	163 breasts	Free TRAM flap (n = 143) DIEP flap (n = 20)	TRAM flap, 9.8% "mild" DIEP flap, 10% "mild"	Weight, age, smoking, muscle sparing	Patient weight is significant ($P < .001$) No other significant factors
Erdmann,[86] 2002	76 breasts	TRAM flap with vascular delay	6.6% partial flap or fat necrosis	Smoking, obesity, RT, chemotherapy	Smoking, obesity significant
Schusterman,[87] 1992	68 breasts	Pedicled or free TRAM flap	23% of pedicled, 0 free	Free vs. pedicled	Free ↓ incidence of fat necrosis ($P = .015$)

DBR, delayed breast reconstruction; DIEP flap, deep inferior epigastric perforator; IBR, immediate breast reconstruction; LD flap, latissimus dorsi flap; RT, radiation therapy; TRAM flap, transverse rectus abdominis musculocutaneous flap.

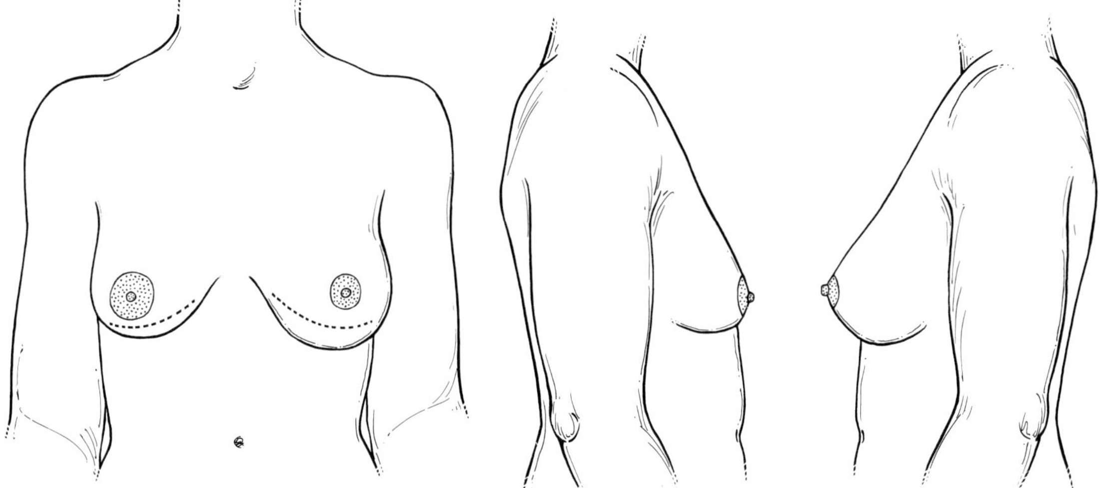

FIGURE 150-20. Contour problem: implant reconstruction with inadequate size and inferior mound fullness (ptosis).

width and projection, to a great extent the contour of the breast mound will be determined by the overlying preserved skin envelope and avoidance of muscle tightness overlying the implant (Fig. 150-20).

Unfortunately, an implant alone will often not correct the infraclavicular hollowness resulting from mastectomy without use of an additional flap. This deficiency is not always apparent but should be discussed as part of the informed consent with the patient who elects implant or expander-implant reconstruction (Figs. 150-21 and 150-22). A custom implant with superior extension (separate compartment) may improve the superior mound contour, but it is subject to capsular contracture and a resultant step-off deformity (see Chapter 134).

The contour of the reconstructed breast when a flap is used depends on the inset technique (Figs. 150-23 and 150-24). When the TRAM flap is used as either a transposition flap or a free flap, the inset must consider the skin island and the soft tissue of the flap that will provide the volume of the breast parenchyma replacement. In immediate reconstruction, the flap can be accurately designed to fulfill the goals of the reconstruction. In delayed reconstruction, it is often more difficult to accurately determine the requirement for skin island and soft tissue inset. In the delayed reconstruction, it may be helpful to overcorrect the skin envelope and to preserve as much of the territory of the TRAM flap as possible for volume replacement with the possible need for a secondary procedure

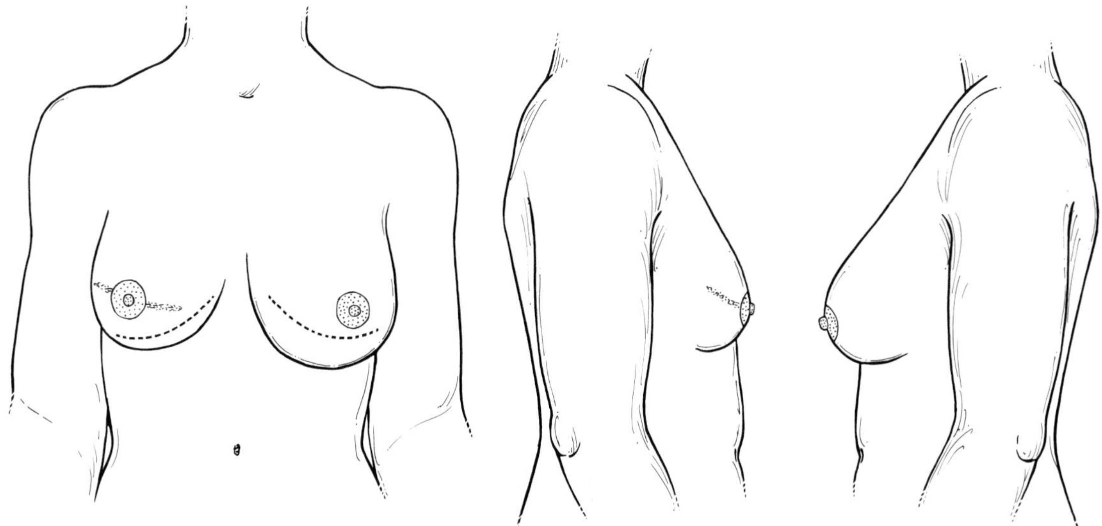

FIGURE 150-21. Contour problem: implant reconstruction with inadequate projection and size.

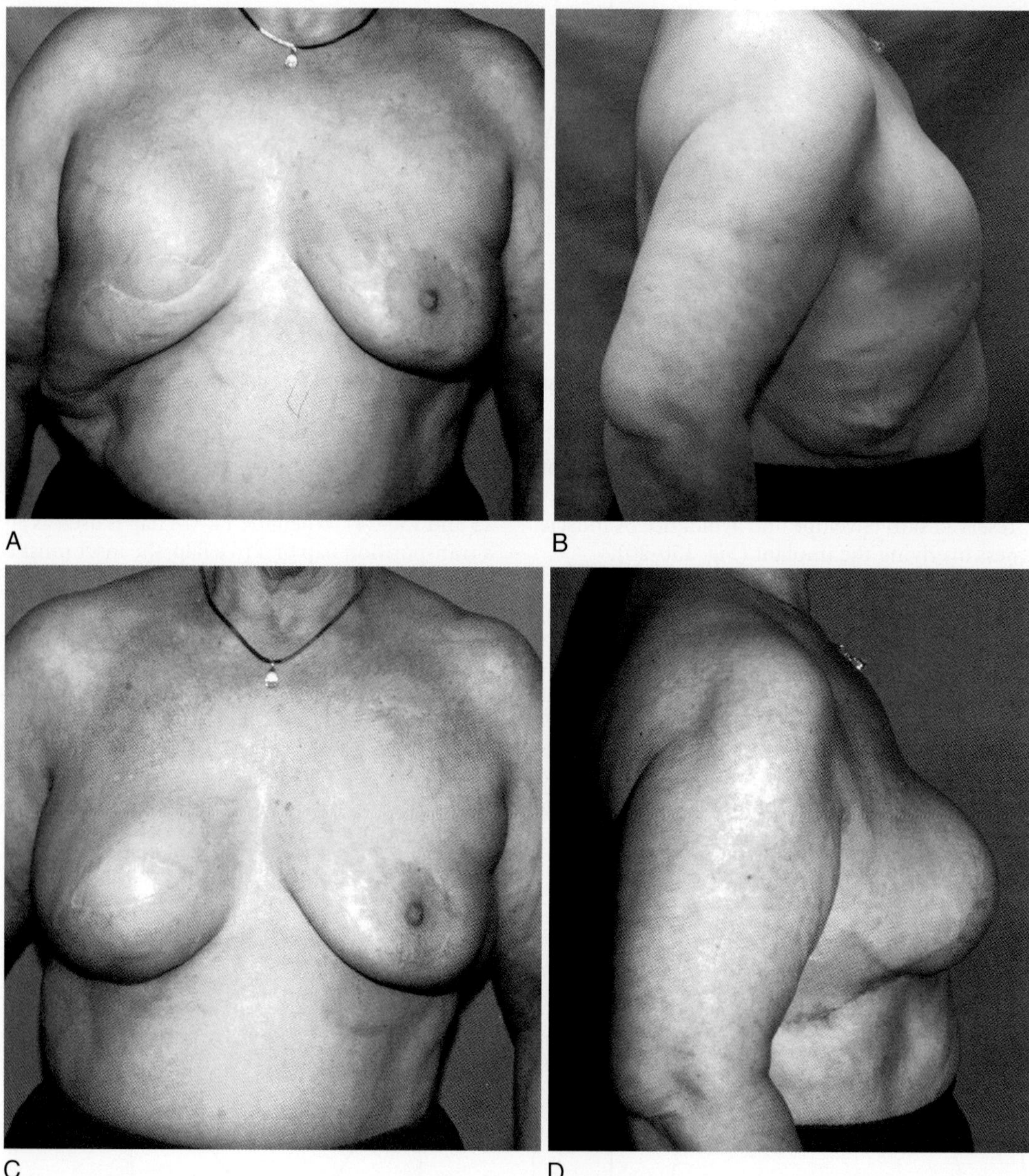

FIGURE 150-22. Contour deficiency. *A*, Anterior view of patient after implant reconstruction of right mastectomy site with inadequate contour. Note excessive fullness in superior mound and inadequate fullness in inferior mound. *B*, Lateral view. Note inadequate fullness in inferior mound. *C*, Postoperative anterior view of secondary reconstruction with implant exchange and positional adjustment. Note that the excessive infraclavicular fullness is corrected. *D*, Lateral view. Note that the skin envelope provides adequate implant coverage. The repositioned implant now provides adequate inferior mound fullness.

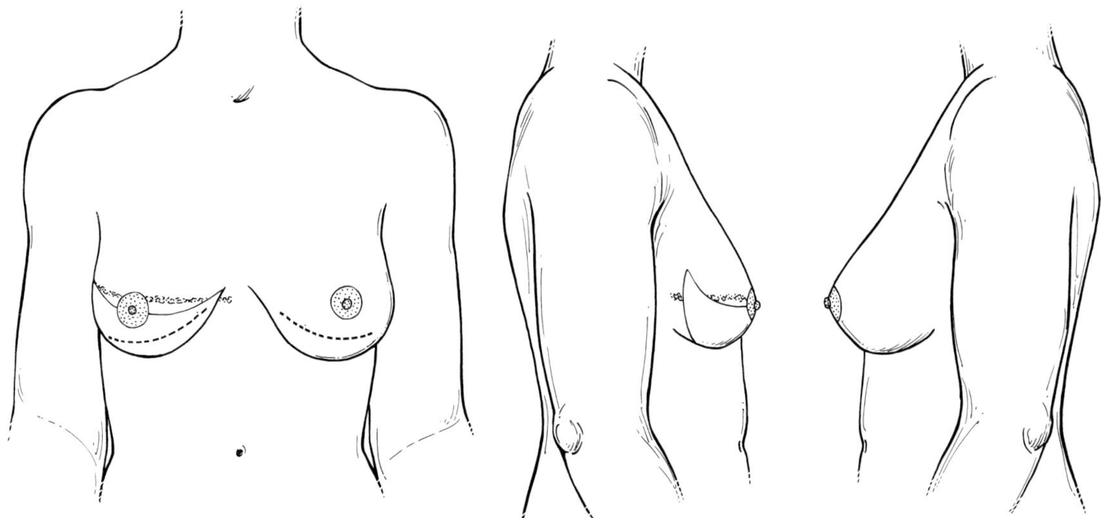

FIGURE 150-23. Contour problem: flap reconstruction with inadequate size.

(Fig. 150-25). This approach may increase the rate of secondary procedures but provides additional tissue in the event it is needed to establish a breast mound pleasing to the patient and meeting the demand of providing symmetry with the contralateral breast.

Maxwell and Andochick[93] suggest that it is preferable to make the reconstructed breast slightly larger than the opposite breast to "allow for volumetric reduction adjustments in the second procedure to enhance the shape." The second procedure should be used to correct any asymmetry of volume or shape, to reposition or to modify the inframammary and anterior axillary folds if necessary, and to design the nipple-areola complex. Fat necrosis may also be excised at this stage. The authors suggest that the ideal time for second-stage revision is around 4 to 6 months, after stabilization of flap maturation. By definition, this additional procedure would be considered a secondary procedure.

In the TRAM flap, contour procedures may improve the reconstructed mound. Liposuction will reduce the volume of the preserved subcutaneous tissue if it is excessive. Adjustment of the skin island may be required if excess skin island was preserved at the initial flap inset. If there is excess ptosis in the reconstructed breast mound, an incision at the superior margin of

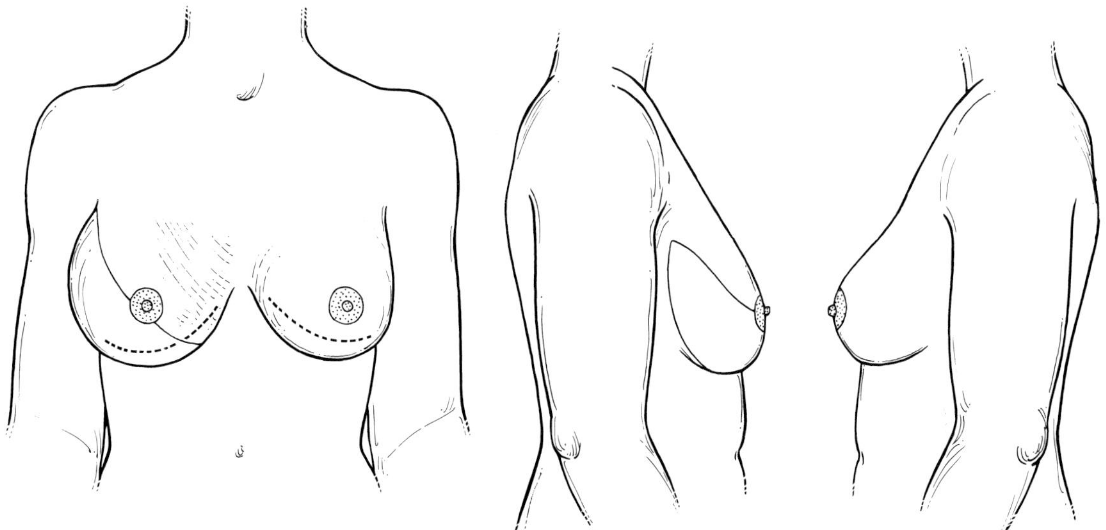

FIGURE 150-24. Contour problem: flap inset provides excess lateral fullness and inadequate medial fullness.

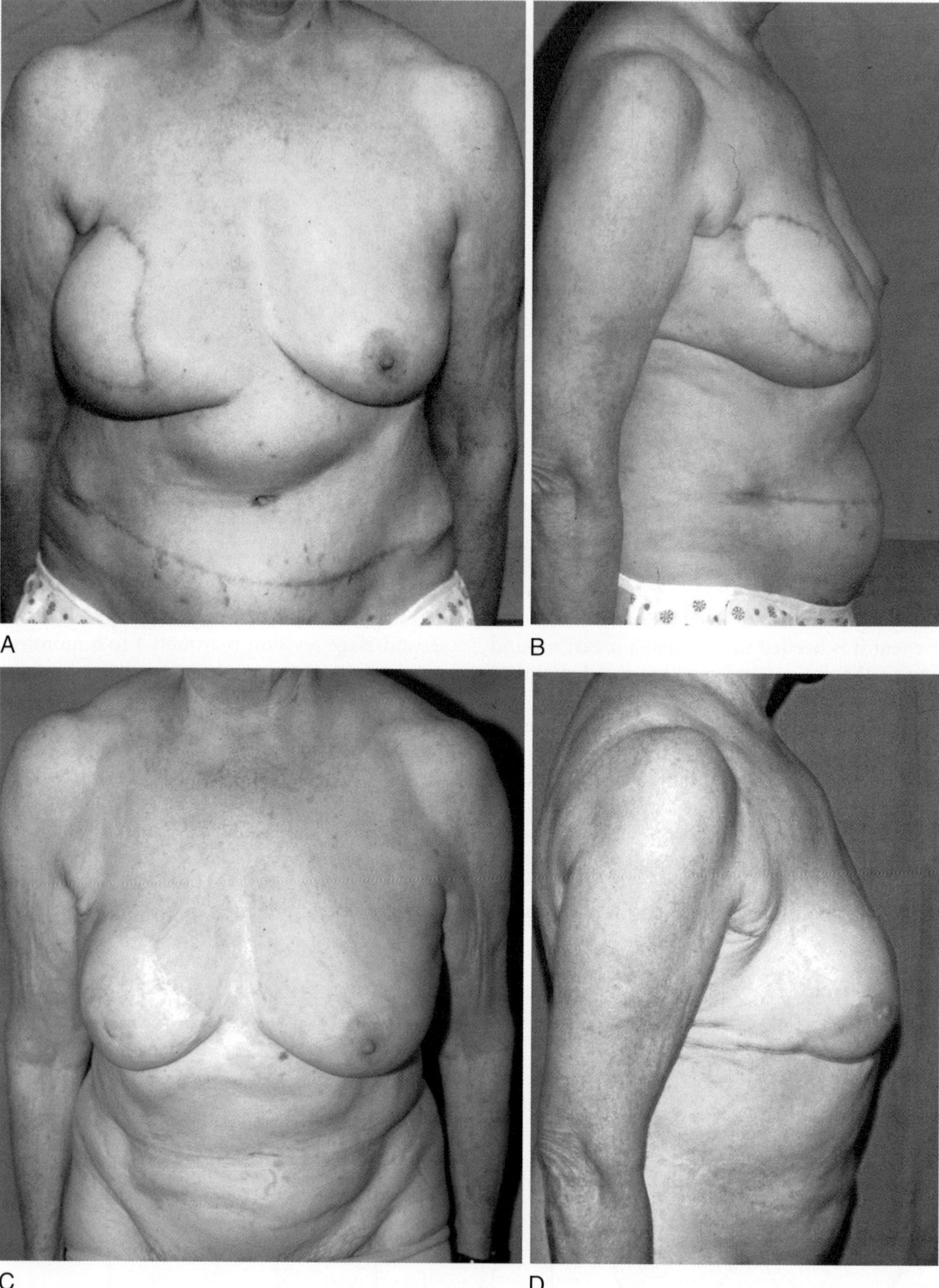

FIGURE 150-25. Contour deficiency. *A,* Anterior view of patient with right TRAM flap breast reconstruction. Reconstructed breast mound is malpositioned with excessive lateral fullness. The patient also presents with abdominal hernia at the donor site. *B,* Lateral view. Note excess lateral and inferior mound fullness and inferior central abdominal hernia. *C,* Postoperative anterior view at 2 years of secondary breast reconstruction and abdominal wall reconstruction. Note that both skin island and soft tissue of the TRAM flap have been modified to improve breast mound contour. *D,* Lateral view: excess lateral and inferior fullness corrected. The abdominal hernia has been repaired with bilateral external and internal oblique advancement flaps and intraperitoneal Prolene mesh.

the inset site with reduction of the excess flap skin will improve the contour of the inferior quadrants of the reconstructed breast mound and at the same time preserve the mastectomy skin at the superior aspect of the breast. If there are areas of deficiency in the reconstructed breast mound, it is also possible to elevate a portion of the flap tissue as a small turnover flap to fill such defects and to restore a normal contour.

The latissimus dorsi musculocutaneous flap primarily replaces the deficient skin envelope, and then the implant is used to restore the breast mound.[94,95] The skin island must have adequate dimensions to replace the missing skin and must be inset to release scar contracture particularly related to the mastectomy scar in delayed reconstruction. In general, the incision for inset of the skin island is located at the designated inframammary line; the skin island is transversely inset, with the medial and lateral inset curving superiorly and crossing the mastectomy scar to eliminate a constriction band across the center of the reconstructed breast mound. Preservation of most of the existing skin envelope is helpful if slight ptosis is desired in the breast mound reconstruction. The true inframammary line will descend with an incision because of tightness within the preserved skin envelope, so it is advisable to elevate the incision from the desired inframammary line 1 to 2 cm as this location will descend on surgical release to the appropriate position. If the mastectomy site has been irradiated before the reconstruction, an expander is recommended until healing is complete and tissues are overexpanded; the permanent implant can then be inserted in 2 to 3 months after the flap inset.

In immediate reconstruction, the latissimus dorsi musculocutaneous flap is ideally suited for inset in skin-sparing mastectomy; the skin island is used to replace only the site of the resected nipple-areola, and the muscle is used for both implant coverage and soft tissue replacement between the clavicle and superior portion of the breast where the implant will not provide contour correction. In modified radical mastectomy, the skin island must be inset at the site of skin resection. Careful skin island design and inset will ensure adequate replacement of the resected skin envelope and minimize the appearance of the different skin consistency in the center of the reconstructed breast mound.

When the latissimus dorsi musculocutaneous flap is designed to provide both skin envelope and autogenous tissue for the breast mound, the flap dissection must include maximal skin island dimension and should include subcutaneous tissue in proximity to the posterior surface of the muscle. Inset is more difficult because the skin island and underlying subcutaneous tissue are the source of the autogenous breast mound. The skin island designed in the inferior posterior trunk will generally incorporate the area where the patient has an increased layer of subcutaneous tissue. Design of an oblique skin island in which the posterior aspect is superior in relation to the anterior aspect following skin lines will yield well-vascularized skin island and the most soft tissue from the posterior trunk (see Chapter 138).

Associated Contour Defects

Axillary Fullness. Axillary fullness is frequently observed after mastectomy and breast reconstruction. With sentinel node or axillary dissection, support for axillary tissue may be lost with resultant fullness in the anterior axilla. Also, in the mildly obese patient, the thicker axillary subcutaneous tissue becomes more prominent after the mastectomy. Even after breast reconstruction, this redundant tissue affects brassiere use and is a source of dissatisfaction for the patient.

With the latissimus dorsi musculocutaneous flap, there may be more fullness in the axilla, depending on the location of the tunnel and level of arc of rotation. If this fullness relates to a tunnel low in the axilla or inadequate mobilization of the muscle flap, the quality of the breast mound reconstruction is adversely affected. Gerber[96] reviewed 60 patients with immediate latissimus dorsi musculocutaneous flap transposition. To minimize the axillary fullness, 48% of patients were randomized for cutting of the insertion; 52% were left intact. The teres major muscle was left intact in all patients. In postoperative evaluation of the aesthetic result, 90% of all patients reported a good result; with the surgeon's analysis of the results, 67.7% without tendinous transection were thought to be good results as opposed to 84% with tendinous transection ($P = .091$). The author stated that the difference seen in the aesthetic outcomes between the two groups was mostly due to the presence of the lateral bulge in patients with intact latissimus dorsi tendon. An "unsatisfactory laterocranial shape" to the breast was noted in 32.3% of patients with intact tendon, compared with 6.9% of patients with the tendon transected ($P = .014$).

If the muscle is fully mobilized, leaving the tendon intact will not result in an abnormal bulge due to the muscle. However, the muscle must have a straight arc from the axilla through the anterior axillary fold to the site of inset at the mastectomy defect. Division of the muscle insertion leaves the pedicle vulnerable to excess tension and potential vascular compromise.

When the patient presents with excess axillary fullness, it is generally located close to the level of the inframammary line. Excision of excess skin and soft tissue with a transverse excision between the anterior and posterior axillary lines will usually provide better definition to the reconstructed breast mound and provide more comfort to the patient when wearing her bra (see Fig. 150-22*B* and *C*).

DEFECTS AFTER LUMPECTOMY AND RADIATION THERAPY. Lumpectomy and radiation therapy have allowed many patients with stage I breast cancer to preserve their breasts without an effect on long-term survival. If local recurrence should develop, a completion mastectomy will provide effective treatment without jeopardizing survival rates (see Chapter 138). The advantage of lumpectomy with radiation therapy is that the breast is saved with its sensation intact. The disadvantage is the potential for shortening of the supporting ligamentous structure as a consequence of the radiotherapy with gradual superior migration of the breast mound, which may accentuate asymmetry if there is mild ptosis on the contralateral breast (Fig. 150-26). The combination of lumpectomy and radiation therapy may also affect the contour of the breast, with less fullness in the breast in the region of the lumpectomy. Improvements in tumor localization, precise lumpectomy, and radiotherapy techniques have allowed excellent results in regard to survival rates and breast preservation. When there are contour irregularities after lumpectomy and radiation therapy, the patient may request secondary surgery to improve breast contour. The use of an implant to correct a contour deformity is associated with increased incidence of capsular contracture related to the effect of prior radiation therapy. For this reason, the use of a flap to release scar contracture and to provide well-vascularized soft tissue for autogenous reconstruction is recommended. The latissimus dorsi musculocutaneous transposition flap is most useful for this purpose because it provides skin to release the contracture with the breast parenchyma, allows the breast to descend to its normal position for the patient's age, and provides adequate soft tissue to fill the segmental contour deformity (Fig. 150-27). The alternative flap, the rectus abdominis musculocutaneous flap (TRAM flap), is also available but generally provides more tissue than is really required for this limited deformity. Furthermore, the TRAM flap should be available in the future should the patient develop local recurrence and require completion mastectomy and reconstruction or develop a contralateral breast cancer that requires a mastectomy. There are, however, instances when the deformity is extensive as a result of lumpectomy and radiation therapy and a TRAM flap may be required to provide a reasonable breast reconstruction (Figs. 150-28 and 150-29).

In a prospective series of 265 patients presenting for follow-up after lumpectomy and breast irradiation, Deutsch and Flickinger[97] examined a variety of aesthetic outcomes, including skin pigmentation, breast distortion, asymmetry, and size discrepancy, and recorded the overall appearance as excellent, good, fair, or poor. All outcomes were determined by a single surgeon. The authors found that 10.2% of patients had a fair or poor result, with the rest of the patients having a good (41.5%) or excellent result. Factors associated with a better aesthetic outcome (good or excellent) included white race ($P = .0056$), smaller breasts (implied by a smaller separation between tangential fields, $P = .01$), the use of a boost dose ($P = .0025$), no use of doxorubicin ($P = .0154$), and no use of tamoxifen ($P = .025$). The authors suggested that the counterintuitive finding of a better aesthetic outcome associated with a boost dose may be explained by more extensive surgical resection in those patients not receiving a boost dose. The authors concluded that the majority of women treated with lumpectomy and

Text continued on p. 1147

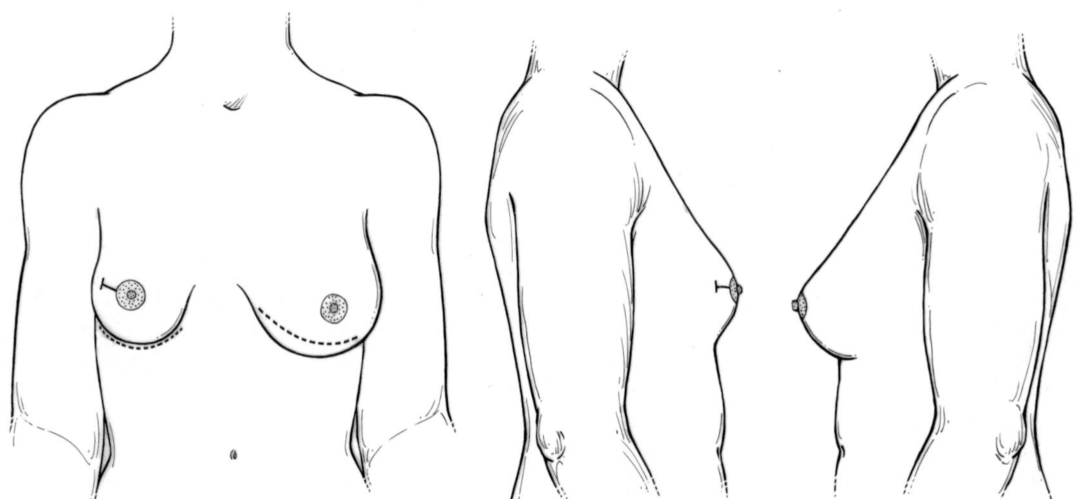

FIGURE 150-26. Lumpectomy and radiation therapy. Positional and volume changes may occur with follow-up. Note loss of volume and superior retraction of breast mound.

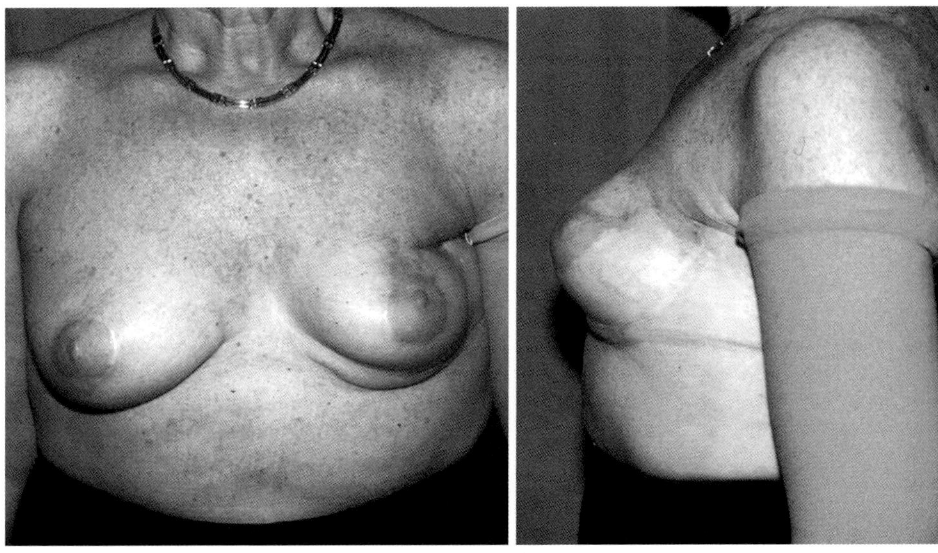

A B

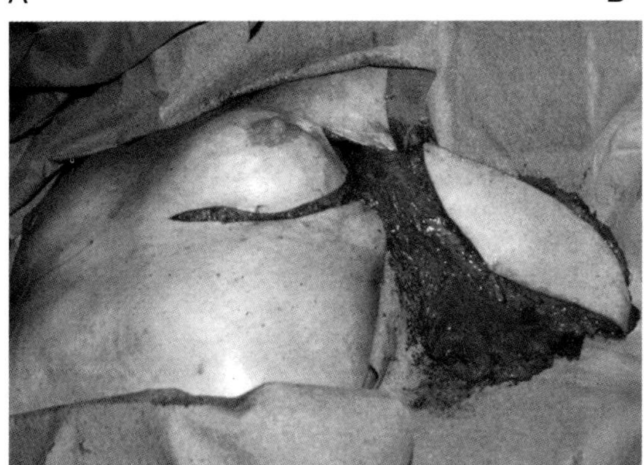

C

FIGURE 150-27. Contour deficiency. *A,* Anterior postoperative view of patient after a left lumpectomy and radiation therapy with concerns about lateral contour deformity and loss of natural inferior breast fullness. *B,* Lateral view. Note superior contraction of breast mound. *C,* Intraoperative view. Latissimus dorsi musculocutaneous flap is ready for inset after release of contracture at inferior lateral breast mound. *D,* Anterior view: postoperative secondary reconstruction with scar release and insertion of ipsilateral latissimus dorsi musculocutaneous transposition flap. *E,* Lateral view. Note that the flap provides fullness in inferior lateral breast mound and release of scar contracture at site of lumpectomy.

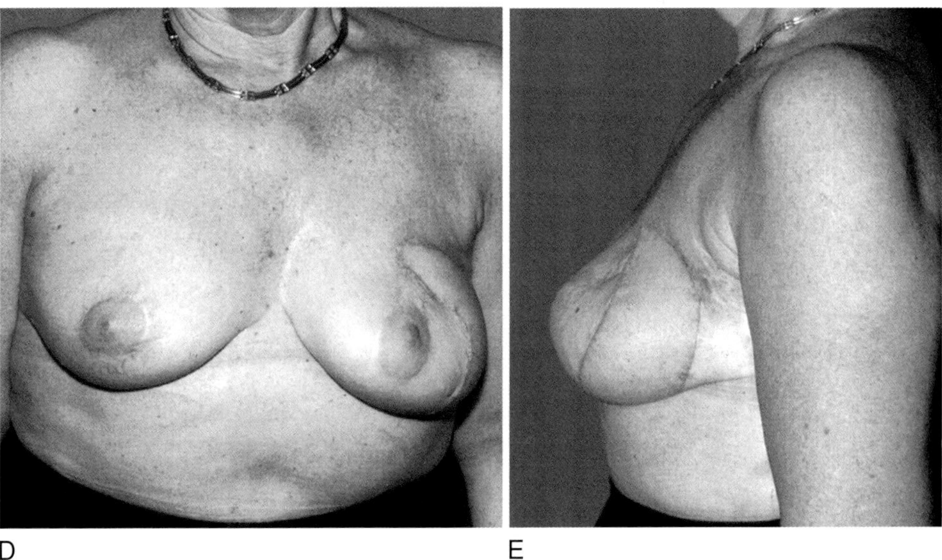

D E

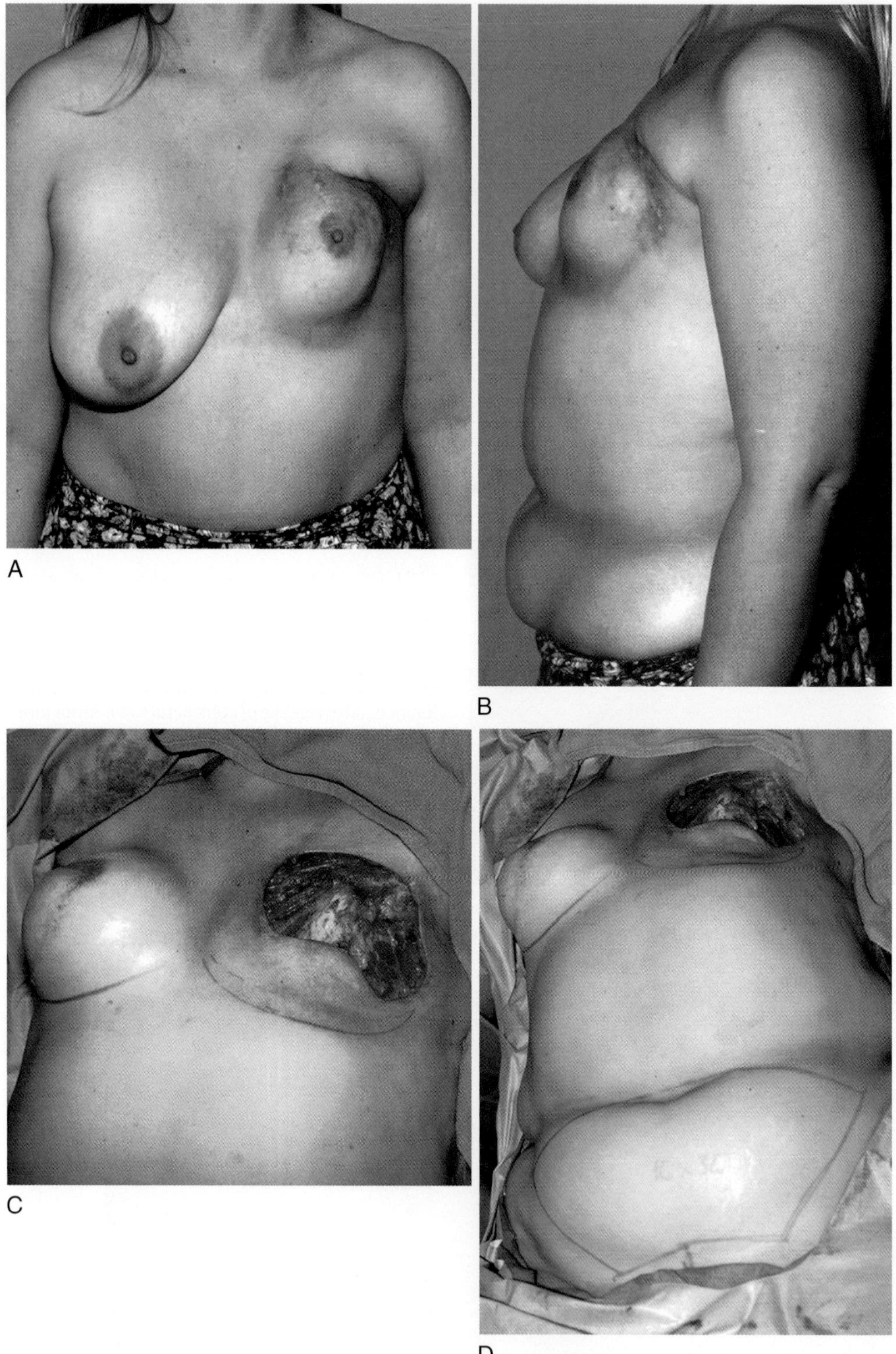

FIGURE 150-28. Contour and position deficiencies. *A,* Anterior postoperative view of right lumpectomy followed by radiation therapy. *B,* Lateral view. Note loss of inferior fullness. *C,* Intraoperative view of completion mastectomy of left breast due to extensive breast mound fibrosis. *D,* Intraoperative view of design of transverse rectus abdominis musculocutaneous (TRAM) flap.

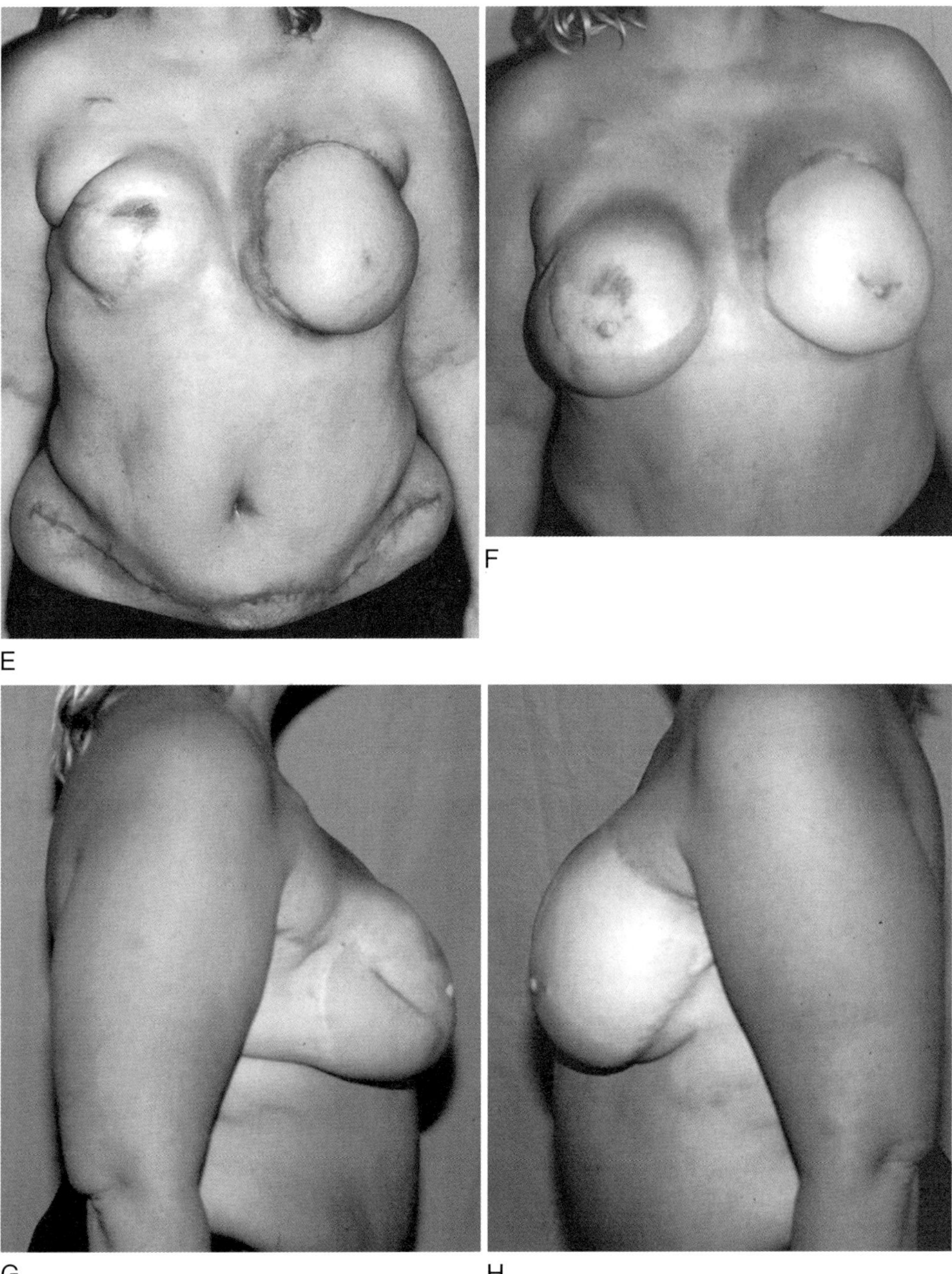

FIGURE 150-28, cont'd. *E,* Postoperative anterior view after secondary reconstruction of left breast. Note that before secondary reconstruction, the patient had undergone a right modified radical mastectomy with expander-implant sequence. The right breast reconstruction site now exhibits envelope deficiency. *F,* Postoperative anterior view after secondary reconstruction of right breast with latissimus dorsi musculocutaneous flap for skin envelope deficiency and coverage of a permanent implant. The right breast mound demonstrates adequate fullness with improved skin envelope. Autogenous reconstruction on left side and flap plus implant on right side provided a natural breast mound bilaterally. *G* and *H,* Postoperative lateral views.

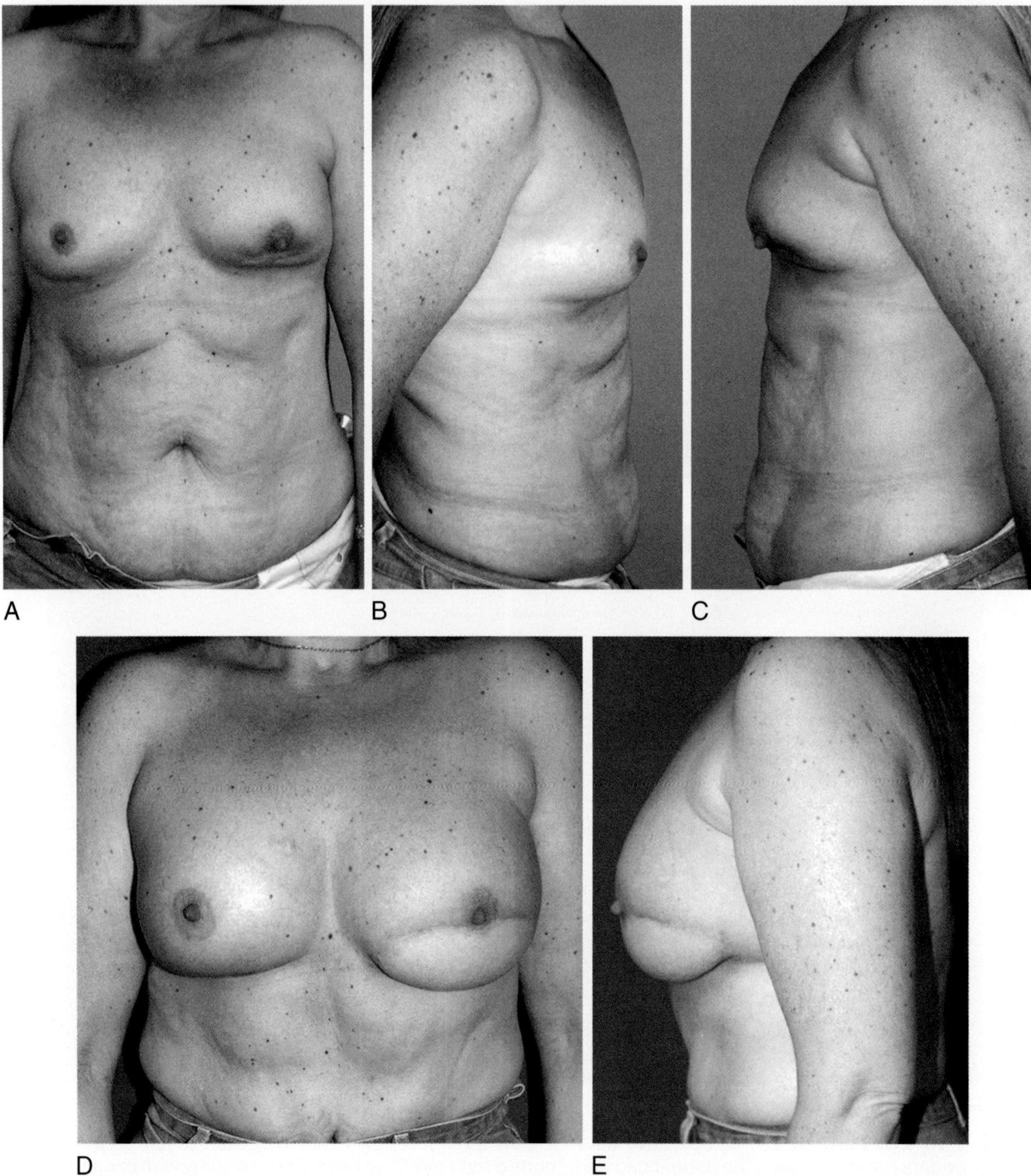

FIGURE 150-29. Skin envelope and contour deficiency. *A*, Anterior view of patient after lumpectomy and radiation therapy. The patient presented for secondary reconstruction after a plastic surgeon used a latissimus flap to correct breast deformity. *B*, Lateral view of normal breast. *C*, Lateral view of latissimus flap that failed to correct skin envelope deficiency or contour abnormality. *D*, Anterior postoperative view 3 months after secondary reconstruction with right rectus abdominis musculocutaneous flap (TRAM flap). *E*, Lateral view of skin envelope and contour deficiency corrected by TRAM flap with autogenous reconstruction.

radiotherapy will have a satisfactory aesthetic outcome and stated that the use of tamoxifen or doxorubicin, black race, and larger breasts are associated with poorer aesthetic outcome.

In a smaller, retrospective series of 32 patients undergoing either lumpectomy with radiation therapy (n = 21) or no treatment to the breast (n = 11, control group), Bajaj et al[98] used subjective evaluation of patient photographs and a patient questionnaire to measure the aesthetic changes after breast conservation surgery and considered 2 standard deviations above the mean for asymmetry scores (range, 1 to 9) as significant. They found that 86% of breast conservation patients were satisfied with their aesthetic outcome, although 35% of patients did note a significant change in the appearance of the breast after treatment. The average treatment-related asymmetry score was 1.93 for lumpectomy-radiation therapy patients compared with 0.93 for the control group (no *P* value given). On the basis of their findings of significant asymmetry in 35%, the authors concluded that plastic surgery consultation should be routinely offered as part of the treatment protocol for patients undergoing breast conservation therapy.

EPIGASTRIC FULLNESS. Epigastric fullness may occur at the site of the tunnel between the abdomen and the reconstructed breast mound. This fullness may detract from the quality of the breast reconstruction and result in dissatisfaction of the patient. In general, this problem can be avoided by two steps in the initial flap transposition procedure:

1. It is important to completely denervate the rectus muscle during its elevation. The superior segmental motor nerve enters the lateral deep muscle at the costal margin, and this branch should be divided if the entire muscle is used in the flap base. Failure to divide this nerve will result in visible contractions of the muscle and prevent desirable muscle atrophy. If muscle-preserving techniques are used, it is helpful to fully separate the lateral muscle, which will be left in place, from the medial muscle that will support the flap.
2. In completing the dissection between the mastectomy defect and the abdominal donor site, it is helpful to resect the subcutaneous tissue from the tunnel to eliminate excess fullness with the addition of the muscle flap passing through this space.

Nahabedian et al[99] compared the epigastric fullness in 155 patients who underwent pedicled TRAM, free TRAM, and DIEP flaps for breast reconstruction. The problem of epigastric fullness occurred in 5 of 37 (13.5%) patients reconstructed with the pedicled TRAM flap and none of the free flaps (as expected). The authors suggest that "upper abdominal fullness after pedicled TRAM reconstruction can be reduced by the tangential excision of subcutaneous fat in the upper abdominal skin flap."

EXPLANTATION

Reoperation after breast reconstruction may be indicated in the absence of postoperative complications or aesthetic problems. The patient may request removal of a silicone prosthesis because of fear of a potential link between silicone and systemic illness. Despite a growing body of evidence that shows no causal relationship between silicone and either breast cancer[100-102] or connective tissue diseases,[102-106] patients may still request removal of silicone implants. It may be possible in some patients to replace the silicone prosthesis with a saline-filled implant, but a significant number of patients may be unhappy with the prospect of another prosthetic device and prefer conversion to autologous tissue reconstruction.

After implant reconstruction, many patients present with a combined concern related to a possible implant leak (implant failure) and the long-term effect of exposure to silicone gel. These patients also may present with the problem of capsular contracture as an additional cause of dissatisfaction with the results of breast reconstruction. Although implant exchange and capsulectomy may provide improved result, some of these patients wish to eliminate the implant with no further interest in reconstruction or switch to autogenous reconstruction (Fig. 150-30 and Table 150-46).

Roberts[107] reviewed 55 women with requests for explantation who had implant placement (72% augmentation and 28% reconstruction—13 prophylactic mastectomies and 2 cancer mastectomies). The most common reason (59%) for request for implant removal was breast health problems (pain, rupture, contracture, connective tissue disorders) (Table 150-47). Some patients were convinced but others were unsure as to a relationship between connective tissue disorder and implants. Twenty-eight patients hoped to enjoy better general health after explantation; 12 wanted relief from generalized pain, and 6 wanted relief from local breast pain.

Slavin[108] reviewed 46 patients who underwent 74 silicone gel implant explantations; 20 of these patients had undergone postmastectomy reconstruction. Average durations of placement were 7.1 years for reconstructed patients and 10.3 years in the augmented group. Indications for explantation were fear of

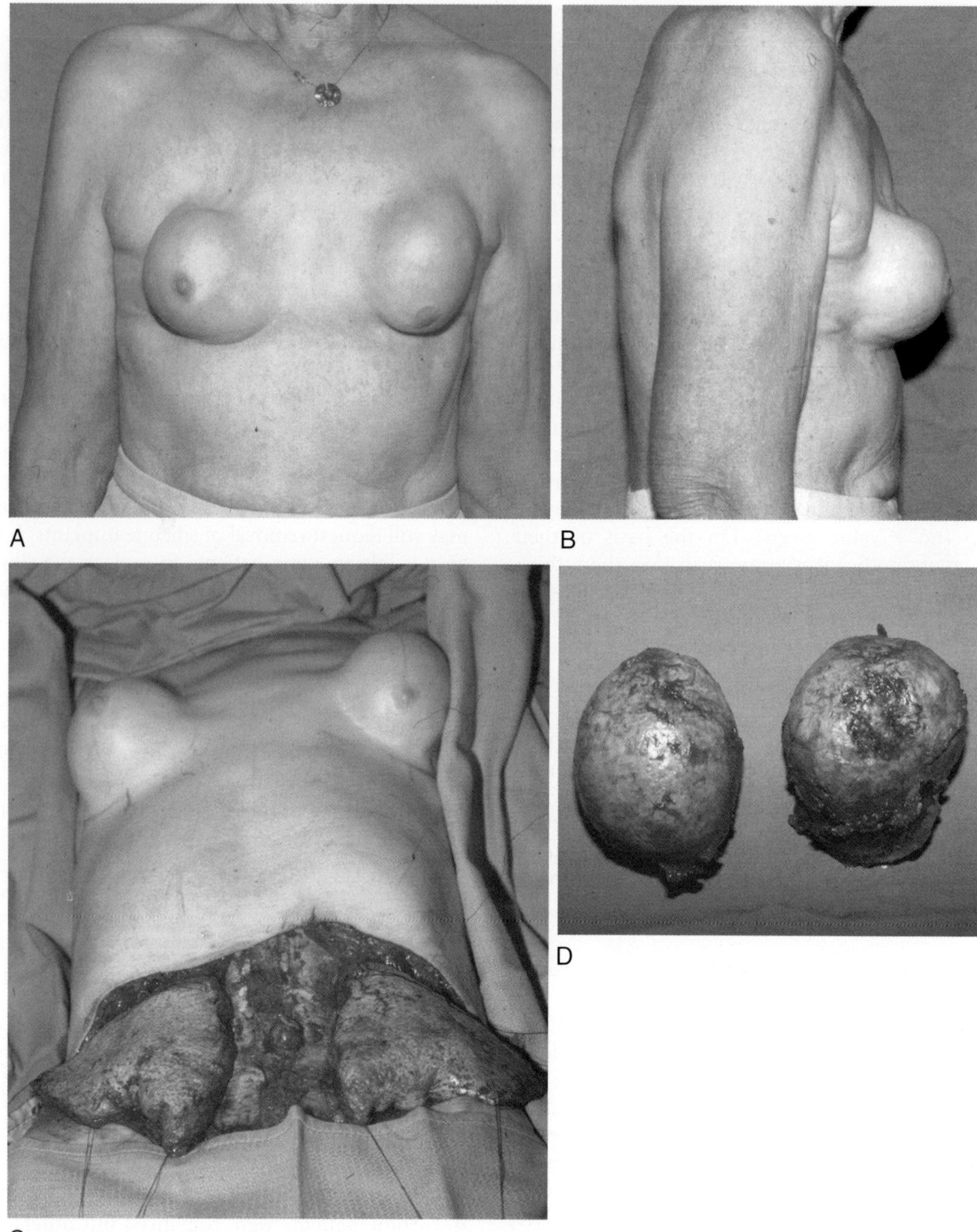

FIGURE 150-30. Explantation. *A,* Anterior view of patient with concerns about polyurethane implants 15 years after bilateral subcutaneous mastectomy. Note Baker grade IV capsular contracture with adequate skin envelope. The patient requested implant removal and autogenous reconstruction. *B,* Lateral view. *C,* Anterior intraoperative view of bilateral de-epithelialized rectus abdominis musculocutaneous flaps ready for transposition to anterior chest for autogenous bilateral mound reconstruction. *D,* Intraoperative view. Note entire capsule with implant removed.

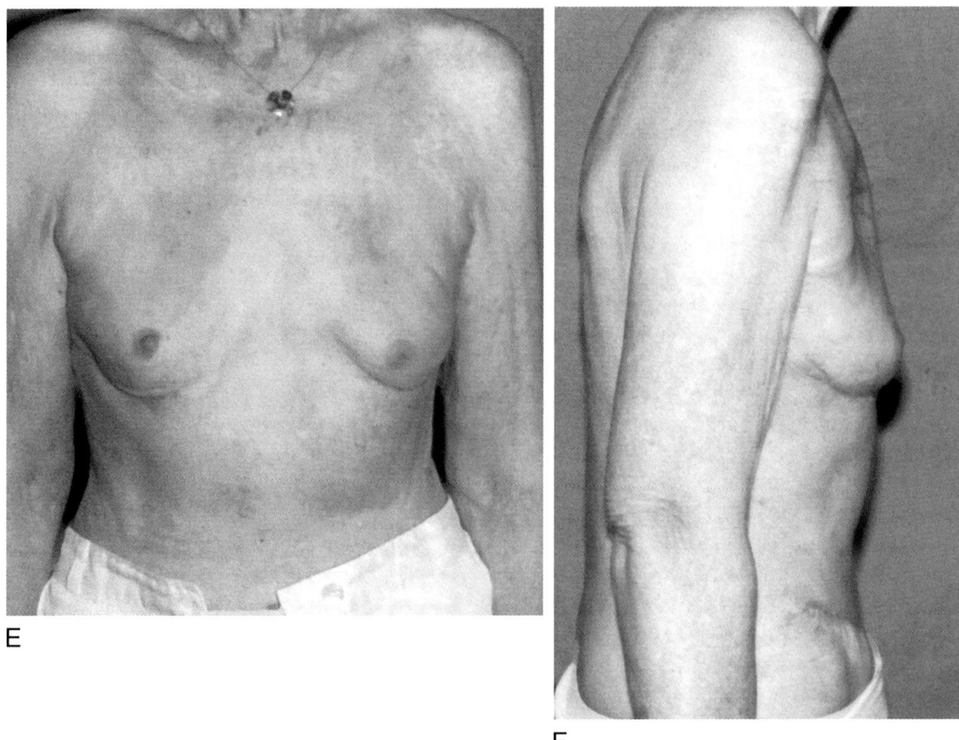

FIGURE 150-30, cont'd. *E,* Postoperative anterior view at 1 year of bilateral secondary breast reconstruction with explantation, total capsulectomy, and bilateral TRAM flaps. *F,* Lateral view. Note natural contour with adequate skin envelope and TRAM autogenous flap for mound.

TABLE 150-46 ✦ SURGICAL OPTIONS AFTER EXPLANTATION

Problem	Surgical Options
Explantation	Reassurance Explantation without replacement or further reconstruction Implant exchange (silicone → saline) ± capsulectomy Conversion to flap reconstruction

TABLE 150-47 ✦ REASONS FOR WANTING IMPLANTS REMOVED

	Number	Percentage*
Breast health problems (pain, rupture, contractures)	26	59
General health problems	21	48
Diagnosed with connective tissue disease	11	25
Fear of long-term effects	8	18
Poor cosmetic results	2	5
Breast cancer	1	2

*Some subjects gave more than one reason; the percentage total exceeds 100.

From Roberts CS, Wells KE, Walden K: Toward understanding women who request removal of silicone breast implants. Breast J 1999;5:246–251.

consequences of silicone gel (n = 17); capsular contracture causing aesthetic problems (n = 14); systemic symptoms, including headaches, arthralgia, fatigue, cough, and recurrent infections (n = 8); mammographic evidence of rupture (n = 7); and fear of interference with mammography or examination for breast cancer (n = 4). Capsulectomy was performed in 34 of 46 patients (74%). Mammography correctly predicted rupture in seven of eight patients. The authors state that patients undergoing explantation for fear of the health effects of silicone will be pleased despite aesthetic limitations. Satisfaction of patients is related to the initial reason for explantation, as patients who are anxious about the health effects of silicone implants will invariably feel more at ease after explantation and aesthetic concerns will be of lesser import (the authors cite Gilboa et al[109]).

Patients who have had implants placed for reconstruction are less likely to seek explantation because of fear of silicone-related health problems compared with augmentation patients. The authors suggest the following reasons:

1. Relative absence of breast tissue may lead patients to believe that they are less at risk for silicone-related health problems.
2. "Familiarity with serious disease—breast cancer—had either insulated them from that concern or had decreased that worry."
3. A few patients stated that the risk of dying of breast cancer was far higher than that of health problems related to silicone.

Schusterman[110] reported a prospective study comparing the incidence of autoimmune disease in various reconstructions (603 patients with silicone gel implant, latissimus dorsi musculocutaneous flap with or without implant, or TRAM flap reconstructions). Follow-up, expressed as person-years, was 615.8 and 663.4 for implant and nonimplant cohorts, respectively. One patient from each cohort developed mild autoimmune disease requiring treatment with steroids, which were subsequently discontinued in both instances. The authors concluded that the incidence of autoimmune disease was not increased in patients receiving silicone gel implants.

Duffy and Woods[106] reported on a retrospective review of 200 patients (681 implants) explanted from 1962 to 1992 for augmentation (n = 27) or reconstruction (n = 173) to evaluate relative incidence of immune-related disorders, siliconoma, acquired nonbreast malignant neoplasms, metachronous breast cancer, and recurrent breast carcinoma between those patients with failed implants and those with intact implants. Results of this analysis showed that 85% of all implants (67.5% of patients) were intact at explantation and that 15% of implants had failed in 65 (32.5%) of the patients. These 65 patients were found to have no increased incidence of any of the abovementioned health problems.

Position

PLACEMENT

The placement of the reconstructed breast mound will determine the success of the procedure. Parameters include the site of the skin envelope resection, shape of the chest wall, and technique of expander-implant insertion or flap inset. The breast mound should be centered on the midclavicular line with maximal fullness located at the medial and lateral inferior quadrants of the breast mound. Failure to achieve an optimal position at the time of the reconstruction is likely to require future revisions as secondary procedures (Table 150-48; see Fig. 150-24).

When an expander-implant sequence is used, the expander must have its inferior shell located at the inframammary line or below this line if advancement flaps are planned after the expansion process. Both medial and lateral skin envelope expansion is required, which may necessitate the wider base expander as opposed to the permanent adjustable implant, particularly in delayed reconstruction. When expansion is asymmetric, the second procedure during expander removal and implant insertion allows adjustment of the breast implant pocket.

The flap inset must again allow greatest skin island dimensions to be located at the midclavicular line and extend laterally to the anterior axillary line. In delayed reconstruction, if skin is unstable laterally or medially, inset of the majority of the flap in an asymmetric position may not provide appropriate positioning of the breast mound. In this situation, options include flap inset for stable chest wall skin, with an expander positioned for the site of the future breast mound, and later use of a second flap for breast reconstruction after the initial flap is used to provide stable chest wall

TABLE 150-48 ✦ SURGICAL OPTIONS FOR PLACEMENT AND INFRAMAMMARY LINE PROBLEMS

Problem	Surgical Options
Placement and inframammary line	No treatment Revision: repositioning of inframammary line Revision: pocket repositioning Revision: reinset of tissue flap Addition of implant Addition of flap Contralateral symmetry procedures: mastopexy, reduction

coverage. When the flap is designed for both skin envelope and autogenous mound, the area of the best vascularized soft tissue with associated skin island should be located in the area of the central and inferior breast mound (zones 1 and 2 of the TRAM flap, area over the perforator in a perforator flap, central third of the latissimus dorsi skin island). Later thinning of the flap can be accomplished in the periphery of the flap inset, but if adequate central fullness is not present, a secondary procedure with use of an implant or an additional flap may be required to provide adequate positioning of the breast mound (Fig. 150-31).

INFRAMAMMARY LINE

Correct positioning of the inframammary line can be difficult to accomplish in both immediate and delayed breast reconstruction (Fig. 150-32 and Table 150-48). In immediate reconstruction, identification of the inframammary line before the surgery and preservation of the skin attachment will help in positioning the expander-implant or subsequent inset of a flap for autogenous reconstruction. In the rectus abdominis musculocutaneous flap (TRAM flap), the inferior pull after the donor site closure has a tendency to lower the inframammary line on the mastectomy site because of release of a portion of the inframammary region for the tunnel for flap transposition. Therefore, the site for the flap inset to define the inframammary line must be 1 to 2 cm superior to the planned location of the inframammary line. Similarly, in delayed reconstruction with the latissimus dorsi musculocutaneous flap when the skin island inset site is planned to coincide with the inframammary line, the incision should be 1 to 2 cm superior to the actual desired location as the inferior skin after release will retract inferiorly.

In delayed reconstruction with a tissue expander, placement of an expander below the desired location of the inframammary line may be helpful to later incorporate expander skin below the inframammary line into the skin envelope. With this approach, the inframammary line must be re-established with either internal or external sutures (Figs. 150-33 to 150-36). Various techniques have been described to establish a well-placed and well-defined inframammary line, including skin de-epithelialization under the implanted breast with fixation of dermis to pectoralis fascia,[111] de-epithelialization on both sides of a crescent-shaped incision with fixation of the flap to perichondrium or intercostal fascia,[112] and lower pole capsulotomy with undermining of the skin under the new inframammary line and suturing of the distal dermis to proximal fascia and periosteum.[113] These techniques emphasize the importance of establishing a well-defined inframammary line. With the use of the textured expander and preservation of the inframammary line at the time of mastectomy, a well-defined and appropriately located inframammary line should be maintained until the permanent implant is inserted. In delayed implant reconstruction or in secondary reconstruction in which the inframammary line is ill-defined or malpositioned, modification of the Pennisi-Ryan techniques may be helpful to relocate and define the inframammary line.

Text continued on p. 1157

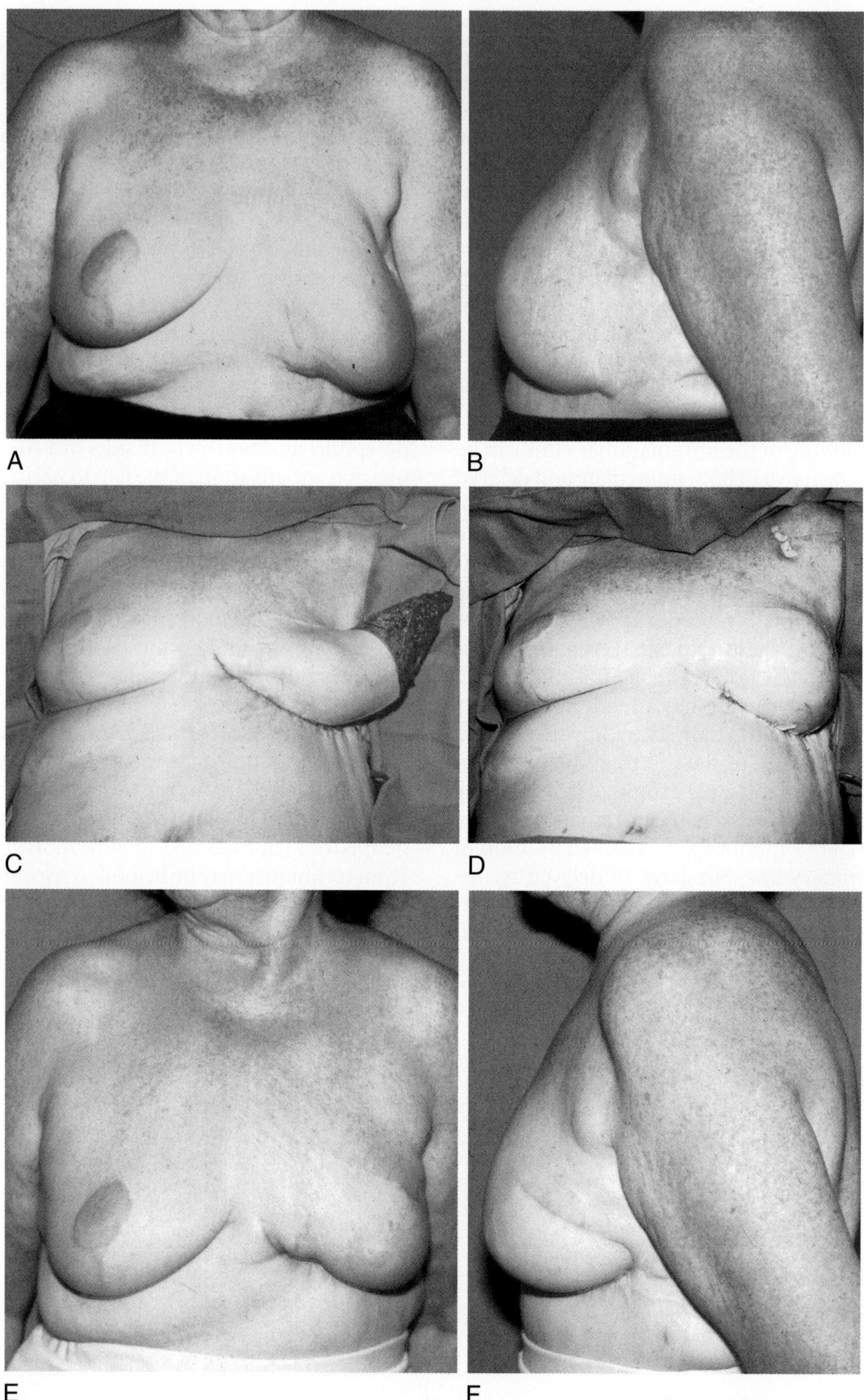

FIGURE 150-31. Placement problem: malposition. *A,* Anterior view of patient after autogenous reconstruction with lateral chest fasciocutaneous flap. The mound is malpositioned laterally and inferiorly without definition of inframammary line. *B,* Lateral view. Note adequate skin envelope and mound contour. *C,* Anterior intraoperative view. The flap is re-elevated as a tubed pedicled flap and inset to provide new inframammary line and decreasing lateral chest fullness. *D,* Anterior intraoperative view after flap reinset. *E,* Anterior postoperative view 6 months after secondary breast reconstruction with flap reinset to reposition flap over the central left hemithorax and to establish correct location for inframammary line. *F,* Lateral view. Note that the breast has definition laterally and does not extend into the lateral hemithorax between the anterior and posterior axillary lines.

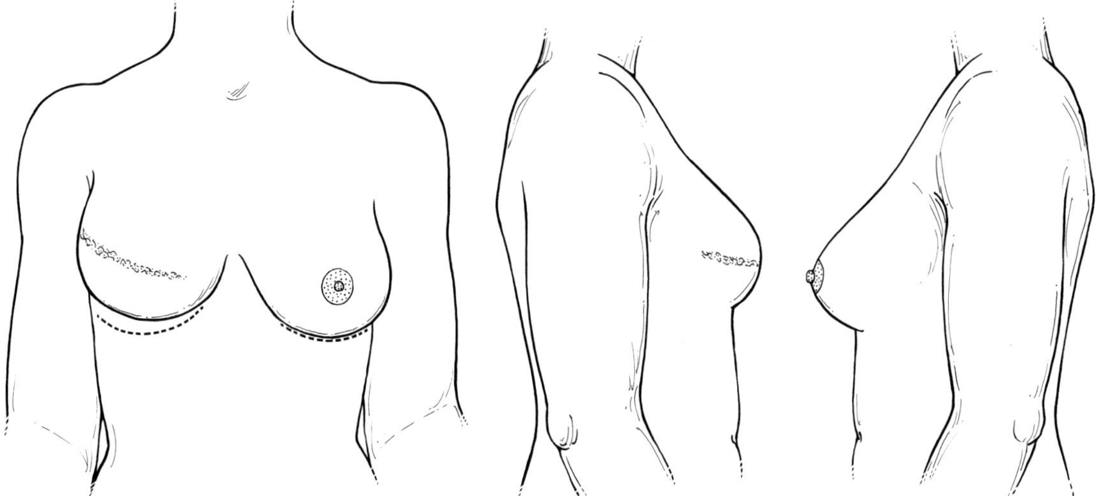

FIGURE 150-32. Inframammary line malposition: implant reconstruction with inferior implant displaced superiorly.

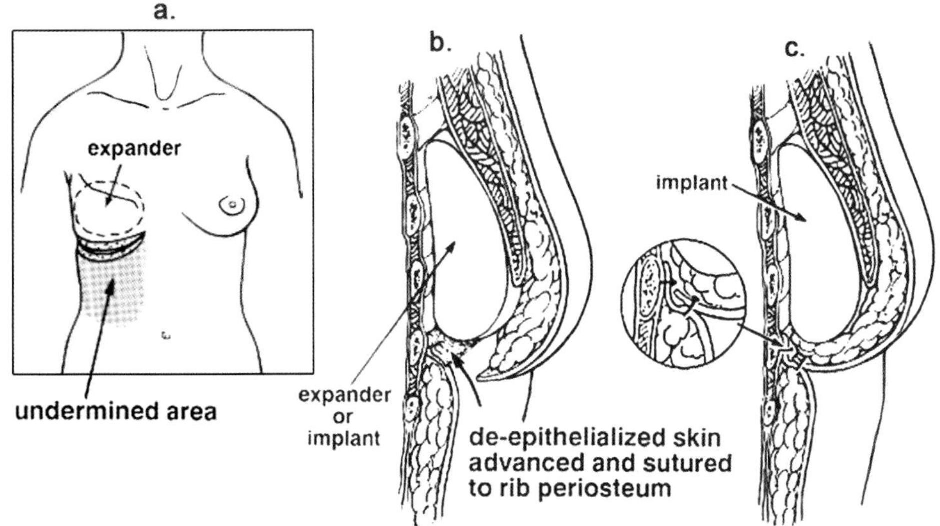

FIGURE 150-33. *A* to *C*, External approach to re-establish incorrectly positioned mammary line by use of local abdominal advancement flap. (From Oliva A, Mathes SJ: Technique of breast reconstruction. Prob Gen Surg 1989;6:564.)

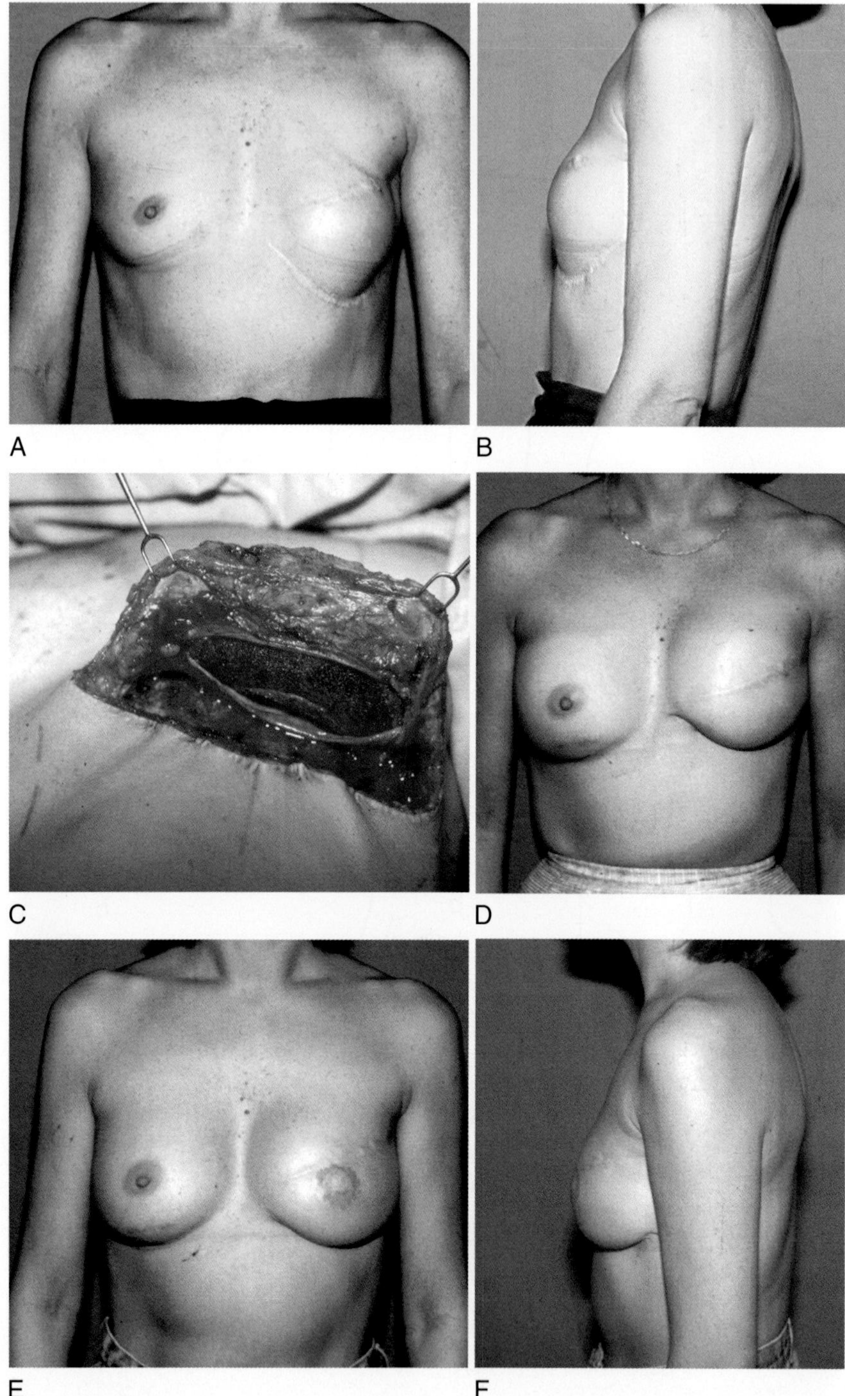

FIGURE 150-34. Inframammary line malposition. *A,* Anterior view of patient after delayed breast reconstruction with permanent implant. Note implant placement below normal position for inframammary line. *B,* Lateral view. Note prior inframammary incision and implant located below level of the sixth intercostal space. *C,* Intraoperative view with inset of the inferior-based abdominal advancement flap at the correct location for the inframammary line. *D,* Anterior view: early postoperative view after secondary breast reconstruction with reconstruction of inframammary line with abdominal advancement flap, capsulectomy, and implant exchange. *E,* Postoperative anterior view 2 years after secondary reconstruction. Note that bilateral implants have improved breast mound contour (right breast augmentation); the abdominal advancement flap has improved inferior skin envelope and defined appropriately located inframammary line. *F,* Lateral view. Note that the inframammary line is well defined and positioned.

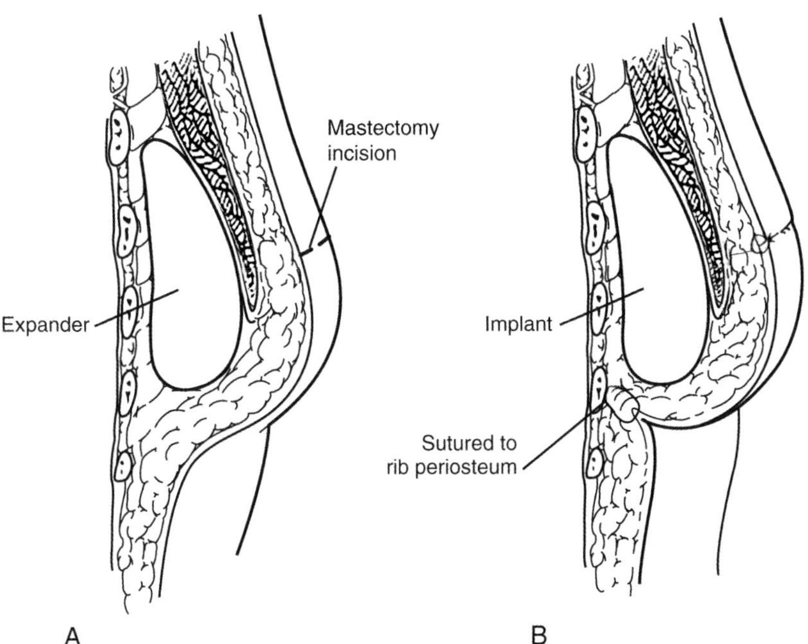

FIGURE 150-35. *A* and *B*, Internal approach to re-establish correctly positioned inframammary line with internal capsular-chest wall suture. (From Oliva A, Mathes SJ: Technique of breast reconstruction. Prob Gen Surg 1989;6:564.)

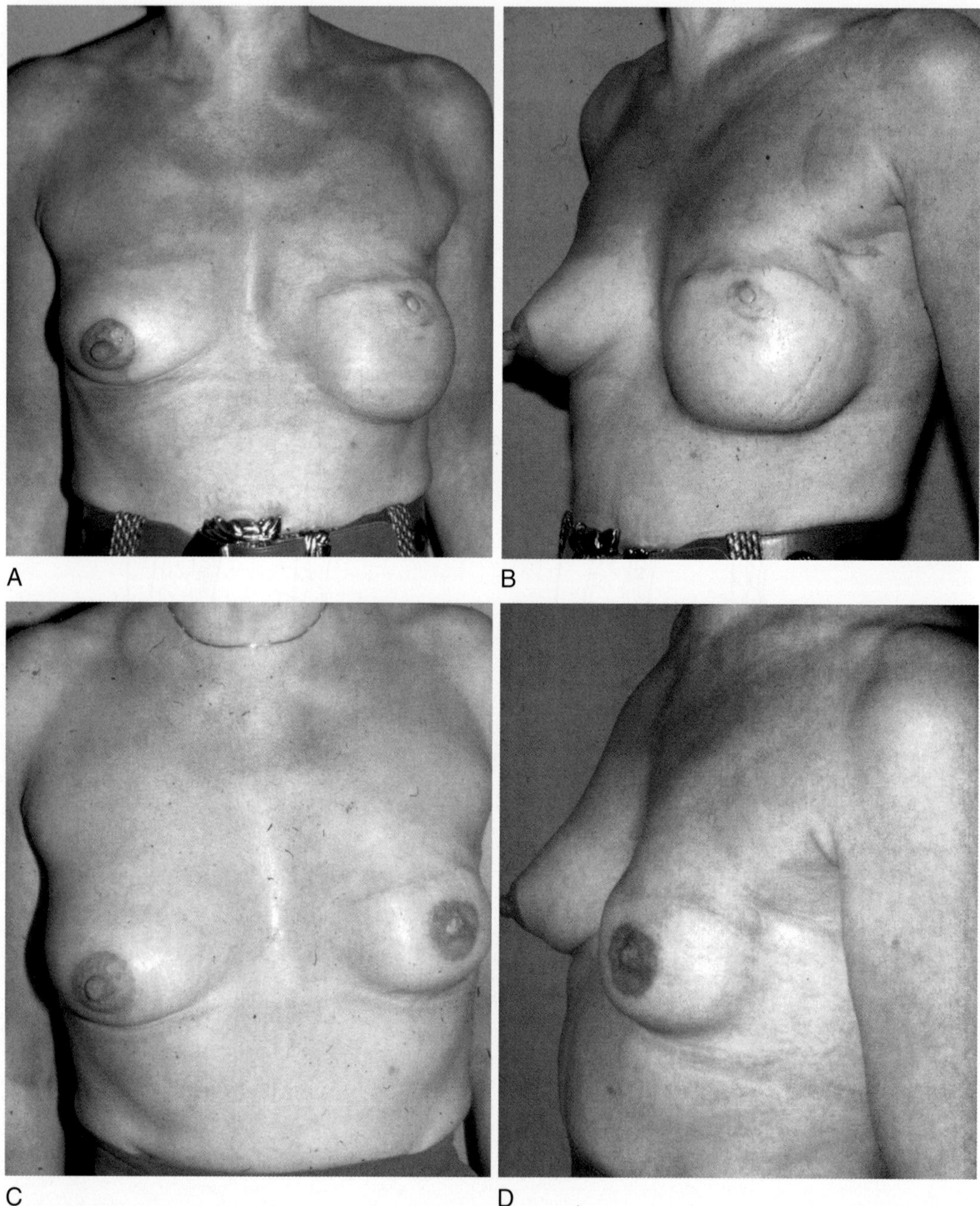

FIGURE 150-36. Inframammary line malposition. *A,* Anterior view of patient after left delayed breast reconstruction with permanent implant. Note implant placement below normal position for inframammary line. *B,* Oblique view. Note implant positioned too lateral and inferior to central anterior left hemithorax. *C,* Postoperative anterior view 1 year after secondary breast reconstruction with inframammary line (internal) reconstruction. *D,* Postoperative lateral view at 1 year. Note that the inframammary line is well defined and positioned.

Scar

POSITION

Scar represents a source of problems that may lead to dissatisfaction and request for secondary reconstruction (Figs. 150-37 and 150-38 and Table 150-49). Mentor's SPS study[3] reported a 5% rate of complications related to scarring after saline breast implant reconstruction (see Table 150-39). INAMED's R95 study[5] reported a 6% rate of complications related to scarring at 3 and 5 years after saline breast implant reconstruction (see Table 150-38). Position of a scar is related primarily to the inset site of a flap used for envelope reconstruction. The initial scar used for mastectomy does influence the inset site for both expander-implant and flap. Toth[114] advocates the need for plastic surgical input in determining the mastectomy incision. The surgical oncologist must obtain appropriate skin margins, depending on tumor size and location (see Chapter 138), but when possible, it is preferable to limit incision to inferior to the superior margin of the areola and lateral to the medial margin of the areola. The most favorable approach, as described by Bensimon and Bergmeyer,[115] is possible with skin-sparing mastectomy. With the flap inset involving only the area of the former site of the nipple-areola, later nipple reconstruction and areola tattoo will essentially eliminate visible scars. Areola or nipple-areola sparing (total skin envelope preservation) is now used in selected patients and also will eliminate positional scar problems. However, ischemia and subsequent loss of the nipple or nipple and areola may necessitate secondary nipple-areola reconstruction with possible introduction of new scar problems.

With delayed reconstruction by the expander-implant sequence, the mastectomy scar will be used for exposure for implant insertion. The lateral aspect of the scar is used, and the medial portion of the scar will continue the maturation process. If the scar is excessively tight, a Z-plasty may be helpful when the permanent implant is inserted. When a flap is used, the inferior aspect of the skin island used to re-establish the skin envelope should be inset at the inframammary line. Unstable and scarred skin should be removed if the dimensions of the skin island are adequate. When the central area of the preserved mastectomy skin is unstable or excessively scarred, it may be necessary to use the skin island at this area despite the patch appearance of the skin island inserted between preserved superior and inferior mastectomy skin. When a large area of the mastectomy skin must be resected because of scarring and instability, the TRAM flap provides a larger skin island and allows replacement of unstable skin, and the skin island may extend to the re-established inframammary line. When a flap is used, it is helpful to have part of the skin island intersect the mastectomy scar. The intersection of the flap with the mastectomy scar avoids a contracted segment in the middle of the reconstructed breast mound (Fig. 150-38).

When the lower mastectomy skin flap is compromised, Restifo[116] recommends replacement of all the retained mastectomy skin down to the inframammary fold as a subunit with use of the TRAM flap skin island. Hidalgo[117] has similarly stressed the importance of establishing a larger defect to hide transitions between retained breast skin envelope and the skin island of the flap. Spear and Davison,[118] in a retrospective series reviewing 264 patients with autologous tissue reconstructions during 10 years, have determined the favorable patterns of skin flap inset and note that "dividing the breast into reconstructive subunits that are to be replaced as a whole rather than as a patch gives superior results." The authors also found that the most desirable subunits are those that are naturally bounded by changes in tissue, color, or texture. These include the transition from breast skin to areola, areola to nipple, inframammary line (breast to chest wall skin), anterior axillary line, and breast to sternal skin (Fig. 150-39).

HYPERTROPHIC SCAR

After re-entry through the mastectomy scar for implant insertion or flap inset, scar hypertrophy can occur. If the patient is susceptible to scar hypertrophy or

TABLE 150-49 ✦ SURGICAL OPTIONS FOR CORRECTION OF UNACCEPTABLE SCARS

Problem	Surgical Options
Scar	No treatment Intralesional steroids after scar maturation Revision: flap reinset to follow aesthetic subunits Addition of flap to reduce skin tension or to alter scar position Resection of unstable skin or scar

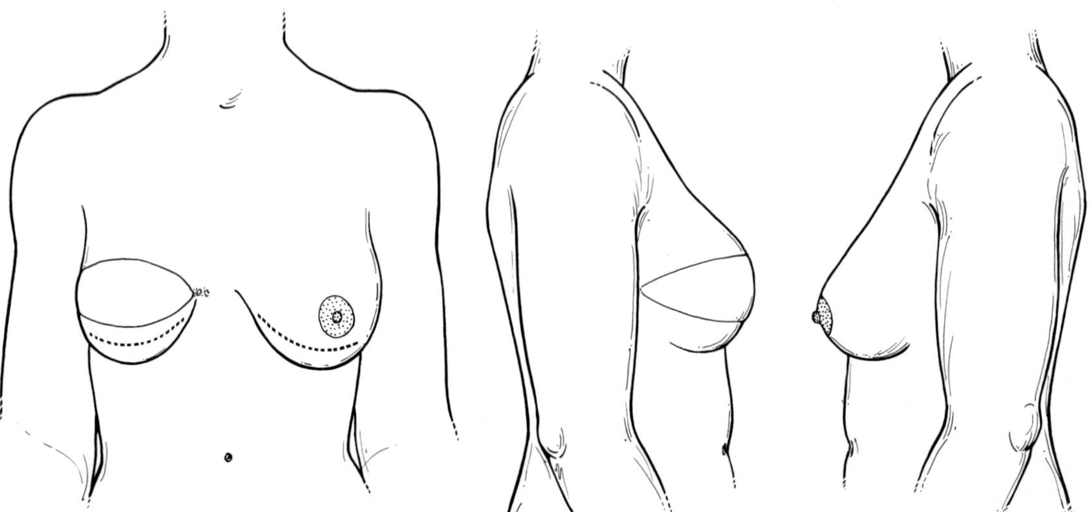

FIGURE 150-37. Position problem. Skin island of flap inset directly into mastectomy scar results in inadequate release of scar and patch-like appearance of flap skin.

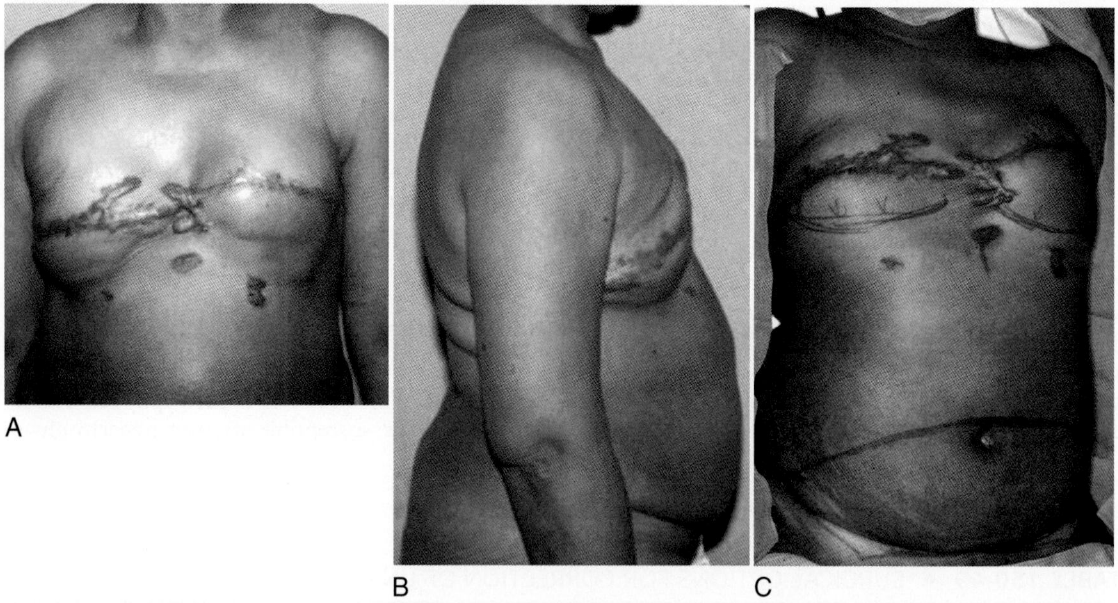

FIGURE 150-38. Scar. *A,* Anterior view of patient with bilateral delayed breast reconstruction with permanent implant. Transverse scar hypertrophy has distorted both skin envelopes and impairs mound contour. *B,* Lateral view. Note hypertrophic scar and inadequate breast mound definition. *C,* Intraoperative view: design of bilateral rectus abdominis musculocutaneous flaps for autogenous breast reconstruction.

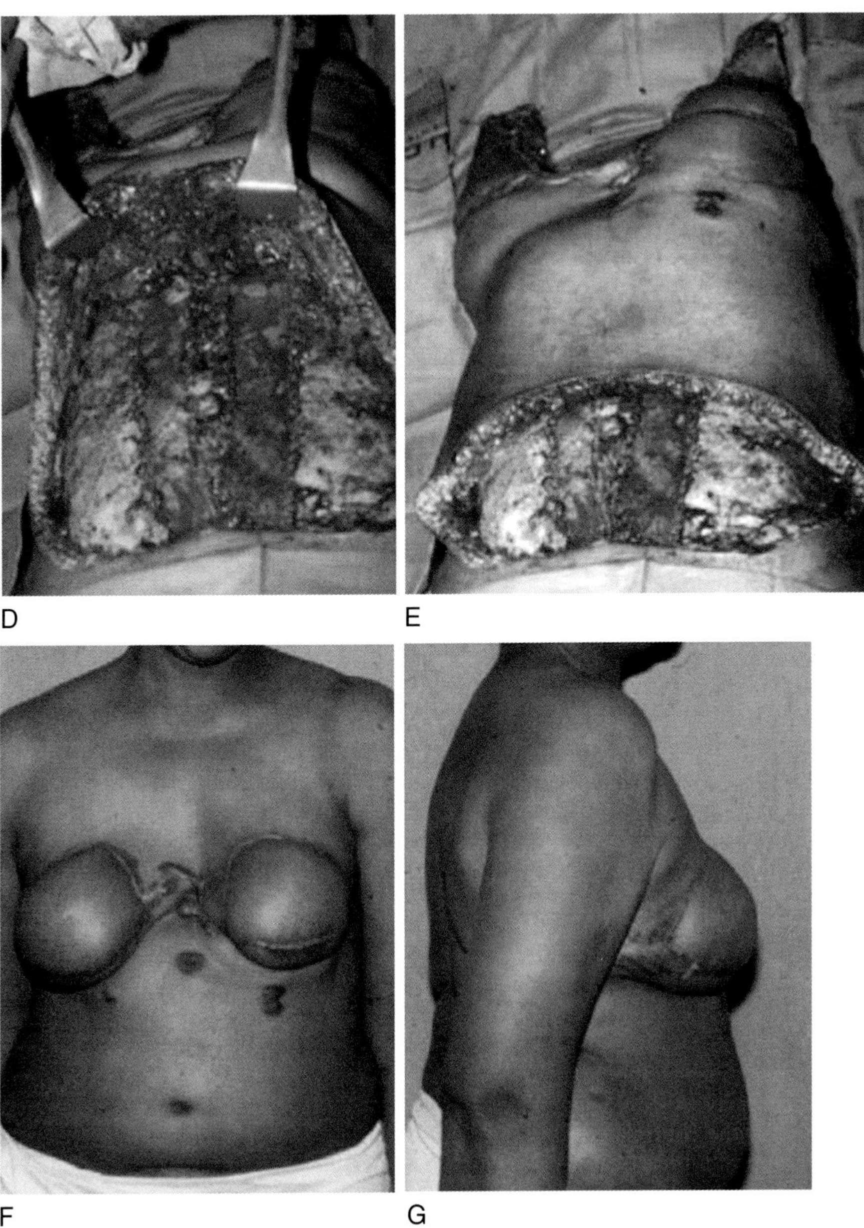

FIGURE 150-38, cont'd. *D,* Intraoperative view of donor site closed with interpositional Prolene mesh. *E,* Intraoperative view of TRAM flaps transposed onto respective chest wall defects. Skin islands of the bilateral TRAM flaps will reduce chest wall tightness and allow resection of hypertrophic scars. *F,* Postoperative anterior view at 1 year of bilateral secondary reconstruction with scar resection, explantation, and bilateral autogenous reconstruction with bilateral TRAM flaps. *G,* Lateral view. Note that the skin envelope with the addition of the skin islands of the TRAM flaps provides stable coverage over the autogenous mound and has reduced the tendency for hypertrophic scar formation.

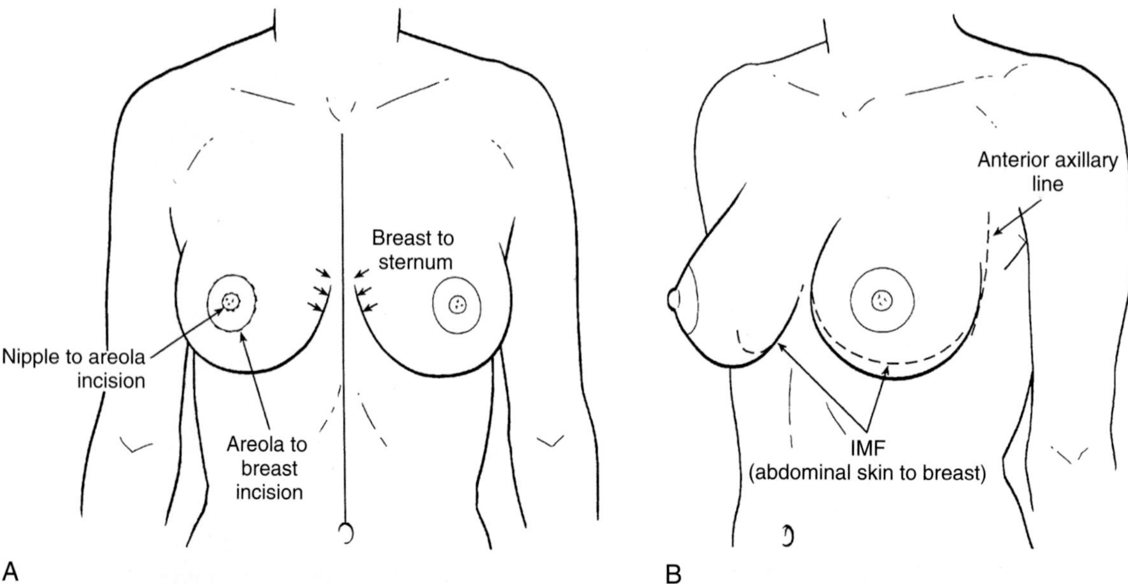

FIGURE 150-39. *A* and *B*, The limited transition lines around the breast include the nipple, areola, inframammary fold (IMF), and anterior axillary line, which can camouflage breast reconstruction. (From Spear SL, Davison SP: Aesthetic subunits of the breast. Plast Reconstr Surg 2003;112:440.)

keloid, an implant or expander-implant sequence may result in skin tension and propensity for hypertrophic or keloid scar (see Fig. 150-38). In this circumstance, flap use to improve the dimensions of the skin envelope may reduce the scar problem. With any incision, scar hypertrophy is possible. Intralesional steroid therapy after a suitable period of postoperative observation to allow scar maturation may reduce the hypertrophic scar at the mastectomy scar or site of flap inset (see Chapter 12).

Symmetry

POSITION AND MOUND

The reconstructed breast ideally should match the opposite breast either in its existing shape or in a planned modification of the contralateral breast. In many instances, the opposite breast cannot realistically be matched by the reconstructive technique selected by the patient. In general, the patient will request modification of the opposite breast as a result of the mastectomy. The opposite breast may require augmentation, mastopexy, augmentation mastopexy, or reduction mammaplasty. When there is high risk for bilateral cancer (see Chapter 138), the patient may request contralateral prophylactic mastectomy. The contralateral breast surgery should be planned as part of the discussion of the reconstruction of the mastectomy site. Use of a flap will certainly assist in achieving symmetry when the opposite breast has mild to severe ptosis or hypertrophy and the patient does not want opposite breast surgery. Despite plans for modification of the opposite breast for symmetry or prophylactic mastectomy, the two sites are likely to undergo slight to major differences in technique, so variations in the bilateral breast position and mound shape must be expected. It is helpful to delay modification of the opposite breast until the mastectomy site reconstruction is completed, when a single-stage procedure (adjustable permanent implant or flap) is used, or at least until the first stage in the reconstructive process (expander-implant sequence) is completed. This delay allows the patient to request secondary procedures on the mastectomy reconstruction before the opposite breast undergoes a procedure to match the reconstructed breast. However, many patients will request bilateral surgery to reduce treatment time and expense. The patient must be informed that the outcome of the reconstruction and the opposite breast modification may vary according to variations in technique and the wound healing process (Table 150-50).

Despite these precautions, dissatisfaction in regard to lack of symmetry is one of the most common reasons for secondary breast reconstruction. The incidence of concern for symmetry in published series ranges from 2.8% to 39% (Table 150-51).[3,5,8,15,18,22,25,37,60,119] Losken et al[120] reviewed 1394 patients undergoing breast reconstruction with prosthetic or autologous techniques and described the use of contralateral procedures to achieve symmetry in 67% of delayed reconstruction patients and 22% of immediate reconstruction patients

TABLE 150-50 ✦ SURGICAL OPTIONS FOR CORRECTION OF ASYMMETRY

Problem	Surgical Options
Symmetry	No treatment Revision: pocket repositioning Revision: flap reinset Implant exchange: size adjustment Liposuction or resection of excess tissue Addition of implant Addition of flap Conversion to flap reconstruction Contralateral symmetry procedures: augmentation, reduction, mastopexy, or mastopexy-augmentation

(*P* = .001). Procedures on the contralateral breast were performed most commonly for implant reconstructions (89% of delayed breast reconstruction patients, 57% of immediate breast reconstructions) and least for TRAM flap reconstructions (59% of delayed breast reconstruction patients, 18% of immediate breast reconstructions). The most common procedure performed with implant reconstructions was augmentation mammaplasty (41%); TRAM flap reconstructions were most commonly combined with contralateral reduction mammaplasty (57%). Skin-sparing mastectomy was also associated with a decreased need for contralateral symmetry procedures in TRAM flap patients. Both immediate reconstruction and autogenous flap reconstruction have reduced the need for contralateral procedures for breast symmetry.

A study by Asplund and Svane[121] looked specifically at patients who underwent symmetry procedures on the opposite breast at a separate operation after postmastectomy prosthetic reconstruction. In this study, 64 of 100 patients underwent a surgical procedure on the contralateral breast (1 to 2 months after primary breast reconstruction). The indications for the opposite breast surgery included correction of size or shape asymmetry and cancer prophylaxis. Mean follow-up was 23 months, with a range of 6 to 48 months. The authors asked the patients to retrospectively evaluate the necessity of the symmetry procedure and found that 96% thought that the procedure was either necessary or very necessary. Postoperative symmetry between the breasts was also evaluated subjectively by the patients and categorized as equal, asymmetric but not disturbing, or asymmetric and disturbing to the patient. The authors found that 14 of 63 patients thought that postoperative size asymmetry was still disturbing, and 13 of 63 patients were disturbed by persistent shape asymmetry. One early complication was encountered in the form of a postoperative hematoma after reduction mammaplasty, and six late capsular contractures occurred after augmentation of the contralateral breast. Another procedure was requested by three patients to improve persistent asymmetry.

Clough[15] evaluated 360 immediate reconstructions with a variety of implants (49.7% saline, 35.6% Becker inflatable implants, 7.2% expander-implant sequence, 7.5% silicone gel) in regard to morbidity and aesthetic outcome with a mean follow-up of 4.2 years (range, 1 to 9 years). Irradiated patients were not included in this study. Early complication rate (within 2 months) is reported at 9.2%, with 1.7% requiring explantation. Late complications occurred in 23%; pathologic capsular contracture occurred in 11% at 2 years and 15% at 5 years. Incidence of implant rupture increased linearly with time (2.7% at 2 years, 8.5% at 5 years). Late implant removal was 7%. Revision surgery was required in 30.2% of patients, and contralateral symmetry procedures were carried out in 92.5% (70.5% immediate, 22% later). The authors evaluated the cosmetic outcome by an objective 5-point global scale, grading each patient at every clinic visit. Despite a high rate of revision surgery, overall aesthetic result was found to deteriorate linearly with time (86% acceptable at 2 years, 54% at 5 years). The authors used Cox model analysis and found that capsular contracture was the only significant contributing factor to poor cosmesis ($P < .0001$; relative risk, 6.3). Mastectomy type, implant volume or type, and age of the patient were not significant risk factors for poor cosmesis. The authors propose that the poor late aesthetic results of implant reconstruction in this series may be due to failure of both breasts to undergo symmetric ptosis with aging.

Nahabedian[21] reviewed 382 patients who underwent autologous reconstruction (n = 217 patients, 277 breasts) and implant (n = 117 patients, 154 breasts) with regard to the need for secondary reconstruction to improve symmetry. This study, with mean follow-up of 21 months, found that final volume symmetry and contour symmetry were more often achieved with autologous reconstructions compared with implant reconstructions (84% versus 75% volume symmetry, and 78% versus 60% contour symmetry). Despite these findings, secondary reconstructions were more often performed in autologous reconstructions (59% versus 39%). The types of ipsilateral secondary reconstructions carried out in this study included skin or fat excision (95%), implant exchange (3%), and implant augmentation (2%). Contralateral breast procedures included reduction mammaplasty (46%), mastopexy (43%), and augmentation (11%). The authors noted that ipsilateral procedures were far more common than contralateral procedures for symmetry (42% versus 10.5%).

Use of a flap to improve the skin envelope generally allows better opportunity to match the

TABLE 150-51 ✦ INCIDENCE OF ASYMMETRY AFTER BREAST RECONSTRUCTION

Author, Year	N	Technique	Asymmetry Incidence	Asymmetric Size	Asymmetric Shape	Asymmetric Position	Lack of Ptosis
Guthrie,[119] 1980	229 breasts	Implants	—	9.6% (5.7% too small, 3.9% too large)	Figures not stated	8.4% (5.2% too high, 3.2% too low)	—
Gabriel,[25] 1997	1454 breasts	Prosthetic augmentation or reconstruction	3.8% reoperation for cosmetic reasons (4.8% of patients)	—	—	—	—
Alderman,[18] 2002	79	Immediate or delayed E/I	—	—	—	"Implant shift" in 1.3%	—
Camilleri,[37] 1996	120	Becker (23% immediate)	5.8% "unfavorable cosmesis"	—	—	1.6% too high	2.5%
Gutowski,[22] 1997	504	Saline implants (6.2% reconstruction)	2.8% reoperation	—	—	—	—
Dickson,[60] 1987	75	Immediate or E/I delayed	—	—	—	1.3%	—
Clough,[15] 2001	334	Immediate E/I or implant	Cosmetic results deteriorate with time (86% acceptable at 2 years, 54% at 5 years). See text for more details.				
Worseg,[8] 1995	167 implants	Reconstruction or augmentation with inflatable implants		2.4% reoperation for change of implant size		1.2% "dislocation"	
Mentor SPS[3]	416	Saline implants, 3-year follow-up	28%	—	—	1%	—
McGhan R95[5]	237	Saline implants, 3- and 5-year follow-up	33% (3-year) 39% (5-year)	—	—	12% (3-year) 17% (5-year)	—

E/I, expander-implant.

contralateral breast. Clough[16] reviewed the results in 171 consecutive patients undergoing TRAM flap reconstruction (unipedicled: n = 75, 43.9%; bipedicled: n = 17, 9.9%; supercharged: n = 65, 38%; free: n = 14, 8.2%). Immediate reconstruction was carried out in 25 patients (14.6%). In this series, the incidence of early complications was 37.4%, late complications (fat necrosis) were seen in 13.5%, and contralateral procedures to establish symmetry were required in 33.9% of patients. In the evaluation of the aesthetic outcome, the authors described acceptable results in 96.4% of patients at 2 years and 94.2% at 5 years.

Tschopp et al[62] reviewed the results in 92 patients undergoing a latissimus dorsi musculocutaneous flap for breast reconstruction with follow-up of 7 to 10 years. Most of the patients were noted to have a natural-appearing ptosis, which will assist in achieving symmetry with the opposite breast. In an earlier report by McCraw and Maxwell,[122] lack of ptosis due to late capsular contracture was observed. In Tschopp's series, significant capsular contracture (grade III/IV) had occurred in 30% of patients by 7 to 10 years, although only 4% required capsulotomy (see Table 150-34). The authors acknowledged capsular contracture as the major problem after latissimus dorsi flap reconstruction with implant but stated that the results in the majority of patients are "very acceptable." It is common to observe late capsular contracture in reconstruction with latissimus dorsi musculocutaneous flap with underlying implant. The contracture around the implant elevates the implant in relation to the reconstructed skin envelope with resultant asymmetry to the opposite breast. Secondary procedures are often required to release the implant to return it to the area of the inferior quadrants of the reconstructed breast mound (Fig. 150-40).

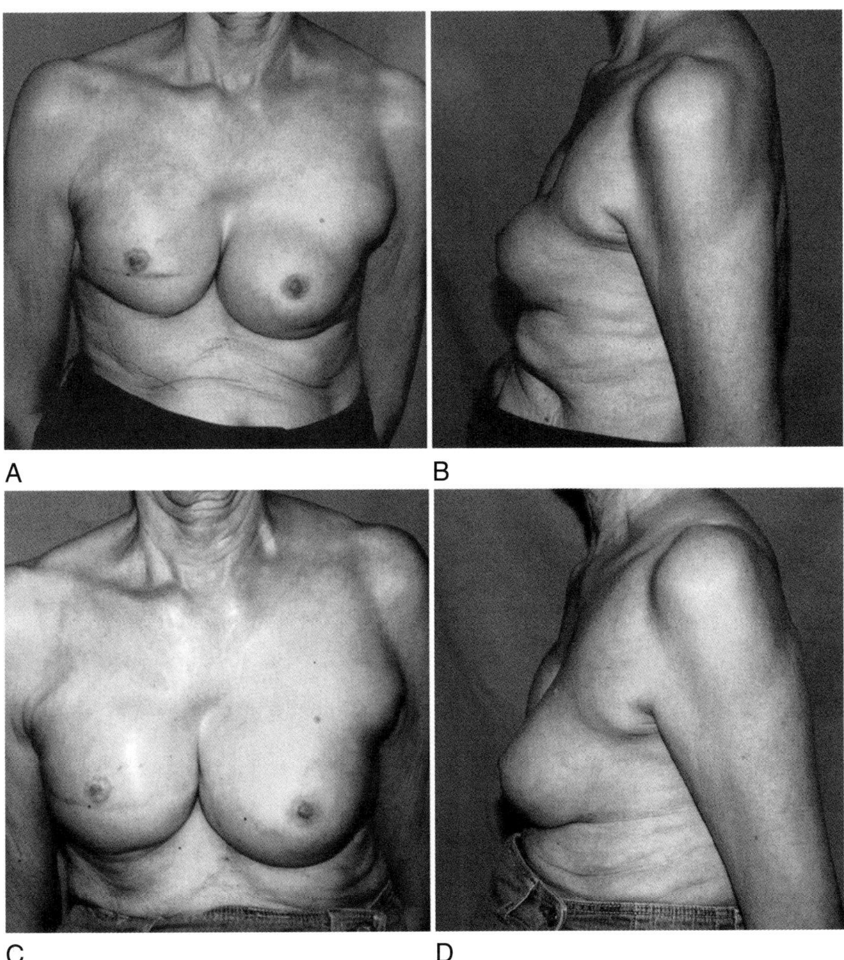

FIGURE 150-40. Asymmetry: position and mound problems. *A*, Anterior view of patient presenting with dissatisfaction related to asymmetry after bilateral implant reconstruction. Note that the right breast lacks contour and the left breast has inferior malposition. *B*, Lateral view. Note inferior position of implant. *C*, Anterior view of postoperative secondary bilateral reconstruction with bilateral implant exchange, capsulectomy, and implant repositioning. *D*, Lateral view. Note improved fullness in superior breast mound.

Nipple-Areola

With its Montgomery tubercles, multiple shades of color, slight elevation on the breast mound, high level of sensitivity, and erectile properties, the nipple-areola complex is not well reproduced by a local flap or graft and tattooing.

—Jabor et al[123]

Reconstruction of the nipple-areola complex is an important part of the complete reconstruction. Patients may not feel that the reconstruction is complete until the nipple-areola complex is present, providing a breast that looks as similar as possible to the contralateral side.

Nipple reconstruction is discussed as part of the informed consent during the planning of the mastectomy reconstruction. The nipple-areola reconstruction is generally delayed until the completion of the breast mound reconstruction and is then performed either at the time of contralateral breast surgery or electively when the patient desires, after the reconstructed mound is fully healed (see Chapter 139). With skin-sparing mastectomy and autogenous reconstruction, the skin island inset into the nipple-areola site may also undergo immediate nipple reconstruction. The nipple-areola complex reconstruction is subject to complications that may require secondary procedures for correction. Major complications are rare, although high-risk patients such as smokers and patients who have undergone radiation therapy are subject to nipple flap loss due to ischemic necrosis. Aesthetic problems are more common and include loss of projection, malposition, and problems with color, size, or texture.

The main problems leading to secondary reconstruction of the nipple-areola complex are loss of projection, malposition, size mismatch, color mismatch or fading, and nipple necrosis or loss. Of these, loss of projection and color problems are the most commonly reported and have received the most attention in the literature (Table 150-52).[124-134]

Jabor et al[123] reviewed 105 patients who underwent a variety of techniques for nipple-areola complex reconstruction (star flap, 36%; nipple sharing, 10%; keyhole flap, 9%; skate flap, 9%; S flap, 8%; full-thickness skin graft, 6%; or other techniques, 22%). The number of procedures required to complete the nipple-areola reconstruction was one in 66%, two in 32%, and three or more in 2%. Repeated tattooing represented 85% of additional procedures. Revision of the nipple accounted for 15% of secondary procedures. Nipple necrosis, occurring in 11%, was the major complication reported. Infection was the other main complication and was treated by systemic antibiotics. In analysis of satisfaction with the result, patients stated that the following aspects of the nipple-areola could be improved: lack of projection (>50%), color match (≈45%), shape (≈30%), size (≈15%), texture (≈12%), and position (≈2%). Approximately 15% of patients stated that they would not make any changes to their reconstructed nipple. Reported satisfaction with the nipple-areola reconstruction was excellent or good in 64%, fair in 22%, and poor in 14%. The authors noted that overall satisfaction with the breast mound reconstruction was higher than overall satisfaction with the nipple reconstruction ($P = .0001$). The interval between breast mound reconstruction and nipple reconstruction was found to have a significant impact on the degree of satisfaction with the nipple-areola reconstruction, with longer intervals leading to lower satisfaction (0.003).

PROJECTION

Multiple procedures have been described in the literature with one inevitable factor in common—loss of nipple projection. The large selection of surgical approaches available is testimony to the fact that long-term results have not yet approached complete surgeon satisfaction, and there is no universal favorite when it comes to nipple reconstruction.

—Losken et al[132]

Shestak et al[126] reviewed 74 nipple-areola reconstructions in 68 patients who underwent a bell, skate, or modified star flap technique with 1-year follow-up. Decisions in regard to selection of technique were based on required projection to match the contralateral nipple. Patients with minimal (<5 mm) nipple projection were treated with the bell flap or modified star flap, whereas the skate flap was used

TABLE 150-52 ✦ INCIDENCE OF NIPPLE COMPLICATIONS FOR VARIOUS RECONSTRUCTIVE TECHNIQUES

Author, Year	N	Technique	Nipple Necrosis or Loss	Loss of Projection	Malposition	Color	Size	Texture
Eskenazi,[124] 1993	100	Modified star	1%	8% of patients	—	—	—	—
Bogue,[125] 2003	31 nipples	Modified skate	3.2%	—	—	—	—	—
Shestak,[126] 2002	74 nipples	Modified star, skate, or bell flap	—	Average loss (all patients): Skate, 41% Star, 43% Bell, 74%	—	—	—	—
Few,[127] 1999	93 nipples	Modified star dermal fat flap	—	Average loss (all patients): 59%	—	—	—	—
Banducci,[128] 1999	32 nipples	Modified Anton-Hartrampf star flap	—	Average shrinkage: Autologous, 64.3% E/I, 76.7%	—	—	—	—
Tanabe,[129] 1997	14	Bilobed or trilobed dermal fat flaps + rolled auricular cartilage	0	Average loss (all patients): Bilobed, 6% Trilobed, 71%	—	—	—	—
Guerra,[130] 2003	454	Arrow flap and rib cartilage	"Exposure of cartilage" in 4%	—	—	—	—	—
Woods,[131] 1989	165 breasts	Subcutaneous mastectomy with nipple preservation	9% (4% when smokers excluded)	—	—	—	—	—
Losken,[132] 2001	14 nipples	C-V with intradermal tattoo	—	—	—	14% requested re-tattoo	—	—
Spear,[133] 1995	151	Intradermal tattoo	—	—	—	60% "lighter than opposite"; 10% required re-tattoo		—
Bhatty,[134] 1997	32 nipples	Nipple sharing + intradermal tattoo	0%	—	—	Re-tattoo in 12.5%	—	—

E/I, expander-implant.

when more projection was required. Evaluations of late projection revealed that the skate and modified star flap techniques were equally effective in maintaining projection (41% versus 43% loss, not significant), whereas the degree of both nipple and areola projection loss (74%) seen with the bell flap has led the authors to discourage its use. The majority of projection loss was seen in the first 3 months, and projection was stable after 6 months. The type of breast reconstruction had no effect on projection of the nipple.

POSITION

Although at one time I advocated a one-stage breast and nipple reconstruction, I soon found that it was difficult to get the site of the nipple correct and, when the breast mound needed to be modified, this could displace the nipple. I have found that the best time for nipple reconstruction is when the breast mound is at its best and the patient can help the reconstructive surgeon select the proper position for it.

—*Bostwick (discussion of Kroll[135])*

It is difficult to predict the correct location of the nipple at the time of breast mound reconstruction with the exception of the skin-sparing mastectomy with immediate replacement of the nipple complex defect with the skin island of a flap (latissimus dorsi, TRAM, or perforator free flap). Even with the predetermined position of the nipple-areola complex in immediate reconstruction, there are often changes in the shape of the breast mound during the initial postoperative period. Because the local flap for nipple reconstruction can be performed under local anesthesia as an outpatient procedure, the patient is generally better served to delay her nipple reconstruction. It is important also to let the patient have input into the location of the nipple-areola complex. A picture of the selected site can be reviewed by the patient and family to ascertain agreement for the selected site before proceeding with the actual reconstruction.

SIZE

The size of the nipple can best be determined by observation of the opposite nipple. When bilateral reconstruction is required, the patient should have input into the size of the nipple. Similarly, the circumference of the areola should be based on the opposite side and can be accurately made by outlining the areola on the opposite breast and transferring the outline to the reconstructed breast mound. If the skin island inset into the nipple-areola defect has stretched, it is preferable to resect excess skin island at the time of the nipple flap and then to proceed with the tattoo process after the nipple-areola incisions have healed.

COLOR

Nipple-areola tattooing done with iron oxide and titanium dioxide pigments thus appears to be a reasonably safe and effective procedure in most patients but may require one or more subsequent touch-ups for appropriate color match.

— *Spear and Arias[133]*

In our patients, the quality of nipple-areola reconstruction, in particular its pigmentation, is seen as inferior to that of the rest of the breast reconstruction in the eyes of patients, their partners and independent observers. The poor color match and fading of reconstructed nipple-areola skin are phenomena that can be measured using color analysis.

—*Dean et al[136]*

The color of the reconstructed nipple is an important determinant of the final aesthetic result, both in unilateral reconstructions (when a match with the normal contralateral breast is desirable) and in bilateral reconstructions (when the color must be appropriate to the patient's skin tone and the same in both breasts).

Spear and Arias[133] reviewed 151 patients undergoing intradermal tattooing with use of iron oxide and titanium dioxide. The results of their survey for color match, complications, and satisfaction include the following:

- color match: 10% required repeated tattooing for excessive fading, 60% were eventually lighter than the opposite side;
- complications: infection was observed in 3 of 151 (5%), rash in 1 of 151 (0.6%), and skin slough in 1 of 151 (0.6%);
- satisfaction: 84% of patients reported satisfaction with the result, 86% of patients studied would repeat the same procedure, and 57% said that the tattoo was "similar to the other areola."

Traditional techniques for achieving a pigmented areola involve free tissue grafting from the inner thigh or labia. These techniques have largely been replaced by the technique of intradermal tattooing. Although tattoo pigments do not provide the texture and projection observed with full-thickness skin grafts, the technique is quick and effective and does not require the use of an additional donor site. Problems with the color of the reconstructed nipple may be related to an initial failure to achieve a color match, failure of the pigment to "take," fading of the pigment after intradermal tattooing, and problems with the size or shape of the tattooed region.[133]

Dean et al[136] reviewed 57 patients undergoing nipple-areola tattooing in which fading of the nipple-areola tattoos and other aspects of the color match between nipple-areola complexes were measured objectively (with a custom software package) and subjectively in a series of 57 patients, 32 partners, and 4 independent observers. The color of reconstructed nipple-areola complexes was significantly different from that of the opposite side, and this difference was related to the time elapsed since reconstruction. This observation corresponds to the fading phenomenon previously described.

NECROSIS OR LOSS

The problem of nipple necrosis or loss is not a frequent one. It is more common after subcutaneous mastectomy or when thin preserved skin envelope is selected for a nipple flap. Because the mastectomy scar is often located in proximity to the appropriate site for nipple flap design, the base of the flap may have to be altered to avoid ischemic necrosis of the flap. Eskenazi[124] reviewed 100 nipple-areola reconstructions by the modified star flap. Only 8% of patients required a revision of the reconstruction, with one requiring correction of partial flap loss and the remaining seven undergoing boost procedures to correct loss of projection. Bogue[125] reviewed the results of 31 nipple-areola reconstructions by a variation of the skate flap technique and noted excellent results with partial skate flap loss in only one patient. This partial flap loss healed secondarily without need for revision. The authors also stated that projection is maintained at 2-year and 3-year follow-up.

ADJUVANT TREATMENT: EFFECT ON OUTCOMES

Radiation Therapy

Radiation therapy is associated with an increased risk for complications, particularly for prosthetic reconstructions. Radiotherapy before reconstruction and radiotherapy to the reconstructed breast have both been shown to increase the risk for complications in prosthetic reconstructions, most notably capsular contracture (see "Capsular Contracture" in the section "Mound"). Irradiation of a transferred TRAM flap may lead to more complications due to increased rate of fat necrosis. Transfer of a TRAM flap to a previously irradiated chest site may also be associated with increased risk for complications; however, there is some disagreement between series.[44,52,137]

The detrimental effects of radiation therapy have traditionally been attributed to microvascular damage.[138,139] However, it has been shown that tissue hypoxia is transient and microvessels are patent at 11 weeks after irradiation, when radiation changes are typically manifested.[140] Radiation-induced chromosomal damage has been shown to inhibit DNA replication and produces abnormalities of collagen synthesis and fibroblast activity, which may lead to some of the changes seen in breasts after radiation therapy.[141,142]

Spear and Onyewu[143] retrospectively reviewed 40 consecutive patients undergoing two-stage saline implant breast reconstruction with postoperative radiotherapy and 40 randomly selected patients undergoing two-stage saline implant reconstruction without radiotherapy. Of the 40 patients who were irradiated after implant insertion, 19 (47%) who received postoperative radiation therapy ultimately needed a second reconstructive procedure with a flap as the result of inadequate contour (poor aesthetic result), capsular contracture, and threatened extrusion. The authors suggest that when secondary reconstruction is required for post–radiation therapy contracture, the latissimus dorsi musculocutaneous flap is an excellent technique, but they caution against its use before radiation therapy.

Chawla et al[137] reviewed 48 patients who underwent either expander-implant sequence (18) or TRAM flap (30) and received radiotherapy before or after reconstruction. A significantly higher total complication rate was observed in the expander-implant group (53% versus 12% in the TRAM flap group; $P = .01$), with a significantly higher reoperation rate in the expander-implant group (48% at 2 years) compared with the TRAM flap group (8%). The timing of radiotherapy was not found to be an important factor in the observed complications. Similarly, the study by Krueger,[78] as part of the Michigan Breast Reconstruction Outcome Study, reviewed 105 expander-implant reconstructions in 81 patients. Complications occurred in 68% (13 of 19) of the radiotherapy group compared with 31% (19 of 62) of the no radiotherapy group ($P = .006$). Reconstruction failure was significantly associated with the use of radiotherapy (37% versus 8%; $P = .005$).

Williams et al[52] reviewed 699 patients who underwent reconstruction with the rectus abdominis musculocutaneous transposition flap (TRAM flap); 108 patients received preoperative adjuvant radiotherapy and 19 received postoperative radiotherapy for locally advanced disease or tumor recurrence. No radiation therapy was required in 572 patients. Mean follow-up in this study was 47.6 months. More than 32% of the irradiated flaps developed a degree of fibrosis. Overall complication rates were marginally significant between the preoperative radiotherapy and nonirradiated groups ($P = .072$) and between the irradiated TRAM flap group and the patients with preoperative radiotherapy followed by TRAM flap reconstruction (31% versus 25%; $P = .749$). Of the individual complications, fat necrosis was found to be statistically significant ($P = .032$). Of the 19 patients with postoperative radiotherapy, 10 patients had 12 flap complications, and 6 of 19 (31.6%) required reoperation for fat necrosis (>10% of the flap).

In a study by Tran et al,[45] 32 immediate breast reconstructions with free TRAM flaps with postoperative radiation therapy were compared with 70 delayed breast reconstructions with prior radiotherapy, with minimum follow-up of 1 year after delayed breast reconstruction or 1 year after completion of radiotherapy for immediate breast reconstruction. In this series, mean follow-up was 3 years for immediate reconstruction and 5 years for delayed breast reconstruction. Incidence of early surgical complications did not differ between the groups. Incidence of late surgical complications was significantly higher in the immediate breast reconstruction group (87.5% versus 8.6%; P = .000), and nine immediate breast reconstruction patients (28%) required an additional flap (secondary breast reconstruction) to correct contour problems. The authors suggest that candidates for free TRAM flap reconstruction should wait until adjuvant radiotherapy is completed to avoid the increased risk of complications (Fig. 150-41).

Once the expander-implant reconstruction is planned, it is preferable to proceed with expander insertion. For advanced tumors or preoperative staging greater than stage I, the patient generally requires a larger skin envelope resection and is not a suitable candidate for the expander-implant sequence. If the patient does require radiation therapy postoperatively, the expander will allow maintenance of the skin envelope during the radiation process. After radiation therapy is completed, the patient may proceed with implant insertion after recovery from adjuvant therapy or will be a candidate for autogenous reconstruction with a flap. The expander will serve in this instance as a device to preserve the skin envelope for later use to assist in the flap reconstruction. The other option is to complete rapid expansion and to insert the permanent implant before onset of radiotherapy.

Cordeiro et al[144] reported a retrospective series of 142 patients, 68 of whom underwent tissue expansion during postoperative chemotherapy, implant exchange 4 weeks after chemotherapy, and chest wall irradiation 4 weeks after exchange. Mean follow-up was 34 months. The authors recorded aesthetic outcomes, capsular contracture incidence, and satisfaction of patients. They found that capsular contracture was more common in the radiation therapy group (68% versus 40%; P = .025), whereas the aesthetic outcome was not significantly different between the groups (80% and 88% rating their outcome as good to excellent, respectively). The authors concluded that "tissue expander-implant reconstruction is an acceptable surgical option even when followed by postoperative radiotherapy and should be considered in the reconstruction algorithm for all patients, particularly those who may not be candidates for autogenous reconstruction."[144]

When a flap is planned for immediate reconstruction, if the sentinel node is positive or the tumor larger or more invasive that anticipated, delay of flap use may be preferable because the radiation therapy will adversely affect the quality of the flap reconstruction. Again, in this instance, expander insertion may be used to allow expansion during the subsequent radiotherapy, to be replaced by an autogenous flap electively after adjuvant therapy is completed.

Adjuvant Chemotherapy

Adjuvant chemotherapy is an important aspect of the management of the breast cancer patient. However, it should not impair the reconstructive process if it is properly managed. Furey et al[29] reviewed 112 patients with 120 reconstructions with immediate tissue expander-implant sequence or silicone gel implant; 36 patients received chemotherapy. Tissue expansion was delayed until completion of chemotherapy. Total wound complications were reported at 20.8% (27.8% versus 17.9% for chemotherapy and no chemotherapy groups, respectively; P = .13). Between the groups, there were statistically significant differences in age (chemotherapy group was an average of 8 years younger, P < .001), mastectomy type (chemotherapy group had more modified radical mastectomies, P < .01), and stage of disease (chemotherapy group had more advanced disease, P < .001). No distinction was made between the severity of complications or which ones required reoperation. The authors concluded that the administration of adjuvant chemotherapy does not significantly alter the incidence of wound complications in patients undergoing immediate breast reconstruction. The slightly increased rate of complications observed may be explained by the more extensive surgical resection, as the chemotherapy group had significantly more axillary nodes harvested. Similarly, Caffo et al[145] retrospectively reviewed 166 patients who underwent immediate breast reconstruction with chemotherapy (n = 52) or without chemotherapy (n = 51) or mastectomy with chemotherapy and without reconstruction (n = 63). All reconstructed patients received an expander-implant, and the timing of inflation was not influenced by chemotherapy. No statistical difference in distribution of complications was noted between the immediate breast reconstruction with chemotherapy group and the immediate breast reconstruction without chemotherapy group. Alderman[18] did note problems with chemotherapy and breast reconstruction. In a review of 326 patients who underwent reconstruction (implants, n = 79; pedicled TRAM flap, n = 179; and free TRAM flap, n = 67) with follow-up of 2 years, chemotherapy was

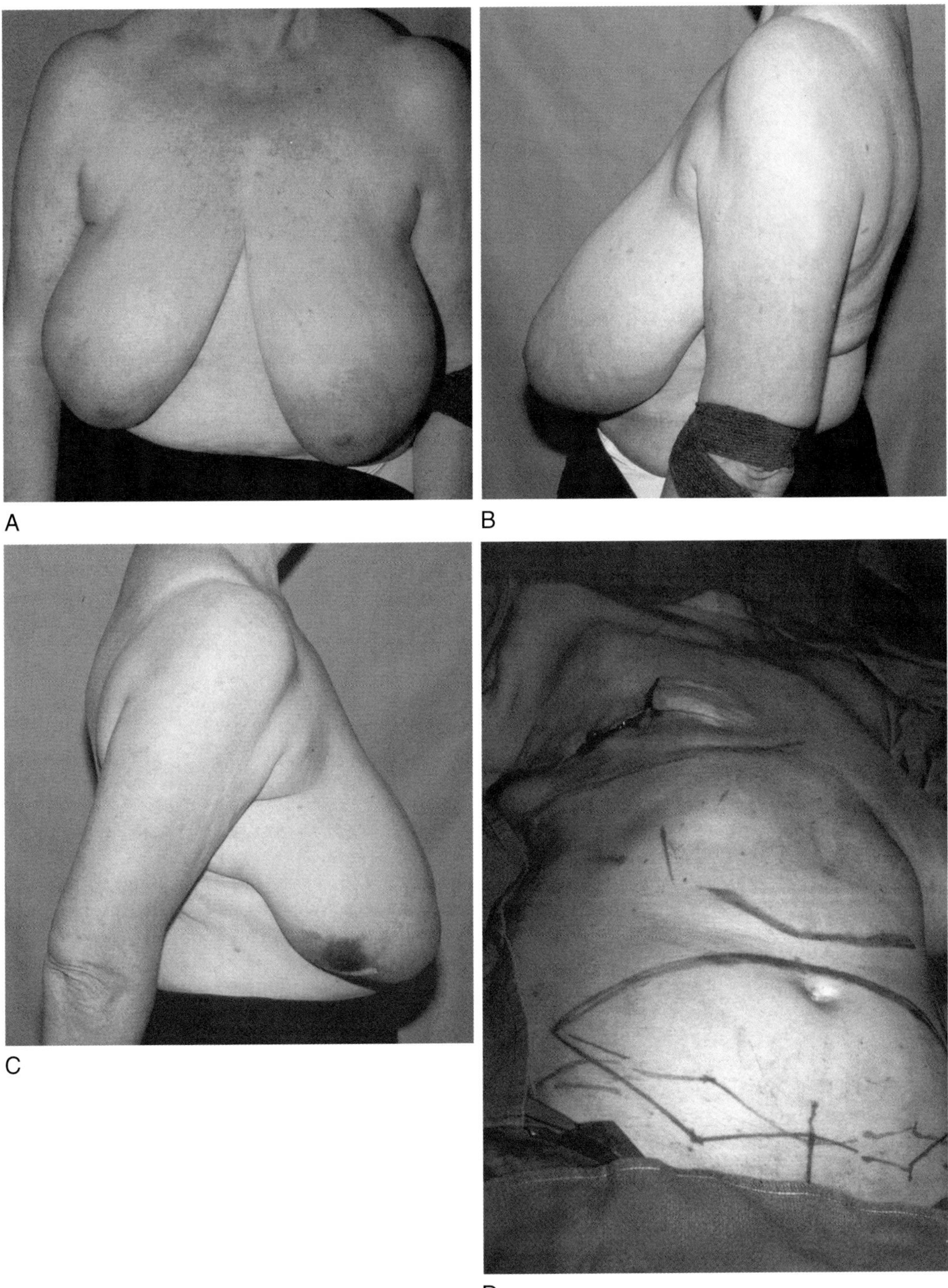

FIGURE 150-41. Delayed flap reconstruction after radiation therapy. *A,* Anterior view of patient after right modified radical mastectomy. *B,* Lateral view. *C,* Lateral view. Note biopsy site for invasive breast cancer. *D,* Intraoperative view. The patient has completed radiation therapy for the right breast. Note design of rectus abdominis musculocutaneous flap (TRAM flap) for right breast reconstruction. *Continued*

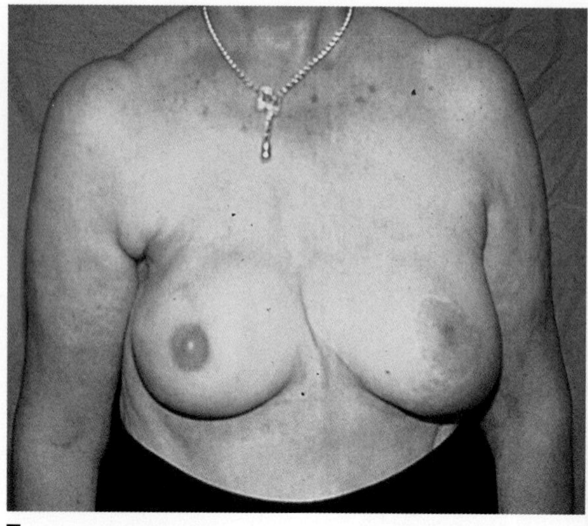

E

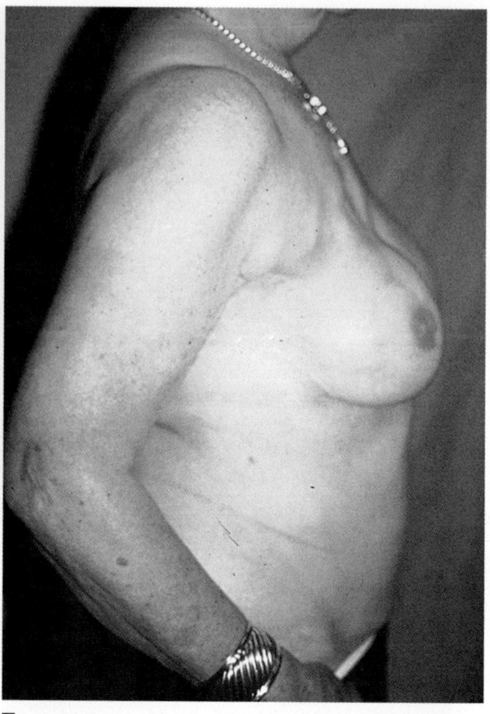

F

FIGURE 150-41, cont'd. *E,* Postoperative anterior view at 1 year of right autogenous breast reconstruction and left reduction mammaplasty for symmetry. *F,* Lateral view. No complications are observed at the site of autogenous reconstruction.

associated with a significantly increased risk for major complications in patients undergoing TRAM flap reconstruction (*P* = .03). Major complications were defined as those requiring reoperation, rehospitalization, or non-perioperative intravenous antibiotic treatment.

As soon as healing is complete after primary breast reconstruction, chemotherapy should be completed. If an expander has been inserted, inflation may be timed between chemotherapy schedules or delayed pending the patient's, plastic surgeon's, and oncologist's preferences. If wound healing problems are delaying the onset of adjuvant therapy, surgical management of the wound problem may be required. In autogenous flap breast reconstruction, minor areas of skin loss may be treated concurrently with chemotherapy.

SUMMARY

With the transition from radical mastectomy to skin-sparing techniques, the opportunities to restore a natural breast have significantly improved. Rather than concentrating on providing stable chest wall skin overlying a breast mound, the plastic surgeon may now use the various techniques for breast reconstruction to provide a breast with appropriate size, projection, and inferior fullness and proper positioning with minimal scarring. Each patient presents with different reconstructive requirements based on extent of skin envelope resection and required adjuvant treatment that may affect the chest wall, configuration of the opposite breast, and preferences for technique selection. Problems may be related to technique failure, inherent procedural complications, and dissatisfaction due to failure to meet the preoperative expectations. Analysis of the unsatisfactory result should include careful analysis of the components of the reconstruction, including envelope, mound, position, scar, and symmetry. Surgical procedures have been described for each of these components of secondary breast reconstruction. When the secondary procedures are carefully selected with informed consent, with the patient understanding the limitations of each technique and emphasis on continued risk of procedural complications, the patient can expect a predictable and satisfying outcome. With familiarity with the incidence of risk factors leading to secondary reconstruction, the plastic surgeon will be able to provide better consultation for primary reconstruction and avoid many of the problems that require subsequent correction.

REFERENCES

1. Kroll SS, Freeman P: Striving for excellence in breast reconstruction: the salvage of poor results. Ann Plast Surg 1989;22:58-64.
2. Malyon AD, Husein M, Weiler-Mithoff EM: How many procedures to make a breast? Br J Plast Surg 2001;54:227-231.
3. Saline-Filled Breast Implant Surgery: Making an Informed Decision. Santa Barbara, Calif, Mentor Corporation, January 2004. Saline Prospective Study.
4. Saline-Filled Breast Implant Surgery: Making an Informed Decision. Santa Barbara, Calif, Mentor Corporation, January 2004. Post Approval Survey Study.
5. Making an Informed Decision [patient brochure]. Santa Barbara, Calif, INAMED Aesthetics, January 2005. R95 Study.
6. Making an Informed Decision [patient brochure]. Santa Barbara, Calif, INAMED Aesthetics, January 2005. Post Approval Survey Study.
7. Gui GP, Tan SM, Faliakou EC, et al: Immediate breast reconstruction using biodimensional anatomical permanent expander implants: a prospective analysis of outcome and patient satisfaction. Plast Reconstr Surg 2003;111:125-138, discussion 139-140.
8. Worseg A, Kuzbari R, Tairych G, et al: Long term results of inflatable mammary implants. Br J Plast Surg 1995;48:183-188.
9. Bailey MH, Smith JW, Casas L, et al: Immediate breast reconstruction: reducing the risks. Plast Reconstr Surg 1989;83:845-851.
10. Hartrampf CR Jr, Bennett GK: Autogenous tissue reconstruction in the mastectomy patient. A critical review of 300 patients. Ann Surg 1987;205:508-519.
11. Trabulsy PP, Anthony JP, Mathes SJ: Changing trends in postmastectomy breast reconstruction: a 13-year experience. Plast Reconstr Surg 1994;93:1418-1427.
12. Kroll SS, Baldwin B: A comparison of outcomes using three different methods of breast reconstruction. Plast Reconstr Surg 1992;90:455-462.
13. Yeh KA, Lyle G, Wei JP, Sherry R: Immediate breast reconstruction in breast cancer: morbidity and outcome. Am Surg 1998;64:1195-1199.
14. Rosen PB, Jabs AD, Kister SJ, Hugo NE: Clinical experience with immediate breast reconstruction using tissue expansion or transverse rectus abdominis musculocutaneous flaps. Ann Plast Surg 1990;25:249-257.
15. Clough KB, O'Donoghue JM, Fitoussi AD, et al: Prospective evaluation of late cosmetic results following breast reconstruction: I. Implant reconstruction. Plast Reconstr Surg 2001;107:1702-1709.
16. Clough KB, O'Donoghue JM, Fitoussi AD, et al: Prospective evaluation of late cosmetic results following breast reconstruction: II. Tram flap reconstruction. Plast Reconstr Surg 2001;107:1710-1716.
17. McCraw JB, Horton CE, Grossman JA, et al: An early appraisal of the methods of tissue expansion and the transverse rectus abdominis musculocutaneous flap in reconstruction of the breast following mastectomy. Ann Plast Surg 1987;18:93-113.
18. Alderman AK, Wilkins EG, Kim HM, Lowery JC: Complications in postmastectomy breast reconstruction: two-year results of the Michigan Breast Reconstruction Outcome Study. Plast Reconstr Surg 2002;109:2265-2274.
19. Lin KY, Johns FR, Gibson J, et al: An outcome study of breast reconstruction: presurgical identification of risk factors for complications. Ann Surg Oncol 2001;8:586-591.
20. Losken A, Carlson GW, Schoemann MB, et al: Factors that influence the completion of breast reconstruction. Ann Plast Surg 2004;52:258-261, discussion 262.
21. Nahabedian MY: Symmetrical breast reconstruction: analysis of secondary procedures after reconstruction with implants and autologous tissue. Plast Reconstr Surg 2005;115:257-260.
22. Gutowski KA, Mesna GT, Cunningham BL: Saline-filled breast implants: a Plastic Surgery Educational Foundation multicenter outcomes study. Plast Reconstr Surg 1997;100:1019-1027.
23. Ramon Y, Ullmann Y, Moscona R, et al: Aesthetic results and patient satisfaction with immediate breast reconstruction using tissue expansion: a follow-up study. Plast Reconstr Surg 1997;99:686-691.
24. Crespo LD, Eberlein TJ, O'Connor N, et al: Postmastectomy complications in breast reconstruction. Ann Plast Surg 1994;32:452-456.
25. Gabriel SE, Woods JE, O'Fallon WM, et al: Complications leading to surgery after breast implantation. N Engl J Med 1997;336:677-682.
26. Pusic AL, Cordeiro PG: An accelerated approach to tissue expansion for breast reconstruction: experience with intraoperative and rapid postoperative expansion in 370 reconstructions. Plast Reconstr Surg 2003;111:1871-1875.
27. Disa JJ, Ad-El DD, Cohen SM, et al: The premature removal of tissue expanders in breast reconstruction. Plast Reconstr Surg 1999;104:1662-1665.
28. O'Brien W, Hasselgren PO, Hummel RP, et al: Comparison of postoperative wound complications and early cancer recurrence between patients undergoing mastectomy with or without immediate breast reconstruction. Am J Surg 1993; 166:1-5.
29. Furey PC, Macgillivray DC, Castiglione CL, Allen L: Wound complications in patients receiving adjuvant chemotherapy after mastectomy and immediate breast reconstruction for breast cancer. J Surg Oncol 1994;55:194-197.
30. Slavin SA, Schnitt SJ, Duda RB, et al: Skin-sparing mastectomy and immediate reconstruction: oncologic risks and aesthetic results in patients with early-stage breast cancer. Plast Reconstr Surg 1998;102:49-62.
31. Schuster DI, Lavine DM: Nine-year experience with subpectoral breast reconstruction after subcutaneous mastectomy in 98 patients utilizing saline-inflatable prostheses. Ann Plast Surg 1988;21:444-451.
32. Spear SL, Majidian A: Immediate breast reconstruction in two stages using textured, integrated-valve tissue expanders and breast implants: a retrospective review of 171 consecutive breast reconstructions from 1989 to 1996. Plast Reconstr Surg 1998;101:53-63.
33. Noone RB, Murphy JB, Spear SL, Little JW 3rd: A 6-year experience with immediate reconstruction after mastectomy for cancer. Plast Reconstr Surg 1985;76:258-269.
34. Contant CM, van Geel AN, van der Holt B, et al: Morbidity of immediate breast reconstruction (IBR) after mastectomy by a subpectorally placed silicone prosthesis: the adverse effect of radiotherapy. Eur J Surg Oncol 2000;26:344-350.
35. Miller AP, Falcone RE: Breast reconstruction: systemic factors influencing local complications. Ann Plast Surg 1991;27:115-120.
36. Cooper GG, Webster MH, Bell G: The results of breast reconstruction following mastectomy. Br J Plast Surg 1984;37:369-372.
37. Camilleri IG, Malata CM, Stavrianos S, McLean NR: A review of 120 Becker permanent tissue expanders in reconstruction of the breast. Br J Plast Surg 1996;49:346-351.
38. Pennisi VR: Long-term use of polyurethane breast prostheses: a 14-year experience. Plast Reconstr Surg 1990;86:368-371.
39. Berry MG, al-Mufti RA, Jenkinson AD, et al: An audit of outcome including patient satisfaction with immediate breast reconstruction performed by breast surgeons. Ann R Coll Surg Engl 1998;80:173-177.
40. Menke H, Erkens M, Olbrisch RR: Evolving concepts in breast reconstruction with latissimus dorsi flaps: results and follow-up of 121 consecutive patients. Ann Plast Surg 2001;47:107-114.

41. Roy MK, Shrotria S, Holcombe C, et al: Complications of latissimus dorsi myocutaneous flap breast reconstruction. Eur J Surg Oncol 1998;24:162-165.
42. de la Torre JI, Fix RJ, Gardner PM, Vasconez LO: Reconstruction with the latissimus dorsi flap after skin-sparing mastectomy. Ann Plast Surg 2001;46:229-233.
43. Chang DW, Youssef A, Cha S, Reece GP: Autologous breast reconstruction with the extended latissimus dorsi flap. Plast Reconstr Surg 2002;110:751-759, discussion 760-761.
44. Chang DW, Reece GP, Wang B, et al: Effect of smoking on complications in patients undergoing free TRAM flap breast reconstruction. Plast Reconstr Surg 2000;105:2374-2380.
45. Tran NV, Chang DW, Gupta A, et al: Comparison of immediate and delayed free TRAM flap breast reconstruction in patients receiving postmastectomy radiation therapy. Plast Reconstr Surg 2001;108:78-82.
46. Paige KT, Bostwick J 3rd, Bried JT, Jones G: A comparison of morbidity from bilateral, unipedicled and unilateral, unipedicled TRAM flap breast reconstructions. Plast Reconstr Surg 1998;101:1819-1827.
47. Tse R, Ross D, Gan BS: Late salvage of a free TRAM flap. Br J Plast Surg 2003;56:59-62.
48. Kroll SS: Fat necrosis in free transverse rectus abdominis myocutaneous and deep inferior epigastric perforator flaps. Plast Reconstr Surg 2000;106:576-583.
49. Kroll SS: The early management of flap necrosis in breast reconstruction. Plast Reconstr Surg 1991;87:893-901.
50. Kroll SS, Schusterman MA, Reece GP, et al: Breast reconstruction with myocutaneous flaps in previously irradiated patients. Plast Reconstr Surg 1994;93:460-469, discussion 470-471.
51. Moran SL, Serletti JM: Outcome comparison between free and pedicled TRAM flap breast reconstruction in the obese patient. Plast Reconstr Surg 2001;108:1954-1960, discussion 1961-1962.
52. Williams JK, Carlson GW, Bostwick J 3rd, et al: The effects of radiation treatment after TRAM flap breast reconstruction. Plast Reconstr Surg 1997;100:1153-1160.
53. Banic A, Boeckx W, Greulich M, et al: Late results of breast reconstruction with free TRAM flaps: a prospective multicentric study. Plast Reconstr Surg 1995;95:1195-1204, discussion 1205-1206.
54. Cunningham BL, Lokeh A, Gutowski KA: Saline-filled breast implant safety and efficacy: a multicenter retrospective review. Plast Reconstr Surg 2000;105:2143-2149, discussion 2150-2151.
55. Handel N, Jensen JA, Black Q, et al: The fate of breast implants: a critical analysis of complications and outcomes. Plast Reconstr Surg 1995;96:1521-1533.
56. Asplund O: Capsular contracture in silicone gel and saline-filled breast implants after reconstruction. Plast Reconstr Surg 1984;73:270-275.
57. Woods JE, Irons GB Jr, Arnold PG: The case for submuscular implantation of prostheses in reconstructive breast surgery. Ann Plast Surg 1980;5:115-122.
58. Wickman M, Jurell G: Low capsular contraction rate after primary and secondary breast reconstruction with a textured expander prosthesis. Plast Reconstr Surg 1997;99:692-697.
59. Thuesen B, Siim E, Christensen L, Schroder M: Capsular contracture after breast reconstruction with the tissue expansion technique. A comparison of smooth and textured silicone breast prostheses. Scand J Plast Reconstr Surg Hand Surg 1995;29:9-13.
60. Dickson MG, Sharpe DT: The complications of tissue expansion in breast reconstruction: a review of 75 cases. Br J Plast Surg 1987;40:629-635.
61. Spear SL, Baker JL Jr: Classification of capsular contracture after prosthetic breast reconstruction. Plast Reconstr Surg 1995;96:1119-1123, discussion 1124.
62. Tschopp H: Evaluation of long-term results in breast reconstruction using the latissimus dorsi flap. Ann Plast Surg 1991;26:328-340.
63. Ersek RA: Rate and incidence of capsular contracture: a comparison of smooth and textured silicone double-lumen breast prostheses. Plast Reconstr Surg 1991;87:879-884.
64. Gylbert L, Asplund O, Jurell G: Capsular contracture after breast reconstruction with silicone-gel and saline-filled implants: a 6-year follow-up. Plast Reconstr Surg 1990;85:373-377.
65. Massiha H: Scar tissue flaps for the correction of postimplant breast rippling. Ann Plast Surg 2002;48:505-507.
66. Dowden RV: Detection of gel implant rupture: a clinical test. Plast Reconstr Surg 1993;91:548-550.
67. Brown SL, Pennello G, Berg WA, et al: Silicone gel breast implant rupture, extracapsular silicone, and health status in a population of women. J Rheumatol 2001;28:996-1003.
68. Brown SL, Silverman BG, Berg WA: Rupture of silicone-gel breast implants: causes, sequelae, and diagnosis. Lancet 1997;350:1531-1537.
69. Young VL, Watson ME: Breast implant research: where we have been, where we are, where we need to go. Clin Plast Surg 2001;28:451-483.
70. Safety outcomes for the Core Study. Santa Barbara, Calif, INAMED Aesthetics, 2003.
71. Nahabedian MY, Galdino G: Symmetrical breast reconstruction: is there a role for three-dimensional digital photography? Plast Reconstr Surg 2003;112:1582-1590.
72. Freedman AM, Jackson IT: Infections in breast implants. Infect Dis Clin North Am 1989;3:275-287.
73. Courtiss EH, Goldwyn RM, Anastasi GW: The fate of breast implants with infections around them. Plast Reconstr Surg 1979;63:812-816.
74. Becker H, Hartman J: Do saline breast implants harbor microbes? Ann Plast Surg 1996;36:342-344.
75. Brown MH, Markus YM, Belchetz B, et al: Microbial growth in saline breast implants and saline tissue expanders. Plast Reconstr Surg 2002;109:2242-2244, discussion 2245-2246.
76. Chen NT, Butler PE, Hooper DC, May JW Jr: Bacterial growth in saline implants: in vitro and in vivo studies. Ann Plast Surg 1996;36:337-341.
77. Young VL, Hertl MC, Murray PR, et al: Microbial growth inside saline-filled breast implants. Plast Reconstr Surg 1997;100:182-196.
78. Krueger EA, Wilkins EG, Strawderman M, et al: Complications and patient satisfaction following expander/implant breast reconstruction with and without radiotherapy. Int J Radiat Oncol Biol Phys 2001;49:713-721.
79. Kraemer O, Andersen M, Siim E: Breast reconstruction and tissue expansion in irradiated versus not irradiated women after mastectomy. Scand J Plast Reconstr Surg Hand Surg 1996;30:201-206.
80. Yule GJ, Concannon MJ, Croll G, Puckett CL: Is there liability with chemotherapy following immediate breast construction? Plast Reconstr Surg 1996;97:969-973.
81. Contant CM, van Geel AN, van der Holt B, et al: Morbidity of immediate breast reconstruction (IBR) after mastectomy by a subpectorally placed silicone prosthesis: the adverse effect of radiotherapy. Eur J Surg Oncol 2000;26:344-350.
82. Armstrong RW, Berkowitz RL, Bolding F: Infection following breast reconstruction. Ann Plast Surg 1989;23:284-288.
83. Brand KG: Infection of mammary prostheses: a survey and the question of prevention. Ann Plast Surg 1993;30:289-295.
84. Yii NW, Khoo CT: Salvage of infected expander prostheses in breast reconstruction. Plast Reconstr Surg 2003;111:1087-1092.
85. Scevola S, Youssef A, Kroll SS, Langstein H: Drains and seromas in TRAM flap breast reconstruction. Ann Plast Surg 2002;48:511-514.
86. Erdmann D, Sundin BM, Moquin KJ, et al: Delay in unipedicled TRAM flap reconstruction of the breast: a review of 76 consecutive cases. Plast Reconstr Surg 2002;110:762-767.

87. Schusterman MA, Kroll SS, Weldon ME: Immediate breast reconstruction: why the free TRAM over the conventional TRAM flap? Plast Reconstr Surg 1992;90:255-261, discussion 262.
88. Serletti JM, Moran SL: Free versus the pedicled TRAM flap: a cost comparison and outcome analysis. Plast Reconstr Surg 1997;100:1418-1424, discussion 1425-1427.
89. Kroll SS, Gherardini G, Martin JE, et al: Fat necrosis in free and pedicled TRAM flaps. Plast Reconstr Surg 1998;102:1502-1507.
90. Keller A: Fat necrosis in free rectus abdominis and deep inferior epigastric perforator flaps. Plast Reconstr Surg 2001; 107:1611-1612.
91. Jewell RP, Whitney TM: TRAM fat necrosis in a young surgeon's practice: is it experience, technique, or blood flow? Ann Plast Surg 1999;42:424-427.
92. Nahabedian MY, Momen B, Galdino G, Manson PN: Breast reconstruction with the free TRAM or DIEP flap: patient selection, choice of flap, and outcome. Plast Reconstr Surg 2002;110:466-475, discussion 476-477.
93. Maxwell GP, Andochick SE: Secondary shaping of the TRAM flap. Clin Plast Surg 1994;21:247-253.
94. Wolf LE, Biggs TM: Aesthetic refinements in the use of the latissimus dorsi flap in breast reconstruction. Plast Reconstr Surg 1982;69:788-793.
95. Millard DR Jr: Breast aesthetics when reconstructing with the latissimus dorsi musculocutaneous flap. Plast Reconstr Surg 1982;70:161-172.
96. Gerber B, Krause A, Reimer T, et al: Breast reconstruction with latissimus dorsi flap: improved aesthetic results after transection of its humeral insertion. Plast Reconstr Surg 1999;103: 1876-1881.
97. Deutsch M, Flickinger JC: Patient characteristics and treatment factors affecting cosmesis following lumpectomy and breast irradiation. Am J Clin Oncol 2003;26:350-353.
98. Bajaj AK, Kon PS, Oberg KC, Miles DA: Aesthetic outcomes in patients undergoing breast conservation therapy for the treatment of localized breast cancer. Plast Reconstr Surg 2004;114:1442-1449.
99. Nahabedian MY, Dooley W, Singh N, Manson PN: Contour abnormalities of the abdomen after breast reconstruction with abdominal flaps: the role of muscle preservation. Plast Reconstr Surg 2002;109:91-101.
100. Deapen DM, Pike MC, Casagrande JT, Brody GS: The relationship between breast cancer and augmentation mammaplasty: an epidemiologic study. Plast Reconstr Surg 1986;77:361-368.
101. Bryant H, Brasher P: Breast implants and breast cancer—reanalysis of a linkage study. N Engl J Med 1995;332:1535-1539.
102. Deapen DM, Brody GS: Augmentation mammaplasty and breast cancer: a 5-year update of the Los Angeles study. Plast Reconstr Surg 1992;89:660-665.
103. Gabriel SE, O'Fallon WM, Kurland LT, et al: Risk of connective-tissue diseases and other disorders after breast implantation. N Engl J Med 1994;330:1697-1702.
104. Englert HJ, Brooks P: Scleroderma and augmentation mammaplasty—a causal relationship? Aust N Z J Med 1994;24:74-80.
105. Sanchez-Guerrero J, Colditz GA, Karlson EW, et al: Silicone breast implants and the risk of connective-tissue diseases and symptoms. N Engl J Med 1995;332:1666-1670.
106. Duffy MJ, Woods JE: Health risks of failed silicone gel breast implants: a 30-year clinical experience. Plast Reconstr Surg 1994;94:295-299.
107. Roberts CS, Wells KE, Walden K: Toward understanding women who request removal of silicone breast implants. Breast J 1999;5:246-251.
108. Slavin SA, Goldwyn RM: Silicone gel implant explantation: reasons, results, and admonitions. Plast Reconstr Surg 1995;95:63-69.
109. Gilboa D, Borenstein A, Floro S, et al: Emotional and psychosocial adjustment of women to breast reconstruction and detection of subgroups at risk for psychological morbidity. Ann Plast Surg 1990;25:397-401.
110. Schusterman MA, Kroll SS, Reece GP, et al: Incidence of autoimmune disease in patients after breast reconstruction with silicone gel implants versus autogenous tissue: a preliminary report. Ann Plast Surg 1993;31:1-6.
111. Pennisi VR: Making a definite inframammary fold under a reconstructed breast. Plast Reconstr Surg 1977;60:523-525.
112. Ryan JJ: A lower thoracic advancement flap in breast reconstruction after mastectomy. Plast Reconstr Surg 1982;70:153-160.
113. Dowden RV: Achieving a natural inframammary fold and ptotic effect in the reconstructed breast. Ann Plast Surg 1987;19:524-529.
114. Toth BA, Lappert P: Modified skin incisions for mastectomy: the need for plastic surgical input in preoperative planning. Plast Reconstr Surg 1991;87:1048-1053.
115. Bensimon RH, Bergmeyer JM: Improved aesthetics in breast reconstruction: modified mastectomy incision and immediate autologous tissue reconstruction. Ann Plast Surg 1995;34:229-233, discussion 233-235.
116. Restifo RJ: The "aesthetic subunit" principle in late TRAM flap breast reconstruction. Ann Plast Surg 1999;42:235-239.
117. Hidalgo DA: Aesthetic refinement in breast reconstruction: complete skin-sparing mastectomy with autogenous tissue transfer. Plast Reconstr Surg 1998;102:63-70, discussion 71-72.
118. Spear SL, Davison SP: Aesthetic subunits of the breast. Plast Reconstr Surg 2003;112:440-447.
119. Guthrie RH Jr, Cucin RL Jr: Breast reconstruction after mastectomy: problems in position, size, and shape. Plast Reconstr Surg 1980;65:595-602.
120. Losken A, Carlson GW, Bostwick J 3rd, et al: Trends in unilateral breast reconstruction and management of the contralateral breast: the Emory experience. Plast Reconstr Surg 2002;110:89-97.
121. Asplund O, Svane G: Adjustment of the contralateral breast following breast reconstruction. Scand J Plast Reconstr Surg 1983;17:225-232.
122. McCraw JB, Maxwell GP: Early and late capsular "deformation" as a cause of unsatisfactory results in the latissimus dorsi breast reconstruction. Clin Plast Surg 1988;15:717-726.
123. Jabor MA, Shayani P, Collins DR Jr, et al: Nipple-areola reconstruction: satisfaction and clinical determinants. Plast Reconstr Surg 2002;110:457-463, discussion 464-465.
124. Eskenazi L: A one-stage nipple reconstruction with the "modified star" flap and immediate tattoo: a review of 100 cases. Plast Reconstr Surg 1993;92:671-680.
125. Bogue DP, Mungara AK, Thompson M, Cederna PS: Modified technique for nipple-areolar reconstruction: a case series. Plast Reconstr Surg 2003;112:1274-1278.
126. Shestak KC, Gabriel A, Landecker A, et al: Assessment of long-term nipple projection: a comparison of three techniques. Plast Reconstr Surg 2002;110:780-786.
127. Few JW, Marcus JR, Casas LA, et al: Long-term predictable nipple projection following reconstruction. Plast Reconstr Surg 1999;104:1321-1324.
128. Banducci DR, Le TK, Hughes KC: Long-term follow-up of a modified Anton-Hartrampf nipple reconstruction. Ann Plast Surg 1999;43:467-469, discussion 469-470.
129. Tanabe HY, Tai Y, Kiyokawa K, Yamauchi T: Nipple-areola reconstruction with a dermal-fat flap and rolled auricular cartilage. Plast Reconstr Surg 1997;100:431-438.

130. Guerra AB, Khoobehi K, Metzinger SE, Allen RJ: New technique for nipple areola reconstruction: arrow flap and rib cartilage graft for long-lasting nipple projection. Ann Plast Surg 2003;50:31-37.
131. Woods JE, Meland NB: Conservative management in full-thickness nipple-areolar necrosis after subcutaneous mastectomy. Plast Reconstr Surg 1989;84:258-264, discussion 265-266.
132. Losken A, Mackay GJ, Bostwick J 3rd: Nipple reconstruction using the C-V flap technique: a long-term evaluation. Plast Reconstr Surg 2001;108:361-369.
133. Spear SL, Arias J: Long-term experience with nipple-areola tattooing. Ann Plast Surg 1995;35:232-236.
134. Bhatty MA, Berry RB: Nipple-areola reconstruction by tattooing and nipple sharing. Br J Plast Surg 1997;50:331-334.
135. Kroll SS: Nipple reconstruction with the double-opposing tab flap. Plast Reconstr Surg 1999;104:511-514, discussion 515-517.
136. Dean NR, Neild T, Haynes J, et al: Fading of nipple-areolar reconstructions: the last hurdle in breast reconstruction? Br J Plast Surg 2002;55:574-581.
137. Chawla AK, Kachnic LA, Taghian AG, et al: Radiotherapy and breast reconstruction: complications and cosmesis with TRAM versus tissue expander/implant. Int J Radiat Oncol Biol Phys 2002;54:520-526.
138. Mansfield C: Effects of radiation therapy on wound healing after mastectomy. Clin Plast Surg 1979;6:19-26.
139. Hopewell JW, Calvo W, Jaenke R, et al: Microvasculature and radiation damage. Recent Results Cancer Res 1993;130:1-16.
140. Aitasalo K, Aro H: Irradiation-induced hypoxia in bones and soft tissues: an experimental study. Plast Reconstr Surg 1986;77:256-267.
141. Rudolph R: Complications of surgery for radiotherapy skin damage. Plast Reconstr Surg 1982;70:179-185.
142. Rudolph R, Vande Berg J, Schneider JA, et al: Slowed growth of cultured fibroblasts from human radiation wounds. Plast Reconstr Surg 1988;82:669-677.
143. Spear SL, Onyewu C: Staged breast reconstruction with saline-filled implants in the irradiated breast: recent trends and therapeutic implications. Plast Reconstr Surg 2000;105:930-942.
144. Cordeiro PG, Pusic AL, Disa JJ, et al: Irradiation after immediate tissue expander/implant breast reconstruction: outcomes, complications, aesthetic results, and satisfaction among 156 patients. Plast Reconstr Surg 2004;113:877-881.
145. Caffo O, Cazzolli D, Scalet A, et al: Concurrent adjuvant chemotherapy and immediate breast reconstruction with skin expanders after mastectomy for breast cancer. Breast Cancer Res Treat 2000;60:267-275.
146. Mansel RE, Horgan K, Webster DJT, et al: Cosmetic results of immediate breast reconstruction post-mastectomy: a follow-up study. Br J Surg 1986;73:813.
147. Schuster RH, Rotter S, Boonn W, Efron G: The use of tissue expanders in immediate breast reconstruction following mastectomy for cancer. Br J Plast Surg 1990;43:413.
148. Mandrekas AD, Zambacos GJ, Katsanton PN: Immediate and delayed breast reconstruction with permanent tissue expanders. Br J Plast Surg 1995;48:572.
149. Hunter-Smith DJ, Laurie SWS: Breast reconstruction using permanent tissue expanders. Aust N Z J Surg 1995;65:492.
150. McGeorge DD, Mahdi S, Tsekouras A: Breast reconstruction with anatomical expanders and implants: our early experience. Br J Plast Surg 1996;49:352.
151. Slavin SA, Schnitt SJ, Duda RB, et al: Skin-sparing mastectomy and immediate reconstruction: oncologic risks and aesthetic results in patients with early-stage breast cancer. Plast Reconstr Surg 1998;102:49.
152. Al-Ghazal SK, Blamey RW: Subcutaneous mastectomy with implant reconstruction: cosmetic outcome and patient satisfaction. Eur J Surg Oncol 2000;26:137.
153. Peyser PM, Abel JA, Straker VF, et al: Ultra-conservative skin-sparing "keyhole" mastectomy and immediate breast and areola reconstruction. Ann R Coll Surg Engl 2000;82:227.

CHAPTER

151

Reconstruction of the Abdominal Wall

MOTOHIRO NOZAKI, MD ✦ KENJI SASAKI, MD ✦ TED T. HUANG, MD, FACS

The abdominal wall encompasses the body's largest cavity and contains various viscera. Structural integrity of the wall is not only essential in supporting visceral functions such as micturition, defecation, and expectoration but also necessary in initiating body movements such as walking, bending, and posture maintenance. Functional integrity may be compromised as the result of an injury or as a consequence of cancer extirpation procedures. The basic principle of abdominal wall reconstruction has traditionally centered on the idea of "converting an open wound to a closed wound." Mobilization of abdominal tissues from an adjacent area to close a defect has been the traditional technique of reconstruction; an alloplastic material may be added to provide structural strength and support. Although the outcome of surgery regardless of techniques used is generally satisfactory, especially when a wall defect is small, restoration of abdominal wall function in patients with an extensive defect can be difficult if not impossible. The basic approach to reconstruction of an abdominal wall defect must therefore aim to restore structural continuity or components of the abdomen to regain functions.

SURGICAL ANATOMY

Topographically, the abdominal wall is bounded superiorly by the costal structures; the inguinal ligaments and the pubic symphysis form the inferior boundary. Although the iliac crest and the spinous processes of the lower thoracic and lumbar vertebrae are the landmarks to denote the posterolateral limit of the abdominal wall, the thoracolumbar fascia that encompasses the erector spinae, quadratus lumborum, longissimus thoracis, and transverse spinal muscles is the integral component of the posterior and the posterolateral abdominal wall.

Anterior-Anterolateral Abdominal Wall

The anterior-anterolateral section of the abdominal wall is bounded superiorly by the xiphoid process and the costal cartilage of the seventh rib and the twelfth rib. The inguinal ligament and the pubic tubercle denote the inferolateral and the inferomedial limit of the wall. The abdominal extension of the midaxillary line through the most prominent point of the iliac crest is generally regarded as the lateral border of the wall. The anterior-anterolateral abdominal wall therefore typically assumes a diamond configuration.

MUSCULOCUTANEOUS STRUCTURES

Structurally, the skin, subcutaneous tissues, five muscles and three fascial layers, extraperitoneal adipose tissues, and peritoneum compose the anterior-anterolateral abdominal wall. Integrity of these structures is essential to provide proper function (Fig. 151-1).

Peritoneum

The peritoneum is a serous membrane that not only covers the entire inner surface of the abdominal wall but also invests on the abdominal viscera. The serous

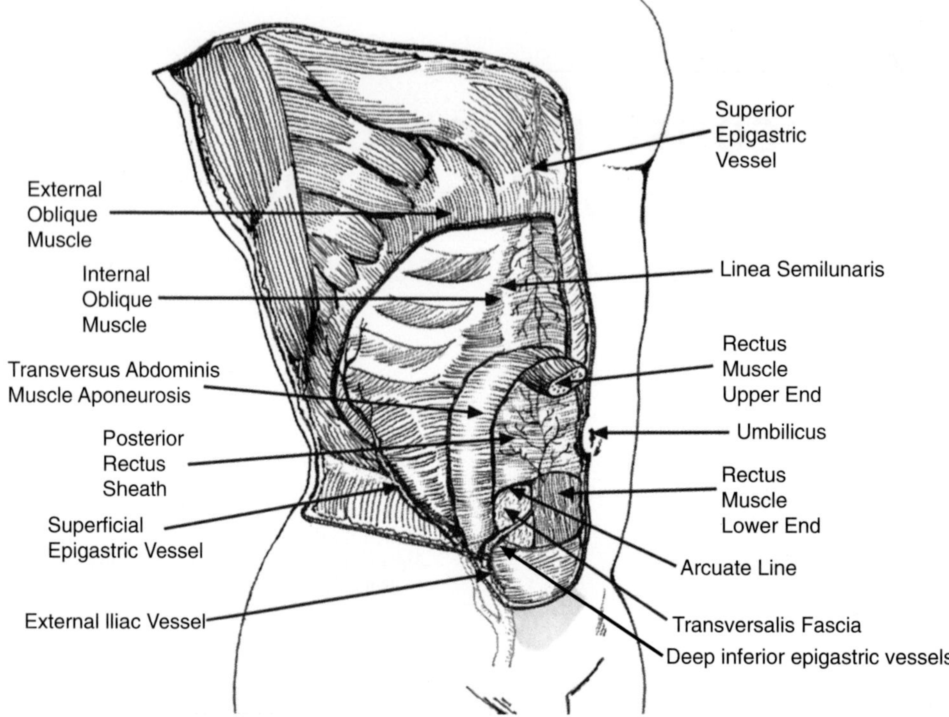

FIGURE 151-1. A schematic drawing illustrating the musculoaponeurotic layers of the anterior and anterolateral abdominal wall. Two major vascular supplies to the abdominal wall, the superficial and the deep epigastric vessels, are shown.

covering allows the viscera to glide smoothly within the cavity; alteration to the surface structure of the peritoneal membrane will lead to cicatricial adhesion. Surgical restoration of the surface continuity of the peritoneum is therefore essential to minimize the consequence of visceral adhesion.

Transversalis Fascia

The transversalis fascia is a firm membranous sheet that lines the entire abdominal cavity. Anteriorly, it is vested on the posterior wall of the transversus abdominis muscle. Located below the arcuate line (or linea semicircularis), the transversalis fascia is the principal layer of the posterior wall of the rectus sheath (see Fig. 151-1). Understanding the anatomic relationship of this fascial layer to the posterior wall of the rectus sheath is important, especially in designing a muscle or a muscle-skin flap that involves the rectus muscle or the rectus sheath. The abdominal wall is weakened by the removal of the rectus muscle and its anterior sheath. The integrity of vascular supply to the flap may be compromised if the inferior epigastric vessel, usually situated posterior to the fascia and entering the muscle at the junction of the linea semilunaris and arcuate line, is injured with flap dissection.

Rectus Sheath

The aponeurotic structures of the transversus abdominis and the internal and external oblique muscles contribute to the formation of this structure. The extent of contribution, however, varies (Fig. 151-2).

The anterior layer of the rectus sheath in the upper three fourths of the abdominal wall caudad to the level of T8 rib cartilage is formed by the aponeurotic extensions of two muscles, namely, the external oblique muscle and the internal oblique muscle, and the anterior leaf of the internal oblique aponeurosis. The posterior leaf of the internal oblique aponeurosis and the transversus abdominis muscle, in contrast, form the posterior layer of the rectus sheath.

The anterior layer of the rectus sheath in the lower fourth of the abdomen is formed by the aponeurosis of the external oblique muscle, the internal oblique muscle, and the transversus abdominis muscle. The transversalis fascia is the sole structure forming the posterior layer of the sheath below the arcuate line (linea semicircularis).

Transversus Abdominis Muscle

Of the five muscles of the anterior abdominal wall, the transversus abdominis muscle is the innermost

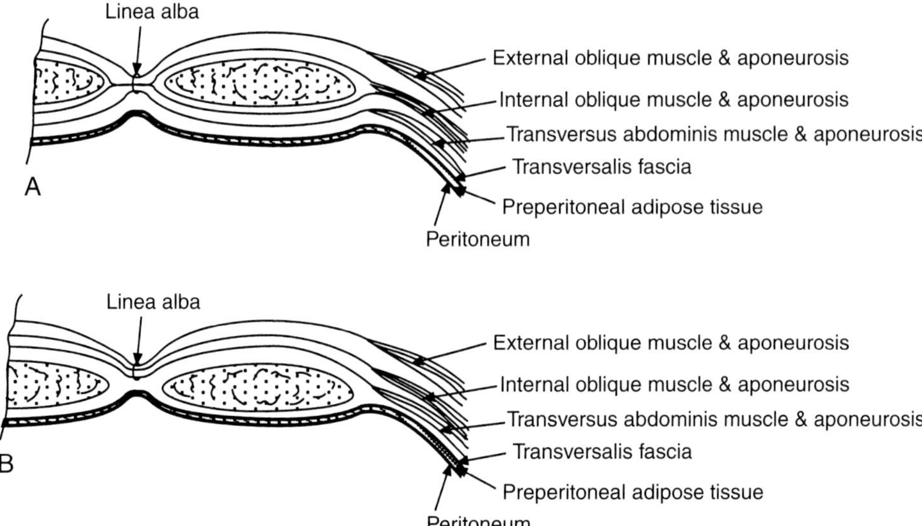

FIGURE 151-2. A schematic drawing illustrating a cross section of the anterior abdominal wall at the level of the umbilicus *(A)* and below the arcuate line (or linea semicircularis) *(B)*. The musculoaponeurotic structures forming the rectus sheath differ above and below the arcuate line.

muscle layer. The muscle fibers originate in the costal cartilage of the sixth through twelfth ribs, the thoracolumbar fascia, the anterior iliac crest, and the inguinal ligament. It ends as an aponeurosis and forms the rectus sheath. The aponeurosis, combined with the posterior leaf of the internal oblique aponeurosis, forms the posterior layer of the rectus sheath in the upper three fourths of the abdomen. The sheath extends from the xiphoid process to the level midway between the umbilicus and the pubic symphysis. In the lower fourth of the abdomen, the aponeurosis contributes to the formation only of the anterior rectus sheath.

Internal Oblique Muscle

The internal oblique muscle is a thin muscle with its fibers originating in the thoracolumbar fascia, the iliac crest, and the inguinal ligament. Superomedially, the fibers insert into the costal margin. Medially and inferomedially, they become the rectus sheath. In the upper three fourths of the abdomen, the aponeurosis splits into two leaves at the semilunaris line, thus contributing to the formation of the anterior and posterior rectus sheath. In the lower fourth of the abdomen, the aponeurosis remains intact and passes to the median line anterior to the rectus abdominis muscle. The arcuate line is the anatomic landmark denoting the change of internal oblique muscle aponeurosis in the formation of the rectus sheath.

External Oblique Muscle

The external oblique muscle is the most superficial muscle of the anterior abdominal wall musculature. Its fibers originate from the outer surface and the lower border of the lower eight ribs. The anteromedial portion of the muscle is aponeurotic and contributes to the formation of the anterior layer of the rectus sheath.

Rectus Abdominis Muscle

The rectus abdominis muscle is the vertical component of the abdominal wall musculature and is located in the middle of the anterior abdominal wall situated on either side of the linea alba. The fibers originate in the superior ramus of the pubis and in the ligaments of the pubic symphysis. They insert into the anterior surface of the xiphoid process and into the cartilages of the fifth, sixth, and seventh ribs. The muscle bundle is thick and narrow at the lower abdomen and thin and broad superiorly.

Pyramidalis Muscle

The pyramidalis muscle, a small triangular muscle, lies anterior to the lower part of the rectus abdominis muscle and is contained within the rectus sheath. It is absent in many and is considered to be functionally insignificant.

Arcuate Line

The arcuate line (linea semicircularis), located at the level midway between the umbilicus and the pubic symphysis, is an anatomic demarcation denoting the change in structural composition of the rectus sheath, specifically the posterior layer. The posterior rectus sheath in the upper abdomen is made mostly of aponeurotic tissues from the transversus abdominis and the internal oblique muscles; the transversalis fascia forms the posterior wall of the rectus sheath in the lower quarter of the lower abdomen. Structural integrity of the lower abdomen is weakened with removal of the anterior lamina of the rectus sheath and the inferior segment of the rectus muscle (see Figs. 151-1 and 151-2).

Linea Semilunaris

The linea semilunaris denotes the lateral margin of the rectus muscle. The line begins inferiorly at the pubic tubercle and ends superiorly at the ninth costal cartilage. The inferior epigastric vessel enters the rectus sheath through the transversalis fascia at a point where the line intersects the arcuate line (see Fig. 151-1).

VASCULAR SUPPLY

The branches of the internal mammary vessel, aorta, femoral vessel, and internal and external iliac vessels form the vascular supply network to the abdominal wall:

1. the superior epigastric vessel, the branch of the internal mammary vessel;
2. the lower two intercostal vessels, the subcostal vessels, and the four lumbar vessels arising from the aorta;
3. the superficial epigastric, superficial circumflex iliac, and superficial external pudendal vessels, all branches of the femoral vessel;
4. the inferior epigastric and deep circumflex iliac vessels, the branches of the external iliac vessel; and
5. the iliolumbar branch of the internal iliac vessel.

Although the path of these vessels varies, they are interconnected through terminal branch anastomoses. Because of the pattern of vascular supply and the rich vascular network, various skin flaps, skin-muscle flaps, and muscle flaps may be mobilized from the abdominal wall for reconstruction.

Generally speaking, the superficial inferior epigastric vessel (see Fig. 151-1) is the primary vascular system that can be used to design an axial skin flap in the lower abdomen. The vessel originates from the common femoral vessel. It pierces through Scarpa fascia just below the inguinal ligament, 8 to 10 cm lateral to the midline. There are several branches off the main trunk that course diagonally toward the costal margin. It joins with branches from the lumbar and intercostal vessels as well as the perforating branches from the deep inferior epigastric vessel. An axial skin flap may therefore be designed in the area extending from the groin to the costal margin. Similarly, an axial skin flap may be designed in the lower abdomen with its vascular supply based on the anastomosis between the superficial inferior epigastric and the deep inferior epigastric vessels.

The deep inferior epigastric vessel (see Fig. 151-1), a branch of the external iliac vessel, pierces through the transversalis fascia and enters the rectus sheath at a point close to the arcuate line. Within the rectus sheath, the vessel is contained within areolar tissues behind the muscle belly. It ascends cephalad and then penetrates into the muscle. Branches extend from the vessel at various levels through anastomotic networks with the costal, lumbar, and deep circumflex iliac vessels to provide blood supply to the medial as well as to the lateral abdominal wall. An axial skin flap or a muscle-skin flap may be designed in the midabdominal, inferior abdominal, and lateral abdominal area.

The superior epigastric vessel (see Fig. 151-1), the medial branch of the internal mammary vessel, penetrates the rectus sheath as it passes behind the seventh costal cartilage. The vessel enters the muscle almost immediately. The vessel connects with the deep inferior epigastric vessel to form the epigastric vascular arcade. A skin island can be harvested in the lower abdominal area and transferred to the upper abdomen or the chest area by incorporating the rectus muscle that contains the epigastric vascular arcade.

NERVE SUPPLY

The muscles of the abdominal wall are innervated by ventral rami of the spinal nerves T7 through L4, including the thoracoabdominal intercostal, subcostal, iliohypogastric, and ilioinguinal nerves.

Thoracoabdominal Intercostal Nerves

The ventral rami of the intercostal nerves enter the wall by passing dorsal to the costal cartilages and course between the transversus abdominis and the internal oblique muscles. The terminal branch of these nerves pierces through the posterior rectus sheath and innervates the rectus muscle; the perforating branches are responsible for skin innervation.

Iliohypogastric and Ilioinguinal Nerves

The iliohypogastric and ilioinguinal nerves originate in the lumbar plexus. They course through the layer between the transversus abdominis and the internal oblique muscles. The terminal branches of these nerves innervate the skin over the suprapubic area, the root of the penis, the mons pubis, the scrotal wall, and the labia.

Posterior-Posterolateral Abdominal Wall

In addition to the iliac wing and the transverse processes of the lower thoracic and lumbar vertebrae, the erector spinae, quadratus lumborum, longissimus thoracis, and transverse spinal muscles are the muscular structures surrounded by the thoracolumbar fascia composing the posterior and the posterolateral boundary of the abdominal wall. The nerve supplies to these muscles are provided by the dorsal rami of the corresponding spinal nerve.

Clinically, the posterior and posterolateral abdominal wall seldom requires reconstruction. Instead, the muscles are used to reconstruct spinal defects in individuals with congenital or, on rare occasions, acquired defects.

ACQUIRED ABDOMINAL WALL DEFECTS

Although the functional impairment experienced by an individual after abdominal surgery is usually limited, extensive tissue loss due to trauma or cancer extirpation procedures can cause a significant degree of impairment in body functions. These circumstances may lead to tissue loss. The extent of tissue loss must be delineated to formulate a regimen to reconstruct the defect.

Clinical Considerations

EVALUATION OF THE PATIENT

In addition to delineation of the extent of the abdominal wall defect, the patient's medical history must be ascertained. Nutritional status of the patient must be assessed to ensure uneventful recovery from ensuing surgical intervention.

The extent and components of the abdominal wall defect should be ascertained to select an appropriate reconstructive procedure. Whereas a defect with limited tissue damage and structural loss may be repaired by means of primary closure, mobilization of tissues with structural components similar to the defect may be necessary to reconstruct a large defect.

EVALUATION OF STRUCTURAL DEFECT

The exact extent and the nature of tissue loss or damage must be delineated. This information is essential to understand the basis of functional impairment observed.

Although a detailed medical history and physical examination findings are useful, other ancillary laboratory studies, such as myographic and radiographic imaging studies, may be required to ascertain the exact extent of the structural defect.

Etiologic Considerations

Trauma and cancer extirpational procedures are the most common causes of abdominal wall defects requiring reconstruction. Ancillary treatments, especially in patients with cancer, may frequently extend the tissue damage. Delineation and complete removal of devitalized tissues are therefore essential steps to restore abdominal wall continuity.

SURGICAL MANAGEMENT OF ABDOMINAL WALL DEFECTS

Functional integrity of the abdominal wall is frequently compromised by structures that are either congenitally defective or deformed from trauma or surgical intervention. Infection, irradiation, or diseases that required repetitive surgical intervention could further aggravate the structural deformities. Restoration of deformed wall structures is essential to preserve the functions of the abdominal wall. This is ideally accomplished by restoring the musculofascial continuity of the abdominal wall and the skin coverage. Availability of thick and vascularized musculofascial tissues and the skin is essential in achieving this goal. Reconstruction of a defective abdominal wall can be difficult in practice, however, especially when the loss of tissue is extensive. In instances in which mobilization of the tissues from the adjacent area to repair the defect is not possible, transfer of soft tissues from other sites will be necessary.

General Considerations

TIMING OF RECONSTRUCTION

To minimize surgical morbidities, immediate and one-stage reconstruction of a wall defect is the approach of choice for patients undergoing abdominal wall herniorrhaphy or tumor extirpation that requires concomitant abdominal wall resection (Table 151-1). Delay of definitive repair is recommended if the condition of the patient is unstable and the injury is extensive. Frequent wound dressing changes, prosthetic mesh, and skin grafts may be used to manage the wound.[1-4] More recently, a technique using a suction device (i.e., vacuum-assisted closure) has been shown to be effective in providing temporary closure of an abdominal wall defect.[5]

TABLE 151-1 ✦ TIMING FOR ABDOMINAL WALL RECONSTRUCTION

Timing of Reconstruction	No. of Patients
Immediate	43
Delayed	1
Total	44

MANAGEMENT OF AN INFECTED ABDOMINAL WOUND

The regimen of wet-to-dry gauze dressing changes or 0.25% acetic acid is used to manage an infected wound. The dressing should be changed frequently to maintain wound moisture and protect the wound. Necrotic tissue should be surgically removed to gain control of infection. Closure of the wound may be considered once it becomes sufficiently clean and bacteriologically "balanced." The defect may be closed primarily. If primary closure of the wound is not possible, skin grafting techniques should be considered despite ensuing consequences of hernia, abdominal wall bulge, and possible trauma to the viscera.[6] Reconstructive intervention for these problems should be delayed for a minimum of 6 months.[2-4]

STATIC RECONSTRUCTION

Static reconstruction of the abdominal wall defect is defined as abdominal wall reconstruction with autologous tissues or alloplastic materials that contain no dynamically functioning muscle structures. The procedure will therefore include the use of a pedicled or free fascial graft, a local or free skin flap, or prosthetic materials. Dynamic movements of the abdominal wall are often preserved despite static repair procedures if the major bulk of the abdominal wall musculature, including the rectus abdominis, internal and external oblique, and iliopsoas muscles, are left undisturbed.

Repair of an abdominal incisional hernia and closure of a transverse rectus abdominis muscle (TRAM) flap donor defect in breast mound reconstruction are procedures that illustrate the principle of static abdominal wall reconstruction. Incorporation of a prosthetic material or autogenous tissue such as a fascial graft may strengthen the abdominal surgical result.[7-10] The efficacy of various static abdominal wall restoration procedures, however, remains controversial. Whereas reports by Chen et al[11] indicate that static reconstruction of the abdominal wall defect after a double-pedicle TRAM flap breast mound reconstruction did not affect subsequent pregnancy in several women, removal of the rectus abdominis muscles substantially limits daily physical activities in some patients.[12-14]

It is established that abdominal hernia, abdominal wall laxity, persistent chronic back pain, and scoliosis are problems commonly associated with loss or absence of abdominal wall muscle structures.[15,16] Scoliosis, for example, is a well-recognized skeletal abnormality associated with a congenital absence of the abdominal wall, also known as the prune-belly syndrome.[12] Similarly, loss of abdominal wall strength is the sequel of a TRAM flap breast reconstruction procedure. Mizgala et al[8] reported loss of abdominal wall strength and a decrease in exercise tolerance in 46% and 25%, respectively, of their 150 patients studied. Similarly, Lejour and Dome[7] indicated that impairment of abdominal wall strength was common in their patients. According to Blondeel et al,[13,14] problems related to daily activities of their patients because of backache after a TRAM flap procedure were more common than in the control group.

FUNCTIONAL RECONSTRUCTION

The abdominal wall not only provides a mechanical barrier for the viscera to trauma and infection but also participates in a variety of body functions. In addition to movements of the trunk and the lower limbs, an intact abdominal wall is essential in controlling respiratory effort and in sustaining sufficient intra-abdominal pressure to initiate bowel movements, coughing, and micturition. An ideal method of abdominal wall reconstruction should restore muscle activities. It should, furthermore, cause minimal or no cicatricial adhesions of the viscera. Pless and Pless[17] reported that dynamic restoration of the abdominal layers effectively reduced the incidence of abdominal wall pain in 27 of 32 patients treated (84%); the lower back pain was cured in 18 patients (56%). By separating the components of the anterior abdominal wall musculature at surgery to repair an abdominal wall defect (i.e., the component musculature separation technique of abdominal wall repair), Ramirez et al[16] were able to cure chronic, disabling back pain associated with a large abdominal hernia.

Although it is essential to identify and separate all muscle components in dynamic repair of an abdominal wall defect, coaptation of the external oblique muscle continuity must be included. In patients with extensive skin loss, prior tissue expansion should be included in the surgical plan. If identification of muscle layers is difficult and primary coaptation of muscle layers is not possible, a pedicled rectus femoris muscle flap or a latissimus dorsi muscle flap or tensor fascia lata muscle flap transferred by microsurgical technique may be considered. A prosthetic material may be incorporated in this type of repair, provided a synthetic material can be firmly attached to innervated musculofascial structures that surround the defect.

Restoration of Muscle Function

It has been shown that dynamic activities of the abdominal wall may be restored by use of a layered wound closure method. That is, functional restoration may require either tissue expansion or a musculoaponeurotic component technique.[16,18] In 1983, Ger and Duboys[19] showed that transfer of a pedicled rectus femoris muscle flap restored contractile activities in the abdomen.

When the length of neural pedicle is insufficient for primary transfer, the nerve continuity may be re-established by microsurgical means. In 1998, Sasaki et al,[20] with a tensor fascia lata muscle flap, and Ninkovic et al,[21] with a latissimus dorsi muscle flap, were able to provide contractile activities in the reconstructed abdominal wall.

Restoration of Sensory Function

Providing sensation in the abdominal wall is important to minimize further trauma to the abdomen.[22] The techniques of component separation and layered closure with or without concomitant skin expansion, a sensate tendon fascia lata musculocutaneous flap, or a sensate anterior thigh fasciocutaneous flap transferred primarily or microsurgically are useful to provide sensation in a reconstructed abdominal wall.[23,24] Preservation of the lateral cutaneous branch of the T7 and L1 intercostal, ilioinguinal, and iliocostal nerves is important in design of a local flap for sensory innervation.

Prevention of Cicatricial Adhesions

Cicatricial adhesion between the inner surface of a reconstructed abdominal wall and the viscera underneath is often blamed for enterocutaneous fistula formation and intestinal obstruction and makes the task of secondary abdominal surgery difficult. Consideration of a material that is less "adhesive" to the viscera is, in this sense, important in flap design and material selection. The materials reported to be relatively inert to cicatricial adhesion include Dacron sheets, Gore-Tex, silicone polymer, and autogenous fascial materials. In 1974, Rayner[25] demonstrated in laboratory animals that a "peritonealization" process takes place over the surface of Dacron mesh (Mersilene) while it is simultaneously converting fibrous tissues contained within the coagulum surrounding the mesh. Matloub et al[26] reported in 1992 that combining an autologous piece of fascia and Gore-Tex prevented visceral peritoneal adhesion, whereas Marlex mesh alone did not. In human subjects, Mansberger et al[27] showed neoperitoneum formation without adherence to the viscera beneath an abdominal wound closed with a piece of silicone sheet. Intra-abdominal adhesions were found to be less extensive if the abdominal wound closure had incorporated a segment of autologous tensor fascia lata with or without areolar tissue underneath.[9,20]

AESTHETIC CONSIDERATIONS

Aesthetic reconstruction of the abdominal wall mostly concerns contour deformity, mismatch of skin color, and scar deformity. Surgery should be considered only if the objectives of functional restoration of the abdominal wall can be maintained. Aesthetic reconstruction may also be aimed at reducing the cicatricial deformities around the abdominal wall. This is accomplished by revising the scarred area and replacing the grafted area with unscarred skin mobilized from an adjacent area. The skin and soft tissues may be expanded if existing tissue is insufficient to cover the defect.

Surgical Techniques

The fundamental principle of abdominal wall restorative surgery follows the basic teaching of reconstructive surgery. A technique must not only be the most effective in restoring structural continuity and functional integrity but also cause the least amount of morbidity (Table 151-2). In practice, selection of an appropriate technique to reconstruct an abdominal wall defect is governed by factors such as the size and location of the defect, the availability of tissue material for reconstruction, and the clinical status of the patient.

PRIMARY DIRECT AND LAYERED CLOSURE TECHNIQUE

Primary direct and layered closure techniques are useful in closing a defect that is no larger than 7 cm.

TABLE 151-2 ✦ SURGICAL TECHNIQUES TO RECONSTRUCT AN ABDOMINAL WALL DEFORMITY

- Primary direct and layered closure technique
  - Relaxing incision technique
  - Layered closure after tissue expansion
- Free skin, fascial graft, or prosthetic material
  - Free skin graft
  - Free fascial graft
  - Prosthetic materials
- Flaps
  - Local pedicled flaps
    - Cutaneous or fasciocutaneous flaps
      - Groin skin flap or anterior thigh fasciocutaneous flap
      - Anterior rectus abdominis fasciocutaneous flap
      - Ilioinguinal skin flap
    - Musculocutaneous flaps
      - Rectus abdominis musculocutaneous flap: superiorly based flap (lower TRAM flap, VRAM flap); inferiorly based flap (upper TRAM flap + "flag flap"; VRAM flap; extended DIE flap)
      - Extended oblique musculocutaneous flap
  - Distant pedicled or free composite tissue transfer
    - Anterolateral thigh fasciocutaneous flap
    - Tensor fascia lata flap
    - Combined free tensor fascia lata musculocutaneous flap and anterolateral thigh flap
    - Rectus femoris flap
    - Latissimus dorsi flap
    - Gracilis flap

DIE, deep inferior epigastric; TRAM, transverse rectus abdominis muscle; VRAM, vertical rectus abdominis muscle.

Components of the abdominal wall, including the peritoneum, muscles, fascia, and skin, are dissected and individually identified. They are coapted in layers without the use of intervening materials such as a mesh or a fascial flap. When a defect is closed with tension, it will lead to wound edge separation and tissue necrosis. Furthermore, pressure on the abdominal cavity caused by tightness of wound closure may interfere with ventilatory effort. Abdominal compartment syndrome is not an uncommon sequel of a tight abdominal wound closure.[4] Relief of tension may be provided by a relaxing incision made in the muscle layers, for example, by use of an external oblique muscle layer-releasing incision, and prior tissue expansion.

Relaxing Incision Technique

In 1990, Ramirez et al[16] were the first to advocate a technique that requires separation of structural components of the abdominal wall to mobilize the musculofascial tissue for closure of a midline abdominal wall defect (Fig. 151-3*A*). The anterior rectus sheath is separated from the external oblique aponeurosis by making a longitudinal relaxing incision along the linea semilunaris (Fig. 151-3*B*). This allows medial mobilization of the anterior rectus sheath and rectus muscle while continuity with the internal oblique and transverse abdominis muscle aponeuroses is preserved. Posteriorly, the rectus muscle is separated from the posterior sheath, but the lateral border is left undisturbed. The muscle belly, with the anterior rectus sheath, is mobilized to cover the structural defect (Fig. 151-3*C*).

Separation of pleural peritoneum is necessary if the structural composition of the posterior rectus sheath cannot be clearly defined. That is, in instances in which separation of the transversus abdominis muscle from the rectus muscle is not possible, the pleural peritoneum is separated from the posterior layer of the rectus muscle. A longitudinal releasing incision is added from within to free the rectus muscle for mobilization. Care is exercised to preserve the segmental neurovascular supply to the rectus muscle as well as the branches of sensory nerves to the abdomen that are passing through the rectus sheath to maintain muscle mobility and skin sensation. Generally speaking, 10 to 12 cm of muscle-fascia mobility in the epigastric level, 20 cm in the midabdomen, and approximately 6 cm in the lower abdomen is possible by use of the technique that combines the separation of abdominal musculature components and fascial release. Lowe et al[28] advocated an endoscopic technique to carry out the task. They reported that the midline perforating vessels to the skin can easily be preserved, and surgical morbidities were minimal.

Thomas et al[29] in 1993 and DiBello et al[30] in 1996 modified Ramirez's technique by making an incision only in the external oblique muscle aponeurosis.

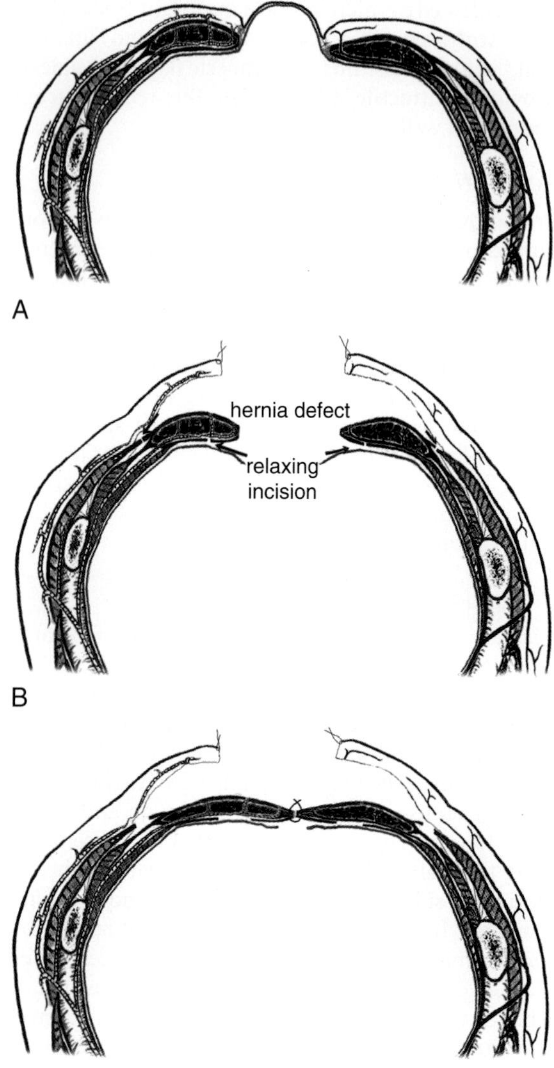

FIGURE 151-3. *A,* A schematic drawing illustrating an anterior midline abdominal wall defect. *B,* A schematic drawing illustrating an anterior rectus sheath separated from the external oblique aponeurosis. Longitudinal relaxing incisions are made anteriorly along the linea semilunaris and posteriorly in the posterior rectus sheath. *C,* Relaxing incisions made in both the anterior and the posterior rectus sheath allow stretching of the rectus muscle as the anterior rectus wall is pulled medially to correct the defect.

Although they claimed to have attained a similar result, almost half of their patients required the use of prosthetic mesh to buttress the fascial defect.[30]

Girotto et al[31] advocated an algorithmic approach in an attempt to define the indication for the procedures. The algorithmic path goes as follows:

The skin-subcutaneous coverage of the abdominal wall is separated to expose the anterior rectus sheath to define the lateral border of the rectus abdominis muscle once the structural defect is defined.

- If the defect cannot be repaired primarily without undue tension, the external oblique muscle is separated from the internal oblique muscle by an incision made in the external oblique muscle aponeurosis on one side just lateral to the anterior rectus sheath.
- If closure of the defect is not possible with unilateral release, the external oblique muscle is separated on the opposite side.
- Additional release is obtained by releasing the posterior rectus sheath to gain rectus muscle mobility.

Layered Closure After Tissue Expansion

The technique of skin–subcutaneous tissue expansion to close a skin–subcutaneous tissue defect resulted from temporary wound closure with skin grafting techniques.[32] The height of skin bulge with an expander fully expanded must be equal to or more than the length of an intended flap to make up the tissue defect and to cover the donor defect. Expansion of the skin is most effective in the area over the rib or the lumbar fascia. The expander is placed between the abdominal musculature and subcutaneous fatty tissues.[33] The expander is removed, and the stretched skin and subcutaneous tissue are advanced to cover the defect. A nonabsorbable mesh may be used if primary concomitant closure of the musculofascial defect is not feasible.[34-36]

The tissue expansion technique is not only useful in reconstructing the structural defect but also effective in attaining aesthetic results. The morbidities are usually minimal. The procedure, on the other hand, requires a staged approach and is not useful in management of an infected wound. Placement of an expander in an infected wound inevitably leads to expander extrusion.

The principle of tissue expansion now includes the expansion of muscles and fascia. Hobar and Byrd[18,37] claimed that they were able to reconstruct a large abdominal wall defect by expanding both the external and the internal oblique muscle layers. An expander is placed between the internal oblique muscle and the transversus abdominis muscle through an incision made in the rectus sheath. Jacobsen et al[38] reported that they were able to place an expander endoscopically in a space made between the external and internal oblique muscles.

SKIN GRAFTS, FREE FASCIAL GRAFTS, AND PROSTHETIC MATERIALS

The indication for the use of skin grafts, free fascial grafts, and prosthetic materials is limited to partial abdominal skin defect or musculofascial defect.

Skin Grafts

Covering an open wound with a skin graft is technically simple and may be accomplished with minimal morbidity. It is the treatment of choice for management of an abdominal wound provided the vascular supply to the wound bed and underlying musculofascial support are adequate.

A partial-thickness skin graft can be transplanted successfully onto the visceral surface even though the area may be potentially contaminated.[39-41] Because the graft does not provide support or mechanical protection of the viscera, it must be considered a temporary measure. This modality is especially useful in patients with massive trauma to the abdomen with bouts of sepsis.[42]

Reconstruction of a grafted area may be considered once the patient is fully recovered from the insult of injury. The task of removing the skin graft densely adherent to the bowel wall or a prosthetic mesh can be difficult. Any attempt to remove an adherent skin graft can lead to excessive bleeding or bowel perforation. Removal of the epithelial layer, leaving a deep dermal layer adherent to the bowel wall or the mesh, is preferred.[21]

Free Fascial Grafts

For a free fascial graft, a sheet of autologous fascial material harvested from the tensor fascia lata or the anterior rectal sheath may be used to close a fascial defect if the skin coverage is adequate.

The tensor fascia lata is considered the preferred source for fascial grafting material. The tissue strength is sufficient to keep the viscera in the abdominal cavity. Harvesting of the material is technically easy, and donor site morbidity is low. It elicits essentially no foreign body reaction and seldom adheres to intra-abdominal viscera.

Many investigators have reported the usefulness of tensor fascia lata as a free fascial grafting material in clinical practice. Hamilton[43] reported the failure rate among patients with ventral hernia repair by use of a fascia obtained from the tensor fascia lata to be 6.4%. Disa et al[9] stated that a free fascial graft of a moderate size, 10 cm × 17 cm, was a reliable alternative for reconstruction of large, contaminated abdominal wounds in patients in whom the use of alloplastic materials was contraindicated. They noted a recurrence rate of hernia with fascial graft to be less than 10%. In an animal study, Matloub et al[26] noted that there was no adhesion between the fascia and the bowel when it was used to line the peritoneal cavity.

A freeze-dried or lyophilized fascial graft, although convenient, has been shown to have a lack of structural strength and has not been useful in practice.[44]

Technique of Graft Harvesting. The fascia is exposed by a skin incision made along the midlateral line of the thigh. Both the anterior and posterior border of the tensor fascia lata may be exposed through this incision once the overlying skin is elevated. The amount of graft needed for reconstruction is then determined. Whereas the superior incision may be made at the level of the trochanter, 5 to 7 cm of the distal iliotibial tract should be left undisturbed to maintain lateral knee stability. An endoscopic technique may be used to minimize the morbidity from a lengthy incision.[45]

The graft is placed in the defect with its fibers in a transverse direction and the posterior surface against the peritoneum. The graft is anchored to the bed by nonabsorbable sutures with a mattress stitch technique to obtain maximal immobilization. The skin is mobilized to cover the graft, and the wound edge is closed primarily. Other techniques of wound closure may be used if primary closure of the resultant wound is not possible.

Prosthetic Materials

A variety of prostheses made of various alloplastic materials are available on the market. These materials are used to augment the fascial strength of the abdomen as well as suture line strength. The prosthetic material is usually classified as meshed or nonmeshed as well as absorbable or nonabsorbable. There are advantages and disadvantages for each prosthetic type, and the indications vary. A nonmeshed material is said to be impermeable to bacteria. Fibrous ingrowth is less likely, thus minimizing cicatricial adhesion between the prosthesis and the viscera. Reopening of the abdominal cavity through the nonmeshed material is said to be easier. Alternatively, a meshed material is said to allow efficient effusion of body and purulent fluids. It also allows ingrowth of granulation tissues through the mesh, thus enhancing tissue strength.[4] The preferred prosthetic material is therefore meshed. A nonabsorbable mesh material generally remains permanently in place. An absorbable mesh material may be used if the repair is temporary. A soft tissue defect over the prosthetic material is covered with skin in the usual manner.

Among various prosthetic materials, polypropylene mesh (Marlex) is the material used most often. It is not only strong but also durable with good tissue tolerance and adequate porosity. It is, furthermore, highly resistant to bacterial contamination.[46,47] Although the material elicits a mild degree of tissue reaction, it promotes fibrous tissue ingrowth between the interstices. The fibrous ingrowth in the interstitial spaces provides tissue strength needed for fascial support. However, extrusion of mesh material and development of an enterocutaneous fistula can be a problem for individuals with intra-abdominal infection. This complication occurs frequently in individuals with thin overlying skin and subcutaneous tissues. Extrusion may be managed with placement of a piece of tensor fascia lata graft or a piece of thick tissue with adequate vascular supply.[17,46-48]

Folds and wrinkles formed in a piece of mesh may exert pressure against the bowel wall. Continuous pressure of mesh against the bowel wall is thought to cause erosion and, consequently, enterocutaneous fistula formation. To minimize this complication, the size of mesh needed must be determined carefully, and it should be anchored to the fascial defect precisely under slight tension. By inference, interposition of a piece of soft tissue, such as omentum or peritoneal tissue, between the mesh and the bowel would conceivably minimize the possibility of bowel erosion.[48]

Prolene mesh, made of polypropylene fiber, has a smoother surface. It is more pliable and easily removable. Erosion of Prolene mesh into bowel is uncommon.[49]

Expanded polytetrafluoroethylene patch (PTFE, Gore-Tex) is another material frequently used as a prosthetic graft in clinical practice. It is soft and causes less adhesion to the visceral surface. It is said to be less adherent for bacteria.[25,27] In addition, PTFE allows essentially no fibrous tissue ingrowth; removal is therefore easy.[47] Although it is often used with an indication similar to that of polypropylene mesh, this material does not allow effusion of fluid from the peritoneal cavity. Many surgeons believe that PTFE is not an appropriate material for abdominal wall reconstruction, especially in a contaminated wound.[50]

An absorbable mesh made of polyglycolic acid (Dexon) or polyglactin 910 (Vicryl) is intended to last for a period not to exceed 3 to 4 months. The mesh will disappear as it becomes hydrolyzed. This type of mesh may be used safely as a temporary means of wound coverage, even if the wound is heavily contaminated.[2,4] The skin opening may be managed later with a piece of skin graft. Because of hydrolytic disintegration of the material, structural strength around the site of repair will diminish with time. Delayed appearance of hernia or abdominal wall weakness is a common sequel of this type of repair. However, a surgeon may not be plagued with the difficulty of removing the prosthetic material 6 to 12 months later in a patient undergoing definitive repair of the defect.

SURGICAL TECHNIQUE. A prosthesis, according to the surgeon's choice, is used to make up the musculofascial defect or to reinforce an area of weakness in the abdominal wall.

There are three approaches in use of prosthetic materials for musculofascial defect repair. For an inlay graft, a piece of prosthetic material is cut into the same size as the fascial defect. It is placed in the defect and anchored to the edges with interrupted stitches. The graft tends to move with contraction of the abdomen. Herniation through a weakened site of graft-fascia

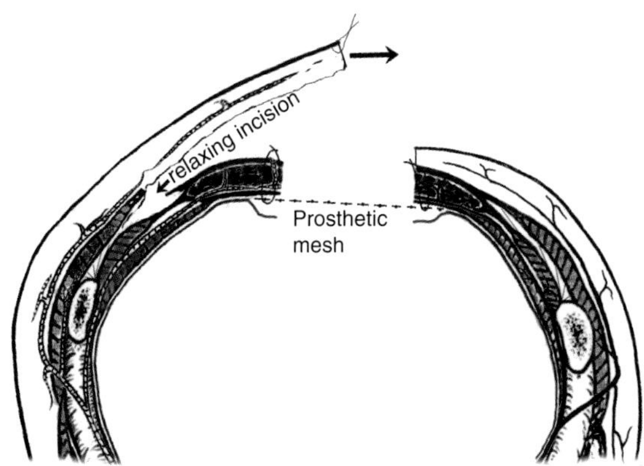

FIGURE 151-4. A schematic drawing illustrating an underlay technique to place prosthetic material between the peritoneum and the rectus sheath or muscle to enhance structural strength of the posterior wall.

coaptation is therefore not uncommon. For an onlay graft, a piece of graft is cut slightly larger than the fascial defect. The graft is placed on the top of the anterior rectus sheath. The edges are anchored to the sheath with interrupted sutures under normal tension. Edges of the graft are flattened and smoothed out with additional stitching. Contact of the graft with the viscera is not possible because of the location. The underlay graft is placed intraperitoneally in the deep surface of the defect. It is commonly placed in a space made between the peritoneum and the posterior rectus sheath or the rectus muscle and the posterior rectus sheath. The location of graft placement is sufficiently deep to prevent hernia formation because the pressure exerted from within helps to anchor the graft (Fig. 151-4).[49,51] Care, however, is needed to avoid direct contact of the graft with the viscera to prevent direct trauma to the viscera. In practice, wrinkling or folding of the graft is inevitable because of abdominal muscle movement associated with respiratory effort.

FLAPS

There are several skin flaps, skin-fascia flaps, and skin-muscle flaps that could be harvested from the abdomen or the upper thigh areas to reconstruct a defect.

Local Flaps

Local flaps are defined as flaps planned and elevated in the area adjacent to the defect.

CUTANEOUS AND FASCIOCUTANEOUS FLAPS. A cutaneous flap is a common flap used to repair a partial defect of the skin and subcutaneous tissue. It is also used with a prosthetic patch to repair a full-thickness wall defect.

Groin Flap and Anterior Thigh Fasciocutaneous Flap. The groin and anterior thigh fasciocutaneous flaps receive their blood supply from the superficial circumflex iliac vessels. They are commonly used to repair abdominal wall defects on the same side.[24,52,53] They may also be used in conjunction with the tensor fascia lata to incorporate fascial support.[54,55] The anterior thigh fasciocutaneous flap, located superficial to the rectus femoris and the sartorius muscle, can provide cutaneous sensation to the reconstructed area as long as the anterior femoral cutaneous nerve is included in the fabrication of the flap.[24]

Anterior Rectus Abdominis Fasciocutaneous Flap. The anterior rectus abdominis fasciocutaneous flap receives its blood supply from the inferior or superior epigastric vessels. It can be used to close an abdominal defect as a transposition or advancement flap.[56]

Iliolumbar Flap. The iliolumbar bipedicle flap is nourished by the superficial circumflex iliac vessels and the perforating cutaneous branches of the lumbar vessels. The flap is commonly used to reconstruct a defect in the middle third of the lateral abdominal wall.[57]

MUSCULOCUTANEOUS FLAPS. Musculocutaneous flaps are used to reconstruct a full-thickness defect of the abdomen.

Rectus Abdominis Musculocutaneous Flap. The rectus abdominis musculocutaneous flap may be harvested from the same side of the defect or from the opposite side. The flap receives its blood supply from the inferior or superior epigastric vessels. A vertical rectus musculocutaneous flap based superiorly is commonly used to reconstruct a wall defect in the upper half of the abdomen. Conversely, a flap based inferiorly is used to reconstruct a defect in the lower half of the abdomen, the groin, and the perineum.[58-60] Restoration of dynamic abdominal wall function with the rectus abdominis musculocutaneous flap may not be possible, however, because the muscle is easily denervated during flap fabrication.

Taylor et al[61] reported the technique of designing a flap in the area covering the lateral aspect of the middle-upper abdomen. This flap, termed an extended deep inferior epigastric flap, bases its blood supply on the paraumbilical perforators of the inferior epigastric vessels. The flap is used to reconstruct a defect in the upper and lower abdomen (Fig. 151-5).[62] A modification of the same flap, a bilobed variant, may be used to cover any defect in the upper abdomen.[3] An upper transverse rectus abdominis flap, more commonly known as a flag flap, may be used to reconstruct a defect in the same area.[63] The rectus muscle, completely freed from the posterior rectus sheath attachment, is turned over and based medially to cover the midline defect of the upper abdomen.[64] The rectus muscle is used as soft tissue coverage; the anterior rectus sheath is attached to the muscle belly to restore the fascial defect and provide structural strength.

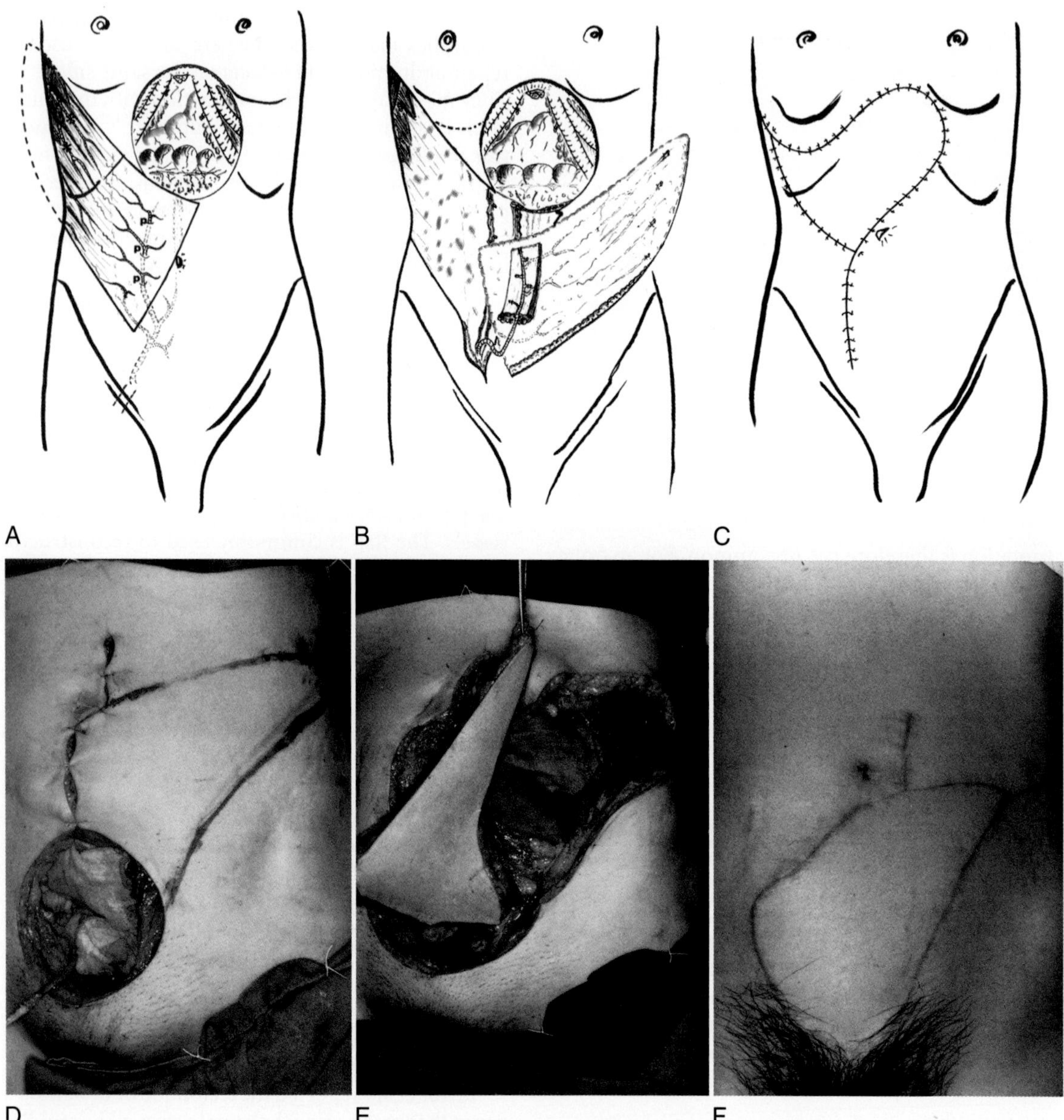

FIGURE 151-5. *A,* A schematic drawing illustrating an extended rectus abdominis musculocutaneous flap that can be used to reconstruct a full-thickness wall defect in the upper abdomen and, in some instances, the lower abdomen. A skin paddle located in the flank extending into the area around the angle of the scapula may be added to the flap. The flap is based on the paraumbilical perforators of the deep inferior epigastric vessels. p, perforating branch; *, lateral cutaneous branch. *B,* The skin island receives its blood supply through the capillary anastomoses existing between the paraumbilical perforators of the deep inferior epigastric vessels and the intercostal perforators. A small segment of the rectus muscle at the umbilical level ensures the vascular supply to an island of skin flap. *C,* The flap is rotated cephalad or caudad to make up the defect. *D,* A 52-year-old woman who underwent an abdominal wall resection because of complications resulting from an ovarian cancer extirpation procedure followed by irradiation treatment. A left rectus abdominis musculocutaneous flap with superolateral extension was used to reconstruct the defect. *E,* The musculocutaneous flap designed as an island flap was rotated inferomedially for reconstruction of the wall defect. *F,* The appearance of the wound 9 months after surgery. Healing of the wound was satisfactory.

External Oblique Musculocutaneous Flap. This flap was described by Hershey and Butcher[65] in 1964. The flap is rotational and based on the external oblique muscle and anterior rectus sheath with a small segment of skin attached (Fig. 151-6). It is used to reconstruct an upper abdominal wall defect in one stage. With modification, the flap is useful in correction of deformities in the upper two thirds of the abdomen.[56,66-68]

Distant Composite Tissue Transfer

ANTEROLATERAL THIGH FASCIOCUTANEOUS FLAP. In 1984, Song et al[69] were the first to describe this flap

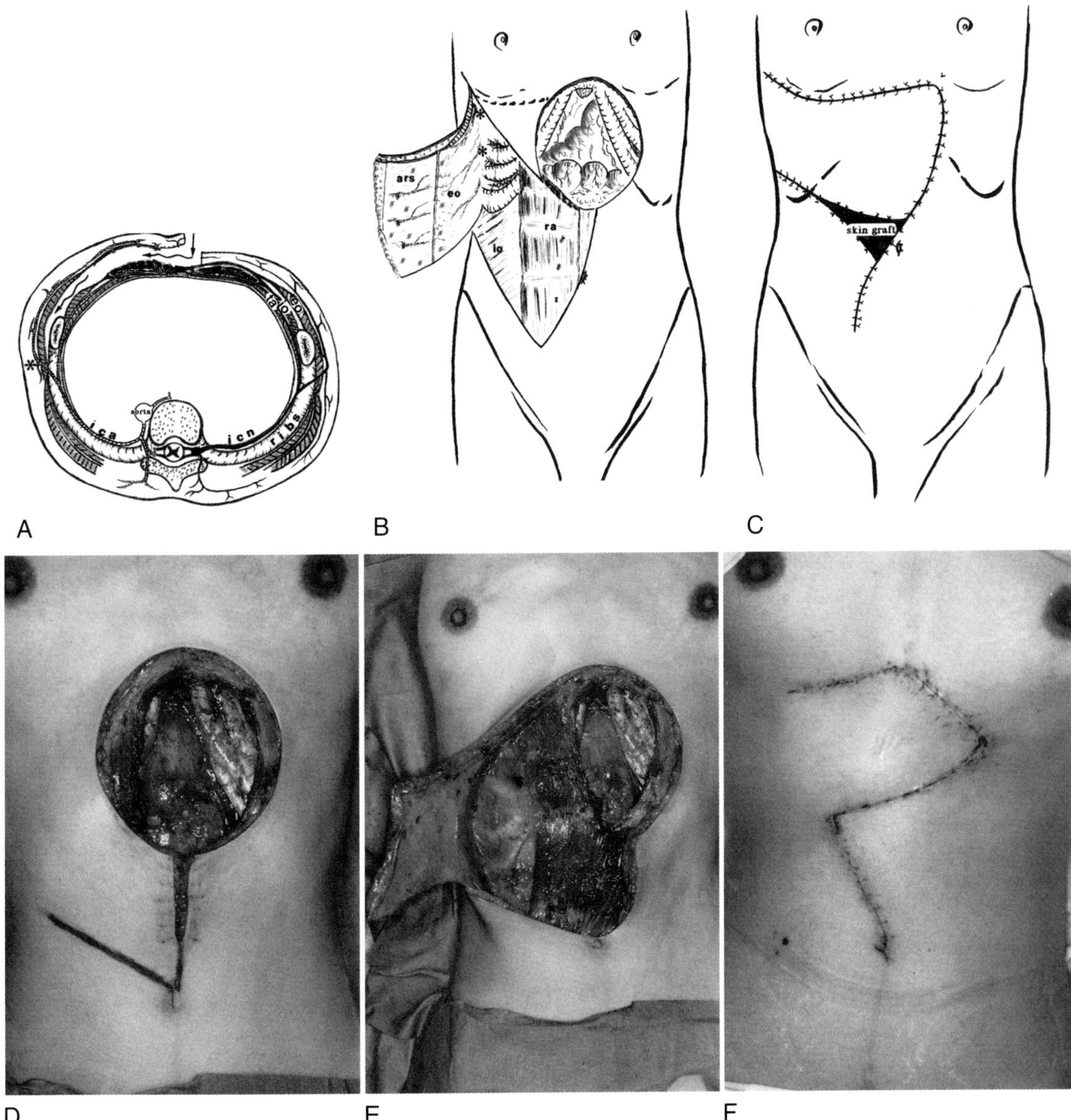

FIGURE 151-6. *A,* A schematic drawing illustrating a musculocutaneous flap designed in the anterior abdomen. The flap includes the external oblique muscle and anterior rectus sheath harvested as a single unit. eo, external oblique; ica, intercostal artery; icn, intercostal nerve; io, internal oblique; ta, transversus abdominis; *, lateral cutaneous branch. *B,* The flap is rotated cephalad. The anterior rectus sheath (ars) attached to the flap may be used to line the peritoneal surface and make up the fascial defect. eo, external oblique; io, internal oblique; ra, rectus abdominis. *C,* The donor site defect may be closed primarily or grafted with a partial-thickness skin graft. *D,* A 32-year-old woman who underwent resection of a desmoid lesion that originated in the rectus sheath. She underwent a wide area of excision that included full-thickness abdominal wall. An external oblique musculocutaneous flap was used to reconstruct the defect. *E,* The upper section of the anterior rectus sheath was included in flap fabrication. The flap was rotated cephalad to cover the defect. *F,* Appearance of the abdominal wound 3 weeks after the surgery indicated proper healing of the wound.

designed in the anterior thigh. The flap receives its blood supply from the septocutaneous branches of the transverse and descending branches of the lateral circumflex femoral artery. This flap can be transferred as a free composite flap or as a pedicled flap. According to Kimata et al,[70] it may be useful in reconstruction of large defects in the abdomen.

PEDICLED TENSOR FASCIA LATA FLAP. In 1934, Wangensteen[71] demonstrated that the tensor fascia lata flap was suitable as a pedicled flap mobilized from the lower leg to reconstruct an abdominal wall defect in 17 patients. The usefulness of this flap was confirmed 50 years later.[23,72,73]

A tensor fascia lata flap may be designed on the anterolateral aspect of the thigh as a muscle flap, a fascial flap, or a fasciocutaneous flap (Fig. 151-7). The vascular territory of a tensor fascia lata fasciocutaneous flap is believed to be quite large. It can theoretically be as large as 40 cm in length and 15 cm in width. Although the vascular supply to the muscle and fascia is believed to extend down to the patella, the vascular territory of the corresponding dermatome is much less if the graft is designed as a pedicled flap or as a fasciocutaneous flap.[23,74,75] The flap dissected as a pedicle will reach a few centimeters above the umbilicus superiorly and the midline of the abdomen medially.

Although the flap may be harvested through a long incision made in the midlateral area of the thigh, the morbidity due to a long incision has been curtailed with the use of an endoscopic technique.[76,77]

FREE TENSOR FASCIA LATA FLAP. Limitation in the arc of rotation due to excessive muscle thickness curtails the usefulness of the tensor fascia lata flap when it is dissected out as a pedicled musculocutaneous or fasciocutaneous flap. Clinical use of the flap is less predictable, furthermore, because of difficulty in ascertaining the exact amount of skin that may safely be included.

Hill et al[78] were the first to use a tensor fascia lata musculocutaneous flap, dissected as a free flap, to reconstruct leg deformities. The free tensor fascia lata flap is now commonly used to reconstruct abdominal wall defects (Fig. 151-8).[72,75,79]

COMBINED FREE TENSOR FASCIA LATA MUSCULOCUTANEOUS FLAP AND ANTEROLATERAL THIGH FLAP. A free tensor fascia lata musculocutaneous flap is not only useful for surface coverage but also effective in restoring musculofascial continuity.[20] The vascular territory of a tensor fascia lata musculocutaneous flap is said to be about 40 cm × 15 cm[73,78]; the size that can be harvested in clinical use, however, is much smaller. Limitation in the arc of rotation further restricts the use of this flap, especially if it is harvested as a pedicled composite flap to reconstruct a defect larger than 25 cm × 10 cm and in the midabdominal area.

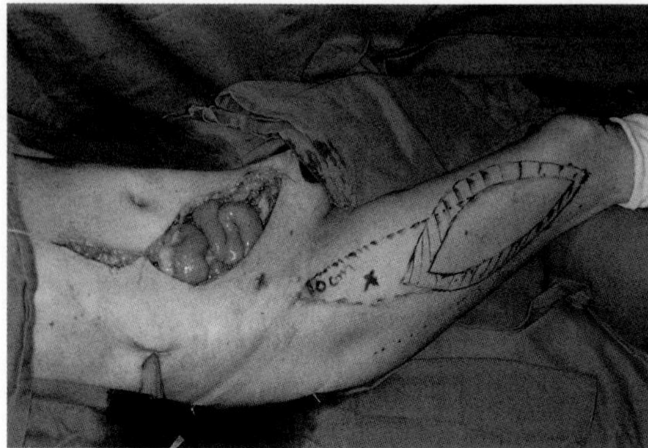

A

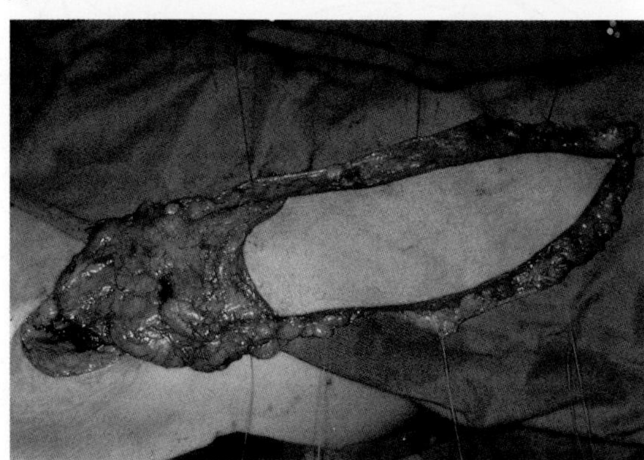

B

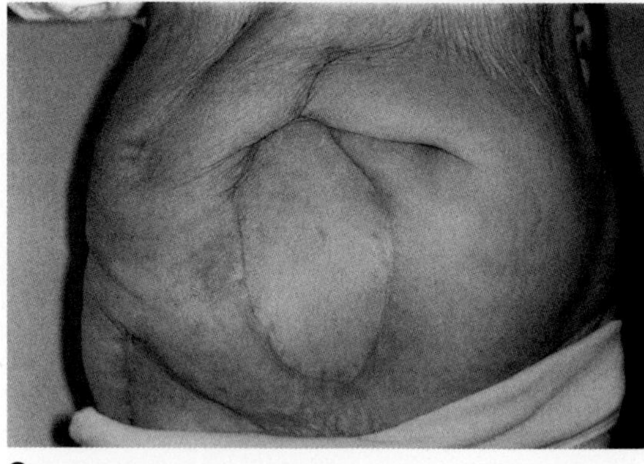

C

FIGURE 151-7. *A,* A 62-year-old woman underwent resection for a urinary bladder cancer that resulted in a full-thickness abdominal wall defect of 25 cm × 15 cm. A tensor fascia lata musculocutaneous flap, designed on the right thigh, was used to reconstruct the resultant defect. *B,* The skin paddle of 30 cm × 15 cm was left attached to the lower section of the muscle. The pedicle was sufficiently long to allow transposition of the musculocutaneous flap to cover the defect. *C,* The appearance of the wound 12 months after the surgery.

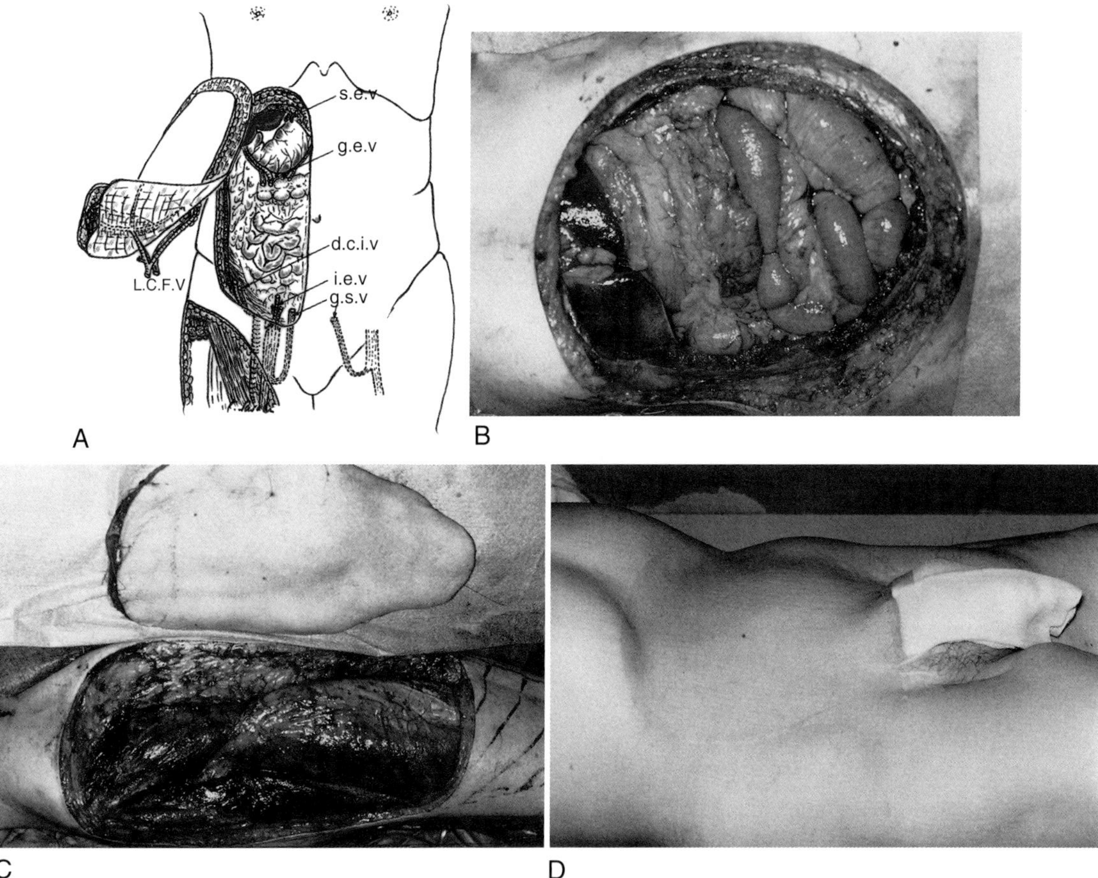

FIGURE 151-8. *A,* A limitation in the arc of rotation caused by thick muscle fibers frequently precludes the use of a tensor fascia lata musculocutaneous flap as a pedicle flap. Instead, the flap can be harvested as a free musculocutaneous flap and transferred to the recipient site by microvascular technique. The inferior epigastric artery and greater saphenous vein are the recipient vessels for the flap. dciv, deep circumflex iliac vessels; gev, gastroepiploic vessels; gsv, great saphenous vein; iev, inferior epigastric vessels; LCFV, lateral circumflex femoral vessels; sev, superior epigastric vessels. *B,* This 68-year-old woman underwent an extensive abdominal wall resection because of squamous cell carcinoma that involved the abdominal wall. A large section of the abdomen was removed. *C,* A tensor fascia lata musculocutaneous flap was harvested from the left thigh to reconstruct the wall defect. *D,* Appearance of reconstructed abdomen 4 years after the surgery.

The advent of the microsurgical technique of flap transfer has made flap transfer relatively easy and uneventful. Despite efficacy of tissue transfer by a microvascular surgical technique, flap survival can be uncertain if not incomplete. This is especially true if a segment of skin is added randomly at the periphery close to the knee area to increase flap dimension.

The skin and subcutaneous tissue in the anterolateral aspect of the upper thigh receive their blood supplies from the septocutaneous perforators of the transverse and descending branches of the lateral circumflex femoral artery. A tensor fascia lata musculocutaneous flap, in this sense, can be harvested in combination with the anterolateral thigh skin to form a composite tissue graft of 30 to 35 cm × 20 cm (Fig. 151-9*A*).

Flap Design. Flap design includes localization of arterial supplies to the proposed tensor fascia lata musculocutaneous flap and the anterolateral thigh flap. The skin pattern marked over the tensor fascia lata and the anterolateral thigh areas should coincide with the abdominal wall defect and encompass the feeding vessels to the two flaps. The tensor fascia lata muscle-iliotibial tract is included in the design of the flap because it is essential in providing strength to the fascial repair (Fig. 151-9*A* and *B*).

Technical Considerations in Flap Harvesting. The musculoseptal perforators supplying the anterolateral thigh skin (their location should be marked before surgery; Fig. 151-9*C*) are confirmed as the dissection continues cephalad. The vessels, branches of the

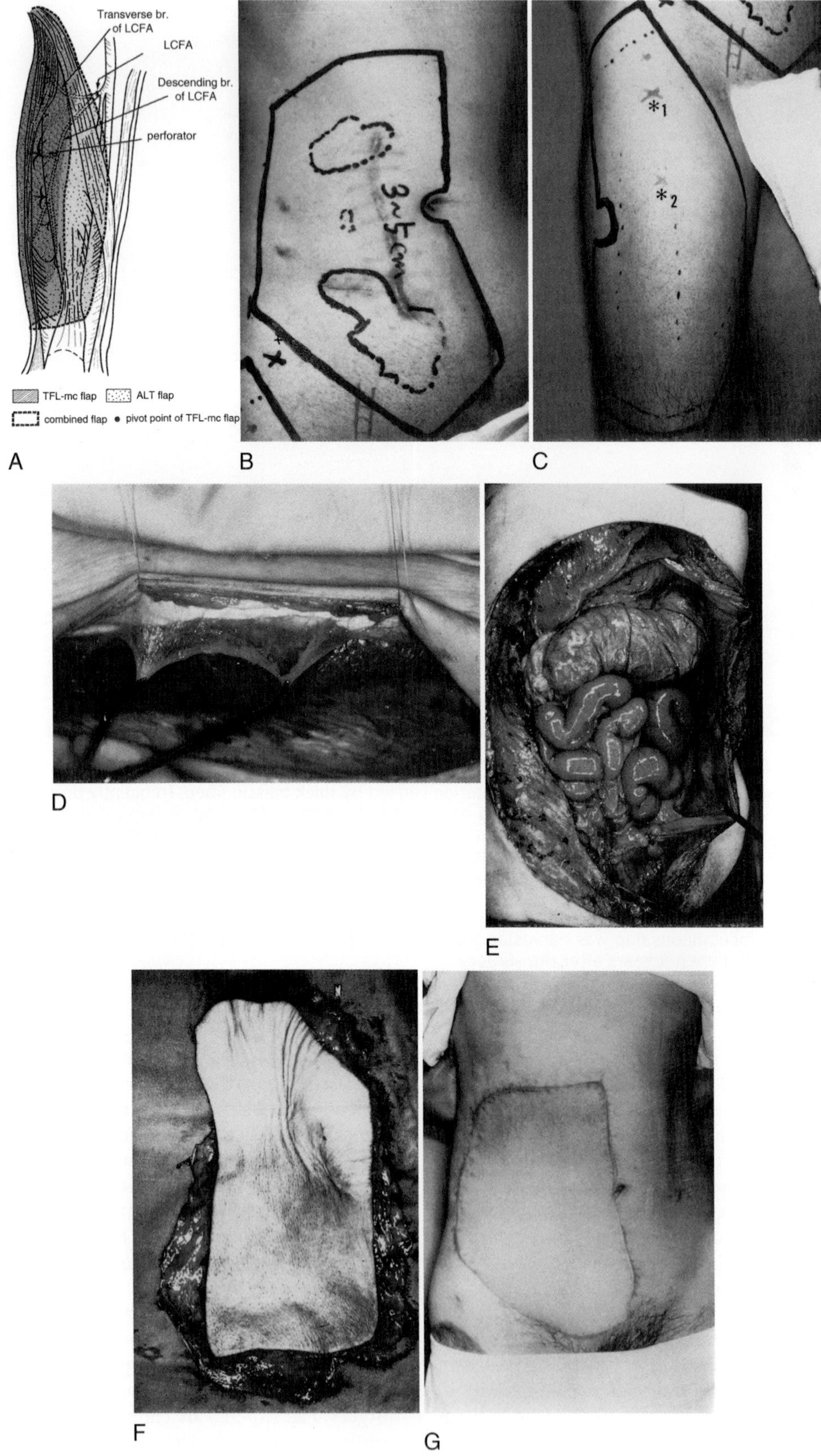
Transverse br. of LCFA
LCFA
Descending br. of LCFA
perforator
TFL-mc flap
ALT flap
combined flap
pivot point of TFL-mc flap
3~5cm
*1
*2
A
B
C
D
E
F
G

FIGURE 151-9. *A,* A schematic drawing illustrating the areas commonly designated for a tensor fascia lata musculocutaneous (TFL-mc) flap and anterolateral thigh (ALT) skin flap. The combined flap is encircled with a dotted line. LCFA, lateral circumflex femoral artery. *B,* A 37-year-old man with metastatic tumor to the abdominal wall after ileocecal resection 9 months earlier. The solid line marks the extent of abdominal wall resection. *C,* The markings indicate the area in which to harvest a flap combining a tensor fascia lata musculocutaneous flap and an anterolateral thigh flap. Skin perforator vessels of the transverse and septocutaneous perforator vessels of the descending branch of the lateral circumflex femoral artery are marked 1 and 2, respectively. *D,* Areolar tissues adherent to the undersurface of the tensor fascia lata are included in the flap. The membrane of loose connective tissues, when interposed between the fascia and the visceral peritoneum, may conceivably reduce cicatricial adhesion. *E,* A full-thickness defect of 30 to 35 cm × 20 to 25 cm resulted from tumor resection. *F,* A harvested combined flap. A fascial sleeve of 2 to 3 cm in width is included in the design of the flap for overlapping closure. *G,* The appearance of the wound 4 months after the surgery. (From Sasaki K, Nozaki M, Nakazawa H, et al: Reconstruction of a large abdominal wall defect using combined free tensor fasciae latae musculocutaneous flap and anterolateral thigh flap. Plast Reconstr Surg 1998;102:2244.)

descending branch of the lateral circumflex femoral artery, typically emerge between the rectus femoris and the vastus lateralis muscles.

The areolar tissues adherent to the undersurface of the tensor fascia lata are included in the graft (Fig. 151-9*D*). A thin membrane of areolar tissues interposed between the fascia and the visceral peritoneum serves as a shield, conceivably minimizing cicatricial adhesion between the two structures.

The superior gluteal nerve innervating the tensor fascia lata can be located in the posteroinferior aspect of the muscle. This is included in the flap dissection to provide motor function to the flap. The nerve stump is coapted with an appropriate intercostal nerve at the site of flap transfer.

The inferior epigastric, deep circumflex iliac, or gastroepiploic artery is chosen as the recipient vessel for the graft. The vena comitantes and great saphenous vein are used as the recipient veins. The proximal segment of the great saphenous vein is brought into the abdominal cavity by rerouting it beneath the inguinal ligament. Fibrin glue may be used to facilitate adhesion of the vascular pedicle against the flap to minimize the possibility of vessel injury at the anastomotic site caused by inadvertent intertwining with bowel (Fig. 151-9*E* to *G*).

RECTUS FEMORIS FLAP. In 1977, McCraw et al[80] described a technique of reconstructing a lower abdominal wall defect with a musculocutaneous flap based on the rectus femoris muscle. Ger and Duboys[19] reported a similar experience of repairing a large abdominal wall defect involving the upper abdomen. They modified the flap design by using only the muscle and fascia covering the wound to gain the length needed. The muscle and fascia were later covered with a partial-thickness skin graft. Numerous small stabbing incisions may be made in the posterior sheath to widen it to stretch the muscle and increase the width of the muscle belly.

Anatomic features of the rectus femoris muscle are sufficiently versatile to allow surgeons to use this tissue either as a musculofascial flap or as a musculofasciocutaneous flap, depending on the location and extent of the defect.[6,19,81-84] The rectus femoris flap receives its blood supply from the lateral femoral circumflex vessels. It enters into the deep surface of the muscle lateral to the sartorius muscle 6 to 8 cm below the pubis. The muscle originates in the anteroinferior iliac spine and inserts on the patellar tendon inferiorly. The primary function of this muscle is to provide 10 to 15 degrees of knee extension. Although functional impediment resulting from use of this muscle for repair is said to be significant, it can be minimized by suturing the distal end to the vastus medialis and lateralis muscles.[6]

In an attempt to elongate the flap, Dibbell et al[6] modified the dissection of this flap by extending the skin portion of the flap to the patella. This was achieved by incorporating a large "mutton chop" of the distal posterolateral iliotibial tract. This extension in the skin pedicle is sufficient to cover a defect in the upper abdomen. Although the muscle is only 6 cm in width, the accompanying fascia lata is sufficiently sturdy to cover a fascial defect of 15 to 20 cm. Despite modifications, lack of arcing mobility remains the major limiting factor when the flap is designed as a pedicled flap.

LATISSIMUS DORSI MUSCULOCUTANEOUS FLAP. The latissimus dorsi musculocutaneous flap, which receives its blood supply from the thoracodorsal vessels, can be harvested either as a pedicled flap or as a free flap. The flap is useful in reconstruction of any defect in the upper lateral abdomen. As a pedicled flap, the extent of mobilization may be limited because of the arc of flap rotation.[85] It is suitable to reconstruct a defect in the upper lateral abdomen, especially when mobilization of conventional flaps from the abdomen or the upper thigh areas is not feasible.

The arc of rotation and the area of coverage for this flap may be increased by incorporating the lumbar dorsal and pregluteal fascia into the flap design.[85] Viability of the skin in the extended area, however, remains uncertain.

In 1979, Bostwick et al[86] reported the use of this flap, dissected out as a free composite flap and transferred by microvascular technique, to repair a large abdominal wall defect. Almost 2 decades later, Ninkovic et al[21] reported their experience in use of the same flap as an innervated flap to provide dynamic restoration of abdominal wall function.

GRACILIS MUSCULOCUTANEOUS FLAP. The gracilis muscle is a thin, narrow, expendable muscle. It tapers into a tendinous extension distally. The gracilis musculocutaneous flap receives its blood supply from the medial circumflex femoral vessels. This flap may be used to repair a defect in the lower third of the abdomen. The vascular territory of the skin overlying the distal segment of the muscle is uncertain.[87]

Postoperative Care

Proper metabolic, hemodynamic, and nutritional status of patients must be maintained throughout the recovery phase of injury and reconstruction. A physiotherapy program is instituted as soon as possible to regain muscle strength.

An effective plan to manage an abdominal wall defect requires that the surgeon have a full grasp of the problems involved. The surgical treatment is made effective only if it is executed properly and based on sound principles of surgical anatomy, physiology, and nutrition.

Clinical Experience

Between 1986 and 2000, various techniques of abdominal wall reconstruction were used in treatment of 44 patients with abdominal wall defect at the Tokyo Women's Medical University (Table 151-3). The tensor fascia lata musculocutaneous flap, dissected as a pedicled flap, was used more frequently during the early years of reporting. Partial necrosis of the flap was encountered in four individuals. The subsequent fascial defect resulted as hernia or bulging of the abdominal wall in seven patients. The use of microvascular transfer technique in recent years appears to have ameliorated the problems of flap necrosis and structural weakening of the reconstructed site. Of six instances of tensor fascia lata musculocutaneous flaps, with or without an anterior thigh flap attached, used to reconstruct various abdominal wall defects, no complications were encountered. Microvascular techniques for flap transfer, although indications may vary, are therefore the most reliable means of tissue transfer.

Although the use of tensor fascia lata musculocutaneous flaps has decreased the need for fascia or alloplastic materials to provide fascial support, a free fascial graft and an alloplastic mesh were used for indicated patients. Outcomes indicate that an alloplastic mesh may provide structural strength superior to that of autologous fascia. However, infection may be a problem. Infection occurred in two of nine patients in whom alloplastic materials were used to provide fascial support to the abdominal wall defect.

Algorithmic Approach to Abdominal Wall Reconstruction

The following regimen is recommended.

PREOPERATIVE EVALUATION OF THE PATIENT. Understanding the cause leading to an abdominal wall defect, assessing the extent of structural involvement, and evaluating the metabolic status of the patient are

TABLE 151-3 ✦ THE TECHNIQUES USED TO RECONSTRUCT THE ADBOMINAL WALL DEFECT (>7 cm) AT TOKYO WOMEN'S MEDICAL UNIVERSITY BETWEEN 1986 AND 2000

		No. of Patients with Various Complications Encountered					
Technique	No. of Patients	*Flap Tip Necrosis*	*Infection*	*Fistula*	*Seroma*	*Hernia*	*Abdominal Wall Weakening*
Pedicled TFL MC flap	12	4				3	4
Free flap							
TFL MC flap + ALT flap	4						
TFL MC flap	2						
LD MC flap	1						
Rectus abdominis MC flap	4						
External oblique MC flap	2						
Groin flap	2						
Free fascial graft	8					2	4
Alloplastic prosthesis							
Marlex mesh	6			1		1	
Gore-Tex mesh	3		2		2		
Total	44	4	2	1	2	6	8

ALT flap, anterolateral thigh skin flap; LD MC flap, latissimus dorsi musculocutaneous flap; TFL MC flap, tensor fascia lata musculocutaneous flap.

the three most important factors in formulating the regimen of treatment. The information concerning the cause of the abdominal wall defect is needed to form the surgical plan; the status of the wound and metabolic status of the patient are extremely important in deciding the priority in management.

PREOPERATIVE MANAGEMENT OF THE PATIENT. The metabolic and nutritional regimen of treatment should aim to correct nutritional abnormalities and blood volume deficit before and after surgery. Whereas medical treatment of infection is essential, early surgical intervention may be necessary to control wound sepsis. Bacteriologic assessment of an open wound is therefore an essential and integral part of the care regimen.

SURGICAL TREATMENT. The surgical treatment regimen varies according to status of the patient and the wound. Grafting of the wound with a partial-thickness skin graft is useful for wound control in individuals whose general condition precludes an elaborate reconstructive procedure. That is, definitive closure of the wound or reconstruction of the wall defect is considered only if the patient's metabolic, hemodynamic, and nutritional status is proper and the patient is able to withstand surgical intervention.

The surgical approach to correction of a wall defect, in practice, is governed by the extent of tissue loss as well as by the size and location of the defect.

Defect ≤ 7 cm

1. Soft tissue loss only. The wound can frequently be closed primarily. Skin grafting is strongly recommended as an initial step for wound control, especially for a contaminated wound. The scarred area is managed secondarily once the patient's condition improves. The technique of tissue expansion may be included.
2. Soft tissue and musculofascial loss. In addition to soft tissue replacement, the fascial defect should be repaired to restore structural integrity of the abdominal wall. Autologous fascial graft or alloplastic mesh and a local flap or musculocutaneous flap mobilized from the adjacent area may be used for wound closure. The exact technique of reconstruction may vary, depending on the location of the defect.
   - Upper abdomen. The component musculoaponeurotic flap of the internal and external oblique muscles or the latissimus dorsi musculocutaneous flap is useful.
   - Midabdomen. The component musculoaponeurotic flap of the internal and external oblique muscles or the vertical rectus abdominis musculocutaneous flap is useful. The iliolumbar skin flap is useful for a wound in the lateral aspect of the midabdomen.
   - Lower abdomen. The component musculoaponeurotic flap, the vertical rectus abdominis musculocutaneous flap, the tensor fascia lata musculocutaneous flap, the anterior thigh flap, and the rectus femoris musculocutaneous flap are useful.

Defect > 7 cm

1. Soft tissue loss *without* musculofascial loss. Despite the size of defect, the initial approach should be autologous skin grafting for wound control. The tissue expansion technique is useful as a secondary procedure for scarred tissue removal. A skin flap harvested from an adjacent area may be considered if the extent of soft tissue loss is extensive.
2. Soft tissue loss *with* musculofascial loss. The exact technique of wound coverage and wall defect reconstruction is governed by the location of the defect. The choice of flap that can be harvested as a pedicled flap is limited. Transfer of a flap designed and harvested as a composite flap therefore requires the use of microvascular surgical technique.
   - Upper abdomen. The lower vertical rectus abdominis musculocutaneous flap and the latissimus dorsi musculocutaneous flap harvested as a pedicled flap may be used. The tensor fascia lata musculocutaneous flap with or without concomitant inclusion of the anterior thigh skin flap transferred by microsurgical technique may be considered if the defect is large.
   - Midabdomen. The musculoaponeurotic component technique of wound closure may be useful in patients in whom the defect is limited to 12 to 15 cm. The lower vertical rectus abdominis musculocutaneous flap may be used to cover the defect. A large defect will require the use of tensor fascia lata musculocutaneous flap with or without concomitant inclusion of the anterior thigh flap. Transference by microsurgical technique is preferred.
   - Lower abdomen. The use of musculocutaneous flaps that can be mobilized from the lower extremity should be considered. A large defect will require the tensor fascia lata musculocutaneous flap with or without concomitant inclusion of the anterior thigh flap. Transference by microsurgical technique is the method of choice if the defect is large.

SUMMARY

The structural integrity of the abdominal wall is frequently altered by direct trauma or surgical intervention because of trauma, infection, or cancer extirpation.

Deformity of the abdominal wall can impair physical movements such as walking, bending, and maintenance of body posture. Abdominal wall defects may also impair physiologic activities such as coughing, sneezing, defecation, and micturition.

Although the objective of reconstructing an abdominal wall deformity is centered on restoration of abdominal wall continuity, the formulated procedure must include a comprehensive plan of preoperative and postoperative care of the patient and aim toward restoration of abdominal structural integrity.

REFERENCES

1. Schmitt HJ, Grinnon GL: Use of Marlex mesh in infected abdominal wall wounds. Am J Surg 1967;113:825.
2. Gottlieb JR, Engrav LH, Walkinshaw MD, et al: Upper abdominal wall defects: immediate or staged reconstruction? Plast Reconstr Surg 1990;86:281.
3. Cormack GC, Quaba AA: Bilobed modification of the deep inferior epigastric artery flap for abdominal wall defect reconstruction. Br J Plast Surg 1991;44:541.
4. Fabian TC, Croce MA, Pritchard FE, et al: Planned ventral hernia: staged management for acute abdominal wall defects. Ann Surg 1994;219:643.
5. Argenta LC, Morykwas MJ: Vacuum-assisted closure: a new method for wound control and treatment: clinical experience. Ann Plast Surg 1997;38:563.
6. Dibbell DJ, Mixter RC, Dibbell DS: Abdominal wall reconstruction (the "mutton chop" flap). Plast Reconstr Surg 1991; 87:60.
7. Lejour M, Dome M: Abdominal wall function after rectus abdominis transfer. Plast Reconstr Surg 1991;87:1054.
8. Mizgala CL, Hartrampf CR, Bennett GK: Assessment of the abdominal wall after pedicled TRAM flap surgery: 5- to 7-year follow up of 150 consecutive patients. Plast Reconstr Surg 1994;93:988.
9. Disa JJ, Goldberg NH, Carlton JM, et al: Restoring abdominal wall integrity in contaminated tissue deficient wounds using autologous fascial graft. Plast Reconstr Surg 1998;101:979.
10. Moscona RA, Ramon Y, Toledano H, et al: Use of synthetic mesh for the entire abdominal wall after TRAM flap transfer. Plast Reconstr Surg 1998;101:706.
11. Chen L, Hartrampf CR, Bennett GK: Successful pregnancies following TRAM flap surgery. Plast Reconstr Surg 1993;91:69.
12. Randolph J, Cavett C, Eng G: Surgical correction and rehabilitation for children with "prune belly" syndrome. Ann Surg 1981;193:757.
13. Blondeel N, Boeckx WD, Vanderstraeten GG, et al: The fate of the oblique abdominal muscles after free TRAM flap surgery. Br J Plast Surg 1997;50:315.
14. Blondeel N, Vanderstraeten GG, Monstrey SJ: The donor site morbidity of free DIEP flaps and free TRAM flap for breast reconstruction. Br J Plast Surg 1997;50:322.
15. Toranto IR: Resolution of back pain with the wide abdominal rectus plication abdominoplasty. Plast Reconstr Surg 1988;81:777.
16. Ramirez OM, Ruas E, Dellon AL: "Component separation" method for closure of abdominal-wall defects: an anatomic and clinical study. Plast Reconstr Surg 1990;86:519.
17. Pless TK, Pless JE: Giant ventral hernias and their repair. A 10-year follow-up study. Scand J Plast Reconstr Surg Hand Surg 1993;27:311.
18. Hobar PC, Rohrich RJ, Byrd HS: Abdominal-wall reconstruction with expanded musculofascial tissue in a post-traumatic defect. Plast Reconstr Surg 1994;94:379.
19. Ger R, Duboys E: The prevention and repair of large abdominal wall defects by muscle transposition: a preliminary communication. Plast Reconstr Surg 1983;72:170.
20. Sasaki K, Nozaki M, Nakazawa H, et al: Reconstruction of a large abdominal wall defect using combined free tensor fasciae latae musculocutaneous flap and anterolateral thigh flap. Plast Reconstr Surg 1998;102:2244.
21. Ninkovic M, Kronberger P, Harpf C, et al: Free innervated latissimus dorsi musculocutaneous flap for reconstruction of full-thickness abdominal wall defects. Plast Reconstr Surg 1998;101:971.
22. Mathes SJ, Buchanan RT: Tensor fasciae latae: neurosensory musculocutaneous free flap. Br J Plast Surg 1979;32:184.
23. O'Hare PM, Leonard AG: Reconstruction of major abdominal wall defects using the tensor fasciae latae myocutaneous flap. Br J Plast Surg 1982;35:361.
24. Koshy CE, Kumar MV, Evans J: Lower abdominal wall reconstruction using the anterior thigh fasciocutaneous flap. Br J Plast Surg 1999;52:667.
25. Rayner CR: Repair of full-thickness defects of the abdominal wall in rats avoiding visceral adhesions. Br J Plast Surg 1974;27:130.
26. Matloub HS, Jensen P, Grunert BK, et al: Characteristics of prosthetic mesh and autologous fascia in abdominal wall reconstruction after prolonged implantation. Ann Plast Surg 1992;29:508.
27. Mansberger A, Kang JS, Beebe HJ, et al: Repair of massive acute abdominal wall defects. J Trauma 1973;13:766.
28. Lowe JB, Garza LR, Bowman JL, et al: Endoscopically assisted "components separation" for closure of abdominal wall defects. Plast Reconstr Surg 2000;105:720.
29. Thomas WO, Parry SW, Rodning CB: Ventral/incisional abdominal herniorrhaphy by fascial partition/release. Plast Reconstr Surg 1993;91:1080.
30. Dibello JN, Moore JH: Sliding myofascial flap of the rectus abdominis muscles for the closure of recurrent ventral hernias. Plast Reconstr Surg 1996;98:464.
31. Girotto JA, Ko MJ, Redett R, et al: Closure of chronic abdominal wall defects: a long-term evaluation of the components separation method. Ann Plast Surg 1999;42:385.
32. Argenta LC, Marks MW, Pasyk KA: Advances in tissue expansion. Clin Plast Surg 1985;12:159.
33. Livingston D, Sharma P, Galntz A: Tissue expanders for abdominal wall reconstruction following severe trauma: technical note and case report. J Trauma 1992;32:82.
34. Okuski WL, Sonntag BV, Murphy RX: Staged reconstruction of abdominal wall defects after intra-abdominal catastrophes. Ann Plast Surg 1996;36:475.
35. Paletta CF, Huang DB, Dehghan K, Kelly C: The use of tissue expanders in staged abdominal wall reconstruction. Ann Plast Surg 1999;42:259.
36. Carlson GW, Elwood E, Loskin A, et al: The role of tissue expansion in abdominal reconstruction. Ann Plast Surg 2000;44:147.
37. Byrd HS, Hobar G: Abdominal wall expansion in congenital defects. Plast Reconstr Surg 1989;84:347.
38. Jacobsen WM, Potty PM, Bite U, et al: Massive abdominal wall hernia reconstruction with expanded external/internal oblique and transversalis musculofascia. Plast Reconstr Surg 1997; 100:326.
39. Millard R, Pigott R, Zies P: Free skin grafting of full-thickness defects of abdominal wall. Plast Reconstr Surg 1969;43: 569.
40. Mladick RA, Pickrell KL, Royer JR, et al: Skin graft reconstruction of a massive full-thickness abdominal wall defect. Plast Reconstr Surg 1969;43:587.
41. Horton C, Georgiade N, Campbell F, et al: The behaviors of split thickness and dermal skin grafts in peritoneal cavity: an experimental study. Plast Reconstr Surg 1953;12:269.

42. Dumanian GA, Llull R, Ramasastry SS, et al: Postoperative abdominal wall defects with enterocutaneous fistulae. Am J Surg 1996;172:332.
43. Hamilton JE: The repair of large or difficult hernias with mattressed onlay grafts of fascia lata: a 21-year experience. Ann Surg 1968;167:85.
44. Shaw WW, Aston SJ, Zide SM: Reconstruction of the trunk. In McCarthy JG, ed: Plastic Surgery. Philadelphia, WB Saunders, 1990:3755.
45. Eaves FF, Price CI, Bostwick J, et al: Subcutaneous endoscopic plastic surgery using a retractor-mounted endoscope system. Perspect Plast Surg 1993;7:1.
46. Voyles CR, Richardson JD, Bland KI, et al: Emergency abdominal wall reconstruction with polypropylene mesh: short term benefits versus long term complications. Ann Surg 1981;194:219.
47. Brown GL, Richardson JD, Malangoni MA, et al: Comparison of prosthetic materials for abdominal wall reconstruction in the presence of contamination and infection. Ann Surg 1985;201:705.
48. Bloom WF, Koops HS, Vermey A, et al: Abdominal wall resection and reconstruction with the aid of Marlex mesh. Br J Surg 1982;69:1982.
49. Mathes SJ, Steinwald PM, Foster RD, et al: Complex abdominal wall reconstruction: a comparison of flap and mesh closure. Ann Surg 2000;232:586.
50. Bleinchrodt RP, Simmermacher RK, van der Lei B, et al: Expanded polytetrafluoroethylene patch versus polypropylene mesh for the repair of contaminated defects of the abdominal wall. Surg Gynecol Obstet 1993;176:18.
51. Mathes SJ, McGrath MH, Nance FC, O'Leary JP: Symposium: abdominal wall reconstruction. Contemp Surg 1999;54:238.
52. Bogart JN, Rowe DS, Parsons RW: Immediate abdominal wall reconstruction with bilateral groin flaps after resection of a large desmoid tumor: case report. Plast Reconstr Surg 1976;58:716.
53. Earle AS, Blackburn WW: Closure of an abdominal hernia with a groin flap lined with a dermal graft. Plast Reconstr Surg 1975;56:447.
54. Sasaki S, Soeda S, Uchida A, et al: Use of a combined groin-tensor fasciae latae flap for reconstruction of a full-thickness defect of the abdominal wall. Br J Plast Surg 1985;38:492.
55. Terashi H, Hashimoto H, Takayasu S, et al: Use of groin flap and anterolateral thigh adipofascial flap of tensor fasciae latae for reconstruction of a wide lower abdominal wall defect. Ann Plast Surg 1995;35:320.
56. Iwahira Y, Maruyama Y, Shiba T: One stage abdominal wall reconstruction with oblique abdominal fasciocutaneous flaps. Ann Plast Surg 1992;19:475.
57. Ohtsuka, H, Ochi K, Seike H: Reconstruction of a large lateral abdominal defect with an ilio-lumbar bi-pedicled flap. Br J Plast Surg 1984;37:327.
58. Mathes SJ, Bostwick J: A rectus abdominis myocutaneous flap to reconstruct abdominal wall defects. Br J Plast Surg 1977; 30:282.
59. Bostwick J, Hill HL, Nahai F: Repairs in the lower abdomen, groin, or perineum with myocutaneous or omental flaps. Plast Reconstr Surg 1979;63:186.
60. Parkash S, Palepu J: Rectus abdominis myocutaneous flap: clinical experience with ipsilateral and contralateral flaps. Br J Surg 1983;70:68.
61. Taylor GI, Corltee R, Boyd JB: The extended deep inferior epigastric flap: a clinical technique. Plast Reconstr Surg 1983;72:751.
62. Gottlieb ME, Chandrasekhar B, Terz JJ, et al: Clinical applications of the extended deep inferior epigastric flap. Plast Reconstr Surg 1986;78:782.
63. Vasconez HC, Sengezer M, MacGrath P: Flap coverage of a large defect after excision of a massive dermatofibrosarcoma protuberance. Plast Reconstr Surg 1995;95:136.
64. DeFranzo AJ, Kingman GJ, Sterchi JM, et al: Rectus turnover flaps for the reconstruction of large abdominal wall defects. Ann Plast Surg 1996;37:18.
65. Hershey FB, Butcher HR: Repair of defects after partial resection of the abdominal wall. Am J Surg 1964;107:586.
66. Fisher J: External oblique fasciocutaneous flap for elbow coverage. Plast Reconstr Surg 1985;75:51.
67. Meland NB, Ivy EJ, Wood JE: Coverage of chest wall and pelvic defects with external oblique musculocutaneous flap. Ann Plast Surg 1988;21:297.
68. Bogossian N, Chaglassian T, Rosenberg PH, et al: External oblique myocutaneous flap coverage of large chest-wall defects following resection of breast tumors. Plast Reconstr Surg 1996;97:97.
69. Song YG, Chen GZ, Song YL: The free thigh flap: a new free flap concept based on the septocutaneous artery. Br J Plast Surg 1984;37:149.
70. Kimata Y, Uchiyama K, Sekido M, et al: Anterolateral thigh flap for abdominal wall reconstruction. Plast Reconstr Surg 1999;103:1191.
71. Wangensteen H: Repair of recurrent and different hernias and other large defects of abdominal wall employing the iliotibial tract of fascia lata as a pedicled flap. Surg Gynecol Obstet 1934;59:766.
72. Caffee HH: Reconstruction of the abdominal wall by variations of the tensor fasciae latae flap. Plast Reconstr Surg 1983;71: 348.
73. Nahai F, Hill L, Hester TR: Experience with the tensor fascia lata flap. Plast Reconstr Surg 1979;63:788.
74. Williams JK, Carlson GW, Howell RL, et al: The tensor fascia lata free flap in abdominal wall reconstruction. J Reconstr Microsurg 1997;13:83.
75. Williams JK, Carlson GW, de Chalain T, et al: Role of tensor fasciae latae in abdominal wall reconstruction. Plast Reconstr Surg 1998;101:713.
76. Onishi K, Maruyama Y, Yakata M: Endoscopic harvest of tensor fasciae latae muscle flap. Br J Plast Surg 1997;50:58.
77. Kara IG, Erdem E, Nessar M, et al: Reconstruction of large abdominal wall defects. Eur J Plast Surg 1999;22:394.
78. Hill HL, Nahai F, Vasconez LO: The tensor fascia lata myocutaneous free flap. Plast Reconstr Surg 1978;61:517.
79. Sekido M, Yamamoto Y, Sugihara T, et al: Microsurgical reconstruction of chest and abdominal wall defects associated with intraperitoneal vessels. J Reconstr Microsurg 1996;12:425.
80. McCraw JB, Dibbell DG, Carraway JH: Clinical definition of independent myocutaneous vascular territories. Plast Reconstr Surg 1977;60:341.
81. Bhagwat BM, Pearl RM, Laub DR: Uses of the rectus femoris myocutaneous flap. Plast Reconstr Surg 1978;62:698.
82. Caulfield WH, Curtsinger L, Powell G, et al: Donor leg morbidity after pedicled rectus femoris muscle flap transfer for abdominal wall and pelvic reconstruction. Ann Plast Surg 1994;32:377.
83. Freedman AM, Gayle LB, Vaughan ED, Hoffman LA: One-stage repair of the anterior abdominal wall using bilateral rectus femoris myocutaneous flap. Ann Plast Surg 1990;25:299.
84. Peters W, Cartotto R, Morris S, et al: The rectus femoris myocutaneous flap for closure of difficult wounds of the abdomen, groin, and trochanteric areas. Ann Plast Surg 1991;26:572.
85. Houston GC, Drew GS, Vasquez B, et al: The extended latissimus dorsi flap in repair of anterior abdominal wall defects. Plast Reconstr Surg 1988;81:917.
86. Bostwick J, Nahai F, Wallace JG, et al: Sixty latissimus dorsi flaps. Plast Reconstr Surg 1979;63:31.
87. Venugopalan S: Repair of midline abdominal incisional hernia by gracilis muscle transfer. Br J Plast Surg 1980;33:43.

CHAPTER

152

Reconstruction of Male Genital Defects: Congenital and Acquired

DAVID A. GILBERT, MD, FRCSC, FACS ✦ GERALD H. JORDAN, MD, FACS

Male genital reconstruction has enjoyed a renaissance in the past 25 years, and it is important that plastic surgery continue to maintain a prominent presence in this evolution. Plastic surgery techniques and traditions have expanded the reconstructive armamentarium of all who aim to repair genital defects, particularly in the context of a genitourinary reconstructive team including plastic surgeons, urologists, colorectal surgeons, gynecologists, and orthopedic surgeons. The essence of a reconstructive team is reflected in this chapter, which is the collaborative work of a plastic surgeon and a urologist.

Microsurgical instrumentation and techniques have been applied to genitourinary reconstruction. Who would have ever conceptualized the use of a forearm flap to help repair or replace an absent penis 30 years ago? Today, microsurgical composite tissue transplantation has made total penile reconstruction a state-of-the-art procedure. However, microsurgery still has a more limited use in the field of genital reconstruction compared with extremity reconstruction. As a result, there are limited reports of microsurgical applications in genital reconstruction and relatively few large or sustained series. In fact, it is refreshing to hear of successful applications of microsurgery and other techniques for challenging reconstructions. Recent experience in microsurgical hypospadias repair has demonstrated that microsurgical magnification and instrumentation contributed to a significant improvement in surgical results.[1] Genital replantation surgery,[2,3] testicular autotransplantation,[4-6] and penile revascularization[7] have all benefited from the application of microsurgical principles. Finally, the use of microsurgery for total "phallic" construction represents an area of unprecedented improvement in form and function, which might be genital microsurgery's greatest legacy at present.[8]

On an independent but parallel path, new local and regional flaps were designed or adapted for genital reconstruction. Led by McCraw,[9] many plastic surgeons described new flaps that were successfully applied to genital reconstruction. Musculocutaneous, fasciocutaneous, and muscle flaps were recognized on the basis of body angiosomes[10] and localization of vascular pedicles to the cutaneous territories. As microsurgical techniques and musculocutaneous principles developed—often parallel, sometimes combined—the applications to genital surgery seemed limitless. In fact, the formation of the Society of Genitourinary Reconstructive Surgeons recruited surgeons from many surgical specialties with a common interest in this field. To accomplish successful genital reconstruction, the surgeon must have a thorough understanding of the following areas: (1) scope and anatomy of congenital and acquired genital deformities, (2) reconstructive options, and (3) past and current techniques that may be used to accomplish reconstructive goals.

GENITAL EMBRYOLOGY

Genetic Sex

Genetic sex of the embryo is established at conception. The ovum, containing 22 autosomes and an X chromosome, is penetrated by one of the surrounding spermatozoa, half of which have an X chromosome and the other half of which have a Y chromosome. The sperm donates either an X or Y chromosome, thereby establishing genetic sexual assignment.

The embryos of both sexes develop identically for approximately 6 weeks of gestation, known as the indifferent stage. During this time, the embryo becomes tubularized as the primitive gut is formed to terminate in the cloacal membrane. At the sixth week, the urorectal septum begins to grow downward and inward from the sides into the cloacal cavity, thereby separating the cloaca into the bladder and rectum.

Externally, a mound of mesoderm with a midline groove develops cephalocaudal to the cloacal membrane. This is known as the indifferent genital tubercle. As the midline mesenchyme progressively fuses in a caudal direction from the umbilicus, the genital primordia fuse to form a genital eminence.

Gonadal Sex

Gonadal sex (differentiated stage) begins at the seventh week of intrauterine life. Evidence suggests that a locus on the Y chromosome (H-Y antigen) induces testicular development by causing differentiation of the seminiferous tubules. There are three endocrine hormones produced that explain the male differentiation. The first is müllerian-inhibiting factor produced transiently by the Sertoli cells in the seminiferous tubules, causing regression of the müllerian duct system (9 to 11 weeks). At the same time, Leydig cells in the seminiferous tubules begin to produce a hormone analogous to testosterone. Testosterone plays two roles: (1) completion of maturation of the seminiferous tubules, epididymis, vas deferens, and seminal vesicles and (2) extratesticular male development by irreversible reduction to dihydrotestosterone made possible by the enzyme 5α-reductase. Dihydrotestosterone is responsible for the virilization of the external genitalia and the anterior urethra.

Phenotypic Sex

Phenotypic sex is "determined" by whether the genital tubercle develops into a male or female pattern. In the male, urogenital swellings migrate ventrally and anteriorly to form the scrotum. The genital tubercle develops by elongation and cylindrical growth. At the same time, urethral folds close over the urethral groove, thereby establishing a urethra and a midline raphe. Mesenchymal tissue coalesces to surround the urethra and form the corpus spongiosum. This development is entirely under the influence (or absence) of testosterone, testosterone derivatives (i.e., dihydrotestosterone), and 5α-reductase and occurs between 6 and 13 weeks of gestation (Fig. 152-1). The prepuce grows to cover the penile glans but is not influenced by dihydrotestosterone.

In the female embryo, the lack of testosterone-influenced virilization holds the urogenital sinus and the genital tubercle in a fixed perineal position. The urethral groove remains unclosed (folds develop into labia minora), and the genital tubercle remains static in size but bends ventrally. The labia majora enlarge, migrate caudally, and fuse to form the posterior fourchette. It is this lack of closure of the ventral urethra (a "nonevent") that causes the female perineum to be shorter and the introitus to be located in a more caudal position.

GENITAL ANATOMY

Male genital anatomy is unique in the human body and evolved phylogenetically as a means of protection from trauma and disease. This evolution has proved essential for the human race to continue procreation and elimination. The expression "anatomy is destiny" is more poignant here than in any other anatomic system.

Genital Fascia

Perhaps the most obvious protective mechanism is the testicular (and penile) withdrawal on exposure to "fight or flight" stresses. Physical stress, such as hypothermia or blunt trauma, causes the unique cremasteric muscles to contract, thereby withdrawing the testicles and shrinking the scrotum as close to the body as possible. Otherwise, the testicles hang free, ostensibly to provide the best milieu for sperm development. At the same time, the penile corporal bodies and the urethra also retract and shrink in size, although the penile skin

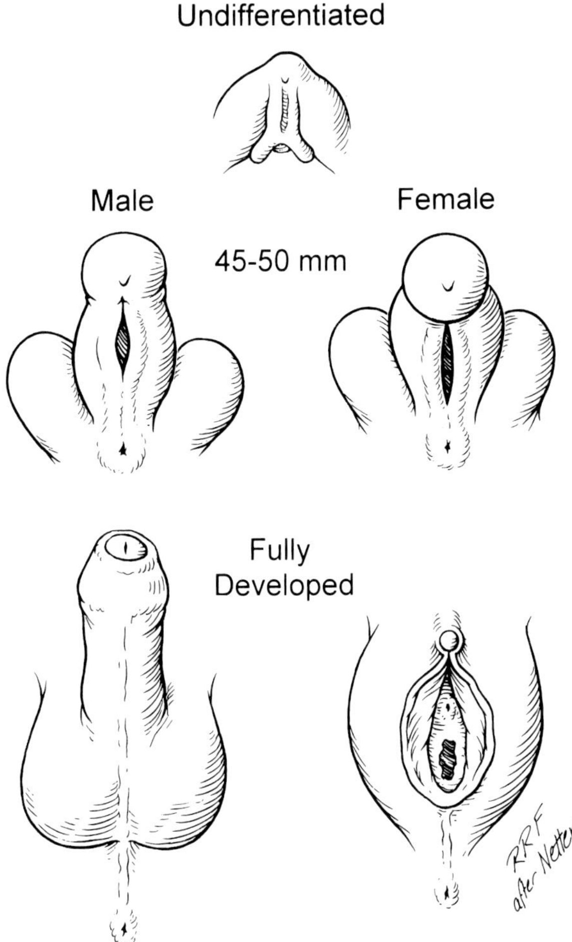

FIGURE 152-1. The definitive phenotypic external genital growth that occurs in utero under the influence (or absence) of testosterone, dihydrotestosterone, and 5α-reductase. The influence of these virilizing hormones causes the genital tubercle to enlarge, the urethral folds to meet and close ventrally, and the scrotum to migrate medially and posteriorly. Any hormone deficit or receptor site inadequacy leads to an external female genitalia tendency ("phenotype by default").

does not have the same retraction properties that the scrotal skin does. Both the penis and the scrotum have redundant skin coverage with their own separate blood supply and underlying supportive superficial fascial system.

The penis contains specially designed tunical tissues that surround the penile corporal bodies and have the ability to expand and hold the inflow of blood and to prevent, along with venous valve mechanisms, the egress of blood during erections. The tunica albuginea fascia envelops the corporal bodies tightly but is perforated by an intercavernosal membranous septum that allows blood flow between the corpora cavernosa. The tunical tissues are thick over the dorsal and lateral aspects of each corporal body but thin out in the ventral sulcus where the urethra and corpus spongiosum are located. The tunica also thins out beneath the glans penis cap where it has direct vascular contact with the glans.

Overlying the tunica is the deep penile fascia (Buck fascia), a strong laminar structure that tightly surrounds and binds the corpora cavernosa together and, in the case of the corpus spongiosum, envelops these tissues into a single-functioning entity. The urethra and its overlying corpus spongiosum are also protected proximally by surrounding muscles and by their location within the intercorporal groove distally. Buck fascia carries important neurovascular structures to the glans penis, including the deep dorsal vein and arteries, the deep dorsal nerves of the penis, the circumflex arteries and veins, and the penile lymphatics (Fig. 152-2).[11]

The penile glans itself is a vascular spongiosum containing unique sensory endings that are erogenous and tactile. The glans epithelium is a unique uroepithelium that contains sensory cells, particularly around the corona. The glans is naturally covered and protected by a prepuce that consists of inner and outer laminae. The inner lamina consists of uroepithelium that is similar to that of the glans and, in fact, developmentally separates from the glans in the last trimester and after birth. The outer lamina consists of epithelium that is consistent with the glabrous skin of the penile shaft. Superficial to Buck fascia but beneath the penile shaft skin and prepuce lies the superficial fascial system, defined by dartos fascia. This fascial layer is a continuation of the Scarpa fascia superiorly and the Colles fascia inferiorly and surrounds the penis from the penoscrotal and penopubic angles to the prepuce.

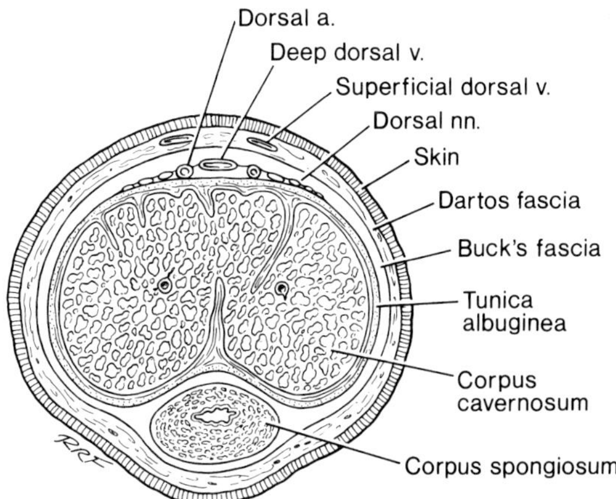

FIGURE 152-2. A cross section of the penile shaft illustrates the superficial and deep fascial layers and their relationships to the corporal bodies and neurovascular structures. (From Quartey JKM: Microcirculation of penile and scrotal skin. Atlas Urol Clin North Am 1997;5:1-9.)

Dartos fascia contains its own vascular plexus that allows overlying skin islands to be elevated on its independent blood supply.

Colles fascia is a deep, tight, triangular fascial system that arises laterally from the inferior pelvic rami and posteriorly from the perineal membrane to protect the genitalia from toxins, trauma, and infections (and envelops both testicles circumferentially, as the tunica dartos). Colles fascia is analogous to the dartos fascia on the penis, and thus skin island flaps can be elevated on the vascular plexus carried on this fascia (Fig. 152-3).[12]

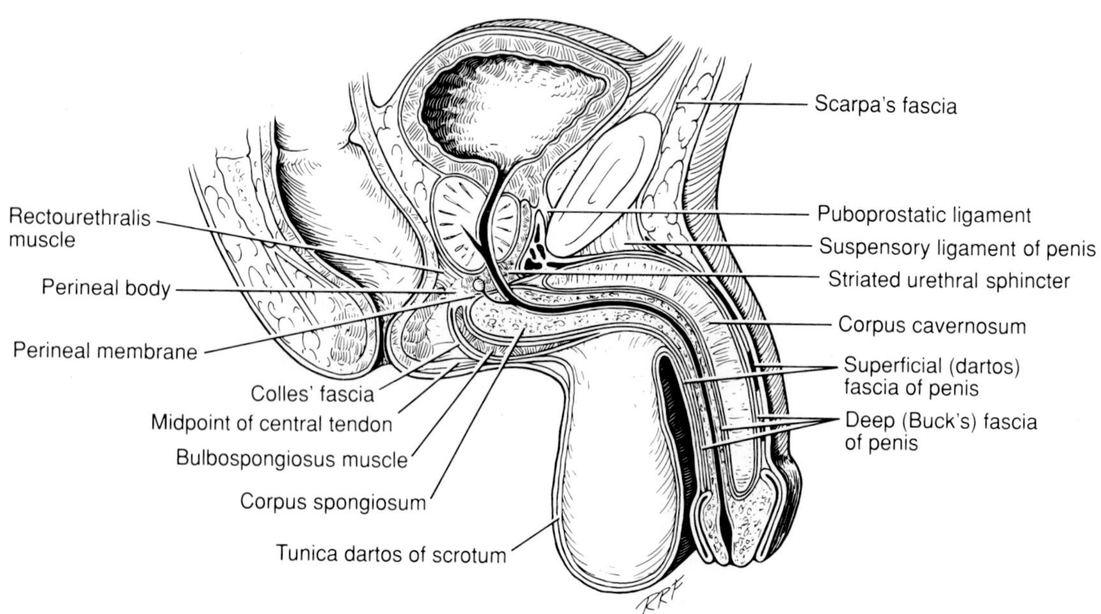

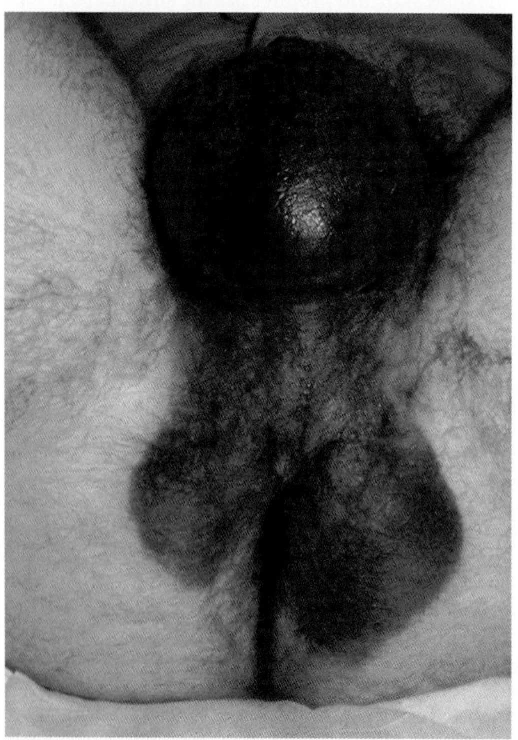

FIGURE 152-3. *A,* A sagittal illustration of the male genitalia illustrates the central location of Colles fascia and its inferior support role. *B,* After perineal trauma, this patient illustrates a hematoma confined to Colles space. (From Jordan GH, Gilbert DA: Male genital trauma. Clin Plast Surg 1988; 15:405-409.)

Overlying both testicles, the epididymis, and the cord structures is a loose, well-vascularized superficial fascial layer. The tunica vaginalis invests the testicles, and the parietal tunica vaginalis acts as the "vaginal space," which can be likened to the peritoneal cavity. Although the testicles are anchored within the scrotum, they move separately and independently on their cremasteric systems. The neurovascular supply to the testicles is dedicated to the viability of the testicles, epididymis, and cord structures (vas deferens) as well as to continued sperm production.

Genital Blood Supply

The genitalia have two separate arterial sources. The first is the deep vascular system originating from the deep internal pudendal artery. The paired pudendal arteries originate from the internal iliac arteries, pass along the borders of the inferior pelvic rami, and then give off the perineal and scrotal branches before continuing as the common penile arteries. After exiting from Alcock canal, a split in the obturator fascia that runs from the lesser sciatic foramen to the ischial tuberosity along the sidewall of the ischiorectal fossa, each common penile artery gives off four named branches. The artery to the bulb is the first branch to enter the penile urethra at its base. This artery has no specifically defined fascial layer of intervention. The second branch is the urethral artery, which passes within the corpus spongiosum to vascularize the urethra proximally. However, the spongiosum may also be supplied by other arteries more distally. The urethral artery and its branches are also considered to pass in and supply the ventral penile tissue layers. The third branch is the deep artery of the penis (a. cavernosus), which enters the ipsilateral corpus cavernosum to supply the corporal bodies bilaterally. The cavernosal arteries communicate through the thin filmy intracavernosal membrane, which helps maintain a complementary pressure between the respective corporal bodies and the corpus spongiosum. The cavernosal arteries pass in the deep layers of the penis. Finally, the common penile artery terminates in the dorsal artery of the penis, which runs within Buck fascia distally to terminate in the balanitic arteries. Although the dorsal arteries of the penis usually run in tandem over the dorsal penile fascia, arterial symmetry is present only one third of the time.[13] Within Buck fascia, the dorsal penile arteries are coiled and tortuous compared with the deep dorsal vein, which is linear and straight. This anatomy may have something to do with erectile function (Fig. 152-4).[14]

The perineal branch of the pudendal artery is just superficial to Colles fascia and has an unpredictable length, but its central location and strong collateral supply make it a mainstay of genitourinary flap reconstruction. The scrotal branch of the perineal artery passes along the fold between the lateral scrotum and medial thigh and arborizes within the tunica dartos (Fig. 152-5).

The second blood supply of the penis is the superficial external pudendal system—branches of the femoral arteries. The femoral artery typically gives off a superficial external pudendal artery and a deep external pudendal artery. The superficial external pudendal artery supplies vascularity to the dartos fascia and genital skin. The deep external pudendal artery arises as a separate branch and passes into the genital skin as the lateral inferior pudendal artery, which then separates into a dorsolateral branch supplying the

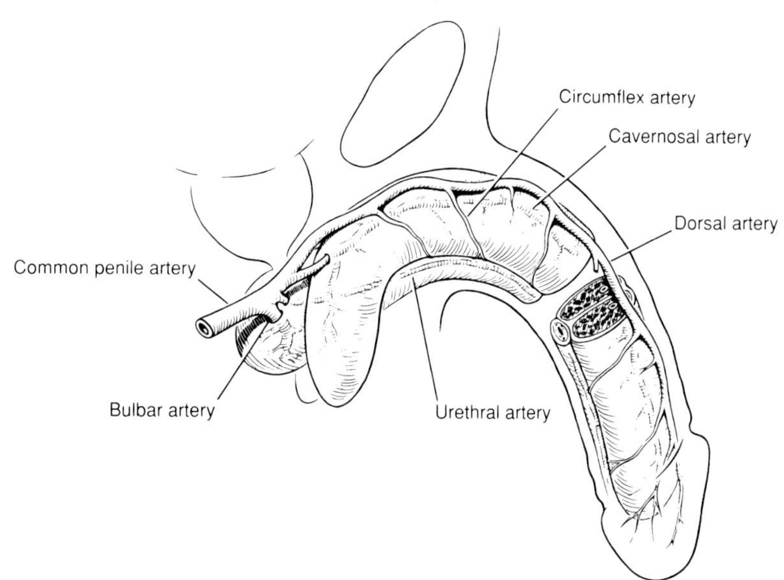

FIGURE 152-4. The deep arterial vascularization to the penis arises from branches of the common penile arteries. Proximal isolated obstruction of a cavernosal artery may be an indication for penile revascularization. (From Quartey JKM: Microcirculation of penile and scrotal skin. Atlas Urol Clin North Am 1997;5:1-9.)

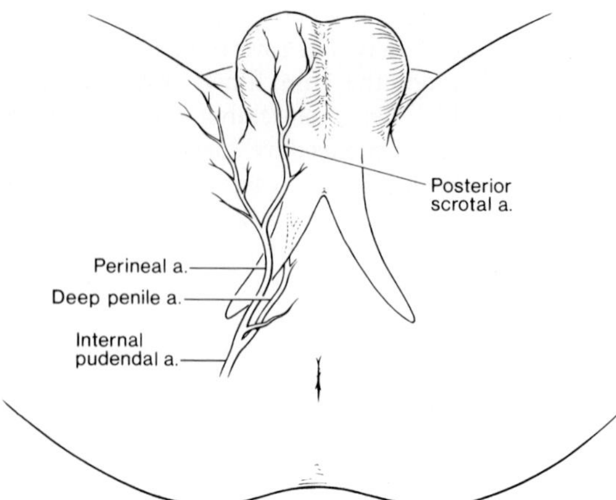

FIGURE 152-5. The internal pudendal artery exits Alcock canal and then divides into the posterior scrotal and perineal arteries. The perineal artery closely follows the crural reflection of Colles fascia. This anatomy is favorable to dissection, elevation, and transposition of fasciocutaneous flaps that can be rotated into the perineum. (From Jordan GH, Stack RS: General concepts concerning the use of genital skin islands for anterior urethral reconstruction. Atlas Urol Clin North Am 1997;5:23-44.)

dorsal and lateral penile shaft skin and an inferior branch supplying the ventral penile skin and the anterior plane of the scrotum (the anterior scrotal artery) (Figs. 152-6 and 152-7). This arrangement allows surgeons to elevate long axial and transverse flaps with relative safety and still cover the shaft donor site with the adjacent skin. This anatomic fact is the basis for the many named fasciocutaneous axial flaps, including Blandy,[15] Quartey,[16] Orandi,[17] and Jordan[18] (Fig. 152-8).

The penile venous system also has an accompanying dual blood supply. The superficial system arises from the distal penile shaft and passes to the superficial dorsal vein within the dartos fascia to drain the penile shaft skin. In approximately 70% of anatomic studies, the superficial dorsal vein empties into the left saphenous vein. Other vascular patterns include connections into the right saphenous vein (10%), left femoral vein (7%), and inferior epigastric vein (3%); in 10%, the deep dorsal vein runs as a dual supply and empties into the saphenous veins bilaterally.[19] These collateral veins are usually of different caliber and are asymmetric in their course (Fig. 152-9).

The deep venous system originates in the retrocorporal plexus and assembles as three or more large tributaries forming the deep dorsal vein in the Buck fascia. This vessel then runs proximally in the fascia, picking up perforators including the periurethral veins from the corpus spongiosum and circumflex veins from the corpora cavernosa as it passes proximally. The vein bifurcates as it reaches the separate proximal corporal bodies and passes through the deep Colles fascia into Santorini plexus. The deep system also consists of cavernosal and medial crural veins that drain into Santorini plexus. The lateral crural veins drain into the femoral system (Fig. 152-10).

Knowledge of the vascularity is important for testicular replantation, autotransplantation, and relocation in the scrotum. The left testicle is inferior to the right in the scrotum and has a longer spermatic cord. The testis is enclosed in a thick fibrous layer of tunica albuginea that contains the seminiferous tubules within lobules. Efferent ductules emerge through the tunica albuginea and converge into the ductus epididymis, which becomes the epididymal head (globus

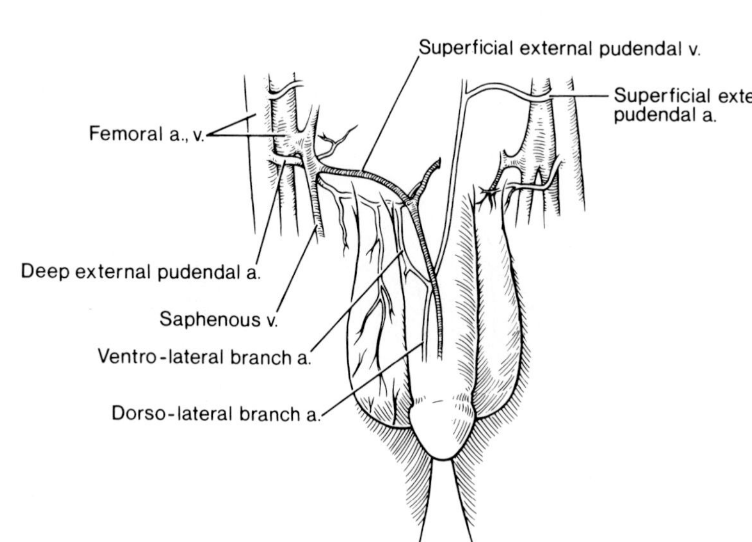

FIGURE 152-6. The deep external pudendal vascular system arises from the femoral artery and empties into the saphenous vein. The vessel passes onto the penile shaft and anterior scrotum to vascularize the skin and dartos fascia. (From Jordan GH, Stack RS: General concepts concerning the use of genital skin islands for anterior urethral reconstruction. Atlas Urol Clin North Am 1997;5:23-44.)

major). The lobular ducts then converge to form an epididymal duct that passes inferiorly down the outside of the testis in a highly convoluted fashion to the inferior pole of the testis. Here the duct enlarges to become the globus minor and then evolves into the vas deferens.

The vas deferens, epididymis, and testes are vascularized from the retroperitoneal blood supply—primarily the spermatic artery, which originates from the aorta, and the deferential artery, which supplies the vas deferens. In addition, collateral blood supply from the retroperitoneal cremasteric artery follows the vas to become the vasal artery. As the spermatic artery and its venae comitantes approach the testis, it divides into the internal testicular artery (which supplies the testis and the adjacent epididymal head and body) and the inferior testicular artery, which passes within the testis. The epididymal tail is supplied by branches of the epididymal, vasal, and testicular arteries.[20]

The veins form in the pampiniform plexus, which coalesces around the testis and epididymis to flow into the testicular veins. The testicular veins then pass in a retroperitoneal plane to empty into the inferior vena cava on the right side and the left renal vein on the left side.

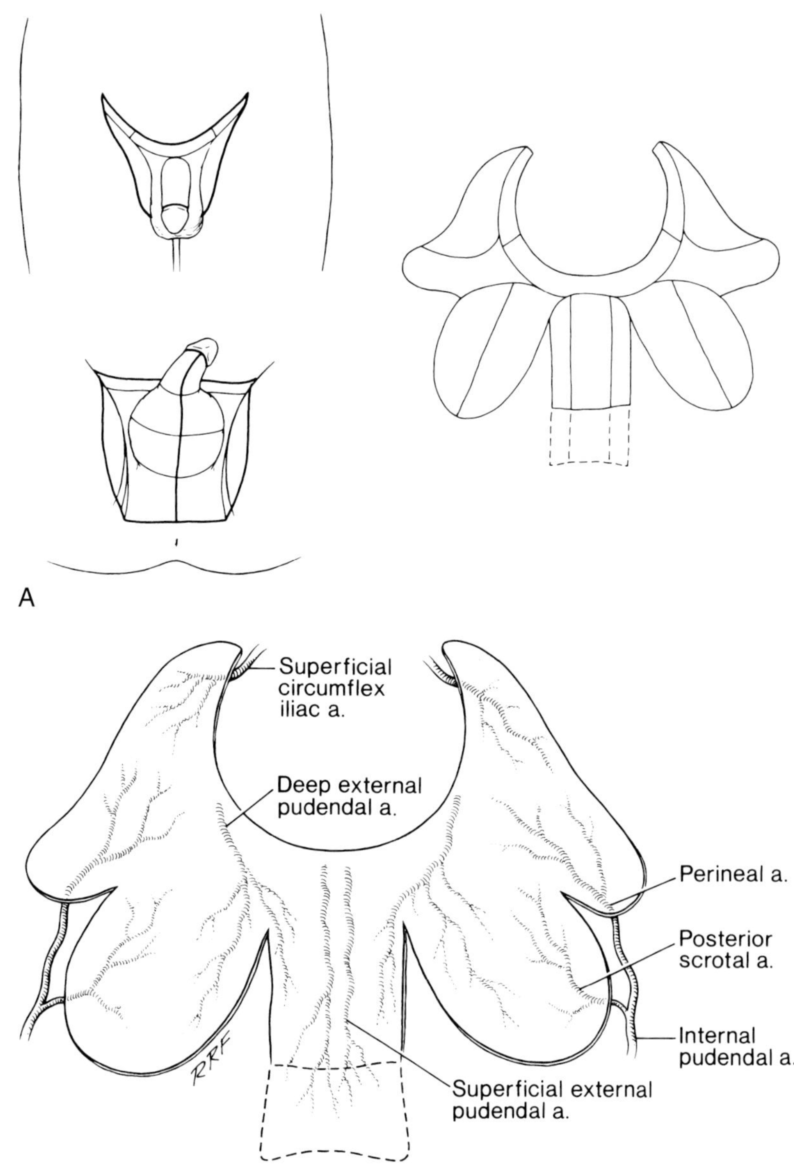

FIGURE 152-7. *A,* When the skin and dartos fascia are dissected and reflected, the deep external pudendal arteries and their vascular patterns are exposed. *B,* These vascular patterns are schematically illustrated. Note the centrifugal pattern that vascularizes all of the skin and dartos fascia—the basis of most male genital fasciocutaneous flaps. *Continued*

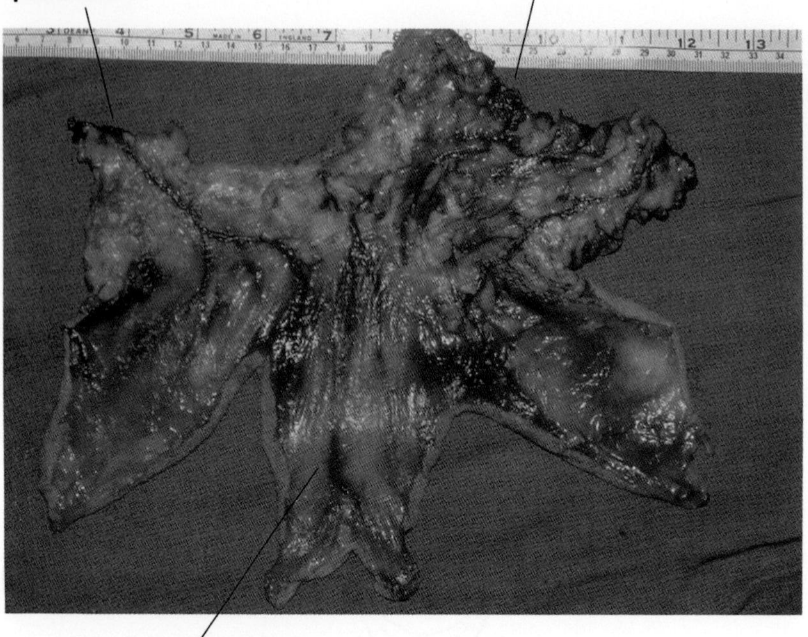

FIGURE 152-7, cont'd. *C,* This injection study demonstrates the vascular territories of the deep external pudendal arteries. Note patches of dye over the distal penile shaft, prepuce, and anterior scrotum bilaterally.

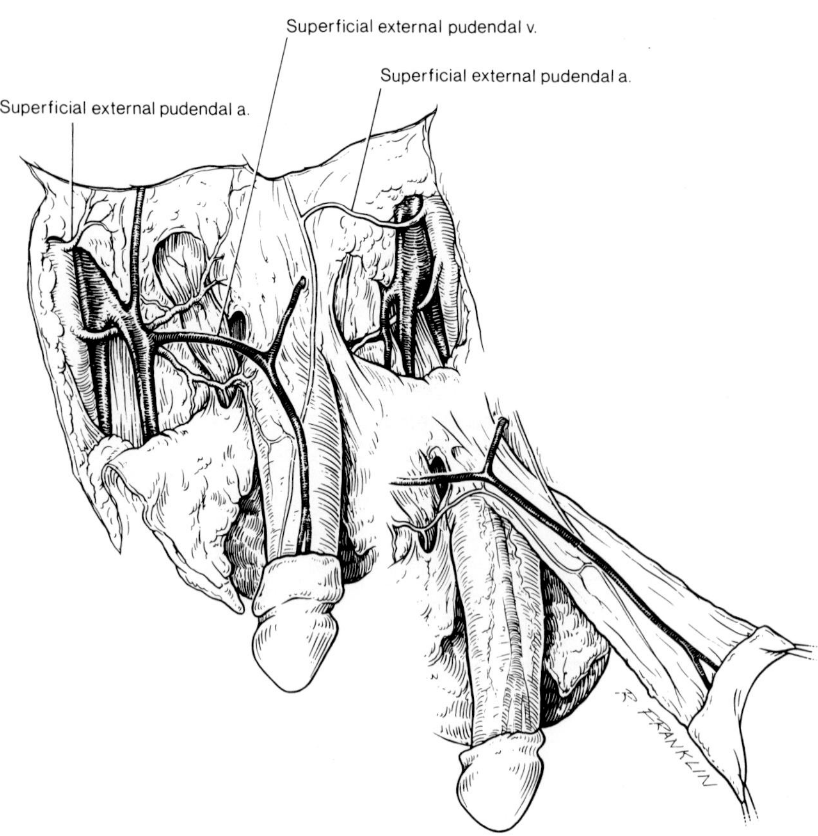

FIGURE 152-8. Although the genital arteries and veins do not run together, their axial patterns make a favorable milieu for long, narrow, and untethered fasciocutaneous flaps. (From Jordan GH, Stack RS: General concepts concerning the use of genital skin islands for anterior urethral reconstruction. Atlas Urol Clin North Am 1997;5:23-44.)

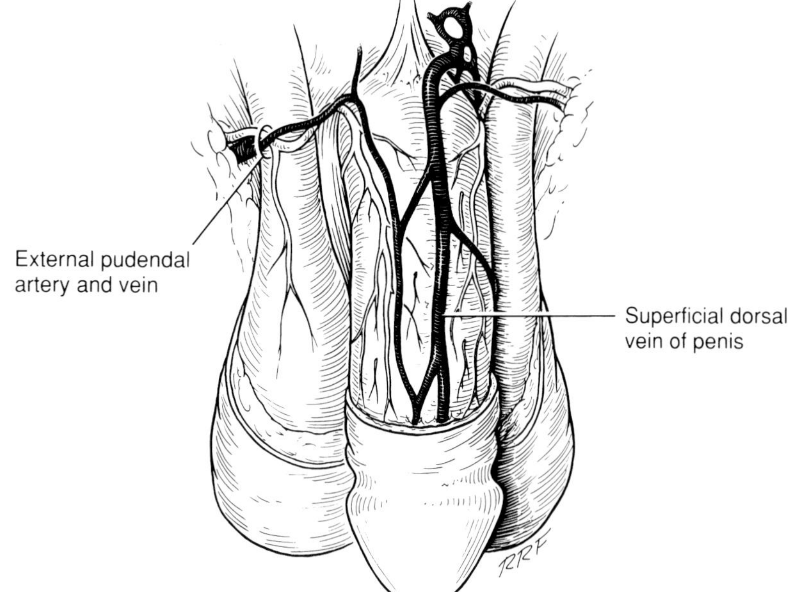

FIGURE 152-9. The superficial dorsal vein of the penis usually empties into the left saphenous system—an anatomic fact that must be taken into account in planning fasciocutaneous flaps. (From Jordan GH, Stack RS: General concepts concerning the use of genital skin islands for anterior urethral reconstruction. Atlas Urol Clin North Am 1997;5:23-44.)

Genital Nerve Supply

The nerve supply of the genitalia also arises from a dual source and runs concurrently with the arterial supply. The major sensory supply to the penis arises from the pudendal nerve in the perineum. The pudendal nerve is a mixed motor, sensory, and autonomic nerve that originates from the sacral roots (S2-4). The nerve passes through the greater sciatic foramen and then courses anteriorly across the pelvic floor to enter the pudendal canal. Within the pelvis, the nerve gives off the inferior rectal nerve, supplying the rectal sphincter and anal skin and conducting the cavernosal reflex before entering Alcock (pudendal) canal. As the nerve exits Alcock canal and passes close to the crural tips of the corporal bodies, it divides into the perineal nerve and the dorsal nerve of the penis. The perineal nerve supplies the perineal muscles, deep structures of the urogenital region, and posterior scrotal skin. The dorsal nerve of the penis gives off a proximal nerve to the urethra before arborizing into its penile branches. Branches of the nerve pass around the penile shaft

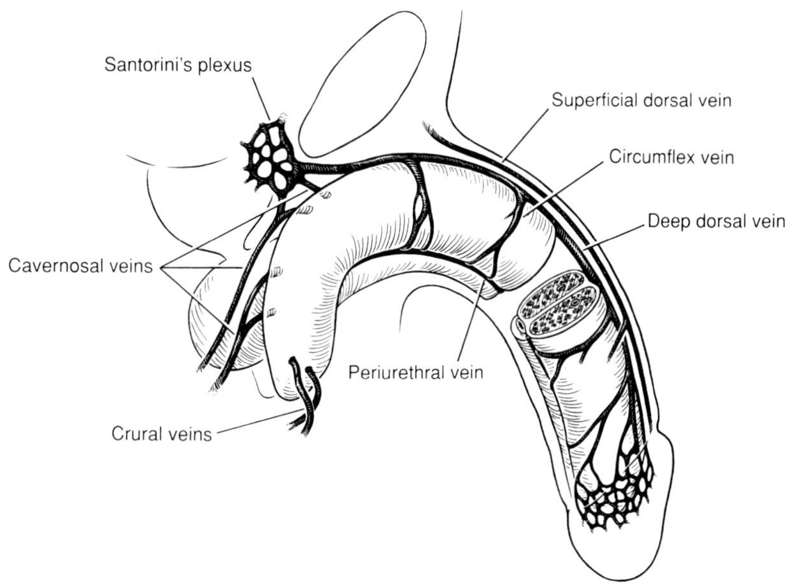

FIGURE 152-10. Knowledge of the deep penile vascular system is important in addressing erectile dysfunction and associated venous leaks. (From Jordan GH, Stack RS: General concepts concerning the use of genital skin islands for anterior urethral reconstruction. Atlas Urol Clin North Am 1997;5:23-44.)

within Buck fascia to innervate the distal shaft and inner lamina of the prepuce as well as pass directly into the glans as the major tactile and erogenous source of the penis (Fig. 152-11).

The dorsal nerves of the penis do not provide sensation to the penile shaft. The shaft is innervated by ancillary erogenous nerves, including the ilioinguinal nerves, which exit through the external inguinal rings and then branch to innervate the anterior scrotum and the penile shaft skin circumferentially to the level of the prepuce, and branches of the genitofemoral nerves. The internal plate of the prepuce does contain branches of the dorsal nerve of the penis.

The scrotum has the advantage of multiple nerve supplies. In addition to the anterior scrotal branches of the ilioinguinal nerve, the anterior scrotum is also supplied by the genital branches of the genitofemoral nerve. The posterior scrotum is innervated by the posterior scrotal branch of the pudendal nerve.

Genital Lymphatic Supply

Lymphatics of the glans and urethra form a plexus on the ventral side before passing around to the deep vein, passing proximally to the superficial inguinal nodes. Some lymphatics also pass to the deep inguinal nodes. The distal urethral lymphatics likewise drain to the deep dorsal vein and the superficial inguinal nodes. The proximal spongy and membranous urethra drains into the external iliac nodes. The lymphatics of the testicles are contained in the spermatic cord and empty into the aortocaudal nodes.

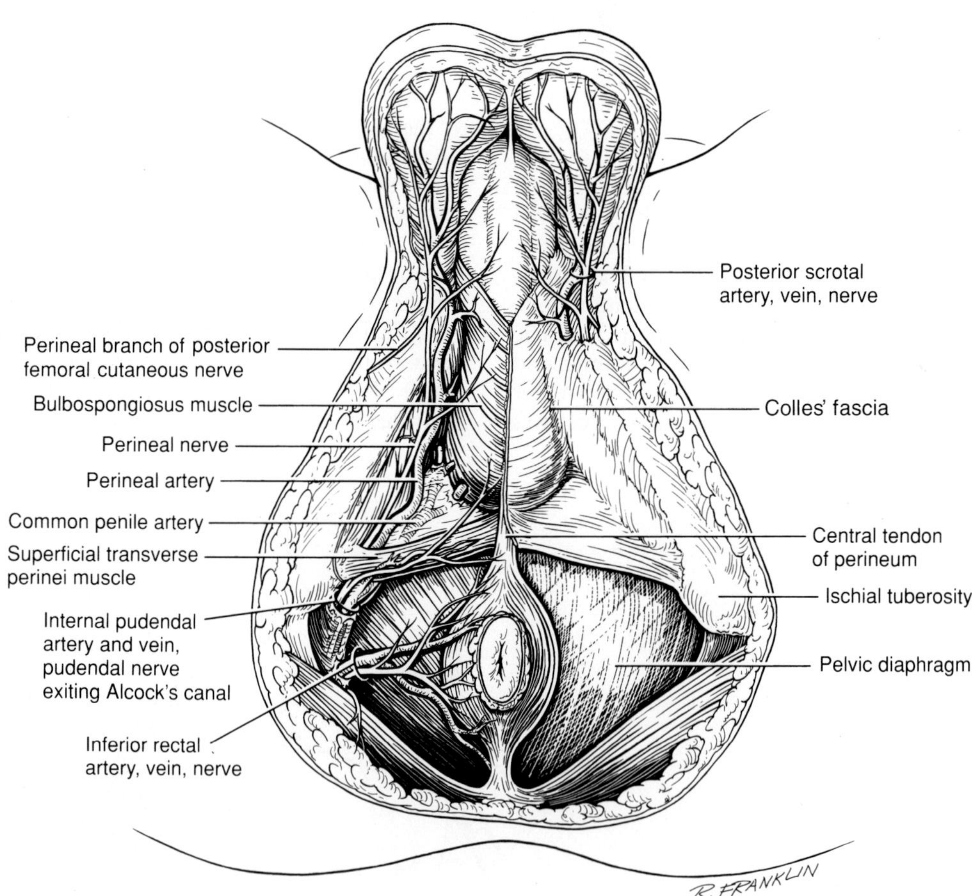

FIGURE 152-11. The superficial perineal anatomy. Note the lateral location of Alcock canal with its important neurovascular structures. Centrally, the perineum is suspended by the superficial transverse perinei muscles and the overlying Colles fascia, which reinforces the central tendon of the perineum. The deep perineal anatomy illustrates the muscle support provided by the bulbospongiosus, ischiocavernosus, deep transverse perinei, and levator muscles. (From Jordan GH, Stack RS: General concepts concerning the use of genital skin islands for anterior urethral reconstruction. Atlas Urol Clin North Am 1997;5:23-44.)

CONGENITAL GENITAL DEFECTS

Exstrophy and Epispadias

Exstrophy of the bladder is an uncommon condition that occurs in approximately 1 of every 30,000 live births, of which boys predominate in a 3 : 1 ratio. The defining features of epispadias and exstrophy are an open and protruding bladder, an open urethra, and a foreshortened epispadiac penis. However, the associated spectrum of anomalies may extend to involve the musculoskeletal structures and the gastrointestinal tract. Classic exstrophy—defined by bladder exstrophy, epispadias, diastasis recti, absence of fusion of the pubic symphysis, and deformed pubic escutcheon—occurs in 60% of cases; epispadias alone occurs in 30% of cases, and 10% of cases are more extensive dysmorphias including cloacal exstrophy.[21]

The etiology of exstrophy-epispadias is controversial, but it does not represent an arrest of a normal fetal developmental stage. It occurs in early gestation between the third and ninth weeks. The anomaly is associated with the formation and normal retraction of the cloacal membrane. In the normal fetus, a mesodermal layer of tissue spreads medially to replace the thin cloacal membrane by the ninth week in utero. According to Muecke's theory,[22] the cloacal membrane persists and resists any medial migration of mesoderm. The membrane then ruptures, thereby producing a lack of mesodermal tissue to form the anterior abdominal wall and endodermal tissue to form the anterior wall of the bladder. This lack of mesodermal migration also has a profound effect on the musculoskeletal system. The pubic rami are widely separated, and the inferior pubic rami are consequently laterally rotated. This defect produces a widened and foreshortened urethra and bladder neck. It also produces an incompletely formed penis that remains rudimentary and, by definition, is a phallus. According to Mitchell,[23] the anomaly is that of a fetal abdominal wall hernia and can be recreated in the laboratory in chickens because they have a persistent cloaca by induction of a localized vascular accident.[24]

The defining features of exstrophy-epispadias are an open urinary tract with protruding bladder and foreshortened epispadiac penis. The crural bodies are attached to the splayed pubic tubercles, producing a penis that is short, wide, and with dorsal chordee. Unlike in the normal anatomy, corporal bodies are independent of each other with no communication through the intercorporal septum. The neurovascular structures to the glans are laterally displaced but move medially at the distal end of the foreshortened penis; the glans is spade shaped and incompletely formed, and each side is totally dependent on the respective dorsal neurovascular supply for its viability. Little circulation passes through the corporal bodies into the glans, as opposed to a penis with normal development. The separated pelvic ring also produces a widened scrotum and lack of competent pelvic musculature. Therefore, the perineum is short and the anus can be patulous and anteriorly displaced. The rectus muscles are widely separated, and inguinal hernias are the rule.

Although the initial postnatal diagnosis and treatment of bladder exstrophy and epispadias remain in the realm of the urologist and orthopedic surgeon, it is important that the plastic surgeon be prepared, if consulted, to help reconstruct such a child. The goals of initial closure are to reconstruct a functional genitourinary system, to reduce the risk of bladder squamous metaplasia, and to close the pelvic ring. This is carried out by direct closure of the bladder and reconstitution of the pelvic ring. If the child undergoes reconstruction within 48 hours of birth, pelvic ring closure is accomplished by the placement of sutures directly through the obturator foramen, which brings the splayed pubic tubercles into coaptation. This can be facilitated by a number of osteotomy techniques.[21,25,26] If the pelvic ring closure is delayed, pelvic osteotomies are necessary. These include an anterior horizontal, innominate osteotomy and diagonal innominate osteotomies. It is at this point that the plastic surgeon is most often consulted for participation in further reconstruction.

Phallic length depends on antenatal development and the results of prior surgery. Penile reconstruction begins by closure of the pelvic ring and release of the penopubic suspensory ligaments to release the corporal bodies. Aggressive but not total detachment of the corporal bodies from the pubis is the goal. This dissection must be carried out subperiosteally to protect the laterally based neurovascular bundles.

Reconstruction of the urethra is then addressed. The penile disassembly technique, well described by both Mitchell[23] and Perovic,[27] has drastically improved the results of the urethral closure and release of the chordee. The urethra is vascularized by ventral dartos fascia, which sends a "mesentery" to the corpus spongiosum. Distally, the urethra, which lays on top of the splayed and epispadiac glans, is detached. The urethra is then released from the dorsal penile corpora with parallel strip incisions. With preservation of the underlying corpus spongiosum mesentery, the urethra is then tubularized and placed on the ventral shaft. Bilateral corporoplasties are then carried out to join the corporal bodies dorsally. This is achieved by incising the dorsomedial aspects of each corporal body and then suturing them together centrally. It is necessary to evaluate any potential dorsal chordee with serial bilateral artificial erections to complete as much penile release as possible. On occasion, dermal grafts must be placed over the corporal bodies to complete straightening of the penis. The distal glans is then closed with a dorsal suture line. The glans, which has been divided, is now resutured with the meatus placed in an anatomically correct position (Figs. 152-12 and 152-13).[25]

Where possible, a low abdominal W flap is dissected and elevated to reconstruct the bifid and laterally displaced escutcheon. After dissection and elevation, these flaps are brought together centrally to cover the pubic imbrication and the proximal penile shaft.

As mentioned, penile length is often dependent on antenatal development more than on surgical expertise. In the past, most of these patients underwent a great number of surgical procedures before they reached puberty. Newer techniques have changed this pattern. The number of children born with exstrophy has decreased, possibly because of a decreasing prevalence of the anomaly and also because of the perinatologists who suggest subtraction when exstrophy is noted on antenatal ultrasonography.

There is a certain population of patients with exstrophy and epispadias who will require further penile reconstruction as they pass through their postadolescent period. These young men have small and undeveloped penises, despite the concerted and continued best efforts of their treating surgeons. To this group we can now offer phallic construction or further penile reconstruction with use of microsurgical tissue transplantation techniques. Most of these patients have some form of urinary diversion and therefore have a nonfunctional urethra. Although the verumontanum and ejaculatory ducts are often intact, they are often abnormally positioned as a prepubic fistula. These anatomic facts create unpredictable sperm production, and most of these patients are unable to procreate naturally. For these reasons, the urethral reconstruction may be a moot point in this group of patients (Fig. 152-14).

Congenital Curvature (Chordee without Hypospadias)

Penile chordee without the pathologic development of the urethra is an uncommon but not rare genital anomaly. The curvature usually does not have any

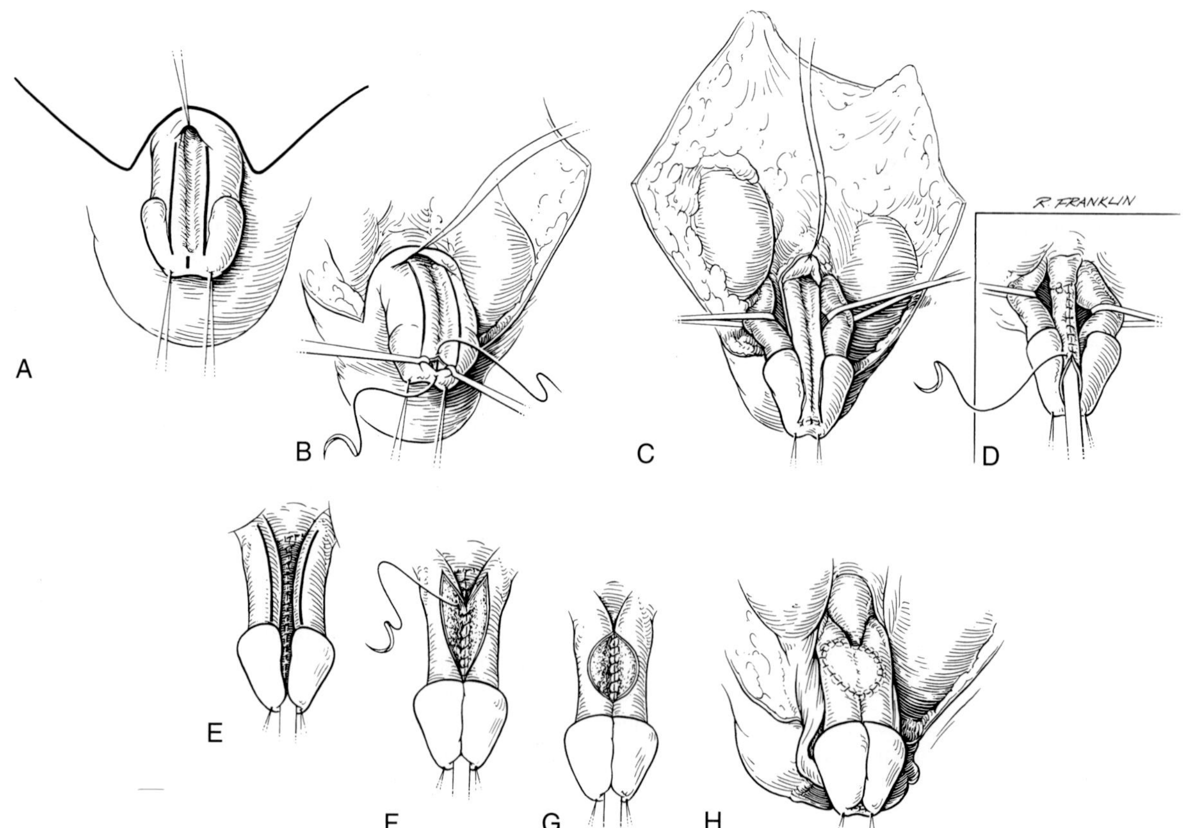

FIGURE 152-12. Typical secondary exstrophy-epispadias reconstruction. *A,* First, elevation of a lower abdominal W flap and release of the penopubic ligaments (not pictured here) release all of the attendant scarring. *B* to *D,* Second, urethral advancement and closure follow disassembly from the corporal bodies. The urethra is then transposed to an anatomically ventral position. *E* and *F,* Third, corporal union is completed by first bivalving the corporal bodies, then conjoining them. *G* and *H,* Fourth, corporal body length is augmented with the dermal graft. (Dorsal penile shaft skin coverage with the W flap is not pictured here.)

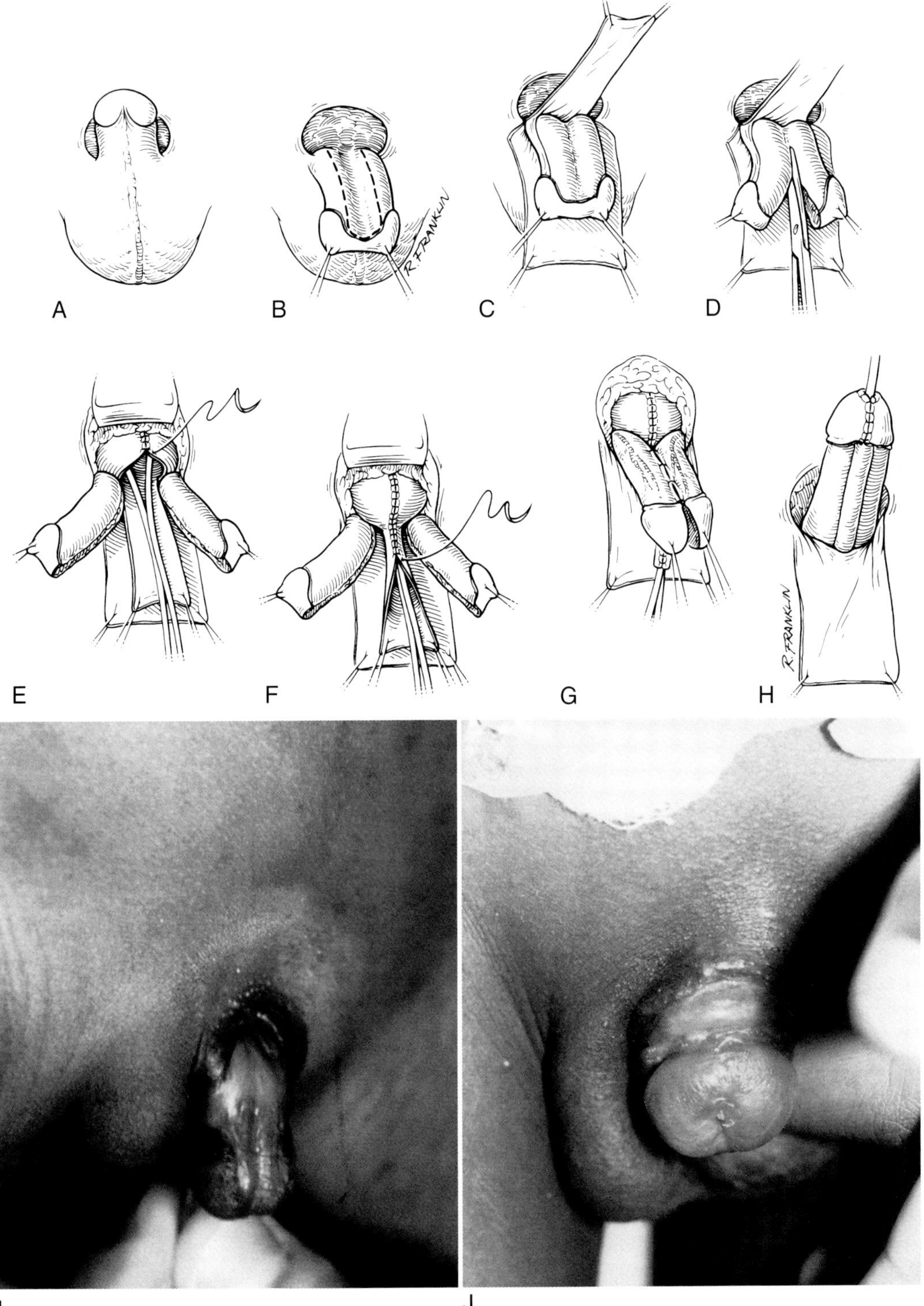

FIGURE 152-13. *A* and *B,* A 12-year-old was born with epispadias without exstrophy. Note the proximal penopubic urethral meatus, the dorsally located urethra with a ventral plate remnant, and dorsal chordee. *C,* With use of a disassembly technique popularized by Mitchell, the ventral urethral plate is initially elevated off the corporal bodies in a retrograde direction. *D,* The corporal bodies are separated. *E,* The corporal bodies are released from the penopubic ligaments, ureteral stents are located, and urethral closure is begun. *F,* Urethral tubing is continued distally. *G,* The urethral tube is closed completely and passed ventrally beneath the corporal bodies. *H,* Bilateral corporoplasties and midline glans fusion are completed, and all chordee is corrected. *I,* A preoperative illustration depicting the challenges of epispadias repair. *J,* The final result after removal of the urethral stent 3 weeks postoperatively.

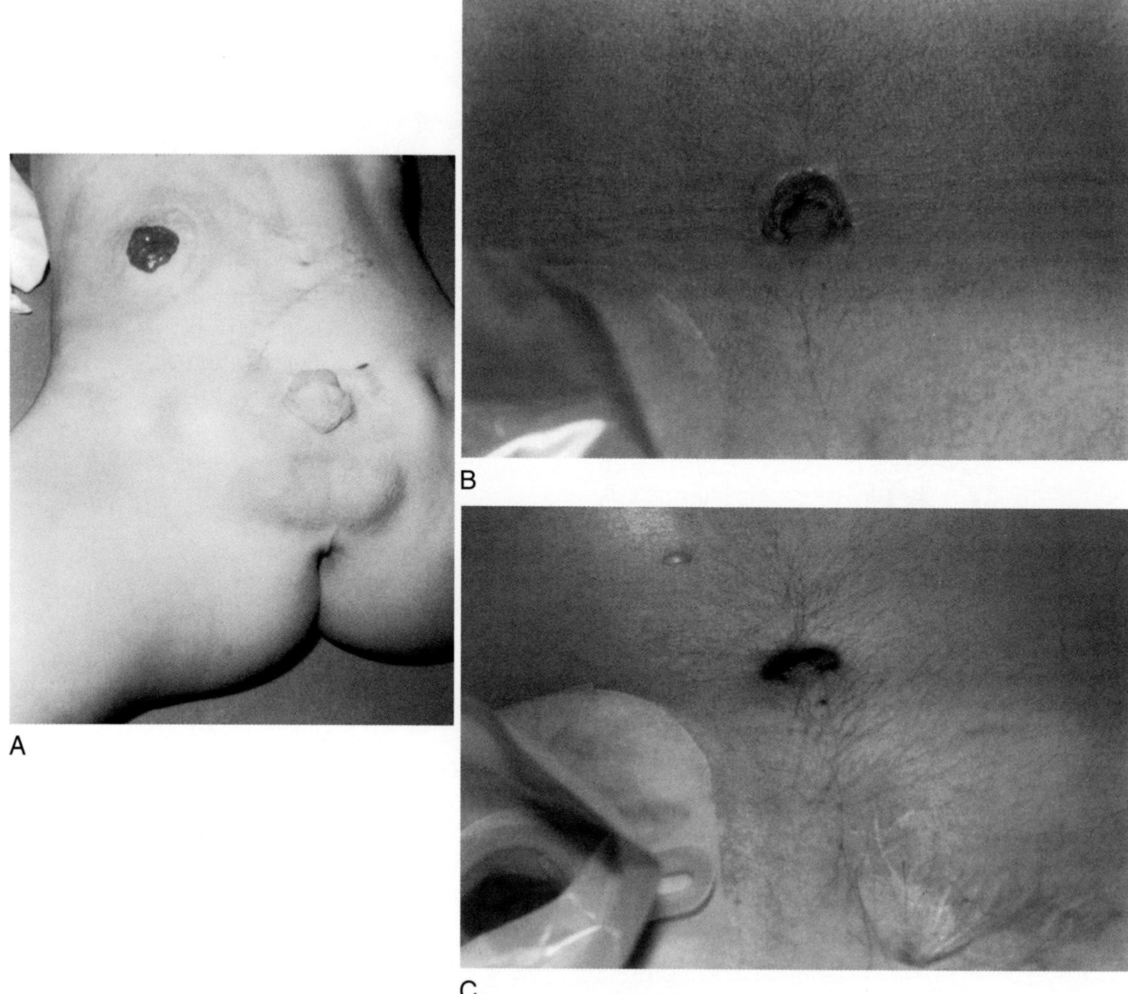

FIGURE 152-14. Umbilicoplasty is often requested by exstrophy patients when they pass through puberty. Depending on the bladder reconstruction, urologists may locate the ileal conduit on the abdominal skin as a catheterizable stoma at the site of a normal umbilicus. *A,* In this patient, the ileal stoma is in the right upper quadrant of the abdominal wall. The umbilicus is located in the abdominal midline at the horizontal plane of the iliac crease. *B,* An inferiorly based flap is dissected, elevated, and sutured to the abdominal wall. The superior defect is then covered with a split-thickness skin graft. *C,* One year later, the skin graft has constricted, creating the appearance of an umbilicus tethered by the falciform ligament.

urinary sequelae—it is strictly a bend to the penis of 45 to 60 degrees. The ventral chordee may be associated with a bend to one side or the other (usually to the left) or a twist of the penile shaft. On occasion, the curvature is recognized by the parents or a treating physician before puberty, but it is usually the patient, in his late teens or early 20s, who recognizes and reveals the presence of a bend (Fig. 152-15).

The cause of such a curvature is unclear. The patient typically complains of a progressive ventral bend of the penis, which is usually painless but makes successful sexual intromission difficult if not impossible. There is no neurovascular compromise of the glans penis, but the patient may have some difficulty directing his urinary stream. A photograph of an erection in the physician's office or a Polaroid provided by the patient is usually adequate documentation of the deformity. The treatment is surgical and includes a stepwise approach. Through a circumcising incision, the penile shaft skin and dartos fascia are sharply separated from the underlying corporal bodies. Dysgenetic tissue layers including the dartos fascia, Buck fascia, tunica albuginea, and corpus spongiosum are recognized and resected sequentially until all of the tethering tissues are released. A foreshortened normal urethra as the primary cause of chordee is rare, if it occurs at all. If

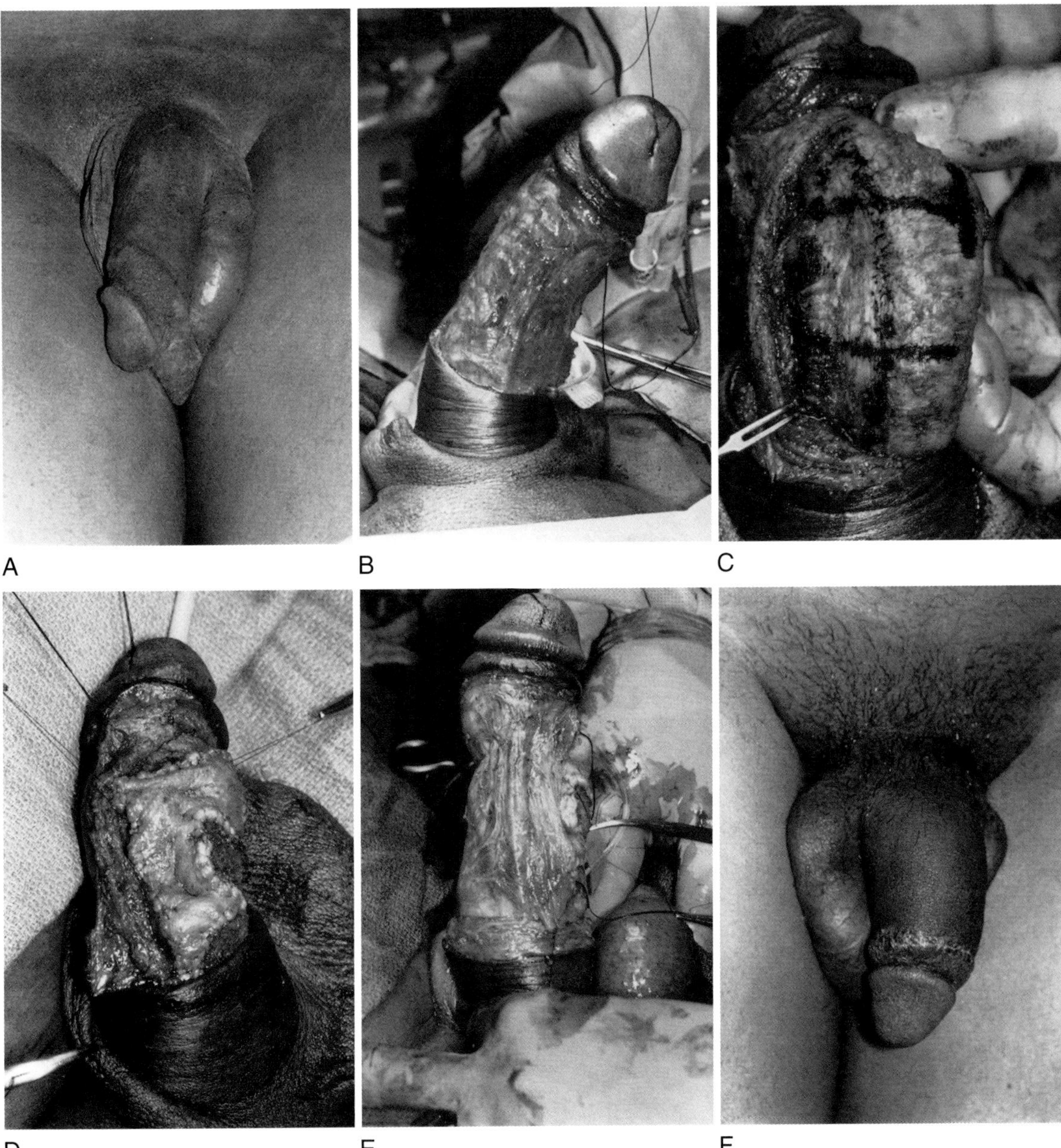

FIGURE 152-15. *A,* This 20-year-old man complained of a penile bend of 45 degrees to the right side and an anticlockwise rotation of 90 degrees. *B,* After release of skin and dartos fascia, an initial artificial erection confirms a right-sided chordee. *C,* In this particular case, a dermal graft is used to correct the defect. The chordee is released by incising but not resecting the right corporal tunica. *D,* A dermal graft is harvested and inset into the corporal defect. *E,* An artificial erection after repair confirms penile straightening. *F,* Postoperatively, the penis is straight and the rotation corrected. Although tunical plication is usually preferred to dermal grafting, some patients decline plication because they fear loss of the penile length.

there are formes frustes of hypospadias (i.e., inadequate development of the corpus spongiosum), the finding is classified as chordee without hypospadias.

Once the ventral surface has been released, a decision must be made by the surgeon either to release the corporal bodies ventrally and reconstruct with a dermal inlay graft or to proceed with elevation of the Buck fascia and dorsally or laterally plicate ellipses of the tunica until the penis is straight (Nesbit tucks).[28] The latter technique is preferred for several reasons. First, several plications (usually two or three) allow the surgeon to more accurately straighten the penis.

Second, when an incision is made in the corporal bodies and a reconstructive "patch" is placed on the corporal bodies to maintain or to exaggerate length, there is always a risk of loss of distal penile turgidity and length. Dorsal plications are not susceptible to these sequelae. In fact, most penises that have congenital chordee are usually longer than average, and therefore plication plays a minimal role in the "perceived" shortening of the penis postoperatively.[29] In young men, plication alone is not recommended because plication sutures frequently tear out.

After a confirming erection, the plications are marked out and the tunica albuginea is placed on traction with 4-0 polypropylene sutures. The plication ellipse is incised and then oversewn with a 4-0 or 5-0 polydioxanone suture. After the final erection, the dartos fascia and skin are sutured, and a small suction drain is placed into the subcutaneous tissues for 24 hours. The surgery is usually successful and the complication rate is low (Fig. 152-16).

Intersex

FEMALE PSEUDOHERMAPHRODITISM

Female pseudohermaphroditism occurs when a 46 XX female is exposed to androgens in utero, usually at about 11 weeks of gestation. For example, there may be an overproduction of the androgenic intermediary metabolites, resulting in internal anatomy that is normally female but external anatomy that is virilized. These adrenogenital syndromes include clitorimegaly and labioscrotal fusion. Pigmented ambiguous

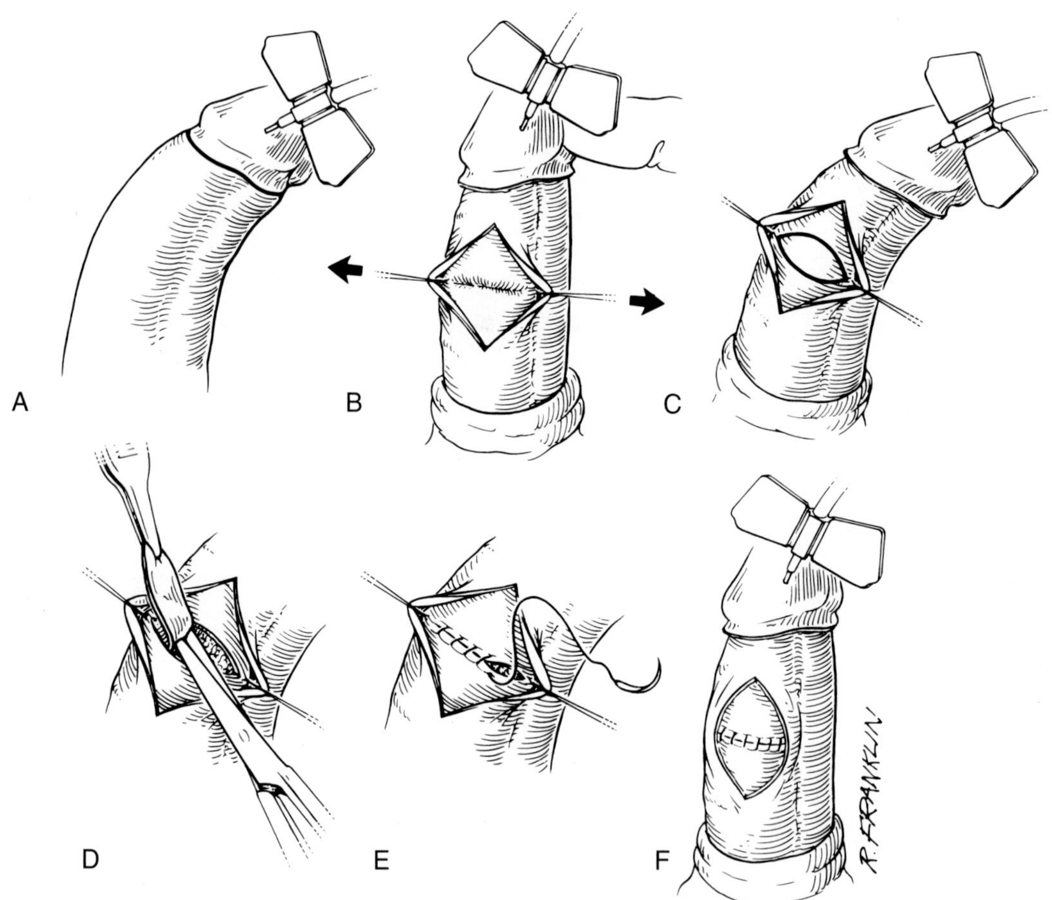

FIGURE 152-16. The Nesbit technique to correct congenital chordee is straightforward and relatively predictable. *A,* In the case of a congenital ventral chordee, an initial artificial erection establishes the location, extent, and degree of the bend. *B,* After initial dissection, Buck fascia is released to expose the contralateral corporal body to the affected side. With temporary sutures producing lateral traction, a second artificial erection is performed. *C,* The limits of the proposed plication are marked out. If the proposed transverse plication is extended or if the chordee persists despite the proposed excision, further excisions may be performed. *D,* An ellipse of corporal tunica is removed (as shown) or plicated without excision. *E,* The corporal tunica is sutured with a running suture. *F,* A final artificial erection confirms that the penis has been straightened.

genitalia may be a clue to the diagnosis. Depending on the level of the enzyme defect, salt washing can be noted. Elevated urinary 17-hydroxyprogesterone levels confirm the diagnosis.

MALE PSEUDOHERMAPHRODITISM

Male pseudohermaphrodites are genetic males with a normal 46 XY karyotype who have incomplete masculinization due to environmental influences such as placental insufficiency or end-organ unresponsiveness due to inheritable gene disorders. These include autosomal recessive defects in testosterone biosynthesis and can include failure of elaboration of cortisol leading to adrenal insufficiency. Congenital adrenal hyperplasia may include hypertension, depending on the level of enzyme defect. Other causes are insufficient testosterone production and a decrease in mRNA nuclear-binding protein. 5α-Reductase deficiency is also associated with inadequate virilization. Hypospadias, although not always an intersex state, is always a sign of arrested virilization. The place of early intersex surgery has been called into question and is the focus of study of the National Task Force on Intersex.

TRUE HERMAPHRODITISM

True hermaphroditism is rare in North America. The presence of well-differentiated male and female gonadal tissue in the same individual is required for the diagnosis. There is asymmetry of gonadal tissue. Most patients are 46 XX but contain an H-Y antigen that induces morphogenesis of the female gonad to a testis. The evaluation of intersex can include visual inspection, chromosome karyotyping, cystoscopy, laparoscopy or laparotomy, urethrography, gonadal biopsy, and buccal smear. Other tests may include evaluation of 17-OH steroids, serum enzyme studies, and fluorescein studies.[30] In the past, the most important factor for gender assignment was the appearance of the external genitalia. Anatomy, not chromosomes, dictated gender choice. In most patients, the diagnosis should be made within 24 hours. However, as mentioned before, the place for early intersex surgery is not defined.

Buried Penis

The buried penis deformity is present in both the pediatric and adult populations. A buried penis is defined as a penis that is of normal size for age but hidden within the peripenile fat and subcutaneous tissues. In the pediatric population, the fat deposit is often part of the constellation of poor virilization. The abnormal mons fat pad (gynecoid mons pubis) may become associated with a generalized obesity in the adolescent patient, and the buried penis must be differentiated from a micropenis in this group. In adults, the problem is almost always associated with obesity and the development of pubic, scrotal, and peripubic ptosis, which must be addressed to correct the problem (hidden penis).

Once the etiology of buried penis has been established, a surgical treatment plan is implemented. In children, direct resection of the suprapubic and peripenile fat is carried out through an adjacent W flap or a low transverse Pfannenstiel-type incision. In this group, fatty tissues are generally "liposuction unfriendly," and open lipectomy is usually indicated. In addition to the abnormal mons, there appears to be a foreshortened dartos fascia that joins superiorly with the Scarpa fascia and tethers the corporal bodies, resulting in the appearance of abundant shaft skin and prepuce.[31] The tethered dartos fascia may be associated with adequate penile shaft skin or, in the patient with an aggressive circumcision, inadequate shaft skin that further tethers and engulfs the penile corporal bodies.[32] Care must be taken to leave adequate subcutaneous tissue beneath the peripenile skin so that plication sutures will not produce overlying dimpling. The lipectomy includes resection of fat superficial and deep to Scarpa fascia and around the cord structures where lipomas are frequent. The dysgenetic dartos fascia is released from Scarpa fascia; if indicated, the penopubic suspensory ligaments are also partially released. If necessary, penoscrotal tethering may be released with a Z-plasty or VY-plasty. To further redefine the penoscrotal junction, tacking sutures from the released dartos fascia to the lateral tunica bodies may be placed bilaterally (Fig. 152-17).

One of the adult hidden penis subgroups is the post-traumatic, obese patient in whom the penis become retrussed after an accident, trauma, or circumcision. Not unusually, patients are circumcised to "expose the penis."[33] During healing, the ptotic pannus skin lies on the genitalia and the circumcision scar contracts, thereby incarcerating the penis. Other recognized causes of penile incarceration are balanitis xerotica obliterans and Fournier disease. The combination of local genital disease and comorbid obesity, diabetes mellitus, panniculitis, and hypertension makes this group of patients a challenge to genitourinary reconstruction (Fig. 152-18).[34]

Micropenis

Micropenis is defined as a penis that is more than two standard deviations smaller than a normal-sized penis for age (Table 152-1).[35] Although a micropenis may be associated with generalized obesity, the treatment is quite different and requires that the penile length be addressed with much more extensive surgery. One of the most controversial areas of genital reconstruction is preadolescent phallic construction and the philosophic treatment of children born with intersex

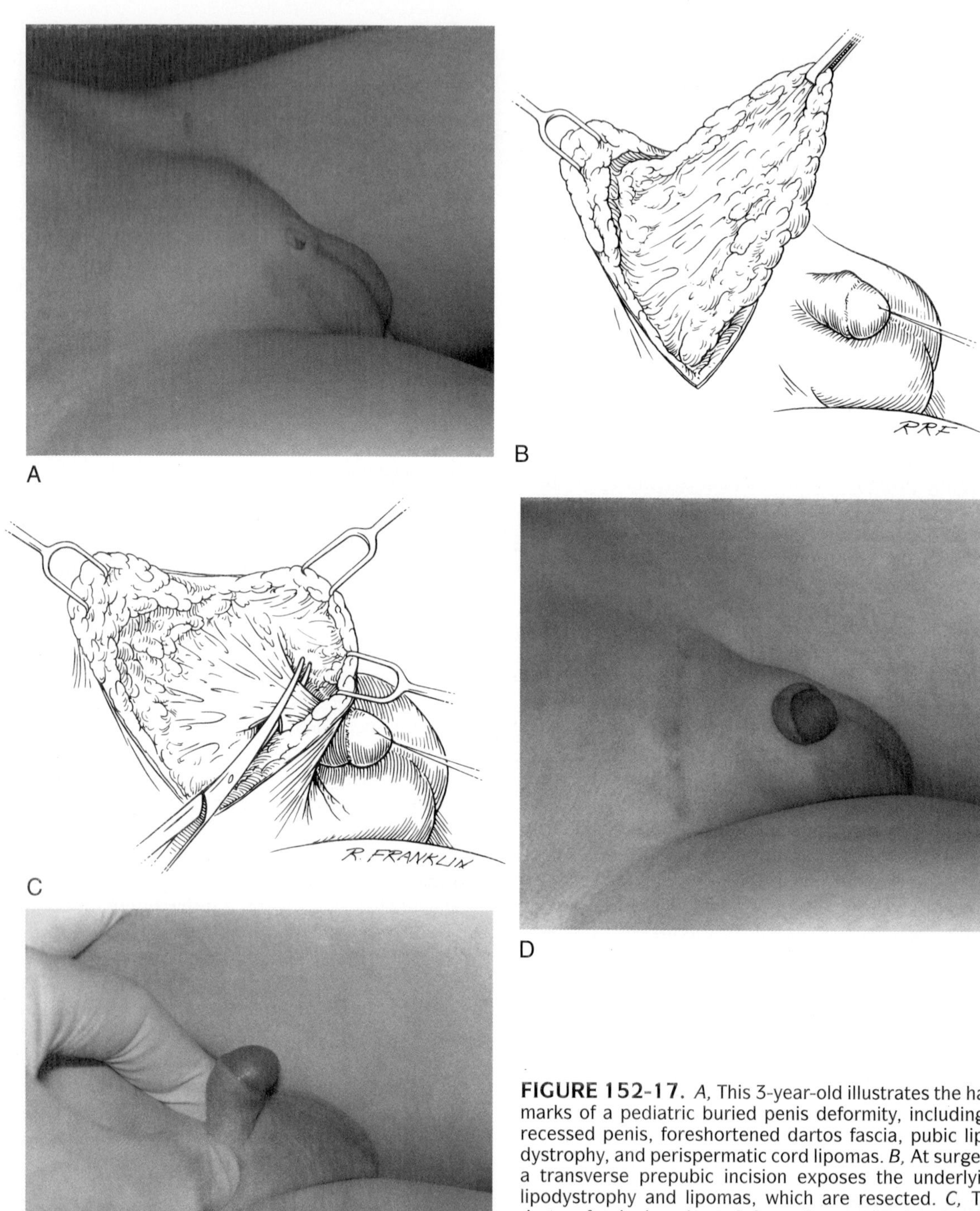

FIGURE 152-17. *A,* This 3-year-old illustrates the hallmarks of a pediatric buried penis deformity, including a recessed penis, foreshortened dartos fascia, pubic lipodystrophy, and perispermatic cord lipomas. *B,* At surgery, a transverse prepubic incision exposes the underlying lipodystrophy and lipomas, which are resected. *C,* The dartos fascia is released from Scarpa fascia, thereby extending the penile shaft skin. The penopubic ligaments are also released. *D,* Postoperatively, the penis is exposed in a recumbent position so that the child will be able to stand and void. *E,* However, penile shaft tacking sutures may be required to produce the best penile exposure. Note that a previous circumcision has potentially foreshortened the penile skin.

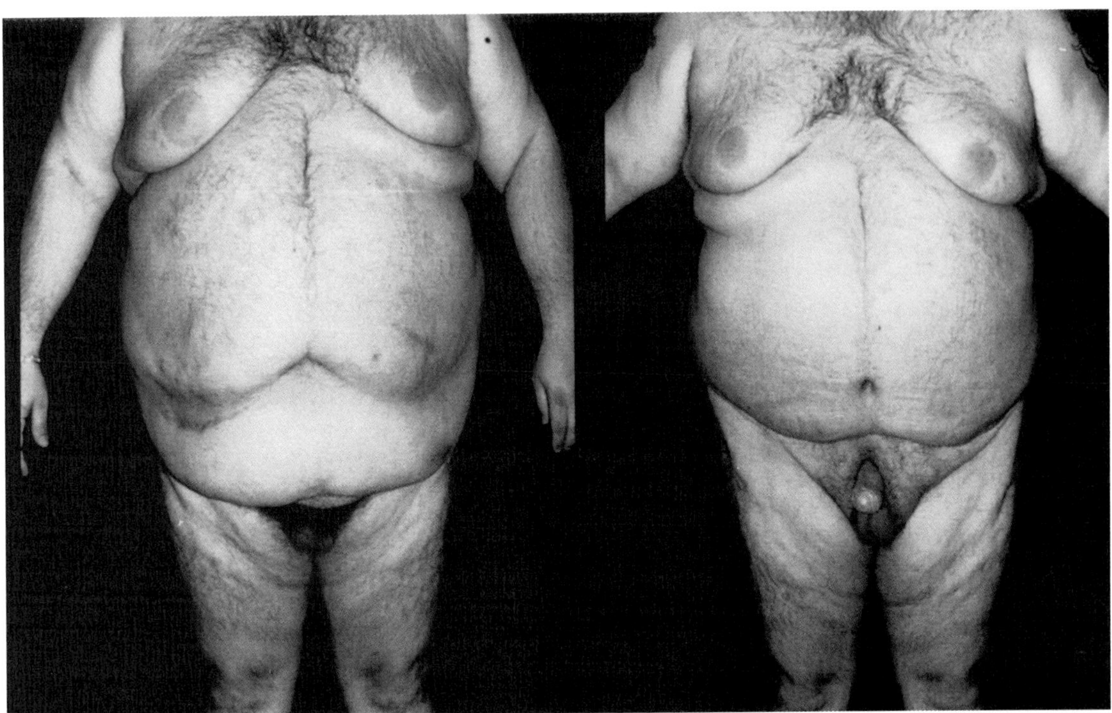

A

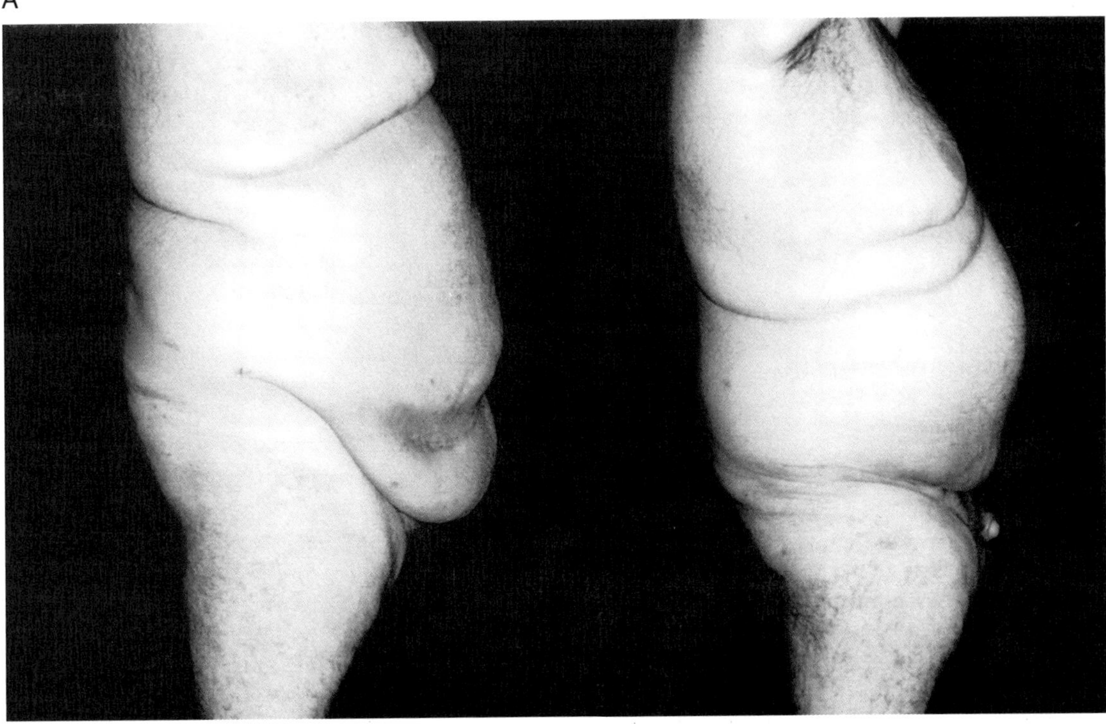

B

FIGURE 152-18. Buried penis in the adult is often a complex, multifactorial problem that is best served with a sound reconstructive algorithm. Although the triggering event is often trauma, infection, or surgery to the genitalia, comorbid factors often play a major role in enabling pain, delayed healing, scarring, and poor hygiene to propagate this disease process. A successful reconstruction must account for all of these factors. *A* to *C,* These preoperative and postoperative photographs illustrate an obese 29-year-old man who underwent a circumcision to improve hygiene. Unfortunately, the circumcision scar healed slowly because of pressure of the overlying abdominal pannus, thereby causing a painful and hypertrophic penile scar, a retrussed penile glans, and a pseudophimosis. *Continued*

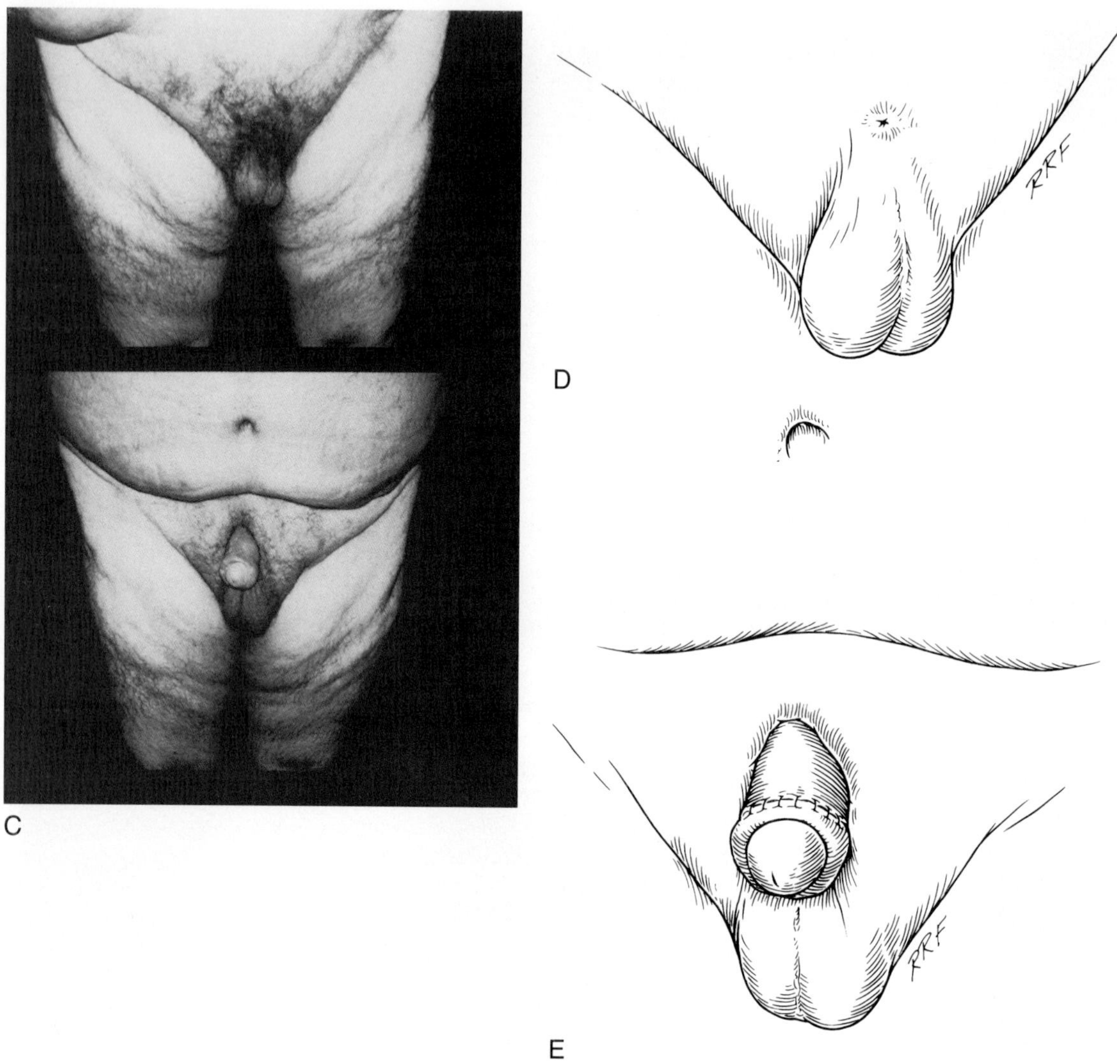

FIGURE 152-18, cont'd. *D* and *E,* Surgery to correct this problem included penile shaft release, split-thickness skin grafting of the penile shaft, aggressive prepubic lipectomy, and abdominal panniculectomy.

or genital dysmorphias, penile loss after circumcision, and prepubertal genital trauma.[36,37] Before the mid-1980s, there was little debate about the management of neonatal intersex problems after the initial diagnosis and establishment of the genotypic sex. In essence, all of these infants were encouraged to be raised female and at the appropriate time would undergo surgical reconstruction to "correct their genitalia." For a neonate with indefinite genitalia, both parents, the consulting physicians, and the treating surgeons all needed to be in accord. The goals of surgery were to remove all vestiges of male anatomy and to reconstruct a vagina. In many patients, there was minimal follow-up of the surgical results and the child's ability to adapt to an arbitrary gender assignment.

The advent of microsurgery provided the medical community with a viable alternative to arbitrary female reassignment and presented the opportunity to construct a phallus for genotypic XY patients. Although prepubertal and adolescent phalloplasties are not ideal, this surgery offers hope to the child, his family, and the treating physicians. Mounting pressure on the family and physicians to make a definitive neonatal gender assignment can be delayed pending further testing, and a viable alternative can still be provided for correct assignment.

Prepubertal phallic construction surgery will continue until it is able to provide predictable optimal results for these unfortunate patients. This progress will be measured generation by generation, and it will

TABLE 152-1 ✦ FIRST AND NINTH DECILES FOR LENGTH AND CIRCUMFERENCE OF THE PENIS, AND FOR VOLUME OF THE TESTIS, BY AGE*

	Stretched Penis				Volume of Testis (mL)	
	Length (cm)		*Circumference (cm)*			
Age (yr)	*First decile*	*Ninth decile*	*First decile*	*Ninth decile*	*First decile*	*Ninth decile*
<1	2.7	5.2	3.1	4.2	0.33	0.86
1-2	3.6	6.1	3.4	4.5	0.59	1.2
3-4	4.1	7.0	3.6	4.6	0.61	1.1
5-6	4.7	7.3	3.7	4.7	0.59	1.1
7-8	4.9	7.6	3.8	5.0	0.60	1.1
9-10	4.9	7.6	3.9	5.1	0.68	1.5
11	4.7	8.7	4.1	6.2	0.82	5.1
12	4.9	11.3	4.3	7.5	0.94 }	11.1 (12-13)
13	6.1	12.2	4.5	8.3	1.6 }	
14	6.6	13.5	4.9	8.5	2.0	14.4
15	9.1	14.8	6.1	9.2	5.7 }	18.3 (15-16)
16 }	10.8 (16-17)	15.3 (16-17)	{ 6.8	9.3	9.7 }	
17 }			{ 6.9	10.0 }	10.4 (17-19)	21.3 (17-19)
18-19	10.8	15.5	6.9	10.1 }		
20-25	11.3	15.5	7.2	9.8	10.8	21.5

* The growth variations of the male genitalia from birth to maturity are recorded. The authors validated that the stretched penile length and circumference closely approximate the penile length and circumference during erection. We frequently quote the table in discussing patients' reconstructive goals and expectations.

From Schonfeld W, Beebe GW: Normal growth and variation in the male genitalia from birth to maturity. J Urol 1942;48:759.

take time to adequately assess the results of phallic construction compared with arbitrary reassignment surgery for intersex patients. Although microsurgical contributions have provided forward philosophic thinking, several nagging problems continue to persist. First, the reconstructed organ is an artificial phallus, not a natural penis. Second, the issue of phallic growth through puberty and into adulthood has not been completely answered. It is still unclear whether a prepubertal phallic reconstruction is adequate or whether further reconstructive surgery is necessary as the patient passes into his adult years (Fig. 152-19).[38] Third, the problem of consent for a minor patient has raised many ethical questions that relate to the paucity of information on this subject and the lack of studies to present to inquiring parents. Fourth, the need for hormonal support also raises many questions in prepubertal and adolescent boys.

Perhaps one of the most intriguing stories of neonatal gender assignment occurred in the mid-1980s when two unrelated, genotypic XY boys were circumcised consecutively and both suffered total necrosis of

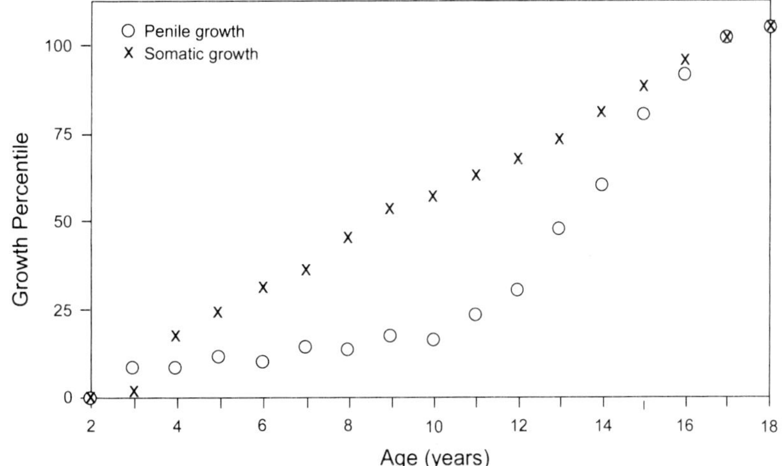

FIGURE 152-19. Phallic growth through puberty. (From Gilbert D, Jordan G, Devine C Jr, et al: Phallic construction in prepubertal and teenage boys. J Urol 1993;149:1521.)

their anterior penises. Both boys were subsequently referred for possible microsurgical phallic reconstructions. Both sets of parents were counseled on the possibilities of penile growth, total phallic reconstruction, gender reassignment, and possible outcomes as they passed through puberty into adulthood. The parents of one of the boys elected to proceed with gender reassignment, and her progress has been reported elsewhere.[39] The other couple elected to continue with the male phenotype, and during the past 15 years, this child has grown into a normal teenage boy. In fact, approximately 70% of his penis was preserved and has grown through puberty. He has undergone penile release, skin grafting of the penile shaft, and glansplasty in anticipation of possible microsurgical phalloplasty surgery, which he has not yet required. Although this story is not yet complete, this child has not demonstrated any obvious psychological sequelae from this accident (Fig. 152-20).

Penile Agenesis (Aphallia)

Genital dysmorphias are rare and are often associated with other anomalies that are incompatible with life. Penile agenesis (aphallia) occurs in 1 of 10 to 30 million live births. The anomaly includes complete absence of the penis and may be associated with severe defects in the development of the caudal axis, distal gastrointestinal deformities, and severe musculoskeletal anomalies but normal testicular and scrotal presence. An occasional patient will have some vestiges of rudimentary penile structures.

According to Skoog,[40] aphallia should be classified according to the relationship of the urethral meatus to the external sphincter (postsphincteric, presphincteric, urethral atresia), with urethral atresia having the poorest prognosis. Although other authors have advocated immediate female sex reassignment[41,42] (bilateral orchiectomy, urethral transposition, and labial construction) to reduce the effect of the early testosterone surge, we have provided a surgical alternative for these patients. A staged reconstruction is recommended that includes separation of the urethral meatus from the rectal verge, urethral transposition, and subsequent phallic construction. These constructions are particularly challenging because of hypoplastic development of the genital and pudendal nerves (Fig. 152-21).

Penoscrotal Transposition

Complete penoscrotal transposition is a rare anomaly that can be helped by surgical correction. It is not at all unusual to see some degree of penoscrotal transposition in all male intersex states and in association with hypospadias. Surgical correction can vary from technically simple excisions of the "surrounding scrotum" to the need for phallic construction (Fig. 152-22).

ACQUIRED GENITAL DEFECTS

Post-Trauma

Post-traumatic genital repair is an uncommon but special chapter in surgical reconstruction. A reconstructive algorithm based on the etiology, an assessment of the extent of injury, and an anatomic inventory includes several goals and observations. First, the anatomically protected position of the genitalia implies that patients who have genital injuries often have large concomitant injuries as well and are often very ill. Resuscitation and life support of the patient take precedent over any reconstruction. However, genital reconstruction is of prime relevance, and only eyelid and lip reconstruction are considered more important in the reconstructive hierarchy. Second, aesthetics are foremost in genital reconstruction. Although it is not often articulated, the appearance of the genitalia is important to the self-esteem of a patient who is recovering from trauma. What is frivolous to one person may be a lifelong obsession to another, and genital aesthetics are as valued as other cosmetic areas such as the face, nose, and breasts. Third, the genitalia appear to be a "privileged site" such that the usual postreconstructive sequelae of scarring and contracture are often spared in genital reconstruction. This may be due to the fact that the average adult man has five to eight nocturnal erections every night, thereby inherently stretching scars or skin grafts on the penile shaft. This stretching may combat and overcome the tendency of myofibroblasts to contract a skin graft or scar. Fourth, both grafts and flaps are used together to complete reconstruction.

Before post-trauma genital reconstruction is discussed, it is necessary to introduce plastic surgeons to two intraoperative procedures that are essential to a successful outcome—an artificial erection and placement of a suprapubic tube.

An artificial erection during the time of genital reconstructive surgery can be very useful. Specifically, one uses an artificial erection to assess the presence of curvature (chordee) and the results of corrective reconstructive techniques. An artificial erection can be produced by a number of means. In pediatric surgery, an artificial erection is produced by placement of a butterfly needle into the corporal bodies, application of a tourniquet at the base of the penis or digital pressure on the corporal bodies with the surgeon's fingertips, and instillation of saline through a syringe. Care must be taken to make sure that the intracorporal pressures do not exceed approximately 110 mm Hg. In adults, the syringe technique is often insufficient, and therefore high-volume pumps are used. The

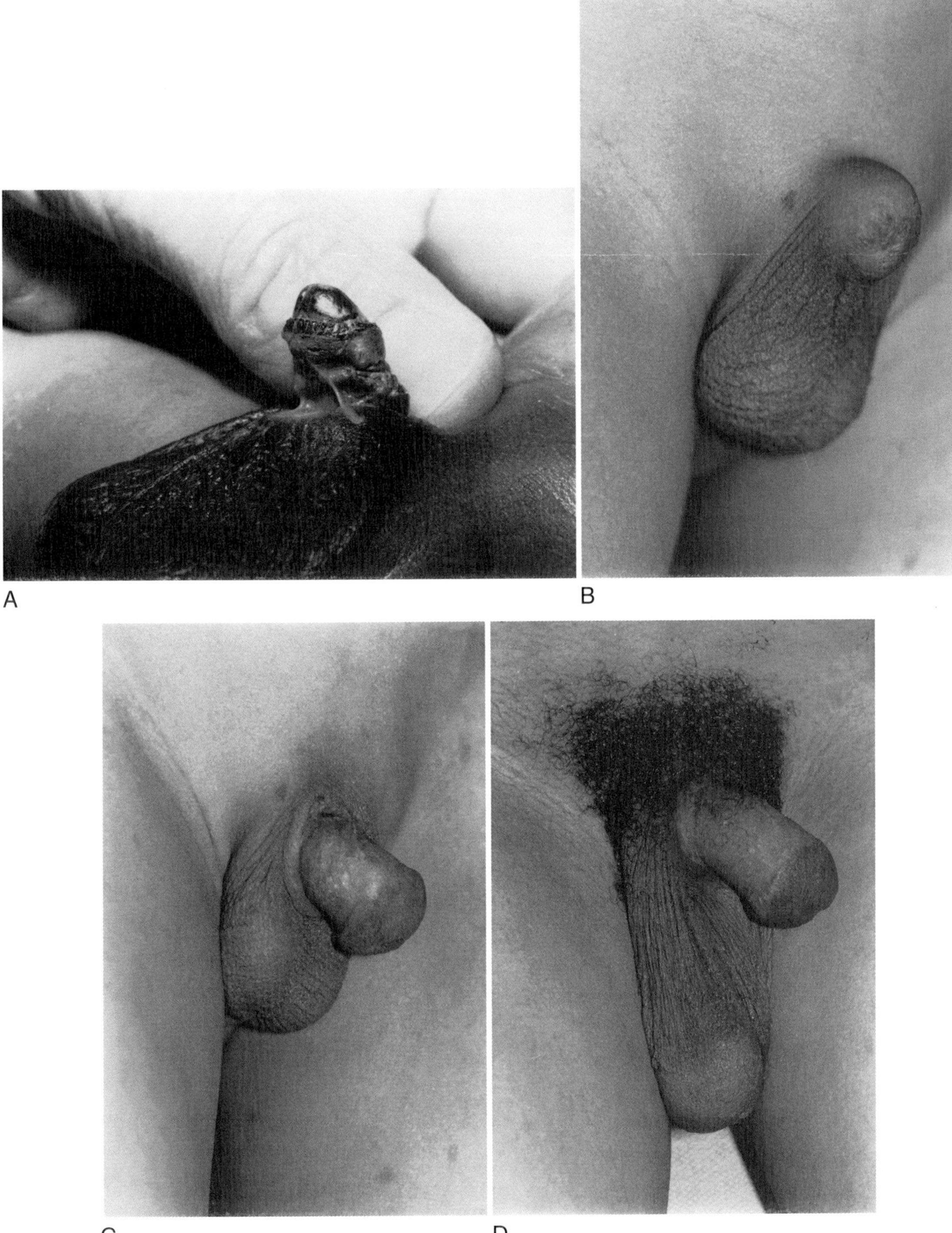

FIGURE 152-20. *A,* This newborn child suffered a circumcision accident at birth. Although all of the anterior penis appeared necrotic, his parents elected to raise him as a boy. *B,* At age 3 years, his penis began to grow in a normal genital growth profile. *C,* At age 7 years, he underwent an anterior penile release, full-thickness skin grafts to the penile shaft, and a composite graft from the groin to form a pseudoglans. *D,* At age 15 years, the penis has begun to grow through puberty.

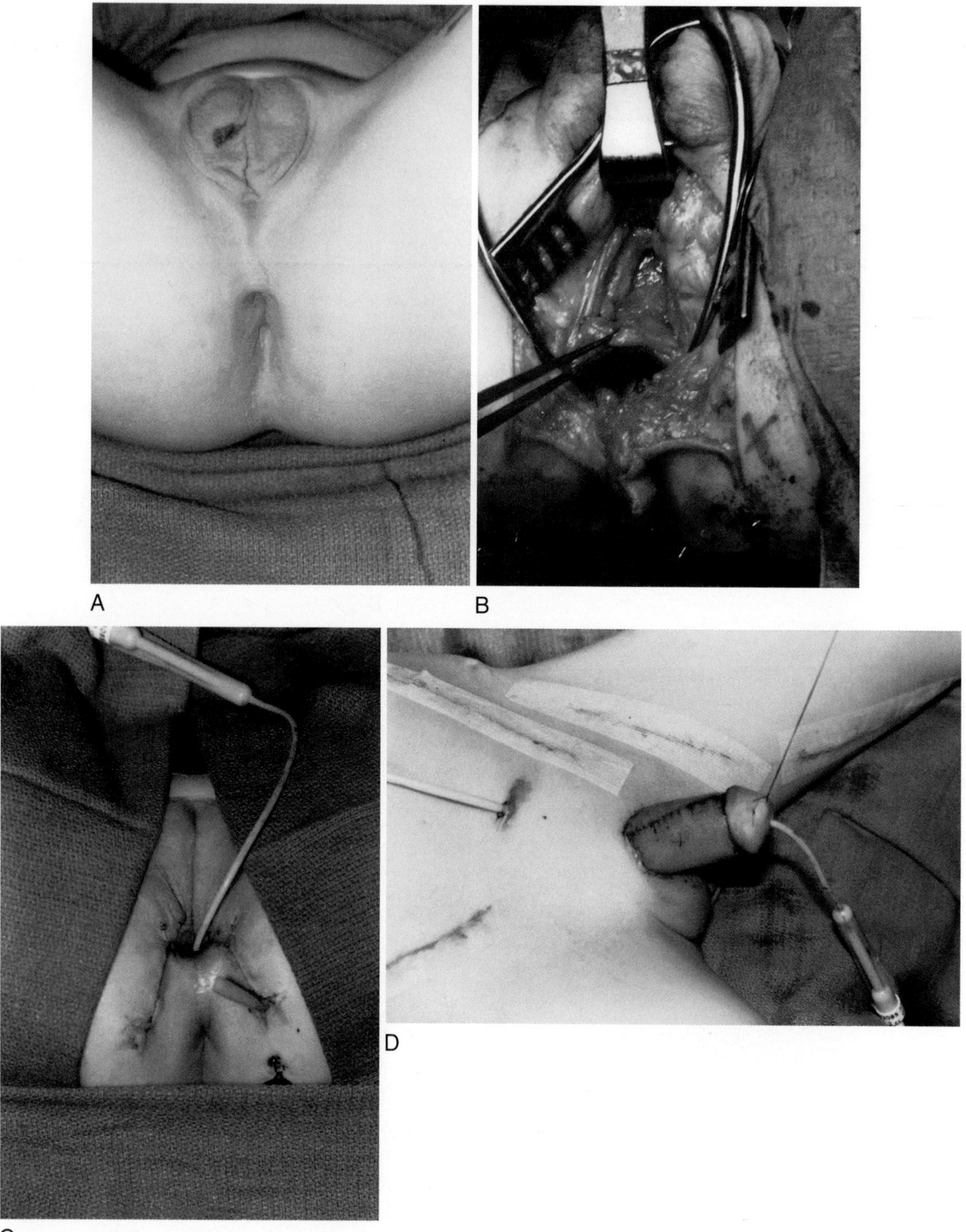

FIGURE 152-21. *A,* Aphallia is a rare congenital deformity that demands immediate consideration of early gender reassignment to preclude the effects of a premature testosterone surge. In this case, a genotypic 46 XY boy had not been reassigned and had not undergone an orchiectomy. *B,* This boy's urethral meatus was caudal to the rectal verge. At age 5 years, the patient underwent perineal relocation of the urethra and closure of the rectum. *C,* The resultant perineal meatus location was then prepared for a phallic construction that included the urethroplasty. *D,* One year later, the patient underwent a definitive microsurgical phallic construction to satisfy the goals of gender confirmation.

CAVROPUMP (manufactured by Life-Tech) is very useful. Again, a butterfly needle is placed into the corporal bodies or through the glans mucosa into the tip of the corporal bodies. The pump is then set on manual infusion with the pressure at 110 mm Hg. With use of a tourniquet at the base of the penis or by digital pressure on the corporal bodies, the pump is used to infuse saline until an artificial erection is achieved. One word of caution—the tourniquet at the base of the penis can conceal proximal ventral curvature. If one is correcting ventral curvature, the surgeon must be extremely careful not to obscure the proximal aspects of the ventral curvature with the placement of the tourniquet.

In some cases, it is beneficial to cause an erection by use of vasodilatory agents. The agent of choice is prostaglandin E_1. The dose is generally 5 to 10 μg of prostaglandin E_1 diluted to 1 mL. The agent is injected into the corporal bodies; within 7 to 10 minutes, an erection is usually achieved. In some plication techniques, surgeons have found it beneficial for the patient to have an erection during the performance of the plication. In cases other than these, the preferred technique in the authors' opinion is to produce an artificial erection by the infusion of saline.

A suprapubic tube is useful for diversion of urine, especially in urethral reconstructive surgery. A number of techniques are used to place the suprapubic tube in a minimally invasive fashion. In a patient with a lower abdomen that has not been operated on, the punch cystostomy techniques are preferred. A number of manufacturers have products on the market for punch cystostomy placement. Almost always, these products use a trocar system with either a peel-away sheath or a removable hub system. Surgeons should check with their operating room and become familiar with those systems. Before the use of trocar cystostomy, the surgeon should place the patient in approximately 15 to 20 degrees of Trendelenburg position. Likewise, the bladder should be well distended, and every effort should be made to place the cystostomy in the dome of the bladder. In the thin individual, the dome can be located with palpation if the bladder is sufficiently distended. In the more corpulent individual, a useful landmark is to place the cystostomy approximately two fingerbreadths above the crest of the pubis. If one is using a trocar cystostomy system, it is useful to establish the depth of the distended bladder. This can be done with an 18-gauge spinal needle attached to a syringe. As the spinal needle is advanced, aspiration pressure is maintained, and as the needle enters the bladder, one gets urine aspirate. In general, the resistance that the surgeon feels as the needle passes through the bladder wall is suddenly lost, and so by palpation the entry into the bladder is confirmed.

The Hurwitz cystostomy trocars are useful for placing a Foley catheter into the bladder as a suprapubic tube. The trocars come in sizes for placement of a 12 French Foley catheter, a 16 French Foley catheter, and a 20 French Foley catheter. In adults, the 16 French size is useful. In children, the 12 French size suffices. The Hurwitz trocar system is an adaptation of the peel-away sheath system. Placement is as with the other percutaneous modalities.

Once the cystostomy tube is placed, a retaining balloon should be seated at the dome and moved slightly into the bladder, and the tube is sutured to the patient's abdominal skin. By relieving the tension of the balloon against the dome of the bladder, spasms are decreased. The packaged cystostomy systems are often marked as to the amount of tube that needs to be placed into the bladder. However, some packaged cystostomy tubes use a Malecot tip; with these systems, the surgeon is cautioned not to seat the tube against the bladder wall. As the bladder decompresses, these small Malecot tubes can be displaced through the bladder wall. In all cases, newly placed cystostomy tubes should be firmly attached to the patient's abdominal skin.

GENITAL RECONSTRUCTION

Genital Skin Grafts

Genital skin loss occurs from burns, avulsion injuries, infections, and gangrene. Every patient has his own story of the accompanying pain, shame, anxiety, and suffering. Burns result in either full-thickness or partial-thickness skin loss from thermal, electrical, radiotherapy, and iatrogenic causes. Burn reconstructive algorithms resemble any other treatment plan. Where possible, direct closure is the most appropriate treatment followed by skin grafting (either split thickness or full thickness), local random-pattern flaps, musculocutaneous flaps, fasciocutaneous flaps, distal flaps, and microsurgical composite tissue transfer.

As a rule, total excision of the necrotic genital tissues followed by early skin grafting produces the best results. Care should be taken to remove all remnants of distal shaft tissue to reduce the risk of postoperative lymphedema. When the wound is contaminated or infected, adequate débridement of necrotic tissues combined with the application of mechanical débriding devices may be indicated.

The thick split-thickness skin graft is a mainstay of penile reconstruction. The graft should be pliable, placed onto a flat bed, and secured with a tie-over bolus pressure dressing to reduce the risk of hematoma or seroma formation. Successful skin graft "take" is directly related to meticulous hemostasis, control of erections, infection-free environment, and adequate immobilization.

The donor site should be close to the genitalia, large enough to produce a sheet skin graft and be well hidden. Ideally, the skin graft should be at least 0.018

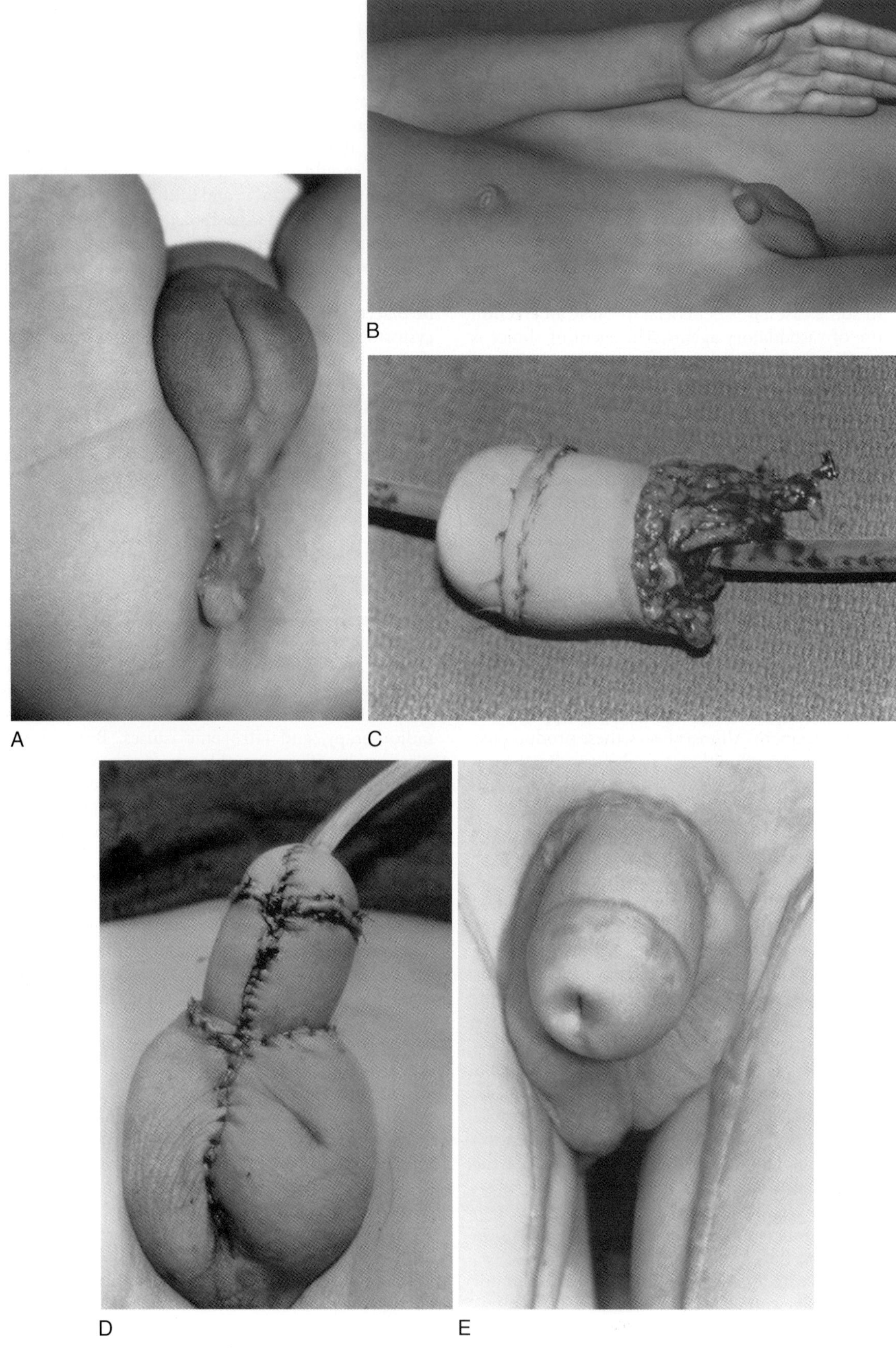
A
B
C
D
E

FIGURE 152-22. *A,* This 7-year-old genotypic male was born with penoscrotal transposition. A phallic remnant was present in the perineum but totally nonfunctional. In this case, the urethral meatus was distal to the anal verge and connected to the phallic remnant. *B,* At the first stage, the phallic remnant is filleted, inverted, and tubed to produce a vascularized urethra that is passed intrascrotally to the pubis. *C,* A left forearm cricket bat flap is dissected, elevated, and transformed into a phallus. *D,* This illustration depicts the closure of the ventral suture line. *E,* One year later, the phallus has healed well, albeit with a urethral fistula. Note the hypertrophic thigh scars.

to 0.02 inch in thickness and large enough to cover the whole breadth of the penile shaft or scrotum. The skin graft should be sutured circumferentially around the penile shaft with a ventral suture line. As a rule, this suture line will not contract (because of the privileged site), but a Z-plasty may often be incorporated to reduce the risk of contracture. The graft is then fixed to the surrounding skin, the underlying Buck fascia, and the tunica with dissolving sutures. Extended bed rest is important in the postoperative period to reduce the risk of graft shearing or movement. Amyl nitrate and diazepam (Valium) are administered to discourage erections in the early postoperative period. However, erections, massage, and stimulation are recommended for all patients after grafting as soon as the bolus dressing is removed on the fifth postoperative day (Fig. 152-23).

Meshed split-thickness skin grafts on the penile shaft are mentioned here only to be condemned. They scar poorly, and they are aesthetically second rate. McAninch[43] has described the use of meshed split-thickness skin grafts for scrotal reconstruction and in situations in which the penis has no erectile function. Meshed grafts in these situations may produce "good aesthetic results," but they will never measure up to the functional capacity of sheet grafts. (Note that nonexpanded meshed split-thickness grafts have become a mainstay of complicated, staged urethral reconstruction.[44,45])

Full-thickness skin grafts also have a place in genital reconstruction, but care must be taken to reduce any risk of lymphatic swelling or distal edema. These skin grafts are used extensively in phallic reconstructions to maintain harmony and stability between the flap skin and adjacent tissues. Full-thickness grafts are particularly useful for coronal sulcus design to prevent "coronal washout."

Scrotal reconstruction adheres to the same reconstructive principles. Where possible, primary closure is the procedure of choice, particularly in partial or hemilateral injuries. However, in the case of total scrotal loss, split-thickness skin grafts are effective if they are placed and immobilized carefully. There is a place for meshed, nonexpanded skin grafts in scrotal and perineal reconstruction because of the uneven and often biconcave contours of this region. In addition, there is an aesthetic dividend in that meshed grafts on the scrotum often emulate the scrotal rugae.

Genital Flaps

Post-traumatic penile, scrotal, and perigenital anatomy dictates flap design to a great degree. Most of the serviceable flaps in genital reconstruction depend on the predictable anatomy of the superficial vascular system and, in some cases, the deep system and are designed on tissues that have recognized arterial names and vascular territories. Such territories include the flaps of the superficial external pudendal system that are the basis for penile shaft and anterior urethral reconstruction (Fig. 152-24). Distally based penile flaps that incorporate the balanitic arteries and internal lamina of the prepuce are based on the internal pudendal vascular system. These include the single-pedicled and bipedicled preputial flaps that can be employed for glans and coronal reconstruction (Figs. 152-25 and 152-26).[18,46] Proximal penile flaps that are vascularized from the lower abdomen and pubis are recognized but are less practical for male genitalia reconstruction.

Scrotal flaps have also been employed in genital reconstruction but have limited application with the exception of hemiscrotal reconstruction. Although the scrotum has a wealth of well-vascularized skin and subcutaneous tissue that it can logically lend to its hemiscrotal twin or the adjacent penis, in fact it is ill-suited for genital reconstruction because of its rigorous and nonglabrous nature. A centrally located scrotal flap designed along the medial raphe has also been described as a reconstructive flap option for proximal urethral repair.[15] However, the unpredictable nature of scrotal hair distribution often dictates presurgical epilation of the flap. This flap is based on the posterior scrotal artery and can be difficult to mobilize extensively. In addition, when the flap has been dissected, elevated, and transferred, there can be the sequela of scrotal tethering, even after successful transfer. A free buccal mucosal graft is often a better choice for proximal urethral reconstruction.[47]

There is a significant need for frequent use of muscle flaps. The gracilis muscle flap is considered "the workhorse of the perineum," acting as the perineal "watchdog" much like the omentum in the abdomen. The gracilis muscle is used extensively to cover and vascularize urethral anastomoses, to cover exposed pelvic bones, to reduce the risk of osteomyelitis, to fill the perineum after exenteration, to vascularize the perineum in postirradiation injuries, and to help shape and support microsurgical phallic reconstructions.[48]

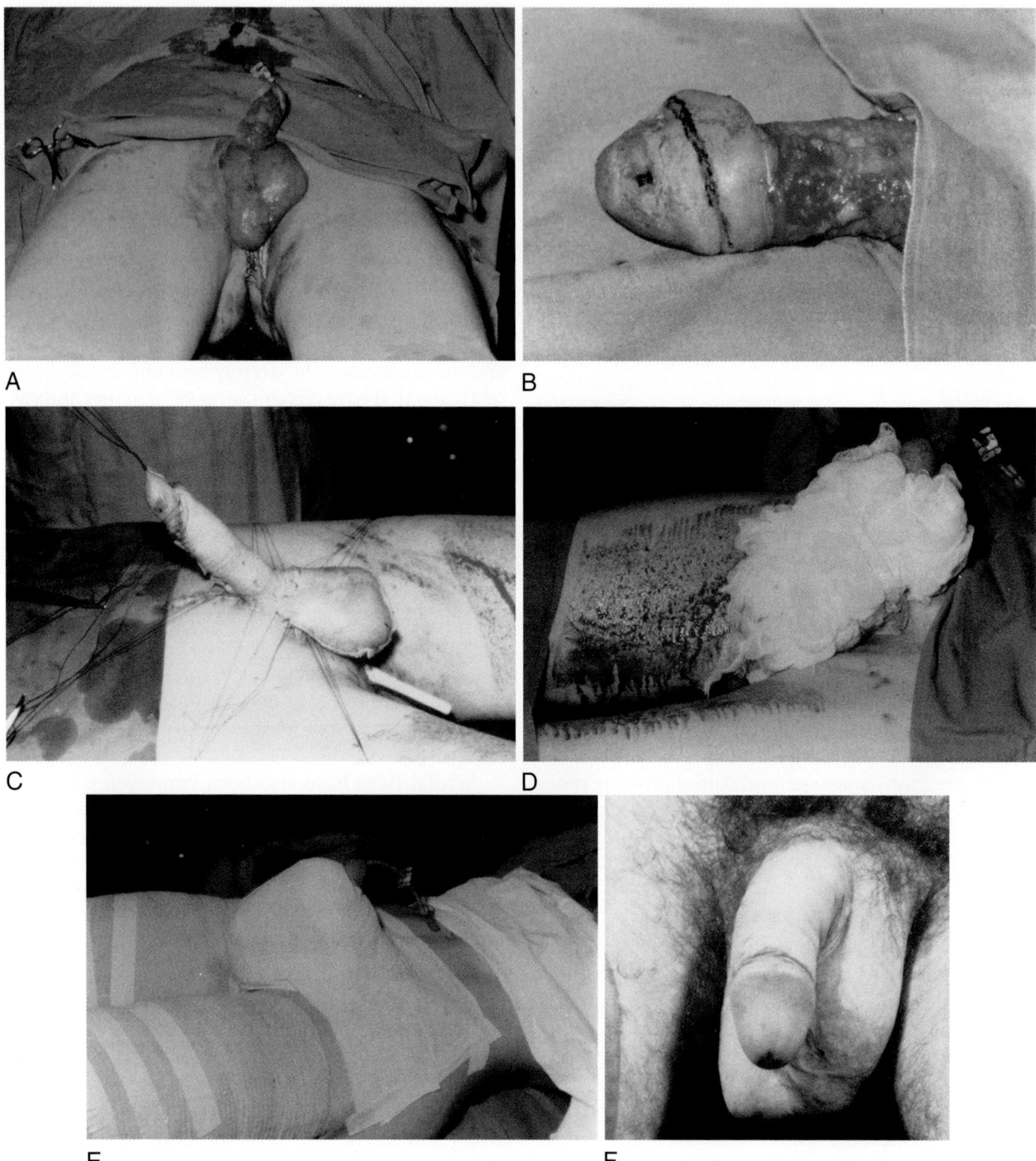

FIGURE 152-23. *A,* This patient suffered almost complete avulsion of the penile and scrotal skin in a tractor "power takeoff" injury. Reconstruction included débridement of all avulsed tissue and apposition of the testicles. *B,* A ring of distal shaft skin is débrided to reduce the risk of penile shaft edema. *C,* Thick split-thickness skin grafts are inlaid onto the penis and scrotum. *D,* A soft bolus dressing is applied and maintained with tie-over sutures. *E,* The dressing is stabilized with bulky outer dressings and tape. *F,* One year later, the grafts healed well with evidence of the "privileged" healing of the genitalia. (Courtesy of J.D.M. Alton, MD.)

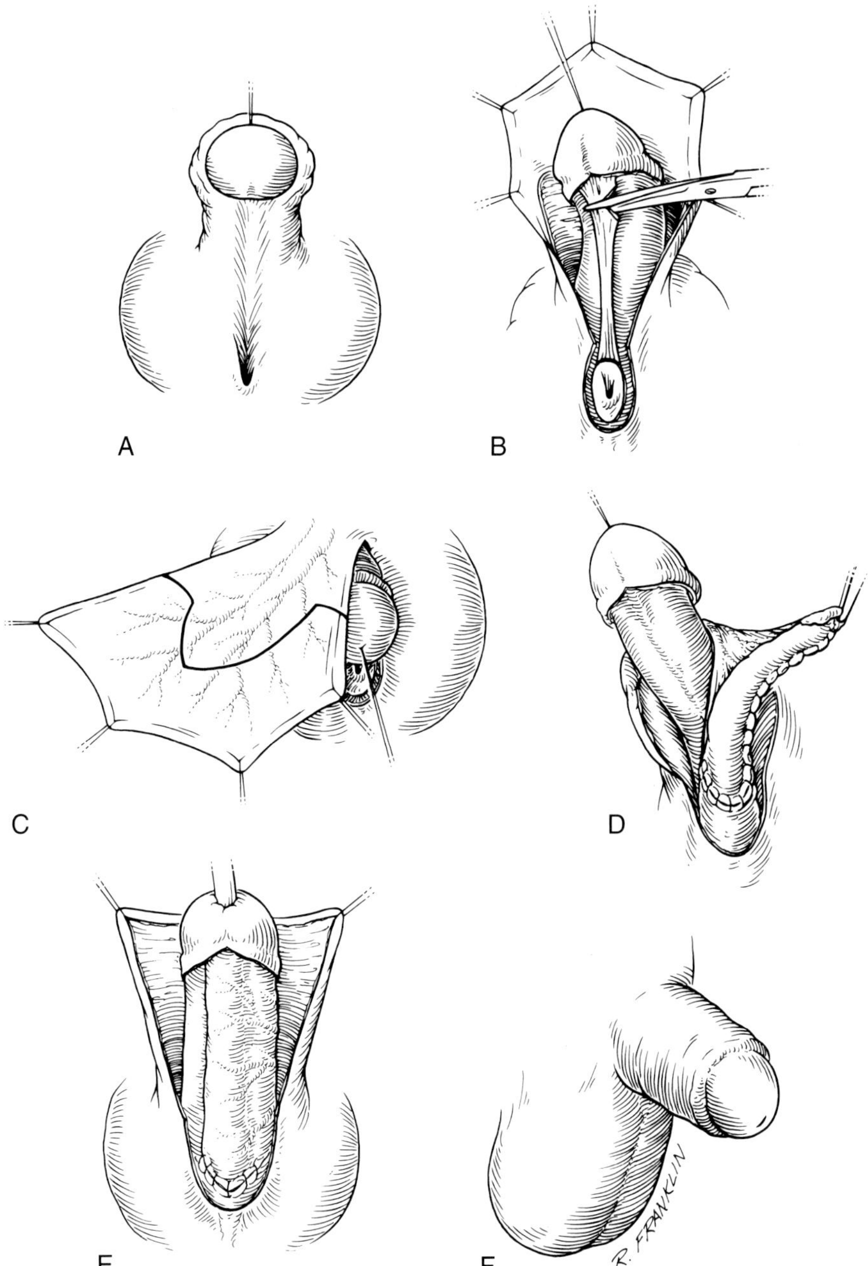

FIGURE 152-24. *A,* This penoscrotal hypospadias repair demonstrates the potential of untethered penile shaft and transverse preputial island flaps. Until these flaps were described, urethral repair depended on full-thickness skin grafts for construction of a viable neourethra. *B,* After chordee release, the penile shaft skin and prepuce are dissected and unfurled to produce enough vascularized tissue to construct a neourethra and to cover the penile shaft. *C,* Microscopic techniques encourage preservation of the vascularity in the remaining penile skin used to cover the penis. *D,* The urethra is tubed and transposed to the penile ventrum, where it is anastomosed to the foreshortened proximal native urethra. *E,* The tube is then drawn through an incision in the glans penis. *F,* One year later, the penis is straight with an intact urethra that extends to the glans tip. The bifid scrotum has also been transposed and closed in the midline.

Continued

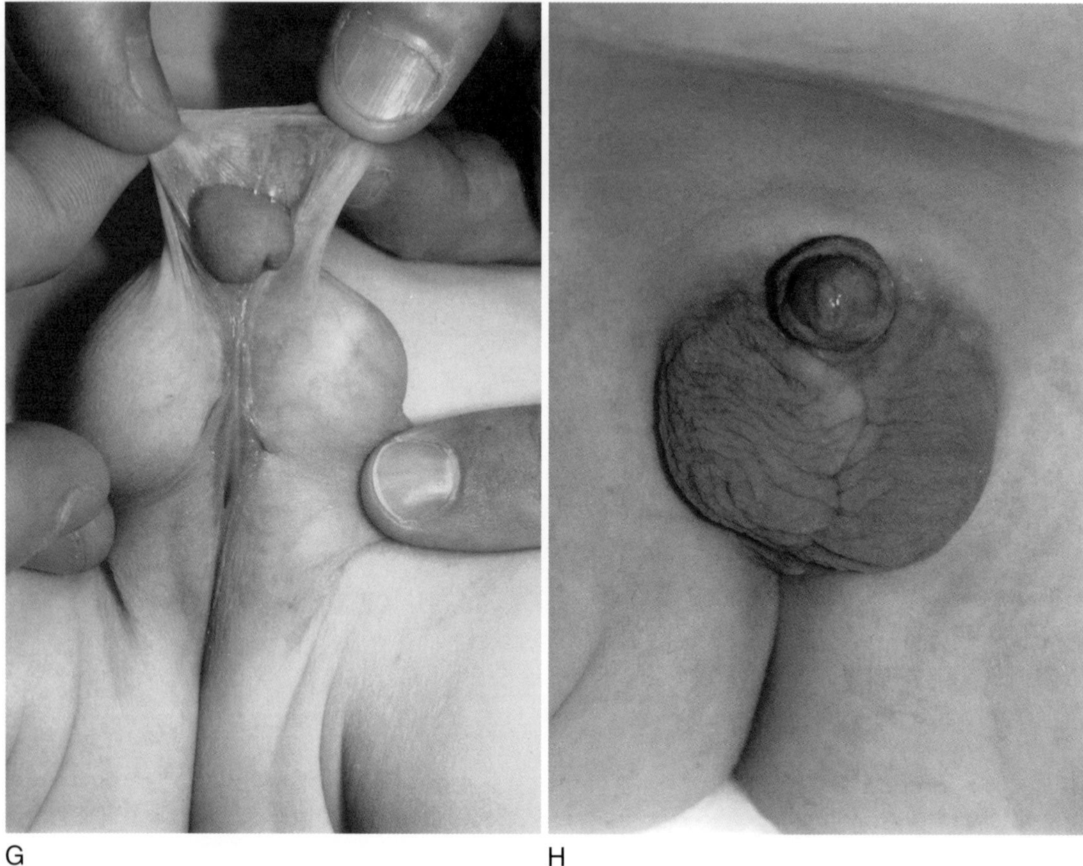

G H

FIGURE 152-24, cont'd. *G* and *H,* Preoperative and postoperative photographs illustrate the successful result.

The rectus abdominis muscle flap may also be employed to help suspend, cover, and vascularize the penile shaft. Release of the muscle's pelvic insertion often promotes flap length and improves configuration. This flap has predictable vascularity, is easy to dissect and transfer, but has a variable size and a theoretical problem of donor site hernia formation postoperatively.

Fasciocutaneous paragenital flaps that have been used, often with limited application, are the superficial circumflex iliac flap,[49] the deep circumflex iliac flap (often combined with an osseous component),[50] the superficial epigastric flap,[51] the double-pedicled composite groin flap,[52] the anteromedial thigh flap,[53] the anterolateral thigh flap,[54] and the pudendal thigh flap.[55,56] The superficial groin flap is based on the superficial circumflex artery system, a branch of the femoral artery, and has an unpredictable origin, direction, and size. The flap must often be delayed, attached or "waltzed" into a central midline position by a secondary procedure to be used as a genital flap. For these reasons, the groin flap has limited primary genital use and is considered only a "plan B" flap.

During the past 10 years, most articles on genital reconstruction have been modifications or attempted improvements of local perigenital arterialized flap design. Several authors have tried to incorporate osseous components into their flap design in an attempt to bring inherent autologous stiffness to their phalloplasties.[51,52,57] At this time, it is unknown what the final results will be.

Medial thigh flaps may be based inferiorly on the perineal artery system or superiorly on the external pudendal system and branches of the profunda femoris artery. The inferiorly based flap has been called by several names, including the Singapore flap[55] and the pudendal thigh flap.[58] Originally described to correct vesicovaginal fistulas, the flap is based posteriorly within the crural fold between the scrotum and the medial wall of the thigh and extends from the posterior crural fold to the medial groin area anteriorly. Although most flap descriptions have focused on vaginal reconstruction and the correction of vesicovaginal and rectovaginal fistulas, this flap has been successfully used for male genital construction by combining a unilateral posteriorly based perineal

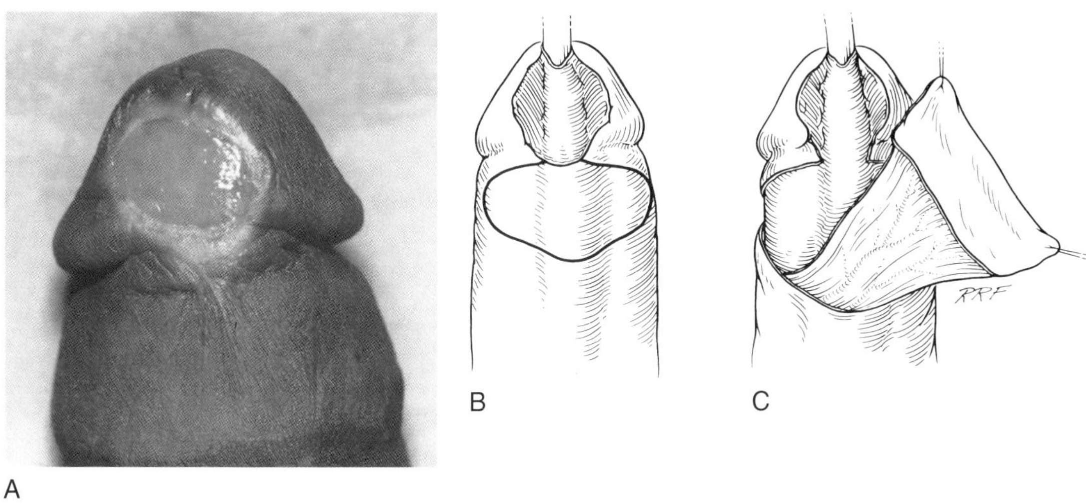

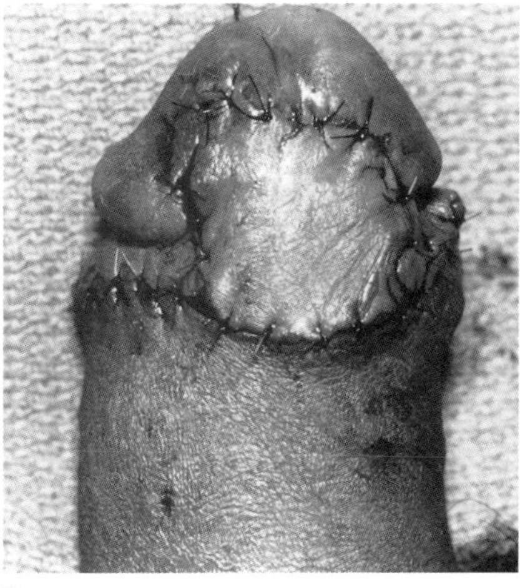

FIGURE 152-25. Glanular reconstruction continues to be a challenge to the reconstructive surgeon. Ideally, the tissues used for reconstruction should mimic the normal genital epithelium in bulk, consistency, feel, and sensation. The scope of this definition obviously limits available tissues to the adjacent glans and the internal and external preputial plates. That said, glanular replacement tissue has also been derived from other autogenous sources. Where possible, excess prepuce can be transferred and even de-epithelialized and rolled to form a glanular mass. *A,* A decubitus ulcer over the ventral glans. *B,* A local rotation flap from the internal lamina of the prepuce is drawn out. *C,* The flap, based on the external pudendal vascular system, is dissected and elevated. *D,* The flap is then inset onto the ventral glans.

artery flap with a contralateral gracilis flap (Fig. 152-27).

To complete the catalogue of fasciocutaneous flaps, the gluteal-posterior thigh flap must also be included.[59,60] This flap is based on the inferior descending branch of the inferior gluteal artery. This vessel and its venae comitantes branch from the inferior gluteal artery and then run inferiorly beneath the muscle fascia down the posterior thigh in a "stocking seam" distribution. This flap can be dissected, elevated, and transferred into the perineum and can even be rolled on itself to form a phallus.

Distant flaps that have been employed in genitourinary reconstruction lack the usual genital attributes and have limited use. Musculocutaneous flaps including the vertical and transverse rectus abdominis flap (based on the deep inferior epigastric artery),[8] the gracilis musculocutaneous flap,[61] the rectus femoris musculocutaneous flap,[62] and the tensor fascia lata musculocutaneous flap[63] have all found occasional favor with some authors seeking to simplify genital reconstruction. Unfortunately, the skin and subcutaneous tissues associated with these usually reliable flaps are nonglabrous, thick, and totally dependent on their tethered blood supply with little chance for aesthetic design once the flap has been transferred to the genitalia. Nevertheless, they are an important part of the surgeon's armamentarium in addressing genital injuries after trauma, infection, and cancer and for patients with comorbid health problems. These flaps are often the *only* tissues available for genital reconstruction. The trauma, cancer, infection, and comorbid disease that originally contributed to genital tissue loss may also preclude sophisticated microsurgical reconstruction. Thus, these flaps are the only hope for functional, albeit suboptimal, genital reconstruction.

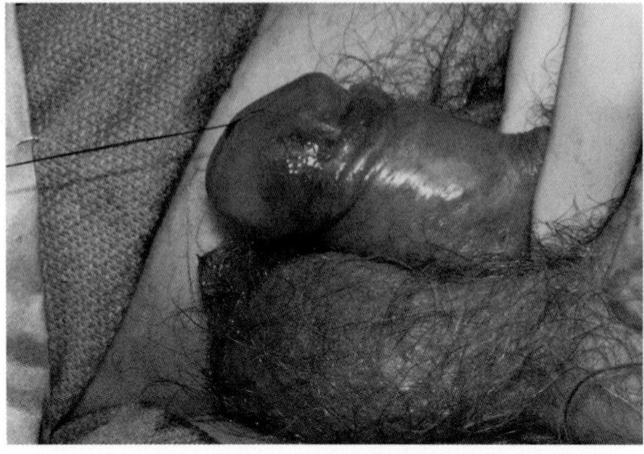

A

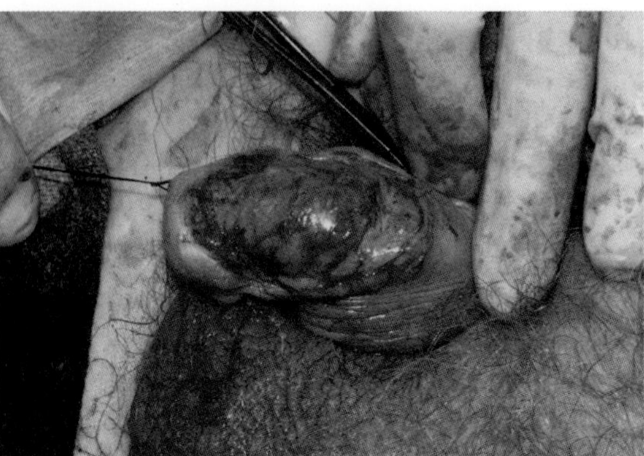

B

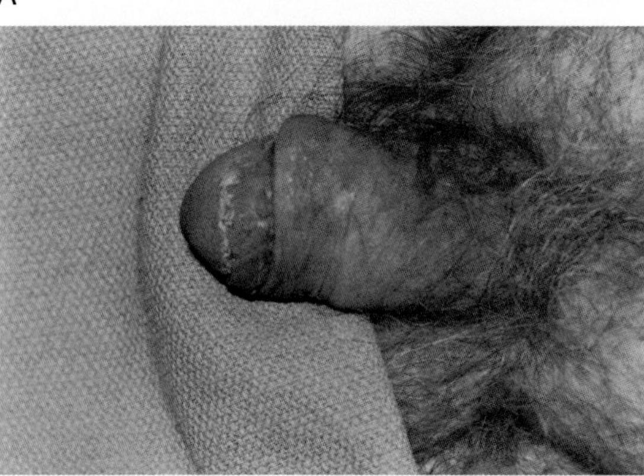

C

FIGURE 152-26. *A,* An 83-year-old man presented with a residual squamous cell carcinoma in situ of the glanular uroepithelium. *B,* After local excision and frozen section confirmation of clear margins, the prepuce is unfurled. *C,* An axial flap designed on the internal preputial lamina is dissected, elevated, transferred, and contoured into the glans corona. Circumcision is also completed.

Microsurgical Genital Reconstruction

GENITAL REPLANTATION

Microsurgical techniques and microsurgical composite tissue transplantation have become the state-of-the-art treatment for many reconstructive problems. The first uses of the microscope in genital reconstruction for penile reattachment after amputation were reported independently by Cohen[2] and Tamai[3] in 1977. However, the first account of successful reattachment long predated the introduction of microsurgical techniques. In 1929, Ehrich[64] first reported a successful penile attachment by opposing and anastomosing the lacerated corporal bodies and repairing the overlying tunica only. This technique was occasionally successful but usually associated with loss of the overlying skin, glans, sensation, and erectile and voiding function. McRoberts modified Ehrich's principles,[65] and the technical nuance significantly improved the results of microsurgical reattachment. Most reports of successful reattachment in the Western world represented solitary patients or small series of patients; the usual etiology was a sharp amputation due to self-mutilation or industrial farm accidents with crush or avulsion injuries.[66-70]

However, it came to our attention that in the 1970s, surgeons in Thailand were exposed to an epidemic of penile amputations perpetrated by the wives of philandering men; these women would cut off their husband's penis while he slept and then often throw the amputated organ out the window. Bhanaganada[71] reported reattaching a series of 18 penises by tunica and urethral repair only. Reports of successful reattachment describe the recruitment of the ventral, deep, and dorsal planes of penile vascularity at various times—all with successful results.[72] It appears that any of these arterial planes are able to provide adequate penile vascularity independently. Likewise, venous repair can also incorporate available venous systems and be successful. Associated morbidity notwithstanding, how do so many of these "macroreplantations" survive despite the lack of state-of-the-art reattachment techniques? It seems that these reattachments somehow act on a "non-flap" fashion in that plasmatic imbibition, vascular inosculation, and capillary ingrowth are all accelerated in time so that the attached part acts "more like a graft than flap physiology." The apparent totality of success is due to communication between the proximal vessels through the corporal spaces. In fact, not only does the penis survive, but urethral function, erectile function, ejaculation,

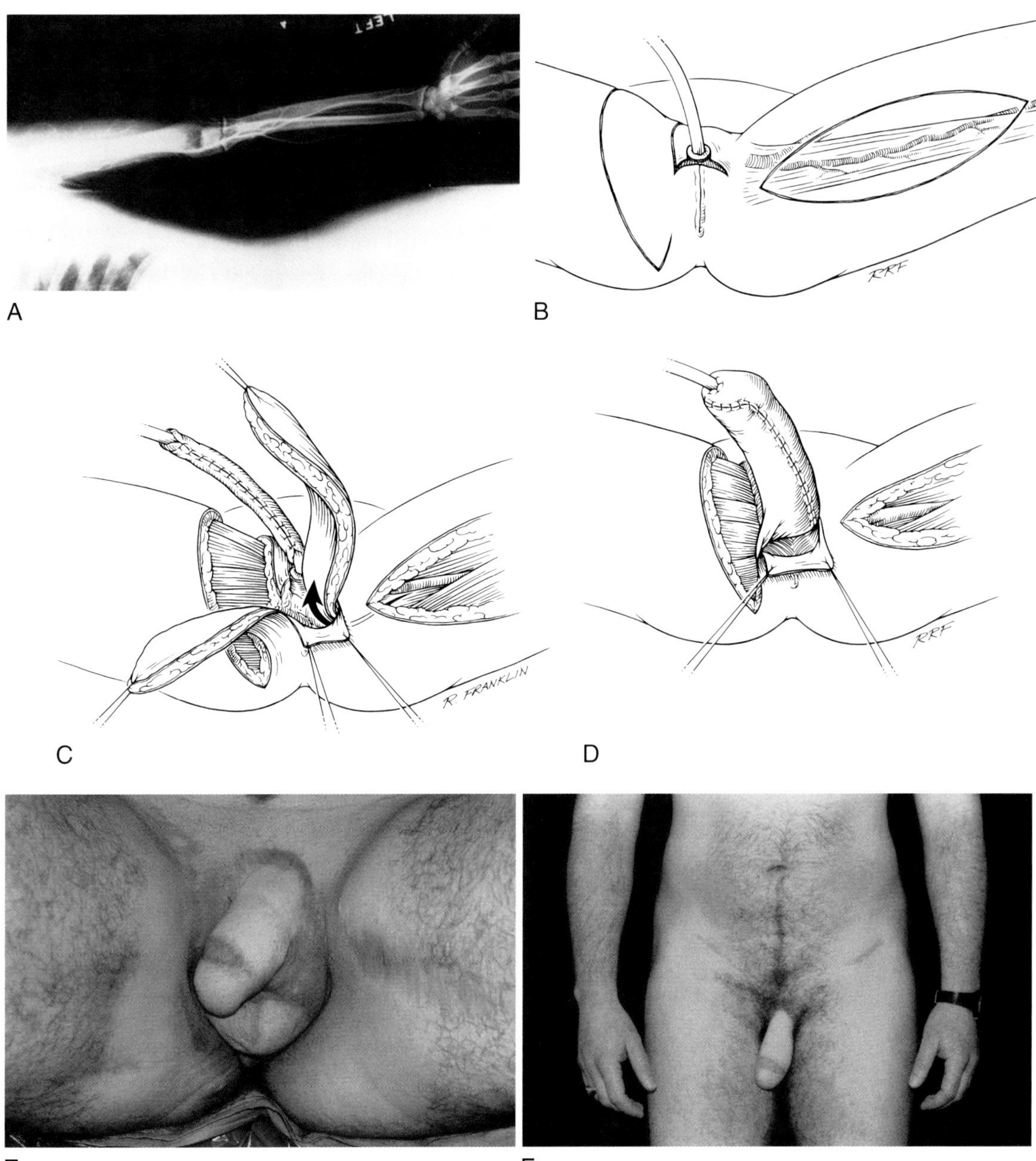

FIGURE 152-27. *A,* A 23-year-old female-to-male transgendered patient presented for definitive genital transformation. A bilaterally abnormal Allen test result and subsequent upper extremity angiograms confirmed bilateral absence of the ulnar arteries, thereby precluding a microsurgical forearm phalloplasty. A first-stage vaginectomy, hysterectomy, bilateral salpingo-oophorectomy, and urethra lengthening were completed without incident. *B,* In this case, a right perineal arterialized flap (Singapore flap) and a left gracilis musculocutaneous flap are dissected, elevated, and transposed to the perineum. *C,* The flaps are sutured together to nourish a full-thickness skin graft neourethra. *D,* The flaps are then waltzed into a normal perineal position. *E,* A skin graft coronaplasty completes the reconstruction. Note the scrotal bulk provided by the gracilis muscle transfer. *F,* The effects of male hormones and flank lipoplasty help confirm a male body habitus.

and tactile and erogenous sensibility are occasionally preserved.[73]

The optimum penile reattachment begins with a "bag-in-a-bag" technique to transfer the amputated part to a replantation center. The patient is also transferred, kept normothermic and well perfused hemodynamically (Fig. 152-28).

After the induction of anesthesia, the proximal and distal ends of the amputated penis are examined microscopically. Minimal débridement is followed by mechanical stabilization of the urethra and reapproximation of the tunica albuginea of the corpora cavernosa.

Revascularization is completed by use of microsurgical magnification, instrumentation, and 9-0 and 10-0 nylon sutures to reanastomose the deep dorsal arteries, the deep dorsal vein, and the superficial dorsal vein. Multiple nerve coaptations are meticulously completed with 10-0 and 11-0 nylon sutures. The dartos fascia and skin are then loosely approximated to complete the reattachment. A suprapubic tube is inserted to divert the urinary flow for 2 to 3 weeks, and the patient is prescribed bed rest in a warm room (Figs. 152-29 and 152-30).

Testicular reattachment has also been reported but requires a sharp amputation etiology for successful anastomosis of the thin-walled arteries and veins that surround and vascularize the testicle, seminiferous tubules, and vas deferens.[74,75] Unfortunately, most testicular amputations are of the avulsion or crush type and therefore are not reattachable. Clinically, the only vessel that has adequate caliber is the testicular artery

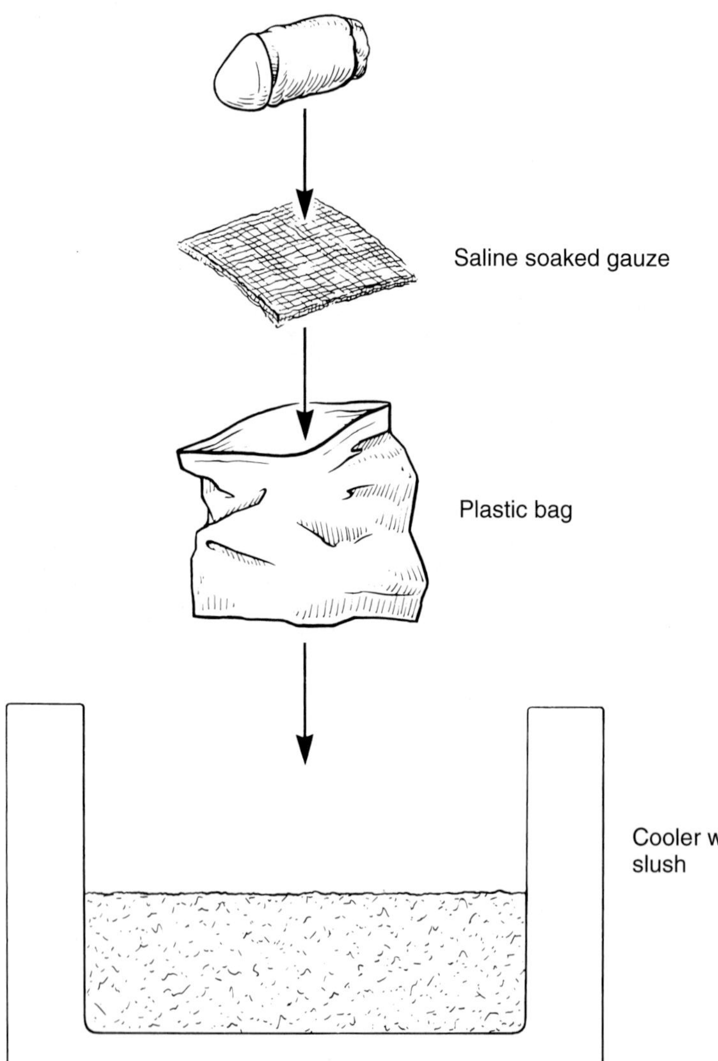

FIGURE 152-28. Penile replantation often mimics the algorithms of other amputated extremities that are candidates for reattachment. The penis is initially wrapped in a saline-soaked gauze and placed into a plastic bag, which in turn is placed in a bag or cooler of ice with water. Because genital amputations are often self-inflicted, it is important to obtain a psychiatric consultation before restorative surgery. Although many patients are diagnosed to be psychotic at the time of their amputation, most have a good or guarded prognosis, and therefore surgery is approved by the psychiatric service. This intervention may also protect the surgeon in the postoperative period when a deranged patient may accuse the surgeon of causing the amputation. (From Jordan GH: Initial management and reconstruction of male amputation injuries. In McAninch JW, ed: Traumatic and Reconstructive Urology. Philadelphia, WB Saunders, 1996: 673-681.)

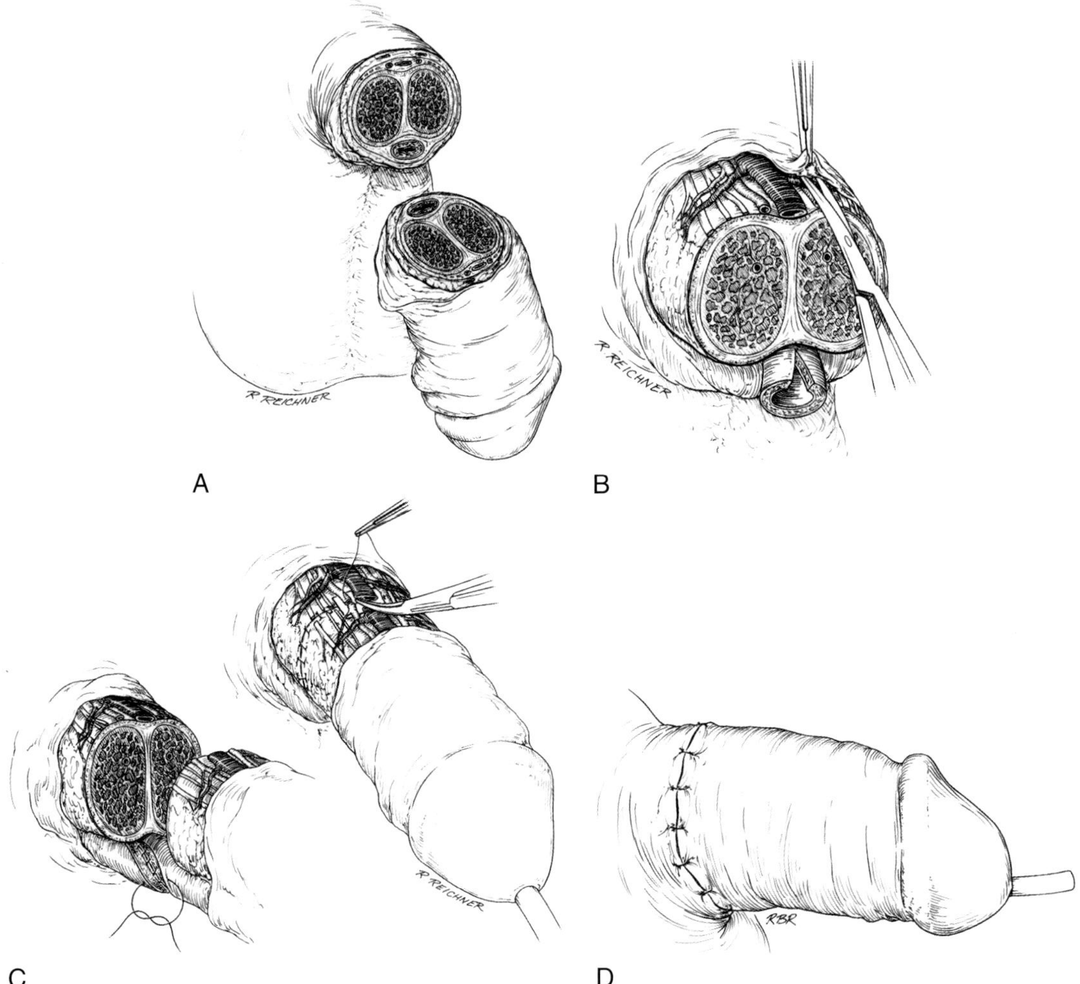

FIGURE 152-29. *A,* The ideal candidate for genital replantation is a patient with a clean, sharp cut in which the amputated part has been cooled. *B,* Both edges of the amputation are dissected and prepared for reattachment. *C,* The urethra and its underlying corpus spongiosum are anastomosed with a two-layer repair and the insertion of a silicone stent. Urethral diversion through a suprapubic tube may be indicated. The corporal bodies are then anastomosed by opposing the edges of the tunica circumferentially. Identification and anastomoses of the corporal arteries are usually forgone. Once the penis is stabilized, arteriovenous anastomosis is completed by use of microsurgical magnification, instrumentation, and sutures. In this illustration, the deep dorsal vein and the parallel dorsal arteries are anastomosed. In addition, the branches of the dorsal nerve of the penis are also coapted. *D,* The postoperative appearance is illustrated. (From Jordan GH: Initial management and reconstruction of male amputation injuries. In McAninch JW, ed: Traumatic and Reconstructive Urology. Philadelphia, WB Saunders, 1996:673-681.)

with its venae comitantes. The artery enters the testicle in its body and then divides into a superior branch that vascularizes the testicular body, its superior pole, and the overlying head (globus major) of the epididymis. An inferior branch supplies the tail of the epididymis (globus minor).

Two other arteries are also involved in testicular vascularization: the deferens artery, which arises from the inferior vesicular artery and vascularizes the epididymis, and the cremasteric artery, which arises from the inferior epigastric artery and vascularizes the cremasteric muscle and the other cord structures. Both of these arteries are small, filmy, and often unrecognizable in reattachment circumstances.

There are five factors to be considered before proceeding with testicular reattachment. First, it is important to understand the three different testicular blood supplies when a candidate is considered for possible reattachment. Second, the venous presence, pattern, and vascular stability may all play into the appropriateness of reattachment. Third, a devascularized testicle has only about 4 to 6 hours of ischemia before

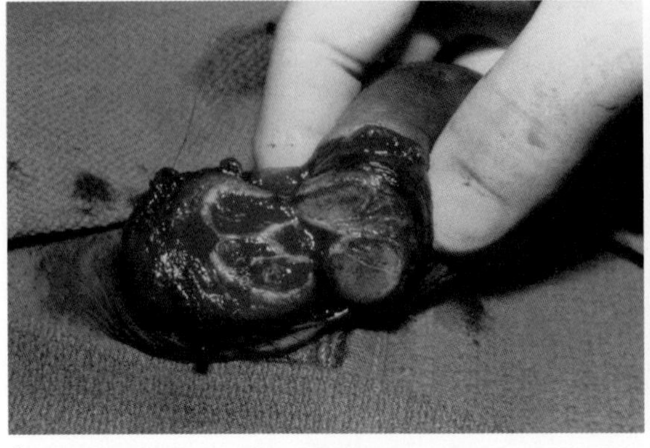

A

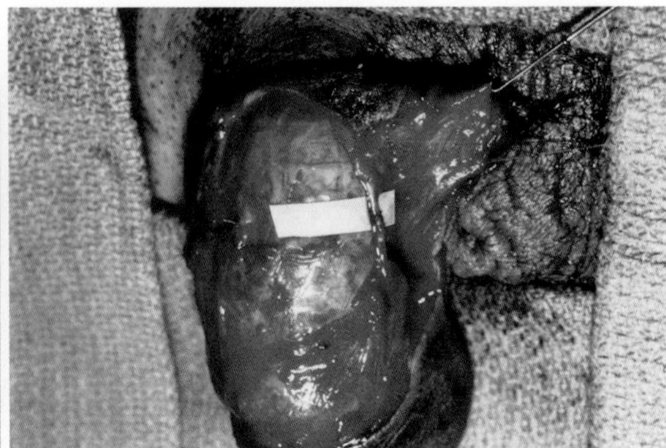

B

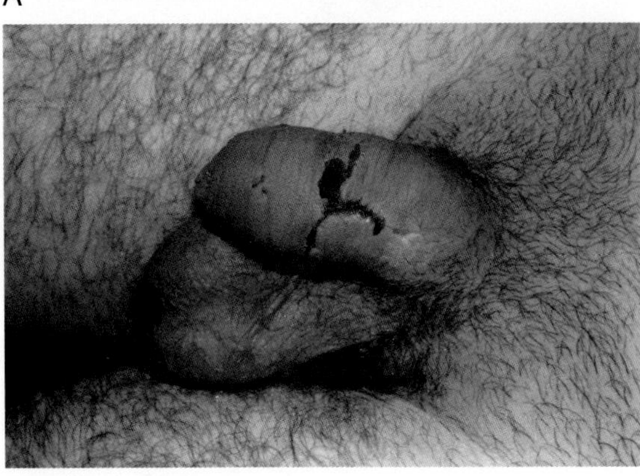

C

FIGURE 152-30. *A,* A self-inflicted penile amputation illustrates the corporal bodies and the corpus spongiosum. *B,* Reattachment includes urethral anastomosis, corporal body anastomosis, unilateral deep penile artery anastomosis, dorsal penile nerve coaptation, and superficial and deep dorsal vein anastomoses. *C,* The final result 3 weeks later illustrates preservation of all penile tissues.

losing its reattachment value. A reattached testicle cannot be expected to recover its sperm-producing function, and even if it does, the sperm count is often too low to be effectual. Fourth, there is the technical issue of vas deferens anastomosis and the maintenance of patency in the face of traumatic amputation. Fifth, the post-reattachment psychological well-being of the patient (particularly in self-mutilation patients) must be considered. When all of these points are considered together, the best that can be hoped for with a reattached testicle is the maintenance of testosterone secretion (Fig. 152-31).

PENILE REVASCULARIZATION

It would be convenient to be able to correct erectile dysfunction with a simple microsurgical procedure. Unfortunately, experience has borne out the restricted place of penile revascularization for erectile dysfunction. The procedure is usually limited to young men (younger than 45 years) who have a hemodynamically specific area of proximal pudendal-penile artery occlusive disease. These problems are usually related to penile injuries or pelvic fractures. In addition, veno-occlusive dysfunction and comorbid diseases such as diabetes mellitus, neuropathies, and proximal atherosclerosis must also be absent. These criteria obviously limit the population of potential patients.

Evaluation of a patient begins by confirming that any potential candidate has a strong sexual libido. Further evaluation must identify a focal cause of erectile dysfunction that is based on demonstrable arterial insufficiency. Evaluation should demonstrate the following: (1) rigidity reduced during sexual activity but relatively maintained by a normal veno-occlusive phase; (2) stronger nocturnal erectile dysfunction than sexual stimulation erectile dysfunction; and (3) poor spontaneity of erections. These symptoms may present immediately after genital trauma or may develop over time after a traumatic event. Erectile function evaluation includes an endocrine evaluation, a nocturnal penile tumescent test, color flow duplex ultrasonography, peak flow velocity in the cavernosal artery, cavernosal artery opening pressure, dynamic cavernosography-cavernosometry, pharmacocavernosometry, and pharmacocavernosography.

Studies at the authors' institution have been aimed at the common penile circulation as it relates to erectile function and reconstructability. Over the years, some interesting findings have been observed. It has

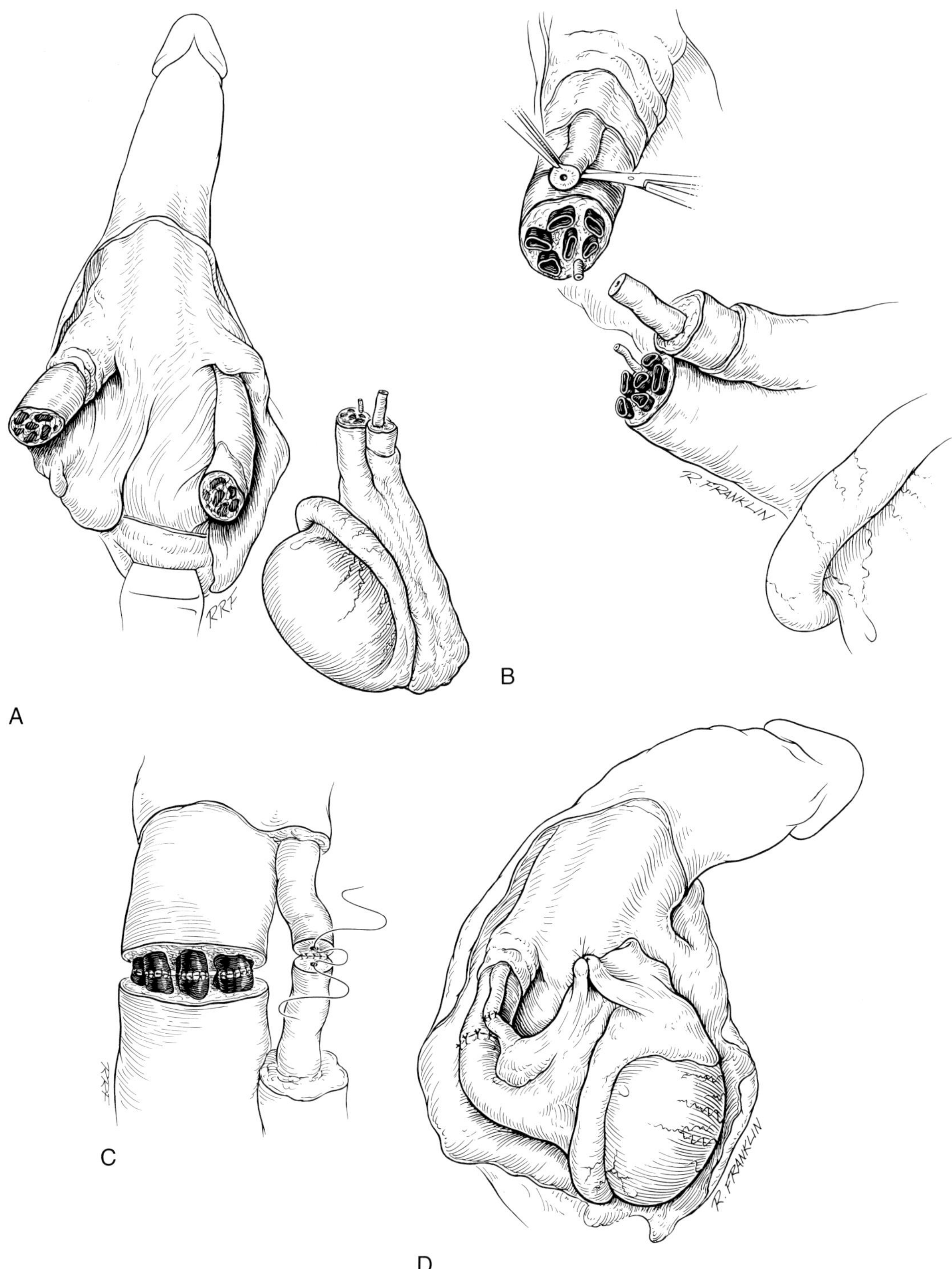

FIGURE 152-31. *A,* Testicular amputation presents the treating surgeon with some special challenges. Although testicular amputation is usually self-inflicted, the goals of the replantation are less clearly defined than for penile reattachment. Testicular replantation must be carried out in an expeditious manner to preserve both spermatogenesis and hormone production. In fact, spermatogenesis is only rarely preserved after reattachment. In this case, the left testicle and the right spermatic cord were the only structures considered to be replantable. *B,* The spermatic cord, the associated testicular artery branches, and the pampiniform plexus are identified both proximally and distally. *C,* The anastomoses of the vasal artery, several pampiniform veins, and a two-layer repair of the spermatic cord are depicted. In most cases, the anastomoses are completed with 11-0 nylon suture. *D,* The final result is illustrated with the left testicle transposed to the right scrotum. (From Jordan GH: Initial management and reconstruction of male amputation injuries. In McAninch JW, ed: Traumatic and Reconstructive Urology. Philadelphia, WB Saunders, 1996:673-681.)

been noted that an intact internal pudendal common penile arterial supply must exist on at least one side for erectile function to be normal or for there to be a normal tumescence response to pharmacologic treatment. On the other hand, for the purposes of urethral reconstruction, only reconstitution is necessary.

To determine these criteria, duplex ultrasonography has been successfully employed. Duplex ultrasonography evaluates arterial parameters through velocity. The systolic velocity should be greater than 25 cm/sec. End-diastolic velocity should be zero with an erection. Resistive index is calculated against end-diastolic velocity. Systolic rise time should be less than 0.1 second. Thus, if one has a normally intact internal pudendal common penile system on one side, then the inflow parameters, peak systolic velocity, and systolic rise time should be normal compared with the norms just quoted. If they are not, that does not mean, however, that there is not reconstitution. Reconstitution is an arteriographic entity. Reconstruction merely implies reconstitution of the internal common pudendal arterial system through multiple collaterals.

Pharmacologic therapy for impotence is aimed at either initiation or facilitation of the intracellular chemical pathways leading to smooth muscle relaxation. These pathways are mediated by the cyclic guanosine monophosphate (cGMP) and cyclic adenosine monophosphate (cAMP) systems. Stimulators of the cGMP system are nitric oxide synthase mediated. For the most part, the pharmacologic agents associated with the cGMP reaction are papaverine and sildenafil. Vasoactive intestinal polypeptide stimulates the cAMP system. Vasoactive intestinal polypeptide is not commercially available in the United States. The prostacyclin system also stimulates the cAMP system; alprostadil is the commercially available preparation of prostaglandin E_1.

Flaccidity is maintained by constant sympathetic tone exerted on the intracavernosal smooth muscle. This tone is maintained by α agonists. α-Blockade thus facilitates erection. With regard to intracavernosal injection agents, phentolamine is the agent most commonly used. Oral preparation of phentolamine has not yet successfully completed clinical trials.

Thus, pharmacotherapy for erectile dysfunction is selected on the basis of the patient's desire and pathophysiologic process. All factors aside, a logical starting point is with oral pharmacotherapy, which at this time means phosphodiesterase type 5 (PDE5) inhibitors. In cardiac patients receiving nitrates, the use of PDE5 inhibitors is contraindicated. Likewise, the American Heart Association has defined criteria for the safe use of PDE5 inhibitors in patients who have recently had coronary artery bypass grafting, angioplasty, or angioplasty with stent. If oral pharmacotherapy fails, one could consider intracavernosal injection therapy. MUSE is a system for delivery of alprostadil. It has been noted that drugs can be absorbed through the urethra, theoretically to enter directly into the corpora cavernosa. However, in reality, alprostadil absorbed through the urethra becomes systemic medication. The MUSE system delivers alprostadil intraurethrally. Because extremely high doses of alprostadil are required, more than 40% of MUSE patients will have a measurable drop in their blood pressure. Only a small percentage will have a symptomatic drop in the blood pressure, but it is a factor that must be considered.

With regard to intracavernosal injection therapy, most individuals would start with prostaglandin E_1. If prostaglandin E_1 therapy is unsuccessful, one can move to a combination of papaverine, α-blockade, and alprostadil (Trimix). A number of formulations of these medications have been proposed. If intracavernosal injection therapy fails, one could propose prosthetic placement. One must not forget, however, the vacuum erection device. The vacuum erection device is a modality that has been successfully employed in motivated patients. For the most part, all of the agents described can be used for the management of erectile dysfunction in the patient with Peyronie disease. The curvature sometimes makes it difficult to place the chamber of the vacuum erection device.

Any potential surgical candidate must have an intact deep dorsal artery to cavernosal artery communication distal to the arterial lesion and intact inferior epigastric artery within the abdominal wall. The preferred surgical procedure offers an evolution of choices. Originally described by Michal,[7] the first described procedure was an anastomosis of the inferior epigastric artery directly into the tunica albuginea (Michal I). More recently, an anastomosis retrograde into the deep dorsal artery (Michal II), an anastomosis into the deep dorsal vein,[76,77] and a combined deep dorsal artery and vein anastomosis have been described.[78] At present, an end-to-side anastomosis from the inferior epigastric artery into the proximal end of the deep dorsal artery adjacent to its cavernosal artery branches is used. This surgery is performed by use of microsurgical magnification and instrumentation and 10-0 interrupted nylon sutures.

The surgery includes a genital incision, through either an inguinal scrotal approach or a dorsal penile approach. This dissection is carried through the skin subcutaneous dartos fascia to the underlying Buck fascia. The Buck fascia is incised dorsally, and the deep dorsal arteries are identified and isolated from the surrounding tissues. Care is taken to maintain their patency by use of microsurgical techniques and vasodilation solutions. Care is also taken to preserve the proximal penile support structures, including the suspensory and fundiform ligaments.

After adequate identification of the genital recipient vessels, attention is turned to the lower abdominal wall. A perimedian incision is made within the lower abdominal wall, and dissection proceeds beneath the rectus abdominis muscle to the ipsilateral inferior epigastric artery and its vena comitans. These vessels are followed from their origin at the external iliac artery up to their arborization and insertion into the ipsilateral rectus abdominis muscle. The artery and its vena comitans are then isolated, skeletonized, and transposed from the abdominal wall subfascially into the perineum. At this point, the recipient and donor arteries are prepared under magnification and microsurgical instrumentation. An arterial anastomosis is then carried out. All incision sites are then closed.

Postoperative evaluation has revealed an increased potency in approximately 25% to 80% of patients. Complications include arterial anastomotic thrombosis, arterial or emissary runoff, and possible hemorrhage due to sexual trauma within the first 6 weeks of the procedure (patients are admonished not to indulge in any sexual activity for 6 weeks after the surgery). Long-term complications may include postoperative numbness, penile lengthening or shortening if the suspensory ligaments are disrupted, and possible glanular hyperemia (reported in 5% of cases) if an anastomosis is performed with a deep dorsal vein.

PHALLIC CONSTRUCTION

Early techniques for reconstruction of the penis were developed to repair penile injuries. In 1936, Bogoraz[79] presented a case report of a war-injured patient and described a technique for phallic construction with use of an abdominal flap. Frumkin[80] followed with another series from the Soviet Union. Gillies,[81] who was aware of the Russians' experience, reported on series of patients in whom he had reconstructed the penis. His paper described patients with congenital absence of the penis; however, much of his experience also resulted from treatment of war injuries. All procedures initially involved the delayed formation and transfer of tubed abdominal flaps. These tubes were developed from random flaps of abdominal skin with their attendant tenuous blood supply. They were formed in surgical stages with a "delay" between the stages to allow new vascular patterns to become established. In the "tube-within-a-tube" design, the inner tube allowed placement of a baculum for intercourse; the outer tube provided skin coverage.[82,83] Patients generally voided through a proximal urethrostomy. This was "state-of-the-art" penile reconstruction until the early 1970s, when Orticochea[61] described total reconstruction of the penis by use of a gracilis musculocutaneous flap.

Once microsurgery established a foothold in genital construction, plastic surgeons began to explore and map out the genital neurovascular supply and to consider expanding the applications of microsurgery to elective reconstruction of the genitalia. Microsurgical composite tissue transplantation for the repair of partial penile injuries and total phallic reconstructions were considered, attempted, and often discarded in searching for the "perfect" donor flap. The early 1980s were a testing ground when surgeons searched for ideal donor flaps that could predictably deliver the seven goals of penile reconstruction and phallic construction. These goals included the following challenges: (1) a one-stage procedure that could be predictably reproduced, (2) a phallus that had both tactile and erogenous sensibility, (3) a phallus with a competent neourethra to allow voiding while standing, (4) enough phallic bulk to tolerate the insertion of a prosthetic stiffener, (5) a phallus that was aesthetically acceptable to the patient and his consort, (6) a phallus that would grow through childhood to full adult size in pediatric patients, and (7) due consideration to the donor site.

Puckett's experience with the groin flap produced a report of the first free flap phalloplasty in 1982.[84] In his two cases, free groin flaps were elevated, de-epithelialized proximally, inset into the crura, and revascularized to recipient branches of the femoral artery and saphenous veins. These flaps underwent subsequent sculpturing and prostheses implantation.

After Puckett's initial description, both Chang and Gilbert described their experiences with microsurgical phallic construction. Chang[85] described a one-stage technique in seven post-trauma patients with use of an ingenious adaptation of the tube-in-tube concept into a free tissue transfer. In his design, the neourethra was constructed from a skin island on the most ulnar aspect of the radial forearm flap originally described by Song.[86] A de-epithelialized strip between the ulnar skin island and the radial part of the flap allowed the ulnar paddle to be wrapped inwardly to form the neourethra; a larger radial paddle was wrapped around the neourethra to form the outer phallic shaft (Chinese flap). In two patients, the flap's medial antebrachial cutaneous nerve was coapted to the nonerogenous femoral or saphenous nerve. A rib cartilage stiffener was placed by introduction of a K-wire and then placement of the cartilage in the space between the two paddles (Fig. 152-32).

In 1987, Gilbert et al[8] reported their phallic construction experience based on 12 total phallic constructions in which several donor sites were cited and rejected as potential suitors for this surgery. All patients had undergone microsurgical transfer of the flap (five radial forearm flaps, one upper lateral arm flap, two dorsalis pedis flaps, one deltoid flap, one saphenous flap, and two upper medial arm flaps) to the perineum. All patients had neourethral construction (eight were full-thickness skin grafts), but none had insertion of autologous cartilage, bone, or prosthetic stiffeners during the primary procedure. It was the authors' belief that no prosthesis should be inserted until there was

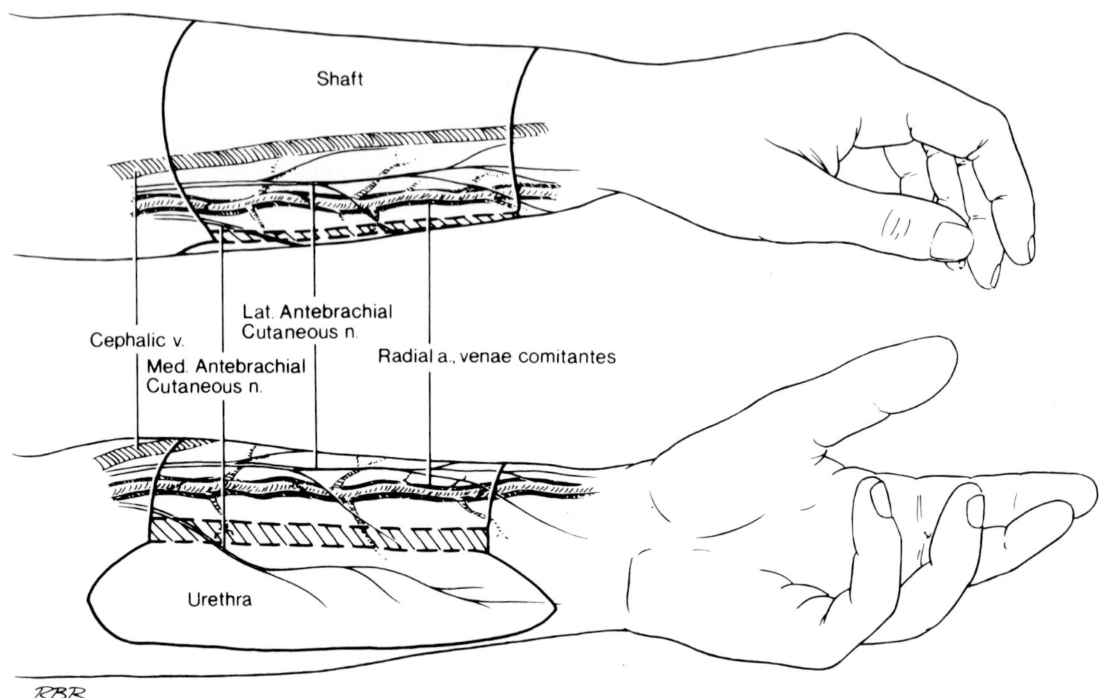

FIGURE 152-32. The Chinese forearm flap design for phallic construction. (From Gilbert DA, Winslow B, Gilbert DM, et al: Transsexual surgery in the genetic female. Clin Plast Surg 1988;15:471-487.)

measurable sensory return to the phallus. Most important, the authors coapted the donor flap nerve to the pudendal nerve in the last 10 cases. This group of patients all reported the return of erogenous sensibility and the ability to masturbate to orgasm (Fig. 152-33).[87]

Boyd's modification of the forearm flap departed from the "skin island wrap" concept.[88] In his "cricket bat" design, the neourethra and shaft were located in tandem over the vascular pedicle with the urethra distal to the flap. The urethra was tubed under and enclosed by the shaft flap. However, the shaft design could be widened to accommodate "double-barreled" penile implants that often provided a more stable reconstruction. Despite the potential limitations of phallic length, this flap provides excellent results in total and subtotal penile amputations (Fig. 152-34).[89] In particular, the cricket bat flap is probably the best design for the reconstruction of exstrophy and foreshortened epispadiac patients.

Biemer[90] modified the Chang design by centering the neourethral skin island over the radial artery and breaking up the phallic shaft into two separate periurethral paddles. The proximity of the neourethra to the flap blood supply had two implications: first, any urethral breakdown due to ischemia was minimized as a result of the optimally located blood supply; and second, the design allowed the neourethra to be extended proximally and distally along the shaft length. This design concept allowed a tension-free anastomosis to the native urethra and construction of a distal neoglans. Unfortunately, centering the urethra over the radial artery pedicle placed it on the most hairy part of the forearm. Final closure of the skin island around the neourethra results in two longitudinal suture lines, which occasionally produces an aesthetic

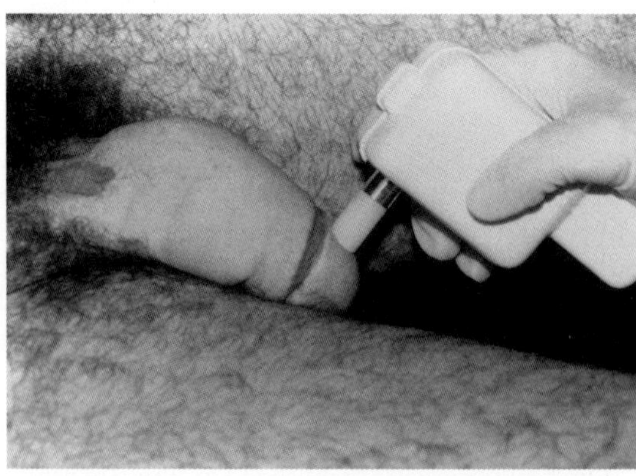

FIGURE 152-33. The most accurate technique to measure genital sensibility is the vibratory bioesthesiometer. Standard measurements of somatic sensation (i.e., two-point discrimination, von Frey hairs) have proved to be inaccurate for genital sensation.

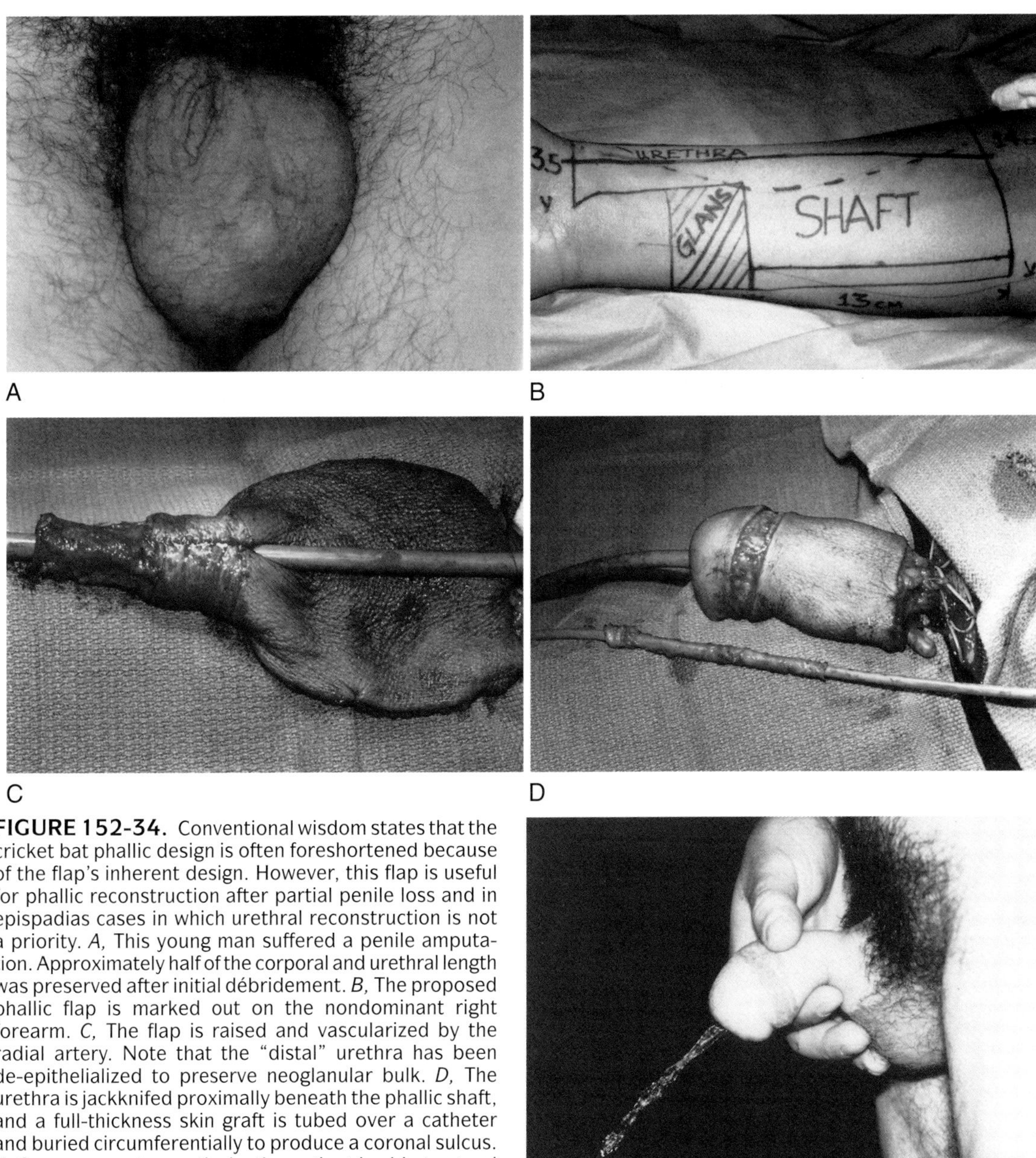

FIGURE 152-34. Conventional wisdom states that the cricket bat phallic design is often foreshortened because of the flap's inherent design. However, this flap is useful for phallic reconstruction after partial penile loss and in epispadias cases in which urethral reconstruction is not a priority. *A,* This young man suffered a penile amputation. Approximately half of the corporal and urethral length was preserved after initial débridement. *B,* The proposed phallic flap is marked out on the nondominant right forearm. *C,* The flap is raised and vascularized by the radial artery. Note that the "distal" urethra has been de-epithelialized to preserve neoglanular bulk. *D,* The urethra is jackknifed proximally beneath the phallic shaft, and a full-thickness skin graft is tubed over a catheter and buried circumferentially to produce a coronal sulcus. *E,* One year postoperatively, the patient is able to stand and void. (From Gilbert D, Jordan G, Devine C Jr, Winslow B: Microsurgical forearm "cricket bat-transformer phalloplasty." Plast Reconstr Surg 1992;90:711-716.)

deformity. Although microsurgical forearm tissue transfers are classically based on the radial artery, the flap can also be raised on the ulnar artery as described by Lovie.[91] The relative paucity of hair on the ulnar forearm and the longer ulnar vascular pedicle make this flap more suitable for phallic construction (Figs. 152-35 and 152-36 and Table 152-2).[92]

In a departure from the forearm design, Sadove[93] described the microsurgical osteocutaneous fibula flap as a potential donor site alternative. However, this flap appears restricted in its urethroplasty potential and may require neourethral prefabrication,[94] has an unpredictable nerve supply, and is difficult to fix to the underlying tissue.[95,96]

Unfortunately, many phalloplasty papers present limited experiences for one of plastic surgery's toughest reconstructive challenges. Only Cheng et al[54] have presented a large series (136 cases) and have reviewed

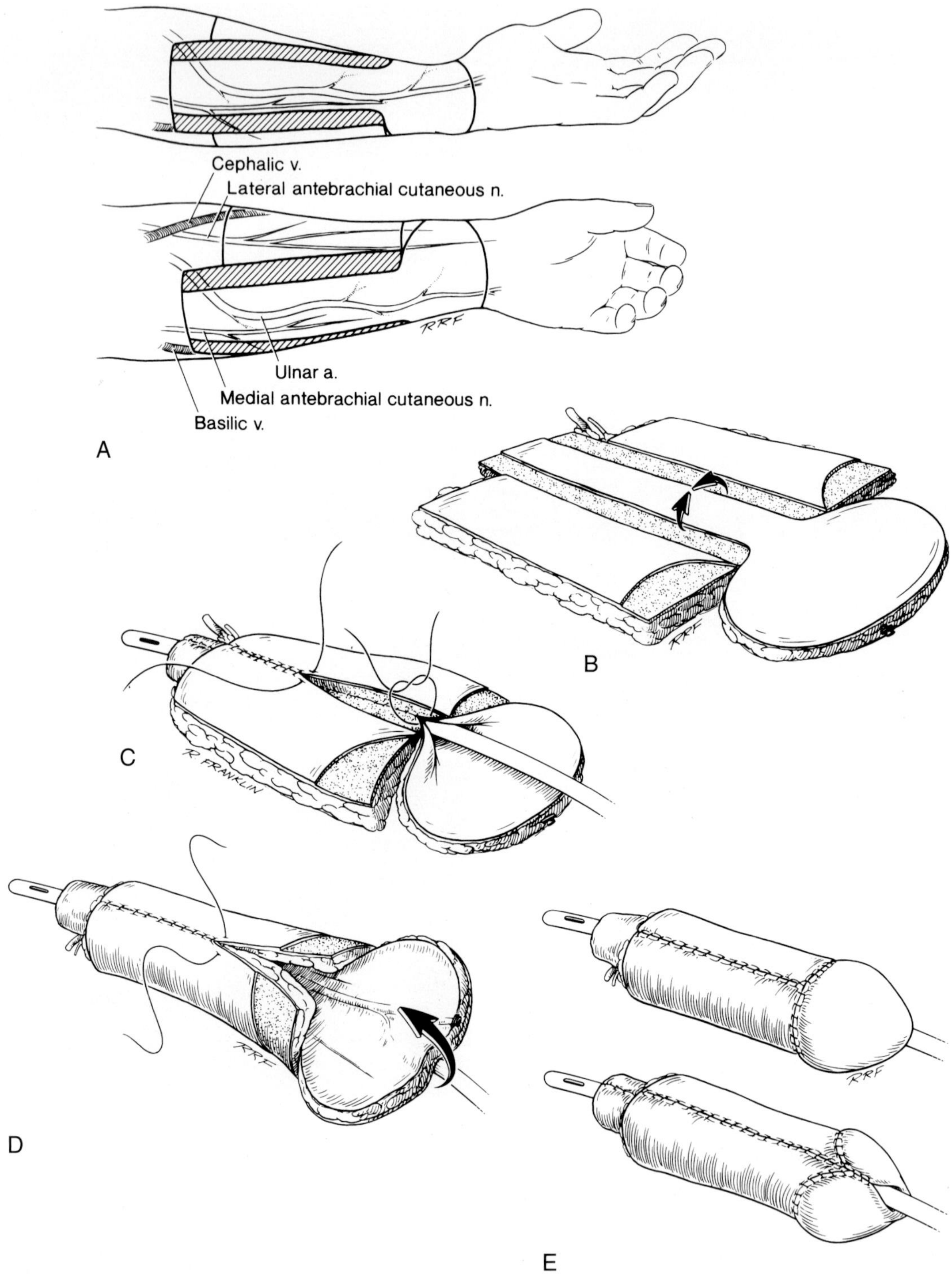

FIGURE 152-35. *A,* During the past 2 decades, the microsurgical forearm phallic flap has evolved into an ulnar-based flap that includes a central urethra (3 × 12 cm) bordered by paraurethral de-epithelialized strips (1.5 × 12 cm) and bilateral shaft swatches (7 × 12 cm). Distally, the neoglans (4 × 8 cm) is a continuation of the distal neourethra. *B* and *C,* Once the flap is dissected and elevated, transformation is begun. The urethra is tubed over a 30 French catheter with four layers of sutures between the neourethral lumen and the ventral skin. *D,* The flap is then flipped or rolled on the proximal forearm to close the dorsal shaft, and the neoglans is reflected proximally over the distally de-epithelialized shaft. *E,* The phallus is ready for microsurgical transfer. (From Gilbert DA, Schlossberg SM, Jordan GH: Ulnar forearm phallic construction and penile reconstruction. Microsurgery 1995;16:314-321.)

TABLE 152-2 ✦ PHALLIC CONSTRUCTION THEN AND NOW

Then	Now
Radial forearm flap	Ulnar forearm flap
"Chinese" design	"Biemer" design
Poorly vascularized urethra	Well-vascularized urethra
Shorter urethra	Longer urethra
Hairy urethra	Less hairy urethra
Good sensation	Good sensation
Shorter vascular pedicle	Longer vascular pedicle
No nerve injury	Theoretical injury to nerves (ulnar n., ant. interosseous n.)
STSG coverage of forearm	FTSG coverage of forearm

STSG, split-thickness skin graft; FTSG, full-thickness skin graft.

several reconstructive methods in an impartial manner. These authors discuss phallic atrophy, delayed urethral reconstruction, and sensory return, and they compare satisfaction between patients who have never had a normal penis (transgendered, micropenis) and those who have lost the penis (trauma, malignant disease). After successful penile reconstruction, the patients with congenital absence or abnormality of the penis reported greater acceptance and satisfaction compared with the patients undergoing reconstruction for trauma or iatrogenic injury.

Urethral Reconstruction

The goal of constructing a patent stable urethra remained elusive. Urethrocutaneous fistulas, stenoses, strictures, diverticula, and hairy urethras all plagued urethral construction. Unfortunately, there have been few long-term series following urethroplasty, probably because of the lack of noteworthy success. Even well-intentioned surgeons have ignored urethral construction completely. Our initial urethroplasty results reflected the relative failure of skin grafts and the need for flap urethras—wisdom that the Russians and Gillies understood. Two recent developments have influenced phallic urethroplasties. First, incorporating a vascularized urethra within a free flap and locating it over the vascular leash increase the blood supply to the native urethra-neourethra anastomosis. Second, routinely transferring a gracilis muscle flap and wrapping it around the urethral anastomosis increase the extrinsic blood supply. By incorporating these trends, we have improved our results (Fig. 152-37). In post-phalloplasty patients who were urethral "cripples," the staged, meshed split-thickness skin graft urethroplasty was the best technique to salvage a functioning urethra.

Phallic Sensation

Historically, little has been written on the subject of penile sensation. The standard sensory measurements (two-point discrimination, von Frey hairs) were inadequate to measure penile sensation. A vibratory bioesthesiometer is the most accurate instrument to measure penile tactile sensation.[87,97] Some attempts were made to innervate phallic flaps with nonerogenous nerves, thereby fostering poor results. Following a suggestion by Terzis,[98] we began to coapt the pudendal nerve or its terminal branches to the medial and lateral antebrachial cutaneous nerves of the forearm. Not only did these neural coaptations preserve tactile sensory return to the phallus, but a strong erogenous component was also augmented when branches of the pudendal nerve were incorporated into the reconstruction. Almost all of our patients regained tactile sensation and were able to masturbate to orgasm. The cortical adaptation of the brain to crude microsurgical techniques may be due to a preordained "love map" that the brain maintains in its enormous plasticity and need for sensibility. Certainly, pressure receptors within the corporal stumps remain as a source of erotic sensation, but the innervated flaps also contain erogenous and tactile sensibility. This finding provided promise to many patients who had no penile sensation and allowed us to proceed with the final definitive step in penile reconstruction—the insertion of penile prostheses (see Fig. 152-33).

Penile Prostheses

It is in the area of penile stiffeners that phalloplasty controversy continues (Table 152-3).[99,100] Although our post-phallic reconstructive patients were able to stand and void, reacquired the return of erogenous and tactile function, and had enough bulk to retain bilateral prostheses, no biomedical company was willing to proceed with the development of a *phallic* prosthesis.

Ideally, a prototype phallic implant requires a built-in double-barreled design for "I beam" stability, some form of fuzzy covering to reduce peri-implant capsule formation, an attachment to surrounding tissues to control pistoning, and a fixation mechanism to attach the implant to the pubic rami. The implant requires a predictable stiffening mechanism (by a semirigid rod, hydraulic inflation, or a series of intercalated joints joined together by a wire), a low infection rate, and replacement potential. All potential patients must have adequate phallic tip sensation before proceeding with the implantation.

Necessity is the mother of invention, and Jordan began to place the penile prosthesis into a sleeve of Gore-Tex vascular graft, which was then inserted into the penis or phallus. Gore-Tex has a strong propensity to facilitate the ingrowth of granulation tissue into its interstices, which makes a stable, relatively sterile

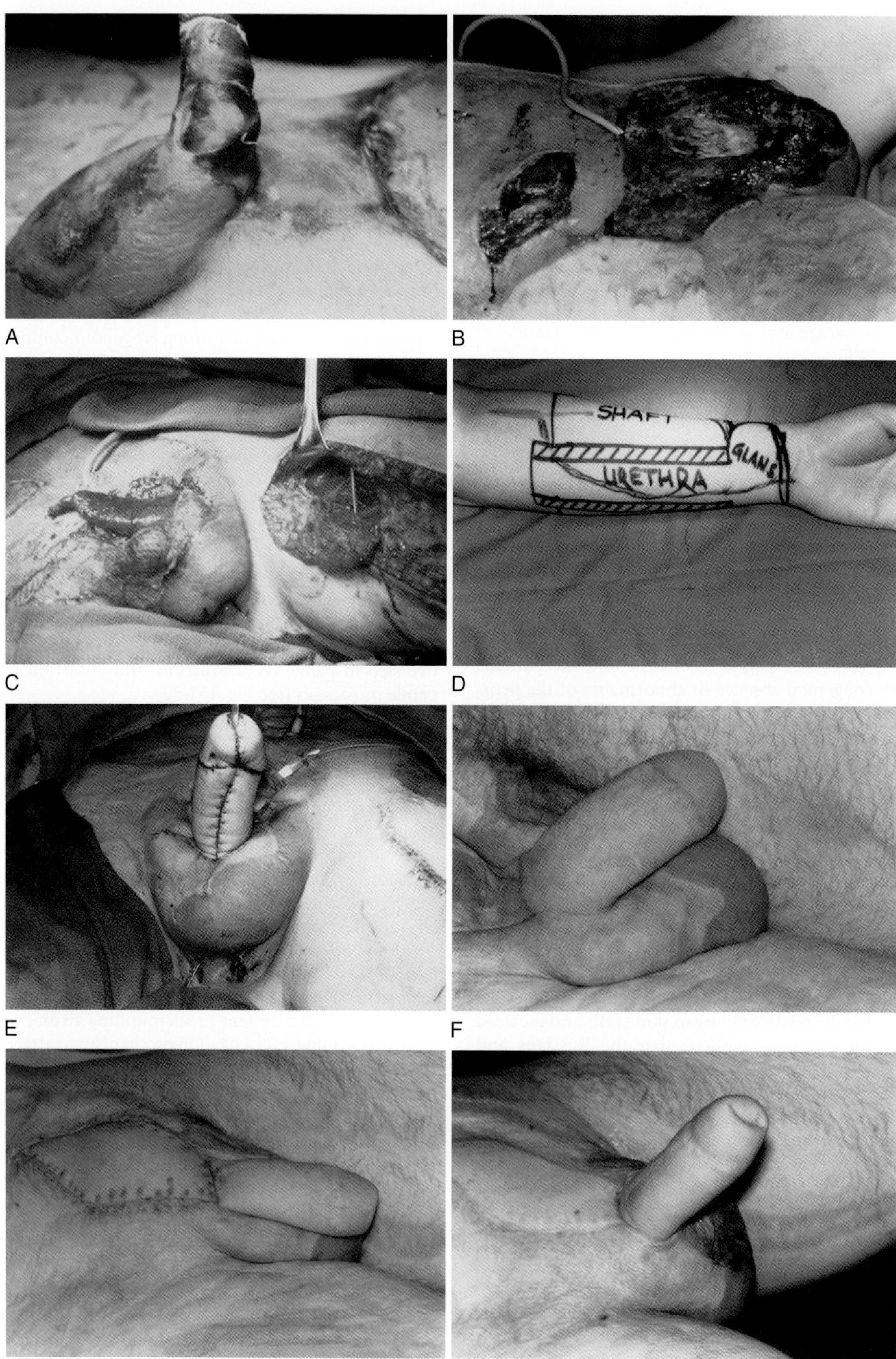
SHAFT
GLANS
URETHRA

FIGURE 152-36. Fourth-degree burns that included total penile loss, left testicular loss, and underlying pubic bone osteomyelitis. *A,* Full-thickness skin loss of the penis, urethra, scrotum, and surrounding penile tissues. The patient had previously undergone débridement of the chest, abdomen, and right thigh. *B,* After complete débridement of all necrotic tissues, the patient is left with an exposed pubis and potential osteomyelitis. *C,* A left gracilis flap is transposed to protect and nourish the infected pubis. *D,* A left nondominant ulnar forearm flap is dissected, elevated, and microsurgically transferred to the perineum. *E,* The flap is well vascularized. *F,* Several months later, the phallus is healed but reflects a continuing defect over the pubis, which discouraged the insertion of penile prostheses. *G,* One year later, a scapular free flap is transferred to the pubis to provide adequate coverage for the insertion of penile prostheses. *H,* After the return of adequate tactile and erogenous sensation, the patient underwent the insertion of DuraPhase penile prostheses.

environment in which the prosthesis could exist. In addition to fenestration of the Gore-Tex sleeve to promote capillary ingrowth, either the sleeve was inserted into the existing crural bodies and sutured to the overlying tunica (in the case of penile reconstruction) or the Gore-Tex base was directly sutured to the inferior pelvic rami periosteum (in the case of total phallic construction).[99,100] By suturing the prosthetic covering to the inferior rami, the natural corporal anatomy was emulated and the prosthesis was adequately fixed to reduce the pistoning effect. In addition, fixation of the dual implant coverings to each other at the phallic base also supported the bidirectional demands of phallic prostheses in sexual intromission, voiding, sports activities, and seating in male clothing (Fig. 152-38).

TABLE 152-3 ✦ PHALLIC PROSTHESES CLASSIFICATION*

	N	Result	Follow-up
Permanent Internal Devices			
Autologous grafts			
Free cartilage grafts			
Bogoraz	1	Success	5 mo
Mukhin	12	?	?
Evans	7	Success	5 yr
Arneri	12	Success	?
Song	11	?	?
Chang	93	?	?
Free bone grafts			
Mutaf	5		
Vascularized bone grafts			
Koshima	1	Success	10 mo
Sun	11	Partial loss	?
Byam	5	Partial loss	?
Endo	5	?	?
Papadopulos	17	Success	12 yr
Biomedical devices			
Hydraulic devices			
Puckett	15	Failure 15 times	?
Wilson	12	Failure 12 times	?
Nonhydraulic implants—rigid			
Pryor/Gill	5	Failure 5 times	?
Exner	32	Infection, one	?
Jordan/Gilbert	30	Failure 5 times	20 yr
Temporary insertable devices			
Laub	?	?	?
External Devices			
External splints	?	?	?
Phallic-base rings	?	?	?
Vacuum devices	?	?	?

* This table depicts the paucity of long-term follow-up for phallic prostheses. Only reviews of five or more patients are cited to eliminate single case reports or small survey numbers. However, even in the larger surveys, there is a lack of postoperative documentation of implant success (viability and intercourse). The Jordan[99] series is the only one that cites prosthesis viability and successful intercourse during a sustained period. Papadopulos[94] cites elegant studies of long-term phallic bone viability.

Modified from Hage JJ, Bloem JJ, Bouman FG: Obtaining rigidity in the neophallus of female-to-male transsexuals: a review of the literature. Ann Plast Surg 1993;30:327.

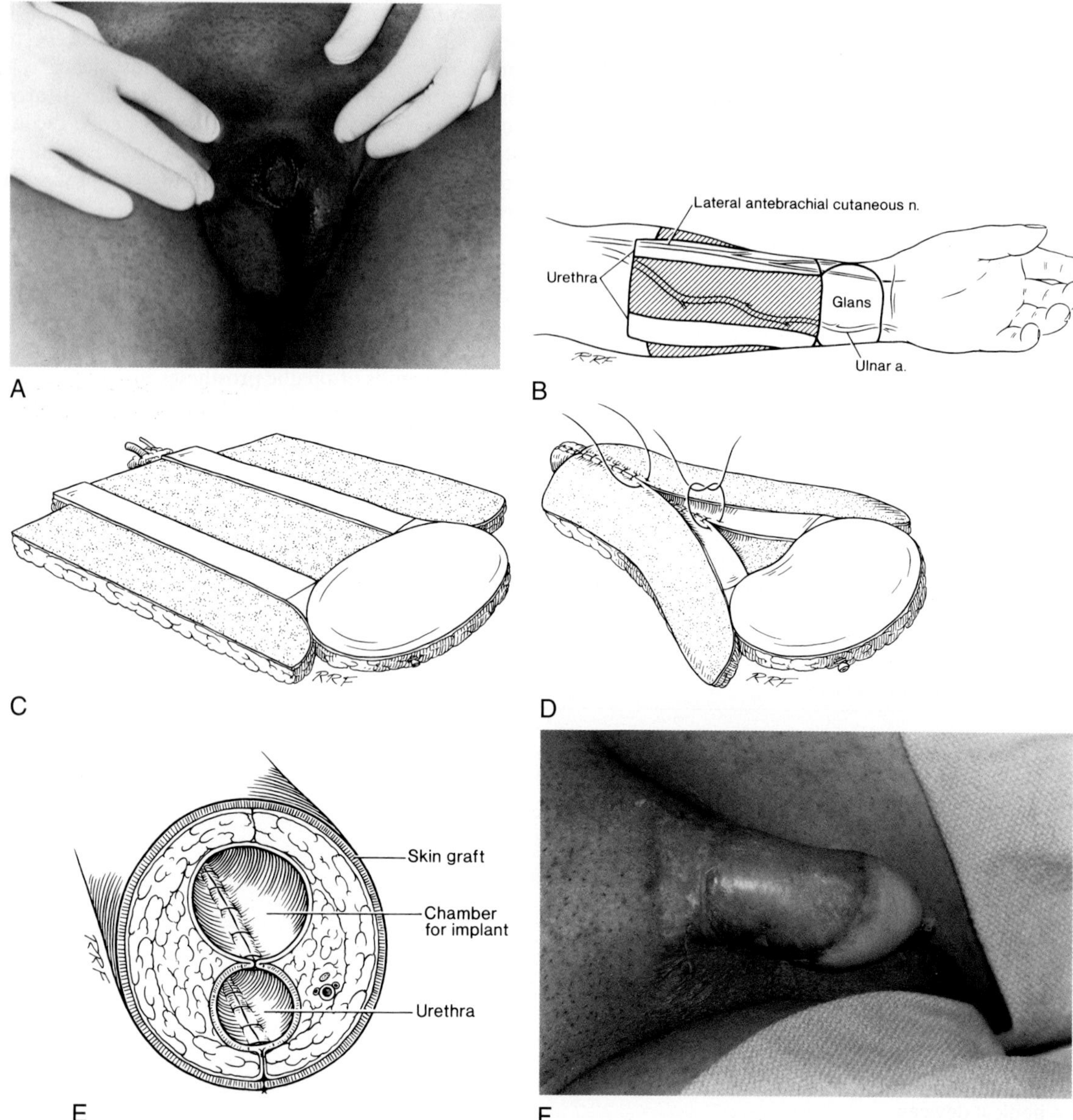

FIGURE 152-37. Phallic reconstruction in a heavy-set adult requires thoughtful planning to avoid a phallus that may be too bulky. *A,* This 29-year-old man has a micropenis, although the scrotum and testicles exhibit normal male development. *B,* A modified ulnar forearm microsurgical flap has been drawn out. Note the bifid neourethra, which is to be sutured to itself in a "clamshell" fashion with use of two suture lines. The central de-epithelialized space between the urethral components is recessed dorsally to provide a sheath for anticipated insertion of a penile prosthesis. *C,* Elevation of this design allows de-epithelialization of the lateral skin flaps, thereby reducing phallic bulk. *D,* The flap is tubed around a urethral catheter. The neoglans is reflected onto the phallic shaft. *E,* The phallic shaft is covered with a thick split-thickness skin graft. Note the dorsal prosthetic "neosheath." *F,* One year postoperatively, the flap has maintained its shape and contour without being too bulky.

Aesthetic Considerations

Phallic construction had become predictable enough to refine its aesthetic goals.[101] The postmodern microsurgical phalloplasty borrowed from previous phallic designs. Distal flaps (Biemer design[90]) and circumferential full-thickness skin grafts are used to define the neoglans and pseudocorona. Nevertheless, all of these designs fall victim to a loss of definition (coronal washout) over time. To reduce the loss of coronal definition, tattoo pigments have been employed to emulate a viable glans color for phallic constructions.

The ulnar artery–based forearm flap provides a hairless portion of the forearm for urethral construction.

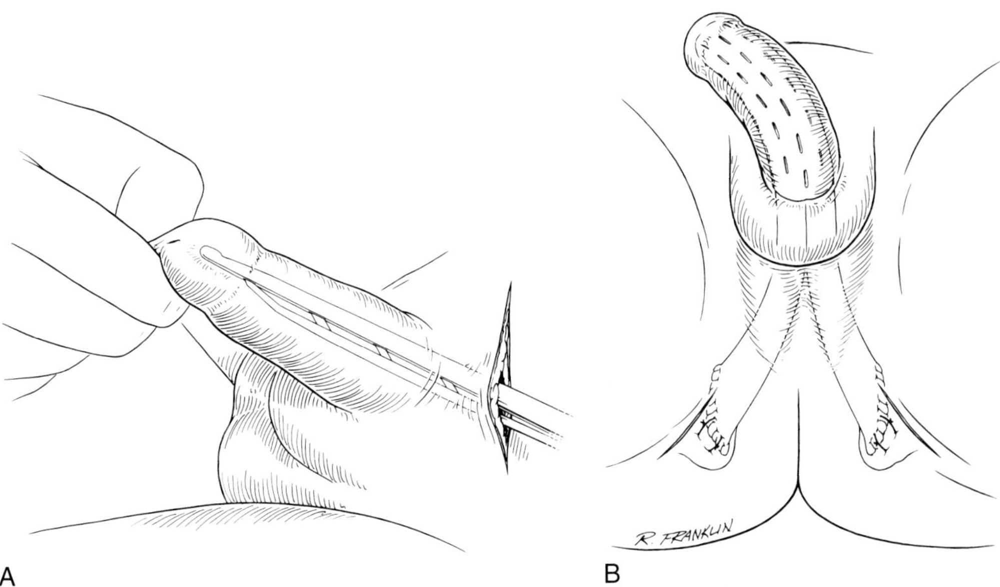

FIGURE 152-38. Implantation of penile prostheses is considered only after there is evidence of anterior urethral competence and return of tactile sensation to the phallic tip. Ignoring these principles will increase the risks of phallic infection and implant extrusion. *A,* Initially, a transverse incision is made in the prepubic subcutaneous space. This location allows access to the phallic shaft and inferior pelvic rami. Care is taken to avoid injury to the phallic blood supply and the urethra. An Otis urethrotome is employed to enlarge the phallic tunnels. *B,* Bilateral DuraPhase penile prostheses are incorporated into Gore-Tex sleeves, advanced subcutaneously to the phallic tip, and fixed to the inferior pelvic rami. (From Alter GJ, Gilbert DA, Schlossberg SM, Jordan GH: Prosthetic implantation after phallic reconstruction. Microsurgery 1995;16:314-321.)

However, many patients are advised to undergo epilation before definitive surgery.

Finally, some flap dimensions are designed to make the phallus as long as possible. These extended phalluses may suit patients' and surgeons' fantasies but are subject to increased urethrocutaneous fistulas, poor sensory return, and difficulty inserting penile prostheses. There is a need for aesthetic responsibility when the patient and his surgeon discuss phallic length preoperatively.

Donor Site Morbidity

Donor site morbidity must be considered in flap selection for penile reconstruction. The forearm donor site, notwithstanding its utilitarian potential to produce the most optimal and autologous phallus, remained a major concern to many patients. Although major loss or compromise of the donor forearm or hand is rare in series of phalloplasty performed by experienced microsurgeons, the transfer of a forearm flap may include nerve injury, cold intolerance, joint stiffness, and chronic edema. Unfortunately, the potential forearm scar often distracted patients. Some patients became so concerned by the potential scar that they chose a much lesser procedure with a poor chance of achieving phalloplasty goals to avoid a forearm scar. Of course, there are other patients who have no problem whatsoever and think that a forearm donor site scar is a small price to pay for a phallus. During the past 10 years, we have dissected and elevated forearm flaps in a prefascial plane to retain forearm muscle integrity. In addition, we routinely employ *full-thickness skin grafts,* harvested from the groins bilaterally, to produce the best possible forearm scars. These two modifications have allayed some patients' concerns (Fig. 152-39).

Growth Through Puberty

Phallic construction in children follows the same goals and guidelines as in adults with one added requirement—growth through puberty to adulthood. Because the phallus is constructed of somatic tissues but replaces a penis that is formed by genital tissues, the growth rates are temporally and quantitatively different.[35] Care must be taken to accurately predict the anticipated growth rate and to design a phallic model of appropriate size and length. Inaccurate forecasting leads to the need for secondary surgery, including a second microsurgical procedure to keep up with the normal adolescent penile growth. Penile length is an important aspect in satisfaction of the patient and continues to be so until the patient is convinced that his phallus is of adequate length.

We developed a graph that compared normal penile growth from birth until the age of 20 years with

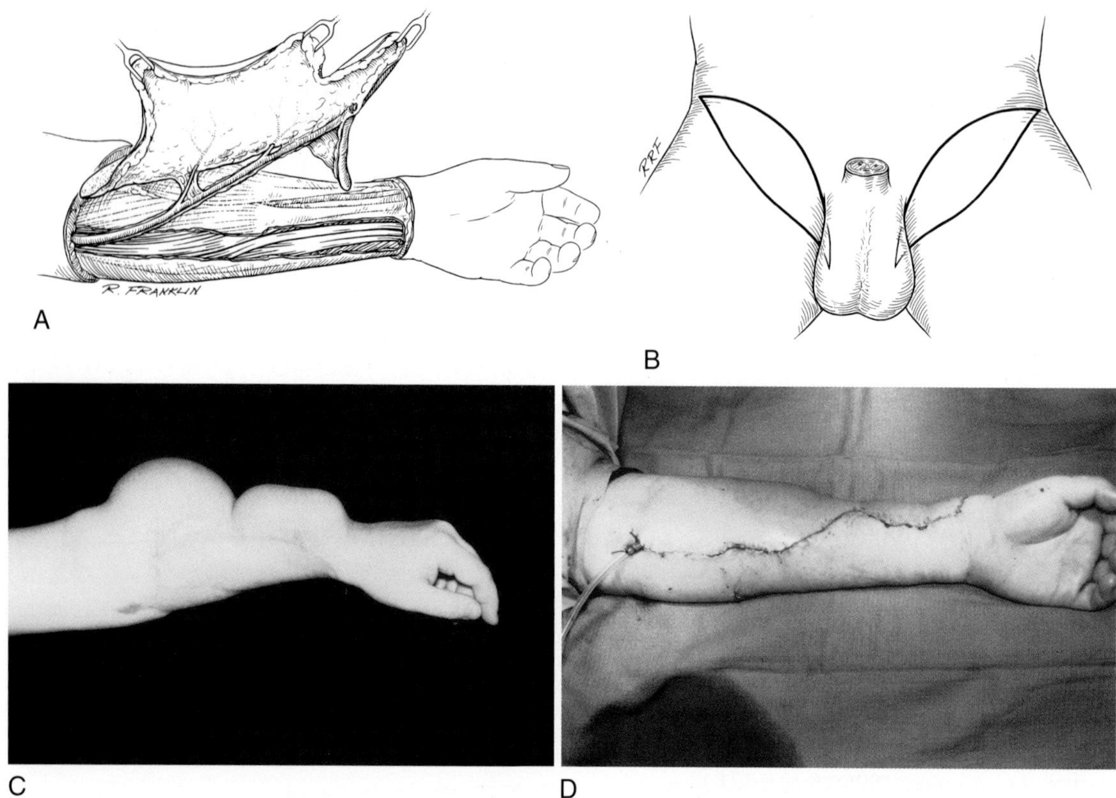

FIGURE 152-39. *A,* A phallic flap is elevated, leaving the deep lamina of the superficial fascia on the forearm. The superficial lamina is carried with the flap. *B,* The donor sites for full-thickness skin grafts are illustrated for donor site closure. *C,* This patient underwent reconstruction of his left nondominant forearm donor site with paired full-thickness skin grafts harvested from the flanks. One year postoperatively, the donor site has healed well. However, the patient sought removal of the skin graft from the radial aspect of the forearm. Two tissue expanders were inserted and sequentially expanded. *D,* The tissue expanders were removed and approximately 50% of the skin graft was removed and closed directly. (*A* and *B* from Gilbert DA, Schlossberg SM, Jordan GH: Ulnar forearm phallic construction and penile reconstruction. Microsurgery 1995;16:314-321.)

nongenital tissue growth through the same time frame. It is well known that genital growth takes the form of an exponential curve as the child passes through puberty. This growth is due to the rapid rise in serum testosterone and the development of testosterone in the testicles that stimulates the genital tissues to activate 5α-reductase, which converts testosterone to dihydrotestosterone. This rapid growth continues until late teens. The normal growth of nongenital tissues in childhood is linear in nature, not withstanding modest growth spurts at the ages of 2 and 6 years and in adolescence. When both graphs are transposed and compared, it is easy to see that the prepubertal phallic construction must be larger and longer than normal genital size for that cohort age group. Our initial impression is that these prepubertal phalluses will grow to normal adult size, but we do not have enough long-term follow-up for an unbiased answer yet. However, there is one aspect that is evident from this experience. Boys who are obese will have obese phalluses that may require serial debulking until their obesity has been controlled (see Fig. 152-18).[36]

Another issue that we are just now beginning to address is the "correct" age at which to proceed with the insertion of penile prostheses. Once these boys have reached 18 years and the age for majority, they must be physically and psychologically prepared to manage a phallus that has previously been erectionless.

There is another nagging problem with operating on children—the lack of informed consent. Although the child's best interest and surgery's best intentions are usually served by early reconstruction, there are no long-term studies that have evaluated the results of this surgery over a lifetime or even a generation.

Finally, it comes as no surprise that the large majority of these genitally compromised boys require prolonged psychological therapy to deal with genital loss, surgical trauma, inadequacy, and scarring. These psychological issues are often closely commingled with the need for secondary surgery to complete reconstruction. Nowhere in surgery is there a stronger need for parental and family support than with these late teenage boys who have essentially undergone years of "surgical" abuse.

Testicular Autotransplantation

Cryptorchidism is present in 20% of all premature and 16% of all full-term infant boys. Approximately 5% to 14% of cryptorchid testes are intra-abdominal.[102-104] High abdominal cryptorchidism is also associated with prune-belly syndrome.

First presented by Silber in 1976,[4] testicular autotransplantation has been described as a technique to microsurgically transfer intra-abdominal testes into the anatomic scrotum. The technique is predicated on revascularization of the testes through the normal spermatic artery and its venae comitantes, which "supercharge" the testes compared with the standard Fowler-Stephens transfer that depends on the deferential vascular supply.[105]

Testicular autotransplantation is indicated in cases of bilateral abdominal cryptorchidism, unilateral abdominal cryptorchidism with a contralateral atrophic testis, concern for malignant degeneration, and prune-belly syndrome.

The diagnosis is made by human chorionic gonadotropin stimulation to establish the presence of a testis and laparoscopy to identify the location of intra-abdominal testes. The laparoscopy will identify high abdominal cryptorchidism versus true anorchism and, if an orchiectomy is performed, will reduce the risk of testicular malignancy. It has been estimated that approximately 0.075% of all cryptorchid testes will become malignant. An orchiectomy presumes that the other testis is normal.

Surgical alternatives for intra-abdominal cryptorchidism include orchiectomy, orchiopexy, multistaged testicular advancement, and testicular autotransplantation. Orchiopexy may include clamping the spermatic vessels and then performing biopsy of the testis to establish collateral flow through the deferential system. If adequate collateral flow is established, the testis is then transferred into the scrotum (Fowler-Stephens procedure).[105]

Another alternative is a multistage procedure in which the testis is advanced first to the pelvic ring after separation of the spermatic vessels and from the pelvic rim into the scrotum (within 6 to 12 months). This surgery has a high percentage of testicular atrophy.

Testicular autotransplantation represents a surgical advance by use of microsurgical techniques. The surgery includes initial exploration of the abdominal and retroperitoneal cavities through a laparoscopy incision. Intra-abdominal testes are established, and a testis is isolated from its surrounding tissues. The spermatic artery and its venae comitantes are then ligated high from their aortic artery, right inferior vena cava, or left renal vein origins. The testis, vas deferens, and deferential plexus are then released carefully into the pelvis, through the external inguinal ring, and then into the scrotum. Before the surgical transposition, the ipsilateral inferior epigastric artery and its venae comitantes are dissected up to the level of the first large intra-abdominal muscle branch. This vascular leash is then transposed into the pelvis and prepared for microsurgical anastomoses.

When the testis has been transposed, microsurgery is initiated with use of microsurgical magnification and instrumentation and 10-0 interrupted nylon sutures. An arterial anastomosis (end-to-end or end-to-side) is performed between the inferior epigastric artery and the spermatic artery. A venous anastomosis is performed between an inferior epigastric vena comitans and the spermatic vein. After completion of the venous anastomosis and confirmation of good blood flow in and out of the testis, the testis is transposed into a sub-dartos pouch within the ipsilateral scrotum (Fig. 152-40).

Care is taken to proceed with all of the non-microsurgical dissection before any microsurgical ischemia. It appears that microsurgical ischemia has a profound and direct effect on spermatogenesis. The success of the transfer depends on both spermatogenesis and the inherent production of testicular hormones. Testicular autotransplantation has a worldwide 87% success rate in a review of 295 cases.[106] This appears to be an improvement over the Fowler-Stephens technique, which has a 73% to 80% success rate.[105] It is

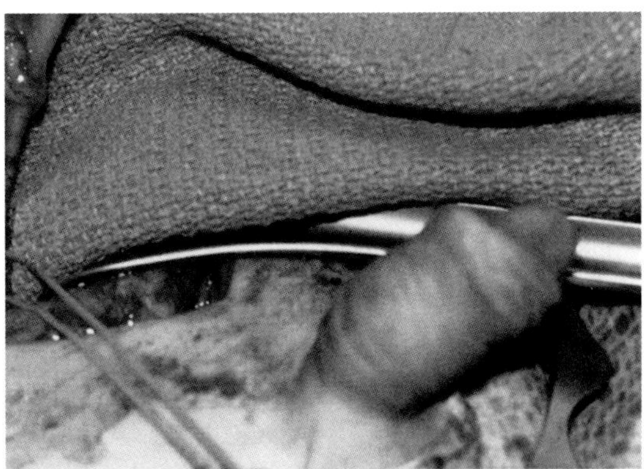

FIGURE 152-40. This photograph illustrates the challenges of testicular autotransplantation. In this particular case, the left intra-abdominal testis was rudimentary—producing serum testosterone but not spermatogenic. The vas deferens was foreshortened and required an aggressive release of perivascular tissues to seat the testis into the scrotal-dartos pouch.

important to carry out venous as well as arterial anastomoses to produce the best result.

The surgical prognosis is dependent on the degree of anoxia or avascular time, the length of the vas deferens and its associated cord structures, and the need to complete the surgery before the age of 2 years if possible.[75]

Reconstruction of the Genitourinary Cripple

One of the greatest challenges to genitourinary surgery is the patient who has had four or more surgical procedures to correct a congenital or acquired deformity without achieving a successful outcome. The surgical sequelae most commonly associated with reconstructive morbidity include residual chordee, foreshortened penis, urethral fistula, urethral stenosis, panurethral stricture, insensate penis, penoscrotal tethering, and aesthetic deformities. After several surgical attempts, the patient often tends to withdraw into a life of silent desperation. Many of these patients are hypospadias repair failures who recall that they spent many of their childhood summers undergoing surgical procedures that minimally, if incrementally, changed their penile function. To many of these patients, this was no more than a form of institutionalized and condoned child abuse, and many required perioperative and postoperative psychological therapy to proceed with this frustrating process.

Fortunately, the advent of new and improved flap designs, the movement away from full-thickness skin grafts and toward onlay buccal mucosal grafts, the acceptance of meshed nonexpanded split-thickness skin grafts for urethral repair, and the use of microsurgical techniques including neurosensory composite tissue transplantation and nerve grafts have all provided new ideas and relief for these moribund patients. As experience has grown, algorithms have been developed to organize and stratify these reconstructive methods (Table 152-4). At a tertiary referral center, teenage boys and men present who give a history of multiple reconstructive surgical procedures to correct genitourinary problems.

Each patient should be approached with specific repair principles associated with the disorder (see Table 152-4). The application of these principles will lead to the successful conversion of a crippled patient to one who has a successfully functioning genitourinary system. Certainly, one of the central reconstructive principles during the past 2 decades has been the meshed split-thickness graft urethroplasty first described by Schreiter.[44,45] On first analysis, this procedure appeared to contradict all reconstructive dogma claiming that tubed full-thickness skin grafts are the only correct answer for urethral reconstruction. However, split-thickness skin grafts are soft and supple, are better contoured to the recipient bed, obviate the risk of intraluminal hair growth, mature faster than full-thickness grafts do, and have a much higher percentage of success (Figs. 152-41 to 152-43). At the same time, it is obvious that primary tubed grafts of any kind are susceptible to stricture, stenoses, and fistulas. Onlay grafts that are placed onto a bed of residual urethral plate and a urethra reconstructed from a local fasciocutaneous flap have a much lower incidence of fistulas despite the incorporation of two suture lines.

TABLE 152-4 ✦ PRINCIPLES FOR SURGICAL RECONSTRUCTION OF THE GENITOURINARY SYSTEM

Panurethral stricture or absence	
First stage	Cystoscopy Release total strictured expanse and extend dissection both proximally and distally; release penile chordee beyond area of local disease (zone of injury) Split-thickness skin grafts, meshed graft to defect
Second stage	Return in 9-12 months for secondary closure of urethra
Urethral absence associated with insensate phallus	
First stage	Release penile/phallic curvature; meshed split-thickness skin graft for urethral defect Sural nerve grafts coapted proximally to pudendal nerve branches and distally to cutaneous tips of the glans or dermal tissue to neurotize the distal phallus
Second stage	Secondary closure 9-12 months later
Penile foreshortening	Release offending tissue layer (corpus spongiosum, dartos fascia, Buck fascia, tunica albuginea) and reconstruct with a dermal graft and/or contralateral plication[107,108]
Penile fistula	See above
Urethral fistula	Cystoscopy to establish the urethral pattern Repair with local fasciocutaneous flaps and possible buccal onlay graft[109]
Urethral stenosis	Cystoscopy to establish urethral pattern Repair with local fasciocutaneous flaps, meshed split-thickness skin grafts, and buccal onlay graft

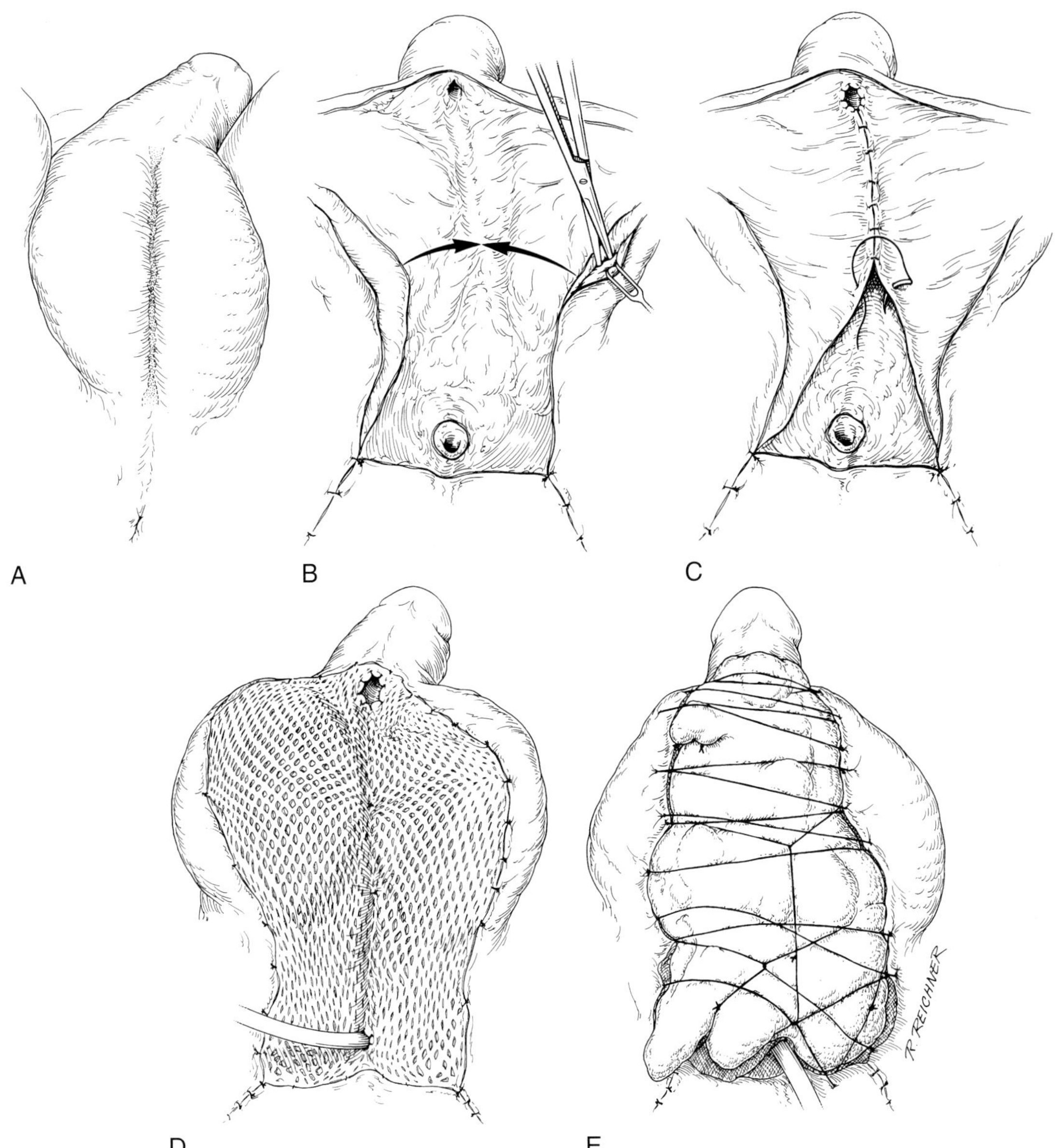

FIGURE 152-41. Historically, full-thickness skin graft urethral reconstruction has been fraught with a high rate of fistulas, stenoses, strictures, residual chordee, hairy urethra, and heavy scarring. In 1989, Schreiter described a two-stage meshed split-thickness skin graft urethroplasty that has become a mainstay in urethral reconstruction and the main exhibit of urology's adaptation of plastic surgery techniques. *A,* The first stage is the cornerstone on which urethral reconstruction is based. *B,* Initially, complete release of any residual chordee is confirmed by artificial erection, and the dartos fascia is dissected from the overlying skin. In this case, the patient has urethral stenosis and panurethral stricture disease. The scrotal skin is elevated at the future site of the planned urethral reconstruction. He requires a total urethral reconstruction. *C,* The graft bed is reinforced with dartos fascia. *D,* A meshed split-thickness skin graft is meticulously inset and carpeted over the bed. *E,* The first stage is completed with judicious placement of a tie-over bolus dressing.

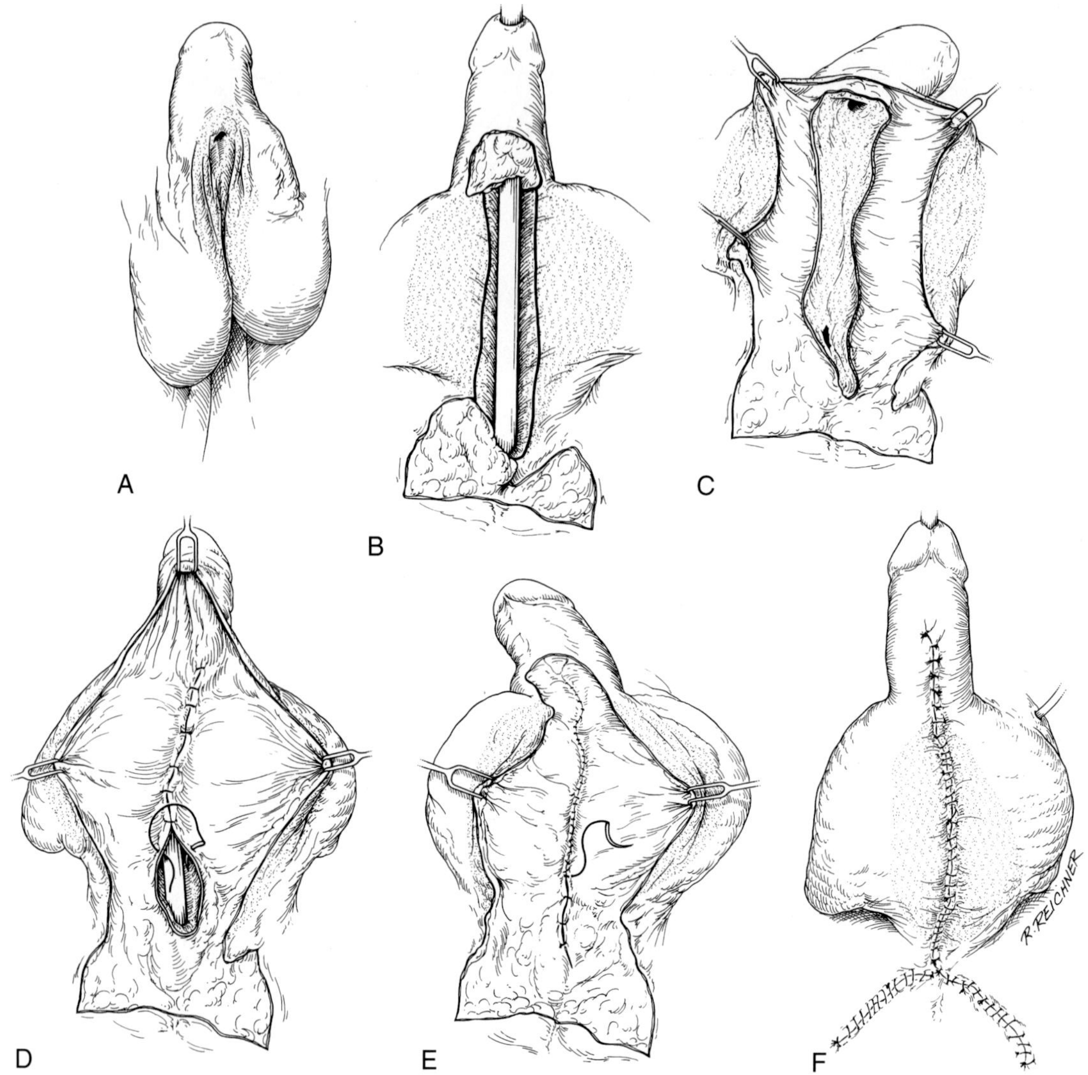

FIGURE 152-42. *A,* Second stage. Nine months later, the meshed skin graft has matured and an erection without chordee is present. *B,* The second stage is initiated by bivalving but not undermining the borders of the proposed urethroplasty. *C,* Panurethral tissues and dartos fascia are undermined. *D,* The urethra is tubed with a layer of interrupted buried intraluminal sutures. *E,* The subcutaneous dartos fascia is then closed over the urethra. *F,* Finally, the ventral skin is opposed, providing a three-layer closure for the urethral reconstruction.

MANAGEMENT AND RECONSTRUCTION FOR SPECIFIC CONDITIONS

Peyronie Disease

Peyronie disease was first reported by Fallopius in 1561 and then popularized in 1743 by François de la Peyronie.[110] Since then, the disease has borne his name. In Europe, it tends to be known as plastic induration of the penis. It is characterized by the formation of fibrous nodules within the tunica albuginea of the corpora cavernosa. These plaques impede tunica expansion during erection and result in a number of deformities. Peyronie disease is incurable, but fortunately most patients benefit from medical attention and few require surgery. For some, reassurance is sufficient; for others, medical therapy may promote stabilization or improvement. A physician may misinform a patient that "nothing can be done." On the other hand, indiscriminate surgery may be worse. Thus, the surgeon's challenge is to develop a plan between these two extremes.

Peyronie disease symptomatically affects about 1 of 100 adult men. In a cadaver study by Smith, a pathologist at the Armed Forces Institute of Pathology, the prevalence appeared to be 22 of 100.[111] The disease peaks

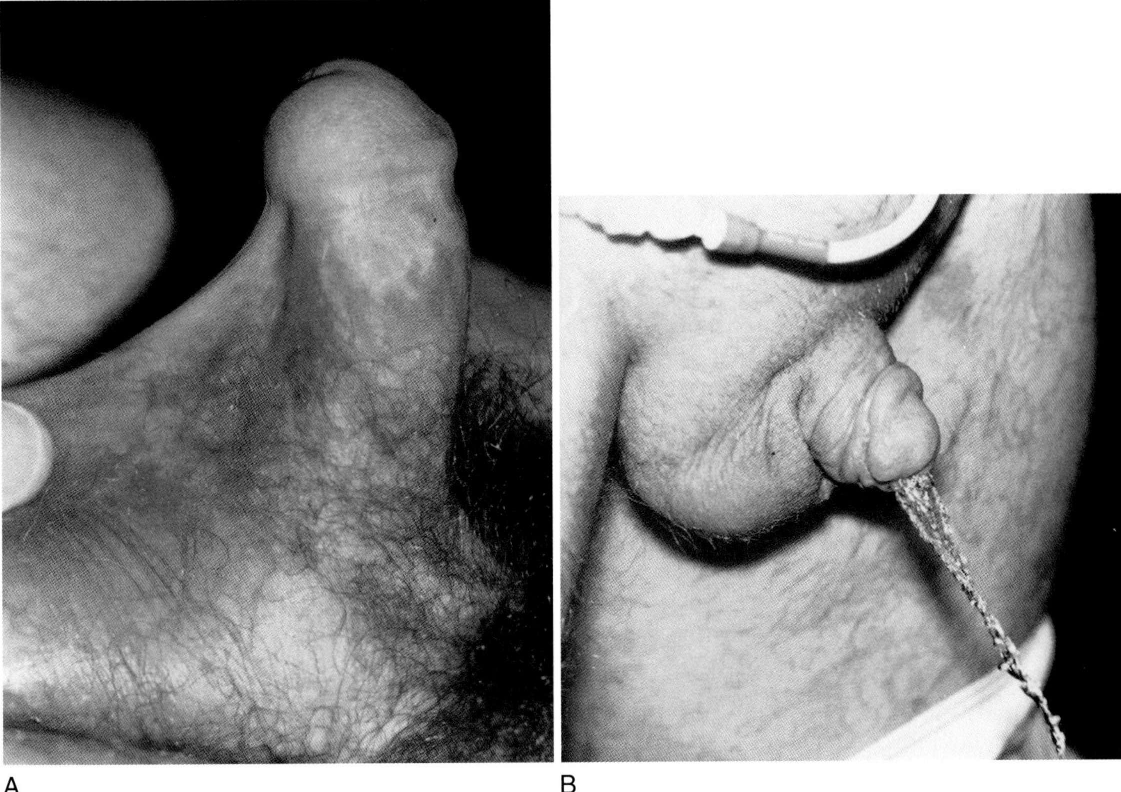

FIGURE 152-43. *A,* This man demonstrates many of the sequelae of attempted hypospadias repair—strictured and foreshortened urethra, residual chordee, lack of penile shaft skin that has produced resultant penoscrotal tethering, and encroachment of nonglabrous pubic skin onto the penile shaft. *B,* Completed healing over the ventral penile shaft is demonstrated. Note that the penis is straight and without chordee, the urethral reconstruction is intact, and some of the residual meshed skin graft has been used on the proximal penile shaft to help release the penoscrotal tethering. Three weeks after the second-stage repair, a voiding trial reveals a competent urethra.

in the mid-50s, coinciding with other age-related generalized losses of tissue elasticity. Although physicians are seeing more patients complaining of Peyronie disease in their office, there is no good evidence to suggest that the epidemiology of the disease is changing. However, the clinical incidence clearly is increasing.

Peyronie disease is thought to represent a localized aberration in wound healing. After trauma to the insertion of the midline septal fibers of the corpora cavernosa, there is an inflammatory response beginning with phagocytosis, proceeding quickly to the secretion of many vasoactive factors. Some of these factors govern the formation of fibrosis, and if these factors are not cleared, further fibrosis occurs, often autoinducing the further secretion of growth factors that govern the formation of fibrosis. It has been proposed that the injured area acts as if the "inflammation is trapped," and the growth factor response is euphemistically described as the "dark side" of wound healing.

The disease is marked by palpable nodularity and scarring in the tunica albuginea. This scarring develops over time. In most cases, onset is associated with an active phase consisting of painful erections and a changing configuration of plaque and deformity. About 30% of patients present with sudden onset of painless curvature. After 12 to 18 months, the disease inevitably passes into quiescent secondary phase, which is characterized by a painless, stable deformity and pathologically by mature scar, albeit "hypertrophic." Peyronie disease is a self-limited disease, and hence difficulty arises in assessing response to various trials, particularly pharmacologically based maneuvers.

The relationship of erectile dysfunction to Peyronie disease has been frequently noted but difficult to quantify. Discussions of erectile dysfunction after the surgery occurred with the very first report of surgery for Peyronie disease by Lowsley in the 1940s.[112,113] Since that time, postoperative erectile dysfunction has been mentioned in passing by most patients. Few papers, however, stratify patients preoperatively with regard to erectile dysfunction, and all series make mention of patients who clearly have erectile dysfunction after surgery. What is clear is that many patients perioperatively complain of the psychological impact of Peyronie disease that continues to plague good surgical results. Jones,[114] a sex therapist who interviewed 2000 patients with Peyronie disease, described the process of counseling men with Peyronie disease as like counseling one dealing with a death.

The medical history should include all aspects of a normal history and physical examination with an emphasis on risk factors for erectile dysfunction and a detailed psychosexual history. During genital examination, stretching the penis demonstrates the plaque. Most surgeons think that radiographic studies such as ultrasonography, magnetic resonance imaging, and computed tomography offer little to the diagnosis. However, the place for vascular testing is still a matter of much discussion and ranges from those who offer vascular testing (cavernosometry, cavernosography) to all patients to others who do not use vascular testing at all. However, most centers would agree that at least all patients who are offered surgery should have vascular testing preoperatively to define their erectile function.

In spite of various treatment options, Peyronie disease continues to present many dilemmas to the treating surgeon. A patient is a surgical candidate when the deformity precludes intercourse or there is erectile dysfunction. As mentioned, most surgeons agree that patients offered surgery should have their erectile function determined by vascular testing preoperatively. Reconstructive surgery is not recommended during the acute phase of the disease. It is imperative that patients give true informed consent; surgery, at best, is palliative, and the patient with unreasonable expectations will not be satisfied by even the best surgical result.

Nesbit[28] described the correction of genital curvature by contralateral plication. The use of plication was applied to Peyronie disease by Pryor.[115] Since then, plication techniques, corporoplasty techniques, and excision with suturing techniques have been proposed. It is clear that the surgeon consulting a patient with Peyronie disease must be prepared to offer these options to the appropriate patient. Lowsley first proposed excision of plaque with fat grafting. Since that time, a number of substances have been proposed as grafts. Few are enthusiastic about the use of nonautologous material; autologous grafts currently used are dermis, vein, and more recently pericardium. Plication or corporoplasty techniques essentially shorten the long or outer side of the curve (excision or incision), and grafting operations lengthen the more involved or foreshortened side.

There is increased enthusiasm about the use of incision and grafting techniques. Because most plaques are dorsal, the surgery begins with a circumscribing incision at the site of the prior circumcision. The penile shaft is degloved in the layer immediately superficial to the superficial lamina of Buck fascia. The dorsum of the penis is then examined, the path of the dorsal vein determined, and the superficial lamina of Buck fascia opened over the dorsal vein. This exposure allows dissection of the dorsal vein, which is excised from the level of the retrocoronal plexus to the penopubic junction. The deep lamina of Buck fascia is then opened and the fascia is elevated in concert with the dorsal neurovascular structures, allowing exposure of the plaque. When the fascia is released, an artificial erection is performed to identify the point of maximal curvature, which is then carefully marked. An H-shaped incision is then made at that point; the flaps of the H are detached from the septal fibers, releasing the curved aspect of the penis. These flaps are allowed to slide and are then sutured in place. The edges of the flaps are darted to preclude indentation. This establishes a roughly circular corporotomy defect, which can be filled with either autologous or nonautologous grafts. The grafts should be reattached to the midline septal fibers. A second artificial erection is then performed. In some patients, there may be some small amount of residual deformity, and if it is judged to be potentially troublesome for the patient, a "touch up plication" procedure is performed. In this situation, the Yachia technique, which consists of a Heineke-Mikulicz corporoplasty maneuver, has been effective.[116] As mentioned, there is probably no graft material that is perfect for replacing tunica albuginea (Figs. 152-44 and 152-45).[117]

Penile prosthesis placement is clearly overused in certain types of patients with Peyronie disease. The implantation of a penile prosthesis with or without grafting is the treatment of choice for men with Peyronie disease *and* erectile dysfunction. The literature shows excellent results with the use of prostheses in association with proper preoperative counseling.

Peyronie disease remains an enigma. The pathogenesis has not been clearly determined, the response to medical treatments is unpredictable, and research concerning the etiology of Peyronie disease continues. The surgeon confronted with a patient with Peyronie disease must adhere to a strict protocol. The patient with Peyronie disease will try to rush himself to the operating room, and the couple requires a great deal of reassurance and counseling. Fortunately, most patients do not require surgery. However, with proper evaluation and counseling, those that do require surgery can usually be offered a result that they consider reasonable.

Fournier Disease

Fournier in 1883 recognized a "fulminant gangrene" of the penis and scrotum that (1) developed suddenly in previously healthy young men, (2) progressed

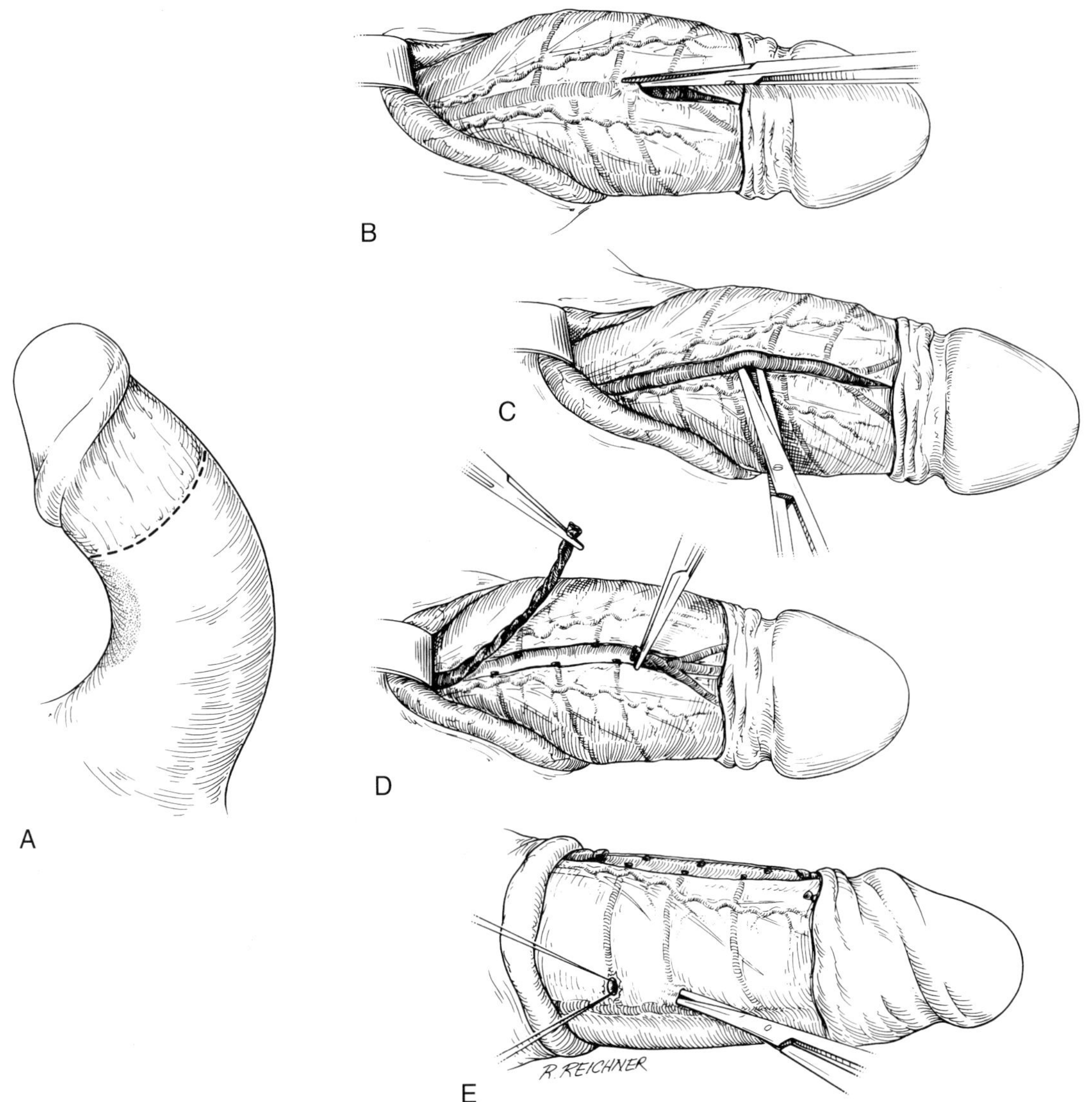

FIGURE 152-44. *A,* Peyronie disease is hallmarked by a dorsal penile chordee of 30 to 90 degrees and associated veno-occlusive dysfunction. The curvature is caused by a plaque of scar in the subtunical space of Smith depicted by the stippled area. *B,* The surgery is initiated by reflecting the penile shaft skin and underlying dartos fascia by a circumferential circumcising incision. Buck fascia is then incised to expose the deep dorsal vein with its distal subglanular tripartite source. *C* to *E,* The vein is dissected out to the penopubic junction, and all tributaries are either cauterized or tied off. Extensive circumferential veins are also followed and tied off at their ventral cavernosal source.

rapidly, and (3) was idiopathic. Since Fournier's original description, an etiologic factor has been identified in most cases, and the disease that bears his name has now been expanded to include a wider age range, male and female patients, and a more indolent course in which an etiologic agent and bacteriologic phaging can be identified. As Eke stated, "The specific pathological process, necrotizing fasciitis, in the specific region of the perineum and genitalia should be termed Fournier's gangrene, the etiology with or without proven infection not withstanding."[118]

Fournier disease is rare but represents a true genitourinary emergency when it is identified. Today, the etiology is identified in about 95% of cases. Common sources of infection include urogenital disease and trauma (renal abscess); urethral stone; urethral stricture; iatrogenic misadventure by the unrecognized rupture of the urethra when penile prostheses are inserted; colorectal (ruptured appendicitis); colon cancer; diverticulitis; perirectal, retroperitoneal, and subdiaphragmatic abscesses; and local trauma.[119]

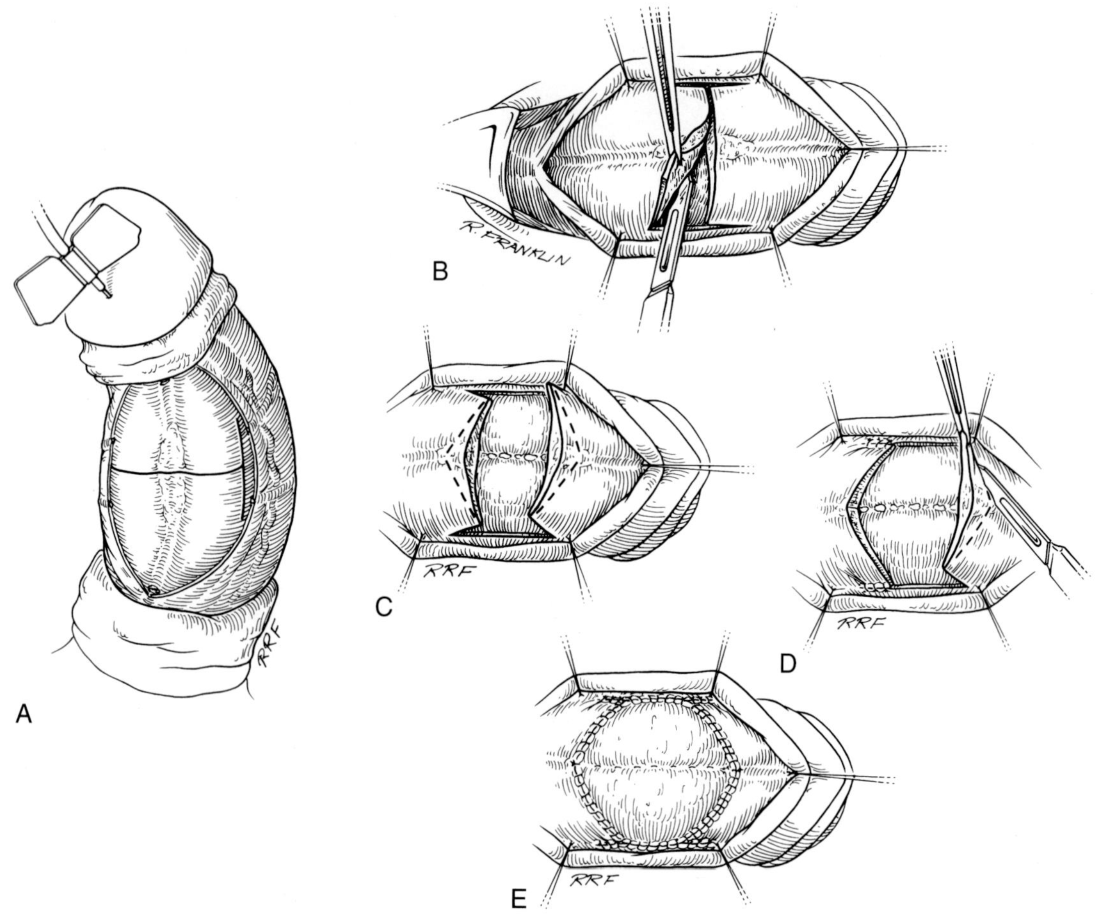

FIGURE 152-45. Surgical treatment of the Peyronie penile plaque has evolved over time. *A,* Total excision of the plaque may exacerbate the veno-occlusive erectile dysfunction and therefore has been replaced with plaque incision and dermal grafting. *B,* The plaque is undermined minimally to reduce venous disruption. *C* and *D,* After penile straightening, the edges of the plaque are sutured to the surrounding tunica. *E,* The dermal graft is then harvested and sutured to the surrounding skin-plaque interface. Note that great care is taken to fix the graft to the underlying intercorporal septum to form a watertight seal with the surrounding tissues.

Several systemic conditions have also been associated with Fournier gangrene and may predispose patients to its development: diabetes mellitus, alcoholism, heavy smoking (more than one pack per day), human immunodeficiency virus infection and acquired immunodeficiency syndrome, and leukemia. There are several theories to explain the increased incidence of the disease in diabetic patients: first, diabetic microvascular disease leads to increased tissue ischemia; second, defective white blood cell phagocytosis leads to increased bacterial spread; and third, diabetic neuropathy in patients with bladder outlet obstruction may result in increased urinary tract infections. Increased incidence of Fournier gangrene in patients with alcoholism can be attributed to immunosuppression and poor hygiene. Immunosuppression associated with human immunodeficiency virus infection, acquired immunodeficiency syndrome, and leukemia is also thought to account for the increased incidence in these patients. Finally, heavy smoking increases capillary vasoconstriction, thereby reducing vascularity to compromised tissues.

Fournier disease is considered a synergistic necrotizing fasciitis that often includes gram-positive organisms, gram-negative organisms, and *Clostridium perfringens* anaerobes in the cultures. The disease often begins as a cellulitis adjacent to the portal of entry. The affected area is swollen, erythematous, and tender as the infection begins to include the deep fascia. There is prominent pain as well as fever and systemic toxicity. Scrotal swelling and crepitus quickly increase with the appearance of dark purple areas that become gangrenous. Specific urinary symptoms include dysuria, urethral discharge, and obstructed voiding. Gram-negative sepsis is probable if symptoms include a change in mental status, tachypnea, tachycardia, and hyperthermia or hypothermia.

Cystoscopy, retrograde urethrography, and sigmoidoscopy are useful tools in the initial diagnosis and management of Fournier disease. Most patients undergo urgent urinary diversion with suprapubic cystotomy and fecal diversion with a proximal colostomy. In addition, ultrasound examination of the scrotum is also used to help diagnose Fournier disease by locating subcutaneous gas.

A high degree of suspicion is crucial to an early diagnosis. A clinical differentiation between necrotizing fasciitis and simple cellulitis may be difficult initially because the initial signs of pain, edema, and erythema are not distinctive. However, the presence of marked systemic toxicity out of proportion to the local findings should alert the surgeon.

Once the disease is identified, intravenous hydration and triple antibiotic therapy should be deployed in preparation for surgical débridement. Antibiotic regimens may include combinations of (1) ampicillin plus sulbactam or a third-generation cephalosporin such as ceftriaxone, (2) gentamicin, and (3) clindamycin or metronidazole (piperacillin). Once culture results are available, antibiotic coverage can be tailored to the specific organisms obtained. However, anaerobic coverage should be continued regardless of culture results because of the difficulty in culturing these organisms. The immediate surgical débridement is critical and is the definitive treatment. Initial débridement should be aggressive and continue along fascial plains until all of the devitalized tissues have been removed and viable tissue borders the wound. The presence of Colles fascia and the unique genital blood supply often restrict the gangrene to the perineum, scrotum, penile shaft, and lower abdominal wall. Buck fascia inherently protects corporal bodies and corpus spongiosum; the external spermatic fascia protects the testicles. Because there are often small distal perforators between the deep and superficial penile blood supply, distal shaft skin may be preserved initially but requires débridement before skin grafting to avoid distal shaft edema. Such vascular idiosyncrasies do not exist in the scrotum, where there is no communication between the testicular and the scrotal blood supply. Because the testicles have their own blood supply, orchiectomy is rarely required.

Hyperbaric oxygen therapy in conjunction with débridement and antibiotics has shown promise in speeding up preparation for reconstructive skin grafting and decreasing hospital stay, increasing wound healing, and minimizing the gangrenous spread, particularly in patients with *C. perfringens* infection. In addition to hyperbaric oxygen, mechanized wound débridement tools (i.e., the Wound VAC) have promoted granulation wound contracture and the reduction of bacterial colonization before reconstruction.

Reconstruction of the genitalia includes release of the penis and testicles from surrounding granulation tissue; release of scar contracture; and split-thickness sheet grafts on the penile shaft and peripenile tissues and nonexpanded meshed split-thickness grafts of the scrotum, perineum, and crural folds. Both musculocutaneous and muscle flaps have also been described to cover and nourish the testicles followed by definitive scrotoplasty. The most common of these flap alternatives is the lateral thigh pocket flap, which is most probably vascularized by branches of the external pudendal, obturator, and medial circumflex blood vessels. The pocket is then converted to a proximal superomedial-based thigh flap that is easily raised and transferred medially to be sutured at the midline to the contralateral flap. The flap donor sites are usually closed directly.

The mortality rate in Fournier disease averages approximately 20% but can range from 7% to 75%. Higher mortality rates are found in diabetics, alcoholics, and those with colorectal sources of infection, who often have a greater delay in diagnosis and more widespread extension. To reduce morbidity and mortality, the key is early diagnosis, aggressive treatment with antibiotics, and surgical débridement.

Balanitis Xerotica Obliterans

Balanitis xerotica obliterans is one of the most misunderstood of all genital diseases and one in which the treatment endpoint is poorly defined.[120] Balanitis xerotica obliterans is the genital form of lichen sclerosus et atrophicus. It has been suggested that lichen sclerosus et atrophicus is infectious in origin and related to the organism *Borrelia burgdorferi*.[121] This organism is a spirochete and is sensitive as most spirochetes are to tetracyclines, penicillins, and fluoroquinolones.

The disease is a destructive skin condition in which a sharply marginated white patch develops on the glans penis. In time, the glans and outer preputial plates become fibrotic, keratotic, acanthotic, and atrophic. Through some poorly understood pathologic mechanism, the disease spreads to the remaining glans, the meatus, the fossa navicularis, and the urethra, thereby causing meatal stenosis and intractable urethral stricture that may then spread down the urethra in a retrograde fashion. There are rare reports of malignant degeneration.

The etiology of balanitis xerotica obliterans is uncertain, but trauma, autoimmune diseases, and infections diseases have been associated. The disease appears to be predominant in diabetic patients and patients with poor immune response.

Perhaps the most important aspect of treatment is a high index of suspicion to avoid exacerbating and irritating the disease process. For example, the treating physician may initially be consulted by a patient with phimosis or another form of strictured prepuce.[122] A circumcision may produce initial relief of symptoms, but the disease process often spreads and continues onto the glans uroepithelium. Once meatal stenosis and urethral stricture occur, continuous urethral dilation usually exacerbates the process (Fig. 152-46).[122]

In patients in whom balanitis xerotica obliterans is active on the glans and distal urethra, it may be beneficial to treat the patient with a chronic course of antibiotics and to use steroid creams including not only glucocorticoids but also AndroGel. Depasquale[123] has recommended dermabrasion of the involved tissue on the glans with reconstruction of the glans by a split-thickness graft. Rather amazing cosmetic results can be achieved in some patients.

Surgical treatment in the past has centered on circumcision, glanular resection, and, where necessary, urethroplasty. Even so, the disease may persist and continue to produce penile foreshortening and scarring. Some of the surgical reconstructions have focused on genital and extragenital skin reconstruction by use of circular penile skin onlay flaps, epilated midline genital skin flaps, and meshed split-thickness extragenital skin grafts.

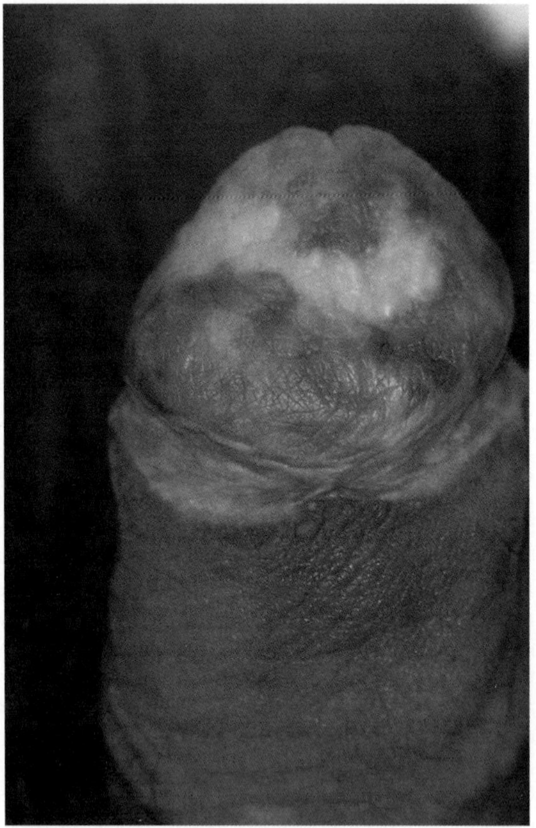

FIGURE 152-46. The diagnosis of balanitis xerotica obliterans is often clouded by a differential diagnosis and comorbid disease. Without treatment, this disease process will spread over the penile glans, the internal lamella of the prepuce, the urethral meatus, the fossa navicularis, and eventually the urethral lumen itself. Uroepithelial scarring highlights the physical examination.

There is enthusiasm now for the return to staged reconstructive techniques and for the use of buccal mucosa. Buccal mucosa grafts can be used for staged urethral reconstruction, and initial results would suggest that this is a superior way of dealing with the problem. In some cases, with the eventual reconstruction of approximately 18 to 20 cm of urethra required, the mouth as a donor site is limited. For early cases (e.g., balanitis xerotica obliterans confined to the perimeatal area only), patients can be treated with a single-stage reconstruction. Jordan[18] has advocated the use of a ventral transverse skin island flap technique. The success rate in this highly selected group of patients has been excellent, with no recurrences and with no fistulas complicating the immediate reconstructive course. These patients, however, are prescribed long courses of antibiotics (the authors use doxycycline when possible) and steroid applications to the area of the glans. Clobetasol cream 0.05% is a useful glucocorticoid cream for many of these patients, and as already mentioned, AndroGel has been used in some patients.

The surgeon involved with only occasional reconstruction of the urethra should not attempt urethral reconstruction for patients with balanitis xerotica obliterans. These are clearly the most challenging patients that most reconstructive surgeons will face, and many patients will require the use of both cheeks as well as the lower lip donor sites.

The Europeans have raised concerns about the lower lip donor site. The authors have used the lower lip donor site in a number of patients without adverse sequelae; however, adverse events have been seen by certain individuals in the European reconstructive surgical community.

Penile Skin Cancers

In the past, treatment of penile cancer ranged from techniques of local excision to emasculation. Classically, penile cancer involving the redundant preputial and penile skin could be adequately treated with circumcision. Superficial penile cancer involving the glans was in recent years treated by laser excision. As penile cancer invaded the glans, the standard of care became partial penectomy; and as the deep structures were invaded, the excision amounted to subtotal or total penectomy. In recent years, it has been appreciated that penile cancer involving the spongy erectile tissue of the glans could be treated by "glansectomy." In other words, excision did not necessarily have to involve the underlying corpora cavernosa. Thus, reconstructive surgery after these techniques often was limited to a redefinition procedure or coverage procedure of the distal corporal bodies. Often, just grafting the tips of the corporal bodies provided an excellent functional as well as cosmetic result.

Another surgical method of treating penile cancer involves Mohs surgery. In Mohs surgery, sequential excisions are accomplished until clean margins in all quadrants are achieved. In classic Mohs surgery, the defect is then left to granulate and close. However, reconstruction of the glans can be facilitated by the use of local flap techniques. The ventral transverse penile skin island may be used as a method of achieving both bulk and definition.

In these patients, a transversely oriented penile skin island is outlined on the ventral surface of the penis and elevated on the ventral dartos fascia. The fascia can be mobilized well down beyond the penoscrotal junction, thus allowing the skin island to be transposed to the dorsum of the glans. The fascial flap is buttonholed in the midline, the buttonhole being oriented in the longitudinal plane, thus interfering minimally with the fascial blood supply. The skin island can then be distributed into the Mohs defect; a subsequent touch up operation can be done at about 6 months. This technique has been used in a number of patients with nice functional and cosmetic results. The resulting defect on the ventral surface of the penis is usually easily closed primarily. In an occasional patient, the penoscrotal junction can be somewhat tethered with that closure, but again with the touch up surgery of the glans at 6 months, the penoscrotal junction can be redefined (see Fig. 152-26).[46]

In patients in whom a true partial penectomy has been performed, reconstructive efforts were directed toward an augmented reconstruction. In these patients, either local flaps or microvascular transplanted flaps were appended to lengthen the penis. The hope was then to incorporate prostheses at a later date. These techniques, however, were found to lack both in cosmetic and functional considerations. However, it is better to sacrifice some superficial penile tissue, saving the remaining corporal bodies, and to accomplish a true phallic construction. The corporal bodies are incorporated in the base of the microvascular free transfer flap. In patients requiring total penectomy, observation for 1 year confirms adequate tumor margins without recurrence. After clearance by the oncologic surgeon, a total phallic reconstruction is planned by microvascular composite tissue. In patients who have had extensive superficial lymph node dissections, there are considerations with regard to recipient vessels. In these patients, angiography is performed to define the deep inferior epigastric vessels, to define the iliofemoral system, and to use delayed films to attempt to define the venous anatomy of the groin. In addition, in cases in which reconstruction is envisioned, if possible, at the time of the extensive exenterative surgery, it is preferable to place intravenous and arterial lines in the dominant forearm, saving the vascularity of the nondominant forearm for subsequent use in phallic construction. Many surgical oncologists are consulting reconstructive surgeons before the exenterative surgery to ensure that these considerations are recognized.

Reconstructive surgery other than in the case of Mohs surgery is best accomplished in delayed fashion, often a year after the extirpative surgery, thus ensuring that the reconstruction will not mask recurrence.

Lymphedema

Genital lymphedema is rarely encountered as an isolated problem. It can be part of the constellation of idiopathic lower extremity lymphedema; it is often seen in the postirradiation patient; and in some patients, idiopathic occurrence of lymphedema is patchy in nature and frequently associated with cellulitis. In fact, cellulitis of the genital skin may be a predisposing event to "idiopathic" genital lymphedema as well as a late complicating event to the other causes of lymphedema.

In patients with spotty occurrence of genital lymphedema, the authors have employed a course of prolonged antibiotics (in some cases 6 to 9 months). In these patients, fluoroquinolones are used in a relatively high dose and for long periods. Interestingly, many of these patients will respond favorably to these long courses of antibiotics without recurrence when the antibiotics are stopped. In most patients presenting for reconstruction for lymphedema, it is advisable to prescribe a course of antibiotics for a number of months before undertaking the reconstruction for lymphedema.

In reconstruction for lymphedema, the edematous tissue must be completely excised. In the case of the penis, the excision should be taken to the level of the superficial lamina of Buck fascia; in the scrotum, the testicles are left covered only by the external spermatic fascia. It is our practice to open the testicular vaginal space as if one were doing a hydrocelectomy. In many patients, accompanying hydroceles are seen. The testicles must be fixed in an anatomically appropriate position before proceeding with graft coverage. If they are not, because of the cremasteric reflex, there will be migration of the gonads beneath the skin grafts. It is our practice to use mesh skin grafts for the area of the scrotal reconstruction and sheet graft to cover the penis. The excision of the lymphatic tissue on the penile shaft should extend to the level of coronal margin. If one leaves a preputial cuff, it often remains edematous, interfering with both the cosmetic appearance and function. Should the lymphedema involve the tissues immediately adjacent to the scrotum, the lymphedematous subcutaneous tissues can be excised, leaving the skin itself. It is helpful to do this because the adjacent skin can then be sutured up around the gonads. These grafts become redundant over time, and cosmetic results in these cases are excellent. Care must be taken to harvest these grafts as thinly as possible. A buttocks donor site is routinely used, and the grafts are harvested at about 0.014-inch thickness. By harvesting the grafts thinly, one carries as little of the reticular dermis as possible, and recurrence rates are much lower. If thick grafts are used, edema can accumulate in the reticular dermis that is carried, and patients can have striking recurrence of lymphedema. Patients should be cautioned that after reconstruction, sensation would be deep sensation. These skin grafts do not readily reinnervate; however, there is no need whatsoever to interfere with the dorsal neurovascular structures of the penis, and thus glans sensation should be unaffected.

Patients will occasionally be seen in other lymphedematous conditions. In patients who have had attempted bulking to increase penile girth with either fat injections or the injection of lipid- or silicone-containing materials, one encounters sclerosing lipoid lymphogranulomas. The lymphedematous process is striking; in addition to the lymphedema, one is confronted with a significant inflammatory granulomatous reaction. In these patients, reconstruction is best accomplished after a course of antibiotics to settle the acute inflammatory phases of these conditions. In that the deeper tissues are often involved, and the skin itself many times is spared, excision of the involved areas can be done with primary closure of the scrotum accomplished. If that is possible, there is no question that the patient's operative course is facilitated, and the eventual cosmetic result is far superior. However, it is seldom possible to spare the penile skin. Fortunately, the lymphogranulomatous process usually does not penetrate the Buck fascia. Thus, with the process excised to the level of Buck fascia, shaft reconstruction can be accomplished as already described. If the penile skin can be spared, unquestionably that would be the best. This approach would then be comparable to the Charles procedure, one of the original techniques for dealing with edematous problems of the extremities as well as of the genitalia.

REFERENCES

1. Gilbert D, Devine C, Winslow B, et al: Microsurgical hypospadias repair. Plast Reconstr Surg 1986;77:460.
2. Cohen BE, May JW, Daly JS, et al: Successful clinical replantation of an amputated penis by microneurovascular repair. Plast Reconstr Surg 1977;59:276.
3. Tamai S, Nakamura Y, Motomiya Y: Microsurgical replantation of a completely amputated penis and scrotum. Plast Reconstr Surg 1977;60:287.
4. Silber SJ, Kelly J: Successful autotransplantation of an intraabdominal testis to the scrotum by microvascular techniques. J Urol 1976;115:452.
5. Wacksman J, Dinner M, Handler M: Results of testicular autotransplantation using the microvascular technique: experience with eight intra-abdominal testes. J Urol 1982;128:1319.
6. Boeckx W, Vereecken R, Depuydt K: Microsurgery for intraabdominal testicular retention. Eur J Obstet Gynecol Reprod Biol 1998;81:191.
7. Michal V, Kramar R, Popischal J, et al: Direct arterial anastomosis on corporal cavernosa penis in the therapy of erective impotence. Rozhl Chir 1973;52:587.
8. Gilbert DA, Horton CE, Terzis JK, et al: New concepts in phallic reconstruction. Ann Plast Surg 1987;18:128.
9. McCraw JB, Dibbell DG: Experimental definition of independent myocutaneous vascular territories. Plast Reconstr Surg 1977;60:212.
10. Manchot C: The Cutaneous Arteries of the Human Body. New York, Springer-Verlag, 1983.
11. Quartey JKM: Microcirculation of penile and scrotal skin. Atlas Urol Clin North Am 1997;5:1.
12. Jordan GH, Gilbert DA: Male genital trauma. Clin Plast Surg 1988;15:405.
13. Juskiewenski S, Vaysse P, Moscovici J: A study of the arterial blood supply to the penis. Anat Clin 1982;4:101.
14. Jordan GH, Stack RS: General concepts concerning the use of genital skin islands for anterior urethral reconstruction. Atlas Urol Clin North Am 1997;5:23.
15. Blandy JP, Singh M, Tresidder GC: Urethroplasty by scrotal flap for long urethral strictures. Br J Urol 1968;40:261.
16. Quartey JKM: One-stage penile/preputial island flap urethroplasty for urethral stricture. J Urol 1985;134:474.
17. Orandi A: One-stage urethroplasty: 4 year follow up. J Urol 1972;107:977.
18. Jordan GH: Reconstruction of the fossa navicularis. J Urol 1987;138:102.
19. Kodos AB: The vascular supply of the penis. Arkh Anat Embriol 1967;43:525.
20. Hinman F Jr: Anatomy of the external genitalia. In Ehrlich RM, Alter GJ, eds: Reconstructive and Plastic Surgery of the External Genitalia. Philadelphia, WB Saunders, 1999:chapter 2.
21. Jordan GH, Shaffer B, Sumfest J, et al: Reconstruction for exstrophy of the bladder and epispadias. In Libertino JA: Reconstructive Urologic Surgery, 3rd ed. St. Louis, Mosby, 1998:chapter 49.
22. Muecke EC: Exstrophy, epispadias and other anomalies of the bladder. In Harrison JH, Gittes RF, Perlmutter AD, et al, eds: Campbell's Urology, vol 2, 4th ed. Philadelphia, WB Saunders, 1979:1443-1468.
23. Mitchell ME, Bagli DJ: Complete penile disassembly for epispadias repair: the Mitchell technique. J Urol 1996;155:300.
24. Sumfest J: Personal communication, 2002.
25. Gearhart JP, Leonard MP, Burgers JK, Jeffs RD: The Cantwell-Ransley technique for repair of epispadias. J Urol 1992;148:851.
26. Gearhart JP, Peppas DS, Jeffs RD: Complications of paraexstrophy skin flaps in the reconstruction of classical bladder exstrophy. J Urol 1993;150:627.
27. Perovic S, Scepanovic D, Sremcevic D, Vukadinovic V: Epispadias surgery—Belgrade experience. Br J Urol 1992;70:647.
28. Nesbit RM: Congenital curvature of the phallus: report of three cases with description of corrective operation. J Urol 1965;93: 230.
29. Devine CJ Jr, Blackley SK, Horton CE, Gilbert DA: The surgical treatment of chordee without hypospadias in men. J Urol 1991;146: 325.
30. Donahoe PK, Hendreh WH: Intersex abnormalities in the newborn infant. In Holder TM, Ashcroft KW, eds: Pediatric Surgery. Philadelphia, WB Saunders, 1980:chapter 66.

31. Maizels M, Zaontz M, Donovan J, et al: Surgical correction of the buried penis: description of a classifications system to correct the disorder. J Urol 1986;136(pt 2):268.
32. Ehrlich RM, Alter GJ: Buried penis. In Ehrlich RM, Alter GJ, eds: Reconstructive and Plastic Surgery of the External Genitalia. Philadelphia, WB Saunders, 1999.
33. Alter GJ, Horton CE, Horton CE Jr: Buried penis as a contraindication for circumcision. J Am Coll Surg 1994; 178:487.
34. Adham MW, Teimourian B, Mosca P: Buried penis release in adults with suction lipectomy and abdominoplasty. Plast Reconstr Surg 2000;106:840.
35. Schonfeld W, Beebe GW: Normal growth and variation in the male genitalia from birth to maturity. J Urol 1942;48: 759.
36. Gilbert D, Jordan G, Devine C Jr, et al: Phallic construction in prepubertal and teenage boys. J Urol 1993;149:1521.
37. Gilbert DA, Jordan GH, Schlossberg SM, Winslow BH: Forearm free flap for pediatric phallic construction. In Ehrlich RM, Alter GJ, eds: Reconstructive and Plastic Surgery of the External Genitalia. Philadelphia, WB Saunders, 1999.
38. Hamill PV, Drizd TA, Johnson CL, et al: Physical growth: National Center for Health Statistics percentiles. Am J Clin Nutr 1979;32:607.
39. Gearhart JP, Rock JA: Total ablation of the penis after circumcision with electrocautery: a method of management and long-term follow-up. J Urol 1989;42:799.
40. Skoog SJ, Belman AB: Aphallia: its classification and management. J Urol 1989;141:589.
41. Stolar CJH, Wiener ES, Hersle TW, et al: Reconstruction of penile agenesis by a posterior sagittal approach. J Pediatr Surg 1987;22:1076.
42. Oesch IL, Pinter A, Ransley PG: Penile agenesis: a report of six cases. J Pediatr Surg 1987;22:172.
43. McAninch JW: Management of genital skin loss. Urol Clin North Am 1989;16:387.
44. Schreiter F, Noll F: Mesh graft urethroplasty. World J Urol 1987;5:41.
45. Schreiter F, Noll F: Mesh graft urethroplasty using split thickness skin graft for foreskin. J Urol 1989;142:1223.
46. Jordan GH, Gilbert DA, Devine CJ Jr: Penile reconstruction following Mohs' micrographic surgery. Presented at American Urological Association 86th annual meeting, Toronto, Ontario, June 3, 1991.
47. Burger RA, Muller SC, el-Damanhoury H, et al: The buccal mucosal graft for urethral reconstruction: a preliminary report. J Urol 1992;147:662.
48. McCraw JB, Arnold PG, eds: Atlas of Muscle and Musculocutaneous Flaps. Norfolk, Va, Hampton Press, 1986;389-421.
49. McGregor IA, Jackson IT: The groin flap. Br J Plast Surg 1972;25:3.
50. Sun G, Huang J: One-stage reconstruction of the penis with composite iliac crest and lateral groin skin flap. Ann Plast Surg 1985;15:519.
51. Sun GC, Zhong AG, He W, et al: Reconstruction of the external genitals and repair of skin defects of the perineal region using three types of lateral groin flap. Ann Plast Surg 1990;24:328.
52. Akoz T, Kargi E: Phalloplasty in female-to-male transsexual using a double pedicle composite groin flap. Ann Plast Surg 2002;48:423.
53. Ustuner TE, Mutaf M, Sensoz O: Anteromedial thigh: a source for phallic reconstruction. Ann Plast Surg 1994;32:426.
54. Cheng KX, Hwang WY, Eid AE, et al: Analysis of 136 cases of reconstructed penis using various methods. Plast Reconstr Surg 1995;95:1070.
55. Woods JE, Alter G, Meland B, Podratz K: Experience with vaginal reconstruction utilizing the modified "Singapore" flap. Plast Reconstr Surg 1992;90:270.
56. Monstrey S, Blondeel P, VanLanduyt K, et al: The versatility of the pudendal thigh fasciocutaneous flap used as an island flap. Plast Reconstr Surg 2001;107:19.
57. Mutaf M: Nonmicrosurgical use of the radial forearm flap for penile reconstruction. Plast Reconstr Surg 2001;107:80.
58. Martius H, McCall J, Bolster KA, eds: Operative Gynecology. Boston, Little, Brown, 1956.
59. Hurwitz DJ, Swartz WM, Mathes SJ: The gluteal thigh flap: a reliable, sensate flap for the closure of buttock and perineal wounds. Plast Reconstr Surg 1981;68:521.
60. Walton RL, Hurwitz DJ, Bunkis J: Gluteal thigh flap for reconstruction of perineal defects. In Strauch B, Vasconez LO, Hall-Findlay EJ, eds: Grabb's Encyclopedia of Flaps, 2nd ed. Philadelphia, Lippincott-Raven, 1998:1499.
61. Orticochea M: A new method of total reconstruction of the penis. Br J Plast Surg 1972;25:347.
62. Horton CE, McCraw JB, Devine CJ, et al: Secondary reconstruction of the genital area. Urol Clin North Am 1977; 4:133.
63. Santanelli F, Scuderi N: Neophalloplasty in female-to-male transsexuals with the island tensor fasciae latae flap. Plast Reconstr Surg 2000;105:1990.
64. Ehrich WS: Two unusual penile injuries. J Urol 1929;21:239.
65. McRoberts JW, Chapman WH, Ansell JS: Primary anastomosis of the traumatically amputated penis: case report and summary of literature. J Urol 1968;100:751.
66. Lidman D, Danielsson P, Abdiu A, Fahraeus B: The functional result two years after a microsurgical penile replantation: case report. Scand J Plast Reconstr Surg Hand Surg 1999;33: 325.
67. Sanger JR, Matloub HS, Yousif NJ, Begun FP: Penile replantation after self-inflicted amputation. Ann Plast Surg 1992;29:579.
68. Matloub HS, Yousif NJ, Sanger JR: Temporary ectopic implantation of an amputated penis. Plast Reconstr Surg Hand Surg 1999;33:325.
69. Greilheimer H, Groves JE: Male genital self-mutilation. Arch Gen Psychiatry 1991;36:441.
70. Szasz UG, McLoughlin MG, Warren RJ: Return of sexual functioning following penile replant surgery. Arch Sex Behav 1990;19:343.
71. Bhanaganada K, Chayavatana T, Pongnumkul C, et al: Surgical management of an epidemic of penile amputations in Siam. Am J Surg 1983;146:376.
72. Tuerk M, Weir WH Jr: Successful replantation of a traumatically amputated glans penis. Plast Reconstr Surg 1971;48:499.
73. Jordan GH: Initial management and reconstruction of male amputation injuries. In McAninch JW, ed: Traumatic and Reconstructive Urology. Philadelphia, WB Saunders, 1996:673-681.
74. Janecka IP, Romas NA: Microvascular free transfer of the human testes. Plast Reconstr Surg 1979;63:42.
75. Martinis FG, Nagler HM: Testicular autotransplantation. Atlas Urol Clin North Am 1996;4:95.
76. Virag R, Zwang G, Dermange H, et al: Vasculogenic impotence: a review 92 cases with 54 surgical operations. Vasc Surg 1981;121:774.
77. Furlow WL, Knoll LD, Benson RC: Deep dorsal vein arterialization: application of the Furlow-Fisher modification in 156 patients with vasculogenic impotence. Int J Impot Res 1992;4:2.
78. Hauri D: A new operative technique in vasculogenic erectile dysfunction. World J Urol 1986;4:237.
79. Bogoraz NA: Plastic restoration of the penis. Sov Khir 1936;8:303.
80. Frumkin AP: Reconstruction of the male genitalia. Am Rev Soviet Med 1944;2:214.
81. Gillies HD, Harrison RJ: Congenital absence of the penis. Br J Plast Surg 1948;1:8.
82. Goodwin WE, Scott WW: Phalloplasty. J Urol 1952;68:903.

83. Evans AJ: Reconstruction of the penis. In Horton CE, ed: Plastic and Reconstructive Surgery of the Genital Area. Boston, Little, Brown, 1973:467-476.
84. Puckett CL, Reinisch JF, Montie JE: Free flap phalloplasty. J Urol 1982;128:294.
85. Chang TS, Hwang YW: Forearm flap in one-stage reconstruction of the penis. Plast Reconstr Surg 1984;74:251.
86. Song R, Gao Y, Song Y, et al: The forearm flap. Clin Plast Surg 1982;9:21.
87. Gilbert DA, Williams MW, Horton CE, et al: Phallic reinnervation via the pudendal nerve. J Urol 1988;140:295.
88. Farrow GA, Boyd JB, Semple JL: Total reconstruction of the penis employing the "cricket bat flap" single stage forearm free graft. AUA Today 1990;3:7.
89. Gilbert D, Jordan G, Devine C Jr, Winslow B: Microsurgical forearm "cricket bat–transformer phalloplasty." Plast Reconstr Surg 1992;90:711.
90. Biemer E: Penile reconstruction by the radial arm flap. Clin Plast Surg 1988;15:425.
91. Lovie MJ, Duncan GM, Glasson DW: The ulnar artery forearm flap. Plast Surg 1984;37:486.
92. Gilbert DA, Schlossberg SM, Jordan GH: Ulnar forearm phallic construction and penile reconstruction. Microsurgery 1995;16:314.
93. Sadove RC, Sengezer M, McRoberts JW, Wells MD: One-stage total penile reconstruction with a free sensate osteocutaneous fibula flap. Plast Reconstr Surg 1993;92:1314.
94. Papadopulos NA, Schaff J, Biemer E: Long-term fate of the bony component in neophallus construction with free osteofasciocutaneous forearm or fibula flap in 18 female-to-male transsexuals. Plast Reconstr Surg 2002;109:1025.
95. Hage JJ, Winters HA, Van Lieshout J: Fibula free flap phalloplasty: modifications and recommendations. Microsurgery 1996;17:358.
96. Hage JJ, Bloem JJ, Bouman FG: Obtaining rigidity in the neophallus of female-to-male transsexuals: a review of the literature. Ann Plast Surg 1993;30:327.
97. Newman HF: Vibratory sensitivity of the penis. Fertil Steril 1970;21:791.
98. Terzis JK: Personal communication, 1982.
99. Jordan GH, Alter GJ, Gilbert DA, Horton CE: Penile prosthesis implantation in total phalloplasty. J Urol 1994;152:410.
100. Alter GJ, Gilbert DA, Schlossberg SM, Jordan GH: Prosthetic implantation after phallic reconstruction. Microsurgery 1995;16:314.
101. Hage JJ: A unique case of secondary microvascular glansplasty: the last genitoreconstructive frontier? Ann Plast Surg 2000;45:422.
102. Pasky L, Albert DJ: Staged orchiopexy. Surg Gynecol Obstet 1971;132:43.
103. McMahon RA, O'Brien B, Cussen LJ: The use of microsurgery in the treatment of the undescended testis. J Pediatr Surg 1976;11:521.
104. Giuliani L, Carmignani G: Autotransplantation of the testicle. In Wagenknecht LV, ed: Microsurgery in Urology. New York, Thieme, 1985:chapter 32.
105. Fowler RJ, Stephens FD: The role of testicular vascular anatomy in the salvage of high, undescended testis. Aust N Z J Surg 1959;29:92.
106. Oesterwitz H, Fahlenkamp D: Microsurgical technique and results of testicular autotransplantation in children—essential venous anastomosis. Int Urol Nephrol 1993;25:587.
107. Horton CE, Devine CJ Jr: Hypospadias cripples. In Horton CE, ed: Plastic and Reconstructive Surgery of the Genital Area. Boston, Little, Brown, 1973:392.
108. Secrest CL, Jordan GH, Winslow BH, et al: Repair of the complications of hypospadias surgery. J Urol 1993;150:1415.
109. Angermeier KW, Jordan GH, Schlossberg SM: Complex urethral reconstruction. Urol Clin North Am 1994;21:567.
110. Peyronie F de la: Sur quelques obstacles qui s'opposent a l'ejaculation naturelle de la semence. Mem Acad Chir 1743;1:318.
111. Smith BH: Peyronie disease. Am J Clin Pathol 1966;45:670.
112. Lowsley O, Gentile A: An operation for the cure of certain cases of plastic induration (Peyronie disease) of the penis. J Urol 1947;57:552.
113. Lowsley OS, Boyce WH: Further experience with an operation for the cure of Peyronie disease. J Urol 1950;63:888.
114. Jones WJ Jr, Horton CE, Stecker JF Jr, Devine CJ Jr: The treatment of psychogenic impotence after dermal graft repair for Peyronie disease. J Urol 1984;131:286.
115. Pryor JP, Fitzpatrick JM: A new approach to the correction of the penile deformity in Peyronie disease. U Urol 1979;122:622.
116. Yachia D: Modified corporoplasty for the treatment of penile curvature. J Urol 1990;143:80.
117. Jordan GH: Treatment of Peyronie disease with plaque incision or excision and dermal graft. In Ehrlich RM, Alter GJ, eds: Reconstructive and Plastic Surgery of the External Genitalia. Philadelphia, WB Saunders, 1999:chapter 82.
118. Eke N: Fournier's gangrene: a review of 1726 cases. Br J Surg 2000; 87:718.
119. Vick R, Carson C: Fournier's disease. Urol Clin North Am 1999;26:841.
120. Akporiaye LE, Jordan GH, Devine CJ Jr: Balanitis xerotica obliterans (BXO). AUA Update Series Lesson 21, vol 16. Houston, Texas, American Urological Association, Office of Education, 1997.
121. Dillon WI, Saed GM, Fivenson DP: *Borrelia burgdorferi* DNA is undetectable by polymerase chain reaction in skin lesions of morphea, scleroderma, or lichen sclerosus et atrophicus of patients from North America. J Acad Dermatol 1995;33:617.
122. Boinbridge DR, Whitaker Rh, Chir M, Shepheard BGF: Balanitis xerotica obliterans and urinary obstruction. Br J Urol 1971;43:487.
123. Depasquale I, Park AJ, Bracka A: The treatment of balanitis xerotica obliterans. BJU Int 2000;86:459.

CHAPTER

153

Hypospadias

DAVID J. COLEMAN, MS, FRCS (Plast) ✦ PAUL E. BANWELL, BSc, FRCS

Hypospadias, one of the most common congenital anomalies, affects in excess of 1 in 300 boys. Its surgical correction has a reputation for being problematic, with countless operative procedures described. In hypospadias, the urethral meatus fails to reach the tip of the glans penis. The penile fascia and skin fail to develop correctly on the ventral surface of the penis, resulting in a ventral curvature and a hooded prepuce. This represents a partial feminization of the male genitalia. The extent of these clinical features varies. Most hypospadias is relatively mild with a meatus at the distal shaft, corona, or glans penis (Fig. 153-1). Patients with mild hypospadias will not usually have a ventral curvature. In more proximal hypospadias, there is a proximal shaft, penoscrotal, scrotal, or perineal meatus and a severe ventral shortage of tissue (Fig. 153-2). These varied manifestations of the condition have driven the development of multiple surgical procedures. Most bear the eponymous name of the author and most have proved unreliable in spite of the initial enthusiasm of their originators. The best approach to hypospadias is appropriate evaluation and subsequent development of a treatment algorithm.

EPIDEMIOLOGY

Incidence

Reported incidence varies between 1 in 400 and 1 in 100 live male births.[1] In general, more recent studies suggest the true incidence is increasing, although part of this is probably due to improved reporting and increasing recognition and referral of mild and minimal hypospadias (Fig. 153-3).

Etiology

The majority of patients present with hypospadias of unknown etiology. However, many authors believe there is a multifactorial process involving a variety of environmental factors. In addition, there may be a genetic component because a small percentage of instances of hypospadias have been shown to arise from single-gene mutations.[2] The most common associations reported in the literature include increasing maternal age,[3] endocrine factors associated with fertility drugs,[4] antiepileptic medication,[5] low birth weight,[6] preeclampsia,[7] and other environmental causes.[8]

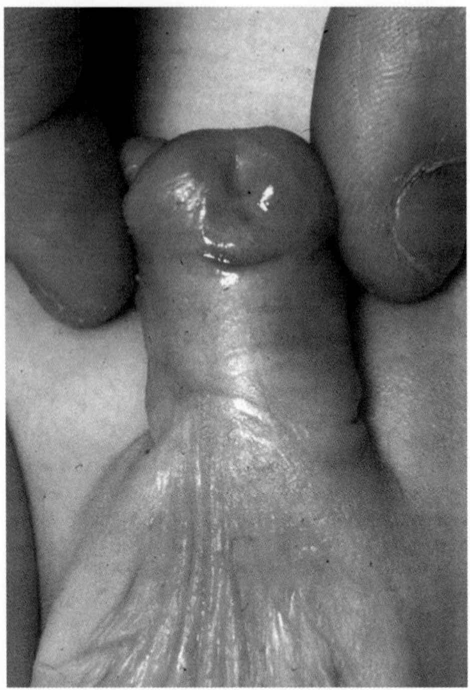

FIGURE 153-1. Distal shaft hypospadias.

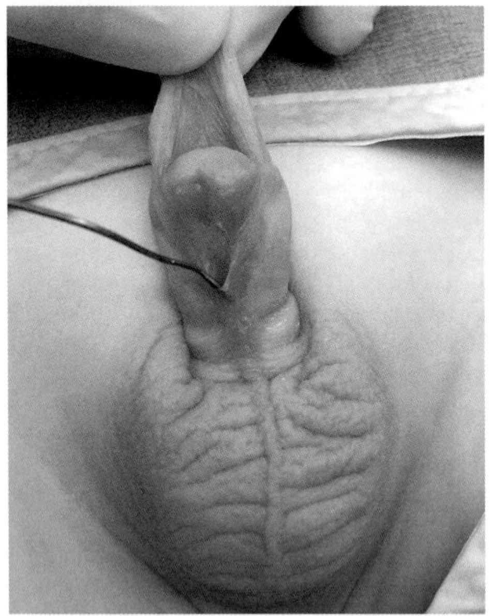

FIGURE 153-2. Proximal hypospadias. The meatus appears to be at midshaft, but ventral tissues are aplastic. After chordee release and meatoplasty, it will be more proximal.

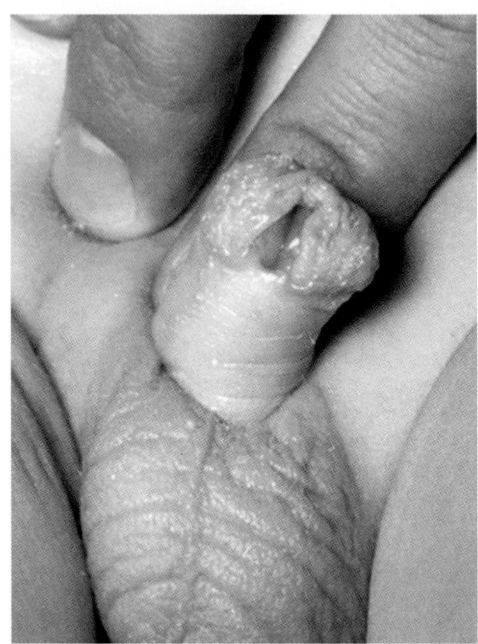

FIGURE 153-3. Minimal hypospadias. Note glanular meatus and ventral failure of fusion of foreskin.

CLINICAL PRESENTATIONS

Hypospadias Classification

Traditional classifications of hypospadias are based on the position of the meatus on the penis or scrotum-perineum, that is, glanular, coronal, penile, penoscrotal, or perineal. However, it is important that patients be assessed according to the new location of the meatus after correction of the associated chordee.[9] By this classification, 60% to 75% are glanular, coronal, or distal shaft; 15% are midshaft; and the remainder are proximal shaft, penoscrotal, scrotal, or perineal.[10]

Chordee

Chordee describes the abnormal ventral curvature of the penis. This results from hypoplasia and longitudinal shortening of ventral tissues. In most patients, mesenchymal tissue that would normally form the corpus spongiosum and fascial layers in the normal penis manifests as fibrous tissue. However, curvature of the penis may also be due to ventral shortage of the skin, the urethra, the fascial layers, or the corpora themselves.

Chordee without hypospadias is a rare condition and may not present until later in childhood as downward-curved erections.[11] The urethral meatus is situated normally at the glans tip, but the foreskin may be incomplete and predominantly dorsal. Ventrally, the corpus spongiosum and urethra are hypoplastic, but other ventral tissues are often also deficient.

Associated Conditions

The most common associations with hypospadias are cryptorchidism, inguinal hernia, and renal tract malformations.[7,12-13] Khuri et al[14] found an incidence of 9.3% of undescended testes and 9.1% of inguinal hernia in patients with hypospadias. The reported incidence of renal tract problems is approximately 1% to 3%.[2] It is recommended that all patients presenting with hypospadias in combination with cryptorchidism or a hernia proceed to screening of their renal tract.[15]

ANATOMY

Penile Anatomy[16]

The shaft of the penis is surrounded by five layers of tissue: skin, superficial penile fascia, tela subfascialis, deep layer of the penile fascia, and tunica albuginea. Penile skin is pliable and expandable and has an extensive vascular network, making it suitable for urethral reconstruction. The superficial penile fascia (dartos fascia) is part of the membranous layer of the superficial fascia of the groin and perineum (Colles fascia). It contains an abundant vascular supply to the skin (superficial penile arteries and superficial dorsal vein). Beneath the dartos fascia lies a thin connective tissue layer, the tela subfascialis of Eberth; it covers the extracorporeal segments of the cavernous arteries, veins, and nerves. The deep penile fascia is otherwise more commonly known as Buck fascia. This heavy, elastic layer covers the corpora cavernosa and corpus spongiosum. It also envelops the deep dorsal vein and the dorsal arteries and nerves. Last, the tunica albuginea encloses the corpora cavernosa in two layers.

Urethral Anatomy

The urethra has three segments, the prostatic, membranous, and spongy parts. The prostatic and membranous parts are collectively known as the posterior urethra clinically. The spongy or penile urethra (anterior urethra) lies within the corpus spongiosum and can further be divided into the bulbous and pendulous parts. The posterior portion of the corpus spongiosum, attached to the undersurface of the perineal membrane, is dilated and enlarged as the bulb. The urethra enters the bulb having first pierced the perineal membrane and then curves forward in a right-angled fashion. Beyond the root of the penis, the urethra continues as the pendulous part. The urethra is lined by transitional epithelium except in the navicular fossa (just proximal to the external urethral meatus), which is lined by stratified squamous epithelium.

EMBRYOLOGY

Sexual differentiation is a function of the sex-determining zone of the Y chromosome. In the absence of this zone, the undifferentiated gonad will become an ovary and the embryo assumes the default female status. In its presence, a testis develops, and by a combination of the secretions of the Leydig cells and Sertoli cells, development of male internal and external genitalia can be expected (Fig. 153-4). Failures along this pathway can lead to various intersex states. Hypospadias is thought to result from failure of the dihydrotestosterone stimulation of the genital tubercle and penis (Fig. 153-5).[17] The urethra develops as an endodermal outgrowth from the cloaca on the ventral surface of the genital tubercle called the urethral plate. Genital folds progressively fuse to advance the meatus from proximal to distal. Mesodermal tissue follows urethral development to make corpora and penile fascia. The glanular urethra forms from an ectodermal ingrowth that meets the tubularized urethral plate at coronal level. The skin then fuses ventrally to make a prepuce.[18] A failure along this sequence can cause varying degrees of hypospadias; the earlier the failure, the more proximal the meatus and the more severe the genital abnormality. Most hypospadias is relatively distal and involves only the last step in this pathway.

TREATMENT GOALS

The reason for correction of the deformity is to allow micturition while standing, to achieve a natural appearance, and to allow normal sexual function. The surgical steps to achieve this involve a combination of orthoplasty, urethroplasty, glansplasty, and skin cover. The ideal hypospadias repair should be readily mastered by any surgeon of average technical ability. It should be reasonably quick and simple in both execution and aftercare and preferably completed in one stage. The outcome should be a straight, symmetric penis with a natural terminal meatus. Normal function and appearance should be maintained with growth. Most of the available techniques fall short of this ideal. The normal meatus is slit shaped and does not have visible suture marks. It may be acceptable in some countries to complete the reconstruction by discarding the prepuce to give a circumcised appearance; but in many countries, most boys are not circumcised, and a preputial reconstruction will be needed. A variety of techniques are needed to deal with the varied manifestations of the deformity.

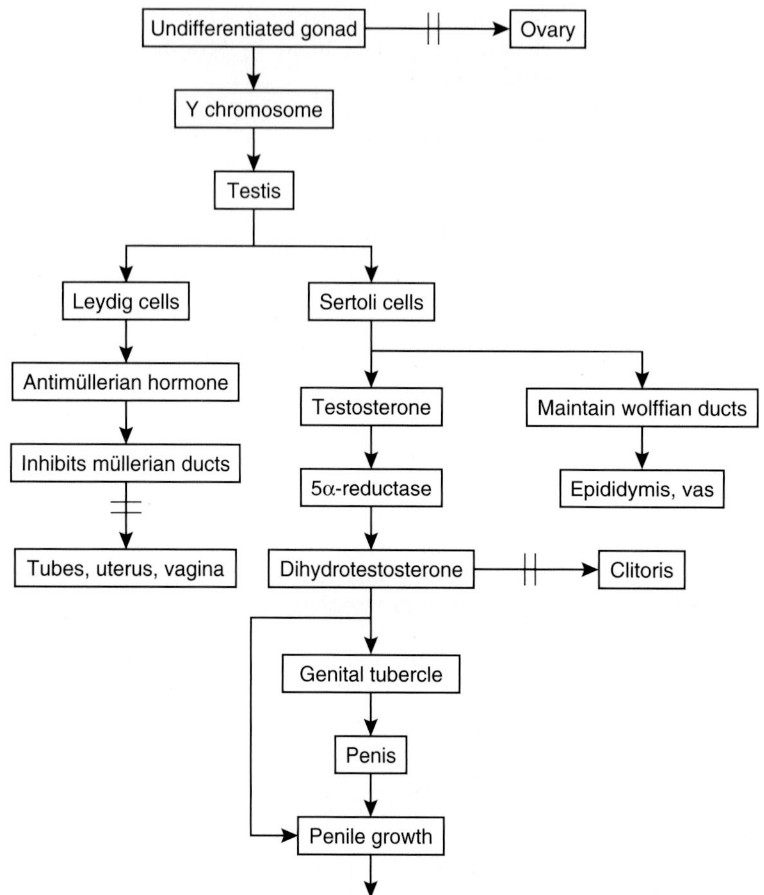

FIGURE 153-4. Embryology of the testis.

SURGICAL TECHNIQUES

The large number of available techniques for correction of hypospadias predicts that many will not achieve the desired aims outlined before. It is helpful to divide these procedures into three categories: historical procedures, textbook operations, and modern techniques.

The historical techniques are generally known by the name of the author; they fail to achieve a slit-shaped terminal meatus without suture marks and often give poor aesthetic results. The most common operations in most plastic surgery and urologic textbooks during the past 2 decades are the meatoplasty and glanuloplasty (MAGPI) operation for coronal and glanular hypospadias, the flip-flap for distal shaft hypospadias, and the inner preputial island flaps for more proximal hypospadias.[19,20] All of these techniques are single staged, but none gives a slit-shaped terminal meatus, and complication rates are unacceptably high for more proximal hypospadias. These operations have been widely used but are now superseded by modern techniques based on tubularization of the remaining urethral plate or replacement of the urethral plate with a graft in a two-stage correction. Published outcomes from the more commonly used operations are discussed later in this chapter. The operative steps of three modern techniques to repair varying degrees of hypospadias, with reference to the textbook operations that they have largely replaced, are discussed.

Distal Hypospadias

In minimal hypospadias, the meatus is on the glans penis and positioned to allow micturition while standing. In this situation, the indications for surgery are aesthetic. There is usually an abnormality of the foreskin; the meatus is sometimes an unusual shape and may be ventral to the tip of the glans. It is usually possible to reconstruct the prepuce. Surgery to the urethral opening should have the aim of giving a slit-shaped meatus. When the meatus is at the coronal sulcus or distal shaft, it is likely that some form of urethroplasty will be needed to allow micturition while standing. When possible, operations that tubularize the existing urethral plate are preferred. In many patients, it will still be possible to do a glans reapproximation procedure. When the proximal portion of the glans sulcus is too shallow or a bar exists between the sulcus and the meatus, a glans reapproximation

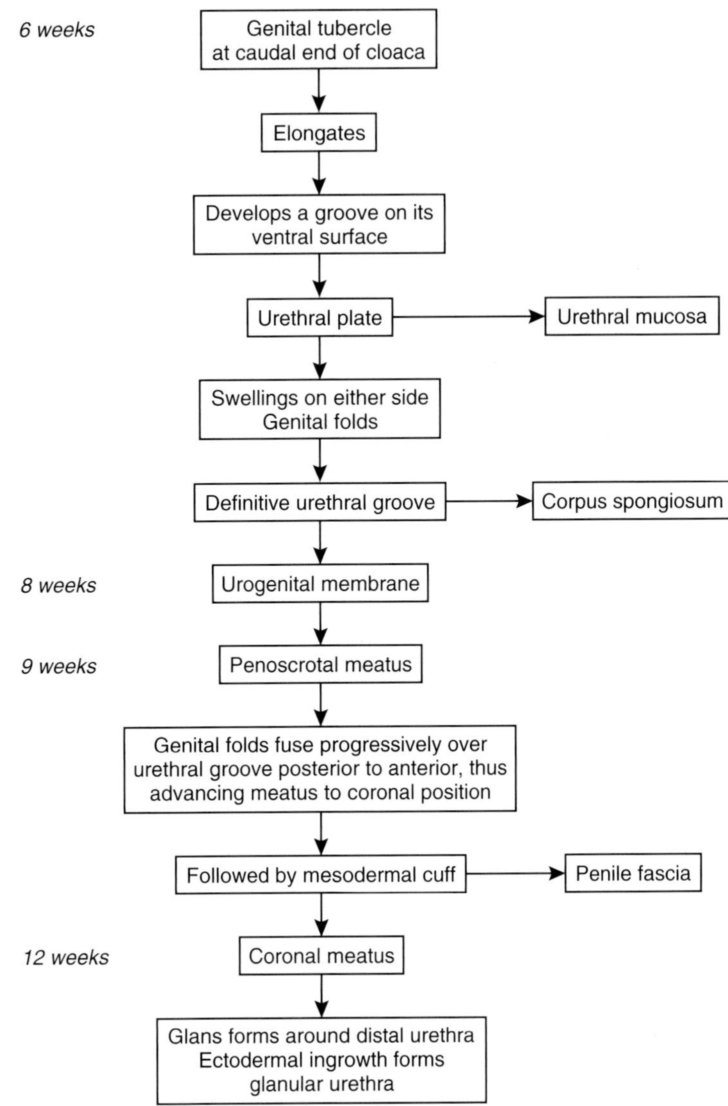

FIGURE 153-5. Embryology of urethra and penis.

procedure is not possible and the urethral plate must be incised.

GLANS REAPPROXIMATION PROCEDURES

Glans reapproximation procedures (GAP and GRAP) are suitable for children with distal hypospadias with a groove in the glans (Fig. 153-6). The glans approximation procedure (GAP) shares its fundamental operative steps with the glanular reconstruction and preputioplasty (GRAP).[21,22] All patients have a general and a caudal anesthetic. A tourniquet is applied to the base of the penis, and an erection test is performed to look for chordee (Fig. 153-7). Provided no gross curvature is present, one can proceed with the single-stage repair.

The incisions are planned and marked (Fig. 153-8). The glans sulcus will be tubularized to establish the neourethra. Glans flaps will close ventral to the neourethra. The incisions on the prepuce will allow foreskin reconstruction to reconstitute the median raphe (Fig. 153-9). An 8FG silicone catheter is inserted, and the incisions are made. Some mobilization of the glans flaps is required (Fig. 153-10). After the glans flaps have been raised, the neourethra is formed by tubularization of the midline tissue around the catheter (Fig. 153-11). The first suture is made distally and is crucial in determining the ventral extent of the meatus. This first layer of interrupted sutures is then buried by a continuous layer of sutures (Fig. 153-12). This closure in turn is covered ventrally if possible by a waterproofing flap raised from the adjacent subcutaneous tissue. The glans flaps are then approximated

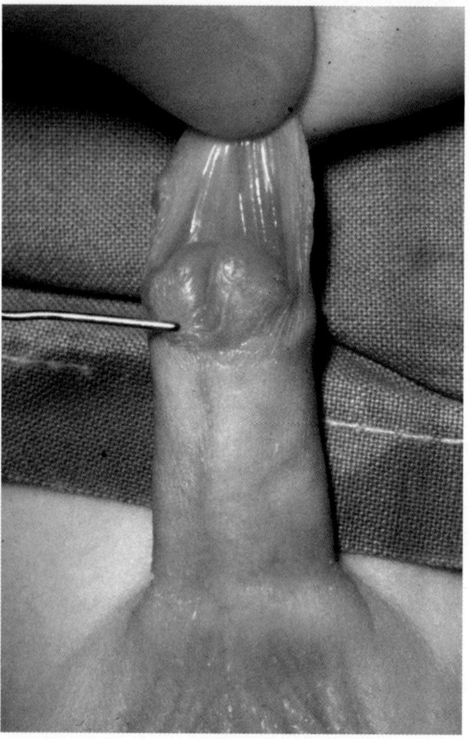

FIGURE 153-6. Hypospadias with coronal meatus and glans groove suitable for single-stage repair.

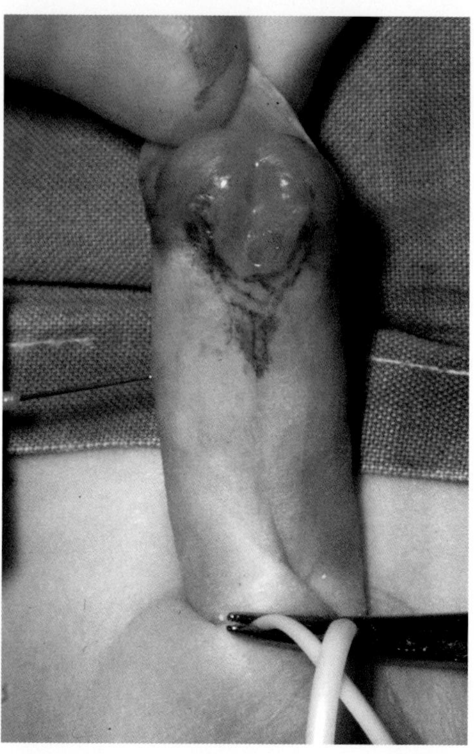

FIGURE 153-8. Markings for glans tubularization of glans sulcus.

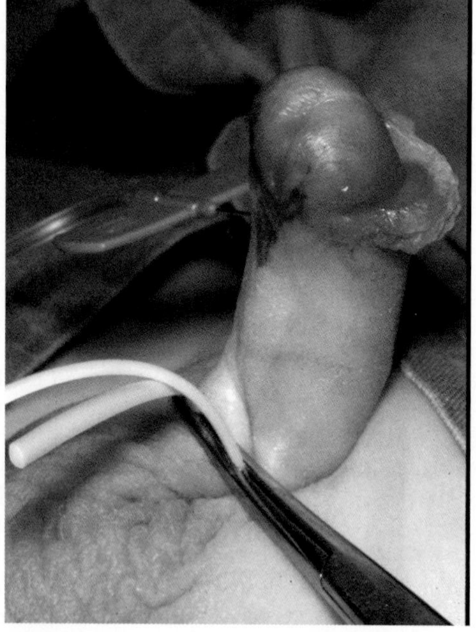

FIGURE 153-7. Artificial erection test showing a straight penis.

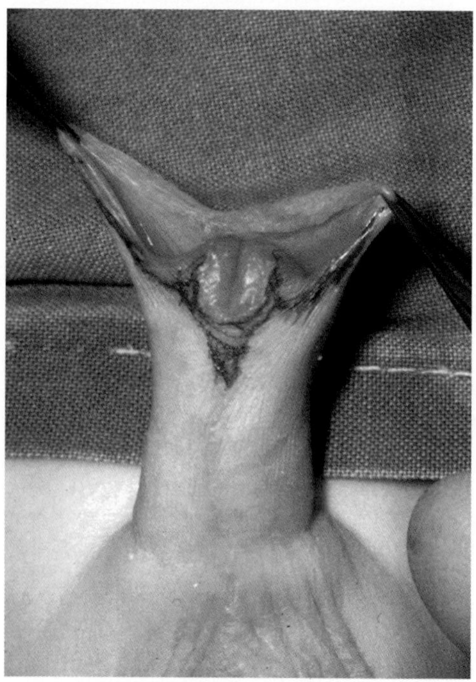

FIGURE 153-9. Incisions on prepuce marked.

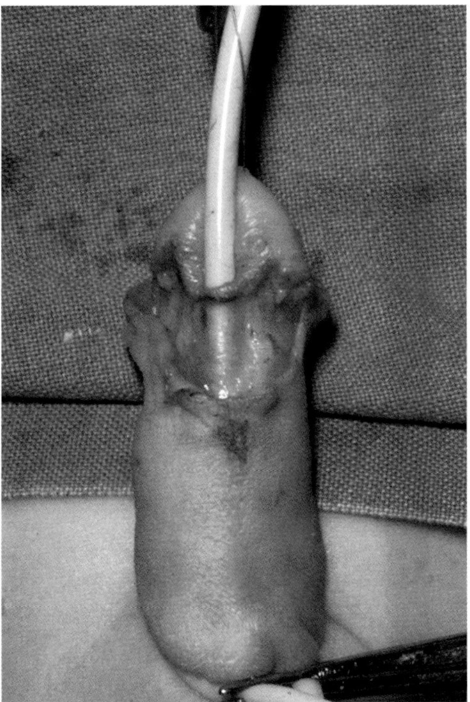

FIGURE 153-10. Incisions have been made. Urethra and glans flaps are shown.

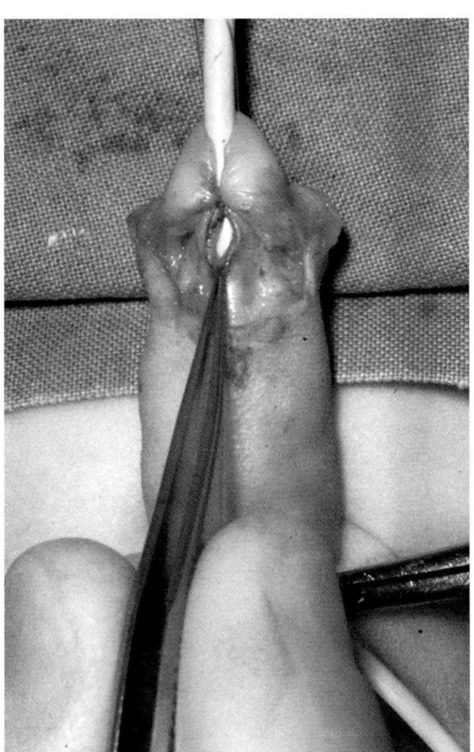

FIGURE 153-11. The first suture has been placed at the ventral margin of the new meatus.

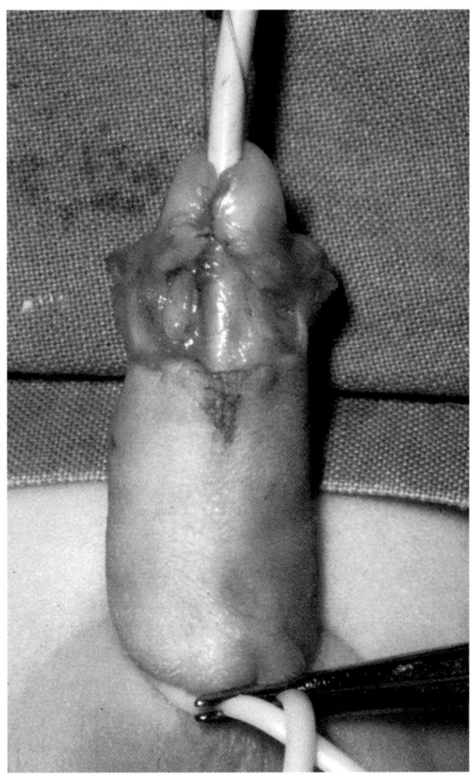

FIGURE 153-12. The remainder of the ventral urethroplasty is closed.

ventral to the neourethra and sutured in place (Fig. 153-13). The tourniquet is then removed and hemostasis secured. The foreskin is then reconstructed. The inner and outer layers of the foreskin are reconstructed separately (Figs. 153-14 and 153-15). There is little bruising or swelling postoperatively, and a hospital stay of 48 hours is usually all that is required. Postoperative results demonstrate a satisfactory meatus and foreskin reconstruction (Figs. 153-16 to 153-19).

MEATOPLASTY AND GLANULOPLASTY PROCEDURE (MAGPI)

The MAGPI (meatoplasty and glanuloplasty incorporated) was originally reported in 1981 by Duckett,[23] who described 200 patients with only one fistula (Fig. 153-20).

TUBULARIZED INCISED PLATE REPAIR

The tubularized incised plate repair extends the principle of hinging the urethral plate[24] by incising the entire urethral plate in the midline from the meatus distally; this incision widens the urethral plate, allowing tubularization without the need for additional flaps. The technique results in a vertically oriented neourethra at the tip of the glans with a normal

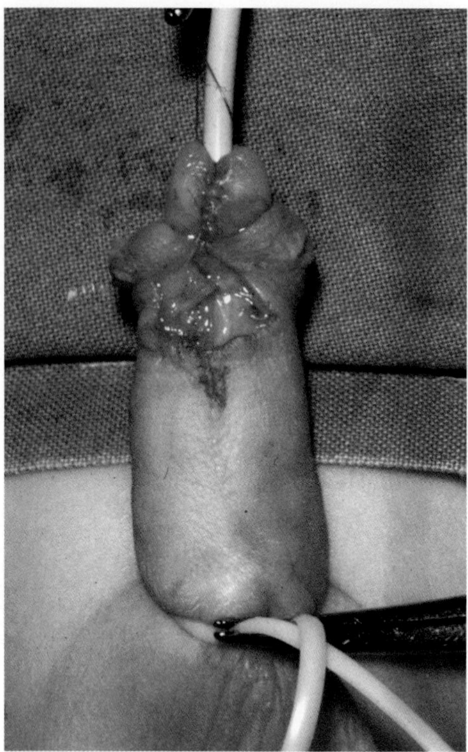

FIGURE 153-13. Completion of glans closure.

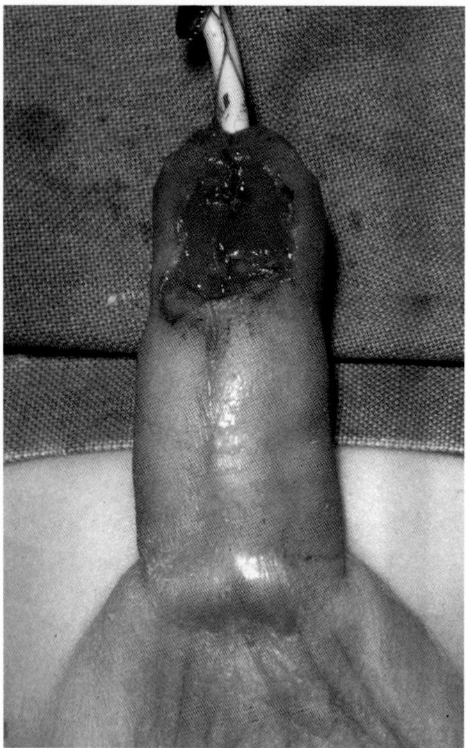

FIGURE 153-14. Inner layer of prepuce has been closed.

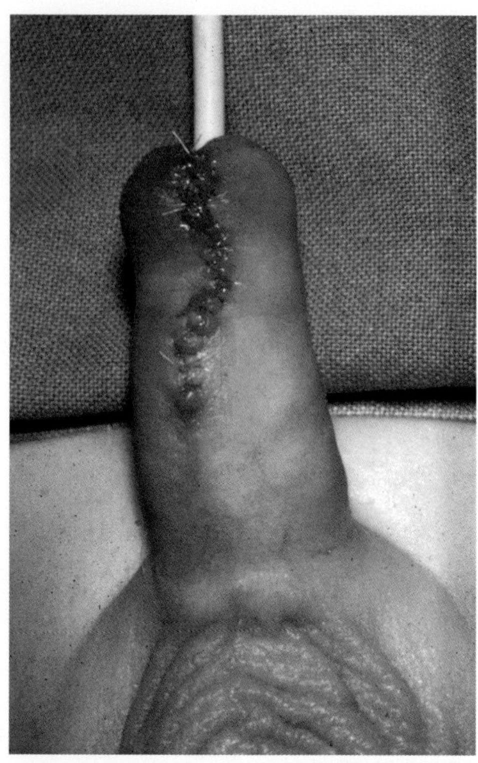

FIGURE 153-15. Repair is completed with closure of outer preputial layer.

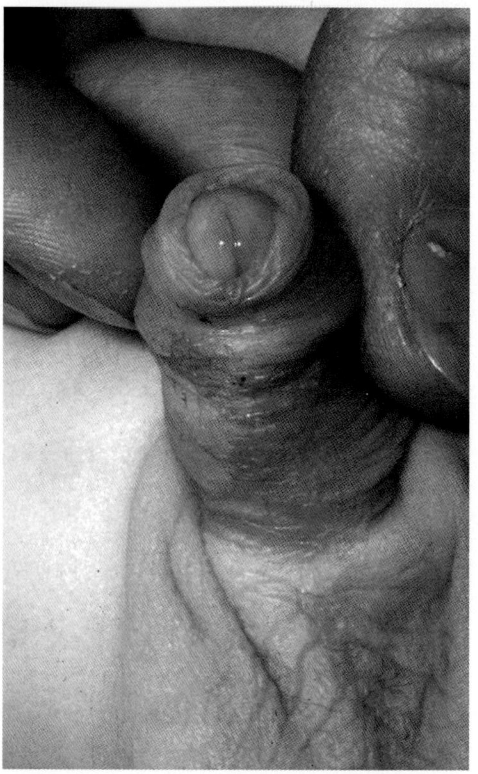

FIGURE 153-16. Result after glans repair showing slit-like terminal meatus without suture marks.

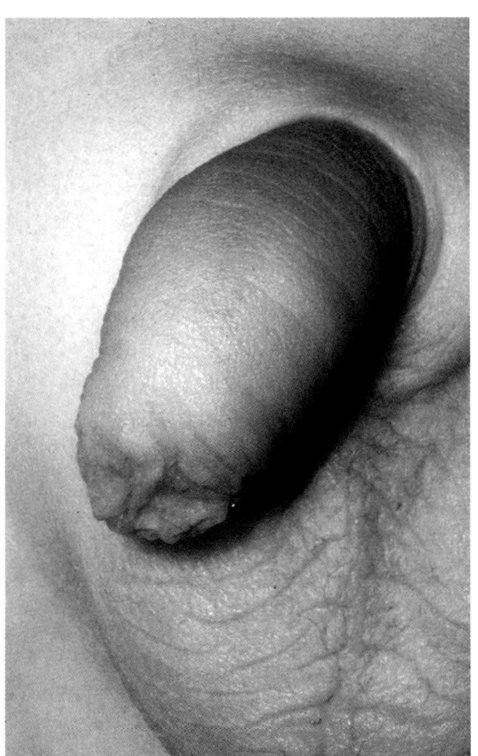

FIGURE 153-17. The reconstructed prepuce after single-stage repair.

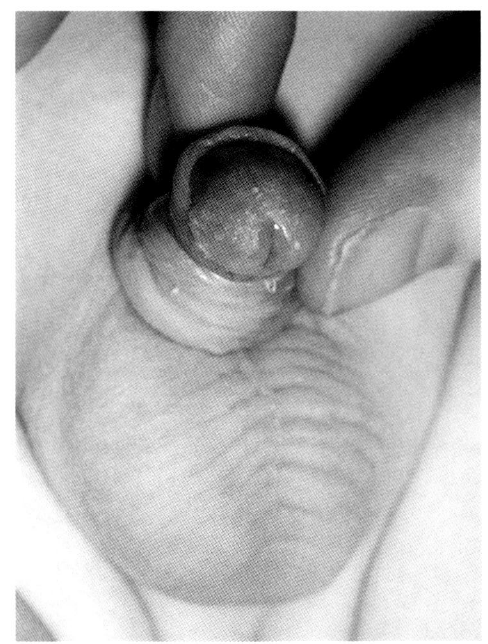

FIGURE 153-18. Slit-shaped meatus at tip of the glans after single-stage repair.

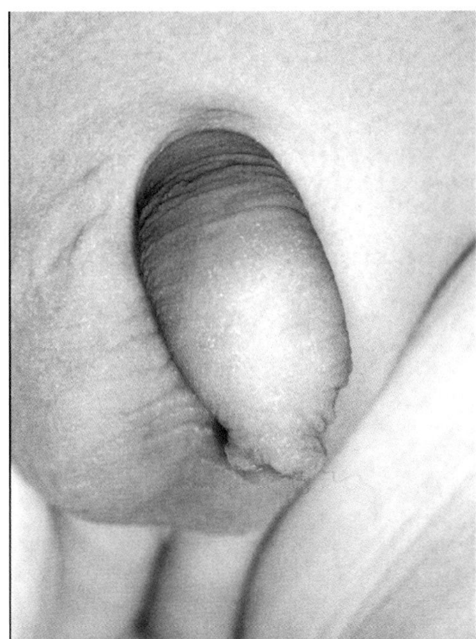

FIGURE 153-19. Symmetric foreskin reconstruction.

diameter. It was originally described for distal hypospadias, but reports have since demonstrated its adaptation for midshaft and even penoscrotal repair. In this technique, the edges of the urethral plate are incised from the hypospadiac meatus distally to the end of the plate (Fig. 153-21). This step results in division of the urethral plate into two epithelial strips. The mobile lateral edges of the urethral plate are then closed over a catheter with absorbable sutures. The dorsal incision into the urethral plate is not sutured and heals spontaneously. The remainder of the repair is completed as in the glans reapproximation technique.

FLIP-FLAP PROCEDURE

The flip-flap procedure was described by Mathieu[25] in 1932 and has since been modified by several authors (Fig. 153-22).

Proximal Hypospadias

In proximal and distal hypospadias where there is a flat glans or severe chordee, it is often only possible to achieve a straight penis with a slit-shaped terminal meatus by a two-stage technique. This operation sets the standard in aesthetic and functional results that other techniques must match.

TWO-STAGE GLANS-SPLITTING BRACKA TECHNIQUE[26, 27]

At the first operation, an axial line is drawn on the ventral glans, starting at the proposed dorsal limit of

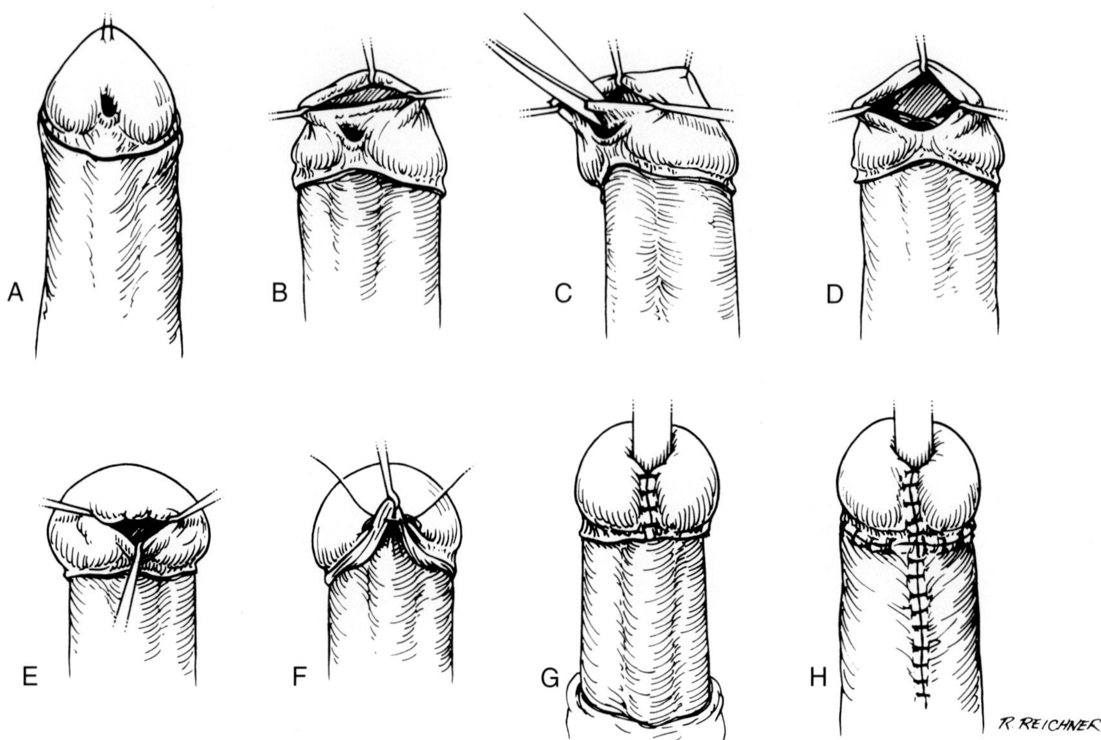

FIGURE 153-20. *A* to *H,* Meatal advancement and glansplasty. (From Horton CE, Sadove RC, Devine CJ Jr: Reconstruction of male genital defects. In McCarthy JG, ed: Plastic Surgery. Philadelphia, WB Saunders, 1990:4153.)

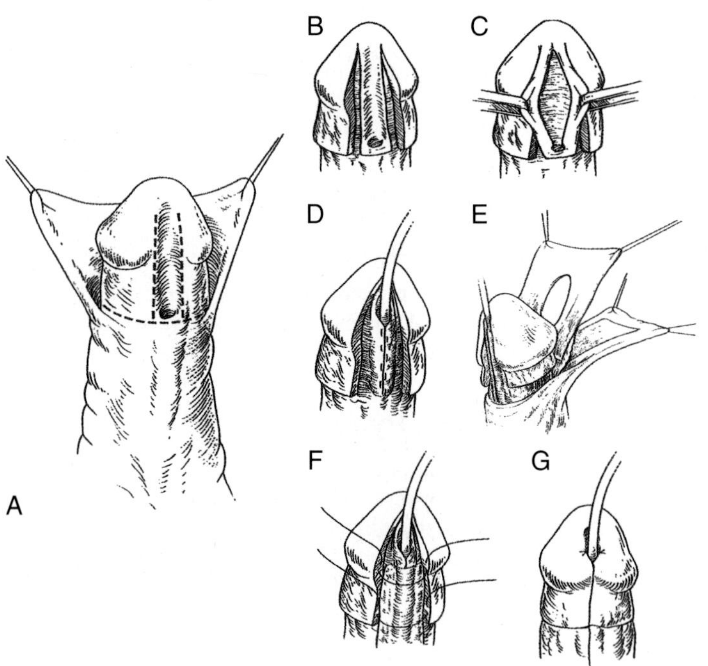

FIGURE 153-21. *A* to *G,* Tubularized incised plate repair. (From Snodgrass W: Tubularized incised plate [TIP] hypospadias repair. Urol Clin North Am 2002;29:285-290.)

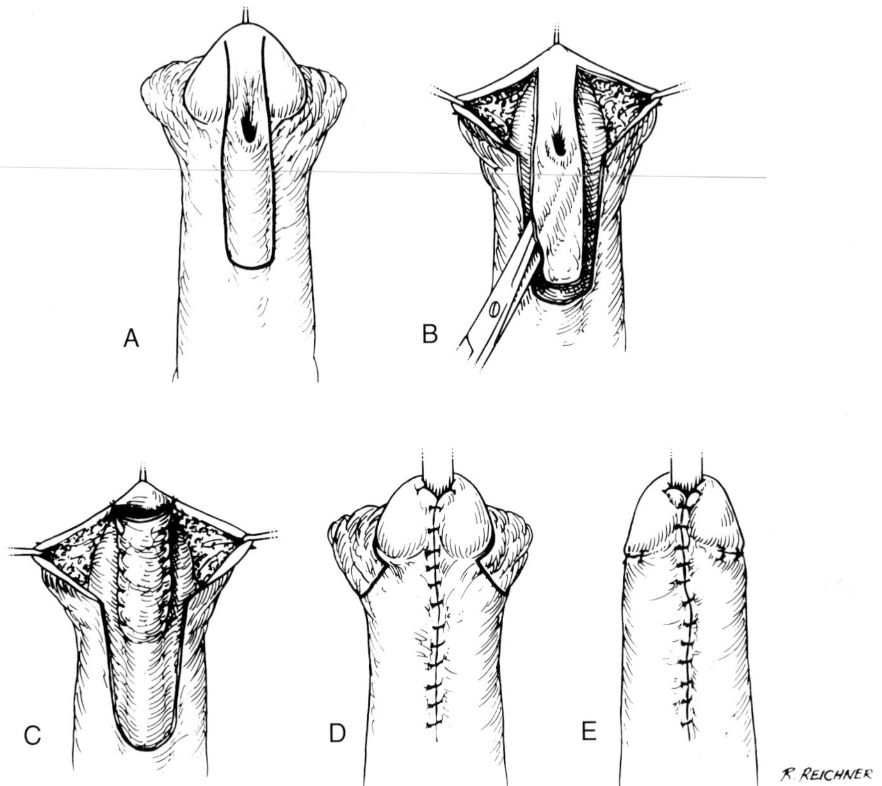

FIGURE 153-22. *A* to *E,* Flip-flap hypospadias repair. (From Horton CE, Sadove RC, Devine CJ Jr: Reconstruction of male genital defects. In McCarthy JG, ed: Plastic Surgery. Philadelphia, WB Saunders, 1990:4153.)

the new meatus and extending proximally down to the ectopic meatus on the shaft. Lateral incision lines are drawn from the midline at a subcoronal level, and these are continued as far around the shaft as is necessary for access and release of chordee. A stay suture in the dorsal glans helps provide traction. Further stay sutures are placed either side of midline just below the ventral limit of the proposed new meatus (Fig. 153-23). The glans is incised in the midline, and chordee is released. The release should be deep enough so that the distal ends of the two corpora cavernosa are clearly demarcated. Release of chordee may require excision of dystopic fibrous tissue (Fig. 153-24). A full-thickness skin graft of the appropriate dimensions is then harvested from the inner prepuce and thinned. The graft is then accurately tailored into the defect with an absorbable suture (Fig. 153-25). A firm tie-over dressing holds the graft snugly in place and prevents any hematoma (Fig. 153-26). This can be removed safely on day 5 postoperatively.

The patient is readmitted 6 months after the first operation. This delay allows maturation of the graft (Fig. 153-27). A preliminary erection test should confirm whether the chordee has been corrected. A U-shaped strip of skin is then marked out from the ventral limit of the new meatus. It should be 15 mm

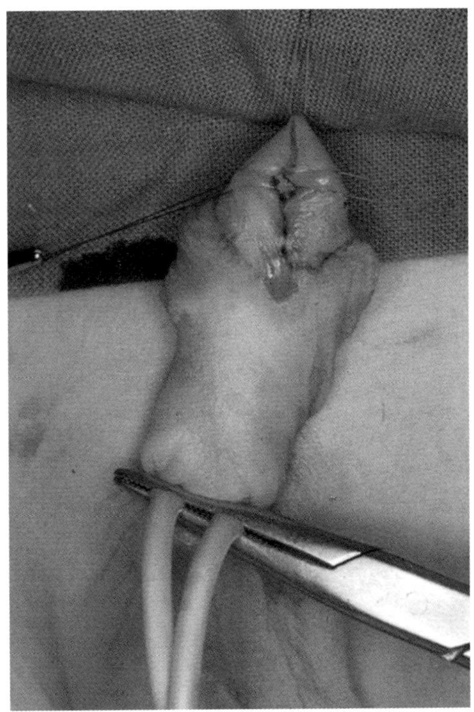

FIGURE 153-23. Incisions for two-stage glans-splitting hypospadias repair.

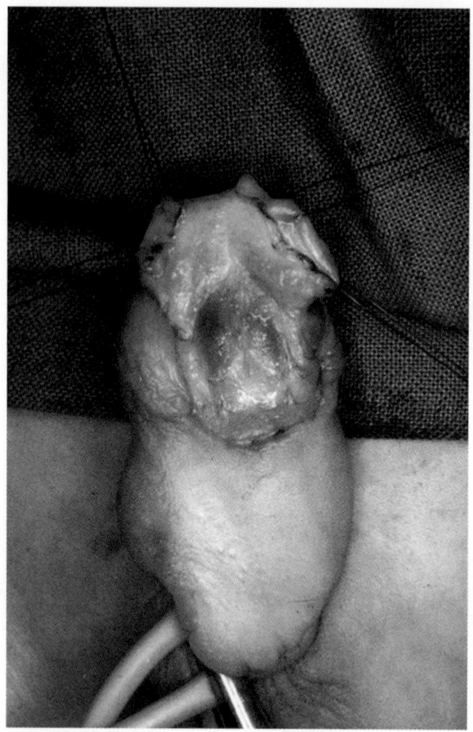

FIGURE 153-24. Glans split and chordee release showing distal corpora cavernosa.

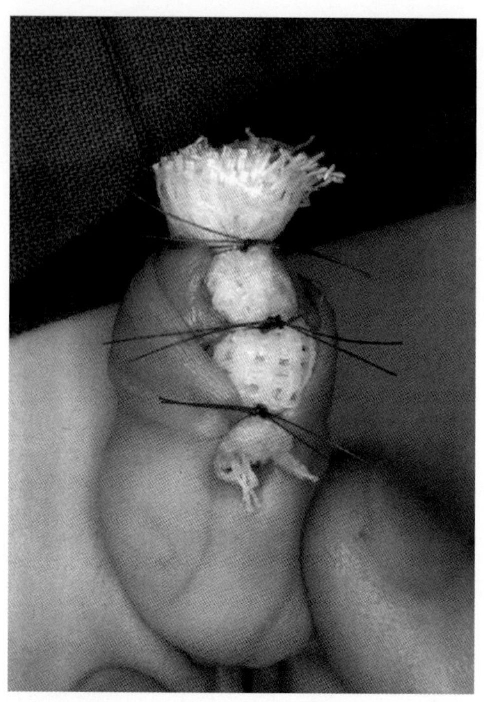

FIGURE 153-26. Tie-over dressing to secure skin graft within glans split.

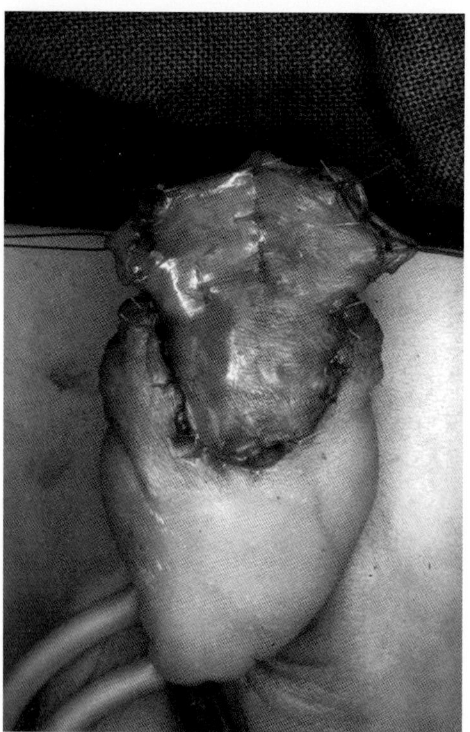

FIGURE 153-25. Full-thickness graft sutured into glans split.

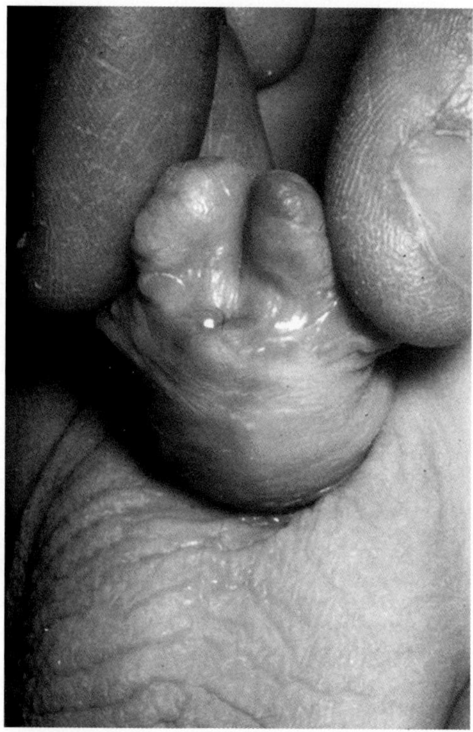

FIGURE 153-27. Skin-grafted glans split 6 months after stage 1 procedure.

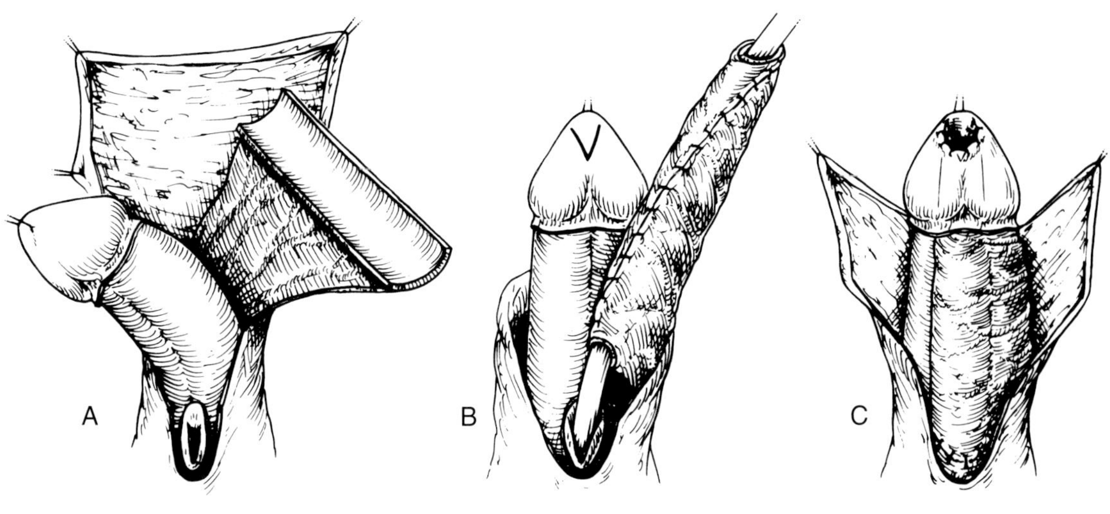

FIGURE 153-28. *A* to *C*, Inner preputial island flap hypospadias repair. (From Horton CE, Sadove RC, Devine CJ Jr: Reconstruction of male genital defects. In McCarthy JG, ed: Plastic Surgery. Philadelphia, WB Saunders, 1990:4153.)

wide in a child. The tubularization of this urethroplasty strip, glansplasty, and foreskin reconstruction are exactly as in the glans reapproximation procedure. In a patient with a more proximal defect, further attempts are made to provide a waterproofing layer to cover the urethroplasty before glans and skin closure. Some authors would use a dorsal degloving incision to allow access for this flap.[28,29] In the preferred approach, incisions are restricted to the ventral surface of the penis because adequate waterproofing of the flap of adjacent subcutaneous tissue can always be established by a ventral approach alone. The avoidance of a dorsal incision also allows preputial reconstruction.

INNER PREPUTIAL ISLAND FLAP

Numerous modifications of the inner preputial island flaps have been described. These depend on independent vascularity from the fascial layers of the penis separate from the vascularization of the skin (Fig. 153-28). This flap can be used as a complete tube or as an onlay flap or sutured to the urethral plate to augment another technique.

SUTURES, DRESSINGS, URINARY DIVERSION, CATHETERS

In general, absorbable sutures are used. In pediatric practices, 7-0 and 8-0 polyglactin (Vicryl) is used. Numerous dressing techniques have been described, but there is no objective evidence that any technique is of benefit over any other. It is preferable to use no dressings (Fig. 153-29); if a technique relies on a dressing for its effect, one should have reservations about its use.

For distal hypospadias repairs with little interference with the urethra, no urinary diversion may be required. However, when a substantial length of urethra is reconstructed, most surgeons would use some form of diversion. The choice is between a dripping stent, a Foley catheter, and a suprapubic catheter.

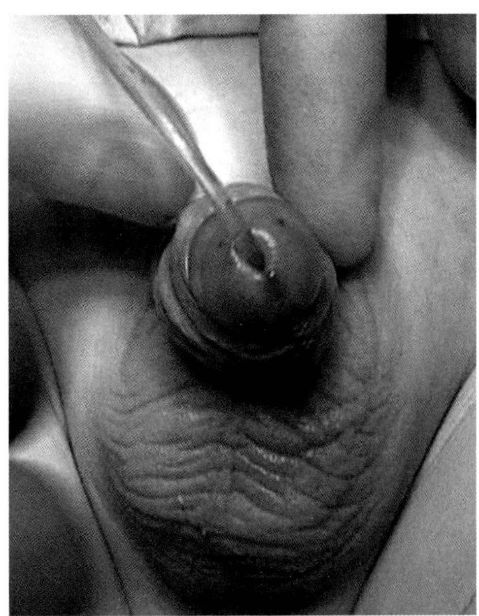

FIGURE 153-29. A completed hypospadias repair. No dressing is required.

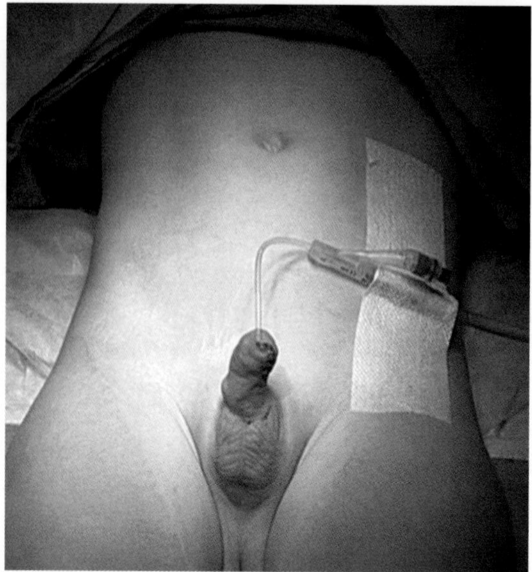

FIGURE 153-30. A silicone Foley catheter and drainage bag attached by tape to the abdomen.

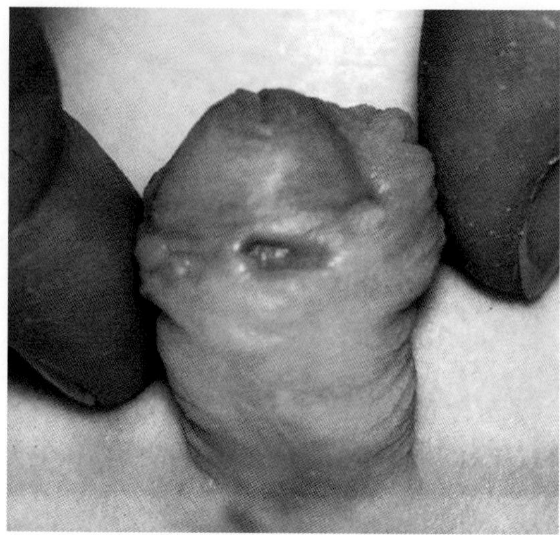

FIGURE 153-31. A large coronal fistula after hypospadias repair.

A short length of silicone or polyethylene tube can be used as a stent through the repair and allowed to drain into the diaper. Such a stent has to be secured to the penis with either a dressing or a retaining suture. Dressings may become dislodged; a glans stitch holding a stent will leave suture marks that many may consider unacceptable. A self-retaining balloon catheter that is simply taped to the abdomen is preferred (Fig. 153-30). The disadvantage is that the deflated balloon must be withdrawn through the repair at the time of catheter removal. It is important, therefore, to select a technique of urethral reconstruction that is sufficiently robust to permit this. In pediatric patients, an 8FG silicone-only catheter is used. Rubber catheters should be avoided because they have a much smaller internal diameter for a given external diameter compared with silicone catheters and are likely to become blocked. A fine-bore tubing drainage bag that works on a siphon principle is used. Ketoconazole may be useful to control erections, and oxybutynin may be prescribed for bladder spasm.

COMPLICATIONS

Fistula

The most troublesome complication of hypospadias repair is urethral fistula (Fig. 153-31). The incidence of fistula for the various operations is outlined later; in general, the more proximal the original meatus, the greater the risk. Fistulas can readily be corrected, provided the remainder of the urethral reconstruction is of adequate caliber distal to the leak. If this is not present, it is better to take down the reconstructed urethra and redo it (Fig. 153-32).

Meatal Problems

Meatal stenosis is a risk in any technique that involves a circumferential suture line at the meatus. It cannot occur in the glans reapproximation technique or two-stage glans-splitting technique (Fig. 153-33), but it can happen after the urethral plate is incised if the incision extends onto the glans skin. If the meatal stenosis is minor, it may be possible to treat it with dilatation. A more significant stenosis will require meatoplasty. Meatal stenosis and a meatus that has an unusual shape will often cause spraying on micturition. This is not a simple problem to correct because most techniques of meatoplasty do not restore a slit-shaped meatus (Figs. 153-34 and 153-35). In many

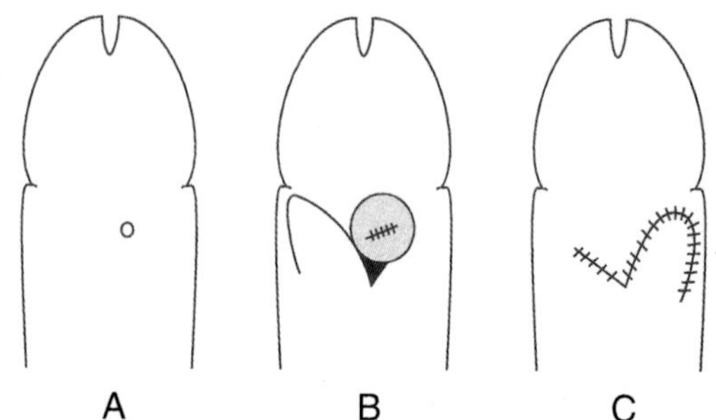

FIGURE 153-32. *A* to *C*, A simple technique for correction of hypospadias fistula. The fistula is dissected out and oversewn. The surrounding skin is de-epithelialized, and a transposition flap is used to cover the repair.

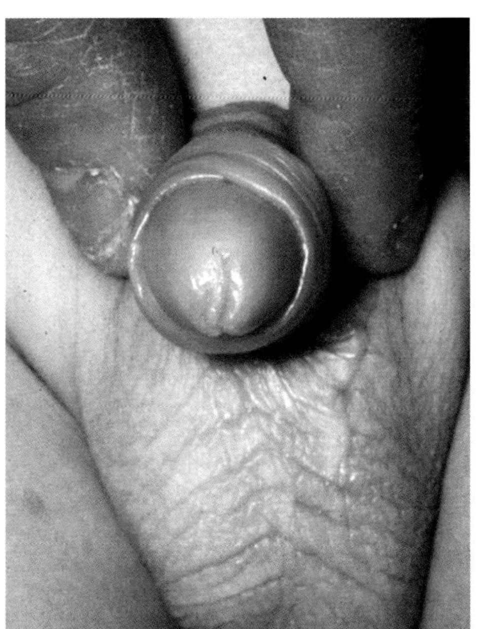

FIGURE 153-33. Slit-shaped urethral meatus without suture marks after two-stage glans-splitting repair.

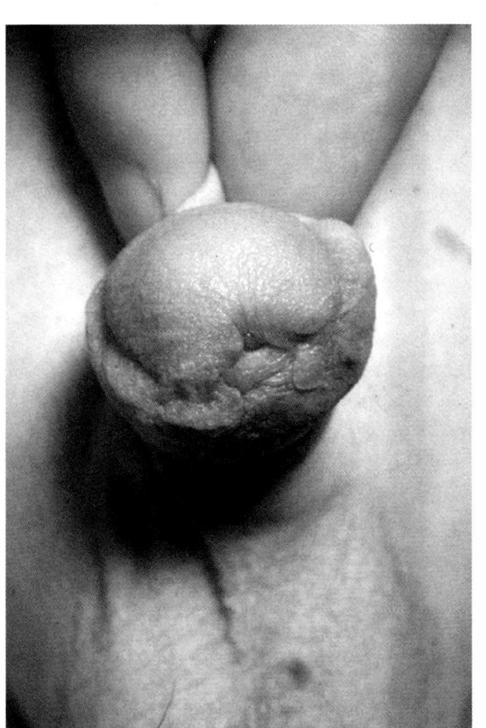

FIGURE 153-34. Glanular meatus after flip-flap repair.

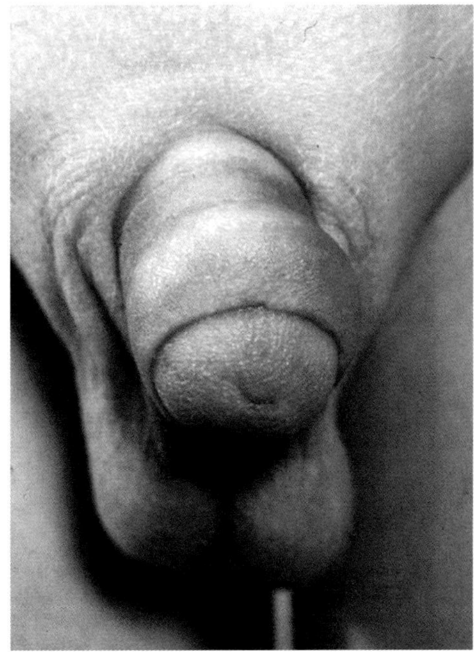

FIGURE 153-35. Horizontal slit-shaped meatus after inner preputial island flap repair.

patients, it may be necessary to redo the urethroplasty, usually in two stages.

Stricture

Strictures can occur at the junction of the native urethra and neourethra or may involve the entire urethral reconstruction. If a stricture occurs early, it will often respond to one or two dilatations. A more severe stricture or one occurring late will usually require another urethroplasty.

Skin Problems

After hypospadias correction, some patients will have minor skin asymmetries that may require further adjustments for aesthetic reasons. On occasion, boys who have had hypospadias repairs will develop lichen sclerosus et atrophicus (balanitis xerotica obliterans).[30] This can cause phimosis or, if it affects the urethral reconstruction, meatal problems or strictures. Patients with mild lichen sclerosus can be treated with topical steroids; but when the reconstruction becomes narrow, it must be taken down and all the affected skin discarded. The reconstruction is redone by a two-stage grafting technique. Skin cannot be used because it has been found that lichen sclerosus will recur in skin from either the penis or extragenital sites. In these patients, grafts of buccal mucosa are used because it appears resistant to the condition.

OUTCOMES AND ASSESSMENT AFTER HYPOSPADIAS REPAIR

The outcomes associated with hypospadias repair have usually been assessed by the incidence of fistula, meatal stenosis, urethral stricture, and residual penile curvature and the reoperation rates to correct these problems. With these traditionally accepted outcomes, complication rates are generally quoted on the order of 5% to 15%.[31] However, it has been suggested that the literature addresses only these immediate results or early complications, and scant attention has been paid to longer term results.[32,33] In particular, follow-up rates after hypospadias surgeries vary enormously, ranging from months[34,35] to years.[32,33,36] Furthermore, the surgeon should also take into account the consideration of cosmetic appearance and the assessment of normal sexual function. Several reports suggest criticism by patients of the appearance of the penis in later life[32,33,36]; photographic documentation may become an essential tool in assessing both the surgeon's and patient's satisfaction.[37] This observation supports the assumption we have made that the only acceptable outcome is a slit-shaped terminal meatus without stitch marks and a symmetric skin arrangement. Although the majority of adult hypospadiacs will have a normal sex life,[38] up to 40% of patients in one study believed personal relationships had been affected during their lives.[39] In patients who have had historical procedures performed, dissatisfaction with outcome correlated with technically unsatisfactory surgical results.[39,40]

The huge diversity of procedures and follow-up times after hypospadias surgery also makes effective comparison and meta-analysis difficult. There is no generally accepted system for the objective assessment of the surgical results of hypospadias repair,[41] although various authors have reported practical preoperative and postoperative classification systems.[42-44] The two-stage Bracka technique or the preferred one-stage technique can be used by trainees or the inexperienced surgeon with reproducible results in the presence of minimal complications.[22,45]

COMPARISON OF MAJOR TECHNIQUES IN HYPOSPADIAS REPAIR

Meatal Advancement and Glansplasty

The aim of the MAGPI procedure is to advance the location of the hypospadiac meatus, without the need for urethral tubularization, to the most distal glans and to refashion the glans beneath. Although this technique has been widely used to correct glanular and coronal hypospadias, there has been a misconception that it is a simple operation that can be applied to all forms of distal hypospadias.[46] Meatal retraction, meatal stenosis, and a fish-mouth appearance of the external meatus have been reported as complications of this procedure.[47-52] Hastie et al[49] reported meatal regression and stenosis rates at 3.5%, although meatal retraction rate at long-term follow-up was 95%. On cumulative analysis of 16 series of patients undergoing this procedure (N = 3064 patients), the overall complication rate was 15.9%, with a fistula rate of 4.3%. Meatal retraction was seen in 10.2% of patients, and stenosis was reported in 0.76%.[53]

As pointed out before, the purpose of surgery in very distal hypospadias is largely aesthetic. No incidence of fistula or stenosis is acceptable. The meatoplasty is nonanatomic and does not result in a slit-shaped meatus. The incidence of meatal regression and retraction further reduces the value of this operation in hypospadias.

Glans Reapproximation Procedures

Tubularization of the urethral plate for distal hypospadias was popularized by several authors following its first description by Thiersch[54-56] in 1869. Techniques based on tubularization of the glans sulcus produce a slit-shaped meatus without suture marks and are more anatomic in their concept than is the MAGPI repair. This principle is met with superior aesthetic results and apparently low complication rates. Although the number of published series is small, the results are universally excellent.[57,58] In a total of 132 patients, the overall complication rate was 6.1% with a fistula rate of 5.9%. There were no meatal retractions and an overall stenosis rate of 1.25%, although this was seen in only one series.[59] Mean follow-up was 18 months. In the author's series of 93 consecutive patients, 85 patients had no postoperative problems. There were no meatal stenoses or iatrogenic phimosis. One adult patient developed a fistula. Seven patients required an adjustment of their foreskin reconstruction.[60]

Tubularized Incised Plate Repair

In 1989, Rich et al[24] described the use of an incision in the glanular urethral plate to obtain a cosmetically acceptable slit-shaped meatus. Snodgrass[61] subsequently adapted this approach along the entire length of the urethral plate as a complement to the Thiersch-Duplay urethroplasty. There is now considerable experience of the Snodgrass procedure reported in the literature. The initial report by Snodgrass[61] of his first 16 patients demonstrated the absence of complications. A subsequent multicenter study of 164 children reported a superior cosmetic result compared

TABLE 153-1 ✦ EXPERIENCE WITH THE TUBULARIZED INCISED PLATE HYPOSPADIAS REPAIR

Authors	No. of Patients	Complications			
		Total	*Stenosis*	*Stricture*	*Fistula*
Snodgrass (1994)	16	0	0	0	0
Multicenter (1996)	164	13	4	0	6
Steckler and Zaontz (1997)	33	0	0	0	0
Ross and Kay (1997)	15	0	0	0	0
Sugarman (1999)	32	2	0	0	1
Retik and Borer (1998)	51	1	0	0	1
Snodgrass (1999)	74	3	0	0	1
Holland and Smith (2000)	46	10	4	0	6
Elbakry (1999)	27	4	4	0	0
Oswald (2000)	30	1	0	0	0
Samuel (2002)	170	6	0	0	6
Cheng (2002)	514	45	14	0	27
Total	1172	85	26	0	48
%	100%	7.7%	2.3%	0	4.3%

with flip-flaps or onlay preputial flaps and an overall complication rate of 7%.[62]

A reported total of 1172 patients have undergone this procedure with an overall complication rate of 7.7%. A total of 48 fistulas (4.3%) and 26 meatal stenoses (2.3%) have been reported (Table 153-1). These favorable published results have led to widespread adoption of the Snodgrass technique. It has replaced a flip-flap and can be used in many situations in which an inner preputial island flap might otherwise be used. The dorsal incision cannot be continued into the glans up to the dorsal margin of the meatus. If this is attempted, stenosis will result.[63] For this reason, this technique is not suitable when the glans is flat. Because the urethral plate is preserved longitudinally, its use is limited if there is severe chordee with a short urethral plate. In some such patients, a dorsal plication may be appropriate; but in others, it may be preferable to divide the plate and revert to a staged technique.

The Snodgrass technique does rely on epithelialization of the raw dorsal strip without contraction. Enthusiasts for the technique claim this wound does heal in a unique fashion[64-66] without stenosis. Skeptics await the results of longer term studies to see whether the initial enthusiasm for this technique is justified.

Inner Preputial Island Flap Repairs

The construction of a vascularized tube of inner prepuce that is then tunneled through the glans in proximal hypospadias, which has probably required a substantial dissection for chordee release, is asking a lot of a surgical technique. There is considerable potential for perioperative complications such as hemorrhage and flap necrosis. There are two circumferential suture lines at the meatus and the junction of the native urethra and neourethra. These technical limitations have resulted in a high incidence of complications, and there can be little justification for use of this method to form a tube. Complication rates are reduced when the island flap is used as an onlay[67,68] or in a hybrid procedure using the flap to supplement a tubularizing repair where the urethral plate is narrow.

TREATMENT ALGORITHM

The analysis in the previous sections allows the development of an algorithm for selection of the most appropriate operation for individuals with hypospadias (Fig. 153-36). The proposed algorithm is based on use of only the glans reapproximation, tubularized incised plate, and two-stage glans-splitting techniques. Most of this assessment can be done at the first outpatient consultation, but in some patients, the final decision concerning the operative technique must be made intraoperatively.

The first assessment is determination of the presence of a glans sulcus. If this is absent and the glans is flat (Fig. 153-37), it will only be possible to achieve a slit-shaped terminal meatus without suture marks by a two-stage glans-splitting technique.

If there is a reasonable glans sulcus, the next assessment is the presence of chordee. If there is significant ventral curvature, the choice will be between dorsal plication and reversion to a two-stage repair. Dorsal plication will have a shortening effect on the phallus

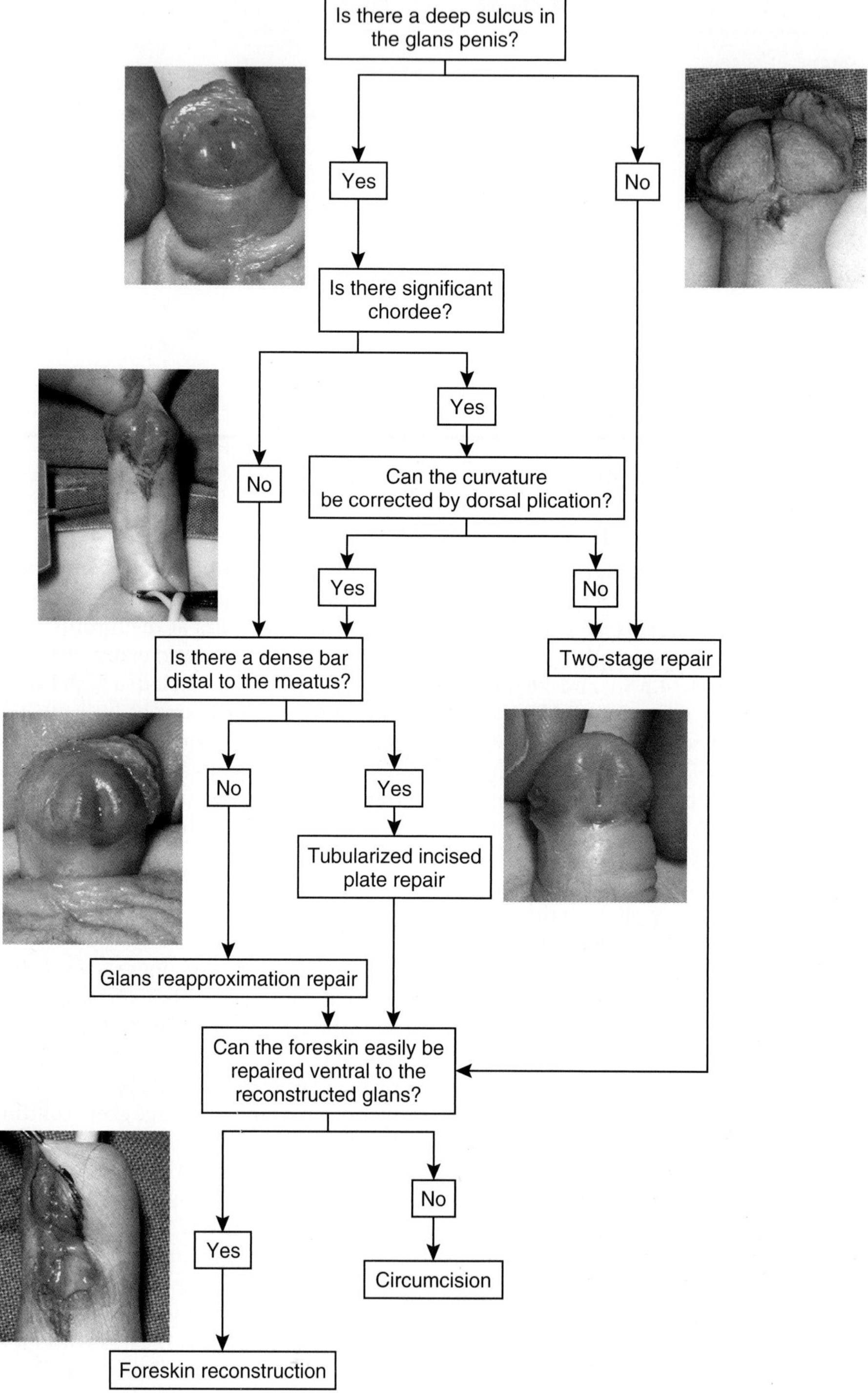

FIGURE 153-36. An algorithm for hypospadias repair.

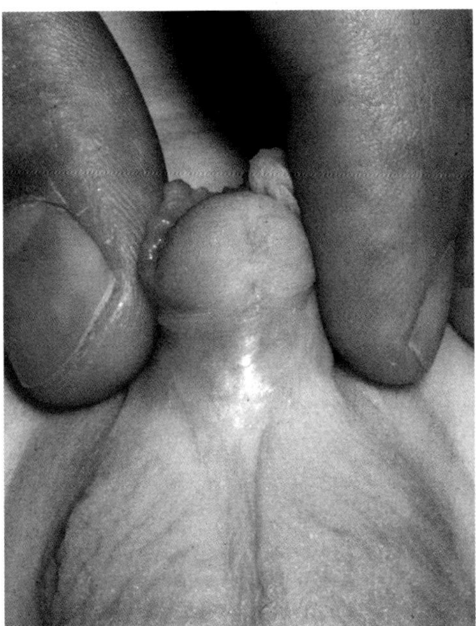

FIGURE 153-37. Hypospadias with a flat glans.

and is not appropriate when there is severe curvature or marked ventral hypoplasia. If the decision is made to proceed with a single-stage operation, an assessment must be made of the glans sulcus and its relation to the meatus. If the two are adjacent with the meatus opening into the sulcus as in a megameatus variant (Fig. 153-38), the patient is ideally suited to a glans reapproximation procedure. If there is a bar between the meatus and the sulcus, this must be incised as in a tubularized incised plate repair.

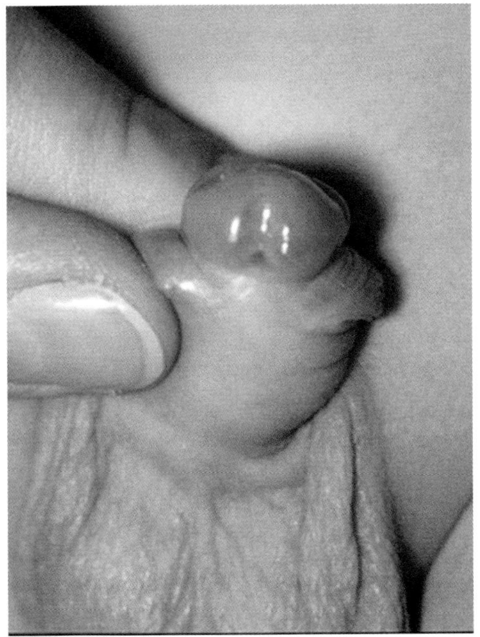

FIGURE 153-38. Megameatus variant of distal hypospadias.

After the urethra and glans penis have been reconstructed, attention is turned to the foreskin. If it can be readily approximated and retracted and the parents request reconstruction, the prepuce should be reconstructed. If the prepuce is too deficient to allow repair or the parents prefer to discard the foreskin, the boy is circumcised.

A HYPOSPADIAS SERVICE

Hypospadias surgery is performed by pediatric urologists and by plastic surgeons. It is sensible to see children within weeks of birth to explain the problem to parents and to make a plan for surgical intervention. The assistance of a pediatric nurse is invaluable to provide a point of contact and family support. Surgery is usually planned for patients approximately 1 year of age. The timing of surgery seems to have little effect on penile size. There is little evidence to suggest that children recall any surgery before 4 years of age. Children can be particularly uncooperative between the ages of 2 and 3 years. One year of age seems a reasonable compromise between safe anesthesia and a desire to get the problem dealt with before the child is aware of it. All patients have a general anesthetic supplemented by caudal epidural or penile block. When it is possible, a penile tourniquet is used. Loupe magnification is employed.

THE FUTURE

One of the most challenging reconstructive problems involves the correction of hypospadias where there is deficient tissue. In this regard, tissue engineering technology has been proposed as a potential strategy for urethral reconstruction.[69] During the last 2 decades, reliable systems for urothelial cell harvest and culture have been developed, allowing expansion in sufficient quantities for reconstructive purposes. Two classes of biomaterials have been used for the engineering of urethral tissues, acellular tissue matrices (e.g., bladder submucosa and small intestinal submucosa) and synthetic polymers (e.g., polyglycolic acid). Encouraging results in a clinical setting[70] suggest that improved techniques in the development of cell-seeded constructs may indeed lead to their routine use in the future.

REFERENCES

1. Roberts CJ, Lloyd S: Observations on the epidemiology of simple hypospadias. Br Med J 1973;1:768-770.
2. Avellan L: On aetiological factors in hypospadias. Scand J Plast Reconstr Surg 1977;11:115-123.
3. Fisch H, Golden RJ, Libersen GL, et al: Maternal age as a risk factor for hypospadias. J Urol 2001;165:934-936.

4. Klip H, Verloop J, van Gool JD, et al, OMEGA Project Group: Hypospadias in sons of women exposed to diethylstilbestrol. Lancet 2002;359:1102-1107.
5. Arpino C, Brescianini S, Robert E, et al: Teratogenic effects of antiepileptic drugs: use of an International Database on Malformations and Drug Exposure (MADRE). Epilepsia 2000;41:1436-1443.
6. Hussain N, Chaghtai A, Herndon CD, et al: Hypospadias and early gestation growth restriction in infants. Pediatrics 2002;109:473-478.
7. Akre O, Lipworth L, Cnattingus S, et al: Risk factor patterns for cryptorchidism and hypospadias. Epidemiology 1999;10:364-369.
8. Dolk H, Vrijheid M, Armstrong B, et al: Risk of congenital anomalies near hazardous-waste landfill sites in Europe: the EUROHAZCON study. Lancet 1998;352:423-427.
9. Barcat J: Current concepts of treatment. In Horton CE, ed: Plastic and Reconstructive Surgery of the Genital Area. Boston, Little, Brown, 1973:249-263.
10. Juskiewenski S, Vaysse P, Guitard J, et al: Traitement des hypospadias anterieurs. Chir Paediatr 1983;24:75-79.
11. Kramer SA, Aydin G, Kelalis PP: Chordee without hypospadias in children. J Urol 1982;128(pt 1):559-561.
12. Weidner IS, Moller H, Jensen TK, Skakkebaek NE: Risk factors for cryptorchidism and hypospadias. J Urol 1999;161:1606-1609.
13. Moller H, Weidner IS: Epidemiology of cryptorchidism and hypospadias. Epidemiology 1999;10:352-354.
14. Khuri FJ, Hardy BE, Churchill BM: Urologic anomalies associated with hypospadias. Urol Clin North Am 1981;8:565-571.
15. Cerasaro TS, Brock WA, Kaplan GW: Upper urinary tract anomalies associated with congenital hypospadias: is screening necessary? J Urol 1986;135:537-542.
16. Hinman F: Anatomy of the external genitalia. In Ehrlich RM, Alter GJ, eds: Reconstructive and Plastic Surgery of the External Genitalia. Philadelphia, WB Saunders, 1999:7-12.
17. Bellinger MF: Embryology of the male external genitalia. Urol Clin North Am 1981;8:375-382.
18. Rowsell AR, Morgan BDG: Hypospadias and embryogenesis of the penile urethra. Br J Plast Surg 1987;40:201-206.
19. Devine CJ, Horton CE, Gilbert DA, Winslow BH: Hypospadias. In Mustarde JC, Jackson IT, eds: Plastic Surgery in Infancy and Childhood, 3rd ed. Edinburgh, Churchill Livingstone, 1988:493-570.
20. Hodgson NB: History of hypospadias repair. In Ehrlich RM, Alter GJ, eds: Reconstructive and Plastic Surgery of the External Genitalia. Philadelphia, WB Saunders, 1999:13-17.
21. Gilpin D, Clements WD, Boston VE: GRAP repair: single-stage reconstruction of hypospadias as an outpatient procedure. Br J Urol 1993;71:226-229.
22. Johnson D, Coleman DJ: The selective use of a single-stage and a two-stage technique for hypospadias correction in 157 consecutive cases with the aim of normal appearance and function. Br J Plast Surg 1998;51:195-201.
23. Duckett JW: MAGPI (meatoplasty and glanuloplasty): a procedure for subcoronal hypospadias. Urol Clin North Am 1981;8:513.
24. Rich MA, Keating MA, Snyder HM: Hinging the urethral plate in hypospadias meatoplasty. J Urol 1989;142:1551-1554.
25. Mathieu P: Traitment en un temps de l'hypospadias balanique ou justabalanique. J Chir 1932;39:481-484.
26. Bracka A: Hypospadias repair: a two-stage alternative. Br J Urol 1995;76:31-41.
27. Bracka A: A versatile two-stage hypospadias repair. Br J Plast Surg 1995;48:345-352.
28. Telfer JR, Quaba AA, Kwai Ben I, Peddi NC: An investigation into the role of waterproofing in a two-stage hypospadias repair. Br J Plast Surg 1998;51:542-546.
29. Khan U, Zic N, Boorman J: Waterproofing in hypospadias: a refinement of the two-stage reconstruction. Br J Plast Surg. 2001;54:528-531.
30. Kumar MVK, Harris DL: Balanitis xerotica obliterans complicating hypospadias repair. Br J Plast Surg 1999;52:69-71.
31. Baskin L, Duckett JW: Hypospadias: long term outcomes. In Mouriquand PDE, ed: Pediatric Surgery and Urology: Long-term Outcome. Philadelphia, WB Saunders, 1998:559-567.
32. Sommerlad BC: A long-term follow-up of hypospadias patients. Br J Plast Surg 1989;42:153-156.
33. Bracka A: A long-term view of hypospadias. Br J Plast Surg 1989;42:251-255.
34. Duckett JW, Snyder HM: The MAGPI hypospadias repair in 1111 patients. Ann Surg 1991;213:620-625.
35. Hinderer UT, Duran FR, Caravaca MP: Hypospadias repair. In Goldwyn RM, ed: Long-term Results in Plastic and Reconstructive Surgery, vol 1, 2nd ed. Boston, Little, Brown, 1978:378-410.
36. Aho MO, Tammela OKT, Tammela TLJ: Aspects of adult satisfaction with the result of surgery for hypospadias performed in childhood. Eur Urol 1997;32:218-222.
37. Baskin L: Hypospadias: a critical analysis of cosmetic outcomes using photography. BJU Int 2001;87:534-539.
38. Aho MO, Tammela OKT, Somppi EMJ, Tammela TLJ: Sexual and social life of men operated in childhood for hypospadias and phimosis. Eur Urol 2000;37:95-101.
39. Bracka A: Sexuality after hypospadias repair. BJU Int 1999;83(suppl 3):29-33.
40. van der Werff JFA, Ultee J: Long-term follow-up of hypospadias repair. Br J Plast Surg 2000;53:588-592.
41. Smith ED: The history of hypospadias. Pediatr Surg Int 1997;12:81-85.
42. Mouriquand PDE, Persad R, Sharma S: Hypospadias repair: current principles and procedures. Br J Urol 1995;76(suppl 3):9-22.
43. Horton CE, Devine CJ, Graham JK: Fistulas of the penile urethra. Plast Reconstr Surg 1980;66:407-418.
44. Holland AJA, Smith GHH, Ross FI, Cass DT: HOSE: an objective scoring system for evaluating the results of hypospadias surgery. BJU Int 2001;88:255-258.
45. Titley OG, Bracka A: A 5-year audit of trainees experience and outcomes with two-stage hypospadias surgery. Br J Plast Surg 1998;51:370-375.
46. Zaontz MR, Dean GE: Glanular hypospadias repair. Urol Clin North Am 2002;29:291-298.
47. Arap S, Mire AI, De Goes GM: Modified meatal advancement and glanuloplasty repair of distal hypospadias J Urol 1984; 131:1140-1141.
48. Duckett JW, Snyder HMcC: The MAGPI hypospadias repair in 1111 patients. Ann Surg 1991;213:620-626.
49. Hastie KJ, Deshpande SS, Moisey CU: Long term follow-up of the MAGPI operation for distal hypospadias. Br J Urol 1989;63:320-322.
50. Duckett JW, Snyder HM III: Meatal advancement and glanuloplasty hypospadias repair after 1,000 cases: avoidance of meatal stenosis and regression. J Urol 1992;147:665-669.
51. Issa MM, Gearheart JP: The failed MAGPI: management and prevention. Br J Urol 1989;64:169-171.
52. Ozen HA, Whitaker RH: Scope and limitations of the MAGPI hypospadias repair. Br J Urol 1987;59:81-83.
53. Unler ES, Miroglu C, Ozdiler E, Ozturk R: Long-term results of the MAGPI (meatal advancement and glanuloplasty) operations in distal hypospadias. Int Urol Nephrol 1991;213:581-587.
54. Thiersch C: On the origin and operative treatment of epispadias. Arch Heilk 1869;10:20-28.
55. King LR: Hypospadias. A one-stage repair without skin graft based on a new principle—chordee is sometimes produced by skin alone. J Urol 1970;103:660-663.

56. Van Horn AC, Kass EJ: Glanuloplasty and in-situ tubularization of the urethral plate: a simple reliable technique for the majority of boys with hypospadias. J Urol 1995;154:1505-1509.
57. Zaontz MR: The GAP (glans approximation procedure) for glanular/coronal hypospadias. J Urol 1989;141:359-361.
58. Gittes GK, Snyder CL, Murphy JP: Glans approximation procedure urethroplasty for the wide deep meatus. Urology 1998;52:499-500.
59. Hoebeke P, De Sy W: The GAP (glans approximation procedure) for distal hypospadias. Technical aspects. Ann Urol (Paris) 1996;30:167-169.
60. Crick A, Coleman DJ: Experience of a single stage technique for correction of distal hypospadias: 93 consecutive cases. Presented at British Association of Plastic Surgeons Winter Meeting, London, November 2001.
61. Snodgrass W: Tubularized, incised plate urethroplasty for distal hypospadias. J Urol 1994;151:464-465.
62. Snodgrass W, Koyle M, Manzoni G, et al: Tubularized incised plate urethroplasty: result of a multicenter experience. J Urol 1996;156:839-841.
63. Elbakry A: Tubularised incised plate urethroplasty: is regular dilatation necessary for success? Br J Urol Int 1999;84:683-688.
64. Elbakry A: Re: mechanism of healing following the Snodgrass repair. J Urol 2001;166:1837-1838.
65. Bleustein CB, Esposito MP, Soslow RA, et al: Mechanism of healing following the Snodgrass repair. J Urol 2001;165:277-279.
66. Erol A, Baskin LS, Li YW: Anatomical studies of the urethral plate: why preservation of the urethral plate is important in hypospadias surgery. BJU Int 2000;85:728-734.
67. Hollowell JG, Keating MA, Snyder HM, et al: Preservation of the urethral plate in hypospadias repair: extended applications and further experience with the onlay island flap urethroplasty. J Urol 1990;143:98-100.
68. Baskin LS, Duckett JW, Ueoka K, et al: Changing concepts of hypospadias curvature lead to more onlay island flap procedures. J Urol 1994;151:191-196.
69. Atala A, Guzman L, Retik AB: A novel inert collagen matrix for hypospadias repair. J Urol 1999;162:1148-1151.
70. Atala A: Experimental and clinical experience with tissue engineering techniques for urethral reconstruction. Urol Clin North Am 2002;29:485-492.

CHAPTER

154

Reconstruction of Female Genital Defects: Congenital

MALCOLM ALAN LESAVOY, MD, FACS ✦ EUGENE J. CARTER, MD

Reconstruction of the female perineum is indicated for congenital absence of the vagina, lymphedema, vaginal defects, previous ablative surgery for various perineal malignant neoplasms, relief of pain after radiation therapy, and, if indicated, repair of labial hypertrophy. Vaginal reconstruction has become a standard procedure performed by plastic surgeons, gynecologists, and urologists. The most common indication for vaginal reconstruction is congenital absence of the vagina.

In general, the results of vaginal reconstruction are satisfactory. However, potential problems can include inadequate genital wound coverage due to foreshortened graft or flap harvest, fecal contamination if preoperative bowel preparation has not been adequate, adjacent urethral injuries during dissection of the new vaginal pocket, and difficult immobilization of the patient in the postoperative period.

Counseller[1] reported that congenital absence of the vagina occurs in approximately 1 in every 4000 births and that these abnormalities usually coexist with uterus and urinary tract abnormalities. The ovaries are usually not affected, however, and the secondary sex characteristics develop normally. Because the cervix and vagina initially form a solid unit embryologically, the reason for vaginal agenesis is the lack of cavitation and cell death needed to form a vagina.[1] However, the hormonal factors that stimulate cavitation are not known.

Patients with labial hypertrophy undergo labioplasty for functional, aesthetic, and social reasons. Hypertrophy of the labia minora or labia majora may be congenital or acquired. Patients with this condition may experience inflammation and poor hygiene as well as self-consciousness during sexual activity and when wearing tight pants. Reduction of the labia minora or labia majora is a relatively minor outpatient procedure that yields satisfactory results for many patients.

VAGINAL RECONSTRUCTION

History

In 1573, a student of Vesalius, Realdus Columbus, first reported vaginal agenesis; it was not until 1872 that Heppner[2] described vaginal reconstruction with use of the labia. However, the true landmark report for vaginal reconstruction is credited to Abbe[3] in 1898. In one patient, Abbe described dissecting a canal and lining it with split-thickness skin grafts. These skin grafts were placed over a rubber stent packed with gauze. After 10 days, the stent was removed, and the skin grafts were found to be completely vascularized. The patient was asked to wear a vaginal conformer postoperatively, and evidently intercourse was possible. However, Abbe's report was lost for almost 40 years until McIndoe[4] popularized the Abbe technique by lining the new vaginal canal with partial-thickness skin grafts. McIndoe[5] reported an impressive array of 63 repairs, and subsequently Counseller[1] in 1948 reported 70.

Other methods of vaginal reconstruction have been attempted, but most have had undesirable effects, specifically when segments of the gastrointestinal tract have been used for lining the new vaginal canal. Conway and Stark[6] in 1953 described use of the rectum (Sneguireff,[7] Popow,[8] and Schubert[9] had earlier described the same thing). Baldwin[10] in 1904 even described use of a loop of ileum. However, obvious difficulties occurred with bowel transposition, such as necrosis, infection, and abscess formation. If the procedure was successful, the type of secretions arising from the bowel lining were mostly inappropriate and unwanted. The added morbidity of an intra-abdominal procedure, various bowel anastomoses, possibility of vascular compromise, and undesired mucosal secretions account for the lack of popularity of these procedures.

The Frank procedure, a nonoperative technique, has been successful in some instances of incomplete vaginal atresia. In 1927, Frank and Geist[11] demonstrated the use of intermittent pressure at the perineal dimple between the anus and the urethra in the normal location of the vagina. This pressure is applied until the patient feels mild discomfort by a series of graduated obturators in the form of increasing sizes of test tubes. The pressure is relieved and then reapplied. The patient gradually stretches this skin inward in the same way that a skin expander works with an outward force. This process continues for weeks until the largest dilator can be introduced within the neovagina and worn comfortably. This procedure requires a compliant and persistent patient and an anatomy that is consistent with incomplete vaginal agenesis. Obviously, the skin lining the new vagina is cutaneous squamous epithelium and must be lubricated externally to allow intercourse.

FIGURE 154-1. Congenital vaginal aplasia with an enlarged urethral meatus below the clitoris. (From Lesavoy MA, Carter EJ: Vaginal reconstruction. In Raz S, ed: Female Urology, 2nd ed. Philadelphia, WB Saunders, 1996:605-616.)

Surgical Techniques

ABBE-McINDOE PROCEDURE

Over the years, the Abbe-McIndoe procedure evolved to become the easiest and most successful method of vaginal reconstruction, avoiding the risks and disadvantages of laparotomy (Figs. 154-1 and 154-2). The procedure must be performed under general or spinal anesthesia. A Y incision is made along the median raphe between the urethra and the anus. A catheter is placed in the urethra, and dissection is carried cephaloposteriorly. This dissection can be done relatively bluntly, and safety is ensured by keeping a gloved finger in the rectum for tactile ease of dissection. The Y incision allows three cutaneous flaps to be enfolded into the vaginal canal so that circumferential scar contraction can be avoided. The depth of dissection should be somewhat exaggerated and is in the range of 10 to 14 cm in the adult. The surgeon must overcorrect somewhat because of the expected subsequent contraction (Fig. 154-3).

After the vaginal canal has been bluntly dissected, a partial-thickness skin graft is harvested from the buttock-hip area. Obviously, one must keep in mind the subsequent scar that will definitely ensue from this partial-thickness skin graft, and one should avoid harvesting the graft from an area low on the thigh just for the surgeon's convenience. The skin graft can be taken with any type of dermatome, and two or three sheets of skin are frequently needed to achieve a total dimension of approximately 14 by 7 cm.

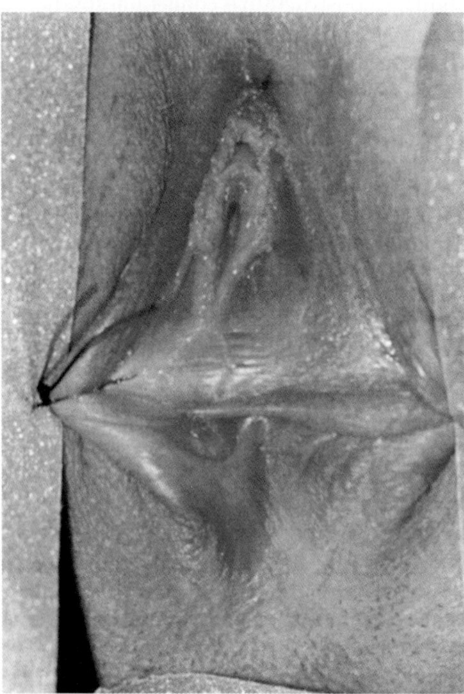

FIGURE 154-2. Sutures holding the labia majora. (From Lesavoy MA, Carter EJ: Vaginal reconstruction. In Raz S, ed: Female Urology, 2nd ed. Philadelphia, WB Saunders, 1996:605-616.)

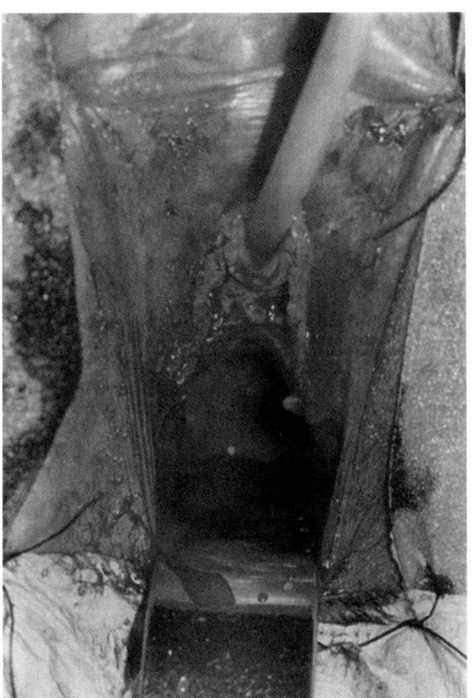

FIGURE 154-3. Catheter in the urethra and dissection of the neovaginal canal. (From Lesavoy MA, Carter EJ: Vaginal reconstruction. In Raz S, ed: Female Urology, 2nd ed. Philadelphia, WB Saunders, 1996:605-616.)

A number of techniques have been developed to apply the skin graft to the vaginal canal. Historically, candle wax, carved balsa wood, gauze packing, syringe casing, dental wax, and hard plastic conformers have been used. The Heyer-Schulte Company has recently produced a soft, pliable, and expandable vaginal conformer that works very well in our opinion. This stent has a central semirigid foam core and a surrounding silicone envelope that can be expanded with air or saline (Fig. 154-4). There is also a central drain site through the core of the stent. Once the graft has been harvested, the vaginal stent should be inflated with air and lubricated with mineral oil.

The skin graft sheets are then sutured to each other and placed over this stent with the raw dermal sides *out* (Fig. 154-5). This means that the epidermal side of the skin is adjacent to the stent. Subsequently, hemostasis is checked in the neovaginal canal, and the now-deflated stent and overlying skin grafts are eased into the canal (Fig. 154-6). It may be necessary to deflate the vaginal stent while slowly rotating and pushing the stent and skin graft into the vaginal canal; but once the stent is seated to the depth of the dissection, it should again be inflated to spread out the skin graft, to ensure direct apposition to the raw walls, and to provide an excellent bolster for the ensuing neovascularization of the skin graft.

FIGURE 154-4. Heyer-Schulte inflatable vaginal stent. (From Lesavoy MA, Carter EJ: Vaginal reconstruction. In Raz S, ed: Female Urology, 2nd ed. Philadelphia, WB Saunders, 1996:605-616.)

After this, the flaps from the Y incision are sutured to the superficial ends of the skin graft in a tacking fashion with absorbable sutures. Fluff gauze is then packed around the perineum under compression, and the labia majora are sutured to each other to ensure that the stent does not slide out of the canal.

Postoperatively, the patient remains in bed for a minimum of 5 days and is medically constipated (a lower bowel preparation is required preoperatively). On the fifth or sixth postoperative day, the patient is sedated in bed, and the labial sutures are removed. The skin graft can then be checked by aspirating the outer lumen of the Heyer-Schulte vaginal stent and actually deflating it, gently removing the stent and leaving the skin graft intact within the vaginal vault. If there is any difficulty with this maneuver, mineral oil can be injected between the stent and the skin graft by use of a soft rubber catheter. This allows lubrication of the interface between the stent and the skin graft so that disruption and shearing of the skin graft are avoided when the stent is removed. The perineum can then be cleaned, and the stent can be washed and replaced immediately. Subsequently, a perineal binder can be applied, and the patient can be allowed to ambulate; the constipating medicine is then discontinued.

The vaginal stent is checked every other day, and the patient is usually discharged on the seventh or eighth day postoperatively. The patient should be fully aware of the mechanics of the stent so that she can remove, wash, and reintroduce the stent daily while at home.

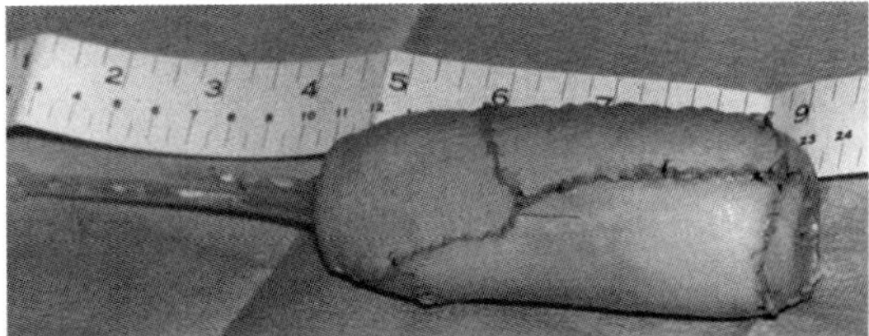

FIGURE 154-5. Split-thickness skin graft sutured around the vaginal stent with the epithelial side inward next to the stent and the raw side out. (From Lesavoy MA, Carter EJ: Vaginal reconstruction. In Raz S, ed: Female Urology, 2nd ed. Philadelphia, WB Saunders, 1996:605-616.)

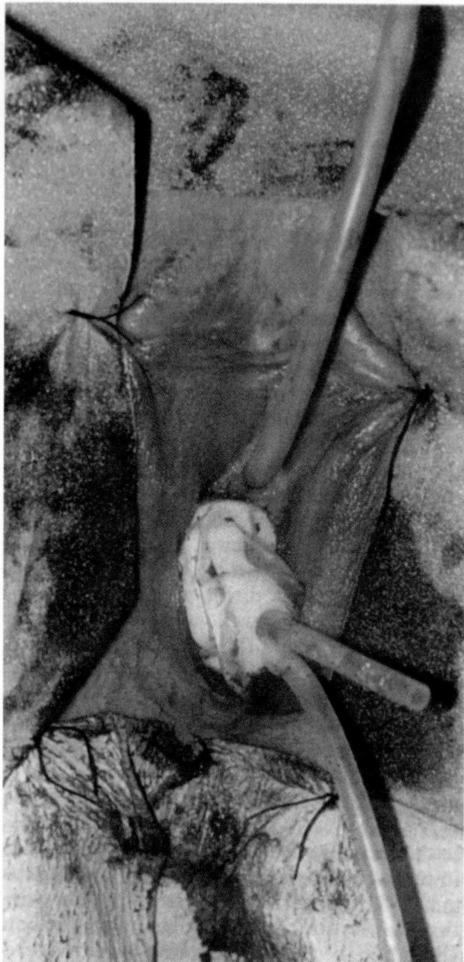

FIGURE 154-6. Vaginal stent with the skin graft invaginated into the neovaginal canal. (From Lesavoy MA, Carter EJ: Vaginal reconstruction. In Raz S, ed: Female Urology, 2nd ed. Philadelphia, WB Saunders, 1996:605-616.)

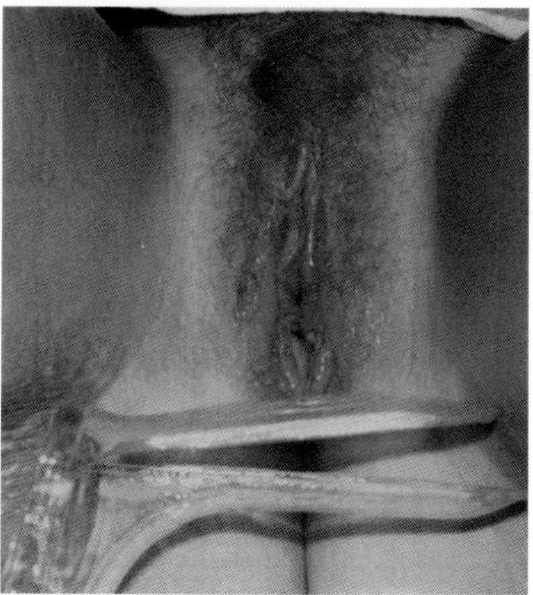

FIGURE 154-7. Photograph taken 3 months postoperatively showing the normal-looking vulva and the size of the speculum that can be inserted into the vagina. (From Lesavoy MA, Carter EJ: Vaginal reconstruction. In Raz S, ed: Female Urology, 2nd ed. Philadelphia, WB Saunders, 1996:605-616.)

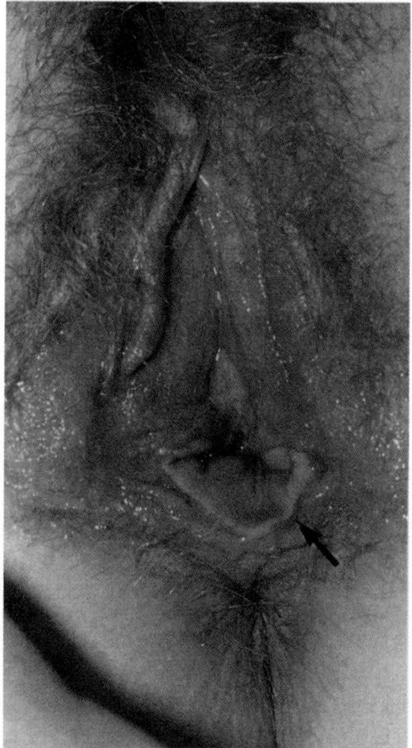

FIGURE 154-8. The discrepancy in the skin graft color of the neovagina. (From Lesavoy MA, Carter EJ: Vaginal reconstruction. In Raz S, ed: Female Urology, 2nd ed. Philadelphia, WB Saunders, 1996:605-616.)

It is extremely important in vaginal reconstruction for the patient to be fully aware that a conformer must be worn for a minimum of 6 months postoperatively. If this is not done, contraction of the vaginal vault will definitely ensue. After 3 or 4 months, as the skin graft matures, vaginal intercourse should be encouraged. As a matter of fact, this procedure should not be done unless intercourse is anticipated. Intercourse, obviously, is an excellent obturator and conformer. After 6 months, the conformer can be eliminated during the day but should be worn at night. If the patient is active sexually and has intercourse two or three times per week, the conformer can be eliminated. However, if there is a time when intercourse is not anticipated for weeks or months, the conformer should be worn at night (Figs. 154-7 to 154-10). Because the skin grafts do not have the same properties as normal vaginal mucosa and do not have secretory abilities, most

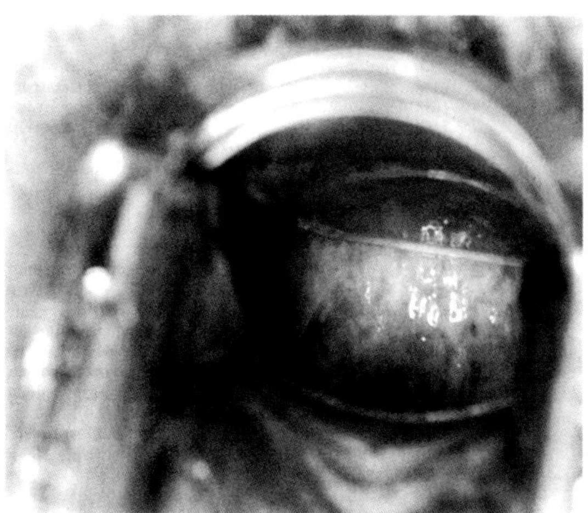

FIGURE 154-9. Depth of the neovagina as seen through the plastic speculum. (From Lesavoy MA, Carter EJ: Vaginal reconstruction. In Raz S, ed: Female Urology, 2nd ed. Philadelphia, WB Saunders, 1996:605-616.)

patients require the application of lubricants before intercourse.

FULL-THICKNESS SKIN GRAFTS

Full-thickness skin grafts are important for certain types of vaginal reconstruction (i.e., vaginal aplasia, vaginal stenosis, intersex conditions, and iatrogenic disease). One advantage of these grafts is that they allow reconstruction at an earlier age (anytime after puberty), providing psychological reassurance as the child develops that she is normal. They also reduce postoperative stenting time and minimize vaginal stenosis by decreasing postoperative vaginal contraction. They improve the cosmesis of the donor site, and a full-thickness skin graft grows with the body proportionately.[12,13] Inguinal donor sites are used for full-thickness skin grafts, and the donor site closure occurs primarily.

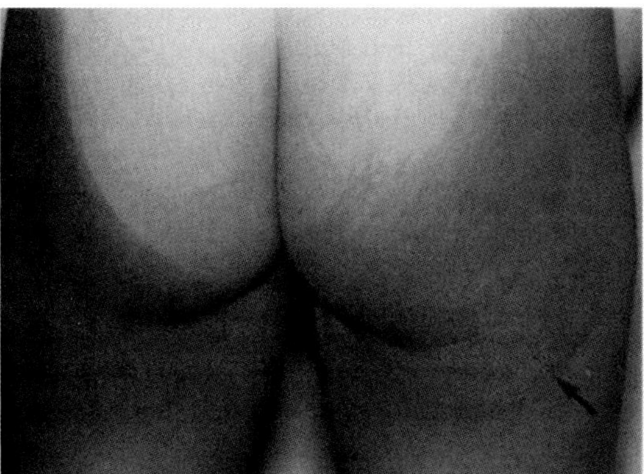

FIGURE 154-10. Donor site on the right buttock (*arrow*). (From Lesavoy MA, Carter EJ: Vaginal reconstruction. In Raz S, ed: Female Urology, 2nd ed. Philadelphia, WB Saunders, 1996:605-616.)

FLAPS

Vulvobulbocavernosus Myocutaneous Flap

The vulvobulbocavernosus myocutaneous flap was described by Knapstein et al[14] in 1990. This flap is based on the skin fat and underlying vulvobulbocavernosus erectile muscle and tissue and is useful because of its low axis. It is not easily used for transfer into the upper pelvis, but it is best for reconstruction of the vagina after a pelvic exenteration that removes the perineal body and the anus (i.e., a lower pelvic defect). This is a relatively new procedure and should be considered especially for patients with anterior or total exenteration with low rectal anastomosis.

In general, the vulvobulbocavernosus myocutaneous flap is not large enough to form a complete vaginal canal. The anterior edges of the flap are sewn together to form the anterior margins of the newly formed vaginal cylinder. Its disadvantage is the retention of vulvar hair, which results in vaginal discharge and strong odor. The blood and nerve supply comes from the pudendals.[15]

Gracilis Myocutaneous Flaps

The gracilis muscle is the most commonly used flap after pelvic exenteration for vaginal reconstruction.[16,17] After pelvic exenteration, abdominoperineal resection, or vaginal irradiation (Fig. 154-11), the patient is usually left with a large vaginal defect. A gracilis island myocutaneous flap can enhance vaginal reconstruction. It also provides adequate vaginal length, and the muscle is expendable for the most part.

The gracilis myocutaneous flap provides sufficient bulk to fill the empty pelvic space and simultaneously brings its own new blood supply, leading to a softness and pliability not achievable with skin graft techniques. The disadvantage of the gracilis may be a loss of approximately 10% to 20% of the flap due to vascular compromise of the flap resulting from potential tension of its small-caliber vascular pedicle when it is transposed into the pelvic defect. Residual scarring on the legs may also be a common source of minor complaints.[18-20]

The principle of employing muscle with its overlying skin, vascularized by the muscle perforators, has been well documented in the plastic and reconstructive surgical literature by Owens,[21] Bakamjian,[22] Hueston and McConchie,[23] and McCraw et al.[24] McCraw and associates were the first to describe the principle of the "skin island" over the muscle unit, and this principle is applicable to vaginal reconstruction. Interestingly, McCraw's paper on vaginal reconstruction was one of the landmark works in the plastic surgery literature that opened the floodgate to the revived use of myocutaneous flaps.

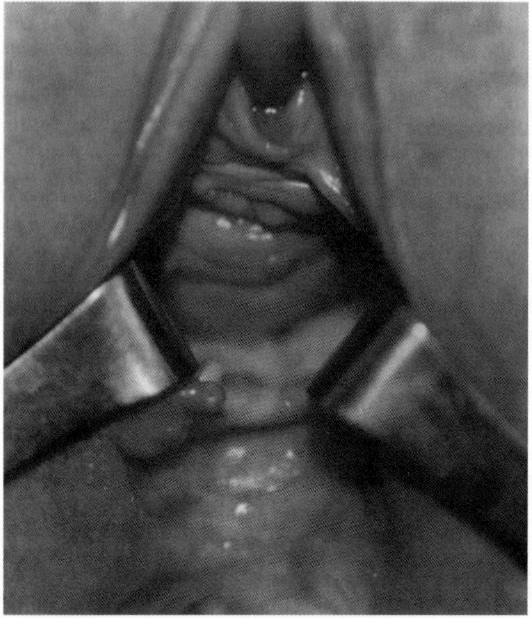

FIGURE 154-11. Patient with radiation vaginitis with severe pain, drainage, fibrosis, and contraction. (From Lesavoy MA, Carter EJ: Vaginal reconstruction. In Raz S, ed: Female Urology, 2nd ed. Philadelphia, WB Saunders, 1996:605-616.)

The operation begins with the patient in the lithotomy position (Fig. 154-12). Either unilateral or bilateral island gracilis myocutaneous flaps are harvested (Fig. 154-13), based on their superior neurovascular pedicles (Fig. 154-14). The flap can then be tunneled (Fig. 154-15) under intact perineal skin (Fig. 154-16) and "invaginated" into the neovaginal canal. A conformer is not needed, and the donor sites are closed in a linear fashion with primary approximation along the medial thigh area (see Fig. 154-15).

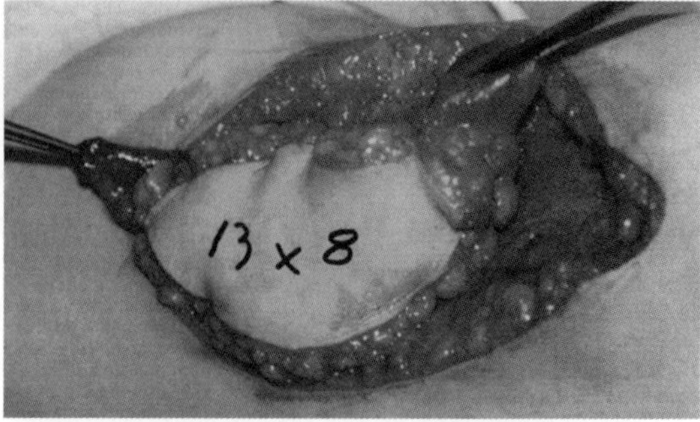

FIGURE 154-13. The gracilis muscle and island skin flap are isolated. (From Lesavoy MA, Carter EJ: Vaginal reconstruction. In Raz S, ed: Female Urology, 2nd ed. Philadelphia, WB Saunders, 1996:605-616.)

A unilateral gracilis myocutaneous flap may be used for radiation contracture and pain of the vaginal vault. Sensibility of the skin of the gracilis myocutaneous island is maintained by way of the sensory branches of the obturator nerve as described by Lesavoy et al.[25] However, sensitivity of the transposed skin is not the same as that of a normal vagina. Sensitivity to pressure is excellent, but tactile sensitivity is diminished.[26] (Sexual sensitivity is mostly cerebral.)

Rectus Abdominis Myocutaneous Flap

Because of its success in breast reconstruction, the rectus abdominis myocutaneous flap can also be used for vaginal reconstruction. Its major and primary arterial blood supply is the inferior epigastric vessels. Two island flaps can be harvested, the horizontally oriented lower abdominal myocutaneous flap[27] and the vertically

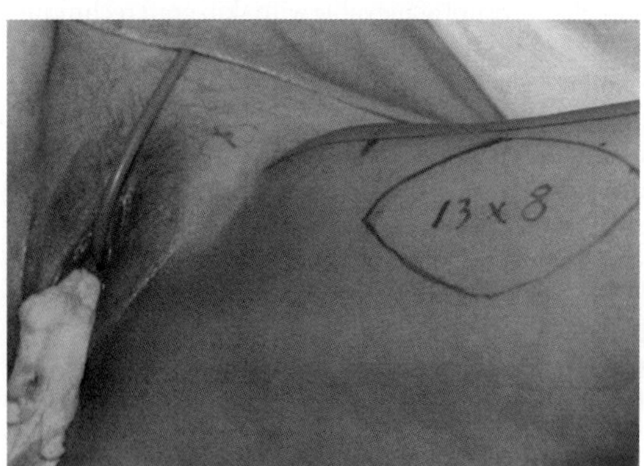

FIGURE 154-12. After excision of radiation-damaged tissue and a pack in the vaginal vault, a 13- × 8-cm gracilis myocutaneous island flap is outlined on the left medial thigh. (From Lesavoy MA, Carter EJ: Vaginal reconstruction. In Raz S, ed: Female Urology, 2nd ed. Philadelphia, WB Saunders, 1996:605-616.)

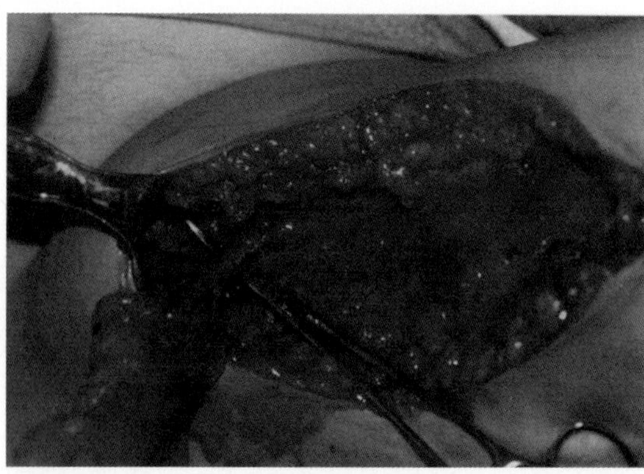

FIGURE 154-14. The undersurface of the gracilis myocutaneous island flap and its neurovascular bundle. (From Lesavoy MA, Carter EJ: Vaginal reconstruction. In Raz S, ed: Female Urology, 2nd ed. Philadelphia, WB Saunders, 1996:605-616.)

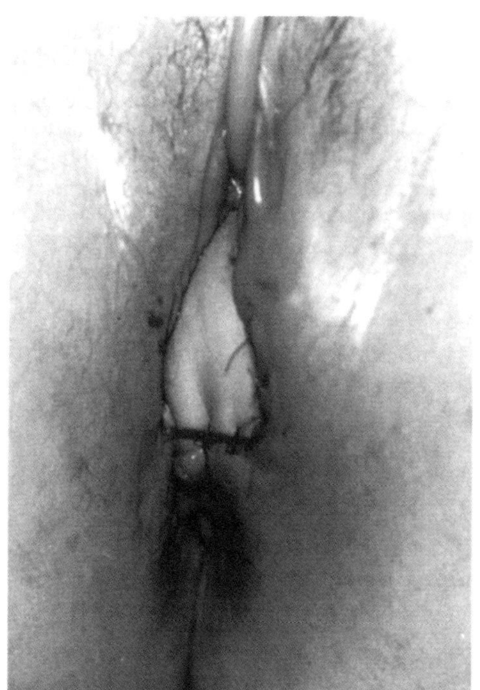

FIGURE 154-15. Inset of the flap into the vaginal defect. The donor site is closed primarily.

oriented upper abdominal myocutaneous flap.[28] The transverse rectus abdominis myocutaneous (TRAM) and vertical rectus abdominis myocutaneous (VRAM) flaps, because of the extended length of their vascular pedicles, allow a high arc of rotation. The axis is determined by the vascular supply and is transferred intra-abdominally through the posterior rectus sheath. This need for laparotomy is one of the obvious negative aspects of this procedure. A vertically oriented flap may be preferred when it is necessary to maintain an intact lower abdominal rectus muscle for exit sites of stomas on the contralateral side.

Among the many advantages of this flap are a reliable blood supply[19] and the ability to resurface a defect with a single flap. This flap also provides ease of mobilization without tension and a low incidence of vascular compromise.[18,29] In a series of 22 patients, there was little tissue loss and an acceptable donor site, and return to sexual activity was possible in 80% of patients.[28]

After completion of the exenteration procedure, attention is directed toward harvesting of the myocutaneous flap from the abdomen. Centered just to the left or right of the umbilicus, a TRAM flap measuring approximately 9 cm long by 12 cm wide is harvested. The flap should include skin, subcutaneous tissue, a strip of anterior rectus sheath, and the rectus muscle itself (Fig. 154-17). The initial incision should commence at the lateral apex of the TRAM flap (which corresponds to the anterior axillary line) and extend medially to include all of the flap components. The rectus muscle is identified and carefully dissected lateral to the region of the deep inferior epigastric perforating vessels, with identification of the inferior epigastric vascular pedicle at its origin on the external iliac vessels. This ensures adequate flap mobilization when the flap is isolated. At this point, the superior and inferior margins of the rectus muscle are divided (Fig. 154-18). A vaginal tube is then formed from the flap by means of continuous and interrupted sutures to approximate the superior and inferior margins of skin and muscle with the raw side out (Fig. 154-19).

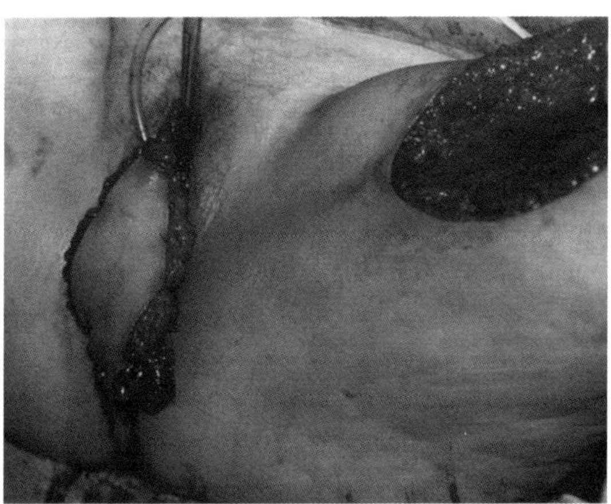

FIGURE 154-16. The myocutaneous island flap is transferred subcutaneously to be inset. (From Lesavoy MA, Carter EJ: Vaginal reconstruction. In Raz S, ed: Female Urology, 2nd ed. Philadelphia, WB Saunders, 1996:605-616.)

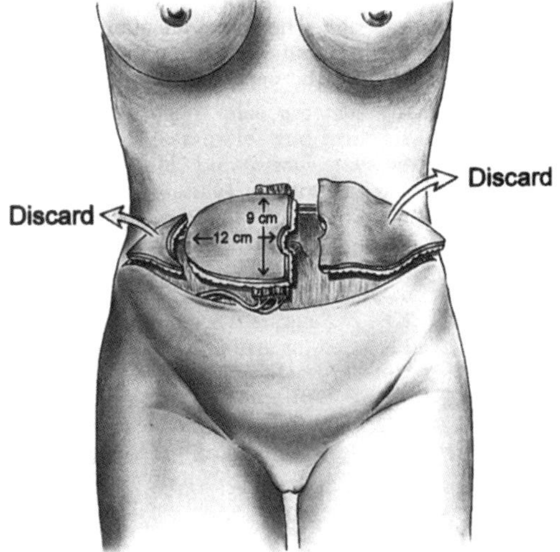

FIGURE 154-17. Harvesting of right rectus abdominis myocutaneous flap for vaginal reconstruction.

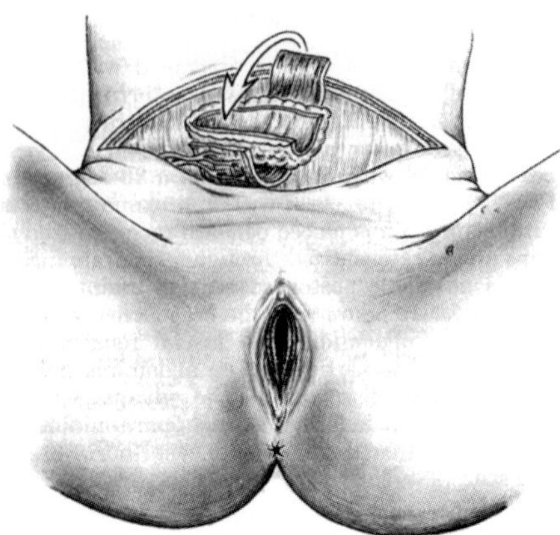

FIGURE 154-18. The flap is mobilized and formed into a tube. (From Lesavoy MA, Carter EJ: Vaginal reconstruction. In Raz S, ed: Female Urology, 2nd ed. Philadelphia, WB Saunders, 1996:605-616.)

The manually formed vaginal cone is then mobilized and transferred through the posterior rectus sheath after a laparotomy incision is made through the peritoneum at the origin of the deep inferior epigastric vessels into the pelvis to reach the vaginal defect (Fig. 154-20). The most lateral portion of the flap becomes the apex of the vagina. Care must be taken in placing the flap to ensure that no tension is put on the vascular pedicle. The neovagina is then attached to the introitus with interrupted sutures (Fig. 154-21).[15,18] An estrogen cream is spread on the mold, which is placed in the vagina and sutured in place.[18] On day 5, the mold is removed, and a vaginal dilator is worn three times per week for 3 months in conjunction with estrogen cream.[18]

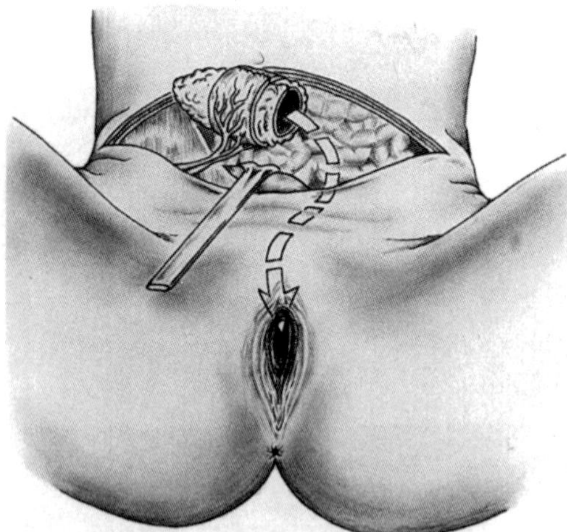

FIGURE 154-19. The mobilized myocutaneous flap is sutured together to form a blind tube of sufficient length and diameter to serve as a functional vagina. It is then transferred through the posterior rectus sheath to reach the vaginal defect. (From Lesavoy MA, Carter EJ: Vaginal reconstruction. In Raz S, ed: Female Urology, 2nd ed. Philadelphia, WB Saunders, 1996:605-616.)

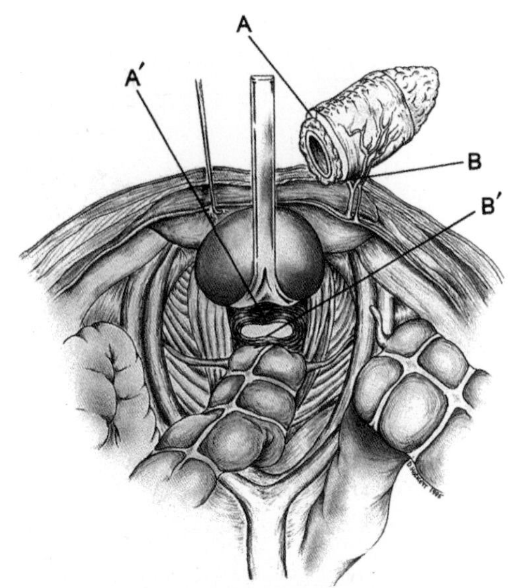

FIGURE 154-20. View after a laparotomy incision is made through the peritoneum at the origin of the deep inferior epigastric vessels into the pelvis to reach the vaginal defect. (From Lesavoy MA, Carter EJ: Vaginal reconstruction. In Raz S, ed: Female Urology, 2nd ed. Philadelphia, WB Saunders, 1996:605-616.)

The initial procedure is concluded—with primary closure of the fascial defect with interrupted or continuous permanent sutures. The closure of subcutaneous tissue after a horizontal (TRAM flap) harvest is best achieved with the patient in a 30-degree semi-Fowler position to assist with approximation. A subcutaneous drain is placed beneath the mobilized skin flaps and externalized through a separate incision.

It is advisable postoperatively to maintain strict bed rest for 48 hours with the hips flexed 30 degrees to decrease abdominal wall fascial tension at the repair

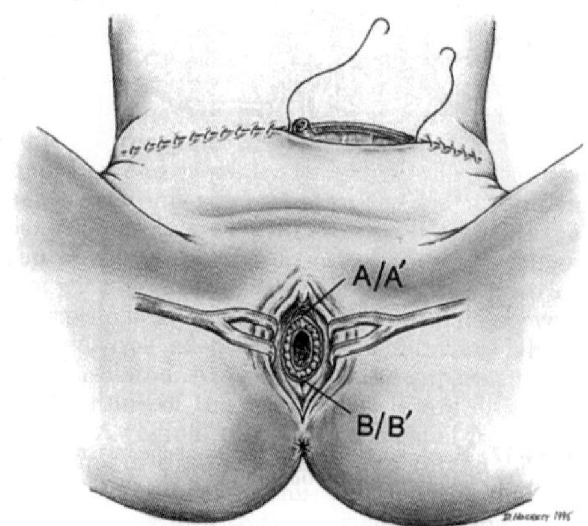

FIGURE 154-21. The myocutaneous flap is transposed into the pelvis and sutured to the perineal (introital) incision.

site. The VRAM flap has all the advantages of the TRAM flap, but it leaves a single paramidline scar at closure rather than the additional horizontal lateral scar.

Intestinal Flaps

For the sake of completeness, other methods of vaginal reconstruction, such as flaps of small intestine, ascending colon, sigmoid colon, and sigmoid and lower rectum, may be briefly described here, since they have been used with varying degrees of success for vaginal reconstruction. The patient requires hospitalization 2 days before the operation to allow time to prepare and sterilize the bowel adequately. With the patient in the lithotomy position, a vaginal tract is first dissected from the perineum into the peritoneum, and the tract is widened laterally. When hemostasis is satisfactory, the vaginal tract is packed and the abdomen opened. The sigmoid is generally mobile enough to allow a satisfactory vascular pedicle to be developed. With proper planning, an adequate length of intestine (12 to 15 cm) can be isolated, an oblique end-to-end anastomosis performed, and the bowel segment drawn through the vaginal tract. The patient is returned to a lithotomy position. The end of the bowel is incised on an angle to gain additional room and then attached to the introitus.

Advantages of the intestinal neovagina include the absence of a need for frequent dilatation or stent wearing. However, the disadvantages include excessive mucus formation, especially when the small intestine is used, and a mortality rate between 1% and 2%.[12]

Summary

Vaginal reconstruction can be an uncomplicated and straightforward procedure when attention to detail is maintained.[30,31] The Abbe-McIndoe procedure of lining the neovaginal canal with split-thickness skin grafts has become the standard. Use of the inflatable Heyer-Schulte vaginal stent provides comfort for the patient and ease for the surgeon in maintaining skin graft approximation.

For large vaginal and perineal defects, myocutaneous flaps such as the gracilis island flap have been extremely useful for correction of radiation-damaged tissue to the perineum and for the reconstruction of large ablative defects. Minimal morbidity and scarring ensue because the donor site can be closed primarily.

The gracilis has sufficient bulk to fill the pelvis, thus decreasing the incidence of herniation or possible obstruction. It also provides vaginal length, is an expendable muscle, and generally is out of the irradiated field. A limitation may be its 10% to 20% incidence of vascular compromise due to the vessel's small caliber, which results in tension as the flap is moved into the pelvic defect.

The TRAM flap is used to form a functional vagina. Its advantage over the gracilis is its variable vascular pedicle caliber and length. Of paramount importance are its extremely reliable blood supply and its potentially long vascular pedicle, which provides flap versatility with a resulting low incidence of vascular compromise. This flap augments the surgical options available for pelvic and vaginal reconstruction.

An absolute contraindication to rectus harvest is a history of potential vascular disruption of the inferior epigastric vessels. Obesity may be a relative contraindication because the thick subcutaneous tissue prohibits flap flexibility and mobilization into the pelvic space.

There remain a wide range of procedures from which to choose for the correction of congenital absence of the vagina; unfortunately, no consensus has been reached about which of these is best. Each patient must be evaluated on an individual basis.

With all vaginal reconstructions, a compliant patient is a necessity. The patient must wear a vaginal obturator for a minimum of 3 to 6 months postoperatively and is encouraged to use intercourse as an excellent obturator. In general, vaginal reconstruction can be an extremely gratifying procedure that enhances the functional and emotional well-being of these patients. In short, vaginal reconstruction can be successful in patients with either congenital or ablative vaginal absence, and it can be a functional and emotional plus for all concerned. Attention to detail and support are necessary for all patients.

LABIAL REDUCTION (LABIOPLASTY)

In some women, the labia minora or the labia majora may be enlarged for congenital, traumatic, or neoplastic reasons. Excision is relatively straightforward for neoplastic concerns, and it is beyond the purview of this chapter. However, congenital hypertrophy of the labia minora is an increasing problem for a number of women. Labia minora that protrude past the labia majora are both functionally and aesthetically unsatisfactory. Patients may experience irritation from clothing and during athletics, interference with sexual intercourse due to both functional and cosmetic concerns, and self-consciousness when wearing tight pants.[32,33]

The procedure for reduction of the labia minora is straightforward and performed on an outpatient basis.[34,35] The labia minora are contoured to the patient's desire. However, in general, the excisions should be tailored to remove more of the mucosal surface than of the external squamous epithelium. In this way, the scars are inconspicuous, and mucosal irritation from eversion does not occur. The protuberant area is excised, and the remaining edge is oversewn with a running suture. Sutures are removed in approximately 1 week (Figs. 154-22 to 154-24).

Reduction of the labia minora will often improve the physical comfort and sexual satisfaction of patients.

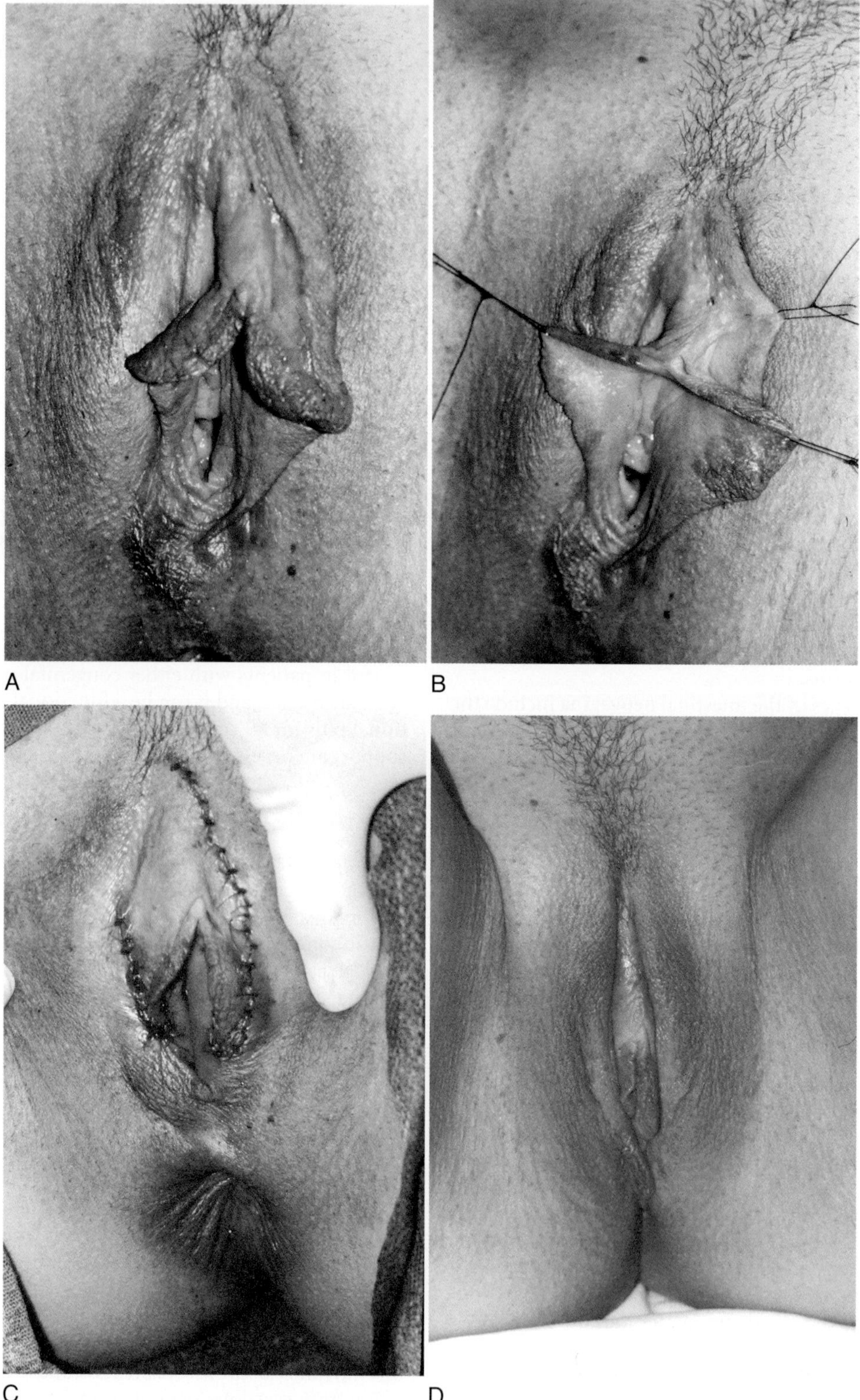

FIGURE 154-22. *A,* Preoperative view of large and patulous labia minora exhibiting symptoms of irritation from sports, clothing, and aggressive sexual activity. *B,* Intraoperative retraction of labia minora. *C,* Immediate postoperative indications of asymmetric resection and closure of labia minora. *D,* Postoperative result.

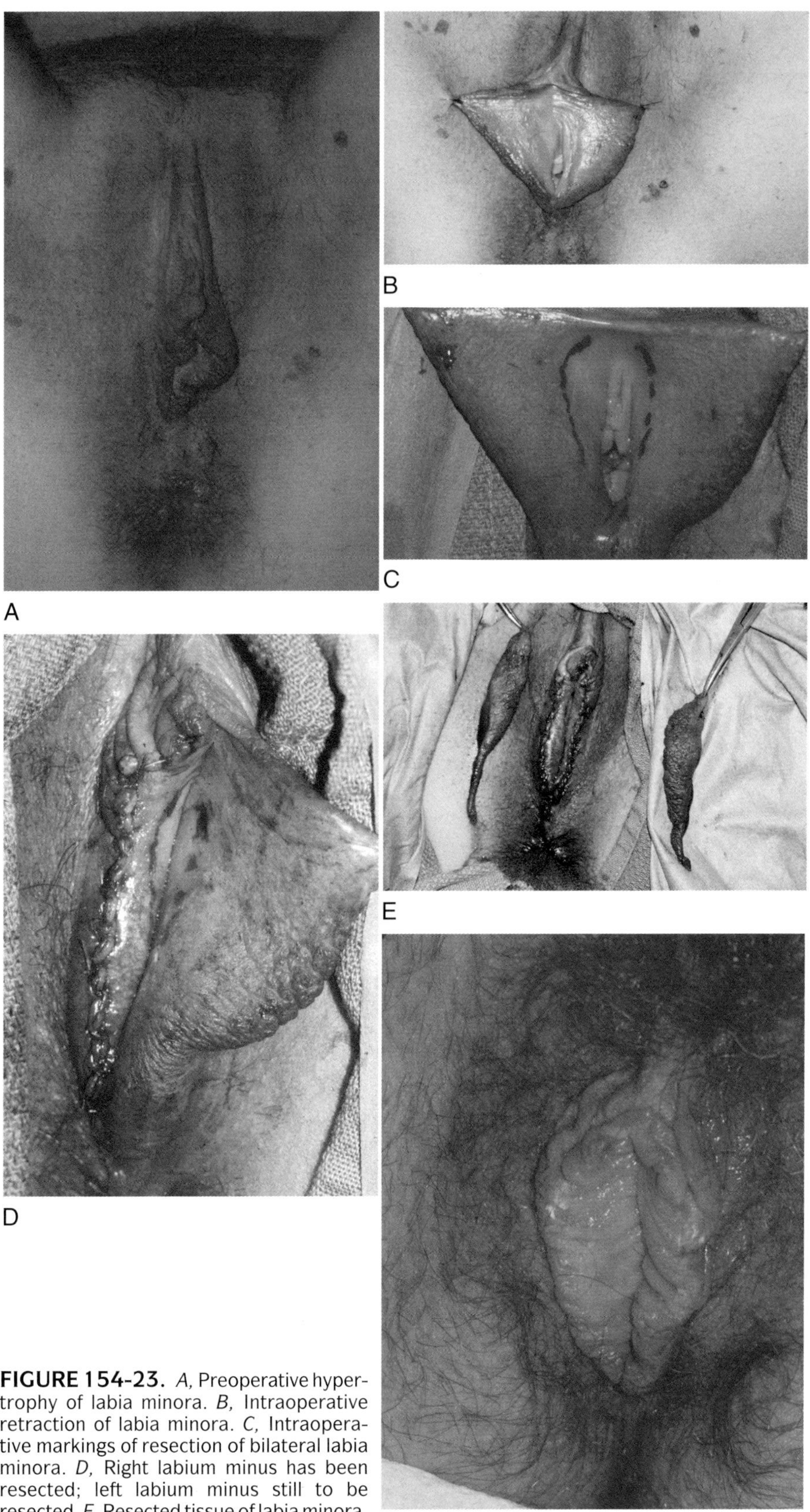

FIGURE 154-23. *A,* Preoperative hypertrophy of labia minora. *B,* Intraoperative retraction of labia minora. *C,* Intraoperative markings of resection of bilateral labia minora. *D,* Right labium minus has been resected; left labium minus still to be resected. *E,* Resected tissue of labia minora. *F,* Postoperative result.

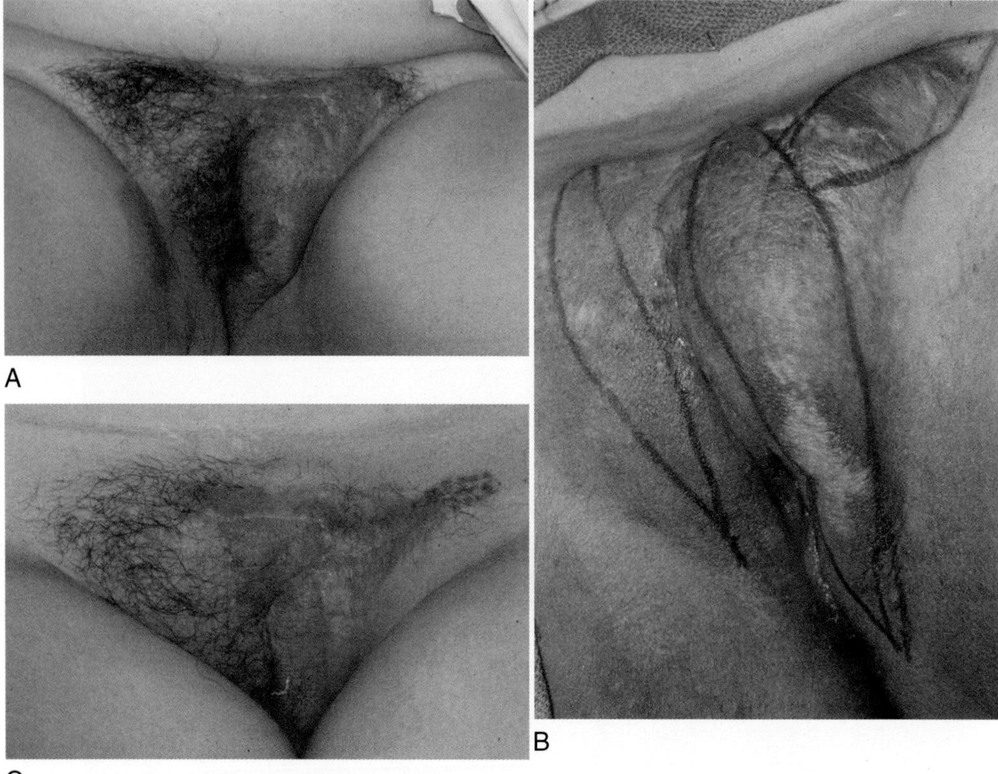

FIGURE 154-24. *A,* Hemangioma of left labium majus and suprapubic area with previous biopsies. *B,* Markings for excision of bilateral labia majora hemangioma. *C,* Postoperative result.

In conclusion, patients undergoing labia minora reduction are generally pleased with the aesthetic and functional results.

REFERENCES

1. Counseller VS: Congenital absence of the vagina. JAMA 1948;136:861.
2. Heppner, 1872. Cited by Paunz A: Formation of an artificial vagina to remedy a congenital defect. Zentralbl Gynakol 1923;47:833.
3. Abbe R: New method of creating a vagina in a case of congenital absence. Med Rec 1898;Dec 10.
4. McIndoe A: The application of cavity grafting. Surgery 1937;1:535.
5. McIndoe A: The treatment of congenital absence and obliterative conditions of the vagina. Br J Plast Surg 1950;2:254.
6. Conway H, Stark RB: Construction and reconstruction of the vagina. Surg Gynecol Obstet 1953;97:573.
7. Sneguireff WF: Zwei neu Falle von Restitutio Vaginiae per Transplantationen Ani et Recti. Zentralbl Gynakol 1904;28:772.
8. Popow DD, 1910. Cited by Meyer HW: Kolpo-plastik. Zentralbl Gynakol 1918;37:639.
9. Schubert G: Concerning the formation of a new vagina in the case of congenital malformation. Surg Gynecol Obstet 1914;193:376.
10. Baldwin JF: The formation of an artificial vagina by intestinal transplantation. Ann Surg 1904;40:398.
11. Frank RT, Geist SH: Formation of an artificial vagina by a new plastic technique. Am J Obstet Gynecol 1927;14:712.
12. Horton CE, Sadove RC, McCraw JB: Reconstruction of female genital defects. Plast Surg 1990;6:4203-4212.
13. Sadove RC, Horton CE: Utilizing full-thickness skin grafts for vaginal reconstruction. Clin Plast Surg 1988;15:443-448.
14. Knapstein PG, Friedberg V, Sevin BU: Reconstructive Surgery in Gynecology. New York, Thieme, 1990:30-32.
15. Hatch KD: Construction of a neovagina after exenteration using the vulvobulbocavernosus myocutaneous graft. Obstet Gynecol 1984;63:110-114.
16. Wee JT, Joseph VT: A new technique for vaginal reconstruction using neurovascular pudendal thigh flaps: a preliminary report. Plast Reconstr Surg 1989;83:701-709.
17. Soper JT, Berchuck A, Creasman WT, Clarke-Pearson DL: Pelvic exenteration: factors associated with major surgical morbidity. Gynecol Oncol 1989;35:93-98.
18. Carlson JW, Soisson AP, Fowler JM, et al: Rectus abdominis myocutaneous flap for primary vaginal reconstruction. Gynecol Oncol 1993;51:323-329.
19. Benson C, Soisson AP, Carlson J, et al: Neovaginal reconstruction with a rectus abdominis myocutaneous flap. Obstet Gynecol 1993;81(pt 2):871-875.
20. Lacey CG, Stern JL, Feigenbaum S, et al: Vaginal reconstruction after exenteration with use of gracilis myocutaneous flaps. The University of California, San Francisco experience. Am J Obstet Gynecol 1988;158(pt 1):1278-1284.
21. Owens N: A compound neck pedicle designed for the repair of massive facial defects. Plast Reconstr Surg 1955;15:369.

22. Bakamjian V: A technique for primary reconstruction of the palate after radical maxillectomy for cancer. Plast Reconstr Surg 1963;31:103.
23. Hueston JJ, McConchie IH: A compound pectoral flap. Aust N Z J Surg 1968;38:61.
24. McCraw J, Massey F, Shankin K, Horton C: Vaginal reconstruction using gracilis myocutaneous flaps. Plast Reconstr Surg 1976;58:176.
25. Lesavoy MA, Dubrow TJ, Korn HN, et al: "Sensible" flap coverage for pressure sores in patients with meningomyelocele. Plast Reconstr Surg 1990;85:390-394.
26. Hatch KD: Neovaginal reconstruction. Cancer 1993;71(suppl): 1660-1663.
27. McCraw J, Kemp G, Givens F, Horton CE: Correction of high pelvic defects with the inferiorly based rectus abdominis myocutaneous flap. Clin Plast Surg 1988;15:449-454.
28. Pursell SH, Day TG Jr, Tobin GR: Distally based rectus abdominis flap for reconstruction in radical gynecologic procedures. Gynecol Oncol 1990;37:234-238.
29. Tobin GR, Day TG: Vaginal and pelvic reconstruction with distally based rectus abdominis myocutaneous flaps. Plast Reconstr Surg 1988;81:62-73.
30. Lesavoy MA: Vaginal reconstruction. Clin Obstet Gynecol 1985;12:515-525.
31. Lesavoy MA: Vaginal reconstruction. Urol Clin North Am 1985;12:369-379.
32. Caparo VJ: Congenital anomalies. Clin Obstet Gynecol 1971;14:988.
33. Radman HM: Hypertrophy of the labia minora. Clin Obstet Gynecol 1976;48(suppl 1):78S.
34. Hodgkinson DJ, Hait G: Aesthetic vaginal labioplasty. Plast Reconstr Surg 1984;74:414.
35. Alter GJ: A new technique for aesthetic labia minora reduction. Ann Plast Surg 1998;40:287.

CHAPTER

155

Reconstruction of Acquired Vaginal Defects

PETER G. CORDEIRO, MD, FACS ✦ ANDREA L. PUSIC, MD, MHS, FRCSC

IDENTIFICATION OF THE PROBLEM

Acquired vaginal defects most commonly result from resection of pelvic malignant neoplasms. Advanced colorectal carcinomas frequently involve the posterior vaginal wall, and carcinoma of the bladder may extend into the anterior vaginal wall. Primary sarcomas of the vaginal wall may result in any number of vaginal defects; local extension or recurrence of uterine or cervical malignant neoplasms can necessitate pelvic exenteration and total vaginal resection. Whereas trauma and burns may also result in vaginal distortion and defects, these are much less common causes given the relatively protected position of the vagina.

Irrespective of their etiology, vaginal defects may range from small mucosal defects to total circumferential loss. In addition, tumor ablation may necessitate resection of vulvar and perineal soft tissue, further complicating reconstruction. Although reconstruction is frequently performed at the time of the oncologic resection, delayed procedures are not uncommon. Scarring and soft tissue contracture may then add to the technical difficulty of the reconstruction.

SCOPE AND COMPONENT PARTS OF THE PROBLEM

Whereas small partial vaginal defects are common and usually repaired primarily, larger defects requiring flap reconstruction are most often treated at oncology referral centers. Two recent trends have affected the nature of pelvic reconstruction after ablative surgery. Gynecologic malignant neoplasms are now being diagnosed at earlier stages in a progressively younger population of patients.[1,2] Maintenance of sexual function and prevention of the psychological sequelae of surgery are vital to these younger patients. In addition, more frequent use of adjuvant radiation and chemotherapy has led to increased early survival.[3,4] A percentage of these patients will ultimately have local recurrence of their disease. Further resection and reconstruction are then complicated by the previous surgery and irradiation.

When pelvic exenteration was first performed in the 1940s, the operative mortality was greater than 20%.[5] Today, perioperative mortality is 3% to 5%.[6,7] Notwithstanding this decrease in operative mortality, pelvic exenteration continues to be a major physiologic and anatomic insult. From a hemodynamic perspective alone, the defect has been equated to a 20% body surface burn and can lead to significant fluid sequestration.[8] In addition, postoperative complications continue to be common. Crowe et al[6] reported significant morbidity in more than 50% of patients. Even with flap reconstruction to improve vascularity and to decrease dead space, infection may occur in 9% to 11% and delayed wound healing in up to 46%. Intestinal adhesions, fistulas, and pelvic herniation are additional significant problems.[9] Preoperative and perioperative irradiation further increases the likelihood of these complications.

Although poor tissue vascularity, dead space, and loss of pelvic support are the main causes of problems in the early postoperative period, long-term issues relating to sexual function and body image are also considerable. After pelvic exenteration, 5-year survival among patients with gynecologic cancer is 40% to 60%.

Among colorectal patients, 5-year survival is 25% to 40%.[6] For this group of patients who do well with their disease, sexual function and body image are fundamental quality of life issues.

ANATOMY

Pelvic Anatomy

The close anatomic relationship between the bladder, vagina, and rectum needs to be well appreciated by the reconstructive surgeon. Ligamentous support of these organs is interrelated, and surgical dissection of any one structure may lead to prolapse and herniation of the remaining components. In addition, pelvic exenteration may disrupt or devascularize the pelvic floor musculature. The pelvic sidewalls define a fixed anatomic space that, once it is cleared of the pelvic organs, will either delineate a dead space or invite small bowel prolapse and adhesions.

The vagina is essentially a distensible cylindrical pouch (Fig. 155-1). Normal length is 6 to 7.5 cm along its anterior wall and 9 cm along the posterior wall.[10] It is constricted at the introitus, dilated in the middle, and narrowed near its uterine extremity. In its normal anatomic position, the vagina tilts posteriorly as it extends up into the pelvis, forming a 90-degree angle with the uterus. Careful orientation of the neovagina is important to successful reconstruction and ultimate sexual function. The introitus is a frequent site of contracture after reconstruction, and any distortion of its normal position relative to other structures such as the urethral orifice, perineal body, and anus should be addressed. If no resection of the external vulva and perineum is required, great care must be taken to avoid their distortion because this may also have an impact on sexual function and body image.

Classification of Defects Based on Anatomy

The classification of acquired vaginal defects is based on their anatomic location (see Fig. 155-1). This classification will ultimately guide reconstructive efforts. There are two basic types of defect, partial (type I) and circumferential (type II). These can be further subclassified. Type IA defects are partial and involve the anterior or lateral wall. Such defects result from resection of urinary tract malignant neoplasms or primary malignant neoplasms of the vaginal wall. Type IB defects are also partial but involve the posterior vaginal wall. These defects result primarily from extension of colorectal carcinomas and are perhaps the most common defects with which the reconstructive surgeon will be asked to deal. Type IIA defects are circumferential defects involving the upper two thirds of the vagina. Uterine and cervical diseases are frequently the cause. Type IIB defects represent circumferential, total vaginal resection and are generally the result of pelvic exenteration. In addition to the considerable soft tissue loss and dead space, the introitus can also be distorted by this defect.

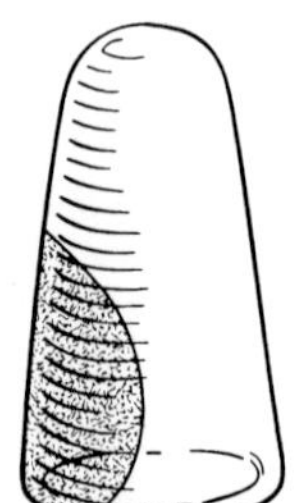

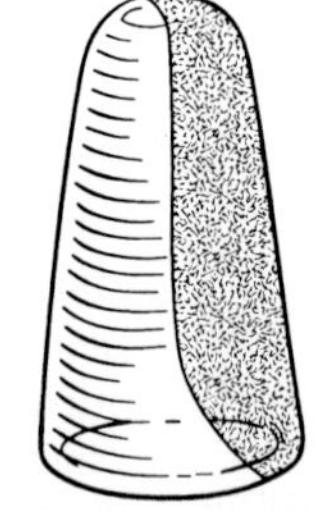

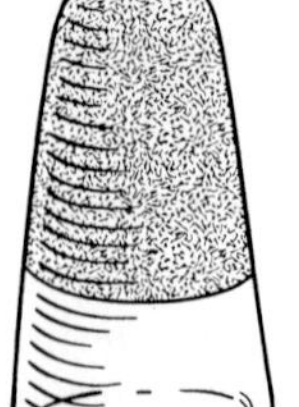

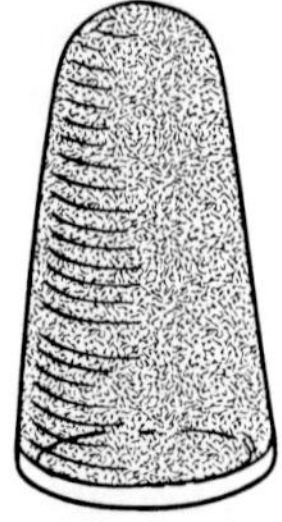

FIGURE 155-1. Classification of acquired vaginal defects. The vagina is essentially a cylindrical pouch. Defects are either partial (type I) or circumferential (type II).

APPROPRIATE CONSULTATIONS

Successful management of patients undergoing vaginal reconstruction is clearly dependent on a multidisciplinary approach. The oncologic and reconstructive surgeons need to communicate well in terms of both the expected defect and the possible reconstructive options. Both the anesthesia and critical care teams need to be well advised of the nature of the procedure and the hemodynamic stress that can be expected.

The radiation oncologist is an important participant in the overall treatment plan. Many patients have had previous radiation therapy, and it is important to be aware of the previous radiation portals. In addition, intraoperative irradiation and occasionally brachytherapy catheter placement can occur at the time of tumor resection. This has important implications for choice of flap because both recipient and donor sites can be affected by radiation injury. The medical oncologist is also involved with decision-making because patients may receive both preoperative and postoperative chemotherapy. Surgical procedures should be optimally timed to minimize chemotherapy effects on wound healing.

Most important to the ultimate success of the reconstruction is the full and informed involvement of the patient and her family. Despite the most anatomic reconstruction, vaginal resection can have significant psychological morbidity. Ratliff et al[11] investigated sexual adjustment after vaginal reconstruction with gracilis myocutaneous flaps and found that although 70% of patients were judged to have physically adequate vaginas, less than 50% resumed sexual activity. Absence of pleasure (37%), problems with vaginal dryness (32%), excess secretions (27%), self-consciousness about ostomies (40%), and nudity (30%) were all considerable concerns. Preoperative and postoperative sexual counseling has been suggested as the most likely way of positively influencing these outcomes and giving patients the best hope of functional and psychological recovery. The psychologist should thus be an integral part of the ablative-reconstructive team. In addition, at most tertiary care institutions, specialized nursing teams help the patient and her family prepare for and adjust to the significant perioperative psychosocial distress that they experience.

TABLE 155-1 ✦ THE GOALS OF VAGINAL RECONSTRUCTION

To promote rapid wound healing, facilitating postoperative radiation therapy and chemotherapy
To decrease pelvic dead space, thus decreasing fluid loss, metabolic demands, and infection
To restore the pelvic floor, preventing herniation and small bowel fistula
To re-establish normal sexual function and body image

TREATMENT

There are four basic goals in vaginal reconstruction (Table 155-1). Selection of the optimal reconstructive method to achieve these goals is based on the type of defect and characteristics of the patient. Small defects that can be closed without tension will ideally be closed primarily. In the case of an irradiated wound, however, one must proceed cautiously with primary closure. Rarely is skin grafting alone an adequate alternative in oncology patients.

Proceeding along the reconstructive ladder, regional flaps continue to be the most frequently used and effective of procedures. Many flaps have been described, none of which is ideal for all defect types. To simplify surgical decision-making, a reconstructive algorithm can be developed on the basis of defect type (Fig. 155-2).

Type IA defects, which involve only the anterior or lateral vaginal walls, usually require little tissue bulk and small to moderate surface coverage. The modified

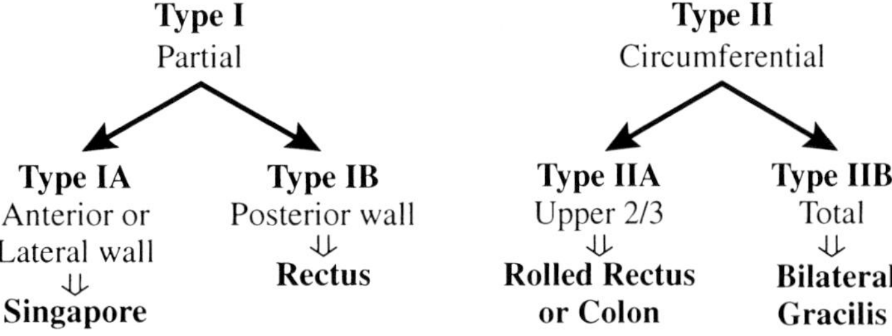

FIGURE 155-2. Algorithm for reconstruction of the vagina based on defect type.

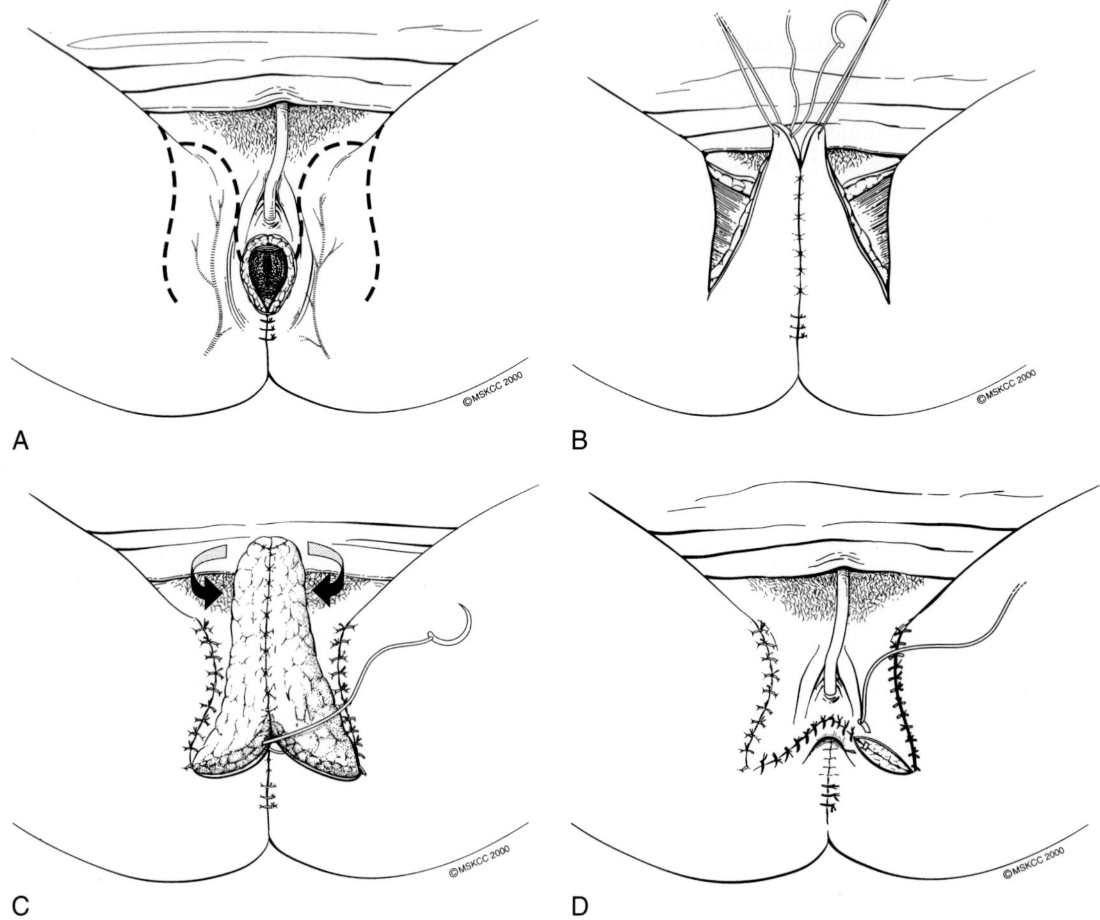

FIGURE 155-3. *A,* Modified Singapore flap design within groin creases. Note location of posterior labial arteries. Unilateral flap can be designed to reconstruct lateral or anterior defects. *B,* Bilateral fasciocutaneous flap elevated and sutured together in the midline. Note flap elevation at the level of the adductor muscles. *C,* Flaps sutured together to form neovaginal pouch. Note primary closure of donor site within the groin creases. *D,* Final inset of flap to reconstruct the introitus.

Singapore (vulvoperineal or pudendal thigh) fasciocutaneous flap is ideal in this setting. It provides a highly vascularized, reliable, thin, and pliable flap that conforms well to the surface of the vaginal cylinder. This flap is based on the posterior labial arteries and innervated by posterior labial branches of the pudendal nerve as well as by perineal branches of the posterior cutaneous nerve of the thigh.[12] The flaps are raised in the thigh crease, lateral to the hair-bearing labia majora, and may be designed to measure 9 × 4 cm to 15 × 6 cm.[13,14] The posterior skin margin is marked at the level of the posterior fourchette (Fig. 155-3*A*). The skin, subcutaneous tissue, deep fascia of the thigh, and epimysium of the adductor muscles are raised (Fig. 155-3*B*). Posteriorly, the base of the flap is undermined at the subcutaneous level to facilitate rotation and insetting. Depending on the defect, unilateral or bilateral flaps may be developed (Fig. 155-3*C*). The flaps may be inset by tunneling under the labia majora or by division of the labia at the level of the fourchette. The donor site is closed primarily (Figs. 155-3*D* and 155-4).

Type IB defects, which encompass the posterior vaginal wall, frequently require greater soft tissue bulk to fill the dead space made by resection of the rectum. Here, the pedicled rectus myocutaneous flap is a preferred choice. This highly reliable flap provides both a large surface area and volume. The skin can easily replace the entire posterior vaginal wall. The healthy muscle and subcutaneous tissue bring well-vascularized tissue to the pelvis, obliterate dead space, and separate the contents of the abdominal cavity from the zone of injury. When it is used for vaginal reconstruction, the flap is based on the deep inferior epigastric vessels that arise from the common femoral arteries and enter the rectus muscle along its

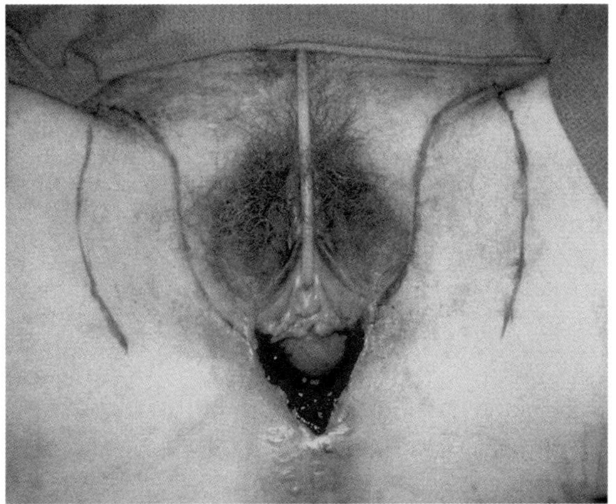

A

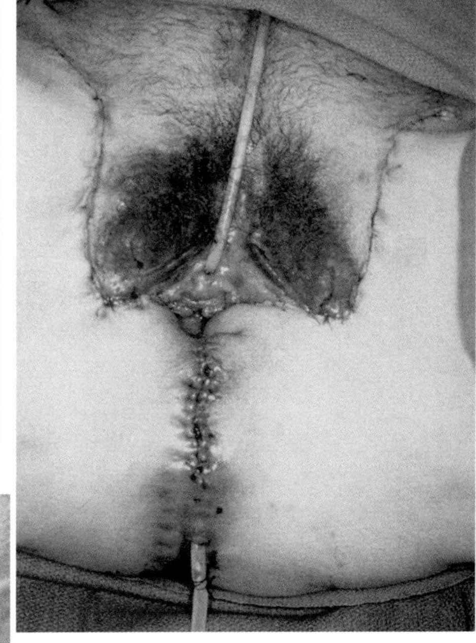

C

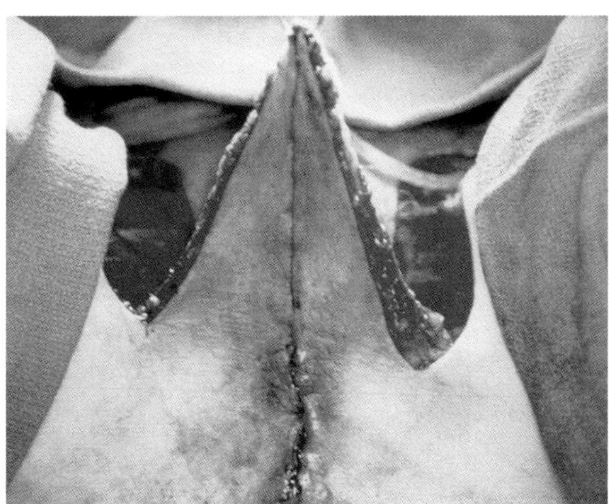

B

FIGURE 155-4. *A*, Bilateral modified Singapore flaps designed to reconstruct a posterior vaginal defect. *B*, Flaps elevated and sutured together in midline. *C*, Flaps inset into the perineal defect.

posterolateral surface 6 to 7 cm above its insertion on the pubis (Fig. 155-5*A*).[8] In planning the flap, one must ensure that these vessels are not divided as part of the cancer resection. Musculocutaneous perforators within an 8-cm radius of the umbilicus predominantly perfuse the skin overlying the muscle. Either the vertical or transverse skin island design may be used, depending on the size of the defect and the characteristics of the patient's abdominal wall. For posterior wall reconstruction, the vertical rectus abdominis myocutaneous (VRAM) design is preferable because it maximizes blood supply by centering the skin island over the muscle and does not interfere with the contralateral muscle and stoma placement. Both the vertical and transverse rectus abdominis myocutaneous flaps can generally be designed up to 10 × 20 cm in size with easy donor site closure. When the flap is inset into a posterior wall defect, care must be taken to avoid any constriction or tension on the vascular pedicle because this is the principal cause of flap failure (Fig. 155-5*B* to *D*).

Type IIA defects are circumferential defects involving the upper two thirds of the vagina, and like type IB defects, they are well reconstructed with the pedicled rectus myocutaneous flap. The myocutaneous flap again provides the necessary skin and soft tissue bulk. It is preferred to bilateral gracilis flaps because the intervening vulvar and pelvic floor musculature prohibits transfer of muscles from the thigh. In this situation, the cutaneous portion of the flap is "tubed." A transverse skin island is easier to manipulate and leaves a slightly longer muscle pedicle than does the VRAM (Fig. 155-6*A*). A flap width of 12 to 15 cm will provide a neovagina with a 4-cm diameter (Fig. 155-6*B*).[15] Once tubed, the flap is then sutured to the remaining vaginal cuff from above (Fig. 155-6*C*).

Sigmoid colon may also be used to reconstruct type IIA defects for patients in whom a rectus flap cannot

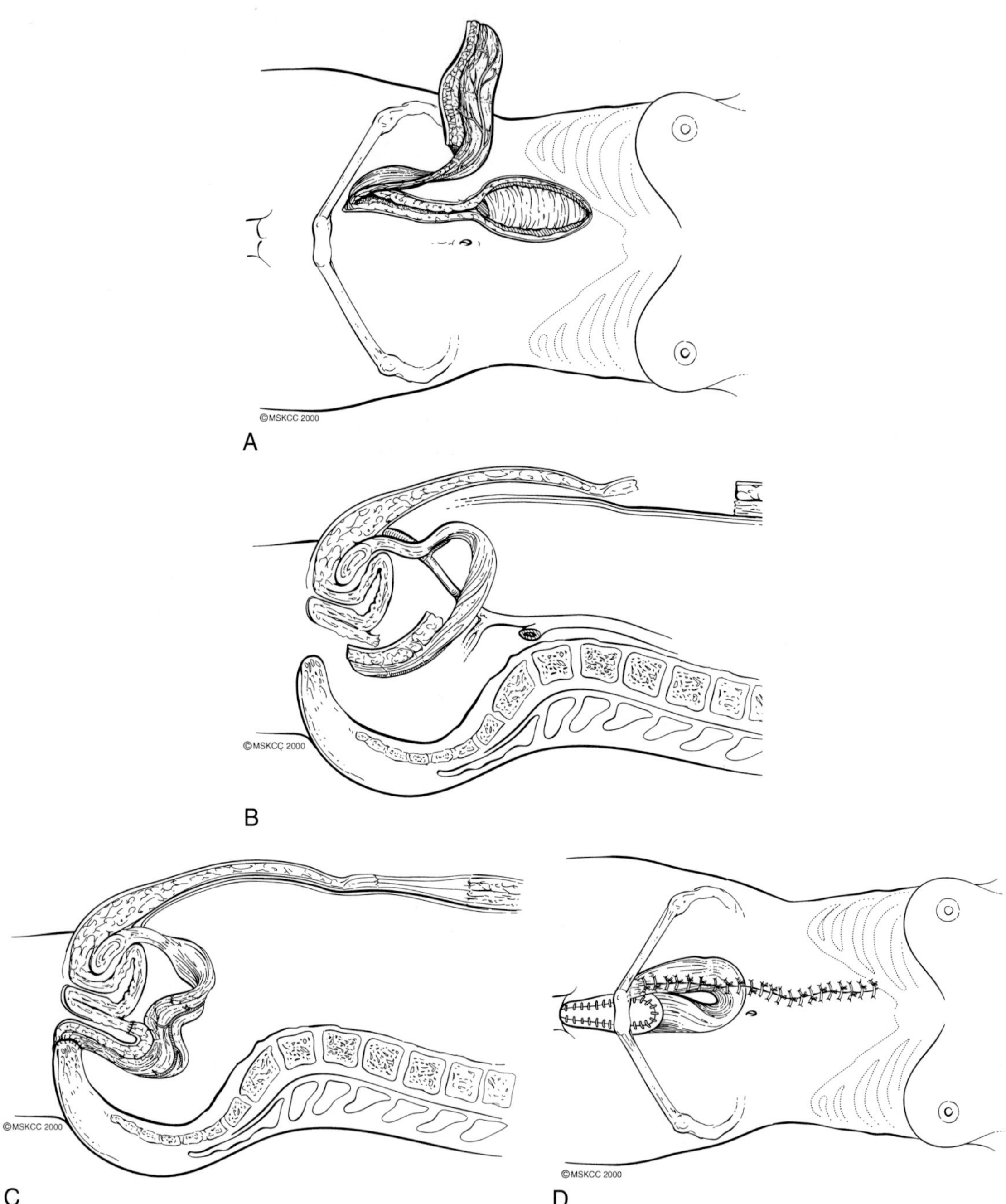

FIGURE 155-5. *A,* The vertical rectus myocutaneous flap designed and elevated on the right rectus muscle. Note cephalad location of skin island, which allows a longer muscle pedicle. *B,* VRAM flap rotated into posterior pelvis. *C,* VRAM flap inset. Note the skin island used to reconstruct posterior vaginal wall and the muscle and subcutaneous tissue used to fill pelvis. *D,* Anterior view showing flap inset and donor site closure.

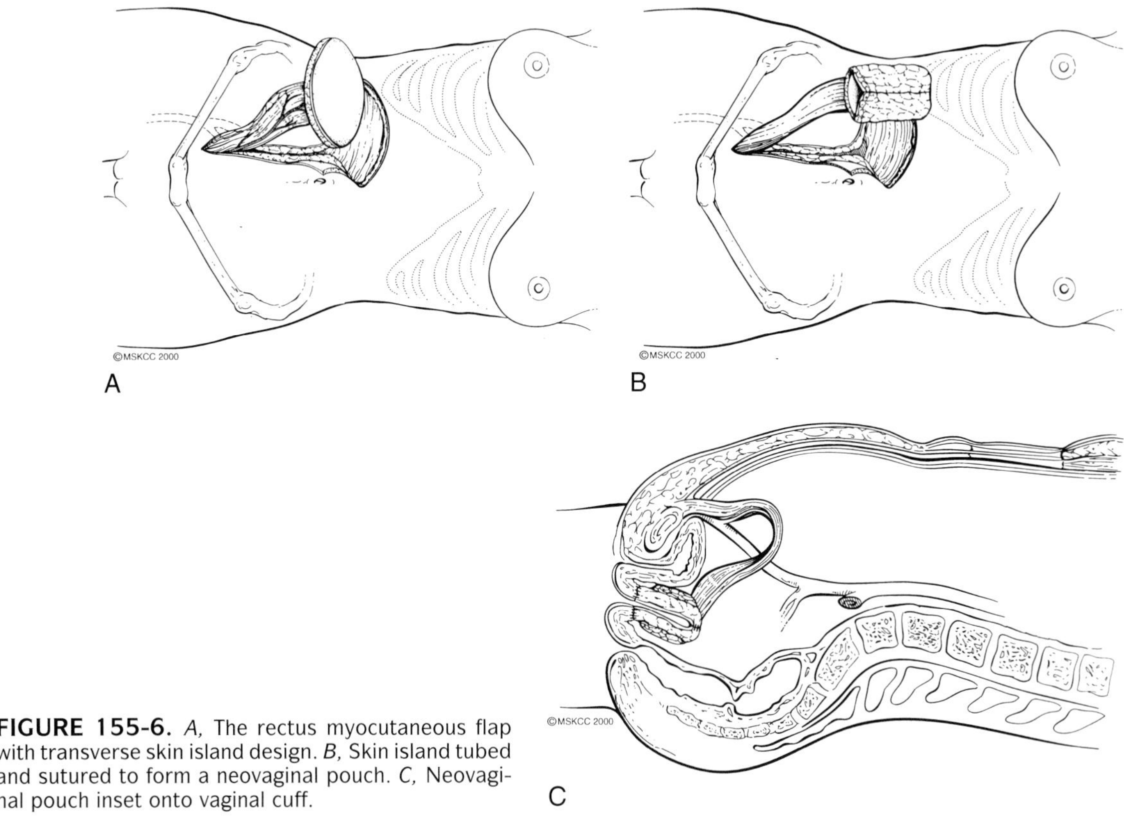

FIGURE 155-6. *A,* The rectus myocutaneous flap with transverse skin island design. *B,* Skin island tubed and sutured to form a neovaginal pouch. *C,* Neovaginal pouch inset onto vaginal cuff.

be performed. A segment of the colon is isolated and pedicled on a branch of the inferior mesenteric artery.[16] This portion is then stapled closed superiorly and sutured inferiorly to the vaginal cuff. Excessive secretions and unpleasant odor persist as common complaints of patients and limit the usefulness of this technique.[17]

Type IIB defects are circumferential defects involving the entire vagina and frequently the introitus. These are usually total pelvic exenteration defects. Given the need for a large skin island, bilateral gracilis flaps are an excellent reconstructive choice. The subcutaneous tissue and muscle of the two conjoined flaps will also provide a large volume of soft tissue that completely fills the pelvis. The vascular supply of the flap is the medial femoral circumflex artery, which enters the gracilis muscle 7 to 10 cm below the pubic tubercle (Fig. 155-7*A*).[9] An elliptical skin island 6 × 20 cm can be designed over the proximal two thirds of the muscle, with the anterior border of the incision lying on a line between the pubic tubercle and the semitendinosus tendon. Once elevated, the flaps are tunneled subcutaneously into the vaginal defect (Fig. 155-7*B* and *C*). The flaps are then sutured together in the midline, and a neovaginal pouch is formed (Fig. 155-7*D* and *E*). This pouch is then inserted into the defect, and the proximal flap edges are sutured to the introitus (Fig. 155-7*F*). The flaps can maintain some pressure sensibility through branches of the obturator nerve (Fig. 155-8).[17]

Flap selection is based on both the type of defect and the individual patient's characteristics. Whereas the majority of patients can be reconstructed by use of the algorithm based on the type of defect, a few may require a modified approach. Obesity, for example, has been shown to be a significant risk factor for poor wound healing after rectus flap reconstruction because of decreased reliability of the skin paddle.[9] Therefore, in obese patients, type IB defects are sometimes better reconstructed with thin, bilateral Singapore flaps (see Fig. 155-4). Alternatively, for a type IIA defect, the rectus flap may be raised without its cutaneous portion and a skin graft applied directly to the muscle over a vaginal stent. This, however, should be considered only in rare cases. In heavily irradiated patients, the rectus flap may be desirable even for small defects because its muscle bulk will aid pelvic revascularization. In elderly patients or patients with significant comorbid conditions who are unlikely to resume intercourse after reconstruction, a full reconstruction of the vaginal vault may be omitted. Placement of the rectus flap into the pelvis without its skin paddle may, however,

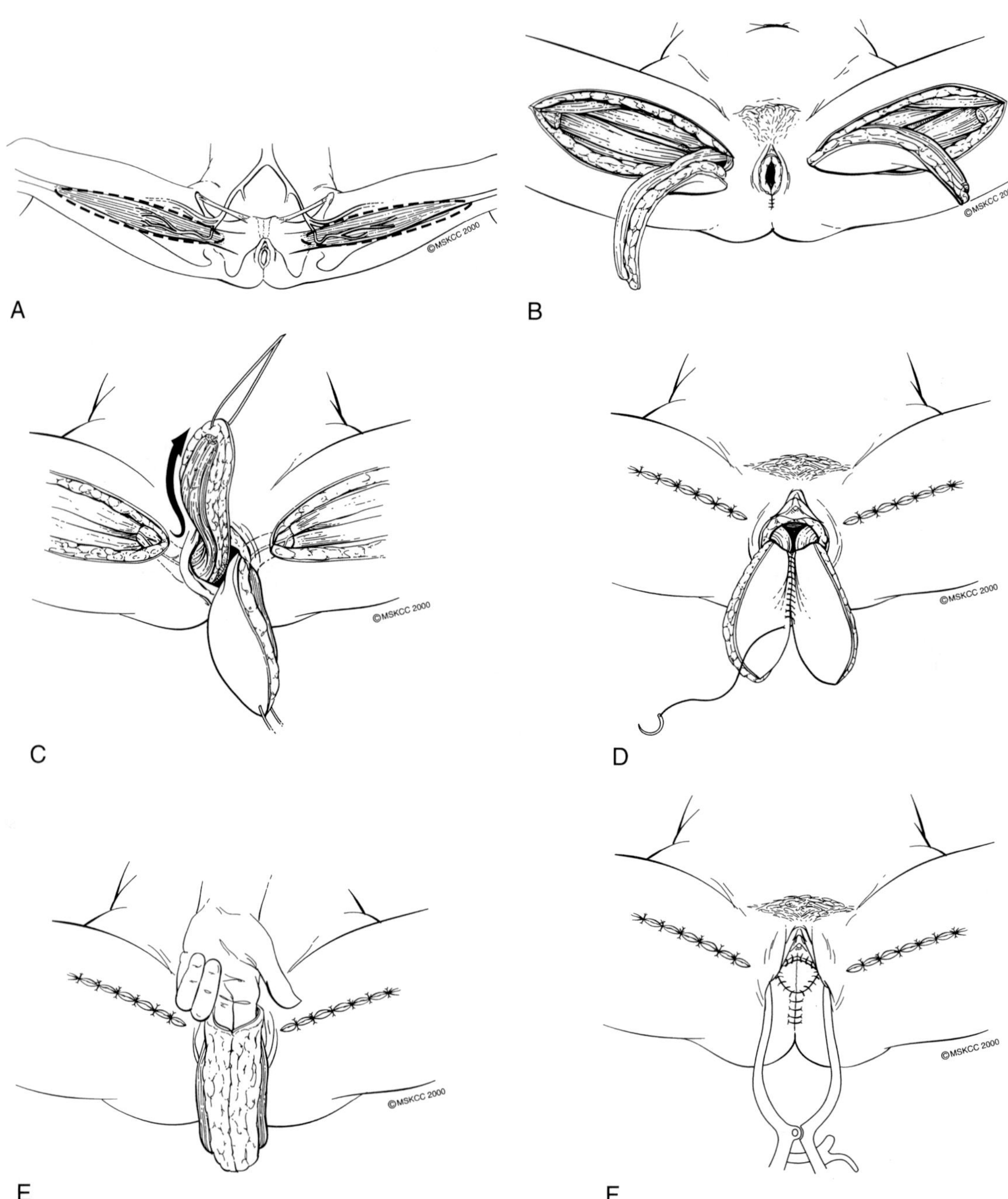

FIGURE 155-7. *A,* Bilateral gracilis myocutaneous flap design for a total pelvic exenteration defect. *B,* Gracilis myocutaneous flaps elevated. *C,* Myocutaneous flaps rotated into perineal defect. Note point of rotation at the medial femoral circumflex vessels. *D,* Posterior borders of skin islands sutured together in the midline. *E,* Anterior borders of flaps sutured together to complete formation of neovaginal pouch. Note the substantial bulk of the two conjoined flaps. *F,* Final inset of neovaginal pouch to reconstruct introitus.

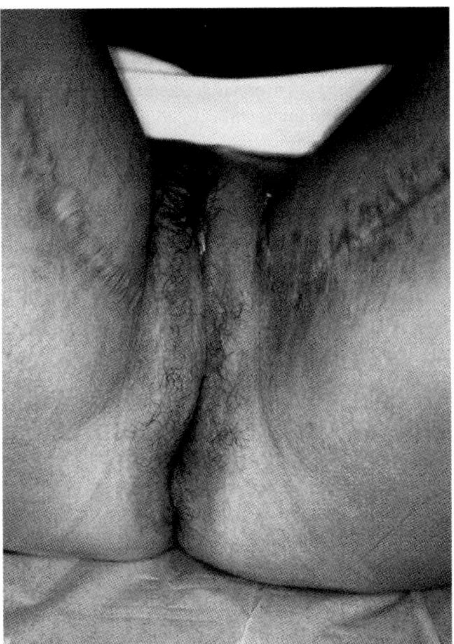

A

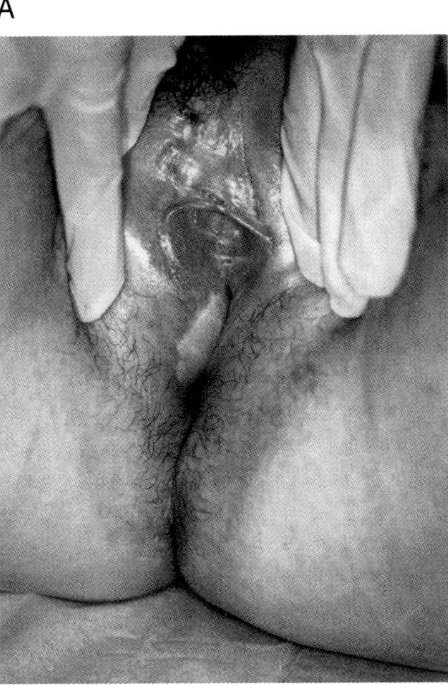

B

FIGURE 155-8. *A,* Final external appearance of bilateral gracilis flap reconstruction of a total pelvic exenteration defect. Note the nearly normal appearance of the perineum. Unsightly donor site scars are not uncommon with this type of reconstruction. *B,* Appearance of the introitus. Note junction of proximal right skin island with labia majora and adequate introital diameter.

still be beneficial as a means of decreasing dead space and infection. In patients with previous vaginal reconstruction and recurrent disease, the choice of regional flaps may be extremely limited. In this situation, free flap reconstruction may be considered.

COMPLICATIONS AND THEIR MANAGEMENT

The principal early complications after vaginal reconstruction include infection, delayed wound healing, and flap loss. Whereas the risk of infection and pelvic abscess is decreased when flap reconstruction is performed after vaginal resection, it still remains significant at approximately 10%.[7,18] Perioperative antibiotics, adequate irrigation, and careful drain placement are all important preventive measures. Once a pelvic infection is established, percutaneous or operative drainage is generally necessary to prevent worsening sepsis.

The incidence of delayed wound healing varies widely in the literature, ranging up to 46% of patients.[19] Radiotherapy, obesity, and smoking are all risk factors that should be considered preoperatively.[19] The most common location for wound separation is at the posterior perineal closure site, and this usually responds to conservative management. In rare cases, surgical revision may be needed.

Flap loss, both partial and complete, is a major postoperative problem that will delay adjuvant therapy and increase morbidity of the patient. The incidence of flap loss depends on the type of flap used, surgical technique, and characteristics of the patient. When it is used for vaginal reconstruction, the vertical rectus flap is highly reliable with a less than 5% incidence of total flap loss; gracilis myocutaneous flaps are less reliable and have a 10% to 20% incidence of skin loss.[20] The success rate with both these flaps depends on careful attention to design and surgical technique. The modified Singapore flap is susceptible to apical necrosis, but complete loss occurs in less than 15%.[12] Partial flap loss may occasionally be managed by débridement and local wound care. In the setting of irradiated tissue or complete flap loss, full débridement and reconstruction with an alternative flap are required.

There are many potential late complications described; however, these are infrequent and minor, and they tend to be functional in nature. These include inadequate or excessive vaginal secretions, inadequate or excessive vaginal size, flap prolapse, vaginal or donor site dysesthesia, hypertrophic donor site scarring, urinary and bowel complaints, and, in the case of rectus reconstruction, abdominal wall hernias. In a review of 44 patients who had undergone bilateral gracilis flap reconstruction, Ratliff et al[11] found that 33% of patients suffered from vaginal dryness, whereas 28% complained of excess secretions. Twenty percent thought that their neovagina was too small, whereas 5% found it to be too large. Eighteen percent had flap prolapse, and a further 18% had pain with intercourse. Late bowel strictures and fistula occurred in 16% of patients in one series.[7] The incidence of abdominal wall hernia can be expected to be less than 10%.[21,22]

Even with careful reconstruction, women who undergo vaginal resection and reconstruction have a significant diminution in sexual function and body image. More than 70% of women can be expected to have anatomically functional vaginas.[11] In spite of this, less than 50% will resume sexual activity.[11] Self-consciousness about ostomies and donor site incisions, lack of pleasure, and anatomic complaints related to vaginal size and secretion are all considerable. In addition, these women must deal with the psychological stress of their primary diagnoses, adjuvant therapy, and fear of recurrence. To improve these outcomes, preoperative and postoperative counseling is essential.[9,23] Patients and their partners need to be well informed not only about the risks and complications of the reconstruction but also about the psychological struggle that lies ahead. A supportive, multidisciplinary health care team, which includes a psychologist or sexual therapist, is key to achieving an optimal outcome.

REFERENCES

1. Mody DR, Davey DD, Branca M, et al: Quality assurance and risk reduction guidelines. Acta Cytol 2000;44:496-507.
2. Yamada SD, McGonigle KF: Cancer of the endometrium and corpus uteri. Curr Opin Obstet Gynecol 1998;10:57-60.
3. Eifel PJ: Chemoradiation for carcinoma of the cervix: advances and opportunities. Radiat Res 2000;154:229-236.
4. Lai CH, Hong JH, Hsueh S, et al: Preoperative prognostic variables and the impact of postoperative adjuvant therapy on the outcomes of stage IB or II cervical carcinoma patients with or without pelvic lymph node metastases: an analysis of 891 cases. Cancer 1999;85:1537-1546.
5. Brunschwig A: Complete excision of pelvic viscera for advanced carcinoma. A one-stage abdominoperineal operation with end colostomy and bilateral ureteral implantation. Cancer 1948; 1:177-183.
6. Crowe PJ, Temple WJ, Lopez MJ, Ketcham AS: Pelvic exenteration for advanced pelvic malignancy [review]. Semin Surg Oncol 1999;17:152-160.
7. Jakowatz JG, Porudominsky D, Riihimaki DU, et al: Complications of pelvic exenteration. Arch Surg 1985;120:1261-1265.
8. McCraw J, Kemp G, Given F, Horton CE: Correction of high pelvic defects with the inferiorly based rectus abdominis myocutaneous flap. Clin Plast Surg 1988;15:449-454.
9. Small T, Friedman DJ, Sultan M: Reconstructive surgery of the pelvis after surgery for rectal cancer. Semin Surg Oncol 2000; 18:259-264.
10. Gray H: Anatomy of the Human Body, 20th ed. Lewis W, ed. Philadelphia, Lea & Febiger, 2000.
11. Ratliff CR, Gershenson DM, Morris M, et al: Sexual adjustment of women undergoing gracilis myocutaneous flap vaginal reconstruction in conjunction with pelvic exenteration. Cancer 1996; 78:2229-2235.
12. Gleeson NC, Baile W, Roberts WS, et al: Pudendal thigh fasciocutaneous flaps for vaginal reconstruction in gynecologic oncology. Gynecol Oncol 1994;54:269-274.
13. Woods JE, Alter G, Meland B, Podratz K: Experience with vaginal reconstruction utilizing the modified Singapore flap [see comments]. Plast Reconstr Surg 1992;90:270-274.
14. Wee JT, Joseph VT: A new technique of vaginal reconstruction using neurovascular pudendal-thigh flaps: a preliminary report. Plast Reconstr Surg 1989;83:701-709.
15. Tobin GR, Pursell SH, Day TG Jr: Refinements in vaginal reconstruction using rectus abdominis flaps. Clin Plast Surg 1990; 17:705-712.
16. Hendren WH, Atala A: Use of bowel for vaginal reconstruction. J Urol 1994;152(pt 2):752-755.
17. Martello JY, Vasconez HC: Vulvar and vaginal reconstruction after surgical treatment for gynecologic cancer [review]. Clin Plast Surg 1995;22:129-140.
18. Shibata D, Hyland W, Busse P, et al: Immediate reconstruction of the perineal wound with gracilis muscle flaps following abdominoperineal resection and intraoperative radiation therapy for recurrent carcinoma of the rectum [see comments]. Ann Surg Oncol 1999;6:33-37.
19. de Haas WG, Miller MJ, Temple WJ, et al: Perineal wound closure with the rectus abdominis musculocutaneous flap after tumor ablation. Ann Surg Oncol 1995;2:400-406.
20. Soper JT, Rodriguez G, Berchuck A, Clarke-Pearson DL: Long and short gracilis myocutaneous flaps for vulvovaginal reconstruction after radical pelvic surgery: comparison of flap-specific complications. Gynecol Oncol 1995;56:271-275.
21. Kroll SS, Marchi M: Comparison of strategies for preventing abdominal-wall weakness after TRAM flap breast reconstruction. Plast Reconstr Surg 1992;89:1045-1051.
22. Reece GP, Kroll SS: Abdominal wall complications. Prevention and treatment. Clin Plast Surg 1998;25:235-249.
23. Gleeson N, Baile W, Roberts WS, et al: Surgical and psychosexual outcome following vaginal reconstruction with pelvic exenteration. Eur J Gynaecol Oncol 1994;15:89-95.

CHAPTER

156

Surgery for Gender Identity Disorder

David Kaufman, MD ✦ Judy Van Maasdam, MA ✦ Donald R. Laub, Sr., MD, FACS

BACKGROUND

Gender identity disorder (DSM-IV 302.85) is a unique human condition that is classified behaviorally but treated medically by hormones and surgery. Treatment is self-rehabilitation through a multidisciplinary team approach, with the final step of the traditional triadic sequence being sex reassignment surgery. Plastic and reconstructive surgeons most familiar with body image change surgery and its psychology often provide the ultimate step in this complete human transformation. Plastic and reconstructive surgical applications in this field are far-reaching, encompass the entire body, and in effect provide the mechanism for total body transformation for sex to meet body image. Improved function and appearance in accordance with the patient's perceived gender enhance dignity, self-confidence, productivity, and overall happiness. Data suggest that properly selected patients who participate in a well-organized gender dysphoria program demonstrate significant improvements in lifestyle, social relationships, sense of self-esteem, body image, employment status, and sexual adjustment.[1]

HISTORY

History is replete with evidence of transsexualism and its treatment. Venus Castina, a Greek goddess, was portrayed to respond with sympathy and understanding to the yearnings and misunderstandings of female souls locked in male bodies.[2] Greek mythology also dramatized myths of sex change. Tiresias, a Theban soothsayer, was changed from a man to a woman for punishment, only later to be returned to male form when he reported a 10-fold increase in female pleasure during intercourse. The Romans were the first historically to record sex change surgery. Sporus, an ex-slave, underwent gender reassignment and subsequently became the wife of Nero, the last Caesar.[3]

Many of the modern techniques used in gender confirmation surgery were born of reconstructive surgery for traumatic and congenital deformities. In 1832, a young girl with vaginal agenesis was treated with repeated strong digital pressure on the vesicorectal septum to create a passage. Refinements in treatment of ambiguous genitalia states, such as congenital adrenal hyperplasia and severe hypospadias, have significantly contributed to our body of knowledge. Further advancements in microsurgery have allowed free tissue transfer to play a vital role in these complex reconstructions. Surgery for gender identification disorder is founded on the fundamental principles of patient management and plastic surgery theory.

Before the 1950s, isolated case reports of this type of surgery were published but were largely relegated to medical journals. However, in the early 1950s, transsexualism aroused widespread interest in the United States when the story of Christina Jorgensen made national news. Christina (formerly George) Jorgensen was a male-to-female transsexual who had undergone a gradual transformation from man to woman. She had completed a trial of cross-living and had been taking female hormones. To the outside world, she was a woman. She went to Denmark in 1953 and underwent surgical gender confirmation by Paul Fogh-Andersen, a Danish plastic surgeon. The report of the operation and other aspects of treatment of gender identity disorder were published in the *Journal of the American Medical Association*.[4] She subsequently returned to the United States, and her publicity generated significant medical and public interest in treatment of gender identity disorder.

In 1963, The Johns Hopkins University was first to establish a multidisciplinary center for the treatment and management of this unique phenomenon. It was recognized that treatment of such a complex, multifactorial process must be addressed with specialists working in harmony, and this laid the foundation for treatment of gender identity disorder today.

In 1966, Harry Benjamin wrote the landmark book *The Transsexual Phenomenon*, wherein he delineated the clinical aspects of transsexualism. His groundbreaking effort is still respected today and forms the basis for the understanding of the clinical behavior of persons with gender identity disorder. He chronicled four pervasive characteristics: (1) lifelong conviction of being a member of the opposite sex, psychologically and behaviorally; (2) gender behavior of the opposite sex and early and persistent cross-dressing without erotic feeling; (3) repugnance and disgust for one's genitalia without deriving pleasure from it; and (4) disdain for homosexual behavior. He was honored in the founding of the professional organization that deals with gender identity disorders, the Harry Benjamin International Gender Dysphoria Association.

To further organize and standardize management of gender identity disorder, the Harry Benjamin International Gender Dysphoria Association developed Standards of Care to formally "articulate the organization's professional consensus about the psychiatric, psychological, medical, and surgical management of gender identity disorders." The treatment goal, through use of psychotherapeutic, endocrine, or surgical therapies, is for people with gender identity disorder to achieve lasting comfort with their perceived gender and to maximize well-being and fulfillment.

INCIDENCE AND PREVALENCE

It is difficult to ascertain the extent and scope of gender identity disorder, primarily because of difficulty in obtaining correct estimates of incidence and prevalence. Most transsexuals claim they have felt that they were of the opposite sex for as long as they can remember. Most specialists believe, from clinical experience, that conversion of a transsexual back to his or her biologic sex is almost impossible.[5] This suggests that the psychological sex "wins" over the biologic sex.

European literature suggests that the incidence of transsexualism has remained constant during the last 30 years, whereas the prevalence figures have increased. This indicates an increased acceptance of the phenomenon. Interestingly, the incidence between sexes appears the same, yet the prevalence was 3:1 male-to-female to female-to-male. This indicates that more biologic men undergo transformation. This does not necessitate surgery, however, because surgery is not requisite for transsexualism.

In the United States, the prevalence of transsexualism is approximately 1 : 100,000 men and 1 : 400,000 women. Current estimates suggest that there are between 6,000 and 10,000 transsexuals in the United States. Although these numbers are not completely consistent, the *Diagnostic and Statistical Manual of Mental Disorders* (fourth edition) states that approximately 1 : 30,000 men and 1 : 100,000 women will seek sex reassignment surgery.

MEDICAL MANAGEMENT

Management of patients with gender identity disorder involves many different aspects of medical care. It should be undertaken in a stepwise, planned fashion for which the Harry Benjamin International Gender Dysphoria Association's Standards of Care may serve as a guide. A team approach should be taken to properly address and manage the wide diversity of medical and psychological issues these patients confront. Reference is made to a triadic treatment sequence. This is the trial of cross-living and hormone treatment or manipulation followed by surgical transformation.

The first step in treatment of this behavioral condition is confirming the diagnosis. Gender dysphoria syndrome is the condition in which one has distress or discomfort with his or her gender. It is a broadly reaching diagnosis. It may include those individuals with "nonconformity to stereotypical sex role behaviors," transvestic fetishism, schizophrenia, or other conditions, including gender identity disorder. Patients with gender identity disorder are a subgroup of patients with gender dysphoria, and it is only the trained behavioral health care professional who establishes this diagnosis. The first step in treatment is extensive and sometimes continuous psychological evaluation and treatment of the patient. However, actual "treatment" is largely self-rehabilitation under professional guidance. Recent trends in the treatment of gender identity disorder, however, have focused on the individual needs of each patient. Whereas completion of a strict sequence was once mandated, there is much greater flexibility in treatment plans today. Experts in the field recognize that not all patients need psychotherapy. In the same manner, it is no longer emphasized that a person must go through the entire transformation to be completely "male" or "female." Each patient is individually assessed and may be comfortable with just hormone manipulation, just surgery, or any combination of the traditional triadic sequence.

For those individuals with gender identity disorder who wish to go forward with transformation, a trial of cross-living may be undertaken. Successful psychological functioning while cross-living in the gender of choice for a period of 1 to 2 years is the goal. This period can be both diagnostic and therapeutic in that the patient undergoing the trial will express either satisfaction or dissatisfaction during this test.

Hormone therapy may be undertaken, although the timing is not absolute, once three readiness criteria are satisfied: (1) consolidation of gender identity disorder has occurred during the cross-living trial; (2) other factors have been improved, leading to stable mental health; and (3) hormones will be taken in a responsible fashion. Sometimes, however, this therapy is given before the trial of cross-living. This actually helps individuals during this period in that they are more "passable" as the other sex. Trends in Europe are toward treatment of patients at earlier ages if the diagnosis is appropriately established. This may be begun with blocking agents that temporarily suppress pubertal transformation. Secondary sexual trait suppression allows much more successful gender transformation.

Hormone treatment is used to suppress secondary sexual characteristics of the biologic sex and to induce those of the opposite sex. Once instituted, this therapy should continue lifelong. Complications from this therapy exist, and their risk should be thoroughly understood by the patient before therapy is begun. Hyperprolactinemia, lipid dyscrasia, acne, sleep apnea, liver toxicity, and hypertension are just some of the potential side effects.

The final phase of triadic therapy is surgical gender confirmation. Surgical management differs from patient to patient and is thoroughly discussed in the following sections. Long-term results after gender confirmation surgery demonstrate successful life conversion in this unique population of patients.

ANATOMY AND EMBRYOLOGY

A detailed understanding of the anatomy and embryology of sexual development is necessary to apply the surgical principles involved in surgery for gender identity disorder. Sex is determined by a number of different factors. Chromosomes, gonads, internal and external genitalia, sex hormone patterns, patterns of behavior, rearing, and differentiation all play a role in sexual development (Color Plate 156-1). The embryos of both sexes develop identically until approximately 40 days of gestation. Each has an undifferentiated gonad, müllerian and wolffian ducts, and a urogenital sinus. Gonads then differentiate on the basis of the presence or absence of a Y chromosome protein product, testis-determining factor. With testis-determining factor, the undifferentiated gonad will develop into a testis. In the absence of testis-determining factor, an ovary will develop (Table 156-1).

Subsequent male phenotypic development is predicated on hormone secretions of the differentiating gonad. The müllerian duct atrophies, and the wolffian duct becomes the ductus deferens. The urogenital sinus evolves to the prostate and seminal vesicle. The genital tubercle and urogenital fold become the glans and shaft of the penis, respectively.

Female development results from transformation of the müllerian duct into the fallopian tube with degeneration of the wolffian duct. The clitoris results from the genital tubercle, the labia minora from the urethral fold and groove.

It is important to understand the analogous structures of development. Whereas the internal genitalia, with the exception of the gonads, evolve from two separate embryologic tissues (wolffian and müllerian

TABLE 156-1 ✦ CRITERIA FOR DETERMINATION OF SEX

Parameter	Time	Criteria
Chromosomal sex	Moment of conception	XX or XY chromosome
Gonads	45 days	H-Y antigen
Internal genitalia	First 3 months	Testosterone + müllerian duct inhibitor
External genitalia	First 6 months	Tissue receptors, 5-dihydromethyl testosterone
Sex hormone patterns	Fetal life and up to menarche	Pulsatile FSH and LH vs. nonpulsatile
Pattern of behavior centers	Prenatally or perinatally	Sex-dimorphic differentiation
Sex of assignment and rearing	Imprinting by the environment	Sex-dimorphic differentiation
Psychosexual differentiation	Lifelong	Gender identity

FSH, follicle-stimulating hormone; LH, luteinizing hormone.

ducts), the external genitalia are derived from the same tissues—the urogenital sinus and grooves. One might consider female external anatomy as "growth-arrested" male anatomy.

When sexual identity is in question, a medical evaluation must rule out disorders of sexual differentiation. These include Klinefelter syndrome, gonadal dysgenesis, congenital adrenal hyperplasia, and others. Although much research has been undertaken to determine a genetic cause of gender identity disorder, no studies to date have identified a genetic linkage, hereditary pattern of inheritance, or other causative factor to explain this behavioral phenomenon. Some studies have implicated changes in the brain found on magnetic resonance imaging and autopsy as possible causative factors. One wonders whether exogenous hormones during the individual's lifetime played a role.

SURGICAL MANAGEMENT: FEMALE TO MALE

The surgical treatment of female-to-male transsexuals may be viewed in components. The goals of the surgeon must be congruent with those of the patient for a successful outcome. Female-to-male patients seeking surgery first and foremost want a sense of wholeness. The surgeon must deeply understand this universal desire. It may be achieved by mastectomy alone or may not be complete until the many components of phalloplasty are attained. Other goals of female-to-male gender confirmation surgery are the following:

- Development of an aesthetic phallus
- Testicle construction with a normal-appearing scrotum
- Maintenance of erogenous sensitivity
- Development of a phallus capable of sexual penetration
- Ability to void in a standing position

There are many phalloplasty and scrotoplasty techniques. This section discusses many options with indications, advantages, disadvantages, and complications of each.

Mastectomy

One of the first surgical procedures performed in female-to-male patients undergoing gender confirmation surgery is mastectomy. This is often done concurrently with hysterectomy and oophorectomy.[5] The surgical goals of this procedure are to remove all breast tissue, to contour the chest wall to the male configuration, and to masculinize the nipple-areola complex. Preservation of nipple viability is not essential but may be achieved through the use of various pedicle techniques. Incision selection is based on the size of the breast. For smaller breasts, periareolar incisions are all that may be necessary. For larger breasts, elliptical excision and even Wise pattern mastectomies may be required to remove larger amounts of excess skin. With Wise pattern or similar pedicles, it may be difficult to achieve complete gland tissue removal. Elliptical excision causes little distortion, and free graft of the 2.8-cm circle of the areola with a mammilla designed by use of a skate flap or star flap carries the bonus of instant nipple sensitivity, although it is not really erogenous. This Laub technique has been performed more than 100 times with success. Some female-to-male patients undergo only mastectomy and hysterectomy-oophorectomy and are satisfied with this as the only surgical procedure.

Phalloplasty

The design of a neophallus is a remarkable surgical undertaking. It encompasses many fundamental principles of plastic and reconstructive surgery. It may use local tissue that has become hypertrophic, such as the clitoris in a metoidioplasty, or it may involve the microvascular transfer of sensate, tubed flaps. The use of local flaps, such as pedicled lower abdominal and groin flaps, is an alternative technique. The decision as to which one to use involves many factors. The surgeon's comfort, the patient's wishes, cost, potential complications, and donor morbidities must be weighed in making such a decision. Overall, surgical development of a functional phallus is often disappointing compared with the excellent results of neocolporrhaphy because of the unique erectile tissue of the penis.[1] Yet, patients undergoing the operation are usually pleased with the result. Most techniques used in phalloplasty have been developed from skills learned in treatment of traumatic loss or used in hypospadias reconstruction.

Metoidioplasty (Greek: *meta,* toward; *oidio,* male genitals; and *plasty,* to form)[6] uses existing tissue to make the neophallus. Male and female external genitalia are of the same embryologic origin, in contradistinction to the internal genitalia. If exposed to the appropriate hormones (specifically testis-determining factor and tissue receptors) during development, the external surface of the labia minora becomes the ventral penis shaft; the internal surface becomes the pendulous urethra and corpus spongiosum. In the same fashion, the clitoris is analogous to glans and ventral penis. When female-to-male patients undergo hormone therapy, these changes occur to some degree.

Surgical completion of this transformation is called metoidioplasty. This requires posterior transposition of the labia majora, fusing them in the midline, and filling them with testicular implants or expanders. The clitoris is moved to a more anterior position by

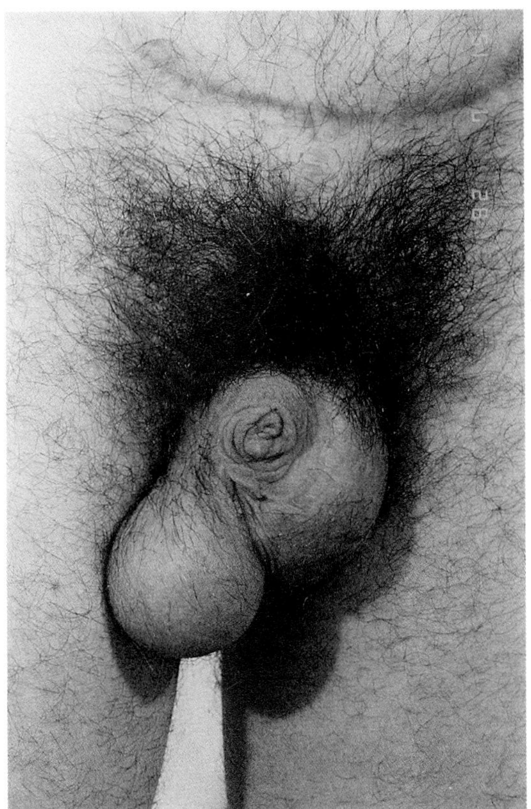

FIGURE 156-1. Postoperative metoidioplasty without urinary extension. In metoidioplasty, the female external genitalia form the male external genitalia according to the embryologic homologues. The labia majora are formed into scrotum, the labia minora are made into ventral penis shaft and pendulous urethra, and the clitoris is formed into the dorsal penis and glans, just as in severe hypospadias. These structures are "transposed." The labia are moved to the midline and paired. The clitoris is moved in the anterior direction after release of the chordee, and the clitoris is "completed" with the intubation of the labia minora for the urethra. They are moved into place and form the urethral tube. The testicular tissue expanders are placed with good soft tissue cover and are partially filled.

releasing the chordee and forming the ventral surface of the penis from the labia minora and the pendulous urethra from the internal surfaces of the labia minora (Fig. 156-1). To allow voiding in an upright position, an anterior vaginal flap is developed and forms a perineal urethroplasty to extend the urinary channel.

Advantages of this technique are that the phallus is aesthetic and sensation is preserved, there is little donor site morbidity, the recovery period is not protracted, and it may be accomplished in a single stage. A disadvantage of metoidioplasty is the small phallus.

NEOSCROTUM

In metoidioplasty, the vagina is not closed off because secretions will collect; also, the vagina becomes a diverticulum for urine. An anterior vaginal flap is formed into a tube to become the perineal urethra, and the vagina donor site is repaired; an opening is allowed to remain for the drainage. Alternatively, vaginectomy can be performed through an endoscopically assisted abdominal approach, or an external vaginectomy can be performed with the argon beam coagulator helping to control what otherwise might be significant blood loss.

LOCAL FLAPS

Adequate local tissue is present to develop an aesthetic, functional phallus. Many authors have reported their techniques in this regard.[7-10] Whereas there are differences in each author's technique, the fundamentals of reconstruction are maintained. In planning the reconstruction, the surgeon must ascertain what elements are missing and what assets are present for reconstruction. In the biologic female, the entire phallus is missing. From a component viewpoint, a soft tissue tube, an area of erogenous sensitivity, a penile urethra, and erectile tissue are absent.

Local flaps are used in the reconstruction of the phallic soft tissue tube. Two primary types of local flaps are employed. Again, variations in approaches are seen, but understanding the principles of reconstruction is the most important feature. The superficial external pudendal artery lower abdominal flap (also called the Stanford flap) and the lateral groin flap are the two most frequently employed local tissue phalloplasty flaps.

The Stanford superficial external pudendal artery flap is a two-stage procedure involving design of a bipedicled fasciocutaneous flap on the superficial external pudendal artery. At the first stage, a bipedicled fasciocutaneous flap is raised at the level of Scarpa fascia. The abdominal skin serves as an internal conduit but cannot become a permanent urethra because it is not glabrous skin. The tube is inside-out, and the exposed Scarpa fascia is skin grafted. The defect made from tube formation is then closed by local fasciocutaneous advancement flaps advanced from each side. At the second stage, the superior pedicle is divided, and a glans is developed. Urethroplasty with a forearm flap previously prepared with tissue expanders leaves only a linear scar (Fig. 156-2) and brings the lateral or medial antebrachial cutaneous nerve to anastomose with the erotic internal pudendal nerve. Stiffening may be done at a later surgical procedure or with a removable prosthesis,[11] or an implant is tolerated because the penis has sensitivity to protect from extrusion of the foreign body. An alternative phalloplasty technique is the lateral groin flap based on the superficial circumflex iliac artery. This again is fashioned by a medially based inside-out tube. The outer surface is covered with split-thickness skin grafts (Fig. 156-3). The inner tube

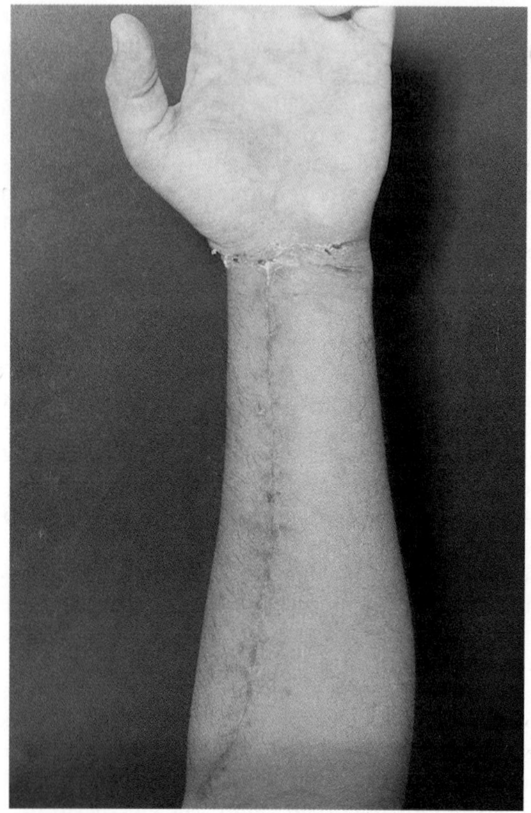

FIGURE 156-2. Donor site of forearm.

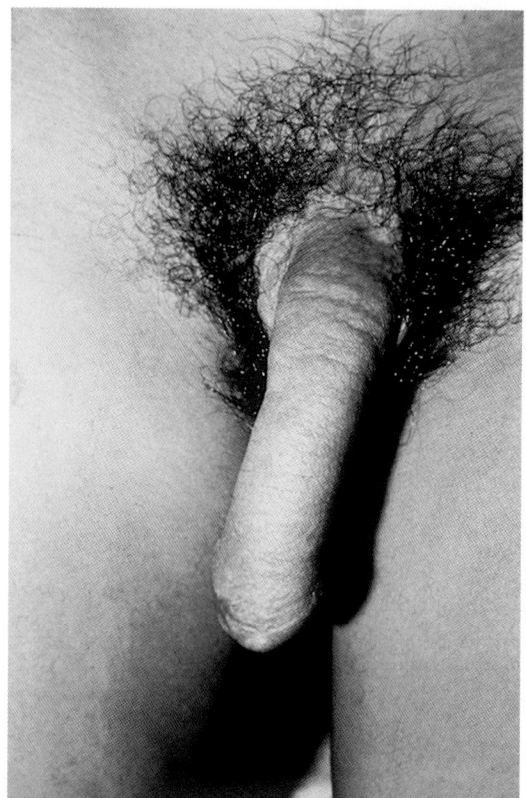

FIGURE 156-3. Postoperative simple phalloplasty without forearm flap.

serves as the tunnel for the baculum (Fig. 156-4). This axial flap may be performed in a single stage, but many stages may be employed.

FREE TISSUE TRANSFER PHALLOPLASTY

Phalloplasty may also be performed by use of distant tissue with microvascular transfer (Color Plate 156-2). This technique is considered by many to be the treatment of choice for gender identity disorder in the female-to-male patient. A fasciocutaneous radial forearm flap is used to preconstruct the phallus on the forearm. The tubed free flap may then be transferred to the groin, and the radial artery and cephalic vein or smaller venae comitantes are coapted to the deep inferior epigastric arteries or the femoral vessels. The medial antebrachial cutaneous nerve is coapted to the internal pudendal nerves, conferring erogenous sensitivity to the neophallus. The urethra is made at the time of the first stage with use of forearm epithelium. This flap has been termed the Chinese flap. In a single procedure, it forms a sensate, aesthetic phallus capable of voiding. There are several disadvantages of this technique, however. The conspicuous donor site left from the flap harvest and the complexity and duration of the procedure must be carefully considered (Fig. 156-5).

Other free tissue transfers have been described in the phalloplasty literature. Lateral arm flaps, periscapular flaps, fibula flaps, and fibula flap with bone have been successfully performed by several brilliant surgeons. Use of tissue expanders in the forearm will provide more tissue, sometimes precluding the large scar on the forearm.

Coronoplasty

The coronoplasty is a commonly requested adjunct surgery. Horton's technique is the most used and is usually performed during a second operation. The corona is formed by doubling up distal shaft skin, holding it in place with mattress sutures, and then covering the donor site with a skin graft.

Scrotoplasty

An aesthetic scrotum with the appearance of testes complements the phalloplasty. The scrotum is formed from the same embryologic tissue as the labia majora. The labia majora, however, are slightly more posterior than

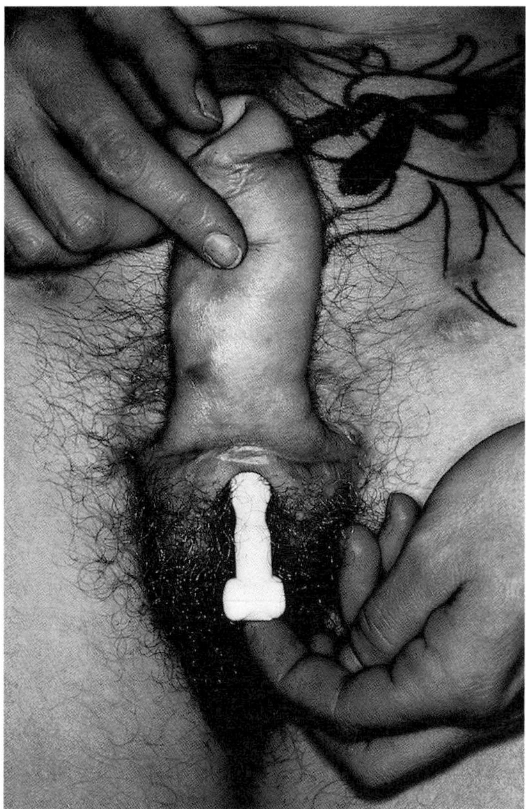

FIGURE 156-4. Teflon baculum custom-made as a stiffening device. It is placed in the tunnel lined with thick and durable abdominal skin.

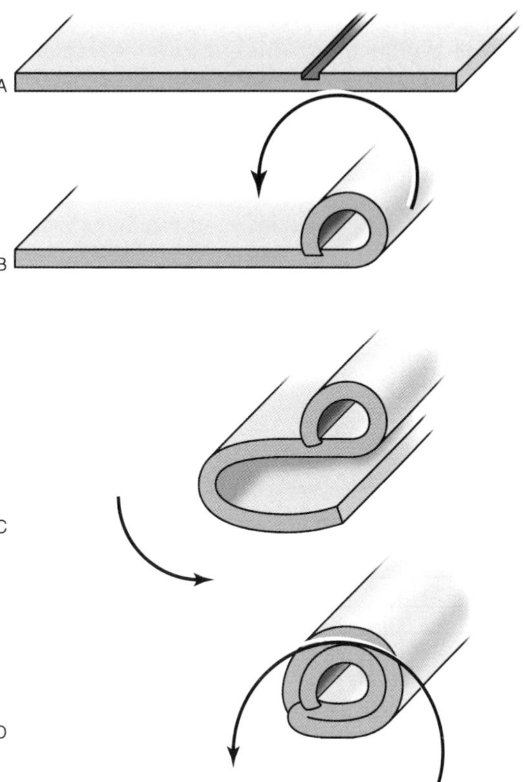

FIGURE 156-5. In a classic radial forearm flap, a glabrous urethral tube is formed within a skin tube. Internal pudendal neurorrhaphy with lateral antebrachial cutaneous nerve or medial endobrachial cutaneous nerve is done. Bone is occasionally included in the innovative flap.

the male counterpart, the scrotum. Tissue expansion is required to obtain sufficient tissue for scrotoplasty, and local tissue rearrangement is generally necessary to advance the tissues anteriorly. Several authors have described variations to a basic principle. In general, the labia majora are divided near the labia minora. The flaps are sutured together in the midline, and a V-Y type advancement is performed to mobilize the neoscrotum anteriorly. Expansion then occurs by subcutaneous placement of saline tissue expanders. Once expansion is completed, usually through remote port injection, the expanders are removed and replaced with silicone testicular implants if available.

Penile Stiffening Techniques

The methods for phalloplasty address formation of the soft tissue phallus and the conduit for urination; however, they do not address the unique erectile tissue of the penis. There are a variety of surgical methods for achieving rigidity, to a varied degree of success. The implantable, semirigid prosthesis is probably the most common, straightforward option available for erection. The problem with this as well as with many of the other techniques is that most flaps are insensate, and hence there is no protective sensation to the flap. Extrusion, infection, and loss are therefore common complications. Other options include the implantable, inflatable devices. These have the benefit of not being constantly rigid. The same risks are present as in the insensate flaps. The literature also reports use of autologous bone and cartilage for rigidity.

In each of these techniques, the implant is permanent. An alternative method is the removable baculum. A rod is inserted into an epithelial (skin) tunnel in the soft tissue penis and removed when not in use. The baculum transmits motion and pressure to the remaining clitoris, providing erogenous sensation. The advantages of this device are limited flap stress and simplicity.

Vaginectomy and Hysterectomy

Removal of the uterus and ovaries is common in the female-to-male patient. There is nothing unique in this regard in the female-to-male patient. However, if it is possible to perform an endoscopically assisted vaginal hysterectomy, this preserves the midline lower abdominal flap without scar. A Pfannenstiel incision divides the blood supply of the Stanford phalloplasty flap in half and development of the phallus is of higher risk, requiring at a minimum a delay procedure.

Endoscopic vaginectomy is surgically possible to perform and is helpful because it avoids the bloody "external" operation and risk of injury to bowel and bladder. Expert use of the argon beam coagulator dramatically reduces blood loss in vaginectomy (colpectomy). Most patients are content without this procedure.

SURGICAL MANAGEMENT: MALE TO FEMALE

Treatment of male-to-female transsexuals may also be viewed in components. The primary goal of surgery in male-to-female transsexuals is the surgical completion of wholeness. This pervasive trait cannot be overstated. It may be accomplished surgically by removal of the penis and testis and development of a vagina. The goal of vaginoplasty is formation of a vagina normal in appearance that has the functional ability to have active intercourse and has its own erotic sensibility and lubrication. There are several techniques for vaginoplasty and clitoroplasty. Each is discussed with indications, advantages, disadvantages, and complications (Color Plates 156-3 and 156-4).

Vaginoplasty

SKIN GRAFT

Abbe,[12] in the late 1800s, first described design of a neovagina in the case of congenital absence by use of skin grafting. This free graft was placed around a rubber pouch and placed into an iatrogenically formed cavity to make the neovagina. Abraham,[13] Skoog,[14] and others[15,16] have described modifications to this basic technique of skin graft vaginoplasty. The source of skin may be either distant nongenital skin or penis and scrotum. Penis skin has the advantage of being hairless and does not leave a donor site scar. Skin graft vaginoplasty is a single-stage technique that entails harvest of the skin graft and placing it inside-out over a mold. A cavity is then made, and the mold is placed and secured. Whereas its advantages include simplicity and the ability to accomplish the procedure in a single stage, there are some inherent disadvantages. Skin graft vaginoplasty without the use of local flaps results in a circular scar at the introitus. This scar ring tends to contract and become stenotic. One technique used to manage this problem is to place a medium-sized pedicled flap in the introitus, eliminating the circular scar and its inherent contractile property. Secondary contracture must also be managed, and patients who undergo this type of procedure are required to perform daily postoperative dilation for a period of approximately 6 months as well as to use nighttime stents. Finally, skin grafts do transfer sebaceous glands, and a peculiar transudation "sweating" occurs; as such, natural lubrication is not a component of this technique. This technique is largely of historical interest; it is not normally used in transsexual patients because of donor site scar but reserved as an alternative technique for patients with vaginal agenesis.

PENILE INVERSION

Penile inversion vaginoplasty is currently the most commonly applied technique for male-to-female transsexuals. Sir Harold Gillies[17] first reported the use of pedicled penile skin for vaginoplasty in 1957. The penile skin may be used solely as the source of vaginal lining as an inside-out skin tube, based on an abdominal pedicle, or this tissue may be supplemented with a scrotal flap to eliminate the circular scar of the introitus. Alternatively, the penile skin can be split to form a rectangular flap. The vaginal vault is then fashioned with the penile skin as the anterior wall, and a scrotal flap of equal size is developed and turned in to form the posterior wall.[18,19] Presurgical epilation is helpful in removing hair that would eventually be transferred into the neovagina. A contribution from Perovic to this technique is the urethra as a flap to the anterior wall. This not only increases the size of the vaginal vault but also confers an extra degree of erotic sensitivity.

The advantage of penile flap vaginoplasty is that there is limited risk of contracture and no donor site morbidity. Postoperative care, however, still requires frequent dilation. A disadvantage of this technique is the limited vault size that may be obtained with penile skin alone (Color Plate 156-5). Adding the posteriorly based scrotal flap to enlarge the vault introduces hair-bearing tissue into a nonphysiologic location. Furthermore, this addition leads to a transverse posterior wall of the introitus.

LOCAL FLAPS

An alternative technique for vaginoplasty is local flap use. This technique may be employed when other techniques, such as inversion, have failed. This may also be used in combination with penile inversion in the primary operation. For example, Huang and others described bilateral fasciocutaneous groin neurovascular island flaps with a pedicled penile flap to design a neovagina (Singapore flap) in a male-to-female transsexual[20] (Color Plate 156-6). An advantage of using local nongenital flaps is decreased contracture of the flaps compared with grafts.

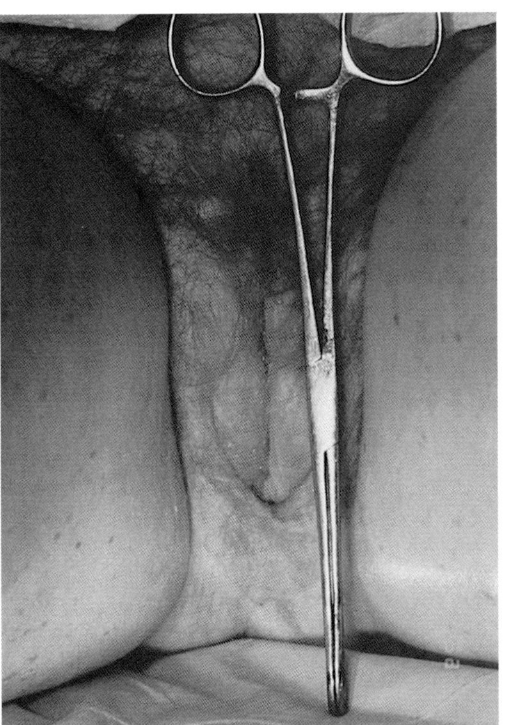

FIGURE 156-6. Rectosigmoid neocolporrhaphy with a long sponge forceps.

RECTOSIGMOID TECHNIQUE

Pedicled intestinal transposition vaginoplasty is a single-stage procedure used to form a self-lubricating vaginal vault of unlimited length (Figs. 156-6 and 156-7). This technique involves isolating a segment of rectosigmoid colon on its vascular pedicle. Intestinal continuity is restored by an end-to-end anastomosis with an EEA stapler. The sigmoid is then closed proximally, and the distal end is brought out to form the introitus. Large local flaps are required to break the circular ring and to prevent vaginal stenosis secondary to scar contracture (Figs. 156-8 and 156-9). Hage has reported endoscopic harvest of the sigmoid with EEA stapling to restore intestinal continuity (Color Plate 156-7).

Advantages of the procedure include long vaginal and vault length, self-lubrication, and sensibility. Disadvantages include complications associated with the intestinal anastomosis, such as leak or stricture, and the increased complexity of adding an intra-

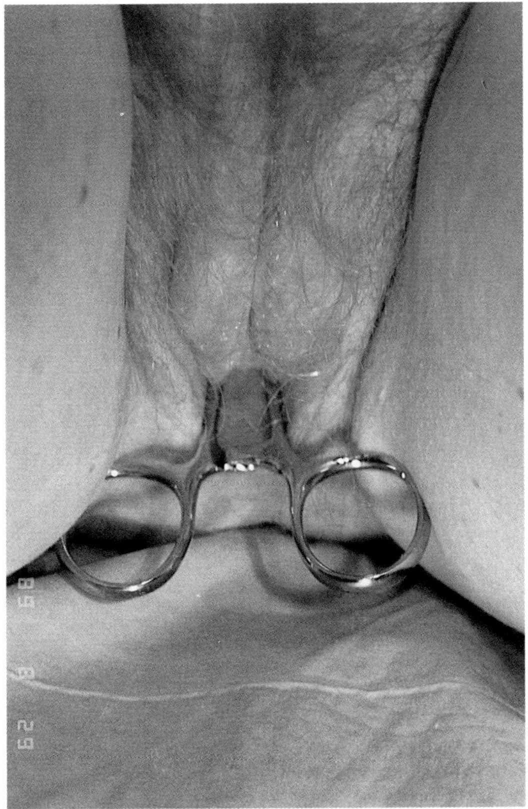

FIGURE 156-7. A very long vaginal depth.

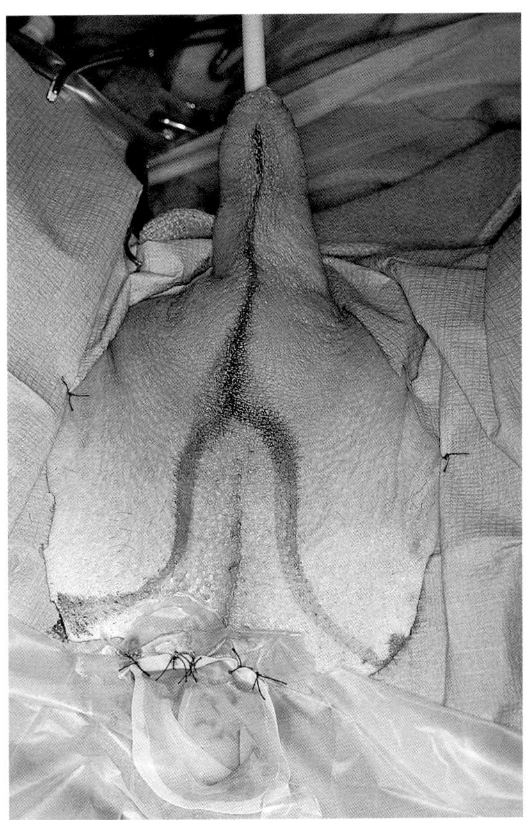

FIGURE 156-8. An intraoperative view of the penile inversion showing posteriorly based scrotal flap that prevents the inevitable stricture if it is not included in the rectosigmoid version, local tissue, or skin graft McIndoe vaginal construction. The flap gives needed diameter.

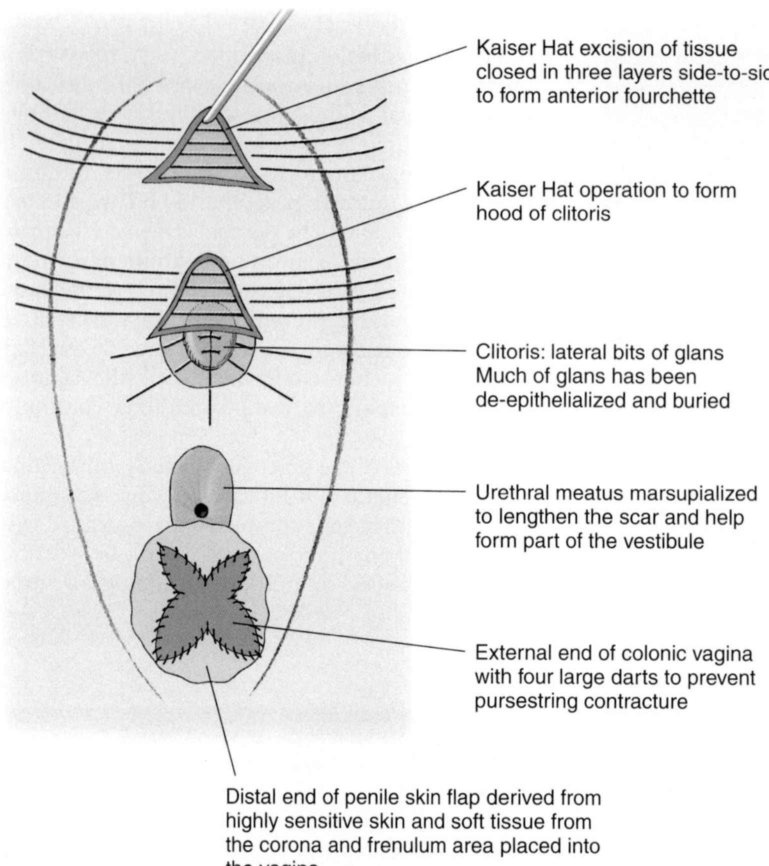

FIGURE 156-9. The wide anterior aspect of the labia is often a telltale mark of a transsexual. The space that was previously occupied by the insertion of the penis separates the labia majora, and simple tension does not approximate them. Biber cleverly devised the double Z-plasty. The excision of this area, named the Kaiser Hat procedure because of the shape of the excision, will help; it actually removes the dog-ear at the time of excision. Closure makes a little cave, which requires hygiene attention. Part of the urethral wall, part of the area near the corona, and the frenulum—all erogenous—become the anterior vagina and vestibule.

abdominal component to the surgery. These complications are uncommon. Excess mucorrhea is not noted if rectosigmoid is used. (This area of intestine absorbs fluid rather than secretes fluid.) Our group has reported the largest series to date and documented the safety and efficacy of this technique (Fig. 156-10).

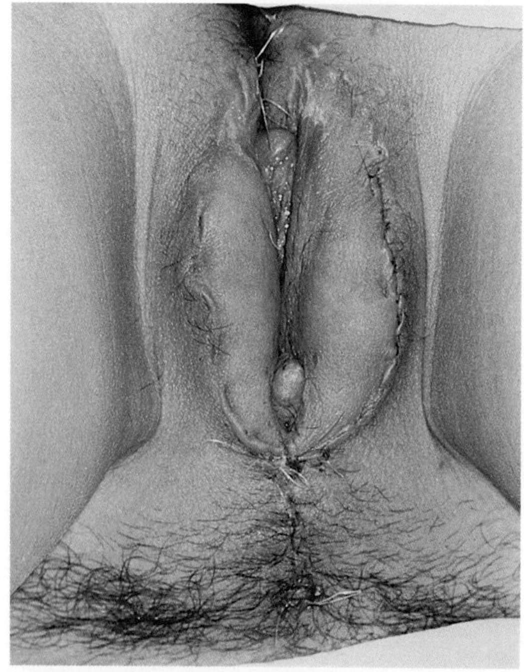

FIGURE 156-10. Completed vaginoplasty, clitoroplasty, and labioplasty with good approximation of labia majora as a cleft and a clitoroplasty with local tissue.

Clitoroplasty

For a successful outcome to be achieved in male-to-female transsexuals, a functional and aesthetic perineum must be formed. A natural-appearing clitoris with maintenance of erogenous sensation is the usual surgical aim. There are several clitoroplasty techniques. Each is discussed.

GRAFT OR LOCAL FLAP NEOCLITOROPLASTY

Erogenous sensation is supplied by the pudendal nerves that enter the dorsal penis superior to the urethra arising from posterior to the pubis. In graft or local flap clitoroplasty, these nerves are identified and transsected at the base of the neoclitoris. A local flap from the urethral mucosa[21] or vaginal skin[22] is transposed to the apex of the vaginal orifice and formed into a small tube. Alternatively, penile glans skin may be used as a free graft to form the neoclitoris.[23] A small amount of corpus spongiosum is left to provide for erotic sensation.[24] These nerves may regrow rapidly into superjacent free graft. Tissue from around this area may be used to form a clitoris just as a skate flap is designed in nipple construction.

PEDICLED NEOCLITOROPLASTY

The male embryologic tissue analogous to the clitoris is the glans. Brown[25] first reported use of pedicled dorsal glans to form a functional clitoris in 1976. Brown's original report of 65 patients had a high incidence of necrosis (33%), and surgical technique modifications were subsequently adopted to reduce this complication (Color Plate 156-8).[26]

The penile skin is dissected off the erectile corporal tissue, following which two incisions are made through Buck fascia, one on each side of the dorsal neurovascular bundles. A portion of the glans is then dissected. The urethra and glans are surgically and gently lifted from the corpus cavernosum; the plane of dissection of the neurovascular bundle can be identified. Once skeletonized, the glans can be inset, with care taken not to kink the neurovascular bundle, occasionally including a portion of the albuginea (Color Plate 156-9).

A high rate of erogenous sensibility is maintained with this technique. Karim[24] reported that 57 of 59 patients retained erogenous sensibility, and of those patients, 47 were able to reach orgasm.

Labioplasty, done with the Kaiser Hat procedure, closes the labia to form the fourchette (Fig. 156-11).

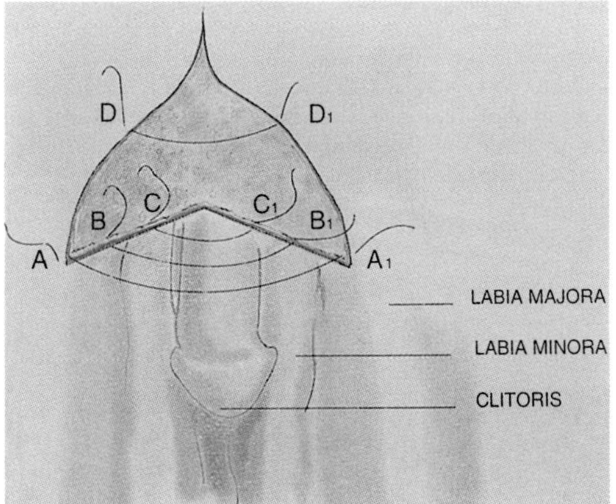

FIGURE 156-11. Plans for narrowing anterior fourchette and covering part of neoclitoris with tissue. The clitoris was fabricated from local tissue by the skate flap technique. No erotic sensitivity is present.

Adjunctive Surgical Procedures

To complete the transformation to the desired sex, additional adjunctive procedures are sometimes indicated.

AUGMENTATION MAMMAPLASTY. Hormone manipulation in the male-to-female transsexual results in varied breast development, just as genetic females' breasts are varied. In many cases, this development is sufficient for the patient. Augmentation mammaplasty is different in the male-to-female patient. In the broader male chest, a wider based implant is helpful to produce a more natural result.[27] Submuscular placement of the implants results in a more natural appearance in the male-to-female patient in whom significant overlying soft tissue growth has not resulted with hormones.

RHINOPLASTY. A prominent, masculine nose (especially those with dorsal humps) decreases a patient's ability to pass as a female. Rhinoplasty can feminize the nose and improve the feminine image. This procedure is often performed during the cross-living period and aids the individual in passing this trial. Whereas some male-to-female patients request this operation, few female-to-male patients appear to be as invested in their nasal appearance.

MENTOPLASTY. Similar to the nose, a masculine chin makes passing as a woman difficult. The chin may be feminized by an intraoral approach, thereby leaving no external scars. Gonzales-Ulloa and Stevens[28] offer guidelines for shaping the profile.

REDUCTION THYROID CHONDROPLASTY. A prominent "Adam's apple" will interfere with acceptance as a woman. Reduction thyroid chondroplasty reduces the ala of the thyroid cartilage, feminizing the appearance. There is some surgical risk in that the insertion of the cords is near the area of resection. A qualified head and neck surgeon should be sought for such a procedure. A horizontal neck incision is performed in lines of resting skin tension. Exposure of the thyroid cartilage is obtained through lateral retraction of the strap muscles. A submucosal dissection of the thyroid cartilage is performed, and the offending cartilage is subperichondrially shaved. This technique has been described by several authors.[29,30]

FACIAL SKELETON FEMINIZATION. Ousterhout[31] noted three craniofacial characteristics used by anthropologists to differentiate male from female. Nasal takeoff angle, chin dimensions, and forehead topography were characteristically different between the sexes. Ousterhout has feminized the male-to-female forehead by sculpting the frontal bone, reducing the characteristic male bossing. In female-to-male patients, a more male-appearing forehead may be obtained with onlay cranioplasty, using cranial bone graft or synthetic bone substitutes, although this is done infrequently.

RIB RESECTION. Prominence of the lower male rib cage helps form the characteristic male habitus. Resection of ribs in the male-to-female patients results in a more feminine relationship between ribs, waist, and hips, the so-called hourglass figure.

VOICE ALTERATION PROCEDURES. In the developmental stage are the voice-altering procedures because they depend on shortening the vocal cords themselves. Alternatively, many transsexuals use a voice coach to assist in the transformation. Word selection and mannerisms are also carefully studied to effect better acceptance in the chosen sex.

CONCLUSION

Surgery for gender identity disorder is one component of the multidisciplinary approach to this fascinating behavioral phenomenon. By following fundamental principles of plastic and reconstructive surgery, safe and successful human gender confirmation may be accomplished in this special population of patients.

REFERENCES

1. Laub DR, Dubin BJ: Gender dysphoria. In Grabb WC, Smith JW, eds: Plastic Surgery, 3rd ed. Boston, Little, Brown, 1979:chapter 56.
2. Bulliet C: Venus Castina: Famous Female Impersonators: Celestial and Human. New York, Covici, Friede, 1928.
3. Durant W: Caesar and Christ. New York, Simon & Schuster, 1944.
4. Hamburger C, Sturup GK, Dahl-Iversen E: Transvestism. Hormonal, psychiatric, and surgical treatment. JAMA 1953; 152:391.
5. Gilbert DA, Winslow BH, Gilbert DM, et al: Transsexual surgery in the genetic female. Clin Plast Surg 1988;15:471.
6. Laub DR: Metoidioplasty. Presented to the Harry Benjamin International Gender Dysphoria Association (HBIGDA) Meeting, Bordeaux, France, 1982.
7. Song RY: Reconstruction of the male genitalia. Chin Med 1954;72:446.
8. Song RY: Total reconstruction of the male genitalia. Chin Plast Surg 1982;9:97.
9. Mukherjee GD: On reconstruction of the penis with urethra and a dorsal skin-lined socket for a removable prosthesis: a new approach. Plast Reconstr Surg 1982;69:377.
10. Sun G, Huang J: One-stage reconstruction of the penis with composite iliac crest and lateral groin flap. Ann Plast Surg 1985;15:519.
11. Noe J, Birdsell D, Laub D: The surgical construction of male genitalia for the female-to-male transsexual. Plast Reconstr Surg 1974;53:511.
12. Abbe R: New method of creating a vagina in a case of congenital absence. Med Rec 1898;54:836.
13. Abraham F: Genitalumwandlung an zwei männlichen Transvestiten. Z Sexualwissenschaft Sexualpolitik 1931;18:223.
14. Ohlsen L, Vedung S: Skoog's technique for constructing female genitalia in the male transsexual developed in 24 operated cases. Chir Plastica 1981;6:1.
15. Foerster DW, Reynolds CL: Construction of natural appearing female genitalia in the male transsexual. Plast Reconstr Surg 1979;64:306.
16. Hore BD, Nicolle FV, Calnan JS: Male transsexualism in England: sixteen cases with surgical intervention. Arch Sex Behav 1975;4:81.
17. Gillies H, Millard RD Jr: Genitalia. In The Principles and Art of Plastic Surgery. London, Butterworth, 1957:369–388.
18. Edgerton MT, Bull J: Surgical construction of the vagina and labia in male transsexuals. Plast Reconstr Surg 1970;46:529.
19. Cairns TS, de Villiers W: Vaginoplasty. S Afr Med J 1980;57:50.
20. Huang TT: Twenty years of experience in managing patients with gender dysphoria: I. Surgical management of the male transsexual. Plast Reconstr Surg 1995;96:921.
21. Laub DR, Laub DR II, Biber S: Vaginoplasty for gender confirmation. Clin Plast Surg 1988;15:463.
22. Wesser DR: A single stage operative technique for castration, vaginal construction and perineoplasty in transsexuals. Arch Sex Behav 1978;7:309.
23. Eicher W, Schmitt B, Bergner CM: Transformationsoperation bei Mann-zu-Frau-Transsexuellen. Z Sexualforschung 1991;4:119.
24. Karim RB: Vaginoplasty in Transsexuals. Amsterdam, VU University Press, 1996.
25. Brown J: Creation of a functional clitoris and aesthetically pleasing introitus in sex conversion. In Marchac D, Hueston JT, eds: Tansactions of the Sixth International Congress of Plastic and Reconstructive Surgery. Paris, Masson, 1976:654–655.
26. Hage JJ, Karim RB, Bloem JJ, et al: Sculpturing the neoclitoris in vaginoplasty for the male-to-female transsexuals. Plast Reconstr Surg 1994;93:358.
27. Laub DR, Laub DR II, Van Maasdam JV: Gender dysphoria syndrome. In Smith JW, Aston S, eds: Grabb and Smith's Plastic Surgery, 4th ed. Boston, Little, Brown, 1991:1393–1412.
28. Gonzales-Ulloa M, Stevens E: The role of chin correction in profileplasty. Plast Reconstr Surg 1968;41:477.
29. Good R: Thyroid cartilage shaved. Proceedings of the Second Interdisciplinary Symposium on Gender Dysphoria Syndrome. Palo Alto, Stanford University School of Medicine, 1973.
30. Wolfort F, Pany R: Laryngeal chondroplasty for appearance. Plast Reconstr Surg 1975;56:371.
31. Ousterhout DK: Feminization of the forehead: contour changing to improve female aesthetics. Presented at the Facial Sculpture Symposium, Washington, DC, 1984, and the American Society for Aesthetic Plastic Surgery, Boston, 1985.

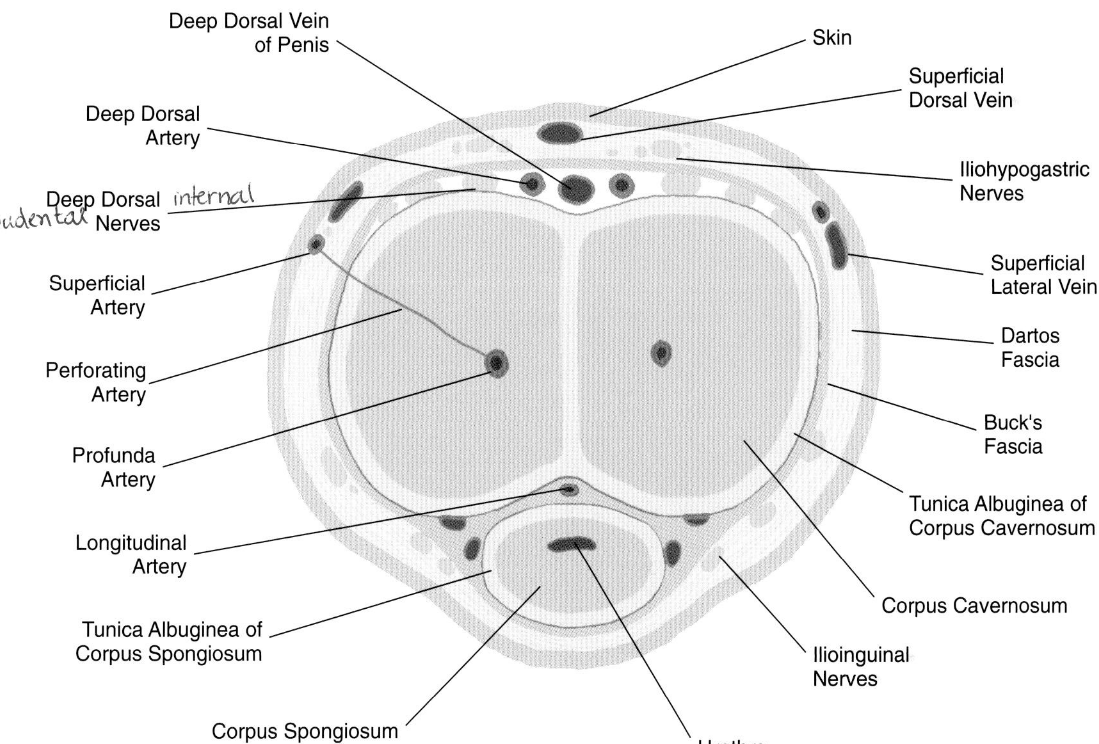

COLOR PLATE 156-1. The penis is a collage of parts. From the abdominal wall, the contributions are made up of skin; superficial fascia and panniculus carnosus remnant, which make up Buck and dartos fasciae; and the vessels and nerves to this skin and fascia. The contributions for urinary function and the sexual apparatus do collage with these but go inside the abdominal wall structures. Sexual and urinary function structures are derived from posterior to the symphysis pubis: the urethra, its spongiosum, corpora cavernosa, internal pudendal artery and nerve. These structures—the abdominal wall structures and the urinary and sexual structures—form two independent blood and nerve supplies that can be surgically separated from each other according to how they were embryologically engineered or put together.

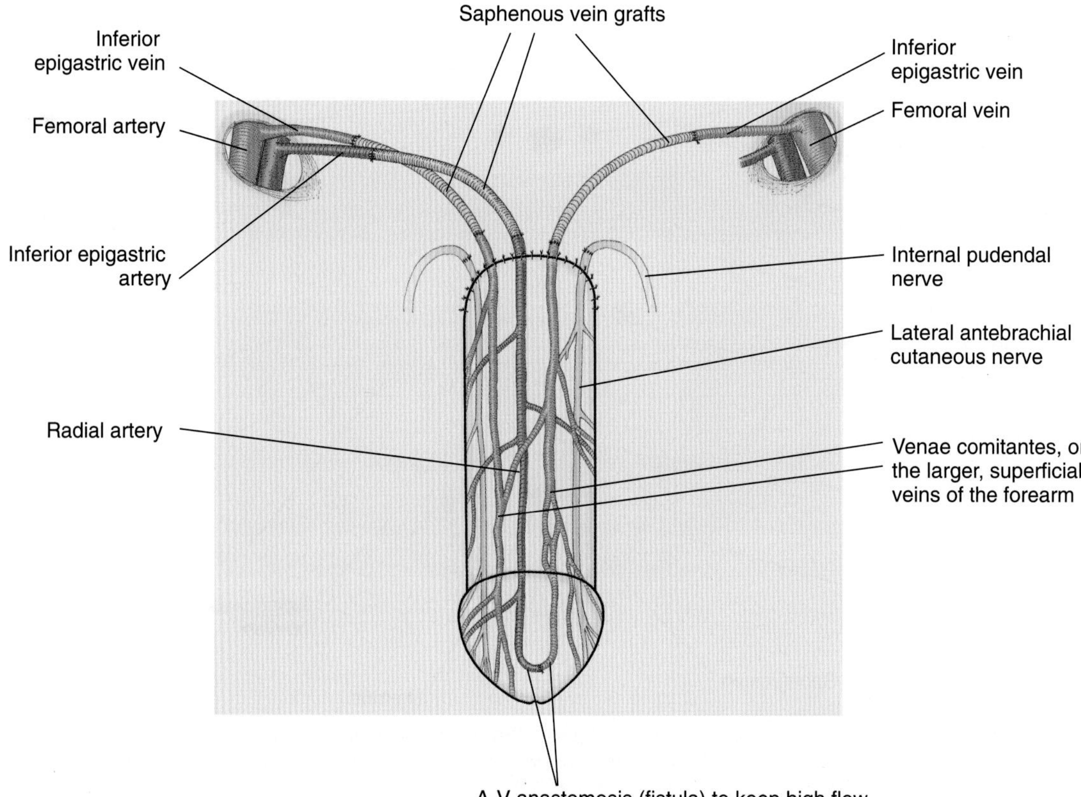

COLOR PLATE 156-2. Completed free forearm phalloplasty with Hage's arteriovenous fistula to produce a high flow rate. Vein grafts are not always necessary.

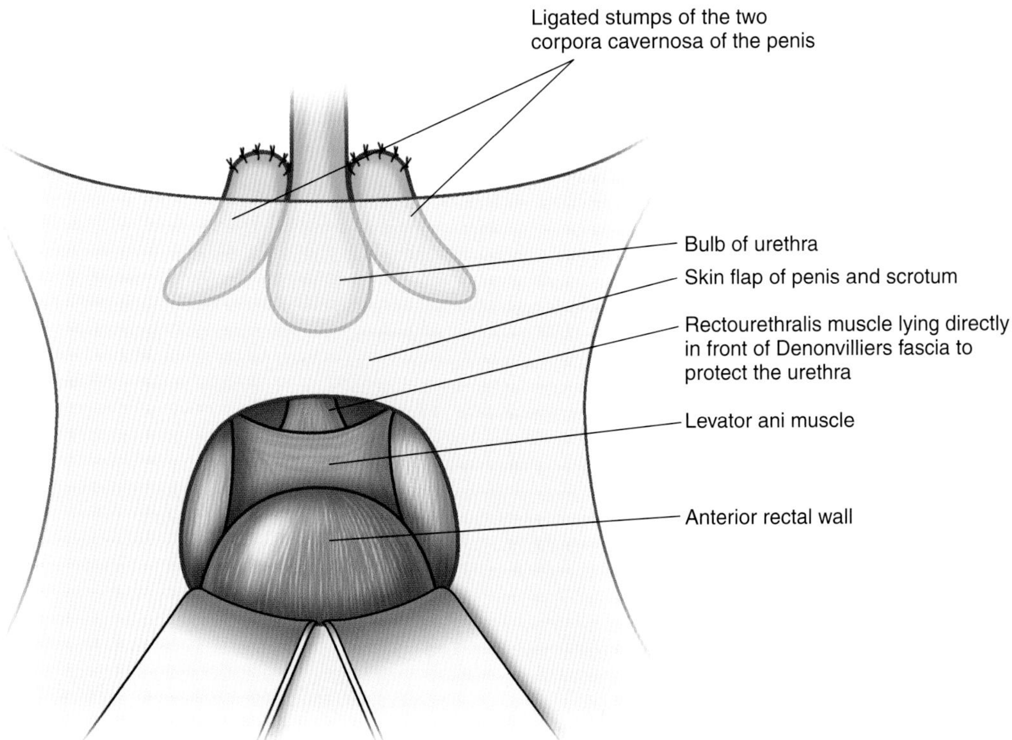

COLOR PLATE 156-3. The dissection of the vaginal cavity in gender cases is really separation of adherent, almost fused structures, whereas the dissection of the vaginal cavity for vaginal atresia in a genetic female is in a potential space, and it is relatively easy to dissect levator ani muscles. See diagram for position of these. Rectourethralis muscle and bulb of the urethra are structures preventing expansion of the cavity. The prostate is behind the Denonvilliers fascia, a structure to be incised. It cannot be safely dissected bluntly. To make room for a functioning vagina, the bulb of the urethra, its investing muscle and erectile tissue, the urogenital diaphragm, and at times the corpora cavernosa are candidates for excision. The prostate is chemically shriveled to a barely recognizable structure; it is the homologue to the female Skene gland, which is the site of Gräfenberg's G-spot, the area of the usual female cystitis and an erogenous spot.

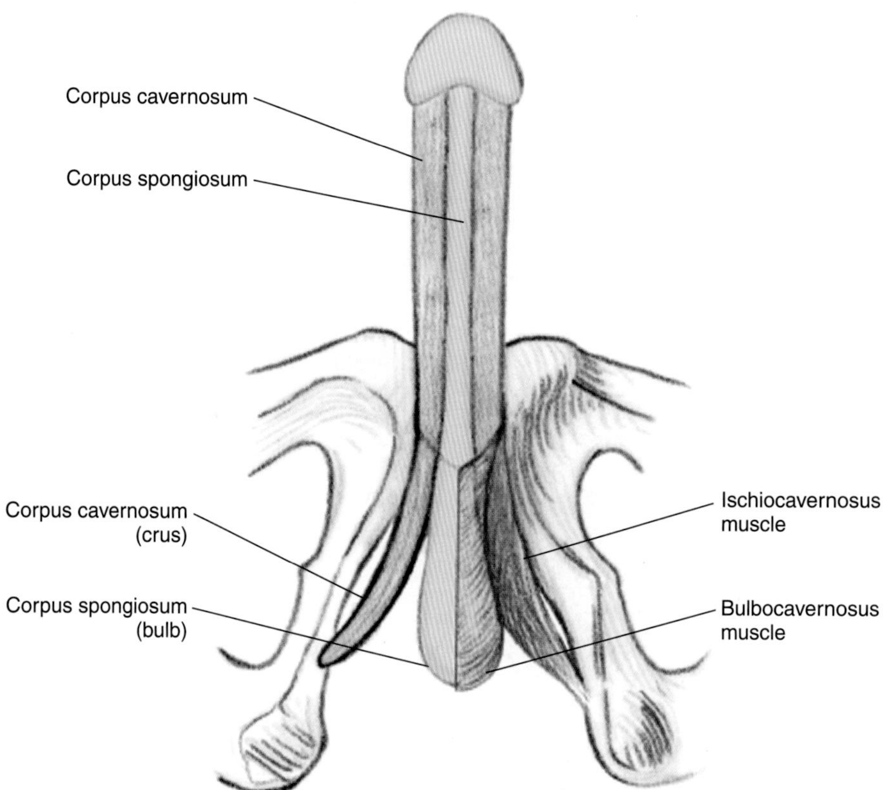

COLOR PLATE 156-4. The cutaway view of the penis helps to show the layers of muscle and erectile tissue. Surgical removal of these muscles investing the corporal bodies is helpful because the underlying structures become much smaller and more easily managed surgically. Some surgeons remove all of these erectile bodies of the perineum but not the pendulous urethra. Muscle and corporal tissue excision have advantages and disadvantages and are carried out at the surgeon's preference. Hemostasis in erectile tissue is achieved with over-and-over locked sutures.

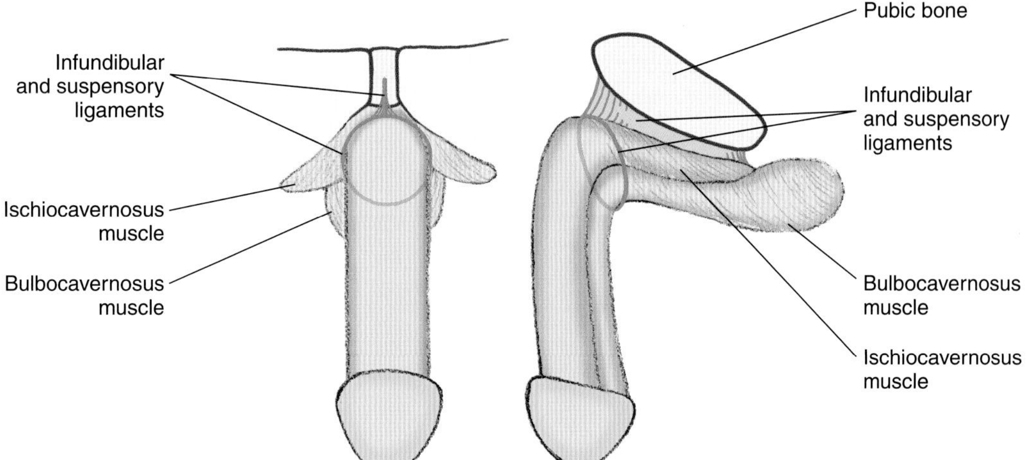

COLOR PLATE 156-5. In penile inversion, note that the suspensory ligament of the penis goes circumferentially around the base of the penis and forms a relatively tight stricture for the neovagina. The infundibular ligament also has the same relative function, and both of these must be completely released to achieve sufficient vaginal diameter.

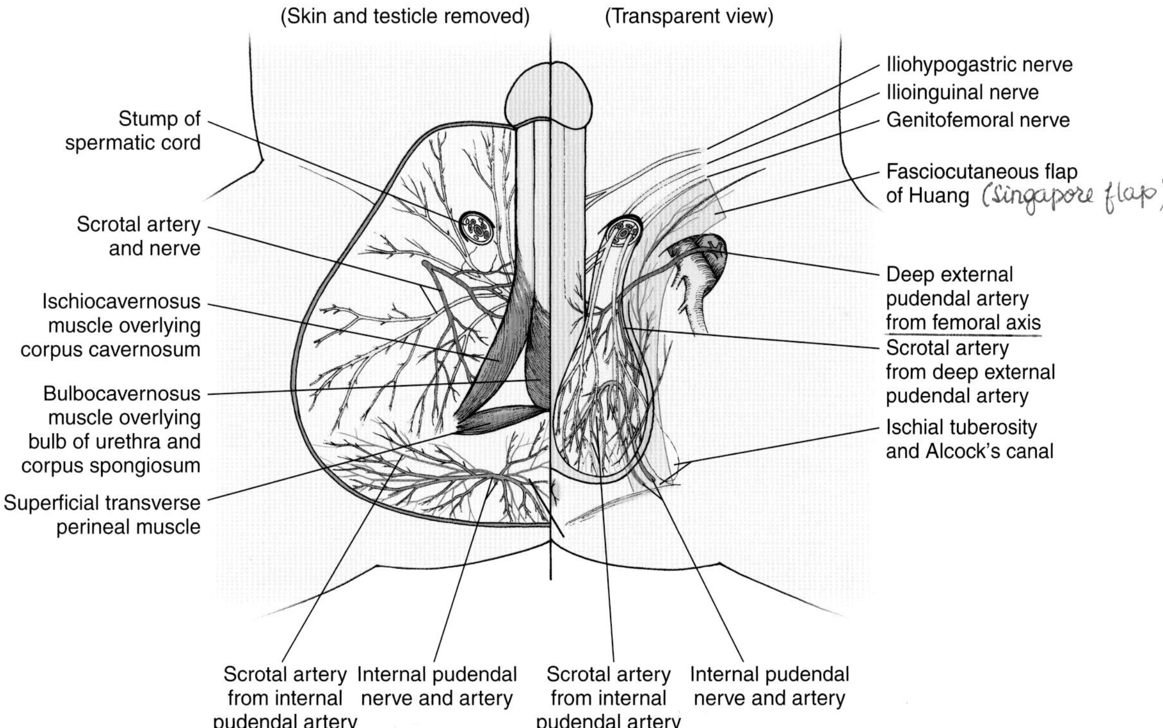

COLOR PLATE 156-6. Important surgical anatomy. These structures demonstrate nerve supply and blood supply. In the genitalia, nerves and vessels do not always follow identical routes. The nerve supply to the skin of the scrotum from the internal pudendal and from the abdominal wall is shown. The vascular supply to the scrotum is from two directions: first, from the abdominal wall by segmental arteries and from the femoral axis; and second, from the internal pudendal from inferior to superior direction. The blood supply to the skin of the scrotum is not entirely collateralized; that is, it will be difficult for the skin to survive if one of the two suppliers is severed and one pedicle is asked to nourish both ends of the new labia. Note that the internal pudendal has a branch nourishing the skin and fascia of the groin crease area. The internal pudendal is able to support a fasciocutaneous flap 12 × 4 cm or larger. Two of these (bilateral) flaps can provide a large surface area to be used in surfacing the major part of the neovaginal cavity. Huang of University of Texas and the Singapore flap are names attached to this flap. They are particularly helpful in treatment of complications, such as surfacing after a vaginal stenosis release.

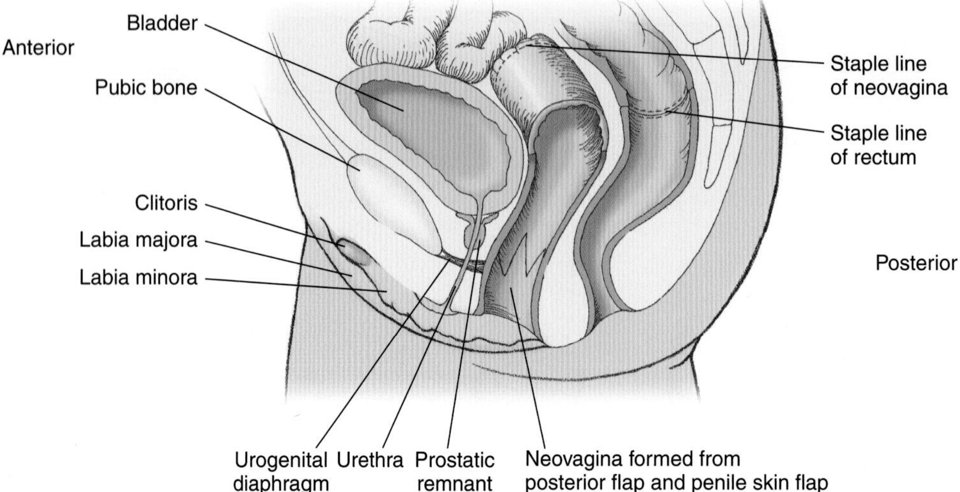

COLOR PLATE 156-7. Completed construction of vagina and vulva using rectosigmoid donor tissue. Note effective breaking up of the circular healing at skin-colon junction. The vagina may be of very long length. The staple line in the rectum is about 10 cm from the anal verge, and it is located propitiously between two "headwaters" of arterial supply of middle rectal and superior rectal. The prostatic remnant becomes Gräfenberg's place. Urogenital diaphragm and levator ani should be loosened. The urethral meatus in this case is marsupialized to become the vestibule but may be turned into the vagina in the manner of Perovic. The clitoris is nourished by deep dorsal vein, artery, and nerve.

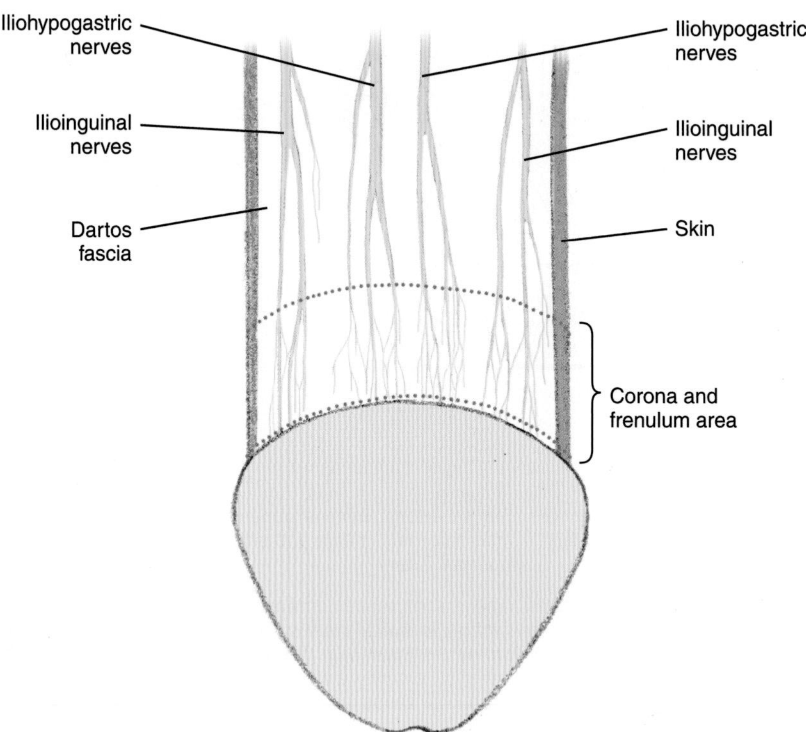

COLOR PLATE 156-8. Important surgical anatomy for pedicled clitoroplasty.

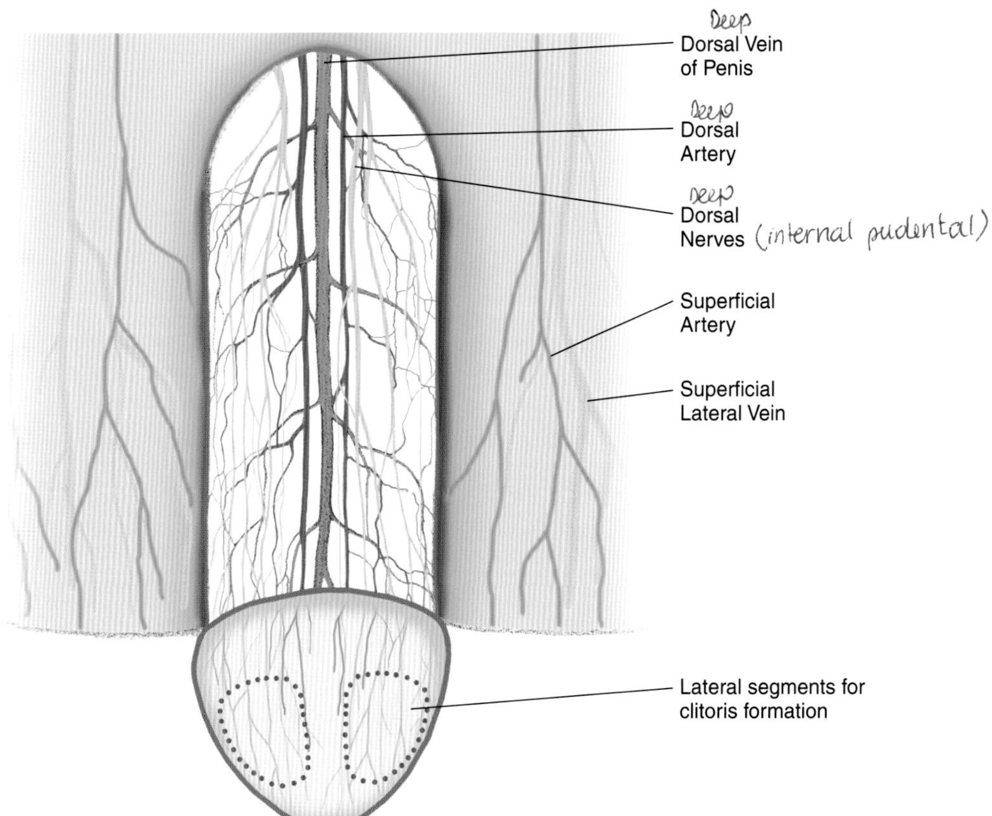

COLOR PLATE 156-9. The superficial abdominal wall nerves end at the distal penile shaft, the skin of which commonly forms the fundus of the vagina in the inversion technique or the area of the "hymen" in the rectosigmoid technique. One central vein, two parasagittal arteries, and, further laterally, the splayed-out deep dorsal internal pudendal nerve are shown. Using midline tissue of the glans penis to make the clitoris and discarding the lateral glans may involve cutting this nerve; therefore, lateral tissue is preferred for clitoroplasty.

CHAPTER

157

Pressure Sores

ROBERT D. FOSTER, MD, FACS

Pressure sores are wounds that result from ischemic tissue loss due to pressure against a bone prominence. With the best of care, pressure sores are preventable. However, despite the best of efforts, pressure sore recurrence rates in patients with spinal cord injuries exceed 50% during the long term. With the number of permanent spinal injuries averaging 2 million worldwide, the management of patients with pressure sores remains an important and significant challenge.[1]

SPINAL CORD INJURY

The following data are generated from the University of Alabama at Birmingham's National Spinal Cord Injury Statistical Center.[1] Developed in 1973, it supervises and directs the collection, management, and analysis of the world's largest spinal cord injury database.

INCIDENCE. It is estimated that the annual incidence of spinal cord injuries in the United States is approximately 40 patients per million Americans or 11,000 new patients each year. On average, a new injury occurs every 49 minutes.

PREVALENCE. The estimated number of people in the United States with spinal cord injury is between 200,000 and 250,000. Internationally, spinal cord injuries affect approximately 2 million people worldwide.

AGE AT INJURY. Since 1973, there has been an increase in the mean age at time of injury. Fifty-three percent of spinal cord injuries occur among persons 16 to 30 years of age. The overall average age at injury is 32.6 years.

ETIOLOGY. Since 1990, motor vehicle crashes accounted for 40.9% of the patients with spinal cord injury. The next largest contributor is falls (22.4%), followed by acts of violence (21.6%, primarily gunshot wounds). Interesting trends show that motor vehicle accidents and sporting accidents leading to spinal cord injuries have declined while injuries from falls have steadily increased since 1973. Acts of violence peaked in the mid-1990s but have subsequently decreased.

LIFE EXPECTANCY. Life expectancies for persons with spinal cord injuries, although they continue to increase, remain below the national average for persons without spinal cord injuries. Life expectancy decreases on the basis of the severity of the injury and the age at the time of the injury (Table 157-1).

CAUSES OF MORTALITY. In years past, renal failure was the leading cause of death for persons with spinal cord injuries. However, advances in urologic management have resulted in a dramatic decrease in the number of kidney complications related to pressure sores. Currently, the leading causes of death in this population are pneumonia, pulmonary emboli, and septicemia.

PRESSURE SORE ETIOLOGY

Pressure

The single most important factor in the development of pressure sores is excessive and prolonged pressure. If external pressure is greater than end-capillary bed pressure (32 mm Hg), tissue perfusion will be impaired and ischemia will result. In 1974, Dinsdale,[2] conduct-

TABLE 157-1 ✦ LIFE EXPECTANCY (YEARS) AFTER INJURY BY SEVERITY OF INJURY AND AGE AT INJURY

		For Persons Who Survive the First 24 Hours					For Persons Surviving at Least 1 Year Post-Injury				
Age at Injury	No Spinal Cord Injury	*Motor Functional at Any Level*	*Para*	*Low Tetra (C5-C8)*	*High Tetra (C1-C4)*	*Ventilator Dependent at Any Level*	*Motor Functional at Any Level*	*Para*	*Low Tetra (C5-C8)*	*High Tetra (C1-C4)*	*Ventilator Dependent at Any Level*
20	57.8	52.9	45.3	40.5	36.0	16.3	53.4	46.0	41.8	38.2	23.3
40	38.9	34.4	27.7	23.7	20.1	7.0	34.9	28.3	24.7	21.8	11.1
60	21.6	17.8	12.7	10.0	7.7	1.3	18.2	13.2	10.7	8.8	2.9

From National Spinal Cord Injury Statistical Center (NSCISC), Birmingham, Alabama: Facts and Figures at a Glance—December 2003. Available at: http://www.spinalcord.uab.edu.

ing pressure studies in animals, concluded that constant pressure equal to twice the end-capillary arterial pressure (70 mm Hg) applied for 2 hours produces irreversible tissue ischemia. If external pressure is kept at levels that are less than the end-capillary arterial pressure, tissue necrosis is unlikely to occur.

In 1965, Lindan et al[3] documented the distribution of pressure throughout the body in the supine, prone, and sitting positions. Pressures were found to be greatest over bone. In the supine position, the sacrum, heels, and occiput are subject to the greatest pressures, ranging from 40 to 60 mm Hg. In the prone position, the knees and chest develop approximately 50 mm Hg of pressure. In the sitting position, pressures up to 75 mm Hg develop over the ischial tuberosities. Tissue ischemia and necrosis of intervening tissues develop first at the deepest tissue, next to the bone. Therefore, pressure sores are typically sizable by the time skin breakdown is apparent. Interestingly, altering pressures for as short as 5 minutes can preserve tissue viability for longer periods and under greater pressures.[4]

Nutritional Status

Although extreme changes in the overall nutritional status of an individual can play a role in the formation of pressure sores,[5] a healthy nutritional state alone does not protect against the development of a pressure wound. Decreased serum protein level, anemia, and vitamin deficiencies are markers that should be further evaluated if a patient's nutritional status is in question.

Muscle Spasticity

In paraplegic patients, muscle spasms can lead to the development of pressure ulcers and subsequent complications of their surgical treatment, such as flap dehiscence. Although the presence of spasms cannot be reliably predicted, the level of spinal cord injury seems to significantly influence their incidence. Patients with cervical or high thoracic lesions are much more likely to be affected than are patients with lumbar lesions (95% incidence above T8 level, 40% below T12).[6] Diminished inhibition of spinal cord reflex arcs is one explanation for this phenomenon. Because the spinal cord ends at the level of L1, injury below this level will result in nerve root damage and therefore interrupt the reflex arc, causing flaccid paralysis.

CLINICAL CONSIDERATIONS

Anatomic Distribution

In 1964, Dansereau and Conway[7] published what is, to this day, the largest series of patients with pressure sores (649 patients with 1604 pressure sores) (Table 157-2). The most common site of occurrence, confirmed by other studies, is the ischium. It is the area

TABLE 157-2 ✦ FREQUENCY OF PRESSURE SORES BY ANATOMIC AREA (N = 1604)

Location of Ulcer	No. of Lesions	Occurrence (%)
Ischial tuberosity	447	28
Trochanter	310	19
Sacrum	278	17
Heel	138	9
Malleolus	85	5
Pretibial	76	5
Patella	65	4
Total	1399	87
Other sites	205	13

Modified from Dansereau JG, Conway H: Closure of decubiti in paraplegics. Plast Reconstr Surg 1964;33:474.

of the body that sustains the greatest amount of pressure with a person in the sitting position. The occiput, sacrum, and heel bear the weight of the patient in the supine position. Sacral pressure sores are common; however, because the majority of patients with spinal cord injuries have sensation over the occiput and can move their heads, occipital pressure ulcers are not particularly common. The trochanteric region bears the body's weight when a person lies on the side. Like pressure sores of the sacrum and heel, pressure ulcers over the trochanter occur most commonly in people who lie in bed for an extended time. They occur most frequently in patients with severe contractures who are forced to lie in the lateral position.

Classification

In 1975, Darrell Shea, an orthopedic surgeon at the University of Miami, published a method for classifying pressure sores.[8] Each stage was defined simply by the anatomic depth of soft tissue damage; the etiology of the ulcer, the presence of osteomyelitis, and the rates of recurrence were not considered. With minor changes during the years, it remains the grading system most commonly used to classify pressure ulcers (Table 157-3). This staging system serves to communicate information between physicians and health care workers about the nature of the patient's wounds and allows more accurate comparisons of similar lesions in experimental studies.

Prevention

Preventing pressure sores is a never-ending process for individuals with spinal cord injuries. Anyone can get a pressure sore. There are several factors that place one at particular risk (Table 157-4). Persons at risk should have the skin carefully inspected for damage or redness, particularly over bone prominences; by the time of skin breakdown, a significantly wider area of permanent tissue damage is already present beneath the skin. Skin should be checked twice daily, once in the morning and once in the evening. In addition, the proper equipment for pressure relief should be provided and maintained, particularly wheelchair cushions and mattresses. The seat cushion needs to properly conform to the body and wheelchair. Cushion material consists most commonly of an air-fluid flotation system (ROHO cushion), but foam and gel are also commonly used. Pressure point mapping can be performed (Fig. 157-1) to custom fit the cushion, minimizing pressure throughout the surface of the seat.

TABLE 157-3 ✦ SHEA PRESSURE SORE GRADING SYSTEM[8]

Grade I	The ulcer is confined to the epidermis and superficial dermis
Grade II	The ulcer extends through the skin and into the subcutaneous fat
Grade III	The ulcer extends into the underlying muscle
Grade IV	The ulcer has invaded bone or joint structures

TABLE 157-4 ✦ RISKS ASSOCIATED WITH PRESSURE SORES

Limited mobility and prolonged bed rest: most common in persons with spinal cord injury or patients with altered mental status; extended pressure is placed on common pressure points (supine: ischium, sacrum, heels, occiput; lateral: trochanter; prone: chest, knees).

Decreased skin sensation: skin breakdown can go unnoticed, and patients are unable to sense discomfort from prolonged pressure in a single position; a cut or scratch can quickly develop into a large problem if it is not recognized and properly treated.

Moisture from bladder or bowel accidents can cause skin to break down more quickly.

Spasticity or improper transfer of patients in and out of chairs or beds can result in skin shearing and injury.

The mattress needs to provide proper support and protection. Specialized beds include air mattresses and air-fluidized beds (e.g., Clinitron or KinAir bed). In 1969, Hargest and Artz[9] developed the air-fluidized bed, which is still the basis for the beds most commonly used to treat patients with pressure sores. The "fluid" supporting the body consists of air and ceramic spheres. The concept is that any size object can be supported on a stream of air if the volume and pressure of stream are adequate. By use of numerous spheres, the density of the supporting medium is increased and the volume of air necessary to support the body is markedly decreased.[10] Warmed and humidified air provides optimal temperature and humidity for the patient. As a result, the bed surface pressures are less than on a foam mattress or waterbed. Patients should also frequently shift their weight at least every 10 minutes when they are sitting and every 1 to 2 hours while lying in bed.

The skin should be kept clean and dry. It should be washed and dried immediately after any bowel movement or occurrence of urinary incontinence. The patient should be treated medically for spasticity when it is present. The drug of choice for spasticity and reflex spasms is baclofen, a γ-aminobutyric acid receptor agonist; however, diazepam and dantrolene are effective alternatives or adjunctive treatments (Table 157-5).[11] When spasticity is refractory to pharmacologic treatment, surgical release of flexion contractures and neurosurgical means (i.e., cordotomy or rhizotomy) have been considered.

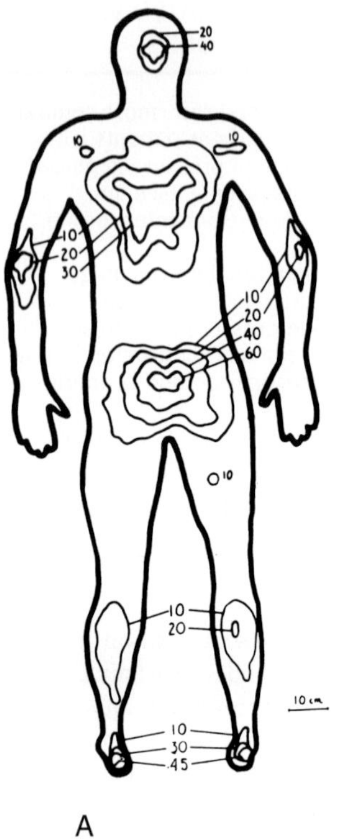

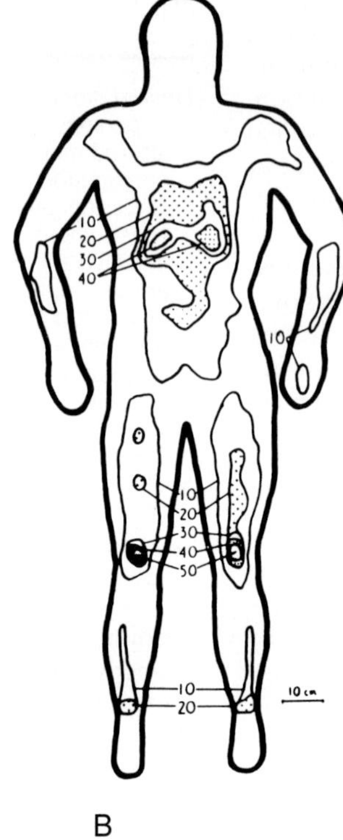

FIGURE 157-1. Comparison of pressure distribution in a healthy adult man supine *(A)* and prone *(B)* with his feet hanging over the edge of the bed. Values in millimeters of mercury. (From Linden O, Greenway RM, Piazza IM: Pressure distribution on the surface of the human body. Arch Phys Med Rehabil 1965;46:378. Reprinted with permission from American Congress of Rehabilitation Medicine and the American Academy of Physical Medicine and Rehabilitation.)

PRESSURE SORE TREATMENT

Evaluation of the Patient

If a pressure sore develops, one should make every effort to determine the cause. The patient can then be educated in ways to modify his or her environment and lifestyle to prevent pressure sore recurrence in the future. Questions that should be asked include the following:

Is there any change in job or activities that would cause a change in routine?
Is there any new equipment or change to any existing equipment?
Have there been any changes in the medical condition?

TABLE 157-5 ✦ TREATMENT OF SPASTICITY FOR SPINAL CORD INJURIES

Drugs
Diazepam, 10-40 mg
Baclofen, 15-100 mg
Dantrolene sodium, 50-800 mg
Mephenesin carbonate, 3-15 mg
Dimethothiazine, 300-500 mg
Orciprenaline, 40 mg
Intrathecal phenol
Operations
Neurosurgical ablation
Amputation
Contracture release and proximal femorectomy

Data from Reuler JB; Cooney TG: The pressure sore: pathophysiology and principles of management. Ann Intern Med 1981;94:661.

WILLINGNESS TO ALTER LIFESTYLE

One of the most important considerations during evaluation of the patient is determining a patient's willingness to alter lifestyle. It could reasonably be argued that if a person is unwilling to correct bad habits that risk pressure sore development, surgery to reconstruct the pressure sore site may be contraindicated because the risk of recurrence in this situation approaches 100%.[12]

OSTEOMYELITIS

Not uncommonly, a patient will be referred for evaluation of a pressure sore as either an inpatient or an outpatient with the diagnosis of osteomyelitis, determined by technetium Tc 99m bone scan or computed tomographic scan. Invariably, many of these patients have received or will go on to receive needless and potentially toxic antibiotic therapy based on this diagnosis. Although a normal bone scan rules out osteomyelitis, an abnormal scan is not diagnostic. Any patient with a grade IV pressure sore can have positive findings on bone scan because inflammation (osteitis) commonly affects the bone at the base of the wound. Likewise, although computed tomographic scan can identify disruption in the cortex of the bone, it cannot accurately diagnose bone infection. Lewis et al,[13] as corroborated by other studies, demonstrated that the single most useful test is a bone biopsy.

Nonsurgical Treatment

In the rare instance when a patient presents with a shallow, newly formed pressure sore (grade I or grade II), nonsurgical measures can be used to optimize conditions for wound healing without the need for surgical reconstruction. The primary objective is to secure a clean wound with beefy red granulation tissue at the base and to take steps to prevent sustained pressure over the wound site. Frequent dressing changes with wet-to-dry saline-soaked gauze dressings combined with daily sharp débridement at the bedside of any devitalized tissue and transfer of the patient to an air-fluidized bed or air mattress are the mainstays of treatment. Wound cultures can be helpful in instances of localized infection in trying to decide on topical therapy (e.g., silver sulfadiazine versus mafenide acetate [Sulfamylon]) or in tailoring the treatment of a systemic infection related to the pressure sore.

Surgical Treatment

The fundamental surgical principles for the management of pressure sores remain essentially unchanged since the report of Conway and Griffith[14] in 1956. Débridement of the ulcer, underlying bursa, and involved bone followed by soft tissue coverage remains the standard approach. The flap used for coverage should be designed as large as possible, with placement of the suture line away from the area of direct pressure; to preserve all future options for coverage, the flap design should not violate adjacent flap territories.

The development of musculocutaneous flaps in the 1970s significantly altered the approach to and success of pressure sore reconstruction.[15] However, despite high rates of flap survival, not all flaps are equally reliable in achieving coverage of the débrided pressure sore wound. Therefore, the most important step for early treatment success is appropriate flap selection. Because pressure sores that fail to heal while the patient is hospitalized virtually never heal after discharge, the immediate postoperative results will dictate future outcomes. Furthermore, the third or fourth option for flap coverage is as important as the primary choice; despite the best of efforts, recurrence rates after pressure sore reconstruction (>50% in the long term) have remained largely unchanged during the past 40 years. Therefore, a rationale for flap coverage designed to treat a patient during the long term is necessary from the time of initial evaluation.

DEFECT ANALYSIS

Location

The ischium is the most frequent site of pressure sore occurrence, due in part to increased pressure exerted on the region during sitting and to motion over the ischial area. The sacrum and trochanter are slightly less common sites of occurrence, followed by pressure sores to the heel (calcaneus).

Size and Depth

In evaluation of most pressure sores, the wound is frequently underestimated before surgical débridement. Failure to débride the pressure sore site adequately is a significant factor in the overall morbidity that follows attempted flap reconstruction. Injection of a mixture of methylene blue and hydrogen peroxide directly into the wound cavity is helpful in defining the wound dimensions and determining the extent of débridement necessary. The peroxide aids in mechanical cleaning of the wound.

With a few exceptions, the flaps described in this chapter can generally cover most pressure sores. Rarely, two different flaps are required to fill a defect. For all insensate patients (e.g., paraplegics, quadriplegics), the bone prominence at the base of the wound is a significant source of pressure sore recurrence; therefore, partial ostectomy is considered in all ischial, sacral, and trochanteric sores. A total unilateral ischiectomy, in an ischial pressure sore, is contraindicated because of the subsequent shift in maximum pressure to the contralateral ischial tuberosity from such an ischial resection (resulting in a high incidence of contralateral ischial pressure sores).[16] Furthermore, bilateral total ischiectomies place the patient flat on the perineum, which may give rise to urethral fistulas and diffuse perineal ulcerations.[17-19]

In long-standing pressure sores, osteomyelitis may be present within the bone at the base of the wound. Therefore, care must be taken to débride all nonviable bone tissue before the reconstruction. Bone biopsy is indicated at the time of débridement if osteomyelitis is suspected to aid in diagnosis and to direct systemic antibiotic therapy. Bone viability is determined most accurately by active bleeding at the bone surface during operative débridement.

Associated Problems

SPINAL CORD INJURY. In the patient with congenital or acquired spinal cord injury, muscle denervation results in muscle fiber atrophy of the flaps used for pressure sore coverage. Therefore, the muscle fibers are often difficult to identify, and care must be taken not to inadvertently divide the muscle during flap elevation.

Prior Surgery. Patients have frequently had multiple procedures to treat a pressure sore wound. A careful surgical history (by examination of the prior skin incisions) and discussion with the patient's previous surgeon are necessary and can often alter the reconstructive plan (Fig. 157-2). Other operative procedures related to the vascular supply of the region should be noted. When the patient has had surgery possibly affecting vascular supply, preoperative angiographic studies may need to be considered. For example, selective arteriography to confirm the patency of the medial circumflex femoral artery is recommended when a gracilis flap is being considered for coverage if the patient has previously undergone aortic or lower extremity revascularization procedures.

Infection. Any sign of local or systemic infection should be evaluated and treated before definitive reconstruction. Localized infection at the pressure sore site is an indication to stage or to delay reconstruction until the infection is treated.

RECONSTRUCTIVE GOALS

Problem Evaluation

The defect must be assessed in terms of its impact on the patient's survival and quality of life. The primary goal of pressure sore reconstruction is reliable soft tissue coverage. Adequate coverage usually entails more than a local skin flap. Although muscle is more sensitive to pressure necrosis than skin is,[20] in the reconstruction of pressure sores, muscle serves an important function both in eliminating the dead space associated with most pressure ulcers and in improving the vascularity of the wound itself.[21] It should also be appreciated, though, that thick muscle flaps may not always be the best choice (e.g., inferior gluteal thigh flap for ischial sore coverage).

Form and Function

When pressure sores develop in ambulatory patients, both postoperative function and body contour need to be considered in planning the reconstruction. For these patients, standard flaps can be modified.[22] For example, one can preserve the inferior half of the gluteus maximus muscle when a gluteus maximus myocutaneous advancement flap is elevated for sacral coverage, preserve the superior half of the gluteus maximus muscle when an ischial sore is covered with the inferior gluteus maximus island flap, or use the transverse back flap or the inferior gluteal thigh flap for sacral coverage. All these flaps provide coverage without compromising function.

RECONSTRUCTIVE OPTIONS

Pedicled Flaps

Local flap transposition is the mainstay of treatment for pressure sore reconstruction. The options for coverage include musculocutaneous flaps, principally to provide adequate tissue bulk and to enhance perfusion, and tissue coaptation in the depths of the pressure sore defect. Several fasciocutaneous flaps, however, have proved to be useful for pressure sore coverage (e.g., the inferior gluteal thigh flap for ischial coverage).

Microvascular Tissue Transplantation

Microvascular tissue transplantation for pressure sore reconstruction is reserved for those instances when local sources of donor tissue are no longer available (due to recurrent prior use) or when extensive and complex wounds are present. The limited flaps available for microvascular transplantation are characterized by long, anatomically constant vascular pedicles with relatively large lumen diameters. The success of these types of flaps depends on the availability of reliable, adequately sized recipient vessels close to the defect. In addition, when one considers that a significant number of patients treated for pressure sores are paraplegic and therefore depend on their upper body strength for mobility (e.g., latissimus dorsi), the list of available free flaps for pressure sore coverage becomes more limited.

SYSTEMATIC APPROACH

Preoperative Planning

The medical and functional status of the patient must be thoroughly evaluated preoperatively. Every attempt should be made to optimize the patient hemodynamically. Respiratory and neurologic function should be stable and adequate enough to tolerate the stress of an operation. Patients with pressure sores, particularly those with permanent spinal cord deficits, are often significantly debilitated, including poor nutritional status (in long-standing ulcers, protein loss through the wound results in a nitrogen imbalance with a lowering of serum protein level, anemia, and vitamin deficiency), localized and systemic infection, and other functional problems directly related to the impaired neurologic state (e.g., neurogenic bladders with recurrent urinary infections). These problems pose a serious risk for impaired wound healing. Twenty-nine percent of patients can be expected to have one risk factor for impaired wound healing,[23,24] and another 15% can be expected to have two risk factors (Table 157-6). All efforts should be made preoperatively to optimize the patient's condition and to decrease the risk of postoperative wound breakdown.

Most pressure sores can be débrided and flap coverage provided in a single operation. Healing rates, in

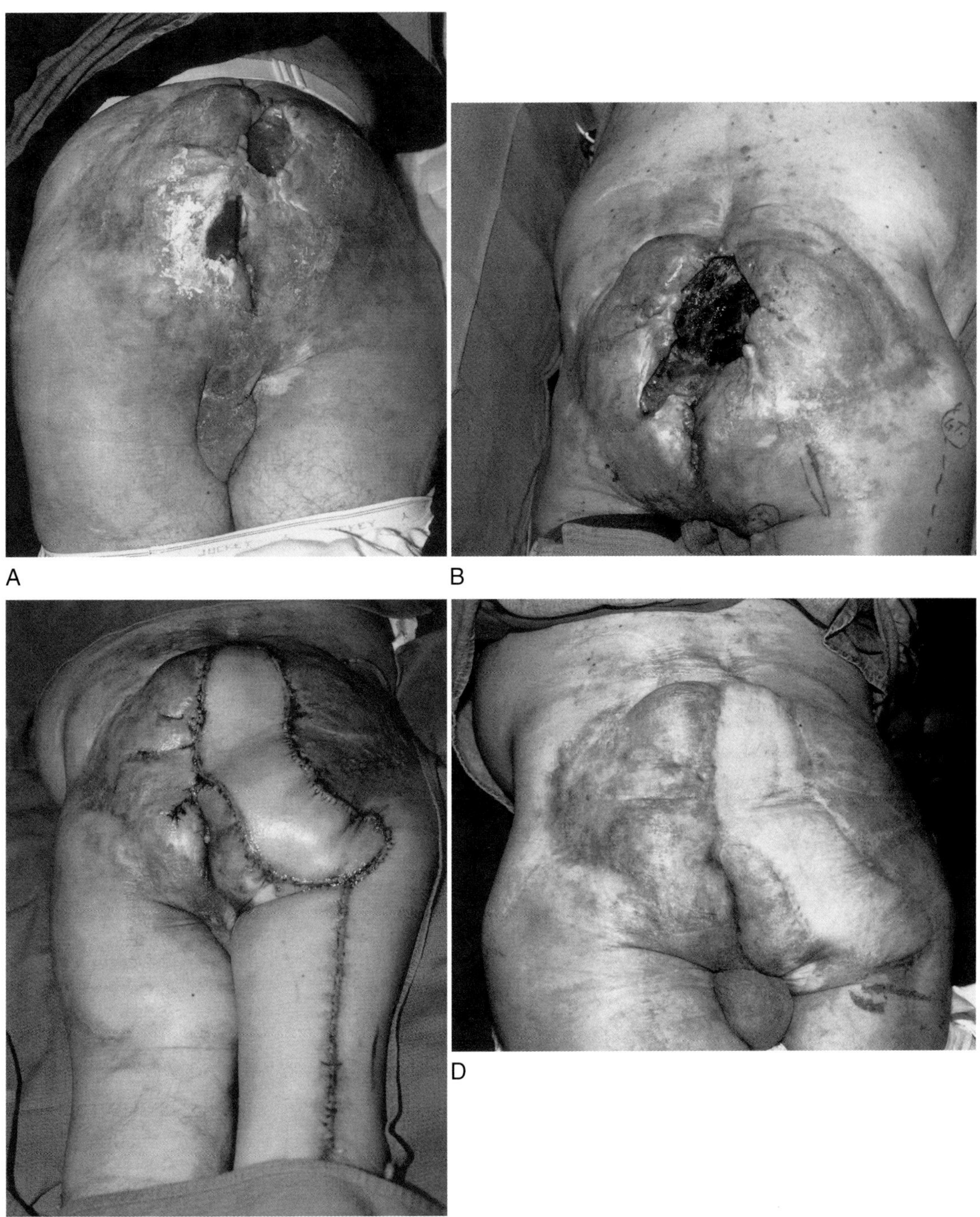

FIGURE 157-2. *A,* A 42-year-old paraplegic with an extensive sacral pressure sore. Examination of prior surgical incision and medical chart review revealed that all local options from the gluteal region had already been used, necessitating a more innovative solution for reconstruction. *B,* Sacral wound after operative débridement. *C,* An extended gluteal thigh flap sutured into position. *D,* Stable wound coverage at 6 months postoperatively.

TABLE 157-6 ✦ RISK FACTORS FOR IMPAIRED WOUND HEALING

Age > 65 yr
Smoking
Diabetes
Renal failure
Wound infection
Local irradiation
Systemic infection
Immunosuppressive agents
Hemodynamic instability
Prolonged hyperalimentation
Low total protein

Data from Parry SW, Mathes SJ: Bilateral gluteus maximus myocutaneous advancement flaps: sacral coverage for ambulatory patients. Ann Plast Surg 1982;8:443; and Riou JP, Cohen JR, Johnson H Jr: Factors influencing wound dehiscence. Am J Surg 1992;163:324.

general, are similar for single-staged and multiple-staged reconstructions. This is true regardless of the patient's age, the size of the pressure sore, or even the number of prior attempts at coverage. In fact, contraindications to performance of immediate flap reconstruction involve only those patients in whom local infection is not fully under control or whose ability to physiologically tolerate the operative procedure is in question (e.g., severe cardiopulmonary disease, sepsis). In patients with local or severe systemic infections, staged débridement should be performed until the infection is cleared and the patient is medically stable enough to withstand the reconstructive procedure.

Once the decision to reconstruct the pressure sore site is made, flap design should be considered. Reliable flap design and transfer depend on a thorough knowledge of the basic features of a flap and its potential modifications and applications. Design of the flap should often begin after operative débridement is complete so that the size of the defect to be filled is not underestimated.

Flap Selection

Forming a rationale for reconstructive selection is based on flap reliability (successful healing rates), reusability, and need to preserve as many future flap options as possible. Flap selection and the appropriate short- and long-term sequence of flap use significantly improve pressure sore coverage success rates. In an effort to devise an algorithm for flap selection in the long term, it is clear that certain flaps are more reliable than others for primary pressure sore coverage. Defining a flap's reliability is, in part, influenced by several factors, including the site of the pressure sore, the design of the flap for a given coverage site, and the location of the flap relative to the site of coverage. On the basis of these criteria, primary, secondary, and tertiary flap choices can be determined for each pressure sore site (Table 157-7).

Ischium

Several characteristics of the selected flaps for ischial pressure sore coverage differentiate in their effectiveness relative to one another. The inferior gluteus maximus island flap provides a large skin island to cover virtually any sore while still allowing primary donor site closure. Because the skin island can be so large, it is always planned to be larger than the débrided ischial defect, thereby ensuring tension-free ischial closure without the suture line's running along the prior sore location. In fact, the suture lines joining the inferior gluteus island flap to the ischial area tend to be superior and inferior to the margins of the prior ischial sore. This extra soft tissue and skin also allow this flap to be re-elevated or rotated for use again in a local sore recurrence. In comparison with other possible flaps for ischial coverage, the inferior gluteus maximus flap places the maximum amount of muscle and soft tissue bulk into the débrided sore. Of equal importance, the harvest of the gluteus maximus does not preclude the future use of any of the other flaps for ischial coverage. Careful gluteal harvest spares the inferior gluteal vessels, preserving the inferior gluteal thigh, biceps

TABLE 157-7 ✦ FLAP SELECTION FOR PRESSURE SORE COVERAGE

	Sacrum	Ischium	Trochanter
1	V-Y gluteus maximus	Inferior gluteus maximus island flap	Tensor fascia lata (TFL) ± V-Y
2	V-Y gluteus maximus (contralateral)	Inferior gluteus thigh flap (IGT)	Readvance TFL
3	Readvance bilateral V-Y gluteus maximus Other gluteal flap Transverse back flap	Readvance IGT V-Y hamstring Gracilis TFL (expanded or delayed) Rectus abdominis	Vastus lateralis Rectus femoris IGT Rectus abdominis

Modified from Foster RD, Anthony JP, Mathes SJ, et al: Flap selection as a determinant of success in pressure sore coverage. Arch Surg 1997;132:868.

femoris, and hamstring flaps. Perhaps also important to its success, the gluteus maximus, like the ischial sore itself, is confined to the pelvis. Both the flap and the ischial area move together as a unit and are thus less susceptible to tension, particularly with leg flexion or extension.

The inferior gluteal thigh flap, although providing no muscle and lacking bulk, is effective for ischial coverage. Like the inferior gluteus maximus flap, the inferior gluteal thigh flap preserves other flap options, although a subsequent hamstring flap would require a skin graft for coverage once the inferior gluteal thigh flap had been used. In contrast to the inferior gluteus maximus island flap, it is subject to slightly more shearing and tension forces because of its location on the mobile leg. The inferior gluteal thigh flap is rotated 90 degrees medially to cover the ischium, thereby distributing any tension across a much longer suture line while simultaneously avoiding placement of a suture line across the center of the ischial sore as a V-Y flap would do.

In patients in whom the inferior gluteus maximus and inferior gluteal thigh flaps are not available, the gracilis flap and the V-Y hamstring flap are viable options. However, whereas V-Y flaps do well for sacral and trochanteric sore coverage (the V-Y gluteus maximus flap and the V-Y tensor fascia lata flap, respectively), all V-Y flaps are intrinsically limited in their advancement by the length of the supplying pedicle, which seems to significantly limit the use of the V-Y hamstring flap. The expanded or delayed tensor fascia lata flap and the rectus abdominis flap (tunneled through the groin) (Fig. 157-3)[25] are additional options that should be pursued before leg amputation or thigh (or other) flap coverage is considered. The tensor fascia lata flap is simply not reliable enough in the distal 6 to 8 cm of the flap (the area adjacent to the knee), and this distal portion of the flap is critical to ischial coverage. Thus, if a tensor fascia lata flap must be used for ischial sore coverage, it should be delayed or an expander used to enhance the vascularity of the distal tip.

Inferior Gluteus Maximus Island Flap.[26,27] The origin of the inferior gluteus maximus island flap is the gluteal line of ilium and sacrum. Its insertion is at the greater tuberosity of the femur and the iliotibial band of the fascia lata. The blood supply is derived from the inferior gluteal artery and venae comitantes (Fig. 157-4). The pedicle runs along the deep surface of the gluteal muscle, below the level of the piriformis muscle.

Flap Elevation

Landmarks. To position the skin paddle over the gluteal muscle, a line is drawn along the medial border of the muscle, from the lower edge of the sacrum to the gluteal tuberosity of the femur, just below the greater tuberosity. The medial edge of the gluteal muscle can usually be identified along the lateral edge of the ischial pressure sore during wound débridement (Fig. 157-5). The skin island of the flap should be centered over the gluteal crease between the ischial tuberosity medially and the greater trochanter laterally.

Flap Design. The medial edge of the skin island usually abuts the lateral edge of the ischial sore (Fig. 157-5*B*), and therefore no skin bridge is necessary. The skin island should not simply be the size of the cutaneous ischial defect but as large as possible (Fig. 157-6) without involving the area over the trochanter. The skin island should also be positioned slightly distal to the ischial sore to compensate for the shortening of the axis of the flap as the muscle is rotated medially.

Flap Elevation and Inset. The skin is incised and the muscle is divided deep distally, several centimeters beyond the skin island of the flap (see Fig. 157-5*B* and *C*). The additional muscle is used to help obliterate the débrided ulcer cavity. Care should be taken to preserve the extension of the inferior gluteal artery and the sciatic nerve as they course onto the thigh. Division of the muscle continues laterally and then superiorly, mobilizing only the inferior half of the gluteus muscle (see Fig. 157-6*C* and *D*). The piriformis muscle, deep to the gluteus maximus muscle, is a reliable landmark for determining the midportion of the gluteus muscle (see Fig. 157-4). Care should be taken to avoid injury to the inferior gluteal artery as it emerges beneath the piriformis muscle onto the undersurface of the gluteal muscle. The muscle is divided just to the point at which the flap can rotate easily into the defect. Proximal to the skin island, the anterior surface of the muscle is exposed and dissected from distal to proximal. The flap is inset over drains, and the donor site is closed primarily.

Technical Considerations. In patients with longstanding paralysis, the muscle can be significantly atrophied to the extent that the color of the muscle is difficult to distinguish from the subcutaneous fat surrounding it. In this instance, it is helpful to widely expose the anterior surface of the muscle first when the flap is elevated because it is easier to distinguish the striations of the muscle from the subcutaneous fat.

Gluteal Thigh Flap.[28] The blood supply for the gluteal thigh flap is the descending terminal branch of the inferior gluteal artery (see Fig. 157-4).

Flap Elevation

Landmarks. A line drawn vertically, midway between the greater trochanter and the ischial tuberosity and perpendicular to the gluteal crease, represents the central axis of the flap as well as the course of the

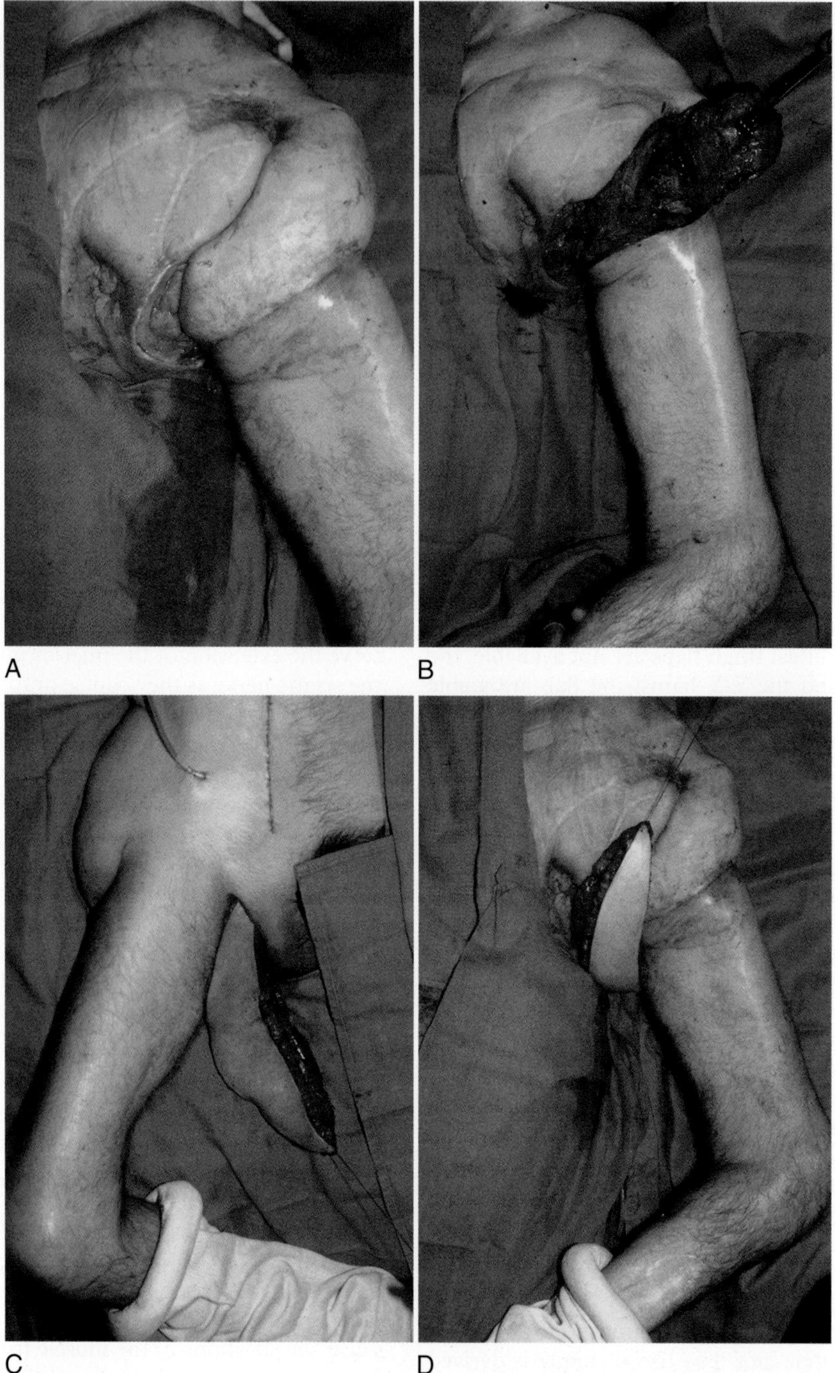

FIGURE 157-3. *A,* Right ischial pressure sore after multiple attempts at flap reconstruction. *B,* After pressure sore débridement and elevation of prior tensor fascia lata flap. *C,* Patient in supine position with right rectus abdominis musculocutaneous flap rotated down into the groin before repositioning of the patient and flap inset. *D,* Patient back in the prone position with rectus flap rotated into the pressure sore site.

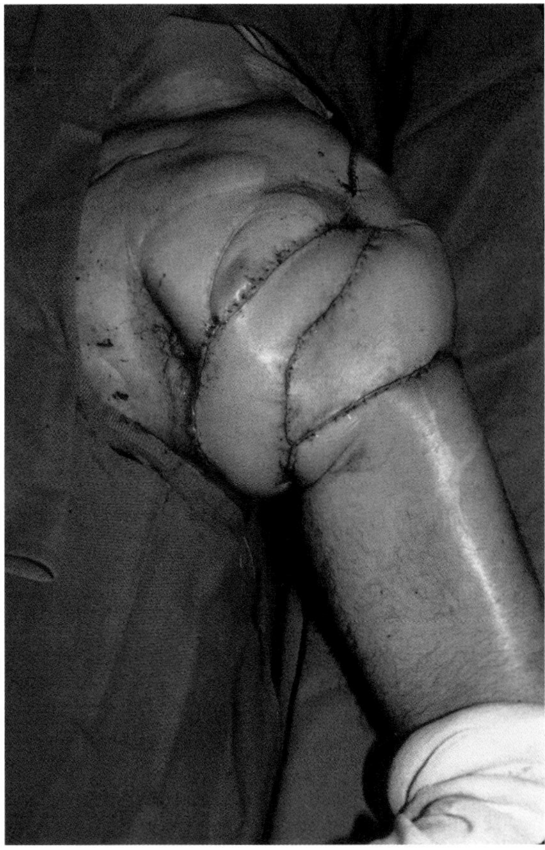

E

FIGURE 157-3, cont'd. *E*, Rectus flap inset and tensor fascia lata flap reinset laterally.

inferior gluteal artery as it continues on to the posterior thigh (Figs. 157-7 and 157-8).

Flap Design. The flap is centered over the posterior thigh and designed less than 12 cm in width to allow direct donor site closure (Fig. 157-8*C*). The distal tip of the flap can extend to within 8 cm of the popliteal fossa. The key anatomic structures during the dissection are the sciatic nerve, the posterior cutaneous nerve (S1-3), and the inferior gluteal artery, which travel together (medial to lateral) around the ischial tuberosity as they exit the gluteal space. On the thigh, the sciatic nerve is the deepest structure, lying on the adductor magnus muscle. The sciatic nerve is crossed obliquely by the long head of the biceps femoris. The posterior cutaneous nerve lies in the subcutaneous tissue (next to the inferior gluteal artery), just below the fascia lata and superficial to the biceps femoris muscle.

Flap Elevation and Inset. The skin incision over the distal third of the flap is made down through the deep fascia on the posterior thigh. The posterior femoral cutaneous nerve should be easily identified at the distal midline tip of the flap; if it is not, the rest of the skin incisions are adjusted so that the flap is centered over the course of the nerve. The descending branch of the inferior gluteal artery is ligated adjacent to the nerve, and the flap is elevated to the level of the gluteal crease (inferior edge of the gluteus maximus muscle) along the plane deep to the fascia. The flap should be easily rotated into the ischial defect at this level of dissection and inset over drains (Fig. 157-8*C*).

Technical Considerations. Flap elevation should begin with the distal skin incision to confirm that the flap is centered over the vascular pedicle. Blood flow Doppler study can be used to trace the course of the descending branch of the inferior gluteal artery during the flap design.

GRACILIS FLAP.[29] The origin of the gracilis flap is the pubic symphysis. The insertion point is the medial condyle of the tibia. The blood supply is derived from the ascending branch of the medial circumflex femoral artery and venae comitantes (Fig. 157-9). The anterior femoral cutaneous nerve (L2-3) provides sensory innervation to the majority of the anterior medial thigh. A small cutaneous branch of the anterior obturator nerve provides sensory innervation to the superior skin territory of the gracilis muscle. The pedicle passes posterior to the adductor longus muscle, crossing in front of the deeper adductor magnus muscle to enter the gracilis muscle. The pedicle can be visualized by medial retraction of the adductor longus muscle.

Flap Elevation

Landmarks. The dominant pedicle enters the posterior medial muscle belly approximately 10 cm inferior to the pubic tubercle.

Flap Design. A line is drawn between the pubic tubercle and the medial condyle of the femur. The muscle is located 2 to 3 cm posterior and parallel to this line. The skin island (8 × 15 cm) is centered over the proximal third of the muscle, the source of the majority of musculocutaneous perforating vessels, but it can extend over the middle third of the muscle.

Flap Elevation and Inset. First, a small incision is made distal to the skin island, over the medial condyle of the knee. Care must be taken to properly identify the tendon of insertion of the gracilis muscle. Several muscles insert in this region (Fig. 157-10). The sartorius muscle and the saphenous vein insert superiorly to the gracilis muscle; the tendons of the semimembranosus and semitendinosus muscles insert directly posterior. A Penrose drain is placed around the gracilis tendon, and upward traction is placed to visualize the course of the muscle throughout the thigh and to confirm the skin island position. The skin island is redrawn if it is not correctly placed over the center of the muscle belly. The skin incisions are completed, and the muscle edge is identified superior and inferior to the skin island dissection. Temporary sutures are placed

Text continued on p. 1334

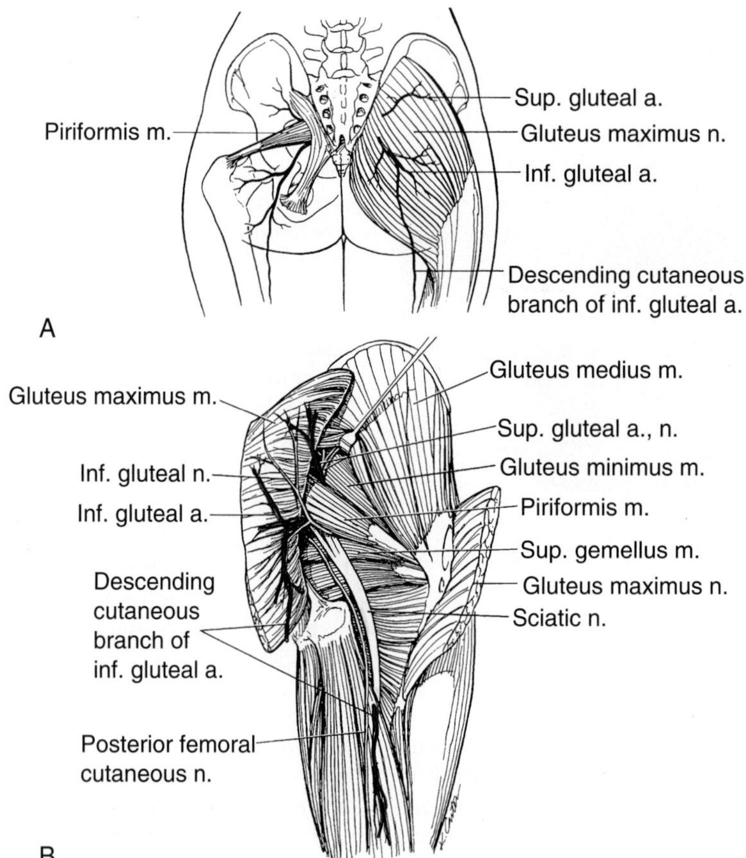

FIGURE 157-4. *A*, Anatomy of the buttock region showing the relationship of the superior and inferior gluteal vessels to the piriformis muscle. *B*, Structures deep to the gluteus maximus muscle.

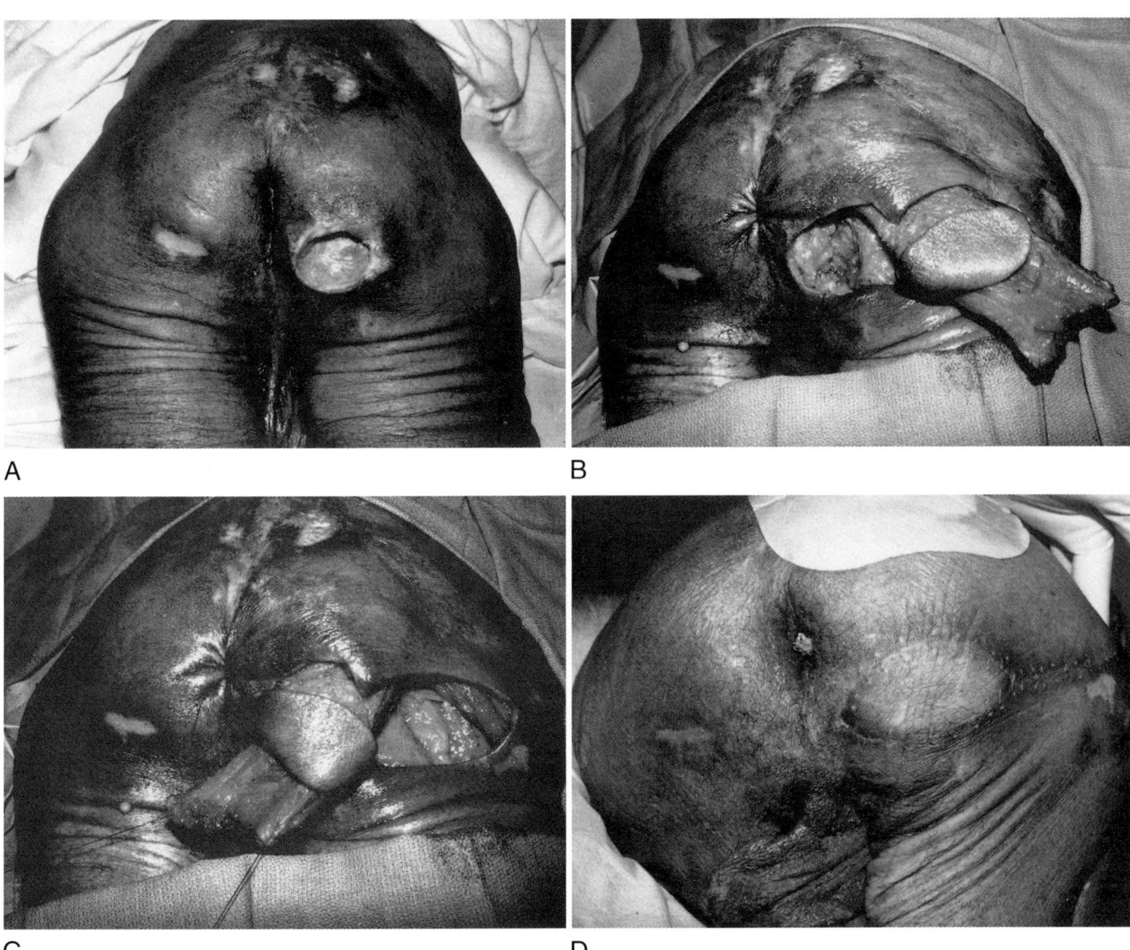

FIGURE 157-5. *A,* A 56-year-old with a stage IV right ischial pressure sore. *B,* Right inferior gluteus maximus island flap raised after ischial sore débridement and partial ostectomy. Note that the muscle is divided distal to the skin island and that the skin island is designed just distal to the level of the pressure sore to compensate for the shortened axis of rotation during flap transposition. The medial edge of the muscle can be identified as it runs along the lateral border of the pressure sore. *C,* Rotation of the flap into the ulcer site. *D,* Healed flap 4 weeks postoperatively.

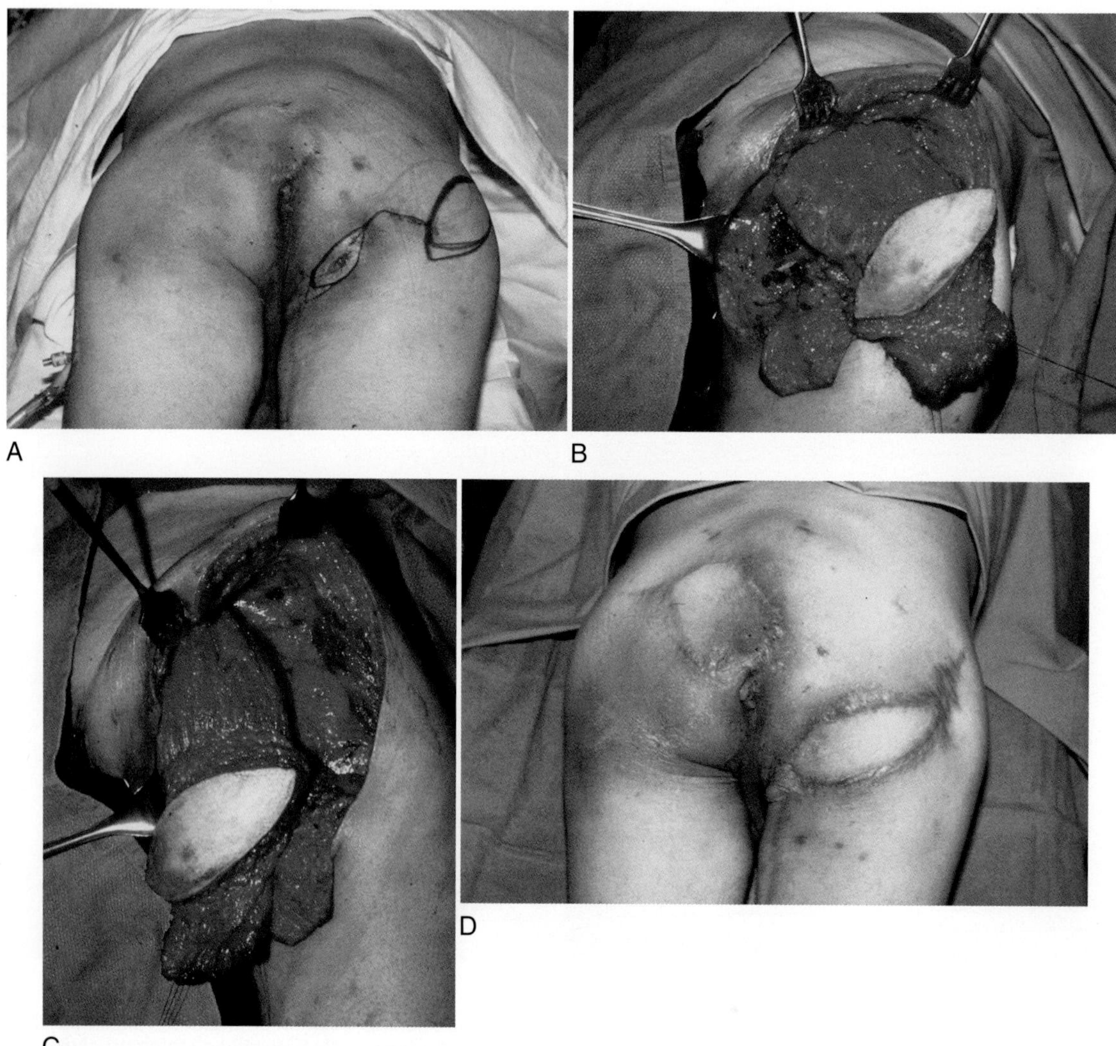

FIGURE 157-6. *A,* Right inferior gluteus maximus island flap for right ischial sore coverage. Note the size of the skin island relative to the size of the cutaneous opening over the ischium. *B,* Flap elevation. *C,* Flap rotation. Note the superior extent of the inferior muscle division to allow flap rotation without tension. *D,* Flap healed 6 weeks postoperatively.

GLUTEAL THIGH FLAP (posterior thigh flap)

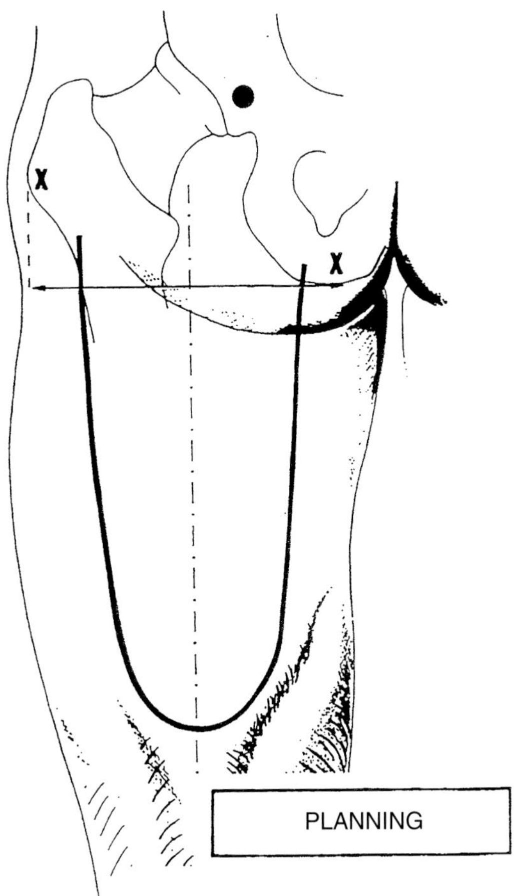

FIGURE 157-7. Flap design. The point of rotation of the flap is marked 5 cm above the ischial tuberosity. The central axis is midway between the greater trochanter and the ischial tuberosity and perpendicular to the gluteal crease. The flap can be extended from the midgluteal region to within 8 cm of the popliteal fossa. (From Hurwitz DJ, Swartz WM, Mathes SJ: The gluteal thigh flap: a reliable, sensate flap for the closure of buttock and perineal wounds. Plast Reconstr Surg 1981;68:521.)

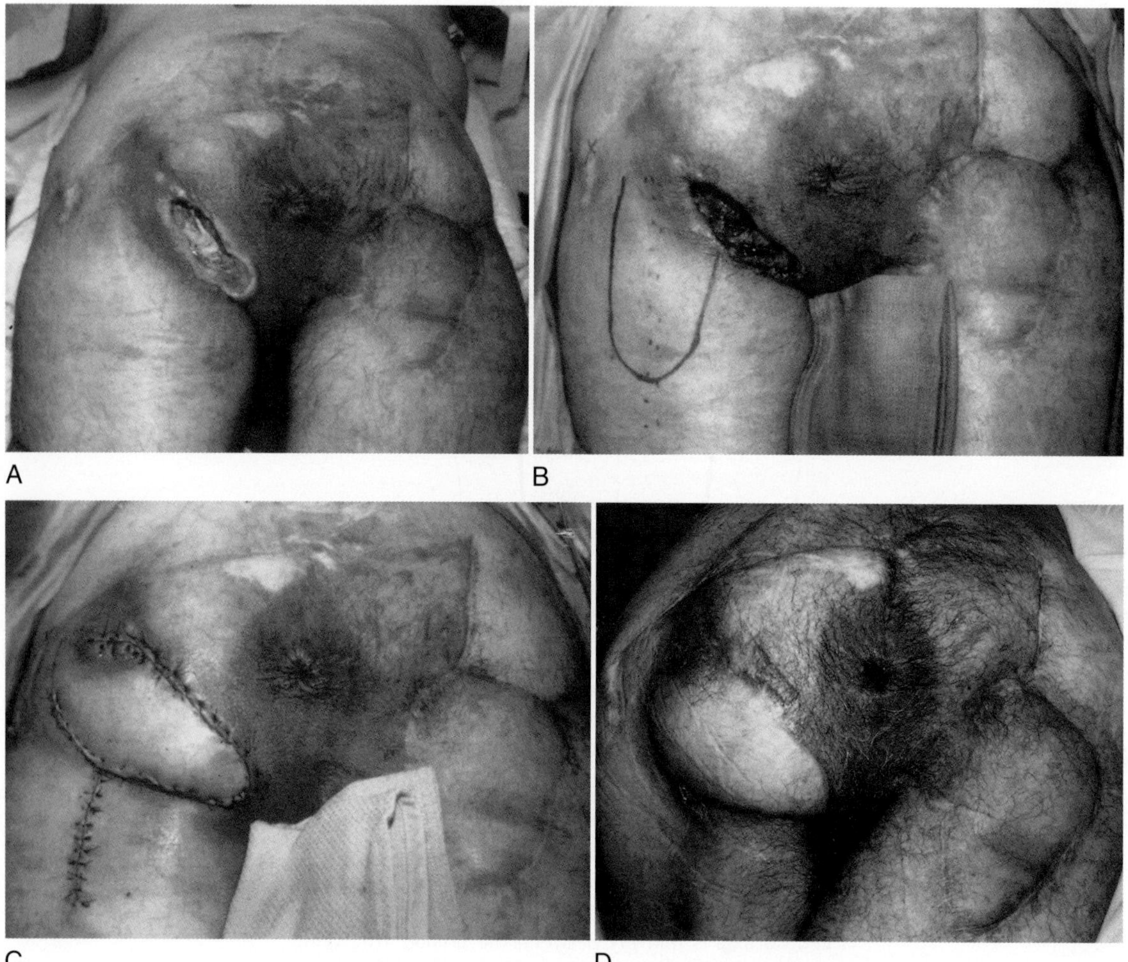

FIGURE 157-8. *A,* Left grade IV ischial pressure sore. *B,* Design of gluteal thigh flap. X marks the trochanter. The dotted line marks the course of the inferior gluteal artery that was confirmed by Doppler examination intraoperatively. *C,* After flap inset and direct donor site closure. *D,* Stable coverage 1 year postoperatively.

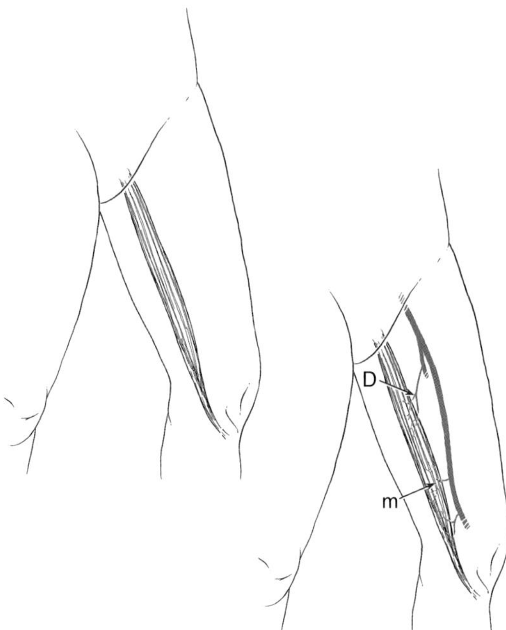

FIGURE 157-9. Dominant pedicle: ascending branch of medial circumflex femoral artery (D). Minor pedicle: one or two branches of superficial femoral artery (m). (From Mathes SJ, Nahai F: Reconstructive Surgery: Principles, Anatomy, and Technique. New York, Churchill Livingstone, 1997:1174.)

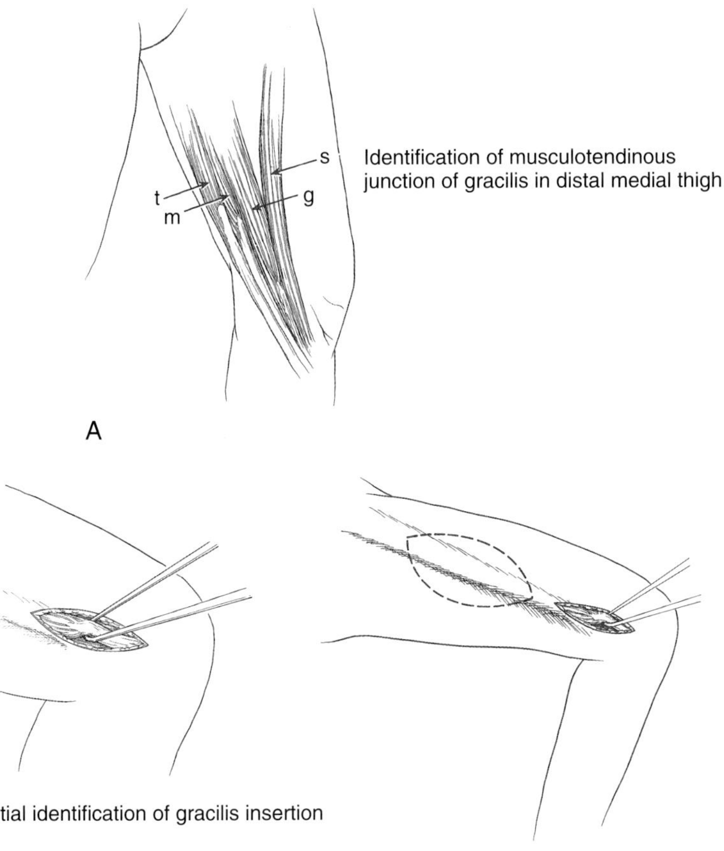

FIGURE 157-10. *A,* Identification of musculocutaneous junction of gracilis in distal medial thigh. *B,* Initial identification of gracilis insertion. *C,* Vertical skin island design with interior traction on muscle insertion. g, gracilis; m, semimembranosus; s, sartorius; t, semitendinosus. (From Mathes SJ, Nahai F: Reconstructive Surgery: Principles, Anatomy, and Technique. New York, Churchill Livingstone, 1997:1185.)

between the muscle and the skin island to maintain the position of the skin over the muscle as it is being elevated. The tendon of insertion of the gracilis muscle is divided; the flap is elevated from distal to proximal, and branches from the superficial femoral artery (see Fig. 157-9) are ligated as necessary. Careful retraction of the adductor longus muscle medially will reveal the dominant blood supply to the flap as it passes over the adductor magnus muscle approximately 10 cm inferior to the pubic tubercle. Every attempt should be made to keep the proximal skin of the thigh intact rather than to design the skin overlying the gracilis muscle as an island. This will maintain further blood supply to the medial thigh skin from the external pudendal vessels. The muscle is rotated (Fig. 157-11) and sutured into the defect (bolster sutures are helpful for flap insetting), followed by suturing of the skin island into the skin defect edges (Fig. 157-11*D*). The distal end of the flap can be de-epithelialized and used to obliterate the deep space beyond the cutaneous defect (Fig. 157-11*C*).

Technical Considerations. To confirm the proper placement of the skin island over the muscle, it is imperative to identify the gracilis tendon distally first, by the insertion at the knee. The skin island over the distal gracilis is not reliable. To maximize the blood supply to the skin over the proximal and middle muscle, the proximal skin territory should remain intact if possible and not be incised as a skin island. This will maintain branches from the external pudendal vessels to the medial thigh.

Sacrum

Relative to the choices for flap coverage of the ischium, there is a decreased variability in flap success rates between the different types of flaps used for sacral coverage. The V-Y gluteus maximus flap and other variations using the gluteus maximus muscle (Fig. 157-12) are the mainstays of treatment for sacral reconstruction. The unilateral V-Y flap design is reliable, and if a large enough skin island is used, it can be readvanced one or more times. Bilateral V-Y advancement is reserved as a tertiary choice or for larger sacral defects. In addition, for managing sacral defects in ambulatory patients, the V-Y gluteus maximus flap provides coverage without loss of function or hip instability by preserving the origin and insertion of the inferior half of the muscle.[22] The transverse back flap is primarily an alternative flap for sacral coverage because of its limited size.[30] It is recommended for small sacral defects.

V-Y Gluteus Maximus Advancement Flap. The origin of the gluteus maximus is the gluteal line of ilium and sacrum. The insertion point is the greater tuberosity of the femur and the iliotibial band of the fascia lata. The blood supply is the superior gluteal artery and venae comitantes. The pedicle courses along the deep surface of the gluteal muscle after emerging above the piriformis muscle (see Fig. 157-4).

For ambulatory patients, the course of the motor and sensory nerves is important to the dissection. Motor innervation is provided by the inferior gluteal nerve (L5 to S1-2) that courses through the sciatic foramen, entering the deep surface of the gluteus maximus muscle at the level of the piriformis muscle. The skin territory of the gluteus maximus muscle receives sensory innervation from the nerve branches of the posterior division of S1-3 medially and the posterior division of L1-3 laterally. A neurosensory musculocutaneous flap can be transposed if the medial skin island is elevated and these nerves are preserved.

Flap Elevation

Landmarks. The bone landmarks, lateral edge of the sacrum and greater trochanter, identify the origin and insertion, respectively, of the muscle. The posterior superior iliac crest and the ischial tuberosity mark the superior and inferior margins of the muscle, respectively.

Arc of Rotation. The point of rotation is at the lateral border of the sacrum where the dominant vascular pedicle enters the muscle. Division of the muscle fibers of origin from the sacrum with mobilization of the vascular pedicle allows better rotation of the muscle and will increase the arc of rotation. It should also be appreciated how extensively the skin alone can be mobilized and advanced (Fig. 157-13).

Flap Design. The skin island is centered over the medial muscle, adjacent to the sacral wound. In patients with an increased risk of pressure sore recurrence (e.g., paraplegics, quadriplegics, patients with altered mental status or decreased local sensation), it is important to design the skin island as large as possible (Fig. 157-14) so that readvancement is an option in the future. For patients who are ambulatory and with normal sensation, the flap needs to be only as large as the defect (Fig. 157-15).

Flap Elevation and Inset. Division of the entire fibers of insertion or of the superior or inferior half of these fibers is performed, depending on whether the flap design is a segmental or a complete muscle advancement flap. The fibers of origin are divided at the lateral edge of the sacrum. The piriformis muscle is key to correct division of the muscle in its midportion for segmental elevation of either the superior or inferior half, and it is also a guide to the location of the point of entry of the superior and inferior gluteal vessels into the deep surface of the muscle. Initial exposure of the pedicle will avoid injury during the muscle division into its superior and inferior halves. The muscle is then elevated over the sacral edge. The unilateral flap can reach beyond the midline as well as be rotated

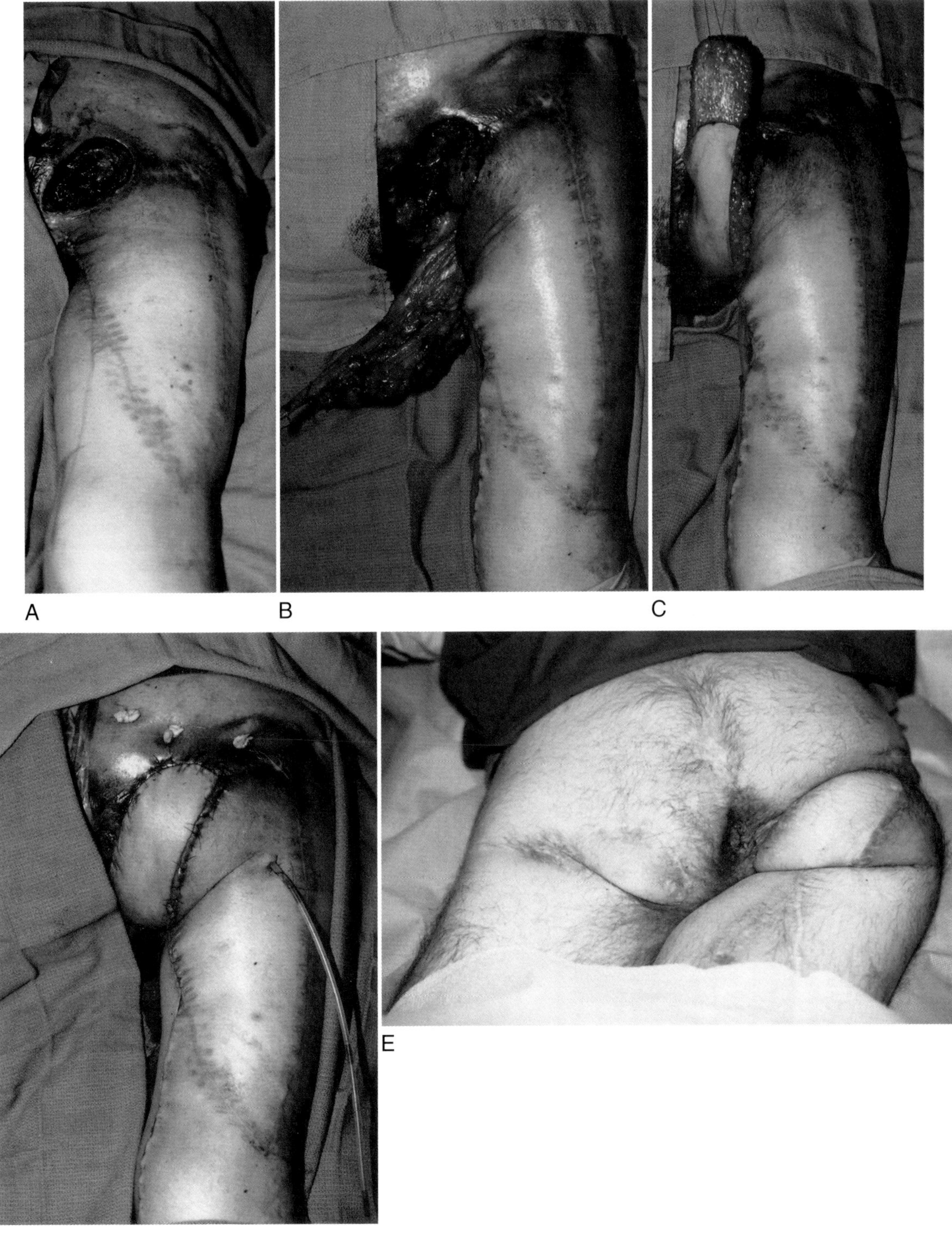

FIGURE 157-11. *A,* Recurrent grade IV right ischial pressure sore after previous V-Y hamstring flap. Note that the inferior gluteal thigh flap and the inferior gluteus maximus island flap are no longer options and that the superior suture line of the hamstring flap lies right along the point of maximum pressure in the area of the ischium. *B,* After pressure sore débridement and elevation of a right gracilis musculocutaneous flap. *C,* Gracilis musculocutaneous flap rotated superiorly. Note that the distal edge of the flap has been de-epithelialized to be used to obliterate the deep superior cavity beyond the cutaneous defect. *D,* Flap inset with bolster sutures superiorly to secure the deep superior portion of the flap. *E,* One year postoperatively with stable coverage.

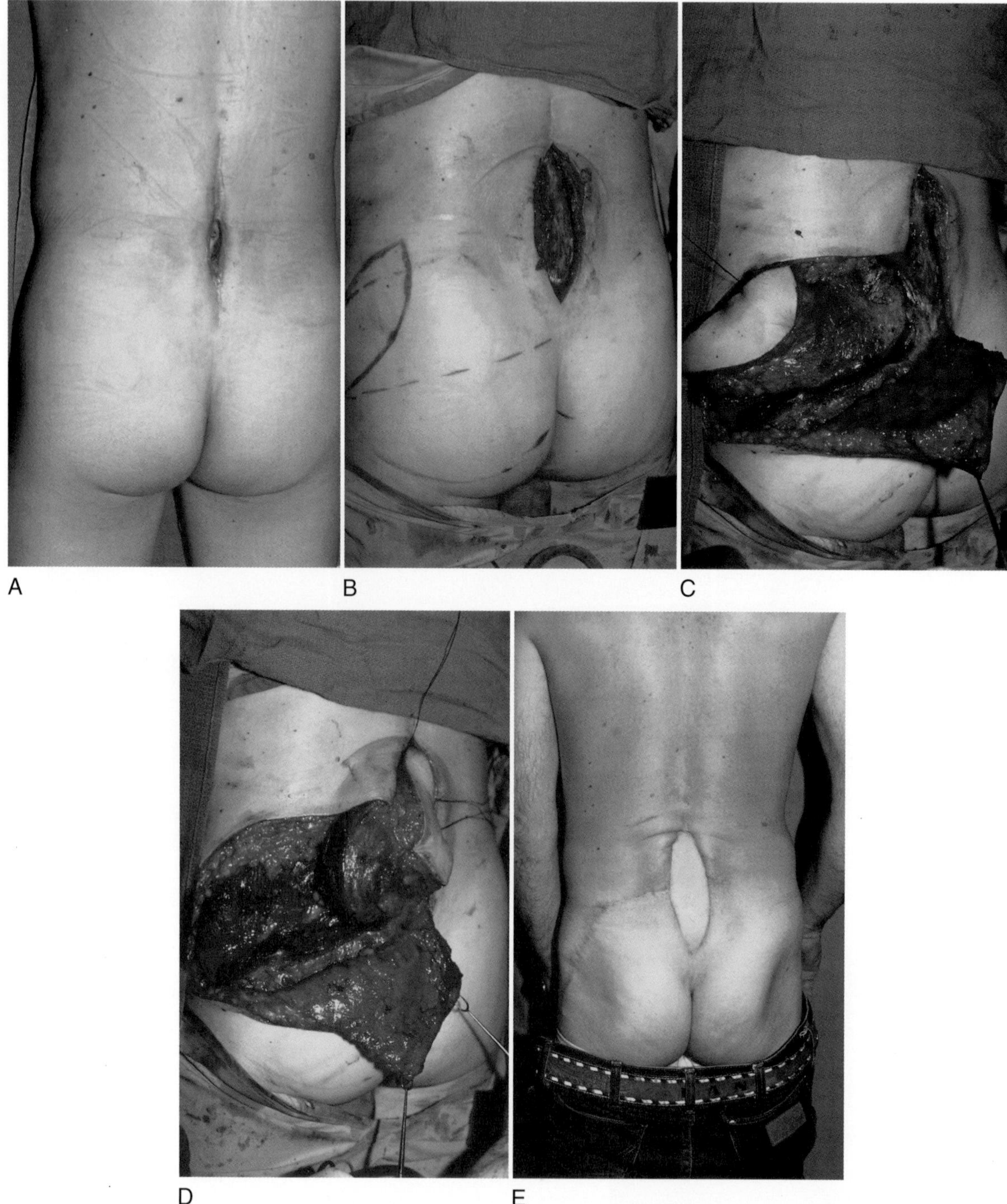

FIGURE 157-12. *A,* Chronic sacral wound in an ambulatory patient. *B,* Design of a superior gluteal island rotational flap after wound débridement. *C,* Flap elevation of the superior half of the gluteal muscle. *D,* Flap rotation to fill the defect. *E,* Stable coverage and good donor site contour with no functional impairment as a result of segmental muscle sacrifice.

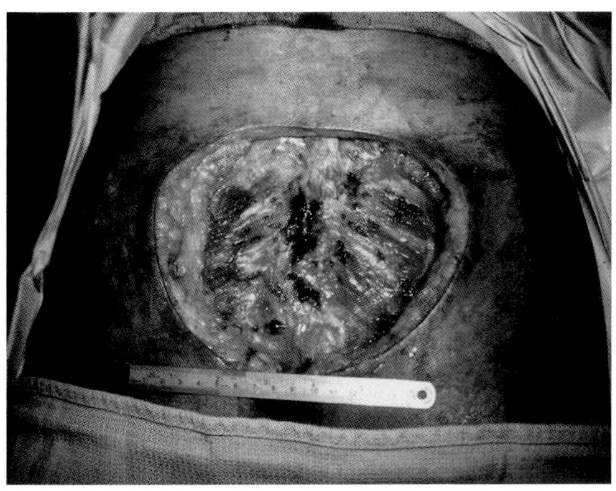

A

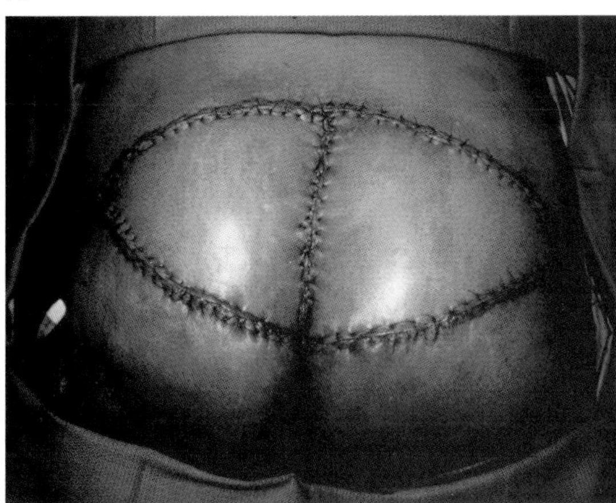

B

FIGURE 157-13. An illustration of the extent that the skin can be advanced when muscle advancement is not necessary. *A,* Sacral defect. *B,* V-Y skin advancement flaps.

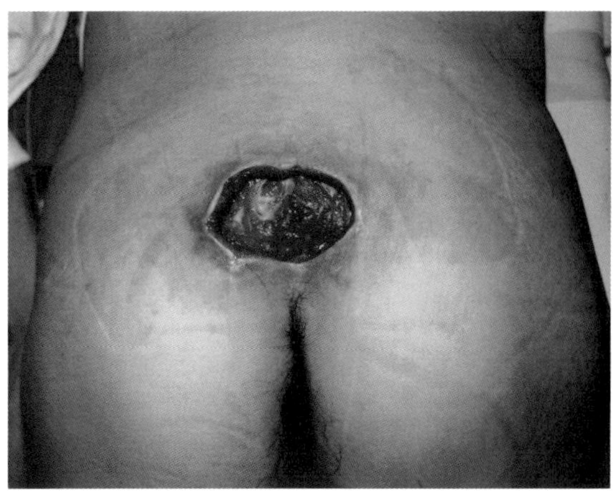

A

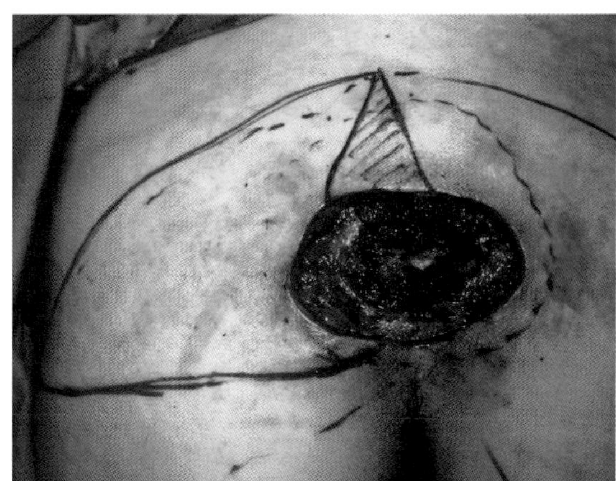

B

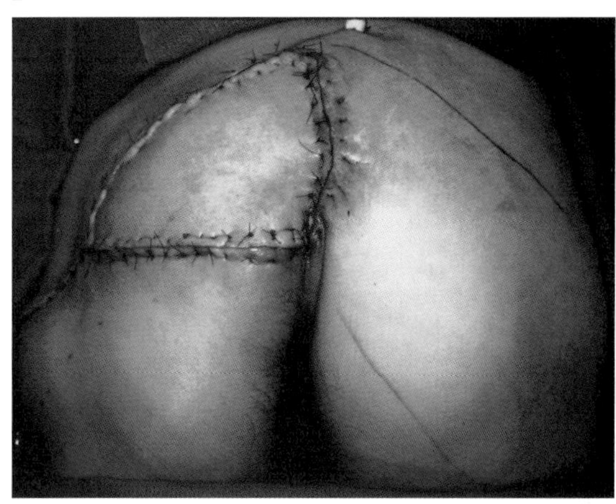

C

FIGURE 157-14. *A,* Grade IV sacral pressure sore in a 38-year-old paraplegic. *B,* A V-Y left gluteus maximus advancement flap designed after wound débridement. Note that the large flap design will more readily allow readvancement of the flap if it is necessary in the future. *C,* Flap inset and donor site closure.

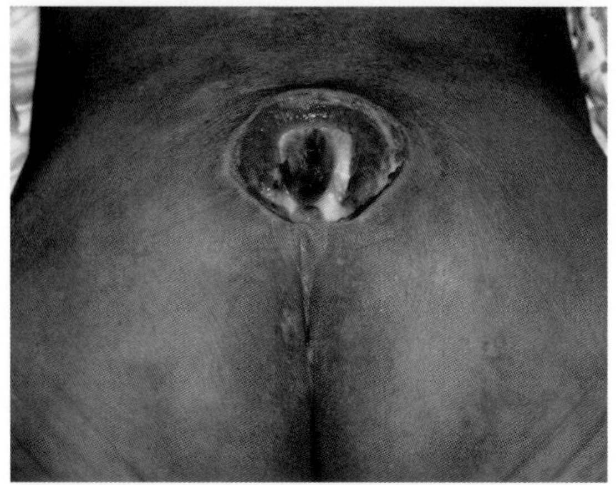

A

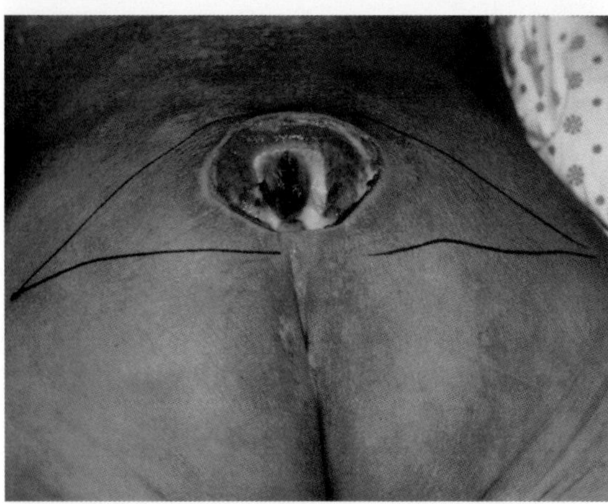

B

C

FIGURE 157-15. *A,* Sacral pressure sore in an ambulatory patient. *B,* Bilateral V-Y gluteus maximus advancement flap design. *C,* Six months postoperatively.

inferiorly if necessary (Fig. 157-16). Bilateral V-Y advancement flaps are generally approximated at the midline of the sacrum. The muscle layer is sutured to the contralateral gluteus maximus muscle, followed by suturing of the skin island into the skin defect edges. The donor site is closed in a V-Y fashion.

Trochanter

Trochanteric pressure sores typically present with minimal skin involvement and extensive bursa formation. The mobile nature of the trochanter, particularly when spasm is poorly controlled, predisposes these ulcerations to extensive undermining. Bone resection, when necessary, typically involves removal of the greater trochanter of the femur.

The tensor fascia lata flap, either as it is classically described (Fig. 157-17) or with a V-Y modification (Fig. 157-18), is reliable and considered the workhorse for trochanteric sore coverage. The V-Y modification of the tensor fascia lata flap provides more proximal and better vascularized tissue than in the classic tensor fascia lata design (Fig. 157-19) as well as a more muscular portion of the flap to fill the area of the débrided pressure sore. Perhaps more important, readvancement, or rotation when necessary, is easier and can be done reliably more than once (Fig. 157-20). The vastus lateralis muscle may be used in conjunction with the tensor fascia lata flap when a deep cavity needs to be filled, or it can be used independently either as a muscle flap alone or as a myocutaneous unit. The rectus femoris (Fig. 157-21), with or without a skin island, and the gluteal thigh flap (Fig. 157-22) are additional secondary options. The rectus abdominis flap (Fig. 157-23) remains a tertiary choice.

V-Y TENSOR FASCIA LATA FLAP.[31-33] The origin of the tensor fascia lata is at the anterior superior iliac spine. The insertion point is the iliotibial tract of the fascia lata. The dominant blood supply is the ascending branch of the lateral circumflex femoral artery and venae comitantes, a branch of the profunda femoris vessels (Fig. 157-24). T12 innervates the upper skin territory over the muscle origin. The lateral femoral cutaneous nerve of the thigh (L2-3) innervates the remaining skin territory.

Flap Elevation

Landmarks. A line drawn from the anterior superior iliac spine to the knee represents the anterior extent of the skin island of the flap that can be designed (see Fig. 157-19*B*). The pedicle is located approximately 10 cm below the line drawn from the anterior superior iliac spine to the knee (see Fig. 157-19*B*). It enters the flap on the medial aspect of the deep surface of the muscle.

Flap Design. A line is drawn from the anterior superior iliac spine to the midportion of the lateral thigh,

Text continued on p. 1345

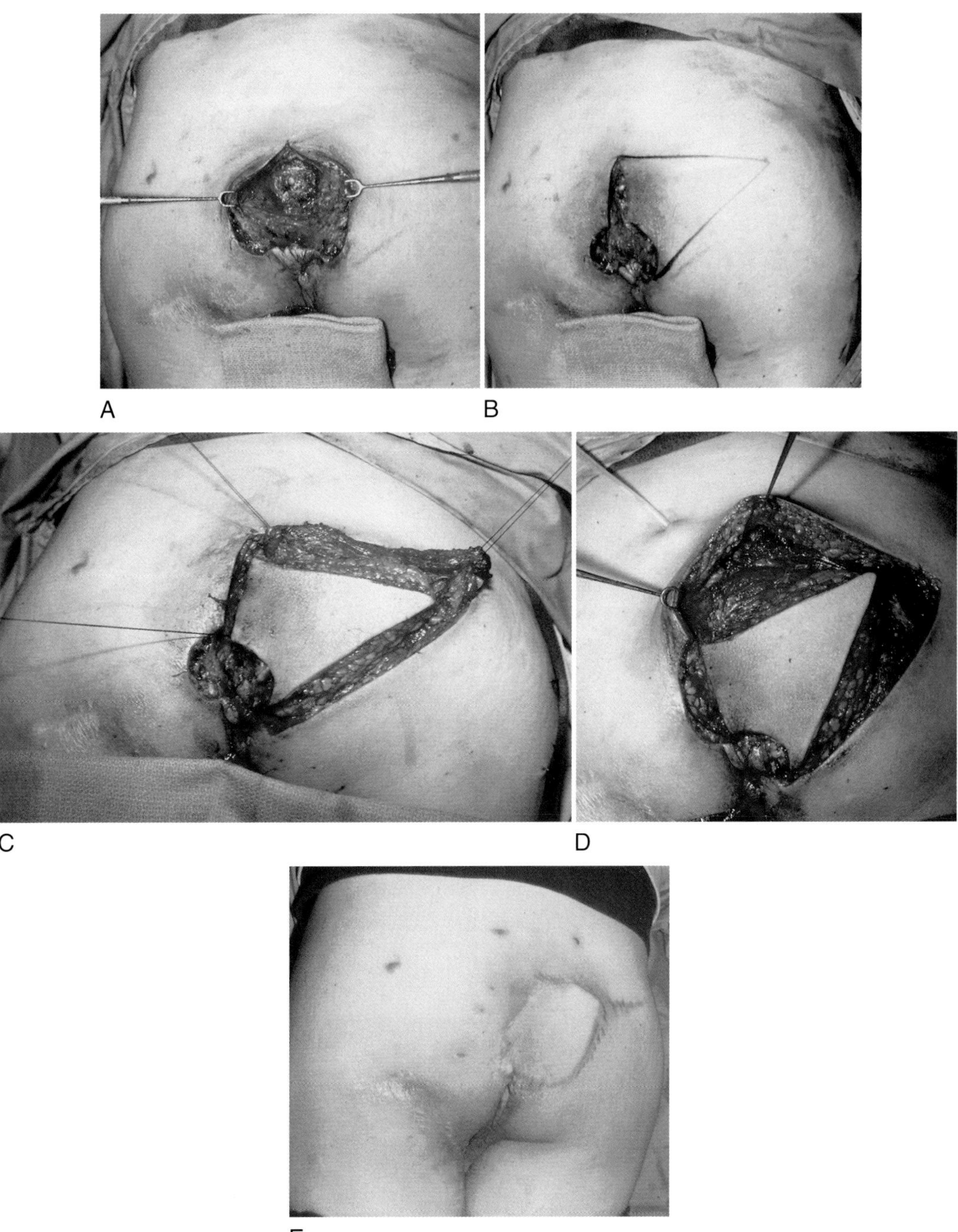

FIGURE 157-16. *A,* Grade IV sacral pressure sore in a 36-year-old paraplegic. *B,* Skin island design for unilateral gluteus maximus V-Y advancement flap. *C* and *D,* Flap advancement after muscle division and separation of the muscle from the sacrum. Note that the flap can be advanced past the midline and rotated *(D)* into the defect. *E,* Healed flap 4 weeks postoperatively.

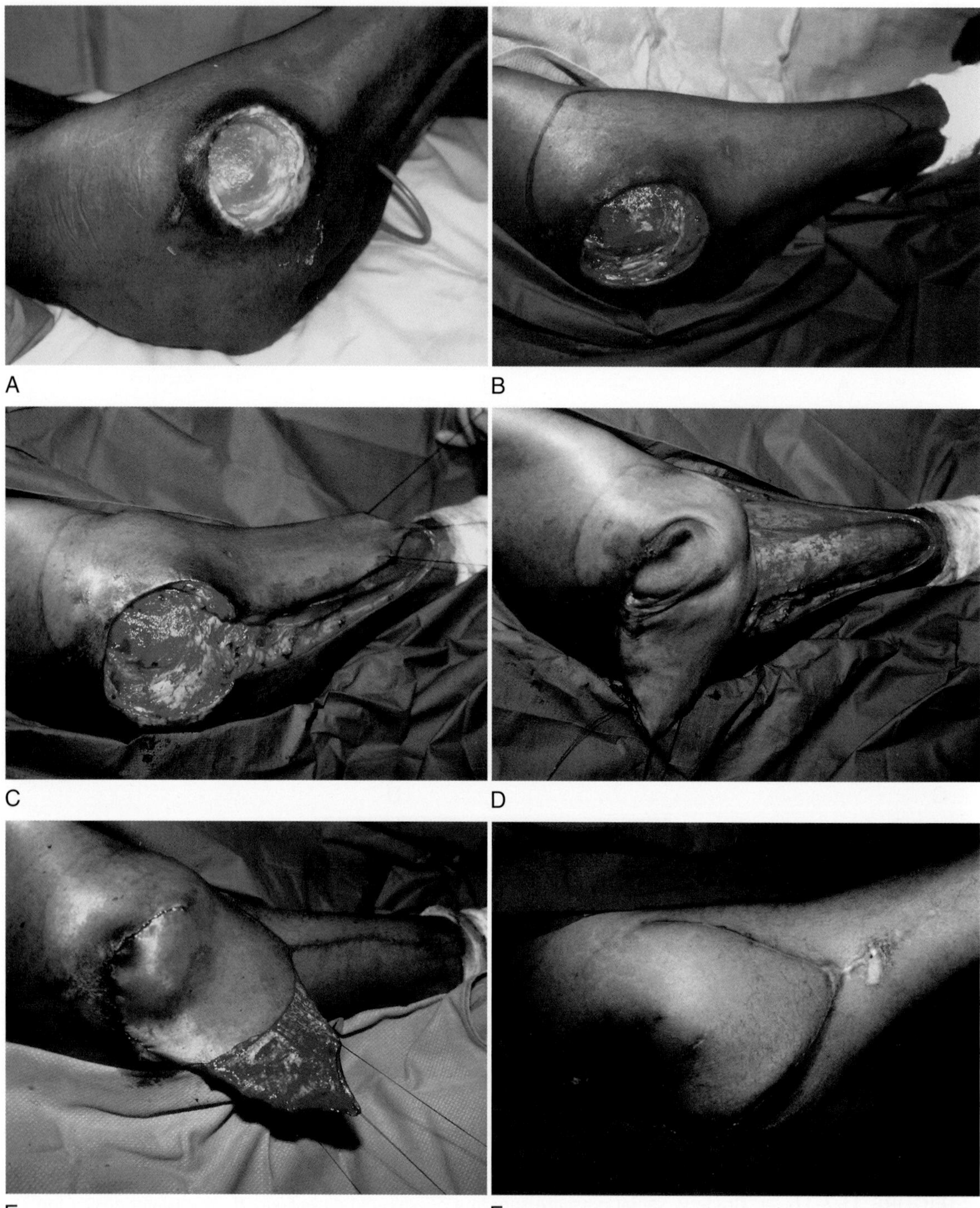

FIGURE 157-17. *A,* Right trochanteric pressure sore. *B,* Wound débridement and standard tensor fascia lata flap design. *C,* Flap elevation. *D,* Flap rotation. Note that the distal portion of the flap is used to reconstruct the defect. The proximal flap has a significant dog-ear that needs to be revised. *E,* Distal flap de-epithelialization. *F,* Healed flap 3 months postoperatively.

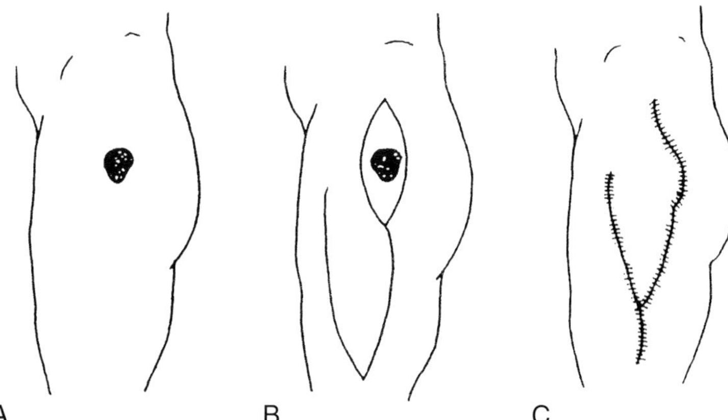

FIGURE 157-18. *A* to *C*, The tensor fascia lata V-Y retroposition flap. (From Siddiqui A, Wiedrich T, Lewis VI Jr: Tensor fascia lata V-Y retroposition myocutaneous flap: clinical experience. Ann Plast Surg 1993;31:313.)

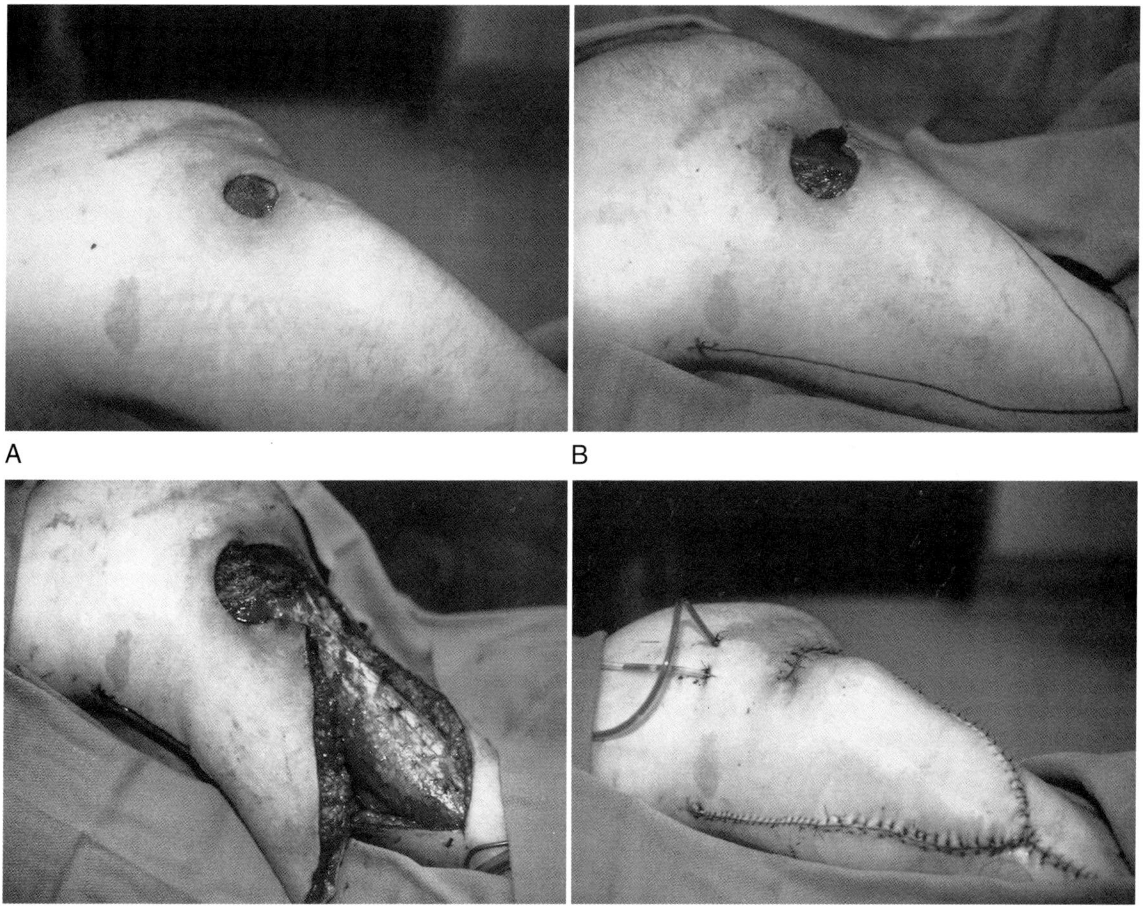

A B

C D

FIGURE 157-19. *A*, Left trochanteric pressure sore in a 36-year-old paraplegic. *B*, Design of the V-Y tensor fascia lata flap after wound débridement. X marks the point 10 cm inferior to the anterior superior iliac spine. *C*, Elevation of the flap. *D*, After inset and V-Y donor site closure.

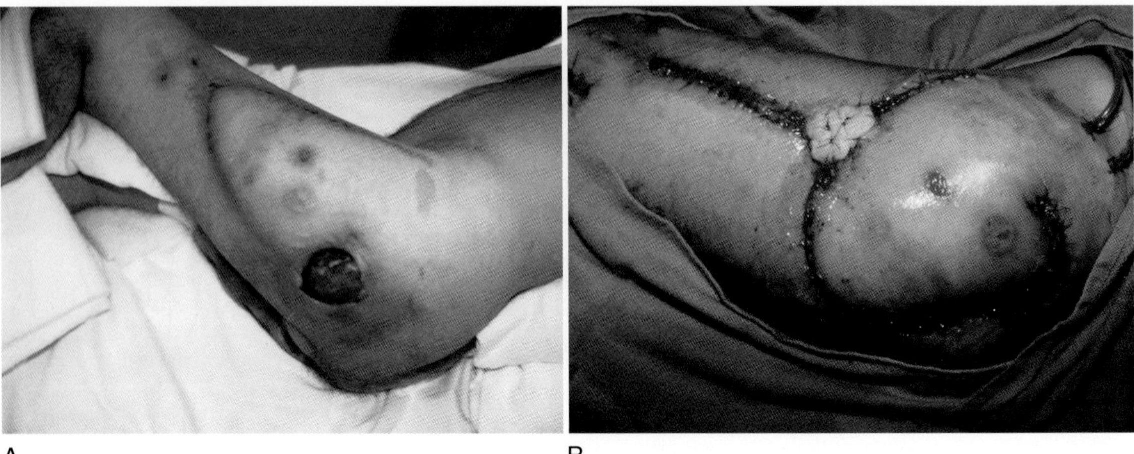

A B

FIGURE 157-20. *A,* Recurrence of left trochanteric pressure sore 3 years after the first reconstruction. *B,* V-Y tensor fascia lata flap rerotated and inset. Bolster dressing covers a small skin graft necessary because of excessive tension during donor site closure.

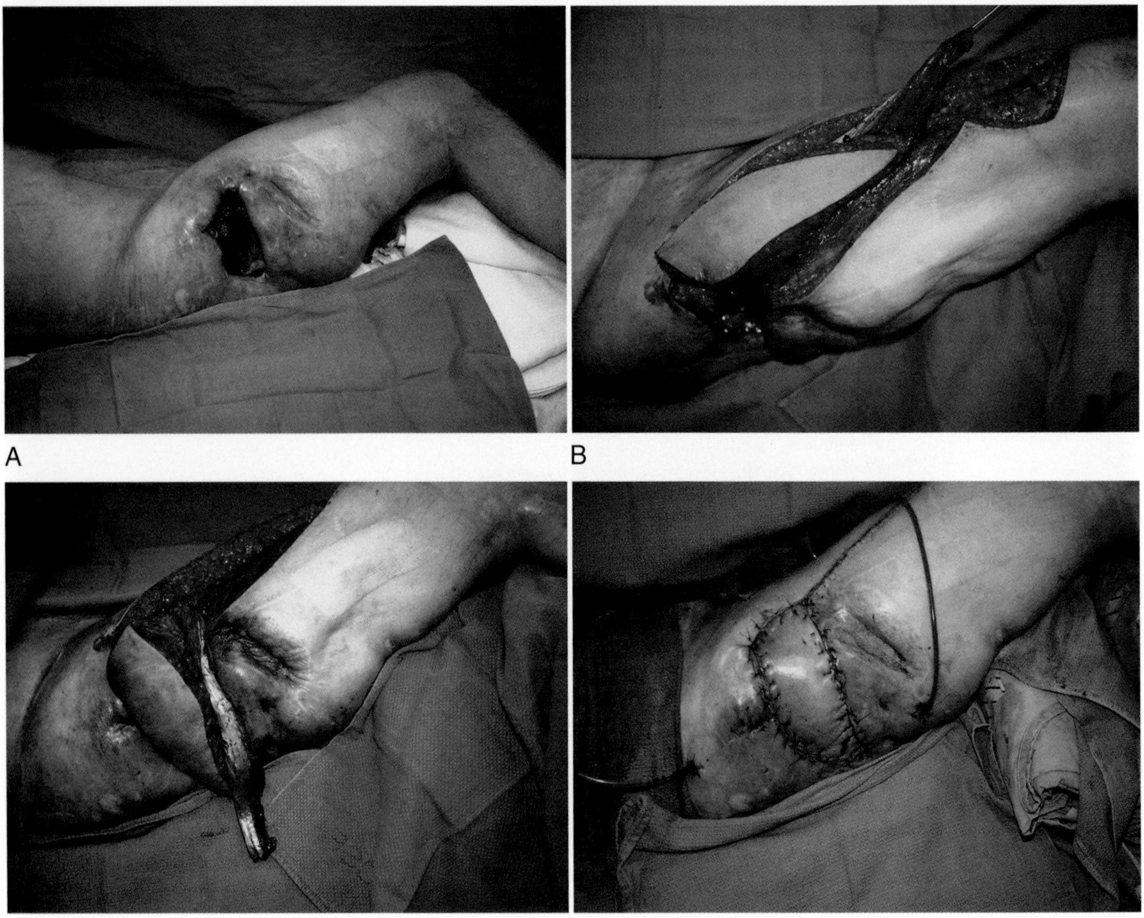

A B

C D

FIGURE 157-21. *A,* Chronic right trochanteric pressure sore. *B,* Elevation of a rectus femoris flap with a skin paddle. *C* and *D,* Flap rotated and inset with direct donor site closure.

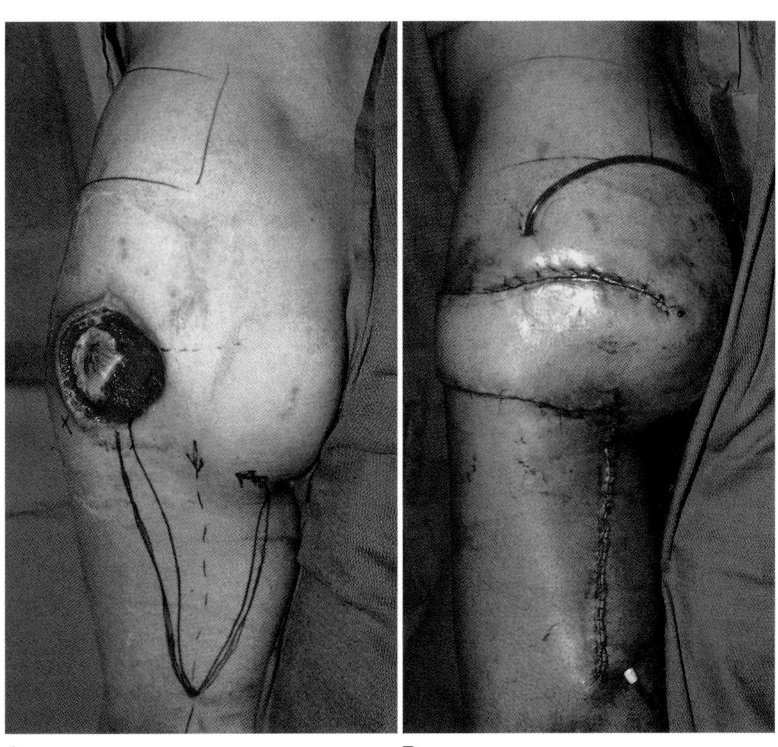

A B

FIGURE 157-22. Large left trochanteric pressure sore. *A,* Left gluteal thigh flap is designed (dotted line marks the course of the descending branch of the inferior gluteal artery). *B,* Gluteal thigh flap rotated into the wound site.

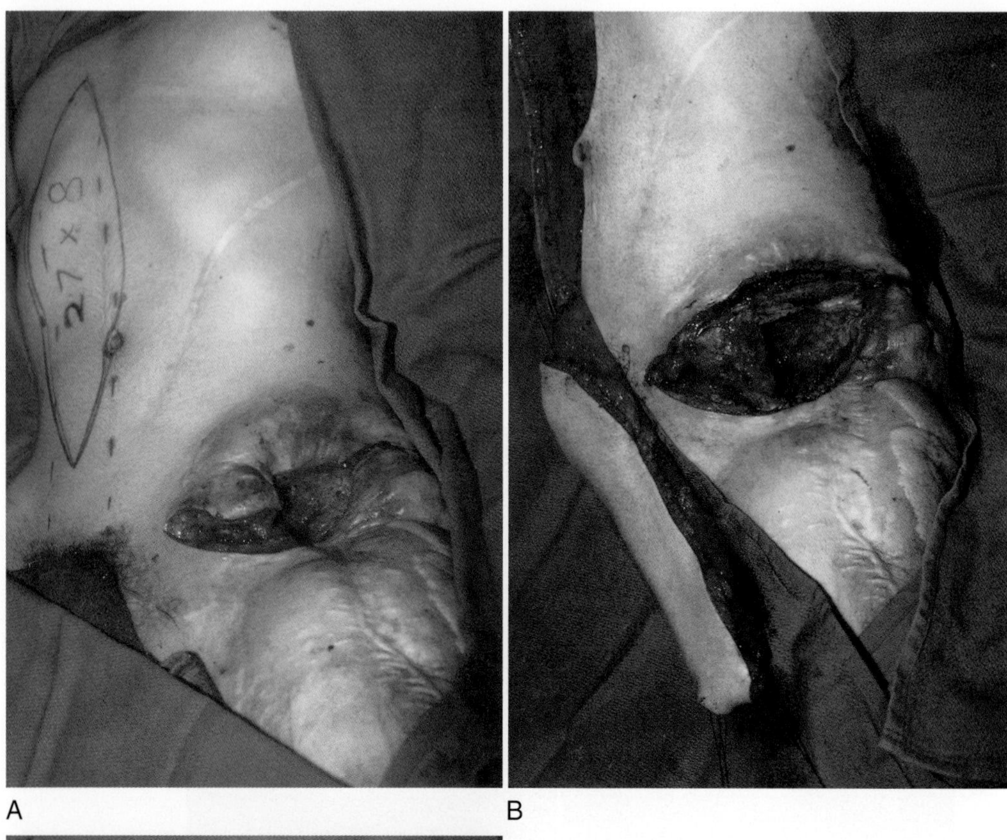

A B

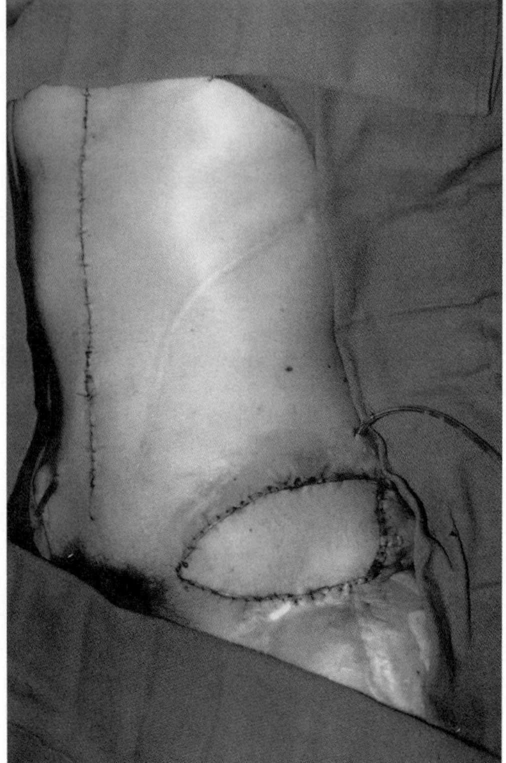

C

FIGURE 157-23. *A,* Left deep chronic hip wound after multiple attempts at flap coverage. A rectus abdominis flap with a large skin paddle is designed. *B,* Left hip wound after wound débridement and rectus flap elevation. Note the significant skin paddle, part of which can be de-epithelialized and used to obliterate the depth of the cavity. *C,* After flap inset and donor site closure.

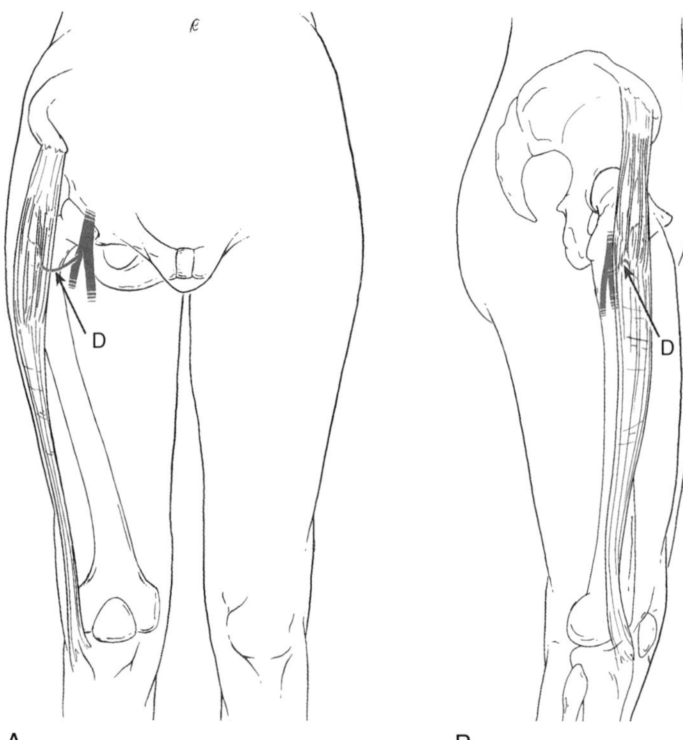

FIGURE 157-24. *A* and *B*, Dominant pedicle: ascending branch of lateral circumflex artery (D). (From Mathes SJ, Nahai F: Reconstructive Surgery: Principles, Anatomy, and Technique. New York, Churchill Livingstone, 1997:1273.)

at least two thirds of the length of the thigh. Although the length of the flap may seem to vary with the size of the defect, a large flap design will increase the ability to rerotate the flap if the pressure sore recurs (see Fig. 157-20). The flap can be designed up to 15 cm in width extending posteriorly from the anterior line and still allow primary closure of the skin. The distal limit of the flap extends to 10 cm above the knee. Beyond this, the flap is best delayed. To complete the flap design, the posterior line is then drawn from the base of the V to the posterior rim of the trochanteric defect (see Fig. 157-19*B*).

Flap Elevation and Inset. The flap is raised by incising the skin, subcutaneous tissue, and fascia from distal to proximal on the thigh. Absorbable sutures between the skin and underlying fascia can be used to prevent shearing of the flap during dissection. The lateral intermuscular septum of the thigh represents the posterior extension of the flap. Violation of this septum can be disorienting, resulting in entrance to the posterior compartment of the thigh. A distinct plane exists between the tensor fascia lata above and the vastus lateralis muscle below, which should expedite the dissection. Superiorly, care should be taken to dissect the muscular portion of the tensor fascia lata from the adherent gluteus medius. After dissection to the level of the vascular pedicle, the flap is rotated superiorly and posteriorly to cover the trochanteric defect. Compared with a standard tensor fascia lata flap, the rotation point and the dog-ear are eliminated. It also places the thickest and best vascularized portion of the flap over the bone defect. This flap is not a true V-Y advancement in the traditional sense because the flap is rotated posteriorly; however, the design and closure follow essentially the same principles as for a V-Y flap. The point of maximum tension during the skin closure is most commonly at the junction of the V-Y advancement. Closure under tension should be avoided because it may lead to a compartment compression syndrome within the thigh. Excessive tension can be alleviated by placement of a skin graft over the vastus lateralis at this juncture point (see Fig. 157-20*B*).

Technical Considerations. The gluteus minimus muscle is firmly adherent to the tensor fascia lata flap posteriorly. Care should be taken to identify the correct plane of dissection during the dissection of the superior half of the flap. The lateral femoral cutaneous nerve is located along the medial border of the flap and should be identified during the initial dissection of the flap if a sensory flap is planned.

Vastus Lateralis Flap.[34-36] The origin of the vastus lateralis flap is the intertrochanteric line, greater trochanter, gluteal tuberosity of the femur, and intermuscular septum. The insertion point is at the patella. The main blood supply consists of the descending and transverse branches of the lateral circumflex femoral artery and venae comitantes. Both branches of the lateral circumflex femoral artery enter the deep surface of the muscle within its superior third (10 to 15 cm

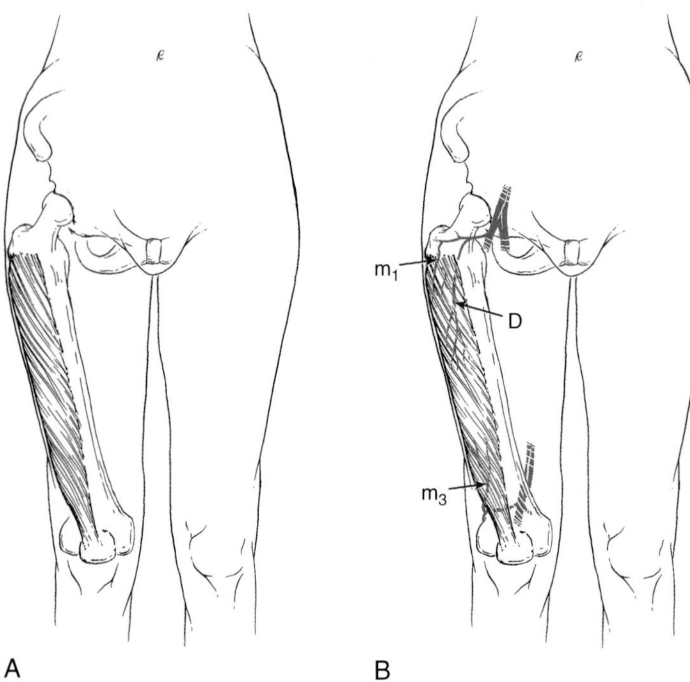

FIGURE 157-25. *A* and *B*, Dominant pedicle: descending branch of lateral circumflex femoral artery (D). Minor pedicles: transverse branch of lateral circumflex femoral artery (m_1); superficial branch of lateral superior genicular artery (m_3). (From Mathes SJ, Nahai F: Reconstructive Surgery: Principles, Anatomy, and Technique. New York, Churchill Livingstone, 1997:1294.)

below the anterior superior iliac spine). The descending branch courses inferiorly along the medial border of the muscle (Fig. 157-25).

Flap Elevation

Landmarks. A line is drawn from the point 10 cm below the anterior superior iliac spine at the level of the greater trochanter to the lateral condyle of the femur.

Flap Design. Most commonly, the vastus lateralis flap is elevated without a skin island. In such instances, the skin incision is made along the line drawn from the level of the greater trochanter to the lateral condyle of the femur. A skin island can be incorporated and de-epithelialized if further tissue bulk is necessary to obliterate the wound cavity or if stable cutaneous coverage is required. The muscle supplies the skin territory over the anterolateral thigh along its middle and distal thirds and between the lateral edge of the rectus femoris and the medial portion of the iliotibial tract. The skin dimensions should not exceed 10 × 15 cm.

Flap Elevation and Inset. The skin incision extends through deep fascia at the medial edge of the tensor fascia lata muscle in the proximal fourth of the leg and the iliotibial tract distally. The rectus femoris muscle is retracted medially to expose the adjacent vastus lateralis in the proximal leg, and distally the vastus lateralis is exposed immediately superior to the lateral condyle of the knee. Because the borders of the vastus intermedius and lateralis muscles are indistinct in the proximal three fourths of the thigh, it is helpful to examine the muscles distally where the two muscles separate before forming their respective tendons of insertion. The muscle fibers of insertion are divided, and the muscle is elevated proximally. In the distal posterior muscle, multiple branches from the superior lateral genicular artery and associated veins are encountered and divided. The muscle is elevated from the underlying femur to the level of the greater trochanter. At this level, care is taken to visualize and preserve the descending branch of the lateral circumflex femoral artery that passes beneath the rectus femoris and enters the medial aspect of the vastus lateralis muscle. The muscle is rotated upward and inset directly into the trochanteric defect. In the Girdlestone arthroplasty, in which the space to be filled is deep, a bolster suture placed through the tip of the flap once it is in the cavity and brought out through the overlying skin helps ensure obliteration of the space. The suture is taken out when the other skin sutures are removed.

Donor Site. The donor site is closed directly. If the vastus lateralis muscle is used in conjunction with the tensor fascia lata musculocutaneous flap, it is essential to achieve direct donor site closure to avoid placement of skin grafts directly on the exposed shaft of the femur.

Technical Considerations. It may be difficult to distinguish the vastus lateralis from the vastus intermedius along the proximal thigh because the muscles are often fused. Determination of an arbitrary line of separation must be made carefully. For this purpose, it is helpful to examine the two muscles where they separate distally, near their respective tendons of insertion, before the muscle is divided.

Acetabular Fossa

The long-term sequelae of untreated ischial or trochanteric pressure sores can include hip joint communication, a diagnosis that is difficult to make and frequently missed. Inadequate treatment of associated pyarthrosis or osteomyelitis of the joint leads to failure of any attempt at related pressure sore flap reconstruction, resulting in persistent draining sinuses and poor wound healing. Experience derived from the orthopedic literature in treatment of septic hip joints secondary to hematogenous spread of tuberculosis or, more recently, after total hip arthroplasty for osteoarthritis or rheumatoid arthritis of the hip demonstrates the efficacy of proximal femoral head resection (Fig. 157-26) and acetabular curettage in promptly eradicating the infection. Obliteration of the resultant cavity after débridement can be achieved by use of one or more local flaps (Table 157-8 and Fig. 157-27; see also Fig. 157-26).

In 1993, Evans et al[37] reported on a group of 15 paraplegic or quadriplegic patients who underwent Girdlestone arthroplasty for septic hips with osteomyelitis. Soft tissue reconstruction to the hip included the vastus lateralis (40%), V-Y tensor fascia lata (33%), and rectus femoris (20%). With a mean follow-up of 20 months, 77% of patients remained healed. The most significant concern after femoral head resection and flap reconstruction is the stabilization of the femur while the flap is healing. Girdlestone, in 1943, highlighted the importance of preventing pistoning of the residual femur for wound healing success.[38] Techniques have included external fixation,[39] leg traction, body casts, and abduction pillows[40] with variable success. Patients in Evans' study received no specific treatment to stabilize the leg. In many patients, the extensive scar tissue from the chronic wound seems to stabilize the femur adequately.

Calcaneus

Whereas the area around the pelvis (ischium, sacrum, trochanter) remains the most common site of pressure sore occurrence, Conway[14] in his large series of treated pressure sores identified the heel (9%) as the next most common site.

For superficial wounds, adequate soft tissue débridement followed by split-thickness skin grafting may be all that is necessary. Even for deeper wounds, primary excision and closure or skin grafting should be considered in paraplegics or quadriplegics where the function of exposed tendons or bone at the base of the pressure sore is less critical. In these situations, serious consideration must also be given to amputation.

When flap reconstruction is considered, every attempt should be made to use local tissue for coverage. Microvascular transfer is also an option, but only as a last resort. Particularly in patients with spinal cord injuries, valuable flap options for coverage around the pelvis (i.e., gracilis for ischial coverage) should not be sacrificed for heel coverage (Table 157-9).

TABLE 157-8 ✦ FLAP OPTIONS AFTER FEMORAL HEAD (GIRDLESTONE) RESECTION

Vastus lateralis
Rectus femoris
Tensor fascia lata

TABLE 157-9 ✦ FLAP OPTIONS FOR HEEL PRESSURE ULCERS

Local tissue
Lateral calcaneal artery flap
Medial plantar flap
Sural artery flap
Microvascular
Radial forearm
Serratus

Pelvis

First described in 1956 by Georgiade et al[41] for the treatment of large trochanteric pressure sores with associated pyarthrosis of the adjacent hip joint, the "total thigh" flap (one of the first musculocutaneous flaps described) is currently reserved for coverage of large recalcitrant or recurrent sacral, ischial, or trochanteric pressure sore wounds (involving one or more pressure sore sites).[42] It is a flap of last resort (Fig. 157-28). A modification, the anterior thigh flap, makes use of multiple muscle units (rectus femoris, sartorius, vastus lateralis, vastus medialis, and vastus intermedius) and provides the arc of rotation necessary to cover all three pressure sore sites reliably.

Anterior Thigh Flap

Location of Incision. The patient is placed on the operating table prone, in a jackknife position. A posterior longitudinal skin incision is made along the lateral border of the long head of the biceps femoris muscle, in the lower third of the thigh. The incision is extended proximally over the lateral intermuscular septum up to the inferior border of the gluteus maximus muscle insertion. At this point, the skin incision is completed proximally by encircling the area of the pressure sore. The distal margin of the flap depends on the area overlying the pelvis that needs to be covered. A circumferential incision is usually made at the distal end of the femur across the popliteal space, but it can be extended below the knee for additional flap length to cover sacral defects.

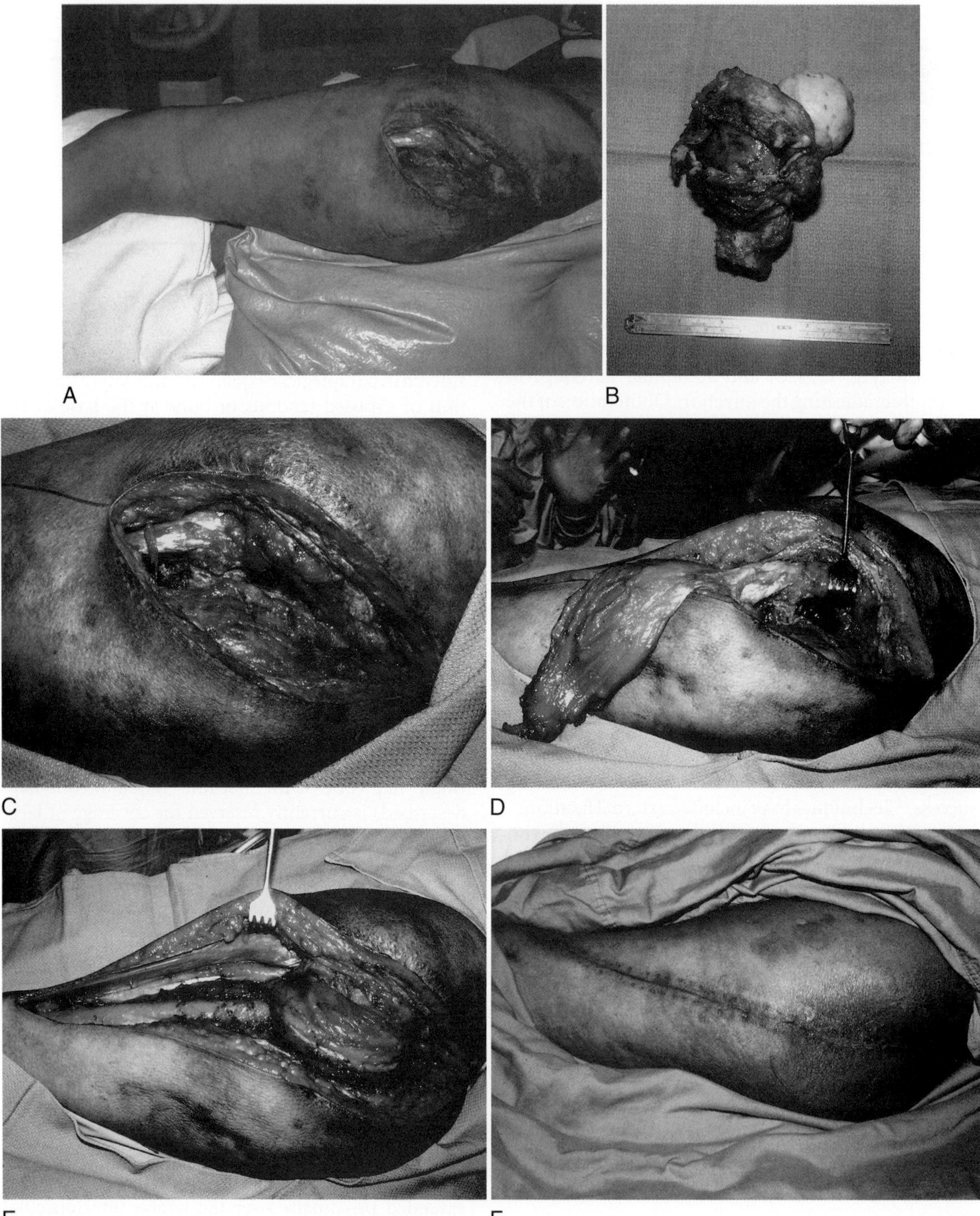

FIGURE 157-26. *A,* Chronic left hip wound after femoral head resection *(B). C,* Close-up view of the wound after débridement. A line is drawn from the wound edge to the vastus lateralis. *D* and *E,* The flap is elevated and inset deep into the wound. *F,* Healed wound and stable coverage 1 year postoperatively.

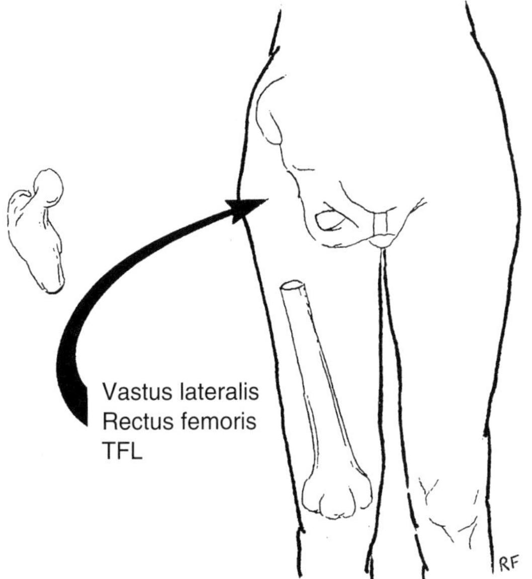

FIGURE 157-27. Local flap options for reconstruction after Girdlestone arthroplasty. TFL, tensor fascia lata.

Flap Elevation. The lateral intermuscular septum, a relatively avascular plane between the short head of the biceps femoris muscle and the vastus lateralis muscle, serves as a direct approach to the femur. The femur is dissected from the muscle attachments and removed. Care is taken not to injure branches from the profunda femoris artery during the amputation. The anterior muscle units preserved for flap rotation include the rectus femoris, vastus lateralis, vastus medialis, vastus intermedius, and sartorius muscles. The flap is tailored to the defect and inset (Fig. 157-29).

Sensory Flap Reconstruction

Much has been written about the use of sensate flaps to treat pressure sores in paraplegic patients.[43-45] The concept is that sensibility can return to an area with no sensation if the flap chosen for reconstruction originates from a region of the body above the level of the original spinal cord injury. Not all flaps can be designed with a skin island that will provide sensation (Table 157-10). The largest experience is with the tensor fascia lata flap.[46,47] Other sensory flaps include descriptions of intercostal flaps for sacral pressure sore coverage.[48]

Postoperative Management

The following principles should be adhered to postoperatively for avoidance of complications and to ensure primary healing at both the recipient and donor sites.

POSITIONING

Pressure on the flap should be avoided during the initial postoperative period. The area of flap inset lacks

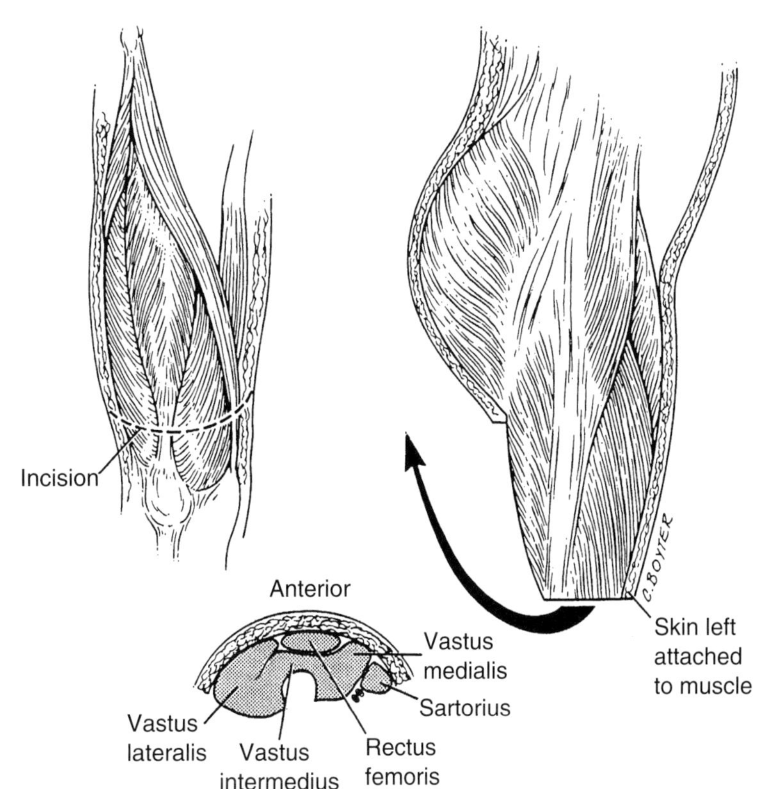

FIGURE 157-28. Illustration of anterior thigh lift.

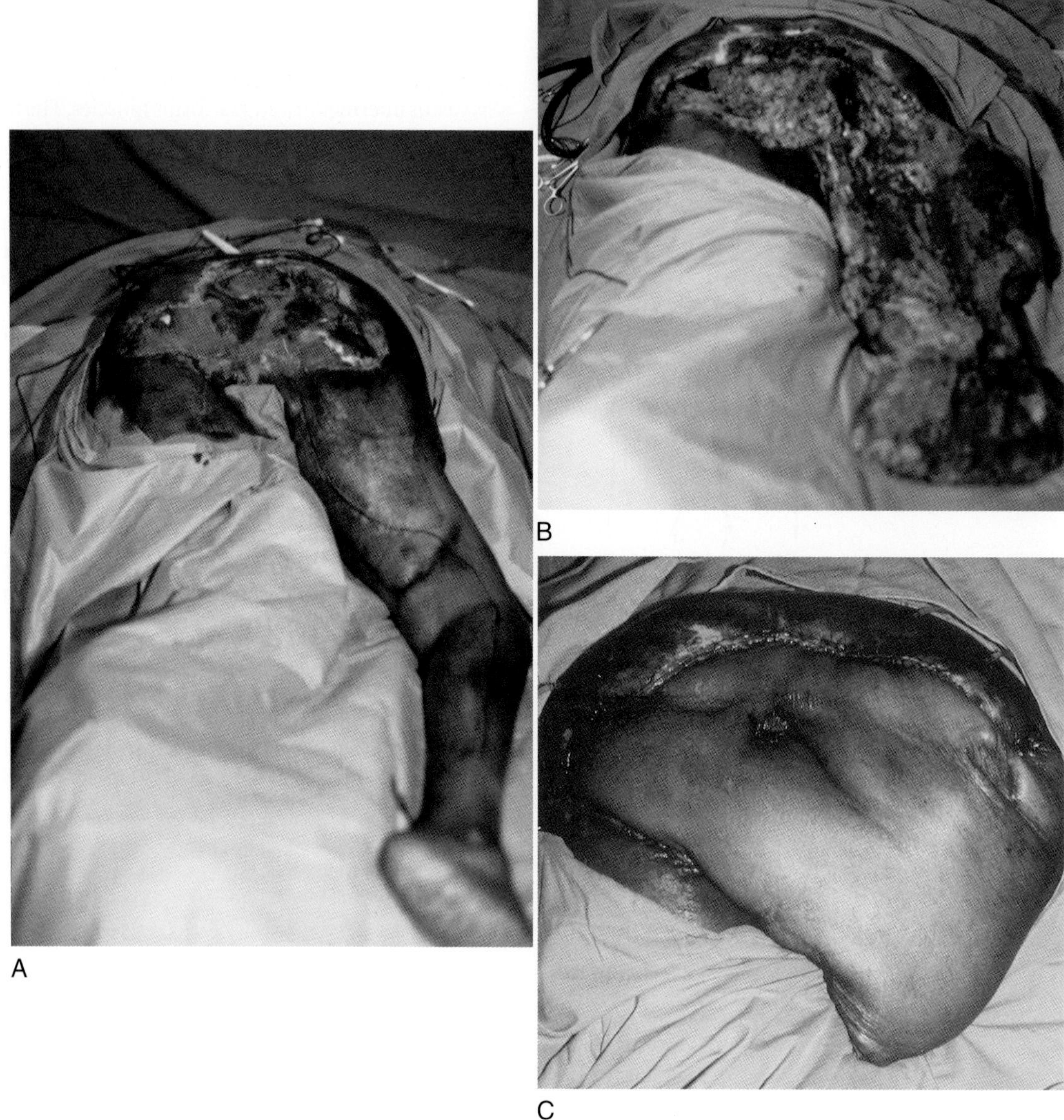

FIGURE 157-29. *A,* Complex and diffuse pressure sore development after multiple attempts at coverage. *B,* Right leg amputation with dissection of an anterior thigh flap. Note that the femur has already been resected. *C,* Flap rotated and inset to cover the entire buttock region.

TABLE 157-10 ✦ SENSORY FLAP INNERVATION

Flap	Level of Cutaneous Innervation
Tensor fascia lata	T12, L2-3
Gluteal thigh or V-Y hamstring	S1-3
Gracilis	—
Vastus lateralis	—

protective sensation, and therefore most patients are placed in the prone or lateral decubitus position postoperatively unless an air-fluidized bed is available. An essential part of the normal postoperative routine is frequent repositioning and turning.

DRESSINGS

Constrictive bandages are avoided, particularly in the area of the flap base where pressure on the flap pedicle can compromise flap circulation. Excessive motion in the area of the flap inset is avoided by padding the areas adjacent to the flap inset site and controlling for local muscle spasms as discussed previously.

SUCTION DRAINS

A closed suction drain system is used for all patients who receive flap coverage for pressure sores. The drains are left in place until serous fluid drainage decreases to 20 to 30 mL in a 24-hour period, which is generally 7 to 10 days postoperatively but may extend up to 4 weeks. Of note, beyond day 10, significant wound contamination through the drain exit site can manifest, resulting in an increased incidence of wound infection and breakdown.

ANTIBIOTICS

Perioperative antibiotics are used in reconstruction because all of the wounds are, at the very least, considered contaminated. Cultures of the wound preoperatively and intraoperatively will guide the choice of culture-specific antibiotic agents. In general, antibiotic therapy is continued for 7 to 10 days postoperatively or longer if signs of infection become evident.

MOBILIZATION

After pressure sore reconstruction, as opposed to reconstructive surgery to other regions of the body, patients are kept on prolonged bed rest. Weight bearing at the site of flap inset is avoided for 3 to 4 weeks, followed by a program of gradually increased weight bearing (sitting) on the pressure sore area.

REHABILITATION

Because of the significant risk of pressure sore recurrence, patients with spinal cord injury require instruction in avoidance of pressure and shear forces at the site of the flap reconstruction. They also need assistance in obtaining specialized equipment (e.g., wheelchair with appropriate padding) to avoid future skin injury.

Complications

SLIGHT WOUND SEPARATION

Slight wound separation is a common complication after flap reconstruction of a pressure sore, particularly in the debilitated patient, when the flap is sutured under pressure, or when the patient is noncompliant with postoperative body positioning. When debilitation is a factor, extra efforts should be made preoperatively to improve the patient's nutritional status. Wound tension generally indicates improper flap design or an attempt to close a donor site when a skin graft may be indicated. Any significant flap suture line breakdowns or nonhealing areas that do not close within a few days should be promptly treated with operative débridement and flap readvancement because these wounds are relatively unlikely to heal otherwise.

HEMATOMA

Hematomas can occur after pressure sore reconstruction. Their presence often predisposes to other complications including wound infection, bursa formation, flap necrosis, and subsequent pressure sore recurrence. When hematomas are recognized, they should be immediately evacuated.

SEROMA

Seromas are relatively common after flap coverage of pressure sores, usually because of residual dead space and inadequate immobilization of the patient postoperatively with resultant shearing forces. Inadequate resection of the bursae can also predispose to seroma formation. Suction drainage should be used for all patients undergoing pressure sore reconstruction. If a seroma develops because of inadequate drainage or after removal of the drains, percutaneous drainage should be performed initially.

WOUND INFECTION

Despite appropriate preoperative wound cultures and antibiotic therapy, wound infection remains a significant postoperative complication. Most often it is due to inadequate wound débridement intraoperatively. When it is diagnosed, it should be treated with wide drainage and appropriate antibiotics.

PARTIAL FLAP NECROSIS

For the majority of flaps used for pressure sore coverage, flap necrosis is a rare complication. However, certain flaps are more susceptible to partial flap loss from a tenuous blood supply to a portion of the flap (e.g., the distal edge of the tensor fascia lata or gracilis flap for ischial coverage). It is important to recognize the size limits to the various rotational flaps because partial flap loss is usually related to incorrect flap design. Modifications of the flaps, by delay of the flap or use of tissue expansion, can help prevent this complication. If the necrotic portion of the flap is small enough, conservative local therapy is warranted to achieve secondary healing.

Outcome

Since the introduction of musculocutaneous flaps, the literature on the surgical management of pressure sores has consisted predominantly of initial flap descriptions, reporting a limited experience with high primary healing rates. Few studies have attempted critical analysis of flap selection to compare the efficacy of one flap with another and to apply this to a model of long-term surgical management.

A 17-year retrospective study analyzing 280 pressure sore reconstructions[49] found that in fact, not all flaps used for pressure sore coverage are equally successful in achieving primary coverage in the immediate postoperative period. From 1979 to 1995, 280 unselected pressure sore reconstructions were performed in 201 patients (113 ischial, 94 sacral, and 73 trochanteric sores) at a single institution. There were 130 men and 71 women; age range was 16 to 90 years (mean, 50 years). Ninety percent of the patients had severe spinal cord injuries (paraplegic or quadriplegic). Forty-one percent of the wounds were chronic (present longer than 3 months). Preoperative risk factors, prior flap history, flap success, complication rates, and length of hospitalization were evaluated. Flap success was defined as a completely healed wound. Average follow-up was 11.8 months (range, 1 month to 9 years). Overall, 89% of the flaps healed primarily: ischium, 94 of 113 (83%); sacrum, 86 of 94 (91%); and trochanter, 68 of 73 (93%). Eighty-eight percent of the patients (201 of 228) treated in a single stage (débridement and flap reconstruction) healed primarily. Although the overall complication rate was 28%, reoperation or prolonged hospital stay was required in only 17% of patients. It is evident, therefore, that reconstruction can reliably be performed in a single stage with a relatively short hospitalization. Furthermore, flap selection and the appropriate short- and long-term sequence of flap use significantly improve success rates for pressure sore coverage.

MALIGNANT DEGENERATION

Any chronic wound, if it is present long enough, has the potential to develop a malignant neoplasm. In 1828, Marjolin[50] described the development of carcinoma within a burn scar. Currently, Marjolin ulcer is a term used to describe malignant degeneration within a burn scar or any chronic wound. Malignant degeneration in a pressure sore, presenting almost exclusively as a squamous cell carcinoma, is associated with a poor prognosis,. In one study of 18 patients (the largest single study to date), the 2-year mortality rate was greater than 60% with a high rate of metastasis, almost double that seen with burns or other variants of scar carcinoma.[51] The average latent period between the diagnosis of a pressure sore and the diagnosis of a related wound carcinoma is 20 years, significantly shorter than with other chronic wounds or burn scars.[52] Therefore, pathologic evaluation of all débrided pressure sore wounds should be a routine practice for any surgeon caring for patients with chronic pressure sores.

SUMMARY

Successful management of pressure sores requires a comprehensive approach to each individual patient. Patients must be carefully evaluated and prepared preoperatively, and nutritional deficiency, muscle spasticity, and coexisting infection must be corrected. In addition, adequate social resources, proper equipment for pressure relief, and a compliant attitude are important factors in successful pressure sore management.

With suitable flap selection and the appropriate short- and long-term sequence of flap use, reconstruction can reliably be performed in a single stage with relatively short-term hospitalization. Furthermore, improved success rates occur when these principles are used. In caring for patients with pressure sores, flap procedures must be planned carefully and social resources must be provided to reduce the risk of a negative outcome.

REFERENCES

1. National Spinal Cord Injury Statistical Center (NSCISC), Birmingham, Alabama: Facts and Figures at a Glance—December 2003. Available at: http://www.spinalcord.uab.edu.
2. Dinsdale SM: Decubitus ulcers: role of pressure and friction in causation. Arch Phys Med Rehabil 1974;55:147.
3. Lindan O, Greenway RM, Piazza JM: Pressure distribution on the surface of the human body: I. Evaluation in lying and sitting positions using a "bed of springs and nails." Arch Phys Med Rehabil 1965;46:378.
4. Husain T: An experimental study of some pressure effects on tissues, with reference to the bed-sore problem. J Pathol Bacteriol 1953;66:347.
5. Hubay CA, Kiehn CC, Drucker WR: Surgical management of decubitus ulcers in the post-traumatic patient. Am J Surg 1957;93:205.
6. Pollock LJ, Boshes B, Finkelman I, et al: Spasticity, pseudospontaneous spasms, and other reflex activities late after injury to the spinal cord. Arch Neurol Psychiatry 1951;66:537.
7. Dansereau JG, Conway H: Closure of decubiti in paraplegics. Plast Reconstr Surg 1964;33:474.
8. Shea JD: Pressure sores: classification and management. Clin Orthop 1975;112:89.
9. Hargest TS, Artz CP: A new concept in patient care: the air-filled fluidized bed. AORN J 1969;10:59.
10. Allman RM, Walker JM, Hart MK, et al: Air-fluidized beds or conventional therapy for pressure sores. Ann Intern Med 1987;107:641.
11. Reuler JB, Cooney TG: The pressure sore: pathophysiology and principles of management. Ann Intern Med 1981;94:661.
12. Evans GRD, Dufresne CR, Manson PN: Surgical correction of pressure ulcers in an urban center: is it efficacious? Adv Wound Care 1994;7:40.
13. Lewis VL Jr, Bailey MH, Pulawski G, et al: The diagnosis of osteomyelitis in patients with pressure sores. Plast Reconstr Surg 1988;81:229.
14. Conway H, Griffith BH: Plastic surgery for closure of decubitus ulcers in patients with paraplegia: based on experience with 1000 cases. Am J Surg 1956;91:946.
15. Ger R, Levine SA: The management of decubitus ulcers by muscle transposition—an eight year review. Plast Reconstr Surg 1976;58:419.
16. Arregui J, Cannon B, Murray JE, O'Leary JJ Jr: Long-term evaluation of ischiectomy in the treatment of pressure ulcers. Plast Reconstr Surg 1965;36:583.

17. Hackler RH, Zampieri TA: Urethral complications following ischiectomy in spinal cord injury patients: a urethral pressure study. J Urol 1987;137:253.
18. Karaca AR, Binns JH, Blumenthal FS: Complications of total ischiectomy for the treatment of ischial pressure sores. Plast Reconstr Surg 1978;62:96.
19. Bors E, Comarr E: Perineal urethral diverticulum complication of removal of ischium. JAMA 1958;168:2000.
20. Nola GT, Vistnes LM: Differential response of skin and muscle in the experimental production of pressure sores. Plast Reconstr Surg 1980;66:728.
21. Daniel RK, Faibisoff B: Muscle coverage of pressure points: the role of myocutaneous flaps. Ann Plast Surg 1982;8:446.
22. Parry SW, Mathes SJ: Bilateral gluteus maximus myocutaneous advancement flaps: sacral coverage for ambulatory patients. Ann Plast Surg 1982;8:443.
23. Riou JP, Cohen JR, Johnson H Jr: Factors influencing wound dehiscence. Am J Surg 1992;163:324.
24. Evans JM, Andrews KL, Chutka DS, et al: Pressure sores: prevention and management. Mayo Clin Proc 1995;70:789.
25. Bunkis J, Fudem GM: Rectus abdominis flap closure of ischiosacral pressure sore. Ann Plast Surg 1989;23:447.
26. Stevenson TR, Pollock RA, Rohrich RJ, VanderKolk CA: The gluteus maximus musculocutaneous island flap: refinements in design and application. Plast Reconstr Surg 1987;79:761.
27. Hurteau JE, Bostwick J, Nahai F, et al: Treatment of ischial pressure sores with an inferior gluteus maximus musculocutaneous flap for coverage of ischial pressure sores. Plast Reconstr Surg 1981;68:539.
28. Hurwitz DJ, Swartz WM, Mathes SJ: The gluteal thigh flap: a reliable, sensate flap for the closure of buttock and perineal wounds. Plast Reconstr Surg 1981;68:521.
29. Wingate GB, Friedland JA: Repair of ischial pressure ulcers with gracilis myocutaneous island flaps. Plast Reconstr Surg 1978;62:245.
30. Hill HL, Brown RG, Jurkiewicz MJ: The transverse lumbosacral back flap. Plast Reconstr Surg 1978;62:177.
31. Lewis VL Jr, Cunningham BL, Hugo NE: The tensor fascia lata V-Y retroposition flap. Ann Plast Surg 1981;6:34.
32. Paletta CD, Freedman B, Shehadi SJ: The VY tensor fasciae latae musculocutaneous flap. Plast Reconstr Surg 1989;83:852.
33. Siddiqui A, Wiedrich T, Lewis VL Jr: Tensor fascia lata V-Y retroposition myocutaneous flap: clinical experience. Ann Plast Surg 1993;31:313.
34. Minami TR, Hentz VR, Vistnes LM: Use of vastus lateralis muscle flap for repair of trochanteric pressure sores. Plast Reconstr Surg 1977;60:364.
35. Bovet JL, Nassif TM, Guimberteau JC, Baudet J: The vastus lateralis musculocutaneous flap in the repair of trochanteric pressure sores: technique and indications. Plast Reconstr Surg 1982;69:830.
36. Hauben DJ, Smith AR, Sonneveld GJ, Van der Meulen JC: The use of the vastus lateralis musculocutaneous flap for the repair of trochanteric pressure sores. Ann Plast Surg 1983; 10:359.
37. Evans GR, Lewis VL Jr, Manson PN, et al: Hip joint communication with pressure sore: the refractory wound and the role of Girdlestone arthroplasty. Plast Reconstr Surg 1993; 91:288.
38. Girdlestone GR: The classic acute pyogenic arthritis of the hip: an operation giving free access and effective drainage, 1943. Clin Orthop 1982;170:3.
39. Klein NE, Luster S, Green S, et al: Closure of defects from pressure sores requiring proximal femoral resection. Ann Plast Surg 1988;21:246.
40. Rubayi S, Pompan D, Garland D: Proximal femoral resection and myocutaneous flap for treatment of pressure ulcers in spinal injury patients. Ann Plast Surg 1991;27:132.
41. Georgiade N, Pickrell K, Maguire C: Total thigh flaps for extensive decubitus ulcers. Plast Reconstr Surg 1956;17:220.
42. Royer J, Pickrell K, Georgiade N, et al: Total thigh flaps for extensive decubitus ulcers. A 16-year review of 41 total thigh flaps. Plast Reconstr Surg 1969;44:109.
43. Dibbell DG, McCraw JB, Edstrom LE: Providing useful and protective sensibility to the sitting area in patients with meningomyelocele. Plast Reconstr Surg 1979;64:796.
44. Lesavoy MA, Dubrow TJ, Korn HN, et al: "Sensible" flap coverage of pressure sores in patients with meningomyelocele. Plast Reconstr Surg 1990;58:390.
45. Daniel RK, Terzis JK, Cunningham DM: Sensory skin flaps for coverage of pressure sores in paraplegic patients. A preliminary report. Plast Reconstr Surg 1976;58:317.
46. Nahai F, Silverton JS, Hill HL, Vasconez LO: The tensor fascia lata musculocutaneous flap. Ann Plast Surg 1978;1:372.
47. Luscher NJ, de Roche R, Krupp S, et al: The sensory tensor fasciae latae flap: a 9-year follow-up. Ann Plast Surg 1991; 26:306.
48. Spear SL, Kroll SS, Little JW 3rd: Bilateral upper-quadrant (intercostal) flaps: the value of protective sensation in preventing pressure sore recurrence. Plast Reconstr Surg 1987;80:734.
49. Foster RD, Anthony JP, Mathes SJ, et al: Flap selection as a determinant of success in pressure sore coverage. Arch Surg 1997;132:868.
50. Marjolin J-N: Ulcere. Dictionnaire de medicine, vol 21. Paris, Bechet, 1828.
51. Mustoe T, Upton J, Marcellino V, et al: Carcinoma in chronic pressure sores: a fulminant disease process. Plast Reconstr Surg 1986;17:116.
52. Berkwits L, Yarkony GM, Lewis V: Marjolin's ulcer complicating a pressure ulcer: case report and literature review. Arch Phys Med Rehabil 1986;67:831.

CHAPTER

158

Reconstructive Surgery: Lower Extremity Coverage

DOUGLAS J. MACKENZIE, MD ✦ ALAN E. SEYFER, MD, FACS

HISTORY

The history of lower extremity reconstruction before World War I is essentially the history of amputation and generally centers on war injuries and their management. However, the advances in wound care and fracture management, sterile technique, anesthesia, and applied anatomy that occurred before World War I laid the groundwork for the modern era of lower extremity reconstruction, that of limb salvage and functional restoration.

Advances in wound care achieved in the ancient world were lost with the fall of the Roman Empire, and the galenic theory of wound suppuration as necessary for healing ruled the next millennium. With the Renaissance, science and medicine again began to advance, and Ambroise Paré (1509-1590) made significant surgical advances through his experience as a war surgeon, including refinement of amputation by amputating through viable tissue, revision of an amputation for better prosthetic fitting, and planning of the amputation with consideration of the prosthetic fitting.[1] He also reintroduced the use of the hemostatic ligature developed by Celsus (25 BC-AD 50) but long abandoned. Andreas Vesalius published the anatomy text *De Humani Corporis Fabrica* in 1543, and William Harvey published *Exercitatio Anatomica de Motu Cordis et Sanguinis in Animalibus (Anatomical Exercise on the Movement of the Heart and Blood in Animals)* in 1628. These laid the foundation for future studies on the functional anatomy of the vascular system.

John Hunter (1728-1793) was a pioneer in experimental physiology that favored primary amputation only for severe injuries, such as massive crush, partial amputation, and uncontrolled bleeding. On the basis of vascular surgical principles he developed in animals in 1785, he successfully treated four of five popliteal aneurysms by proximal ligation of the superficial femoral artery in the subsartorial canal that still bears his name. The previous technique of ligating the popliteal artery above and below the aneurysm met with a high mortality. His achievement highlighted the appreciation of vascular functional anatomy and the importance of anastomotic vessels around the knee; it was perhaps the first description of a surgical delay.[2]

Pierre-Joseph Desault (1744-1795) of the Hôtel-Dieu in Paris coined the term *débridement* and was the first to advocate it in traumatic wounds; Ollier

(1830-1900) introduced the concept of immobilization and developed the plaster cast.[3] Baron Dominique-Jean Larrey (1766-1842), Napoleon's chief surgeon, advanced the wound management practices of Desault and Ollier and avoided primary closure of all wounds except facial wounds.[1] He was a strong proponent of early amputation, as opposed to Hunter's support of delayed amputation.

Robert Liston (1794-1847) performed the first major operation under ether anesthesia in 1846, amputating a leg for tibial osteomyelitis. Although the Crimean War (1854-1856) and American Civil War (1861-1865) provided a wealth of experience with extremity injury and amputation and served to further define indications for amputation, earnest reconstructive efforts on the lower extremity would have to wait until the modern era of surgery began, the era marked by the development of aseptic technique. It was Joseph Lister (1827-1912) who in 1867 successfully treated 11 patients with compound fractures with dressings soaked in carbolic acid. Alexis Carrel, who pioneered vascular surgical techniques that a half-century later would be put to use in the developing fields of cardiovascular surgery and microsurgery, also developed the Carrel-Dakin method of wound irrigation, the use of which was popularized in World War I.

World War I marked a turning point in wound management and trauma surgery; aseptic surgery was being used, injured soldiers were being evacuated with ambulances, and the past practice of amputating all compound fractures was abandoned. The reconstructive experience of World War I also gave rise to modern orthopedic surgery and the specialty of plastic surgery. H. Winnett Orr revived the method of plaster cast immobilization of fractured extremities, incising wounds before cast application; Josep Trueta took Orr's method one step further in the Spanish Civil War (1936-1939) with the addition of thorough wound débridement.

A better understanding of shock, improved casualty evacuation, use of blood transfusions, and availability of sulfa drugs and penicillin helped decrease wound mortality from 8% in World War I to 4.5% in World War II (1939-1945).[1,4] However, owing to the advances in weaponry, the incidence of amputation rose from 2% in World War I to 5.3% in World War II, still only a tenth of the incidence of amputation in the Civil War. Major arterial injuries were still largely treated with ligation during World War II, but a sharp fall in amputation rates with arterial repair of these injuries was shown during the Korean Conflict (1950-1953).

Vascular surgical techniques were applied to small vessels in 1960 with the use of a microscope, thus sparking the modern era of microvascular reconstruction that continues to this day. With the ability to transplant various tissues, including compound flaps, digits, and large flaps previously unavailable with local techniques, soft tissue reconstruction was able to complement the evolving techniques of bone fixation, joint reconstruction, and vascular surgery. Currently, we are witnessing profound developments in tissue engineering, genetic engineering, and limb transplantation. While expanding the possibilities for limb reconstruction, these developments will add new complexity to the field by imparting ethical questions not previously considered in evaluation of the seriously injured extremity.

PRINCIPLES

The evaluation and subsequent treatment of a lower extremity wound only begin with a thorough examination of the wound and leg. An evaluation of the patient as a whole allows treatment to be planned within the context of coexisting morbidity, socioeconomic considerations, and rehabilitative potential.

Whether the wound is an acute injury or the result of tumor ablation, treatment of the wound and the patient is usually a multidisciplinary endeavor. Optimal results are best expected when there is full cooperation and communication between physicians, other health professionals, patient, and family.

The patient must be treated as an individual, with reconstructive planning often influenced by the patient's needs and desires. The direct and indirect costs of surgery and months of rehabilitation can be enormous. Thus, the 35-year-old sole breadwinner in a household of five may be better served by amputation with a functional prosthesis, whereas the 20-year-old college student with an identical injury may warrant an intensive reconstruction effort with an 18-month rehabilitation regimen.

The primary goal of surgical reconstruction of the lower extremity wound is to restore or to maintain function. Functionality first demands a stable skeleton capable of supporting the patient's weight, with a stable surrounding soft tissue envelope. The presence or rehabilitative potential of muscles and joints along with proprioception and plantar sensibility will determine functional level. Profound detriments to a good outcome include chronic pain and the development of infection, particularly osteomyelitis. The patient's motivation and compliance and the family's support will be critical during the rehabilitative phase and should be considered in choosing salvage procedures. Finally, the aesthetic outcome of reconstructive options should be considered, but never at the expense of functionality.

The Reconstructive Ladder

For every complicated problem there is a simple answer. And it is wrong.

—H. L. Mencken

This quotation especially suits the reconstructive ladder as it is applied to the lower extremity wound. Although the classic reconstructive ladder ("simple" primary closure through "complicated" microvascular free tissue transplantation) serves a pedantic role, the consequences of failed techniques in lower extremity reconstruction are often devastating, leading to greater tissue loss, functional deficits, osteomyelitis, or amputation. It is best to choose the initial procedure with the best chance of success and avoidance of morbidity. The proven success with free tissue transplantation has made this technique the cornerstone in the management of complex lower extremity wounds.

Less complex wounds, or those wounds not susceptible to disastrous consequences in the event of reconstructive failure, may be treated with more expedient techniques, including the time-honored techniques of primary closure and skin graft (Fig. 158-1). Other techniques that may be indicated in select patients include tissue expansion (Fig. 158-2), skin stretching, and vacuum-assisted closure.[5] Free tissue transplantation has largely supplanted the cross-leg flap, although it remains an option in selected patients, primarily children. Pharmacologic manipulation of the healing wound remains in its infancy but is likely to assume a significant future role in the management of difficult wounds.

ANATOMY

The human being is unique in having developed two relatively large legs capable of supporting balanced upright ambulation and two relatively small arms that mainly serve to position the hands, which are key to interacting with the immediate environment. The reconstructive needs of the lower extremity are fundamentally simpler than those of the hand and upper extremity; replacement of soft tissue coverage is the primary goal rather than replacement of soft tissue function.

The anatomy of the lower leg and the pattern of common injuries and wounds present certain unique problems for the reconstructive surgeon. Blunt high-speed injury to the leg often inflicts complex damage to the mid and distal tibia, a bone with minimal soft tissue coverage anteriorly and limited local tissue for use in distal reconstruction. Atherosclerosis may compromise distal blood supply, causing wounds to develop de novo or complicating reconstructive efforts after trauma. The dependency of the leg contributes to venous disease, which can lead to venous stasis ulcers or make flaps more susceptible to postoperative venous congestion. The need for plantar sensibility makes rehabilitation delayed or impossible after repair of proximal nerve injury and influences salvage attempts.

Knowledge of arterial anatomy with respect to muscles, fascia, and skin combined with an appreciation of tissue angiosomes will allow known flaps to be raised safely and unknown flaps to be developed.

Vascular Anatomy

The external iliac and common femoral arteries supply a rich network of "deep" vessels above the inguinal ligament and "superficial" vessels below the ligament (Fig. 158-3). This radiating pattern of vessels has been likened to the spokes of a wheel. The deep inferior epigastric artery and deep circumflex iliac artery off the internal iliac supply the rectus abdominis and iliac bone, respectively. The superficial inferior epigastric artery exits the femoral canal from the common femoral artery to supply a territory over the lower abdomen that may extend to the costal margin; the superficial circumflex iliac artery extends laterally across the inguinal region and supplies the groin flap.[6]

The common femoral artery becomes the superficial femoral artery after it gives off its biggest branch, the profunda femoris. The profunda femoris supplies most of the muscles of the thigh, dividing medially and inferiorly. The first branch of the profunda femoris supplies anastomoses with the inferior gluteal, which continues down the posterior thigh to within 8 cm of the popliteal fossa. The lateral femoral circumflex comes off as the third branch of the profunda as it enters the adductor compartment and supplies the sartorius, rectus femoris, and tensor fascia lata. The medial femoral circumflex also branches from the profunda to supply the gracilis. The superficial femoral artery continues inferiorly and gives off the superior geniculate artery at the adductor hiatus, where it then becomes the popliteal artery. The superior geniculate passes along the medial knee and leg and sends off a saphenous branch, which descends with the saphenous nerve and supplies the saphenous flap.[7] The inferior geniculate comes from the popliteal and along with the superior geniculate forms a rich anastomotic network around the knee.

In addition to the geniculate arteries, the popliteal artery supplies paired sural arteries, which supply the medial and lateral gastrocnemius muscles. It then bifurcates into the tibioperoneal trunk and anterior tibial

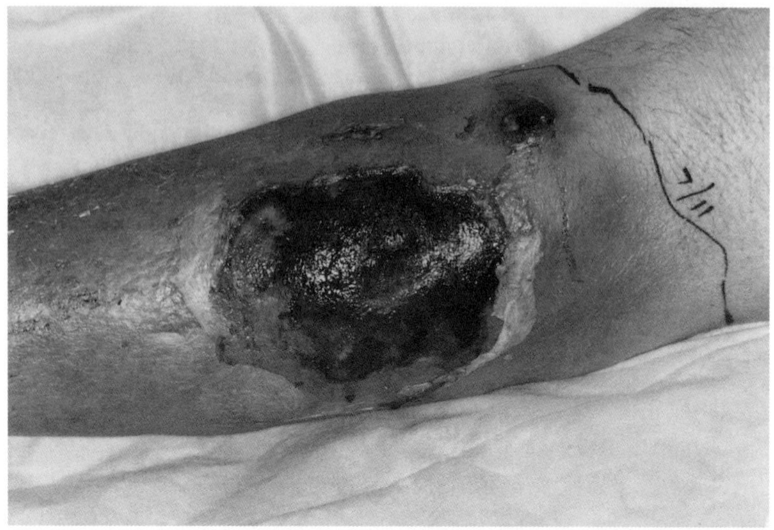

A

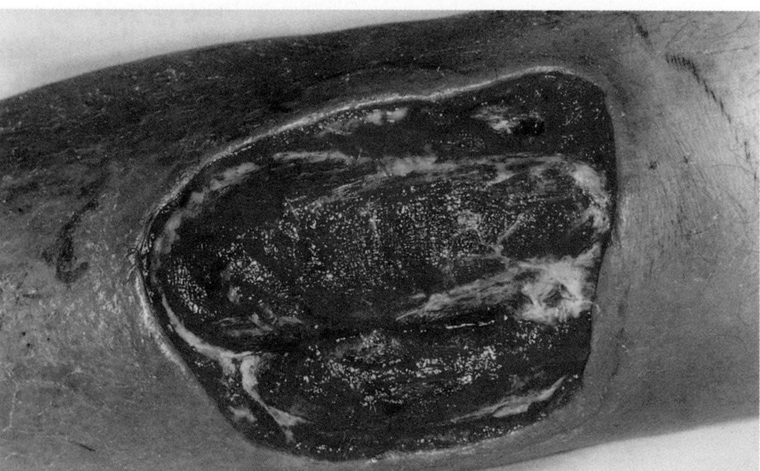

B

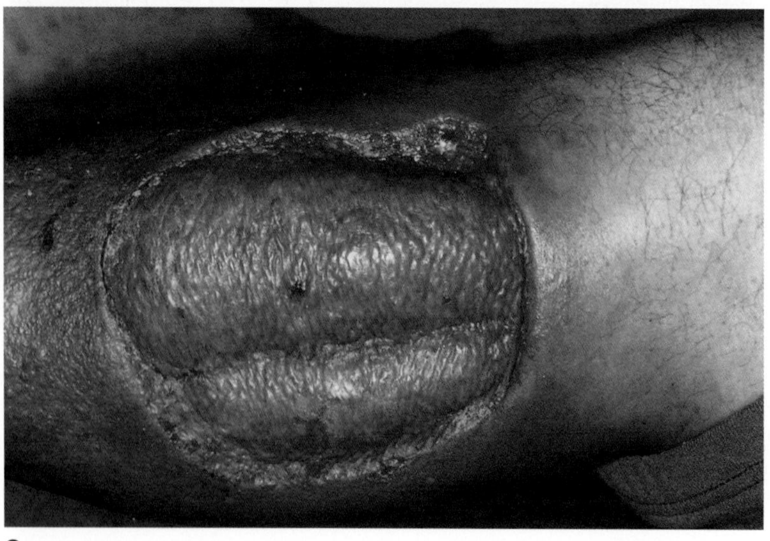

C

FIGURE 158-1. *A* to *C,* Skin graft. After débridement of this necrotic wound, the extent of the tissue damage and contamination was unclear. Granulation tissue was allowed to develop, indicating a wound bed ready for grafting. Before application of the graft, granulation tissue should be thoroughly débrided to minimize contamination and scar tissue beneath the graft.

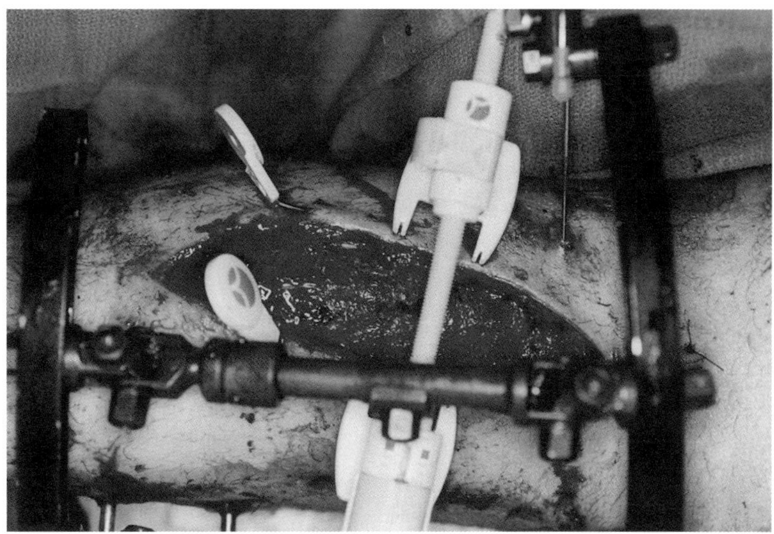

A

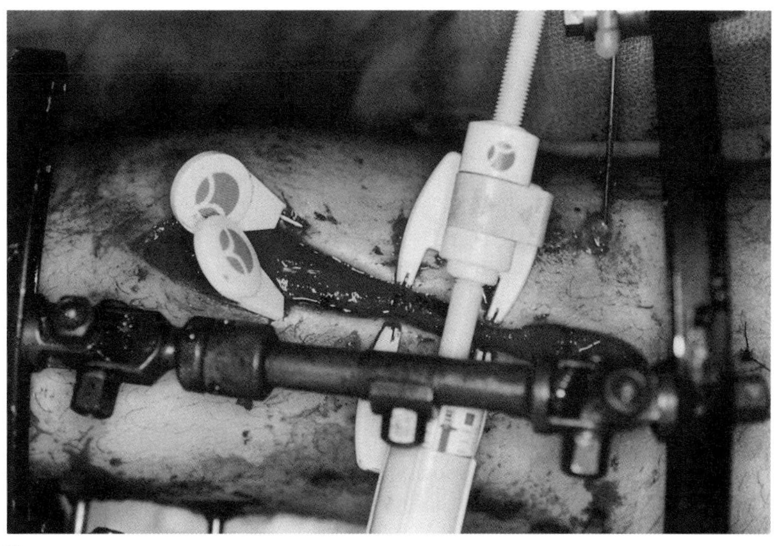

B

FIGURE 158-2. *A* and *B*, Wound closure device. When swelling is allowed to subside and the wound is advanced with a wound closure device, skin grafts or other procedures can often be avoided because there is no skin loss with which to contend.

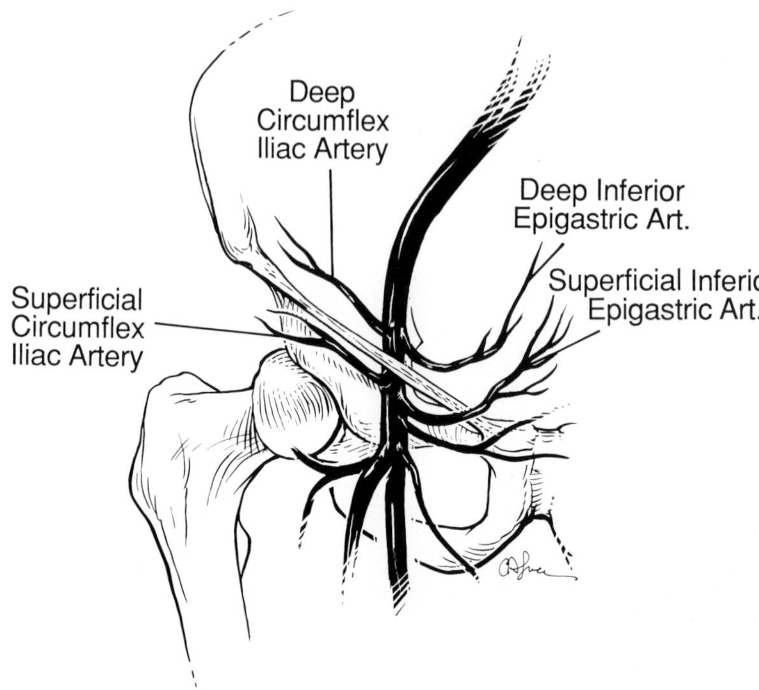

FIGURE 158-3. Arterial anatomy of the inguinal region. The "deep" branches arise proximal and the "superficial" branches arise distal to the inguinal ligament. Arterial branches are numerous in this region and are oriented in all directions like the spokes of a wheel. Fasciocutaneous flaps need not be designed according to classically described flaps (such as the groin flap) but rather can be based over the femoral vessels and oriented in any direction. (From Thorne CHM, Siebert JW, Grotting JC, et al: Reconstructive surgery of the lower extremity. In McCarthy JG, ed: Plastic Surgery. Philadelphia, WB Saunders, 1990:4029-4092.)

artery (Fig. 158-4). The anterior tibial artery supplies the muscles of the anterior compartment of the lower leg after passing over the interosseous membrane and becomes the dorsalis pedis artery on the dorsum of the foot. The tibioperoneal trunk bifurcates into the peroneal and posterior tibial arteries. The peroneal descends posterior to the interosseous membrane, medial to the fibula, nourishing the fibula and supplying the overlying skin through perforators through the posterior crural septum. Its terminal branch is the lateral calcaneal artery of the foot, supplying the versatile lateral calcaneal flap.[8] The posterior tibial artery provides the nutrient artery to the tibia as well as the adjacent muscles in the deep posterior compartment. It divides into the medial and lateral plantar arteries in the foot. Variations in origin of the three dominant lower leg arteries and single-artery supply (the so-called peroneus magnus) are examples of anatomic variations the surgeon should be aware of in planning reconstruction.

Because of the large muscle mass of the thigh, blood supply of the skin tends to be from musculocutaneous perforators. In the proximal lower leg, more fasciocutaneous perforators are seen, with vessels traveling along the fascia, supplying muscle, bone, and skin. Distally, arteries travel more directly to the overlying skin while supplying the subcutaneous tissues along the way. Axial vessels lying along fascia provide sources for vascularized fascial and fasciocutaneous flaps, especially in the lower leg and foot.

Compartments and Angiosomes

The lower extremity has been divided into several compartments bound by fascial or bony walls: three compartments in the thigh and four in the lower leg. The lower leg compartments are clinically significant, whereas the thigh compartments are rarely so. Tissue blood flow is impaired when trauma, ischemia, or even overuse causes swelling of the tissues within the unyielding compartment. This compartment syndrome may lead to muscle necrosis and sepsis and is a surgical emergency when it is diagnosed. Sequelae of delayed intervention include sensorimotor dysfunction and muscle fibrosis and contracture from nerve and muscle injury. Chronic compartment syndrome may also occur and is also treated by operative release of the fascial envelope. On the basis of the clinical examination and supplemented with measured compartment pressures when the examination findings are equivocal, evolving, or limited by the patient's mental status, operative intervention serves to release the fascial envelope.

The lower extremity is usually divided into four compartments (Fig. 158-5). All compartments of the lower leg can be released with medial and lateral incisions, through skin and outer fascia of the superficial posterior and lateral compartments, followed by dissection and release of the anterior and posterior intermuscular septa to release the anterior and deep posterior compartments. Without loss of tissue, the

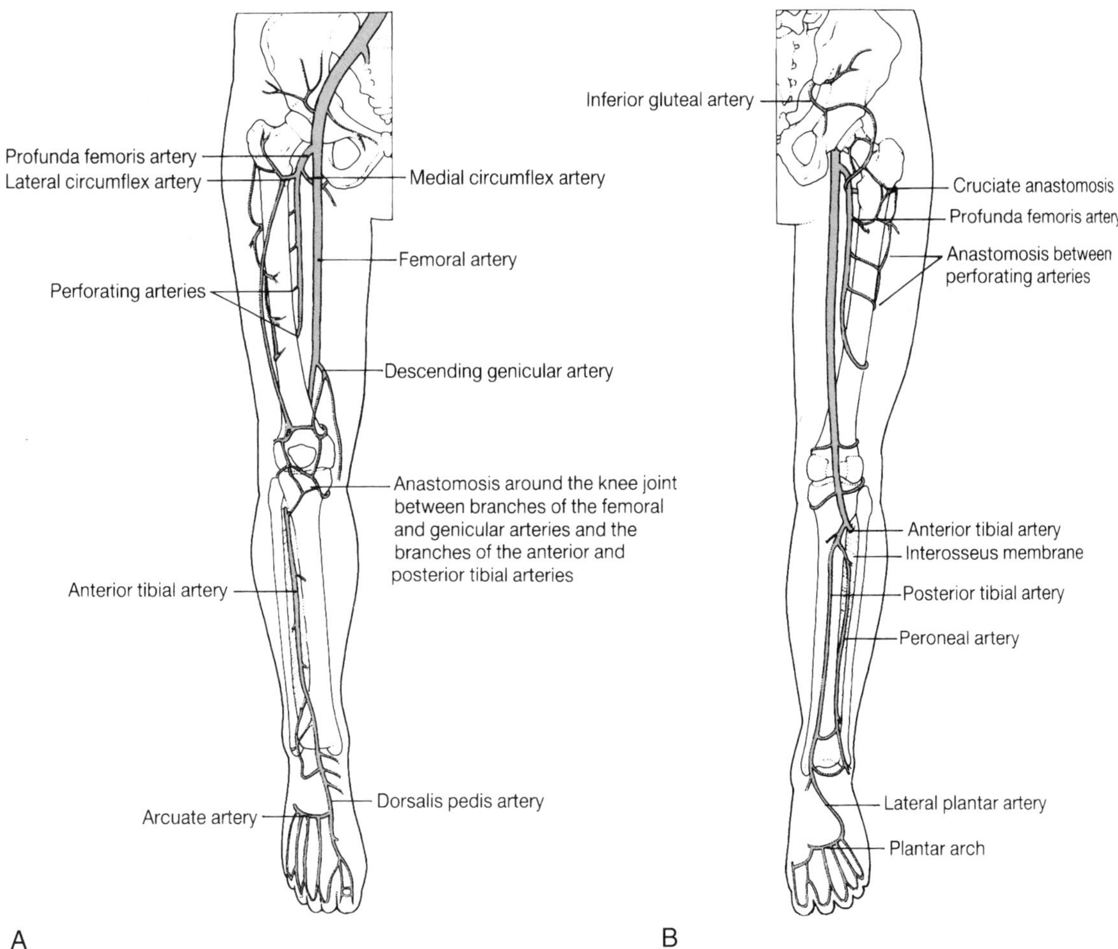

FIGURE 158-4. Summary diagram showing the arteries of the lower limb. *A,* Anterior view. *B,* Posterior view. (From Rogers AW: Textbook of Anatomy. Edinburgh, Churchill Livingstone, 1992:624.)

resulting fasciotomy wounds may be allowed to contract and close through secondary intention. They may also be closed by delayed primary closure, sometimes with the help of a skin-stretching device, once swelling begins to abate, generally 1 week after fasciotomy. Skin grafting of fasciotomy wounds is generally unnecessary unless skin loss has occurred.

Arterial injection studies have elucidated the pattern of blood perfusion between tissues in the body, including the leg.[2,9] Source arteries and veins supplying a three-dimensional volume of tissue from skin to bone have been identified, and these regions have been termed angiosomes. Vascular connections between adjacent angiosomes generally occur within tissues, not between adjacent tissue types. Typically, anastomotic pathways allow an area of skin, muscle, or bone to receive branches from two or more angiosomes; however, the anterior compartment of the leg is somewhat unique in that it receives blood supply only from the anterior tibial artery.[2] Many clinical problems can be better understood by coupling knowledge of the anatomy of the rigid osseofascial compartments of the leg with the angiosome concept of blood supply. In addition, the harvesting of composite flaps, the development of new flaps, and the avoidance of iatrogenic vascular compromise during surgical interventions can be enhanced with an appreciation of tissue angiosomes.

Nerves

The lower extremity muscles are supplied by motor fibers carried through the obturator, femoral, and sciatic nerves. The obturator and femoral nerves come from the lumbar plexus, which is derived from nerve roots L2, L3, and L4. The femoral nerve travels on the anterior surface of the iliopsoas muscle, passing under the inguinal ligament just lateral to the femoral artery, and serves knee extension by innervating the quadriceps and sartorius muscles. The obturator nerve accompanies the obturator artery and exits through

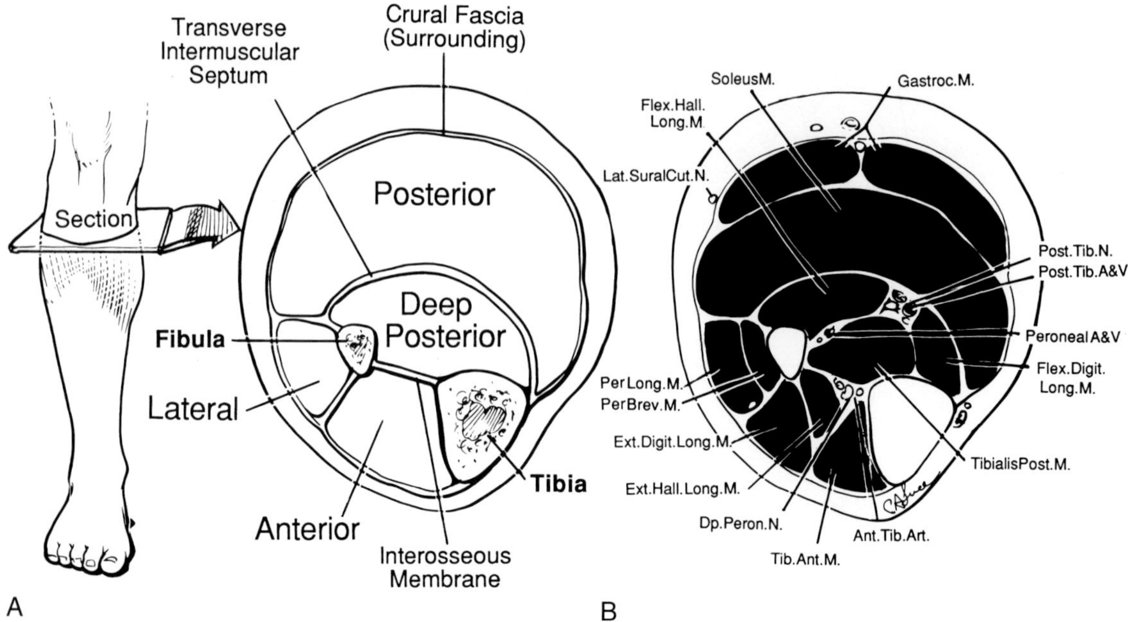

FIGURE 158-5. Compartmental anatomy of the leg. *A,* Fascial septa separate the calf into four compartments. *B,* The peroneal and posterior tibial arteries are located in the deep posterior compartment, which must be included in any fasciotomy. (From Thorne CHM, Siebert JW, Grotting JC, et al: Reconstructive surgery of the lower extremity. In McCarthy JG, ed: Plastic Surgery. Philadelphia, WB Saunders, 1990:4029-4092.)

the bony obturator canal, supplying the muscles that adduct the thigh, including the gracilis and adductor magnus. The sciatic nerve, which is the largest nerve of the body, exits the pelvis through the sciatic foramen lateral to the ischial tuberosity and carries the tibial and common peroneal nerves. The tibial nerve supplies the knee flexors in the thigh before the sciatic divides into separate tibial and common peroneal nerves above the popliteal space. The tibial nerve courses adjacent to the posterior tibial vessels in the deep posterior compartment of the leg, supplying the flexors in the deep and superficial posterior compartments. After traveling posterior to the medial malleolus and giving off the calcaneal nerve to supply sensibility to the heel skin, it divides into the medial and plantar nerves. The common peroneal nerve crosses the popliteal fossa and travels around the fibular head, where it is vulnerable to blunt injury and iatrogenic injury during fibular harvest. It then bifurcates into superficial and deep peroneal nerves; the superficial supplies muscles of the lateral compartment, and the deep supplies muscles of the anterior compartment. The superficial also sends sensory fibers to the lateral leg and dorsum of the foot; the deep sends sensory fibers to a small area over the dorsal first web space.

Sensibility of the thigh is provided by the anterior femoral cutaneous from the femoral nerve and lateral femoral cutaneous nerves from the lumbar plexus, both supplied by L2 and L3 nerve roots. The lateral femoral cutaneous nerve is susceptible to painful neuroma from compression or injury as it passes underneath the inguinal ligament. The medial thigh is supplied by the ilioinguinal nerve proximally and the obturator nerve distally; the posterior thigh is supplied by the posterior femoral cutaneous nerve from the sacral plexus (S1-3) (Fig. 158-6).

In addition to the peroneal nerve, the saphenous nerve supplies the lower leg over its medial half, and the sural nerve that branches from the tibial nerve supplies the posterolateral leg and lateral foot. Sensibility to the plantar surface of the foot is critical for function.

SOFT TISSUE EXPANSION

The use of tissue expansion in the lower extremity has not been embraced by plastic surgeons as it has in other areas of the body, such as the breast and scalp. The potential advantages of using expanded skin in the lower extremity over other reconstructive methods include improved contour, coverage with like tissue, and improved aesthetic result. However, implant placement and subsequent expansion are not forgiving of errors in planning or impatience during expansion. Wound infection and dehiscence are the most common complications, but seroma, implant displacement, neurapraxia, hematoma, and contour defects can also occur. The technique is generally useful

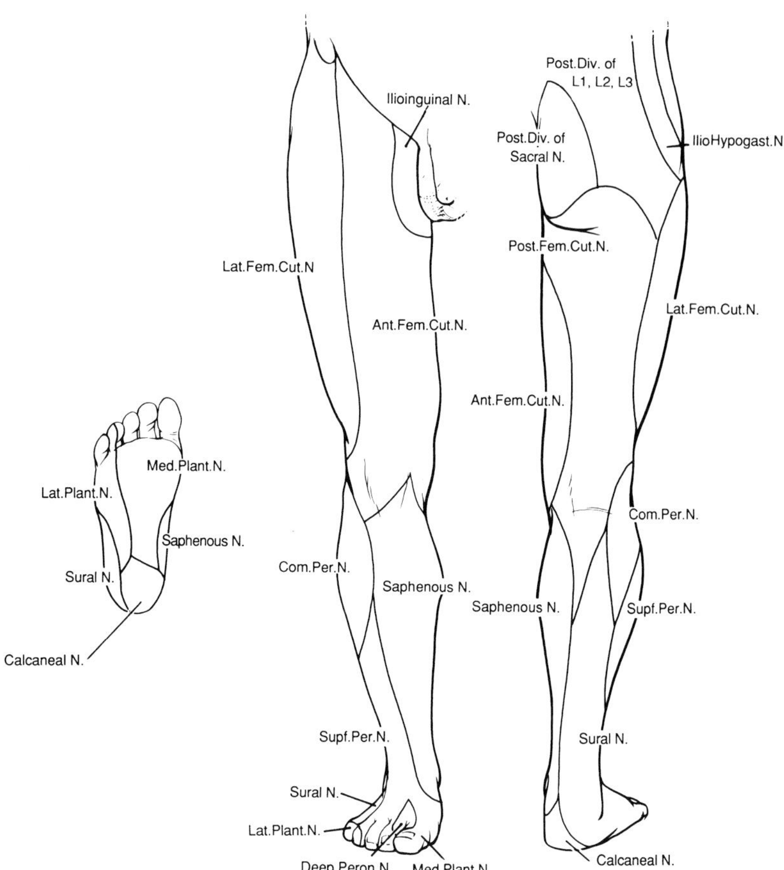

FIGURE 158-6. Sensory innervation of the lower extremity. (From Thorne CHM, Siebert JW, Grotting JC, et al: Reconstructive surgery of the lower extremity. In McCarthy JG, ed: Plastic Surgery. Philadelphia, WB Saunders, 1990: 4029-4092.)

for healed, chronic defects, and placement near open wounds results in more complications. Placement planning should consider that extremity skin is best expanded lateral to the defect, as skin will tend to advance transversely but not longitudinally. Rectangular or crescent-shaped expanders generally work best; hemispheric expanded flaps do not advance as well. For avoidance of wound dehiscence, neurapraxia, and fat necrosis, expansion should proceed slowly, stopping before the onset of pain or, if it is measured, before intraexpander pressure exceeds 40 mm Hg.[10]

Flap prefabrication with tissue expansion may have a role in select reconstructions of the lower extremity including free tissue transplantation[11] and expansion of the medial side of the opposite leg before cross-leg transfer.[12]

TRAUMATIC LOWER EXTREMITY WOUNDS

Evaluation of the patient with a significant lower extremity injury should first focus on the patient as a whole, with assessment and treatment following standard guidelines for multisystem trauma. Although associated life-threatening injuries take priority in treatment, severe injuries to the lower extremities must also be respected as life-threatening injuries, typically due to blood loss and the sequelae of inadequate resuscitation such as hypothermia, coagulopathy, and adult respiratory distress syndrome. Emergency department evaluation of the extremity itself can be brief and focused, especially if the patient will soon be going to the operating room. Most important is the neurovascular examination, particularly the distal blood supply, the presence of compartment syndrome, and the sensibility of the plantar surface of the foot if the patient is conscious. Thorough examination of the injury is deferred to the operating room, where illumination, sterility, and anesthesia are optimal. To expedite treatment of the devascularized leg, on-table femoral angiography can also be performed in the operating room.

Evaluation begins after removal of any dressings, with the surgical preparation done by the physician under proximal tourniquet control. Thorough débridement of all devitalized tissue including smaller bone fragments is performed with care to avoid stripping periosteum off larger bone fragments. Degloved areas requiring débridement may be sources of skin graft to be used immediately or stored for subsequent surgery. Fasciotomies are performed as necessary, usually through medial and lateral incisions on the lower leg. Crushed muscle is débrided, with care to preserve and assess adjacent neurovascular structures. The wound is pulse irrigated, and the tourniquet is then released to allow hemostasis and evaluation of tissue perfusion; additional devitalized tissues are débrided. Angiography before reconstruction is not generally necessary in young patients with at least one palpable distal pulse, but it should be considered in older patients in whom vascular disease may coexist. Posterior knee dislocations or distal femur fractures may require preoperative evaluation of the popliteal artery with duplex ultrasonography or angiography. Orthopedic stabilization of fractures commences unless distal vascular compromise dictates revascularization or temporary shunting before bone fixation. Although definitive wound coverage is best done early, it is usually prudent to defer the reconstruction briefly to allow complete resuscitation and further evaluation of questionably viable tissues (Fig. 158-7).

Timing of Soft Tissue Coverage

The loss of soft tissue cover over a fracture, particularly when interrupted endosteal blood supply is combined with periosteal damage, demands coverage of the exposed bone with vascularized tissue after thorough débridement of devitalized tissue.[13] Soft tissue coverage of severe, type III and type IV open fractures of the leg diminishes the rate of infection, nonunion, and secondary amputation when it is performed early. Byrd et al[14] described acute, subacute, and chronic phases of an open tibial fracture. Ideally, the wound is covered in the first 5 to 6 days after injury, the so-called acute phase. In severe type III (IIIB) and all type IV (IIIC) injuries, free muscle transplantation obtained the best results. Colonized wounds and a higher propensity to infections and flap failures characterized the subacute phase between 1 and 6 weeks after injury. Between 4 and 6 weeks, the wound enters a chronic phase characterized by robust granulation tissue, adherent soft tissue, and clear demarcation between viable and nonviable bone. Supporting even earlier soft tissue reconstruction, the concept of emergency free tissue transplantation was developed in the 1980s by Marko Godina.[15,16] Godina reported 0.75% incidence of flap failure, 1.5% incidence of infection, and 6.8 months to union in a group reconstructed within 72 hours. This compared with 12% flap failure, 17.5% infection, and 12.3 months to union in a group reconstructed between 72 hours and 3 months of injury. Those reconstructed beyond 3 months had slightly better flap failure and infection rates (9.5% and 6%, respectively) but even longer time to union (29 months).[16] Series with larger proportions of more severe leg injuries have noted that definitive coverage may need to be delayed on the basis of the overall condition of the patient and that good results can still be expected when coverage occurs within 15 days of injury. More important is thorough débridement with removal of all questionable bone fragments.[17,18] Also, a radical débridement may be difficult to perform in the early period after injury if the extent of the wound remains ill-defined.[19]

The "gold standard" for coverage of severe lower extremity injuries is free tissue transplantation. In one large study comparing complication rates between severe ASIF/OTA type C injuries, 44% of rotational flaps had complications versus 23% with free tissue transplantation.[20] Ideal free flaps for the lower extremity include the latissimus dorsi, rectus abdominis, serratus anterior, and gracilis. The first three provide flaps with long pedicles to reach out of the zone of injury and can be chosen on the basis of size demands, donor site considerations, and positioning of the patient (Fig. 158-8). Although smaller and supplying a shorter pedicle, the gracilis is ideal for smaller wounds to avoid bulk and to improve recipient and donor site appearance. These muscle flaps should be covered with an immediate skin graft, and the temptation to harvest musculocutaneous free flaps for the lower extremity should be avoided. The skin paddles are invariably too small and too bulky, rarely preclude a skin graft, and commonly lead to the wise decision to remove the unhelpful tissue immediately rather than later. However, free fasciocutaneous flaps, such as the scapular, lateral thigh, and radial forearm, are suitable for many lower extremity applications and often provide for excellent contour reproduction and appearance.

The planning for a free tissue reconstruction of the lower extremity ideally includes two teams, one for wound preparation and one for harvesting and donor site closure. Unless the reconstruction is performed in the acute setting when the trauma surgeons and orthopedic surgeons are also intimately involved in the patient's care, the reconstructive surgeon will have likely assumed the role of "captain of the ship" and should ensure that all necessary specialists and ancillary professionals are prepared and available for the procedure. These may include orthopedic surgeons to remove and replace hardware and physical therapists or prosthetists to apply splinting or orthotics postoperatively.

Once the wound has been thoroughly débrided, suitable vessels are dissected, most commonly the anterior tibial or posterior tibial. These vessels should be out of the zone of injury, which demands some subjective assessment on the part of the microsurgeon. Although performing the anastomosis proximal to the zone of injury is preferred, distal vessels are often easier to dissect, with easier access for anastomosis, and anastomoses distal to the zone of injury have comparable

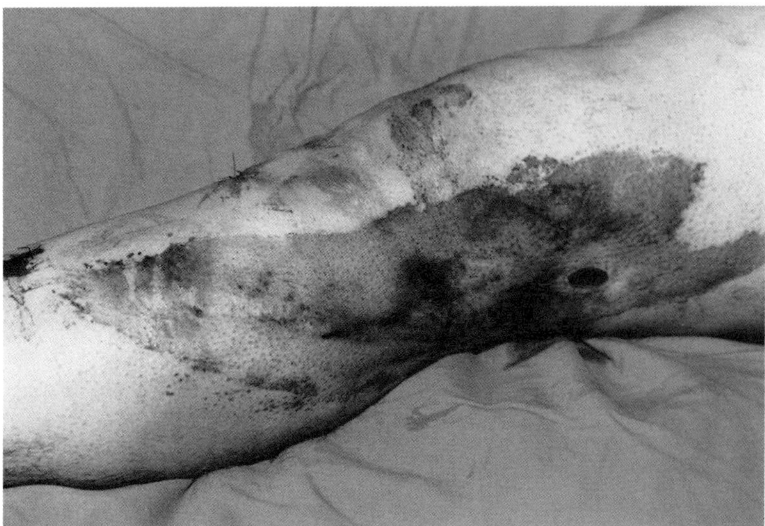

A

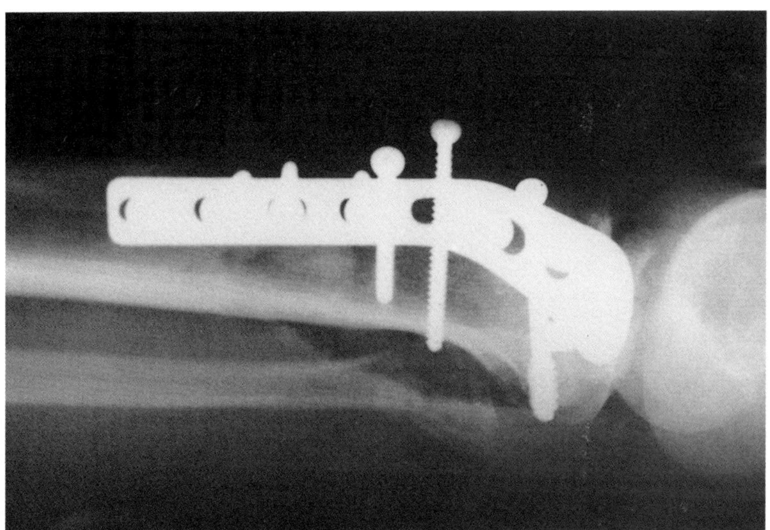

B

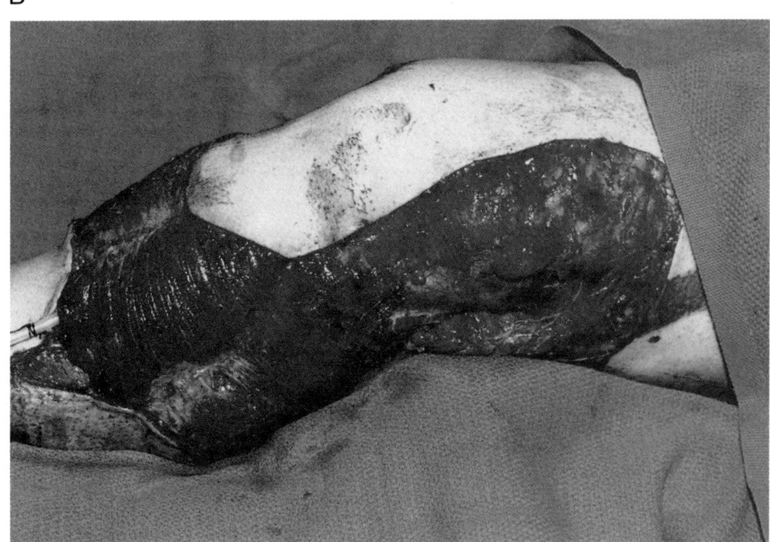

C

FIGURE 158-7. *A* to *C*, Rectus free flap. Compromise of the soft tissue envelope over this complex knee injury required débridement of questionably viable soft tissue and coverage of joint and hardware with free tissue transplantation.

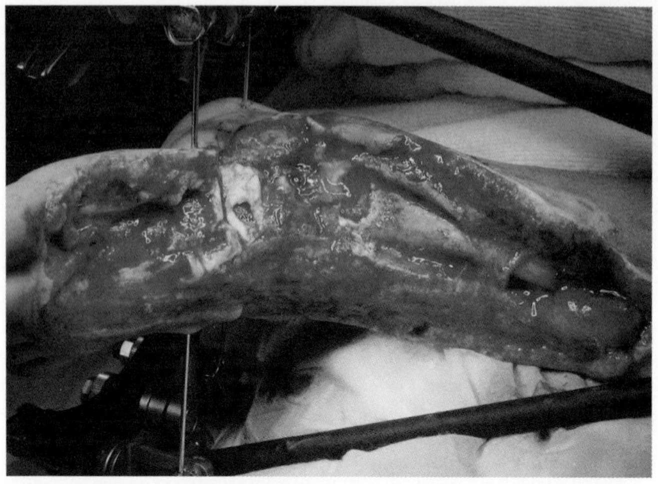

A

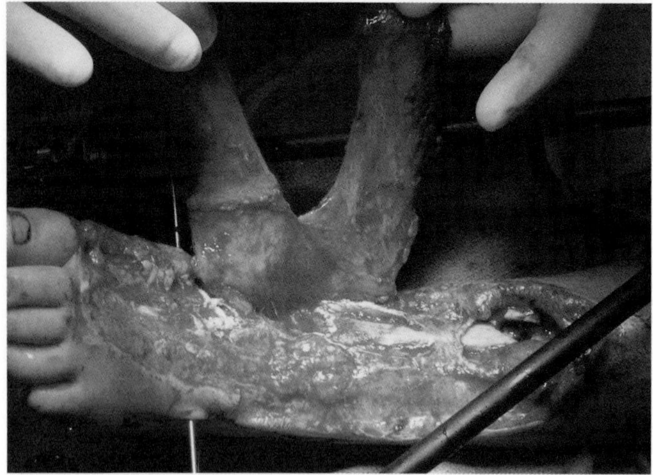

B

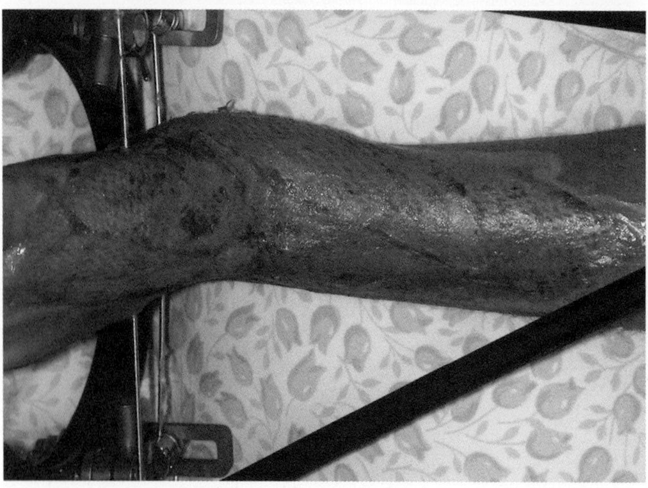

C

FIGURE 158-8. *A* to *C*, Latissimus flap. Knowledge of the vascular anatomy allows customization of flaps to suit the defect. This patient was dragged under a vehicle and sustained this complex avulsion wound of the dorsal foot and lower leg. A latissimus flap split between its two main vascular territories allowed coverage of this entire wound with no need for secondary debulking.

outcomes in select patients.[21,22] The arterial anastomosis enjoys more success when it is performed end-to-side,[23,24] whereas the venous anastomosis is usually performed end-to-end to one of the venae comitantes. The superficial veins are more susceptible to vasospasm and are avoided if possible. The flap is tacked into place, and the microscope is brought in. Details of the microscopic technique and adjuvant pharmacologic practices can be found in another chapter. Following the anastomoses, the vein clamps should be released first to avoid hypertension in the flap when the arterial clamps are released. Hemostasis is achieved, the flap is inset over drains, and a split-thickness skin graft is applied. Dressings should be tailored to allow easy inspection of the flap; no monitoring technique duplicates the accuracy of the assessment of the experienced examiner.

A failing free flap demands emergent exploration because prompt intervention will give the best chance of salvage. Most series of lower extremity free tissue transplantations report failure rates below 10%; yet this remains higher than for other sites, such as breast or head and neck, primarily because of the frequently associated vascular injuries in these patients.[19] Extremity salvage is likely even with complete failure of the flap, although the mean number of subsequent procedures to save the limb after flap failure in one series was 3.3, and approximately one third of the tibia-fibula fractures required amputation.[25]

Postoperative management is best coordinated with a physical therapy team to provide for graduated dependent positioning of the limb before weight bearing and ambulation and to provide appropriate foot and leg orthotics. Compressive wraps help reduce flap edema and perhaps assist muscle atrophy to shrink the flap, but it is best to plan and execute the flap to provide optimal contour at the initial operation, since postoperative contour change is often minimal.[26]

Salvage Versus Amputation

The decision to amputate is one that is not always clear-cut and must often be made on a patient by patient basis, considering not only the extremity wound but also the associated injuries, age, and socioeconomic situation of the patient. Recovery and rehabilitation can be a long and arduous process for the patient who has had attempted salvage of a severely injured lower extremity. Amputation often expedites recovery, lessens financial hardship from loss of work, and can often offer patients a functional extremity with the appropriate prosthesis. Heroic attempts to salvage many type IIIB injuries or those with proximal tibial nerve disruption often lead to problems with chronic pain, ulcers, and osteomyelitis, with secondary amputation seen by the surgeon and patient alike as a frustrating failure. Because of the importance of plantar sensibility to a successful outcome, most would regard disruption of the posterior tibial nerve as a contraindication to salvage.[4,27]

Various scoring systems have been devised in an attempt to predict ultimate amputation in severe lower extremity injuries and to guide surgeons in their decision to primarily amputate or attempt salvage of these limbs. The use of any of these systems should be as a guide only, never as the sole determinant of whether to amputate. The Mangled Extremity Severity Score (MESS) remains the most common scoring system and claimed 100% accuracy in predicting amputation in both 25 retrospective and 26 prospective patients in its original description.[28] The MESS is derived from scoring in categories of skeletal or soft tissue injury, limb ischemia, shock, and age. Among other shortcomings, it has been criticized for requiring subjective analysis of degree of energy imparted in the soft tissue category and for excluding nerve injuries. A modified MESS with improved sensitivity and specificity was devised to include nerve injury and to separate soft tissue and bone injuries.[29] However, several investigators have found limited or no predictive utility of the MESS system or others and have had successful outcomes of patients who would have otherwise been predicted to benefit from initial amputation.[27,30-32]

OSTEOMYELITIS

Osteomyelitis often follows severe open leg fractures with massive contamination or devascularized soft tissue and bone. Inadequate débridement or delayed coverage of the wound markedly increases the chances for development of this dreaded complication. Chronic osteomyelitis has been described as having evidence of endosteal and cortical infection of more than 6 months' duration and as having "one or more foci in bone that contains pus, infected granulation tissue, sequestra, a draining sinus, and resistant cellulitis. The inflammatory foci are surrounded by sclerotic bone with poor blood supply and are covered by a thick, relatively avascular periosteum and scarred muscle and subcutaneous tissue."[33,34]

The most important step in the surgical treatment of osteomyelitis is thorough débridement of all devascularized and contaminated tissue, including bone, granulation tissue, and the scarred surrounding soft tissue. Timidity in resection of questionably infected bone will not be rewarded with success; a large segmental defect is easier to treat than a persistent or recurrent osteomyelitis. Subsequent management of the bone defect may be achieved with bone grafting, vascularized free bone transplantation, bone distraction lengthening, or a combination of these techniques. Antibiotic-impregnated beads may be fashioned and placed within or on bone defects and open fractures

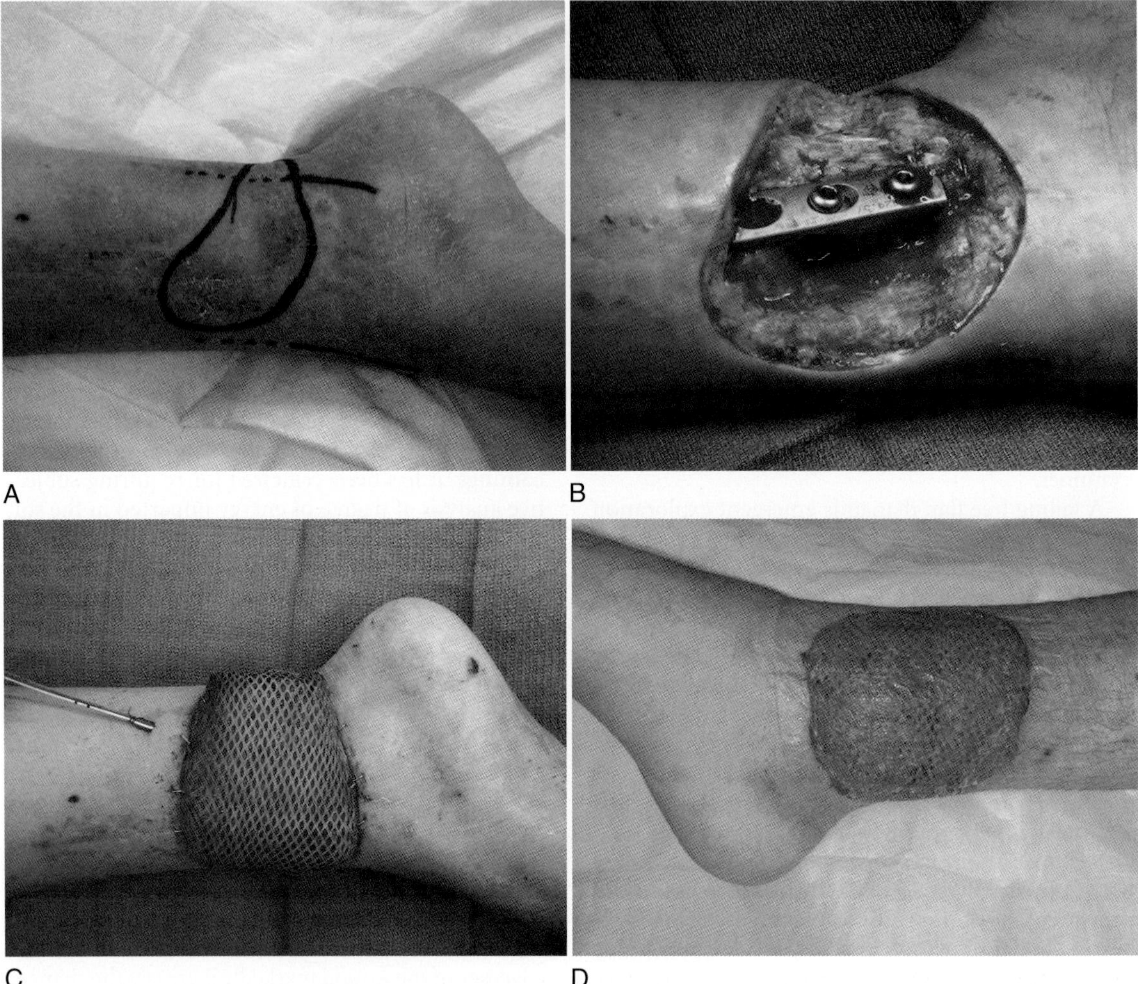

FIGURE 158-9. Osteomyelitis. *A*, Months of intravenous antibiotics and hyperbaric oxygen before referral to a plastic surgeon failed to cure this tibial osteomyelitis. *B*, The hardware was preserved in place after débridement of the soft tissue envelope and offending bone. *C*, Gracilis free muscle transfer and skin grafting allowed expeditious recovery. *D*, Partially healed wound.

when significant contamination is suspected or as an interim measure before definitive flap treatment.

The coverage of the resulting wound after débridement of osteomyelitis is generally best served with vascularized muscle, a technique begun by Stark[35] and advanced by Ger and others.[36-39] Microsurgical muscle transplantation has revolutionized treatment of osteomyelitis by allowing generous débridement to be covered by sufficient tissue previously unavailable from local sites (Fig. 158-9).[40] Credence was given to the clinical practice of using muscle flap reconstructions on these difficult wounds when it was demonstrated experimentally that inoculated wounds covered with muscle had improved oxygen tension and decreased bacterial counts.[41]

SOFT TISSUE RECONSTRUCTION AFTER TUMOR ABLATION

Techniques of soft tissue and bone reconstruction are often necessary to salvage lower extremities after oncologic resection. The development of techniques of tumor excision combined with adjuvant radiation therapy that claimed survival rates equal to amputation popularized limb salvage surgery and demanded increasingly complex reconstructive techniques. The extirpation of lower extremity tumors, typically sarcomas, often necessitates wide or radical margins, leading to segmental bone or joint loss and large defects that require filling of dead space and stabilization of adjacent joints.

Patients with lower extremity malignant neoplasms often have the additional complicating factors of adjuvant radiation therapy or chemotherapy that may render the wound less hospitable and the patient immunocompromised. Well-vascularized flaps with adequate bulk to avoid dead space and suture line tension will be the best defense against dehiscence and infection, which could jeopardize postoperative chemotherapy. These defects are best served by well-vascularized muscle, often in the form of a free tissue transplantation, to provide the bulk to fill dead space as well as to provide the optimum coverage for bone grafts and endoprostheses. In addition, the use of a muscle flap offers the possibility of functional restoration in selected patients.[42] Most patients having primary reconstructions with musculocutaneous flaps have good success and do not seem to have increased complications despite adjuvant therapy, which is most commonly given as preoperative irradiation.[43,44] Overall success rate was shown to be 96.6% in a series of 59 free flaps in 57 patients undergoing lower extremity reconstruction after tumor ablation, with 12% major and 7% minor complications.[43]

Patients who undergo joint replacement for degenerative or rheumatologic joint disease or after tumor ablation are at risk for wound breakdown and prosthetic exposure. The soft tissue coverage may be tenuous from a variety of causes: compromise of the blood supply to the skin during joint removal, previous scar tissue, adjuvant therapy, steroids, tobacco abuse, diabetes, and obesity. Soft tissue complications may be manifested as persistent aseptic wound drainage, soft tissue necrosis and dehiscence, hematoma, and infection. The incidence of infection after total joint replacement ranges from 0.25% to 12%, and it is important to distinguish superficial breakdown and contamination over the prosthesis from deep infection.[45] Early superficial infection with imminent exposure of the implant may be treated with aggressive débridement, irrigation, and flap coverage of the implant; deep exposures and prolonged infections generally require removal of the implant, débridement and irrigation, and management of the resulting segmental gap. Options include two-staged reconstruction with an initial antibiotic-impregnated spacer, resection arthroplasty, arthrodesis, and amputation.

REPLANTATION

Only in rare circumstances will a patient with an amputated lower extremity benefit from reimplantation. Lower extremity prostheses often afford the patient a high level of functionality, with a significantly shorter and less complicated rehabilitation period. In addition to the severe local trauma of the amputated limb, patients with lower extremity amputations often need lifesaving treatment for severe associated injuries, preventing timely reimplantation.

Replantation of the lower extremity may be considered if a durable, sensate, and painless foot is deemed possible. Contraindications to replantation include severe associated injuries, crush or multilevel injuries of the amputated part, and prolonged ischemia.[46] The limit of excessive warm ischemia depends on many factors that must be judged in each individual patient, but it should generally be no longer than 8 hours; cooling extends this significantly. Leg length discrepancy of more than 10 cm in an adult is probably a contraindication to replantation.[47] Mobilization of two skilled teams is desirable to expedite the replantation and to minimize ischemic time. Early placement of an arterial shunt is desirable, especially in more proximal injuries, and serves not only to perfuse the ischemic tissue but also to assist in the delineation of nonviable tissue, the removal of toxic metabolites, and the identification of veins for anastomosis.

In patients in whom reconstruction of a functional lower extremity is not possible, consideration may be given to use of portions of the amputated part as free tissue transplantations to the remaining limb. This may help preserve stump length or avoid a more proximal completion amputation, and it may also help avoid subsequent flap surgery and donor site morbidity.[48,49]

MUSCULOCUTANEOUS FLAPS

Muscle and musculocutaneous flaps are generally the most versatile flaps for lower extremity reconstruction and often the flaps first mastered by the plastic surgeon in training. The use of transplanted muscle in various forms has achieved wide success, which is mirrored by the rich body of literature on the subject.[13,35,36,41,50,51]

Gluteus Maximus

FEATURES. The gluteus maximus is the largest muscle in the body. As the most powerful extensor of the hip, it also serves to stabilize the pelvis and hip during the important functions of ambulation, rising from a sitting position, and ascending stairs (Fig. 158-10). Its two dominant and two minor pedicles allow versatility in flap design for reliable and well-vascularized coverage of areas over the buttock, coccyx, hip, and upper thigh.

ANATOMY. It originates from a wide area, including the posterior iliac crest and ilium, sacrum, coccyx, and sacrotuberous ligament. The deepest fibers insert into the gluteal tuberosity of the femur; a greater portion inserts into the iliotibial tract. The circulatory pattern is type III, with two dominant pedicles (the superior and inferior gluteal vessels) and two minor pedicles (the first perforator of profunda

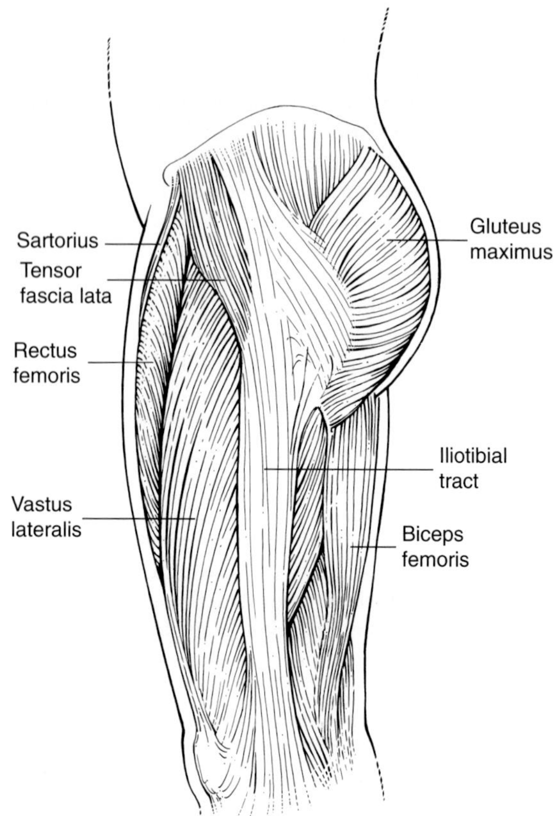

FIGURE 158-10. Thigh musculature.

femoris and two or three intermuscular branches of the lateral femoral circumflex vessels). Motor innervation derives from the inferior gluteal nerve. Skin sensation is from the posterior branches of S1-3 and L1-3.

FLAP DESIGN. For the standard flap, the arc of rotation centers on the dominant vascular pedicles at the margin of the sacrum. The insertion may be divided, allowing the muscle to be mobilized to cover the sacrum or ipsilateral ilium. The muscle may also be split to mobilize the cranial segment on the superior gluteal artery or to mobilize the caudal portion on the inferior gluteal artery. In either instance, the remaining, undisturbed segment can preserve function.[52] For the gluteal thigh flap, it may encompass the skin of the posterior thigh as a fasciocutaneous unit, and the inferior half of the muscle can also be incorporated to increase the area of coverage. The flap may be rotated anteriorly to reach the groin, trochanter, and scrotum; posterior rotation will reach the sacrum, perineum, and contralateral ischium. For the reversed flap, the origin and inferior gluteal vessels are divided, and the inferior half of the muscle is transposed to the posterior thigh on the perforators of the lateral femoral circumflex artery.

SURGICAL TECHNIQUE. A skin island over the muscle is designed according to the needs of the defect to be covered, and the incision is carried to the deep fascia of the gluteus muscle. The direction of the fibers is followed, dissecting between them to the underside of the muscle. In the thigh flap, the dissection is performed in the subfascial plane, centered over the posterior cutaneous nerve of the thigh, until the inferior edge of the gluteus is encountered. At this point, with each type of flap design, the submuscular plane is entered, and the dissection is advanced toward the pedicle with blunt technique where possible. When the pedicle is reached, the flap is rotated onto the defect.

Tensor Fascia Lata

FEATURES. The tensor fascia lata has a short muscle belly but a long fascial extension down the lateral aspect of the thigh (Fig. 158-11). Its flat shape, excellent length, and reliable vascularity make it useful in many reconstructive scenarios, both as a pedicled flap for local and regional coverage and as a free, composite unit that incorporates skin, muscle, and iliac bone. One of its most common applications is to provide closure of trochanteric pressure sores. It is an expendable muscle unit.

ANATOMY. The muscle arises just subjacent to the external lip of the anterior superior iliac crest, passing downward and backward to insert into and blend with the iliotibial tract. It abducts, medially rotates, and flexes the hip, acting to tighten the fascia lata and iliotibial tract. This allows the thigh musculature to act with increased power during ambulation and standing. The circulatory pattern is type I; the dominant pedicle is the ascending branch of the lateral femoral circumflex artery. Motor innervation is from the superior gluteal nerve. Sensation is derived from T12 (upper skin area) and the lateral femoral cutaneous nerve (L2-3) lower skin area.

FLAP DESIGN. The arc of rotation centers on a point 8 to 10 cm below the anterior superior iliac spine. From this center, a flap can be designed to rotate anteriorly to reach the paraumbilical and lower abdominal areas, groin, and perineum. Rotated posteriorly, it can reach the greater trochanter, ischium, perineum, and sacrum.[53,54] The flap can also be advanced superiorly as a V-Y flap to cover trochanteric wounds.[55] The skin overlying the muscle and fascia lata can be harvested as a unit with the flap and can extend to within 10 cm above the knee; it can incorporate a strip of skin 10 × 40 cm.

SURGICAL TECHNIQUE. A line is drawn from the anterior superior iliac spine straight down the thigh to a point 10 to 12 cm above the knee joint, anterior to the lateral epicondyle of the knee. A parallel line is

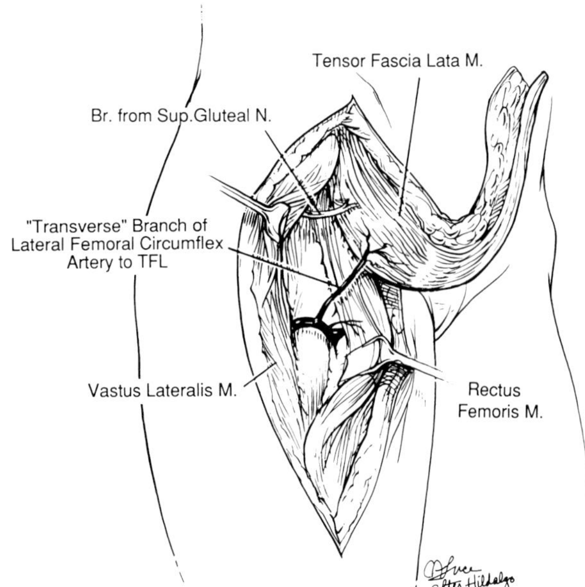

FIGURE 158-11. Tensor fascia lata free flap. The arterial pedicle and the motor nerve enter the muscle from different directions. The muscle itself is small and composes a small portion of the overall flap area. (From Thorne CHM, Siebert JW, Grotting JC, et al: Reconstructive surgery of the lower extremity. In McCarthy JG, ed: Plastic Surgery. Philadelphia, WB Saunders, 1990:4029-4092.)

drawn 12 to 15 cm posterior to the first line, straight down the thigh, curving anteriorly as it crosses posterior to the lateral epicondylar area to meet at the same point. The skin island can be designed within this long strip, according to the needs and distance to the recipient defect. The distal margin of the flap is entered, carrying the incision through the fascia lata and dissecting deep to the fascia lata and iliotibial tract. This bloodless plane can be easily and swiftly swept upward, extending the skin and fascial incisions proximally to completely liberate the flap. The pedicle and its associated branches can be seen entering medially along the underside of the muscle; this is visible 10 to 12 cm from its origin. For added mobility, the origin can also be divided.

Rectus Femoris

FEATURES. The rectus femoris, located on the anterior thigh, is suited for coverage of certain defects of the lower abdominal area. It serves as one of the four "heads" of the quadriceps femoris group of muscles and acts to extend the leg at the knee. It is important in stabilizing the weight-bearing knee in almost all positions, such as ambulation, rising from or gaining a seated position, stair-climbing, and fully extending the knee. As such, the rectus femoris is not considered totally expendable.

ANATOMY. The muscle arises from the ilium by two heads, one from the anterior inferior iliac spine and one from just cephalad to the edge of the acetabulum. These join to give rise to a bulky, fusiform, and lengthy muscle belly that coalesces with the others to form the quadriceps tendon complex. However, by virtue of its origins, the rectus femoris is the only member of this group that acts on the hip as well as on the knee. The circulatory pattern is type II; the dominant pedicle is the descending branch of the lateral circumflex femoral artery, with minor pedicles from the ascending branch of the same vessel as well as from muscle branches of the superficial femoral artery. Motor innervation is from the femoral nerve, and muscle branches enter adjacent to the dominant pedicle. The intermediate anterior femoral cutaneous nerve (L2-3) provides sensation.

FLAP DESIGN. The arc of rotation for the standard, proximally based flap is approximately 8 to 10 cm distal to the anterior inferior iliac spine and represents the region where the major pedicle enters the muscle. Once mobilized, the flap will reach the lower (infraumbilical) abdominal wall, perineum, and trochanteric areas.[56,57] The skin perforators are most reliable over the muscle itself in the central strip (12 × 20 cm) of midanterior thigh, but an island can be extended over the proximal and distal portions as well.

SURGICAL TECHNIQUE. A longitudinal incision is marked from 3 cm below the anterior superior iliac spine to just above the superior margin of the patella. The skin island is centered over this axis, and the incision is begun at the distal edge of the skin island, along the axis itself. The rectus femoris muscle is identified and separated from the vastus medialis and lateralis while ensuring that the skin island is centered over the rectus. The skin island is then incised circumferentially down to the fascia of the muscle and tacked with temporary sutures to the fascia of the muscle. The rectus is elevated from distal to proximal and from medial to lateral so that the pedicle and nerve can be identified and protected medially along the underside of the muscle. The muscle may be tunneled under a bridge of skin and fat, but it may be safest to open a trough for the flap. There should be no tension on the pedicle. The donor area should be repaired by careful suturing of the tendinous fascia of the vastus medialis and lateralis together above the patella in an effort to preserve full knee extension.

Biceps Femoris

FEATURES. This large, well-vascularized posterior muscle of the mid and lateral thigh is well suited for the coverage of ischial pressure sores, and its bulk allows filling of the cavitary defects that often characterize these wounds. It can be employed as either a musculocutaneous or muscle flap. Although it includes a robust blood supply, its short pedicle limits its use to a relatively small range encompassing the posterior upper thigh and hip regions. As a powerful knee flexor, it is not considered expendable in the ambulatory patient.

ANATOMY. The muscle has, as its name implies, two heads, one long head that originates on the ischial tuberosity and one short head that originates on the femur. Its rounded tendon is easily palpable at the lateral edge of the popliteal fossa as it passes the knee to insert into the fibular head. Its long head extends the hip, and both heads flex the leg at the knee. The circulatory pattern is type II; the long head has dominant and minor pedicles from the first and second perforating branches of the profunda femoris artery, respectively, and the short head receives the second (or third) perforating branch of the profunda and a minor source from the lateral superior geniculate artery. The long head derives its motor innervation from the tibial division of the sciatic nerve, the short head from the peroneal division of the sciatic nerve.

FLAP DESIGN. The most common application is a V-Y advancement of a musculocutaneous unit incorporating a large triangle of overlying skin, the base of which is horizontally marked along the buttock crease (usually the edge of the ischial defect) and the apex just above the popliteal fossa. The relatively short pedicles make the flap unsuitable for wide rotation flaps but serve well in sliding the muscle proximally along the femur toward the pelvis. The medial thigh skin may also be left uncut, preserving skin as a rotation-advancement modification of the flap.[58]

SURGICAL TECHNIQUE. The skin is incised around the flap, which can be 10 cm wide and 35 cm in length, before the tendon is isolated distally. The tendon is sectioned, and the dissection proceeds from the distal thigh toward the ischium, freeing the muscle on its deep aspect from the femur and from the adductor group of muscles medially until enough mobility is attained so that the defect can easily be filled.

Gracilis

FEATURES. As a pedicled flap, the versatile gracilis muscle or musculocutaneous flap provides an excellent source for perineal reconstruction as well as for ischial coverage (Fig. 158-12). It also serves as a reliable free tissue transplantation, capable of providing functional restoration as an innervated flap. It serves as an excellent free tissue transplantation for lower extremity reconstruction; its smaller size tends to improve its contour compared with other popular free

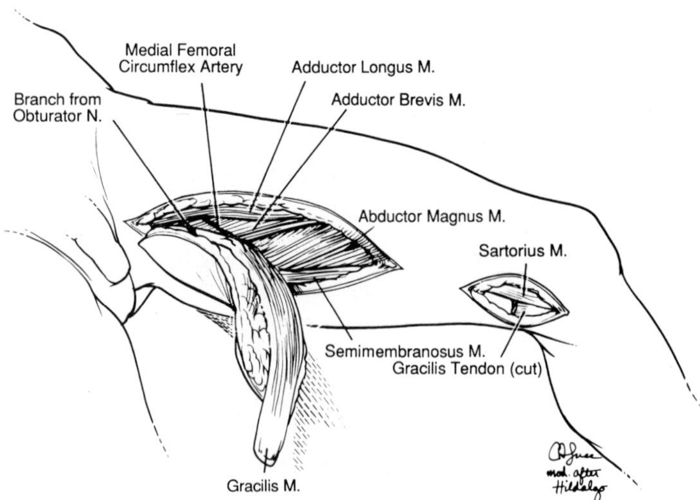

FIGURE 158-12. Gracilis free flap. The arterial pedicle and the motor nerve enter the muscle close to each other. A small distal incision allows identification of the gracilis tendon. The tendon is put on traction, permitting identification of the skin, which lies over the gastrocnemius belly. (From Thorne CHM, Siebert JW, Grotting JC, et al: Reconstructive surgery of the lower extremity. In McCarthy JG, ed: Plastic Surgery. Philadelphia, WB Saunders, 1990:4029-4092.)

muscle sources, it allows epidural anesthesia in the operative and postoperative period, and it causes no donor site functional deficit.[59]

ANATOMY. The gracilis muscle originates on the pubic symphysis and inserts onto the medial tibial condyle; it is innervated by the anterior branch of the obturator nerve. The adductor longus and magnus muscles duplicate the thigh adduction it provides. The muscle is a type II muscle. The dominant pedicle is the terminal branch of the medial circumflex femoral artery and its venae comitantes; these vessels enter the proximal third of the muscle. One or two minor pedicles arise as branches of the superficial femoral artery and enter the distal half of the muscle.

FLAP DESIGN. When skin is harvested with the gracilis muscle, the flap is generally oriented longitudinally, centered over the proximal third of the muscle, where the majority of the musculocutaneous perforators are located. A proximal transversely oriented skin flap is optional, and injection studies showing transverse flow in the perforators to the skin support the logic of this approach.[60] The longitudinal flap averages 15 cm in length and 8 cm in width and is best marked with the patient in lithotomy position. A slight extension of the knee allows the gracilis to be seen and felt, and it tends to be more posterior than expected. For elevation of the muscle only, an incision is made 2 to 3 cm posterior to a line drawn from the symphysis pubis to the medial condyle of the knee.

SURGICAL TECHNIQUE. Because the inner thigh skin tends to be loose and falls posteriorly while the patient is in lithotomy, care must be taken to orient the skin island to include skin well vascularized by the musculocutaneous perforators. In all but the thinnest of patients, this is best done by starting the dissection distally. The distal gracilis tendon should be identified and encircled above the knee; traction on the tendon will highlight the proximal outline of the muscle. Encircling muscle tissue above the knee is a common mistake and indicates identification of the sartorius muscle. The adductor longus can also be palpated and helps guide design and elevation of the flap. Dissection of the anterior and posterior skin borders then proceeds proximally approximately half the length of the muscle, whereby the distal tendon is divided and the distal muscle is likewise dissected. Minor perforators are identified and ligated, and retraction of the adductor longus muscle identifies the major pedicle passing over the adductor magnus approximately 10 cm below the pubic symphysis.

Soleus

FEATURES. The soleus is a well-vascularized muscle flap best suited for defects of the middle third of the lower leg.[51] Its bipennate morphology and dual blood supply allow distally based flaps, particularly when the muscle is split as a hemisoleus flap.[61] The soleus is the largest muscle below the knee and not only contributes significant force to ankle flexion but also contributes to venous return to the heart through compression of numerous valved veins in its substance. For these reasons, its use as a flap has been criticized,[2] and consideration should be given to alternative reconstructive options such as free flaps for the middle and distal thirds of the leg.

ANATOMY. The medial and lateral heads of the soleus arise from the posterior tibia and fibula and insert into the calcaneus through the Achilles tendon. A midline intramuscular septum divides the distal half of the muscle. The circulation pattern is type II, with dominant pedicles from the popliteal, posterior tibial, and peroneal arteries. Minor pedicles from posterior tibial and peroneal arteries supply the distal medial and lateral bellies, respectively, providing the basis for distally based hemisoleus flaps. Innervation is from the posterior tibial and popliteal nerves.

FLAP DESIGN. The arc of rotation for a proximally based soleus flap centers on the junction between proximal and middle thirds of the leg. Through fasciocutaneous perforators, overlying skin may be harvested to extend the length and arc of rotation of the flap, but a skin-grafted muscle flap is generally more suited for middle third defects. Hemisoleus flaps may improve the arc of rotation and preserve soleus function while sacrificing flap coverage area. The medial reversed hemisoleus pivots around the most superior distal minor perforator of the posterior tibial artery, approximately 7 cm above the malleolus; the lateral reversed hemisoleus has a tenuous blood supply through minor perforators from the peroneal and a limited arc of rotation.

SURGICAL TECHNIQUE. Access is through a longitudinal incision placed 2 cm medial to the tibia or laterally along the fibula. Subcutaneous neurovascular structures are identified and preserved, and the posterior compartment fascia is opened. The plane between the soleus and gastrocnemius is usually well defined superiorly, but scalpel dissection distally may be necessary to separate the tendons, with care taken to avoid cutting the gastrocnemius contributions to the Achilles tendon. For proximally based flaps, distal perforators are divided in the deep plane, and the tendon is divided distally. Identification and dissection of the midline raphe allow a hemisoleus flap to be developed. Distally based flaps demand identification of the most proximal perforator to be preserved, and the muscle harvest is limited to no more than the distal two thirds of the muscle.

Gastrocnemius

Features. The muscle has two heads, medial and lateral, that form the distal boundary of the popliteal space. Each head can be used as a separate muscle or musculocutaneous unit, based on its own pedicle, to provide reliable coverage to the upper third of the tibia, suprapatellar thigh, and knee regions (Fig. 158-13).[62] Anastomotic vessels that course across the muscular raphe allow its use as a distally based flap; after transection of the proximal muscle origins, it can be advanced a short distance to cover areas over the Achilles tendon or rotated to close defects in the area of the mid tibia. Because of its participation in ambulation, the gastrocnemius should not be employed unless the soleus remains intact.

Anatomy. This most superficial muscle of the posterior compartment forms most of the prominence of the calf. The larger, medial head arises from the popliteal surface of the femur superior to the medial condyle; the lateral head arises from the lateral surface of the lateral femoral condyle. The muscle heads unite in a midaxial raphe that courses distally to establish a tight adherence with the fascia of the soleus, forming the calcaneal (Achilles) tendon that inserts into the calcaneus. The circulatory pattern is type I; the medial muscle is supplied by the medial sural artery, and the lateral muscle is supplied by the lateral sural artery. Both heads receive a minor source across the raphe that joins them as anastomotic vessels within the muscle substance. Motor innervation derives from branches of the tibial nerve. Sensation to the skin overlying the medial head is from the saphenous nerve; that to the lateral and distal skin overlying the lateral head is from the sural nerve.

Flap Design. A skin island of 10 × 15 cm over the medial muscle and of 8 × 12 cm over the lateral muscle can be designed. However, depending on the depth of the recipient defect, it may be preferable to harvest the unit as a muscle flap and cover the muscle with grafted skin. In doing so, the thick tendinous layer can be removed sharply, and the underlying fresh muscle forms an excellent and well-vascularized recipient bed for the graft.

Surgical Technique. If the muscle alone is employed, a midline posterior incision affords excellent access to both heads. If a skin island is used, the skin is incised to the muscle fascia, and the muscle head is exposed. The midline muscular raphe is located, and with finger dissection, the underlying soleus muscle is separated from the gastrocnemius proximally and distally. The musculotendinous raphe is then separated sharply or with the cautery. Care is taken to protect the neurovascular structures, especially the more superficial saphenous and sural nerves. Distally, the thick tendinous layer is sharply dissected free from the remaining calcaneal tendon. Proximally, especially if added freedom for rotation is required for the distal thigh or suprapatellar area, the muscle origin can be transected while the sural vessels are protected.[63] The flap is rotated into place without tension on the pedicle, either through an ample subcutaneous tunnel to the defect or by opening the tunnel and insetting the flap directly.

FASCIOCUTANEOUS FLAPS

Fasciocutaneous flaps expand on the applicability of random flaps by providing larger and longer vascularized flaps and are suitable for many defects of the lower extremity that do not require the bulk of a free muscle transplantation. Ponten noted that the survival of posterior calf skin in a boy with an electrical injury correlated with an angiogram showing only one unoccluded small superficial posterior central artery arising from the popliteal artery. This inspired him to perform a proximally based flap on the calf, including the deep fascia with sural nerves and vessels.[64] His landmark description of a proximally pedicled fasciocutaneous transposition flap prompted numerous varieties of fasciocutaneous flaps to be developed.[65] More alternatives have been provided to the reconstructive surgeon with the evolving appreciation and study of cutaneous circulation; these include distally based fasciocutaneous flaps that are especially useful as an alternative to free tissue transplantation in coverage of the distal third of the leg and ankle.[66,67] Examples of several useful lower extremity fasciocutaneous flaps follow.

Groin

Features. The groin flap enjoys a long history as one of the early fasciocutaneous axial flaps and has been used as a free flap and a pedicled flap (Fig. 158-14).[6] It provides a large amount of skin and soft tissue, which can also be a detriment because these flaps tend to be bulky, often requiring subsequent debulking. The donor site is well tolerated and well hidden, but the pale skin and frequent hair growth of the donor site make for a poor match, particularly with head and neck reconstructions. Vessels are short and often variable in size and configuration, making the free groin flap a riskier option than many alternatives.

Anatomy. The lateral groin is nourished by the superficial inferior epigastric artery, the deep circumflex iliac artery, and the superficial circumflex iliac artery, which is typically chosen to support the groin flap. The superficial circumflex iliac artery pedicle is 2 to 3 cm long after arising from the common femoral artery, then splits into superficial and deep branches, with the superficial coursing laterally

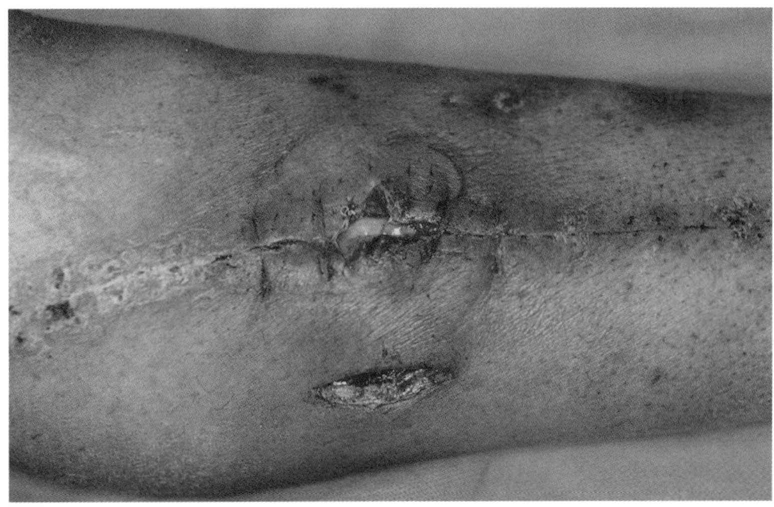

A

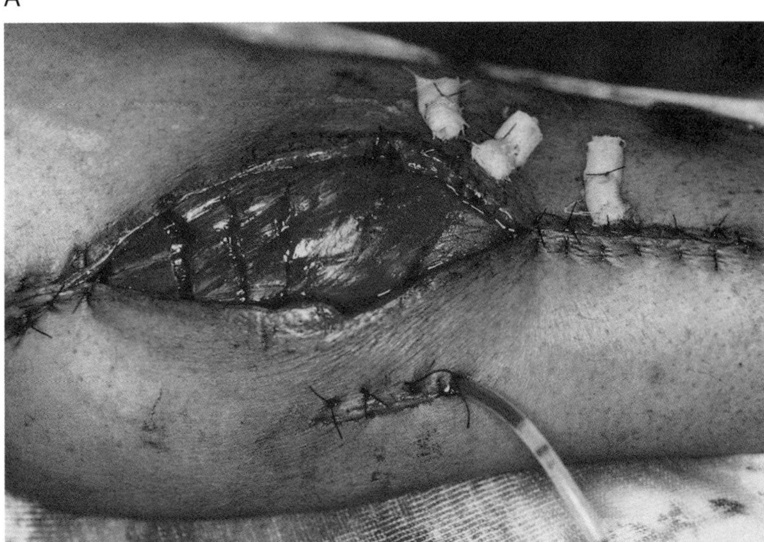

B

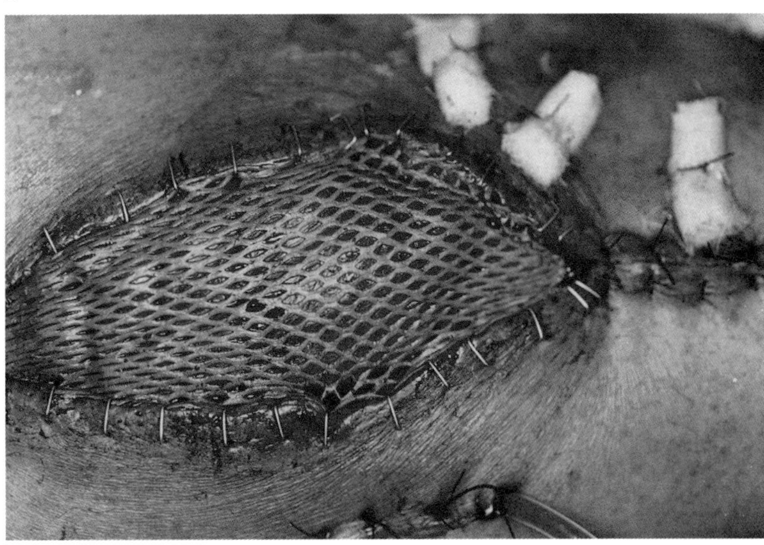

C

FIGURE 158-13. Gastrocnemius flap. *A,* A timid attempt at a bipedicled flap by the vascular surgeon failed to provide coverage over this exposed saphenous vein bypass graft. *B* and *C,* Reliable coverage was obtained with a medial gastrocnemius flap and skin graft.

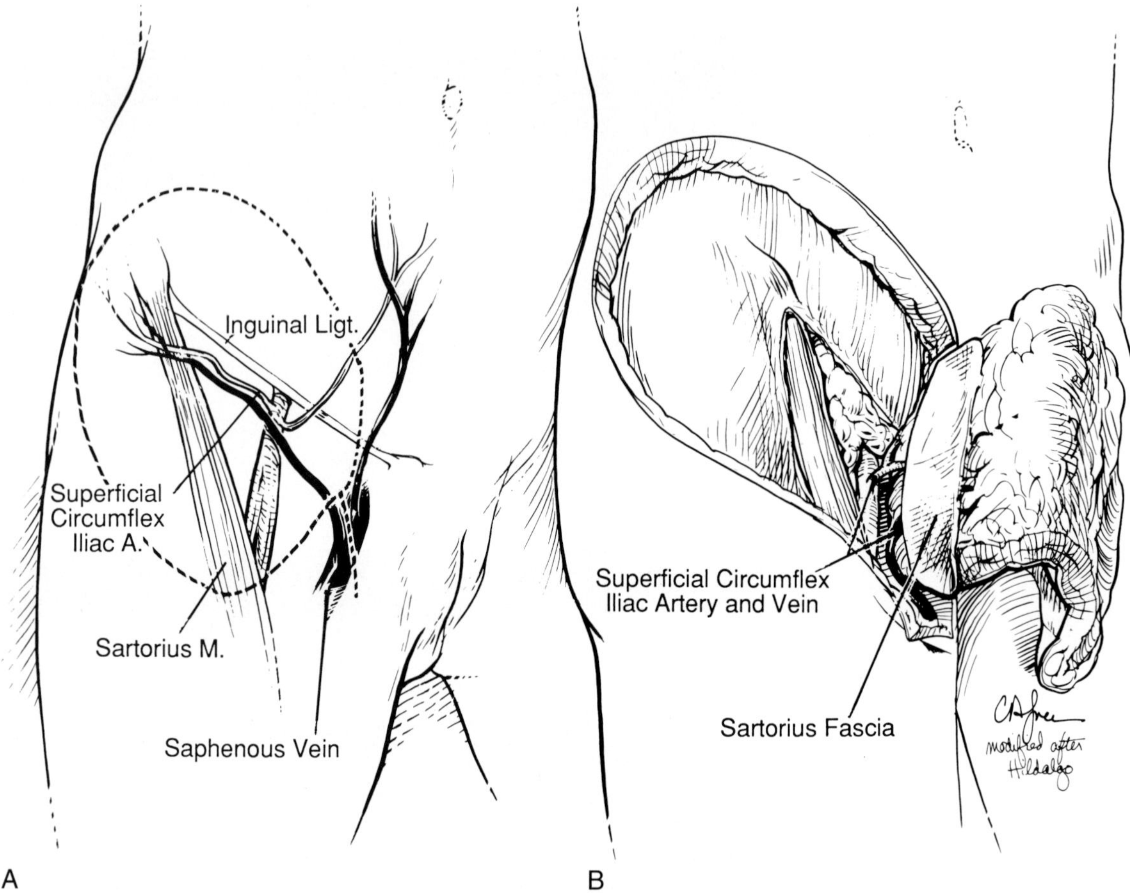

FIGURE 158-14. The groin free flap. *A,* The flap is centered on the arterial pedicle, which is parallel and caudal to the inguinal ligament. *B,* The flap is dissected lateral to medial. When the lateral border of the sartorius is reached, the dissection is carried deep to the sartorius fascia so as not to injure the arterial pedicle. (From Thorne CHM, Siebert JW, Grotting JC, et al: Reconstructive surgery of the lower extremity. In McCarthy JG, ed: Plastic Surgery. Philadelphia, WB Saunders, 1990:4029-4092.)

parallel to the inguinal ligament. The veins draining the flap are generally larger and more numerous than the arteries. Drainage is by deep venae comitantes along the superficial circumflex iliac artery, which drain into the femoral vein, and more superficially through the typically larger superficial circumflex iliac vein, which drains into the saphenous vein. The T12 sensory innervation is at the lateral margin of the flap away from the pedicle, precluding use as a sensate flap.

Flap Design. The groin flap is oriented along a line 2 to 3 cm below the inguinal ligament between the anterior superior iliac spine and the femoral vessels. In general, two thirds of the flap is harvested from above this line and one third from below. Flaps as large as 20 × 10 cm may be harvested with primary closure of the donor site; flaps as large as 35 × 20 cm will require skin grafting of the donor site.

Surgical Technique. For pedicled flaps, dissection should proceed from lateral to medial; initial dissection of the medial side with assessment of the vasculature is recommended for free flap harvest. If an unsuitable superficial circumflex iliac artery is encountered, the flap may be elevated over the superficial inferior epigastric artery; or dissection of the opposite groin may be done, as 66% of patients have asymmetric anatomy. Dissection of the flap is above the deep fascia laterally and makes the transition to include the deep fascia over the sartorius to preserve the overlying vessels.

Medial Thigh

Features. The medial thigh flap is useful for defects of the perineum, groin, lower abdomen, and thigh; it can be raised as a free flap also (Fig. 158-15).[68] Taken with the medial anterior cutaneous nerve of the thigh (L2-3), it can serve as a neurosensory flap. The saphenous vein may be elevated with the flap for improved venous drainage.

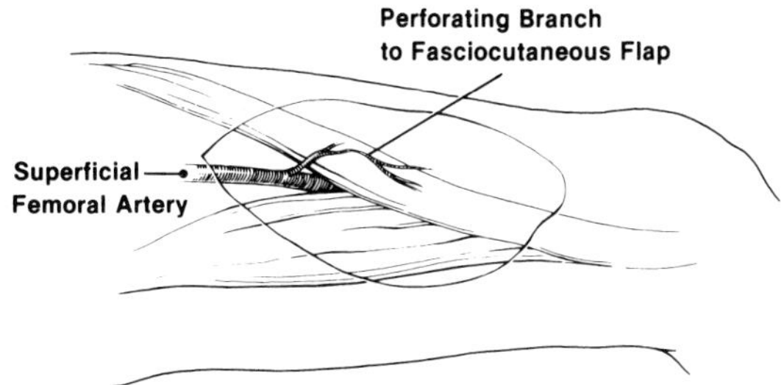

FIGURE 158-15. Medial thigh fasciocutaneous flap. (From Thorne CHM, Siebert JW, Grotting JC, et al: Reconstructive surgery of the lower extremity. In McCarthy JG, ed: Plastic Surgery. Philadelphia, WB Saunders, 1990:4029-4092.)

Anatomy. Although variable, the dominant blood supply of this type B fasciocutaneous flap is typically the anterior septocutaneous artery and venae comitantes from the superficial femoral artery and vein at the apex of the femoral triangle. When the flap is based more anteriorly, it is termed the anteromedial thigh flap and is based on a branch of the lateral femoral circumflex artery emerging from the lateral border of the sartorius. Minor pedicles are contributed by musculocutaneous perforating vessels of the sartorius and gracilis muscles.

Flap Design. A flap up to 10 × 20 cm is designed over the middle third of the proximal medial thigh. Approximately 6 to 8 cm below the inguinal ligament, the dominant pedicle is typically located at the apex of the femoral triangle, bordered medially by the adductor longus and laterally by the sartorius.

Surgical Technique. A proximal incision is made to locate the vessels at the apex of the femoral triangle; if they are absent, dissection proceeds distally and lateral to the sartorius to identify the vessels supplying the anteromedial flap. The remainder of the skin and fascia is then incised and elevated, generally leaving the proximal tissues intact unless the flap is being harvested for microvascular transplantation.

Lateral Thigh

Features. Flaps along the lateral aspect of the thigh can be based on the three perforating branches of the profunda femoris (Fig. 158-16).[68] The first and third are generally used; the first is used for proximally based flaps to the trochanteric and ischial areas, and the third is for use as a microvascular transplantation because of the long pedicle available.

Anatomy. The flap is a type B fasciocutaneous flap with innervation from the lateral cutaneous nerve of the thigh (L2-3) and blood supply from perforators of the profunda femoris that travel through the lateral intermuscular septum. The first perforator arises just below the insertion of the gluteus maximus; the third perforator arises between the vastus lateralis and biceps femoris muscles, midway between the greater trochanter and lateral condyle of the femur.

Flap Design. A longitudinally oriented flap up to 7 × 20 cm is centered over the perforator of choice. For the first perforator flap, two thirds of the flap is designed anterior to a line joining the greater trochanter and lateral femoral condyle.

Surgical Technique. The anterior border is incised down to the fascia lata, and dissection proceeds posteriorly above the fascia lata, which is left undisturbed. The vessels are identified in the lateral intermuscular septum between the vastus lateralis and the biceps femoris. The remainder of the flap is elevated, and for free tissue harvesting, retraction of the vastus lateralis allows dissection of the third perforator to its origin at the profunda femoris, providing a generous pedicle.

Sural

Features. The sural flap provides for potentially the longest fasciocutaneous flap of the lower leg, based

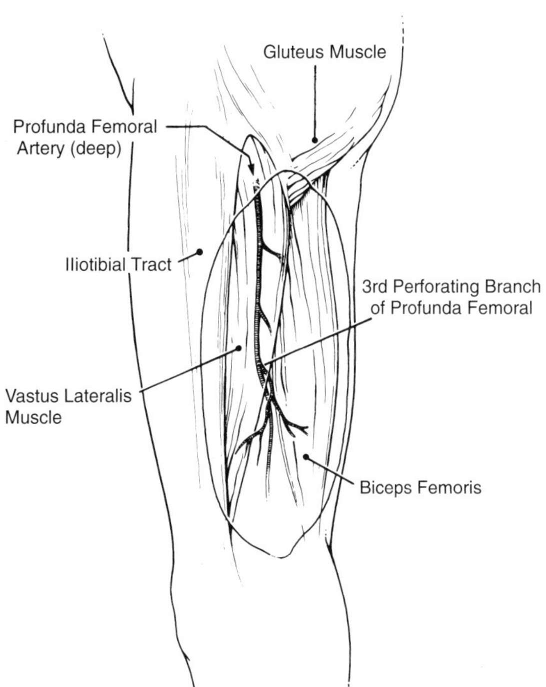

FIGURE 158-16. Lateral thigh fasciocutaneous flap. (From Thorne CHM, Siebert JW, Grotting JC, et al: Reconstructive surgery of the lower extremity. In McCarthy JG, ed: Plastic Surgery. Philadelphia, WB Saunders, 1990: 4029-4092.)

on the sural artery in the upper central calf and extending to the Achilles tendon distally.[69,70] It is useful for defects of the knee, popliteal fossa, and upper third of the leg and as a free tissue transplantation. It can be distally based and used as a reversed sural fascial or fasciocutaneous flap (Fig. 158-17).

ANATOMY. This type A fasciocutaneous flap is innervated by the medial sural cutaneous nerve (S1-2). Its dominant vascular supply is a direct cutaneous sural artery branch that arises in the distal popliteal fossa between the two heads of the gastrocnemius muscle and minor musculocutaneous perforators from the gastrocnemius muscle. The lesser saphenous vein provides venous drainage.

FLAP DESIGN. The flap is generally centered between the popliteal fossa and the midposterior leg with a width of up to 12 cm, but the length can be extended 20 cm to the Achilles tendon. For the proximally based flap, only enough skin to afford rotation is divided.

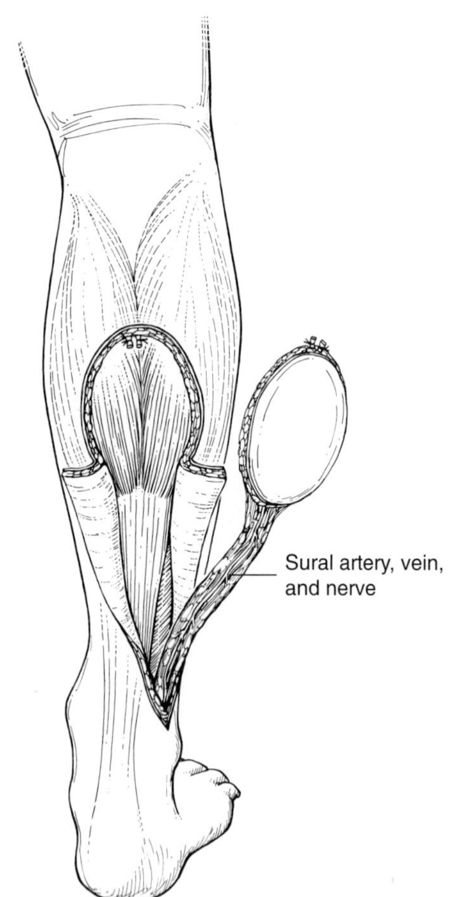

FIGURE 158-17. Reversed sural artery flap.

SURGICAL TECHNIQUE. The flap is raised from distal to proximal, in the plane beneath the deep fascia and above the gastrocnemius muscles. The sural nerve and lesser saphenous vein are divided distally and elevated with the flap. The pedicle should be visualized and protected in the popliteal fossa, with continued dissection of the pedicle for free tissue harvesting. For free tissue transplantation, proximal superficial veins should be dissected and preserved for possible anastomosis because the venae comitantes are small.

Saphenous

FEATURES. This flap provides options for knee coverage as well as being a good source for free tissue transplantation (Fig. 158-18). The vascular anatomy is variable, making the dissection of this flap more difficult than most. A reversed flap may be based on ascending vessels communicating with the saphenous branches, and an osseofasciocutaneous flap can be elevated with a portion of the medial femoral condyle based on the articular branch of the descending genicular artery.[71]

ANATOMY. This type A fasciocutaneous flap is innervated by the anterior femoral cutaneous nerve (L2-3) superiorly and the saphenous nerve (L3-4) inferiorly. The blood supply is from the saphenous branch of the descending genicular artery, which variably sends dominant fasciocutaneous perforators anterior or posterior to the sartorius muscle. Venous drainage is from both venae comitantes and the greater saphenous vein running superficially posterior to the artery.[7]

FLAP DESIGN. The skin island is designed on the inner aspect of the knee and distal thigh, with typical dimensions of up to 7 × 20 cm. A line from the anterior superior iliac spine to the medial condyle of the tibia outlines the sartorius and guides orientation of the flap.

SURGICAL TECHNIQUE. The dissection is begun proximal and anterior, with identification of the anterior border of the sartorius. The medial femoral cutaneous nerve and saphenous vein are identified, and the sartorius is then dissected off the vastus medialis. The saphenous artery lies beneath the sartorius and is traced distally to determine whether the dominant vessels to the skin proceed anterior or posterior to the muscle. The skin island may then be modified accordingly. A portion of the muscle may be dissected and included in the flap if necessary to preserve flap blood supply. The remainder of the skin is incised, the distal saphenous vein is ligated, and the proximal pedicle is dissected for up to 15 cm of length.

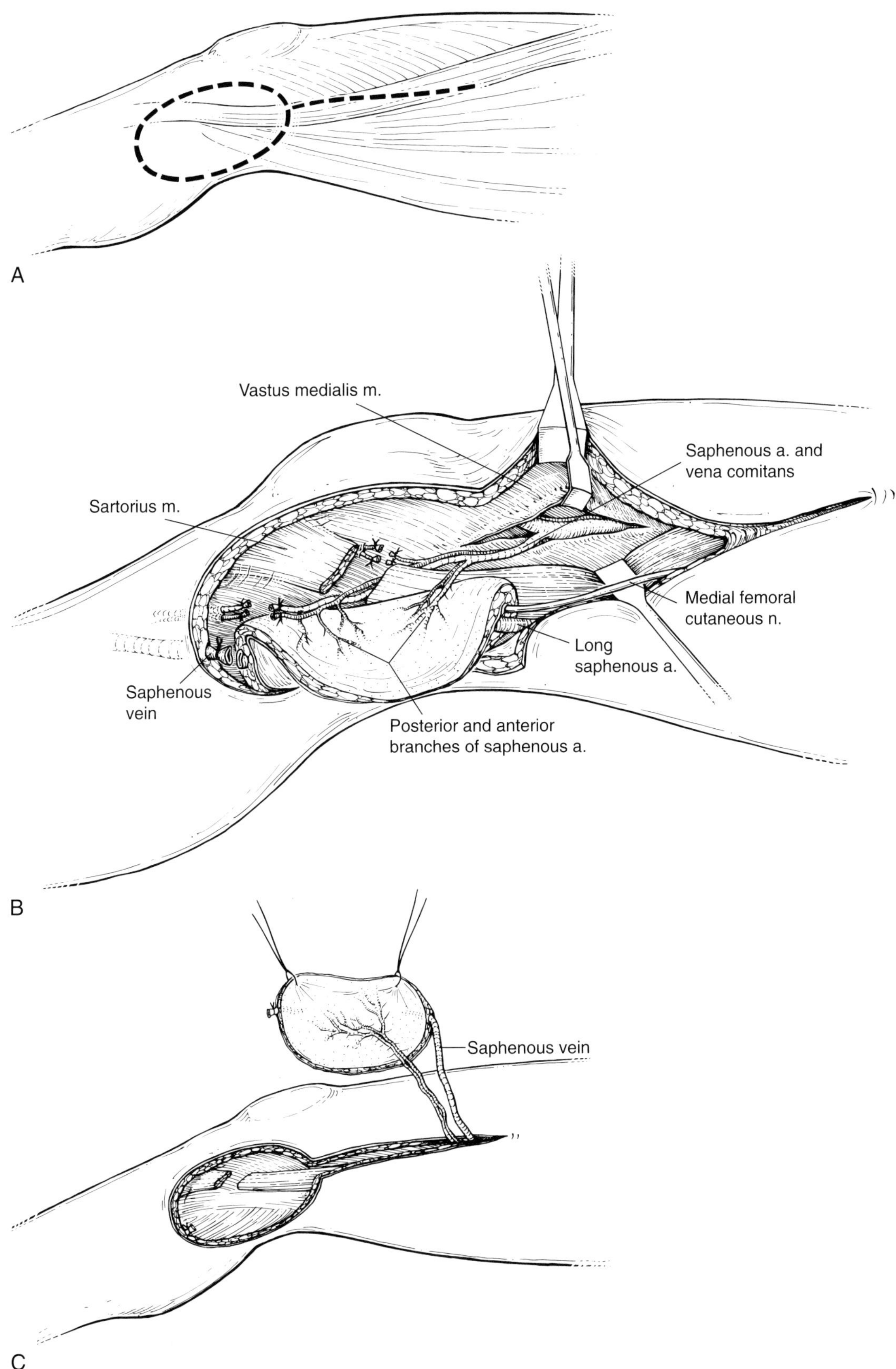

FIGURE 158-18. Saphenous flap. The sartorius muscle is divided to maintain continuity of the saphenous branches.

REFERENCES

1. Aldea PA, Shaw WW: The evolution of the surgical management of severe lower extremity trauma. Clin Plast Surg 1986;13:549-569.
2. Taylor GI, Pan WR: Angiosomes of the leg: anatomic study and clinical implications. Plast Reconstr Surg 1998;102:599-616, discussion 617-618.
3. Thorne CHM, Siebert JW, Grotting JC, et al: Reconstructive surgery of the lower extremity. In McCarthy JG, ed: Plastic Surgery. Philadelphia, WB Saunders, 1990:4029-4092.
4. Lange RH, Bach AW, Hansen ST, Johansen KH: Open tibial fractures with associated vascular injuries: prognosis for limb salvage. J Trauma 1985;25:203-208.
5. DeFranzo AJ, Argenta LC, Marks MW, et al: The use of vacuum-assisted closure therapy for the treatment of lower-extremity wounds with exposed bone. Plast Reconstr Surg 2001;108: 1184-1191.
6. McGregor IA, Jackson IT: The groin flap. Br J Plast Surg 1972;25:3-16.
7. Acland RD, Schusterman M, Godina M, et al: The saphenous neurovascular free flap. Plast Reconstr Surg 1981;67:763-774.
8. Grabb WC, Argenta LC: The lateral calcaneal artery skin flap (the lateral calcaneal artery, lesser saphenous vein, and sural nerve skin flap). Plast Reconstr Surg 1981;68:723-730.
9. Taylor GI, Palmer JH: The vascular territories (angiosomes) of the body: experimental study and clinical applications. Br J Plast Surg 1987;40:113-141.
10. Borges Filho PT, Neves RI, Gemperli R, et al: Soft-tissue expansion in lower extremity reconstruction. Clin Plast Surg 1991;18:593-599.
11. Furukawa H, Yamamoto Y, Kimura C, et al: Clinical application of expanded free flaps based on primary or secondary vascularization. Plast Reconstr Surg 1998;102:1532-1536.
12. Magalon G: Extremities. In Nordstrom REA, ed: Tissue Expansion. Boston, Butterworth-Heinemann, 1996:131-135.
13. Ger R: The management of open fracture of the tibia with skin loss. J Trauma 1970;10:112-121.
14. Byrd HS, Spicer TE, Cierney G: Management of open tibial fractures. Plast Reconstr Surg 1985;76:719-728.
15. Arnez ZM: Immediate reconstruction of the lower extremity—an update. Clin Plast Surg 1991;18:449-457.
16. Godina M: Early microsurgical reconstruction of complex trauma of the extremities. Clin Plast Surg 1986;13:619-620.
17. Francel TJ, Vander Kolk CA, Hoopes JE, et al: Microvascular soft-tissue transplantation for reconstruction of acute open tibial fractures: timing of coverage and long-term functional results. Plast Reconstr Surg 1992;89:478-487, discussion 488-489.
18. Yaremchuk M, Brumback R, Manson P, et al: Acute and definitive management of traumatic osteocutaneous defects of the lower extremity. Plast Reconstr Surg 1987;80:1-14.
19. Khouri RK, Shaw WW: Reconstruction of the lower extremity with microvascular free flaps: a 10-year experience with 304 consecutive cases. J Trauma 1989;29:1086-1094.
20. Pollak AN, McCarthy ML, Burgess AR: Short-term wound complications after application of flaps for coverage of traumatic soft-tissue defects about the tibia. The Lower Extremity Assessment Project (LEAP) Study Group. J Bone Joint Surg Am 2000;82:1681-1691.
21. Kolker AR, Kasabian AK, Karp NS, Gottlieb JJ: Fate of free flap microanastomosis distal to the zone of injury in lower extremity trauma. Plast Reconstr Surg 1997;99:1068-1073.
22. Stompro BE, Stevenson TR: Reconstruction of the traumatized leg: use of distally based free flaps. Plast Reconstr Surg 1994;93:1021-1025.
23. Godina M: Preferential use of end-to-side arterial anastomoses in free flap transfers. Plast Reconstr Surg 1979;64:673-682.
24. Serafin D, Sabatier RE, Morris RL, Georgiade NG: Reconstruction of the lower extremity with vascularized composite tissue: improved tissue survival and specific indications. Plast Reconstr Surg 1980;66:230-241.
25. Benacquista T, Kasabian AK, Karp NS: The fate of lower extremities with failed free flaps. Plast Reconstr Surg 1996;98:834-840.
26. Isenberg JS: What you see is what you get: lack of significant postoperative contour change in muscle transplants to the lower leg. Ann Plast Surg 1997;38:46-49.
27. Bonanni F, Rhodes M, Lucke JF: The futility of predictive scoring of mangled lower extremities. J Trauma 1993;34:99-104.
28. Johansen K, Daines M, Howey T, et al: Objective criteria accurately predict amputation following lower extremity trauma. J Trauma 1990;30:568-572, discussion 572-573.
29. McNamara MG, Heckman JD, Corley FG: Severe open fractures of the lower extremity: a retrospective evaluation of the Mangled Extremity Severity Score (MESS) [see comments]. J Orthop Trauma 1994;8:81-87.
30. Lin CH, Wei FC, Levin LS, et al: The functional outcome of lower-extremity fractures with vascular injury. J Trauma 1997;43:480-485.
31. O'Sullivan ST, O'Sullivan M, Pasha N, et al: Is it possible to predict limb viability in complex Gustilo IIIB and IIIC tibial fractures? A comparison of two predictive indices. Injury 1997;28:639-642.
32. Durham RM, Mistry BM, Mazuski JE, et al: Outcome and utility of scoring systems in the management of the mangled extremity. Am J Surg 1996;172:569-573, discussion 573-574.
33. Moore JR, Weiland AJ: Vascularized tissue transfer in the treatment of osteomyelitis. Clin Plast Surg 1986;13:657-662.
34. Weiland AJ, Moore JR, Daniel RK: The efficacy of free tissue transfer of osteomyelitis. J Bone Joint Surg Am 1983;66:181-193.
35. Stark WJ: The use of pedicled muscle flaps in the surgical treatment of chronic osteomyelitis resulting from compound fractures. J Bone Joint Surg Am 1946;28:343-350.
36. Ger R, Efron G: New operative approach in the treatment of chronic osteomyelitis of the tibial diaphysis. A preliminary report. Clin Orthop 1970;70:165-169.
37. Ger R: Muscle transposition for treatment and prevention of chronic post-traumatic osteomyelitis of the tibia. J Bone Joint Surg Am 1977;59:784-791.
38. Anthony JP, Mathes SJ, Alpert BS: The muscle flap in the treatment of chronic lower extremity osteomyelitis: results in patients over 5 years after treatment. Plast Reconstr Surg 1991;88:311-318.
39. May JW Jr, Gallico GG, Jupiter J, Savage RC: Free latissimus dorsi muscle flap with skin graft for treatment of traumatic chronic bony wounds. Plast Reconstr Surg 1984;73:641-649.
40. May JW Jr, Jupiter JB, Gallico GG 3rd, et al: Treatment of chronic traumatic bone wounds. Microvascular free tissue transfer: a 13-year experience in 96 patients. Ann Surg 1991;214:241-250, discussion 250-252.
41. Chang N, Mathes SJ: Comparison of the effect of bacterial inoculation in musculocutaneous and random-pattern flaps. Plast Reconstr Surg 1982;70:1-9.
42. Nichter LS, Menendez LR: Reconstructive considerations for limb salvage surgery. Orthop Clin North Am 1993;24:511-521.
43. Cordeiro PG, Neves RI, Hidalgo DA: The role of free tissue transfer following oncologic resection in the lower extremity. Ann Plast Surg 1994;33:9-16.
44. Evans GR, Black JJ, Robb GL, et al: Adjuvant therapy: the effects on microvascular lower extremity reconstruction. Ann Plast Surg 1997;39:141-144.
45. Chandrasekhar B, Brien W: Coverage strategies in total joint replacement. Orthop Clin North Am 1993;24:523-529.
46. Gayle LB, Lineaweaver WC, Buncke GM, et al: Lower extremity replantation. Clin Plast Surg 1991;18:437-447.

47. Chen ZW, Zeng BF: Replantation of the lower extremity. Clin Plast Surg 1983;10:103-113.
48. Jupiter JB, Tsai TM, Kleinert HE: Salvage replantation of lower limb amputations. Plast Reconstr Surg 1982;69:1-8.
49. Colen SR, Romita MC, Godfrey NV, Shaw WW: Salvage replantation. Clin Plast Surg 1983;10:125-131.
50. Pers M, Medgyesi S: Pedicle muscle flaps and their applications in the surgery of repair. Br J Plast Surg 1973;26:313-321.
51. Ger R: The technique of muscle transposition and the operative treatment of traumatic and ulcerative lesions. J Trauma 1971;2:502-510.
52. Ramirez OM, Swartz WM, Futrell JW: The gluteus maximus muscle: experimental and clinical considerations relevant to reconstruction in ambulatory patients. Br J Plast Surg 1987;40: 1-10.
53. Nahai F, Silverton JS, Hill HL, Vasconez LO: The tensor fascia lata musculocutaneous flap. Ann Plast Surg 1978;1:372-379.
54. Nahai F, Hill L, Hester TR: Experiences with the tensor fascia lata flap. Plast Reconstr Surg 1979;63:788-799.
55. Lewis VL, Cunningham BL, Hugo NE: The tensor fascia lata V-Y retroposition flap. Ann Plast Surg 1981;6:34-37.
56. Bhagwat BM, Pearl RM, Laub DR: Uses of the rectus femoris myocutaneous flap. Plast Reconstr Surg 1978;62:699-701.
57. Ger R: The surgical management of decubitus ulcers by muscle transposition. Surgery 1971;69:106-110.
58. Tobin GR, Sanders BP, Man D, Weiner LJ: The biceps femoris myocutaneous advancement flap: a useful modification for ischial pressure ulcer reconstruction. Ann Plast Surg 1981;6: 396-401.
59. Zukowski M, Lord J, Ash K, et al: The gracilis free flap revisited: a review of 25 cases of transfer to traumatic extremity wounds. Ann Plast Surg 1998;40:141-144.
60. Yousif NJ, Matloub HS, Kolachalam R, et al: The transverse gracilis musculocutaneous flap. Ann Plast Surg 1992;29: 482-490.
61. Tobin GR: Hemisoleus and reversed hemisoleus flaps. Plast Reconstr Surg 1985;76:87-96.
62. McCraw JB, Fishman JH, Sharzer LA: The versatile gastrocnemius myocutaneous flap. Plast Reconstr Surg 1978;62:15-23.
63. Arnold PG, Mixter RC: Making the most of the gastrocnemius muscles. Plast Reconstr Surg 1983;72:38-48.
64. Ponten B: Events leading to the rediscovery of the fasciocutaneous flap. In Hallock GG, ed: Fasciocutaneous Flaps. Boston, Blackwell Scientific Publications, 1992:10-12.
65. Ponten B: The fasciocutaneous flap: its use in soft tissue defects of the lower leg. Br J Plast Surg 1981;34:215-220.
66. Hallock GG: Clinical scrutiny of the de facto superiority of proximally versus distally based fasciocutaneous flaps. Plast Reconstr Surg 1997;100:1428-1433.
67. Erdmann MWH, Court-Brown CM, Quaba AA: A five year review of islanded distally based fasciocutaneous flaps on the lower limb. Br J Plast Surg 1997;50:421-427.
68. Baek S: Two new cutaneous free flaps: the medial and lateral thigh flaps. Plast Reconstr Surg 1983;71:354-363.
69. Lamberty BGH: Use of fasciocutaneous flaps in lower extremity reconstruction. Perspect Plast Surg 1990;4:146-162.
70. Walton RL, Bunkis J: The posterior calf fasciocutaneous free flap. Plast Reconstr Surg 1984;74:76-85.
71. Martin D, Bitonti-Grillo J, De Biscop J, et al: Mandibular reconstruction using a free vascularized osteocutaneous flap from the internal condyle of the knee. Br J Plast Surg 1991;44: 397-402.

CHAPTER

159

Reconstructive Surgery: Skeletal Reconstruction

EDWARD J. HARVEY, MD, MSc ✦ L. SCOTT LEVIN, MD, FACS

The surgeon undertaking delayed skeletal reconstruction has many factors to consider for a successful outcome. Treatment of open fractures and associated soft tissue injuries during the last 400 years has made the necessary evolution from the use of hot oil to amputation, from open wound packing to stable internal fixation and soft tissue coverage.

Although the principles of open reduction and internal fixation have been accepted and promoted, the resultant postoperative complications of infection and soft tissue deficits have risen in number. The trauma surgeon has to adhere to the tenet of orthoplastic reconstruction to ensure the maximal outcome for the patient. Surgical reconstructive skeletal problems—after tumor, trauma, or infection—follow the same rules and pose many of the same problems. This chapter deals with reconstruction of the skeletal system, with particular attention to the infected patient whom the plastic surgeon is often asked to treat.

COMPLEX MUSCULOSKELETAL INJURIES

Complex musculoskeletal injuries occur in the context of polytrauma and are often complicated by other injuries. The patient is taken through several, sometimes disparate, treatment protocols. The acute phase of therapy is composed of Advanced Trauma Life Support protocols, treatment of the open wounds with repeated débridement, appropriate antibiotic and tetanus coverage, soft and hard tissue reconstruction, and initialization of rehabilitation. The reconstruction phase includes the management of soft tissue and bone defects, sepsis, malunions, and nonunions. Rehabilitation is conceptually the final phase. For maximal results to be achieved, these three phases are instituted concurrently by a multiteam approach to care of the patient. Care of these patients without a dedicated trauma management plan is often disastrous. Special care must be served to the soft tissue envelope (Table 159-1). Surgery through a severely injured soft tissue layer may yield a disastrous result.[1] Recognition of soft tissue injury, for example, the effect of an expanding hematoma from a fracture to an already tenuous vascular supply of overlying skin, is also important. The use of simple reconstructive regimens allows appropriate orthoplastic reconstruction (Fig. 159-1).[2]

OPEN FRACTURES

Fractures with soft tissue opening have been classified to allow some prognostic and operative indicators (Table 159-2). The rate of infection for fractures ranges from 1% of type I fractures to 25% of type III fractures.[3] The goal of treatment is to have a healed fracture with a closed wound in a nearly normal functioning limb. The treatment of the limb includes radical débridement, antibiotic therapy, antibiotic beads (if needed), maintenance of fracture stability, delayed closure of the wound at secondary débridement, soft

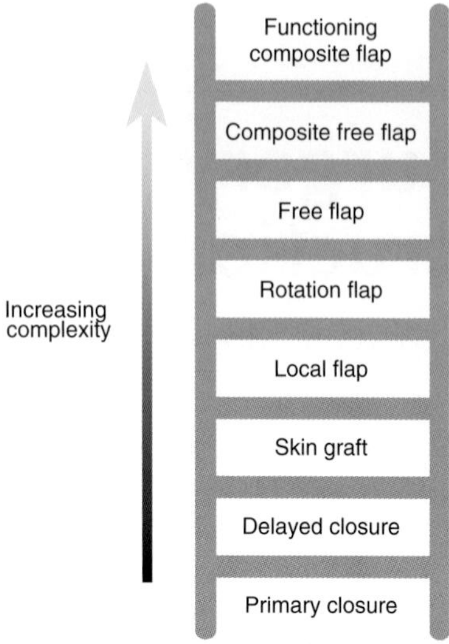

FIGURE 159-1. Orthoplastic ladder. Reconstruction of soft tissue–skeletal defects is often a complicated procedure. There is a greater ease of reconstruction and speed of rehabilitation if the approach to the musculoskeletal defect starts at simple solutions and progresses to the more complicated.

tissue coverage, and cancellous or bridging bone graft.

Débridement of the fracture is carried out by the surgeon. All free fragments of bone (if they are not part of the joint) are removed. Joint pieces should be assessed for cleanliness and functionality; if they are not salvageable, they may just be used for piecing together the "puzzle" and then removed before definitive fixation. Bone fragments in the wound can be assessed by laser Doppler flowmetry,[4] although the authors have had difficulty with the use of this device. Removal of all avascular tissue is the goal at the first operation, and the failure to eventually remove all dead tissue is the prime reason that osteomyelitis occurs.

TABLE 159-1 ✦ SOFT TISSUE INJURY CLASSIFICATION OVER CLOSED FRACTURES

Grade 0	Minimal damage, simple fracture patterns (spiral tibia fracture—torsional)
Grade 1	Superficial abrasion or contusion caused by pressure from within, mild-moderate fracture pattern (fracture of ankle)
Grade 2	Deep abrasion with localized muscle contusion, possible compartment syndrome (high-velocity tibia fracture)
Grade 3	Extensive contusion or crush, degloving, vascular injury

After Tscherne H, Gotzen L: Fractures with Soft Tissue Injuries. New York, Springer-Verlag, 1984.

TABLE 159-2 ✦ CLASSIFICATION OF OPEN FRACTURES

Type I	Open fracture with a clean wound <1 cm in length
Type II	Open fracture with a laceration >1 cm long and without extensive soft tissue damage, flaps, or avulsion
Type III	An open fracture with extensive soft tissue laceration, damage, or loss; an open segmental fracture; or a traumatic amputation
	High-velocity gunshot injuries; open fractures caused by farm injuries; open fractures requiring vascular repair; open fractures older than 8 hours
Type III subtype (1984)	
A	Adequate periosteal cover of a fractured bone despite extensive soft tissue laceration or damage; high-energy trauma irrespective of size of wound
B	Extensive soft tissue loss with periosteal stripping and bone exposure; usually associated with massive contamination
C	Associated with arterial injury requiring repair, irrespective of degree of soft tissue injury

From Gustilo R, Merkow R, Templeman D: The management of open fractures. J Bone Joint Surg Am 1990;72:299-304. Reprinted with permission from The Journal of Bone and Joint Surgery.

The patient is prescribed broad-spectrum antibiotics appropriate to the grade of fracture. These can be modified at a later date to cover any pathogens that are grown from deep cultures taken at subsequent débridement. Antibiotic-impregnated cement bead pouches are left in the wound for 48 to 72 hours until the time of secondary débridement.[5] Meticulous débridement of contaminated soft tissues is regarded as one of the most important initial steps in the management of open fractures.[6] The advent of pulsatile lavage has further improved the removal of bacteria from soft tissues. The use of high-pressure pulsatile lavage of soft tissues has been extrapolated to débridement of bone. The increased use of high-pressure pulsatile lavage for fracture débridement may result in complications. In an in vivo study of rabbits, Dirschl et al[7] found that high-pressure pulsatile lavage resulted in visible damage at the fracture site and delayed healing. It has been found that high-pressure irrigation resulted in macroscopic damage to bone and carried surface bacteria into the intramedullary canal.[8] The optimal techniques for bone débridement should remove the maximal number of adherent bacteria yet preserve the structure and function of bone. Low-pressure pulsatile lavage has obvious potential advantages over high-pressure lavage in terms of decreasing the degree of damage to bone, but it may remove adherent bacteria less effectively. In a subsequent study,

Bhandari et al[9] showed that low-pressure lavage results in significantly less damage to bone ($P < .001$) and that it is as effective as high-pressure lavage in removing bacteria within 3 hours after contamination. However, when irrigation was delayed for more than 3 hours, low-pressure lavage was ineffective in removing bacteria.

External fixation devices are usually employed for stabilization of lower extremity fractures, although intra-articular fractures should be fixed at the first operation with an aim of early mobilization. Unless the wound is grossly contaminated, forearm fractures and hand fractures can be treated with definitive open reduction with rigid internal fixation. External fixation can be exchanged for intramedullary rods if it is done in the first 10 days.[10] Access to the wound by the nursing staff, ease of application, and ability for secondary procedures to be performed with the fixator left in position are benefits of external fixation, and the soft tissue stripping of bone is kept to a minimum. Potential disadvantages include pin site infections (5% to 50%); internal fixation after pin site contamination may cause infection; and careful planning must be made for flap coverage with the new small wire fixators to avoid impingement on the vascular pedicle. Traction is rarely used as definitive therapy because it is difficult to care for the wound and there is no inherent stability. Closed suction irrigation around the fracture site is associated with a high rate of recurrence of drainage and should not be used for this problem.

MANAGEMENT OF INFECTIONS

Osteomyelitis

The plastic surgeon is often called on to eradicate infection in the soft tissues or bone. Infection of bone is resistant to nonoperative treatment. Bone is a relatively acellular collagen matrix containing hydroxyapatite crystals. This inherently results in a potential area of decreased immune response in which bacteria can multiply. Trauma surgery has seen the development of a large number of implantable devices. The advent of implanted biomaterials has revolutionized the treatment of arthritis and trauma. However, foreign material is a predisposing factor to infection and an impediment to treatment once infection has occurred.

Duration and mechanism define osteomyelitis. Inoculation is the primary colonization before a histologic response has occurred. Acute osteomyelitis has come to refer to the first 6 weeks of the infectious course. This definition is arbitrary because there are components of acute infection in chronic osteomyelitis. Chronic osteomyelitis includes components such as fistulas and long-term radiographic changes. May et al[11,12] defined five criteria for the diagnosis of chronic infection: presence of exposed bone with drainage of more than 6 weeks, positive culture from wound at débridement, positive bone histologic response, consistent radiographic findings, and bone scan consistent with chronic infection. In the initial infection, the inflammatory phase increases the blood flow to the bone, after which the blood flow decreases to below normal levels. Even with the use of antibiotics and surgery, the blood flow never returns to normal.[13] Osteomyelitis is therefore an ischemic disease of bone as well as an infectious problem. Histologic study of chronic osteomyelitis reveals dense fibrous tissue with minimal vascular tissue. Oxygen tensions are reduced at the infected area.

Mechanisms of infection are either exogenous or hematogenous. Hematogenous spread is from another primary source of infection. The immunologic deficiency in acute hematogenous infection is a malfunction at the level of the tissue-based phagocytes. Exogenous seeding is the more common mechanism of infection in adult patients. Organisms are directly inoculated into the injury zone by penetrating or iatrogenic trauma. Bone is a relatively acellular matrix in which damaged tissue without an appropriate immunologic response provides ligands for bacterial binding. This inability to mount a timely immunologic response results in osteomyelitis.

Hematogenous osteomyelitis is more widespread in the pediatric population. It is seen in childhood and adolescent infections (patients aged 1 to 16 years), less commonly in the neonatal period (0 to 1 year), and even less commonly in the adult. These infections are seen primarily in the metaphyseal section of long bones secondary to the vascular anatomy of the bone, which permits deposition of bacteria at these sites. Other theories include traumatically induced vulnerable zones in the metaphysis that result in decreased immunologic response.[14] The adult patients have a higher predilection for flat bone hematogenous osteomyelitis (vertebral bodies, pelvis, and skull). Most of these infections are caused by *Staphylococcus aureus* species,[13] but other organisms, and multiple organisms,[15,16] have been described. The phagocytic cellular infiltration eventually breaches the thin metaphyseal cortex in long bones if the infection is not controlled. In the child, subperiosteal elevation and abscess formation cause increased vascular compromise with periostitis and sequestrum formation. In the adult, the periosteum is tightly bound to the bone surface, and infection tracks along the long bone but not through the cortex.

Exogenous osteomyelitis in the adult is the result of colonization of wounds. The most commonly traumatized areas are the areas most often involved with osteomyelitis (i.e., tibia). Diaphyseal bone is more often involved. The signs of acute trauma might mask nascent infection. The bacteria are inoculated into a milieu of poorly vascularized bone and soft tissue with abundant ligands for bonding and lacking sufficient local immunologic response.

Leukocytes can reach an area of infection within hours and are responsible for suppurative reaction. Pus forming under pressure can increase the local area of avascularity. Cytokine-driven mechanisms then act to increase the host defense mechanisms. The host defenses attempt to wall off the infection from normal tissue, resulting in a sequestrum, in which bacteria can multiply in isolation from host defense mechanisms. Bacteria secrete a broad range of toxins to benefit their reproduction and thus decrease the host immunologic response. Glycocalyx is a specialized mucopolysaccharide film. This aids in bacterial adherence to bone or implants. It also presents a barrier to host defenses and antibiotics.[17]

Depending on bacterial virulence, the extent of local compromise, and the host response, several outcomes are possible. Chronic latent infection is the result of a walled off sequestrum. Chronic osteomyelitis results in a chronic abscess or sinus track formation.

The treatment of acute osteomyelitis includes judicious use of antibiotics and surgical decompression with thorough débridement. Reconstruction after acute osteomyelitis is delayed until the infection is cleared. Reconstruction after chronic osteomyelitis is more difficult. The treatment is more radical because of the inherent chronicity and immunologic compromise in the local area of the infection. Unfortunately, patients with this type of infection need extensive surgery to optimize rehabilitation return to normal daily activities.

DIAGNOSIS

The diagnosis of infection can be difficult because of underlying medical conditions (previous infection, sequelae of trauma, arthritis, and vascular disease) and the presence of implants (prostheses, internal fixation devices). Inherent difficulties in differentiating any active musculoskeletal process make diagnosis of osteomyelitis with a single test extremely difficult. Most authors in the literature recommend a broader approach with the correlation of several tests.

In a normal patient without previous disease, a normal bone scan rules out osteomyelitis. A scan will detect infection 1 to 2 weeks before radiographic changes are apparent. Technetium 99m is the principal radioisotope used. Osteomyelitic regions are seen as hot spots on the scan. Photopenic or cold lesions are less common and can represent early osteomyelitis at dysvascular areas due to pus under pressure, vasospasm, or soft tissue swelling. Sensitivity is reported to be 32% to 100%, but it is probably in the 90% range.

Gallium scans are less specific because of the generalized uptake of gallium by all bone. The gallium scan can be matched to the bone scan for greater sensitivity. Not all sequestra will be diagnosed with this method, but Cierny[16] has found that false-negative results are usually obtained in the severely ill patient and that the general examination is enough to diagnose infection in these patients.

Labeled white blood cell studies are expensive and time demanding. The sensitivity and specificity are 83% and 94%, which is significantly better than with combined gallium and technetium scans. The uptake by normal bone marrow can mask early infection. Indium-labeled immunoglobulins have been studied but not in a sufficient number of patients for their efficacy to be evaluated.

Magnetic resonance imaging changes are consistent with the replacement of marrow with water in the form of exudate and edema. Images have decreased T1 signal and increased T2 brightness. Sensitivity and specificity are both in the 90% to 100% range, but only in patients without other musculoskeletal diseases such as tumor or prosthesis in the scan area.[18]

Arteriography is often ordered for these patients to evaluate their inherent vasculature because the treatment of chronic osteomyelitis includes free tissue transfer. Computed tomographic scans or tomograms are useful in the identification of sequestra and sinus tracks. Old and new radiographs are particularly useful in the identification of avascular segments or regions at risk for infection. In conjunction with the method of fixation and the approach to the area, particular areas at risk for sequestra or necrosis can be identified.

Biopsy remains the "gold standard" for diagnosis of infection.

CLASSIFICATION OF OSTEOMYELITIS

The Cierny classification of adult chronic osteomyelitis is divided into four categories: I, medullary; II, superficial; III, localized; and IV, diffuse (Fig. 159-2). Medullary osteomyelitis is an endosteal disease. Superficial osteomyelitis is a periosteal problem that is initiated by an initial trauma coupled with inadequate soft tissue coverage. This focal disease does not breach the cortical bone. Localized osteomyelitis is a full-thickness defect in the cortical bone, but the bone retains its mechanical integrity. It can be the progression of either medullary or superficial osteomyelitis. Diffuse osteomyelitis is also a full-thickness cortical breach of the bone, but the mechanical integrity of the bone is insufficient or is sacrificed if the infection is removed.

The anatomic classification of chronic osteomyelitis is modified by the condition of the host. In class A, patients are normal with normal physiologic reactions to trauma. In class B, patients are compromised by predisposing medical conditions that affect the immunologic response; these are subdivided into

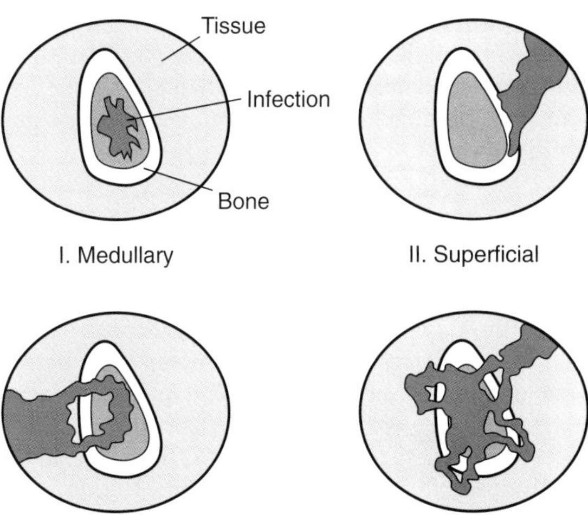

FIGURE 159-2. Classification of osteomyelitis. Four types of osteomyelitis as described by Cierny are represented in cross section through the infectious process, illustrating different locations and bone involvement. (From Cierny G: Chronic osteomyelitis: results of treatment. Instr Course Lect 1990;39:495-508.)

local and systemic causes of compromise. Local factors that cause compromise are chronic lymphedema, venous stasis, major vascular disease, extensive scarring, and radiation fibrosis. Systemic factors are malnutrition, immune deficiency, chronic hypoxia, malignant disease, diabetes mellitus, age, renal or liver failure, and tobacco abuse. Local conditions limit perfusion and oxygen delivery at the tissue level, and systemic factors affect the immunologic, hematopoietic, and metabolic capabilities of the host. In class C, the final category, the patients are not surgical candidates because the surgical risks outweigh the benefits of treatment.[16]

Each infectious process needs to be evaluated individually with optimization of the patient as the final goal. In some instances, this may require an amputation rather than a free tissue transfer. Cierny has found that 24% of patients assigned to stage IVA had wound complications as opposed to 62% in stage IVB. By use of the classification system, the patient can receive the best treatment option.

Acute, Subacute, and Chronic Infections

The clinical scenario of reconstruction in the presence of infection will be manifested by acute, subacute, or chronic infection. Acute infection refers to infected fractures; subacute, to the infected implant or prosthesis; and chronic, to a more prolonged clinical course. Recognition of the underlying temporal relationship of infection will make the treatment planning more facile. Contamination of open fractures with the resultant infection still poses a problem for the orthopedic surgeon. Depending on the grade of the fracture, the energy of the wounding object, the time to operative management, and the treatment protocol, the outcome of the patient can vary. Traditional treatment of pins and plaster, or traction, with antibiotic therapy to sterilize the wound has no place in today's surgical options. Acute management is discussed earlier in the section on open fractures. Prophylactic antibiotics have been shown to decrease infection rates during surgery, but a small percentage of prostheses and a larger number of allografts and fixation devices become infected.

Treatment of infected nonunion encompasses the same principles as treatment of infected fractures. The differences are that the patient has often undergone multiple procedures, sinus tracks complicate the operative area, osteomyelitis results in avascular bone with scar tissue, and the patient can be infected with a drug-resistant organism. The zone of injury results in a fibrotic, relatively ischemic area around the osteomyelitic wound.[19] Mathes pointed out that typically 3 to 11 attempts at treatment fail. The organisms in the wound become multiple or resistant with the iatrogenic trauma and repeated surgeries. The goals of treatment are to establish fracture stability, to initiate a favorable vascular environment, to obtain soft tissue coverage, and to guarantee adequate bone stock through grafting.

AMPUTATION VERSUS SALVAGE PROCEDURES

Modern methods of open fracture management, skeletal fixation, and soft tissue and bone reconstruction have dramatically improved the potential for limb salvage. The surgeon's judgment still remains a large portion of the decision process. The absence of adequate objective parameters on which to base the decision for salvage results in delayed amputations in some instances. The role of scoring systems as predictors of amputation and functional outcome in severe blunt extremity trauma has been examined.[20] Mangled Extremity Syndrome Index, Mangled Extremity Severity Score, Predictive Salvage Index, and Limb Salvage Index were compared by evaluation of 23 upper extremity and 51 lower extremity injuries. For each system, there were no differences between patients with good and poor functional outcomes. All of the scoring systems were able to identify the majority of patients who required amputation. However, prediction in individual patients was problematic. None of the scoring systems was able to predict functional outcome.

Bondurant[21] described 263 patients with grade III open tibia fractures, 43 of whom ultimately had amputations. All patients were taken to surgery for consideration of limb salvage procedures, including débridement, fasciotomy, revascularization, or rigid fixation. The standard subjective criteria of color, consistency, bleeding, and contractility were used to determine muscle viability at the time of débridement. If substantial muscle mass was found to be nonviable, amputation was considered. Of these patients, 14 (32.6%) had primary amputations. They averaged 22.3 days of hospitalization, 1.6 surgical procedures to the involved lower extremity, and $28,964 in hospital costs (range, $5344 to $81,282). The 29 patients with delayed amputations had an average of 53.4 days of hospitalization, 6.9 surgical procedures, and $53,462 in hospital costs (range, $14,574 to $102,434). Of the patients with delayed amputation, 6 (20.7%) developed sepsis secondary to their involved lower extremity and died; no patient in the primary amputation group developed sepsis or died.

Quirke et al[22] described patients who required primary amputation and patients who underwent vascular, orthopedic, and delayed soft tissue reconstruction. They had a 93% success rate in the 14 patients with type IIIC injuries who were successfully revascularized. Their initial management approach to the devascularized lower limb included immediate revascularization with temporary shunts to minimize ischemia time, followed by revascularization with vein grafts beyond the zone of injury and external fixation. Subsequent management included liberal use of microsurgical free transplantation to overcome soft tissue defects, bone grafting as soon as infection and soft tissue coverage permitted, and delayed wound closure. Their approach differed in that definitive wound closure was avoided for 4 to 6 weeks to allow resolution of myonecrosis secondary to initial ischemia and subsequent reperfusion injury.

Hertel et al[23] compared patients who underwent complex microvascular reconstruction with patients receiving amputations. The mean number of interventions was 3.5 for amputation and 8 for reconstruction ($P < .009$). Total rehabilitation time was 12 months for amputation and 30 months for reconstruction ($P < .009$). Changes in lifestyle were consistently more important in the amputee group. The mean annual hospital cost for amputated patients was 15,112 Swiss francs for the first 4 years. The mean annual hospital cost for reconstructed patients was 17,365 Swiss francs for the first 4 years. Fifty-six percent of the amputees and 19% of the reconstructed patients were retrained to a different profession ($P < .025$). Fifty-four percent of the amputees and 16% of the reconstructed patients were drawing an extremely costly and lifelong invalidity pension ($P < .02$). They concluded that for potentially salvageable legs, reconstruction is advisable because the functional outcome is better than for amputation and there is no permanent social disintegration due to the long treatment.

Indications for amputation are probably poor health of the patient before injury, completely severed limb, segmental tibial loss greater than 8 cm, ischemia time longer than 6 hours, and severance of the posterior tibial nerve.

RECONSTRUCTIVE LADDER

Evaluation of the Patient

Evaluation of the patient for skeletal reconstruction includes many factors. General work-up must determine nutritional status and baseline metabolic, electrolyte, and hematologic values. General conditions must allow classification into type A, B, or C host. C-reactive protein and erythrocyte sedimentation rates may be needed. For reconstructions after tumor or nerve damage, the underlying function of the limb should be outlined before a procedure is planned. If muscle or nerve transfers are needed around a damaged joint, reconstruction is often simpler with fusion of the joint (e.g., shoulder reconstruction after brachial plexus injury).

CLASSIFICATION OF SOFT TISSUE INJURY

For the acute injury associated with a skeletal defect or fracture, the classification popularized by Tscherne[24] has been adopted (see Table 159-1). This classification really serves only to heighten the physician's awareness of underlying soft tissue injuries in the event of fracture.

CLASSIFICATION OF BONE INJURY

Classification by initial injury as described by Gustilo et al for tibia fractures (see Table 159-2) has been adopted as the standard of reporting for all open fractures. However, this classification does not have the same prognostic relevance to some fractures (i.e., hand fractures) as it had to Gustilo's original group of tibia fractures.[25]

Débridement

Surgical treatment by débridement is the only accepted treatment for chronic osteomyelitis of class A or class B. Antibiotic coverage, nutrient supplementation, and hyperbaric therapy are only adjuncts to the adequate débridement of the sequestrum. The operative treatment of all osteomyelitis includes adequate surgical débridement, attempts at identification of the organism, closure of all dead space caused by débridement, revascularization of the area, antibiotic coverage, and usually skeletal reconstruction.

Débridement is the most important step in the treatment of this problem.[2] Even with apparently successful eradication of infection, the osteomyelitis can recur.[26] The planning of all procedures necessary for the rehabilitation of the patient is crucial before the first débridement is undertaken. The approach to the infection must take into consideration vasculature, expanse of excision, and future coverage with soft tissue and bone reconstruction. The entire area of osteomyelitis should be resected like a marginal excision of a tumor. Débridement protocol must take into consideration skeletal stability and bone involvement of the infection. If adequate débridement will leave an unstable extremity, an external fixator should be applied before débridement occurs. The approach to the infection as a combined soft tissue and skeletal tissue malignant neoplasm will result in the best rate of obliteration of the osteomyelitis. This approach is the conservative approach to infection. Returning the patient to the operating room multiple times because of an inadequate initial débridement slows the patient's rehabilitation and increases costs to the patient and the hospital (Fig. 159-3). An adequate resection by use of modern reconstructive hard and soft tissue techniques should be implemented rather than relying on antibiotics and adjuvant therapies to eradicate infection in marginal areas.

The area of infection is initially débrided under tourniquet control. The obviously sclerotic and involved bone is taken down by a power burr with copious irrigation to avoid further cell death at the margins. Pinpoint bleeding (paprika sign) is the endpoint for bone removal. Some investigators[4] have had success with the laser Doppler flowmeter for evaluation of blood flow to the bone in both traumatic injuries and osteomyelitis. The Doppler device is used to determine when viable bone is reached in the débridement. This device might be limited to use after débridement is thought to be finished because the threshold detection thickness for cortical and cancellous bone is 2.1 mm and 2.7 mm, respectively.

The soft tissue envelope is removed with the contiguous infection. Any involved soft tissue will remain as scar tissue and promote a local environment of low oxygen tension. Vasculature and neural structures can be dissected free of the infection and left in the wound. Attention must be given to the vasculature to ensure that the vessels are not coagulated from their proximity to the infection. Any limb with questionable blood supply or blood return should be evaluated with flow studies before débridement. The tourniquet is released only after the osteomyelitic area has been débrided. The wound is then further débrided, and major bleeding is stopped. This treatment protocol demands sacrifice of some viable tissue to ensure that the infection has been extirpated. The posterior cortex of bone, particularly in the tibia, is sometimes still viable after débridement because of remaining blood supply from the periosteum. If this viable bone interferes with the osseous reconstruction plans, it too is excised. Ilizarov treatment can be accomplished with acute shortening rather than retaining a mechanically unstable piece of bone. Single-stage reconstructions have led to a higher incidence of wound complications in all except type IIA wounds.[27] The patient is taken back to the operating room at day 3 to day 5 for second-look débridement and possible secondary reconstruction (i.e., flap transfers). This allows a sufficient delay for species-specific cultures to be analyzed. Longer delays to reconstruction have not been shown to decrease complications and merely prolong the rehabilitation process.[13] The well-demarcated osteomyelitic sequestrum with good excision margins is probably an exception to this school of thought[28] and can be reconstructed in a single stage.

Adequate débridement is the cornerstone of eradicating infection. Planning of the overall procedure with attention to postoperative soft and hard tissue

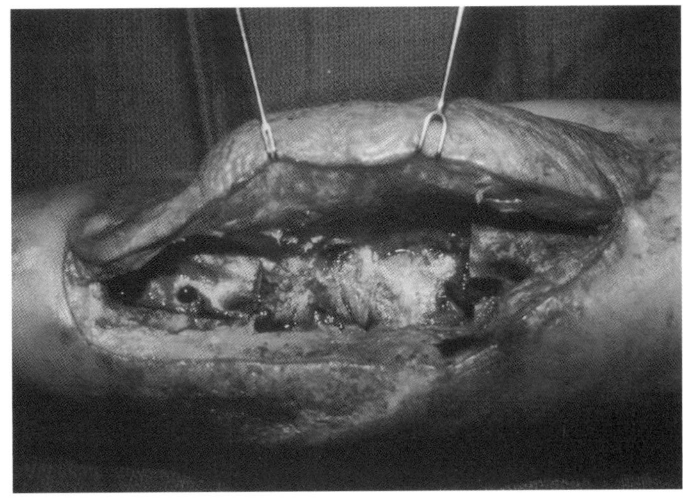

FIGURE 159-3. Infected tibia. Even with soft tissue coverage, this tibia continues to have chronic osteomyelitis. This is an example of inadequate débridement. The original treating physician relied on the tissue flap to cleanse the area rather than destabilizing the tibia with an extensive excision. A 10-cm débridement was required with necessary destabilization of the tibia for the area to be adequately débrided. This illustrates the need for a team approach to these complicated multitissue defects; the plastic surgeon collaborates with an orthopedic team to maximize resection of avascular and infected tissue while still maintaining skeletal stability.

reconstruction allows the surgeon to minimize the number of procedures and the time to recovery.

Preparation for Definitive Skeletal Reconstruction

WOUND DRESSING

With the goal of early definitive coverage, complex wound dressing is not usually needed. Early débridement occurs, and if there is a need for delay to definitive closure (24 to 48 hours), a temporary dressing is applied. The dressing most commonly applied is a simple bead pouch or string of antibiotic-laden polymethyl methacrylate beads placed in the wound. The area is then sealed with an adhesive occlusive plastic sheet, augmented with skin staples to hold it in place. This not only theoretically adds to sterility in the fields but both keeps the soft tissues open for definitive débridement and closure and maintains a moist environment.

ANTIBIOTIC BEADS

Antibiotics alone are not sufficient for the treatment of chronic osteomyelitis.[29] Antibiotics are only an important adjuvant to débridement in chronic osteomyelitis. An attempt at isolation of an organism by superficial biopsy is often unsuccessful or misleading. Deep biopsies of affected cortical and cancellous bone are more helpful. Antibiotics should be started at the time of surgery. The expected serum concentration of the antibiotic should be six to eight times more than the minimal inhibitory concentration and minimal bactericidal concentration.[29] Antibiotics are started empirically postoperatively if the organism has not been recognized. *S. aureus, Pseudomonas,* and anaerobic bacteria are the most common causes of chronic osteomyelitis; if empirical treatment has to be implemented, these organisms must be covered.[16] The antibiotics are continued for 6 weeks in a compromised host or if inert material (hardware, bone graft) has been left in the wound. One week of coverage is used for a clean wound with definitive treatment of the infection or if antibiotic beads have been left in the wound.

When immediate reconstruction is not safe, staged management of dead space is recommended. After débridement, wound coverage is secured, but the dead space is maintained with customized antibiotic beads. Antibiotic beads have had success in animal models,[30] although clinical results have been mixed.[31] Beads are used with gentamicin powder added. They are formed into a doughy polymethyl methacrylate mixture and then strung onto a 20-gauge wire to completely fill the dead space (Fig. 159-4). Antibiotic cement should never be poured into the bone defect and allowed to fill all the exposed interstices of bone. The antibiotics used in the cement can be tailored to the sensitivities of the bacteria present in the wound; however, most institutions use an aminoglycoside such as gentamicin. The overall success rate reported by Cierny[16] with this delayed dead space management protocol was 92%, indicating that the delayed technique is a reasonable alternative to immediate management. The indications for use of beads (compromised hosts, staging cancellous grafts larger than 50 mL, future internal fixation, and complex wound closures) are reflections of the aspects of coverage and the physiologic status of the at-risk host.[32] Class B hosts are at risk for graft resorption and failure if the wound is grafted primarily. These wounds are first covered and sterilized with beads, and the patients are brought back at a later date when their wound healing ability and local vascularity are restored. New research in the field of biodegradable antibiotic-laden cement or polyanhydrides may further refine the treatment method.[33,34] The first laboratory studies in rats have shown this type of delivery to be significantly more efficient than nondegradable cement.[33] Enthusiasm must be reserved until after evaluation of the effect on the reticuloendothelial system in mammalian studies.

Duration of infection, classification, association with fractures or nonunion, and immune status of the patient affect the antibiotic treatment. Acute infection may resolve with antibiotics combined with drainage of the site, but rarely are antibiotics sufficient in a chronic situation. The class C host may be left with sustained antibiotic coverage because of the inability to be helped by surgical intervention. Attention must be paid to the underlying medical condition that has resulted in the patient's being assigned to class C. Some end-stage organ disease will affect the more common antibiotic clearance curves (end-stage liver and renal disease). Normally safe doses could result in damage to other organs or exacerbation of the underlying condition. The association with fractures, particularly if there is an implant in the infected area, will result in a need for prolonged antibiotic therapy. Underlying immunodeficiencies that can affect the wound, such as diabetes or human immunodeficiency virus infection, will require prolonged antibiotics or more extensive surgery (amputation), which in these patients is a more conservative approach because of the morbidity of other conventional therapy.

HYPERBARIC OXYGEN

Hyperbaric oxygen is merely an adjunct to the surgical treatment of infection. Hyperbaric oxygen does augment the normal cellular defenses that are affected by the local hypoxia at the infected area and may be useful in the more advanced osteomyelitis that is slow to recover. An oxygen tension in infected bone of 23 mm Hg can be increased up to 1200 mm Hg.[35] The

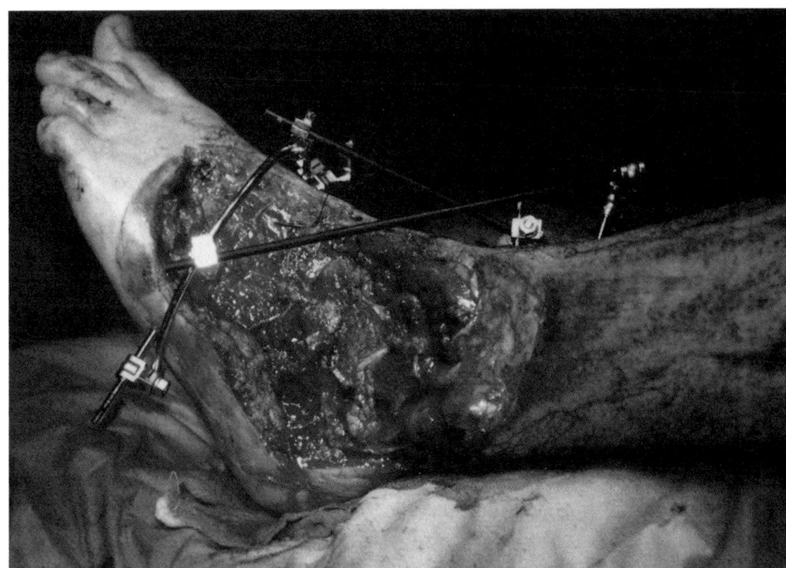

A

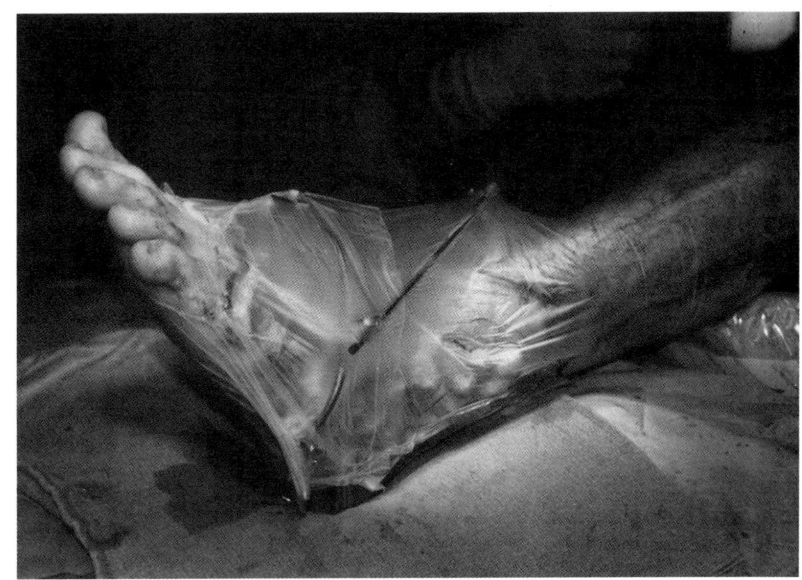

B

FIGURE 159-4. Management of the complex acute injury. *A,* There is definitely a desire to retain as much bone structure as possible, especially in this patient with an injured foot. In a motorcycle accident, this patient incurred injury to all the foot articulations. All bones and joints of the foot were open and abraded. Extensive débridement was carried out; however, any more extensive resection would have resulted in destabilization of the foot and subsequent amputation. *B,* After initial débridement, antibiotic beads were placed beneath an occlusive dressing for 48 hours. Stabilization of the foot and ankle was accomplished with an external fixator construct. Secondary débridement of all marginal tissue was then accomplished at the time of free tissue transfer. The patient at 5-year follow-up has full ankle range of motion and has returned to jogging and some sports.

increased oxygen tension has a direct bactericidal effect on anaerobes and clostridial species. It also inhibits the formation of clostridial toxin. Hyperbaric oxygen augments the oxygen-dependent intercellular killing mechanisms of leukocytes as well as the bactericidal effects of aminoglycosides and vancomycin. There is no direct deleterious effect on aerobic bacteria.[36]

NUTRITION

Malnutrition will play a role in augmenting the infectious process.[37] The orthopedic patient is often in a catabolic phase because of trauma or incipient poor nutrition, and therefore the added insult of rampant infection may be too much for the patient's reserves. Nutritional status can be measured by levels of serum proteins and circulating lymphocytes, antibody reaction to antigens in skin testing, and wound tensile strength measurements as well as by observation of calorie intake and weight changes. Total lymphocyte count and the serum albumin level are the most predictive and reproducible of these tests and are used in concert to determine nutritional status. Patients with a serum albumin level below 3.5 g/dL will have more complications than will those patients with a higher level (83.3% versus 17.5%). Total lymphocyte count below 1500/mm³ increases the risk of complication.[37] These values should be verified for the patient who appears to be at risk to minimize complications.

VACUUM-ASSISTED CLOSURE

Despite numerous advances, chronic and other difficult to manage wounds continue to be a treatment challenge. A subatmospheric pressure technique, vacuum-assisted closure, has been explored.[38] The technique entails placement of an open-cell foam into the wound, sealing of the site with an adhesive drape, and application of subatmospheric pressure (125 mm Hg below ambient) that is transmitted to the wound in a controlled manner.

A series of basic animal studies with use of this technique to expedite wound healing were reviewed.[39] With a pig model, four studies were undertaken to determine the effect of subatmospheric pressure on laser Doppler-measured blood flow in the wound and adjacent tissue, rate of granulation tissue formation, clearance of bacteria from infected wounds, and nutrient flow by random-pattern flap survival. Blood flow levels increased fourfold when subatmospheric pressure of 125 mm Hg was applied. Significantly increased rates of granulation tissue formation occurred. Tissue bacterial counts significantly decreased ($P \leq .05$) after 4 days of application. Random-pattern flap survival significantly increased ($P \leq .05$) by 21% compared with controls. Argenta[40] published results of 300 wounds (175 chronic wounds, 94 subacute wounds, and 31 acute wounds) treated with vacuum-assisted closure; 296 wounds responded favorably to subatmospheric pressure treatment, with an increased rate of granulation tissue formation. The technique removed chronic edema, leading to increased localized blood flow, with enhanced formation of granulation tissue. Vacuum-assisted closure seems to be an efficacious modality for treatment of chronic and difficult wounds. This technique has promise and may become a gold standard for closure of mild to moderate wounds. It should certainly be an element of any microsurgeon's surgical armamentarium.

Timing of Reconstruction

When free tissue transfers are available, early radical débridement is possible even in the largest wounds. This combined osseous and cutaneous reconstruction technique has decreased rates of infection and improved bone healing without increasing flap mortality.[28] There are several advantages to obtaining wound closure within 72 hours of injury. Vessels adjacent to the wound have not yet become fibrotic; there is no granulation tissue with attendant superficial infection; and desiccation and progressive necrosis of exposed bone and tendon have not yet occurred. Further, the surgeon need not deal with poorly perfused scar and colonized or infected areas of the wound. Godina's retrospective historical study[41] evaluating free tissue transfers in the treatment of extremity trauma clearly revealed the advantages of radical débridement and early (within 72 hours) wound closure with vascularized tissue. With use of this technique for limb salvage, the percentage of patients with nonunion and osteomyelitis decreased. In addition, the number of hospitalizations and of anesthetics and the time to fracture healing were substantially reduced.[41] Care must be taken in interpreting these results because of the wide variety of flap types used in this study. Byrd[42] compared classic open wound care of type III tibial fractures with the early débridement and wound closure by use of vascularized muscle on a prospective basis. The number of procedural complications in both these studies rose markedly if wounds were not closed in the early phase (defined by Byrd et al[42] as the first 6 days from injury and by Godina[41] as the first 72 hours from injury). Each study noted that the inflammatory nature of the wound, as it remained open, led to greater chance of continuing infection and increased thrombosis rate at the time of delayed flap closure.[43] Yaremchuk et al[44] showed good results despite the longer periods between initial injury and ultimate closure. They pointed out that their success was dependent on meticulous débridement.

Free tissue transfer is accomplished at the first or second débridement. If there is a potential dead space at any time in the staged procedure, this space is filled with antibiotic beads. After the tissue transfer, local or distant, bone graft is considered. The bone graft is usually placed at 6 weeks, which permits time for the tissue transfer to sterilize the wound. Grafts are either cancellous autograft or vascularized transfers. The size and function of the bone deficit will determine the type of graft to be used.

Cierny[16] uses the loss of 30% to 50% of volume as a requirement for a structural graft. Patients who receive cancellous bone grafts at the time of delayed primary closure (5 to 7 days after the débridement) have a success rate of 93%. The long-term success rate was 95%. In contrast, patients who receive a graft an average of 34 days after an implant of antibiotic beads had an initial success rate of 86% and an overall rate of 92%. There was no significant difference between these two techniques. However, we believe that the advantages of early closure (within 3 to 5 days) for rehabilitation and management dictate that the surgeon not delay definitive closure.

Adjuvant therapies in patients undergoing resection for malignant disease can affect the outcome of a reconstruction. Patients may receive preoperative or postoperative chemotherapy. Wound healing in the immediate postoperative period and host-allograft healing may both be delayed. Not infrequently, there is little evidence of bone healing as the patient finishes the chemotherapy protocol postoperatively. Cancellous bone graft may be required when chemotherapy is completed. Patients sometimes undergo external beam irradiation as a primary means of local disease control. Radiation can affect the healing potential of the soft tissue envelope and the bone host-graft junction. Although radiation does not preclude allograft reconstruction,[45] it may make it necessary to consider vascularized soft tissue transfer at the time of surgery for wound closure. This technique has been shown to lower the postoperative complication rate and the incidence of graft infection.[46]

Types of Fixation in Preparation for Bone Reconstruction

Radical débridement is the first step of the operation. If solid fracture fixation is already in place, the device can remain; the bone is grafted, and antibiotic therapy is initiated. Even if solid fixation is in place, there are some instances when acute shortening with or without later lengthening will allow better bone contact and therefore increase the likelihood of healing. If the infected area is diaphyseal and a rod is already in place, removal of the rod with reaming of the intramedullary cavity and placement of an external fixator is the preferred treatment. This helps re-establish the vasculature to the bone and removes the infected and scarred endosteal surface. Fracture stability is the most important principle because an infected nonunion will heal if the fracture is stable.[47] The benefit of metal plates in the wound far outweighs the risk of increasing the infection. Recent work from McGill University and Harborview Medical Center has shown that rigid internal fixation with a custom blade plate, even in the face of infection and large bone defects, allows 100% healing (Fig. 159-5). Although the use of a plate has not been shown clinically to be a detriment to fracture healing or eradication of infection (83% to 93% good results[48,49]), many authors have shown that an external fixator will give the same good results as a plate,[15,50-52] without an implant remaining in the wound. Patzakis[52] had 91% success at 3 months postoperatively with 32 grade IIIA/B tibias treated with external fixation.

Infected fractures fixed with an intramedullary rod need revision if the rod is loose. Reaming to larger size and placing a new rod can rectify the problem, but most surgeons choose to ream the intramedullary cavity and use an external fixator to stabilize the fracture. Replacement intramedullary nails were used by MacAusland and Eaton[53] for femur fractures. There is risk of massive osteomyelitis, but they obtained 100% union rates without progression of infection. This study has not been reproduced. There is no place for traction in the management of this problem because of the instability.

Bone Reconstruction

DEAD SPACE MANAGEMENT OF BONE DEFECTS

It is often difficult to close the infected or severely traumatized wound after adequate débridement. If it is closed, there is a dead space that represents a potential nidus for infection.[54] The wound often has a dead space left after removal of all questionable tissue. The principles of management of the dead space in chronic osteomyelitis are dictated by more than one school of thought. The methods of dead space management are generally limited to healing by second intention, local approximation with a myoplasty and possible skin grafting, or closure with a vascularized tissue transfer. Bone grafts may be required to restore form and to reconstruct bone defects.[16]

Open wound management of defects in osteomyelitis is no longer in favor, but this may be the only viable option in some patients. The disadvantages of open wound treatment are that selection of patients is limited to class A hosts, the defects treated should be small, the wounds require the patient's cooperation and continuous care, and the success rates are moderate. No publications in the current literature support treatment protocols that propose wound healing by second intention alone. This would leave a chronic wound with, in the best situation, friable tissue covering the underlying bone. Granulation tissue is a good culture medium and may lead to further infection. The series of Shannon[55] illustrates that treatment of the wound by skin grafting on freshly débrided surfaces allows a long-term success rate of 60% to 70%. The skin grafts prevent the accumulation of dense scar tissue on the bone surface. This method does not address the need for revascularization to combat infection or help eliminate contamination. Bacteria may persist in the exposed interstitial lamellae and small fissures. The same problems exist if these defects are closed without dead space obliteration by use of closed irrigation systems. The 70% or lower success rates occur because scar and granulation tissue accumulate on the surface, where they temporarily entrap organisms that are fostered to grow in the local ischemic environment. Washing the dead space with high doses of antibiotics or detergents has not changed the prognosis of this treatment protocol.

The open cancellous grafting technique of Papineau[56] is one method used to obliterate defects. The débridement is followed by a brief waiting period of 10 to 14 days. When the wound surfaces develop granulation tissue, autogenous, cancellous grafts are compressed into the defect slightly above the bone surface. Once the grafts are revascularized from the

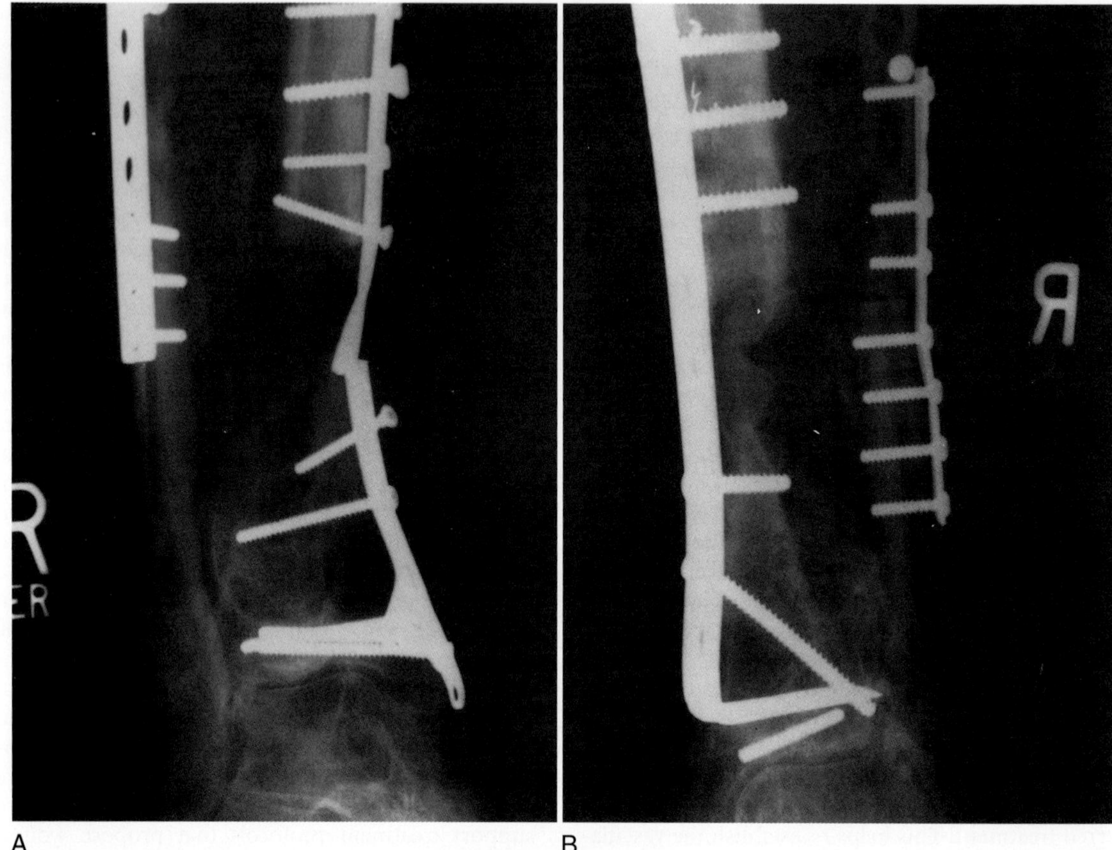

FIGURE 159-5. *A,* Blade plate reconstruction of large skeletal defect. Combined soft tissue defect and open fracture had been treated with inadequate internal fixation. *B,* Resulting macromotion had established an infected and malaligned extremity with constant pain. The treatment for this problem is excision of the infected pseudarthrosis. After removal of the avascular tissue and pursuant bone reconstruction as dictated by the orthoplastic ladder, adequate skeletal stability is required. Infection is not a contraindication to internal fixation. Adequate stability has allowed healing of the tibia and improved functional outcome.

bone below, split-thickness skin is applied only if the spontaneous re-epithelialization is insufficient to seal the wound. This type of management differs from the previous open methods because the cancellous grafts induce a permanent revascularization of the defect. However, the patient should be a class A host with an adequate supply of autogenous cancellous grafts to fill the defect. The Papineau procedure will heal large defects; however, its reliance on secondary epithelialization and granulation tissue results in a thin epithelial layer that is susceptible to breakdown with minimal trauma. The success of the graft relies on many factors, such as host response, reliability of the patient, and frequent hospital visits. Class B hosts cannot support the metabolic requirement of revascularization, graft incorporation, and wound consolidation in the face of persistent bacterial contamination. Multiple operations make this a less desirable option for closure. The method itself is successful in 70% to 80% of uncomplicated cases only. This graft should be thought of for the patient in whom any other method is impossible.

Simple approximation of the wound is often not an option in subcutaneous areas or where there is a large defect after adequate débridement. Flap coverage by either transposition or transplantation is required for these patients. In 1946, Stark[57] reported the use of pedicled flaps for osteomyelitis; 84% of patients (27 of 32) were successfully treated with débridement and muscle flap closure compared with 43% with débridement and closure. Perhaps because of the advent of antibiotic therapy, his work was ignored for decades. Since 1980, many authors have reported success rates of 80% to 100% with the use of pedicled flaps. Koval et al[58] looked at 25 infected tibias in 25 patients who were treated by one of three methods. They used muscle flap coverage, primary closure with suction irrigation, or open cancellous bone graft. Their success rates were 80%, 45.5%, and 40%, respectively. In another study, 42 consecutive patients[50] with osteomyelitis of the tibia were treated after débridement and antibiotic therapy with Papineau procedure, bypass posterolateral graft, or soft tissue transfer. After exclusion of patients, the success rate was 66% with open cancellous graft, 87.5% with soft tissue transfer, and 87.5% with grafting.

If the underlying structure of the bone is intact, simple closure of the dead space with a myoplasty brings a good vascular supply to the area. This not only closes the wound but also affords treatment of the infection locally with wound healing and restoration of the form and possibly function of the area. Myoplasty is followed at 6 weeks by cancellous grafting if the underlying skeleton needs reconstruction. Consideration is given to larger vascularized bone grafts, but these are usually done after the vascularized muscle flap to allow control of the infection. Potential dead space under a flap is managed with prolonged treatment with antibiotic-impregnated cement beads acting as a placeholder until final osseous reconstruction can take place.

When the débridement defect can be obliterated with live tissues, these problems are overcome. The best results for infection come from techniques in which muscle is used as either a transposition or a free flap to completely obliterate the dead space. The overall success rates of these two methods are comparable. However, the perfusion of transferred tissue with a microvascular anastomosis is often superior to that with a local transposition because it is harvested and perfused from outside the zone of injury. Furthermore, a free flap may be used anywhere in the body, but transpositions are limited to their anatomic arc of rotation.

APPLICATION OF THE ILIZAROV TECHNIQUE

Bone transport mechanisms, such as the Ilizarov apparatus, provide an attractive alternative to free bone flaps and large cancellous grafts.[59-63] Distraction osteogenesis and bone union with compression at the docking site are successful even in the face of infection and systemic or local compromise. The method is suitable for patients unable to have conventional treatment because of a lack of autogenous graft reserves, suitable vessels, or adequate length. Shortened extremities can be simultaneously lengthened with this technique.

This technique is not dependent on microvascular surgery, although the combination of the Ilizarov device and free tissue transfer has shown some promising early results.[51,63] There are four categories of Ilizarov implementation with concomitant microsurgery.[63] Some of these combinations are useful in reconstruction of osteomyelitis. The type I case is exemplified by a distal third tibia fracture with an open wound. The juxta-articular location precludes the use of an unreamed nail, and the inherent soft tissue stripping around the joint associated with a plate makes that option less desirable. The small pin fixator is a more physiologic construct. A type II combination is the application of the Ilizarov device after flap placement for correction of an evolving deformity. Typically, this is after a plate in place has resulted in nonunion, malunion, or infection. A free tissue transfer done earlier in the clinical course has healed, but the bone defect or osteomyelitis needs to be addressed. The defect can be treated by the application of an external fixator, allowing transport and compression at the area of concern, with or without additional bone graft. The type III combination is immediate corticotomy and transport through a recent free flap. This can involve either transport through a maturing flap or acute shortening of smaller defects and corticotomy distant to the flap and area of docking. The last combination, type IV reconstruction, is the use of the Ilizarov as an immediate fixation device for a bone flap. This is particularly useful in the patient with associated osteopenia of the affected bone. The Ilizarov type of fixator is better tolerated in these patients. It also allows solid fixation of the free bone flap and compression at both ends of the graft. This may help with incorporation and avoid the large number of failures seen in earlier studies.

The method of Ilizarov is not without its problems. The operations are relatively bloodless, limited to the extremity, and usually percutaneous, and they can be done by one surgeon. However, the surgeries are complicated, many outpatient adjustments are required, and the daily adjustments are painful. The results of treatment are difficult to assess. Union can be achieved in 74% to 100% of patients. Various problems, including deformities at joints, iatrogenic neuropathies, dystrophies, nonunion, and pin track infections, occur in 28% to 38% of patients.[16] However, this complication rate is similar to that of Cierny with use of conventional techniques. Thus, the Ilizarov method compares favorably and could become the treatment of choice for bone defects.

BONE GRAFT OPTIONS

Allograft Versus Autograft

Late reconstruction after trauma is possible with an allograft. However, the use of allograft is usually reserved for tumor or pathologic bone conditions (e.g., multiple hip revisions).[64] The use of large allograft replacements has been associated with a high infection rate, although some centers have had good results.[65] The cellular, molecular, and histologic sequence is similar in both allograft and autograft incorporation (and fracture healing). After implantation, the graft becomes immersed in a hematoma that contains elements of both a humoral and a cellular inflammatory response. Any viable cells within the graft survive by diffusion of nutrients from the hematoma. The hematoma organizes, and a healing response is initiated by a release of cytokines that results in pluripotential stem cell recruitment and differentiation. Cells differentiate into chondroblastic and osteoblastic lines, leading to endochondral and intramembranous bone formation across the graft-host junction. If an allograft has rigid fixation, there can be healing and subsequent revascularization. Cancellous and cortical allografts undergo two distinctly different mechanisms of revascularization. Cancellous allografts undergo creeping substitution; cortical allografts undergo resorption through existing Volkmann and haversian canals, which is then followed by deposition of new bone. The revascularization process does not extend into the interstitial lamellar bone and occurs over a limited distance into the allograft. Frequently, new periosteal bone is formed over the surface of the graft, which promotes soft tissue reattachment. Coupled with revascularization, a specific immune response to antigens within the graft takes place. In a dog model,[66] genetic disparity between donor and recipient was associated with reduced bone incorporation and an increased fibrous reaction. The immune components explain, at least in part, the clinical situation in which the allograft resorbs over time. Regardless, particularly after large en bloc resection (i.e., devastating trauma, tumor surgery), allografts are a good option for regaining bone stock and maintaining the functional soft tissue envelope.

It is important that tumor resection not be compromised by the preoperative planning. The involvement of muscle groups by the malignant process may require resection that precludes active motion across a joint. In such patients, an arthrodesis may be a better option than an osteoarticular reconstruction. A patient's recreational and expected vocational activities should also be considered. Under heavy functional demands, an arthrodesis is more durable than an osteoarticular allograft. Conversely, a patient who requires dexterity without high functional loads would benefit from preservation of joint motion with an osteoarticular allograft. However, it is difficult to decide this in children with tumors because future demands are generally unclear. Thus, it is worthwhile to attempt to restore anatomy and to preserve joint motion whenever possible.

The use of allografts to reconstruct defects in the child is limited primarily to intercalary defects and arthrodesis. Juxta-articular defects in children are complicated by disruption of growth. Intercalary defects arise infrequently and most often result from trauma or a diaphyseal Ewing sarcoma. A structural allograft can be selected on the basis of the required length and diameter of the host-graft junction and used to span such a defect. Hardware needed to secure the allograft must avoid constraining the adjacent physis. An allograft arthrodesis can be used to reconstruct a defect that includes an epiphysis, such as the proximal humerus or the distal radius. This method of reconstruction provides a structurally sound upper extremity that requires host-graft junction healing across both a diaphyseal and a metaphyseal subchondral surface. Arthrodesis is a particularly appropriate choice when tumor resection requires sacrifice of adjacent stabilizing muscle groups. In the proximal humerus, for example, the loss of rotator cuff muscles requires arthrodesis for functional stability to be achieved.

In children who are either at or near skeletal maturity, the indications for allograft reconstruction are the same as in younger patients. In addition, osteoarticular allografting becomes an option in this age group because the contiguous articular surface will undergo little further growth and development. Such grafts may be used in the proximal humerus and the distal radius if the tumor resection allows one to reconstruct a joint capsule. Although there is usually some loss of motion, functional outcomes of osteoarticular allografts at these sites are satisfactory.

PEDICLE BONE FLAPS IN LOWER EXTREMITY

Transfer of the fibula to reconstruct a defect in the tibia after fracture, nonunion, or tumor resection is a technically simple one-stage procedure. The site of the pseudarthrosis is not exposed with a theoretical decreased risk of recurrent infection. Consolidation was achieved in 75% of patients in one study.[67] Functional results revealed that knee mobility was normal in most patients, and ankle mobility was only slightly decreased.

One author[68] has discussed cross-leg pedicled fibular grafts. The flap can be raised in two fashions, depending on blood flow direction in the pedicle. In the case of regular flow, up to 18 cm of fibula is available; in reversed pedicular flow, more than 20 cm of fibula can be harvested. An arc of rotation of the flap reaches midthigh and peripheral part of the lower extremity. Cross-leg pedicled fibular graft can be used for concomitant soft tissue defect reconstruction as well. Crossing with immobilization of both lower extremities is necessary for 4 weeks. No microsurgical procedure is required. A skin island of the fibular flap or a narrow muscle cuff left around the fibular vessels is sufficient to protect the pedicle. The cross-leg pedicled fibular flap is mainly indicated for patients with major lower extremity injury with axial vessel damage or with history of previous trauma and thrombosis and for patients after bone tumor resection who had chemotherapy or radiotherapy. The indications may be markedly broadened, especially in centers with no access to microsurgery. In general, cross-leg flaps are not considered in trauma patients because of other injuries and required therapy.

FREE VASCULARIZED BONE FLAPS

Biologic reconstruction for large intercalary segments that are resected in the treatment of bone tumors establishes a requirement for similar bone that will be incorporated into the extremity and function like the resected part. Fresh, nonvascularized autografts avoid the risk of disease transmission and optimize biologic and immunologic considerations but involve donor site morbidity and have limited utility. Cancellous autograft is used primarily to fill cavitary defects and to supplement osteosynthesis sites. Structural cortical autografts are limited in terms of donor site and include the fibula and iliac crest. Fibular autograft can be useful in benign lesions such as fibrous dysplasia, in which cortical interstitial bone provides long-term structural support because it is not remodeled. Vascularized fibular autografts have been popular since their introduction in 1970, when Ian Taylor successfully transplanted one for a long bone reconstruction. The fibula has since then been a "workhorse" for vascularized bone grafting.[69]

Another choice for a vascularized bone graft is the deep circumflex artery flap, which supplies vascularized iliac crest as the bone graft.[70] Owing to the presence of the iliac apophysis, the length and dimensions of iliac bone, and the arc of curvature of the ilium, the iliac crest is not particularly suited for an intercalary long bone reconstruction even in children. The lateral border of the scapula with overlying skin, the so-called osteocutaneous scapular flap, has provided bone for mandible reconstruction and metacarpal reconstruction, but the volume of bone is not sufficient for major reconstructions. The metatarsal with overlying osteocutaneous dorsalis pedis composite flap has also been used as a source of vascularized bone. However, the inherent structural deformity to the foot that this flap causes makes this a difficult choice unless other options are unavailable. Rib grafts have an advantage in that they have a contour similar to that of skull, they can be shaped easily to fit many defects, long grafts (14 cm) can be harvested to bridge large defects, and regeneration occurs at the donor site if periosteum is left intact. The disadvantages are the possibility of pneumothorax, postoperative pain, second scar, and resorption.

The most common membranous bone graft is the calvarial graft. This bone graft has minimal donor site pain, and its harvest can typically be incorporated into incisions made for the primary reconstruction (i.e., bicoronal incision). The donor site defect can often be hidden by the hair; it has a useful gradual curvature, and minimal resorption occurs.[71] The disadvantages of calvarial grafts include the risk of epidural hematoma from damage to the sagittal or other dural sinuses, dural tears, limited shaping because of bone rigidity, and limited amount of cancellous bone. Use of split calvarial instead of full-thickness bone grafts can minimize the risks of intracranial complications and donor site deformity. The skull as a donor site has another advantage in that skull chips or shavings as well as bone dust can be harvested to fill certain defects that do not require a formal graft or can be used to augment a bone graft.

Other flaps available include the radial forearm and lateral arm, but these are for small bone volume reconstructions. Periosteal flaps based on the geniculate artery or the deep circumflex iliac artery have been used to re-establish bone defects and are filled with cancellous bone that ultimately reconstitutes into intercalary segments. Other flaps continue to be described and offer their own special applications.[72]

The fibula, however, in its many forms as a free or pedicled transfer, is the most important flap for the plastic surgeon to use. It is employed in basic anatomic free flap design as described by Taylor et al[69]; as a "shotgun" configuration, folded on its periosteal sleeve to reconstruct shorter large-volume defects[73]; as a multiple osteotomized transfer for reconstruction of curved defects, such as of the mandible[74]; as a flap with a functioning epiphysis for growing bones after tumor resection[75]; as a split transfer with longitudinal coronal haloing for long, thin defects without need for great structural strength; and as a mixed flap with a combination of skin, muscle, and bone for reconstruction of complex wounds.[76-78] It has great strength and provides a length of bone with dimensions similar to the long bones in the extremities.[79] The graft has excellent potential to hypertrophy.[80] The versatility of the fibula is based on the availability of a long vascular pedicle (peroneal artery and its venae comitantes) and the ability to osteotomize and fold the fibula to increase cross-sectional area and promote interface healing. Donor site morbidity is slight, provided sufficient distal fibula is left.[81]

The procurement of the flap with the skin paddle left in place is the most challenging of these several techniques. If careful attention is paid to the anatomic layers as the dissection is done, this flap is actually facile to harvest. An oval paddle, approximately 10 × 12 cm, is designed directly over the middle of the fibula. Normally, for a plain fibular harvest, the dissection is through a longitudinal line over the fibula. This technique was illustrated by Urbaniak and Harvey.[82] The dissection for the osteocutaneous flap lies first along the longitudinal line and then along the posterior portion of the paddle back to the longitudinal line of the fibula. This dissection is straight from the skin to the muscle fascia without any undermining. The soft tissues are reflected gently anteriorly, and the peroneal muscles are visualized. Several vascular leashes are

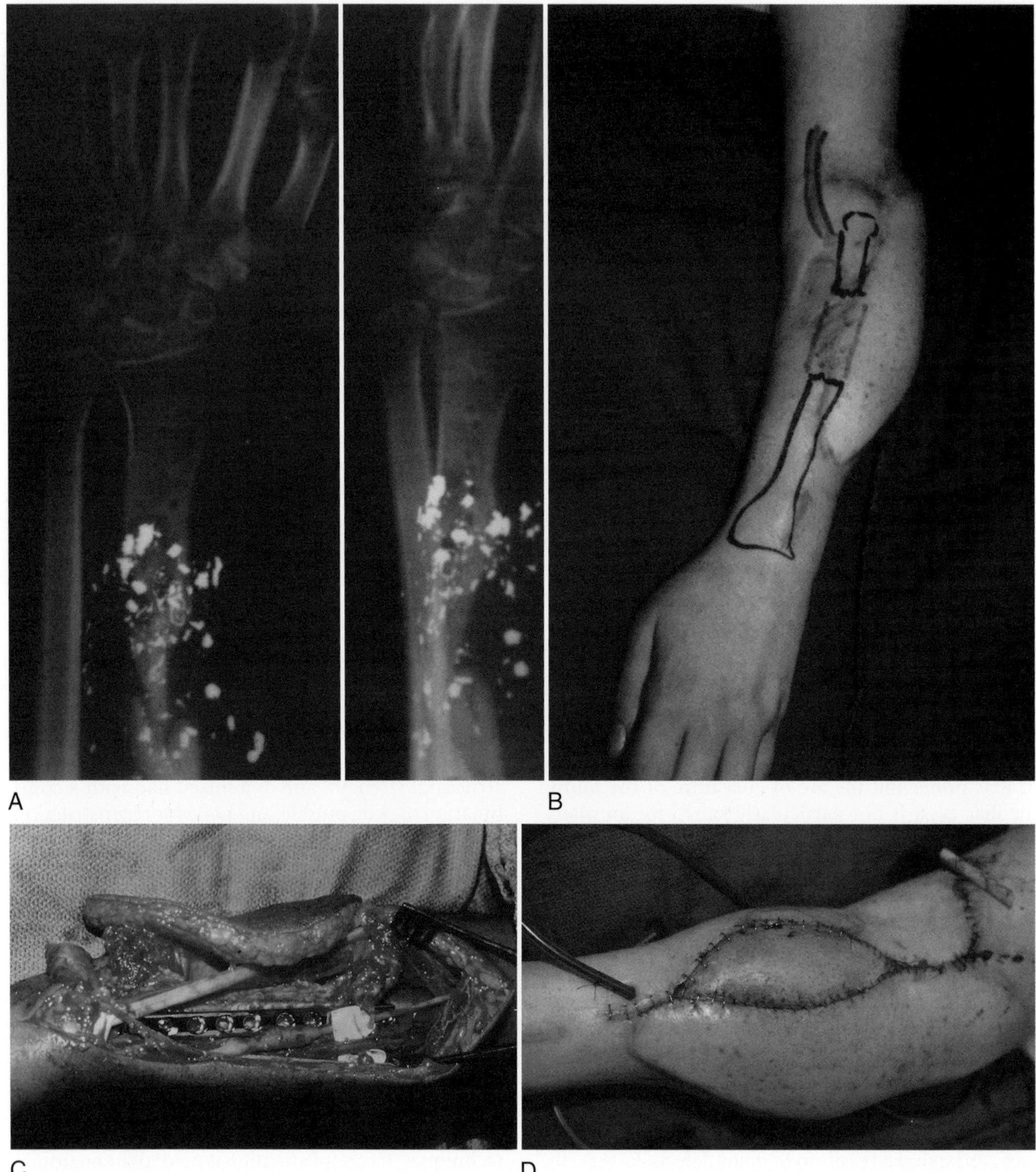

FIGURE 159-6. Free vascularized fibula transfer with or without the soft tissue pedicle has become the workhorse flap for reconstruction of the forearm and other long bone defects.[76,79] This is an example of compound soft tissue and bone defect after gunshot wound treated with staged reconstruction. *A,* Large defects in both the radius and the overlying soft tissue envelope were restricting recovery. *B,* Soft tissue and tendon-muscle deficits were addressed at an earlier surgery with free tissue transfer. A 6-cm defect still existed in the radius. *C,* Instability and contracted soft tissue envelope were treated with an osteoseptocutaneous free fibula graft. The paddle is laid into place after the fibula is secured in its anatomic position. This is accomplished with a bridge plate that has two unicortical screws to hold the actual fibula while purchase is obtained both proximally and distally with bicortical screws. The fibula is keyed into position with notches cut in the native radius to accept the donor fibula. *D,* The paddle is held in place with skin staples. A drain is brought out through a separate incision away from the pedicle.

visualized lying on the peroneal vessels in the anterior part of the wound. These vary somewhat in number, but usually two to three supply the overlying skin paddle. If these vascular structures are maintained throughout the rest of the dissection, the skin paddle remains attached to the fibula with a fascial layer. This affords a limited mobility to the paddle, but no attempts at tensioning the fascial layer to the paddle should be made because the dermal blood supply is more tenuous than the supply of the fibula itself. If these steps are observed, large complex multisystem wounds can be reconstructed with expectations of a gliding skin envelope overlying a hypertrophying skeletal replacement to allow nearly anatomic reconstitution (Fig. 159-6).[79]

FUTURE OPTIONS IN SKELETAL RECONSTRUCTION

With the development of improved methods of tissue management, new treatment options are becoming available in orthopedics to aid in the healing capacity of musculoskeletal tissues. Current techniques in gene therapy and tissue engineering based on the use of muscle- or fat-derived stem cells will apply in improving the healing of the musculoskeletal system, including muscle injuries, bone injuries, and damage to intra-articular structures (such as ligament, cartilage, and meniscus). Starting with a building material (e.g., extracellular matrix, biodegradable polymer), a bone or structure will be formed, seeded with living cells, and bathed with growth factors. When the cells multiply, they fill up the scaffold and grow into three-dimensional tissue, and once implanted in the body, the cells recreate their intended tissue functions. Blood vessels attach themselves to the new tissue, the scaffold dissolves, and the newly grown tissue eventually blends in with its surroundings.[83]

REFERENCES

1. Hak D, Olson S, Matta J: Diagnosis and management of closed internal degloving injuries associated with pelvic and acetabular fractures: the Morel-Lavallee lesion. J Trauma 1997;42:1046-1051.
2. Levin L: The reconstructive ladder—an orthoplastic approach. Orthop Clin North Am 1993;24:393-409.
3. Gustilo R, Anderson J: Prevention of infection in the treatment of one thousand and twenty-five open fractures of long bones—retrospective and prospective analysis. J Bone Joint Surg Am 1976;58:453-458.
4. Swiontkowski M: Criteria for bone débridement in massive lower limb trauma. Clin Orthop 1989;243:41-47.
5. Keating J, Blachut P, O'Brien P, et al: Reamed nailing of open tibial fractures: does the antibiotic bead pouch reduce the deep infection rate? J Orthop Trauma 1996;10:298-303.
6. Hamer M, Robson M, Krizek T, Southwick W: Quantitative bacterial analysis of comparative wound irrigations. Ann Surg 1975;181:819-822.
7. Dirschl D, Duff GP, Dahners LE, et al: High pressure pulsatile lavage irrigation of intraarticular fractures: effects on fracture healing. J Orthop Trauma 1998;12:460-463.
8. Bhandari M, Schemitsch E, Adili A, et al: High and low pressure pulsatile lavage of contaminated tibial fractures: an in vitro study of bacterial adherence and bone damage. J Orthop Trauma 1999;13:526-533.
9. Bhandari M, Adili A, Schemitsch E: The efficacy of low-pressure lavage with different irrigating solutions to remove adherent bacteria from bone. J Bone Joint Surg Am 2001;83:412-419.
10. Blachut P, Meek R, O'Brien P: External fixation and delayed intramedullary nailing of open fractures of the tibial shaft. A sequential protocol. J Bone Joint Surg Am 1990;72:729-735.
11. May J, Gallico G, Lukash F: Microvascular transfer of free tissue for closure of bone wounds of the distal lower extremity. N Engl J Med 1982;306:253-257.
12. May J, Gallico G, Jupiter J, Savage R: Free latissimus dorsi muscle flap with skin graft for treatment of traumatic chronic bony wounds. Plast Reconstr Surg 1984;73:641-651.
13. Fitzgerald R, Whalen J, Peterson S: Pathophysiology of osteomyelitis and pharmacokinetics of antimicrobial agents in normal and osteomyelitic bone. In Esterhai JL, Gristina AG, Poss R, eds: Musculoskeletal Infection. Park Ridge, Ill, American Academy of Orthopaedic Surgeons, 1992:387-400.
14. Morrissy R, Haynes D, Nelson C: Acute hematogenous osteomyelitis: a model with trauma as an etiology. J Pediatr Orthop 1989;9:447-456.
15. Toh CL, Jupiter J: The infected nonunion of the tibia. Clin Orthop 1995;315:176-191.
16. Cierny G: Chronic osteomyelitis: results of treatment. Instr Course Lect 1990;39:495-508.
17. Gristina A, Costerton J: Bacterial adherence and the glycocalyx and their role in musculoskeletal infection. Orthop Clin North Am 1984;15:517-535.
18. Wegener W, Alavi A: Diagnostic imaging of musculoskeletal infection. Orthop Clin North Am 1991;22:401-418.
19. Mathes S, Alpert B, Chang N: Use of the muscle flap in chronic osteomyelitis: experimental and clinical considerations. Plast Reconstr Surg 1982;69:815-829.
20. Durham R, Mistry B, Mazuski J, et al: Outcome and utility of scoring systems in the management of the mangled extremity. Am J Surg 1996;172:569-573.
21. Bondurant F, Cotler H, Buckle R, et al: The medical and economic impact of severely injured lower extremities. J Trauma 1988;28:1270-1273.
22. Quirke T, Sharma P, Boss W, et al: Are type IIIC lower extremity injuries an indication for primary amputation? J Trauma 1996;40:992-996.
23. Hertel R, Strebel N, Ganz R: Amputation versus reconstruction in traumatic defects of the leg: outcome and costs. J Orthop Trauma 1996;10:223-229.
24. Tscherne H, Gotzen L: Fractures with Soft Tissue Injuries. New York, Springer-Verlag, 1984.
25. Swanson T, Szabo R, Anderson D: Open hand fractures: prognosis and classification. J Hand Surg Am 1991;16:101-107.
26. Gallie W: First recurrence of osteomyelitis eighty years after infections. J Bone Joint Surg Br 1951;33:110-111.
27. Damholt V: Treatment of chronic osteomyelitis. Acta Orthop Scand 1982;53:715-720.
28. Wood M, Cooney W, Irons G: Lower extremity salvage and reconstruction by free-tissue transfer: analysis of results. Clin Orthop 1985;201:151-161.
29. Waldvogel F, Medoff G, Swartz M: Osteomyelitis: a review of clinical features, therapeutic considerations and unusual aspects. Parts I, II, and III. N Engl J Med 1970;282:198-206, 260-266, 316-322.

30. Fitzgerald R: Experimental osteomyelitis: description of a canine model and the role of depot administration of antibiotics in the prevention and treatment of sepsis. J Bone Joint Surg Am 1983;65:371-380.
31. Anthony J, Mathes S: Update on chronic osteomyelitis. Clin Plast Surg 1991;18:515-523.
32. Cierny G, Mader J, Couch L: Adjunctive local antibiotics in the management of contaminated orthopaedic wounds. Orthop Transcripts 1986;10:465.
33. Laurencin C, Gerhart T, Witschger P, et al: Bioerodible polyanhydrides for antibiotic drug delivery: in vivo osteomyelitis treatment in a rat model system. J Orthop Res 1993;11:256-262.
34. Gerhart T, Roux RD, Hanff PA, et al: Antibiotic loaded biodegradable bone cement for prophylaxis and treatment of experimental osteomyelitis in rats. J Orthop Res 1993;11:250-255.
35. Sheffield P: Tissue oxygen measurements with respect to soft tissue wound healing with normobaric and hyperbaric oxygen. Hyperbaric Oxygen Rev 1985;6:18-46.
36. Calhoun J, Cobos J, Mader J: Does hyperbaric oxygen have a place in the treatment of osteomyelitis? Orthop Clin North Am 1991;22:467-471.
37. Smith T: Nutrition: its relationship to orthopaedic infections. Orthop Clin North Am 1991;22:373-377.
38. DeFranzo A, Marks M, Argenta L, Genecov D: Vacuum-assisted closure for the treatment of degloving injuries. Plast Reconstr Surg 1999;104:2145-2148.
39. Morykwas M, Argenta L, Shelton-Brown E, McGuirt W: Vacuum-assisted closure: a new method for wound control and treatment: animal studies and basic foundation. Ann Plast Surg 1997;38:553-562.
40. Argenta L, Morykwas M: Vacuum-assisted closure: a new method for wound control and treatment: clinical experience. Ann Plast Surg 1997;38:563-576.
41. Godina M: Early microsurgical reconstruction of complex trauma of the extremities. Plast Reconstr Surg 1986;78:285-292.
42. Byrd H, Cierny G, Tebbetts J: The management of open tibial fractures with associated soft-tissue loss: external pin fixation with early flap coverage. Plast Reconstr Surg 1981;68:73-82.
43. Sherman R, Ecker J: Soft tissue coverage. In Browner BD, Jupiter JB, Levine AM, Trafton PG, eds: Skeletal Trauma. Philadelphia, WB Saunders, 1992:337-365.
44. Yaremchuk M, Brumback RJ, Manson PN, et al: Acute and definitive management of traumatic osteocutaneous defects of the lower extremity. Plast Reconstr Surg 1987;80:1-14.
45. Barwick W, Goldberg J, Scully S, Harrelson J: Vascularized tissue transfer for closure of irradiated wounds after soft tissue sarcoma resection. Ann Surg 1992;216:591-595.
46. Teknos T, Myers L: Surgical reconstruction after chemotherapy or radiation. Problems and solutions. Hematol Oncol Clin North Am 1999;13:679-687.
47. Gustilo R: Management of infected fractures. In Evarts C, ed: Surgery of the Musculoskeletal System. New York, Churchill Livingstone, 1990:4429-4453.
48. Meyer S, Weiland A, Willenegger H: The treatment of infected nonunion of fractures of long bones. J Bone Joint Surg Am 1975;57:836-842.
49. Muller M, Thomas R: Treatment of nonunion in fractures of long bones. Clin Orthop 1979;138:141-153.
50. Esterhai J, Sennett B, Gelb H, et al: Treatment of chronic osteomyelitis complicating nonunion and segmental defects of the tibia with open cancellous bone graft, posterolateral bone graft, and soft tissue transfer. J Trauma 1990;30:49-54.
51. Feibel R, Oliva A, Jackson R, et al: Simultaneous free tissue transfer and Ilizarov distraction osteosynthesis in lower extremity salvage. J Trauma 1994;37:322-327.
52. Patzakis M, Scilaris T, Chon J, et al: Results of bone grafting for infected tibial nonunion. Clin Orthop 1995;315:192-198.
53. MacAusland W, Eaton R: Sepsis following fixation of fractures of the femur. J Bone Joint Surg Am 1963;45:1647-1653.
54. Irons G, Fisher J, Schmitt E: Vascularized muscular and musculocutaneous flaps for management of osteomyelitis. Orthop Clin North Am 1984;15:473-480.
55. Shannon J, Woolhouse F, Eisinger P: The treatment of chronic osteomyelitis by saucerization and immediate skin grafting. Clin Orthop 1973;96:98-107.
56. Papineau L, Alfageme A, Dalcourt J, Pilon L: Chronic osteomyelitis: open excision and grafting after saucerization. Int Orthop 1979;3:165-176.
57. Stark W: The use of pedicled muscle flaps in the surgical treatment of chronic osteomyelitis resulting from compound fractures. J Bone Joint Surg Am 1946;28:343-350.
58. Koval K, Meadows S, Rosen H, et al: Posttraumatic tibial osteomyelitis: a comparison of three treatment approaches. Orthopedics 1992;15:455-460.
59. Ilizarov G: The tension-stress effect on the genesis and growth of tissues. Part II. The influence of the rate and frequency of distraction. Clin Orthop 1989;239:263-285.
60. Ilizarov G: The tension-stress effect on the genesis and growth of tissues. Part I. The influence of stability of fixation and soft-tissue preservation. Clin Orthop 1989;238:249-281.
61. Green S: Osteomyelitis—the Ilizarov perspective. Orthop Clin North Am 1991;22:515-522.
62. Green S: The Ilizarov method. In Browner BD, Jupiter JB, Levine AM, Trafton PG, eds: Skeletal Trauma. Philadelphia, WB Saunders, 1992:543-570.
63. Levin L: The Ilizarov method and microsurgery. Reconstr Microsurg 1996;6:6-7.
64. Blackley H, Davis A, Hutchison C, Gross A: Proximal femoral allografts for reconstruction of bone stock in revision arthroplasty of the hip. A nine to fifteen-year follow-up. J Bone Joint Surg Am 2001;83:346-354.
65. Dean G, Holliger E, Urbaniak J: Elbow allograft for reconstruction of the elbow with massive bone loss. Long term results. Clin Orthop 1997;341:12-22.
66. Stevenson S, Li X, Martin B: The fate of cancellous and cortical bone after transplantation of fresh and frozen tissue-matched and mismatched osteochondral allografts in dogs. J Bone Joint Surg Am 1991;23:143-156.
67. De Meulemeester C, Verdonk R, Bongaerts W: The fibula pro tibia procedure in the treatment of nonunion of the tibia. Acta Orthop Belg 1992;58:187-189.
68. Molski M: Cross-leg pedicled fibular graft—a new reconstructive method with vascularized bone graft [in Polish]. Chir Narzadow Ruchu Ortop Pol 1999;64:539-545.
69. Taylor G, Miller G, Ham F: The free vascularized bone graft: a clinical extension of microvascular techniques. Plast Reconstr Surg 1975;55:533-544.
70. Salibian A, Anzel S, Salyer W: Transfer of vascularized grafts of iliac bone to the extremities. J Bone Joint Surg Am 1987;69:1319-1327.
71. Jackson I, Pellett C, Smith J: Skull as a bone graft donor site. Ann Plast Surg 1983;11:527-532.
72. Chen HC, Demirkan F, Wei FC, et al: Free fibula osteoseptocutaneous-pedicled pectoralis major myocutaneous flap combination in reconstruction of extensive composite mandibular defects. Plast Reconstr Surg 1999;103:839-845.
73. Yajima H, Tamai S: Twin-barrelled vascularized fibular grafting to the pelvis and lower extremity. Clin Orthop 1994;303:178-184.
74. Hidalgo D: Fibula free flap: a new method of mandible reconstruction. Plast Reconstr Surg 1989;84:71-79.
75. Millesi H, Piza-Katzer H: Free transplantation of a fibula with epiphysis. Handchirurgie 1978;10:115-119.
76. Harvey EJ, Levin L: The use of the osteoseptocutaneous free fibula transfer in the upper extremity [videotape]. Rosemont, Ill, American Society for Surgery of the Hand, 1996.

77. Chuang D, Chen H, Wei F, Noordhoff M: Compound functioning free muscle flap transplantation (lateral half of soleus, fibula, and skin flap). Plast Reconstr Surg 1992;89:335-339.
78. Beppu M, Hanel D, Johnston G, et al: The osteocutaneous fibula flap: an anatomic study. J Reconstr Microsurg 1992;8:215-223.
79. Jupiter J, Gerhard H, Guerrero J, et al: Treatment of segmental defects of the radius with use of the vascularized osteoseptocutaneous fibular autogenous graft. J Bone Joint Surg Am 1997;79:542-550.
80. Mathoulin C, Gilbert A, Azze R: Congenital pseudarthrosis of the forearm: treatment of six cases with vascularized fibular graft and a review of the literature. Microsurgery 1993;14:252-259.
81. Babovic S, Johnson C, Finical S: Free fibula donor-site morbidity: the Mayo experience with 100 consecutive harvests. J Reconstr Microsurg 2000;16:107-110.
82. Urbaniak JR, Harvey EJ: Revascularization of the femoral head in osteonecrosis. J Am Acad Orthop Surg 1998;6:44-54.
83. Shea L, Wang D, Franceschi R, Mooney D: Engineered bone development from a pre-osteoblast cell line on three-dimensional scaffolds. Tissue Eng 2000;6:605-617.

CHAPTER

160

Foot Reconstruction

LAWRENCE B. COLEN, MD, FACS ✦ THEODORE UROSKIE, Jr., MD, FACS

The human foot is an important part of the body in that it supports the body's weight on standing and provides a stable interface between the body and the ground during ambulation. Its function depends on many factors that may be adversely affected by a wide variety of pathologic processes and trauma. The mechanical interactions of the numerous small bones, the pain-free articulation of the small joints, an intact and durable soft tissue envelope, and appropriate sensory feedback are essential to the proper function required for normal ambulation. Aging, peripheral vascular disease, diabetes mellitus, and rheumatoid arthritis are just a few of the many disease processes that may adversely affect this "balance" of foot function.

Plastic surgeons must often treat the foot ravaged by disease or trauma. The goal of reconstruction with return to function is the standard for successful care. Therefore, factors that could lead to loss of function (soft tissue loss, soft tissue contracture, joint adhesions, malunion, nonunion, neurologic or vascular injury) as well as dystrophic changes need special attention. Success can be achieved only through the multidisciplinary, coordinated efforts of plastic, orthopedic, and vascular surgeons as well as podiatrists and rehabilitation specialists. The key to any reconstructive effort is an adequate preoperative evaluation and preparation, a well-executed support program, and a closely supervised postoperative routine.

A thorough understanding of the anatomy and pathophysiology of the foot "injury" is necessary for restoration of both form and function. Although the reconstructive surgeon is influenced by the successes and failures of past endeavors, it is imperative to perform ongoing re-evaluation of one's results and to modify one's approach accordingly.

ANATOMY

A proper understanding of the anatomy of the foot, the weight-bearing interface for ambulation, is essential to the successful reconstruction of foot injuries. The reconstructive surgeon must have a complete knowledge of the bone architecture, the longitudinal and transverse arches, the compartments, and the role that each plays during this process.

Dorsal Soft Tissue

The structures of the dorsum of the foot are continuous with those of the anterior compartment of the leg. As in the hand, the skin is thin and pliable and has little subcutaneous fat. The deep fascia overlies the paratenon of the extensor tendons and is contiguous with the retinaculum proximally and the plantar fascia medially and laterally. As in the leg, a network of vessels is located in the deep fascial plane; the vessels originate from the anterior tibial artery, perforate the extensor retinaculum, and then travel on the deep surface of the fascia. Over the instep, small vessels course longitudinally just superficial to the fascia.

The muscles in this region include the extensor digitorum brevis and the extensor hallucis brevis, often considered one thin, broad muscle with four tendons originating from the distal superior and lateral surface of the calcaneus and inserting into the base of the proximal phalanx of each of the medial four toes through the extensor expansion. The deep peroneal nerve innervates these muscles, and the lateral tarsal artery provides the blood supply. Both the motor nerve and vascular pedicle enter the muscle proximally.

The dorsalis pedis artery is the continuation of the anterior tibial artery at the ankle (Fig. 160-1). The dorsalis pedis artery and its branches supply the dorsum of the foot and ankle as well as the first web space.[1] It courses deep to the extensor digitorum brevis muscle toward the first metatarsal base. There it divides into the arcuate artery, the first dorsal metatarsal artery, and the deep plantar artery. The dorsalis pedis artery lies against the bones and ligaments of the dorsum, with the deep peroneal nerve and venae comitantes adjacent to it. The lateral and medial tarsal arteries are the most proximal branches of the dorsalis pedis artery after the vessel crosses the ankle joint. In the 3.7% of patients with congenital absence of the dorsalis pedis artery, lateral tarsal vessels are greatly enlarged through vascular connections with the peroneal artery.[2] After giving off branches to the extensor digitorum brevis muscle, the lateral tarsal artery interconnects with branches of the arcuate artery, the anterior lateral malleolar artery, and the perforating branch of the peroneal

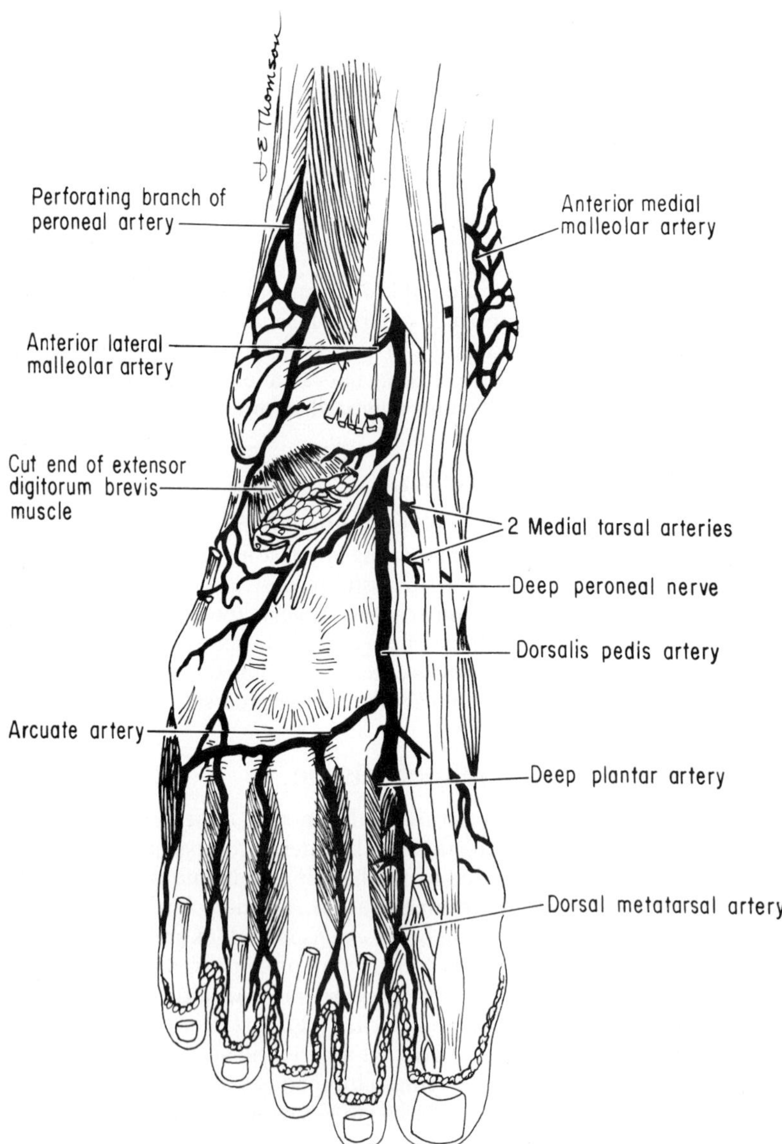

FIGURE 160-1. Arterial anatomy of the dorsum of the foot.

artery. The medial tarsal vessels consist of two or three small arteries that ramify over the medial foot dorsum and anastomose with the medial malleolar arteries. The arcuate artery arises at the bases of the metatarsals, courses laterally, and interconnects with the lateral tarsal and lateral plantar vessels. The dorsal metatarsal arteries arise from the arcuate artery and ultimately branch into dorsal digital arteries to the adjacent toes. Anterior and posterior perforating branches anastomose with corresponding plantar metatarsal arteries. The deep plantar artery passes between the two heads of origin of the first dorsal interosseous muscle to contribute to the plantar arch.

The deep peroneal nerve divides into medial and lateral branches just distal to the ankle joint. The lateral component innervates the extensor digitorum brevis and extensor hallucis brevis muscles, and the medial component is sensory to the first web space. The remainder of the foot dorsum is innervated by branches of the superficial peroneal nerve and sural nerve, which lie in the subcutaneous plane.

Plantar Soft Tissue

The skin on the plantar aspect of the foot varies from region to region, being thickest (up to 3.5 mm) over the heel and metatarsal heads and thinner over the toes and instep. A moderate amount of subcutaneous fat is intermingled with fibrous connective tissue, providing a cushion for weight bearing. The plantar fascia is continuous with the deep fascia of the foot's dorsum after attachments to the sides of the first and fifth metatarsals. Thinner membranous sheets lie medially and laterally to enclose the compartments of the great and small toes; a thickened plantar aponeurosis is found centrally. This thickened aponeurosis consists of longitudinally arranged bands of fibrous connective tissue that originate from the medial process of the calcaneus and diverge as "slips" toward the five toes. Deeper transverse fibers form the superficial transverse metatarsal ligament in the region of the metatarsal heads. Additional components, oriented in the anteroposterior direction, tether the longitudinal elements to the underlying metatarsals (Fig. 160-2).[3]

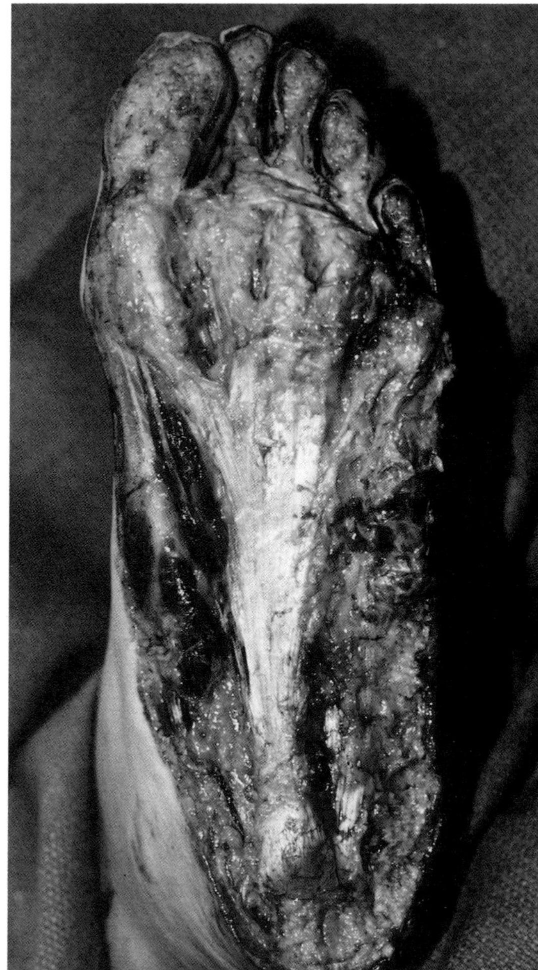

FIGURE 160-2. Plantar foot with the skin and subcutaneous tissue removed showing the course of the plantar fascia.

The compartments of the sole of the foot are similar to those of the palm of the hand. Knowledge of these compartments facilitates their decompression when it is clinically indicated. There is a compartment associated with the great toe and its intrinsic musculature, another for the small toe, a central compartment, and an interosseous-adductor compartment. The muscles and tendons may also be considered "layers" in the foot. The most superficial layer consists of the abductor hallucis, flexor digitorum brevis, and abductor digiti minimi muscles. The second layer is composed of the quadratus plantae muscle, the lumbrical muscles, and the extrinsic tendons of the long flexors. The flexor hallucis brevis, adductor hallucis, and flexor digiti minimi brevis muscles compose the third layer. The interosseous muscles form the last layer (Fig. 160-3).

SUPERFICIAL LAYER

All three muscles in the superficial layer arise primarily from the calcaneus but also have attachments to adjacent fascial layers (Fig. 160-4). The abductor hallucis muscle inserts into the medial side of the base of the great toe's proximal phalanx, blending with the medial head of the flexor hallucis brevis and sharing with it the tibial sesamoid of the great toe. Innervated by branches of medial plantar nerve, the abductor hallucis muscle abducts the great toe. The medial plantar neurovascular bundle emerges from the undersurface of the muscle proximally before coursing onto the plantar surface of the foot.

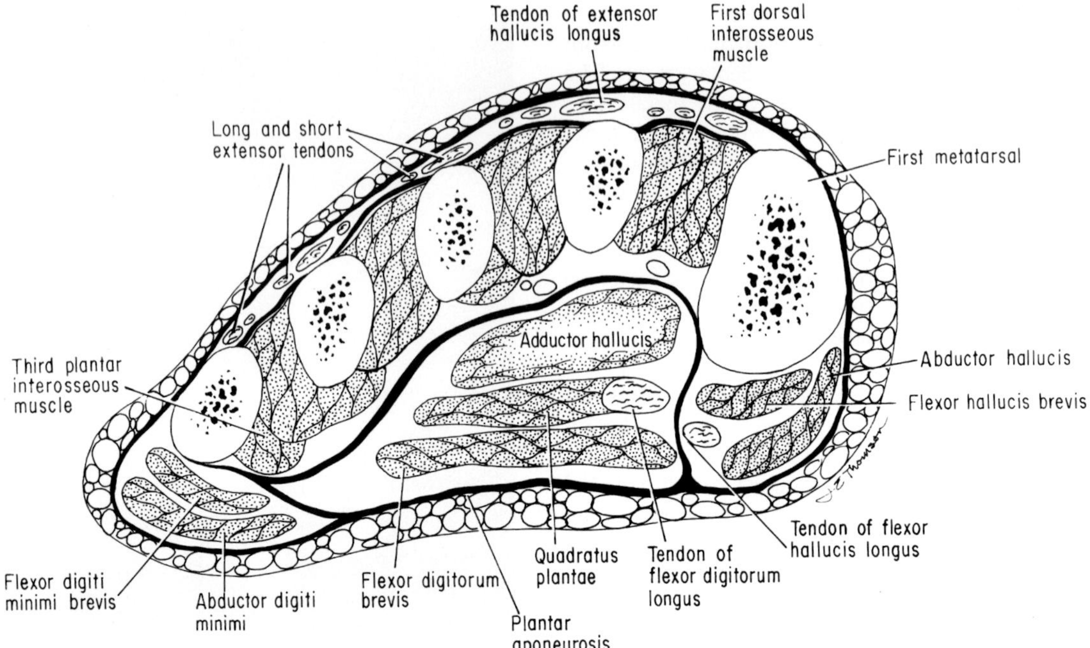

FIGURE 160-3. The four compartments of the foot.

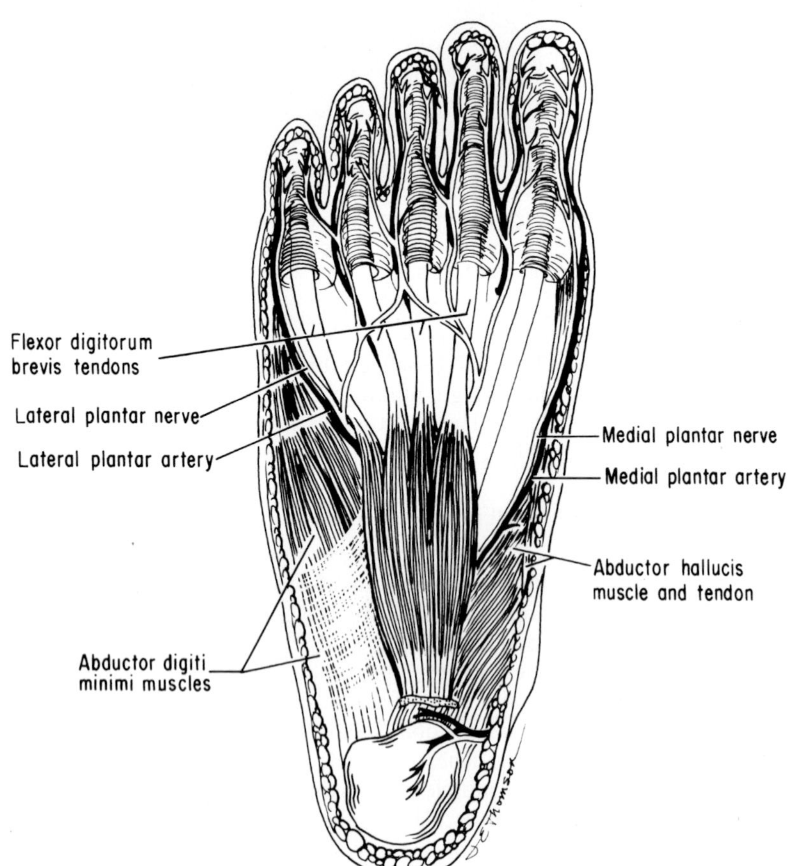

FIGURE 160-4. Superficial layer of the plantar foot.

The flexor digitorum brevis muscle is the pedal equivalent of the flexor digitorum superficialis muscle in the upper extremity. It gives rise to four small tendons that pass distally to enter the digital tendon sheaths with the long flexor tendons of the lateral four toes. They insert into the middle phalanges of the toes after dividing into two slips. Innervated by branches of the medial plantar nerve, the muscle flexes the middle phalanges of the four lateral toes. The lateral plantar neurovascular structures pass beneath the abductor hallucis, penetrate the medial intermuscular septum, continue deep to the flexor digitorum brevis, and penetrate the lateral intermuscular septum.

The abductor digiti minimi muscle becomes tendinous in the forefoot and lies on the surface of the flexor digiti minimi brevis. The abductor inserts on the lateral side of the proximal phalanx of the small toe. Innervated by a branch of the lateral plantar nerve, this muscle abducts the small toe.

SECOND LAYER

The tendon of the flexor digitorum longus muscle passes into the sole of the foot deep to the abductor hallucis muscle, where it crosses superficial to the flexor hallucis longus tendon to enter the central compartment. Within this compartment, the flexor digitorum longus becomes associated with one muscle (quadratus plantae) and one set of muscles (lumbricals) to form the second layer of the sole of the foot (Fig. 160-5).

The quadratus plantae arises by two heads from the medial and lateral sides of the calcaneus (plantar surface). The two heads join to form a short, flattened muscle belly that inserts into the tendon of the flexor digitorum longus at the point where it divides into four slips. The muscle is innervated by a branch of the lateral plantar nerve and assists the long flexors in flexion of the toes. The lateral plantar neurovascular bundle passes between this muscle and the more superficial flexor digitorum brevis.

Located more distally in the foot are the lumbrical muscles. The first of these, the most medial, arises from the medial side of the long flexor tendon to the second toe. The others arise from the adjacent sides of the long flexor tendons. The lumbricals course medial to the long flexor tendons of the toes with which they are associated, become tendinous, pass superficial to the deep transverse metatarsal ligament, and insert into the extensor expansion of the proximal interphalangeal joints. The medial plantar nerve innervates the first

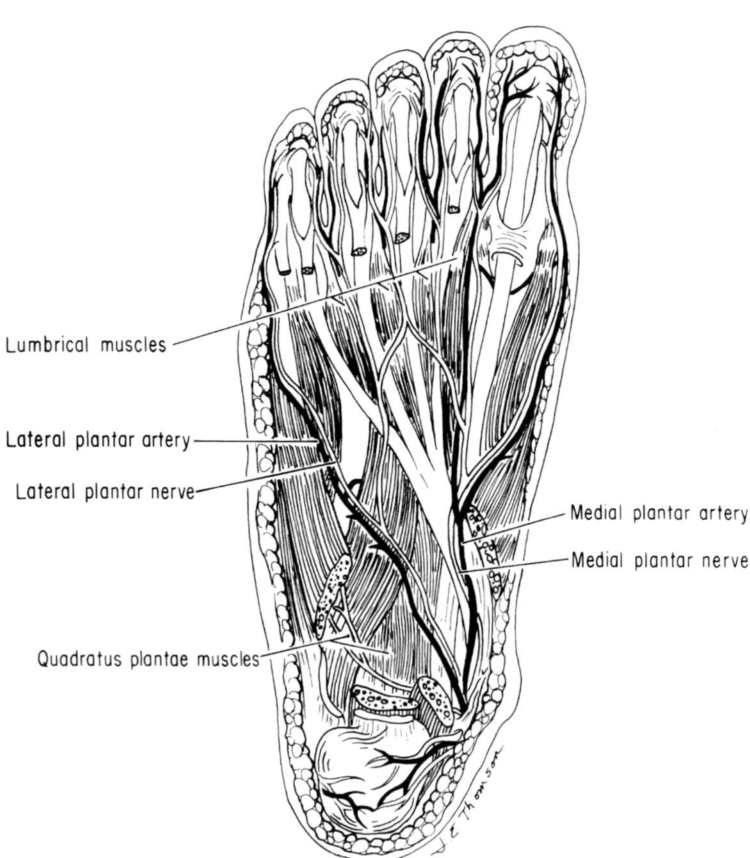

FIGURE 160-5. Second layer of the plantar foot.

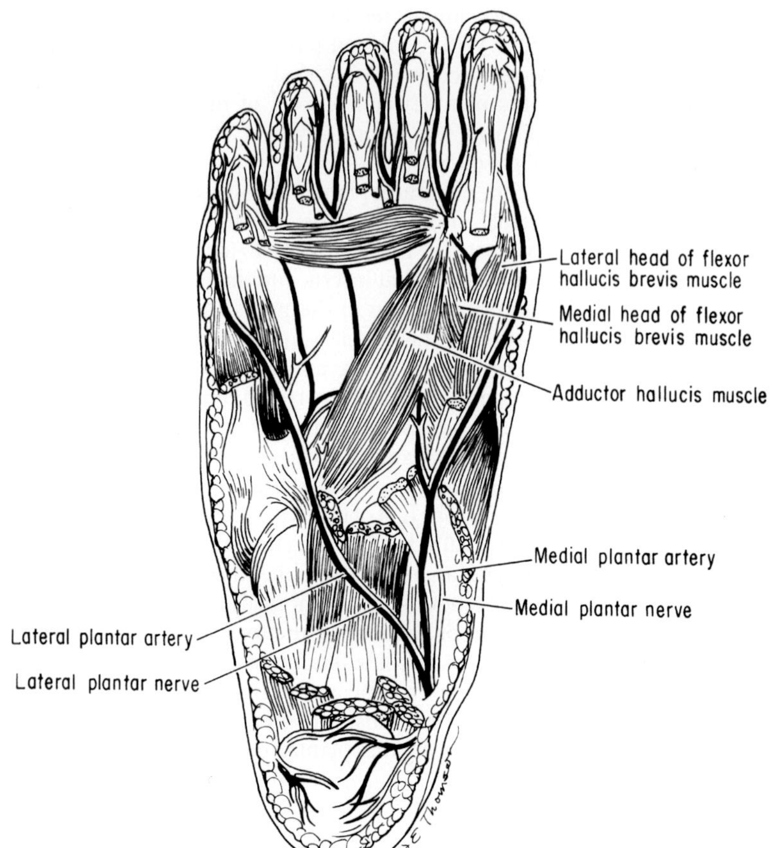

FIGURE 160-6. Third layer of the plantar foot.

lumbrical, whereas branches of the lateral plantar nerve innervate the lateral three muscles. They flex the metatarsophalangeal joints and extend the proximal interphalangeal joints.

THIRD LAYER

Three muscles compose this layer of the foot: the flexor hallucis brevis, the adductor hallucis, and the flexor digiti minimi brevis (Fig. 160-6). The most medial, the flexor hallucis brevis, arises from the medial border of the cuboid. The muscle belly lies on the plantar surface of the first metatarsal, is grooved proximally, and divides distally to form separate tendons of insertion. The medial component blends with the abductor hallucis to insert into the proximal phalanx of the great toe and contains the tibial sesamoid bone. The lateral component blends with the tendon of the adductor hallucis, inserts on the lateral aspect of the great toe's proximal phalanx, and contains the fibular sesamoid bone. The tendon of the long flexor to the great toe lies on the groove formed by the two components of this muscle belly proximally and between the two tendon insertions distally. The muscle is innervated by a branch of the medial plantar nerve and helps flex the metatarsophalangeal joint of the great toe.

The adductor hallucis muscle comprises a larger oblique head that arises from the plantar surface of the lateral four metatarsal bases and a smaller transverse head that arises from the plantar metatarsophalangeal ligaments of the lateral three toes as well as the associated deep transverse metatarsal ligament. The tendons of both heads insert into the lateral side of the base of the great toe's proximal phalanx. The two heads are supplied by branches of the lateral plantar nerve (deep branch); they assist in adduction of the great toe and maintenance of the transverse arch of the foot.

The flexor digiti minimi brevis is the most lateral muscle in the third layer. It arises from the base of the fifth metatarsal, passes distally on the plantar surface of the fifth metatarsal, and inserts as a tendon into the lateral side and flexor side of the small toe's proximal phalanx in association with the abductor digiti minimi. Innervated from branches of the lateral plantar nerve (superficial branch), the muscle flexes the metatarsophalangeal joint of the small toe.

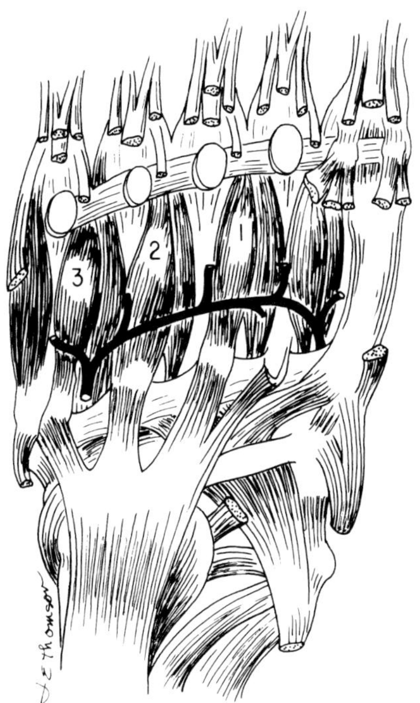

FIGURE 160-7. Fourth layer of the plantar foot.

FOURTH LAYER

The deepest layer of the sole is formed by the interosseous muscles. There are four dorsal and three plantar interosseous muscles. The midline of the foot is considered the second ray, and it is around this ray that these muscles are arranged (Fig. 160-7).

Each plantar interosseous muscle arises from a single metatarsal, whereas dorsal interossei arise from the metatarsals they lie between. The tendons of all the interossei pass along the deep transverse metatarsal ligament to insert into the base of the proximal phalanx of the toes with which they are associated. The plantar interossei adduct the three lateral toes toward the midline, help flex the metatarsophalangeal joints, and may assist in interphalangeal joint extension. Innervation is from the lateral plantar nerve. The four dorsal muscles abduct the second, third, and fourth toes and are also supplied by branches of the lateral plantar nerve.

The arteries of the sole of the foot are the medial and lateral plantar vessels that arise from the posterior tibial artery just deep to the abductor hallucis muscle. The medial plantar artery is the smaller vessel (Fig. 160-8). After giving off branches to the abductor hallucis muscle, it continues distally between this muscle and the flexor digitorum brevis, to which it also supplies minor vascular pedicles. Its largest terminal branch passes distally on the surface of the flexor hallucis brevis (medial head) to join a digital branch of the first plantar metatarsal artery to the medial side of the great toe. Its other branches include several small cutaneous vessels that supply the overlying instep skin and subcutaneous tissue.[4-7] The larger lateral plantar artery courses laterally and obliquely between the flexor digitorum superficially and the quadratus plantae deeply. Continuing distally between the abductor digiti minimi and the flexor digitorum brevis, it then pierces the plantar interosseous fascia and turns medially across the plantar surface of the interossei to form the plantar arch. In its course, the plantar artery supplies vessels to the quadratus plantae, the abductor digiti minimi, the flexor digiti minimi brevis, the skin overlying the lateral sole of the foot, and the digital artery to the lateral side of the small toe. The plantar arch courses across the width of the foot. Lying on the proximal ends of the interosseous muscles, it is deep to the other intrinsic and extrinsic musculature of the foot. It is completed medially by the deep plantar branch of the dorsalis pedis artery that courses between the first and second metatarsals (Fig. 160-9). In approximately 80% of fresh cadaver foot dissections, the deep plantar branch of the dorsalis pedis artery is the chief contributor to the plantar arch (Fig. 160-10).[8] From the arch, the plantar metatarsal arteries arise and send branches to the lumbrical muscles, the flexor hallucis brevis muscle, the adductor hallucis muscle, and the plantar interosseous muscles. Before dividing at the adjacent web spaces to supply the plantar digital arteries of the two adjacent toes between which the vessel lies, several perforating branches course dorsally to communicate

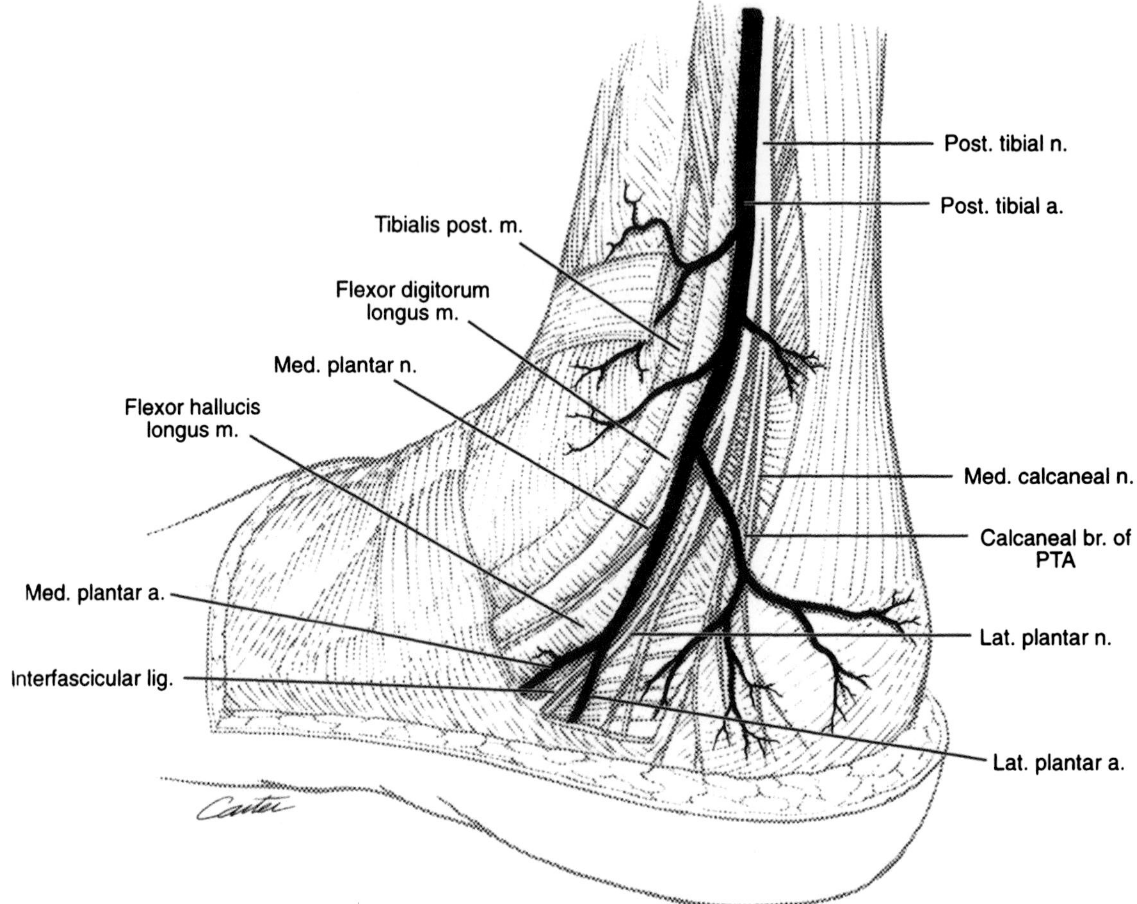

FIGURE 160-8. The terminal branches of the posterior tibial artery (PTA) are shown as the vessel travels within the tarsal tunnel. (From Attinger CE, Cooper P, Blume P: Vascular anatomy of the foot and ankle. Operative Techniques Plast Reconstr Surg 1997;4:183.)

with the corresponding dorsal metatarsal vessel (Fig. 160-11).

The medial and lateral plantar nerves follow the course of their vascular counterparts into the intrinsic musculature of the foot and the plantar skin and toes. These neurovascular structures branch from the parent posterior tibial vessels and nerve and course through two distinct tunnels (medial and lateral plantar tunnels) beneath the origin of the abductor hallucis muscle.

Bone

A general overview of the bone anatomy and the normal pattern of weight distribution is essential to the plastic surgeon treating complex foot wounds. The bone architecture is similar to that of the hand, with modifications that have evolved because of the weight-bearing duties of the foot. Thus, the bones of the ankle and foot consist of the talus and calcaneus posteriorly as well as the tarsals, metatarsals, and phalanges more distally (Fig. 160-12). The five tarsal bones are arranged in two rows, with one bone traversing the two rows. The posterior row consists of the navicular and cuneiform, which articulate with the calcaneus proximally and the distal tarsal row distally. In the distal row, the cuneiforms (medial, intermediate, and lateral) and the cuboid lie side by side with the navicular between the two rows on the medial side. The talus is the only bone that articulates with the long bones of the leg; therefore, all of the weight on the foot is transmitted onto the talus. The calcaneus and the five metatarsal heads are the weight-bearing points of the foot, with an arched skeleton in between (higher medially than laterally). Although generally larger, the foot's metatarsals and phalanges closely resemble the metacarpals and phalanges of the hand.

The foot is arched longitudinally, and in the midfoot where the metatarsal bases articulate with the distal tarsal row, a transverse arch is evident. The concept of

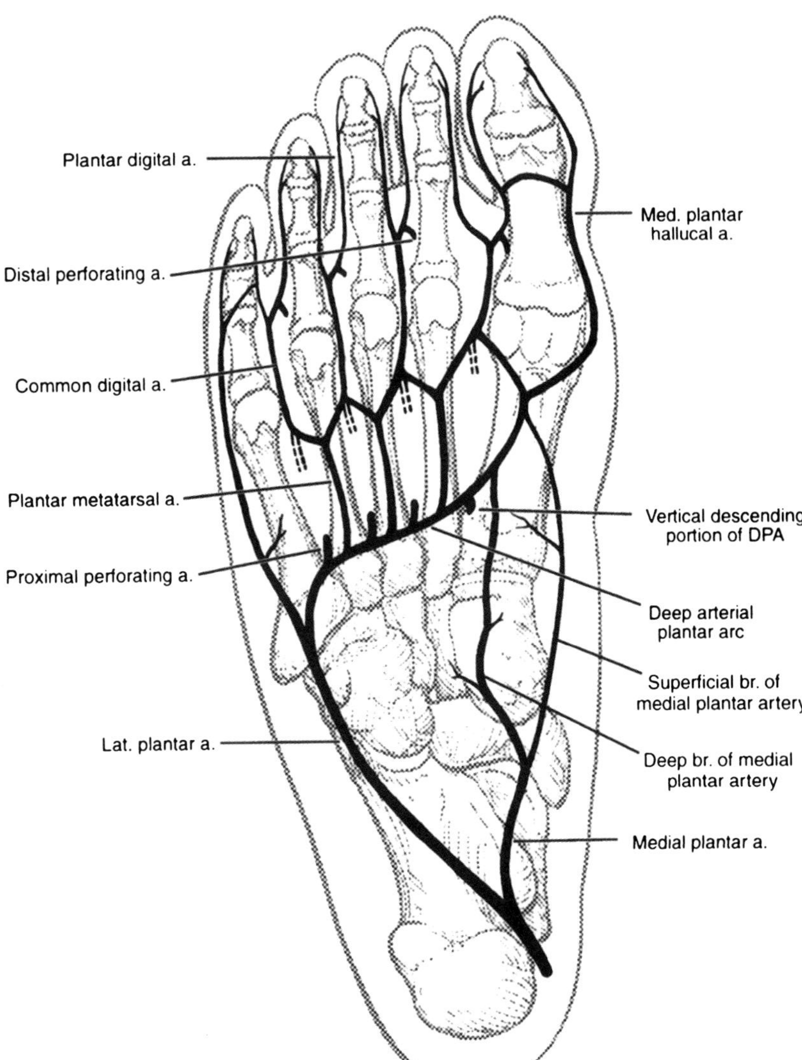

FIGURE 160-9. The most common pattern of the medial and lateral plantar branches of the posterior tibial artery. DPA, dorsalis pedis artery. (From Attinger CE, Cooper P, Blume P: Vascular anatomy of the foot and ankle. Operative Techniques Plast Reconstr Surg 1997;4:183.)

a transverse arch at the heads of the metatarsals with the forefoot bearing weight only on the first and fifth metatarsal heads has not been observed.[9]

In normal standing, half of the weight on the extremity is transferred to the calcaneus and the other half to the five metatarsals. Weight distributes across the forefoot in a ratio of 2:1:1:1:1, with the first metatarsal bearing one third of all the weight to the forefoot.[10] Support of the arch is derived from heavy plantar ligaments, the plantar aponeurosis, and the short plantar muscles. The long muscles of the leg, which position the foot through contraction to effectively bear weight, afford some protection.

CLINICAL EVALUATION

All foot injuries should be evaluated in conjunction with assessment of the entire lower extremity. In acute trauma, especially with crush injuries, one should look for compartment syndromes. A thorough examination of the bone structures, the gait pattern, the sensory status, and the nature of the blood supply is of paramount importance.

Vascular Evaluation

Particular attention should be paid to the vascular status of the limb, since the foot is the "end organ." Multiple segmental arterial stenoses exert a cumulative effect on the foot that is of a much greater magnitude than the effect seen on more proximal regions of the lower extremity.

The presence or absence of pedal pulses should be noted on physical examination. Induration, edema, pain, and mild peripheral vascular disease may make it difficult to assess the circulation adequately in this

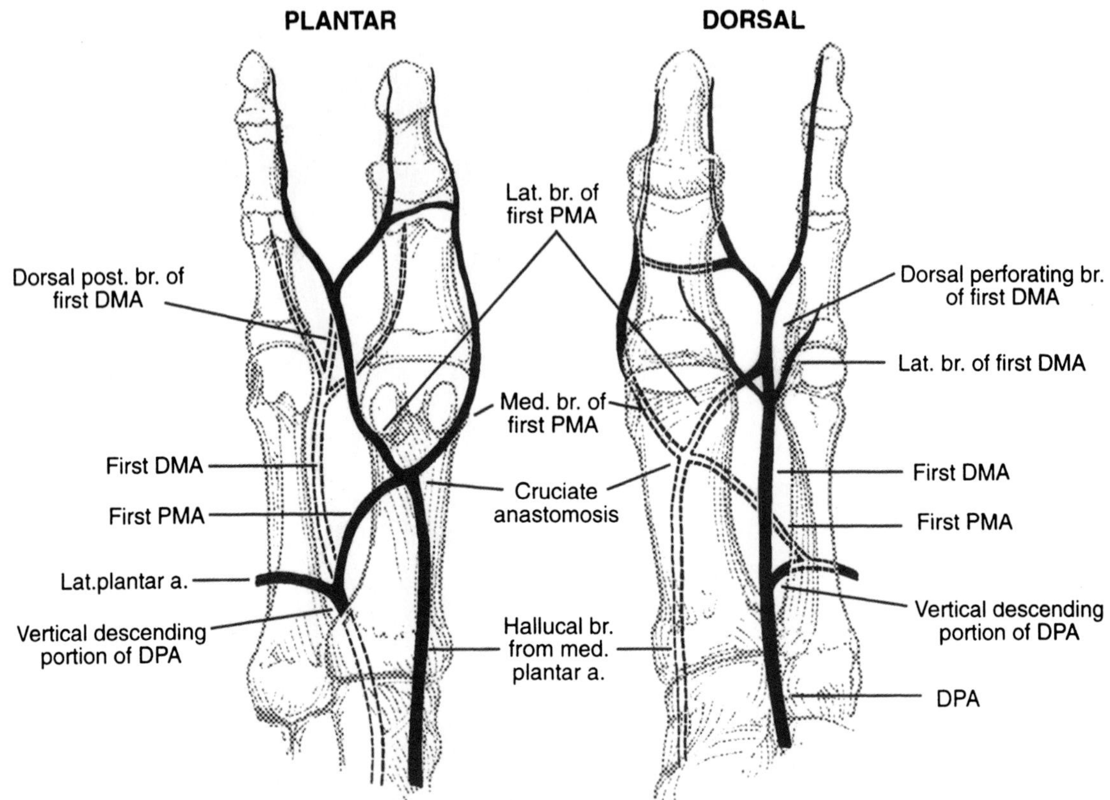

FIGURE 160-10. The relationship between the dorsal and plantar circulations. Notice how the vertical descending portion of the dorsalis pedis artery contributes to the plantar arch. DMA, dorsal metatarsal artery; DPA, dorsalis pedis artery; PMA, plantar metatarsal artery. (From Attinger CE, Cooper P, Blume P: Vascular anatomy of the foot and ankle. Operative Techniques Plast Reconstr Surg 1997;4:183.)

manner. In these situations, it becomes important to use the noninvasive vascular laboratory.

ANKLE/BRACHIAL INDICES

Brachial artery systolic pressure generally serves as a reference for determining the ankle/brachial index and gives an indication of the relative degree of ischemia. In addition, the absolute pressure measured at the ankle correlates well with the healing potential of most soft tissue wounds. A pressure cuff 12 cm in width may be placed at the ankle level. By listening with the handheld 10-MHz Doppler probe over the dorsalis pedis and posterior tibial vessels, the examiner can record the pressure at which the flow is occluded and compare it with the brachial artery occlusion pressure. In general, a normal index is 1.0 or slightly greater. Ankle/brachial indices exceeding 0.7 have been thought to be "acceptable" for most reconstructive techniques. Patients with indices of 0.3 or lower have rest pain, nonhealing wounds, or both. One review of patients with vascular disease suggested that an ankle/brachial index of less than 0.5 indicates the need for a revascularization procedure before a complex reconstruction is undertaken. The decision, however, is multifactorial and generally requires a complete extremity evaluation.[11]

Absolute pressure measurements of less than 50 mm Hg signify severe arterial disease with a poor prognosis for healing[12]; however, neither the absolute pressure nor the ankle/brachial index is always accurate.[13] Noncompressible arterial walls are seen in 5% to 30% of patients with diabetes mellitus and are caused by medial calcification, which falsely elevates the values for both tests.

TOE PRESSURES

Holstein et al[13] demonstrated that absolute toe pressures provide a highly accurate method for determining the likelihood of healing in the affected foot. Barnes[14] and others[15] agree that toe pressures in diabetic patients predict healing potential. A toe pressure of 20 to 30 mm Hg seems to represent severe ischemia that requires vascular bypass surgery.[16]

DIRECTIONAL DOPPLER FLOW STUDIES

Directional Doppler flow studies are extremely important in assessing the status of the peripheral

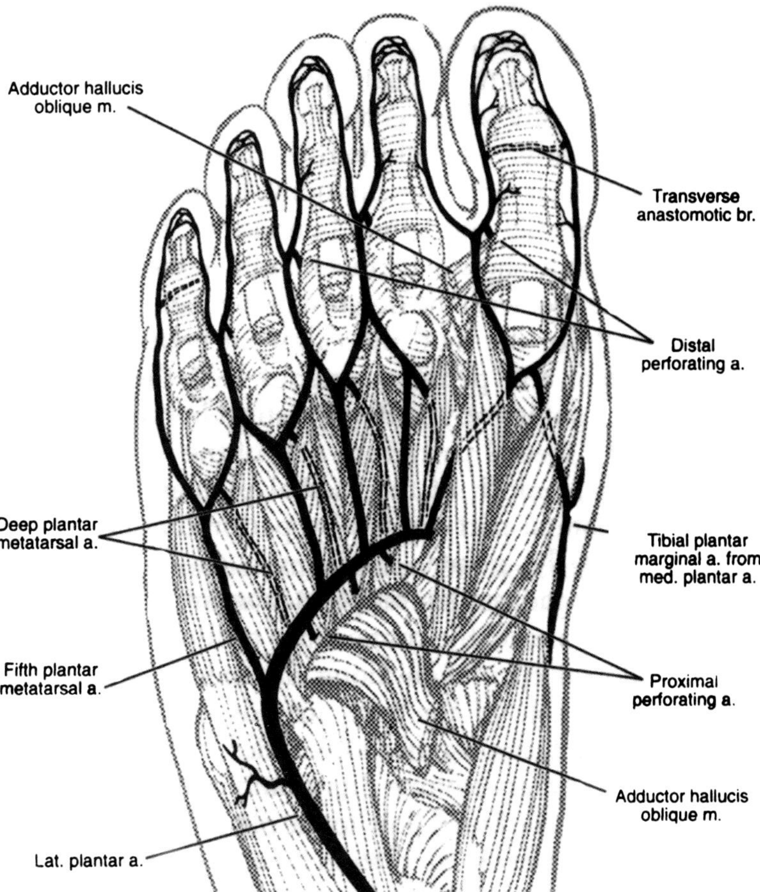

FIGURE 160-11. The plantar metatarsal arteries arise from the lateral plantar artery. The superficial vessels lie between the flexor digitorum brevis and interosseous muscles. The deep vessels lie directly on the metatarsal bone, deep to the interossei. (From Attinger CE, Cooper P, Blume P: Vascular anatomy of the foot and ankle. Operative Techniques Plast Reconstr Surg 1997;4:183.)

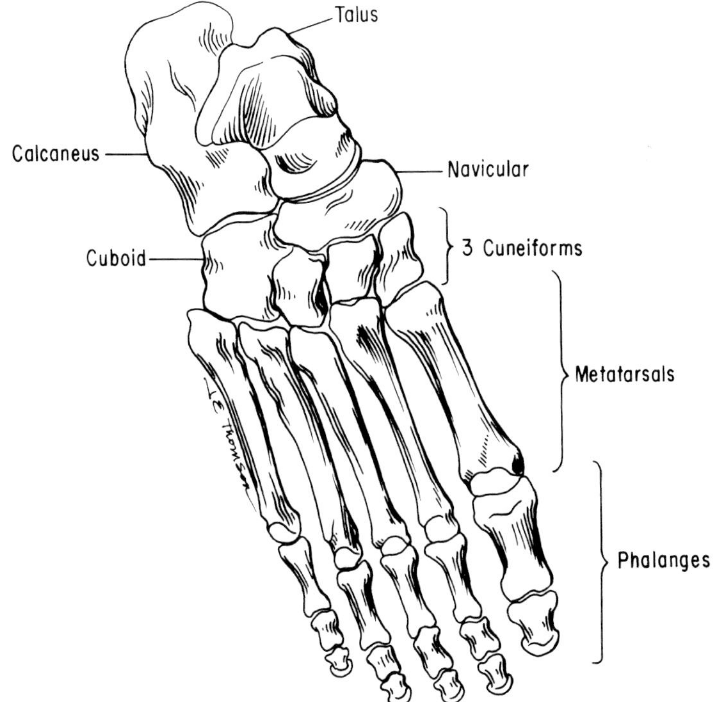

FIGURE 160-12. The osseous anatomy of the foot.

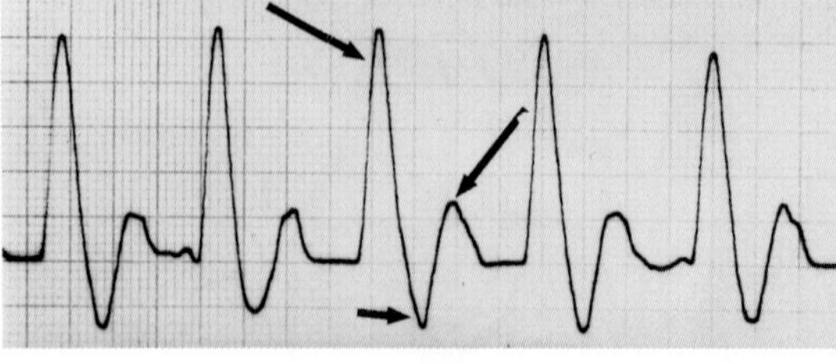

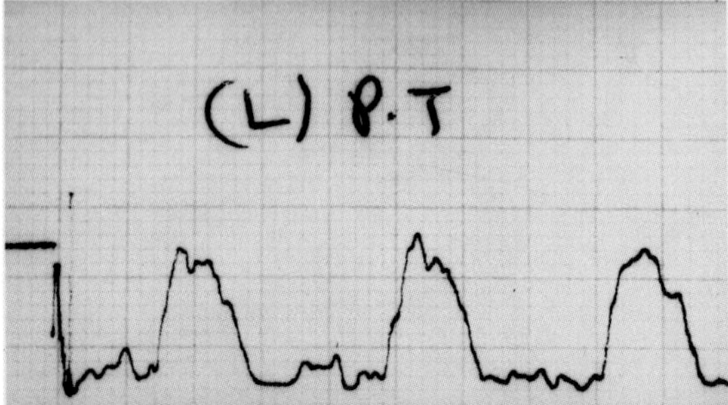

FIGURE 160-13. *Top,* Normal analogue Doppler waveform with a forward flow component, a reversed flow component, and a second forward flow component. *Bottom,* With obstruction, the waveform becomes dampened and is characterized by low velocity and an attenuated or absent reversed flow component.

circulation. Although many approaches to quantitative analysis of waveforms have been suggested, adequate assessment of waveforms is provided by qualitative evaluation.[17] The normal triphasic waveform becomes abnormal distal to an obstructing vascular lesion. As the obstruction becomes more significant, the waveform may deteriorate from triphasic to biphasic with a reversed flow component, to biphasic, to monophasic, to aphasic (Fig. 160-13). All patients with aphasic waveforms and foot wounds should undergo vascular surgery before attempts at reconstruction. Patients with triphasic or either of the two forms of biphasic flow generally do not require vascular reconstructive procedures. Limbs with monophasic flow require further study, depending on the location of the wound and the complexity of the proposed reconstruction. If microvascular composite tissue transplantation is required for wound closure, one should attempt to obtain at least biphasic or "good" monophasic flow in the recipient vessel before the reconstruction. A narrow complex with a sharp upstroke and good amplitude characterizes good monophasic signals. If local flap or skin grafting techniques are employed, additional information about skin blood flow is needed before vascular surgical intervention can be deemed necessary.

DUPLEX IMAGING

This technique has been a component of the noninvasive vascular laboratory for more than 2 decades. It is most useful in the evaluation of patients with peripheral vascular disease as well as of any patient who will need microvascular composite tissue transplantation (free flap) techniques in the reconstruction of soft tissue loss. Through the use of a real-time B-mode imaging system combined with a pulsed Doppler unit, it is possible to obtain a combination of anatomic, geometric, and velocity data as well as blood flow measurements from most desired locations within the vascular system.

A two-dimensional image may be "stored" digitally on a monitor to obtain accurate measurements and is updated continuously or by request while the transducer is used in the pulsed Doppler mode. The position of the incident Doppler beam with respect to the vessel axis may be displayed on the B-mode imager, and the computed angle of the sound beam can then be used to provide measurements of blood flow and red cell velocity within the discrete region where flow is being measured, referred to as the sample volume. The data can be stored and reviewed at a later time or printed on film. The B-mode image is used to identify the vessel of interest and to recognize anatomic variants, localized stenoses or occlusions, and atherosclerotic plaques. The image allows accurate placement of the sample volume and ensures a constant angle of the incident Doppler beam with respect to the vessel axis.

The directional Doppler signals are analyzed both audibly and by spectral analysis. In patients with peripheral arterial disease, the degree of involvement can be classified by the pulsed Doppler signal because the changes seen in the overall waveform contour, peak systolic velocity, and spectral width are characteristic. In patients without significant vascular disease, the technique is useful to determine the best location for microvascular arterial anastomosis as well as to give both anatomic and functional data on the superficial and deep venous systems.[11]

REGIONAL TISSUE PERFUSION MEASUREMENTS

More recent investigations of peripheral ischemic conditions by noninvasive methods have centered on the microcirculation. Transcutaneous oxygen tension ($TcPO_2$) measurement recordings, laser Doppler velocimetry, and quantitative fluorometry with sodium fluorescein and a digital dermofluorometer are currently available techniques to better predict whether local flap procedures, skin grafts, or secondary closure techniques will be successful in patients with monophasic waveforms on Doppler examination.[18-22]

$TcPO_2$ monitors contain a chemical electrode that is placed both in the area in question (referred to as peripheral) and over the left side of the chest just inferior to the clavicle (referred to as the central or the reference position). The electrode is heated to 44°C to activate a local vasodilatory response within the surface of the skin. Resting measurements are obtained with the patient standing after a 10- to 15-minute equilibration interval. In studies performed on patients with foot ulcers, the ulcers healed in nearly all patients with $TcPO_2$ of 25 mm Hg or greater. The measurements are simple and reproducible, with little procedural risk.

ANGIOGRAPHY

If either vascular surgical intervention (bypass or angioplasty) or free flap reconstruction is necessary, angiographic delineation of the blood supply about the ankle and foot is often mandatory. Angiography provides important anatomic information about vessel patency, direction of blood flow, and location of arterial stenoses (which may be overestimated or underestimated, depending on the plane of the radiograph). The qualitative and quantitative physiologic effects of these diseased segments are best enumerated by the techniques already noted. Duplex imaging also supplements the data obtained in the vascular laboratory.

Sensory Evaluation

In patients with neurotrophic ulceration of the foot, it is important to evaluate the distribution of the sensory loss. Spotty sensory loss over the plantar aspect of the foot as a result of prior lumbosacral spine problems may lead to neurotrophic ulceration, which may be treated with neurovascular island flaps from sensate areas. If a similar patient has sensory loss in the tibial nerve distribution but has intact sural or peroneal nerve sensibility, nerve transfer surgery may help restore protective sensation to the weight-bearing sole of the foot. Nerve conduction studies have been helpful in clarifying some of these issues and should be performed as part of the diagnostic evaluation.

Compartment Pressure Measurement

Compartment syndrome of the foot, like that in the leg, must be evaluated and treated if necessary. The signs and symptoms of compartment syndrome of the foot are similar to those of compartment syndrome in general. Pain that is out of proportion to the clinical examination is often the first symptom. Weakness of the toe flexors and extensors and pain with passive dorsiflexion of the toes represent important physical signs. Pallor, paresthesia, a palpably tense compartment, and absent digital pulses on Doppler assessment eventually occur. Compartment pressure recordings should be obtained by a physician who understands the compartmental anatomy of the foot.

Gait Analysis

Abnormalities of gait can be detected in most patients evaluated for soft tissue repair. Midfoot and forefoot ulceration will be accompanied by shortening of the Achilles tendon with resultant increases in weight-bearing pressures over these regions during ambulation, especially in patients with diabetes mellitus. Patients with prior transmetatarsal amputations and recurrent forefoot ulceration are a second group of patients with biomechanical disturbances accounting for their wounds. These problems are usually related to equinus deformity as well as varus abnormalities. Soft tissue repair should be accompanied by Achilles tendon lengthening or tibialis anterior tendon transfer. Finally, patients with chronic heel ulceration will often be found to bear excessive weight on this area during gait. This may be a result of a prior Achilles tendon lengthening procedure that was done to excess or a previously undetected injury to the Achilles tendon. Reconstruction should include some method of shortening or strengthening of this important musculotendinous unit.

Preoperative evaluation of gait should include a measure of ankle dorsiflexion as well as an F-scan analysis. In evaluation for equinus deformity, the leg must be held in complete extension in an effort to keep the gastrocnemius muscles at their full resting length. F-scan gait analysis uses multiple pressure-sensing surface probes that record pressures on the sole of the foot during all phases of gait. Areas of excessive compression during weight bearing can be displayed in graphic format to help plan the biomechanical components of the required reconstruction (Fig. 160-14). The changes that occur with tendon transfer or lengthening procedures may be documented as well with this technique.

Bone Assessment

Plain films should be obtained before any surgical intervention on the foot is planned. Bone spurs, bone prominences, malunion, nonunion, and other deformities or abnormalities are readily identified with these simple studies. This information is extremely useful in the formation of an operative plan.

The presence of osteomyelitis in conjunction with an open wound of the foot is *not* common when plain radiographs are normal. Whenever abnormalities on plain films suggest osteomyelitis, it is important to obtain additional studies before committing the patient to a prolonged course of parenteral antibiotics. The proper approach to the evaluation of the bone structures of the foot is detailed later in this chapter in the discussion of the diabetic foot. If osteomyelitis is suspected, a bone biopsy should be performed in a separate approach rather than by obtaining tissue

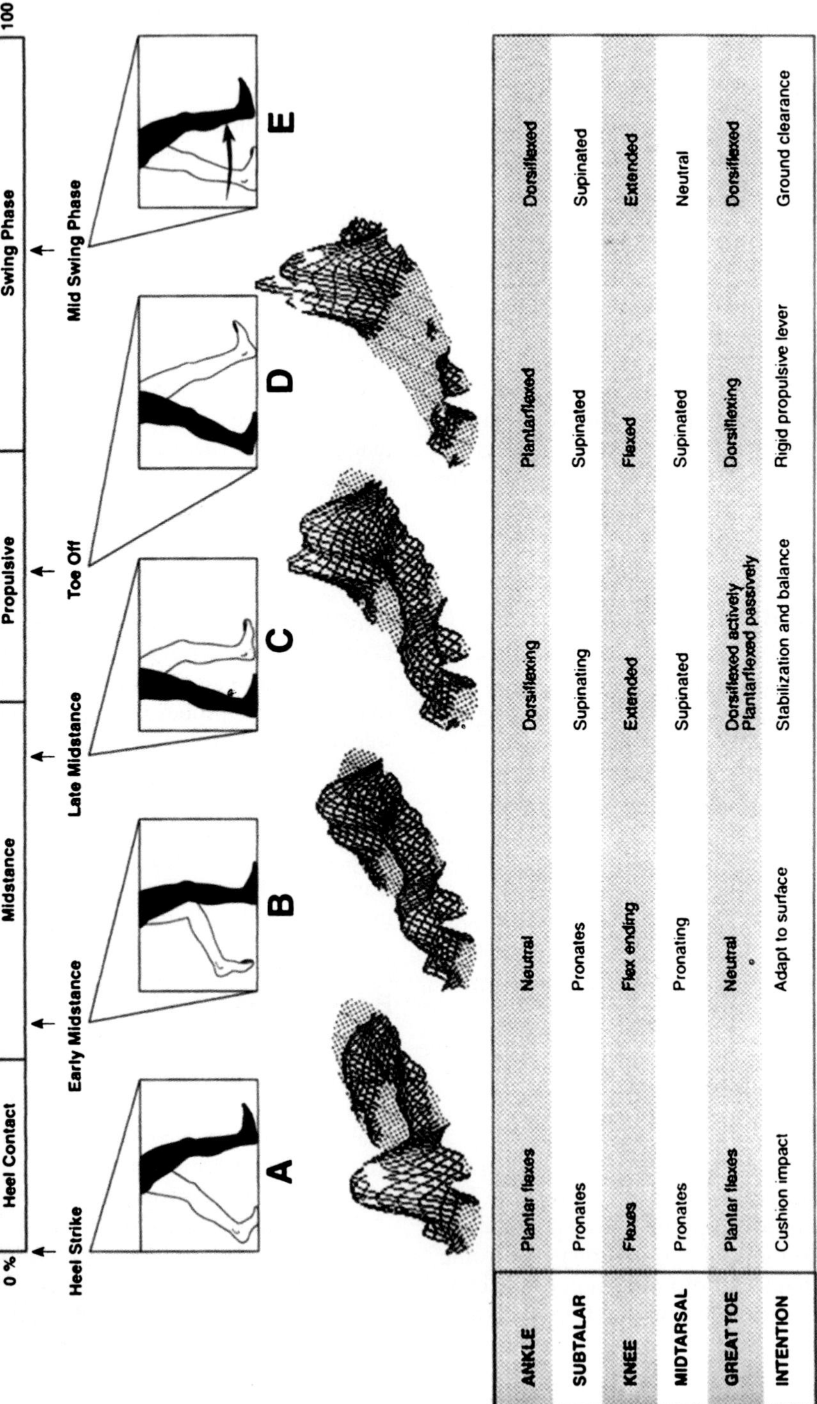

	A	B	C	D	E
ANKLE	Plantar flexes	Neutral	Dorsiflexing	Plantarflexed	Dorsiflexed
SUBTALAR	Pronates	Pronates	Supinating	Supinated	Supinated
KNEE	Flexes	Flex ending	Extended	Flexed	Extended
MIDTARSAL	Pronates	Pronating	Supinated	Supinated	Neutral
GREAT TOE	Plantar flexes	Neutral	Dorsiflexed actively Plantarflexed passively	Dorsiflexing	Dorsiflexed
INTENTION	Cushion impact	Adapt to surface	Stabilization and balance	Rigid propulsive lever	Ground clearance

FIGURE 160-14. The normal gait cycle with representative F-scan pressure mapping and joint function.

directly through the ulcerated wound. Most often, however, bone is sampled through the operative site because it is often present at the base of the débrided wound. In these instances, medullary tissue should be obtained with a previously unused curet and submitted for both decalcification (in formalin) and culture and sensitivity (in a few drops of normal saline solution). On the basis of the results of these studies, accurate selection of antibiotics may be performed.

The precise evaluation of the extent of sequestra in patients with chronic osteomyelitis can be a formidable problem. Isosulfan blue dye may be used to help distinguish viable from nonviable bone. This dye has been administered either systemically[23] or regionally through a superficial vein.[24] The regional technique allows one to use a lower total dose of the dye and a lower concentration. An intravenous catheter is placed through a superficial vein on the dorsum of the foot. An ankle tourniquet is then inflated and 10 mL of 0.1% isosulfan blue dye is injected, followed by catheter removal. During a period of minutes, the bone and soft tissues of the foot become stained with the dye. The contrast between unstained, avascular bone and soft tissue and the stained tissue is readily apparent, thus facilitating precise débridement techniques.

MANAGEMENT

Initial evaluation involves a thorough examination of the patient, with attention to wound location, involvement of contiguous structures, and vascular status of the limb. Crush injuries or ischemic insults to the foot can elevate pressures within the myofascial compartments. In measuring the compartment pressures of the foot, it may be difficult to determine the compartment in which the pressure is actually being recorded. If clinical indications are present, a four-compartment release should be performed.[25]

Compartment Release

The medial approach to the foot, as advocated by Henry,[26] allows decompression of all four compartments with a single incision. Mubarek and Hargens[27] have advocated two longitudinal incisions on the dorsum of the foot through which the interosseous compartments may be decompressed (as in the hand). Whitesides[28] anecdotally described compartment syndrome of the foot secondary to burns and direct trauma and recommended decompression by the medial approach of Henry.

For compartment decompression, a curvilinear incision is made on the medial side of the foot, beginning at the first metatarsal head and extending to the heel. Both the skin and fascia are divided and the flap is then reflected plantarly to permit visualization of the abductor hallucis muscle and its tendon, thus decompressing the medial compartment. The abductor hallucis is retracted toward the plantar surface and the medial intermuscular septum is opened, providing for release of the central compartment. The small toe compartment may be released next by a linear incision along the lateral aspect of the foot from the level of the fifth metatarsal head to the calcaneus. This approach adequately releases the fascia enveloping the small-toe compartment. Decompression of the interosseous compartment is best achieved through two linear incisions on the foot dorsum overlying the second and fourth metatarsals. The fascia overlying the four interosseous spaces may be opened (Fig. 160-15).

Patients with chronic ulceration of the foot may require initial débridement to obtain soft tissue and bone cultures and to determine the full extent of the wound. The care of a thoroughly débrided wound requires the use of topical agents that maintain a moist environment as well as bacteriologic control. Subatmospheric pressure dressings may achieve these goals while simplifying the nursing care required. Special emphasis should be placed on the use of compressive elastic wrap support and non-weight-bearing ambulation before definitive wound closure is performed.

Soft Tissue Reconstruction

Reconstruction of soft tissue defects of the foot remains a complex and challenging undertaking despite advances in the transfer of fasciocutaneous, musculocutaneous, and composite tissue flaps. The plantar skin is a unique weight-bearing surface. The glabrous epidermis and dermis are much thicker than in other areas of the body, including the hands, and measure up to 3.5 mm. The vertical fibrous septa tend to resist the shearing forces of ambulation and produce numerous "shock absorbers" by enclosing the subcutaneous fat into discrete compartments. In planning a plantar foot reconstruction, three principles should be observed to achieve an optimal result. First, the underlying cause of the wound must be investigated because it will have implications for the reconstruction. Second, the underlying bone architecture and its dispersion of weight must be thoroughly evaluated because a bone resection, osteotomy, or other procedure may be necessary to help provide durability to the soft tissue repair. Third, if possible, the reconstruction should provide some degree of protective sensation.

Many of the local flaps discussed in this chapter depend largely on antegrade blood flow in their parent vessels (posterior tibial artery and its branches). The presence or absence of peripheral vascular disease, therefore, greatly affects the type of reconstruction to be performed. On the foot dorsum and in the Achilles region, the skin is thinner and more mobile; reconstructive techniques employed for the plantar

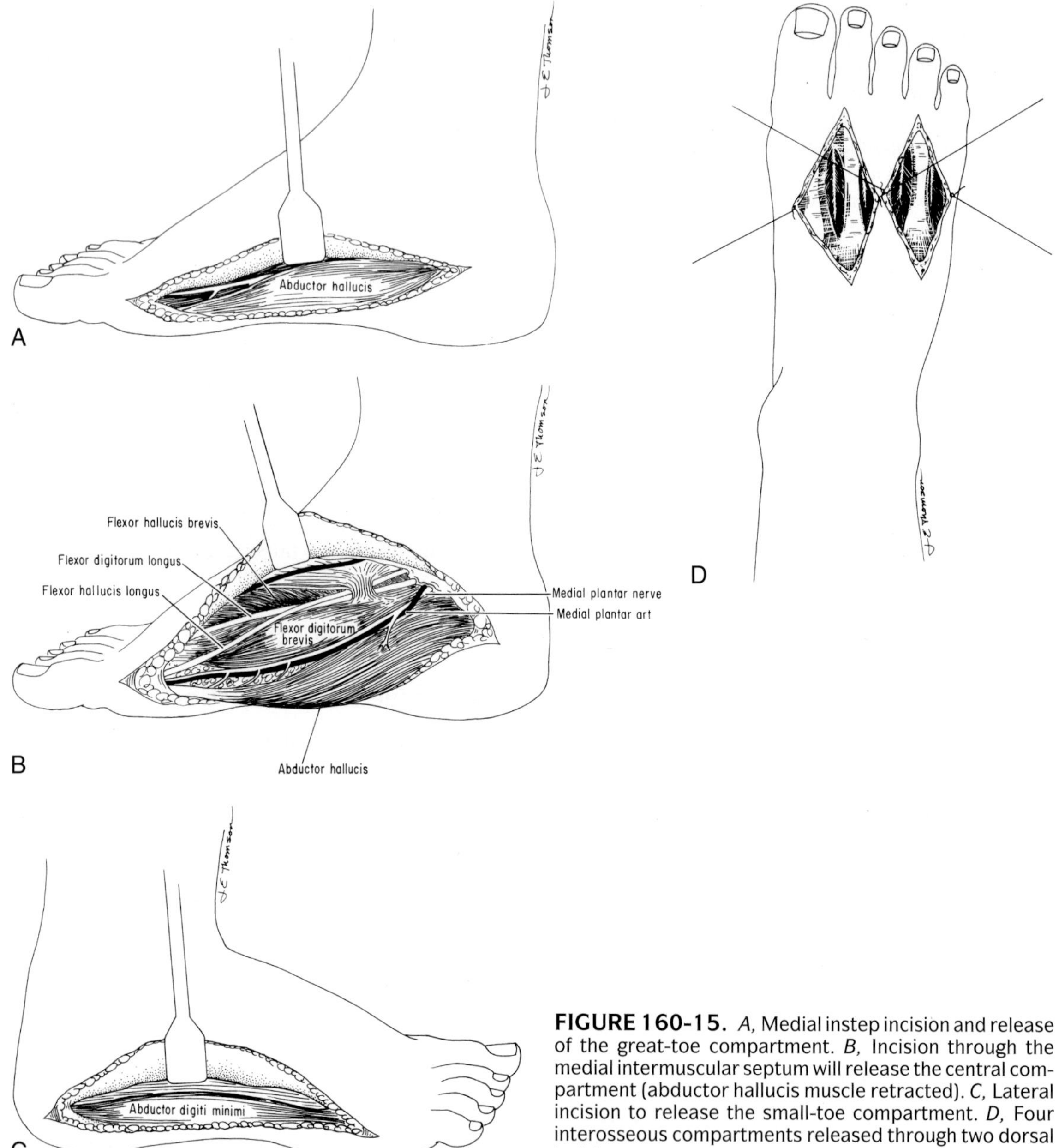

FIGURE 160-15. *A,* Medial instep incision and release of the great-toe compartment. *B,* Incision through the medial intermuscular septum will release the central compartment (abductor hallucis muscle retracted). *C,* Lateral incision to release the small-toe compartment. *D,* Four interosseous compartments released through two dorsal incisions.

surface may be entirely inappropriate for these two locations.

In general, skin grafting techniques are appropriate for shallow defects, especially on non-weight-bearing surfaces. On the plantar surface, however, split-thickness skin grafts are usually unstable for prolonged periods, and about 50% of patients require additional reconstructive procedures.[29,30] Innervated full-thickness skin grafts have been employed in selective patients by use of a defatted skin flap in the sural nerve territory, leaving the nerve intact,[31] or by the transfer of grafts from the great toe or forearm, with nerve repair being performed between donor and recipient tissues.[32] Although somewhat useful, this latter form of reconstruction requires a healthy soft tissue bed to permit graft "take." Bone devoid of periosteum or tendon without paratenon will not accept a skin graft; hence, flap closure must be considered. Large defects or "unfavorable" local tissues require flaps from distant locations. Because the reconstructive options vary according to location, it is best to differentiate between four distinct locations: the Achilles area, ankle, and foot dorsum; the plantar forefoot; the plantar midfoot; and the plantar hindfoot.

ANKLE AND FOOT DORSUM

Most shallow wounds on the foot dorsum may be safely closed with a split-thickness skin graft. Often, as a result of infection, the wound causes exposure of devitalized extensor tendons. When exposure occurs, these structures may be excised and a skin graft applied to the periosteum of the underlying bones. Depending on the patient's associated medical problems, excision of viable tendon devoid of paratenon may be preferable to composite tissue transplantation for dorsal foot wounds (Fig. 160-16). In general, however, large areas of exposed bone or tendon will require flap coverage.

Abductor Hallucis–Abductor Digiti Minimi Muscle Flaps

The abductor hallucis muscle, with or without the medial head of the flexor hallucis brevis, and the abductor digiti minimi muscle have been useful for closing small proximal dorsal foot wounds.[33] Because these muscles are most often used for closure of plantar hindfoot wounds, they are discussed more thoroughly in that section.

Extensor Digitorum Brevis Muscle Flap

The extensor digitorum brevis muscle may be transposed proximally to cover the ankle, the dorsal foot, and malleolar wounds, provided the anterior tibial-dorsalis pedis artery has antegrade blood flow. The blood supply to the muscle is derived from the lateral tarsal artery, which is a branch of the dorsalis pedis artery at the level of the distal edge of the extensor retinaculum. Exposure is obtained through a curvilinear incision on the foot dorsum that communicates with the wound to be closed. The entire dorsalis pedis pedicle is divided distally to the origin of the lateral tarsal vessels to provide the needed arc of rotation for muscle transposition. The long extensors are then dissected off the underlying short extensor muscle slips, and then the dorsalis pedis artery and its associated veins are divided distal to the extensor digitorum brevis. The medial tarsal branches are ligated as the dissection proceeds proximally. The lateral tarsal vessels are elevated with the muscle while the origin and tendinous extensions of the muscle are divided. The four slips of the muscle are broad and thin, measuring 4.5×6 cm in the adult, making the flap useful for relatively small wounds (Fig. 160-17).[34]

Sural Neurocutaneous Flap

Although the sural flap works well for coverage of the anterior ankle and the malleoli (Fig. 160-18), it is more frequently used for hindfoot and Achilles soft tissue repair. The details of elevation and transposition of this flap are discussed in that section.

Lateral Supramalleolar Flap

The lateral supramalleolar flap has been most useful in the coverage of bone defects that accompany loss of soft tissue over the lateral malleolus and anterior ankle. The flap should be distally based because the blood supply is derived from the perforating branch of the peroneal artery as it pierces the interosseous membrane 5 cm proximal to the tip of the lateral malleolus. Cutaneous vessels then course upward, anterior to the fibula, and anastomose with the vascular network that accompanies the superficial peroneal nerve.

The perforating branch of the peroneal artery may be located with the hand-held Doppler probe. The base of the flap should be centered at this point. Flap width includes the tissue between the fibula and tibia. The length should be adequate to reach the malleolus (6 to 8 cm) or more distally as dictated by wound location.[35] Most often, the tissue is developed as a fascial flap, turned over like a page of a book, and its surface skin grafted. When the flap is designed in this manner, the donor site may be closed directly.

The skin incision is made so that skin flaps may be elevated off the underlying deep fascia. The fascia is then incised along its anterior margin and progressively reflected until the perforating branch is seen. Branches of the superficial peroneal nerve course within the fascia and must be divided to permit safe elevation and rotation. Final release of the flap will require incision through the posterior margin and release of its attachments to the septum that separates the anterior and lateral muscle compartments (Fig. 160-19).

PLANTAR FOREFOOT

The area from the midshaft of the metatarsals distally is referred to as the forefoot. Local flaps play a major role in the reconstruction of deep wounds of the distal third of the foot. Severe injury or infection of a single toe may be managed best by toe or ray amputation. Plantar or dorsal flaps of the proximal toe skin may usually be fashioned for simple closure. If additional skin is necessary, an adjacent toe may be filleted and transposed for closure. Ray amputation (digit plus associated metatarsal) may be necessary, especially if the associated metatarsal is severely infected, devascularized, or otherwise irreparable (Fig. 160-20).

Transposition of local tissues may take many forms. Metatarsal head ulceration is extremely common in patients with peripheral neuropathy and associated arthropathy. Numerous techniques have been described, some of which are discussed here. First introduced by Moberg[36] in 1964, the neurovascular island flap of a filleted toe remains a useful technique today for forefoot repair.[37,38] When a metatarsal head wound is closed with the soft tissue from an associated toe, flap dissection as an island is not necessary because

Text continued on p. 1424

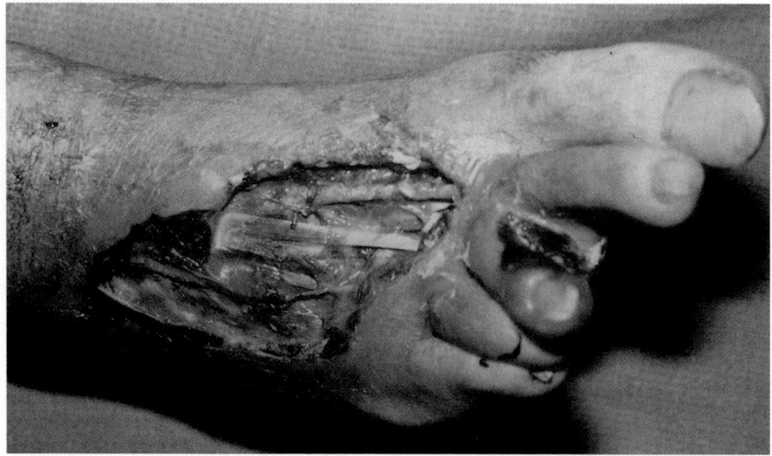

A

B

C

FIGURE 160-16. *A,* Ischemic foot with extensive dorsal soft tissue loss. *B,* After revascularization and débridement of nonviable tendons and third toe. *C,* Several months after split-thickness skin grafting.

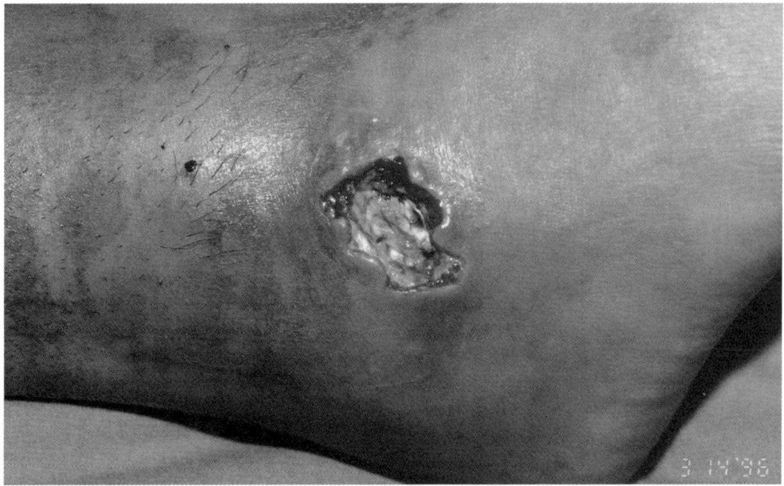

A

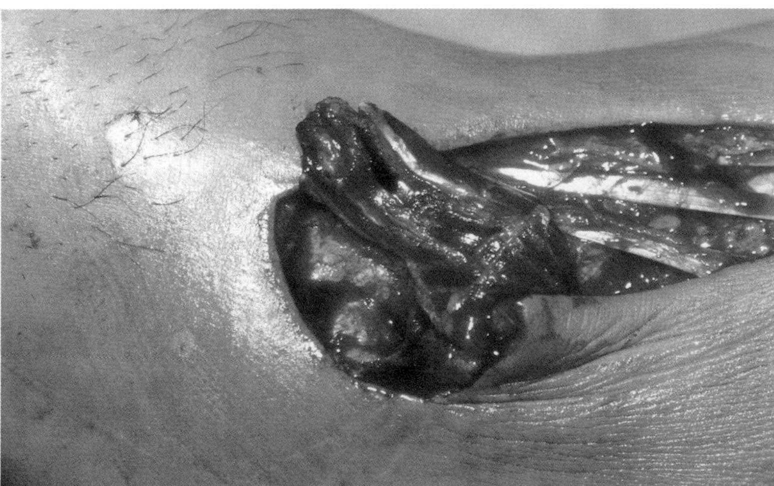

B

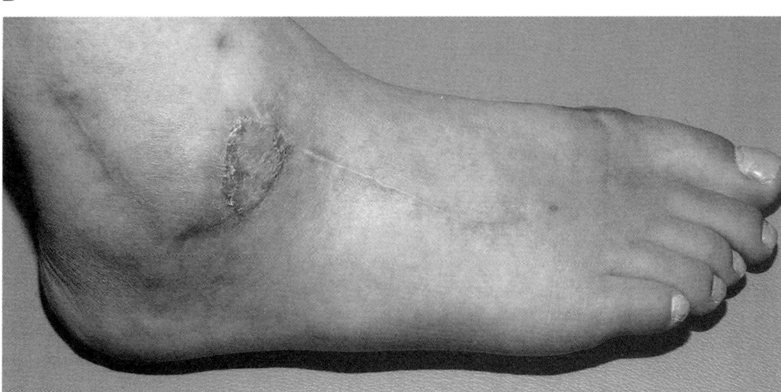

C

FIGURE 160-17. *A,* Chronic anterolateral ankle wound. *B,* The wound has been débrided and the extensor digitorum brevis muscle flap has been transposed. *C,* Three months after skin grafting of the muscle flap.

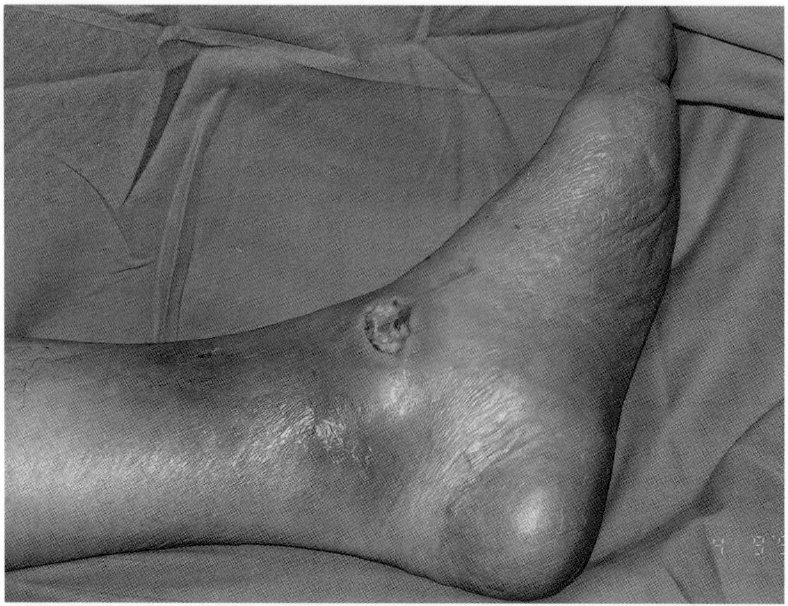

A

B

FIGURE 160-18. *A,* Anterolateral ankle wound after open reduction and internal fixation. *B,* Closure after screw removal and sural flap transfer.

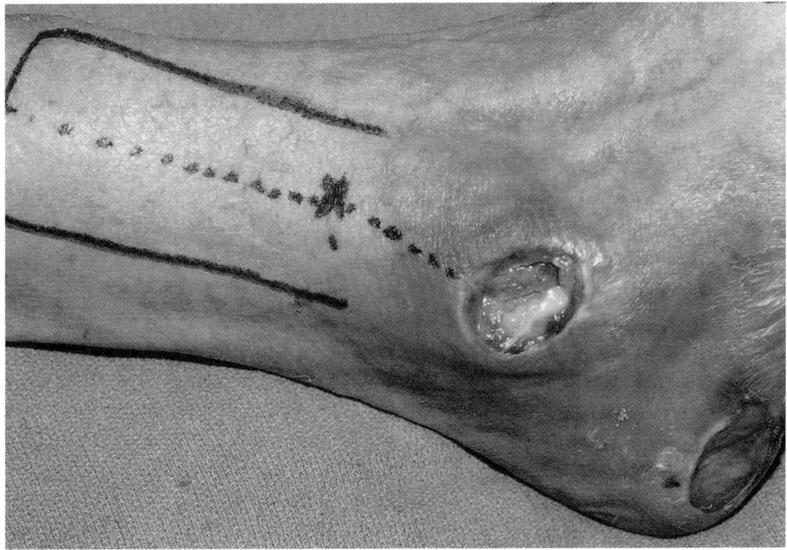

A

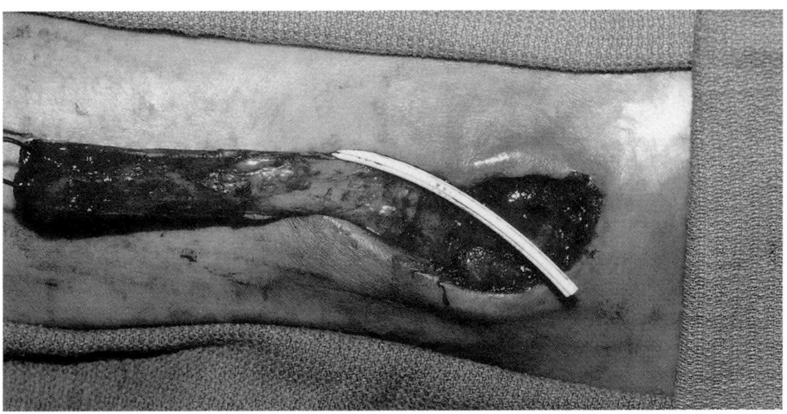

B

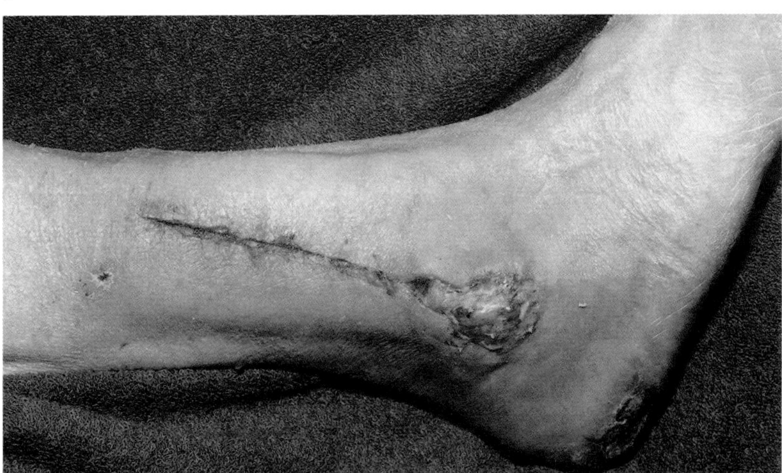

C

FIGURE 160-19. *A,* Lateral malleolar ulcer with bone exposure; outline of fascial flap to be elevated. *B,* After flap elevation. A drain has been placed. *C,* Healed after being covered with a split-thickness skin graft.

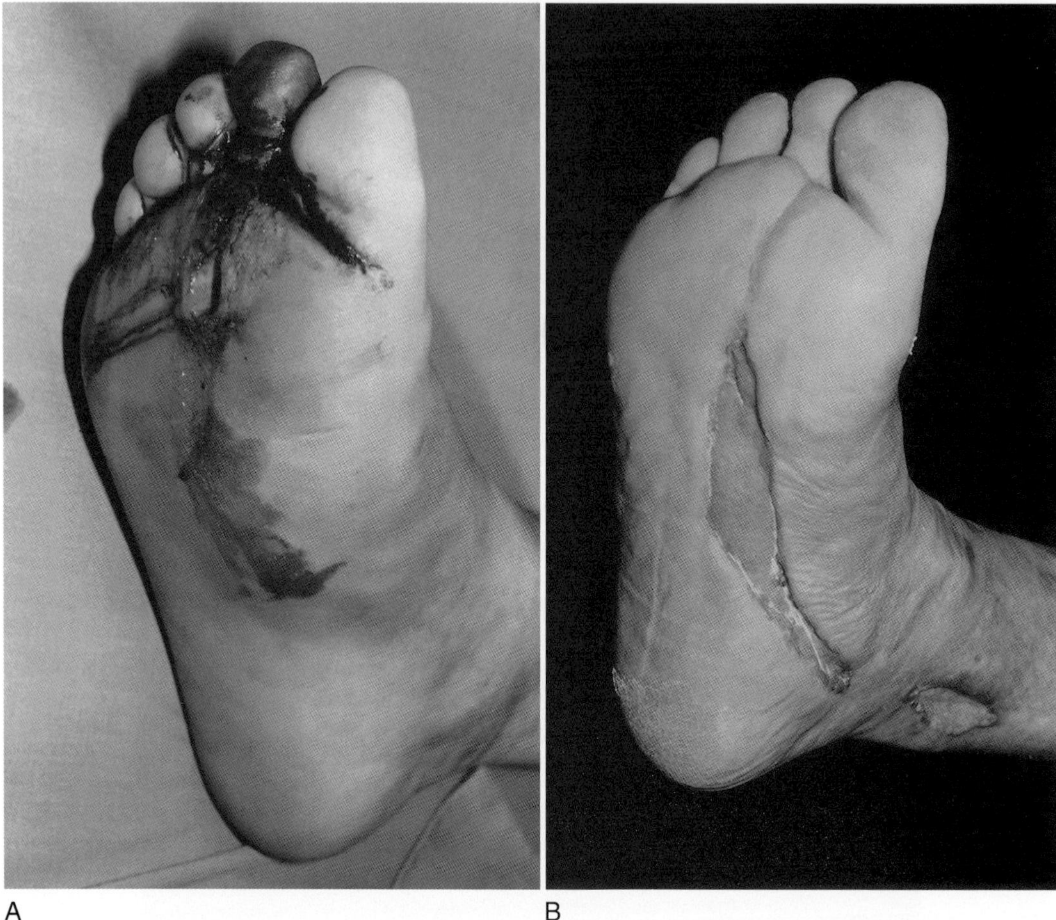

FIGURE 160-20. *A,* Chronic second metatarsal head ulcer with acute infection. Note associated toe gangrene and plantar abscess. *B,* After serial débridement, ray amputation, and split-thickness skin grafting to the instep.

the mobilization obtained by removal of the bone framework is often enough to permit effective wound closure.[39-41]

Toe Fillet Flap

This island flap is dissected most easily with the patient in the supine position under tourniquet control.[38] The plantar wound is débrided, and the flap of adjacent toe soft tissues is outlined. The flap is elevated, beginning distally, off the distal phalanges and flexor tendons. The medial and lateral neurovascular bundles are identified in the associated web spaces. A connecting incision is made between the flap and the wound to permit transposition and safe placement of the neurovascular structures. The remnant toe is then disarticulated at the metatarsophalangeal joint level, and the dorsal skin is used for donor site closure (Fig. 160-21). As with other neurovascular island flaps, no discrete venous drainage is obvious. The tourniquet is deflated, hemostasis is obtained, and the wounds are closed. If necessary, more proximal dissection of the plantar neurovascular structures may extend the flap's arc of rotation to more proximal locations. When the great-toe pulp is the chosen donor site, a dominant first dorsal metatarsal artery may make the dissection more tedious and require division of the superficial and deep transverse metatarsal ligaments to permit flap transfer.

Neurovascular Island Flap

Alternatively, a neurovascular island flap from the fibular side of the great toe may be used without sacrificing the entire toe. Depending on flap size, the donor site is closed either directly or with a split-thickness skin graft.[42,43] The flap is centered over the area of the Doppler pulse of the fibular neurovascular bundle of the great toe. As in the island toe flap procedure, the use of a tourniquet as well as magnifying loupes facilitates the safe completion of the procedure. The flap is outlined and then elevated on the

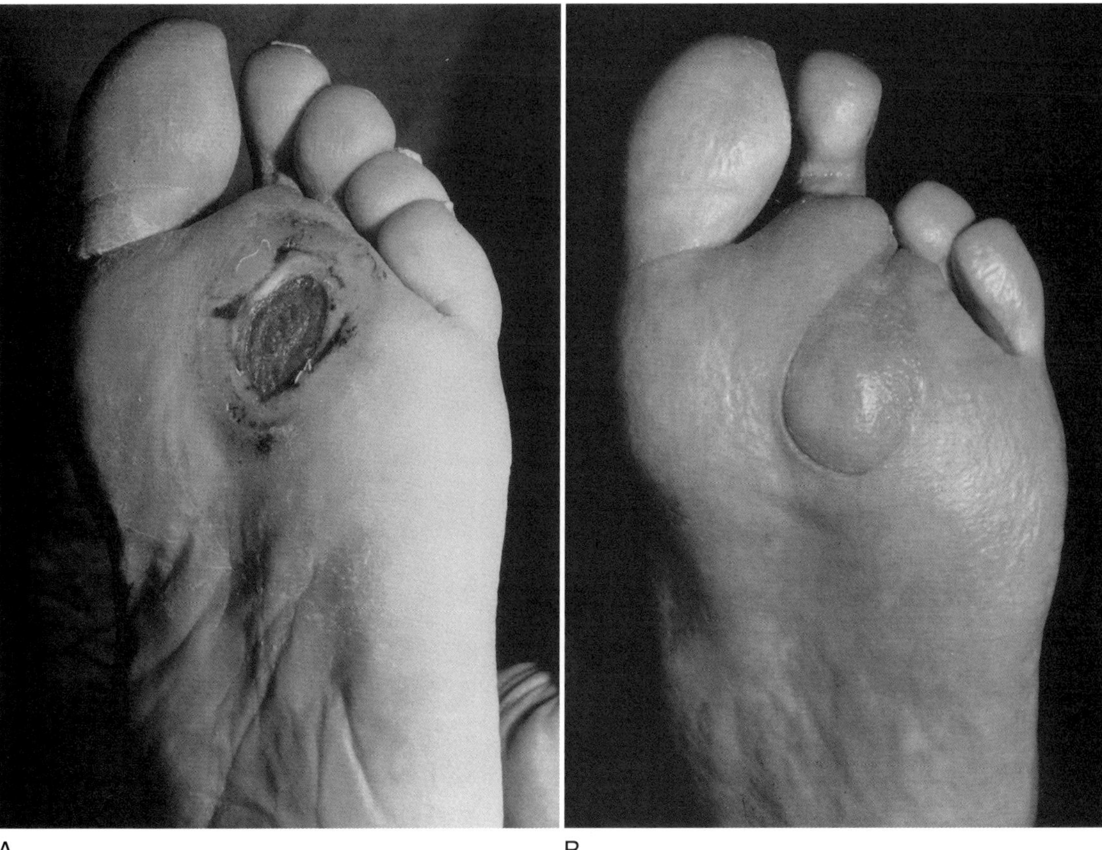

A B

FIGURE 160-21. *A,* Neuropathic ulceration of the third metatarsal head region. *B,* Closure obtained with an adjacent toe fillet flap.

lateral plantar aspect of the great toe at the level of the phalangeal periosteum. Identification of the digital neurovascular bundle in the web space permits a more proximal dissection if necessary. A connecting incision is made from the web space to the débrided wound to transpose the flap. These techniques are effective for wounds up to 2 to 3 cm in diameter. The preoperative work-up must include assessment of the vascular status of the extremity (Fig. 160-22).

V-Y Plantar Flap

Forefoot skin, fat, and fascia may be advanced in a V-Y fashion either singly or in pairs to close wounds up to 4 to 5 cm^3. Anatomic studies of fresh cadavers and latex (Microfil) injections have revealed numerous vertical perforating vessels throughout the plantar aspect of the foot. The location of these perforators facilitates the design of many different V-Y advancement flaps (Fig. 160-23). Under tourniquet control, the wound is débrided and an adjacent V-Y flap is outlined and incised. The plantar fascia about the circumference of the flap must be completely incised as well. Careful division of the septal attachments to the underlying metatarsal may further aid in flap advancement. After release of the tourniquet, hemostasis is obtained and the wound is closed (Fig. 160-24). Wounds too large to be managed with one flap may be reconstructed with two opposing flaps without difficulty.

Suprafascial Flaps

Medially or laterally based flaps of plantar skin and fat may be advanced to cover wounds of the forefoot, with skin graft applied, if necessary, to the non-weight-bearing instep donor site.[44,45] Although popular in the 1970s, this technique has been largely supplanted by the other procedures already discussed. It is still useful in plantar hindfoot repair because the instep donor site may be closed in a V-Y fashion (see section on the plantar hindfoot).

Forefoot Amputations

Reconstructive surgeons managing patients with foot ulceration should be well versed in the options available for forefoot amputation; these procedures will often be the simplest way to provide stable soft tissue closure and bipedal ambulation. Transmetatarsal

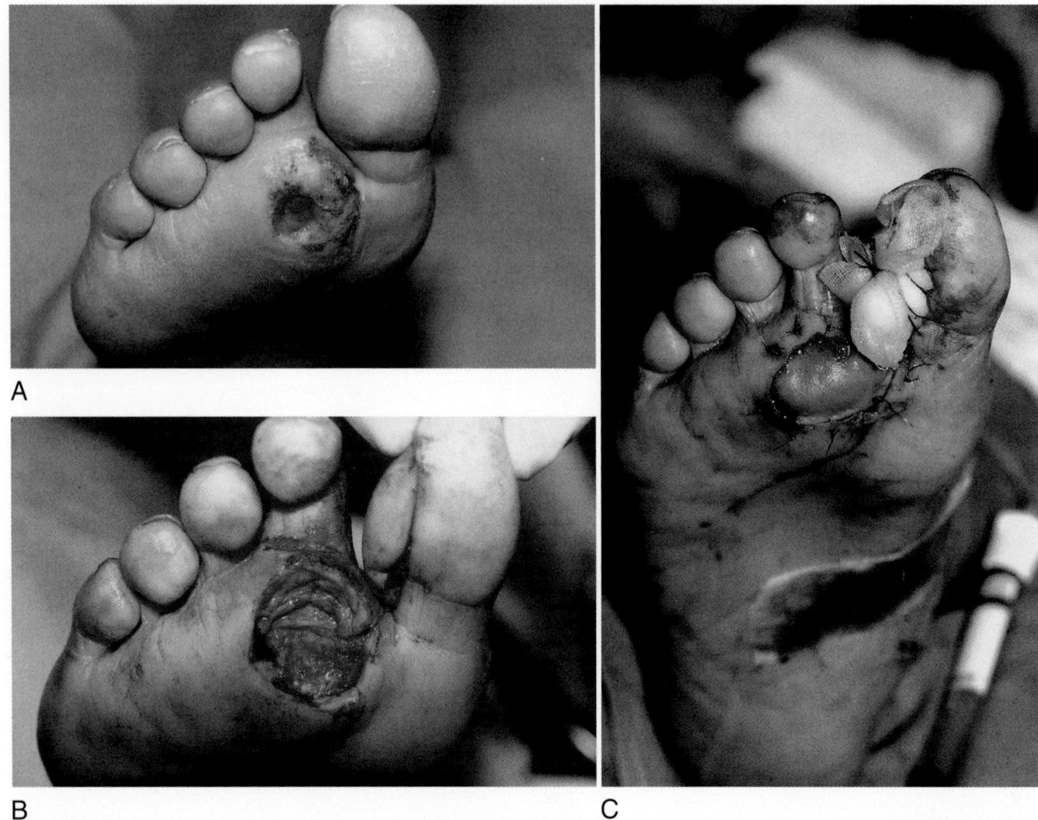

FIGURE 160-22. *A,* Chronic ulceration of the plantar forefoot. *B,* The wound has been débrided and the neurovascular island flap elevated. *C,* After flap inset and release of the tourniquet. A skin graft from the instep was used to close the donor site.

amputation is indicated when three or more rays have been deleted. This is usually accomplished by advancement of a plantar flap of skin, subcutaneous tissue, and fascia over the metatarsal stumps. With significant plantar ulceration, however, one may have to use dorsal soft tissues for this purpose. The key is to preserve as much soft tissue as possible (both dorsal and plantar) so that length may be maintained and suture lines are free of tension. More proximal applications of the transmetatarsal amputation may be necessary in some patients. In these situations, care should be exercised to avoid injury to the vertical descending branch of the dorsalis pedis artery. This vessel courses between the first and second metatarsal bases and is at risk for injury when bone resection is necessary nearby. In patients with significant stenoses in the posterior tibial artery, the vertical descending branch of the dorsalis pedis artery may be the only blood supply to the plantar forefoot.

Transmetatarsal amputation provides an excellent functional level for post-traumatic, ischemic, or neuropathic patients as long as the blood supply is adequate, the patient is nutritionally sound, and any infection or necrosis has been thoroughly eradicated.[46] No formal prosthetic or orthotic device is necessary, and the patient may wear normal shoes with a small, distal insert. Attention should be paid to avoiding equinus deformity, which will often lead to recurrent stump ulceration. If necessary, Achilles tendon lengthening should be recommended to avoid this complication (Fig. 160-25).

PLANTAR MIDFOOT

The midfoot is defined as the region between the proximal tarsal row and the midshaft of the metatarsals. It comprises the medial non-weight-bearing arch as well as the more lateral weight-bearing soft tissues. Small wounds in this region may be closed by any of the options discussed previously for the forefoot. Split-thickness skin grafts may be adequate, provided the transverse arch of the foot has been maintained. This implies that the midfoot remains largely a non-weight-bearing region.

Neurovascular Island Flaps

The neurovascular island procedures discussed previously are useful for the repair of 2- to 3-cm defects.

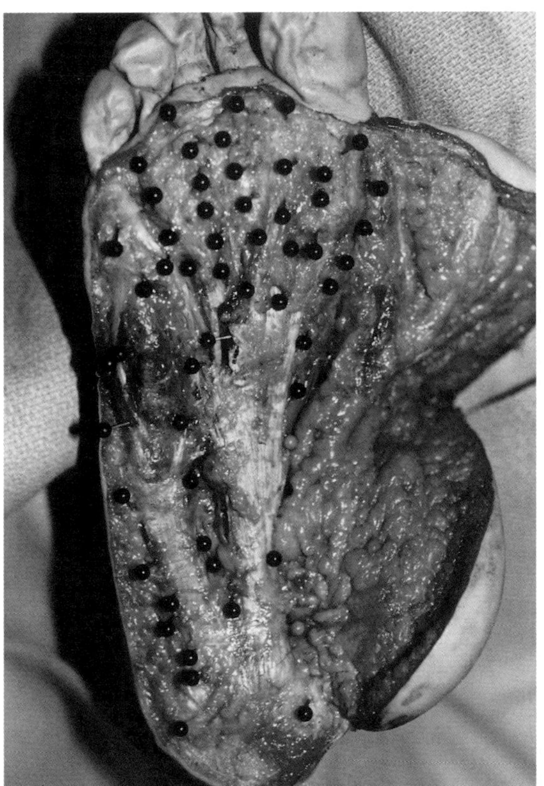

FIGURE 160-23. Location of multiple cutaneous vascular perforating vessels on the plantar aspect of the foot.

This repair necessitates a more proximal dissection of the vessels and nerves from the plantar surface of the foot. If the dominant circulation is from the first dorsal metatarsal artery, division of the deep transverse metatarsal ligament will be necessary to permit flap transfer and inset (Fig. 160-26).

V-Y Advancement Flap

V-Y advancement flaps are also helpful in this region. The anatomic studies discussed earlier provide a basis for such techniques. Adequate mobilization requires complete release of the plantar fascia about the perimeter of the flap. Any underlying bone prominences should be managed with ostectomy, osteotomy, or fusion as indicated by the specifics of the defect (Fig. 160-27).

Suprafascial Flaps

Medially or laterally based plantar flaps have been described and appear to be another reconstructive alternative.[47] Tourniquet control allows a bloodless dissection. Medially based flaps are raised by incising laterally and elevating the subcutaneous tissues off of the abductor digiti minimi muscle and plantar fascia from lateral to medial. The medial dissection allows identification and preservation of the cutaneous branches of the medial plantar nerve as they emerge from the cleft between the abductor hallucis and the plantar fascia. With continued elevation of the flap off of the plantar fascia, branches of the medial plantar artery and nerve are seen coursing into the flap from the cleft between the plantar fascia and the abductor hallucis muscle. When the flap is elevated in a proximal dissection, the medial and lateral branches of the plantar nerve are separated from the main trunk for a short distance to preserve flap sensation without sacrificing flap motility. For the laterally based flap, a similar dissection may be performed; however, all branches of the medial plantar artery are sacrificed to permit flap rotation.

Microvascular Composite Tissue Transplantation (Free Flaps)

Wounds larger than 4 to 5 cm generally require either free flap reconstruction or midfoot amputation for stable soft tissue coverage to be obtained. Microvascular composite tissue transplantation is extremely useful in trying to maintain foot length in patients with "guillotine" type midfoot amputation. As such, it is an alternative to more proximal Syme or below-knee amputations. Adequate soft tissue coverage may be provided without additional bone resection (Fig. 160-28). Because the use of free flaps is more common in the hindfoot, a more detailed discussion follows in that section.

Midfoot Amputations

Deformities at the tarsometatarsal junctions (Lisfranc joint) occur when a shortened gastroc-soleus complex alters normal ankle motion. The inability to fully dorsiflex at the ankle puts undue strain across Lisfranc joint during gait. Over time, the inability to fully dorsiflex the ankle leads to increased compensatory motion at the midfoot level with breakdown of Lisfranc joint and resultant midfoot deformity. Soft tissue ulceration is inevitable and commonly seen in diabetic patients as well as in others with peripheral neuropathy.

Patients who are not candidates for the reconstructive procedures previously discussed may be best served with a midfoot amputation. Midfoot amputations may be the preferred "repair" because the procedure is simple and may be performed relatively rapidly without the significant morbidity associated with more complex reconstructions. If patients are appropriately chosen and the procedure is executed properly, one may be able to salvage a limb that provides a stable platform for ambulation without increasing the energy expenditure involved. The two most common forms of midfoot amputation are the Lisfranc amputation and the Chopart amputation.

The Lisfranc amputation involves removal of all metatarsal remnants. Amputation at the

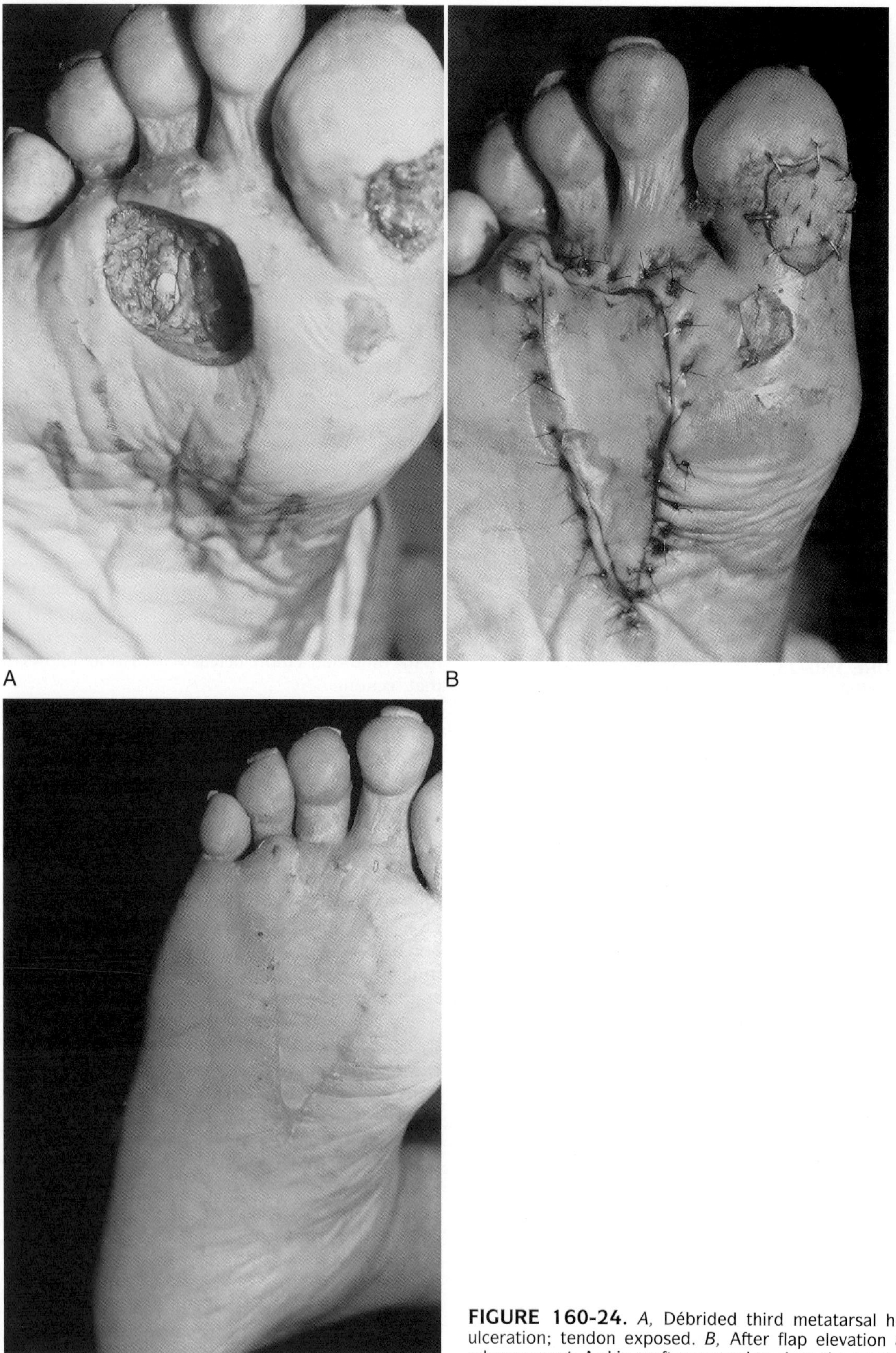

A

B

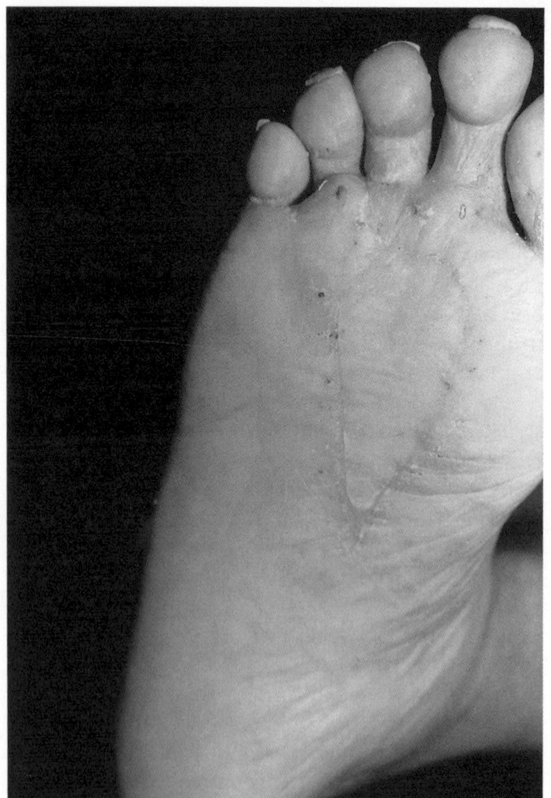

C

FIGURE 160-24. *A,* Débrided third metatarsal head ulceration; tendon exposed. *B,* After flap elevation and advancement. A skin graft was used to close the great-toe wounds. *C,* Appearance at 2 months after surgery.

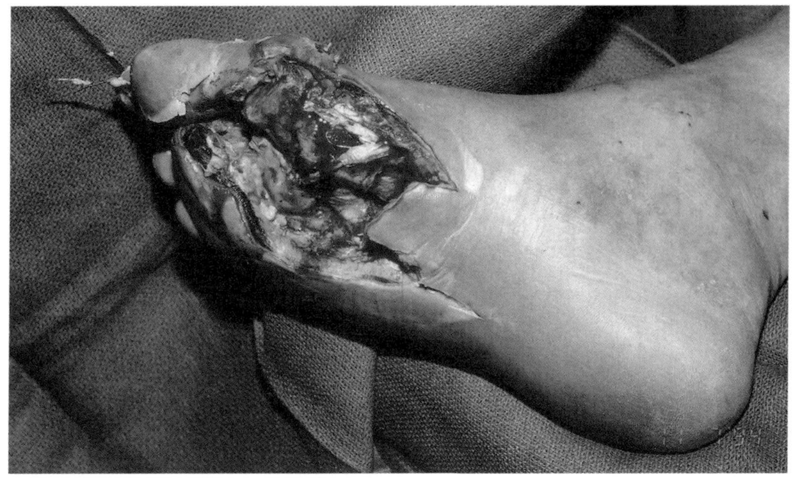

A

B

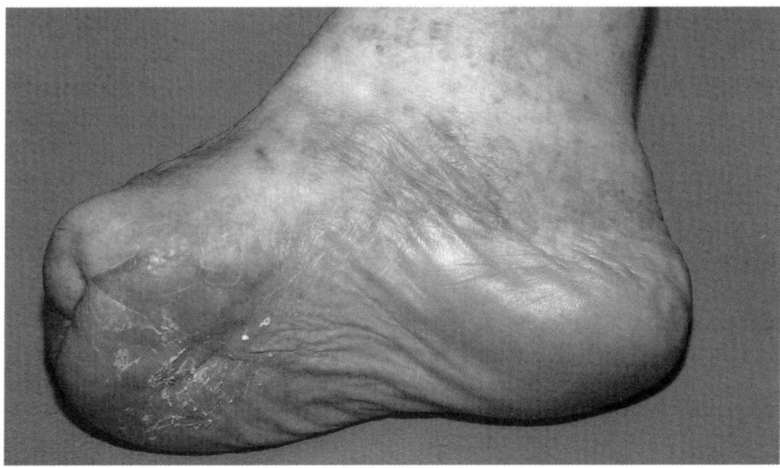

C

FIGURE 160-25. *A,* Complex forefoot wound with significant tissue loss. *B,* After débridement as a "fillet" of forefoot procedure. The laterally based flap will close the wound. *C,* Six months postoperatively.

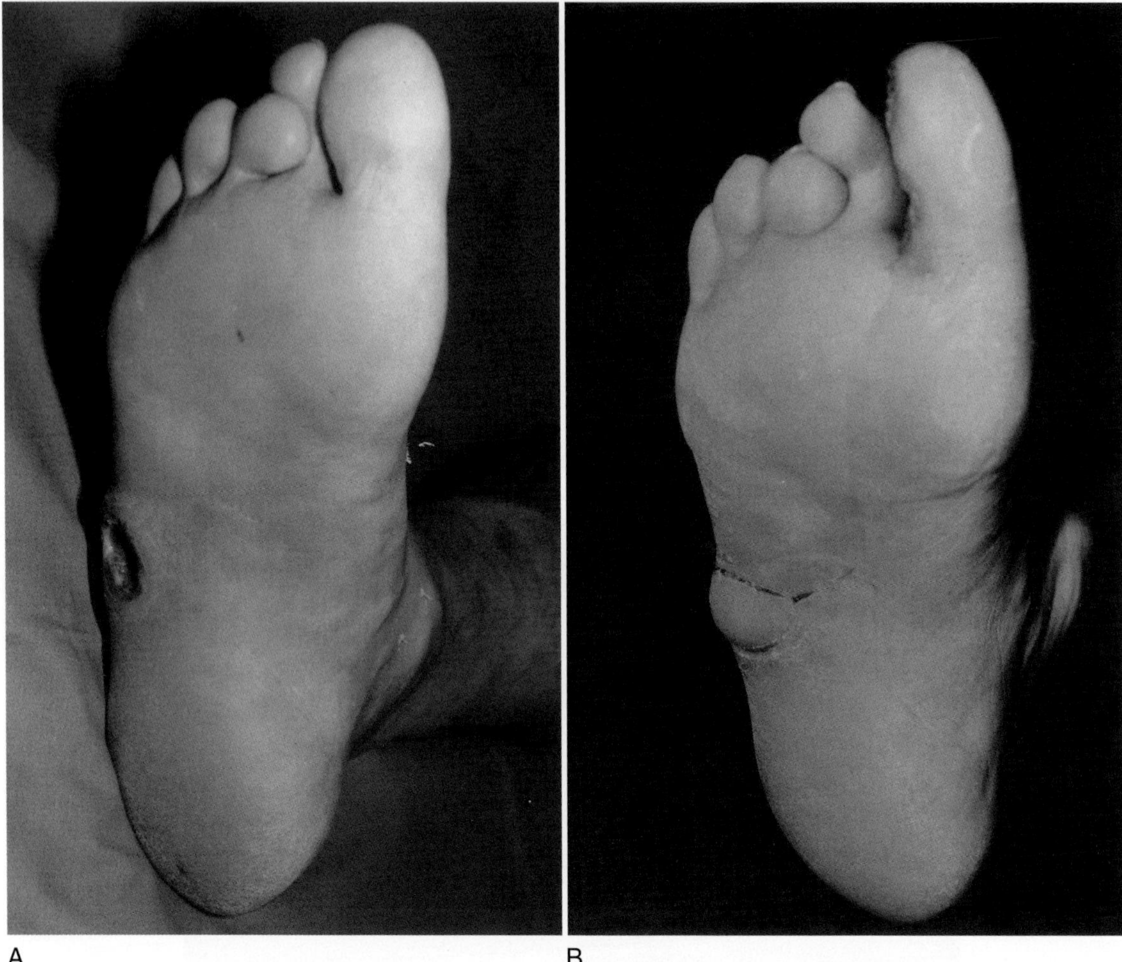

FIGURE 160-26. *A,* Lateral midfoot wound in a patient with intact medial plantar nerve sensibility but absent lateral plantar nerve function. *B,* After neurovascular island flap transfer from the lateral side of the great toe. Because of a dominant dorsal circulation, mobilization required division of the deep transverse metatarsal ligament and dissection of the first dorsal metatarsal artery.

tarsometatarsal joint (Lisfranc level) is associated with a high rate of equinovarus deformity. Although some would argue that tendon transfers and joint stabilization are necessary to prevent this late deformity, others have found that a simple, transcutaneous Achilles tendon lengthening, performed at the time of the midfoot amputation, effectively prevents these late changes. Patients have little need for custom footwear and generally return to their previous ambulatory level with little if any increase in energy expenditure (Fig. 160-29).[48]

The Chopart procedure requires an intertarsal resection and is therefore a more proximal amputation, just distal to the cuboid and navicular. Like the Lisfranc amputation, the Chopart procedure will affect the patient's ability to dorsiflex and evert the involved foot because the insertions of the peroneal tendons as well as the tibialis anterior tendon will be disrupted as a result of the amputation. Lengthening of the Achilles tendon and repositioning of the tibialis anterior tendon more laterally on the foot dorsum will greatly assist the reconstruction and help prevent recurrence. Postoperatively, the limb is cast in dorsiflexion for 4 to 6 weeks.[49]

PLANTAR HINDFOOT

Hindfoot soft tissue repair provides the greatest challenge to the reconstructive surgeon. The hindfoot is a specialized location, with specific requirements for its repair. In addition to the thick, durable heel pad and the underlying calcaneus, the Achilles tendon and its thin, pliable soft tissue envelope must be managed appropriately. Reconstruction should provide durable soft tissues for safe weight bearing while permitting nearly normal ankle motion. More than in any other

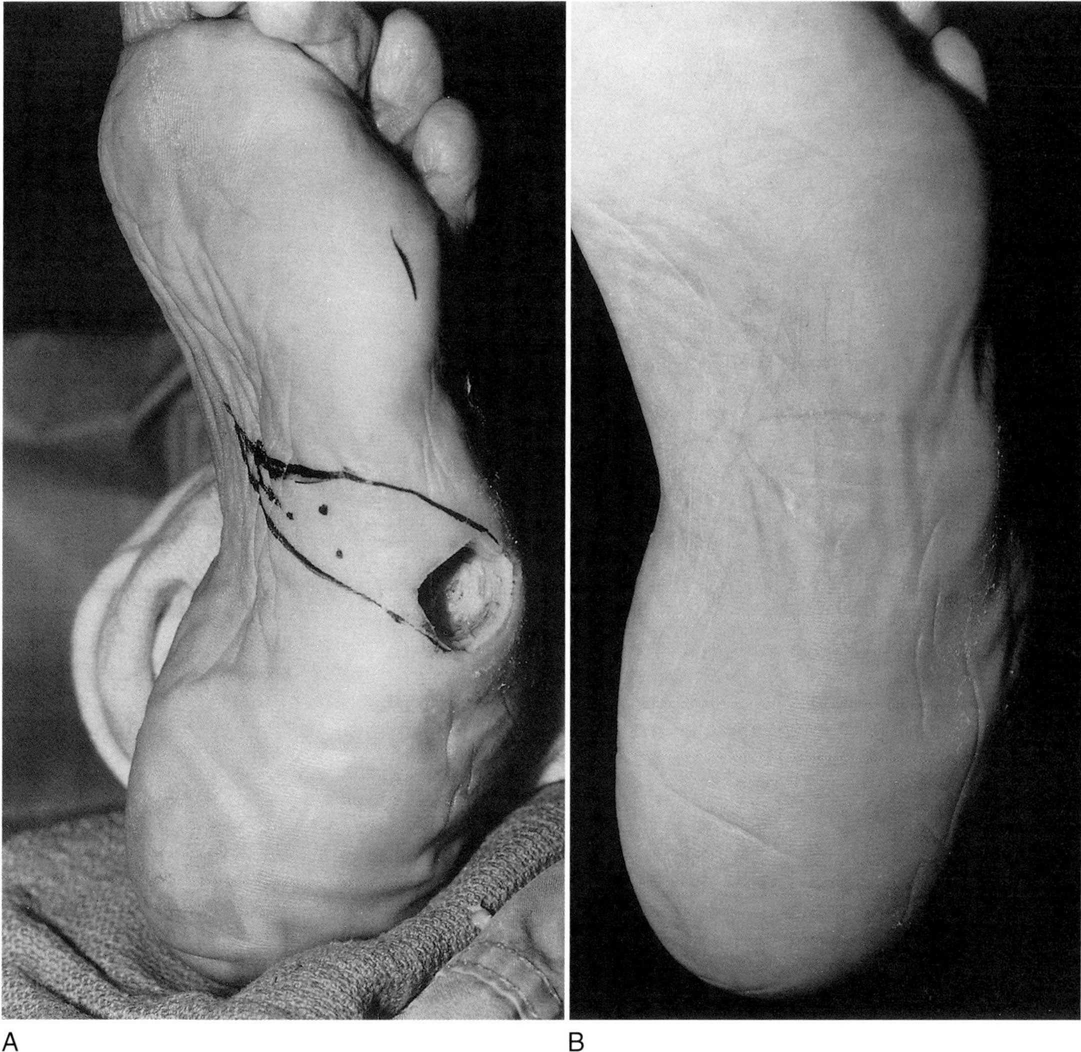

FIGURE 160-27. *A,* Lateral midfoot wound secondary to severe Charcot midfoot deformity. *B,* After débridement of the cuboid, subtalar fusion, and soft tissue repair with a V-Y advancement flap.

region of the foot, the surgeon must consider both form and function when managing wounds in this area.

Tendons from the muscles of the posterior, deep posterior, and lateral compartments of the leg traverse this region as they enter the foot. One of the most important and frequently injured is the Achilles tendon. The posterior tibial artery and tibial nerve lie between the flexor digitorum longus and the flexor hallucis longus tendons, posterior to the medial malleolus. These structures, along with the tibialis posterior tendon, travel beneath the laciniate ligament (flexor retinaculum) to enter the foot. The sural nerve and the lateral leg compartment musculature also pass posterior to the lateral malleolus to enter the foot. Loss of tissue in this location, whether through trauma or disease, is a catastrophe that may cripple the patient permanently or mandate a below-knee amputation.

During the past 4 decades, numerous local flaps have been described to facilitate wound closure in the hindfoot. All of the techniques discussed for more distal locations may be used in heel reconstruction, although they are probably not first-choice options. The following discussion includes those procedures that have withstood "the test of time" and are commonly used today.

Intrinsic Muscle Flaps

Three intrinsic foot muscles may be used to close defects of the hindfoot. The abductor hallucis, flexor digitorum brevis, and abductor digiti minimi muscles may be used individually or together to repair small

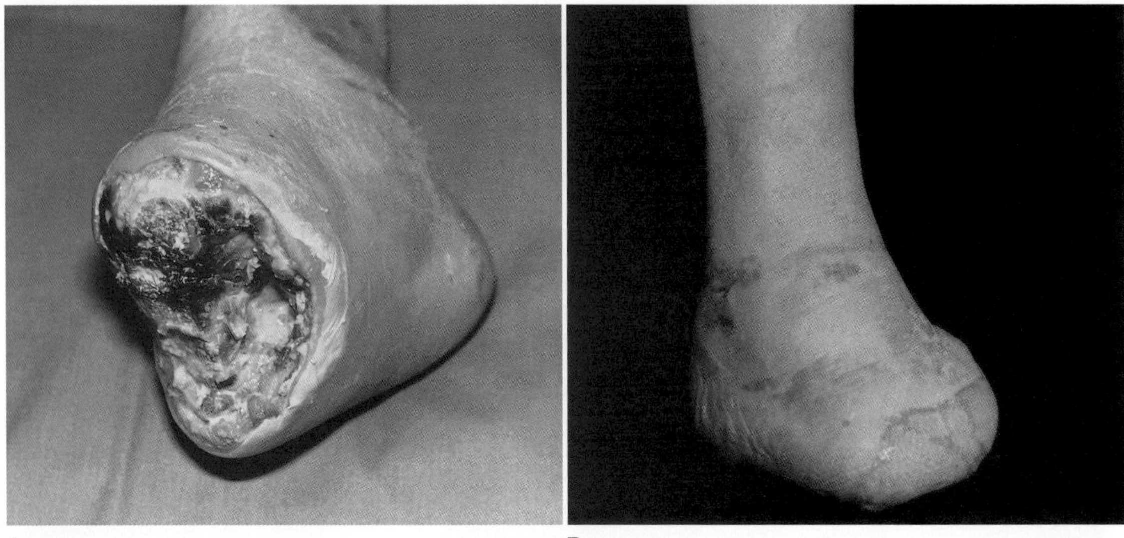

FIGURE 160-28. *A*, Guillotine midfoot amputation after embolization to the foot. *B*, After revascularization, a serratus anterior free flap and skin graft maintain limb length.

wounds in the hindfoot region.[50-55] The abductor hallucis muscle is elevated through a medial foot incision on the non-weight-bearing surface.[54] The tendon is divided distally, and the muscle is separated from the medial head of the flexor hallucis brevis, although this may be raised with the abductor if additional tissue is needed. The blood supply enters the muscle proximally as branches from the medial plantar artery. If an increase in the arc of rotation is needed, the medial plantar artery may be ligated and divided distal to the branches of the abductor, and more proximal dissection of the medial plantar artery to its origin from the posterior tibial artery can be accomplished. The muscle will cover small defects about the heel and medial malleolus (Fig. 160-30).

The flexor digitorum brevis muscle is the largest of the three muscles and is useful for heel pad reconstruction.[52] Its blood supply comes from branches of both the medial and lateral plantar arteries, with the lateral usually being dominant. The lateral plantar artery courses deep to the proximal muscle belly, where small arterial branches course into the muscle. A midline plantar foot incision is used to expose the muscle for elevation. The skin is elevated medially and

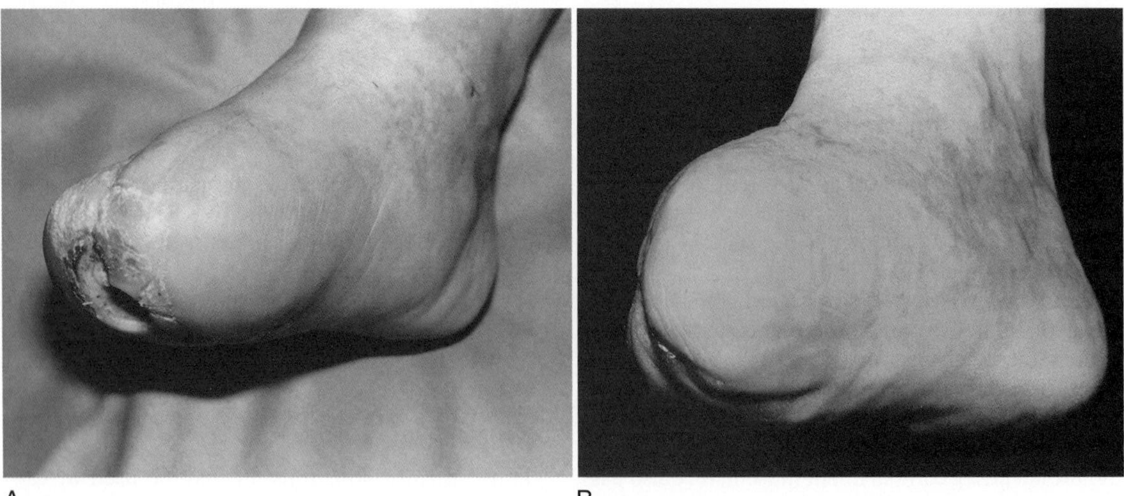

FIGURE 160-29. *A*, Recurrent ulceration of the transmetatarsal stump. *B*, Stable closure after revision to the Lisfranc level.

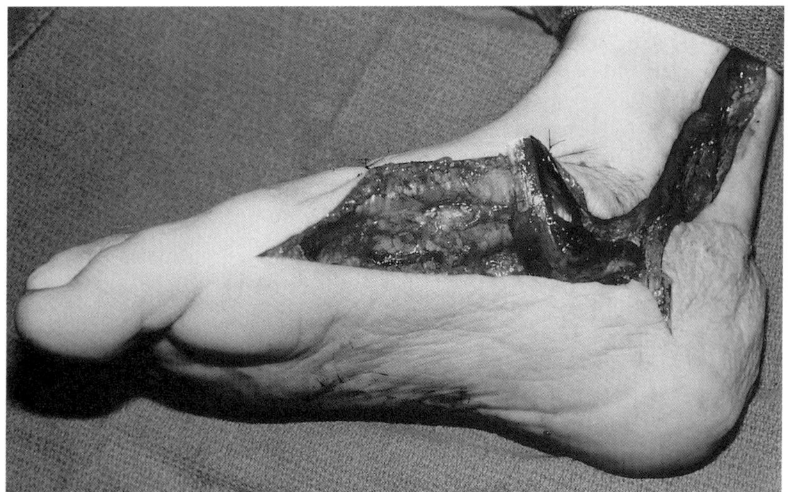

A

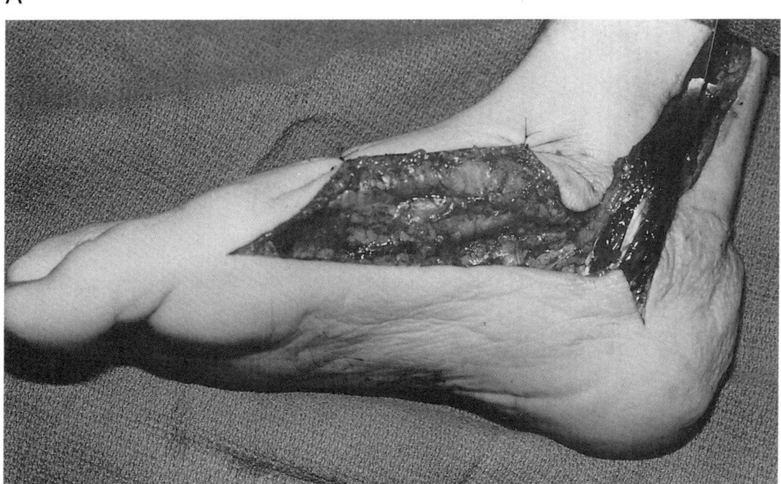

B

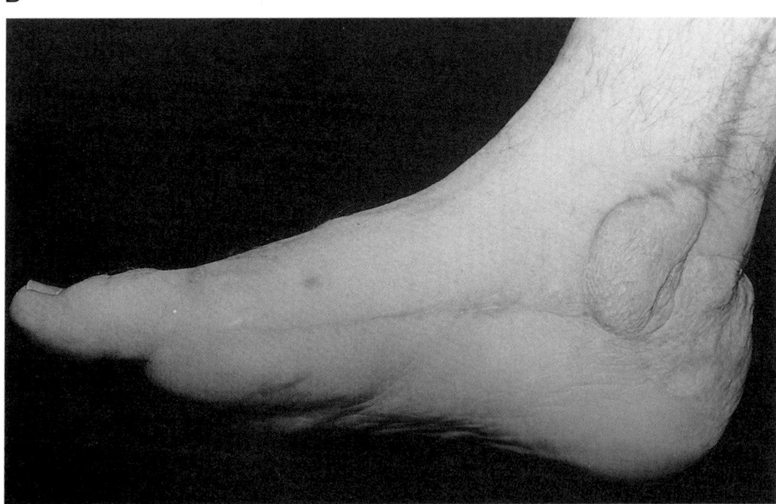

C

FIGURE 160-30. *A,* Elevation of the abductor hallucis muscle for management of persistent calcaneal osteomyelitis. *B,* More posterior mobilization is achieved by making the flap into an island based on the medial plantar artery. *C,* Two years after the procedure. The muscle was covered by a split-thickness skin graft. (A previously performed gracilis free flap is over the posterior calcaneus.)

laterally off the underlying plantar fascia. The fascia is usually elevated with the muscle to simplify the procedure and to add bulk to the flap. The four tendons are divided distally and then the muscle is turned on itself as it is dissected off the quadratus plantae muscle. Further mobilization is possible to permit the use of this flap for posterior hindfoot reconstruction.[55] This requires ligation of the lateral plantar artery after it passes beneath the muscle and proximal dissection of the lateral plantar artery to its origin from the posterior tibial artery. The division of the origin of the abductor hallucis simplifies this modification and increases the arc of rotation of the muscle flap (Fig. 160-31). A neurosensory musculocutaneous variant of this flap is possible but has been replaced largely with the use of the medial plantar island flap.

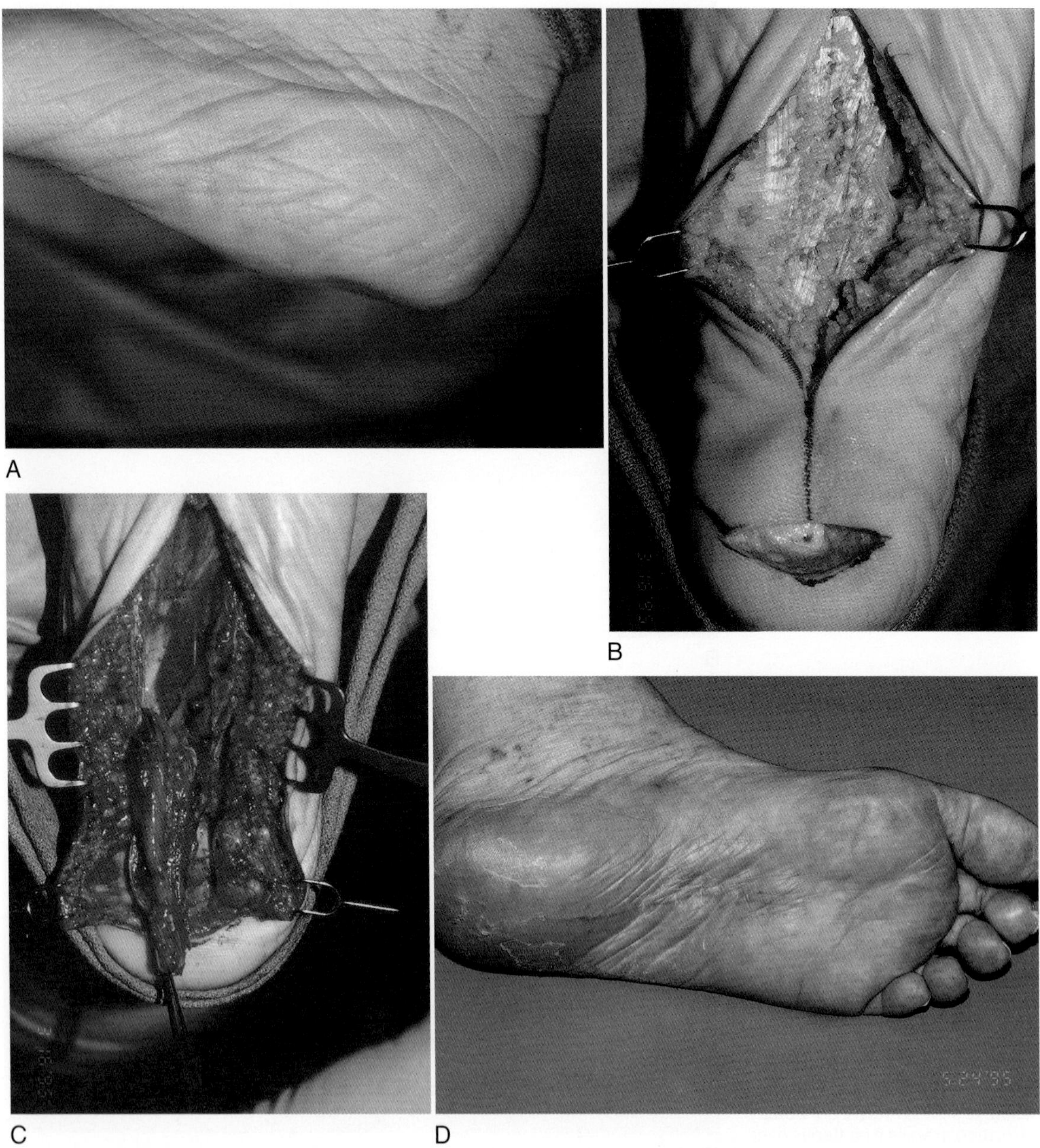

FIGURE 160-31. *A,* Lateral view of the heel with loss of the subcutaneous padding secondary to trauma. *B,* The flexor digitorum brevis muscle flap is elevated, with the plantar fascia, through a midline plantar foot incision. *C,* Posterior transposition, leaving its proximal attachments to the calcaneus intact. *D,* Two months postoperatively with good restoration of the plantar heel pad and relief of pain.

The abductor digiti minimi, the smallest of the three muscles, may be mobilized with a lateral foot incision through the non-weight-bearing skin. Both motor innervation and blood supply are derived from the lateral plantar neurovascular bundle through branches entering the proximal portion of the muscle. The muscle is detached from the fifth metatarsal and the tendinous insertion divided, allowing posterior rotation of the flap. Further rotation may be obtained by ligation of the lateral plantar artery distal to the branches to the muscle and dissection of the vessel proximally by dividing the flexor digitorum brevis and abductor hallucis muscles.[55] Use of the abductor digiti minimi muscle is not recommended. Its small size and arc of rotation significantly impair its ability to assist in wound repair. It may, however, be used in combination with the other intrinsic muscle flaps already discussed.

Medial Plantar Artery Flap

This flap is useful for heel pad reconstruction provided the instep is not a weight-bearing surface, as can occur with Charcot midfoot collapse. The donor site must be skin grafted; hence, when instep collapse is present, a relative contraindication to this procedure exists.

The instep of the foot may be elevated as a fasciocutaneous flap based on the medial plantar artery and transposed posteriorly to cover the heel.[5,7,56] If the lateral plantar artery is divided, pedicle length is increased, thus allowing its use for closure of ankle and heel wounds.[4] The great appeal of this procedure originates from the goal of reconstructing the sole of the foot with tissue from the plantar surface as was originally described almost 40 years ago.[57,58] Mir y Mir[57] used a cross-foot flap from the instep of the opposite extremity for coverage of heel defects. The flap is outlined over the medial instep of the foot centered on the medial plantar artery as isolated with the hand-held Doppler probe. The extremity is exsanguinated, and a thigh tourniquet is inflated. The distal extent of the flap is incised first, through the skin and plantar fascia. The medial plantar neurovascular bundle is readily found in the cleft between the abductor hallucis and the flexor digitorum brevis muscles. The vessels are divided and elevated with the flap. An intraneural dissection of the medial plantar nerve is performed so that the cutaneous fascicles from the plantar nerve are preserved with the flap. The dissection plane is superficial to the muscles, just deep to the plantar fascia. The deep fascial septa in the clefts between the muscles must be divided. For most reconstructions, the dissection may stop where the vessels emerge from the lateral border of the abductor hallucis muscle. However, further mobilization is possible by dividing this muscle and the laciniate ligament and tracing the medial plantar artery to its origin from the posterior tibial artery (Fig. 160-32).

Heel Pad Flaps

Small wounds over the weight-bearing and posterior heel may be closed with a suprafascial flap of heel pad based either medially or laterally.[44,50] After the flap is outlined, an incision is made and the flap is elevated off of the underlying calcaneus and the plantar fascial attachments. If the flap is based medially, the branches of the lateral plantar vessels may need to be ligated. If the flap is based laterally, the same holds true for the perforators from the medial plantar vessels (Fig. 160-33). Such flaps may be accompanied by calcanectomy, which will remove bone prominences as well as simplify the closure. Generous calcanectomy (up to one third or more of the calcaneus) may “free up” enough soft tissue to close rather large wounds without resorting to more complex reconstructive procedures. This technique is especially useful in patients with significant comorbid factors rendering them poor candidates for free flap repair (Fig. 160-34).

Sural Artery Flap

The blood supply to this flap is derived from the small arteries that accompany the sural nerve along its course just superficial to the deep fascia in the posterior aspect of the distal two thirds of the lower leg. In most patients, this will be a “vascular network,” although one may occasionally see a well-defined median superficial sural artery accompanying the nerve. There are numerous anastomoses between this network and the peroneal artery. The most important of these is the most distal one approximately 5 cm cephalad to the lateral malleolus. The vessel is usually audible with the Doppler probe, which may be useful in mapping the flap preoperatively. The flap should be outlined over the central third of the calf. Efforts to extend pedicle length by designing the skin island cephalad to this point will jeopardize flap perfusion as the sural nerve and its accompanying vessels course subfascially toward the popliteal fossa. The pedicle consists of a 2-cm-wide strip of subcutaneous tissue and fascia containing the sural nerve, its associated arteries, and the lesser saphenous vein.[59]

The flap is outlined over the raphe between the two heads of the gastrocnemius muscle. A line is drawn from the inferior edge of the flap to the pivot point for the pedicle approximately 5 cm above the lateral malleolus. Flap elevation is begun along its cephalic perimeter. Through this incision, the sural nerve and the lesser saphenous vein are identified just superficial to the deep fascia and ligated so that they may be elevated along with the overlying soft tissue. The deep fascia should be elevated with the flap to protect the aforementioned structures. The flap pedicle is formed by elevating a medial and lateral skin flap and then developing a 1.5- to 2.0-cm-wide “strip” of subcutaneous fat and fascia that harbors the sural nerve and

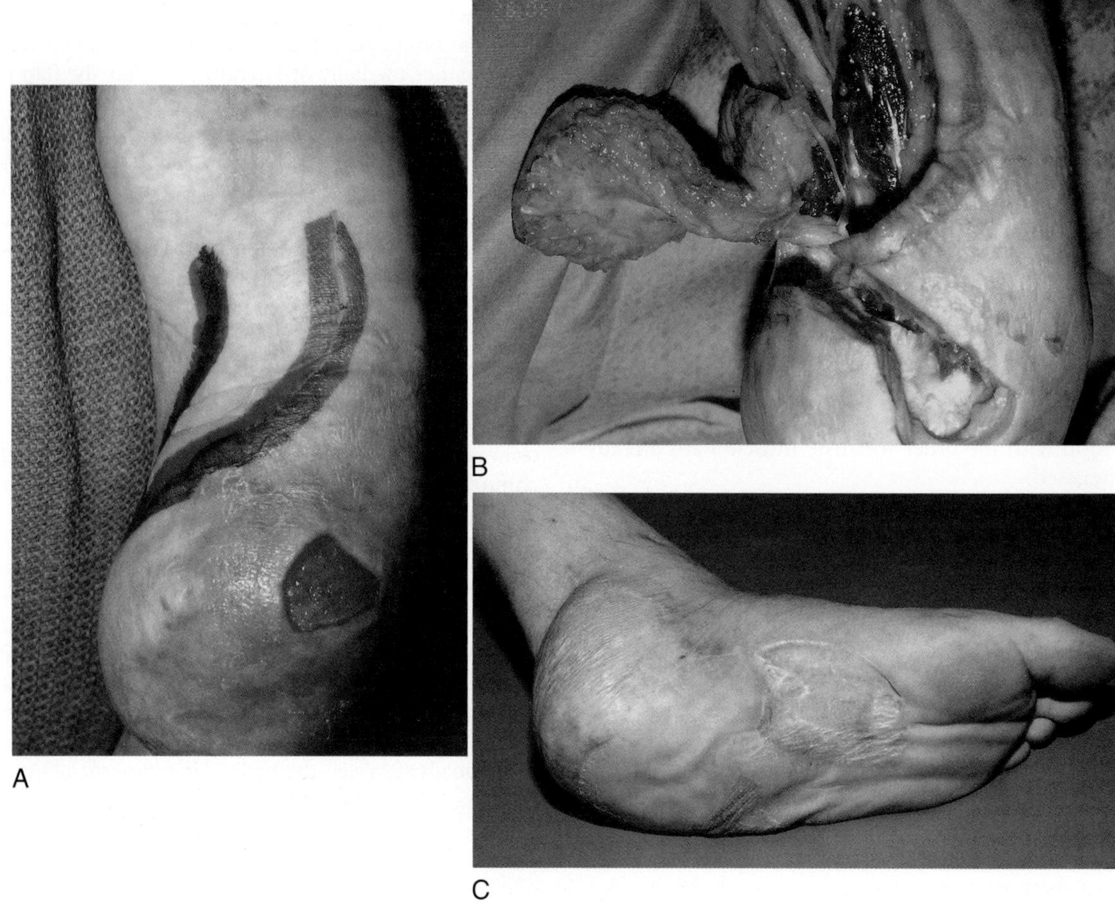

FIGURE 160-32. *A,* Chronic plantar heel ulceration through a previous latissimus free flap and skin graft after a degloving injury to the foot. *B,* The flap has been mobilized on the medial plantar vessels and is ready to be inset. *C,* Three years postoperatively.

lesser saphenous vein. The flap and pedicle may then be separated from the underlying muscle and paratenon layers. The arc of rotation will provide coverage of the posterior heel-Achilles and anterior ankle. The donor site may be closed primarily if it is small or with a split-thickness skin graft if it is larger (Fig. 160-35).

Microvascular Composite Tissue Transplantation (Free Flaps)

Large hindfoot wounds (>6 cm), defects in patients devoid of the posterior tibial vessels (from either trauma or disease), and patients who have been revascularized to the distal anterior tibial-dorsalis pedis artery by long saphenous vein grafts should be considered for reconstruction that uses microsurgical techniques. With the exception of the sural artery flap, all of the regional flaps described for hindfoot repair require antegrade blood flow in the posterior tibial artery and its branches (medial and lateral plantar arteries). As will be discussed, these procedures are often not possible in dealing with patients with significant peripheral vascular disease.

Many neurosensory flaps have been described for microvascular transplantation in an effort to provide sensation to the plantar reconstruction. Two useful donor sites are the deltoid and the lateral arm flaps.[60-62] Although the donor site scar may be undesirable, these flaps have reliable neurovascular anatomy and are relatively thin. If a suitable recipient nerve is available in proximity to the flap inset, both coverage and flap sensation are possible after microneurovascular transfer.

May[63] and others reviewed their experience with patients who underwent free muscle transplantation and split-thickness skin grafting to the weight-bearing portions of the foot and concluded that cutaneous sensibility did not appear to be necessary to maintain a functional and well-healed extremity. In a similar report, Stevenson and Mathes[64] also noted successful

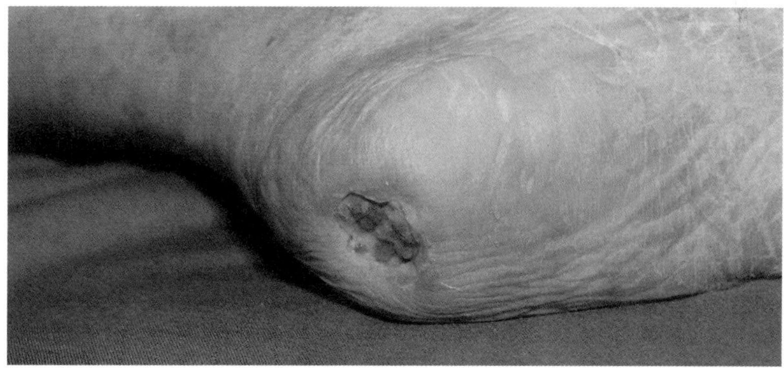

A

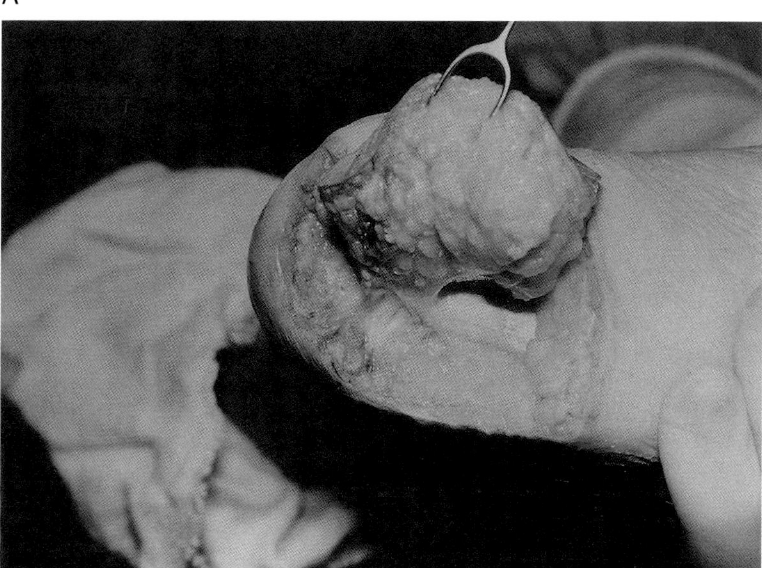

B

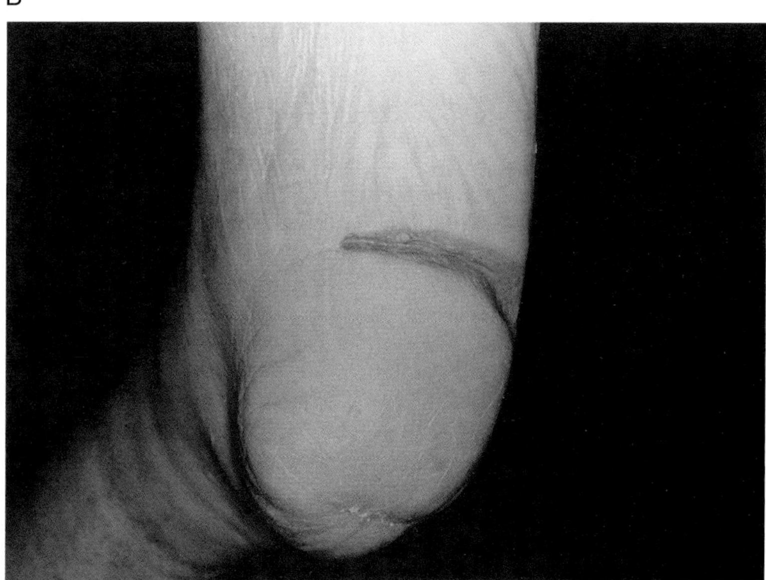

C

FIGURE 160-33. *A,* Chronic posterior heel ulcer. *B,* Heel pad mobilized on the medial perforators. *C,* The donor site has been grafted with unmeshed skin.

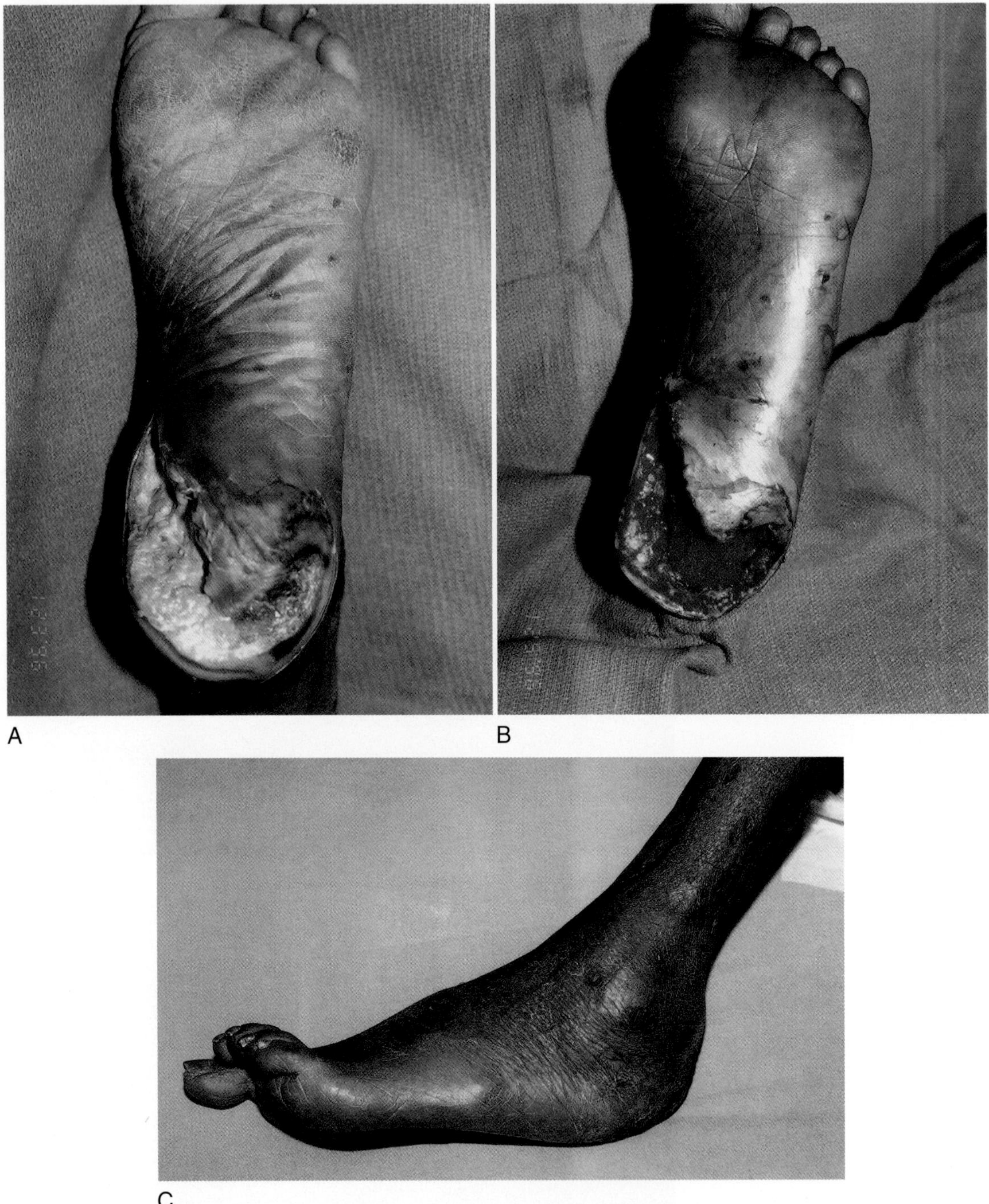

FIGURE 160-34. *A,* Large posterior heel wound. *B,* Appearance after soft tissue débridement and 30% calcanectomy. *C,* Seven months after "simple" closure of the available soft tissue.

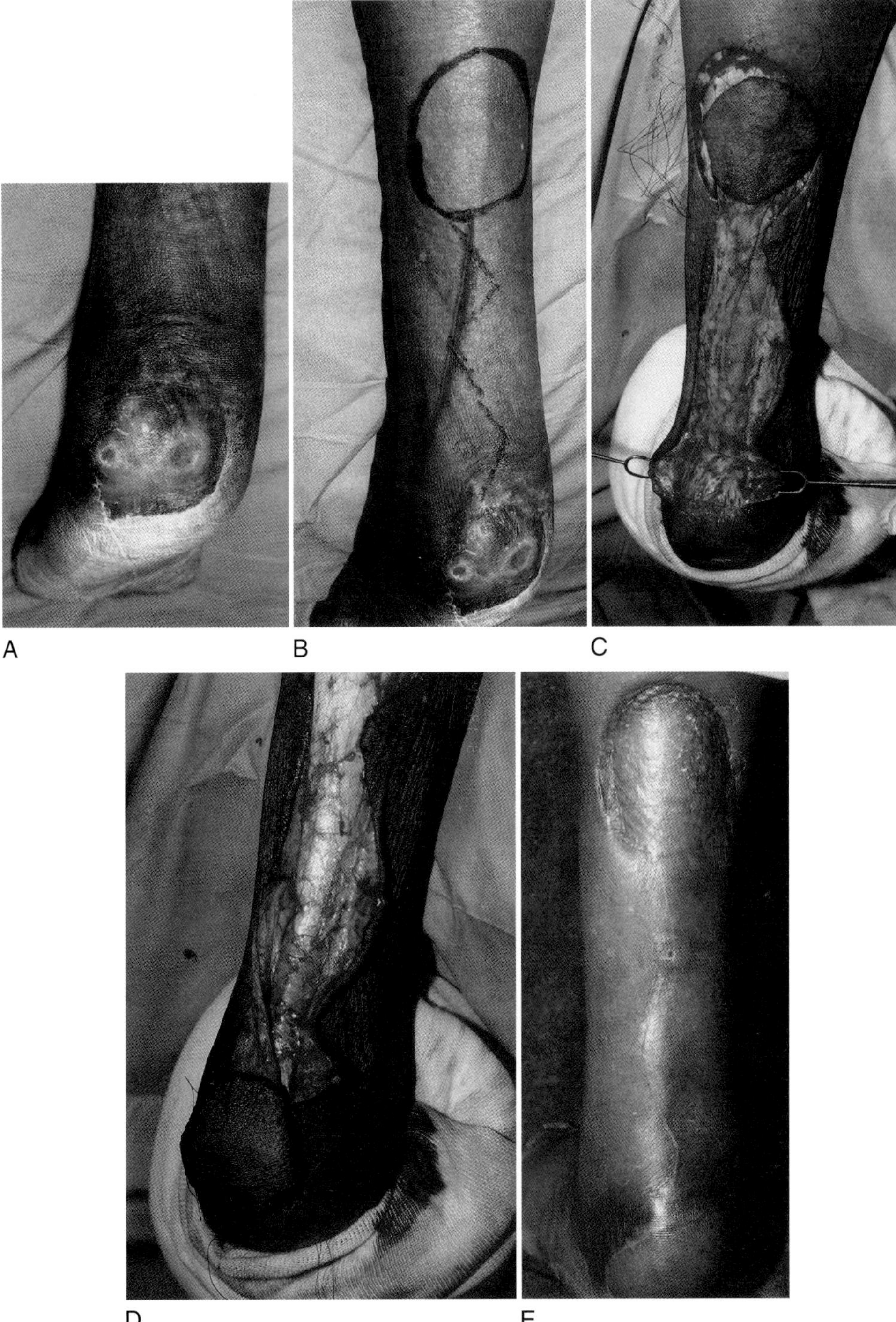

FIGURE 160-35. *A,* Unstable skin graft directly on the posterior calcaneus. *B,* Sural flap centered over the visible lesser saphenous vein. *C,* The flap has been elevated to include the lesser saphenous vein and the sural nerve. A 2-cm width of fascia containing these structures composes the "pedicle." *D,* The flap is inset over the defect and the donor site is skin grafted. *E,* Appearance 3 months after the reconstruction.

coverage of a weight-bearing plantar defect after microvascular transplantation of muscle with skin graft coverage. Others have also found that the presence of sensation did not correlate with successful reconstruction.[30] Importance should be placed on meticulous flap inset, removal of underlying bone prominences, education of the patient, and frequent follow-up. Additional reports assessing sensory nerve repair to the motor nerves of free muscle transplants and the implantation of sensory nerves directly between the muscle surface and the skin graft have been published[65]; however, large prospective studies have never been reported, and the routine use of these neurotization techniques has not been recommended.

As in other locations, the use of muscle to obliterate dead space and to aid in delivering both neutrophils and parenteral antibiotics to regions of chronic osteomyelitis is particularly effective (Fig. 160-36).[66,67] When performing bone débridement, one may administer 5 mL of isosulfan blue dye through a superficial vein on the dorsum of the foot while the limb tourniquet is inflated. “Healthy” bone will stain intensely blue, making the débridement more straightforward. More often than not, this requires free muscle transplantation because the “local” muscles of the foot are often too small to fulfill the reconstructive requirements. Free flap repair is equally of value in the immediate or early repair of post-traumatic and postablative foot wounds (Fig. 160-37). In these clinical situations, the defects are commonly large and complex, and the blood supply to the available local flap alternatives is often compromised. The posterior hindfoot region presents additional challenges. Its anatomy includes a high concentration of various structures essential to normal foot function. There are five principles that must be observed in repairing wounds in this unique location: one should maintain the function of the Achilles tendon and avoid contractures, attempt to restore the normal anatomy, reconstruct tissue deficiencies, re-establish normal foot contour, and select donor tissues by the specific requirements of the wound. Although the sural flap has largely supplanted microvascular composite tissue transplantation in this anatomic location, the selective use of free flaps may be the only suitable technique that adequately fulfills these requirements.[68]

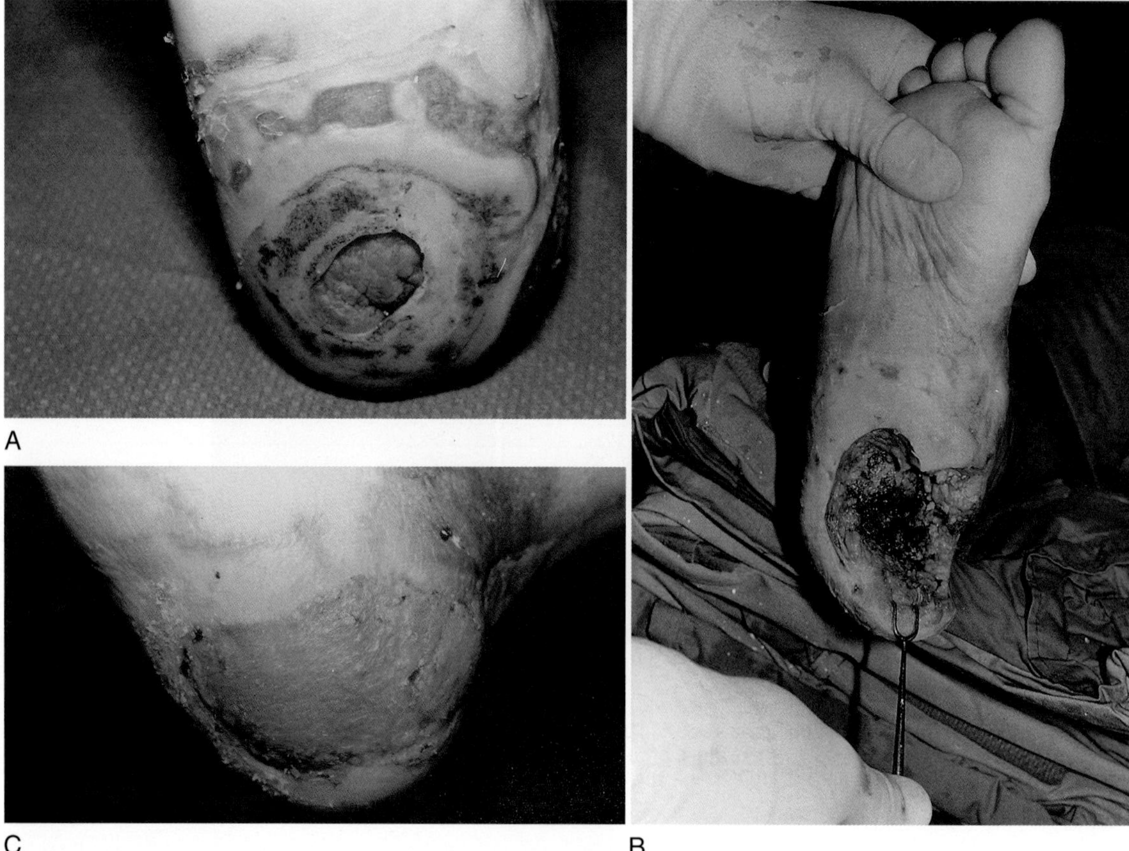

FIGURE 160-36. *A,* Chronic osteomyelitis of the calcaneus. *B,* After débridement with the assistance of isosulfan blue dye. Only “healthy” calcaneus remains. *C,* One month after serratus anterior free flap and skin graft.

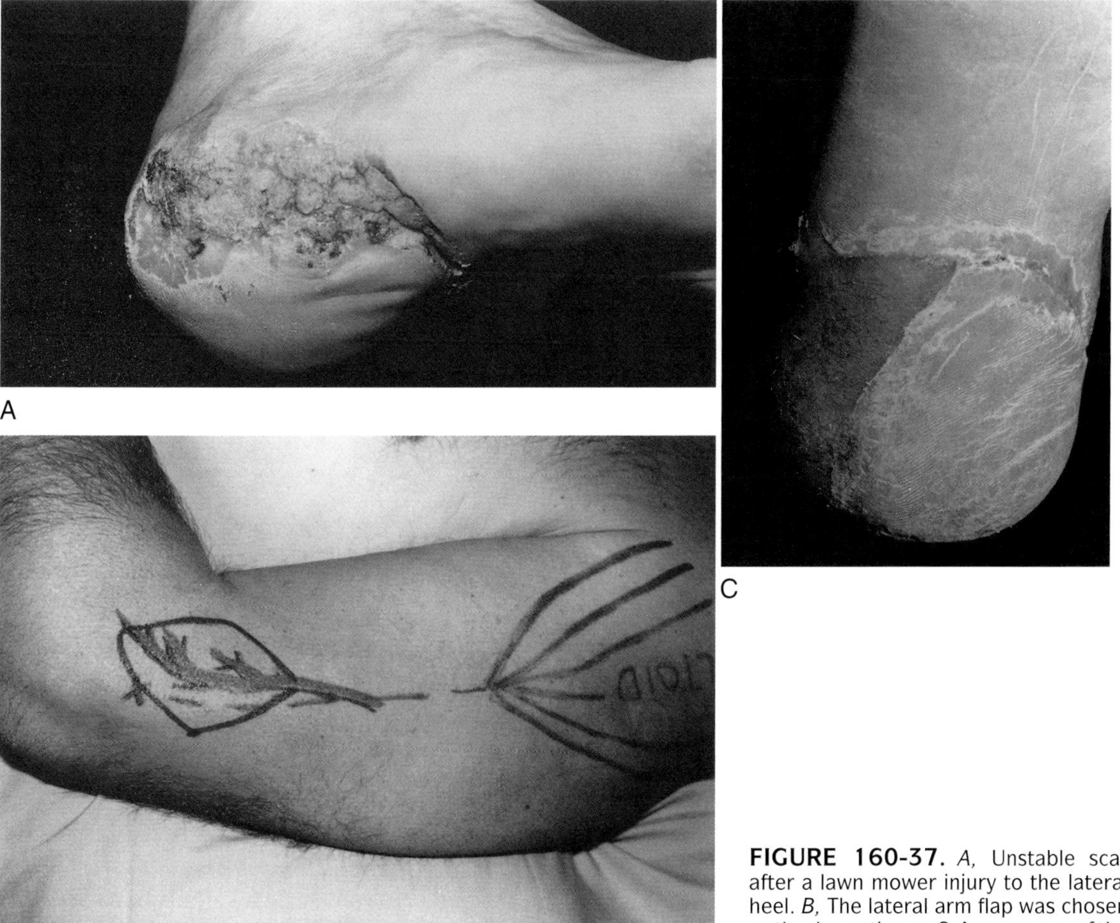

FIGURE 160-37. *A,* Unstable scar after a lawn mower injury to the lateral heel. *B,* The lateral arm flap was chosen as the donor tissue. *C,* Appearance of the heel 6 months after the reconstruction.

Because of its proximity to the wound margin, the posterior tibial artery is the preferred recipient vessel. If the recipient artery is either a dorsally placed bypass graft or the anterior tibial artery, a long donor pedicle becomes of paramount importance. For these patients, the serratus anterior muscle is usually an excellent choice. Venous outflow is usually through the deep system, which should be thoroughly mapped preoperatively by a duplex imaging system (Fig. 160-38).

Hindfoot Amputations

Syme[69] first described amputation at the ankle in 1843, and arguments continue now, as then, as to its merits. The Syme amputation has a definite role in the reconstruction of difficult hindfoot problems, especially in the diabetic patient. The procedure involves use of the heel pad as a soft tissue cover over the distal end of the osteotomized tibia and fibula. Amputation is preferred through the distal tibia and fibula at the level of the medial and lateral malleoli. "Fillet" of the heel pad must be performed at the level of the calcaneal and talar periosteum so that "buttonholing" of the thin soft tissues just distal to the ankle is avoided. It is recommended that the approach to this amputation be modified by leaving a 1-cm-thick "slice" of the plantar cortex of the calcaneus attached to the heel pad and performing osteosynthesis between this structure and the osteotomized distal tibia. Incisional closure should always avoid tension. This usually means that medial and lateral "dog-ears" are left and revised during a second operative procedure. Significant wounds that involve the plantar heel will require the use of dorsal soft tissues as a "flap" that is turned down to provide closure over the bone ends.

For the diabetic patient with prior contralateral amputation, Syme amputation permits weight bearing and allows the patient to ambulate. These patients generally require no physical therapy for gait training, and energy expenditure (oxygen uptake, velocity of cadence, and stride length) is consistently better than that measured for below-knee and above-knee amputees.[70] It is in this specific population of patients

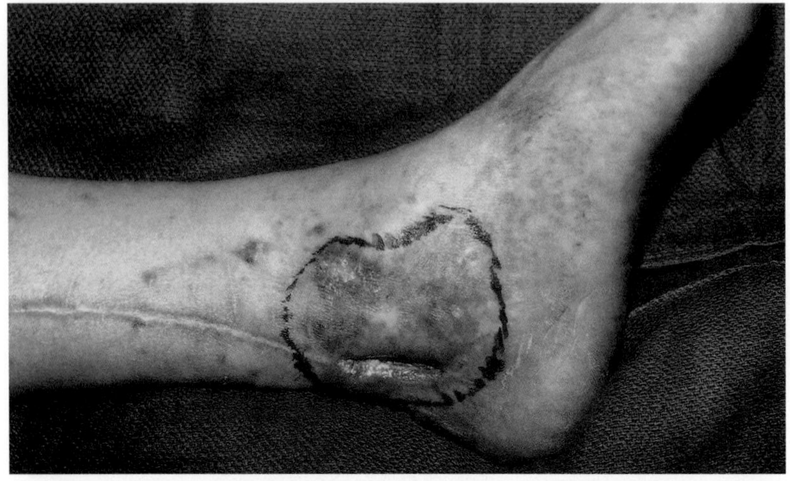

A

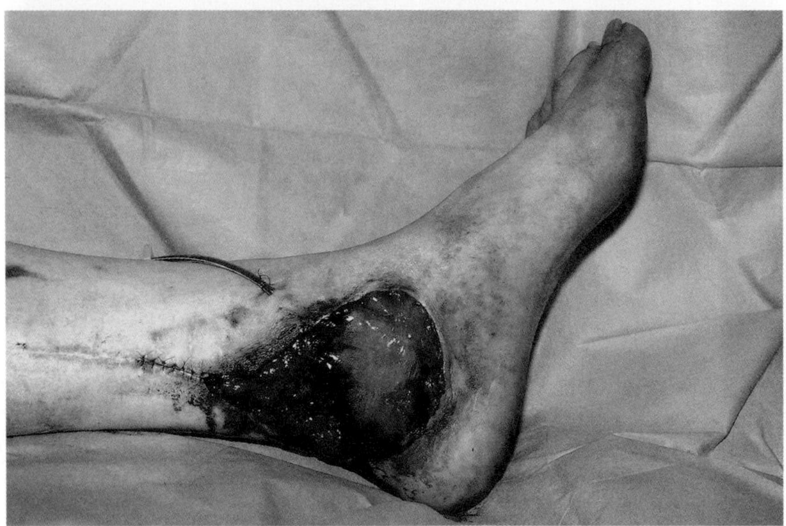

B

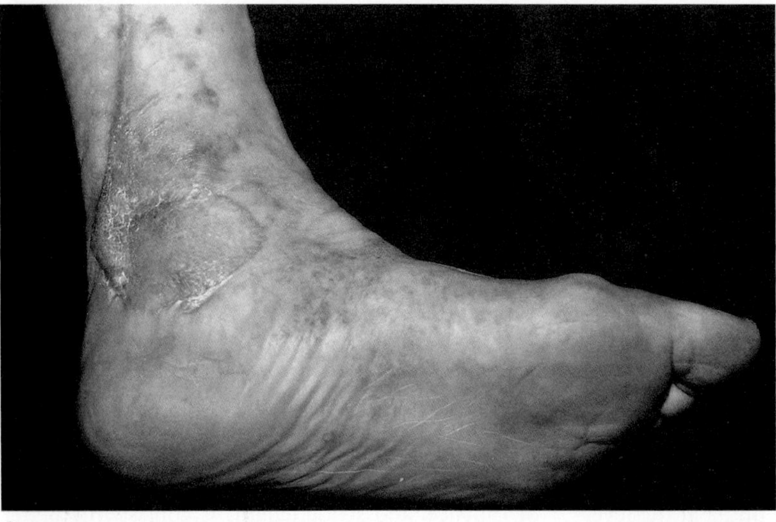

C

FIGURE 160-38. *A,* Chronic hindfoot wound with Achilles tendon exposure. *B,* Inset of a peritoneal-posterior sheath free flap based on the deep inferior epigastric vascular pedicle. The tissue was surfaced with a skin graft. *C,* Foot appearance 5 months postoperatively.

(the diabetic with contralateral below- or above-knee amputation) that the Syme amputation is the most useful.

Postoperative Care

All patients who have undergone reconstructive foot surgery require a structured, well-planned, multidisciplinary recovery program to ensure success. All patients are maintained on a non-weight-bearing regimen for at least 3 weeks after procedures that place suture lines on the plantar surface of the foot. This is of paramount importance to ensure uneventful healing. The use of strict bed rest and wheelchairs after reconstruction varies with the nature of the procedure performed. Local flaps generally require a day of elevation; skin grafts, 3 to 5 days; and free flaps, up to 2 weeks. Control of pedal edema is important and may be accomplished with bed rest and elevation followed by the careful use of elastic wraps once the patient is permitted to place the limb in a dependent position. During the bed rest phase, the use of low-molecular-weight heparin significantly reduces the risk of deep venous thrombosis.

Postoperative antibiotic use should be dictated by the surgical findings. Patients who present without acute infection and normal findings on bone biopsy usually require only 5 days of broad-spectrum antimicrobials (parenteral while they are in the hospital, enteral once they have been discharged). Patients who present with acute infection will require a 2-week course of culture-specific antibiotics. These are usually started intravenously and continued orally after discharge from the hospital. Patients who have biopsy-proven osteomyelitis are a bit more complex. If the débridement procedure completely removes the offending bone, a 2-week course of culture-specific antibiotics should be prescribed; otherwise, a 6-week course is standard therapy.

The L'Nard splint has been a useful tool in keeping the posterior heel off the surface of the bed while providing the necessary immobilization of the foot and ankle. It is lightweight and therefore useful when the patient begins non-weight-bearing ambulation with crutches or a walker. The CAM walker boot is often used to protect foot repairs and tendon transfers or lengthenings when the patient begins to bear weight. A heavy device (similar to a cast), it comfortably and effectively immobilizes the foot and ankle while allowing adjustment of the degree of equinus required at the ankle level.

Sutures are generally removed just before the patient is permitted to begin weight-bearing ambulation. Sutures will often incite callus formation on the plantar surface of the foot, and trimming of the callus is extremely important. Local care may be necessary for 7 to 10 days before weight bearing is allowed.

Follow-up should be frequent and performed in a multidisciplinary manner. Plastic surgery, vascular surgery, orthopedic surgery, podiatry, and prosthetics-orthotics should all be available to participate in the patient's care and follow-up. Experienced nursing personnel adept at all aspects of wound assessment and care contribute as well.

DIABETIC AND ISCHEMIC FOOT RECONSTRUCTION

No discussion of foot reconstruction would be complete without a thorough review of the diabetic patient. These individuals present specific challenges to the reconstructive surgeon. Any surgeon with interests in reconstruction of the foot will necessarily have significant numbers of diabetic patients in his or her practice. Eighty percent to 85% of amputations are preceded by nonhealing ulcers in patients with neuropathy.[71,72] Despite attempts to decrease the number of amputations in the United States by various strategies from better glucose control to monitoring screening examinations for impaired sensibility, the number of amputations has continued to increase from 54,000 in 1990 to 92,000 in 1999.[73,74] The need for a better understanding of the pathogenesis and treatment of diabetic foot ulceration is strongly supported by the literature and this depressing statistic: trends in amputation have not shown any tendency toward improvement in recent years, and foot ulceration remains the most common cause of hospitalization for diabetic subjects in the United States.[75,76]

Foot ulceration is much more common in those patients with neuropathy and vascular disease; the annual incidence rises from less than 1% in patients who do not have neuropathy, for example, to more than 7% in those with established neuropathy.[77,78] The average cost of an ulceration was $27,500 in 1997, and the cost of an amputation ranged from $22,702 for a toe to $51,281 for a leg; the annual cost for diabetic neuropathy and its complications in the United States is between $4.6 and $13.7 billion.[79,80] More than 10 million Americans have diabetes mellitus, and more than 1.5 million, or 15%, will have foot problems during their lifetime.[81] In fact, 20% of all hospitalizations for diabetic patients are for the management of their foot disease.[82] Diabetics battle numerous complications related to their underlying disease, but none is more devastating, both psychologically and economically, than gangrene of an extremity and its associated risk of amputation. Yearly, 50% to 70% of all lower extremity amputations performed for nontraumatic indications are due to diabetes.[83,84]

The cost of managing "the diabetic foot" in the United States is enormous. Recent data suggest that 5% to 6% of the U.S. population is diabetic; their annual health care cost exceeds $20 billion, of which $1.5 billion is directly related to amputations secondary to infection.[85] Once an amputation has been performed, the incidence of a second amputation in the contralateral limb approaches 50% within 2 years.[86-88] One randomized sample of more than 700 diabetic patients revealed that only 30% were free of diabetic foot symptoms.[89] Prudent surgical intervention has substantially reduced the morbidity in these patients and should have a positive impact on the economics of their care. Numerous advances during the past 2 decades have permitted the salvage of extremities in patients with diabetes and peripheral vascular disease who previously underwent below-knee amputation. With their predominance of infrapopliteal arterial occlusive disease, distal tibial arterial revascularizations have particularly benefited diabetic patients.

Several misconceptions have perpetuated a "fatalistic" approach toward the management of the diabetic foot, resulting in numerous amputations over the years. The first is that all diabetic foot problems are due to "small-vessel disease." Specifically, the presumption is that distal arteriolar occlusive disease can cause ischemic wounds even in the presence of normal pedal pulses. This misconception dates to the work of Goldenberg more than 40 years ago.[90] Amputation specimens from both diabetic and nondiabetic patients were examined by light microscopy. Periodic acid-Schiff staining in the arterioles of the diabetic specimens was interpreted as a diabetic-specific vascular occlusive disease. More recent studies, including a blinded study by Strandness[91] performed in a prospective fashion, did not corroborate this retrospective analysis. Other prospective evaluations by arterial casting techniques also failed to show diabetic-specific arterial occlusions.[92] Blood flow studies in diabetic patients undergoing femoral-popliteal bypass have shown no difference in the responsiveness of the runoff bed to papaverine vasodilatation compared with the same measurements made in nondiabetic patients, indicating normal activity of the resistance vessels (the arterioles).[93] The second misconception is that endothelial cell proliferation occurs within the small vessels of diabetic patients and thereby results in small-vessel occlusions. Prospective studies have failed to show an increase in the incidence of intimal hyperplasia in the small vessels of these individuals.[94] Thickening of the capillary basement membrane has been well documented, but capillary narrowing or occlusion has not.

Although the infrapopliteal arterial occlusive disease present in diabetic patients often results in distal vascular insufficiency, it is now well accepted that peripheral neuropathy is the primary cause of foot wounds in the diabetic population.[95] The lack of a PO_2 gradient between arterial blood and foot skin among diabetic patients without ulceration, diabetic patients with ulceration, and nondiabetic patients with normal transcutaneous oxygen tension further implicates a nonischemic cause.[96]

Neuropathic Changes

The neuropathic changes observed in the diabetic foot are a direct result of the abnormalities in the motor, sensory, and autonomic nervous systems. The loss of sudomotor function from autonomic neuropathy leads to anhidrosis and hyperkeratosis. Fissuring of the skin results and facilitates bacterial entry and subsequent infection. The lack of sensibility over bone prominences and between the toes often delays the detection of these small breaks in the skin.

Charcot deformities (neuroarthropathy) of the small joints of the foot occur in 0.1% to 2.5% of the diabetic population.[97-100] When they are present, the tarsometatarsal joints are involved in 30%, the metatarsophalangeal joints in 30%, the intertarsal joints in 24%, and the interphalangeal joints in 4%.[92] The widely accepted explanation for these degenerative changes is neurotraumatic, that is, joint collapse as a result of damage that has accumulated because of insensitivity to pain, although small-fiber functions may be preserved.[101] The destructive changes that occur in the Charcot foot cause a collapse of the medial longitudinal arch, which alters the biomechanics of gait. The normal calcaneal pitch is distorted, which in turn causes severe strain to the ligaments binding the metatarsal, cuneiform, navicular, and other small bones that form the long arch of the foot.[102] These degenerative changes further alter the gait, resulting in abnormal weight-bearing stress, causing a collapse of the foot. Unfortunately, ulceration, infection, gangrene, and limb loss are frequent outcomes if the process is not halted in its early stages.

The process probably begins with a ligamentous soft tissue injury accompanied by synovitis and effusion. In the absence of pain perception, continued use of the extremity exacerbates the inflammatory process. Eventually, distention of the joint capsule leads to ligament distortion, resulting in joint instability. Further activity causes articular cartilage erosion, with debris being trapped within the synovium. Heterotopic bone formation and eburnation of load-bearing surfaces frequently exist.

The motor component of the neuropathy further contributes to Charcot deformities as the intrinsic foot musculature atrophies and becomes fibrotic. The resulting metatarsophalangeal joint extension and interphalangeal joint flexion produce excessive pressure on the metatarsal heads and the ends of phalanges. The loss of both the transverse and longitudinal arches with the foot exacerbates the unfavorable weight distribution across the midfoot and metatarsal heads.

Some evidence suggests that diabetic neuropathy may be vascular in origin; however, specific changes in the endoneural vessels of diabetic and nondiabetic patients do not differ significantly.[103,104] In addition, the electrodiagnostic changes seen in diabetic neuropathy do not parallel those seen in ischemic nerves.[105] Current studies suggest that endoneural edema resulting from the osmotic effects of sorbitol (derived from glucose through the aldose reductase pathway) may play the most important etiologic role.[106-110] As edema within the nerve fascicle occurs, endoneural pressure increases, causing compression of the microvasculature and reduction of blood flow.[111-113] In animals with streptozotocin-induced diabetes, the neural changes correlate with reduced nerve conduction velocities, which are reversible by aldose reductase inhibition therapy (sorbinil).[114] An increase of up to 54% in the hydration of sural nerves of "untreated" type I diabetic patients with symptomatic polyneuropathy has been observed. Selected patients treated with sorbinil have "normal" sural nerve hydration as determined by magnetic resonance spectroscopy.[115]

Histologic similarities between chronically entrapped nerves and those seen in diabetic neuropathy provide substantial evidence that diabetic patients are unusually susceptible to peripheral nerve compression.[116,117] Several authors suggest that nerve compression (subclinical) in concert with early diabetic nerve changes (subclinical) may give rise to a clinical picture of diabetic neuropathy (the "double crush" hypothesis) and therefore advocate peripheral nerve release at known anatomic sites of compression.[118,119]

Hemorheologic Abnormalities

Although "small-vessel disease" has not been anatomically confirmed in diabetic patients, recent evidence suggests that a functional alteration in capillary blood flow probably exists. This hemorheologic abnormality may be responsible for much of the clinical picture now defined as "diabetic complications," that is, retinopathy, nephropathy, microangiopathy, and neuropathy.[120] Increases in blood and serum viscosity and flow abnormalities in leukocytes, erythrocytes, platelets, and plasma proteins have been reported in diabetic patients.[121] Many investigators describe these hemorheologic impairments as the functional equivalent of diabetic microangiopathy.[122-125]

The increase in blood viscosity noted in diabetic patients appears to have its origin in a stiffened red blood cell membrane as well as an increase in erythrocyte aggregation.[126-128] Because red blood cells must deform to pass through capillary beds, stiffened cells may resist passage and even traumatize the endothelium. The nonenzymatic glycosylation of the red blood cell membrane protein spectrin is responsible for the membrane stiffening and the increased aggregation that occurs.[129] Both of these result in an increase in blood viscosity. The mechanism of this glycosylation is similar to that seen with hemoglobin and is directly proportional to serum glucose levels.[130,131]

The altered flow characteristics that result from changes in viscosity trigger a compensatory rise in perfusion pressure, causing an increase in transudation across capillary beds and further increases in viscosity. Ischemia to the peripheral tissues is further exacerbated by the increased affinity of glycosylated hemoglobin for the oxygen molecule. The detrimental effects of hyperglycemia on blood flow and tissue perfusion are significant (Fig. 160-39).

Fortunately, many of these effects may be reversed by establishing good metabolic control of the diabetes.[129] Juhan et al[132] found that the stiff red blood cell in the uncontrolled diabetic could be reversed to normal within 24-hours of a controlled insulin infusion. In addition, pharmacologic means are now available to help reduce blood viscosity in diabetic patients. Serum fibrinogen levels, commonly elevated in diabetic patients,[133] may be lowered and measured improvement in red blood cell aggregation accomplished by the administration of ancrod, a purified protein derivative of Malayan pit viper venom. Although its use has been beneficial in Europe, it is not available in the United States.[134,135] Pentoxifylline, a trisubstituted methylxanthine derivative, improves the deformability of erythrocytes and may be of considerable benefit to diabetic patients with extremity wounds. Pentoxifylline increases adenosine triphos-

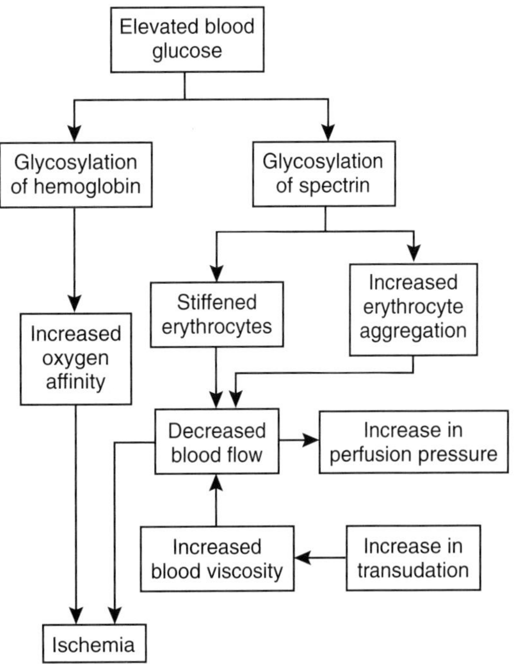

FIGURE 160-39. Effects of serum glucose elevation on blood flow and tissue perfusion.

phate (ATP) levels within red blood cells. Because erythrocyte deformability is ATP dependent,[136] the net result is a more flexible erythrocyte. Both in vitro and in vivo studies have documented measurable improvements in blood viscosity, as well as in extremity blood flow, in diabetic patients with peripheral vascular disease treated with pentoxifylline.[129,137-140] The salutary effects of long-term administration of pentoxifylline to patients with type I and type II diabetes with microvascular (retinopathy and nephropathy) and macrovascular (ischemic heart disease and peripheral vascular disease) complications have been well documented.[141]

Preoperative Evaluation

The unique nature of the wounds found with diabetes and vascular disease requires the use of additional techniques for preoperative evaluation. Because neuropathy in the diabetic may involve a single nerve, a complete sensory examination of the foot is warranted. If a patient has hypesthesia in the tibial nerve distribution but has intact sural or peroneal nerve sensibility, the surgeon may consider nerve transfer to help restore protective sensation in the weight-bearing sole of the foot.[142] Nerve conduction studies may help find sites of tibial nerve compression, such as tarsal tunnel syndrome, a condition amenable to surgical decompression. The improvement of plantar sensibility after tarsal tunnel release may prevent further wound development after reconstructive surgery has been completed.[143]

Wound Management

The basic wound management principles outlined earlier in this chapter apply to the care of diabetic foot ulcers. Strict bed rest and elevation of the extremity are essential to eliminate edema and help control infection. Adequate surgical débridement of necrotic tissue and drainage of purulent cavities are mandatory. Plantar space infection should be suspected in any patient who has cellulitis and a plantar ulcer, especially if palpation of the instep reveals tenderness or swelling. Aspiration with a 3-mL syringe and an 18-gauge needle helps confirm the presence of such a problem. The liberal use of antibiotics and subcutaneous heparin will help eradicate infection while providing deep venous thrombosis prophylaxis. The role of hyperbaric oxygen remains controversial, although most would agree that in the treatment of anaerobic infections, adjuvant hyperbaric oxygen use should be considered.[144]

Although x-ray studies and bone scans are not helpful in the diagnosis of bone infection, they are useful for detection of bone spurs, prominences, and other osseous abnormalities.[145] The "gold standard" for the diagnosis of osteomyelitis remains bone biopsy of the suspected segment.[146]

In the diabetic patient, the diagnosis of osteomyelitis can usually be made with plain films. Osteomyelitis occurs from the direct extension of the pressure ulcer through the soft tissues into bone. This will show as cortical irregularities on these films, although most patients will have additional studies. After plain film evaluation, most patients will have nuclear scans ordered. These studies are often misleading and unnecessary. These studies are often "positive" at the level of the ankle, midfoot, and forefoot in patients with diabetes who have no associated foot ulceration. The neuroarthropathy that these patients have will usually give rise to false-positive scans. The use of Ceretec scans (technetium-labeled white blood cell studies) is presently being investigated; however, the magnetic resonance imaging scan remains the noninvasive study of choice for diagnosis of osteomyelitis.

Patients who have had recent distal vascular bypass procedures to either the anterior tibial or peroneal vessels in the region of the ankle or foot or who have occlusion of the posterior tibial artery may not be candidates for local arterialized flap coverage of hindfoot wounds because these procedures require antegrade flow in the posterior tibial artery and its plantar branches to ensure adequate flap viability. These special circumstances mandate the use of microvascular composite tissue transplantation (Fig. 160-40). When long distal bypass surgery has been performed, direct arterial anastomosis to the bypass graft is always preferable. If the revascularization is performed proximally, however, the distal vessels must be re-evaluated for their suitability as recipient vessels for the transplanted flaps. In this circumstance, duplex imaging of the pedal vessels is useful. This method helps the surgeon choose the "ideal" location for performing a microvascular anastomosis.[11]

Free flap donor sites should be located in the chest or upper extremity, where the incidence of atherosclerosis in the donor flap pedicles is decreased.[147] The serratus anterior muscle is an excellent choice; the long vascular pedicle permits the reconstruction of large hindfoot wounds in patients who have undergone revascularization to the anterior tibial artery. Direct end-to-side anastomosis is possible without the need for interposition vein grafting.

Adjunctive techniques alluded to earlier in this chapter are extremely important in preventing ulcer recurrence in patients with neuropathic wounds. The important role of osseous manipulation at the time of soft tissue reconstruction cannot be overemphasized. Bone spurs, joint dislocations, and other causes of improper weight dispersion on the sole of the foot must be corrected to help maintain a stable soft tissue envelope. Charcot deformities of the midfoot are often heralded by mild effusions, joint instability, crepitus, and

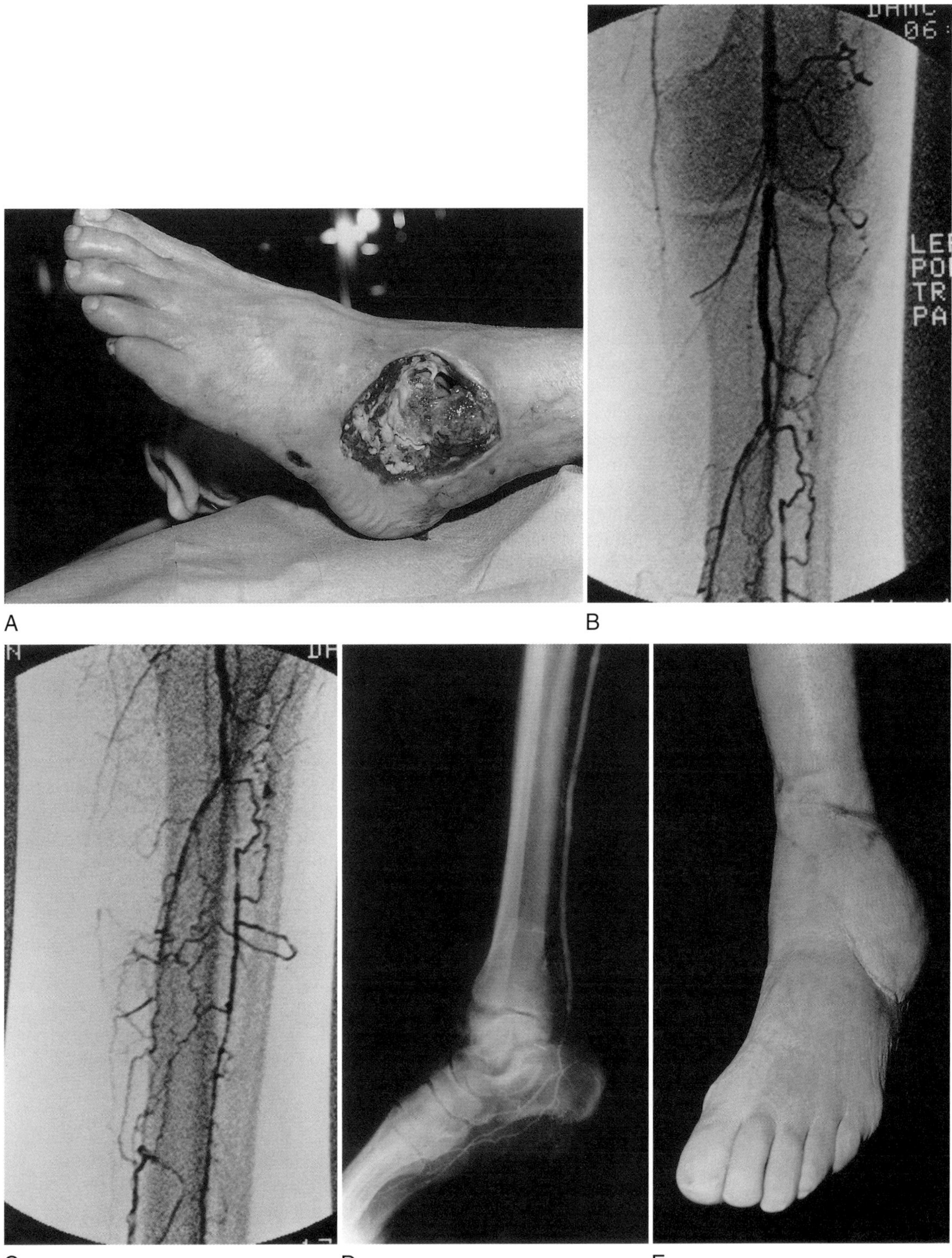

FIGURE 160-40. *A,* Hindfoot-lateral ankle wound in an ischemic limb. *B* and *C,* Angiogram shows tight popliteal stenosis and trifurcation disease. *D,* Intraoperative angiogram shows the saphenous vein bypass from the distal popliteal artery to the posterior tibial artery. *E,* Six months after serratus anterior free flap and skin graft with arterial anastomosis directly to the bypass graft (end-to-side).

soft tissue swelling before a fixed deformity appears. If these symptoms are identified early, casting may prevent permanent deformity.[148] When forefoot ulceration occurs over the fifth metatarsal head, resection through the metatarsal neck is recommended. This may be accomplished either through the débrided wound, if the ulcer penetrates deeply, or through a linear tendon-splitting incision dorsally. The first metatarsal is débrided only if it is involved with the ulcer base. Complete resection is not recommended because this procedure will result in excessive weight transfer to the adjacent metatarsal head. Rather, resection of the plantar flare of the metatarsal head makes the most sense. Frequently, the medial or lateral sesamoid bones are the source of the ulceration. These small bones may be excised through the wound at the time of flap closure. With ulceration over the second, third, and fourth metatarsal heads, perform a "floating" metatarsal neck osteotomy at the time of wound closure.[149] As with fifth metatarsal head resection, a linear dorsal approach may be used. This procedure allows the prominent metatarsal head to move dorsally without transfer of excessive weight bearing to the adjacent metatarsals. Address bone prominences associated with midfoot wounds with judicious resection. The medial instep wound results from deformity about the first metatarsal base, medial cuneiform, and navicular bones. The more lateral wounds are usually secondary to prominence of the fifth metatarsal base and cuboid bones. Limited midfoot fusions should be strongly considered when they will prevent subluxation of joints and thereby provide for more uniform weight distribution.

Recent evidence indicates that the "stocking-glove" pattern of peripheral neuropathy associated with diabetes mellitus may be caused, in part, by known sites of anatomic compression of the major peripheral nerves.[111,137] Release of the tibial nerve as it courses through the tarsal tunnel has benefited many diabetic patients.

After sterile preparation, exsanguinate the extremity and inflate a thigh tourniquet. Begin the incision 3 cm proximal to the medial malleolus and 3 cm posterior to it to prevent injury to saphenous nerve branches. The incision is extended distally, following the course of the nerve, toward the instep. After deepening of the incision, the nerve is identified proximally and dissected distally. The flexor retinaculum is divided under direct vision. The medial calcaneal nerve branch from the posterior tibial nerve is identified and protected. The origin of the abductor hallucis muscle is divided both to expose and to release the medial and lateral plantar branches from their respective tunnels. The nerve is carefully inspected, at which time it is decided whether an epineurectomy or internal neurolysis should be performed. For most patients, this is not necessary because it excessively traumatizes the nerve. It is more important to make certain that separate release of the medial and lateral plantar tunnels is achieved (Fig. 160-41).

Amputation Alternatives

Some of the prevailing myths among surgical disciplines are that midfoot or hindfoot amputations are unsatisfactory because of tendon imbalance and that the Syme amputation has a high failure rate rendering below-knee amputation safer. In determining the amputation level, several factors must be considered: the age of the patient, the cause of the problem, the blood supply and soft tissue quality to the area,

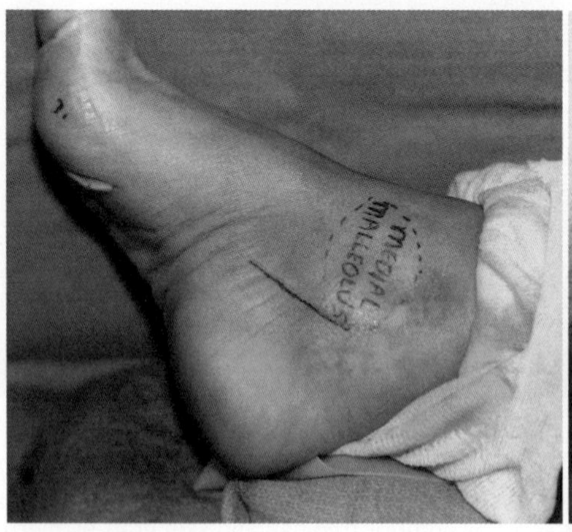

A

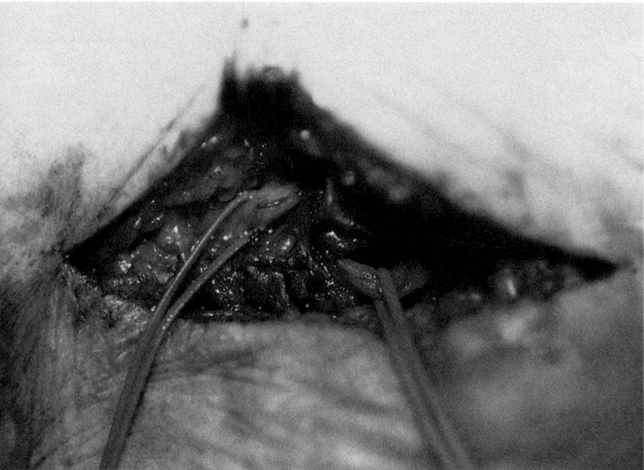

B

FIGURE 160-41. *A,* Skin incision for tarsal tunnel release. *B,* Complete division of the abductor hallucis origin and release of the medial and lateral plantar tunnels. The septum between the tunnels will be resected as well.

the associated medical or surgical illnesses, and the status of the contralateral limb. As noted earlier, the diabetic patient with a foot ulceration or infection requiring amputation will often have contralateral foot disease. For these patients, all efforts should be directed at salvaging the remaining foot so that prosthetic-free bipedal ambulation may be maintained. The young person amputated because of trauma may be managed differently from the geriatric amputee. A major surgical effort should be made to form a "stump" that is pain free and able to tolerate partial end bearing.[150]

In an effort to maintain bipedal ambulation, the conservation of tissue is paramount. Toe amputation leaves little disability, and its clinical indications are obvious. Ray resection of the toe and associated metatarsal is equally effective when it is clinically indicated. When three or more toe rays are resected, the forefoot becomes narrow, tends to develop an equinus deformity, and is extremely difficult to fit into a shoe. The function of the resultant foot does not exceed that of the midfoot or forefoot amputee; hence, amputation revision to the transmetatarsal or midfoot level should be strongly considered.

The vacuum-assisted closure device has often simplified the management of complex foot wounds. Its use has served as an adjunct by expediting closure of a wound while decreasing local wound care intensity and duration. It can effectively be used for foot wounds when surgery is contraindicated, for wounds with partial surgical failure, or for wounds that are being prepared for surgical closure. Wounds that may have required free flap closure initially may be "converted" into ones that can be reconstructed with simpler techniques (see Fig. 160-25).

Outcomes

Only recently have there been data available regarding the outcomes from a closely supervised multidisciplinary approach to the management of a diabetic foot. Review of the literature suggests that limb salvage is improved when certain management schemes are followed. Because of the many variables that exist within the few studies published, it is difficult to determine exactly which variables account for the improved outcomes. For example, reports that deal with surgical interventions compare groups of patients who have undergone certain procedures with "controls." The improved outcomes after surgery are often attributed to the procedure itself, without acknowledging the importance of frequent multidisciplinary follow-up that attends the surgical procedure.

Several groups have reported their experience by use of a multidisciplinary approach within a "diabetic foot clinic." A study from the University of Louisville compared two groups of patients. One group developed ulcers while receiving prophylactic care at a multidisciplinary clinic (group I); the other, identical group was referred to the clinic after ulceration had already occurred (group II). The sites and sizes of the lesions were no different between the two groups. Despite similarities between the two groups, group I had significantly better prognosis than group II did. The study concluded that the establishment of a dedicated diabetic foot care clinic and regular patient review can reduce the morbidity associated with diabetic foot ulceration. New ulceration, when it occurs, will be detected earlier and lead to management that is more effective in attaining limb preservation.[151]

The role of early, aggressive revascularization surgery in the long-term outcome of diabetic foot management is addressed in several studies as well. Researchers from the University of California, San Francisco, have shown that a multidisciplinary wound care program including vascular surgery and adjuvant hyperbaric oxygen therapy can provide limb salvage that is both cost-effective and durable. Sixty-three percent of their patients healed their wounds and remained healed during the 5 years of follow-up.[152] The vascular surgery section at New England Deaconess Hospital similarly showed the beneficial effects of revascularization surgery in the outcome of diabetic foot management. They compared the outcomes of patients during two different time intervals. The "modern" approach included distal bypass arterial grafting and led to improved outcomes as evidenced by a decrease in major and minor amputation rates, a reduced length of hospital stay, and a reduced cost for care. In spite of this, however, they pointed out that reimbursement through Medicare remained insufficient with an average loss of $7480 per admission.[153]

Studies that have specifically looked at frequent multidisciplinary wound care and its effect on the healing of diabetic foot ulceration are numerous. They repeatedly show that foot wounds will heal when pressure points are off-loaded and wound management is properly attended to at frequent intervals.[146,154] However, it is difficult to properly maintain off-loading with the use of orthoses alone. In the author's study,[155] the outcomes of patients treated with plantar wound closure surgery (flap repairs) were compared with those of patients who underwent identical surgical procedures combined with the removal of bone prominences, repair of Charcot midfoot deformities, and Achilles tendon lengthening surgery. The first group of patients was operated on from 1983 to 1990. The second group was treated between 1990 and 1997. All patients were observed a minimum of 2 years, although average follow-up was 5 years. All patients were fitted with footwear appropriate for the procedure performed. When wounds were closed without attention to correction of the biomechanical abnormalities, ulcer recurrence rates were 25%. With the addition of the aforementioned procedures, recurrence dropped to 2%.[155]

The authors have also studied the long-term outcome in the management of 68 patients who required both arterial revascularization surgery and microvascular composite tissue transplantation procedures to obtain limb salvage.[156] Seventy limbs required 78 free flap procedures. Follow-up averaged 48 months, at which time 52% of patients had died. Cardiac events were the main cause of mortality, and patients with diabetes of more than 10 years' duration correlated with a higher mortality at follow-up. Early limb salvage rates were 95%, with late preservation in 91% of extremities. Perioperative myocardial infarction occurred in 24% of patients. Operative mortality rates were 5% per patient and 1.3% per procedure. Post-reconstructive function was rated good in 35%, intermediate in 50%, and poor in 15%. This was related to wound location as well as to the status of the contralateral extremity. On the basis of these data, a selective approach to the management of these problems is advocated.[156]

UNSOLVED PROBLEMS

Although much progress has been made in the salvage and reconstruction of the foot, many difficult challenges continue to exist. Research efforts exploring the microcirculation should provide additional insight into the problems seen in patients with neuropathic extremities and severe peripheral vascular disease. Prosthetic management of the foot and lower extremity has made remarkable progress during the past decade, and this should be considered in evaluating reconstructive procedures versus the use of a prosthesis alone.

Reinnervation has long been thought to be the limiting factor in foot and lower extremity reconstruction; however, evidence suggests that well-contoured soft tissue repair of the plantar surface of the foot is the most important element in providing a successful, durable reconstruction.[30,149] Most agree that the shear forces between the flap and the underlying bone architecture and between the flap and the overlying shoe must be minimized to eliminate the problems of recurrent ulceration. The current use of heat-molded plastizote orthoses has been helpful but has not entirely eliminated the problems associated with shear forces. Similarly, the ideal tissue with which to reconstruct the plantar surface of the foot has not been agreed on. Further work in these areas is needed.

Newer approaches to patients with vascular impairment and peripheral neuropathy have been promising. The technique of in situ saphenous vein reconstruction of the infrapopliteal arteries has set the stage for the bone and soft tissue procedures dictated by the clinical problem. What about the patient with "non-reconstructible" peripheral vascular disease? Can foot revascularization be accomplished exclusively through the use of microsurgical composite (free) flaps revascularized from the groin or popliteal fossa? Some authors have had limited success with such techniques, but others have been disappointed.[157,158] The healing potential of the area to be reconstructed must be accurately determined before embarking on sophisticated reconstructive procedures. The laser Doppler velocitometer or measurements of transcutaneous oxygen tension can assess cutaneous blood flow and accurately predict which patients may benefit from these combined vascular and plastic surgical techniques. For a flap to "revascularize" an extremity, the flap must first successfully "incorporate" into the involved foot. This demands a certain level of perfusion in the foot at the time of the flap transfer.

The improved understanding of the hemorheologic abnormalities in diabetes mellitus should permit pharmacologic manipulation of the erythrocyte and improve capillary blood flow. The effect of stiffened red cells in the microcirculation may be amplified by the special circumstances existing in various tissues and organs. The influence of intraocular pressure on retinal blood flow, the influence of gravity and hydrostatic pressure on the return of blood from the feet to the heart, and the effects of the pressure of weight bearing on the microcirculatory flow in the lower extremity are a few examples of this concept. The resistance of stiffened red cells to passage through the capillaries within the foot is compounded by the compressive effects of weight bearing and elevated hydrostatic forces. Poiseuille's law predicts that the effects of pressure should be most severe on the smaller vessels, and it is these vessels that are most affected in the diabetic patient.

As noted earlier, the problem of peripheral neuropathy in the diabetic patient is being approached in a more rational and physiologic manner. Studies have shown the salutary effects of aldose reductase inhibition on the changes that are usually seen in the peripheral nerves of diabetic patients, and further refinement of this approach to the treatment of peripheral neuropathy appears promising. Ongoing research protocols currently under way are looking at new and exciting pharmaceuticals in the treatment and prevention of peripheral neuropathy. As soft tissue reconstruction has become commonplace in the foot, new avenues to combat the pathophysiologic mechanism that leads to instability and recurrent wound problems should be explored.

REFERENCES

1. Cormack GC, Lamberty BG: The Arterial Anatomy of Skin Flaps. Edinburgh, Churchill Livingstone, 1986.

2. Grant JCB: An Atlas of Anatomy, 6th ed. Baltimore, Williams & Wilkins, 1972.
3. Colen LB, Replogle SL, Mathes SJ: The V-Y plantar flap for reconstruction of the forefoot. Plast Reconstr Surg 1988; 81:220.
4. Baker GL, Newton ED, Franklin JD: Fasciocutaneous island flap based on the medial plantar artery: clinical applications for leg, ankle, and forefoot. Plast Reconstr Surg 1990;85:47.
5. Morrison WA, Crabb DM, O'Brien BM, Jenkins A: The instep of the foot as a fasciocutaneous island and as a free flap for heel defects. Plast Reconstr Surg 1983;72:56.
6. Reiffel RS, McCarthy JG: Coverage of heel and sole defects: a new subfascial arterialized flap. Plast Reconstr Surg 1980;66:250.
7. Shanahan RE, Gingrass RP: The medial plantar sensory flap for coverage of heel defects. Plast Reconstr Surg 1979;64:295.
8. Vann HM: A note on the formation of the plantar arterial arch of the human foot. Anat Rec 1943;85:269.
9. Manter JT: Distribution of compression forces in the joints of the human foot. Anat Rec 1946;96:313.
10. Elftman H: A cinematic study of the distribution of pressure in the human foot. Anat Rec 1934;59:481.
11. Colen LB, Musson A: Preoperative assessment of the peripheral vascular disease patient for free tissue transfer. J Reconstr Microsurg 1987;4:1.
12. Lassen NA, Tonnesen KH, Holstein P: Distal blood pressure. Scand J Clin Lab Invest 1976;36:705.
13. Holstein P, Noer I, Tonnesen KH, et al: Distal blood pressure in severe arterial insufficiency. In Bergan J, Yao J, eds: Gangrene and Severe Ischemia of the Lower Extremities. New York, Grune & Stratton, 1978.
14. Barnes RW, Thornhill B, Nix L, et al: Prediction of amputation wound healing: roles of Doppler ultrasound and digit photoplethysmography. Arch Surg 1981;116:80.
15. Vincent D, Salles-Cunha SX, Bernhard VM, Towne JB: Noninvasive assessment of toe systolic pressures with special references to diabetes mellitus. J Cardiovasc Surg 1983;24:22.
16. Faris I, Duncan H: Skin perfusion pressure in the prediction of healing in diabetic patients with ulcers or gangrene of the foot. J Vasc Surg 1985;2:536.
17. Fronek A, Coel M, Bernstein EF: Quantitative ultrasonic studies of lower extremity flow velocities in health and disease. Circulation 1976;53:957.
18. Rhodes G, Skudder P: Salvage of ischemic feet: roles of transcutaneous oxygen mapping and multiple configurations of in-situ bypass. Am J Surg 1986;152:165.
19. Tagagi-Smith M, et al: The measurement of transcutaneous oxygen tension and its application in the vascular laboratory. Bruit 1984;8:213.
20. Graham BH, Walton RL, Elings VB, Lewis FR: Surface quantification of injected fluorescein as a predictor of flap viability. Plast Reconstr Surg 1983;71:826.
21. Matsen FA 3rd, Wyss CR, Robertson CL, et al: The relationship of transcutaneous PO_2 and laser Doppler measurements in a human model of arterial insufficiency. Surg Gynecol Obstet 1984;11:418.
22. Winsor T, Haumschild DJ, Winsor DW, et al: Clinical application of laser Doppler fluorometry for measurement of cutaneous circulation in health and disease. Angiology 1987;38:727.
23. van Dooren J, Verdonk R, Uyttendaele D, et al: Disulphine blue as a diagnostic aid in the demarcation of bone sequestra. Acta Orthop Belg 1978;44:797.
24. Mayor MB, Caulkins M, Colen LB: Regional assessment of bone perfusion using isosulfan blue dye. J Bone Joint Surg; submitted.
25. Bonutti PM, Bell GR: Compartment syndrome of the foot: a case report. J Bone Joint Surg Am 1986;68:1449.
26. Henry AK: Extensile Exposure, 2nd ed. Baltimore, Williams & Wilkins, 1957.
27. Mubarak SJ, Hargans AR: Compartment Syndromes and Volkmann's Contracture. Philadelphia, WB Saunders, 1981.
28. Whitesides TE: Compartment syndromes. In Jahss MH, ed: Disorders of the Foot. Philadelphia, WB Saunders, 1982:1201.
29. Maisels DO: Repair of the heel. Br J Plast Surg 1961;14:117.
30. Sommerlad BC, McGrouther DA: Resurfacing the sole: long-term follow-up and comparison of techniques. Br J Plast Surg 1978;31:107.
31. Lister GD: Use of an innervated skin graft to provide sensation to the reconstructed heel. Plast Reconstr Surg 1978;62:157.
32. Maquira NO: An innervated full-thickness skin graft to restore sensibility to fingertips and heels. Plast Reconstr Surg 1974;53:568.
33. Ger R: The management of chronic ulcers of the dorsum of the foot by muscle transposition and skin grafting. Br J Plast Surg 1976;29:199.
34. Leitner DW, Gordon L, Buncke HJ: The extensor digitorum brevis as a muscle island flap. Plast Reconstr Surg 1985;76:777.
35. Masquelet AC, Beveridge J, Romana MC, Gerber C: The lateral supramalleolar flap. Plast Reconstr Surg 1988;81:74.
36. Moberg E: Evaluation and management of nerve injuries in the hand. Surg Clin North Am 1964;44:1019.
37. Snyder GB, Edgerton MT: The principle of the island neurovascular flap in the management of ulcerated anesthetic weight bearing areas of the lower extremity. Plast Reconstr Surg 1965;36:518.
38. Morain WD: Island toe flaps in neurotrophic ulcers of the foot and ankle. Ann Plast Surg 1984;13:1.
39. Giannini JT: Surgical treatment of plantar warts, callosities, and ulcers. Plast Reconstr Surg 1954;13:130.
40. Greeley PW: Plastic repair of radiation ulcers of the sole. US Naval Med Bull 1945;45:827.
41. Pangman WJ, Gurdin M: The treatment of uncomplicated plantar lesions. Plast Reconstr Surg 1950;5:516.
42. Buncke HJ, Colen LB: An island flap from the first web space of the foot to cover plantar ulcers. Br J Plast Surg 1980;33:242.
43. Colen LB, Buncke HJ: Neurovascular island flaps from the plantar vessels and nerves for reconstruction. Ann Plast Surg 1984;12:327.
44. Curtin JW: Functional surgery for intractable conditions of the sole of the foot. Plast Reconstr Surg 1977;59:806.
45. Hidalgo DA, Shaw WW: Anatomic basis of plantar flap design. Plast Reconstr Surg 1986;78:627.
46. McKittrick LS, McKittrick BM, Risley TS: Transmetatarsal amputation for infection of gangrene in patients with diabetes mellitus. J Clin Invest 1974;53:1071.
47. Shaw WW, Hidalgo DA: Anatomic basis of plantar flap design: clinical applications. Plast Reconstr Surg 1986;78:637.
48. Pinzur, Kaminsky M, Sage R, et al: Amputations at the middle level of the foot. J Bone Joint Surg Am 1986;68:1061.
49. Wagner FW: Amputations of the foot and ankle. Clin Orthop 1977;122:62.
50. Bostwick J: Reconstruction of the heel pad by muscle transposition and split skin graft. Surg Gynecol Obstet 1976;143:972.
51. Ger R: The surgical management of ulcers of the heel. Surg Gynecol Obstet 1975;140:909.
52. Hartrampf CR, Scheflan M, Bostwick J: The flexor digitorum brevis muscle island pedicle flap: a new dimension in heel reconstruction. Plast Reconstr Surg 1980;66:264.
53. Ikuta Y, Murakami T, Yoshioka K, Tsugo K: Reconstruction of the heel pad by flexor digitorum brevis musculocutaneous flap transfer. Plast Reconstr Surg 1984;74:86.
54. Scheflan M, Nahai F, Hartrampf CR: Surgical management of heel ulcers: a comprehensive approach. Ann Plast Surg 1981;7:385.
55. Attinger CE, Ducic I, Cooper P, et al: The role of intrinsic muscle flaps of the foot for bone coverage in foot and ankle defects in diabetic and nondiabetic patients. Plast Reconstr Surg 2002;110:1047.

56. Harrison DH, Morgan BD: The instep island flap to resurface plantar defects. Br J Plast Surg 1981;34:315.
57. Mir y Mir L: Functional graft of the heel. Plast Reconstr Surg 1954;14:444.
58. Taylor GA, Hopson WL: The cross-foot flap. Plast Reconstr Surg 1975;55:677.
59. Masquelet AC, Romana MC, Wolf G: Skin island flap supplied by the vascular axis of the sensitive superficial nerves: anatomic study and clinical experience in the leg. Plast Reconstr Surg 1992;89:1115.
60. Franklin JD: The deltoid flap: anatomy and clinical applications. In Buncke HJ, Furnas DW, eds: Symposium on Clinical Frontiers in Reconstructive Microsurgery, vol 24. St. Louis, CV Mosby, 1984.
61. Russell RC, Guy RJ, Zook EG, Merrell JC: Extremity reconstruction using the free deltoid flap. Plast Reconstr Surg 1985;76:586.
62. Katsaros J, Schusterman M, Beppu M, et al: The lateral upper arm flap: anatomy and clinical applications. Ann Plast Surg 1969;22:143.
63. May JW, Halls MJ, Simon SR: Free microvascular muscle flaps with skin graft reconstruction of extensive defects of the foot: a clinical and gait analysis study. Plast Reconstr Surg 1985;75:627.
64. Stevenson TR, Mathes SJ: Management of foot injuries with free muscle flaps. Plast Reconstr Surg 1986;78:665.
65. Chang KN, DeArmond SJ, Buncke HJ: Sensory reinnervation in microsurgical reconstruction of the heel. Plast Reconstr Surg 1986;78:652.
66. Mathes SJ, Alpert BS, Chang N: Use of the muscle flap in chronic osteomyelitis: experimental and clinical correlation. Plast Reconstr Surg 1982;69:815.
67. Mathes SJ, Feng LG, Hunt TK: Coverage of the infected wound. Ann Surg 1983;198:420.
68. Colen LB, Reus WF, Kalus R: Posterior hindfoot reconstruction. J Reconstr Microsurg 1990;6:143.
69. Syme J: Amputation at the ankle joint. London and Edinburgh Monthly J Med Sci 1843;2:93.
70. Waters RL, Campbell J, Thomas L, et al: Energy costs of walking of amputees: the influence of level of amputation. J Bone Joint Surg Am 1976;58:42.
71. Pecoraro RE, Reiber GE, Burgess EM: Pathways to diabetic limb amputation: basis for prevention. Diabetes Care 1990; 13:513.
72. Ollendorf D, Kotsanos J, Wishner W: Potential economic benefits of lower-extremity amputation prevention strategies in diabetes. Diabetes Care 1998;21:1240.
73. Centers for Disease Control and Prevention: Diabetes Surveillance, 1993. Atlanta, Georgia, U.S. Department of Health and Human Services, 1993.
74. Bloomgarden ZT: American Diabetes Association 60th Scientific Sessions, 2000: the diabetic foot. Diabetes Care 2001;24:946.
75. Mayfield JA, Reiber GE, Maynard C, et al: Trends in lower limb amputation in the Veterans Health Administration, 1989-1998. J Rehab Res Dev 2000;37:23-30.
76. Boulton AJM, Vileikyte L: Diabetic foot problems and their management around the world. In Bowker JH, Pfeifer MA, eds: Levin and O'Neal's The Diabetic Foot. St. Louis, Mosby, 2001.
77. Young MJ, Breddy JL, Veves A, Boulton AJ: The prediction of diabetic foot ulceration using vibration perception thresholds. Diabetes Care 1994;17:557.
78. Abbott CA, Vileikyte L, Williamson SH, et al: Multicenter study of the incidence and predictive factors for diabetic foot ulceration. Diabetes Care 1998;231:1071.
79. Ramsey SD, Newton K, Blough D, et al: Incidence, outcomes and cost of foot ulcers in patients with diabetes. Diabetes Care 1999;22:382.
80. Gordois A, Oglesby A, Scuffhamn P, et al: The health care costs of diabetic peripheral neuropathy in the U.S. Diabetes Care 2003;26:1790.
81. Palumbo PJ, Melton LJ: Peripheral vascular disease and diabetes. In Harris MI, Hamman RF, eds: Diabetes in America. Bethesda, Md, U.S. Department of Health and Human Services, National Institutes of Health, National Institute of Arthritis, Diabetes and Digestive and Kidney Diseases, 1985. NIH publication 85-1468.
82. Block P: The diabetic foot ulcer: a complex problem with a simple treatment approach. Milt Med 1981;146:644.
83. Report of the National Diabetes Advisory Board. Bethesda, Md, National Diabetes Advisory Board, 1980. NIH publication 81-2284.
84. Warren R, Kihn RB: A survey of lower extremity amputations for ischemia. Surgery 1988;63:107.
85. Holzer SES, Camerota A, Martinez L, et al: Costs and duration of care for lower extremity ulcers in patients with diabetes. Clin Ther 1998;20:518.
86. Ecker ML, Jacobs BS: Lower extremity amputation in diabetic patients. Diabetes 1970;19:189.
87. Goldner MG: The fate of the second leg in the diabetic amputee. Diabetes 1960;9:100.
88. Kucan JO, Robson MC: Diabetic foot infections: fate of the contralateral foot. Plast Reconstr Surg 1986;77:439.
89. Rosenqvist U: An epidemiological survey of diabetic foot problems in the Stockholm County, 1982. Acta Med Scand Suppl 1984;687:55.
90. Maeda N, Kon K, Imaizumi K, et al: Alteration of rheological properties of human erythrocytes by cross linking of membrane proteins. Biochem Biophys Acta 1983;735:104.
91. Strandness DE, Priest RE, Gibbons GE: Combined clinical and pathological study of diabetic and nondiabetic peripheral arterial disease. Diabetes 1964;13:366.
92. Conrad NC: Large and small artery occlusion in diabetics and non-diabetics with severe vascular disease. Circulation 1967;36:83.
93. Barnes HB, Kaiser GC, William VL: Blood flow in the diabetic leg. Circulation 1971;43:391.
94. Banson BB, Lacy PE: Diabetic microangiopathy in human toes: with emphasis on ultrastructural change in dermal capillaries. Am J Pathol 1964;45:41.
95. LoGerfo FW, Coffman JD: Vascular and microvascular disease of the foot in diabetes. N Engl J Med 1984;311:1615.
96. Krahenbuhl B, Mossang A: On vascular non-disease of the foot in diabetes [letter]. N Engl J Med 1985;312:1190.
97. Frykberg RG, Kozak GP: Neuropathic arthropathy in the diabetic foot. Am Fam Physician 1978;17:105.
98. Kristiansen B: Ankle and foot fractures in diabetics provoking neuropathic joint changes. Acta Orthop Scand 1980;51:975.
99. Lippman HJ, Perotto A, Ferrar R: The neuropathic foot of the diabetic. Bull N Y Acad Med 1976;52:1159.
100. Sinha CS, Munichoodappa I, Kozak GP: Neuroarthropathy (Charcot joints) in diabetes mellitus. Medicine (Baltimore) 1972;51:191.
101. Brower AC, Allman RM: Pathogenesis of the neuropathic joint: neurotraumatic vs. neurovascular. Radiology 1981;9:349.
102. Hoeldtke RD, Cavanaugh ST: Treatment of orthostatic hypotension with dihydroergotamine and caffeine. Ann Intern Med 1996;105:168.
103. Dolman CL: Morbid anatomy of diabetic neuropathy. Neurology 1955;13:135.
104. Eames RA, Long LS: Clinical and pathological study of ischemic neuropathy. J Neurol Neurosurg Psychiatry 1964;30:215.
105. Chopra JS, Hurwitz LG, Montgomery DA: Pathogenesis of sural nerve changes in diabetes mellitus. Brain 1969;92:391.
106. Clements RA: Diabetic neuropathy: new concepts of its etiology. Diabetes 1987;28:604.

107. Gabbay KH: The sorbitol pathway and the complications of diabetes. N Engl J Med 1973;288:831.
108. Gabbay KH, O'Sullivan JB: The sorbitol pathway in diabetes and galactosemia: enzyme and substrate localization. Diabetes 1968;17:300.
109. Jakobsen J: Peripheral nerve in early experimental diabetes: expansion of the endoneural space as a cause of increased water content. Diabetologia 1978;14:113.
110. Stewart MA, Passoneau JV, Lowry OH: Substrate changes in peripheral nerve during ischemia and wallerian degeneration. J Neurochem 1965;12:719.
111. Low PA, Dyck PJ, Schmelzer JD: Chronic elevation of endoneural fluid pressure is associated with low-grade fiber pathology. Muscle Nerve 1982;5:162.
112. Myers RR, Powell HC: Galactose neuropathy: impact of chronic endoneural edema on nerve blood flow. Ann Neurol 1984;126:587.
113. Tuck RR, Schmelzer JD, Low PA: Endoneural blood flow and oxygen tension in the sciatic nerves of rats with experimental diabetic neuropathy. Brain 1984;107:935.
114. Cameron NE, Leonard MB, Roos IS: The effects of sorbinil on peripheral nerve conduction velocity polyol concentrations, and morphology in streptozotocin-diabetic rat. Diabetologia 1986;29:168.
115. Griffey RH, Eaton RP, Sibbett RR, et al: Diabetic neuropathy: structural analysis of nerve hydration by magnetic resonance spectroscopy. JAMA 1988;260:2872.
116. Mackinnon SE, Dellon AL, Hunter D: Chronic nerve compression: an experimental model in the rat. Ann Plast Surg 1984;13:112.
117. Waltman HW, Wilde RM: Diabetes mellitus: pathological changes in the spinal cord and peripheral nerves. Arch Intern Med 1929;44:576.
118. Dellon AL, Seiler WA, Mackinnon SE: Susceptibility of the diabetic nerve to chronic compression. Ann Plast Surg 1988;20:117.
119. Upton AR, McComas AJ: The double crush in nerve entrapment syndromes. Lancet 1973;2:359.
120. Simpson LO: Intrinsic stiffening of red blood cells as the fundamental cause of diabetic nephropathy and microangiopathy: a new hypothesis. Nephron 1985;396:344.
121. Jones RL, Peterson CM: Hematologic alterations in diabetes mellitus. Am J Med 1981;70:339.
122. Ditenfass L: Blood viscosity factors in severe nondiabetic and diabetic retinopathy. Biorheology 1980;17:355.
123. McMillan DE, Utterback NG, Stocki J: Low shear rate blood viscosity in diabetes. Biorheology 1977;14:151.
124. McMillan DE: Disturbance of serum viscosity in diabetes mellitus. J Clin Invest 1974;53:1071.
125. Skovborg F, Nielsen AV, Schlichtkrull J, Ditzel J: Blood viscosity in diabetic patients. Lancet 1966;1:129.
126. Ditzel J: The nature of the intravascular erythrocyte aggregation in disease with particular reference to diabetes mellitus. Acta Med Scand 1955;152:372.
127. Schmid-Schonbein H: Microrheology of erythrocytes, blood viscosity, and the distribution of blood flow in microcirculation. In Guyton AL, ed: Cardiovascular Physiology II. Baltimore, Md, University Park Press, 1976.
128. Karuda T, Otsuki S: Lower levels of erythrocyte membrane fluidity in diabetic patients: a spin level study. Diabetes 1983;32:585.
129. Schmid-Schonbein H, Wells R, Goldstone J: Influence of deformability of human red cells upon viscosity. Circ Res 1969;25:131.
130. Bridges JM, Dalby AM, Hadden DR, et al: An effect of D-glucose on platelet stickiness. Lancet 1965;1:75.
131. McMillan DE, Utterback NG, LaPuma J: Reduced erythrocyte deformability in diabetes. Diabetes 1982; 31(suppl):64.
132. Juhan L, Vague P, Buonocore M, et al: Abnormalities of erythrocyte deformability and platelet aggregation in insulin-dependent diabetes corrected by insulin in vivo and in vitro. Lancet 1982;1:535.
133. Chien S, et al: Influence of fibrinogen and globulins on blood rheology at low shear rates. In Hartet HH, Copley AL, eds: Theoretical and Clinical Hemorheology. New York, Springer-Verlag, 1971.
134. Ehrly AM: Influence of Arwin on the flow properties of human blood. Biorheology 1973;10:543.
135. Reid HA, Chan KE, Theare PC: Prolonged coagulation defect (defibrination syndrome) in Malayan viper bite. Lancet 1963;1:621.
136. Stefanovich V: Effect of pentoxifylline on erythrocyte adenine nucleotide levels in rats: IRCS medical science. Biochem Hematol Pharmacol 1975;3:91.
137. Ehrly AM: The effect of plasma substitutes on erythrocyte aggregation and blood viscosity. Bibl Haematol 1969; 33:302.
138. Ehrly AM, Kohler HJ: Altered deformability of erythrocytes from patients with chronic occlusive arterial disease. Vasa 1976;5:319.
139. Roeren T, LeVeen R, Nugent L: Photoplethysmographic documentation of improved microcirculation after pentoxifylline therapy. Angiology 1988;39:929.
140. Schwartz RW, Logan NM, Johnston PJ, et al: Pentoxifylline increases extremity blood flow in diabetic atherosclerotic patients. Arch Surg 1989;124:434.
141. Ferrari E, Fioravante M, Patti AL, et al: Effects of long-term treatment (4 years) with pentoxifylline on haemorheologic changes and vascular complications in diabetic patients. Pharmatherapeutica 1987;5:26.
142. Gordon L, Buncke HJ: Restoration of sensation to the sole of the foot by nerve transfer. J Bone Joint Surg Am 1981; 63:828.
143. Dellon AL: A cause for optimism in diabetic neuropathy. Ann Plast Surg 1988;20:103.
144. Cianci P: Adjunctive HBO therapy in the treatment of the diabetic foot. Wounds 1992;4:158.
145. Shults DW, Hunter GC, McIntyre KE, et al: Value of radiographs and bone scans in determining the need for therapy in diabetic patients with foot ulcers. Am J Surg 1989;158:525.
146. Boulton AJ, Meneses P, Ennis WJ: Diabetic foot ulcers: a framework for prevention and care. Wound Repair Regen 1999;7:7.
147. Colen LB: Limb salvage in the patient with severe peripheral vascular disease: the role of microsurgical free-tissue transfer. Plast Reconstr Surg 1987;79:389.
148. Cohn BT, Brahms MA: Diabetic arthropathy of the first metatarsal cuneiform joint: introduction of a new surgical fusion technique. Orthop Rev 1987;16:465.
149. Martin WJ, Weil LS, Smith SD: Surgical management of neurotrophic ulcers in the diabetic foot. J Am Podiatr Med Assoc 1975;65:365.
150. Kostiuk JP, ed: Amputation Surgery and Rehabilitation: The Toronto Experience. New York, Churchill Livingstone, 1981.
151. Gibbons GW, Marcaccio EJ, Burgess AM, et al: Improved quality of diabetic foot care, 1984 vs 1990. Reduced length of stay and costs, insufficient reimbursement. Arch Surg 1993;128:576.
152. Cianci P, Hunt T: Long-term results of aggressive management of diabetic foot ulcers suggest significant cost effectiveness. Wound Repair Regen 1997;5:141.
153. Edmonds ME, Blundell MP, Morris ME, et al: Improved survival of the diabetic foot: the role of a specialized foot clinic. Q J Med 1986;60:763.
154. Sibbald RG, Kensholme A, Carter L: Special foot clinics for patients with diabetes. J Wound Care 1996;5:238.
155. Colen LB: Unpublished data, 2003.

156. Colen LB, Reus WF, Sasmor MT: Long-term follow-up of patients undergoing vascular bypass procedures and free tissue transfer for limb salvage. Plast Reconstr Surg; submitted.
157. Shestak KC, Fitz DG, Newton ED, Swartz WM: Expanding the horizons in treatment of severe peripheral vascular disease using microsurgical techniques. Plast Reconstr Surg 1990;85:406.
158. Cronenwett JL, McDaniel MD, Zwolak RM, et al: Limb salvage despite extensive tissue loss: free tissue transfer combined with distal revascularization. Arch Surg 1989;124:609.

CHAPTER

161

Vascular Insufficiency of the Lower Extremity: Lymphatic, Venous, and Arterial

ELISABETH K. BEAHM, MD, FACS ✦ ROBERT L. WALTON, MD, FACS ✦ ROBERT F. LOHMAN, MD, FACS

LYMPHEDEMA

Lymphedema describes a clinical condition in which there is accumulation of interstitial fluid. The pathologic collection of fluid may stem from either a congenital maldevelopment of the lymphatic system (primary) or an acquired condition (secondary).[1] Lymphedema primarily affects the extremities, although visceral lymphatic abnormalities have also been reported.[2] The disease may have a devastating impact on quality of life. There may be pain, mobility, hygiene, and body image issues as well as difficulty in vocational, domestic, and social settings. Patients with lymphedema manifest clinical anxiety, depression, and adjustment disorders.[3-7]

Anatomy and Pathophysiology

The functional unit of the lymphatic circulation is the lymphangion, which is segmentally contractile (Color Plate 161-1).[8] Blood vessels and lymphatics are anatomically similar, distinguished primarily by the structure of their basement membranes. The basement membrane in blood vessels is well defined, whereas in lymphatics it exhibits numerous intercellular gaps that permit diffusion of fat and protein into the lymphatic capillaries (Color Plate 161-2). Anatomic studies have delineated superficial and deep lymphatic systems, which ramify throughout the body and are contiguous with but separate from the adjacent venous system.[9] Muscle, although highly vascular, does not contain lymphatics. Direct communication between the lymphatic and venous systems normally occurs only in the major neck veins, at which point the thoracic and cervical lymphatic channels drain. Lymphatic vessels in the superficial and intermediate dermis, which lack valves, drain into the valved deep dermal and subdermal plexuses. The deep subfascial system is composed of much larger paired channels separate from the superficial system, connecting only at the supratrochlear, inguinal, and popliteal lymph nodes. The barriers between these separate and distinct systems may be broken down with the onset of lymphatic obstruction, resulting in communications between the superficial and deep lymphatics and between the lymph and venous channels.[10,11]

The lymphatic system is a high-volume transport system that functions to clear protein and lipids from the interstitial space to the vasculature by use of differential pressures (Color Plate 161-3). The intralymphatic pressure is low. Muscle contractions and the differential of abdominal and intrathoracic pressures occurring with respiratory effort propel lymph. In a functional state, the lymphatic system is so efficient that it is able to clear nearly half of the circulating albumin from the interstitium every day.[12] When this system breaks down, the disease state of lymphedema occurs. The pathophysiology and natural history of lymphedema have been well delineated in animal models.[13] In these studies, mechanical interruption of lymphatic vessels first leads to lymphangiographic changes, without overt interstitial abnormalities. Edema occurs only after the lymphatic channels become fibrotic, with junctional incompetence of the skin lymph capillaries. The chronic lymphedematous state is characterized by a decrease in lymphatic support as opposed to lymphatic hypertension or overproduction of lymph as might be suggested by models of venous hypertension. In the pathologic lymphedematous state, lymphatic load exceeds capacity, intralymphatic pressure builds, flow stagnates, and valvular incompetence occurs.[14] Dermal backflow (the reversal of flow into the dermal plexus) occurs as the intralymphatic pressure rises. As the capability of impaired lymphatic transport is overwhelmed, protein-rich fluid accumulates in the extracellular space.[15] Macromolecular protein and hyaluronan deposition leads to increased tissue colloid osmotic pressure, resulting in the influx of water and increased interstitial hydraulic pressure.[16,17] Fibroblasts, monocytes, adipocytes, and keratinocytes increase in the tissues, and brawny, nonpitting edema occurs from fibrovascular proliferation.[18,19] The elastic fibers degenerate and thicken, and the basement membrane of the lymphatic channels becomes thickened and eventually obliterated as ground substance, inflammatory cells, and fibroblasts proliferate (Color Plate 161-4). Collagen deposition outstrips the rate of phagocytosis, leading to further fibrosis and tissue overgrowth.[16,17,20]

Classification

The classification of lymphedema relies on a distinction between primary and secondary causes of the disease state. Primary lymphatic obstruction may be caused by several anatomic abnormalities, including lymphatic hypoplasia and functional insufficiency or absence of lymphatic valves (Fig. 161-1).[1] In addition, the lymphangion may fail to be contractile. Primary lymphedema is further classified by the age at onset of the lymphedema. Secondary lymphedema is far more common and may result from surgical, infectious-inflammatory, neoplastic, or traumatic compromise of the lymphatic pathways.

PRIMARY LYMPHEDEMA

Congenital lymphedema is noted within the first 2 years of life and is often apparent at birth. It may involve multiple limbs, the genitalia, and even the face. The lower extremity is involved three times more often than the upper extremity. Bilateral lower extremity edema is the most common presentation of congenital lymphedema, and the involvement of both lower extremities is far more likely in this condition than in other forms of primary lymphedema. Girls are affected twice as often as are boys. Fortunately, the majority of patients require no specific therapy, and a number of patients demonstrate some spontaneous improvement of the edema over time.[21] Certain chromosome abnormalities have been associated with intrauterine and congenital lymphatic dysfunction. Genes for lymphedema-distichiasis have been elucidated.[22] Genetic mapping of familial cohorts with a few of the lymphedema-related syndromes, such as cholestasis-lymphedema, has successfully identified a disease locus.[23] An autosomal dominant etiology is often noted with familial clusters of lymphedema.[24,25] The autosomal dominant form of hereditary lymphedema (Milroy disease) has been attributed to a mutation that inactivates the VEGFR3 tyrosine kinase mechanism specific to lymphatic vessels.[26,27] However, the most common inheritance pattern of congenital lymphedema is isolated and sporadic.

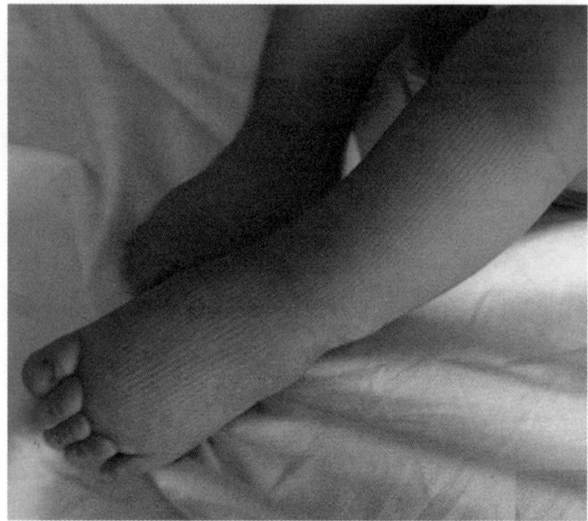

FIGURE 161-1. Primary lymphedema is often apparent at birth. It may result from lymphatic hypoplasia, absence or insufficiency of the valves, or failure of lymphangions to contract. (Courtesy of BSN-Jobst, Inc.)

Lymphedema praecox, also known as early lymphedema or Meige disease, is the most common form of primary lymphedema, accounting for more than 90% of patients with primary lymphedema with an estimated incidence of approximately 1 in 100,000.[21] Lymphedema praecox is usually diagnosed during puberty but may appear as late as the third decade of life.[16] The edema is usually unilateral and limited to the foot and calf. There is a strong female predominance of this disorder (4:1 up to 10:1), suggesting an estrogenic effect.[26] Lymphedema tarda, which usually presents after the age of 35 years, is relatively rare, accounting for less than 10% of patients with primary lymphedema.[16]

Lymphedema has also been classified by the morphologic characteristics of the affected lymphatics as seen on lymphangiography.[21,26] Aplastic lymphedema (representing approximately 15% of patients) is the pattern most commonly seen in congenital lymphedema. Patients suffering from aplastic lymphedema demonstrate a normal dermal plexus with total absence of the subcutaneous lymphatics. Hypoplastic lymphedema is most often seen in lymphedema praecox. Distal hypoplasia of the lymphatics is clinically associated with bilateral peripheral edema of the lower extremities, which is indolent and progressive. It demonstrates a female predominance and familial clustering. Hypoplastic lymphedema is further divided into obstructive and nonobstructive patterns. Obstructive lymphedema represents a decrease in the number of proximal lymphatics; nonobstructive lymphedema represents an adequate number but inadequate caliber of vessels. Proximal obstructive hypoplasia usually manifests an aggressive clinical pattern of rapidly worsening edema refractory to treatment and involving the entire affected extremity. Lymphatic hyperplasia with megalymphatics (an increase in both size and number) most often presents with unilateral edema of the entire lower extremity. It is seen in late-onset lymphedema and is the least common of the anatomic variants.[16,26]

SECONDARY LYMPHEDEMA

Secondary lymphedema results from the disruption of normal lymphatic channels and is far more common than primary lymphedema. World wide, filariasis is the leading cause of secondary lymphedema, affecting more than 90 million people (Fig. 161-2).[27,28] In the Western Hemisphere, secondary lymphedema is commonly the result of surgery or radiotherapy.[29] Upper extremity edema after surgical treatment of breast cancer affects the greatest number of patients with a reported incidence of 6% to 80%.[29,30] Lower extremity edema is usually associated with neoplasm and its surgical treatment (Fig. 161-3). The incidence of secondary lymphedema after inguinal or pelvic lymph node dissection is increased after radiotherapy and has an incidence reported to be between 1% and 47%.[31,32]

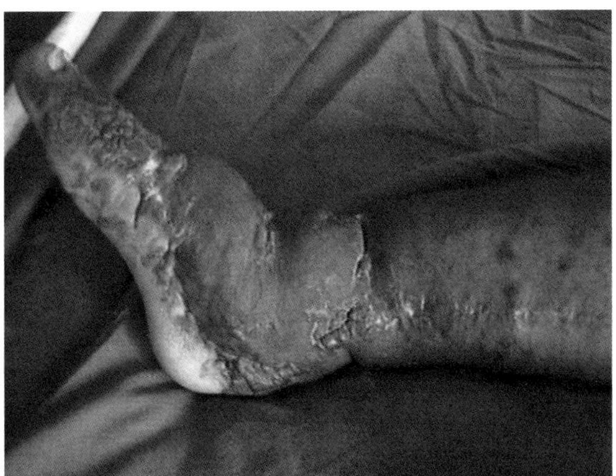

FIGURE 161-2. Lower extremity lymphedema resulting from the parasitic filarial worm. Filariasis is the most common cause of secondary lymphedema worldwide, currently affecting more than 90 million people. (Courtesy of BSN-Jobst, Inc.)

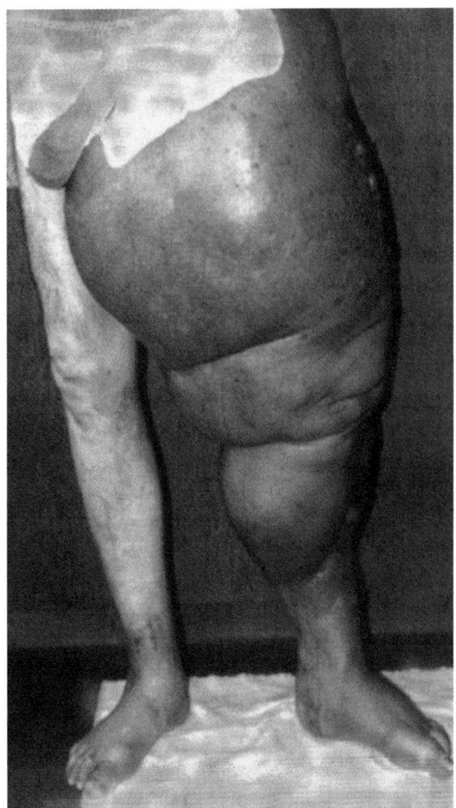

FIGURE 161-3. In the Western Hemisphere, secondary lymphedema is most often the result of neoplasm and its treatment. As evidenced by this patient, the combination of pelvic or inguinal node dissection and radiation therapy carries a greatly increased risk for lower extremity lymphedema, which may reach massive proportions if it is untreated. (Courtesy of BSN-Jobst, Inc.)

Natural History

The timing of the clinical onset of lymphedema is uncertain in both acquired and primary forms of the disease. There may be a prolonged latent phase in either situation, and the precipitating factors for the appearance of lymphedema are uncertain. Clinical lymphedema begins with mild swelling of the involved extremity. Initially, the involved extremity becomes edematous and soft. Fibrotic changes develop with chronicity. Recurrent soft tissue infection is one of the most problematic aspects of lymphedema. Lymphatic dysfunction stifles the local immune responses and immunosurveillance. The accumulated tissue fluid and proteins encourage microbial growth. Infections may be mild or severe. Recurrent infections result in progressive damage to the lymphatic capillaries, worsen the skin quality, and aggravate the edema.[33,34]

Diagnosis

The diagnosis of lymphedema is usually determined by a thorough history and physical examination, although other disease states may mimic lymphedema.[35] Ascertaining the precise onset of the lymphedema is less accurate because the patient's report may be flawed. Clinical detection may also be variable and is highly dependent on the examiner. Circumferential limb measurements have been the most commonly used objective test (Fig. 161-4). Differences of more than 2 cm between sides are generally considered clinically significant. It has been demonstrated that extremity volume estimated by circumferential measurements is nearly as accurate as water displacement.[36] The classic diagnostic signs of lower extremity lymphedema include peau d'orange changes in the skin (the result of fibrosis), the Stemmer sign (inability to tent the skin over the toes), and the blunted appearance of the digits of the involved extremity (Fig. 161-5).[35,36]

Chronic venous insufficiency may be confused with lymphedema of the legs, but it can be distinguished by chronic pruritus, pigmentary changes due to hemosiderin deposits, varicosities, and ulceration if it is advanced.[37] Thyroid disease may lead to myxedema, in which the edema results from deposition of hyaluronic acid-rich proteins in the dermis. In thyrotoxicosis, this process is localized to the pretibial region, whereas it is more diffuse in hypothyroidism.[38] Myxedema may be distinguished from lymphedema by the accompanying findings of dry or roughened skin (especially the palms, soles, elbows, and knees), dry and thinning hair, reduced sweat production, and yellowish tinge of the skin.[39] Lipedema is an abnormal accumulation of subcutaneous fat between the pelvis and ankle (usually affecting the hips and thighs) that may be confused with lymphedema (Fig. 161-6). The cause is unclear, but abnormalities in the subcutaneous adipocytes and local dermal vascular structure have been noted. Lipedema usually arises within several years after puberty and affects women and men with feminizing disorder. There is associated pain and easy bruising. Lipedema spares the feet and thus may be distinguished from lymphedema by absence of the Stemmer sign.[40]

Lymphoscintigraphy and magnetic resonance imaging (MRI) have become helpful tools in evaluating fluid accumulation. Diagnostic studies may be useful in establishing the diagnosis in early stages of lymphedema, such as in patients with mild or intermittent edema. They may also be used to confirm or

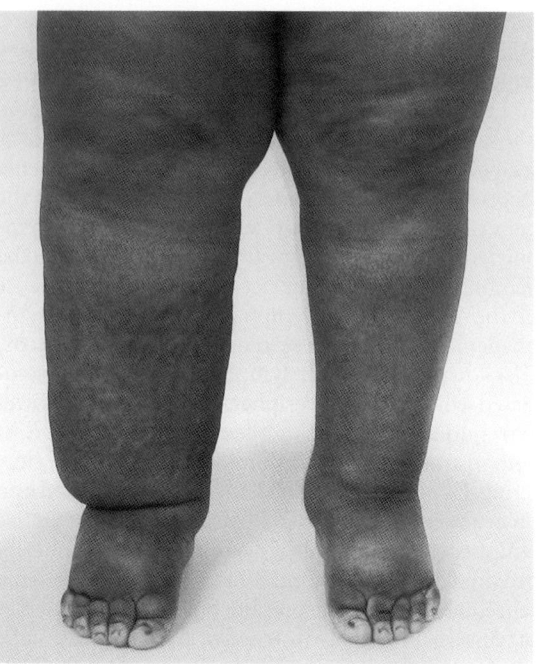

FIGURE 161-5. Classic diagnostic signs in lower extremity lymphedema demonstrated by this patient include not only edema but also peau d'orange changes in the skin and a blunted appearance of the digits.

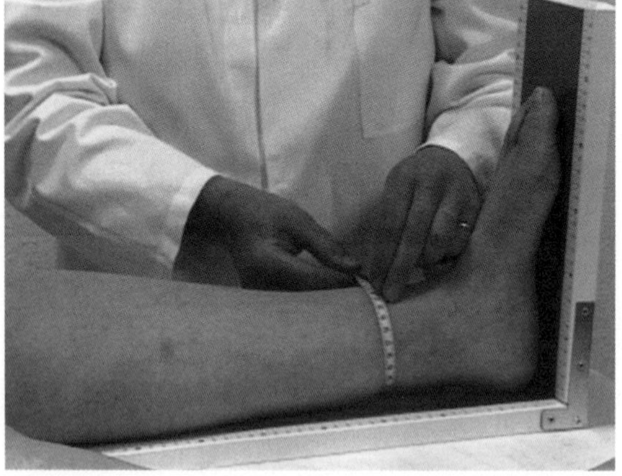

FIGURE 161-4. Circumferential limb measurements are the most commonly used objective measure for the diagnosis and longitudinal evaluation of efficacy of treatment of lymphedema. Extremity volume estimated by this method is thought to be as accurate as more complex and cumbersome techniques such as volume displacement. (Courtesy of BSN-Jobst, Inc.)

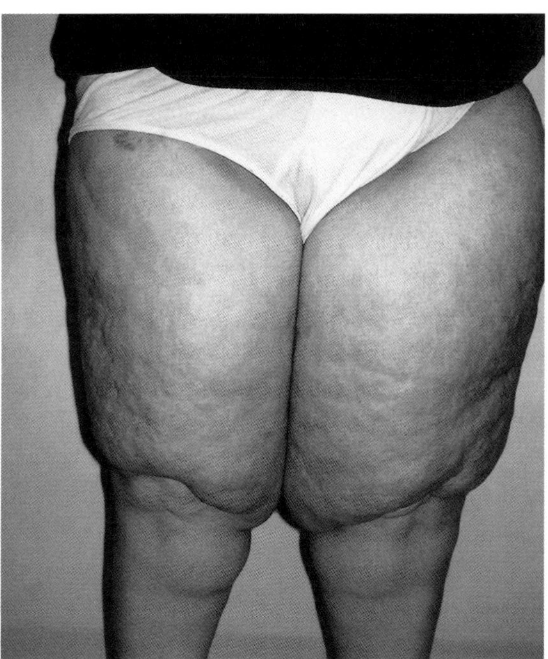

FIGURE 161-6. This patient demonstrates lipedema, which is manifested by an abnormal deposition of subcutaneous fat localized between the pelvis and ankle. Whereas lipedema may coexist or be confused with lymphedema, lipedema most commonly affects the hips and thighs and spares the feet, thus distinguishing it from lymphedema.

quantify the impaired lymphatic flow, to characterize the pattern of fluid distribution in the tissues, and to identify potential operative candidates.[41,42]

DIAGNOSTIC STUDIES

Contrast Lymphography

Historically, radiologic evaluation of the lymphatic system was performed with direct injection of contrast medium into the lymphatic channels, each of which was identified for cannulation by the subcutaneous injection of patent blue dye.[43,44] The procedure is technically difficult and tedious. It may be associated with progressive fibrosis and worsening of the lymphedema due to pooling of the lipid-soluble contrast medium. In addition, there is the potential for significant reactions to the contrast agent. For these reasons, direct lymphography is rarely used today except to visualize anatomy before reconstructive lymphatic surgery, and lymphoscintigraphy has emerged as the primary diagnostic tool for the assessment of lymphatic function.

Indirect Lymphangiography

Indirect lymphangiography uses water-soluble iodinated contrast material, which is injected intradermally. Xeroradiography is used to image the lymphatics. It may be useful in visualization of local skin lymphatics, in patients with localized or complex presentations of lymphedema, and in preoperative study for reconstructive surgery of the lymphatics. However, this technique is infrequently used because of the need for radiation exposure and the potential for reactions to the contrast agent.[45,46]

Isotopic Lymphoscintigraphy

Lymphoscintigraphy uses a nonionizing contrast agent injected into the interstitial space. It provides reasonable elucidation of the anatomy of the major lymphatic trunks as well as of the severity of the lymphatic obstruction.[45,47-50] A radiolabeled macromolecule (technetium Tc 99m–labeled antimony sulfide colloid, rhenium sulfate, or human serum albumin nanocolloid [^{99m}Tc-HSA, ^{99m}Tc-dextran]) is injected into the dermis (subdermally or intradermally) in the interdigital space of the affected limb. A gamma camera is used to follow transport of the macromolecule, providing both static, anatomic information and dynamic assessment of lymph flow. The rate of tracer disappearance and accumulation of counts in the inflow lymph node are quantified. Static lymphoscintigraphy is most sensitive for moderate or severe forms of lymphedema. It defines the number of lymph vessels and collaterals, the presence or absence of backflow, and the location of regional lymph nodes. Dynamic lymphoscintigraphy is useful in the evaluation of mild or transient forms of lymphedema. Stress tests with passive and active physical activity are thought to improve the reliability of the results. Some authors contend that evaluation of both the epifascial and subfascial lymphatic compartments (through subdermal and intradermal injections, respectively) is necessary for accurate assessment of lymphatic transport in the lower extremity.[45]

Lymphoscintigraphy is the most common diagnostic method currently used for the evaluation of lymphedema. It does not require the tedious cannulation of the lymphatic channels and provides useful anatomic and functional evaluation of the lymphatic system. However, the type and amount of tracer, the site of injection (intradermal or subdermal), and the stress protocol used in these studies require standardization for accurate data comparison. In addition, lymphoscintigraphy may not readily delineate lymphatics and lymph nodes distal to a point of obstruction because the tracer diffuses into the subcutaneous tissues or stagnates at the injection site.

Magnetic Resonance Imaging

MRI provides detailed anatomic information of the lymphatic trunks and nodes as well as of any obstructing lesions in secondary edema that may not be well elucidated by lymphoscintigraphy.[51-54] MRI may be used to complement the functional data obtained from lymphoscintigraphy and may be useful to distinguish lymphedema from other similar conditions. In chronic lymphedema, edema occurs in the epifascial compartment and exhibits a characteristic honeycomb pattern on MRI with reticular lymphangiectasis and lakes demonstrating a marked increase on T2-weighted imaging. In contrast, venous edema affects both the epifascial and subfascial compartments; lipedema is characterized by fat accumulation without fluid. MRI is recognized as a safe, nonionizing method for quantifying water content in tissues. High-resolution MRI is able to demonstrate thickening of all skin layers. The major tissue changes that result from lymphedema occur in the dermis, including marked fluid retention in the interlobular spacing just above the superficial fascia. MRI may be useful in distinguishing hyperplastic lymphedema and cavernous lymphangiomatosis, which exhibit characteristic T1 and T2 patterns.[54]

Computed Tomography

Computed tomography also identifies the characteristic honeycomb pattern of the subcutaneous tissue in lymphedema and permits identification of the anatomic distribution of the edema (subfascial or epifascial). Computed tomography may also be used to follow (through cross-sectional area) the limb volume and response to therapy, but it does not provide the functional data of lymphoscintigraphy or the anatomic precision offered by MRI.[55-57]

Ultrasonography

Ultrasonography is a valuable noninvasive method to quantify the volume of an edematous extremity. High-frequency ultrasonography can demonstrate characteristic patterns of fluid localization in various types of extremity edema and has been of particular benefit in observing women with postmastectomy lymphedema. Doppler studies can quickly and safely allow serial assessment of volumetric changes or venous compromise of the affected limb.[52-58]

Treatment

MEDICAL MANAGEMENT

Treatment of lymphedema may be divided into medical and surgical approaches. The majority of patients with lymphedema are treated successfully with medical therapy alone. The principles of conservative lymphedema treatment focus on the avoidance of infection and the application of compression to maintain or to improve limb volume. A number of specific treatment protocols have been studied, and although the majority of the experience has been with the upper extremity (because of its increased incidence), the principles of therapy are comparable. These protocols include various combinations of extremity elevation with massage and exercise (with and without compression garments), standard elastic sleeve (with and without electrically stimulated lymphatic drainage), uniform pneumatic compression, sequential compression by hydrostatic pressure, complex physical therapy, and sequential pneumatic compression.[16,28,59-62] Elevation alone is ineffective, but it may be used as an adjunct to other therapies. Simple elastic compression garments have been shown to be effective with a 30% to 40% reduction of edema in a range of ages.[28,63,64] More vigorous compression techniques, such as the use of compression pumps, have also been shown to be efficacious in the improvement of lymphedema.[35,62,64,65] The pumps are pneumatic and provide intermittent uniform or sequential pressure to the edematous limb. Treatments are lengthy (daily use for up to 1.5 to 6 hours per day for up to 4 weeks), and patients may complain about the period of immobilization required for treatment. Pneumatic compression has been shown to be effective, although the optimal pressure, duration, frequency of treatment, and amount of therapeutic maintenance necessary are unclear. In addition, compression pumps are most effective in the more distal extremities, and the base of each limb must be treated with manual compression. Complex physical therapy (also known as complex decongestive therapy, complex lymphedema therapy, multimodal physical therapy, complex decongestive physiotherapy, and complete decongestive physiotherapy) incorporates skin care, manual lymphedema treatment, exercises, and compression wrapping followed by a maintenance program and psychosocial rehabilitation.[59-63] This modality has been recommended by a number of consensus panels as a primary treatment of lymphedema refractory to more conventional therapy or compression (Figs. 161-7 and 161-8). Initially, an intense 4-week period of manual drainage is undertaken. This is a specialized massage technique intended to enhance lymphatic contractility and redirect flow into the nonobstructed lymphatics. The acute-phase therapy is then followed by wrappings and elastic support, which continue as maintenance. High-grade compression garments (40 to 80 mm Hg) are recommended to prevent reaccumulation of fluid. To be effective, compression garments must be fitted carefully and replaced when they lose their elasticity (every 3 to 6 months). In upper extremity edema, this approach has resulted in reduction of the lymphedema in 97% of patients, and a greater than 50% reduction in arm volume in more than half the patients was maintained at 3 years.[64,65] Most series demonstrate a 15% to 75% reduction in limb circumference.[61-65] To evaluate the efficacy of each therapeutic component, optimization of timing, and length of treatment, larger randomized studies will be necessary. Most authors recommend a

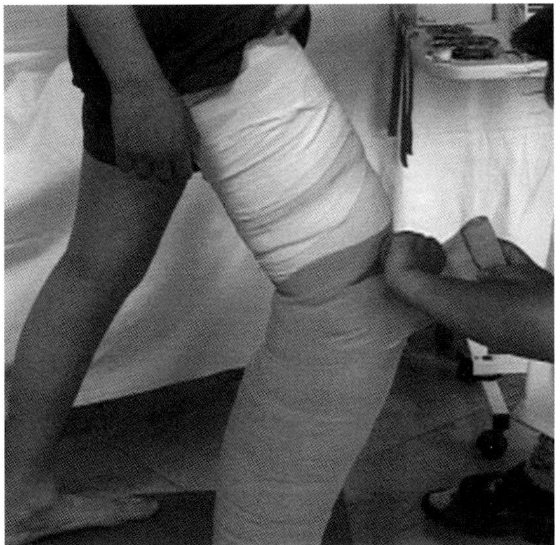

FIGURE 161-7. Surgical therapy for lymphedema is largely disappointing. Outcome after operative intervention in the lower extremity is significantly less favorable than in the upper extremity. As such, compression therapy is the current mainstay for treatment of lymphedema. The careful application of a firm compression wrap, which is demonstrated here, is used during the manual drainage and decompression phase of complex physical therapy, an intense and comprehensive program of massage and compression currently recommended by most authorities for the treatment of refractory lymphedema. (Courtesy of BSN-Jobst, Inc.)

multidisciplinary program for effective lymphedema management, incorporating therapies that address issues of mobility and body image as well as specific edema treatments.[28]

Ultrasound therapy and localized hyperthermia have demonstrated subjective improvement in certain select patients with lymphedema.[66,67] Intra-arterial injection of autologous lymphocytes, which is postulated to lead to greater expression of L-selectin, a lymphocyte-specific adhesion molecule, has shown some promise in initial studies.[68-70]

Pharmacotherapy and Dietary Therapy

Pharmacologic intervention has been used as primary and adjunctive therapy for lymphedema. A number of agents have been used, including benzopyrones, flavonoids, antibiotics, and diuretics. Coumarin (a benzopyrone) has been credited with improvement in lymphedema. This is thought to occur through protein resorption and proteolysis, induced by stimulation of cutaneous macrophages and an enhanced general immune system response in patients with upper and lower extremity edema and filariasis.[71,72] Oral coumarin is, however, associated with a doubling of serum aminotransferases and idiosyncratic hepatitis and was removed from the U.S. market after several deaths during one trial.[73,74] Diuretics do not improve interstitial edema but act only to cause hemoconcentration and thus have no efficacy in the treatment of lymphedema. Antibiotics are best reserved for treatment of bouts of cellulitis and are not recommended for prophylaxis.

Dietary manipulation has been proposed as a treatment of lymphedema. The flavonoids (specifically the rutin derivatives) are believed to have a protective effect on the vascular endothelium and to improve the microcirculation. Daflon, a flavonoid, demonstrated a nonsignificant improvement in arm edema in a double-blind study. Dietary restriction of long-chain triglycerides has also shown some benefit in one report.[74,75]

SURGICAL OPTIONS

The efficacy of surgical interventions for lymphedema is, in general, so poor that they should be considered only when aggressive conservative measures have failed. Classically, surgical procedures for lymphedema are categorized as excisional, in which involved tissue is removed, and physiologic, in which an attempt is made to restore or to improve lymphatic flow.

Excisional Techniques

In the early 1900s, Charles lent his name to a treatment of filariasis involving radical excision of all involved lymphedematous tissue including skin, subcutaneous tissues, and fascia, covering the resultant wound with split- or full-thickness skin grafts.[76] Several reviews of patients treated with this technique demonstrated good functional results if compression garments were diligently used.[77-80] Cosmetic results were highly unfavorable, however, and in some patients were worse than the original lymphedematous appearance. In addition, there was a high incidence of wound breakdown and contracture, hyperkeratosis, and ulcerations as well as aggravation of foot edema.

Kondoleon[81] subsequently advocated staged excision of the subcutaneous tissues. This technique, which was modified by Sistrunk[82] and popularized by Miller[83,84] and Homans,[85] has been the mainstay of excisional techniques.[86] These procedures result in an approximate 50% reduction in extremity volume, with improvement not only in the size of the extremity but also in the symptoms and incidence of cellulitis. Careful follow-up and conscientious use of elastic support stockings are necessary for maintenance of postoperative results.

Suction-Assisted Lipectomy

Suction-assisted lipectomy has also been used in the treatment of lymphedema and has demonstrated some benefit.[87-89] Suction-assisted lipectomy is most often used in combination with another treatment

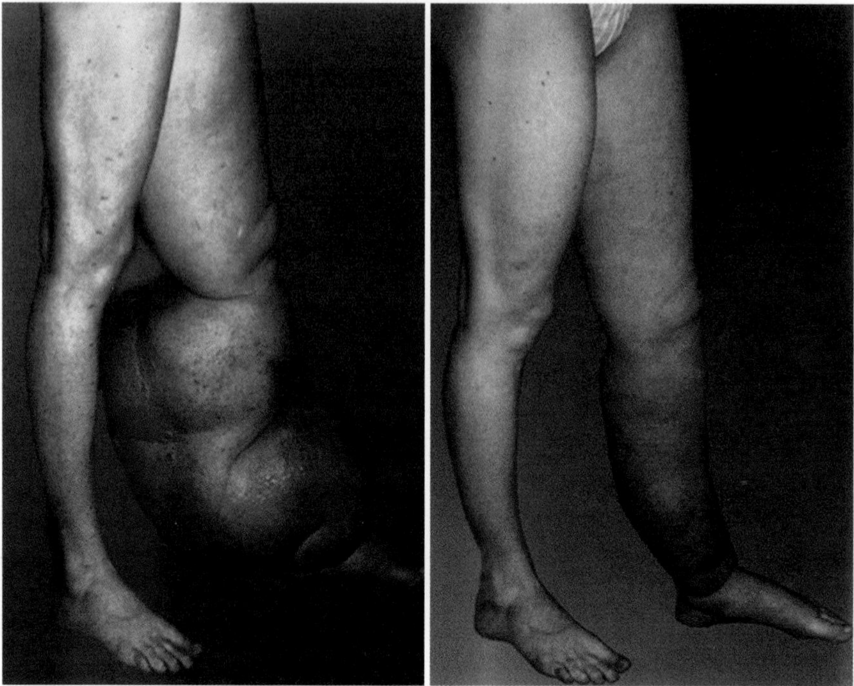

FIGURE 161-8. Conservative therapies, which incorporate compression wrapping and complex physical therapy, require a high level of compliance by the patient and a lifetime of use of some sort of compression treatment to avoid recurrence. The efficacy of this treatment approach, even for advanced cases of lymphedema, is demonstrated by the photographs of this patient with secondary lymphedema before and after treatment. (Courtesy of BSN-Jobst, Inc.)

modality, such as extremity compression, surgical excision, or lymphatic-venous shunt. As such, the effectiveness of suction alone is unclear. One study noted an average of 106% reduction in limb volume at 1 year after suction-assisted lipectomy; however, all of these patients also received manual lymphatic drainage or pneumatic compression therapy.[87] A prospective study of liposuction alone or in combination with controlled compression therapy was performed in the upper extremity and demonstrated that liposuction was significantly more effective than compression therapy alone (average reduction of 113% versus 47%, respectively).[88,89] However, removal of the compression garment for only 1 week, a full year after the liposuction, resulted in a marked increase in arm edema. Fortunately, the arm volume was restored with reapplication and continued use of the garment.

Physiologic Techniques

Lymphangioplasty. Handley[90] theorized that placement of a silk suture into the subcutaneous tissues of lymphedematous extremities would act by capillary force to promote lymphatic flow and the regeneration of lymphatic channels. Unfortunately, these attempts were ineffective and complicated by infection and extrusion. Subsequently, a number of materials (both autogenous and alloplastic) have been inset to establish drainage channels. These modifications of Handley's approach have met with similar failure.[91]

Bridging Techniques. Disruption of the underlying fascial barrier has been undertaken in an effort to establish functional lymphatic communication between the superficial and deep systems. Kondoleon[81] attempted to allow drainage of the superficial lymphatics through the deep system by excision of strips of fascia. However, the fascial barrier was noted to re-form, and the operation was thus rendered ineffective.

Along a similar line of reasoning, bridging techniques that interpose normal tissue into a lymphadenomatous area to enhance drainage of the obstructed superficial system into the deep subfascial compartment have been advocated.[17,91] In the modified Charles procedure, the buried tissue, usually dermis, is postulated to enhance lymph drainage by leading to the formation of connecting channels between the superficial and deep dermal lymphatic systems. Unfortunately, this approach had results comparable to those of the original Charles technique.[91] Thompson[17,92] used a buried dermal flap in an attempt to improve lymphatic flow through dermal lymphatics. He combined this technique with excision of the lymphedematous subcutaneous tissues and obtained good or satisfactory results in more than 90% of patients. The mechanism of edema reduction is unknown, but volume reduction appears to closely correlate with the amount of tissue excised. Radioisotope studies of buried dermal flaps failed to confirm any new lymphatic-lymphatic or lymphatic-venous communications, and at 2 years postoperatively, lymphatic size returned to normal.[93] Other bridging techniques have also been undertaken. The enteromesenteric bridge is a segment of ileum with its intact mesentery that is coapted to an inguinal lymph node to bypass occluded pelvic lymphatics. Used in patients with primary pelvic lymphedema, this method demonstrated good results in six of eight patients.[94] Omental transfer, however, has been fraught with difficulties, mainly stemming from fibrosis of the transferred omentum. Despite promising results with omental flaps in animal models, only a few clinical reports of omental flap transfer with lymphatic nodal-venous anastomoses have demonstrated salutary results.[95-99] Musculocutaneous and fasciocutaneous flaps to improve edema have also been proposed but are limited to a few animal models and some anecdotal clinical applications, which are not well studied.[97,100-102]

In summary, a number of flaps have been used as a physiologic bridge in the treatment of lymphedema. Because this approach has been largely employed in combination with other techniques, the results are difficult to interpret. These methods have demonstrated only variable success, carry the potential for significant morbidity, and clearly require further study before widespread clinical use is advocated.

LYMPHATIC ANASTOMOSES. Lymphatic-lymphatic, lymphatic-venous, lymphatic-venous-lymphatic, and lymph node-venous anastomoses have all been used in an attempt to relieve obstructive lymphedema. Lymphatic-venous shunts were introduced by Nielubowicz,[103] who coapted a sectioned lymph node to an adjacent vein, theorizing that the high pressure in the lymphatics would drive drainage into the venous system. O'Brien[104] performed microlymphatic-venous (end-to-end) anastomoses (MLVA) between lymphatic vessels and veins with good results. His experience with this technique, both alone and in conjunction with excisional techniques, led him to recommended the combination of these methods because of improved results in the resection group. Long term, the initial 83% to 90% reduction in limb edema had fallen to 60% improvement in the combined groups (excision and MLVA) and a 42% improvement with MLVA only. In addition, a concerning 45% of patients undergoing MLVA had worsening of lymphedema.[105] O'Brien[104,105] found that the number of anastomoses performed did not correlate with the success of MLVA; Gloviczki,[106] using a similar technique, found the reverse. Both authors concluded that the results of MLVA, although encouraging in early stages of lymphedema, were disappointing overall because of at least some recurrence of edema long term. More recently, MLVA has been evaluated in a number of centers and has demonstrated a similarly modest long-term outcome.[107,108] Animal models have shown a similar pattern, with lymphatic-venous anastomoses demonstrating a high early patency rate and a subsequent fall by 3 weeks, which is clinically accompanied by a return of edema. This recurrence may be due to valvular dysfunction. It has been postulated that once the pressure in the lymphatic system is reduced, the incompetent valves cause reversal of flow from the venous side and eventual obstruction.[109]

Lymphatic-lymphatic grafting was initially studied by Baumeister[110] in dogs with highly favorable results. The technique was subsequently used in patients with upper and lower limb edema with an impressive 60% to 80% volume reduction and 30% improvement in lymphatic flow at 3 years, which was assessed by lymphoscintigraphy.[111] Interestingly, whereas many authors claim that surgical intervention for the treatment of lymphedema should be undertaken within the first 2 years after onset, Baumeister has noted success in patients up to 20 years after mastectomy.[112] The criteria used by this group to select patients for lymphatic grafting include the presence of adequate donor lymphatics (studied by lymphoscintigraphy), continued use of conservative measures, waiting a minimum of 6 months for postoperative edema to stabilize, and ensuring that tumor recurrence is not an issue. Most of the patients in these studies had secondary postmastectomy arm edema, which tends to respond more favorably to all types of treatment than do other forms of lymphedema.

Interposition lymphatic-venous-lymphatic anastomoses have shown promising results.[113] Vein grafts are placed between lymphatic channels both proximal and distal to the site of obstruction. Significant reduction in edema (>75%) was seen in more than 60% of patients. The technique may be of greatest utility in patients with chronic lymphedema who have not responded well to conservative measures or in those whose venous disease contraindicates a lymphatic-venous procedure.

Lymph node–venous anastomoses in lower extremity edema appear to be most beneficial in patients who have a postsurgical cause. Long-term follow-up (10 years) suggested an overall 80% improvement in patients after surgery, 50% improvement in patients with hyperplastic lymphedema, and less than 10% improvement in patients with postinflammatory lymphedema.[113,114]

All anastomotic techniques have demonstrated some efficacy early on, but long-term results are less impressive, and a combination of therapeutic approaches is usually required for maximal efficacy. Patients with postinflammatory and primary lymphedema are rarely candidates for a microsurgical technique because the lymphatic ducts are often not patent distal to the area of obstruction, a requirement for this technique. Patients with these types of lymphedema are best treated with a combined approach incorporating excisional techniques.

Specific Lymphatic Disorders and Treatment

GENITAL LYMPHEDEMA

Lymphedema of the genitalia may be a disfiguring disorder characterized by progressive swelling of the penis or scrotum. Genital lymphedema is comparable to extremity edema in its classification and presentation but differs in its improved response to surgery. In addition, it is often relentlessly progressive, evolving from mild lymphatic ectasis to severe dermal fibrosis, lymphangiomas, and ulceration.[115-117] In children with primary lymphedema, the intrinsic lymphatic dysfunction does not appear to be limited to the genitalia. Extremity involvement (upper or lower) and even distant manifestations such as pleural effusions are seen in many patients. In infant girls, primary genital lymphedema may result in pseudosexual ambiguity. These patients often reveal a family history of extremity edema, such as Nonne-Milroy disease.[118]

Excision of all lymphedematous tissue is the most commonly employed treatment of genital lymphedema. All involved tissues above the deep fascia are removed, including the skin, superficial lymphatics, and subcutaneous tissue.[115-123] The posterior scrotal skin is often uninvolved and is used as a source of skin flaps for reconstruction of the scrotum. Several large series have demonstrated good success with this approach.[117-119] Penile coverage is more problematic. Whereas some authors have recommended use of uninvolved preputial skin, the penile skin appears to be invariably involved, and use of local tissue has led to a tendency for recurrence of the edema. As such, split-thickness skin grafts are usually recommended for reconstruction of penile cover, and results appear to be satisfactory with this approach.[121] Although recurrence may not be an issue with grafting, skin grafts invariably contract, and the experience with this technique has been largely in adults with limited follow-up (1 to 5 years).[119,122] Several authors have suggested that skin graft contraction could potentially limit penile growth in children, and this should be considered in early interventions for genital lymphedema.[117,119] Genital lymphedema in women is most commonly associated with pelvic malignant neoplasia, and management focuses on treatment of the underlying condition.

LYMPHANGIOSARCOMA

Lymphangiosarcoma is a rare but aggressive and deadly lesion. Unfamiliarity with this disease and its innocuous appearance (presenting with bruising, increased swelling, or multiple blue-red subcutaneous nodules in the affected extremity) often leads to a delay in diagnosis. The cause of the tumor is not yet well understood. On histologic examination, lymphangiosarcoma arises from vascular endotheliocytes. All vascular sarcomas originating in the setting of a chronic lymphedema are categorized as lymphangiosarcoma. Lymphangiosarcoma has only recently been described in association with late-onset hereditary lymphedema. Because of a high association (10%) of multiple primary tumors with lymphangiosarcoma, a hereditary predisposition is thought to underlie the development of lymphedema-associated lymphangiosarcoma. The occurrence of lymphangiosarcoma after mastectomy is coined the Stewart-Treves syndrome, after the original description in 1948.[124] The incidence of Stewart-Treves syndrome ranges from 0.07% to approximately 0.5%, with a latency after breast cancer treatment of approximately 10 years (range, 5 to 21 years).[125-128] Local recurrence after treatment and metastasis are common. Survival after diagnosis, however, is only 8 to 15 months on average. There is no standard treatment of lymphangiosarcoma. Treatment is usually multimodality incorporating radical surgical resection, chemotherapy, and radiotherapy if it was not primarily employed in the breast cancer therapy. There have been several reported long-term survivors who appeared to benefit from early detection and aggressive treatment.[129]

VENOUS INSUFFICIENCY

Lower extremity ulceration and swelling are the most common complaints of patients seeking medical attention. Venous ulcers, which have historically (and inaccurately) been referred to as stasis ulcers, represent most of these lesions (80% to 90%).[130,131] Venous insufficiency, although it is less likely than arterial disease to lead to limb threat, carries a significant impact on the patient's quality of life and economic productivity. In both Europe and the United States, chronic venous insufficiency (CVI) has a prevalence of 0.1% to 2%.[132-134] It is estimated that at any given time, approximately 1 in 1000 people in the United States has an unhealed venous leg ulcer.[135] The annual cost of caring for these ulcers is estimated at more than $2 billion.[133-138]

A number of factors contribute to venous ulceration. A history of prior trauma or phlebitis will increase the risk for development of CVI, as will a family history of varicose veins or CVI, suggesting a genetic component to the disease.[139] The incidence of venous disease and leg ulcers increases with obesity, diabetes, heart failure, hypertension, renal disease, and rheumatoid arthritis and is slightly more common in women (1.6 : 1).[131-140] Venous ulceration appears to seriously affect the quality of life, and these patients often harbor feelings of anger, depression, and fear, conditions that appear to resolve with healing of the ulcer.[132,133] Chronic pain is a complaint of two thirds of the patients with venous ulceration. Whereas the incidence of CVI and ulceration increases with increasing age (peak occurrence at 60 to 80 years), it is not solely a disease of the elderly. More than 70% of patients have their first ulcer before the age of 60 years and 20% before the age of 40 years.[131] The average duration of most ulcers is longer than 1 year, and in a significant subset of patients (up to 34%), ulceration lasts more than 5 years.[133] In addition, the recurrence rate of ulceration is nearly 75%. The summation of these factors illuminates the potential negative impact of lower extremity venous disease on work productivity, lost wages, lost hours, and forced early retirement. An estimated 2 million workdays are lost annually in the United States because of leg ulcers alone.[136-138]

Anatomy and Pathophysiology

Superficial, deep, and perforating veins are the three distinct networks of venous drainage of the lower extremity. The superficial venous system, composed of the greater and lesser saphenous veins and their tributaries, lies in the subcutaneous plane and does not have an arterial counterpart.

The deep veins of the leg lie in the subfascial muscle compartments (intramuscular and intermuscular) of the leg. These vessels are accompanied by a named artery and include the three sets of tibial veins that coalesce into the popliteal vein. The popliteal vein, which becomes the superficial femoral vein at the level of the adductor canal, joins the deep femoral vein in the femoral triangle to form the common femoral vein. These veins account for 85% to 90% of venous drainage of the leg. In the thigh, a single vein accompanies each artery; distally, two or more draining veins accompany each arterial branch. The perforating veins connect the superficial and deep venous systems.

Venous drainage of the lower extremity is accomplished by a series of one-way valves and is propelled by differential pressures in the various systems. All leg veins have bicuspid valves that permit only unidirectional flow. Valves in the superficial and deep systems provide for cephalic directional blood flow; the perforating veins transport blood from the superficial into the deep system. Hydrostatic pressure in the standing posture is approximately 80 mm Hg at rest. During ambulation, the deep veins are compressed by the contraction of the leg musculature. The pressure in the deep veins thus rises, and blood is propelled proximally, primarily by the pumping action of the leg musculature. Retrograde flow into the superficial system is prevented by closure of the venous valves. Once the deep veins empty and the pressure in the deep system falls, the flow from the superficial into the deep system recurs, and the cycle is repeated.

Any breakdown in the mechanisms promoting venous drainage, either a diseased venous system or a compromised muscle pump, can lead to venous insufficiency. Valvular dysfunction may be due to congenital absence, congenital or acquired incompetence, injury, or deep venous outflow obstruction. Pump disjunction may arise from compromise of the leg musculature or joints.[141] In the diseased state with valvular incompetence, the venous pressure in the deep system remains high during all phases of ambulation. The tissues are exposed to continually elevated venous pressures ("venous hypertension" or "chronic venous insufficiency").[142] Eventually, hypertension in the deep system is transmitted to the superficial veins, and edema results.[143] Lipodermatosclerosis develops with chronic venous hypertension, a sequence of changes in the skin and subcutaneous tissues that may occur in CVI.[144] Initially, the leg may exhibit inflammation in which diffuse, tender, erythematous induration is noted proximal to the malleolus (usually medial) (Fig. 161-9). Subsequently, the induration of the medial leg

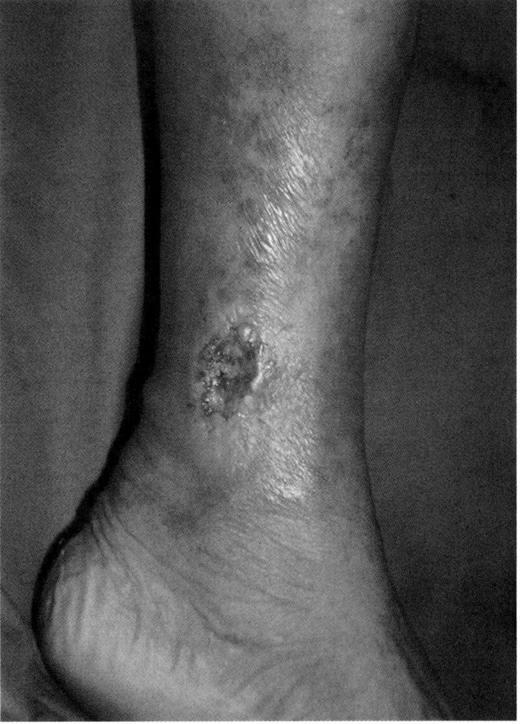

FIGURE 161-9. This patient demonstrates diffuse erythema of the distal lower extremity with induration and ulceration near the malleolus typical of early venous stasis disease.

becomes more clearly demarcated from the surrounding normal skin. The epidermis develops pigmentary changes and atrophy, and progressive fibrosis is noted in the subcutaneous tissues. Lipodermatosclerosis frequently precedes the development of venous ulceration, although ulcerations may occur in its absence, highlighting the multifactorial cause of ulceration.[145] The degree of lipodermatosclerosis directly correlates with the impairment of wound healing in the wounded extremity.[146]

The mechanisms that lead from venous hypertension to ulceration are not entirely clear. Edema may be a factor. However, patients with congestive heart failure, hepatic congestion, and lymphedema do not routinely develop the skin changes and ulcerations typical of venous disease. Several theories have been promoted to explain the changes seen in the limb exposed to chronically elevated venous pressures.

FIBRIN CUFF THEORY

The fibrin cuff theory is based on histologic studies of lipodermatosclerotic skin.[144] It is postulated that elevated venous pressures are transmitted to the capillary circulation, leading to dilatation of the capillary bed and an increase in the size of the interstitial pores. This in turn leads to leakage of macromolecules (such as fibrinogen) into the dermis that polymerize to fibrin. This fibrin then forms a cuff around the capillaries, which may pose an impediment to oxygen and nutrient diffusion and potentially trap growth factors necessary for healing.[147] This fibrin cuff is theorized to lead to local tissue deprivation and hypoxia, compromising the adjacent tissue enough that even minor trauma to this area could be expected to lead to ulceration.[148] Support for this theory is derived from direct immunofluorescent studies demonstrating pericapillary fibrin cuffs in lipodermatosclerotic skin and venous ulcers. It does appear that pericapillary fibrin deposits precede the development of skin changes in venous disease, and fibrin sheets have been shown to interfere with oxygen transport into tissue.[147] However, the premise that the fibrin cuff leads to hypoxia through interruption of diffusion is far from certain. The amount of fibrin deposition does not correlate with the severity of the ulceration or venous insufficiency or the severity of the lipodermatosclerosis.[149,150] The fibrin cuffs are often discontinuous around dermal capillaries, suggesting that they may not form a true barrier.[141,142,151,152] In addition, oxygen pressure in these tissues improves with administration of oxygen, which does not support the premise of a true diffusion barrier.[153,154]

Increased fibrin deposition may also play a role in tissue breakdown and poor wound healing through an alternative mechanism. Extravasation into the interstitial space is markedly increased with venous insufficiency, which not only leads to a greater degree of local fibrin deposition but also contributes to systemic fibrinolytic and coagulation abnormalities.[155] Altered euglobin lysis time, increased protein C, D-dimer, D-monomer, fibrin monomer, elevated plasma fibrinogen, and reduced factor XIII have all been observed in patients with venous ulcers.[156-158] It is unclear whether these abnormalities are primary or secondary to the venous disease. Fibrin and fibrinogen additionally have a direct down-regulatory effect on collagen synthesis by fibroblasts. Fibrin may also lead to fibrosis through the release of fibrinopeptides and contribute to the inflammatory process in liposclerosis.[159] Alternatively, fibrinogen, α_2-macroglobulin, and other macromolecules that diffuse into the extravascular space may act as a "growth factor trap" by binding with growth factors and rendering then unavailable to the tissues.[142] It is well known that α_2-macroglobulin acts as a scavenger of transforming growth factor-β, and these substances have been found in high numbers within the fibrin cuffs of venous ulcer beds.[160]

WHITE CELL TRAPPING

It has been postulated that venous ulceration in CVI results from an inflammatory reaction. The reduced pressure gradient between the arterial and venous systems in venous hypertension is theorized to lead to leukocyte entrapment in the capillary endothelial wall, erythrocyte aggregation, and leukocyte plugging of the capillaries.[161] The aggregation of white cells may act as a physical barrier, but it may also become activated through attachment to intracellular adhesion molecules, resulting in the release of a cascade of cytokines, free radicals, and proteolytic enzymes such as collagenase. This could exacerbate fibrin deposition because of increased vascular permeability and inflammation with resultant injury to venous valves and adjacent tissue, which might in turn predispose to ulceration.[162]

Diagnosis

CVI may be recognized by classic signs and symptoms. Patients will complain of heaviness and pain in the affected limb, which characteristically worsen toward the end of the day. Edema, varicosities, and areas of hyperpigmentation due to the deposition of hemosiderin (which stimulates melanin production) will be present.[163] Eczematous changes with erythema, scaling, and pruritus ("venous dermatitis") may be exacerbated by sensitization to topical medications used to treat the condition.[13] Atrophie blanche, smooth white plaques of sclerosis speckled with telangiectases, is noted in nearly 40% of patients with CVI and often leads to painful ulceration.[164-167]

Venous ulcers are most commonly located over the medial malleolus where the long saphenous vein is superficial and has the greatest curvature. These ulcers may be single or multiple and may involve the entire circumference of the leg.[142] The borders of the ulcer are irregular. The wound bed of a venous ulcer is shallow, often with an exudate or granulation (Fig. 161-10).[168] Whereas most leg ulcers are due to venous insufficiency, ulcers may also be due to arterial insufficiency and altered sensibility or be multifactorial in origin. Venous ulceration may usually be distinguished from other confounding causes by physical findings. Arterial ulcers are typically more distal on the extremity than are venous ulcers, often over a bone prominence, and present with a round shape, sharp border, necrotic base, and scant granulation.[164] Tendon exposure or a deep wound, especially in association with trophic findings such as hair loss, shiny thin skin, abnormal toenails, cool feet, compromised pulses, and prolonged capillary refill, is suggestive of an arterial cause. In contrast, neuropathic ulceration, which is most commonly seen in patients with diabetes, usually develops in the face of adequate blood supply. These ulcers are commonly due to inadvertent trauma or pressure injury. Thickened callus at a pressure point may break down, leading to ulceration and eventual osteomyelitis.[164] Pyoderma gangrenosum presents with an ulcer that is blue-purple and has an undermined border with a cribriform base. The majority of these lesions are associated with autoimmune disorders, such as inflammatory bowel diseases or rheumatoid arthritis, or with hematologic malignant neoplasms.[169] Vasculitis may lead to acute or chronic ulceration. Infectious organisms may also colonize and cause leg ulcers. Quantitative bacteriology from tissue culture is an invaluable tool in ulcer diagnosis and management. Biopsy of a long-standing ulcer is recommended to rule out basal cell or squamous cell carcinoma, which may look remarkably like exuberant granulation tissue adjacent to the wound edges. Biopsy has been recommended of those ulcers that persist for more than 6 weeks after control of edema and infection has been achieved.[170]

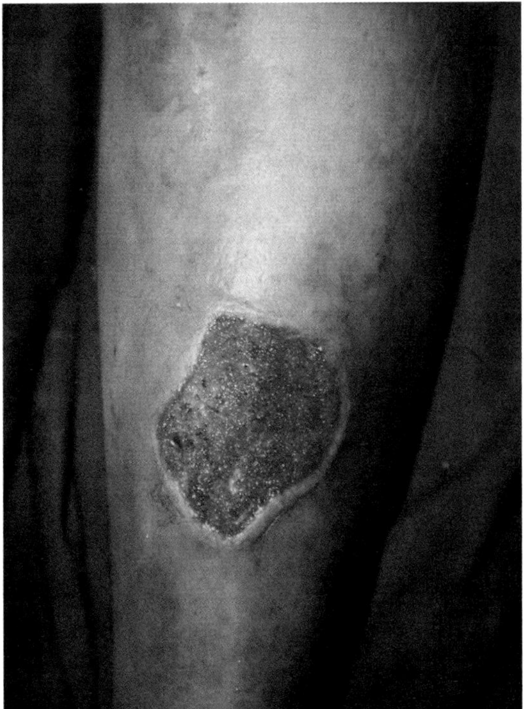

FIGURE 161-10. In contrast to the early venous ulcer seen in Figure 161-9, this case illustrates the typical appearance of a chronic venous ulcer demonstrating an irregular border and shallow granulating base.

DIAGNOSTIC STUDIES

The diagnosis of CVI can be made on clinical grounds alone in the majority of patients.[171] Noninvasive vascular assessment may help evaluate alternative pathologic conditions that may mimic venous disease and also identify the presence of venous obstruction or reflux. The degree of reflux has been correlated with the chronicity and size of the venous ulcer. The primary role for these studies is to assess the patient's suitability for venous surgery.

The ankle/brachial index by Doppler ultrasonography is a useful test for patients with lower extremity ulceration to exclude concomitant arterial disease, which contraindicates use of compression therapy. The ankle/brachial index is unreliable in the face of diabetes or stiff, calcific noncompressible arteries. In these conditions, a high clinical suspicion for arterial disease must be maintained.[172] Continuous wave Doppler studies provide useful anatomic information on the level of obstruction or valvular dysfunction but do not distinguish superficial from deep venous insufficiency well.[173,174] Color flow duplex ultrasound scanning provides the most accurate, reproducible, noninvasive assessment of venous disease currently available. Individual segments of the deep and superficial systems may be delineated, and the presence of reflux, obstruction, or a combination of both can be determined. Alternative pathologic entities, such as soft tissue masses or vascular malformations, may also be well visualized by this technique.[175,176]

Photoplethysmography and air plethysmography can measure the degree of venous reflux and the efficiency of the calf muscle pump at rest and after exercise. Occlusion of the superficial system with a tourniquet will allow assessment of deep venous obstruction with these simple tests.[177]

Immunofluorescence studies may be used to detect pericapillary fibrin but are of limited practical utility.

Computed tomography, MRI, and bone scans are reserved for evaluation of soft tissue or bone lesions such as osteomyelitis.[178] Invasive phlebography is usually reserved for patients who may be considered candidates for valvular surgery.[179]

Classification

In an effort to provide greater standardization in the reporting of venous disease, a clinical scoring system has been promoted by the executive council of the American Venous Forum.[180,181] This system uses categories of clinical presentation, etiology, anatomy, and pathophysiology to describe the severity of CVI. The clinical category has six gradations of increasing severity, from telangiectasia to active ulceration. Etiology is described as congenital, primary, and secondary (traumatic and post-thrombotic) in this system. The anatomic distribution of venous insufficiency is divided into superficial, deep, and communicating veins, with a subscript for specific anatomic locations. Pathophysiology is divided into reflux, obstruction, or a combination of both.

Treatment

The treatment of CVI is directed toward the correction of venous hypertension and its adverse effects. A range of approaches have been used to provide for relief of pain, reduction in edema, control of infection, improvement of lipodermatosclerosis, healing of any ulceration, and prevention of recurrence.[145]

MEDICAL TREATMENT

Compression Therapy

The simplest method to counteract the effects of venous hypertension is complete bed rest with leg elevation. Beyond the confines of a hospital setting, however, this treatment is difficult to enforce. Elevation of the affected extremity to above the level of the heart for 30 minutes, three or four times per day, may be a reasonable alternative outpatient protocol for improvement of edema in patients with early venous insufficiency. Leg elevation alone is inadequate for patients with more advanced venous disease or ulceration. In these patients, compression therapy is indicated. The application of pressure to treat venous insufficiency was known to Hippocrates and practiced in ancient Greece and Rome.[182] Compression is postulated to improve venous hypertension through a mechanical effect that improves the venous pump and facilitates lymphatic drainage. Compression raises the local hydrostatic pressure and decreases the superficial venous pressure, thereby reducing edema and the interstitial spillage of macromolecules. By decreasing the extravasation of macromolecules into the extravascular space, the inflammatory response is reduced. Stifling of the inflammatory response may limit the release of mediators detrimental to the process of wound healing. Compression of a normal limb decreases cutaneous blood flow. In contrast, in an edematous extremity, cutaneous blood flow and blood flow in the superficial and deep veins are actually increased by compression because of the reduction in edema. This may explain why transcutaneous oxygen pressure increases after compression treatment.[140,183] Lymphatic flow and fibrinolysis also improve with compression, and exercise improves the efficacy of this treatment.[184,185] Compression also leads to an improvement in reflux in the deep venous system. Compression allows approximation of valve leaflets, rendering once incompetent valves functional. Unfortunately, the hemodynamic benefits of compression stockings are lost once they are removed.[186,187]

Compression therapy plays a significant role in the management of CVI and ulceration. Patients who are diligent with their compression therapy have a significantly improved ulcer healing rate and decreased rate of recurrence.[156,188-190] The success of compression therapy is directly related to the patient's compliance. Two widely cited university-based studies noted more than 90% healing of venous ulceration with a strict regimen of cleansing and elastic compression.[188,191] Nearly half (44%) of the patients in one of the studies required hospitalization to achieve control of the wound, and slightly more than 70% of the limbs were ulcer free at 5 years.[188] Whereas compliance in the two studies was measured differently (defined solely by the use of compression garments in one study and by clinic appointment attendance in the other), patients with poor compliance demonstrated a 70% recurrence by 24 months and 100% recurrence at 36 months in both groups.[188,191] Unfortunately, the general community experience is even worse, with only about one third of patients remaining ulcer free at 5 years in both the United States and Europe.[192]

In compression therapy for CVI, two phases of treatment are generally involved. The therapy is initially aimed at edema reduction and treatment of any ulceration, usually necessitating rigid or elastic bandages. Ideally, the dressings supply a high working pressure (pressure when the patient walks) and a relatively low resting pressure (when the legs swing back in relaxation).[193] The second (or maintenance) phase is best maintained with graded compression stockings, which supply pressure that is maximal at the ankle and minimal at the thigh. The optimal pressure necessary to overcome venous hypertension is not well defined, but it is generally agreed that an external pressure of 35 to 40 mm Hg at the ankle is necessary to prevent capillary exudation.[183]

A number of bandaging systems (rigid, elastic, and multilayered) are currently available to treat venous hypertension, and each has its indications, limitations, and ardent supporters. Dressings are, of course, only as effective as the care with which they are applied. Bandages must be adapted to account for the variation in ankle and extremity sizes. Extra padding and attention must be paid to pressure points. An effort must be made to apply even, graduated compression to the "inverted champagne bottle" extremity, especially along the concave areas adjacent to the malleolus where venous ulcers typically occur.

The first modern application of this treatment was the Unna boot, a zinc paste bandage introduced in 1885.[183] The Unna boot is the prototype of a rigid inelastic bandage. Rigid bandages primarily provide support at rest. These bandages supply high pressure with muscle contraction (working pressures), and therefore they are effective only in ambulatory patients. Modified short-stretch bandages* have similar properties. These bandages do not accommodate changes in limb volume and must be frequently reapplied by a skilled caregiver to be effective.

Long-stretch (elastic) bandages provide adequate working pressures and higher resting pressures than rigid bandages do and are therefore more effective after the initial stage of edema treatment.[183,193] Effective use of these bandages requires careful attention to proper application. Varying the degree of overlap may increase pressure markedly, and although a loose application is ineffective, an unduly tight bandage may be detrimental. There are three classes of elastic bandages characterized by increasing degrees of compression.[194] Class I (lightweight) and class II bandages are light support bandages used in mild edema and ankle sprains and are relatively inelastic and rigid. Class III bandages are compression bandages that may provide up to 40 mm Hg of ankle pressure and are used in the treatment of severe varicosities and severe edema. Multilayered (three and four layers) bandage systems† have been introduced.[164,195] These bandages are easily adapted to legs of various sizes and provide sustained pressures of 40 to 45 mm Hg at the ankle, graded down to 17 mm Hg below the knee. These multilaminate systems are more expensive than traditional bandages but appear to be effective in healing recalcitrant ulcerations and may therefore be more cost-effective because of faster healing rates.[189]

Pneumatic compression devices have also been used for venous insufficiency. These devices provide intermittent compression and were initially developed for the treatment of lymphedema and deep venous prophylaxis. Unfortunately, they require multiple treatments and sedentary periods (to which many active patients object). As a result, this approach appears to be most effective in those patients who are bedridden or inactive.[196,197]

Once venous ulcers are healed, compression stockings become the mainstay of therapy. Graded compression stockings are available in four classes (a classification similar to that used for elastic bandages), depending on the pressure.[194] Class I stockings exert 20 to 30 mm Hg at the ankle and are useful for mild edema or fatigue. Class II stockings (30 to 40 mm Hg) are useful for severe varicosities and moderate edema. Class III stockings (40 to 50 mm Hg) and class IV stockings (>60 mm Hg) are recommended for severe edema and CVI. Elasticity decreases with time and laundering. For optimal effectiveness, compression stockings should be replaced every 6 months. Most important, stockings must be worn to be effective. This may be difficult in patients who are infirm, arthritic, or obese and may find application of the stockings to be a challenge.[198] Compliance with below-knee garments may be slightly better because they are easier to apply. A number of commercially available aids‡ can facilitate application of the stockings in these patients and enhance compliance with treatment.

Occlusive Dressings

Wet-to-dry dressings have traditionally been the mainstay of ulcer care, primarily because of their ease of application and low cost. However, this technique is painful, causes desiccation of the wound, and results in nondiscriminatory removal of viable tissue along with necrotic tissue. Occlusive dressings are less painful to the patient and provide a moist environment, which permits more rapid wound healing.[199-203] Several types of occlusive dressings are currently available. These include hydrogels (Nu-Gel, Vigilon), alginates (Kaltostat, AlgiDerm), hydrocolloids (DuoDERM, Restore), foams (Allevyn, Curafoam), and films (OpSite, Tegaderm). Lysis of the perivascular fibrin cuff has been demonstrated with hydrocolloid dressings, but the significance of this is not yet clear. Whereas each type of dressing has its proponents, none is likely to be adequate without compression therapy. In addition, several studies suggest that no currently available occlusive dressing is superior to a simple, nonadherent dressing placed properly under a compression bandage.[204-206]

Pharmacologic Therapy

Diuretics. Diuretics are probably the most commonly used drugs in the treatment of CVI. These medications may be of assistance in fluid mobilization, but they are effective only if they are used in conjunction with compression therapy.

*UnnaFlex, ConvaTec, Princeton, New Jersey; Comprilan, Beiersdorf-Jobst, Hamburg, Germany.

†Dynaflex, Johnson & Johnson Medical, Arlington, Texas; Profore, Smith & Nephew, New York, New York.

‡Easy Slide stocking donner, Beiersdorf-Jobst, Hamburg, Germany; Sigvaris stocking donner, Ganzoni & Cie, St. Gallen, Switzerland.

ANTIBIOTICS. Antimicrobials have been used extensively in the treatment of venous ulceration, despite the fact that these wounds are not typically infected. Topical antimicrobial agents should be administered only sparingly. Routine use of these compounds will not only select out resistant organisms but also induce hypersensitivity because of an increased susceptibility to the development of contact dermatitis in patients with venous insufficiency.[207] Tissue quantitative bacteriology is the most accurate means to determine whether an ulcer is infected or simply colonized, and it will also identify the most appropriate antimicrobial therapy. The presence of greater than 10^5 bacteria per gram of tissue is correlated with infection that may impede wound healing.[208-210] Topical antiseptic compounds such as povidone-iodine have also been used to treat venous ulcers. The majority of these substances are tissue toxic in commercially available concentrations; their routine use is not recommended because it will retard wound healing.[211] Several studies suggest that cadexomer iodine preparations (which exhibit antimicrobial efficacy without cellular toxicity) may decrease ulcer size and healing.[212,213] Systemic antibiotics have not been demonstrated to be efficacious in the treatment of venous ulcers and should be reserved for use in those patients who have disease complicated by cellulitis.[214]

SYSTEMIC HEMORHEOLOGIC AND ANTI-INFLAMMATORY AGENTS. Treatment approaches to venous ulcers have included systemic correction of the fibrinolytic abnormalities, reduction of inflammation, and dissolution of the pericapillary fibrin deposits associated with venous disease and ulceration.

Stanozolol is an androgenic steroid with fibrinolytic properties. It has been studied in conjunction with compression therapy. Use of stanozolol has resulted in improvement of lipodermatosclerosis, but it has not been demonstrated to increase healing rates of ulcers.[215,216] Stanozolol is considered safe for clinical use; however, sodium retention, hypertension, hirsutism, and liver and lipid abnormalities may occur, and patients must be carefully monitored if this treatment is contemplated. Although rare, peliosis, hepatitis, and hepatocellular carcinoma have been reported with its use.[216,217]

Some reports suggest that pentoxifylline may be efficacious for the treatment of venous ulceration.[210,218] Pentoxifylline mediates cytokine production, which results in antithrombotic effects and a reduction in white cell adhesion to the vascular endothelium. It also exerts fibrinolytic activity. Any or all of these actions may be responsible for the effects of pentoxifylline on venous ulcers.[219-223] Study suggests, however, that higher doses of pentoxifylline (800 mg three times daily) are necessary in the treatment of ulceration because lower doses (400 mg three times daily) were no more effective than placebo.[218,219,223]

Alternative substances such as a dietary flavonoid (Daflon, 100 mg daily) have also been studied in the treatment of venous disease. Daflon decreases white cell adhesion and plugging and should therefore theoretically increase red cell velocity and decrease capillary permeability. Although it has shown some promise in the treatment of small venous ulcerations, further study is needed.[224]

Theoretically, the inhibition of inflammation by inhibition of thromboxane or other compounds on the arachidonic acid pathway should enhance ulcer healing. A clinical study using ifetroban, a thromboxane receptor antagonist, has, however, not demonstrated any increased effects over compression therapy alone.[225] Conversely, aspirin (enteric, 300 mg daily) has been associated with an increased rate of ulcer healing.[226]

Débridement

Débridement is the cornerstone of management of surgical infection and may be employed to remove nonviable tissue. However, venous ulcers rarely have considerable necrotic debris, and unfortunately, débridement serves primarily to enlarge these wounds. The efficacy of mechanical and enzymatic débridement techniques in venous ulcers has not been elucidated. As such, the routine débridement of venous stasis ulcers is not recommended. It appears that unless the wound is infected, débridement may actually aggravate the condition.[227-229]

SURGICAL

Surgical treatment may be divided into treatment of the ulcer with a skin graft, treatment of the venous incompetence, and introduction of well-vascularized tissue by microsurgical transfer.

Skin Grafts

Skin grafting should be considered with large (>4 cm) nondiseased or refractory ulcers. Skin grafts may markedly reduce pain and enhance wound healing even if there is only partial take of the graft. Split-thickness skin grafts have been the most common graft used in the treatment of chronic leg ulcers with a healing rate of 50% to 78% in long-term (17 years) follow-up (Fig. 161-11).[230-232] Poor graft take has been associated with noncompliance, local fibrin abnormalities preventing adhesion to the wound bed, and microthrombi in the wound leading to ischemia.[230-232] Trauma, infection, or recurrent edema can result in skin graft loss. It appears that a critical 3-month period follows grafting, after which the graft tends to remain. Split-thickness grafts are more commonly used for closure of refractory venous ulcers. These grafts are readily available but have a tendency to be unstable in trauma

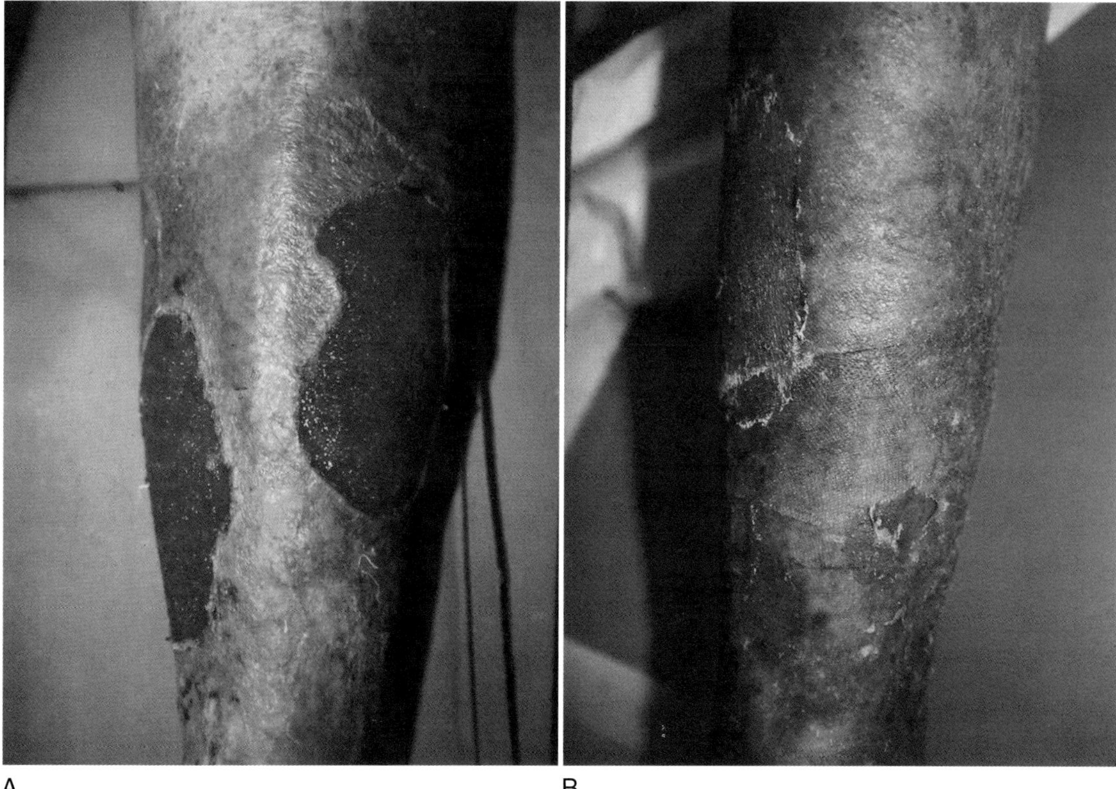

FIGURE 161-11. *A,* Refractory venous ulcers in a woman with chronic venous insufficiency. *B,* These wounds were successfully closed with the application of split-thickness skin grafts in conjunction with elastic stocking therapy. The patient's surgical result is seen 6 months postoperatively.

and have a proclivity to contract. Full-thickness skin grafts demonstrate better contour, durability, and sensibility but require a more meticulous inset and a longer period of immobilization and elevation postoperatively to ensure graft take. Although they are considered to be superior to split-thickness grafts, full-thickness grafts have the disadvantage of limited donor sites. Meshed split-thickness skin grafts have been advocated to permit drainage of exudate from the bed.[233] However, these interstices seal quickly on placement of the graft, preventing true "drainage." In addition, meshed grafts provide a poor cosmetic result, are unstable, and are of lesser utility in this setting.

Venous Surgery

The benefits of surgery to correct venous valvular incompetence are somewhat difficult to interpret because these procedures are usually performed after healing of the ulcer is achieved. Surgical success is thus quantified in terms of prevention of recurrent ulceration and improvement in hemodynamics rather than by healing of ulceration. Saphenous incompetence is a common factor contributing to ulceration in CVI. Whereas perforator incompetence alone is rarely a cause of ulceration, ligation of these vessels may be an important adjunct to therapy. Surgical ablation of superficial and perforating veins is generally well tolerated and may provide clinical and hemodynamic improvement. Endoscopic subfascial vein ligation has greatly improved the morbidity of the procedure. Minimally invasive techniques permit accurate ligation of communicating veins from a small, remote incision and reduce complications compared with open subfascial ligation (which carries a 20% to 55% infection rate, prolonged hospitalization, pain, and a long medial or posterior incision on the leg).[187,234-237] Superficial or saphenous incompetence is a common contributing factor leading to ulceration in CVI, and hemodynamic improvement has been seen in ulcerative venous disease with saphenofemoral ligation and stripping alone.[238-245] It is difficult to separate the hemodynamic and clinical benefits of superficial versus perforator ligation. Several studies of traditional subfascial perforator ligation demonstrated an initial rate of ulcer healing of 88%, which fell to a disappointing 53% to 59% ulcer-free status at 5 years.[234,237] Although the hemodynamic benefit of subfascial perforator ligation is difficult to establish, large perforating veins are often associated with lipodermatosclerosis and ulceration.[187,246]

The majority of limbs with severe CVI have incompetence in at least two of the three systems, suggesting concurrent correction of all affected venous pathways to be most prudent.[239,247-249] These findings have prompted a consensus panel to recommend ligation of perforating veins less than 4 mm in diameter.[239,240] Ligation of communicating veins in combination with "clinically indicated" superficial veins has demonstrated improvement in both leg hemodynamics and ulceration.[247,250] Using this technique, Bradbury et al[250] noted that 79% of patients were free of ulceration at 42 months. In this study, deterioration in the hemodynamic status preceded the onset of ulceration (popliteal or saphenous incompetence) in the affected limbs.[251] Duplex evaluation has demonstrated improvement in CVI with the treatment of incompetent superficial and perforating veins even in the presence of deep venous insufficiency.[177,236,246,247,251] These observations have led most authors to preferentially employ ligation of the perforating and superficial systems in the face of deep system disease before embarking on the more complex techniques required for intervention in the deep venous system.

The original surgical repair of incompetent femoral valves has been updated regularly and appears to result in an ulcer-free period of approximately 6 years.[240,248,249] Unfortunately, after 7 years, venous ulceration appears to recur.[252] Patients with primary deep valvular incompetence seem to have the best results, but this is a rare pathologic entity. Deep venous reconstruction appears safe, with minimal complications and no evidence of thrombosis in treated limbs.[240,243,248,249,252] Critical evaluation of the procedure is confounded by the variable incidence of prior thrombosis and concurrent superficial or perforating vein ligation as well as by the difficulty in assessing a hemodynamic improvement after deep vein reconstruction in these studies. Currently, the use of cryopreserved valves for deep venous reconstruction is being studied in a controlled trial.[253]

Venous bypass for obstruction has been successfully employed. Venous obstruction, however, is a rare cause (3% to 5%) of CVI and is usually accompanied by some degree of reflux.[254] Sclerotherapy as a treatment of CVI has been well studied. Randomized prospective study demonstrates that sclerotherapy is equivalent to surgical treatment only in the saphenous tributaries. CVI due to saphenofemoral, saphenopopliteal, or communicating veins is best treated with conventional techniques.[239,255]

Free Tissue Transfer

Free tissue transfer has been employed to treat CVI. Study patients who underwent free tissue transfer all demonstrated severe venous insufficiency with prior failed attempts at surgical correction, and many had prior episodes of thrombosis. All treated limbs remained free of ulceration for the duration of the observation, which ranged from 2 to 10 years (Figs. 161-12 and 161-13).[256,257] Hemodynamic improvement in the treated limbs has been attributed to the addition of competent veins within the transplanted tissue. The role of both the excision of the ulcer, with its surrounding fibrotic tissue and incompetent veins, and the addition of well-vascularized tissue, venous valvular competent tissue having its own blood supply, must be considered in the efficacy of this procedure. Microsurgical reconstruction in the lower extremity, although challenging, has provided a stable healed wound and relief of ulceration in patients with the most severe venous insufficiency.

EVOLVING TECHNOLOGIES

Growth Factors

The use of growth factors appears theoretically to have great potential in enhancing the healing of venous ulcerations. However, experimental and clinical results have been inconsistent. Application of a growth factor inhibitor (suramin) to experimental occluded wounds has been shown to slow epithelialization by 20%.[258] Topically applied recombinant tissue plasminogen activator has also been used to remove the pericapillary fibrin cuff in an effort to enhance wound healing.[259] Topical application of human recombinant epidermal growth factor has not been found to significantly speed or promote healing of venous ulcers in clinical trials.[260] Becaplermin, human platelet-derived growth factor, is approved by the U.S. Food and Drug Administration as a topical agent for use in diabetic ulcers, but its efficacy in venous lesions has not been demonstrated.[260]

Human Skin Equivalents

Graftskin (Apligraf) is a bilaminate human skin equivalent composed of an epidermal layer with live keratinocytes and a dermal layer that delivers growth factors and cytokines to the wound bed.[261,262] Apligraf is approved by the Food and Drug Administration, and a prospective randomized study has demonstrated improved healing of venous ulcers with a shorter time to wound closure in patients treated with it than in those patients treated with compression alone.[263] Apligraf appears to be particularly effective in the healing of small ulcers of more than 6 months' duration.[263] Durability of the healed ulcers over time has not been clearly evaluated.

Others

Topical application of granulocyte-macrophage colony-stimulating factor has been shown to improve ulcer healing and relapse rate for venous ulceration in

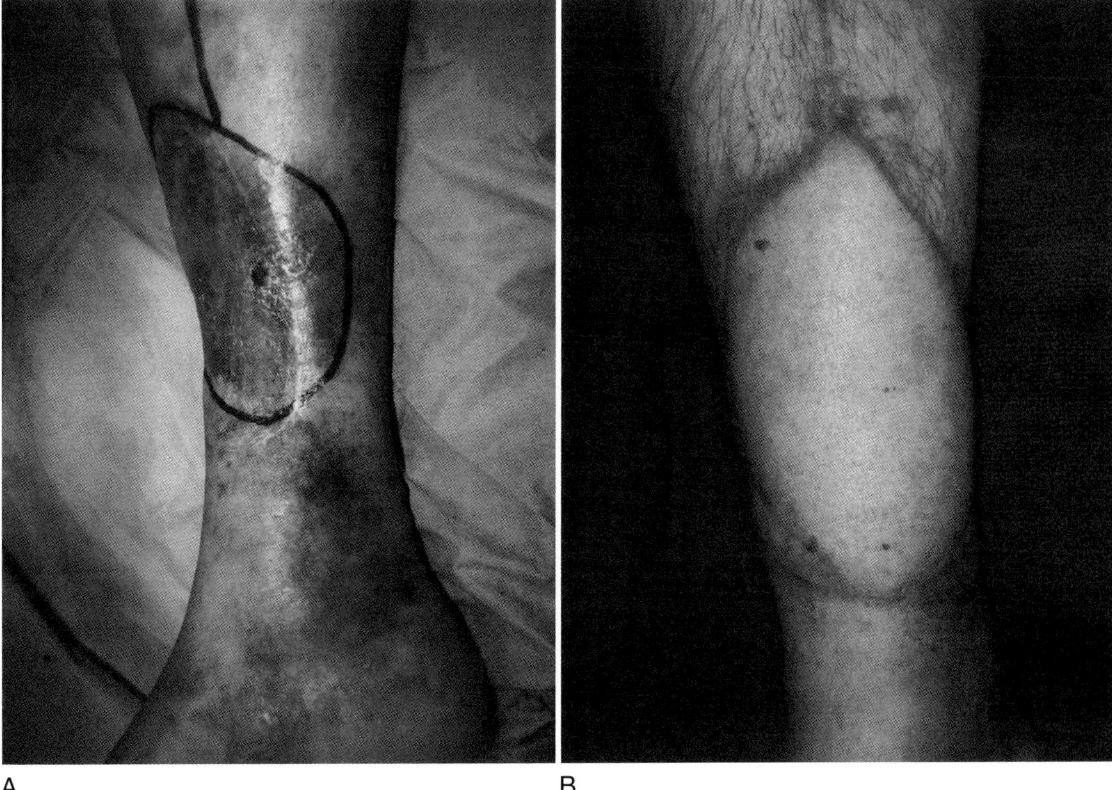

FIGURE 161-12. *A,* Patient with a history of venous insufficiency and recurrent skin ulcers that were refractory to prior attempts of skin grafting. *B,* After excision of the diseased skin and subcutaneous tissue, the wound was closed with a free scapular flap. The wound has remained stable with the demonstrated result on follow-up of just more than 5 years.

limited clinical studies.[264] A radiant heat bandage* has been used in refractory ulcers.[265] A monochromatic infrared energy has also been applied to leg ulcers. Evaluation of the efficacy of these treatments awaits controlled study.[266]

ARTERIAL INSUFFICIENCY

Chronic arterial insufficiency of the lower extremity initially causes intermittent claudication and occurs in about 5% of men and 2.5% of women older than 60 years.[267] Most patients with intermittent claudication remain asymptomatic for long periods, but 15% to 20% will eventually develop critical ischemia.[268,269] Critical ischemia is defined as arterial disease with threatened tissue loss requiring vascular reconstruction or amputation. Population studies have demonstrated that only 2% to 3% of patients with arterial insufficiency ever require amputation.[270] The risk factors identified for the development of lower extremity ischemia are similar to those identified for coronary artery and cerebrovascular ischemia. These risk factors include age older than 50 years, male sex, hypertension, hyperlipidemia, diabetes, and smoking. Lower extremity arterial disease can therefore be "viewed as a sign of potentially diffuse and significant arterial disease."[271] In a 1992 review, Vogt et al[272] reported that 28% of patients with lower extremity arterial disease had concurrent coronary disease and 10% had concurrent cerebrovascular disease. Whereas patients with lower extremity ischemia are at increased risk for death compared with the general population, this is largely due to events caused by cardiac or cerebral ischemia.

Diagnosis

Critical ischemia of the lower limb classically presents with nonhealing ulcers or rest pain. Venous ulcers are the most common cause of lower extremity ulceration, but the differential diagnosis of nonhealing lower extremity ulcers is extensive. Patients with ischemic ulcers and tissue loss involving the foot

*Warm Up Active Wound Therapy, Augustine Medical, Eden Prairie, Minnesota.

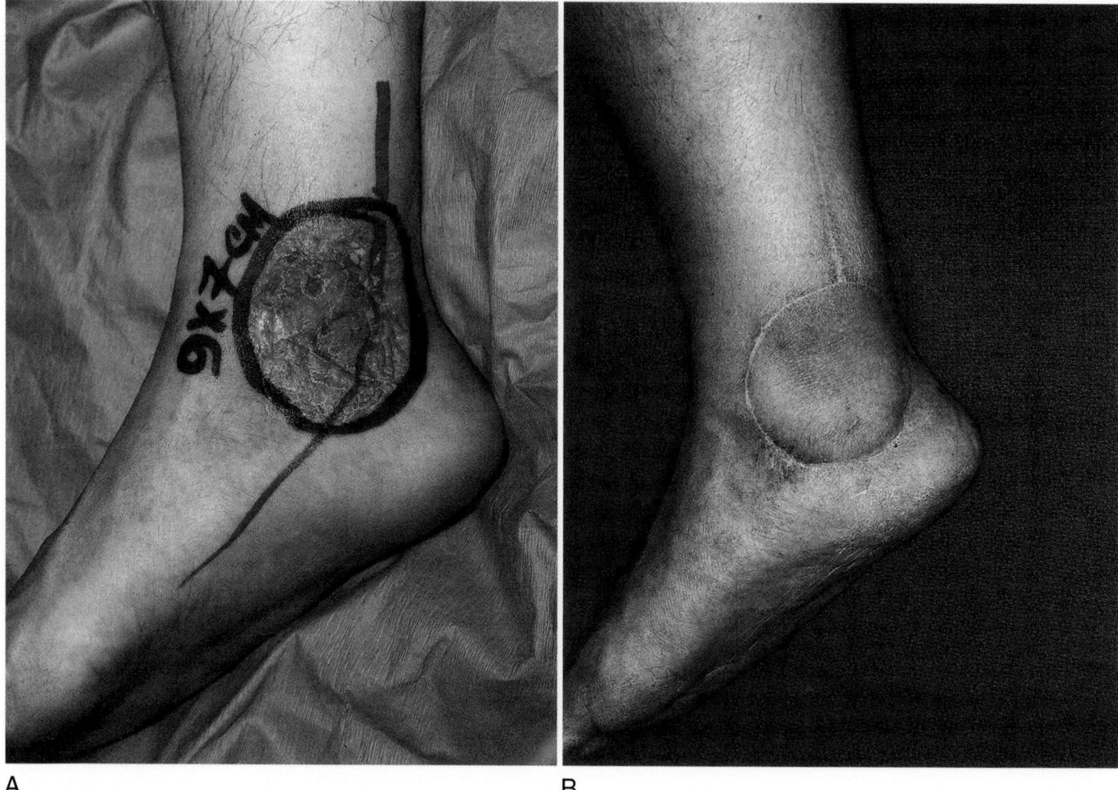

FIGURE 161-13. *A,* A man with refractory chronic venous insufficiency and ulceration. *B,* After surgical excision of involved tissue and closure of the resultant defect with a free posterior calf flap, the patient has remained ulcer free for the past 16 years, with the stable long-term result demonstrated here.

warrant an urgent, multidisciplinary evaluation to minimize the risk for limb loss. According to the Trans-Atlantic Inter-Society Consensus report, "the leisurely investigation of these patients in a nonspecialized primary care setting is quite inappropriate."[273] Tissue loss is usually the result of multisystem disease, and as such, evaluation of the cardiac, renal, endocrine, and vascular systems is usually indicated (Fig. 161-14).

The diagnosis of arterial insufficiency is primarily clinical. The classic physical findings associated with limb ischemia include atrophy of skin appendages and thickening of the toenails. The skin is cool, shiny, and often cyanotic. Capillary refill time is usually delayed (beyond 3 or 4 seconds) but may be rapid because of acute inflammation around ulcers or chronic dilatation of pericapillary vessels. Elevation of the extremity may lead to worsening cyanosis, and dependency causes rubor. Tissue loss from chronic ischemia usually occurs in the toe pulp. "Kissing ulcers" occur in adjacent toes and are also common. Severe ischemia of the lower extremity may lead to tissue loss involving the forefoot. Wounds in other areas of the foot are typically preceded by minor episodes of trauma but may also be associated with pressure injury, most commonly caused by ill-fitting shoes in neuropathic patients. Arterial ulcers are usually irregular, pale, and often surrounded by a rim of hyperkeratotic skin. In the absence of infection, the involved areas become covered with a dry eschar. Ischemia leading to tissue death is often complicated by infection that may range from superficial cellulitis to invasive abscess formation. Invasive infections can result in local capillary thrombosis, progressive tissue necrosis, and osteomyelitis. Bacterial spread along fascial planes may lead to widespread tissue destruction.[274]

DIFFERENTIAL DIAGNOSIS

Venous Disease

Venous ulcers usually occur just proximal to the medial malleolus and are generally painless, whereas arterial ulcers are painful and located more distally on the extremity. Fifteen percent of patients with venous ulcers also have concurrent arterial occlusive disease and often have wounds that are increasingly refractory to standard therapy.[274] These patients may ultimately develop a combination of medial malleolar ulcers and lesions involving the toes or forefoot.

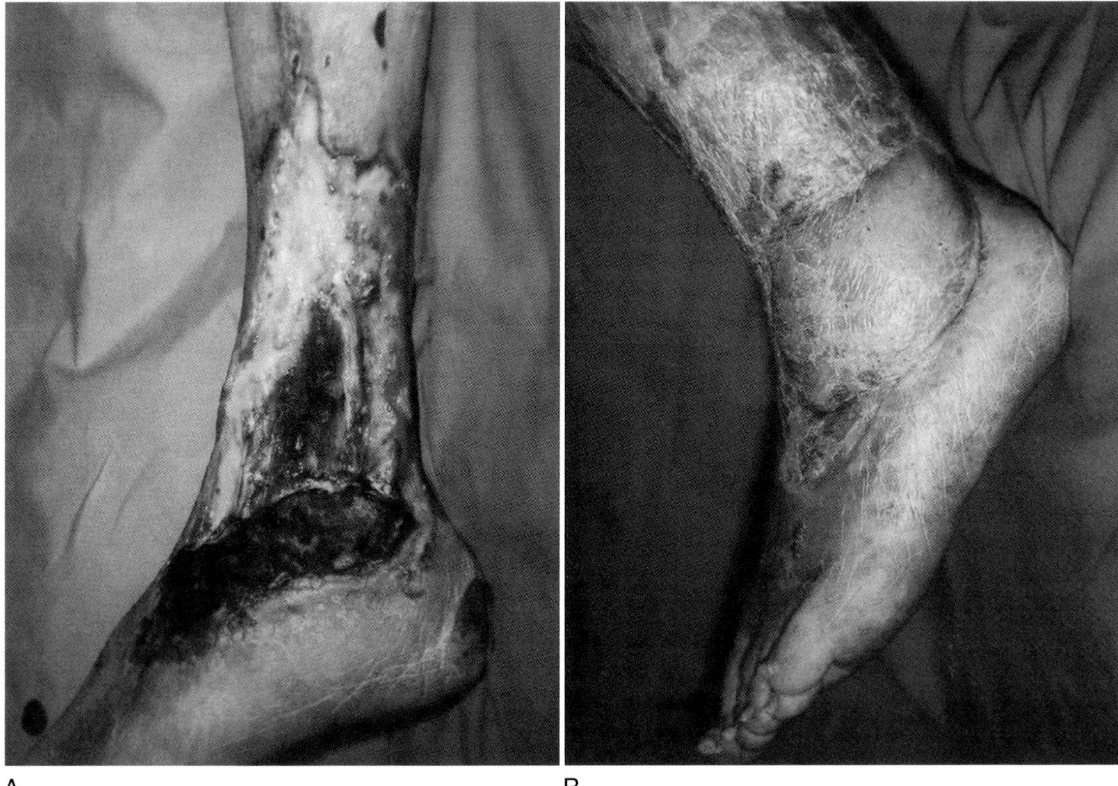

FIGURE 161-14. *A,* Patient with Sturge-Weber syndrome and severe peripheral vascular disease demonstrates a large, deep ulcer involving the distal leg and foot with exposed tendon, necrotic debris, and eschar. *B,* After débridement, the wound was closed with a free latissimus flap repaired to the revascularized tibial artery and vein. Partial loss of the latissimus flap necessitated completion closure with a free gracilis muscle flap and skin grafting 1 week later. The patient was rehabilitated to full ambulation with the aid of a walker and is shown 1 year postoperatively.

Buerger Disease

Buerger disease, or thromboangiitis obliterans, is thought to result from an inflammatory response of the small arteries and veins to chronic tobacco use. The larger arteries are not involved. The presenting signs of Buerger disease include ulceration of the fingertips and toes, without claudication. Raynaud phenomenon is common in these individuals. Patients are typically male and younger than 40 years. Angiography reveals an absence of stenotic lesions in the proximal vessels and "corkscrew" collaterals. The only known effective treatment of this condition is the cessation of smoking.[275]

Diabetes

Diabetic patients may present with either ischemic or neuropathic ulcers. In pure neuropathic ulcers, the proximal circulation is normal, and pulses are likely to be palpable in the foot. Among diabetic patients with foot ulcers, the underlying causes are evenly divided: approximately one third are purely neuropathic, one third are purely ischemic, and another third are mixed.[276]

Diabetic sensory neuropathy impairs protective sensation, promoting both acute and chronic foot trauma. Sympathetic neuropathy impairs skin integrity, promoting microtrauma and infection. Neuropathic ulcers typically occur on the sole of the foot, are surrounded by calluses, and are painless. Loss of vibratory sensation indicates neuropathy and loss of protective sensation. Skeletal abnormalities and abscess formation are frequently associated with neuropathic ulcers. They usually heal once devitalized tissue is débrided and the foot is protected by off-loading techniques, such as total contact casting.

Collagen Vascular Disease

Lower extremity ulcers may also occur with a variety of collagen vascular diseases. Multiple, painful ulcers frequently complicate systemic lupus erythematosus. Patients with systemic lupus erythematosus may also present with thrombotic complications and limb-threatening ischemia. Most patients with collagen vascular disease will have other systemic evidence of disease, but antibody testing may be indicated for patients with nonhealing ulcers in whom no obvious explanation can be found (Fig. 161-15).

Hematologic Diseases

Hematologic diseases, such as polycythemia vera, thrombocythemia, and sickle cell disease, may also cause nonhealing lower extremity ulcers; these can be ruled out with an appropriate, specific test. Pyoderma gangrenosum presents with small, painful lesions that coalesce and over time become an undermined ulcer with a cribriform base. Pyoderma is commonly associated with inflammatory bowel disease or rheumatoid arthritis but may also occur with other conditions, such as colorectal cancer and hematologic malignant neoplasm. Vasculitic ulcers usually have a typical "punched out" appearance. Treatment of these lesions should be targeted toward control of the primary disease process because débridement often results in exacerbation and a larger wound (Fig. 161-16).

Metastatic Disease

Processes such as primary and metastatic cancer, although less common than the aforementioned conditions, may also occur in the foot. Accordingly, any long-standing ulceration should prompt biopsy.

DIAGNOSTIC STUDIES

In patients with soft tissue necrosis of the foot, palpable pulses at the ankle suggest an absence of significant occlusive arterial disease. However, palpable pulses do not absolutely rule out ischemia as a factor contributing to ulcer formation, and more detailed investigation is required. This evaluation should include a bedside Doppler examination, measurement of ankle pressures, and calculation of the ankle/brachial index. An absolute ankle pressure less than 40 mm Hg or an ankle/brachial index of less than 0.5 implies severe ischemia caused by proximal arterial occlusive disease.[277-279] These measurements are of limited value in diabetic patients. Calcium deposition in the arterial media of vessels near the ankle causes them to become stiff and noncompressible and may yield a spuriously high ankle/brachial index. In these patients, measurement of toe pressures may be more accurate. If the physical examination does not suggest arterial occlusive disease, abnormalities of capillary function interfering with oxygen delivery may be responsible for tissue necrosis. Capillary function can be assessed with various nuclide perfusion studies and transcutaneous oxygen measurements. These studies, although interesting, are rarely helpful in directing clinical practice.

If operative therapy is considered for patients with ischemic tissue loss, imaging of the lower extremity vascular system is indicated. Duplex scanning and magnetic resonance angiography have become increasingly popular because they are noninvasive and avoid use of ionic, potentially nephrotoxic contrast agents. These studies help define the location of arterial occlusion and are particularly useful in evaluating the vascular system proximal to the knee. Angiography is often still indicated, especially when occlusive disease is present below the knee, because it more precisely defines arterial anatomy. This facilitates detailed preoperative planning before vascular reconstruction is undertaken. Imaging of the coronary and cerebrovascular systems may also be required before operation, depending on the patient's complaints and physical findings. Computed tomography and MRI of the foot have gained popularity to define the extent of abscess formation and osteomyelitis. These studies are rarely justified; the extent of soft tissue infection is best defined by operative exploration, and osteomyelitis is best diagnosed by bone biopsy and culture.

Treatment

MEDICAL MANAGEMENT

Arterial disease that does not cause critical ischemia is usually treated conservatively. In the absence of occlusive arterial disease (i.e., patients with palpable pulses at the ankle or normal findings on angiographic and noninvasive studies), local wound care is the mainstay of therapy for lower extremity ulcers.[277,278] This situation occurs most often in the neuropathic diabetic, in whom most of the wounds will heal by secondary intent.[276] Treatment includes débridement of all devitalized tissue, off-loading, and patience. Wound healing is slow but generally progresses to closure. Topical wound healing factors (e.g., Regranex, Apligraf) are reported to reduce healing time and have found great utility in the treatment of venous ulcers.[280-282] Currently, the precise role these agents might play in the treatment of arterial lesions of the lower extremity is less clear. In the absence of infection, topical antimicrobial preparations are generally not warranted because they may lead to hypersensitivity reactions or selective bacterial colonization, which may stall wound healing. Wounds colonized with bacteria should be treated with topical agents demonstrating reactivity to the offending organism. Systemic antibiotics are reserved for the treatment of cellulitis or osteomyelitis. Invasive wound infections are treated by incision, drainage, and débridement of all nonviable elements in concert with appropriate topical and systemic antibiotic therapy.

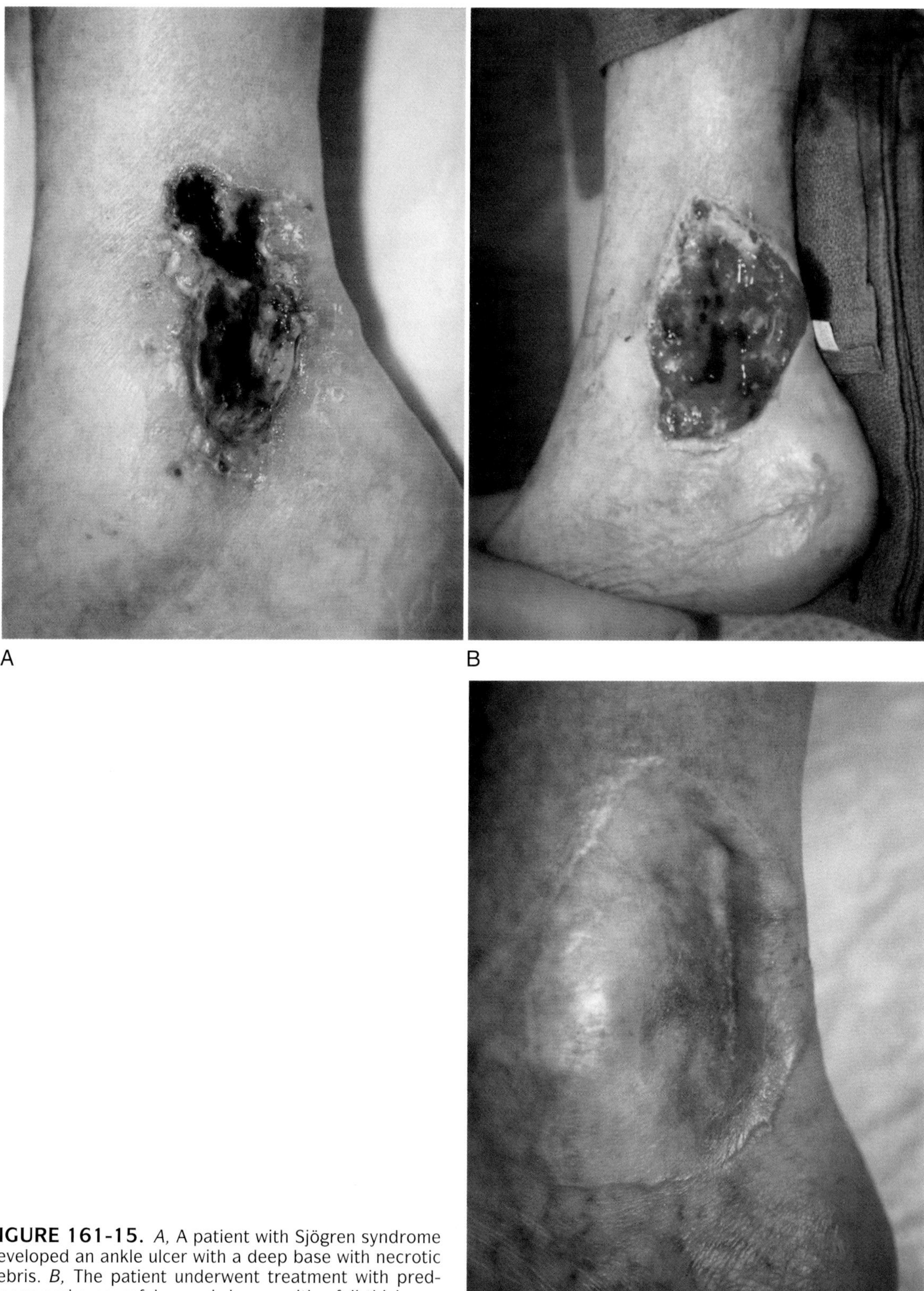

FIGURE 161-15. *A,* A patient with Sjögren syndrome developed an ankle ulcer with a deep base with necrotic debris. *B,* The patient underwent treatment with prednisone and successful wound closure with a full-thickness skin graft. *C,* Her result is demonstrated 2 years postoperatively.

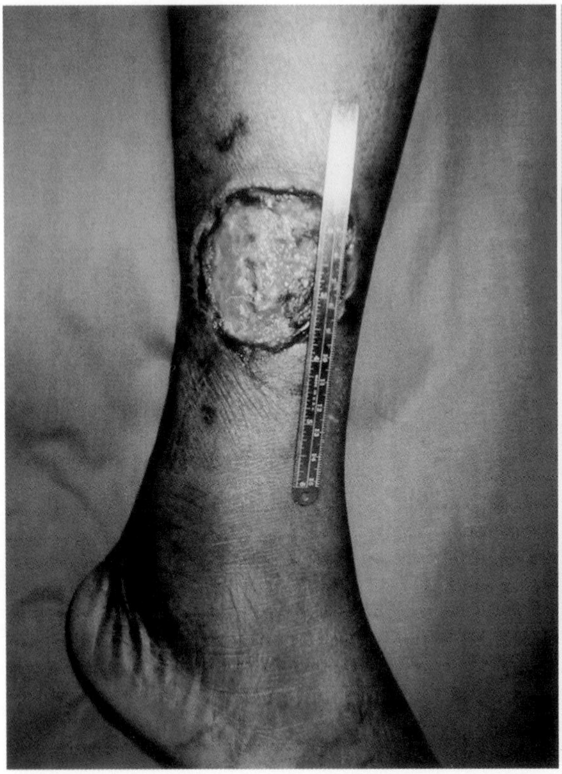

A

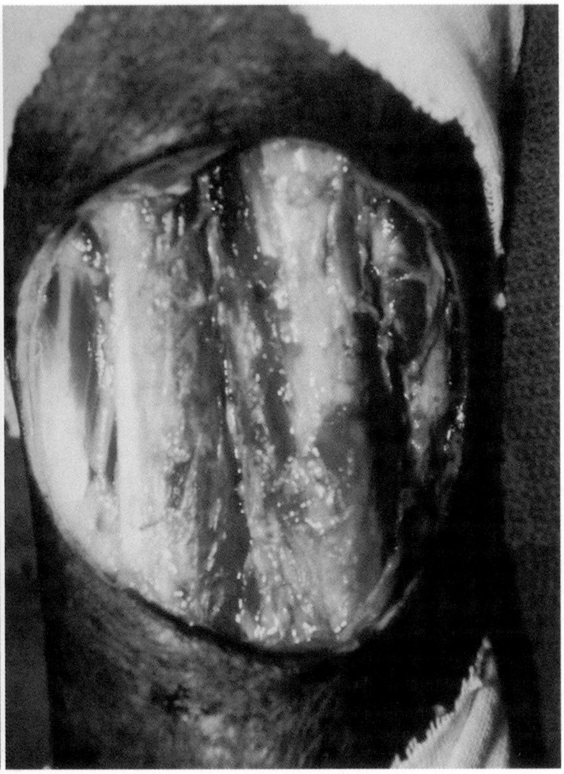

B

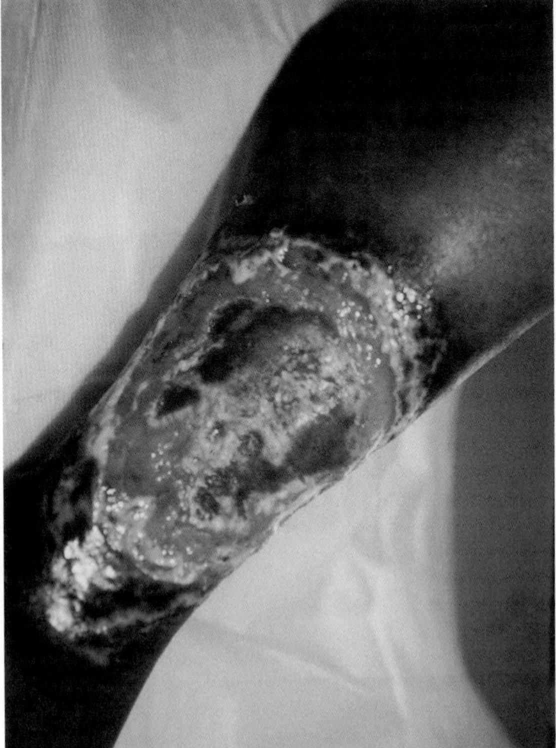

C

FIGURE 161-16. *A,* A patient presented with a long-standing lower extremity lesion with a "punched out" appearance. *B* and *C,* She underwent débridement and subsequent skin grafting of the lesion, which resulted in progressive loss of the débrided edges and exacerbation of the wound. Subsequent work-up revealed a vasculitic origin of the lesion.

INDICATIONS FOR LIMB SALVAGE

Limb salvage relates to the successful treatment of critical ischemia (gangrene, nonhealing ulcer, rest pain) and is defined as retention of a limb useful for ambulation without a prosthesis. Amputations proximal to the foot typically require a prosthesis for ambulation. The indications for operative therapy of lower extremity ischemia are clinical and defined by symptoms rather than by diagnostic tests such as angiography or Doppler studies. Arterial reconstruction is indicated for rest pain, exclusion of sources of arterial emboli, gangrene, and treatment of nonhealing ischemic ulcers.[271] The Ad Hoc Committee on Reporting Standards of the Society for Vascular Surgery and the International Society for Cardiovascular Surgery has suggested that outcome after vascular reconstruction be reported in terms of operative mortality, morbidity, survival of patients, patency, and limb salvage.[283]

Lower extremity reconstruction for critical ischemia is fraught with complications and carries a high morbidity and mortality. These patients are at increased risk for death, largely due to the cerebrovascular and cardiac comorbidity. The 5-year mortality for patients undergoing vascular reconstruction for critical ischemia may be as high as 62%.[284] This rises to 88% for patients with failed operations for vascular reconstruction.[285] Given these figures, it may seem inappropriate to use scarce and often costly medical resources for treatment of lower extremity critical ischemia. However, in combination with careful follow-up, arterial reconstruction leads to limb salvage rates of about 90% and operative mortality rates of less than 5%.[286,287] A number of patients undergo one operation that allows them to retain the extremity for life. Compared with amputation, arterial reconstruction has a reduced operative mortality, reduced hospital stay, and improved long-term survival.[287,288] The long-term cost of successful arterial reconstruction is also less than the cost of amputation.[289]

However, the benefits of vascular reconstruction for limb salvage may not extend to all patients with critical ischemia. Patients must be selected carefully in terms of their medical status and anatomic disease. They must be prepared for repeated operative procedures, complications, and failure necessitating amputation. In an analysis by Farkouh et al,[290] 26% of patients with lower extremity arterial reconstruction required at least one operation to revise the graft, and 20% ultimately underwent ipsilateral amputation. Infrainguinal reconstruction was more likely to lead to amputation compared with aortoiliac reconstruction.

SURGICAL OPTIONS

The most appropriate therapeutic option for each patient with an ischemic limb must take into account the realistic chance for surgical salvage of the limb, weighed against the risk of operative morbidity. This reconstructive paradigm may be simplified by dividing these patients into five categories. First, there are patients who are not candidates for complex limb salvage because of a prohibitive medical risk. Second, there are patients with an acceptable risk for surgery, but they do not have a realistic expectation for surgical salvage of the affected extremity. The third category consists of those patients who are medically stable with an extremity that can be salvaged by vascular reconstruction alone. The fourth group consists of medically stable patients who can be managed by soft tissue reconstruction alone. The fifth clinical category encompasses medically stable patients who require both soft tissue and vascular reconstruction of the ischemic extremity. Differentiating between the last three categories is particularly important for the plastic surgeon.

Amputation

Patients with severe, untreatable coronary or carotid disease (category 1) are excluded from consideration for extremity salvage operations. The risk of operative mortality outweighs the potential benefit of limb salvage. Patients chronically debilitated by stroke, paralysis, and advanced age (category 2) are also poor surgical candidates. Limb salvage may be feasible, but ambulation is not. Patients with lower extremity wounds caused by pressure sores frequently fall into this group. These patients may have coexisting arterial insufficiency, and their wounds may appear similar to those of patients with peripheral arterial disease and threatened limb loss. Pressure sores of the foot and ankle can be treated by combined vascular and soft tissue reconstruction (vascular reconstruction alone is rarely adequate). However, durable limb salvage is impossible and should not be undertaken unless the principal cause of the wound (i.e., unrelieved pressure) is eliminated. Return to ambulation is unlikely. Accordingly, primary amputation is a reasonable option in nonambulatory or invalid patients with extensive pressure sores distal to the knee.

Revascularization

Vascular reconstruction alone (category 3) is indicated for patients with arterial occlusive disease causing ischemic rest pain, for those with threatened tissue loss, and for those with small uncomplicated ulcers, such as gangrene of a toe. Reliable healing can be expected after vascular reconstruction and simultaneous or staged débridement. Frequent follow-up, meticulous wound care, and strict non-weight-bearing status of the involved foot are of the utmost importance. The wound should be kept clean, moist, and free of any necrotic tissue. A wide variety of topical wound care products are available. Spray gel and alginate preparations are especially useful for their efficacy, ease of application, and degree of comfort for the patient.

Soft Tissue Procedures

The most common foot wound in the neuropathic patient occurs over the metatarsal heads.[291] Neuropathic patients are also subject to repeated microtrauma and gross trauma involving their feet, which may lead to abscess formation requiring wide débridement and drainage. In these patients, samples of underlying bone should be harvested for pathologic analysis and culture to rule out osteomyelitis. These wounds will usually heal without soft tissue reconstruction, provided they are brought into bacteriologic balance. Options for local flap reconstruction on the foot are limited. In limited situations, local flaps may be employed for smaller leg or foot wounds. Delayed healing or complication with local flap reconstruction should prompt the surgeon to search for a missed septic focus (undrained abscess, osteomyelitis, or foreign body) or underlying ischemia. Dellon et al[292] suggest that neuropathic patients may benefit from tarsal tunnel release as a measure to improve sensation of the foot and potentially reduce the incidence of ulcer formation.

Combined Vascular-Microvascular Reconstruction

Extensive, gangrenous wounds with exposed bone, tendons, or joints suggest a component of ischemia. Limb salvage for this group of patients involves combining revascularization with soft tissue reconstruction by use of well-perfused flaps (category 5). This most commonly requires well-vascularized tissue to be transferred microsurgically from remote sites (Fig. 161-17).[293] Local flaps are likely to be complicated by partial or total flap necrosis in patients with arterial disease and are of little utility in this setting. Wound size per se is not the primary indication for free flap reconstruction. A major determinant is the location of the wound and how this might affect the ability to ambulate. A relatively small wound, therefore, may require aggressive measures for soft tissue reconstruction if it is critical for ambulation. Patients who might otherwise be considered appropriate for primary amputation may be candidates for limb salvage with combined soft tissue and vascular reconstruction if they have large wounds or if it is expected that they will have difficulty using a prosthesis. Several series[294,295] have supported this position, suggesting that free flaps in conjunction with vascular reconstruction are indicated for wounds larger than 15 cm^2. This is especially true for patients with preexisting contralateral amputations or blindness, for whom the morbidity of bilateral amputations may be unacceptable.

Salvage of the ischemic extremity with combined vascular and microvascular techniques requires three stages to bring the reconstruction to a successful conclusion. These steps may be carried out in a sequential or simultaneous fashion. The initial procedure must prepare the wound bed for coverage. All necrotic tissue should be excised, and bone and soft tissue biopsy samples should be sent for culture to ensure a healthy wound base. Wound preparation may involve an open transmetatarsal or other type of limited amputation. Ideally, as much of the glabrous, weight-bearing skin of the sole of the foot should be preserved. Débridement frequently leads to additional edge necrosis and may establish a continually enlarging wound in patients with significant ischemia. For this reason, simultaneous wound preparation and vascular-soft tissue reconstruction may be advisable. Negative-pressure wound therapy (vacuum-assisted closure) has been shown to be beneficial in the interim management of these wounds. This approach holds promise, but indications are not yet clearly defined. Vascular and soft tissue reconstruction should be delayed if abscess or infection is encountered at the time of débridement. Local wound sepsis may increase the risk for thrombosis of both the vascular graft and the microvascular anastomosis.

After adequate wound preparation, vascular reconstruction is carried out, usually with translocated or in situ vein grafts. Large studies have shown that autogenous vein grafts to the popliteal artery are more likely to remain patent for longer periods compared with other grafts (polytetrafluoroethylene, Dacron, cryopreserved vein); this difference is more significant when autogenous vein grafts are compared with prosthetic grafts distal to the popliteal artery. Use of autogenous vein grafts does not appear to influence rates of operative mortality, morbidity, or limb salvage.[296] Whereas there is little experience of combining free tissue transfer with Teflon or Dacron arterial grafts, extrapolation from the experiences in revascularization suggests that this option should probably be avoided. The authors have successfully treated one patient by use of cryopreserved vein for distal arterial reconstruction followed by free tissue transfer because of a paucity of suitable donor tissue, but this is not recommended as a standard option. Vascular reconstruction may precede or be carried out simultaneously with microvascular soft tissue reconstruction. With simultaneous vascular and soft tissue reconstruction, the flap can usually be harvested while the bypass is completed, which may avoid an additional lengthy operative procedure. The microvascular anastomoses and insetting of the flap do not dramatically prolong the operation, and overall complication rates are comparable to those of a staged approach.[293,294]

CONSIDERATIONS IN THE USE OF FREE FLAPS. Not only are microvascular considerations such as the optimal pedicle, pedicle drape, and positioning

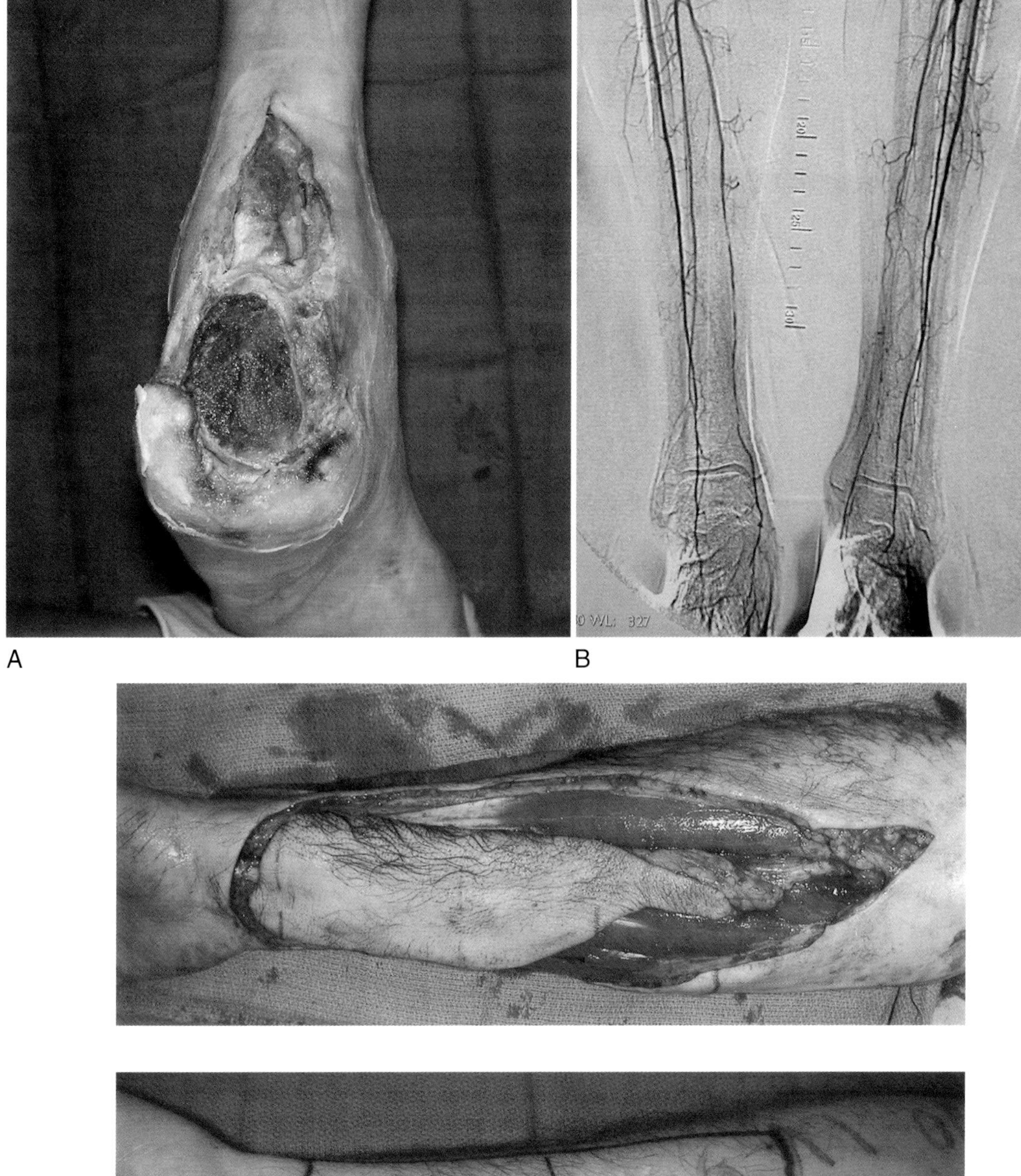

FIGURE 161-17. *A,* A large posterior heel and distal leg ulcer in a patient with severe arterial insufficiency. *B,* Angiographic evaluation of the lower extremities demonstrates the extent of the distal arterial disease and the segmental defect in the posterior tibial artery *(right)*. This was repaired with a femoral–distal tibial saphenous vein bypass graft. *C,* A 13- × 7-cm radial forearm free flap was harvested from the patient's nondominant hand and revascularized by an end-to-side anastomosis to the saphenous bypass graft. *Continued*

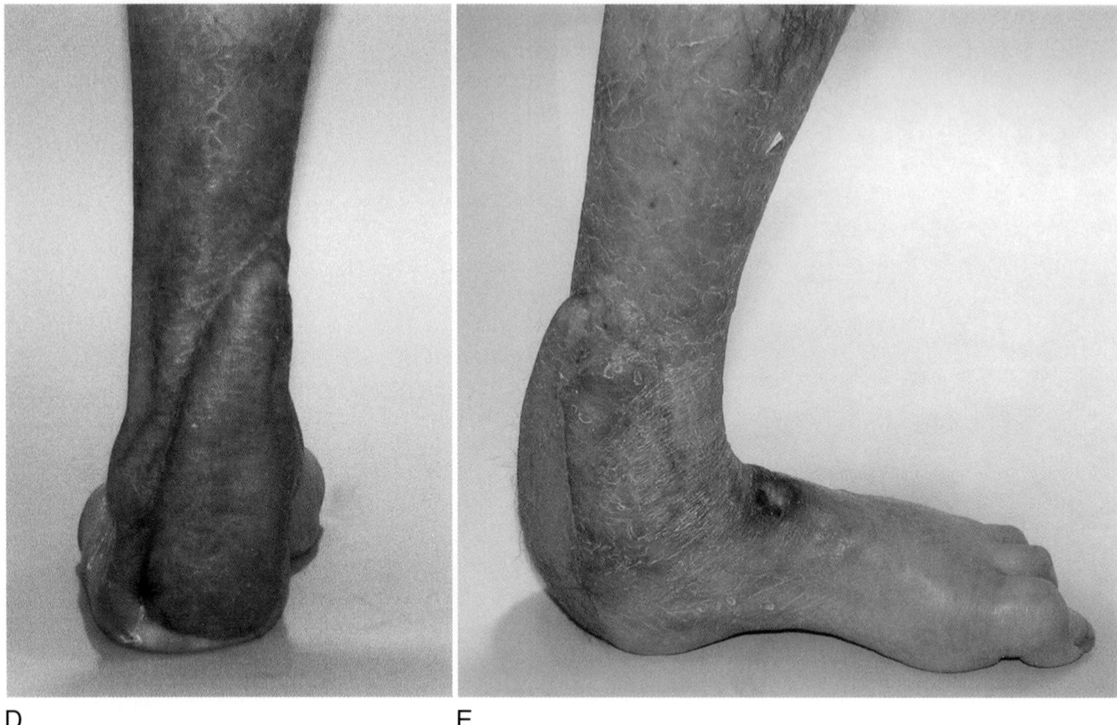

FIGURE 161-17, cont'd. *D* and *E,* Postoperatively, the patient was able to ambulate and demonstrated no further ulceration at 2-year follow-up.

critical to success of these procedures, but also the surgeon must contend with the existing vascular status of the limb as well as the strategy employed for revascularization. Extensive undermining is best avoided. The setup and lie of the microvascular anastomosis must be carefully considered in the ischemic limb. End-to-side anastomoses are generally preferred to preserve distal perfusion. The donor artery of the free flap can be anastomosed to either the vein graft used for the revascularization or the native artery. An end-to-side anastomosis to the vein graft allows the microsurgeon to work with a soft, large-caliber vessel. The potential disadvantage of this approach is that flow in the vein graft must be interrupted while the anastomosis is completed. It is advantageous to fully anticoagulate the patient with heparin and to occlude the vein graft with vessel loops during this portion of the operation. An aortic punch can be inserted through a small incision in the graft to establish a uniform aperture for anastomosis. Alternatively, the donor vessels can be anastomosed directly to the native arteries of the foot, usually distal to the distal anastomosis of the vein graft. In this instance, it is not necessary to interrupt flow in the vein graft, but the recipient vessels are often sclerotic, making the microvascular anastomosis difficult.

With single-vessel runoff, it is acceptable to use the sole patent artery as the recipient vessel (in an end-to-side fashion).[295] With a blind popliteal segment (i.e., zero vessel runoff), some authors have recommended anastomosis of the donor vessels of the flap to the vein graft in an end-to-end fashion, forming a "nutrient flap."[297] The nutrient flap is essentially a free flap fed by long vein grafts and sutured to an otherwise ischemic foot without distal revascularization. Mimoun et al[298] think that the supplementary blood supply from the flap leads to "progressive development of a new distal capillary bed." Furthermore, they state that long-term patency of the vein graft is not essential for limb salvage.[298] Other authors have employed the ingenious solution of the cross-leg free flap in this situation and used recipient vessels from the contralateral leg to supply the flap.[299,300] These techniques appear promising but are not at this time considered standard therapy.

It may be a challenge to find a suitable recipient vein. The venae comitantes traveling with the major arteries of the leg are often of poor quality in patients with advanced arterial disease. These veins can sometimes be injured during the arterial reconstruction. They should be carefully inspected at the distal anastomosis of the vein graft before use. An end-to-end venous anastomosis may be advantageous because of the technical ease and speed. The greater or lesser saphenous veins are usually of larger caliber than the vena comitans and are usually better candidates for draining the free flap. These veins are often not available because they may have been used as in situ grafts during the revascularization. Preoperative vein mapping with ultrasonography can help identify both the location and size of potential recipient veins at the foot and ankle. The radial forearm flap and the rectus abdominis muscle flap with a skin graft are most frequently used for reconstruction of lower extremity wounds. Both of these flaps are relatively easy to raise, allow simultaneous harvest with the revascularization, and are dependable. The radial forearm flap is ideal for smaller defects. Its long pedicle usually allows the microvascular anastomosis to be remote from the wound and also permits a high degree of flexibility in flap design and positioning. In addition, significant atherosclerotic disease, which is often seen in the inferior epigastric vessels of these patients, is rarely seen in the radial artery (with the exception of dialysis patients). The skin paddle can be designed so that it extends over the radial vessels toward the cubital fossa. This negates the need for skin grafting over the vascular pedicle, which is sometimes required near the ankle. There has been criticism of the aesthetic quality of the radial forearm donor site. This site is quite acceptable when it is treated with a full-thickness skin graft harvested from the inguinal crease.

For larger lower extremity wounds, the rectus abdominis muscle flap with a skin graft is often employed. The rectus flap has the disadvantage of being somewhat bulky and has a shorter vascular pedicle than the radial forearm flap. In addition, the donor site, although hidden in clothes, has the potential for abdominal hernia or bulge. A number of flaps, including the serratus, latissimus, scapular, and omental and a spectrum of fascial flaps, have been successfully employed for lower extremity reconstruction.[301,302] However, no one flap has proved to be more durable or associated with fewer complications.[301,302] Flap selection is usually dictated by donor availability and the surgeon's preference, including considerations to limit operative time and morbidity by avoiding flaps requiring lengthy harvest or repositioning of the patient.

ADJUVANT DRUG THERAPY

Adjuvant drug therapy is frequently used in the perioperative and postoperative period. Several perioperative regimens have been recommended, for example, antiplatelet therapy with aspirin starting in the recovery room and administered indefinitely. Bolus heparin and dextran alternatively given intraoperatively, followed by continuous heparin for 5 days, continuous heparin for 5 days in combination with continuous dextran for 7 days, and aspirin for 2 to 3 weeks, have all been used.[303-308] Low-molecular-weight heparin is as effective as nonfractionated heparin and may reduce the risk of bleeding complications during vascular operations.[303] At present, there are no randomized, controlled trials suggesting that any specific intraoperative anticoagulation protocol is superior to any of the others. On the other hand, antiplatelet therapy with daily aspirin has been demonstrated to reduce vascular events in patients with peripheral arterial disease. In addition, evidence from Europe suggests that daily aspirin improves both survival and graft patency.[307] Oral coumarin has also been shown to improve survival in patients with peripheral arterial disease as well as graft patency and limb salvage rates.[308] Therapy with oral coumarin, however, results in bleeding complications in approximately 12% of patients. To date, there have been no studies that specifically evaluated patients undergoing combined vascular and soft tissue reconstruction. Intraoperative anticoagulation with heparin, followed by lifelong therapy with either oral coumarin or aspirin, seems a reasonable approach until more definitive data are available.

POSTOPERATIVE MANAGEMENT

Careful attention to postoperative management is crucial for success of limb salvage. The patient is kept on strict bed rest for 5 to 7 days after the operation. The leg is initially placed in a supportive dressing. The dressing must give light compression to avoid undue edema or compromise of the free flap and be carefully padded to avoid any pressure points. After the first dressing change, the leg is wrapped attentively in a light compressive elastic bandage. Patients should be allowed to dangle the foot at the bedside. If there is any evidence of flap congestion, dangling should be delayed. After 2 days of dangling for 15 to 20 minutes four times a day, the patient may begin to ambulate with crutches or a walker. If the flap covers any of the weight-bearing portions of the foot, strict non–weight-bearing status is maintained for 6 weeks. Gradual weight bearing is introduced under the supervision of a physical therapist. Any wound complication, such as hematoma, skin graft loss, or separation of incisions, merits delay of weight-bearing ambulation until it has resolved. The soft tissue flaps used to reconstruct wounds of the foot and leg usually remain insensate but may develop sensation to deep pressure over time. Patients must be carefully coached to avoid pressure ulceration of these flaps. As the patient begins to bear weight, frequent inspection of the flap for signs of pressure is recommended. Consultation with a prosthetist skilled in shoe modification and the manufacture of partial foot prostheses can be especially helpful in these patients.

Outcome

When free flaps are combined with revascularization for limb salvage, 90% to 95% of flaps may be expected to survive.[302,309] In this setting, flap loss usually leads to amputation. Complications are common and may be significant. Illig et al[310] reported a 5% perioperative mortality risk and "major complications" in 16% of patients, including nonfatal myocardial infarction, congestive heart failure, and bypass graft infection, comparable to previous reports. Complications at the recipient site are also common and have been reported in up to 47% of patients. These complications usually involve partial flap necrosis, skin graft problems, wound separation, and hematoma. Prolonged hospital stay is common and is related to both the complexity of the operative treatment and concurrent medical problems in these patients. Combined vascular and soft tissue reconstruction can be expected to yield long-term limb salvage (at least 18 months) in about 60% of patients. About 40% of patients return to ambulation, although often not independently. In their excellent analysis, Illig et al[310] identified diabetes and end-stage renal failure as the two most important preoperative factors correlated with poor outcome. They found that only 56% of patients with diabetes, 25% of patients with end-stage renal failure, and 14% with both were alive with an intact limb by 1 year after operation. This same report found that no other factor, including age, sex, timing of operation (simultaneous or staged), location of the flap, weight-bearing status, type of bypass graft, or presence of osteomyelitis, had any bearing on the outcome.

Soft tissue wounds of the ischemic lower extremity pose a challenging problem. These patients often have other serious medical problems, and a careful systematic approach coupled with a clear understanding of the issues associated with vascular reconstruction is required for their care.

REFERENCES

1. Szuba A, Rockson S: Lymphedema: anatomy, physiology and pathogenesis. Vasc Med 1997;2:321-326.
2. Schirger A, Harrison EG, Janes JM: Idiopathic lymphedema. Review of 131 cases. JAMA 1962;182:124-132.
3. Velanovich V, Szymanski W: Quality of life of breast cancer patients with lymphedema. Am J Surg 1999;177:184-188.
4. Passik S, Newman M, Brennan M, et al: Psychiatric consultation for women undergoing rehabilitation for upper-extremity lymphedema following breast cancer treatment. Psycho-oncology 1995;4:255-263.
5. Zeissler RH, Rose GB, Nelson PA: Postmastectomy lymphedema: late results of treatment in 385 patients. Arch Phys Med Rehabil 1972;53:159-166.
6. Woods M, Tobin M, Mortimer P: The psychosocial morbidity of breast cancer patients with lymphoedema. Cancer Nurs 1995;18:467-471.
7. Hewitt M, Breen N, Devesa S: Cancer prevalence and survivorship issues: analyses of the 1992 National Health Interview Survey. J Natl Cancer Inst 1999;91:1480-1486.
8. Browse NL, Stewart G: Lymphedema: pathophysiology and classification. J Cardiovasc Surg 1985;26:91-106.
9. Crockett DJ: Lymphatic anatomy and lymphedema. Br J Plast Surg 1965;18:12.
10. Wallace S, Jackson L, Dodd GD, et al: Lymphatic dynamics in certain abnormal states. Am J Roentgenol Radium Ther Nucl Med 1964;91:1187.
11. Stone EJ, Hugo NE: Lymphedema. Surg Gynecol Obstet 1972;135:625.
12. Witte MH, Honto D, Witte CL: Clinical and experimental techniques to study the lymphatic system. Vasc Surg 1977; 11:20.
13. Olszewski WL: Pathophysiological and clinical observations of obstructive lymphedema of the limbs. In Clodius L, ed: Lymphedema. Stuttgart, Thieme, 1977:79-102.
14. Foldi E, Foldi M, Clodius L: The lymphedema chaos: a lancet. Ann Plast Surg 1989;22:505.
15. Reed RK, Laurent TC, Taylor AE: Hyaluronan in prenodal lymph from skin: changes with lymph flow. Am J Physiol 1990;259:H1097-H1100.
16. Kobayashi MR, Miller TA: Lymphedema. Clin Plast Surg 1987;14:303.
17. Foldi J: Physiology and pathophysiology of lymph flow. In Clodius L, ed: Lymphedema. Stuttgart, Thieme, 1977:1-11.
18. Schirger A, Harrison EG, Janes JM: Idiopathic lymphedema. Review of 131 cases. JAMA 1962;182:124-132.
19. Piller NB: Macrophage and tissue changes in the developmental phases of secondary lymphoedema and during conservative therapy with benzopyrone. Arch Histol Cytol 1990;53:209-218.
20. Ryan T, de Berker D: The interstitium, the connective tissue environment of the lymphatic, and angiogenesis in human skin. Clin Dermatol 1995;13:451-458.
21. Smeltzer DM, Stickler GB, Schirger A: Primary lymphedema in children and adolescents: a follow-up study and review. Pediatrics 1985;76:206-218.
22. Mangion J, Rahman N, Mansour S, et al: A gene for lymphedema-distichiasis maps to 16q24.3. Am J Hum Genet 1999;65:427-432.
23. Bull LN, Roche E, Song EJ, et al: Mapping of the locus for cholestasis-lymphedema syndrome (Aagenaes syndrome) to a 6.6-dM interval of chromosome 15q. Am J Hum Genet 2000;67:994-999.
24. Ferrell RE, Levinson KL, Esman JH, et al: Hereditary lymphedema: evidence for linkage and genetic-heterogeneity. Hum Mol Genet 1998;7:2073-2078.
25. Milroy WF: An undescribed variety of hereditary oedema. N Y Med J 1892;56:505.
26. Wolfe JHN, Kinmonth JB: The prognosis of primary lymphedema of the lower limbs. Arch Surg 1981;116:1157-1160.
27. Lymphatic filariasis—tropical medicine's origin will not go away [editorial]. Lancet 1987;1:1409.
28. Anonymous: Lymphatic Filariasis. Fourth report of the WHO Expert Committee on Filariasis. WHO Tech Rep Ser 1984;702: 3-112.
29. Segerstrom K, Bjerle P, Graffman S, et al: Factors that influence the incidence of brachial oedema after treatment of breast cancer. Scand J Plast Reconstr Surg Hand Surg 1992;26:223-227.
30. Erickson V, Pearson M, Ganz L, et al: Arm edema in breast cancer patients. J Natl Cancer Inst 2001;93:96-111.
31. Soisson AP, Soper JT, Clarke-Pearson DL, et al: Adjuvant radiotherapy following radical hysterectomy for patients with stage IB and IIA cervical cancer. Gynecol Oncol 1990;37:390-395.
32. Fiorica JV, Roberts WS, Greenberg H, et al: Morbidity and survival patterns in patients after radical hysterectomy and postoperative adjuvant pelvic radiotherapy. Gynecol Oncol 1990;36:343-347.

33. Clodius L: Secondary arm lymphedema. In Clodius L, ed: Lymphedema. Stuttgart, Thieme, 1977:147-174.
34. Mallon E, Powell S, Mortimer P, et al: Evidence for altered cell-mediated immunity in postmastectomy lymphoedema. Br J Dermatol 1997;137:928-933.
35. Rockson SG, Miller LT, Senie R, et al: American Cancer Society lymphedema workshop. Workgroup III: diagnosis and management of lymphedema. Cancer 1998;83(suppl 12):2882-2885.
36. Stemmer R: Ein klinisches Zeichen zur früh und differential Diagnose des Lymphödems. [A clinical symptom for the early and differential diagnosis of lymphedema.] Vasa 1976;5:261-262.
37. Bergan J, Yao J, Flinn W, et al: Surgical treatment of venous obstruction and insufficiency. J Vasc Surg 1986;3:174-181.
38. Bull RH, Coburn PR, Mortimer PS: Pretibial myxoedema: a manifestation of lymphoedema? Lancet 1993;341:403-404.
39. Holt P, Lazarus J, Marks R: The epidermis in thyroid disease. Br J Dermatol 1976;95:513-518.
40. Ryan T, Curri S: Hypertrophy and atrophy of fat. Clin Dermatol 1989;7:93-106.
41. Cambria RA, Gloviczki P, Naessens JM, et al: Noninvasive evaluation of the lymphatic system with lymphoscintigraphy: a prospective, semiquantitative analysis in 386 extremities. J Vasc Surg 1993;18:773-782.
42. Case TC, Witte CL, Witte MH, et al: Magnetic resonance imaging in human lymphedema: comparison with lymphangioscintigraphy. Magn Reson Imaging 1992;10:549-558.
43. Servelle M: La lymphographic, moyen d'etude de la physiopathologic des grosses jambes. Rev Chir 1944;82:251-258.
44. Kinmonth JB, Taylor GW, Tracy GD, et al: Primary lymphoedema. Clinical and lymphangiographic studies of a series of 107 patients in which the lower limbs were affected. Br J Surg 1957;45:1-10.
45. Partsch H: Assessment of abnormal lymph drainage for the diagnosis of lymphedema by isotopic lymphangiography and by indirect lymphography. Clin Dermatol 1995;13:445-450.
46. Gan JL, Zhang DS, Fu KD, et al: Indirect lymphography with Isovist-300 in various forms of lymphedema. Clin Med J (Engl) 1991;104:49-53.
47. Cambria RA, Gloviczki P, Naessens JM, et al: Noninvasive evaluation of the lymphatic system with lymphoscintigraphy: a prospective, semiquantitative analysis in 386 extremities. J Vasc Surg 1993;18:773-782.
48. Ter SE, Alavi A, Kim CK, et al: Lymphoscintigraphy. A reliable test for the diagnosis of lymphedema. Clin Nucl Med 1993;18:646-654.
49. Weissleder R, Thrall JH: The lymphatic system: diagnostic imaging studies. Radiology 1989;172:315.
50. Intenzo CM, Desai AG, Kim SS, et al: Lymphedema of the lower extremities: evaluation by microcolloidal imaging. Clin Nucl Med 1989;14:107.
51. Duewell S, Hapspiel KD, Zuber J, et al: Swollen lower extremity: role of MR imaging. Radiology 1992;184:227-231.
52. Haaverstad R, Nilsen G, Myhre HO, et al: The use of MRI in the investigation of leg oedema. Ear J Vasc Surg 1992;6:124-129.
53. Vassalloo P, Matei C, Heston W, et al: AMU-227 enhanced MR lymphography: usefulness for differentiating reactive from tumor-bearing lymph nodes. Radiology 1994;193:501-506.
54. Ilana I, Bittoun J, Alliot F, et al: Lymphedematous skin and subcutis: in vivo high resolution magnetic resonance imaging evaluation. J Invest Dermatol 1998;111:782-787.
55. Hadjis NS, Carr DH, Banks L, et al: The role of CT in the diagnosis of primary lymphedema of the lower limb. AJR Am J Roentgenol 1985;144:361.
56. Vaughan BF: CT of swollen legs. Clin Radiol 1990;41:24.
57. Collins CD, Mortimer PS, D'Ettorre H, et al: Computed tomography in the assessment of response to limb compression in unilateral lymphoedema. Clin Radiol 1995;50:541-544.
58. Gniadecka M: Localization of dermal edema in lipodermatosclerosis, lymphedema, and cardiac insufficiency. J Am Acad Dermatol 1996;35:37-41.
59. Morgan RG, Casley-Smith JR, Mason MR, et al: Complex physical therapy for the lymphoedematous arm. J Hand Surg Br 1992;17:437-441.
60. Foldi M: Treatment of lymphedema [editorial]. Lymphology 1994;27:1-5.
61. Foldi E, Foldi M, Weissleder H: Conservative treatment of lymphedema of the limbs. Angiology 1985;36:171-180.
62. Britton RC: Management of peripheral edema, including lymphedema of the arm after radical mastectomy. Cleve Clin Q 1959;26:53.
63. Foldi E, Foldi M, Clodius I: The lymphedema chaos: a lancet. Am Plast Surg 1989;22:505-515.
64. Svensson WE, Mortimer PS, Tohno E, et al: Colour Doppler demonstrates venous flow abnormalities in breast cancer patients with chronic arm swelling. Eur J Cancer 1994;30A:657.
65. Richmond DM, O'Donnell TF, Zelikowski A: Sequential pneumatic compression for lymphedema. Arch Surg 1985;120:1116-1119.
66. Liu NF, Olszewski W: The influence of local hyperthermia on lymphedema and lymphedematous skin of the human leg. Lymphology 1993;26:28-37.
67. Chang T, Han L, Gan J, et al: Microwave, an alternative to electric heating in the treatment of peripheral lymphedema. Lymphology 1989;22:20-24.
68. Katoh I, Harada K, Tsuda Y, et al: Intra-arterial lymphocytes injection for treatment of lymphedema. Jpn J Surg 1984;14:331-334.
69. Egawa Y, Sato A, Katoh I, et al: Reduction in arm swelling and changes in protein components of lymphedema fluid after intra-arterial injection of autologous lymphocytes. Lymphology 1993;26:169-176.
70. Nagata Y, Murata R, Mitsumori M, et al: Intra-arterial infusion of autologous lymphocytes for the treatment of refractory lymphoedema. Preliminary report. Eur J Surg 1994;160:105-109.
71. Casley-Smith JR, Wang CT, Casley-Smith JR, Zi-hai C: Treatment of filarial lymphoedema and elephantiasis with 5,6-benzo-alpha-pyrone (coumarin). BMJ 1993;307:1037-1041.
72. Casley-Smith JR, Jamal S, Casley-Smith J: Treatment of filarial lymphoedema and elephantiasis with 5,6-benzo-alpha-pyrone (coumarin) and the effects of diethylcarbamazine (DEC). Ann Trop Med Parasitol 1993;87:247-258.
73. Egan D, O'Kennedy R, Moran E, et al: The pharmacology, metabolism, analysis, and applications of coumarin and coumarin-related compounds. Drug Metab Rev 1990;22:503-529.
74. Piller NB, Morgan RG, Casley-Smith JR: A double-blind, crossover trial of O-(beta-hydroxyethyl)-rutosides (benzopyrones) in the treatment of lymphoedema of the arms and legs. Br J Plast Surg 1988;41:20-27.
75. Soria P, Cuesta A, Romero H, et al: Dietary treatment of lymphedema by restriction of long-chain triglycerides. Angiology 1994;45:703-707.
76. Charles RH: Elephantiasis scroti. In Latham A, English TC, eds: A System of Treatment. London, Churchill, 1912:vol III.
77. Dellon AL, Hoopes JE: The Charles procedure for primary lymphedema. Plast Reconstr Surg 1977;60:589.
78. Mavili ME, Naldoken S, Safak T: Modified Charles operation for primary fibrosclerotic lymphedema. Lymphology 1994;14:20.
79. Kim DI, Huh S, Lee SJ, et al: Excision of subcutaneous tissue and deep muscle fascia for advanced lymphedema. Lymphology 1998;31:190-194.

80. Poth E, Barnes S, Ross G: A new operative treatment for elephantiasis. Surg Gynecol Obstet 1947;84:642-644.
81. Kondoleon E: Ultimate results of Kondoleon operation for elephantiasis edema. Arch Fr Belg Chir 1924;27:104.
82. Sistrunk WE: Experiences with the Kondoleon operation for elephantiasis. JAMA 1918;71:800.
83. Miller TA: A surgical approach to lymphedema. Am J Surg 1977;134:191.
84. Miller TA: Surgical management of lymphedema of the extremity. Ann Plast Surg 1978;1:184.
85. Homans J: Treatment of elephantiasis of the legs. A preliminary report. N Engl J Med 1936;215:1099.
86. Gloviczki P: Principles of surgical treatment of chronic lymphoedema. Int Angiol 1999;18:42-46.
87. Brorson H, Svensson H: Complete reduction of lymphoedema of the arm by liposuction after breast cancer. Scand J Plast Reconstr Surg Hand Surg 1997;31:137-143.
88. Brorson H, Svensson H: Skin blood flow of the lymphedematous arm before and after liposuction. Lymphology 1997;30:165-172.
89. Brorson H, Svensson H: Liposuction combined with controlled compression therapy reduces arm lymphedema more effectively than controlled compression therapy alone. Plast Reconstr Surg 1998;102:1058-1068.
90. Handley WS: Lymphangioplasty. Lancet 1908;1:783.
91. Gillies HD, Fraser FR: Treatment of lymphedema by a plastic operation: a preliminary report. Br Med J 1935;1:96.
92. Thompson N: Buried dermal flap operation for chronic lymphedema of the extremities. Ten-year survey of results in 79 cases. Plast Reconstr Surg 1970;45:541.
93. Sawhney CP: Evaluation of Thompson's buried dermal flap operation for lymphedema of the limbs: a clinical and radioisotopic study. Br J Plast Surg 1974;27:278.
94. Hurst PA, Stewart G, Kinmonth JB, et al: Long term results of the enteromesenteric bridge operation in the treatment of primary lymphoedema. Br J Surg 1985;72:272-274.
95. Goldsmith HS, De Los Santos R: Omental transposition for the treatment of chronic lymphedema. Rev Surg 1966;23:303.
96. Goldsmith HS: Long term evaluation of omental transposition for chronic lymphedema. Ann Surg 1974;180:847.
97. Savage RC: The surgical management of lymphedema. Surg Gynecol Obstet 1985;160:283-289.
98. O'Brien BM, Hickey MJ, Hurley JV, et al: Microsurgical transfer of the greater omentum in the treatment of canine obstructive lymphoedema. Br J Plast Surg 1990;43:440-446.
99. Egorov YS, Abalmasov KG, Ivanov VV, et al: Autotransplantation of the greater omentum in the treatment of chronic lymphedema. Lymphology 1994;27:137-143.
100. Kambayashi J, Ohshiro T, Mori T: Appraisal of myocutaneous flapping for treatment of postmastectomy lymphedema. Case report. Acta Chir Scand 1990;156:175-177.
101. Chitale VR: Role of tensor fascia lata musculocutaneous flap in lymphedema of the lower extremity and external genitalia. Ann Plast Surg 1989;23:297-304.
102. Medgyesi SA: Successful operation for lymphoedema using a myocutaneous flap as a "wick." Br J Plast Surg 1983;36:64.
103. Nielubowicz J, Olszewski W, Sokolowski J: Surgical lymphovenous shunts. J Cardiovasc Surg 1968;9:262-267.
104. O'Brien BM, Sykes P, Threlfall GN, Browning FS: Microlymphaticovenous anastomoses for obstructive lymphedema. Plast Reconstr Surg 1977;60:197-211.
105. O'Brien BM, Mellow CG, Khazanchi RK, et al: Long-term results after microlymphaticovenous anastomoses for the treatment of obstructive lymphedema. Plast Reconstr Surg 1990;85:562-572.
106. Gloviczki P, Fisher J, Hollier LH, et al: Microsurgical lymphovenous anastomosis for treatment of lymphedema: a critical review. J Vasc Surg 1988;7:647-652.
107. Campisi C: The autologous grafts in reconstructive microsurgery for lymph stasis. In Olszewski WL, ed. Lymph Stasis: Pathophysiology, Diagnosis and Treatment. Boca Raton, Fla, CRC Press, 1991:554-573.
108. Filipetti M, Santoro E, Graziano F, et al: Modern therapeutic approaches to postmastectomy brachial lymphedema. Microsurgery 1994;15:604-610.
109. Puckett CL: Microlymphatic surgery for lymphedema. Clin Plast Surg 1983;10:133.
110. Baumeister RG, Seifert J, Wiebecke B, Hahn D: Experimental basis and first application of clinical lymph vessel transplantation of secondary lymphedema. World J Surg 1981;5:401-407.
111. Baumeister RG, Siuda S: Treatment of lymphedemas by microsurgical lymphatic grafting: what is proved? Plast Reconstr Surg 1990;85:64.
112. Baumeister RG: Microsurgical autologous lymph-vessel grafting. In Olszewski WL, ed: Lymph Stasis: Pathophysiology, Diagnosis and Treatment. Boca Raton, Fla, CRC Press, 1991:545-552.
113. Campisi C, Boccardo F, Tacchella M: Reconstructive microsurgery of lymph vessels: the personal method of lymphatic-venous-lymphatic (LVL) interpositioned grafted shunt. Microsurgery 1995;16:161-166.
114. Olszewski WL: Surgical lympho-venous anastomoses for treatment of lymphedema. In Olszewski WL, ed: Lymph Stasis: Pathophysiology, Diagnosis and Treatment. Boca Raton, Fla, CRC Press, 1991:526-536.
115. Das S, Tuerk D, Amar AD, et al: Surgery of male genital lymphedema. J Urol 1983;129:1240.
116. Dijkstra JW, Bergfeld WF, Kay R: Congenital lymphedema of genitalia and extremities. Cleve Clin Q 1984;51:553-557.
117. Ross JH, Kay R, Yetman RJ, et al: Primary lymphedema of the genitalia in children and adolescents. J Urol 1998;160:1485-1489.
118. Sarda P, Jalaguier J, Montoya F, et al: Hereditary congenital lymphedema with pseudosexual ambiguity. J Genet Hum 1988;36:353-360.
119. Tapper D, Eraklis AJ, Colodny AH, et al: Congenital lymphedema of the penis: a method of reconstruction. J Pediatr Surg 1980;15:481.
120. Vaught SK, Litvak AS, McRoberts JW: The surgical management of scrotal and penile lymphedema. J Urol 1975;113:204.
121. Dandapat MC, Mohapatro SK, Patro SK: Elephantiasis of the penis and scrotum. A review of 350 cases. Am J Surg 1985;149:686.
122. Ollapallil JJ, Watters DA: Surgical management of elephantiasis of male genitalia. Br J Urol 1995;76:213.
123. Sauer PF, Bueschen AJ, Vasconez LO: Lymphedema of the penis and scrotum. Clin Plast Surg 1988;15:507.
124. McConnell AH, Haslam P: Angiosarcoma in postmastectomy lymphedema: a report of five cases and a review of the literature. Br J Surg 1959;46:322.
125. Tomita K, Yokogawa A, Oda Y, Terahata S: Lymphangiosarcoma in postmastectomy lymphedema (Stewart-Treves syndrome): ultrastructural and immunohistologic characteristics. J Surg Oncol 1988;38:275.
126. Janse AJ, van Coevorden F, Peterse H, et al: Lymphedema-induced lymphangiosarcoma. Eur J Surg Oncol 1995;21:155.
127. Chung KC, Kim HJ, Jeffers LL: Lymphangiosarcoma (Stewart-Treves syndrome) in postmastectomy patients. J Hand Surg Am 2000;25:1163-1168.
128. Andersson HC, Parry DM, Mulvihill JJ: Lymphangiosarcoma in late-onset hereditary lymphedema: case report and nosological implications. Am J Med Genet 1995;56:72-75.
129. Heitmann C, Ingianni G: Stewart-Treves syndrome: lymphangiosarcoma following mastectomy. Ann Plast Surg 2000;44:72-75.

130. Baker SR, Stacey MC, Jopp-McKay AG, et al: Epidemiology of chronic venous ulcers. Br J Surg 1991;78:864-867.
131. Nelzen O, Bergqvist D, Lindhagen A: Venous and non-venous leg ulcers: clinical history and appearance in a population study. Br J Surg 1994;81:182-187.
132. Krasner D: Painful venous ulcers: themes and stories about their impact on quality of life. Ostomy Wound Manage 1998;44:38-49.
133. Phillips T, Stanton B, Provan A, Lew R: A study of the impact of leg ulcers on quality of life: financial, social and psychological implications. J Am Acad Dermatol 1994;31:49-53.
134. Collum M: Prevalence of chronic leg ulceration and severe chronic venous disease in western countries. Phlebology 1992;suppl:6-12.
135. Capeheart JK: Chronic venous insufficiency: a focus on prevention of venous ulceration. J Wound Ostomy Continence Nurs 1996;23:227-234.
136. Ruckley CV: Socioeconomic impact of chronic venous insufficiency and leg ulcers. Angiology 1997;48:67-69.
137. Lazarus GS, Cooper DM, Knighton DR, et al: Definitions and guidelines for assessment of wounds and evaluation of healing. Arch Dermatol 1994;130:489-493.
138. Olin JW, Beusterien KM, Childs MB, et al: Medical costs of treating venous stasis ulcers: evidence from a retrospective cohort study. Vasc Med 1999;4:1-7.
139. Scott TE, LaMorte WW, Gorin DR, Menzoian JO: Risk factors for chronic venous insufficiency: a dual case-control study. J Vasc Surg 1995;22:622-628.
140. Nelson O, Bequest D, Lindhagen A: Leg ulcer: a cross sectional population study. J Vasc 1991;14:557-564.
141. Falanga V: Venous ulceration. J Dermatol Surg Oncol 1993;19:764-771.
142. Falanga V, Eaglstein WH: The trap hypothesis of venous ulceration. Lancet 1993;341:1006-1008.
143. Burnand KG, O'Donnell TF, Thomas ML, Browse NL: The relative importance of incompetent communicating veins in the production of varicose veins and venous ulcers. Surgery 1977;82:9-14.
144. Browse NL, Burnand KG: The cause of venous ulceration. Lancet 1982;2:243-245.
145. Alguire PC, Mathes BM: Chronic venous insufficiency and venous ulceration. J Gen Intern Med 1997;12:374-383.
146. Greenberg A, Hasan A, Montaivo BM, et al: Acute lipodermatosclerosis is associated with venous insufficiency. J Am Dermatol 1996;35:566-568.
147. Burnand KG, Whimster I, Naidoo A, Browse NL: Pericapillary fibrin in the ulcer-bearing skin of the lower leg: the cause of lipodermatosclerosis and venous ulceration. Br Med J (Clin Res Ed) 1982;285:1071-1072.
148. Franzeck UK, Bollinger A, Huch R, Huch A: Transcutaneous oxygen tension and capillary morphologic characteristics and density in patients with chronic venous incompetence. Circulation 1984;70:806-811.
149. Stacey MC, Burnand KG, Bhogal BS, Black MM: Pericapillary fibrin deposits and skin hypoxia precede changes of lipodermatosclerosis in limbs at increased risk of developing a venous ulcer. Cardiovasc Surg 2000;8:372-380.
150. Mani R, White JE, Barret DF, Weaver PW: Tissue oxygenation, venous ulcers and fibrin cuffs. J R Soc Med 1989;82:345-346.
151. Pardess JD, Tonneson MG, Talaya V, et al: Skin capillaries surrounding chronic venous ulcers demonstrate smooth muscle hyperplasia and increased laminin type IV collagen. J Invest Dermatol 1987;94:563-568.
152. Falanga V, Moose HH, Nemeth AJ, et al: Dermal pericapillary fibrin in venous disease and venous ulceration. Arch Dermatol 1987;123:620-623.
153. Parsch H: Hyperaemic hypoxia in venous ulceration. Br J Dermatol 1983;109:249-250.
154. Roszinski S, Schmeller W: Differences between intracutaneous and transcutaneous skin oxygen tension in chronic venous insufficiency. J Cardiovasc Surg 1995;36:407-413.
155. Speiser DE, Bollinger A: Microangiopathy in mild chronic venous incompetence (CVI): morphological alterations and increased transcapillary diffusion detected by fluorescence videomicroscopy. Int J Microcirc Clin Exp 1991;10:55-66.
156. Erickson CA, Lanza DJ, Karp DL, et al: Healing of venous ulcers in an ambulatory care program: the role of chronic venous insufficiency and patient compliance. J Vasc Surg 1995;22:629-636.
157. Falanga V, Bontempo FA, Eaglstein WH: Protein C and protein S plasma levels in patients with lipodermatosclerosis and venous ulceration. Arch Dermatol 1990;126:1195-1197.
158. Paye M, Nusgens BV, Lapiere CM: Factor XIII of blood coagulation modulates collagen biosynthesis by fibroblasts in vitro. Haemostasis 1989;19:274-283.
159. Stacey MC, Burnand KG, Pattison M, et al: Changes in the apparently normal limb in unilateral venous ulceration. Br J Surg 1987;74:936-939.
160. Higley HR, Ksander GA, Gerhardt CO, Falanga V: Extravasation of macromolecules and possible trapping of transforming growth factor-β in venous ulceration. Br J Dermatol 1995;132:79-85.
161. Zuccarelli F, Taccoen A, Razavian M, Chabanel A: Increasing erythrocyte aggregability with the progressive grades of chronic venous insufficiency: importance and mechanisms. J Cardiovasc Surg 1995;36:387-391.
162. Thomas PR, Nash GB, Dormandy JA: White cell accumulation in dependent legs of patients with venous hypertension: a possible mechanism for trophic changes in the skin. Br Med J (Clin Res Ed) 1988;296:1693-1695.
163. Kirsner RS, Pardes JB, Eaglstein WH, Falanga V: The clinical spectrum of lipodermatosclerosis. J Am Acad Dermatol 1993;28:623-627.
164. Phillips TJ: Successful methods of treating leg ulcers: the tried and true, plus the novel and new. Postgrad Med 1999;105:159-179.
165. Moll B: Vasculitis and atrophie blanche. Hautartzt 1969;20:474-475.
166. Sadick NS, Allen SL: Atrophie blanche in chronic myelogenous leukemia. Cutis 1988;42:206-209.
167. Falanga V: Venous ulceration. J Dermatol Surg Oncol 1993;19:764-771.
168. Callen JP: Pyoderma gangrenosum. Lancet 1998;351:581-585.
169. Harris B, Eaglstein WH, Falanga V: Basal cell carcinoma arising in venous ulcer and mimicking granulation tissue. J Dermatol Surg Oncol 1993;19:150-152.
170. Scriven JM, Hartshorne T, Bell PR, et al: Single-visit venous ulcer assessment clinic: the first year. Br J Surg 1997;84:334-336.
171. McGuckin M, Stineman M, Goin J, Williams S: Draft guideline: diagnosis and treatment of venous leg ulcers. Ostomy Wound Manage 1996;42:48-78.
172. Araki CT, Back TL, Padberg FT, et al: Refinements in the detection of popliteal vein reflux. J Vasc Surg 1993;18:742-748.
173. Falanga V, Eaglstein WH, Bucalo B, et al: Topical use of human recombinant epidermal growth factor (h-EGF) in venous ulcers. J Dermatol Surg Oncol 1992;18:604-606.
174. Van Bemellen PS, Bedford G, Beach K, Strandness DE: Quantitative segmental evaluation of venous valvular reflux with duplex ultrasound scanning. J Vasc Surg 1989;10:425-431.
175. Labropoulos N, Leon M, Geroulakos G, et al: Venous hemodynamic abnormalities in patients with leg ulceration. Am J Surg 1995;169:72-74.
176. Thibault PK: Duplex examination. Dermatologica 1995;21:77-82.
177. Pearce WH, Ricco JB, Queral LA, et al: Hemodynamic assessment of venous problems. Surgery 1983;93:715-721.

178. Raju S, Fredericks R: Valve reconstruction procedures for nonobstructive venous insufficiency: rationale, techniques and results in 107 procedures with 2- to 8- year follow-up. J Vasc Surg 1988;7:301-310.
179. Padberg FT, Hobson RW, Lee B: Femoral pseudoaneurysm from drugs of abuse: ligation or reconstruction. J Vasc Surg 1992;15:642-648.
180. Porter J, Moneta G: Reporting standard in venous disease: an update. J Vasc Surg 1995;21:635-645.
181. Statement of the International Consensus Committee on Chronic Venous Diseases: Classification and grading of chronic venous disease in the lower limbs. In Gloviczki P, Yao JST, eds: Handbook of Venous Disorders. London, Chapman & Hall, 1996:652-660.
182. Negus D: Leg Ulcers: A Practical Approach to Management. Boston, Butterworth Heinemann, 1991:3.
183. Partsch H: Compression therapy of the legs: a review. J Dermatol Surg Oncol 1991;17:799-808.
184. Partsch H: Dermal lymphangiopathy in chronic venous incompetence. In Bollinger A, Partsch H, Wolfe JHN, eds: The Initial Lymphatics. New York, Thieme Stratton, 1985: 178-187.
185. Allenby F, Boardman L, Pflug JJ, Calnan JS: Effect of external pneumatic intermittent compression on fibrinolysis in man. Lancet 1973;2:1412-1414.
186. Christopoulos D, Nicolaides AN, Szendro G: Venous reflux: quantification and correlation with the clinical severity of chronic venous disease. Br J Surg 1988;75:352-356.
187. Stacey MC, Burnand KG, Layer GT, Pattison M: Calf pump function in patients with healed venous ulcers is not improved by surgery to the communicating veins or by elastic stockings. Br J Surg 1988;75:436-439.
188. Mayberry JC, Moneta GL, Taylor LMJ, Porter JM: Fifteen-year results of ambulatory compression therapy for chronic venous ulcers. Surgery 1991;109:575-581.
189. Blair SD, Wright DD, Backhouse CM, et al: Sustained compression and healing chronic venous ulcers. BMJ 1988;297: 1159-1161.
190. Fletcher A, Sheldon TA: A systematic review of compression treatment for venous leg ulcers. BMJ 1997;315:576-580.
191. Erickson CA, Lanza DJ, Karp DL, et al: Healing of venous ulcers in an ambulatory care program: the roles of chronic venous insufficiency and patient compliance. J Vasc Surg 1995;22:629-636.
192. Callam MJ, Harper DR, Dale JJ, Ruckley CV: Chronic ulcer of the leg: clinical history. Br Med J 1987;294:1389-1391.
193. Kunimoto BT: Compression therapy: theory and practice. Dermatol Ther 1999;9:63-68.
194. Nelson EA: Compression bandaging in the treatment of venous leg ulcers: a guide to the evidence for the effective selection of bandages. J Wound Care 1996;125:415-418.
195. Buchbinder D, McCullough GM, Melick CF: Patients evaluated for venous disease may have other pathological conditions contributing to symptomatology. Am J Surg 1993;166:211-215.
196. Richmond DM, O'Donnell T, Zelikovski A: Sequential pneumatic compression for lymphedema. Arch Surg 1985;20:1116-1119.
197. Zelikovski A, Deutsch A, Reiss A: The sequential pneumatic compression device in surgery for lymphedema of the limbs. J Cardiovasc Surg 1983;24:122-126.
198. Choucair M, Phillips T: Compression therapy. Dermatol Surg 1998;24:141-148.
199. Margolis DJ, Berlin JA, Strom BL: Risk factors associated with the failure of a venous ulcer to heal. Arch Dermatol 1999;135:920-926.
200. Alvarez O, Rozin T, Wiseman D: Moist environment for healing: matching the dressing to the wound. Wounds 1989; 1:35-51.
201. Friedman S, Su WPD: Hydrocolloid occlusive dressing management of leg ulcers. Arch Dermatol 1984;120:1329-1331.
202. Mertz PM, Marshall DA, Eaglstein WH: Occlusive wound dressings to prevent bacterial invasion and wound infection. J Am Acad Dermatol 1985;12:662-668.
203. Helfman T, Ovington L, Falanga V: Occlusive dressings and wound healing. Clin Dermatol 1994;12:121-127.
204. Blair SD, Backhouse CM, Wright DD, et al: Do dressings influence the healing of chronic venous ulcers? Phlebology 1988;3:129-134.
205. Freak L, Simon DA, Edwards AT, McCollum CN: Comparative study of three primary dressings in the healing of chronic venous ulcers. Br J Surg 1992;79:1235.
206. Kikta MJ, Schuler JJ, Meyer JP, et al: A prospective, randomized trial of Unna's boots versus hydroactive dressings in the treatment of venous stasis ulcers. J Vasc Surg 1988;7:478-483.
207. Lineaweaver W, Howard R, Soucy D, et al: Topical antibiotic therapy. Arch Surg 1985;120:267-270.
208. Dagher FJ, Algoni SV, Smith A: Bacterial studies of leg ulcers. Angiology 1987;29:641-653.
209. Mertz PM, Eaglstein WH: The effect of a semiocclusive dressing on the microbial population in superficial wounds. Arch Surg 1984;119:641-653.
210. Colgan MP, Dormandy JA, Jones PW, et al: Oxpentifylline treatment of venous ulcers of the legs. BMJ 1990;300:972-975.
211. Foresman PA, Payne DS, Becker D, et al: The relative toxicity index for wound cleansers. Wounds 1993;5:226-231.
212. Hillstrom L: Iodosorb compared to standard treatment in chronic venous leg ulcers—a multicenter study. Acta Chir Scand Suppl 1988;544:53-56.
213. Holloway GA, Johansen KH, Barnes RW, Pierce GE: Multicenter trial of cadexomer iodine to treat venous stasis ulcers. West J Med 1989;151:35-38.
214. Alinovi A, Bassissi P, Pini M: Systemic administration of antibiotics in the management of venous ulcers: a randomized clinical trial. J Am Acad Dermatol 1986;15:186-191.
215. Falanga V, Kirsner RS, Eaglstein WH, et al: Stanozolol in treatment of leg ulcers due to cryofibrinogenemia. Lancet 1991;338:347-348.
216. Glazer G: Atherogenic side effects of anabolic steroids on serum lipid levels. Arch Intern Med 1991;151:1925-1933.
217. Soe KL, Soe M, Gluud C: Liver pathology associated with the use of anabolic-androgenic steroids. Liver 1992;12:73-79.
218. Falanga V, for the Trental Collaborative Group: Pentoxifylline (Trental) accelerates the healing of venous ulcers in a double blind randomized study. Proceedings from the European Tissue Repair Society, Cologne, Germany, August 25, 1997.
219. Falanga V, Sabolinski M: A bilayered skin construct (Apligraf) accelerates complete closure of hard-to-heal venous ulcers. Wound Repair Regen 1999;7:201-207.
220. Bertocchi F, Proserpio P, Lampugnal MG, Dejana E: The effect of pentoxifylline on polymorphonuclear cell adhesion to cultured endothelial cells. In Mandell GL, Novici WJ, eds: Pentoxifylline and Leukocyte Function. Somerville, NJ, Hoechst-Roussel Pharmaceuticals, 1988:68-74.
221. Weithmann KU: The influence of pentoxifylline on interactions between blood vessel wall and platelets. IRCS Med Sci 1980;8:293-294.
222. Zabel P, Wolter DT, Schonharting MM, Schade UF: Oxpentifylline in endotoxaemia. Lancet 1998;2:1474-1477.
223. Dale JJ, Ruckley CV, Harper DR, et al: Randomized, double blind placebo controlled trial of pentoxyphilline in the treatment of venous leg ulcers. BMJ 1999;319:875-878.
224. Guilhou JJ, Dereure O, Marzin L, et al: Efficacy of Daflon 500 mg in venous leg ulcer healing: a double-blind, randomized, controlled versus placebo trial in 107 patients. Angiology 1997;48:77-85.

225. Lyon RT, Veith FJ, Bolton L, Machado F: Clinical benchmark for healing of chronic venous ulcers. Am J Surg 1998;176:172-175.
226. Layton AM, Ibbotson SH, Davies JA, Goodfield MJ: Randomised trial of oral aspirin for chronic venous leg ulcers. Lancet 1994;344:164-165.
227. Eaglstein WH, Falanga V: Chronic wounds. Surg Clin North Am 1997;77:689-700.
228. Falabella AF: Débridement and management of exudative wounds. Dermatol Ther 1999;9:36-43.
229. Westerhof W: Future prospects of proteolytic enzymes and wound healing. In Westerhof W, Vanscheidt W, eds: Proteolytic Enzymes and Wound Healing. New York, Springer-Verlag, 1994:99-102.
230. Trier WC, Peacock EE, Madden JW: Studies on the effectiveness of surgical management of chronic leg ulcers. Plast Reconstr Surg 1970;45:20-23.
231. Teh BT: Why do skin grafts fail? Plast Reconstr Surg 1979;49:323-330.
232. Kirsner RS, Matta SM, Falanga V, Kerdel FA: Split thickness skin grafting of leg ulcers. J Dermatol Surg 1995;21:701-703.
233. Tanner JC, Vandeput J, Olley JF: The mesh skin graft. Plast Reconstr Surg 1964;34:287.
234. Johnson WC, O'Hara ET, Corey C, et al: Venous stasis ulceration: effectiveness of subfascial ligation. Arch Surg 1985;120:797-800.
235. Pierik EG, Wittens CHA, Van Urk H: Subfascial endoscopic ligation in the treatment of incompetent perforator veins. Eur J Vasc Endovasc Surg 1997;25:654-657.
236. Negus D, Friedgood A: The effective management of venous ulceration. Br J Surg 1983;70:623-627.
237. Linton R: John Homans' impact on diseases of the veins of the lower extremity, with special references to deep thrombophlebitis and the post-thrombotic syndrome with ulceration. The John Homans Lecture, Society for Vascular Surgery, 1976. Surgery 1977;81:1-11.
238. Sarin S, Scurr JH, Smith PD: Medial calf perforators in venous disease: the significance of outward flow. J Vasc Surg 1992;16:40-46.
239. Alexander House Group Consensus Statement: Consensus paper on venous leg ulcers. Phlebology 1992;7:48-58.
240. Kistner RL: Definitive diagnosis and definitive treatment in chronic venous disease: a concept whose time has come. J Vasc Surg 1996;24:703-710.
241. Gloviczki P, Bergan JJ, Menawat SS: Safety, feasibility, and early efficacy of subfascial endoscopic perforator surgery: a preliminary report from the North American registry. J Vasc Surg 1997;25:94-105.
242. Burnand KG, O'Donnell TF, Thomas M, Browse NL: The relative importance of incompetent communicating veins in the production of varicose veins and venous ulcers. Surgery 1977;82:9-14.
243. Lees TA, Lambert D: Patterns of venous reflux in limbs with skin changes associated with chronic venous insufficiency. Br J Surg 1993;80:725-728.
244. Shami SK, Sarin S, Cheatle TR, et al: Venous ulcers and the superficial venous system. J Vasc Surg 1993;17:487-490.
245. Sethia KK, Darke SG: Long saphenous incompetence as a cause of venous ulceration. Br J Surg 1994;71:754-755.
246. Akesson H, Brudin L, Cwikiel W, et al: Does the correction of insufficient superficial and perforating veins improve venous function in patients with deep venous insufficiency? Phlebology 1992;5:113-123.
247. Padberg FT, Pappas PJ, Araki CJ, et al: Hemodynamic and clinical improvement after superficial vein ablation in primary combined venous insufficiency with ulceration. J Vasc Surg 1996;24:711-718.
248. Masuda EM, Kistner RL: Long-term results of venous valve reconstruction: a four- to twenty-one-year follow-up. J Vasc Surg 1994;19:391-403.
249. Kistner R: Surgical repair of incompetent femoral vein valve. Arch Surg 1975;110:1336-1142.
250. Bradbury AW, Stonebridge PA, Callam MJ, et al: Foot volumetry and duplex ultrasound after saphenous and perforating vein ligation. Br J Surg 1993;80:845-848.
251. Walsh JC, Bertan JJ, Beeman S, Comer T: Femoral venous reflux is abolished by greater saphenous stripping. Ann Vasc Surg 1994;8:566-570.
252. Raju S, Fredricks RK, Neglen PN, Bass JD: Durability of venous valve reconstruction techniques for "primary" and post-thrombotic reflux. J Vasc Surg 1996;23:357-367.
253. Burkhart HM, Fath SW, Dalsing MC, et al: Experimental repair of venous valvular insufficiency using a cryopreserved venous valve autograft aided by a distal arteriovenous fistula. J Vasc Surg 1997;26:817-822.
254. Halliday P, Harris J, May J: Femoro-femoral crossover grafts (Palma operation): a long-term follow-up study. In Bergan JJ, Yao JST, eds: Surgery of the Veins. Orlando, Fla, Grune & Stratton, 1985:241-254.
255. Hobbs JT: Surgery and sclerotherapy in the treatment of varicose veins: a random trial. Arch Surg 1974;109:793-796.
256. Dunn RM, Fudem GM, Walton RL, et al: Free flap valvular transplantation for refractory venous ulceration. J Vasc Surg 1994;19:525-531.
257. Weinzweig N, Schuler J: Free tissue transfer in treatment of the recalcitrant chronic venous ulcer. Ann Plast Surg 1997;38:611-619.
258. Cazzsamoga AL, Helfman T, Falanga V, et al: Suramin application decreases epithelialization of porcine partial thickness wounds: blockage of wound growth factor as a possible mechanism of action [abstract]. J Invest Dermatol 1991;96:574A.
259. Falanga V, Carson P, Greenberg A: Topically applied recombinant tissue plasminogen activator for the treatment of venous ulcers. Dermatol Surg 1996;22:822-827.
260. Bello YM, Phillips TJ: Recent advances in wound healing. JAMA 2000;283:716-718.
261. Choucair M, Faria D, Fivenson D: Use of human skin equivalent in the successful treatment of chronic venous leg ulcers. Wounds 1998;10:97-104.
262. Falanga V, Margolis D, Alvarez O, et al: Rapid healing of venous ulcers and lack of clinical rejection with an allogeneic cultured human skin equivalent. Arch Dermatol 1998;134:293-300.
263. Schonfeld WH, Villa KF, Fastenau JM, et al: An economic assessment of Apligraf (Graftskin) for the treatment of hard-to-heal venous leg ulcers. Wound Repair Regen 2000;8:251-257.
264. Jaschke E, Zabernigg A, Gattringer C: Recombinant human granulocyte-macrophage colony-stimulating factor applied locally in low doses enhances healing and prevents recurrence of chronic venous ulcers. Int J Dermatol 1999;38:380-386.
265. Santilli SM, Valusek PA, Robinson C: Use of non-contact radiant heat bandage for the treatment of chronic venous stasis ulcers. Adv Wound Care 1999;12:89-93.
266. Horwitz LR, Burke TJ, Carnegie D: Augmentation of wound healing using monochromatic infrared energy. Adv Wound Care 1999;12:35-40.
267. Jelnes R, Gaardsting O, Hougaard Jensen K, et al: Fate in intermittent claudication: outcome and risk factors. Br Med J 1986;293:1137-1140.
268. Cronenwett JL, Warner KG, Zelenock GB, et al: Intermittent claudication: current results of nonoperative management. Arch Surg 1984;119:430-436.
269. Imparato AM, Kim GE, Davidson T, et al: Intermittent claudication: its natural course. Surgery 1975;78:795-799.
270. Peabody CN, Kannel WB, McNamara PM: Intermittent claudication: surgical significance. Arch Surg 1974;109:693-697.

271. Weitz JI, Byrne J, Claggett GP, et al: Diagnosis and treatment of chronic arterial insufficiency of the lower extremities: a critical review. Circulation 1996;94:3026-3049.
272. Vogt MT, Wolfson SK, Kuller LH: Lower extremity arterial disease and the aging process: a review. J Clin Epidemiol 1992;45:529-542.
273. TransAtlantic Inter-Society Consensus: Management of peripheral arterial disease. J Vasc Surg 2000;31:S1-S296.
274. Baker SR, Stacey MC, Singh G, et al: Aetiology of chronic leg ulcers. Eur J Vasc Surg 1992;6:245-251.
275. Colburn MD, Moore WS: Buerger's disease. Heart Dis Stroke 1993;2:424-432.
276. Standl E, Hillebrand B, Stiegler H: Microangiopathy in the context of diabetic foot problems: fact or fiction? Vasa Suppl 1992;35:25-26.
277. Rosenbloom MS, Flanigan DP, Schuler JJ, et al: Risk factors affecting the natural history of intermittent claudication. Arch Surg 1988;123:867-870.
278. Dormandy JA, Murray GD: The fate of the claudicant: a prospective study of 1969 claudicants. Eur J Vasc Surg 1991;5:131-133.
279. Jonason T, Ringqvist I: Changes in peripheral blood pressures after five years of follow-up in non-operated patients with intermittent claudication. Acta Med Scand 1986;220:127-132.
280. Choucair M, Faria D, Fivenson D: Use of human skin equivalent in the successful treatment of chronic venous leg ulcers. Wounds 1998;10:97-104.
281. Falanga V, Margolis D, Alvarez O, et al: Rapid healing of venous ulcers and lack of clinical rejection with an allogeneic cultured human skin equivalent. Arch Dermatol 1998;134:293-300.
282. Schonfeld WH, Villa KF, Fastenau JM, et al: An economic assessment of Apligraf (Graftskin) for the treatment of hard-to-heal venous leg ulcers. Wound Repair Regen 2000;8:251-257.
283. The Ad Hoc Committee on Reporting Standards, Society for Vascular Surgery/North American Chapter, International Society for Cardiovascular Surgery: Suggested standards for reports dealing with lower extremity ischemia. J Vasc Surg 1986;4:80-94.
284. Taylor LM, Hamre D, Dalman RL, et al: Limb salvage vs amputation for critical ischemia: the role of vascular surgery. Arch Surg 1991;126:1251-1258.
285. Edwards JE, Taylor LM, Porter JM: Treatment of failed lower extremity bypass grafts with new autogenous vein bypass grafting. J Vasc Surg 1990;11:136-144.
286. Veith FJ, Gupta SK, Wengerter KR, et al: Changing arteriosclerotic disease patterns and management strategies in lower-limb-threatening ischemia. Ann Surg 1990;212:402-414.
287. Ouriel K, Fiore WM, Geary JE: Limb-threatening ischemia in the medically compromised patient: amputation or revascularization? Surgery 1988;104:667-672.
288. De Frang RD, Taylor LM, Porter JM: Basic data related to amputations. Ann Vasc Surg 1991;5:202-207.
289. Mackey WC, McCullough JL, Conlon TP, et al: The costs of surgery for limb-threatening ischemia. Surgery 1986;99:26-35.
290. Farkouh ME, Rihal CS, Gersh BJ, et al: Influence of coronary heart disease on morbidity and mortality after lower extremity revascularization surgery: a population based study in Olmsted County Minnesota (1970-1987). J Am Coll Cardiol 1994;25:1290-1296.
291. Mathes SJ, Nahai F: Foot. In Mathes SJ, Nahai F: Reconstructive Surgery: Principles, Anatomy, and Technique, vol II. New York, Churchill Livingstone, 1997:1513-1592.
292. Aszmann OC, Kress KM, Dellon AL: Results of decompression of peripheral nerves in diabetics: a prospective, blinded study. Plast Reconstr Surg 2000;106:816-822.
293. Shestak KC, Fitz DG, Newton ED, et al: Expanding the horizons in treatment of severe peripheral vascular disease using microsurgical techniques. Plast Reconstr Surg 1990;85:406-411.
294. Cronenwett JL, McDaniel MD, Zwolak RM, et al: Limb salvage despite extensive tissue loss. Arch Surg 1989;124:609-615.
295. Serletti JM, Hurwitz SR, Jones JA, et al: Extension of limb salvage by combined vascular reconstruction and adjunctive free-tissue transfer. J Vasc Surg 1993;18:972-980.
296. Van Damme H, Creemers E, Limet R: Venous allografts for critical limb ischaemia. Acta Chir Belg 1995;95:14-20.
297. Oishi SN, Levin LS, Pederson WC: Microsurgical management of extremity wounds in diabetics with peripheral vascular disease. Plast Reconstr Surg 1993;92:485-492.
298. Mimoun M, Hilligot P, Baux S: The nutrient flap: a new concept of the role of the flap and application to the salvage of arteriosclerotic lower limbs. Plast Reconstr Surg 1989;84:458-467.
299. Ninkovic MM, Schwabeggar AH, Hausler JW, et al: Limb salvage after fulminant septicemia using a free latissimus dorsi cross-leg flap. J Reconstr Microsurg 2000;16:603-607.
300. Tvrdek M, Pros Z, Nejedly A, et al: Free cross leg flap as a method of reconstruction of soft tissues defects. Acta Chir Plast 1995;37:12-16.
301. Karp NS, Kasabian AK, Siebert JW, et al: Microvascular free-flap salvage of the diabetic foot: a 5-year experience. Plast Reconstr Surg 1994;94:834-840.
302. Ciresi KF, Anthony JP, Hoffman WY, et al: Limb salvage and wound coverage in patients with large ischemic ulcers: a multidisciplinary approach with revascularization and free tissue transfer. J Vasc Surg 1993;18:648-655.
303. Wahlberg E, Olofsson P, Swedenborg J, et al: Changes in post-occlusive reactive hyperaemic values as measured with laser Doppler fluxmetry after infrainguinal arterial reconstructions. Eur J Vasc Endovasc Surg 1995;9:197-203.
304. Edmondson RA, Cohen AT, Das SK, et al: Low-molecular-weight heparin versus aspirin and dipyridamole after femoropopliteal bypass grafting. Lancet 1994;344:914-918.
305. Violi F, Balsano F: Rationale for the use of antiplatelet drugs in patients with peripheral vascular disease. Clin Trials Metaanal 1994;29:81-87.
306. Brothers TE, Vincent CK, Darvishian D, et al: Effects of duration of acetylsalicylic acid administration on patency and anastomotic hyperplasia of ePTFE grafts. ASAIO Trans 1989;35:558-560.
307. Neilipovitz DT, Bryson GL, Nichol G: The effect of perioperative aspirin therapy in peripheral vascular surgery: a decision analysis. Anesth Analg 2001;93:573-580.
308. Ranke C, Creutzig A, Luska G, et al: Controlled trial of high- versus low-dose aspirin treatment after percutaneous transluminal angioplasty in patients with peripheral vascular disease. Clin Invest 1994;72:673-680.
309. Arfvidsson B, Lundgren F, Drott C, et al: Influence of coumarin treatment on patency and limb salvage after peripheral arterial reconstructive surgery. Am J Surg 1990;159:556-560.
310. Illig KA, Moran S, Serletti J, et al: Combined free tissue transfer and infrainguinal bypass graft: an alternative to major amputation in selected patients. J Vasc Surg 2001;33:17-23.

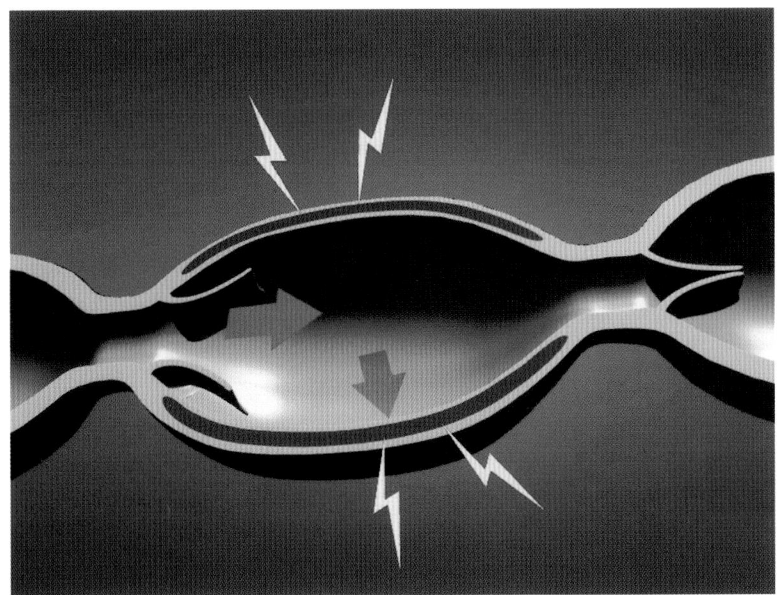

COLOR PLATE 161-1. The lymphangion is the functional unit of the lymphatic circulation. Although lymphatic flow is determined primarily by filling pressure, each lymphangion has proximal and distal valves that work in concert to direct the proximal flow of lymph. (Courtesy of BSN-Jobst, Inc.)

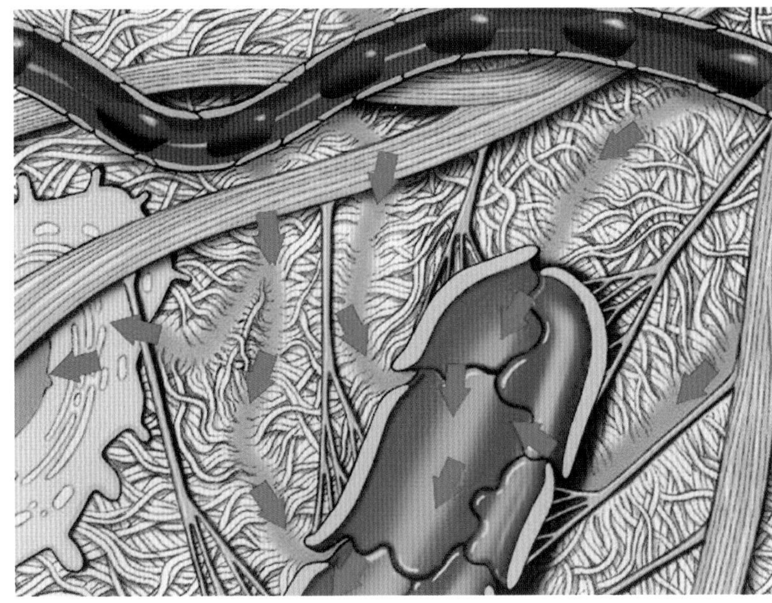

COLOR PLATE 161-2. The numerous intercellular gaps that characterize the structure of the basement membrane of the lymphatic system permit flow of fluid, fat, and protein *(arrows)* into the lymphatic capillaries. (Courtesy of BSN-Jobst, Inc.)

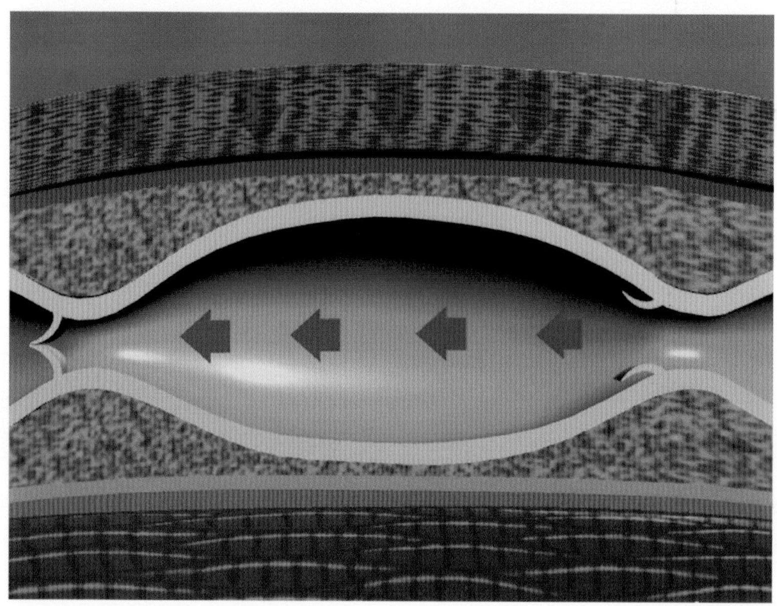

COLOR PLATE 161-3. Lymphatic flow is driven by muscle contractions that produce a pressure differential to propel lymph fluid *(arrows)* through the system. (Courtesy of BSN-Jobst, Inc.)

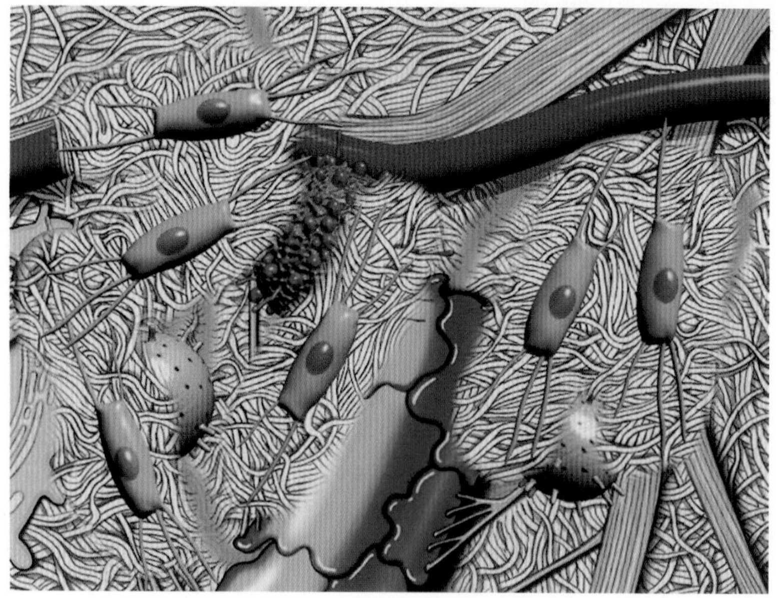

COLOR PLATE 161-4. In chronic lymphedema, lymph flow is stifled. Macromolecular protein deposition increases and fibroblasts accumulate in the interstitium. Fibrovascular proliferation results in worsening brawny edema, obliteration of elastic fibers, increased collagen deposition, and fibrosis. (Courtesy of BSN-Jobst, Inc.)

Index

*Note: **Boldface** roman numerals indicate volume. Page numbers followed by f refer to figures; page numbers followed by t refer to tables.*

B

D

F

G

H

M

O

T

V

W